P9-BHY-503

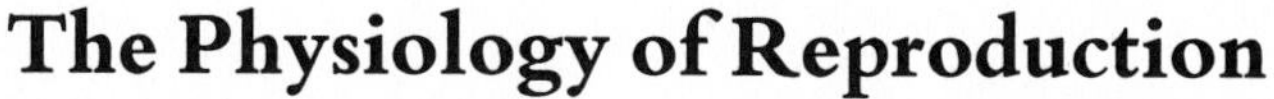

The Physiology of Reproduction

The PHYSIOLOGY of REPRODUCTION

Volume 1

Editors-in-Chief

Ernst Knobil
The H. Wayne Hightower Professor
in the Medical Sciences and
Director, Laboratory for Neuroendocrinology
The University of Texas
Health Science Center at Houston—Medical School
Houston, Texas

Jimmy D. Neill
Professor and Chairman
Department of Physiology and Biophysics
The University of Alabama at Birmingham
Birmingham, Alabama

Associate Editors

Larry L. Ewing
Professor, Division of Reproductive Biology
Department of Population Dynamics
The Johns Hopkins University
School of Hygiene and Public Health
Baltimore, Maryland

Clement L. Markert
University Research Professor
Department of Animal Sciences
North Carolina State University
School of Agriculture and Life Sciences
Raleigh, North Carolina

Gilbert S. Greenwald
Distinguished Professor and Chairman
Department of Physiology
University of Kansas Medical Center
Kansas City, Kansas

Donald W. Pfaff
Professor
Laboratory of Neurobiology and Behavior
Rockefeller University
New York, New York

Raven Press New York

Raven Press, 1185 Avenue of the Americas, New York, New York 10036

Made in the United States of America

Library of Congress Cataloging-in-Publication Data

The Physiology of reproduction.
Includes bibliographies and index.
1. Reproduction. 2. Mammals—Physiology. I. Knobil, Ernst. II. Neill, Jimmy D. [DNLM: 1. Reproduction. WQ 205 P5784]
QP251.P525 1988 Vol. I 599'.016 85-42819
ISBN 0-88167-281-5

The material contained in this volume was submitted as previously unpublished material, except in the instances in which credit has been given to the source from which some of the illustrative material was derived.

Great care has been taken to maintain the accuracy of the information contained in the volume. However, neither Raven Press nor the editors can be held responsible for errors or for any consequences arising from the use of the information contained herein.

9 8 7 6 5 4 3 2 1

Preface

This work was undertaken, after much deliberation, in an attempt to fill a need for a comprehensive, scholarly treatise on the physiology of mammalian reproduction. A major inspiration for this effort has been the volume, *Sex and Internal Secretions*, a factual and conceptual beacon which guided generations of reproductive biologists from the time of its first publication in 1932 to the appearance of its last edition over a quarter of a century ago.

The book is divided into five major sections, and these, in turn, are loosely arrayed in two domains. The first covers the components of the reproductive system, and the second discusses reproductive processes and their physiological control. In the latter, we have included reproductive behavior in the conviction that this fundamental aspect of reproduction clearly belongs in the physiological realm and will remain a demanding challenge long after all the other mysteries in the field have been resolved.

In our discussion of reproductive systems, we have been aware of the profound differences among mammals in the way some fundamental processes, such as the ovarian cycle, are controlled. We have addressed this issue, in part, by providing separate coverage of major mammalian groups where this seemed appropriate. It has been left to the reader to ascertain the similarities and differences among them. In any case, we must ever be mindful in considering reproductive processes, from the control of ovulation to the initiation of parturition, not to extrapolate from one species to another without due reflection.

It is hoped that this book will be useful to all serious students of reproductive physiology be they scientists, teachers, or physicians.

THE EDITORS

Contents

VOLUME 1

The Gametes, Fertilization and Early Embryogenesis

The Reproductive Systems

The Female

VOLUME 2

Reproductive Behavior and Its Control

Reproductive Processes and Their Control

Contributors

Miriam Altstein *Laboratory of Neurochemistry and Neuroimmunology, National Institute of Child Health and Human Development, National Institutes of Health, Bethesda, Maryland 20892*

David T. Armstrong *Medical Research Council Group in Reproductive Biology, Department of Physiology and Obstetrics and Gynaecology, The University of Western Ontario, London, Ontario, Canada N6A 5A5*

C. Wayne Bardin *The Population Council, New York, New York 10021*

Donald H. Barron *Department of Obstetrics and Gynecology, University of Florida College of Medicine, Gainesville, Florida 32601*

George S. Benson *Professor of Surgery (Urology), The University of Texas Health Science Center, Houston, Texas 77225*

C. Beyer *Centro de Investigacíon en Reproduccíon Animal, CINVECTAVUAT Panothla, Tlaxacala, Mexico*

Robert D. H. Boyd *Action Research Placental and Perinatal Unit, Department of Child Health, University of Manchester, St. Mary's Hospital, Manchester M13 0JH, United Kingdom*

Robert M. Brenner *Division of Reproductive Biology and Behavior, Oregon Regional Primate Research Center, Beaverton, Oregon 97006*

F. H. Bronson *Institute of Reproductive Biology, Department of Zoology, University of Texas, Austin, Texas 78712*

D. E. Brooks (*Deceased*) *Department of Animal Sciences, Waite Agricultural Research Institute, University of Adelaide, Adelaide, South Australia*

Anne Grete Byskov *Laboratory of Reproductive Biology II, Rigshospitalet, University of Copenhagen, DK-2100 Copenhagen, Denmark*

J. R. G. Challis *Departments of Obstetrics and Gynaecology and Physiology, The Research Institute, St. Joseph's Health Centre, University of Western Ontario, London, Ontario, Canada N6A 4V2*

C. Yan Cheng *The Population Council, New York, New York 10021*

James H. Clark *Department of Cell Biology, Baylor College of Medicine, Houston, Texas 77030*

G. Clarke *Department of Anatomy, Medical School, University of Bristol, Bristol, BS8 1TD, United Kingdom*

Donald S. Coffey *Department of Urology, The Johns Hopkins University, School of Medicine, Baltimore, Maryland 21205*

D. M. de Kretser *Department of Anatomy, Monash University, Melbourne, Victoria 3168, Australia*

E. M. Eddy *Gamete Biology Section, Laboratory of Reproductive and Developmental Toxicology, National Institute of Environmental Health Sciences, National Institutes of Health, Research Triangle Park, North Carolina 27709*

Ransome N. Etindi *Department of Physiology, Wayne State University, School of Medicine, Detroit, Michigan 48201*

John W. Everett *Department of Anatomy, Duke University School of Medicine, Durham, North Carolina 27710*

Caleb E. Finch *Andrus Gerontology Center, Department of Biological Sciences, University of Southern California, Los Angeles, California 90081*

Paul R. Findell *Department of Obstetrics, Gynecology, and Reproductive Sciences, University of California at San Francisco, School of Medicine, San Francisco, California 94143*

George Fink *MRC Brain Metabolism Unit, University Department of Pharmacology, Edinburgh EH8 9JZ, United Kingdom*

Douglas L. Foster *Associate Professor of Obstetrics and Gynecology, and Biological Sciences and Associate Research Scientist of Developmental and Reproductive Biology, The University of Michigan, Ann Arbor, Michigan 48106*

Marc E. Freeman *Department of Biological Science, Florida State University, Tallahassee, Florida 32306*

Harold Gainer *Laboratory of Neurochemistry and Neuroimmunology, National Institute of Child Health and Human Development, National Institutes of Health, Bethesda, Maryland 20892*

Fredrick W. George *Department of Cell Biology and Anatomy, University of Texas Health Science Center at Dallas, Southwestern Medical School, Dallas, Texas 75235*

Thomas J. Gill III *Department of Pathology, University of Pittsburgh, School of Medicine, Pittsburgh, Pennsylvania 15261*

Robert L. Goodman *Department of Physiology, West Virginia University, Morgantown, West Virginia 26506*

Robert E. Gore-Langton *Medical Research Council Group in Reproductive Biology, Department of Physiology and Obstetrics and Gynaecology, The University of Western Ontario, London, Ontario, Canada N6A 5A5*

Gilbert S. Greenwald *Department of Physiology, University of Kansas Medical Center, Kansas City, Kansas 66103*

Roy O. Greep *Director of the Laboratory of Human Reproduction and Reproductive Biology, Professor of Anatomy, Emeritus, Harvard Medical School, Boston, Massachusetts 02115*

Glen L. Gunsalus *The Population Council, New York, New York 10021*

Peter F. Hall *Department of Medicine, Prince of Wales Hospital, Randwick, New South Wales 2301, Australia*

Michael J. K. Harper *Departments of Obstetrics and Gynecology and Physiology, The University of Texas Health Science Center at San Antonio, San Antonio, Texas 78284*

Louis Hermo *Centre for the Study of Reproduction, Department of Anatomy, McGill University, Montreal, Quebec, Canada H3G 1Y6*

Gary D. Hodgen *The Jones Institute for Reproductive Medicine and Department of Obstetrics and Gynecology, Eastern Virginia Medical School, Norfolk, Virginia 23507*

Julane Hotchkiss *Laboratory for Neuroendocrinology, The University of Texas Health Science Center at Houston, The University of Texas Medical School, Houston, Texas 77225*

Poul Erik Høyer *Institute of Medical Anatomy A, The Panum Institute, University of Copenhagen, DK-2200 Copenhagen, Denmark*

Joseph Itskovitz *Department of Obstetrics and Gynecology, Technion, Israel Institute of Technology, Faculty of Medicine, Rambam Medical Center, Haifa, Israel 31096*

J. B. Kerr *Department of Anatomy, Monash University, Melbourne, Victoria 3168, Australia*

Ernst Knobil *Laboratory for Neuroendocrinology, The University of Texas Health Science Center at Houston, The University of Texas Medical School, Houston, Texas 77225*

Claude Kordon *Unité de Neuroendocrinologie, INSERM U159, 75014 Paris, France*

Harry Lipner *Department of Biological Sciences, Florida State University, Tallahassee, Florida 32306*

Barry M. Markaverich *Department of Cell Biology, Baylor College of Medicine, Houston, Texas 77030*

Peter Marler *The Rockefeller University, Field Research Center, Millbrook, New York 12545*

Ila A. Maslar *Division of Reproductive Biology and Behavior, Oregon Regional Primate Research Center, Beaverton, Oregon 97006*

Alan S. McNeilly *MRC Reproductive Biology Unit, University of Edinburgh, Centre for Reproductive Biology, Edinburgh EH3 9EW, United Kingdom*

Robert L. Meisel *Department of Psychological Sciences, Purdue University, West Lafayette, Indiana 47907*

James Metcalfe *Heart Research Laboratory, Department of Medicine, Oregon Health Sciences University, Portland, Oregon 97201*

Frank H. Morriss, Jr. *Department of Pediatrics, University of Iowa Hospitals and Clinics, Iowa City, Iowa 52242*

Neil A. Mustow *The Population Council, New York, New York 10021*

Jimmy D. Neill *Department of Physiology and Biophysics, University of Alabama at Birmingham, Birmingham, Alabama 35294*

Terry M. Nett *Department of Physiology and Biophysics, Colorado State University, Fort Collins, Colorado 80532*

Gordon D. Niswender *Department of Physiology and Biophysics, Colorado State University, Fort Collins, Colorado 80532*

Michael Numan *Department of Psychology, Boston College, Chestnut Hill, Massachusetts 02167*

John P. Ofenstein *Department of Physiology, Wayne State University, School of Medicine, Detroit, Michigan 48201*

Linda Ogren *Biology Board of Studies, Thimann Laboratories, University of California, Santa Cruz, California 95064*

Sergio R. Ojeda *Department of Physiology, The University of Texas Health Science Center at Dallas, Dallas, Texas 75235-9040*

D. M. Olson *Departments of Paediatrics and Physiology, The Research Institute, St. Joseph's Health Centre, University of Western Ontario, London, Ontario, Canada N6A 4V2*

Robert B. Page *Professor of Neurosurgery and Anatomy, Chairman, Neuroscience Program, Milton S. Hershey Medical Center, The Pennsylvania State University, Hershey, Pennsylvania 17033*

Roger A. Pedersen *Laboratory of Radiobiology and Environmental Health (LR-102), University of California at San Francisco, San Francisco, California 94143*

Donald W. Pfaff *Laboratory of Neurobiology and Behavior, The Rockefeller University, New York, New York 10021*

John G. Pierce *Department of Biological Chemistry, UCLA School of Medicine, Los Angeles, California 90024*

Tony M. Plant *Department of Physiology, University of Pittsburgh, Pittsburgh, Pennsylvania 15261*

Victor D. Ramirez *Department of Physiology and Biophysics, University of Illinois at Urbana-Champaign, Urbana, Illinois 61801*

James A. Rillema *Department of Physiology, Wayne State University, School of Medicine, Detroit, Michigan 48201*

Bernard Robaire *Centre for the Study of Reproduction, Departments of Pharmacology and Therapeutics, and Obstetrics and Gynecology, McGill University, Montreal, Quebec, Canada H3G 1Y6*

Benjamin D. Sachs *Department of Psychology, University of Connecticut, Storrs, Connecticut 06268*

Susan Schwartz-Giblin *Laboratory of Neurobiology and Behavior, The Rockefeller University, New York, New York 10021*

B. P. Setchell *Department of Animal Sciences, Waite Agricultural Research Institute, University of Adelaide, Adelaide, South Australia*

O. David Sherwood *University of Illinois, College of Medicine and Department of Physiology and Biophysics, University of Illinois, Urbana, Illinois 61801*

Ann-Judith Silverman *Department of Anatomy and Cell Biology, Columbia University, College of Physicians and Surgeons, New York, New York 10032*

S. Solomon *Departments of Medicine and Obstetrics and Gynecology, McGill University and the Royal Victoria Hospital, Montreal, Quebec H3A 1A1, Canada*

Anna Steinberger *Department of Obstetrics, Gynecology and Reproductive Sciences, The University of Texas Medical School at Houston, Houston, Texas 77030*

Michael K. Stock *Heart Research Laboratory, Department of Medicine, Oregon Health Sciences University, Portland, Oregon 97201*

A. J. S. Summerlee *Department of Anatomy, Medical School, University of Bristol, Bristol, BS8 1TD, United Kingdom*

Frank Talamantes *Biology Board of Studies, Thimann Laboratories, University of California, Santa Cruz, California 95064*

Paul F. Terranova *Department of Physiology, University of Kansas Medical Center, Kansas City, Kansas 66103*

Andrée Tixier-Vidal *Groupe de Neuroendocrinologie Cellulaire et Moléculaire, Collège de France, ll, Place Marcelin Berthelot, 75231 Paris Cédex 05, France*

Claude Tougard *Groupe de Neuroendocrinologie Cellulaire et Moléculaire, Collège de France, ll, Place Marcelin Berthelot, 75231 Paris Cédex 05, France*

Alex Tsafriri *Department of Hormone Research, The Weizmann Institute of Science, Rehovot 76100, Israel*

H. Allen Tucker *Department of Animal Science, Michigan State University, East Lansing, Michigan 48824*

Fred W. Turek *Department of Neurobiology and Physiology, Northwestern University, Evanston, Illinois 60201*

Henryk F. Urbanski *Department of Physiology, The University of Texas Health Science Center at Dallas, Dallas, Texas 75235-9040*

Eve Van Cauter *Institute of Interdisciplinary Research, Free University of Brussels, B-1070 Brussels, Belgium and Department of Medicine, University of Chicago, Chicago, Illinois 60637*

John G. Vandenbergh *Department of Zoology, North Carolina State University, Raleigh, North Carolina 27695*

Frederick S. vom Saal *Division of Biological Sciences, John M. Dalton Research Center, University of Missouri, Columbia, Missouri 65211*

J. B. Wakerley *Department of Anatomy, Medical School, University of Bristol, Bristol, BS8 1TD, United Kingdom*

Darrell N. Ward *Department of Biochemistry and Molecular Biology, The University of Texas, M.D. Anderson Hospital and Tumor Institute, Houston, Texas 77030*

Paul M. Wassarman *Department of Cell Biology, Roche Institute of Molecular Biology, Roche Research Center, Nutley, New Jersey 07110*

Steven B. Waters *Department of Physiology, Wayne State University, School of Medicine, Detroit, Michigan 48201*

Richard I. Weiner *Department of Obstetrics, Gynecology, and Reproductive Sciences, University of California, San Francisco, School of Medicine, San Francisco, California 94143*

H. M. Weitlauf *Department of Cell Biology and Anatomy, Texas Tech University Health Sciences Center, Lubbock, Texas 79430*

Mark H. Whitnall *Laboratory of Neurochemistry and Neuroimmunology, National Institute of Child Health and Human Development, National Institutes of Health, Bethesda, Maryland 20892*

H. G. Williams-Ashman *Ben May Institute, and Departments of Biochemistry and Molecular Biology and Pharmacological and Physiological Sciences, University of Chicago, Chicago, Illinois 60637*

Jean D. Wilson *Department of Internal Medicine, University of Texas Health Science Center at Dallas, Southwestern Medical School, Dallas, Texas 75235*

John C. Wingfield *The Rockefeller University, Field Research Center, Millbrook, New York 12545*

Susan Wray *Laboratory of Neurochemistry and Neuroimmunology, National Institute of Child Health and Human Development, National Institutes of Health, Bethesda, Maryland 20892*

R. Yanagimachi *Department of Anatomy and Reproductive Biology, University of Hawaii School of Medicine, Honolulu, Hawaii 96822*

Foreword

I am pleased and honored to have been asked to prepare the Foreword to this volume of work depicting the progress in research on the physiology of reproduction as well as the resulting gains in understanding made over the past few years. The expertise that is represented by the numerous contributors to this work is so impressive that I am humbled even to contemplate adding anything of note. It is only by virtue of the perspective garnered from my vantage point of having personally witnessed a very large segment of twentieth century research on reproduction that I am emboldened to reflect on the byways and the trail blazings that have brought this field to its present proud state of enlightenment with regard to the long sought-after means of controlling the procreative process in humankind. Clearly, there are many important and knotty problems yet to be resolved, but the pace of progress over the past several years has quickened to the extent that one is left in expectant wonderment as to where and when the next revolutionizing development will occur.

The experimental method of studying reproduction was initiated in 1849 with Berthold's discovery of a blood-borne activity that came from the testis and stimulated growth of distant organs such as the comb and wattles. In so doing he utilized one of the most fundamental means of demonstrating the function of an endocrine organ, namely, surgical removal to determine what deficiencies follow, coupled with implantation or transplantation to ascertain whether the deficiencies were repaired. At that time it was not possible to take the next step, namely, preparation of an active extract of the testes, because nothing was known about the chemical nature of the bioactivity. Forty years later, Brown-Sequard claimed to have prepared an active extract of dog testes; however, as is well known, his enthusiastic claims for restoration of his own sexual activity at an advanced age were not substantiated. Actually, these simple means of studying reproductive physiology persisted well into the twentieth century, including the studies of such pioneering stalwarts as Marshall, Heape, Prenant, Bouin, Ancel, Loeb, Cushing, and Aschner. Observations otherwise were limited to cyclic and seasonal changes in sexual behavior among common laboratory and small domestic animals. This type of eyeball research remained in vogue through the early 1920s and overlapped the extension of visualization to the microscopic level. The latter revealed, for the first time, the precise timing of events in the ovarian cycle through microscopically observable cellular changes in the vaginal fluid. My point in mentioning these early studies is to emphasize that although the tools and techniques were inordinately primitive by present standards, the results established a firm base of knowledge on which to build.

The study of cyclic changes in the vaginal smear in rats and the finding of estrogenic activity in follicular fluid during the early 1920s led to an explosion of interest in the study of reproduction. The field was fortunate in attracting to its ranks a small band of exceedingly able biologists and biochemists who were to become authors of the classic compendium, the first edition, in 1932, of *Sex and Internal Secretions*, overwhelmingly devoted to reproductive endocrinology. It was this landmark of progress that finally gave propriety to the study of reproduction and put it on a par with the study of other major bodily systems. Incredible as it may seem, it was only a decade earlier that a distinguished panel of the National Research Council had declared that sex research was not a fitting topic for scientific study.

Lest our pride in today's spectacular pace of progress unduly bedazzle the mind, it should not be overlooked that the developments recorded in the 10-year span from 1926 to 1936 may never be equaled. Among those monumental achievements, all of the native sex steroid hormones were brought to light, their structures were determined, their functions were defined, and they were made available in pure form for research and therapy. Similarly, all of the pituitary, placental, and urinary tropic hormones were identified, and their functions were defined. Like today's competition for priority rights, publicity, and potential financial gain, these earlier periods also were times of intense rivalries, but rarely with prospects for financial rewards. It would be difficult to overstate the boost that was given to basic and clinical research in reproduction as a result of having available estradiol-17β, testosterone, and progesterone in pure form and of known potency. The replacement of homemade extracts and such elastic entities as rat units, mouse units, capon units, etc., with micrograms of pure hormone was revolutionizing and allowed the study of reproduction to be on a quantitative basis.

Prior to World War II the thrust of research on reproduction dealt predominantly with the steroid hormones. This was the heyday of steroid biochemistry. After World War II the emphasis shifted to the protein and peptide hormones, where it still remains strong. This prolonged and difficult effort yielded many biochemical triumphs. Most notable among these were the isolation of the pituitary, placental, and urinary gonadotropins as well as the determination of their primary structure as glycoproteins comprised of two dissimilar and covalently bonded subunits, the isolation and synthesis of the gonadotropin-releasing hormone (GnRH) of hypothalamic origin, and the isolation and structural characterization of relaxin.

The availability of pure protein and polypeptide hormones made possible the production of hormone-specific antibodies as well as the application of immunological techniques to the study of reproduction. An outcome of great consequence was the development of radioimmunoassay as a new means of measuring all of the hormones relating to reproduction. The sensitivity of this new technique was so great that it made possible, for the first time, the measurement of all these hormones in the body fluids. It had the further distinct advantage of requiring such a small amount of fluid that the monitoring of blood levels of the hormones of reproduction could be done throughout an estrous or menstrual cycle by close serial sampling. This revealed still another and most unexpected finding, the pulsatile pattern of secretion.

Identifying the homeostatic mechanism(s) responsible for maintaining a steady state in various physiologic systems of the body has been fraught with many challenging problems, but these pale in comparison with the difficulties encountered in trying to elucidate the mechanisms maintaining a constantly changing system, a characteristic of the reproductive system of female mammals. The earliest piece of evidence suggested the existence of a "push-pull" mechanism that later came to be known as *negative feedback*. It was based on the demonstration that an estrogenic extract administered to immature rats would maintain the ovaries in an infantile state. This was quickly followed by conclusive evidence that estrogen acted to inhibit pituitary follicle-stimulating hormone (FSH) stimulation of follicular growth and maturation; however, the effect on luteinizing hormone (LH), ovulation, and luteinization remained unsettled. Gaps continued to exist in all proposed explanations of reproductive cycles. None of these explanations took account of the influence of photoperiodicity on seasonal breeders, nor did they account for the stimulus of mating in nonspontaneous ovulators. Following the discovery of the hypothalamic control of pituitary function, estrogen was shown to exert its action on both the pituitary and the hypothalamus; however, the problem of accounting for cyclicity remained. Adding to the complexity, radioimmunoassay revealed an unexpectedly high level of blood estrogen just prior to ovulation—an event not in keeping with the negative feedback concept.

Finally, after many years of searching for a way out of this frustrating situation, a glimmer of light appeared at the end of this long dark tunnel—light that soon turned to brilliance. In 1969, Goding and associates found that the administration of large doses of estrogen to ewes at the time of estrus did not block, but instead entrained, ovulation. Shortly thereafter, in more elaborate examination of the relationship of blood estrogen levels and ovulation in rhesus monkeys in Knobil's laboratory, it was revealed that elevated estrogen levels preceded and appeared to trigger ovulation. On further examination, Knobil and colleagues found that when blood estrogen reached a critical level the feedback mechanism switched from a negative to a positive, or stimulative, action. This utterly new finding greatly advanced our understanding of the endocrine mechanism governing reproductive cycles. There still remain, however, some uncertainties: Why does the switch in feedback action occur; to what extent and at what stage of the cycle does estrogen act at the level of the pituitary or the hypothalamus, or both; and lastly, what role, if any, do the ovarian peptides, especially inhibin, play in controlling reproductive cycles?

The progress of research on reproduction has been chronicled in numerous review articles by individual authors. Many have appeared in *Recent Progress in Hormone Research, Volumes 1 to 42*. Other major sources include the multiple editions of such titles as: *Marshall's Physiology of Reproduction*, now being produced in its fourth edition; *Sex and Internal Secretions*, whose third and last edition was issued in 1981; two volumes on the *Female Reproductive System* (1973), and one on the *Male Reproductive System* (1975) in *Section 7 of the Handbook of Physiology*, published by the American Physiological Society; and four serial volumes on reproductive physiology in the *International Review of Physiology*, the last one being issued in 1983. The present volume will provide comprehensive coverage and meet the current needs of the field of reproductive physiology, a field that is rapidly gathering momentum from the application of new and highly sophisticated tools and techniques.

In viewing the vast literature dealing with research on the male and female reproductive systems and considering the rate at which it is accumulating, one might ask whether this staggering proliferation of books and articles is essential to progress; the answer is an emphatic "yes." The yardstick by which progress is measured in this or any other field is not in number of articles published or amount of financial support but in improved understanding. Such gains are generally marked by sharp peaks at indeterminate intervals, separated by avalanches of incremental gains, as recorded in an ever-growing list of journals. The point to remember is that without this persistent chipping away at a major problem there would be no solutions and no quantum leaps forward. In research very little comes from out of the blue. Part of the driving force in research is its adventuresome nature and the ever-present possibility that one's efforts will pay off in an important manner. It may not be entirely fair, but in research (as in most human activities), the spoils go to the victor in the form of kudos, prizes, awards, public attention, and, increasingly in the present technological age, monetary gains—sometimes of great magnitude. What effect this latter may have, if any, on the long-cherished sanctity of science has not been determined, but it has become a matter of concern.

This volume bears the title *The Physiology of Reproduction*. Physiology, by traditional consensus, is that branch of science which studies the functions of a living organism or any of its parts and includes the basic underlying processes. It will be understood that most of the studies reviewed here will be based more on holistic research than on research at the submicroscopic or molecular level. It is unfortunate that the excitement generated by recent fantastic advances in molecular biology and development has tended to downgrade the value of whole-animal research, and physiology in particular is sometimes looked upon as passé. Actually, the two categories of research are complementary, and both are essential for maximal advancement of knowledge. Whole-animal research cannot become outdated because it is the quintessence of biological relevance and the means by which molecular findings must ultimately be evaluated.

In this same vein, no one immersed in reproductive endocrinology can be unaware of the current tendency to regard research at the molecular level as representative of exceptional scientific talent. This is a common consequence of the opening of a new arena of investigation. I recall an incident that happened at a scientific meeting back in the 1930s. The first three papers in a session chaired by an eminent embryologist were on endocrine topics—mine was the third. That being ended, the chairman took pains to assure the audience that the meeting could now turn to considerations of more fundamental nature. One of the other three papers was given by Herbert M. Evans, who bristled noticeably but held his fire. There was also an earlier period when one either worked on steroid biochemistry or something of lesser appeal like biology. Anyone who remembers the 1950s will recall a flash-in-the pan ignited by cybernetics, a study of automatic control systems both neural and physical. The gurus of cybernetics captured the attention of the press and of audiences throughout the land, but eventually this obsession suffered the fate of other passing preoccupations. My own observation is that the closer one approaches the molecular level of research, the more one becomes dependent on highly sophisticated instrumentation to make the observations and to read out results that are often quite free of extraneous variables. Toward the obverse situation, one's dependence on an extensive background of experience and physiological insight increases as does the unavoidable complex of *in vivo* variables that must be taken into account. In either case we have today the availability of far more diverse approaches to a given problem in any field of biomedical research than has ever existed before. In Berthold's day there was only one experimental method available; today's number is untold but is probably in the hundreds, perhaps thousands. That is an exceedingly promising situation and one to which investigators of all persuasions must adjust. Open minds will experience exhilaration over substantive achievements at any point on this observational spectrum.

One of the major factors influencing research on reproduction has been the availability of funds or lack thereof. Prior to the institution of federal funding (i.e., prior to the middle of the twentieth century), reproductive research was sparsely supported by university departmental funds, industry, small grants from the Committee for Research in Problems of Sex within the National Research Council, and some aid from the Rockefeller Foundation. The National Institutes of Health were slow in providing significant support of research on reproduction because of restrictions on the support of work related in any way to birth control. This occurred despite the simultaneous postwar baby boom. What kept research afloat during this critical period was major support by the Ford Foundation plus lesser contributions by other major foundations. It was not until the establishment in 1968 of the Center for Population Research in the NICHD that major governmental funding in this area became available, but the boost was short-lived. As a result of the imposition of fiscal restraints in the early 1970s, federal support dwindled and has remained at a minimal level ever since. Support from all sources is woefully incommensurate with the distressing expansion of the human population and the need for safe, effective, economical, and readily available means of limiting human fertility.

The physiology of reproduction is predominantly under hormonal control. The first essential step in studying reproduction was identification of the hormones involved and the functions they serve. This having been accomplished, efforts turned to a detailed analysis as to how hormones act within the body. During the past decade there has been a rising tide of interest in the binding of steroid, protein, or peptide hormones to receptors on specific target cells. Much effort is currently being directed toward the isolation and chemical characterization of these receptors. They are known to be composed of a protein or proteins, and some information has already been gained as to their partial or provisional structure. This, however, is only a preliminary step in the complex process whereby hormone action results in an end response such as growth, secretion of a target cell hormone, or altered behavior. The curtain has already been raised on the climactic and final chapter of the story on how hormones act. This involves linkage of the hormone-receptor complex with the nuclear genetic apparatus leading through a now well-defined series of processes to the manifestation of a physiological response in the living organism. Genes that bring about the expression of certain hormonal signals are being isolated, modified, transferred between species, and also inserted into bacteria where they direct the biosynthesis of specific hormones in large quantity. Thus genes are being manipulated in ways that raise the potential of altering the reproductive process. It is largely as a result of developments in endocrinology at the molecular level that bewildering possibilities loom on the horizons of reproductive research—they are within reach; they are science, not fiction; and they stagger the imagination.

ROY O. GREEP

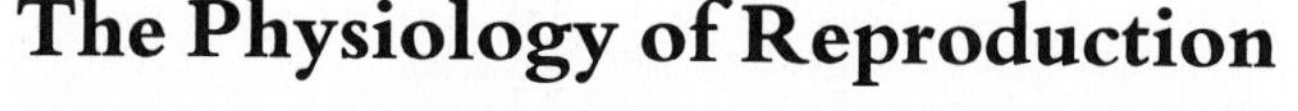

The Gametes, Fertilization and Early Embryogenesis

The Physiology of Reproduction,
edited by E. Knobil and J. Neill *et al.*
Raven Press, Ltd., New York © 1988.

CHAPTER 1

Sex Determination and Differentiation

Fredrick W. George and Jean D. Wilson

Sexual differentiation is a sequential process beginning with the establishment of chromosomal sex at the time of fertilization, followed by the development of gonadal sex, and culminating in the formation of the sexual phenotypes (Fig. 1). Each step in this process is dependent on the preceding one, and, under normal circumstances, chromosomal sex agrees with the phenotypic sex. Occasionally, however, chromosomal sex and phenotypic sex do not agree, or the sexual phenotype may be ambiguous. Abnormalities of sexual development are usually not life threatening and occur at many levels. They encompass clinical consequences that range from defects in the terminal phases of male development (cryptorchidism and microphallus) to more fundamental abnormalities that result in conditions of intersex. In many cases, disorders of sexual differentiation are inherited as single gene mutations, and the analysis of these disorders has been especially informative in defining the molecular and genetic determinants involved in the normal process of sexual development. Although the principal focus of this chapter is on human sexual determination, many aspects of the process have been best studied in other species.

CHROMOSOMAL SEX

The chromosomal basis for sex determination was established between 1910 and 1916, largely by T. H. Morgan and his colleagues. The nature of the genetic information responsible for sexual differentiation has, however, remained largely enigmatic. The pioneering work in this field, performed in *Drosophila,* suggested that sex is determined by the number of X chromosomes. Flies with a single X chromosome (XY, XO) are male, whereas the presence of two or more X chromosomes (XX, XXX, or XXY) confers a female phenotype (reviewed in ref. 248). The mammalian Y chromosome was also originally believed to be a null chromosome without genetic information, with the possible exception of some factor that promoted fertility in males (227). However, with the development of techniques for the karyotyping of the mammalian chromosome in the early 1960s, it became apparent that in humans (and other mammalian species) the Y chromosome specifies the development of the testis. That is, no matter how many X chromosomes are present, a testis will develop as long as a Y chromosome is present (as in XXY, XXYY, XXXY, XXXXY, etc.) (47). The phenotype of the 45,X human is female, although ovarian development is incomplete, implying that X chromosomes do participate in human ovarian differentiation. Nevertheless, the presence of a second X chromosome (as in XXY or XX_{Sxr}) does not appear to affect sexual differentiation at the gonadal level; e.g., either a Y chromosome or a critical fragment of a Y chromosome that contains the testis-determining genes is capable of inducing testicular development, no matter how many X chromosomes are present. However, if two X chromosomes are present, spermatogenesis is impaired (except in XX true

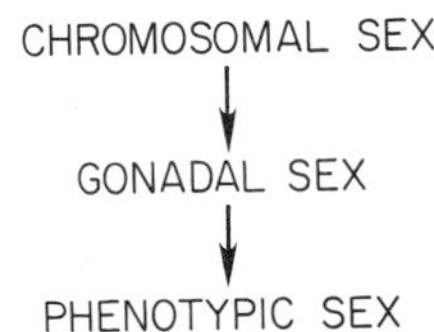

FIG. 1. The Jost paradigm.

hermaphroditism). The most likely explanation for the infertility in the XXY state is that inactivation of the X chromosome in the formation of the XY body (see below) during normal spermatogenesis is essential for fertility. In other words, some X-coded gene product must prevent male germ development (172). This concept is in keeping with the fact that some balanced translocations of X chromosomes to autosomes in mice (76) and in humans (163) are associated both with male infertility and with incomplete inactivation of X chromosomal genes. Furthermore, if the situation in the creeping vole (193), in which the X chromosome is eliminated from the testicular germ line, is applicable to other species, then it can be assumed that function of an X chromosome is not essential for either testicular differentiation or spermatogenesis.

The Y Chromosome

The Y chromosome is the third smallest human chromosome, on average just larger than chromosomes 20 and 21 (248). The short arm is invariable in size whereas, among normal men, the long arm can vary considerably in length. The distal portion of the long arm exhibits brilliant fluorescence after quinacrine staining, with two or three separate fluorescent bands being visible in interphase nuclei (Fig. 2).

The Y chromosomes of all species, like many other chromosomes, contain satellites that are only visible under certain staining conditions. In the human Y chromosome, satellite DNAs are present both within a distal heterochromatin segment and in the centromeric region. The satellite DNA on the human Y chromosome, whose function is unknown, does not cross-hybridize with Y-chromosome-associated satellite DNA of other species (248).

Pairing of the X and Y Chromosomes

The two X chromosomes in females pair at the centromere and segregate during the first meiotic division of oogenesis by a mechanism analogous to the pairing of the autosomes. The X and Y chromosomes, like homologous autosomes, must also pair during meiosis to ensure that they segregate properly. However, the pairing of X and Y does not occur at the centromere but apparently occurs at a small region of homology between the short arm of the X and the short arm of the Y (30) (Fig. 3). In this way, they duplicate and partition evenly on the spindle. Thus at the second meiotic

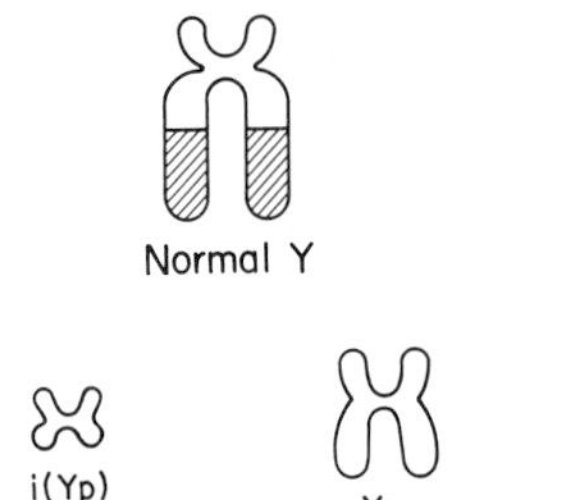

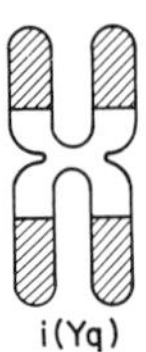

FIG. 2. Diagrams of normal and variant Y chromosomes. Cross-hatching indicates quinacrine-bright region of the long arm (Yq). Three abnormal types are depicted: i(Yp), isochrome of the short arm; i(Yq), isochrome of the long arm; Yq⁻, fragment arising as a result of loss of the distal long arm.

division, only two types of sperm are produced, those containing X and those containing Y chromosomes (227).

In some instances the pairing has been described as being "side by side"; in other instances, "end to end." In the hamster, where this has been studied extensively, there is considerable variability among strains (225). In any event, the net effect is the formation, during spermatogenesis, of the XY body (i.e., the condensed chromatin of the fused X and Y chromosomes), which is identifiable between zygotene and mid-pachytene (207,225).

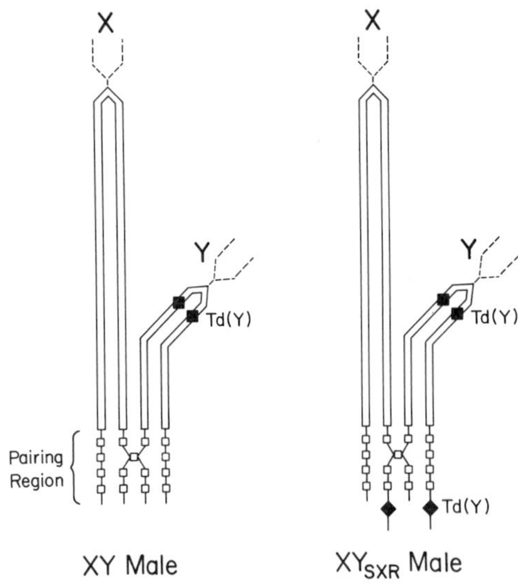

FIG. 3. Pairing of the X and Y chromosomes, and pseudoautosomal inheritance of the testis-determining region of the Y chromosome [Td(Y)].

Testis-Determining Genes

For the reasons mentioned above, the primary gene (or genes) that controls testicular differentiation is thought to be located on the Y chromosome. Analyses of structural abnormalities of the Y chromosome in humans have suggested that the short arm of the Y carries the responsible genes. Loss of the fluorescent segment of the long arm of the Y (Yq^-) (Fig. 2) or the formation of a Y "ring" chromosome (which requires loss of the distal-most segments of both the long and the short arms) does not interfere with the formation of a normal testis (47). An abnormal Y chromosome consisting of a duplicated short arm [$i(Y_p)$] also has no effect on male development. However, several examples of isochromosomes for the long arm of the Y [i(Yq)] (Fig. 2) have been observed to result in failure of testicular development, with subsequent formation of a female phenotype (18,102,129). It is therefore likely that the testis-determining gene(s) is located on the short arm of the Y near the centromere (243). Additional gene(s) on the short or long arms may be essential for normal spermatogenesis (64,100).

Homologous single-copy regions of the DNA of the human X and Y chromosomes have been identified with the use of restriction endonuclease techniques. These fragments appear to be unique to the human (e.g., different than the homologous regions in other species), and hence these regions, like the major repeat segments, are not thought to play a role in sexual differentiation (195). More importantly, some of the homologous regions appear to be on the tips of the short arms of the X and Y chromosomes (100) and are presumed to be the segments responsible for pairing of the two chromosomes during meiosis rather than to contain genes that specify gonadal development (Fig. 3). These pairing sequences are highly polymorphic; indeed almost every family appears to have unique segments (41).

About 70% of the DNA of the human Y chromosome consists of repeated sequences of DNA located on the long arm (41). These sequences are related, in an evolutionary sense, to sequences on the human X. Hence no detectable phenotypic effect results when the long arm of the Y becomes translocated onto autosomes. These long repetitive fragments of DNA of the Y chromosome in *Drosophila,* the mouse, and the human are composed of two repeating base quadruplets (GATA and GACA). In the human these repetitive fragments are believed to be responsible for fluorescence of the distal long arm of the Y and for much of the variability in length among normal Y chromosomes.

Sex-specific DNA was originally described in the W chromosomes of snakes and is now known to be conserved in many vertebrate species (69,132). In the mouse these sequences are concentrated on the short arm of the Y chromosome (e.g., near the site thought to contain the determinants of testicular differentiation), and these regions of DNA are transcribed into a male-specific RNA of 1,250 to 1,400 bases (70,223). However, there is considerable variability in the location and organization of these sequences among species, and it is thus unlikely that they are involved in sex determination (64).

The molecular basis by which a gene (or genes) on the Y chromosome promotes testicular differentiation is not known. A leading theory, based on a male-specific transplantation antigen, proposes that the Y chromosome specifies, or regulates, the production of a differentiative, cell-surface antigen that mediates transformation of the sexually indifferent gonad into a testis. This male-specific transplantation antigen was identified in certain inbred strains of mice in 1955 by Eichwald and Silmser (66). Female mice rejected skin grafts from male mice of the same strain. However, in the same strains, males do not reject skin grafts from females. The graft rejection in females was attributed to a transplantation antigen present only in the males. Presumably the only source of genetic incompatibility between males and females of this inbred strain of mouse was the Y chromosome. Therefore it was deduced that male-to-female skin graft rejection was caused by a Y-situated histocompatibility gene. This gene is termed the histocompatibility-Y (H-Y) gene (13).

In the early 1970s, male-specific antibodies were detected in the serum of female mice with male skin grafts, and serologic assays were developed for measuring the male antigen (94). Using these assays it was found that the presence of a testis is usually associated with the presence of serologically detected male antigen. Furthermore, the widespread phylogenetic conservation of H-Y antigen suggested that the antigen has an important biological function. Based on this evidence, it was proposed that the H-Y gene is, in fact, the testis-determining gene (250).

However, the H-Y antigen was originally defined on the basis of rejection of skin transplantation, e.g., a transplantation antigen, whereas the serological tests examine for the presence of an antigen on the surface of cells. It is difficult in most instances to be certain whether the two assays measure the same property; therefore the gene that determines the H-Y plasma membrane antigen may, in fact, not be identical to the gene that specifies H-Y transplantation antigen (219).

Subsequently, questions have also arisen as to whether the relationship between H-Y antigen and testicular development is actually one of cause and effect (42,103, 131,262,265). One of the complicating features of the thesis is that in birds, in which the female rather than the male is the heterogametic sex (e.g., ZW/ZZ species), the female is H-Y antigen positive (249,264). As pointed out by Ohno (190), it would be more straightforward to suppose that any testis inducer conserved throughout evolution would be present in all testis-bearing males, whether homogametic or heterogametic. The presence of H-Y antigen in female chickens is even more puzzling in view of the fact that administration of estradiol to ZZ male chicks causes a change in phenotype from $H\text{-}Y^-$ to $H\text{-}Y^+$ (249). A second problem is that some 45,X women with gonadal dysgenesis are H-

Y antigen positive (249), a finding that also does not fit with the original thesis. Furthermore, studies in the Sxr mouse have been interpreted as indicating that the testis-determining (Tdy) gene and the H-Y antigen gene are separate (174), although it is possible that the H-Y antigen gene codes for a factor essential for spermatogenesis (31). Even if the structural gene that specifies H-Y antigen (or a regulatory gene that controls expression of the antigen) is not the testis determinant, its location on the short arm of the Y chromosome may be so near the Tdy gene that accurate measurement of the H-Y antigen would be clinically useful, since its presence would correspond, in most instances, to the presence of the testis determinant.

Ovary-Determining Genes

Eicher and Washburn (63) have reported that genotypic males that carry a Y chromosome derived from a *Mus domesticus* strain on the genetic background of an inbred *Mus musculus* strain (C57BL/6J) develop ovaries or ovotestes. Sex reversal in these animals is apparently due to interaction between an autosomal recessive gene carried by C57BL/6J and the Y chromosome of *Mus domesticus*. Other autosomal testis-determining loci have subsequently been identified (64). Based on these results, Eicher and Washburn have proposed that, in addition to the testis-determining gene on the Y chromosome, autosomal genes are also necessary for normal gonadal differentiation and that there are also ovary-determining genes. According to their hypothesis, in XY individuals the testis-determining genes are activated prior to, and inactivate, ovary-determining gene(s). XX individuals lack the initial testis-determining gene, and hence the ovary-determining genes dominate. Mutations of the testis-determining loci that interfere with the timely and coordinated expression of these genes may result in failure of suppression of ovarian determinants, with subsequent development of ovarian tissue in XY individuals.

X-Chromosome Inactivation During Spermatogenesis

Soon after implantation of the eutherian embryo, X chromosomes in excess of one are randomly inactivated in somatic cells (81,158,160). The X-chromosome inactivation in somatic cells is associated with chemical modification of the DNA (263) and the formation of a heterochromatin body in cells of the female (9,192).

The formation, during spermatogenesis, of the XY body in pachytene is associated with features typical of X-chromosome inactivation, namely, late replication of the X chromosome (and presumably late replication of the Y chromosome as well) (189) and decreased incorporation of radioactive uridine into messenger-like RNA (181). The concept that a functional X chromosome is not essential for testicular differentiation is supported by the finding that, in the creeping vole, the X chromosome is eliminated (by nondisjunction) during spermatogenesis so that the germ cell lines in the male are OY in composition (193). This also suggests that an X chromosome is not necessary for the formation of fertile sperm. Additional evidence in support of this view has come from studies of translocations of X chromosomes to autosomes in the mouse. Some of these translocations impair spermatogenesis, presumably by impairing X inactivation in primary spermatocytes (76,77, 153,154,212). The mechanism of X-chromosome inactivation during spermatogenesis appears to be fundamentally different than the random X-chromosome inactivation that occurs in the autosomes of XX females. The latter type of X-inactivation is associated with chemical modification of the DNA (263), whereas the X-chromosome DNA from sperm is functional in *in vitro* transcriptional assays and is presumably not modified (241).

Development of a Testis in the Absence of a Y Chromosome

Study of several disorders that result from the alteration of the number or structure of the X and Y chromosomes has provided insight into the control of sexual differentiation. Disorders in which a testis develops in the apparent absence of a Y chromosome have been particularly informative in this regard.

The XX Male

The sex-reversal mutation in the mouse (Sxr), which causes XX genotypic females to develop as phenotypic (albeit infertile) males (38), was originally assumed to be inherited as an autosomally linked gene; subsequent linkage studies in several laboratories failed to substantiate this view.

In 1982, Singh and Jones (222) detected a Y-specific DNA fragment on the distal end of an X chromosome in XX_{Sxr} metaphase chromosomes. This finding, coupled with the formulation of Burgoyne (29) that crossing over can occur in the pairing region of the X and Y chromosome during meiosis, provides an explanation for the apparent (pseudo) autosomal inheritance of the Sxr mutation. In support of this interpretation, an additional fragment has been identified at the distal end of the Y chromosome in XY_{Sxr} carrier males and at the distal end of one X chromosome in XX_{Sxr} males (71).

Thus, it is now possible to explain testicular development in the Sxr mouse in the absence of a Y chromosome (171). The testis-determining portion of the Y chromosome is present as a duplicated element on the distal pairing region of the Y chromosome in XY_{Sxr} male mice. Translocation of this duplicated testis-determining region to an X chromosome during meiosis can cause testicular differentiation in XX males (Fig. 3). Nevertheless, fertility does not occur on the background of an XX chromosome composition. In this sense, this disorder is a phenocopy of the 47,XXY Klinefelter's syndrome, involving a Y fragment rather than an intact Y chromosome (see above).

A disorder similar to that of the Sxr mouse occurs in humans. The incidence of the 46,XX karyotype in phenotypic men is approximately 1 in 20,000 to 24,000 male births (49,50). Clinical features include small, firm testes (generally less than 2 ml in volume), normal male wolffian duct derivatives, and male external genitalia. Azoospermia and hence infertility are invariably present (197,215). 46,XX men resemble Klinefelter's syndrome subjects (209).

Four theories were proposed to explain the pathogenesis of the human disorder: (i) mosaicism for a Y-containing cell line or early loss of a Y chromosome in an individual who was originally 47,XXY; (ii) an autosomal gene mutation that acts independently of a Y chromosome; (iii) deletion or inactivation of an X-chromosome gene that normally has a negative regulatory effect on testis development; or (iv) interchange of a Y-chromosome fragment with the X chromosome, analogous to the situation in the Sxr mouse (50). Most cases in the human appear to be a result of the latter mechanism because most XX males, like the XX_{Sxr} mouse, contain Y-specific DNA on the tip of the X chromosome (4,51,111,243). Additional genes encoded on the human X and Y chromosomes are also inherited in a pseudoautosomal fashion (40,211,220), and at least one of these pseudoautosomal genes, *MIC2,* is located sufficiently close to the testis-determining gene(s) on the short arm of the Y to be a potential marker for the testis determinant(s) (101). The human testis determinant(s) also maps to the short arm of the Y chromosome (243).

True Hermaphroditism

True hermaphroditism is a condition in which both an ovary and a testis, or a gonad with histologic features of both ovary and testis (ovotestis), are present (238–240). To justify the diagnosis in the human, both types of gonadal epithelium must be present. The presence of ovarian stroma without oocytes is not sufficient. True hermaphroditism is actually several different disorders (221). About two-thirds of human subjects have a 46,XX karyotype, one-tenth have a 46,XY karyotype, and the remainder are chromosomal mosaics, i.e., either 46,XX/46,XY or 45,X/46,XY chimeras. Instances of true hermaphroditism associated with mosaicism are generally assumed to be clonal in origin, with the X- or XX-containing cells giving rise to ovarian cell lines and the Y-containing cell lines giving rise to testicular elements. XY true hermaphroditism is assumed to be caused by a mutation in the testis-determining gene(s) that impairs suppression of the ovarian determinants in some cells (63–65).

Hermaphroditism in the presence of an XX karyotype, like the XX male syndrome, is an apparent contradiction to the axiom that a Y chromosome is necessary for testicular differentiation. Possible explanations include (a) undetected loss of a Y chromosome after initiation of testicular development or undetected chromosomal mosaicism or chimerism, (b) translocation of testicular determinants from the Y to the X chromosome or to an autosome, or (c) a single gene mutation. In all instances reported to date, 46,XX true hermaphrodites are H-Y antigen positive, including the XX form of true hermaphroditism in the dog (19,213,217). Although several family aggregates of 46,XX true hermaphroditism have been reported (6,39,80,156,185,210), most are sporadic in nature. The available data in the familial cases are compatible with either autosomal recessive inheritance, new autosomal dominant mutations, or translocation of a fragment of a Y chromosome in a paternal line. In addition, two families have been reported in which one affected member was a 46,XX male and the other was a 46,XX true hermaphrodite (11,140).

Insight into the pathogenesis of the XX true hermaphrodite has come from studying the Sxr mouse. According to the Lyon hypothesis, extragonadal cells in the female have only one active X chromosome; additional X chromosomes are inactivated and form the sex chromatin bodies characteristic of the nuclei of female cells (159). In normal females, X inactivation is random and occurs early in embryonic life so that, in individual cells, either the maternal- or paternal-derived X chromosome remains active (159). This random inactivation is believed to be operative in all somatic cells of the female; however, in the ovary, X inactivation differs from that in other tissues. By studying women heterozygous for electrophoretic variants of the X-linked enzyme glucose-6-phosphate dehydrogenase, it was shown that oocytes both from adult and from fetal ovaries (82,83) express both X-linked alleles. Furthermore, both X chromosomes appear to be active in germ cells prior to entering meiosis (178). However, Kratzer and Chapman (149) have shown that, up to day 10 of embryogenesis, only one X chromosome is active in the embryonic mouse ovary and that the inactive X is reactivated as germ cells enter meiosis. Thus, random X inactivation occurs in ovarian development, as in other tissues of the female, and reactivation of the inactivated X subsequently occurs in the oogonia. To summarize: In testicular development the single X chromosome appears to be inactivated as a part of the XY body; in oogenesis, however, one of two X chromosomes is active during organogenesis of the ovary, and both X chromosomes are active during oogenesis itself. Random X-chromosome inactivation of the Lyon type involves chemical modification of the DNA and hence is thought to occur by a different mechanism than that responsible for X-chromosome inactivation in the XY body (241,263).

X-autosome translocations have been described in mice in which the normal X chromosome (i.e., those not undergoing autosomal translocation) is preferentially inactivated (191). When XY_{Sxr} mice are crossed with female mice carrying such an X-autosome translocation trait (216) (the translocated X is designated X_T), the $X_{Sxr}X_T$ offspring develop as sterile males, fertile females, or hermaphrodites (37,173). This finding can most simply be explained by assuming that the region of the X chromosome that carries the Sxr and the Tdy genes is inactivated in some cells but not others.

Inactivation is conceived as spreading to a variable extent from the inactive X chromatin to the Sxr fragment, and it is assumed that the extent of inactivation is transmittable to progeny cells after the time of X-chromosome inactivation during embryogenesis. In effect, such 46,XX individuals are mosaics, with some cell lines expressing Sxr and some not. The sex of the gonads (and hence the aggregate sex of the individual) depends on the proportion of cells expressing Sxr in the gonad primordia. If 30% of the cells in a gonadal primordia are XY, a normal testis will develop. When the X chromosome containing the Sxr gene is paired with an X_T, X_TX_{Sxr} females and hermaphrodites will occur at a low, but measurable, frequency. However, when the X chromosome to which Sxr is attached is paired with a normal X chromosome, half of the cells will express Sxr; hence, the majority of individuals will be sterile males, and females and hermaphrodites are rare.

At a theoretical level, the same type of disorder, namely duplication of the male-determining gene(s) on the Y chromosome and translocation of these genes onto the X chromosome, could explain the development of either the XX male or the XX true hermaphrodite, depending on the *completeness* and *frequency* of the inactivation of such testis-determining genes during the embryogenesis of the XX individual carrying such a translocation trait. (It has yet to be proven that this model can explain the potential fertility of the XX true hermaphrodite.) This model has two implications for the human disorder: (i) It implies that testis-determining genes, and hence Y-chromosome fragments, will be detectable in cells from 46,XX true hermaphrodites as well as from 46,XX men, and (ii) if the translocation is to an X chromosome (as in the case of the mouse Sxr) and not to an autosome, it explains why the XX male is more common than the XX true hermaphrodite.

GONADAL SEX

Embryonic Development

The gonad develops as a stratification of the coelomic epithelium on the medial aspect of the mesonephric kidney (the urogenital ridge) around the fourth week of gestational development in the human. Most of the cell types of the gonads are derived from the mesoderm cells of the urogenital ridges. The primordial germ cells originate, however, outside the area of the presumptive gonad and are initially identifiable in the entoderm of the yolk sac. The germ cells, which are derived from primitive ectodermal cells of the inner cell mass (81), are distinguished from other cells of the developing embryo because of their large size as well as their large round nuclei and clear cytoplasm. Histochemically, they are characterized by high alkaline phosphatase activity and glycogen (169). The mechanism by which the germ cells differentiate from other cell types is not understood, but the process must commence early in embryogenesis because primordial germ cells have been recognized in the $4\frac{1}{2}$-day-old human blastocyst (114). At the beginning of the fourth week of development the germ cells commence to migrate by ameboid movement (15,78,261) through the gut entoderm and into the mesoderm of the mesentery, finally ending up in the coelomic epithelium of the gonadal ridges. It is not known what entices the primordial germ cells to migrate to this area. However, once there, the primitive gonocytes move from the epithelium into the gonadal parenchyma, and lose their motile characteristics (60). Closely attached epithelial cells move with them into the underlying mesenchyme. The formation of the gonadal blastema is completed by weeks 5 to 6 of gestation in human embryos. At this time the primitive ("indifferent") gonad is composed of three distinct cell types: (i) germ cells, (ii) supporting cells of the coelomic epithelium of the gonadal ridge that give rise to the Sertoli cells of the testis and the granulosa cells of the ovary, and (iii) stromal (interstitial) cells derived from the original mesenchyme of the gonadal ridge.

Histological Differentiation of the Fetal Gonad

The first morphological sign of sexual dimorphism in the gonads is the development of the primordial Sertoli cells and their aggregation into spermatogenic cords in the fetal testis (139). In the human this occurs between weeks 6 and 7 of gestational development (130). In contrast to the early development of the fetal testis, the fetal ovary shows no characteristic development until months later in embryogenesis and initially is identified histologically early only by exclusion. At weeks 6 to 7 of gestation in the human, the ovarian epithelial components form irregular groups of cells around the primordial germ cells. At about the sixth month, the primitive granulosa cells organize around the dividing oocytes to form a single layer of follicular cells, thus establishing the primordial follicle (93). In general, gonadogenesis in other mammalian species is similar to that in humans in that histologic differentiation of the fetal testis precedes that of the fetal ovary by days to weeks.

The Role of the Germ Cells in Gonadal Development

It seems unlikely that gonadal development or differentiation is dependent on the presence or type of germ cell that migrates into the coelomic epithelium of the gonadal ridge. Neither selective destruction of germ cells with drugs (175) nor surgical excision of primordial germ cells in the anterior germinal crest before they reach the gonadal primordium (168) inhibits gonadal development. Furthermore, mutant mice homozygous for the atrichosis gene are genetically deficient in germ cells, yet Sertoli cells differentiate and aggregate into tubules that are devoid of germ cells (112). Thus, it appears that the somatic cells can organize into an ovary or a testis irrespective of the presence or absence of the germ cells.

Endocrine Differentiation of the Testis

By demonstrating that castration of sexually indifferent rabbit embryos invariably results in female development of embryos of both sexes (Fig. 4), Jost (136,138) established that the induced phenotype in mammals is male and that secretions from the fetal testes are necessary for male development. Development of the female urogenital tract occurs in the absence of gonads and apparently does not require secretions from the fetal ovaries. Furthermore, Jost deduced that two substances from the fetal testes are essential for male development: (i) a nonsteroid hormone that acts ipsilaterally to cause regression of the mullerian duct (mullerian-inhibiting substance) and (ii) an androgenic steroid responsible for virilization of the wolffian duct, urogenital sinus, and urogenital tubercle.

Mullerian-Inhibiting Substance

Mullerian-inhibiting substance is a large (~140,000 daltons) dimeric glycoprotein formed by the Sertoli cells of the fetal and newborn testis (56,58,202,203,234,247). It is thought to act locally to suppress mullerian duct development rather than as a circulating hormone (238; however, see ref. 119). Monoclonal antibodies to mullerian-inhibiting substance (186,246) block mullerian duct regression in a species-specific manner in *in vitro* bioassays (245), as well as *in vivo* (235). Although mullerian duct regression begins in the male embryo shortly after formation of the spermatic cords in the fetal testis (14) the secretion of mullerian-inhibiting substance is independent of spermatogenic tubule formation in the testis (166).

Even though they are not primarily responsible for mullerian duct regression, androgens and estrogens appear to influence the process. For example, regression of rat mullerian ducts in organ culture is enhanced by testosterone, although testosterone alone is inactive (74,124). Interestingly, neither dihydrotestosterone nor estradiol affects mullerian duct regression in this system. In other systems, estrogens interfere with mullerian duct regression (120, 122,144,170,228,232). Thus, although mullerian-inhibiting substance is required for mullerian duct regression, steroid hormones appear to influence its action.

The concept that mullerian duct regression in male development is an active process is supported by studies of the persistent mullerian duct syndrome in the human (5,20,21,224). In this disorder, genetic and phenotypic males have fallopian tubes and a uterus (in addition to normal wolffian-duct-derived structures) as the result of either an autosomal or an X-linked gene defect. The pathogenesis of the disorder is uncertain, but is probably due to either a failure of production of mullerian-inhibiting substance by the fetal testis or a failure of the tissue to respond to the hormone.

Persistence of the mullerian ducts is usually accompanied by failure of the testes to descend (133). Furthermore, mullerian-inhibiting activity is lower in biopsied testicular cells from newborn boys with cryptorchidism than from normal newborns (57). Therefore, it is conceivable that mullerian-

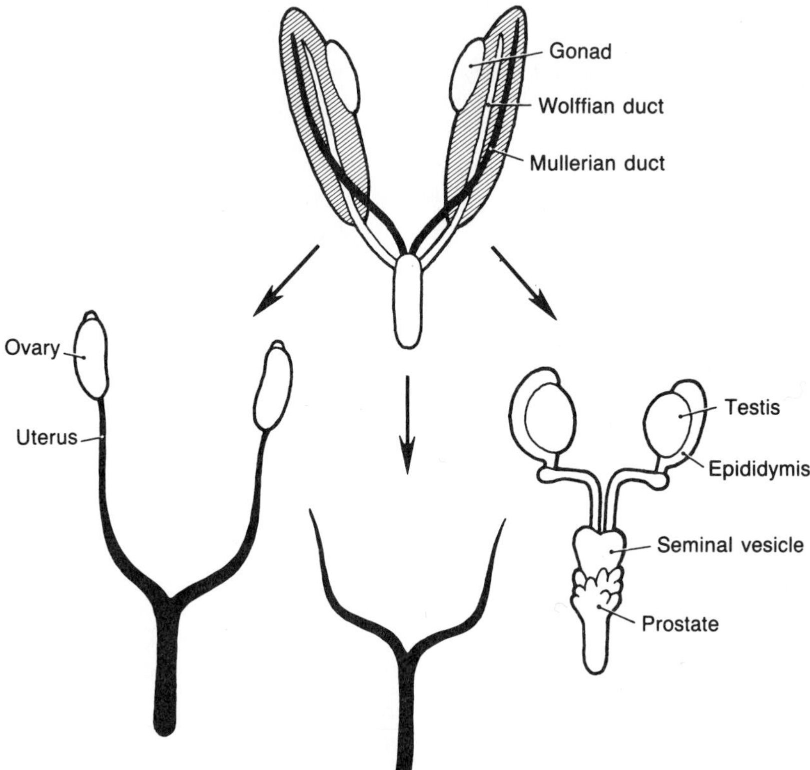

FIG. 4. Fetal castration experiment of Jost. The indifferent urogenital tract (*top*) undergoes male differentiation (*bottom right*) if a testis develops, or female differentiation (*bottom left*) if an ovary develops. Embryos castrated prior to sexual differentiation develop as phenotypic females (*bottom middle*). (Adapted from ref. 138.)

inhibiting substance plays a role in testicular descent, possibly by influencing the cranial anchoring of the testis to the peritoneal fold.

Androgen

The second developmental hormone of the fetal testis was identified by Jost as an androgenic steroid (136). Testosterone, the principal testicular androgen formed in postnatal life, is also the androgenic steroid formed by the testes of rabbit and human embryos during male phenotypic development (155,218,259). Testosterone formation in the testis begins shortly after the onset of differentiation of the spermatogenic cords and is concomitant with the histological differentiation of the Leydig cells (38,98).

The critical role of testosterone in the development of the male urogenital tract was deduced from three types of embryologic and endocrinologic evidence. First, as shown in Fig. 5, the fact that testosterone synthesis immediately precedes the initiation of virilization of the urogenital tract in a variety of species suggested a cause-and-effect relationship between the two events (7,155,208,218,259). Second, the administration of androgens to female embryos at the appropriate time in fetal development causes male development of the internal and external genitalia (214). And third, administration of pharmacologic agents that inhibit the synthesis or action of androgens in embryogenesis impairs male development (95,187).

This concept, furthermore, has been substantiated on genetic grounds. In the human, five single-gene defects in androgen synthesis are known to cause inadequate testosterone synthesis and incomplete virilization of the male embryo (107,257). Severely affected males may develop as phenotypic women, with complete failure of virilization of the wolffian ducts, urogenital sinus, and external genitalia. At the other extreme, mildly affected men appear normal, except for developmental abnormalities such as hypospadias. The fact that the fallopian tubes and uterus are absent in such patients indicates that regression of the mullerian ducts takes place normally during embryogenesis and that mullerian regression is not primarily dependent on testosterone biosynthesis and action.

Regulation of testosterone synthesis in the fetal testis. Many questions concerning the regulation of testosterone synthesis and secretion by the fetal testis are not resolved. The enzymatic differentiation of the fetal gonads that underlies the onset of endocrine function has been characterized in detail in the rabbit embryo. Enzymatic differentiation of fetal ovaries and testes in this species is apparent by day 18 of gestation and is manifested by an increase in the rate of 3β-hydroxysteroid dehydrogenase activity in the fetal testis and by an increase in aromatase activity in the fetal ovary (179). At this time of development, activities of all other enzymes in the pathway of steroid hormone synthesis are similar in the ovaries and testes (Fig. 6) (90).

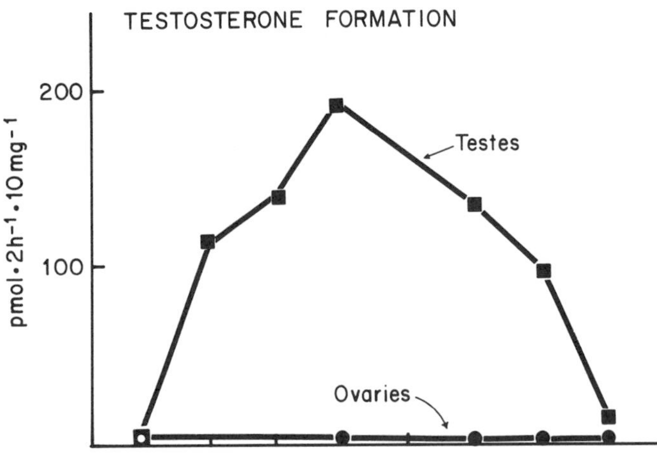

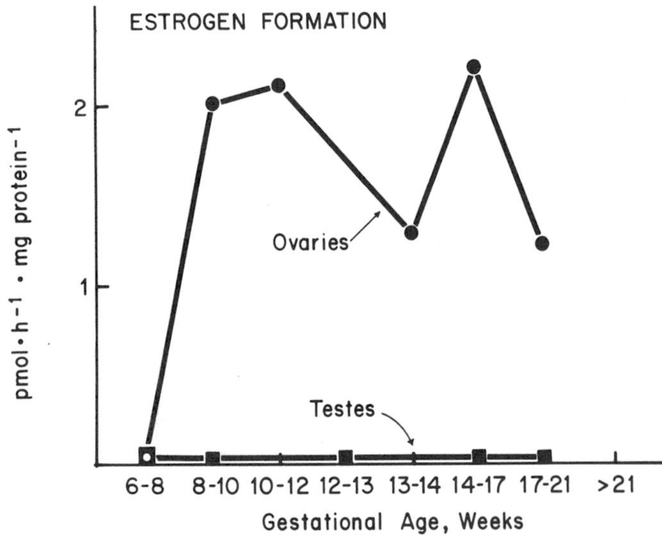

FIG. 5. Enzymatic differentiation of the human fetal gonad. (Adapted from refs. 86 and 218.)

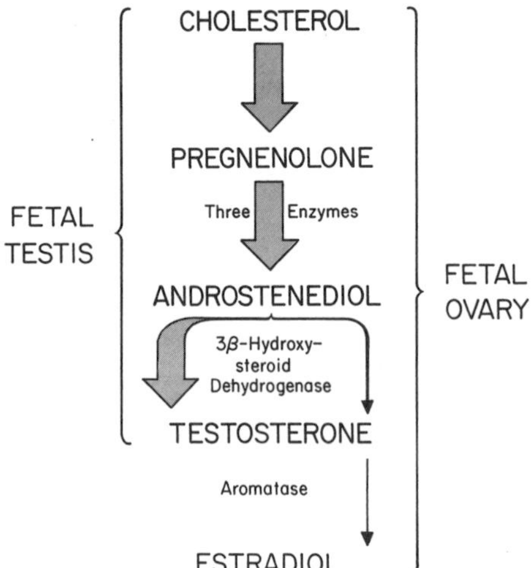

FIG. 6. Enzymatic differentiation of fetal rabbit ovaries and testes on day 18 of gestation.

Thus, in the rabbit, changes in the rates of only a few enzymatic reactions in the gonads at a critical time in embryonic development have profound consequences for sexual differentiation. Furthermore, this enzymatic differentiation appears to be an autonomous function of the steroidogenic cells, because it occurs at the appropriate time in fetal testes cultured in defined medium without hormones (88,89) as well as in testes that fail to develop spermatogenic cords (196).

Whether the actual rate of testosterone production in the rabbit fetal testis is regulated by fetal and/or placental gonadotropins at the onset of testosterone synthesis is not clear. On the one hand, receptors for luteinizing hormone (LH) are present in fetal rabbit testes at the time of initial testosterone synthesis (36); furthermore, these LH receptors are functional, as evidenced by the enhancement of testicular cyclic AMP formation (89) and cholesterol side-chain cleavage activity (90) by human chorionic gonadotropin. On the other hand, basal, unstimulated cholesterol side-chain cleavage activity in fetal rabbit testes in the absence of gonadotropin stimulation appears to be sufficient to provide enough steroid substrate to support testosterone synthesis at a maximum rate during the initial period of male phenotypic development. Later in embryogenesis, when sexual differentiation is far advanced, testosterone synthesis is enhanced by gonadotropin treatment (90). As a consequence, we believe that in rabbits the onset of testosterone synthesis and the resulting differentiation of the male urogenital tract are independent of gonadotropin control.

It is uncertain whether a similar situation exists in embryonic sexual differentiation in humans. LH receptors are present in human fetal testes as early as the twelfth week of gestation (117,180), and human fetal testes respond to human chorionic gonadotropin stimulation by exhibiting increased testosterone synthesis at this time (117). It is not known what happens between weeks 8 and 11, when the major portion of male phenotypic differentiation takes place. Because testosterone synthesis is gonadotropin dependent during the latter two-thirds of gestation, analogous to the situation in the rabbit embryo, it follows that those aspects of male sexual development that take place during this time—growth of the penis and descent of the testes—are probably gonadotropin-dependent in all species (206).

Endocrine Differentiation of the Ovary

In many if not most species, endocrine differentiation of the fetal ovary, as evidenced by the appearance of the capacity to synthesize estrogen, occurs simultaneously with the development of the ability of the fetal testis to synthesize testosterone (Fig. 5) (86,179). Although estrogen formation is not essential for normal female phenotypic development (136), estrogen may play a role in the development of the ovary itself. The change in the developing ovary that correlates with the onset of estrogen synthesis is the accumulation of lipid in the primitive granulosa cells (99).

Possible Role of Steroid Hormones in Gonadal Differentiation

In some species it is possible to influence gonadal differentiation with sex hormones (reviewed in ref. 33). For example, in the embryonic male (ZZ) bird, treatment with estrogens during embryonic development leads to the development of an ovotestis. In amphibians and fish, treatment with steroid hormones of the opposite sex can lead to sex reversal of the gonads. In contrast with the striking effects of sex hormones on the differentiation of the gonads of birds and amphibians is the apparent failure to obtain comparable effects in mammalian embryos (25,104,135,237,252,253). Nevertheless, the bipotentiality of the indifferent mammalian gonad is suggested by transplantation experiments. Although it is felt that the testicular primordium represents remarkable stability in its development, fetal ovarian development appears to be more malleable. For example, several investigators have reported that fetal rodent ovaries develop "testis-like" structures when transplanted into male hosts (34,116,167,182,230,233), and these grafted fetal ovaries secrete testosterone *in vitro* (231). Thus in some situations, mammalian gonadal differentiation also appears to be influenced by the endocrine environment.

PHENOTYPIC SEX

Urogenital Tract Development During the Indifferent Phase

Prior to the eighth week of human development, the urogenital tract is identical in the two sexes. The internal accessory organs of reproduction develop from a dual duct system (wolffian and mullerian) that forms within the mesonephric kidney early in embryogenesis (Fig. 7). Within the substance of the mesonephros, tubules connect primitive capillary networks with a longitudinal mesonephric (wolffian) duct. The wolffian duct extends caudally to the primitive urogenital sinus. At about 6 weeks the development of the paramesonephric (mullerian) ducts begins in embryos of both sexes as an evagination in the coelomic epithelium, just lateral to the wolffian ducts. This evagination develops into a tubular structure, the caudal end of which becomes intimately associated with the wolffian duct (i.e., no basement membrane separates their epithelia) (110). Whether the mullerian duct "splits off" from the wolffian duct in its later caudal development to become an independent duct system emptying into the urogenital sinus or whether the wolffian duct simply acts as a guide for the subsequent evolution of the mullerian duct from the coelomic epithelium is uncertain. However, mullerian duct development cannot take place in the absence of the wolffian duct (110). At the

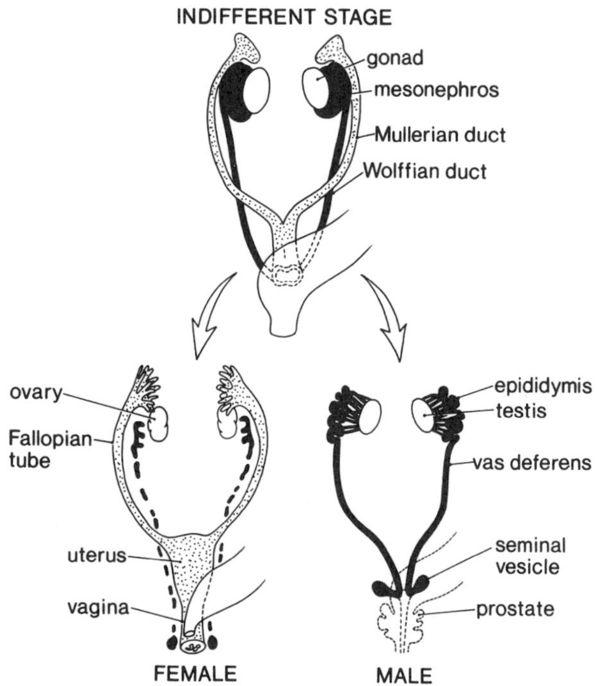

FIG. 7. Differentiation of the internal genitalia. (From ref. 256.)

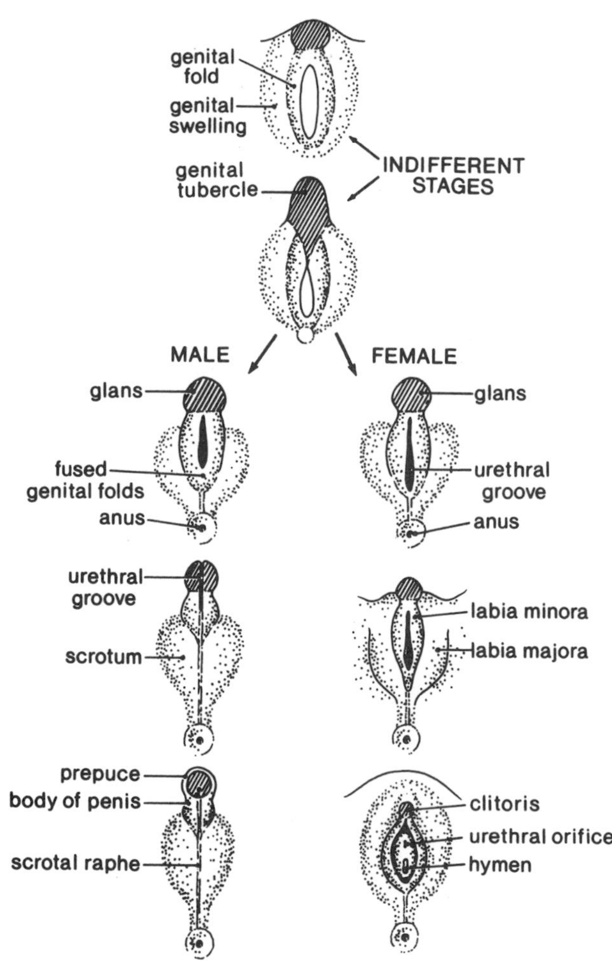

FIG. 8. Differentiation of the external genitalia. (From ref. 256.)

end of the indifferent phase of phenotypic sexual differentiation (prior to week 8 of gestation), a dual duct system (wolffian and mullerian) constitutes the anlagen of the internal accessory organs of reproduction (Fig. 7). The termination of the mesonephric ducts in the urogenital sinus divides the sinus into an upper and a lower portion. The upper portion, the vesicourethral canal, is involved in the development of the bladder and the upper urethra. The lower portion contributes to the development of the external genitalia.

Prior to week 6 of gestation, the anlagen of the external genitalia are also indistinguishable in the two sexes. The genital eminence is a rounded mass between the umbilicus and the tail (226) and is composed of a genital tubercle flanked by prominent genital swellings. The opening of the urogenital sinus between the genital swellings (the urethral groove) is surrounded by genital folds (Fig. 8). At week 7 of gestation in the human, the genital tubercle begins to elongate; a shallow, circular depression defines the glans of the tubercle. At this stage of development, there are no remarkable differences between the external genitalia of male and female embryos.

Male Development

The first sign of male differentiation of the urogenital tract is degeneration of the mullerian ducts adjacent to the testes, a process that begins just after formation of the spermatogenic cords in the testes. Eventually, the mullerian ducts of the male undergo almost complete regression.

The transformation of the wolffian ducts into the male reproductive tract begins subsequent to the onset of mullerian duct regression. The portion of the wolffian duct adjacent to the testis becomes convoluted to form the epididymis; the central portion of the duct becomes the muscular vas deferens. The seminal vesicles develop as buds off the lower portions of the wolffian ducts just before they enter into the urogenital sinus. The prostatic and membranous portions of the male urethra develop from the pelvic portion of the urogenital sinus. The prostate originates as a series of endothermal buds off this portion of the urogenital sinus (10,143,157).

The external genitalia of the male begin to develop shortly after the onset of virilization of the wolffian ducts and urogenital sinus (Fig. 8). The genital tubercle elongates, and the urethral folds begin to fuse over the urethral groove from posterior to anterior. The two urogenital swellings move posterior to the genital tubercle and eventually fuse to form the scrotum. The elongated urogenital cleft becomes closed to form the penile urethra (Fig. 8). These events in male development are completed relatively early (during the first trimester) in human fetal development and are dependent on hormonal secretions from the testis.

Two aspects of male phenotypic development take place during the late phases of virilization. The first involves growth of the male phallus. Just after closure of the male urethra is complete, there is little difference in the size of the genital tubercle in the two sexes. However, under the influence of androgens from the fetal testis, the male phallus grows during the latter phases of fetal development and by the time of birth is much larger than the urogenital tubercle of the female.

Testicular descent also takes place during later stages of fetal development (92). Testicular descent is both complex and incompletely understood. For didactic purposes, the process can be divided into three phases. The first phase (transabdominal movement) involves, at a minimum, degeneration of the portion of the peritoneal fold that anchors the cranial part of the gonad to the abdominal wall, shortening of the caudal gonadal ligament (gubernaculum), and rapid growth of the abdominal-pelvic region of the fetus. As a result, the testis comes to rest against the anterior abdominal wall in the inguinal region. The second phase involves formation of the processus vaginalis and development of the inguinal canal and scrotum. Increasing intraabdominal pressure is believed to cause a herniation in the abdominal wall (the processus vaginalis) along the course of the inguinal portion of the gubernaculum. Continued pressure causes enlargement of the processus vaginalis around the gubernaculum and leads to formation of the inguinal canal. The gubernaculum increases in size until the diameter of the inguinal canal approaches that of the testis. In the final stage of testicular descent the abdominal testis traverses the inguinal canal and comes to rest in the scrotum. Descent of the testis into the scrotum probably involves a progressive degeneration of the proximal portion of the gubernaculum. Although the process is at least, in part, androgen dependent (206), the early stages (e.g., transabdominal movement) of testicular descent may be the result of other factors (118).

Female Development

The internal reproductive tract of the female is formed from the mullerian ducts; the wolffian ducts persist only in remnant form. The cephalic ends of the mullerian ducts (the portions derived from coelomic epithelium) are the anlagen of the fallopian tubes, whereas the caudal portions fuse to form the uterus (Fig. 7). Contact of the mullerian ducts with the urogenital sinus induces formation of the uterovaginal plate (an intense proliferation of endodermal cells) between the mullerian ducts and the urogenital sinus (194). Although it is felt that both the mullerian ducts and wolffian ducts contribute to the formation of the uterovaginal plate, the relative degree to which they contribute is unknown (16,28,110). The cells of the uterovaginal plate proliferate, thus increasing the distance between the uterus and the urogenital sinus (Fig. 9). Later, the central cells of this plate break down to form the lumen of the vagina.

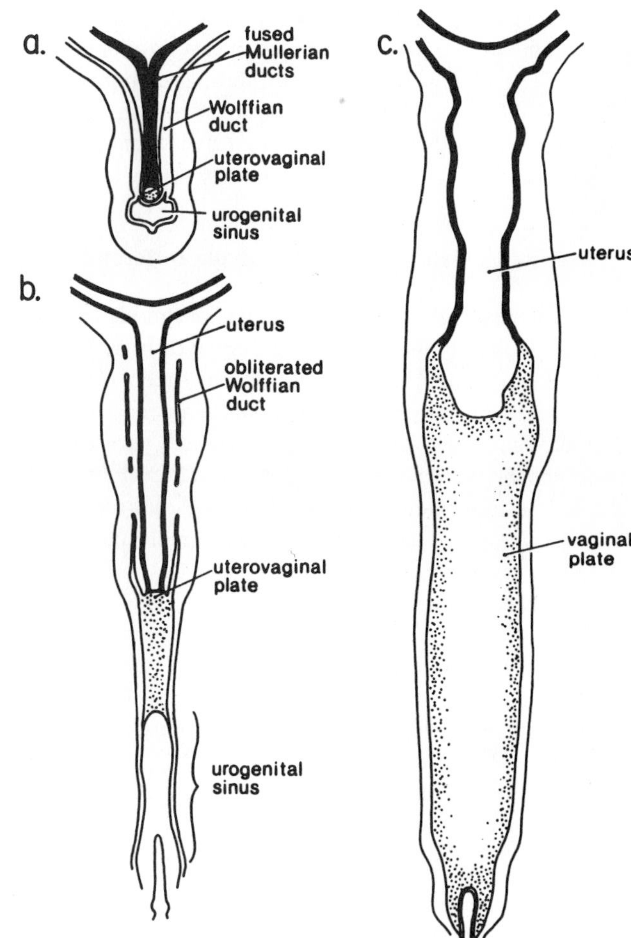

FIG. 9. Development of the uterus and vagina. (From ref. 256.)

In contrast to the male, in which the phallic and pelvic portions of the urogenital sinus are enclosed by fusion of the genital swellings, most of the urogenital sinus of the female remains exposed on the surface as a cleft into which the vagina and urethra open (Fig. 8). The urogenital tubercle in the female undergoes limited growth and development to form the clitoris.

Breast Development in Both Sexes

Breast development occurs along "mammary lines," which are bilateral epidermal thickenings that extend from the forelimbs to the hindlimbs on the ventral surface of the embryo. In human development, these "mammary lines" largely disappear except for a small portion on each side of the thoracic region that condenses and penetrates the underlying mesenchyme. This single pair of mammary buds undergoes little change until the fifth month of human development, when secondary epithelial buds appear and nipples develop. Proliferation of the ductules occurs throughout the remainder of gestation so that, by the time of birth, 15 to 25 separate glands are present, each of which is connected to the exterior through the nipple. In some species, breast development in males is inhibited by androgens during embryogenesis (96,126,147), but this does not occur in humans; the development of the breast in boys and girls is identical prior to puberty (200).

Endocrine Control of Male Phenotypic Differentiation

As a consequence of experiments demonstrating that castration of sexually indifferent rabbit embryos invariably results in female development (Fig. 4), Jost recognized that the induced phenotype in mammalian embryos was male and that secretions from the fetal testis were necessary for male phenotypic development (136,137). Development of the female urogenital tract apparently does not require secretions from the fetal ovaries, since female phenotypic development occurs in the absence of gonads. Furthermore, Jost deduced that two substances from the fetal testes are essential for male development: (i) a polypeptide that acts ipsilaterally to cause regression of the mullerian ducts and (ii) an androgenic steroid, testosterone, responsible for virilization of the wolffian duct, urogenital sinus, and genital tubercle.

Mechanism of Action of Mullerian-Inhibiting Substance

The initial endocrine function of the fetal testis is probably secretion of the protein hormone that causes regression of the mullerian ducts, namely, mullerian-inhibiting substance. Although mullerian-inhibiting substance has been purified and much is known about the structure of the protein itself (26,54,134) and about the genes that code for the protein in humans and cows (35,201), the mechanism of action of the hormone is poorly understood. Dissolution of the basement membrane and condensation of the mesenchymal cells around the ducts is an early event in mullerian duct regression (62,113,204,236). Mullerian-inhibiting substance may act by modulating cell-surface protein phosphorylation in a manner similar to the mechanism of action of epidermal growth factor (57,121).

The finding that partially purified mullerian-inhibiting substance is cytotoxic to a human ovarian-cancer-derived cell line, but not to cell lines derived from an adenocarcinoma of the colon, raises the possibility that mullerian-inhibiting substance may also inhibit growth of malignant tumors of the female genital tract (55,59,79).

Mechanism of Androgen Action

Basic model. The current concept of how androgens act within target cells is schematically depicted in Fig. 10. Testosterone, the major androgen secreted by the testis and circulating in plasma, is thought to enter target tissues by a passive diffusion process. In some cells, testosterone is converted to dihydrotestosterone by a 5α-reductase enzyme present within the cells. In androgen target tissues, testosterone or dihydrotestosterone binds to a specific high-affinity, intracellular receptor protein. Subsequently the hormone-receptor complex undergoes a poorly understood transformation process in which the hormone-receptor complex acquires the capacity to bind to DNA and other anionic substances. It is not clear whether the primary hormone-receptor interaction takes place in the nucleus or the cytoplasm. However, the transformed nuclear hormone-receptor complexes are presumed to interact with specific acceptor sites on the chromosomes. The nature of the acceptor sites within the nucleus (i.e., whether protein or DNA) and their number are not clear, but the consequence of the interaction of the hormone-receptor complexes with chromatin is to increase the transcription of tissue-specific structural genes, with the subsequent appearance of new messenger RNAs and new proteins in the cytoplasm of the cell. If the androgen-receptor system is analogous to other steroid hormone systems, it is likely that the androgen-receptor complexes bind to DNA at specific regulatory sites near the structural genes under regulatory control by the hormones (48,199). On the basis of a variety of evidence (see below), it is now felt that testosterone-receptor complexes mediate fetal wolffian duct virilization and that dihydrotestosterone-receptor complexes mediate differentiation of the male external genitalia.

The androgen receptors from fetal urogenital sinus and urogenital tubercles appear to be identical to those of adult prostate (84), so that the hormone is presumed to act by the same mechanism in embryonic as in postnatal life. 5α-Dihydrotestosterone binds to the androgen receptor of most species with greater affinity than does testosterone (84,146, 165,254), and the dihydrotestosterone-receptor complex is

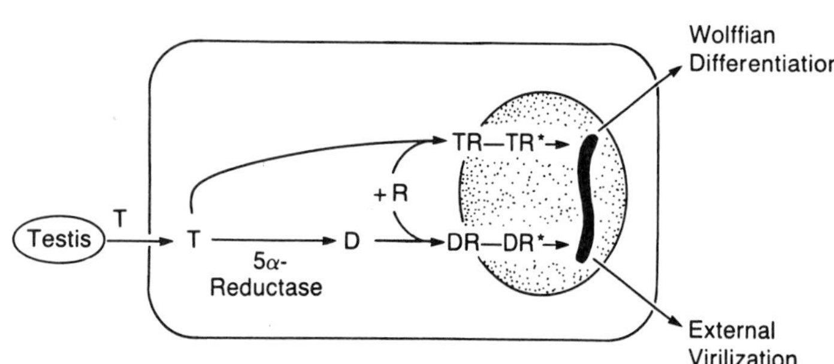

FIG. 10. Androgen action. (T) Testosterone; (D) dihydrotestosterone; (R) androgen receptor; (R*) transformed androgen receptor.

more readily transformed to the DNA-binding state than is the testosterone-receptor complex (145). The net consequence is that dihydrotestosterone formation generally amplifies the androgenic signal. Since only one receptor appears to mediate the action of both androgens, a central, as yet unresolved, issue of androgen physiology is concerned with the mechanism by which testosterone and dihydrotestosterone exert different actions during embryogenesis. One possibility is that the two hormones act in exactly the same manner to promote virilization. By this schema, dihydrotestosterone, although amplifying the hormonal signal within most androgen target cells, is not absolutely required for androgen action, provided that the intracellular concentration of testosterone is sufficiently high and that sufficient time is available to allow registration of the weaker hormonal signal produced by testosterone. Alternatively, testosterone may promote virilization of the wolffian ducts by an indirect means, analogous to the involvement of erythropoietin in androgen-mediated control of erythropoiesis (72). In some tissues (e.g., hypothalamus), testosterone can be aromatized to estradiol, and androgen action is, paradoxically, mediated by an estrogen.

Role of dihydrotestosterone in virilization. Separate roles for testosterone and dihydrotestosterone in male differentiation were postulated on the basis of studies of androgen metabolism in embryos (218,255,258). In rat, rabbit, guinea pig, and human embryos, 5α-reductase activity is maximal in the urogenital sinus and urogenital tubercle prior to virilization; however, the enzyme is virtually undetectable in the wolffian duct derivatives until after virilization is advanced (Fig. 11). Therefore, it was deduced that testosterone mediates virilization of the wolffian ducts, whereas dihydrotestosterone is responsible for differentiation of the male urethra, prostate, and external genitalia (258).

This hypothesis was substantiated by studies of patients with 5α-reductase deficiency, a rare autosomal recessive mutation causing abnormal sexual development in affected men (75,198,251). Affected persons are 46,XY males who have predominantly female external genitalia in association with bilateral testes. The internal genitalia (epididymis, vas deferens, seminal vesicle, and ejaculatory duct) that are derived from the wolffian ducts are virilized normally, however, and terminate in a pseudovagina. At the time of expected puberty, testosterone production increases into the male range, and the external genitalia may virilize to a limited extent. Gynecomastia does not develop; axillary and pubic hair develop normally.

There is considerable heterogeneity in the mutant 5α-reductase among different families with the disorder (75,127,260). The most common defect appears to be a marked deficiency in the amount of a catalytically active 5α-reductase enzyme (183,184). Some patients, however, have structural abnormalities of the enzyme that affect cofactor (NADPH) and/or steroid binding (128,151).

Because a mutation that causes decreased dihydrotestosterone formation has not yet been described in an animal

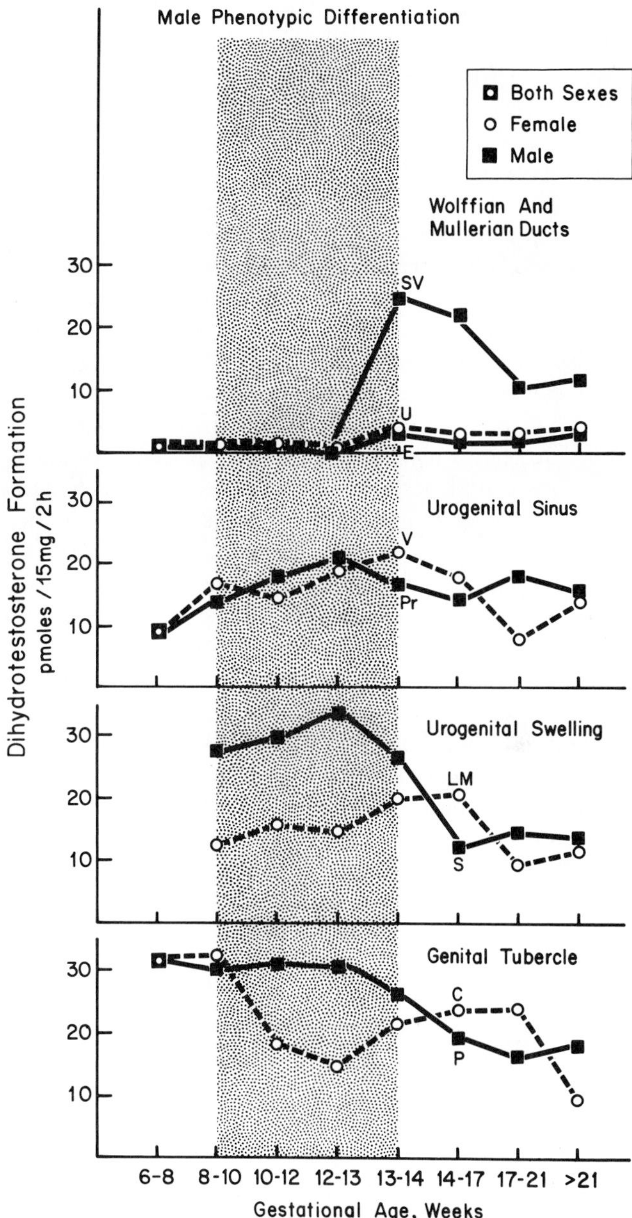

FIG. 11. Developmental study of 5α-reductase activity in urogenital tracts of human fetuses. (Adapted from ref. 218.)

species, direct characterization of the separate roles for testosterone and dihydrotestosterone in formation of the male phenotype has been difficult (22,23,152). However, the administration of 5α-reductase inhibitors to pregnant rats during the period of embryonic sexual differentiation reproduces many of the characteristics of the 5α-reductase-deficiency phenotype in the male offspring. Virilization of the external genitalia is impaired, whereas no effect on the male differentiation of wolffian-duct-derived structures is apparent (23,125). Since the androgen receptor system of the wolffian duct derivatives, like other androgen receptors, appears to bind dihydrotestosterone preferentially (85), it has been difficult to understand why testosterone can mediate wolffian differentiation but cannot virilize the urogenital sinus and external genitalia. It is conceivable that the local concentration of testosterone in the wolffian ducts is exceptionally high because it is secreted directly from the testis into the lumen of the wolffian duct; it is also possible that this high concentration of testosterone compensates for its relative ineffectiveness as an androgen. Two types of evidence are in keeping with this theory. First, active immunization of pregnant rabbits against testosterone reduces circulating androgen and causes pseudohermaphroditism in male offspring similar to the phenotype described for human males with 5α-reductase deficiency (12,244), suggesting that androgens that are not exposed to antibody (androgens within the lumen of the wolffian ducts) may remain effective. Second, a heritable trait in the rat causes unilateral hypoplasia of the testis in 50% of males (123). Hypoplasia of the testis is accompanied by ipsilateral aplasia of the epididymis and vas deferens despite the fact that prostate development and virilization of the external genitalia are normal, presumably mediated by plasma androgens derived from the normal testis. This finding is consistent with the concept that a noncirculating factor from the testis (testosterone?) causes virilization of the adjacent wolffian duct.

A perplexing aspect of 5α-reductase deficiency is the partial virilization that occurs in some patients at the time of expected puberty (198,205). Late virilization in these patients may be caused by the combination of (a) higher levels of plasma testosterone at puberty than during embryogenesis and (b) the presence of some residual 5α-reductase activity in all patients with this defect who have been characterized to date.

Role of androgen receptor in male development. A specific, high-affinity receptor protein mediates the action of both testosterone and dihydrotestosterone in all androgen-dependent tissues. Androgen receptors in fetal urogenital tissues have characteristics similar to those in adult androgen-dependent tissues, and they probably mediate virilization of the fetus by the same mechanisms as in postnatal life (85). Studies of single-gene mutations that impair androgen receptor function are in keeping with this concept.

The first disorder of the androgen receptor to be characterized in molecular terms was the testicular feminization (*Tfm*) mutation in the mouse, an X-linked disorder in which affected males have testes and normal testosterone production but differentiate as phenotypic females (8,97,161). The mullerian-inhibiting function of the fetal testis is presumed to be normal because no mullerian duct derivatives (uterus or fallopian tubes) are present in affected males. Dihydrotestosterone formation is normal. However, profound resistance to androgen action results in failure of all androgen-mediated aspects of male development in the wolffian duct, urogenital sinus, and external genitalia. Functional cytoplasmic androgen receptors are not detectable (27,84,242) (Fig. 12). Consequently, the hormone cannot reach the nucleus of the cell and interact with the chromosomes.

Studies of subjects with the human counterpart of the *Tfm*

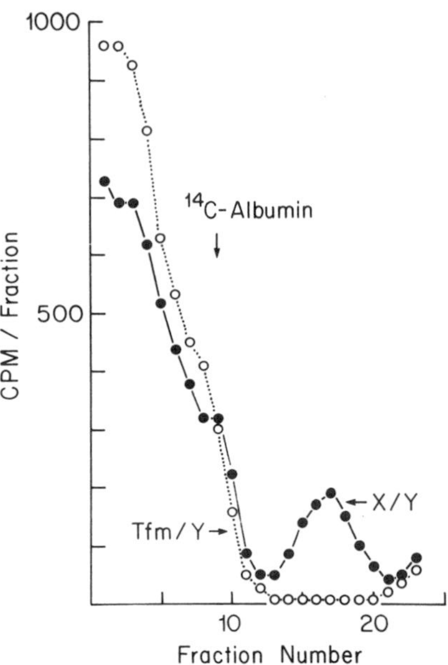

FIG. 12. Sucrose density gradient analysis of [^{3}H]dihydrotestosterone binding in kidney cytosol from normal (X/Y) and androgen-resistant (*Tfm*/Y) male mice. (Adapted from ref. 242.)

mouse have provided additional insight into the role of the androgen receptor in embryonic virilization (260). Defects in the human androgen receptor cause a spectrum of abnormalities that vary in severity, ranging from men with mild defects in androgen action to phenotypic women with testicular feminization. Women with testicular feminization usually come to the attention of the physician when they are evaluated for primary amenorrhea. The karyotype is 46,XY, but the general habitus is female. Axillary, facial, and pubic hair is absent or scanty. The external genitalia are unambiguously female, and the vagina is short and blind-ending. All internal genitalia are absent except testes, which may be located in the abdomen, along the course of the inguinal canal, or in the labia majora. Female breast development occurs at the time of expected puberty and is probably due to increased estrogen synthesis by the testis (162). A small percentage of patients with the phenotype of testicular feminization have axillary and pubic hair as well as a modest degree of virilization (164). These patients are designated as having an "incomplete" form of testicular feminization. Patients with Reifenstein syndrome (most commonly with hypospadias, azoospermia, and gynecomastia; see ref. 260) and phenotypically normal men with infertility (1,2) complete the spectrum of individuals with disorders of the androgen receptor.

The molecular defect in some patients is similar to that in the *Tfm* mouse (i.e., no high-affinity androgen receptor can be detected; see refs. 109 and 142). It is not known whether the absence of binding in these instances is due to absence of the receptor protein or to a defect in the protein that precludes its ability to bind androgen. Other patients with testicular feminization have either a diminished amount or a qualitative abnormality of the receptor. Qualitative abnormalities of the androgen receptor were initially identified in studies of thermolability of androgen receptors in skin fibroblasts cultured from patients with phenotypic androgen resistance (105). Subsequently, other mutations have been identified in which the cytosolic androgen receptor is unstable in molybdate-containing buffers (106). Studies of the process by which androgen-receptor complexes are "transformed" to the DNA-binding state have identified yet another subset of patients with qualitatively abnormal androgen receptors in whom the abnormality of the receptor becomes manifest during transforming conditions (145,146). Qualitative abnormalities of the androgen receptor that have been described in other laboratories include altered affinity of binding (24), impaired nuclear retention (67), and impaired augmentation of receptor binding following prolonged incubation with ligand (141). Since some patients with qualitatively abnormal receptors have androgen resistance as profound as that observed in patients in whom androgen binding cannot be detected, it appears that such structural abnormalities can totally prevent function of the receptor. The normal gene that codes for the androgen receptor and the mutant gene that causes absence of the receptor are X-linked (176,177); mutations that cause qualitative abnormalities of the receptor are probably allelic mutations of the same gene (68).

In some patients, androgen resistance occurs despite apparently normal androgen receptors. It was originally postulated that androgen resistance in these patients was caused by defects in the later phases of androgen action, the so-called "postreceptor androgen resistance" (3). Individuals from 10 such families that have been analyzed in our laboratory span a phenotypic spectrum ranging from testicular feminization to the infertile male syndrome (108). As more sensitive techniques for characterizing qualitative abnormalities in the androgen receptor have been developed, many of these subjects, including those in the original family described by Amrhein et al. (3), are known to have subtle functional alterations of the androgen receptor.

Role of the mesenchyme in androgen action. In many tissues the embryonic mesenchyme (stroma) appears to control the differentiation of the associated epithelium (reviewed in ref. 46). A compelling case for stromal-epithelial interactions in androgen action comes from studies of tissue recombinants in the development of the urogenital sinus. When mesenchyme from the urogenital sinus of embryonic mice is recombined with homotypic urogenital sinus epithelium and grown as intraocular grafts in male animals, the epithelium acquires the characteristics of the glandular epithelium of the prostate (43,44). In contrast, heterotypic recombinants of epithelium from urogenital sinus and mesenchyme of integumental origin are incapable of glandular (prostatic) development, but form keratinized epithelium characteristic of skin under similar circumstances (Fig. 13). Furthermore, mesenchyme derived from the urogenital sinus of androgen-resistant (*Tfm*/Y) mice is incapable of mediating prostatic growth when recombined with normal urogenital sinus epithelium and exposed to androgen. However, when reciprocal recombinants (*Tfm*/Y epithelium with normal mesenchyme) are made, prostate development occurs (45,150).

Autoradiographic studies of androgen binding in the urogenital sinus of developing rats (229) provide additional insight into the role of the mesenchyme in morphogenesis of the prostate. At the time of prostatic bud formation, androgen-binding sites are located predominantly over the nuclei of mesenchymal cells that surround the developing buds. The urogenital sinus of female embryos also has androgen-binding sites in the nuclei of mesenchymal cells. In contrast, no labeling was detected in the epithelia of fetal urogenital sinuses. After postnatal day 10, androgen binding

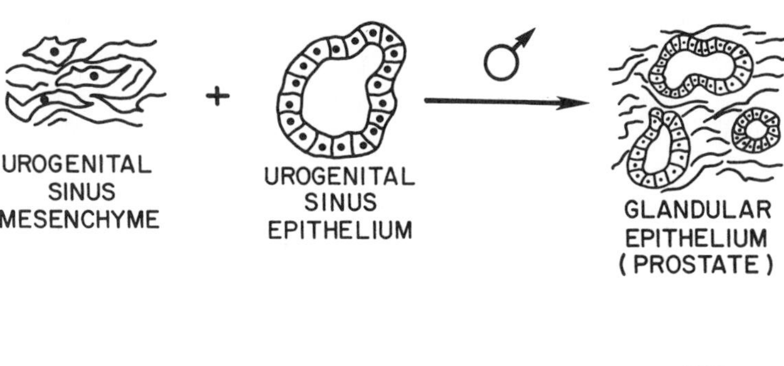

FIG. 13. Diagram of tissue recombinant experiments of Cunha. (Adapted from ref. 46.)

was present in the epithelial cells of the prostate, and labeling in mesenchymal cells became less prominent. These results suggest that, during morphogenesis of the male urogenital tract, androgen action is initiated through mesenchymal cells, whereas androgen responses of the prostate after differentiation are mediated by interaction with epithelium and mesenchyme.

A similar system is responsible for the androgen-mediated regression of the embryonic mammary bud in the mouse (61,148). However, in this tissue the response to androgen requires specific interaction of the mesenchyme with mammary epithelium (115), suggesting that in some cases the epithelium may also play a role in the differentiation process. There are also indications that epithelium of mesodermal origin, when recombined with androgen-responsive mesenchyme, responds differently than does epithelium of endoderm (46). Elucidating the nature of these mesenchymal-epithelial interactions is of critical importance in understanding androgen-mediated differentiative processes.

Despite the fact that a great deal of information has been accumulated about the hormones involved in differentiation of the urogenital tract and about the cellular sites of their initial actions, little is known about the specific gene products that are synthesized in response to the hormones or how such products direct cellular organization during embryogenesis.

Effects of androgens in female embryos. Female embryos have the same androgen receptor system in the urogenital tract as do male embryos (85). For example, androgen receptors are as readily detectable in the same regions of the female and male urogenital tracts (Fig. 14). Therefore, it is not surprising that exposure to androgens during the time of sexual differentiation causes profound virilization of female offspring (214). The anatomical consequences of such an experiment in rats are demonstrated in Fig. 15. Figure 15A and B show urogenital tracts dissected from female and male newborn rats whose mothers had been treated with oil (control) from day 14 through day 21 of gestation. Figure 15C shows a urogenital tract from a newborn female exposed *in utero* to an inactive androgen analog (5β-dihydrotestosterone). Figure 15D shows a urogenital tract from a female exposed to 5α-dihydrotestosterone. Exposure to this active androgen caused differentiation of the wolffian ducts in this female embryo into prominent epididymides, vasa deferentia, and seminal vesicles. Furthermore, the urogenital sinuses from female rats exposed *in utero* to 5α-dihydrotestosterone contain prostatic buds and a male-type urethra and exhibited no vaginal development (F. W. George, *unpublished observations*). The fact that females virilize when exposed to androgens indicates that differences in anatomical development between males and females depend on differences in the hormonal signals themselves and not on differences in the hormone receptors in target tissues. It also follows that the sexual fate of the normal embryo is determined largely by whether testosterone production commences in the fetal testis at the precise time in embryonic development.

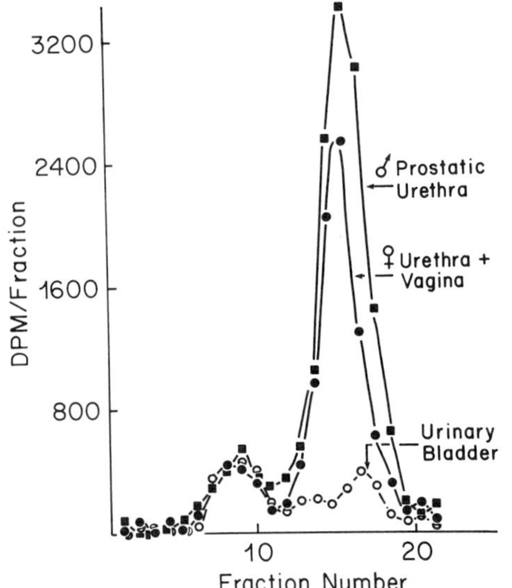

FIG. 14. Sucrose gradient analysis of [^{3}H]dihydrotestosterone binding in cytosol of urogenital sinuses and bladder of fetal rabbits on the 28th day of gestation.

The most common cause of virilization of human female embryos is congenital adrenal hyperplasia (188). Inherited mutations that result in decreased synthesis of cortisol in the adrenal gland lead to a compensatory increase in ACTH secretion by the pituitary. This, in turn, leads to an increase in adrenal androgen secretion. The adrenal androgens then virilize the external genitalia of the female. The internal genitalia are, however, not virilized, and wolffian duct remnants are no more prominent in women with congenital adrenal hyperplasia than in normal women. Therefore, it is likely that the degeneration of the wolffian ducts precedes the onset of adrenal androgen synthesis or that the wolffian ducts are insensitive to the predominant androgens formed in affected females.

DO HORMONES PLAY A ROLE IN FEMALE PHENOTYPIC DEVELOPMENT?

In the eutherian mammal, embryogenesis takes place in a "sea" of hormones (steroidal and nonsteroidal) derived from the placenta, the maternal circulation, the fetal adrenal gland, the fetal testis, and possibly from the fetal ovary. It is not known whether any of these substances influence female phenotypic differentiation or development. It is conceivable that estrogens or progestogens, or both, are involved in the growth and maturation of the female urogenital tract during the latter part of embryonic development, even if they are not required for their differentiation. Presumably, fetal castration experiments [such as those performed by Jost (136) to elucidate the role of the fetal testis in male development in the rabbit] would be uninformative, since

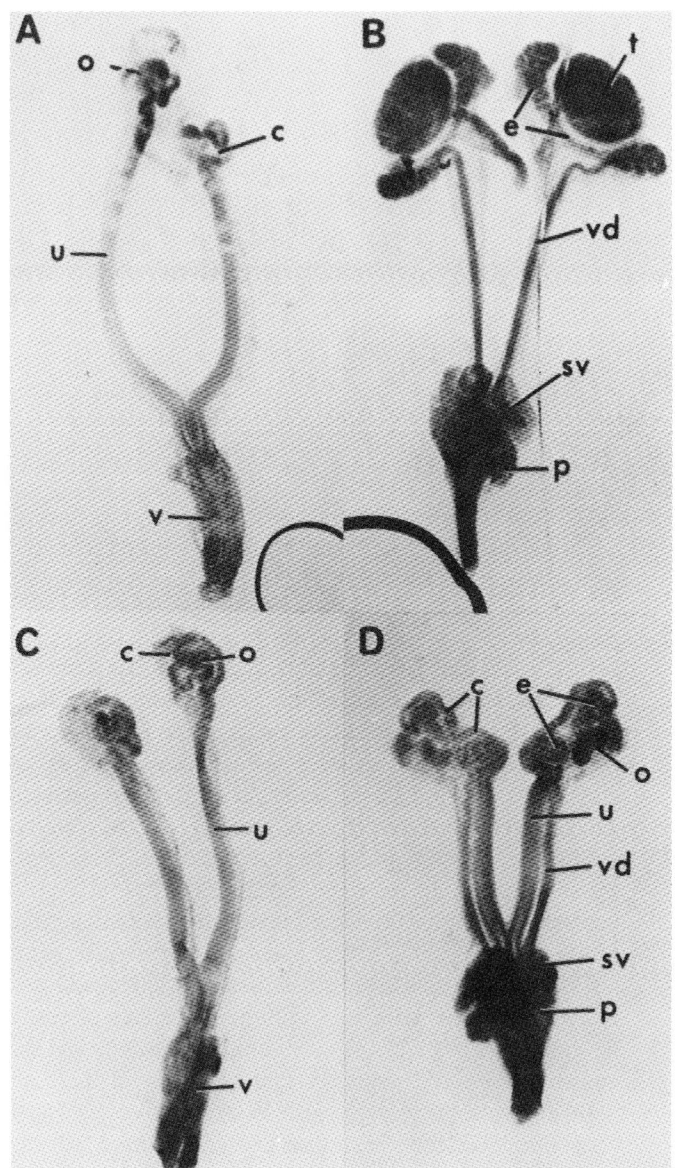

FIG. 15. Virilization of the female rat urogenital tract caused by 5α-dihydrotestosterone administration to the mother. **A** and **B,** respectively: Female and male urogenital tracts of newborn rats from a mother given oil from days 14–21 of gestation. **C:** Female urogenital tract following administration of 16 mg/day of 5β-dihydrotestosterone. **D:** Female urogenital tract following administration of 16 mg/day of 5α-dihydrotestosterone. (o) Ovary; (u) uterus; (c) coils of oviduct; (v) vagina; (t) testis; (e) epididymis; (vd) vas deferens; (sv) seminal vesicle; (p) prostate. (From ref. 214.)

removal of fetal ovaries would not remove the major source of female hormones. Experimental agents that block estrogen synthesis or action interfere with placental function and precipitate abortion. Furthermore, no mutations have been identified that result in either deficient estrogen synthesis or resistance to estrogen action. This is in contrast to the situation in regard to testosterone synthesis and action where single-gene mutations that interfere with both processes have been characterized in many species (260). In the rabbit, estrogen synthesis is temporarily activated in both male and female embryos at the time the blastocyst implants in the uterine wall between days 6 and 7 of gestation (87) (Fig. 16). Later in the embryogenesis of the rabbit, estrogen synthesis (aromatase activity) is activated in placenta (transiently), brain, and ovary, but specific activity of aromatase in these tissues is never as high as in the implanting blastocyst (Fig. 16). Estrogens may be necessary for implantation and survival of the blastocyst (52,53), suggesting that estrogen action is essential for life in eutherian mammals. If this is true, mutations that prevent either the synthesis of, or the response to, estrogens may be lethal at an early stage of development by preventing implantation of the blastocyst.

In many species, estradiol formation is initiated in the ovary before definitive histological differentiation has occurred; it is possible that cellular organization of the ovary may be mediated, in part, by estrogens formed locally (99), analogous to the postulated role of testosterone in maturation of the spermatogenic cords of the testis.

In contrast to eutherian mammals in which sexual differentiation occurs *in utero,* marsupial young are born sexually indifferent. Development of the sexual phenotypes takes place in the pouch, independent of the maternal milieu, and the pouch young are accessible for experimentation

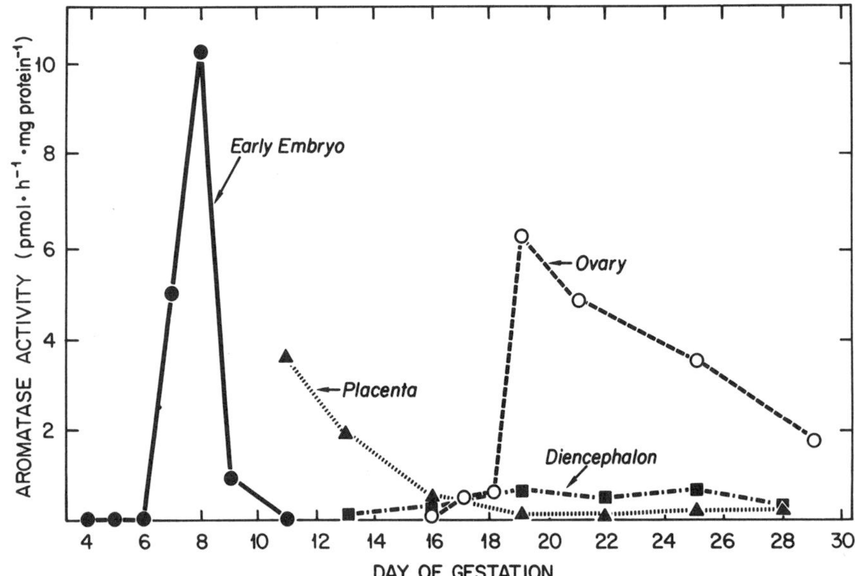

FIG. 16. Distribution of aromatase activity in the developing rabbit embryo. (Composite of data in refs. 87, 91, and 179.)

throughout sexual development. Marsupials therefore represent an important model system for studying the hormonal factors controlling sexual differentiation. Burns (32) studied the effects of the administration of androgen or estrogen on the development of the sexual phenotypes in newborn opossums (*Didelphis virginiana*). Testosterone administration caused a marked hypertrophy and male differentiation of the phallus in both male and female pouch young. In contrast, estrogen caused female-type development of the phallus and cloacal region in both sexes. Similar effects have been reported in the gray opossum (*Monodelphis domestica*) (73). Thus, estrogens appear to play a role in the development of the female external genitalia in these marsupial species.

The development of the pouch in female, and of the scrotum in male, opossums occurs 10 days after birth, and the two structures are thought to derive from common anlage (17). Pouch development is the earliest evidence of sexual dimorphism that can be identified grossly. Interestingly, in the opossum pouch young that Burns treated with androgen or estrogen, some of which were treated soon after entering the pouch, the development of the pouch or scrotum was not influenced.

Thus, phenotypic differentiation in this marsupial appears to be an exception to Jost's formulation for sexual differentiation in eutherian mammals in that (a) estrogens may play a role in development of the female urogenital tract and (b) some aspects of the sexual phenotype (scrotum and pouch development) appear to be independent of hormonal control.

SUMMARY

Jost's formulation has proved to be a powerful paradigm for understanding normal and abnormal sexual differentiation. Chromosomal sex determines gonadal sex, and gonadal sex determines phenotypic sex. A minimum of 19 genes have been implicated in sexual differentiation in humans (257). Some of these genes are located on the sex chromosomes, some on the autosomes. Thus, the relatively simple mechanism that imposes male development on the indifferent embryo requires the participation of many genes common to both the male and female embryo. Much of our understanding of the process of sexual differentiation is due to the fact that, unlike many other congenital defects, abnormalities of sexual differentiation are not lethal, and such individuals, even those with mild abnormalities of sexual development, come to the attention of physicians and scientists and are systematically studied. Many of these abnormalities are due to single-gene defects, and detailed analyses of these disorders in humans and animals have provided a great deal of insight into the endocrine, molecular, and genetic determinants that regulate sexual differentiation.

Determinants on the Y chromosome cause the indifferent gonad to develop into a testis. Two hormonal secretions from the fetal testis, namely mullerian-inhibiting substance and testosterone, then transform the indifferent urogenital tract into one that is characteristic of the male. Mullerian-inhibiting substance, secreted by the Sertoli cells, causes regression of the female (mullerian) duct system. Testosterone, secreted by the Leydig cells, is responsible for the remainder of male development, including stabilization and differentiation of the wolffian ducts into the male accessory organs of reproduction as well as differentiation of the male external genitalia and prostate.

The role of hormones in female development is less clear. In the opossum, ovarian hormones may play a role in the differentiation of the female urogenital tract and development of the pouch. However, in the eutherian mammal it has not been possible to design experiments to determine whether hormones from the placenta, the maternal circulation, or the fetal ovary play an essential role in female development.

A major portion of androgen action in the fetus and in postembryonic life is mediated by 5α-reduced metabolites of testosterone rather than by testosterone itself. Thus, a genetic deficiency in the 5α-reductase enzyme that catalyzes the formation of dihydrotestosterone from testosterone impairs androgen action and can cause male pseudohermaphroditism. Although wolffian duct development is apparently normal in these individuals, other aspects of male development are defective.

Testosterone and dihydrotestosterone act via a common receptor to virilize male fetuses. Consequently, normal phenotypic sexual development is determined by the presence (in males) or the absence (in females) of specific hormonal signals at the critical time in embryonic development. At the time of sexual differentiation, differences in the activity of only a few enzymes involved in steroid biosynthesis in the gonads have profound consequences on the character of the hormones secreted and thus on the sexual development of the fetus.

Although we now understand, in considerable detail, the hormonal and genetic factors that are responsible for mammalian sexual differentiation, many fundamental issues in the embryonic development of the urogenital tract remain poorly understood. What, for instance, is the mechanism by which the same hormonal signal is translated into different physiologic effects in different tissues? What are the molecular and cellular changes that cause these diverse differentiative events? Ultimately, these fundamental issues of embryogenesis will have to be clarified before it will be possible to understand the entire program by which the myriad of genetic determinants and hormones interact to cause the development of phenotypic sex.

REFERENCES

1. Aiman, J., and Griffin, J. E. (1982): The frequency of androgen receptor deficiency in infertile men. *J. Clin. Endocrinol. Metab.*, 54:725–732.
2. Aiman, J., Griffin, J. E., Gazak, J. M., Wilson, J. D., and MacDonald, P. C. (1979): Androgen insensitivity as a cause of infertility in otherwise normal men. *N. Engl. J. Med.*, 300:223–227.
3. Amrhein, J. A., Meyer, W. J. III, Jones, H. W. Jr., and Migeon, C. J. (1976): Androgen insensitivity in man: Evidence for genetic heterogeneity. *Proc. Natl. Acad. Sci. USA*, 73:891–894.
4. Andersson, M., Page, D. C., and de la Chapelle, A. (1986): Chromosome Y-specific DNA is transferred to the short arm of X chromosome in human XX males. *Science*, 233:786–788.
5. Armendares, S., Buentello, L., and Frenk, S. (1973): Two male sibs with uterus and fallopian tubes. A rare, probably inherited disorder. *Clin. Genet.*, 4:291–296.
6. Armendares, S., Salamanca, F., Cantu, J. M., del Castillo, V., Nava, S., Dominguez-de-la-Piedra, E., Cortes-Gallegos, V., Gallegos, A., Cervantes, C., and Parra, A. (1975): Familial true hermaphrodism in three siblings. Clinical, cytogenetic, histological and hormonal studies. *Humangenetik*, 29:99–109.
7. Attal, J. (1969): Levels of testosterone, androstenedione, estrone and estradiol-17β in the testes of fetal sheep. *Endocrinology*, 85:280–289.
8. Bardin, C. W., Bullock, L. P., Sherins, R. J., Mowszowisz, I., and Blackburn, W. R. (1973): Androgen metabolism and mechanism of action in male pseudohermaphroditism: A study of testicular feminization. *Recent Prog. Horm. Res.*, 29:65–105.
9. Barr, M. L., and Bertram, L. F. (1949): A morphological distinction between neurones of the male and female and the behavior of the nucleolar satellite during accelerated nucleoprotein synthesis. *Nature*, 163:676–677.
10. Bengmark, S. (1958): *The Prostatic Urethra and Prostate Glands*. Berlingska Boktryckeriet, Lund, Sweden.
11. Berger, R., Abonyi, D., Nodot, A., Vialatte, J., and Lejeune, J. (1970): Hermaphrodisme vrai et "Garcon XX" dans une fratrie. *Rev. Eur. Etud. Clin. Biol.*, 15:330–333.
12. Bidlingmaier, F., Knorr, D., and Neumann, F. (1977): Inhibition of masculine differentiation in male offspring of rabbits actively immunized against testosterone before pregnancy. *Nature*, 266:647–648.
13. Billingham, R. E., and Silvers, W. K. (1960): Studies on tolerance of the Y chromosome antigen in mice. *J. Immunol.*, 85:14–26.
14. Blanchard, M. G., and Josso, N. (1974): Source of the anti-mullerian hormone synthesized by the fetal testis: Mullerian-inhibiting activity of the fetal bovine Sertoli cells in tissue culture. *Pediatr. Res.*, 8:968–971.
15. Blandau, R. J., White, B. J., and Rumery, R. E. (1963): Observations on the movements of the living primordial germ cells in the mouse. *Fertil. Steril.*, 14:482–489.
16. Bok, G., and Drews, U. (1983): The role of the wolffian ducts in the formation of the sinus vagina; an organ culture study. *J. Embryol. Exp. Morphol.*, 73:275–295.
17. Bolliger, A. (1944): An experiment on the complete transformation of the scrotum into a marsupial pouch in *Trichosurus vulpecula*. *Med. J. Aust.*, 2:56–58.
18. Böök, J. A., Eilon, B., Halbrecht, I., Komlos, L., and Shabtay, F. (1973): Isochromosome Y [46,X,i(Yq)] and female phenotype. *Clin. Genet.*, 4:410–414.
19. Boucekkine, C., Menasria, A., Choutier, A., Benelkadi, N., and Benmiloud, M. (1981): H-Y positive 46 XX true hermaphroditism with intrascrotal uterus. *Clin. Endocrinol.*, 15:529–535.
20. Brook, C. G. D. (1981): Persistent mullerian duct syndrome. *Pediatr. Adolesc. Endocrinol.*, 8:100–104.
21. Brook, C. G. D., Wagner, H., Zachmann, M., Prader, A., Armendares, S., Frenk, S., Abeman, P., Najjar, S. S., Slim, M. S., Genton, N., and Bozic, C. (1973): Familial occurrence of persistent mullerian structures in otherwise normal males. *Br. Med. J.*, 1:771–773.
22. Brooks, J. R., Baptista, E. M., Berman, C., Ham, E. A., Hichens, M., Johnston, D. B. R., Primka, R. L., Rasmusson, G. H., Reynolds, G. F., Schmitt, S. M., and Arth, G. E. (1981): Response of rat ventral prostate to a new and novel 5α-reductase inhibitor. *Endocrinology*, 109:830–836.
23. Brooks, J. R., Berman, C., Hichens, M., Primka, R. L., Reynolds, G. F., and Rasmusson, G. H. (1982): Biological activities of a new steroidal inhibitor of Δ^4-5α-reductase (41309). *Proc. Soc. Exp. Biol. Med.*, 169:67–73.
24. Brown, T. R., Maes, M., Rothwell, S. W., and Migeon, C. J. (1982): Human complete androgen insensitivity with normal dihydrotestosterone receptor binding capacity in cultured genital skin fibroblasts. Evidence for a qualitative abnormality of the receptor. *J. Clin. Endocrinol. Metab.*, 55:61–69.
25. Bruner, J. A., and Witschi, E. (1946): Testosterone-induced modifications of sex development in female hamsters. *Am. J. Anat.*, 79:293–320.
26. Budzik, G. P., Powell, S. M., Kamagata, S., and Donahoe, P. K. (1983): Mullerian-inhibiting substance fractionation by dye affinity chromatography. *Cell*, 34:307–314.
27. Bullock, L. P., Bardin, C. W., and Ohno, S. (1971): The androgen insensitive mouse: Absence of intranuclear androgen retention in the kidney. *Biochem. Biophys. Res. Commun.*, 44:1537–1543.
28. Bulmer, D. (1957): The development of the human vagina. *J. Anat.*, 91:490–509.
29. Burgoyne, P. S. (1982): Genetic homology and crossing over in the X and Y chromosomes of mammals. *Hum. Genet.*, 61:85–90.
30. Burgoyne, P. S. (1986): Mammalian X and Y crossover. *Nature*, 319:258–259.
31. Burgoyne, P. S., Levy, E. R., and McLaren, A. (1986): Spermatogenic failure in male mice lacking H-Y antigen. *Nature*, 320:170–172.

32. Burns, R. K. (1945): The differentiation of the phallus in the opossum and its reaction to sex hormones. *Contrib. Embryol.*, 31:147–162.
33. Burns, R. K. (1961): Role of hormones in the differentiation of sex. In: *Sex and Internal Secretions*, edited by W. C. Young, pp. 76–158. Williams & Wilkins, Baltimore.
34. Buyse, A. (1935): The differentiation of transplanted mammalian gonad primordia. *J. Exp. Zool.*, 70:1–41.
35. Cate, R. L., Mattaliano, R. J., Hession, C., Tizard, R., Faber, N. M., Cheung, A., Ninfa, E. G., Frey, A. Z., Gash, D. J., Chow, E. P., Fisher, R. A., Bertonis, J. M., Torres, G., Wallner, B. P., Ramachandran, K. L., Ragin, R. C., Manganaro, T. F., MacLaughlin, D. T., and Donahoe, P. K. (1986): Isolation of the bovine and human genes for mullerian inhibiting substance and expression of the human gene in animal cells. *Cell*, 45:685–698.
36. Catt, K. J., Dufau, M. L., Neaves, W. B., Walsh, P. C., and Wilson, J. D. (1975): LH-hCG receptors and testosterone content during differentiation of the testis in the rabbit embryo. *Endocrinology*, 97:1157–1165.
37. Cattanach, B. M., Evans, E. P., Burtenshaw, M. D., and Barlow, J. (1982): Male, female and intersex development in mice of identical chromosome constitution. *Nature*, 300:445–446.
38. Cattanach, B. M., Pollard, C. E., and Hawkes, S. G. (1971): Sex-reversed mice XX and XO males. *Cytogenetics*, 10:318–337.
39. Clayton, G. W., Smith, J. D., and Rosenberg, H. S. (1958): Familial true hermaphroditism in pre- and postpubertal genetic females. Hormonal and morphologic studies. *J. Clin. Endocrinol. Metab.*, 18:1349–1358.
40. Cooke, H. J., Brown, W. R. A., and Rappold, G. A. (1985): Hypervariable telomeric sequences from the human sex chromosomes are pseudoautosomal. *Nature*, 317:687–692.
41. Cooke, H. J., Fantes, J., and Green, D. (1983): Structure and evolution of human Y chromosome DNA. *Differentiation*, 23:S48–S55.
42. Crichton, D. N., and Steel, C. M. (1985): Serologically detectable H-Y ('male') antigen: Mr or myth? *Immunol. Today*, 6:202–203.
43. Cunha, G. R. (1972): Epithelial-mesenchymal interactions in primordial gland structures which become responsive to androgenic stimulation. *Anat. Rec.*, 172:179–196.
44. Cunha, G. R. (1972): Tissue interactions between epithelium and mesenchyme of urogenital and integumental origin. *Anat. Rec.*, 172:529–542.
45. Cunha, G. R., and Chung, L. W. K. (1981): Stromal-epithelial interactions. I. Induction of prostatic phenotype in urothelium of testicular feminized (Tfm/Y) mice. *J. Steroid Biochem.*, 14:1317–1321.
46. Cunha, G. R., Chung, L. W. K., Shannon, J. M., and Reese, B. A. (1980): Stromal-epithelial interactions in sex differentiation. *Biol. Reprod.*, 22:19–42.
47. Davis, R. M. (1981): Localisation of male determining factors in man: A thorough review of structural anomalies of the Y chromosome. *J. Med. Genet.*, 18:161–195.
48. Dean, D. C., Gope, R., Knoll, B. J., Riser, M. E., and O'Malley, B. W. (1984): A similar 5′-flanking region is required for estrogen and progesterone induction of ovalbumin gene expression. *J. Biol. Chem.*, 259:9967–9970.
49. De la Chapelle, A. (1972): Nature and origin of males with XX sex chromosomes. *Am. J. Hum. Genet.*, 24:71–105.
50. De la Chapelle, A. (1981): The etiology of maleness in XX men. *Hum. Genet.*, 58:105–116.
51. De la Chapelle, A., Tippett, P. A., Wetterstrand, G., and Page, D. (1984): Genetic evidence of X-Y interchange in a human XX male. *Nature*, 307:170–171.
52. Dickmann, Z., and Dey, S. K. (1976): A new concept: Control of early pregnancy by steroid hormones originating in the preimplantation embryo. *Vitam. Horm.*, 34:215–242.
53. Dickmann, Z., Gupta, J. S., and Dey, S. K. (1977): Does "blastocyst estrogen" initiate implantation? *Science*, 195:687–688.
54. Donahoe, P. K., Budzik, G. P., Trelstad, R., Mudgett-Hunter, M., Fuller, A. Jr., Hutson, J. M., Ikawa, H., Hayashi, A., and MacLaughlin, D. (1982): Mullerian-inhibiting substance: An update. *Recent Prog. Horm. Res.*, 38:279–326.
55. Donahoe, P. K., Fuller, A. F. Jr., Sailly, R. E., Guy, S. R., and Budzik, G. P. (1981): Mullerian inhibiting substance inhibits growth of a human ovarian cancer in nude mice. *Ann. Surg.*, 194:472–480.
56. Donahoe, P. K., Ho, Y., Morikawa, Y., and Hendren, W. H. (1977): Mullerian inhibiting substance in human testes after birth. *J. Pediatr. Surg.*, 12:323–330.
57. Donahoe, P. K., Hutson, J. M., Fallat, M. E., Kamagata, S., and Budzik, G. P. (1984): Mechanism of action of mullerian inhibiting substance. *Annu. Rev. Physiol.*, 46:53–65.
58. Donahoe, P. K., Ito, Y., Price, J. M., and Herndon, W. H. III (1977): Mullerian inhibiting substance activity in bovine fetal, newborn and prepubertal testes. *Biol. Reprod.*, 16:238–243.
59. Donahoe, P. K., Swann, D. A., Hayashi, A., and Sullivan, M. D. (1979): Mullerian duct regression in the embryo correlated with cytotoxic activity against human ovarian cancer. *Science*, 205:913–915.
60. Donovan, P. J., Stott, D., Cairns, L. A., Heasman, J., and Wylie, C. C. (1986): Migratory and postmigratory mouse primordial germ cells behave differently in culture. *Cell*, 44:831–838.
61. Drews, U., and Drews, U. (1977): Regression of mouse mammary gland anlagen in recombinants of Tfm and wild-type tissues: Testosterone acts via the mesenchyme. *Cell*, 10:401–404.
62. Dyche, W. J. (1979): A comparative study of the differentiation and involution of the mullerian duct and wolffian duct in the male and female fetal mouse. *J. Morphol.*, 162:175–210.
63. Eicher, E. M., and Washburn, L. L. (1983): Inherited sex reversal in mice: Identification of a new primary sex-determining gene. *J. Exp. Zool.*, 228:297–304.
64. Eicher, E. M., and Washburn, L. L. (1986): Genetic control of primary sex determination in mice. *Annu. Rev. Genet.*, 20:327–360.
65. Eicher, E. M., Washburn, L. L., Whitney, J. B. III, and Morrow, K. E. (1982): *Mus poschiavinus* Y chromosome in the C57BL/6J murine genome causes sex reversal. *Science*, 217:535–537.
66. Eichwald, E. J., and Silmser, C. R. (1955): Untitled communication. *Transplant. Bull.*, 2:148–149.
67. Eli, C. (1983): Familial incomplete male pseudohermaphroditism associated with impaired nuclear androgen retention. *J. Clin. Invest.*, 71:850–858.
68. Elawady, M. K., Allman, D. R., Griffin, J. E., and Wilson, J. D. (1983): Expression of a mutant androgen receptor in cloned fibroblasts derived from a heterozygous carrier for the syndrome of testicular feminization. *Am. J. Hum. Genet.*, 35:376–384.
69. Epplen, J. T., Cellini, A., Shorte, M., and Ohno, S. (1983): On evolutionarily conserved simple repetitive DNA sequences: Do "sex-specific" satellite components serve any sequence dependent function? *Differentiation*, 23:S60–S63.
70. Epplen, J. T., McCarrey, J. R., Sutou, S., and Ohno, S. (1982): Base sequence of a cloned snake W-chromosome DNA fragment and identification of a male-specific putative mRNA in the mouse. *Proc. Natl. Acad. Sci. USA*, 79:2798–3802.
71. Evans, E. P., Burtenshaw, M. D., and Cattanach, B. H. (1982): Meiotic crossing-over between the X and Y chromosomes of male mice carrying the sex-reversing (Sxr) factor. *Nature*, 300:443–445.
72. Evens, R. P., and Amerson, A. B. (1974): Androgens and erythropoiesis. *J. Clin. Pharmacol.* 14:94–101.
73. Fadem, B. H., and Tesoriero, J. V. (1986): Inhibition of testicular development and feminization of the male genitalia by neonatal estrogen treatment in a marsupial. *Biol. Reprod.* 34:771–776.
74. Fallat, M. E., Hutson, J. M., Budzik, D. P., and Donahoe, P. K. (1984): Androgen stimulation of nucleotide pyrophosphatase during mullerian duct regression. *Endocrinology*, 114:1592–1598.
75. Fisher, L. K., Kogut, M. D., Moore, R. J., Goebelsmann, U., Weitzmann, J. J., Isaacs, H. Jr., Griffin, J. E., and Wilson, J. D. (1978): Clinical, endocrinological, and enzymatic characterization of two patients with 5α-reductase deficiency. Evidence that a single enzyme is responsible for the 5α-reduction of cortisol and testosterone. *J. Clin. Endocrinol.*, 47:653–664.
76. Forejt, J. (1979): Meiotic studies of translocations causing male sterility in the mouse. II. Double heterozygotes for Robertsonian translocations. *Cytogenet. Cell Genet.*, 21:163–170.
77. Forejt, J., and Gregorova, S. (1977): Meiotic studies of translocations causing male sterility in the mouse. I. Autosomal reciprocal translocation. *Cytogenet. Cell Genet.*, 19:159–179.
78. Fujimoto, T., Miyayama, Y., and Fuyuta, M. (1977): The origin, migration and fine morphology of human primordial germ cells. *Anat. Rec.*, 188:315–330.
79. Fuller, A. F. Jr., Guy, S., Budzik, G. P., and Donahoe, P. K. (1982): Mullerian-inhibiting substance inhibits colony growth of a human ovarian carcinoma cell line. *J. Clin. Endocrinol. Metab.*, 54:1051–1055.
80. Gallegos, A. J., Guizar, E., Cortes-Gallegos, V., Cervantes, C., Bedolla, N., and Parra, A. (1976): Familial true hermaphrodism in

three siblings: Plasma hormonal profile and *in vitro* steroid biosynthesis in gonadal structures. *J. Clin. Endocrinol. Metab.*, 42:653–660.
81. Gardner, R. L., Lyon, M. F., Evans, E. P., and Burtenshaw, M. D. (1985): Clonal analysis of X-chromosome inactivation and the origin of the germ line in the mouse embryo. *J. Embryol. Exp. Morphol.*, 88:349–363.
82. Gartler, S. M., Liskay, R. M., Campbell, B. K., Sparkes, R., and Gant, N. (1972): Evidence for two functional X chromosomes in human oocytes. *Cell Differ.* 1:215–218.
83. Gartler, S. M., Liskay, R. M., and Gant, N. (1973): Two functional X chromosomes in human fetal oocytes. *Exp. Cell Res.*, 82:464–465.
84. Gehring, U., Tomkins, G. M., and Ohno, S. (1971): Effect of the androgen-insensitivity mutation on a cytoplasmic receptor for dihydrotestosterone. *Nature (New Biol.)*, 232:106–107.
85. George, F. W., and Noble, J. F. (1984): Androgen receptors are similar in fetal and adult rabbits. *Endocrinology,* 115:1451–1458.
86. George, F. W., and Wilson, J. D. (1978): Conversion of androgen to estrogen by the human fetal ovary. *J. Clin. Endocrinol. Metab.*, 47:550–555.
87. George, F. W., and Wilson, J. D. (1978): Estrogen formation in the early rabbit embryo. *Science,* 199:200–202.
88. George, F. W., and Wilson, J. D. (1980): Endocrine differentiation of the fetal rabbit ovary in culture. *Nature,* 283:861–863.
89. George, F. W., Catt, K. J., Neaves, W. B., and Wilson, J. D. (1978): Studies on the regulation of testosterone synthesis in the rabbit fetal testis. *Endocrinology,* 102:106–107.
90. George, F. W., Simpson, E. R., Milewich, L., and Wilson, J. D. (1979): Studies on the regulation of steroid hormone biosynthesis in fetal rabbit gonads. *Endocrinology,* 105:1100–1106.
91. George, F. W., Tobleman, W. T., Milewich, L., and Wilson, J. D. (1978): Aromatase activity in the developing rabbit brain. *Endocrinology,* 102:86–91.
92. Gier, H. T., and Marion, G. B. (1969): Development of the mammalian testis and genital ducts. *Biol. Reprod.*, 1:1–23.
93. Gillman, J. (1948): The development of the gonads in man, with a consideration of the role of fetal endocrines and the histogenesis of ovarian tumors. *Carnegie Contrib. Embryol.*, 32:83–131.
94. Goldberg, E. H., Boyse, E. A., Bennett, D., Scheid, M., and Carswell, E. A. (1971): Serological demonstration of H-Y (male) antigen on mouse sperm. *Nature,* 232:478–480.
95. Goldman, A. S. (1971): Production of hypospadias in the rat by selective inhibition of fetal testicular 17α-hydroxylase and $C_{17\text{-}20}$-lyase. *Endocrinology,* 88:527–531.
96. Goldman, A. S., Shapiro, B. H., and Neuman, F. (1976): Role of testosterone and its metabolites in the differentiation of the mammary gland in rats. *Endocrinology,* 99:1490–1495.
97. Goldstein, J. L., and Wilson, J. D. (1972): Studies on the pathogenesis of the pseudohermaphroditism in the mouse with testicular feminization. *J. Clin. Invest.*, 51:1647–1658.
98. Gondos, B. (1980): Development and differentiation of the testis and male reproductive tract. In: *Testicular Development, Structure, and Function,* edited by A. Steinberger and E. Steinberger, pp. 3–20. Raven Press, New York.
99. Gondos, B., George, F. W., and Wilson, J. D. (1983): Granulosa cell differentiation and estrogen synthesis in the fetal rabbit ovary. *Biol. Reprod.*, 29:791–798.
100. Goodfellow, P., Darling, S., and Wolfe, J. (1985): The human Y chromosome. *J. Med. Genet.*, 22:329–344.
101. Goodfellow, P. J., Darling, S. M., Thomas, N. S., and Goodfellow, P. N. (1986): A pseudoautosomal gene in man. *Science,* 234:740–743.
102. Gordon, J. W., and Ruddle, F. H. (1981): Mammalian gonadal determination and gametogenesis. *Science,* 211:1265–1271.
103. Gore-Langston, R. E., Tung, P. S., and Fritz, I. B. (1983): The absence of specific interaction of Sertoli-cell-secreted proteins with antibodies directed against H-Y antigen. *Cell,* 32:289–301.
104. Greene, R. R. (1942): Hormonal factors in sex inversion: The effects of sex hormones on embryonic sexual structures of the rat. *Biol. Symp.*, 9:105–123.
105. Griffin, J. E. (1979): Testicular feminization associated with a thermolabile androgen receptor in cultured human fibroblasts. *J. Clin. Invest.*, 64:1624–1631.
106. Griffin, J. E., and Durrant, J. L. (1982): Qualitative receptor defects in families with androgen resistance: Failure of stabilization of the fibroblast cytosol androgen receptor. *J. Clin. Endocrinol. Metab.*, 55:465–474.
107. Griffin, J. E., and Wilson, J. D. (1978): Hereditary male pseudohermaphroditism. *Clin. Obstet. Gynaecol.*, 5:457–479.
108. Griffin, J. E., Kovacs, W. J., and Wilson, J. D. (1985): Characteristics of androgen resistance. In: *Regulation of Androgen Action,* edited by N. Bruchovsky, A. Chapdelaine, and F. Neumann, The Proceedings of an International Symposium, pp. 127–131. Congressdruck R. Brückner, Berlin.
109. Griffin, J. E., Punyashthiti, K., and Wilson, J. D. (1976): Dihydrotestosterone binding by cultured human fibroblasts. Comparison of cells from control subjects and from patients with hereditary male pseudohermaphroditism due to androgen resistance. *J. Clin. Invest.*, 57:1342–1351.
110. Gruenwald, P. (1941): The relation of the growing müllerian duct to the wolffian duct and its importance for the genesis of malformation. *Anat. Rec.*, 81:1–19.
111. Guellaen, G., Casanova, M., Bishop, C., Geldwerth, D., Andre, G., Fellous, M., and Weissenbach, J. (1984): Human XX males with Y single-copy DNA fragments. *Nature,* 307:172–173.
112. Handel, M. A., and Eppig, J. J. (1979): Sertoli cell differentiation in the testes of mice genetically deficient in germ cells. *Biol. Reprod.*, 20:1031–1038.
113. Hayashi, A., Donahoe, P. K., Budzik, G. P., and Trelstad, R. L. (1982): Periductal and matrix glycosaminoglycans in rat mullerian duct regression. *Dev. Biol.*, 92:16–26.
114. Hertig, A. T., Adams, E. C., McKay, D. G., Rock, J., Mulligan, W. J., and Menkin, M. (1956): A description of 34 human ova within the first 17 days of development. *Am. J. Anat.*, 98:435–493.
115. Heuberger, B., Fritzka, I., Wasner, G., and Kratochwil, K. (1982): Induction of androgen receptor formation by epithelium-mesenchyme interaction in embryonic mouse mammary gland. *Proc. Natl. Acad. Sci. USA,* 79:2957–2961.
116. Holyoke, E. A. (1949): The differentiation of embryonic gonads transplanted to the adult omentum in the albino rat. *Anat. Rec.*, 103:675–699.
117. Huhtaniemi, I. T., Korenbrat, C. C., and Jaffe, R. B. (1977): hCG binding and stimulation of testosterone biosynthesis in the human fetal testis. *J. Clin. Endocrinol. Metab.*, 44:963–967.
118. Hutson, J. M. (1985): A biphasic model for the hormonal control of testicular descent. *Lancet,* 2:419–421.
119. Hutson, J. M., and Donahoe, P. K. (1983): Is mullerian-inhibiting substance a circulating hormone in the chick-quail chimera? *Endocrinology,* 113:1470–1475.
120. Hutson, J. M., Donahoe, P. K., and MacLaughlin, D. T. (1985): Steroid modulation of mullerian duct regression in the chick embryo. *Gen. Comp. Endocrinol.*, 57:88–102.
121. Hutson, J. M., Fallat, M. E., Kamagata, S., Donahoe, P. K., and Budzik, G. P. (1984): Phosphorylation events during mullerian duct regression. *Science,* 223:586–588.
122. Hutson, J. M., Ikawa, H., and Donahoe, P. K. (1982): Estrogen inhibition of mullerian inhibiting substance in the chick embryo. *J. Pediatr. Surg.*, 17:953–959.
123. Ikadai, H., Sakuma, Y., Suzuki, K., and Imamichi, T. (1985): Congenital abnormalities of the male genital organs in the newly established TW rat strain. *Cong. Anom.*, 26:65–71.
124. Ikawa, H., Hutson, J. M., Budzik, D. P., MacLaughlin, D. T., and Donahoe, P. K. (1982): Steroid enhancement of mullerian duct regression. *J. Pediatr. Surg.* 17:453–458.
125. Imperato-McGinley, J., Binienda, Z., Arthur, A., Mininberg, D. T., Vaughan, D. Jr., and Quimby, F. W. (1985): The development of a male pseudohermaphroditic rat using an inhibitor of the enzyme 5α-reductase. *Endocrinology,* 116:807–812.
126. Imperato-McGinley, J., Binienda, Z., Gedney, J., and Vaughan, E. D. (1986): Nipple differentiation in fetal male rats treated with an inhibitor of the enzyme 5α-reductase: Definition of a selective role for dihydrotestosterone. *Endocrinology,* 118:132–137.
127. Imperato-McGinley, J., Guerrero, L., Gautier, T., and Peterson, R. E. (1974): Steroid 5α-reductase deficiency in man: An inherited form of male pseudohermaphroditism. *Science,* 186:1213–1215.
128. Imperato-McGinley, J., Peterson, R. E., Leshin, M., Griffin, J. E., Cooper, G., Draghi, S., Berenyi, M., and Wilson, J. D. (1980): Steroid 5α-reductase deficiency in a 65 year old pseudohermaphrodite: The natural history, ultrastructure of the testis and evidence for inherited enzyme heterogeneity. *J. Clin. Endocrinol. Metab.*, 50:15–22.
129. Jacobs, P. A., and Ross, A. (1966): Structural abnormalities of the Y chromosome in man. *Nature,* 210:352–354.

130. Jirasek, J. E. (1976): Principles of reproductive embryology. In: *Disorders of Sexual Differentiation,* edited by J. L. Simpson, pp. 51–110. Academic Press, New York.
131. Jones, H. W. Jr., Rary, J. M., Rock, J. A., and Cummings, D. (1979): The role of H-Y antigen in human sexual development. *Johns Hopkins Med. J.,* 145:33–43.
132. Jones, K. W. (1983): Evolutionary conservation of sex specific DNA sequences. *Differentiation,* 23:S56–S59.
133. Josso, N., Fekete, C., Cachin, O., Nezelof, C., and Rappaport, R. (1983): Persistence of mullerian ducts in male pseudohermaphroditism, and its relationship to cryptorchidism. *Clin. Endocrinol.,* 19:247–258.
134. Josso, N., Picard, J.-Y., and Tran, D. (1977): The anti Mullerian hormone. *Recent Prog. Horm. Res.,* 33:117–167.
135. Jost, A. (1947): Recherches sur la différenciation de l'embryon de lapin. II. Action des androgénes synthèse sur sur l'histogénsès génitale. *Arch. Anat. Microsc. Morphol. Exp.,* 36:242–270.
136. Jost, A. (1953): Problems in fetal endocrinology: The gonadal and hypophyseal hormones. *Recent Prog. Horm. Res.,* 8:379–418.
137. Jost, A. (1961): The role of fetal hormones in prenatal development. *Harvey Lect.,* 55:201–226.
138. Jost, A. (1972): A new look at the mechanisms controlling sexual differentiation in mammals. *Johns Hopkins Med. J.,* 130:38–53.
139. Jost, A., and Magre, S. (1984): Testicular development phases and dual hormonal control of sexual organogenesis. In: *Sexual Differentiation: Basic and Clinical Aspects,* edited by M. Serio et al., pp. 1–15. Raven Press, New York.
140. Kasdan, R., Nankin, H. R., Troen, P., Wald, N., Pan, S., and Yanaihara, T. (1973): Paternal transmission of maleness in XX human beings. *N. Engl. J. Med.,* 288:539–545.
141. Kaufman, M., Pinsky, L., Hollander, R., and Bailey, J. D. (1983): Regulation of the androgen in normal and androgen resistant genital skin fibroblasts. *J. Steroid Biochem.,* 18:383–390.
142. Keenan, B. S., Meyer, W. J. III, Hadjian, A. J., Jones, H. W., and Migeon, C. J. (1974): Syndrome of androgen insensitivity in man: Absence of 5α-dihydrotestosterone binding protein in skin fibroblasts. *J. Clin. Endocrinol. Metab.,* 38:1143–1146.
143. Kellokumpo-Lehtinen, P., Santti, R., and Pelliniemi, L. J. (1980): Correlation of early cytodifferentiation of the human fetal prostate and Leydig cells. *Anat. Rec.,* 196:263–273.
144. Kobayashi, S. (1984): Induction of mullerian duct derivatives in testicular feminized (Tfm) mice by prenatal exposure to diethylstilbestrol. *Anat. Embryol.* 169:35–39.
145. Kovacs, W. J., Griffin, J. E., and Wilson, J. D. (1983): Transformation of human androgen receptors to the deoxyribonucleic acid-binding state. *Endocrinology,* 113:1574–1581.
146. Kovacs, W. J., Griffin, J. E., Weaver, D. D., Carlson, B. R., and Wilson, J. D. (1984): A mutation that causes lability of the androgen receptor under conditions that normally promote DNA-binding state. *J. Clin. Invest.,* 73:1095–1104.
147. Kratochwil, K. (1971): *In vitro* analysis of the hormonal basis for the sexual dimorphism in the embryonic development of the mouse mammary gland. *Embryol. Exp. Morphol.,* 25:141–153.
148. Kratochwil, K., and Schwartz, P. (1976): Tissue interaction in androgen response of embryonic mammary rudiment of mouse: Identification of target tissue for testosterone. *Proc. Natl. Acad. Sci. USA,* 73:4041–4044.
149. Kratzer, P. G., and Chapman, V. M. (1981): X chromosome reactivation in oocytes of *Mus caroli. Proc. Natl. Acad. Sci. USA,* 78:2093–2097.
150. Lasnitzki, I., and Mizuno, T. (1980): Prostatic induction: Interaction of epithelium and mesenchyme from normal wild-type and androgen insensitive mice with testicular feminization. *J. Endocrinol.,* 85:423–428.
151. Leshin, M., Griffin, J. E., and Wilson, J. D. (1978): Hereditary male pseudohermaphroditism associated with an unstable form of 5α-reductase. *J. Clin. Invest.,* 62:685–691.
152. Liang, T., and Heiss, C. E. (1981): Inhibition of 5α-reductase, receptor binding, and nuclear uptake of androgens in the prostate by a 4-methyl-4-aza-steroid. *J. Biol. Chem.,* 256:7998–8005.
153. Lifschytz, E. (1971): X-chromosome inactivation: An essential feature of normal spermiogenesis in male heterogametic organisms. In: *The Genetics of the Spermatozoon,* edited by R. A. Beatty and S. Gluecksohn-Waelsch, pp. 223–232. Bogtrykkenèt Forum, Copenhagen.
154. Lifschytz, E., and Lindsley, D. L. (1972): The role of X-chromosome inactivation during spermatogenesis. *Proc. Natl. Acad. Sci.. USA,* 69:182–186.
155. Lipsett, M. B., and Tullner, W. W. (1965): Testosterone synthesis by the fetal rabbit gonad. *Endocrinology,* 77:273–277.
156. Lowry, R. B., Honore, L. H., Arnold, W. J. D., Johnson, H. W., Kliman, M. R., and Marhsall, R. H. (1975): Familial true hermaphroditism. *Birth Defects,* 11:105–113.
157. Lowsley, O. S. (1912): The development of the human prostate with reference to the development of other structures of the neck of the urinary bladder. *Am. J. Anat.,* 13:299–349.
158. Lyon, M. F. (1961): Gene action in the X-chromosome of the mouse. *Nature,* 190:372–373.
159. Lyon, M. F. (1962): Sex chromatin and gene action in the mammalian X-chromosome. *Am. J. Hum. Genet.,* 14:135–148.
160. Lyon, M. F. (1968): Chromosomal and sub-chromosomal inactivation. *Annu. Rev. Genet.,* 2:31–52.
161. Lyon, M. F., and Hawkes, S. G. (1970): X-Linked gene for testicular feminization in the mouse. *Nature,* 227:1217–1219.
162. MacDonald, P. C., Madden, J. D., Brenner, P. F., Wilson, J. D., and Siiteri, P. K. (1979): Origin of estrogen in normal men and in women with testicular feminization. *J. Clin. Endocrinol. Metab.,* 49:905–916.
163. Madan, K. (1983): Balanced structural changes involving the human X: Effect on sexual phenotype. *Hum. Genet.,* 63:216–221.
164. Madden, J. D., Walsh, P. C., MacDonald, P. C., and Wilson, J. D. (1975): Clinical and endocrinological characterization of a patient with the syndrome of incomplete testicular feminization. *J. Clin. Endocrinol. Metab.,* 40:751–760.
165. Maes, M., Sultan, C., Zerhouni, N., Rothwell, S. W., and Migeon, C. J. (1979): Role of testosterone binding to the androgen receptor in male sexual differentiation of patients with 5α-reductase deficiency. *J. Steroid Biochem.,* 11:1385–1390.
166. Magre, S., and Jost, A. (1984): Dissociation between testicular organogenesis and endocrine cytodifferentiation of Sertoli cells. *Proc. Natl. Acad. Sci. USA,* 81:7831–7834.
167. Mangoushi, M. A. (1975): Scrotal allografts of fetal ovaries. *J. Anat.,* 120:595–599.
168. McCarrey, J. R., and Abbott, U. K. (1978): Chick gonad differentiation following excision of primordial germ cells. *Dev. Biol.,* 66:256–265.
169. McKay, D. G., Hertig, A. T., Adams, E. C., and Danziger, S. (1953): Histochemical observation on the germ cells of the human embryos. *Anat. Rec.,* 117:201–220.
170. McLachlan, J. A. (1977): Prenatal exposure to diethylstilbestrol in mice: Toxicological studies. *J. Toxicol. Environ. Health,* 2:527–537.
171. McLaren, A. (1983): Sex reversal in the mouse. *Differentiation* 23:S93–S98.
172. McLaren, A., and Monk, M. (1981): X chromosome activity in the germ cells of *sex-reversed* mouse embryos. *J. Reprod. Fertil.,* 63:533–537.
173. McLaren, A., and Monk, M. (1982): Fertile females produced by inactivation of an X chromosome of *'sex-reversed'* mice. *Nature,* 300:446–448.
174. McLaren, A., Simpson, E. Tomonari, K., Chandler, P., and Hogg, H. (1984): Male sexual differentiation in mice lacking H-Y antigen. *Nature,* 312:552–555.
175. Merchant, H. (1975): Rat gonadal and ovarian organogenesis with and without germ cells. An ultrastructural study. *Dev. Biol.,* 44:1–21.
176. Meyer, W. J. III, Migeon, B. R., and Migeon, C. J. (1975): Locus on human X chromosome for dihydrotesterone receptor and androgen insensitivity. *Proc. Natl. Acad. Sci. USA,* 72:1469–1472.
177. Migeon, B. R., Brown, T. R., Axelman, J., and Migeon, C. J. (1981): Studies of the locus for androgen receptor: Localization on the human X chromosome and evidence for homology with the *Tfm* locus in the mouse. *Proc. Natl. Acad. Sci. USA,* 78:6339–6343.
178. Migeon, B. R., and Jelalian, K. (1977): Evidence for two active X chromosomes in germ cells of female before meiotic entry. *Nature,* 269:242–243.
179. Milewich, L., George, F. W., and Wilson, J. D. (1977): Estrogen formation by the ovary of the rabbit embryo. *Endocrinology,* 100:187–196.

180. Molsberry, R. L., Carr, B. R., Mendelson, C. R., and Simpson, E. R. (1982): Human chorionic gonadotropin binding to human fetal testes as a function of gestation age. *J. Clin. Endocrinol. Metab.*, 55:791–794.
181. Monesi, V. (1965): Synthetic activities during spermatogenesis in the mouse. RNA and protein. *Exp. Cell Res.*, 39:197–224.
182. Moore, C. R., and Price, D. (1942): Differentiation of embryonic gonads transplanted into post-natal hosts. *J. Exp. Zool.*, 90:229–265.
183. Moore, R. J., and Wilson, J. D. (1976): Steroid 5α-reductase in cultured human fibroblasts: Biochemical and genetic evidence for two enzyme activities. *J. Biol. Chem.*, 251:5895–5900.
184. Moore, R. J., Griffin, J. E., and Wilson, J. D. (1975): Diminished 5α-reductase activity in extracts of fibroblasts cultured from patients with familial incomplete male pseudohermaphroditism, type 2. *J. Biol. Chem.*, 250:7168–7172.
185. Mori, Y., and Mitzutani, S. (1968): Familial true hermaphroditism in genetic females. *Jpn. J. Urol.*, 59:857–864.
186. Mudgett-Hunter, M., Budzik, G. P., Sullivan, M., and Donahoe, P. K. (1982): Monoclonal antibody to mullerian inhibiting substance. *J. Immunol.*, 128:1327–1333.
187. Neumann, F., von Berswordt-Wallrabe, R., Elger, W., Steinbeck, H., Hahn, J. D., and Kramer, M. (1970): Aspects of androgen-dependent events as studied by antiandrogens. *Recent Prog. Horm. Res.*, 26:337–405.
188. New, M. I., Dupont, B., Grunback, K., and Levine, L. S. (1983): Congenital adrenal hyperplasia and related conditions. In: *The Metabolic Basis of Inherited Disease*, 5th ed., edited by J. B. Stanbury, J. B. Wyngaarden, D. S. Fredrickson, J. L. Goldstein, and M. S. Brown, pp. 973–1000. McGraw-Hill, New York.
189. Odartchenko, N., and Pavillard, M. (1970): Late DNA replication in male mouse meiotic chromosomes. *Science*, 167:1133–1134.
190. Ohno, S. (1978): The role of H-Y antigen in primary sex determination. *J. Am. Med. Assoc.*, 239:217–220.
191. Ohno, S., and Lyon, M. F. (1965): Cytological study of Searle's X-autosome translocation in *Mus musculus*. *Chromosoma*, 16:90–100.
192. Ohno, S., and Makino, S. (1961): The single-X nature of sex chromatin in man. *Lancet*, 1:78–79.
193. Ohno, S., Jainchill, J., and Stenius, C. (1963): The creeping vole (*Microtus oregoni*) as a gonosomic mosaic. The OY/XY constitution of the male. *Cytogenetics*, 2:232–239.
194. O'Rahilly, R. (1977): The development of the vagina in the human. In: *Morphogenesis and Malformation of the Genital System*, edited by R. J. Blandua and D. Bergsma. *Birth Defects*, 13:123–136.
195. Page, D., de Martinville, B., Barker, D., Wyman, A., White, R., Francke, U., and Botstein, D. (1982): Single-copy sequence hybridizes to polymorphic and homologous loci on human X and Y chromosomes. *Proc. Natl. Acad. Sci. USA*, 79:5352–5356.
196. Patsavoudi, E., Magre, S., Castanier, M., Scholler, R., and Jost, A. (1985): Dissociation between testicular morphogenesis and functional differentiation of Leydig cells. *J. Endocrinol.*, 105:235–238.
197. Perez-Palacios, G., Medina, M., Ullao-Aguirre, A., Chavez, B. A., Villareal, G., Dutrem, M. T., Cahill, L. T., and Wachtel, S. (1981): Gonadotropin dynamics in XX males. *J. Clin. Endocrinol. Metab.*, 53:254–257.
198. Peterson, R. E., Imperato-McGinley, J., Gautier, T., and Sturla, E. (1977): Male pseudohermaphroditism due to steroid 5α-reductase deficiency. *Am. J. Med.*, 62:170–191.
199. Pfahl, M. (1982): Specific binding of the glucocorticoid-receptor complex to the mouse mammary tumor proviral promotor region. *Cell*, 31:475–482.
200. Pfaltz, C. R. (1949): Das embryonale und postnatale Verholten der mannlichen Brust drüse beim menschen. II. Das mammarorgan im Kindes-, Jünglings-, Mannes-und Greisenalter. *Acta Anat.*, 8:293–328.
201. Picard, J. Y., Benarous, R., Guerrier, D., Josso, N., and Kahn, A. (1986): Cloning and expression of cDNA for anti-Mullerian hormone. *Proc. Natl. Acad. Sci. USA*, 83:5464–5468.
202. Picard, J. Y., Tran, D., and Josso, N. (1978): Biosynthesis of labelled anti-müllerian hormone by fetal testes: Evidence for the glycoprotein nature of the hormone and for its disulfide-bonded structure. *Mol. Cell. Endocrinol.*, 12:17–30.
203. Price, J. M. (1979): The secretion of mullerian inhibiting substance by cultured isolated Sertoli cells of the neonatal calf. *Am. J. Anat.*, 156:147–157.
204. Price, J. M., Donahoe, P. K., Ito, Y., and Hendren, W. H. III (1977): Programmed cell death in the mullerian duct induced by mullerian inhibiting substance. *Am. J. Anat.*, 149:353–376.
205. Price, P., Wass, J. A. H., Griffin, J. E., Leshin, M., Savage, M. O., Large, D. M., Bu'Lock, D. E., Anderson, D. C., Wilson, J. D., and Besser, G. M. (1984): High dose androgen therapy in male pseudohermaphroditism due to 5α-reductase deficiency and disorders of the androgen receptor. *J. Clin. Invest.*, 74:1496–1508.
206. Rajfer, J., and Walsh, P. C. (1977): Hormonal regulation of testicular descent: Experimental and clinical observations. *J. Urol.*, 118:985–990.
207. Rasmussen, S. W., and Holm, P. B. (1980): Mechanics of meiosis. *Hereditas*, 93:187–216.
208. Rigaudiere, N. (1979): The androgens in the guinea-pig foetus throughout the embryonic development. *Acta Endocrinol.*, 92:174–186.
209. Roe, T. F., and Alfi, O. S. (1977): Ambiguous genitalia in XX male children: Report of two infants. *Pediatrics*, 60:55–59.
210. Rosenberg, H. S., Clayton, G. W., and Hsu, T. C. (1963): Familial true hermaphrodism. *J. Clin. Endocrinol. Metab.*, 23:203–206.
211. Rouyer, F., Simmler, M. C., Johnsson, C., Vergnaud, G., Cooke, H. J., and Weissenbach, J. (1986): A gradient of sex linkage in the pseudoautosomal region of the human sex chromosomes. *Nature*, 319:291–295.
212. Russell, L. B., and Montgomery, C. S. (1969): Comparative studies on X-autosome translocations in the mouse. I. Origin, viability, fertility, and weight of five *T(X,I)'S*. *Genetics*, 63:103–120.
213. Saenger, P., Levine, L. S., Wachtel, S. S., Korth-Schutz, S., Doberne, Y., Koo, G. C., Lavengood, R. W. Jr., German, J. L. III, and New, M. I. (1976): Presence of H-Y antigen and testis in 46,XX true hermaphroditism, evidence of Y-chromosomal function. *J. Clin. Endocrinol. Metab.*, 43:1234–1239.
214. Schultz, F. M., and Wilson, J. D. (1974): Virilization of the wolffian duct in the rat fetus by various androgens. *Endocrinology*, 94:979–986.
215. Schweikert, H. U., Weissbach, L., Leyendecker, G., Schwinger, E., Wartenberg, H., and Kruck, F. (1982): Clinical, endocrinological, and cytological characterization of two 46,XX males. *J. Clin. Endocrinol. Metab.*, 54:745–752.
216. Searle, A. G. (1962): Is sex-linked *Tabby* really recessive in the mouse? *Heredity*, 17:297.
217. Selden, J. R., Wachtel, S. S., Koo, G. C., Haskins, M. E., and Patterson, D. F. (1978): Genetic basis of XX male syndrome and XX true hermaphroditism: Evidence in the dog. *Science*, 201:644–646.
218. Siiteri, P. K., and Wilson, J. D. (1974): Testosterone formation and metabolism during male sexual differentiation in the human embryo. *J. Clin. Endocrinol. Metab.*, 38:113–125.
219. Silvers, W. K., Gasser, D. L., and Eicher, E. M. (1982): H-Y antigen, serologically detectable male antigen and sex determination. *Cell*, 28:439–440.
220. Simmler, M. C., Rouyer, F., Vergnaud, G., Nystrom-Lahti, M., Ngo, K. Y., de la Chapelle, A., and Weissenbach, J. (1985): Pseudoautosomal DNA sequences in the pairing region of the human sex chromosomes. *Nature*, 317:692–697.
221. Simpson, J. L. (1978): True hermaphroditism: Etiology and phenotypic considerations. *Birth Defects*, 14:9–35.
222. Singh, L., and Jones, K. W. (1982): Sex reversal in the mouse (*Mus musculus*) is caused by a recurrent non-reciprocal crossover involving the X and the aberrant Y chromosome. *Cell*, 28:205–216.
223. Singh, L., Purdom, I. F., and Jones, K. W. (1980): Sex chromosome associated satellite DNA: Evolution and conservation. *Chromosoma* 79:137–157.
224. Sloan, W. R., and Walsh, P. C. (1976): Familial persistent müllerian duct syndrome. *J. Urol.*, 115:459–461.
225. Solari, A. J. (1974): The behavior of the XY pair in mammals. *Int. Rev. Cytol.*, 38:273–317.
226. Spaulding, M. H. (1921): The development of the external genitalia in the human embryo. *Carnegie Contrib. Embryol.*, 13:67.
227. Stern, C. (1957): The problem of complete Y-linkage in man. *Am. J. Hum. Genet.*, 9:147–165.
228. Suzuki, Y., Ishii, H., Furuya, H., and Arai, Y. (1982): Developmental changes of the hypogastric ganglion associated with the differentiation of the reproductive tracts in the mouse. *Neurosci. Lett.*, 32:271–276.
229. Takeda, H., Mizuno, T., and Lasnitzki, I. (1985): Autoradiographic studies of androgen-binding sites in the rat urogenital sinus and postnatal prostate. *J. Endocrinol.*, 104:87–92.

230. Taketo, T., Merchant-Larios, H., and Koide, S. S. (1984): Induction of testicular differentiation in the fetal mouse ovary by transplantation into adult male mice. *Proc. Soc. Exp. Biol. Med.*, 176: 148–153.
231. Taketo-Hosotani, T., Merchant-Larios, H., Thau, R. B., and Koide, S. S. (1985): Testicular differentiation in fetal mouse ovaries following transplantation into adult male mice. *J. Exp. Zool.*, 236:229–237.
232. Teng, C. S., and Teng, C. T. (1979): Prenatal effect of the estrogenic hormone on embryonic genital organ differentiation. In: *Ontogeny of Receptors and Reproductive Hormone Action*, edited by T. H. Hamilton, J. H. Clark, and N. A. Sadler, pp. 421–440. Raven Press, New York.
233. Torrey, T. W. (1950): Intraocular grafts of embryonic gonads of the rat. *J. Exp. Zool.*, 115:37–38.
234. Tran, D., and Josso, N. (1982): Localization of antimullerian hormone in the rough endoplasmic reticulum of the developing bovine Sertoli cell using immunocytochemistry with a monoclonal antibody. *Endocrinology*, 111:1562–1567.
235. Tran, D., Picard, J. Y., Vigier, B., Berger, R., and Josso, N. (1986): Persistence of müllerian ducts in male rabbits passively immunized against bovine anti-müllerian hormone during fetal life. *Dev. Biol.*, 116:160–167.
236. Trelstad, R. L., Hayashi, A., Hayashi, K., and Donahoe, P. K. (1982): The epithelial-mesenchymal interface of the male mullerian duct: Basement membrane integrity and ductal regression. *Dev. Biol.*, 92:27–40.
237. Turner, C. D. (1940): The influence of testosterone proprionate upon sexual differentiation in genetic female mice (etc.). *J. Exp. Zool.*, 83:1–31.
238. van Niekerk, W. A. (1974): *True Hermaphroditism. Clinical Morphologic and Cytogenetic Aspects*. Harper and Row, New York.
239. van Niekerk, W. A. (1981): True hermaphroditism. *Pediatr. Adolesc. Endocrinol.*, 8:80–99.
240. van Niekerk, W. A., and Retief, A. E. (1981): The gonads of human true hermaphrodites. *Hum. Genet.*, 58:117–122.
241. Venolia, L., Cooper, D. W., O'Brien, D. A., Millette, C. F., and Gartler, S. M. (1984): Transformation of the *Hprt* gene with DNA from spermatogenic cells. *Chromosoma*, 90:185–189.
242. Verhoeven, G., and Wilson, J. D. (1976): Cytosol androgen binding in submandibular gland and kidney of the normal mouse and the mouse with testicular feminization. *Endocrinology*, 99:79–92.
243. Vergnaud, G., Page, D. C., Simmler, M. C., Brown, L., Rouyer, F., Noel, B., Botstein, D., de la Chapelle, A., and Weissenbach, J. (1986): A deletion map of the human Y chromosome based on DNA hybridization. *Am. J. Hum. Genet.*, 38:109–124.
244. Veyssière, G., Corre, M., Berger, M., Jean-Faucher, Ch., de Turikheim, M., and Jean, Cl. (1980): Androgènes circulants etorganogenèse sexuelle mâle chez le foetus de lapin. Etude après immunisation active delamère contre la testostèrone. *Arch. Anat. Microsc. Morphol. Exp.*, 69:17–28.
245. Vigier, B., Picard, J-Y., and Josso, N. (1982): A monoclonal antibody against bovine anti-mullerian hormone. *Endocrinology*, 110:131–137.
246. Vigier, B., Legali, L., Picard, J.-Y., and Josso, N. (1982): A sensitive radioimmunoassay for bovine anti-müllerian hormone, allowing its detection in male and freemartin fetal serum. *Endocrinology*, 111:1409–1411.
247. Vigier, B., Picard, J.-Y., Champargue, J., Forest, M. G., Heyman, Y., and Josso, N. (1985): Secretion of anti-mullerian hormone by immature bovine Sertoli cells in primary culture studied by a competition-type radioimmunoassay: Lack of modulation by either FSH or testosterone. *Mol. Cell. Endocrinol.*, 43:141–150.
248. Vogel, F., and Motulsky, A. G. (1979): *Human Genetics*. Springer-Verlag, Berlin.
249. Wachtel, S. S. (1983): *H-Y Antigen and the Biology of Sex Determination*. Grune and Stratton, New York.
250. Wachtel, S. S., Ohno, S., Koo, G. C., and Boyse, E. A. (1975): Possible role of H-Y antigen in the primary determination of sex. *Nature*, 257:235–236.
251. Walsh, P. C., Madden, J. D., Harrod, M. J., Goldstein, J. L. MacDonald, P. C., and Wilson, J. D. (1974): Familial incomplete male pseudohermaphroditism, type 2. Decreased dihydrotestosterone formation in pseudovaginal perineoscrotal hypospadias. *N. Engl. J. Med.*, 291:944–949.
252. Wells, L. J., and van Wagenen, G. (1954): Androgen-induced female pseudohermaphroditism in the monkey (*Macaca mulatta*); anatomy of the reproductive organs. *Contrib. Embryol. Carnegie Inst.* (*Wash.*), 35:93–106.
253. White, M. R. (1949): Effects of hormones on embryonic sex differentiation in the golden hamster. *J. Exp. Zool.*, 110:153–181.
254. Wilbert, D. M., Griffin, J. E., and Wilson, J. D. (1983): Characterization of the cytosol androgen receptor of the human prostate. *J. Clin. Endocrinol. Metab.*, 56:113–120.
255. Wilson, J. D. (1971): Testosterone metabolism in skin. *Symp. Dtsch. Ges. Endokrinol.*, 17:11–18.
256. Wilson, J. D. (1979): Embryology of the genital tract. In: *Urology, Vol. 2*, 4th ed., edited by J. H. Harrison, R. F. Gittes, A. D. Perlmutter, T. A. Stamey, and P. C. Walsh, Chapter 41, pp. 1469–1483. W. B. Saunders, Philadelphia.
257. Wilson, J. D., and Goldstein, J. L. (1975): Classification of hereditary disorders of sexual development. *Birth Defects*, 11:1–16.
258. Wilson, J. D., and Lasnitzki, I. (1971): Dihydrotestosterone formation in fetal tissues of the rabbit and rat. *Endocrinology*, 89:659–668.
259. Wilson, J. D., and Siiteri, P. K. (1973): Developmental pattern of testosterone synthesis in the fetal gonad of the rabbit. *Endocrinology*, 92:1182–1191.
260. Wilson, J. D., Griffin, J. E., Leshin, M., and MacDonald, P. C. (1983): The androgen resistance syndromes: 5α-reductase deficiency, testicular feminization, and related disorders. In: *The Metabolic Basis of Inherited Disease*, edited by J. B. Stanbury, J. B. Wyngaarden, D. S. Fredrickson, J. L. Goldstein, and M. S. Brown, pp. 1001–1026. McGraw-Hill, New York.
261. Witschi, E. (1948): Migration of the germ cells of human embryos from the yolk sac to the primitive gonadal folds. *Contrib. Embryol. Carnegie Inst.* (*Wash.*), 32:67–80.
262. Wolfe, J., and Goodfellow, P. N. (1985): The elusive testis determining factor. *Trends Genet.*, 1:3–4.
263. Yen, P. H., Patel, P., Chinault, A. C., Mohandas, T., and Shapiro, L. J. (1984): Differential methylation of hypoxanthine phosphoribosyltransferase genes on active and inactive human X chromosomes. *Proc. Natl. Acad. Sci. USA*, 83:1759–1763.
264. Zaborski, P. (1985): H-Y antigen in nonmammalian vertebrates. *Arch. Aust. Microsc. Morphol. Exp.*, 74:33–37.
265. Zenzes, M. T., and Reed, T. E. (1984): Variability in serologically detected male antigen titer and some resulting problems: A critical review. *Hum. Genet.*, 66:103–109.

The Physiology of Reproduction,
edited by E. Knobil and J. Neill *et al.*
Raven Press, Ltd., New York © 1988.

CHAPTER 2

The Spermatozoon

E. M. Eddy

The spermatozoon is the end product of the process of gametogenesis in the male, occurring within the seminiferous tubules of the testis. This involves a series of mitotic division of spermatogonial stem cells, two meiotic divisions by spermatocytes, extensive morphological remodeling of the spermatid during spermiogenesis, and the release of the free cell into the lumen of the seminiferous tubule by spermiation. It is an interesting paradox that the process of spermatogenesis produces a cell that is highly differentiated in structure and function, while at the same time is developmentally totipotent, being able to combine with the egg and thereby begin the process that gives rise to a new individual.

The mammalian spermatozoon has two main components, the head and the tail or flagellum (Fig. 1). The head consists of the acrosome, the nucleus, and lesser amounts of cytoskeletal structures and cytoplasm. The acrosome is a large secretory granule that closely surrounds and overlies the anterior end of the nucleus. The sperm nucleus is haploid, containing only one member of each chromosome pair, and the chromatin becomes highly condensed during the latter part of spermatogenesis. The tail contains a centrally placed axoneme, which is a highly ordered complex of microtubles surrounded by dense fibers extending from the head to near the posterior end of the axoneme. In addition, the anterior part of the flagellum contains mitochondria wrapped in a tight helix around the dense fibers, and the most posterior part of the tail contains the fibrous sheath surrounding the dense fibers. The dense fibers and the fibrous sheath form the cytoskeleton of the flagellum. These cytoskeletal features appear to have evolved with the development of internal fertilization (1). The tail, like the head, is closely wrapped by the plasma membrane and contains little cytoplasm. Although all mammalian spermatozoa have these general characteristics, there are species-specific differences in the size and shape of the head as well as the length and relative size of the components of the flagellum. Nonmammalian species show greater variation in sperm structure; although sperm in most invertebrates and nonmammalian vertebrates have an acrosome, they often contain few mitochondria, and their flagellum consists only of an axoneme. In some species, spermatozoa are amoeboid cells lacking an acrosome and a flagellum (2,3).

The specialized structural features of the spermatozoon are a reflection of its unique functional activities. The acrosome contains enzymes essential for fertilization, while the flagellum contains the energy sources and machinery necessary to produce spermatozoon motility. The roles of these components are to ensure delivery of the genetic material contained in the nucleus to the egg, where combination of the haploid male and female pronuclei occurs, ending the process of reproduction and initiating the process of development. In most vertebrates, the sex chromosome carried in the haploid sperm nucleus determines the gender of the resulting individual (4). Both a maternal and a paternal genome are required for development to proceed to term, probably because differential imprinting of gamete genomes occurs during gametogenesis in males and females (5).

This chapter examines the structure and function of the mammalian spermatozoon, with an emphasis on the molecules currently known to be involved. The major topics considered are: the organization of the sperm plasma mem-

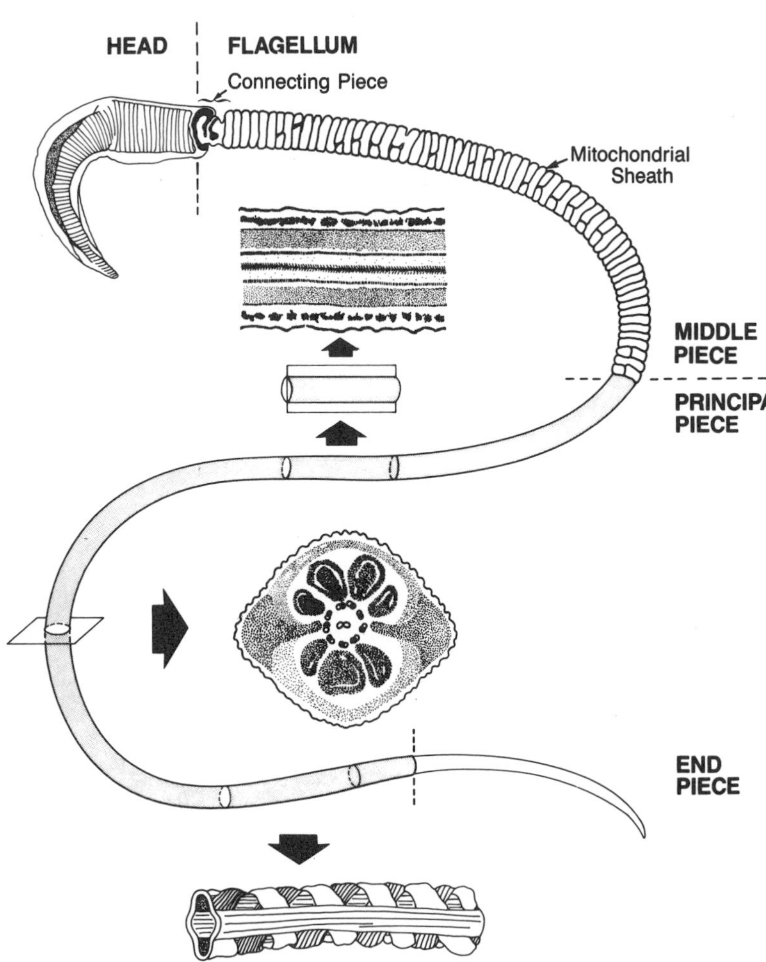

FIG. 1. General features of the mammalian sperm. The head of the spermatozoon is attached to the connecting piece of the flagellum. The other regions of the flagellum are the middle piece, the principal piece, and the end piece. The middle piece contains the mitochondrial sheath, while the principal piece contains the fibrous sheath. Longitudinal and cross-sectional views of the principal piece and a segment of fibrous sheath are indicated by arrows; the internal components of the flagellum are identified in Fig. 9.

brane into domains, changes in the composition and function of the domains during the life of the cell, the structural components of the head of the sperm, and the features of the flagellum. Other chapters are concerned with the formation of the male gamete (6), participation of the spermatozoon in fertilization (7), and the subsequent development of a new individual (8). They contain additional information that is important for understanding the structure and function of the spermatozoon and its role in the reproductive process.

THE PLASMA MEMBRANE

Surface Domains

A unique feature of the spermatozoon is that the plasma membrane is subdivided into sharply delineated regional domains that differ in composition and function. The heterogeneous nature of the sperm surface first became apparent from studies of surface charge, lectin binding to specific sugar moieties, freeze-fracture patterns, and antibody labeling. The evidence that the organization and composition of the plasma membrane varied between different regions of the sperm surface led to the concept that the sperm plasma membrane is a mosaic of restricted domains that reflect the specialized functions of surface and cytoplasmic components of the spermatozoon (9). Subsequent studies have supported this and have further demonstrated that the domains are dynamic features that undergo changes in organization and composition during the life of the cell.

The major domains of the head region of the sperm surface in most mammals (Fig. 2) are (a) the *anterior acrosome* (acrosomal cap) and *equatorial segment* (posterior acrosome) overlying the acrosome and (b) the *postacrosomal region* (postacrosomal sheath, postnuclear sheath) covering the portion of the head posterior to the acrosome. In addition, the less well-defined *anterior band* is situated between the anterior acrosome and the equatorial segment (10), and a *serrated band* girdles the sperm head at the posterior margin of the equatorial segment. The *posterior ring* (nuclear ring, striated ring) lies at the junction between head and tail and apparently forms a tight seal between the cytoplasmic compartments of the two main portions of the spermatozoon. The plasma membrane of the flagellum is

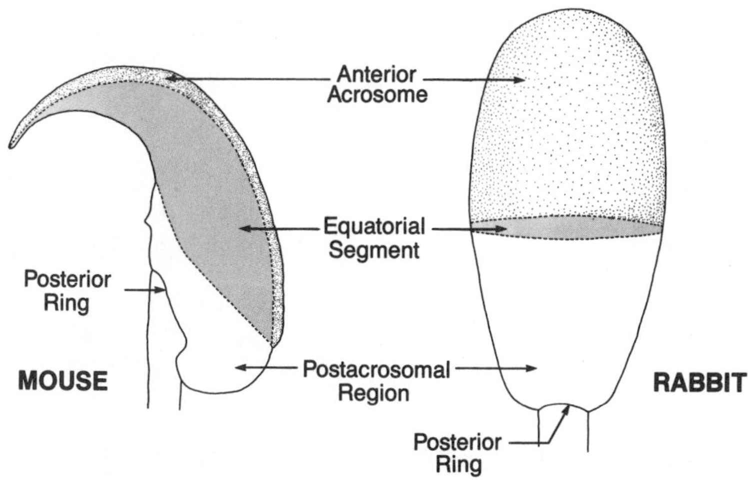

FIG. 2. Plasma membrane domains on the surface of the head of mouse and rabbit spermatozoa. The anterior acrosome domain is more extensive on sperm containing a spatulate head, such as that of the rabbit, whereas the equatorial segment domain overlying the posterior part of the acrosome is larger on sperm containing a falciform head. The posterior ring forms a boundary between the postacrosomal domain of the head and the middle piece domain of the flagellum. The distribution of the domains on the heads of sperm of these and other species are compared in Fig. 3.

separated into domains overlying the *middle piece* and *posterior tail* (distal tail) by the *annulus,* a fibrous ring that surrounds the components of the axoneme and is firmly attached to the membrane.

The Mosaic Sperm Surface

The first studies to suggest the heterogeneity of the sperm plasma membrane were those that examined regional differences in surface charge (Table 1). When spermatozoa from the ram, rabbit, or bull were suspended between oppositely charged electrodes, they were found to be drawn tail first by electrophoresis toward the anode. This suggested that sperm have a net negative charge and that more of this charge is on the tail than at the head (11–13). Other studies indicated that at least some of the moieties responsible for sperm net negative charge were on the surface and that there were regional differences in this surface charge. Electron microscopy was used to show that binding of positively charged colloidal iron hydroxide to the surface of rabbit sperm was greater on the flagellum than on the head (14,15).

Lectins have relatively specific affinities for particular saccharide molecules (16,17). They are often multimeric and can bind simultaneously to more than one saccharide ligand on a given cell or can cause agglutination by linking adjacent cells. Lectins can be tagged with fluorescent markers, enzymes, radioactive labels, or materials visible in the electron microscope. Agglutination assays carried out with spermatozoa from different species have demonstrated regional differences in the location and amount of specific saccharides on the sperm surface (Table 1). An early study with soybean agglutinin (SBA; recognizing α-D-GalNAc, D-Gal) indicated that it caused predominantly tail-to-tail agglutination of ejaculated bull sperm (18). Other studies indicated that hamster sperm agglutinated more readily by the tail than the head, following treatment with concanavalin A (Con A; recognizing α-D-Glc, α-D-Man) or wheat-germ agglutinin (WGA; recognizing [β(1-4)D-GalNAc]2) (19). However, it has been noted that there are discrepancies between the number of lectin-binding sites and the agglutination of treated cells (20,21). Quantitative studies using iodinated lectins indicated that there are 1 to 3 $\times$ 10^7 Con-A- and WGA-binding sites per rabbit or hamster epididymal spermatozoon, but fewer RCA-binding sites (22). When expressed on the basis of surface area, the average density of binding sites was similar between sperm from those species. However, when the data on Con-A binding were recalculated on the basis of square-micrometer surface area, the sperm head possessed approximately 10 times more sites than the flagellum (21). The greater surface area and motion of the tail, compared to the head, apparently lead to tail-to-tail agglutination, even though the tail has a lower number of lectin-binding sites.

The use of lectins conjugated with fluorescent labels or ultrastructural markers has confirmed the regional heterogeneity of distribution of saccharides on the sperm surface (Table 1). However, they have given somewhat different results than were seen in agglutination studies. With fluorescent lectins, Con A was found to bind predominantly to the acrosome region of mouse sperm (23,24), WGA was found to bind to the head of mouse sperm and over the acrosome of guinea-pig sperm (25,26), SBA was found to bind over the anterior acrosome of guinea-pig sperm (21), and peanut agglutinin (PNA; recognizing D-Gal, β[1-3]-GalNAc) was found to bind over the anterior acrosome of mouse sperm (27). A peroxidase histochemical method was used to show that Con-A binding is more intense on the head than on the tail of rabbit sperm (28). Other ultrastructural studies used ferritin-conjugated castor-bean agglutinin (RCA; recognizing β-D-Gal, D-GalNAc) on rabbit sperm (29) and used ferritin- and hemocyanin-labeled Con A on hamster sperm (30) and also noted greater binding on the head than on the tail. These studies confirmed that lectin-binding sites are generally present in higher density on the head than on the tail of the sperm. However, the surface domains recognized by lectins are often not well defined, and different binding patterns have been observed for the

TABLE 1. *Regional heterogeneity of the sperm plasma membrane*

Characteristic	References
Surface charge distribution	
Sperm drawn tail-first toward the anode in electrophoretic field	11–13
Positively charged colloidal iron hydroxide particle binding greater on the tail than on the head	14, 15
Surface saccharide distribution	
Sperm agglutinated tail-to-tail following lectin treatment	18, 19
Different lectins bind to specific regions of the sperm surface	21, 23–30
Intramembranous particle distribution	
Hexagonal arrays of particles in the plasma membrane overlying the acrosome	31–33
Dense populations of intramembranous particles in the plasma membrane overlying the postacrosomal region	26, 31, 34, 38, 41
Oblique strands of particles in plasma membrane of middle piece overlying mitochondria	31, 38, 40, 49, 51
Localized surface features	
Serrated band at posterior margin of equatorial segment of acrosome	31, 33–36, 38, 39
Palisades of prominent particles at posterior margin of postacrosomal region	31, 41–43
Belt of fine periodicities in plasma membrane over the posterior ring	31, 34, 37, 38, 49
Close array of fine particles in plasma membrane over annulus	31, 49
Staggered row of large particles running longitudinally on principal piece	31, 49, 51, 55, 56, 58
Membrane intercalating agents	
Filipin-induced complexes with sterols frequent in plasma membrane over acrosome	40, 43, 56, 59–61
Polymyxin B binds anionic phospholipids in plasma membrane over anterior acrosome	60, 62–64
Fluorescent lipid analog integrates preferentially into plasma membrane over acrosome	65
Sperm plasma membrane antigens recognized by antisera	
Antigens shared with other cells in restricted domains on sperm surface	
Equatorial segment	67
Potacrosomal region	68
Anterior acrosome	69
Antigens in single domains recognized by antisera to male germ cells	
Anterior acrosome	70
Postacrosomal region	71
Principal piece	72
Antigens in multiple domains recognized by antisera to male germ cells	
Equatorial segment and postacrosomal region	73
Acrosome and midpiece	72
Head and midpiece	74
Head and tail	75
Entire sperm surface	76–78

same lectin on sperm from the same species (see, e.g., refs. 21 and 24).

Freeze-fracture, freeze-etch, and surface replica studies have shown differences in the number and patterns of distribution of intramembranous particles and in membrane-associated structures in different regions of the sperm plasma membrane (Table 1). Although there are significant species differences, these studies have demonstrated characteristic features of the plasma membrane associated with the anterior region of the acrosome, the equatorial segment, the posterior margin of the equatorial segment, and the postacrosomal area. Other regions of the sperm plasma membrane showing structural specialization are (a) the posterior ring at the junction between head and tail and (b) the annulus situated between the midpiece region and the more distal part of the tail.

In most species, the plasma membrane overlying the anterior acrosome and equatorial segment contains randomly distributed intramembranous particles, but numerous hexagonal arrays of particles are present in guinea-pig sperm stacked closely together in the epididymis, and small patches of similarly organized particles are seen occasionally in rat sperm (31). These particle arrays have been noted by other investigators studying rat (32) and boar sperm (33). The posterior margin of the equatorial segment usually has a saw-toothed pattern, formed of rows of closely packed particles (Table 1). The location and general topography of this serrated band can be seen as a surface feature on whole spermatozoa by light microscopy (34), scanning electron microscopy (34–36), and transmission electron microscopy of surface replicas (37–39).

The plasma membrane of the postacrosomal area of the sperm head usually contains a more dense population of intramembranous particles (26,31,34,39–41) than does the acrosomal area, and the particles are sometimes in clusters (Table 1). The basal part of the postacrosomal area contains prominent cords or bands of particles (31,41–43), which often lie in palisades (Table 1). They lie adjacent to the posterior ring, which is a belt of fine periodicities or cords of small particles in the plasma membrane at the junction between head and tail of the spermatozoon (31,34,37,44). This structure was first reported by light microscopists (45,46), and its presence was confirmed by electron microscopists studying sections (47) and replicas (48) of spermatozoa. The posterior ring is formed by plasma membrane being closely applied to a belt of dense fibrous material lying upon the nuclear envelope (31,34,37,38,44,48) and appears to produce a seal between head and tail compartments of the spermatozoon. The posterior ring of mammalian spermatozoa may allow substantially different ionic and metabolic conditions to be maintained in the cytoplasmic compartments of the head and flagellum (49).

The plasma membrane of the midpiece region of the flagellum in some species contains strands of particles, which run in diagonal arrays that coincide in pitch with the underlying helically wound mitochondria (Table 1). The particle strands appear to be present only when the plasma membrane is closely applied to mitochondria; these strands are usually not present in cytoplasmic droplets (31,38,40,41,50,51). It has been suggested (52) that the particle strands might be homologous to the necklace of particles at the base of cilia (see, e.g., ref. 53). The strands are particularly prominent in guinea-pig sperm; in other species, however, patches of hexagonally packed particles are present in the midpiece plasma membrane and tend to follow the contour of the mitochondrial helix (49). A different pattern has been reported in opossum spermatozoa, where intramembrane particles are present in parallel longitudinally arranged aggregates (54).

The annulus is a dense fibrous ring surrounding the axonemal complex at the junction between the middle piece and the principal piece of the flagellum. Upon use of freeze-fracture techniques, the plasma membrane in this area appears to have a rough texture or to contain a close array of small particles, sometimes in circumferential strands (31). The plasma membrane is closely applied to the annulus, and these features may represent anchoring of the annulus into the membrane (49).

The intramembranous particles in the plasma membrane of the principal piece posterior to the annulus appear larger than those in the middle piece. In addition, sperm of some species have a staggered double row of yet larger particles (31,51), resembling a zipper coursing longitudinally over the ribs of the fibrous sheath, opposite outer dense fiber number 1 (31). The zipper-like structure terminates before reaching the posterior end of the principal piece of the flagellum. The large particles that form this structure are seen on surface replicas and are probably part of a transmembrane complex (49,55). The particles appear to be slightly oval and to have a depression in their center, possibly indicative of a pore. This feature has led to the suggestion that zipper particles may be sites of ion transport (56). It has also been postulated that the zipper is a membrane-anchoring device for some of the axonemal components (55). Treatment of guinea-pig sperm with digitonin, a detergent that disrupts cholesterol-rich plasma membrane (57), does not remove the zipper. However, the zipper particles can be removed by subsequent treatment with Triton X-100 (55). The zipper binds the lectins Con A, RCA, and WGA, and the Triton-X-100-soluble fraction includes four polypeptides ranging from 24,000 to 110,000 daltons (58).

Freeze-fracture techniques used in conjunction with membrane intercalating agents has provided evidence of compositional differences between sperm surface membrane domains (Table 1). Treatment of guinea-pig sperm with filipin, a polyene that complexes β-hydroxysterols with sterol, indicated that the regions between the plaques of intramembranous particles in the plasma membrane over the anterior acrosome and equatorial segment are sterol-rich (43,59). The sterols (cholesterol and dermosterol) appear to be present in higher concentration in the inner half than in the outer half of the membrane leaflet (60). However, filipin fluorescence indicates that sterols may exist throughout the entire plasma membrane of the anterior acrosome, not just between the plaques (10). The plasma membrane of the postacrosomal region has less than one-fourth as many filipin-induced complexes as that of the anterior acrosome and equatorial segment, with a pattern suggesting that they are present mainly in the outer half of the bilayer (10,60). These studies also indicated that the anterior acrosome is separated from the equatorial segment by an anterior band, a subdomain that, in guinea-pig sperm, often contains circles of membrane cleared of sterols and intramembranous particles (56,61).

The antibiotic polymyxin B binds anionic phospholipids, producing crenulations of anionic phospholipid-rich membranes (62,63). Treatment of guinea-pig sperm with polymyxin B indicated that the plasma membrane over the anterior acrosome has a high anionic lipid concentration (64). In sperm from the epididymis, the concentration of anionic lipids appears to be greatest at the anterior tip of the acrosome. The high anionic lipid concentration is not seen in the anterior band or posterior to the equatorial segment (60,62,64).

The fluorescent lipid analog, 1,1′-dihexadecyl-3,3′-tetramethyl-indocarbocyanine perchlorate (C_{16}dil), intercalates into the outer leaflet of the sperm plasma membrane, and it was found that the anterior part of the head of ram sperm was labeled more intensely than the posterior head with this agent (65). The differences in affinity of the probe for these regions of the sperm apparently result from interactions of the probe with lipids and proteins heterogeneously distributed within the plane of the membrane.

Sperm-Surface Antigens

Antibodies to spermatozoa, germ cells, other cell types, or isolated molecules have identified more distinct surface regions on living sperm than those seen with other methods (Table 1). Antibodies can be conjugated directly with various labels or detected indirectly with second antibodies (66) that carry labels visible by light or electron microscopy. Antibodies can also be used to isolate and identify specific molecules and to test their roles in bioassays. In some cases, it has been found that antigens shared with other cell types are restricted to specific regions of the sperm surface. With mouse sperm, (a) an antiserum to the H-Y antigen has been found to react with the plasma membrane over the equatorial segment (67), (b) an antiserum to F9 teratocarcinoma cells to bind to the postacrosomal region (68), and (c) an antiserum to galactosyltransferase to bind to the anterior acrosome (69). In addition, some antisera to sperm or spermatogenic cells react with specific regions, such as anterior acrosome (70), postacrosomal region (71), or principal piece (72). Other antisera to germ cells react with multiple regions of the sperm surface, such as equatorial segment and postacrosomal region (73), acrosome and midpiece (72), head and midpiece (74) or whole tail (75), or even with the entire sperm surface (76–78). The molecules recognized by these antisera have not been identified in most cases. It is tempting to speculate that antisera reacting with specific regions may recognize one or a few antigens, whereas those reacting with the whole surface recognize multiple antigens. However, binding to the whole sperm surface has been seen with both an antiserum to a single antigen (77) and one to multiple antigens (78).

The multiple and variable specificities of antisera to whole cells or mixtures of antigens limit their usefulness for dissecting the distribution of sperm-surface components and defining the biochemical characteristics and functional roles of such components. Monoclonal antibodies have been produced against spermatozoa to overcome some of these limitations (Table 2). Although monoclonal antibodies are often specific to particular molecules, they may also recognize epitopes shared by many molecules (see, e.g., ref. 79). Furthermore, monoclonal antibodies, which label only one domain on the sperm surface, may immunoprecipitate proteins of more than one molecular weight from that domain (see, e.g., ref. 80). It is possible that these proteins are either subunits of a membrane complex that coprecipitate under such conditions or are not associated but share a common epitope recognized by the antibody. Studies with monoclonal antibodies have been carried out most frequently in mouse, rat, guinea pig, and human, but less often in boar, hamster, and rabbit. In some cases, the monoclonal antibody recognizes the whole sperm surface (81–83), the whole head (80,83,84,86,100,101), or the whole tail (80,84,87–93). Other monoclonal antibodies bind specifically to anterior acrosome, equatorial segment, postacrosomal region, middle piece, or posterior tail of living sperm (79,80,84,85,94–108) (Table 2). Other patterns have been reported on air-dried or fixed sperm, but these treatments can expose internal antigens (see, e.g., ref. 82). In addition, some monoclonal antibodies recognize variable patterns or apparent subdomains on spermatozoa, possibly as a result of shedding of sperm-surface components during processing, partial masking of components by extrinsic molecules, or relocalization of components due to membrane fluidity (see, e.g., ref. 109). However, a variety of studies have used monoclonal antibodies against sperm from different species to confirm that the sperm surface consists of well-defined domains and that different proteins and glycoproteins may be either confined to individual domains or shared by multiple domains (Table 2).

TABLE 2. *Sperm-surface domains recognized with monoclonal antibodies*

Antibodies	Species	Mass (kilodaltons)	References
Antigens restricted to single domains			
Anterior acrosome			
HS 1A.1	Human	ND[a]	79
MA 1	Human	84	94
MA 2	Human	ND	94
MA 3	Human	240	94
D81, G112, G176, G225[b]	Human	ND	95
SMA1	Mouse	ND	84
MS-1	Mouse	69	96
1B3	Mouse	28	97
AMSIV-33[b]	Mouse	200	92
—	Mouse	ND	98
J1, C6	Mouse	ND	27
M5	Mouse	54	99
M41	Mouse	21, 35, 60	99
M42	Mouse	220–240	85, 99
AH-1	Guinea pig	52	80, 100, 101
AH-2	Guinea pig	18, 25, 46, 62, 70	100, 101
AH-3	Guinea pig	38, 52, 62	100, 101
AH-4	Guinea pig	16, 38	100, 101
AH-5	Guinea pig	ND	100, 101
8C10.5	Rabbit	63	102
Equatorial segment			
D3	Human	ND	95
M2[c]	Mouse	36, 44	103
M29[c]	Mouse	40	103
Postacrosomal region			
HS 1E.1	Human	53, 56, 73	79
PH-1	Guinea pig	60	100, 101
PH-2	Guinea pig	41, 48, 66	100, 101
PH-3	Guinea pig	48, 58	100, 101
PH-4	Guinea pig	ND	100, 101
1B6	Rat	ND	93
WS 35.22	Hamster	ND	104
Middle piece			
MA 4	Human	30	94
HSA-1	Human	ND	88
AMSIV-25[b]	Mouse	ND	92
Posterior tail			
PT-1	Guinea pig	ND	80, 100, 101
Antigens present in multiple domains			
Whole head			
SMA3	Mouse	ND	84
OBF13	Mouse	ND	86
WH-1	Guinea pig	42	80
WH-2	Guinea pig	45, 89	80, 100, 101
WH-3	Guinea pig	ND	80, 100, 101
HMS3.1	Hamster	ND	83

(continued)

TABLE 2. *(Continued)*

Antibodies	Species	Mass (kilodaltons)	References
Acrosome and midpiece			
G177	Human	ND	95
WH 97.25	Hamster	>500	104
Equatorial segment and middle piece			
bF4	Human	ND	95
HS 2M.1	Human	32, 83	79
HS 2N.1	Human	26–105	79
Equatorial segment and principal piece			
M2	Mouse	36, 44	103
Equatorial segment and whole tail			
MA 5	Human	71	94
MA 6	Human	ND	94
Postacrosomal region and middle piece			
HS-4	Human	130	105
Postacrosomal region and whole tail			
MA-24[b]	Human	23	106
XT-1	Mouse	ND	107, 108
Neck and middle piece			
MS 76.11	Hamster	ND	104
Middle piece and end piece			
WS 64.23	Hamster	23	104
Whole tail			
YWK-1	Human	84	87
HSA-1	Human	ND	88
SP1D1, AP7A7	Human	ND	89
SMA4	Mouse	54	84, 90
T21	Mouse	31	91
AMSIV-54[b], AMSIV-75[b]	Mouse	ND	92
WT-1	Guinea pig	ND	80
2B1	Rat	40	93
Whole sperm			
2D6	Rat	23	81, 82
HMS1.0, HMS2.0	Hamster	ND	83

[a]ND, not determined.
[b]Determined by indirect immunofluorescence on fixed or air-dried sperm.
[c]Determined by indirect immunofluorescence on acrosome-reacted sperm.

Formation of Domains

It is likely that most sperm-surface domains are established during spermiogenesis, while the round spermatid is being remodeled into the spermatozoon. However, spermatozoa of some species undergo shape changes in the epididymis, and their surface domains reach final distribution and form after spermiogenesis. Probably most affected are the middle piece and the acrosome. The cytoplasmic droplet migrates from the anterior to the posterior end of the middle piece and is usually shed as the sperm transits the epididymis. The acrosome can undergo a reduction in size (110,111) and, in some species, most notably the guinea pig, a substantial change in shape (112). New surface antigens also appear in specific domains during maturation, but they probably arise through modification or unmasking of preexisting molecules or by attachment of new molecules to acceptor sites already segregated into domains (see, e.g., ref. 113). It has also been reported that a monoclonal antibody reacts with the whole head of testicular sperm in the guinea pig, but only with the postacrosomal region of sperm from the tail of the epididymis (101). Such a change could occur by lateral migration of that antigen in the plasma membrane or by loss of an antigen from one domain and appearance of another antigen with the same epitope in a different domain (101).

The mechanisms responsible for establishing sperm-surface domains during spermiogenesis have not been defined. However, most of the surface domains overlie distinct cytoplasmic organelles or features. Some of the mechanisms that establish the shape and organization of the spermatozoon may also be involved in determining the location of surface domains. Morphogenetic processes that shape the sperm are probably carried out by cytoskeletal components of the germ cell. Transmembrane proteins that are stabilized by attachment through linkage proteins to cytoskeletal structures (114) may define the boundary and contents of different domains.

An *actin*-specific monoclonal antibody was used in conjunction with biochemical procedures to show that testicular spermatozoa of the rabbit contain filamentous actin in a sheath around the nucleus and throughout the equatorial segment and postacrosomal region (115). This study also confirmed an earlier report that actin is present in the postacrosomal region of rabbit epididymal spermatozoa (116). In addition, actin has been reported to be present in the subacrosomal space of testicular spermatozoa of the rat (116); in the posterior region of the head and in the connecting piece, midpiece, and principal piece of the tail of human sperm (116–118); and in the postacrosomal region of spermatozoa from boar (119,120). One study has reported that myosin is present in the acrosomal region of mammalian spermatozoa (116). Filamentous structures have been observed associated with the plasma membrane on the concave margin of the acrosome in vole spermatozoa (121). These may correspond to a cytoskeletal structure recently identified lying between the plasma membrane and the acrosome in hamster sperm (122).

Spectrin is a major actin-binding protein and usually is associated closely with the cytoplasmic surface of the plasma membrane (123,124). It is also a main calmodulin-binding protein and a structural component of the cytoskeleton (124). It was present in the cytoplasm overlying the acrosome of round spermatids and elongating spermatids as well as in that of some testicular spermatozoa in the mouse, but was not detected in epididymal spermatozoa (125). Guinea-pig spermatozoa are reported to lack spectrin (126), but human spermatozoa apparently contain spectrin in the anterior acrosome and principal piece regions (127). This suggests that spectrin and possibly other actin-binding proteins might be involved in establishing sperm-surface domains.

Microtubules have been shown to play an important role in determining the cell shape, and it has been suggested that microtubules in the manchette may be responsible for the elongation and shaping of the spermatid nucleus (128). The manchette is a sheath of microtubules that assemble as spermatid elongation begins. It attaches to a deposition of dense fibrillar material on the plasma membrane which migrates from the anterior to the caudal end of the nucleus during spermiogenesis (129). This attachment site later becomes the posterior ring lying at the junction between head and tail, which serves to separate the domains of the postacrosomal region and the middle piece. This suggests that the manchette contributes to the definition of the boundary between these two surface domains. However, a comparative study of morphogenetic factors influencing the shape of the sperm head concluded that its form is probably a consequence of the aggregation of DNA and protein during condensation of chromatin rather than due to forces external to the nucleus (129). In addition, microtubule-like components have been observed in close association with the plasma membrane overlying the postacrosomal region of the spermatozoon of the bull (130) and vole (121). However, they have not been shown to contain tubulin. Such features may represent the periodic densities seen in the postnuclear dense lamina (130,132).

The annulus also appears during spermiogenesis, encircling the axonemal complex at the distal end of the basal body, where the plasma membrane is reflected onto the forming flagellum of the elongating spermatid (133). The annulus remains firmly adherent to the plasma membrane as it moves down the flagellum to take up its final position, late in spermiogenesis, at the posterior end of the mitochondrial sheath and the anterior end of the fibrous sheath. At this location it also serves to separate the plasma membrane domains of middle piece and posterior tail.

The Sertoli cells may influence the establishment of domains, particularly those on the sperm head. Junctional structures, referred to as Sertoli-cell "ectoplasmic specializations," maintain a tight association between Sertoli cells and spermatids (134). The ectoplasmic specializations appear to grasp the head of spermatids and are present in large amounts facing cells undergoing the elongation and maturation phases of spermiogenesis (135). This association is maintained until near the time of sperm release (136), apparently holding the spermatid in a recess extending deeply into the Sertoli cell. The ectoplasmic specialization consists of bundles of actin or actin-like filaments and more deeply placed saccules of endoplasmic reticulum within the Sertoli cell (134); this might aid in shaping the sperm head or in maintaining cell polarity necessary for domain formation.

Another specialized relationship between Sertoli cells and spermatids appears during an even later part of spermiogenesis. The "tubulobulbar complexes" form as spermatids begin to move from deep recesses in the Sertoli-cell plasma membrane toward the lumen of the seminiferous tubule (137). The tubulobulbar complexes arise around the spermatid head as the ectoplasmic specialization begins to dissociate (134). Successive generations of complexes extend from spermatids into Sertoli cells, where they are actively phagocytosed (138). This process continues until the time of spermiation and morphometric data indicate that as much as 70% of the cytoplasm of spermatids may be eliminated by this mechanism (138). This process also has the potential to substantially alter the composition and organization of the plasma membrane and could serve a role in defining the nature and organization of proximate surface domains.

Maintenance of Domains

It has been suggested that sperm-surface domains might be maintained by restriction of mobility of surface molecules in their final domain, by the existence of a membrane barrier to surface component movement at the domain boundary, or through thermodynamic partitioning of molecules into a specific region (101). Restriction of mobility might occur through interactions of intramembranous components with molecules outside or inside the membrane. Although there is no direct evidence that external constraints can be imposed on domains by molecules applied to the sperm surface, capacitation involves loss of extrinsic components and a concomitant increase in membrane mobility in some domains (discussed below). Also, the glycocalyx between closely stacked sperm heads in the guinea pig has a septate structure (139) that may be congruent with the quilted pattern of intramembranous particles in that area of the plasma membrane (31). This quilted pattern is diminished by treatments that remove the cell coat (60,61). Furthermore, there is a correlation between the loss of the quilted pattern and changes in the rat sperm glycocalyx in the epididymis (32).

Internal constraints seem likely to play a major role in maintaining domains in the plasma membrane. The regions of plasma membrane over the posterior ring and the annulus hardly deserve to be called domains, but cytoplasmic components are involved in the formation and stabilization of these specialized regions. Furthermore, the transmembrane particles that comprise the zipper-like structure of the flagellum appear to be held in place by attachments to the ribs of the fibrous sheath (31). Also, the oblique strands of intramembranous particles in the middle piece are associated with the underlying mitochondria (31). In addition, the plasma membrane of the postacrosomal region is underlaid by long rod-like structures that form the postnuclear dense lamina (34,140) and that may stabilize the plasma membrane of this domain. Finally, a cytoplasmic tuft underlies the particle-bare filipin-complex sparse region of the anterior band, between the anterior acrosome and equatorial segment (10,64).

Barriers within the plane of the plasma membrane may restrict the movement of surface components between domains. Such potential barriers are present between the domains of the equatorial segment and the postacrosomal region (serrated band), the postacrosomal region and the middle piece (posterior ring), and the midpiece and the distal tail (annulus). For example, a surface antigen (PT-1) has been found to exhibit free diffusion within the plasma membrane of the distal tail domain, but apparently is prevented from migrating into the midpiece by the annulus (141). Also, two antigens (2B1, 2D6) present over the whole surface of the flagellum of rat sperm show antibody-induced patching, but the patches do not migrate onto the head (81). In addition, the lectin RCA caused clustering of binding sites within the postacrosomal region of rabbit sperm, but additional lectin-binding sites did not appear to migrate into this area from the acrosome (29). Finally, an antigen (RSA-1) over the entire surface of rabbit sperm undergoes antibody-induced clustering over the acrosome, but not in other regions of the plasma membrane (77). It appears that even though sperm-surface antigens may be mobile within their own domain, they are unable to migrate into other domains. However, this does not appear to be the case for all membrane components. Using fluorescence recovery after photobleaching, it was observed that there is free exchange of a lipid analog by lateral diffusion between plasma membrane of head and midpiece and between plasma membrane of midpiece and distal tail (65).

Plasma Membrane Composition

The membranes of human spermatozoa are said to be similar to the plasma membrane of the erythrocyte with regard to lipid composition (142). However, many earlier studies were carried out on whole spermatozoa from the cauda epididymis or ejaculates. More accurate determinations can be made with purified plasma membranes. Using this approach, it was found that phospholipids make up about 70% of the total plasma membrane lipid in boar sperm, with the major phospholipids being phosphatidylcholine, phosphatidylethanolamine, sphingomyelin, phosphatidylserine, phosphatidylinositol, and lysophosphatidylcholine (143). Sterols are the next most abundant lipid, with a cholesterol/phospholipid molar ratio of about 0.12. Glycolipids are less abundant, and this lipid class consists mainly of sulfatoxygalactosylacylalkylglycerol (SGG) (144). Free fatty acid makes up a relatively small amount of the lipid in boar spermatozoa, whereas diacylglycerols are present in about the same amounts as glycolipids (143).

SGG is a major component of the germ-cell plasma membrane in mammals (144). This glycolipid is synthesized in primary spermatocytes (145,146) and remains a stable component without turnover throughout the life of the cell. SGG is present in both the head and tail fractions of spermatozoa (144). It was detected with an antiserum on spermatogenic cells but not on spermatozoa (147). However, a monoclonal antibody to SGG (148) reacts with the equatorial segment and midpiece of living mouse spermatozoa. SGG binds three proteins of 68,000, 34,000, and 24,000 daltons isolated from rat spermatogenic cells (146) and is believed to be tightly associated with those proteins in the sperm plasma membrane.

The phospholipid/protein ratio is approximately 0.68 on a weight basis in plasma membranes isolated from boar spermatozoa (143), suggesting that the amounts of total lipid and protein in the sperm plasma membrane are about the same. However, this is for the whole plasma membrane, and the amount and type of lipids and the lipid/protein ratios are probably different in various domains. Freeze-fracture studies with filipin suggest that the amount of sterol in the anterior acrosome is about four times that present in the postacrosomal region in guinea-pig and bull spermatozoa (43,60,61). The postacrosomal region apparently contains few sterols or anionic lipids in guinea-pig spermatozoa (64), but the cytoplasmic droplet of the middle piece is probably rich in both (10,60). Also, cholesterol sulfate makes up only a small fraction of the total sterol but is a major component of the plasma membrane over the acrosome of human sperm (149). However, changes in the lipid content of the spermatozoal plasma membrane occur during maturation and capacitation, and these may have substantial effects on the composition and function of the membrane in different domains.

Modification of the Sperm Plasma Membrane During Epididymal Maturation

Spermatozoa undergo changes during transit through the epididymis that give them the ability to fertilize. Functional modifications that have been identified include alterations in metabolism (150), changes in the pattern and effectiveness of flagellar activity (see, e.g., refs. 151 and 152), and acquisition of ability to bind to the zona pellucida (153,154). The sperm plasma membrane is modified in composition during epididymal maturation (Table 3), and some of these changes appear to be required for the functional modifications to occur. Changes have been reported in surface charge, lectin binding, intramembranous particle distribution, membrane fluidity, lipid composition, protein composition, and antibody binding as sperm travel through the epididymis.

Changes in Surface Charge and Intramembranous Particle Distribution

The net negative surface charge has been found to be greater on spermatozoa from the cauda than on those from the caput epididymidis in several species (13,155,156). Furthermore, the density of colloidal iron particles bound to the tail, and to a lesser extent those bound to the head, was greater on rabbit sperm from the cauda epididymidis than on sperm that has not undergone epididymal maturation (14,15). It has been suggested that an increase in sialic acid moieties may be responsible for the change in surface charge

TABLE 3. *Sperm-surface modifications during epididymal maturation*

Modification	References
Increase in net negative surface charge	13, 14, 155, 156
Increase in binding of cationic colloidal iron	14, 15, 158, 159, 284
Changes in lectin-binding properties	28, 157, 160–164, 187, 284
Changes in intramembranous particle distribution	32, 33
Changes in membrane fluidity	65
Changes in lipid composition	143
Decreases in cholesterol, phosphatidylethanolamine, phosphatidylserine, phosphotidylinositol	
Increases in diacylglycerol, cholesterol sulfate, dermosterol, phosphatidylcholine, sphingomyelin, polyphosphoinositides	
Changes in protein and glycoprotein composition	
New surface components detected with vectorial labels	186–193
New surface components detected by gel electrophoresis	194–201
New surface components detected with antisera	193, 202–219, 222–224
New surface components detected with monoclonal antibodies	81, 82, 90, 97, 207, 208, 225–227
Loss of surface components	27, 97, 189, 190, 221

during maturation (157). One cytochemical study using neuraminidase treatment and colloidal iron staining of ram sperm during epididymal maturation supported this hypothesis (158), but other similar studies did not (15,159). Such changes in saccharides also have been detected with lectins. One study found that WGA and RCA binding to rabbit sperm decreased as the sperm proceeded from caput to cauda epididymidis, although Con-A binding did not change (157). Other investigators reported a decrease in WGA binding to hyrax sperm (160); they also reported decreased binding of RCA (161) and Con A (162) to ram sperm. However, another study found that washed rabbit sperm from the caput bound Con A poorly, while washed sperm from the cauda bound substantially more Con A than did unwashed sperm, particularly over the head (28). It was concluded that sperm-coating substances from the seminal fluid were masking lectin-binding sites on unwashed sperm. Additional studies indicated that Con-A binding to rat spermatozoa increased over the acrosome during maturation (163) and that the total amount of rat sperm surface material that will bind to a Con-A-affinity column approximately doubled during this process (164).

Boar sperm studied using freeze-fracture techniques transiently showed regular geometric arrays of intramembranous particles in the plasma membrane over the anterior acrosome as they passed through the distal region of the caput epididymis. A different hexagonal array developed as spermatozoa approached the cauda epididymis, appearing initially at the margin of the acrosome and then extending to the postacrosomal region, but disappearing almost completely upon ejaculation (33). In rat spermatozoa, plaques of parallel rows of particles appeared in the plasma membrane of the head at the distal end of the proximal caput epididymis, but largely disappeared by the proximal cauda epididymis (32). It has been suggested that these changes in patterns of intramembranous particles reflect changes in the nature of the sperm glycocalyx during epididymal transit (32).

Changes in Lipid Content

The lipid content of whole sperm has been reported to decrease during epididymal maturation in boar, bull, ram, and rat (165–171); the cholesterol content of whole sperm has been reported to decrease in ram, rat, and hamster (172–174). The cholesterol/phospholipid ratio and the concentration of phosphatidylserine, phosphatidylethanolamine, cardiolipin, and ethanolamine plasmalogen has also been reported to decrease in the ram (166,172). However, increases have been reported in the amount of sulfoconjugated sterols in hamster and human spermatozoa (173,175) as well as in unsaturated fatty acids in ram spermatozoa (172). When similar studies were carried out using plasma membranes isolated from boar spermatozoa, they confirmed that the amount of lipid in the plasma membrane decreased during epididymal maturation (143). Although there was a decrease in cholesterol, no significant change was seen in the cholesterol/phospholipid ratio. These studies also found decreases in phosphatidylethanolamine and phosphatidylinositol, as well as increases in dermosterol, cholesterol sulfate, phosphatidylcholine, and polyphosphoinositides. There was a decrease in the level of fatty acids and an increase in diacylglycerol, but no change in the degree of unsaturation of fatty acids. Preparations enriched for plasma membrane from the anterior head region of ram sperm were particularly rich in ethanolamine and choline phosphoglycerides (176). The amount of dermosterol and ethanolamine in this region of the plasma membrane was reported to decrease, while the cholesterol to phospholipid ratio increased, during epididymal maturation.

Changes in the amount and composition of lipids in the plasma membrane of spermatozoa during maturation are thought to explain why ejaculated sperm are more sensitive to cold shock than are testicular sperm (177–179). These changes may also account for the maturation-dependent decrease in charge density at the phospholipid-water interface of ram spermatozoa, detected by electron spin resonance (177), and the decrease in membrane fluidity of bull spermatozoa, seen by fluorescence polarization spectroscopy (180). Analysis of testicular and ejaculated ram spermatozoa by fluorescence recovery after photobleaching indicated that there are regional differences in the decrease of plasma membrane fluidity (65). During maturation, the diffusion rate of a fluorescent lipid analog increased in all regions of the sperm except the midpiece.

Changes in Protein Composition

The sperm plasma membrane also undergoes major changes in protein composition during epididymal maturation (181–185). These changes occur by addition of new components to the sperm surface, by unmasking or modification of preexisting sperm surface moieties, or by loss of sperm-surface components. They have been identified using biochemical approaches and antibodies to sperm-surface components or epididymal fluid components (Table 3). These changes are probably responsible for most of the previously described modifications in sperm-surface charge and lectin binding that occur during epididymal maturation, although changes in glycolipid composition could also be involved. Changes involving a particular component often occur within specific regions of the epididymis, suggesting that specializations of epididymal function in these regions play important roles in modifications of the sperm surface during epdidymal maturation.

New components that appear on the sperm surface have been detected in biochemical studies using vectorial labeling of sperm from different regions of the epididymis. For example, the galactose-oxidase–tritium-borohydride procedure was used to label accessible D-galactose or *N*-acetyl-D-galactosamine and to detect a 37,000-dalton glycoprotein present on sperm from the cauda, but not on sperm from the corpus epididymidis of the rat (186). Similar results were seen when lactoperoxidase-catalyzed iodination was used to label surface tyrosine residues or when fluorescein-conjugated Con-A lectin was used to identify glycoprotein-containing bands on polyacrylamide gels (187). Other studies using similar approaches have reported that the major change during rat sperm maturation is the increase in a 31,000- (188), a 32,000- (189), a 34,000- (190–192), or a 37,500-dalton (193) surface glycoprotein. In addition, biochemical approaches have been used to identify changes during maturation in spermatozoa from ram (194–197), bull (198), rabbit (199), boar (200), and chimpanzee (201).

Changes in Sperm-Surface Antigens

Immunological approaches have also proven to be effective for identifying differences in the surface composition of spermatozoa which arise during maturation (Table 3). Studies using these approaches have complemented biochemical studies, and the two procedures have frequently been used together. Antisera raised against either spermatozoa or epididymal fluid have often reacted with both, suggesting that an epididymal fluid component binds to the sperm surface. This has given rise to the term "sperm-coating antigens" for components found both in the fluid and on sperm (202–206). It is also possible that spermatozoa might shed components into the epididymal fluid during maturation which would be recognized by antisera to sperm or components in the fluid. However, several studies have identified components that are secreted by the epididymis and become bound to the sperm surface (see below).

An antiserum to a 33,000-dalton acidic epididymal glycoprotein (AEG) purified from the rat epididymis was used in immunohistochemical studies to demonstrate that AEG was secreted by principal cells in the epithelium of the caput and corpus epididymis and bound to sperm as they left the initial segment of the caput epididymis (207). AEG was found to have a slight stimulatory effect on sperm motility, but bovine serum albumin and rabbit serum were equally effective (208). Another study used an antiserum to partially purified specific epididymal proteins (SEP) in the rat (209) to confirm the organ specificity of SEP (210). The SEP were found by gel electrophoresis to be a complex mixture of proteins, including the PAS-positive glycoproteins "C" (22,400 daltons and pI 5.35–5.79) and "D" and "E" (37,000 daltons and pI 5.13 and 4.95, respectively) (210). The main region of synthesis was determined to be the caput epididymis, and sperm were coated with SEP as they left the initial segment of the caput epididymis (211). Proteins D and E apparently bound weakly and could be removed from sperm by a modest increase in ionic strength of the medium (212). The antiserum bound to the head of mature sperm and inhibited fertilization in artificially inseminated animals (213).

In another series of studies, different proteins isolated and purified from the rat caput epididymis were designated proteins "B" and "C" (16,000 daltons "D" (30,000 daltons), and "E" (32,000 daltons) (214–216). By using antisera and surface labeling methods, it was found that proteins D and E were absent from testis sperm but present on cauda sperm, whereas proteins B and C showed little, if any, binding to sperm (217,218). Antisera to D and E (redesignated as 27,000-

and 28,000-dalton glycoproteins, respectively) bound to the head of sperm from the cauda, but not to sperm from the testis (218). Proteins B and C were biosynthetically labeled, along with a new protein "G" (37,000 daltons), and were found to bind to sperm from testis and cauda epididymis and to erythrocytes to a similar degree, suggesting that the binding was not specific to epididymal sperm (217).

A sialoprotein, designated "SP" (37,500 daltons and pI 4.7), was also purified from rat epididymis and shown by immunohistochemistry to be present on the apical surface of cells in the caput and corpus epididymides, in the cytoplasm of certain epididymal epithelial cells, and on sperm in the lumen of the epididymis (193). The antiserum did not cross-react with supernatants of epididymal homogenates from dog, rabbit, guinea pig, or human. Two extrinsic glycoproteins of 50,000 and 100,000 daltons were extracted from cauda sperm in the rat by washing with a high-ionic-strength buffer (219). Antisera to these glycoproteins reacted with the "periacrosomal" region of the head of cauda sperm, and immunohistochemical studies indicated that the antigen first appeared in the cytoplasm of principal cells in the proximal region of the cauda epididymis. Peptide maps suggested that the two glycoproteins had very similar composition and that the larger molecule may be a dimer of the smaller molecule. Both glycoproteins bound lectins on Western blots, which indicated that their glycoconjugates contained mannose and *N*-acetylglucosamine (219).

It is possible that the same sperm-surface maturation glycoprotein has been identified in some of the different biochemical and immunological studies in the rat (217,220). It is the major glycoprotein present on sperm from the cauda epididymis, has sialic acid or galactose and tyrosine accessible to surface labels, and has an estimated mass between 24,000 and 37,000 daltons (186,187,189,190,192,220,221). It has been suggested that this molecule is present on caput sperm and that glycosylation during movement through the epididymis changes its pI from a range of 5.5 to 5.6 to a range of 5 to 5.5 and makes it more readily labeled by tritium borohydride (220). This molecule may be the α-lactalbumin that regulates galactosyl-transferase activity on the sperm surface (220).

Although epididymal secretory products that become associated with the sperm surface have been studied most extensively in the rat, studies in other species have shown that this is a general phenomenon. In the rabbit, epididymal glycoproteins first become associated with spermatozoa in the distal caput and proximal corpus epididymis (222); in the hamster, however, epididymal glycoproteins first become associated with the sperm in the proximal caput region (222). Other studies in the hamster also identified epididymal glycoproteins that became deposited on the spermatozoa during maturation (223). In the human, an antiserum to ejaculated spermatozoa reacted specifically with epididymal fluid and with epididymal sperm, but not testicular sperm, and apparently identified an epididymal secretory product that binds to sperm (224).

A few studies have used monoclonal antibodies to examine sperm-surface changes during maturation. The advantages of these probes are that they are highly specific and often identify antigens restricted to specific domains on the sperm surface. Two rat sperm-surface antigens that first appear in the caput epididymis were identified; one was present on the postacrosomal portion of the head (identified with monoclonal antibody 1B6), and the other was uniformly distributed over the entire sperm surface (identified with antibody 2D6) (81). The latter antigen was susceptible to antibody-induced patching and was observed to be inserted into the egg surface upon fertilization (207). Two antigens were also identified on hamster spermatozoa that were modified during maturation (208). One was over the head at an apparently higher concentration and on a greater percentage of cauda than on testicular sperm (recognized by antibody HM 3.1). The other was over the entire tail and appeared to be present in higher concentration on corpus sperm than on caput or cauda sperm (recognized by antibody HM 5.8). Antibody HM 3.1 blocked fertilization *in vitro,* whereas HM 5.8 reduced fertilization *in vitro* due to sperm agglutination. A 28,000-dalton antigen (identified with monoclonal antibody 1B3) was present over the entire surface of spermatozoa from the testis or caput epididymis in the mouse, but was present only on the tip of the head of sperm from the cauda epididymidis (97). Other studies used monoclonal antibodies to identify four sperm-maturation antigens (SMA) in the mouse which were restricted to the anterior acrosome (SMA 1), posterior acrosome and midpiece (SMA 2), whole head (SMA 3), and whole tail (SMA 4) (84). SMA 4 was secreted by the epithelium in the distal-caput–proximal-corpus region of the epididymis as an 85,000-dalton component and was trimmed to a 54,000-dalton component upon attachment to the surface of the flagellum (90,225,226). Another monoclonal antibody was used to show, in the mouse, that an antigen carrying the fucosylated lactosaminoglycan SSEA-1 was secreted by the caput epididymis and absorbed by sperm (227).

The appearance of new antigens on the sperm surface during epididymal maturation might also occur because of unmasking or alteration of preexisting sperm-surface proteins. Although there do not appear to be well-documented examples of appearance due to unmasking, a possible case of this has been seen in the mouse. A monoclonal antibody was used to identify a 31,000-dalton antigen on the surface of the flagellum of spermatozoa from the cauda epididymis (91). The antigen gradually appeared on sperm as they passed through the mid-corpus region of the epididymis. It apparently was present first in higher-molecular-weight forms that were converted to the final protein, suggesting that the unmasking involved removal of moieties by limited proteolysis. Proteases (150,228,229) and glycosidases (230–232) are present in the epididymis, and β-galactosidase and β-glucoronidase are secreted in substantial amounts by rat epididymal cells in culture (233). In addition, the secretion of glycosidases in the epididymis is reported to be androgen dependent (234,235). Such enzymes might be responsible for unmasking of sperm-surface maturation components by partial degradation of surface glycoproteins. A proteinase inhibitor has been isolated from the epididymis in the mouse (236), and such molecules might be involved in regulating or limiting enzyme-mediated sperm-surface modifications in the epididymis.

Changes in Sperm-Surface Carbohydrates

Another way that sperm-surface components are altered in the epididymis is by glycosylation. Epididymal homogenates are rich in glycosyltransferases; dolichol, the polyisoprenoid carrier of oligosaccharide side chains used in assembly of *N*-glycosylated glycoproteins, is present in high concentration in the caput and corpus epididymis in the rat (237). The rat epididymis contains androgen-dependent glucosyl and mannosyl transferases (238), and the corpus has the highest β-*N*-glucosaminidase, β-*N*-acetyl-galactosaminidase, and β-*N*-galactosidase activities in the epididymis (232). Also, *N*-acetylneuraminyl transferase activity is higher in caput than cauda epididymidis (239), although some sialoglycoproteins in the epididymal fluids are produced only in the cauda (188). There is evidence that the increase in negative surface charge by ram and bull spermatozoa in the epididymis is due to the addition of sialic acid groups to the sperm surface (9). Other studies have suggested that lactosaminoglycans present on the surface of testicular spermatozoa are fucosylated by an epididymal fucosyltransferase (240).

UDP-galactose:*N*-acetylglucosamine galactosyltransferase activity has been detected in fluids from the vas deferens of mice and rats (241–243) and in the rete testis fluid of rats (244). The galactosyltransferase appeared to be produced in the testis and concentrated in the caput epididymi (244). Rat spermatozoa were capable of incorporating galactose from UDP-[^{14}C]galactose into surface glycoproteins, and the addition of rete testis fluid increased the amount incorporated (245). The major incorporation was into 37,000- and 23,000-dalton proteins, suggesting that sperm-surface components are altered during maturation by galactosylation of exposed *N*-acetylglucosamine residues (245). The 37,000-dalton glycoprotein may have been the same maturation-dependent sperm-surface glycoprotein identified in earlier surface-labeling studies (186).

There is also galactosyltransferase activity on the sperm surface (69,247,248) which may be involved in sperm-surface modifications during epididymal maturation. This enzyme appears to be different from the one in epididymal fluid (249). The galactosyltransferases may be regulated by α-lactalbumin, which is apparently present in epididymal fluid (246) and on the surface of the sperm flagellum (250,251) and is produced by the epididymis (252). Galactosyltransferase interacts with α-lactalbumin to form lactose synthetase, which catalyzes the transfer of galactose from UDP-galactose to glucose, forming lactose (253).

It has also been hypothesized that the sperm-surface galactosyltransferase binds to *N*-acetylglucosamine on the zona pellucida as part of the fertilization process (249,254). The evidence for this comes from studies on a strain of mice that have a genetic predisposition for increased fertilizing ability and have elevated sperm-surface galactosyltransferase activity (248). However, sperm from recombinant strains of these mice did not show elevated galactosyltransferase activity or increased fertilizing ability (249); competitive substrates for the enzyme, α-lactalbumin, and enzyme substrate analogs inhibited sperm binding to the zona pellucida (249,254). Also, enzymatic removal or unmasking of terminal *N*-acetylglucosamine residues produced coincident inhibition or stimulation, respectively, of binding (249,254). Other studies have shown (a) that purified galactosyltransferase produced a dose-dependent inhibition of sperm binding to the zona pellucida and caused sperm bound to the zona pellucida to be released and (b) that monospecific antiserum to the enzyme produced a dose-dependent inhibition of sperm binding to the zona pellucida and concomitantly blocked sperm galactosyltransferase activity (69). The enzyme was shown to be localized to the plasma membrane over the dorsal surface of the mouse-sperm acrosome (69).

Loss of Sperm-Surface Components

Sperm-surface proteins also are apparently lost during epididymal maturation. A 110,000-dalton glycoprotein was the major surface component of rat testicular spermatozoa labeled with the glucose-oxidase–tritium-borohydride procedure, but it was not labeled on spermatozoa from the cauda epididymis (189,190). In other studies on the rat, 94,000-, 72,000-, and 59,000-dalton components were iodinated on caput sperm but not on cauda sperm (221). In a study of mouse spermatozoa, a 28,000-dalton antigen was seen to be present over the entire surface of spermatozoa from the testis and caput epididymis, whereas those from the cauda epididymidis were labeled only over the anterior acrosome (97). However, it was not determined in these studies whether the components were (a) shed from the sperm surface, (b) modified in molecular weight because of processes such as limited proteolysis or addition of new moieties, or (c) still present but no longer accessible to surface labeling because of masking by other moieties. Immunological studies have suggested that terminal *N*-acetylglucosamine on testicular spermatozoa was lost during epididymal transit, probably as a result of galactosylation (27).

Modification of the Sperm Plasma Membrane During Ejaculation and Capacitation

Other alterations of sperm-surface composition may occur upon ejaculation (Table 4). These include: changes in surface charge (155,255–257) and in lectin binding (19,157); and possibly changes in lipid composition (142,256). In addition, there is absorption of blood-group antigens (259,260), histocompatibility antigens (261), and immunosuppressive factors (262). Sperm also become coated with proteins produced by accessory glands and absorbed from the seminal plasma. Human spermatozoa have been reported to be coated with lactoferrin (263,264), ferrisplan (265), PP5 (266), HSP-5 (267), pg12 (268), and a basic 140,000-dalton protein (269), all produced by the seminal vesicles. The latter protein cross-reacted immunologically with rat seminal-vesicle protein-IV (RSV-IV), a 17,000-dalton seminal-vesicle protein found in the rat (270). Another rat seminal-vesicle protein (50,000 dalton) was present in ejaculated, but not in epididymal, rat sperm (271). Similarly, a 20,000-dalton protein was present in ejaculated, but not in epididymal, sperm from the rabbit (272), and a 40,000-dalton collagen-binding protein was present in ejaculated, but not in epididymal, rabbit sperm (273). It has been reported that 25,000- and 14,000-dalton proteins bind to bull sperm during ejaculation (198). Also, a 34,000-dalton component was present in ejaculated mouse sperm, in seminal-vesicle fluid, and in sperm from the distal vas deferens, but not in epididymal sperm (78).

Some of the proteins that bind to sperm upon ejaculation have been localized to specific sperm-surface domains. A 6,400-dalton proteinase inhibitor produced by mouse seminal vesicles was bound to a 15,000-dalton plasma-membrane component on the acrosome of ejaculated mouse sperm (274). A 30,000-dalton prostate protein found in the dog was shown to be a proteolytic enzyme and to be present on the tail and postacrosomal region of ejaculated dog sperm (275). Some of the components in the seminal plasma also appear to interact with each other and the sperm surface. Transglutaminase promoted covalent linking of spermidine to RSV-IV *in vitro,* and the protein was then able to bind to rat sperm (276). During ejaculation, a calcium-dependent transglutaminase from the prostate may modify the seminal-vesicle protein to enhance its binding to the sperm surface (276).

The plasma membrane undergoes additional modifications in the female reproductive tract as spermatozoa gain the capacity to fertilize the ovum. Although the initial observations were on changes that occurred *in vivo* (277,278), subsequent studies found that, in most species, comparable changes could be produced *in vitro* in defined media (279–283). This allowed experimental studies to be carried out which identified modifications in sperm-surface charge (255,284), lectin binding (21,25,28,30,285), intramembranous particle distribution (10,30,50,51,61,286,287), membrane fluidity (77,288–290), lipid composition (61,286–289,291,292), protein composition (272,273, 293–299), and antibody binding (206,226,298,300,301) during capacitation (Table 5). These membrane modifications occur concomitantly with essential functional changes involving sperm motility, ion fluxes, and metabolism (7). Capacitation is a multistep process, but one aspect of it appears to be removal or modification of extrinsic components added to the sperm surface in the male reproductive tract. An example of this type of change is the loss of a mouse-sperm maturation antigen (SMA 4). This antigen is secreted by the epididymal epithelium and bound to the surface of the flagellum, but is shed by sperm as they approach the surface of the egg (226). Another type of change with capacitation is the apparent release of constraints forming domain boundaries. An antigen present on the posterior tail of guinea-pig spermatozoa (PT-1) migrates onto the middle piece following capacitation, indicating that it is no longer constrained by the annulus (141). Following the acrosome reaction, another antigen (PH-20) migrates from the postacrosomal region to the inner acrosomal membrane (302).

TABLE 4. *Alterations of sperm surface upon ejaculation*

Alteration	References
Changes in sperm surface charge	155, 255–257
Changes in lectin binding	19, 157
Changes in lipid composition	142
Integration of lipoproteins	258
Absorption of blood group antigens	259, 260
Absorption of histocompatibility antigens	261
Absorption of immunosuppressive factors	262
Absorption of accessory gland secretions	78, 263–276

TABLE 5. *Alteration of sperm plama membrane during capacitation*

Alteration	References
Reduction in negative surface charge	255, 284
Modification in lectin-binding ability	21, 25, 28, 30, 285
Changes in intramembranous particle distribution	10, 30, 50, 51, 61, 286, 287
Changes in membrane fluidity	77, 288–290
Changes in lipid composition	61, 286–292
Changes in protein composition	226, 272, 273, 293–299
Changes in antibody binding	206, 226, 298, 300, 301
Release of constraints forming domain boundaries	141, 302

The serrated band at the posterior margin of the equatorial segment apparently does not pose a barrier to lateral diffusion at that time, but the antigen does not migrate to the midpiece, suggesting that the posterior ring remains a barrier to lateral diffusion.

THE SPERM HEAD

The head of the mammalian spermatozoon is occupied mostly by the nucleus and acrosome, but also contains cytoskeletal components and a small amount of cytoplasm (Figs. 3–6). The acrosome lies at the anterior end of the head, just beneath the plasma membrane, and is deeply indented posteriorly by the nucleus. Cytoskeletal components lie in the narrow space between the inner acrosomal membrane and the nuclear membrane and also just below the plasma membrane. Spermatozoa in most species have a spatulate head (Fig. 3), and the nucleus and acrosome are flattened in the plane of the anterior-posterior axis. The acrosome and nucleus are usually symmetrical structures; however, in some animals, protrusions of the acrosome extend perpendicularly to the flattened plane of the sperm head (Fig. 4). In rodent spermatozoa, which have a falciform-shaped head, the acrosome overlies the convex margin of the nucleus. Although spermatozoa are uniform in size and shape in most species, in the human there is often variability in the size and shape of the head of some sperm, even in fertile individuals (303,304).

The Sperm Nucleus

The volume of the sperm nucleus is less than that of somatic cells, and its chromatin is highly condensed. The sperm nucleus is unique, both in the amount of DNA present and in the composition of its nucleoproteins. The two meiotic divisions that occur during spermatogenesis produce a haploid genome, with only one member of each chromosome pair being present in the sperm nucleus.

Nuclear Proteins

The major nuclear proteins associated with sperm DNA are protamines (305). These are relatively small (27–65 amino acids) highly basic proteins rich in arginine and cysteine (306,307). The mRNA encoding for mouse protamines are synthesized in spermatids, indicating that protamines are products of the haploid genome (308). The highly condensed protamine-DNA complex is stabilized by disulfide bonds between the protamines. Most mammals have only one protamine, but mice and humans are reported to have two (309–311). There are two general models showing how protamines associate with DNA (312). One suggests that protamines are present in an extended configuration and lie in the major or minor groove of the DNA double helix. They are presumed to cross-link the chromatin by forming covalent disulfide linkages with protamines on nearby DNA (313). The other model suggests that protamine is packaged into α-helical cylinders (314). These are thought to lie in the major or minor DNA groove and to facilitate orderly DNA condensation and subsequently to cross-link with neighboring cylinders to effect stabilization. Although both models are based on physical data and presume the lack of nucleosomes in sperm nuclei, some morphological studies have suggested that nucleosomes are present (315,316). In addition, studies using freeze-fracture (31,34,37), birefringence (317), and physical methods (318) have suggested

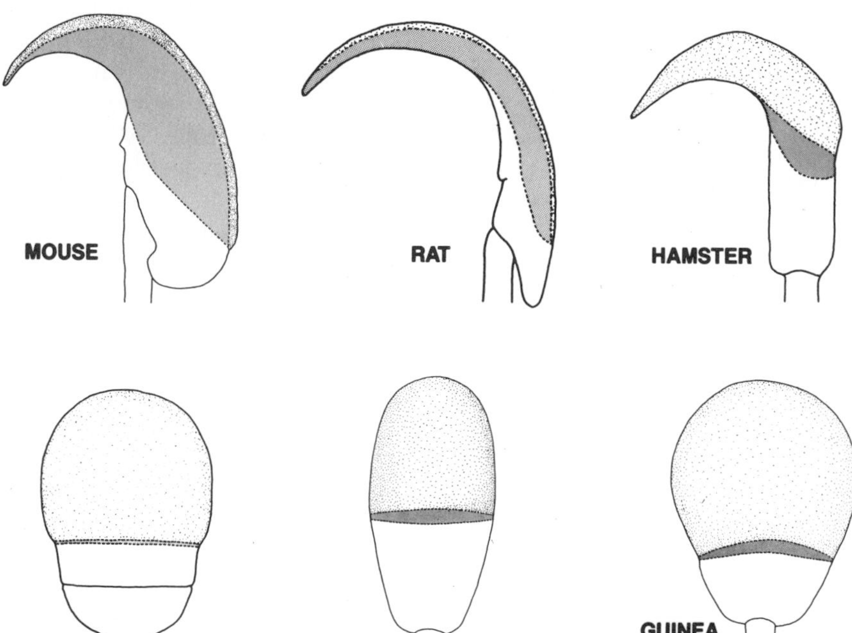

FIG. 3. Shape of the head of spermatozoa from different species. The falciform heads of mouse, rat, and hamster sperm are viewed laterally, whereas the spatulate heads of human, rabbit, and guinea-pig sperm are viewed dorsoventrally. (Adapted from ref. 184.)

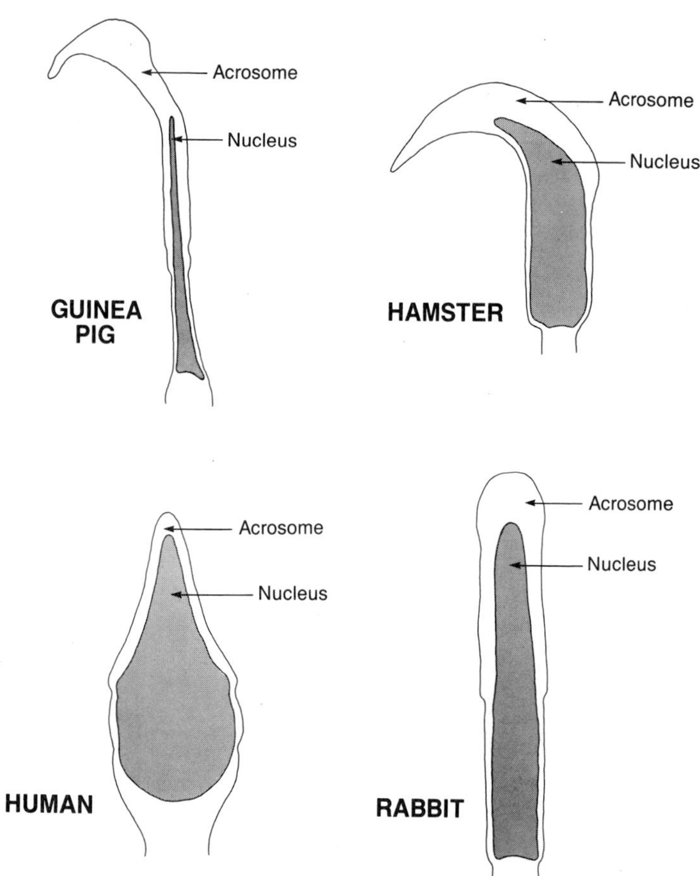

FIG. 4. Cross-sectional views of the heads of spermatozoa from different species. Guinea pig, rabbit, and human sperm heads are seen in the sagittal plane, whereas the hamster sperm head is seen in the coronal plane. The acrosome and nucleus of rabbit and human spermatozoa are symmetrical, but those of guinea pig and hamster are asymmetrical in these planes.

that the chromatin in the spermatozoa of some mammals is stacked in lamellar plates. However, the chromatin of mouse and human spermatozoa appears to have a random fibrogranular pattern (44,319). Additional studies will be required to fully understand how protamines and other nucleoproteins (305,312) interact with DNA in sperm nuclei.

Nuclear Envelope

The sperm nucleus is enclosed by an unusual nuclear envelope. Over most of the nucleus, nuclear pores are absent and the two membranes of the nuclear envelope lie only 7 to 10 nm apart. However, caudal to the posterior ring, in the so-called "redundant nuclear envelope," nuclear pores are abundant and arranged in a hexagonal pattern; the two membranes are 40 to 60 nm apart as in most other cells (31,34,44,52,348). The membranes of the anterior part of the nuclear envelope contain a rich array of random intramembranous particles (320), whereas the closely apposed membranes of the nuclear envelope in the implantation fossa contain large closely packed particles surrounding particle-free areas (31).

Nuclear Lamina

The nuclear lamina is a protein meshwork lining the inner surface of the nuclear envelope. It is thought to form the skeletal framework of the nuclear envelope and to serve as an anchoring site for chromatin (321–325). The nuclear lamina contains three closely related proteins: lamins A, B, and C. Lamins A (70,000 dalton) and C (60,000 dalton) have similar peptide maps but different antigenic epitopes. However, some antibodies recognize lamin B (67,000 dalton) as well as lamins A and C (326–328), indicating that all three share sequence homologies. Earlier immunohistochemical studies indicated that mouse spermatozoa did not contain proteins recognized by antibodies to lamins (329,330). However, a more recent study found that several other antibodies to lamins did react with nuclei of mouse spermatozoa (331). Immunostaining patterns were variable and were dependent on fixation and extraction conditions. The results indicated that an epitope recognized by antibody to lamin B was present over most of the sperm nucleus, that epitopes of lamin G (identified with an antibody to clam nuclei) were present on the convex margin of the nucleus, and that an epitope of lamins A and C was present on the convex margin, the anterior part of the concave margin, and adjacent to the implantation fossa (331). It was established recently that the lamins have extensive sequence homology with intermediate filament proteins (332,333) and apparently belong to the same family of structural proteins. A male germ-cell-specific lamin has been identified in Xenopus (334), and it has been suggested that a germ-cell-specific lamin may be present in mouse sperm (331). Al-

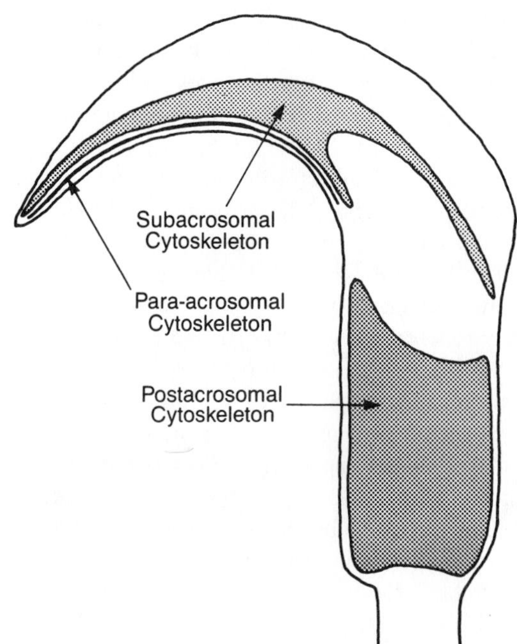

FIG. 5. Cytoskeleton of head of the hamster spermatozoon. The subacrosomal cytoskeleton (perforatorium) lies between the acrosome and the anterior part of the nucleus and extends to the tip of the falciform head. The para-acrosomal cytoskeleton lies between the plasma membrane and the acrosome on the concave margin of the sperm head. The postacrosomal cytoskeleton surrounds the posterior part of the nucleus, lying between the nuclear envelope and the plasma membrane of the postacrosomal domain.

though biochemical evidence for the presence of lamins in the mammalian sperm nucleus is lacking, it appears likely that lamins or related proteins contribute to the structure of the sperm nucleus.

Cytoskeleton of Sperm Head

Some cytoskeletal components of spermatogenic cells were discussed earlier in this chapter. Other cytoskeletal structures have been identified in the head of mammalian spermatozoa (Table 6) lying between the nucleus and the acrosome (subacrosomal cytoskeleton), between the plasma membrane and the postacrosomal portion of the nucleus (postacrosomal cytoskeleton), and between the plasma membrane and the anterior tip and convex surface of the acrosome of falciform sperm (para-acrosomal cytoskeleton) (Fig. 5). The subacrosomal and postacrosomal cytoskeletons can be isolated together (319) and have been referred to as the *perinuclear theca* (312). This complex resembles the nuclear matrix that has been isolated from somatic cells, but, unlike the nuclear matrix, it lies external to the nuclear envelope (319). The isolated perinuclear theca contains a diverse population of proteins ranging from 8,000 to 80,000 daltons, but the major proteins present were 13,000, 15,000, 16,500 and 25,000 daltons (319). The isolated perinuclear theca retains the shape of the sperm nucleus in the absence of DNA and the acrosome. It has been suggested that the perinuclear theca may be an extrinsic determinant of nuclear shape (312).

The *subacrosomal cytoskeleton* (subacrosomal material, perinuclear material, perforatorium) is composed of amor-

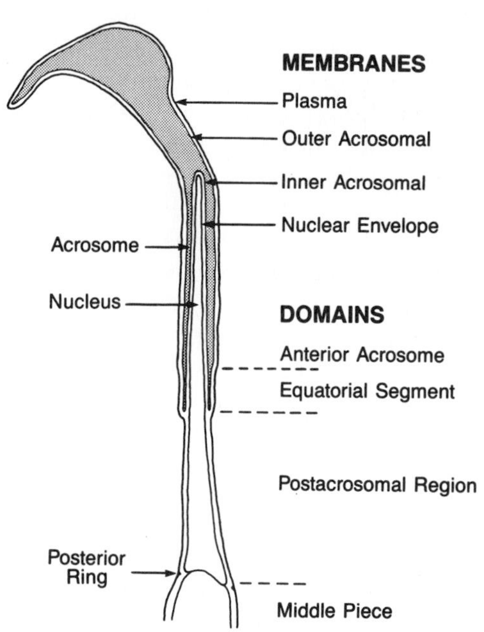

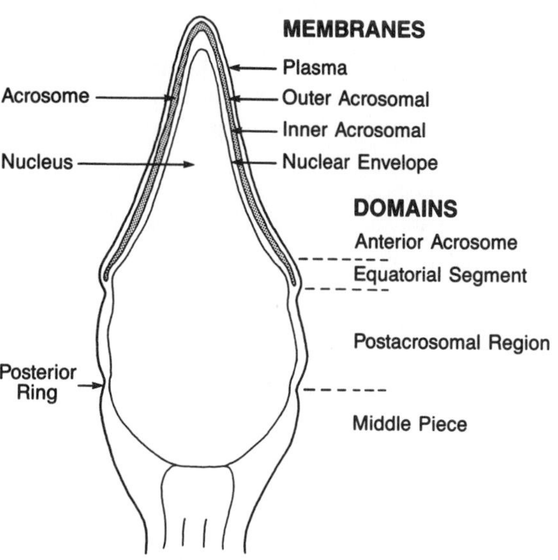

FIG. 6. Structure of the head of guinea-pig and human spermatozoa. The plasma membrane in the anterior acrosomal and equatorial segment domains overlies the outer acrosomal membrane. The inner acrosomal membrane, in turn, overlies the nuclear envelope. The acrosome is thinner in the equatorial segment region than in the anterior acrosome region. The posterior ring separates the postacrosomal domain of the head from the middle-piece domain of the flagellum.

TABLE 6. *Sperm cytoskeletal components*

Component	References
Head	
Subacrosomal cytoskeleton (perforatorium)	335–346
Postacrosomal cytoskeleton (postacrosomal sheath, postnuclear sheath, postacrosomal dense lamina, postnuclear cap, postnuclear body)	34, 37, 41, 42, 44, 52, 121, 131, 319, 336, 346–352
Para-acrosomal cytoskeleton (filamentous cytoskeletal complex)	121, 122, 341, 342, 349, 352
Connecting piece	
Capitulum	52, 425, 426, 429
Segmented columns	52, 418, 429
Tail	
Axoneme	308, 433, 434, 436, 437
Outer dense fibers	52, 337, 362, 425, 429, 450, 454–465, 467–472
Satellite fibers	52, 336, 459, 474, 476
Fibrous sheath	2, 303, 336, 337, 344, 457, 458, 473, 477–486

phous, electron-dense material situated in the narrow space between the inner acrosomal membrane and the outer membrane of the nuclear envelope (335). It is an extensive feature in rodents such as the rat, mouse, and hamster, which possess falciform sperm heads (336), but is a minor component in sperm heads of other mammalian species (337,338). It has been referred to as the *perforatorium* in rodents because of its similarity in appearance to a structure in toads (339) and birds (340), thought to have a mechanical role in egg penetration (341,342). Earlier studies determined that the subacrosomal cytoskeleton was highly resistant to solubilization (343), apparently because of extensive disulfide bond formation (337). Advantage was taken of the insolubility of the subacrosomal cytoskeleton to devise a procedure for its isolation from rat spermatozoa (335,344). This allowed confirmation of earlier findings that the subacrosomal cytoskeleton became more resistant to solubilization during epididymal transit (335,337). It also allowed the isolated subacrosomal cytoskeleton to be characterized biochemically, and it was found to consist of a 13,000-dalton protein containing 6.5% cysteine (335). The subacrosomal cytoskeleton is first visible in early spermatids as a dense layer between the forming acrosomal granule and the nuclear envelope. It extends peripherally over the anterior pole of the nucleus, just ahead of the advancing acrosome, as the sperm head elongates during spermiogenesis (345,346).

The *postacrosomal cytoskeleton* (postacrosomal sheath, postnuclear sheath, postacrosomal dense lamina, postnuclear cap, postnuclear body) lies between the nuclear envelope and the plasma membrane of the postacrosomal segment of the sperm head (34,52,336,347,348). It abuts the posterior end of the subacrosomal cytoskeleton anteriorly, at the posterior margin of the acrosome, and extends caudally to the posterior ring. It has a periodic substructure (34,39,121,131,348,349) and, in bull sperm, is composed of closely associated 10- to 12-nm filamentous elements aligned parallel to the long axis of the head (350). In addition, the basal region contains coarse striations, formed by short rows of large particles (31,34,37,41,42,44,52,131). The basal region corresponds to a zone of close adhesion between the plasma membrane, the postacrosomal cytoskeleton, and the nuclear envelope (350). Postacrosomal cytoskeleton formation begins in late spermiogenesis (346), with dense material appearing just caudal to the posterior margin of the acrosome, coincident with the formation of the manchette (351). The postacrosomal cytoskeleton appears to assemble as the manchette moves caudally to form the posterior ring (352). This portion of the sperm-head cytoskeleton has not been isolated successfully, but it presumably contains some of the perinuclear theca proteins that have been identified (319).

The *para-acrosomal cytoskeleton* (filamentous cytoskeletal complex) has been identified recently in hamster sperm as a tripartite structure, consisting of a cone at the anterior tip and a bifurcated sheet on the convex surface of the head, lying between the acrosome and the plasma membrane (122). It is formed of filaments similar in size to intermediate filaments. Filaments have also been seen along the convex side of the acrosome of vole sperm (121), and striations were noted along the ventral surface of the acrosome of rat sperm (349), suggesting that the para-acrosomal cytoskeleton may be present in these species.

Sperm-head cytoskeletal structures have been suggested to have mechanical (341,342) and functional roles (350,352) in fertilization, and other roles are possible. The subacrosomal and para-acrosomal cytoskeletons are well developed in sperm possessing a falciform head and might serve as scaffolding to form or maintain this shape. However, the postacrosomal cytoskeleton is slightly more prominent in sperm containing a spatulate head and may provide stiffening and support for the posterior part of the sperm head and prevent its flexure during sperm motion. The function of the sperm-head cytoskeletal structures may be better understood once their composition is better defined. The major proteins forming cytoskeletal structures include tubulin, actin, and intermediate filament proteins. Microtubules are not present in these structures and although actin has been identified with antibodies in the postacrosomal region of testicular sperm, it was not detected in epididymal sperm (115,116,119,120). Structures similar in appearance to intermediate filaments have been identified in the postacrosomal (350) and the paracrosomal (122) cytoskeleton. However, antibodies to intermediate filaments do not react with these regions of the sperm head (127,350). This suggests that the sperm-head cytoskeletal structures are composed of unique proteins or of germ-cell-specific isoforms of cytoskeletal proteins that lack antigenic determinants present on related proteins in somatic cells. However, sperm-head cytoskeletal proteins may be related to flagellar cytoskeletal proteins. In sterile mutant mice, it is often the case that both the head and flagellum of sperm are defectively formed (353,354).

The Acrosome

The acrosome originates from the Golgi complex in the spermatid and contains enzymes necessary for the sperm to penetrate to and/or fuse with the plasma membrane of the egg to achieve fertilization. This membranous structure sits as a cap over the nucleus in the anterior part of the sperm head.

Structure of Acrosome

The *inner acrosomal membrane* is closely applied to the anterior part of the nuclear envelope; the *outer acrosomal membrane* underlies the plasma membrane. The acrosome consists of two segments, the *anterior acrosome* (acrosomal cap) and the *equatorial segment* (posterior acrosome), which immediately underlie the plasma membrane domains with the same names (Fig. 6). During the acrosome reaction the outer acrosomal membrane and the plasma membrane fuse and vesiculate, and most of the acrosomal contents are discharged. The inner acrosomal membrane and the equatorial segment persist until sperm-egg fusion in most species (7). The acrosome varies widely in size and shape in different species (Figs. 3 and 4), and the distribution and relative prominence of these two segments differ accordingly (336).

The equatorial segment forms a band that approximately overlies the equator of the head of spatulate spermatozoa. In sperm possessing a falciform head, the equatorial segment may cover much of the lateral surface of the head. However, in species containing a discoid sperm head flattened in the plane perpendicular to the axis of the tail ("carpet tack-shaped head"), such as the wooly opossum (355), an equatorial segment may not be identifiable. The portion of the anterior acrosome which extends beyond the anterior margin of the nucleus has been referred to as the *apical segment,* and the portion overlying the nucleus has been referred to as the *principal segment* (52). In the human, monkey, bull, boar, rabbit, and bat the acrosome is relatively small, with no appreciable extension beyond the nucleus, whereas in guinea pig, chinchilla, and ground squirrel the acrosome has a large apical segment (112,140,336,356).

Electron microscopy revealed (a) that the acrosome, particularly the apical segment, often has a much more complex shape than is obvious by examining sperm smeared onto a slide and (b) that the shape of the acrosome is characteristic of the species (336,356). The final shape of the acrosome may be influenced by (a) extrinsic forces generated by cytoskeletal elements in the spermatid and/or Sertoli-cell cytoplasm (122,134) or (b) by forces intrinsic to the nucleus (357). However, in some species, it also appears that forces intrinsic to the acrosome may be involved. Acrosomes of guinea-pig and chinchilla sperm continue to undergo morphological differentiation after spermatogenesis, and the definitive shape is not achieved until sperm reaches the distal portion of the epididymis (112,356). As might be expected from species differences, genetic factors also influence acrosome formation and shape. Structurally defective acrosomes form in pink-eyed sterile mutant mice (358,359), whereas acrosomes fail to form in blind sterile mutant mice, even though proacrosomal granules, the manchette, and flagellar structures form and some nuclear elongation and chromatin condensation occurs (354).

The acrosome sometimes shows an internal lamellar or crystalline structure (31), an ordered substructure (360), or a cobblestone-like pattern (42,131). A 4.2-nm periodicity was present in the cortical region of the acrosome of rat sperm, lying just deep to the outer acrosomal membrane on the convex surface (31,361). A similar pattern was also reported in the acrosome of human sperm (362). Other evidence that the acrosome has a substructure comes from studies on hamster spermatozoa disrupted by nitrogen cavitation. This treatment resulted in loss of much of the acrosomal matrix, but components immediately underlying the outer acrosomal membrane remained intact (122). These components were present in two areas: One was a larger and looser layer of fibrous material over the dorsal and lateral surfaces of the acrosome, whereas the other was a more compact fibrous layer adjacent to the anterior margin of the acrosome.

The membrane of the acrosome, particularly the equatorial segment, contains particles that form a crystalline array, giving the membrane a highly regular, granular appearance. These may be an indication of ordered structure in the underlying acrosomal components. Such features have been reported in rabbit (34), bull (39,131), human (44), rat (31,363), mouse (320), guinea pig (31,39,363), degu (39), and rhesus monkey (39). This pattern has been seen by freeze-etch, by freeze-fracture, and on replicas of air-dried and critical-point-dried spermatozoa. Although the outer acrosomal membrane appears to be fragile and easily displaced or disrupted at the time of the acrosome reaction, it also has a thickened appearance because of an electron-dense coating on the inner surface (364–368). This inner surface coat of the outer acrosomal membrane has been isolated from bull sperm and shown to be composed of three high-molecular-weight glycoproteins (290,000, 280,000 and 260,000 daltons) as well as 115,000-, 81,000-, 58,000-, and 46,000-dalton proteins. In addition, there was a set of proteins between 34,000 and 12,000 daltons (368). Lectins were found to bind to the inner surface of the membrane; WGA was observed to bind to the 46,000-dalton component. It was suggested that glycosylated molecules at this site may help to stabilize the membrane or play a functional role in the membrane fusion events of the acrosome reaction (368). The 200,000- and 58,000-dalton components were phosphorylated in a cAMP-independent manner, whereas the proteins between 34,000 and 12,000 daltons appeared to include calmodulin-binding proteins (368).

Inner acrosomal membrane development begins in early spermatids when the membrane of the proacrosomal granule abuts and then flattens against the nuclear envelope. This attachment spreads over the apical end of the nucleus during acrosomal development and nuclear elongation (369,370). The inner acrosomal membrane becomes exposed at the sperm surface and continuous with the plasma membrane when the acrosome reaction occurs. The inner acrosomal membrane in mouse and rabbit spermatozoa is quite resistant to chemical and physical disruption, including treatment with nonionic detergents and sonication (371,372). However, boar-sperm inner acrosomal membrane is sensitive to proteinase treatment (373), and lectins bind to the inner acrosomal membrane of sperm from hamster (30,374) and guinea pig (25), indicating that glycoproteins are present. Bridges 7 nm wide and with 7-nm center-to-center spacing were reported to be present between the inner and outer acrosomal membranes in boar sperm, apparently holding these structures together (373). However, the inner acrosomal membrane appears to be fluid because antigens recognized by monoclonal antibody PH-20 migrate from the plasma membrane of the postacrosomal region of the guinea-pig sperm head to the inner acrosomal membrane following the acrosome reaction (302,375). It has been suggested that the inner acrosomal membrane is associated with an extensive scaffolding network, possibly transmembrane in nature, in the equatorial segment (338).

Contents of Acrosome

The acrosome is a large zymogen-secreting granule whose contents are discharged during the acrosome reaction. However, it also contains enzymes typically found in primary lysosomes (Table 7). It has been described as a specialized lysosome (150,376), even though it apparently does not serve the usual lysosomal role of breaking down materials scavenged from the cytoplasm or entering the cell. The enzymes that are unique to the mammalian sperm acrosome are acrosin and hyaluronidase, and both are major constituents of the acrosome.

Acrosin is a trypsin-like serine proteinase, but it differs from similar enzymes in other tissues in molecular weight, substrate, and inhibitor specificities, indicating that it is probably a spermatogenic cell-specific isozyme (377–381). It was observed that fertilization was decreased by soybean trypsin inhibitor (382) and that pancreatic and seminal plasma trypsin inhibitors block fertilization *in vitro* (383), indicating that acrosin is required for fertilization. The enzyme is present in the acrosome as proacrosin, which is converted to the active form during the acrosome reaction (377–379,381,384). Immunolocalization studies have suggested that acrosin is present mainly in the anterior acrosome in human, boar, bull, and rabbit spermatozoa (385), but others have reported that it is localized to the inner acrosomal membrane (386–388). However, acrosin is rapidly released following the acrosome reaction, and it has been suggested that the bulk of the acrosin may be in the soluble acrosomal matrix (184).

TABLE 7. *Enzymes in the acrosome*

Enzyme	References
β-*N*-Acetylglucosaminadase	416
Acid phosphatase	415
Acrosin	184, 377–398
Arylamidase	412
Arylsulfatase A	414
Aspartylamidase	413
Calpain II	409
Cathepsin-D-like protease	408
Collagenase-like peptidase	407
Esterases, nonspecific	411
β-Glucuronidase	417
Hyaluronidase	399–406
Neuraminidase	410
Phospholipase A	376

Although acrosins from various species are quite similar functionally (389–391), there are species differences in proacrosin and acrosin at the molecular level. Boar proacrosin was present in 55,000- and 53,000-dalton forms; acrosin was present in 49,000-, 34,000-, and 25,000-dalton forms (377,392). Hamster-sperm proacrosin was present in forms between 56,000 and 51,000 daltons acrosin was present in multiple forms in two groups between 56,000 and 49,000 daltons and between 40,000 and 30,000 daltons (393). Rabbit proacrosin was present as a 27,300-dalton dimer (381), and a 38,000-dalton acrosin has been isolated from ram sperm (394). A monoclonal antibody (C 11 H) to human-sperm acrosin reacted with a 50,000-dalton protein and with several other proteins in the 34,000 to 24,000-dalton range extracted from human sperm (395). The antibody also reacted with the 55,000- and 53,000-dalton forms of acrosin isolated from boar sperm and was used to determine that acrosin is first detectable in step-9 spermatids during mouse spermatogenesis (396). Other studies have indicated that acrosin first appears in spermatids during spermatogenesis in the bull, ram, rabbit, boar, and human (395,397,398).

The hyaluronidase present in the acrosome has been reported to be distinct from the common lysosomal form and, like acrosin, appears to be a spermatogenic cell-specific isozyme (399–401). This glycosidase is abundant in acrosomes (402) and is located predominantly in the anterior acrosome in bull (403,404) and ram sperm (405). However, ram sperm denuded of the plasma membrane and outer acrosomal membrane still have half the hyaluronidase of an intact acrosome (406), and it has been suggested that some of the enzyme may be bound to the inner acrosomal membrane (405). Ram-sperm hyaluronidase was found to be a 62,000-dalton protein (400), whereas bull-sperm hyaluronidase was a 60,000-dalton protein and had a pH optimum of 3.8 (399).

Other hydrolytic enzymes have been detected in the acrosome (Table 7). Proteinases reported include a 110,000-dalton collagenase-like peptidase, with a pH optimum of 7.5 (407), and a cathepsin D-like protease (408). Antiserum to a calcium-activated neutral proteinase, calpain II, reacted with porcine-sperm acrosomes by indirect immunofluorescence and recognized an 80,000-dalton subunit of the enzyme on immunoblots (409). A neuraminidase (410), nonspecific esterases (411), arylamidase (412), aspartylamidase (413), arylsulfatase A (414), acid phosphatase (415), β-*N*-acetylglucosaminidase (416), β-glucuronidase (417), and phospholipase A (376) have also been reported to be present in the acrosome.

THE FLAGELLUM

The flagellum of the mammalian spermatozoon consists of four distinct segments: the *connecting piece* (neck), the *middle piece,* the *principal piece,* and the *end piece* (Fig. 1). The main structural features of the flagellum of the mammalian spermatozoon are the *axoneme,* the *mitochondrial sheath,* the *outer dense fibers,* and the *fibrous sheath* (Table 6). The axoneme is composed of a "9 + 2" complex of microtubules which extends the full length of the flagellum. The middle-piece segment contains the mitochondrial sheath, while the principal-piece segment contains the fibrous sheath. The mitochondria underlie the plasma membrane in the middle piece, while the fibrous sheath underlies the plasma membrane in the principal piece. The outer dense fibers extend from the connecting piece into the posterior part of the principal piece and are situated between the mitochondria and the axoneme in the middle piece, and between the fibrous sheath and the axoneme in the principal piece. The base of the flagellum abuts the nucleus at the junction between connecting piece and head (140,418,419).

The flagellum provides the motile force necessary for the sperm to reach the egg surface and achieve fertilization. The different elements of the flagellum are involved (a) in generating and shaping the waves of bending that produce this force and (b) in propagating the waves from the base to the tip. The flagellum contributes most of the length of the mammalian spermatozoon. For example, the spermatozoon of the human is about 60 μm long, and the head is only 4 to 5 μm of this length (303). However, the length of the spermatozoon varies considerably between species. The spermatozoon in the rabbit is 46 μm long; that in the mouse is 120 μm long, that in the rat is 190 μm long, and that in the Chinese hamster is 250 μm long (420). The human-sperm flagellum, which is more than 1 μm in diameter in the connecting-piece segment, tapers progressively toward its posterior tip (303).

Connecting Piece

The main structural components of the connecting piece (Fig. 7) are the *capitulum* (a dense fibrous plate-like structure that conforms to the shape of the *implantation fossa*) and the *segmented columns* (52). The implantation fossa is formed by a specialized region of the nuclear envelope and a dense plaque of material on the cytoplasmic surface of the nuclear envelope, the *basal plate.* The interspace between the two membranes of the nuclear envelope in this region is traversed by regular periodic densities 6 nm wide and 6 nm apart (52). Freeze-fracture studies indicated that the membrane of the nuclear envelope lining the implantation fossa contains a dense population of large regularly spaced intramembranous particles surrounding a particle-free region of membrane (31). Fine filaments traversing the narrow region between capitulum and basal plate presumably are responsible for attaching the capitulum of the flagellum to the basal plate of the head (320,362). This region between capitulum and basal plate appears to be the site of cleavage of heads from tails following trypsin treatment (23,421), but decapitation of sperm with primary amines or sodium dodecyl sulfate usually results in cleavage between inner and outer nuclear membranes, next to the basal plate (422). Heads and tails can also be separated by sonication, but the cleavage site is not predictable (423,424). The basal plate and capitulum are composed of proteins that are soluble in ionic detergent containing a disulfide-bond reducing agent (425,426). Although the composition of these structures has not been determined, they may be related to ciliary rootlets (52), which contain a 250,000- and 230,000-dalton protein dimer called *ankyrin* (303). A genetic defect is sometimes seen in bulls in which the flagella of most mature sperm are detached from the heads (427). Detachment begins during late spermatogenesis and continues in the epididymis; the resulting detached flagella are motile, metabolically active, and able to penetrate cervical mucus (428).

Extending posteriorly from the capitulum are two major and five minor segmented columns 1 to 2 μm in length. The two major columns split into two columns each and, along with the other columns, fuse to the nine outer dense fibers extending throughout much of the remaining length of the flagellum (Fig. 9). However, the segmented columns and outer dense fibers have different origins, and the continuity between them develops late in spermiogenesis (418,429). The segmented columns of the connecting piece are cross-striated, with a periodicity of 6.65 nm between segments; and each segment, in turn, has nine or 10 hori-

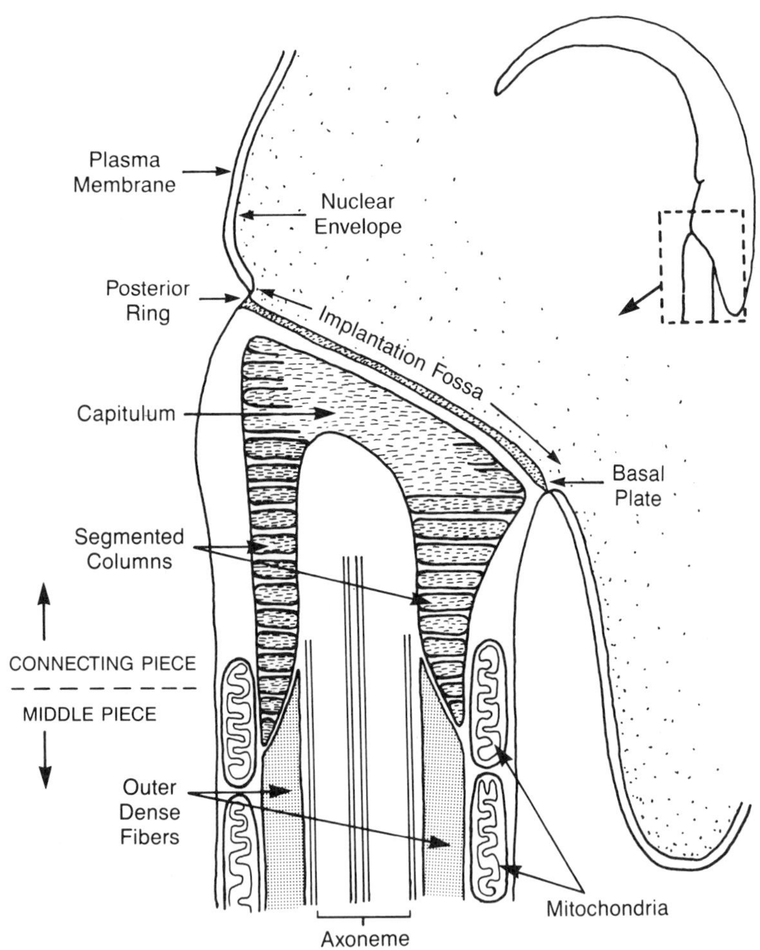

FIG. 7. Connecting piece of the flagellum. The basal plate is adherent to the nuclear envelope, defining the implantation fossa and forming the site of attachment of the flagellum to the sperm head. The connecting piece is topped by the capitulum, with the segmented columns extending from it caudally to fuse with the outer dense fibers. (Modified from ref. 432.)

zontal bands (429). During development of the flagellum, a transversely or obliquely oriented proximal centriole lies between the longitudinally oriented distal centriole and a depression in the capitulum (429). The distal centriole is continuous with the axoneme and is surrounded by other accessory structures of the connecting piece. In many species, the distal centriole disintegrates late in spermatogenesis and the proximal centriole is retained (140,362,418,430,431). It has been suggested that the proximal centriole is the center of sperm motility (418). However, the proximal centriole disintegrates during the latter part of spermiogenesis in some species with normal motility (429,432), indicating that it is not required for generation of the flagellar beat. It appears that the centrioles serve as organizing centers for the formation of the axoneme and segmented columns, but are not required for initiation or propagation of waves of bending along the tail (52). The connecting piece joins the middle piece distally at the beginning of the mitochondrial sheath.

Axoneme

The axoneme or axial filament complex of the mammalian sperm tail (Fig. 8) has the same organization as that in cilia and flagella, present in most plants and animals. It consists of two central microtubules surrounded by nine microtubule doublets (433). Each doublet consists of a complete A microtubule, onto which is attached a "C-shaped" B microtubule. Two arms extend from the A microtubule toward the B microtubule of the adjacent doublet. When axonemes are viewed from base to tip, the arms project clockwise (434). In the rat spermatozoon, the central pair of microtubules extend into the connecting piece to the capitulum, whereas the other microtubules appear to end on the remnants of the base of the distal centriole (432,435). Spokes radiate from the central pair of microtubules to the outer doublets in a double helix around the central tubules (436). The doublets are numbered one through nine, with number one being the doublet situated on a plane perpendicular to that bisecting both microtubules of the central pair. Doublet number two is adjacent to the arms of doublet number one, and so on.

The microtubules are composed of "α-tubulin" and "β-tubulin," closely related proteins of approximately 56,000- and 54,500 daltons respectively (437). At least one new form of both α- and β-tubulin first appears during spermatogenesis in spermatids (437,438), indicating that postmeiotic tubulin gene expression occurs in these haploid cells (308). A cDNA for α-tubulin appears to differ in sequence from other α-tubulin genes, suggesting that a unique sper-

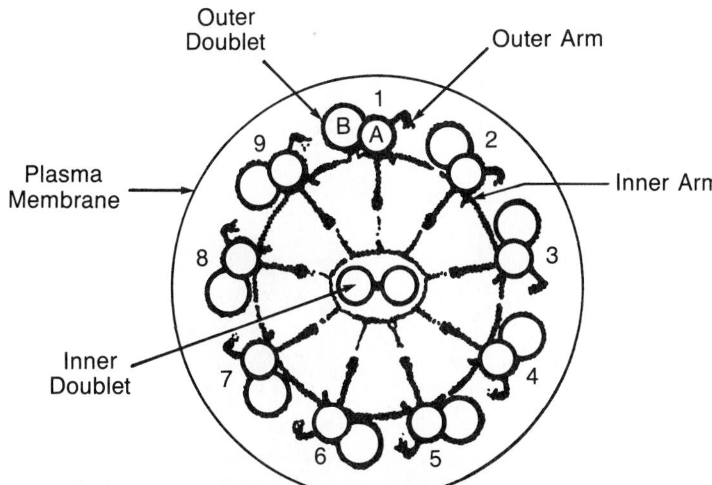

FIG. 8. The axoneme in the end-piece of the sperm flagellum. Nine outer doublets of microtubules surround an inner doublet of microtubules. The outer doublets consist of A and B microtubules. Inner and outer dynein arms extend from the A microtubule toward the B microtubule of the adjacent pair.

matogenic cell α-tubulin isoform is present in spermatids (438). It has not yet been determined whether this tubulin is present in the microtubules of the flagellum and might be involved in determining some of the special properties of the sperm axoneme. "Kinesin" is another interesting protein associated with microtubules that has been identified recently (439). It is a 600,000-dalton complex, composed of 110,000- and 65,000- to 70,000-dalton subunits, which interacts with the surface of microtubules to effect movement. Isolated microtubules move over the surface of a slide coated with kinesin, and latex beads are moved along microtubules in the presence of the protein. Kinesin has been shown to cause anterograde translocation of cell organelles along axonal microtubules, and recently a retrograde translocator was characterized partially (440). Both translocators require ATP, but differ from myosin or dynein in their structural and enzymatic characteristics (439,440). It will be interesting to learn whether kinesin is present in the mammalian sperm flagellum and whether it has a role in generating or propagating the flagellar wave.

Other proteins originally identified in the axoneme of sea urchin sperm are probably also present in mammalian sperm. The arms of the microtubule doublets contain "dynein," an approximately 500,000-dalton protein with ATPase activity (441). The ATPase activity is believed to be responsible for the sliding forces generated between adjacent doublets of microtubules during flagellar movement (442). ATPase has been extracted from mammalian spermatozoa, and ATPase activity has been identified by histochemistry on the arms of the doublets and at the junction between radial spokes and central tubules in human sperm (303,443).

The links between adjacent microtubule doublets in sea urchin sperm contain "nexin," a 165,000- to 150,000-dalton protein thought to constitute about 2% of the axonemal proteins (444). In addition, the sperm doublet microtubules of the sea urchin sperm flagellum can be dissociated with various treatments to produce ribbons of two to four protofilaments (445) that have been further fractionated with chemical agents (446). The ribbons contain proteins that have been named "tektins," and the filaments that they form are 2 to 3 nm in diameter, highly insoluble, and have physical and chemical properties similar to intermediate filaments (447,448). The filaments contain 55,000-, 51,000-, and 47,000-dalton proteins, and an antiserum to this set of proteins reacted with the entire length of the axoneme (449). They also appear to be laterally associated with the doublet microtubules, are probably structural components of the A microtubule wall, and may be involved in assembly or function of microtubules (449).

Mitochondrial Sheath

The mitochondria are helically wrapped around the outer dense fibers in the middle piece of the sperm tail (Fig. 1). They are generally arranged end-to-end, but the number of parallel helices, the number of gyres, and the length of the middle piece vary between species. In the mouse, the mitochondria are usually arranged in two parallel helices, with an average of 87 windings around the flagellum (450). The morphogenesis of this arrangement in the spermatid was found to occur by: (a) the migration of the annulus from the connecting piece down the flagellum to the beginning of the fibrous sheath, (b) the formation of a dextral helix of elongated mitochondria around the flagellum, (c) the division of these mitochondria into spherical mitochondria, and (d) finally the elongation and end-to-end apposition of these mitochondria into two tight sinestral helices (450). In the mouse, the mitochondria are usually of variable length and abut end-to-end at random along the helix. It was possible by a genetic selection program to produce strains of mice with sperm midpieces longer and shorter than the 21-μm average midpiece length (451).

In some species there is a precise order in the mitochondrial sheath. In the common brown bat, there are two mitochondria of identical size in each turn of the gyre, and their ends always meet on a plane passing through the central pair of microtubules in the axoneme (132). Mitochondrial sheaths composed of a precise number of mitochondria of identical size and shape are present in the little brown bat (132), woolly opossum (452), and Chinese hamster (453). In rhesus monkey sperm there is a tendency for the demarcation between mitochondria to occur in longitudinal register in alternate gyres (453).

The length of the middle piece and the disposition of mitochondria in spermatozoa was determined for several species using surface replica methods (453). The middle piece in bull sperm was 12 μm long, the number of mitochondrial gyres was about 64, and there were usually three helices. Some mitochondria were found to extend parallel with the long axis of the flagellum into the connecting piece. The rabbit sperm midpiece was 8.5 μm long and contained about 41 gyres of mitochondria in a quadruple or quintuple helix. The middle piece of rhesus monkey spermatozoa was about 10 μm long with 40 gyres of mitochondria arranged in a single or double helix. The middle piece of rat sperm was 64 μm long and contained about 362 mitochondrial gyres. The large outer dense fibers in rat sperm produced a broad middle piece, and the gently spiraling mitochondria fitted together in intricate patterns. The middle piece in Chinese hamster sperm was about 100 μm long, with the mitochondria apparently disposed in a double helix, each wrapping one-third the circumference of the quite broad middle piece. The degu sperm middle piece was 7 μm long, with about 33 gyres of mitochondria in concentric rows of single or double helices. Finally, the guinea-pig spermatozoan middle piece was determined to be 9 μm long, and the mitochondria were found to be arranged in irregular concentric patterns (453).

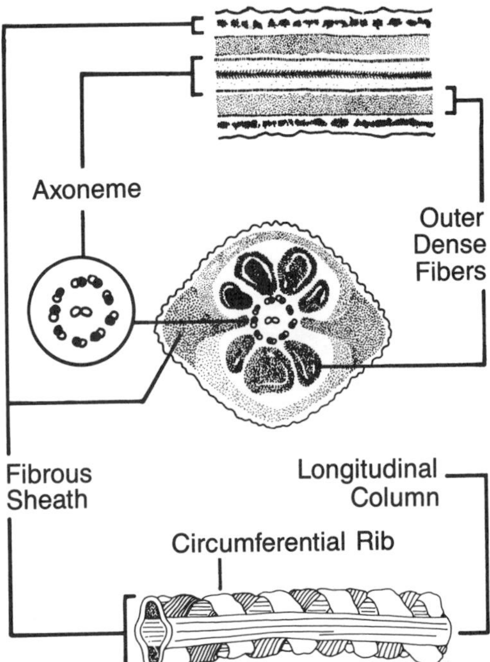

FIG. 9. Cytoskeletal components of the sperm flagellum. The axoneme extends from the connecting piece of the flagellum to the distal tip. In the principal piece of the flagellum, the axoneme is surrounded by the fibrous sheath, composed of longitudinal columns connected by circumferential ribs. The outer dense fibers extend from the connecting piece to the posterior part of the principal piece. They lie between the mitochondrial sheath and the axoneme in the middle piece and between the fibrous sheath and the axoneme in the principal piece.

Outer Dense Fibers

The outer dense fibers surround the axoneme, forming a "9 + 9 + 2" complex throughout the length of the middle piece and throughout most or all of the principal piece of the flagellum of mammalian spermatozoa (Figs. 1 and 9). Although similar structures are present in spermatozoa of nonmammalian species (2), it has not been determined whether they are related in composition or function to the outer dense fibers in mammalian spermatozoa. The basic structural plan of the sperm flagellum shows little variation in mammals, but the outer dense fibers differ considerably in size and shape between species. The fibers are often tear-drop shaped in cross section, with a rounded outer contour and an inner margin tapering toward a doublet of the axoneme (52). The dense fibers also differ among themselves in shape and size, with fibers 1, 5, and 6 (and sometimes 9) being larger than the others. They are numbered corresponding to the adjacent microtubule doublet. The fibers are thickest in the proximal part of the middle piece and gradually taper in thickness toward the distal tip. They terminate in the proximal half of the principal piece in the human, macaque, and bat, but extend farther in the principal piece in the rat, hamster, guinea pig, and ground squirrel (52). In the human (454), bull, and rat (455), the dense fibers occupy 60% of the length of the principal piece. In most species, fibers 3 and 8 terminate in the first part of the principal piece, and their place is taken by inward extensions of the longitudinal columns of the fibrous sheath. The larger fibers (1, 5, and 6) are usually the last to terminate (456).

The formation of the outer dense fibers begins in spermatids, with the appearance of a small dense fiber immediately adjacent to the outer aspect of each microtubule doublet (429,457,458). In the rat, fibers first appear in the most proximal part of the future middle piece in step 8 and extend into the principal piece by step 14 (459). During step 15 of spermiogenesis the outer dense fibers increase in diameter and change shape, with fibers 1, 5, and 6 developing ahead of the other fibers. During step 16 the fibers enlarge rapidly along their entire length and take on their nearly final form, with slight growth continuing during steps 17 to 19 (459). Radioautography following incorporation of labeled proline and cysteine suggested that rapid protein synthesis accompanied the rapid growth of the outer dense fiber during step 16 (459).

On electron micrographs the fibers usually appear dense, with a slightly less dense cortical layer. This cortical layer stained intensely with phosphotungstic acid (460) and tannic acid (52) and, when fixed in the presence of ruthenium red, appeared to be composed of a single lamina of 6- to 7-nm globular particles (461). Surface replicas of rat- and mouse-sperm outer dense fibers showed striations in the outer contour of the cortex, with a periodicity of 40 nm (461,462); these striations had the same 70 to 80° "sinistral obliquity" as the mitochondrial helix in the middle piece (450). On replicas each striation appeared to be composed of a double linear array of 6- to 8-nm diameter globular subunits (461), and a central depression in each striation probably accounts for an apparent periodicity of 20 nm seen on negatively stained specimens (461,463). In the bull, 20-nm (464) and 50-nm (465) periodicity has been reported, and a 16-nm repeat was reported for human-sperm outer dense fibers (362). Studies on the rat have indicated that the periodic substructure is confined to the cortex (461); however, this substructure is reported to be present in both cortical and medullary elements in human and bull sperm (362,465).

It has been possible to take advantage of the relative insolubility of fibrous components of the flagellum in the absence of disulfide bond-reducing agents to isolate outer dense fibers for biochemical analysis. Early studies reported that tail components contain keratin-like proteins rich in cysteine (466) and that disulfide bond cross-linking of proteins in the outer dense fiber increased during epididymal maturation (337,425). Initial studies on outer dense fibers isolated from rat sperm and analyzed by gel electrophoresis in the presence of disulfide-bond-reducing agents indicated that they contained 40,000-, 25,000-, 12,000-, and 11,000-dalton proteins (467). A subsequent study indicated that the main proteins in the rat were 75,000, 35,000, 25,000, and 15,000 daltons (468). Another study reported that rat outer dense fibers contained major proteins of 87,000, 25,000, 19,000, and 12,000 daltons, as well as minor proteins of 71,000, 64,000, and 55,000 daltons (461). A more recent study indicated that the major proteins in the rat outer dense fibers were 87,000, 30,400, 26,000, 18,400, 13,000, and 11,500 daltons (469). Similar studies on bull-sperm outer dense fibers identified 55,000-, 30,000-, and 15,000-dalton proteins (465), later revised to be 75,000- to 72,000-, 57,000- to 54,000-, and 27,000- to 24,000-dalton proteins (463).

Several studies have confirmed that the outer dense fibers have a high cysteine content (461,463,469). In addition, it has been shown that there are differences between individual outer dense fiber proteins in amino acid composition, amino-terminal amino acid, net charge, and phosphorylation (461,463,469). The 87,000-dalton protein in rat outer dense fibers contained relatively large amounts of glutamic acid, lysine, alanine, and leucine, but had relatively small amounts of serine, glycine, and cysteine. However, the 30,400-, 26,000-, 18,400-, and 11,500-dalton proteins contained high amounts of cysteine, tyrosine, and proline plus glycine, but less glutamic acid. The 13,000-dalton component had a high content of glutamic acid and no histidine (469). The 30,400- and 26,000-dalton proteins had similar amino acid composition, histidine in the amino-terminal position, and similar peptide maps, suggesting that they share a common peptide chain (469).

Other differences have been reported for the proteins that compose the outer dense fibers. Infrared spectrum analysis suggested that the higher-molecular-weight components have an alpha-helical configuration (463), whereas other studies indicated that the lower-molecular-weight components are capable of binding zinc to sulfhydryl groups (468). Zinc is required for spermatogenesis (470), is incorporated into the flagellum in late spermatids (471), and is localized in the outer dense fibers (463). Isoelectric focusing indicated that the proteins have large charge heterogeneities, indicative of posttranslational modifications (469,472). Some studies have suggested that the outer dense fiber proteins are glycosylated (465), but other studies indicated that carbohydrates were either absent (461) or barely detectable, suggesting that they may be present as contaminants (469). All of the major polypeptides contained appreciable amounts of phosphate bound as phosphoserine, which could account for the charge heterogeneities, particularly in the higher-molecular-weight polypeptides (469). Early studies also suggested that triglycerides may be associated with the outer dense fibers (465,467).

Satellite fibers are present in the flagellar matrix between the outer dense fibers (52,336,476). These fibers form in step 19 of spermiogenesis in the rat, just before spermatozoa are released from the seminiferous epithelium (459). They are present in limited numbers in most species, but are highly developed in the ground squirrel (336) and bandicoot (474), which have thick sperm tails (336). It has been suggested that they may be accessory tensile elements of the motor apparatus (336). The satellite fibers appear to arise by exfoliation from the free edge of the cortex on the sides of the outer dense fibers and have the same resistance to solubilization as the outer dense fibers (52). However, they have not been isolated separately from the outer dense fibers, and their composition is not known.

An early speculation was that the outer dense fibers might be contractile because of their close association with the axoneme, their coincident appearance during phylogeny with internal fertilization, and a concomitant increase in the size of the mitochondrial sheath (336). This appeared to be supported by (a) a report that the outer dense fibers were antigenically similar to actin (475) and (b) histochemical studies that suggested that an ATPase was associated with the outer dense fibers (460). However, subsequent biochemical studies did not indicate a similarity between the composition of outer dense fibers and actin, myosin, or tubulin (461); also, other investigators did not detect ATPase activity in outer dense fibers (465,476). It now appears unlikely that the outer dense fibers play an active role in flagellar motion. However, stabilization of outer dense fiber proteins by abundant disulfide cross-linking may give them significant passive elastic properties that serve to stiffen or provide elastic recoil for the sperm tail (52). By use of high-speed cinematography, spermatozoa of mouse, human, rabbit, and opossum appeared relatively flexible, and as they beat they formed arcs with a small radius of curvature. Spermatozoa of rat and Chinese hamster appeared very stiff while beating and had a large radius of curvature (420). There was a correlation between the radius of curvature and the size of the dense fibers in these species, suggesting that the dense fibers might influence the form of the beat by determining the elastic properties of the sperm tail (420).

Fibrous Sheath

The fibrous sheath defines the extent of the principal piece (Figs. 1 and 9), which is the longest segment of the flagellum and is the most effective in locomotion (336). It appears to be a cytoskeletal structure of the flagellum that is unique to spermatozoa in mammals and some birds. It closely underlies, but is not attached to, the plasma membrane (2). The fibrous sheath is a tapering cylinder formed by two *longitudinal columns* connected by *circumferential ribs* (Fig. 9). The columns are formed by longitudinally oriented, loosely packed filamentous structures 15 to 20 nm in diameter. The longitudinal columns run peripheral to microtubule doublets 3 and 8 of the axoneme and are attached to outer dense fibers 3 and 8 in the proximal part of the principal piece (473). Distal to the termination of these two dense fibers, the tapered central edges of the longitudinal columns attach to ridges projecting from microtubule doublets 3 and 8 (336). The columns lie approximately in the plane of the central pair of axoneme microtubules throughout the principal piece segment and have been referred to as *dorsal* and *ventral columns* in sperm containing a falciform head (336). The size and shape of the longitudinal columns vary between species. They are narrow and inconspicuous in the common brown bat and guinea pig, but in the Chinese hamster and opossum they are large and result in prominent ridges that give the principal piece an elliptical profile in cross section (336).

The ribs of the fibrous sheath are composed of closely packed, circumferentially oriented filaments (336). The ribs broaden toward their ends, where they merge with the longitudinal columns and with each other. They are closely spaced and may bifurcate to anastomose with adjacent ribs. This occurs frequently in the mouse, resulting in broad bands instead of slender separate ribs. The ribs may also vary in shape and size, being broad and flat in the bat and greatly expanded at their ends in the opossum. The thickness of the ribs diminishes toward the distal end of the principal piece, and the ribs end abruptly at the posterior margin of the principal piece (52,336). In human spermatozoa, the ribs are 10 to 20 nm apart and about 50 nm thick (303).

A study using electron microscopy and radioautography indicated that formation of the fibrous sheath takes place throughout much of spermiogenesis in the rat and proceeds in a distal to proximal direction (477). The longitudinal columns appeared in the distal end of the flagellum in step 2 of spermiogenesis, as thin rods joined to microtubule doublets 3 and 8. The columns increased in length during steps 2 to 10; in step 11, evenly spaced and circumferentially arranged pairs of spines formed against the plasma membrane in the distal part of the flagellum. During steps 12 to 14, these structures associated with the columns in a distal to proximal direction. In early step 15, additional material was deposited between the pairs of spines to form the definitive ribs, and the longitudinal columns became thickened. During steps 15 to 17, additional ribs were formed from posterior to anterior, along the remaining proximal segment of the principal piece (477). Radioautography following injection of labeled amino acids indicated that the fibrous sheath proteins were synthesized during the entire 15-day period of fibrous sheath formation (477). These studies supported earlier suggestions that filamentous material present in the cytoplasm of step-11 to -15 spermatids was rib precursor in human and marmoset sperm (457,478,479). They confirmed and extended the general understanding of fibrous sheath formation that had come from earlier studies on bandicoot sperm (458). A monoclonal antibody that reacts with the mouse sperm fibrous sheath (480) was used in an immunohistochemical study on fibrous sheath formation (481). The antigen was first detected in the cytoplasm of stage-14 spermatids, and staining intensity increased at stage 15. The positive reaction was observed first in the proximal portion of the principal piece and was present throughout the fibrous sheath by step 16 (481). This proximal-to-distal appearance of the antigen was opposite to that reported previously in the rat (477).

Early studies indicated that the fibrous sheath was highly resistant to acid solubilization (482) and that the proteins of the fibrous sheath are stabilized by disulfide bonds (337). More recent studies took advantage of these characteristics to devise a differential solubilization procedure for isolating the fibrous sheath of rat spermatozoa (344,483). Isolated fibrous sheaths were analyzed by polyacrylamide gel electrophoresis under disulfide-bond-reducing conditions and were found to consist of a major protein of 80,000-daltons and minor proteins of 90,000-, 25,000-, and 11,000-daltons (483). In another study, the major insoluble tail component synthesized during spermiogenesis in the mouse was a 74,000-dalton protein (484), which may be a fibrous sheath component. Monoclonal antibodies to the fibrous sheath which have been reported recently should be useful for further defining its composition (481,485,486). The antigens recognized by two of the antibodies have not yet been identified, but one antibody appears to recognize a 67,000-dalton protein in the mouse, a 65,000-dalton protein in the rat, and a 66,000-dalton protein in the hamster (486). This antibody also reacted with late spermatids in all three species, but did not react with spermatids or the fibrous sheath in rabbit and guinea pig.

It has been suggested that a function of the fibrous sheath might be to modulate the plane of the flagellar beat. The attachment of doublets 3 and 8 to the longitudinal columns might restrict their participation in microtubule sliding and axoneme bending during flagellar motion. The longitudinal columns themselves might also limit bending of the flagellum in this same plane, whereas flagellar bending perpendicular to this plane would not be restricted by these features (52). Although sperm appear to swim with a planar effective stroke and recovery stroke somewhat like cilia, they also rotate (420), and the propagated waves have a three-dimensional component in the distal portion of the tail (52). However, it is not known how the fibrous sheath might influence flagellar movement in the female reproductive tract.

Abnormal Flagella

Spermatozoa with abnormal flagella are present in low numbers in most, or perhaps all, mammals but are relatively common in humans. One study indicated that 12.5 ± 5.5% of sperm from 20 fertile men had abnormal flagella and that an even higher number of sperm (24.4 ± 7.7%) had abnormal axonemes; 41.6 ± 15.3% of sperm were motile (487). Infertile men have been reported to have 18% (488) or over 30% (489) sperm with abnormal tails. It is generally assumed that abnormal sperm have little chance of achieving fertilization. However, completely immotile human spermatozoa have been reported to undergo capacitation, the acrosome reaction, and fusion with the vitelline membrane of zona-free hamster oocytes *in vitro* (490). Also, a sperm tail lacking four doublets and the outer dense fibers has been observed in the cytoplasm of a fertilized mouse egg (491).

Anecdotal reports of infertile men with sperm that are immotile or have abnormal flagella are not uncommon (492–495). Although the causes of these abnormalities are seldom known, a hereditary condition has been identified, referred to as *immotile-cila syndrome* or *Kartagener's syndrome,* which results in male sterility, situs inversus in 50% of cases, and chronic respiratory problems (496). It appears that these problems are directly or indirectly a consequence of an autosomal recessive trait for inability of cilia and flagella to move or to perform normal and coordinated movements (497). The sperm from 12 males who have the syndrome had defective axonemes with a partial or complete lack of dynein arms, a lack of outer dynein arms but a presence of the inner arms, a disorganized axoneme lacking inner arms, or abnormal short spokes and a lack of the central sheath (498). Because of the different types of defects seen in sperm and cilia, the failure to locate a single gene by linkage analysis, and the relatively high prevalence of the condition, it has been suggested that many genes, when mutated, may produce the syndrome (496).

Several mutations that affect formation of the flagellum have been identified in mice. All of the mutations described so far are pleiotropic, affecting processes in addition to spermatogenesis, and most affect formation of the sperm head as well as the flagellum (353,354). Homozygous mice with the Wobbler mutation apparently produced normal numbers of sperm, but few sperm were motile (499). The sperm appeared to have tails of normal length, and they formed heads of normal appearance, but 70% of sperm in the ductus deferens had ultrastructural defects in the flagellum. These defects included the absence of from one to four outer doublets and their corresponding dense fibers, most commonly those from position 4 through 7. Other defects seen less frequently were supernumerary tubules or absence of central pair tubules (499). Defective sperm were common in T/t mice, with the most frequent flagellar defects seen in sterile mice being a lack of four outer dense fibers and doublets (500). The male-sterile mutation, hydrocephalic-polydactyl (*hpy*), resulted in an absence of flagella or in partially assembled axonemal structures and/or poorly organized aggregates of other tail components (501). The axoneme was usually absent or abnormally formed; the outer dense fibers and fibrous sheath were morphologically atypical, when present. It was suggested that this axoneme dysgenesis might be due to failure to form stabile structures because of defective subunits (501).

The sperm from four infertile men with flagellar dyskinesia had normal axonemes, but abnormal periaxonemal structures. These included abnormal extension of individual dense fibers along the axoneme, altered order of termination of these structures, and a modified number and location of longitudinal columns of the fibrous sheath (502). The outer dense fibers were found to have abnormal positions with respect to each other, being placed symmetrically with respect to a plane that passes through microtubular doublet 1 and between doublets 5 and 6. The most common defect of the longitudinal columns of the fibrous sheath was the presence of only one column adjacent to doublet 3 or 8 (502). It was suggested that these abnormalities might be due to a defect of the components of the wall of A microtubules of the outer nine doublets, at the site of formation or assembly of the outer dense fibers and longitudinal columns (503).

A defect common to abnormal or degenerating flagella is the absence of microtubule doublets and dense fibers 4 through 7 (499,500,504). The same alteration has been produced by adding ATP to detergent-extracted rat sperm tails; doublets and fibers 8 through 3 appear to remain firmly attached to the fibrous sheath, while doublets 4 through 7 are extruded from the sperm tail (505). This suggests that some sperm seen with this defect may be undergoing degeneration. It has also been noted in some studies that the flagellar axoneme may appear to form normally and then become progressively disorganized. This appears to occur during spermiogenesis in quaking (506) and in *hpy*/*hpy* mice (501). However, in Wobbler mice, the percentage of abnormal sperm increases along the male tract. Only about 5% of sperm tails were abnormal in the testis, while nearly 70% of sperm from the ductus deferens were abnormal (499).

Flagellar Motion

The flagellar wave is reported to propagate in a plane perpendicular to the central pair of microtubules of the axoneme and to pass through doublet 1 and between doublets 5 and 6, with the active stroke being toward doublet 1 (507). The flagellum appears to twist during bend propagation (508,509), with the plane of bending moving toward doublet 2 (508). It has been suggested that the part of the axoneme containing doublets 1 through 5 is active during this phase of flagellar motion (508,510). The outer dense fibers and fibrous sheath appear to play a passive role in flagellar motion (511–514). It has been suggested that the tapering of the dense fibers results in decreasing local resistance to bending (454,502) and might explain the progressive increase in the amplitude of curvature observed during flagellar wave propagation (513,515,516). The small flagellar amplitude observed in certain abnormal human sperm (517) may be due to the constraint imposed by the abnormal arrangement of dense fibers in those sperm (502).

Sperm acquire the capacity for progressive motility during epididymal maturation. Sperm from the cauda epididymis are immotile in epididymal fluid, and it is not until they are diluted into physiological medium that the capacity for motility is expressed. It is likely that in most species, immotility is enforced by the viscoelastic drag produced by a high-molecular-weight glycoprotein (immobilin) present in epididymal fluid (518,519). However, rabbit sperm show motility in their native fluid (520), and epididymal fluid in the bull is not particularly viscous (521). Sperm from the caput epididymis in most mammals have a vibratory or slow and ineffective beat that often results in circular swimming patterns (183). In contrast, sperm from the cauda epididymis usually move with a vigorous motion that results in rapid forward movement. In correlation with this change in swimming pattern, the flagellum appears to become more rigid and to beat with a reduced arc of curvature (183). This may be due to the increased disulfide bond formation that occurs in outer dense fibers and the fibrous sheath during epididymal maturation (337). However, cauda sperm from different species show different patterns of motility, flagellar beat, and flagellar rigidity (420). Sperm undergo additional changes in the pattern of motility in the female reproductive tract. They become hyperactivated as capacitation proceeds, moving with a vigorous whip-like beating of the flagellum at the time of fertilization (7,184).

A variety of factors appear to be involved in the initiation and regulation of sperm motility (Table 8), but a unifying hypothesis for how these factors interact to accomplish this is lacking. It is generally accepted that cyclic adenosine monophosphate (cAMP) mediates sperm motility, because cAMP levels increase in sperm during epididymal transit (522,523). Also, a number of cAMP phosphodiesterase inhibitors that elevate levels of cAMP in sperm induce a poorly coordinated pattern of motility in caput sperm (524). This pattern is converted to the effective pattern comparable to that seen in caudal sperm by addition of a "forward motility protein" present in epididymal fluid (525,526). Another change that occurs as sperm transit the epididymis is an increase in internal pH; bicarbonate ions, in the presence of calcium, markedly elevate cAMP levels in cauda sperm

TABLE 8. *Factors involved in initiation and regulation of sperm motility*

Factor	References
ATP required for sperm motility	530–532
ATP interacts with dynein ATPase to promote sliding of outer doublets of axoneme	529
Calcium-dependent and calmodulin-regulated adenyl cyclase converts ATP to cAMP	534–537
cAMP levels in sperm increase during epididymal transit	522, 523
Phosphodiesterse inhibitors elevate cAMP levels and induce partial motility in caput sperm	524
Increase in internal pH and cAMP induces motility	527, 528
cAMP-dependent protein kinases present	536–538
cAMP stimulates phosphorylation of sperm proteins	533, 542, 554–556
Phosphoprotein phosphatase present	539
cAMP phosphodiesterase present	540
Inhibitor of cAMP-dependent protein kinase present	542
Low-molecular-weight factor in seminal plasma stimulates sperm adenyl cyclase	544
Adenosine elevates cAMP levels and initiates motility in caput sperm	545
High levels of adenosine inhibit sperm adenyl cyclase activity	546–548
Adenosine increases level of *S*-adenosylhomocysteine, which inhibits sperm motility	562–564
Adenyl cyclase inhibitory guanine-nucleotide-binding protein present	551
Inhibitor of cAMP-independent protein kinase present in seminal plasma	558, 559
Inhibitor of calcium uptake present in seminal plasma	560, 561
Forward motility protein in epididymal fluid modulates pattern of sperm motility	525, 526
Motility inhibitor present in seminal plasma	557
pH-dependent sperm motility quiescence factor present in epididymal fluid	521, 565
Immotility of epididymal sperm enforced by viscoelastic drag produced by high-molecular-weight glycoprotein in epididymal fluid	578, 579

(527), and conditions that elevate both pH and cAMP in caput sperm cause them to swim like cauda sperm (528). ATP is required for motility, and one of its roles is to interact with ATPases associated with the dynein arms to promote sliding of the outer doublets (529). Sperm that have been permeabilized by detergent treatment are immotile but can be reactivated with ATP, and addition of cAMP causes an increase in motility (530–532).

The major role of cAMP in sperm is probably to mediate cAMP-stimulated phosphorylation of proteins essential for initiation or maintenance of motility (533). ATP is converted to cAMP in sperm by a calcium-dependent adenylate cyclase that may be controlled partly by calmodulin (534,535). The 55,000- and 49,000-dalton RI and RII regulatory subunits as well as the 40,000-dalton catalytic (C) subunits of cAMP-dependent protein kinase are present in sperm, and most of the cAMP-binding activity is in the tail (536,537). Some investigators have suggested that protein kinase may exist on the surface of the sperm and that cAMP may be a first message (537), but others report that the enzyme is internal (536,538). Other enzymes needed for protein phosphorylation and dephosphorylation are also present in sperm, including phosphoprotein phosphatase (539) and cAMP phosphodiesterase (540,541). In addition, sperm have been reported to contain an inhibitor of cAMP-dependent protein kinase (542), and a 32,000-dalton calmodulin-binding protein that inhibits phosphodiesterase has been identified in the testis (543).

Seminal plasma is rich in prostaglandins and steroid hormones known to alter cAMP levels in other tissues, but until recently no external regulators had been shown to affect sperm cAMP levels, adenylate cyclase activity, or motility (533). However, it has been reported that a low-molecular-weight factor in porcine seminal plasma stimulates sperm adenylate cyclase activity (544). In addition, adenosine and its analogs have been shown to elevate cAMP levels and to initiate motility in immature caput sperm in a pH-dependent manner (545). Some of the analogs used do not appear to enter cells, suggesting that adenosine may act on sperm through external adenosine receptors. There have also been reports that high levels of adenosine inhibit sperm adenylate cyclase activity, possibly through an inhibitory "P" site associated with the adenylate cyclase catalytic subunit (546–548). Earlier studies indicated that sperm adenylate cyclase is unaffected by fluoride, guanine nucleotides, forskolin, or cholera toxin plus NAD (533,549), suggesting that the enzyme is not regulated by guanidine-nucleotide-binding regulatory proteins. Although stimulatory (G_s) and inhibitory (G_i) guanine-nucleotide-binding regulatory proteins for adenylate cyclase were not detected in sperm in one recent study (550), another study identified the 41,000-dalton α_i subunit and the 35,000-dalton β-subunit of G_i in detergent extracts of mouse, bovine, and human sperm (551). However, G_s was not found and adenylate cyclase did not reconstitute with exogenous G_s regulatory protein (551), suggesting that adenylate cyclase may have unique regulatory properties in sperm (550). Receptor-mediated regulation of guanylate cyclase activity by a peptide released from eggs has been reported in invertebrate sperm (552), but a comparable system has not been identified in vertebrate sperm.

Adenylate cyclase activation in most cells results in phosphorylation of specific proteins by cAMP-dependent protein kinases (553). It has been reported that radioactive phosphate was incorporated into a 55,000-dalton protein in sperm from the cauda but not into those from the caput epididymis in the rat (554). In addition, a 55,000-dalton protein in bull sperm was more heavily phosphorylated in motile than in nonmotile sperm (555). Another study reported that sperm tubulin was phosphorylated in a cAMP-dependent manner and that the amount of phosphorylation was correlated with an increase in sperm motility (542). Tubulin is approximately 55,000 daltons, but the phosphorylated protein in bull sperm did not bind colchicine (555). A more recent study reported that the stimulatory effect of cAMP on reactivation of detergent-extracted dog, human, and sea-urchin sperm required the phosphorylation of a soluble 56,000-dalton protein, "axokinin" (556). Axokinin was present in extracts of immature testis, indicating that it was synthesized during spermatogenesis.

Other modulators of sperm motility have been reported. A motility inhibitor in seminal plasma was highest in the fluid from the seminal vesicles, but was also present in prostatic fluid from bull, rat, and rabbit (557). This 15,000-dalton modulator inhibited the reactivation of motility in detergent-extracted sperm and reduced the motility of previously reactivated sperm and may itself be regulated by a dialyzable activator (557). An inhibitor of cAMP-independent protein kinase was also present in human seminal plasma (558,559). It was a high-molecular-weight, heat-labile, trypsin-insensitive protein. It did not appear to act via an enzymatic mechanism and was present in seminal plasma of vasectomized men, indicating that it was produced by one of the male accessory organs. Seminal plasma has also been reported to contain low-molecular-weight components that inhibit the pattern (560) or uptake of calcium by sperm (561), and calcium is important for sperm motility (531–533). Adenosine has been shown to increase the level of *S*-adenosylhomocysteine, a competitive inhibitor of *S*-adenosylmethionine protein carboxymethylation (562). Carboxymethylation occurs in motile sperm (563,564), and agents that elevate *S*-adenosylhomocysteine inhibit sperm motility (562). Finally, a pH-dependent sperm motility quiescence factor has been reported to be present in cauda epididymal fluid but has not been characterized (521,565).

SUMMARY

There recently has been a considerable increase in knowledge about the sperm surface and the composition, organization, and function of the plasma membrane. Proteins, glycoproteins, and lipids, which make up the plasma membrane, have been identified and characterized. However, the most important advance has been the realization that sperm-surface components often are segregated into specific regions or domains of the plasma membrane. The regional differentiation in composition of the sperm surface results in components associated with specialized functions being located in specific domains. For example, molecules involved in the acrosome reaction are present over the anterior acrosome (85), molecules involved in fusion of the sperm and egg are present over the posterior acrosome (103), and molecules involved in flagellar activity are associated with the plasma membrane of the flagellum (551).

It also has been found that the composition of the plasma membrane is modified after spermatozoa leave the testis. Changes in the sperm surface occur during maturation in the epididymis and exposure to accessory gland secretory products during ejaculation. The sperm surface is further modified in the female reproductive tract. During capacitation, some sperm-surface components are lost and others migrate laterally out of their domains. These changes in composition and organization indicate that although the domains are constant in distribution, the components of the sperm surface are dynamic features of the cell.

These are exciting discoveries, but much remains to be learned about the composition, organization, and function of the sperm surface. Some proteins present in specific domains have been identified, but their amino acid sequences and native structures remain to be determined. The definition of the primary structure of functionally significant sperm-surface molecules in laboratory animals may allow comparable proteins and their genes to be identified in humans. Knowing the secondary and tertiary structures of these proteins will help to determine how they associate with other molecules in the cytoplasm and plasma membrane, as well as how they participate in sperm functions. In addition, the lipids present in the sperm plasma membrane are being characterized (143), but how specific lipids are distributed among different domains remains to be determined. Although it is generally accepted that the sperm surface is organized in domains, little is known about how and when domains are established, what mechanisms are responsible for targeting or segregating molecules into specific domains, and how the boundaries of domains are maintained.

The morphology of spermatozoa from different species has been thoroughly described, and the main structural features of the head and flagellum have been well characterized. Although the time and sequence of formation of different cytoplasmic structures during spermatogenesis are known, much remains to be learned about the mechanisms of morphogenesis of spermatozoa, the regulation of these mechanisms, and the composition and function of sperm-specific structures. Perhaps a good example of this is the cytoskeletal architecture of the head and flagellum (Table 6). The cytoskeleton of the sperm head includes structures lying between the acrosome and the nucleus, between the acrosome and plasma membrane, and surrounding the nucleus posterior to the acrosome. Some of these structures are more distinguishable in sperm containing a falciform head, whereas others are more obvious in sperm possessing a spatulate head. Several of the proteins in these structures have been partially characterized, but we do not know when they are synthesized or how they interact to form the cytoskeleton of the sperm head. It can only be hypothesized that the role of these features is to help determine or maintain the shape of the sperm head. The cytoskeleton of the flagellum includes the axoneme, outer dense fibers, fibrous sheath, and satellite fibers. The microtubules of the axoneme contain tubulin, but little is known about the composition and function of other parts of the complex and highly organized flagellum. Work is just beginning on the identification of the proteins in this structure, but the time of synthesis, distribution, organization, and function of specific proteins remain to be determined. Because the individual components of the flagellum are not well characterized, there is little understanding of how they function together to produce the effective flagellar beat.

Similar observations can be made about other components and activities of the spermatozoon. Some of the enzymes of the acrosome have been well characterized *in vitro,* but their function *in vivo* is not well understood. Surprisingly little is known about the nature and role of most of the other enzymes in the acrosome. The acrosome reaction to release these enzymes occurs at the end of capacitation, a process involving poorly understood metabolic changes in the sperm and in the structure and function of the plasma membrane (7). Other such changes during epididymal maturation give sperm the ability to perform coordinated flagellar motion. This is likely to involve components of the cAMP-dependent second message system in spermatozoa that are used in other cells to respond to hormonal first message stimuli (533). However, neither the first message(s) that influences flagellar motion nor the sperm receptor for the message(s) has been identified (551).

These specialized features of the spermatozoon serve a common purpose of delivering new genetic material to the egg. It remains to be determined how chromatin is organized in the mammalian spermatozoon, how paternally derived genes required during development are imprinted in sperm, and whether sperm have other roles in initiation of development besides awakening the egg and donating a haploid genome to the next generation.

It is clear that substantial questions remain about the composition, organization, and function of the spermatozoon. However, many of them may be answered with new research methods now available that are leading to rapid progress in knowledge in cell and molecular biology. Monoclonal antibodies already have proven to be valuable tools for studying the structure and function of sperm-surface domains, because of their specificity, sensitivity, and usefulness as morphological, biochemical, and physiological probes. It is likely that they will be equally useful for dissecting the nature and role of the cytoskeleton of the spermatozoon. The advances of molecular genetics are having profound effects on the understanding of the structure and function of genes and cells. Probes for genes identified in other cells are being used to determine when these genes are active in spermatogenesis (see, e.g., ref. 437) and can be used to study their regulation. As more functionally significant sperm-specific proteins are identified, the approaches of molecular genetics can be used to identify and characterize the nature and function of their genes. In addition, genetic mutations that affect spermatogenesis and sperm function may provide valuable clues for identifying genes important to spermatozoa (353). Furthermore, it is likely that there will soon be a better understanding of the regulation of sperm function. There have been substantial gains in understanding the components and activities of the second message system, and this knowledge is beginning to be applied to spermatozoa (551). Other powerful physical and chemical approaches that have not been used to study sperm before, such as use of fluorescent membrane-intercalating agents and fluorescence redistribution after photobleaching, are now providing important new insights into the properties of the plasma membrane (65) and the behavior of specific surface antigens (141). Because the spermatozoon is highly polarized and can be studied *in vitro,* it is proving to be the cell type of choice for such investigations. The use of these and other new approaches should provide a substantially better understanding of the composition, organization, and function of the spermatozoon in the near future.

REFERENCES

1. Baccetti, B. (1986): Evolutionary trends in sperm structure. *Comp. Biochem. Physiol.,* 85A:29–36.
2. Baccetti, B., and Afzelius, B. A. (1976): *The Biology of the Sperm Cell, Monographs in Developmental Biology, Vol. 10,* edited by A. Wolsky. S. Karger, Basel.
3. Roosen-Runge, E. (1977): *The Process of Spermatogenesis in Mammals, Developmental and Cell Biology Series, Vol. 10,* edited by M. Abercrombie, D. R. Newth, and J. G. Torrey. Cambridge University Press, Cambridge.
4. Segal, S. (1985): Sexual differentiation in vertebrates. In: *The Origin and Evolution of Sex, MBL Lectures in Biology, Vol. 7,* edited by H. O. Halvorson and A. Monroy, pp. 263–270. Alan R. Liss, New York.
5. Anderegg, C., and Markert, C. L. (1986): Successful rescue of microsurgically produced homozygous uniparental mouse embryos via production of aggregation chimeras. *Proc. Natl. Acad. Sci. USA,* 83:6509–6513.
6. de Kretser, D. M., and Kerr, J. B. (1987): Cytology of spermatogenesis. Chapter 20, *this volume.*
7. Yanagimachi, R. (1987): Fertilization. Chapter 5, *this volume.*
8. Pedersen, R. A. (1987): Early embryogenesis. Chapter 6, *this volume.*
9. Holt, W. V. (1984): Membrane heterogeneity in the mammalian spermatozoon. In: *International Review of Cytology, Vol. 87,* edited by G. H. Bourne and J. F. Danielli, pp. 159–194. Academic Press, New York.
10. Friend, D. S. (1984): Membrane organization and differentiation in the guinea-pig spermatozoon. In: *Ultrastructure of Reproduction,* edited by J. Van Blerkom and P. M. Motta, pp. 75–85. Martinus Nijhoff, The Hague.
11. Bangham, A. D. (1961): Electrophoretic characteristics of ram and rabbit spermatozoa. *Proc. R. Soc. Lond. (Biol.),* 155:292–305.
12. Nevo, A. C., Michaeli, I., and Schindler, H. (1961): Electrophoretic properties of bull and of rabbit spermatozoa. *Exp. Cell Res.,* 23:69–83.
13. Bedford, J. M. (1963): Changes in the electrophoretic properties of rabbit spermatozoa during passage through the epididymis. *Nature,* 200:1178–1180.
14. Cooper, G. W., and Bedford, J. M. (1971): Acquisition of surface charge by the plasma membrane of mammalian spermatozoa during epididymal maturation. *Anat. Rec.,* 169:300–301.
15. Yanagimachi, R., Noda, Y. D., Fujimoto, M., and Nicholson, G. (1972): The distribution of negative surface charges on mammalian spermatozoa. *Am. J. Anat.,* 135:497–520.
16. Sharon, N., and Lis. H. (1974): Use of lectins for the study of membranes. In: *Methods in Membrane Biology, Vol. 3,* edited by E. D. Korn, pp. 147–199. Academic Press, New York.
17. Nicolson, G. (1974): The interactions of lectins with animal cell surfaces. In: *International Review of Cytology, Vol. 39,* edited by G. H. Bourne and J. F. Danielli, pp. 89–190. Academic Press, New York.
18. Kashiwahara, T., Tanaka, R., and Matsomoto, T. (1965): Tail to tail agglomeration of bull spermatozoa by phytoagglutinins present in soy beans. *Nature,* 207:831–832.
19. Nicolson, G., and Yanagimachi, R. (1972): Terminal saccharides on sperm plasma membranes. Identification by specific agglutinins. *Science,* 177:276–279.
20. Nicolson, G., Poste, G., and Ji, T. H. (1977): The dynamics of cell membrane organization. In: *Dynamic Aspects of Cell Surface Organization,* edited by G. Poste and G. Nicolson, pp. 1–73. North-Holland, Amsterdam.
21. Koehler, J. K. (1981): Lectins as probes of the spermatozoon surface. *Arch. Androl.,* 6:197–217.
22. Nicolson, G., Lacorbiere, M., and Yanagimachi, R. (1972): Quantitative determination of plant agglutinin membrane sites on mammalian spermatozoa. *Proc. Soc. Exp. Biol. Med.,* 141:661–663.
23. Edelman, G. M., and Millette, C. F. (1971): Molecular probes of spermatozoon structures. *Proc. Natl. Acad. Sci. USA,* 68:2436–2440.
24. Millette, C. F. (1977): Distribution and mobility of lectin binding sites on mammalian spermatozoa. In: *Immunobiology of Gametes,* edited by M. Edidin and M. H. Johnson, pp. 51–71. Cambridge University Press, Cambridge.
25. Schwarz, M. A., and Koehler, J. K. (1979): Alterations in lectin binding to guinea pig spermatozoa accompanying *in vitro* capacitation and the acrosome reaction. *Biol. Reprod.,* 21:1295–1307.
26. Koehler, J. K. (1982): The mammalian sperm surface: An overview of structure with particular reference to mouse spermatozoa. In: *Prospects for Sexing Mammalian Sperm,* edited by R. P. Amann and G. E. Seidel, Jr., pp. 23–42. Colorado Associated University Press, Boulder.
27. Fenderson, B. A., O'Brien, D. A., Millette, C. F., and Eddy, E. M. (1984): Stage-specific expression of three cell surface carbohydrate antigens during murine spermatogenesis detected with monoclonal antibodies. *Dev. Biol.,* 103:117–128.
28. Gordon, M., Dandekar, P. V., and Bartoszewicz, W. (1975): The surface coat of epididymal, ejaculated and capacitated sperm. *J. Ultrastruct. Res.,* 50:199–207.
29. Nicolson, G., and Yanagimachi, R. (1974): Mobility and restriction of mobility of plasma membrane lectin-binding components. *Science,* 184:1294–1296.
30. Kinsey, W. H., and Koehler, J. K. (1976): Fine structural localizations of concanavalin A binding sites on hamster spermatozoa. *J. Supramol. Struct.,* 5:185–189.
31. Friend, D. S., and Fawcett, D. W. (1974): Membrane differentiations in freeze-fractured mammalian sperm. *J. Cell Biol.,* 63:641–664.
32. Suzuki, F., and Nagano, T. (1980): Epididymal maturation of rat spermatozoa studied by thin sectioning and freeze-fracture. *Biol. Reprod.,* 22:1219–1231.
33. Suzuki, F. (1981): Changes in intramembranous particle distribution in epididymal spermatozoa of the boar. *Anat. Rec.,* 199:361–376.

34. Koehler, J. K. (1970): A freeze-etch study of rabbit spermatozoa with particular reference to head structures. *J. Ultrastruct. Res.*, 33:598–614.
35. Schulte-Wrede, S., and Wetzstein, R. (1972): Raster-Elektronenmikroskopie von Spermien des Hausschaufs (*Ovis ammon aries*, L.), *Z. Zellforsch.*, 134:105–127.
36. Eddy, E. M., and Koehler, J. K. (1982): Restricted domains of the sperm surface. In: *Scanning Electron Microscopy, Vol. 3,* edited by O. Johari, pp. 1313–1323. SEM Inc., Chicago.
37. Koehler, J. K. (1966): Fine structure observations in frozen-etched bovine spermatozoa. *J. Ultrastruct. Res.*, 16:359–375.
38. Koehler, J. K. (1978): The mammalian sperm surface: Studies with specific labeling techniques. In: *International Review of Cytology, Vol. 54,* edited by G. H. Bourne and J. F. Danielli, pp. 73–108. Academic Press, New York.
39. Phillips, D. M. (1977): Surface of the equatorial segment of mammalian acrosome. *Biol. Reprod.*, 16:128–137.
40. Toshimori, K., Higashi, R., and Ōura, C. (1986): Distribution of intramembranous particles and filipin-sterol complexes in mouse sperm membranes: Polyene antibiotic filipin treatment. *Am. J. Anat.*, 174:455–470.
41. Koehler, J. K. (1973): Studies on the structure of the postnuclear sheath of water buffalo spermatozoa. *J. Ultrastruct. Res.*, 44:355–368.
42. Fléchon, J.-E. (1974): Freeze-fracturing of rabbit spermatozoa. *J. Submicrosc. Cytol.*, 19:59–64.
43. Bradley, M. P., Ryans, D. G., and Forrester, I. T. (1980): Effects of filipin, digitonin, and polymyxin B on plasma membrane of ram spermatozoa—An EM study. *Arch. Androl.*, 4:195–204.
44. Koehler, J. K. (1972): Human sperm head ultrastructure: A freeze-etching study. *J. Ultrastruct. Res.*, 39:520–539.
45. Gresson, R. A. R., and Zlotnik, I. (1945): A comparative study of the cytoplasmic components of the male germ-cells of certain mammals. *Proc. R. Soc. Edinb. B*, 62:137–170.
46. Hancock, J. L., and Trevan, D. J. (1957): The acrosome and post-nuclear cap of bull spermatozoa. *J. R. Microsc. Soc.*, 76:77–83.
47. Pikó, L. (1969): Gamete structure and sperm entry in mammals. In: *Fertilization, Vol. 2,* edited by C. B. Metz and A. Monroy, pp. 325–403. Academic Press, New York.
48. Woolley, D. M. (1970): A posterior ring in the spermatozoa of species of muridae. *J. Reprod. Fertil.*, 23:361–363.
49. Koehler, J. K. (1983): Structural heterogeneity of the mammalian sperm flagellar membrane. *J. Submicrosc. Cytol.*, 15:247–253.
50. Friend, D. S., and Rudolf, I. (1974): Acrosomal disruption in sperm. Freeze-fracture of altered membranes. *J. Cell. Biol.*, 63:466–479.
51. Koehler, J. K., and Gaddum-Rosse, P. (1975): Media induced alterations of the membrane associated particles of the guinea pig sperm tail. *J. Ultrastruct. Res.*, 51:106–118.
52. Fawcett, D. W. (1975): The mammalian spermatozoon. *Dev. Biol.*, 44:394–436.
53. Gilula, N. B., and Satir, P. (1972): The ciliary necklace: A ciliary membrane specialization. *J. Cell Biol.*, 53:494–509.
54. Olson, G. E., Lifsics, M., Hamilton, D. W., and Fawcett, D. W. (1977): Structural specializations in the flagellar plasma membrane of opossum spermatozoa. *J. Ultrastruct. Res.*, 59:207–221.
55. Friend, D. S., Elias, P. M., and Rudolf, I. (1979): Disassembly of the guinea-pig sperm tail. In: *The Spermatozoon,* edited by D. W. Fawcett and J. M. Bedford, pp. 157–168. Urban and Schwarzenberg, Baltimore.
56. Friend, D. S., and Heuser, J. E. (1981): Orderly particle arrays on the mitochondrial outer membrane in rapidly-frozen sperm. *Anat. Rec.*, 159:198–199.
57. Elias, P. M., Gorke, J., and Friend, D. S. (1978): Freeze-fracture identification of sterol-digitonin complexes in cell and liposome membrane. *J. Cell Biol.*, 78:577–596.
58. Enders, G. C., Werb, Z., and Friend, D. S. (1983): Lectin binding to guinea-pig sperm zipper particles. *J. Cell Sci.*, 60:303–329.
59. Elias, P. M., Friend, D. S., and Goerke, J. (1979): Membrane sterol heterogeneity. Freeze-fracture detection with saponins and filipin. *J. Histochem. Cytochem.*, 27:1247–1260.
60. Friend, D. S. (1982): Plasma-membrane diversity in a highly polarized cell. *J. Cell Biol.*, 93:243–249.
61. Friend, D. S. (1980): Freeze-fracture alterations in guinea-pig sperm membrane preceding gamete fusion. In: *Membrane-Membrane Interactions,* edited by N. B. Gilula, pp. 153–165. Raven Press, New York.
62. Bearer, E. L., and Friend, D. S. (1980): Anionic lipid domains: Correlation and functional topography in a mammalian cell membrane. *Proc. Natl. Acad. Sci. USA,* 77:6601–6605.
63. Friend, D. S., and Bearer, E. L. (1981): β-Hydroxysterol distribution as determined by freeze-fracture cytochemistry. *Histochem. J.*, 13:535–546.
64. Bearer, E. L., and Friend, D. S. (1982): Modifications of anionic lipid domains preceding membrane fusion in guinea pig sperm. *J. Cell Biol.*, 92:604–615.
65. Wolf, D. E., and Voglmayr, J. K. (1984): Diffusion and regionalization in membranes of maturing ram spermatozoa. *J. Cell Biol.*, 98:1678–1684.
66. Sternberger, L. A. (1979): *Immunocytochemistry,* John Wiley & Sons, New York.
67. Koo, G. C., Stackpole, C. W., Boyse, E. A., Hammerling, U., and Lardis, M. P. (1973): Topographical location of H-Y antigen on mouse spermatozoa by immunoelectronmicroscopy. *Proc. Natl. Acad. Sci. USA,* 70:1502–1505.
68. Fellous, M., Gachelin, G., Buc-Caron, M.-H., Dubois, P., and Jacob, F. (1974): Similar location of an early embryonic antigen on mouse and human spermatozoa. *Dev. Biol.*, 41:331–337.
69. Lopez, L. C., Bayna, E. M., Litoff, D., Shaper, N. L., Shaper, J. H., and Shur, B. D. (1985): Receptor function of mouse sperm surface galactosyltransferase during fertilization. *J. Cell Biol.*, 101:1501–1510.
70. O'Rand, M. G., and Romrell, L. J. (1980): Appearance of regional surface autoantigens during spermatogenesis: Comparison of anti-testis and anti-sperm antisera. *Dev. Biol.*, 75:431–441.
71. Koehler, J. K. (1974): Studies on the distribution of antigenic sites on the surface of rabbit spermatozoa. *J. Cell Biol.*, 67:647–659.
72. Millette, C. F., and Bellvé, A. R. (1977): Temporal expression of membrane antigens during mouse spermatogenesis. *J. Cell Biol.*, 74:86–97.
73. Koehler, J. K., and Perkins, W. D. (1974): Fine structure observations on the distribution of antigenic sites on guinea pig spermatozoa. *J. Cell Biol.*, 60:789–795.
74. Tung, K. S. K., Han, L.-B. P., and Evan, A. P. (1979): Differentiation autoantigen of testicular cells and spermatozoa in the guinea pig. *Dev. Biol.*, 68:224–238.
75. Tung, P. S., and Fritz, I. B. (1978): Specific surface antigens on rat pachytene spermatocytes and successive classes of germinal cells. *Dev. Biol.*, 64:297–315.
76. Koo, G. C., Boyse, E. A., and Wachtel, S. S. (1977): Immunogenetic techniques and approaches in the study of sperm and testicular cell surface antigens. In: *Immunobiology of Gametes,* edited by M. Edidin and M. H. Johnson, pp. 73–80. Cambridge University Press, Cambridge.
77. O'Rand, M. J. (1977): The presence of sperm-specific isoantigens on the egg following fertilization. *J. Exp. Zool.*, 202:267–273.
78. Herr, J. C., and Eddy, E. M. (1980): Identification of mouse sperm surface antigens by a surface labeling and immunoprecipitation approach. *Biol. Reprod.*, 22:1263–1274.
79. Villarroya, S., and Scholler, R. (1986): Regional heterogeneity of human spermatozoa detected with monoclonal antibodies. *J. Reprod. Fertil.*, 76:435–447.
80. Primakoff, P., and Myles, D. G. (1983): A map of the guinea pig sperm surface constructed with monoclonal antibodies. *Dev. Biol.*, 98:417–428.
81. Gaunt, S. J., Brown, C. R., and Jones, R. (1983): Identification of mobile and fixed antigens on the plasma membrane of rat spermatozoa using monoclonal antibodies. *Exp. Cell Res.*, 144:275–284.
82. Jones, R., Brown, C. R., von Glós, K. I., and Gaunt, S. J. (1985): Development of a maturation antigen on the plasma membrane of rat spermatozoa in the epididymis and its fate during fertilization. *Exp. Cell Res.*, 156:31–44.
83. Moore, H. D. M., and Hartman, T. D. (1984): Localization by monoclonal antibodies of various surface antigens of hamster spermatozoa and the effect of antibody on fertilization *in vitro*. *J. Reprod. Fertil.*, 70:175–183.
84. Feuchter, F. A., Vernon, R. B., and Eddy, E. M. (1981): Analysis of the sperm surface with monoclonal antibodies: Topographically

restricted antigens appearing in the epididymis. *Biol. Reprod.*, 24:1099–1110.
85. Saling, P. M. (1986): Mouse sperm antigens that participate in fertilization. IV. A monoclonal antibody prevents zona penetration by inhibition of the acrosome reaction. *Dev. Biol.*, 117:511–519.
86. Okabe, M., Katsuaki, T., Adachi, T., Kohama, T., and Mimura, T. (1986): Inconsistent reactivity of an anti-sperm monoclonal antibody and its relationship to sperm capacitation. *J. Reprod. Immunol.*, 9:67–70.
87. Yan, C. Y., Wang, L. F., Sato, E., and Koide, S. S. (1983): Monoclonal antibody inducing human sperm agglutination. *Am. J. Reprod. Immunol.*, 4:111–115.
88. Herr, J. C., Fowler, J. E., Howards, S. S., Sigman, M., Sutherland, W. M., and Koons, D. J. (1985): Human antisperm monoclonal antibodies constructed postvasectomy. *Biol. Reprod.*, 32:695–712.
89. Glassy, M. C., Surh, C. D., and Sarkar, S. (1984): Murine monoclonal antibodies that identify antigenically distinct subpopulations of human sperm. *Hybridoma*, 3:363–371.
90. Vernon, R. B., Muller, C. H., and Eddy, E. M. (1987): Further characterization of a secreted epididymal glycoprotein in mice that binds to sperm tails. *J. Androl.* 8:123–128.
91. Toshimori, K., and Eddy, E. M. (1987): Epididymal maturation produces a 31,000 molecular weight antigen on the surface of flagellum of the mouse spermatozoon (*submitted*).
92. Schmell, E. D., Gulyas, B. J., Yuan, L. C., and August, J. T. (1982): Identification of mammalian sperm surface antigens: II. Characterization of an acrosomal cap protein and a tail protein using monoclonal anti-mouse sperm antibodies. *J. Reprod. Immunol.*, 4:91–106.
93. Gaunt, S. J., Brown, C. R., and Jones, R. (1983): Identification of mobile and fixed antigens on the plasma membrane of rat spermatozoa using monoclonal antibodies. *Exp. Cell Res.*, 144:275–284.
94. Isahakia, M., and Alexander, N. J. (1984): Interspecies cross-reactivity of monoclonal antibodies directed against human sperm antigens. *Biol. Reprod.*, 30:1015–1026.
95. Hinrichsen-Kohane, A. C., Hinrichsen, M. J., and Schill, W.-B. (1985): Analysis of antigen expression on human spermatozoa by means of monoclonal antibodies. *Fertil. Steril.*, 43:279–285.
96. Crichton, D. N., and Cohen, B. B. (1983): Analysis of the murine sperm surface with monoclonal antibodies. *J. Reprod. Fertil.*, 68:497–505.
97. Gaunt, S. J. (1982): A 28K-dalton cell surface autoantigen of spermatogenesis: Characterization using a monoclonal antibody. *Dev. Biol.*, 89:92–100.
98. Lee, G., C.-Y., Wong, E., and Teh, C.-Z. (1984): Analysis of mouse sperm isoantigens using specific monoclonal antibodies. *Am. J. Reprod. Immunol.*, 6:37–43.
99. Saling, P. M., and Lakoski, K. A. (1985): Mouse sperm antigens that participate in fertilization. II. Inhibition of sperm penetration through the zona pellucida using monoclonal antibodies. *Biol. Reprod.*, 33:527–536.
100. Myles, D. G., Primakoff, P., and Bellvé, A. R. (1981): Surface domains of the guinea pig sperm defined with monoclonal antibodies. *Cell*, 23:433–439.
101. Myles, D. G., and Primakoff, P. (1985): Sperm surface domains. In: *Hybridoma Technology in the Biosciences and Medicine*, edited by T. A. Springer, pp. 239–250. Plenum Press, New York.
102. Naz, R. N., Saxe, J. M., and Menge, A. C. (1983): Inhibition of fertility in rabbits by monoclonal antibodies against sperm. *Biol. Reprod.*, 28:249–254.
103. Saling, P. M., Irons, G., and Waibel, R. (1985): Mouse sperm antigens that participate in fertilization. I. Inhibition of sperm fusion with the egg plasma membrane using monoclonal antibodies. *Biol. Reprod.*, 33:515–526.
104. Ellis, D. H., Hartman, T. D., and Moore, H. D. M. (1985): Maturation and function of the hamster spermatozoon probed with monoclonal antibodies. *J. Reprod. Immunol.*, 7:299–314.
105. Wolf, D. P., Sokoloski, J. E., Dandekar, P., and Bechtol, K. B. (1983): Characterization of human sperm surface antigens with monoclonal antibodies. *Biol. Reprod.*, 29:713–723.
106. Naz, R. K., Alexander, N. J., Isahakia, M., and Hamilton, M. S. (1984): Monoclonal antibody to a human germ cell membrane glycoprotein that inhibits fertilization. *Science*, 225:342–344.
107. Bechtol, K. B., Brown, S. C., and Kennett, R. H. (1979): Recognition of differentiation antigens of spermatogenesis in the mouse by using antibodies from spleen cell-myeloma hybrids after syngeneic immunization. *Proc. Natl. Acad. Sci. USA*, 76:363–367.
108. Bechtol, K. B. (1984): Characterization of a cell-surface differentiation antigen of mouse spermatogenesis: Timing and localization of expression by immunohistochemistry using a monoclonal antibody. *J. Embryol. Exp. Morphol.*, 81:93–104.
109. Saxena, N. K., Russell, L. D., Saxena, N., and Peterson, R. N. (1986): Immunofluorescence antigen localization on boar sperm plasma membranes: Monoclonal antibodies reveal apparent new domains and apparent redistribution of surface antigens during sperm maturation and at ejaculation. *Anat. Rec.*, 214:238–252.
110. Bedford, J. M. (1963): Morphological changes in rabbit spermatozoa during passage through the epididymis. *J. Reprod. Fertil.*, 5:169–282.
111. Jones, R. C. (1971): Studies of the structure of the head of boar spermatozoa from the epididymis. *J. Reprod. Fertil.* (*Suppl.*), 13:51–64.
112. Fawcett, D. W., and Hollenberg, R. D. (1963): Changes in the acrosomes of guinea pig spermatozoa during passage through the epididymis. *J. Reprod. Fertil.* (*Suppl.*), 6:276–292.
113. Eddy, E. M., Vernon, R. B., Muller, C. H., Hahnel, A. C., and Fenderson, B. A. (1985): Immunodissection of sperm surface modifications during epididymal maturation. *Am. J. Anat.*, 174:225–237.
114. Burridge, K., and Feramisco, J. R. (1982): α-Actinin and vinculin from nonmuscle cells: Calcium-sensitive interactions with actin. In: *Cold Spring Harbor Symposia on Quantitative Biology, Vol. XLVI, Part 2*, pp. 587–597. Cold Spring Harbor, New York.
115. Welch, J. E., and O'Rand, M. G. (1985): Identification and distribution of actin in spermatogenic cells and spermatozoa of the rabbit. *Dev. Biol.*, 109:411–417.
116. Campanella, C., Gabbiani, G., Baccetti, B., Burrini, A. G., and Pallini, V. (1979): Actin and myosin in the vertebrate acrosomal region. *J. Submicrosc. Cytol.*, 11:53–71.
117. Clarke, G. N., Clarke, F. M., and Wilson, S. (1982): Actin in human spermatozoa. *Biol. Reprod.*, 26:319–327.
118. Talbot, P., and Kleve, M. G. (1978): Hamster sperm cross-react with antiactin. *J. Exp. Zool.*, 204:131–136.
119. Peterson, R. N., Russell, L. D., Bundman, D., and Freund, M. (1978): Presence of microfilaments and tubular structure in chemically induced acrosome reactions of boar spermatozoa. *Biol. Reprod.*, 19:459–465.
120. Tamblyn, T. M. (1980): Identification of actin in boar epididymal spermatozoa. *Biol. Reprod.*, 22:727–734.
121. Koehler, J. K. (1978): Observations on the fine structure of vole spermatozoa with particular reference to cytoskeletal elements in the mature sperm head. *Gamete Res.*, 1:247–257.
122. Olson, G. E., and Winfrey, V. P. (1985): Substructure of a cytoskeletal complex associated with the hamster sperm acrosome. *J. Ultrastruct. Res.*, 92:167–179.
123. Goodman, S. R., and Schiffer, K. (1983): The spectrin membrane skeleton of normal and abnormal human erythrocytes: A review. *Am. J. Physiol.*, 244:C121–C141.
124. Lazerides, E., and Moon, R. T. (1984): Assembly and topogenesis of the spectrin-based membrane skeleton in erythroid development. *Cell*, 37:354–356.
125. Damjanov, I., Damjanov, A., Lehto, V.-P., and Virtanen, I. (1986): Spectrin in mouse gametogenesis and embryogenesis. *Dev. Biol.*, 114:132–140.
126. Repasky, E. A., Granger, B. L., and Lazarides, E. (1982): Widespread occurrence of avian spectrin in nonerythroid cells. *Cell*, 29:821–833.
127. Virtanen, I., Badley, R. A., Paasivuo, R., and Lehto, V.-P. (1984): Distinct cytoskeletal domains revealed in sperm cells. *J. Cell Biol.*, 99:1083–1091.
128. McIntosh, J. R., and Porter, K. R. (1967): Microtubules in the spermatids of the domestic fowl. *J. Cell Biol.*, 35:153–173.
129. Fawcett, D. W., Anderson, W. A., and Phillips, D. M. (1971): Morphogenetic factors influencing the shape of the sperm head. *Dev. Biol.*, 26:220–251.
130. Blom, E., and Birch-Anderson, A. (1965): The ultrastructure of the bull sperm. *Nord, Vet. Med.*, 17:193–212.

131. Plattner, H. (1971): Bull spermatozoa: A re-investigation by freeze etching using widely different cryofixation procedures. *J. Submicrosc. Cytol.*, 3:19–32.
132. Fawcett, D. W., and Ito, S. (1965): The fine structure of bat spermatozoa. *Am. J. Anat.*, 116:567–610.
133. Fawcett, D. W., Eddy, E. M., and Phillips, D. M. (1970): Observations on the fine structure and relationships of the chromatoid body in mammalian spermatogenesis. *Biol. Reprod.*, 2:129–153.
134. Russell, L. D. (1980): Sertoli-germ cell interactions: A review. *Gamete Res.*, 3:179–202.
135. Russell, L. D. (1984): Spermiation—The sperm release process: Ultrastructural observations and unresolved problems. In: *Ultrastructure of Reproduction*, edited by J. Van Blerkom and P. M. Motta, pp. 46–66. Martinus Nijhoff, The Hague.
136. Ross, M. H., and Dobler, J. (1975): The Sertoli cell junctional specializations and their relationship to the germinal epithelium as observed after efferent ductule ligation. *Anat. Rec.*, 183:267–292.
137. Russell, L. D., and Clermont, Y. (1976): Anchoring device between Sertoli cells and late spermatids in rat seminiferous tubules. *Anat. Rec.*, 185:259–278.
138. Russell, L. D. (1979): Spermatid-Sertoli tubulobulbar complexes as devices for elimination of cytoplasm from the head region of late spermatids of the rat. *Anat. Rec.*, 194:233–246.
139. Burgos, M. H., Blaquier, J., Cameo, M. S., and Gutierrez, L. (1972): Morphological maturation of spermatozoa in the epididymis. In: *Biology of Reproduction, Symposium III, Pan American Congress of Anatomy*, edited by J. T. Vilardo and B. A. Kasprow, pp. 367–371. Pan American Association of Anatomy, New Orleans.
140. Fawcett, D. W. (1965): The anatomy of the mammalian spermatozoon with particular reference to the guinea pig. *Z. Zellforsch.*, 67:279–296.
141. Myles, D. G., Primakoff, P., and Koppel, D. E. (1984): A localized surface protein of guinea pig sperm exhibits free diffusion in its domain. *J. Cell Biol.*, 98:1905–1909.
142. Langlais, J., and Roberts, K. D. (1985): A molecular membrane model of sperm capacitation and the acrosome reaction of mammalian spermatozoa. *Gamete Res.*, 12:183–224.
143. Nikolopoulau, M., Soucek, D. A., and Vary, J. C. (1985): Changes in the lipid content of boar sperm plasma membranes during epididymal maturation. *Biochem. Biophys. Acta*, 815:486–498.
144. Murry, R. K., Narasimhan, R., Levine, M., Shirley, M., Lingwood, C. A., and Schachter, H. (1980): Galactoglycerolipids of mammalian testis, spermatozoa and nervous tissues. In: *Cell Surface Glycolipids, ACS Symposium Series, No. 128*, edited by C. Sweeley, pp. 105–125. American Chemical Society Press, Washington D.C.
145. Kornblatt, M. J., Knapp, A., Levine, M., Schachter, H., and Murray, R. K. (1974): Studies on the structure and formation during spermatogenesis of the sulfoglycerogalactolipid of rat testis. *Can. J. Biochem.*, 52:689–697.
146. Lingwood, C. A. (1985): Protein-glycolipid interactions during spermatogenesis. Binding of specific germ cell proteins to sulfatoxygalactosylacylalkylglycerol, the major glycolipid of mammalian male germ cells. *Can. J. Biochem. Cell Biol.*, 63:1077–1085.
147. Lingwood, C. A., and Schachter, H. (1981): Localization of sulfatoxygalactosylacylalkylglycerol at the surface of rat testicular germinal cells by immunocytochemical techniques: pH dependence of a nonimmunological reaction between immunoglobulin and germinal cells. *J. Cell Biol.*, 89:621–630.
148. Eddy, E. M., Muller, C. H., and Lingwood, C. A. (1985): Preparation of monoclonal antibody to sulfatoxygalactosylglycerolipid by *in vitro* immunization with a glycolipid-glass conjugate. *J. Immunol. Methods*, 81:137–146.
149. Langlais, J., Zollinger, M., Plante, L., Chapdelaine, A., Bleau, G., and Roberts, K. D. (1981): Localization of cholesteryl sulfate in human spermatozoa in support of a hypothesis for the mechanism of capacitation. *Proc. Natl. Acad. Sci. USA*, 78:7266–7270.
150. Mann, T., and Lutwak-Mann, C. (1981): *Male Reproductive Function and Semen*, Springer-Verlag, New York.
151. Acott, T. S., Katz, D. F., and Hoskins, D. D. (1983): Movement characteristics of bovine epididymal spermatozoa: Effects of forward motility protein and epididymal maturation. *Biol. Reprod.*, 29:389–399.
152. Cooper, T. G., Waites, G. M. H., and Nieschlag, E. (1986): The epididymis and male fertility. A symposium report. *Int. J. Androl.*, 9:81–90.
153. Saling, P. M. (1982): Development of the ability to bind zonae pellucidae during epididymal maturation: Reversible immobilization of mouse spermatozoa by lanthanum. *Biol. Reprod.*, 26:429–436.
154. Orgebin-Crist, M.-C., and Fournier-Delpech, S. (1982): Sperm-egg interaction. Evidence for maturational changes during epididymal transit. *J. Androl.*, 3:429–433.
155. Moore, H. D. M. (1979): The net negative surface charge of mammalian spermatozoa as determined by isoelectric focusing. Changes following sperm maturation, ejaculation, incubation in the female tract, and after enzyme treatment. *Int. J. Androl.*, 2:244–262.
156. Bedford, J. M., Calvin, H. I., and Cooper, G. W. (1973): The maturation of spermatozoa in the human epididymis. *J. Reprod. Fertil. (Suppl.)*, 18:199–213.
157. Nicolson, G. L., Usui, N, Yanagimachi, R., Yanagimachi, H., and Smith, J. R. (1977): Lectin-binding sites on the plasma membranes of rabbit spermatozoa. Changes in surface receptors during epididymal maturation and after ejaculation. *J. Cell Biol.*, 74:950–962.
158. Holt, W. V. (1980): Surface-bound sialic acid on ram and bull spermatozoa: Deposition during epididymal transit and stability during washing. *Biol. Reprod.*, 23:847–857.
159. Fléchon, J. E. (1975): Ultrastructural and cytochemical modifications of rabbit spermatozoa during epididymal transport. In: *The Biology of Spermatozoa. Transport, Survival and Fertilizing Ability*, edited by E. S. E. Hafez and C. G. Thibault, pp. 36–45. Karger, Basel.
160. Bedford, J. M., and Millar, R. P. (1978): The character of sperm maturation in the epididymis of the ascrotal hyrax, Procavia capensis, and armadillo, Dasypus novemcinctus. *Biol. Reprod.*, 19:396–406.
161. Hammerstedt, R. H., Hay, S. R., and Amann, R. P. (1982): Modification of ram sperm membranes during epididymal transit. *Biol. Reprod.*, 27:745–754.
162. Fournier-Delpech, S., and Courot, M. (1980): Glycoproteins of ram sperm plasma membrane. Relationship of protein having affinity for Con A to epididymal maturation. *Biochem. Biophys. Res. Commun.*, 96:756–761.
163. Lewin, L. W., Weissenberg, R., Sobel, J. S., Marcus, Z., and Nebel, L. (1979): Differences in Con-A-FITC binding to rat spermatozoa during epididymal maturation and capacitation. *Arch. Androl.*, 2:279–281.
164. Fournier-Delpech, S., Danzo, B. J., and Orgebin-Crist, M.-C. (1977): Extraction of concanavalin A affinity material from rat testicular and epididymal spermatozoa. *Ann. Biol. Anim. Biochem. Biophys.*, 17:207–213.
165. Dawson, R. M. C., and Scott, T. W. (1964): Phospholipid composition of epididymal spermatozoa prepared by density gradient centrifugation. *Nature*, 202:292–293.
166. Quinn, P. J., and White, I. G. (1967): Phospholipid and cholesterol content of epididymal and ejaculated ram spermatozoa and seminal plasma in relation to cold shock. *Aust. J. Biol. Sci.*, 20:1205–1215.
167. Grogan, D. E. Mayer, D. T., and Sikes, J. D. (1966): Quantitative differences in phospholipids of ejaculated spermatozoa and spermatozoa from three different levels of the epididymis of the boar. *J. Reprod. Fertil.*, 12:431–436.
168. Poulos, A., Voglmayr, J. K., and White, I. G. (1973): Phospholipid changes in spermatozoa during passage through the genital tract of the bull. *Biochim. Biophys. Acta*, 306:194–202.
169. Poulos, A., Brown-Woodman, P. D. C., White, I. G., and Cox, R. I. (1975): Changes in phospholipids of ram spermatozoa during migration through the epididymis and possible origin of prostaglandins $F_{2\alpha}$ in testicular and epididymal fluid. *Biochim. Biophys. Acta*, 388:12–21.
170. Terner, C., MacLaughlin, J., and Smith, B. R. (1975): Changes in lipase and phospholipase activities of rat spermatozoa in transit from the caput to the cauda epididymis. *J. Reprod. Fertil.*, 45:1–8.
171. Evans, R. W., and Setchell, B. P. (1979): Lipid changes in boar spermatozoa during epididymal maturation with some observations on the flow and composition of boar rete testis fluid. *J. Reprod. Fertil.*, 57:189–196.
172. Scott, T. W., Voglmayr, J. K., and Setchell, B. P. (1967): Lipid composition and metabolism in testicular and ejaculated ram spermatozoa. *Biochem. J.*, 102:456–461.
173. Bleau, G., and VandenHeuvel, W. J. A. (1974): Desmosteryl sulfate and desmosterol in hamster epididymis. *Steroids*, 24:549–556.

174. Legault, Y., Bouthillier, M., Bleau, G., Chapdelaine, A., and Roberts, K. D. (1979): The sterol and sterol sulfate content of the male hamster reproductive tract. *Biol. Reprod.,* 20:1213–1219.
175. Lalumiere, G., Bleau, G., Chapdelaine, A., and Roberts, K. D. (1976): Cholesterol sulfate and sterol sulphatase in the human reproductive tract. *Steroids,* 27:247–260.
176. Parks, J. E., and Hammerstedt, R. H. (1985): Developmental changes occurring in the lipids of ram epididymal spermatozoa plasma membrane. *Biol. Reprod.,* 32:653–668.
177. Hammerstedt, R. H., Keith, A. D., Hay, S., Deluca, N., and Amann, R. P. (1979): Changes in ram sperm membranes during epididymal transit. *Arch. Biochem. Biophys.,* 196:7–12.
178. Voglmayr, J. K., Scott, T. W., Setchell, B. P., and Waites, G. M. H. (1967): Metabolism of testicular spermatozoa and characteristics of testicular fluid collected from conscious rams. *J. Reprod. Fertil.,* 14:87–99.
179. Scott, T. W., Voglmayr, J. K., and Setchell, B. P. (1967): Lipid composition and metabolism in testicular and ejaculated ram spermatozoa. *Biochem. J.,* 102:456–461.
180. Vijayasarathy, S., and Balaram, P. (1982): Regional differentiation in bull sperm plasma membranes. *Biochem. Biophys. Res. Commun.,* 108:760–764.
181. Orgebin-Crist, M.-C., Danzo, B. J., and Davies, J. (1975): Endocrine control of the development and maintenance of sperm fertilizing ability in the epididymis. In: *Handbook of Physiology, Vol. 5, Endocrinology, Section 7, Male Reproductive System,* edited by R. O. Greep, pp. 319–338. American Physiological Society, Washington D.C.
182. Hamilton, D. W. (1975): Structure and function of the epithelium lining the ductuli efferentes, ductus epididymis, and ductus deferens in the rat. In: *Handbook of Physiology, Vol. 5, Endocrinology, Section 7, Male Reproductive System,* edited by R. O. Greep, pp. 259–301. American Physiological Society, Washington D.C.
183. Bedford, J. M. (1975): Maturation, transport and fate of spermatozoa in the epididymis. In: *Handbook of Physiology, Vol. 5, Endocrinology, Section 7, Male Reproductive System,* edited by R. O. Greep, pp. 303–317. American Physiological Society, Washington D.C.
184. Yanagimachi, R. (1981): Mechanisms of fertilization in mammals. In: *Fertilization and Embryonic Development in Vitro,* edited by L. Mastroianni and J. D. Biggers, pp. 81–182. Plenum Press, New York.
185. Austin, C. R. (1985): Sperm maturation in the male and female genital tracts. In: *Biology of Fertilization, Vol. 2, Biology of the Sperm,* edited by C. B. Metz and A. Monroy, pp. 121–155. Academic Press, Orlando, Florida.
186. Olson, G. E., and Hamilton, D. W. (1978): Characterization of the surface glycoproteins of rat spermatozoa. *Biol. Reprod.,* 19:26–35.
187. Olson, G. E., and Danzo, B. J. (1981): Surface changes in rat spermatozoa during epididymal transit. *Biol. Reprod.,* 24:431–443.
188. Toowicharanount, P., and Chulavatnatol, M. (1983): Characterization of sialoglycoproteins of rat epididymal fluid and spermatozoa by periodate-tritiated borohydride. *J. Reprod. Fertil.,* 67:133–141.
189. Brown, C. R. von Glós, K. I., and Jones, R. (1983): Changes in plasma membrane glycoproteins of rat spermatozoa during maturation in the epididymis. *J. Cell Biol.,* 96:256–264.
190. Jones, R., Phorpramool, C., Setchell, B. P., and Brown, C. R. (1981): Labelling of membrane glycoproteins on rat spermatozoa collected from different regions of the epididymis. *Biochem. J.,* 200:457–460.
191. Jones, R., von Glós, K. I., and Brown, C. R. (1981): Characterization of hormonally regulated secretory proteins from the caput epididymidis of the rabbit. *Biochem. J.,* 196:105–114.
192. Zaheb, R., and Orr, G. A. (1984): Characterization of a maturation-associated glycoprotein on the plasma membrane of rat caudal epididymal sperm. *J. Biol. Chem.,* 259:839–848.
193. Faye, J. C., Duguet, L., Mazzuca, M., and Bayard, F. (1980): Purification, radioimmunoassay, and immunohistochemical localization of a glycoprotein produced by the rat epididymis. *Biol. Reprod.,* 23:423–432.
194. Voglmayr, J. K., Fairbanks, G., Jakowitz, M. A., and Colella, J. R. (1980): Post-testicular developmental changes in the ram sperm cell surface and their relationship to luminal fluid proteins of the reproductive tract. *Biol. Reprod.,* 22:655–667.
195. Voglmayr, J. K., Fairbanks, G., Vespa, D. B., and Colella, J. R. (1982): Studies on mechanisms of surface modifications in ram spermatozoa during the final stages of differentiation. *Biol. Reprod.,* 26:483–500.
196. Voglmayr, J. K., Fairbanks, G., and Lewis, R. G. (1983): Surface glycoprotein changes in ram spermatozoa during epididymal maturation. *Biol. Reprod.,* 29:767–775.
197. Dacheaux, J. L., and Voglmayr, J. K. (1983): Sequence of sperm cell surface differentiation and its relationship to exogenous fluid proteins in the ram epididymis. *Biol. Reprod.,* 29:1033–1046.
198. Vieurla, M., and Rajaniemi, H. (1980): Radioiodination of surface proteins of bull spermatozoa and their characterization by sodium dodecyl sulfate-polyacrylamide gel electrophoresis. *J. Reprod. Fertil.,* 58:483–489.
199. Nicolson, G. L., Bronginski, A. B., Beattie, G., and Yanagimachi, R. (1979): Cell surface changes in the proteins of rabbit spermatozoa during epididymal passage. *Gamete Res.,* 2:153–162.
200. Russell, L. D., Peterson, R. N., Hunt, W., and Strack, L. E. (1984): Post-testicular surface modifications and contributions of reproductive tract fluids to the surface polypeptide composition of boar spermatozoa. *Biol. Reprod.,* 30:959–978.
201. Young, L. G., Hinton, B. T., and Gould, K. G. (1985): Surface changes in chimpanzee sperm during epididymal transit. *Biol. Reprod.,* 32:399–412.
202. Hunter, A. G. (1969): Differentiation of rabbit sperm antigens from those of seminal plasma. *J. Reprod. Fertil.,* 20:413–418.
203. Barker, L. D. S., and Amann, R. P. (1970): Epididymal physiology. I. Specificity of antisera against bull spermatozoa and reproductive fluids. *J. Reprod. Fertil.,* 22:441–452.
204. Barker, L. D. S., and Amann, R. P. (1971): Epididymal physiology. II. Immunofluorescent analysis of epithelial secretion and absorption, and of bovine sperm maturation. *J. Reprod. Fertil.,* 26:319–332.
205. Killian, G. J., and Amann, R. P. (1973): Immunoelectrophoretic characterization of fluid and sperm entering and leaving the bovine epididymis. *Biol. Reprod.,* 9:489–499.
206. Dravland, E., and Joshi, M. S. (1981): Sperm-coating antigens secreted by the epididymis and seminal vesicle of the rat. *Biol. Reprod.,* 25:649–658.
207. Lea, O. A., Petrusz, P., and French, F. (1978): Purification and localization of acidic epididymal glycoprotein (AEG): A sperm coating protein secreted by the rat epipidymis. *Int. J. Androl. (Suppl.),* 2:592–607.
208. Cameo, M. S., and Blaquier, J. A. (1976): Androgen-controlled specific protein in rat epididymis. *J. Endocrinol.,* 69:47–55.
209. Pholpramol, C., Lea, O. A., Burrow, P. V., Dott, H. M., and Setchell, B. P. (1983): The effects of acidic epididymal glycoprotein (AEG) and some other proteins on the motility of rat epididymal spermatozoa. *Int. J. Androl.,* 6:240–248.
210. Garberi, J. C., Kohane, A. C., Cameo, M. S., and Blaquier, J. A. (1979): Isolation and characterization of specific rat epididymal proteins. *Mol. Cell. Endocrinol.,* 13:73–82.
211. Kohane, A. C., Gonzáles Echeverría, F. M. C., Piñeiro, L., and Blaquier, J. A. (1980): Distribution and site of production of specific proteins in rat epididymis. *Biol. Reprod.,* 23:181–187.
212. Kohane, A. C., Gonzáles Echeverría, F. M. C., Piñeiro, L., and Blaquier, J. A. (1980): Interactions of proteins of epididymal origin with spermatozoa. *Biol. Reprod.,* 23:737–742.
213. Cuasnicú, P. S., Gonzáles Echeverría, F., Piazza, A., Cameo, M. S., and Blaquier, J. A. (1984): Antibodies against epididymal glycoproteins block fertilizing ability in rat. *J. Reprod. Fertil.,* 72:461–471.
214. Brooks, D. E., and Higgins, S. J. (1980): Characterization and androgen-dependence of proteins associated with luminal fluid and spermatozoa in the rat epididymis. *J. Reprod. Fertil.,* 59:262–375.
215. Brooks, D. E. (1981): Secretion of proteins and glycoproteins by the rat epididymis: Regional differences, androgen-dependence, and effects of protease inhibitors, procaine, and tunicamycin. *Biol. Reprod.,* 25:1099–1117.
216. Brooks, D. E. (1981): Metabolic activity in the epididymis and its regulation by androgens. *Physiol. Rev.,* 61:515–555.
217. Brooks, D. E. (1983): Selective binding of specific rat epididymal secretory proteins to spermatozoa and erythrocytes. *Gamete Res.,* 4:367–376.

218. Brooks, D. E., and Tiver, K. (1983): Localization of epididymal secretory proteins on rat spermatozoa. *J. Reprod. Fertil.*, 69:651–657.
219. Rifkin, J., and Olson, G. E. (1985): Characterization of maturation-dependent extrinsic proteins of the rat sperm surface. *J. Cell Biol.*, 100:1582–1591.
220. Hamilton, D. W., Wenstrom, J. C., and Baker, J. B. (1986): Membrane glycoproteins from spermatozoa: Partial characterization of an integral $M_r = \sim 24,000$ molecule from rat spermatozoa that is glycosylated during spididymal maturation. *Biol. Reprod.*, 34:925–936.
221. Olson, G. E., and Orgebin-Crist, M.-C. (1982): Sperm surface changes during epididymal maturation. In: *The Cell Biology of the Testis, Vol. 383, Annals of the New York Academy of Sciences*, edited by C. W. Bardin and R. J. Sherins, pp. 372–390. New York Academy of Sciences, New York.
222. Moore, H. D. M. (1980): Localization of specific glycoproteins secreted by the rabbit and hamster epididymis. *Biol. Reprod.*, 22:705–718.
223. Gonzáles Echiverriá, F., Cuasnicú, P. S., and Blaquier, J. A. (1982): Identification of androgen-dependent glycoproteins in the hamster epididymis and their association with spermatozoa. *J. Reprod. Fertil.*, 64:1–7.
224. Tezón, J. G., Ramella, R., Cameo, M. S., Vazquez, M. H., and Blaquier, J. A. (1985): Immunochemical localization of secretory antigens in the human epididymis and their association with spermatozoa. *Biol. Reprod.*, 32:591–597.
225. Vernon, R. B., Muller, C. H., Herr, J. C., Feuchter, F. A., and Eddy, E. M. (1982): Epididymal secretion of a mouse sperm surface component recognized by a monoclonal antibody. *Biol. Reprod.*, 26:523–535.
226. Vernon, R. B., Hamilton, M. S., and Eddy, E. M., (1985): Effects of *in vivo* and *in vitro* fertilization environments on the expression of a surface antigen of the mouse sperm tail. *Biol. Reprod.*, 32:669–680.
227. Fox, N., Damjanov, I., Knowles, B. B., and Solter, D. (1982): Teratocarcinoma antigen is secreted by epididymal cells and coupled to maturing sperm. *Exp. Cell Res.*, 137:485–488.
228. Jones, R. (1978): Comparative biochemistry of mammalian epididymal plasma. *Comp. Biochem. Physiol. (B)*, 61:365–370.
229. Zaneveld, L. J. D., and Chatterton, R. T. (1982): *Biochemistry of Mammalian Reproduction*. John Wiley & Sons, New York.
230. Conchie, J., Findlay, J., and Levvy, G. A. (1959): Mammalian glycosidases. Distribution in the body. *Biochem. J.*, 71:318–325.
231. Kemp, W. R., and Killian, G. J. (1978): Glycosidase activity in epididymal epithelial cells isolated from normal and α-chlorohydrin treated male rats. *Contraception*, 17:93–101.
232. Chapman, D. A., and Killian, G. J. (1984): Glycosidase activities in principal cells, basal cells, fibroblasts and spermatozoa isolated from the rat epididymis. *Biol. Reprod.*, 31:627–636.
233. Skudlarek, M. D., and Orgebin-Christ, M.-C. (1986): Glycosidases in cultured rat epididymal cells: Enzyme activity, synthesis and secretion. *Biol. Reprod.*, 35:167–178.
234. Grandmont, A.-M., Chapdelaine, P., and Tremblay, R. R. (1983): Presence of α-glucosidases in the male reproductive system of the rat and hormonal influences. *Can. J. Biochem. Cell Biol.*, 61:764–769.
235. Jones, R. (1974): Absorption and secretion in the cauda epididymidis of the rabbit and the effects of degenerating spermatozoa on epididymal plasma after castration. *J. Endocrinol.*, 63:157–165.
236. Poirier, G. R., and Jackson, J. (1981): Isolation and characterization of two proteinase inhibitors from the male reproductive tract of mice. *Gamete Res.*, 4:555–569.
237. Wenstrom, J. C., and Hamilton, D. W. (1980): Dolichol concentration and biosynthesis in rat testis and epididymis. *Biol. Reprod.*, 23:1054–1069.
238. Iusem, N. B., de Larminant, M. A., Tezón, Blaquier, J. A., and Belocopitow, E. (1984): Androgen dependence of protein *N*-glycosylation in rat epididymis. *Endocrinology*, 114:1448–1458.
239. Bernal, A., Torres, J., Reyes, A., and Rosada, A. (1980): Presence and regional distribution of sialyl transferase in the epididymis of the rat. *Biol. Reprod.*, 23:290–293.
240. Cossu, G., and Boitani, C. (1984): Lactosaminoglycans synthesized by mouse male germ cells are fucosylated by an epididymal fucosyltransferase. *Dev. Biol.*, 102:402–408.
241. Letts, P. J., Meistrich, M. R., Bruce, W. R., and Schachter H. (1974): Glycoprotein glycosyltransferase levels during spermatogenesis in mice. *Biochim. Biophys. Acta*, 343:192–207.
242. Reddy, P. R. K., Tadolini, B., Wilson, J., and Williams-Ashman, H. G. (1976): Glycoprotein glycosyltransferase in male reproductive organs and their hormonal regulations. *Mol. Cell. Endocrinol.*, 5:23–31.
243. Tadolini, B., Wilson, J., Reddy, P. R. K., and Williams-Ashman, H. G. (1977): Characteristics and hormonal control of some glycoprotein glycosyltransferase reactions in male reproductive organs. *Adv. Enzymol. Regul.*, 15:319–336.
244. Hamilton, D. W. (1980): UDP-galactose: *N*-acetylglucosamine glalctosyltransferase in fluids from rat testis and epididymis. *Biol. Reprod.*, 23:377–385.
245. Hamilton, D. W., and Gould, R. P. (1982): Preliminary observations on enzymatic galactosylation of glycoproteins on the surface of rat caput epididymal spermatozoa. *Int. J. Androl. (Suppl.)*, 5:73–80.
246. Hamilton, D. W. (1981): Evidence for α-lactalbumin-like activity in reproductive tract fluids of the male rat. *Biol. Reprod.*, 25:385–392.
247. Durr, R., Shur, B., and Roth, S. (1977): Sperm-associated sialyltransferase activity. *Nature*, 265:547–548.
248. Shur, B. D., and Bennett, D. (1979): A specific defect in galactosyltransferase on sperm bearing mutant alleles of the T/t locus. *Dev. Biol.*, 71:243–259.
249. Shur, B. D., and Hall, N. G. (1982): Sperm surface galactosyltransferase activities during *in vitro* capacitation. *J. Cell Biol.*, 95:567–573.
250. Klinefelter, G. R., and Hamilton, D. W. (1985): Synthesis and secretion of proteins by perfused caput epididymal tubules, and association of secreted proteins with spermatozoa. *Biol. Reprod.*, 33:1017–1027.
251. Ensrude, K., Wenstrom, J. C., Baker, J. B., and Hamilton, D. W. (1985): A monoclonal antibody against rat epididymal α-lactalbumin-like 24Kd polypeptide recognizes rat cauda sperm surface. *J. Androl. (Suppl.)* 6:54.
252. Quasba, P. K., Hewlett, I. K., and Byers, S. (1983): The presence of the milk protein, α-lacatalbumin and its mRNA in the rat epididymis. *Biochem. Biophys. Res. Commun.*, 117:306–312.
253. Brobek, U., Denton, W. L., Tanahashi, N. and Ebner, K. E. (1967): The isolation and identification of the B protein of lactose synthetase as α-lactalbumin. *J. Biol. Chem.*, 242:1391–1397.
254. Shur, B. D., and Hall, N. G. (1982): A role for mouse sperm surface galactosyltransferase in sperm binding to the egg zona pellucida. *J. Cell Biol.*, 95:574–579.
255. Vaidya, R. A., Glass, R. W., Dandekar, P., and Johnson, K. (1971): Decrease in electrophoretic mobility of rabbit spermatozoa following intra-uterine incubation. *J. Reprod. Fertil.*, 24:299–301.
256. Rosado, A., Valezquez, A., and Lara-Ricalde, R. (1973): Cell polarography. II. Effect of neuraminidase and follicular fluid upon the surface characteristics of human spermatozoa. *Fertil. Steril.*, 24:349–354.
257. Moore, H. D. M., and Hibbits, K. G. (1975): Isoelectric focusing of boar spermatozoa. *J. Reprod. Fertil.*, 44:329–332.
258. Clegg, E. D., and Foote, R. H. (1973): Phospholipid composition of bovine sperm fractions, seminal plasma and cytoplasmic droplet. *J. Reprod. Fertil.*, 34:379–383.
259. Edwards, R. G., Ferguson, L. C., and Coombs, R. R. A. (1964): Blood group antigens on human spermatozoa. *J. Reprod. Fertil.*, 7:153–161.
260. Boettcher, B. (1968): Correlation between human ABO blood group antigens in seminal plasma and on seminal spermatozoa. *J. Reprod. Fertil.*, 16:49–54.
261. Kerek, G., Biberfeld, P., and Afzelius, B. A. (1973): Demonstration of HL-A antigens, "species," and "semen"-specific antigens on human spermatozoa. *Int. J. Fertil.*, 18:145–155.
262. James, K., and Hargreave, T. B. (1984): Immunosuppression by seminal plasma and its possible clinical significance. *Immunol. Today*, 5:357–363.
263. Hekman, A., and Rumke, P. (1969): The antigens of human seminal plasma with special reference to lactoferrin, a spermatozoa coating antigen. *Fertil. Steril.*, 20:312–323.
264. Roberts, T. K., and Boettcher, B. (1969): Identification of human sperm coating antigen. *J. Reprod. Fertil.*, 18:347–350.
265. Koyama, Y., Takuda, Y., Takamura, T., and Isojima, S. (1983): Localization of human seminal plasma No. 7 antigen (ferrisplan) in accessory glands of the male genital tract. *J. Reprod. Immunol.*, 5:135–143.
266. Wahlstrom, T., Bohn, H., and Seppala, M. (1982): Immunohistochemical demonstration of placental protein 5 (PP5)-like material in

the seminal vesicle and the ampullar part of the vas deferens. *Life Sci.*, 31:2723–2725.

267. Evans, R. J., and Herr, J. C. (1986): Immunohistochemical localization of the MHS-5 antigen in principal cells of human seminal vesicle epithelium. *Anat. Rec.*, 214:372–377.
268. Saji, J., Minagawa, Y., Ohashi, K., Negoro, T., and Tanizawa, O. (1986): Further characterization of a human sperm coating antigen (gp12). *Am. J. Reprod. Immunol.*, 12:13–16.
269. Abrescia, P., Lombardi, G., De Rosa, M., Quagliozzi, L., Guardiola, J., and Metafora, S. (1985): Identification and preliminary characterization of sperm-binding protein in normal human semen. *J. Reprod. Fertil.*, 73:71–77.
270. Ostrowski, M. C., Kistler, M. K., and Kistler, W. S. (1979): Purification and cell-free synthesis of a major protein from rat seminal vesicle secretion. *J. Biol. Chem.*, 254:4007–4021.
271. Draveland, E., and Joshi, M. S. (1981): Sperm-coating antigens secreted by the epididymis and seminal vesicle of the rat. *Biol. Reprod.*, 25:649–658.
272. Oliphant, G., and Singhas, C. A. (1979): Iodination of rabbit sperm plasma membrane: Relationship of specific surface proteins to epididymal function and sperm capacitation. *Biol. Reprod.*, 21:937–944.
273. Koehler, J. K., Nudelman, E. D., and Hakomori, S. (1980): A collagen-binding protein on the surface of ejaculated rabbit spermatozoa. *J. Cell Biol.*, 86:529–536.
274. Irwin, M., Nicholson, N., Haywood, J. T., and Pourier, G. R. (1983): Immunoflourescent localization of a murine seminal vesicle proteinase inhibitor. *Biol. Reprod.*, 28:1201–1206.
275. Isaacs, W., and Coffey, D. S. (1984): The predominant protein of canine seminal plasma is an enzyme. *J. Biol. Chem.*, 259:11520–11526.
276. Paonessa, G., Metafora, G., Tajana, G., Abrescia, P., De Santis, A., Gentile, V., and Porta, R. (1984): Transglutaminase-mediated modifications of the rat sperm surface *in vitro*. *Science*, 226:852–855.
277. Chang, M. C. (1951): Fertilizing capacity of spermatozoa deposited into fallopian tubes. *Nature*, 168:697–698.
278. Austin, C. R. (1951): Observations on the penetration of the sperm into the mammalian egg. *Aust. J. Sci. Res. B*, 4:581–596.
279. Bedford, J. M. (1972): Sperm transport, capacitation and fertilization. In: *Reproductive Biology*, edited by H. Balin and S. Glasser, pp. 338–392. Excerpta Medica, Amsterdam.
280. Barros, C. (1974): Capacitation of mammalian spermatozoa. In: *Physiology and Genetics of Reproduction, Part B*, edited by E. M. Coutinho and F. Fuchs, pp. 3–24. Plenum Press, New York.
281. Chang, M. C., and Hunter, R. H. F. (1975): Capacitation of mammalian sperm: Biological and experimental aspects. In: *Handbook of Physiology, Vol. 5, Endocrinology, Section 7, Male Reproduction*, edited by R. O. Greep, pp. 339–351. American Physiological Society, Washington D.C.
282. Rogers, B. J. (1978): Mammalian sperm capacitation and fertilization *in vitro:* A critique of methodology. *Gamete Res.*, 1:165–223.
283. O'Rand, M. J. (1979): Changes in sperm surface properties correlated with capacitation. In: *The Spermatozoon*, edited by D. W. Fawcett and J. M. Bedford, pp. 195–204. Urban & Schwarzenberg, Baltimore.
284. Courtens, J. L., and Fournier-Delpech, S. (1979): Modifications in the plasma membranes of epididymal ram spermatozoa during maturation and incubation *in utero*. *J. Ultrastruct. Res.*, 68:136–148.
285. Talbot, P., and Franklin, L. E. (1978): Surface modification of guinea pig sperm during *in vitro* capacitation: An assessment using lectin-induced agglutination of living sperm. *J. Exp. Zool.*, 203:1–14.
286. Friend, D. S. (1977): The organization of the sperm membrane. In: *Immunobiology of Gametes*, edited by M. Edidin and M. H. Johnson, pp. 5–30. Cambridge University Press, Cambridge.
287. Friend, D. S., Orci, L., Perrelet, A., and Yanagimachi, R. (1977): Membrane particle changes attending the acrosome reaction in guinea pig spermatozoa. *J. Cell Biol.*, 74:561–577.
288. Davis, B. K. (1980): Interaction of lipids with the plasma membrane of sperm cells. I. The antifertilization action of cholesterol. *Arch. Androl.*, 5:249–254.
289. Davis, B. K., Byrne, R., and Hungund, B. (1979): Studies on the mechanism of capacitation. II. Evidence for lipid transfer between plasma membrane of rat sperm and serum albumin during capacitation *in vitro*. *Biochim. Biophys. Acta*, 558:257–266.
290. O'Rand, M. J. (1979): Changes in sperm surface properties correlated with capacitation. In: *The Spermatozoon*, edited by D. W. Fawcett and M. J. Bedford, pp. 195–204, Urban & Schwarzenberg, Baltimore.
291. Clegg, E. D., Morre, D. J., and Lunstra, D. D. (1975): Porcine sperm membrane: *In vivo* phospholipid changes, isolation and electron microscopy. In: *The Biology of Male Gametes*, edited by J. G. Duckett and P. A. Racey, pp. 321–335. Academic Press, London.
292. Snider, D. R., and Clegg, E. D. (1975): Alteration of phospholipids in procine spermatozoa during *in vivo* uterus and oviduct incubation. *J. Anim. Sci.*, 40:269–274.
293. Oliphant, G., and Brackett, B. G. (1973): Capacitation of mouse spermatozoa in media with elevated ionic strength and reversible decapacitation with epididymal extracts. *Fertil. Steril.*, 24:948–955.
294. Aonuma, S., Mayumi, T., Suzuki, K., Noguchi, T., Iwai, M., and Okabe, M. (1973): Studies on sperm capacitation. I. The relationship between a guinea-pig sperm-coating antigen and a sperm capacitation phenomenon. *J. Reprod. Fertil.*, 35:425–432.
295. Brackett, B. G., and Oliphant, G. (1975): Capacitation of rabbit spermatozoa *in vitro*. *Biol. Reprod.*, 12:260–274.
296. Johnson, M. H. (1975): The macromolecular organization of membranes and its bearing on events leading up to fertilization. *J. Reprod. Fertil.*, 44:167–184.
297. Schill, W. B., Heimburger, N., Schiessler, H., Stolla, R., and Fritz, H. (1975): Reversible attachment and localization of acid-stable seminal plasma acrosin-trypsin inhibitors on boar spermatozoa as revealed by the indirect immunofluorescent staining technique. *Biol. Chem. Hoppe Seyler*, 356:1473–1476.
298. Koehler, J. K. (1976): Changes in antigenic site distribution on rabbit spermatozoa after incubation in "capacitating" media. *Biol. Reprod.*, 9:444–456.
299. Eng, L. A., and Oliphant, G. (1978): Rabbit sperm reversible capacitation by membrane stabilization with a highly purified glycoprotein from seminal plasma. *Biol. Reprod.*, 19:1083–1094.
300. Johnson, W. L., and Hunter, A. G. (1972): Seminal antigens: Their alteration in the genital tract of female rabbits and during partial *in vitro* capacitation with beta amylase and beta glucuronidase. *Biol. Reprod.*, 7:332–340.
301. Oliphant, G., and Brackett, B. G. (1973): Immunological assessment of surface changes of rabbit sperm undergoing capacitation. *Biol. Reprod.*, 9:404–414.
302. Myles, D. G., and Primakoff, P. (1984): Localized surface antigens of guinea pig sperm migrate to new regions prior to fertilization. *J. Cell Biol.*, 99:1634–1641.
303. Baccetti, B. (1984): The human spermatozoon. In: *Ultrastructure of Reproduction*, edited by J. Van Blerkom and P. M. Motta, pp. 110–126. Martinus Nijhoff, The Hague.
304. Wyrobek, A. J., Gordon, L. A., Burkhart, J. G., Francis, M. W., Kapp, R. W. Jr., Letz, G., Malling, H. V., Topham, J. C., and Whorton, M. D. (1983): An evaluation of human sperm as indicators of chemically induced alterations of spermatogenic function. A report of the U.S. Environmental Protection Agency Gene-Tox Program. *Mutat. Res.*, 115:73–148.
305. Grimes, S. R. Jr. (1986): Nuclear proteins in spermatogenesis. *Comp. Biochem. Physiol.*, 83D:495–500.
306. Coelingh, J. P., Monfoort, C. H., Rozijin, T. H., Gevers-Leuven, J. A., Shiphof, R., Steyn-Parve, E. P., Brauntizer, G., Shrank, B., and Ruhfus, A. (1972): The complete amino acid sequence of the basic nuclear protein of bull spermatozoa. *Biochim. Biophys. Acta*, 285:1–14.
307. Kistler, W. S., Keim, P. S., and Heinrickson, R. L. (1976): Partial structural analysis of the basic chromosomal protein of rat spermatozoa. *Biochim. Biophys. Acta*, 427:931–954.
308. Hecht, N. B., Bower, P. A., Waters, S. H., Yelick, P. C., and Distel, R. J. (1986): Evidence for haploid expression of mouse testicular genes. *Exp. Cell Res.*, 164:183–190.
309. Bellvé, A. R., and Carraway, R. (1978): Characterization of two basic chromosomal proteins isolated from mouse spermatozoa. *J. Cell Biol.*, 79:177a.
310. Mayer, J. F., Chang, T. S. K., and Zirkin, B. R. (1981): Spermatogenesis in the mouse. 2. Amino acid incorporation into basic nucleoproteins of mouse spermatids and spermatozoa. *Biol. Reprod.*, 25:1041–1051.
311. Balhorn, R., Weston, S., Thomas, C., and Wyrobek, A. J. (1984): DNA packaging in mouse spermatids. Synthesis of protamine variants and four transition proteins. *Exp. Cell Res.*, 150:298–308.

312. Bellvé, A. R., and O'Brien, D. A. (1983): The mammalian spermatozoon: Structure and temporal assembly. In: *Mechanisms and Control of Animal Fertilization,* edited by J. F. Hartmann, pp. 55–137. Academic Press, Orlando, Florida.
313. Balhorn, R. (1982): A model for the structure of chromatin in mammalian sperm. *J. Cell Biol.,* 93:298–305.
314. Warrent, R. W., and Kim. S.-H. (1978): α-Helix-double helix interaction shown in the structure of a protamine-transfer RNA complex and a nucleoprotamine model. *Nature,* 271:130–135.
315. Gusse, M., and Chevaillier, P. (1980): Electron microscopic evidence for the presence of globular structures in different sperm chromatins. *J. Cell Biol.,* 87:280–284.
316. Tsanev, R., and Avramova, Z. (1981): Nonprotamine nucleoprotein ultrastructures in mature ram sperm nuclei. *Eur. J. Cell Biol.,* 24:139–145.
317. Bendet, I. J., and Bearden, J., Jr. (1972): Birefringence of bull sperm. II. Form birefringence of bull sperm. *J. Cell Biol.,* 55:501–510.
318. Sipski, M. R., and Wagner, T. E. (1977): The total structure and organization of chromosomal fibers in eutherian sperm nuclei. *Biol. Reprod.,* 16:428–440.
319. Bellvé, A. R. (1982): Biogenesis of the mammalian spermatozoon. In: *Prospects for Sexing Mammalian Sperm,* edited by R. P. Amann and G. E. Seidel, Jr., pp. 69–102. Colorado Associated University Press, Boulder.
320. Stackpole, C. W., and Devorkin, D. (1974): Membrane organization in mouse spermatozoa revealed by freeze-etching. *J. Ultrastruct. Res.,* 49:167–187.
321. Gerace, L., Comeau, C., and Benson, M. (1984): Organization and modulation of nuclear lamina structure. *J. Cell Sci. (Suppl.),* 1:137–160.
322. Krohne, G., and Benavente, R. (1986): The nuclear lamins. A multigene family of proteins in evolution and differentiation. *Exp. Cell Res.,* 162:1–10.
323. Gerace, L., Blum, A., and Blobel, G. (1978): Immunocytochemical localization of the major polypeptides of the nuclear pore complex lamina fraction. Interphase and mitotic distribution. *J. Cell Biol.,* 79:546–566.
324. Hancock, R., and Baulikis, T. (1982): Functional organisation of the nucleus. In: *International Review of Cytology, Vol. 79,* edited by G. H. Bourne and J. F. Danielli, pp. 165–214. Academic Press, New York.
325. Lebkowski, Y. S., and Laemmli, U. K. (1982): Non-histone proteins and long-range organization of HeLa interphase DNA. *J. Mol. Biol.,* 156:121–141.
326. Gerace, L., and Blobel, G. (1980): The nuclear envelope lamina is reversibly depolymerized during mitosis. *Cell,* 34:13–23.
327. Burke, B., Tooze, J., and Warren, G. (1983): A monoclonal antibody which recognizes each of the nuclear lamin polypeptides in mammalian cells. *EMBO J.,* 1:1621–1628.
328. Krone, G., Debus, E., Osborn, W., and Franke, W. W. (1984): A monoclonal antibody against nuclear lamina proteins reveals cell type-specificity in *Xenopus laevis. Exp. Cell Res.,* 150:47–59.
329. Stick, R., and Schwarz, H. (1982): The disappearance of the nuclear lamina during spermatogenesis: An electron microscopic and immunofluorescence study. *Cell Differ.,* 11:235–243.
330. Hogner, D., Telling, A., Lepper, K., and Jost, E. (1984): Patterns of nuclear lamins in diverse animal and plant cells and in germ cells as revealed by immunofluorescence microscopy with polyclonal and monoclonal antibodies. *Tissue Cell,* 16:693–703.
331. Maul, G. G., French, B. T., and Bechtol, K. B. (1986): Identification and redistribution of lamins during nuclear differentiation in mouse spermatogenesis. *Dev. Biol.,* 115:68–77.
332. McKeon, F. D., Kirschner, M. W., and Caput, D. (1986): Homologies in both primary and secondary structure between nuclear envelope and intermediate filament proteins. *Nature,* 319:463–468.
333. Fisher, D. Z., Chaudhary, N., and Blobel, G. (1986): cDNA sequencing of nuclear lamins A and C reveals primary and secondary structural homology to intermediate filament proteins. *Proc. Natl. Acad. Sci. USA,* 83:6450–6454.
334. Benavente, R., and Krohne, G. (1985): Changes of karyoskeleton during spermatogenesis of Xenopus: Expression of lamin LIV, a nuclear lamina protein specific for the male germ line. *Proc. Natl. Acad. Sci, USA,* 82:6176–6180.
335. Olson, G. E., Hamilton, D. W., and Fawcett, D. W. (1976): Isolation and characterization of the perforatorium of rat spermatozoa. *J. Reprod. Fertil.,* 47:293–297.
336. Fawcett, D. W. (1970): A comparative view of sperm ultrastructure. *Biol. Reprod. (Suppl.)* 2:90–127.
337. Calvin, H. I., and Bedford, J. M. (1971): Formation of disulfide bonds in the nucleus and accessory structures of mammalian spermatozoa during maturation in the epididymis. *J. Reprod. Fertil. (Suppl.),* 13:65–75.
338. Huang, T. T. F., and Yanagimachi, R. (1985): Inner acrosomal membrane of mammalian spermatozoa: Its properties and possible functions in fertilization. *Am. J. Anat.,* 174:249–268.
339. Burgos, M. H., and Fawcett, D. W. (1956): An electron microscopic study of spermatid differentiation in the toad, *Bufo arenarum Hensel. J. Biophys. Biochem., Cytol.,* 2:223–240.
340. Nagano, T. (1962): Observations on the fine structure of the developing spermatid in the domestic chicken. *J. Cell Biol.,* 14:193–205.
341. Clermont, Y., Einberg, E., Leblond, C. P., and Wagner, S. (1955): The perforatorium—An extension of the nuclear membrane of the rat spermatozoon. *Anat. Rec.,* 121:1–12.
342. Yanagimachi, R., and Noda, Y. D. (1970): Ultrastructural changes in the hamster sperm head during fertilization. *J. Ultrastruct. Res.,* 31:465–485.
343. Austin, C. R., and Bishop, M. W. H. (1958): Some features of the acrosome and perforatorium in mammalian spermatozoa. *Proc. R. Soc. Lond. (Biol.),* 149:234–240.
344. Olson, G. E. (1979): Isolation of the fibrous sheath and perforatorium of rat spermatozoa. In: *The Spermatozoon,* edited by D. W. Fawcett and J. M. Bedford, pp. 395–400. Urban & Schwarzenberg, Baltimore.
345. Courtens, J. L., Courot, M., and Fléchon, J. E. (1976): The perinuclear substance of boar, bull, ram and rabbit spermatozoa. *J. Ultrastruct. Res.,* 57:54–64.
346. Lalli, M., and Clermont, Y. (1981): Structural changes in the head component of the rat spermatid during late spermatogenesis. *Am. J. Anat.,* 160:419–434.
347. Nicander, L., and Bane, A. (1966): Fine structure of the sperm head in some mammals with particular reference to the acrosome and subacrosomal substance. *Z. Zelforsch.,* 72:496–515.
348. Pedersen, H. (1972): The postacrosomal region of man and *Macaca artoides. J. Ultrastruct. Res.,* 40:366–377.
349. Phillips, D. M. (1975): Cell surface structure of rodent sperm heads. *J. Exp. Zool.,* 191:1–8.
350. Olson, G. E., Noland, T. D., Winfrey, V. P., and Garbers, D. L. (1983): Substructure of the postacrosomal sheath of bovine spermatozoa. *J. Ultrastruct. Res.,* 85:204–218.
351. Maxwell, W. L. (1982): The acrosomal zonule. *Tissue Cell,* 14:283–288.
352. Czaker, R. (1985): Morphogenesis and cytochemistry of the postacrosomal dense lamina during mouse spermiogenesis. *J. Ultrastruct. Res.,* 90:26–39.
353. Searle, A. G. (1982): The genetics of sterility in the mouse. In: *Genetic Control of Gamete Production and Function,* edited by P. G. Crosignai, B. L. Rubin, and M. Fraccaro, pp. 93–114. Grune & Stratton, New York.
354. Sotomayor, R. E., and Handel, M. A. (1986): Failure of acrosome assembly in a male sterile mutant. *Biol. Reprod.,* 34:171–182.
355. Phillips, D. M. (1970): Development of spermatozoa in the woolly opossum with special reference to the shaping of the sperm head. *J. Ultrastruct. Res.,* 33:369–380.
356. Fawcett, D. W., and Phillips, D. M. (1969): Observations on the release of spermatozoa and on changes in the head during passage through the epididymis. *J. Reprod. Fertil., (Suppl.),* 6:405–418.
357. Fawcett, D. W., Anderson, W. A., and Phillips, D. M. (1971): Morphogenetic factors influencing the shape of the sperm head. *Dev. Biol.,* 26:220–251.
358. Hunt, D. M., and Johnson, D. R. (1971): Abnormal spermiogenesis in two pink-eyed sterile mutants in the mouse. *J. Embryol. Exp. Morphol.,* 26:111–121.
359. Bryan, J. H. D. (1977): Spermatogenesis revisited: III. The course of spermatogenesis in a male-sterile pink-eyed mutant type in the mouse. *Cell Tissue Res.,* 180:173–186.
360. Wooding, F. B. P. (1973): The effect of Triton X-100 on the ultrastructure of ejaculated bovine sperm. *J. Ultrastruct. Res.,* 42:502–516.
361. Phillips, D. M. (1972): Substructure of the mammalian acrosome. *J. Ultrastruct. Res.,* 38:591–604.
362. Pedersen, H. (1972): Further observations on the fine structure of the human spermatozoon. *Z. Zellforsch.,* 123:305–315.

363. Koehler, J. K. (1975): Periodicities in the acrosome or acrosomal membrane: Some observations on mammalian spermatozoa. *Biol. J. Linnean Soc. (Suppl.)*, 1:337–342.
364. Zahler, W. L., and Doak, G. A. (1975): Isolation of the outer acrosomal membrane from bull spermatozoa. *Biochim. Biophys. Acta*, 406:479–488.
365. Russell, L., Peterson, R., and Freund, M. (1979): Direct evidence for formation of hybrid vesicles by fusion of plasma and outer acrosomal membranes during the acrosome reaction in boar spermatozoa. *J. Exp. Zool.*, 208:41–56.
366. Noland, T. D., Olson, G. E., and Garbers, D. L. (1983): Purification and partial characterization of plasma membranes from bovine spermatozoa. *Biol. Reprod.*, 29:987–998.
367. Topfer-Petersen, E., and Schill, W. B. (1981): A new separation method of subcellular fractions of boar spermatozoa. *Andrologia*, 13:174–176.
368. Olson, G. E., Winfrey, V. P., Garbers, D. L., and Noland, T. D. (1985): Isolation and characterization of a macromolecular complex associated with the outer acrosomal membrane of bovine spermatozoa. *Biol. Reprod.*, 33:761–779.
369. Burgos, M. H., and Fawcett, D. W. (1955): Studies on the fine structure of the mammalian testis. I. Differentiation of the spermatids in the cat (*Felis domestica*). *J. Biophys. Biochem. Cytol.*, 1:287–299.
370. Hermo, L., Rambourg, L. A., and Clermont, Y. (1980): Three-dimensional architecture of the cortical region of the Golgi apparatus in rat spermatids. *Am. J. Anat.*, 157:357–373.
371. Thakkar, J. K., East, J., Seyler, D., and Fanson, R. C. (1983): Surface-active phospholipase A_2 in mouse spermatozoa. *Biochim. Biophys. Acta*, 754:44–50.
372. Rahi, H., Sheikhnejade, G., and Srivastava, P. N. (1983): Isolation of the inner acrosomal-nuclear membrane complex from rabbit spermatozoa. *Gamete Res.*, 7:215–225.
373. Russell, L., Peterson, R. N., and Freund, M. (1980): On the presence of bridges linking the inner and outer acrosomal membranes of boar spermatozoa. *Anat. Rec.*, 198:449–459.
374. Yanagimachi, R. (1977): Specificity of sperm-egg interaction. In: *Immunobiology of Gametes*, edited by M. Edidin and M. H. Johnson, pp. 255–296. Cambridge University Press, London.
375. Cowen, A. E., Primakoff, P., and Myles, D. G. (1986): Sperm exocytosis increases the amount of PH-20 antigen on the surface of guinea pig sperm. *J. Cell Biol.*, 103:1289–1297.
376. Allison, A. C., and Hartree, E. F. (1970): Lysosomal enzymes in the acrosome and their possible role in fertilization. *J. Reprod. Fertil.*, 21:501–515.
377. Polakoski, K. L., and Parrish, R. F. (1977): Boar proacrosin. Purification and preliminary activation studies of proacrosin isolated from ejaculated boar sperm. *J. Biol. Chem.*, 252:1888–1894.
378. Tobias, P. S., and Schumacher, G. F. B. (1977): Observation of two proacrosins in extracts of human spermatozoa. *Biochem. Biophys. Res. Commun.*, 74:434–439.
379. Brown, C. R., and Harrison, R. A. P. (1978): The activation of proacrosin in spermatozoa from ram, bull and boar. *Biochim. Biophys. Acta*, 526:202–217.
380. Mukerji, S. K., and Meizel, S. (1979): Rabbit testis proacrosin. Purification, molecular weight estimation, and amino acid and carbohydrate composition of the molecule. *J. Biol. Chem.*, 254:11721–11728.
381. Müller-Esterl, W., and Fritz, H. (1981): Sperm acrosin. In: *Methods in Enzymology, Vol. 80*, edited by L. Lorand, pp. 621–632. Academic Press, New York.
382. Stambaugh, R., and Buckley, J. (1969): Identification and subcellular localization of the enzymes effecting penetration of the zona pellucida by rabbit spermatozoa. *J. Reprod. Fertil.*, 19:423–432.
383. Zaneveld, L. J. D., Robetson, R. T., Kessler, M., and Williams, W. L. (1971): Inhibition of fertilization *in vivo* by pancreatic and seminal plasma trypsin inhibitors. *J. Reprod. Fertil.*, 25:387–392.
384. Mukerji, S. K., and Meizel, S. (1975): The molecular transformation of rabbit testis proacrosin into acrosin. *Arch. Biochem. Biophys.*, 168:720–721.
385. Garner, D. L., and Easton, M. P. (1977): Immunofluorescent localization of acrosin in mammalian spermatozoa. *J. Exp. Zool.*, 200:157–162.
386. Morton, D. B. (1975): Acrosomal enzymes: Immunochemical localization of acrosin and hyaluronidase in ram spermatozoa. *J. Reprod. Fertil.*, 45:375–378.
387. Morton, D. B. (1977): Lysosomal enzymes in mammalian spermatozoa. In: *Immunobiology of Gametes*, edited by M. Edidin and M. H. Johnson, pp. 115–155. Cambridge University Press, London.
388. Green, D. P. L., and Hockaday. A. R. (1978): The histochemical localization of acrosin in guinea-pig sperm after the acrosome reaction. *J. Cell Sci.*, 32:177–184.
389. McRorie, R. A., and Williams, W. L. (1974): Biochemistry of mammalian fertilization. *Ann. Rev. Biochem.*, 43:777–803.
390. Stambaugh, R. (1978): Enzymatic and morphological events in mammalian fertilization. *Gamete Res.*, 1:65–85.
391. Meizel, S. (1978): The mammalian sperm acrosome reaction. In: *Development in Mammals, Vol. 3*, edited by M. H. Johnson, pp. 1–62. North-Holland, Amsterdam.
392. Parrish, R. F., and Polakoski, K. L. (1979): Mammalian sperm proacrosin-acrosin system. *Int. J. Biochem.*, 10:391–395.
393. Siegel, M. S., Bechtold, D. S., Kopta, C. I., and Polakoski, K. L. (1986): Quantification and partial characterization of the hamster sperm proacrosin-acrosin system. *Biol. Reprod.*, 35:485–491.
394. Brown, C. R., and Hartree, E. F. (1978): Studies on ram acrosin. Activation of proacrosin accompanying the isolation of acrosin from spermatozoa and purification of the enzyme by affinity chromatography. *Biochem. J.*, 175:227–238.
395. Kallojoki, M., and Suominen, J. (1984): An acrosomal antigen of human spermatozoa and spermatogenic cells characterized with a monoclonal antibody. *Int. J. Androl.*, 7:283–296.
396. Kallojoki, M., Parvinen, M., and Suominen, J. J. O. (1986): Expression of acrosin during mouse spermatogenesis: A biochemical and immunocytochemical analysis by a monoclonal antibody C 11 H. *Biol. Reprod.*, 35:157–165.
397. Phi-van, L., Müller-Esterl, W., Florke, S., Schmid, M., and Engel, W. (1983): Proacrosin and the differentiation of the spermatozoa. *Biol. Reprod.*, 29:479–486.
398. Florke, S., Phi-van, L., Müller-Esterl, W., Scheuber, H.-P., and Engel, W. (1983): Acrosin in the spermiohistogenesis of mammals. *Differentiation*, 24:250–256.
399. Zaneveld, L. J. D., Polakoski, K. L., and Schumacher, G. F. B. (1973): Properties of acrosomal hyaluronidase from bull spermatozoa. Evidence for its similarity to testicular hyaluronidase. *J. Biol. Chem.*, 248:564–570.
400. Yang, C.-H., and Srivastava, P. N. (1975): Purification and properties of hyaluronidase from bull sperm. *J. Biol. Chem.*, 250:79–83.
401. Goldberg, E. (1977): Isozymes in testes and spermatozoa. In: *Isozymes: Current Topics in Biological and Medical Research, Vol. 1*, edited by M. Ratazzi, J. Scandalios, and G. Whitt, pp. 79–124. Alan R. Liss, New York.
402. Brown, C. R. (1981): Distribution of hyaluronidase in the ram spermatozoon. *J. Reprod. Fertil.*, 45:537–539.
403. Mancini, R. E., Alonso, A., Barquet, J., and Nemirovski, B. (1964): Histo-immunological localization of hyaluronidase in bull testis. *J. Reprod. Fertil.*, 8:325–330.
404. Gould, S. F., and Bernstein, M. H. (1975): Localization of bovine sperm hyaluronidase. *Differentiation*, 3:123–132.
405. Morton, D. B. (1975): Acrosomal enzymes: Immunological localization of acrosin and hyaluronidase in ram spermatozoa. *J. Reprod. Fertil.*, 45:375–378.
406. Brown, C. R. (1975): Distribution of hyaluronidase in the ram spermatozoa. *J. Reprod. Fertil.*, 45:537–539.
407. Koren, E., and Milkovíc, S. (1973): "Collagenase-like" peptidase in human, rat and bull spermatozoa. *J. Reprod. Fertil.*, 32:349–356.
408. Erickson, R. P., and Martin, S. R. (1974): The relationship of mouse spermatozoal to mouse testicular cathepsins. *Arch. Biochem. Biophys.*, 165:114–120.
409. Schollmeyer, J. E. (1986): Identification of calpain II in porcine sperm. *Biol. Reprod.*, 34:721–731.
410. Srivastava, P. N., and Abou-Issa, H. (1977): Purification and properties of rabbit spermatozoal acrosomal neuraminidase. *Biochem. J.*, 161:193–200.
411. Bryan, J. H. D., and Unithan, R. R. (1972): Non-specific esterase activity in bovine acrosomes. *Histochem. J.*, 4:413–419.
412. Meizel, S., and Cotham, J. (1972): Partial characterization of a new bull sperm arylaminidase. *J. Reprod. Fertil.*, 28:303–307.
413. Bhalla, V. K., Tillman, W. L., and Williams, W. L. (1973): Presence of β-aspartyl *N*-acetylglucosamine amido hydrolase in mammalian spermatozoa. *J. Reprod. Fertil.*, 34:137–139.

414. Dudkiewicz, A. B. (1984): Purification of boar acrosomal arylsulfatase A and possible role in the penetration of cumulus cells. *Biol. Reprod.*, 30:1005–1014.
415. Gonzales, L. W., and Meizel, S. (1973): Acid phosphatases of rabbit spermatozoa. II. Partial purification and biochemical characterization of the multiple forms of rabbit spermatozoan acid phosphatase. *Biochim. Biophys. Acta.*, 320:180–194.
416. Stambaugh, R., and Buckley, J. (1970): Comparative studies of the acrosomal enzymes of rabbit, rhesus monkey and human spermatozoa. *Biol. Reprod.*, 3:275–282.
417. Bhattacharyya, A. K., and Zaneveld, L. J. D. (1982): The sperm head. In: *Biochemistry of Mammalian Reproduction*, edited by L. J. D. Zaneveld and R. T. Chatterton, pp. 119–152. John Wiley & Sons, New York.
418. Zamboni, L., and Stefanini, M. (1971): The fine structure of the neck of mammalian spermatozoa. *Anat. Rec.*, 169:155–172.
419. Ōura, C. (1971): The ultrastructure and development of the neck region of the golden hamster spermatozoon. *Monitore Zool. Ital.*, 5:253–264.
420. Phillips, D. M. (1972): Comparative analysis of mammalian sperm motility. *J. Cell Biol.*, 53:561–573.
421. Millette, C. F., Spear, P. G., Gall, W. E., and Edelman, G. M. (1973): Chemical dissection of mammalian spermatozoa. *J. Cell Biol.*, 58:662–675.
422. Young, R. J., and Cooper, G. W. (1979): Separation of the head and tail of mammalian spermatozoa by primary amines: Evidence for their junction by Schiff bases. In: *The Spermatozoon*, edited by D. W. Fawcett and J. M. Bedford, pp. 391–394. Urban & Schwarzenberg, Baltimore.
423. Calvin, H. I. (1976): Isolation and subfractionation of mammalian sperm heads and tails. In: *Methods in Cell Biology, Vol. 13*, edited by D. M. Prescott, pp. 85–104. Academic Press, New York.
424. Calvin, H. I. (1979): Isolation of stable structures from rat spermatozoa. In: *The Spermatozoon*, edited by D. W. Fawcett and J. M. Bedford, pp. 387–389. Urban & Schwarzenberg, Baltimore.
425. Bedford, J. M., and Calvin, H. I. (1974): Changes in the -S-S- linked structures of the sperm tail during epididymal maturation with comparative observations in sub-mammalian species. *J. Exp. Zool.*, 187:181–204.
426. Bellvé, A. R., Anderson, E., and Hanley-Bowdoin, L. (1975): Synthesis and amino acid composition of basic proteins in mammalian sperm nuclei. *Dev. Biol.*, 47:349–365.
427. Mann, T. (1964): *The Biochemistry of Semen and of the Male Reproductive Tract*, Methuen, London.
428. Blom, E., and Birch-Anderson, A. (1970): The ultrastructure of decapitated sperm defect in Guernsey bulls. *J. Reprod. Fertil.*, 23:67–72.
429. Fawcett, D. W., and Phillips, D. W. (1969): The fine structure and development of the neck region of the mammalian spermatozoon. *Anat. Rec.*, 165:153–184.
430. Nicander, L., and Bane, A. (1962): Fine structure of boar spermatozoa. *Z. Zellforsch.*, 57:390–405.
431. Illison, L. (1966): Fine structure of the mature spermatozoan head and neck of the mouse. *J. Anat.*, 100:949–950.
432. Woolley, D. M., and Fawcett, D. W. (1973): The degeneration and disappearance of the centrioles during the development of the rat spermatozoon. *Anat. Rec.*, 177:289–302.
433. Fawcett, D. W., and Porter, K. R. (1954): A study of the fine structure of ciliated epithelia. *J. Morphol.*, 94:221–281.
434. Gibbons, I. R., and Grimstone, A. V. (1960): On flagellar structure in certain flagellates. *J. Biophys. Biochem. Cytol.*, 7:697–716.
435. Olson, G. E., and Linck, R. W. (1977): Observations of the structural components of flagellar axonemes and central pair microtubules from rat sperm. *J. Ultrastruct. Res.*, 61:21–43.
436. Bryan, J., and Wilson, L. (1971): Are cytoplasmic microtubules heteropolymers? *Proc. Natl. Acad. Sci. USA*, 8:1762–1766.
437. Hecht, N. B., Kleene, K. C., Distel, R. J., and Silver, L. M. (1984): The differential expression of the actins and tubulins during spermatogenesis in the mouse. *Exp. Cell Res.*, 153:275–280.
438. Distel, R. J., Kleene, K. C., and Hecht, N. B. (1984): Haploid expression of a mouse testis α-tubulin gene. *Science*, 224:68–70.
439. Vale, R. D., Reese, T. S., and Sheetz, M. P. (1985): Identification of a novel force generating protein, kinesin, involved in microtubule-based motility. *Cell*, 42:39–50.
440. Vale, R. D., Schnapp, B. J., Mitchison, T., Steuer, E., Reese, T. S., and Sheetz, M. P. (1985): Different axoplasmic proteins generate movement in opposite directions along microtubules *in vitro*. *Cell*, 43:623–632.
441. Gibbons, I. R., and Rowe, A. J. (1965): Dynein: A protein with ATPase activity from cilia. *Science*, 149:424–426.
442. Gibbons, I. R., and Fronk, E. (1972): Some properties of bound and soluble dynein from sea urchin flagella. *J. Cell Biol.*, 54:365–381.
443. Baccetti, B., Burrini, A. G., Pallini, V., and Renieri, T. (1981): Human dynein and sperm pathology. *J. Cell Biol.*, 88:102–107.
444. Stephens, R. E. (1974): Enzymatic and structural proteins of the axoneme. In: *Cilia and Flagella*, edited by M. A. Sleigh, pp. 39–76. Academic Press, New York.
445. Linck, R. W. (1976): Flagellar doublet microtubules: Fractionation of minor components and α-tubulin from specific regions of the A-tubule. *J. Cell Sci.*, 20:405–539.
446. Linck, R. W., and Langevin, G. L. (1982): Structure and chemical composition of insoluble filamentous components of sperm flagellar microtubules. *J. Cell Biol.*, 58:1–22.
447. Linck, R. W. (1982): The structure of microtubules. *Ann. N.Y. Acad. Sci.*, 383:98–121.
448. Linck, R. W., Albertini, D. F., Kenny, D. M., and Langevin, G. L. (1982): Tektin filaments: Chemically unique filaments of sperm flagellar microtubules. *Cell Motil. (Suppl.)*, 1:127–132.
449. Linck, R. W., Amos, L. A., and Amos, W. B. (1985): Localization of tektin filaments in microtubules of sea urchin flagella by immunoelectron microscopy. *J. Cell Biol.*, 100:126–135.
450. Woolley, D. M. (1970): The midpiece of the mouse spermatozoon: Its form and development as seen by surface replication. *J. Cell Sci.*, 6:865–879.
451. Woolley, D. M. (1970): Selection for the length of the spermatozoan midpiece in the mouse. *Genet. Res.*, 16:225–228.
452. Phillips, D. M. (1970): Ultrastructure of spermatozoa of the woolly opossum *Caluromys philander*. *J. Ultrastruct. Res.*, 33:381–397.
453. Phillips, D. M. (1977): Mitochondrial disposition in mammalian spermatozoa. *J. Ultrastruct. Res.*, 58:144–154.
454. Serres, C., Escalier, D., and David, G. (1983): Ultrastructural morphometry of human spermatozoa flagellum with a sterological analysis of the lengths of the dense fibers. *Biol. Cell*, 49:153–162.
455. Lindemann, C. B., Fentie, I., and Rikmenspoel, R. (1980): A selective effect of Ni^{2+} on wave initiation in bull sperm flagella. *J. Cell Biol.*, 87:420–426.
456. Telkka, A., Fawcett, D. W., and Christensen, A. K. (1961): Further observations on the structure of the mammalian sperm tail. *Anat. Rec.*, 141:231–246.
457. de Kretser, D. M. (1969): Ultrastructural features of human spermiogenesis. *Z. Zellforsch.*, 98:229–236.
458. Sapsford, C. S., Rae, C. A., and Cleland, K. W. (1970): Ultrastructural studies on the development and form of the principal piece sheath of the Bandicoot spermatozoon. *Aust. J. Zool.*, 8:21–48.
459. Irons, M. J., and Clermont, Y. (1982): Formation of the outer dense fibers during spermiogenesis in the rat. *Anat. Rec.*, 202:463–471.
460. Gordon, M., and Bensch, K. G. (1968): Cytochemical differentiation of the guinea pig sperm flagellum with phosphotungstic acid. *J. Ultrastruct. Res.*, 24:33–50.
461. Olson, G. E., and Sammons, D. W. (1980): Structural chemistry of outer dense fibers of rat sperm. *Biol. Reprod.*, 22:319–332.
462. Woolley, D. M. (1971): Striations in the peripheral fibers of rat and mouse spermatozoa. *J. Cell Biol.*, 49:936–939.
463. Baccetti, B., Pallini, V., and Burrini, A. G. (1976): The accessory fibers of the sperm tail. III. High-sulfur and low-sulfur components in mammals and cephalopods. *J. Ultrastruct. Res.*, 57:289–308.
464. Pihlaja, D. J., and Roth, L. E. (1973): Bovine sperm fractionation. II. Morphology and chemical analysis of tail segments. *J. Ultrastruct. Res.*, 44:293–309.
465. Baccetti, B., Pallini, V., and Burrini, A. G. (1973): The accessory fibers of the sperm tail. I. Structure and chemical composition of the bull coarse fibers. *J. Submicrosc. Cytol.*, 5:237–256.
466. Zittle, C. W., and O'Dell, R. A. (1941): Chemical studies of bull spermatozoa. Lipid, sulfur, cystine, nitrogen, phosphorus, and nucleic acid content of whole spermatozoa and of the parts obtained by physical means. *J. Biol. Chem.*, 140:899–907.
467. Price, J. M. (1973): Biochemical and morphological studies of outer dense fibers of rat spermatozoa. *J. Cell Biol.*, 59:272a.
468. Calvin, H. I. (1979): Electrophoretic evidence for the identity of the major zinc-binding polypeptides in the rat sperm tail. *Biol. Reprod.*, 21:873–882.

469. Vera, J. C., Brito, M., Zuvic, T., and Burzio, L. O. (1984): Polypeptide composition of rat sperm outer dense fibers. *J. Biol. Chem.*, 259:5970–5977.
470. Gunn, S. A., and Gould, T. C. (1970): Cadmium and other mineral elements. In: *The Testis, Vol. III,* edited by A. D. Johnson, W. R. Gomes, and N. L. Vandemark, pp. 377–481. Academic Press, New York.
471. Miller, M. J., Vincent, N. R., and Mawson, C. A. (1961): An autoradiographic study of the distribution of zinc-65 in rat tissues. *J. Histochem. Cytochem.*, 9:111–125.
472. Bradley, F. M., Meth, B. M., and Bellvé, A. R. (1981): Structural proteins of the mouse spermatozoan tail: An electrophoretic analysis. *Biol. Reprod.*, 24:691–701.
473. Fawcett, D. W., and Phillips, D. M. (1970): Recent observations on the ultrastructure and development of the mammalian spermatozoon. In: *Comparative Spermatology,* edited by B. Baccetti, pp. 13–28. Academic Press, New York.
474. Cleland, K. W., and Lord Rothschild (1959): The bandicoot spermatozoon: An electron microscopic study of the tail. *Proc. R. Soc. B,* 150:24–42.
475. Nelson, L. (1958): Cytochemical studies with the electron microscope. I. Adenosine triphosphatease in the rat spermatozoa. *Biochem. Biophys. Acta,* 27:634–641.
476. Nagano, T. (1965): Localization of adenosine triphosphatase activity in the rat sperm tail as revealed by electron microscopy. *J. Cell Biol.*, 25:101–112.
477. Irons, M. J., and Clermont, Y. (1982): Formation of the outer dense fibers during spermiogenesis in the rat. *Anat. Rec.*, 202:463–471.
478. Rattner, J. B., and Brinkley, B. R. (1970): Ultrastructure of mammalian spermiogenesis. I. A tubular complex in developing sperm of the cottontop marmoset *Sequinus oedipus*. *J. Ultrastruct. Res.*, 32:316–322.
479. Wartenberg, H., and Holstein, A. F. (1975): Morphology of the "Spindle-shaped body" in the developing tail of human spermatids. *Cell Tissue Res.*, 159:435–443.
480. Koyama, Y., Shinomiya, T., Sakai, Y., Shiba, T., and Yanagisawa, K. O. (1984): Identification of sperm antigenic determinants with phylogenetically diverse and limited distribution using monoclonal antibodies. *J. Reprod. Immunol.*, 6:141–150.
481. Sakai, Y., Koyama, Y.-I., Fujimoto, H., Nakamoto, T., and Yamashina, S. (1986): Immunocytochemical study of fibrous sheath formation in mouse spermiogenesis using a monoclonal antibody. *Anat. Rec.*, 215:119–126.
482. Bradfield, J. R. G. (1955): Fibre patterns in animal flagella and cilia. *Symp. Soc. Exp. Biol.*, 9:306–334.
483. Olson, G. E., Hamilton, D. W., and Fawcett, D. W. (1976): Isolation and characterization of the fibrous sheath of rat epididymal spermatozoa. *Biol. Reprod.*, 14:517–530.
484. O'Brien, D. O., and Bellve, A. R. (1980): Protein constituents of the mouse spermatozoon. II. Temporal synthesis during spermatogenesis. *Dev. Biol.*, 75:405–418.
485. Jones, R., Brown, C. R., Cran, D. G., and Gaunt, S. J. (1983): Surface and internal antigens of rat spermatozoa distinguished using monoclonal antibodies. *Gamete Res.*, 8:255–265.
486. Fenderson, B. A., Toshimori, K., Muller, C. H., Lane, T. F., and Eddy, E. M. (1987): Identification of a protein in the fibrous sheath of the sperm flagellum. *Biol. Reprod.* (submitted for publication).
487. Hunter, D. G., and Kretzer, F. L. (1986): Abnormal axonemes in sperm of fertile men. *Arch. Androl.*, 16:1–12.
488. Pelfrey, J. J., Overstreet, J. W., and Lewis, E. L. (1982): Abnormalities of sperm morphology in cases of persistent infertility after vasectomy reversal. *Fertil. Steril.*, 33:160–166.
489. Escalier, D., and David, G. (1984): Pathology of the cytoskeleton of the human sperm flagellum: Axonemal and peri-axonemal anomalies. *Biol. Cell,* 50:37–52.
490. Aitken, R. J., Ross, A., and Lees, M. M. (1983): Analysis of sperm function in Kartagener's syndrome. *Fertil. Steril.*, 40:696–698.
491. Smith, D., Ōura, C., and Zamboni, L. (1970): Fertilizing ability of structurally abnormal spermatozoa. *Nature,* 227:79–80.
492. Baccetti, B., Burrini, A. G., and Pallini, V. (1980): Spermatozoa and cilia lacking axoneme in an infertile man. *Andrologia,* 12:525–532.
493. Ross, A., Christie, S., and Edmond, P. (1973): Ultrastructural tail defects in the spermatozoa from two men attending a subfertility clinic. *J. Reprod. Fertil.*, 32:243–251.
494. Williamson, R. A., Koehler, J. K., and Smith, W. D. (1984): Ultrastructural sperm tail defects associated with sperm immotility. *Fertil. Steril.*, 41:103–107.
495. Sauvalle, A., Le Bris, C., and Izard, J. (1983): Supernumerary microtubules and prolongation of the middle piece in two infertile patients. *Int. J. Fertil.*, 28:173–176.
496. Afzelius, B. A. (1981): Genetical and ultrastructural aspects of the immotile-cilia syndrome. *Am. J. Hum. Genet.*, 33:852–864.
497. Afzelius, B. A. (1976): A human syndrome caused by immotile cilia. *Science,* 193:317–319.
498. Afzelius, B. A., and Eliasson, R. (1979): Flagellar mutants in man: On the heterogeneity of the immotile-cilia syndrome. *J. Ultrastruct. Res.*, 69:43–52.
499. Leestma, J. E., and Sepsenwol, S. (1980): Sperm tail axoneme alterations in the Wobbler mouse. *J. Reprod. Fertil.*, 58:267–270.
500. Olds, P. J. (1971): Effect of the T locus on sperm ultrastructure in the house mouse. *J. Anat.*, 109:31–37.
501. Bryan, J. H. D. (1977): Spermatogenesis revisited. IV. Abnormal spermiogenesis in mice homozygous for another male-sterility-inducing mutation, hpy (hydrocephalic-polydactyl). *Cell Tissue Res.*, 180:187–201.
502. Serres, C., Feneux, D., and Jouannet, P. (1986): Abnormal distribution of the periaxonemal structures in a human sperm flagellar dyskinesia. *Cell Motil. Cytoskel.*, 6:68–76.
503. Escalier, D., and Serres, C. (1985): Aberrant distribution of the periaxonemal structures in the human spermatozoon: Possible role of the axoneme in the spatial organization of the flagellar components. *Biol. Cell,* 53:239–250.
504. Cooper, T. G., and Hamilton, D. W. (1977): Observations on destruction of spermatozoa in the cauda epididymides and proximal vas deferens of non-seasonal male animals. *Am. J. Anat.*, 149:93–110.
505. Olson, G. E., and Linck, R. W. (1977): Observations of the structural components of flagellar axonemes and central pair microtubules from rat sperm. *J. Ultrastruct. Res.*, 61:21–43.
506. Bennett, W. I., Gall, A. M. Southard, J. L., and Sidman, R. L. (1971): Abnormal spermiogenesis in quaking. A myelin-deficient mutant mouse. *Biol. Reprod.*, 5:30–58.
507. Woolley, D. M. (1977): Evidence for twisted plane undulation in golden hamster sperm tails. *J. Cell Biol.*, 67:159–170.
508. Yeung, C. H., and Woolley, D. M. (1984): Three-dimensional bend propagation in hamster sperm models and the direction of roll in free-swimming cells. *Cell Motil.*, 4:215–226.
509. Woolley, D. M., and Osborn, I. W. (1984): Three-dimensional geometry of motile hamster spermatozoa. *J. Cell Sci.*, 67:159–170.
510. Mohri, H., and Yano, Y. (1982): Reactivation and microtubules sliding in rodent spermatozoa. *Cell Motil.* (*Suppl.*), 1:143–147.
511. Phillips, D. M., and Olson, G. E. (1975): Mammalian sperm motility. Structure in relation to function. In: *The Functional Anatomy of the Spermatozoon,* edited by B. A. Afzelius, pp. 117–126. Pergamon Press, New York.
512. Lindemann, C. B. (1980): Requirements for motility in mammalian sperm. In: *Testicular Development, Structure and Function,* edited by A. Steinberger and E. Steinberger, pp. 473–479. Raven Press, New York.
513. Yeung, C. H., and Woolley, D. M. (1983): A study of bend formation in locally reactivated hamster sperm flagella. *J. Muscle Res. Cell Motil.*, 4:625–645.
514. Rikmenspoel, R. (1984): Movements and active moments of bull sperm flagella as a function of temperature and viscosity. *J. Exp. Biol.*, 108:205–230.
515. Gray, J. (1958): The movement of the spermatozoa of the bull. *J. Exp. Biol.*, 35:96–108.
516. Serres, C., Feneux, D., Jouannet, P., and David, G. (1984): Influence of the flagellar wave development and progagation on the human sperm movement in seminal plasma. *Gamete Res.*, 9:183–195.
517. Feneux, D., Serres, C., and Jouannet, P. (1985): Sliding spermatozoa: A dyskinesia responsible for human infertility? *Fertil. Steril.*, 44:508–511.
518. Turner, T. T., and Giles, R. D. (1982): A sperm motility inhibiting factor in the rat epididymis. *Am. J. Physiol.*, 242:R199–R203.
519. Usselman, M. C., and Cone, R. A. (1983): Rat sperm are mechanically immobilized in the cauda epididymidis by "immobilin," a high molecular weight glycoprotein. *Biol. Reprod.*, 29:1241–1253.
520. Turner, T. T., and Reich, G. W. (1985): Cauda epididymal sperm motility: A comparison among five species. *Biol. Reprod.*, 32:120–128.

521. Carr, D. W., and Acott, T. S. (1984): Inhibition of bovine spermatozoa by cauda epididymidal fluid: I. Studies of a sperm motility quiescence factor. *Biol. Reprod.*, 30:913–925.
522. Hoskins, D. D., Stephens, D. T., and Hall, M. L. (1974): Cyclic adenosine 3′,5′-monophosphate and protein kinase levels in developing bovine spermatozoa. *J. Reprod. Fertil.*, 37:131–133.
523. Amann, R. P., Hay, S. R., and Hammerstedt, R. H. (1982): Yield, characteristics, motility and cAMP content of sperm isolated from seven regions of ram epididymis. *Biol. Reprod.*, 27:723–733.
524. Hoskins, D. D., Hall, M. L., and Munsterman, D. (1975): Induction of motility in immature bovine spermatozoa by cyclic AMP phosphodiesterase inhibitors and seminal plasma. *Biol. Reprod.*, 13:168–176.
525. Brandt, H., Acott, T. S., Johnson, D. J., and Hoskins, D. D. (1978): Evidence for the epididymal origin of bovine sperm forward motility protein. *Biol. Reprod.*, 19:830–835.
526. Acott, T. S., Katz, D. F., and Hoskins, D. D. (1983): Movement characteristics of bovine epididymal spermatozoa: Effects of forward motility protein and epididymal maturation. *Biol. Reprod.*, 29:389–399.
527. Garbers, D. L. Tubb, D. J., and Hyne, R. V. (1982): A requirement of bicarbonate for Ca^{2+}-induced elevation of cyclic AMP in guinea pig spermatozoa. *J. Biol. Chem.*, 257:8980–8984.
528. Vijayaraghavan, S., Critchlow, L. M., and Hoskins, D. D. (1985): Evidence for a role for cellular alkalinization in the cyclic adenosine 3′,5′-monophosphate-mediated initiation of motility in bovine caput spermatozoa. *Biol. Reprod.*, 32:489–500.
529. Gibbons, I. R. (1981): Cilia and flagella of eukaryotes. *J. Cell Biol.*, 91:107s–124s.
530. Lindemann, C. B. (1978): A cAMP-induced increase in the motility of demembranated bull sperm models. *Cell*, 13:9–18.
531. Mohri, H., and Yanagimachi, R. (1980): Characteristics of motor apparatus in testicular, epididymal and ejaculated spermatozoa. A study using demembranated sperm models. *Exp. Cell Res.*, 127:191–196.
532. White, I. G., and Voglmayr, J. K. (1986): ATP-induced reactivation of ram testicular, cauda epididymal, and ejaculated spermatozoa extracted with Triton X-100. *Biol. Reprod.*, 34:183–193.
533. Garbers, D. L., and Kopf, G. S. (1980): The regulation of spermatozoa by calcium and cyclic nucleotides. In: *Advances in Cyclic Nucleotide Research,* edited by P. Greengard and G. A. Robison, pp. 251–306. Raven Press, New York.
534. Hyne, R. V., and Garbers, D. L. (1979): Regulation of guinea pig sperm adenylate cyclase by calcium. *Biol. Reprod.*, 21:1135–1142.
535. Wasco, W. M., and Orr, G. A. (1984): Function of calmodulin in mammalian sperm: Presence of a calmodulin-dependent cyclic nucleotide phosphodiesterase associated with demembranated rat caudal epididymal sperm. *Biochem. Biophys. Res. Commun.*, 188:632–642.
536. Horowitz, J. A., Toeg, H., and Orr, G. A. (1984): Characterization and localization of cAMP-dependent protein kinases in rat caudal epididymal sperm. *J. Biol. Chem.*, 259:832–838.
537. Atherton, R. W. Khatoon, S., Schoff, P. K., and Haley, B. E. (1985): A study of rat epididymal sperm adenosine 3′,5′-monophosphate-dependent protein kinases: Maturation differences and cellular location. *Biol. Reprod.*, 32:155–171.
538. Noland, T. D., Corbin, J. D., and Garbers, D. L. (1986): Cyclic AMP-dependent protein kinase isozymes of bovine epididymal spermatozoa: Evidence against the existence of an ectokinase. *Biol. Reprod.*, 34:681–689.
539. Tang, F. Y., and Hoskins, D. D. (1976): Phosphoprotein phosphatase of bovine epididymal spermatozoa. *Biochem. Biophys. Res. Commun.*, 62:328–335.
540. Tash, J. S. (1976): Investigations on adenosine 3′,5′-monophosphate phosphodiesterase in ram semen and initial characterization of a sperm-specific enzyme. *J. Reprod. Fertil.*, 47:63–67.
541. Stephens, D. T., Wang, J. L., and Hoskins, D. D. (1979): The cyclic AMP phosphodiesterase of bovine spermatozoa: Multiple forms, kinetic properties, and changes during development. *Biol. Reprod.*, 20:483–491.
542. Tash, J. S., and Means, A. R. (1982): Regulation of protein phosphorylation and motility of sperm by cyclic adenosine monophosphate and calcium. *Biol. Reprod.*, 26:745–763.
543. Ono, T., Koide, Y., Arai, Y., and Yamashita, K. (1985): Establishment of an efficient purification method and further characterization of 32K calmodulin-binding protein in testis. *J. Biochem.*, 98:1455–1461.
544. Okamura, N., and Sugita, Y. (1983): Activation of spermatozoan adenylate cyclase by a low molecular weight factor in porcine seminal plasma. *J. Biol. Chem.*, 258:13056–13062.
545. Vijayaraghavan, S., and Hoskins, D. D. (1986): Regulation of bovine sperm motility and cyclic adenosine 3′,5′-monophosphate by adenosine and its analogues. *Biol. Reprod.*, 34:468–477.
546. Hyne, R. V., and Lopata, A. (1982): Calcium and adenosine affect human sperm adenylate cyclase activity. *Gamete Res.*, 6:81–89.
547. Brown, M. A., and Casillas, E. R. (1984): Bovine sperm adenylate cyclase inhibition by adenosine and adenosine analogs. *J. Androl.*, 5:361–368.
548. Henry, D., Ferino, F., Tomova, S., Ferry, N., Stengel, D., and Hanoune, J. (1986): Inhibition of the catalytic subunit of ram sperm adenylate cyclase by adenosine. *Biochem. Biophys. Res. Commun.*, 137:970–977.
549. Forte, L. R., Bylund, D. B., and Zahler, W. L. (1983): Forskolin does not activate sperm adenylate cyclase. *Mol. Pharmacol.*, 24:42–47.
550. Hildebrandt, J. D., Codina, J., Tash, J. S., Kirchick, H. J., Lipschultz, L., Sekura, R. D., and Birnbaumer, L. (1985): The membrane-bound spermatozoal adenyl cyclase system does not share coupling characteristics with somatic cell adenyl cyclases. *Endocrinology,* 116:1357–1366.
551. Kopf, G. S., Woolkalis, M. J., and Gerton, G. L. (1986): Evidence for a guanine nucleotide-binding regulatory protein in invertebrate and mammalian sperm. Identification by islet-activating protein-catalyzed ADP-ribosylation and immunochemical methods. *J. Biol. Chem.*, 261:7327–7331.
552. Ramarao, C., and Garbers, D. L. (1985): Receptor-mediated regulation of guanylate cyclase activity in spermatozoa. *J. Biol. Chem.*, 260:8390–8396.
553. Krebs, E. G., and Beavo, J. A. (1979): Phosphorylation-dephosphylation of enzymes. *Annu. Rev. Biochem.*,48:923–956.
554. Chulavatnatol, M., Panyim, S., and Wititsuwannakul, D. (1982): Comparison of phosphorylated proteins in intact rat spermatozoa from caput and cauda epididymidis. *Biol. Reprod.*, 26:197–207.
555. Brandt, H., and Hoskins, D. D. (1980): A cAMP-dependent phosphorylated motility protein in bovine epididymal sperm. *J. Biol. Chem.*, 255:982–987.
556. Tash, J. S., Kakar, S. S., and Means, A. R. (1984): Flagellar motility requires the cAMP-dependent phosphorylation of a heat-stable NP-40-soluble 56 kd protein, axokinin. *Cell,* 38:551–559.
557. de Lamirande, E., and Gagnon, C. (1984): Origin of a motility inhibitor within the male reproductive tract. *J. Androl.*, 5:269–276.
558. Freedman, M. F., and Kopf, G. S. (1985): Characterization of a seminal plasma-associated inhibitor of human seminal plasma protein kinase. *Biol. Reprod.*, 32:322–332.
559. Pliego, J. F., Van-Arsdalen, K., and Kopf, G. S. (1986): Distribution of a seminal plasma-associated protein kinase inhibitor in normal, oligozoospermic, and vasectomized men. *Biol. Reprod.*, 34:885–893.
560. Byrd, W., Sodoloski, J. E., and Wolf, D. P. (1983): Analysis of calcium uptake during incubation of human spermatozoa. *Biol. Reprod. (Suppl.)*, 28:103.
561. Rufo, G. A., Singh, J. P., Babcock, D. F., and Lardy, H. A. (1982): Purification and characterization of a calcium transport inhibitor from bovine seminal plasma. *J. Biol. Chem.*, 257:4627–4632.
562. Goh, P., and Hoskins, D. D. (1985): The involvement of methyl transfer reactions and *S*-adenosylhomocysteine in the regulation of bovine sperm motility. *Gamete Res.*, 12:399–409.
563. Bouchard, P., Penningroth, S. M., Cheung, A., Gagnon, C., and Bardin, C. W. (1981): Erythro-9-[3-(2-hydroxynonyl)] adenine is an inhibitor of sperm motility that blocks dynein ATPase and protein carboxymethylase activities. *Proc. Natl. Acad. Sci. USA,* 78:1033–1036.
564. Gagnon, C., Sherins, R. J., Phillips, D. M., and Bardin, C. W. (1982): Deficiency of protein carboxymethylase in immotile spermatozoa of infertile men. *N. Engl. J. Med.*, 306:821–825.
565. Acott, T. S., and Carr, D. W. (1984): Inhibition of bovine spermatozoa by cauda epididymal fluid: II. Interaction of pH and a quiescence factor. *Biol. Reprod.*, 30:926–935.

The Physiology of Reproduction,
edited by E. Knobil and J. Neill *et al.*
Raven Press, Ltd., New York © 1988.

CHAPTER 3

The Mammalian Ovum

Paul M. Wassarman

The mammalian ovum, or egg, is the link between one generation and the next. In 1880, Nussbaum (187) recognized that "The fertilized egg, accordingly, divides into cells that constitute the individual and cells for maintenance of the species." This concept was expanded insightfully by Wilson (285) in 1925 while explaining that the differences in form and function between sperm and egg are attributable to "a physiological division of labor between the gametes of the two sexes." Continuing this theme, Wilson explains: "The ovum has to supply most of the material for the body of the embryo, and often also to provide for its protection and maintenance during development. For this service it prepares by extensive growth, accumulating a large amount of protoplasm, commonly laden with reserve food-matter (yolk or deutoplasm), and in many cases becoming surrounded by membranes or other protective envelopes. During its early history, therefore, the ovum is characterized by predominance of the constructive or anabolic process of metabolism." Herein lies the origin of the concept that there is not only a genetic but also a biochemical basis for the phrase *embryogenesis begins during oogenesis*. Today, there is overwhelming experimental evidence that the zygote inherits from the egg an extensive reserve of macromolecules and organelles that, to varying degrees, supports the nutritional, synthetic, energetic, and regulatory requirements of the early embryo (10,55,89). This is as true for mammals as it is for lower vertebrates and invertebrates, despite the obvious enormous differences in both reproductive and developmental behavior of mammals and nonmammals.

Here, many of the features of mammalian egg development are reviewed. Although emphasis is placed on mouse egg development in order to increase the clarity of the presentation, most of the principles discussed can be applied to other mammals. Furthermore, in the interest of clarity and brevity, some important contributions are not cited and specific points of view are adopted on issues that may be the subject of some controversy among workers in the field. It is hoped that because of these and other shortcomings, the reader will be stimulated to refer to other detailed accounts of research on mammalian egg development (9,11,35,55,144,149,197,269,291,293), as well as technical aspects of this research (87,88,144,217).

THE MAMMALIAN OVUM: A CHRONOLOGICAL PERSPECTIVE

Although the ovary was recognized as an anatomical entity by Herophilus of Alexandria in ca. 300 B.C. and described in some detail by Soranus of Ephesus in ca. 50 A.D., the mammalian ovum or egg was not identified until early in the 19th century A.D. by Karl Ernst von Baer. Earlier, De Graaf (ca. 1670) had recognized that eggs came from the ovary, but concluded incorrectly that the entire follicle (Graafian follicle) was an egg. This misconception was rectified somewhat by Cruickshank (ca. 1795) and others; however, it remained for von Baer (ca. 1825) to elucidate the exact anatomical relationship between egg and follicle in mammals (Fig. 1). Therefore, nearly 150 years separated identification of spermatozoa by Leeuwenhoek (ca. 1675) and eggs by von Baer.

Waldeyer (ca. 1870) is credited with championing the concept that, in mammals, the sexually mature female possesses a finite stock of oocytes that is drawn upon throughout her reproductive life. However, the alternative view, that generation of oocytes is a continual process throughout a female's reproductive life (i.e., similar to spermatogenesis), although based on subjective interpretation of relevant observations, prevailed during the first half of this century. Not until the early 1950s was this controversial issue finally put to rest and Waldeyer's tenet accepted, due essentially to the work of Zuckerman and colleagues.

Goette (ca. 1875) and Nussbaum (ca. 1880) were among the first to recognize that primordial germ cells, destined to give rise to oocytes and eggs, arise from undifferentiated cells located some distance away from, and appearing before the formation of, the genital ridges. Appreciation for the subsequent organogenesis of the mammalian ovary came about primarily as a result of the work of de Winiwarter and Sainmont in ca. 1910, and by the 1920s, a great deal of cytological information about oocyte development was already available. In the 1920s it was recognized that the ovary is under functional control of the anterior hypophysis and, by the late 1920s and early 1930s, the relationship between oocyte and follicle development began to be appreciated as a result of work by Brambell, Parkes, Zuckerman, Pincus, and colleagues. Particularly important work during this period, primarily from Pincus's laboratory, involved comparison of mammalian egg behavior *in vivo* and *in vitro*. In the late 1930s the principal ovarian steroids were isolated and characterized, and by the early 1950s much of the endocrinological basis of pituitary-ovarian interaction affecting oogenesis and ovulation was appreciated. By the 1960s, *in vitro* culture of mammalian eggs and biochemical investigation of their metabolism became a reality as a result of work by Mintz, Biggers, McLaren, Epstein, Brinster, Graham, Piko, and others.

This brief history has been drawn from discussions found in refs. 8,187,219,241,285,292, and 294.

DEVELOPMENT OF THE OVUM

Oogenesis: From Primordial Germ Cells to Eggs

In mammals, oogenesis begins relatively early in fetal development and ends, months to years later, in the sexually mature adult (23,24,50–52,119,130,144,149,197,202, 224,242,292,294). Oogenesis begins with primordial germ cell formation and encompasses a series of cellular transformations, from primordial germ cells to oogonia (fetus), from oogonia to oocytes (fetus), and from oocytes to eggs (adult) (Fig. 2). This exquisitely orchestrated process results in a cell uniquely able to give rise to a new individual that expresses and maintains characteristics of the species. A description of oogenesis in mammals follows.

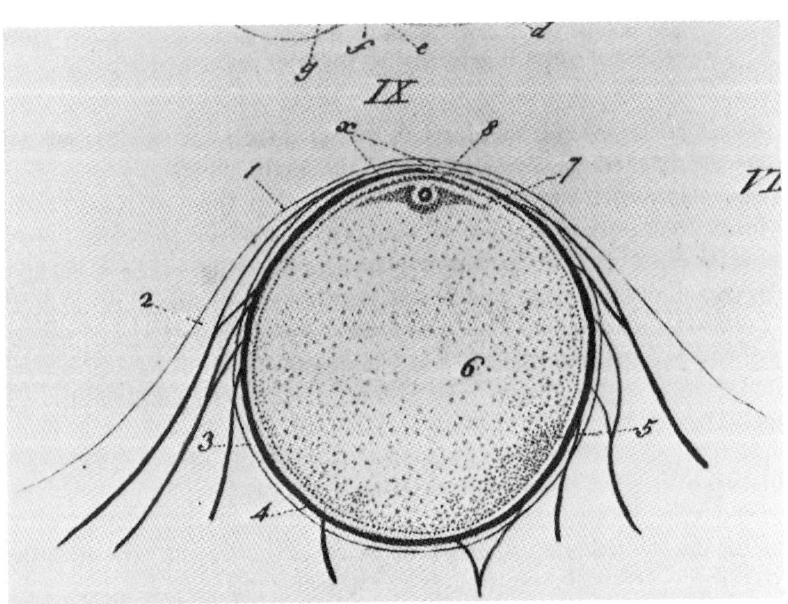

FIG. 1. Drawing of the mammalian egg within the Graafian follicle by von Baer, *De Ovi Mammalium et Hominis Genesi* (1827). Vesicula Graafiana (mediae magnitudinis) scrofae, decies aucta ad axin dissecta (IX). (*1*) Epithelium peritoneale; (*2*) tela formativa (stroma); (*3*) stratum externum (thecae); (*4*) stratum internum (thecae); (*5*) membrana granulosa (nuclei); (*6*) fluidum contentum; (*7*) discus proligerus (nuclei); (*8*) ovulum (nuclei); (*x*) stigma. (From ref. 241.)

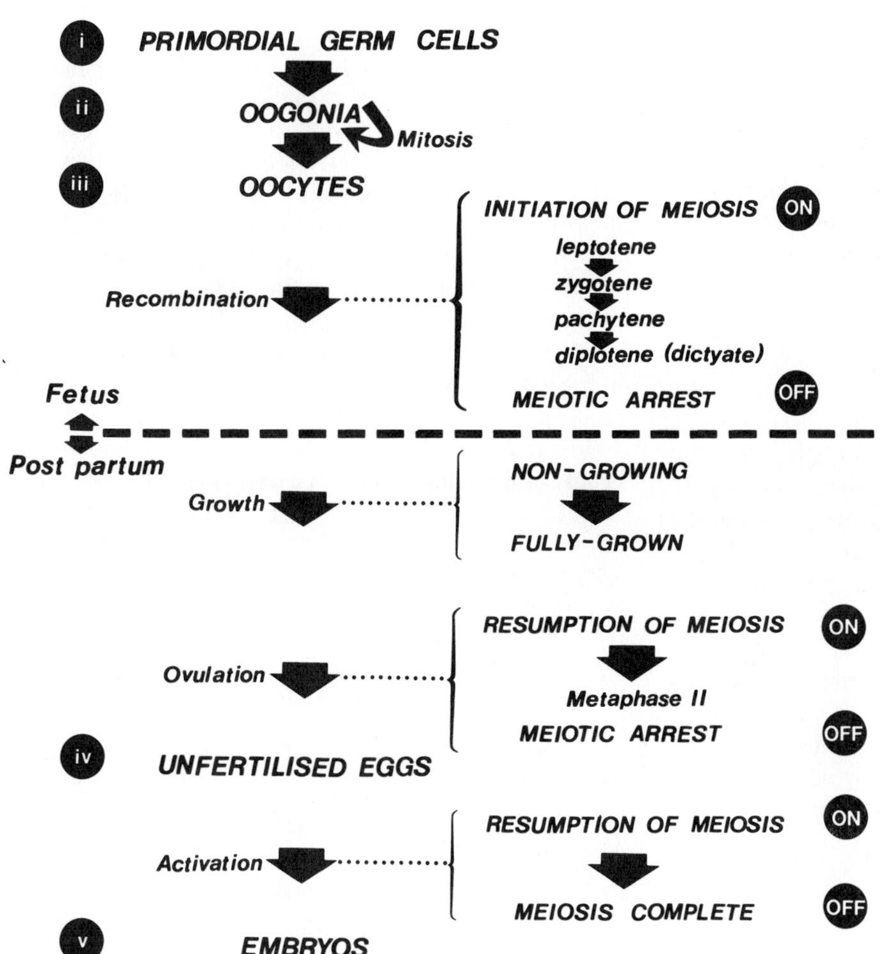

FIG. 2. Landmarks of oogenesis in the mouse. Progression from primordial germ cells to nongrowing oocytes during fetal development, as well as from nongrowing oocytes to fertilized eggs in sexually mature adults.

Origin and Behavior of Primordial Germ Cells

Eggs originate from a small number of stem cells, the *primordial germ cells,* that have an extragonadal origin (62,72,78,103,104,119,130,137,144,149,174,224). Formation of these cells in presomite embryos signals the beginning of oogenesis. In 8-day mouse embryos (4 pairs of somites), as few as 15 and as many as 100 primordial germ cells are recognizable because of their size, distinctive morphology, and characteristic cytochemical staining properties. These large cells (~12 μm in diameter) are found in the yolk-sac endoderm and in that region of the allantois arising from the primitive streak. Several lines of evidence suggest that the embryonic rudiment of the allantois and caudal end of the primitive streak may be considered regions of primordial germ cell formation. In this context, it has been found that primitive ectoderm, taken from the caudal end of 7-to 7.5-day egg cylinders and cultured *in vitro,* differentiates into cells having properties characteristic of primordial germ cells. Subsequently, primordial germ cells migrate, first by passive transfer into the endodermal epithelium of the hindgut (170–350 primordial germ cells are found in or near the hindgut epithelium in 9-day embryos) and then by ameboid movement along the dorsal mesentery of the genital ridges (present in 10- to 11-day embryos) found in the roof of the coelom; the site of gonad development. It appears likely that chemotactic mechanisms operate during migration of primordial germ cells from extraembryonic sites to the presumptive gonad. As a result of continuous mitotic activity, the number of primordial germ cells increases to approximately 5,000 in 11- to 12-day embryos and to more than 20,000 by the time genital ridges of 13- to 14-day embryos are fully colonized (Note: This represents a doubling of the number of primordial germ cells every 18 hr or so, between day 8 and day 14 of embryogenesis; it is estimated that they divide seven to eight times during the 4-day migration period). Primordial germ cells proliferate for only 2 to 3 days after migrating to the genital ridges; less than 1% of the germ cells exhibit an S phase in 16- to 17-day embryos. These primordial germ cells are the sole source of adult germ cells. It is noteworthy that the origin and migration of primordial germ cells to the genital ridges is the same in males and females; gonadal sex differentiation, to either testis or ovary, occurs in the 12- to 13-day embryo.

In summary, the germ cell line originates before or during primitive streak formation (~7-day embryo), but precisely where, when, and how is still not clear. Mouse primordial germ cells are found sequentially in four different sites as embryogenesis proceeds: (i) First, they appear in the extraembryonic tissues of the yolk sac and allantois of 8- to 9-day embryos. (ii) Then they appear in the hindgut epithelium of 9- to 10-day embryos. (iii) Then they are found in the dorsal mesentery of the gut of 10- to 12-day embryos. (iv) Finally they are found in the developing gonads of 10.5- to 11-day embryos. These primordial germ cells are the sole source of adult germ cells.

From Primordial Germ Cells to Oogonia

Upon reaching the surface epithelium of the gonad, primordial germ cells move into the cortex and, together with supporting epithelial cells, give rise to the cortical sex cords (119,129,149,293). The somatic components of the ovary arise from coelomic epithelium and mesenchyme of the dorsal body wall, and the mesonephros probably makes a contribution. In 13-day mouse embryos (52–60 pairs of somites), containing a differentiated ovary, migration of primordial germ cells is complete, with virtually all of the cells converted to actively dividing *oogonia* in the sex cords. Oogonia exhibit a characteristic morphology (including the presence of intercellular bridges connecting adjacent germ cells) and a high frequency of mitotic division.

From Oogonia to Nongrowing Oocytes

As early as day 12 of embryogenesis, a few oogonia (~5%) enter the preleptotene, and then leptotene, stage of the first meiotic prophase (23,24,62,119,129,149,202,293). Once meiotic prophase commences, apparently there is no endocrine requirement for continued meiotic progression. Furthermore, since germ cells, either cultured *in vitro* or located at ectopic sites, enter and progress through meiosis, a gonadal environment is not required for the progress of meiosis (90,264). It is during preleptotene (interphase following the last mitotic division of oogonia) that the final DNA replication takes place in preparation for *meiosis*. This synthetic activity signals transformation of oogonia into *oocytes*. It is possible that a factor originating from the rete ovarii, or simply contact with the rete ovarii, induces oogonia to enter meiosis. In 14-day mouse embryos (61–62 pairs of somites), the germ cell population is about equally divided between oogonia and oocytes, and by day 17 (full quota of 65 pairs of somites) the ovary contains only oocytes at various stages of the first meiotic prophase (17,23,24, 26–30,118,135,249). Oocytes progress through leptotene in 3 to 6 hr and then take 12 to 40 hr to complete zygotene. During zygotene, homologous chromosomes pair and synapse to form what appear to be single chromosomes but are actually bivalents composed of four chromatids. In 16-day embryos nearly all oocytes are in pachytene of the first meiotic prophase, a stage that lasts about 60 hr and involves genetic crossing-over and recombination. Therefore, it takes approximately 4 days to complete nuclear progression from leptotene through pachytene. By day 18 of embryogenesis, the first oocytes are seen in diplotene of the first meiotic prophase, with their chromosomes exhibiting chiasmata that result from crossing-over. By parturition, a majority of oocytes have entered late diplotene ("diffuse diplotene"), or the so-called dictyate stage, and by day 5 postpartum, nearly all oocytes have reached the dictyate stage, where they will remain until stimulated to resume meiosis at the time of ovulation. This pool of small (~12–15 μm in diameter), nongrowing oocytes is the sole source of unfertilized eggs in the sexually mature adult.

From Nongrowing to Fully Grown Oocytes

Shortly after birth, the mouse ovary is populated with approximately 8,000 nongrowing oocytes arrested in meiosis and enclosed within several squamous follicular cells (23,24,52,149,202,293). Approximately 50% of these oocytes are lost during the first 2 weeks following birth; this is attributable, in large measure, to oocytes leaving the ovary through the surface epithelium. However, during this same period, more oocytes begin to grow (~5%) than at any other period in the lifetime of the mouse. Commencement of oocyte growth is apparently regulated within the ovary, with the number of oocytes entering the growth phase being a function of the size of the pool of nongrowing oocytes (153). The oocyte and its surrounding follicle grow coordinately, progressing through a series of definable morphological stages (198–203). In sexually mature mice, oocytes complete growth before formation of a follicular antrum; consequently, the vast majority of follicle growth occurs after the oocyte has stopped growing. Growth is continuous, ending in either ovulation of a matured oocyte (unfertilized egg) or degeneration (atresia) of the oocyte and its follicle.

Completion of oocyte growth in the mouse takes 2 to 3 weeks, a relatively short period of time in comparison to the months or years required for completion of oocyte growth in many nonmammalian species (9,11,24,89,149,200, 202,208,273,292,294). The oocyte grows from a diameter of about 12 μm (volume ~ 0.9 pl) to a final diameter of about 80 μm (volume ~270 pl), not including the zona pellucida (discussed in the sections on structural and biochemical aspects of oocyte growth). Therefore, during its growth phase, while continually arrested in dictyate of the first meiotic prophase, the mouse oocyte undergoes a 300-fold increase in volume and becomes one of the largest cells of the body.

Each oocyte is contained within a cellular follicle (~17 μm in diameter) that grows concomitantly with the oocyte, from a single layer of a few flattened cells to three layers of cuboidal *granulosa cells* (~ 900 cells; ~125-μm-diameter follicle) by the time the oocyte has completed its growth (7,24,38,52,61,119,142,143,145,149,191,198–203,273,292–294). The *theca* is first distinguishable, outside of and separated by a basement membrane from the granulosa cells, when the granulosa region is two cell-layers thick (~400 cells; ~100-μm-diameter follicle). During a period of several days, while the oocyte remains a constant size, the follicular cells undergo rapid division, increasing to more than 50,000 cells and resulting in a *Graafian follicle* greater than 600 μm in diameter. The follicle exhibits an incipient *antrum* when it is several layers thick (~6,000 cells; ~250-μm-diameter follicle) and, as the antrum expands, the oocyte takes up an acentric position surrounded by two or more layers of granulosa cells. The innermost layer of granulosa cells becomes columnar in shape and constitutes the *corona radiata;* these cells form specialized intercellular junctions, called *gap junctions,* with the oolemma.

From Fully Grown Oocytes to Unfertilized Eggs

In sexually mature mice, fully grown oocytes in Graafian follicles resume meiosis and complete the first meiotic reductive division just prior to ovulation (discussed in the sections on structural, regulatory, and biochemical aspects of oocyte maturation). Resumption of meiosis can be mediated by a hormonal stimulus *in vivo* or simply by the release of oocytes from their ovarian follicles into a suitable culture medium *in vitro* (23,24,110,256,257,281). Oocytes undergo nuclear progression from dictyate of the first meiotic prophase (four times the haploid DNA complement) to metaphase II (two times the haploid DNA complement). They remain at this stage of meiosis in the oviduct, or in culture, until stimulated to complete meiosis when either fertilization or parthenogenetic activation occurs. Progression from the dictyate stage (*oocyte*) to metaphase II (*egg*) of meiosis is called *meiotic maturation*. Meiotic maturation is characterized by dissolution of the oocyte's nuclear (germinal vesicle) membrane, condensation of chromatin into distinct bivalents, separation of homologous chromosomes, emission of the first polar body, and arrest of meiosis with chromosomes aligned on the metaphase II spindle (discussed in the section on structural aspects of oocyte maturation). These ovulated eggs complete meiosis, with separation of chromatids and emission of a second polar body (second reductive division), upon fertilization.

Summary

It should be apparent that the process of oogenesis in mammals includes several noteworthy features, including: (a) extraembryonic and extragonadal origin of germ cells; (b) migration of germ cells to presumptive gonads; (c) sexual differentiation of germ cells into oogonia or spermatogonia; (d) cessation of mitosis (oogonia) and initiation of meiosis (oocytes); (e) prolonged cessation of meiosis in the dictyate stage; (f) oocyte growth; (g) reinitiation of meiosis (meiotic maturation; first meiotic reduction) and ovulation (eggs); and (h) completion of meiosis (second meiotic reduction) in response to fertilization. From the appearance of primordial germ cells during fetal development until ovulation of unfertilized eggs in sexually mature adults, oogenesis represents one of the most highly specialized and regulated biological processes in mammals.

GROWTH OF THE OOCYTE: STRUCTURAL ASPECTS

Oocyte Growth: General Features

Throughout the reproductive life of mammals, their ovaries contain pools of nongrowing and growing oocytes arrested in dictyate of the first meiotic prophase. Only fully grown oocytes resume meiosis and are ovulated during each reproductive (estrous) cycle. Recruitment of oocytes into the growing pool is apparently under control of pituitary gonadotropins, although oocyte growth, without follicle development, does occur in hypophysectomized animals and during culture *in vitro* in the absence of hormones.

The volume of a mouse oocyte increases nearly 300-fold during its 2-3 week growth phase. This tremendous enlargement of the cell is indicative of a period of intense metabolic activity (discussed in the section on biochemical aspects of oocyte growth) which, in turn, is reflected in marked changes in oocyte ultrastructure, including the appearance (biogenesis) of some novel organelles (2,12,37,149,190,248,252, 270,276,282,289,290). For example, cortical granules and the zona pellucida, both involved in regulating fertilization, first appear in oocytes during their growth phase. A description of certain of the ultrastructural changes accompanying oocyte growth follows.

Nucleus (Germinal Vesicle)

The nucleus, or germinal vesicle (GV), of growing mouse oocytes increases in diameter, from 9 to 10 μm in small (~20 μm) oocytes to 20 to 22 μm in fully grown (~80 μm) oocytes (77,276). Consequently, growth of mouse oocytes results in a marked change in the ratio of cytoplasmic to nucleoplasmic volume, increasing from about 8 to 1 in small oocytes to about 64 to 1 in fully grown oocytes. Concomitant with nuclear enlargement, the nucleolus and extranucleolar bodies undergo progressive, characteristic ultrastructural changes, while chromosomes remain as highly diffuse bivalents.

Nucleolus

The nucleus (GV) of growing mouse oocytes contains a single large nucleolus and, frequently, one or two smaller nucleoli. Throughout oocyte growth the nucleolus enlarges, increasing in diameter from 2 to 3 μm in small (~20 μm) oocytes to 9 to 10 μm in fully grown (~80 μm) oocytes

(75,76,276) (Fig. 3). This enlargement is accompanied by progressive changes in nucleolar fine structure, indicative of a period of intense ribosomal-RNA synthesis (25,75,76,138,176,177,189,196). The nucleolus undergoes a transition during oocyte growth, from a diffuse, reticulated type of structure, composed primarily of a fibrillogranular network (small oocytes), to a dense, uniform mass, exclusively fibrillar in nature (fully grown oocytes).

Mitochondria

Oocyte growth is accompanied not only by a substantial increase in the number of mitochondria present, but also by marked changes in mitochondrial ultrastructure (250,252,276,286,290) (Fig. 4). Small (~20 μm) oocytes contain elongated (~1.5 μm long) mitochondria with numerous transversely oriented cristae in the so-called orthodox configuration and, in most cases, contain a single vacuole. Continued oocyte growth is accompanied by accumulation of round- and oval-shaped mitochondria, which are vacuolated and beginning to display columnar-shaped arched cristae. Throughout this growth period, mitochondria are closely associated with smooth endoplasmic reticulum and are present in increasing numbers. Many dumbbell-shaped mitochondria are found, indicative of extensive mitochondrial growth and division. Fully grown oocytes (~80 μm) contain round or oval (~0.5 μm diameter), highly vacuolated mitochondria (~10^5 per oocyte) (175,207) that have arched and concentrically arranged cristae. Consequently, the morphology of mitochondria in fully grown oocytes is radically different than that of mitochondria in nongrowing and small oocytes.

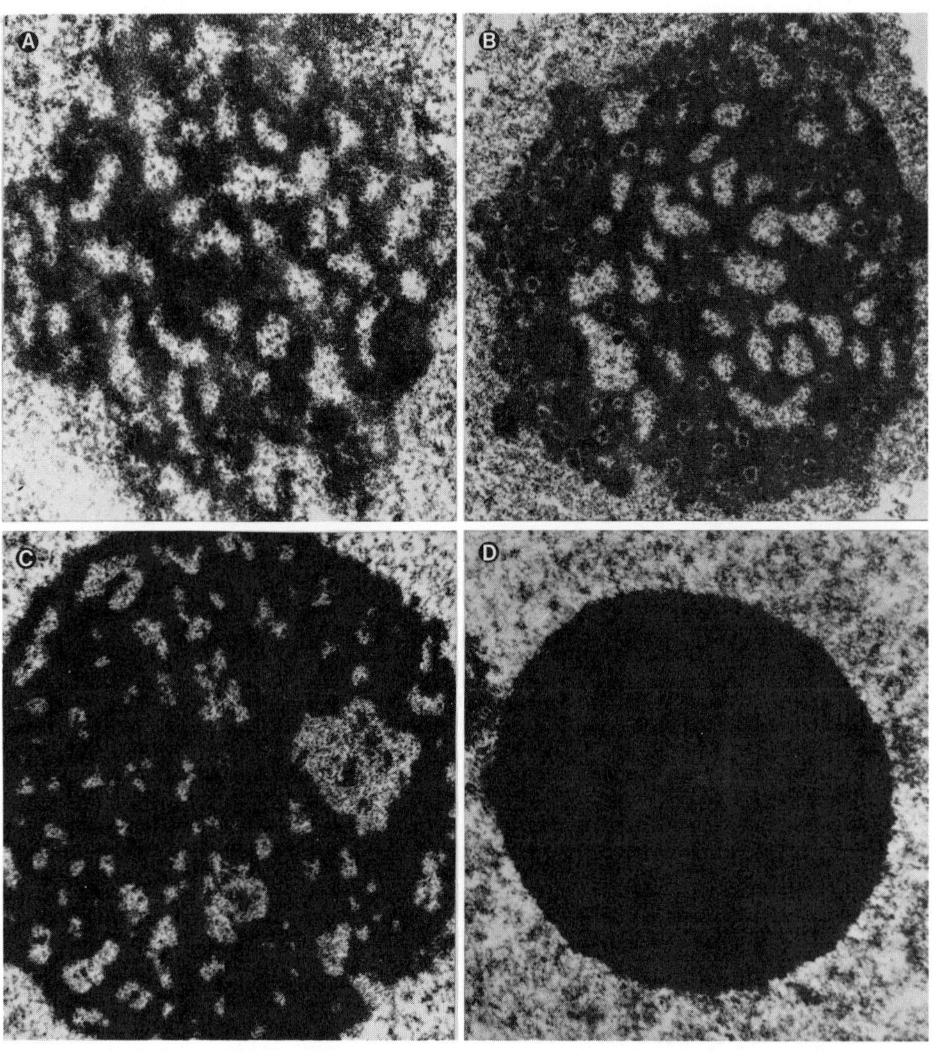

FIG. 3. Transmission electron micrographs comparing nucleolar ultrastructure during growth of the mouse oocyte. Oocytes are isolated from 3- (**A**), 5- (**B**), 10- (**C**), and 14-day-old (**D**) animals and range in diameter from about 20 μm (3 days) to 60 μm (14 days). Note the marked change from a sparse, fibrillogranular (A) to a dense (D) nucleolus during oocyte growth. (From ref. 276.)

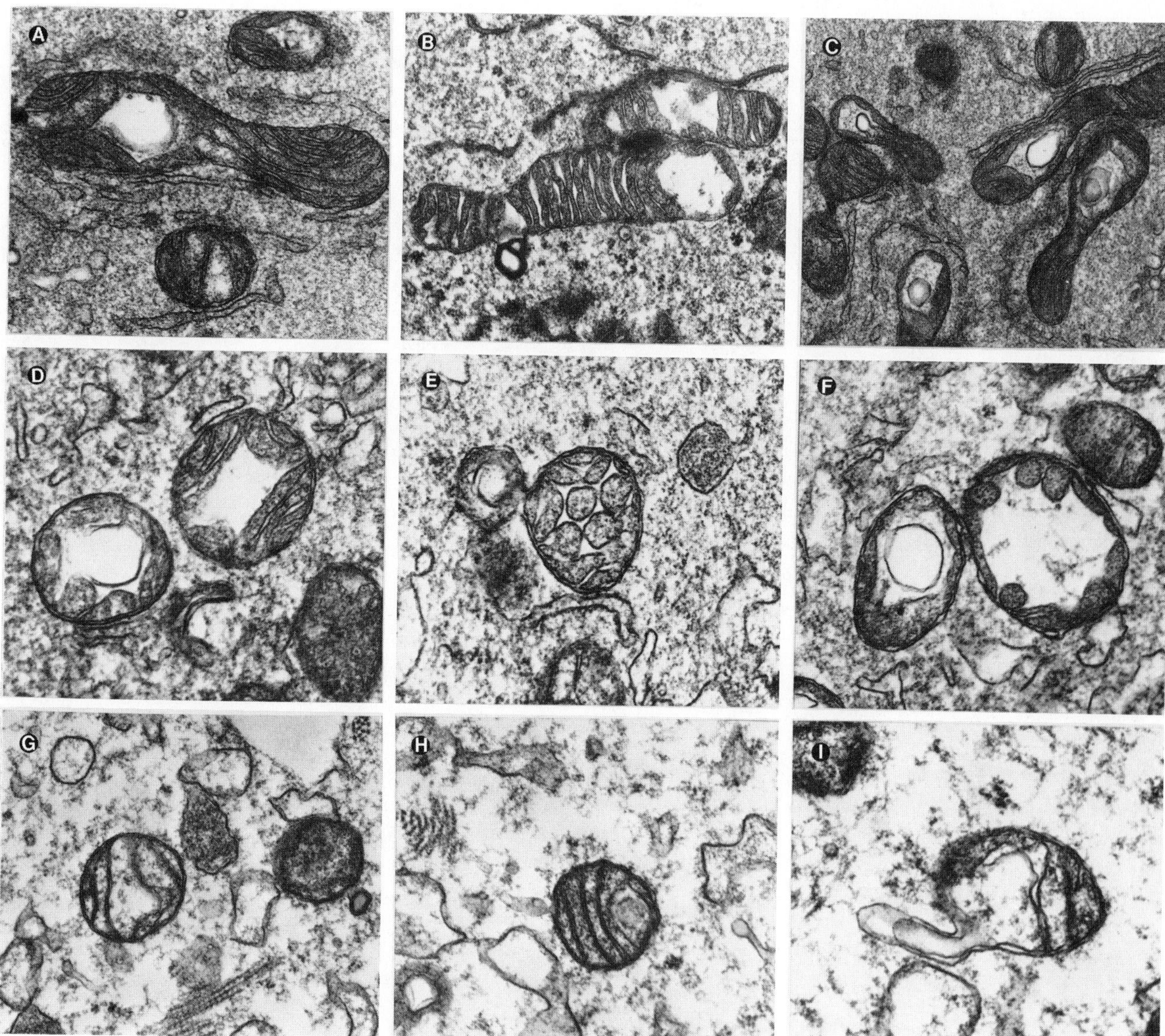

FIG. 4. Transmission electron micrographs comparing mitochondrial ultrastructure during growth of the mouse oocyte. Oocytes are isolated from 5- (**A**), 3- (**B**), 5- (**C**), 10- (**D–F**), and 21-day-old (**G–I**) animals and range in diameter from about 20 μm (3 days) to 85 μm (21 days). Note the marked change from elongated mitochondria with transverse cristae ("orthodox configuration") (A–C) to round or oval mitochondria with concentric cristae ("unorthodox configuration") (D–I) during oocyte growth. (From ref. 276.)

Golgi Complex

As in the case of mitochondria, the Golgi complex undergoes dramatic ultrastructural changes during oocyte growth; these changes are indicative of increasing Golgi activity (252,276,290) (Fig. 5). In small (~20 μm) oocytes, Golgi membranes appear as flattened stacks of arched lamellae and are associated with few, if any, vacuoles or granules. During early stages of oocyte growth, Golgi membranes become more active, as evidenced by lamellae that are spaced further apart (swelling at termini of lamellae), by the appearance of vacuoles, and by the proximity of numerous lipid vesicles. In the middle to late stages of oocyte growth, Golgi membranes exhibit increased numbers of very swollen, stacked lamellae that are associated with numerous vacuoles, granules, coated vesicles, and lipid vesicles. These changes are consistent with increased participation of the Golgi in processing and concentration of secretory products (e.g., zona pellucida glycoproteins) and cortical granule formation during oocyte growth. It is noteworthy that, concomitant with the conversion of fully grown oocytes to fertilized eggs, there is a dramatic decrease in the amount of recognizable Golgi membrane and an increase in the number of small membrane vesicles.

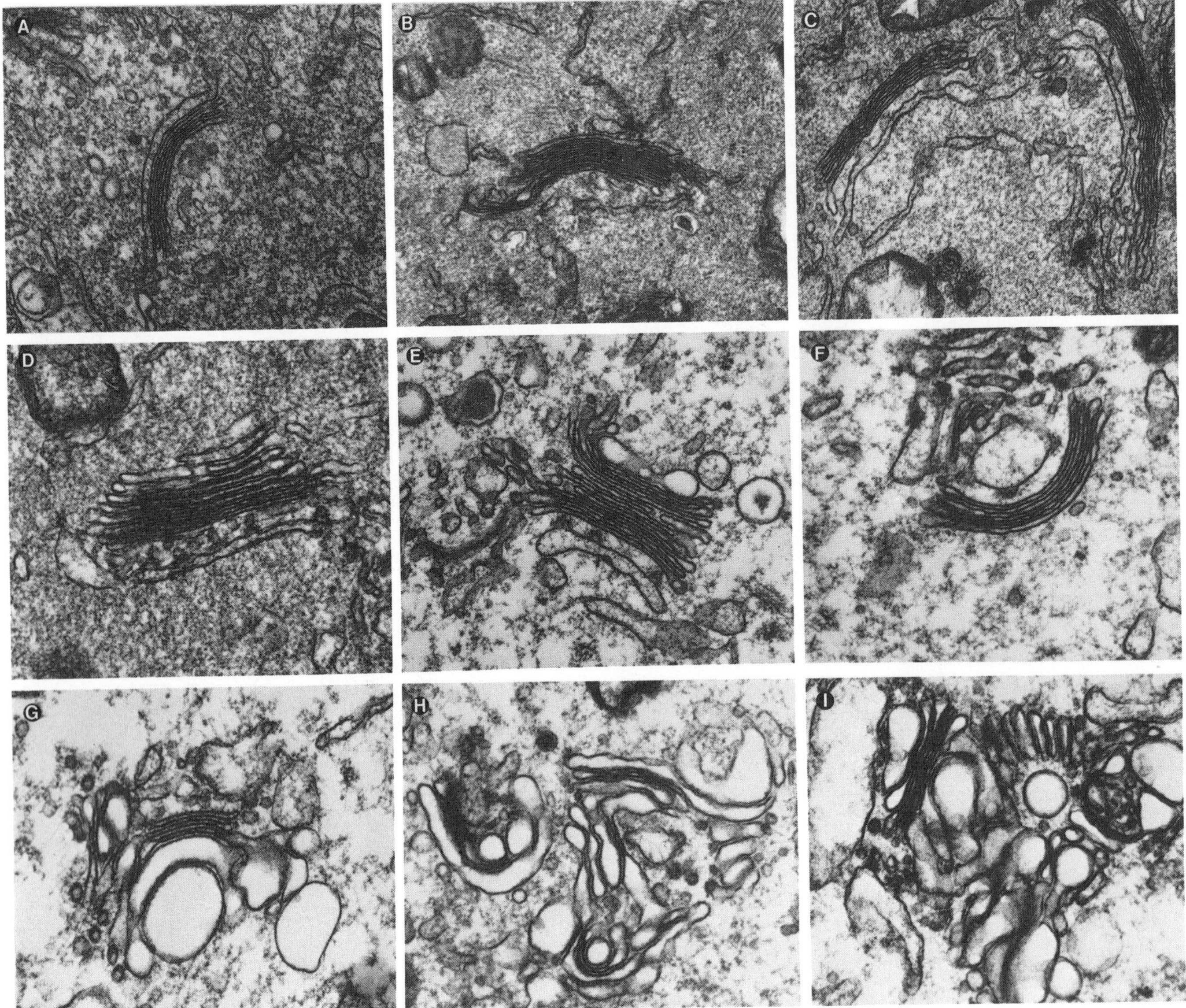

FIG. 5. Transmission electron micrographs comparing Golgi complex ultrastructure during growth of the mouse oocyte. Oocytes isolated from 3- (**A**), 5- (**B**), 8- (**C**), 10- (**D**), 14- (**E,F**), and 21-day-old (**G–I**) animals and ranging in diameter from about 20 μm (3 days) to 85 μm (21 days). Note the marked change from flattened stacks of parallel lamellae (A–D) to swollen, highly vacuolated, granular lamellae (E–I) during oocyte growth. (From ref. 276.)

Cortical Granules

Cortical granules are small, spherical, membrane-bound organelles that are found in the cortical region of unfertilized eggs and thought to resemble lysosomes (133,230). These granules fuse with the oolema at fertilization and, by releasing their contents (including proteinases) into the perivitelline space, alter functional properties of the zona pellucida (secondary block to polyspermy). Mouse eggs contain approximately 4,500 cortical granules (ranging in diameter from 200 to 600 μm) within about 2 μm of the plasma membrane (188). Cortical granules first appear during oocyte growth, associated with an expanding Golgi that has moved to the subcortical region of growing oocytes. Although it is clear that cortical granules are derived from Golgi, certain evidence suggests that there is a contribution from multivesicular bodies as well as from granular endoplasmic reticulum. Morphological studies suggest that the cortical-granule population is heterogeneous with respect to contents, with some granules even containing ordered crystalline arrays. It is unclear whether this heterogeneity of cortical-granule contents reflects functional differences or simply different extents of granule maturation. In any case, it is clear that oocyte growth is accompanied by formation and accumulation of increasing numbers of cortical granules in anticipation of ovulation and fertilization.

Zona Pellucida

The *zona pellucida,* a relatively thick extracellular coat that surrounds all mammalian eggs, appears during oocyte growth, increasing in width as oocytes increase in diameter (40,55,73,102,136,150,273,276) (Fig. 6). In mice, the zona pellucida of fully grown oocytes is about 7 μm thick, contains about 3 ng of protein, and is permeable to both large macromolecules and small viruses. The protein components of zonae pellucidae are synthesized and secreted by growing oocytes, representing a major metabolic activity of the oocyte during this period (discussed in the section on biochemical aspects of oocyte growth). Appearance of zona pellucida material in the perivitelline space correlates with initiation of oocyte growth; nongrowing oocytes do not have a zona pellucida. In early stages of oocyte growth, zona pellucida material appears as patches of fine filaments between the oocyte and follicle cells (Fig. 7). These filaments are of uniform width, can be several microns in length, and exhibit a structural periodicity (132). As growth continues, the zona pellucida becomes a denser and thicker meshwork of interconnected filaments completely surrounding the oocyte and largely separating it from follicle cells. However, contact between the oocyte and the innermost layer of follicle cells continues via junctional complexes formed between oocyte microvilli and follicle cell extensions that penetrate the zona pellucida (discussed in the section on the role of intercellular communication). As in the case of cortical granules, the zona pellucida is laid down during oocyte growth in anticipation of its roles during and after fertilization (11). The zona pellucida contains sperm receptors that mediate sperm-egg interaction as a prelude to fertilization; it also participates in a secondary block to polyspermy following fertilization of eggs (41,42,115,116).

Ribosomes

Ribosomal RNA accumulates through much of mouse oocyte growth (discussed in the section on biochemical aspects of oocyte growth), consistent with changes in nucleolar morphology during this period. It is estimated that the number of ribosomes present in the cytoplasm increases three- to fourfold as the oocyte diameter increases from 20 to 65 μm (122). In view of the enormous change in oocyte volume during this period of growth, this suggests that ribosome density (i.e., number of ribosomes per square micron of cytoplasm) decreases as much as 10-fold. The number of ribosomes present in polysomes also increases severalfold during oocyte growth, with the number of single polysomes, which are abundant in small oocytes (>70% of total), decreasing dramatically (<10% of total) in large oocytes. These changes in the ribosome population during oocyte growth are consistent with changes in overall rates of protein synthesis during this period. For, while the rate of protein synthesis per oocyte increases dramatically, the

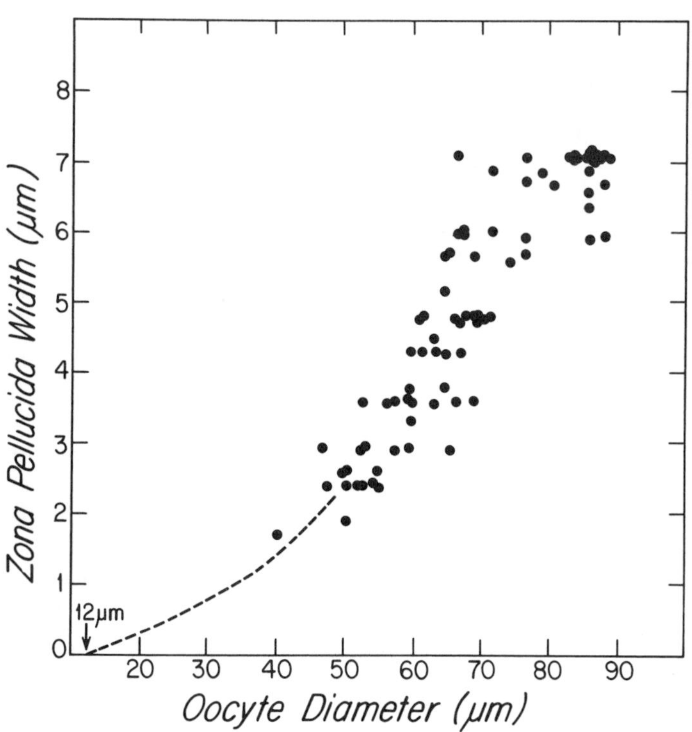

FIG. 6. Relationship between width of zona pellucida and diameter of oocytes during growth of mouse oocytes. Note that as oocytes increase in diameter from about 40 μm to 85 μm the zona pellucida increases in width from about 1.6 to 7 μm (i.e., about 4.5 times). (Data taken from J. M. Greve and P. M. Wassarman, *unpublished results.*)

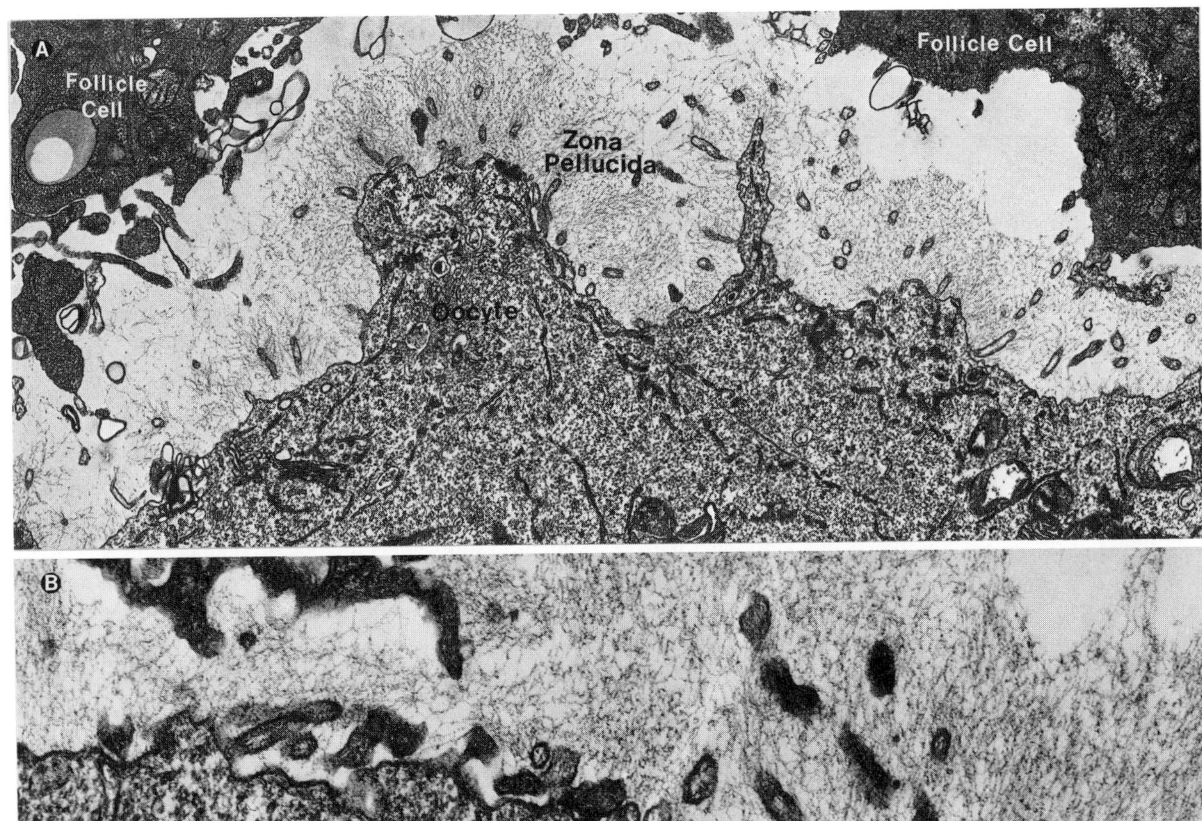

FIG. 7. Transmission electron micrographs of mouse zona pellucida filaments during the early stages of oocyte growth. Shown are stained and sectioned growing oocytes (about 20 μm in diameter) with associated follicle cells and developing zona pellucida (**A,B**). Note the filamentous nature of the nascent zona pellucida and its close apposition to the surface of the growing oocyte.

rate per picoliter of cytoplasm actually decreases during oocyte growth (discussed in the section on biochemical aspects of oocyte growth).

Cytoplasmic Lattices

Lattice-like structures (placques, lamellae, fibrillar arrays) are found in the cytoplasm of both fully grown mouse oocytes and unfertilized eggs (60,252,282–284,290). Although not present in nongrowing oocytes, these lattices increase in number dramatically throughout oocyte growth and become a dominant feature of the fully grown oocyte. In some cases, the lattices appear as highly ordered aggregates of individual chains (60) (Fig. 8). The chains, in turn, are composed of particles that are connected by bridges, giving rise to a structural periodicity. The individual chains themselves are interconnected, so that lattices appear to form layers of interconnected sheets. The function of this extremely abundant cytoplasmic component is not known, although the possibility that it serves either as yolk (252) or as a storage form of ribosomes (18,21,58,60,205), since it completely disappears during the cleavage stages of early embryogenesis, has been considered.

OOCYTE MATURATION: STRUCTURAL ASPECTS

Meiotic Maturation: General Features

Meiotic maturation specifically refers to the conversion of fully grown oocytes (present in antral follicles) into unfertilized eggs just prior to ovulation, following the preovulatory gonadotropin [follicle-stimulating hormone (FSH) and luteinizing hormone (LH)] surge. In particular, meiotic maturation involves nuclear progression, from dictyate of the first meiotic prophase (late G_2) to metaphase II (first meiotic reduction), as well as metabolic changes necessary for activation of the egg at fertilization. Isolated, fully grown oocytes undergo meiotic maturation spontaneously during culture *in vitro* in the absence of hormones (70,209,255), thus providing an advantageous experimental system for structural and biochemical studies. The timing of cytological events (e.g., nuclear membrane breakdown, spindle formation, etc.) observed with maturing oocytes *in vitro* resembles that observed *in vivo*. Only oocytes that have undergone successful meiotic maturation are capable of being fertilized and developing normally. Mammalian oocytes matured and fertilized *in vitro* exhibit normal preimplantation development *in vitro* (180,269) and develop into vi-

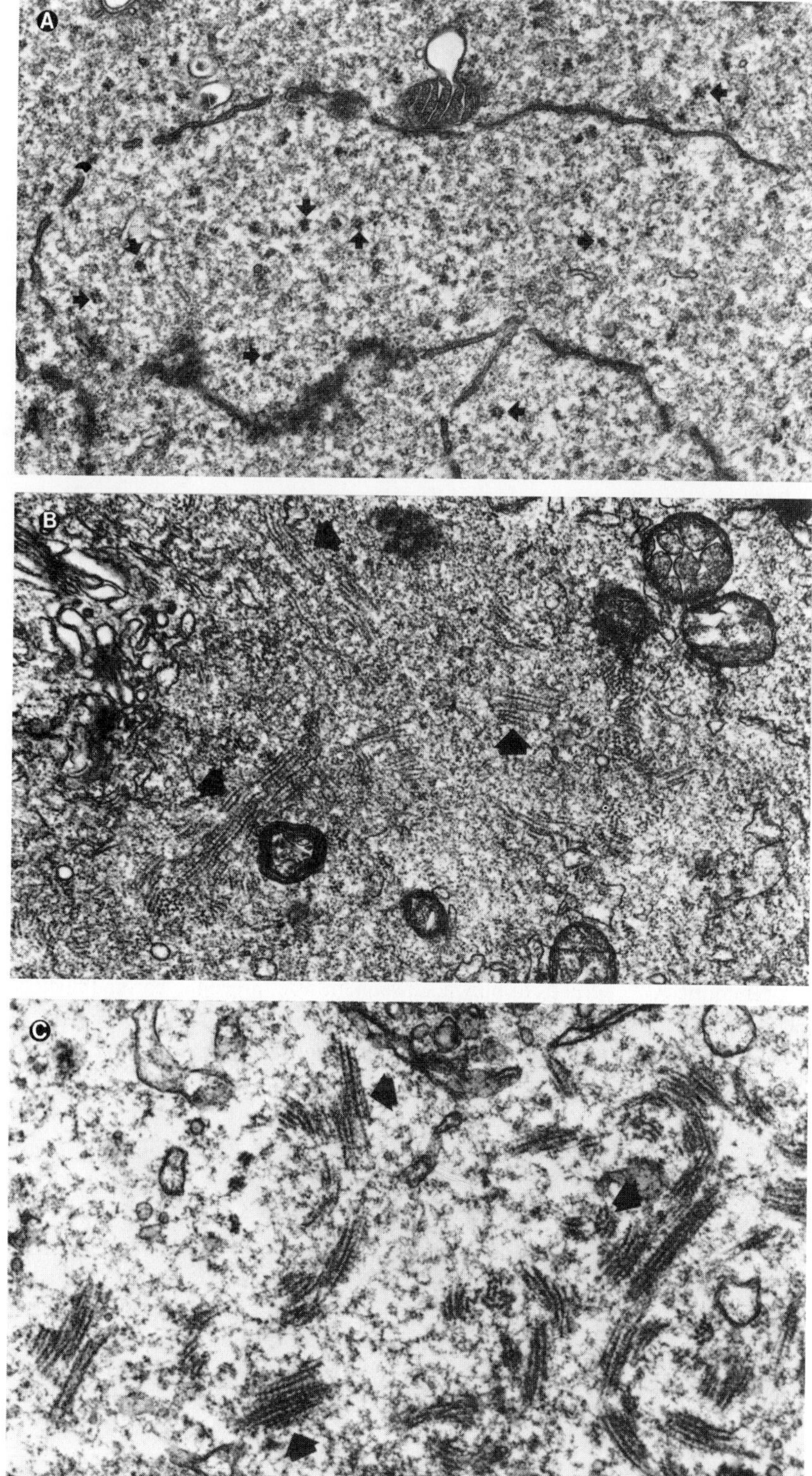

FIG. 8. Transmission electron micrographs comparing oocyte cytoplasm during growth of the mouse oocyte. Oocytes are isolated from 3- (**A**), 10- (**B**), and 21-day-old (**C**) animals and range in diameter from about 20 μm (3 days) to 85 μm (21 days). Note the abundance of clustered ribosomes during the early stages of oocyte growth (A: *arrows*), the appearance of lattice structures during the middle stages of oocyte growth (B: *arrows*), and the considerable accumulation of lattice structures during the late stages of oocyte growth (C: *arrows*). (From ref. 276.)

able fetuses following transplantation to the uteri of foster mothers (85,186,229).

Acquisition of Meiotic Competence

Dictyate-stage oocytes acquire the ability to undergo meiotic reduction (*meiotic competence*) during oocyte growth (247,254,256,257). This applies to oocytes *in vivo* as well as to those grown under *in vitro* conditions. Only mouse oocytes larger than about 60 μm in diameter mature *in vitro;* smaller oocytes remain arrested at the dictyate stage (Fig. 9). However, small meiotically incompetent oocytes are able to mature *in vitro* following fusion with large meiotically competent oocytes (31,32,121). The acquisition of

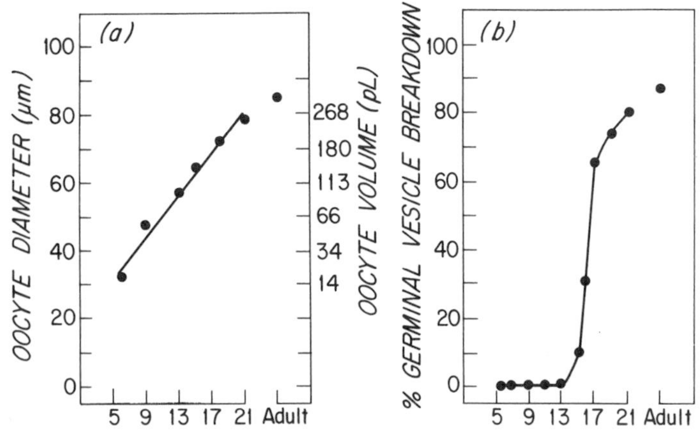

FIG. 9. Relationship between mouse oocyte diameter and ability of oocytes to undergo meiotic maturation *in vitro.* (**a**) Diameter (in microns) of isolated oocytes as a function of the age (days *post-partum*) of the donor mice. (**b**) Percent of isolated oocytes undergoing germinal vesicle breakdown *in vitro* as a function of the age (days *post-partum*) of the donor mice. (Data taken from ref. 247.)

meiotic competence apparently occurs in two steps; growing oocytes first acquire the ability to undergo nuclear (GV) envelope breakdown with progression to metaphase I, followed by acquisition of the ability to progress from metaphase I to metaphase II (247). Certain evidence suggests that the acquisition of meiotic competence is time dependent, but independent of the presence of follicle cells, heterologous cell contacts, and cell growth (65). In this context, it is evident that mouse oocytes should be included among those meiotic and mitotic cell types for which the transition from G_2 to M phase of the cell cycle is regulated by a cytoplasmic factor, the so-called maturation-promoting factor (MPF). MPF activity appears during meiotic maturation of mouse oocytes (31,246). Finally, a role for hypophyseal hormones (especially FSH) in the acquisition of meiotic competence has been suggested, with their effect mediated by follicular steroids (estrogen).

Nuclear (Germinal Vesicle) Breakdown

Within a few hours of culture *in vitro,* fully grown mouse oocytes undergo complete nuclear (GV) breakdown or dissolution (64,99,245) (Fig. 10). This process begins with slight undulation of the nuclear envelope a few minutes after placing oocytes in culture, which continues with increasing intensity during the next 1 to 2 hr. These undulations may be related to chromosome condensation that is initiated during this period. Nuclear pores disappear within 1 hr or so of culture; breaks in the nuclear envelope are visible after about 2 hr, on average. After 3 hr of culture, on average, the nuclear envelope is completely dispersed into membrane doublets that apparently join the endoplasmic reticulum pool, perhaps to play a subsequent role in pronuclear and nuclear envelope formation (253). The mean time for complete breakdown of the nuclear envelope, measured from the first

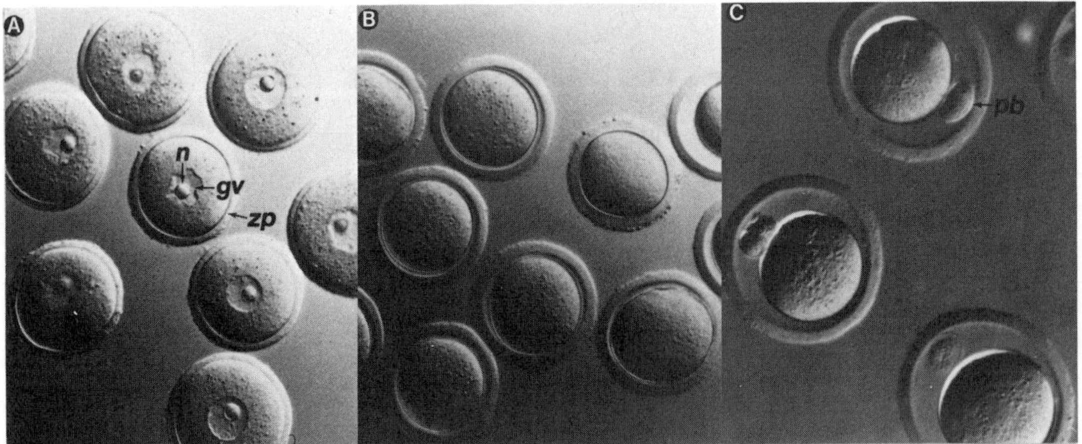

FIG. 10. Light photomicrographs of fully grown mouse oocytes during culture *in vitro.* Photographs were taken using Nomarski differential interference contrast microscopy. **A:** Isolated oocytes arrested in dictyate of the first meiotic prophase. **B:** Isolated oocytes that have undergone germinal vesicle breakdown and chromosome condensation during culture. **C:** Isolated oocytes that have completed meiotic maturation in culture and become unfertilized eggs. Note that they have emitted a polar body and have arrested at metaphase II. (gv) Germinal vesicle; (n) nucleolus; (zp) zona pellucida.

sign of membrane disintegration to disappearance of the nucleolus, is 11 min. Disappearance of the nucleolus occurs shortly after contacting invading cytoplasm (Fig. 11).

Chromosome Condensation

During meiotic maturation, oocyte chromosomes (bivalents) pass through metaphase I, anaphase I, and telophase I, arresting at metaphase II without an intervening prophase II (Fig. 12). Diffuse dictyate-stage chromosomes (resembling "lampbrush" chromosomes) undergo significant condensation along the inner margin of the nuclear envelope, concomitant with the envelope's undulatory behavior (64,277). During this period, chiasmata move to the ends of the chromosomes. The chromatin becomes heterochromatic and contains dense granules that increase in number with increasing chromosome condensation. Chromosome condensation occurs within the agranular vestige of the nucleus within 20 min of nucleolar dissolution. After 2 to 3 hr of culture, on average, when chromosome condensation is nearly complete (with "lampbrush" loops withdrawn), the bivalents are V-shaped and telocentric and are often associated with fragments of nuclear envelope. Shortly thereafter, highly condensed chromosomes become circularly arranged in the center of the egg, lose their contacts with nuclear envelope fragments, and then (after 6–9 hr of culture) line up on the equator of the metaphase-I spindle.

Spindle Formation

During the period of nuclear envelope breakdown and chromosome condensation, kinetochores with associated microtubules, as well as other microtubule organizing centers, appear; microtubules extend from these centers, through breaks in the nuclear envelope, into the nucleoplasm (63,64). Apparently, there is a kinetochore associated with each chromatid of each chromosomal homolog. A small but morphologically identifiable meiotic spindle appears after about 6 hr of culture and is clearly recognizable by 9 hr (Fig. 13). Unlike the situation in most cells, the poles of the oocyte spindle lack centrioles and are composed solely of bands of so-called pericentriolar material. The size of the spindle increases progressively, with a fully formed, barrel-shaped metaphase-I spindle present within 9 to 10 hr of culture (99,245,275). The pole-to-pole distance of the spindle is about 40 μm, and its width is about 25 μm. One of the spindle's poles is located near the cortex of the cell; the spindle is surrounded by a dense area composed of mitochondria, vacuoles, and granules. As meiosis proceeds to anaphase, bivalents move toward the opposite ends of the spindle, and the spindle rotates through 90°; these movements apparently involve microfilaments. It is noteworthy that maturing oocytes spend about 6 hr in prometaphase I (period from initial chromosome condensation to line up of bivalents on the metaphase I plate) and about 4 hr in me-

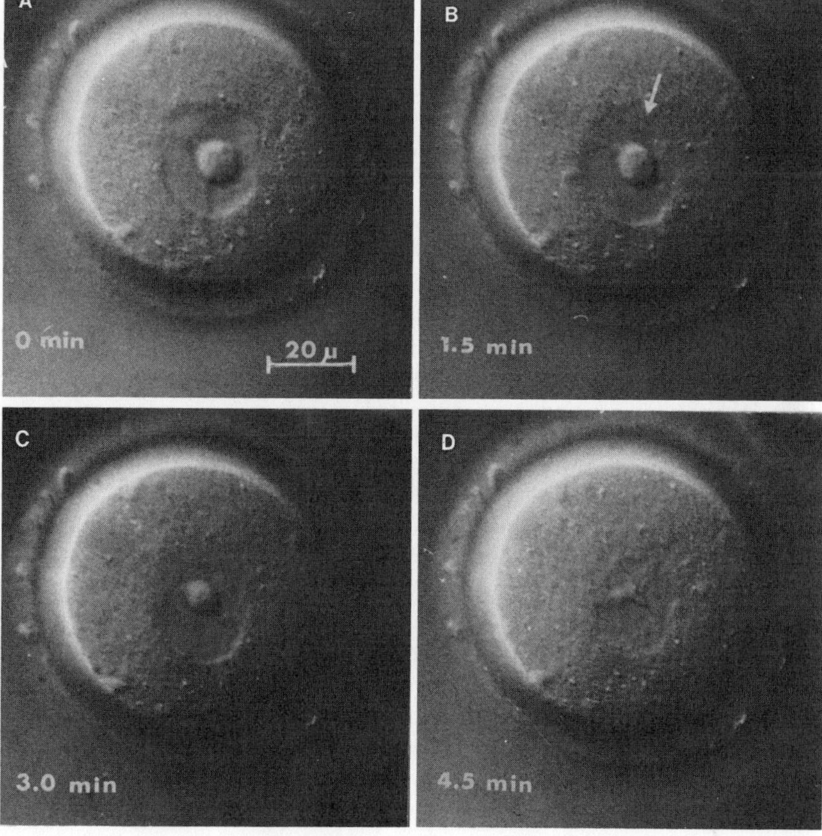

FIG. 11. Light photomicrographs of a fully grown mouse oocyte undergoing germinal vesicle breakdown during culture *in vitro.* Photographs were taken from a cinefilm made using Nomarski differential interference contrast microscopy. Actual time elapsed (in minutes) is recorded. **A:** Intact germinal vesicle with a single prominent nucleolus. **B:** Incipient disintegration of the germinal vesicle membrane with invasion of cytoplasm into the germinal vesicle. **C:** Vestiges of germinal vesicle remain and the nucleolus begins to shrink in size. **D:** Complete dissolution of the germinal vesicle membrane with only a small remnant of the nucleolus remaining; the region occupied by the germinal vesicle remains granular. (From ref. 245.)

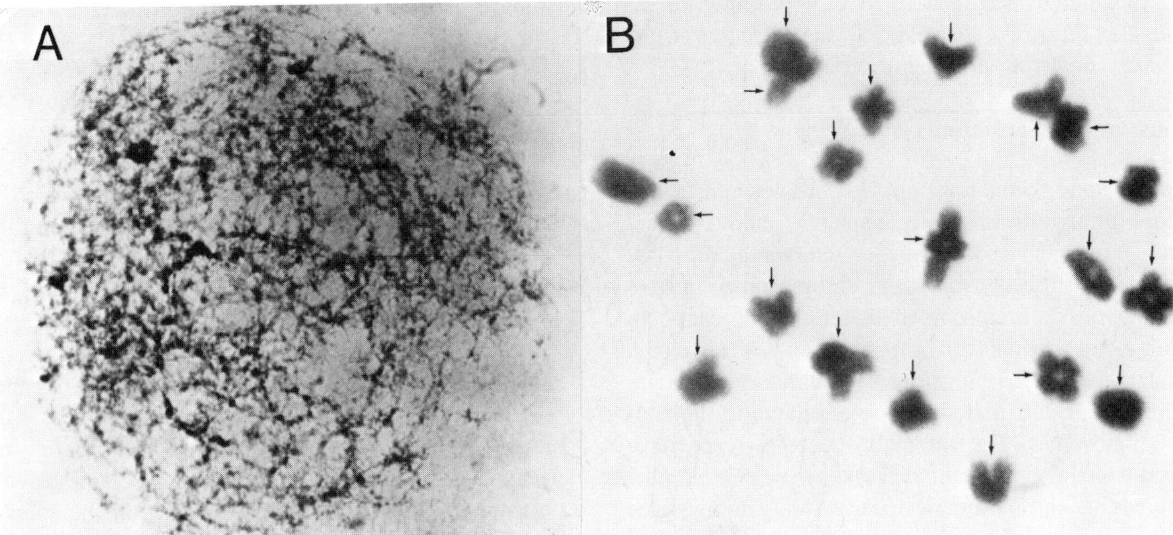

FIG. 12. Chromosome spreads from fully grown mouse oocytes during culture *in vitro*. Shown are Geimsa-stained chromosome spreads from oocytes before (**A**) and after (**B**) germinal vesicle breakdown (i.e., the early stages of meiotic maturation). Note the diffuse state of chromosomes prior to germinal vesicle breakdown (dictyate of the first meiotic prophase) as compared to after germinal vesicle breakdown. Arrows (in part B) indicate 20 bivalents.

taphase I; this long period probably reflects the time necessary to synthesize and assemble the spindle apparatus.

Polar-Body Emission

Anaphase and telophase figures predominate by 10 to 13 hr of culture *in vitro*, and it is during this period that a bulge, destined to become the first polar body, appears (Fig. 14). During telophase the midbody (a membranous and vacuolar basophilic ring around the central region of the telophase spindle) is formed, and pinching-off of the polar body is initiated (99,245,275). Separation of homologous chromosomes takes place, together with an asymmetric cleavage of oocyte cytoplasm containing one-half of the original chromosomal complement (late telophase). In addition to chromosomes, the first polar body contains a variety of organelles, including mitochondria, ribosomes, and cortical granules, as well as the midbody (289). Although a spindle is occasionally found in the first polar body, it is rarely a well-defined structure, and polar body chromosomes begin to degenerate in late telophase I. An area deficient in organelles, but rich in submembranous microfilamentous actin, overlies the metaphase-II spindle of unfertilized eggs. Furthermore, plasma membrane overlying the spindle is relatively smooth, whereas the remainder of the egg surface is highly microvillous. Microtubule organizing centers, not associated with the spindle, are found in the cytoplasm near the cell's cortex. Progression beyond metaphase II, with separation of chromatids and emission of a second polar body, awaits fertilization or parthenogenetic activation of the egg.

OOCYTE MATURATION: REGULATORY ASPECTS

Meiotic Maturation: General Considerations

Mammalian oocytes have the unusual ability to undergo meiotic maturation spontaneously when released from follicles and cultured *in vitro* (110,168,169,208,209,256,257, 281). Unlike oocytes from nonmammalian species, no hormonal stimulus is needed for mammalian oocytes to reinitiate meiotic progression and reach metaphase II (i.e., to undergo the transition from oocyte to egg) *in vitro*. It is in this context that regulation of meiotic maturation, including prolonged arrest of oocytes at the dictyate stage and reentry of oocytes into meiotic progression just prior to ovulation, have been considered experimentally.

Inhibitors of Meiotic Maturation

A variety of agents prevent spontaneous meiotic maturation of mouse oocytes *in vitro* at specific stages of nuclear progression. Nuclear (GV) breakdown, the initial morphological feature characteristic of meiotic maturation, is inhibited by dibutyryl cyclic adenosine monophosphate (dbcAMP) and agents that increase intracellular levels of cyclic adenosine monophosphate (cAMP) (110,256,257) (discussed in the section on the role of cAMP). However, even in the presence of dbcAMP, the nuclear membrane becomes extremely convoluted, and chromosome condensation is initiated but aborts at a stage short of compact bivalents (277). Complete chromosome condensation re-

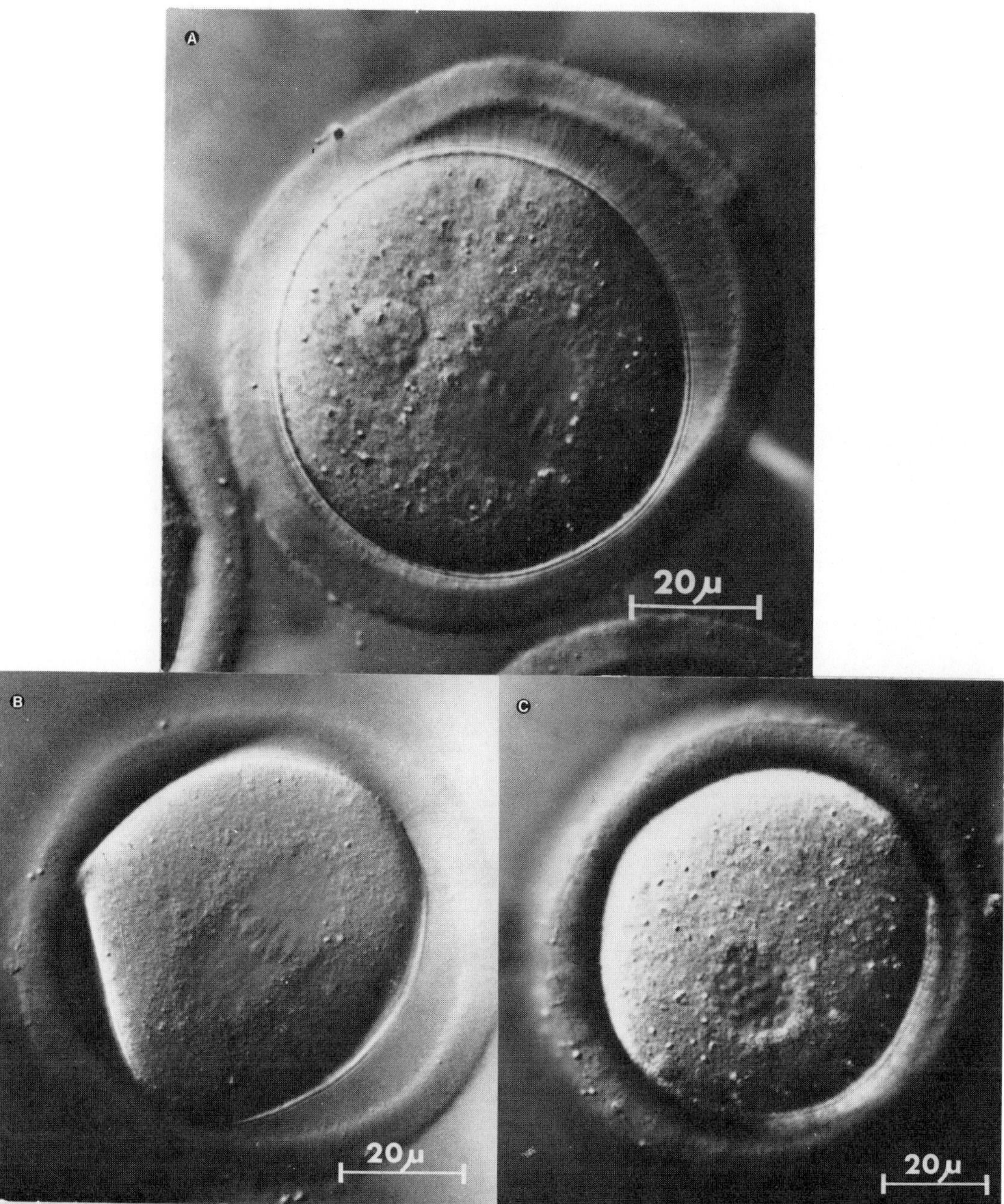

FIG. 13. Light photomicrographs of fully grown mouse oocytes at metaphase I during culture *in vitro.* Photographs were taken from a cinefilm made using Nomarski differential interference contrast microscopy. **A:** Early metaphase-I oocyte with a short, almost spherical, spindle. **B:** Late metaphase-I oocyte with an elongated spindle. Note that the oocyte plasmalemma is still attached to the zona pellucida at one point, causing distortion of the oocyte's shape. **C:** Polar view of a late metaphase-I oocyte with 17 or 18 bivalents seen clearly in the plane of focus. (From ref. 245.)

quires breakdown of the nuclear envelope, probably attributable to the multiple associations of dictyate chromosomes with the nuclear envelope (64,253,277). In the presence of puromycin (protein synthesis inhibitor), colcemid (microtubule assembly inhibitor), or cytochalasin B (microfilament assembly inhibitor), nuclear membrane breakdown and chromosome condensation occur in an apparently normal manner (277,281). However, nuclear progression is blocked at the circular bivalent stage when oocytes are cultured continuously in the presence of either puromycin or colcemid, whereas oocytes cultured in the presence of cytochalasin B proceed to metaphase I, form a normal spindle, and arrest (243,277,281). Although this suggests that nascent protein synthesis is not required for nuclear (GV) breakdown and chromosome condensation, it is possible that spontaneous resumption of meiosis *in vitro* is, in fact, de-

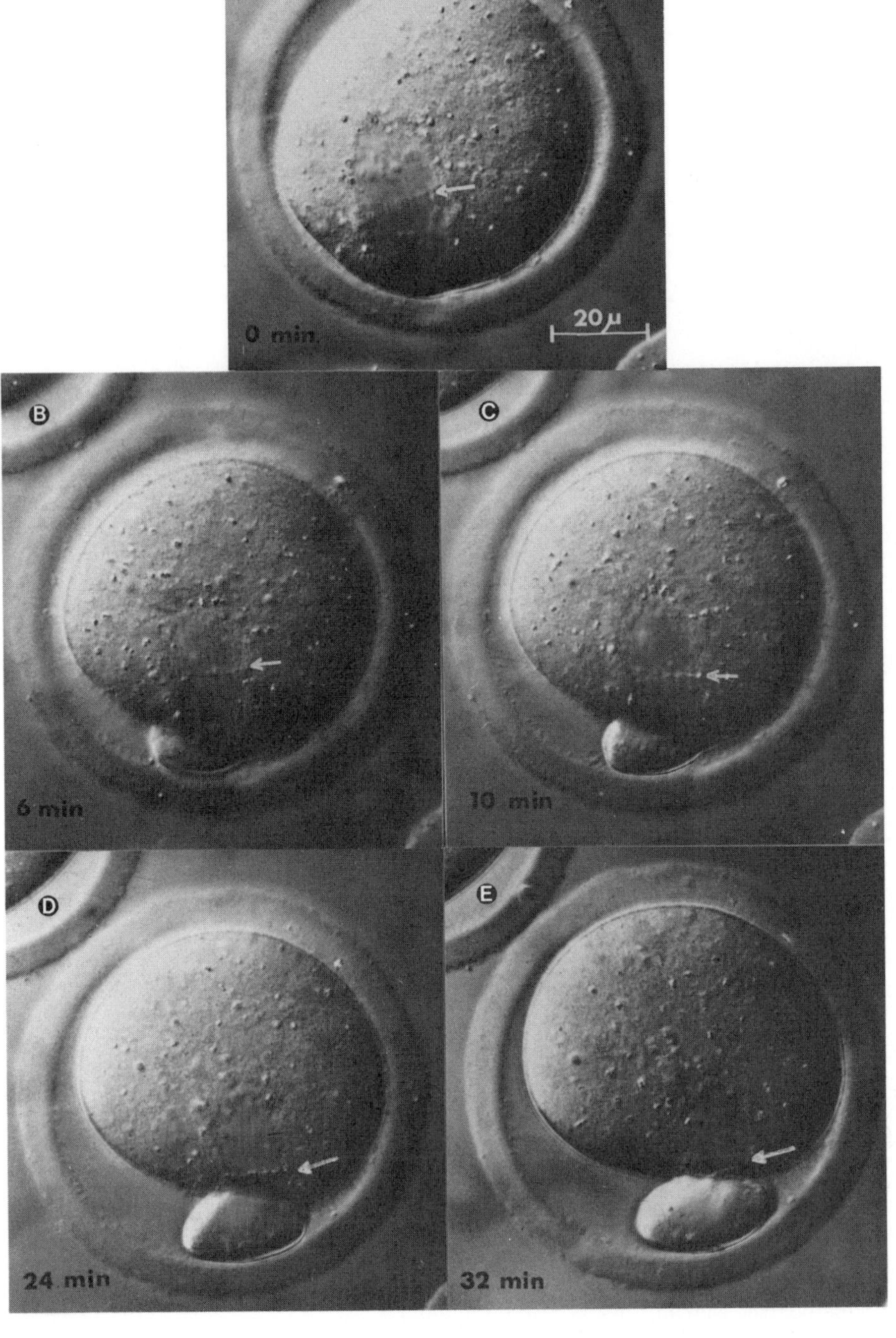

FIG. 14. Light photomicrographs of a fully grown mouse oocyte at anaphase I and telophase I during culture *in vitro.* Photographs were taken from a cinefilm made using Nomarski differential interference contrast microscopy. Actual time elapsed (in minutes) is recorded. **A:** Early anaphase-I oocyte with the midbody forming between the separating groups of chromosomes (*arrow*). Note the slight outpocketing of the oocyte membrane well in advance of the migrating polar-body chromosomes. **B:** Late anaphase I. **C:** Late anaphase I–early telophase I with polar-body chromosomes in the polar body. **D:** Telophase I with the entire spindle moving toward the polar body. **E:** Telophase I with the midbody reaching the boundary separating the oocyte and polar body. (From ref. 245.)

on some oocyte proteins with very high turnover rates (105). The effect of cytochalasin on meiotic maturation suggests that microfilaments are involved in events following metaphase-I spindle formation (e.g., separation of homologous chromosomes). Emission of a polar body is inhibited by all of these drugs, suggesting that cytokinesis is blocked when any one of the earlier events of maturation fails to take place (277,281). In this context, it has been found that activators of protein kinase-C (e.g., phorbol esters; see below), but not dbcAMP, inhibit polar-body emission by oocytes that had already undergone nuclear (GV) breakdown *in vitro* (46).

Role of cAMP

Spontaneous maturation of mouse oocytes does not occur *in vitro* when oocytes are cultured in the presence of either membrane-permeable analogs of cAMP, such as dbcAMP and 8-bromo-cAMP, or inhibitors of cyclic nucleotide phosphodiesterase (PDE), such as isobutyl methylxanthine (IBMX) and theophylline (74,93,164,236,238,277). Similarly, other agents that increase intracellular cAMP levels by activation of adenyl cyclase, such as forskolin, also prevent sponta neous maturation of mouse oocytes *in vitro* (47,92, 193,212,228,236,265). Furthermore, microinjection of PDE into oocytes cultured in the presence of IBMX overcomes the inhibitory effect of IBMX on meiotic maturation (45). An oocyte PDE activity has been identified and characterized and has been shown to be membrane-bound and modulated by calmodulin; a calmodulin-dependent step occurs subsequent to, or concurrently with, the decrease in oocyte cAMP levels (see below) during spontaneous maturation (49). The behavior of oocytes under these conditions suggests that cAMP is involved in the maintenance of meiotic arrest at the dictyate stage; a fall in intracellular cAMP levels could signal reentry of oocytes into meiotic progression. In fact, a significant decrease in cAMP levels of oocytes does occur just prior to nuclear envelope (GV) breakdown, both *in vitro* and *in vivo* (94,236,271). Therefore, just as cAMP is involved in regulating the G_2-to-M transition during the mitotic cell cycle, it appears to be involved in the reentry of oocytes into meiotic progression. It should be noted that exposure of oocytes to dbcAMP following nuclear envelope (GV) breakdown has no effect on subsequent events of meiotic maturation; polar-body emission with arrest at metaphase II occurs in a normal manner (277,281).

Involvement of cAMP in meiotic maturation implies that, as in many other biological situations, it acts via cAMP-dependent protein kinase (PK), an enzyme consisting of catalytic (C) and regulatory (R) subunits (165). While the R:C complex is enzymatically inactive, binding of cAMP to the R (inhibitory) subunit results in dissociation of the complex and activation of the C-subunit kinase activity. Assuming that continuous phosphorylation of an oocyte protein(s) by PK is essential for maintenance of meiotic arrest, cAMP levels could thereby regulate meiotic maturation by determining the amount of free C subunit available. Under conditions of low levels of free C subunit (low cAMP), the relevant oocyte phosphoprotein(s) would be dephosphorylated and the meiotic maturation would be initiated. In this context, mouse oocytes microinjected with the C subunit of PK fail to undergo spontaneous meiotic maturation during culture *in vitro* in the absence of dbcAMP and IBMX (45,46). Furthermore, changes in the phosphorylation patterns of oocyte proteins, under a variety of experimental conditions, are consistent with this proposed regulatory scheme (45,236). However, other evidence suggests that cAMP is only one of the components of a complex system employed in the maintenance of oocytes in the dictyate stage of the first meiotic prophase (discussed in the sections on the roles of calcium, intercellular communication, steroids, and oocyte maturation inhibitor). In particular, it is noteworthy that increasing the levels of cAMP in cumulus cells, in the presence of FSH or cholera toxin, results in inhibition of meiotic maturation without a detectable rise in oocyte cAMP levels (111,237). This suggests the possibility that an inhibitory factor other than cAMP is transferred from cumulus cells to oocytes, resulting in inhibition of meiotic maturation *in vitro* (discussed in the section on the role of oocyte maturation inhibitor).

Finally, phorbol esters and diacylglycerol, known activators of calcium/phospholipid-dependent protein kinase (PK-C), also inhibit spontaneous maturation of oocytes *in vitro* without a decrease in oocyte cAMP levels (46). These PK-C activators also inhibit the changes in oocyte phosphoprotein metabolism associated with spontaneous maturation, suggesting that PK-C activators inhibit resumption of meiosis by acting distal to a decrease in cAMP-dependent PK activity, prior to changes in oocyte phosphoprotein metabolism that are necessary for resumption of meiosis.

Role of Calcium

Involvement of calmodulin during meiotic maturation implies that there is a role for calcium (49,91,159,258). Verapamil and tetracaine, two inhibitors of transmembrane calcium transport, transiently prevent breakdown of the nuclear envelope *in vitro* (195). Furthermore, increasing extracellular calcium concentrations decreases the effectiveness of dbcAMP as an inhibitor of meiotic maturation, whereas verapamil and tetracaine (which decrease intracellular calcium concentration) increase its effectiveness (210). Therefore, intracellular levels of calcium and cAMP may act synergistically, through a calmodulin-dependent step, to regulate meiotic maturation of mammalian oocytes.

Role of Intercellular Communication

Gap junctions represent regions of physical continuity between cellular membranes. As such, in many biological systems they serve as mediators of intercellular communication and metabolic coupling by permitting passage of small molecules between cells; in this manner, one type of cell can influence the function of another (124,157). Fully grown mouse oocytes are coupled with surrounding cumulus cells by gap junctions (3–6,123). They are found at areas of contact between the oocyte's plasma membrane and processes that emanate from cumulus cells and traverse the zona pellucida. Furthermore, an extensive network of gap junctions interconnect all follicle cells with the cumulus and, consequently, with the oocyte.

Throughout oocyte growth and folliculogenesis, both *in vivo* and *in vitro,* gap junctions mediate intercellular communication between the oocyte and follicle cells. The cells are both metabolically and ionically coupled, and iontophoretically injected dye is transferred between cumulus cells and oocyte (123,216). However, just prior to ovulation there is a significant decrease in the number of gap junctions, together with a decrease in the extent of ionic coupling, and following ovulation the oocyte and surrounding cumulus cells are no longer coupled as a result of mucification and cumulus expansion (96,123,140,156,179) (Fig. 15). In the latter state, cumulus-cell processes are retracted away from the oocyte surface. This behavior suggests that spontaneous meiotic maturation takes place *in vitro* as a result of removing oocytes from the inhibitory influence of follicle cells. In this context, it has been demonstrated that either grafting oocytes to follicle walls or co-culture of oocytes with granulosa cells prevents spontaneous maturation *in vitro*.

Between 2 and 3 hr following administration of an ovulatory stimulus (hCG), there is about a 15-fold decrease in the net area of cumulus-cell gap-junction membrane (i.e., about 90% of the total gap-junction membrane per cumulus cell is lost within an hour) (156) (Fig. 16). The loss of cumulus-cell gap junctions is temporally correlated with nuclear envelope breakdown and cumulus expansion (109,156,226). In this context, the inhibitory effects of both FSH and suboptimal concentrations of dbcAMP are lost when intercellular communication between cumulus cells and the oocyte is disrupted *in vitro*. However, although the coupling of cumulus cells and the oocyte terminates before ovulation, it is not completed until after nuclear envelope breakdown. Therefore, while it is tempting to attribute the onset of meiotic maturation exclusively to termination of intercellular communication between cumulus cells and the oocyte (e.g., cessation of transfer of an "inhibitory factor" from cumulus cells to the oocyte via gap junctions), there is evidence to the contrary.

Role of Steroids

Although LH induces both maturation of oocytes and progesterone production in intact follicles *in vitro*, LH apparently does not induce maturation via progesterone synthesis (95,97,256,257). Furthermore, it remains problematic whether or not other steroid hormones, such as estradiol and testosterone, play a role in regulation of meiotic maturation: Whereas a number of steroid hormones potentiate the FSH-induced inhibition of meiotic maturation of cumulus-cell-enclosed oocytes *in vitro* [without an increase in oocyte cAMP levels; see section on nuclear (germinal vesicle) breakdown], they only inhibit maturation of denuded oocytes when their cAMP levels are elevated by exposure to dbcAMP or forskolin (110,111,213,237). On the other hand, at very high nonphysiological concentrations, testosterone, progesterone, pregnenolone, as well as other steroids, inhibit meiotic maturation, either alone or in conjunction with dbcAMP or agents that affect intracellular cAMP levels (112,120,158,170,178,215,218,244).

Role of Oocyte Maturation Inhibitor

It has been suggested that oocyte maturation inhibitor (OMI), a product of granulosa cells, maintains oocytes in the dictyate stage of first meiotic prophase (256,257,

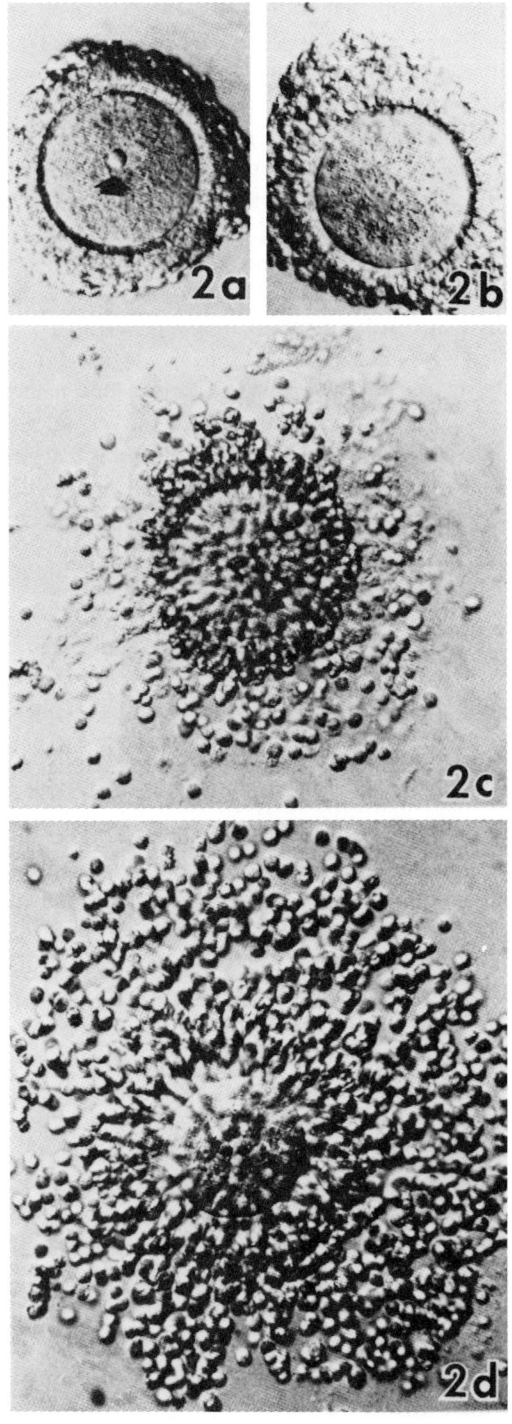

FIG. 15. Light photomicrographs of oocyte–cumulus-cell complexes isolated from control and hCG-injected mice. (**a**) Control; (**b–d**) 3, 6, and 9 hr post-hCG injection. The germinal vesicle is clearly seen (*arrow*) in the oocytes from control mice (a). At 3 hr post-hCG, the germinal vesicle has broken down, but cumulus cells are still tightly packed around the oocytes (b). At 6 hr post-hCG injection, cumulus expansion includes only the outer cumulus cell, while those adjacent to the oocyte are still tightly packed (c). Cumulus expansion appears complete by 9 hr post-hCG (d), and these oocytes show a reduction in intercellular coupling as compared to controls. (From ref. 109.)

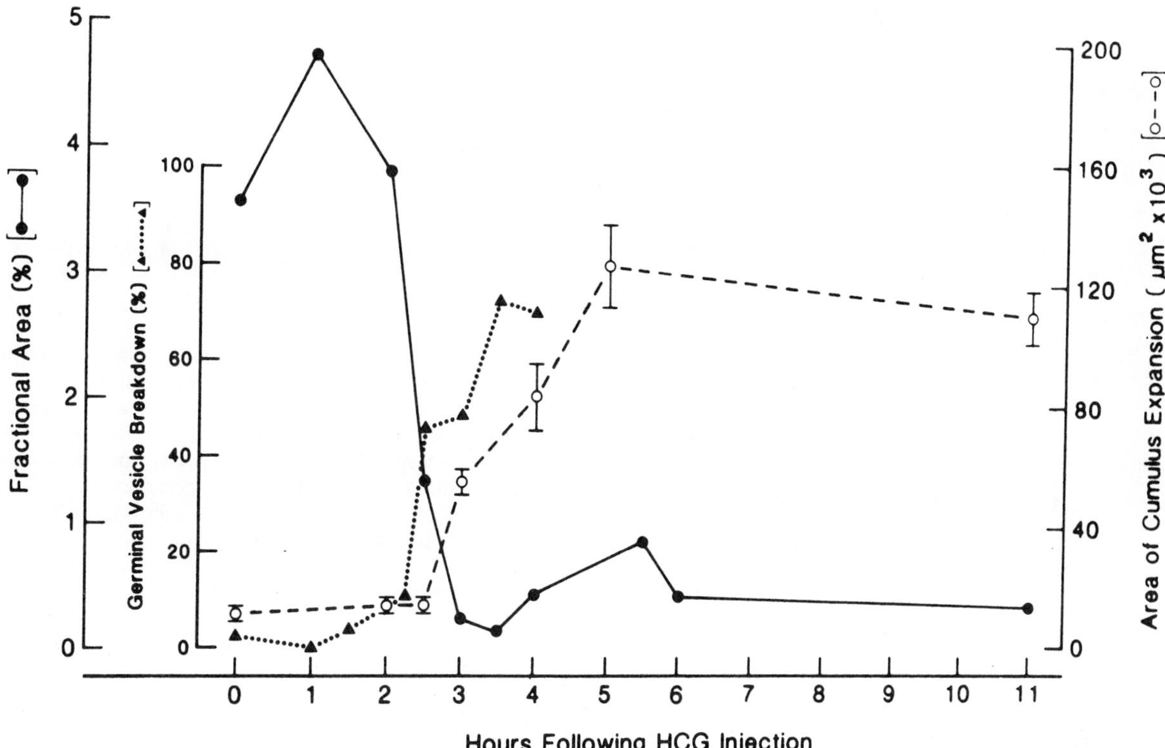

FIG. 16. Changes in gap-junction fractional area, projected cumulus-oocyte area, and fraction of rat oocytes showing no germinal vesicle at varying times after an ovulatory stimulus. (From ref. 156.)

259,261,262). This is consistent with the relatively old observation that follicular fluid inhibits oocyte maturation *in vitro* (69,71,134,260,261,263). OMI is a polypeptide that has a molecular weight of about 1 to 2 kilodaltons, is found in follicular fluid from ovaries of a variety of mammals, and prevents oocytes from undergoing spontaneous meiotic maturation when cultured *in vitro*. However, OMI apparently exerts its inhibitory action via cumulus cells, since it prevents maturation of oocytes cultured within their cumulus cells but does not interfere with maturation of completely denuded oocytes; in this context, it is likely that OMI is small enough to pass through gap junctions between cumulus cells and the oocyte (256,257,259). Preovulatory follicles have relatively low concentrations of OMI, consistent with its proposed role in regulating meiotic maturation. It is possible that the inhibitory action of OMI is potentiated by cAMP, suggesting that OMI could account for some of the effects of cAMP on cumulus-enclosed oocytes observed *in vitro* (48,101,111,237) (discussed in the section on regulatory aspects of oocyte maturation). However, it should be noted that the existence of OMI has been seriously questioned in some quarters and, in the absence of additional biochemical support, remains a highly controversial subject (114,160,161,214). Furthermore, recent evidence suggests that hypoxanthine and/or adenosine (inhibit cAMP phosphodiesterase) are, in fact, the low-molecular-weight components of follicular fluid that prevents spontaneous meiotic maturation of oocytes *in vitro* (100,113).

Summary

Many factors potentially influence the maintenance of mammalian oocytes in the dictyate stage of first meiotic prophase. These include cAMP, as well as enzyme systems involved in regulating intracellular levels of cAMP, calcium, calmodulin, steroids, hypophyseal hormones, purine bases, putative polypeptide inhibitors, and intercellular communication between cumulus cells and between cumulus cells and the oocyte, in the form of gap junctions. At present, the interplay between these factors in regulating meiotic maturation both *in vivo* and *in vitro* is not precisely understood, precluding formulation of a detailed regulatory pathway that satisfies all relevant observations. However, it is clear that such a pathway would include many of the features thought to be involved in regulation of meiotic maturation of amphibian oocytes (165) and would undoubtedly involve cAMP (Fig. 17). Finally, it is apparent that, overall, it is the integrity of the follicle that maintains mammalian oocytes in meiotic arrest.

GROWTH OF THE OOCYTE: BIOCHEMICAL ASPECTS

Oocyte Growth *In Vitro*

The ability to isolate and culture growing mouse oocytes *in vitro* has resulted in significant advances in our understanding of various aspects of the metabolism of oocyte

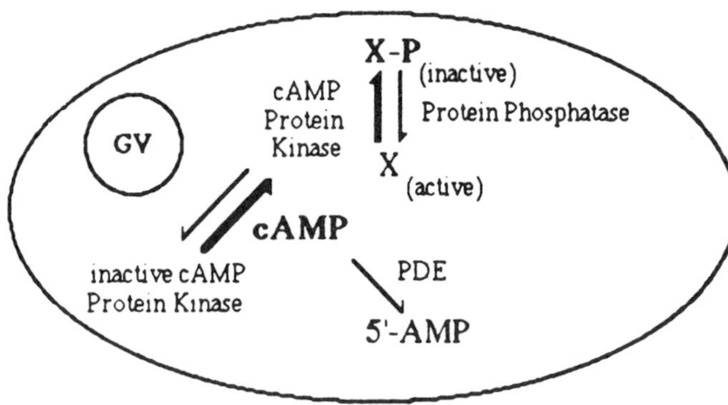

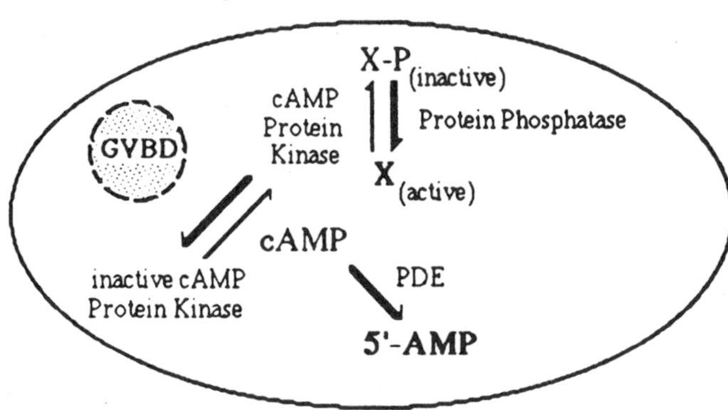

FIG. 17. Model of regulation of meiotic arrest and resumption of meiosis. The model proposes that a phosphoprotein, X-P, maintains meiotic arrest; the dephosphorylated form, X, promotes resumption of meiosis. X is phosphorylated by protein kinase, and X-P is dephosphorylated by phosphoprotein phosphatase; these two enzyme activities determine the steady-state levels of X-P and X in the oocyte. Resumption of meiosis is initiated by a decrease in cAMP, which leads to a decrease in protein kinase activity. Assuming that phosphoprotein phosphatase activity is unchanged, this decrease in protein kinase activity would induce a net dephosphorylation of X-P, triggering resumption of meiosis. It should be noted that although X is depicted as actively promoting GVBD (germinal vesicle breakdown), X-P could just as well actively maintain meiotic arrest; this would not alter the model significantly. Boldface type indicates the putative predominant species. (From ref. 45.)

growth. Improving upon earlier methods for obtaining growing oocytes from juvenile animals, at least two reliable culture systems are now available that support oocyte growth *in vitro*. In one, follicles obtained from collagenase-treated juvenile ovaries rapidly attach to culture dishes and, although some granulosa cells leave the follicles, oocytes remain surrounded by at least one layer of granulosa cells (106–108,139). These oocytes increase in size at a rate comparable to that observed *in vivo*. In the other system, follicles obtained from Pronase-treated juvenile ovaries rapidly attach to culture dishes and then follicle cells migrate away, liberating oocytes that rest on a monolayer of ovarian cells (16,33). These oocytes grow, but at a rate lower than that observed *in vivo* (16). In both of these systems, oocyte growth is assessed to be normal in that oocytes (a) display increasing levels of CO_2 production from exogenous pyruvate, (b) exhibit appropriate changes in size, morphology, and ultrastructure, (c) express growth-specific, differential regulation of certain alloenzyme activities (59), (d) exhibit a progressively thickening zona pellucida, and (e) become competent to undergo meiotic maturation during prolonged culture *in vitro*.

Intercellular communication between the oocyte and granulosa cells, via gap junctions, apparently is necessary for oocyte growth *in vitro* (16,108,141). In the absence of gap junctions, oocytes grow very little, if at all, and, after several days in culture, undergo necrosis. It is likely that denuded oocytes will become necrotic because they normally depend on granulosa cells to meet certain of their nutritional demands. In this connection, gap-junction-mediated metabolic cooperativity between oocytes and cumulus cells has been demonstrated in several ways. For example, cumulus-enclosed fully grown oocytes take up significantly more leucine, uridine, choline, and inositol from culture medium than do denuded, fully grown oocytes (86,140, 179,278) (Figs. 18 and 19).

Similarly, follicle-enclosed growing oocytes take up significantly more uridine, guanosine, choline, and deoxyglucose from culture medium than do denuded, growing oocytes (139). Furthermore, differences in the distribution of phosphorylated metabolites of ribonucleosides in oocytes have been noted when comparing denuded with either cumulus or follicle-enclosed oocytes cultured *in vitro* (57,139). The evidence suggests, for example, that oocytes derive most of their ribonucleosides and ribonucleotides from granulosa cells; denuded oocytes are poorly able to take up ribonucleosides and metabolize them to ribonucleotides. In addition, since growing oocytes lack the energy-dependent so-called A-transport system for uptake of certain amino acids, it is likely that follicle cells provide these amino acids, routing them to oocytes through gap junctions (83). These and other observations strongly suggest that intercellular

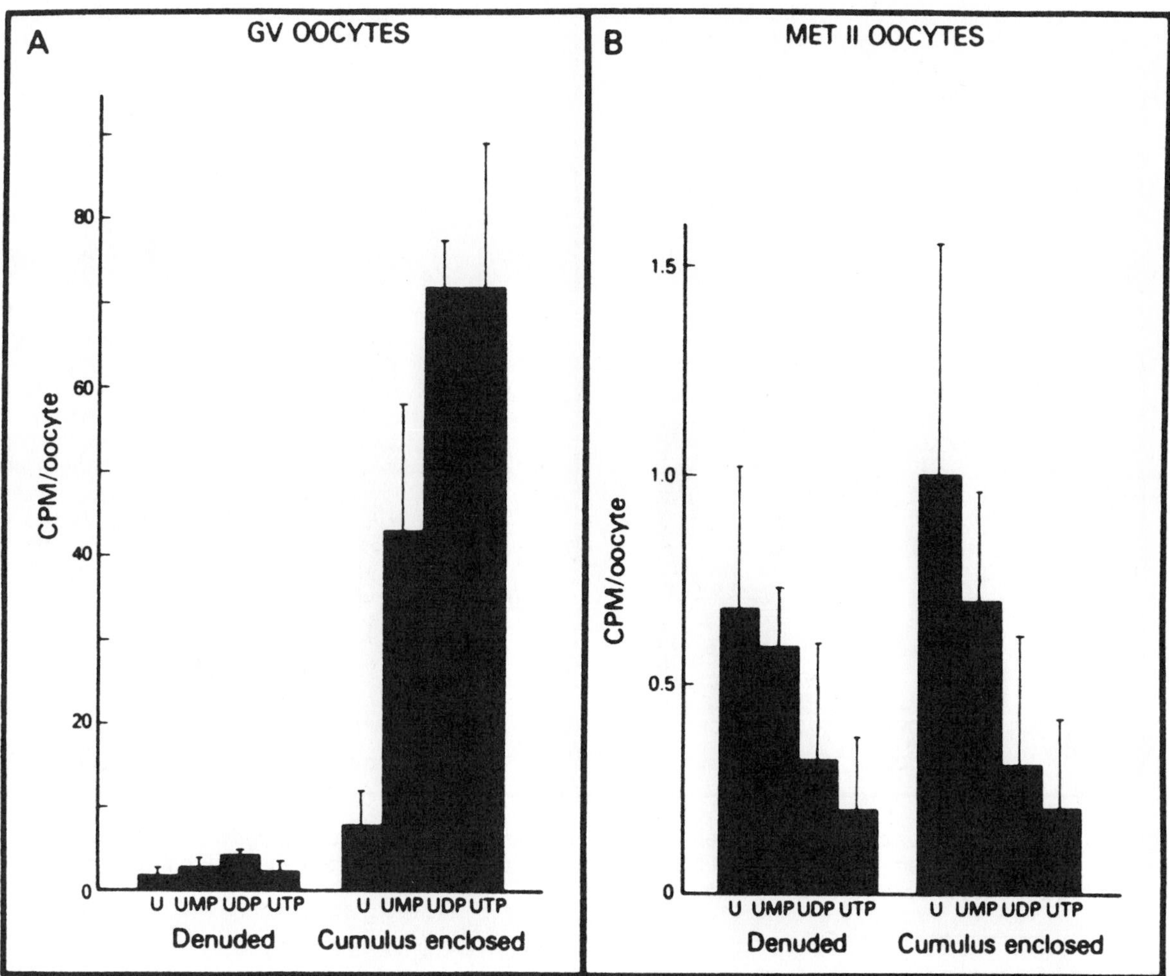

FIG. 18. Distribution of uridine, UMP, UDP, and UTP in denuded and cumulus-enclosed mouse oocytes at two stages of nuclear progression. **A:** Oocytes arrested at the dictyate stage of the first meiotic prophase. **B:** Oocytes arrested at metaphase II (unfertilized eggs). (From ref. 140.)

communication between follicle cells and oocytes plays a vital nutritional role during oocyte growth. Consistent with this role, the extent of metabolic cooperativity increases during oocyte growth *in vivo* and *in vitro,* and the rate of oocyte growth *in vitro* is positively correlated with the extent of intercellular communication (gap junction formation) (57) (Fig. 20). Perhaps the relationship between oocyte growth and intercellular communication reflects "an economization and compartmentalization of metabolic function, thereby liberating the oocyte from numerous house-keeping functions" (57). Such a division of labor between oocytes and follicle cells would emulate the situation in most nonmammals.

Overall RNA Synthesis

Fully grown mouse oocytes contain about 500 to 600 pg of RNA, or about 200 times the amount found in typical somatic cells (15,151,192,251,273). Of the total, approximately 10% to 15% is polyadenylated RNA (informational RNA), 20% to 25% is transfer RNA, and 60% to 65% is ribosomal RNA (15,273). Virtually all of this RNA is synthesized during the 2 to 3 week period of oocyte growth (discussed in the section on structural aspects of oocyte growth). The RNA content of oocytes increases dramatically during their growth phase, with RNA accumulation exhibiting biphasic kinetics with respect to oocyte volume (151,251). During early and midgrowth stages, changes in nucleolar ultrastructure and in levels of RNA polymerase activity are consistent with high rates of transcription of ribosomal DNA (117,156,181–185). Although the rate of RNA synthesis during this period is high with respect to some somatic cells, it does not approach the rates estimated for growing amphibian oocytes, which have *bone fide* "lampbrush chromosomes", leading some, but not all, investigators to conclude that "true lampbrush chromosomes do not exist at any point in development of mouse oocytes" (15).

When oocytes reach about three-quarters of their final volume, they contain nearly as much RNA as is found in

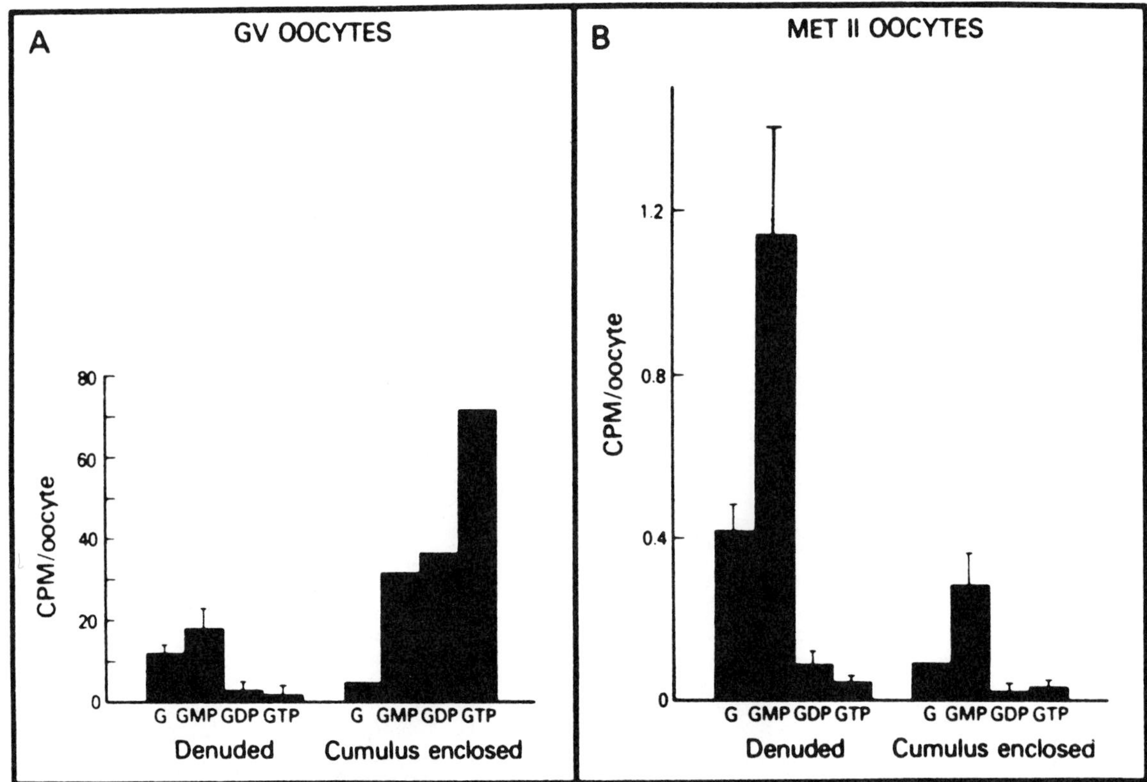

FIG. 19. Distribution of guanosine, GMP, GDP, and GTP in denuded and cumulus-enclosed mouse oocytes at two stages of nuclear progression. **A:** Oocytes arrested at the dictyate stage of the first meiotic prophase. **B:** Oocytes arrested at metaphase II (unfertilized eggs). (From ref. 140.)

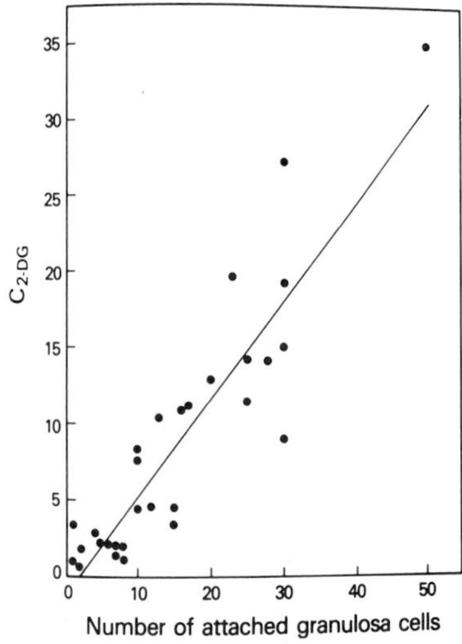

FIG. 20. Intercellular communication as monitored by metabolic cooperativity between granulosa cells and oocytes. Value of $C_{2\text{-DG}}$ (2-deoxyglucose), indicative of intercellular communication, is plotted as a function of the number of granulosa cells attached to oocytes. *C,* a metabolic cooperativity ratio, is defined as $(A - B)/B$, where *A* is the number of cpm/granulosa cell-enclosed oocyte and *B* is the number of cpm/denuded oocyte. Values of *C* greater than 0 indicate the existence of metabolic cooperativity. Each point represents a determination made with a single oocyte–granulosa-cell complex. Note that *C* increases with increasing numbers of attached granulosa cells. (From reference 57.)

fully grown oocytes (251) (Fig. 21). It can be estimated that, overall, there is a 300-fold increase in the RNA content of oocytes during their growth phase, consistent with changes in nuclear and nucleolar sizes as well as in levels of RNA synthesis during this period. Similarly, measurements of endogenous levels of RNA polymerase during oocyte growth are consistent with progressively increasing extents of RNA synthesis until oocytes reach about three-quarters of their final volume (181,184). RNA continues to be synthesized in fully grown oocytes, although at a diminished rate compared to midgrowth oocytes, declining to barely detectable levels only after the onset of meiotic maturation (ovulation) (43,221,278).

Specific RNA Synthesis

Several experimental approaches have been used to assess synthesis of specific classes of RNA during oocyte growth in mice:

1. A radiolabeled RNA precursor, such as ^{3}H-uridine/adenosine, is injected into the ovarian bursa. Analyses of radiolabeled RNA in ovulated eggs is then carried out 1 to 24 days after the injection. Since the major growth phase of oocytes occurs between 20 and 6 days prior to ovulation, these analyses provide information about kinds of RNA synthesized and their stability *in vivo* (13,15,19,98,147).

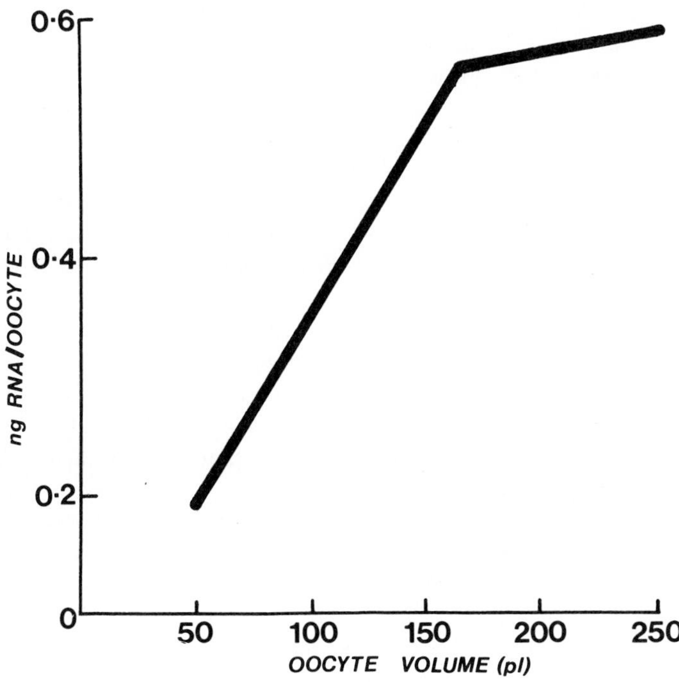

FIG. 21. Relationship between mouse oocyte growth and accumulation of oocyte RNA. Note that, overall, there is nearly a 300-fold increase in RNA content during growth of mouse oocytes, from about 12 to 85 μm in diameter. Here, the smallest oocytes examined were about 40 μm in diameter; the change in RNA content during growth of oocytes from 12 to 40 μm was not determined. (From ref. 251.)

The time course of RNA labeling, following injection of [^{3}H]uridine/adenosine into the ovarian bursa, indicates that significant levels of RNA synthesis occur in growing oocytes during the 2 weeks prior to ovulation. Furthermore, about three-quarters of nascent RNA, synthesized 19 to 43 hr after bursal injection of radiolabel, is retained until ovulation 10 to 20 days later, suggesting that RNA synthesized in growing oocytes is extremely stable. Analyses of the RNA on sucrose gradients and gels indicate that about 65%, 20%, and 15% of the radiolabel is in ribosomal RNA, 5S- and transfer RNA, and heterogeneous RNA, respectively, throughout oocyte growth. The average rate of ribosomal-RNA synthesis is 15 fg/min during oocyte growth. It is not necessary to propose extensive amplification of the mouse oocyte's ribosomal genes in order to account for this level of ribosomal-RNA synthesis, although a fourfold amplification may occur in oocytes from other mammals (287,288). At any time during oocyte growth, from 7 to 19 days prior to ovulation, approximately 10% of radiolabel present in nascent RNA is associated with polyadenylated RNA. Furthermore, 9 to 12% of RNA synthesized at each stage of oocyte growth and conserved in unfertilized eggs is polyadenylated RNA. From such information, one can calculate (a) that enough polyadenylated RNA is made during oocyte growth to account for about 6% to 8% of the mass of egg RNA (~30–45 pg) and (b) that enough polyadenylated RNA is produced to account for virtually all polysomal informational RNA present in mouse eggs. The relatively large amount of informational RNA in eggs is attributable to both high rates of synthesis during oocyte growth and unusual stability of the RNA.

2. Denuded oocytes, cumulus-oocyte complexes, or follicle-enclosed oocytes are incubated in the presence of a radiolabeled RNA precursor in an appropriate culture medium *in vitro*. Analyses of radiolabeled RNA in oocytes is then carried out after various times of culture (14,15,44,56).

Total RNA synthesized by follicle-enclosed growing oocytes is unusually stable (having a half-life of about 28 days) as long as oocytes continue growing *in vitro* (the half-life decreases to about 4 days when oocytes are viable, but the oocytes do not grow *in vitro*). Under conditions of oocyte growth, turnover of ribosomal, 5S-, and transfer RNA is barely detectable. On the other hand, polyadenylated RNA turns over slowly (with a half-life of about 10 days) and exhibits kinetics suggestive of a relatively unstable species of high-molecular-weight heterogeneous RNA. As much as one-half of RNA synthesized by follicle-enclosed growing oocytes, 35 to 65 μm in diameter, is polyadenylated; decreasing to as little as one-fifth of the nascent RNA of fully grown oocytes.

The behavior of heterogeneous RNA has been well characterized in denuded oocytes cultured in the presence of ovarian somatic cell monolayers, under conditions that permit oocyte growth *in vitro*. In these growing oocytes, heterogeneous RNA is synthesized at the relatively high rate of 0.6 pg/min and turns over rapidly, with a half-life of 20 min. As a result of the high rate of synthesis, the steady-state amount of nuclear, heterogeneous RNA present in these oocytes is quite large, approximating 15 pg. About 2% of this RNA is conserved, reaches the cytoplasm, and accumulates at the rate of approximately 0.01 pg/min. All of these values are based on the assumption that ribosomal RNA is synthesized at the rate of 0.2 ng/week and is completely stable during the measurements.

3. ^{3}H-labeled poly(U) is hybridized *in situ* to ovarian sections or fixed oocytes, followed by autoradiography, to

estimate relative amounts, as well as intracellular localization, of polyadenylated RNA (15,22,205,251).

By this method, the kinetics of accumulation of polyadenylated RNA are similar to the biphasic kinetics of accumulation of total RNA during oocyte growth. Nearly 95% of the polyadenylated RNA present in fully grown oocytes is found in growing oocytes that have reached about three-quarters of their final volume. There is as much as a two-fold reduction in the amount of cytoplasmic polyadenylated RNA during the interval between completion of oocyte growth and ovulation; however, the relative concentration of polyadenylated RNA in the nucleus remains about two times that in the cytoplasm, suggesting that polyadenylated-RNA synthesis continues following completion of oocyte growth. Solution-hybridization experiments suggest that, just prior to ovulation, fully grown oocytes contain about 26 pg of polyadenylated RNA but that this falls to about 19 pg in unfertilized eggs.

Finally, it would appear that growing mouse oocytes also synthesize an RNA species resembling U1-RNA; a small nuclear RNA thought to play a role in processing of heterogeneous nuclear RNA (hnRNA) (152). Similarly, growing oocytes contain intracisternal A-particle-related RNA sequences (IAP-RNA), which are found at high levels in fully grown oocytes (~ 17,000 molecules/oocyte; 61 fg) but at much lower levels in unfertilized eggs (~1,000 molecules/egg; 4 fg) (206). On the other hand, surprisingly, mouse-egg RNA is not enriched in Alu-like repetitive sequence transcripts, as compared to cytoplasmic RNA from various mammalian tissues (152).

RNA Synthesis: Summary

From the preceding, it should be apparent that RNA synthesis and accumulation are major activities of growing mammalian oocytes. On a per-cell basis, the fully grown mouse oocyte contains about 200 times more RNA and 1,000 times more ribosomes than does a typical mammalian somatic cell. Especially noteworthy is the large amount of informational RNA in fully grown oocytes, large even in comparison with amphibian oocytes (on a percentage of total RNA basis). It should be realized, however, that on a volume (per picoliter) basis, mouse oocytes are not unlike somatic cells with respect to RNA and ribosome concentration. Therefore, to some extent, it is simply the failure of growing oocytes to undergo cytokinesis that results in unusually large stores of RNA and ribosomes.

Overall Protein Synthesis

Electrophoretic analyses of proteins synthesized by growing and fully grown mouse oocytes reveal a remarkable degree of constancy at the qualitative level (128,238,273). Several hundred discrete species are detected on fluorograms of high-resolution two-dimensional gels containing proteins radiolabeled with ^{35}S-methionine during culture of oocytes *in vitro*. The most intensely radiolabeled proteins are also the most abundant, based on patterns of comparable silver-stained gels. Although changes in overall patterns of protein synthesis occur during oocyte growth, most, but not all, of these can be characterized as quantitative changes. In other words, overall, these analyses suggest that the same proteins are synthesized throughout oocyte growth, but at different relative rates at different times in the growth phase. It is almost certain that stage-specific synthesis of particular proteins occurs during oocyte growth (e.g., proteins involved in regulation of meiotic maturation); however, thus far, these proteins have not been identified. Analysis of cDNA libraries, prepared from messenger RNA purified at different stages of oocyte growth, should lead to identification and characterization of such proteins.

The sizes of endogenous methionine pools and absolute rates of protein synthesis in growing and fully grown mouse oocytes have been determined using isolated oocytes that are denuded of follicle cells and cultured *in vitro* (234,235,273) (Fig. 22). As the oocyte undergoes about a 300-fold increase in volume during its growth phase, a corresponding increase occurs in the size of the oocyte's endogenous methionine pool, from 0.16 to 56 fmole/oocyte. Therefore, each doubling of oocyte volume is accompanied by a doubling of the size of the methionine pool, such that the concentration of intracellular free methionine remains fairly constant at about 170 μM throughout oocyte growth. These analyses also suggest that the entire intracellular methionine pool, not just a smaller compartment of the pool, serves as precursor for protein synthesis. On the other hand, although the absolute rate of protein synthesis increases markedly during oocyte growth, from 1.1 to 41.8 pg/hr per oocyte, the increase is only about 38-fold as compared to the 300-fold increase in oocyte volume. Consequently, the absolute rate of protein synthesis, expressed on a volume (per picoliter) basis, actually decreases during oocyte growth. As a result, it takes about 10 pl of cytoplasm from a fully grown oocyte to synthesize as much as 1 pl of protein from a nongrowing oocyte. Considering that 90% of the cytoplasmic volume of amphibian oocytes consists of yolk platelets, leaving only 10% as active cytoplasm, the absolute rate of protein synthesis in fully grown mouse oocytes (~0.17 pg/hr per pl) compares quite favorably with that of amphibian oocytes (0.34 pg/hr per pl).

Calculations using values for absolute rates of protein synthesis, given above, indicate that only about one-half of the protein present in fully grown mouse oocytes can be accounted for by protein synthesis during oocyte growth (235). This apparent discrepancy may be accounted for by errors in one (or more) of the measurements or by the presence of a yolk-like component in oocytes that is synthesized elsewhere and taken up by endocytosis (analogous to the situation in amphibians). The former possibility should be considered seriously in view of the fact that these measurements were made with denuded oocytes. In the presence

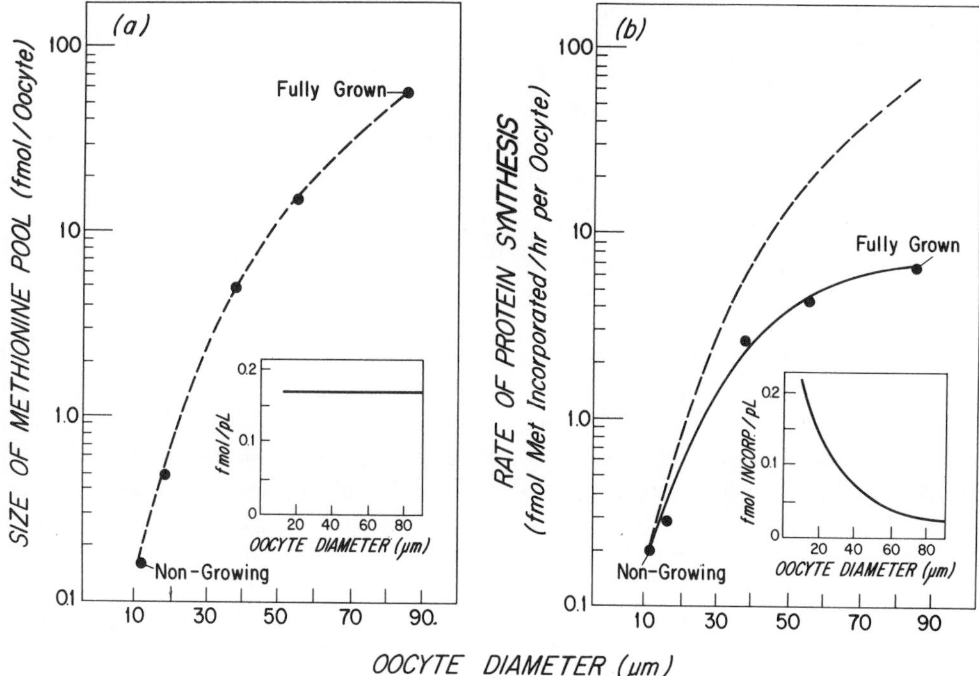

FIG. 22. Relationship between mouse oocyte diameter, sizes of intracellular methionine pools, and absolute rates of protein synthesis. (**a**) Methionine pool sizes as a function of oocyte diameter. (●) Experimentally determined values for methionine pool sizes. (– – –) Theoretical curve constructed by assuming a simple linear relationship between methionine pool size and oocyte volume, using a value of 56 fmole of methionine per oocyte for the fully grown oocyte. (*Inset*) Data converted to femtomoles of methionine per picoliter as a function of oocyte diameter. (**b**) Absolute rates of protein synthesis as a function of oocyte diameter. (●) Experimentally determined values for absolute rates of protein synthesis. (– – –) Theoretical curve constructed by assuming a simple linear relationship between absolute rates of protein synthesis and oocyte volume, using a value of 41.8 pg/hr per oocyte for the fully grown oocyte. (*Inset*) Data converted to femtomoles of methionine incorporated per picoliter as a function of oocyte diameter. (From ref. 235.)

of follicle cells *in vivo,* the absolute rates of protein synthesis in growing oocytes may be substantially higher than reported for the *in vitro* situation (66,225). Similarly, the presence of a yolk-like component in mouse oocytes should be considered seriously, since mammalian oocytes have the capacity to accumulate such a component from the blood (125–127). Therefore, whether or not growing oocytes synthesize all of the protein found in fully grown oocytes remains an open question.

Specific Protein Synthesis

At least three different experimental approaches have been used to identify specific oocyte proteins and examine their synthesis during oocyte growth in mice (273): (i) immunoprecipitation of metabolically radiolabeled proteins with antisera directed against specific proteins; (ii) coelectrophoresis of metabolically radiolabeled proteins with purified proteins on high-resolution two-dimensional gels; (iii) specific inhibition of the synthesis of particular proteins. Used in combination with absolute rates of protein synthesis, these approaches permit determination of rates of synthesis of specific proteins during oocyte growth.

Mitochondrial Proteins: Growing and fully grown oocytes synthesize several proteins encoded by the mitochondrial genome (67,204). Overall, mitochondrial protein synthesis represents 1% to 2% of total protein synthesis during oocyte growth, not unlike the percentage estimated for other eukaryotic cells. It is noteworthy that the same spectrum of mitochondrial proteins is synthesized as the mitochondria undergo morphological transformations during oocyte growth (discussed in the section on structural aspects of oocyte growth).

Ribosomal Proteins: Synthesis of ribosomal proteins occurs throughout oocyte growth and in fully grown oocytes (154,155). It is estimated that ribosomal protein synthesis accounts for 1.5% of total protein synthesis during oocyte growth, resulting in the accumulation of about 200 pg of ribosomal protein in fully grown oocytes. This large store of ribosomal protein reflects the large number of ribosomes (~ 10^8) assembled during oocyte growth (discussed in the section on structural aspects of oocyte growth). It is noteworthy that different ribosomal proteins are synthesized at different rates (i.e., not under tight coordinate control) during oocyte growth, even though the proteins are present in equimolar amounts in ribosomes.

Zona Pellucida Glycoproteins: The mouse oocyte's zona pellucida is composed of three different glycoproteins, all of which are synthesized and secreted by growing oocytes

(39,40,131,223,227,240). Synthesis of zona pellucida glycoproteins represents as much as 5% to 10% of total protein synthesis in growing oocytes. Furthermore, zona pellucida glycoproteins are the major class of proteins glycosylated and secreted during oocyte growth. One of the zona pellucida glycoproteins, called ZP3, functions as both *sperm receptor* and *acrosome reaction inducer* during fertilization of ovulated eggs (41,42,115,116).

Histones: Histone H4 is synthesized by growing and fully grown oocytes, accounting for about 0.07% and 0.05% of total protein synthesis, respectively (279). It is estimated that synthesis of all four types of histone (h2A, H2B, H3, and H4) represents 0.2% to 0.3% of total protein synthesis during oocyte growth, resulting in the accumulation of about 60 pg of histone in fully grown oocytes.

Tubulin: The α and β subunits of tubulin are synthesized throughout oocyte growth and are among the most abundant proteins in mouse oocytes (234,235). Tubulin synthesis represents 1.5% to 2.0% of total protein synthesis during oocyte growth, resulting in the accumulation of as much as 300 pg of tubulin in fully grown oocytes. Presumably, this tubulin store is recruited to form the relatively large spindles observed during meiotic maturation of fully grown oocytes (discussed in the section on structural aspects of oocyte maturation).

Actin: Synthesis of actin occurs throughout oocyte growth, representing about 1% of total protein synthesis during this period (273). The distribution of synthesis (percent of total) among α (muscle type), β (cytoplasmic type), and γ (cytoplasmic type) actin during oocyte growth is approximately 5%, 80%, and 15%, respectively.

Calmodulin: Although rates of synthesis are not available, it is clear that calmodulin is synthesized and accumulates during oocyte growth, accounting for as much as 0.3% of the total oocyte protein (49).

Lactate Dehydrogenase: "Heart-type" lactate dehydrogenase (LDH-H_4) is synthesized throughout oocyte growth, representing 2% to 5% of total protein synthesis during this period (68,166,167). As a result, 200 to 400 pg of lactate dehydrogenase accumulates in fully grown oocytes.

Creatine Kinase: Although rates of synthesis are not available, it is clear that creatine kinase is synthesized and accumulates throughout oocyte growth, accounting for as much as 1.4% of the total protein in fully grown mouse oocytes (146). Presumably, this relatively large store of creatine kinase is used to maintain the high level of ATP found in fully grown oocytes.

Glucose-6-phosphate Dehydrogenase: Although rates of synthesis are not available, it is clear that glucose-6-phosphate dehydrogenase is synthesized and accumulates throughout oocyte growth, since its specific activity (units/picoliter) remains constant during this period (166). Presumably, the relatively large store of glucose-6-phosphate dehydrogenase is required to produce NADPH-reducing equivalents.

Finally, it is clear that synthesis of certain proteins is regulated in a posttranscriptional manner during oocyte growth; an example of this is the synthesis of the *fertilization proteins* (53,68). Messenger RNA for the fertilization proteins is synthesized throughout oocyte growth but is translated at extremely low rates, in view of its abundance, during this period (2 to 3 weeks). It is only subsequent to fertilization that this particular class of proteins is synthesized at high rates, apparently utilizing mRNA transcribed days to weeks earlier during oocyte growth.

Protein Synthesis: Summary

Fully grown mouse oocytes contain about 25 ng of protein, exclusive of the zona pellucida, or about 50 to 60 times more protein than a mammalian liver cell (54,163,238,273). since the volume of a fully grown oocyte is about 50 to 60 times greater than that of a liver cell, the concentration of protein (picograms/picoliter) is about the same in both cell types. Therefore, as in the case of RNA and ribosomes (discussed in the section on biochemical aspects of oocyte growth), it is apparently the failure of growing oocytes to undergo cytokinesis that results in an unusually large store of protein. Whether or not the growing oocyte itself synthesizes all of this protein remains an open question; the possibility remains that some proteins are synthesized elsewhere and taken up into growing oocytes by endocytosis. It is clear that both structural proteins and enzymes are synthesized and stored throughout oocyte growth. Turnover of nascent protein in growing mouse oocytes, like nascent RNA, occurs at a relatively low rate, partly accounting for the large stores inherited by unfertilized eggs. Some proteins synthesized by growing oocytes, such as zona pellucida and some cortical granule proteins, are essential for development beyond the unfertilized egg stage and may be unique to mammalian oocytes. Regulatory proteins involved in stage-specific transcription and translation, as well as in control of meiosis, undoubtedly are synthesized during oocyte growth and should be identified and characterized in the near future by application of recombinant DNA and immunological technology. Finally, it would appear that translation of some oocyte mRNAs is regulated such that translation rates during oocyte growth do not reflect mRNA abundance (posttranscriptional control).

OOCYTE MATURATION: BIOCHEMICAL ASPECTS

Meiotic Maturation *In Vitro*

A discussion of morphological and regulatory events that are characteristic of meiotic maturation *in vitro* is presented above (see sections on fully grown oocytes and unfertilized eggs, on structural aspects of oocyte maturation, and on regulatory aspects of oocyte maturation). In particular, it is important to reiterate that mammalian oocytes matured *in vitro,* under appropriate culture conditions, undergo normal development following insemination. Therefore, it is reasonable to assume that biochemical measurements made during this period *in vitro* are physiologically meaningful.

RNA Synthesis

Although RNA continues to be synthesized in fully grown oocytes (discussed in the section on biochemical aspects of oocyte growth), RNA synthesis is barely detectable after breakdown of the nuclear envelope and chromosome condensation, i.e., after meiotic maturation is initiated (194, 221,278). Cessation of ribosomal-RNA synthesis apparently is associated with dissolution of the nucleolus upon mixing of nucleoplasm and cytoplasm. Furthermore, as much as one-half of the polyadenylated RNA accumulated during oocyte growth is either degraded or deadenylated during meiotic maturation (15,20). Therefore, during a period when certain maternal messages are utilized for the first time (see below), there is an overall decrease in levels of total and polyadenylated RNA inherited by the unfertilized egg from the fully grown oocyte.

Protein Synthesis

The sizes of the methionine pool and absolute rates of protein synthesis during meiotic maturation of mouse oocytes *in vitro* have been determined (232,273). As meiotic maturation progresses from the dictyate stage to metaphase II, the size of the intracellular methionine pool decreases from about 56 (~170 μM) to 35 fmole per oocyte (~138 μM), and the absolute rate of protein synthesis decreases from about 42 to 33 pg/hr per oocyte. The decrease in absolute rate of protein synthesis during this period is not simply due to the decrease in size of the intracellular methionine pool. Because the absolute rate of protein synthesis in ovulated eggs is nearly identical to that in oocytes matured *in vitro,* the decrease observed during meiotic maturation apparently is of physiological significance. Since the rate of RNA synthesis decreases dramatically following breakdown of the nuclear envelope and chromosome condensation, it is likely that the modest decrease in absolute rate of protein synthesis during meiotic maturation reflects turnover of oocyte RNA (see above) and/or translational control mechanisms.

The decrease in overall protein synthesis during meiotic maturation of oocytes is reflected in the behavior of a variety of specific proteins (267,268,273). For example, the rates of synthesis of tubulin, actin, histones, and ribosomal proteins decrease by 30% to 50%, and the rate of synthesis of lactate dehydrogenase decreases by 80% to 90% during meiotic maturation. Synthesis of zona pellucida glycoproteins decreases to extremely low levels during meiotic maturation. In this context, electrophoretic analyses of nascent proteins have revealed many changes in the overall pattern of protein synthesis during meiotic maturation of oocytes (84,171,172,220,222,233,239,266,272,280). Both the appearance and disappearance of particular protein species have been noted. Virtually all of the changes observed in protein synthesis occur subsequent to nuclear envelope dissolution but are not dependent on other events such as spindle formation or polar-body emission. Oocytes that remain arrested at the dictyate stage, with an intact nuclear envelope, either in the presence or absence of drugs, do not exhibit these changes in protein synthesis. Therefore, it is likely that many of the changes in protein synthesis accompanying meiotic maturation result from mixing of the oocyte's nucleoplasm and cytoplasm.

Summary

Meiotic maturation represents the final stage of preparation of eggs for fertilization and early development (discussed in the sections on fully grown oocytes and unfertilized eggs, on structural aspects of oocyte maturation, and on regulatory aspects of oocyte maturation). Accordingly, biochemical changes occur during this period that are essential for meiotic progression, as well as for further development. However, at present, the nature of these changes is appreciated only at a superficial level, i.e., as the appearance and disappearance of proteins on gels.

THE UNFERTILIZED EGG: MACROMOLECULAR STORES

The unfertilized mammalian egg, like nonmammalian eggs, contains an extensive store of materials poised to be mobilized following fertilization (15,34,36,79–82,148,162, 211,231,273,274). The mouse egg contains about 40 pg of DNA (not including polar body), 500 pg of RNA, 20 to 25 ng of protein (not including zona pellucida), and 150 pg of glycogen. In addition, the egg inherits about 100,000 mitochondria, 100,000,000 ribosomes, 4,500 cortical granules, and a zona pellucida. Each egg has about 800 fmole of ATP, as compared to about 15 to 25 fmole found in a typical somatic cell. Finally, the egg inherits substantial pools of tubulin (~250 pg) and actin (~100 pg), as well as unusually high levels of a variety of enzymes involved in macromolecular biosynthesis and energy metabolism. Since the unfertilized mouse egg is 60 to 70 times larger (volume) than a typical somatic cell, accumulation of this impressive store is attributable, at least in part, to growth without cytokinesis.

Although cleavage of mouse embryos is extremely slow, relative to amphibian and echinoderm embryos, the mass of nascent proteins synthesized during this period is very small compared to that contributed by the unfertilized egg. For example, during the transition from a 1- to 8-cell mouse embryo (~ 60 hr), about 50 pg of tubulin is synthesized by the cleaving embryo (~6 pg/blastomere); this represents only about 20% of the tubulin pool (~ 250 pg) inherited by the embryo from the unfertilized egg (1,234,235). A similar situation applies for many of the structural proteins and enzymes examined during oogenesis and early embryogenesis in mammals. Furthermore, it is clear that certain organelles, such as cortical granules, zona pellucida, and mitochondria, are made during oogenesis for use during fertilization and early embryogenesis. It is also likely that the large store of ribosomes inherited by the embryo functions during the first two to three cleavage divisions, at which time the rates of synthesis of ribosomal RNA and ribosomal proteins achieve relatively high levels. Finally, unfertilized eggs inherit a store of histones sufficient to support the first few cleavage divisions.

Thus, in the egg, oogenesis achieves several objectives: an increase in genotypic variation, production of a haploid cell, biogenesis of macromolecules and organelles involved in fertilization, and establishment of a store of materials to support and regulate development of the preimplantation embryo. In all of these respects, mammalian eggs resemble their nonmammalian counterpart.

A FINAL WORD

It is hoped that this presentation has conveyed the theme that *animal development is rooted in oogenesis,* the process by which eggs are produced. This is as true for mammals as it is for nonmammals. Research in this particular area has a long, illustrious history and continues to reveal principles that underlie not only animal development but also cellular mechanisms in general. Research on molecular aspects of mammalian egg and embryo development, in particular, has made impressive strides in recent years; this has been made possible largely by important conceptual and technological advances. In many instances, the paucity of biological material available from mammals, a factor that inhibited research on mammalian oogenesis for so long, is no longer as serious a consideration. Perhaps, most exciting, is the prospect that one will soon be able to carry out and investigate the entire process of mammalian oogenesis, from primordial germ cells to unfertilized eggs, in culture *in vitro*. The technology required to fertilize such eggs *in vitro* and produce viable offspring is already available. Consequently, it is to be expected that expanded research on egg and embryo development in mammals during the next decade will achieve a more complete understanding of molecular mechanisms involved in our own development from a single cell. This knowledge undoubtedly will have far-reaching consequences and great impact on both medical and social issues in ensuing years. These issues should be addressed with reason, not emotion.

ACKNOWLEDGMENTS

The author is delighted to take this opportunity to acknowledge the members of his laboratory who, through the years, have provided a stimulating, productive, and cordial environment in which to work. He also thanks the Rockefeller Foundation, National Institute of Child Health and Human Development, and National Science Foundation, who supported much of the research on mammalian development carried out in his laboratory.

REFERENCES

1. Abreu, S., and Brinster, R. (1978): Synthesis of tubulin and actin during the preimplantation development of the mouse. *Exp. Cell Res.*, 114:135–141.
2. Adams, E., and Hertig, A. (1964): Studies on guinea pig oocytes. I. Electron microscopic observations on the development of cytoplasmic organelles in oocytes of primordial and primary follicles. *J. Cell Biol.*, 21:397–427.
3. Albertini, D., and Anderson, E. (1974): The appearance and structure of the intercellular connections during the ontogeny of the rabbit ovarian follicle with special reference to gap junctions. *J. Cell Biol.*, 2:234–250.
4. Albertini, D., Fawcett, D., and Olds, P. (1975): Morphological variations in gap junctions of ovarian granulosa cells. *Tissue Cell,* 7:389–405.
5. Amsterdam, A., Josephs, R., Lieberman, M., and Lindner, H. (1976): Organization of intramembrane particles in freeze-cleaved gap junctions of rat graafian follicles: Optical diffraction analysis. *J. Cell Sci.*, 21:93–105.
6. Anderson, E., and Albertini, E. (1976): Gap junctions between the oocyte and companion follicle cells in the mammalian ovary. *J. Cell Biol.*, 71:680–686.
7. Anderson, E., Wilkinson, R., Lee, G., and Meller, S. (1978): A correlative microscopical analysis of differentiating ovarian follicles of mammals. *J. Morphol.*, 156:339–366.
8. Asdell, A. (1969): Historical introduction. In: *Reproduction in Domestic Animals,* edited by H. Cole and P. Cupps, pp. 1–14. Academic Press, New York.
9. Austin, C. (1961): *The Mammalian Egg*. Blackwell Science Publications, Oxford.
10. Austin, C. (1982): The egg. In: *Reproduction in Mammals, Vol. 1,* edited by C. Austin and R. Short, pp. 46–62. Cambridge University Press, Cambridge.
11. Austin, C., and Short, R., editors (1982): *Reproduction in Mammals, Vol. 1, Germ Cells and Fertilization*. Cambridge University Press, Cambridge.
12. Baca, M., and Zamboni, L. (1967): The fine structure of human follicular oocytes. *J. Ultrastruct. Res.*, 19:354–381.
13. Bachvarova, R. (1974): Incorporation of tritiated adenosine into mouse ovum RNA. *Dev. Biol.*, 40:52–58.
14. Bachvarova, R. (1981): Synthesis, turnover, and stability of heterogeneous RNA in growing mouse oocytes. *Dev. Biol.*, 86:384–392.
15. Bachvarova, R. (1985): Gene expression during oogenesis and oocyte development in mammals. In: *Developmental Biology: A Comprehensive Synthesis, Vol. 1, Oogenesis,* edited by L. Browder, pp. 453–524. Plenum Press, New York.
16. Bachvarova, R., Baran, M., and Tejblum, A. (1980): Development of naked growing mouse oocytes *in vitro*. *J. Exp. Zool.*, 211:159–169.
17. Bachvarova, R., Burns, J., Speigelman, I., Choy, J., and Chaganti, R. (1982): Morphology and transcriptional activity of mouse oocyte chromosomes. *Chromosoma,* 86:181–196.
18. Bachvarova, R., and De Leon, V. (1977): Stored and polysomal ribosomes of mouse ova. *Dev. Biol.*, 58:248–254.
19. Bachvarova, R., and De Leon, V. (1980): Polyadenylated RNA of mouse ova and loss of maternal RNA in early development. *Dev. Biol.*, 74:1–8.
20. Bachvarova, R., De Leon, V., Johnson, A., Kaplan, G., and Paynton, B. (1985): Changes in total RNA, polyadenylated RNA, and actin mRNA during meiotic maturation of mouse oocytes. *Dev. Biol.*, 108:325–331.
21. Bachvarova, R., De Leon, V., and Spiegelman, I. (1981): Mouse egg ribosomes: Evidence for storage in lattices. *J. Embryol. Exp. Morphol.*, 62:153–164.

22. Bachvarova, R., and Moy, K. (1985): Autoradiographic studies on the distribution of labeled maternal RNA in early mouse embryos. *J. Exp. Zool.*
23. Baker, T. (1972): Oogenesis and ovarian development. In: *Reproductive Biology,* edited by H. Balin and S. Glasser, pp. 398–437. Excerpta Medica, Amsterdam.
24. Baker, T. (1982): Oogenesis and ovulation. In: *Reproduction in Mammals, Vol. 1,* edited by C. Austin and R. Short, pp. 17–45. Cambridge University Press, Cambridge.
25. Baker, T., Beaumont, H., and Franchi, L. (1969): The uptake of tritiated uridine and phenylalanine by the ovaries of rats and monkeys. *J. Cell Sci.,* 4:655–675.
26. Baker, T., and Franchi, L. (1967): The fine structure of oogonia and oocytes in human ovaries. *J. Cell Sci.,* 2:213–224.
27. Baker, T., and Franchi, L. (1967): The structure of the chromosomes in human primordial oocytes. *Chromosoma,* 22:358–377.
28. Baker, T., and Franchi, L. (1967): The fine structure of chromosomes in bovine primordial oocytes. *J. Reprod. Fertil.,* 14:511–513.
29. Baker, T., and Franchi, L. (1972): The fine structure of oogonia and oocytes in the rhesus monkey (*Macaca mulatta*). *Z. Zellforsch. Mikrosk. Anat.* 126:53–74.
30. Bakken, A., and McClanahan, M. (1978): Patterns of RNA synthesis in early meiotic prophase oocytes from fetal mouse ovaries. *Chromosoma,* 67:21–40.
31. Balakier, H. (1978): Induction of maturation in small oocytes from sexually immature mice by fusion with meiotic or mitotic cells. *Exp. Cell Res.,* 112:137–141.
32. Balakier, H., and Czolowska, R. (1977): Cytoplasmic control of nuclear maturation in mouse oocytes. *Exp. Cell Res.,* 110:466–469.
33. Baran, M., and Bachvarova, R. (1977): *In vitro* culture of growing mouse oocytes. *J. Exp. Zool.,* 202:283–289.
34. Biggers, J. (1971): Metabolism of mouse embryos. *J. Reprod. Fertil.* (*Suppl.*), 14:41–54.
35. Biggers, J., and Schuetz, A., editors (1973): *Oogenesis.* University Park Press, Baltimore.
36. Biggers, J., and Stern, S. (1973): Metabolism of the preimplantation mammalian embryo. *Adv. Reprod. Physiol.,* 6:1–59.
37. Blanchette, E. (1961): A study of the fine structure of the rabbit primary oocyte. *J. Ultrastruct. Res.,* 5:349–363.
38. Blandau, R. (1970): Growth of the ovarian follicle and ovulation. *Prog. Gynecol.,* 5:58–76.
39. Bleil, J., and Wassarman, P. (1980): Synthesis of zona pellucida proteins by denuded and follicle-enclosed mouse oocytes during culture *in vitro. Proc. Natl. Acad. Sci. USA,* 77:1029–1033.
40. Bleil, J., and Wassarman, P. (1980): Structure and function of the zona pellucida: Identification and characterization of the proteins of the mouse oocyte's zona pellucida. *Dev. Biol.,* 76:185–202.
41. Bleil, J., and Wassarman, P. (1980): Mammalian sperm-egg interaction: Identification of a glycoprotein in mouse egg zonae pellucidae possessing sperm receptor activity. *Cell,* 20:873–882.
42. Bleil, J., and Wassarman, P. (1986): Autoradiographic visualization of the mouse egg's sperm receptor bound to sperm. *J. Cell Biol.,* 102:1363–1371.
43. Bloom, A., and Mukherjee, B. (1972): RNA synthesis in maturing mouse oocytes. *Exp. Cell Res.,* 74:577–582.
44. Boreen, S., Gizang, E., and Schultz, R. (1983): Biochemical studies of mammalian oogenesis: Synthesis of 5S and 4S RNA during growth of the mouse oocyte. *Gamete Res.,* 8:379–383.
45. Bornslaeger, E., Mattei, P., and Schultz, R. (1986): Involvement of cAMP-dependent protein kinase and protein phosphorylation in regulation of mouse oocyte maturation. *Dev. Biol.,* 114:453–462.
46. Bornslaeger, E., Poueymirou, W., Mattei, P., and Schultz, R. (1986): Effects of protein kinase C activators on germinal vesicle breakdown and polar body emission of mouse oocytes. *Exp. Cell Res.,* 165:507–517.
47. Bornslaeger, E., and Schultz, R. (1985): Adenylate cyclase activity in zona-free mouse oocytes. *Exp. Cell Res.,* 156:277–281.
48. Bornslaeger, E., and Schultz, R. (1985): Regulation of mouse oocyte maturation: Effect of elevating cumulus cell cAMP on oocyte cAMP levels. *Biol. Reprod.,* 33:698–704.
49. Bornslaeger, E., Wilde, M., and Schultz, R. (1984): Regulation of mouse oocyte maturation: Involvement of cyclic AMP phosphodiesterase and calmodulin. *Dev. Biol.,* 105:488–499.
50. Brambell, F. (1927): The development and morphology of the gonads of the mouse. Part I. The morphogenesis of the indifferent gonad and of the ovary. *Proc. R. Soc. Lond.* (*Biol.*), 101:391–409.
51. Brambell, F. (1928): The development and morphology of the gonads of the mouse. Part III. The growth of the follicles. *Proc. R. Soc. Lond.* (*Biol.*), 103:258–272.
52. Brambell, F. (1956): Ovarian changes. In: *Marshall's Physiology of Reproduction, Vol. 1,* edited by A. Parkes, pp. 397–542. Longmans, Green, New York.
53. Braude, P., Pelham, H., Flach, G., and Lobatto, R. (1979): Post-transcriptional control in the early mouse embryo. *Nature,* 282:102–105.
54. Brinster, R. (1967): Protein content of the mouse embryo during the first five days of development. *J. Reprod. Fertil.,* 10:227–240.
55. Browder, L., editor (1985): *Developmental Biology: A Comprehensive Synthesis, Vol. 1, Oogenesis.* Plenum Press, New York.
56. Brower, P., Gizang, E., Boreen, S., and Schultz, R. (1981): Biochemical studies of mammalian oogenesis: Synthesis and stability of various classes of RNA during growth of the mouse oocyte *in vitro. Dev. Biol.,* 86:373–383.
57. Brower, P., and Schultz, R. (1982): Intercellular communication between granulosa cells and mouse oocytes: Existence and possible nutritional role during oocyte growth. *Dev. Biol.,* 90:144–153.
58. Brower, P., and Schultz, R. (1982): Biochemical studies of mammalian oogenesis: Possible existence of a ribosomal and poly(A)-containing RNA-protein supramolecular complex in mouse oocytes. *J. Exp. Zool.,* 220:251–260.
59. Buehr, M., and McLaren, A. (1985): Expression of glucose-phosphate isomerase in relation to growth of the mouse oocyte *in vivo* and *in vitro. Gamete Res.,* 11:271–281.
60. Burkholder, G., Comings, D., and Okada, T. (1971): A storage form of ribosomes in mouse oocytes. *Exp. Cell Res.,* 69:361–371.
61. Byskov, A. (1969): Ultrastructural studies on the preovulatory follicle in the mouse ovary. *Z. Zellforsch. Mikrosk. Anat.,* 100:285–299.
62. Byskov, A. (1982): Primordial germ cells and regulation of meiosis. In: *Reproduction in Mammals, Vol. 1,* edited by C. Austin and R. Short, pp. 1–16. Cambridge University Press, Cambridge.
63. Calarco, P. (1972): The kinetochore in oocyte maturation. In: *Oogenesis,* edited by J. Biggers and A. Schuetz, pp. 65–86. University Park Press, Baltimore.
64. Calarco, P., Donahue, R., and Szollosi, D. (1972): Germinal vesicle breakdown in the mouse oocyte. *J. Cell Sci.,* 10:369–385.
65. Canipari, R., Palombi, F., Riminucci, M., and Mangia, F. (1984): Early programming and maturation competence in mouse oogenesis. *Dev. Biol.,* 102:519–524.
66. Canipari, R., Pietrolucci, A., and Mangia, F. (1979): Increase of total protein synthesis during mouse oocyte growth. *J. Reprod. Fertil.,* 57:405–413.
67. Cascio, S., and Wassarman, P. (1981): Program of early development in the mammal: Synthesis of mitochondrial proteins during oogenesis and early embryogenesis in the mouse. *Dev. Biol.,* 83:166–172.
68. Cascio, S., and Wassarman, P. (1982): Program of early development in the mammal: Post-transcriptional control of a class of proteins synthesized by mouse oocytes and early embryos. *Dev. Biol.,* 89:397–408.
69. Centola, G., Anderson, L., and Channing, C. (1981): Oocyte maturation inhibition activity in porcine granulosa cells. *Gamete Res.,* 4:451–462.
70. Chang, M. (1955): The maturation of rabbit oocytes in culture and their maturation, activation, fertilization, and subsequent development in the fallopian tubes. *J. Exp. Zool.,* 128:378–405.
71. Chari, S., Hillensjo, T., Magnusson, C., Sturm, G., and Daume, E. (1983): *In vitro* inhibition of rat oocyte meiosis by human follicular fluid fractions. *Arch. Gynecol.,* 233:155–164.
72. Chiquoine, A. (1954): The identification, origin and migration of the primordial germ cells in the mouse embryo. *Anat. Rec.,* 118:135–146.
73. Chiquoine, A. (1960): The development of the zona pellucida of the mammalian ovum. *Am. J. Anat.,* 106:149–170.
74. Cho, W.-K., Stern, S., and Biggers, J. (1974): Inhibitory effect of dibutyryl cAMP on mouse oocyte maturation *in vitro. J. Exp. Zool.,* 187:383–386.
75. Chouinard, L. (1971): A light- and electron-microscope study of the nucleolus during growth of the oocyte in the prepubertal mouse. *J. Cell Sci.,* 9:637–663.

76. Chouinard, L. (1973): An electron-microscope study of the extranucleolar bodies during growth of the oocyte in the prepubertal mouse. *J. Cell Sci.*, 12:55–69.
77. Chouinard, L. (1975): A light- and electron-microscope study of the oocyte nucleus during development of the antral follicle in the prepubertal mouse. *J. Cell Sci.*, 17:589–615.
78. Clark, J., and Eddy, E. (1975): Fine structural observations on the origin and association of primordial germ cells of the mouse. *Dev. Biol.*, 47:136–155.
79. Clegg, K., and Piko, L. (1977): Size and specific activity of the UTP pool and overall rates of RNA synthesis in early mouse embryos. *Dev. Biol.*, 58:76–95.
80. Clegg, K., and Piko, L. (1982): RNA synthesis and cytoplasmic polyadenylation in the one-cell mouse embryo. *Nature*, 295:342–345.
81. Clegg, K., and Piko, L. (1983): Poly(A) length, cytoplasmic adenylation and synthesis of poly(A)$^+$ RNA in early mouse embryos. *Dev. Biol.*, 95:331–341.
82. Clegg, K., and Piko, L. (1983): Quantitative aspects of RNA synthesis and polyadenylation in 1-cell and 2-cell mouse embryos. *J. Embryol. Exp. Morphol.*, 74:169–182.
83. Colonna, R., Cecconi, S., Buccione, R., and Mangia, F. (1983): Amino acid transport systems in growing mouse oocytes. *Cell Biol. Int. Rep.*. 7:1007–1015.
84. Crosby, I., Osborn, J., and Moor, R. (1984): Changes in protein phosphorylation during the maturation of mammalian oocytes *in vitro*. *J. Exp. Zool.*, 229:459–466.
85. Cross, P., and Brinster, R. (1970): *In vitro* development of mouse oocytes. *Biol. Reprod.*, 3:298–307.
86. Cross, P., and Brinster, R. (1974): Leucine uptake and incorporation at three stages of mouse oocyte maturation. *Exp. Cell Res.*, 86: 43–46.
87. Daniel, J., editor (1971): *Methods in Mammalian Embryology*, W. H. Freeman. San Francisco.
88. Daniel, J., editor (1978): *Methods in Mammalian Reproduction*. Academic Press, New York.
89. Davidson, E. (1976): *Gene Activity in Early Development*. Academic Press, New York.
90. De Felici, M., and McLaren, A. (1982): Isolation of mouse primordial germ cells. *Exp. Cell Res.*, 142:476–482.
91. De Felici, M., and Siracusa, G. (1982): Survival of isolated, fully grown mouse ovarian oocytes is strictly dependent on external Ca^{2+}. *Dev. Biol.*, 92:539–543.
92. Dekel, N., Aberdam, E., and Sherizly, I. (1984): Spontaneous maturation *in vitro* of cumulus-enclosed rat oocytes is inhibited by forskolin. *Biol. Reprod.*, 31:244–250.
93. Dekel, N., and Beers, W. (1978): Rat oocyte maturation *in vitro:* Relief of cyclic AMP inhibition with gonadotropins. *Proc. Natl. Acad. Sci. USA*, 75:4369–4373.
94. Dekel, N., and Beers, W. (1980): Development of the rat oocyte *in vitro:* Inhibition and induction of maturation in the presence or absence of the cumulus oophorus. *Dev. Biol.*, 75:247–254.
95. Dekel, N., Hillensjo, T., and Kraicer, P. (1979): Maturational effects of gonadotropins on the cumulus-oocyte complex of the rat. *Biol. Reprod.*, 20:191–197.
96. Dekel, N., Kraicer, P., Phillips, D., Sanchez, R., and Segal, S. (1978): Cellular associations in the rat oocyte-cumulus cell complex: Morphology and ovulatory changes. *Gamete Res.*, 1:47–57.
97. Dekel, N., Lawrence, T., Gilula, N., and Beers, W. (1981): Modulation of cell-to-cell communication in the cumulus-oocyte complex and the regulation of oocyte maturation by LH. *Dev. Biol.*, 80:356–362.
98. De Leon, V., Johnson, A., and Bachvarova, R. (1983): Half-lives and relative amounts of stored and polysomal ribosomes and poly(A)$^+$ RNA in mouse oocytes. *Dev. Biol.*, 98:400–408.
99. Donahue, R. (1968): Maturation of the mouse oocyte *in vitro*. I. Sequence and timing of nuclear progression. *J. Exp. Zool.*, 169:237–250.
100. Downs, S., Coleman, D. Ward-Bailey, P., and Eppig, J. (1985): Hypoxanthine is the principal inhibitor of murine oocyte maturation in a low molecular weight fraction of porcine follicular fluid. *Proc. Natl. Acad. Sci. USA*, 82:454–458.
101. Downs, S., and Eppig, J. (1984): Cyclic adenosine monophosphate and ovarian follicular fluid act synergistically to inhibit mouse oocyte maturation. *Endocrinology*, 114:418–427.
102. Dunbar, B., Wardrip, N., and Hedrick, J. (1980): Isolation, physiochemical properties, and macromolecular composition of zona pellucida from porcine oocytes. *Biochemistry*, 19:356–365.
103. Eddy, E., Clark, J., Gong, D., and Fenderson, B. (1981): Origin and migration of primordial germ gells in mammals. *Gamete Res.*, 4:333–362.
104. Eddy, E., and Hahnel, A. (1983): Establishment of the germ line in mammals. In *7th Symposium of British Society for Developmental Biology*, edited by A. McLaren and C. Wylie, pp. 41–69. Cambridge University Press, Cambridge.
105. Ekholm, C., and Magnusson, C. (1979): Rat oocyte maturation: Effects of protein synthesis inhibitors. *Biol. Reprod.*, 21:1287–1293.
106. Eppig, J. (1976): Analysis of mouse oogenesis *in vitro*. Oocyte isolation and the utilization of exogenous energy sources by growing oocytes. *J. Exp. Zool.*, 198:375–382.
107. Eppig, J. (1977): Mouse oocyte development in vitro with various culture systems. *Dev. Biol.*, 60:371–388.
108. Eppig, J. (1979): A comparison between oocyte growth in coculture with granulosa cells and oocytes with granulosa cell-oocyte junctional contact maintained *in vitro*. *J. Exp. Zool.*, 209:345–353.
109. Eppig, J. (1982): The relationship between cumulus cell-oocyte coupling, oocyte meiotic maturation, and cumulus expansion. *Dev. Biol.*, 89:268–272.
110. Eppig, J. (1985): Oocyte-somatic cell interactions during oocyte growth and maturation in the mammal. In: *Developmental Biology: A Comprehensive Synthesis, Vol. 1, Oogenesis,* edited by L. Browder, pp. 313–347. Plenum Press, New York.
111. Eppig, J., Freter, R., Ward-Bailey, P., and Schultz, R. (1983): Inhibition of oocyte maturation in the mouse: Participation of cAMP, steroid hormones, and a putative maturation-inhibitory factor. *Dev. Biol.*, 100:39–49.
112. Eppig, J., and Koide, S. (1978): Effects of progesterone and oestradiol-17β on the spontaneous meiotic maturation of mouse oocytes. *J. Reprod. Fertil.*, 53:99–101.
113. Eppig, J., Ward-Bailey, P., and Coleman, D. (1985): Hypoxanthine and adenosine in murine ovarian follicular fluid: Concentrations and activity in maintaining oocyte meiotic arrest. *Biol. Reprod.*, 33:1041–1049.
114. Fleming, A. Khalil, W., and Armstrong, D. (1983): Porcine follicular fluid does not inhibit maturation of rat oocytes *in vitro*. *J. Reprod. Fertil.*, 69:665–670.
115. Florman, H., Bechtol, K., and Wassarman, P. (1984): Enzymatic dissection of the functions of the mouse egg's receptor for sperm. *Dev. Biol.*, 106:243–255.
116. Florman, H., and Wassarman, P. (1985): *O*-Linked oligosaccharides of mouse egg ZP3 account for its sperm receptor activity. *Cell*, 41:313–324.
117. Fourcroy, J. (1982): RNA synthesis in immature mouse oocyte development. *J. Exp. Zool.*, 219:257–266.
118. Franchi, L., and Mandl, A. (1962): The ultrastructure of oogonia and oocytes in the foetal and neonatal rat. *Proc. R. Soc. Lond. (Biol.)*, 157:99–114.
119. Franchi, L., Mandl, A., and Zuckerman, S. (1962): The development of the ovary and the process of oogenesis. In: *The Ovary, Vol. 1*, edited by S. Zuckerman, pp. 1–88. Academic Press, New York.
120. Freter, R., and Schultz, R. (1984): Regulation of murine oocyte maturation: Evidence for a gonadotropin-induced, cAMP-dependent reduction in a maturation inhibitor. *J. Cell Biol.*, 98:1119–1128.
121. Fulka, J., Motlik, J., Fulfa, J., and Crozet, N. (1985): Inhibition of nuclear maturation in fully grown porcine and mouse oocytes after their fusion with growing porcine oocytes. *J. Exp. Zool.*, 235:255–259.
122. Garcia, R., Pereyra-Alfonso, S., and Sotelo, J. (1979): Protein-synthesizing machinery in the growing oocyte of the cyclic mouse. *Differentiation (Berl.)*, 14:101–106.
123. Gilula, N., Epstein, M., and Beers, W. (1978): Cell-to-cell communication and ovulation: A study of the cumulus cell-oocyte complex. *J. Cell Biol.*, 78:58–75.
124. Gilula, N., Reeves, O., and Steinbach, A. (1972): Metabolic coupling, ionic coupling, and cell contacts. *Nature*, 235:262–265.
125. Glass, L. (1961): Localization of autologous and heterologous serum antigens in the mouse ovary. *Dev. Biol.*, 3:797–804.
126. Glass, L. (1971): Transmission of maternal proteins into oocytes. *Adv. Biosci.*, 6:29–58.

127. Glass, L., and Cons, J. (1968): Stage-dependent transfer of systematically injected foreign protein antigen and radiolabel into mouse ovarian follicles. *Anat. Rec.*, 162:139–156.
128. Golbus, M., and Stein, M. (1976): Qualitative patterns of protein synthesis in the mouse oocyte. *J. Exp. Zool.*, 198:337–342.
129. Gondos, B. (1978): Oogonia and oocytes in mammals. In: *The Vertebrate Ovary,* edited by R. Jones, pp. 83–120. Plenum Press, New York.
130. Green, E., editor (1975): *Biology of the Laboratory Mouse,* Dover Publications, New York.
131. Greve, J., Salzmann, G., Roller, R., and Wassarman, P. (1982): Biosynthesis of the major zona pellucida glycoprotein secreted by oocytes during mammalian oogenesis. *Cell,* 31:749–759.
132. Greve, J. and Wassarman, P. (1985): Mouse egg extracellular coat is a matrix of interconnected filaments possessing a structural repeat. *J. Mol. Biol.*, 181:253–264.
133. Gulyas, B. (1980): Cortical granules of mammalian eggs. *Int. Rev. Cytol.* 63:357–392.
134. Gwatkin, R., and Andersen, O. (1976): Hamster oocyte maturation *in vitro:* Inhibition by follicular components. *Life Sci.*, 19:527–536.
135. Habibi, B., and Franchi, L. (1978): Fine-structural changes in the nucleus of primordial oocytes in immature hamsters. *J. Cell. Sci.*, 34:209–223.
136. Haddad, A., and Nagai, E. (1977): Radioautographic study of glycoprotein biosynthesis and renewal in the ovarian follicles of mice and the origin of the zona pellucida. *Cell Tissue Res.*, 177:347–369.
137. Hardisty, M. (1978): Primordial germ cells and the vertebrate germ line. In: *The Vertebrate Ovary,* edited by R. Jones, pp. 1–82. Plenum Press, New York.
138. Hartung, M., and Stahl, A. (1978): Autoradiographic study of RNA synthesis during meiotic prophase in the human oocyte. *Cytogenet. Cell Genet.*, 20:51–58.
139. Heller, D., Cahill, D., and Schultz, R. (1981): Biochemical studies of mammalian oogenesis: Metabolic cooperativity between granulosa cells and growing mouse oocytes. *Dev. Biol.*, 84:455–464.
140. Heller, D., and Schultz, R. (1980): Ribonucleoside metabolism by mouse oocytes: Metabolic cooperativity between the fully-grown oocyte and cumulus cells. *J. Exp. Zool.*, 214:355–364.
141. Herlands, R., and Schultz, R. (1984): Regulation of mouse oocyte growth: Probable nutritional role for intercellular communication between follicle cells and oocytes in oocyte growth. *J. Exp. Zool.*, 229:317–325.
142. Hertig, A., and Adams, E. (1967): Studies on the human oocyte and its follicle. Ultrastructural and cytochemical observations on the primordial follicle stage. *J. Cell Biol.*, 34:647–675.
143. Hisaw, F. (1947): Development of the Graafian follicle and ovulation. *Physiol. Rev.*, 27:95–119.
144. Hogan, B., Costantini, F., and Lacy, E., editors (1986): *Manipulating the Mouse Embryo. A Laboratory Manual.* Cold Spring Harbor Laboratory, Cold Spring Harbor.
145. Hope, J. (1965): The fine structure of the developing follicle of the rhesus ovary. *J. Ultrastruct. Res.*, 12:592–610.
146. Iyengar, M., Iyengar, C., Chen, H., Brinster, R., Bornslaeger, E., and Schultz, R. (1983): Expression of creatine kinase isoenzyme during oogenesis and embryogenesis in the mouse. *Dev. Biol.*, 96:263–268.
147. Jahn, C., Baran, M., and Bachvarova, R. (1976): Stability of RNA synthesized by the mouse oocyte during its major growth phase. *J. Exp. Zool.*, 197:161–172.
148. Johnson, M., McConnell, J., and Van Blerkom, J. (1984): Programmed development in the mouse embryo. *J. Embryol. Exp. Morphol. (Suppl.)*, 83:197–231.
149. Jones, R., editor (1978): *The Vertebrate Ovary.* Plenum Press, New York.
150. Kang, Y. (1974): Development of the zona pellucida in the rat oocyte. *Am. J. Anat.*, 139:535–566.
151. Kaplan, G., Abreu, S., and Bachvarova, R. (1982): rRNA accumulation and protein synthetic patterns in growing mouse oocytes. *J. Exp. Zool.*, 220:361–380.
152. Kaplan, G., Jelinek, W., and Bachvarova, R. (1985): Repetitive sequence transcripts and U1 RNA in mouse oocytes and eggs. *Dev. Biol.*, 109:15–24.
153. Krarup, T., Pedersen, T., and Faber, M. (1969): Regulation of oocyte growth in the mouse ovary. *Nature,* 224:187–188.
154. LaMarca, M., and Wassarman, P. (1979): Program of early development in the mammal: Changes in absolute rates of synthesis of ribosomal proteins during oogenesis and early embryogenesis in the mouse. *Dev. Biol.*, 73:103–119.
155. LaMarca, M., and Wassarman, P. (1984): Relationship between rates of synthesis and intracellular distribution of ribosomal proteins during oogenesis in the mouse. *Dev. Biol.*, 102:525–530.
156. Larsen, W., Wert, S., and Brunner, G. (1986): A dramatic loss of cumulus cell gap junctions is correlated with germinal vesicle breakdown in rat oocytes. *Dev. Biol.*, 113:517–521.
157. Lawrence, T., Beers, W., and Gilula, N. (1978): Transmission of hormonal stimulation by cell-to-cell communication. *Nature,* 272:501–506.
158. Lawrence, T., Ginzberg, R., Gilula, N., and Beers, W. (1979): Hormonally induced cell shape changes in cultured rat ovarian granulosa cells. *J. Cell Biol.*, 80:21–36.
159. Leibfried, L., and First, N. (1979): Effects of divalent cations on *in vitro* maturation of bovine oocytes. *J. Exp. Zool.*, 210:575–580.
160. Leibfried, L., and First, N. (1980): Follicular control of meiosis in the porcine oocyte. *Biol. Reprod.*, 23:705–709.
161. Leibfried, L., and First, N. (1980): Effect of bovine and porcine follicular fluid and granulosa cells on maturation of oocytes *in vitro. Biol. Reprod.*, 23:699–704.
162. Levey, I., Stull, G., and Brinster, R. (1978): Poly(A) and synthesis of polyadenylated RNA in the preimplantation mouse embryo. *Dev. Biol.*, 64:140–148.
163. Lowenstein, J., and Cohen, A. (1964): Dry mass, lipid content, and protein content of the intact and zona-free mouse ovum. *J. Embryol. Exp. Morphol.*, 12:113–121.
164. Magnusson, C., and Hillensjo, T. (1977): Inhibition of maturation and metabolism of rat oocytes by cyclic AMP. *J. Exp. Zool.*, 201:138–147.
165. Maller, J. (1985): Oocyte maturation in amphibians. In: *Developmental Biology: A Comprehensive Synthesis, Vol. 1, Oogenesis,* edited by L. Browder, pp. 289–311. Plenum Press, New York.
166. Mangia, F., and Epstein, C. (1975): Biochemical studies of growing mouse oocytes: Preparation of oocytes and analysis of glucose-6-phosphate dehydrogenase and lactic dehydrogenase activities. *Dev. Biol.*, 45:211–220.
167. Mangia, F., Erickson, R., and Epstein, C. (1976): Synthesis of LDH-1 during mammalian oogenesis and early development. *Dev. Biol.*, 54:146–150.
168. Masui, Y. (1985): Meiotic arrest in animal oocytes. In: *Biology of Fertilization, Vol. 1,* edited by C. Metz and A. Monroy, pp. 189–220. Academic Press, New York.
169. Masui, Y., and Clark, H. (1979): Regulation of oocyte maturation. *Int. Rev. Cytol.*, 57:185–282.
170. McGaughey, R. (1977): The culture of pig oocytes in minimal medium, and the influence of progesterone and estradiol-17β on meiotic maturation. *Endocrinology,* 100:39–45.
171. McGaughey, R., Montgomery, D., and Richter, J. (1979): Germinal vesicle configuration and patterns of polypeptide synthesis of porcine oocytes from antral follicles of different size, as related to their competency for spontaneous maturation. *J. Exp. Zool.*, 209:239–254.
172. McGaughey, R., and Van Blerkom, J. (1977): Patterns of polypeptide synthesis of porcine oocytes during maturation *in vitro. Dev. Biol.*, 56:241–254.
173. McLaren, A. (1982): The embryo. In: *Reproduction in Mammals, Vol. 2,* edited by C. Austin and R. Short, pp. 1–25. Cambridge University Press, Cambridge.
174. McLaren, A., and Wylie, C., editors (1983): Current problems in germ cell differentiation. In: *7th Symposium British Society of Developmental Biology,* Cambridge University Press, Cambridge.
175. Michaels, G., Hauswirth, W., and Laipis, P. (1982): Mitochondrial DNA copy number in bovine oocytes and somatic cells. *Dev. Biol.*, 94:246–251.
176. Mirre, C., and Stahl, A. (1978): Ultrastructure and activity of the nucleolar organizer in the mouse oocyte during meiotic prophase. *J. Cell Sci.*, 31:79–100.
177. Mirre, C., and Stahl, A. (1981): Ultrastructural organization, sites of transcription and distribution of fibrillar centers in the nucleolus of the mouse oocyte. *J. Cell Sci.*, 48:53–64.
178. Moor, R., Osborn, J., Cran, D., and Walters, D. (1981): Selective effect of gonadotrophins on cell coupling, nuclear maturation and

protein synthesis in mammalian oocytes. *J. Embryol. Exp. Morphol.*, 61:347–365.

179. Moor, R., Smith, M., and Dawson, R. (1980): Measurement of intercellular coupling between oocytes and cumulus cells using intracellular markers. *Exp. Cell Res.*, 126:15–29.
180. Moor, R., and Trounson, A. (1977): Hormonal and follicular factors affecting maturation of sheep oocytes *in vitro* and their subsequent developmental capacity. *J. Reprod. Fertil.*, 49:101–109.
181. Moore, G. (1978): RNA synthesis in fixed cells by endogenous RNA polymerase. *Exp. Cell Res.*, 111:317–326.
182. Moore, G., and Lintern-Moore, S. (1974): A correlation between growth and RNA synthesis in the mouse oocyte. *J. Reprod. Fertil.*, 39:163–166.
183. Moore, G., and Lintern-Moore, S. (1978): Transcription of the mouse oocyte genome. *Biol. Reprod.*, 18:865–870.
184. Moore, G., and Lintern-Moore, S. (1979): Stimulation of endogenous RNA polymerase I activity in the mouse oocyte after PMSG treatment. *Biol. Reprod.*, 21:373–377.
185. Moore, G., Lintern-Moore, S., Peters, H., and Faber, M. (1974): RNA synthesis in the mouse oocyte. *J. Cell Biol.*, 60:416–422.
186. Mukherjee, A. (1972): Normal porgeny from fertilization *in vitro* of mouse oocytes matured in culture and spermatozoa capacitated *in vitro*. *Nature*, 237:397–398.
187. Needham, J. (1959): *A History of Embryology*. Cambridge University Press, Cambridge.
188. Nicosia, S., Wolf, D., and Inoue, M. (1977): Cortical granule distribution and cell surface characteristics in mouse eggs. *Dev. Biol.*, 57:56–74.
189. Oakberg, E. (1968): Relationship between stage of follicular development and RNA synthesis in the mouse oocyte. *Mutat. Res.*, 6:155–165.
190. Odor, D. (1960): Electron microscopic studies on ovarian oocytes and unfertilized tubal ova in the rat. *J. Biophys. Biochem. Cytol.*, 7:567–574.
191. Odor, D. (1965): The ultrastructure of unilaminar follicles of the hamster ovary. *Am. J. Anat.*, 116:493–522.
192. Olds, P. Stern, S., and Biggers, J. (1973): Chemical estimates of the RNA and DNA contents of the early mouse embryo. *J. Exp. Zool.*, 186:39–46.
193. Olsiewski, P., and Beers, W. (1983): cAMP synthesis in the rat oocyte. *Dev. Biol.*, 100:287–293.
194. Osborn, J., and Moor, R. (1983): Time-dependent effects of α-amanitin on nuclear maturation and protein synthesis in mammalian oocytes. *J. Embryol. Exp. Morphol.*, 73:317–338.
195. Paleos, G., and Powers, R. (1981): The effect of calcium on the first meiotic division of the mammalian oocyte. *J. Exp. Zool.*, 217:409–416.
196. Palombi, F., and Viron, A. (1977): Nuclear cytochemistry of mouse oogenesis. I. Changes in extranuclear ribonucleoprotein components through meiotic prophase. *J. Ultrastruct. Res.*, 61:10–20.
197. Parkes, A., editor (1956): *Marshall's Physiology of Reproduction, Vol. 1, Part 1*. Longmans, Green, New York.
198. Pedersen, T. (1969): Follicle growth in the immature mouse ovary. *Acta Endocrinol. (Copenh.)*, 62:117–132.
199. Pedersen, T. (1970): Follicle kinetics in the ovary of the cyclic mouse. *Acta Endocrinol. (Copenh.)*, 64:304–323.
200. Pedersen, T. (1972): Follicle growth in the mouse ovary. In: *Oogenesis*, edited by J. Biggers and A. Schuetz, pp. 361–367. University Park Press, Baltimore.
201. Pedersen, T., and Peters, H. (1968): Proposal for the classification of oocytes and follicles in the mouse ovary. *J. Reprod. Fertil.*, 17:555–557.
202. Peters, H. (1969): The development of the mouse ovary from birth to maturity. *Acta Endocrinol. (Copenh.)*, 62:98–116.
203. Peters, H. (1978): Folliculogenesis in mammals. In: *The Vertebrate Ovary*, edited by R. Jones, pp. 121–144. Plenum Press, New York.
204. Piko, L., and Chase, D. (1973): Role of the mitochondrial genome during early development in mice. *J. Cell Biol.*, 58:357–378.
205. Piko, L., and Clegg, K. (1982): Quantitative changes in total RNA, total poly(A) and ribosomes in early mouse embryos. *Dev. Biol.*, 89:362–378.
206. Piko, L., Hammons, M., and Taylor, K. (1984): Amounts, synthesis, and some properties of intracisternal A particle-related RNA in early mouse embryos. *Proc. Natl. Acad. Sci. USA*, 81:488–492.
207. Piko, L., and Matsumoto, L. (1976): Number of mitochondria and some properties of mitochondrial DNA in the mouse egg. *Dev. Biol.*, 49:1–10.
208. Pincus, G. (1936): *The Eggs of Mammals*. Macmillan, New York.
209. Pincus, G., and Enzmann, E. (1935): The comparative behavior of mammalian eggs *in vivo* and *in vitro*. I. The activation of ovarian eggs. *J. Exp. Med.*, 62:665–675.
210. Powers, R., and Paleos, G. (1982): Combined effects of calcium and dibutyryl cAMP on germinal vesicle breakdown in the mouse oocyte. *J. Reprod. Fertil.*, 66:1–8.
211. Pratt, H., Bolton, V., and Gudgeon, K. (1983): The legacy from the oocyte and its role in controlling early development of the mouse embryo. *CIBA Found. Symp.*, 98:197–227.
212. Racowsky, C. (1985): Effect of forskolin on the spontaneous maturation and cyclic AMP content of hamster oocyte-cumulus complexes. *J. Exp. Zool.*, 234:87–96.
213. Racowsky, C. (1985): Antagonistic actions of estradiol and tamoxifen upon forskolin-dependent meiotic arrest, intercellular coupling, and the cAMP content of hamster oocyte-cumulus complexes. *J. Exp. Zool.*, 234:251–260.
214. Racowsky, C., and McGaughey, R. (1982): Further studies of the effects of follicular fluid and membrana granulosa cells on the spontaneous maturation of pig oocytes. *J. Reprod. Fertil.*, 66:505–512.
215. Racowsky, C., and McGaughey, R. (1982): In the absence of protein, estradiol suppresses meiosis of porcine oocytes *in vitro*. *J. Exp. Zool.*, 224:103–110.
216. Racowsky, C., and Satterlie, R. (1985): Metabolic, fluorescent dye and electrical coupling between hamster oocytes and cumulus cells during meiotic maturation *in vivo* and *in vitro*. *Dev. Biol.*, 108:191–202.
217. Rafferty, K. (1970): *Methods in Experimental Embryology of the Mouse*. Johns Hopkins Press, Baltimore.
218. Rice, C., and McGaughey, R. (1981): Effect of testosterone and dibutyryl cAMP on the spontaneous maturation of pig oocytes. *J. Reprod. Fertil.*, 62:245–256.
219. Richards, J. (1980): Maturation of ovarian follicles: Actions and interactions of pituitary and ovarian hormones on follicular cell differentiation. *Physiol. Rev.*, 60:51–89.
220. Richter, J., and McGaughey, R. (1981): Patterns of polypeptide synthesis in mouse oocytes during germinal vesicle breakdown and during maintenance of the germinal vesicle stage by dibutyryl cAMP. *Dev. Biol.*, 83:188–192.
221. Rodman, T., and Bachvarova, R. (1976): RNA synthesis in preovulatory mouse oocyts. *J. Cell. Biol.*, 70:251–257.
222. Rodman, T., and Barth, A. (1979): Chromosomes of mouse oocytes in maturation: Differential trypsin sensitivity and amino acid incorporation. *Dev. Biol.*, 68:82–95.
223. Roller, R., and Wassarman, P. (1983): Role of asparagine-linked oligosaccharides in secretion of glycoproteins of the mouse egg's extracellular coat. *J. Biol. Chem.*, 258:13243–13249.
224. Rugh, R. (1968): *The Mouse: Its Reproduction and Development*. Burgess, Minneapolis.
225. Salustri, A., and Martinozzi, M. (1983): A comparison of protein synthetic activity in *in vitro* cultured denuded and follicle-enclosed oocytes. *Cell Biol., Int. Rep.*, 7:1049–1055.
226. Salustri, A., and Siracusa, G. (1983): Metabolic coupling cumulus expansion and meiotic resumption in mouse cumuli oophori cultured *in vitro* in the presence of FSH or dbcAMP, or stimulated *in vivo* by hCG. *J. Reprod. Fertil.*, 68:335–341.
227. Salzman, G., Greve, J., Roller, R., and Wassarman, P. (1983): Biosynthesis of the sperm receptor during oogenesis in the mouse. *EMBO J.*, 2:1451–1456.
228. Sato, E., and Koide, S. (1984): Forskolin and mouse oocyte maturation *in vitro*. *J. Exp. Zool.*, 230:125–129.
229. Schroeder, A., and Eppig, J. (1984): The developmental capacity of mouse oocytes that matured spontaneously *in vitro* is normal. *Dev. Biol.*, 102:493–497.
230. Schuel, H. (1985): Functions of egg cortical granules. In: *Biology of Fertilization*, edited by C. Metz and A. Monroy, *Vol. 3*, pp. 1–44. Academic Press, New York.
231. Schultz, G. (1975): Polyadenylic acid-containing RNA in unfertilized and fertilized eggs of the rabbit. *Dev. Biol.*, 44:270–277.
232. Schultz, R., LaMarca, M., and Wassarman, P. (1978): Absolute rates of protein synthesis during meiotic maturation of mammalian oocytes *in vitro*. *Proc. Nat. Acad. Sci. USA*, 75:4160–4164.

233. Schultz, R., Letourneau, G., and Wassarman, P. (1978): Meiotic maturation of mouse oocytes *in vitro:* Protein synthesis in nucleate and anucleate oocyte fragments. *J. Cell Sci.*, 30:251–264.
234. Schultz, R., Letourneau, G., and Wassarman, P. (1979): Program of early development in the mammal: Changes in patterns and absolute rates of tubulin and total protein synthesis during oogenesis and early embryogenesis in the mouse. *Dev. Biol.*, 68:341–359.
235. Schultz, R., Letourneau, G., and Wassarman, P. (1979): Program of early development in the mammal: Changes in the patterns and absolute rates of tubulin and total protein synthesis during oocyte growth in the mouse. *Dev. Biol.*, 73:120–133.
236. Schultz, R., Montgomery, R., and Belanoff, J. (1983): Regulation of mouse oocyte meiotic maturation: Implication of a decrease in oocyte cAMP and protein dephosphorylation in commitment to resume meiosis. *Dev. Biol.*, 97:264–273.
237. Schultz, R., Montgomery, R., Ward-Bailey, P., and Eppig, J. (1983): Regulation of oocyte maturation in the mouse: Possible roles of intercellular communication, cAMP, and testosterone. *Dev. Biol.*, 95:294–304.
238. Schultz, R., and Wassarman, P. (1977): Biochemical studies of mammalian oogenesis: Protein synthesis during oocyte growth and meiotic maturation in the mouse. *J. Cell Sci.*, 24:167–194.
239. Schultz, R., and Wassarman, P. (1977): Specific changes in the pattern of protein synthesis during meiotic maturation of mammalian oocytes *in vitro*. *Proc. Natl. Acad. Sci. USA*, 74:538–541.
240. Shimuzu, S., Tsuji, M., and Dean, J. (1983): In vitro biosynthesis of three sulfated glycoproteins of murine zonae pellucidae by oocytes grown in follicle culture. *J. Biol. Chem.*, 258:5858–5863.
241. Short, R. (1977): The discovery of the ovaries. In: *The Ovary, Vol. 1*, edited by S. Zuckerman and B. Weir, pp. 1–41. Academic Press, New York.
242. Siracusa, G., De Felici, M., and Salustri, A. (1985): The proliferative and meiotic history of mammalian female germ cells. In: *Biology of Fertilization, Vol. 1*, edited by C. Metz and A. Monroy, pp. 253–298. Academic Press, New York.
243. Siracusa, G., Whittingham, D., Molinaro, M., and Vivarelli, E. (1978): Parthenogenetic activation of mouse oocytes induced by inhibitors of protein synthesis. *J. Embryol. Exp. Morphol.*, 43:157–166.
244. Smith, D., and Tenney, D. (1980): Effect of steroids on mouse oocyte maturation *in vitro*. *J. Reprod. Fertil.*, 60:331–338.
245. Sorenson, R. (1973): Cinemicrography of mouse oocyte maturation utilizing Nomarski differential-interference microscopy. *Am. J. Anat.*, 136:265–276.
246. Sorensen, R., Cyert, M., and Pedersen, R. (1985): Active maturation-promoting factor is present in mature mouse oocytes. *J. Cell. Biol.*, 100:1637–1640.
247. Sorensen, R., and Wassarman, P. (1976): Relationship between growth and meiotic maturation of the mouse oocyte. *Dev. Biol.*, 50:531–536.
248. Sotelo, J., and Porter, K. (1959): An electron microscope study of the rat ovum. *J. Biophys. Biochem. Cytol.*, 5:327–341.
249. Speed, R. (1982): Meiosis in the foetal mouse ovary. I. An analysis at the light microscope level using surface-spreading. *Chromosoma*, 85:427–437.
250. Stern, S., Biggers, J., and Anderson, E. (1971): Mitochondria and early development of the mouse. *J. Exp. Zool.* 176:179–192.
251. Sternlicht, A., and Schultz, R. (1981): Biochemical studies of mammalian oogenesis: Kinetics of accumulation of total and poly(A)-containing RNA during growth of the mouse oocyte. *J. Exp. Zool.*, 215:191–200.
252. Szollosi, D. (1972): Changes of some cell organelles during oogenesis in mammals. In: *Oogenesis*, edited by J. Biggers and A. Schuetz, pp. 47–64. University Park Press, Baltimore.
253. Szollosi, D., Calarco, P., and Donahue, R. (1972): The nuclear envelope: Its breakdown and fate in mammalian oogonia and oocytes. *Anat. Rec.*, 174:325–340.
254. Szybek, K. (1972): *In vitro* maturation of oocytes from sexually immature mice. *J. Endocrinol.*, 54:527–528.
255. Thibault, C. (1972): Final stages of mammalian oocyte maturation. In: *Oogenesis*, edited by J. Biggers and A. Schuetz, pp. 397–411. University Park Press, Baltimore.
256. Tsafriri, A. (1978): Oocyte maturation in mammals. In: *The Vertebrate Ovary*, edited by R. Jones, pp. 409–442. Plenum Press, New York.
257. Tsafriri, A. (1985): The control of meiotic maturation in mammals. In: *Biology of Fertilization, Vol. 1*, edited by C. Metz and A. Monroy, pp. 221–252. Academic Press, New York.
258. Tsafriri, A., and Bar-Ami, S. (1978): Role of divalent cations in the resumption of meiosis in rat oocytes. *J. Exp. Zool.*, 205:293–300.
259. Tsafriri, A., Bar-Ami, S., and Lindner, H. (1983): Control of the development of meiotic competence and of oocyte maturation in mammals. In: *Fertilization of the Human Egg In Vitro*, edited by H. Beier and H. Lindner, pp. 3–17. Springer-Verlag, Berlin.
260. Tsafriri, A., and Channing, C. (1975): An inhibitory influence of granulosa cells and follicular fluid upon porcine oocyte meiosis *in vitro*. *Endocrinology*, 96:992.
261. Tsafriri, A., Channing, C., Pomerantz, S., and Lindner, H. (1977): Inhibition of maturation of isolated rat oocytes by porcine follicular fluid. *J. Endocrinol.*, 75:258–291.
262. Tsafriri, A., Dekel, N., and Bar-Ami, S. (1982): The role of oocyte maturation inhibitor in follicular regulation of oocyte maturation. *J. Reprod. Fertil.*, 64:541–551.
263. Tsafriri, A., Pomerantz, S., and Channing, C. (1976): Inhibition of oocyte maturation by porcine follicular fluid: Partial characterization of the inhibitor. *Biol. Reprod.*, 14:511–516.
264. Upadhyay, S., and Zamboni, L. (1982): Ectopic germ cells: Natural model for the study of germ cell sexual differentiation. *Proc. Natl. Acad. Sci. USA*, 79:6584–6588.
265. Urner, F., Herrmann, W., Baulieu, E., and Schorderet-Slatkine, S. (1983): Inhibition of denuded mouse oocyte maturation of forskolin, an activator of adenylate cyclase. *Endocrinology*, 113:1170–1172.
266. Van Blerkom, J. (1981): Structural relationship and posttranslational modification of stage-specific proteins synthesized during early preimplantation development in the mouse. *Proc. Natl. Acad. Sci. USA*, 78:7629–7633.
267. Van Blerkom, J. (1985): Protein synthesis during oogenesis and early embryogenesis in the mammal. In: *Biology of Fertilization, Vol. 3*, edited by C. Metz and A. Monroy, pp. 379–401. Academic Press, New York.
268. Van Blerkom, J., and McGaughey, R. (1978): Molecular differentiation of the rabbit ovum. I. During oocyte maturation *in vivo* and *in vitro*. *Dev. Biol.*, 63:139–150.
269. Van Blerkom, J., and McGaughey, R. (1978): Molecular differentiation of the rabbit ovum. II. During the preimplantation development of *in vivo* and *in vitro* matured oocytes. *Dev. Biol.*, 63:151–164.
270. Van Blerkom, J., and Motta, P. (1979): *The Cellular Basis of Mammalian Reproduction*. Urban & Schwarzenberg, Baltimore.
271. Vivarelli, E., Conti, M., De Felici, M., and Siracusa, G. (1983): Meiotic resumption and intracellular cAMP levels in mouse oocytes treated with compounds which act on cAMP metabolism. *Cell Differ.*, 12:271–276.
272. Warnes, G., Moor, R., and Johnson, M. (1977): Changes in protein synthesis during maturation of sheep oocytes *in vivo* and *in vitro*. *J. Reprod. Fertil.*, 49:331–335.
273. Wassarman, P. (1983): Oogenesis: Synthetic events in the developing mammalian egg. In: *Mechanism and Control of Animal Fertilization*, edited by J. Hartmann, pp. 1–54. Academic Press, New York.
274. Wassarman, P., Bleil, J., Cascio, S., LaMarca, M., Letourneau, G., Mrozak, S., and Schultz, R. (1981): Programming of gene expression during mammalian oogenesis. In: *Bioregulators of Reproduction*, edited by G. Jagiello and H. Vogel, pp. 119–150. Academic Press, New York.
275. Wassarman, P., and Fujiwara, K. (1978): Immunofluorescent antitubulin staining of spindles during meiotic maturation of mouse oocytes *in vitro*. *J. Cell Sci.*, 29:171–188.
276. Wassarman, P., and Josefowicz, W. (1978): Oocyte development in the mouse: An ultrastructural comparison of oocytes isolated at various stages of growth and meiotic competence. *J. Morphol.*, 156:209–235.
277. Wassarman, P., Josefowicz, W., and Letourneau, G. (1976): Meiotic maturation of mouse oocytes *in vitro:* Inhibition of maturation at specific stages of nuclear progression. *J. Cell Sci.*, 22:531–545.
278. Wassarman, P., and Letourneau, G. (1976): RNA synthesis in fully-grown mouse oocytes. *Nature*, 361:73–74.
279. Wassarman, P., and Mrozak, S. (1981): Program of early development in the mammal: Synthesis and intracellular migration of histone H4 during oogenesis in the mouse. *Dev. Biol.*, 84:364–371.

280. Wassarman, P., Schultz, R., and Letourneau, G. (1979): Protein synthesis during meiotic maturation of mouse oocytes *in vitro*. Synthesis and phosphorylation of a protein localized in the germinal vesicle. *Dev. Biol.*, 69:94–107.
281. Wassarman, P., Schultz, R., Letourneau, G., LaMarca, M., and Bleil, J. (1979): Meiotic maturation of mouse oocytes *in vitro*. In *Ovarian Follicular and Corpus Luteum Function,* edited by C. Channing, J. Marsh, and W. Sadler, pp. 251–268. Plenum Press, New York.
282. Weakley, B. (1966): Electron microscopy of the oocyte and granulosa cells in the developing ovarian follicles of the golden hamster (*Mesocricetus auratus*). *J. Anat.*, 100:503–534.
283. Weakley, B. (1967): Investigations into the structure and fixation properties of cytoplasmic lamellae of hamster oocytes. *Z. Zellforsch. Mikrosk. Anat.*, 81:91–99.
284. Weakley, B. (1968): Comparison of cytoplasmic lamellae and membranous elements in oocytes of five mammalian species. *Z. Zellforsch. Mikrosk. Anat.*, 85:109–123.
285. Wilson, E. (1925): *The Cell in Development and Heredity*. Macmillan, New York.
286. Wischnitzer, S. (1967): Intramitochondrial transformations during oocyte maturation in the mouse. *J. Morphol.*, 121:29–46.
287. Wolgemuth, D., Jagiello, G., and Henderson, A. (1979): Quantitation of ribosomal RNA genes in fetal human oocyte nuclei using rRNA : DNA hybridization in situ. Evidence for increased multiplicity. *Exp. Cell Res.*, 118:181–190.
288. Wolgemuth, D., Jagiello, G., and Henderson, A. (1980): Baboon late diplotene oocytes contain micronucleoli and a low level of extra rDNA templates. *Dev. Biol.*, 78:598–604.
289. Zamboni, L. (1970): Ultrastructure of mammalian oocytes and ova. *Biol. Reprod.* (*Suppl.*), 2:44–63.
290. Zamboni, L. (1972): Comparative studies on the ultrastructure of mammalian oocytes. In: *Oogenesis,* edited by J. Biggers and A. Schuetz, pp. 5–46. University Park Press, Baltimore.
291. Zamboni, L., and Mastroianni, L. (1966): Electron microscopy studies on rabbit ova. I. The follicular oocyte. *J. Ultrastruct. Res.*, 14:95–117.
292. Zuckerman, S., editor (1962): *The Ovary, Vol. 1*. Academic Press, New York.
293. Zuckerman, S., and Baker, T. (1977): The development of the ovary and the process of oogenesis. In: *The Ovary, Vol. 1,* edited by S. Zuckerman and B. Weir, pp. 42–68. Academic Press, New York.
294. Zuckerman, S., and Weir, B., editors (1977): *The Ovary*. Academic Press, New York.

The Physiology of Reproduction,
edited by E. Knobil and J. Neill *et al.*
Raven Press, Ltd., New York © 1988.

CHAPTER 4

Gamete and Zygote Transport

Michael J. K. Harper

Gametes are properly defined as mature germ cells possessing a haploid chromosome set capable of initiating formation of a new individual by fusion with another gamete (1). Thus, at the moment of ovulation, the ovum is a gamete because it has already undergone the first meiotic division with extrusion of the first polar body and has reached the metaphase stage of the second meiotic division, where it is arrested until activation occurs. This is generally induced by penetration of a spermatozoon through the vitelline membrane of the ovum, although it can also occur rarely parthenogenetically. The spermatozoon at the moment of ejaculation is also a gamete because it has been produced through the two meiotic divisions that result in four spermatozoa being produced from each primary spermatocyte. Therefore, strictly speaking, the term *gamete* is applicable only up to fertilization. Fertilization is a process that begins with sperm penetration and is completed at syngamy, which is defined as the union of the two sets of haploid chromosomes to form a new diploid fertilized ovum (or egg). Strictly speaking, the correct term for this new structure is *zygote*.

Hence the title of this chapter is somewhat misleading because, although initial transport of sperm and egg deals with them as gametes, after fertilization the further transport should be referred to as *zygote transport*. In modern usage, one finds the terms *ovum, egg,* and *zygote* used interchangeably and qualified as fertilized or unfertilized, two-cell, etc. Because an ovum, by definition, is unfertilized, this qualification should be unnecessary. In this chapter, the term *gamete* (ovum or spermatozoon) is used to refer to the haploid chromosomal state, and the term *zygote* is used to refer to the diploid chromosomal state resulting from the union of the two gametes. The term *oviduct(s)* is preferred over the more correct term *fallopian tube(s)* [named after their discoverer, Gabrielle Fallopius, who described them in 1561 (2)] solely because of brevity.

Much of gamete transport takes place in the oviduct, since spermatozoa are transported upward to the site of fertilization and ova are transported downward from the ovarian (or distal) end of the oviduct to the uterine (or proximal) end, during which time fertilization and early development as a zygote occur. However, before ova, which enter the oviduct only following ovulation, and spermatozoa, after ejaculation and deposition in the vagina (in primates; in some other species spermatozoa are deposited into the uterus) can meet, the spermatozoa have to transverse the cervix, the uterus, and the uterotubal junction before reaching the oviduct. Each of these barriers reduces the population of spermatozoa such that, theoretically, only the fittest and most normal ones have the opportunity of fertilize an ovum. This is one way in which natural selection operates to ensure the survival of the optimal genetic combinations from generation to generation. In this chapter, each of these various events will be discussed. There may be some overlap with other chapters; in those cases the discussion of these duplicated events will be limited here to the information necessary to understand the integration of the system.

SPERM TRANSPORT

Sperm Transport in the Male

Following the process of spermatogenesis, the spermatozoa, which are almost completely immotile, are transported passively from the seminiferous tubules to the rete testis. The rete testis is a branched reservoir into which both ends of each seminiferous tubule open. The rete testis is linked to the epididymis by the 10 to 20 vasa efferentia that are located near the upper pole of the testis. These efferent ducts become highly convoluted as they reach the epididymis.

The epididymis is a single, long, highly convoluted duct on the posterior border of the testis. It has usually been divided into three regions—the head, the body, and the tail (caput, corpus, and cauda)—but these are rather arbitrary divisions, and the exact proportions of the epididymis contributing to each segment vary between species. In the human, the caput region is comprised largely of the extensive efferent duct system, and unlike in other species, the cauda is inconspicuous.

Sperm transport into and through the epididymis is not due to sperm motility, but is thought to be a passive process due initially to secretions flowing from the testis and also assisted by ciliary activity of the luminal epithelium and contractile activity of the smooth-muscular elements of the efferent duct walls (3). Regular peristaltic contractions of the epididymal duct wall propel the spermatozoa from the caput to the cauda. The rate of transport through this organ is not influenced by ligation of the vasa efferentia (4,5), reinforcing the notion of epididymal transport being a local phenomenon. These peristaltic contractions have been observed in both rats and rabbits (6,7) and seem likely to be a general phenomenon. The cauda epididymidis and the vas deferens are richly innervated with sympathetic neurons lying in association with smooth-muscle cells, whereas in the caput of the epididymis, the adrenergic nerve terminals are sparse and are more associated with blood vessels (8–10). As in the female, these neurons are short and postganglionic, originating from ganglia lying near the effector organ (8), and are of special significance in the process of ejaculation.

Sperm transit through the epididymis is relatively slow and fairly constant among different species. In the human, the mean epididymal transport time has been estimated to be 12 days (11), but owing to mixing of epididymal contents of younger and older spermatozoa, the actual transport time of any one sperm may be considerably different from the mean value (12). Time of transport of spermatozoa through the epididymis can be decreased about 10% to 20% by increased frequency of ejaculation (13). It has also been noted that although surgical diversion of the epididymis into the abdomen raises the temperature to which spermatozoa are exposed, spermatozoal maturation in the epididymis is not compromised. Transit time through the epididymides is, however, accelerated by 4 to 7 days (14). This lack of effect on spermatozoal maturation is surprising, since intraabdominal placement of both testis and epididymis rapidly leads to sterility (15) that is, however, accompanied by only minor changes in epididymal secretions (16).

In the normal state, spermatozoa are transported from the epididymis to the vas deferens by a steady flow of secretion through the epididymis and the contractile activity of the lower portion of the epididymis. Although it has been generally held that up to 50% of spermatozoa not ejaculated are reabsorbed by the male reproductive tract, this now seems to be less certain. The current view is that, in many species, excess spermatozoa are voided in the urine and that constant leakage of spermatozoa occurs (17–19). In the human, retrograde ejaculation due to weak bladder neck function, spinal cord injury, or prostate surgery is well documented, but whether spermatozoa are normally voided in the urine is not certain. It is known that, after vasectomy or in men with bilateral obstruction of the epididymides, macrophages are involved in phagocytosis of spermatozoa (20). The likelihood is that the human behaves like other species and that excess sperm are lost gradually via leakage down the vas deferens and voiding during urination.

During transport through the epididymis the sperm undergo certain maturational changes, so that at ejaculation fully functional spermatozoa are released. In some species, spermatozoa derived from the caput are unable to fertilize ova, but a proportion of spermatozoa taken from the corpus can fertilize ova. Spermatozoa from the cauda or vas deferens are almost always fully fertile (21). The majority of the changes occurring in the epididymis relate to the acquisition of motility. This has been studied extensively in a variety of species (3), but is somewhat different in the human than in rodents, in that there is no circling phase of sperm activity (22). Sperm from the caput epididymis exhibit varied patterns of motility, ranging from immotility to a vigorous flexing movement of the tail. Rapid forward progression occurs only with a reduced flexing of the tail; this appears first in a few spermatozoa in the corpus and is the general pattern in those from the cauda and vas deferens (22). Thus, acquisition of progressive motility may be largely a function of aging of the spermatozoa. There is evidence from the rabbit, in which species sperm motility, but not fertility, can be achieved after ligation of the lower region of the corpus epididymidis, that motility is not necessarily synonymous with fertilizing capacity (23).

Although, in the rabbit, fertilizing capacity is acquired during transport through the epididymis, this does not seem to be so clear-cut in the human. In men subjected to epididymovasovasotomy (where the vas is joined to the caput region of the epididymis to bypass an epididymal blockage), fertility, at least in a proportion of individuals, is restored (24). However, reversal of a simple vasectomy by microsurgical vasovasotomy also leads to restored fertility in only a percentage of men (25), so that the low incidence of fertility after epididymovasovasotomy may relate to factors other than lack of sperm maturation. Nevertheless, the restoration of fertility after epididymovasovasotomy may indicate that maturation of spermatozoa can occur in the vas or that epididymal maturation is not important.

Ejaculation

The process of ejaculation and orgasm in the male can be divided into two component parts—seminal emission and a central excitatory state (26). It is suggested that for orgasm there is a "buildup of excitation in specific centers in the central nervous system" and that when there is a neuroelectrical discharge, the excitation spreads to adjoining regions of the central nervous system (26). The so-called "ejaculation" can itself be subdivided into seminal emission and ejaculation proper. Seminal emission is defined as a leakage or oozing of spermatozoa from the penis without any pulsatile properties, whereas ejaculation indicates the emission of semen in spurts. Ejaculation usually occurs only in tandem with orgasm.

It is well known from a variety of experimental evidence that α-adrenergic neurons are intimately involved in the process of seminal emission. Patients who have been subjected to surgery to remove lymph glands in the thorax and abdomen as part of the treatment of testicular tumors do not experience seminal emission. That is, they can experience orgasm, but have a so-called "dry" ejaculation. Erection is, however, normal. Semen is not even voided retrogradely into the bladder. This type of surgery unavoidably involves extensive damage to sympathetic nerves from T12 to L3. In contrast, removal of T2 to T11 ganglia by transthoracic sympathectomy does not disturb ejaculation (27,28). As noted above, the male reproductive tract is mainly innervated by short adrenergic neurons, and these are located in the cauda epididymidis and vas deferens (8). Thus stimulation of these neurons leads to movement of the spermatozoa from the cauda of the epididymis, but not from the caput or the corpus. It has been found that repeated ejaculation of rats, which reduced sperm numbers in the ejaculate almost to zero, did not deplete sperm numbers in the upper portions of the epididymis (29).

Parasympathetic fibers also innervate the male genital tract, but they probably do not participate in the motor innervation of the longitudinal musculature of the vas deferens (30,31). Further evidence that the motor innervation of the ductus deferens is largely α-adrenergic is provided by *in vitro* studies on the human vas deferens (32) and from patients receiving drugs that produce chemical sympathectomy, e.g., guanethidine (28,33). Similar findings have been reported following treatment with the α-adrenergic blocking drug, phenoxybenzamine (34), and with the psychoactive drug thioridazine hydrochloride (a moderate α-adrenergic blocker) (35–37). Indeed, phenoxybenzamine has been recommended as a treatment for premature ejaculation (38). These findings provide convincing evidence for the role of the α-adrenergic system in seminal emission.

The pulsatile forces producing the ejaculatory discharge are partly caused by the contractile waves along the vas deferens produced by the α-adrenergic stimulation, but are mainly caused by the rhythmic muscular contractions of the striated-muscle groups, the ischiocavernosus and bulbospongiosus, which surround the urethra in the penis (26). This pumping action in the penis gives rise to ejaculation, which is closely associated with orgasm—the characteristic ejaculatory inevitability which, once started, is hard to stop even with use of the squeeze technique (39).

During the process of seminal emission and ejaculation, the mature spermatozoa from the epididymis, already suspended in secretions from the testis and epididymis, are, during their transport through the vas deferens and urethra, further joined by the secretions of the various accessory glands, i.e., the ampullary glands, the seminal vesicles, the prostate, and the bulbourethral (Cowper's) and urethral (Littré's) glands (see Fig. 1). Analysis of the various portions of the ejaculate reveals considerable differences in sperm density and biochemical characteristics, which can be used to determine the accessory gland from which the major proportion of that sample is derived (40,41). The highest sperm density is usually seen in the third and fourth fractions, with a progressive decline in subsequent fractions. In most men the ejaculate cannot be subdivided into more than six fractions. Interestingly, sperm motility is significantly lower in the fractions from the second half of the total ejaculate (41).

The bulk of the seminal plasma (fluid portion of the ejaculate) is derived from the seminal vesicles (60%) and the prostate (30%) (42). The pH of semen is basic, lying between 7.2 and 7.8, and reflects the relative contributions of acidic prostatic fluid (pH 6.5) and the alkaline seminal vesicular secretion. Prostatic fluid is rich in citric acid, acid phosphatase, zinc, and magnesium, whereas the seminal

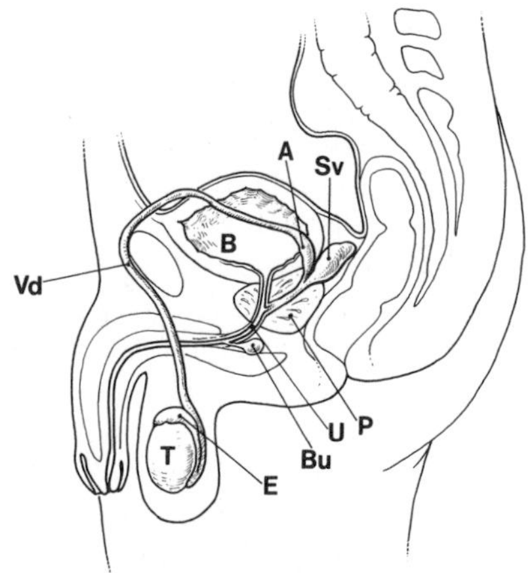

FIG. 1. Lower part of the trunk in a man, showing the reproductive tract and neighboring organs. (A) Ampulla; (B) bladder; (Bu) bulbourethral glands; (E) epididymis; (P) prostate; (Sv) seminal vesicle; (T) testis; (U) urethra; (Vd) vas deferens. (Reprinted from ref. 390.)

vesicular secretion is rich in fructose (3.2 mg/ml) and 19-hydroxylated prostaglandins (long-chain unsaturated fatty acids derived mainly from arachidonic acid) and contains smaller amounts of inositol and sorbitol (40,43). The normal volume of the ejaculate in the human male is between 2 and 6 ml, and a sperm concentration of 40 million to 250 million spermatozoa/ml has been considered normal (44). More recently, these parameters have been revised, and sperm counts of 10 million/ml or 25 million/ejaculate, provided other factors are not abnormal (e.g., motility or presence of abnormal forms), are considered perfectly compatible with normal fertility (45,46). Indeed, normal pregnancies have occurred in partners of men whose ejaculates had sperm counts of less than 1 million/ml, the sperm counts being depressed by hormonal therapy (depomedroxyprogesterone acetate and testosterone) to produce a contraceptive effect (47). Thus, if motility and shape are normal, even very low numbers of spermatozoa can induce pregnancy in a fertile partner. The presence of poor motility and/or the presence of many abnormally formed spermatozoa is usually associated with infertility.

In the human, the ejaculated semen is deposited into the vagina close to the external cervical os. In some other species, notably the rodents, pigs, and horses, spermatozoa are ejaculated directly into the uterine cavity, and thus the cervical canal and its mucoid secretion are not barriers to sperm transport. The vagina is very acid, with a pH of less than 5.0 in normal women. This acidity is maintained by the presence of lactic acid formed by the action of *Doederlein bacilli* on the vaginal secretions. The spermatozoa find this a hostile environment and those that are not rapidly entrapped in the cervical mucus or have progressed to the upper portions of the reproductive tract die and are voided to the exterior. In one normally fertile couple, an immediate change (within 8 sec) in vaginal pH from 4.3 to 7.2 was seen after deposition of the seminal plasma, which has buffering capacity. This provides a temporarily more favorable environment for the spermatozoa. However, vaginal pH reverts to normal within 4 min of ejaculation (48).

Immediately following ejaculation in primates, seminal plasma coagulates (within 1 min); this coagulum is broken down by proteolytic enzymes in the ejaculate within the next 20 to 30 min. Within 1 hr, all material should be liquefied and all spermatozoa should be fully motile (44). The coagulum probably acts to retain spermatozoa in the vagina close to the cervical canal, thus permitting maximal access for the spermatozoa to become entrapped in the cervical mucus.

Coitus in the human is relatively rapid, usually occurring within 10 min (or less) of intromission (49). In other species, the process can be very prolonged (camels and pigs) or very rapid (rabbits, rats, and bulls). During intercourse, intravaginal pressure is negative during intromission and male orgasm, but becomes positive to 40 cm H_2O during female orgasm, followed by a sharp fall after orgasm to a negative pressure of 26 cm H_2O (50). This may lead to sucking of spermatozoa into the cervical canal. Testosterone levels in men have been found not to vary immediately before and after intercourse (51), and thus are not directly involved in the ejaculatory process. Inhibition of androgenic activity, however, with an antiandrogenic drug such as cyproterone acetate, causes atrophy of accessory structures and sexual organs, partial failure of spermatogenesis, and loss of libido and potency (52,53). Thus a continued normal plasma level of androgenic stimulation is essential for the correct functioning of the reproductive tract, sperm maturation, and spermiogenesis.

Sperm Transport Through the Cervix

The role of vaginal and uterine contractions in the transport of spermatozoa from the vagina to the uterus has been well reviewed by Fox and Fox (49). Although there seems to be good evidence that, in other species (e.g., the rabbit), fluids placed in the vagina can enter the uterus in detectable amounts and relatively rapidly, the situation is much less clear in the human. Particulate material placed in the vagina has been claimed to enter the uterus (54–56). In the best-documented case, carbon particles suspended in 30% dextran were used, but 10 U of oxytocin was given intramuscularly at the same time (56). In contrast, radio-opaque fluid failed to enter the uterus from a cervical cap during either coitus or clitoral stimulation (57,58).

It is now well known that human semen contains large quantities of various prostaglandins, mainly the 19-hydroxylated series (59,60). These prostaglandins are less biologically active than the related prostaglandins E_2 or $F_{2\alpha}$; substantial quantities of the prostaglandin (PG) E series are also present in the seminal plasma of fertile men. Given that prostaglandins stimulate uterine contractility and thus cause uterine pain, as for example in dysmenorrhea (61), it seems unlikely that much seminal fluid per se enters the uterus. However, spermatozoa can pass rapidly to the oviducts; within 5 min of artificial insemination, spermatozoa were found within the oviducts of women, but the numbers were small, ranging from 4 to 53 within 5 to 45 min after insemination (62). Spermatozoa migrate through midcycle cervical mucus at a rate of only 2.0 to 3.0 mm/min (63). It is clear that sperm motility alone would be unable to cause sperm passage to the oviducts within 5 min. This suggests that the negative vaginal pressure recorded after orgasm, coupled with the associated increased vaginal and uterine contractions (50), immediately propel the small proportion of the ejaculated spermatozoa not trapped in the coagulum between the cervical mucus and cervical epithelium into the uterus; along with these spermatozoa may be carried a small quantity of seminal fluid. Although prostaglandins are known to cause contractions of both uterine and oviductal musculature, the relationship between levels of seminal plasma prostaglandins and male fertility is tenuous or nonexistent (64). Nonetheless, if prostaglandin $F_{2\alpha}$ is added to midcycle cervical mucus at a concentration of 250 ng/ml and the mucus is incubated for 1 hr at 37°C, sperm motility and sperm penetration through the mucus are increased significantly (65).

Since the majority of spermatozoa that reach the oviducts do so at much longer times after insemination than those recorded above, it seems probable that sperm motility is important in the progression through the cervical mucus lying in the cervical canal. The cervical canal has very thick walls comprised mainly of connective tissue and is lined with many deep crypts. These crypts are pockets of columnar epithelium of the cervical mucosa which extend in many different directions and can even be branched (66). The cervical epithelium is comprised of both ciliated and nonciliated (presumably secretory) cells covered with microvilli. The secretory cells are filled with cytoplasmic granules, and the intensity of reaction with the periodic acid-Schiff (PAS) reagent is related to the number of these granules. The release of secretory granules seems to be caused by rupture of the cell membrane rather than by an apocrine mechanism (66). Ciliary action does not appear to be important in sperm transport through the cervix, but may assist passage of the cervical secretions (mucus) to the vagina. The consensus is that "the rate of mucus secretion is a function of (a) the number of mucus-secretory units in the cervical canal, (b) the percentage of mucus-secreting cells per unit, and (c) the secretory activity and the responsiveness of secretory cells to circulating hormones" (66). There are approximately 100 such mucous-secretory units in the cervical canal, and the mucous secretion varies from 600 mg/day at midcycle to 20 to 60 μg/day at other times in the cycle in normal women of reproductive age (66).

Cervical mucus is comprised of two main elements: cervical mucin and soluble components. The mucin is a glycoprotein rich in carbohydrates (more than 40%), with a fibrillar system of glycoproteins linked either directly by disulfide bonds or through cross-linking polypeptides. Cervical mucin has a polypeptide core rich in hydroxyl amino acids (i.e., threonine and serine), and these constitute one-third of the total polypeptides. Considerable quantities of proline and alanine are also present, but there are only small amounts of basic (e.g., lysine and arginine), sulfur-containing (e.g., cysteine and methionine), and aromatic (e.g., tyrosine and phenylalanine) amino acids. About 70% to 80%, of the molecular weight is contributed by the carbohydrate side chains, including galactose (30%), sialic acid (10–20%), glucosamine (7–10%), galactosamine (7–10%), and fucose (5%) (66).

The soluble components of the mucus consist of inorganic salts (e.g., NaCl), proteins, and low-molecular-weight organic compounds (e.g., glucose, mannose, maltose, amino acids, peptides, and lipids). The soluble proteins are dispersed throughout the aqueous phase of the mucous gel. The consistency of this hydrogel (cervical mucus contains 95% water at midcycle) changes in relation to the balance between the secretion of ovarian hormones, mainly estradiol and progesterone. At midcycle, which is under estrogenic dominance, mucus is thin and watery and is composed of macromolecular fibrils arranged to form micelles (parallel chains) with spaces between the micelles large enough to permit the passage of spermatozoa. In contrast, under the dominance of progesterone (i.e., during the luteal phase of the cycle), cervical mucus contains less water (90%), is thicker, and lacks the micellar structure, and hence is unsuitable for sperm migration (66).

The consistency of the mucus has been assessed in terms of consistency, crystallization (ferning), and spinnbarkeit (fibrosity). Observation of these changes in cervical mucus by the individual woman forms the basis for the ovulation method (Billings) of natural family planning (67,68). In one large-scale trial, over 94% of women of different ethnic backgrounds and economic circumstances were successfully taught this method (69). Unfortunately, the overall cumulative net probability of discontinuation because of pregnancy was 19.6%, although this was mainly a matter of inaccurate application of instructions or lack of motivation, since the modified Pearl index for method failure was only 2.8 (70). Thus, the physical changes in the mucus at midcycle (fertile period) are definitive and easily recognized. Spermatozoa can begin to penetrate cervical mucus as early as the ninth day of the cycle; the rate of penetration then increases gradually, reaching a peak at or just before ovulation (the time of the estradiol peak), and is inhibited within 1 to 2 days after ovulation as progesterone levels rise (71) (see Fig. 2).

Spermatozoa, after entry into the cervical mucus, are not uniformly distributed throughout the mucus, but tend to be in the vicinity of the mucosal surface (72). Many spermatozoa are lodged in the cervical crypts, from which they are subsequently released to continue their journey upward through the reproductive tract. Apparently only motile spermatozoa are lodged in these crypts, where they are separated from the leukocytes in the central mass of mucus and thus protected from phagocytosis (72). Dead spermatozoa are eliminated from the tract either by phagocytosis or by the movement of the cervical mucus to the vagina. Thus it is likely that the cervical crypts act as reservoirs to permit a continued release of viable spermatozoa over a period of hours (73). The cervix clearly provides a major barrier to sperm ascent to the uterus. In experiments in rabbits in which about 280 million spermatozoa were deposited in the vagina at coitus, only 0.6% were found in the uteri 2 hr later, and this increased to a maximum of only 1.74% at 12 hr (74). Similar data are not available for women.

Sperm transport through the cervix can therefore be separated into three distinct phases: initial rapid transport, sperm storage in the crypts, and a final prolonged phase. The extent of the final phase is not known precisely, but in well-documented studies, motile spermatozoa have been found in the mucus up to 2 to 3 days after coitus (see ref. 75 for further references). Claims of motile sperm being found up to $3\frac{1}{2}$ weeks after coitus seem less believable (75).

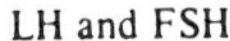

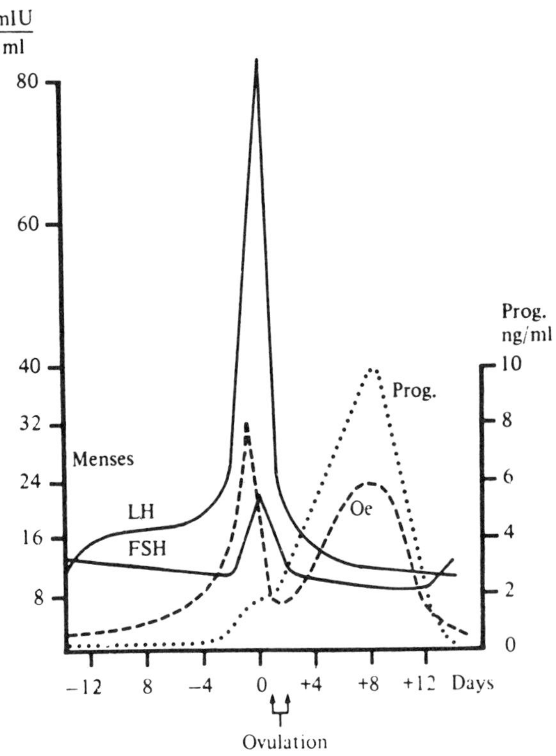

FIG. 2. Plasma levels of gonadotrophins (—), oestradiol (---), and progesterone (· · ·) during the human menstrual cycle. The cycle is centered on day 0, the day of the mid-cycle peak of LH. [Adapted from Speroff, L. and Vande Wiele, R. L. (1971): Regulation of the human menstrual cycle. *Am. J. Obstet. Gynecol.*, 109:234–247. Reprinted from ref. 152.]

In summary, it seems that four major factors are involved with sperm passage through the cervix: (a) spermatozoal motility; (b) muscular activity of the vagina, cervix, and uterus; (c) structure of the cervical mucus; and lastly, (d) the cervical crypts. All play a major role, but in the absence of sperm motility, it seems that few, if any, spermatozoa will reach the uterus.

Sperm Transport Through the Uterus

From the foregoing discussion it is clear that, if spermatozoa can be found in the oviducts within 5 min of insemination, they cannot have reached there solely through their own motility. This indicates that contractions of the uterine smooth musculature (myometrium) are extremely important in ensuring this rapid propulsion from the internal cervical os to the uterotubal junction. It may be that smooth-muscle contractility is stimulated by substances released at coitus or present in the semen. Oxytocin has been detected in the peripheral plasma of women after orgasm (76), but the nonpregnant uterus is not responsive to oxytocin (77). Excretion of catecholamines increases in humans during increased emotional and sexual (noncoital) excitement (78).

The presence of prostaglandins in the ejaculate has already been noted (59,60,64). Even if the prostaglandins do not enter the uterus directly, they can be readily absorbed through the vaginal wall (79–81). Prostaglandins can stimulate uterine activity both *in vitro* (82,83) and *in vivo* (84). However, it has been estimated that, on balance, the composition of seminal fluid prostaglandins, if applied directly to uterine strips *in vitro*, would lead to an inhibition of uterine contractility (83). On the other hand, administration of pharmacological doses of prostaglandins *in vivo* usually stimulates endogenous production of prostaglandins, which are known to cause uterine contractions (85). It seems, therefore, that prostaglandins are the most likely candidates for stimulation of uterine contractility.

When spermatozoa are suspended in uterine fluid, there is no known mechanism to ensure that they will always swim toward the uterotubal junction, so that, in the absence of an external force propelling them in that direction, sperm movement in the uterine cavity is likely to be random. Inert particles have also been shown to be rapidly transported from one end of the uterus to the other (61).

Sperm numbers in the uterus increase with time (up to 6 hr) after mating, then remain more or less constant up to 18 hr, at least in the rabbit. During this time period, the percentage of nonviable sperm in the uterus does not change greatly (86). In contrast, it has been shown that when large numbers of spermatozoa are placed in a rabbit uterine horn with both ends ligated, only 20% of the spermatozoa can be recovered 6 hr later. This destruction of spermatozoa is caused by an influx of leukocytes that phagocytose the spermatozoa (74,87). This is one major mechanism by which dead, damaged, or immotile spermatozoa are removed from the reproductive tract.

In some species, especially the bat, spermatozoa can become lodged in a uterine gland and thus perhaps remain protected from phagocytosis for long periods of time (88). However, this is probably not the case in humans. Sperm are found in the uterus consistently up to 24 hr after intercourse, but only a few are found thereafter (89). Intensive efforts to locate sperm in the uterus between 25 and 41 hr after coitus, at a time when many sperm are still present in cervical mucus, were also relatively unsuccessful (90). This suggests that destruction or removal of spermatozoa from the uterus increases after 24 hr.

Spermatozoa in the uterus have the greatest flagellar activity $1\frac{1}{2}$ to 16 hr after mating in rabbits. The swimming trajectories of the majority of spermatozoa, which have progressive motility, are linear, but circular movement has also been seen (91). Progressive motility appears to be related to the ability to fertilize ova.

At the time of ovulation, the human endometrium is characterized by the following: Epithelial glands increased in length and tortuosity, the individual columnar epithelial cells at their greatest height, and maximal pseudostratification of the nuclei. There is also less edema in the stroma than was present during the few days earlier, but there are still many mitoses. It is only after ovulation that intraluminal secretion from these epithelial cells becomes exceptionally abundant (92). At the time of ovulation, endometrial secretions have been found to contain a variety of proteins: In particular, albumin, prealbumin, transferrin, and post-transferrin have been identified (93,94). Zones of precipitation that are not present in serum have also been found in the β-globulin region in uterine washings (95). Total uterine protein, uncontaminated by sperm or blood, is greatest just prior to ovulation (96). Osmolarity of uterine fluid is about 284 mosm/liter and does not differ throughout the cycle. Total cation concentration and that of albumin are lower in uterine fluid than in serum. The concentration of potassium is high and that of sodium and calcium is low compared to those of serum. Only potassium and calcium vary throughout the cycle, being lowest at midcycle (97). Uterine fluid volumes are greatest at midcycle, about 83 to 180 μl (98). Changes in the composition of uterine fluid by the presence of a copper-releasing intrauterine device (IUD) may be responsible for the reduced rate of fertilization seen in women wearing such a device (99). Studies on the epithelial cells of the endometrium indicate that, at midcycle, material staining with PAS is present and that ribonucleoprotein and alkaline phosphatase are maximal (100). Lastly, there will be a mixture of cells in uterine fluid, representing the following: migratory cells such as neutrophils, macrophages, and lymphocytes; exfoliated epithelial cells; foreign cells such as bacteria; and non-nucleated portions of epithelial cells. The number of cells present is variable, but, in the absence of an IUD, ranges between 10,000 and 100,000 (101). The function of these cells, except for the phagocytosis of dead spermatozoa, is unknown.

In summary, sperm transport through the uterus depends mainly on uterine contractions and not on sperm motility. The spermatozoa are suspended in the uterine secretions. Owing to the difficulties of collecting human uterine fluid without altering its properties during the collection process, information on composition of such fluid is limited, but this fluid certainly acts to suspend and maintain spermatozoa during the transport process and contains macrophages that remove dead and nonviable spermatozoa.

Sperm Transport Through the Uterotubal Junction

Although the cervical canal acts as a major barrier to sperm ascent, substantial numbers still reach the uterus. In those species in which intrauterine insemination occurs, clearly the numbers in the uterus are very large. Nonetheless, the number of spermatozoa that actually enter the oviduct remains remarkably constant. It seems that the uterotubal junction forms a further barrier to sperm ascent (Table 1). The anatomical complexity of the junction, which is very complex in some species, such as the pig, and comparatively simple in others, such as the carnivores, does not seem to be related to its ability to impair sperm transport.

Woodruff and Pauerstein (102) reviewed many morphological studies and concluded that no anatomic sphincter

TABLE 1. *Species variation in number of spermatozoa ejaculated and site of deposition in different animals*[a]

Animal	Average number of sperm sperm/ejaculate (millions)	Site of sperm deposition	Number of sperm in ampulla of oviduct
Mouse	50	Uterus	<100
Rat	58	Uterus	500
Rabbit	280	Vagina	250–500
Ferret	—	Uterus	18–1,600
Guinea pig	80	Vagina and uterus	25–50
Cattle	3,000	Vagina	A few
Sheep	1,000	Vagina	600–700
Pig	8,000	Uterus	1,000
Man	280	Vagina	200

[a]Data from various sources. Reprinted from ref. 390.

could be demonstrated at the uterotubal junction of the human oviduct. Furthermore, there is no mucosal or capillary structure acting as a valve. The intramural portion of the human oviduct is convoluted and varies in length from 1 to 2 cm. Owing to its tortuosity, it is impossible to pass a probe through the interstitial portion of the human oviduct. The diameter of the lumen in this portion of the oviduct is approximately 0.1 to 1 mm (Fig. 3). The oviductal epithelial folds may continue all the way to the uterine cavity or terminate a few millimeters short of this. Ciliated mucosa has been found lying between the endometrial and oviductal epithelia. The inner longitudinal smooth muscle layer of the interstitial portion disappears in the isthmus approximately 2.5 cm from the uterotubal junction. The outer smooth-muscle layer continues into the broad ligament (103). Despite the tortuosity of the human interstitial region of the oviduct, it has been stated that the passage of inert small particles can occur in either direction and at all times in the cycle (102). This is not the case in other species, especially the rodents and rabbits, in which (a) only motile spermatozoa can ascend to the oviduct and (b) passage of fluid from the uterus to the oviduct or oviduct to the uterus is prevented except at the time of ovum passage through the uterotubal junction some 3 days after ovulation (104).

Although the numbers of spermatozoa found in the oviducts are very similar in different species, despite the differing numbers of spermatozoa ejaculated and the different sites of deposition of the ejaculate, there is evidence, from studies on rabbits, that when inseminations with very small numbers of sperm are done, fewer spermatozoa reach the oviduct. Inseminations with normal numbers of spermatozoa (200+ million), or even 10 times less, have no effect in this regard, but insemination with only 0.5% of the total ejaculate (1.21 million spermatozoa) reduced sperm in the oviduct about 60 times (5,000–6,000 down to an average of 88) (105). In the human, where there is no apparent barrier to passage of inert particles through the uterotubal junction (56,102), it is not clear why only a thousand or so spermatozoa reach the oviduct (106–108), but there is a relationship between the number of spermatozoa inseminated and the number reaching the oviduct during the first 45 min after insemination (109).

Thus, it is clear that, whatever the mechanism, a certain selective filtering of spermatozoa does occur at the utero-

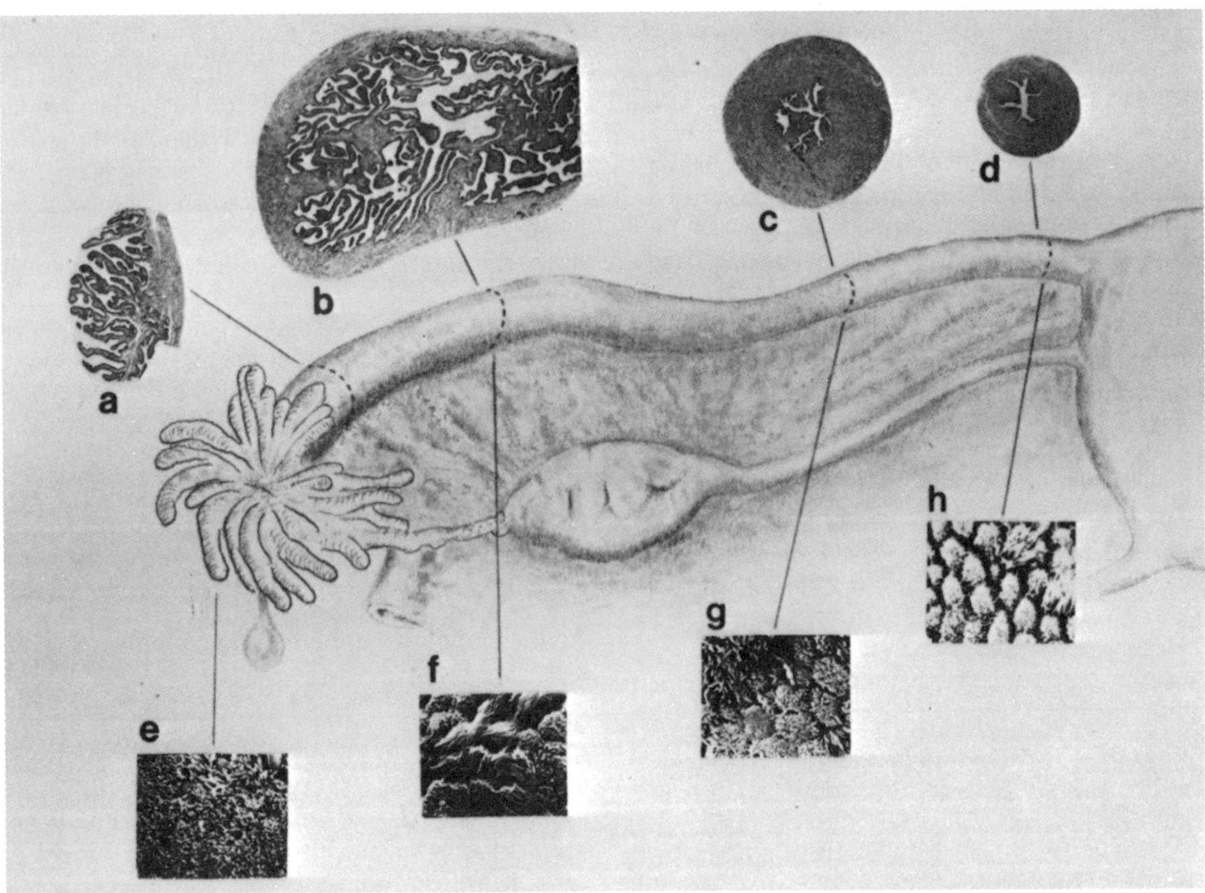

FIG. 3. Anatomy and morphology of the human oviduct. (a–d) Light microscopy photomicrographs depicting cross-sections taken at the level of the distal ampulla, midampulla, distal isthmus and proximal isthmus, respectively. (e–h) Scanning electron microscopy photomicrographs depicting surface ultrastructure of the oviductal lumen at the level of the fimbriae, midampulla, distal isthmus, and proximal isthmus, respectively. (Reprinted from refs. 103 and 391.)

tubal junction, presumably to permit the fittest to survive to fertilize the ova in the ampullar region of the oviduct.

Sperm Transport Through the Oviduct

It might seem that the title to this section is a misnomer in the sense that "through" denotes an onward progression of spermatozoa in one direction. However, it is now known that spermatozoa do not stop when they reach the site of fertilization, but progress onward out of the infundibular end of the oviduct into the peritoneal cavity. This is clearly shown by the pioneering work of Ahlgren (106), in which sperm numbers in the ampullar region of normal human oviducts did not exceed 200 during the period of 2 to 34 hr after intercourse; however, in women with oviduct pathology, which involves occlusion of the infundibulum and causes hydrosalpinx, many thousands were seen.

A review, by Ahlgren and collaborators, of the numerous reports on sperm migration in women shows that in cases where examination of peritoneal fluid was done, spermatozoa were usually found (110). These reports were confirmed by Ahlgren's own observations. Interestingly, the percentage of spermatozoa with normal morphology, which averaged 84% (n = 8 patients examined 10–60 hr post-intercourse) in the ejaculate, was much higher in the uterus (96%; n = 3 at 11–60 hr) and oviduct (93%; n = 8 at 10–60 hr) (110). Furthermore, up to 85 hr after intercourse, motile spermatozoa could be recovered from the cervix, the uterine cavity, the ampullar region of the oviduct, and the abdominal cavity (106,110). An earlier report had indicated that motile spermatozoa could be found up to at least 60 hr after intercourse (111), and there have been many reports of motile sperm in the oviducts at shorter times after intercourse. It is likely that 85 hr may be the upper limit of maintenance of sperm motility in the human. Whether this is also the upper limit for fertilizing capacity is not known; but if motility is still present, there would seem to be a chance for fertilization to occur. Thus, when natural family planning methods are to be used, an allowance of up to 4 days for sperm survival should be made.

It was originally thought that spermatozoa moved up the oviduct in a constant progression, with the numbers reaching the ampullar region rising progressively until a constant number was achieved after a few hours (112). This is now known to be incorrect. Spermatozoa, after entry into the oviduct, are distributed in two ways. A few spermatozoa are rapidly transported to the ampullar region, and these are the ones observed by various investigators shortly after mating or intercourse (Table 2). These are not the spermatozoa that generally fertilize ova in species in which mating takes place before ovulation. In species like the human, in which intercourse may occur before, after, or at the same time as ovulation, it cannot be definitively stated that the first spermatozoa do not normally fertilize the ovum. However, in view of the similarity of the second phase of sperm transport

TABLE 2. *Time between coitus or artificial insemination and arrival of spermatozoa in the oviduct*[a]

Animal	Time	Region of tube
Mouse	15 min	Ampulla
Rat	15–30 min	Ampulla
Hamster	2–60 min	Ampulla
Rabbit	A few minutes	Ampulla
Guinea pig	15 min	Ampulla
Dog	2 min to a few hours	Oviducts
Sow	15 min	Ampulla
Cow	2–13 min	Ampulla
Ewe	6 min to 5 hr	Ampulla
Woman	5–68 min	Oviducts

[a]Data from various sources. Reprinted from ref. 390.

in the oviduct in many species, it is likely that generally the same trend holds true.

The second phase of sperm distribution and transport was first observed in small animals, e.g., the mouse (113) and the rabbit (114). It was found that, after sperm entry into the oviduct, the majority of the spermatozoa remained in the proximal isthmus until about the time of ovulation. Initial experiments suggested that upward movement was again initiated by the presence of the products of ovulation (ova, follicular fluid, or ovum investments) entering the oviduct (115). It is now known that this congregation of spermatozoa in the isthmus occurs in pigs (116), sheep (117), and cows (118). Similarly, the recent studies of Croxatto and collaborators (107) document that the same trend is seen in the human. They flushed whole oviducts and recovered considerably larger numbers of spermatozoa than had Ahlgren (106), who had flushed only the ampullar region.

One of the major reasons that spermatozoa remain in the isthmus has to do with their motility. This has been extensively studied in the rabbit (91). In the lower isthmus the percentage of spermatozoa with activated motility was minimal up to 4 hr post coitum, then increased to about 3% at 6 hr and remained relatively constant up to 16 hr. In contrast, in the ampulla the percentage of spermatozoa with activated motility was minimal up to 6 hr, then rose rapidly and more or less continuously up to 16 hr when it was 35%. In the lower isthmus, flagellar activity and thus progressive movement was low. In contrast, the "activated motility" seen in the ampulla beginning at 6 hr post coitum was characterized by alternating patterns of linear progressive and vigorous nonprogressive movement (91). In the nonprogressive mode, the spermatozoa swam in a tight circle and exhibited whiplike activity of the tail, whereas in the progressive mode they often appeared to "crawl" in the presence of cellular debris, as described by Phillips (119).

It has been noted that many of the motile spermatozoa had cilia attached to their heads, thus suggesting a close apposition to epithelial cells of the isthmus (91), which is perhaps caused by oviductal mucus (120). By flushing human oviducts with oil and collecting the aqueous material extruded before the oil, Croxatto calculated that the volume of oviductal secretions at midcycle ranges from 20 to 40 μl (108). On this basis he has estimated that the *concentration* of spermatozoa in the oviduct can range from 5,000 to 50,000/ml. Even these concentrations are two orders of magnitude lower than those used in *in vitro* fertilization (IVF) programs, and it is not surprising that excessive numbers of spermatozoa attached to the zona pellucida are common in such *in vitro* fertilized ova (121). This phenomenon is not seen in normally fertilized ova, but, provided that polyspermy does not occur, is apparently not deleterious to zygote development.

The structure of the oviduct has been the subject of extensive investigation for at least 400 years. A short description is included here to place in perspective the various component parts and structures that play a role in both sperm and, as described below, ovum transport (see Fig. 3) (102). The intramural portion (also called *interstitial portion*), which includes the uterotubal junction, has already been described. The isthmus begins at the junction between the uterus and oviduct (uterotubal junction) and extends distally for 2 to 3 cm, ending at the ampullar-isthmic junction. The wall of this segment consists of a very thick layer of smooth musculature, encompassing a narrow lumen of approximately 0.4 mm. Since the musculature is better developed in this region than in the adjacent ones, it can perhaps be classified as a sphincter and is certainly a major factor in controlling ovum transport to the uterus.

The ampulla is the longest portion of the human oviduct and extends from the ampullar-isthmic junction to the infundibulum, a distance of about 5 to 8 cm. The lumen of the ampulla is wider than that of the isthmus, ranging from 1 cm at the infundibular end to 1 mm at the ampullar-isthmic junction. The wall is relatively thin in this region, with a thin musculature and well-developed mucosal surface with many branched folds.

The infundibulum is the trumpet-shaped organ which comprises the most distal portion of the oviduct and which opens into the peritoneal cavity. It has very thin walls and is covered with densely ciliated, petal-like structures known as *fimbriae*. The fimbriae are partially attached to the ovarian surface, and this arrangement helps to maintain close apposition of the ovary and oviduct, thus facilitating ovum "pick-up" at the time of ovulation.

There are two main types of cells in the oviductal epithelium: ciliated and secretory. The ciliated cells are much more numerous on the fimbriae and in the ampulla. The secretory cells predominate in the isthmus. Both types of cells undergo changes in structure and function under the influence of the ovarian hormones secreted during the menstrual cycle (see Fig. 2). These changes have been recently reviewed by Jansen (122). At midcycle the epithelium reaches maximal height (30–35 μm), and both ciliated and secretory cells are of equal height. The secretory cells form domes among the tufts of cilia, but shortly after ovulation, as the secretory cells shrink in height due to discharge of secretion, the cilia become more prominent. Then the whole epithelium becomes shorter due to broadening and flattening of the ciliated cells.

At midcycle the secretory cells of the isthmus appear to be most active with an apocrine secretion occurring. Serous granules also appear in the apical portion of these secretory cells. The isthmus can be fully filled with secretion at this time. Apocrine secretion does not appear to occur in the ampulla. This secretion continues through the ovulatory period, and some can also be seen in the ampulla.

The fluid in the oviduct is comprised partly of the secretions from these epithelial cells, but the major portion is from mucosal transudation. This transudation is stimulated by estrogen (123) and is maximal at midcycle (124,125). Protein concentration is maximal at the time of ovulation and consists predominantly of albumin (33.8%), β-globulin (44.4%), and γ-globulin (11.8%) (125). Potassium and chloride are present in oviductal fluid in higher concentrations than in serum, but calcium concentration is lower. Sodium and magnesium concentrations are similar to those in serum (126). This balance gives rise to a negative potential and can be expected to maintain acidic high-molecular-weight proteoglycans and glycoproteins in an expanded state (122). The enzymes amylase and lactate dehydrogenase, which are abundant in oviductal fluid (124), can convert the large quantities of glycogen present to pyruvate and glucose. Pyruvate is an essential substrate for early zygote cleavage and growth (127), whereas spermatozoa and later stages of zygote development can utilize the glucose as an energy source (40,128). In addition, bicarbonate ion concentration is high at midcycle and is accompanied by an increase in the pH of oviductal fluid, from 7.1 to 7.3 in the follicular phase to 7.5 to 7.8 at ovulation, in the monkey (129).

It appears that the secretion in the ampulla will be more watery because of the greater transudation due to the larger surface area of epithelium, whereas in the isthmus the secretion will have more mucous consistency for the reverse reasons and because of the larger number of secretory cells in this region (122). The endosalpinx in the ampulla is highly plicated and the branched folds tend to occlude the lumen, whereas in the isthmus the endosalpinx is much less plicated and the individual folds are much shorter and broader. The cilia on the epithelial surface all beat toward the uterus, do not differ in rhythm among the different portions of the oviduct and exhibit no greater activity at the time of ovulation than earlier in the cycle (130). This abovarian beat causes a current of oviductal fluid flow over the epithelium in the same direction. Owing to the thicker consistency of the isthmic secretions, the thicker muscular wall not permitting distention, the narrower lumen, and the edema of the wall itself (131), fluid passage through the isthmus and into the uterus is not permitted or only minimal (at least not until the time of ovum passage into the uterus after ovulation). Consequently, the direction of fluid flow is reversed

(132), and a flow of fluid in the less-ciliated mucosal crypts develops toward the infundibulum. In this way, excess oviductal secretion is voided through the infundibulum to the peritoneal cavity, carrying with it those spermatozoa that have reached the ampullar region. This is a constant process until all spermatozoa have left the oviduct, or the ovum and oviductal fluid are transported into the uterus.

During the periovulatory period the oviductal musculature is not quiescent. Electrophysiological recording of rabbit oviducts has shown that there are bursts of electrical activity propagating in each direction, with some indication of more propagating toward the ovary at ovulation (133,134). Similar activity has been seen in human oviducts (135). *In vitro,* annular segments and longitudinal strips of human oviduct also show high spontaneous activity in the periovulatory phase (136). The consequence of this muscular activity is to ensure a thorough mixing of the luminal contents, which increases the chance of spermatozoon and ovum meeting and may also hasten sperm transport through the ampulla and into the peritoneal cavity.

During the transport through the reproductive tract, the spermatozoa undergo certain maturational changes, which are a prerequisite for fertilization. Freshly ejaculated sperm are incapable of fertilization; during their brief stay in the uterus and oviduct, they undergo a process known as *capacitation,* which prepares them for the final change before fertilization can begin. Capacitation involves a destabilization of the plasma membrane of the sperm head without any visible morphological changes (137). Capacitation was first described by Austin and Chang independently (138,139). The necessity for capacitation of human sperm has been debated, because fertilization of human ova can be achieved *in vitro* in defined media containing follicular fluid, human blood serum, or fetal cord blood (140–143). If it exists, the process must be rapid and easily accomplished *in vitro*. This is not the case for other species, such as the rabbit (144), where the optimal conditions involve sequential exposure to uterus and oviduct. After capacitation and when the spermatozoa come into close contact with the investments of the ovum (cumulus oophorus and corona radiata cells) in the ampullar region of the oviduct, a final maturational change occurs. This is known as the *acrosome reaction* and involves the fusion of the outer acrosomal membrane and the plasma membrane, thereby permitting release, through the pores thus formed, of certain enzymes involved in the fertilization process, notably hyaluronidase and acrosin (137). If spermatozoa die in the oviduct, the acrosome reaction as described does not occur; instead, the acrosome is lost intact.

In most species, fertilization occurs only in the oviduct, but experimentally one can demonstrate that, in limited cases, fertilization can take place in the uterus (e.g., in the rabbit; see ref. 145), but this is not the case in the hamster (146). In the human, uterine fertilization can occur, at least in a limited number of cases (147–149), and this re-emphasizes the ease with which capacitation and the acrosome reaction must occur in humans. The detailed process of fertilization is dealt with in another chapter and is not discussed further here.

In summary, sperm transport through the oviduct consists of a rapid phase and a slow phase. Sperm remaining in the isthmus are less motile and only gradually move up to the site of fertilization. Sperm movement is caused by a combination of sperm motility, fluid flow, and muscular activity of the oviductal musculature.

OVULATION AND OVUM "PICK-UP"

The process of ovulation is discussed in another chapter and so will not be dealt with here, except insofar as it relates to the entry of the ovum into the oviduct. In some species, ovulation is triggered by the act of coitus, as in the rabbit, and in others it is causally linked to a defined estrous period during which the female is receptive to the male. In both of these situations, mating antedates ovulation by a number of hours, and capacitated spermatozoa are already waiting in the oviduct by the time the ovum arrives. The situation can often be different in the human, since intercourse takes place throughout the cycle, not just around the time of ovulation at midcycle. Consequently, spermatozoa may be present in the oviducts at the time of ovulation, or may only arrive there after ovulation and ovum "pick-up" has occurred. Thus, there is a greater possibility of an aged ovum being fertilized.

It is known that, in many species, aging of the ovum before fertilization as a result of delaying insemination progressively diminishes the number of young born as the delay increases and also increases the percentage of abnormally developing embryos (150). Direct observations of this phenomenon have not been made in the human, but its occurrence is all the more probable, given the potential for desynchronization of insemination and ovulation mentioned above. The fertilizable life of the human ovum has been estimated as approximately 24 hr, but apparently the ova remain fertilizable for longer than they remain capable of producing normal young (151).

Ovulation occurs a number of hours after the release of a surge of luteinizing hormone (LH) from the anterior pituitary gland. LH induces a great many changes in the follicle, and among these is the resumption of meiosis in the oocyte. Thus, at ovulation, ovum development has reached the metaphase stage of the second meiotic division and remains at this stage until fertilization begins. The time between the LH surge and ovulation varies among species, being only about 12 to 15 hr in rodents, but as long as 42 hr in the pig (152). In the human, ovulation occurs between 40 and 63 hr after the estradiol peak in peripheral serum (153), and the estradiol peak antedates the LH peak by about 24 hr (154). This indicates that ovulation occurs between 16 and 39 hr after the LH surge. Peters and McNatty (155) have given a figure of 28 to 36 hr after the LH surge for the human. As a result of the hormonal changes taking place around the time of ovulation (Fig. 2), changes also occur in the cellular investments surrounding the ovum.

At ovulation, the ovum is surrounded by two distinct arrangements of follicle cells (the cumulus cells). Closely attached to the zona pellucida are the coronal cells, arranged radially and two to three cells thick—the so-called *corona radiata*. Surrounding the corona radiata are more cells—the cumulus oophorus—a sticky gelatinous matrix containing many cumulus cells. The presence of a normally developed cumulus oophorus is important for normal ovum pick-up and may be important for the early stages of ovum transport.

In animals without a closed bursa at the infundibular end of the oviduct, follicular rupture and extrusion of the ovum are not an explosive process; instead, there is an immediate protrusion of a portion of the cumulus containing the ovum from the ruptured follicle followed by a slow oozing of the remainder of this cumulus oophorus in a strand-like manner (156). It seems that there are three possible mechanisms involved in transfer of the ovum from the ovarian surface across the fimbriae into the oviduct. It has been suggested that there is a region of negative pressure caused by local contractions of the oviductal musculature in the infundibular region (157). Negative pressures within the oviduct have been detected by means of intraluminal catheters (158). Whether these negative pressures do exert any suction effect is questionable, because the soft-walled ampulla would collapse, thereby closing the lumen, and because, at least in the rabbit, ovum "pick-up" can occur despite the presence of a ligation just below the infundibulum (159). On balance, Blandau (156) feels that it is unlikely that such a phenomenon is involved in ovum "pick-up."

A second possibility is that integrated contractions of the oviduct and its accessory membranes, the fimbriae and the ovary, contribute to ensure the mechanical "pick-up" of the ovum in its cumulus mass. It is known that these structures are active during ovulation in the human (160,161), and similar observations have been made in many other species (156). The smooth musculature of the oviductal and ovarian ligaments contracts, so that these structures are brought into close apposition. They then contract rhythmically so that the folds of fimbriae are swept across the ovarian surface. The fimbriae become engorged with blood and themselves also contract rhythmically (156,162).

Lastly, it has already been noted that the fimbriae are covered with cilia, which are all beating toward the uterotubal junction. Intimate contact of these cilia with the cumulus mass is held to be critical to the process of ovum "pick-up." The cilia become attached to the cumulus mass and draw it out into long streamers as they attempt to propel the ovum and its investments into the ostium of the oviduct (162). Thus it is likely that ovum "pick-up" is caused by a combination of factors, the most important being the ciliary beat and the rhythmic sweeping of the ovarian surface by the fimbriae. However, microsurgical removal of the infundibulum and fimbriae and the first 2 cm of the ampulla does not cause infertility in rabbits (163).

These observations have been best documented in the rabbit by the pioneering studies of Blandau (156), but it is likely, given the anatomical similarities, that the mechanisms are the same in primates. However, it should be noted that, despite the efficiency of this process under optimal circumstances, the close apposition of ovarian surface and fimbriae is not essential for ovum "pick-up." Transperitoneal migration of ova is known to occur in women with only one ovary and the contralateral oviduct (164). Similarly, inert particles or spermatozoa placed in the peritoneal cavity can be found in the oviduct (165–169), but, owing to their smaller size, this "pick-up" can probably be accomplished by ciliary action alone. Further evidence as to the efficiency of the "pick-up" process is provided by experiments in which silastic hoods were placed over the infundibulum in monkeys in an attempt to prevent ovum "pick-up." These hoods were anchored by six inert sutures, but it was found that even small gaps in the suturing of the hood permitted ovum "pick-up" and pregnancy (170,171). Similar findings were recorded in limited studies in women when plastic hoods were used (172).

In summary, ovum "pick-up" is an efficient process in which ciliary activity on the fimbriae as well as the rhythmic contractions of the fimbriated folds, the ampullar smooth musculature, and the ligaments supporting the ovary and the oviduct all participate to differing degrees.

OVUM TRANSPORT

Although the overall transport time is remarkably constant for most mammalian species (3 to 4 days), there are differences in the detailed pattern of transport through the different regions of the oviduct. In most species, the transport time remains the same whether the ova are fertilized or not: This is not true, however, for the horse, whose unfertilized ova remain in the oviducts and the zygote derived from a fertile mating at a subsequent estrous period bypasses the unfertilized ova and enters the uterus at the normal time (173). Furthermore, in some species, zygotes can survive in the oviduct after fertilization at a time when they cannot survive in the uterus (174). Thus, in these species, although not necessarily in the human, a correct programming of the oviduct to retain the ova until they are capable of survival in the uterine environment is essential.

OVUM SURVIVAL

Secretions of the oviductal epithelial cells are important in maintaining growth and well-being of the developing embryo. In nonprimates, premature entry of the ova into the uterus is detrimental to their further development, suggesting either that uterine secretion is hostile at this time or that it lacks some essential nutrient (174). In primates, this seems not to be the case, in that, following Estes' operation (147,149,175), ova ovulated into the uterine cavity can become fertilized and undergo complete development without exposure to oviductal secretions. The collected material has been summarized by Adams (176), and, although firm data are absent in many reports, it seems that approximately 11% of patients can eventually become pregnant after this procedure (i.e., 29 of 270 patients operated in 11 series). In many reports there is no indication as to the length of time elapsing between operation and pregnancy. However, in the best-documented cases, Adams (176) estimates that 14 pregnancies in eight patients may have occurred over a period of 267 menstrual cycles. If these estimates are correct, this indicates a pregnancy rate of only 6.78 per 100 women years. Of course, in this situation, not only does the zygote have to survive in the uterus, but also the ovum must be fertilized in the uterus and, as noted above, in other species this process is not optimal (145,146). Thus, a large proportion of the failures to become pregnant may be a reflection of lack of fertilization rather than interference with embryonic survival.

This supposition is made more plausible by the experiments of Marston and collaborators (177) in rhesus monkeys. They transferred two freshly fertilized zygotes from one oviduct to another, which resulted in two successful live births. Six other successful live births also resulted from autotransfers of seven 2- to 6-cell zygotes from one oviduct to the other, but the transfer of a 22-cell morula failed. In these experiments, the success rate for transfers from one oviduct to another was an astonishing 80% (8 of 10 transfers). In these same experiments, autotransfers of two 7- to 8-cell zygotes from the oviduct to the uterus resulted in only a chemical pregnancy (positive pregnancy test). This preliminary work was then continued; successful live births were achieved following transfer of oviductal zygotes at early stages (2–6 cells) to the uterus of the same animals, 24 hr earlier than they would normally have arrived there without the intervening culture period (178).

Early development in embryos of most species appears to take place largely under the control of the maternal genome (see ref. 179 for further references), with the sequential activation and utilization of components from the oocyte (180). In mouse embryogenesis, DNA replication takes place over a 1- to $1\frac{1}{2}$-hr period after the first cleavage division. Two bursts of putative transcription occur immediately before and after DNA replication, and translation products are detectable within 3 to 4 hr (181). The entire first cell cycle, from cleavage to the two-cell stage in the mouse, the second round of DNA replication, and the loss of maternal mRNA are all regulated at a post-transcriptional level and are independent of the expression of the embryonic genome (181). A similar sequence of events appears to take place in the human zygote after fertilization, although the exact stage of development at which expression of the embryonic genome occurs is still not certain (182). The timing of development through this first two-cell stage is controlled by an event associated with sperm penetration rather than germinal vesicle breakdown (183). It is postulated that, following ovulation, development is controlled at two levels. An endogenous program, initiated by oocyte maturation, may regulate the "housekeeping" functions of the zygote, while sperm penetration activates a further endogenous program that initiates embryogenesis (183).

The early one-cell mouse zygote requires pyruvate or oxaloacetate as an energy source; at the two-cell stage it can also utilize phosphoenolpyruvate and lactate, and it is only at the eight-cell stage that glucose can be utilized (see ref. 184 for further references). Thus, the mouse embryo is very dependent on the correct composition of the culture medium for *in vitro* development. In the human, a variety of different media, ranging from simple to complex (e.g., Krebs-Ringer bicarbonate, Ham's F10, Earle's, Modified Whitten's, Whittingham's modified, Tyrode's and Menezeo's B2), have all been used by *in vitro* fertilization programs (121,143,185–188). Many of these media are then supplemented with a serum source, either fetal cord serum or heat-inactivated serum from the ovum donor. Serum can, however, apparently be eliminated, and the bovine serum albumin can be replaced with human serum albumin, with no effect on cleavage *in vitro* or on subsequent survival *in vivo* of *in-vitro*-fertilized human ova (187). Thus, it seems that the human zygote is much less dependent on a critical composition of the surrounding medium either *in vivo* or *in vitro* than are those of the mouse and other species.

In-vitro-cultured human zygotes reach the one-cell (pronuclear) stage at 12 to 31 hr after insemination, the two-cell stage between 27 and 43 hr, the four-cell stage between 36 and 65 hr, the eight-cell stage between 45 and 73 hr, and the 16-cell stage between 68 and 85 hr (121). Compaction of the blastomeres occurs between 96 and 120 hr at the morula stage of 32 cells, and a blastocoele is visible between 120 and 144 hr. Fully expanded blastocysts and those hatched from the zona pellucida have been observed at 140 to 160 hr after *in vitro* insemination (121).

The numerous reports of successful human pregnancies following intrauterine deposition of oocytes fertilized *in vitro* and at an early stage of development confirm that oviductal secretions are not essential for ovum development (121,143,188). In the human, oviductal secretions may, as noted above, be important for sperm transport and maintenance of sperm viability. Their role in ovum transport is questionable. Even their importance in sperm transport may be overstated, since in experiments in which the isthmic region of the oviduct is resected, fertilization and early cleavage of the zygotes proceed normally. The only abnormality seen is an increased incidence of polyspermy, presumably due to the loss of filtering function of the isthmus (189,190).

PHYSIOLOGICAL CONTROL MECHANISMS

When considering mechanisms that control the function of the oviduct and consequently the transportation of ova and zygotes, it is necessary to consider the contractility of the smooth musculature, the activity of the cilia, and the flow of oviductal secretion. The nature and extent of oviductal secretions have already been described in the section entitled "Sperm Transport Through the Oviduct." It was noted that, owing to the larger diameter of the lumen and the thin expandable wall of the ampulla, more secretion remains in the ampulla than in the isthmus, and thus ampullar secretion tends to be more watery.

Steroid Hormones

It is known that receptors for steroid hormones are present in oviductal tissue (191–195) and that steroid concentrations in oviductal tissue are higher than in peripheral plasma (196,197). Both estradiol and progesterone receptor concentrations are highest in the proliferative phase of the cycle (193); whether there are differences in receptor concentrations between different regions of the oviduct is debatable (192,193). It is still not certain that the known actions of estrogens and progestins on gamete transport (198–201) are caused by transduction via a receptor-activated mechanism. These latter reports all deal with a variety of laboratory rodents, and the exact actions of estrogens and progestins on the human oviduct are not known. However, an emergency postcoital contraceptive treatment based on the administration of estrogen (diethylstilbestrol or ethinyl estradiol) (202,203) or a combination of ethinyl estradiol and *dl*-norgestrel (204) is known to prevent pregnancy reliably, provided that treatment is started within 72 hr of the unprotected coitus. Since the first 72 hr after ovulation is the time that ovum transport is occurring, this suggests that estrogens interfere with ovum transport in the same manner as in animals, although whether this is by acceleration into the uterus or retardation in the oviduct is not known. Given the propensity for ectopic pregnancies in the human (102), it seems probable that these steroid treatments cause accelerated transport, because ectopic pregnancy rates are unchanged; they must also accelerate the zygote out of the uterus, or else an intrauterine pregnancy would occur. However, *large* doses of estrogen given during the period of ovum transport can cause an increased incidence of ectopic pregnancies (205,206). The closest approximation that can be achieved with regard to examining the effects of progestins on the human oviduct is provided by studies in which megestrol acetate was given continuously from an implant, thus causing delayed transport of ovum surrogates (207). In women using such implants for contraception, there was a significant increase in the incidence of ectopic pregnancy (208). Again, this is a result dissimilar to that seen in nonprimates, but the dosing schedule also differed significantly. Continuous low-dose progestins given for oral contraception similarly increase the incidence of ectopic pregnancy (209). These findings definitely imply a delay in zygote transport.

Thus, it is likely that ovarian steroidal hormones and their synthetic analogs do affect the human oviduct and do in some manner disrupt transport. It is known that, in the pig, a correlation between changes in estradiol and progesterone plasma levels and oviductal steroid hormone receptors exists (210). Consideration of the time that elapses between steroid administration and changes in oviductal function suggest that transduction via hormone receptors is most likely.

Experiments in rabbits have shown that, in the absence of ovarian steroid hormones (e.g., after ovariectomy), ovum transport is extremely irregular, with many ova or ovum surrogates retained in the oviducts (211–213). In such animals deprived of hormonal support, progesterone alone has little effect on transport of ovum surrogates (213), whereas estrogen alone causes either "locking" of ova in the oviduct or premature expulsion to the uterus, depending on dose and timing of administration relative to entry of ova into the oviducts (200,212,213). Administration of constant combinations of estrogen and progesterone are not more successful in regularizing transport when compared to administration of each one alone (213,214). More normal results have been achieved in long-term ovariectomized animals by use of a regimen of decreasing estrogen and increasing progesterone treatments (215).

In summary, the correct programming of ovum or zygote transport through the oviduct is very dependent on the support provided by the ovarian hormones—estradiol and progesterone—and, more importantly, on the secretion of these hormones in the correct balance during the first few days after ovulation. These hormones probably exert their action via steroid hormone receptors located in the oviductal tissue.

Catecholamines

There are many agents known to stimulate or relax the musculature of the oviduct. These include the catecholamines, prostaglandins, and peptides. Norepinephrine is the main catecholamine present in the sympathetic nerve endings of the oviduct (136,216,217). The oviduct is supplied with both "long" and "short" adrenergic neurons, and it is the short ones that are important in innervation of the oviductal smooth musculature (136). Both α- and β-adrenergic receptors in smooth musculature have been described (218,219). The distribution of this innervation in the human oviduct has been described as follows: The thin muscle layer in the ampulla contains relatively few nerves, and these are mainly vasomotor fibers. In the isthmus the innervation is greatly increased, especially the number of fibers supplying the circular muscle layer. The number of fluorescent nerves then decreases in the portion of the isthmus adjacent to the uterotubal junction and is further decreased in the intramural portion (136). In *in vitro* studies, norepinephrine contracts the longitudinal muscle layer of the isthmus, and this activity is particularly intense just before ovulation. The circular muscles contract only at ovulation; otherwise they relax upon administration of norepinephrine (136). These findings could be considered *prima facie* evidence for the existence of an isthmic spincter that would retain the zygotes in the oviduct for 2 to 3 days after ovulation.

However, destruction of these neurons, either by a chemical agent (6-hydroxydopamine) or by surgical denervation, had little disruptive effect on ovum transport in rabbits (220). An alternative approach has been to deplete endogenous stores of norepinephrine with reserpine or to increase them with iproniazid, an inhibitor of monoamine oxidase. Such treatments in rabbits were again ineffective in disrupting transport (221). α-Adrenergic blockade by phenoxybenzamine (222,223) as well as β-adrenergic blockade with propranolol (223) similarly had little effect on transport. When the parameter examined was fertility rather than ovum transport, neither reserpine in rabbits nor 6-hydroxydopamine in mice affected the number of live young born (224,225).

It must be concluded that, despite the extensive innervation of the isthmic region of the oviduct, the adrenergic system is not a primary control pathway for modulation of ovum transport. Finally, the oviduct is only sparsely innervated by cholinergic fibers, and the parasympathetic system probably plays little role in regulation of ovum transport (102,226).

Prostaglandins

Prostaglandin concentrations in oviductal tissue have been shown to vary with the stage of pregnancy in rabbits (227,228) and in hamsters (229). Prostaglandins have also been identified by immunohistology in human oviducts (230) and in oviductal tissue extracts subjected to thin layer chromatography (231). In these latter experiments it was suggested that, while $PGF_{2\alpha}$ was consistently found in the isthmic extracts, the ampullar extracts contained mainly only PGE_1. Such regional differences in prostaglandin content were not seen in rabbits (227,228), and, in view of the relatively insensitive methods used, may not be correct in the human.

Despite the variations in prostaglandin concentrations seen in the various portions of the oviduct—ampulla, distal isthmus, and proximal isthmus—it is hard to relate these changes directly to changes in ovum transport. In addition, tissue measurements of prostaglandins are notoriously subject to artifact (232). However, it is known that PGF- and PGE-series prostaglandins can have differing effects on oviductal musculature *in vitro* and *in vivo*. In the human, PGE_1 and PGE_2 relax the circular muscle layers of the isthmus *in vitro*, but contract the longitudinal muscle. $PGF_{2\alpha}$ causes a powerful stimulation of both these muscular layers (233). In contrast, PGI_2 has only a weak stimulatory effect on both layers (234). That these differences are not just artifacts of the recording technique has been shown in later experiments, since a high degree of agreement between electrical and mechanical signals was observed (235). It is still not clear which of the two muscle layers provides the driving force for ovum transport or whether both are equally important.

In vivo recording poses many more problems than the *in vitro* system because it usually entails placing the recording device into the lumen of the oviduct, thus possibly altering the system response as a result of the foreign body. Nonetheless, some idea of the integrated activity of the system can be obtained by use of intraluminal balloons or open-ended catheters. Limited studies in the human have shown that intravenous or topical administration of PGE_2 is inhibitory and that $PGF_{2\alpha}$, administered similarly, stimulates oviductal contractility (236). More extensive *in vivo* studies can only be done in experimental animals, such as the rabbit. In this species, it was found that intravenous $PGF_{1\alpha}$ and $PGF_{2\alpha}$ increased spontaneous oviductal activity, whereas PGE_1 and PGE_2 suppressed it (237). Injection of high doses of PGEs often caused an initial contraction, which was then followed by relaxation (237). This had previously been reported also in the sheep (238). In the rabbit, the actions of one series of prostaglandins can counteract the actions of the other series, but the second prostaglandin must be administered intravenously at least 2 min after the first one (239). Similarly, a stimulation of activity caused by norepinephrine can be suppressed by PGEs, and the relaxation induced by β-stimulation (isoproterenol) can be overcome by PGFs (239). However, the actions of the prostaglandins are not mediated through the adrenergic system, since the prostaglandins still exert their characteristic effects in the face of α- or β-adrenergic blockade (239). Subcutaneous administration of the prostaglandins produced qualitatively similar results, but with a longer period of action than by the intravenous route (237). There are also limited data available from studies in rhesus monkeys. Intravenous administration of PGEs had little effect on spontaneous activity during the preovulatory period, but some suppression of bursts of activity after ovulation was seen. $PGF_{2\alpha}$ only caused an increase in amplitude of contractions just prior to ovulation (240).

Thus there is considerable evidence, obtained from several species, that oviductal tissue contains prostaglandins and is sensitive to their actions. It is tempting to hypothesize that the balance between the PGEs and PGFs could provide a control mechanism for the activity of the smooth musculature. If this is the case, then one would expect to find distinct binding sites for $PGF_{2\alpha}$ and for PGE_2. Preparations of single smooth muscle cells have been made from ampulla and distal and proximal isthmic segments from rabbits at different times after an ovulating injection or mating. The binding affinity (equilibrium dissociation constant) for $PGF_{2\alpha}$ was 0.19 nM; that for PGE_2 was 0.55 nM (241). These affinities did not differ at different stages of pregnancy or pseudopregnancy, but the actual number of binding sites/cell was changed (242). The numbers of PGE_2-binding sites measured increases in the distal isthmus at 48 hr and in the proximal isthmus at 48 and 72 hr after the ovulating injection. The concentration of $PGF_{2\alpha}$-binding sites is high in the distal isthmus up to 48 hr and then falls, whereas that in the proximal isthmus does not change between the estrous and 72-hr pregnant or pseudopregnant condition (241,242). Furthermore, uptake of radiolabeled calcium [^{45}Ca] was increased when such cells were exposed to 1 nM $PGF_{2\alpha}$, but was decreased after exposure to 1 nM PGE_2. Calcium uptake by the smooth-muscle cells thus paralleled the contractile activity (243). However, there was no correlation between the numbers of binding sites and oviductal prostaglandin concentrations measured previously.

In addition, treatment of rabbits with a variety of inhibitors of prostaglandin synthesis, release, or metabolism during the first 24 hr after ovulation had only modest effects on the rate of ovum transport, the most effective compound being benzydamine, an inhibitor of thromboxane synthesis; classical inhibitors of cyclooxygenase (e.g., indomethacin and sodium meclofenamate) were without effect (244). No greater effect was seen if reserpine treatment to deplete catecholamines and sodium meclofenamate treatment to deplete prostaglandins were combined (244). Indomethacin treatment was similarly ineffective in hamsters (229). In other experiments in rabbits in which indomethacin was given 11 times during the period of ovum transport, no effect on numbers of implantations was seen (245). Suppression of the cyclooxygenase enzyme will, of course, inhibit production of PGE-, PGF-, and PGI-series prostaglandins; thus the actual balance between the prostaglandins with opposing actions may not be changed. Alternatively, ovum transport is not controlled by prostaglandins.

Investigations into the role of prostaglandins on ovum transport have also examined the actions of exogenously administered prostaglandins. In general, systemic administration of such prostaglandins as PGE_1, PGE_2, and $PGF_{2\alpha}$ has not been very effective (see ref. 240 for further references), perhaps because of rapid metabolism (246,247), except when given in large pharmacological doses (240). When effects were seen, they depended on the species, the time of administration relative to ovulation and the dose; thus, generally, an acceleration of transport was seen with both PGE and PGF series compounds, but occasionally a delay of transport was recorded. More predictable effects were seen following intraperitoneal administration in hamsters when the prostaglandin could act directly on the oviduct. $PGF_{2\alpha}$ usually caused accelerated transport (229), but even in these experiments a luteolytic action on the corpora lutea of pregnancy was seen and a reduction of progesterone secretion may also have been implicated in the results observed.

As a result of the observations on differences in binding sites for prostaglandins on smooth-muscle cells of the oviduct, it has been suggested that changing sensitivity to prostaglandins during ovum transport may be the result of a phase-dependent variation in the number of specific binding sites in the myosalpinx (242). The equivocal results obtained with inhibition of prostaglandin synthesis and pharmacological treatments with exogenous prostaglandins suggest that this control system may be of only limited importance, and significant interaction with the adrenergic system also seems unlikely (239,244).

Peptides

Peptidergic neurons have now been described in the female genital tract of a variety of species, including the cat, guinea pig, and rat (248). Vasoactive intestinal peptide (VIP), a 28-amino-acid peptide first isolated from porcine duodenum (249,250), has been identified by immunofluorescence in such nerves in uterus, cervix, and prostate (248). Moderate numbers of fine-varicose fibers were found in the oviduct of the cat, but not in that of the guinea pig or rat (248). In the human, a moderate number of VIP-containing nerves have been found in the isthmic region of the oviduct. These are localized primarily beneath the epithelium, but also to a lesser extent in the lamina propria of the mucosa and the smooth musculature (251).

In vitro experiments with the isthmic region of the human oviduct showed that electrical field stimulation reduced the motor activity of the circular muscle layer. This effect was blocked by tetrodotoxin, suggesting neural involvement. It was deduced that VIP was the neural transmitter responsible for this inhibition of activity (252). VIP is also known to be a potent inhibitor of spontaneous motor activity of the isthmic region of the oviduct, the ED_{50} falling between 25 and 200 ng/ml in the bath fluid (253). Further studies revealed that there was good agreement between immunohistochemical and immunochemical measurements of VIP location and concentration, and VIP was found to inhibit spontaneous activity of the ampulla (both circular and longitudinal muscle layers) and of the isthmus (both circular and longitudinal muscle layers). The ED_{50} for inhibition of circular muscle activity of the isthmus was approximately 10^{-8} M (254). It was suggested that this peptidergic innervation might play a role in control of the sphincter function of the oviduct. To test this hypothesis, experiments were done in which rabbits were given estrogen alone or in combination with progesterone, and the content of VIP in the oviducts was measured by radioimmunoassay (255). Estrogen treatment increased VIP, but addition of progesterone for the last 3 days of estrogen treatment returned VIP levels to control values. Reduction of both circular and longitudinal muscular spontaneous activity was seen in this species also, with ED_{50} values similar to those for the human (254,255). These experiments therefore were felt to support the hypothesis of relaxation of a sphincter in the isthmic region. It had been previously shown, using doughnut-shaped intraluminal pressure transducers, that the isthmic lumen of the rabbit oviduct is constricted after ovulation (256) and relaxes by 56 hr after ovulation, a time when ova normally pass through this region (257).

These data provided significant evidence that VIP indeed could act as an important control mechanism for oviductal function. However, when rabbits were infused with VIP at a rate of 75 pmole/kg/min for 1 hr at the time of the preovulatory progesterone surge (i.e., between 2 and 3 hr after mating) or for 4 hr at the time of ovulation (i.e., 9–13 hr after mating), no effects on ovum transport were seen. Similarly, fertility was unaffected. This dose of VIP was sufficient to increase plasma progesterone levels, although its action on oviductal musculature was not studied (258). It is likely that the dose administered was not optimal, since *in vitro* no effects on human oviductal musculature were seen at 10^{-10} M (255), and in previous experiments in the rabbit, only modest *in vivo* inhibition of isthmic motility had been observed at a dose of 7.5×10^{-11} M/kg/min (which equals 1 μg/min) (259).

The presence of other peptides in the oviduct has also been reported. Neuropeptide Y, a 36-amino-acid neuropeptide with a COOH-terminal tyrosine (260), has been described in the rat reproductive tract (261). Fluorescence immunocytochemistry revealed its presence in the ovary, oviduct, uterus, and cervix. The most prominent supply was found in the cervix (261). However, further work revealed that peptide Y immunoreactivity was found in nerve fibers around blood vessels and in the muscle layers of the human oviduct. A few fibers were connected to the isthmic epithelium, but the remaining ones were distributed in a pattern similar to that of adrenergic fibers (262). Radioimmunoassay measurements showed that, in the oviducts of rat, mouse, and guinea pig, neuropeptide Y concentrations were always the highest of these peptides. In the rat and mouse, VIP was the next most abundant peptide, but, in the guinea pig, large quantities of substance P were seen (263). Neuropeptide Y inhibited the adrenergic contractile response and [^{3}H]norepinephrine release to field stimulation in the longitudinal muscle layer of the isthmus. This suggests that the peptide acts through prejunctional adrenergic inhibition (262).

Very few enkephalin-immunoreactive nerve fibers have been found in the cat female reproductive tract, except in the region of the cervix (264). Neither met- nor leu-enkephalin had a stimulatory or inhibitory action on human ampullar or isthmic oviductal contractility (265). Similar findings were recorded in experiments using the same tissues from cats and rabbits. It was, however, observed that leu-enkephalin increased myometrial blood flow in cats (266).

Substance P was first described in 1931 (267) and identified as an undecapeptide in 1971 (268). Substance-P-like immunoreactivity has been described in the female genitourinary tract of guinea pigs and cats, but not in the rat. Although such fibers are frequent in the vagina, they are sparse in the uterus and oviducts (269). More recent studies using radioimmunoassay showed that substance P was low in the mouse oviduct, but relatively more abundant in that of the guinea pig. In this latter species, the concentrations in the uterus, oviduct, and ovary were similar, whereas in the mouse the highest concentration was in the vagina. In these experiments, the stage of the estrous cycle was not stated (263). Both human and rabbit oviducts have been shown to be sensitive to the action of substance P. The ED_{50} for causing contraction in the human oviduct *in vitro* is only 57 nM (270,271). Further studies revealed that the stimulation of the human oviduct by substance P at a concentration of 10^{-6} M could be antagonized by addition of VIP at a concentration of 6×10^{-7} M (265).

When radioimmunoassay measurements of substance P were made in different portions of the human oviduct, the concentrations were as follows: 3.09 ± 1.40, 1.08 ± 0.30, and 0.74 ± 0.30 pmole/g wet weight of tissue in the uterotubal junction, ampullar-isthmic junction, and ampulla, respectively (272). Both circular and longitudinal muscle preparations from the human ampullar-isthmic junction responded to substance P at 10^{-6} M, but at 10^{-7} M the longitudinal muscle layer showed a greater stimulation than did the circular layer (272). Removal of calcium from the medium inhibited this stimulation, and VIP (10^{-7} M) significantly decreased the response (272). Substance P also increased uterine blood flow in the cat (266). This peptidergic system seems not to involve either the adrenergic or cholinergic nervous systems, since neither cholinergic nor adrenergic (α- or β-) blockade inhibited the responses of the oviduct to substance P or VIP (266,272).

It is clear that several peptides exert actions on the oviduct, and in view of the opposing activities of VIP and substance P, it has been suggested that these functional antagonists could provide a peptidergic control mechanism (272). Whether this is indeed the case remains to be determined by further work.

Cyclic nucleotides have been thought to be involved in the control of smooth-muscle contractions. Increases in cAMP have been associated with relaxation, whereas increases in cGMP have been associated with contraction (273,274). In the oviduct, cAMP levels are increased by PGE_2 and decreased by $PGF_{2\alpha}$ (275), which fits the general theory regarding cyclic nucleotides and contraction. Such changes could provide a mechanism for regulation of myogenic activity, but in the same series of experiments it was found that altered tissue cAMP levels were not essential for the actions of adrenergic agonists to be manifest on the oviduct (275). Furthermore, cGMP levels were not decreased, nor were cAMP levels increased, in the isthmic region of rabbit oviducts at 68 hr after an ovulating injection and injection of a dose of estrogen that would normally decrease muscular activity. Levels of both cyclic nucleotides were, however, higher in the isthmus than in the ampulla (276).

Cyclic nucleotides are known to exert direct effects on oviducts *in vitro* (277). Dibutyryl cAMP induces relaxation of the isthmus and ampulla in rabbits, guinea pigs, and humans. It also reduces the response to norepinephrine and $PGF_{2\alpha}$. Similarly, theophylline, a phosphodiesterase inhibitor, increases cAMP levels in oviduct tissue and inhibits spontaneous and $PGF_{2\alpha}$-induced activity. Conversely, imidazole, an activator of phosphodiesterase, increases oviductal contractility. Lastly, in these same experiments, cAMP concentration was found to decrease in the rabbit oviductal isthmus during the first 3 days after ovulation. PGE_2 restored these values to control levels and inhibited isthmic contractions. However, the cAMP values recorded (277) were about five to six times lower than those found by others (276). Thus, whether the changes in cyclic nucleotides are directly responsible for changes in contractility or are simply associated with such changes is not clear. It seems unlikely that, in themselves, the cyclic nucleotides can provide the major control mechanism.

Gamma-aminobutyric acid (GABA) is a major inhibitory neurotransmitter in the brain, and recently it has been found in higher concentrations in the oviduct than in the brain of the rat (278,279). Similarly, GABA has been found in the human oviduct, and a single population of high-affinity binding sites identified (K_D = 40 nM; B_{max} = 690 fmole/mg protein; nonspecific binding < 20%) (280). In the rat oviduct, similar specific binding was observed (K_D = 52 nM), but the maximum binding-site concentration was very low (B_{max} = 17 fmole/mg protein) and nonspecific binding was very high (~50%) (281). For this reason and because of the irreproducibility of the binding studies, others have concluded that GABA binding in this tissue is nonexistent or dependent on an uncontrolled critical variable (282). The enzyme that catalyzes the synthesis of GABA is L-glutamate-1-decarboxylase, which has been found in oviduct homogenates. This enzyme appears in two types, depending on whether it is in neural or non-neural tissue; the enzyme in the oviduct is similar to that in the brain neurons, thus suggesting that GABA may act as a neurotransmitter in the oviduct (283). In the human oviduct, GABA levels are higher in the ampulla than in the isthmus (280,283), but binding capacity is greater in the isthmus and GABA can influence isthmic contractility (280). *In vitro* studies with estrous rabbit oviducts showed that high concentrations of GABA (10^{-5} M) increased contraction frequency and elevated basal tone in both longitudinal and circular muscle from ampulla and isthmus. This action was not inhibited by bicuculline, suggesting a $GABA_B$ receptor system. Neither α- nor β-adrenergic blockade inhibited the actions of GABA on the oviduct, thus eliminating involvement of the sympathetic nervous system (284). There is no information available as to the effects of GABA or its inhibition on ovum transport, so the significance of this neurotransmitter system is still not certain. (See note 1 on p. 134.)

Oxytocin has been shown to stimulate oviductal contractility in sheep (285) and in the human (286). However, the stimulatory effect of oxytocin is maximal during menstruation and only minimal at ovulation. In contrast, vasopressin is more effective during the preovulatory period (286). In rats, binding sites for oxytocin have been observed in oviduct homogenates with an apparent K_D of 1.8×10^{-9} M. Binding capacity was 215 fmole/mg protein (287). When oxytocin was infused into the peripheral circulation of ewes in a pulsatile fashion, no significant relationships were observed between plasma concentrations of oxytocin and motility of the cervix or uterus. No observations were made on oviductal contractility in these studies (288). Given that, in the human at least, oviductal response to oxytocin is lowest at midcycle, it seems unlikely that oxytocin is involved in control of ovum transport.

CONTRACTILITY OF THE SMOOTH MUSCULATURE

The section entitled "Physiological Control Mechanisms" identified at least three systems that exhibit positive and negative effects on oviductal contractility and that might be implicated as control systems: the adrenergic system, the prostaglandins, and a peptidergic system (VIP and substance P). Which, if any, is the control system remains unclear, although they all affect contractility. It has always been assumed that change in contractility is the major factor promoting ovum transport to the uterus. Studies on the rapid phase of ovum transport through the ampullar region have certainly demonstrated that waves of contraction are correlated with the movement of the cumulus mass containing the ova (289,290). In the rabbit, the phase of ampullar transport is rapid (291), whereas in other species, such as the human or the rhesus monkey, it can take up to 24 hr or longer (292,293). Ova usually pass into the uterus between 96 and 120 hr after the LH peak in women, so that the actual total time of transport is about 80 hr (294).

It may be that this progression toward the uterus is a result of intrinsic activity of the oviductal musculature. Talo and Brundin (295) devised a technique for recording, in detail, muscular activity of the rabbit oviduct. Spontaneous electrical activity and intraluminal pressure were simultaneously recorded *in vitro* by means of suction electrodes and perfusion at constant flow rates of 1.4, 2, or 5.8 μl/min. Suction electrodes were used to map electrical activity throughout the whole oviduct (296). Using such techniques, it has been reported that the electrical activity of the oviduct varies from that of other structures of the reproductive tract, at least in duration. The duration of bursts is short (a few seconds) and the contractions are of a short phasic type (133). The rabbit oviduct normally exhibits multipacemaker activity with shifting pacemaker location, being highest in the distal isthmus or at the ampullar-isthmic junction. In the isthmus and ampullar-isthmic junction of postovulatory rabbit oviducts, all regions can initiate electrical activity, but certain pacemaker regions may predominate statistically. The frequency of generation may vary in a short segment. Electrical activity often propagates in both directions, but over shorter distances in the isthmus than in the ampulla. The speed of propagation is normally low, only a few millimeters per second, but reaches nearly 20 mm/sec in the isthmus of castrated, estrogen-treated rabbits (133). In the human, pacemaker activity seems to be higher in the ampulla than in the isthmus (135).

A hypothesis regarding ovum transport, in which ova are propelled by circular muscular contractions whose direction approaches randomness, has been developed (134). In these studies, ova were usually located in a region of inactivity, proximal to the uterus. At the time of uterine entry, this inactive region was short (less than 10% of oviductal length) (128). It is not certain whether uterine entry involves activation of the entire isthmus (which could be brief if contractions are unidirectional) or whether other mechanisms also operate at the uterotubal junction. A computer model of ovum transport suggests that these changes in bias and propagation would promote propulsion toward the uterotubal junction (297).

It has been suggested that over the 3-day period of transport, a net directional bias toward the uterus develops which causes the ultimate appearance of the ovum or zygote in the uterus (297,298). In the ampulla, this bias is associated with differences in distance traveled by the cumulus masses in each direction, rather than with the number of movements (299). Associated with this bias in movement toward the uterus is a constriction of the circular muscle layer of the isthmus after ovulation, thus producing its sphincter action (257).

All these conflicting data have been recently reviewed *in extenso* (122), and the most probable conclusion is that the myogenic activity of the oviductal musculature and the random walk theory provide the most likely explanation for the net movement of ova toward the uterus. However, what actually controls this myogenic activity is still obscure.

CILIARY ACTIVITY

As discussed in the sections entitled "Sperm Transport Through the Oviduct" and "Ovulation and Ovum Pick-Up," the endosalpinx is lined with an epithelial surface that has a variable number of ciliated cells, this number being greatest in the fimbria and least in the isthmus. These cells undergo changes in structure with the cyclic changes in steroid hormone levels. Under progestational influence, ciliated cells tend to de-differentiate and so be reduced in number (300). Ciliogenesis takes place during the proliferative phase of the cycle, and mature cilia are seen at midcycle (301). In contrast, ciliary activity seems to be increased during the luteal phase of the cycle (302). A similar increase in ciliary activity has been seen in the rabbit oviduct by the third day after mating (303). By this time the ova or zygotes would be in the sparsely ciliated isthmus, so the significance of this change is unknown.

It has been suggested that ciliary activity can provide some, or perhaps all, of the propulsive force that is required to transport ova along the ampullar region of the oviduct. If a 1-cm (or larger) segment of the oviduct is surgically reversed in rabbits, then ova are not transported across the reversed segment in which cilia now beat toward the ovary rather than in the usual orientation toward the uterus (304,305). Similarly, if a polyethylene tube is inserted into the ampulla of the rabbit oviduct, ova can pass through tubes up to 10 mm long, but not through those of 15 mm or longer (306). Ciliary activity was clearly not involved in ovum movement through the 10 mm tube. In the human, a correlation has been made between a reduction in the percentage of ciliated cells present on the fimbriae and in fertility (307), but this failure to become pregnant may be more a reflection of problems with ovum "pick-up" after ovulation than with subsequent transport. It has also been recorded that women suffering from the immotile cilia syndrome, in which cilia throughout the body are nonfunctional, are normally fertile (308,309). Although in these particular patients the absence of ciliary activity in the oviduct was not specifically confirmed, the implication remains that ciliary activity is not essential for ovum transport in the human. (See note 2 on p. 134.) It may, however, be a contributing factor, since in experiments with ovum surrogates in rabbits, it was found that the rate of transport through the ampullar region was abnormally slow in the absence of the cumulus oophorus (290,310). Retarded or inhibited transport of similar ovum surrogates has also been seen in sheep (311). This suggests that an important interaction between the cumulus and the cilia may occur in these species. In the human, ovum surrogates appear to be transported more readily, and actual size is not so critical until sizes of 600 μm or larger are used (168).

On balance, it must be concluded that in the human, at least, ciliary activity plays little, if any, role in the process of ovum transport through the ampulla, and it plays no role in transport through the isthmus. It is likely to be important in ensuring normal "pick-up" of ova from the ovarian surface or from the peritoneal cavity at ovulation.

OVIDUCTAL SECRETIONS

The nature of the oviductal secretion has already been described in the section entitled "Sperm Transport Through the Oviduct" in connection with its role in sperm transport and in the section entitled "Ovum Survival." Whether it plays any major role in ovum transport per se is questionable. The experiments mentioned above on reversal of ampullar segments and placement of tubes in the ampulla suggest that fluid flow alone is insufficient to transport ova along the ampulla (304–306).

However, it is known that fluid will accumulate in the rabbit oviduct if the fimbriated end is ligated (312) and that this accumulation disappears only at the time the ova usually enter the uterus, approximately 60 to 72 hr after mating (104). If a plastic tube is inserted through the ampullar-isthmic junction, the fluid flows through the tube and carries the ova with it into the uterus inappropriately early (312). A similar sphincter mechanism has been shown to operate at the uterotubal junction in the cow (313), sheep (314), and human (315). Yet it has also been claimed that there is no evidence for a functional sphincter at the uterotubal junction in the human and that small particles pass in either direction through the interstitial portion of the oviduct at any time in the cycle (102). It may be that there is a functional occlusion occurring for only a limited period of 2 to 3 days after ovulation.

It is unusual to find ova in the final 10% of the isthmic region of the oviduct; usually they are clumped just above this final portion and then pass rapidly *en masse* into the uterus (153,214,310). There is little circular muscular activity in this region (104). Recording of electrical activity of the oviduct confirmed that there was a region of inactivity in the isthmus which was reduced to less than 10% of the oviductal length at the time of entry of ova into the uterus (134). Edema of the isthmus occurring around the time of ovulation has been observed in rabbits (131), pigs (316), and humans (130). Reduction of this edema can be produced by progesterone treatment in pigs (317,318), and a similar reduction occurs normally about 68 hr after ovulation in the rabbit (131,319).

Thus, the reduction in length of the inactive segment (134), combined with relaxation of isthmic constriction (257) and reduction of edema under the action of progesterone, may be sufficient to permit fluid flow to carry the ova into the uterus.

Oviductal secretions have been claimed to play a role in maintaining ova at the ampullar-isthmic junction for a considerable period during the transport process. Koester (320) has proposed that the isthmic constriction is such that fluid flow, back up the ampulla to the infundibulum and thence into the peritoneal cavity, is sufficiently strong so as to prevent the denuded ova from entering the isthmus until this constriction starts to relax. Whether this is the case or whether the isthmic constriction alone is sufficient to prevent ovum entry is not certain.

In summary, apart from maintaining an environment conducive to zygote survival, oviductal secretions may be important for ovum and zygote transport in two ways. Firstly, they may prevent entry into the isthmus because of the force of the reverse flow, and secondly they can assist ovum or zygote entry into the uterus at the appropriate time when the uterotubal junction is relaxed under the influence of progesterone.

TIME OF OVUM TRANSPORT THROUGH THE OVIDUCT

I and others have shown that, in the rabbit, ovum transport through the ampullar region takes only a few minutes—approximately 4 to 15 min (289–291,321–323). This process takes somewhat longer in the pig—about 45 min (324). Transport through the ampulla is much slower in the sheep (311). The situation in primates is not so clear, since observation of transport of newly ovulated or transferred ova to the ampullar region has not been studied, except in *Macaca nemestrina* (the pig-tailed macaque), where a transit time of 22 min has been recorded (162).

In the rabbit, ova are retained at the ampullar-isthmic junction for approximately 24 hr before passing on into the isthmus (214,310). The situation is much different in primates. In baboons (*Papio anubis*), the ova remain in the ampulla for approximately 36 hr (half the total transport time) (325); however, in rhesus monkeys (*Macaca mulatta*), ova are found in the ampulla until 48 hr after ovulation (two-thirds of total transport time) (293), and in women ova can be confined to the ampulla for up to 72 hr (nine-tenths of total transport time) (292). Ova first appear in the uterus in women about 80 hr after ovulation (292). An earlier article had indicated that ova could be found in the uterus as early as 2 days after ovulation, whereas zygotes were observed there on only the fourth and fifth days after ovulation (326). However, timing of ovulation was not so precise in these experiments as in subsequent ones. Whether there is really a significant difference in the transport of zygotes compared with ova is not certain, but the difference, if any, is small. The zygotes in the human enter the uterus in a relatively immature state compared to those in some other mammals (Table 3). A 12-cell zygote was the youngest one that has been recovered from the human uterus (327), and a seven-cell zygote was the oldest one still found in the human oviduct (207). Thus, uterine entry of zygotes occurs approximately at the 7- to 12-cell stage. This agrees well with the cleavage rates recorded *in vitro* following *in vitro* fertilization, where eight-cell zygotes are seen between 45 and 73 hr and 16-cell ones are seen between 68 and 85 hr after insemination (121).

TABLE 3. *Time of egg denudation, time of entry into uterus, and cell stage at entry, in relation to ovulation*[a]

Animal	Denudation of eggs after ovulation (hr)	Entry into uterus after ovulation (hr)	Cell stage at entry
Opossum	—	24	Pronuclear
Shrew	—	87–95	Late morula
Rat	Rapid	95–100	8–16
Mouse	12	72	16–32
Guinea pig	24+	80–85	8
Rabbit	6 8–10[b]	60	Morula
Dog	48 or more	168–192	16–32
Ferret	19½–40	88½–108½	16–32
Cat	48 or more	121–161½	Late morula
Horse	<24	98+[c]	16
Pig	<24	24–48	4
Cow	9–14	72	8–16
Goat	<30½	85–98	12
Sheep	0–5	70–80	8–16
Rhesus monkey	24 48[b]	72 ± 12	16
Baboon	48[b]	72	—
Human	?24	80	7–12

[a]Data from various sources. Reprinted from ref. 390.
[b]Unmated.
[c]Except unfertilized eggs.

During the process of transport through the oviduct, the ova lose the cumulus oophorus. This can occur mechanically in unmated animals or by the action of hyaluronidase released from the sperm heads in mated animals. Usually, denudation occurs faster in mated than in unmated animals (see Table 3). Whether this is also true of the human is not certain; however, an unfertilized ovum with the corona radiata cells still attached has been recorded at the ampullar-isthmic junction at 72 hr after the LH peak (i.e., approximately 56 hr after ovulation) (292). In contrast, a two-cell zygote almost completely denuded of cumulus and corona cells was recovered from the oviduct by Hertig and collaborators (327). The age of this latter zygote was presumed to be between $1\frac{1}{2}$ and $2\frac{1}{2}$ days, but dating was estimated from endometrial morphology and menstrual history, so it is only approximate. Nonetheless, this two-cell zygote is unlikely to be older than the unfertilized ovum described by Croxatto et al. (292). In some species, such as the rabbit, the corona radiata cells do not disperse as readily as the cumulus oophorus and may remain attached even after sperm penetration of the ovum has occurred (328). Persistence of the corona cells has also been reported for human ova, even though the cumulus mass has dispersed (329). The corona radiata also persists in the rhesus monkey. One unfertilized ovum still had corona cells present up to approximately 24 to 48 hr after ovulation, whereas another ovum was denuded at 12 to 24 hr after ovulation. A fertilized two-cell ovum, recovered 23 hr after mating (but ovulation had occurred previous to mating), was totally denuded (330). In other studies, six unfertilized monkey ova still were in cumulus at 36 ± 12 hr after ovulation (determined by laparoscopy), whereas one 7- to 8-cell zygote, recovered at the same time interval, was denuded. All four zygotes that were recovered at 48 ± 12 hr were denuded (331). The importance of these cellular investments for normal ovum transport in the human is not certain, since transport through the ampulla is slow and denudation has already occurred before passage through the isthmus usually commences.

In summary, ovum transport in the human consists of slow transit through the ampulla, with retention at the ampullar-isthmic junction until 72 hr after ovulation, followed by transport through the isthmus and uterotubal junction into the uterus during the subsequent 8 hr.

PHARMACOLOGICAL ACTIONS ON THE OVIDUCT AND CONTRACEPTIVE POTENTIAL

In the section entitled "Physiological Control Mechanisms" a great many agents that affect oviductal motility and sperm transport were described. These included steroids, cyclic nucleotides, prostaglandins, catecholamines, and assorted peptides. It is clear that when excessive amounts of these drugs are administered exogenously, interference with ovum transport can result. Consequently, synthetic estrogens, antiestrogens, synthetic progestins, and assorted prostaglandins have all been used to accelerate transport of ova through the oviduct in a variety of mammals (see refs. 332–334 for further references). Apart from the use of estrogens and/or progestin combinations for contraceptive purposes (202–204), there is little good evidence for such actions occurring in the human.

Again, in small animals, a variety of substances have been shown to stimulate oviductal contractility. These include angiotensin, bradykinin, epinephrine, norepinephrine, and phenylephrine. Others induce a relaxation of activity, e.g., butanephrine, isoproterenol, and vasopressin (see ref. 335 for further references). Other substances, such as $PGF_{2\alpha}$ and substance P (which cause contraction) as well as PGE_2 and VIP (which cause relaxation), have already been discussed (see sections entitled "Prostaglandins" and "Peptides"). Unfortunately the correlation between increased oviductal motility and accelerated transport is not well established. Reduction of oviductal motility is unlikely to be useful, since the possibility of ectopic pregnancy in the human is always a hazard. Despite the fact that in the human the action of many of these stimulating agents is similar to that observed in nonprimates, their contraceptive potential seems limited.

It has been reported that an ergot alkaloid, ergonovine maleate, which is not active in rabbits, has a potent stimulatory action on the human oviduct at a dose of 10 μg intravenously. Repeated administration at 4- to 6-hr intervals maintained contractility (336). It has been claimed that a daily oral dose of 0.02 mg of ergonovine maleate provides some contraceptive effect, but six pregnancies in 48 women over 262 months of use were nonetheless observed (336). When this drug was given only pre- or post-coitally, pregnancies also occurred. It was therefore suggested that it was necessary to combine ergonovine treatment (to stimulate oviductal contractility) with sparteine sulfate (to stimulate uterine contractility). Sparteine sulfate at a single oral dose of 100 to 200 mg maintains uterine activity for up to 3 hr, and, given at the same dose every 4 hr for 3 days, causes abortion (336). Preliminary clinical trials suggested that the combination could be acceptable and effective (336,337).

Further successful application of this method has not been reported, and there appear to be no other suitable candidates for a contraceptive that would act exclusively by altering oviductal transport time. The difficulties inherent in this approach in the human have already been discussed; briefly, they involve the possibility of ectopic pregnancy when transport is delayed, and the possibility of normal pregnancy even when transport is accelerated, unless the uterus is also evacuated. Because uterine evacuation can be more reliably achieved once pregnancy is established (at the time of a missed menses), either by prostaglandins alone (338,339) or combined with an antiprogestin such as RU486 (340,341), the attraction of a post-coital contraceptive acting only 1 to 2 days immediately after ovulation is minimal, especially since the time of ovulation cannot be reliably and easily predicted.

PATHOLOGY OF THE OVIDUCT

The normal functioning of the oviduct can be disrupted by a variety of pathological causes. Many of these have been dealt with extensively by Woodruff and Pauerstein (102) and will not be discussed in detail here. One of the most common is salpingitis, i.e., inflammation of the oviduct. This can arise from an ascending infection through the cervix and endometrium, as a result of puerperal or post-traumatic endometritis, or from adjacent or distant inflammation.

The ascending infection is usually associated with a sexually transmitted disease, such as gonorrhea or chlamydial infection. Where the salpingitis becomes chronic, the oviduct can fill with pus (pyosalpinx) or fluid secretion (hydrosalpinx). In either case, fertility will be severely compromised or abolished. Genital tuberculosis, secondary to systemic infection, may be one of the greatest causes of infertility in developing countries. Although the result can resemble salpingitis or chronic nontuberculous salpingitis, typically there are granulomatous changes. Last, a variety of oviductal tumors, both benign and neoplastic, that cause luminal occlusion have been recorded (102).

Infertility can be caused by obvious pathological conditions that occlude the reproductive tract and so prevent normal gamete transport or by more subtle conditions that result in so-called unexplained infertility. In these latter conditions, disruption of oviduct function may occur, but if it does, there seems to be no dominant factor in the etiology of this disease. It has been estimated that, world wide, 5% to 10% of all married couples may be infertile (342). It was found as a result of further world wide studies that in 26% of couples enrolled with no demonstrable cause of infertility, but in which the cause was subsequently diagnosed, only the female partner was affected, and in 19.4% both partners were affected. An oviductal factor was identified in 44.6% and 29.6% of these two subsets, respectively (343). A later report indicated that bilateral oviductal occlusion was diagnosed in 14.2% of cases overall, ranging from 42% in Africa to 16% in other developing countries and to 9% in developed countries (344). These differences were ascribed to different levels of sexually transmitted diseases and the occurrence of postpartum or postabortal infections in these areas. In all countries, the incidence of bilateral occlusion always increased with number of pregnancies, previous abortion, or previous live birth. The usual methods of diagnosis of oviductal occlusion are hysterosalpingography, insufflation, or laparoscopy, with hysterosalpingography being the most reliable.

Repair of occluded oviducts can be successful, but skilled microsurgical procedures are required to give the best results (345,346). Obviously, where infection is the predisposing cause of the oviductal pathology, its cure must antedate any attempt at reconstructive surgery. It is only relatively recently in developed countries that the role of infection with *Chlamydia trichomatis* has been recognized as a cause of oviductal sterility and failure of tuboplastic repair procedures. In a series of 69 women with oviductal obstruction, 18.8% were found to have positive cultures for *Chlamydia* compared to only 2% in 49 normal controls (347).

An increased risk of pelvic inflammatory disease has been reported associated with the use of an intrauterine device (IUD) (348,349), and, at least in nulliparous women, an association with an increased risk for subsequent infertility is also associated with IUD use (350,351). Endometriosis, which involves the implantation of endometrial cells in ectopic locations such as the peritoneal surface or the ovaries, is found in approximately 50% of women presenting with infertility and in about 38% with unexplained infertility (352,353). In many cases, salpingitis can be clinically confirmed in association with histologically proven endometriosis, and, in these women, this alone could be the cause of the resulting infertility (354). However, in many instances, no obvious pathology of the oviduct can be seen. In such cases, it has been suggested that inappropriate production of prostaglandins from the endometriotic implants on the peritoneum or ovary could disrupt oviductal function. Excessive prostaglandin concentrations have been found in the abdominal fluid of such women (355) and in monkeys with artificially induced endometriosis (356). However, in other studies, prostaglandin levels have not been elevated (357–359) or were not associated with endometriosis in infertile patients (360). Thus, if there is any effect of endogenous prostaglandins on oviductal function in infertile patients with endometriosis, the association seems very tenuous.

The incidence of ectopic pregnancy has been reported to vary from 1 in 30 to 1 in 300 live births, depending on the population surveyed (361). Its incidence in the United States is increasing; the incidence over the last decade has risen from 4.8/1,000 live births in 1970 to 14.5/1,000 in 1980 (362). Ectopic pregnancy does not seem to be associated with coexisting salpingitis (361), although prior salpingitis may given rise to salpingitis isthmica nodosa, which may be associated with this increased incidence (363). Usually there is no obvious reason why, in some women, the developing embryo implants in an extrauterine site, especially in the oviduct. Certainly, when the oviductal lumen is partially occluded at the uterotubal junction, as when hysteroscopic sterilization using cautery is performed, then the incidence of ectopic pregnancy can be greatly increased (364). Conversely, a markedly decreased incidence of ectopic pregnancies has been noted in patients who were treated with prostaglandins for termination of first-trimester pregnancies (365).

Although IUD use is associated with an increase in the relative incidence of ectopic pregnancies as a result of the prevention of the intrauterine ones, there is actually no increase in absolute numbers of ectopic pregnancies for most IUDs (366–368). However, IUDs releasing progesterone have been associated with a positive increased ectopic pregnancy rate (368,369). Similarly, previous abortion (370) or use of large doses of estrogen as an interceptive agent (205,206) can increase the incidence of ectopic pregnancy. Ovarian hyperstimulation caused by exogenous gonadotrophin treatment (371) or use of chronic low-dose progestins for contraception (208,209) has been reported to have a similar effect. All of these factors suggest that when an interference with the balance of ovarian steroids required for normal zygote transport occurs, a failure of the transport mechanism can occur.

Since ectopic pregnancy does not occur naturally in nonprimates, and even when it is induced artificially in sites outside the reproductive tract it gives rise to growth of only trophoblast, no small animal model is available for experimental manipulation. Even in nonhuman primates, the incidence of ectopic pregnancy is extremely rare (102,372,373). The most common locations for pregnancies in the oviduct are the ampulla (60%) and isthmus (30%) (363); preseumably the zygotes are trapped either at the ampullar-isthmic or uterotubal junctions. In view of the lack of a suitable animal model, further work on the causality of this condition can only be achieved retrospectively in case control studies or in prospective large-scale epidemiological studies.

TRANSPORT AND SPACING OF ZYGOTES IN THE UTERUS

Once the developing embryo enters the uterus, it is transported to the site of implantation primarily by muscular activity of the uterine wall. The position that the blastocyst achieves within the uterus is not random, but is the same within any major taxonomic group (374). This leads to a fixed placental position. In the simplex uterus of the human, the uterine lumen is dorsoventrally flattened, and implantation occurs most often on the surface of the midportion of the posterior wall of the uterus (375). The regularity of positioning of blastocysts in the uterus suggests that there must be some underlying mechanism.

In those polytocous species with multiple embryos within a single uterine horn, the regular spacing along the horn, except in the case of overcrowding, can be explained mainly by muscular activity of the myometrium. In the rabbit, whose blastocysts swell to about 5 mm at implantation (376), the blastocysts act as a focal point for the initiation of waves of muscular contraction. This results in uniform spacing of the blastocysts (377). It is now known that rabbit blastocysts contain and produce prostaglandins (378–380), which can be transported from the uterine lumen to the myometrium (381). Prostaglandins can be accumulated by the rabbit blastocyst and released in a site-directed manner (382,383). The release of these prostaglandins could be the trigger to initiate regular spacing in the uterus in this species. Prostaglandin synthesis has also been reported for blastocysts of sheep (384), cows (385), pigs (386), and mice (387). Thus it may be that this is a common mechanism inducing regular spacing. In mice, uterine contractility has been shown to be the overriding cause of blastocyst spacing (388). In monotocous species, such as the human, the situation is not so clear. In the luminal epithelium, ciliated cells that might contribute to the orientation in the endometrial cavity have been described in the human (389). In the absence of other evidence, it seems likely that myometrial contractions triggered by the presence of the blastocyst play a major role in blastocyst placement in this species also.

CONCLUSIONS

This review has attempted to highlight various processes that have been proposed as control mechanisms for gamete transport. The role of the oviduct is very central in this phase of the reproductive process: It ensures an environment for maturation of sperm and ovum and for fertilization and subsequent zygote development. It is clear that there are many mechanisms that exert actions on oviductal function, but none appears to be the crucial controlling factor. Under appropriate circumstances they can all be shown to play some role. It seems that there is a redundancy of mechanisms, which can substitute one for another. This redundancy may be important because of the crucial role of the oviduct during early preimplantation stages of pregnancy in most species.

This may not be the case in the human, since, as noted above, pregnancy can occur in the absence of the oviduct or when many of these various mechanisms are suppressed. This should not be construed to indicate that the incidence of pregnancy in such cases is normal, only that it is possible. In his recent extensive review, Jansen (122) concluded that the oviduct "has much redundancy in its repertoire of gamete transporting properties," and, specifically with regard to ovum transport, that there is a lack of convincing empirical evidence that any one of the mechanisms predominates.

One may therefore conclude that the oviduct remains an enigma and that the concerted efforts of many scientists from different disciplines over the last 40-odd years, while advancing our knowledge about individual processes, have contributed little to our understanding of the integration of the whole system. Indeed, we know in good detail what occurs, as well as the timing, the changes in sperm and ovum, and the changes in morphology of the reproductive tract, but we still cannot be certain what controls (a) sperm transport to the site of fertilization and (b) zygote transport through the oviduct to the uterus. The most likely explanations are those indicated toward the end of the various sections, but it must be recognized that new information could change these views dramatically. It seems certain to this observer that the approaches of the past have failed to provide us with the correct blueprint for integration of function of this system and that new approaches are required.

ACKNOWLEDGMENTS

The writing of this chapter and some of the work described herein was supported by NIH grant HD14048. Grateful thanks are due to Beverly Evans for typing the first draft and to Gretta Small for production and editorial assistance of the finished version.

REFERENCES

1. Woolf, H. B., editor (1977): *Webster's New Collegiate Dictionary*, p. 472. G. & C. Merriam Co., Springfield, Mass.
2. Fisher, G. J. (1880): Historical and biographical notes: V. Gabrillo Fallopio, 1523–1562. *Ann. Anat. Surg. Soc.*, 2:200–204.
3. Bedford, J. M. (1975): Maturation, transport and fate of spermatozoa in the epididymis. In: *Handbook of Physiology, Section 7: Endocrinology, Vol. 5, Male Reproductive System*, edited by D. W. Hamilton, and R. O. Greep, pp. 303–317. American Physiological Society, Washington, D.C.
4. MacMillan, E. W. (1957): The mechanical influence of the vasa efferentia on the transport of radiopaque medium through the ductus epididymidis of the rat. *Stud. Fertil.*, 9:65–71.
5. MacMillan, E. W., and Aukland, J. (1960): The transport of radiopaque medium through the initial segment of the rat epididymis. *J. Reprod. Fertil.*, 1:139–145.
6. Risley, P. L. (1963): Physiology of the male accessory organs. In: *Mechanisms Concerned with Conception*, edited by C. G. Hartman, pp. 73–133. Macmillan, New York.
7. Cross, B. A. (1959): Hypothalamic influences on sperm transport in the male and female genital tract. In: *Recent Progress in the Endocrinology of Reproduction*, edited by C. W. Lloyd, pp. 167–177. Academic Press, New York.
8. Sjöstrand, N. O. (1965): The adrenergic innervation of the vas deferens and the accessory male genital glands. *Acta Physiol. Scand.*, 65 (Suppl. 257): 82 pp.
9. El-Badawi, A., and Schenk, E. A. (1967): The distribution of cholinergic and adrenergic nerves in the mammalian epididymis. *Am. J. Anat.*, 121:1–14.
10. Baumgarten, H. G., Holstein, A. F., and Rosengren, E. (1971): Arrangement, ultrastructure, and adrenergic innervation of smooth musculature of the ductuli efferentes, ductus epididymidis and ductus deferens of man. *Z. Mikrosk. Anat. Forsch.*, 120:37–79.
11. Rowley, M., Teshima, J. F., and Heller, C. G. (1970): Duration of transit of spermatozoa through the human male ductular system. *Fertil. Steril.*, 21:390–396.
12. Orgebin-Crist, M. C. (1965): Passage of spermatozoa labelled with thymidine-^{3}H through the ductus epididymidis of the rabbit. *J. Reprod. Fertil.*, 10:241–251.
13. Amir, D., and Ortavant, R. (1968): Influence de la fréquence des collectes sur la durée du transit des spermatozoides dans le canal epididymaire du belier. *Ann. Biol. Anim. Biochim. Biophys.*, 8:195–207.
14. Bedford, J. M. (1978): Influence of abdominal temperature on epididymal function in the rat and rabbit. *Am. J. Anat.*, 152:509–522.
15. Cummins, J. M., and Glover, T. D. (1970): Artificial cryptorchidism and fertility in the rabbit. *J. Reprod. Fertil.*, 23:423–433.
16. Jones, R. (1975): The effects of artificial cryptorchidism on the composition of epididymal plasma in the rabbit. *Fertil. Steril.*, 25:432–438.
17. Orbach, J. (1961): Spontaneous ejaculation in the rat. *Science*, 134:1072–1073.
18. Lino, B. F., Braden, A. W. H., and Turnbull, E. K. (1967): Fate of unejaculated spermatozoa. *Nature*, 213:594–595.
19. Martan, J. (1969): Epididymal histochemistry and physiology. *Biol. Reprod. (Suppl.)*, 1:134–154.
20. Phadke, A. M. (1964): Fate of spermatozoa in case of obstructive azoospermia and after ligation of vas deferens in man. *J. Reprod. Fertil.*, 7:1–12.
21. Orgebin-Crist, M. C. (1967): Maturation of spermatozoa in the rabbit epididymis. Fertilizing ability and embryonic mortality in does inseminated with epididymal spermatozoa. *Ann. Biol. Anim. Biochim. Biophys.*, 7:373–389.
22. Bedford, J. M., Calvin, H., and Cooper, G. W. (1973): The maturation of spermatozoa in the human epididymis. *J. Reprod. Fertil. (Suppl.)*, 18:199–213.
23. Bedford, J. M. (1967): Effect of duct ligation on the fertilizing ability of spermatozoa from different regions of the rabbit epididymis. *J. Exp. Zool.*, 166:271–282.
24. Young, D. H. (1970): Surgical treatment of male infertility. *J. Reprod. Fertil.*, 23:541–542.
25. Silber, S.J. (1980): Reversal of vasectomy and the treatment of male infertility. *J. Androl.*, 1:261–268.
26. Bancroft, J. (1980): Human sexual behaviour. In: *Reproduction in Mammals, Vol. 8: Human Sexuality*, edited by C. R. Austin and R. V. Short, pp. 34–67. Cambridge University Press, Cambridge, U.K.
27. Whitelaw, G. P., and Smithwick, R. H. (1951): Some secondary effects of sympathectomy with particular reference to disturbance of sexual function. *N. Engl. J. Med.*, 245:121–130.
28. Kedia, K. R., and Markland, C. (1976): The ejaculatory process. In: *Human Semen and Fertility Regulation in Men*, edited by E. S. E. Hafez, pp. 497–503. C. V. Mosby, St. Louis.
29. Bedford, J. M. (1986): Personal communication.
30. Ambache, N., and Zar, M. A. (1971): Evidence against adrenergic motor transmission to the guinea-pig vas deferens. *J. Physiol. (Lond.)*, 216:359–389.
31. Furness, J. B., and Iwayama, T. (1972): The arrangement and identification of axons innervating the vas deferens of the guinea pig. *J. Anat.*, 113:179–196.
32. MacLeod, D. G., Reynolds, D. G., and Demaree, G. E. (1973): Some pharmacologic characteristics of the human vas deferens. *Invest. Urol.*, 10:338–341.
33. Bauer, G. E., Hull, R. D., Stokes, G. S., and Raftos, J. (1973): The reversibility of side effects of guanethidine therapy. *Med. J. Aust.*, 1:930–933.
34. Green, M., and Berman, S. (1954): Failure of ejaculation produced by dibenzyline. *Conn. State Med. J.*, 18:30–33.
35. Singh, H. (1961): A case of inhibition of ejaculation as a side effect of mellaril. *Am. J. Psychiatry*, 117:1041–1042.
36. Freyhan, F. A. (1961): Loss of ejaculation during mellaril treatment. *Am. J. Psychiatry*, 118:171–172.
37. Heller, J. (1961): Another case of inhibition of ejaculation as a side effect of mellaril. *Am. J. Psychiatry*, 118:173.
38. Shilon, M., Paz, G. F., and Homonnai, Z. T. (1984): The use of phenoxybenzamine treatment in premature ejaculation. *Fertil. Steril.*, 42:659–661.
39. Masters, W. H., and Johnson, V. E. (1970): Premature ejaculation. In: *Human Sexual Inadequacy*, pp. 92–115, Little, Brown and Co., Boston.
40. Mann, T. (1964): *The Biochemistry of Semen and of the Male Reproductive Tract*. Methuen & Co., Ltd., London.
41. Eliasson, R., and Lindholmer, C. (1972): Distribution and properties of spermatozoa in different fractions of split ejaculates. *Fertil. Steril.*, 23:252–256.
42. Lundquist, F. (1949): Aspects of the biochemistry of human semen. *Acta Physiol. Scand.* 19 (Suppl. 66):108 pp.
43. Cavazos, L. F. (1977): The mammalian accessory sex glands: A morphological and functional analysis. In: *Frontiers in Reproduction and Fertility Control. A Review of the Reproductive Sciences and Contraceptive Development*, edited by R. O. Greep and M. A. Koblinsky, pp. 402–410. MIT Press, Cambridge, Mass.
44. Eliasson, R. (1973): Parameters of male fertility. In: *Human Reproduction. Conception and Contraception*, edited by E. S. E. Hafez and T. N. Evans, pp. 39–51. Harper & Row, Hagerstown, Md.
45. Nelson, C. M. K., and Bunge, R. G. (1974): Semen analysis: Evidence for changing parameters of male fertility potential. *Fertil. Steril.*, 25:503–507.
46. Zuckerman, Z., Rodriguez-Rigau, L. J., Smith, K. D. and Steinberger, E. (1977): Frequency distribution of sperm counts in fertile and infertile males. *Fertil. Steril.*, 28:1310–1313.
47. Barfield, A., Melo, J., Coutinho, E., Alvarez-Sanchez, F., Faundes, A., Brache, V., Leon, P., Frick, J., Bartsch, G., Weiske, W. H., Brenner, P., Mishell, D. Jr., Bernstein, G., and Ortiz, A. (1979): Pregnancies associated with sperm concentrations below 10 million/ml in clinical studies of a potential male contraceptive method, monthly depot medroxyprogesterone acetate and testosterone esters. *Contraception*, 20:121–127.
48. Fox, C. A., Meldrum, S. J., and Watson, B. W. (1973): Continuous measurement by radio-telemetry of vaginal pH during human coitus. *J. Reprod. Fertil.*, 33:69–75.

49. Fox, C. A., and Fox, B. (1971): A comparative study of coital physiology with special reference to the sexual climax. *J. Reprod. Fertil.*, 24:319–336.
50. Fox, C. A., Wolff, H. S., and Baker, J. A. (1970): Measurement of intra-vaginal and intra-uterine pressures during human coitus by radio-telemetry. *J. Reprod. Fertil.*, 22:243–251.
51. Fox, C. A., Ismail, A. A. A., Love, D. N., Kirkham, K. E., and Loraine, J. A. (1972): Studies on the relationship between plasma testosterone levels and human sexual activity. *J. Endocrinol.*, 52:51–58.
52. Neumann, F., Von Berswoldt-Wallrabe, R., Elger, W., Steinbeck, H., Hahn, J. D., and Kramer, M. (1970): Aspects of androgen-dependent events as studied by antiandrogens. *Recent Prog. Horm. Res.*, 26:337–405.
53. Morse, H. C., Leach, D. R., Rowley, M. J., and Heller, C. G. (1973): Effect of cyproterone acetate on sperm concentration, seminal fluid volume, testicular cytology and levels of plasma and urinary ICSH, FSH and testosterone in normal men. *J. Reprod. Fertil.*, 32:365–378.
54. Amersbach, R. (1930): Sterilität und Frigidität. *Münch. Med. Wochenschr.*, 77:225–227.
55. Trapl, J. (1943): Neue Anschauungen über den Ei- und Samentransport in den inneren Geschlechtsteilen der Frau. *Zentralbl. Gynakol.*, 67:547–550.
56. Egli, G. E., and Newton, M. (1961): The transport of carbon particles in the human female reproductive tract. *Fertil. Steril.*, 12:151–155.
57. Grafenberg, E. (1950): The role of urethra in female orgasm. *Int. J. Sex*, 3:145–148.
58. Masters, W. H., and Johnson, V. E. (1966): *Human Sexual Response*, 366 pp. Little, Brown & Co., Boston.
59. Bygdeman, M., and Samuelsson, B. (1966): Analysis of prostaglandins in human semen. Prostaglandins and related factors 44. *Clin. Chim. Acta*, 13:465–474.
60. Bygdeman, M., Fredericsson, B., Svanborg, K., and Samuelsson, B. (1970): The relation between fertility and prostaglandin content of seminal fluid in man. *Fertil. Steril.*, 21:622–629.
61. Wiqvist, N., Widholm, O., Nillius, S. J., and Nilsson, B. (1979): Dysmenorrhea and prostaglandins. *Acta Obstet. Gynecol. Scand. (Suppl.)*, 87:117 pp.
62. Settlage, D. S. F., Motoshima, M., and Tredway, D. R. (1973): Sperm transport from the external cervical os to the Fallopian tubes in women: A time and quantitation study. *Fertil. Steril.*, 24:655–661.
63. Moghissi, K. S. (1972): Sperm migration through the human cervix. In: *Cervical Mucus in Human Reproduction*, edited by M. Elstein, K. S. Moghissi, and R. Borth, pp. 128–152. Scriptor, Copenhagen.
64. Templeton, A. A., Cooper, I., and Kelly, R. W. (1978): Prostaglandin concentrations in the semen of fertile men. *J. Reprod. Fertil.*, 52:147–150.
65. Eskin, B. A., Azarbal, S., Sepic, R., and Slate, W. G. (1973): *In vitro* responses of the spermatozoa-cervical mucus system treated with prostaglandin $F_{2\alpha}$. *Obstet. Gynecol.*, 41:436–439.
66. Elstein, M., Moghissi, K. S., and Borth, R., editors (1972): *Cervical Mucus in Human Reproduction*, 163 pp. Scriptor, Copenhagen.
67. Billings, E. L., Billings, J. J., Brown, J. B., and Burger, H. G. (1972): Symptoms and hormonal changes accompanying ovulation. *Lancet* 1:282–284.
68. Flynn, A. M., and Lynch, S. S. (1976): Cervical mucus and identification of the fertile phase of the menstrual cycle. *Br. J. Obstet. Gynaecol.*, 83:656–659.
69. World Health Organization (1981): A prospective multicentre trial of the ovulation method of natural family planning. 1. The teaching phase. *Fertil. Steril.*, 36:152–158.
70. World Health Organization (1981): A prospective multicentre trial of the ovulation method of natural family planning. II. The effectiveness phase. *Fertil. Steril.*, 36:591–598.
71. Moghissi, K. S. (1966): Cyclic changes of cervical mucus in normal and progestin-treated women. *Fertil. Steril.*, 17:663–675.
72. Mattner, P. E. (1968): The distribution of spermatozoa and leucocytes in the female genital tract in goats and cattle. *J. Reprod. Fertil.*, 17:253–261.
73. Hafez, E. S. E. (1973): The comparative anatomy of the mammalian cervix. In: *The Biology of the Cervix*, edited by R. J. Blandau and K. S. Moghissi, pp. 23–56. University of Chicago Press, Chicago.
74. Chang, M. C. (1956): Reaction of the uterus on spermatozoa in the rabbit. *Ann. Ostet. Ginecol.*, 78:74–86.
75. Hafez, E. S. E. (1973): Gamete transport. In: *Human Reproduction. Conception and Contraception*, edited by E. S. E. Hafez and T. N. Evans, pp. 85–118, Harper & Row, Hagerstown, Md.
76. Fox, C. A., and Knaggs, G. S. (1969): Milk-ejection activity (oxytocin) in peripheral venous blood in man during lactation and in association with coitus. *J. Endocrinol.*, 45:145–146.
77. Kumar, D. (1967): Hormonal regulation of myometrial activity: Clinical implications. In: *Cellular Biology of the Uterus*, edited by R. M. Wynn, pp. 449–474. Appleton-Century-Crofts, New York.
78. Levi, L. (1965): The urinary output of adrenalin and noradrenalin during pleasant and unpleasant emotional states. A preliminary report. *Psychosom. Med.*, 27:80–85.
79. Sparks, M., and Lee, C. M. (1973): Clinical use of PGs in fertility control. *Popul. Rep. (G)*,1–15.
80. Bygdeman, M., and Bergström, S. (1976): Clinical use of prostaglandins for pregnancy termination. *Popul. Rep. (G)*, 65–75.
81. Gréen, K., and Bygdeman, M. (1976): Plasma levels of the methyl ester of 15-methyl $PGF_{2\alpha}$ in connection with intravenous and vaginal administration. *Prostaglandins*, 11:879–892.
82. Bygdeman, M., and Eliasson, R. (1963): The effect of prostaglandin from human seminal fluid on the motility of the non-pregnant human uterus *in vitro*. *Acta Physiol. Scand.*, 59:43–51.
83. Bygdeman, M., Hamberg, M., and Samuelsson, B. (1976): The content of different prostaglandins in human seminal fluid and their threshold dose on the human myometrium. *Mem. Soc. Endocrinol.*, 14:49–63.
84. Karim, S. M. M., and Sharma, S. D. (1971): Therapeutic abortion and induction of labour by the intravaginal administration of prostaglandins E_2 or $F_{2\alpha}$. *J. Obstet. Gynaecol. Br. Commonw.*, 78:294–300.
85. Gréen, K., and Svanborg, K. (1979): On the mechanism of action of 15-methyl $PGF_{2\alpha}$ as an abortifacient. *Prostaglandins*, 17:277–282.
86. Overstreet, J. W., Cooper, G. W., and Katz, D. F. (1978): Sperm transport in the reproductive tract of the female rabbit. II. The sustained phase of transport. *Biol. Reprod.*, 19:115–132.
87. Howe, G. R. (1967): Leukocytic response to spermatozoa in ligated segments of the rabbit vagina, uterus and oviduct. *J. Reprod. Fertil.*, 13:563–566.
88. Austin, C. R. (1960): Fate of spermatozoa in the female genital tract. *J. Reprod. Fertil.*, 1:151–156.
89. Rubinstein, B. B., Strauss, H., Lazarus, M. L., and Hankin, H. (1951): Sperm survival in women. Motile sperm in the fundus and tubes of surgical cases. *Fertil. Steril.*, 2:15–19.
90. Moyer, D. L., Rimdusit, S., and Mishell, D. R. Jr. (1970): Sperm distribution and degradation in the human female reproductive tract. *Obstet. Gynecol.*, 35:831–840.
91. Cooper, G. W., Overstreet, J. W., and Katz, D. F. (1979): The motility of rabbit spermatozoa recovered from the female reproductive tract. *Gamete Res.*, 2:35–42.
92. Wynn, R. M. (1977): Histology and ultrastructure of the human endometrium. In: *Biology of the Uterus*, edited by R. M. Wynn, pp. 341–376. Plenum Press, New York.
93. Beier, H. M., and Beier-Hellwig, K. (1973): Specific secretory protein of the female genital tract. *Acta Endocrinol. (Suppl.)*, 180:404–422.
94. Beier, H. M. (1974): Oviducal and uterine fluids. *J. Reprod. Fertil.*, 37:221–237.
95. Bernstein, G. S., Aladjem, F., and Chen, S. (1971): Proteins in human endometrial washings—A preliminary report. *Fertil. Steril.*, 22:722–726.
96. Maathius, J. B., and Aitken, R. J. (1978): Cyclic variation in concentrations of protein and hexose in human uterine flushings collected by an improved technique. *J. Reprod. Fertil.*, 52:289–295.
97. Casslén, B., and Nilsson, B. (1984): Human uterine fluid examined in undiluted samples for osmolarity and the concentrations of inorganic ions, albumin, glucose and urea. *Am. J. Obstet. Gynecol.*, 150:877–881.
98. Casslén, B. (1986): Uterine fluid volume. Cyclic variations and possible extrauterine contributions. *J. Reprod. Med.*, 31:506–510.
99. Alvarez, F., Diaz, S., and Croxatto, H. B. (1985): Personal communication.

100. Wilborn, W. H., and Flowers, C. E. (1979): Histoenzymology of human endometrium during the proliferative and secretory phases. In: *The Biology of the Fluids of the Female Genital Tract*, edited by F. K. Beller and G. F. B. Schumacher, pp. 73–87. Elsevier/North Holland, New York.
101. Moyer, D. L., El Sahwi, S., Macaulay, L., and Shaw, S. T. Jr. (1979): Cells of the uterine fluid. In: *The Biology of the Fluids of the Female Genital Tract*, edited by F. K. Beller and G. F. B. Schumacher, pp. 59–71. Elsevier/North Holland, New York.
102. Woodruff, J. D., and Pauerstein, C. J. (1969): *The Fallopian Tube. Structure, Function, Pathology, and Management*, 361 pp. Williams & Wilkins, Baltimore.
103. Eddy, C. A., and Pauerstein, C. J. (1978): Tubal reproductive function and the development of reversible sterilization techniques. In: *Reversal of Sterilization*, edited by J. J. Sciarra, G. I. Zatuchni, and J. J. Speidel, pp. 100–116. Harper & Row, Hagerstown, Md.
104. Black, D. L., and Asdell, S. A. (1959): Mechanism controlling entry of ova into rabbit uterus. *Am. J. Physiol*, 197:1275–1278.
105. Chang, M. C. (1951): Fertilization in relation to the number of spermatozoa in the Fallopian tubes of rabbits. *Ann. Ostet. Ginecol.*, 73:918–925.
106. Ahlgren, M. (1975): Sperm transport to and survival in the human Fallopian tube. *Gynecol. Invest.*, 6:206–214.
107. Croxatto, H.B., Faundes, A., Medel, M., Avendaño, S., Croxatto, H.D., Vera, C., Anselmo, J., and Pastene, L. (1975): Studies on sperm migration in the human female genital tract. In: *The Biology of Spermatozoa*, edited by E. S. E. Hafez and C. G. Thibault, pp. 56–62. Karger, Basel.
108. Croxatto, H. B. (1985): Personal communication.
109. Settlage, D. S. F., Motoshima, M., and Tredway, D. (1975): Sperm transport from the vagina to the Fallopian tubes in women. In: *The Biology of Spermatozoa*, edited by E. S. E. Hafez and C. G. Thibault, pp. 74–82. Karger, Basel.
110. Ahlgren, M., Boström, K., and Malmqvist, R. (1973): Sperm transport and survival in women with special reference to the Fallopian tube. In: *The Biology of Spermatozoa*, edited by E. S. E. Hafez and C. G. Thibault, pp. 63–73. Karger, Basel.
111. Horne, H. W. Jr., and Audet, C. (1985): "Spider cells," a new inhabitant of peritoneal fluid. A preliminary report. *Obstet. Gynecol.*, 11:421–423.
112. Braden, A. W. H. (1953): Distribution of sperms in the genital tract of the female rabbit after coitus. *Aust. J. Biol. Sci.*, 6:693–705.
113. Zamboni, L. (1972): Fertilization in the mouse. In: *Biology of Mammalian Fertilization and Implantation*, edited by K. S. Moghissi and E. S. E. Hafez, pp. 213–262. Charles C Thomas, Springfield, Ill.
114. Harper, M. J. K. (1973): Relationship between sperm transport and penetration of eggs in the rabbit oviduct. *Biol. Reprod.*, 8:441–450.
115. Harper, M. J. K. (1973): Stimulation of sperm movement from the isthmus to the site of fertilization in the rabbit oviduct. *Biol. Reprod.*, 8:369–377.
116. Hunter, R. H. F. (1975): Physiological aspects of sperm transport in the domestic pig, *Sus scrofa*. II. Regulation, survival and fate of cells. *Br. Vet. J.*, 131:681–690.
117. Hunter, R. H. F., Barwise, L., and King, R. (1982): Sperm transport, storage and release in the sheep oviduct in relation to the time of ovulation. *Br. Vet. J.*, 138:225–232.
118. Hunter, R. H. F., and Wilmut, I. (1983): The rate of functional sperm transport into the oviducts of mated cows. *Anim. Reprod. Sci.*, 5:167–173.
119. Phillips, D. M. (1972): Comparative analysis of mammalian sperm motility. *J. Cell Biol.*, 53:561–573.
120. Jansen, R. P. S. (1978): Fallopian tube isthmic mucus and ovum transport. *Science*, 201:349–351.
121. Trounson, A. E., Mohr, L. R., Wood, C., and Leeton, J. F. (1982): Effect of delayed insemination on *in vitro* fertilization, culture and transfer of human embryos. *J. Reprod. Fertil.*, 64:285–294.
122. Jansen, R. P. S. (1984): Endocrine response in the Fallopian tube. *Endocr. Rev.*, 5:525–551.
123. Hammar, M., and Larsson-Cohn, U. (1978): Massive enlargement of occluded tubes after postmenopausal treatment with natural estrogens. *Acta Obstet. Gynecol. Scand.*, 57:189–190.
124. Lippes, J., Enders, R. G., Pragay, D. A., and Bartholomew, W. R. (1972): The collection and analysis of human fallopian tube fluid. *Contraception*, 5:85–103.
125. Lippes, J., Kramer, J., Alfonso, L. A., Dacalos, E. D., and Lucero, R. (1981): Human oviductal fluid proteins. *Fertil. Steril.*, 36:623–629.
126. Borland, R. M., Biggers, J. D., Lechene, C. P., and Taymor, M. L. (1980): Elemental composition of fluid in the human Fallopian tube. *J. Reprod. Fertil.*, 58:479–482.
127. Brinster, R. L. (1965): Studies on the development of mouse embryos *in vitro*. II. The effect of energy source. *J. Exp. Zool.*, 158:59–68.
128. Brinster, R. L. (1968): *In vitro* culture of mammalian embryos. *J. Anim. Sci.*, 27(Suppl. 1):1–14.
129. Maas, D. H. A., Storey, B. T., and Mastroianni, L. Jr. (1977): Hydrogen ion and carbon dioxide content of the oviductal fluid of the Rhesus monkey (*Macaca mulatta*). *Fertil. Steril.*, 28:981–985.
130. Weström, L., Mårdh, P.-A., Mecklenberg, C., and Håkansson, C. H. (1977): Studies on ciliated epithelia of the human genital tract. II. The mucociliary wave pattern of Fallopian tube epithelium. *Fertil. Steril.*, 28:955–961.
131. Hodgson, B. J. (1978): Post-ovulatory changes in the water content and inulin space of the rabbit oviduct. *J. Reprod. Fertil.*, 53:349–351.
132. Blake, J. R., Vann, P. G., and Winet, H. (1983): A model of ovum transport. *J. Theor. Biol.*, 102:145–166.
133. Talo, A. (1976): Electrophysiology of the oviduct. In: *Ovum Transport and Fertility Regulation*, edited by M. J. K. Harper, C. J. Pauerstein, C. E. Adams, E. M. Coutinho, H. B. Croxatto, and D. M. Paton, pp. 161–167. Scriptor, Copenhagen.
134. Talo, A., and Hodgson, B. J. (1978): Spike bursts in rabbit oviduct. 1. Effect of ovulation. *Am. J. Physiol.*, 234:E430–E438.
135. Talo, A., and Pulkkinen, M. O. (1982): Electrical activity in the human oviduct during the menstrual cycle. *Am. J. Obstet. Gynecol.*, 142:135–147.
136. Owman, C. L., Falck, B., Johansson, E. D. B., Rosengren, E., Sjöberg, N.-O., Sporrong, B., Svensson, K.-G., and Walles, B. (1976): Autonomic nerves and related amine receptors mediating motor activity in the oviduct of monkey and man. Histochemical, chemical and pharmacological study. In: *Ovum Transport and Fertility Regulation*, edited by M. J. K. Harper, C. J. Pauerstein, C. E. Adams, E. M. Coutinho, H. B. Croxatto, and D. M. Patton, pp. 256–275. Scriptor, Copenhagen.
137. Chang, M. C., Austin, C. R., Bedford, J. M., Brackett, B. G., Hunter, R. H. F., and Yanagimachi, R. (1977): Capacitation of spermatozoa and fertilization in mammals. In: *Frontiers in Reproduction and Fertility Control. A Review of the Reproductive Sciences and Contraceptive Development*, edited by R. O. Greep and M. A. Koblinsky, pp. 434–451. MIT Press, Cambridge, Mass.
138. Austin, C. R. (1951): Observations on the penetration of sperm into the mammalian egg. *Aust. J. Sci. Res. B*, 4:581–596.
139. Chang, M. C. (1951): Fertilizing capacity of spermatozoa deposited into the Fallopian tubes. *Nature*, 168:697–698.
140. Brackett, B. G., Seitz, H. M. Jr., Rocha, G., and Mastroianni, L. Jr. (1972): The mammalian fertilization process. In: *Biology of Mammalian Fertilization and Implantation*, edited by K. S. Moghissi and E. S. E. Hafez, pp. 165–184. Charles C Thomas, Springfield, Ill.
141. Edwards, R. G., Bavister, B. D., and Steptoe, P. C. (1969): Early stages of fertilization *in vitro* of human oocytes matured *in vitro*. *Nature*, 221:632–635.
142. Edwards, R. G., Steptoe, P. C., and Purdy, J. M. (1970): Fertilization and cleavage *in vitro* of preovulatory human oocytes. *Nature*, 227:1307–1309.
143. Ahuja, K. K., Smith, W., Tucker, M., and Craft, I. (1985): Successful pregnancies from the transfer of pronucleate embryos in an outpatient *in vitro* fertilization program. *Fertil. Steril.*, 44:181–184.
144. Harper, M. J. K., and Chang, M. C. (1971): Some aspects of the biology of mammalian eggs and spermatozoa. *Adv. Reprod. Physiol.*, 5:167–218.
145. Chang, M. C. (1955): Développement de la capacité fertilisatrice des spermatozoïdes du lapin à l'intérieur du tractus génital femelle et fécondabilité des oeufs de lapine. In: *La Fonction Tubaire et Ses Troubles: Physiologie, Explorations, Pathologie, Thérapeutique*, pp. 40–52, Masson & Cie, Paris.
146. Hunter, R. H. F. (1968): Attempted fertilization of hamster eggs following transplantation into the uterus. *J. Exp. Zool.*, 168:511–516.
147. Estes, W. L. Jr., and Heitmeyer, P. L. (1934): Pregnancy following ovarian implantation. *Am. J. Surg.*, 24:563–580.

148. Preston, P. G. (1953): Transplantation of the ovary into the uterine cavity for the treatment of sterility in women. *J. Obstet. Gynaecol. Br. Emp.*, 60:862–864.
149. Iklé, F. A. (1961): Schwangerschaft nach Implantation des Ovars in den Uterus. *Gynaecologia*, 151:95–99.
150. Austin, C. R. (1970): Ageing and reproduction: Post-ovulatory deterioration of the egg. *J. Reprod. Fertil. (Suppl.)*, 12:39–53.
151. Austin, C. R. (1982): The egg. In: *Reproduction in Mammals. I. Germ Cells and Fertilization*, 2nd ed., edited by C. R. Austin and R. V. Short, pp. 46–62. Cambridge University Press, Cambridge, U.K.
152. Baker, T. G. (1982): Oogenesis and ovulation. In: *Reproduction in Mammals. I. Germ Cells and Fertilization*, edited by C. R. Austin and R. V. Short, 2nd ed, pp. 17–45. Cambridge University Press, Cambridge, U.K.
153. Cheviakoff, S., Díaz, S., Carril, M., Patritti, N., Croxatto, H. D., Llados, C., Ortíz, M. E., and Croxatto, H. B. (1976): Ovum transport in women. In: *Ovum Transport and Fertility Regulation*, edited by M. J. K. Harper, C. J. Pauerstein, C. E. Adams, E. M. Coutinho, H. B. Croxatto, and D. M. Paton, pp. 416–424. Scriptor, Copenhagen.
154. Ferin, J. Thomas, K., and Johansson, E. D. B. (1973): Ovulation detection. In: *Human Reproduction. Conception and Contraception*, edited by E. S. E. Hafez and T. N. Evans, pp. 260–283. Harper & Row, Hagerstown, Md.
155. Peters, H., and McNatty, K. P. (1980): *The Ovary: A Correlation Between Structure and Function*. University of California Press, Berkeley.
156. Blandau, R. J. (1969): Gamete transport—Comparative aspects. In: *The Mammalian Oviduct. Comparative Biology and Methodology*, edited by E. S. E. Hafez and R. J. Blandau, pp. 129–162. University of Chicago Press, Chicago.
157. Westman, A. (1937): Investigations into the transit of ova in man. *J. Obstet. Gynaecol. Br. Emp.*, 44:821–838.
158. Maia, H. S., and Coutinho, E. M. (1970): Peristalsis and antiperistalsis of the human Fallopian tube during the menstrual cycle. *Biol. Reprod.*, 2:305–314.
159. Clewe, T. H., and Mastroianni, L. Jr. (1958): Mechanisms of ovum pickup. I. Functional capacity of rabbit oviducts ligated near the fimbriae. *Fertil. Steril.*, 9:13–17.
160. Doyle, J. B. (1951): Exploratory culdotomy for observation of tubo-ovarian physiology at ovulation time. *Fertil. Steril.*, 2:475–484.
161. Doyle, J. B. (1954): Ovulation and the effects of selective uterotubal denervation. Direct observations by culdotomy. *Fertil. Steril.*, 5:105–129.
162. Blandau, J. R., and Verdugo, P. (1976): An overview of gamete transport—Comparative aspects. In: *Ovum Transport and Fertility Regulation*, edited by M. J. K. Harper, C. J. Pauerstein, C. E. Adams, E. M. Coutinho, H. B. Croxatto, and D. M. Paton, pp. 138–146. Scriptor, Copenhagen.
163. Beyth, Y., and Winston, R. M. L. (1981): Ovum capture and fertility following microsurgical fimbriectomy in the rabbit. *Fertil. Steril.*, 35:464–466.
164. First, A. (1954): Transperitoneal migration of ovum or spermatozoon. *Obstet. Gynecol.*, 4:431–434.
165. Heil, K. (1893): Der Fimbrienstrom und die Überwanderung des Eies vom Ovarium zur Tube. *Arch. Gynaekol.*, 43:503–533.
166. Lode, A. (1894): Experimentelle Beiträge zur Lehre der Wanderung des Eies von Ovarium zur Tube. *Arch. Gynaekol.*, 45:293–322.
167. Gyarmati, E. (1934): Sulla eliminazione transtubarica di sostanze estranee introdotte nella cavità peritoneale. *Riv. Ital. Ginecol.*, 16:721–735.
168. Díaz, J., Vásquez, J., Díaz, S., Díaz, F., and Croxatto, H. B. (1976): Transport of ovum surrogates by the human oviduct. In: *Ovum Transport and Fertility Regulation*, edited by M. J. K. Harper, C. J. Pauerstein, C. E. Adams, E. M. Coutinho, H. B. Croxatto, and D. M. Paton, pp. 404–415. Scriptor, Copenhagen.
169. Van Pelt, L. F. (1970): Intraperitoneal insemination of *Macaca mulatta*. *Fertil. Steril.*, 21:159–162.
170. Laufe, L. E., Eddy, C., Brosens, I., and Boeckx, W. (1980): Reversible methods of fimbrial closure. In: *Research Frontiers in Fertility Regulation*, edited by G. I. Zatuchni, M. H. Labbok, and J. J. Sciarra, pp. 287–301. Harper & Row, Hagerstown, Md.
171. Laufe, L. E. (1985): Personal communication.
172. El Kady, A. A., Sami, G., Lawrence, K. A., and Badawi, S. (1978): The Tubal hood: A potentially reversible sterilization technique. In: *Reversal of Sterilization*, edited by J. J. Sciarra, G. I. Zatuchni, and J. J. Speidel, pp. 232–240. Harper & Row, Hagerstown, Md.
173. Van Niekerk, C. H., and Gerneke, W. H. (1966): Persistence and parthogenetic cleavage of tubal ova in the mare. *Onderstepoort J. Vet. Res.*, 33:195–232.
174. Adams, C. E. (1976): Egg survival relative to maternal endocrine status. In: *Ovum Transport and Fertility Regulation*, edited by M. J. K. Harper, C. J. Pauerstein, C. E. Adams, E. M. Coutinho, H. B. Croxatto, and D. M. Paton, pp. 425–440. Scriptor, Copenhagen.
175. Estes, W. L. Jr. (1924): Ovarian implantation. The preservation of ovarian function after operation for disease of the pelvic viscera. *Surg. Gynecol. Obstet.*, 38:394–398.
176. Adams, C. E. (1979): Consequences of accelerated ovum transport, including a re-evaluation of Estes' operation. *J. Reprod. Fertil.*, 55:239–246.
177. Marston, J. H., Penn, R., and Sivelle, P. C. (1979): Successful autotransfer of tubal eggs in the rhesus monkey (*Macaca mulatta*). *J. Reprod. Fertil.*, 49:175–176.
178. World Health Organization (1978): Special Programme of Research, Development and Research Training in Human Reproduction. *Seventh Annual Report*, p. 88. WHO, Geneva.
179. Pratt, H. P. M., Bolton, V. N., and Gudgeon, K. A. (1983): The legacy from the oocyte and its role in controlling early development of the mouse embryo. In: *Molecular Biology of Egg Maturation*, Ciba Symposium 98, edited by R. Porter and J. Whelan, pp. 197–227. Pitman, London.
180. Davidson, E. H. (1976): *Gene Activity in Early Development*, 2nd ed. 452 pp. Academic Press, New York.
181. Bolton, V. N., Oades, P. J., and Johnson, M. H. (1984): The relationship between cleavage, DNA replication, and gene expression in the mouse 2-cell embryo. *J. Embryol. Exp. Morphol.*, 79:139–163.
182. Bolton, V. N. (1985): Embryo viability and function. *Presentation at the Fifth World Congress on Human Reproduction, Athens*. Personal communication.
183. Howlett, S. K., and Bolton, V. N. (1985): Sequence and regulation of morphological and molecular events during the first cell cycle of mouse embryogenesis. *J. Embryol. Exp. Morphol.*, 87:175–206.
184. Biggers, J. D., and Borland, R. M. (1976): Physiological aspects of growth and development of the preimplantation mammalian embryo. *Annu. Rev. Physiol.*, 38:95–119.
185. Wentz, A. G., Torbit, C. A., Daniell, J. F., Fleischer, A. C., Garner, C. H., Pittaway, D. E., Christianson, C. D., Repp, J. E., and Maxson, W. S. (1983): Combined screening laparoscopy and timed follicle aspiration for human *in vitro* fertilization. *Fertil. Steril.*, 39:270–276.
186. Mahadevan, M. M., Trounson, A. O., and Leeton, J. F. (1983): Successful use of human cryobanking for *in vitro* fertilization. *Fertil. Steril.*, 40:340–343.
187. Menezeo, Y., Testart, J., and Perrone, D. (1984): Serum is not necessary in human *in vitro* fertilization, early embryo culture, and transfer. *Fertil. Steril.*, 42:750–755.
188. Veeck, O. L., Wortham, J. W. E. Jr., Witmyer, J., Sandow, B. A., Acosta, A. A., Garcia, J. E., Jones, G. S., and Jones, H. W. Jr. (1983): Maturation and fertilization of morphologically immature human oocytes in a program of *in vitro* fertilization. *Fertil. Steril.*, 39:594–602.
189. Hunter, R. H. F., and Léglise, P. C. (1971): Tubal surgery in the rabbit: Fertilization and polyspermy after resection of the isthums. *Am. J. Anat.*, 132:45–52.
190. Hunter, R. H. F., and Léglise, P. C. (1971): Polyspermic fertilization following tubal surgery in pigs, with particular reference to the role of the isthmus. *J. Reprod. Fertil.*, 24:233–246.
191. Verhage, H. G., Akbar, M., and Jaffe, R. C. (1980): Cyclic changes in cytosol progesterone receptor of human Fallopian tube. *J. Clin. Endocrinol. Metab.*, 51:776–780.
192. Punnonen, R., and Lukola, A. (1981): Binding of estrogen and progestin in the human Fallopian tube. *Fertil. Steril.*, 36:610–614.
193. Pollow, K., Inthraphuvasak, J., Manz, B., Grill, H.-J., and Pollow, B. (1981): A comparison of cytoplasmic and nuclear estradiol and progesterone receptors in human Fallopian tube and endometrial tissue. *Fertil. Steril.*, 36:615–622.

194. Pollow, K., Inthraphuvasak, J., Grill, H. J., and Manz, B. (1982): Estradiol and progesterone binding components in the cytosol of normal human Fallopian tubes. *J. Steroid Biochem.*, 16:429–435.
195. Pino, A. M., Devoto, L., Soto, E., Castro, O., and Sierralta, W. (1982): Changes in cytosolic and nuclear estradiol receptors of normal Fallopian tube throughout the menstrual cycle. *J. Steroid Biochem.*, 16:193–197.
196. Batra, S., Helm, G., Owman, C., Sjöberg, N.-O., and Walles, B. (1980): Female sex steroid concentrations in the ampullary and isthmic regions of the human fallopian tube and their relationship to plasma concentrations during the menstrual cycle. *Am. J. Obstet. Gynecol.*, 136:986–991.
197. Devoto, L., Soto, E., Magofke, A. M., and Sierralta, W. (1980): Unconjugated steroids in the Fallopian tube and peripheral blood during the normal menstrual cycle. *Fertil. Steril.*, 33:613–617.
198. Burdick, H. O., and Pincus, G. (1935): The effect of oestrin injections upon the developing ova of mice and rabbits. *Am. J. Physiol.*, 111:201–208.
199. Chang, M. C., and Harper, M. J. K. (1966): Effects of ethinyl estradiol on egg transport and development in the rabbit. *Endocrinology*, 78:860–872.
200. Greenwald, G. S. (1967): Species differences in egg transport in response to exogenous estrogen. *Anat. Rec.*, 157:163–172.
201. Chang, M. C. (1967): Effects of progesterone and related compounds on fertilization, transportation and development of rabbit eggs. *Endocrinology*, 81:1251–1260.
202. Kuchera, L. (1974): Postcoital contraception with diethylstilbestrol. *JAMA*, 218:562–563.
203. Haspels, A. A. (1976): Interception: Postcoital estrogens in 3016 women. *Contraception*, 14:375–381.
204. Yuzpe, A. A., Smith, R. P., and Rademaker, A. W. (1982): A multicenter clinical investigation employing ethinyl estradiol combined with dl-norgestrel as a postcoital contraceptive agent. *Fertil. Steril.*, 37:508–513.
205. Morris, J. M., and van Wagenen, G. (1973): Interception: The use of postovulatory estrogens to prevent implantation. *Am. J. Obstet. Gynecol.*, 15:101–106.
206. Coutinho, E. M. (1971): In Discussion of paper. Tubal and uterine motility. In: *Control of Human Fertility, Nobel Symposium 15,* edited by E. Diczfalusy and U. Borell, pp. 97–115. John Wiley & Sons, New York.
207. Croxatto, H. B. (1974): The duration of egg transport and its regulation in mammals. In: *Physiology and Genetics of Reproduction, Part B*, pp. 159–166, edited by E. M. Coutinho and F. Fuchs. Plenum Press, New York.
208. Croxatto, H. B., Díaz, S., Atria, P., Cheviakoff, S., Rosatti, S., and Oddó, H. (1971): Contraceptive action of megestrol acetate implants in women. *Contraception*, 4:155–167.
209. Liukko, P., Erkkola, R., and Laakso, L. (1977): Ectopic pregnancies during the use of low-dose progestogens for oral contraception. *Contraception*, 16:575–580.
210. Stanchev, Ph., Rodriguez-Martinez, H., Edqvist, L. E., and Eriksson, H. (1985): Oestradiol and progesterone receptors in the pig oviduct during the oestrous cycle. *J. Steroid Biochem.*, 22:115–120.
211. Adams, C. E. (1958): Egg development in the rabbit: The influence of post-coital ligation of the uterine tube and of ovariectomy. *J. Endocrinol.*, 16:283–293.
212. Noyes, R. W., Adams, C. E., and Walton, A. (1959): The transport of ova in relation to the dosage of oestrogen in ovariectomized rabbits. *J. Endocrinol.*, 18:108–117.
213. Harper, M. J. K. (1964): The effects of constant doses of oestrogen and progesterone on the transport of artificial eggs through the reproductive tract of ovariectomized rabbits. *J. Endocrinol.*, 30:1–19.
214. Greenwald, G. S. (1961): A study of the transport of ova through the rabbit oviduct. *Fertil. Steril.*, 12:80–95.
215. Harper, M. J. K. (1965): The effects of decreasing doses of oestrogen and increasing doses of progesterone on the transport of artificial eggs through the reproductive tract of ovariectomized rabbits. *J. Endocrinol.*, 31:217–226.
216. Owman, Ch., Rosengren, E., and Sjöberg, N.-O. (1967): Adrenergic innervation of the human female reproductive organs: A histochemical and chemical investigation. *Obstet. Gynecol.*, 30:763–773.
217. Bodkhe, R. R., and Harper, M. J. K. (1973): Mechanism of egg transport: Changes in amount of adrenergic transmitter in the genital tract of normal and hormone treated rabbits. In: NIH Symposium, *The Regulation of Mammalian Reproduction*, edited by S. J. Segal, R. Crozier, P. A. Corfman, and P. G. Condliffe, pp. 364–374. Charles C Thomas, Springfield, Ill.
218. Brundin, J. (1965): Distribution and function of adrenergic nerves in the rabbit Fallopian tube. *Acta Physiol. Scand.* 66(Suppl. 259):57 pp.
219. Marshall, J. M. (1970): Adrenergic innervation of the female reproductive tract: Anatomy, physiology and pharmacology. *Ergeb. Physiol.*, 62:6–67.
220. Pauerstein, C. J., Hodgson, B. J., Fremming, B. D., and Martin, J. E. (1974): Effects of sympathetic denervation of the rabbit oviduct on normal ovum transport and on transport modified by estrogen and progesterone. *Gynecol. Invest.*, 5:121–132.
221. Bodkhe, R. R., and Harper, M. J. K. (1972): Changes in the amount of adrenergic neurotransmitter in the genital tract of untreated rabbits, and rabbits given reserpine or iproniazid during the time of egg transport. *Biol. Reprod.*, 6:288–297.
222. Pauerstein, C. J., Fremming, B. D., and Martin, J. E. (1970): Estrogen-induced tubal arrest of ovum: Antagonism by alpha adrenergic blockade. *Obstet. Gynecol.*, 35:671–675.
223. Polidoro, J. P., Howe, G. R., and Black, D. L. (1973): The effects of adrenergic drugs on ovum transport through the rabbit oviduct. *J. Reprod. Fertil.*, 35:331–337.
224. Hodgson, B. J., and Eddy, C. A. (1975): The autonomic nervous system and its relationship to tubal ovum transport—A reappraisal. *Gynecol. Invest.*, 6:162–185.
225. Johns, A., Chlumecky, J., and Paton, D. M. (1974): Role of adrenergic nerves in ovulation and ovum transport. *Lancet*, 2:1079.
226. Jordan, S. M. (1970): Adrenergic and cholinergic innervation of the reproductive tract and ovary in the guinea-pig and rabbit. *J. Physiol. (Lond.)*, 210:115P–117P.
227. Saksena, S. K., and Harper, M. J.K. (1975): Relationship between concentration of prostaglandin F (PGF) in the oviduct and egg transport in rabbits. *Biol. Reprod.*, 13:68–76.
228. Rajkumar, K., Garg, S. K., and Sharma, P. I. (1979): Relationship between concentration of prostaglandins E and F in the regulation of ovum transport in rabbits. *Prostaglandins Med.*, 2:445–454.
229. Thomas, C. M. G. (1978): "Steroid Hormones, Prostaglandins and Ovum Transport: A Study in the Golden Hamster, *Mesocricetus auratus* (Waterhouse)." Ph.D. Thesis, Catholic University of Nijmegen, Janssen, Nijmegen, 96 pp.
230. Ogra, S. S., Kirton, K. T., Tomasi, T. B. Jr., and Lippes, J. (1974): Prostaglandins in the human Fallopian tube. *Fertil. Steril.*, 25:250–255.
231. Vastik-Fernandez, J., Gimeno, M. F., Lima, F., and Gimeno, A. L. (1975): Spontaneous motility and distribution of prostaglandins in different segments of human Fallopian tubes. *Am. J. Obstet. Gynecol.*, 122:663–668.
232. Granström, E., and Samuelsson, B. (1978): Quantitative measurement of prostaglandins and thromboxanes: General considerations. *Adv. Prostaglandin Thromboxane Leukotriene Res.*, 5:1–13.
233. Lindblom, B., Hamberger, L., and Wiqvist, N. (1978): Differentiated contractile effects of prostaglandins E and F on the isolated circular and longitudinal smooth muscle of the human oviduct. *Fertil. Steril.*, 30:553–559.
234. Lindblom, B., Wilhelmsson, L., and Wiqvist, N. (1979): The action of prostacyclin (PGI_2) on the contractility of the isolated circular and longitudinal muscle layer of the human oviduct. *Prostaglandins*, 17:99–104.
235. Lindblom, B., and Wikland, M. (1982): Simultaneous recording of electrical and mechanical activity in isolated smooth muscle of the human oviduct. *Biol. Reprod.*, 27:393–398.
236. Coutinho, E. M., and Maia, H. S. (1971): The contractile response of the human uterus, Fallopian tubes and ovary to prostaglandins *in vivo*. *Fertil. Steril.*, 22:539–543.
237. Spilman, C. H., and Harper, M. J. K. (1973): Effect of prostaglandins on oviduct motility in estrous rabbits. *Biol. Reprod.*, 9:36–45.
238. Horton, E. W., Main, I. H. M., and Thompson, C. J. (1965): Effects of prostaglandins on the oviduct, studied in rabbits and ewes. *J. Physiol. (Lond.)*, 180:514–528.
239. Spilman, C. H., and Harper, M. J. K. (1974): Comparison of the effects of adrenergic drugs and prostaglandins on rabbit oviduct motility. *Biol. Reprod.*, 10:549–554.

240. Spilman, C. H., and Harper, M. J. K. (1976): Effects of prostaglandins on oviductal motility and egg transport. *Gynecol. Invest.*, 6:186–205.
241. Riehl, R. M., and Harper, M. J. K. (1981): Preparation of smooth muscle cell suspensions from the rabbit oviduct and prostaglandin binding analysis. *Endocrinology*, 108:18–26.
242. Riehl, R. M., and Harper, M. J. K. (1981): Changes in prostaglandin binding capacity of single oviductal smooth muscle cells after ovulation in the rabbit. *Endocrinology*, 109:1011–1016.
243. Riehl, R. M. (1980): "Prostaglandin Binding Sites in the Rabbit Oviduct: A Dissertation." Ph.D. Thesis, University of Texas Graduate School of Biomedical Sciences at San Antonio, 90 pp.
244. Velenzuela, G., Ross, H. D., Hodgson, B. J., Harper, M. J. K., and Pauerstein, C. J. (1977): Effect of inhibitors of prostaglandin synthesis and metabolism on ovum transport in the rabbit. *Fertil. Steril.*, 28:992–997.
245. Hodgson, B. J. (1976): Effects of indomethacin and ICI 46,474 administered during ovum transport on fertility in rabbits. *Biol. Reprod.*, 14:451–457.
246. Ångåard, E., and Samuelsson, B. (1967):The metabolism of prostaglandins in lung tissue. In: *Prostaglandins. Nobel Symposium 2*, edited by S. Bergström and B. Samuelsson, pp. 97–105. Interscience, New York.
247. Samuelsson, B., Granström, E., Gréen, K., and Hamberg, M. (1971): Metabolism of prostaglandins. *Ann. NY Acad. Sci.*, 180:138–161.
248. Alm, P., Alumets, J., Håkanson, R., Owman, Ch., Sjöberg, N.-O., Sundler, F., and Walles, B. (1980): Origin and distribution of VIP (vasoactive intestinal polypeptide) nerves in the genito-urinary tract. *Cell Tissue Res.*, 205:337–347.
249. Said, S. I., and Mutt, V. (1970): Polypeptide with broad biological activity: Isolation from small intestine. *Science*, 169:1217–1218.
250. Mutt, V., and Said, S. I. (1974): Structure of the porcine vasoactive intestinal octosapeptide. *Eur. J. Biochem.*, 42:581–589.
251. Alm, P., Alumets, J., Håkanson, R., Helm, G., Owman, C., Sjöberg, N.-O., and Sandler, F. (1980): Vasoactive intestinal polypeptide nerves in the human female genital tract. *Am. J. Obstet. Gynecol.*, 136:349–351.
252. Helm, G., Håkanson, R., Leander, S., Owman, C., Sjöberg, N.-O., and Sporrong, B. (1982): Neurogenic relaxation mediated by vasoactive intestinal polypeptide (VIP) in the isthmus of the human Fallopian tube. *Regul. Pept.*, 3:145–153.
253. Walles, B., Håkanson, R., Helm, G., Owman, Ch., Sjöberg, N.-O., and Sundler, F. (1980): Relaxation of human female genital sphincters by the neuropeptide vasoactive intestinal polypeptide. *Am. J. Obstet. Gynecol.*, 138:337–338.
254. Helm, G., Ottesen, B., Fahrenkrug, J., Larsen, J.-J., Owman, C., Sjöberg, N.-O., Stolberg, B., Sundler, F., and Walles, B. (1981): Vasoactive intestinal polypeptide (VIP) in the human female reproductive tract: Distribution and motor effects. *Biol. Reprod.*, 25:227–234.
255. Helm, G., Ekman, R., Rydhstöm, H., Sjöberg, N.-O., and Walles, B. (1985): Changes in oviductal VIP content induced by sex steroids and inhibitory effect of VIP on spontaneous oviductal contractility. *Acta Physiol. Scand.*, 125:219–224.
256. Blair, W. D., and Beck, L. (1976): A system for measurement of oviductal motility and contractility and chronic changes in luminal diameter. In: *Ovum Transport and Fertility Regulation*, edited by M. J. K. Harper, C. J. Pauerstein, C. E. Adams, E. M. Coutinho, H. B. Croxatto, and D. M. Paton, pp. 41–74. Scriptor, Copenhagen.
257. Blair, W. D., and Beck, L. (1976): Demonstration of postovulatory sphincter action by the isthmus of the rabbit oviduct. *Fertil. Steril.*, 27:431–441.
258. Fredericks, C. M., Lundquist, L. E., Mathur, R. S., Ashton, S. H., and Landgrebe, S. C. (1983): Effects of vasoactive intestinal polypeptide upon ovarian steroids, ovum transport and fertility in the rabbit. *Biol. Reprod.*, 28:1052–1060.
259. Fredericks, C. M., and Ashton, S. H. (1982): Effects of vasoactive intestinal polypeptide (VIP) on the *in vitro* and *in vivo* motility of the rabbit reproductive tract. *Fertil. Steril.*, 37:845–850.
260. Tatemoto, K. (1982): Neuropeptide Y: Complete amino acid sequence of the brain peptide. *Proc. Natl. Acad. Sci. USA*, 79:5485–5489.
261. Stjernqvist, M., Emson, P., Owman, Ch., Sjöberg, N.-O., Sundler, F., and Tatemoto, K. (1983): Neuropeptide Y in the female reproductive tract of the rat. Distribution of nerve fibers and motor effects. *Neurosci. Lett.*, 39:279–284.
262. Samuelson, U. E., and Dalsgaard, C.-J. (1985): Action and localization of neuropeptide Y in the human Fallopian tube. *Neurosci. Lett.*, 58:49–54.
263. Huang, W.M., Gu, J., Blank, M. A., Allen, J. M., Bloom, S. R., and Polak, J. M. (1984): Peptide-immunoreactive nerves in the mammalian female genital tract. *Histochem. J.*, 16:1297–1310.
264. Alm, P., Alumets, J., Håkanson, R., Owman, Ch., Sjöberg, N.-O., Stjernqvist, M., and Sundler, F. (1981): Enkephalin-immunoreactive nerve fibers in the feline genito-urinary tract. *Histochemistry*, 72:351–355.
265. Ottesen, B., Söndergaard, F., and Fahrenkrug, J. (1983): Neuropeptides in the regulation of female genital smooth muscle contractility. *Acta Obstet. Gynecol.*, 62:591–592.
266. Ottesen, B., Gram, B. R., and Fahrenkrug, J. (1983):Neuropeptides in the female genital tract: Effect on vascular and non-vascular smooth muscle. *Peptides*, 4:387–392.
267. von Euler, U. S., and Gaddum, J. H. (1931): An unidentified depressor substance in certain tissue extracts. *J. Physiol.* (*Lond.*), 72:74–87.
268. Chang, M. M., Leeman, S. E., and Niall, H. D. (1971): Amino-acid sequence of substance P. *Nature* (*New Biol.*), 232:86–87.
269. Alm, P., Alumets, J., Brodin, E., Håkanson, R., Nilsson, G., Sjöberg, N.-O., and Sundler, F. (1978): Peptidergic (substance P) nerves in the genito-urinary tract. *Neuroscience*, 3:419–425.
270. Zetler, G., Mönkemeier, D., and Wiechell, H. (1969): Stimulation of Fallopian tubes by prostaglandin $F_{2\alpha}$, biogenic amines and peptides. *J. Reprod. Fertil.*, 18:147–149.
271. Zetler, G., Mönkemeier, D., and Wiechell, H. (1969): Peptid-Receptoren für Tachykinine in der Tuba uterina des Menschen. *Naunyn Schmiedebergs Arch. Pharmacol.*, 262:97–111.
272. Forman, A., Andersson, K.-E., Maigaard, S., and Ulmsten, U. (1985): Concentrations and contractile effects of substance P in the human ampullary-isthmic junction. *Acta Physiol. Scand.*, 124: 17–23.
273. Schultz, G., Schultz, K., and Hardman, J. G. (1975): Effects of norepinephrine on cyclic nucleotide levels in the ductus deferens of the rat. *Metabolism*, 24:429–437.
274. Johansson, S., and Andersson, R. G. G. (1975): Variations of cyclic nucleotide monophosphate levels during spontaneous uterine contractions. *Experientia*, 31:1314–1315.
275. Lindblom, B., and Hamberger, L. (1980): Cyclic AMP and contractility of the human oviduct. *Biol. Reprod.*, 22:173–178.
276. Valenzuela, G., Antonini, R., Hodgson, B. J., Jones, D. J., and Harper, M. J. K. (1977): Cyclic nucleotides and prostaglandins (PGs) produced by the rabbit oviduct: Effects of estrogen treatment. *Res. Commun. Chem. Pathol. Pharmacol.*, 17:361–364.
277. Maia, H. Jr., Barbosa, I., and Coutinho, E. M. (1976): Relationship between cyclic AMP levels and oviductal contractility. In: *Ovum Transport and Fertility Regulation*, edited by M. J. K. Harper, C. J. Pauerstein, C. E. Adams, E. M. Coutinho, H. B. Croxatto, and D. M. Paton, pp. 168–181. Scriptor, Copenhagen.
278. Martin del Rio, R. (1981): γ-Aminobutyric acid system in rat oviduct. *J. Biol. Chem.*, 256:9816–9819.
279. Erdö, S. L., Rosdy, B., and Szporny, L. (1982): Higher GABA concentrations in Fallopian tube than in brain of the rat. *J. Neurochem.*, 38:1174–1176.
280. Erdö, S. L., László, A., Szporny, L., and Zsolnai, B. (1983): High density of specific GABA binding sites in the human Fallopian tube. *Neurosci. Lett.*, 42:155–160.
281. Erdö, S. L., and Lapis, E. (1982): Presence of GABA receptors in rat oviduct. *Neurosci. Lett.*, 33:275–279.
282. Orensanz, L. M., and Fernández, I. (1985): On the binding of γ-[^{3}H]aminobutyric acid to the rat oviduct. *Neurosci. Lett.*, 57:213–214.
283. Erdö, S. L., Kiss, B., and Szporny, L. (1984): Comparative characterization of glutamate decarboxylase in crude homogenates of oviduct, ovary and hypothalamus. *J. Neurochem.*, 43:1532–1537.
284. Erdö, S. L., Riese, M., Kärpäti, E., and Szporny, L. (1984): $GABA_B$ receptor-mediated stimulation of the contractility of isolated rabbit oviduct. *Eur. J. Pharmacol.*, 99:333–336.
285. Noonan, J. J., Adair, R. L., Halbert, S. A., Ringo, J. A., and Reeves, J. J. (1978): Quantitative assessment of oxytocin-stimulated oviduct contractions of the ewe by optoelectronic measurements. *J. Anim. Sci.*, 47:914–918.

286. Coutinho, E. M., and Maia, H. (1970): The influence of the ovarian steroids on the response of the human Fallopian tubes to neurohypophyseal hormones *in vivo*. *Am. J. Obstet. Gynecol.*, 108:194–202.
287. Soloff, M. S. (1975): Oxytocin receptors in rat oviduct. *Biochem. Biophys. Res. Commun.*, 66:671–677.
288. Garcia-Villar, R., Toutain, P. L., Schams, D., and Ruckebusch, Y. (1983): Are regular activity episodes of the genital tract controlled by pulsatile releases of oxytocin? *Biol. Reprod.*, 29: 1183–1188.
289. Harper, M. J. K. (1961): Egg movement through the ampullar region of the Fallopian tube of the rabbit. In: *Proceedings of the IVth International Congress on Animal Reproduction, The Hague*, pp. 375–380.
290. Harper, M. J. K. (1961): The mechanisms involved in the movement of newly ovulated eggs through the ampulla of the rabbit Fallopian tube. *J. Reprod. Fertil.*, 2:522–524.
291. Harper, M. J. K. (1965): Transport of eggs in cumulus through the ampulla of the rabbit oviduct in relation to day of pseudopregnancy. *Endocrinology*, 77:114–123.
292. Croxatto, H. B., Ortiz, M. E., Díaz, S., Hess, R., Balmaceda, J., and Croxatto, H.-D. (1978): Studies on the duration of egg transport by the human oviduct. II. Ovum location at various intervals following the luteinizing hormone peak. *Am. J. Obstet. Gynecol.*, 132:629–634.
293. Eddy, C. A., Garcia, R. G., Kraemer, D. C., and Pauerstein, C. J. (1975): Detailed time course of ovum transport in the rhesus monkey (*Macaca mulatta*). *Biol. Reprod.*, 13:363–369.
294. Díaz, S., Ortiz, M. E., and Croxatto, H. B. (1980): Studies on the duration of ovum transport by the human oviduct. III. Time interval between the luteinizing hormone peak and recovery of ova by transcervical flushing of the uterus in normal women. *Am. J. Obstet. Gynecol.*, 137:116–121.
295. Talo, A., and Brundin, J. (1971): Muscular activity in the rabbit oviduct: A combination of electric and mechanic recordings. *Biol. Reprod.*, 5:67–77.
296. Talo, A., and Hodgson, B. J. (1976): Effect of time after ovulation and estrogen and progesterone on electrical activity of the rabbit oviduct. *Pharmacologist*, 18:181 (abstract No. 377).
297. Portnow, J., Talo, A., and Hodgson, B. J. (1977): A random walk model of ovum transport. *Bull. Math. Biol.*, 39:349–357.
298. Hodgson, B. J., Talo, A., and Pauerstein, C. J. (1977): Oviductal ovum surrogate movement: Interrelation with muscular activity. *Biol. Reprod.*, 16:394–396.
299. Verdugo, P., Blandau, R. J., Tam, P. Y., and Halbert, S. A. (1975): Stochastic elements in the development of deterministic models of egg transport. In: *Ovum Transport and Fertility Regulation*, edited by M. J. K. Harper, C. J. Pauerstein, C. E. Adams, E. M. Coutinho, H. B. Croxatto, and D. M. Paton, pp. 126–137. Scriptor, Copenhagen.
300. Brenner, R. M., Carlisle, K. S., Hess, D. L., Sandow, B. A., and West, N. B. (1983): Morphology of the oviducts and endometria of cynomolgus macaques during the menstrual cycle. *Biol. Reprod.*, 29:1289–1302.
301. Verhage, H. G., Bareither, M. L., Jaffe, R. C., and Akbar, M. (1979): Cyclic changes in ciliation, secretion and cell height of the oviductal epithelium in women. *Am. J. Anat.*, 156:505–511.
302. Critoph, F. N., and Dennis, K. J. (1977): Ciliary activity in the human oviduct. *Br. J. Obstet. Gynaecol.*, 84:216–218.
303. Borell, U., Nilsson, O., and Westman, A. (1957): Ciliary activity in the rabbit Fallopian tube during oestrus and after copulation. *Acta Obstet. Gynecol. Scand.*, 36:22–28.
304. Eddy, C. A., Flores, J. J., Archer, D. R., and Pauerstein, C. J. (1978): The role of cilia in fertility: An evaluation by selective microsurgical modification of the rabbit oviduct. *Am. J. Obstet. Gynecol.*, 132:814–820.
305. McComb, P. F., Halbert, S. A., and Gomel, V. (1980): Pregnancy, ciliary transport, and the reversed ampullary segment of the rabbit Fallopian tube. *Fertil. Steril.*, 34:386–390.
306. Dickmann, Z. (1961): The role of the cumulus oophorus and tubal factors in the process of fertilization of the rabbit egg. In: *Proceedings of the IVth International Congress on Animal Reproduction, The Hague*, pp. 731–735.
307. Brosens, I. A., and Vasquez, G. (1976): Fimbrial microbiopsy. *J. Reprod. Med.*, 16:171–178.
308. Afzelius, B. A., Camner, P., and Mossberg, B. (1978): On the function of cilia in the female reproductive tract. *Fertil. Steril.*, 29:72–74.
309. Bleau, G., Richer, C.-L., and Bousquet, D. (1978): Absence of dynein arms in cilia of endocervical cells in a fertile woman. *Fertil. Steril.*, 30:362–363.
310. Harper, M. J. K., Bennett, J. P., Boursnell, J. C., and Rowson, L. E. A. (1960): An autoradiographic method for the study of egg transport in the rabbit Fallopian tube. *J. Reprod. Fertil.*, 1:249–267.
311. Bennett, J. P., and Rowson, L. E. A. (1961): The use of radioactive artificial eggs in studies of egg transfer and transport in the female reproductive tract. In: *Proceedings of the IVth International Congress on Animal Reproduction, The Hague*, pp. 360–366.
312. Black, D. L., and Asdell, S.A. (1958): Transport through the rabbit oviduct. *Am. J. Physiol.*, 192:63–68.
313. Black, D. L., and Davis, J. (1962): A blocking mechanism in the cow oviduct. *J. Reprod. Fertil.*, 4:21–26.
314. Edgar, D. G., and Asdell, S. A. (1960): The valve-like action of the utero-tubal junction of the ewe. *J. Endocrinol.*, 21:315–320.
315. Rauscher, H. (1969): Rundfischgespräch zum III. Hauptthema. Von der Ovulation zur Implantation. *Arch. Gynakol.*, 207:181–182.
316. Hunter, R. H. F. (1973): Polyspermic fertilization in pigs after tubal deposition of excessive numbers of spermatozoa. *J. Exp. Zool.*, 183:57–64.
317. Day, B. N., and Polge, C. (1968): Effects of progesterone on fertilization and egg transport in the pig. *J. Reprod. Fertil.*, 17:227–230.
318. Hunter, R. H. F. (1972): Local action of progesterone leading to polyspermic fertilization in pigs. *J. Reprod. Fertil.*, 31:433–444.
319. Seki, K., Rawson, J. M. R., and Hodgson, B. J. (1978): Postovulatory changes in cell contacts and intercellular space of rabbit oviductal smooth muscle. *Biol. Reprod.*, 18:679–685.
320. Koester, H. (1970): Ovum transport. In: *Mammalian Reproduction: 21 Colloquium der Geselleschaft für Biologische Chemie*, edited by H. Gibian and E. J. Plotz, pp. 189–228. Springer-Verlag, Heidelberg.
321. Harper, M. J. K. (1966): Hormonal control of transport of eggs in cumulus through the ampulla of the rabbit oviduct. *Endocrinology*, 78:568–574.
322. Blandau, R. J. (1970): Observing ovulation and egg transport. In: *Methods in Mammalian Embryology*, edited by J. C. Daniel, Jr., pp. 1–14. W.H. Freeman, San Francisco.
323. Boling, J. F., and Blandau, R. J. (1971): Egg transport through the ampullae of the oviducts of rabbits under various experimental conditions. *Biol. Reprod.*, 4:174–184.
324. Hunter, R. H. F. (1974): Chronological and cytological details of fertilization and early embryonic development in the domestic pig, *Sus scrofa*. *Anat. Rec.*, 178:169–186.
325. Eddy, C. A., Turner, T. T., Kraemer, D. C., and Pauerstein, C. J. (1976): Pattern and duration of ovum transport in the baboon (*Papio anubis*). *Obstet. Gynecol.*, 47:658–664.
326. Croxatto, H. B., Díaz, S., Fuentalba, B., Croxatto, H. D., Carrillo, D., and Fabres, C. (1972): Studies on the duration of egg transport in the human oviduct. 1. The time interval between ovulation and egg recovery from the uterus in normal women. *Fertil. Steril.*, 23:447–458.
327. Hertig, A. T., Rock, J., and Adams, E. C. (1956): A description of 34 human ova within the first 17 days of development. *Am. J. Anat.*, 98:435–493.
328. Chang, M. C., and Bedford, J. M. (1962): Fertilizability of rabbit ova after removal of the corona radiata. *Fertil. Steril.*, 13:421–425.
329. Allen, E., Pratt, J. P., Newell, Q. U., and Bland, L. J. (1930): Human tubal ova; related early corpora lutea and uterine tubes. *Contrib. Embryol. Carnegie Inst.*, 22:45–76.
330. Lewis, W. H., and Hartman, C. G. (1941): Tubal ova of the rhesus monkey. *Contrib. Embryol. Carnegie Inst.*, 29:7–14.
331. Eddy, C. A. (1986): Personal communication.
332. Harper, M. J. K. (1968): Pharmacological control of reproduction in women. *Prog. Drug Res.*, 12:47–136.
333. Harper, M. J. K. (1972): Agents with antifertility effects during preimplantation stages of pregnancy. In: *Biology of Mammalian Fertilization and Implantation*, edited by K. S. Moghissi and E. S. E. Hafez, pp. 431–492. Charles C Thomas, Springfield, Ill.

334. Harper, M. J. K. (1977): Contraception—Retrospect and prospect. *Prog. Drug Res.*, 21:293–407.
335. Black, D. L. (1974): Neural control of oviduct musculature. In: *The Oviduct and Its Functions*, edited by A. D. Johnson and C. H. Foley, pp. 65–118. Academic Press, New York.
336. Coutinho, E. M. (1976): Interference with ovum transport: Implications for fertility control. In: *Ovum Transport and Fertility Regulation*, edited by M. J. K. Harper, C. J. Pauerstein, C. E. Adams, E. M. Coutinho, H. B. Croxatto, and D. M. Paton, pp. 544–556. Scriptor, Copenhagen.
337. Coutinho, A. M., Maia, H., and Nascimento, L. (1976): The response of the human Fallopian tube to ergonovine and methylergonovine *in vivo*. *Am. J. Obstet. Gynecol.*, 126:48–54.
338. Bygdeman, M., Bremme, K., Christensen, N., Lundström, V., and Gréen, K. (1980): A comparison of two stable prostaglandin E analogues for termination of early pregnancy and for cervical dilatation. *Contraception*, 22:471–483.
339. Bygdeman, M., Christensen, N., Gréen, K., and Zheng, S. (1981): Self-administration of prostaglandin for termination of early pregnancy. *Contraception*, 24:45–52.
340. Kovacs, L., Sas, M., Resch, B. A., Ugocsai, G., Swahn, M. L., Bygdeman, M., and Rowe, P. J. (1984): Termination of very early pregnancy by RU486—An antiprogestational compound. *Contraception*, 29:399–410.
341. Swahn, M. L., Cekan, S., Wang, B., Lundström, V., and Bygdeman, M. (1985): Pharmacokinetic and clinical studies of RU486 for regulation of fertility. In: *The Antiprogestin Steroid RU486 and Human Fertility Control*, edited by E.-E. Baulieu and S. J. Segal, pp. 249–258. Plenum Press, New York.
342. World Health Organization (1979): Special Programme of Research, Development and Research Training in Human Reproduction. *Eighth Annual Report*, 126 pp. WHO, Geneva.
343. World Health Organization (1982): Special Programme of Research, Development and Research Training in Human Reproduction. *Eleventh Annual Report*, 152 pp. WHO, Geneva.
344. World Health Organization (1984): Special Programme of Research, Development and Research Training in Human Reproduction. *Thirteenth Annual Report*, 152 pp. WHO, Geneva.
345. Winston, R. M. L. (1980): Microsurgery of the Fallopian tube: From fantasy to reality. *Fertil. Steril.*, 34:521–533.
346. Wallach, E. E. (1980): Tubal reconstructive surgery—1980. *Fertil. Steril.*, 34:531–533.
347. Henry-Suchet, J., Catalan, F., Loffredo, V., Sanson, M.J., Debache, C., Pigeau, F., and Coppin, R. (1981): *Chlamydia trachomatis* associated with chronic inflammation in abdominal specimens from women selected for tuboplasty. *Fertil. Steril.*, 36:599–605.
348. Faulkner, W. L., and Ory, H. W. (1976): Intrauterine devices and acute pelvic inflammatory disease. *JAMA*, 235:1851–1853.
349. Weström, L., Bengtsson, L. P., and Mårdh, P. (1976): The risk of pelvic inflammatory disease in women using intrauterine contraceptive devices as compared to non-users. *Lancet*, 2:221–224.
350. Daling, J. R., Weiss, N. S., Metch, B. J., Chow, W. H., Soderstrom, R. M., Moore, D. E., Spadoni, L. R., and Stadel, B. V. (1985): Primary tubal infertility in relation to the use of an intrauterine device. *N. Engl. J. Med.*, 312:937–941.
351. Cramer, D. W., Schiff, I., Schoenbaum, S. C., Gibson, M., Belisle, S., Albrecht, B., Stillman, R. J., Berger, M. J., Wilson, E., Stadel, B. V., and Seibel, M. (1985): Tubal infertility and the intrauterine device. *N. Engl. J. Med.*, 312:941–947.
352. Ben-Nun, I., and Greenblatt, R. B. (1982): Infertility associated with endometriosis. In: *Genital Endometriosis in Infertility*, edited by K. Semm, R. B. Greenblatt, and L. Mettler, pp. 1–10. Thieme-Stratton, New York.
353. Friedman, J. (1982): The incidence of endometriosis in unexplained infertility. In: *Genital Endometriosis in Infertility*, edited by K. Semm, R. B. Greenblatt, and L. Mettler, pp. 28–31. Thieme-Stratton, New York.
354. Czernobilsky, B., and Silverstein, A. (1978): Salpingitis in ovarian endometriosis. *Fertil. Steril.*, 30:45–49.
355. Drake, T. S., O'Brien, W. F., Ramwell, P. W., and Metz, S. A. (1981): Peritoneal fluid thromboxane B_2 and 6-ketoprostaglandin $F_{1\alpha}$ in endometriosis. *Am. J. Obstet. Gynecol.*, 141:401–404.
356. Schenken, R. S., Asch, R. H., Williams, R. F., and Hodgen, G. D. (1984): Etiology of infertility in monkeys with endometriosis: Measurement of peritoneal fluid prostaglandins. *Am. J. Obstet. Gynecol.*, 150:349–353.
357. Rock, J. A., Dubin, N. H., Ghodgaonkar, R. B., Bergquist, C. A., Erozan, Y. S., and Kimball, A. W. Jr. (1982): Cul-de-sac fluid in women with endometriosis: Fluid volume and prostanoid concentration during the proliferative phase of the cycle—days 8 to 12. *Fertil. Steril.*, 37:747–750.
358. Sgarlata, C. S., Hertelendy, F., and Mikhail, G. (1983): The prostanoid content in peritoneal fluid and plasma of women with endometriosis. *Am. J. Obstet. Gynecol.*, 147:563–565.
359. Damon, M., Thaler, H., Mercklein, L., Denjean, R., Hedon, B., and Crastes de Paulet, A. (1984): Prostanoids in the peritoneal fluids of infertile women. In: *Medical Management of Endometriosis*, edited by J.-P. Raynaud, T. Ojasoo, and L. Martini, pp. 107–124. Raven Press, New York.
360. Badawy, S. Z. A., Marshall, L., Gabel, A. A., and Nusbaum, M. L. (1982): The concentration of 13,14-dihydro-15-keto prostaglandin $F_{2\alpha}$ and prostaglandin E_2 in peritoneal fluid of infertile patients with and without endometriosis. *Fertil. Steril.*, 38:166–170.
361. Pauerstein, C. J. (1974): *The Fallopian Tube: A Reappraisal*, 196 pp. Lea & Febiger, Philadelphia.
362. Centers for Disease Control (1984): Ectopic pregnancies—United States, 1979–1980. Centers for Disease Control. *M.M.W.R.*, 33:201–202.
363. Persaud, V. (1970): Etiology of tubal ectopic pregnancy. Radiologic and pathologic studies. *Obstet. Gynecol.*, 36:257–263.
364. Israngkun, C., and Phaosavasdi, S. (1976): Hysteroscopic sterilization: Complications in 296 cases. In: *Advances in Female Sterilization Techniques*, edited by J. J. Sciarra, W. Droegemueller, and J. J. Speidel, pp. 148–152. Harper & Row, Hagerstown, Md.
365. Borten, M., and Friedman, E. A. (1985): Ectopic pregnancy among early abortion patients: Does prostaglandin reduce the incidence? *Prostaglandins*, 30:891–905.
366. Lehfeldt, H., Tietze, C., and Gorstein, F. (1970): Ovarian pregnancy, and the intrauterine device. *Am. J. Obstet. Gynecol.*, 108:1005–1009.
367. Seward, P. H., Israel, R., and Ballard, C. A. (1972): Ectopic pregnancy and intrauterine contraception. A definite relationship. *Obstet. Gynecol.*, 40:214–217.
368. Tatum, H. J., and Schmidt, F. H. (1977): Contraceptive and sterilization practices and extrauterine pregnancy: A realistic perspective. *Fertil. Steril.*, 28:407–421.
369. Díaz, S., Croxatto, H. B., Pavez, M., Quinteros, E., Carrillo, D., Simonetti, L., Croxatto, H.-D., and Rosati, S. (1980): Ectopic pregnancies associated with low dose progestagen-releasing IUDs. *Contraception*, 22:259–269.
370. Panayotou, P. P., Kaskarelis, D. B., Miettinen, O.S., Trichopoulos, D. B., and Kalandidi, A. K. (1972): Induced abortion and ectopic pregnancy. *Am. J. Obstet. Gynecol.*, 114:507–510.
371. McBain, J. C., Pepperell, R. J., Robinson, H. P., Smith, M. A., and Brown, J. B. (1980): An unexpectedly high rate of ectopic pregnancy following the induction of ovulation with human pituitary and chorionic gonadotrophin. *Br. J. Obstet. Gynaecol.*, 87: 5–9.
372. Thibault, C. (1972): Some pathological aspects of ovum maturation and gamete transport in mammals and man. *Acta Endocrinol. (Copenh)*, 70(Suppl. 166):59–66.
373. Jerome, C. P., and Hendrickx, A. G. (1982): A tubal pregnancy in a rhesus monkey (*Macaca mulatta*). *Vet. Pathol.*, 19:239–245.
374. Mossman, H. W. (1971): Orientation and site of attachment of the blastocyst: A comparative study. In: *The Biology of the Blastocyst*, edited by R. J. Blandau, pp. 49–57. University of Chicago Press, Chicago.
375. Tuchmann-Duplessis, H., David, G., and Haegel, P. (1972): *Illustrated Human Embryology, Vol. 1, Embryogenesis*, 110 pp. Springer-Verlag, New York.
376. Beatty, R. A. (1958): Variation in the number of corpora lutea and in the number and size of 6-day blastocysts in rabbits subjected to superovulation treatment. *J. Endocrinol.*, 17:248–260.
377. Böving, B. G. (1956): Rabbit blastocyst distribution. *Am. J. Anat.*, 98:403–434.
378. Dickmann, Z., and Spilman, C. H. (1975): Prostaglandins in rabbit blastocysts. *Science*, 190:997–998.

379. Dey, S. K., Chien, S. M., Cox, C. L., and Crist, R. D. (1980): Prostaglandin synthesis in the rabbit blastocyst. *Prostaglandins*, 19:449–453.
380. Harper, M. J. K., Norris, C. J., and Rajkumar, K. (1983): Prostaglandin release by zygotes and endometria of pregnant rabbits. *Biol. Reprod.*, 28:350–362.
381. Cao, Z.-D., Jones, M. A., and Harper, M. J. K. (1984): Prostaglandin translocation from the lumen of the rabbit uterus *in vitro* in relation to day of pregnancy or pseudopregnancy. *Biol. Reprod.*, 31:505–519.
382. Jones, M. A., and Harper, M. J. K. (1984): Rabbit blastocysts accumulate [^{3}H] prostaglandins *in vitro*. *Endocrinology*, 115:817–824.
383. Jones, M. A., Anderson, W., Turner, T. G., and Harper, M. J. K. (1985): Storage *in vivo* of [^{3}H]-prostaglandins by rabbit blastocysts. *Endocrinology*, 116:993–997.
384. Hyland, J. H., Manns, J. G., and Humphrey, W. D. (1982): Prostaglandin production by ovine embryos and endometrium *in vitro*. *J. Reprod. Fertil.*, 65:299–304.
385. Lewis, G. S., Thatcher, W. W., Bazer, F. W., and Curl, J. S. (1982): Metabolism of arachidonic acid *in vitro* by bovine blastocysts and endometrium. *Biol. Reprod.*, 27:431–439.
386. Davis, D. L., Pakrasi, P. L., and Dey, S. K. (1983): Prostaglandins in swine blastocysts. *Biol. Reprod.*, 28:1114–1118.
387. Chepenik, K. P., and Smith, J. B. (1980): Synthesis of prostaglandins by mouse embryos. *IRCS J. Med. Sci.*, 8:783.
388. McLaren, A., and Michie, D. (1959): The spacing of implantation in the mouse uterus. *Mem. Soc. Endocrinol.*, 6:65–75.
389. Hafez, E. S. E., and Ludwig, H. (1977): Scanning electron microscopy of the endometrium. In: *Biology of the Uterus*, edited by R. M. Wynn, pp. 309–340. Plenum Press, New York.
390. Harper, M. J. K. (1982): Sperm and egg transport. In: *Reproduction in Mammals. I. Germ Cells and Fertilization*, 2nd ed., edited by C. R. Austin and R. V. Short, pp. 102–127. Cambridge University Press, Cambridge, U.K.
391. Eddy, C. A., and Harper, M. J. K. (1980): Gamete transport, fertilization, and implantation. In: *Fertility Control. Biologic and Behavioral Aspects*, edited by R. N. Shain and C. J. Pauerstein, pp. 32–48. Harper & Row, Hagerstown, Md.
392. Erdö, S. L., Kiss, B., Riesz, M., and Szporny, L. (1986): Stimulus-evoked efflux of GABA from preloaded slices of the rabbit oviduct. *Eur. J. Pharmacol.*, 130:295–303.
393. Erdö, S. L., and Amenta, F. (1986): Characterization and localization of high-affinity GABA uptake in slices of the rabbit oviduct. *Eur. J. Pharmacol.*, 130:287–294.
394. McComb, P., Langley, L., Villalon, M., and Verdugo, P. (1986): The oviductal cilia and Kartagener's syndrome. *Fertil. Steril.*, 46:412–416.

NOTES ADDED IN PROOF

1. Recent studies show that stimulus-evoked GABA efflux from rabbit oviduct differs from that of neuronal release (392) and that uptake of [^{3}H] GABA is localized in the oviductal epithelium (393). These findings do not support the presence of a neuronal GABA uptake system or of a GABAergic innervation of the oviduct.

2. This has recently been refuted on the basis of one woman with Kartagener's syndrome who had *absolutely immotile* cilia in both the respiratory and reproductive tracts (394). In previously reported cases, respiratory ciliary activity was usually abnormal rather than absent, suggesting the possibility of some ciliary motility in the reproductive tract.

The Physiology of Reproduction,
edited by E. Knobil and J. Neill *et al.*
Raven Press, Ltd., New York©1988.

CHAPTER 5

Mammalian Fertilization

R. Yanagimachi

Fertilization in mammals normally represents the beginning of life for a new individual. Since I last reviewed the processes and mechanisms of mammalian fertilization in 1981 (530), there has been a considerable increase of our knowledge in this area. Because recently many excellent reviews have covered various aspects of mammalian fertilization (see, e.g., refs. 7,22,53,104,137,144,154,178,218, 316,329,359,370,468,507,663), I have deliberately cited relatively few articles published before 1980. This does not mean that I consider the uncited publications outdated. On the contrary, many of them are of the utmost importance and will continue to retain their value for many years to come. I would hope that readers, especially young students, do not overlook at least the key references when reading the review articles of the past. Because of the recent deluge of literature, few young students may have read such classic reviews as those by Chang (99), Austin and Walton (26), Austin (20), Bishop (60), Blandau (63), and Piko (396). They are still "treasure chests" of basic information about mammalian gametes and fertilization.

EPIDIDYMAL MATURATION OF SPERMATOZOA

Mammalian spermatozoa leaving the testis do not have the ability to fertilize eggs. They gain this ability while making the slow passage through the epididymis. This process is called the *epididymal maturation* (for recent reviews, see refs. 22,53,111,122,144,227,233,362,374, and 376). The site where the spermatozoa begin to acquire their fertilizing ability varies from species to species. In some species (e.g., the boar), it is the distal segment of the caput epididymis, whereas in others (e.g., the rat) it is the distal segment of the corpus epididymis (cf. ref. 122). It is unlikely that all the spermatozoa gain their fertilizing capacity simultaneously. Some spermatozoa apparently become fertile much faster (or in a more proximal region of the epididymis) than others. However, as a rule, it is not until they enter the cauda epididymis that the great majority of spermatozoa attain their full fertilizing potential.

One of the most prominent changes in spermatozoa during the epididymal maturation is the development of sperm's ability to move. Testicular spermatozoa are either motionless or very weakly motile. This is true not only within the testis, but also when these spermatozoa are suspended in physiological salt solutions. Fully mature spermatozoa isolated from the cauda epididymis, on the other hand, initiate active, progressive movement upon exposure to physiological salt solutions. The inability of testicular spermatozoa to move is probably due, at least in part, to the "immaturity" of the plasma membrane because they can move almost as actively as mature cauda epididymal spermatozoa if they are demembranated and exposed to ATP, cAMP, and Mg^{2+} (252,326,512). Transfer of several substances, such as a forward motility protein (2,3), carnitin (95,96), and glycerophosphocholine (250) from the epididymal fluid to the spermatozoa, is believed to be important for the development of sperm's ability to move.

In some species (e.g., the guinea pig, bush baby, and pig-tailed monkey), the gross morphology and internal structure of the acrosome change during the epididymal maturation (44a,151,230). The gross morphology of the sperm nucleus does not change drastically during maturation, but its chromatin is steadily stabilized by disulfide bonds (47,273,386). Tail components (e.g., the coarse outer fibers and fibrous sheath) are also stabilized by disulfide bonds during maturation (48).

The epididymis has a very high fluid-absorbing and -secreting activity. The osmolality (123) and chemical composition (81,236,286,290) of the fluid secreted by the epididymis vary from one segment to another. Therefore, it would be expected that the sperm plasma membrane, which is exposed directly to the epididymal fluid, is altered step by step as spermatozoa pass through the different regions of the epididymis. There is no doubt that the plasma membrane is one of the most prominent sites of change during epididymal maturation (for reviews, see refs. 144,153,234, and 362). The steady increase in the ability of the sperm head to adhere to the egg zona pellucida as the spermatozoa pass through the epididymis (117,375,390,424), for instance, clearly indicates a chemical alteration of the sperm plasma membrane. Another indication of chemical modifications of the sperm plasma membrane is the change in net negative surface charge of spermatozoa during maturation (37,147,232,328,544).

The sperm plasma membrane is already "coated" with several macromolecules (antigens) when spermatozoa leave the testis (for further references, see refs. 53,370, and 418). During the passage of spermatozoa through the epididymis, these preexisting molecules are either lost or altered; furthermore, new macromolecules of epididymal origin are adsorbed onto, or integrated into, the plasma membrane (53,144). The most prominent of these macromolecules are *glycoproteins* (for further references, see refs. 84,144, 271,391,421, and 550). The alteration in the characteristics of preexisting glycoproteins and the addition of new glycoproteins to the sperm plasma membrane seem to be mediated, at least in part, by such enzymes as galactosyltransferase and sialytransferase in the epididymal fluid (56,207,210) as well as an alpha-lactoalbumin-like substance (208,258) that regulates glycosylation of sperm surface glycoproteins. The synthesis and secretion of various glycoproteins by the testis and the different regions of the epididymis (Fig. 1), as well as the integration of these glycoproteins onto/into different regions of the sperm plasma membrane, have been well documented (143b,412,478,517). The change in lectin-binding ability of the sperm plasma membrane during epididymal maturation (147,211,351,361) indicates that certain terminal saccharide residues of sperm membrane glycoproteins are altered (removed, masked, or added) during the maturation.

Glycoproteins are not the only membrane molecules that change during the maturation. Membrane lipids also undergo change in their chemical and physical characteristics (352,384,434). The fact that the epididymis, particularly the corpus epididymis, has a high cholesterol synthesis activity (206,209) may suggest that cholesterol is one of the lipid molecules integrated in the sperm plasma membrane during sperm maturation. The change in the distribution pattern of protein (glycoprotein) particles in the plasma membrane during sperm maturation (360,407,464) seems

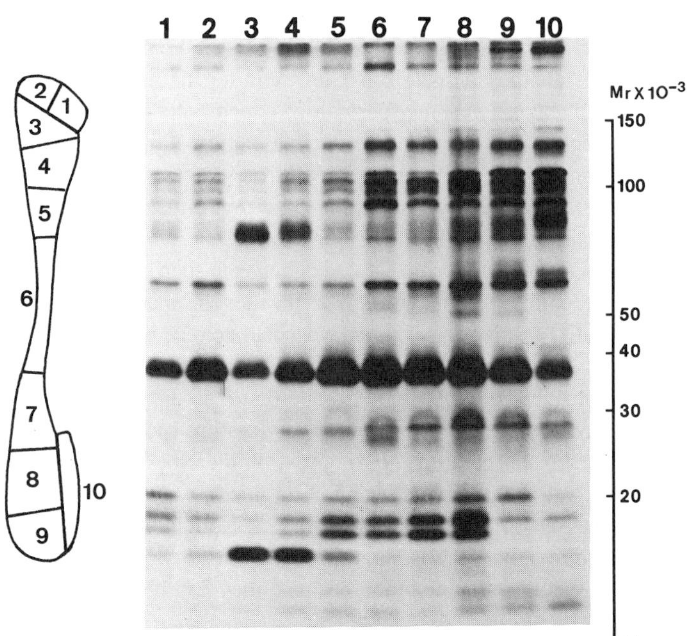

FIG. 1. Polyacrylamide gel electophoresis of proteins secreted by various segments of the rat epididymis. The epididymis is subdivided into 10 arbitrary segments: 1–2 is the initial segment, 3–5 is the caput epididymis, 6–7 is the corpus epididymis, and 8–10 is the cauda epididymis. (From ref. 82.)

to reflect chemical alterations of both protein and lipid molecules of the sperm plasma membrane.

The adsorption and/or integration of a variety of glycoproteins onto/into the plasma membrane covering the sperm head is very prominent during the epididymal maturation (for further references, see refs. 85,112,412, and 478). Figure 2 is an electron micrograph of a Chinese hamster spermatozoon in the corpus epididymis. Many vesicular and tubular structures can be seen on and near the plasma membrane over the acrosome, but not on the plasma membrane of other regions (538). These vesicular and tubular structures begin to appear on the sperm surface when the spermatozoa reach the distal caput epididymis, where the spermatozoa begin to gain the ability to move. The number of vesicles and tubules accumulated on the plasma membrane reaches the maximum in the proximal cauda epididymis, where spermatozoa gain the full ability to move and fertilize eggs. Interestingly, these vesicles and tubules disappear from the sperm surface as the spermatozoa proceed through the cauda epididymis. Although the origin and chemical nature of these vesicular and tubular structures remain to be determined, their selective accumulation on the plasma membrane of the acrosomal region is impressive. The plasma membrane over the acrosome must have a specific affinity to the vesicles and tubules. In almost all other mammalian species, we do not see such distinctly visible structures on the surface of maturing spermatozoa. However, there seems to be no doubt that the plasma membrane of the sperm head interacts specifically with luminar components of the epididymis.

It is important to note that the plasma membrane over the sperm head is not the only part of the membrane that undergoes chemical modification during sperm maturation. Absorption and/or integration of several specific glycoproteins and peptides on/in the plasma membrane of tail regions during sperm maturation have been reported (83,88,363,478). In other words, the entire sperm plasma membrane, from the anterior end of the sperm head to the distal end of the sperm tail, is likely to change its chemical characteristics during epididymal maturation.

It is generally believed that the maturation of spermatozoa is completed when the spermatozoa reach the distal segment of the cauda epididymis. This is probably true for most mammals. However, in species in which spermatozoa are stored in the vas deferens for some time before they are released (ejaculated), the maturation may continue, or even be completed, in the vas deferens. In the Chinese hamster, a large number of spermatozoa are stored in the vas deferens before they are ejaculated. When we inseminated Chinese hamster eggs *in vitro* with cauda epididymal and vas deferens spermatozoa, 100% of the eggs were fertilized. All of the eggs fertilized by cauda epididymal spermatozoa were monospermic, whereas about 30% of the eggs inseminated with vas deferens spermatozoa were polyspermic (538). The conditions of insemination and the time of examination of the eggs following insemination were constant in this ex-

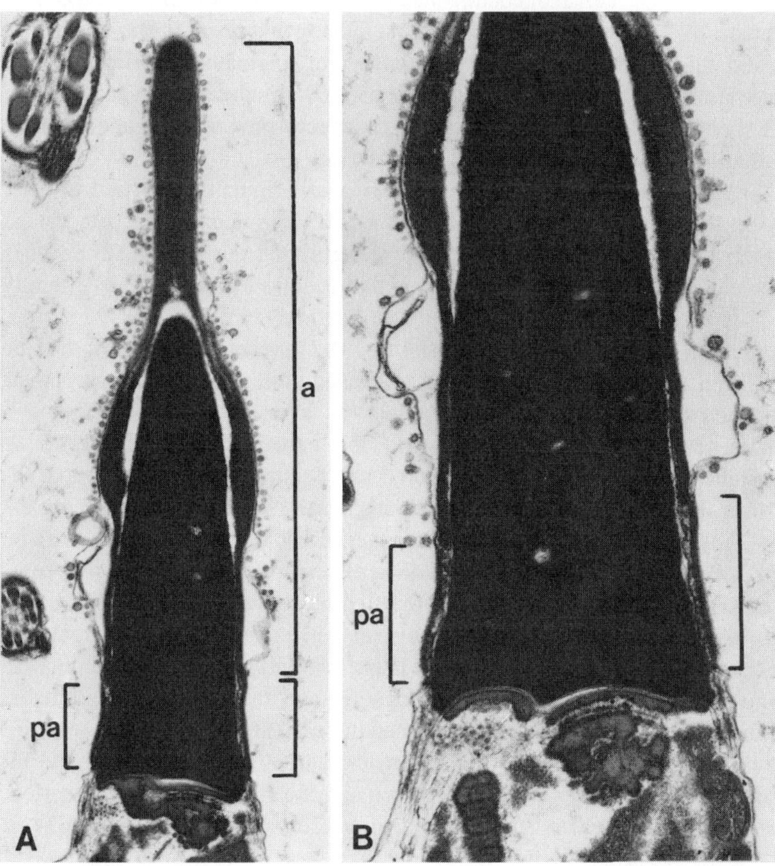

FIG. 2. Longitudinal sections through the heads of Chinese hamster spermatozoa in the proximal cauda epididymis. Note many vesicles on, or in the vicinity of, the plasma membrane over the acrosome, but not on the membrane of other areas. (a) Acrosomal region; (pa) postacrosomal region. (From ref. 539.)

periment. Therefore, it seems that spermatozoa from the vas deferens were capacitated either more quickly or in larger proportions than epididymal spermatozoa, so that more of them were able to penetrate the eggs during the interval before the block to polyspermy was established. In other words, the spermatozoa from the vas deferens, as a whole, must be more competent for fertilization than epididymal spermatozoa. Thus, it is quite possible that Chinese hamster spermatozoa continue their maturation even after they have entered the vas deferens.

CAPACITATION OF SPERMATOZOA

Mammalian spermatozoa, matured in the epididymis and ejaculated, are not yet ready to fertilize eggs. They must reside in the female genital tract for some time before gaining the ability to fertilize the eggs. Apparently, spermatozoa undergo some physiological (functional) changes in the female genital tract. These changes, which render the spermatozoa capable of fertilization, are collectively called *capacitation*.

Even today, 36 years since the discovery of capacitation by Chang (98) and Austin (17), some investigators still cast doubt on the necessity of sperm capacitation, because epididymal or freshly ejaculated spermatozoa, which have never been exposed to the female genital tract, are capable of fertilizing eggs in artificial media without the presence of any contributions from the female genital tract. If we define capacitation as a phenomenon that takes place only in the female genital tract, their doubt is justifiable. However, it would seem more appropriate to consider that the artificial media they used for inseminating the eggs mimicked the sperm-capacitating action of the female tract. If capacitation is not required, then freshly ejaculated spermatozoa should be able to fertilize the eggs immediately upon insemination. In reality, there is always some delay between insemination and the beginning of fertilization. This delay can be less than 1 hr or more than several hours, depending on the species. It must represent the approximate time for capacitation.

The time required for capacitation can be determined in various ways. One of them is to mate or artificially inseminate recently ovulated females and determine the time of fertilization. If there is a delay of 2 hr between mating (or insemination) and the onset of fertilization, for instance, this interval (2 hr) is considered the minimum time for capacitation. This method has an inherent problem, however. The 2 hr may represent the minimum time of sperm transport to the site of fertilization. The spermatozoa may be capacitated sooner. An alternate approach is to preincubate spermatozoa in either the female genital tract or artificial media for various periods of time, depositing them in the oviducts of recently ovulated females (or mixing the spermatozoa with eggs *in vitro*), and determine the time of fertilization. If the spermatozoa have not been capacitated at all or have been capacitated only partially, they will either fail to fertilize the eggs or fertilize the eggs a number of hours later. On the other hand, if the spermatozoa have been fully capacitated, they will fertilize the eggs without delay (at least within 30 to 60 min after insemination, taking into consideration the time needed for sperm passage through the egg investments). Using such methods, minimum capacitation times for rabbit, golden hamster, and mouse spermatozoa, for examples, were estimated to be about 5 to 6 hr, about 2 hr, and about 1 hr, respectively (cf. ref. 22). It is important to note that capacitation time for each species is by no means fixed. It is significantly influenced, for example, by the strain of animals (cf. ref. 235), hormonal state of females (cf. refs. 101,224, and 499), and the composition of the medium to which spermatozoa are exposed (cf. ref. 530). The contact of spermatozoa with the seminal plasma seems to affect capacitation time very significantly (see below).

What is capacitation, then? We still do not know exactly what it is, but it seems to be very certain that the removal or alteration of substances adsorbed on, or integrated in, the sperm plasma membrane during epididymal maturation, and upon contact of spermatozoa with the seminal plasma, constitutes a very important part of capacitation (for recent reviews, see refs. 22,104, and 359). The removal or alteration of a "protective coat" from the surface of sperm plasma membrane could "sensitize" the membrane to the specific milieu of fertilization and more important, to the target of spermatozoa, the eggs. I quote here the statement made by Piko (396) in 1969: ". . . capacitation consists, at least in part, in the gradual removal of coating material from the sperm surface, especially in the acrosome region. This would result in an exposure of sperm receptor sites allowing spermatozoa to interact specifically with egg receptors, or with substances emanating from the egg, and to undergo the acrosome reaction upon contact with the outer coats of the egg."

The term *capacitation* was originally proposed to refer to physiological changes in spermatozoa that render the spermatozoa capable of fertilizing the eggs (18). Because the acrosome reaction that follows capacitation is definitely needed for normal fertilization, some investigators (see, e.g., ref. 100) insist that the acrosome reaction should be considered as a part of capacitation. Although I respect their opinion, I am personally in favor of the opinion of Austin (21) and Bedford (41), that capacitation and the acrosome reaction be considered two separate phenomena; capacitation is a series of changes that makes the spermatozoa capable of undergoing the acrosome reaction (this will be discussed later). The acrosome reaction is a widely occurring phenomenon throughout the animal kingdom. Capacitation, on the other hand, is a rather unique phenomenon in mammals and perhaps in relatively few nonmammalian animals. Both capacitation and the preceding epididymal maturation of mammalian spermatozoa may be a result of evolutional adaptation to internal fertilization. For the biological and evolutional significance of sperm capacitation, readers are referred to an interesting article by Bedford (46).

Capacitation *In Vivo*

Capacitation normally takes place in the genital tract of the estrous female. The sites where capacitation begins and is completed may vary, depending on the site of sperm deposition at coitus. In species in which the spermatozoa are deposited in the vagina at coitus (e.g., the rabbit and human), capacitation may start while the spermatozoa are passing through the cervix or cervical mucus (for studies in the human, see refs. 190 and 279). Although there is no doubt that rabbit spermatozoa, for instance, can complete their capacitation within the uterus (4), it is unknown whether fertilizing spermatozoa complete their capacitation in the uterus before migrating into the oviduct. According to Overstreet et al. (381), the rabbit spermatozoa that participate in fertilization stay in the isthmic region of the oviduct for a number of hours until ovulation commences. Therefore, it is possible that the rabbit spermatozoa that are destined to fertilize eggs are capacitated partially in the uterus, then they migrate into the oviduct where they complete capacitation. It is interesting to note that capacitation of rabbit spermatozoa is accomplished most efficiently when the spermatozoa are sequentially exposed to the uterus and the oviduct (40).

In species in which semen is deposited directly in the uterus at coitus (e.g., many rodents and pig), the principal site of capacitation is most likely the oviduct. Here again, the spermatozoa destined to fertilize eggs stay in the isthmic region of the oviduct for some time before moving to the ampulla, where they fertilize the eggs (for further references, see ref. 244). Not all the spermatozoa in the isthmus are transported to the ampulla. In fact, only a very small fraction of isthmic spermatozoa are released and reach the ampulla to effect fertilization (cf. ref. 120). It is unknown, at the moment, when and where the spermatozoa in the oviduct complete their capacitation.

Virtually nothing is known about the conditions or factors directly controlling capacitation of spermatozoa within the female genital tract. A variety of substances have been suggested as possible candidates for the sperm-capacitating or capacitation-controlling factors within the tract. They include such enzymes as beta-amylase and beta-glucuronidase (cf. ref. 199), proteinase and neuraminidase (cf. refs. 255 and 444), arylsulfatase, fucosidase and acetylhexosaminidase (403,404), carbonic anhydrase (105), and steroid sulfatase (283,289), glycosaminoglycans (214), catecholamine (223), and taurine and hypotaurine (319). Further studies are definitely needed to determine whether such substances are really involved in capacitation of spermatozoa *in vivo*. Whatever the native sperm-capacitating conditions or factors are, they are apparently not extremely species-specific because the spermatozoa and eggs of one species can effect fertilization in the female genital tract (oviducts) of another species (cf. refs. 130,177,229,405, and 425).

In vitro sperm capacitation and fertilization are certainly possible without any contributions from the female genital tract (see below). Apparently, no special substances of female tract origin are essential to support or induce capacitation of spermatozoa, at least in the many species that have been studied. However, this does not necessarily imply that the conditions supporting or inducing capacitation *in vitro* are identical with those *in vivo*. What can happen *in vitro* and what is taking place *in vivo* (naturally) could well be different. There are several claims that the spermatozoa capacitated *in vivo* fertilize eggs far more efficiently than those capacitated *in vitro* (see, e.g., refs. 446 and 500). Mother nature has done her job for millions of years, whereas we have started to mimic her job rather recently. There are many things we still have to learn from nature.

Capacitation *In Vitro*

In 1963, Yanagimachi and Chang (535) first reported that mammalian spermatozoa can be capacitated *in vitro*. We collected unfertilized eggs of golden hamster by breaking the oviducts of recently ovulated females. When the eggs were inseminated with cauda epididymal spermatozoa (suspended in either Tyrode's solution or a tissue culture medium TC 199) and examined several hours later, 55% of the eggs were penetrated by spermatozoa. Although successful *in vitro* fertilization surely indicates successful *in vitro* capacitation of spermatozoa, the system we used was too crude to analyze what caused capacitation of spermatozoa. It could be the medium itself, cumulus oophorus, or oviduct fluid. In the early stage of investigation, oviduct fluid, follicular fluids, or blood serum, all having very complicated compositions, were used to induce *in vitro* capacitation of spermatozoa. Since Toyoda et al. (486) first reported successful *in vitro* fertilization of the mouse eggs using a "chemically defined" medium, media for *in vitro* fertilization (*in vitro* sperm capacitation as well) have been greatly simplified. This has made the analysis of capacitation mechanisms considerably easier than before. The media commonly used today for *in vitro* fertilization (*in vitro* sperm capacitation) are modified Tyrode's and Krebs-Ringer's solution supplemented with proper energy sources (e.g., glucose, lactate, and pyruvate) and albumin. Commercially available tissue culture media (e.g., Ham F-10) supplemented with blood serum are also used commonly, particularly for the human. So far, there is no single medium that can support *in vitro* fertilization (*in vitro* sperm capacitation) in every species. The medium that is excellent for gametes of one species is not necessarily suitable for the gametes of other species. Spermatozoa and eggs of each species seem to demand their own specific environment to perform their functions most efficiently.

The prime goal of many investigators who engaged in the study of *in vitro* fertilization was to fertilize eggs, not to analyze the mechanism of sperm capacitation. Although information obtained by these investigators is very valuable, we must be cautious in citing their conclusions, at least in terms of sperm capacitation. For instance, many investigators concluded that certain reagents blocked sperm capacitation completely because no fertilization took place *in vitro* in the presence of these reagents. Their conclusions may or may not be correct, because capacitation is not the only process spermatozoa must undergo to fertilize the eggs successfully. To fertilize the eggs, the spermatozoa must be, at least, highly motile as well as being capable of undergoing the acrosome reaction, penetrating through the egg investments, and fusing with the egg proper. Successful fertilization *in vitro* certainly implies that the spermatozoa underwent capacitation successfully. Unsuccessful *in vitro* fertilization, on the other hand, does not necessarily mean that the spermatozoa failed to undergo capacitation.

It is very common to take the acrosome reaction as an indicator of the completion of capacitation. Because the spermatozoa do not undergo the acrosome reaction unless they have been capacitated, the acrosome reaction can be used as a reliable indicator of successful capacitation. We must be careful, however, because unusual conditions or special reagents may induce the acrosome reaction, bypassing capacitation. The absence of the acrosome reaction does not necessarily mean that the spermatozoa failed to undergo capacitation. These spermatozoa may well be capacitated, but merely prevented from undergoing the acrosome reaction. Keeping these facts in mind, I will make a brief summary of what we have learned about conditions or factors that have significant influence on capacitation *in vitro*. I do not intend to make a complete literature survey here. For more information about capacitation, see the following reviews: refs. 22,41,42,45,50,104,170,227,283, 329,369,410,415, and 530.

Some Factors Controlling or Affecting Capacitation, as Revealed by *In Vitro* Studies

Temperature

Sperm capacitation is temperature dependent (157,309). The incubation temperature of 37 to 38°C, used in most laboratories, is apparently adequate to support capacitation *in vitro* in most cases. However, it is interesting to note that *in vitro* fertilization of pig and sheep eggs, which has proven to be rather difficult in the past, can now be achieved very efficiently by preincubating spermatozoa at 39°C and/ or mixing the eggs and freshly ejaculated (washed) spermatozoa at this temperature (cf. refs. 102 and 113). At least in the case of the sheep and pig, capacitation might proceed much more efficiently at the temperature slightly higher than 37 to 38°C.

Individual Variations

We do not expect that all the spermatozoa in the same cauda epididymis or in the same ejaculate are capacitated at the same rate. Some might be capacitated much faster than others, even under the same conditions. Spermatozoa from some males might be capacitated considerably faster (or more easily) than those from some other males of the same species. Interindividual variation within any given species is considerable (cf. refs. 436 and 534 for the rat and the human, respectively).

Epididymal Spermatozoa Versus Ejaculated Spermatozoa

Although both cauda epididymal and ejaculated spermatozoa are considered fully mature, these two types of spermatozoa do not necessarily behave in the same way *in vitro*. According to Shalgi et al. (436), who compared the fertilizing ability (*in vitro*) of the cauda epididymal and ejaculated spermatozoa from the same male rat, epididymal spermatozoa fertilize more eggs (average: 59%) than ejaculated spermatozoa (average: 21%) under identical experimental conditions. There are some reports that both epididymal and ejaculated spermatozoa fertilize eggs *in vitro* at the same rate (see, e.g., ref. 487), but, in general, epididymal spermatozoa appear to be able to fertilize eggs *in vitro* much more easily than can ejaculated spermatozoa. According to Nagai et al. (349), 71% to 75% of pig eggs are fertilized *in vitro* by cauda epididymal spermatozoa, whereas none are fertilized by ejaculated spermatozoa. Interestingly, epididymal spermatozoa become infertile once they are exposed to the seminal plasma.

The cat is extremely interesting in terms of sperm capacitation. According to Niwa et al. (353), cat spermatozoa, freshly collected from the cauda epididymis, are apparently capable of penetrating eggs as early as 20 min after insemination. By 30 min after insemination, 100% of the eggs are penetrated. This is the fastest egg penetration by fresh epididymal spermatozoa ever recorded. One may wonder if cat spermatozoa even require capacitation. According to Hammer et al. (213), washed cat ejaculated spermatozoa are unable to fertilize eggs *in vitro*. However, they become capable of fertilizing the eggs consistently when they are incubated in the uteri of estrous females for 2 hr or more. Brief intrauterine sperm incubation ($\frac{1}{2}$ hr) is not enough to ensure successful fertilization *in vitro*. Obviously, ejaculated spermatozoa (the spermatozoa exposed to the seminal plasma) and the epididymal spermatozoa (those not exposed to the seminal plasma) are not identical physiologically. Cat epididymal spermatozoa may be in a capacitated state in the cauda epididymis. The seminal plasma may decapacitate the spermatozoa. Decapacitated (ejaculated) spermatozoa must be recapacitated, of course, before they become capable of fertilizing eggs.

Why are ejaculated spermatozoa more resistant to *in vitro* capacitation than are epididymal spermatozoa? Perhaps the plasma membrane of ejaculated spermatozoa is more stable than that of epididymal spermatozoa. Although the plasma membrane of the epididymal spermatozoa is already stabilized, to some extent, by adsorption and/or integration of epididymal glycoproteins, it seems to be further "stabilized" upon its contact with the seminal plasma. There is ample evidence that some of the seminal plasma components (e.g., glycoproteins, polypeptides, and fibronectin-like proteins) bind very firmly to the surface of ejaculated spermatozoa (1,243,269,330,359,420,433,502,509). The binding is so firm that they cannot readily be removed from the sperm surface by repeated washings with ordinary physiological solutions (420,509). As already stated, the removal or alteration of sperm surface-coating materials is most likely an essential part of capacitation. Apparently, the genital tract of the estrous female is capable of capacitating both epididymal and ejaculated spermatozoa equally (378). It must have some very efficient mechanisms to remove or alter sperm surface-coating materials originating from the epididymis (the "primary" surface coat) and from the seminal plasma (the "secondary" surface coat). Since the primary surface coat is less stable than the secondary coat (420), the primary coat on the epididymal spermatozoa must be removed or altered easily in the so-called "sperm-capacitating media." Some of the capacitation media currently available are probably not very effective in removing or altering the stable secondary coat on the ejaculated spermatozoa. Whether or not the ejaculated spermatozoa of a given species are capacitated easily in artificial media (*in vitro*) may depend on the stability of the secondary coat.

Cumulus Oophorus

Fully mature eggs released from the ovary are each surrounded by the cumulus oophorus. In most mammals, the cumulus persists around the eggs *in vivo* not only during fertilization, but also for some time after the eggs have been fertilized (Fig. 3). The presence of cumulus oophorus around the eggs is not essential for fertilization *in vitro* (28,307,530), but its presence may facilitate fertilization (28,446), particularly when the medium is lacking or deficient in albumin (33,171). Some components of the cumulus seem to promote the acrosome reaction of spermatozoa (33,477,511).

According to Gwatkin et al. (200), hamster cumulus cells can capacitate spermatozoa *in vitro* without any contributions from the female genital tract. Although the cumulus cells may indeed capacitate spermatozoa under the experi-

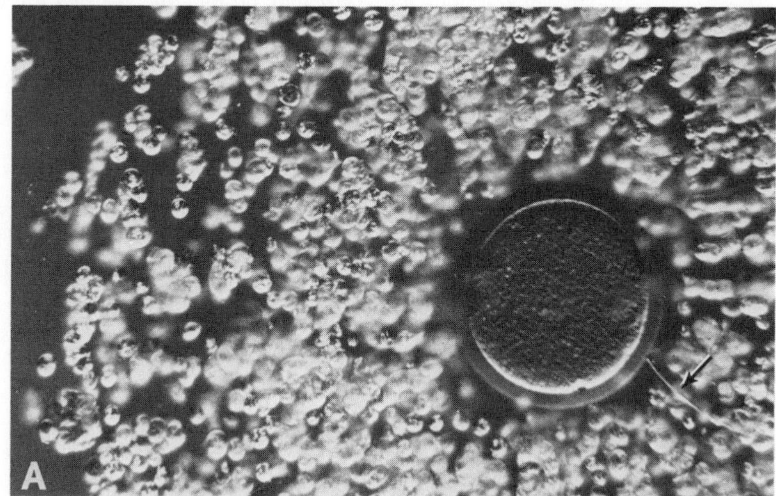

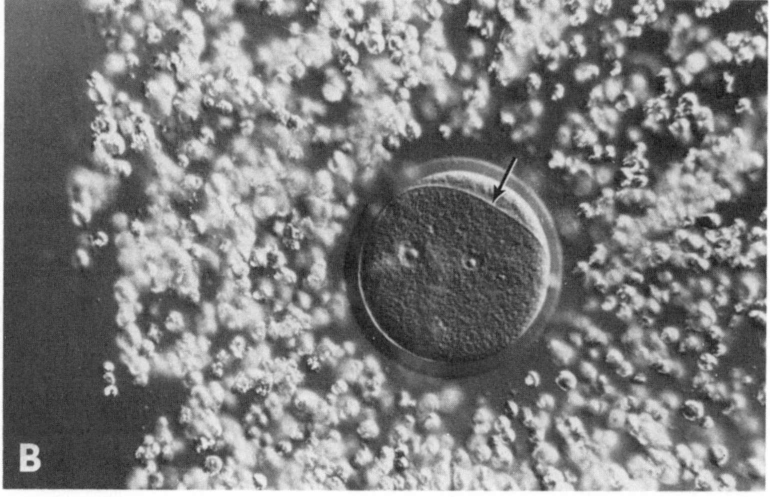

FIG. 3. Photomicrographs showing that the cumulus oophorus continues to surround the egg during (**A**) and after (**B**) fertilization in the Chinese hamster. Arrows indicate sperm tails.

mental conditions that these investigators employed, it is unlikely that these cells are primarily responsible for sperm capacitation *in vivo*. Hamster spermatozoa that are about to enter the cumulus oophorus *in vivo* are apparently capacitated already (cf. refs. 120 and 545). This would suggest that the secretory products of the female genital tract, not the cumulus components, are primarily responsible for capacitation of spermatozoa *in vivo*.

Composition of the Medium

Table 1 shows the composition of a modified Krebs-Ringer's solution which is known to support *in vitro* capacitation of mouse spermatozoa. The ionic composition of the sheep oviduct fluid is also shown in this table for comparison.

All of the components in sperm-capacitating media must be contributing, directly or indirectly, to capacitation. If a particular component in the medium is absolutely necessary for capacitation, deleting this component should render the medium completely incapable of capacitating spermatozoa. It is somewhat surprising to learn that there is no such component. Media free of (strictly speaking, deficient in) K^+ are known to capacitate spermatozoa (62,169,338). Capacitation can proceed in media free of or deficient in: Ca^{2+} (168,547), HCO_3^- (288), exogenous energy substrates (172,430), albumin (158,171), or even Na^+ and Cl^- (A. Bhattacharyya and R. Yanagimachi, *unpublished data*). Thus, the presence or absence of a particular component in the medium may not be critical for capacitation. As long as other medium components and endogenous energy can support the survival of spermatozoa, capacitation seems to proceed.

TABLE 1. *Concentrations (mM) of the components of a modified Krebs-Ringer's solution[a] and of sheep oviductal fluid[b]*

Components	Modified Krebs-Ringer's solution	Oviductal fluid in Ampulla	Oviductal fluid in Isthmus
Cation			
Na	141.50	135.00	141.00
K	6.77	8.12	6.90
Ca	1.71	3.80	2.98
Mg	1.19	0.59	0.54
Anion			
Cl	98.63	122.00	120.00
HCO_3	25.07	23.70	27.30
PO_4	1.19	1.11[c]	
SO_4	1.19	N.D.[d]	N.D.
Energy substrate			
Lactate	25.00	5.60	3.40
Pyruvate	1.00	N.D.[e]	N.D.
Glucose	5.56	N.D.[e]	N.D.
Other			
Albumin	0.33	N.D.	N.D.

[a]For *in vitro* capacitation of mouse spermatozoa; cited from Inoue and Wolf (251).
[b]Of estrous ewe; cited from Table 2 of Restall and Wales (409).
[c]Site of fluid collection, not identified; cited from Table 1 of Restall and Wales (408).
[d]N.D., no data.
[e]The presence of pyruvate and glucose in oviduct fluids of other species has been reported (cf. refs. 170 and 212).

Spermatozoa of many mammals can survive and capacitate in artificial media similar to a modified Krebs-Ringer's solution shown in Table 1. The spermatozoa of the golden hamster are unique in this regard. They simply die in such media within a few hours. Capacitation is not possible unless the medium is supplemented with additional sperm survival factors. These factors are heat-stable, low-molecular-weight substances present in follicular fluid and blood serum (524–526) and very rich in the extracts of adrenal gland (35). Following up on this lead, Meizel and his associates reached the conclusion that the factors (which they called *sperm motility factors*) are catecholamines (e.g., epinephrine) and taurine or hypotaurine (110,342). Thanks to this discovery, we are now able to capacitate hamster spermatozoa in "chemically defined" media (32,291,306,531). No one knows exactly how the sperm motility factors assist the survival of hamster spermatozoa. They may prolong the sperm's life by slowing down peroxidation of membrane lipids (12) or by reducing the activity of membrane-bound Na^+/K^+-ATPase (340). Alternatively, they may serve as membrane-stabilizing osmoregulators (494).

Why is it that golden hamster spermatozoa cannot survive in artificial media without sperm motility factors, whereas spermatozoa of most other species can do without them? Since the spermatozoa of hamster, guinea pig, and human all contain the factors capable of supporting hamster's sperm survival (34), the species difference could be due to the stability of the factors within cells. Hamster spermatozoa probably are unable to hold the factors within cells unless they are surrounded by the same factors. Spermatozoa of other species, on the other hand, must be able to hold in the factors fairly (or very) well, regardless of the presence or absence of the factors in surrounding media.

Events That Occur in Spermatozoa During Capacitation

Changes in Adenylate Cyclase/Protein Kinase Systems

Ejaculated spermatozoa move very actively. Although fertilizing spermatozoa may reduce or lose their motility temporarily while they are in certain segments of the female genital tract (380), they are vigorously motile at least at the beginning and end of capacitation. There is no doubt that both adenylate cyclase and cAMP-dependent protein kinase systems play vital roles in the initiation and maintenance of motility (for reviews, see refs. 216,312, and 475). Are these systems functioning just to sustain the motility of spermatozoa? It is highly probable that these systems are also actively involved in capacitation. There is evidence that sperm adenylate cyclase increases its activity during capacitation (55,333,457,458). Increased adenyl cyclase activity probably increases cAMP availability and turnover rate (457), which, in turn, would stimulate cAMP-dependent protein kinase. Stimulated protein kinase may alter the tertiary and quarternary structure of the sperm membranes through phosphorylation of membrane proteins (237,246), resulting in changes in the physiological properties (e.g., ion permeability) of membranes.

Changes in Metabolism

There have been many articles reporting that spermatozoa exhibit increased metabolism (e.g., glycolytic activity and oxygen consumption) after being incubated in the female genital tract or in media containing uterine, oviductal, or follicular fluids—treatments that lead to capacitation (for further references, see ref. 72). According to Boell (72), mouse spermatozoa incubated in a capacitating medium (a modified Krebs-Ringer's solution containing albumin and energy substrates) exhibit a constantly high level of respiration from the beginning to the end of a $2\frac{1}{2}$-hr incubation period. Since the spermatozoa consume oxygen at the same rate in "noncapacitating" media (e.g., albumin-free Krebs-Ringer's solution or phosphate-buffered sucrose, both containing energy substrates), Boell concluded that "the increased respiration of sperm in a capacitating medium is due to the presence of oxidizable substrates and, as such, is an accompaniment of the process of capacitation rather than a factor in bringing it about." Although it appears to be certain that mouse spermatozoa do not change their respiration rate before and after capacitation, I am not entirely sure that the media Boell called "noncapacitating" are really noncapacitating. They could be "capacitating." As was pointed out earlier, it might be the acrosome reaction, not capacitation, that fails to occur in these media. In many species, spermatozoa begin to exhibit very vigorous movement, called *hyperactivation* (530), sometime before they initiate the acrosome reaction. Capacitation might bring about some changes in the sperm plasma membrane (phosphorylation?) such that energy becomes more accessible to the sperm's motor apparatus. An increase in metabolic rate during and after capacitation is still a distinct possibility.

Changes in Intracellular Ions

Live spermatozoa efficiently keep up ionic gradients across the plasma membrane, the concentration of K^+ inside the spermatozoa being higher than outside, whereas the reverse is true of Na^+ (312). This ionic gradient is believed to be maintained by an ATPase-mediated Na^+/K^+ exchange pump (401,402,488). According to Babcock (27), intracellular concentrations of K^+ and Na^+ in bovine (cauda epididymal) spermatozoa are about 120 and 14 mM, respectively. Are the intracellular concentrations of K^+ and Na^+ maintained constant during the entire course of capacitation? According to Hyne et al. (247), guinea pig spermatozoa incubated in a capacitating medium (consisting of 106 mM NaCl, 1 mM $MgCl_2$, 25 mM $NaHCO_3$, 20 mM Na-lactate, and 0.25 mM Na-pyruvate), reduce their intracellular K^+ concentration significantly (from 3 to 5 μg to 0.6 μg/10^8 sperm) by the end of 2 hr of incubation, when the spermatozoa are ready for the acrosome reaction. Intracellular Na^+ concentration, on the other hand, increases dramatically (from 0.2 to 0.4 μg to 11 to 12 μg/10^8 sperm) during the same period. Although there is no doubt that intracellular concentrations of K^+ and Na^+ are altered in the medium Hyne et al. used, it should be noted that the medium they used was lacking, or at least deficient in, K^+. The drastic ion changes reported by Hyne et al. could be due, in part, to a gradual inactivation of sperm Na^+,K^+-ATPase in a K^+-free (or deficient) environment. According to Mrsny et al. (341), Na^+,K^+-ATPase activity of hamster spermatozoa increases significantly during 2 hr of incubation in a normal (K^+-containing) capacitating medium. Whether intracellular concentrations of Na^+ and K^+ remain unchanged or are altered during capacitation was not reported by these investigators.

Although it is well established that a massive influx of extracellular Ca^{2+} through the sperm head plasma membrane triggers the acrosome reaction (cf. ref. 530), little is known about the kinetics of intracellular Ca^{2+} during capacitation. It is generally accepted that the concentration of intracellular Ca^{2+} in spermatozoa is rather low, at both head and tail regions, because of the presence of an ATPase-mediated Ca^{2+} pumping mechanism and a Na^+/Ca^{2+} antiporter in the plasma membrane (for further references, see refs. 75–80,448, and 497). According to Singh et al. (448), guinea-pig spermatozoa pick up radioactive Ca^{2+} during 1 hr of incubation in a capacitating medium. Singh et al. have considered that this is caused by a loose association of Ca^{2+} to sperm surface, rather than by its penetration into the spermatozoa. Using quin-2, a calcium-selective fluorescent indicator, Mahanes et al. (308) have found that the concentration of intracellular free Ca^{2+} in rabbit spermatozoa does not change as the result of *in vitro* capacitation. Since the technique these investigators used allowed them to measure Ca^{2+} in sperm mass, rather than in individual spermatozoa, they have suggested that Ca^{2+} concentration might change in discrete, localized regions of the spermatozoon. It is an attractive hypothesis that an increase in intracellular Ca^{2+} concentration during capacitation stimulates sperm adenylate cyclase, allowing the expression of cAMP-dependent events that are a prerequisite for fertilization (327).

Changes in the Acrosome

In most species, the structure of the acrosome does not change noticeably during capacitation of spermatozoa (cf. refs. 38,115,465,481, and 547). The acrosome of the golden hamster may be exceptional. Its contour and the texture of the acrosomal matrix change soon after the spermatozoa are exposed to capacitating media (cf. Fig. 4; see also ref. 536). The reason for this is unknown, but it could be due to a slight influx or efflux of some small molecules through the plasma and outer acrosomal membranes, which does not seem to occur in mouse spermatozoa until the acrosome reaction begins (287). According to Wincek et al. (513), enzymatically inactive proacrosin in the boar sperm acrosome is converted to enzymatically active acrosin by glycosaminoglycans in uterine fluid. There is no doubt that glycosaminoglycans stimulate the conversion of proacrosin to acrosin in test tubes (385), but how do such large molecules like glycosaminoglycans penetrate into the acrosome through both the plasma and acrosomal membranes of spermatozoa? Whether acrosomal enzymes remain in inactive forms (185) or are converted to an active form during capacitation is still an open question.

Changes in the Nucleus

The nuclei of spermatozoa of most eutherian mammals are very stable structures owing to extensive cross-linkings of nuclear proteins by -S-S- bonds (94). Their stability is maintained throughout capacitation (273,324). The nuclear proteins of human spermatozoa are cross-linked by -S-S- bonds (49), but less extensively than those of most other species (65). In the seminal plasma, Zn^{2+} (of prostatic gland origin) binds to the free -SH radicals of the nuclear proteins of spermatozoa upon ejaculation (276), thus causing a temporary stabilization of nuclear proteins (275,411). During capacitation, the nuclei lose Zn^{2+} and increase in stability, probably by oxidation of released -SH radicals in disulfide bonds (292).

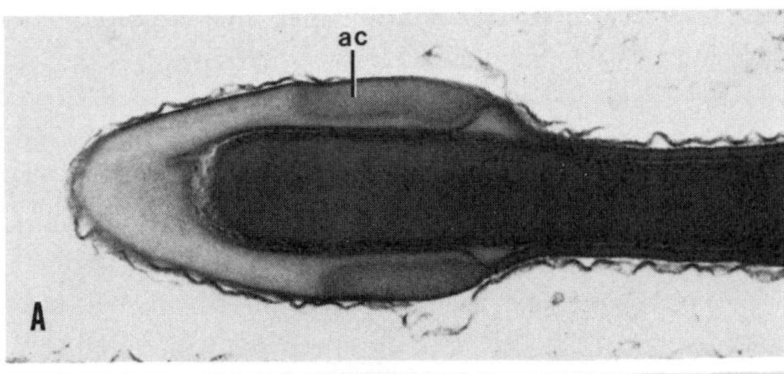

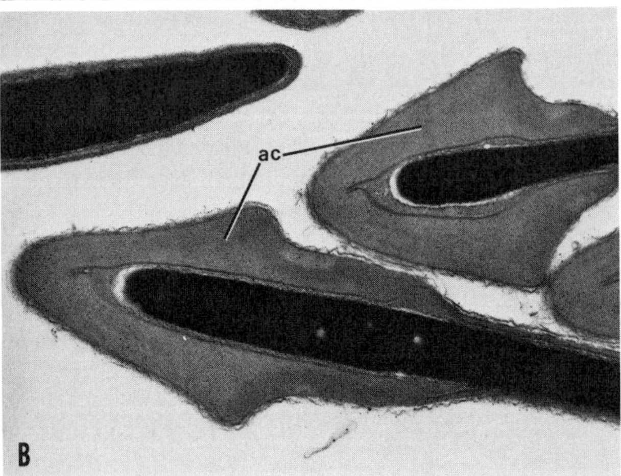

FIG. 4. Longitudinal sections through the anterior region of the heads of golden hamster spermatozoa, showing that the shape of the acrosomal cap (ac) changes during *in vitro* capacitation. Five minutes (**A**) and 1 hr (**B**) after the start of sperm incubation in a capacitating medium.

Changes in the Plasma Membrane

Because the plasma membrane is directly exposed to the capacitating environment, it is not surprising that very prominent changes take place in this membrane during capacitation. Since Weinman and Williams (510) and Piko (395) postulated that the removal or alteration of coating materials from the sperm surface constitutes an important part of capacitation, the evidence supporting this view has accumulated (for further references, see refs. 104,266,267,359, and 530) (cf. Fig. 5). Instead of compiling a complete list of publications here, I will cite a few recent articles confirming and/or adding new information about the removal or alteration of the sperm surface materials during capacitation.

According to Okabe et al. (356), an antigen (which specifically binds to monoclonal antibody TSC4) is on the plasma membrane over the entire acrosome of cauda epididymal spermatozoa of the mouse. This antigen, of corpus epididymal origin, cannot be removed easily from the sperm surface by repeated washings. It disappears (or becomes unreactive with the antibody) by the time spermatozoa enter the perivitelline space of the egg. This antigen must be either removed or altered (masked?) during capacitation. Okabe et al. (357) have reported an interesting behavior of another mouse sperm antigen. This antigen, which specifically binds to monoclonal antibody OBF13, is not detectable on cauda epididymal spermatozoa. It becomes detectable on the head plasma membrane when the spermatozoa are capacitated *in vitro*. This antigen must be hidden (masked) in fresh epididymal spermatozoa and exposed during capacitation (Fig. 6). Sperm surface antigens that are removed or altered during capacitation are not restricted to the head region. They are on the sperm tail as well. A rat sperm antigen, SMA 4, is an example. This antigen of caput epididymal origin (496) is localized on the entire tail surface of fresh epididymal spermatozoa. It disappears (or becomes nonreactive with antibody) from tail surfaces as the spermatozoa are capacitated either *in vitro* or *in vivo* (Fig. 7; 495). According to Voglmayr and Sawyer (503), ejaculated ram spermatozoa incubated in uterine fluid release three different glycosylated proteins (65, 41, and 24 kilodaltons) from their surfaces into the fluid. At the same time, they adsorb a 16-kilodalton protein from the fluid. In the oviduct fluid, the spermatozoa release 97- and 41-kilodalton proteins from their surfaces.

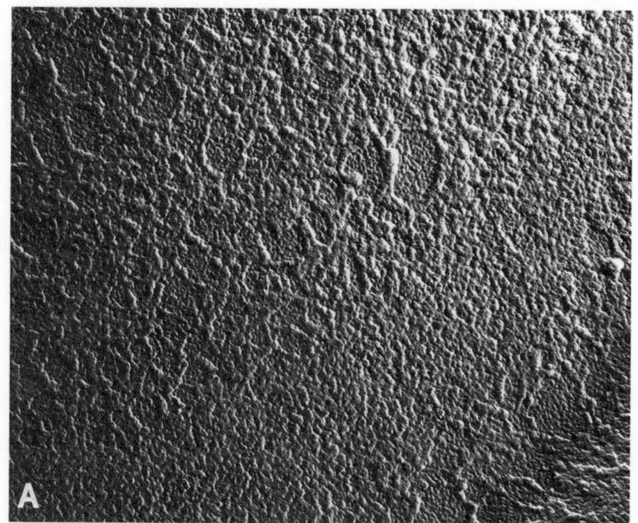

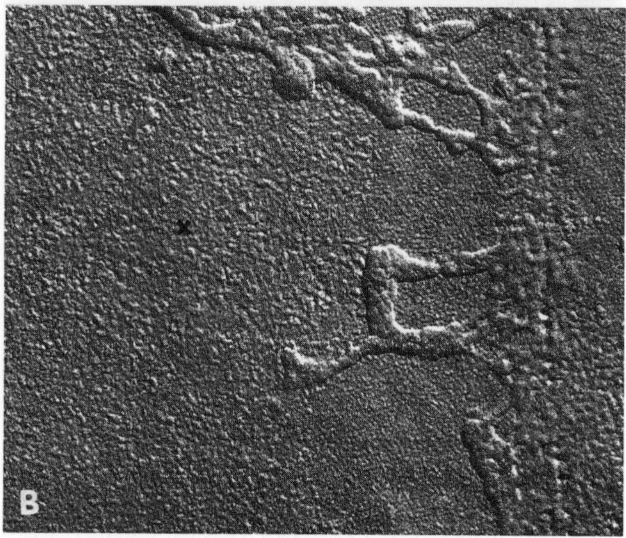

FIG. 5. Surface replicas of the acrosomal region of guinea-pig spermatozoa. During incubation in a sperm-capacitating medium, the surface "coat" is removed or modified, exposing the plasma membrane surface (x). Thirty minutes (**A**) and 24–26 hr (**B**) after the start of sperm incubation in Ca^{2+}-free (deficient) TS medium. (Provided by Dr. Daniel S. Friend.)

Interestingly, spermatozoa exposed first to uterine fluid then to oviduct fluid adsorb several components (13–190 kilodaltons) from the latter. Although Voglmayr and Sawyer did not evaluate how the oviductal and uterine fluids they used were effective in capacitating spermatozoa *in vitro,* their findings certainly indicate the possibility that the release of sperm surface components and the absorption of exogenous fluid components are integral parts of *in vivo* capacitation.

According to the widely accepted "fluid mosaic" model of biological membranes (447), proteins (or glycoproteins) are noncovalently associated with the lipid bilayers that form the matrix of the membrane. Intrinsic proteins, which are firmly embedded in the bilayer, can be removed only by harsh treatments (e.g., treatment with detergent), whereas peripheral proteins, which are associated with the membrane primarily through electrostatic interactions, can be liberated by merely adding chelating agents or by increasing the pH or ionic strength (186). Thus, proteins or glycoproteins released from and/or added to sperm surfaces during capacitation must be peripheral proteins (or glycoproteins). At the moment, we know very little about the precise nature of the peripheral proteins (or glycoproteins) that are removed or eluted during capacitation. One of them could be a fibronectin or fibronectin-like protein (269). It is very tempting to speculate that molecules like fibronectin "cross-link" intrinsic proteins and "freeze" their lateral movement within lipid bilayers; its detachment from the membrane would allow the intrinsic proteins to move more freely within lipid bilayers.

Freeze-fracture examination of sperm plasma membrane before and after capacitation has revealed that intramembranous particles (IMPs), which are intrinsic proteins within lipid bilayers, change their distributions in both head and tail regions. Figure 8A shows IMPs that are almost evenly distributed in the plasma membrane over the acrosome of an uncapacitated guinea-pig spermatozoon. The membrane of the same area of a capacitated spermatozoon has many small patches that are free of IMPs (Fig. 8B). In human spermatozoa, too, IMP-free zones appear in the plasma membrane during capacitation (476). According to Friend (174) and Bearer and Friend (36), IMP-free areas, unlike the surrounding IMP-rich areas, have no or very few sterols (e.g., cholesterol) and anionic lipids (e.g., cardiolipin). The plasma membrane covering the middle piece of uncapacitated guinea-pig spermatozoa has concentrically arranged IMPs in close apposition to the underlying mitochondrial helix. This unique arrangement of IMPs disappears when spermatozoa are capacitated (268). All of these changes must be the result of physical and/or chemical alteration of lipid bilayers during capacitation.

There have been several articles reporting or suggesting that the phospholipid composition of sperm membrane changes during capacitation. According to Snider and Clegg (450), phosphatidyl inositol, which is absent in freshly ejaculated porcine spermatozoa, is synthesized by spermatozoa during incubation (capacitation?) in the female genital tract. Methylation of phospholipids (e.g., conversion of phosphatidyl ethanolamine to phosphatidyl choline) seems to occur during capacitation of hamster spermatozoa (298). Bearer and Friend (36) have postulated that during capacitation of guinea-pig spermatozoa, intracellular phosphatidic acid is converted to cardiolipin, which is then inserted in the outer leaflet of the lipid bilayers of the plasma membrane.

Recently, much attention has been directed to cholesterol in sperm membrane (for a review, see ref. 182). This is sensible because cholesterol is known to exert a variety of profound effects on the characteristics of all biological membranes (e.g., active and passive ion permeability) by regulating orientation, fluidity, and thickness of membrane lipids (cf. ref. 399). According to Davis et al. (129), rat

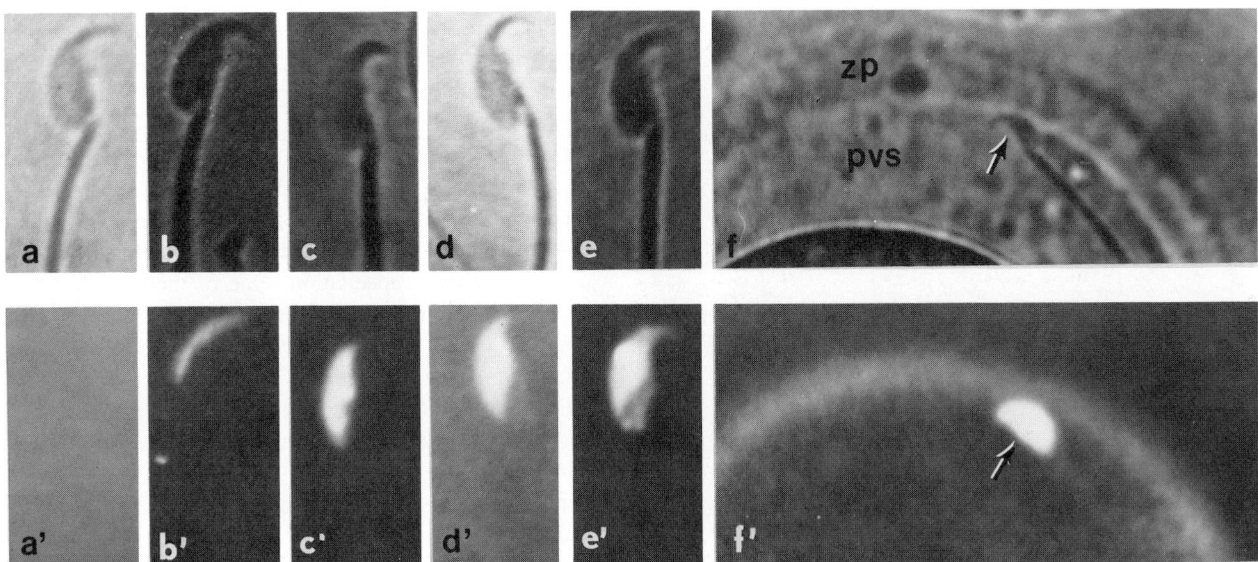

FIG. 6. Photomicrographs of mouse spermatozoa taken at different times, showing that a "surface" antigen of the sperm head is exposed or becomes reactive with a monoclonal antibody (OBF 13) during *in vitro* capacitation. Indirect immunofluorescent microscopy. (pvs) Perivitelline space; (zp) zona pellucida. Arrows indicate sperm heads in the perivitelline space. (From ref. 357.)

spermatozoa in a capacitating medium lose a part of their plasma membrane cholesterol. It is albumin in the medium that picks up the cholesterol. Since *in vivo* capacitated rabbit spermatozoa greatly lose their fertilizing capacity when treated with cholesterol-loaded media (127), Davis (128) has proposed that a gradual removal of sperm membrane cholesterol by albumin (or some other components of female genital tract fluid) is an essential part of capacitation. Although the importance of cholesterol removal from sperm plasma membrane for capacitation has been stressed by Go and Wolf (182,183) and Langlais and Roberts (283), cholesterol depletion may not take place as extensively and uniformly as generally imagined. Only very limited areas of the membrane may become free of cholesterol, as demonstrated by Friend (174). It could be the phase separation of the membrane lipids and cholesterol (lateral migration of these molecules within the lipid bilayers to form domains), not the actual efflux of cholesterol from the membrane, that is more important for capacitation. There are reports that the fluidity of lipids of sperm head and tail plasma membranes changes as the result of capacitation (367,368,451,514). We must be reminded that in these studies, measurements were made at the light microscopic level. Fluidity changes in very small, localized areas, which could be most important, would be

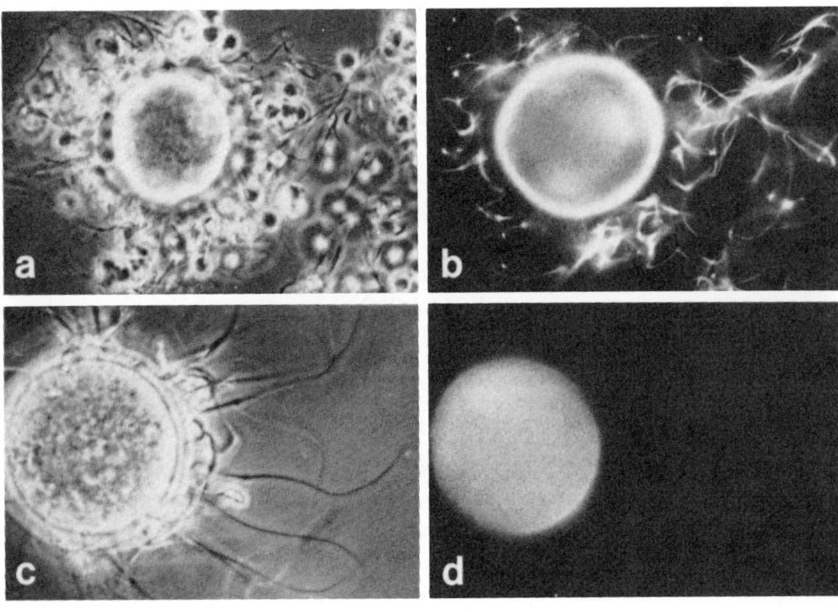

FIG. 7. Photomicrographs of mouse spermatozoa and eggs, showing that a sperm-tail antigen is lost or becomes unreactive with a monoclonal antibody (SMA 4) during capacitation. Indirect immunofluorescent microscopy. Thirty minutes (**a** and **b**) and 4 hr (**c** and **d**) after epididymal spermatozoa were mixed with eggs in a sperm-capacitating medium. (From ref. 495.)

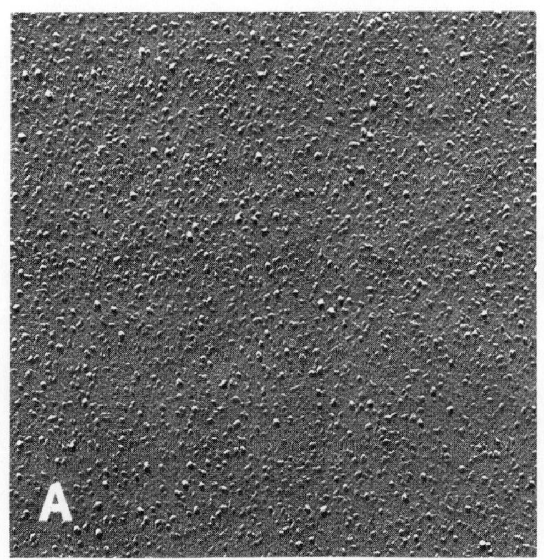

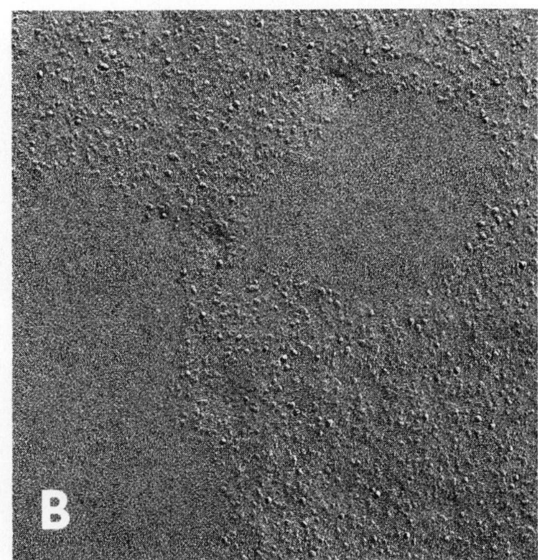

FIG. 8. Intramembranous particles in the plasma membrane of the acrosomal cap region of guinea-pig spermatozoa before (**A**) and after (**B**) capacitation *in vitro*. Note the presence of particle-free patches in the plasma membrane of the capacitated spermatozoon. Capacitated spermatozoa were prepared by incubating cauda epididymal spermatozoa for 17 hr in Ca^{2+}-free (deficient) mT medium. (Provided by Dr. Fumie Suzuki.)

very difficult to detect using the techniques these investigators have employed.

ACROSOME AND THE ACROSOME REACTION

Acrosome and Acrosomal Enzymes

The acrosome is a membrane-bound, cap-like structure covering the anterior portion of the sperm nucleus. Although the size and shape of the acrosome vary considerably from species to species (24,150), its basic structure is the same in all eutherian mammals (cf. ref. 530). The acrosome is believed to be analogous to a lysosome (11) or a zymogen granule of pancreatic cells (173). Indeed, it contains a large array of hydrolytic enzymes (Table 2). Although some of these enzymes may be localized in or on the acrosomal membrane, rather than in the acrosomal matrix, there is no doubt that the acrosome contains powerful hydrolyzing enzymes.

TABLE 2. *Enzymes reported to be of acrosomal origin*

First reported before 1980	First reported after 1980 (references)
Hyaluronidase	β-*N*-Acetylhexosaminidase (454)
Acrosin	β-Galactosidase (454)
Proacrosin	β-Glucuronidase (454)
Acid proteinase	α-L-Fucosidase (454)
Esterase	Phospholipase C (453)
Neuraminidase	Cathepsin D (456)
Phosphatase	Peptidyl peptidase (471b)
Phospholipase A	Ornithin decarboxylase (400)
β-*N*-acetylglucosaminidase	
Arylsulfatase	
Arylamidase	
Collagenase	

Hyaluronidase and acrosin are the two acrosomal enzymes that have been most extensively studied and well characterized. Their presence within acrosomal matrix has been demonstrated convincingly by cytochemical or immunocytochemical techniques at the electron microscopic level (97,192,196,253,440,504). Although several investigators have maintained that a portion of the acrosomal hyaluronidase and acrosin is bound tightly to the inner acrosomal membrane, none of the evidence presented at the electron microscopic level is strong enough to verify this (for discussion, see ref. 241).

Carbohydrate is a distinct component of the acrosomal matrix (231,270,285). A thin layer of glycoprotein covering the inner surface of the outer acrosomal membrane (152) may serve to hold vesiculated (fenestrated) plasma and outer acrosomal membranes together during the acrosome reaction (Fig. 9C). Other glycoproteins or carbohydrate-containing materials within the acrosomal matrix may aid in the conversion of acrosomal enzymes from inactive forms (e.g., proacrosin) to active forms (e.g., acrosin) before or during the acrosome reaction.

Functional Significance of the Acrosome Reaction

The eggs of many animals are surrounded by glycoprotein coats through which spermatozoa must pass before reaching the egg plasma membrane. In some invertebrates, acrosomal "lysins" released by (or carried on the surface of) an acrosome-reacted spermatozoon dissolve the coat locally to produce a "hole" through which the spermatozoon then swims.

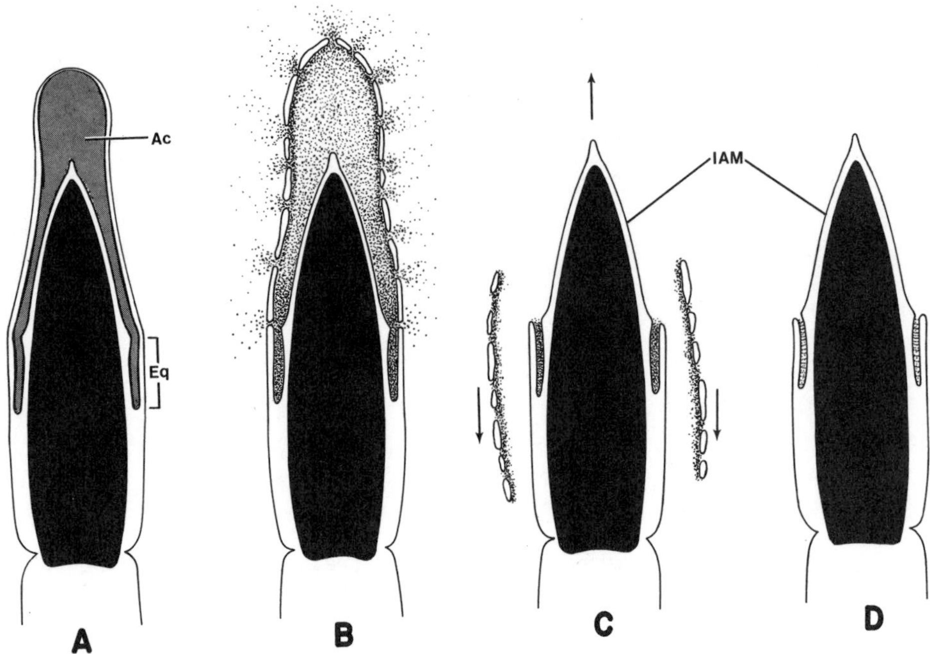

FIG. 9. Diagrams showing the progression of a typical acrosome reaction. (Ac) Acrosomal cap; (Eq) equatorial segment of the acrosome; (IAM) inner acrosomal membrane. (From ref. 530, slightly modified.)

The dissolution of the coat by lysins is either enzymatic (digestion) or stoichiometric (intermolecular hydrophobic interaction) (see ref. 296 for further references).

All mammalian eggs are surrounded by a thick glycoprotein coat, the zona pellucida. In most species, the zona is further surrounded by the cumulus oophorus, which consists of cumulus cells and their matrix. The main component of the cumulus matrix is hyaluronic acid. It has been the general belief that hyaluronidase released from acrosome-reacting spermatozoa digests the cumulus matrix and that acrosin carried on the surface of acrosome-reacted spermatozoa aids in the passage of spermatozoa through the zona. Although this notion must be reevaluated (see below), there is no doubt that acrosome-reacted spermatozoa are capable of passing through the zona and fusing with the egg plasma membrane (cf. ref. 530). In other words, the acrosome reaction has at least two functions: it renders spermatozoa capable of (a) penetrating through the zona and (b) fusing with the egg plasma membrane.

Morphology and Kinetics of the Acrosome Reaction

Distinction Between "True" and "False" Acrosome Reaction

Since the acrosome contains a variety of powerful hydrolyzing enzymes, the acrosome may be "autodigested" in moribund or dead spermatozoa. The relatively unstable outer acrosomal membrane and the overlying plasma membrane may either be destroyed (partially or totally) or become detached from the main body of the spermatozoon. Spermatozoa with such disrupted or missing plasma and outer acrosomal membranes may look like acrosome-reacting or acrosome-reacted spermatozoa when examined under the light microscope. It is very important to distinguish such degenerative acrosomal modifications in moribund and dead spermatozoa from the physiological acrosome reaction that occurs in lively motile spermatozoa. Bedford (41) proposed to call the former the "false" acrosome reaction and the latter the "true" acrosome reactions.

Detection of True (Physiological) Acrosome Reaction by Light Microscopy

The acrosome reaction of the spermatozoa with large acrosomes can be readily detected by light microscopy without any treatment of spermatozoa. Acrosomes of the musk-shrew (107,264) and guinea-pig spermatozoa (528) are so huge that a low-power objective lens would be good enough to detect the reaction. In our laboratory, we routinely use a 4× or 6.3× objective lens, with dark-field (or pseudo-dark-field) illumination, for quick evaluation of the acrosome reaction in living guinea-pig spermatozoa.

Acrosomes of the spermatozoa of the golden hamster (541) and Chinese hamster (539) are considerably smaller than those of guinea-pig spermatozoa. To clearly visualize the acrosome reaction in living hamster spermatozoa, a 40× phase-contrast (or differential interference-contrast) objective lens is needed. With some experience, the acrosome reaction (the presence or absence of acrosomal caps) in moving spermatozoa can be evaluated with ease. However, when the spermatozoa are moving vigorously (e.g., hyperactivated), assessing the acrosome reaction can be very difficult or impossible. This difficulty can be overcome by slowing down the movement of spermatozoa (e.g., by cooling the stage of microscope) or by immobilizing spermatozoa, one by one, by a brief exposure to an ultraviolet (UV) spot (119).

Acrosomes of rabbit and mouse spermatozoa are thin and tightly fitted to the sperm heads. Detecting the acrosome reaction in the living spermatozoa of these species is obviously not as easy as in guinea-pig or hamster spermatozoa. However, detecting the acrosome reaction in rabbit spermatozoa by light (phase-contrast or interference-contrast) microscopy is certainly possible (69,382,461).

Since spermatozoa of many mammals (e.g., the mouse, bull, ram, and human) have either very thin or rather small acrosomes and their acrosome reactions are difficult to detect in the living state, several techniques have been developed to aid in the assessment of the acrosome reaction. They include: the naphthyl-yellow/erythrosine B method (91,224), the acridin orange-UV method (61,77), the chlortetracycline-UV method (287,427), the triple stain technique (135,469), and the pea (*Pisum sativum*) lectin method (114). Monoclonal antibodies against acrosomal contents (516) and polyclonal antibodies against the outer acrosomal membrane (483) have also been used to evaluate acrosome reactions in human or porcine spermatozoa. Although these techniques allow us to evaluate the acrosome reaction much faster than the time-consuming electron microscopic technique, the procedures used in these techniques inevitably kill the spermatozoa (by either chemical fixation or UV irradiation). It is hoped that new techniques will be developed in the near future so that we can assess the acrosome reaction of spermatozoa without killing them.

Exocytotic Nature of the Acrosome Reaction

The typical, true acrosome reaction involves multiple fusions between the outer acrosomal membrane and the overlying plasma membrane, which enables the contents of the acrosome to escape through the fenestrated membranes. Since Barros et al. (29) first demonstrated this clearly in the hamster and rabbit, a number of investigators have confirmed this not only in these species, but also in a variety of other mammalian species (Fig. 9).

The site where the fusion between the plasma and the outer acrosomal membrane first takes place may vary according to species. In the rabbit, it could be the frontal or peripheral margin of the acrosomal cap region (cf. refs. 44b and 530). In the golden hamster (133), ram (154,155, 455,508), and human (348), it could be at or near the border of the acrosomal cap region and the equatorial segment of the acrosome. This is not surprising because in the spermatozoa of many species, the plasma and outer acrosomal membranes in this area are apparently the least stable (179). According to Watson and Plummer (508), the outer acrosomal membrane of this region is very rich in calcium-binding sites.

Figure 10 illustrates the process of the acrosome reaction

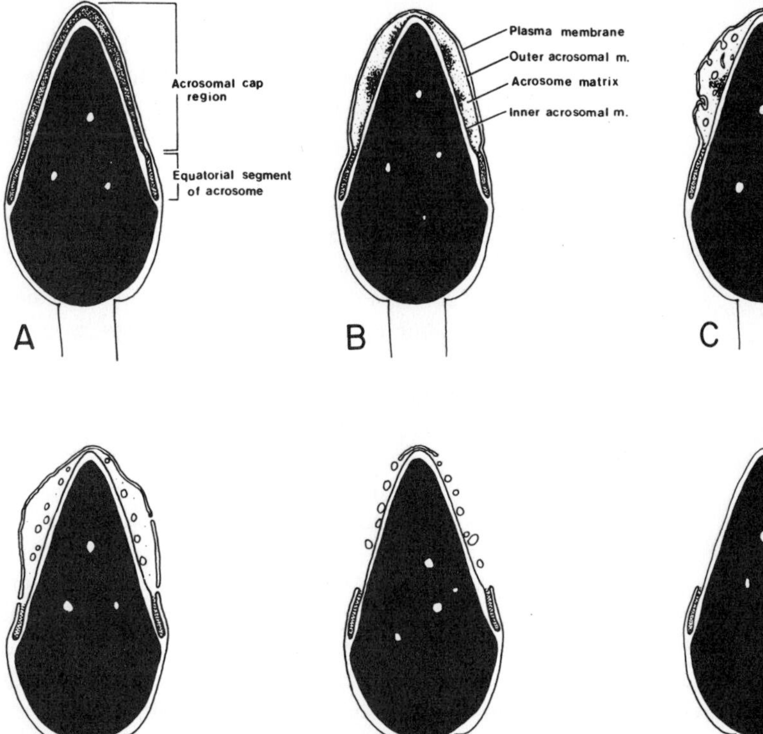

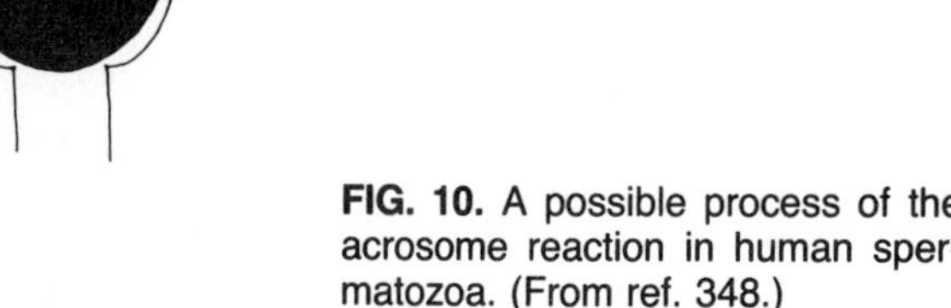

FIG. 10. A possible process of the acrosome reaction in human spermatozoa. (From ref. 348.)

in human spermatozoa, which is somewhat different from that of the "typical" acrosome reaction (compare with Fig. 9), although the end result is the same. Although I am one of the co-authors of the article that originally presented this diagram (348), I am not completely convinced that this reaction pattern represents the true (physiological) acrosome reaction of human spermatozoa. Until we examine the acrosome reaction in human spermatozoa in the act of fertilizing living human eggs, this diagram should be viewed with reservation.

How Fast Is the Acrosome Reaction?

The speed of the acrosome reaction is probably dependent on species as well as sperm's condition and environment. When guinea-pig spermatozoa are capacitated in a Ca^{2+}-deficient medium and then exposed to Ca^{2+}, the acrosome reaction is initiated and completed by many spermatozoa within 2 min (547). When hamster spermatozoa are capacitated in a K^+-deficient medium and then exposed to K^+ and nigericin (K^+/H^+ ionophore), many spermatozoa initiate and complete the acrosome reaction within 15 min (338). Ohzu and Yanagimachi (354) have found that hamster spermatozoa preincubated for 1 to 2 hr in a normal capacitating medium can initiate and complete the acrosome reaction within 2 min of exposure to a low concentration of lysolecithin (50 μg/ml). According to Motomura and Toyoda (335), mouse spermatozoa preincubated in a capacitating medium for 1 hr (presumably capacitated) penetrate through zonae pellucidae of 15% of mouse eggs by 11 min after *in vitro* insemination; by the end of the next 4 and 9 min, zonae pellucidae of 54% and 80% of the eggs are penetrated, respectively. Although Motomura and Toyoda did not examine the status of the acrosomes of these spermatozoa, it is very likely that the spermatozoa had "intact" acrosomes when they first contacted the zona. At least some of spermatozoa must have initiated and completed the acrosome reaction within 10 to 15 min of contact with the zona. Cherr et al. (103) have found that many capacitated hamster spermatozoa complete the acrosome reaction within 10 to 15 min of contact with intact or solubilized zonae pellucidae of the hamster, but not with those of the mouse. All of these facts seem to indicate that once the spermatozoa are capacitated and receive the proper signals or stimuli, they undergo the reaction rather promptly.

Natural Inducer(s) of the Acrosome Reaction

In the sea urchin, the egg is surrounded by a thin glycoprotein coat called the *vitelline layer,* which is further surrounded by a thick jelly coat. The vitelline layer is homologous to the zona pellucida of mammalian eggs. The jelly may correspond to the cumulus oophorus of the mammal. In many species of the sea urchin, the acrosome reaction takes place when spermatozoa contact the jelly or while the spermatozoa are passing through it. Biochemically, the jelly is a mixture of glycoproteins and a fucose sulfate polymer. The acrosome reaction-inducing activity is in the fucose sulfate-rich fraction (see ref. 301 for a review). No one knows exactly how the jelly material triggers the acrosome reaction. Dan et al. (126) proposed that the binding of the active jelly components to the acceptor proteins in the sperm plasma membrane causes a conformational change of the plasma membrane, which allows a temporal increase in membrane permeability to external Ca^{2+}.

In some species of the sea urchin, spermatozoa do not undergo their acrosome reaction while they are swimming in the jelly. Only those that have come into contact with the vitelline layer undergo the reaction (10). Eggs of some other marine invertebrates (e.g., an annelid, *Hyroides,* and an enteropneust, *Saccoglossus*) do not have distinct jelly coats. The acrosome reaction in such species takes place on the surface of the vitelline layer (106). Vitelline layers of these eggs must contain molecules capable of inducing the acrosome reaction.

What is the natural inducer of the acrosome reaction of mammalian spermatozoa? It appears to be the cumulus and/or the zona pellucida. When females are mated (or artificially inseminated) and the spermatozoa are collected from the ampullary region of the oviducts when fertilization is in progress, all or the vast majority of spermatozoa swimming freely in the ampullary fluid have unreacted acrosomes (24,90,120,382,461,545). Spermatozoa swimming within the cumulus have either unreacted, reacting, or reacted acrosomes (24,43,120,461,542,545). Most or all of the spermatozoa on the zona surface have reacting or reacted acrosomes.

There is no doubt that the zona pellucida has the ability to induce the acrosome reaction (see ref. 316 for a review). Even solubilized zona materials can induce the reaction very efficiently (68,103,162,373). According to Bleil and Wassarman (69), one of three mouse zona glycoproteins, ZP3, binds to the plasma membrane over the acrosomal cap. The polypeptide chain in ZP3 molecules seems to function as inducer of the acrosome reaction (506).

Whether the cumulus oophorus has the ability to induce the acrosome reaction is still controversial. The presence of the cumulus is certainly beneficial for fertilization of mouse and hamster eggs in albumin-free media (33,171), but it is not clear whether this is due to the cumulus' ability to induce or stimulate the acrosome reaction. Although there are several reports that cumulus or cumulus components (477,511,539) and glycosaminoglycans (215,293,322) stimulate or support the acrosome reaction, there has been no unequivocal evidence that the cumulus or cumulus components *induce* the acrosome reaction. It is possible that the cumulus components initiate the very early stage of the acrosome reaction, and those components associated with the zona act synergistically with the zona molecules to complete the reaction (103).

Whatever the natural acrosome reaction-inducing substances are, it is obvious that they are not the only substances capable of inducing the acrosome reaction. In the sea urchin, for instance, the acrosome reaction can be induced very efficiently by a variety of physical and chemical agents (124,125,225,428). It is well known that mammalian spermatozoa can undergo the acrosome reaction in the total absence of the egg and egg-associated materials (e.g., the cumulus oophorus and the zona pellucida). Any conditions or agents that directly or indirectly alter the permeability to ions (e.g., Ca^{2+} and Na^{+}) of the plasma membrane over the acrosomal cap of "capacitated" spermatozoa must be able to trigger the acrosome reaction.

Mechanism of the Acrosome Reaction

Since many reviews dealing with the mechanism of the acrosome reaction in mammalian spermatozoa are already available (e.g., refs 104,154,170,194,217,227,283,314, 315,316,329,530), it is unnecessary to present here another comprehensive review.

The mechanism of the acrosome reaction has been studied extensively in marine invertebrates, particularly the sea urchin (for reviews, see refs. 301,428, and 441). The spermatozoa of the sea urchin, unlike those of mammals, do not require capacitation. They are ready to fertilize eggs upon leaving the male's body. In most species of sea urchins, spermatozoa undergo the acrosome reaction in the jelly surrounding the egg. According to a working model presented by Shapiro et al. (441), egg jelly interacts with a putative sperm plasma membrane receptor to initiate two parallel pathways. One of them is a Ca^{2+}-independent pathway leading to an increased intracellular pH via Na^{+} influx and H^{+} efflux. Another pathway is a Ca^{2+}-dependent membrane depolarization. Both the membrane depolarization and the increase in intracellular pH open Ca^{2+} channels, resulting in a massive influx of extracellular Ca^{2+}. The Ca^{2+} that has penetrated through the plasma membrane induces the fusion between the plasma and outer acrosomal membranes, culminating in an exocytosis of acrosomal contents and an elongation of the inner acrosomal membrane (in the case of mammals, the inner acrosomal membrane does not change its gross morphology during and after the acrosome reaction). Although intracellular cAMP concentration of sea urchin spermatozoa increases dramatically under the conditions that allow the acrosome reaction (180), the precise relationship between intracellular cAMP and the acrosome reaction is not clear (301,428). The jelly is the natural inducer of the acrosome reaction of sea-urchin spermatozoa, but it is not the only substance capable of eliciting the reaction. A variety of conditions or reagents can induce the reaction very efficiently (301,428).

Table 3 lists molecules reported to control or influence mammalian sperm acrosome reaction. There is a possibility that some of these molecules affect capacitation rather than the acrosome reaction per se. There have been many articles reporting that certain conditions or reagents enhanced or blocked the acrosome reaction because the incidence of the acrosome reaction was increased or reduced when freshly ejaculated or epididymal spermatozoa were incubated under particular conditions or in the presence of particular reagents. What was affected could have been the acrosome

TABLE 3. *Molecules reported to be involved in the acrosome reaction, excluding components of female genital tract secretory products, cumulus oophorus, and zona pellucida*

Molecules	References[a]
Extracellular[b]	
H^{+}	245, 249, 338, 346, 519
Ca^{2+}	47, 57, 193, 448, 474, 547
Na^{+}	58, 245, 247, 249, 345
K^{+}	62, 245, 247, 338, 519
HCO_3^{-}	70, 245, 288
Glucose/pyruvate/lactate	34, 134, 167, 172, 325, 343
Albumin	183, 255, 283, 303, 304, 325, 377, 526
Sperm membrane	
Intramembranous proteins	36, 155, 176, 546
SS/SH in proteins	156, 537
Anionic phospholipids	36
Cholesterol	36, 129, 158, 183, 284
Fatty acids (including arachidonic)	160, 320, 321
Lysophospholipids	158, 298, 354
Na^{+}, K^{+}-ATPase	15, 78, 339, 341
Ca^{2+}/Mg^{2+}-dependent ATPases	15, 78, 189, 430, 492, 518, 547
Phospholipases A_2 and C	158, 283, 297, 305, 366, 479, 480
Lysophopholipase	282, 442
Intracellular	
Ca^{2+}	57, 508
Cyclic nucleotide/ adenylate cyclase/ protein kinase system	167, 237, 248, 282, 337, 416, 429
Calmodulin	257, 521
Unidentified Ca^{2+}-binding molecule	398, 419, 508
Calpain II	435
Cytoskeletal system (including actin)	364, 435, 473, 501
Intra-acrosomal[c]	
Proteinases (including acrosin)	133, 187, 195, 239, 242, 305, 318, 388
Cathepsin D	456
H^{+}	239, 317
Natural acrosin inhibitors	59, 184, 553

[a]See Meizel (314–316) and Fraser (170) for additional references.

[b]Including influx and efflux through the plasma membrane.

[c]Controlling the proacrosin/acrosin status and the dispersion of acrosomal matrix.

reaction indeed, but it could also have been capacitation, which precedes the acrosome reaction. Readers should keep this in mind when reading these original articles.

There is no doubt that Ca^+ influx is an essential step of mammalian sperm acrosome reaction. However, Ca^{2+} influx alone is not enough to elicit the reaction. It is very likely that almost all components of the plasma and outer acrosomal membranes, as well as materials (including ions) present inside and outside of these membranes, are directly or indirectly involved in the reaction. Diagrams of molecular events of the acrosome reaction, as presented by Yanagimachi (530) and Langlais and Roberts (283), are obviously too simple to explain what is really going on during the reaction. To stimulate readers (and invite criticism), I will present here another working model of the mammalian sperm acrosome reaction.

To undergo the acrosome reaction at the right time and place, spermatozoa must survive long enough. Maintaining a high intracellular K^+ concentration and low intracellular Na^+ and Ca^{2+} concentrations must be important for the survival of spermatozoa as well as protecting spermatozoa from a premature acrosome reaction. This must be accomplished, at least in part, by membrane-bound Na^+-K^+ ATPase (pumping Na^+ out of and K^+ into the cell) and Ca^{2+}-ATPase (pumping Ca^{2+} out of the cell). During capacitation, macromolecular sperm surface coats are either removed or altered so that intrinsic (integral) membrane proteins (including putative "zona or cumulus receptors" in the sperm plasma membrane over the acrosome) are "exposed." Alteration or removal of the coat gives intrinsic membrane proteins the ability to move more freely within lipid bilayers. The lipid bilayers themselves change their molecular organization during capacitation by endogenous and exogenous factors. Albumin could be one of the exogenous factors responsible for the reorganization of membrane lipids. When capacitated spermatozoa come into contact with the cumulus or the zona, the glycosaminoglycans of the cumulus or the glycoproteins of the zona bind to the putative receptors. These "zona or cumulus receptors" could be Ca^{2+}-carrier proteins. Activated receptors facilitate the diffusion of extracellular Ca^{2+}. A massive influx of Ca^{2+} inactivates Na^+-K^+ ATPase, resulting in a rapid increase in intracellular Na^+. This causes an efflux of H^+ (through Na^+/H^+ antiporter), resulting in a rise in intracellular pH. The Ca^{2+} that has penetrated through the plasma membrane acts, with or without participation of calmodulin, on both the plasma membrane (from inside) and the outer acrosomal membrane (from outside). Ca^{2+} facilitates the fusion between two membranes by binding to anionic phospholipids and inducing phase separation of membrane phospholipids. Ca^{2+} also activates membrane phospholipases. Activated phospholipases attack nearby phospholipids to yield fusiogenic products (e.g., arachidonic acid and lysophospholipids). When the membranes are about to fuse or have fused with each other, Ca^{2+} enters and H^+ leaves the acrosome matrix. This causes the conversion of proacrosin to enzymatically active acrosin, which disperses the acrosomal matrix containing other enzymes.

Like sea-urchin spermatozoa, mammalian spermatozoa can undergo the acrosome reaction without any contribution from the egg or egg-associated materials. Spermatozoa of many mammalian species begin the acrosome reaction spontaneously in sperm-capacitating media. This could be due to either (a) spontaneous activation of the putative zona or cumulus receptors or Ca^{2+}-carrier proteins in the sperm plasma membrane or (b) inactivation of Ca^{2+}-pumping mechanism (Ca^{2+}-ATPase). In moribund or dead spermatozoa, intracellular ions would leak out and external ions would penetrate freely into the cells (due to weakened or inactivated ATPases). Proacrosin within the acrosome would be converted to acrosin, which would digest the acrosomal matrix. Acrosin and other acrosomal enzymes would attack sperm membranes, resulting in the partial or total disappearance of acrosomal caps (the so-called "false" acrosome reaction).

Since the acrosome reaction is a membrane fusion event, we must learn much more about the physical and biochemical characteristics of sperm membranes in order to fully understand the mechanisms involved in the reaction. In the past, we have collected a considerably large body of information about the structure and biochemical characteristics of the plasma membrane (for reviews, see refs. 175,265, and 391). In contrast, we know very little about the outer acrosomal membrane, which is obviously as important as (or even more important than) the plasma membrane in the acrosome reaction. Although there were attempts to isolate and characterize the outer acrosomal membranes (see, e.g., refs. 331,344, and 551), it was not until recently that it became possible to obtain fairly pure preparations of the membrane (cf. refs. 365 and 484). What we have learned about the outer acrosomal membrane to date includes: (a) molecular weight of its proteins (365,485), (b) its immunogenicity (226,483), (c) its lectin-binding property (5,365,482), (d) the density and distribution of its anionic sites (5,145), (e) the density and distribution of its sterol (174,498), (f) its fluidity (498), and (g) its Ca^{2+}-binding property (57,398,419,508). We must be aware that most information about the outer acrosomal membrane is still very preliminary. It is hoped that we will have a unified view of the mechanism of the acrosome reaction in the near future by learning more about physical and biochemical properties of the plasma and outer acrosomal membranes as well as of the materials associated with the membranes.

HYPERACTIVATION OF SPERMATOZOA

Spermatozoa of some species begin to move very actively before undergoing the acrosome reaction. I originally called this "activation" of spermatozoa (527), and later proposed to rename it "hyperactivation" (530) because the term "activation" had been already used to refer to the initiation of active movement by epididymal or vas deferens spermatozoa when they come into contact with seminal plasma or physiological salt solutions.

The golden hamster is the species in which the phenomenon of hyperactivation was first recognized (524,526). The spermatozoa of this species, like those of most other species, are either motionless or only very weakly motile when they are in the epididymis and vas deferens. They begin to move actively upon contact with capacitating media. Soon, most of them aggulutinate in a head-to-head fashion (cf. Fig. 6-1a of ref. 531). The spermatozoa remain agglutinated for a few hours, beating their tails actively, but rather stiffly. Then, spermatozoa break free from these agglutinated masses to swim freely. This is when the spermatozoa move much more actively than ever before. At first, they swim in a linear fashion, but soon begin to display a unique movement characterized by very vigorous, whiplash-like beatings of the tail, with the sperm head tracing an erratic figure 8. This nonprogressive ("dancing") movement is intermitted by a brief linear ("dashing") movement. These two types of movements are cumulatively called *hyperactivation*.

The manner of hyperactivated movement is probably not the same in all species. In the golden hamster and guinea pig, the entire tail flexes very vigorously during the dancing movement (cf. Figs. 11 and 12 of ref. 530), but in the case of the Chinese hamster, only the anterior (midpiece) region of the tail flexes, with the posterior part of the tail remaining almost stiff (539). It is unknown at present whether hyperactivation is limited to just certain species or is a general phenomenon in all mammals, but the number of species in which hyperactivation has been recognized is increasing steadily. They include: mouse (14,109,166,167), bat (277), rabbit (108,254,461), dolphin (161), dog (310), sheep (118,439), cattle (449), pig (349), rhesus monkey (70), and human (92,332).

Hyperactivated motility of spermatozoa, as seen *in vitro*, is apparently physiological because spermatozoa displaying hyperactivated motility can be seen through the wall of the oviductal ampulla about the time of fertilization (261, 527). Many hyperactivated spermatozoa have been collected from ampullae of the rabbit (108), guinea pig (540), and sheep (118) about the time of fertilization.

Where do spermatozoa *in vivo* begin their hyperactivated movement? In the rabbit, all the spermatozoa in the oviductal isthmus are weakly motile (93,380), whereas most spermatozoa in the ampulla are hyperactivated (461). Thus, at least in the rabbit, spermatozoa seem to initiate their hyperactivated movement sometime (perhaps soon) after they are released from the isthmus.

This hyperactivated motility obviously provides the spermatozoa with strong thrusting power. It seems to be beneficial, not only for the migration of spermatozoa from the isthmus to the ampulla (383) but also for sperm passage through the egg investments, particularly the relatively "hard" zona pellucida (262,530). The existence of a close correlation between hyperactivated motility of spermatozoa and the sperm's ability to cross the zona has been reported (159,172) (Table 4). The possible relationships between hyperactivation, capacitation, and the acrosome reaction have been discussed (503).

The components of the medium obviously influence the initiation and maintenance of hyperactivated motility of spermatozoa. Ca^{2+}, for example, is essential for initiation of hyperactivation of guinea-pig, hamster, and mouse spermatozoa (14,109,166,168,532,547). HCO_3^- seems to be necessary for hyperactivation of hamster spermatozoa (70). K^+ (93,169), energy substrates (93,109,134,172,530), and albumin (171,527) are all known to control or modulate hyperactivation of mouse, hamster, guinea-pig, and rabbit spermatozoa. There is circumstantial evidence that the level of intracellular cAMP controls hyperactivation of hamster and mouse spermatozoa (71,109,167,326).

We know virtually nothing of the molecular basis of hy-

TABLE 4. *The ability of acrosome-reacted guinea-pig spermatozoa to fertilize zona-intact and zona-free eggs*[a]

Age (hours) of acrosome-reacted sperm at insemination	% Acrosome-reacted sperm (in entire population) which are: Motile	Hyperactivated	% Eggs fertilized: Zona-intact	Zona-free
1	100	95	100	—
2	96	66	98	—
3	92	39	33	—
4	90	6	0	100
6	57	0	0	—
8	—	—	—	94
10	0	0	—	0

[a]From Flemming and Yanagimachi (159). Guinea-pig spermatozoa were induced to undergo a synchronous acrosome reaction. A population of 100% acrosome-reacted spermatozoa was isolated and incubated for up to 10 hr before they were mixed with zona-intact or zona-free guinea-pig eggs. Note that (a) there is a close correlation between hyperactivated motility of spermatozoa and the ability of spermatozoa to fertilize zona-intact eggs (to cross the zona) and (b) spermatozoa retain their ability to fuse with zona-free eggs for many hours after losing their ability to cross the zona.

peractivation. Since some macromolecules covering the surface of tail plasma membrane are removed or altered during capacitation (495), we can expect that the physical and chemical characteristics of the tail plasma membrane change as capacitation progresses. According to Koehler and Gaddum-Rosse (268) and Friend (173), intramembranous protein particles in the tail plasma membrane of hyperactivated guinea-pig spermatozoa are less orderly arranged than those in prehyperactivated spermatozoa. The tail plasma membrane of hyperactivated mouse spermatozoa has a higher "fluidity" than that of prehyperactivated spermatozoa (514). This indicates that there are alterations of the physical and chemical characteristics of the tail membrane lipids during capacitation of spermatozoa. Methylation of membrane phospholipids could be one of the membrane lipid alterations occurring during capacitation (298). Methylation of membrane phospholipids is known to facilitate the entry of Ca^{2+} into cells (228). An increased Ca^{2+} entry into the sperm plasma membrane may stimulate membrane-bound adenylate cyclase, resulting in an increased intracellular concentration of cAMP. Both intracellular Ca^{2+} and cAMP are known to be important regulators of sperm tail movement (475). As mentioned already, prehyperactivated spermatozoa beat their tails rather stiffly, whereas hyperactivated spermatozoa flex their tails very pliantly. Apparently, hyperactivated spermatozoa are relieved from the rigidity (stiffness) of the tail. This could be due to "softening" of the outer coarse fibers by Mg-ATP (413). The fact that hyperactivated spermatozoa repeat the "dancing" (pliant) and "dashing" (less pliant) movements alternately may be explained by attachment of Mg-ATP to the fibers (softening the fibers) and its detachment from the fibers (stiffening the fibers).

SPERM PENETRATION THROUGH THE EGG INVESTMENTS

All mammalian eggs are surrounded by investments through which spermatozoa must pass before fusing with the egg proper (vitellus). The zona pellucida, the innermost investment lying immediately above the vitellus, is a relatively thick, elastic coat composed of several major glycoproteins (for reviews, see refs. 137 and 141). In most eutherian mammals, the zona is surrounded by the cumulus oophorus during natural fertilization *in vivo*. The cumulus is composed of both cellular and acellular components. Carbohydrates (including hyaluronic acid) and proteins are major constituents of the acellular component (matrix) of the cumulus (74,396). In some ungulates (e.g., sheep and cow), monotremes, and marsupials, the cumulus is shed either shortly before or after ovulation (63,414). In such cases, the zona is (or could be) the only egg investment the spermatozoa must pass through before reaching the egg plasma membrane.

How do spermatozoa pass through the cumulus and the zona? Since the acrosome of mammalian spermatozoa contains powerful enzymes capable of hydrolyzing the cumulus matrix and the zona pellucida, it has been the most common belief that spermatozoa utilize these enzymes during their passage through these structures. It is now clear that we must reevaluate the roles of acrosomal enzymes in this biological process very carefully (for discussion, see refs. 197,329, and 468).

Sperm Penetration Through the Cumulus Oophorus

It was once thought that many spermatozoa swam around each egg in order to loosen or disperse the cumulus, so that one of the spermatozoa could penetrate into the egg. Although this can happen when we inseminate eggs *in vitro* with many spermatozoa, perhaps this is not the way spermatozoa fertilize the eggs *in vivo*. Under ordinary *in vivo* conditions, very few spermatozoa are present near the eggs during fertilization (for references, see ref. 533). In many mammals, the eggs are fertilized *after*, not before, the cumulus disperses from egg surfaces (16,63). Zamboni (552), who studied fertilization of mouse eggs *in vivo*, stated that ". . . the number of sperm at the site of fertilization is always lower than the total number of eggs and that it is only after all the eggs have been penetrated that it becomes equal to or slightly higher than the latter." This is true for the golden hamster (120). During the early phase of *in vivo* fertilization of hamster eggs, we often do not see spermatozoa within the ampullary lumen or the cumulus oophorus, yet we see spermatozoa *within* some of the eggs (T. Smith and R. Yanagimachi, *unpublished observation*). Sperm-egg encounter in the ampulla is obviously very efficient.

Austin (19) was the first to report that spermatozoa must be capacitated to penetrate into the cumulus. Uncapacitated spermatozoa (of the rabbit, rat, and mouse) may attach to the surface of the cumulus, but they fail to penetrate into it. Capacitated spermatozoa, on the other hand, move freely within the cumulus. This has been confirmed in the hamster (121,462,467,468). Interestingly, spermatozoa that have completed their acrosome reactions before meeting the cumulus stick to the surface of the cumulus and do not penetrate into it (121,462,468). Only capacitated spermatozoa that retain their acrosomal caps are able to enter the cumulus.

How do the capacitated spermatozoa pass through the cumulus to reach the surface of the zona pellucida? Are the acrosome reaction and acrosomal enzymes involved in this process? According to recent studies by Talbot (467) and Cherr et al. (103), most capacitated hamster spermatozoa penetrate through the cumulus without undergoing the acrosome reaction. According to Talbot et al. (472), sea-urchin and frog spermatozoa, which do not possess any hyaluronidase, penetrate the hamster cumulus with great ease. I have observed that rooster spermatozoa (known to be lacking in hyaluronidase; cf. ref. 311) penetrate through the hamster cumulus without any difficulties (R. Yanagimachi, *unpublished observation*). Do these observations indicate that spermatozoa pass through the cumulus without any aid from acrosomal enzymes? What about hyaluronidase, which has been thought to be the "cumulus lysin" for many years? Is the cumulus penetration by spermatozoa purely mechanical? Talbot (468) and Talbot et al. (472) are of the opinion that hyaluronidase is not essential for cumulus penetration, but that it does facilitate it. Talbot (468) and Zao et al. (554) speculate that the surface (the plasma membrane) of hamster spermatozoa carries hyaluronidase, which, in part, originates from the male genital tract, and that this surface hyaluronidase, not acrosomal hyaluronidase, aids in sperm passage through the cumulus oophorus. The notion that hyaluronidase that is bound to the sperm or sperm surface assists cumulus penetration by spermatozoa is not new (13,260,294,295,323). It is an intriguing notion, but to date there is no unequivocal evidence to support this. The possibilities that part of the acrosomal enzymes escape through the outer acrosomal and plasma membranes prior to their fenestration (348,465) and that enzymes other than hyaluronidase are part of the cumulus lysins (148) should not be ignored.

It is somewhat surprising that the exact function of hyaluronidase in fertilization is still the subject of controversy today. This was the first sperm enzyme identified and characterized more than 40 years ago. Lorton and First (302) maintain that bovine sperm hyaluronidase has no biological function because (a) hyaluronidase is unable to disperse the bovine cumulus oophorus surrounding ovarian eggs, and (b) oviductal eggs shed the cumulus spontaneously within a few hours after ovulation. These investigators inferred that "this acrosomal enzyme is not functional in this species, but is a remnant of evolutional changes." I do not agree with this inference. The inability of hyaluronidase to disperse the cumuli around ovarian eggs is not unique to this species. The cumuli of ovarian eggs of many other species are resistant to hyaluronidase. The expansion of the cumulus (synthesis and assembly of hyaluronic acid complex) may not be completed until shortly before ovulation (cf. ref. 146). According to Brackett et al. (73), oviductal bovine eggs, immediately after ovulation, are surrounded by the cumulus oophorus. Since bovine eggs are probably fertilized immediately after ovulation, sperm hyaluronidase might function in depolymerizing hyaluronic acid of the cumulus matrix. Hyaluronidase may also play a role in zona penetration by spermatozoa (see below).

Inhibition of fertilization by antihyaluronidase antibodies (139,259,323,387,406) has been reported. Although the site of action of the antibodies and inhibitors could be the zona rather than the cumulus in some cases (387), it might be the cumulus in other cases (259,406). Cummins and Yanagimachi (121) have found that Myocrisin (= Na-aurothiomalate, a hyaluronidase inhibitor) inhibits cumulus-dispersing action of hyaluronidase and prevents the entry of capacitated hamster spermatozoa into the cumulus, without apparent effect on the motility of spermatozoa. In the presence of this inhibitor, capacitated spermatozoa were very "sticky" to the cumulus surface and unable to enter the cumulus. Although Myocrisin may not be an inhibitor specific to hyaluronidase, there is still a strong possibility that hyaluronidase is involved in cumulus penetration by spermatozoa. Hyaluronidase may serve as a "lubricant" for spermatozoa entering and passing through the cumulus matrix. Whether this lubricant is on the plasma membrane, escaping through the membrane over the acrosome, or being released through fenestrated membranes is a matter of conjecture. According to Kusan et al. (274), rabbit spermatozoa recovered from the perivitelline space of fertilized eggs (believed to be acrosome-reacted) are able to penetrate cumuli and zonae of other eggs. If hyaluronidase is needed for cumulus penetration, it could be the hyaluronidase bound to the surface of acrosome-reacted spermatozoa which renders the spermatozoa capable of penetrating the cumulus.

Sperm Attachment to, and Penetration into, the Zona Pellucida: Background

Chemical Characteristics of the Zona Pellucida

The zona pellucida is a sulfated glycoprotein. The overall chemical composition of the pig zona, for example, includes 71% protein, 19% neutral hexose, 2.7% sialic acid, and 2.4% sulfate (140). Several different families of glycoproteins have been identified in zonae of various species. The pig zona, for example, has four different families of glycoproteins: ZP 1 (82,000 MW), ZP 2 (61,000 MW), ZP 3 (55,000 MW), and ZP 4 (21,000 MW) (cf. ref. 422). The mouse zona has three: ZP 1 (200,000 MW), ZP 2 (120,000 MW), and ZP 3 (83,000 MW) (cf. ref. 198). The hamster zona also has three; ZP 1 (240,000 MW), ZP 2 (150,000 MW), and ZP 3 (80,000 MW) (cf. ref. 8). It should be noted that different molecular weights for each glycoprotein have been reported, even by investigators working on the zona of same species. Discrepancies could be a result of the different techniques employed. The structural integrity of the zona seems to be maintained by noncovalent forces (67,141,198,347,443), although there are some intermolecular disulfide bonds (198). How different glycoprotein families are distributed in the zona is not completely known, but ZP 2 glycoprotein of mouse zona, for example, is known to be distributed throughout the thickness of the zona (143a). In the pig, ZP 1, ZP 2, and ZP 3 glycoproteins are all on the external surface of the zona (221). When examined by scanning electron microscopy, the outer surfaces of the zona has a fenestrated, lattice-like appearance, whereas the inner surface of the zona has an irregular particulated appearance (392). Hyaluronic acid, the major component of the cumulus oophorus, is inserted into the outer fenestrated region of the zona (cf. ref. 470).

It has been the general belief that the chemical composition of the zona does not change throughout oocyte maturation or even after ovulation. According to Fowler and

Grainge (164), however, the zona (of mouse eggs) loses glycosaminoglycans several hours before ovulation. There is convincing evidence that glycoproteins of the oviductal origin are added to zonae of pig and hamster eggs after the eggs are transported from the ovary to the oviduct (87,165, 222,355,459,505).

It is well known that in many species the properties of the zona pellucida change drastically upon fertilization such that excess spermatozoa are unable to penetrate through it. This is the so-called *zona reaction* (23,515). It is a cortical granule-mediated modification of zona material (31,203). In the mouse, partial hydrolysis of ZP 2 and ZP 3 glycoproteins by cortical granule proteinase is believed to be responsible for this reaction (66,506,507). It is important to note that the strong zona reaction does not occur in all mammalian species. In some species (e.g., rabbit, pika, and mole), the zona remains penetrable by excess spermatozoa for many hours after the first spermatozoon has entered the egg (20), although some chemical properties of the zona are altered, possibly by cortical granule materials, after fertilization (191).

Time Course of Sperm Attachment to, and Penetration into, the Zona

When eggs are collected from oviducts of naturally mated females while fertilization is in progress, one seldom encounters eggs with spermatozoa within the zona pellucida. Sperm passage through the zona must be a very rapid process (17,64). Austin (17) estimated that the rat spermatozoon probably takes no more than a few minutes to pass through the zona. According to Sato and Blandau (432), who continuously observed sperm penetration through the zona pellucida of the mouse inseminated *in vitro,* spermatozoa took an average of 20 min (ranging from 15 min to 26 min) to cross the zona. This cannot be considered fast. If spermatozoa *in vivo* take more than 15 min to cross the zona, one should be able to see spermatozoa within zonae rather frequently when eggs are examined about the time of fertilization. Since this is not the case, it is possible that the *in vitro* conditions Sato and Blandau employed were not completely comparable to *in vivo* conditions.

The point in time when spermatozoa begin to penetrate eggs *in vitro* seems to be influenced greatly by the physiological state of spermatozoa. For instance, when golden hamster spermatozoa are collected from the cauda epididymis and mixed immediately with eggs in capacitation medium, many acrosome-intact spermatozoa are seen firmly attached to zona surface soon after insemination. The acrosome reaction of these spermatozoa begins sometime thereafter, and sperm penetration into the eggs occurs commonly between 3 and 4 hr after insemination (542). When hamster spermatozoa are "precapacitated" prior to mixing with the eggs, sperm penetration into the zona can be seen as early as 10 min after insemination, but most spermatozoa do not begin to penetrate into the zona earlier than 30 min after insemination (524). In other words, most spermatozoa spend 30 min or more before they begin to enter the zona. According to Yang et al. (548), who examined hamster spermatozoa within cumuli of eggs collected from oviducts about the time of fertilization, spermatozoa took an average of only 7 min and 3 sec from the moment of their attachment to the zona surface to completion of sperm-head penetration through the zona. Apparently, hamster spermatozoa capacitated *in vivo* penetrate the zona much faster than those capacitated *in vitro*. According to Storey et al. (460), "capacitated" mouse spermatozoa mixed with cumulus-intact eggs *in vitro* remain attached to the surface of the zonae for at least 2 hr without undergoing the acrosome reaction. Zona penetration seldom takes place before 2 hr after insemination. According to Motomura and Toyoda (335), however, "capacitated" mouse spermatozoa penetrate the zona much faster. According to them, heads of some spermatozoa are already within the zona by 5 min after insemination. The zonae of 15% of the eggs are completely penetrated by sperm heads at 11 min after insemination. By 20 min after insemination, the zonae of 80% of the eggs have been penetrated completely. Thus, the speed of sperm penetration into and through the zona seems to be influenced greatly by the condition of spermatozoa (how well they are capacitated) as well as the condition of external milieu of the gametes. At least in the hamster and mouse, well-capacitated spermatozoa do not seem to spend much time on or in the zona as long as they are in the most favorable environment.

Sperm Attachment to the Zona Pellucida

Zona's Sperm Receptor

Fertilizing spermatozoa attach firmly (bind) to the surface of the zona pellucida before penetrating into it. That this strong sperm-zona binding is mediated by the interaction between zona and sperm surface molecules was demonstrated first by Gwatkin and Williams (202), who reported that the presence of solubilized zonae pellucidae (of the hamster) in the fertilization medium prevents capacitated spermatozoa from binding to the surface of native zonae. The solubilized zonae apparently do not affect the motility of spermatozoa. Why are the spermatozoa unable to bind to the zona in the presence of solubilized zonae? It would be reasonable to assume that the surface of spermatozoa carries receptors for zona molecules and that saturation of these receptors with zona molecules renders the spermatozoa incapable of binding to ("recognizing") native zonae. There is no doubt that sperm membranes carry proteins (or glycoproteins) with strong affinity to zona molecules (372,463).

The chemical nature of zona molecules responsible for sperm-zona binding has been studied most extensively in the mouse. According to Wassarman and his associates (for further references, see refs. 69,507, and 508), it is the glycoproteins ZP 3 and ZP 2, not ZP 1, that have sperm-binding (sperm-receptor) activities. ZP 3 is the "primary" sperm receptor, which binds to spermatozoa prior to the acrosome reaction. ZP 2 is the "secondary" sperm receptor, which binds to spermatozoa after the acrosome reaction. ZP 3 has both sperm-receptor and acrosome reaction-inducing activities. The O-linked saccharide moiety of ZP 3 is responsible for the sperm-receptor activity, whereas its polypeptide moiety is apparently involved in the acrosome reaction-inducing function of this glycoprotein.

Sperm's Zona Receptor

There have been many articles reporting that freshly ejaculated spermatozoa, or spermatozoa collected from the epididymis, bind to zonae of eggs of homologous or heterologous species (see ref. 218 for further references). Apparently, uncapacitated spermatozoa and, in some cases, even immature spermatozoa from the epididymis are able to attach firmly to zonae. Does this mean that sperm's zona receptors are assembled on the sperm surface and ready to interact with the zona long before spermatozoa are ready to fertilize eggs? As stated previously, at least some of sperm-surface-coating materials are removed or modified extensively during capacitation. Under natural *in vivo* conditions, perhaps only fully capacitated spermatozoa meet the zona. Therefore, until it becomes clear that the zona receptors of uncapacitated spermatozoa are identical with those of capacitated spermatozoa, we should be cautious in interpreting the results of experiments using uncapacitated spermatozoa to detect, isolate, and identify sperm's zona receptors.

There is no reason to believe that the sperm surface becomes completely free of the glycoprotein coat after completion of capacitation. The presence of lectin-binding materials on the head plasma membrane of capacitated spermatozoa (188,263) and on the plasma and inner acrosomal membranes of acrosome-reacted spermatozoa (263,529) indicates that the plasma and inner acrosomal membranes retain at least some of the peripheral glycoproteins (and perhaps most of the integral glycoproteins) during capacitation and the acrosome reaction. It is unknown at the present time whether sperm's zona receptors are protein, glycoprotein, or components of glycoprotein. Some investigators (6,7,278,280) maintain that the glycoprotein's terminal saccharides (e.g., *N*-acetyl-D-glucosamine, mannose, fucose, galactose, and sialic acid) have receptor activities. Some other investigators maintain that sperm membrane proteins have zona-receptor activities (372,389,463). A fucose-binding protein on the plasma membrane of boar spermatozoa (482) could be one of such zona-receptor proteins. Others have suggested that proteins with glycotransferase activities (7,300,445) or with proteinase activities (136,201,423) may serve as sperm's zona receptors. Urch and Hedrick (489) have proposed that peptides produced by autocatalysis of acrosin may serve as sperm's zona receptors.

Where are the sperm's zona receptors located? Before answering this question, we must discuss the structure with which spermatozoa make their contact with the zona. Storey and his associates maintain that in the mouse it is the plasma membrane over the acrosome (162,426,427). According to Saling and Storey (427), only acrosome-intact spermatozoa can attach firmly (bind) to zona surfaces. Acrosome-reacted spermatozoa, which have lost the plasma membrane over the acrosomal cap, are unable to bind the zona. In other words, the plasma membrane over the acrosomal cap is the likely site of the zona receptors. However, one must be aware that the assay method Saling and Storey used ("washing" eggs through Dextran gradient using centrifugal force) may have removed acrosome-reacted spermatozoa that were weakly bound to zona surfaces. In the golden hamster, both acrosome-intact and acrosome-reacted spermatozoa can attach to the zona surface (462,530). In other words, zona receptors of hamster spermatozoa must not only be on the plasma membrane over the acrosomal cap, but also on the plasma membrane of other areas of the sperm head and/or the inner acrosomal membrane. In the guinea pig, the acrosome-reacted spermatozoa, not the acrosome-intact ones, firmly bind to the zona (238). In this species, the principal site of the zona receptor could be on both the inner acrosomal membrane and the plasma membrane over the equatorial segment (240). Yanagimachi (530) has suggested the possibility that an insoluble, "sticky" component of the acrosomal matrix, which holds the fenestrated membranes of acrosome-reacted mammalian spermatozoa, could be analogous to the "bindin" (301,493) of sea urchin spermatozoa. Both sea urchins' bindin and the sticky components of mammalian sperm acrosomal matrix serve for holding acrosome-reacted or -reacting spermatozoa to the vitelline coat (see Figs. 4–6 of ref. 336) or to the zona pellucida (Figs. 18 and 19 of ref. 545).

Is the site of the zona receptors different from species to species? In this context, a recent study by Bleil and Wassarman (69), using the mouse, is of particular interest. According to these investigators, sperm's zona receptors for the zona glycoprotein ZP 3 are on the plasma membrane over the entire acrosome of capacitated spermatozoa; they are hardly detectable on the same membrane of acrosome-reacted spermatozoa. Receptors for another zona glycoprotein, ZP 2, are hardly detectable on the plasma membrane of acrosome-intact spermatozoa. Once the spermatozoa undergo the acrosome reaction, however, ZP 2 receptors can be detected very clearly on the plasma membrane over the equatorial segment as well as on the inner acrosomal membrane. These results indicate that, at least in some species, there is more than one type of zona receptor on the sperm surface, and these different receptors become active or inactive (unmasked or masked) at different times during sperm-zona interactions. The notion that spermatozoa have at least two types of zona receptors in different regions of the spermatozoon is sensible. If spermatozoa have only one type of zona receptor exclusively on the plasma

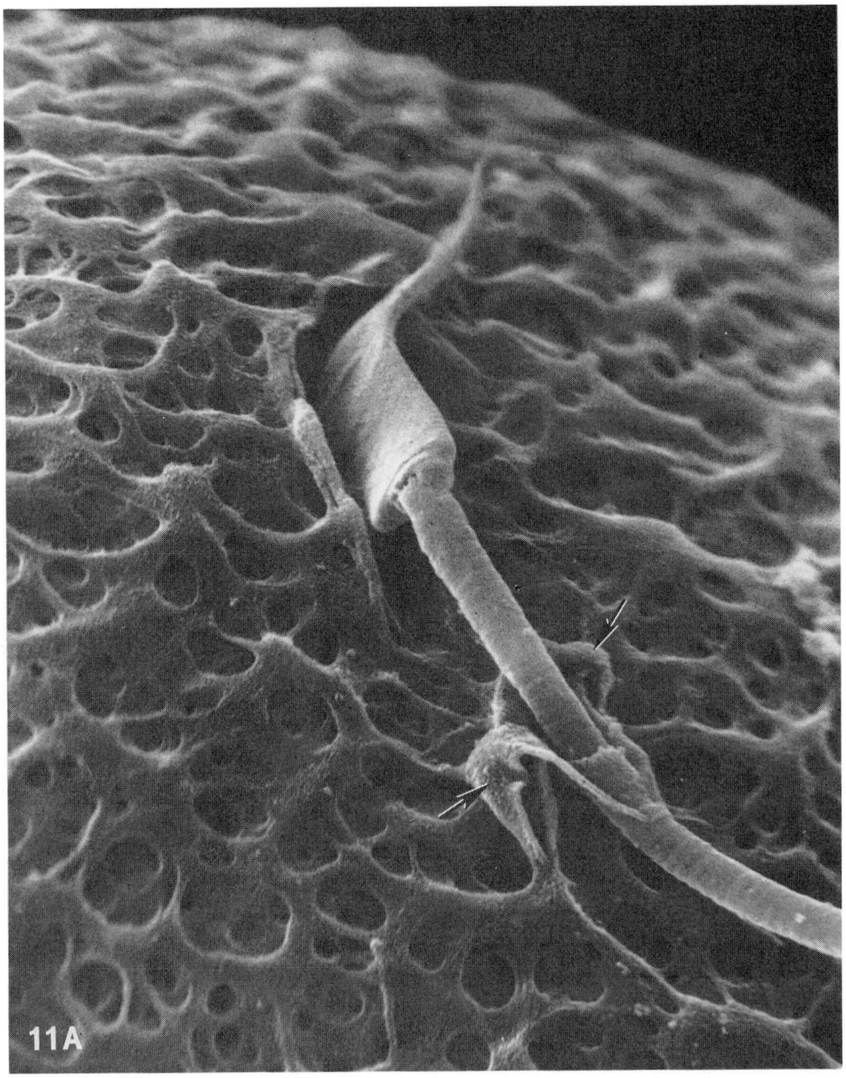

FIG. 11A. A scanning electron micrograph of a golden hamster spermatozoon about to enter the zona pellucida. The acrosomal ghost (*arrows*), stuck to the zona, is seen encircling the midpiece of the spermatozoon. (From ref. 545.)

membrane over the acrosomal cap, spermatozoa that have undergone the acrosome reaction of the zona (i.e., those which have lost the plasma membrane over the acrosomal cap) would swim away from the surface of the zona instead of penetrating into it. Since this is not the case, zona receptors must also be located somewhere on the surface of acrosome-reacted spermatozoa. One should not expect the binding between acrosome-related spermatozoa and zona molecules to be very strong. If it were too strong, acrosome-reacted spermatozoa would stay on the zona surface forever.

The rabbit represents an interesting example of sperm-zona interaction. The plasma membrane over the entire head of the capacitated rabbit spermatozoon has zona receptors. After the acrosome reaction, these zona receptors can be detected at the anterior margin of the equatorial segment and the anterior region of the postacrosomal area (371). During normal fertilization, rabbit spermatozoa must use the zona receptors on the plasma membrane over the acrosome first, then those on plasma membrane of the posterior half of the sperm head, to bind to the zona. According to Kusan et al. (274), rabbit spermatozoa collected from the perivitelline space (most probably acrosome-reacted) are able to repenetrate zonae of other eggs. These spermatozoa must use the zona receptors located on the plasma membrane of the posterior half of the sperm head to bind to the zona.

How Do the Zona's Sperm Receptors and the Sperm's Zona Receptors Interact with (Recognize) Each Other?

The zona's sperm receptors and the sperm's zona receptors must be complementary to each other. According to Florman and Wassarman (163), sperm-receptor activity resides in *O*-linked oligosaccharides in one of the zona glycoproteins, ZP 3. Circumstantial evidence suggests that oligosaccharides containing *N*-acetyl-D-glucosamine, sialic acid, fucose, and/or galactose constitute the active sites of the sperm receptors of the zona (300,445,466,520).

It is tempting to speculate that the sperm's zona receptors are lectin-like proteins with saccharide-binding activity. Some proteins isolated from spermatozoa are known to have the ability to bind to zona molecules, but it is not clear whether

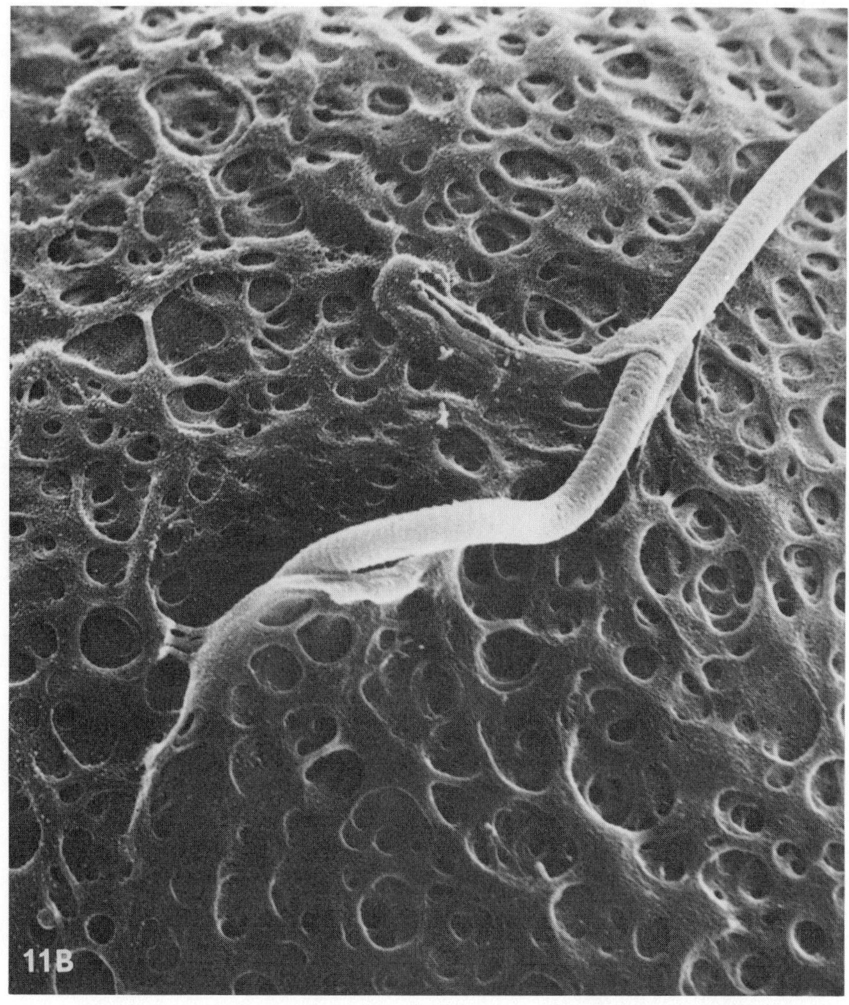

FIG. 11B. Same as Fig. 11A, but the head of this spermatozoon is deep inside the zona. Note the sharply defined border of the penetration slit. (From ref. 545.)

zona receptors are pure proteins or conjugated proteins. Although there is the possibility that the sperm's zona-receptor activity resides in the saccharide moiety of glycoprotein, the activity may reside in the protein moiety as well. Shur and his associates (300,445) maintain that galactosyltransferase is the sperm's zona receptor and that the terminal *N*-acetyl-D-glucosamine is the complementary sperm receptor of the zona. Sperm-zona binding, according to them, takes place in an enzyme-substrate fashion. Sperm's sialyltransferase (142) and zona's sialic acid may interact in this fashion to participate in sperm-zona binding.

Hartmann and Hutchison (219) and Saling (423) have suggested the possible involvement of trypsin-like activity in sperm-zona binding after observing the failure of hamster and mouse spermatozoa to bind zonae strongly in the presence of proteinase inhibitors. According to Benau and Storey (54), the sperm's zona-binding sites have an affinity to proteinase inhibitors (share some common characteristics with serine proteinases), but are lacking in proteolytic activity. These proteinase-like, nonenzymic molecules could be the ones that bind to the zona. The exact location of these molecules is unknown. They may be on the plasma membrane. Since capacitated spermatozoa bound to the zona surface soon initiate or complete the acrosome reaction, some components of the acrosomal matrix, particularly the insoluble "sticky" acrosomal material that holds fenestrated membranes, could be the molecules in question.

Sperm Penetration Through the Zona Pellucida

Spermatozoa must complete the acrosome reaction before entering the zona (Figs. 11A and 11B). This was first noticed by Austin and Bishop (25) and confirmed by all subsequent investigators (for reviews, see refs. 41, 329, and 530). The acrosome-reacted spermatozoon, in the act of passing through the zona, loses all of its acrosomal components except for the equatorial segment and the inner acrosomal membrane. The inner acrosomal membrane, which covers the anterior "half" of the head of the acrosome-reacted spermatozoon, is in direct contact with zona material (Fig. 12). The spermatozoon passing through the zona beats its tail vigorously. Apparently, vigorous sperm tail movement is essential for successful zona penetration, which is accomplished by a "slicing" side-to-side motion and a backward-and-forward movement of the sperm head (178,523). The fertilizing sper-

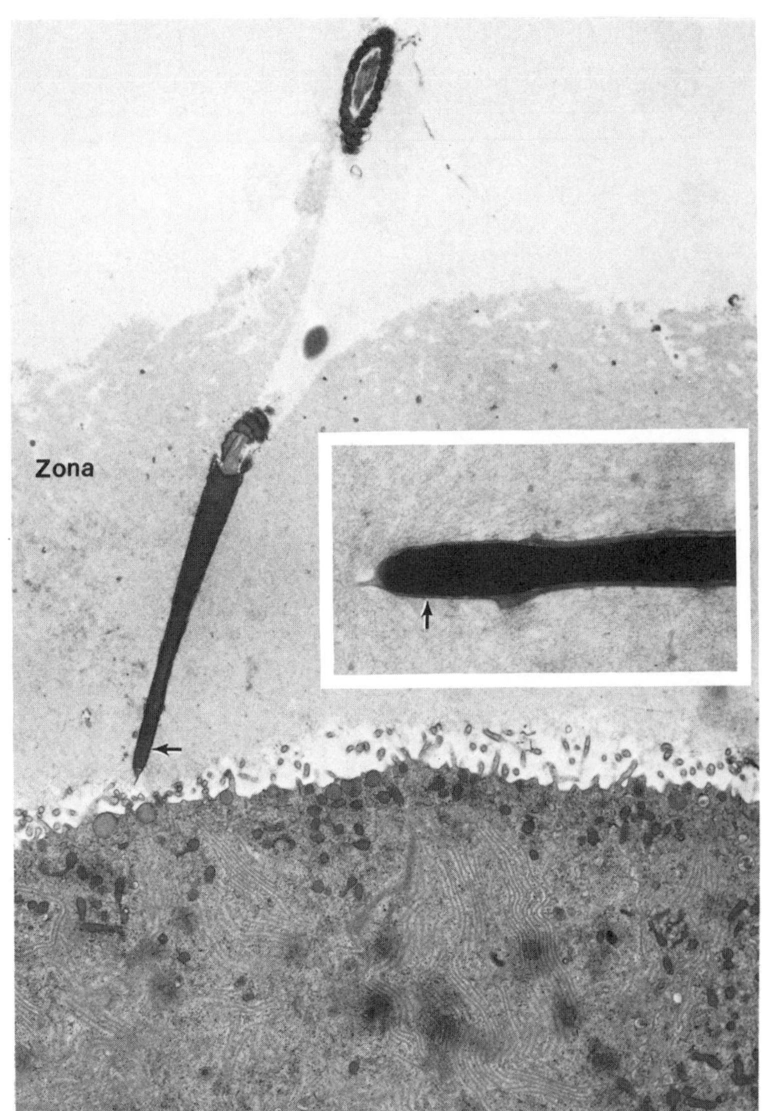

FIG. 12. Longitudinal sections of golden hamster spermatozoa in the act of passage through the zona pellucida. Arrows indicate the inner acrosomal membrane, which is in direct contact with the zona material. Note the distortion of zona material around the head of a spermatozoon in the inset. (From ref. 241.)

matozoon always leaves a thin, sharply defined penetration slit in the zona. Spermatozoa of many species take curved paths through the zona (25,131,132), but vertical penetration is certainly possible (178).

How do the spermatozoa penetrate the zona? In birds and marsupials, acrosomal contents released by an acrosome-reacted spermatozoon dissolve the zona locally to produce a "hole" through which the spermatozoon then swims (358,414). The major zona lysins in these species are most probably trypsin-like enzymes (281,414,471a).

Despite our continuing endeavor, we still do not know how the spermatozoa of eutherian mammals pass through the zona (for recent reviews, see refs. 241,329, and 468). For the sake of discussion, let us consider two hypotheses.

(*a*) *Mechanical hypothesis*. Sperm penetration through the egg investment is purely mechanical. The only function of acrosomal enzymes is to initiate or assist the acrosome reaction. Acrosomal enzymes have nothing to do with sperm penetration through egg investments. The sole purpose of the acrosome reaction is to expose the *perforatorium* (the inner acrosomal membrane underlined by the subacrosomal material). The sharply pointed perforatorium cuts open the zona mechanically as the spermatozoon beats its tail vigorously.

(*b*) *Enzymatic hypothesis*. In contrast to the hypothesis above, every step of sperm passage through the egg investments is enzyme dependent. Surface hyaluronidase and/or acrosomal hyaluronidase released during sperm passage through the cumulus serves as a lubricant for the spermatozoon swimming through the cumulus. Some other enzymes on the sperm surface mediate sperm adhesion (binding) to the zona surface (423,445). The bulk of the acrosomal enzymes are released by the spermatozoon on the zona surface. Some of the acrosomal hyaluronidase released digests the hyaluronic acid in the outer region of the zona (554). Acrosin does not dissolve the zona per se, but hydrolyzes specific zona glycoproteins to "soften" the zona

(138,490,491). Some of the acrosin and possibly some other acrosomal enzymes remain bound on the inner acrosomal membrane. These membrane-bound enzymes cleave zona molecules as the inner acrosomal membrane is pushed against the zona by vigorous movement of the spermatozoon. Probable candidates for the membrane-bound zona lysins include acrosin (89,334), nonacrosin proteinases (452), hyaluronidase (13,86,334,387), arylsulfatase (148), glycosulfatase (9), and *N*-acetylhexosaminidase (149).

The mechanical hypothesis has both strong and weak points. Some of the arguments that have been considered favorable to this hypothesis are as follows. (a) Theoretically, the force exerted by the spermatozoon can be as great as 100 pN. This is strong enough to induce stress relaxation of noncovalently associated zona glycoproteins, which can behave as a viscoelastic fluid (197). (b) The penetration slit the fertilizing spermatozoon leaves in the zona has very sharply defined borders (25,39,43). It looks as if the spermatozoon "cut" the zona rather than "dissolved" it. (c) Rabbit zonae treated with wheat germ lectin become resistant to trypsin and acrosin digestion, yet they remain readily penetrable by spermatozoa (51). (d) Proteinase inhibitors block binding of spermatozoa to the zona surface, but once the binding is established, they cannot prevent spermatozoa from passing through the zona (220,423).

One may argue that the sharply defined borders of the penetration slit are a result of the digestion of the zona by sperm enzymes tightly bound on the inner acrosomal membrane. Although no one has ever presented unequivocal evidence for the presence of membrane-bound proteinases on the surface of zona-penetrating spermatozoa (cf. ref. 241), it is possible that we have looked for the wrong enzyme. An enzyme (or enzymes) other than proteinase could be the one we are looking for. It is possible that zona lysins are unique proteins that can break up zona glycoproteins stoichiometrically, not enzymatically or catalytically. Such nonenzymatic zona lysins have been isolated and characterized in invertebrates (204,205,296).

If mammalian spermatozoa can pass through the egg investments without any assistance from enzymes, why do they have acrosomes loaded with such powerful enzymes as hyaluronidase and acrosin, which are capable of hydrolyzing the matrix of cumulus and the zona? If the acrosome and acrosomal enzymes are relics of evolution, we should encounter at least some mammalian species in which the spermatozoa totally lack acrosomes or acrosomal enzymes. Since this is not the case, acrosome and its enzymes must exist to perform very important functions.

The enzymatic hypothesis has its weak points too. If cumulus penetration by spermatozoa depends completely on hyaluronidase, spermatozoa lacking in this enzyme (e.g., sea-urchin and rooster spermatozoa) should not be able to penetrate into the cumulus, which is not the case (cf. ref. 472). Some investigators speculate that the spermatozoa of eutherian mammals, like those of marsupials and birds, release acrosomal enzymes (including hyaluronidase and acrosin) on the zona surface to "soften" the zona before spermatozoa enter it. This speculation sounds sensible if the zona is very thin (e.g., 1–2 μm, like the zonae of marsupials and birds). The enzyme released by a spermatozoon on the zona surface will "soften" the entire depth of the zona. However, in reality, the zonae of eutherian mammals are rather thick (5–27 μm; cf. ref. 137). It is difficult to visualize that the acrosomal enzymes released by the fertilizing spermatozoon on the zona surface could affect the sperm's entire future path through the zona. This is particularly evident in cases where the relative size of the sperm head (acrosome) is small compared to the thickness of the zona and where the fertilizing spermatozoon takes a curved path through the zona.

Acrosomal enzymes may play important roles in the initial stage of sperm entry into the zona. According to Overstreet et al. (379), human spermatozoa penetrate into cervical mucus much more efficiently when spermatozoa are in seminal plasma than when they are in artificial salt solution. Modification of the semen-mucus interface by seminal enzymes seems to facilitate sperm entry into the mucus. By the same token, acrosomal enzymes released by the spermatozoon on the zona surface may aid in the entry of the spermatozoon into the zona. The amount of acrosomal enzymes needed for this initial entry may vary according to species. If a relatively large amount of acrosomal enzymes is needed, spermatozoa will have to undergo the acrosome reaction on the zona surface. If not, spermatozoa need not undergo the reaction on the zona surface, and those that have undergone the reaction before meeting zonae should be able to penetrate into zonae. The mouse and hamster (30,427) might be examples of the former. The guinea pig and rabbit may represent the latter (238,274).

Most probably, spermatozoa use both mechanical and enzymatical means in passing through the zona. Obviously, spermatozoa could never penetrate thick zonae if they were immotile or weakly motile. Spermatozoa must possess strong thrusting power to successfully pass through the zona. However, strong motility alone is apparently not enough for successful sperm passage through the zona. Acrosomal materials (including enzymes) seem to pave the way for sperm passage. Some of the acrosomal materials released may alter zona molecules ("soften" the zona?) prior to sperm penetration, whereas other acrosomal materials, which remain bound to the spermatozoa, may actively break up zona molecules either enzymatically or stoichiometrically.

O'Rand et al. (373) have proposed a "binding-releasing" hypothesis of sperm-zona interaction. According to this hypothesis, the zona molecules (ZP) and sperm's zona-binding proteins (ZBP) first undergo a high-affinity binding. This is followed by degradation and release of bound ZP by sperm enzymes. The sperm's ZBP then becomes available to bind to new ZP. This is when sperm movement plays its role. Without the forward movement of the spermatozoon, no new substrate (ZP) would be available for the next binding step, and penetration would not occur. If the sperm's enzymatic activity or its ability to turn over the bound ligand is blocked (i.e., inhibitor added), the bound ZP would not be degraded, the ZBP would remain saturated with receptors, and penetration would not occur. O'Rand et al. think that this hypothesis could explain the species specificity of zona penetration by spermatozoa.

SPERM-EGG FUSION

Upon passing through the zona pellucida, the sperm head crosses the perivitelline space, becomes attached to the vitellus, and is gradually incorporated into it. This dynamic process can be observed continuously under carefully controlled *in vitro* conditions (for a recent review, see ref. 178).

In the opossum (a marsupial), sperm-egg fusion begins between the inner acrosomal membrane and the egg plasma membrane (414), as in the case of the bird (358), amphibian (394,549), lamprey (350), and marine invertebrate (106). The situation is different in the eutherian mammal. It is sperm-head plasma membrane, not the inner acrosomal membrane, that fuses first with the egg plasma membrane. This was first discovered in the rat by Piko and Tyler (397) (Fig. 13) and has been confirmed by others in various other species. With a few exceptions, the entry of the sperm head into the egg is followed by the gradual incorporation of the entire sperm tail (for a recent review, see ref. 178).

Sites of the Initiation of Sperm-Egg Fusion

Although Piko and Tyler (397) did not mention this specifically, diagrams presented by them (Fig. 13) gave readers the impression that the fusion begins between the plasma membrane of the postnuclear cap (= postacrosomal) region of the spermatozoon and the egg plasma membrane. Yanagimachi and Noda (543a), who examined the fusion between zona-free hamster eggs and acrosome-reacted spermatozoa, concluded that the plasma membrane of the postacrosomal region fuses first with the egg plasma membrane. This notion must be abandoned. Careful examination of spermatozoa in the act of fertilizing zona-intact eggs has revealed that it is the plasma membrane above the equatorial segment that fuses first with the egg plasma membrane (52,329) (Fig. 14).

It is important to note that the plasma membrane above the equatorial segment becomes capable of fusing with the egg plasma membrane only after the spermatozoon has undergone its acrosome reaction. The acrosome-intact spermatozoon, regardless of whether it is capacitated or not, is unable to fuse with the egg, even if it is brought directly on the egg surface, bypassing the zona pellucida (530,543b). An important physiological change must take place in the plasma membrane over the equatorial segment concurrent with (or as the result of) the acrosome reaction. Exactly what is happening in this membrane is not yet clear.

Figures 15 and 16 are scanning electron micrographs of hamster spermatozoa fusing with eggs. As seen in Fig. 15, the surface of the egg has numerous microvilli except for the area above the metaphase spindle of the second meiotic division. The cytoplasm of this microvilli-free area is known to be rich in polymerized actin (299,313). Sperm-egg fusion does not occur, or seldom occurs, in this "bald" area (256,393,437,438). Although the sperm head "lands on a meadow of microvilli," some investigators maintain that it is the plasma membrane of the intermicrovillar regions, not the plasma membrane of the microvilli, that is destined to fuse with the spermatozoon (50,329).

Intermingling of Sperm and Egg Plasma Membrane During Fertilization

Although there is no doubt that the sperm plasma membrane becomes part of the egg plasma membrane during fertilization (530), no one has proven this as clearly as Gaunt (181). He prepared an FITC-conjugated monoclonal antibody that binds specifically to surface antigen(s) of rat spermatozoa. This antibody stained the entire surface of the

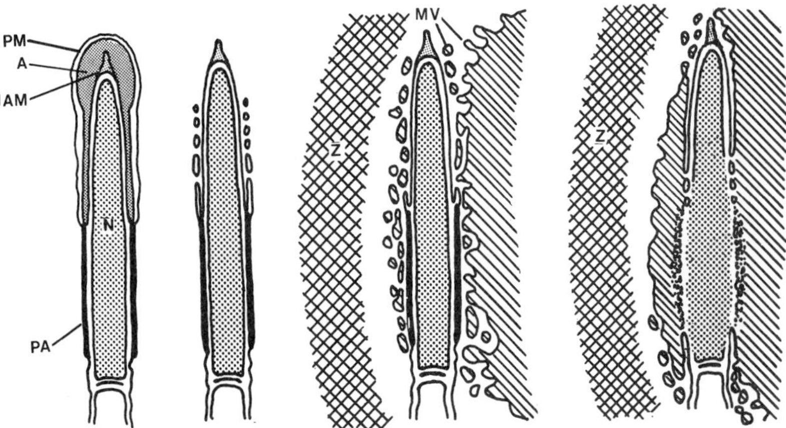

FIG. 13. Diagram of the acrosome reaction and sperm-egg fusion in the rat. (A) Acrosome; (IAM) inner acrosomal membrane; (MV) egg microvilli; (PA) postacrosomal region; (PM) sperm plasma membrane; (N) nucleus; (Z) zona pellucida. (From refs. 395 and 397, rearranged and relabeled.)

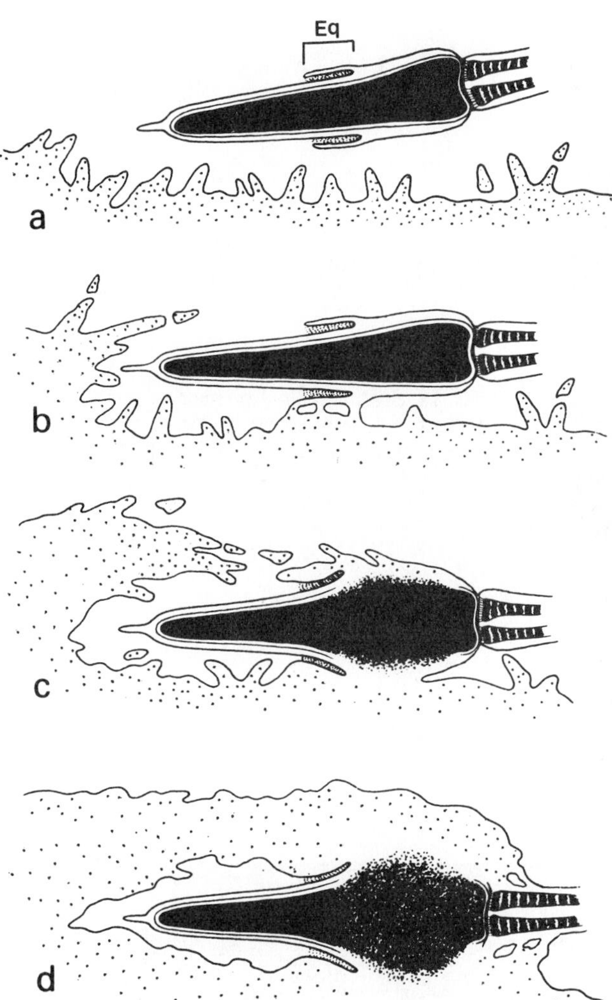

FIG. 14. Diagrams of the sequence of events through which the fertilizing spermatozoon fuses and is believed to be incorporated by the vitellus. (Eq) Equatorial segment of the acrosome. (From ref. 50, with an added label.)

spermatozoa, but not the surface (plasma membrane) of the unfertilized egg. When recently fertilized eggs were stained with this antibody, the presence of the sperm antigen in the egg plasma membrane was evident. The antigen was seen dispersing gradually from the point of sperm-egg fusion to the remaining surface of the egg. By the time the egg reached the pronuclear stage, the entire egg surface was seen labeled by the antibody. Interestingly, the antigen was no longer detectable on the surface of two-cell embryos. The antibody, in the presence of guinea-pig complement, caused lysis of fertilized eggs, but not unfertilized eggs and two-cell embryos. Although Gaunt (181) was unable to detect sperm antigens on the surface of two-cell embryos, some antigens must persist on/in the plasma membrane of the developing embryos, because another anti-rat sperm-surface antibody (272) markedly impairs *in vitro* development of rat morulae to blastocysts in the presence of complement. For more details of the process and mechanism of sperm-egg fusion, readers are referred to a recent review article by the author (660).

POSTFUSION EVENTS

Upon fusion with the spermatozoon, the metabolically quiescent egg "awakens" to initiate a series of morphological and biochemical events that lead to differentiation and the formation of a new individual. This awakening of the egg is referred to as *activation*. The most easily recognizable visible indication of egg activation in mammals is the exocytosis of cortical granules (Fig. 17a–d) and the resumption of meiosis. The egg nucleus, which was arrested at metaphase of the second meiosis before fertilization, resumes the meiosis upon sperm-egg fusion (Fig. 17e–g). The resulting haploid nucleus then transforms into the egg (female) pronucleus (Fig. 17h–j). Meanwhile, the sperm nucleus decondenses and transforms into the sperm (male) pronucleus (Fig. 17f–j). DNA synthesis (chromosome duplication) in both the egg and sperm pronuclei is more or less synchronous with the development of the pronuclei. The fully developed sperm and egg pronuclei come into close approximation at the center of the egg, their nuclear envelopes disintegrate, and their chromosomes mingle (Fig. 17k–n) for the first mitotic division (cleavage). The mingling of chromosomes can be considered as the end of fertilization and the beginning of embryonic development. In many invertebrates and nonmammalian vertebrates, the interval between sperm-egg fusion and the initiation of the first cleavage is a few hours or less, whereas in mammals it usually takes 12 hr or more, despite the high temperature (30–40°C) of the female's body in which fertilization takes place. The reason for this is not clear, but it could be related partly to differences in the nature of the maternal messenger RNA (mmRNA) stored in the egg cytoplasm during oogenesis. For example, sea urchins may already have transcribed mmRNA important for the cleavage program (648); this may include "cyclins" (580), which are postulated to be involved in control of embryonic mitosis. Although mammals also have mmRNAs (563), cleavage and early development appear to be relatively more sensitive to transcription inhibitors such as alpha-amanatin (581). Thus, in mammals, *de novo* mRNA transcription, in addition to mRNA translation, may be rate limiting to cleavage division.

Egg Activation

The physiology and biochemistry of egg activation have been studied extensively in nonmammalian vertebrates (e.g., fishes and amphibians) and invertebrates, particularly the sea urchin (for review, see refs. 578,579,594,595,618,652, and 653); however, even for the sea urchin, the mechanism of egg activation is not fully understood. It is generally believed that sperm-egg fusion somehow causes an explo-

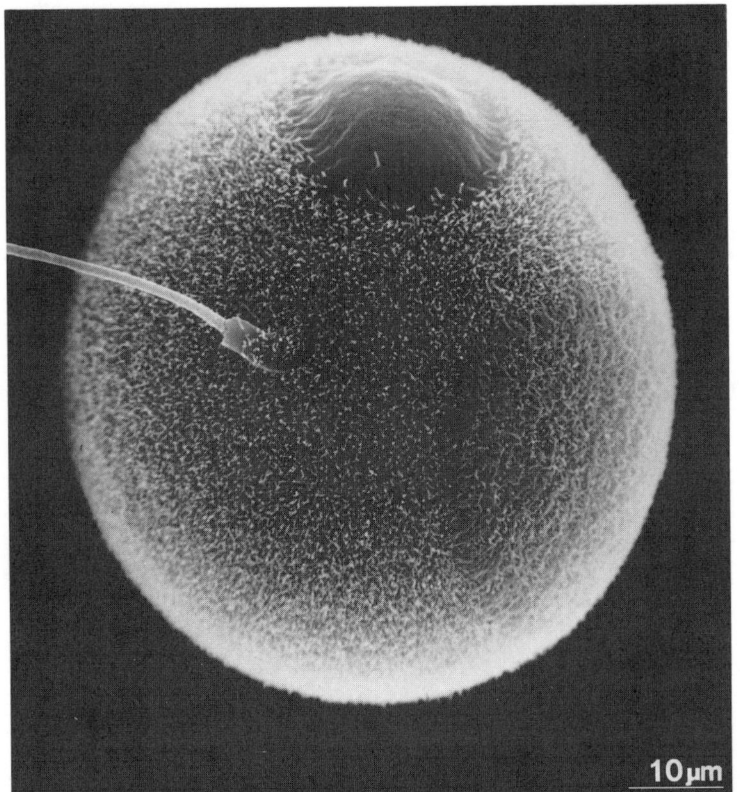

FIG. 15. Scanning electron micrograph of a golden hamster spermatozoon fusing with the vitellus. (From ref. 530.)

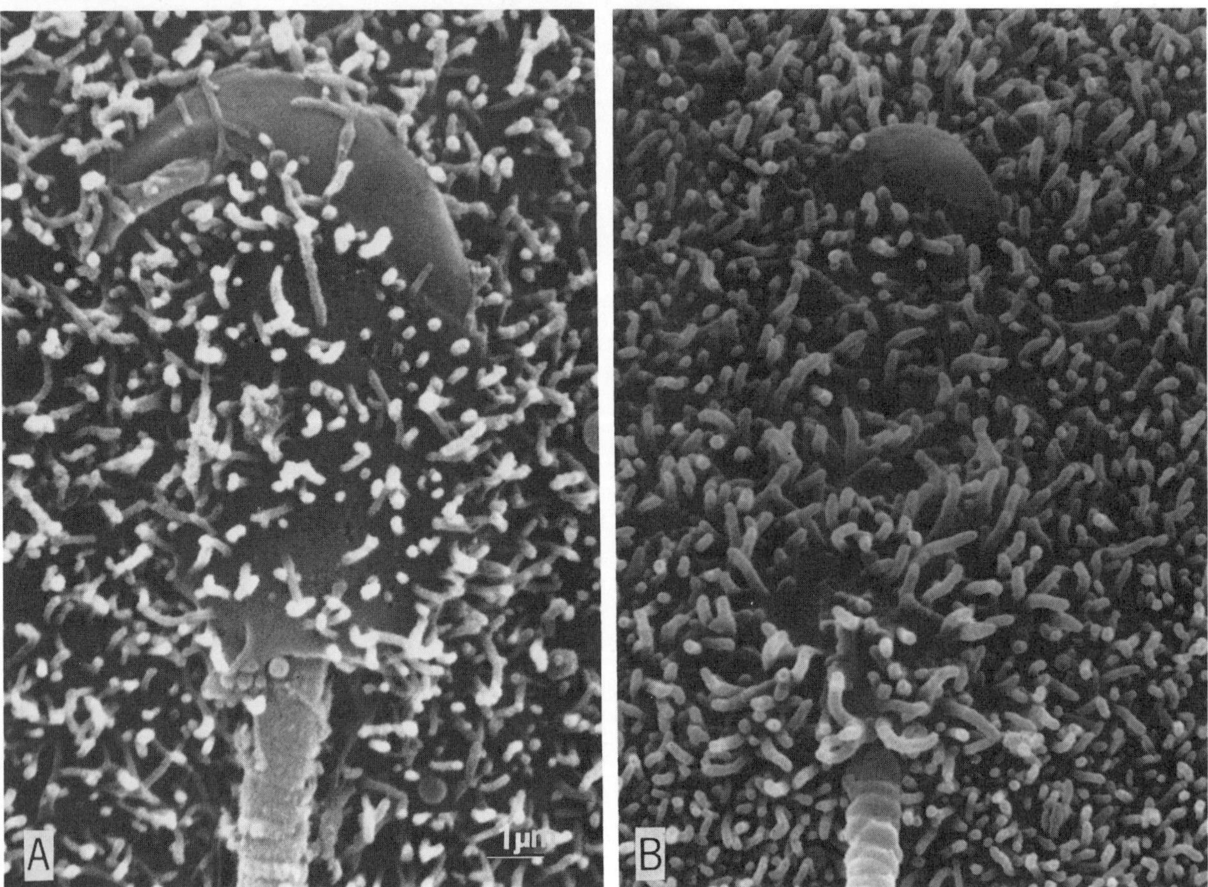

FIG. 16. Scanning electron micrographs of hamster spermatozoa fusing with eggs. (From ref. 530.)

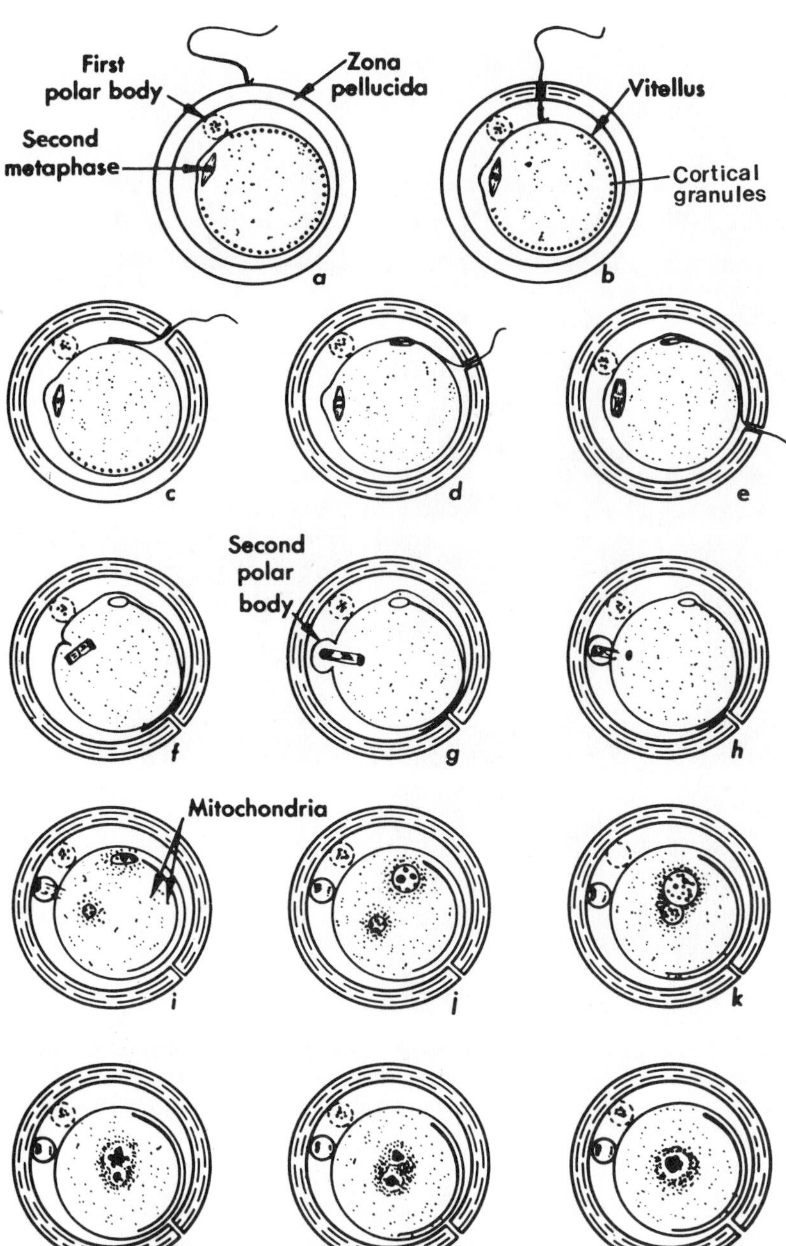

FIG. 17. Diagram of egg activation and pronuclear development in the rat. (**a–d**) Sperm-egg fusion and cortical granule exocytosis. The shading of the zona pellucida denotes the occurrence of the cortical-granule-mediated zona reaction. (**d–h**) Completion of the second meiosis. (**i–k**) Pronuclear development. (**l–m**) Reappearance of sperm and egg chromosomes. (**n**) Prometaphase of the first cleavage. (From ref. 556, with slight modifications.)

sive release of Ca^{2+} from intracellular storage sites (e.g., endoplasmic reticulum) (594). This temporal intracellular Ca^{2+} increase triggers an Na^+/H^+ exchange through the egg plasma membrane, resulting in a transient increase in intracellular pH. This temporal pH increase seems to remove or mask inhibitory proteins in the egg cytoplasm, resulting in irreversible activation of the egg's oxidative pathways, lipid metabolism, nicotinamide nucleotide reduction, and protein and DNA syntheses (cf. refs. 578 and 653).

Very little is known about the mechanism of egg activation in mammals. According to Miyazaki et al. (617), an explosive release of intracellular Ca^{2+} occurs in the hamster egg 10 to 30 sec after attachment of the fertilizing spermatozoon to the egg plasma membrane. The Ca^{2+} release begins near the sperm attachment site. It spreads throughout the egg within 4 to 7 sec and ends 15 to 20 sec later (Fig. 18). Interestingly, the Ca^{2+} explosion occurs repeatedly, at more or less regular intervals (3 min or so), for at least 100 min. The biological significance of this recurring Ca^{2+} release is unknown, but it could be related to some activities of cytoskeletal systems (e.g., tubulin depolymerization and polymerization).

According to Leese et al. (604), the concentration of ATP in the unfertilized mouse egg is quite high (1.52 ± 0.15 pmole/egg), whereas the concentration of ADP is very low (0.56 ± 0.15 pmole/egg). Since the availability of ADP is one of the major limiting factors of respiration in cells, its low concentration in the unfertilized egg would certainly result in the depression of cellular respiration. After fertilization (sperm-egg fusion), the concentration of ADP in-

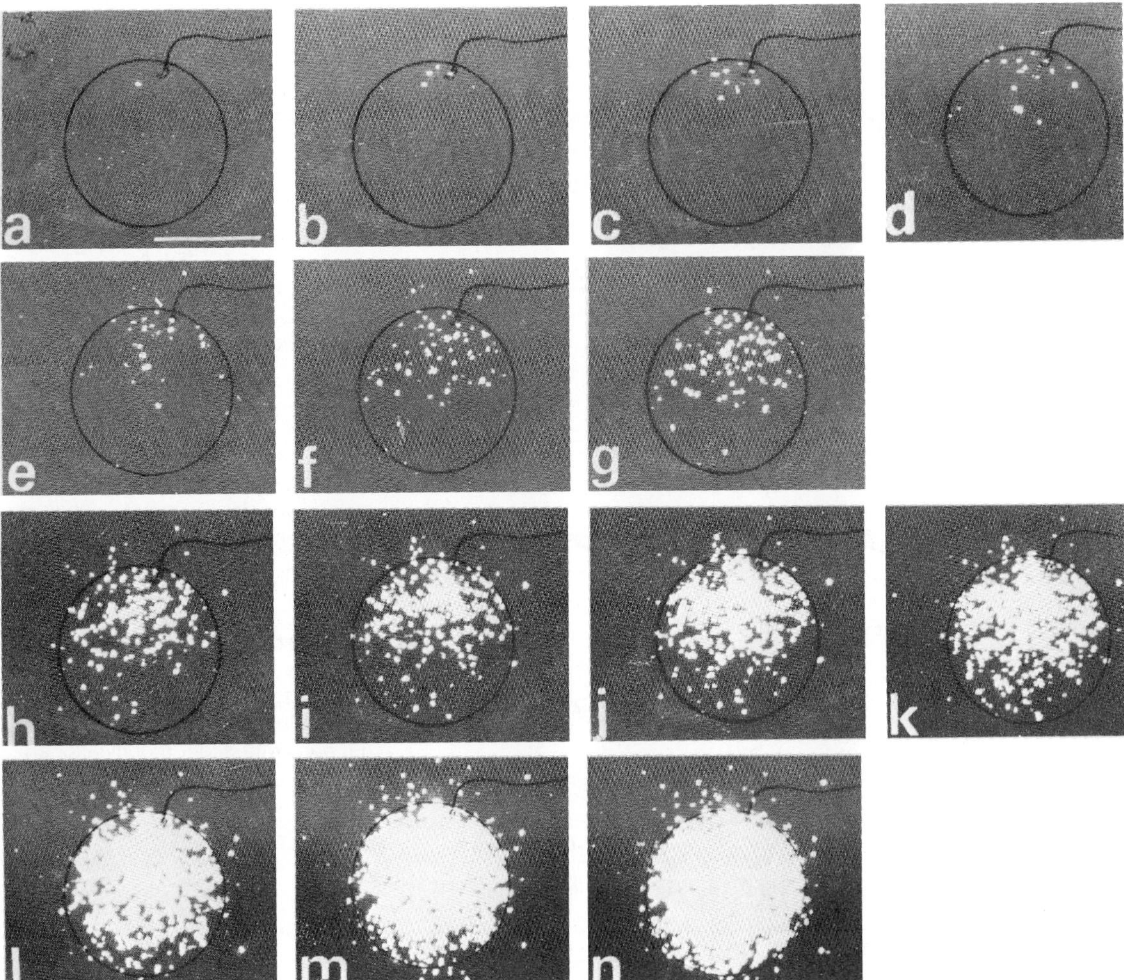

FIG. 18. A series of micrographs showing a release of intracellular Ca^{2+} upon sperm-egg fusion in the hamster. A zona-free egg was injected with aequorin, then inseminated in darkness. Luminescence emitted by the interaction of aequorin with Ca^{2+} was recorded every 0.5 sec. using a high-sensitivity video camera. These micrographs represent continuous accumulation of light spots during the first Ca^{2+} transient. (From ref. 617.)

creases dramatically (1.61 ± 0.38 pmole/egg). So, it would appear that fertilization (activation) releases the egg from a state of depressed respiration and metabolism.

It is most probable that many components of the egg (including the egg plasma membrane) change their physiological and biochemical characteristics upon, or sometime after, egg activation. For instance, the permeability of the mouse egg plasma membrane to glycerol increases dramatically within 3 hr after fertilization (egg activation) (592). The number of votage-gated Ca^{2+} channels in the egg plasma membrane increases significantly during the first hour following egg activation (658). Fertilization, or egg activation, however, seems to have little or no distinct effect on the permeability of the mouse egg plasma membrane to water (605) or amino acids (588). Also, the mobility of lipid molecules in the egg plasma membrane does not change significantly following egg activation (656). It is important to note that most investigators have not examined eggs continuously (or at short regular intervals) from the moment of fertilization or egg activation. By only comparing unfertilized eggs and fertilized eggs at the advanced pronuclear stage, they may have overlooked some temporal, yet very important, changes that occur immediately or soon after egg activation.

Mammalian eggs can be activated by a wide variety of physical and chemical stimuli (cf. refs. 584,600,644, and 654). These activating stimuli all seem to cause a rise in the intracellular Ca^{2+} concentration. Most of these stimuli appear to initiate some response at the level of the egg plasma membrane (654). No one knows exactly how the spermatozoon triggers egg activation. The idea that the spermatozoon brings some specific egg-activating substance into the egg is not new (see, e.g., ref. 631), and the search for such substances has been continued (572). There is no doubt that eggs are capable of activation without spermatozoa. It is well known that some insects, fishes, and lizards reproduce parthenogenetically generation to generation (cf. refs. 616 and 650). The eggs of these animals must activate spontaneously. Although mammalian eggs are potentially capable of initiating development without spermatozoa, this does not imply that the spermatozoon has no function in egg activation. Under normal conditions, it is the spermatozoa that activate the eggs.

How the spermatozoon triggers egg activation is still unclear. The author (660) has postulated that the part of sperm membrane that is destined to fuse with the egg plasma membrane (i.e., the plasma membrane over the equatorial segment of the acrosome-reacted spermatozoon) contains some specific proteins. When inserted into the egg plasma membrane, these proteins cause a local (and perhaps temporal) perturbance of the egg membrane lipids. This could be the primary trigger for egg activation. In both the sea urchin (586) and mouse (582), direct injection of Ca^{2+} into the egg cytoplasm is known to activate eggs very efficiently. Therefore, it does not seem to be unreasonable to assume that the primary trigger for egg activation is the Ca^{2+} that is carried into the egg cytoplasm by the spermatozoa. Jaffe (595) has called this the "detonation Ca^{2+}." In this context, it is interesting to note that the postacrosomal dense lamina of the ram spermatozoon is very rich in calcium (398,508). It is conceivable that Ca^{2+} liberated from the lamina after sperm-egg fusion triggers egg activation. Ca^{2+} is not the only substance capable of causing egg activation. According to Whitaker and Irvine (651) and Slack et al. (641b), inositol triphosphatase microsurgically injected into sea urchin eggs activates the eggs very efficiently. Thus, the "detonating" factors for egg activation could include some of the substances involved in the phosphoinositide cycle.

Exocytosis of Cortical Granules and Block to Polyspermy

Cortical granules are small, spherical, membrane-limited organelles found beneath the plasma membrane of mature unfertilized eggs in most vertebrates and invertebrates (639,640). Using the phase-contrast microscope, Austin (555) discovered these granules in the mammal. He observed many small granules in the cortex of unfertilized hamster egg; these granules subsequently disappeared during fertilization. Austin and Braden (23) correctly inferred that these granules were homologous to the cortical granules (CGs) of the sea urchin (577,619), which play a leading role in the modification of the egg envelope during fertilization. Figure 19 shows CGs of the mouse before and after exocytosis.

In sea urchins and fish, exocytosis of CGs begins near the point of sperm-egg fusion. It rapidly propagates from this point, in a wave-like fashion, to the opposite side of the egg. It has been well established that this wave of CG exocytosis is preceded by a wave of intracellular Ca^{2+} release (cf. ref. 595). There is convincing evidence that CG exocytosis is a Ca^{2+}-dependent process (640,647). In the hamster, the release of intracellular Ca^{2+} begins near the point of sperm-egg fusion (617), but the wave-like propagation of CG exocytosis has not been witnessed.

The CGs of mammalian eggs are known to contain hydrolytic enzymes and saccharide components (cf. ref. 585). In some species, the CG contents, which are released from the egg cortex during fertilization or egg activation, alter the physical and chemical characteristics of the zona pel-

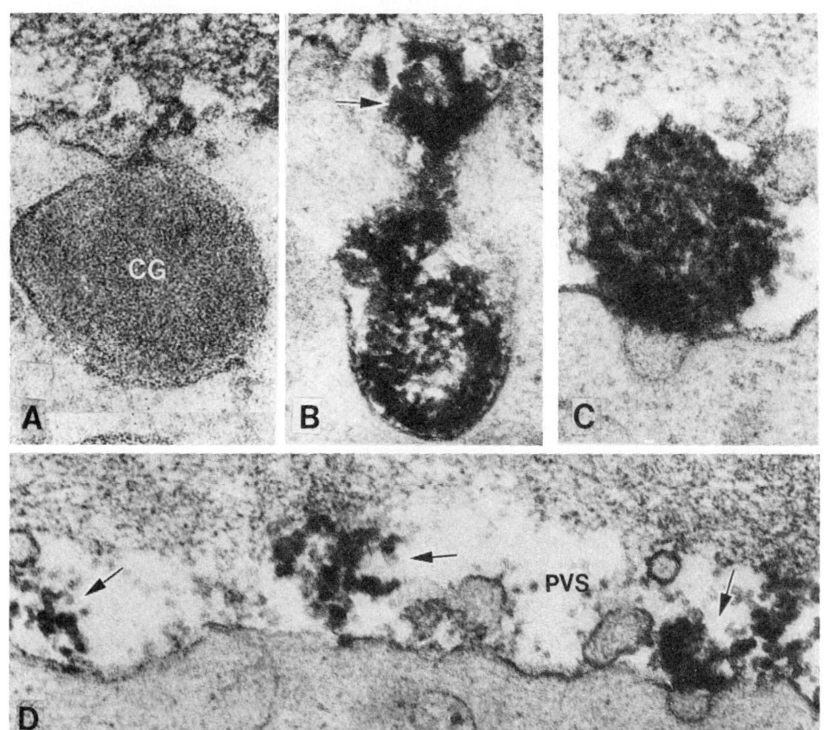

FIG. 19. Exocytosis of the cortical granule (CG) in the mouse. Eggs were fixed with Karnovsky's fixative containing 2% tannic acid. **A:** A CG immediately before its fusion with the egg plasma membrane. **B:** The limiting membrane of the CG immediately following fusion with the egg plasma membrane; part of the contents of CG (*arrow*) has been ejected into the perivitelline space. Note that the CG content has transformed into coarse granular structures with a strong affinity to tannic acid. **C:** Contents of a CG immediately after ejection into the perivitelline space. **D:** Perivitelline space (PVS) with scattering CG materials (*arrows*). (From ref. 643.)

lucida in such a way that the zona becomes "refractory" to sperm penetration. This has been termed the *zona reaction* (23,515). Wassarman and associates (506,649) maintain that, at least in the mouse, the zona reaction is due to a hydrolysis (inactivation) of a zona glycoprotein, ZP3, by a proteinase or glycosidase released from CGs during exocytosis. The ZP3 is primarily responsible for the firm attachment of mouse spermatozoa to the zona (cf. previous section of this chapter). Once the ZP3 is hydrolyzed, the zona can no longer hold spermatozoa firmly. The acrosome-reaction-inducing ability of the zona is also largely diminished. As a consequence, spermatozoa are no longer able to pass through the zona.

The CG-mediated zona reaction is not the only mechanism to block polyspermy. The egg plasma membrane has also the ability to reject excess spermatozoa. This block to polyspermy, at the level of egg plasma membrane, has been called the *vitelline block* (23) or *egg plasma membrane block* (515). Unfortunately, the nature and mechanism of the vitelline block in mammals are poorly understood. Although some investigators have suggested the possible involvement of CG material in establishing the vitelline block, no unequivocal evidence has been presented to support this notion (515,638). In the sea urchin egg, the egg plasma membrane becomes refractory to excess spermatozoa within a few seconds after attachment of the first (fertilizing) spermatozoon to the membrane. This fast block to polyspermy is electrical in nature (for additional reviews, see ref. 593). A sudden increase in membrane potential, caused by the fusion of the first fertilizing spermatozoon with the egg plasma membrane, prevents excess spermatozoa from fusing with it (for additional reviews, see refs. 593 and 595). To date, there has been no convincing evidence that the vitelline block in mammals is achieved by a similar electrical mechanism (593,638).

The relative efficiency of the zona reaction and of the vitelline block can be inferred by studying the numbers of spermatozoa entering the perivitelline space and the egg cytoplasm following natural mating or artificial insemination (20). In this way, the eggs of the hamster, dog, sheep, and field vole were judged to undergo a very strong zona reaction. The eggs of the rabbit, pika, and mole, on the other hand, do not seem to undergo a zona reaction, or they have only a weak reaction under natural conditions. The eggs of the latter species appear to depend almost entirely on the vitelline block to avoid polyspermy (Fig. 20A). The eggs of rat, mouse, guinea pig, cat, and ferret appear to represent an intermediate situation. Human eggs *in vitro* seem to undergo a strong zona reaction (632). Even when human eggs are inseminated with an excessive number of spermatozoa and a large number of spermatozoa are seen bound to the zona surface, supernumerary spermatozoa seldom penetrate beyond the inner region of the zona. It is very likely that the inner zona is the site of the zona reaction (Fig. 20B). Polyspermic fertilization can occur. One possible cause of polyspermy in the human, according to Sathananthan and Trounson (632), is the delayed CG exocytosis and consequent delay in the zona reaction. The immaturity of the egg at the time of sperm penetration, excessive aging of eggs in culture, and/or an inherent zona defect could all be responsible for the ineffective or partial block to polyspermy at the level of the zona.

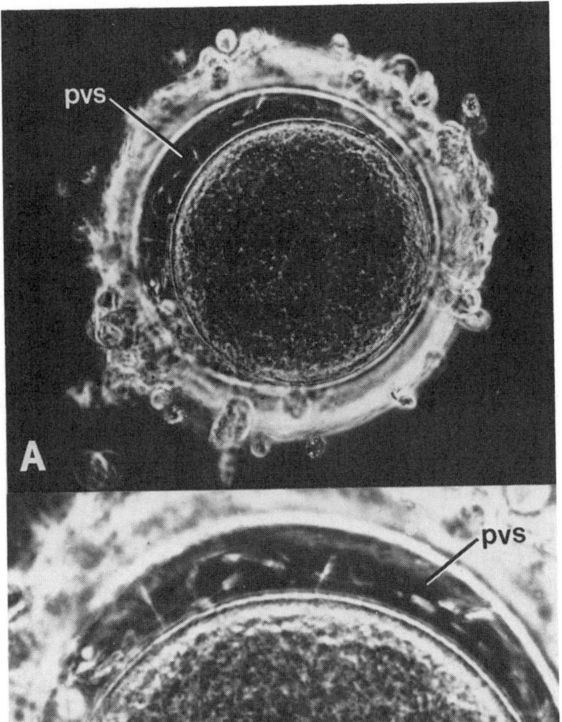

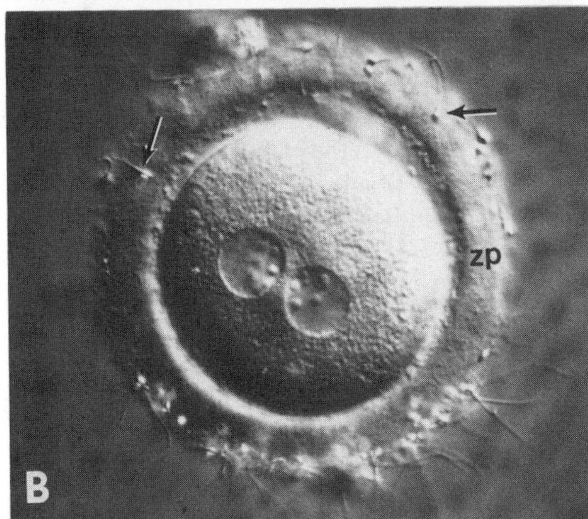

FIG. 20. Fertilizated eggs of the rabbit (**A**) and human (**B**). In the rabbit, many surplus spermatozoa are seen in the perivitelline space (pvs) of a monospermically fertilized egg. In the human, surplus spermatozoa are seldom seen in the perivitelline space of normally fertilized eggs. Micrograph B shows that at least two spermatozoa (*arrows*) have entered deep inside the zona pellucida (zp) but failed to pass through it. [Provided by Dr. J. Michael Bedford (micrograph A) and Dr. Phillip Matson (micrograph B).]

Under physiological conditions, virtually all, or at least the vast majority, of the CGs are released from the egg cortex within several minutes after the initiation of sperm-egg fusion. Therefore, normally fertilized eggs and developing preimplantation embryos possess very few or no CGs. Although CG exocytosis is a good visible indication of egg activation, it is not an absolute necessity for the initiation of normal development of embryo. The initiation of development without CG exocytosis (or with incomplete CG exocytosis) is certainly possible in mammals (585) as well as in sea urchins (640) and fish (597).

According to Cavanagh et al. (568), mouse eggs secrete a factor, termed *ovum factor* (OF), that directly or indirectly stimulates the mother's progesterone production. The OF is not a single molecule. It exists in multiple molecular-weight forms of approximately 160,000, 2,800, and 1,500. The OF is first released by the egg upon fertilization (or parthenogenetic activation) and continues to be produced at least until the blastocyst stage. Although it is tempting to speculate that the OF which is released from the egg upon fertilization is a component of exocytosed CGs, the continuous production of the OF by embryos during their entire preimplantation development seems to suggest that the OF is derived from cell components other than CGs.

The exocytosis of CGs occurs "explosively" upon fertilization (sperm-egg fusion). However, a considerable number of CGs are released while the egg is still in the ovary (625,630,661). A fairly large number of CGs are also released from mature unfertilized eggs before fertilization takes place (622,625). The biological significance of such "premature" CG exocytosis is not clear at the present time. Okada et al. (625) have postulated that the premature CG exocytosis has two functions. First, it may contribute to the formation of the perivitelline space. It is highly probable that the preexistence of the perivitelline space prior to fertilization greatly facilitates sperm-egg fusion in mammals. If the pervitelline space was absent before fertilization, the tip of the acrosome-reacted spermatozoon, which had passed through the zona, might become stuck on the surface of egg cortex. Being prevented from further advancement, the spermatozoon would not fuse with the egg plasma membrane because the inner acrosomal membrane that covers the anterior portion of the acrosome-reacted spermatozoon is nonfusigenic (241). On the other hand, when the perivitelline space is present, the sperm head that has passed through the zona can move freely. The fusigenic sperm plasma membrane over the equatorial segment of the acrosome is able to meet the egg plasma membrane without any difficulties. Secondly, a premature CG exocytosis might slightly modify the physical and chemical characteristics of both the zona pellucida and the egg plasma membrane in such a way that only a very vigorously motile spermatozoon could penetrate the egg. It may be reasonable to speculate that the premature CG exocytosis prior to fertilization and the burst in CG exocytosis during fertilization work synergistically in protecting the egg from the danger of polyspermy and/or fertilization by a "weak" spermatozoon.

Decondensation of Sperm Nucleus in the Egg Cytoplasm

During the terminal stages of spermatogenesis, when compaction of sperm nucleus takes place, all or almost all of the "somatic" histones in the sperm nucleus are replaced by a distinct group of "sperm-specific" histones or protamines that are very rich in arginine, serine, and cysteine (cf. ref. 566). It is believed that the complexing of sperm DNA to these highly charged basic amino acids permits condensation of chromatin and the repression of DNA activities (560,609,657).

One of the unique features of the mammalian sperm nucleus is the extensive SS cross-linking of the nuclear protamines (566), which occurs during sperm passage (maturation) through the epididymis (94). As a result, the nucleus of the fully matured spermatozoon has a prominent elastic "rigidity" (cf. 659). This rigidity appears to be beneficial for the "mechanical" passage of the spermatozoon through the thick, rather tough, zona pellucida (559). Excessive cross-linkings, however, may make it difficult for the nucleus to decondense within egg cytoplasm. In the case of the human, Zn^{2+} (of prostate origin) may serve in the prevention of the formation of excessive SS cross-linkings of the nuclear protein, which could occur during sperm capacitation (275,561,590,603).

One of the first events to occur when the sperm nucleus is incorporated into the cytoplasm of the mature egg is a rapid disintegration of the nuclear envelope. As a result of the breakdown of the sperm nuclear envelope, the sperm chromatin is directly exposed to the egg cytoplasm, and this allows factors within the egg cytoplasm to gain access to the chromatin and thereby alter its composition (609). The nature of the factor (or factors) responsible for this rapid disintegration of the nuclear envelope is not known, but this factor is apparently present in the cytoplasm of immature and fertilized eggs (646).

Once the nuclear envelope has disintegrated, sperm chromatin begins to lose protamines quickly (602), even before the decondensation of chromatin becomes evident (573,576). Although the newly synthesized basic proteins will eventually replace protamines, there is a period of time (i.e., during the late stage of chromatin decondensation) when the sperm chromatin is devoid of both protamines and somatic histones (629). If this is true, it represents a most unique situation, because even in rapidly dividing cells, histones are deposited almost immediately onto the DNA (657). DNA synthesis begins only after protamine removal and chromatin decondensation are completed (for additional references, see ref. 621).

Since Calvin and Bedford (94) reported that the nuclei

of mammalian spermatozoa were decondensed by dithiothreitol (DTT) and sodium dodecyl sulfate, many additional compounds have been shown to decondense sperm nuclei in a more or less similar way (657). All of these compounds have one thing in common in that they break either the SS or the noncovalent bonds of proteins. Although it is most probable that *in vivo* (within the egg) decondensation of the sperm nucleus is mediated by an SS reduction of nuclear proteins, harsh reagents such as DTT could not be the native nucleus-decondensing factor. A probable candidate for this is the reduced form of glutathione (GSH) (610). In fact, artificial reduction of GSH within the egg (by inhibiting GSH synthetase) renders the egg incapable of decondensing sperm nuclei (567,626). However, GSH cannot be the sole factor responsible for *in vivo* nuclear decondensation, because the cytoplasm of both immature (at the germinal vesicle stage) and fully mature eggs of the hamster are rich in GSH (Yanagimachi, *unpublished data*), yet the former, unlike the latter, is unable to decondense sperm nuclei (646). Since DTT-treated nuclei of hamster spermatozoa can decondense within the cytoplasm of immature eggs at the germinal vesicle stage (627,628), it is conceivable that (a) something within the cytoplasm of immature egg is blocking the GSH from acting on the nuclear protein or (b) something other than GSH is missing from the cytoplasm. The nuclei of the frog (598,606,641a), mouse (558), and hamster (646) do not decondense at all, or they decondense only very slightly, without the presence of germinal vesicle (GV) material in the egg cytoplasm. The GV material (or some product of its interaction with the egg cytoplasmic components) must either remove/mask some hypothetical blocking factor or provide the cytoplasm with another factor needed for an efficient decondensation of the sperm nucleus. It is also possible that the sperm-nucleus decondensing factor(s) is gradually accumulated in the cytoplasm during the growth of the egg and is "activated" by the GV material after GV breakdown (530). It is important to note that the egg cytoplasm of some other animals [e.g., the dog (610), the fish (591), the mollusc (575)] can decondense sperm nuclei before GV breakdown or when GV breakdown is inhibited under experimental conditions. Apparently, in the eggs of these animals, the sperm-nucleus decondensing factor(s) is active or becomes active before the GV material mixes with the egg cytoplasm.

It was once thought that a proteinase associated with the sperm nucleus was involved in sperm nuclear decondensation, but later studies have been unable to confirm this (628,662). However, the direct or indirect involvement of proteinases within egg cytoplasm is still a possibility. According to Mumford et al. (620), the unfertilized hamster egg has aminopeptidase and elastase-like activities. Whether such enzymic activities participate in the decondensation of the sperm nucleus remains to be determined. Wiesel and Schultz (655) were able to detect glutathione reductase and protein kinase in the homogenate of rabbit eggs. They postulated (a) that a protein-kinase-mediated phosphorylation of the sperm nuclear protamine facilitates the detachment of protamines from DNA and (b) that GSH, which is produced and maintained by glutathione reductase, reduces the SS bonds of the detached protamine molecules. The isolation of the sperm-nucleus decondensing factor (or factors) from the cytoplasm of mammalian eggs has been hampered by both the small size of the egg and the limited number of eggs available for chemical analysis. We may gain access to fundamental information about the chemical nature of the factor(s) using large eggs such as those from the frog (e.g., *Xenopus*), which possess the ability to decondense the nuclei of mammalian (human) spermatozoa (583,623). Sea urchin eggs, of which a large quantity is readily available, could be useful as well (574).

Development and Association of Sperm and Egg Pronuclei

The decondensed sperm nucleus and the group of chromosomes left within the egg after completion of the meiosis transform into the sperm (male) and egg (female) pronuclei, respectively. A probable source of the membrane material that makes up the nuclear envelopes of the pronuclei is the endoplasmic reticulum (609). However, small portions of the nuclear envelope of the sperm pronucleus may be derived from the intrinsic sperm nuclear envelope. According to Longo (608), the portion of the sperm nuclear envelope just above the acrosomal and centriolar fossae of the sea urchin spermatozoon does not disintegrate during nuclear decondensation, but instead becomes part of the nuclear envelope of the sperm pronucleus. Nuclear lamins, which are known to be a major component of the nuclear envelope, can be detected very clearly on the surface of both the sperm and egg pronuclei (633).

During pronuclear development, active DNA synthesis (621,642) occurs. At least in the mouse, active RNA transcription can be detectable during the pronuclear stage (571,657). The ability of the pronuclear mouse egg to synthesize and secrete new proteins has been recognized (564,569). According to Brandriff and Pedersen (562), DNA damage given to spermatozoa before fertilization can be repaired during the pronuclear stage.

The egg cytoplasmic factors that control the development of the sperm pronucleus and those regulating the development of the egg pronucleus may not be identical (530). The former has been called the *male pronucleus growth factor* (MPGF) (645) or the *sperm pronucleus development factor* (SPDF) (530). Some of the biological characteristics of the SPDF have been revealed. The SPDF, which is apparently less stable than the factor regulating the development of egg (female) pronucleus, is readily "inactivated" or fails to appear within egg cytoplasm when eggs are matured *in vitro* under "suboptimal" conditions (614). The SPDF may appear in the egg cytoplasm independently of the breakdown of the germinal vesicle (GV). According to Iwamatsu and Ohta

(591), fish (*Oryzias*) eggs, which have been matured without GV breakdown, allow sperm nuclei to decondense and transform into normal-looking pronuclei. In these eggs, however, sperm chromosomes degenerate without participating in mitosis (cleavage). The role of the GV material appears to be in the support of the development of functional sperm (and perhaps egg) chromosomes (570,591,614). The amount of the SPDF available in an individual mammalian egg seems to be limited. When very many spermatozoa enter an egg, all of them may begin nuclear decondensation simultaneously, but only a few of them (sometimes none of them) will develop into pronuclei. In the hamster, five spermatozoa per egg appears to be the limit for all of the sperm nuclei to transform into well-developed pronuclei. When more than nine spermatozoa enter one egg, none of the sperm nuclei develop into well-developed pronuclei (587). Apparently, a competition occurs among sperm nuclei for the materials supporting sperm pronuclear development (587,589) and chromosome development (570). Although there seems to be a competition between the sperm and egg nuclei for the "pronucleus development factors" (557), it is not clear whether the sperm and egg nuclei compete for the same factors. Some factors may be needed only for the development of the sperm pronucleus. Whatever the egg and sperm pronuclei development factors are, they are apparently not strictly species-specific (530,657,659). Human sperm nuclei incorporated into the cytoplasm of a hamster egg, for example, can develop into what appear to be normal pronuclei and then transform into at least structurally normal chromosomes (cf. refs. 534 and 596).

The morphological sequence of the migration of sperm and egg pronuclei to the center of the fertilized egg has been studied extensively at both light- (20,26) and electron-microscopic levels (607–609). Recently, our knowledge concerning the behavior of cytoskeletal systems during mammalian fertilization has been expanded considerably thanks to the availability of many specific molecular probes (including various fluorescein-conjugated antibodies against cytoskeletal components) (611–613,634–637). The behavior of microfilaments (actins) and of microtubules during normal fertilization in the mouse is summarized diagramatically in Fig. 21. Microfilaments exist throughout the cortex of the unfertilized egg, but they are most conspicuous in the cortex above the meiotic spindle (599) (Fig. 21, diagram 1). Microfilaments are apparently not involved in sperm-egg fusion but play a crucial role in the polar-body formation and the migration of pronuclei (Fig. 21, diagrams 2–4). Microtubules in the egg are essential for meiosis (including polar-body formation) and the migration of pronuclei. Interestingly, in addition to the spindle microtubules there are 16 cytoplasmic microtubule organizing centers or foci (Fig. 21a). Each centrosomal focus organizes an aster; after sperm incorporation, some foci, along with their asters, begin to associate with the developing pronuclei (Fig. 21b and c). When two pronuclei are closely apposed at the egg center, several foci are found in contact with the pronuclei and typically a pair reside between the adjacent pronuclei (Fig. 21d). Shortly before the nuclear envelopes of sperm and egg pronuclei disintegrate, all the foci condense on the pronuclear surface; also, sheaths of microtubules circumscribe the adjacent pronuclei (Fig. 21e). At the prophase of the first mitosis (cleavage), the centrosomes detach from

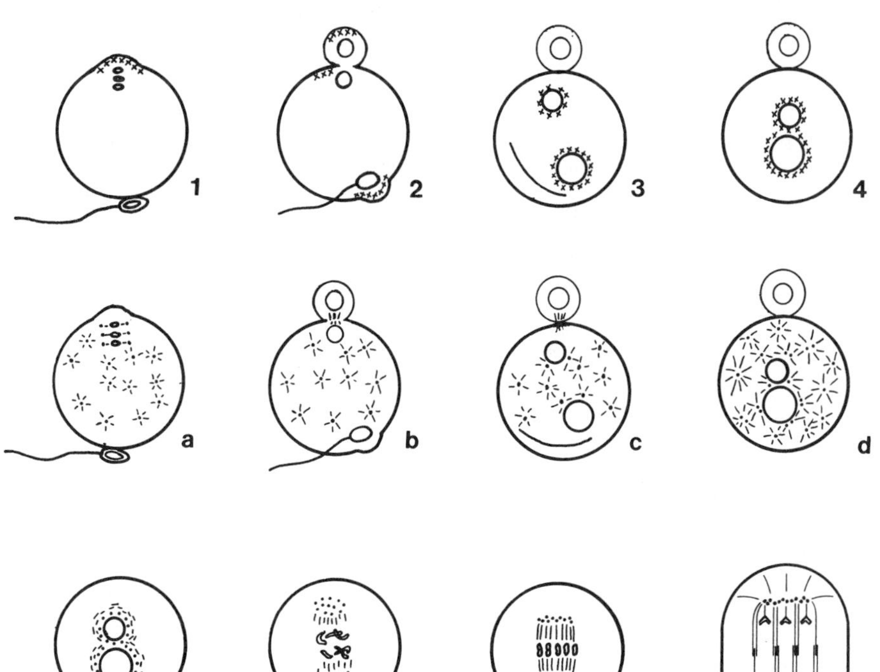

FIG. 21. Behavior of microfilaments (**1–4**) and microbules (**a–h**) during fertilization and first cleavage in the mouse. For explanation, see the text. (×) Microfilaments; (dots) centrosomal foci; (lines) microtubules. (Redrawn based on information from refs. 611 and 637.)

the nuclear region, appearing as two broad clusters (Fig. 21f) that aggregate into irregular bands at the metaphase (Fig. 21g). At the anaphase and telophase the centrosomes widen somewhat (Fig. 21h).

ACKNOWLEDGMENTS

The invaluable assistance of Dr. T. T. F. Huang, Mr. T. Timothy Smith, and Mrs. H. Yanagimachi in the preparation of this chapter is gratefully acknowledged. The author is supported by Grant HD-03402 from the National Institutes of Health.

REFERENCES

1. Abrescia, P., Lombarli, G., DeRosa, M., Quagliozzi, L., Guardiola, J., and Metafora, S. (1985): Identification and preliminary characterization of a sperm-binding protein in normal human semen. *J. Reprod. Fertil.*, 73:71–77.
2. Acott, T. S., and Hoskins, D. D. (1981): Bovine sperm forward motility protein: Binding to epididymal spermatozoa. *Biol. Reprod.*, 24:234–240.
3. Acott, T. S., Katz, D. F., and Hoskins, D. D. (1983): Movement characteristics of bovine epididymal spermatozoa: Effects of forward motility protein and epididymal maturation. *Biol. Reprod.*, 29:389–399.
4. Adams, C. E., and Chang, M. C. (1962): Capacitation of rabbit spermatozoa in the Fallopian tube and in the uterus. *J. Exp. Zool.*, 151:159–165.
5. Aguas, A. P., and Pinto da Silva, P. (1985): The acrosomal membrane of boar sperm: A Golgi-derived membrane poor in glycoconjugates. *J. Cell Biol.*, 100:528–534.
6. Ahuja, K. K. (1982): Fertilization studies in the hamster: The role of cell surface carbohydrates. *Exp. Cell Res.*, 140:353–362.
7. Ahuja, K. K. (1985): Carbohydrate determinants involved in mammalian fertilization. *Am. J. Anat.*, 174:207–223.
8. Ahuja, K. K., and Bolwell, C. P. (1983): Probable asymmetry in the organization of components of the hamster zona pellucida. *J. Reprod. Fertil.*, 69:49–55.
9. Ahuja, K. K., and Giebert, D. J. (1985): Involvement of sperm sulphatase in early sperm-zona interactions in the hamster. *J. Cell Sci.*, 78:247–261.
10. Aketa, K., and Ohta, T. (1977): When do sperm of the sea urchin, *Pseudocentrotus depressus*, undergo the acrosome reaction at fertilization? *Dev. Biol.*, 61:366–372.
11. Allison, A. C., and Hartree, E. F. (1970): Lysosomal enzymes in the acrosome and their possible role in fertilization. *J. Reprod. Fertil.*, 21:501–515.
12. Alvarez, A. C., and Storey, B. T. (1983): Taurine, hypotaurine, epinephrine and albumin inhibit lipid peroxidation in rabbit spermatozoa and protect against loss of motility. *Biol. Reprod.*, 29:548–555.
13. Anand, S. R., Kaur, S. P., and Chaudhry, P. S. (1977): Distribution of b-*N*-acetylglucosamindiase, hyaluronoglucosaminidase and acrosin in buffalo and goat spermatozoa. *Hoppe-Seyler's Z. Physiol. Chem.*, 358:685–688.
14. Aonuma, S., Okabe, M., Kawaguchi, M., and Kishi, Y. (1980): Studies on sperm capacitation IX. Movement characteristics of spermatozoa in relation to capacitation. *Chem. Pharm. Bull. (Tokyo)*, 28:1497–1502.
15. Ashraf, M., Peterson, R. N., and Russell, L. D. (1982): Activity and location of cation-dependent ATPase on the plasma membrane of boar spermatozoa. *Biochem. Biophys. Res. Commun.*, 107: 1273–1278.
16. Austin, C. R. (1948): Function of hyaluronidase in fertilization. *Nature*, 162:63.
17. Austin, C. R. (1951): Observations on the penetration of the sperm into the mammalian egg. *Aust. J. Sci. Res. (B)*, 4:581–596.
18. Austin, C. R. (1952): The "capacitation" of the mammalian sperm. *Nature*, 170:326.
19. Austin, C. R. (1960): Capacitation and the release of hyaluronidase from spermatozoa. *J. Reprod. Fertil.*, 3:310–311.
20. Austin, C. R. (1961): *The Mammalian Egg*. Charles C Thomas, Springfield, Ill.
21. Austin, C. R. (1967): Capacitation of spermatozoa. *Int. J. Fertil.*, 12:25–31.
22. Austin, C. R. (1985): Sperm maturation in the male and female genital tracts. In: *Biology of Fertilization, Vol. 2,* edited by C. B. Metz and A. Monroy, pp. 121–155. Academic Press, New York.
23. Austin, C. R., and Braden, A. W. H. (1956): Early reaction of the rodent egg to spermatozoa penetration. *J. Exp. Biol.*, 33:358–365.
24. Austin, C. R., and Bishop, M. W. H. (1958): Some features of the acrosome and perforatorium in mammalian spermatozoa. *Proc. R. Soc. Lond. (Biol.)*, 149:234–240.
25. Austın, C. R., and Bishop, M. W. H. (1958): Role of the rodent acrosome and perforatorium in fertilization. *Proc. R. Soc. Lond. (Biol.)*, 149:241–248.
26. Austin, C. R., and Walton, A. (1960): Fertilisation. In: *Marshall's Physiology of Reproduction, Vol. 1, Part 2,* edited by A. S. Parkes, pp. 310–416. Longmans, Green, London.
27. Babcock, D. F. (1983): Examination of the intracellular ionic environment and of ionophore action by null point measurements employing the fluorescein chromophore. *J. Biol. Chem.*, 258:6380–6389.
28. Ball, G. D., Leibfried, M. L., Lenz, R. W., Ax, R. L., Bavister, B. D., and First, N. L. (1983): Factors affecting successful *in vitro* fertilization of bovine follicular oocytes. *Biol. Reprod.*, 28:717–725.
29. Barros, C., Bedford, J. M., Franklin, L. E., and Austin, C. R. (1967): Membrane vesiculation as a feature of the mammalian acrosome reaction. *J. Cell Biol.*, 34:C1–C5.
30. Barros, C., Jedliki, A., Bize, I., and Aguirre, E. (1984): Relationship between the length of sperm preincubation and zona penetration in the golden hamster: A scanning electron microscopy study. *Gamete Res.*, 9:31–43.
31. Barros, C., and Yanagimachi, R. (1971): Induction of the zona reaction in golden hamster eggs by cortical granule material. *Nature*, 233:268–269.
32. Bavister, B. D. (1981): Substitution of synthetic polymer for protein in a mammalian gamete culture system. *J. Exp. Zool.*, 217:45–51.
33. Bavister, B. D. (1982): Evidence for a role of post-ovulatory cumulus components in supporting fertilizing ability of hamster spermatozoa. *J. Androl.*, 3:365–372.
34. Bavister, B. D., and Yanagimachi, R. (1977): The effects of sperm extracts and energy sources on the motility and acrosome reaction of hamster spermatozoa *in vitro*. *Biol. Reprod.*, 16:228–237.
35. Bavister, B. D., Yanagimachi, R., and Teichman, R. J. (1976): Capacitation of hamster spermatozoa with adrenal gland extracts. *Biol. Reprod.*, 14:219–221.
36. Bearer, E. L., and Friend, D. S. (1982): Modifications of anionic-lipid domains preceding membrane fusion in guinea pig sperm. *J. Cell Biol.*, 92:604–615.
37. Bedford, J. M. (1963): Changes in the electrophoretic properties of rabbit spermatozoa during passage through the epididymis. *Nature*, 200:1178–1180.
38. Bedford, J. M. (1964): Fine structure of the sperm head in ejaculate and uterine spermaotozoa of the rabbit. *J. Reprod. Fertil.*, 7:221–228.
39. Bedford, J. M. (1968): Ultrastructural changes in the sperm head during fertilization in the rabbit. *Am. J. Anat.*, 123:329–358.
40. Bedford, J. M. (1969): Limitation of the uterus in the development of the fertility (capacitation) of spermatozoa. *J. Reprod. Fertil. (Suppl.)*, 8:19–26.
41. Bedford, J. M. (1970): Sperm capacitation and fertilization in mammals. *Biol. Reprod. (Suppl.)*, 2:128–158.
42. Bedford, J. M. (1970): The saga of mammalian sperm from ejaculation to syngamy. In: *Mammalian Reproduction*, edited by H. Gibian and E. J. Plotz, pp. 124–182. Springer-Verlag, New York.
43. Bedford, J. M. (1972): An electron microscopic study of sperm penetration into rabbit egg after natural mating. *Am. J. Anat.*, 133:213–254.
44a. Bedford, J. M. (1974): Biology of primate spermatozoa. In: *Contributions to Primatology, Vol. 3,* edited by W. P. Luckett, pp. 97–140. S. Karger, Basel.

44b. Bedford, J. M. (1974): Mechanisms involved in penetration of spermatozoa through the vestments of the mammalian egg. In: *Physiology and Genetics of Reproduction, Part B,* edited E. M. Coutinho and F. Fuchs, pp. 55–68. Plenum Press, New York.
45. Bedford, J. M. (1982): Fertilization. In: *Reproduction in Mammals I: Germ Cells and Fertilization,* edited C. R. Austin and R. V. Short, pp. 128–163. Cambridge University Press, London.
46. Bedford, J. M. (1983): Significance of the need for sperm capacitation before fertilization in eutherian mammals. *Biol. Reprod.,* 28:108–120.
47. Bedford, J. M., and Calvin, H. I. (1974): The occurrence and possible functional singificance of -S-S-crosslinks in sperm heads, with particular reference to eutherian mammals. *J. Exp. Zool.,* 188:137–156.
48. Bedford, J. M., and Calvin, H. I. (1974): Changes in -S-S- linked structures of the sperm tail during epididymal maturation, with comparative observation in sub-mammalian species. *J. Exp. Zool.,* 187:181–204.
49. Bedford, J. M., Calvin, H. I., and Cooper, G. W. (1973): The maturation of spermatozoa in the human epididymis. *J. Reprod. Fertil. (Suppl.),* 18:199–213.
50. Bedford, J. M., and Cooper, G. W. (1978): Membrane fusion events in fertilization of vertebrate eggs. In: *Membrane Surface Reviews (Membrane Fusion), Vol. 5,* edited by G. Poste and G. L. Nicolson, pp. 65–125. North-Holland, Amsterdam.
51. Bedford, J. M., and Cross, N. L. (1978): Normal penetration of rabbit spermatozoa through a trypsin and acrosin resistant zona pellucida. *J. Reprod. Fertil.,* 54:385–392.
52. Bedford, J. M., Moore, H. D. M., and Franklin, L. E. (1979): Significance of the equatorial segment of the acrosome of the spermatozoa in eutherian mammals. *Exp. Cell Res.,* 119:119–126.
53. Bellve, A. R., and O'Brien, D. A. (1983): The mammalian spermatozoa: Structure and temporal assembly. In: *Mechanism and Control of Animal Fertilization,* edited by J. F. Hartman, pp. 55–137. Academic Press, New York.
54. Benau, D. A., and Storey, B. T. (1987): Zona-binding site sensitive to trypsin inhibitors. *Biol. Reprod.,* 32:282–292.
55. Berger, T., and Clegg, E. D. (1983): Adenylate cyclase activity in porcine sperm in response to female reproductive tract secretions. *Gamete Res.,* 7:169–177.
56. Bernal, A., Torres, J., Reyes, A., and Rosado, A. (1980): Presence and regional distribution of sialyl transferase in the epididymis of the rat. *Biol. Reprod.,* 23:290–293.
57. Berruti, G., Franchi, E., and Camatini, M. (1986): Ca^{2+} localization in boar spermatozoa by the pyroantimonate technique and X-ray microanalysis. *J. Exp. Zool.,* 237:257–262.
58. Bhattacharyya, A., Roldan, E. R. S., and Yanagimachi, R. (1986): Requirement of monovalent cations in the acrosome reaction of guinea pig spermatozoa. *Gamete Res.,* 15:285–294.
59. Bhattacharyya, A. K., and Zaneveld, L. J. D. (1978): Release of acrosin and acrosin inhibitor from human spermatozoa. *Fertil. Steril.,* 30:70–78.
60. Bishop, D. W. (1961): Biology of spermatozoa. In: *Sex and Internal Secretions, Vol. 2,* edited by W. C. Young, pp. 707–796. Williams & Wilkins, Baltimore.
61. Bishop, M. W. H., and Smiles, J. (1957): Induced fluorescence in mammalian gametes with acridine orange. *Nature,* 176:307–308.
62. Bize, I., and Santander, G. (1985): Epinephrine decreases the potassium requirement of hamster sperm capacitation: Furosemide blocks the effect of epinephrine. *J. Exp. Zool.,* 235:261–267.
63. Blandau, R. J. (1961): Biology of eggs and implantation. In: *Sex and Internal Secretions, Vol. 2,* edited by W. C. Young, pp. 797–882. Williams & Wilkins, Baltimore.
64. Blandau, R. J., and Odor, D. L. (1952): Observations on sperm penetration into the ooplasm and changes in the cytoplasmic components of the fertilizing spermatozoa in the rat ova. *Fertil. Steril.,* 3:13–26.
65. Blazak, W. F., and Overstreet, J. W. (1982): Instability of nuclear chromatin in the ejaculated spermatozoa of fertile men. *J. Reprod. Fertil.,* 65:331–339.
66. Bleil, J. D., Beall, C. F., and Wassarman, P. M. (1981): Mammalian sperm-egg interaction: Fertilization of mouse eggs triggers modification of the major zona pellucida glycoprotein, ZP2. *Dev. Biol.,* 89:189–197.
67. Bleil, J. D., and Wassarman, P. M. (1980): Structure and function of the zona pellucida: Identification and characterization of the proteins of the mouse oocyte's zona pellucida. *Dev. Biol.,* 76:185–202.
68. Bleil, J. D., and Wassarman, P. M. (1983): Sperm-egg interactions in the mouse: Sequence of events and induction of the acrosome reaction by a zona pellucida glycoprotein. *Dev. Biol.,* 95:317–324.
69. Bleil, J. D., and Wassarman, P. M. (1986): Autoradiographic visualization of the mouse egg's sperm receptor bound to sperm. *J. Cell Biol.,* 102:1363–1371.
70. Boatman, D. E., and Bavister, B. D. (1983): Regulation of hamster sperm capacitation by bicarbonate ion-carbon dioxide. *J. Cell Biol.,* 97(5): abstract 40.
71. Boatman, D. E., and Bavister, B. D. (1984): Stimulation of rhesus monkey sperm capacitation by cyclic nucleotide mediators. *J. Reprod. Fertil.,* 71:357–366.
72. Boell, E. J. (1985): Oxygen consumption of mouse sperm and its relationship to capacitation. *J. Exp. Zool.,* 234:105–116.
73. Brackett, B. G., Bousquet, D., Boice, M. L., Donawick, W. J., Evans, J. F., and Dressel, M. A. (1982): Normal development following *in vitro* fertilization in the cow. *Biol. Reprod.,* 27:147–208.
74. Braden, A. W. (1952): Properties of the membranes of rat and rabbit eggs. *Aust. J. Sci. Res.,* 5:460–471.
75. Bradley, M. P., and Forrester, I. T. (1980): A $[Ca^{2+} + Mg^{2+}]$-ATPase and active Ca^{2+} transport in the plasma membranes isolated from ram sperm flagella. *Cell Calcium,* 1:381–390.
76. Bradley, M. P., and Forrester, I. T. (1980): A sodium-calcium exchange mechanism in plasma membrane vesicles isolated from ram sperm flagella. *FEBS Lett.,* 121:15–18.
77. Bradley, M. P., and Forrester, I. T. (1985): Sperm calcium homeostasis during maturation. In: *Male Fertility and Its Regulation,* edited by T. J. Lobl and E. S. E. Hafez, pp. 437–449. MIT Press, Boston.
78. Breitbart, H., Darshan, R., and Rubinstein, S. (1984): Evidence for the presence of ATPase-dependent calcium pump and ATPase activities in bull sperm head membranes. *Biochem. Biophys Res. Commun.,* 122:479–489.
79. Breitbart, H., Rubinstein, S., and Nass-Arden, L. (1985): The role of calcium and Ca^{2+}-ATPase in maintaining motility in ram spermatozoa. *J. Biol. Chem.,* 260:11548–11553.
80. Breitbart, H., Stern, B., and Rubinstein, S. (1983): Calcium transport and Ca^{2+}-ATPase activity in ram sperm plasma membrane vesicles. *Biochim. Biophys. Acta,* 728:349–355.
81. Brooks, D. E. (1979): Biochemical environment of sperm maturation. In: *The Spermatozoa,* edited by D. W. Fawcett and J. M. Bedford, pp. 23–34. Urban and Schwarzenberg, Baltimore.
82. Brooks, D. E. (1982): Purification of rat epididymal proteins 'D' and 'E', demonstration of shared immunological determinant, and identification of regional synthesis and secretion. *Int. J. Androl.,* 5:513–524.
83. Brooks, D. E. (1985): Characterization of a 22 KDa protein with widespread tissue distribution but which is uniquely present in secretions of the testis and epididymis and on the surface of spermatozoa. *Biochim. Biophys Acta,* 841:59–70.
84. Brooks, D. E., Means, A. R., Wright, E. J., Singh, S. P., and Tiver, K. K. (1986): Molecular cloning of the cDNA for two major androgen-dependent secretory proteins of 18.5 kilodaltons synthesized by the rat epididymis. *J. Biol. Chem.,* 261:4956–4961.
85. Brooks, D. E., and Tiver, K. K. (1983): Localization of epididymal secretory proteins on rat spermatozoa. *J. Reprod. Fertil.,* 69:651–657.
86. Brown, C. R. (1975): Distribution of hyaluronidase in the ram spermatozoa. *J. Reprod. Fertil.,* 45:537–539.
87. Brown, C. R., and Cheng, W. K. T. (1986): Changes in composition of the porcine zona pellucida during development of the oocyte to the 2- to 4-cell embryo. *J. Embryol. Exp. Morphol.,* 92:183–191.
88. Brown, C. R., von Glos, K. I., and Jones, R. (1983): Changes in plasma membrane glycoproteins of rat spermatozoa during maturation in the epididymis. *J. Cell Biol.,* 96:256–264.
89. Brown, C. R., and Hartree, E. F. (1974): Distribution of a trypsin-like proteinase in the ram spermatozoa. *J. Reprod. Fertil.,* 36:195–198.
90. Bryan, J. H. D. (1974): Capacitation in the mouse: The response of murine acrosomes to the environment of the female genital tract. *Biol. Reprod.,* 10:414–421.

91. Bryan, J. H. D., and Akruk, S. R. (1977): A naphthol-yellow-S and erythrosin B staining procedure for use in studies of the acrosome reaction of rabbit spermatozoa. *Stain Technol.*, 52:47–50.
92. Burkman, L. J. (1984): Characterization of hyperactivated motility by human spermatozoa during capacitation: Comparison of fertile and oligospermic sperm populations. *Arch. Androl.*, 13: 153–165.
93. Burkman, L. J., Overstreet, J. W., and Katz, D. F. (1984): A possible role for potassium and pyruvate in the modulation of sperm motility in the rabbit oviductal isthmus. *J. Reprod. Fertil.*, 71:367–376.
94. Calvin, H. I., and Bedford, J. M. (1971): Formation of disulfide bonds in the nucleus and accessory structures of mammalian spermatozoa during maturation in the epididymis. *J. Reprod. Fertil. (Suppl.)*, 13:65–75.
95. Casillas, E. R. (1973): Accumulation of carnitin by bovine spermatozoa during maturation in the epididymis. *J. Biol. Chem.*, 248:8227–8232.
96. Casillas, E. R., and Chaipayungpan, S. (1982): Carnitin content of rabbit epididymal spermatozoa in organ culture. *J. Reprod. Fertil.*, 65:247–251.
97. Castellani-Ceresa, L., Berruiti, G., and Colombo, R. (1983): Immunocytochemical localization of acrosin in boar spermatozoa. *J. Exp. Zool.*, 227:297–304.
98. Chang, M. C. (1951): Fertilizing capacity of spermatozoa deposited in Fallopian tubes. *Nature*, 168:997–998.
99. Chang, M. C. (1957): Some aspects of mammalian fertilization. In: *The Beginning of Embryonic Development*, edited by A. Tyler, B. C. Van Bostel, and C. B. Metz, pp. 109–134. American Association for the Advancement of Science, Washington, D.C.
100. Chang, M. C. (1984): The meaning of sperm capacitation. *J. Androl.*, 5:45–50.
101. Chang, M. C., and Hunter, R. H. F. (1977): Capacitation of mammalian sperm: Biological and experimental aspects. In: *Handbook of Physiology, Section 7, Vol. 5*, edited by R. O. Greep, pp. 339–351. American Physiological Society, Washington, D.C.
102. Cheng, W. T. K., Moor, R. M., and Polge, C. (1986): *In vitro* fertilization of pig and sheep oocytes matured *in vivo* and *in vitro*. *Theriogenology*, 25:146a.
103. Cherr, G. N., Lambert, H., Meizel, S., and Katz, D. F. (1986): *In vitro* studies of the golden hamster sperm acrosome reaction: Completion on the zona pellucida and induction by homologous solubilized zonae pellucidae. *Dev. Biol.*, 114:119–131.
104. Clegg, E. G. (1983): Mechanisms of mammalian sperm capacitation. In: *Mechanism and Control of Animal Fertilization*, edited by J. F. Hartmann, pp. 177–212. Academic Press, New York.
105. Collado, M. L., Castro, G., and Hicks, J. J. (1979): Effect of spermatozoa upon carbonyl anhydrase activity of rabbit endometrium. *Biol. Reprod.*, 20:747–750.
106. Colwin, L. H., and Colwin, A. L. (1967): Membrane fusion in relation to sperm-egg association. In: *Fertilization, Vol. 1*, edited by C. B. Metz and A. Monroy, pp. 295–367. Academic Press, New York.
107. Cooper, G. W., and Bedford, J. M. (1976): Asymmetry of spermiation and sperm surface change patterns over the giant acrosome in the musk shrew *Suncus murinus*. *J. Cell Biol.*, 69:415–428.
108. Cooper, G. W., Overstreet, J. W., and Katz, D. F. (1979): The motility of rabbit spermatozoa recovered from the female genital tract. *Gamete Res.*, 2:35–42.
109. Cooper, T. G. (1984): The onset and maintenance of hyperactivated motility of spermatozoa from the mouse. *Gamete Res.*, 9:55–74.
110. Cornett, L. E., and Meizel, S. (1978): Stimulation of *in vitro* activation and the acrosome reaction of hamster spermatozoa by catecholamines. *Proc. Natl. Acad. Sci. USA*, 10:4954–4958.
111. Courot, M. (1981): Transport and maturation of spermatozoa. *Prog. Reprod. Biol.*, 8:67–79.
112. Courtens, J. L., Rozinek, J., and Fournier-Delpech, S. (1982): Binding of epididymal proteins to the spermatozoa of the ram. *Andrologia*, 14:509–514.
113. Cran, D. G., and Cheng, W. T. K. (1986): The cortical reaction in pig oocytes during *in vivo* and *in vitro* fertilization. *Gamete Res.*, 13:241–251.
114. Cross, N. L., Morales, P., and Overstreet, J. W. (1986): Two simple methods for detecting human sperm acrosome reactions. *J. Androl.*, 7:28a.
115. Crozel, N. (1984): Ultrastructural aspects of *in vivo* fertilization in the cow. *Gamete Res.*, 10:241–251.
116. Crozet, N., and Dumont, M. (1984): The site of the acrosome reaction during *in vivo* penetration of the sheep oocyte. *Gamete Res.*, 10:97–105.
117. Cuasnicu, P. S., Echeverria, F. G., Piazza, A., and Blaquier, J. A. (1984): Addition of androgens to cultured hamster epididymus increases zona recognition by immature spermatozoa. *J. Reprod. Fertil.*, 70:541–547.
118. Cummins, J. M. (1982): Hyperactivated motility patterns of ram spermatozoa recovered from the oviducts of mated ewes. *Gamete Res.*, 6:53–63.
119. Cummins, J. M., Fleming, A. D., Crozel, N., Kuehl, T. J., Kosower, N. S., and Yanagimachi, R. (1986): Labeling of live mammalian spermatozoa with the fluorescent thio alkylating agent, monobromobimane (MB): Immobilization upon exposure to ultraviolet light and analysis of acrosomal status. *J. Exp. Zool.*, 237:375–382.
120. Cummins, J. M., and Yanagimachi, R. (1982): Sperm-egg ratios and the site of the acrosome reaction during *in vivo* fertilization in the hamster. *Gamete Res.*, 5:239–256.
121. Cummins, J. M., and Yanagimachi, R. (1986): Development of ability to penetrate the cumulus oophorus by hamster spermatozoa capacitated *in vitro*, in relation to the timing of the acrosome reaction. *Gamete Res.*, 15:187–212.
122. Dacheux, J. L., and Paquignon, M. (1980): Relations between the fertilizing ability, motility and metabolism of epididymal spermatozoa. *Reprod. Nutr. Dev.*, 20:1085–1099.
123. D'Addario, D. A., Turner, T. T., and Howards, S. S. (1980): Effect of vasectomy on the osmolarity of hamster testicular and epididymal intraluminal fluid. *J. Androl.*, 1:167–170.
124. Dan, J. C. (1952): Studies on the acrosome reaction. I. Reaction to egg-water and other stimuli. *Biol. Bull.*, 103:54–66.
125. Dan, J. C. (1956): The acrosome reaction. *Int. Rev. Cytol.*, 5:365–393.
126. Dan, J. C., Hashimoto, S., and Kubo, M. (1975): The fine structure of the acrosome trigger. In: *The Functional Anatomy of the Spermatozoa*, edited by B. J. Afzelins, pp. 39–45. Pergamon Press, New York.
127. Davis, B. K. (1976): Inhibitory effect of synthetic phospholipid vesicles containing cholesterol on the fertilizing capacity of rabbit spermatozoa. *Proc. Soc. Exp. Biol. Med.*, 152:257–261.
128. Davis, B. K. (1981): Timing of fertilization in mammals: Sperm cholesterol/phospholipid ratio as a determinant of the capacitation interval. *Proc. Natl. Acad. Sci. USA*, 78:7560–7564.
129. Davis, B. K., Byrne, R., and Hangund, B. (1979): Studies on the mechanism of capacitation II. Evidence for lipid transfer between plasma membrane of rat sperm and serum albumin during capacitation *in vitro*. *Biochim. Biophys. Acta.*, 558:257–266.
130. DeMayo, F. J., Mizoguchi, H., and Dukelow, W. R. (1980): Fertilization of squirrel monkey and hamster ova in the rabbit oviduct. *Science*, 208:1468–1469.
131. Dickmann, Z. (1964): The passage of spermatozoa through and into the zona pellucida of the rabbit egg. *J. Exp. Biol.*, 41:177–182.
132. Dickmann, Z., and Dziuk, P. J. (1964): Sperm penetration of the zona pellucida of the pig egg. *J. Exp. Biol.*, 41:603–608.
133. Dravland, J. E., Llanus, M. N., Munn, R. J., and Meizel, S. (1984): Evidence for the involvement of a sperm trypsin-like enzyme in the membrane events of the hamster acrosome reaction. *J. Exp. Zool.*, 232:117–128.
134. Dravland, J. E., and Meizel, S. (1981): Stimulation of sperm capacitation and acrosome reaction *in vitro* by glucose and lactate and the inhibition by glycolytic inhibitor alpha-chlorohydrin. *Gamete Res.*, 4:515–523.
135. Dudenhausen, E., and Talbot, P. (1982): Detection and kinetics of the normal acrosome reaction of mouse sperm. *Gamete Res.*, 6:257–265.
136. Dudkiewicz, A. B., and Garrison, G. A. (1982): Substrate preference of boar acrosin in zona pellucida lysis. *J. Cell Biol.*, 95:164.
137. Dunbar, B. S. (1983): Morphological, biochemical and immunochemical characterization of the mammalian zona pellucida. In: *Mechanism and Control of Animal Fertilization*, edited by J. F. Hartmann, pp. 139–157. Academic Press, New York.
138. Dunbar, B. S., Budkiewicz, A. B., and Bundman, D. S. (1985): Proteolysis of specific porcine zona pellucida glycoproteins by boar acrosin. *Biol. Reprod.*, 32:619–630.

139. Dunbar, B. S., Munoz, M. G., Cordle, C. T., and Metz, C. B. (1976): Inhibition of fertilization *in vitro* by treatment of rabbit spermatozoa with univalent isoantibodies to rabbit sperm hyaluronidase. *J. Reprod. Fertil.*, 47:381–384.
140. Dunbar, B. S., Wardrip, N. J., and Hedrick, J. K. (1980): Isolation, physicochemical properties and macromolecular composition of the zona pellucida from porcine oocytes. *Biochemistry*, 19: 356–365.
141. Dunbar, B. S., and Wolgemuth, D. J. (1984): Structure and function of the mammalian zona pellucida, a unique extracellular matrix. In: *Modern Cell Biology, Vol. 3,* edited by B. H. Satier, pp. 77–111. Alan R. Liss, New York.
142. Durr, R., Shur, B., and Roth, S. (1977): Sperm-associated sialyltransferase activity. *Nature*, 265:547–548.
143a. East, I. J., and Dean, J. (1984): Monoclonal antibodies as probes of the distribution of ZP-2, the major sulfated glycoprotein of the mouse zona pellucida. *J. Cell Biol.*, 98:795–800.
143b. Echeverria, F. M. G., Cuasnicu, P. S., and Blaquier, J. A. (1982): Identification of androgen-dependent glycoproteins in the hamster epididymus and their association with spermatozoa. *J. Reprod. Fertil.*, 64:1–7.
144. Eddy, E. M., Vernon, R. B., Muller, C. H., Hahnel, A. C., and Fenderson, B. A. (1985): Immunodissection of sperm surface modifications during epididymal maturation. *Am. J. Anat.*, 174:225–237.
145. Enders, G. C., and Friend, D. S. (1985): Detection of anionic sites on the cytoplasmic surface of the guinea pig acrosomal membrane. *Am. J. Anat.*, 173:241–256.
146. Eppig, J. J. (1982): The relationship between cumulus cell-oocyte coupling, oocyte meiotic maturation, and cumulus expansion. *Dev. Biol.*, 89:268–272.
147. Fain-Maurel, M. E., Danoune, J. P., and Reger, J. F. (1984): A cytochemical study on surface charges and lectin-binding sites in epididymal and ejaculated spermatozoa of *Macaca fascicularis*. *Anat. Rec.*, 208:375–382.
148. Farooqui, A. A., and Srivastava, P. N. (1979): Isolation, characterization and the role of rabbit testicular arylsulfatase A in fertilization. *Biochem. J.*, 181:331–337.
149. Farooqui, A. and Srivastava, P. N. (1980): Isolation of *p-N*-acetylhexosaminidase from rabbit semen and its role in fertilization. *Biochem. J.*, 191:827–834.
150. Fawcett, D. W. (1975): The mammalian spermatozoon. *Dev. Biol.*, 44:394–436.
151. Fawcett, D. W., and Hollenberg, R. D. (1963): Changes in the acrosome of guinea pig spermatozoa during passage through the epididymus. *Zeil. Zellforsch.*, 60:276–292.
152. Flechon, J. E. (1979): Sperm glycoproteins of the boar, bull, rabbit, and ram: Acrosomal glycoproteins. *Gamete Res.*, 2:43–51.
153. Flechon, J. E. (1981): Ultrastructural and cytochemical analysis of the mammalian sperm plasma membrane during epididymal maturation. *Prog. Reprod. Biol.*, 8:90–99.
154. Flechon, J. E. (1985): Sperm surface changes during the acrosome reaction as observed by freeze-fracture. *Am. J. Anat.*, 174:239–248.
155. Flechon, J. E., Harrison, R. A. P., Flechon, B., and Escaig, J. (1986): Membrane fusion events in the Ca^{2+}/ionophore-induced acrosome reaction of ram spermatozoa. *J. Cell Sci.*, 81:43–63.
156. Flemming, A. D., Kosower, N. S., and Yanagimachi, R. (1986): Alteration of sperm thiol-disulfide status and capacitation in guinea pig. *Gamete Res.*, 13:93–102.
157. Flemming, A. D., and Kuehl, T. J. (1985): Effects of temperature upon capacitation of guinea pig spermatozoa. *J. Exp. Zool.*, 233:405–411.
158. Flemming, A. D., and Yanagimachi, R. (1981): Effects of various lipids on the acrosome reaction and fertilizing capacity of guinea pig spermatozoa, with special reference to the possible involvement of lysophospholipid in the acrosome reaction. *Gamete Res.*, 4:253–273.
159. Flemming, A. D., and Yanagimachi, R. (1982): Fertile life of acrosome-reacted guinea pig spermatozoa. *J. Exp. Zool.*, 220:109–115.
160. Flemming, A. D., and Yanagimachi, R. (1984): Evidence suggesting the importance of fatty acids and fatty acid moieties of sperm membrane phospholipids in the acrosome reaction of guinea pig spermatozoa. *J. Exp. Zool.*, 229:485–489.
161. Flemming, A. D., Yanagimachi, R., and Yanagimachi, H. (1981): Spermatozoa of the atlantic bottlenosed dolphin, *Tursiops truncatus*. *J. Reprod. Fertil.*, 63:509–514.
162. Florman, H. M., and Storey, B. T. (1982): Mouse gamete interactions: The zona pellucida is the site of the acrosome reaction leading to fertilization *in vitro*. *Dev. Biol.*, 91:121–130.
163. Florman, H. M., and Wassarman, P. M. (1985): O-linked oligosaccharides of mouse egg ZP-3 account for its sperm receptor activity. *Cell*, 4:313–324.
164. Fowler, R. E., and Grainge, C. (1985): A histochemical study of the changes occurring in the protein-carbohydrate composition of the cumulus-oocyte complex and zona pellucida in immature mice in response to gonadotropin stimulation. *Histochem. J.*, 17:1235–1249.
165. Fox, L. L., and Shivers, C. A. (1975): Immunologic evidence for addition of oviductal components to the hamster zona pellucida. *Fertil. Steril.*, 26:599–608.
166. Fraser, L. R. (1977): Motility patterns in mouse spermatozoa before and after capacitation. *J. Exp. Zool.*, 202:439–444.
167. Fraser, L. R. (1981): Dibutyryl cyclic AMP decreases capacitation time *in vitro* in mouse spermatozoa. *J. Reprod. Fertil.*, 62:63–72.
168. Fraser, L. R. (1982): Ca^{2+} is required for mouse sperm capacitation and fertilization *in vitro*. *J. Androl.*, 3:412–419.
169. Fraser, L. R. (1983): Potassium ions modulate expression of mouse sperm fertilizing ability, acrosome reaction and hyperactivated motility *in vitro*. *J. Reprod. Fertil.*, 69:539–553.
170. Fraser, L. R. (1984): Mechanisms controlling mammalian fertilization. In: *Oxford Review of Reproductive Biology, Vol. 6,* edited by C. A. Finn, pp. 174–225. Clarendon Press, Oxford.
171. Fraser, L. R. (1985): Albumin is required to support the acrosome reaction but not capacitation in mouse spermatozoa *in vitro*. *J. Reprod. Fertil.*, 74:185–196.
172. Fraser, L. R., and Quinn, P. J. (1981): A glycolytic product is obligatory for initiation of sperm acrosome reaction and whiplash motility required for fertilization in the mouse. *J. Reprod. Fertil.*, 61:25–35.
173. Friend, D. S. (1977): The organization of the sperm membrane. In: *Immunobiology of Gametes,* edited by M. Edidin and M. H. Johnson, pp. 5–30. Cambridge University Press, Cambridge.
174. Friend, D. S. (1980): Freeze-fracture alterations in guinea pig sperm membranes preceding gamete fusion. In: *Membrane-Membrane Interactions,* edited by N. B. Gilula, pp. 153–165. Raven Press, New York.
175. Friend, D. S. (1982): Plasma-membrane diversity in a highly polarized cell. *J. Cell Biol.*, 93:243–249.
176. Friend, D. S., Orci, L., Perrelet, A., and Yanagimachi, R. (1977): Membrane particle changes attending the acrosome reaction in guinea pig spermatozoa. *J. Cell Biol.*, 74:561–577.
177. Funaki, Y., Fukushima, M., and Ono, H. (1983): Fertilization and cleavage of bovine follicular oocytes in rabbit reproductive tracts after maturation *in vitro*. *J. Exp. Zool.*, 226:137–142.
178. Gaddum-Rosse, P. (1985): Mammalian gamete interactions: What can be gained from observations on living eggs? *Am. J. Anat.*, 173:347–356.
179. Gaddum-Rosse, P., and Blandau, R. J. (1972): Comparative studies on the proteolysis of fixed gelatin membranes by mammalian sperm acrosomes. *Am. J. Anat.*, 134:133–144.
180. Garbers, D. L. (1981): The elevation of cyclic AMP concentrations in flagella-less sea urchin sperm heads. *J. Biol. Chem.*, 256:620–624.
181. Gaunt, S. J. (1983): Spreading of the sperm surface antigen within the plasma membrane of the egg after fertilization in the rat. *J. Embryol. Exp. Morphol.*, 75:257–270.
182. Go, K. J., and Wolf, D. P. (1983): The role of sterols in sperm capacitation. *Adv. Lipid Res.*, 20:317–330.
183. Go, K. J., and Wolf, D. P. (1985): Albumin-mediated changes in the sperm sterol contents during capacitation. *Biol. Reprod.*, 32:145–153.
184. Goodpasture, J. C., Polakoski, K. L., and Zaneveld, L. J. D. (1980): Acrosin, proacrosin and acrosin inhibitor of human spermatozoa: Extraction, quantitation and stability. *J. Androl.*, 1:16–27.
185. Goodpasture, J. C., Reddy, J. M., and Zaneveld, L. J. D. (1981): Acrosin, proacrosin, and acrosin inhibitor of guinea pig spermatozoa capacitated and acrosome-reacted *in vitro*. *Biol. Reprod.*, 25: 44–55.
186. Gordon, L. M., and Mobley, P. W. (1985): Membrane lipids, membrane fluidity, and enzyme activity. In: *Membrane Fluidity in Biology, Vol. 4,* edited by R. C. Aloia and J. M. Boggs, pp. 1–49. Academic Press, Orlando, Fla.

187. Gordon, M. (1973): Localization of phosphatase activity on membranes of the mammalian sperm head. *J. Exp. Zool.*, 185:111–120.
188. Gordon, M., Dandekar, P. V., and Bartoszewicz, W. (1975): The surface coat of epididymal, ejaculated, and capacitated sperm. *J. Ultrastruct. Res.*, 50:199–207.
189. Gordon, M., Dandekar, P. V., and Eager, P. R. (1978): Identification of phosphatases on the membranes of guinea pig sperm. *Anat. Rec.*, 191:123–133.
190. Gould, J. E., Overstreet, J. W., and Hanson, F. W. (1985): Interaction of human spermatozoa with the human zona pellucida and zona-free hamster oocyte following capacitation by exposure to human cervical mucus. *Gamete Res.*, 12:47–54.
191. Gould, K., Zaneveld, L. J. D., Srivastava, P. N., and Williams, W. L. (1971): Biochemical changes in the zona pellucida of rabbit ova induced by fertilization and sperm enzymes. *Proc. Soc. Exp. Biol. Med.*, 136:6–10.
192. Gould, S. F., and Bernstein, M. H. (1975): The localization of bovine sperm hyaluronidase. *Differentiation*, 3:123–132.
193. Green, D. P. L. (1976): Induction of the acrosome reaction in guinea pig spermatozoa *in vitro* by Ca ionophore A23187. *J. Physiol.*, 260:18–19.
194. Green, D. P. L. (1978): The mechanism of the acrosome reaction. In: *Development in Mammals, Vol. 3*, edited by M. H. Johnson, pp. 65–81. North-Holland, New York.
195. Green, D. P. L. (1978): The activation of proteolysis in the acrosome reaction of guinea pig spermatozoa. *J. Cell Sci.*, 32:153–164.
196. Green, D. P. L., and Hockaday, A. R. (1978): The histochemical localization of acrosin in guinea pig sperm after the acrosome reaction. *J. Cell Sci.*, 32:177–184.
197. Green, D. P. L., and Purves, T. D. (1984): Mechanical hypothesis of sperm penetration. *Biophys. J.*, 45:659–662.
198. Greve, J. M., and Wassarman, P. M. (1985): Mouse egg extracellular coat is a mixture of interconnected filaments possessing a structural repeat. *J. Mol. Biol.*, 181:253–264.
199. Gwatkin, R. B. L. (1977): *Fertilization Mechanisms in Man and Mammals*. Plenum Press, New York.
200. Gwatkin, R. B. L., Andersen, O. F., and Hutchison, C. F. (1972): Capacitation of hamster spermatozoa *in vitro:* The role of cumulus components. *J. Reprod. Fertil.*, 30:389–394.
201. Gwatkin, R. B. L., and Klein, D. (1985): Binding of solubilized zona by porcine sperm as they undergo the acrosome reaction. *J. Androl.*, 6:28a.
202. Gwatkin, R. B. L., and Williams, D. T. (1977): Receptor activity of the hamster and mouse solubilized zona pellucida before and after the zona reaction. *J. Reprod. Fertil.*, 49:55–59.
203. Gwatkin, R. B. L., Williams, D. T., Hartmann, J. F., and Kniazuk, M. (1973): The zona reaction of hamster and mouse eggs. Production *in vitro* of a trypsin-like protease from cortical granules. *J. Reprod. Fertil.*, 32:259–265.
204. Haino, K. (1971): Studies on the egg membrane lysin of *Tegula pfeifferi:* Purification and properties of the egg-membrane lysin. *Biochim. Biophys. Acta*, 229:459–470.
205. Haino-Fukushima, K. (1974): Studies on the egg membrane lysin of *Tegula pfeifferi:* The reaction mechanism of the egg membrane lysin. *Biochim. Biophys. Acta*, 352:459–470.
206. Hamilton, D. W. (1971): Steroid function in the mammalian epididymis. *J. Reprod. Fertil (Suppl.)*, 13:89–97.
207. Hamilton, D. W. (1980): UDP-galactose: *N*-acetylglucosamine galactosyltransferase in fluids from rat testis and epididymis. *Biol. Reprod.*, 23:377–385.
208. Hamilton, D. W. (1981): Evidence for alpha-lactoalbumin-like activity in reproductive tract fluids of the male rat. *Biol. Reprod.*, 25:385–392.
209. Hamilton, D. W., and Fawcett, D. W. (1970): *In vitro* synthesis of cholesterol and testosterone from acetate by rat epididymis and vas deferens. *Proc. Soc. Exp. Biol. Med.*, 133:693–695.
210. Hamilton, D. W., and Gould, R. P. (1980): Galactosyltransferase activity associated with rat epididymis. *Anat. Rec.*, 196:71a.
211. Hammerstedt, R. H., Hay, S. R., and Amann, R. P. (1982): Modification of ram sperm membranes during epididymal transit. *Biol. Reprod.*, 27:745–754.
212. Hammer, C. E., and Fox, S. B. (1969): Biochemistry of oviductal secretions. In: *The Mammalian Oviduct*, edited by E. S. E. Hafez and R. J. Blandau, pp. 333–355. University Chicago Press, Chicago.
213. Hammer, C. E., Jennings, L. L., and Sojka, N. J. (1970): Cat (*Feris catus* L.) spermatozoa require capacitation. *J. Reprod. Fertil.*, 23:477–480.
214. Handrow, R. R., Boehm, S. K., Lenz, R. W., Robinson, J. A., and Aux, R. L. (1984): Specific binding of glycosaminoglycan ^{3}H-heparine to bull, monkey and rabbit spermatozoa *in vitro*. *J. Androl.*, 5:51–63.
215. Handrow, R. R., Lenz, R. W., and Aux, R. L. (1982): Structural comparisons among glycosaminoglycans to promote an acrosome reaction in bovine spermatozoa. *Biochem. Biophys. Res. Commun.*, 107:1326–1332.
216. Harrison, R. A. P. (1975): The metabolism of mammalian spermatozoa. In: *Frontiers in Reproduction and Fertility Control*, edited by R. O. Greep and M. A. Koblinsky, pp. 379–401. MIT Press, Cambridge.
217. Harrison, R. A. P. (1983): The acrosome, its hydrolase, and egg penetration. In: *The Sperm Cell*, edited by J. Andre, pp. 259–273. Martinus Nijhoff, The Hague.
218. Hartmann, J. F. (1985): Mammalian fertilization: Gamete surface interactions *in vitro*. In: *Mechanism and Control of Animal Fertilization*, edited by J. F. Hartmann, pp. 325–364. Academic Press, New York.
219. Hartmann, J. F., and Hutchison, C. F. (1974): Nature of the pre-penetration contact interactions between hamster gametes *in vitro*. *J. Reprod. Fertil.*, 36:49–57.
220. Hartmann, J. F., and Hutchison, C. F. (1976): Is acrosin the lysin of the zona pellucida during fertilization? *Proc. 9th Annu. Soc. Study Reprod. Meet., Philadelphia* (abstract #2).
221. Hedrick, J. L., and Wardrip, N. J. (1982): Topographical radiolabeling of zona pellucida glycoproteins. *J. Cell Biol.*, 95:162a.
222. Hedrick, J. L., Wardrip, N. J., and Berger, T. (1986): Difference in the macromolecular composition of the zona pellucida isolated from pig oocytes, eggs and zygotes. *J. Exp. Zool.*, 241: 257–262.
223. Helm, G., Owman, C. H., Rosengren, E., Sjoberg, N. O. (1982): Regional and cyclic variations in catecholamine concentrations of the human Fallopian tube. *Biol. Reprod.*, 26:553–558.
224. Herz, Z., Northey, D., Lawyer, M., and First, N. L. (1985): Acrosome reaction of bovine spermatozoa *in vitro:* Sites and effects of the stages of the estrous cycle. *Biol. Reprod.*, 32:1163–1168.
225. Hinkley, R. E., Wright, B. D., and Greenberg, C. A. (1986): Induction of the acrosome reaction in sea urchin spermatozoa by the volatile anesthetic halothane. *Biol. Reprod.*, 34:119–125.
226. Hinrichsen, A. C., Topfer-Petersen, E., Dietl, T., Schmoeckel, C., and Schill, W. B. (1985): Immunological approach to the characterization of the acrosomal membrane of boar spermatozoa. *Gamete Res.*, 11:143–155.
227. Hinrichsen-Kohane, A. C., Hinrichsen, M. J., and Schill, W. S. (1984): Molecular events leading to fertilization. *Andrologia*, 16:321–341.
228. Hirata, F., and Axelrod, J. (1980): Phospholipid methylation and biological signal transmission. *Science*, 209:1082–1090.
229. Hirst, P. J., DeMayo, F. J., and Dukelow, W. R. (1981): Xenogenous fertilization of laboratory and domestic animals in the oviduct of the pseudopregnant rabbit. *Theriogenology*, 15:67–75.
230. Hoffer, A. P., Shalev, M., and Frisch, D. H. (1981): Ultrastructure and maturational changes in spermatozoa in the epididymis of the pigtail monkey, *Macaca nemestrina*. *J. Androl.*, 2:140–146.
231. Holt, W. V. (1979): Development and maturation of the mammalian acrosome: A cytochemical study using phosphotungstic acid staning. *J. Ultrastruct. Res.*, 68:58–71.
232. Holt, W. V. (1980): Surface-bound sialic acid on ram and bull spermatozoa: Deposition during epididymal transit and stability during washing. *Biol. Reprod.*, 23:847–857.
233. Holt, W. V. (1982): Functional development of the mammalian sperm plasma membrane. In: *Oxford Review of Reproductive Biology, Vol. 4*, edited by C. A. Finn, pp. 195–240. Clarendon Press, Oxford.
234. Holt, W. V. (1984): Membrane heterogeneity in the mammalian spermatozoa. *Int. Rev. Cytol.*, 87:159–194.
235. Hoppe, P. C. (1980): Genetic influences on mouse sperm capacitation *in vivo* and *in vitro*. *Gamete Res.*, 3:343–349.
236. Howards, S., Lechene, C., and Vigersky, R. (1979): The fluid environment of the maturing spermatozoa. In: *The Spermatozoa*, edited by D. W. Fawcett and J. M. Bedford, pp. 35–41. Urban and Schwarzenberg, Baltimore.

237. Huacuja, L., Delgado, N. M., Merchant, H., Pancardo, R. M., and Rosado, A. (1977): Cyclic AMP induced incorporation of ^{33}Pi into human sperm membrane components. *Biol. Reprod.*, 17: 89–96.
238. Huang, T. T. F., Flemming, A. D., and Yanagimachi, R. (1981): Only acrosome-reacted spermatozoa can bind and penetrate into zona pellucida: A study using guinea pig. *J. Exp. Zool.*, 217:286–290.
239. Huang, T. T. F., Hardy, D., Yanagimachi, H., Teuscher, C., Tung, K., Wild, G., and Yanagimachi, R. (1985): pH and proteinase control of acrosomal content stasis and release during the guinea pig acrosome reaction. *Biol. Reprod.*, 32:451–462.
240. Huang, T. T. F., and Yanagimachi, R. (1984): Fucoidin inhibits attachment of guinea pig spermatozoa to the zona pellucida through binding to the inner acrosomal membrane and equatorial domains. *Exp. Cell Res.*, 153:363–373.
241. Huang, T. T. F., and Yanagimachi, R. (1985): Inner acrosomal membrane of mammalian spermatozoa: Its properties and possible functions in fertilization. *Am. J. Anat.*, 174:249–268.
242. Huneau, D., Harrison, R. A. P., and Flechon, J. E. (1984): Ultrastructural localization of proacrosin and acrosin in ram spermatozoa. *Gamete Res.*, 9:425–440.
243. Hunter, A. G., and Nornes, H. O. (1969): Characterization and isolation of a sperm-coating antigen from rabbit seminal plasm with capacity to block fertilization. *J. Reprod. Fertil.*, 20:419–427.
244. Hunter, R. H. F. (1984): Pre-ovulatory arrest and periovulatory redistribution of competent spermatozoa in the isthmus of the pig oviduct. *J. Reprod. Fertil.*, 72:203–211.
245. Hyne, R. V. (1984): Bicarbonate and calcium dependent induction of rapid guinea pig acrosome reaction by monovalent ionophore. *Biol. Reprod.*, 31:312–323.
246. Hyne, R. V., and Edwards, K. P. (1985): Influence of 2-deoxyl-D-glucose and energy substrates on guinea-pig sperm capacitation and acrosome reaction. *J. Reprod. Fertil.*, 73:59–69.
247. Hyne, R. V., Edwards, K. P., and Smith, J. D. (1985): Changes in guinea pig sperm intracellular sodium and potassium content during capacitation and treatment with monovalent ionophore. *Gamete Res.*, 12:65–73.
248. Hyne, R. V., and Garbers, D. L. (1979): Calcium-dependent increase in adenosin 3′,5′-monophosphate and induction of the acrosome reaction in guinea pig spermatozoa. *Proc. Natl. Acad. Sci. USA*, 76:5699–5703.
249. Hyne, R. V., Higginson, R., Kohlman, D., and Lopata, A. (1984): Sodium requirement for capacitation membrane fusion during the guinea pig acrosome reaction. *J. Reprod. Fertil.*, 70:83–94.
250. Infante, J. P., and Huszagh, V. A. (1985): Synthesis of highly unsaturated phosphatidylcholine in the development of sperm motility: A role for epididymal glycerol-3-phosphorylcholine. *Mol. Cell. Biochem.*, 69:3–9.
251. Inoue, M., and Wolf, D. P. (1975): Fertilization-associated changes in the murine zona pellucida: A time sequence study. *Biol. Reprod.*, 13:546–551.
252. Ishijima, S., McCracken, J. A., and Witman, G. B. (1985): Flagellar movement of intact and demembranated ram spermatozoa. *J. Cell Biol.*, 101:364a.
253. Johnson, L. A., Garner, D. L., Truitt-Gilbert, A. J., and Lessley, A. (1983): Immunocytochemical acrosin on both acrosomal membranes and in the acrosomal matrix of porcine spermatozoa. *J. Androl.*, 4:222–229.
254. Johnson, L. L., Katz, D. F., and Overstreet, J. W. (1981): The movement characteristics of rabbit spermatozoa before and after activation. *Gamete Res.*, 4:275–282.
255. Johnson, M. H. (1975): The macromolecular organization of membranes and its bearing on events leading up to fertilization. *J. Reprod. Fertil.*, 44:167–184.
256. Johnson, M. H., Eager, D., and Muggleton-Harris, A. (1975): Mosaicism in organization of concanavalin A receptors on the surface membrane of mouse eggs. *Nature*, 257:321–322.
257. Jones, H. P., Lenz, R. W., Palevitz, B. A., and Cormier, M. J. (1980): Calmodulin localization in mammalian spermatozoa. *Proc. Natl. Acad. Sci. USA*, 77:2772–2776.
258. Jones, R., and Brown, C. R. (1982): Association of epididymal secretory proteins showing α-lactoalbumin-like activity with plasma membrane of rat spermatozoa. *Biochem. J.*, 206:161–164.
259. Joyce, C. (1982): The antifertility activity of sperm hyaluronidase inhibitors. *Biol. Reprod.*, 26:117a.
260. Joyce, C., Jeyendran, R. S., and Zaneveld, L. J. D. (1985): Release, extraction and stability of hyaluronidase associated with human spermatozoa: Comparison with rabbit. *J. Androl.*, 6:152–161.
261. Katz, D. F., and Yanagimachi, R. (1980): Movement characteristics of hamster spermatozoa within the oviduct. *Biol. Reprod.*, 22:759–764.
262. Katz, D. F., and Yanagimachi, R. (1981): Movement characteristics of hamster and guinea pig spermatozoa upon attachment to the zona pellucida. *Biol. Reprod.*, 25:785–791.
263. Kinsey, W. H. and Koehler, J. K. (1978): Cell surface charges associated with *in vitro* capacitation of hamster sperm. *J. Ultrastruct. Res.*, 64:1–13.
264. Koehler, J. K. (1977): Fine structure of spermatozoa of the Asiatic musk shrew, *Suncus murinus*. *Am. J. Anat.*, 149:135–152.
265. Koehler, J. K. (1978): The mammalian sperm surface: Studies with specific labeling techniques. *Int. Rev. Cytol.*, 54:73–108.
266. Koehler, J. K. (1981): Lectins as probes of the spermatozoa surface. *Arch. Androl.*, 6:197–217.
267. Koehler, J. K. (1981): Surface alterations during the capacitation of mammalian spermatozoa. *Am. J. Primatol.*, 1:131–141.
268. Koehler, J. K., and Gaddum-Rosse, P. (1975): Media induced alterations of the membrane associated particles of the guinea pig sperm tail. *J. Ultrastruct. Res.*, 51:106–118.
269. Koehler, J. K., Nudelman, E. D., and Hakomori, S. (1980): A collagen-binding protein of the surface of ejaculated rabbit spermatozoa. *J. Cell Biol.*, 86:529–536.
270. Kopecny, V., and Flechon, J. E. (1981): Fate of acrosomal glycoproteins during the acrosome reaction and fertilization: A light and electron microscope autoradiographic study. *Biol. Reprod.*, 24: 201–216.
271. Kopecny, V., Flechon, J. E., and Pivko, J. (1984): Binding of secreted glycoproteins to spermatozoa in the mammalian epididymis: A fine-structure autoradiographic study. *Anat. Rec.*, 208:197–206.
272. Koyama, K., Hasegawa, A., and Isojima, S. (1984): Effect of antisperm antibody on the *in vitro* development of rat embryos. *Gamete Res.*, 10:143–152.
273. Krzanowska, H. (1982): Toluidine blue staining reveals changes in chromatin stabilization of mouse spermatozoa during epididymal maturation and penetration of ova. *J. Reprod. Fertil.*, 64:97–101.
274. Kusan, F., Flemming, A. D., and Seidel, G. (1984): Successful fertilization *in vitro* of fresh intact oocytes by perivitelline (acrosome-reacted) spermatozoa in the rabbit. *Fertil. Steril.*, 41:766–770.
275. Kvist, U., and Bjorndahl, L. (1985): Zinc preserves and inherent capacity for human sperm chromatin decondensation. *Acta Physiol. Scand.*, 124:195–200.
276. Kvist, U., Bjorndahl, L., Roomans, C., and Lindholmer, C. (1985): Nuclear zinc in human epididymal and ejaculated spermatozoa. *Acta Physiol. Scand.*, 125:297–303.
277. Lambert, H. (1981): Temperature dependence of capacitation in bat sperm monitored by zona-free hamster ova. *Gamete Res.*, 4:525–533.
278. Lambert, H. (1984): Role of sperm-surface glycoproteins in gamete recognition in two mouse species. *J. Reprod. Fertil.*, 70:281–284.
279. Lambert, H., Overstreet, J. W., Morales, P., Hanson, F. W., and Yanagimachi, R. (1985): Sperm capacitation in the female reproductive tract. *Fertil. Steril.*, 43:325–327.
280. Lambert, H., and Van Le, A. (1984): Possible involvement of a sialyated component of the sperm plasma membrane in sperm-zona interaction in mouse. *Gamete Res.*, 10:153–163.
281. Langford, B. B., and Howarth, B. (1974): A trypsin-like enzyme in acrosomal extracts of chicken, turkey, and quail spermatozoa. *Poult. Sci.*, 53:834–837.
282. Langlais, J., Plante, L., Bleau, G., Chapedelaine, A., and Roberts, K. D. (1982): Metabolism of lysophosphatidylcholine in relation to sperm capacitation. *Fertil. Steril.*, 38:135–136.
283. Langlais, J., and Roberts, K. D. (1985): A molecular membrane model of sperm capacitation and the acrosome reaction of mammalian spermatozoa. *Gamete Res.*, 12:183–224.
284. Langlais, J., Zollinger, M., Plante, L., Chapedelaine, A., Bleau, G., and Roberts, K. D. (1981): Localization of cholesterol sulfate in human spermatozoa in support of a hypothesis of the mechanism of capacitation. *Proc. Natl. Acad. Sci. USA*, 78:7266–7270.
285. Leblond, C. P., and Clermont, Y. (1952): Spermatogenesis of rat, mouse, hamster, and guinea pig as revealed by the periodic acid-fuchsin sulfurous acid technique. *Am. J. Anat.*, 90:167–215.

286. Lechene, C. (1982): Elemental and biochemical microanalysis of the male reproductive tract. *Ann. N.Y. Acad. Sci.*, 383:513–526.
287. Lee, M. A., and Storey, B. T. (1985): Evidence for plasma membrane impermeability to small ions in acrosome intact mouse spermatozoa bound to mouse zonae pellucidae, using aminoacridine fluorescent pH probe. *Biol. Reprod.*, 33:235–246.
288. Lee, M. A., and Storey, B. T. (1986): Bicarbonate is essential for fertilization of mouse eggs: Mouse sperm require it to undergo the acrosome reaction. *Biol. Reprod.*, 34:349–356.
289. Legault, Y., Bleau, G., Chapedelaine, A., and Roberts, K. D. (1980): Steroid sulfatase activity of hamster reproductive tract during the estrous cycle. *Biol. Reprod.*, 23:720–725.
290. Legault, Y., Bouthiller, M., Bleau, G., Chapedelaine, A., and Roberts, K. D. (1979): The sterol and sterol sulfate content of the male hamster reproductive tract. *Biol. Reprod.*, 20:1213–1219.
291. Leibfried, M. L., and Bavister, B. D. (1982): Effects of epinephrine and hypotaurine in *in vitro* fertilization in the golden hamster. *J. Reprod. Fertil.*, 66:87–93.
292. LeLannou, D., Colleu, D., Boujard, D., and Segalin, J. (1985): Stabilization of nuclear chromatin in human spermatozoa during capacitation *in vitro*. In: *Human In Vitro Fertilization,* edited by J. Testart and R. Frydman, pp. 149–152. Elsevier, Amsterdam.
293. Lenz, R. W., Bellin, M. E., and Aux, R. L. (1983): Rabbit spermatozoa undergo an acrosome reaction in the presence of glycoaminoglycans. *Gamete Res.*, 8:11–19.
294. Lewin, L. M., Nevo, Z., Gabsu, A., and Weissenberg, R. (1982): The role of sperm bound hyaluronidase in the dispersal of the cumulus oophrus surrounding the rat ova. *Int. J. Androl.*, 5:37–44.
295. Lewin, L. M., Nevo, Z., and Weissenberg, R. (1981): The role of bound hyaluronidase in rat sperm-cumulus oophorus interaction. *Ann. N. Y. Acad. Sci.*, 383:473–474.
296. Lewis, C. A., Talbot, C. F., and Vacquier, V. D. (1982): A protein from abalone sperm dissolves the egg vitelline layer by a nonenzymatic mechanism. *Dev. Biol.*, 92:227–239.
297. Llanos, M. N., Lui, C. W., and Meizel, S. (1982): Studies of phospholipase A_2 related to the hamster sperm acrosome reaction. *J. Exp. Zool.*, 221:107–117.
298. Llanos, M. N., and Meizel, S. (1983): Phospholipid methylation increases during capacitation of golden hamster sperm *in vitro*. *Biol. Reprod.*, 28:1043–1051.
299. Longo, F. J., and Chen, D. Y. (1985): Development of cortical polarity in mouse eggs: Involvement of the meiotic apparatus. *Dev. Biol.*, 107:382–394.
300. Lopez, L. C., Bayna, E. M., Litoff, D., Shaper, N. L., Shaper, J. H., and Shur, B. D. (1985): Receptor function of mouse sperm surface galactosyltransferase during fertilization. *J. Cell Biol.*, 101:1501–1510.
301. Lopo, A. C. (1983): Sperm-egg interactions in invertebrates. In: *Mechanism and Control of Animal Fertilization,* edited by J. F. Hartmann, pp. 269–324. Academic Press, New York.
302. Lorton, S. P., and First, N. L. (1979): Hyaluronidase does not disperse the cumulus oophorus surrounding bovine ova. *Biol. Reprod.*, 21:301–308.
303. Lui, C. W., Cornett, L. E., and Meizel, S. (1977): Identification of the bovine follicular fluid protein involved in the *in vitro* induction of the hamster sperm acrosome reaction. *Biol. Reprod.*, 17:34–41.
304. Lui, C. W., and Meizel, S. (1977): Biochemical studies of the *in vitro* acrosome reaction inducing activity of bovine serum albumin. *Differentiation,* 9:59–66.
305. Lui, C. W., and Meizel, S. (1979): Further evidence in support of a role for hamster sperm hydrolytic enzymes in the acrosome reaction. *J. Exp. Zool.*, 207:173–186.
306. Lui, C. W., Mrsny, R. J., and Meizel, S. (1979): Procedure for obtaining high percentages of viable *in vitro* capacitated hamster sperm. *Gamete Res.*, 2:207–211.
307. Mahadevan, M. M., and Traunson, A. O. (1985): Removal of the cumulus oophorus from the human oocyte for *in vitro* fertilization. *Fertil. Steril.*, 43:263–267.
308. Mahanes, M. S., Ochs, D. L., and Eng, L. A. (1986): Cell calcium of ejaculated rabbit spermatozoa before and following *in vitro* capacitation. *Biochem. Biophys. Res. Commun.*, 134:664–670.
309. Mahi, C. A., and Yanagimachi, R. (1973): The effect of temperature, osmolality and hydrogen ion concentration on the activation and acrosome reaction of golden hamster spermatozoa. *J. Reprod. Fertil.*, 35:55–66.
310. Mahi, C. A., and Yanagimachi, R. (1976): Maturation and sperm penetration of canine ovarian oocytes *in vitro*. *J. Exp. Zool.*, 196:189–196.
311. Mann, T. (1964): *The Biochemistry of Semen and of the Male Reproductive Tract.* Methuen, New York.
312. Mann, T., and Lutwak-Mann, C. (1981): *Male Reproductive Function and Semen.* Springer-Verlag, New York.
313. Mars, B., Johnson, M. H., Pickering, S. J., and Flach, G. (1984): Changes in actin distribution during fertilization in the mouse egg. *J. Embryol. Exp. Morphol.*, 81:211–237.
314. Meizel, S. (1978): The mammalian sperm acrosome reaction. A biochemical approach. In: *Development in Mammals,* edited by M. H. Johnson, pp. 1–64. North-Holland, New York.
315. Meizel, S. (1984): The importance of hydrolytic enzymes to an exocytotic event, the mammalian sperm acrosome reaction. *Biol. Rev.*, 59:125–157.
316. Meizel, S. (1985): Molecules that initiate or help stimulate the acrosome reaction by their interaction with the mammalian sperm surface. *Am. J. Anat.*, 174:285–302.
317. Meizel, S., and Deamer, D. W. (1978): The pH of the hamster sperm acrosome. *J. Histochem. Cytochem.*, 26:98–105.
318. Meizel, S., and Lui, C. W. (1976): Evidence for a role of a trypsin-like enzyme in the hamster sperm acrosome reaction. *J. Exp. Zool.*, 195:137–144.
319. Meizel, S., Lui, C. W., Working, P. K., and Mrsny, R. J. (1980): Taurine and hypotaurine: Their effects on motility, capacitation and the acrosome reaction of hamster sperm *in vitro* and their presence in sperm and reproductive tract fluids of several mammals. *Dev. Growth Diff.*, 22:483–494.
320. Meizel, S., and Turner, K. O. (1983): Stimulation of an exocytotic event, the hamster sperm acrosome reaction, by cis-unsaturated fatty acids. *FEBS Lett.*, 161:315–318.
321. Meizel, S., and Turner, K. O. (1984): The effects of products and inhibitors of arachidonic acid metabolism on the hamster sperm acrosome reaction. *J. Exp. Zool.*, 231:283–288.
322. Meizel, S., and Turner, K. O. (1986): Glycosaminoglycans stimulate the acrosome reaction of previously capacitated hamster sperm. *J. Exp. Zool.*, 237:137–139.
323. Metz, C. B., Seiguer, A. C., and Castro, A. E. (1972): Inhibition of the cumulus dispersing and hyaluronidase activities of sperm by heterologous and isologous antisperm antibodies. *Proc. Soc. Exp. Biol. Med.*, 140:776–781.
324. Miller, M. A., and Masui, Y. (1982): Changes in the stainability and sulfhydryl level in the sperm nucleus during sperm-oocyte interaction in mice. *Gamete Res.*, 5:167–179.
325. Miyamoto, H., and Chang, M. C. (1973): The importance of serum albumin and metabolic intermediates for capacitation of spermatozoa and fertilization of mouse eggs *in vitro*. *J. Reprod. Fertil.*, 32:193–205.
326. Mohri, H., and Yanagimachi, R. (1980): Characteristics of motor apparatus in testicular, epididymal and ejaculated spermatozoa: A study using demembranated sperm model. *Exp. Cell Res.*, 127:191–196.
327. Monks, N. J., Stein, D. M., and Fraser, L. R. (1985): Mouse sperm adenylate cyclase is stimulated by calcium. *Proc. Annu. Meet. Soc. Study Fertil. London,* 13 (abstract 10).
328. Moore, H. D. M. (1979): The net surface charge of mammalian spermatozoa as determined by isoelectric focusing: Changes following sperm maturation, ejaculation, incubation in the female tract, and after enzyme treatment. *Int. J. Androl.*, 2:449–462.
329. Moore, H. D. M., and Bedford, J. M. (1983): The interaction of mammalian gametes in the female. In: *Mechanism and Control of Animal Fertilization,* edited by J. F. Hartmann, pp. 453–497. Academic Press, New York.
330. Moore, H. D. M., and Hibbitt, K. G. (1976): The binding of labelled basic proteins by boar spermatozoa. *J. Reprod. Fertil.*, 46:71–76.
331. Morre, D. J., Clegg, E. D., Lunstra, D. D., and Mollenhauer, H. H. (1974): An electron-dense stain for isolated fragments of plasma and acrosomal membrane from porcine sperm. *Proc. Soc. Exp. Biol. Med.*, 145:1–6.
332. Mortimer, D., Courtot, A. M., Giovangrandi, Y., Jeulin, C., and David, G. (1984): Human sperm motility after migration into, and incubation in, synthetic media. *Gamete Res.*, 9:131–144.
333. Morton, B., and Albagli, L. (1973): Modification of hamster sperm adenyl cyclase by capacitation *in vitro*. *Biochem. Biophys. Res. Commun.*, 50:695–703.

334. Morton, D. B. (1975): Acrosomal enzymes: Immunological localization of acrosin and hyaluronidase in ram spermatozoa. *J. Reprod. Fertil.*, 45:375–378.
335. Motomura, M., and Toyoda, Y. (1980): Scanning electron microscopic observations on the sperm penetration through the zona pellucida of mouse oocytes fertilized *in vitro*. *Jpn. J. Zootech. Sci.*, 51:595–601.
336. Moy, G. W., and Vacquier, V. D. (1979): Immunoperoxidase localization of binding during the adhesion of sperm to sea urchin eggs. *Curr. Top. Dev. Biol.*, 13:31–44.
337. Mrsny, R. J., and Meizel, S. (1980): Evidence suggesting a role for cyclic nucleotides in acrosome reactions of hamster sperm *in vitro*. *J. Exp. Zool.*, 211:153–158.
338. Mrsny, R. J., and Meizel, S. (1981): Potassium ion influx and Na^+,K^+-ATPase activity are required for the hamster sperm acrosome reaction. *J. Cell Biol.*, 91:77–82.
339. Mrsny, R. J., and Meizel, S. (1983): Initial evidence for the modification of hamster sperm Na^+,K^+-ATPase activity by cyclic nucleotide mediated processes. *Biochem. Biophys. Res. Commun.*, 112:132–138.
340. Mrsny, R. J., and Meizel, S. (1985): Inhibition of hamster sperm Na^+,K^+-ATPase activity by taurine and hypotaurine. *Life Sci.*, 36:271–275.
341. Mrsny, R. J., Siiteri, J. E., and Meizel, S. (1984): Hamster sperm Na^+,K^+-adenosine triphosphatase: Increased activity during capacitation *in vitro* and its relationship to cyclic nucleotides. *Biol. Reprod.*, 30:573–584.
342. Mrsny, R. J., Waxman, L., and Meizel, S. (1979): Taurine maintains and stimulates motility of hamster sperm during capacitation *in vitro*. *J. Exp. Zool.*, 210:123–128.
343. Mujica, A., and Ruiz, M. A. V. (1983): On the role of glucose in capacitation and acrosome reaction of guinea pig sperm. *Gamete Res.*, 8:335–344.
344. Multamaki, S., Pelliniemi, L. J., and Suominen, J. (1975): Ultrastructural study of separated cell and acrosomal membranes of bull spermatozoa. *Fertil. Steril.*, 26:932–938.
345. Murphy, S. J., Roldan, E. R. S., and Yanagimachi, R. (1986): Effects of extracellular cations and energy substrates on the acrosome reaction of precapacitated guinea pig spermatozoa. *Gamete Res.*, 14:1–10.
346. Murphy, S. J., and Yanagimachi, R. (1984): The pH-dependence of motility and the acrosome reaction of guinea pig spermatozoa. *Gamete Res.*, 10:1–8.
347. Nakano, M., Otsuka, M., Akama, K., and Tobita, T. (1984): Predominance of beta-structure in solubilized zona pellucida from porcine ova. *Biochem. Int.*, 9:39–43.
348. Nagae, T., Yanagimachi, R., Srivastava, P. N., and Yanagimachi, H. (1986): Acrosome reaction in human spermatozoa. *Fertil. Steril.*, 45:701–707.
349. Nagai, T. Niwa, K., and Iritani, A. (1984): Effect of sperm concentration during preincubation in a defined medium on fertilization *in vitro* of pig follicular oocytes. *J. Reprod. Fertil.*, 70:271–275.
350. Nicander, L., and Sjoden, I. (1971): An electron microscopical study of the acrosomal complex and its role in fertilization in the river lamprey, *Lampetra fluriatilis*. *J. Submicrosc. Cytol.*, 3:309–317.
351. Nicolson, G. L., Usui, N., Yanagimachi, R., Yanagimachi, H., and Smith, J. R. (1977): Lecitin-binding site on the plasma membranes of rabbit spermatozoa changes in surface receptors during epididymal maturation and after ejaculation. *J. Cell Biol.*, 74:950–962.
352. Nikolopoulou, M., Soucek, D. A., and Vary, J. C. (1985): Changes in the lipid content of boar sperm plasma membranes during epididymal maturation. *Biochim. Biophys. Acta,* 815:486–498.
353. Niwa, K., Ohara, K. Hoshi, Y., and Iritani, A. (1985) Early events of *in-vitro* fertilization of cat eggs by epididymal spermatozoa. *J. Reprod. Fertil.*, 74:657–660.
354. Ohzu, E., and Yanagimachi, R. (1982): Acceleration of acrosome reaction in hamster spermatozoa by lysolecithin. *J. Exp. Zool.*, 224:259–263.
355. Oikawa, T., Kurata, S., and Sendai, Y. (1986): Discovery of a novel zona pellucida glycoprotein (ZP-O) having a sperm binding activity. *J. Reprod. Immunol.*, (1986 suppl.):81.
356. Okabe, M., Takada, K., Adachi, T., Kohama, Y., Miura, T., and Aonuma, S. (1986): Studies on sperm capacitation using monoclonal antibody—Disappearance of an antigen from the anterior part of mouse sperm head. *J. Pharmacol. Dyn.*, 9:55–60.
357. Okabe, M., Takada, K., Adachi, T., Kohama, Y., and Miura, T. (1986): Inconsistent reactivity of an anti-sperm monoclonal antibody and its relationship to sperm capacitation. *J. Reprod. Immunol.*, 9:67–70.
358. Okamura, F., and Nishiyama, H. (1978): The passage of spermatozoa through the vitelline membrane in the domestic fowl, *Gallus gallus*. *Cell Tissue Res.*, 188:497–508.
359. Oliphant, G., Reynolds, A. B., and Thomas, T. S. (1985): Sperm surface components involved in the control of the acrosome reaction. *Am. J. Anat.*, 174:269–283.
360. Olson, G. E. (1980): Changes in intramembranous particle distribution in the plasma membrane of *Didelphis virginiana* spermatozoa during maturation in the epididymis. *Anat. Rec.*, 197:471–488.
361. Olson, G. E., and Danzo, B. J. (1981): Surface changes in rat spermatozoa during epididymal transit. *Biol. Reprod.*, 24:431–443.
362. Olson, G. E., and Orgebin-Crist, M. C. (1982): Sperm surface changes during epididymal maturation. *Ann. N.Y. Acad. Sci.*, 383:372–391.
363. Olson, G. E., Lifsics, M. R., Winfrey, V. P., and Rifkin, J. M. (1986): Association of a 26KD polypeptide with the flagellar plasma membrane of rat spermatozoa during maturation in the epididymis. *J. Androl.*, 7:13a.
364. Olson, G. E., and Winfrey, V. P. (1985): Substructure of a cytoskeletal complex associated with the hamster sperm acrosome. *J. Ultrastruct. Res.*, 92:167–179.
365. Olson, G. E., Winfrey, V. P., Garbers, D. L., and Noland, T. D. (1985): Isolation and characterization of macromolecular complex associated with the outer acrosomal membrane of bovine spermatozoa. *Biol. Reprod.*, 13:761–779.
366. Ono, K., Yanagimachi, R., and Huang, T. T. F. (1982): Phospholipase A of guinea pig spermatozoa: Its preliminary characterization and possible involvement in the acrosome reaction. *Dev. Growth Diff.*, 24:305–310.
367. O'Rand, M. G. (1977): Restriction of a sperm surface antigen's mobility during capacitation. *Dev. Biol.*, 55:260–270.
368. O'Rand, M. G. (1979): Changes in sperm surface properties correlated with capacitation. In: *The Spermatozoa,* edited by D. W. Fawcett and J. M. Bedford, pp. 195–204. Urban and Schwarzenberg, Baltimore.
369. O'Rand, M. G. (1982): Modification of the sperm membrane during capacitation. *Ann. N.Y. Acad. Sci.*, 383:392–404.
370. O'Rand, M. G. (1985): Differentiation of mammalian sperm antigens. In: *Biology of Fertilization, Vol. 2,* edited by C. B. Metz and A. Monroy, pp. 103–119. Academic Press, New York.
371. O'Rand, M. G., and Fisher, S. J. (1987): Localization of zona pellucida binding sites on rabbit spermatozoa and induction of the acrosome reaction by solubilized zonae. *Dev. Biol.*, 119:551–559.
372. O'Rand, M. G., Matthews, J. E., Welch, J. E., and Fisher, S. J. (1985): Identification of zona binding proteins of rabbit, pig, human and mouse spermatozoa on nitrocellulose blots. *J. Exp. Zool.*, 235:423–428.
373. O'Rand, M. G., Welch, J. E., and Fisher, S. J. (1986): Sperm membrane and zona pellucida interactions during fertilization. In: *Molecular and Cellular Aspects of Reproduction,* edited by D. S. Dhindsa and O. P. Bahl, pp. 131–144. Plenum Press, New York.
374. Orgebin-Crist, M. C. (1981): Epididymal physiology and sperm maturation. *Prog. Reprod. Biol,*, 8:80–89.
375. Orgebin-Crist, M. C., and Fournier-Delpech, S. (1982): Sperm-egg interaction: Evidence for maturational changes during epididymal transit. *J. Androl.*, 3:429–433.
376. Orgebin-Crist, M. C., Olson, G. E., and Danzo, B. J. (1981): Factors influencing maturation of spermatozoa in the epididymis. In: *Intragonadal Regulation of Reproduction,* edited by P. Franchimont and C. P. Channing, pp. 393–417. Academic Press, New York.
377. Oshio, S., Kaneko, S., and Mohri, H. (1986): Impurities in commercial preparations of bovine serum albumin inhibits the acrosome reaction of hamster spermatozoa. *Zool. Sci.*, 3:295–299.
378. Overstreet, J. W., and Bedford, J. M. (1974): Transport, capacitation and fertilizing ability of epididymal spermatozoa. *J. Exp. Zool.*, 189:203–214.
379. Overstreet, J. W., Coats, C., Katz, D. K., and Hanson, F. W. (1980): The importance of seminal plasma for sperm penetration of human cervical mucus. *Fertil. Steril.*, 34:569–572.
380. Overstreet, J. W., and Cooper, G. W. (1975): Reduced sperm motility in the isthmus of the rabbit oviduct. *Nature,* 258:718–719.

381. Overstreet, J. W., Cooper, G. W., and Katz, D. F. (1978): Sperm transport in the reproductive tract of the female rabbit II. The sustained phase of transport. *Biol. Reprod.*, 19:115–132.
382. Overstreet, J. W., and Cooper, G. W. (1979): The time and location of the acrosome during sperm transport in the female rabbit. *J. Exp. Zool.*, 209:97–104.
383. Overstreet, J. W., and Cooper, G. W. (1979): Effect of ovulation and sperm motility on the migration of rabbit spermatozoa to the site of fertilization. *J. Reprod. Fertil.*, 55:53–59.
384. Parks, J. E., and Hammerstedt, R. H. (1985): Developmental changes occurring in the lipid of ram epididymal sperm plasma membranes. *Biol. Reprod.*, 32:653–668.
385. Parrish, R. F., Wincek, T. J., and Polakoski, K. L. (1980): Glycosaminoglycon stimulation of the *in vitro* conversion of boar proacrosin into acrosin. *J. Androl.* 1:89–95.
386. Pellicciari, C., Hosokawa, Y., Fukuda, M., and Romanini, M. G. M. (1983): Cytofluorometic study of nuclear sulphydryl and disulphide groups during sperm maturation in the mouse. *J. Reprod. Fertil.*, 68:371–376.
387. Perreault, S., Zaneveld, L. J. D., and Rogers, B. J. (1980): Inhibition of fertilization in the hamster by sodium aurothiomalate, a hydronidase inhibitor. *J. Reprod. Fertil.*, 60:461–467.
388. Perreault, S. D., Zirkin, B. R., and Rogers, B. J. (1982): Effect of trypsin inhibitors on acrosome reaction of guinea pig spermatozoa. *Biol. Reprod.*, 26:343–351.
389. Peterson, R. N., Henry, L., Saxena, W., and Russell, L. D. (1985): Further characterization of boar sperm plasma membrane proteins with affinity for the porcine zona pellucida. *Gamete Res.*, 12:91–100.
390. Peterson, R. N., Hunt, W. P., and Henry, L. H. (1986): Interaction of boar spermatozoa with porcine oocytes: Increase in proteins with high affinity for the zona pellucida during epididymal transit. *Gamete Res.*, 14:57–64.
391. Peterson, R. N., and Russell, L. D. (1985): The mammalian spermatozoon: A model for the study of regional specificity in the plasma membrane organization and function. *Tissue Cell*, 17:769–791.
392. Phillips, D. M., and Shalgi, R. M. (1980): Surface properties of the zona pellucida. *J. Exp. Zool.*, 213:1–8.
393. Phillips, D. M., and Shalgi, R. M. (1982): Sperm penetration into rat ova fertilized *in vivo*. *J. Exp. Zool.*, 221:373–378.
394. Picheral, B., and Charbonneau, M. (1982): Anural fertilization: A morpohological reinvestigation of some early events. *J. Ultrastruct. Res.*, 81:306–321.
395. Piko, L. (1967): Immunological phenomena in the reproductive process. *Int. J. Fertil.*, 12:377–383.
396. Piko, L. (1979): Gamete structure and sperm entry in mammals. In: *Fertilization, Vol. 2*, edited by C. B. Metz and A. Monroy, pp. 325–403. Academic Press, New York.
397. Piko, L., and Tyler, A. (1964): Fine structural studies of sperm penetration in the rat. *Proceedings of the 5th International Congress on Animal Reproduction, Trento, Italy, Vol. 2*, pp. 372–374.
398. Plummer, J. M., and Watson, P. F. (1985): Ultrastructural localization of calcium ions in ram spermatozoa before and after cold shock is demonstrated by a pyroantimonate technique. *J. Reprod. Fertil.*, 75:255–263.
399. Presti, F. T. (1985): The role of cholesterol in regulating membrane fluidity. In: *Membrane Fluidity in Biology, Vol. 4: Cellular Aspects*, edited by R. C. Aloia and J. M. Boggs, pp. 97–146. Academic Press, Orlando, Fla.
400. Quian, Z., Tsai, Y., Steinberg, A., Lu, M., Greenfild, A. R. L., and Haddox, M. K. (1985): Localization of ornithin decarboxylase in rat testicular cells and epididymal spermatozoa. *Biol. Reprod.*, 33:1189–1195.
401. Quinn, P. J., and White, I. G. (1967): Active cation transport in dog spermatozoa. *Biochem. J.*, 104:328–340.
402. Quinn, P. J., and White, I. G. (1968): Distribution of adenosintriphosphatase activity in ram and bull spermatozoa. *J. Reprod. Fertil.*, 15:449–452.
403. Rahi, H., and Srivastava, P. N. (1983): Hormonal regulation of lysosomal hydrolases in the reproductive tract of the rabbit. *J. Reprod. Fertil.*, 67:447–455.
404. Rahi, H., and Srivastava, P. N. (1984): Lysosomal hydrolases in reproductive organs during estrous cycle of the hamster. *Gamete Res.*, 10:57–66.
405. Rao, V. H., Sarmah, B. C., and Bhattacharyya, N. K. (1984): Xenogenous fertilization of goat ova in the rabbit oviduct. *J. Reprod. Fertil.*, 71:377–379.
406. Reddy, J. M., Joyce, C., and Zaneveld, L. J. D. (1980): Role of hyaluronidase in fertilization: The antifertility activity of Myocrisin, a nontoxic hyaluronidase inhibitor. *J. Androl.*, 1:28–32.
407. Reger, J. F., Fain-Maurel, M. A., and Dadoune, J. P. (1985): A freeze-fracture study on epididymal and ejaculate spermatozoa of the monkey (*Macaca fascicularis*). *J. Submicrosc. Cytol.*, 17:49–56.
408. Restall, B. J., and Wales, R. G. (1966): The Fallopian tube of the sheep. III. The chemical composition of the fluid from the Fallopian tube. *Aust. J. Biol. Sci.*, 19:687–698.
409. Restall, B. J., and Wales, R. G. (1968): The Fallopian tube of the sheep. V. Secretion from the ampulla and isthmus. *Aust. J. Biol. Sci.*, 21:491–498.
410. Reyes, A., Chavarria, M. E., and Rosado, A. (1980): Interference with spermatozoa capacitation. In: *Regulation of Male Fertility*, edited by G. R. Cunningham, W. S. Schill, and E. S. E. Hafez, pp. 135–149. Martinus Nijhoff, The Hague.
411. Reyes, R., Magdaleno, V. M., Hernandez, O., Rosado, A., and Delgado, N. M. (1983): Effect of zinc on decondensation of human spermatozoa nuclei by heparine. *Arch. Androl.*, 10:155–160.
412. Rifkin, J. M., and Olson, G. E. (1984): Characterization of maturation-dependent extrinsic proteins of the rat sperm surface. *J. Cell Biol.*, 100:1582–1591.
413. Rikmenspoel, R., Orris, S. E., and Isles, C. A. (1981): Effect of vandate, Mg^{2+} and electric current injection on the stiffness of impaled bull spermatozoa. *J. Cell. Sci.*, 51:53–61.
414. Rodger, J. C., and Bedford, J. M. (1982): Separation of sperm pairs and sperm-egg interaction in the opossum *Didelphis virginiana*. *J. Reprod. Fertil.*, 64:171–179.
415. Rogers, B. J. (1978): Mammalian sperm capacitation and fertilization *in vitro:* A critique of methodology. *Gamete Res.*, 1:165–223.
416. Rogers, B. J., and Garcia, L. (1979): Effect of cAMP on acrosome reaction and fertilization. *Biol. Reprod.*, 21:365–372.
417. Roldan, E. R. S., Shibata, S., and Yanagimachi, R. (1986): Effect of Ca^{2+} channel antagonists on the acrosome reaction of guinea pig and golden hamster spermatozoa. *Gamete Res.*, 13:281–292.
418. Romrell, L. J., O'Rand, M. G., Sandow, P. S., and Porter, J. P. (1982): Identification of surface autoantigens which appear during spermatogenesis. *Gamete Res.*, 5:35–48.
419. Roomans, G. M. (1975): Calcium binding to the acrosomal membrane of human spermatozoa. *Exp. Cell Res.*, 96:23–30.
420. Russell, L. D., Kramper, B., Hunt, W., and Peterson, R. N. (1984): Selective solubilization of major boar sperm plasma membrane (PM) polypeptides (PS) by detergents and buffer of various ionic strength. *Biol. Reprod.*, 30(Suppl. 1):111a.
421. Russell, L. D., Peterson, N. R., Hunt, W., and Strack, L. E. (1984): Posttesticular surface modifications and contributions of reproductive fluids to the surface polypeptide composition of boar spermatozoa. *Biol. Reprod.*, 30:959–978.
422. Sacco, A. G., Yurewicz, E. G., and Subramanian, M. G. (1986): Carbohydrate influences the immunogenic and antigenic characteristics of the ZP3 macromolecule (Mr 55000) of the pig zona pellucida. *J. Reprod. Fertil.*, 76:575–586.
423. Saling, P. M. (1981): Involvement of trypsin-like activity in binding of mouse spermatozoa to zona pellucida. *Proc. Natl. Acad. Sci. USA*, 78:6231–6235.
424. Saling, P. M. (1982): Development of the ability to bind zonae pellucidae during epididymal maturation. *Biol. Reprod.*, 26:429–436.
425. Saling, P. M., and Bedford, J. M. (1981): Absence of species-specificity for mammalian sperm capacitation *in vivo*. *J. Reprod. Fertil.*, 63:119–123.
426. Saling, P. M., Sowinski, J., and Storey, B. T. (1979): An ultrastructural study of epididymal mouse spermatozoa binding to zonae pellucidae *in vitro:* Sequential relationship to the acrosome reaction. *J. Exp. Zool.*, 209:229–238.
427. Saling, P. M., and Storey, B. T. (1979): Mouse gamete interaction during fertilization *in vitro:* Chlorfelracycline as a fluorescent probe for the mouse sperm acrosome reactions. *J. Cell Biol.*, 83:544–555.
428. Sano, K. (1985): Acrosome reaction of echinoderm sperm. In: *Calmodulin Antagonists and Cellular Physiology*, edited by H. Hidaka and D. J. Hartshorne, pp. 117–127. Academic Press, New York.

429. Santos-Sacchi, J., and Gordon, M. (1980): Induction of the acrosome reaction in guinea pig spermatozoa by cGMP analogues. *J. Cell Biol.*, 5:798–803.
430. Santos-Sacchi, J., and Gordon, M. (1982): The effect of ATP deletion open the acrosome reaction in guinea pig sperm. *J. Androl.*, 3:108–112.
431. Santos-Sacchi, J., Gordon, M., and Williams, W. L. (1980): Potentiation of the cGMP-induced guinea pig acrosome reaction by zinc. *J. Exp. Zool.*, 213:289–291.
432. Sato, K., and Blandau, R. J. (1979): Time and process of sperm penetration into cumulus-free mouse eggs fertilized *in vitro*. *Gamete Res.* 2:295–304.
433. Saxena, N. K., Russell, L. D., Saxena, N., and Peterson, R. N. (1986): Immunofluorescence antigen localization on boar sperm plasma membrane: Monoclonal antibodies reveal apparent new redistribution of surface antigens during sperm maturation and at ejaculation. *Anat. Rec.*, 214:238–252.
434. Schlegel, R. A., Hammerstedt, R., Cofer, G. P., and Kozarsky, K. (1986): Changes in the organization of the lipid bilayer of the plasma membrane during spermatogenesis and epididymal maturation. *Biol. Reprod.*, 34:379–391.
435. Schollmeyer, J. E. (1986): Identification of calpain II in porcine sperm. *Biol. Reprod.*, 34:721–731.
436. Shalgi, R., Kaplan, R., Nebel, L., and Kraicer, P. F. (1981): The male factor in fertilization of rat eggs *in vitro*. *J. Exp. Zool.*, 217:399–402.
437. Shalgi, R., and Phillips, D. M. (1980): Mechanics of *in vitro* fertilization in the hamster. *Biol. Reprod.*, 23:433–448.
438. Shalgi, R., and Phillips, D. (1980): Mechanics of sperm entry in cycling hamsters. *J. Ultrastruct. Res.*, 71:154–161.
439. Shams-Borham, G., and Harrison, R. A. P. (1981): Production, characterization, and use of ionophore-induced, calcium-dependent acrosome reaction in ram spermatozoa. *Gamete Res.*, 4:407–432.
440. Shams-Borham, G., Huneau, D., and Flechon, J. E. (1979): Acrosin does not appear to be bound to the inner acrosomal membrane of bull spermatozoa. *J. Exp. Zool.*, 209:143–149.
441. Shapiro, B. M., Schackmann, R. W., Tombes, R. M., and Kazazoglan, T. (1985): Coupled ionic and enzymatic regulation of sperm behavior. *Curr. Top. Cell. Regul.*, 26:97–113.
442. Sheikhnejad, R. G., and Srivastava, P. N. (1986): Isolation and properties of a phospholidylcholine-specific phospholipase C from bull seminal plasma. *J. Biol. Chem.*, 261:7544–7549.
443. Shimizu, S., Tsuji, M., and Dean, J. (1983): *In vitro* synthesis of three sulfated glycoproteins of murine zonae pellucidae by oocytes grown in follicle culture. *J. Biol. Chem.*, 258:5858–5863.
444. Shinohara, H., Yanagimachi, R., and Srivastava, P. N. (1985): Enhancement of the acrosome reaction of hamster spermatozoa by proteolytic enzymes, kallikrein, trypsin and chymotrypsin. *Gamete Res.*, 11:19–28.
445. Shur, B. D., and Hall, N. G. (1982): A role for mouse sperm surface galactosyltransferase in sperm binding to the egg zona pellucida. *J. Cell Biol.*, 95:574–579.
446. Siddiquey, A. K. S., and Cohen, J. (1982): *In vitro* fertilization in the mouse and the relevance of difference sperm/egg concentrations and volumes. *J. Reprod. Fertil.*, 66:237–242.
447. Singer, S. J., and Nicolson, G. L. (1972): The fluid mosaic model of the structure of the cell membrane. *Science*, 175:720–731.
448. Singh, J. P., Babcock, D. F., and Lardy, H. A. (1978): Increased calcium-ion influx is a component of capacitation of spermatozoa. *Biochem. J.*, 172:549–556.
449. Singh, J. P., Babcock, D. F., and Lardy, H. A. (1983): Motility activation, respiratory stimulation, and alteration of Ca^{2+} transport in bovine sperm treated with amine local anesthetic and calcium transport antagonists. *Arch. Biochem. Biophys.*, 221:291–303.
450. Snider, D. R., and Clegg, E. D. (1975): Alteration of phospholipids in porcine spermatozoa during *in vivo* uterus and oviduct incubation. *J. Anim. Sci.*, 40:269–274.
451. Soucek, D. A., Nikolopoulou, M., Vary, J. C., and Zirkin, B. (1985): Fluidity measurements of sperm membranes from *in vitro* capacitated and acrosome reacted boar sperm. *J. Cell. Biol.*, 101:263a.
452. Srivastava, P. N., Akruk, S. R., and Williams, W. L. (1979): Dissolution of rabbit zona by sperm acrosome extract: Effect of calcium. *J. Exp. Zool.*, 207:521–529.
453. Srivastava, P. N., Brewer, J. M., and White, R. A. (1982): Hydrolysis of *p*-nitrophenylphosphorylcholine by alkaline phosphatase and phospholipase c from rabbit sperm acrosome. *Biochem. Biophys. Res. Commun.*, 108:1120–1125.
454. Srivastava, P. N., Farooqui, A. A., and Gould, K. G. (1981): Studies on hydrolytic enzymes of chimpanzee sperm. *Biol. Reprod.*, 25:363–369.
455. Srivastava, P. N., Munnell, J. F., Yang, C. H., and Foley, C. W. (1974): Sequential release of acrosomal membrane and acrosomal enzymes of ram spermatozoa. *J. Reprod. Fertil.*, 36:363–372.
456. Srivastava, P. N., and Ninjour, V. (1982): Isolation of rabbit testicular cathepsin D and its role in the activation of proacrosin. *Biochem. Biophys. Res. Commun.*, 109:63–69.
457. Stein, D. M., and Fraser, L. R. (1984): Cyclic nucleotide metabolism in mouse epididymal spermatozoa during capacitation *in vitro*. *Gamete Res.*, 10:283–299.
458. Stein, D. M., Fraser, L. R., and Monks, N. J. (1986): Adenosine and Gpp(NH)p modulate mouse sperm adenylate cyclase. *Gamete Res.*, 13:151–158.
459. St. Jacques, S., Forget, A., and Roberts, K. D. (1986): Monoclonal antibodies specific for an oviduct component associated with the zona pellucida. *J. Reprod. Immunol.* (1986 Suppl.):52.
460. Storey, B. T., Lee, M. A., Muller, C., Ward, C. R., and Wirtshafter, D. G. (1984): Binding of mouse spermatozoa to the zona pellucida of mouse eggs in cumulus: Evidence that the acrosomes remain substantially intact. *Biol. Reprod.*, 3:1119–1128.
461. Suarez, S. S., Katz, D. F., and Overstreet, J. W. (1983): Movement characteristics and acrosomal status of rabbit spermatozoa recovered at the site and time of fertilization. *Biol. Reprod.*, 29:1277–1287.
462. Suarez, S. S., Katz, D. F., and Meizel, S. (1984): Changes in motility that accompany the acrosome reaction in hyperactivated hamster spermatozoa. *Gamete Res.*, 10:253–265.
463. Sullivan, R., and Bleau, G. (1985): Interaction of isolated components from mammalian sperm and egg. *Gamete Res.*, 12:101–116.
464. Suzuki, F. (1981): Changes in intramembranous particle distribution in epididymal spermatozoa of the boar. *Anat. Rec.*, 199:361–376.
465. Szollosi, D., and Hunter, R. H. F. (1978): The nature and occurrence of the acrosome reaction in spermatozoa of the domestic pig, *Sus scrofa*. *J. Anat.*, 127:33–41.
466. Takahashi, N., and Yamagata, T. (1982): Involvement of sialic acids in fertilization of the mouse. *Dev. Growth Diff.*, 24:407.
467. Talbot, P. (1984): Events leading to fertilization in mammals. In: *Fertility and Sterility: Proceedings of the 11th World Congress on Fertilization and Sterilization*, edited by R. F. Harrison and J. B. W. Thompson, pp. 121–131. MTP Press, Boston.
468. Talbot, P. (1985): Sperm penetration through oocyte investments in mammals. *Am. J. Anat.*, 174:331–346.
469. Talbot, P., and Chacon, R. S. (1980): A triple stain technique for scoring acrosome reaction of human sperm. *J. Exp. Zool.*, 215:201–208.
470. Talbot, P., and DiCarlantonio, G. (1984): The oocyte-cumulus complex: Ultrastructure of the extracellular components in hamster and mice. *Gamete Res.*, 10:127–142.
471a. Talbot, P., and DiCarlantonio, G. (1984): Ultrastructure of opossum oocyte investing coats and their sensitivity to trypsin and hyaluronidase. *Dev. Biol.*, 103:159–167.
471b. Talbot, P., and DiCarlantonio, G. (1985): Cytochemical localization of dipeptidyl peptidase II (DPP-II) in mature guinea pig sperm. *J. Histochem. Cytochem.*, 33:1169–1172.
472. Talbot, P., DiCarlantonio, G., Zao, P., Penkala, J., and Haimo, L. T. (1985): Motile cells lacking hyaluronidase can penetrate the hamster oocyte cumulus complex. *Dev. Biol.*, 108:387–398.
473. Talbot, P., and Kleve, M. G. (1978): Hamster sperm cross react with antiactin. *J. Exp. Zool.*, 204:131–136.
474. Talbot, P. Summers, R. G., Hylander, B. L., Keough, E. M., and Franklin, L. E. (1976): The role of calcium in the acrosome reaction: An analysis using ionophore A23187. *J. Exp. Zool.*, 198: 383–392.
475. Tash, J. S., and Means, A. R. (1983): Cyclic adenosin 3′,5′monophosphate, calcium and protein phosphorylation in flagella motility. *Biol. Reprod.*, 28:75–104.
476. Tesarik, J. (1984): Topographic relations of intramembranal particle distribution patterns in human sperm membranes. *J. Ultrastruct. Res.*, 89:42–55.

477. Tesarik, J. (1985): Comparison of acrosome reaction-inducing activities of human cumulus oophorus, follicular fluid and ionophore A23187 in human sperm populations of proven fertilizing ability *in vitro*. *J. Reprod. Fertil.*, 74:383–388.
478. Tezon, J. G., Ramella, E., Cameo, M. S., Vazquez, M. H., and Blacquier, J. A. (1985): Immunochemical localization of secretory antigens in the human epididymis and their association with spermatozoa. *Biol. Reprod.*, 32:591–597.
479. Thakkart, J. K., East, J., and Franson, R. (1984): Modulation of phospholipase A_2 activity associated with human sperm membranes by divalent cations and calcium. *Biol. Reprod.*, 30:679–689.
480. Thakkart, J. K., East, J., Seyle, D., and Franson, R. C. (1983): Surface-active phospholipase A_2 in mouse spermatozoa. *Biochim. Biophys. Acta*, 754:44–50.
481. Thompson, R. S., Smith, D. M., and Zamboni, L. (1974): Fertilization of mouse ova *in vitro:* An electron microscopic study. *Fertil. Steril.*, 25:222–249.
482. Topfer-Peterson, E., Friess, A. E., Nguyen, H., and Schill, W. S. (1985): Evidence for a fucose-binding protein in boar spermatozoa. *Histochemistry*, 83:139–145.
483. Topfer-Peterson, E., Friess, A. E., Sinowalz, F., Bielz, S., and Schill, W. S. (1985): Immunocytological characterization of the outer acrosomal membrane (OAM) during acrosome reaction in boar. *Histochemistry*, 82:113–120.
484. Topfer-Peterson, E., and Schill, W. B. (1981): A new separation method of subcellular fraction of boar spermatozoa. *Andrology*, 13:174–176.
485. Topfer-Peterson, E., and Schill, W. S. (1983): Characterization of lectin receptors isolated from the outer acrosome membrane of boar spermatozoa. *Int. J. Androl.*, 6:375–392.
486. Toyoda, Y., Yokoyama, M., and Hoshi, T. (1971): Studies on the fertilization of mouse eggs *in vitro*. *Jpn. J. Anim. Reprod.*, 16:147–157.
487. Tsunoda, Y., and Chang, M. C. (1977): *In vitro* fertilization of hamster eggs by ejaculated or epididymal spermatozoa in the presence of male accessory secretions. *J. Exp. Zool.*, 201:445–450.
488. Uesugi, S., and Yamazoe, S. (1966): Presence of sodium-potassium-stimulated ATPase in boar epididymal spermatozoa. *Nature*, 209:403.
489. Urch, U. A., and Hedrick, J. L. (1985): Acrosin derived peptides bind the zona pellucida. *J. Cell Biol.*, 101:378a.
490. Urch, U. A., Wardrip, N. J., and Hedrick, J. L. (1985): Proteolysis of the zona pellucida by acrosin: The nature of the hydrolysis product. *J. Exp. Zool.*, 236:239–243.
491. Urch, U. A., Wardrip, N. J., and Hedrick, J. L. (1985): Limited and specific proteolysis of the zona pellucida by acrosin. *J. Exp. Zool.*, 233:479–483.
492. Usui, N., and Yanagimachi, R. (1986): Cytochemical localization of membrane-bound Mg^{2+}-dependent ATPase activity in guinea pig sperm head before and during the acrosome reaction. *Gamete Res.*, 13:271–280.
493. Vacquier, V. D., and Moy, G. W. (1977): Isolation of bindin: The protein responsible for adhesion of sperm to sea urchin eggs. *Proc. Natl. Acad. Sci. USA*, 74:2456–2460.
494. Velazquez, A., Delgado, N. D., and Rosado, A. (1986): Taurine content and amino acid composition on human acrosome. *Life. Sci.*, 38:991–995.
495. Vernon, R. B., Hamilton, M. S., and Eddy, E. M. (1985): Effects of *in vivo* and *in vitro* fertilization environments on the expression of a surface antigen of the mouse sperm tail. *Biol. Reprod.*, 32:669–680.
496. Vernon, R. B., Muller, C. H., Herr, J. C., Feuchter, F. A., and Eddy, E. M. (1982): Epididymal secretion of a mouse sperm surface component recognized by a monoclonal antibody. *Biol. Reprod.*, 26:523–535.
497. Vijayasarathy, S., and Balarm, P. (1982): Regional differentiation in bull sperm plasma membranes. *Biochem. Biophys. Res. Commun.*, 108:760–769.
498. Vijayasarthy, S., and Shivaji, S. (1982): Bull sperm plasma and acrosomal membrane: Fluorescence studies of lipid phase fluidity. *Biochem. Biophys. Res. Commun.*, 108:585–591.
499. Viriyapanich, P., and Bedford, J. M. (1981): Sperm capacitation in the Fallopian tube of the hamster and its suppression by endocrine factors. *J. Exp. Zool.*, 217:403–407.
500. Viriyapanich, P., and Bedford, J. M. (1981): The fertilization performance *in vivo* of rabbit spermatozoa capacitated *in vitro*. *J. Exp. Zool.*, 216:169–174.
501. Virtanen, I., Bradley, R. A., Paaivuo, R., and Lehto, V. P. (1984): Distinct cytoskeletal domains revealed in sperm cells. *J. Cell Biol.*, 99:1083–1091.
502. Volglmayr, J. K., Fairbanks, G., and Lewis, R. G. (1983): Surface glycoprotein changes in ram spermatozoa during epididymal maturation. *Biol. Reprod.*, 29:767–775.
503. Volglmayr, J. K., and Sawyer, F. R. (1986): Surface transformation of ram spermatozoa in uterus, oviduct and cauda epididymal fluids in vitro. *J. Reprod. Fert.*, 78:315–325.
504. de Vries, J. W. A., Willemsen, R., and Geuze, H. J. (1985): Immunocytochemical localization of acrosin and hyaluronidase in epididymal and ejaculated porcine spermatozoa. *Eur. J. Cell Biol.*, 37:81–88.
505. Wardrip, N. J., Hedrick, J. L., and Berger, T. (1985): Comparison of pig zona pellucida from oocytes, eggs and zygotes. *Fed. Proc.*, 44:1778a.
506. Wassarman, P. M., Bleil, J. D., Florman, H. M., Greve, J. M., Roller, R. J., Salizman, G. S., and Samuels, F. G. (1985): The mouse eggs receptor for sperm: What is it and how does it work? *Cold Spring Harbor Symp. Quant. Biol.*, 50:11–19.
507. Wassarman, P. M., Florman, H. M., and Greve, J. M. (1985): Receptor-mediated sperm-egg interactions in mammals. In: *Fertilization, Vol. 2*, edited by C. B. Metz and A. Monroy, pp. 341–360. Academic Press, New York.
508. Watson, P. F., and Plummer, J. M. (1986): Relationship between calcium binding sites and membrane fusion during the acrosome reaction induced by ionophore in ram spermatozoa. *J. Exp. Zool.*, 238:113–118.
509. Weil, A. J. (1965): The spermatozoa-coating antigen (SCA) of the seminal vesicle. *Ann. N.Y. Acad. Sci.*, 124:267–269.
510. Weinman, D. E., and Williams, W. L. (1964): Mechanism of capacitation of rabbit spermatozoa. *Nature*, 203:423–424.
511. Westrick, J. C., Boatman, D. E., and Bavister, B. D. (1985): Characteristics of acrosome reaction-inducing factor from hamster cumulus and follicular fluid. *Biol. Reprod.* 32:351a.
512. White, I. G., and Volglmayr, J. K. (1986): ATP-induced reactivation of ram testicular, caudal epididymal, and ejaculated spermatozoa extracts with Triton X-100. *Biol. Reprod.*, 34:183–193.
513. Wincek, T. J., Parrish, R. F., and Polakoski, K. L. (1979): Fertilization: A uterine glycosaminoglycan stimulates the conversion of sperm proacrosin to acrosin. *Science*, 203:553–554.
514. Wolf, D. E., Hagopian, S. S., and Isojima, S. (1986): Changes in sperm plasma membrane lipid diffusibility after hyperactivation during *in vitro* capacitation in the mouse. *J. Cell Biol.*, 102:1372–1377.
515. Wolf, D. P. (1981): The mammalian egg's block to polyspermy. In: *Fertilization and Embryonic Development In Vitro*, edited by L. Mastroianni and B. J. Biggers, pp. 183–197. Plenum Press, New York.
516. Wolf, D. P., Boldt, J., Byrd, W., and Bechtol, K. B. (1985): Acrosomal status evaluation in human ejaculate sperm with monoclonal antibodies. *Biol. Reprod.*, 32:1157–1162.
517. Wong, P. Y. D., and Tang, A. Y. E. (1982): Studies on the binding of a 32K rat epididymal protein to rat epididymal spermatozoa. *Biol. Reprod.*, 27:1239–1246.
518. Working, P. K., and Meizel, S. (1982): Preliminary characterization of a Mg^{2+}-ATPase in hamster sperm head membranes. *Biochem. Biophys. Res. Commun.*, 104:1060–1065.
519. Working, P. K., and Meizel, S. (1983): Correlation of increased intraacrosomal pH with the hamster sperm acrosome reaction. *J. Exp. Zool.*, 227:97–107.
520. Yamagata, T., Ito, M., and Takahashi, K. (1983): The involvement of a saccharide-mediated recognition mechanism in the interaction between sperm and the zona pellucida of the egg cells of the mouse. In: *Glycoconjugates*, edited by M. A. Chester, D. Heingard, A. Lundblad, and S. Sevenssen, pp. 623–624. Rahmis i Lund, Lund.
521. Yamamoto, N. (1985): Immunoelectron microscopic localization of calmodulin in guinea pig testis and spermatozoa. *Acta Histochem. Cytochem.*, 18:199–211.
522. Yanagimachi, R. (1964): Sperm penetration into hamster egg *in vitro*. *Proc. 5th Int. Congr. Anim. Reprod. (Trento)*, 3:321–324.

523. Yanagimachi, R. (1966): Time and process of sperm penetration into hamster ova *in vivo* and *in vitro*. *J. Reprod. Fertil.*, 11:359–370.
524. Yanagimachi, R. (1969): *In vitro* capacitation of hamster spermatozoa by follicular fluid. *J. Reprod. Fertil.*, 18:275–286.
525. Yanagimachi, R. (1969): *In vitro* acrosome reaction and capacitation of golden hamster spermatozoa by bovine follicular fluid and its fractions. *J. Exp. Zool.*, 170:269–280.
526. Yanagimachi, R. (1970): *In vitro* capacitation of golden hamster spermatozoa by homologous and heterologous blood sera. *Biol. Reprod.*, 3:147–153.
527. Yanagimachi, R. (1970): The movement of golden hamster spermatozoa before and after capacitation. *J. Reprod. Fertil.*, 23:193–196.
528. Yanagimachi, R. (1972): Fertilization of guinea pig eggs *in vitro*. *Anat. Rec.*, 174:9–20.
529. Yanagimachi, R. (1977): Specificity of sperm-egg interaction. In: *Immunobiology of Gametes*, edited by M. Edidin and M. H. Johnson, pp. 255–295. Cambridge University Press, London.
530. Yanagimachi, R. (1981): Mechanisms of fertilization in mammals. In: *Fertilization and Embryonic Development In Vitro*, edited by L. Mastroianni and J. D. Biggers, pp. 81–182. Plenum Press, New York.
531. Yanagimachi, R. (1982): *In vitro* sperm capacitation and fertilization of golden hamster eggs in a chemically defined media. In: *In Vitro Fertilization and Embryo Transfer*, edited by E. S. E. Hafez and K. Semm, pp. 65–76. MTP Press, Lancaster.
532. Yanagimachi, R. (1982): Requirement of extracellular calcium ions for various stages of fertilization and fertilization related phenomena in the hamster. *Gamete Res.*, 5:323–344.
533. Yanagimachi, R. (1983): Fertilization. In: *In Vitro Fertilization and Embryo Transfer*, edited by P. G. Crosignani and B. L. Rubin, pp. 65–100. Academic Press, London.
534. Yanagimachi, R. (1984): Zona-free hamster eggs: Their use in assessing fertilizing capacity and examining chromosomes of human spermatozoa. *Gamete Res.*, 10:178–232.
535. Yanagimachi, R., and Chang, M. C. (1963): Fertilization of hamster eggs *in vitro*. *Nature*, 200:281–282.
536. Yanagimachi, R., and Cummins, J. M. (1985): Optical changes in the acrosomal caps of golden hamster spermatozoa prior to the acrosome reaction. *Proc. Annu. Conf. Soc. Study Reprod. (Aberdeen):* abstract 20.
537. Yanagimachi, R., Huang, T. T. F., Flemming, A. D., Kosower, N. S., and Nicolson, G. L. (1983): Dithiorestal, a disulfide-reducing agent, inhibits capacitation, acrosome reaction and interaction with eggs by guinea pig spermatozoa. *Gamete Res.*, 7:145–154.
538. Yanagimachi, R., Kamiguchi, K., Mikamo, K., Suzuki, F., and Yanagimachi, H. (1985): Maturation of spermatozoa in the epididymis of the chinese hamster. *Am. J. Anat.*, 172:317–330.
539. Yanagimachi, R., Kamiguchi, K., Sugawara, S., and Mikamo, K. (1983): Gametes and fertilization in the chinese hamster. *Gamete Res.*, 8:97–117.
540. Yanagimachi, R., and Mahi, C. A. (1976): The sperm acrosome reaction and fertilization in the guinea pig: A study *in vivo*. *J. Reprod. Fertil.*, 46:49–54.
541. Yanagimachi, R., and Noda, Y. D. (1970): Fine structure of the hamster sperm head. *Am. J. Anat.*, 128:367–388.
542. Yanagimachi, R., and Noda, Y. D. (1970): Ultrastructural changes in the hamster sperm head during fertilization. *J. Ultrastruct. Res.*, 31:465–485.
543a. Yanagimachi, R., and Noda, Y. D. (1970): Electron microscope studies of sperm incorporation into the hamster egg. *Am. J. Anat.*, 128:429–462.
543b. Yanagimachi, R., and Noda, Y. D. (1970): Physiological changes in the post-nuclear cap region of mammalian spermatozoa: A necessary preliminary to the membrane fusion between sperm and egg cells. *J. Ultrastruct. Res.*, 31:486–493.
544. Yanagimachi, R., Noda, Y. D., Fujimoto, M., and Nicolson, G. L. (1972): The distribution of negative surface charge of mammalian spermatozoa. *Am. J. Anat.*, 135:497–520.
545. Yanagimachi, R., and Phillips, D. M. (1984): The status of acrosomal caps of hamster spermatozoa immediately before fertilization *in vitro*. *Gamete Res.*, 9:1–19.
546. Yanagimachi, R., and Suzuki, F. (1985): A further study of lysolecithin-mediated acrosome reaction of guinea pig spermatozoa. *Gamete Res.*, 11:29–40.
547. Yanagimachi, R., and Usui, N. (1974): Calcium dependence of the acrosome reaction and activation of guinea pig spermatozoa. *Exp. Cell Res.*, 89:161–174.
548. Yang, W. H., Lin, L. L., Wang, J. R., and Chang, M. C. (1972): Sperm penetration through zona pellucida and perivitelline space in hamster. *J. Exp. Zool.*, 179:191–206.
549. Yoshigaki, N., and Katagiri, C. (1982): Acrosome reaction of sperm of the toad, *Bufo bufo japonicus*. *Gamete Res.*, 6:343–352.
550. Young, L. G., Hinton, B. T., and Gould, F. G. (1985): Surface changes in chimpanzee sperm during epididymal transit. *Biol. Reprod.*, 32:399–412.
551. Zahler, W. L., and Doak, G. A. (1975): Isolation of the outer acrosomal membrane from bull sperm. *Biochim. Biophys. Acta*, 406:479–488.
552. Zamboni, L. (1972): Fertilization in the mouse. In: *Biology of Mammalian Fertilization and Implantation*, edited by K. S. Moghissi and E. S. E. Hafez, pp. 213–262. Charles C Thomas, Springfield, Ill.
553. Zaneveld, L. J. D., Polakoski, K. L., and Williams, W. L. (1973): A proteinase and proteinase inhibitor of mammalian sperm acrosomes. *Biol. Reprod.*, 9:219–225.
554. Zao, P. Z. R., Meizel, S., and Talbot, P. (1985): Release of hyaluronidase and beta-acetylhexosaminidase during *in vitro* incubation of hamster sperm. *J. Exp. Zool.*, 234:63–74.
555. Austin, C. R. (1956): Cortical granules in hamster eggs. *Exp. Cell Res.*, 10:533–540.
556. Austin, C. R. (1965): *Fertilization*. Prentice-Hall, Englewood Cliffs, NJ.
557. Austin, C. R., and Braden A. W. H. (1955): Observations on nuclear size and form in living rat and mouse eggs. *Exp. Cell Res.*, 8:163–172.
558. Balakier, H., and Tarkowski, A. K. (1980): The role of germinal vesicle karyoplasm in the development of male pronucleus in the mouse. *Exp. Cell Res.*, 128:79–86.
559. Bedford, J. M. (1983): Oocyte structure and the design and function of the sperm head in eutherian mammals. In: *The Sperm Cell*, edited by J. Andre, pp. 75–89. Academic Press, London.
560. Bellve, A. R. (1979): The molecular biology of mammalian spermatogenesis. In: *Oxford Reviews of Reproductive Biology, Vol. 1*, edited by C. A. Finn, pp. 159–261. Clarendon Press, Oxford.
561. Bjorndahl, L., Kjellberg, S., Roomans, G. M., and Kvist, U. (1986): The human sperm nucleus takes up zinc at ejaculation. *Int. J. Androl.*, 9:77–80.
562. Brandriff, B., and Pedersen, R. A. (1981): Repair of the ultraviolet-irradiated male genome in fertilized mouse eggs. *Science*, 211:1431–1433.
563. Braude, P. R., Pelham, H. R. B., Flach, G., and Lobatto, R. (1979): Post transcriptional control in the early mouse embryo. *Nature*, 282:102–105.
564. Brinster, R. L., Chen, H. Y., Trumbauer, M. E., and Payton, B. V. (1981): Secretion of proteins by the fertilized mouse ovum. *Exp. Cell Res.*, 134:291–296.
565. Calvin, H. I. (1975): Keratinoid proteins in the heads and tails of mammalian spermatozoa. In: *The Biology of the Male Gamete*, edited by J. G. Duckett and P. A. Racey, pp. 257–273. Academic Press, London.
566. Calvin, H. I. (1976): Comparative analysis of the nuclear basic proteins in rat, human, guinea pig, mouse and rabbit spermatozoa. *Biochim. Biophys. Acta*, 434:377–389.
567. Calvin, H. I., Grosshans, K., and Blake, E. J. (1986): Estimation and manipulation of glutathion levels in prepuberal mouse ovaries and ova: Relevance to sperm nucleus transformation in the fertilized egg. *Gamete Res.*, 14:265–275.
568. Cavanagh, A., Morton, H., Roefe, B. A., and Gidley-Baird, A. L. (1982): Ovum factor: A first signal of pregnancy? *Am. J. Reprod. Immunol.*, 2:97–101.
569. Chen, H. Y., Brinster, R. L., and Merz, E. A. (1980): Changes in protein synthesis following fertilization of the mouse ovum. *J. Exp. Zool.*, 212:355–360.
570. Clarke, H. J., and Masui, Y. (1987): Dose-dependent relationship between oocyte cytoplasmic volume and transformation of sperm nuclei to metaphase chromosomes. *J. Cell Biol.*, 104:831–840.

571. Clegg, K. B., and Piko, L. (1982): RNA synthesis and cytoplasmic polyadenylation in the one-cell mouse embryo. *Nature,* 295:342–345.
572. Dale, B., DeFelice, J., and Ehrenstein, G. (1985): Injection of a soluble sperm fraction into sea urchin eggs triggers the cortical reaction. *Experientia,* 41:1068–1070.
573. Da-Yuan, C., and Longo, F. J. (1983): A cytochemical study of nuclear changes in fertilized hamster eggs. *Anat. Rec.,* 207:327–334.
574. Delgado, N. M., Reyes, R., Huacuja, L., Carranco, A., Merchant, H., and Rosado, A. (1982): Decondensation of human sperm nuclei by glycosaminoglycan sulfate from sea urchin egg. *J. Exp. Zool.,* 224:457–460.
575. Dube, F., Dufresne-Duke, L., and Guerrier, P. (1982): Sperm nuclear decondensation in *Barnea candida* (mollusca, pelecypoda) oocytes does not require germinal vesicle breakdown. *J. Exp. Zool.,* 221:383–387.
576. Ecklund, P. S., and Levine, L. (1975): Mouse sperm basic nuclear protein: Electrophoretic characterization and fate after fertilization. *J. Cell Biol.,* 66:251–262.
577. Endo, Y. (1952): The role of the cortical granules in the formation of the fertilization membrane in eggs from Japanese sea urchins. *Exp. Cell Res.,* 3:406–418.
578. Epel, D. (1979): The triggering of development at fertilization. In: *Mechanisms of Cell Change,* edited by J. Ebert and T. Okada, pp. 17–31. John Wiley & Sons, New York.
579. Epel, D. (1982): The physiology and chemistry of calcium during the fertilization of eggs. In: *Calcium and Cell Function, Vol. 2,* edited by W. Y. Cheung, pp. 355–385. Academic Press, New York.
580. Evans, T., Rosenthal, E., Youngblom, J., Distel, D., and Hunt, T. (1983): Cyclin: A protein specified by maternal mRNA in sea urchin eggs that is destroyed at each cleavage division. *Cell,* 33: 389–396.
581. Flach, G., Johnson, M. H., Braude, P. R., Taylor, R. A. S., and Holton, V. N. (1982): The transition from maternal to embryonic control in the 2-cell mouse embryo. *EMBO J.,* 1:681–686.
582. Fulton, B. P., and Whittingham, D. G. (1978): Activation of mammalian oocytes by intercellular injection of calcium. *Nature,* 273:149–151.
583. Gordon, K., Brown, D. B., and Ruddle, F. H. (1985): *In vitro* activation of human sperm induced by amphibian egg extract. *Exp. Cell Res.,* 157:409–418.
584. Graham, C. F. (1974): The production of parthenogenetic mammalian embryos and their use in biological research. *Biol. Rev.,* 49:399–422.
585. Gulyas, B. J. (1980): Cortical granules of mammalian eggs. *Int. Rev. Cytol.,* 63:357–392.
586. Hamaguchi, Y., and Hiramoto, Y. (1981): Activation of sea urchin eggs by microinjection of calcium buffers. *Exp. Cell Res.,* 134:171–179.
587. Hirao, Y., and Yanagimachi, R. (1979): Development of pronuclei in polyspermic eggs of the golden hamster: Is there any limit to the number of sperm heads that are capable of developing into male pronuclei? *Zool. Mag. (Tokyo),* 88:24–33.
588. Holmberg, S. R. M., and Johnson, M. H. (1979): Amino acid transport in the unfertilized and fertilized mouse eggs. *J. Reprod. Fertil.,* 56:223–231.
589. Hunter, R. H. F. (1967): Polyspermic fertilization in pig during the luteal phase of the estrous cycle. *J. Exp. Zool.,* 165:451–460.
590. Huret, J. L. (1986): Nuclear chromatin decondensation of human sperm. *Arch. Androl.,* 16:97–109.
591. Iwamatsu, T., and Ohta, T. (1980): The changes in sperm nuclei after penetrating fish oocytes matured without germinal vesicle material in their cytoplasm. *Gamete Res.,* 3:121–132.
592. Jackowski, S., Leibo, S. P., and Mazur, P. (1988): Glycerol permeability of fertilized and unfertilized mouse ova. *J. Exp. Zool.,* 212:329–341.
593. Jaffe, L. A., and Gould, M. (1985): Polyspermy-preventing mechanisms. In: *Biology of Fertilization, Vol. 3,* edited by C. B. Metz and A. Monroy, pp. 223–250. Academic Press, Orlando, Fla.
594. Jaffe, L. F. (1983): Sources of calcium in egg activation: A review and hypothesis. *Dev. Biol.,* 99:265–276.
595. Jaffe, L. F. (1985): The role of calcium explosions, waves, and pulses in activating eggs. In: *Biology of Fertilization, Vol. 3,* edited by C. B. Metz and A. Monroy, pp. 127–165. Academic Press, Orlando, Fla.
596. Kamiguchi, Y., and Mikamo, K. (1986): An improved, efficient method for analyzing human sperm chromosomes using zona-free hamster ova. *Am. J. Human Genet.,* 38:724–740.
597. Kanoh, Y., and Yanagimachi, R. (1956): Ueber den japonischen Hering (*Clupea pallasii* C. et V.) II. Der beginn der Entwicklung ohne Zerfallen der Kortikalaveoli. *J. Fac. Sci. Hokkaido Univ., Ser. VI (Zool.),* 12:264–272.
598. Katagiri, C., and Moiya, M. (1976): Spermatozoan response to the toad egg matured after removal of germinal vesicle. *Dev. Biol.,* 50:235–241.
599. Karasiewicz, J., and Soltynska, M. S. (1985): Ultrastructural evidence for the presence of actin filaments in mouse eggs at fertilization. *Roux's Arch. Dev. Biol.,* 194:369–372.
600. Kaufman, M. H. (1983): *Early Mammalian Development: Parthenogenetic Studies.* Cambridge University Press, Cambridge.
601. Kay, E. S., and Shapiro, B. M. (1985): The formation of the fertilization membrane of the sea urchin egg. In: *Biology of Fertilization, Vol. 3,* edited by C. B. Metz and A. Monroy, pp. 45–80. Academic Press, Orlando, Fla.
602. Kopecny, V., and Pavlok, A. (1975): Autoradiographic study of mouse spermatozoan arginine-rich nuclear protein in fertilization. *J. Exp. Zool.,* 191:85–96.
603. Kvist, U. (1980): Spermatozoal thiol-disulphide interaction: A possible event underlying physiological sperm nuclear chromatin decondensation. *Acta Physiol. Scand.,* 115:503–505.
604. Leese, H. J., Biggers, J. D., Mroz, E. A., and Lechene, C. (1984): Nucleotides in a single mammalian ovum or preimplantation embryo. *Anal. Biochem.,* 140:443–448.
605. Leibo, S. P. (1980): Water permeability and its activation energy of fertilized and unfertilized mouse ova. *J. Membr. Biol.,* 53:179–188.
606. Lohka, M. J., and Masui, Y. (1983): The germinal vesicle material required for sperm pronuclear formation is located in the soluble fraction of egg cytoplasm. *Exp. Cell Res.,* 148:481–491.
607. Longo, F. J. (1973): Fertilization: A comparative ultrastructural review. *Biol. Reprod.,* 9:149–215.
608. Longo, F. J. (1981): Regulation of pronuclear development. In: *Regulators of Reproduction,* edited by G. Jagiello and C. Vogel, pp. 529–557, Academic Press, New York.
609. Longo, F. J. (1985): Pronuclear events during fertilization. In: *Biology of Fertilization, Vol. 3,* edited by C. B. Metz and A. Monroy, pp. 251–298. Academic Press, Orlando, Fla.
610. Mahi, C. A., and Yanagimachi, R. (1975): Induction of nuclear decondensation of mammalian spermatozoa *in vitro. J. Reprod. Fertil.,* 44:293–296.
611. Maro, B. (1986): Fertilization and the cytoskeleton in the mouse. *Bioessays,* 3:18–21.
612. Maro, B., Howlett, S. H., and Webb, M. (1985): Non-spindle microtubule organization centers in metaphase II-arrested mouse oocytes. *J. Cell Biol.,* 101:1665–1672.
613. Maro, B., Johnson, M. H., Pickering, S. J., and Flach, G. (1984): Changes in actin distribution during fertilization of the mouse egg. *J. Embryol. Exp. Morphol.,* 81:211–237.
614. Masui, Y., and Clarke, H. J. (1979): Oocyte maturation. *Int. Rev. Cytol.,* 57:185–282.
615. McCulloh, D. H., Rexroad, C. E., and Levitan, H. (1983): Insemination of rabbit egg is associated with slow depolarization and repetitive diphasic membrane potentials. *Dev. Biol.,* 95:372–377.
616. Mittwoch, U. (1978): Parthenogenesis. *J. Med. Genet.,* 15:165–181.
617. Miyazaki, S., Hashimoto, N., Yoshimoto, Y., Kishimoto, T., Igusa, Y., and Hiramoto, Y. (1986): Temporal and spatial dynamics of the periodic increase in intercellular free calcium at fertilization of golden hamster eggs. *Dev. Biol.,* 118:259–267.
618. Monroy, A. (1965): *Chemistry and Physiology of Fertilization.* Holt, Rinehart and Winston, New York.
619. Moser, F. (1939): Studies on cortical layer response to stimulating agents in the *Arbacia* eggs. I. Response to insemination. *J. Exp. Zool.,* 80:423–446.
620. Mumford, R. A., Hartmann, J. F., Ashe, B. M., and Zimmerman, M. (1981): Proteinase activities of the golden hamster eggs and cells of the cumulus oophorus. *Dev. Biol.,* 81:332–335.
621. Naish, S. J., Perreault, S. D., Foehner, A. L., and Zirkin, B. R. (1987): DNA synthesis in the fertilizing hamster sperm nucleus:

Sperm template availability and egg cytoplasmic control. *Biol. Reprod.*, 36:245–253.
622. Nicosia, S. V., Wolf, D. P., and Inoue, M. (1977): Cortical granule distribution and cell surface characteristics in mouse eggs. *Dev. Biol.*, 57:56–74.
623. Ohsumi, K., Katagiri, C., and Yanagimachi, R. (1986): Development of pronuclei from human spermatozoa injected microsurgically into frog (*Xenopus*) eggs. *J. Exp. Zool.*, 237:319–325.
624. Oikawa, T., and Maruyama, Y. (1983): Detection of differences in surface carbohydrates of unfertilized and fertilized golden hamster eggs using potato agglutinin. *J. Exp. Zool.*, 227:139–143.
625. Okada, A., Yanagimachi, R., and Yanagimachi, H. (1986): Development of a cortical granule-free area of cortex and the perivitelline space in the hamster oocyte during maturation and following fertilization. *J. Submicrosc. Cytol.*, 18:233–247.
626. Perreault, S. D., and Barbee, R. R. (1986): Sperm nucleus decondensation depends on glutathione synthesis in maturing hamster oocytes. *Dev. Growth Diff.*, 28(Suppl.):53 (Abstract 7).
627. Perreault, S. D., Wolff, R. A., and Zirkin, B. R. (1984): The role of desulfide bond reduction during mammalian sperm nuclear decondensation *in vivo*. *Dev. Biol.*, 101:160–167.
628. Perreault, S. D., and Zirkin, B. R. (1982): Sperm nuclear decondensation in mammals: Role of sperm-associated proteinase *in vivo*. *J. Exp. Zool.*, 224:253–257.
629. Rodman, T. C., Pruslin, F. H., Hoffmann, H. P., and Alfrey, V. G. (1981): Turnover of basic chromosomal protein in fertilized eggs: A cytoimmunochemical study of events *in vivo*. *J. Cell Biol.*, 90:351–361.
630. Rousseau, P., Meda, P., Lecart, C., Haumont, S., and Ferin, J. (1977): Cortical granule release in human follicular oocytes. *Biol. Reprod.*, 16:104–111.
631. Sampson, M. M. (1926): Sperm filtrates and dialyzates: Their action on ova of the same species. *Biol. Bull.*, 50:301–338.
632. Sathananthan, A. H., and Trounson, A. O. (1985): The human pronuclear ovum: Fine structure of monospermic and polyspermic fertilization *in vitro*. *Gamete Res.*, 12:385–398.
633. Schatten, G., Maul, G. G., Schatten, H., Chaly, N., Simery, C., Balczon, R., and Brown, D. L. (1985): Nuclear lamins and peripheral nuclear antigens during fertilization and embryogenesis in mice and sea urchins. *Proc. Natl. Acad. Sci. USA*, 82:4727–4731.
634. Schatten, G., Simerly, C., Cline, H., and Maul, G. (1984): Cytoskeleton and nuclear lamin organization during mammalian fertilization and early development. *J. Embryol. Exp. Morphol.*, 82(Suppl.):74.
635. Schatten, G., Simerly, C., and Schatten, H. (1985): Microtubule configurations during fertilization, mitosis, and early development in the mouse and the requirement for egg microtubule-mediated motility during mammalian fertilization. *Proc. Natl. Acad. Sci. USA*, 82:4152–4156.
636. Schatten, H., and Schatten, G. (1986): Motility and centrosomal organization during sea urchin and mouse fertilization. *Cell Motil. Cytoskel.*, 6:163–175.
637. Schatten, H., Schatten, G., Mazia, D., Balczon, R., and Simerly, C. (1986): Behavior of centrosomes during fertilization and cell division in mouse oocytes and in sea urchin eggs. *Proc. Natl. Acad. Sci. USA*, 83:105–109.
638. Schmell, E. D., Gulyas, B. J., and Hedrick, J. L. (1986): Egg surface changes during fertilization and the molecular mechanism of the block to polyspermy. In: *Mechanism and Control of Animal Fertilization*, edited by J. F. Hartmann, pp. 365–413. Academic Press, New York.
639. Schuel, H. (1978): Secretory function of egg cortical granules in fertilization and development. *Gamete Res.*, 1:299–382.
640. Schuel, H. (1985): Functions of egg cortical granules. In: *Biology of Fertilization, Vol. 3*, edited by C. B. Metz and A. Monroy, pp. 1–43. Academic Press, Orlando, Fla.
641a. Skoblina, M. N. (1976): Role of karyoplasm in the emergency of capacity of egg cytoplasm to induce DNA synthesis in transplanted sperm nuclei. *J. Embryol. Exp. Morphol.*, 36:67–72.
641b. Slack, B. E., Bell, J. E., and Benos, D. J. (1986): Inositol-1,4,5-trisphosphate injection mimics fertilization potentials in sea urchin eggs. *Am. J. Physiol.*, 250:C340–C344.
642. Szollosi, D. (1965): Time and duration of DNA synthesis in rabbit eggs after sperm penetration. *Anat. Rec.*, 154:209–212.
643. Takeuchi, I. K., and Takeuchi, Y. K. (1985): Changes in stainability of cortical granule materials with tannic acid before and after fertilization of ova. *Zool. Sci.*, 2:415–418.
644. Tarkowski, A. K. (1975): Induced parthenogenesis in the mouse. In: *Developmental Biology of Reproduction*, edited by C. L. Markert and J. Papaconstantinon, pp. 107–129. Academic Press, New York.
645. Thibault, C., and Gerard, M. (1973): Cytoplasmic and nuclear maturation of rabbit oocytes *in vitro*. *Ann. Biol. Anim. Biochim. Biophys.*, 13:145–156.
646. Usui, N., and Yanagimachi, R. (1976): Behavior of hamster sperm nuclei incorporated into eggs at various stages of maturation, fertilization and early development. *J. Ultrastruct. Res.*, 57:276–288.
647. Vacquier, V. D. (1975): The isolation of intact cortical granules from sea urchin eggs: Calcium ions trigger granule discharge. *Dev. Biol.*, 43:62–74.
648. Wagenaar, E. B., and Mazia, D. (1978): The effect of emetine on the first cleavage division of the sea urchin, *Stronglyocentrotus purpuratus*. In: *Cell Reproduction*, edited by E. R. Dirksen, D. M. Prescott, and L. F. Fox, pp. 539–545. Academic Press, New York.
649. Wassarman, P. M. (1987): The biology and chemistry of fertilization. *Science*, 235:553–554.
650. Went, D. F. (1982): Egg activation and parthenogenetic reproduction in insect. *Biol. Reprod.*, 57:319–344.
651. Whitaker, M. J., and Irvine, R. F. (1984): Inositol 1,4,5-triphosphate microinjection activates sea urchin eggs. *Nature*, 312:636–639.
652. Whitaker, M. J., and Steinhardt, R. A. (1982): Ionic regulation of egg activation. *Q. Rev. Biophys.*, 15:593–666.
653. Whitaker, M. J., and Steinhardt, R. A. (1985): Ionic signaling in the sea urchin egg at fertilization. In: *Biology of Fertilization, Vol. 3*, edited by C. B. Metz and A. Monroy, pp. 167–221. Academic Press, Orlando, Fla.
654. Whittingham, D. G. (1980): Parthenogenesis in mammals. In: *Oxford Reviews of Reproductive Biology, Vol. 2*, edited by C. A. Finn, pp. 205–231. Clarendon Press, Oxford.
655. Wiesel, S., and Schultz, G. A. (1981): Factors which may affect removal of protamine from sperm DNA during fertilization in rabbit. *Gamete Res.*, 4:25–34.
656. Wolf, D. E., Edidin, M., and Handyside, A. H. (1981): Changes in the organization of the mouse egg plasma membrane upon fertilization and first cleavage: Indications from the lateral diffusion rates of fluorescent lipid analogs. *Dev. Biol.*, 85:191–198.
657. Wolgemuth, D. J. (1983): Synthetic activities of the mammalian early embryos: Molecular and genetic alterations following fertilization. In: *Mechanism and Control of Animal Fertilization*, edited by J. F. Hartmann, pp. 415–452. Academic Press, New York.
658. Yamashita, N. (1982): Enhancement of currents through voltage-gated channels in the mouse oocyte after fertilization. *J. Physiol.*, 329:263–280.
659. Yanagimachi, R. (1978): Sperm-egg association in mammals. In: *Current Topics in Developmental Biology, Vol. 12*, edited by A. A. Moscona and A. Monroy, pp. 83–105. Academic Press, New York.
660. Yanagimachi, R. (1987): Sperm-egg fusion. In: *Current Topics in Membranes and Transport*, edited by F. Bronner and N. Duzgunes. Academic Press, Orlando, Fla. (*in press*).
661. Zamboni, L. (1974): Fine structure of the follicular wall and follicle cell-oocyte association. *Biol. Reprod.*, 10:125–149.
662. Zirkin, B. R., Soucek, D. A., Chang, T. S. K., and Perreault, S. D. (1985): *In vitro* and *in vivo* studies of mammalian sperm nuclear decondensation. *Gamete Res.*, 11:349–365.
663. Hedrick, J. L., ed. (1986): *The Molecular and Cellular Biology of Fertilization*. Plenum Press, New York.

The Physiology of Reproduction,
edited by E. Knobil and J. Neill *et al.*
Raven Press, Ltd., New York © 1988.

CHAPTER 6

Early Mammalian Embryogenesis

Roger A. Pedersen

This chapter is devoted to advances in the field of early mammalian development. During the past decade we have witnessed revolutionary progress in our understanding of preimplantation and early postimplantation differentiation of mammalian embryos. Although much of this work has been carried out in laboratory animals, particularly rodents, the technology has already been extended to livestock species and even to humans, with major economic and clinical benefits. These successes in the areas of embryo transfer in agricultural animals (1–3) and human *in vitro* fertilization (4–7) have drawn widespread attention to the potential for further application of our knowledge of mammalian embryos. Because these successful applications have been extensively reviewed elsewhere, I would prefer to focus here on advancements in basic understanding of early mammalian embryogenesis, because they alone provide the technical and conceptual foundation for any future applications to human health problems. This review addresses morphological, genetic, and biochemical aspects of early embryogenesis. Gametogenesis and fertilization, although closely related to embryogenesis, are not treated here because they are the subjects of other chapters in this volume. A comprehensive review addressing strictly physiological aspects of the preimplantation embryo has recently been published (8).

Laboratory of Radiobiology and Environmental Health (LR-102), University of California, San Francisco, San Francisco, California 94143

HISTORICAL OVERVIEW OF MAMMALIAN EMBRYOLOGY

Since the time of Aristotle, mammalian development has attracted the attention of scholars and healers. In the seventeenth and eighteenth centuries this interest culminated in discovery of the sperm and egg as the cellular components of animal reproduction. Von Baer extended this observation to the mammal with his description of the dog's egg in 1828. The nineteenth century was characterized by intense activity in descriptive embryology, stimulated by Haeckel's germ-layer theory and Wolff's epigenetic philosophy. The technical accomplishment that made these studies possible was the development of histological techniques by His in the middle of the nineteenth century (9,10).

The advent of experimental embryology came in the late nineteenth century with the work of Boveri and his contemporaries, although it was largely confined to invertebrates and amphibians, which yielded abundant embryos for experimental analysis. However, there were early successes with mammalian embryos during this period, including embryo transfer (11) and light-microscopic morphological descriptions of rodent embryos, that are still unsurpassed in their detail (12).

Our modern era of experimental mammalian embryology had its origins in successful attempts to culture mouse embryos by Whitten (13) and by Biggers and Brinster (14–17). Another crucial contribution was the development of methods for increasing the number and controlling the stage of mammalian embryos by superovulation using gonadotropins (18). What followed was an explosion of information about the fate and potency of blastomeres, developmental genetics, biochemical properties, and physiology between fertilization and early organogenesis in the mammalian embryo. This rapid development of the field, initiated by inherent curiosity about our own origins, has been sustained by our social perceptions of the need to gain control over human reproduction and to assess the risks of prenatal exposure to environmental pollutants. It also seems likely that advancements in this field will lead to an understanding of the causes of birth defects.

METHODS USED IN MAMMALIAN EMBRYOLOGY

In some cases, investigators used traditional approaches for experimental mammalian embryology, such as disaggregation or extirpation of blastomeres, but in many cases the mammalian embryo, small and fragile when compared with other vertebrate embryos, demanded new approaches. The most elegant approaches took advantage of the accumulated genetic information about mammals.

The first productive approach unique to mammals was the aggregation chimera, pioneered by Tarkowski (19) and Mintz (20) (Fig. 1). See McLaren (21) for a review of the early work using chimeras. These chimeras were formed by aggregating two 8- to 16-cell-stage mouse embryos after removing their zonae pellucidae. For analytical purposes, the two embryos were obtained from strains that differed in coat or eye color, chromosomal morphology, or biochemical traits. The most commonly used biochemical markers were the isozymes of glucose phosphate isomerase (22), which could be readily resolved on gels prepared from even small amounts of embryonic tissue. As a marker for analyzing chimeras, glucose phosphate isomerase was advantageous because it was present in virtually all tissues of the embryo and the adult, whereas pigmented or rapidly dividing cells were not ubiquitous. But this chimera marker's disadvantage was that the resulting animal's three-dimensional structure was lost in preparing tissue extracts for analysis (21). These limitations spurred a quest for better markers.

The criteria for an ideal marker include cell autonomy (i.e., the marker must not require other cells for its expression), ubiquity, heritability, and ease of detection (23). The methods and concepts involved in mammalian and avian chimeras have recently been extensively reviewed (24).

Development of techniques for introducing individual cells

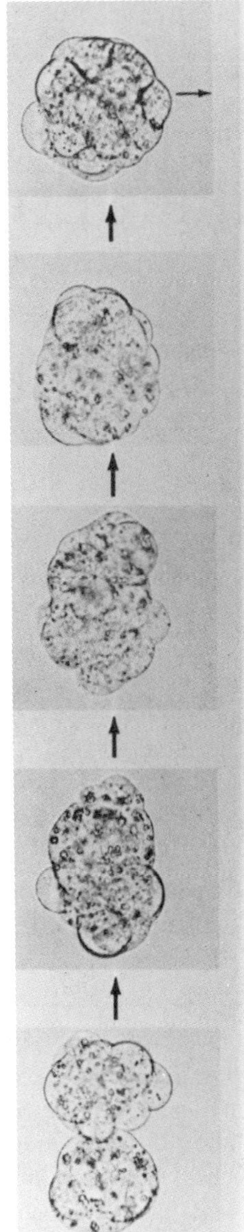

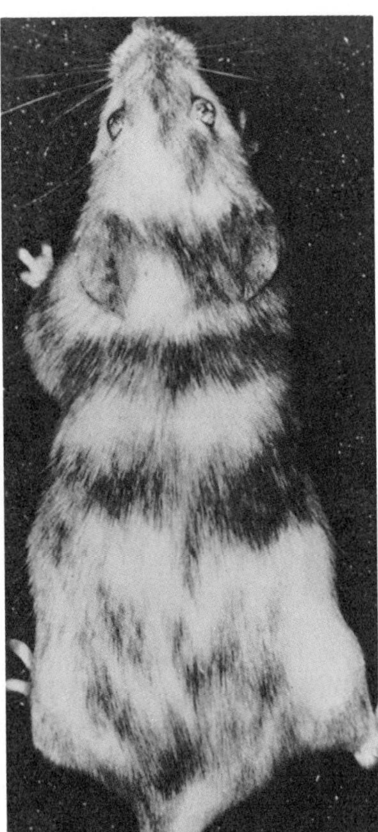

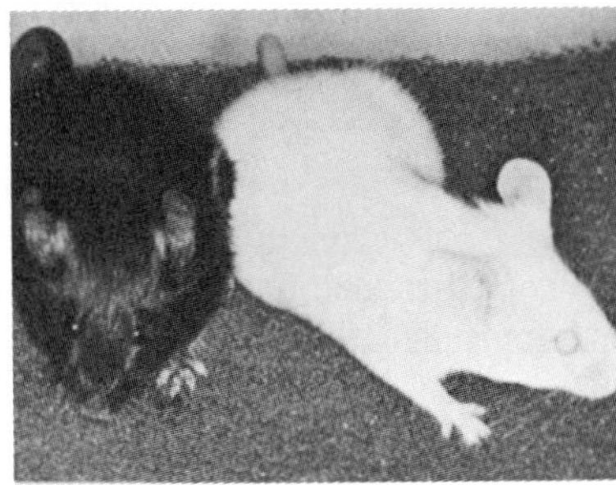

FIG. 1. Lower left: Two cleavage-stage embryos of pigmented (CC) and albino (cc) genotypes, aggregated *in vitro* after zona pellucida removal. Successive photographs show formation of one spherical embryo (CC ↔ cc) from all the blastomeres of two embryos. One of the resultant chimeric mice from these paired genotypes is at the upper right; note transverse clones of black and white in the coat and radiating clones in the eyes. The chimeric mouse was a germinal mosaic female; at the lower right are two of her offspring, one from a genetically pigmented and one from an albino germ cell, after mating with a pure-strain albino male. (From ref. 591.)

into blastocysts (25) led to a new generation of chimera studies that assessed the fate and potency of cells at later stages and with greater resolution than was possible with aggregation chimeras (Fig. 2). In these studies, Gardner and associates generally used the biochemical markers developed for aggregation chimeras and analyzed the progeny either at midgestation or after birth. Taking advantage of

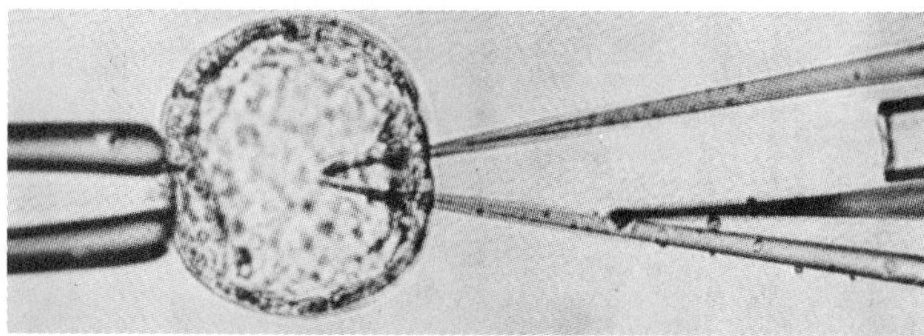

FIG. 2. Injection into the mouse blastocoel through a triangular opening in the trophectoderm to generate chimeras at the blastocyst stage. (From ref. 592.)

the discovery of a mouse mutant lacking cytoplasmic malic enzyme, Gardner (26) recently developed a marker that meets most of the criteria described earlier and used it to study the postimplantation fate of extraembryonic endoderm cells. Also, Rossant and associates have developed a recombinant DNA probe for chimeras between closely related mouse species, using *in situ* hybridization to distinguish donor and host descendants (27).

Immunosurgery, the cytotoxic immune lysis of outer cells by sequential treatment with heat-inactivated antiserum and active complement (28) (Fig. 3), is an allied technique used in making chimeras and reconstructing blastocysts from isolated trophectoderm and inner cell masses. The results of these studies are described in a later section dealing with fate and potency in early development.

Microinjection into cells is another approach that has been widely used in mammalian embryology. Pioneered by Lin (29), this technique provides high-resolution marking with minimal disturbance to the intact embryo. Initially, oil droplets were used to mark cells, but this marker suffered from the propensity to segregate to a single blastomere (30,31). Recently, markers developed for use in amphibian and annelid embryos (32–34) have been successfully applied to the mouse embryo (35,36) (Fig. 4). This latest generation of cell markers relies on the ease of detecting horseradish peroxidase by histochemical staining, making it possible to trace the lineage of marked progenitor cells during early stages of development. Such passively distributed markers are limited, in that they become diluted during embryonic growth and are thus confined to short-term studies.

Until recently, the lack of a reliable procedure for nuclear transfer has made efforts to define the roles of nucleus and cytoplasm in early mammalian development frustrating. The importance of such studies was evident from the earlier work on amphibian embryos by Briggs and King (37), who demonstrated the totipotency of blastula nuclei, and by Gurdon (38), who extended these observations to some tadpole nuclei. The novel nuclear transfer method devised by McGrath and Solter (39) uses Sendai virus to fuse together cytoplast and karyoplast fragments that have been produced microsurgically. Experiments using appropriate genetic markers for donor and host components have revealed unique roles

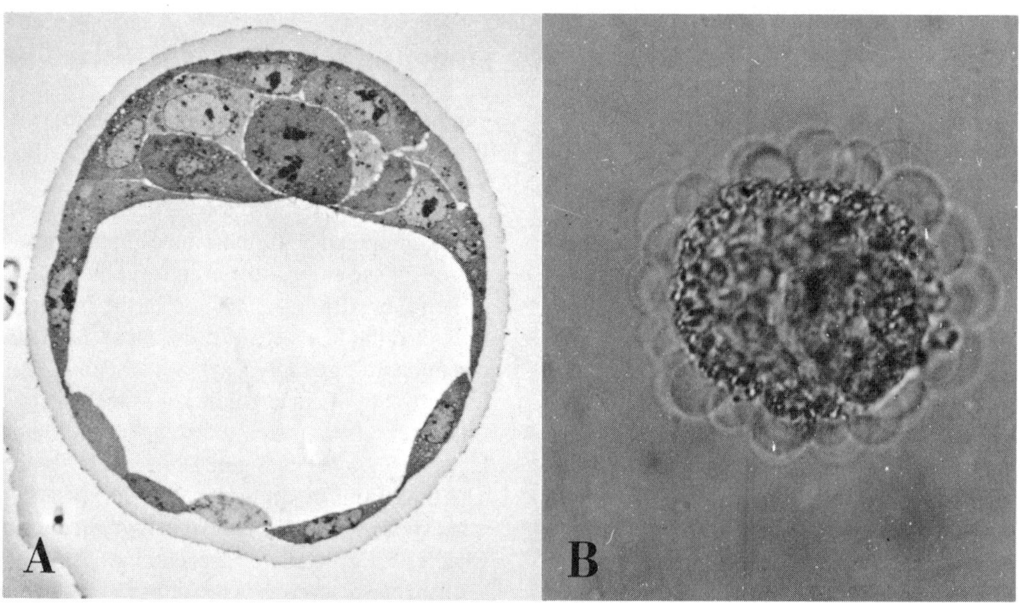

FIG. 3. A: Thick-section scanning electron micrograph of 3.5-d.g. mouse blastocyst showing large rounded cells of inner cell mass and flattened cells of trophectoderm (x595). (From ref. 593.) **B:** Isolation of inner cell mass by immunosurgery. Trophectoderm cells are lysed by successive treatment with antiserum and complement (x850). (Photo provided by Dr. Barry Pierce.)

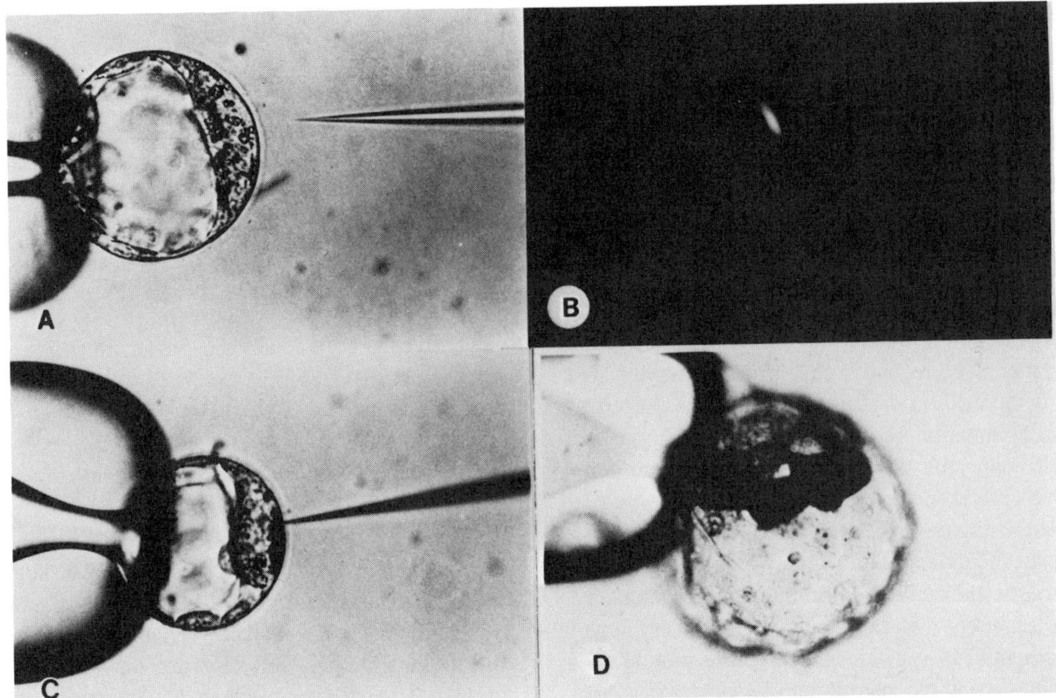

FIG. 4. Fate of polar trophectoderm during mouse blastocyst growth. **A:** Mid-stage blastocyst prepared for microinjection into central trophectoderm cell. **B:** Fluorescence of rhodamine-conjugated dextran immediately after injection. **C:** Staining of injected cell with horseradish peroxidase immediately after injection. **D:** Staining of descendant cells with horseradish peroxidase after 48-hr culture, showing predominantly mural localization of stained trophectoderm cells. (From ref. 122.)

for maternal and paternal pronuclei in early mouse embryogenesis (*vide infra*).

Production of transgenic animals by injecting exogenous DNA into the zygote pronucleus (40) is the most recent and potentially most powerful method for studying mammalian embryogenesis. This method produces genetically novel animals that carry one or more copies of the exogenous DNA integrated into the genome. These integrated genes are inherited as Mendelian traits in subsequent generations and may be expressed in a tissue-specific and temporally correct pattern (41). Like the integration of exogenous genes by P-element-mediated transposition in *Drosophila* (42), production of transgenic mice provides access to the mammalian genome for a wide variety of genetic, biochemical, and physiological studies. The results of this approach are described in a later section.

Miniaturization is the most widely applied method for studying mammalian embryos. In addition to the microscopic techniques used in microinjection studies, many investigators have ingeniously reduced the amounts of tissue required for the biochemical studies described in a later section. This trend is epitomized in the physiological analysis of individual preimplantation mouse embryos, using enzymological recycling techniques (8).

Because amounts of material are often limiting, mammalian embryologists have tended to treat the individual embryo as the experimental unit and to rely on small population sizes. Often a critical conclusion has been based on a few embryos! This should serve as a continual reminder of the delicate condition of our knowledge about mammalian embryogenesis. Despite its revolutionary progress, the field of early mammalian development still promises many revelations.

MORPHOLOGICAL ASPECTS

Timing of Cleavage, Compaction, and Blastocyst Formation

The events of fertilization occur relatively slowly in mammals, compared with most other organisms. The time required for sperm-egg fusion and second polar-body emission is 1 to 2 hr after insemination in the mouse (43,44) and 2 to 5 hr in the hamster (45). Pronuclei form about 6 hr after insemination, and DNA synthesis begins 2 to 4 hr later, in most strains of mice studied (44,46). In the hamster, the time from insemination to pronuclear formation is about 4 hr, and to the beginning of DNA synthesis about 8 hr (47). The time from insemination to sperm penetration varies in other species, depending on the duration of capacitation (see Chapter 5 for details of capacitation).

Cleavage also progresses slowly (Fig. 5). Whereas *Drosophila* embryos undergo cleavage at 10-min intervals, and amphibian embryos cleave at approximately 30-min intervals, mouse embryos undergo their first and second cleavages at 14- to 26-hr intervals *in vivo* in most strains studied

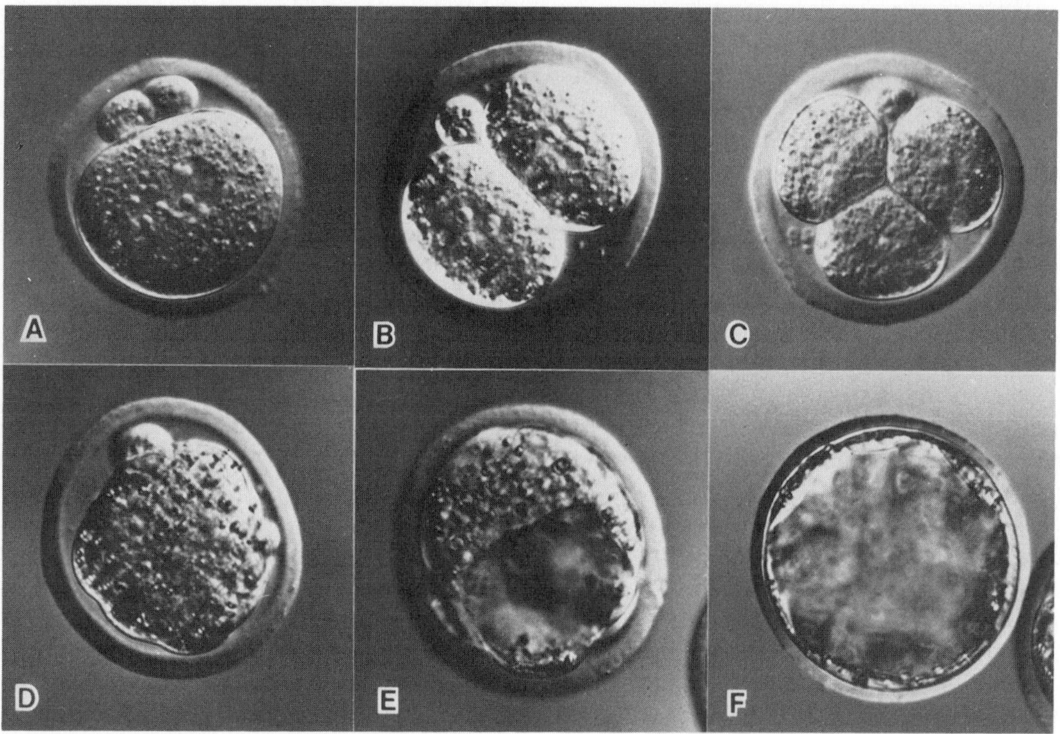

FIG. 5. Preimplantation stages of mouse embryo development: (**A**) zygote; (**B**) 2-cell stage; (**C**) 4-cell stage; (**D**) compacted morula stage (~16 cells); (**E**) early blastocyst stage; (**F**) expanded blastocyst stage; inner cell mass is out of focal plane (~64 cells). x340. (From ref. 54.)

(44). There is a marked effect of genetic background on cleavage time in the first two cycles (48,49). Later cleavages occur at approximately 10-hr intervals in most strains of mice; however, there is an association between certain haplotypes at the H-2 locus and slow versus fast development (50). When mouse embryos are placed in culture, their development is retarded, with cleavage progressing 2 hr or more slower each cycle than *in vivo*, so that the time for development to the blastocyst stage *in vitro* may be an entire day longer than *in vivo* (51,52).

There is now considerable information, also for the mouse embryo, about the cell cycle dynamics at various cleavage stages in the mouse embryo (Fig. 5). In the first cell cycle, the S phase lasts 4 to 8 hr and G_2 + M ranges from 3 to 8 hr. In the second cycle, S takes 4 to 7 hr, and G_2 + M ranges from 12 to 15 hr (44,46,53,54). The comparable values for the third and fourth cycles are 7 hr for S and 1 to 5 hr for G_2 + M (55). The G_1 phase of the cycle is brief at all cleavage stages (1–2 hr). These estimates are valuable when attempting to infer at what point important events in cell determination and differentiation occur. Human embryos also develop as slowly *in vitro* as mouse embryos, dividing at 16- to 24-hr intervals during early cleavages (56,57).

Cleavage is invariably asynchronous in mammalian embryos. Asynchronous division from the 2-cell stage creates a 3-cell embryo. The earlier dividing blastomere of the 2-cell mouse embryo, in turn, has descendants that divide earlier than descendants of the other blastomere (58). The range from the earliest to latest division at late cleavage stages can reach 4 hr or more in culture.

During late cleavage stages for all placental mammals, the blastomeres begin a process of compaction during which individual blastomeres seem to lose their identity, merging into a single coherent mass of cells (59). This early morphogenetic event is marked by junctional differentiation in which gap junctions and incipient tight junctions form between outer blastomeres and initiate the process of epithelial differentiation, culminating in the formation of trophectoderm at the blastocyst stage (60–64). It is interesting that compaction does not occur in marsupial embryos (65). The importance of compaction as one of the first visible signs of embryonic differentiation has motivated extensive analysis of its biochemical aspects (*vide infra*).

The next morphogenetic event in mammalian development is the formation of the blastocyst cavity, also known as the blastocoel, although it is not homologous to the amphibian blastocoel. Blastocyst formation manifests the beginning of fluid transport by the trophectoderm cells, as well as physical partitioning of cells between an inner compartment (the inner cell mass) and an outer epithelium (the trophectoderm) that envelops the inner cells and retains the blastocoel fluid. The mural trophectoderm surrounds the blastocoel, and the polar trophectoderm overlies the inner cell mass (Fig.3). The cell number at the time of blastocyst formation varies considerably among various species of placental mammals (59,66,67). Generally, fluid begins to accumulate in late cleavage: after division to the 16-cell stage in the hamster and pig, the 32-cell stage in the mouse, the 64-cell stage in the sheep, and the 128-cell stage in the rabbit. Some rare species accumulate fluid at earlier stages; for example, the *Elephantulus* embryo accumulates blastocoel fluid at the 4-cell stage (66).

During blastocyst expansion, asynchrony increases between cell divisions in the mouse embryo (68,69). This tendency culminates in giant cell transformation, a process of endoreduplication (DNA synthesis without cell division), which begins in the abembryonic mural trophectoderm—opposite to the inner cell mass—at 4.5 to 6.5 days of gestation (d.g.), depending on the species (67). At 4.0 to 4.5 d.g. in the mouse, hatching commences, and the blastocyst escapes from the zona pellucida. Then the embryo begins to implant in the uterine wall, where it undergoes rapid growth and begins the morphogenetic events that transform it into a recognizably vertebrate individual.

The correlation between specific cleavage divisions and the early morphogenetic events naturally raises the question of what kind of clock regulates the early embryo. This question has been approached experimentally using aggregation chimeras and other techniques. Increasing the number of cells in the mouse embryo, either by aggregating two or more embryos together or by decreasing the cell number by inducing tetraploidy, does not appreciably change the time of cavitation, but simply changes the number of cells in the embryo at the time the cavity forms (70). This observation led to the proposal that nuclear divisions count time in early mammalian development. Contrary to this idea, however, are the results of treating mouse embryos with phorbol esters, aphidicolin (an inhibitor of DNA polymerase alpha), or inhibitors of polyamine biosynthesis. These treatments cause cavitation with fewer cells and at earlier times than in the normal embryo (71–75). Thus, there may be a cytoplasmic component to timekeeping in the mammal, as there is in the amphibian embryo (76), rather than a strictly nuclear clock, as in the ascidian (77). Support for this conclusion comes from the fact that anucleate fragments of mouse zygotes and parthenogenetically activated eggs undergo persistent contractile waves (78).

The nature of cellular clocks is an active topic in considering other cell systems and may ultimately enable us to understand timing in the early mammalian embryo. Cytoplasmic factors regulate the progression of meiosis in amphibian embryos (79). Maturation-promoting factor (MPF), which is abundant in the mature amphibian oocyte, mouse oocyte, and in embryonic and somatic cells at the time of mitosis, induces nuclear breakdown and chromosomal condensation of meiotic as well as mitotic nuclei (80–86). In addition to MPF, the membrane phospholipids, phosphatidyl inositol and diacyl glycerol, together with cytosolic calcium, calmodulin, and oncogene-related protein kinases, are known to be involved in regulating the cell cycle (87,88). These components may act in turn through changes in cytoplasmic pH, which oscillates during the cell cycle (89). Finally, polyamines are known to be required for cell proliferation in the mouse embryo and numerous other cell types (72,90,91). All of these factors are potential candidates for regulating cell proliferation in the early mammalian embryo. Sorting out the mechanistic relationships between cell cycle events and morphogenesis is an even more complex problem that needs to be resolved before we can understand how early development is coordinated.

Potency of Isolated Blastomeres

Developmental biologists have long been interested in determining the potency of early cell types. Prospective potency is defined as the full range of developmental capabilities of an embryonic cell or tissue (92), and as such it can be characterized only by experimental perturbation of the intact embryo. Restriction of potency—that is, determination—indicates that a decisive event has occurred that limits the future capabilities of the cell or tissue. Understanding the molecular mechanisms that underlie this aspect of developmental decision making is a fundamental problem of developmental biology, and assessing the potency of cells during mammalian development has assumed major importance. Tarkowski and Wroblewska (93) found that most individual blastomeres isolated at the 4-and 8-cell stages developed into trophoblast vesicles devoid of inner cells. They proposed that the differentiation into trophectoderm and inner cell mass was determined by the outer or inner position of blastomeres at the morula stage (16 to 32 cells). This "inside-outside" hypothesis predicted that blastomeres would remain totipotent at least until they assume their positions at the morula stage. A substantial body of work confirms this prediction, showing that mouse embryo blastomeres maintain their potency at the 2- to 16-cell stages (94–98). A similar degree of totipotency seems to exist in cleavage-stage rabbit, horse, cow, and sheep embryos (67). Beyond the morula stage, the increasing junctional differentiation of the outer cells that accompanies their incipient differentiation into trophectoderm makes it difficult to disaggregate the embryo and assess their potency (99). Nonetheless, outer cells of the late morula (~30-cell stage) have been shown to be totipotent in mouse embryos, as are the inner cells at this stage (97).

Furthermore, the inner cells of the early mouse blastocyst are also totipotent, because they can form trophectoderm when isolated by immunosurgery and grown in culture, and they can even differentiate into invasive giant cells when transferred to the uteri of foster mothers (100–103). Immunosurgery has also been used to isolate inner cells at later stages of blastocyst development. These studies show that the inner cells lose their totipotency during blastocyst expansion at approximately the time of the division from 32 to 64 cells (100–102). Inner cells isolated from expanded blastocysts either by immunosurgery or by microdissection form an outer layer of primitive endoderm cells, rather than trophectoderm (104). It is difficult, however, to define the precise stage at which this important developmental transition occurs. Cells differentiating from individual inner cell masses isolated at the 32- to 64-cell stages often contain a mixture of trophectoderm and primitive endoderm cells (69, 105). This heterogeneity could arise from asynchrony within the inner cell mass, with cells at their sixth cycle forming trophectoderm and cells at their seventh cycle forming primitive endoderm. Thus, restriction in the potency of inner cells occurs relatively late in preimplantation development.

Cell Allocation in Preimplantation Embryos

The potency of preimplantation mammalian embryos is a characteristic and distinguishing feature that focuses our attention on the timing and mechanisms that allocate some blastomeres to the inner cell mass and others to the trophectoderm lineage. Several studies have made it clear that the position of a blastomere in the early embryo is crucial to its subsequent fate. When totipotent blastomeres of cleavage-stage embryos that had been experimentally marked with [^{3}H]thymidine or that differed in their glucose phosphate isomerase isozyme were placed on the outside of aggregation chimeras, they generally developed into trophectoderm. Conversely, cells on the inside generally developed into inner cell mass (95,96). These results fulfill a major prediction of the inside-outside hypothesis and raise the question of when and how cells acquire their positions in the intact embryo.

The early cleavage stages of mouse embryos have only outer cells, presumably because packing of equal-size round objects requires a minimum number to completely enclose one or more of them. This number ranges from 10 to 17 in modeling studies, depending on the deformability assumed for the objects (106,107). Inside cells are first observed in mouse embryos at the 10- to 16-cell stage, when 1 to 6 cells are enclosed, as determined by time-lapse cinemicrography (107) or by paraffin serial sectioning, immunosurgery, or labeling intact embryos on the outer surface with fluorescent antibodies and then disaggregating them (108). The mean number of enclosed cells increases to 10 to 13 at the early blastocyst-stage (32-cell) mouse embryo (Fig. 3), with some variation according to the method used (69). The ratio of inner cells to total blastocyst cell number decreases from 0.40 in the early mouse blastocyst to 0.25 in the late blastocyst (128–256-cell stage) (68). This decreasing fraction of inner cells has been interpreted as indicating a contribution of inner-cell-mass cells to the trophectoderm during blastocyst growth (100) or an attrition of inner cells owing to cell death (109). (The prospective fate of inner-cell-mass cells is discussed in the next section.) Approximately 10% of blastocyst cells are indeed necrotic during blastocyst expansion, suggesting that programmed cell death may occur at this stage (109).

The distribution of cleavage products into inner cell mass and trophectoderm is not random. First, mixing between regions of cleavage-stage mouse embryos is limited, as shown by aggregating [^{3}H]thymidine-labeled and unlabeled 8-cell embryos and sectioning them for autoradiography at the blastocyst stage. The descendants of the labeled blastomeres tend to remain together in the same quadrant of the resulting chimera, rather than mixing thoroughly (110,111). Moreover, the earlier-dividing blastomere of the 2-cell mouse embryo contributes slightly more cells to the inner cell mass than the later-dividing cell, also indicative of nonrandom contribution (58,112). This attribute of earlier-dividing cells is even more dramatic when 4- and 8-cell mouse embryos are combined, in which case the inner cell mass of the chimera is composed almost entirely of cells from the more advanced component (113). The phenomenon of disproportionate contribution to the inner cell mass by the more advanced blastomeres has been exploited to manufacture sheep-goat chimeras in which the primary fetal component is derived from the goat, but the sheep trophoblast constitution is compatible with development to term in a sheep foster mother (114). The mechanism for this differential contribution may involve the size or cell surface characteristics of the blastomeres, because smaller, advanced blastomeres tend to be engulfed by larger, earlier-stage blastomeres when they are combined in pairs (115,116).

Further evidence for an orderly partitioning of cleavage products into the inner cell mass and trophectoderm has been obtained by reaggregating outer and inner blastomeres of 16-cell mouse embryos. At this stage, the outer blastomeres are slightly larger than the inner ones, and are polarized, having a higher density of microvilli on their free surfaces than on portions of their membranes apposed to other blastomeres. In contrast to this polarized phenotype of the outer cells, inner cells are apolar (117,118). When labeled outer cells are combined in either inner or outer locations with various proportions of unlabeled inner or outer cells, the labeled outer cell invariably contributes at least one descendant to the trophectoderm of the resulting blastocyst. The developmental contributions of inner cells are not as constrained; they give rise to either inner cell mass or trophectoderm, depending primarily on their initial position in the aggregates (119,120).

Microinjection of horseradish peroxidase into individual blastomeres also demonstrates the developmental constraints that appear during early development of the intact mouse embryo. Labeled descendants of 2-cell blastomeres almost always occupy both inner cell mass and trophectoderm. Single 8-cell blastomeres often have descendants in both inner cell mass and trophectoderm, but may have exclusively trophectoderm descendants (35). Outer, 16-cell blastomeres have principally trophectoderm descendants, but may have inner-cell-mass descendants as well (121). However, descendants of outer cells marked at the 32- to 64-cell stages (early and expanding blastocysts) are exclusively trophectodermal (122). Thus, an outer position at late cleavage stages constrains a mouse blastomere to produce at least one outer descendant in subsequent cleavages. This constraint appears to arise together with the polarized phenotype at the time of compaction, and the extent of contribution to trophectoderm coincides with the degree of epithelial differentiation that has occurred at each stage.

Unfortunately, this information does not allow us to make a conclusive statement about what controls differentiation into either trophectoderm or inner cell mass. The predictions of the inside-outside hypothesis about totipotency and the role of position in cell fate are supported by available evidence, but this does not indicate what kind of signals might cause the differentiation of enclosed cells into inner cell mass and outer cells into trophectoderm. It is unlikely that diffusible substances in the blastocoel cavity cause or sustain inner-cell-mass differentiation, because embryos at totipotent stages inserted with intact zonae pellucidae into the blastocoel of giant chimeras develop into morphologically normal blastocysts, rather than into inner-cell-mass-like structures (123).

The polarization hypothesis likewise accounts for many of the events leading to trophectoderm differentiation (124). In this hypothesis, the separation of cleaving blastomeres into two lineages is thought to be the result of the propensity of outer cells to polarize, owing to their asymmetric cell contacts (125). When combined with the constraints of polarization discussed previously, this presumably leads to the allocation of polarized descendants to the trophectoderm at the blastocyst stage and of apolar descendants to the inner cell mass. The polarization hypothesis predicts that polarized blastomeres will maintain the capacity to generate apolar cells and that apolar cells will maintain the capacity to polarize, until the two tissue lineages of the blastocyst become clonally distinct populations. It does not exclude the possibility that inner-cell-mass cells will have outer descendants. The inside-outside hypothesis predicts, however, that cells located on the inside at the morula or blastocyst stage will remain stably located in the inner-cell-mass lineage during subsequent development.

Cell Fate During Postimplantation Development

The prospective fate of embryonic cells is defined as their normal contribution to tissues or organs that arise in subsequent development. It is to be distinguished from prospective potency, which is the full range of developmental capabilities of a cell under any experimental circumstances (92). The prospective fate of blastocyst cells during postimplantation development of the mouse embryo has been studied with injection chimeras and reconstituted blastocysts. These studies have generally been performed with expanded (3.5-d.g.) blastocysts containing approximately 64 cells. Using these approaches, it has been possible to assess the fate of inner-cell-mass cells and trophectoderm cells by combining genetically marked cells at the same stages and assessing their contributions to the conceptus at midgestation or at term. Similarly, it has been possible to determine the fate of the more advanced cells, particularly endoderm and ectoderm obtained from the 4.5-d.g. embryo. The primitive endoderm cells first differentiate as a layer covering the blastocoelic surface of the mouse inner cell mass about 4.5 d.g., whereupon the remaining core cells of the inner cell mass are, by convention, designated the primitive ectoderm (Fig. 6). Primitive endoderm from later-stage embryos (6.5 and 7.5 d.g.) has also been used as a source of cells for blastocyst injection chimeras, but cells identified as primitive ectoderm from these stages have not produced descendants in chimeric blastocysts (126,127).

Cells derived from the trophectoderm layer have been identified in mouse chimeras and reconstituted blastocysts containing genetically marked trophectoderm and inner-cell-mass components. These studies show that the mural trophectoderm gives rise to the giant cells involved in implantation and that polar trophectoderm gives rise to the ectoplacental cone and extraembryonic ectoderm, as well as to secondary giant cells that develop after implantation (128–130). These trophectoderm descendants are confined to the chorioallantoic placenta. Assuming that similar lineage relationships exist in embryos of other placental mammals, trophectoderm thus represents a unique product of vertebrate evolution that is allocated during the earliest morphogenetic events of embryogenesis and makes no subsequent contribution to the fetus or its membranes. There is, nonetheless, some flexibility within the trophectoderm lineage, because diploid trophectoderm cells of the blastocyst can be induced to proliferate by juxtaposing a donor inner cell mass. Moreover, diploid cells of the midgestation extraembryonic ectoderm and ectoplacental cone remain capable of producing trophoblast giant cells either *in vitro* or when transplanted to ectopic sites (103,128,131). Also, extraembryonic ectoderm cells of 5.5- or 6.5-d.g. mouse embryos contribute to ectoplacental cone and trophoblast giant cells after injection into blastocysts (132). These observations also suggest that polar trophectoderm (in preimplantation embryos) and extraembryonic ectoderm (in postimplantation embryos) serve as stem cell populations for the trophectoderm lineage (103,133).

However, polar trophectoderm of the early blastocyst may not itself constitute the stem cell population from which further proliferation of trophectoderm occurs. In their study of reconstituted blastocysts using the *M. musculus–M. caroli* marker system, Rossant and Croy (130) found a small but highly significant incidence of inner-cell-mass descendants in the midgestation trophectoderm lineage of the placenta when early blastocyst inner cell masses were used as donors in the reconstitutions. Analysis of inner cell fate in mouse blastocysts by injecting horseradish peroxidase into single cells and culturing the labeled embryos 24 hr led to a similar finding (G. K. Winkel and R. A. Pedersen, *unpublished observations*). In this case, descendants of labeled

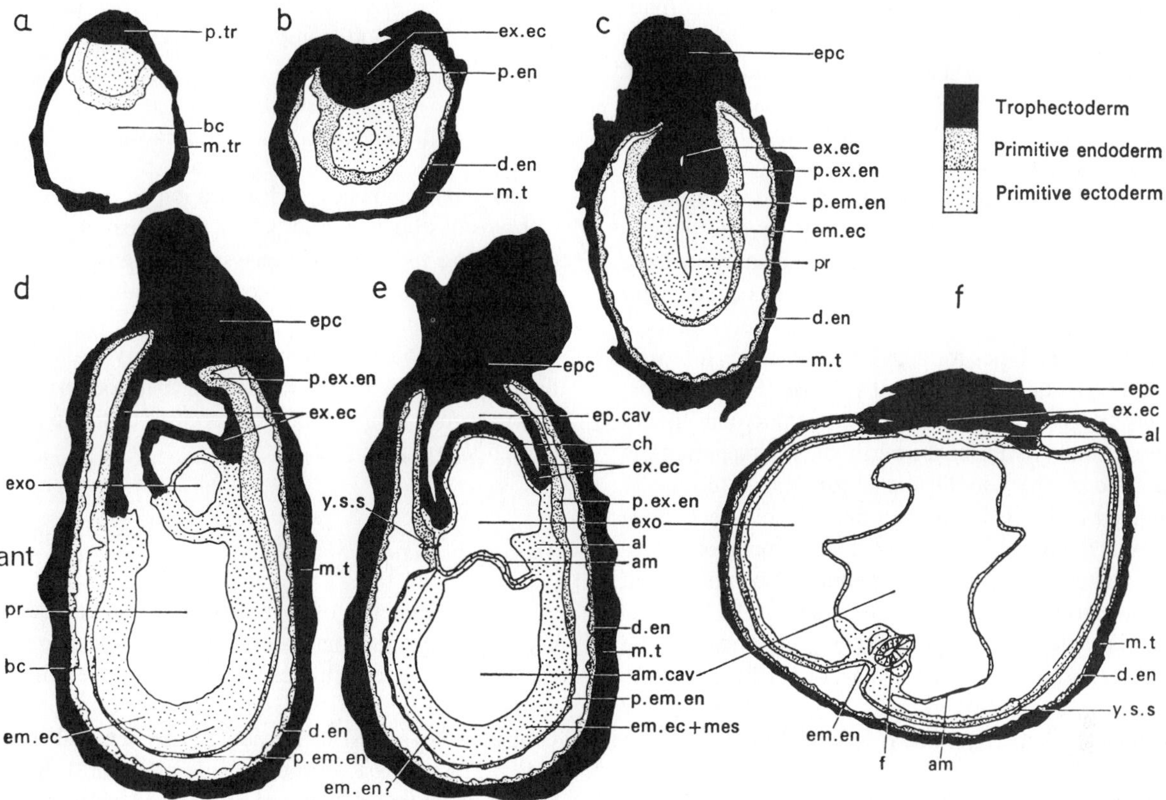

FIG. 6. Tentative fate map of the trophectoderm, primitive endoderm, and primitive ectoderm of the late mouse blastocyst projected onto successive developmental stages; (**a**) 4.5 days; (**b**) 5- or 6-day egg cylinder; (**c**) 5.5 days; (**d**) 7 days; (**e**) 7.5 days; (**f**) 8.5 days. The parts of the figure are drawn to different scales. *al*, allantois; *am*, amnion; *am. cav*, amniotic cavity; *ant*, anterior; *bc*, blastocoel; *ch*, chorion; *d. en*, distal (parietal) endoderm; *em. ec*, embryonic ectoderm; *em. en*, definitive embryonic endoderm; *epc*, ectoplacental cone; *ep. cav*, ectoplacental cavity; *ex. ec*, extraembryonic ectoderm; *exo*, exocoelom; *f*, fetus; *mes*, mesoderm; *m. t*, mural trophoblast; *m. tr*, mural trophectoderm; *p. em. en*, proximal embryonic endoderm; *p. en*, proximal endoderm; *p. ex. en*, proximal extraembryonic (visceral) endoderm; *pr*, proamnion; *p. tr*, polar trophectoderm; *y. s. s*, yolk sac splanchnopleure. (From ref. 594.)

inner cells clearly occupied sites in the polar and mural trophectoderm, despite unambiguous controls showing no labeling in these sites at the outset of culture. These observations and results of marking polar trophectoderm cells with peroxidase (122) led to the proposal that definitive polar trophectoderm is formed only during the later stages of blastocyst growth. Nonetheless, stem cell model for the trophectoderm lineage predicts that there is a time during early development when cells within the inner cell mass become allocated to a strictly inner fate. Although this time has not yet been defined precisely, the preponderance of data from blastocyst injection and reconstitution studies using expanded 3.5-d.g. blastocysts as hosts and donors implies that the segregation of the trophectoderm and inner-cell-mass lineages is complete before the time of implantation (134).

The fate of primitive endoderm cells from 4.5-d.g. blastocysts has been studied by injecting them into 3.5-d.g. hosts; synchronous hosts have not been used, owing to the low rate of development to term after transfer to foster mothers at the late blastocyst stage. These studies have shown that primitive endoderm cells of the mouse embryo produce detectable descendants only in the visceral and parietal yolk sac endoderm during postimplantation development and do not contribute to the fetal gut (134–136). Interestingly, visceral yolk sac endoderm from later-stage embryos (6.5 and 7.5 d.g.) produced a similar pattern of descent, whereas parietal endoderm descendants of any donor age were invariably limited to the parietal yolk sac endoderm. These results suggest that primitive endoderm serves as a stem cell population for visceral and parietal endoderm at the late blastocyst stage, and visceral endoderm or a morphologically indistinguishable cell type serves as the stem cell for both types of extraembryonic endoderm at postimplantation stages (136). This model is supported by observations that visceral endoderm cells of the 7.5-d.g. mouse embryo are able to differentiate into parietal endoderm in culture (137) and that peroxidase-labeled visceral embryonic endoderm cells overlying the most anterior region of the mouse egg cylinder at 7.5 d.g. move into extraembryonic positions during 24 hr of culture (138).

A comparison of these models for trophectoderm and

extraembryonic endoderm fate reveals a similar morphogenetic theme. Both lineages appear to be set aside early in development, before implantation and the period of dramatic growth begin. Once allocated, both lineages seem to emerge from relatively small stem cell populations of 20 to 30 cells. Both yield a pluripotent cell type (extraembryonic ectoderm in the trophectoderm lineage and visceral endoderm in the extraembryonic endoderm lineage). Both have terminally differentiated cell types that accumulate distally, after a period of morphogenetic movement or translocation (trophoblast giant cells and parietal cells, respectively). Indeed, these latter two cell types form an intimate association with each other, constituting the parietal yolk sac (Fig. 6). Thus, the pattern of growth of the major extraembryonic tissues of the mouse embryo during the periimplantation period can be visualized as the coordinated expansion of terminally differentiated cells by distal accretion of cells that move away from actively proliferating stem cell populations. This does not, however, exclude the possibility of continued cell proliferation in the terminally differentiated cells, particularly parietal endoderm. Implicit in this interpretation is a series of bifurcating decisions associated with the successive partitioning of lineages. These can be represented in the form of binary choices, as shown in Fig. 9 (139).

Unfortunately, it is not known to what extent this generalized model for early morphogenesis and decision making applies to the primitive ectoderm lineage. In injection chimeras, primitive ectoderm cells from late blastocysts (4.5 d.g.) contribute descendants to all tissues of the fetus, including the gut. Primitive ectoderm also has descendants in the extraembryonic mesoderm of the visceral yolk sac, the amnionic ectoderm, and the mesoderm of the chorion (135,140). There is evidence from the pattern of X-chromosome inactivation of primitive-ectoderm descendants in mouse chimeras that primordial germ cells are also derived from this tissue (141). Primitive ectoderm has descendants neither in trophectoderm nor in extraembryonic endoderm, demonstrating that primitive ectoderm is a committed cell population by the time of implantation. Gardner (142) has recently demonstrated that pure populations of primitive ectoderm isolated by enzymatic treatment and microdissection do not subsequently generate any cells resembling primitive endoderm, despite earlier reports of endoderm regeneration by immunosurgically isolated ectodermal cores from 4.5-d.g. mouse blastocysts (143–145). This result is consistent with the behavior of primitive endoderm and ectoderm as clonally distinct populations in blastocyst injection chimeras.

Apart from the early allocation of primitive ectoderm as a small cell population, there is simply no basis for comparing decision making in the primitive ectoderm lineage with that in the extraembryonic lineages of trophectoderm and extraembryonic endoderm. It remains to be determined whether primitive ectoderm differentiates into fetal mesoderm, endoderm, and ectoderm by a series of binary decisions or by a more complex scenario.

Potency and Allocation in Postimplantation Embryos

Analysis of potency and allocation in postimplantation embryos has been carried out by four separate approaches: transferring tissues to ectopic sites in adult animals, culturing isolated tissues, generating postimplantation chimeras, and marking cells in intact embryos. Although the information about postimplantation embryos derived from these approaches is still rudimentary, it does permit some general conclusions about the processes of tissue allocation during gastrulation (127,146).

Analysis in Ectopic Sites

Tissue fragments of primitive-streak-stage rodent embryos develop into mature tissue in several ectopic sites, specifically the anterior chamber of the eye, the kidney capsule, and the testis capsule. The pioneering studies of Grobstein (147,148) demonstrated that the embryonic ectoderm, or epiblast, formed a wide range of differentiated tissues, including derivatives of all three germ layers. This finding, which is incompatible with the notion of epiblast as definitive ectoderm, was later confirmed by other investigators, who transferred tissues of rat (149,150) or mouse (151,152) embryos to ectopic sites. When visceral embryonic endoderm from the same stages was transferred to ectopic sites, it was resorbed (149,153) or developed only into parietal endoderm (151). Visceral extraembryonic endoderm likewise developed into tissue with a parietal endoderm phenotype (154). The broad developmental potential of epiblast is even more striking in the demonstration that all regions (anterior, distal, and posterior) of the epiblast (Fig. 6) have the capacity to form derivatives of the three definitive germ layers in ectopic sites (152,155–157). It can be inferred from these results that the epiblast of the primitive-streak-stage rodent embryo contains cells that can differentiate into ectoderm, mesoderm, and endoderm. However, these tissues do not necessarily descend from single progenitor cells within the epiblast. To demonstrate the latter degree of totipotency would require a clonal analysis.

A restriction in the potency of epiblast in rodent embryos can be detected at the headfold stage, when isolated epiblast no longer differentiates into endoderm derivatives, but still forms mesodermal tissues (153). Endoderm isolated from this stage did not survive, but combined with mesoderm developed into both gut and mesoderm derivatives (153). The anterior and posterior fractions of these combined tissues produced complementary derivatives of the gut, suggesting that some regionalization of potential has occurred by the headfold stage.

Analysis In Vitro

A single analysis of explanted embryo fragments indicates that there is regionalization in the embryo before the head-fold stage. In that study, Snow (158) dissected fragments of the intact primitive-streak-stage mouse embryo containing all three germ layers and cultured these for 24 hr. These multilayered fragments produced only a portion of the tissue repertoire of the embryo. Most notably, a region at the posterior end of the primitive streak was the only fragment capable of producing germ cells. The same region is the site where germ cells are first visible by alkaline phosphatase staining in the intact embryo (159). These results, together with the pluripotency of the isolated epiblast layer at comparable stages, imply that regionalized restrictions in the fate of the rodent epiblast occur as the result of tissue interactions at or after the primitive-streak stage and that these limitations are not caused by limited potency of the epiblast.

Analysis in Postimplantation Chimeras

Using an approach developed for the chick embryo (160), Beddington carried out an analysis of donor tissues in chimeric mouse embryos using [^{3}H]thymidine as a marker (161,162). Groups of approximately 20 labeled epiblast cells were grafted into the same or a different site of the primitive-streak-stage embryo, and the tissue contributions of the labeled cells 36 hr later were scored by autoradiography (Fig. 6). Transplanted anterior epiblast formed mainly neuroectoderm and surface ectoderm when placed in anterior and distal sites, and it formed surface ectoderm and loose mesoderm even when placed in a posterior location. Transplanted posterior epiblast formed mainly surface ectoderm when placed in an anterior site and formed only mesoderm when placed into distal or posterior sites. Transplanted distal epiblast formed surface ectoderm, neuroectoderm, and mesoderm when placed in an anterior site, formed only mesoderm when placed in a posterior site, but formed mainly mesoderm and gut endoderm when placed in a distal site. These patterns of contribution indicate that there are regional differences in the fate of cells in the epiblast of postimplantation chimeras, despite the apparent totipotency of the isolated tissue (127,161,162).

Using a similar approach, Copp et al. (163) recently transferred labeled grafts of embryonic epiblast plus mesoderm obtained from the posterior part of the primitive streak to the same site at the base of the allantois, where they formed somatic cells and germ cells (as identified by alkaline phosphatase staining). Grafts of epiblast plus mesoderm from lateral regions into the base of the allantois produced somatic descendants, but failed to produce germ cells. These results appear to reinforce the conclusions that donor epiblast cells in postimplantation chimeras show greater regionalization than their pluripotency in ectopic sites. An alternative possibility is that germ cell and somatic lineages diverge early in development, before somatic cells are allocated to organ rudiments (164,165,171).

Analysis in Intact Embryos

Analysis of cell fate in intact embryos has the advantage that it does not alter the normal tissue relationships within the embryo. Thus, it should be possible to determine the fate of descendants of single marked progenitor cells in their undisturbed environment. Although studying radiation-induced somatic mosaicism has provided enormous insight into *Drosophila* cell lineages, the extreme radiation sensitivity of the mammalian embryo precludes such an approach, except for relatively late in gestation (166). Direct visual observation has been used in *Caenorhabditis elegans* embryos to determine their complete lineage, but this approach cannot be used in the intact early mammalian embryo, which lacks the polarity and cytoplasmic localizations that could serve as landmarks to identify blastomeres reproducibly. It is possible to circumvent these limitations and achieve a clonal analysis of cell lineage in the mouse embryo by using the microinjected lineage tracer, horseradish peroxidase, in postimplantation embryos (138). This analysis indicates that embryonic endoderm at the mid- to late-primitive-streak stage of the mouse embryo is a mixed population consisting of cells that have descendants either in extraembryonic endoderm or in the embryonic gut, but not in both tissues. Further evidence from analysis of pre- and early-primitive-streak stages indicates that progenitors of embryonic foregut endoderm appear in the midline of the endoderm layer near the anterior tip of the primitive streak early in gastrulation (K. A. Lawson and R. A. Pedersen, *unpublished data*). The cells that subsequently appear in this location are progenitors of midgut endoderm and notochord and constitute the head process (138). It can be inferred from these results that the progenitors of the embryonic gut arise from epiblast during gastrulation, replacing primitive endoderm cells, which move into the yolk sac, where they form strictly extraembryonic descendants. The lineage analysis of fate in embryonic ectoderm confirms this conclusion, showing that peroxidase-labeled ectoderm cells can produce descendants in the embryonic endoderm (K. A. Lawson et al., *unpublished observations*). This conclusion is consistent with the observed tissue pluripotency of the rodent epiblast, the fate of tissue grafts in postimplantation chimeras, and the fate of pre- and early-streak-stage embryos of single embryonic ectoderm cells in blastocyst injection chimeras. Moreover, labeled ectoderm cells can have descendants in more than one germ layer, showing that single mouse epiblast cells are indeed pluripotent (K. A. Lawson et al., *unpublished observations*). Finally, the emerging fate map of the mouse epiblast derived from analysis of tissue fragments *in vitro*, postimplantation chimeras, and intact postimplantation embryos is strikingly similar to that of the chick embryo, in which the entire embryo is derived from epiblast (168,169; K. A. Lawson et al., *unpublished observations*). A clonal analysis of tissue fates in organ formation will require further work using long-term markers such as retroviruses (170,171).

Relationship Among Potency, Allocation, and Fate

Although the segregation of potencies and allocation to mutually exclusive lineages in early development clearly imply a binary mode of decision making, at least in the formation of trophectoderm and extraembryonic endoderm lineages, there is no evidence that these decisions are made *a priori* in the egg or in early-cleavage-stage blastomeres. Rather, they seem to occur later, coinciding with gradual morphological changes in phenotype during preimplantation development. Therefore, the concept of determination does not apply to early mammalian embryonic development in the traditional sense of an event that precedes morphological differentiation (172). Rather, commitment emerges during differentiation and, indeed, may not be separable from morphological and biochemical aspects of phenotypic divergence of cells. For example, the trophectoderm cells and inner cells of the early mouse blastocyst are differentiated to the extent that they synthesize some distinct polypeptides, yet the inner cell mass can still undergo molecular differentiation into trophectoderm at the early blastocyst stage (131).

The delayed loss of totipotency in mammalian embryos appears to reflect the plasticity of cell allocation during formation of the early lineages. The inner cell mass is formed by a gradual accumulation of progenitors allocated to internal positions during two cell generations in the mouse embryo, thus utilizing the totipotency of the outer cells at those stages. Inner cells of the mouse blastocyst may also contribute descendants to the polar trophectoderm during early stages of blastocyst growth, thus utilizing the totipotency of the inner population at the early blastocyst stage. Epiblast-derived cells enter the endoderm layer during gastrulation as precursors of the embryonic gut, utilizing the potency of the epiblast. These examples of cell allocation during cleavage, blastocyst formation, and postimplantation growth indicate an active interaction between cells and their environment, which in turn implies a capacity for gene regulation even at early stages. As we shall see in the following section, there is substantial evidence for this conclusion.

GENETIC ASPECTS

Gene Activation and Regulation: Fate of Maternal Messenger RNA

Although mammalian preimplantation development is often compared to the morphologically similar processes of cleavage and blastulation in other vertebrate classes and in invertebrates, these similarities are only superficial, because mammals use a fundamentally different reproductive strategy. Cleavage in nonmammals produces the cells of the blastula, which imminently begins gastrulation. By contrast, the events following cleavage in placental mammals establish the extraembryonic lineages necessary for viviparous survival. Another difference inherent in the mammalian strategy is the reduction of yolk. Only vestiges persist of the large stores of yolk seen in the eggs of amphibians, reptiles, birds, and egg-laying mammalian species. The early embryos of eutherians rely instead on exchange with maternal nutrient sources through the visceral yolk sac and chorioallantoic placenta. Embryos of placental mammals show an early onset of embryonic gene expression, which is necessary for the differentiation of the specialized cells required for intrauterine growth. Because this mammalian reproductive strategy has perhaps resulted in the minimal egg mass for a vertebrate organism, the period from fertilization to implantation is genetically a critical transition from a program of gametogenesis to one of rapid proliferation and diversification. The changes in gene expression that accompany preimplantation development as discussed in this section have been reviewed recently (173–175).

The newly ovulated mouse egg contains approximately 350 pg of "maternal" RNA, of which the majority is ribosomal and transfer RNAs (176) (Table 1). Judging by the quantity of poly(A) tracts in the egg, approximately 20 pg is poly(A)+ messenger RNA (mRNA), assuming average poly(A) tract lengths of 63 nucleotides and mRNA lengths of 2,000 nucleotides (176,177). The quantity of specific mRNAs has been measured using recombinant DNA techniques, showing 431 fg of actin mRNA and 167 fg of histone mRNA per ovulated oocyte (178,179). This maternal mRNA is capable of serving as a template for protein synthesis, as shown by *in vitro* translation (180). Although some of the changes in protein synthetic pattern following fertilization (1–2-cell stage) appear to result from posttranslational modifications (181–183), other changes seem to utilize the stored maternal mRNA (184). In contrast to the situation in *Xenopus* and sea urchin oocytes, cytoplasmic mRNA of mouse oocytes does not contain any excess of the repetitive sequences that indicate unprocessed mRNA (185). Further-

TABLE 1. *RNA content of early mouse embryos*

Stage	Total RNA (ng/embryo)	poly(A)+ (pg/embryo)	rRNA (ng/embryo)
Mature oocyte	0.35	19	0.22
2 cells	0.24	8	0.17
8 cells	0.69	14	0.40
32 cells (early blastocyst)	1.47	37	1.00

Sources: Total RNA (176); poly(A)+ (mRNA) calculated from (177), assuming average length of 2,000 nucleotides; rRNA (176); adapted from (175).

more, growing and fully grown mouse oocytes contain normal amounts of U1 RNA, an essential component of the mRNA splicing machinery. This also contrasts with the fully grown *Xenopus* oocyte and early sea urchin embryo, which are deficient in this regard (186,187).

Despite the apparent normality of the maternal mRNA in mouse eggs, translational efficiencies for actin and histone mRNAs are quite low, less than one-tenth of what occurs in blastocysts (175). Furthermore, the mouse egg has little spare translational capacity, as shown by the injection of mRNA (188) and the fact that the net rate of protein synthesis does not increase within the first 24 hr after fertilization (189,190). A possible explanation for these results is a deficiency in oocyte ribosomes (191). Increases in ribosome content and loading of ribosomes by mRNA accompany subsequent increases in the rate and efficiency of protein synthesis (175,176,192).

During development to the 2-cell stage, the mouse embryo begins to rely on products of the embryonic genome. During this transition, the total amount of mRNA per embryo decreases to less than half that present in the oocyte (Table 1), while the amounts of actin and histone mRNAs decrease to approximately one-tenth the amount in the egg (178,179). Whether this represents an active degradative process or normal rates of mRNA turnover is unclear. When exogenous globin mRNA is injected into embryos, it is available for translation for 15 to 17 hr, but is no longer functional as a template for protein synthesis after 48 hr (193).

In contrast to the transcription-independent events of protein synthesis before the 2-cell stage (180,194), development beyond the 2-cell stage requires mRNA synthesis. This requirement is manifested as two periods of α-amanitin sensitivity just before and after the S phase of the second cell cycle (195,196). Treatment during the first period of sensitivity blocks the appearance of a set of 67- to 70-kD proteins, identified as heat-shock proteins (197). Neither DNA replication nor degradation of maternal mRNA is affected by the α-amanitin treatments. At the 2-cell stage, poly(A)+ mRNA is synthesized at the rate of 0.2 pg per embryo per hour, and ribosomal RNA at the rate of 0.4 pg per embryo per hour (198). The total amount of mRNA accumulated by the 8-cell stage approaches that present in the ovulated egg (Table 1), but amounts of histone and actin mRNAs are still only one-fourth to one-half that of the egg (178,179).

The use of genetic markers for paternal gene expression has made it possible to independently demonstrate embryonic gene expression as early as the 2-cell stage. The paternal isozyme of β-glucuronidase is detected in mouse embryos at late-2-cell to 4-cell stages (199). Similarly, the paternal isoform of β_2-microglobulin first appears in 2-cell embryos (200).

Given the substantial time elapsed between fertilization and the mid- to late-2-cell stage, it remains interesting to question whether any embryonic gene expression occurs at the earlier stages. There is evidence for considerable turnover of poly(A) tracts of mRNA and 3′-terminal AMP of tRNA in both 1- and 2-cell mouse embryos (177,198,201). Also, the mRNAs of both unfertilized and fertilized eggs show normal levels of cap structures (202,203). In addition to labeling of these terminal structures by [^{3}H]adenosine and [^{3}H]guanosine (204), [^{3}H]adenosine labels internal sites in tRNA and in both poly(A)− and poly(A)+ heterogeneous RNA (presumed mRNA) of 1-cell and early-2-cell embryos, but at very low rates; ribosomal RNA synthesis is undetectable before the 2-cell stage (198). Therefore, a modest amount of mRNA synthesis (about one-fifth the 2-cell rate) probably occurs in 1-cell embryos, but its functional significance is unclear.

The morphogenetic events of compaction and blastocyst development require prior embryonic gene expression, as shown by stage-specific sensitivity to α-amanitin (205–207). One consequence of this gene activity is the synthesis of lineage-specific polypeptides in trophectoderm and inner cell mass (208–210). Some of these will be considered in further detail later.

In sum, the available evidence acquired almost exclusively in the mouse indicates that the pattern of gene expression in the preimplantation embryo changes from predominantly posttranscriptional and posttranslational control between fertilization and the 2-cell stage to predominantly transcriptional control in successive stages, transcription being required for all major morphogenetic processes during preimplantation development (207).

Mutations Affecting Early Development

Before direct measurements of gene expression were made on mammalian embryos, the only indication of early involvement of the embryonic genome was the homozygous lethal mutation. Out of approximately 700 known mutations in the mouse, about 20 adversely affect early development (211). None of the early acting mutations will be described in depth here because they have been covered in recent reviews (212–215); see also the reviews of specific genetically complex regions: A locus (216), C locus (217), and T locus (218–220). Rather, this section evaluates the results of studying these mutations and the prospects for producing additional, specific genetic effects on preimplantation and early postimplantation stages. Virtually all this work has been accomplished in the mouse, because few genes affecting early development have been described in other species.

Spontaneous Genetic Abnormalities

The spontaneous genetic abnormalities can be grouped into those visible at (a) cleavage stages, (b) blastocyst formation, (c) periimplantation stages, (d) early postimplantation growth, and (e) early to late gastrula stages (Table 2). Those affecting cleavage stages are c^{25H}, a deletion at

TABLE 2. *Mutations affecting early mouse development*

Stage affected	Mutation	Chromosome	Homozygous phenotype	References
Cleavage	c^{25H}	7	Arrests at 2- to 6-cell stage, but may live for 2 days longer	221,222
	$t^{12}(t^{w32})$	17	Excess lipid synthesis at 2- to 4-cell stage; arrest at morula stage	223
Blastocyst formation	Ovum mutation	?	Poor trophoblast development; affected morula through implantation stage	224
	Tail short	11	Reduced cell number; affected morula through implantation stage	225
	T^{hp}	17	Abnormalities in morula-blastocyst transition	226
Periimplantation period	a^{x}	2	Abnormal blastocyst development, implantation	227
	A^{y}	2	Abnormal blastocyst hatching, implantation	216,228
	Oligosyndactyly	8	Mitotic arrest at 64-cell stage and beyond	229,230
	t^{w73}	17	Aberrant extraembryonic cells, beginning at implantation	231,232
	$t^{wPa\text{-}1}$	17	Disorganized structures at implantation	233
Early postimplantation	Blind	15	Growth retarded at egg cylinder stage	212
	c^{6H}	7	Abnormality of parietal endoderm and retardation, egg cylinder stage	234
	Dickie's Small eye	2	Embryonic ectoderm dies at egg cylinder stage	212
	T^{0}	17	Abnormal differentiation of extraembryonic and embryonic ectoderm	235
	t^{w5}	17	Death of embryonic ectoderm at egg cylinder stage	218
	Velvet coat	15	Abnormal differentiation of extraembryonic and embryonic ectoderm	212
	Waved coat	14	Death of embryonic ectoderm at egg cylinder stage	212
Gastrulation	Fused (kinky)	17	Multiple complete or partial embryonic axes formed at primitive-streak stage	236
	Short ear	9	Overgrowth of extraembryonic tissues, mesoderm deficiency	212
	t^{9}	17	Mesoderm deficiency	218

the albino locus, and t^{12} at the *t* locus. Mutations affecting blastocyst formation are ovum mutant, tail short, and T hairpin. Those affecting periimplantation stages are the *a*-locus mutants, lethal nonagouti (a^{x}), lethal yellow (A^{y}); oligosyndactyly; and three *t*-complex mutants, t^{w73}, t^{wPa-1}, and t^{Orl} (Table 2). Mutations affecting early postimplantation growth include two at the *t* locus, t^{0} and t^{w5}, the albino locus mutant, c^{6H}, and several others. Mutations affecting gastrulation are t^{9}, short ear, and fused (kinky). Most of these mutants have been known for years, owing largely to the pioneering work of L. C. Dunn and associates. The availability of the mutants consistently captures the imagination of developmental geneticists, because they hold the promise of genetic inroads to developmental mechanisms. Yet there is not a single instance in which the basic biochemical defect of a spontaneous mutant affecting early mammalian development has been defined. This could mean that known genetic abnormalities are altering the timing and quantity of essential gene expression, rather than disrupting specific structural genes.

It is difficult to argue from the phenotypes of existing mouse mutants (Table 2) that any of them specifically affects important developmental processes, such as commitment or differentiation, rather than essential metabolic pathways. Clearly, the former case would be more interesting. For example, saturation mutagenesis for processes involved in early developmental decisions has proved enormously useful in understanding *Drosophila* and *C. elegans* (237,238).

Another limitation of the existing recessive lethal mutations is that the homozygotes are generally first recognized as they become retarded and moribund. This complicates attempts to determine the primary causes of developmental arrest. In principle, this problem can be circumvented by using linked genetic markers. One such example is the *t* locus, in which mutant alleles can be recognized by a closely linked polypeptide (239). Another is the A^y allele, which is closely linked with an integrated proviral sequence (240). Mutant embryos can be identified by separating blastomeres at the 2-cell stage (241), then pooling for biochemical determinations at later stages. Even this elegant approach, however, provides only small amounts of material. These limitations should provoke us to consider other means of interfering with gene expression in mammalian embryos.

Other Deleterious Genetic Effects

The lethality of haploidy and aneuploidies illustrates the importance of a balanced chromosome constitution for normal early development. Haploid embryos can be produced by parthenogenesis or by mechanically altering the number of pronuclei in the zygote (242–246). These genetically altered individuals die during cleavage and periimplantation stages. Parthenogenesis often produces diploid embryos as a result of second polar-body suppression. These individuals may develop to midgestation stages, as subsequently discussed. Therefore, it is the loss of an entire chromosome set in haploids, rather than some trauma associated with the experimental procedures, that is responsible for their early death.

The early lethality of all mammalian monosomies also supports the argument that the intact diploid set of chromosomes must be present for normal embryonic development. Mouse embryos nullisomic for the X chromosome begin to die at early cleavage stages (245,247,248). Mouse embryos monosomic for specific autosomes have been produced using the Robertsonian translocation stocks developed by Gropp (215,249). These begin to die during the late cleavage or early blastocyst stages (monosomies for chromosomes 1, 2, 5, and 15) or at later stages in blastocyst development (monosomies 4, 10, 12, 14, 17, 18, and 19). Almost none of these embryos survives beyond implantation (215,250,251). Although cells of monosomic embryos can be sustained in chimeras for a time, there appears to be a progressive reduction in the monosomic component, so that few of the resulting fetuses are chimeric at term (215,251–254). The absence of monosomies in recognized human conceptions argues for a similar early stage of death, because they should be produced by nondisjunction at meiosis in equal frequencies as trisomies, which are frequent among spontaneous abortions during the first trimester of pregnancy (255,256). Trisomies in mice, as in humans, are generally capable of development to relatively advanced stages, but rarely to term (249).

These results indicate that both diploid chromosome sets must be present for normal mammalian development. They do not rule out a deleterious effect of lethal genes in monosomies, although this seems unlikely in inbred strains of mice. Thus, the detrimental effects of monosomy must be due either to the dosage-dependent decrease in gene products from the affected chromosome or to altering patterns of gene function due to failure of normal interactions between homologous chromosomes (257). Differences in stage of death among monosomies indicate that the genes present on different autosomes have distinct roles during early development.

Prospects for Specific Genetic Interference with Development

Given the apparent existence of genes on every autosome whose function is critical for early development, it may be worthwhile to isolate additional mutants using novel genetic and molecular techniques. One possible approach is saturation mutagenesis, as previously done with invertebrate species. The difficulty in this approach is that most autosomal defects will have to be established in homozygous form by multigeneration crosses before their effects are apparent. Although this complicates the analysis, it does not preclude collecting additional mutants for easily assayed phenotypes. This has been done for the *t* region of mouse chromosome 17 (258). In order to apply this approach to the early stages of development, it would be necessary to devise screening criteria for developmentally interesting defects, such as failure to differentiate into inner cell mass and trophectoderm, rather than death, owing to metabolic deficiencies. Another complication is that these new mutants would provide no more molecular accessibility to the affected genes than do currently available mutants.

Molecular accessibility is provided by insertional mutagenesis caused from retrovirus infection or pronuclear DNA injection in transgenics. Endogenous retroviruses are responsible for at least one mutation in mice, the dilute locus. Copeland et al. (259,260) demonstrated that the closely linked proviral sequence was partially excised in two revertants of dilute to wild type. The other mutation that is closely linked to a retrovirus is A^y (240). In this case, the decisive proof for viral integration as the cause of the phenotype might be difficult, because revertants of A^y would not be recognized against the background of wild-type siblings generated in matings between heterozygous A^{y+} parents.

An experimentally induced retrovirus integration has been identified as the cause of the homozygous lethality of Mov-13 mice at 12 to 13 d.g. (261). (The production of transgenic mice by retroviral infection will be discussed in a later section.) The insertional event took place in the first intron of the α1(I) collagen gene, completely blocking transcription of this gene, which is essential for development of blood vessels *in vivo*, but not for epithelial branching of organ rudiments *in vitro* (262–266). Most notably, the unique DNA sequence of the exogenous retrovirus facilitated molecular cloning and identification of the flanking regions surrounding the integration site. This approach has been further refined by incorporating a bacterial tRNA suppressor gene in the retrovirus, which simplifies the cloning process (267). The practical limitation of insertional mutagenesis by retroviruses is the relative rarity of mutations. Although retroviral infection and integration are efficient, there is a relatively low incidence of mutagenesis with this approach (261).

By contrast, the incidence of insertional mutagenesis resulting from pronuclear DNA injection appears to be relatively high. Introducing cloned genes into the mammalian germ line by pronuclear microinjection has been a valuable technique for studying gene regulation and exploring the possibilities of gene therapy, as discussed later. An unexpected by-product of this approach was the discovery that the injected DNA can act as a mutagen, producing developmental mutants at a frequency on the order of 10% (268). In the study by Wagner et al. (268), two of six transgenic lines carried recessive lethal mutations as a result of integration of human growth hormone sequences. In the study by Palmiter et al. (269), one of seven transgenic lines produced by injecting a metallothionein–thymidine kinase fusion gene was unable to transmit the inserted DNA through males, even though these were fertile. This result suggests that the integration event disrupted a function essential during haploid stages of spermatogenesis, thus accounting for the pattern of its transmission. There is also a transgenic line containing a Rous sarcoma virus–chloramphenicol acetyltransferase fusion gene that shows transmission distortion and dominant lethality owing to an induced translocation (270). Another line produced by microinjection of a mammary tumor virus–*myc* fusion gene is characterized by a recessive limb abnormality (271). This latter mutant appears to be allelic to the known spontaneous mutation, limb deformity. A junction fragment has been cloned from the integration site, showing that this approach may yet fulfill the objective of identifying the molecular basis of certain developmentally significant genes. In the transgenic line studied by Woychik et al. (271), however, the integration event caused a deletion of approximately 1 kb of DNA, showing that injected DNA may cause rearrangements in the process of integration. These structural changes could significantly complicate the task of identifying the developmentally significant sequences from the cloned junction fragments. Nevertheless, insertional mutagenesis appears to be a source of molecularly identifiable mutants, some of which are alleles of existing mutations, despite the statistical improbability of such events. Thus, the production and analysis of these mutants could serve two purposes: addition of new mutants and insight into the known ones.

Interference with Development Using Antisense RNA

One additional novel strategy for specific genetic interference is based on blocking translation of mRNA by introducing an excess of the complementary, antisense strand. Tissue culture cells expressing antisense genes show reduced thymidine kinase activity (272). Similarly, microinjection of antisense mRNA directly into the cytoplasm blocks the translation of coinjected globin mRNA in *Xenopus* oocytes (273), although microinjection into fertilized eggs is less successful (274). The 5′ homologous regions of the mRNAs are critical for these effects. Rosenberg et al. (275) injected *Drosophila* embryos with antisense mRNA for the gene that is affected in the Kruppel mutation, thus producing phenocopies of the mild alleles of this locus. As yet, no one has reported using antisense mRNA to interfere with the development of mammalian embryos. Furthermore, problems must be resolved in the choice of promoters and the mode of delivering the antisense mRNA to the embryo. For example, any mRNAs injected into the mouse zygote would probably meet the same fate as endogenous maternal mRNAs, thus precluding this delivery route. Injecting DNA into mouse zygotes often results in mosaicism, which would complicate analysis of such antisense studies (165). Nonetheless, this promising approach deserves scrutiny, because it could potentially provide a means of blocking the function of any gene that has been cloned. This potential clearly does not relieve us of the task of deciding which are developmentally interesting genes. Many of the gene products expressed specifically in the early tissue lineages of mammalian embryos (*vide infra*) could be considered candidates for antisense interference, because a large proportion of these have been or soon will be cloned. Another possible approach is that of creating cDNA libraries at various stages and with specific tissues and exploring the effect of functional ablation of these genes by use of antisense mRNA.

The evidence for differential function of specific maternally and paternally inherited genes in embryonic and extraembryonic tissues makes this an intriguing possibility.

Differential Roles of the Maternal and Paternal Genomes

Parthenogenesis

The phenomenon of virgin birth, or parthenogenesis, occurs in at least one species of every vertebrate class except mammals. There are parthenogenetic birds, reptiles, fish, and amphibians (257,276–279). Although the predominant strategy for reproduction in each of these vertebrate classes involves sexual recombination and mating, the existence of parthenogenetic species is conclusive evidence that development can occur in the absence of a paternal contribution to the genome: In other words, maternal and paternal genomes can be functionally equivalent in every significant way except in mammals (257). Despite claims of successful development of mice both from normal and from parthenogenetic nuclei transferred to normally fertilized egg cytoplasm (281,282), it is now clear that the parthenogenetic genome is incapable of supporting development to term of the individual mammalian embryo (283,284).

Developmental failure of parthenotes does not generally occur at preimplantation stages. Spontaneous parthenogenesis occurs in ovarian oocytes of the LT/Sv strain of mice (285), and experimental parthenogenesis can be induced with a variety of treatments, all of which yield apparently normal activation, cleavage, and blastocyst formation in the diploid individuals that occur as a result of suppression of second polar-body formation (278). Some spontaneous diploidization of haploids also occurs. These diploid parthenogenetic individuals develop until postimplantation stages, with a rare few developing into small 25-somite embryos by day 10 of gestation (286,287).

What makes this delayed death of parthenotes even more intriguing is that parthenogenetic embryos can contribute viable cells to chimeras made by aggregation or by injection of the parthenogenetic inner cell mass into a normal blastocyst; in one case, the parthenote even contributed to the germ line of a fertile chimera (288,289). The parthenotes' capacity to reach advanced developmental stages, but not beyond day 10, indicates that functions not previously required become necessary for development at that stage. Because homozygous blastocysts could be produced by diploidizing a single female or male pronucleus after removal of the other pronucleus from normally fertilized zygotes (290), it appeared possible that the failure of parthenogenetic mammalian development was due to a deficiency of some nonnuclear contribution normally made by the sperm during the process of fertilization. It would be reasonable on this basis to expect development to term by homozygous embryos produced experimentally from fertilized eggs. However, despite an early claim of success (291), several attempts to demonstrate the development to term of homozygous diploid maternal (digynic) or paternal (diandric) pronuclei have failed (257,283,292).

The development of an efficient method for nuclear transfer in mouse embryos using microsurgery and virus-mediated cell fusion (293) has stimulated rapid progress in defining the developmental potential of mouse pronuclei and determining the reasons for developmental arrest of parthenotes. By transferring a normal pronuclear pair to parthenogenetic egg cytoplasm and carrying out the reciprocal transfer, it was possible to show unequivocally that the failure of parthenotes is determined by their nuclear rather than their cytoplasmic condition (294). Furthermore, zygotes containing two maternal pronuclei, even from different strains of mice, manifest a pattern of developmental arrest essentially indistinguishable from that of parthenotes (295,296). These embryos never develop to term, but arrest at early postimplantation stages, sometimes reaching day 10 as a retarded embryo with sparse extraembryonic tissues (296). These results suggest that the genetic basis of developmental arrest in parthenotes is a deficiency in gene expression at postimplantation stages that can be complemented only by a sperm-derived pronucleus, not by one derived from the female. This excludes homozygosity as the cause of death and indicates that the maternal and paternal nuclear contributions to the mammalian embryo are not equivalent. The homozygous cells of diploid, digynic uniparental mouse embryos can contribute to chimeras when aggregated with normal blastomeres at the 8- to 16-cell stage and have even produced viable gametes in a fertile female mouse derived in this way (297). Nonetheless, the low incidence of such contributions indicates that the digynic constitution is extremely detrimental to development.

Differences Between Gynogenones and Androgenones

Diandric mouse embryos can be produced by similar nuclear transfer techniques. Such embryos develop to early postimplantation stages when transferred to the uteri of foster mothers, but never reach term (295,296). The postimplantation diandric embryos analyzed on day 10 of gestation have extremely rudimentary embryonic and yolk sac development, but the extent of trophoblast development is near normal (298) (Fig. 7). The pattern of developmental arrest in experimentally produced diandric embryos is thus strikingly different from that of parthenotes and digynic embryos, which have retarded extraembryonic growth (299). These observations led Surani to hypothesize a complementary relationship between the two parental genetic contributions, the maternal component performing a unique role in embryonic development, and the paternal component a unique role in extraembryonic development (296).

Evidence for Complementary Roles of Maternal and Paternal Genomes

Additional studies provide evidence for the necessary function of specific maternally or paternally inherited genes in mouse development. One of these (300) demonstrates that the defect in T^{hp}, which behaves as a maternal-effect lethal mutation (301,302), is nuclear rather than cytoplasmic. Because the T^{hp} mutation is a deletion, the requirement for maternal origin of the normal allele implies that during embryonic and fetal development, only the maternal allele is active, and presence of a normal paternal allele is inconsequential because it is inactive, as suggested by McLaren (303). The recent characterization in the mouse of a *T*-associated maternal-effect locus (T^{me}) on chromosome 17 (304) will aid in the further analysis of this region.

Cattanach and Kirk (305) used heterozygotes for Rob-

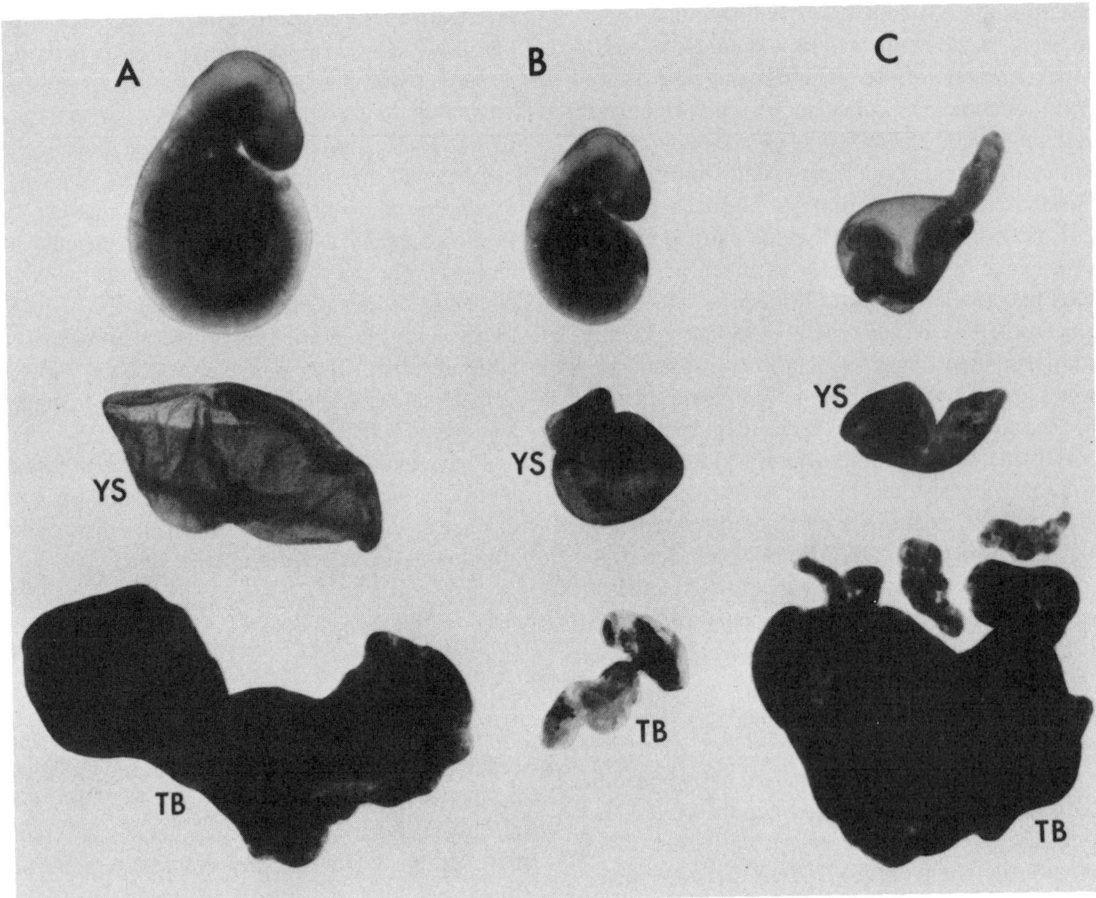

FIG. 7. Development of reconstituted pronuclear-stage mouse embryos (dissected on day 10 of gestation): (**A**) control embryo; (**B**) embryo with two maternal pronuclei (digynic); (**C**) embryo with two paternal pronuclei (diandric). Note differences in the extent of embryonic and extraembryonic tissue development. YS, yolk sac; TB, trophoblast. (From ref. 316.)

ertsonian translocations to generate chromosomally balanced young that had either maternal or paternal duplication for chromosome 11 or for the distal portion of chromosome 2. Using linked genetic markers to distinguish the progeny, they showed that when both copies of chromosome 11 were maternally inherited, the fetuses were consistently smaller than their normal littermates, whereas the fetuses with a paternally inherited pair of chromosome 11 were consistently larger. Using reciprocal translocations, they narrowed the source of this effect to the proximal portion of chromosome 11. These same translocations implicated the distal portion of chromosome 2 in a similar pattern of complementary maternal and paternal genetic effects on development. In this case, maternal duplication/paternal deficiency produced newborn young with long, flat-sided bodies and arched backs; they were hypokinetic and died soon after birth. By contrast, paternal duplication/maternal deficiency gave mice with short, square bodies and flat backs; these were hyperkinetic and survived for several days, but grew poorly. The reciprocal phenotypes of these newborns, sometimes obtained within the same litter, showed that the maternal and paternal chromosomes or genes contained thereon functioned differentially during development (305,306).

Using a similar approach of generating duplications/deficiencies from mice with reciprocal translations, Searle and Beechey (307) examined many of the chromosomes of the mouse genome for their capacity to support development to term as maternal duplications. Additional evidence has been compiled on the effects of paternal duplications (308). This extensive analysis shows that maternal duplication of distal chromosome 2, chromosome 6, distal chromosome 8, and proximal chromosome 11 failed to rescue the reciprocal paternal deficiencies; likewise, paternal duplication of distal chromosome 7 and proximal chromosome 17 failed to rescue the reciprocal maternal deficiencies (Fig. 8). The parental origin of chromosomes 1, 4, 5, 9, 13, 14, and 15 was not restricted (308). Therefore, there is substantial genetic evidence for the existence of specific chromosomal regions that function differentially depending on their parental origin. This implies that some form of selective marking, or imprinting, takes place during gametogenesis (295,296,307). It has not been determined if this imprinting phenomenon is restricted to specific chromosomal regions or if imprinting affects the entire complement, but only manifests itself at specific loci that must be expressed for normal development.

Implications of Imprinting

If such a fundamental process as genomic imprinting occurs during mouse gametogenesis and is the inherent cause of parthenogenetic arrest in this species, then there should be evidence among other mammalian species for a similar phenomenon. Indeed, such distinctions are known, including the mule (produced by mating a jackass and a mare) and the hinny (produced from the mating of a stallion and a female donkey). A more extreme example is the development of hydatidiform mole in the human, the result of fertilization by two spermatozoa (309,310). These embryos become androgenetic, owing to failure of the maternal genome to participate in development, thus producing a 46,XX or 46,XY conceptus in which all of the chromosomes are from sperm. The trophoblastic hyperplasia and embryonic dysgenesis of moles are strongly reminiscent of the development of diandric mouse embryos. This observation is consistent with Surani's hypothesis, showing that as a result of imprinting, the paternal genome preferentially supports development of the extraembryonic tissues and fails to support development of the fetus (296).

Another implication of imprinting during gametogenesis is that the cloning of mammalian embryos by nuclear transfer from later-stage donor cells may be impossible in mammals, in contrast to the situation in frogs (37,38). Attempts to transfer nuclei from preimplantation mouse embryo cells to enucleated zygotes have met with only limited success. Early studies (29) demonstrated the feasibility of microsurgery on zygotes; these were extended by Modlinski (311)

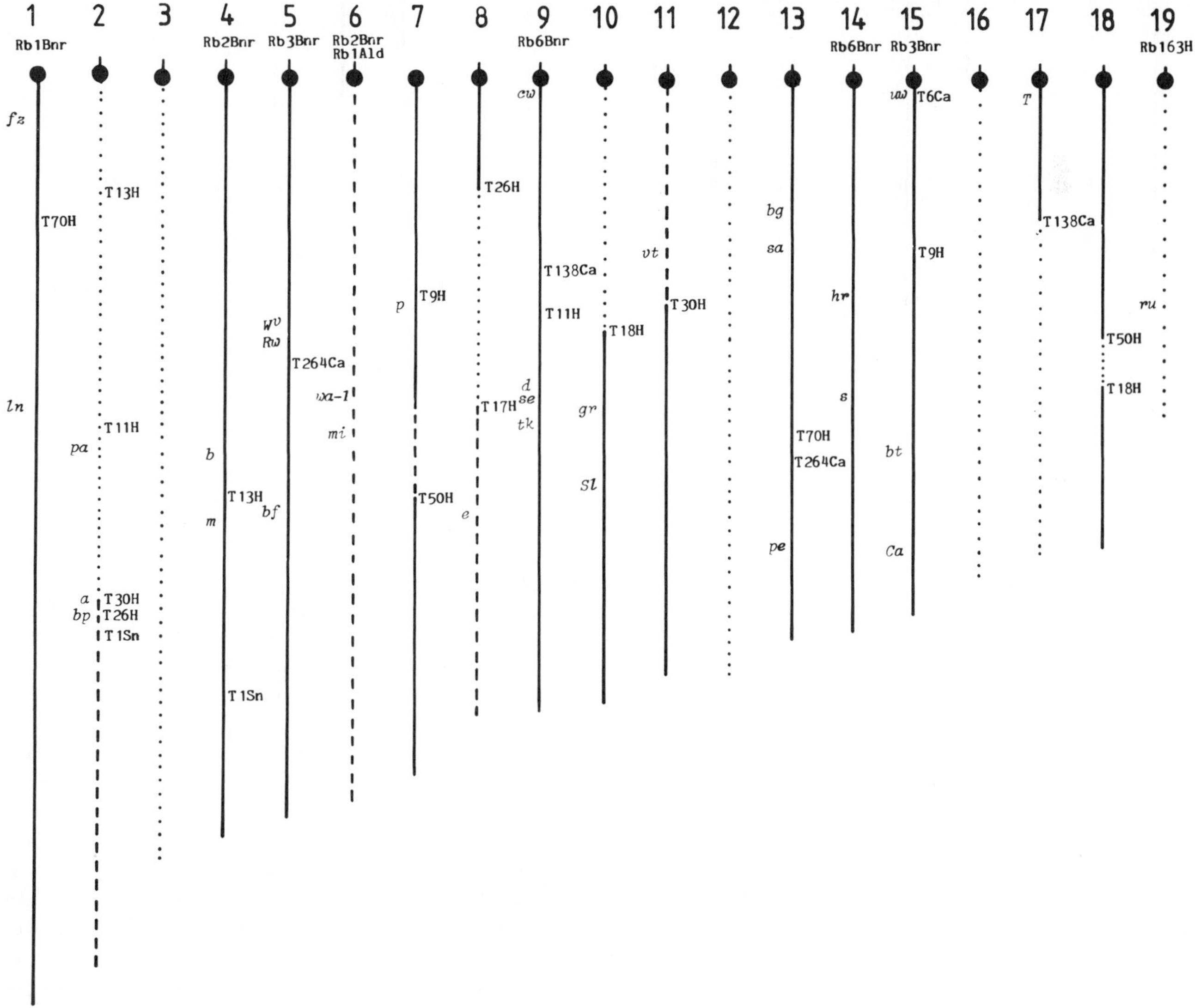

FIG. 8. Diagram of mouse autosomes showing regions resulting in abnormal development (*broken lines*) or normal development (*solid lines*); in some regions, evidence is inconclusive (*dotted lines*): (**A**) maternal duplication with paternal deficiency; (**B**, p. 206) paternal duplication with maternal deficiency. (From ref. 308.)

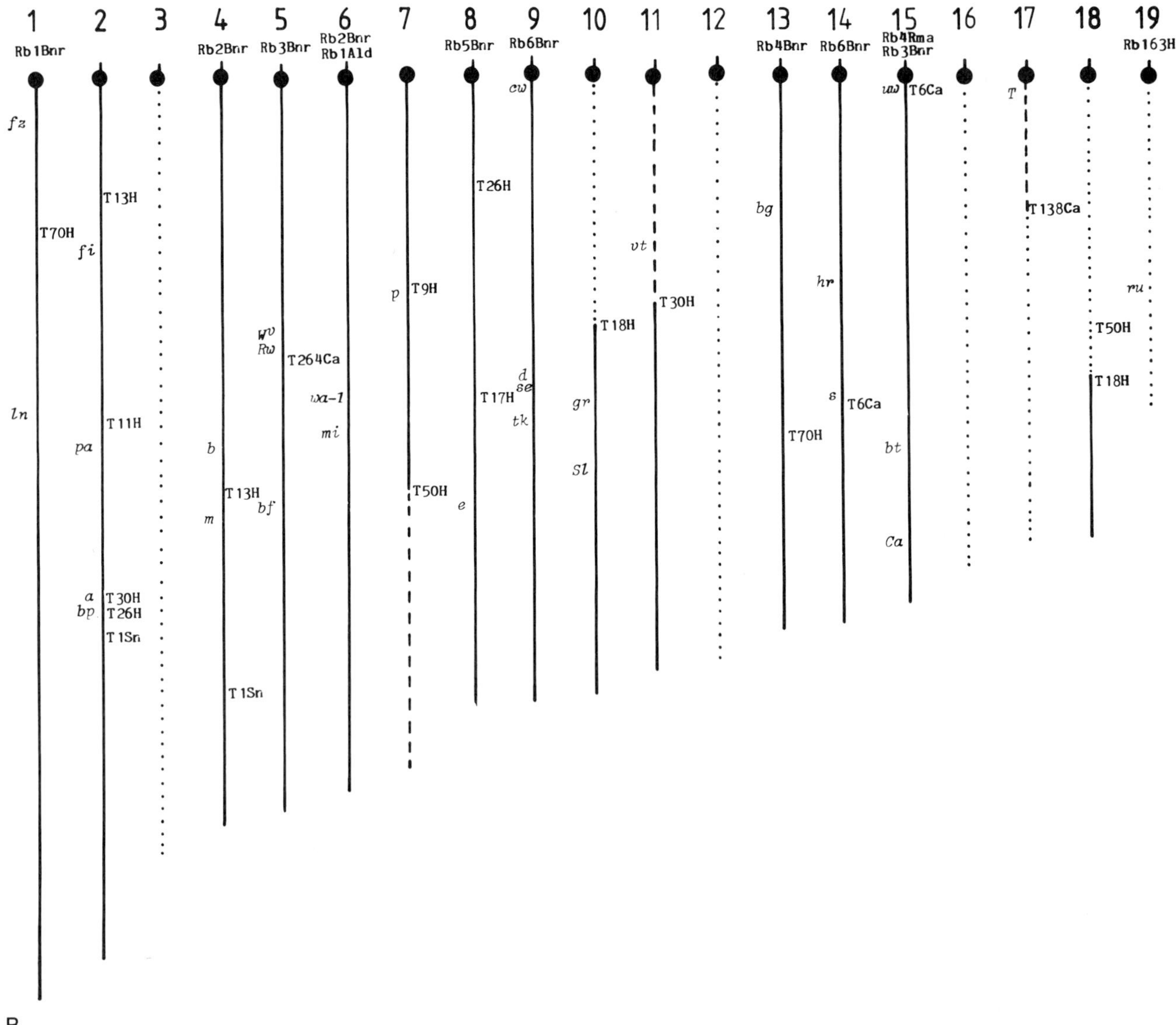

FIG. 8. See legend on previous page.

and Markert and Petters (290), who demonstrated the feasibility of pronuclear removal and subsequent diploidization. Nuclei of inner-cell-mass cells, but not of trophectoderm cells, reportedly supported development to term when transferred to enucleated zygotes (281). Subsequent work has indeed shown that transplantation of trophectoderm nuclei to zygotes in which the maternal and paternal pronuclei remain intact interferes with preimplantation development, but that inner-cell-mass nuclei do not exert this effect (280). However, a carefully controlled attempt to confirm that inner-cell-mass nuclei by themselves support preimplantation development has failed (312), thus casting doubt on the previous claim by Illmensee and Hoppe (281). In the study by McGrath and Solter (312), only nuclei of 2-cell embryos supported development into morphologically normal blastocysts when transferred to enucleated zygotes; nuclei from the 8-cell stage and beyond led to abortive cleavage (313). Robl et al. (314) obtained better development of transferred 8-cell nuclei of mouse embryos by combining them with 2-cell cytoplasm. In this case, half of the embryos formed blastocysts (a small fraction of which developed to early postimplantation stages), but none lived beyond day 12 of gestation (314). Even this limited success of 8-cell-stage mouse nuclei in supporting development of 2-cell cytoplasm indicates the importance of nuclear and cytoplasmic synchrony. Recent experiments with sheep embryos indicate that this species is more amenable to development with donor nuclei from 8-cell embryos. When 8-cell sheep blastomeres were fused with anucleate zygote halves, several developed into full-term, healthy individuals, whereas embryos derived from donor 16-cell nuclei developed to normal fetuses (315). Although the data for a species comparison are sparse, there appears to be a correlation between the cell numbers at which nuclear totipotency is lost and blastocyst formation occurs (*vide supra*). That is, transfer of late-cleavage-stage nuclei was most successful in the species with a high cell number at the time of blastocyst formation (i.e., the sheep).

Whereas the previously described studies establish certain time limits for nuclear totipotency (at least in the mouse), they do not formally address the issue of whether or not genomic imprinting is stable throughout cleavage, because the inability of more advanced nuclei to support early development may be due to asynchrony between donor nucleus and host cytoplasm (or other more trivial reasons). A recent study by Surani et al. (316), however, addresses this point. Experimentally produced haploid gynogenetic or androgenetic embryos were used as a source of donor haploid nuclei between the 2- and 16-cell stages. These were then transferred to haploid gynogenetic or androgenetic zygotes. Re constituted diploids developed normally to term if they contained both maternal and paternal genetic contributions, but not if they were digynic or diandric (successful androgenetic donors were at the 2–4-cell stages; gynogenetic donors were at the 2–8-cell stages). Although several questions still must be resolved in this approach, the results indicate that genomic imprinting acquired during gametogenesis is stable at least through early cleavage.

A final implication of imprinting during gametogenesis is that there must be a mechanism for stable differentiation of the maternal and paternal genetic contributions. X-chromosome inactivation during embryogenesis provides a model for such a process.

X-Chromosome Activity During Development

One X chromosome of female placental mammals is inactivated during development, leading to dosage compensation of X-linked genes (317–320). The process of X-inactivation is a paradigm for gene regulation, because changes in X-chromosome chromatin are correlated with changes in the expression of genes on this chromosome. Furthermore, the activity of the second X chromosome in females changes in a regular, well-documented sequence throughout the life cycle. Finally, the pattern of X-chromosome inactivation in extraembryonic tissues reinforces the idea of imprinting during gametogenesis.

The status of X-chromosome activity has been studied by cytogenetic techniques, ratios of autosomal and X-linked enzymes, and isozymic patterns of polymorphic X-linked genes. Cytogenetic approaches rely on the differential staining of the inactive X chromosome in interphase nuclei or metaphase chromosomes or on its asynchronous replication. The dosage of X-linked gene products is generally deduced from the absolute amounts of one or more gene products [including glucose-6-phosphate dehydrogenase (G6PD), hypoxanthine-guanine phosphoribosyl transferase (HPRT), and phosphoglycerate kinase (PGK)] or from the ratio of these activities to autosomal gene products. Isozymic variants in human and mouse G6PD and mouse HPRT and PGK have been used as qualitative indications of X-chromosome activity. By combining the information from these approaches, we now have a detailed picture of the temporal and spatial aspects of X-chromosome activity, although the mechanistic basis of these patterns remains obscure.

X-Chromosome Activity During Gametogenesis and Embryogenesis

The activity ratios of X-linked enzymes in XX and XO mice indicate that both X chromosomes of normal females are active in the oocyte (321). This is confirmed by the isozyme patterns of G6PD in human ovaries early in gestation (322) and by the patterns of G6PD and HPRT in mice (323). Similar studies of germ cells isolated from various stages of *M. caroli* embryos indicate that onset of activity in the previously inactive X chromosome coincides with meiosis (323). By contrast, the X chromosome of spermatogenic cells appears to be expressed at a low level or not at all (324,325). Thus, X-chromosome reactivation occurs during early stages of meiosis in the female, and this activity persists throughout oocyte growth until the time of ovulation, when transcription ceases (175).

Because of the relative inactivity of the X chromosome during spermatogenesis, it was important to determine whether both X chromosomes are expressed in the early embryo or only that inherited from the egg. Cytogenetic observations made at various stages of embryogenesis first revealed asynchronous X-chromosome replication at the blastocyst stage; before this stage, both chromosomes have the appearance of active chromatin (326,327). Quantitative assays of X-linked gene products demonstrated a bimodal distribution when single embryos were assayed (328–331), presumably indicating the presence of embryos with one active X (males) and two active Xs (females). Epstein and associates accomplished a direct comparison of male and female embryos by separating blastomeres at the 2-cell stage, characterizing the sex of one half of the embryo cytogenetically, and assaying small groups of the other halves of embryos for HPRT levels (241,332). Female embryos had twofold higher levels of HPRT on the average than males. Together, these results demonstrate that the female preimplantation mouse embryo has two active X chromosomes. This has been confirmed in studies of feral mice heterozygous for HPRT isozymes, showing that both X chromosomes are expressed at least from the 8-cell stage (319; V. M. Chapman and G. Johnson, *unpublished observations*). Therefore, the preimplantation embryo, like the egg, is characterized by activation of both X chromosomes.

When does X-inactivation occur? Cytogenetic observations suggest that inactivation begins at the late morula to early blastocyst stage (327) or the late blastocyst stage (326). However, evidence from injection chimera experiments using single inner-cell-mass cells from genetically marked mouse blastocysts (3.5–4.5 d.g.) reveals that both X chromosomes are active in the inner cell mass at these donor stages (333). This implies that the cytogenetic results on blastocysts are derived only from the trophectoderm cells. In addition, biochemical evidence indicates that there are two active X chromosomes in the embryonic ectoderm until day 6 of gestation (330,331,334). However, not all inner-cell-mass derivatives remain active until this time. Cytogenetic observations by Takagi et al. (335) showed that there is an early-replicating X chromosome in the visceral endoderm as early as 5.3 d.g. and that this pattern changes to late replication in the visceral endoderm between 6.0 and 6.5 d.g., and also in the extraembryonic ectoderm and ectoplacental cone. Although the significance of the shift from early to late replication is unknown, both states reflect inactivity of the allocyclic X (336). Thus, X-chromosome inactivation accompanies cellular differentiation, occurring first in trophectoderm and its derivatives, then in primitive endoderm and its derivatives, and finally in the primitive ectoderm and its derivatives, including the germ cells (337). Only in early embryos and oocytes are both X chromosomes of a female individual active (Fig.9).

Perhaps the most intriguing observation about the pattern of X-inactivation in early mouse embryos is that inactivation in the extraembryonic tissue lineages is nonrandom, the paternal X chromosome (X^p) being preferentially inactivated. This was first seen at the cytogenetic level (335) and was confirmed by analyzing PGK isozyme patterns in heterozygous female embryos (335,338–342). These studies demonstrate conclusively that the X^p is preferentially inactivated, whereas the X^m is active in the visceral and parietal endoderm, the ectoplacental cone, and the extraembryonic ectoderm. Of the extraembryonic tissues examined, only visceral yolk sac mesoderm had a mosaic pattern of random X-inactivation. This is another manifestation of heritable imprinting of maternal and paternal chromosomes, presumably acquired during gametogenesis (319). In marsupials, the paternal X chromosome is preferentially inactivated in somatic tissues (320). The similarity between the spatial pattern of paternal X-inactivation and the specific extraembryonic developmental retardation in digynics and parthenotes implies a mechanistic relationship at the level of imprinting.

Mechanisms of X-Inactivation

The alternation of periods of X-chromosome activity and inactivity throughout the life cycle (Fig. 9) implies that there is a mechanism for controlling X-chromosome function. This process can be viewed either as inhibitory inactivation (343) or as stimulatory activation (319,344). Although these models differ in their implications, both involve stage-specific synthesis of chromatin-modifying gene products and their subsequent dilution or degradation. It has not yet been possible to define these products and thus to discriminate between the two models. Cattanach (345) has described a region (*Xce*) modifying X-chromosome expression, but there is no evidence that it directly encodes the putative regulatory factors.

Secondary modification of DNA structure, particularly by methylation, has also been considered likely to be involved in X-chromosome regulation. The methylation of cytosine in CpG sequences often correlates with decreased expression in the affected or adjacent genes (346,347).

Studies of DNA methylation in X-linked genes, however, have suggested a secondary rather than a primary role in X-inactivation (348). This doubt about the role of methylation in the initial events of X-inactivation is heightened by the observation that the first tissues to show X-inactivation are extensively hypomethylated. Initial work on rabbit blastocysts revealed that trophoblast was significantly hypomethylated in comparison with inner-cell-mass derivatives, but not with adult tissues (349). Further work has focused on the extraembryonic tissues of the mouse conceptus and has revealed extensive undermethylation in satellite and dispersed repetitive DNA sequences in all the derivatives of trophectoderm and primitive endoderm, as compared with early inner-cell-mass derivatives or adult tissues (350–352). Recent work shows that unique DNA sequences are also undermethylated in these same extraembryonic tissues (353). The causes and consequences of hypomethylation in the trophectoderm and primitive endoderm lineages are still unclear. However, the hypomethylation pattern provides information about its role in X-chromosome inactivation. DNA from the inactive X chromosome of adult tissues functions poorly in DNA-mediated transformation experiments with cultured HPRT-deficient cells (354). By contrast, DNA from

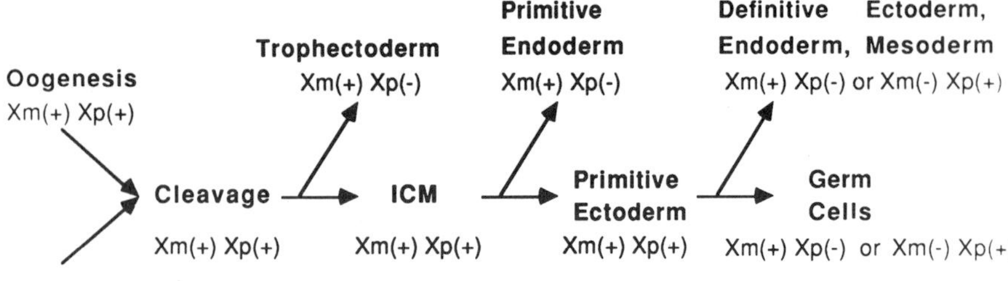

FIG. 9. Hypothesis linking X-chromosome differentiation to cellular differentiation. X-chromosome differentiation is shown as occurring in different cell lineages as they differentiate (m, maternal; p, paternal; +, active; −, inactive). Tissues differentiating early, that is, trophectoderm and primary endoderm, show preferential inactivation of the paternally inherited X chromosome, suggesting some imprinting mechanism for the paternal origin of the two X chromosomes. This mechanism is presumably nullified by the time of gastrulation, when inactivation is random. (Adapted from ref. 337.)

the inactive X chromosome of extraembryonic tissues functions as well as DNA from the active X chromosome (355).

Similar results have recently been obtained with a transgenic mouse line containing an α-fetoprotein minigene integrated into the X chromosome. Unlike the endogenous X-linked genes, the exogenous α-fetoprotein gene was expressed in visceral endoderm even when it was paternally inherited, but it was not expressed on the inactive X chromosome in the fetal liver (356). These results may indicate a role for DNA methylation in stabilizing X-inactivation, because the inactivation is less profound in cells exhibiting low levels of methylation.

As yet, there is no information about the nature of X-chromosome imprinting leading to nonrandom inactivation in the extraembryonic tissues, or about how this terminates before X-inactivation in the primitive ectoderm lineage. The change from early to late replication of the inactive X in the extraembryonic tissues is intriguing because it coincides with the beginning of random X-inactivation between 6.0 and 6.5 d.g. (335,336). This may imply that growth progressively dilutes either the imprint itself or the embryonic gene products that recognize it, with extinction occurring at the time of intense postimplantation growth.

What information serves as the basis for nonrandom inactivation? The extraembryonic tissue lineages are notably all derived from cells that occupy external positions in the late preimplantation embryo, when inactivation of their X chromosome occurs. The pattern of preferential paternal X-inactivation in somatic tissues of the marsupial (320) reinforces this correlation because the unilaminar structure of its blastocyst results in all cells having an external position (65,66). X-inactivation in primitive ectoderm also coincides with epithelial differentiation and formation of the proamniotic cavity. The correlation between embryonic position, epithelial differentiation, DNA hypomethylation, and precocious inactivation of the paternal X chromosome indicates there is an epigenetic source of critical information common to these processes, but it does not provide any hint about its content. The evidence for a contribution from inner cell mass to the polar trophectoderm during mouse blastocyst growth implies that this epigenetic information is present during a period of several cell cycles, rather than occurring as a singular event at a specific early time.

The net result of these early events is a restriction of random X-inactivation to the innermost cells of the periimplantation embryo. These cells are also characterized by levels of DNA methylation similar to those in adult tissues. In light of recent evidence that preimplantation mouse embryos are also hypomethylated in repetitive DNA sequences (J. Sanford, J. Rossant, and V. M. Chapman, *unpublished observations*), it appears that *de novo* methylation may begin shortly after the divergence of the first two cell types that form in the preimplantation embryo. When random X-inactivation occurs in early postimplantation development, it results in stable, permanently heritable patterns of X-linked gene activity, perhaps a secondary consequence of DNA methylation. Another consequence of this capacity for *de novo* methylation is the modification of exogenous DNA sequences introduced into the preimplantation embryo (357).

In summary, X-chromosome inactivation during early development first occurs in extraembryonic tissue lineages as they differentiate (337). The pattern of inactivation in these tissues is nonrandom, resulting in preferential X^p-inactivation, in contrast to the random inactivation occurring slightly later in the primitive ectoderm lineage. Finally, the tissue-specific pattern of DNA methylation suggests a secondary rather than a primary role for these modifications in the X-inactivation process.

Introduction of Exogenous Genes

Probably no single genetic technique has generated more excitement for developmental biologists than the introduction of exogenous genes into the early embryo. This approach has flourished with the availability of recombinant DNA techniques for producing and analyzing DNA sequences. Furthermore, the use of cloned DNA sequences to transform cultured cells (358) was a compelling incentive for studying the fate of these genes throughout the whole of development, when they could potentially be regulated during the growth and differentiation of the intact organism. However, the first attempt at genetically altering mammalian embryos by the introduction of foreign DNA used virus as the DNA source. Jaenisch microinjected SV40 DNA into the blastocoele cavity in mouse embryos and detected the sequences in the adult mice (359,360). Subsequent studies performed with cloned DNA focused on the pronuclear-stage mouse embryo (40) and on the early *Drosophila* embryo (42). When the injected DNA integrates into the host embryo genome, it is subsequently transmitted as a Mendelian trait, and the offspring of these novel individuals become unique strains. The first such mammals were termed transgenic mice (40,361–364). Subsequent similar studies have resulted in transgenic rabbits, sheep, and pigs (365). This approach has been strikingly successful in generating informative integration events (366–372).

Although the earliest transgenic mice produced by injection of pronuclear DNA did not express the exogenous genes, Wagner and associates eventually obtained activity using the herpes simplex virus (HSV) thymidine kinase gene (363), and Brinster and associates also obtained expression with a mouse metallothionein–HSV thymidine kinase fusion gene (361). These results stimulated numerous subsequent studies. The primary objectives of such studies have been to determine the requirements for efficient, tissue-specific expression and to localize the genetic determinants of this specificity. Successful studies of exogenous gene expression have provided numerous insights into the biochemical and physiological aspects of hematopoiesis, immune system development, tumorigenesis, and other subjects. As a consequence of recent results that show a high incidence of efficient expression, gene therapies involving hematopoietic stem cells in humans and gene augmentation in livestock appear to be realistic possibilities.

There are other potential uses for transgenic animals, such as insertional mutagenesis, which provides access to developmentally significant genes (*vide supra*). The remainder of this section focuses on the requirements and consequences of exogenous gene expression in transgenic mice.

Transgenics Produced by Pronuclear Injection

To date, more than 40 cloned gene sequences have been introduced into pronuclear-stage mouse embryos, with at least some degree of expression (Table 3). The major categories of sequences used are intact genomic clones (with their native controlling elements) and cDNA or genomic clones with heterologous controlling elements. The control sequences have most often been the immediate, 5′ (up-

TABLE 3. *Transgenic mice: function of exogenous DNAs*

Exogenous gene	Expression	References
α-Fetoprotein (mouse)	Tissue-specific	376
α-Globin (mouse)	Not specific	401
β-Globin (human)	None	402
	Tissue-specific	382
β-Globin (human-mouse fusion)	Tissue-specific	403,404
β-Globin (rabbit)	Not determined	362
	Not specific	405
	Questionable	364
Collagen α2(I)-chloramphenicol acetyltransferase (fusion)	Tissue-specific	379
αA-crystallin-chloramphenicol acetyltransferase	Tissue-specific	378
*E*α (mouse)	Tissue-specific	391–393
Elastase I (rat)	Tissue-specific	374
Elastase-growth hormone (rat-human fusion)	Tissue-specific	380
Growth hormone (human)	Not expressed	406
Hepatitis B surface antigen	Not specific	400
Herpes simplex virus	Not determined	40
	Not specific	363
Immunoglobulin κ (mouse)	Not specific	386
	Tissue-specific	387
Immunoglobulin κ, μ	Tissue-specific	389
Immunoglobulin μ	Tissue-specific	388
Insulin-SV40 T antigen (fusion)	Tissue-specific	398
Metallothionein-growth hormone (mouse-human fusion)	Not specific	384
Metallothionein-growth hormone (mouse-rat fusion)	Not specific	383
Metallothionein-growth hormone-releasing factor (mouse-human fusion)	Not specific	407
Metallothionein-HPRT (mouse-human fusion)	Semispecific	408
Metallothionein-thymidine kinase	Not specific	361
Metallothionein-somatostatin (mouse-rat fusion)	Not specific	409
Mouse mammary tumor virus-thymidine kinase (fusion)	Semispecific	410
Mouse mammary tumor virus-*myc*	Semispecific	397
Moloney murine leukemia virus	Not specific	411,412
Myosin light chain 2 (rat)	Tissue-specific	375
Rous sarcoma virus-chloramphenicol acetyltransferase	Not specific	379
SV40	Not determined	413
SLA (pig class I major histocompatibility gene)	Tissue-specific	390
SV40 T antigen	Not specific	396
	Semispecific	394
	Tissue-specific	395
SV40 and *v-myc*	Semispecific	414
Transferrin (chicken)	Semispecific	373

Abbreviations: HPRT, hypoxanthine guanine phosphoribosyl transferase; SV40, simian virus 40.

stream) regions adjacent to structural genes. This region includes the promoter and enhancer sequences that are thought to be necessary for tissue-specific expression, based on studies in cultured cells (358). Thus, the major hypothesis being tested in studies with transgenic mice is whether or not the controlling elements used are both necessary and sufficient for normal expression.

Several studies have demonstrated that specific expression can be obtained using genomic DNA. The earliest indication of tissue-specific expression was a study by McKnight et al. (373) demonstrating synthesis of chicken transferrin in the liver of transgenic mice. A subsequent study using the rat elastase I gene showed high levels of tissue-specific synthesis in the mouse pancreas (374). The rat myosin light chain 2 was expressed specifically in the muscles of two transgenic mice (375). Interestingly, the mice varied widely in their levels of specific synthesis, despite similar copy numbers of the exogenous genes. This theme was repeated in mice containing a modified α-fetoprotein minigene; expression was specific to the visceral yolk sac and the fetal liver and gut, but at highly varying levels (376). In studies by Brinster, Palmiter, and associates, the metallothionein promoter was used to obtain gene expression predominantly in the liver of transgenic mice. However, the correlation between levels of expression and number of integrated copies was poor (361,377).

The major conclusions arising from these and other related studies (Table 3) are that genomic sequences located adjacent (generally 5′) to the structural genes studied are indeed necessary and sufficient in many cases for tissue-specific gene expression. Other factors are clearly involved, however, in the specific level of transcription obtained in each case. One possible cause for variable expression between mice is the effect of the local chromatin environment at the site of integration. Another is the number of gene copies integrated, which varies from 1 to about 100, though there is generally little correlation between number of copies and total transcriptional activity. This creates a problem in the quantitative analysis of gene expression in transgenic mice, because it is therefore impossible to determine if transgenic individuals are synthesizing normal amounts of product per active exogenous gene, as compared with the native gene.

Recent studies have demonstrated the effectiveness of using reporter or indicator genes encoding distinctive products to study tissue-specific expression. Fusion genes containing the bacterial structural gene for chloramphenicol acetyltransferase and either the mouse αA-crystallin promoter or the α2(I) collagen promoter have led to tissue- and temporal-specific expression (378,379). A detailed analysis of control by rat elastase promoter using elastase–human growth hormone fusion genes indicated that sequences between 80 and 200 base pairs "upstream" of the 5′ end of the structural gene were responsible for the transcriptional regulation conferred by this enhancer (380). This was the first demonstration of a mammalian gene regulatory sequence by the criteria of tissue specificity in transgenic animals.

Reporter sequences are also valuable in the analysis of gene expression during embryogenesis. They are particularly useful when the expression of the structural gene is detectable in the intact embryo by virtue of a histochemical product. The use of histochemically detectable gene products has been a powerful asset in studies of mouse chimeras (26). The expression of metallothionein promoter-regulated *Escherichia coli* β-galactosidase, can be detected in single embryos after microinjection (M. Stevens, J. J. Meneses, and R. A. Pedersen, *unpublished observations*). Similarly, tissue-specific expression of a γ-crystallin/β-galactosidase fusion gene has recently been observed (381). These observations indicate that structural genes, including some derived from prokaryotes, can be fused with mammalian controlling elements and yield tissue-specific expression.

Although these indicator genes with bacterial structural components were expressed in an apparently normal manner in the transgenic mice described earlier, inclusion of bacterial cloning vector sequences (e.g., pBR322) in the DNA injected into zygote pronuclei resulted in poor or erratic expression. Conversely, expression of human β-globin genes occurred in a tissue- and temporal-specific way if vector sequences were reduced or eliminated entirely (382). Similar observations have been made with the α-fetoprotein gene (376) and with growth hormone genes (368). It is not yet clear what sequences of the bacterial plasmid confer inactivity or what mechanisms are involved in the silencing process.

Although a comprehensive review of the information gained through injection of pronuclear DNA is beyond the scope of this chapter (371,372), several accomplishments are notable because they illustrate the power of this approach in generating novel basic information and possible future practical applications. The dramatic growth of mice carrying metallothionein–growth hormone fusion genes demonstrates the high levels of gene product that can be produced from exogenous genes and their impact on the individual's physiology (383,384). The induction of growth in dwarf mice homozygous for the *little* mutation (deficient for growth hormone) demonstrates the potential for correcting genetic deficiencies with exogenous DNA (385).

Several recent studies have demonstrated the enormous utility of transgenic mice for understanding immune system development. When a functional κ light chain was introduced, the rearrangement of endogenous κ genes was blocked (386,387). Similar results were obtained by injecting rearranged immunoglobulin μ heavy-chain gene (388,389). Other studies have demonstrated the expression of pig major histocompatibility antigen genes in transgenic mice (390) and of exogenous E_α genes. In the latter case, a new immune response resulted from expression of the exogenous gene (391–393). These results should have profound implications for future work in immunology.

A third example is the analysis of oncogene function in

transgenic mice. Expression of the SV40 early-region genes led to tumors of the choroid plexus (394). Tumorigenesis could be attributed to the large-T antigen, although the tissue specificity resided in the SV40 enhancer (395,396). Transgenic mice with the mouse mammary tumor virus promoter driving the *c-myc* proto-oncogene developed mammary adenocarcinomas (397), and mice with the SV40 large-T antigen under the control of the rat insulin promoter developed pancreatic tumors in the islets of Langerhans (398). Finally, transgenic mice expressing genes from human hepatitis B virus have been produced by two groups (399,400) and may be useful as an animal model for this disease.

These examples, though by no means exhaustive (Table 3), confirm the tremendous advantages of generating novel individuals and strains that express defined genetic elements in a tissue-specific manner.

Transgenics Produced by Virus Infection

Although virus DNA was used in the first studies demonstrating that exogenous genes could be integrated into the germ line of mice at embryonic stages (359), only recently have viruses become efficient vectors for producing transgenic animals (371). The primary DNA viruses used for this purpose are the closely related simian virus 40 (SV40) and polyoma virus. These differ in that mouse cells are not permissive for productive infection by SV40, but are for polyoma infection. Recent work shows that preimplantation mouse embryos can support the replication of both viruses (415) and that plasmids containing the polyoma origin of replication can persist without integration into the host chromosomes of transgenic mice (416). The other virus now used widely in transgenic studies is the RNA tumor virus, Moloney murine leukemia virus (MuLV) (417). During their life cycle, the RNA viruses are transformed into a circular DNA that is integrated into the host cell chromosome. The integrated retroviral genome is not expressed in the preimplantation embryo (418), and, moreover, it becomes irreversibly inactivated in most cases, presumably by *de novo* DNA methylation (357,419). An equally persistent block to expression occurs for SV40 virus after infection of early embryonic cells (420). A fraction of mice derived from MuLV-infected embryos become viremic as adults, presumably because the position of integration is close to developmentally regulated genes (421). In recent work (422,423) it has been shown that genes regulated by internal promoters, rather than by the promoters of the MuLV long terminal repeats, can be expressed efficiently in embryonal carcinoma cells, which are closely analogous to embryos (371, 424–426). This, together with the demonstration that MuLV can be used to efficiently transform preimplantation mouse embryos, offers an alternative to pronuclear-DNA injection for introducing exogenous genes in a functional state (427).

Transgenics Produced by Transforming Embryonic Stem Cells

Another means for introducing exogenous genes into the mouse germ line combines viral technology with cell culture and experimental chimerism. This approach is based on the recent ability to culture euploid pluripotent cells (embryonic stem cells) directly from embryos, thereby circumventing the long growth period previously required to adapt embryonal carcinoma cells from tumors to culture (426). The main advantage in using the embryonic stem cells is their euploidy and the attendant high frequency with which they colonize the germ line in chimeras produced by blastocyst injection (428). Using this approach, Stewart et al. (424) have recently introduced genes conferring neomycin resistance into mice. Moreover, it has recently proved to be possible to obtain germ line integration by means of embryonic stem cell transformation, selection, and transfer to host blastocysts (429,430). These efforts have benefited markedly from the availability of dominant selectable markers, such as the bacterial neomycin-resistance gene and guanine phosphoribosyltransferase gene (431,432). These attempts to transform mouse embryos share technologies and goals with current efforts at gene therapy. The benefits of transgenic animals include elucidating the mechanisms of tissue-specific gene regulation, optimizing procedures for introducing exogenous genes into cells, and determining which promoters are effective in a wide variety of target tissues. This information is the necessary background for clinically effective gene therapy to correct biochemical defects in humans.

BIOCHEMICAL ASPECTS

This section emphasizes the lineage-specific biochemical differentiation of the cell types that form in the early mammalian embryo. The reason for this emphasis is that cell-lineage-related products are likely to provide clues to mechanisms of differentiation. In addition, the general aspects of metabolic activities in mammalian embryos have been known for some time or have been adequately reviewed elsewhere (8,433). Because of their potential importance as probes for cell differentiation, many of the genes for products described here have been cloned from one or more mammalian species. Molecular cloning goes hand in hand with analysis of early mammalian embryos, because the use of molecular probes confers such sensitivity and specificity.

Secreted Products

The serum glycoprotein, α-fetoprotein (AFP), is probably the most thoroughly studied lineage-specific product in mammalian embryos. AFP is produced from early postimplantation stages specifically by the visceral endoderm of rat and mouse embryos (434–436). AFP accumulates to high levels in the amniotic fluid, where it appears to function as an embryonic counterpart to albumin, to which it is evolutionarily related and genetically linked (437). The half-life of AFP mRNA is relatively long (30 hr) in the mouse visceral yolk sac (438). There is evidence for independent regulation of AFP and albumin genes in mouse and rat development (439,440). Evidence from studies of AFP-transgenic mice shows that the DNA sequences necessary for temporal- and tissue-specific expression reside in the immediately adjacent 5′ sequences (441,442).

Several other serum proteins are also synthesized and secreted specifically by the visceral yolk sac. These include transferrin, metallothionein, α_1-antitrypsin, and apolipoproteins (443–448). The similarity of products of the rodent visceral yolk sac and fetal liver has prompted the observation that these two organs, albeit derived from independent cell lineages, have homologous functions at early and late stages of intrauterine development, respectively (448).

Extracellular Matrix

The substrates surrounding cells in an intact embryo have a profound impact on their morphology, behavior, and gene expression (449). Mouse embryos begin to synthesize fibronectin at the blastocyst stage, when it accumulates on the basal surfaces of primitive endoderm cells and near the junction of parietal endoderm and trophectoderm (450,451). At later stages, fibronectin is present in the basement membrane of visceral endoderm, trophoblast, and mesoderm. In addition to fibronectin, laminin and type IV collagen are major components of basement membranes in the early mouse embryo (452,453). Although one component of laminin is synthesized in unfertilized eggs, intercellular deposits do not accumulate until the 8- to 16-cell stage (454,455). Type III collagen deposits begin to accumulate at the 16-cell stage (456), but type I collagen does not begin to be synthesized until day 8 of gestation, when it accumulates in several fetal and extraembryonic tissues (453). An essential role for type I collagen in development is evident from the death at 12 d.g. of transgenic mice homozygous for a retrovirus insertion into this gene (457). The most prominent basement membrane in the early rodent embryo is Reichert's membrane, consisting mainly of laminin, type IV collagen, and chondroitin sulfate proteoglycans; it is apparently synthesized by parietal endoderm cells (458,459). The availability of DNA probes to the mRNAs of most of these basement membrane components should facilitate the analysis of the precise location and time of their synthesis (448).

Cell Surface Molecules

The cell surface differentiation of mammalian embryos has been the subject of extensive work (460–466). The purpose of this section is to provide an overview of recent work.

Cell Adhesion Molecules

The compacting morula in placental mammals is unique in its precocious cell adhesiveness and junctional differentiation (125,464). The fact that cleavage-stage embryos of marsupials and embryos in other vertebrate classes do not undergo compaction implies that this process may be integrally involved in the development of trophectoderm. Indeed, removing calcium from the culture medium prevents or reverses compaction of morula-stage mouse embryos and thwarts trophectoderm differentiation (467). Similar results can be obtained by treating early-cleavage-stage embryos with cytochalasin, which dissociates microfilaments, or with certain antibodies to embryonal carcinoma cells (125,465). The common denominator of this disruption of compaction appears to be cell adhesion molecules that are necessary for compaction. Described variously as uvomorulin (468), cadherin (469), and cell adhesion molecule 120/80 (470,471), cell adhesion molecules present on the preimplantation mouse embryo are calcium-dependent surface molecules resembling those present on liver cells (472). Because these cell adhesion molecules are present on mouse embryos even before the beginning of compaction, they cannot, however, be considered sufficient for compaction (473).

Lectins and Their Receptors

The effects of some lectins on preimplantation development suggests a role for lectin-saccharide interactions in compaction and blastocyst formation. Agarose beads coated with concanavalin A (con-A), peanut agglutinin, or wheat germ agglutinin (WGA) induce spreading of 8-cell blastomeres of mouse embryos (474). Moreover, WGA induces compaction and cavitation in 2-cell mouse embryos (474). On the other hand, culturing 4-cell mouse embryos in either WGA or con-A prevents compaction and blastocyst formation and leads to vacuole formation in the blastomeres (476). As would be expected from these results, these three lectins bind to preimplantation mouse embryos (477). There are also receptors for the lectins *Dolichos biflorus* agglutinin and *Ricinus communis* agglutinin in early mouse embryos (478). Although the distribution of con-A on blastomeres is uniform before compaction, it becomes polarized in late-8-cell embryos, and this persists at subsequent stages; this distribution is one component of the polarized phenotype (*vide supra*) that precedes the differentiation of trophectoderm (125). Despite the presence of these lectin receptors, there is no compelling evidence that they have a role in development, because physiological concentrations of various saccharides did not inhibit compaction of 8-cell mouse embryos (474).

Oligosaccharide Antigens

With the advent of monoclonal antibodies, several carbohydrate antigens have been defined on the surfaces of embryonic cells. The best-studied of these, SSEA-1, is a lacto-series carbohydrate that appears on the 8-cell-stage mouse embryo, then segregates to the inner cell mass at the blastocyst stage (479). This antigen is expressed on the surfaces of visceral endoderm and embryonic ectoderm cells in postimplantation mouse embryos (480,481). Other lacto-series carbohydrates expressed on early mouse embryos are the human blood group precursor antigens I and i; I antigens are present at all preimplantation stages, and both antigens are present on parietal and visceral endoderm after day 6 of gestation (482–484). The globo-series carbohydrates recognized by the monoclonal antibodies SSEA-3 and SSEA-4 are present on mouse oocytes, preimplantation embryos, inner cell mass, and first on primitive and then on visceral endoderm at postimplantation stages (485–487); globoside is present on 2-cell- to morula-stage mouse embryos (488); Forssman antigen is present on late-morula- and blastocyst-stage embryos (489). The chemical structures of these carbohydrate antigens have been well defined, so their biosynthetic pathways can be inferred (465). Consistent with these findings, glycosyl transferases are present on the surfaces of early embryo cells and embryonal carcinoma cells (490–492) and appear to have roles in compaction (493) and in the interconversion of the carbohydrate antigens (465).

Other Surface Molecules

Alkaline phosphatase, Na^+,K^+-ATPase, and histocompatibility antigens deserve special mention. Alkaline phosphatase activity appears on the surfaces of 2-cell blastomeres and increases in intensity at the 8- to 16-cell stages, when it is concentrated on apposing cell surfaces; activity in blastocysts is restricted to the inner cell mass and subsequently to its derivatives (494,495). Activity on embryonic ectoderm decreases gradually after gastrulation, but remains associated with the primordial germ cells, which are localized at the base of the allantois in 8-day mouse embryos (159). The activity can be used to localize the primordial germ cells during their migration through hindgut endoderm and mesenteries to the genital ridges during early stages of gonad formation (496,497).

The accumulation of blastocoel fluid in the rabbit and mouse has been shown to depend on Na^+,K^+-ATPase activity, which becomes localized on apposed surfaces of blastomeres, beginning at the morula stage (498). Analysis of the blastocoel fluid composition in rabbit embryos cultured in normal and hyperosmotic medium indicated that Na^+ and Cl^- are transported, with presumed passive movement of water (499). The ionic movements have been attributed to Na^+,K^+-ATPase, which can be identified on the juxtacoelic surfaces of the cells of the rabbit blastocyst by using labeled ouabain as a specific marker (500,501). Mouse blastocysts exposed to ouabain in the culture medium (exposing only outer surfaces of trophectoderm cells) develop normally; however, embryos treated with cytochalasin to cause a collapse of the blastocoel failed to reexpand when they were treated with ouabain, presumably because the drug inhibited the juxtacoelic Na^+,K^+-ATPase (502). An integral role for this enzyme in the polarization of mouse blastomeres at the morula stage has been hypothesized by Wiley (503), who has suggested that it is responsible for osmotic flows leading to a shift in the positions of cytoplasmic organelles and other processes leading to the formation of the blastocoel.

Except for a transient appearance on the outer surfaces of trophectoderm cells at the blastocyst stage (504,505), major histocompatibility antigens are absent from mouse embryos until midgestation (506). However, β_2-microglobulin synthesis begins at the 2-cell stage (507) and continues through preimplantation development (508). Because major histocompatibility antigen synthesis does not occur at early cleavage stages, the function of β_2-microglobulin at these stages may be to anchor the minor histocompatibility antigens, which appear on cleavage-stage embryos and blastocysts (463,509).

Cytoskeletal Elements

The cytoskeleton in early mammalian embryos has been studied using inhibitors of specific cytoskeletal elements and using antibodies or other probes to localize and quantitate the components of the cytoskeleton at various stages. Colchicine, colcemid, and nocodazole have been used to study the role of tubulin in the mouse embryo. These inhibitors cause cleavage arrest and prevent blastocoel formation (510–512). There have been conflicting reports that microtubule inhibitors induce decompaction of 8-cell embryos (513), but that nocodazole, also a microtubule-depolymerizing drug, accelerates compaction at the same stage (514). Cytochalasins, which disrupt microfilaments, cause cleavage arrest and inhibit compaction (510,513,515–517). Mouse embryos treated with cytochalasins during cleavage form aggregates of vacuolated cells at the time the blastocoel normally forms; if the inhibitor is removed before vacuolation occurs, the embryos form trophectoderm vesicles that have polypeptide synthetic profiles similar to that of intact blastocysts (515).

The compound effects of inhibitors that dissociate microtubules or microfilaments on cell division and other morphogenetic events make it difficult to distinguish between effects induced because of cytoskeletal disruption and those resulting from cell cycle arrest. Thus, the inhibitor studies must be interpreted with caution. When the effects of such inhibitors were studied in interphase cells, surface (microvillar) polarization occurred in the absence of microtubules or microfilaments, even though underlying cytoplasmic polarization of the cytoskeleton and of endocytotic organelles was prevented (125,518,519). These results imply that organization of the major cytoskeletal elements derives from the cell surface and cell-cell interactions.

In addition to the microtubules and microfilaments that are evident in cleavage-stage mouse embryos (520–523), several cytoskeletal elements implicated in cytoskeletal–cell surface interaction are present. Their roles in the embryo are inferred from the functions of similar or identical proteins in erythrocytes, muscle cells, and nonmuscle cells (465). These include α-actinin (522) and spectrin (524), which are present at cleavage stages and could anchor actin filaments to the membrane, and myosin (525–527), which would be involved with actin in cell shape changes, mobility, and contractility.

Another category of cytoskeletal elements contained in embryos is intermediate-filament proteins, which are expressed in lineage-specific patterns (448,528). For example, desmins are found in muscle, glial fibrillar acidic protein is found in glial cells and astrocytes, and cytokeratins are found in epithelial cells. Cytokeratins designated as Endo A (TROMA-1) and Endo B first accumulate in the trophectoderm of mouse embryos at the blastocyst stage (529–532). At later stages, both cytokeratins are found also in the primitive-endoderm lineage of mouse embryos (533). The mRNA encoding Endo A can be detected in trophectoderm, but not inner cell mass, at the blastocyst stage; at postimplantation stages, it appears in visceral endoderm and amnion (534). This pair of cytokeratins corresponds to the major pair of cytokeratins in adult mouse liver (Endo A = type II; Endo B = type I), as indicated by DNA cloning and sequencing (535). Although the role of cytokeratins in early mammalian development is not yet understood, their lineage specificity makes them useful as markers for studying differentiation and commitment at late preimplantation and early postimplantation stages.

The potential for interactions between the cytoskeleton and the cell membrane makes the analysis of cytoskeletal elements in mammalian embryos an important area for further work. This is particularly evident from the effects of cell shape and extracellular matrix on proliferation and gene expression in other systems (536–539). Despite the advantages of a reductionist approach to development, the highly regulative nature of the mammalian embryo is a compelling argument for studying cell interactions in intact embryos whenever possible.

Regulatory Elements

Several categories of lineage-related products may be implicated in the regulation of growth and differentiation. These include growth factors and their receptors, heat-shock proteins, and homeobox-containing genes.

Growth Factors and Their Receptors

In addition to the secreted products previously described, early mammalian embryos produce and secrete growth factors; in some cases, they also possess the receptors for these same factors (448,540). Transforming growth factor (TGF) α and β are epidermal-growth-factor-like polypeptides that stimulate anchorage-independent growth of untransformed TGF-α binds to the epidermal growth factor (EGF) receptor, but not to anti-EGF antibodies; using these criteria to assess the quantity of TGF-α reveals a high specific activity in the 7.5-d.g. mouse embryo (541) and in the human placenta (542). Somatomedins, or insulin-like growth factors (IGF), are produced by postimplantation mouse embryo tissues, specifically allantois and amnion (J. Heath, *unpublished observations*), and are present in human amniotic fluid (543). Trophoblast giant cells produce a prolactin-like protein (544,545), and prolactin is present in high concentrations in human amniotic fluid. Human chorionic gonadotropin is produced by the syncytiotrophoblast cells of the placenta and can be detected in the maternal serum as soon as 2 weeks after fertilization (546,547).

The presence of growth factor receptors may be indicative of a developmental function of the relevant factor. Not restricted to a specific lineage, the EGF receptor appears at 11 to 12 d.g. on all cell types except parietal endoderm and is present at high levels on cells of the amnion and various fetal tissues (548,549). Because TGF-α can bind to the EGF receptor, it is plausible that the midgestation embryo can respond to TGF-α in an autocrine fashion. Alternatively, receptors may bind EGF produced in maternal tissues; no embryonic EGF source has been detected (550). The inner cell mass and primitive endoderm of the mouse embryo react with antibodies to the transferrin receptor, as do labyrinthine cells of the placenta, whereas trophoblast giant cells derived by *in vitro* outgrowth do not (E. D. Adamson, *unpublished observation*).

The function of proto-oncogenes during development is of considerable interest because viral oncogenes promote the growth of cells. Moreover, a number of proto-oncogenes are either identical with or homologous with known growth factors or their receptors (551). The class I proto-oncogenes *c-abl* and *c-src* are expressed in a wide variety of tissues in mouse fetuses (448,552). This class is associated with tyrosine protein kinase activity. The class-I-related proto-oncogene *c-erb-A* is maximally expressed at day 14 of mouse gestation, but *c-erb-B*, which is homologous with EGF receptor, is not present in high amounts in any tissue, contrary to expectation (552). Other class-I-related proto-oncogenes, *c-fms* [homologous with the CSF-1 receptor (553)] and *c-mos*, are active in mouse embryos, the former predominantly in the placenta (555,556). Class II proto-oncogenes (mediating GTP binding) are active in fetal tissues throughout development (557). The class III secreted proto-oncogene *v-sis*, homologous with platelet-derived growth factor, reaches its highest levels at 8 days in the mouse (552). Class IV nuclear proto-oncogenes *c-fos* and *c-myc* are actively expressed during development, the former in the amnion and chorion of the mouse, and the latter in the cytotrophoblast of the human placenta (558,559). Although it is not yet possible to identify the role of each of these proto-oncogenes in mammalian development, their functions clearly deserve further analysis, because they may be among the multiple factors regulating embryonic and fetal growth.

Heat-Shock Proteins

Exposure to heat and a variety of other environmental stresses induces the synthesis of a set of proteins known as heat-shock proteins (HSP) (560). Embryos of a wide variety of species, both vertebrate and invertebrate, synthesize HSP constitutively at early developmental stages (175). Mammalian embryos are not exceptional, mouse embryos constitutively synthesizing HSP 68–70 at the 2-cell stage (197). Indeed, this is perhaps the first product of the mouse embryonic genome after division to the 2-cell stage (195,561). The capacity to respond to environmental stress by increased HSP synthesis does not appear until the blastocyst stage in mouse and rabbit embryos (562–564). At postimplantation stages, mouse embryos continue to synthesize HSP 68 constitutively in several extraembryonic tissues, but not in embryonic ectoderm (R. Kothary and J. Rossant, *unpublished observations*). The preimplantation period is the most heat-sensitive time in mammalian development (565), with the most sensitive event in the mouse being activation of gene expression at the 2-cell stage (566). Even though the function of HSP remains obscure, and the acquisition of thermotolerance in mammalian embryos by means of HSP synthesis is still conjectural, the pattern of HSP synthesis suggests that these proteins may have an important role during cleavage and early postimplantation development. Tissue-specific levels of HSP synthesis appear to support this view (567).

Homeobox Genes as Possible Regulatory Elements

Morphogenesis of *Drosophila* is known to require the function of genes that control segment number and polarity and genes that specify segment identity (568–570). The latter group, known as homeotic genes, often possess a conserved sequence of nucleotides known as the "homeobox." Moreover, this family of sequences has remained highly conserved throughout evolution (571). In mammals (primarily the mouse and human have been studied) there is a steadily increasing number of known genes containing sequences homologous with the *Drosophila* homeobox (572–579). Of these, two have been mapped to mouse chromosome 1, one to chromosome 6, and five to chromosome 11. Two of the genes located on mouse chromosome 11 were mapped first to human chromosome 17, implying synteny between regions of these chromosomes (576,581). Although several known morphogenetic mutations also map to these chromosomes in the mouse (215,577), none of them has been identified as a homeobox-containing gene. The homeobox gene on mouse chromosome 11 is expressed beginning at 7.5 d.g. (574), and several others are expressed at later stages, some specifically in the spinal cord and brain and others during spermatogenesis as well (574,578–583). Homeobox genes described in *Xenopus* are also expressed during early development (584,585). The extreme degree of evolutionary conservation of the homeobox sequences and the regulated developmental expression of these genes raise the possibility that they have an integral role in switching differentiative pathways, as they do in *Drosophila*. The relatively small number of homeobox sequences and their restricted tissue expression in spinal cord make it seem unlikely that they regulate metamerism or developmental decision making in any general way. Nonetheless, the high arginine and lysine contents of polypeptides encoded by the conserved homeobox domains and the nuclear location of the product in *Drosophila* suggest that the homeobox sequences themselves may have a DNA-binding function, whatever the role of the remainder of the protein may be (586). It is this intriguing idea that sets homeobox-containing genes apart from those involved in strictly physiological activities for consideration as possible regulatory genes.

CONCLUSION

The Mammalian Embryo *In Vitro:* Advantages and Limitations

The success of experimental approaches to early mammalian embryogenesis is largely attributable to work with cultured embryos. Since the 1950s, most investigators have used *in vitro* methods for part or all of their analyses. The enormous advantage conferred by this approach is the accessibility of the embryo itself for treatment and intervention. During preimplantation stages, the embryo is normally free in the oviduct or uterine lumen anyway, so the task of maintaining the embryo in a normal state is one of approximating the fluid and gas conditions of the native environment. Maintaining normal development *in vitro* throughout the preimplantation period has been accomplished with only a few species, including the mouse, rabbit, and human. In these cases, the successful culture was largely a result of empirically altering the growth conditions to optimize development, rather than mimicking reproductive tract conditions *in vivo*; these latter parameters were largely unknown. Nonetheless, the adequacy of preimplantation culture conditions for any species could be determined by transferring preimplantation-stage embryos to the oviduct or uterus of the natural or a surrogate mother, with development to term as the endpoint (1).

In the case of postimplantation culture, however, returning embryos to the uterus has been marginally successful, without development to term after transfer (587). Thus, despite the advantages of accessibility provided by culture, postimplantation embryos cannot yet be restored to their normal intrauterine potential for growth. The extent of normal growth and morphology *in vitro* for postimplantation embryos is limited to 2 to 3 days for rodents, which have been the subject of most experimental work (588). The alternative approach of culturing preimplantation embryos to postimplantation stages (589,590) yields a low incidence of successful development, and certain features of these embryos do not closely resemble those of the equivalent stages *in vivo*. The main differences are (a) the two-dimensional growth of trophoblast derivatives as a monolayer on the substrate used for culture and (b) the retardation of the embryo proper. These phenomena may be related, in the sense that failure to maintain three-dimensionality *in vitro* may prevent normal cell-cell interactions necessary for placental morphogenesis and therefore embryonic nutrition; alternatively, autocrine factors produced by either placenta or embryo may become diluted by culture medium, thus depriving the embryo of essential growth-promoting substances. Clearly, defining the nature of interactions between mammalian embryonic and maternal cells and tissues through membrane contacts, extracellular matrix, and humoral factors remains one of the major tasks in early mammalian embryology.

Mammalian Embryos as Models for Vertebrate Development

Are laboratory animals justifiable models for vertebrate development? Whatever insights are gained in such model systems will have to be examined closely to verify their relevance to the human or to other vertebrates. This comparison will have to take place at all levels of organization (e.g., cellular as well as molecular). It should be apparent from this review that current experimental approaches to mammalian embryos make them superb systems for many aspects of developmental biology. The body of knowledge obtained from transgenic mice alone attests to the power of these novel approaches. Among higher eukaryotes, mice rival *Drosophila* in their diversity of genetic markers. *In situ* hybridization and other amplification techniques now make it possible to study gene expression in the small tissue samples available from laboratory mammals. Finally, clonal analysis of cell lineages has provided insight into the architectural rules for construction of the mammalian embryo.

Another compelling reason for studying mammals as models for vertebrate development is that development during and after gastrulation appears to be extensively conserved. This conclusion is based on recent work showing the extensive similarity of the gastrula fate map of the mouse to those of the chick and urodele embryo (127,138,169; K. A. Lawson, J. J. Meneses, and R. A. Pedersen, *unpublished observations*). Consequently, it appears that the basic way of establishing the vertebrate body plan has remained essentially unchanged for more than 250 million years. Naturally, this could be an argument for using chicks, frogs, and fish to study mammals, but mammals have some features that justify their use instead. These pertain mainly, but not exclusively, to extraembryonic tissues and structures. They include the precocious differentiation and allocation of the progenitors of the extraembryonic lineages, random X-chromosome inactivation in the fetus, preferential paternal X-chromosome inactivation in placental and yolk sac tissues, and genetic imprinting of genes in the maternal and paternal genomes such that all individuals require both a mother and a father. Thus, mammals are deeply generalized in some aspects of their organogenesis, yet uniquely specialized in other aspects of their early gene expression. This combination makes a compelling case for studying mechanisms of mammalian embryogenesis and organogenesis. Analysis of these mechanisms in mammals should be informative of developmental phenomena among vertebrates in general and should provide numerous opportunities for future beneficial applications to problems of human health.

ACKNOWLEDGMENTS

Work in my laboratory was supported by the Office of Health and Environmental Research, U.S. Department of Energy, contract DE-AC03-76-SF01012. This review was partially written while I was a guest of the Laboratory of Developmental and Reproductive Toxicology of the National Institute of Environmental Health Sciences, Research Triangle Park, North Carolina, under the terms of the Interagency Personnel Act. I thank Drs. John McLachlan and E. Mitchell Eddy for their encouragement and support. I thank Drs. Greg Barsh, Julia Emerson, Kirstie Lawson, and Akiko Spindle for their comments, and Drs. Eileen Adamson, Verne Chapman, John Heath, Kirstie Lawson, and Janet Rossant for allowing me to cite their unpublished work. I am grateful to Michelle Bloom and Leslie Roberts for their assistance with the manuscript.

REFERENCES

1. Adams, C. E. (1982): *Mammalian Egg Transfer*. CRC Press, Boca Raton, Fla.
2. Brackett, B. G., Seidel, G. E., and Seidel, S. M. (editors) (1981): *New Technologies in Animal Breeding*. Academic Press, New York.
3. Hafez, E. S. E., and Semm, K. (editors) (1982): *In Vitro Fertilization and Embryo Transfer*. Alan R. Liss, New York.
4. Beier, H. M., and Lindner, H. R. (editors) (1983): *Fertilization of the Human Egg In Vitro. Biological Basis and Clinical Application*. Springer-Verlag, Berlin.
5. Jones, H. W., Jr., Jones, G. S., Hodgen, G. D., and Rosenwaks, Z. (editors) (1986): *In Vitro Fertilization. Norfolk*. Williams and Wilkins, Baltimore.
6. Seppala, M., and Edwards, R. G. (editors) (1985): *In Vitro Fertilization and Embryo Transfer*. New York Academy of Sciences, New York.
7. Trounson, A., and Woods, C. (editors) (1984): *In Vitro Fertilization and Embryo Transfer*. Churchill Livingstone, Edinburgh.

8. Kaye, P. L. (1986): Metabolic aspects of the physiology of the preimplantation embryo. In: *Experimental Approaches to Mammalian Embryonic Development,* edited by J. Rossant and R. A. Pedersen, pp. 267–292. Cambridge University Press, Cambridge.
9. Bodemer, C. W. (1971): The biology of the blastocyst in historical perspective. In: *Biology of the Blastocyst,* edited by R. J. Blandau, pp. 1–25. University of Chicago Press, Chicago.
10. Horder, T. J., Witkowski, J. A., and Wilie, C. C. (editors) (1986): *A History of Embryology*. Cambridge University Press, London.
11. Heape, W. (1891): Preliminary note on the transplantation and growth of mammalian ova within a uterine foster mother. *Proc. R. Soc. Lond. [Biol.],* 48:457.
12. Rossant, J., and Papaioannou, V. E. (1977): The biology of embryogenesis. In: *Concepts in Mammalian Embryogenesis,* edited by M. I. Sherman, pp. 1–36. MIT Press, Cambridge, Mass.
13. Whitten, W. K. (1956): Culture of tubal mouse ova. *Nature,* 177:96.
14. Brinster, R. L. (1965): Studies on the development of mouse embryos *in vitro*. II. The effect of energy source. *J. Exp. Zool.,* 158:59–68.
15. Biggers, J. D., and Brinster, R. L. (1965): Biometrical problems in the study of early mammalian embryos *in vitro*. *J. Exp. Zool.,* 158:39–48.
16. Biggers, J. D., Whitten, W. K., and Whittingham, D. G. (1971): The culture of mouse embryos *in vitro*. In: *Methods in Mammalian Embryology,* edited by J. C. Daniel, Jr., pp. 86–116. W. H. Freeman, San Francisco.
17. Hogan, B., Costantini, F., and Lacy, E. (1986): *Manipulating the Mouse Embryo. A Laboratory Manual,* pp. 12–15. Cold Spring Harbor Laboratory, Cold Spring Harbor, N.Y.
18. Edwards, R. G., and Gates, A. H. (1959): Timing of the stages of the maturation, divisions, ovulation, fertilization and the first cleavage of eggs of adult mice treated with gonadotrophins. *J. Endocrinol.,* 18:292–304.
19. Tarkowski, A. K. (1961): Mouse chimaeras developed from fused eggs. *Nature,* 190:857–860.
20. Mintz, B. (1964): Formation of genetically mosaic mouse embryos, and early development of "lethal (t^{12}/t^{12})-normal" mosaics. *J. Exp. Zool.,* 157:273–292.
21. McLaren, A. (1976): *Mammalian Chimaeras*. Cambridge University Press, London.
22. Chapman, V. M., Ansell, J. D., and McLaren, A. (1972): Trophoblast giant cell differentiation in the mouse: expression of glucose phosphate isomerase (GPI-1) electrophoretic variants in transferred and chimeric embryos. *Dev. Biol.,* 29:48–54.
23. West, J. D. (1978): Analysis of clonal growth using chimaeras and mosaics. In: *Development in Mammals, Vol. 3,* edited by M. H. Johnson, pp. 413–460. North-Holland, Amsterdam.
24. LeDouarin, N., and McLaren, A. (editors) (1984): *Chimeras in Developmental Biology*. Academic Press, New York.
25. Gardner, R. L. (1968): Mouse chimaeras obtained by the injection of cells into the blastocyst. *Nature,* 220:596–597.
26. Gardner, R. L. (1984): An *in situ* cell marker for clonal analysis of development of the extraembryonic endoderm in the mouse. *J. Embryol. Exp. Morphol.,* 80:251–288.
27. Rossant, J., Vijh, M., Siracusa, L. D., and Chapman, V. M. (1983): Identification of embryonic cell lineages in histological sections of *M. musculus* ↔ *M. caroli* chimaeras. *J. Embryol. Exp. Morphol.,* 73:179–191.
28. Solter, D., and Knowles, B. (1975): Immunosurgery of mouse blastocyst. *Proc. Natl. Acad. Sci. USA,* 72:5099–5102.
29. Lin, T. P. (1971): Egg micromanipulation. In: *Methods in Mammalian Embryology,* edited by J. C. Daniels, Jr., pp. 157–185. W. H. Freeman, San Francisco.
30. Wilson, I. B., Bolton, E., and Cutler, R. H. (1972): Preimplantation differentiation in the mouse egg as revealed by microinjection of vital markers. *J. Embryol. Exp. Morphol.,* 27:467–479.
31. Graham, C. F., and Deussen, Z. A. (1978): Features of cell lineage in preimplantation mouse development. *J. Embryol. Exp. Morphol.,* 48:53–72.
32. Jacobson, M., and Hirose, G. (1978): Origin of the retina from both sides of the embryonic brain: a contribution to the problem of crossing at the optic chiasma. *Science,* 202:637–639.
33. Weisblat, D. A., Sawyer, R. T., and Stent, G. S. (1978): Cell lineage analysis by intracellular injection of a tracer enzyme. *Science,* 202:1295–1298.
34. Gimlich, R. L., and Braun, J. (1985): New fluorescent cell lineage tracers. *Dev. Biol.,* 115:340–352.
35. Balakier, H., and Pedersen, R. A. (1982): Allocation of cells to inner cell mass and trophectoderm lineages in preimplantation mouse embryos. *Dev. Biol.,* 90:352–362.
36. Pedersen, R. A. (1987): Analysis of cell lineage during early mouse embryogenesis. In: *Developmental Toxicology: Mechanisms and Risk,* edited by J. A. McLachlan, R. M. Pratt, and C. L. Markert. Cold Spring Harbor Laboratory, Cold Spring Harbor, N.Y (*in press*).
37. Briggs, R., and King, T. J. (1952): Transplantation of living nuclei from blastula cells into enucleated frogs' eggs. *Proc. Natl. Acad. Sci. USA,* 38:455–463.
38. Gurdon, J. B. (1962): The developmental capacity of nuclei taken from intestinal epithelium cells of feeding tadpoles. *J. Embryol. Exp. Morphol.,* 10:622.
39. McGrath, J., and Solter, D. (1983): Nuclear transplantation in the mouse embryo by microsurgery and cell fusion. *Science,* 220:1300–1303.
40. Gordon, J. W., Scangos, G. A., Plotkin, D. J., Barbosa, J. A., and Ruddle, F. H. (1980): Genetic transformation of mouse embryos by microinjection of purified DNA. *Proc. Natl. Acad. Sci. USA,* 77: 7380–7384.
41. Brinster, R. L., and Palmiter, R. D. (1986): Introduction of genes into the germ line of animals. *Harvey Lect.,* 80:1–38.
42. Rubin, G. M., and Spradling, A. C. (1982): Transposition of cloned P elements into *Drosophila* germ line chromosomes. *Science,* 218:348–353.
43. Gaddum-Rosse, P., Blandau, R. J., Langley, L. B., and Sato, K. (1982): Sperm tail entry into the mouse egg in vitro. *Gamete Res.,* 6:215–223.
44. Howlett, S. K., and Bolton, V. N. (1985): Sequence and regulation of morphological and molecular events during the first cell cycle of mouse embryogenesis. *J. Embryol. Exp. Morphol.,* 87:175–206.
45. Yanagimachi, R. (1966): Time and process of sperm penetration into hamster and ova *in vivo* and *in vitro*. *J. Reprod. Fertil.,* 11:359–370.
46. Molls, M., Zamboglou, N., and Streffer, C. (1983): A comparison of the cell kinetics of preimplantation mouse embryos from two different mouse strains. *Cell Tissue Kinet.,* 16:277–283.
47. Naish, S. J., Perreault, S. D., Foehner, A. L., and Zirkin, B. R. (1987): DNA synthesis in the fertilizing hamster sperm nucleus: sperm template availability and egg cytoplasmic control. *Biol. Reprod.,* (*in press*).
48. Shire, J. G. M., and Whitten, W. K. (1980): Genetic variation in the timing of first cleavage in mice: effect of paternal genotype. *Biol. Reprod.,* 23:363–368.
49. Shire, J. G. M., and Whitten, W. K. (1980): Genetic variation in the timing of first cleavage in mice: effect of maternal genotype. *Biol. Reprod.,* 23:369–376.
50. Goldbard, S. B., and Warner, C. M. (1982): Genes affect the timing of early mouse embryo development. *Biol. Reprod.,* 27:419–424.
51. Harlow, G. M., and Quinn, P. (1982): Development of pre-implantation mouse embryos in vivo and in vitro. *Aust. J. Biol. Sci.,* 35:187–193.
52. Streffer, C., van Beuningen, D., Molls, M., Zamboglou, N., and Schultz, S. (1980): Kinetics of cell proliferation in the preimplanted mouse embryo in vivo and in vitro. *Cell Tissue Kinet.,* 13: 135–143.
53. Sawicki, W., Abramczuk, J., and Blaton, O. (1978): DNA cycles in the second and third cell cycles of mouse preimplantation development. *Exp. Cell Res.,* 112:199–205.
54. Pedersen, R. A. (1986): Potency, lineage and allocation in preimplantation mouse embryos. In: *Experimental Approaches to Mammalian Embryonic Development,* edited by J. Rossant and R. A. Pedersen, pp. 3–33. Cambridge University Press, Cambridge.
55. Smith, R. K. W., and Johnson, M. H. (1986): Analysis of the third and fourth cell cycles of mouse early development. *J. Reprod. Fertil.* 76:393–399.
56. Sundstrom, P., Nilsson, O., and Liedholm, P. (1981): Cleavage rate and morphology of early human embryos obtained after artificial fertilization and culture. *Acta Obstet. Gynecol. Scand.,* 60:109–120.
57. Trouson, A. O., Mohr, L. R., Wood, C., and Leeton, J. F. (1982): Effect of delayed insemination on in-vitro fertilization, culture and transfer of human embryos. *J. Reprod. Fertil.,* 64:285–294.

58. Kelly, S. J., Mulnard, J. G., and Graham, C. F. (1978): Cell division and cell allocation in early mouse development. *J. Embryol. Exp. Morphol.*, 48:37–51.
59. Lewis, W. H., and Wright, E. S. (1935): On the early development of the mouse egg. *Carnegie Instit. Contrib. Embryol.*, 25:113–143.
60. Ducibella, T., Albertini, D. F., Anderson, E., and Biggers, J. (1975): The preimplantation mammalian embryo: characterization of intracellular junctions and their appearance during development. *Dev. Biol.*, 45:231–250.
61. Magnuson, T., Dempsey, A., and Stackpole, C. W. (1977): Characterization of intercellular junctions in the preimplantation mouse embryo by freeze-fracture and thin-section electron microscopy. *Dev. Biol.*, 61:252–261.
62. Magnuson, T., Jacobson, J. B., and Stackpole, C. W. (1978): Relationship between intercellular permeability and junctional organization in the preimplantation mouse embryo. *Dev. Biol.*, 67:214–224.
63. McLachlin, J. R., Caveney, S., and Kidder, G. M. (1983): Control of gap junction formation in early mouse embryos. *Dev. Biol.*, 98:155–164.
64. Goodall, H., and Johnson, M. H. (1984): The nature of intercellular coupling within the preimplantation mouse embryo. *J. Embryol. Exp. Morphol.*, 79:53–76.
65. Selwood, L., and Young, G. J. (1983): Cleavage in vivo and in culture in the dasyurid marsupial *Antechinus stuartii* (Macleay). *J. Morphol.*, 176:43–60.
66. Wimsatt, W. A. (1975): Some comparative aspects of implantation. *Biol. Reprod.*, 12:1–40.
67. Papaioannou, V. E., and Ebert, K. M. (1986): Comparative aspects of embryo manipulation in mammals. In: *Experimental Approaches to Mammalian Embryonic Development,* edited by J. Rossant and R. A. Pedersen, pp. 67–96. Cambridge University Press, Cambridge.
68. Barlow, P., Owen, D. A. J., and Graham, C. (1972): DNA synthesis in the preimplantation mouse embryo. *J. Embryol. Exp. Morphol.*, 27:431–455.
69. Chisholm, J. C., Johnson, M. H., Warren, P. D., Fleming, T. P., and Pickering, S. J. (1985): Developmental variability within and between mouse expanding blastocysts and their ICMs. *J. Embryol. Exp. Morphol.*, 86:311–336.
70. Smith, R., and McLaren, A. (1977): Factors affecting the time of formation of the mouse blastocoel. *J. Embryol. Exp. Morphol.*, 41:79–92.
71. Sawicki, W., and Mystkowska, E. T. (1981): Phorbol ester-mediated modulation of cell proliferation and primary differentiation of mouse preimplantation embryos. *Exp. Cell Res.*, 136:455–458.
72. Alexandre, H. (1979): The utilization of an inhibitor of spermidine and spermine synthesis as a tool for the study of determination of cavitation in the preimplantation mouse embryo. *J. Embryol. Exp. Morphol.*, 53:145–162.
73. Alexandre, H. (1982): Effet de l'inhibition specifique de la replication de l'ADN par l'aphidicoline sur la differentiation primarie de l'oeuf de souris en preimplantation. *C. R. Acad. Sci. (Paris)*, 294:1001–1006.
74. Dean, W. L., and Rossant, J. (1984): Effect of delaying DNA replication on blastocyst formation in the mouse. *Differentiation,* 26:134–137.
75. Spindle, A. I., Nagano, H., and Pedersen, R. A. (1985): Inhibition of DNA replication in preimplantation mouse embryos by aphidicolin. *J. Exp. Zool.*, 235:289–295.
76. Newport, J., and Kirschner, M. (1982): A major developmental transition in early *Xenopus* embryos: II. Control of the onset of transcription. *Cell,* 30:687–696.
77. Mita-Miyazawa, I., Ikegami, S., and Satoh, N. (1985): Histospecific acetylcholinesterase development in the presumptive muscle cells isolated from 16-cell-stage ascidian embryos with respect to the number of DNA replications. *J. Embryol. Exp. Morphol.*, 87: 1–12.
78. Waksmundzka, M., Krysiak, E., Karasiewicz, J., Czolowska, R., and Tarkowski, A. K. (1984): Autonomous cortical activity in mouse eggs controlled by a cytoplasmic clock. *J. Embryol. Exp. Morphol.*, 79:77–96.
79. Masui, Y., and Markert, C. L. (1971): Cytoplasmic control of nuclear behavior during meiotic maturation of frog oocytes. *J. Exp. Zool.*, 117:129–146.
80. Newport, J., and Kirschner, M. (1984): Regulation of the cell cycle during early *Xenopus* development. *Cell,* 37:731–742.
81. Kishimoto, T., Yamazaki, K., Kato, Y., Koide, S. S., and Kanatani, H. (1984): Induction of starfish oocyte maturation by maturation-promoting factor of mouse and surf clam oocytes. *J. Exp. Zool.*, 231:293–295.
82. Sorensen, R. A., Cyert, M. S., and Pedersen, R. A. (1985): Active maturation promoting factor is present in mature mouse oocytes. *J. Cell Biol.*, 100:1637–1640.
83. Balakier, H., and Czolowska, R. (1977): Cytoplasmic control of nuclear maturation in mouse oocytes. *Exp. Cell Res.*, 110:466–469.
84. Balakier, H. (1978): Induction of maturation in small oocytes from sexually immature mice by fusion with meiotic or mitotic cells. *Exp. Cell Res.*, 112:137–141.
85. Balakier, H., and Masui, Y. (1986): Chromosome condensation activity in the cytoplasm of anucleate and nucleate fragments of mouse oocytes. *Dev. Biol.*, 113:155–159.
86. Masui, Y., and Clarke, J. H. (1979): Oocyte maturation. *Int. Rev. Cytol.*, 57:185–283.
87. Berridge, M. J. (1984): Inositol triphosphate and diacylglycerol as second messengers. *Biochem. J.*, 220:345–360.
88. Macara, I. G. (1985): Oncogenes, ions, and phospholipids. *Am. J. Physiol.* (*Cell Physiol.*, 17), 248:C3–C11.
89. Busa, W. B., and Nuccitelli, R. (1984): Metabolic regulation via intracellular pH. *Am. J. Physiol.*, 246:R409–R438.
90. Zwierzchowski, L., Czlonkowska, M., and Guszkiewicz, A. (1986): Effect of polyamine limitation on DNA synthesis and development of mouse preimplantation embryos *in vitro*. *J. Reprod. Fertil.*, 76:115–121.
91. Heby, O. (1981): Role of polyamines in the control of cell proliferation and differentiation. *Differentiation,* 19:1–20.
92. Weiss, P. (1939): *Principles of Development*. Holt, New York.
93. Tarkowski, A. K., and Wroblewska, J. (1967): Development of blastomeres of mouse eggs isolated at the 4- and 8-cell stage. *J. Embryol. Exp. Morphol.*, 18:155–180.
94. Tarkowski, A. K. (1959): Experiments on the development of isolated blastomeres of mouse eggs. *Nature,* 184:1286–1287.
95. Kelly, S. J. (1977): Studies of the developmental potential of 4- and 8-cell stage mouse blastomeres. *J. Exp. Zool.*, 200:365–376.
96. Hillman, N., Sherman, M. I., and Graham, C. F. (1972): The effect of spatial arrangement on cell determination during mouse development. *J. Embryol. Exp. Morphol.*, 28:263–278.
97. Rossant, J., and Vijh, K. M. (1980): Ability of outside cells from preimplantation mouse embryos to form inner cell mass derivatives. *Dev. Biol.*, 76:475–482.
98. Ziomek, C. A., Johnson, M. H., and Handyside, A. H. (1982): The developmental potential of mouse 16-cell blastomeres. *J. Exp. Zool.*, 221:345–355.
99. Stern, M. S. (1972): Experimental studies on the organization of the preimplantation mouse embryo. II. Reaggregation of disaggregated embryos. *J. Embryol. Exp. Morphol.*, 28:255–261.
100. Handyside, A. H. (1978): Time of commitment of inside cells isolated from preimplantation mouse embryos. *J. Embryol. Exp. Morphol.*, 45:37–53.
101. Hogan, B., and Tilly, R. (1978): In vitro development of inner cell masses isolated immunosurgically from mouse blastocysts. II. Inner cell masses from 3.5- to 4.0 day p.c. blastocysts. *J. Embryol. Exp. Morphol.*, 45:107–121.
102. Spindle, A. I. (1978): Trophoblast regeneration by inner cell masses isolated from cultured mouse embryos. *J. Exp. Zool.*, 203:483–489.
103. Rossant, J., and Lis, W. T. (1979): Potential of isolated mouse inner cell masses to form trophectoderm derivatives *in vivo*. *Dev. Biol.*, 70:255–261.
104. Rossant, J. (1975): Investigation of the determinative state of the mouse inner cell mass. II. The fate of isolated inner cell masses transferred to the oviduct. *J. Embryol. Exp. Morphol.*, 33: 991–1001.
105. Nichols, J., and Gardner, R. L. (1984): Heterogeneous differentiation of external cells in individual isolated early mouse inner cell masses in culture. *J. Embryol. Exp. Morphol.*, 80:225–240.
106. Izquierdo, L., and Ortiz, M. E. (1975): Differentiation in the mouse morulae. *Wilhelm Roux's Archiv,* 177:67–74.
107. Daniel, J. C., Jr. (1976): The first potential I.C.M. cell during cleavage of the rabbit ovum. *Wilhelm Roux's Archiv,* 179:249–250.

108. Handyside, A. H. (1981): Immunofluorescence techniques for determining the numbers of inner and outer blastomeres in mouse morulae. *J. Reprod. Immunol.*, 2:339–350.
109. Copp, A. J. (978): Interaction between inner cell mass and trophectoderm of the mouse blastocyst. I. A study of cellular proliferation. *J. Embryol. Exp. Morphol.*, 48:109–125.
110. Garner, W., and McLaren, A. (1974): Cell distribution in chimaeric mouse embryos before implantation. *J. Embryol. Exp. Morphol.*, 32:495–503.
111. Kelly, S. J. (1979): Investigations into the degree of cell mixing that occurs between the 8-cell and the blastocyst stage of mouse development. *J. Exp. Zool.*, 207:121–130.
112. Surani, M. A. H., and Barton, S. C. (1984): Spatial distribution of blastomeres is dependent on cell division order and interactions in mouse morulae. *Dev. Biol.*, 102:335–343.
113. Spindle, A. I. (1982): Cell allocation in preimplantation mouse chimeras. *J. Exp. Zool.*, 219:361–367.
114. Meinecke-Tillmann, S., and Meinecke, B. (1984): Experimental chimaeras—removal of reproductive barrier between sheep and goat. *Nature*, 307:637–638.
115. Surani, M. A. H., Kimbers, S. J., and Barton, S. C. (1981): Differential adhesiveness as a mechanism of cell allocation to inner cell mass and trophectoderm in the mouse blastocyst. In: *Culture Techniques. Applicability for Studies on Prenatal Differentiation and Toxicity*, edited by D. Neubert and H.-J. Merker, pp. 397–412. W. de Gruyter, Berlin.
116. Kimber, S. J., Surani, M. A. H., and Barton, S. C. (1982): Interactions of blastomeres suggest changes in cell surface adhesiveness during the formation of inner cell mass and trophectoderm in the preimplantation mouse embryo. *J. Embryol. Exp. Morphol.*, 58: 231–249.
117. Handyside, A. H. (1980): Distribution of antibody- and lectin-binding sites on dissociated blastomeres from mouse morulae: evidence of polarization at compaction. *J. Embryol. Exp. Morphol.*, 60:99–116.
118. Ziomek, C. A., and Johnson, M. H. (1980): Cell surface interaction induces polarization of mouse 8-cell blastomeres at compaction. *Cell*, 21:935–942.
119. Ziomek, C. A., and Johnson, M. H. (1982): The roles of phenotype and position in guiding the fate of 16-cell mouse blastomeres. *Dev. Biol.*, 91:440–447.
120. Johnson, M. H., and Ziomek, C. A. (1983): Cell interactions influence the fate of mouse blastomeres undergoing the transition from the 16- to the 32-cell stage. *Dev. Biol.*, 95:211–218.
121. Pedersen, R. A., Wu, K., and Balakier, H. (1986): Origin of the inner cell mass in mouse embryos: cell lineage analysis by microinjection. *Dev. Biol.*, 117:581–595.
122. Cruz, Y. P., and Pedersen, R. A. (1985): Cell fate in the polar trophectoderm of mouse blastocysts as studied by microinjection of cell lineage tracers. *Dev. Biol.*, 112:73–83.
123. Pedersen, R. A., and Spindle, A. I. (1980): Role of the blastocoel microenvironment in early mouse embryo differentiation. *Nature*, 284:550–552.
124. Johnson, M. H., Pratt, H. M. P., and Handyside, A. H. (1981): The generation and recognition of positional information in the preimplantation mouse embryo. In: *Cellular and Molecular Aspects of Implantation*, edited by S. R. Glasser and D. W. Bullock, pp. 55–74. Plenum, New York.
125. Johnson, M. H., and Maro, B. (1986): Time and space in the mouse early embryo: a cell biological approach to cell diversification. In: *Experimental Approaches to Mammalian Embryonic Development*, edited by J. Rossant and R. A. Pedersen, pp. 35–65. Cambridge University Press, Cambridge.
126. Rossant, J. (1977): Cell commitment in early rodent development. In: *Development in Mammals, Vol. 2*, edited by M. H. Johnson, pp. 119–150. North-Holland, Amsterdam.
127. Beddington, R. (1986): Analysis of tissue fate and prospective potency in the egg cylinder. In: *Experimental Approaches to Mammalian Embryonic Development*, edited by J. Rossant and R. A. Pedersen, pp. 121–147. Cambridge University Press, Cambridge.
128. Gardner, R. L., Papaioannou, V. E., and Barton, S. C. (1973): Origin of the ectoplacental cone and secondary giant cells in mouse blastocysts reconstituted from isolated trophoblast and inner cell mass. *J. Embryol. Exp. Morphol.*, 30:561–572.
129. Papaioannou, V. E. (1982): Lineage analysis of inner cell mass and trophectoderm using microsurgically reconstituted mouse blastocysts. *J. Embryol. Exp. Morphol.*, 68:199–209.
130. Rossant, J., and Croy, B. A. (1985): Genetic identification of tissue of origin of cellular populations within the mouse placenta. *J. Embryol. Exp. Morphol.*, 86:177–189.
131. Johnson, M. H. (1979): Molecular differentiation of inside cells and inner cell masses isolated from the preimplantation mouse embryo. *J. Embryol. Exp. Morphol.*, 53:335–344.
132. Rossant, J., Gardner, R. L., and Alexandre, H. L. (1978): Investigation of the potency of cells from the postimplantation mouse embryo by blastocyst injections. A preliminary report. *J. Embryol. Exp. Morphol.*, 48:239–247.
133. Copp, A. J. (1979): Interaction between inner cell mass and trophectoderm of the mouse blastocyst. II. Fate of the polar trophectoderm. *J. Embryol. Exp. Morphol.*, 51:109–120.
134. Rossant, J. (1986): Development of extraembryonic cell lineages in the mouse embryo. In: *Experimental Approaches to Mammalian Embryonic Development*, edited by J. Rossant and R. A. Pedersen, pp. 97–120. Cambridge University Press, Cambridge.
135. Gardner, R. L., and Rossant, J. (1979): Investigation of the fate of 4.5 day post-coitum mouse inner cell mass cells by blastocyst injection. *J. Embryol. Exp. Morphol.*, 52:141–152.
136. Gardner, R. L. (1982): Investigation of cell lineage and differentiation in the extraembryonic endoderm of the mouse embryo. *J. Embryol. Exp. Morphol.*, 68:175–198.
137. Hogan, B. L. M., and Tilly, R. (1981): Cell interactions and endoderm differentiation in cultured mouse embryos. *J. Embryol. Exp. Morphol.*, 62:379–394.
138. Lawson, K. A., Meneses, J. J., and Pedersen, R. A. (1986): Cell fate and cell lineage in the endoderm of the presomite mouse embryo, studied with an intracellular tracer. *Dev. Biol.*, 115:325–329.
139. Monk, M., and Harper, M. I. (1979): Sequential X chromosome inactivation coupled with cellular differentiation in early mouse embros. *Nature*, 281:311–313.
140. Rossant, J. (1984): Somatic cell lineages in mammalian chimeras. In: *Chimeras in Developmental Biology*, edited by N. LeDouarin and A. McLaren, pp. 89–109. Academic Press, Orlando, Fl.
141. Gardner, R. L., Lyon, M. F., Evans, E. P., and Burtenshaw, M. D. (1985): Clonal analysis of X-chromosome inactivation and the origin of the germ line in the mouse embryo. *J. Embryol. Exp. Morphol.*, 88:349–363.
142. Gardner, R. L. (1985): Regeneration of endoderm from primitive ectoderm in the mouse embryo: fact or artifact? *J. Embryol. Exp. Morphol.*, 88:303–326.
143. Pedersen, R. A., Spindle, A. I., and Wiley, L. M. (1977): Regeneration of endoderm by ectoderm isolated from mouse blastocysts. *Nature*, 270:435–437.
144. Dziadek, M. (1979): Cell differentiation in isolated inner cell masses of mouse blastocysts *in vitro:* onset of specific gene expression. *J. Embryol. Exp. Morphol.*, 53:367–379.
145. Atienza-Samols, S. B., and Sherman, M. I. (1979): *In vitro* development of core cells of the inner cell mass of the mouse blastocyst: effects of conditioned medium. *J. Exp. Zool.*, 208:67–71.
146. Svajger, A., Levak-Svajger, B., and Skreb, N. (1986): Rat embryonic ectoderm as renal isograft. *J. Embryol. Exp. Morphol.*, 94:1–27.
147. Grobstein, C. (1951): Intraocular growth and differentiation of the mouse embryonic shield implanted directly and following in vitro cultivation. *J. Exp. Zool.*, 116:501–525.
148. Grobstein, C. (1952): Intraocular growth and differentiation of clusters of mouse embryonic shields cultured with and without primitive endoderm and in the presence of possible inductors. *J. Exp. Zool.*, 119:355–380.
149. Levak-Svajger, B., and Svajger, A. (1971): Differentiation of endodermal tissues in homografts of primitive ectoderm from two-layered rat embryonic shields. *Experientia*, 27:683–684.
150. Skreb, N., and Svajger, A. (1975): Experimental teratomas in rats. In: *Teratomas and Differentiation*, edited by D. Solter, pp. 83–97. Academic Press, London.
151. Diwan, S. B., and Stevens, L. C. (1976): Development of teratomas from ectoderm of mouse egg cylinders. *J. Natl. Cancer Inst.*, 57:937–942.

152. Beddington, R. S. P. (1983): Histogenic and neoplastic potential of different regions of the mouse embryonic egg cylinder. *J. Embryol. Exp. Morphol.*, 75:189–204.
153. Levak-Svajger, B., and Svajger, A. (1974): Investigation of the origin of definitive endoderm in the rat embryo. *J. Embryol. Exp. Morphol.*, 32:445–459.
154. Solter, D., and Damjanov, I. (1973): Explantation of extraembryonic parts of 7d mouse egg cylinders. *Experientia,* 29:701–703.
155. Skreb, N., Svajger, A., and Levak-Svajger, B. (1976): Developmental potentialities of the germ layers. In: *Embryogenesis in Mammals,* CIBA Foundation Symposium 40 (new series), pp. 27–39. Elsevier, Amsterdam.
156. Svajger, A., Levak-Svajger, B., Kostovic-Knezevic, L., and Bradamante, Z. (1981): Morphogenetic behaviour of the rat embryonic ectoderm as a renal homograft. *J. Embryol. Exp. Morphol. [Suppl.],* 65:243–267.
157. Tam, P. P. L. (1984): The histogenetic capacity of tissues in the caudal end of the embryonic axis of the mouse. *J. Embryol. Exp. Morphol.*, 82:253–266.
158. Snow, M. H. L. (1981): Autonomous development of parts isolated from primitive-streak-stage mouse embryos. Is development clonal? *J. Embryol. Exp. Morphol. [Suppl.],* 65:269–287.
159. Ozdzenski, W. (1967): Observations on the origin of the primordial germ cells in the mouse. *Zool. Pol.*, 17:367–379.
160. Rosenquist, G. C. (1966): A radioautographic study of labeled grafts in the chick blastoderm. Development from primitive-streak stages to stage 12. *Carnegie Inst. Wash. Contrib. Embryol.*, 38:71–110.
161. Beddington, R. S. P. (1981): An autoradiographic analysis of the potency of embryonic ectoderm in the 8th day postimplantation mouse embryo. *J. Embryol. Exp. Morphol.*, 64:87–104.
162. Beddington, R. S. P. (1982): An autoradiographic analysis of tissue potency in different regions of the embryonic ectoderm during gastrulation in the mouse. *J. Embryol. Exp. Morphol.*, 69:265–285.
163. Copp, A. J., Roberts, H. M., and Polani, P. E. (1986): Chimaerism of primordial germ cells in the early postimplantation mouse embryo following microsurgical grafting of posterior primitive streak cells *in vitro*. *J. Embryol. Exp. Morphol.*, 15:95–115.
164. Soriano, P., and Jaenisch, R. (1986): Retroviruses as probes for mammalian development: allocation of cells to the somatic and germ cell lineages. *Cell,* 46:19–29.
165. Wilkie, T. M., Brinster, R. L., and Palmiter, R. D. (1986): Germline and somatic mosaicism in transgenic mice. *Dev. Biol.*, 118:9–18.
166. Russell, L. B., and Russell, W. L. (1954): Analysis of the changing radiation response of the developing mouse embryo. *J. Cell. Comp. Physiol. [Suppl. 1],* 43:103–147.
167. Pedersen, R. A. (1987): Analysis of cell lineage during early mouse embryogenesis. In: *Developmental Toxicology: Mechanisms and Risk,* edited by J. A. McLachlan, R. M. Pratt, and C. L. Markert. Cold Spring Harbor Laboratory, Cold Spring Harbor, N.Y. (*in press*).
168. Gardner, R. L. (1978): The relation between cell lineage and differentiation in the early mouse embryo. In: *Genetic Mosaics and Cell Differentiation,* edited by W. J. Gehring, pp. 205–241. Springer-Verlag, Berlin.
169. Beddington, R. S. P. (1983): The origin of the foetal tissues during gastrulation in the rodent. In: *Development in Mammals, Vol. 5,* edited by M. H. Johnson, pp. 1–32. Elsevier, Amsterdam.
170. Sanes, J. R., Rubenstein, J. L. R., and Nicolas, J.-F. (1986): Use of a recombinant retrovirus to study post-implantation cell lineage in mouse embryos. *EMBO J.*, 5:3133–3142.
171. Rossant, J. (1987): Cell lineage analysis in mammalian embryogenesis. *Curr. Top. Dev. Biol.*, (*in press*).
172. Johnson, M. H., Handyside, A. H., and Braude, P. R. (1977): Control mechanisms in early mammalian development. In: *Development in Mammals, Vol. 2,* edited by M. H. Johnson, pp. 67–97. North-Holland, Amsterdam.
173. Johnson, M. H. (1981): The molecular and cellular basis of preimplantation mouse development. *Biol. Rev.*, 56:463–498.
174. Schultz, G. A., Clough, J. R., Braude, P. R., Pelham, H. R. B., and Johnson, M. H. (1981): A reexamination of messenger RNA populations in the preimplantation mouse embryo. In: *Cellular and Molecular Aspects of Implantation,* edited by S. R. Glasser and D. W. Bullock, pp. 137–154. Plenum, New York.
175. Schultz, G. A. (1986): Utilization of genetic information in the preimplantation mouse embryo. In: *Experimental Approaches to Mammalian Embryonic Development,* edited by J. Rossant and R. A. Pedersen, pp. 239–265. Cambridge University Press, Cambridge.
176. Piko, L., and Clegg, K. B. (1982): Quantitative changes in total RNA, total poly(A), and ribosomes in early mouse embryos. *Dev. Biol.*, 89:362–378.
177. Clegg, K. B., and Piko, L. (1983): Poly(A) length, cytoplasmic adenylation, and synthesis of polyA + RNA in early mouse embryos. *Dev. Biol.*, 95:331–341.
178. Giebelhaus, D. H., Weitlauf, H. M., and Schultz, G. A. (1985): Actin mRNA content in normal and delayed implanting mouse embryos. *Dev. Biol.*, 107:407–413.
179. Graves, R. A., Marzluff, W. F., Giebelhaus, D. H., and Schultz, G. A. (1985): Quantitative and qualitative changes in histone gene expression during early mouse development. *Proc. Natl. Acad. Sci. USA,* 82:5685–5689.
180. Braude, P. R., Pelham, H., Flach, G., and Lobatto, R. (1979): Post-transcriptional control in the early mouse embryo. *Nature,* 282:102–105.
181. van Blerkom, J. (1981): The structural relation and post-translational modification of stage-specific proteins synthesized during early preimplantation development in the mouse. *Proc. Natl. Acad. Sci. USA,* 78:7629–7633.
182. van Blerkom, J. (1985): Post-translational regulation of early development in the mammal. In: *Differentiation and Proliferations,* edited by C. Venizale, pp. 67–86. Van Nostrand Reinhold, New York.
183. van Blerkom, J., and Runner, M. N. (1984): Mitochondrial reorganization during resumption of arrested meiosis in the mouse oocyte. *Am. J. Anat.*, 171:335–355.
184. Howlett, S. K., and Bolton, V. N. (1985): Sequence and regulation of morphological and molecular events during the first cell cycle of mouse embryogenesis. *J. Embryol. Exp. Morphol.*, 87:175–206.
185. Kaplan, G., Jelinek, W. R., and Bachvarova, R. (1985): Repetitive sequence transcripts and U1 RNA in mouse oocytes and eggs. *Dev. Biol.*, 109:15–24.
186. Forbes, D. J., Kornberg, T. B., and Kirschner, M. W. (1983): Small nuclear RNA transcription and ribonucleoprotein assembly in early *Xenopus* development. *J. Cell Biol.*, 97:62–72.
187. Zeller, R., Nyffenegger, T., and DeRobertis, E. M. (1983): Nucleocytoplasmic distribution of snRNPs and stockpiled snRNA-binding proteins during oogenesis and early development in *Xenopus laevis*. *Cell,* 32:425–434.
188. Ebert, K. M., and Brinster, R. L. (1983): Rabbit α-globin messenger RNA translation by the mouse ovum. *J. Embryol. Exp. Morphol.*, 74:159–168.
189. Brinster, R. L., Wiebold, J. L., and Brunner, S. (1976): Protein metabolism in preimplanted mouse ova. *Dev. Biol.*, 51:215–224.
190. Merz, E. A., Brinster, R. L., Brunner, S., and Chen, H. Y. (1981): Protein degradation during preimplantation development of the mouse. *J. Reprod. Fertil.*, 61:415–418.
191. Bachvarova, R., and De Leon, V. (1977): Stored and polysomal ribosomes of mouse ova. *Dev. Biol.*, 58:248–254.
192. Kidder, G. M., and Conlon, R. A. (1985): Utilization of cytoplasmic poly(A) + RNA for protein synthesis in preimplantation mouse embryos. *J. Embryol. Exp. Morphol.*, 89:223–234.
193. Brinster, R. L., Chen, H. Y., Trumbauer, M. E., and Avarbock, M. R. (1980): Translation of rabbit globin messenger RNA by the mouse ovum. *Nature,* 283:499–501.
194. Petzoldt, U., Hoppe, P. C., and Illmensee, K. (1980): Protein synthesis in enucleated fertilized and unfertilized mouse eggs. *Wilhelm Roux's Arch. Dev. Biol.*, 189:215–219.
195. Flach, G., Johnson, M. H., Braude, P. R., Taylor, R. A. S., and Bolton, V. N. (1982): The transition from maternal to embryonic control in the 2-cell mouse embryo. *EMBO J.*, 1:681–686.
196. Bolton, V. N., Oades, P. J., and Johnson, M. H. (1984): The relationship between cleavage, DNA replication, and gene expression in the mouse 2-cell embryo. *J. Embryol. Exp. Morphol.*, 79:139–163.
197. Bensaude, O., Babinet, C., Morange, M., and Jacob, F. (1983): Heat shock proteins, first major products of zygotic gene activity in the mouse embryo. *Nature,* 305:331–333.
198. Clegg, K. B., and Piko, L. (1983): Quantitive aspects of RNA synthesis and polyadenylation in 1-cell and 2-cell mouse embryos. *J. Embryol. Exp. Morphol.*, 74:169–182.

199. Wudl, L., and Chapman, V. (1976): The expression of β-glucuronidase during preimplantation development of mouse embryos. *Dev. Biol.*, 48:104–109.
200. Sawicki, J. A., Magnuson, T., and Epstein, C. J. (1982): Evidence for expression of the paternal genome in the two-cell mouse embryo. *Nature*, 294:450–451.
201. Young, R. J., and Sweeny, K. (1979): Adenylation and ADP-ribosylation in the mouse 1-cell embryo. *J. Embryol. Exp. Morphol.*, 49:139–152.
202. Young, R. J. (1977): Appearance of 7-methylguanosine-5′-phosphate in the RNA of 1-cell embryos three hours after fertilization. *Biochem. Biophys. Res. Commun.*, 76:32–39.
203. Schultz, G. A., Clough, J. R., and Johnson, M. H. (1980): Presence of cap structures in messenger RNA of mouse eggs. *J. Embryol. Exp. Morphol.*, 56:139–156.
204. Young, R. J., Sweeny, K., and Bedford, J. M. (1978): Uridine and guanosine incorporation by the mouse one-cell embryo. *J. Embryol. Exp. Morphol.*, 44:133–148.
205. Braude, P. R. (1979): Control of protein synthesis during blastocyst formation in the mouse. *Dev. Biol.*, 68:440–452.
206. Braude, P. R. (1979): Time-dependent effects of α-amanitin on blastocyst formation in the mouse. *J. Embryol. Exp. Morphol.*, 52:193–202.
207. Kidder, G. M., and McLachlin, J. R. (1985): Timing of transcription and protein synthesis underlying morphogenesis in preimplantation mouse embryos. *Dev. Biol.*, 112:265–275.
208. van Blerkom, J., Barton, S. C., and Johnson, M. H. (1976): Molecular differentiation in the preimplantation mouse embryo. *Nature*, 259:319–321.
209. Handyside, A. H., and Johnson, M. H. (1978): Temporal and spatial patterns of the synthesis of tissue-specific polypeptides in the preimplantation mouse embryo. *J. Embryol. Exp. Morphol.*, 44:191–199.
210. Howe, C. C., Gmur, R., and Solter, D. (1980): Cytoplasmic and nuclear protein synthesis during *in vitro* differentiation of murine ICM and embryonal carcinoma cells. *Dev. Biol.*, 74:351–363.
211. Green, M. C. (1981): In: *Genetic Variants and Strains of the Laboratory Mouse*, edited by M. C. Green. Gustav Fischer, Stuttgart.
212. McLaren, A. (1976): Genetics of the early mouse embryo. *Annu. Rev. Genet.*, 10:361–388.
213. Magnuson, T., and Epstein, C. J. (1981): Genetic control of very early mammalian development. *Biol. Rev.*, 56:369–408.
214. Magnuson, T. (1983): Genetic abnormalities and early mammalian development. In: *Development in Mammals, Vol. 5*, edited by M. H. Johnson, pp. 209–249. Elsevier, Amsterdam.
215. Magnuson, T. (1986): Mutations and chromosomal abnormalities: How are they useful for studying genetic control of early mammalian development? In: *Experimental Approaches to Mammalian Embryonic Development*, edited by J. Rossant and R. A. Pedersen, pp. 437–474. Cambridge University Press, Cambridge.
216. Pedersen, R. A., and Spindle, A. I. (1981): Cellular and genetic analysis of mouse blastocyst development. In: *Cellular and Molecular Aspects of Implantation*, edited by S. R. Glasser and D. W. Bullock. pp. 91–108. Plenum, New York.
217. Gluecksohn-Waelsch, S. (1979): Genetic control of morphogenetic and biochemical differentiation: lethal albino deletions in the mouse. *Cell*, 16:225–237.
218. Bennett, D. (1975): The *T* locus of the mouse. *Cell*, 6:441–454.
219. Bennett, D. (1980): The *T*-complex in the mouse: an assessment after 50 years of study. *Harvey Lect.*, 74:1–21.
220. Silvers, L. M. (1985): Mouse *t* haplotypes. *Annu. Rev. Genet.*, 19:179–208.
221. Lewis, S. E. (1978): Developmental analysis of lethal effects of homozygosity for the c^{25H} deletion in the mouse. *Dev. Biol.*, 65:553–557.
222. Nadijcka, M. D., Hillman, N., and Gluecksohn-Waelsch, S. (1979): Ultrastructural studies of lethal c^{25H}/c^{25H} mouse embryos. *J. Embryol. Exp. Morphol.*, 52:1–11.
223. Hillman, N., and Hillman, R. (1975): Ultrastructural studies of t^{w32}/t^{w32} mouse embryos. *J. Embryol. Exp. Morphol.*, 33:685–695.
224. Wakasugi, N. (1973): Studies on fertility of DDK mice: reciprocal crosses between DDK and C57BL/6J strains and experimental transplantation of the ovary. *J. Reprod. Fertil.*, 33:283–291.
225. Paterson, H. F. (1980): In vivo and in vitro studies on the early embryonic lethal tail-short (*Ts*) in the mouse. *J. Exp. Zool.*, 211:247–256.
226. Babiarz, B. (1983): Deletion mapping of the *T/t* complex: evidence for a second region of critical embryonic genes. *Dev. Biol.*, 95:342–351.
227. Papaioannou, V. E., and Mardon, H. (1983): Lethal nonagouti (a^x): description of a second embryonic lethal at the agouti locus. *Dev. Genet.*, 4:21–29.
228. Papaioannou, V. E., and Gardner, R. L. (1979): Investigation of the lethal yellow A^y/A^y embryo using mouse chimaeras. *J. Emryol. Exp. Morphol.*, 52:153–163.
229. Paterson, H. F. (1979): In vivo and in vitro studies on the early embryonic lethal oligosyndactylism (*Os*) in the mouse. *J. Embryol. Exp. Morphol.*, 52:115–125.
230. Magnuson, T., and Epstein, C. J. (1984): Oligosyndactyly: a lethal mutation in the mouse that results in mitotic arrest very early in development. *Cell*, 38:823–833.
231. Spiegelman, M., Artzt, K., and Bennett, D. (1976): Embryological study of a *T/t* locus mutation (t^{w73}) affecting trophectoderm development. *J. Embryol. Exp. Morphol.*, 36:373–381.
232. Babiarz, B., Garrisi, G. J., and Bennett, D. (1982): Genetic analysis of the t^{w73} haplotype of the mouse using deletion mutations: evidence for a parasitic lethal mutation. *Genet. Res.*, 39:111–120.
233. Guenet, J., Condamine, H., Gaillard, J., and Jacob, F. (1980): t^{wPa-1}, t^{wPa-2}, t^{wPa-3}: three new *t*-haplotypes in the mouse. *Genet. Res.*, 36:211–217.
234. Lewis, S. E., Turchin, H. A., and Gluecksohn-Waelsch, S. (1976): The developmental analysis of an embryonic lethal (c^{6H}) in the mouse. *J. Embryol. Exp. Morphol.*, 36:363–371.
235. Nadijcka, M. D., and Hillman, N. (1975): Autoradiographic studies of t^n/t^n mouse embryo. *J. Embryol. Exp. Morphol.*, 33:725–730.
236. Gluecksohn-Schoenheimer, S. (1940): The effect of an early lethal (t^0) in the house mouse. *Genetics*, 25:391–400.
237. Nusslein-Volhard, C., Wieschaus, E., and Kluding, H. (1984): Mutations affecting the pattern of the larval cuticle of *Drosophila melanogaster*. I. Zygotic loci on the second chromosome. *Wilhelm Roux's Arch. Dev. Biol.*, 193:267–282.
238. Sternberg, P. W., and Horvitz, H. R. (1984): The genetic control of cell lineage during nematode development. *Annu. Rev. Genet.*, 18:489–524.
239. Silvers, L. M., Uman, J., Danska, J., and Garrels, J. I. (1983): A diversified set of testicular cell proteins specified by genes within the mouse *t* complex. *Cell*, 35:35–45.
240. Copeland, N. G., Jenkins, N. A., and Lee, B. K. (1983): Association of the lethal yellow (A^y) coat-color mutation with an ecotropic murine leukemia virus genome. *Proc. Natl. Acad. Sci. USA*, 80:247–249.
241. Epstein, C. J., Smith, S., Travis, B., and Tucker, G. (1978): Both X-chromosomes function before visible X-chromosome inactivation in female mouse embryos. *Nature*, 274:500–502.
242. Kaufman, M. H., and Gardner, R. L. (1974): Diploid and haploid mouse parthenogenetic development following *in vitro* activation and embryo transfer. *J. Embryol. Exp. Morphol.*, 31:635–642.
243. Kaufman, M. H., and Sachs, L. (1975): The early development of haploid and aneuploid parthenogenetic embryos. *J. Embryol. Exp. Morphol.*, 34:645–655.
244. Modlinski, J. A. (1975): Haploid mouse embryos obtained by microsurgical removal of one pronucleus. *J. Embryol. Exp. Morphol.*, 33:897–905.
245. Tarkowski, A. K. (1977): In vitro development of haploid mouse embryos produced by bisection of one-cell fertilized eggs. *J. Embryol. Exp. Morphol.*, 38:187–202.
246. Tarkowski, A. K., and Rossant, J. (1976): Haploid mouse blastocysts developed from bisected zygotes. *Nature*, 259:663–665.
247. Luthardt, F. W. (1976): Cytogenetic analysis of oocytes and early preimplantation embryos from XO mice. *Dev. Biol.*, 54:73–81.
248. Burgoyne, P. S., and Biggers, J. D. (1976): The consequences of X-dosage deficiency in the germ line: impaired development in vitro of preimplantation embryos from XO mice. *Dev. Biol.*, 51:109–117.
249. Epstein, C. J. (1986): *The Consequences of Chromosome Imbalance: Principles, Mechanisms, Models*. Cambridge University Press, London.
250. Baranov, V. S. (1983): Chromosomal control of early embryonic development in mice. I. Experiments on embryos with autosomal monosomy. *Genetica*, 61:165–177.
251. Magnuson, T., Debrot, S., Dimpfl, J., Zweig, A., Zamora, T., and Epstein, C. J. (1985): The early lethality of autosomal monosomy in the mouse. *J. Exp. Zool.*, 236:353–360.

252. Epstein, C. J., Smith, S. A., Zamora, T., Sawicki, J. A., Magnuson, T. R., and Cox, D. R. (1982): Production of viable adult trisomy 17 ↔ diploid mouse chimeras. *Proc. Natl. Acad. Sci. USA,* 79:4376–4380.
253. Cox, D. R., Smith, S. A., Epstein, L. B., and Epstein, C. J. (1984): Mouse trisomy 16 as an animal model of human trisomy 21 (Down syndrome): production of viable trisomy 16 ↔ diploid mouse chimeras. *Dev. Biol.,* 101:416–424.
254. Epstein, C. J., Smith, S. A., and Cox, D. R. (1984): Production and properties of mouse trisomy 15 ↔ diploid chimeras. *Dev. Genet.,* 4:159–165.
255. Boue, J., Boue, A., and Lazar, P. (1975): Retrospective and prospective epidemiological studies of 1500 karyotyped spontaneous human abortions. *Teratology,* 12:11–26.
256. Hassold, T. J., Matsuyama, A., Newlands, J. M., Matsuura, J. S., Jacobs, P. A., Manuel, B., and Tsuei, J. (1978): A cytogenetic study of spontaneous abortions in Hawaii. *Ann. Hum. Genet.,* 41:443–454.
257. Markert, C. L. (1982): Parthenogenesis, homozygosity, and cloning in mammals. *J. Hered.,* 73:390–397.
258. Bode, V. C. (1984): Ethylnitrosourea mutagenesis and the isolation of mutant alleles for specific genes located in the *t*-region of mouse chromosome 17. *Genetics,* 108:457.
259. Jenkins, N. A., Copeland, N. G., Taylor, B. A., and Lee, B. K. (1981): Dilute (*d*) coat colour mutation of DBA/2J mice is associated with the site of integration of an ecotropic MuLV genome. *Nature,* 293:370–374.
260. Copeland, N. G., Hutchison, K. W., and Jenkins, N. A. (1983): Excision of the DBA ecotropic provirus in dilute coat-color revertants of mice occurs by homologous recombination involving the viral LTRs. *Cell,* 33:379–387.
261. Jaenisch, R., Harbers, K., Schnieke, A., Lohler, J., Chumakov, I., Jahner, D., Grotkopp, D., and Hoffman, E. (1983): Germline integration of Moloney murine leukemia virus at the Mov 13 locus leads to recessive lethal mutation and early embryonic death. *Cell,* 32:209–216.
262. Schnieke, A., Harbers, K., and Jaenisch, R. (1983): Embryonic lethal mutation in mice induced by retrovirus insertion into the $\alpha 1$(I) collagen gene. *Nature,* 304:315–320.
263. Harbers, K., Kuehn, M., Delius, H., and Jaenisch, R. (1984): Insertion of retrovirus into the first intron of $\alpha 1$(I) collagen gene leads to embryonic lethal mutation in mice. *Proc. Natl. Acad. Sci. USA,* 81:1504–1508.
264. Breindle, M., Harbers, K., and Jaenisch, R. (1984): Retrovirus-induced lethal mutation in collagen 1 gene is associated with altered chromatin structure. *Cell,* 38:9–16.
265. Lohler, J., Timpl, R., and Jaenisch, R. (1984): Embryonic lethal mutation in mouse collagen 1 gene causes rupture of blood vessels and is associated with erythropoietic and mesenchymal cell death. *Cell,* 38:597–607.
266. Kratochwil, K., Dziadek, M., Lohler, J., Harbers, K., and Jaenisch, R. (1986): Normal epithelial branching morphogenesis in the absence of collagen 1. *Dev. Biol.,* 117:596–606.
267. Reik, W., Weiher, H., and Jaenisch, R. (1985): Replication competent Moloney leukemia virus carrying a bacterial suppressor tRNA gene: selective cloning of proviral and flanking host sequences. *Proc. Natl. Acad. Sci. USA,* 82:1141–1145.
268. Wagner, E. F., Covarrubias, L., Stewart, T. A., and Mintz, B. (1983): Prenatal lethalities in mice homozygous for human growth hormone gene sequences integrated in the germ line. *Cell,* 35:647–655.
269. Palmiter, R. D., Wilkie, T. M., Chen, H. Y., and Brinster, R. L. (1984): Transmission distortion and mosaicism in an unusual transgenic mouse pedigree. *Cell,* 36:869–877.
270. Mahon, K. A., Overbeek, P. A., and Westphal, H. (1986): Dominant pre-natal lethality in a transgenic mouse line is associated with a chromosomal translocation. *J. Cell Biol.,* 103:146a.
271. Woychik, R. P., Stewart, T. A., Davis, L. G., D'Eustachio, P., and Leder, P. (1985): An inherited limb deformity created by insertional mutagenesis in a transgenic mouse. *Nature,* 318:36–40.
272. Izant, J. G., and Weintraub, H. (1984): Inhibition of thymidine kinase gene expression by anti-sense RNA: a molecular approach to genetic analysis. *Cell,* 36:1007–1015.
273. Melton, D. (1985): Injected anti-sense RNAs specifically block messenger RNA translation in vivo. *Proc. Natl. Acad. Sci. USA,* 82:144–148.
274. Melton, D. A., and Rebogliati, M. R. (1986): Anti-sense RNA injections in fertilized eggs as a test for the function of localized mRNAs. *J. Embryol. Exp. Morphol. [Suppl.],* 97:211–221.
275. Rosenberg, U. B., Preiss, A., Seifert, E., Jackle, H., and Knipple, D. C. (1985): Production of phenocopies by Kruppel antisense RNA injection into *Drosophila* embryos. *Nature,* 313:703–706.
276. Kaufman, M. H. (1981): Parthenogenesis: A system facilitating understanding of factors that influence early mammalian development. In: *Progress in Anatomy,* Vol. 1, edited by R. J. Harrison and R. L. Holmes, pp. 1–34. Cambridge University Press, London.
277. Mittwoch, U. (1978): Parthenogenesis. *J. Med. Genet.,* 15:165–181.
278. Kaufman, M. H. (1983): *Early Mammalian Development: Parthenogenetic Studies.* Cambridge University Press, London.
279. Markert, C. L., and Seidel, G. E., Jr. (1981): Parthenogenesis, identical twins and cloning in mammals. In: *New Technologies in Animal Breeding,* edited by B. G. Brackett, G. E. Seidel, Jr., and S. M. Seidel, pp. 181–200. Academic Press, New York.
280. Modlinski, J. A. (1981): The fate of inner cell mass and trophectoderm nuclei transplanted to fertilized mouse eggs. *Nature,* 292:342–343.
281. Illmensee, K., and Hoppe, P. C. (1981): Nuclear transplantation in *Mus musculus:* developmental potential of nuclei from preimplantation embryos. *Cell,* 23:9–18.
282. Hoppe, P. C., and Illmensee, K. (1982): Full term development after transplantation of parthenogenetic embryonic nuclei into fertilized mouse eggs. *Proc. Natl. Acad. Sci. USA,* 79:1912–1916.
283. Surani, M. A. H. (1986): Evidences and consequences of differences between maternal and paternal genomes during embryogenesis in the mouse. In: *Experimental Approaches to Mammalian Embryonic Development,* edited by J. Rossant and R. A. Pedersen, pp. 401–435. Cambridge University Press, Cambridge.
284. Surani, M. A. H., Reik, W., Norris, M. L., and Barton, S. C. (1986): Influence of germline modifications of homologous chromosomes on mouse development. *J. Embryol. Exp. Morphol., [Suppl.],* 97:123–136.
285. Stevens, L. C. (1975): Teratocarcinogenesis and spontaneous parthenogenesis in mice. In: *Developmental Biology of Reproduction,* edited by C. L. Markert and J. Papaconstantinou, pp. 13–106. Academic Press, New York.
286. Graham, C. F. (1974): The production of parthenogenetic mammalian embryos and their use in biological research. *Biol. Rev.,* 49:399–422.
287. Kaufman, M. H., Barton, S. C., and Surani, M. A. H. (1977): Normal post-implantation development of mouse parthenogenetic embryos to the forelimb bud stage. *Nature (Lond.),* 265:53–55.
288. Stevens, L. C., Varnum, D. S., and Eicher, E. M. (1977): Viable chimaeras produced from normal and parthenogenetic mouse embryos. *Nature (Lond.),* 269:515.
289. Surani, M. A. H., Barton, S. C., and Kaufman, M. H. (1977): Development to term of chimaeras between diploid parthenogenetic and fertilized embryos. *Nature (Lond.),* 270:601–602.
290. Markert, C. L. and Petters, R. M. (1977): Homozygous mouse embryos produced by microsurgery. *J. Exp. Zool.,* 201:295–302.
291. Hoppe, P. C., and Illmensee, K. (1977): Microsurgically produced homozygous-diploid uniparental mice. *Proc. Natl. Acad. Sci. USA,* 74:5657–5661.
292. Modlinski, J. A. (1980): Preimplantation development of microsurgically obtained haploid and homozygous diploid mouse embryos and effects of pretreatment with cytochalasin B on enucleated eggs. *J. Embryol. Exp. Morphol.,* 60:153–161.
293. McGrath, J., and Solter, D. (1983): Nuclear transplantation in the mouse embryo by microsurgery and cell fusion. *Science,* 220: 1300–1303.
294. Mann, J. R., and Lovell-Badge, R. H. (1984): Inviability of parthenogenones determined by pronuclei, not egg cytoplasm. *Nature (Lond.),* 310:66–67.
295. McGrath, J., and Solter, D. (1984): Completion of mouse embryogenesis requires both maternal and paternal genomes. *Cell,* 37:179–183.
296. Surani, M. A. H., Barton, S. C., and Norris, M. L. (1984): Development of reconstituted mouse eggs suggests imprinting of the genome during gametogenesis. *Nature (Lond.),* 308:548–550.
297. Anderegg, C., and Markert, C. L. (1986): Successful rescue of microsurgically produced homozygous, uniparental mouse embryos

via production of aggregation chimeras. *Proc. Natl. Acad. ci. USA,* 83:6509–6513.

298. Barton, S. C., Surani, M. A. H., and Norris, M. L. (1984): Role of paternal and maternal genomes in mouse development. *Nature (Lond.)*, 311:374–376.
299. Barton, S. C., Adams, C. A., Norris, M. L., and Surani, M. A. H. (1985): Development of gynogenetic and parthenogenetic inner cell mass and trophectoderm tissues in reconstituted blastocysts in the mouse. *J Embryol. Exp. Morphol.*, 90:267–285.
300. McGrath, J., and Solter, D. (1984): Maternal (T^{hp}) lethality in the mouse is a nuclear, noncytoplasmic defect. *Nature (Lond.)*, 308:550–551.
301. Johnson, D. R. (1974): Hairpin-tail: a case of post-reductional gene action in the mouse egg. *Genetics,* 76:795–805.
302. Johnson, D. R. (1975): Further observations on the hairpin-tail (T^{hp}) mutation in the mouse. *Genet. Res.*, 24:207–213.
303. McLaren, A. (1979): The impact of pre-fertilization events on post-fertilization development in mammals. In: *Maternal Effects in Development,* edited by D. R. Newth, and M. Balls, pp. 287–320. Cambridge University Press, London.
304. Winking, H., and Silver, L. M. (1984): Characterization of a recombinant mouse *t* haplotype that expresses a dominant lethal maternal effect. *Genetics,* 108:1013–1020.
305. Cattanach, B. M., and Kirk, M. (1985): Differential activity of maternally and paternally derived chromosome regions in mice. *Nature,* 315:496–498.
306. Cattanach, B. M. (1986): Parental origin effects in mice. *J. Embryol. Exp. Morphol. [Suppl.],* 97:137–150.
307. Searle, A. G., and Beechey, C. V. (1978): Complementation studies with mouse translocations. *Cytogenet. Cell Genet.*, 20:282–303.
308. Searle, A. G., and Beechey, C. V. (1985): Non-complementation phenomena and their bearing on non-disjunctional effects. In: *Aneuploidy, Aetiology and Mechanisms,* edited by V. L. Dellarco, P. E. Voytek, and A. Hollaender, pp. 363–376. Plenum, New York.
309. Jacobs, P. A., Wilson, C., Sprenkle, J. A., Rosenshein, N. B., and Migeon, B. R. (1980): Mechanism of origin of complete hydatidiform moles. *Nature (Lond.)*, 286:714–716.
310. Szulman, A. E., and Surti, V. (1984): Complete and partial hydatidiform moles: cytogenetic and morphological aspects. In: *Human Trophoblast and Neoplasms,* edited by R. A. Patillo and R. O. Hussa, pp. 135–146. Plenum, New York.
311. Modlinski, J. A. (1975): Haploid mouse embryos obtained by microsurgical removal of one pronucleus. *J. Embryol. Exp. Morphol.*, 33:897–905.
312. McGrath, J., and Solter, D. (1984): Inability of mouse blastomere nuclei transferred to enucleated zygotes to support development *in vitro. Science,* 226:1317–1319.
313. McGrath, J., and Solter, D. (1986): Nucleocytoplasmic interactions in the mouse embryo. *J. Embryol. Exp. Morphol. [Suppl.],* 97:277–289.
314. Robl, J. M., Gilligan, B., Critser, E. S., and First, N. L. (1986): Nuclear transplantation in mouse embryos: assessment of recipient cell stage. *Biol. Reprod.*, 34:733–739.
315. Willadson, S. M. (1986): Nuclear transplantation in sheep embryos. *Nature,* 320:63–65.
316. Surani, M. A. H., Barton, S. C., and Norris, M. L. (1986): Nuclear transplantation in the mouse: heritable differences between parental genomes after activation of the embryonic genome. *Cell,* 45:127–136.
317. Lyon, M. F. (1961): Gene action in the X-chromosome of the mouse (*Mus musculus* L.). *Nature,* 190:372–373.
318. West, J. D. (1982): X-chromosome expression during mouse embryogenesis. In: *Genetic Control of Gamete Production and Function,* edited by P. G. Crosignani and B. W. Rubin, pp. 49–91. Academic Press, New York.
319. Chapman, V. M. (1986): X-chromosome regulation in oogenesis and early mammalian development. In: *Experimental Approaches to Mammalian Embryonic Development,* edited by J. Rossant and R. A. Pedersen, pp. 365–398. Cambridge University Press, Cambridge.
320. Van de Berg, J. L., Johnston, P. G., Cooper, D. W., and Robinson, E. S. (1983): X-chromosome inactivation and evolution in marsupials and other mammals. In: *Isozymes: Current Topics in Biological and Medical Research, Vol. 9: Gene Expression and Development,* edited by M. C. Ratazzi, J. G. Scandalios, and G. S. Whitt, pp. 201–218. Alan R. Liss, Inc., New York.
321. Epstein, C. J. (1972): Expression of the mammalian X-chromosome before and after fertilization. *Science,* 175:1467–1468.
322. Migeon, B. R., and Jelalian, K. (1977): Evidence for two active X chromosomes in germ cells of female before meiotic entry. *Nature,* 269:242–243.
323. Kratzer, P. G., and Chapman, V. M. (1981): X chromosome reactivation in oocytes of *Mus caroli. Proc. Natl. Acad. Sci. USA,* 78:3093–3097.
324. Lifschytz, E., and Lindsley, D. L. (1974): Sex chromosome activation during spermatogenesis. *Genetics,* 78:323–331.
325. Kramer, J. M., and Erickson, R. P. (1981): Developmental program of PGK-1 and PGK-2 isozymes in spermatogenic cells of the mouse: specific activities and rates of synthesis. *Dev. Biol.*, 87:37–45.
326. Mukherjee, A. B. (1976): Cell cycle analysis and X-chromosome inactivation in the developing mouse. *Proc. Natl. Acad. Sci. USA,* 73:1608–1611.
327. Takagi, N. (1974): Differentiation of X-chromosomes in early female mouse embryos. *Exp. Cell Res.*, 86:127–135.
328. Adler, D. A., West, J. D., and Chapman, V. M. (1977): Expression of α-galactosidase in preimplantation mouse embryos: implications for X-chromosome inactivation. *Nature,* 267:838–839.
329. Monk, M., and Kathuria, H. (1977): Dosage compensation for an X-linked gene in preimplantation mouse embryos. *Nature,* 270:599–601.
330. Monk, M., and Harper, M. (1978): X-chromosome activity in preimplantation mouse embryos from XX and XO mothers. *J. Embryol. Exp. Morphol.*, 46:53–64.
331. Kratzer, P. G., and Gartler, S. M. (1978): HGPRT activity changes in preimplantation mouse embryos. *Nature,* 274:503–504.
332. Epstein, C. J., Travis, B., Tucker, G., and Smith, S. (1978): The direct demonstration of an X-chromosome dosage effect prior to inactivation. In: *Genetic Mosaics and Chimeras in Mammals,* edited by L. B. Russell, pp. 261–267. Plenum, New York.
333. Gardner, R. L., and Lyon, M. F. (1971): X-chromosome inactivation studies by injection of a single cell into the mouse blastocyst. *Nature,* 231:385–386.
334. Kratzer, P. G., and Gartler, S. M. (1978): Hypoxanthine guanine phosphoribosyl transferase expression in early mouse development. In: *Genetic Mosaics and Chimeras in Mammals,* edited by L. B. Russell, pp. 247–260. Plenum, New York.
335. Takagi, N., Sugawara, O., and Sasaki, M. (1982): Regional and temporal changes in the pattern of X-chromosome replication during the early post-implantation development of the female mouse. *Chromosoma (Berl.)*, 85:275–286.
336. Sugawara, O., Takagi, N., and Sasaki, M. (1983): Allocyclic early replicating X chromosome in mice: genetic inactivity and shift into a later replication in early embryogenesis. *Chromosoma (Berl.)*, 88:133–138.
337. Monk, M., and Harper, M. I. (1979): Sequential X-chromosome inactivation coupled with cellular differentiation in early mouse embryos. *Nature,* 281:311–313.
338. West, J. D., Frels, W. I., Chapman, V. M., and Papaioannou, V. E. (1977): Preferential expression of the maternally derived X-chromosome in the mouse yolk sac. *Cell,* 12:873–882.
339. Frels, W. I., Rossant, J., and Chapman, V. M. (1979): Maternal X chromosome expression in mouse chorionic ectoderm. *Dev. Genet.*, 1:123–132.
340. Frels, W. I., and Chapman, V. (1980): Expression of the maternally derived X chromosome in the mural trophoblast of the mouse. *J. Embryol. Exp. Morphol.*, 56:179–190.
341. Papaioannou, V. E., West, D. D., Bucher, T., and Linke, I. M. (1981): Non-random X-chromosome expression early in mouse development. *Dev. Genet.*, 2:305–315.
342. McMahon, A., and Monk, M. (1983): X-chromosome activity in female mouse embryos heterozygous for Pgk-1 and Searle's translocation, T(X;16)16H. *Genet. Res. Camb.*, 41:69–83.
343. Gartler, S. M., and Riggs, A. D. (1983): Mammalian X-chromosome inactivation. *Annu. Rev. Genet.*, 17:155–190.
344. Lyon, M. F. (1974): Mechanisms and evolutionary origins of variable X-chromosome activity in mammals. *Proc. R. Soc. Lond. [Biol.],* 187:243–268.
345. Cattanach, B. M. (1975): Control of chromosome inactivation. *Annu. Rev. Genet.*, 9:1–18.
346. Razin, A., Cedar, H., and Riggs, A. (editors) (1984): *DNA Methylation.* Springer-Verlag, Berlin.

347. Doerfler, W. (1983): DNA methylation and gene activity. *Annu. Rev. Biochem.*, 52:93–124.
348. Wolf, S. F., Jolly, D. J., Lunnen, K. D., Friedman, T., and Migeon, B. R. (1984): Methylation of the hypoxanthine phosphoribosyl transferase locus on the human X-chromosome: implications for X-chromosome inactivation. *Proc. Natl. Acad. Sci. USA*, 81:2806–2810.
349. Manes, C., and Menzel, P. (1981): Demethylation of CpG sites in DNA of early rabbit trophoblast. *Nature*, 293:589–590.
350. Chapman, V., Forrester, L., Sanford, J., Hastie, N., and Rossant, J. (1984): Cell lineage-specific undermethylation of mouse repetitive DNA. *Nature*, 307:284–286.
351. Razin, A., Webb, C., Szyf, M., Ysraeli, J., Rosenthal, A., Naveh-Many, T., Sciaky-Gallili, N., and Cedar, H. (1984): Variations in DNA methylation during mouse cell differentiation *in vivo* and *in vitro*. *Proc. Natl. Acad. Sci. USA*, 81:2275–2279.
352. Young, P. R., and Tilghman, S. M. (1984): Induction of α-fetoprotein synthesis by differentiation of teratocarcinoma cells is accompanied by a genome-wide loss of DNA methylation. *Mol. Cell. Biol.*, 4:898–907.
353. Rossant, J., Sanford, J. P., Chapman, V. M., and Andrews, G. K. (1986): Undermethylation of structural gene sequences in extraembryonic lineages of the mouse. *Dev. Biol.*, 117:567–573.
354. Chapman, V., Kartzer, P. G., Siracusa, L. D., Quarantillo, B. A., Evans, R., and Liskay, R. M. (1982): Evidence from DNA modification in the maintenance of X-chromosome inactivation of adult mouse tissues. *Proc. Natl. Acad. Sci. USA*, 79:5357–5361.
355. Kratzer, P. G., Chapman, V. M., Lambert, H., Evans, R. E., and Liskay, R. M. (1983): Differences in the DNA of the inactive X-chromosomes of fetal and extraembryonic tissues of mice. *Cell*, 33:37–42.
356. Krumlauf, R., Hammer, R. E., Brinster, R., Chapman, V. M., and Tilghman, S. M. (1985): Regulated expression of α-fetoprotein genes in transgenic mice. *Cold Spring Harbor Symp. Quant. Biol.*, 50:371–378.
357. Jahner, D., Stuhlmann, H., Stewart, W. L., Harbers, K., Lohler, J., Simon, J., and Jaenisch, R. (1982): *De novo* methylation and expression of retroviral genomes during mouse embryogenesis. *Nature*, 298:623–628.
358. Pellicer, A., Robins, D., Wold, B., Sweet, R., Jackson, J., Lowy, I., Roberts, J. M., Sim, G. K., Silverstein, S., and Axel, R. (1980): Altering genotype and phenotype by DNA-mediated gene transfer. *Science*, 29:1414–1422.
359. Jaenisch, R. (1974): Infection of mouse blastocysts with SV40 DNA: Normal development of the infected embryos and persistence of SV40 specific DNA sequences in the adult animals. *Cold Spring Harbor Symp. Quant. Biol.*, 39:375–380.
360. Jaenisch, R., and Mintz, B. (1974): Simian virus 40 DNA sequences in DNA of healthy adult mice derived from preimplantation blastocysts injected with viral DNA. *Proc. Natl. Acad. Sci. USA*, 71:1250–1254.
361. Brinster, R. L., Chen, H. Y., Trumbauer, M. E., Denear, A. W., Warren, R., and Palmiter, R. D. (1981): Somatic expression of herpes thymidine kinase in mice following injection of a fusion gene into eggs. *Cell*, 27:223–231.
362. Costantini, F., and Lacy, E. (1981): Introduction of a rabbit β-globin gene into the mouse germ line. *Nature*, 294:92–94.
363. Wagner, E. F., Stewart, T. A., and Mintz, B. (1981): The human β-globin gene and a functional viral thymidine kinase gene in developing mice. *Proc. Natl. Acad. Sci. USA*, 78:5016–5020.
364. Wagner, T. E., Hoppe, P. C., Jollick, J. D., Scholl, D. R., Hodinka, R. L., and Gault, J. B. (1981): Microinjection of a rabbit β-globin gene into zygotes and its subsequent expression in adult mice and their offspring. *Proc. Natl. Acad. Sci. USA*, 78:6376–6380.
365. Hammer, R., Pursel, V. G., Rexroad, C. E., Jr., Wall, R. J., Bolt, D. J., Ebert, K. M., Palmiter, R. D., and Brinster, R. L. (1985): Production of transgenic rabbits, sheep, and pigs by microinjection. *Nature*, 315:680–683.
366. Gordon, J. W., and Ruddle, F. H. (1985): DNA mediated genetic tranformation of mouse embryos and bone marrow—a review. *Gene*, 33:121–136.
367. Palmiter, R. D., and Brinster, R. L. (1985): Transgenic mice. *Cell*, 14:343–345.
368. Brinster, R. L., Chen, H. Y., Trumbauer, M., Yagle, M. K., and Palmiter, R. D. (1985): Factors affecting the efficiency of introducing foreign DNA into mice by microinjecting eggs. *Proc. Natl. Acad. Sci. USA*, 82:4438–4442.
369. Wagner, E. F., Ruther, U., and Stewart, C. L. (1984): Introducing genes into mice and into embryonal carcinoma stem cells. In: *The Impact of Gene Transfer Techniques in Eucaryotic Cell Biology*, edited by J. S. Schell and P. Starlinger, pp. 127–133. Springer-Verlag, Berlin.
370. Wagner, E. F., Ruther, U., and Stewart, C. L. (1986): Gene transfer into mouse stem cells. In: *Dahlem Workshop Report: Biotechnology: Potentials and Limitations. Life Sciences Report No. 35*, edited by S. Silver, pp. 185–196. Springer-Verlag, Cambridge.
371. Wagner, E. F., and Stewart, C. L. (1986): Integration and expression of genes introduced into mouse embryos. In: *Experimental Approaches to Mammalian Embryonic Development*, edited by J. Rossant and R. A. Pedersen, pp. 509–549. Cambridge University Press, Cambridge.
372. Brinster, R. L., and Palmiter, R. D. (1985): Introduction of genes into the germ line of animals. *Harvey Lect.*, 80:1–38.
373. McKnight, G. S., Hammer, R. E., Kuenzel, E. A., and Brinster, R. L. (1983): Expression of the chicken transferrin gene in transgenic mice. *Cell*, 34:335–341.
374. Swift, G. H., Hammer, R. E., McDonald, R. J., and Brinster, R. L. (1984): Tissue-specific expression of the rat pancreatic elastase I gene in transgenic mice. *Cell*, 38:639–646.
375. Shani, M. (1985): Tissue-specific expression of rat myosin light-chain 2 gene in transgenic mice. *Nature*, 314:283–286.
376. Krumlauf, R., Hammer, R., Tilghman, S., and Brinster, R. L. (1985): Developmental regulation of alphafoetoprotein genes in transgenic mice. *Mol. Cell. Biol.*, 5:1639–1648.
377. Palmiter, R. D., Chen, H. Y., and Brinster, R. L. (1982): Differential regulation of metallothionein-thymidine kinase fusion gene in transgenic mice and their offspring. *Cell*, 29:701–710.
378. Overbeek, P. A., Chepelinsky, A., Khillan, J. S., Piatigorsky, J., and Westphal, H. (1985): Lens-specific expression and developmental regulation of the bacterial chloramphenicol acetyltransferase gene driven by the murine αA-cystallin promoter in transgenic mice. *Proc. Natl. Acad. Sci. USA*, 82:7815–7819.
379. Westphal, H., Overbeek, P. A., Khillan, J. S., Chepelinsky, A. B., Schmidt, A., Mahon, K. A., Bernstein, K. E., Piatigorsky, J., and de Crombrugghe, B. (1985): Promoter sequences of murine αA cystallin, murine α2(1) collagen or avian sarcoma virus genes linked to the bacterial CAT gene direct tissue specific patterns of CAT expression in transgenic mice. *Cold Spring Harbor Symp. Quant. Biol.*, 50:411–416.
380. Ornitz, D. M., Palmiter, R. D., Hammer, R. E., Brinster, R. L., Swift, G. H., and McDonald, J. R. (1985): Specific expression of an elastase-human growth hormone fusion gene in pancreatic acinar cells of transgenic mice. *Nature*, 313:600–602.
381. Goring, D. R., Rossant, J., Clapoff, S., Breitman, M. L., and Tsui, L.-C. (1986): *In situ* detection of β-galactosidase activity in lenses of transgenic mice harboring a γ-crystallin/*Lac-z* hybrid gene. *Science* 235:456–458.
382. Townes, T. M., Lingrel, J. B., Chen, H. Y., Brinster, R. L., and Palmiter, R. D. (1985): Erythroid specific expression of human β-globin genes in transgenic mice. *EMBO J.*, 4:1715–1723.
383. Palmiter, R. D., Brinster, R. L., Hammer, R. E., Trumbauer, M. E., Rosenfeld, M. G., Birnberg, N. C., and Evans, R. M. (1982): Dramatic growth of mice that develop from eggs microinjected with metallothionein-growth hormone fusion genes. *Nature*, 300:611–615.
384. Palmiter, R. D., Norstedt, G., Gelinas, R. E., Hammer, R. E., and Brinster, R. L.(1983): Metallothionein-human GH fusion genes stimulate growth of mice. *Science*, 222:809–814.
385. Hammer, R. E., Palmiter, R. D., and Brinster, R. L. (1984): Partial correction of murine hereditary growth disorder by germ line incorporation of a new gene. *Nature*, 311:65–67.
386. Brinster, R. L., Ritchie, K. A., Hammer, R. E., O'Brien, R. L., Arp, B., and Storb, U. (1983): Expression of a microinjected immunoglobulin gene in the spleen of transgenic mice. *Nature*, 306:332–336.
387. Storb, U., O'Brien, R. L., McMullen, M. D., Gollahon, K. A., and Brinster, R. L. (1984): High expression of cloned immunoglobulin κ gene in transgenic mice is restricted to B lymphocytes. *Nature*, 310:238–241.
388. Grosschedl, R., Weaver, D., Baltimore, D., and Costantini, F. (1984): Introduction of a μ-immunoglobulin gene into the mouse germ line:

specific expression in lymphoid cells and synthesis of functional antibody. *Cell,* 38:647–658.
389. Rusconi, S., and Kohler, G. (1985): Transmission and expression of a specific pair of rearranged immunoglobulin μ and κ genes in a transgenic mouse line. *Nature,* 314:330–334.
390. Frels, W. I., Bluestone, J. A., Hodes, R. J., Capecchi, M. R., and Singer, D. S. (1985): Expression of a microinjected porcine class I major histocompatibility complex gene in transgenic mice. *Science,* 228:577–580.
391. Le Meur, M., Gerlinger, P., Benoist, C., and Mathis, D. (1985): Correcting an immune response deficiency by creating E_α gene transgenic mice. *Nature,* 316:38–42.
392. Yamamura, K., Kikutani, H., Folson, V., Clayton, L. K., Kimoto, M., Akira, S., Kashiwamura, S., Tonegawa, S., and Kishimoto, R. (1985): Functional expression of a microinjected E_α^d gene in C57BL/6 transgenic mice. *Nature,* 316:67–69.
393. Pinkert, C. A., Widera, G., Cowing, C., Heber-Katz, E., Palmiter, R. D., Flavell, R. A., and Brinster, R. L. (1985): Tissue-specific, inducible and functional expression of the E_α^d MHC class II gene in transgenic mice. *EMBO J.,* 4:2225–2230.
394. Brinster, R. L., Chen, H. Y., Messing, A., van Dyke, T., Levine, A. J., and Palmiter, R. D. (1984): Transgenic mice harboring SV40 T-antigen genes develop characteristic brain tumors. *Cell,* 37:367–379.
395. Palmiter, R. D., Chen, H. Y., Messing, A., and Brinster, R. L. (1985): SV40 enhancer and large-T antigen are instrumental in development of choroid plexus tumours in transgenic mice. *Nature,* 36:457–460.
396. Messing, A., Chen, H. Y., Palmiter, R. D., and Brinster, R. L. (1985): Peripheral neuropathies, hepatocellular carcinomas, and islet cell adenomas in transgenic mice. *Nature,* 316:461–463.
397. Stewart, T. A., Pattengale, P. K., and Leder, P. (1984): Spontaneous mammary adenocarcinomas in transgenic mice that carry and express MTV/*myc* fusion genes. *Cell,* 23:627–637.
398. Hanahan, D. (1985): Heritable formation of pancreatic β-cell tumors in transgenic mice expressing recombinant insulin/SV40 oncogenes. *Nature,* 315:115–122.
399. Babinet, C., Farza, H., Morello, D., Hadchouel, M., and Pourcel, C. (1985): Specific expression of hepatitis B surface antigen (HBsAg) in transgenic mice. *Science,* 230:160–163.
400. Chisari, F. V., Pinkert, C. A., Milich, D. R., Filippi, P., McLachlan, A., Palmiter, R. D., and Brinster, R. L. (1985): A transgenic mouse model of the chronic hepatitis B surface antigen carrier state. *Science,* 230:1157–1160.
401. Rusconi, S. (1984): Gene transfer in living organisms. In: *The Impact of Gene Transfer Techniques in Eucaryotic Cell Biology,* edited by J. S. Schell and P. Starlinger, pp. 134–152. Springer-Verlag, Berlin.
402. Stewart, T. A., Wagner, E. F., and Mintz, B. (1982): Human β-globin gene sequences injected into mouse eggs, retained in adults, and transmitted to progeny. *Science,* 217:1046–1048.
403. Chada, K., Magram, J., Raphael, K., Radice, G., Lacy, E., and Costantini, F. (1985): Specific expression of a foreign β-globin gene in erythroid cells of transgenic mice. *Nature,* 314:377–380.
404. Magram, J., Chada, K., and Costantini, F. (1985): Developmental regulation of a cloned adult β-globin gene in transgenic mice. *Nature,* 315:338–340.
405. Lacy, E., Roberts, S., Evans, E. P., Burtenshaw, M. D., and Costantini, F. (1983): A foreign β-globin gene in transgenic mice: integration at abnormal chromosomal positions and expresson in inappropriate tissues. *Cell,* 34:343–358.
406. Wagner, E. F., Covarrubias, L., Stewart, T. A., and Mintz, B. (1983): Prenatal lethalities in mice homozygous for human growth hormone gene sequences integrated in the germ line. *Cell,* 35:647–655.
407. Hammer, R. E., Brinster, R. L., Rosenfeld, M. G., Evans, R. M., and Mayo, K. E. (1985): Expression of human growth factor in transgenic mice results in increased somatic growth. *Nature,* 315:413–416.
408. Stout, J. T., Chen, H. Y., Brennand, J., Caskey, C. T., and Brinster, R. L. (1985): Expression of human HPRT in the central nervous system of transgenic mice. *Nature,* 317:250–252.
409. Low, M. J., Hammer, R. E., Goodman, R. H., Habener, J. F., Palmiter, R. D., and Brinster, R. L. (1985): Tissue-specific post-translational processing of pre-prosomatostatin encoded by a metallothionein-somatostatin fusion gene in transgenic mice. *Cell,* 41:211–219.
410. Ross, S. R., and Solter, D. (1985): Glucocorticoid regulation of mouse mammary tumor virus sequences in transgenic mice. *Proc. Natl. Acad. Sci. USA,* 82:5880–5884.
411. Harbers, K., Jahner, D., and Jaenisch, R. (1981): Microinjection of cloned retroviral genomes into mouse zygotes: integration and expression in the animal. *Nature,* 293:540–542.
412. Stewart, C. L., Harbers, K., Jahner, D., and Jaenisch, R. (1983): X chromosome-linked transmission and expression of retroviral genomes microinjected into mouse zygotes. *Science,* 221:760–762.
413. Jaenisch, R., and Mintz, B. (1974): Simian virus 40 DNA sequences in DNA of healthy adult mice derived from preimplantation blastocysts injected with viral DNA. *Proc. Natl. Acad. Sci. USA,* 71:1250–1254.
414. Small, J. A., Blair, D. G., Showalter, S. D., and Scangos, G. A. (1985): Analysis of a transgenic mouse containing SV40 and v-*myc* sequences. *Mol. Cell. Biol.,* 5:642–648.
415. Wirak, D. O., Chalifour, L. E., Wassarman, P. M., Muller, W. J., Hassell, J. A., and De Pamphilis, M. L. (1985): Sequence-dependent DNA replication in preimplantation mouse embryos. *Mol. Cell. Biol.,* 5:2924–2935.
416. Rassoulzadegan, M., Leopold, P., Vailly, J., and Cuzin, F. (1986): Germ line transmission of autonomous genetic elements in transgenic mouse strains. *Cell,* 46:513–519.
417. Kelly, F., and Condamine, H. (1982): Tumor viruses and early mouse embryos. *Biochim. Biophys. Acta,* 651:105–141.
418. Jaenisch, R., Fan, H., and Croker, B. (1975): Infection of preimplantation mouse embryos and of newborn mice with leukaemia virus: tissue distribution of viral DNA and RNA and leukemogenesis in the adult animal. *Proc. Natl. Acad. Sci. USA,* 72:4008–4012.
419. Jaenisch, R., and Jahner, D. (1984): Methylation, expression and chromosomal position of genes in mammals. *Biochim. Biophys. Acta,* 782:1–9.
420. Willison, K., Babinet, C., Boccara, M., and Kelly, F. (1983): Infection of preimplantation mouse embryos with simian virus 40. In: *Cold Spring Harbor Conference, Vol. 10,* edited by L. M. Silver, G. R. Martin, and S. Strickland, pp. 307–317. Cold Spring Harbor Laboratory, Cold Spring Harbor, N.Y.
421. Jaenisch, R., Jahner, D., Nobis, P., Simon, I., Lohler, J., Harbers, K., and Grotkopp, D. (1981): Chromosomal position and activation of retroviral genomes inserted into the germ line of mice. *Cell,* 24:519–529.
422. Rubinstein, J. L. R., Nicolas, J.-F., and Jacob, F. (1984): Construction of a retrovirus capable of transducing and expressing genes in multipotential embryonic cells. *Proc. Natl. Acad. Sci. USA,* 81:7137–7140.
423. Wagner, E. F., Vanek, M., and Vennstrom, B. (1985): Transfer of genes into embryonal carcinoma cells by retrovirus infection: efficient expression from an internal promoter. *EMBO J.,* 4:663–669.
424. Stewart, C. L., Vanek, M., and Wagner, E. F. (1985): Expression of foreign genes from retroviral vectors in mouse teratocarcinoma chimaeras. *EMBO J.,* 4:3701–3709.
425. Stewart, C. L., Ruther, U., Garber, C., Vanek, M., and Wagner, E. F. (1986): The expression of retroviral vectors in murine stem cells and transgenic mice. *J. Embryol. Exp. Morphol. [Suppl.],* 97:263–275.
426. Robertson, E. J., and Bradley, A. (1986): Production of permanent cell lines from early embryos and their use in studying developmental problems. In: *Experimental Approaches to Mammalian Embryonic Development,* edited by J. Rossant and R. A. Pedersen, pp. 475–508. Cambridge University Press, Cambridge.
427. Soriano, P., Cone, R. D., Mulligan, R. C., and Jaenisch, R. (1986): Tissue-specific and ectopic expression of genes introduced into transgenic mice by retroviruses. *Science,* 234:1409–1413.
428. Bradley, A., Evans, M., Kaufman, M. H., and Robertson, E. (1984): Formation of germ line chimaeras from embryo derived teratocarcinoma cell lines. *Nature,* 309:255–256.
429. Gossler, A., Doetschman, T., Korn, R., Serfling, E., and Kemler, R. (1986): Transgenesis via blastocyst-derived embryonic stem cell lines. *Proc. Natl. Acad. Sci. USA,* 83:9065–9069.
430. Robertson, E., Bradley, A., Kuehn, M., and Evans, M. (1986): Germ-line transmission of genes introduced into cultured pluripotential cells by retroviral vector. *Nature,* 323:445–448.

431. Mulligan, R. C., and Berg, P. (1981): Selection for animal cells that express the *Escherichia coli* gene coding for xanthine-guanine phosphoribosyl transferase. *Proc. Natl. Acad. Sci. USA,* 78:2072–2076.
432. Southern, P. J., and Berg, P. (1982): Transformation of mammalian cells to antibiotic resistance with a bacterial gene under control of the SV40 early region promoter. *J. Mol. Appl. Genet.,* 1:327–341.
433. Johnson, M. H. (1981): The molecular and cellular basis of preimplantation mouse development. *Biol. Rev.,* 56:463–498.
434. Dziadek, M., and Adamson, E. D. (1978): Localisation and synthesis of alpha-foetoprotein in post-implantation mouse embryos. *J. Embryol. Exp. Morphol.,* 43:289–313.
435. Dziadek, M. (1978): Modulation of alphafoetoprotein synthesis in the early postimplantation mouse embryo. *J. Embryol. Exp. Morphol.,* 46:135–146.
436. Albrechtsen, R., and Norgaard-Pederson, B. (1978): Immunofluorescent localisation of alpha-fetoprotein synthesis in the endodermal sinus of rat placenta. *Scand. J. Immunol.,* 8:193–199.
437. Ruoslahti, E., and Seppala, M. (1979): α-Fetoprotein in cancer and fetal development. *Adv. Cancer Res.,* 29:275–346.
438. Andrews, G. K., Janzen, R. G., and Tamaski, T. (1982): Stability of α-fetoprotein messenger RNA in mouse yolk sac. *Dev. Biol.,* 89:111–116.
439. Tilghman, S. M., and Belayew, A. (1982): Transcriptional control of the murine albumin/α-fetoprotein locus during development. *Proc. Natl. Acad. Sci. USA,* 79:5254–5257.
440. Sellem, C. H., Frain, M., Erdos, T., and Sala-Trepat, J. M. (1984): Differential expression of albumin and α-fetoprotein genes in fetal tissues of mouse and rat. *Dev. Biol.,* 102:51–60.
441. Krumlauf, R., Hammer, R. E., Tilghman, S. M., and Brinster, R. L. (1985): Developmental regulation of α-fetoprotein genes in transgenic mice. *Mol. Cell. Biol.,* 5:1639–1648.
442. Hammer, R. E., Krumlauf, R., Camper, S., Brinster, R. L., and Tilghman, S. M. (1986): The regulation of α-fetoprotein minigene expression in the germline of mice. *J. Embryol. Exp. Morphol. [Suppl.],* 97:257–262.
443. Renfree, M. B., and McLaren, A. (1974): Foetal origin of transferrin in mouse amniotic fluid. *Nature,* 252:159–160.
444. Adamson, E. D. (1982): The location and synthesis of transferrin in mouse embryos and teratocarcinoma cells. *Dev. Biol.,* 91:227–234.
445. Meek, J., and Adamson, E. D. (1985): Transferrin in fetal and adult mouse tissues: synthesis, storage, and secretion. *J. Embryol. Exp. Morphol.,* 86:205–218.
446. Andrews, G. K., Adamson, E. D., and Gedamu, L. (1984): The ontogeny of expression of murine metallothionein: comparison with the α-fetoprotein gene. *Dev. Biol.,* 103:294–303.
447. Hopkins, B., Sharpe, C. R., Baralle, F. E., and Graham, C. F. (1986): Organ distribution of apolipoprotein gene transcripts in 6-12 week postfertilization human embryos. *J. Embryol. Exp. Morphol.,* 97:177–187.
448. Adamson, E. D. (1986): Cell-lineage-specific gene expression in development. In: *Experimental Approaches to Mammalian Embryonic Development,* edited by J. Rossant and R. A. Pedersen, pp. 321–364. Cambridge University Press, Cambridge.
449. Trelstad, R. L. (editor) (1984): *The Role of Extracellular Matrix in Development, 42nd Symposium of the Society for Developmental Biology.* Alan R. Liss, New York.
450. Wartiovaara, J., Leivo, I., and Vaheri, A. (1979): Expression of the cell surface-associated glycoprotein, fibronectin, in the early mouse embryo. *Dev. Biol.,* 69:247–257.
451. Semoff, S., Hogan, B. L. M., and Hopkins, C. R. (1982): Localisation of fibronectin, laminin-entactin and entactin in Reichert's membrane by immuno-electron microscopy. *EMBO J.,* 1:1171–1175.
452. Adamson, E. D., and Ayers, S. E. (1979): The localization and synthesis of collagen in mouse embryos. *Cell,* 16:953–965.
453. Leivo, I., Vaheri, A., Timpl, R., and Wartiovaara, J. (1980): Appearance and distribution of collagens and laminin in the early mouse embryo. *Dev. Biol.,* 76:100–114.
454. Cooper, A. R., and MacQueen, H. A. (1983): Subunits of laminin are differentially synthesized in mouse eggs and early embryos. *Dev. Biol.,*96:467–471.
455. Wu, T. C., Wan, Y.-J., Chung, A. E., and Damjanov, I. (1983): Immunohistochemical localization of entactin and laminin in mouse embryos and fetuses. *Dev. Biol.,* 100:496–505.
456. Sherman, M. I., Gay, R., Gay, S., and Miller, E. J. (1980): Association of collagen with preimplantation and peri-implantation mouse embryos. *Dev. Biol.,* 74:470–478.
457. Schnieke, A. A., Harbers, K., and Jaenisch, R. (1983): Embryonic lethal mutation in mice induced by retrovirus insertion into the α1(I) collagen gene. *Nature,* 304:315–320.
458. Hogan, B. L. M., Cooper, A. R., and Kurkinen, M. (1980): Incorporation into Reichert's membrane of laminin-like extracellular proteins synthesized by parietal endoderm cells of the mouse embryo. *Dev. Biol.,* 80:289–300.
459. Hogan, B. L. M., Taylor, A., and Cooper, A. R. (1982): Murine parietal endoderm cells synthesize heparan sulphate and 170 K and 145 K sulphated glycoproteins as components of Reichert's membrane. *Dev. Biol.,* 90:210–214.
460. Jacob, F. (1979): Cell surface and early stages of mouse embryogenesis. *Curr. Top. Dev. Biol.,* 13:117–135.
461. Solter, D., and Knowles, B. B. (1979): Developmental stage-specific antigens during mouse embryogenesis. *Curr. Top. Dev. Biol.,* 13:139–165.
462. Wiley, L. M. (1979): Early embryonic cell surface antigens as developmental probes. *Curr. Top. Dev. Biol.,* 13:167–197.
463. Johnson, L. V., and Calarco, P. G. (1980): Mammalian preimplantation development: the cell surface. *Anat. Rec.,* 196:201–219.
464. Johnson, M. H. (1981): Membrane events associated with the generation of a blastocyst. *Int. Rev. Cytol. [Suppl.],* 12:1–37.
465. Richa, J., and Solter, D. (1986): Role of cell surface molecules in early mammalian development. In: *Experimental Approaches to Mammalian Embryonic Development,* edited by J. Rossant and R. A. Pedersen, pp. 293–320. Cambridge University Press, Cambridge.
466. Webb, C. A. G. (1983): Glycoproteins on gametes and early embryos. In: *Development in Mammals, Vol. 5,* edited by M. H. Johnson, pp. 155–185. Elsevier, Amsterdam.
467. Ducibella, T., and Anderson, E. (1975): Cell shape and membrane changes in the eight-cell mouse embryo: prerequisites for morphogenesis of the blastocyst. *Dev. Biol.,* 47:45–58.
468. Hyafil, F., Morello, D., Babinet, C., and Jacob, F. (1980): A cell surface glycoprotein involved in the compaction of embryonal carcinoma cells and cleavage stage embryos. *Cell,* 21:927–934.
469. Yoshida-Noro, C., Suzuki, N., and Takeichi, M. (1984): Molecular nature of the calcium-dependent cell-cell adhesion in mouse teratocarcinoma and embryonic cells studied with a monoclonal antibody. *Dev. Biol.,* 101:19–27.
470. Damsky, C. H., Richa, J., Solter, D., Knudsen, K., and Buck, C. A. (1983): Identification and purification of a cell surface glycoprotein mediating intercellular adhesion in embryonic and adult tissue. *Cell,* 34:455–466.
471. Richa, J., Damsky, C. H., Buck, C. A., Knowles, B. B., and Solter, D. (1985): Cell surface glycoproteins mediate compaction, trophoblast attachment and endoderm formation during early mouse development. *Dev. Biol.,* 108:513–521.
472. Gallin, W. J., Edelman, G., and Cunningham, B. (1983): Characterization of L-CAM, a major cell adhesion molecule from embryonic liver cells. *Proc. Natl. Acad. Sci. USA,* 80:1038–1042.
473. Ogou, S.-I., Okada, T. S., and Takeichi, M. (1982): Cleavage stage mouse embryos share a common cell adhesion system with teratocarcinoma cells. *Dev. Biol.,* 92:521–528.
474. Kimber, S. J., and Surani, M. A. H. (1982): Spreading of blastomeres from eight-cell mouse embryos on lectin coated beads. *J. Cell Sci.,* 56:191–206.
475. Johnson, L. V. (1985): Wheat germ agglutinin induces compaction- and cavitation-like events in 2-cell mouse embryos. *Dev. Biol.,* 113:1–9.
476. Zvzack, J. S., and Tasca, R. J. (1985): Lectin-induced blockage of developmental processes in preimplantation mouse embryos in vitro. *Gamete Res.* 12:275–290.
477. Brownell, A. G. (1977): Cell surface carbohydrates of preimplantation embryos as assessed by lectin binding. *J. Supramol. Struct.,* 7:223–234.
478. Sato, M., and Muramatsu, T. (1985): Reactivity of five *N*-acetylgalactosamine-recognizing lectins with preimplantation embryos, early postimplantation embryos, and teratocarcinoma cells of the mouse. *Differentiation,* 29:29–38.

479. Solter, D., and Knowles, B. B. (1978): Monoclonal antibody defining a stage-specific mouse embryonic antigen (SSEA-1). *Proc. Natl. Acad. Sci. USA,* 75:5565–5569.
480. Solter, D., and Knowles, B. B. (1979): Developmental stage-specific antigens during mouse embryogenesis. *Curr. Top. Dev. Biol.,* 13:139–165.
481. Fox, N., Damjanov, I., Martinez-Hernandez, A., Knowles, B. B., and Solter, D. (1981): Immunohistochemical localization of the early embryonic antigen (SSEA-1) in postimplantation mouse embryos, and fetal and adult tissues. *Dev. Biol.,* 83:391–398.
482. Rastan, S., Thorpe, S. J., Scudder, P., Brown, S. Gooi, H. C., and Feizi, T. (1985): Cell interactions in preimplantation embryos: evidence for involvement of saccharides of the poly-*N*-acetyllactosamine series. *J. Embryol. Exp. Morphol.,* 87:115–128.
483. Knowles, B. B., Rappaport, J., and Solter, D. (1982): Murine embryonic antigen (SSEA-1) is expressed on human cells and structurally related human blood group antigen I is expressed on mouse embryos. *Dev. Biol.,* 93:54–58.
484. Kapadia, A., Feizi, T., and Evans, M. J. (1981): Changes in the expression and polarization of blood group I and i antigens in postimplantation embryos and teratocarcinomas of mouse associated with cell differentiation. *Exp. Cell Res.,* 131:185–195.
485. Shevinsky, L. H., Knowles, B. B., Damjanov, I., and Solter, D. (1982): Monoclonal antibody to murine embryos defines a stage-specific embryonic antigen expressed on mouse embryos and human teratocarcinoma cells. *Cell,* 30:697–705.
486. Kannagi, R., Cochran, N. A., Ishigami, F., Hakomori, S.-I., Andrews, P. W., Knowles, B. B., and Solter, D. (1983): Stage-specific embryonic antigens (SSEA-3 and -4) are epitopes of a unique globo-series ganglioside isolated from human teratocarcinoma cells. *EMBO J.,* 2:2355–2361.
487. Fox, N. W., Damjanov, I., Knowles, B. B., and Solter, D. (1984): Stage-specific embryonic antigen 3 as a marker of visceral extraembryonic endoderm. *Dev. Biol.,* 103:263–266.
488. Willison, K. R., Karol, R. A., Suzuki, A., Kundu, S. K., and Marcus, D. M. (1982): Neutral glycolipid antigens as developmental markers of mouse teratocarcinomas and early embryos: an immunologic and chemical analysis. *J. Immunol.,* 129:603–609.
489. Willison, K. R., and Stern, P. L. (1978): Expression of a Forssman antigenic specificity in the preimplantation mouse embryo. *Cell,* 14:785–793.
490. Muramatsu, H., and Muramatsu, T. (1983): A fucosyltransferase in teratocarcinoma cells. Decreased activity accompanying differentiation to parietal endoderm cells. *FEBS Lett.,* 163:181–184.
491. Shur, B. D. (1983): Embryonal carcinoma cell adhesion: the role of surface galactosyltransferase and its 90K lactosaminoglycan substrate. *Dev. Biol.,* 99:360–372.
492. Sato, M., Muramatsu, T., and Gerger, E. G. (1984): Immunological detection of cell surface galactosyltransferase in preimplantation mouse embryos. *Dev. Biol.,* 102:514–518.
493. Shur, B. D., Oettgen, P., and Bennett, D. (1979): UDP-galactose inhibits blastocyst formation in the mouse. *Dev. Biol.,* 73:178–181.
494. Mulnard, J., and Huygens, R. (1978): Ultrastructural localization of non-specific alkaline phosphatase during cleavage and blastocyst formation in the mouse. *J. Embryol. Exp. Morphol.,* 44:121–131.
495. Johnson, L. V., Calarco, P. G., and Siebert, M. L. (1977): Alkaline phosphatase activity in the preimplantation mouse embryo. *J. Embryol. Exp. Morphol.,* 40:83–89.
496. Eddy, E. M. (1975): Germ plasm and the differentiation of the germ cell line. *Int. Rev. Cytol.,* 43:229–280.
497. Eddy, E. M., Clark, J. M., Gong, D., and Fenderson, B. A. (1981): Origin and migration of primordial germ cells in mammals. *Gamete Res.,* 4:333–362.
498. Vorbrodt, A., Konwinski, M., Solter, D., and Koprowski, H. (1977): Ultrastructural cytochemistry of membrane-bound phosphatases in preimplantation mouse embryos. *Dev. Biol.,* 55:117–134.
499. Borland, R. M., Biggers, J. D., and Lechene, C. P. (1976): Kinetic aspects of rabbit blastocoele fluid accumulation: an application of electron probe microanalysis. *Dev. Biol.,* 50:201–211.
500. Benos, D. J. (1981): Ouabain binding to preimplantation rabbit blastocysts. *Dev. Biol.,* 83:69–78.
501. Benos, D. J., Biggers, J. D., Balaban, R. S., Mills, J. W., and Overstrom, E. G. (1985): Developmental aspects of sodium dependent transport processes of preimplantation rabbit embryos. In: *Regulation and Development of Membrane Transport Processes,* edited by J. S. Graves, pp. 211–235. Wiley, New York.
502. DiZio, S. M., and Tasca, R. J., (1977): Sodium-dependent amino-acid transport in preimplantation mouse embryos. III. Na^+-K^+-ATPase-linked mechanism in blastocysts. *Dev. Biol.,* 59:198–205.
503. Wiley, L. M. (1984): Cavitation in the preimplantation embryo: Na/K-ATPase and the origin of nascent blastocoel fluid. *Dev. Biol.,* 105:330–342.
504. Searle, R. F., Sellens, M. H., Elson, J., Jenkinson, E. J., and Billington, W. D. (1976): Detection of alloantigen during preimplantation development and early trophoblast differentiation in the mouse by immunoperoxidase labeling. *J. Exp. Med.,* 14:348–359.
505. Warner, C. M., and Spannans, D. J. (1984): Demonstration of *H-2* antigens on preimplantation mouse embryos using conventional antisera and monoclonal antibody. *J. Exp. Zool.,* 230:37–52.
506. Kirkwood, K. J., and Billington, W. D. (1981): Expression of serologically detectable H-2 antigens on mid-gestation mouse embryonic tissues. *J. Embryol. Exp. Morphol.,* 61:207–219.
507. Sawicki, J. A., Magnuson, T., and Epstein, C. J. (1982): Evidence for expression of the paternal genome in the two-cell mouse embryo. *Nature,* 294:450–451.
508. Hakansson, S., and Peterson, P. A. (1976): Presence of beta-2-microglobulin on the implanting mouse blastocyst. *Transplantation,* 21:358–360.
509. Heyner, S. (1983): Alloantigen expression on mouse oocytes and early embryos. In: *Immunology of Reproduction,* edited by T. G. Wegmann and J. J. Gill, pp. 79–99. Oxford University Press, London.
510. Pratt, H. P. M., Ziomek, C. A., Reeve, W. J. D., and Johnson, M. H. (1982): Compaction of the mouse embryo: an analysis of its components. *J. Embryol. Exp. Morphol.,* 70:113–132.
511. Ducibella, T. (1980): Divalent antibodies to mouse embryonal carcinoma cells inhibit compaction in the mouse embryo. *Dev. Biol.,* 79:356–366.
512. Wiley, L. M., and Eglitis, M. A. (1980): Effect of colcemid on cavitation during mouse blastocoele formation. *Exp. Cell Res.,* 127:89–101.
513. Surani, M. A. H., Barton, S. C., and Burling, A. (1980): Differentiation of 2-cell and 8-cell mouse embryos arrested by cytoskeletal inhibitors. *Exp. Cell Res.,* 125:275–286.
514. Maro, B., and Pickering, S. J. (1984): Microtubules influence compaction in preimplantation mouse embryos. *J. Embryol. Exp. Morphol.,* 84:217–232.
515. Pratt, H. P. M., Chakraborty, J., and Surani, M. A. H. (1981): Molecular and morphological differentiation of the mouse blastocyst after manipulations of compaction with cytochalasin D. *Cell,* 26:279–292.
516. Petzoldt, U., Burki, K., Illmensee, G. R., and Illmensee, K. (1983): Protein synthesis in mouse embryos with experimentally produced asynchrony between chromosome replication and cell division. *Wilhelm Roux's Arch. Dev. Biol.,* 192:138–144.
517. Petzoldt, U. (1986): Expression of two surface antigens and paternal glucose-phosphate isomerase in polyploid one-cell mouse eggs. *Dev. Biol.,* 113:512–516.
518. Fleming, T. P., Cannon, P. M., and Pickering, S. J. (1986): The cytoskeleton, endocytosis and cell polarity in the mouse preimplantation embryo. *Dev. Biol.,* 113:406–419.
519. Johnson, M. H., Chisholm, J. C., Fleming, T. P., and Houliston, E. (1986): A role for cytoplasmic determinants in the development of the mouse early embryo? *J. Embryol. Exp. Morphol. [Suppl.],* 97:97–121.
520. Ducibella, T., Ukena, T., Karnovsky, M., and Anderson, E. (1977): Changes in cell surface and cortical cytoplasmic organization during embryogenesis in the preimplantation mouse embryo. *J. Cell Biol.,* 74:153–167.
521. Opas, J., and Soltynska, M. S. (1978): Reorganization of the cortical layer during cytokinesis in mouse blastomeres. *Exp. Cell Res.,* 113:208–211.
522. Lehtonen, E., and Badley, R. A. (1980): Localization of cytoskeletal proteins in preimplantation mouse embryos. *J. Embryol. Exp. Morphol.,* 55:211–225.
523. Johnson, M. H., and Maro, B. (1984): The distribution of cytoplasmic actin in mouse 8-cell blastomeres. *J. Embryol. Exp. Morphol.,* 82:97–117.

524. Sobel, J. S., and Alliegro, M. A. (1985): Changes in the distribution of a spectrin-like protein during develoment of the preimplantation mouse embryo. *J. Cell Biol.*, 100:333–336.
525. Sobel, J. S. (1983): Cell-cell contact modulation of myosin organization in the early mouse embryo. *Dev. Biol.*, 100:207–213.
526. Sobel, J. S. (1983): Localization of myosin in the preimplantation mouse embryo. *Dev. Biol.*, 95:227–231.
527. Sobel, J. S. (1984): Myosin rings and spreading in mouse blastomeres. *J. Cell Biol.*, 99:1145–1150.
528. Steinert, P. M., Steven, A. C., and Roop, D. R. (1985): The molecular biology of intermediate filaments. *Cell,* 42:411–419.
529. Brulet, P., Babinet, C., Kemler, R., and Jacob, F. (1980): Monoclonal antibodies against trophectoderm-specific markers during mouse blastocyst formation. *Proc. Natl. Acad. Sci. USA,* 77:4113–4114.
530. Brulet, P., and Jacob, F. (1982): Molecular cloning of a cDNA sequence encoding a trophectoderm-specific marker during mouse blastocyst formation. *Proc. Natl. Acad. Sci. USA,* 79:2328–2332.
531. Oshima, R. G. (1981): Identification and immunoprecipitation of cytoskeletal proteins from murine extra-embryonic endodermal cells. *J. Biol. Chem.*, 256:8124–8133.
532. Oshima, R. G. (1982): Developmental expression of murine extra-embryonic endodermal cytoskeletal proteins. *J. Biol. Chem.*, 257:3414–3421.
533. Oshima, R. G., Howe, W. E., Klier, F. G., Adamson, E. D., and Shevinsky, L. H. (1983): Intermediate filament protein synthesis in preimplantation murine embryos. *Dev. Biol.*, 99:447–455.
534. Duprey, P., Morello, D., Vasseur, M., Babinet, C., Condamine, H., Brulet, P., and Jacob, F. (1985): Expression of the cytokeratin endo A gene during early mouse embryogenesis. *Proc. Natl. Acad. Sci. USA,* 82:8535–8539.
535. Trevor, K., and Oshima, R. G. (1985): Preimplantation mouse embryos and liver express the same type I keratin gene product. *J. Biol. Chem.*, 260:15885–15891.
536. Bissell, M., Hall, H. G., and Parry, G. (1982): How does the extracellular matrix direct gene expression? *J. Theor. Biol.*, 99:31–68.
537. Haeuptle, M.-T., Suard, Y. L. M., Bogenmann, E., Reggio, H., Racine, L., and Kraehenbuhl, J.-P. (1983): Effect of cell shape change on the function and differentiation of rabbit mammary cells in culture. *J. Cell Biol.*, 96:1425–1434.
538. Suard, Y. M. L., Haeuptle, M.-T., Farinon, E., and Kraehenbuhl, J.-P. (1983): Cell proliferation and milk protein gene expression in rabbit mammary cell cultures. *J. Cell Biol.*, 96:1435–1442.
539. Unemori, E. N., and Werb, Z. (1986): Reorganization of polymerized actin: a possible trigger for induction of procollagenase in fibroblasts cultured in and on collagen gels. *J. Cell Biol.*, 103:1021–1031.
540. Adamson, E. D. (1983): Growth factors in development. In: *The Biological Basis of Reproductive and Developmental Medicine,* edited by J. B. Warshaw, pp. 307–336. Elsevier, Amsterdam.
541. Twardzik, D. R. (1985): Differential expression of transforming growth factor-α during prenatal development of the mouse. *Cancer Res.*, 45:5413–5416.
542. Stromberg, K., Pigott, D. A., Ranchalis, J. E., and Twardzik, D. R. (1982): Human term placenta contains transforming growth factors. *Biochem. Biophys. Res. Commun.*, 106:354–364.
543. Merimee, T. J., Grant, M., and Tyson, J. E. (1984): Insulin-like growth factors in amniotic fluid. *J. Clin. Endocrinol. Metab.*, 59:752–767.
544. Tabarelli, M., Kofler, R., and Wick, G. (1983): Placental hormones. I. Immunofluorescence studies of the localization of chorionic gonadotropin placental lactogen and prolactin in human and rat placenta and in the endometrium of pregnant rats. *Placenta,* 4:379–388.
545. Soares, M. J., Julian, J. A., and Glasser, S. R. (1985): Trophoblast giant cell release of placental lactogens: temporal and regional characteristics. *Dev. Biol.*, 107:520–526.
546. Boime, I., Boothby, M., Hoshina, M., Daniels-McQueen, S., and Darnell, R. (1982): Expression and structure of human placental hormone genes as a function of placental development. *Biol. Reprod.*, 26:73–91.
547. Hoshina, M., Boothby, M., and Boime, I. (1982): Cytological localization of chorionic gonadotropin α and placental lactogen mRNAs during development of the human placenta. *J. Cell Biol.*, 93: 190–198.
548. Adamson, E. D., and Meek, J. (1984): The ontogeny of epidermal growth factor receptors during mouse development. *Dev. Biol.*, 103:62–71.
549. Hortsch, M., Schlessinger, J., Gootwine, E., and Webb, C. (1983): Appearance of functional EGF receptor kinase during rodent embryogenesis. *EMBO J.*, 2:1937–1941.
550. Nexo, E., Hollenberg, M. D., Figueroa, A., and Pratt, R. M. (1980): Detection of epidermal growth factor-urogastrone and its receptors during mouse fetal development. *Proc. Natl. Acad. Sci. USA,* 77:2782–2785.
551. Muller, R., and Verma, I. M. (1984): Expression of cellular oncogenes. *Curr. Top. Microbiol.*, 112:73–115.
552. Slamon, D. J., and Cline, M. J. (1984): Expression of cellular oncogenes during embryonic and fetal development of the mouse. *Proc. Natl. Acad. Sci. USA,* 81:7141–7145.
553. Sherr, C. J., Rettenmier, C. W., Sacca, R., Roussel, M. F., Look, A. T., and Stanley, E. R. (1985): The c-*fms* proto-oncogene product is related to the receptor for the mononuclear phagocyte growth factor, CSF-1. *Cell,* 41:665–676.
554. Propst, F., and Vande Woude, G. F. (1985): Expression of c-*mos* proto-oncogene transcripts in mouse tissues. *Nature,* 315:516–518.
555. Muller, R., Slamon, D. J., Adamson, E. D., Tremblay, J. M., Muller, D., Cline, M. J., and Verma, I. M. (1983): Transcription of cellular oncogenes c-ras^{K1} and c-*fms* during mouse development. *Mol. Cell. Biol.*, 3:1062–1069.
556. Muller, R., Tremblay, J. M., Adamson, E. D., and Verma, I. M. (1983): Tissue and cell type-specific expression of two human c-*onc* genes. *Nature,* 304:454–456.
557. Muller, R. (1983): Differential expression of cellular oncogenes during murine development and in teratocarcinoma cell lines. In: *Teratocarcinoma Stem Cells, Vol. 10,* edited by L. M. Silver, G. R. Martin, and S. Strickland, pp. 451–468. Cold Spring Harbor Laboratory, Cold Spring Harbor, N.Y.
558. Muller, R., Verma, I. M., and Adamson, E. D. (1983): Expression of c-*onc* genes: c-*fos* transcripts accumulate to high levels during development of mouse placenta, yolk sac, and amnion. *EMBO J.*, 2:679–684.
559. Pfeifer-Ohlsson, S., Goustin, A. S., Rydnert, J., Wahlstrom, T., Bjersing, L., Stehelin, D., and Ohlsson, R. (1984): Spatial and temporal pattern of cellular *myc* oncogene expression in developing human placenta: implications for embryonic cell proliferation. *Cell,* 38:585–596.
560. Pelham, H. R. B. (1986): Speculations on the functions of the major heat shock and glucose-regulated proteins. *Cell,* 46:959–961.
561. Howlett, S. K. (1986): A set of proteins showing cell-cycle dependent modification in the mouse early embryo. *Cell,* 45:387–396.
562. Wittig, S., Hensse, S., Keitel, C., Elsner, C., and Wittig, B. (1983): Heat shock gene expression is regulated during teratocarcinoma cell differentiation and early embryonic development. *Dev. Biol.*, 96:507–514.
563. Morange, M., Diu, A., Bensaude, O., and Babinet, C. (1984): Altered expression of heat shock proteins in embryonal carcinoma and mouse early embryonic cells. *Mol. Cell. Biol.*, 4:730–735.
564. Heikkila, J. J., and Schultz, G. A. (1984): Different environmental stresses can activate the expression of a heat shock gene in rabbit blastocysts. *Gamete Res.*, 10:45–56.
565. Ulberg, L. C., and Sheean, L. A. (1973): Early development of mammalian embryos in elevated temperatures. *J. Reprod. Fertil. [Suppl.],* 19:155–161.
566. Bellve, A. R. (1976): Incorporation of [^{3}H]uridine by mouse embryos with abnormalities induced by parental hyperthermia. *Biol. Reprod.*, 15:632–646.
567. Kim, K., and Markert, C. L. (1987): Are heat shock proteins involved in development? In: *Developmental Toxicology: Mechanisms and Risk,* edited by J. McLachlan, R. M. Pratt, and C. L. Markert. Cold Spring Harbor Laboratory, Cold Spring Harbor, N.Y. (*in press*).
568. Nusslein-Volhard, C., and Wieschaus, E. (1980): Mutations affecting segment number and polarity in *Drosophila. Nature,* 287:795–801.
569. Garcia-Bellido, A. (1975): Genetic control of wing development in *Drosophila*. In: *Cell Patterning, Ciba Foundation Symposium 29,* pp. 161–178. Associated Scientific, Amsterdam.
570. Lewis, E. B. (1978): A gene complex controlling segmentation in *Drosophila*. *Nature,* 276:565–570.

571. Gehring, W. J. (1975): The homeo box: a key to the understanding of development. *Cell,* 40:3–5.
572. McGinnis, W., Garber, R. L., Wirz, J., Kuroiwa, A., and Gehring, W. J. (1984): A homologous protein-coding sequence in *Drosophila* homeotic genes and its conservation in other metazoans. *Cell,* 37:403–408.
573. Hart, C. P., Awgulewitsch, A., Fainsed, A., McGinnis, W., and Ruddle, F. H. (1985): Homeo box gene complex on mouse chromosome II: molecular cloning, expression in embryogenesis, and homology to a human homeo box locus. *Cell,* 43:9–18.
574. Jackson, I., Schofield, P., and Hogan, B. (1985): A mouse homeo box gene is expressed during embryogenesis and in the adult kidney. *Nature,* 317:745–748.
575. Joyner, A. L., Kornberg, T., Coleman, K. G., Cox, D. R., and Martin, G. R. (1985): Expression during embryogenesis of a mouse gene with sequence homology to the *Drosophila engrailed* gene. *Cell,* 43:29–37.
576. Rabin, M., Hart, C. P., Ferguson-Smith, A., McGinnis, W., Levine, M., and Ruddle, F. H. (1985): Two homeo box loci mapped in evolutionarily related mouse and human chromosomes. *Nature,* 314:175–178.
577. McGinnis, W., Hart, C. P., Gehring, W. J., and Ruddle, F. H. (1984): Molecular cloning and chromosome mapping of a mouse DNA sequence homologous to homeotic genes of *Drosophila. Cell,* 38:675–680.
578. Wolgemuth, D. J., Engelmyer, E., Duggal, R. N., Gizang-Ginsberg, E., Mutter, G. L., Ponzetto, C., Niviano, C., and Zakeri, Z. F. (1986): Isolation of a mouse cDNA coding for a developmentally regulated, testis-specific transcript containing homeo box homology. *EMBO J.,* 5:1229–1235.
579. Rubin, M. R., Toth, L. E., Patel, M. D., D'Eustachio, P., and Nguyen-Huu, M. C. (1986): A mouse homeo box gene is expressed in spermatocytes and embryos. *Science,* 233:663–667.
580. Hauser, C. A., Joyner, A. L., Klein, R. D., Learned, T. K., Martin, G. R., and Tjian, R. (1985): Expression of homologous homeo-box-containing genes in differentiated human teratocarcinoma cells and mouse embryos. *Cell,* 43:19–28.
581. Joyner, A. L., Lebo, R. V., Kan, Y. W., Tjian, R., Cox, D. R., and Martin, G. R. (1985): Comparative chromosome mapping of a conserved homeo box region in mouse and human. *Nature,* 314:173–175.
582. Colberg-Poly, A. M., Voss, S. D., Chowdhury, K., and Gruss, P. (1985): Structural analysis of murine genes containing homeo box sequences and their expression in embryonal carcinoma cells. *Nature,* 314:713–718.
583. Colberg-Poley, A. M., Voss, S. D., Chowdhury, K., Stewart, C. L., Wagner, E. F., and Gruss, P. (1985): Clustered homeo boxes are differentially expressed during murine development. *Cell,* 43:39–45.
584. Carrasco, A. E., McGinnis, W., Gehring, W. J., and DeRobertis, E. M. (1984): A homologous protein-coding sequence in *Drosophila* homeotic genes and its conservation in other metazoans. *Cell,* 37:409–414.
585. Muller, M. M., Carrasco, A. E., and DeRobertis, E. M. (1984): A homeo-box-containing gene expressed during oogenesis in *Xenopus. Cell,* 39:157–162.
586. White, R. A. H., and Wilcox, M. (1984): Protein products of the bithorax complex in *Drosophila. Cell,* 39:163–171.
587. Beddington, R. S. P. (1985): The development of 12th to 14th day foetuses following reimplantation of pre- and early-primitive-streak-stage mouse embryos. *J. Embryol. Exp. Morphol.,* 88:281–291.
588. New, D. A. T. (1978): Whole-embryo culture and the study of mammalian embryos during organogenesis. *Biol. Rev.,* 53:81–122.
589. Wiley, L. M., and Pedersen, R. A. (1977): Morphology of mouse egg cylinder development *in vitro:* a light and electron microscopic study. *J. Exp. Zool.,* 200:389–402.
590. Hsu, Y. C. (1978): *In vitro* development of whole mouse embryos beyond the implantation stage. In: *Methods in Mammalian Reproduction,* edited by J. C. Daniel, Jr., pp. 229–245. Academic Press, New York.
591. Mintz, B. (1971): Allophenic mice of multi-embryo origin. In: *Methods in Mammalian Embryology,* edited by J. C. Daniel, Jr., pp. 186–214. W. H. Freeman, San Francisco.
592. Gardner, R. L. (1971): Manipulations on the blastocyst. In: *Advances in the Biosciences, Vol. 6,* edited by G. Raspe, pp. 279–296. Pergamon, Oxford.
593. Pierce, B. (1983): The cancer cell and its control by the embryo. *Am. J. Pathol.,* 113:117–124.
594. Gardner, R. L. and Papaioannou, V. E. (1975): Differentiation in the trophectoderm and inner cell mass. In: *The Early Development of Mammals, British Society for Developmental Biology, Symp. 2,* edited by M. Balls and A. E. Wild, pp. 107–132. Cambridge University Press, Cambridge.

The Physiology of Reproduction,
edited by E. Knobil and J. Neill *et al.*.
Raven Press, Ltd., New York © 1988.

CHAPTER 7

Biology of Implantation

H. M. Weitlauf

Implantation of embryos in the wall of the uterus is a basic feature of mammalian reproduction. It is the result of a complex series of interactive steps beginning with fixation of the blastocyst in the uterus and ending with formation of a definitive placenta. Details of the intervening steps vary in different species, but the fundamental elements of embryo attachment and penetration of the epithelium with invasion into the endometrium, as well as formation of decidual tissue by the uterus, are features common to many animals. Furthermore, in the species studied so far, it appears the embryos and the uterus must be "synchronized"; typically, this means that the embryos have reached the expanded blastocyst stage and that the endometrium has undergone certain hormone-dependent changes that cause it to become "receptive" to the embryo.

Because of its complexity, the process of implantation is difficult to study *in toto,* and most research has been carried out on those component steps that can be dissected out for description or definition. This approach has been quite successful, and a vast literature has grown up over the last 50 years in which detailed accounts have been compiled describing the processes of embryo attachment, the penetration of the epithelium, the endocrine basis for uterine receptivity, and the chemical and cytological changes associated with initiation of the decidual reaction and differentiation of decidual tissue. On the other hand, because they have focused on selected facets of the process, often in only one species, investigators have sometimes been tempted to look for and champion single mechanisms as the "cause" of implantation. But because implantation is not an isolated event established at a moment in time, or even necessarily involving the same mechanisms in different species, there is no single cause or mechanism and the resulting controversies tend to dominate the literature. Because it is difficult to develop an overview of implantation from the perspective of the conflicts, those findings that are most consistent and that seem to reflect common elements in various species are emphasized in this chapter. Several extensive reviews dealing with specific aspects of implantation should be consulted for further details regarding the controversial issues (1–11).

CELLULAR ASPECTS OF IMPLANTATION

Details of implantation vary in different species. However, in all animals it ultimately involves a direct interaction of the trophoblast with the luminal epithelium of the uterus. This basic step has been described in detail from a morphological perspective and provides a framework upon which physiological and biochemical observations can be organized.

Attachment

For descriptive purposes it has been useful to consider that the attachment of embryos to the uterine epithelium occurs in two phases, apposition and adhesion (8); the processes involved are quite distinct. The term *apposition* denotes the progressively increasing intimacy of contact between the trophoblast and the uterine epithelium. In mice and rats the uterine lumen closes down around the embryos in the earliest phase of implantation and thus the uterus has the appearance of "clasping" the blastocysts (12). On the other hand, in animals such as the rabbit, the blastocyst enlarges to fill the uterine lumen and hence brings the trophoblast into apposition with the epithelium without general obliteration of the lumen (8,13). In either case, investment of embryos with maternal epithelium seems to provide the initial mechanism for their immobilization within the uterus. At this stage the blastocyst can be dislodged without damage by gentle perfusion of the uterus, and hence the earliest fixation of the embryo is functional rather than involving structural connections between the two individuals. During this phase there is a progressive interdigitation of microvilli and an increasingly intimate association between the membranes of the blastocyst and endometrium. The microvilli become shorter, more blunted, and irregular (14–19), and there is the appearance of large bulbous cytoplasmic projections, particularly on the antimesometrial surface (2,20). The obliteration of the uterine lumen with progressively closer apposition of the apical ends of the endometrial epithelial cells and the trophoblast has been referred to as the *attachment reaction* (15).

The mechanisms responsible for the development of apposition, clasping, and the attachment reaction have not been worked out in detail, although in mice, rats, hamsters, and guinea pigs the changes appear to be associated with a more generalized closure of the uterine lumen that is dependent on the endocrine status of the mother (13,16–18, 21–27). For instance, the uterine lumen remains relatively open in ovariectomized mice given no replacement hormones and becomes obliterated only after the animals are injected with progesterone (28,29). Following treatment with progesterone alone, the process of closure tends to be arrested at the stage characterized by simple interdigitation of microvilli and does not show the progressively closer apposition characteristic of normal pregnancy. This "first stage" of closure can be maintained with progesterone for prolonged periods in castrated animals and is induced to progress to the "second stage" only by adding estrogen to the regimen (30). As might be expected then, some degree of closure and clasping has been reported to occur in mice with lactational or experimentally induced delayed implantation (24,31). In those situations, the interaction between uterine epithelium and trophoblast is characterized by simple interdigitation of the microvilli as long as the animals are nursing or are maintained with progesterone. However, after the addition of estrogen the association between the embryo and the uterus becomes more intimate, with a reduction in the microvilli and progression to the typical attachment reaction (29). With the development of more intimate apposition in response to estrogen, there is apparently increased pressure on the blastocysts as their surfaces become marked and distorted by corresponding irregularities in the uterine epithelium (32). There is some degree of clasping of delayed-implanting rat embryos (23), but the preponderance of evidence indicates that, in that species also, estrogen must be added for a typical attachment reaction (33,34).

It is now generally assumed that uterine closure and clasping of embryos or other objects (35,36) involves both endocrine-dependent resorption of fluid from the lumen, presumably by way of the irregular cytoplasmic projections referred to as *pinopods* (37–39), and a mild generalized edema that occurs throughout the endometrium in response to estrogen (40,41). However, associated changes in the apical membranes of the uterine epithelial cells (42) and the occurrence of increased membrane turnover (43) indicate that processes associated with uterine closure are not limited to the removal of luminal fluid. Furthermore, although closure and clasping appear to be primarily hormone-dependent uterine functions, it has been reported that the presence of blastocysts (or oil droplets) in the lumen hastens the second stage of closure and the appearance of the attachment reaction (44), presumably because they provide some additional stimulus to the epithelium.

The significance of closure and the attachment reaction in mice and rats is presumably that a period of stability is provided during which adhesion between the embryo and the uterus can develop. However, in animals such as the rabbit, the mink, or the rhesus monkey, there does not appear to be a typical closure of the uterine lumen or clasping of the embryos (13,45), and it seems to be the expansion of the blastocyst that is primarily responsible for establishing the initial apposition between trophoblast and epithelium. It is interesting in this regard that there is no evidence for pinopod-mediated uptake of fluid from the lumen of the rabbit uterus (46). In large domestic species also, with their strated the exsuperficial epitheliochorial-type implantation, the interdigitation of microvilli is particularly extensive and the embryos appear to be firmly fixed in the uterus even though a typical attachment reaction with progressive loss of microvilli is not observed (47–49).

Adhesion of the trophoblast cells to the apical ends of the uterine epithelial cells develops as the apposition phase progresses. Cytologic evidence most often cited as demonstrating the development of adhesiveness is twofold. First, with tissue taken from progressively later stages in the early phase of implantation, there is an increase in the amount and frequency of distortion of one or both surfaces. This is thought to occur as a normal part of the attachment process and to be exaggerated as a differential shrinkage artifact when the tissues are fixed for microscopy. Second, not only are there extensive areas where closely apposed membranes of trophoblast and apical ends of the uterine cells are parallel and separated by less than 150 to 200 Å, but primitive junctional complexes are established (8,9). Although some descriptions of these regions have indicated the existence of mature septate-type desmosomal junctions and areas of cytoplasmic confluence (18,23), the usual observation is of less specialized and more primitive types of junctional complexes and the absence of cytoplasmic confluence (8,9,12, 24,50). Once the epithelium is penetrated, however, typical mature junctional complexes are often observed to be shared between uterine epithelium and the invading trophoblast (50).

The molecular basis for initial adhesion of trophoblast and uterine epithelium at implantation has not yet been determined. However, the expression of complementary surface glycoproteins and the elaboration of aggregation molecules and extracellular matrix material are known to be involved in cell recognition and adhesion in some simple multicellular organisms, and these mechanisms are thought to be generally applicable to vertebrates as well (51). Therefore, most studies of the acquisition of adhesiveness at implantation have been concerned with documenting the changes in cell-surface molecules during the peri-implantation period. The several changes observed either at the time of normal implantation or after termination of the dormant phase associated with delayed implantation may be relevant to the development of adhesiveness. Thus, Enders and Schlafke (52), using a combination of colloidal thorium, ruthenium red, and concanavalin A-peroxidase, demonstrated the extensive distribution of negative charges and acidic glycoproteins on the surface of mouse uterus during the fourth and fifth days of normal pregnancy and on the seventh day of lactation-delayed implantation. Although those workers were the first to suggest that there is a reduction in the thickness of the glycocalyx at implantation, the methods used were not considered to be quantitative. Others, however, have subsequently reported that there are both a generalized loss of anionic sites and a reduction in thickness of the uterine glycocalyx at implantation: rabbit (53), rat (54), and mouse (55). Interestingly, these changes are apparently not dependent on the presence of embryos, since they occur in pseudopregnant as well as pregnant animals. In the ferret, however, the uterine glycocalyx does appear to be reduced in thickness initially at the specific points of contact between the embryo and uterus, indicating that, in that species at least, the embryo plays a role in the process of modifying the uterine surface (56). A reduction in the thickness of the glycocalyx could be associated with the removal of masking residues and thus be responsible for opening a variety of specific binding sites. Indeed, Chavez and Anderson (55) have reported that binding sites for the *Ricinus communis* lectin (i.e., binds D-galactose) appear at both implantation and interimplantation areas in mouse uterus in the peri-implantation period. They suggest that lectin-like receptors for galactose, appearing on the embryos, could bind to those sites and act as part of the adhesion mechanism at implantation.

Characteristics of surface molecules on the embryos have also been observed to change at the time of attachment. For instance, histocompatibility antigens (H-2) on dormant delayed-implanting mouse blastocysts decrease during reactivation (57,58), suggesting that these glycoprotein factors are either removed or masked; there is a reduction in binding of positively charged colloidal iron to the surface of these blastocysts as well, indicating a decrease in the density of negative charges (59–61). This histochemical finding was confirmed by the results of experiments utilizing free-zone electrophoresis (62,63). Such changes in the embryos are compatible with removal of terminal sialic acid residues or larger moieties of the oligosaccharide components of surface glycoproteins at the time of attachment and at the initiation of implantation.

In related experiments, lectins have been used to probe the glycocalyx of the embryo for changes in the "accessibility" of specific sugars at the time of implantation. Because it appears, in many species, that the initial attachment of embryos occurs on specific limited regions of their surfaces (52,56,64,65), it might be anticipated that those regions would acquire adhesiveness earlier than other areas on the embryos and, therefore, that changes in lectin binding which are relevant to implantation would have corresponding temporal and regional patterns in the peri-implantation period. Although binding of various lectins has been observed by several investigators, in most cases the appropriate temporal and regional changes have not been demonstrated. Thus, it was shown with the electron microscope that concanavalin A-peroxidase binds to the surface of both the embryos and the uterus of mice, but there was no evidence of a change with implantation or of regional differences in distribution on the blastocysts (52,66). Chavez and Enders (67), using ferritin-conjugated lectins on days 5 and 6 of normal pregnancy, as well as during delayed implantation, found stage-specific changes in the binding of peanut agglutinin and the agglutinin from *Ricinus communis* to the surface of blastocysts as they prepared to implant (these lectins bind preferentially to *N*-acetylgalactosamine and D-galactose, respectively), but neither change could be implicated as a factor in the acquisition of adhesiveness because the binding pattern was not different in nonadhesive delayed-implanting embryos. On the other hand, those same workers (68) reported that the lectin from *Dolichos biflorus* (specific for *N*-acetylglucosamine) did bind to delayed-implanting embryos but did not bind to embryos that were reactivated and, although regional differences were not seen, they suggested that the loss of binding sites is associated with the acquisition of adhesiveness. With concanavalin A bound to red blood cells, Sobel and Nebel (69,70) observed increased agglutination over the abembryonic pole of mouse blastocysts and, similarly, concanavalin A attached to latex beads was shown to bind preferentially to the abembryonic end of delayed-implanting blastocysts (71). However, again, there was no change in this regional pattern of binding upon reactivation and subsequent implantation. From such observations it cannot be determined whether changes in the glycocalyx which lead to changes in lectin binding are simply not related to the acquisition of regional adhesiveness or whether the methods used are too insensitive to demonstrate subtle differences in binding. By contrast, it has been observed that binding of molecular [^{3}H]concanavalin A to delayed-implanting embryos decreases in the abembryonic region during the process of reactivation and suggested that there is a regional change in availability of mannose-like sugars, or membrane fluidity, on the embryo that is related to the development of adhesiveness (72). A similar temporal and regional change in the glycocalyx during reactivation of delayed-implanting mouse embryos was inferred from increased staining of the abembryonic pole with Alcian blue (71). Although the precise nature of the changes in the glycocalyx cannot be deduced from such information, the observation of such temporal and regional patterns is compatible with the interpretation that they are related to the acquisition of adhesiveness at implantation.

Pinkser and Mintz (73) are often credited with the first attempts to establish qualitative differences in composition of surface glycoproteins in preimplantation mouse embryos. Those workers labeled two- to four-cell embryos or morula-early blastocysts differentially with [^{3}H]- and [^{14}C]glucosamine, combined them, and removed the glycocalyx with trypsin; the trypsinate was treated with pronase and the digest was subjected to gel filtration. They found more label and generally larger fragments in the material from blastocysts, but were unable to determine whether the change was due to synthesis of qualitatively new glycoproteins or due to differentially regulated expression of those present in the earlier stages. In either case, they did not examine blastocysts at the time they acquire adhesiveness; therefore, their results do not provide information strictly about changes associated with implantation.

The reports that mouse blastocysts are capable of synthesizing a variety of glycoproteins that could be involved in changes in embryo adhesiveness (74), the suggestion that type-III collagen is present on the surface of late blastocysts and may be the material in the intercellular ridges (75), and the report that fibronectin is synthesized by the inner cell mass but not trophoblast of mouse blastocysts (76) have apparently not been followed up. If confirmed, the observations that such extracellular factors are synthesized would have potentially important implications for the acquisition of adhesiveness at implantation (51).

The fact that changes occur in both the thickness of the glycocalyx and the capacity of embryos and uterus to bind specific lectins demonstrates that there are alterations in surface glycoproteins in the peri-implantation period. Although it must be emphasized that the precise nature of the changes cannot be deduced from such information and that it cannot be assumed that the changes are responsible for the acquisition of adhesiveness, it seems probable that they are involved. The further possibility that aggregation factors and secreted extracellular matrix materials are involved in attachment of the embryos remains to be examined critically.

Penetration of the Epithelium

It is clear that, with the exception of those species having a superficial (i.e., epitheliochorial) type of placentation, all mammalian embryos penetrate the uterine epithelium and its associated basal lamina to establish a definitive vascular relationship with the mother. However, the process varies considerably from species to species in terms of both timing and precise cytological features, and the early literature was replete with what appeared to be conflicting observations. Some conceptual order was brought to this complex problem when Schlafke and Enders (9) pointed out that there are really three general strategies for penetrating the uterine epithelium and that various animals have adopted one or another of these approaches. Many of the apparent inconsistencies disappear when comparisons are confined to a single type of penetration. A brief description of the essential cytological details in each of the three categories is useful to demonstrate the various ways in which different species have solved the problem of breaching the epithelial barrier.

Intrusive Penetration

In species that have adopted the intrusive approach to penetration of the epithelium, the embryos are generally considered to be highly "invasive"; the ferret provides an excellent example (56,77). Attachment initially occurs at specialized regions (i.e., ectoplasmic pads) of developing syncytial trophoblast. Whereas the broader regions of syncytial plaque generally follow the contour of the apical end of the epithelial cells, the ectoplasmic pads tend to indent them and appear to provide the initial points of attachment. The first penetration of epithelium is seen as the projection of a thin fold of syncytial trophoblast between adjacent epithelial cells. Initially the processes are ectoplasmic, but as they enlarge and progress to the basal lamina, the cytoplasm is found to contain the usual array of organelles. The trophoblastic membrane is observed to share both apical junctional complexes and punctate desmosomes with the lateral membrane of adjacent epithelial cells. It is not known how the original epithelial apical junctional complexes are breached, but the process typically occurs at many sites that are separated by only a few cells. Although the trophoblast eventually surrounds large numbers of epithelial cells, and there is evidence of cell death and phagocytosis, the overwhelming impression is of apparently undisturbed epithelial cells adjacent to the trophoblast. Indeed, it has been suggested that healthy epithelium is necessary for anchoring the trophoblast as it penetrates deeper into the endometrium (56). The trophoblastic processes pause at the basal lamina and are disposed along it for a brief time, then proceed to invade the stroma where they surround but do not penetrate the basal lamina of the capillaries. Other species having the intrusive type of penetration include the guinea pig (50,78,79) and the rhesus monkey (45). There are subtle but potentially important differences in detail in these animals. For example, the syncytial trophoblastic processes of both the monkey and the ferret typically pause at the epithelial basal lamina; in the monkey, they then go on to invade the basal lamina of endometrial blood vessels, something which is not seen in the ferret.

The intrusion of the cellular trophoblast to form the isolated endometrial cups responsible for secretion of gonadotropin in the horse provides an interesting variation in this form of epithelial penetration that appears to be unrelated to the process of implantation per se (80).

Displacement Penetration

The rat and the mouse provide typical examples of displacement penetration (12,81). As the apposition phase proceeds and the first signs of decidualization appear in the subjacent stroma, there is typically evidence of cell death in the epithelial layer and of detachment of cells either singly or in groups. With the light microscope, these cells occasionally appear as dark masses (W-bodies) between the embryo and the endometrium and were originally thought to reflect the passage of some material from the embryo to the uterus (82). However, it was subsequently shown with the electron microscope that these masses are really dead epithelial cells that are being phagocytized by the trophoblast (81). As the trophoblast comes into contact with the basal lamina, it pauses and sends out processes that undermine adjacent cells and thus extends the epithelial defect and increases the area available for contact with the embryo. The basal lamina is then breached, apparently not by the trophoblast but rather by ectoplasmic processes of underlying decidual cells (83).

The mechanism responsible for death and detachment of the epithelium in this type of implantation is not known. However, it does appear to be intrinsic to the uterus because it occurs in the "implantation chambers" associated with an oil-induced decidual reaction in pseudopregnant mice (84–87) and is blocked by administration of actinomycin D (88). Considerable histochemical evidence has been presented which indicates that the activity of various lysosomal enzymes decreases in the epithelial cells adjacent to an implanting embryo but not in interimplantation areas or in pseudopregnant animals (89–94), and it has been argued on this basis that the cells are undergoing autolysis in response to an embryonic signal (95). When the sloughing of epithelium was prevented by actinomycin D, mouse blastocysts became attached to the epithelium but were unable to penetrate to the basal lamina or stroma and thus could not truly implant (88). Hence, mouse blastocysts seem to be only weakly invasive, and an intact uterine epithelium may be an effective barrier to implantation. Therefore, autolytic destruction of the epithelium seems to be an important precondition for implantation in that species at least, and the finding that mouse blastocysts transferred to the uteri of cyclic females implant only if the epithelium is disrupted (96) supports this suggestion.

Fusion Penetration

The rabbit provides an example of fusion penetration (50,64,97,98). First attachment occurs between syncytial knobs of the abembryonic trophoblast and individual epithelial cells. The apical membrane of the epithelial cell fuses with that of the trophoblastic knob, resulting in cytoplasmic confluency. As the epithelial cell is converted to syncytium, it becomes cytologically distinct from its neighbors and appears, using the light or electron microscope, as a "peg" of trophoblast extending to the basal lamina. The original nucleus is present for some time, and the lateral plasma membrane retains the original junctional complexes with its apparently normal neighboring cells. There may be more than one peg per trophoblastic knob, and after some delay the basal lamina is penetrated at the locations of these pegs and the trophoblastic processes proceed to penetrate the endometrial blood vessels. Subsequently, there is widespread formation of epithelial symplasma, and fusion occurs in areas between the trophoblastic knobs (99).

Localized Changes in the Stroma

In rats and mice the endometrial stroma eventually undergoes dramatic cytological changes to form a decidua in response to the implanting embryo. This process is discussed in detail later, but it should be noted here that subtle changes occur locally in the endometrium as an early part of the decidual response. The most obvious of these are the increases in alkaline phosphatase activity (85) and vascular permeability (100–102), which occur in the stroma immediately adjacent to the embryos even before they have penetrated the epithelium.

It is clear, even from these strictly morphological accounts of early pregnancy, that at least two different sorts of changes occur in the peri-implantation uterus. First, there are certain hormone-dependent changes in the endometrium that make subsequent steps possible. These "enabling" changes, such as closure of the lumen and the acquisition, by epithelium, of the potential for self-destruction, occur throughout the endometrium, apparently without regard to the presence of an embryo. By contrast, there are other changes in the endometrium that must be provoked by a stimulus, from either an embryo or a suitable experimental substitute. These "evoked" responses, such as autolysis of epithelial cells or decidual transformation of stromal cells, are typically localized to the endometrium adjacent to the embryo or the site of experimental stimulation. Although the actual roles of many of these changes have not been established with certainty, it is presumed that they are important for the implantation process; a great deal of work has been directed at defining their molecular and cellular basis. The process of decidual transformation, and the associated enabling changes leading to acquisition of sensitivity by the endometrium, may be the most thoroughly studied of all.

Decidualization

Decidual transformation of the endometrium in response to an implanting embryo results in grossly observable increases in the size and weight of the uterus. This growth is due not only to proliferation and differentiation of the endometrial stromal cells, but also to swelling of the tissue caused by localized increases in vascular permeability and the development of tissue edema. Thus, following attachment the embryo typically becomes embedded in an enlarging mass of decidual tissue, each so-called "nidus" being separated from the others by intervening areas of nontransformed endometrium. Formation of the decidua is a conspicuous part of the process of implantation, and although the function of this specialized tissue has not been determined with certainty, it is generally believed to be a critical component of the mother's response to the embryo.

The discovery by Loeb (103–105) nearly 80 years ago, that a similar transformation of the endometrium could be induced by indifferent stimuli in the uteri of animals that were suitably prepared with ovarian steroid hormones, has led to the development of an experimental model for this maternal response to the implanting embryo. Several investigators have pointed to subtle differences between the "deciduomata" of the experimental model and naturally occurring decidua, particularly with respect to the timing of development and minor morphological details (106–108). However, the basic processes responsible for decidual transformation in response to the embryo appear to be the same as those leading to formation of experimental deciduomata, and the model has come to be widely accepted (109).

One of the most important observations made with the experimental model has been that the decidual response can be obtained only during a limited time in pregnancy or pseudopregnancy (110,111) and that this period varies with the nature of the experimental stimulus. Thus, a grossly traumatic stimulus such as crushing or cutting the uterus was found to be effective during a period of 3 or 4 days early in pseudopregnancy, whereas less traumatic stimuli such as intraperitoneal injection of pyrathiazine or the intraluminal instillation of various chemical substances can elicit a response only during a period of a few hours (84,112–118). Furthermore, this period of maximum sensitivity to the so-called "nontraumatic stimuli" was found to correspond to the period of uterine receptivity for blastocysts as established by asynchronous embryo transfer experiments (119–126).

With this information in hand, it then became possible to determine the endocrine basis for developing uterine sensitivity. In an extensive series of experiments with mice and rats, it was eventually shown that although progesterone alone would support the development of a deciduoma in response to traumatic stimuli, it is estrogen acting on the endometrium after preconditioning with progesterone for at least 2 days that is responsible for entraining the pattern of sensitivity and subsequent refractoriness characteristic of the peri-implantation period (1–3,109,118). As might be anticipated, this endocrine regimen is essentially the same as that necessary to obtain implantation of blastocysts in ovariectomized rats and mice (100,127,128).

Once it was established that formation of this new "decidual organ" (129) was dependent on appropriate hormonal conditioning and the application of a suitable stimulus during a limited time, the emphasis of investigators shifted to defining those chemical and cytological changes within the endometrium that are associated with establishing receptivity and the differentiation of decidual tissue (1–7).

Preparation of the Endometrium

Hormone-dependent changes in cell proliferation and differentiation occur in all compartments of the endometrium and, although it has not been possible to determine how the changes are related to the acquisition of receptivity or to the development of the decidual reaction, it is generally thought that they are essential.

Cell Proliferation

Changes in the rates of proliferation of endometrial components have been examined in intact animals during the estrous cycle and early pregnancy and pseudopregnancy: mice (130–132); rats (133–136); guinea pig (137–139); and hamster (140).

Luminal epithelium. Mitotic activity in luminal epithelium of mice varies during the ovarian cycle, with a peak at about the time of ovulation and a smaller secondary peak 3 days later. The secondary peak falls on the third day of pregnancy if mating has occurred, and there is little or no mitotic activity in the luminal epithelium thereafter (130,131). A similar pattern appears in the rat, with the first peak at about the time of ovulation and a second one 2 days later on the second day of pregnancy or pseudopregnancy (133–135). It has been reported similarly that in guinea pigs there is mitotic activity at about the time of ovulation and a secondary peak 2 to 3 days later (137–139). With hamsters also, mitotic activity is found in the epithelium at the time of ovulation, with a marked increase 2 days later (140).

Synthesis of DNA, as demonstrated by incorporation of [^{3}H]thymidine and autoradiographic or scintillation counting techniques, follows the same pattern. Incorporation of [^{3}H]thymidine increases in luminal epithelium of the mouse on the second day of pseudopregnancy and decreases thereafter (131,141). In rats also, the epithelium is labeled with [^{3}H]thymidine on the second and third days of pseudopregnancy (142).

Glandular epithelium. Proliferation of endometrial glands tends to be low in mice at and before ovulation but shows a marked increase 3 days later, coincident with the second peak of epithelial mitosis (130,132). The pattern appears to be similar in the rat, with a peak on the second day of pregnancy (134,135,143); a corresponding incorporation of [^{3}H]thymidine has been observed on the second day of pregnancy (144). Mitotic activity in the glands of the guinea pig is of relatively greater extent than that in the mouse and the rat and appears somewhat later, with a peak on the fourth day of the estrous cycle (137–139).

Stroma. A small amount of mitotic activity is observed in the stroma of the mouse just before ovulation and is minimal thereafter until a marked increase occurs on the fourth day of pseudopregnancy or pregnancy; the high levels of mitotic activity carry over into the fifth day, when implantation occurs (130,131). There appears to be some preferential distribution of the active cells near the luminal epithelium, although mitosis occurs throughout the endometrium. A similar pattern is observed in the rat, with stromal mitosis appearing late on the third day and peaking on the fourth day, and the active cells appear to be concentrated in the subepithelial antimesometrial stroma (134–136). The pattern in the guinea pig seems to peak between the sixth and seventh days of the cycle (137–139).

Incorporation of [^{3}H]thymidine into DNA is observed in the stroma of mice and rats after epithelial mitosis has ceased. It is maximal on the fourth and fifth days of pseudopregnancy (131,141,142) in the subepithelial cells of the antimesometrial region (145) and appears to be a consequence of estrogen action after preparation by progesterone (146).

The endocrine regulation of cell division in the various tissue compartments of the endometrium has been examined critically using ovariectomized animals given replacement therapy: mice (147–152); rats (136,146,153); guinea pig (137,138); and rabbit (154,155). The relationships between changes in the endocrine milieu and mitotic activity in the luminal epithelium, the glands, and the stroma have been most completely established for mouse endometrium. A description of these relationships in the mouse therefore seems useful as a basis for comparison. The observations on intact mice fit well with what has been discovered about endocrine regulation of these tissues in replacement experiments with ovariectomized animals; these observations also fit well with what is known about the changing levels of ovarian steroid hormones in the estrous cycle and early pregnancy (3,4).

Luminal epithelium. Mitotic activity is nil in the luminal epithelium of ovariectomized mice given no hormone replacement. However, following a single injection of estrogen, there is an increase in mitotic activity; the response is biphasic with peaks at about 24 and 36 hr (147–150, 152,156–160). If estrogen is administered continuously, the effect on mitotic activity in epithelial cells is maintained for 2 days and then drops off (151). Progesterone administered by itself has no stimulatory effect on luminal epithelium but markedly reduces the effect of estrogen if the two hormones are administered simultaneously; typically, the first peak of mitotic activity is reduced and the second peak is blocked completely. The effect of progesterone can be obtained up to about 17 hr after estrogen (161,162). On the other hand, if progesterone is given for 3 days, a subsequent injection of estrogen has no effect on mitotic activity in the epithelium (163). The rat is apparently similar to the mouse in that estrogen stimulates mitotic activity in luminal epithelial cells within 24 hr; pretreatment with progesterone suppresses that effect (136,153). The rabbit seems to respond differently in that estrogen stimulates epithelium only mildly whereas progesterone alone (in sufficiently high doses) is the more effective stimulus; it has been reported, however, that priming with estrogen reduces the amount of progesterone needed for the mitogenic effect (154,155). In the ovariectomized guinea pig, estrogen stimulates epithelial mitosis (137,138); pretreatment with progesterone prevents this effect (137).

Glandular epithelium. A single injection of estrogen has no effect on mitosis in uterine glands of mice (150). However, with continuous administration of estrogen a wave of mitosis is seen in the glands at 72 hr; this is followed by a second wave of mitotic activity 72 hr after terminating treatment (151). Progesterone given beforehand suppresses both waves of activity, whereas progesterone given with the estrogen, or following estrogen treatment, blocks only the second wave. In the rat, estrogen causes an increase in mitosis in the glands within 24 hr and causes a further increase at 48 hr; again, pretreatment with progesterone suppresses that effect (136,153). In rabbits, there is reported to be some mitotic activity in the glands following treatment with estrogen alone, but it is much greater with progesterone (155). There is a question regarding control of mitosis in uterine glands of the guinea pig because some investigators have achieved proliferation with estrogen alone and suggest that the guinea pigs are like mice and rats (137); others have reported that mitotic activity is stimulated by progesterone after estrogen priming and suggest, therefore, that guinea pigs are similar to rabbits (138).

Stroma. Neither estrogen nor progesterone alone appears to have an effect on mitotic activity in stroma in mice. However, progesterone is able to induce stromal mitosis if a priming dose of estrogen has been given previously (164). Furthermore, if progesterone is given for 3 days, the stroma undergoes marked hypertrophy in response to a subsequent injection of estrogen regardless of whether priming estrogen was given (150,163). Priming with estrogen appears to compress the progesterone-induced changes into just 2 days (165). Interestingly, a second injection of estrogen given to progesterone-treated animals at 48 hr will cause a second increase in mitotic activity, but if it is given between 12 and 36 hr after the first injection, the endometrium is refractory and the estrogen is redirected to affect the epithelium (166). In the rat also, estrogen has no effect on stromal mitosis unless there has been pretreatment with progesterone (136,153). In addition, it appears the mitotic activity in the rat is concentrated in the antimesometrial stroma adjacent to the luminal epithelium (153). With the rabbit, estrogen alone causes a modest increase in stromal mitosis (155). Again, there appears to be a question in the guinea pig because some investigators find that progestrone alone stimulates little mitotic activity in the stroma but when estrogen is added it increases dramatically as it does in the mouse (137), whereas others report that progestrone after estrogen priming causes massive increases in stromal mitosis and suggest that the guinea pig is like the rabbit with regard to the regulation of proliferation in the endometrium (138).

Associated with the changes in proliferation during the peri-implantation period there are marked changes in the levels of steroid receptors (167–171). However, it has been difficult to evaluate the significance of the changes with respect to development of endometrial receptivity and mitotic activity, not only because of the heterogeneity within the receptor populations (172,173) but also because in many cases the measurements were made on whole uterus rather than in the various tissue compartments or cell populations of the endometrium. Because the myometrium accounts for as much as 90% of the mass of the uterus, measurements of the whole organ tend to reflect changes in that compartment rather than in the endometrium. The significance of this distinction was demonstrated by Glasser and McCormack (7), who observed that, as measured in whole uterus, both nuclear and cytosol estrogen receptor concentration decreases from the second or third day of pregnancy onward while in stroma the content actually increases. Martel and Psychoyos (174) likewise found differential changes in cytosol estrogen receptor levels in the different uterine compartments in response to progesterone, with increases occurring in stroma after 48 hr accompanied by simultaneous decreases in the epithelium. Although the concentrations of estrogen receptors therefore are correlated with the mitogenic effect of estrogen in the peri-implantation period, levels of receptor do not appear to be the limiting factor (174); also, the acquisition of sensitivity to estrogen after 48 hr of progesterone appears to involve other regulatory factors.

In general, then, estrogen stimulates proliferation of both luminal and glandular epithelium, whereas progesterone inhibits the mitogenic effect of estrogen on epithelium. Furthermore, estrogen given after several days of progesterone treatment causes the stroma, rather than epithelium, to proliferate. Pretreatment of the uterus with estrogen reduces the time necessary for this effect of progesterone to become manifest. The changes in mitotic activity are reflected, as would be expected, by parallel changes in the incorporation of [^{3}H]thymidine into DNA. In light of these findings, the patterns of mitotic activity in cyclic and pregnant mice and rats have led to the hypothesis that it is the estrogen released at about the time of ovulation that initiates the first wave of epithelial proliferation, its withdrawal being responsible for a wave of activity in the glands on the third day of pregnancy. According to this hypothesis, progesterone from the corpus luteum then conditions the stroma, and the nidatory estrogen induces proliferation of the stroma on the fourth and fifth days in preparation for implantation. Thus, the hormone regimen necessary to establish a typical peri-implantation pattern of mitotic activity in the endometrium of ovariectomized mice appears to be the same as that which is required to develop maximum uterine sensitivity to a nontraumatic intraluminal stimulus for decidualization (118). It is not known whether this pattern of proliferative activity enables the endometrium to respond to a decidual stimulus or merely accompanies the acquisition of sensitivity.

Cell Differentiation

Morphological changes. Results of morphological examination of the endometrium in cyclic and pregnant animals, or castrated animals given various hormone replacements, demonstrate clearly again that changes occur in all compartments of the endometrium in response to ovarian steroid hormones. The cytological changes indicate that there are significant differences in overall synthetic activity in the stromal cells as the endometrium moves from presensitivity through the sensitive phase and becomes refractory.

Luminal Epithelium: Uterine luminal epithelium becomes atrophic after removal of the ovaries. The typical high columnar cells quickly change to a more cuboidal shape, with the nucleus located in a middle position. The cytoplasm becomes weakly basophilic, with meager amounts of endoplasmic reticulum, and the Golgi complex is small. Numerous lipid droplets accumulate in the basal regions of the cells; and the apical microvilli become short, with little evidence of surface coat material. Following the injection of estrogen, the cells increase in height, the cytoplasm becomes intensely basophilic, and there is an increase in the amount and prominence of the endoplasmic reticulum. The nuclei come to occupy a more basal position, the Golgi complex increases markedly and may occupy the lateral as well as the supranuclear area of the cells, and the apical microvilli increase in length. It is estimated that the apical surface area of the cells increases by as much as 50% and becomes covered with a "fuzz" (156–158,175). It is generally presumed that this extracellular material is a typical glycocalyx composed of negatively charged acidic glycoproteins (23,24,52,176). Other consistent findings following the administration of estrogen are the rapid dissipation of basal lipid droplets (177–181) and increases in several enzymatic activities, including alkaline phosphatase and nonspecific esterase (182–185).

Progesterone, given by itself to ovariectomized animals, also leads to an increase in cell height. However, the cytoplasm remains pale-staining and there is increased accumulation of lipid in the basal area of the cells (28). Although cathepsin D activity increases in the luminal epithelium upon stimulation with progesterone (186), there is no increase in alkaline phosphatase activity (184). However, probably the most dramatic cytologic change that takes place in epithelium treated for several days with progesterone is the development of extensive interdigitation of the apical microvilli on the apposed luminal surfaces (28–30) and the formation of pinopods (20,65,187,188). It will be recalled that these features are characteristic of the first phase of uterine closure and are, therefore, associated with "presensitive" endometrium.

The addition of estrogen in this situation leads to loss of the lipid droplets, increased prominence of the rough endoplasmic reticulum, and a reduction in the number and size of the microvilli. Subsequently the apical membranes are more closely apposed and the surface becomes irregular, with attainment of the second stage of uterine closure characteristic of postsensitive or refractory endometrium (30). Although the transition from first to second stage of closure appears to be dependent on ovarian steroid hormones, the fact that it occurs more rapidly in the presence of an embryo or oil droplet in the lumen indicates that some additional factors are involved (44). The luminal epithelium of intact cyclic, or pregnant, animals shows corresponding changes in lipid and in the activity of several enzymes, presumably in response to changing levels of ovarian steroid hormones (186,189–193).

Uterine Glands: There is relatively little information about endocrine-dependent cytodifferentiation of the glandular epithelium in ovariectomized animals, and most attention has been directed at the hormonal basis for secretory activity. It is reported that continuous treatment of ovariectomized mice with progesterone (with or without estrogen priming) leads to increased glandular secretion after 8 days; simultaneous injection of progesterone and estrogen leads to more massive secretory activity in just 5 days, whereas injection of estrogen after 3 days of progesterone leads to maximum secretion 48 hr later (194). Cells of the uterine glands in mice are typically more cuboidal in shape than luminal epithelium; they also have less lipid and appear to respond more slowly to ovarian steroid hormones (195). By the fourth day of pregnancy the gland cells are found to have large lucent apical vesicles that disappear on the fifth and sixth day, as the lumen becomes distended (196). With cytochemical methods it has been shown that this material contains carbohydrate and appears first in multivesicular bodies and on the concave, but not the convex, surface of the Golgi complex. The lumen is narrowed during the progesterone domination characteristic of delayed implantation; the Golgi complex is typically located lateral to the nucleus, although there is abundant smooth and rough endoplasmic reticulum (197). The addition of estrogen after several days of progesterone domination leads to the second stage of uterine closure within 24 hr, and the glands start to become distended, although there are no significant ultrastructural changes in the cells. However, by 48 hr the glandular lumen becomes filled with carbohydrate-rich material, and electron-dense granules are found at the apical border of the cells; the Golgi complex is located apical to the nucleus, and rough endoplasmic reticulum is present in increased amounts. That the glands are normally active on the sixth to seventh day of pregnancy or pseudopregnancy (i.e., 48 hr after nidatory estrogen is imposed on progesterone domination) correlates well with the observed changes in endocrine replacement studies.

Stroma: The stromal cells also show hormone-dependent changes, particularly in the nucleoli (198). Tachi et al. (199) demonstrated, with the electron microscope, that following ovariectomy (a) the nucleoli in stromal cells are small and the fibrous component predominates, (b) there is a reduction in the amount of cytoplasm, and (c) the rough endoplasmic reticulum is less prominent. Following treatment with estrogen alone there is only a slight increase in the granular component of the nucleoli and no significant change in cytoplasmic features. By contrast, after treatment with progesterone there is a marked enlargement of the nucleoli, with augmentation of the granular component. There are also increases in the rough endoplasmic reticulum, which becomes distended, and the cytoplasm has many polyribosomes. If estrogen is added after progesterone pretreatment, all aspects of these changes are accentuated. Another prominent hormone-dependent feature in presensitive stroma is the development of a generalized edema that leads, in part, to the first phase of uterine closure (40,41,127,200).

Metabolic changes: The results of extensive studies of uterine metabolism demonstrate that there are hormone-dependent changes at the molecular level which correlate with the changes in proliferation and cytodifferentiation observed in the peri-implantation period.

The metabolism of uterine RNA in early pregnancy has been examined in some detail. Incorporation of [^{3}H]uridine into RNA increases between the second and third day of pregnancy or pseudopregnancy in mice and rats (201–203). In rats the increase is biphasic, with a small peak on the third day and a more sustained increase on the fifth day, which then decreases unless decidualization occurs (204,205). This latter increase appears to be largely in the nuclear fraction, is thought to be associated with increased processing of ribosomal RNA (206,207), and is correlated temporally with the increased numbers of polyribosomes observed in stroma on the fifth day (136). Measurements of DNA template activity with bacterial RNA polymerase *in vitro* generally confirm the biphasic nature of the pattern of RNA synthesis, with the greatest activity in chromatin prepared from uteri on the third and fifth day (6,208). Furthermore, it has been inferred from DNA/RNA competitive hybridization studies that there are species of RNA synthesized on the fifth day of pregnancy that are not present on the second or the seventh day (208). Although increases in the synthesis of RNA were found in all compartments of the endometrium, the greatest increase was in the stroma (209). It is of particular interest that the activity was found to be greater in pregnant horns than in pseudopregnant horns, even at this time before attachment of the embryo.

Ornithine decarboxylase activity increases within 4 hr of estrogen administration, and this change is prevented by cycloheximide (210). There is a biphasic peak in ornithine decarboxylase activity, with increases on the third and fifth day; this persists in implantation sites but not in interimplantation areas (211,212).

Synthesis of uterine proteins, as inferred from the incorporation of labeled amino acids, also has a biphasic pattern in the peri-implantation period. Thus, incorporation of label increases on the third day of pregnancy, decreases on the fourth day, and increases again on the fifth (213,214). The increased rates of synthesis are maintained beyond the fifth day in implantation sites but not in interimplantation areas. With estrogen alone the increases are greatest in epithelium; with progesterone alone the increase is more dramatic in stroma (215). Along with the increase in overall protein synthesis, specific and apparently new proteins appear. These migrate in the post-transferrin region during electrophoresis on polyacrylamide gels (216,217). Interestingly, the pattern in pseudopregnant animals is different in that there is no increase in protein synthesis on the fifth day, again suggesting that the embryos provide some stimulus to the uterus even before attachment (214).

Chemical analysis of endometrium for lipid throughout the peri-implantation period confirms the cytologic observations. There are changes in both total lipid and the relative proportions of neutral triglycerides (218). The studies have been undertaken with both intact cyclic, or pregnant, animals as well as with ovariectomized animals given replacement ovarian steroid hormone therapy. Although there are some species differences, it appears in general that estrogen reduces total lipid, primarily by influencing neutral triglycerides, whereas progesterone causes an increase; progesterone is particularly effective in this regard when it has been preceded by estrogen (219–223). Neutral triglycerides tend to accumulate in the endometrium, both epithelium and stroma, in the first 4 days of pregnancy, presumably because of the effect of luteal progesterone. Interestingly, lipids decrease in the implantation sites, but not interimplantation areas, on days 6 and 7 as decidualization proceeds (224). Although various investigators have suggested that neutral lipids provide an energy source for the developing embryo and that phospholipids may be important for synthesis of such components as cell membrane and prostaglandins during decidualization, it has not been possible to directly relate changes in lipids to regulation of proliferation or differentiation of the endometrium.

Endocrine-dependent changes have also been observed in the intermediary metabolism of the endometrium during the estrous cycle and in the early progestational period in the rat. Attempts have been made to relate differing patterns of intrauterine oxygen tension, activity of glycolytic enzymes, uterine respiration, and glucose utilization to the shift in stromal cells away from mitotic activity and toward cytodifferentiation and the development of progestational sensitivity (5,189,225–233). Although it is clear that hormone-dependent changes in cell proliferation, in cytodifferentiation, and in the various metabolic and synthetic patterns must ultimately be responsible for the development of uterine receptivity, none of the observations has provided a clear understanding of the process at the molecular level.

However, an interesting suggestion has been made recently that may begin to explain the mechanisms of the process. Yochim and his colleagues have shown that the ovarian steroid hormones regulate availability of the pyridine nucleotide cofactor nicotinamide adenine dinucleotide phosphate and thus ultimately control pentose shunt activity in the endometrium (233–236). It is hypothesized by these workers that progestational sensitivity develops in the endometrium because increased levels of cofactor lead to increased pentose shunt activity and thus provide endometrial cells with increased capacity to recycle cofactors for reductive biosynthesis and to provide sugars for nucleic acid synthesis. This situation would facilitate cytodifferentiation, whereas the consequent reduced flux in the nicotinamide adenine dinucleotide salvage path would limit production of ADP-ribose and thus may impair DNA synthesis and cell division (237–239).

Transformation of the Endometrium

Sensitization of the endometrium is essential for the subsequent decidual transformation in response to an appropriate stimulus. Decidualization per se involves profound changes in both morphologic and biochemical characteristics of the endometrial stroma. Although details of timing and of the extent of endometrial involvement vary between species, the basic cytological changes are similar in different animals, and comprehensive descriptions of the process at the light microscopic level are to be found in several early papers (200,240–243).

The precursors, from which decidual tissue forms, are fibroblast-like cells in the stroma (142,145). In rats the process typically begins in compact areas of the subepithelial antimesometrial stroma (153), although this is apparently not critical because the initial changes occur throughout the antimesometrial region in the mouse (244). Among the earliest changes to be observed are the development of edema (26,101,123,124,245) and an increase in alkaline phosphatase activity in the fibroblast-like precursor cells (85). Subsequently, these cells become slightly enlarged, the nuclei become rounded, and there is typically an increase in the prominence of the nucleoli. The cells tend to align themselves into a continuous layer beneath the epithelium (12,18); and while mitotic activity in the central area declines and finally ceases, there is continued proliferation of cells in the areas adjacent to the developing nidus (130,136,246,247). As the process continues, the cells assume an epithelioid appearance (i.e., a characteristically rounded shape) and typically contain two or more polyploid nuclei (248).

At the ultrastructural level, differentiation of decidual cells is characterized by the accumulation of glycogen, often in association with lipid droplets, and progessively increasing amounts of fibrillar material organized into parallel arrays and appearing as bundles in the cytoplasm. There is an increase in the number of polyribosomes, as well as in the amount and distention of rough endoplasmic reticulum; the nucleoli become enlarged, with an increase in the granular component (12,26,108,249–254). It has recently been reported that the amount of fibronectin on the surface of these cells decreases as they undergo differentiation and that this change may be important in the development of their characteristic rounded shape (255). A consistent finding in the various electron microscopic studies of decidualization is that the cells are crowded closely together, with finger-like projections and numerous junctions of the adherens and gap types (12,249,256,257). The temporal aspect of the development of these junctions has been described in detail (250,258).

Localized changes in vascular permeability is one of the earliest responses of the sensitive endometrium to any kind of deciduogenic stimulus and has most often been demonstrated by the extravascular accumulation of intravenously injected macromolecular dye (100,101). The development of fenestrations and gaps in the endothelium of endometrial blood vessels at implantation sites, but not between implantations, has been described and provides an explanation at the ultrastructural level for the so-called "Pontamine Blue reaction" in those areas (252,259). Although Lundkvist and Ljungkvist (250) argue that some cytological changes precede the appearance of overt edema and the Pontamine Blue reaction, it has subsequently been shown, in the rat, that labeled albumin leaks from the vessels within 15 min of a decidualizing stimulus (260). Thus, the development of edema is still one of the earliest changes known to be associated with the endometrial response to a decidualizing stimulus. These changes can occur while blastocysts are still enclosed in the zona pellucida, and thus the signal does not require direct contact between trophoblast and uterine epithelium (102,261).

Development of mature decidual tissue involves both proliferation and differentiation of the stromal cells. It is not surprising, therefore, that significant changes in both the total content and rates of synthesis of DNA, RNA, and protein have been observed. As indicated earlier, the synthesis of DNA can be demonstrated in endometrial stromal cells on the fourth and fifth days of pseudopregnancy or pregnancy by incorporation of [^{3}H]thymidine (131,142,146). This increase in synthetic activity in the stroma follows the decline of proliferation in the epithelium. It occurs in response to the nidatory estrogen and accompanies the transition through the receptive phase and into the refractory phase (141). The synthesis of DNA continues on the sixth day in areas undergoing decidualization, but not in those areas between implantations (144). However, it appears that once the decidual cells have become differentiated they no longer synthesize DNA; rather it is those cells peripheral to the forming nidus that continue to incorporate the labeled thymidine (145). It has been observed in mice that there are two populations of cells that begin DNA synthesis at about 11 to 15 hr after the decidualizing stimulus; one differentiates into mature decidual cells without dividing, the other goes on to divide before differentiating (262). The peak in DNA synthesis occurs about 30 hr after application of the decidual stimulus (263); chemical measurements of total DNA content revealed that changes are substantial, with increases of up to 70% per day in the second and third day after the experimentally applied stimulus (264). As might be expected, this increase in DNA content did not occur when decidualization was prevented by the antiestrogen MER-25 (265).

The decidual cells typically become binucleate and polyploid (246,247). Production of these nuclei, some containing as much as 32n DNA in rats and 64n DNA in mice, involves endoreplication rather than fusion (248) and reaches a maximum at about 96 hr after application of the decidualizing stimulus (266). With rats it has been possible to separate decidual cells on the basis of ploidy by means of differential sedimentation velocity on serum albumin gradients (267). It appears that those cells that are destined to develop the highest ploidy will synthesize DNA on the fourth day of pseudopregnancy, whereas those engaged in synthesis of DNA on the fifth day will typically develop lower ploidy (268,269). On the other hand, it appears that it is those cells that are synthesizing DNA early in the process of transformation which remain in the 2n to 4n population, whereas those synthesizing DNA later tend to end up in the 6n to 8n range. Thus, Moulton (268) finds evidence to support the concept that there are two populations of stromal cells in rats: one population that differentiates without dividing, and a second population that divides before undergoing differentiation. It appears, then, that the rat is similar to the mouse (262) in this regard. The continued synthesis of DNA and RNA by decidual cells in ovariectomized animals is dependent on progesterone replacement, apparently more so in the cells at 4n to 8n DNA than in smaller cells. In contrast, synthesis of proteins is more progesterone-dependent in smaller cells than it is in the 4n to 8n population (268).

The hormone-dependent nature of these various changes led some investigators to examine differences in steroid receptors in the endometrium. Martel and Psychoyos (270) report that the amount of estrogen receptor in implantation sites decreases relative to DNA and protein, and that there is little evidence of receptor in the nucleus. This seems to be compatible with the observation of decreased uptake of [^{3}H]estradiol by implantation versus interimplantation sites (271,272). The conflicting report by Logeat et al. (169), that estrogen receptor increases markedly in implantation sites identified by Trypan Blue dye, appears to be based on the artifactual binding of steroids by the dye (270). Moulton and Koenig (273) have, however, reported that the number of estrogen receptors in cells with high ploidy increases relative to DNA, whereas McConnell et al. (274) report that progesterone receptors in the same cells decrease relative to DNA. These several observations demonstrate that a marked degree of heterogeneity exists in endometrial cells and developing decidual tissue. Although it seems probable that these profound cellular differences are related to various aspects of the process of implantation and the specialized functions of decidual tissue, interpretation of the findings has been difficult and little progress has been made toward determining what role those differences actually play.

Although synthesis of RNA occurs in stroma of pregnant and pseudopregnant mice and rats before the acquisition of sensitivity, further increases are observed with decidual transformation. Synthesis and accumulation of uterine RNA change dramatically upon formation of mature decidual tissue, with increases in content being observed as little as 5 hr after the systemic injection of pyrathiazine as the decidualizing stimulus (242). This early change in RNA was localized, by histochemical means, to the superficial cells of the antimesometrial stroma in rat (243). The increase is limited to decidualizing tissue and is not observed in those areas that fail to become transformed (203–205); it can be detected within 8 hr of the intraluminal application of the decidualizing stimulus (275). The overall increase in RNA content of decidual tissue has been estimated at 95% to 110% on the first day after stimulation (264,275). A corresponding increase in uridine incorporation is observed and thought to reflect largely increased processing of ribosomal RNA (207,208); however, increases in activity of both RNA polymerase types I and III have been reported in the mouse (276), and template activity is significantly increased in decidualizing tissue on the sixth day of pregnancy, suggesting that there are substantial changes in the synthesis of all classes of RNA (6,209).

Ornithine decarboxylase increases in a biphasic manner early in decidual transformation, presumably to support nucleic acid synthesis, and the increases are blocked by cycloheximide, actinomycin D (277), and indomethacin (278). Protein content in the rat deciduoma increases by as much as 70% per day in the second and third days after stimulation (264). In the mouse there is a biphasic increase in the protein content: a two- to threefold increase in the first 24 hr, and a secondary and more sustained increase of four- or fivefold in the third and fourth day (263). Rates of protein synthesis, as measured by incorporation of single radiolabeled amino acids, increase on the third day and fall on the fourth day. A larger and more sustained increase that is localized in implantation sites occurs on the fifth day (214,279). Increases in protein synthesis are dependent on appropriate hormonal preparation of the endometrium as well as on the decidualizing stimulus and can be blocked with antiestrogens (MER-25; 265), tamoxifen (215), and cycloheximide (279). These treatments also block the decidual transformation. Progesterone appears to be necessary for continued high levels of protein synthesis by decidual tissue and may be acting primarily on the smaller stromal cells (i.e., those with 2–4n DNA; 268). Because decidual transformation is associated with significant increases in tissue mass, it is not surprising that there are marked increases in synthesis of DNA, RNA, and protein. However, although it has been essential to document the changes in macromolecular synthesis, the observations have not provided insights into either the nature of this unique process or the potential functional significance of the new tissue.

As it became clear that increases in general protein synthesis accompanied the decidual transformation, efforts were made to determine whether decidual cell-specific proteins could be identified that might provide a clue to the function of this developing organ. Yoshinaga (280) prepared rabbit antiserum to crude extracts of rat deciduomata and found that it would prevent decidualization in both the rat and mouse (280,281); he suggested that some proteins in decidual tissue of these species have similar immunological characteristics. Similarly, Joshi et al. (282) reported the existence of a decidua-specific antigen in the baboon, and Sacco and Mintz (283) reported a uterine-specific antigen on the fourth day of pregnancy in mice. Although none of these antigens has been characterized further, their existence demonstrates the potential for unique function of proteins in this tissue.

Several investigators have demonstrated the existence of unique decidual proteins by resolving dual radiolabeled proteins on polyacrylamide gels (284–290). Again, however, none of these proteins has been described in sufficient detail to determine if they are the same between species. Denari et al. (286) observed a unique protein within 1 hr of the stimulus for decidualization in the rat. In terms of electrophoretic mobility, this protein (protein A) was similar to estrogen-induced uterine protein (i.e., IP; 291–293). However, it (i.e., protein A) was not increased in animals treated with estrogen alone and was not observed in nonstimulated uteri; it seems unlikely that this protein is the IP. Another protein with characteristics similar to those of IP was found to be synthesized maximally on the fourth and sixth days of pregnancy and depressed on the fifth day; the investigators suggested that it is associated with regulation of cell division (290). Although this protein was presumed to be IP because of its electrophoretic mobility, it was found to be greatly increased in deciduomata when there were no concomitant increases in estrogen; and because it was shown that IP is induced by estrogen in all cell layers (294), it seems unlikely that this protein is the IP. In addition, a pregnancy-associated protein was found in the post-transferrin region of the same gels. Its synthesis increased from the fourth through the sixth day of pregnancy and remained elevated in implantation sites but not in interimplantation areas (218,287,288). The significance of these various proteins is obscure.

Two-dimensional polyacrylamide gel electrophoresis has recently been used because of the significant increase in resolution over conventional electrophoresis, and it has been possible to demonstrate in the rat that at least four new peptides appear with decidualization and that several others decrease (295). More recently, with hamster uterus, it has been shown that several decidua-specific nuclear and cytoplasmic proteins are modulated both positively and negatively by progesterone (296), and more significantly, that decidual cells continue to produce these distinctive proteins *in vitro* (297). Because it should now be possible to purify these proteins, there is reason to expect that this approach will provide the breakthrough necessary to determine what the decidual cells are doing.

Initiation

That transformation of sensitized endometrium can be initiated by a variety of stimuli and will proceed in the absence of an embryo implies not only that elements necessary for decidualization are intrinsic to the uterus, but also that events entrained by the various stimuli converge at a common physiological point. It has been proposed that histamine and prostaglandins, released locally in the uterus in response to the various stimuli, provide the common locus and that these factors initiate the vascular and cellular changes of decidualization.

Histamine

The hypothesis that it is histamine released from uterine mast cells by the nidatory surge of estrogen that is responsible for initiating the decidual reaction was formulated over a period of several years by Shelesnyak and his colleagues, based on the following observations: (a) Histamine antagonists instilled into the uterine lumen prevent the formation of deciduomata and reduce the number of implantations in rats (298,299); (b) histamine injected intraluminally, as well as histamine releasers administered systemically, induced decidual reactions in pseudopregnant rats (298–300); and (c) histamine content of rat uteri is reduced at the time of implantation (301), as well as in the uteri of ovariectomized rats following the injection of estrogen (302,303). Several investigators have disputed this hypothesis (109,304) and raise the following objections: (a) Intraluminal stimulators of the decidual response may be nonspecific (114,115,305); (b) systemic antihistamines are not particularly effective in blocking the decidual response (306–308); (c) in the hands of other investigators, instillation of histamine in the uterine lumen has not elicited greater responses than the vehicle alone, nor can a dose-response relationship be demonstrated (304,309,310); (d) depletion of histamine in mast cells with 48/80 does not prevent the decidual reaction (109); and (e) the decidual reaction normally occurs only in the vicinity of the embryo, or as discrete foci following administration of a systemic stimulus, and it would be expected that a generalized release of mast cell histamine in response to nidatory estrogen would result in a response throughout the uterus (109).

Although many of the objections can be argued away, the failure of systemic antihistamines to block decidualization was seen as damaging; thus the hypothesis was not universally accepted. The subsequent finding that there are two types of histamine receptors (H_1 and H_2), and that both may have to be blocked for a complete antihistamine effect, suggested that the early failures (i.e., typically with blockers of H_2 receptors) did not constitute evidence against a role for histamine in implantation. Thus, interest was renewed when Brandon and Wallis (311) reported that implantation and decidualization were reduced in rats treated with a combination of blockers of H_1 and H_2 receptors (pyrilamine and burimamide, respectively). This finding seemed even more significant when coupled with the demonstration that rabbit blastocysts have H_2 receptors whereas endometrium has the H_1 type (312). However, more recently Brandon and Raval (313) were unable to block the attachment of embryos with another specific and more potent blocker of the H_2 receptor (i.e., metiamide), and it has now been questioned whether the earlier effect with burimamide (311) was actually mediated through an effect on H_2 receptors (314).

Although the question of histamine receptors is still open, other evidence seems to support the hypothesis that histamine from mast cells is important in the uterine response. Thus, Ferrando and Nalbandov (315) depleted areas of the endometrium of mast cells by localized freezing and found that although this prevented implantation and decidualization, the effect could be overcome by instillation of histamine into the uterine lumen. Furthermore, Dey et al. (316) found that inhibition of histamine release from mast cells by means of intraluminal instillation of disodium cromoglycate prevented implantation and the decidual reaction in the rabbit and concluded that mast cell histamine plays a critical role in decidualization, and thus in implantation.

From these observations, as well as those of Shelesnyak and his colleagues, it seems probable that histamine has something to do with decidual transformation and implantation. However, many of the objections raised by DeFeo (109) are still relevant, and a role for uterine histamine remains to be clearly defined.

Prostaglandins

The proposition that uterine prostaglandins have an obligatory role in the development of endometrial vascular permeability and subsequent decidual transformation is based on several lines of evidence (317,318). First, it has been shown that blocking the synthesis of prostaglandins with indomethacin during the first few days of pregnancy inhibits or delays implantation in mice (319–322), rats (323–325), hamsters (326), and rabbits (327). It was generally observed in those experiments that, following treatment with indomethacin, the implantation sites appeared later and were smaller than in control animals and that embryonic development was retarded. Furthermore, the expected localized increases in vascular permeability associated with implantation are blocked or delayed by indomethacin in rats (324,328) and rabbits (329,330). In some cases, exogenous prostaglandins partially overcame the effects of indomethacin (320,322,327). That this effect is on the uterus rather than on the embryos, or on the production of steroid hormones by the ovary, was shown by experiments with spayed animals given progesterone and estrogen replacement to achieve uteri with maximum sensitivity to decidualizing stimuli. Again, it was found that indomethacin blocked or greatly attenuated the artificially stimulated decidual response (331–336).

Second, the concentration of prostaglandins is observed to increase in decidualizing tissue in both normal pregnant animals and those with artificially stimulated deciduoma; again, this increase is blocked by indomethacin (324,328,334,337–341). Furthermore, exogenous prostaglandins placed in the lumen of sensitized uteri are able to stimulate an increase in vascular permeability, even when endogenous prostaglandin synthesis is inhibited. There has been some disagreement about which of the prostaglandins is most effective. For example, Kennedy (328) found that prostaglandin E-2 (PGE-2) instilled into the lumen was effective in increasing vascular permeability whereas prostaglandin F-2a (PGF-2α) was not. On the other hand, constant infusion of PGF-2α was as effective as PGE-2 (336). Complete decidual transformation can be elicited by intraluminal application of prostaglandins, with or without suppressing endogenous synthesis with indomethacin; PGF-2α instilled into the lumen is reported to be effective (342), and implants of PGE-2 and PGF-2α are both effective (343). More recently, it has been shown that there are specific receptors for PGE-2 in the stroma of rat endometrium (344) and that their concentration increases with progesterone, reaching a maximum on the fifth and sixth days of pseudopregnancy. There are no receptors for PGF-2α in the rat endometrium (345). It is suggested, therefore, that any effect of PGF-2α on decidual tissues is a result of its conversion to PGE-2 or because PGF-2α cross-reacts with PGE-2 receptors. This could provide an explanation for the effect of PGF-2α after constant infusion, when instillation as a bolus was less effective (328,336). However, the uterus is in a neutral state after several days of progesterone, and there was no change of PGE-2 receptor concentration upon addition of estrogen to develop the sensitive or receptive state (346). It has been reported that progesterone translocation to the nucleus is mediated by prostaglandins (347). Furthermore, production of prostaglandins increases in uterine tissue on the fifth day of pregnancy or pseudopregnancy (325). However, Kennedy (337) did not find such differences in ovariectomized animals treated with ovarian steroid hormones, even though the expected increase in vascular permeability in response to intraluminal PGE-2 (or saline) was present. Thus, the acquisition of endometrial sensitivity does not appear to be directly correlated to the ability of the uterus to produce prostaglandins, and it appears that no simple relationship exists between the condition of endometrial receptivity and the level of prostaglandin production or receptors.

Several observations have been made which suggest that changes in cyclic AMP mediate the decidualizing effects of prostaglandin at the cellular level. Thus, there is a rapid and dramatic increase in cyclic AMP following artificial stimulation of the decidual response (334,348–350), and this is inhibited by indomethacin (334,350). Furthermore, the instillation of cholera toxin causes increases in both vascular permeability and decidualization (349). Although the process of decidualization following cholera toxin may not be identical with that associated with PGE-2 (351), there are at least the typical changes in permeability and steroid receptors (352). On the other hand, intrauterine instillation of cyclic AMP or dibutyryl cyclic AMP does not induce decidualization (343,348,349,353), but will induce implantation if embryos are present (354,355). Thus, it is clear that prostaglandins have some obligatory role in implantation, presumably involving the increase in vascular permeability associated with decidualization, but the importance of their role in the overall decidual transformation and the process of implantation remains unclear.

Embryonic Signals

It has long been suspected that some form of embryonic signaling is necessary for the process of implantation and the "maternal recognition of pregnancy" (356,357). However, the nature of the putative signals, and how they function remains very controversial. There are several problems: First, the localized nature of the uterine response during the apposition phase of implantation implies that some type of embryonic signal acts at short range, whereas systemic changes associated with the maternal recognition of pregnancy, such as maintenance of the corpus luteum and modulation of the immune response, indicate that some are effective at longer range. Therefore, it seems probable that in many cases there are more than one embryonic signal. Second, even when the purpose of embryonic signaling is the same in two species, the mode of action may be quite different. For example, in women and nonhuman primates it is the production of a chorionic gonadotropin that is responsible for "rescuing" the corpus luteum (358), and although there is controversy about whether that embryonic signal is actually synthesized by preimplantation blastocysts, it is clear that it operates as a luteotrophic factor (11). By contrast, in domestic animals such as the sheep, pig, and cow it is the production of an antiluteolysin by the embryo that is essential to neutralize the effect of uterine PGF-2α and thus prevent destruction of the corpus luteum.

Many reports have appeared over the last 25 years that deal with the attempts to demonstrate that various potential signal substances are synthesized and released by preimplantation embryos. At one time or another, carbon dioxide, steroids, histamine, prostaglandins, and proteins of embryonic origin have all been proposed as signals. In addition to diffusible chemical factors, it has even been suggested that physical contact between the embryo and the endometrium provides a signaling mechanism. In reviewing the evidence for these various factors it should be kept in mind that it is unlikely that any one factor will be identified that could be considered as "the" signal for implantation in all animals; furthermore, in most cases there is no reason to suggest that any of the proposed factors are mutually exclusive.

Physical Stimuli

Two observations have been used to support the hypothesis that it is physical contact between the embryo and the epithelium that is responsible for signaling at implantation. The first is the finding that embryo-sized beads of glass, paraffin, or agar produce decidual reactions in pseudopregnant rats (359,360). Although it is interesting, this hypothesis has not been supported by results of other experiments with various kinds of artificial or surrogate embryos. For example, unfertilized rat eggs, two-cell embryos, or mouse or sea-urchin eggs apparently had little or no ability to elicit the reaction in rats (360); McLaren (361) found that beads made of glass or an acrylic polymer did not produce deciduomas in pseudopregnant mice, and Blandau (359) was unable to obtain the reaction in pseudopregnant guinea pigs by using beads made of glass or paraffin. The second proposal is that because microvilli of the trophoblast interdigitate with those of the epithelium, pulsations of the blastocyst at this stage (362,363) might lead to distortion of the epithelium (317,364) and augment a physical signal. However, the finding that localized edema will occur when embryos are still in the zona pellucida (102,262) makes the significance of this mechanism questionable. Although it may eventually be possible to demonstrate that such physical contact results in epithelial distortion and that it is important, the findings to date have not been convincing and none of the observations is clear-cut enough to assign a specific role to contact-mediated signals at implantation.

Carbon Dioxide

The possibility that carbon dioxide (produced as a metabolic by-product of developmentally active blastocysts) is important as a signal for implantation was originally proposed by Boving (365,366). It was hypothesized that carbon dioxide removed from the rabbit embryo as bicarbonate ion is converted to carbonic acid and an alkaline carbonate salt in the uterine epithelium, with the carbonic acid subsequently being converted to carbon dioxide by carbonic anhydrase. It was envisioned that a resulting increase in pH could have local effects on the uterus. Hetherington (116,367) also suggested that embryonic carbon dioxide might be involved in eliciting the decidual reaction, since small bubbles of that gas, or air, were more effective in inducing a decidual response in pseudopregnant mice than was N_2 or O_2. Although there is no direct evidence to support this hypothesis, the observation that ethoxzolamide (an inhibitor of carbonic anhydrase) reduces the number of implantations in pregnant rabbits (366) is difficult to discount, and the question of a role for embryonic carbon dioxide as a unique embryonic signal at implantation remains unresolved.

Steroids

The concept that the embryos synthesize steroid hormones which then play a role in implantation has evolved from the original observation by Huff and Eik-Ness (368) that 6-day-old rabbit blastocysts were not only capable of forming pregnenolone from [^{14}C]acetate, but that they "biotransformed" pregnenolone, 17α-hydroxypregnenolone, progesterone, and androstenedione to other phenolic compounds. The question of synthesis of estrogen by blastocysts and the putative involvement of such "embryonic estrogen" in implantation (369) has been controversial. However, it should be noted that steroid metabolism by preimplantation embryonic tissue has been found in many of the animals that have been studied in detail (356,357,370,371). The observations in various species are summarized as follows.

Pig: It has been known for more than 10 years that 12- to 14-day-old pig trophoblast is capable of synthesizing estrogens from labeled androstenedione, dehydroepiandrosterone, and testosterone and thus that the embryos have aromatase activity (370,372–374). The finding that pig blastocysts convert labeled progesterone and pregnenolone to estrogen, in the presence of a system for generating cofactors, demonstrates functional Δ^5-3β- and 17β-hydroxysteroid dehydrogenase activities as well as those of the steroid C-17-20 lyase (375). Similar results have recently been reported by Fischer et al. (376), who demonstrated that estrogen can be produced from labeled progesterone by pig embryos. Estradiol production was first observed at the large spherical blastocyst stage; estrone and estradiol were synthesized by tubular embryos, with amounts decreasing at the filimentous stage and increasing again between days 16 and 25. The enzymatic activity was demonstrated definitively in these studies by conversion of labeled substrates *in vitro,* as well as recovery and recrystallization (to constant specific activity) of the products. The results confirmed earlier histochemical findings on changing levels of Δ^5-3β- and 17β-hydroxysteroid dehydrogenase in the embryos between days 12 and 16 (377). Furthermore, the blastocysts have relatively high concentrations of estrogen and progesterone *in utero,* and the gradients between mother and embryo make it appear likely that the steroids are of embryonic rather than maternal origin (375,378).

The maternal recognition of pregnancy in the pig occurs between day 10 and 12 (379) and involves an antiluteolytic effect. Bazer and Thatcher (380) have argued that estrogen of embryonic origin is involved as follows: (i) PGF-2α from the uterus is the luteolysin in the pig and is reduced in utero-ovarian blood between days 12 and 20 of gestation (381,382), but its concentration in the uterine lumen is increased at that time (383); (ii) systemic estrogen duplicates this pattern of changes in PGF-2α (381,382); and (iii) it is estrogen from the embryo that is responsible for redirecting the secretion of endometrial prostaglandin from the bloodstream to the uterine lumen and thus spares the corpus luteum. Pig endometrium incubated with an embryo also has the capacity to convert progesterone to estrogen. There is no evidence for endometrial conversion of progesterone to estrogen by pseudopregnant animals and, therefore, the embryo must be responsible for altering the endometrial cells (376). A second possibility has been raised, namely, that estrogen from the embryo is sulfated in the endometrium (356,373,384) and, in the conjugated form, goes to the ovary, where it is luteotrophic (357). A third possibility has recently been raised with the report that pig blastocysts have the capacity for synthesis of catechol estrogens from estradiol (385). Because catechol estrogens have been implicated in regulation of prostaglandin synthesis, and because the transient increase in estrogen 2,4-dioxylase activity occurs at the time of maternal recognition of pregnancy, Mondschein et al. (385) suggested that estrogen synthesized by the embryo as a result of increased aromatase activity, between days 10 and 14 of pregnancy, is used in the formation of catechol estrogen, which acts as a signal in implantation. It is of interest in this regard that catechol estrogens have been reported to cause implantation in delayed-implanting mice (386) and to stimulate production of prostaglandins by preimplantation rabbit embryos and endometrium (387). The endometrium of pig also appears to be responsible for concentrating steroids in the lumen that may act as substrates for embryos (388).

Rabbit: The hypothesis that steroids of embryonic origin are important not only for development of the blastocyst but also locally to induce implantation (389,390) has been controversial. As applied to rabbits, this concept has been attacked on several grounds, including: lack of specificity of the histochemical assay (391); the supposition that high concentrations of steroids in rabbit blastocysts (392,393) are of maternal origin rather than from the embryo (394–396); and the argument that the presence of enzymatic capacity does not necessarily mean that it functions *in vivo* (397). Nevertheless, definitive measurements were eventually made of the conversion of dehydroepiandrosterone to androstenedione by 5-day-old rabbit embryos and of conversion of testosterone to estradiol by 7-day-old embryos (398). Coupled with demonstrations of aromatase activity in cell-free lysates of embryos in the presence of an NADPH-generating system (399) and in whole blastocysts *in vitro* (400), these observations appear to establish that the enzymatic capacity for synthesis of estrogen exists in preimplantation rabbit blastocysts.

The question of a function for steroids associated with the embryos, whether of maternal or embryonic origin, is unresolved. The several observations that implicate estradiol as a factor in preimplantation development and implantation in the rabbit are: (i) incubation of blastocysts with the anti-estrogen CI-628 reduces their ability to implant when transferred to pseudopregnant recipients, and the effect is reversible (401); (ii) instillation of CI-628 into the uterine lumen reduces the number of implantations (402) and prevents the increases in acid phosphatase that are expected in luminal epithelium adjacent to the embryos (403); and (iii) estradiol binds to a soluble cytosolic protein in rabbit blastocysts, and this binding is blocked by CI-628 (401). Although these findings implicate estradiol in development and implantation in the rabbit, they do not prove that it is of embryonic origin. Indeed, the finding that an inhibitor of aromatase (4-hydroxy-4-androstene-3,17-dione) reduces blastocyst production of estradiol from testosterone *in vitro,* but does not interfere with either embryo development or implantation (400), is difficult to reconcile with that premise. The further finding that rabbit endometrium can synthesize labeled estrogen from [^{3}H]progesterone and [^{3}H]androstenedione and that the presence of the embryo influences this metabolic activity complicates this problem further (404).

Rat, Mouse, and Hamster: Enzymatic capacity for steroid metabolism in preimplantation embryos of small laboratory rodents has also been inferred from the histochemical demonstration of Δ^5-3β- and 17β-hydroxysteroid dehydrogenase activities in rats (405–408) and hamsters (409). Dickmann and his colleagues have published an extensive series of articles in which it has been proposed that estrogen of embryonic origin is important for the development of preimplantation stage rat, mouse, and hamster embryos as well as for the initiation of implantation (390,410). The hypothesis is supported largely by the histochemical evidence for changes in enzyme activity at the morula and blastocyst stages and the observation that CI-628 blocks embryo development at the morula stage (411) and interferes with implantation (91,412). Although this concept has now generally been accepted with respect to embryos of pigs and rabbits, largely because it has been possible to demonstrate enzymatic conversion of precursors to estrogen with biochemical techniques in addition to the histochemistry, that has not been the case with the embryos of the smaller laboratory rodents. Indeed, attempts by several investigators to identify transformed products of pregnenolone, progesterone, androstenedione, and dehydroepiandrosterone with preimplantation embryos of mouse and rat by radioimmunoassay (413–415) or chromatographic methods have been unsuccessful (413–416). Although the various studies with CI-628 seem to point to estrogen of embryonic origin (91,403,411,412), a question has been raised as to whether the effects are due to nonspecific toxicity (411); these effects may be difficult to reconcile in light of the conflicting observations that there is little estrogen receptor in the nucleus at implantation sites (270). Levels of enzymatic activity in hamsters do not change with development (417), and inhibitors of aromatase (418) and steroidogenesis (419) do not block implantation, at least in hamsters.

Other Species: Estrogen production by horse blastocysts *in vitro* has been reported (420), and in a comparative study with tissue from sheep, cows, roe deer, ferrets, cats, a plains viscacha, rabbits, and pigs, Gadsby et al. (374) reported observing significant aromatase activity and estrogen synthesis in pig trophoblast, whereas it was appreciably lower in all other species. In that study, labeled estrogens were recovered only from incubations of allantochorionic tissue of roe deer recovered shortly after implantation, as well as from pooled samples of tissue from early bovine embryos.

Histamine

It has been reported that preimplantation embryos of rabbits (421) and mice (422) have the enzymatic capacity to synthesize histamine from histidine *in vitro* (i.e., histidine decarboxylase). In rabbits the activity peaks on the sixth day of pregnancy and intraluminal instillation of low doses of an inhibitor of histidine decarboxylase (α-methylhistidine dihydrochloride) on the fifth day of pregnancy delayed implantation and, at higher doses, interrupted implantation; simultaneous administration of histidine counteracted the inhibitor (423). Blastocyst formation in mice was also inhibited with α-methylhistidine, and again this effect was overcome with histidine (422). These findings, along with the observation that histamine reduces the requirement for estrogen in inducing implantation in hypophysectomized progesterone-treated rats (424), prompted the suggestion that histamine synthesized by the embryo is important for development of the blastocyst and acts as a local signal to the endometrium at the time of implantation. Although the hypothesis that histamine produced by the embryo is involved in causing localized changes in the endometrium at implantation is appealing, it has not been substantiated and is difficult to reconcile with the report that histamine-releasing implants did not induce a significant decidual reaction in pseudopregnant rabbits (329). Furthermore, it is clear that localized decidual reactions will occur without an embryo being present.

Prostaglandins

Several approaches have been taken in evaluating the ability of preimplantation embryos of different species to synthesize prostaglandins and in assessing their role in the process of implantation (425). Thus, it has been possible to demonstrate that some biological processes are suppressed in blastocysts *in vitro* by inhibitors of prostaglandin synthesis; it has been shown *in vitro* that the quantity of prostaglandin within the embryo or released into the medium increases with time; and in some cases it has been possible to demonstrate the synthesis of labeled prostaglandins from radioactive arachidonic acid supplied either exogenously or from endogenous pools. The reported observations made with these various approaches can be summarized as follows.

Rabbit: The presence of prostaglandins in preimplantation blastocysts was first reported by Dickmann and Spilman (426). Prostaglandin of the F and E series was detected by radioimmunoassay in freshly recovered blastocysts on the sixth day of development. An increase in the content of prostaglandin F was also observed in rabbit blastocysts incubated *in vitro* for 24 hr (427), demonstrating that they do have the capacity for prostaglandin synthesis. Dey et al. (427) did not observe the release of prostaglandins into the medium during incubation of rabbit blastocysts. However, more recent studies have demonstrated both synthesis and release of prostaglandins E and F by 6- and 7-day-old rabbit embryos (428). Although it has not been possible to demonstrate the synthesis of labeled prostaglandins by rabbit blastocysts from exogenous arachidonic acid, it has been shown that when the endogenous phospholipid pools were prelabeled *in vitro* with [^{3}H]arachidonic acid and released by a calcium-specific ionophore, labeled prostaglandins were synthesized and released into the medium (425). From these observations it seems clear that rabbit blastocysts have the ability to synthesize and release prostaglandins to influence the endometrium locally. Furthermore, it appears that treatment with indomethacin early in pregnancy reduces the number of implantation sites in rabbits (327) and, therefore, that prostaglandins are involved in the process of implantation in this species. However, it remains unproven as to whether the local changes in endometrium (428) and the increase in concentration of prostaglandins at implantation sites (429) are caused by embryonic prostaglandins.

Cow: Measureable amounts of immunoreactive prostaglandins of E and F series were observed in cow blastocysts recovered on the thirteenth through the sixteenth day of development and incubated for up to 48 hr *in vitro;* the amounts increased in proportion to the ages of the embryos (430). Similarly, increasing amounts of radiolabeled prostaglandins were recovered after incubation of 16- and 19-day-old bovine embryos with radioactive precursors (431). Clearly, cow blastocysts have the capacity to synthesize prostaglandins, and again the suggestion that they (or other metabolites of arachidonic acid) might be important for embryonic development, act as local signals to the uterus, or be involved in maintenance of the corpus luteum (431) remains unproven.

Rat and Mouse: It has not been possible to detect the synthesis of prostaglandins by preimplantation embryos of rat using radioimmunoassay methods, even after incubation of up to 150 embryos for 24 hr (318). Similarly, it has not been possible to demonstrate synthesis of labeled prostaglandins by mouse blastocysts from either exogenous or endogenous [^{3}H]arachidonic acid (425). However, in the case of the mouse at least, there is strong evidence that prostaglandins of embryonic origin are involved in expansion of the blastocyst, because several antagonists suppress the process of hatching *in vitro* (432–434). Although instillation of some of these prostaglandin antagonists into the uterine lumen also interfered with implantation, the degree of their effectiveness was not the same as that for suppression of hatching (435), and it is not clear if they act at the level of the embryo or the endometrium. Because prostaglandins of the E series are often involved in water transport across epithelia, Biggers and his colleagues have suggested that these prostaglandins are important for that function in the blastocyst as well and thus could be involved in implantation by virtue of maintaining the turgidity necessary for apposition and adhesion of the blastocyst and endometrium rather than as local signal factors (432,435). It must be recognized that these possibilities are not mutually exclusive.

Sheep: Sheep blastocysts (at days 12 and 15 of development) were found to synthesize prostaglandins of the E and F series when incubated with labeled arachidonic acid (436), and the total amounts released into the medium in

$8\frac{1}{2}$ hr was 28 times the amount contained in the embryos at the time of recovery (437). Although the concentrations of prostaglandins E and F were shown to be high in both 14- and 23-day-old blastocysts, and synthesis of prostaglandin F in the endometrium increased after day 14, indomethacin had no effect on implantation in this species (438).

Taken together, these findings provide strong evidence for production of prostaglandins by preimplantation embryos of the rabbit, sheep, and cow. The evidence for the mouse is indirect and less compelling, and, as pointed out by Racowsky and Biggers (425), alternative methods will have to be used before the question can be settled with respect to the rat. When embryonic prostaglandins function as local signals to the uterus or are important to the embryo simply for maintaining normal cell function is unclear.

Proteins

It has been known for almost 20 years that proteins of embryonic origin are important for the maternal recognition of pregnancy in sheep. Evidence is now beginning to accumulate which supports the suggestion that such embryonic protein factors are involved in establishing pregnancy in a number of other species as well.

Sheep: The concept that a protein signal of embryonic origin plays a role in maternal recognition of pregnancy in sheep dates back to the observations, by Moor and Rowson (439–442), that luteolysis is prevented if a conceptus is present between days 12 and 13, or if homogenates of 14- to 15-day-old conceptuses are instilled into the uterine lumen. The active principal in the homogenates was heat labile and presumed, therefore, to be a protein. In similar experiments, Martal et al. (443) confirmed this observation and demonstrated that the active material (which they called *trophoblastin*) from 14- to 16-day-old embryos was not only heat labile, but was ineffective after treatment with protease. That extracts from older embryos [i.e., 21 and 23 days old (443) or 25 days old (442)] were ineffective in prolonging the life of the corpus luteum led to the suggestion that the protein was synthesized by the embryos only during the period from day 13 to day 21. This protein factor is presumably of trophoblast origin because transfer of trophoblastic vesicles (from 11- to 13-day-old embryos) to the uteri of nonpregnant ewes (on day 12 of the cycle) prolonged luteal life (444).

Although the signal has not been definitively identified, it has recently been shown *in vitro* that stage-specific proteins are synthesized and secreted by preimplantation sheep blastocysts. Thus, Godkin et al. (445) demonstrated with two-dimensional polyacrylamide gel electrophoresis that the major labeled product of 13-day-old sheep embryos incubated *in vitro* with [^{3}H]leucine was a low-molecular-weight (17,000 dalton), acidic (PI 5.5) protein (initially designated protein X). Although several other proteins were synthesized and secreted by embryos between days 14 and 21, protein X was predominant up to day 23, when it could no longer be detected. This protein is apparently synthesized in trophoblast, as shown by immunocytochemical methods (446), and has been redesignated "ovine trophoblast protein 1" (oTP-1). It binds to receptors in the endometrium with high affinity and apparently changes the pattern of protein synthesis in endometrium *in vitro* (446). This protein is the major translation product of trophoblastic mRNA, in a cell-free wheat-germ lysate system, and its production appears to peak in 13-day-old embryos (447). In addition, instillation of oTP-1 into the uterine lumen of cyclic ewes prolongs the life of the corpus luteum (448). However, this protein does not compete for luteinizing-hormone receptors on the corpus luteum nor does it stimulate progesterone synthesis (446), and thus it is apparently not the luteotrophic factor in conceptus homogenates reported by Godkin et al. (449) and Ellinwood et al. (450). For these reasons it has been suggested that oTP-1 is the embryonic protein factor involved in protecting against luteolysis (trophoblastin), presumably because its interaction with the uterine epithelium leads to altered release or metabolism of endometrial PGF-2α (447). In addition, Masters et al. (451) have reported that the major glucosamine-labeled product, purified by ion-exchange and gel-filtration chromatography of medium from 14- to 16-day-old embryos, is a large glycoprotein (660,000 daltons), consisting of at least 50% carbohydrate (largely *N*-acetylglucosamine and galactose) and relatively resistant to proteolysis. A similar embryonic-secreted factor has been observed in the cow and pig, but no functional significance has been ascribed to this glycoprotein as yet.

Cow: The cow is similar to the sheep and pig in that the presence of conceptus tissues *in utero* (prior to day 17) results in the maintenance of the corpus luteum (452–454). Furthermore, the infusion of homogenates of 17- and 18-day-old embryos has been shown to delay luteal regression, although it is not known if the active principal is sensitive to heat or protease as it is in sheep (454). Preattachment bovine conceptuses have been shown to synthesize and secrete a complex array of stage-specific proteins between days 16 and 24 of development (455). The individual proteins were separated by two-dimensional polyacrylamide gel electrophoresis and ion-exchange and gel-filtration chromatography. The amount of radiolabel incorporated into secreted material increases from day 16 through day 22 and decreases by day 24. Several low-molecular-weight acidic proteins are secreted during this period which are similar to, but not identical with, those secreted by ovine trophoblast. These factors are no longer evident by day 29 and thus are restricted to the period of maternal recognition of pregnancy in the cow. In addition, a large glycoprotein labeled with [^{3}H]glucosamine was secreted by tissue from all stages including postimplantation (day 69) chorion. This may be the same factor isolated earlier by Masters et al. (451) using similar techniques.

Pig: The time of maternal recognition of pregnancy in the pig is day 10 to day 12 and as with the sheep and the cow, a conceptus must be present *in utero* (prior to day 13) if the corpus luteum is to survive (379,456). It has been known for some time that the preattachment pig blastocyst is active in synthesizing and releasing proteins (457–459). Stage-specific proteins have been demonstrated in the pig *in vitro* by incubation of preattachment-stage embryos with radiolabeled precursors and by analysis of the conditioned medium using two-dimensional polyacrylamide gel electrophoresis (460). The major labeled products between $10\frac{1}{2}$ and 12 days appear to be a group of low-molecular-weight acidic proteins similar to those reported for the sheep and the cow. However, between days 13 and 16 the major products are larger and more basic, and after day 18 the major secreted products are a group of serum proteins synthesized by the embryo rather than by the trophoblast. A large glycoprotein labeled with [^{3}H]glucosamine and similar to that observed in sheep and cows was isolated with ion-exchange and gel-filtration chromatography from all stages (451).

Mouse: The concept that proteins secreted by the preimplantation mouse embryo might be involved in signaling at implantation dates back to the observation, by Fishel and Surani (461), that a labeled glycoprotein (approximately 87,000 daltons) could be recovered from the medium after incubating blastocysts with [^{3}H]glucosamine. More recently, it has been demonstrated that a complex array of stage-specific proteins are synthesized and secreted when preimplantation mouse blastocysts are incubated with [^{35}S]methionine (462). The proteins were isolated from conditioned medium and separated with two-dimensional polyacrylamide gel electrophoresis. It was found that synthesis and secretion of labeled proteins increased between days 4 and 5 of pregnancy and, as with embryos of the sheep, pig, and cow, there were several low-molecular-weight acidic proteins released before implantation. Of special interest was the finding that some of the proteins secreted by the mouse embryos were decreased in amount as embryos entered the dormant phase associated with delayed implantation. Those proteins that decreased as embryos became dormant typically increased as the embryos were reactivated. Furthermore, the appearance of these secreted factors was correlated temporally with the appearance of the Pontamine Blue reaction in the uterus. Although these findings are highly suggestive of a signal role for secreted proteins in preimplantation mouse embryos, that function remains to be demonstrated.

Early Pregnancy Factor

Several observations have been reported which indicate that other systemic signals of embryonic origin are involved in the maternal recognition of pregnancy. Of these, the so-called *early pregnancy factor* (EPF) has received the most attention. The existence of EPF was hypothesized after the observation that lymphocytes from pregnant mice had less activity in the rosette inhibition test with a standard anti-lymphocyte serum than did those from nonpregnant animals (463). Subsequently, it was found that the activity was a serum factor that enhanced the ability of rabbit anti-mouse serum to prevent rosette formation with normal red blood cells and spleen cells in the presence of complement (464,465). The amount of activity appeared to vary with the number of fetuses and to drop quickly once the embryos were removed (466). The factor was reported to suppress "adoptive transfer" of contact sensitivity to trinitrochlorobenzene, and it was suggested that it regulates cellular immunity *in vivo* (467). There are at least two types of EPF activity that appear at characteristic times in pregnancy (i.e., pre- and post-implantation). The early form is a large molecule [mice, 180,000 daltons by gel filtration (468); sheep, 250,000 daltons (469)], which can be separated into a nonactive protein fraction and an active factor (50,000 daltons) by ion-exchange chromatography; recombining these fractions returns activity. It appears, then, that the early form of EPF is associated with a normal serum protein carrier. The active principal in the early form of EPF consists of two components, EPF-A and EPF-B. These components can be separated by differential precipitation with 40% NH_4SO_4; neither component alone has any effect, but activity is restored when they are recombined (469–471). In the mouse, EPF-A is secreted by the oviduct in an inactive form and will not alter the rosette inhibition test until EPF-B is added; EPF-B is secreted by the ovary [in the presence of a pituitary factor later shown to be prolactin (472)] in response to a factor secreted by the fertilized or parthenogenically stimulated ovum (473–475). The early form of mouse EPF has been purified by immunoabsorption, electrofocusing, and gel filtration (476); the monomeric form has a molecular weight of 21,000 daltons and can be resolved into peptides of three sizes (i at 10,501 daltons is EPF-A; ii at 7,200 and iii at 3,400 daltons combine to form EPF-B). In mice, the late form of EPF appears to be produced by the embryo as the oviduct and ovary lose the capacity to synthesize components of the early form by about day 7 of pregnancy, but EPF activity can still be detected in the serum and urine in those animals as well as in animals ovariectomized on day 4 of pregnancy (468). Similar activity has been reported in sheep (470,475,477,478), humans (465,479–483), rats (484), pigs (485), and cows (475). It appears that EPF from mice, sheep, pigs, and humans have similar characteristics with respect to the effect on the rosette inhibition test and the appearance of different forms in each stage of pregnancy. Furthermore, there appears to be no species specificity; for example, human and pig ova produce a factor that will work in the mouse after intraperitoneal injection and extracts of fertilized mouse ova (but not unfertilized ova) elicit EPF activity when injected into the sheep oviduct (475).

Whether EPF functions in regulation of the maternal immune system in pregnancy, or exists at all, has been questioned by some investigators (486,487). On the other hand, because it (a) has been detected early in pregnancy in all species studied, (b) requires the presence of a viable embryo (or fetus), and (c) appears to last through at least the first half of pregnancy, some investigators have proposed that it be used as a diagnostic test for pregnancy (488–493).

Other Signals

Several other putative signal-response mechanisms have been reported that may be related to early pregnancy factors. For example, two-cell hamster embryos are reported to release an octapeptide that inhibits ovulation (494–496); fertilized horse ova are transported into the uterus while unfertilized ova are retained in the oviduct (497,498); lactate levels in the mouse oviduct remain elevated longer in animals with viable embryos than in pseudopregnant animals (499); and thrombocytopenia occurs in mice from the first day to the seventh day of pregnancy and does not occur in pseudopregnant mice (500). This latter response can be observed, however, within 3 hr of the transfer of fertilized embryos to pseudopregnant mice and thus seems to be initiated by an embryonic signal. Although the importance of these various signal factors to the biology of implantation and the precise mechanism of their action in various animals remain obscure, the study of embryonic factors is of major importance and will be an important area for research in the next few years.

Influence of the Uterine Environment on Blastocyst Development

In addition to observations which indicate that blastocysts can affect local and systemic changes in the mother during the peri-implantation period, it has become clear that development of the embryos is, in turn, influenced by the uterine environment. The uterine potential for regulating development of preimplantation embryos is dramatically illustrated by the phenomenon of delayed implantation. In that situation, development is arrested at the blastocyst stage for a period of several days, or even months, and resumes only in response to a change in the maternal endocrine status. During this phase of developmental quiescence the blastocysts typically have reduced levels of metabolic and synthetic activity, and cell division actually stops. In some species such a period of embryonic diapause occurs as an obligatory part of pregnancy; in others it may or may not occur depending on conditions in the maternal environment. In either case, following reactivation the "dormant" blastocysts resume development, and the subsequent implantation and fetal development are normal (501,502). It is generally accepted that the uterus is responsible for the embryonic quiescence associated with delayed implantation, because removing blastocysts to extrauterine sites either *in vivo* or *in vitro* leads to their metabolic reactivation (503). The presumed mechanism, as proposed 50 years ago by Brambell (504), is that the uterus regulates development in delayed implantation by either (a) restricting a critical "growth factor" or (b) secreting an "inhibitory substance" into the lumen. Most studies directed at defining the mechanisms responsible for embryonic quiescence in delayed implantation have made use of the fact that the blastocysts become "reactivated" *in vitro* after being removed from the uterus and incubated for a few hours in various tissue culture media. In this case, reactivation is characterized by (a) increases in metabolic activity and macromolecular synthesis, as occurs with reactivation of embryos *in vivo* (503,505–518), and (b) the outgrowth of trophoblast cells, which has been likened to the initial changes associated with implantation *in utero* (519–524).

The observations most often cited to support the concept that restriction of essential factors is a mechanism for delayed implantation can be summarized as follows: Trophoblast outgrowth does not occur *in vitro* in the absence of certain amino acids (521–524), serum factors (521,522), or glucose (523,525,526). It has been suggested from such observations that the uterus might impose developmental quiescence on the embryos by restricting one or more of these factors or even restricting concentrations of various ions (526–532) during delayed implantation. However, the level of amino acids in uterine fluid from delayed-implanting mice appears to be the same as that in normal animals (533), and although deletion of amino acids or serum from the culture medium prevents outgrowth, it apparently does not prevent metabolic activation (516). The suggestion that embryos do not develop beyond the blastocyst stage *in vitro* in the absence of glucose because they are energy deficient and thus that developmental arrest *in vivo* is due to the same cause (534) has not proven tenable. Dormant embryos actually have a higher ATP/ADP ratio than reactivated embryos and, indeed, it appears that reduced utilization of glucose by dormant embryos (514,535) is due to allosteric inhibition of glycolysis because of the high energy state of the cells (512). Furthermore, it has been impossible to maintain metabolic quiescence *in vitro* by restricting the concentrations of various ions in the medium, and it now seems unlikely that this is a mechanism by which the uterus renders the embryos quiescent *in vivo* (513). Several investigators have reported the results of experiments in which embryos were incubated in uterine fluid and examined for changes in metabolic activity or shedding of the zona pellucida (507,508,517,518,536–538). Results indicate that there is a factor present in flushings of uteri from cyclic or pseudopregnant animals that reduces RNA synthesis by blastocysts *in vitro*. The factor is heat stable, dialyzable, and is neutralized in the uteri of pregnant, but not pseudopregnant, animals 6.5 hr after the injection of estrogen (538). The nature of this putative inhibitory factor has not been determined. It is not known if the blastotoxic factor reported by Psychoyos et al. (539) is the same one responsible for these changes, and although these results provide support for the interesting possibility that the uterus can inhibit embryonic growth, this proposal has not been proven conclusively and has not been universally accepted.

SUMMARY

It is obvious from the foregoing presentation that implantation of mammalian embryos is a complex phenomenon in which a variety of interactive processes occur between the conceptus and the mother. It should also be clear that although various facets of the process have been described in much detail, relatively little is known at the molecular or cellular level about the actual mechanisms responsible for implantation in any one species, let alone in a comparative sense. However, in spite of our failure to understand totally this critical aspect of mammalian reproduction, it is possible to develop a general overview of the process in hopes that it will allow the reader to focus on common and, thus, presumably important features.

(a) The embryo and the uterus must be synchronized. From work in mice and rats, this seems to be related largely to the ability of the uterus to respond to an appropriate stimulus from a blastocyst, with changes in both the epithelium and stroma leading to attachment and the formation of a decidua. The period of uterine receptivity is limited, and the changes responsible for this condition are entrained by estrogen in progesterone-conditioned endometrium. The transition from nonsensitivity to receptivity and on to refractoriness is associated with many changes in the endometrium, including altered rates of synthesis of RNA and protein, cell proliferation, and various changes in cytologic characteristics. However, it is not clear, at the cellular or molecular level, what uterine receptivity is; at present, sensitivity is only an operational definition that describes an essential condition for implantation.

(b) In response to a locally effective signal from the embryo, the sensitized endometrial stroma undergoes the process of decidual transformation. This typically involves cellular proliferation and differentiation, including the development of localized increases in vascular permeability, polyploid nuclei, dramatic cytological changes, and synthesis of unique species of RNA and protein. The so-called "decidua" that are formed typically provide a solid mass of cells into which the conceptus is embedded. The process responsible for formation of decidual tissue appears to require an intact epithelium to conduct the embryonic signal to the stroma and may utilize histamine and/or the local release of prostaglandin E-2 to initiate the reaction. Although formation of the decidua is a conspicuous part of the process of implantation in many species, and it seems to represent the development of an entirely new organ at implantation, its actual function remains unknown.

(c) The trophoblast of the embryo and the luminal epithelium of the uterus become adherent, with or without subsequent penetration of the endometrium. Adhesion of embryos to the uterine epithelium presumably involves changes in the glycoprotein molecules on one or both surfaces. Changes in lectin binding may reflect the expression of complementary surface glycoproteins and, thus, might be related to the acquisition of adhesiveness. However, it has not yet been shown that these changes are causally related to attachment and implantation.

(d) In response to a variety of signal factors from preimplantation embryos, there are local and systemic changes in the mother that can be considered to constitute the "maternal recognition of pregnancy." It is generally assumed that implantation and subsequent pregnancy will not be successful unless such recognition takes place.

REFERENCES

1. Psychoyos, A. (1973): Hormonal control of ovoimplantation. In: *Vitamins and Hormones: Advances in Research and Applications, Vol. 31,* edited by R. S. Harris, P. L. Munson, E. Diczfalusy, and J. Grover, pp. 201–256. Academic Press, New York.
2. Psychoyos, A. (1973): Endocrine control of egg implantation. In: *Handbook of Physiology, Section 7: Endocrinology, Vol. II, Part 2,* edited by R. O. Greep and E. B. Astwood, pp. 187–215. American Physiological Society, Washington, D.C.
3. Finn, C. A. (1977): The implantation reaction. In: *Biology of the Uterus,* edited by R. Wynn, pp. 245–308. Plenum Press, New York.
4. O'Grady, J. E., and Bell, S. C. (1977): The role of the endometrium in blastocyst implantation. In: *Development in Mammals, Vol. 1,* edited by M. H. Johnson, pp. 165–243. North-Holland, New York.
5. Yochim, J. M. (1975): Development of the progestational uterus: Metabolic aspects. *Biol. Reprod.,* 12:106–133.
6. Glasser, S. R., and Clark, J. H. (1975): A determinant role for progesterone in the development of uterine sensitivity to decidualization and ovo-implantation. In: *The Developmental Biology of Reproduction,* edited by S. L. Markert and J. Papaconstantinou, pp. 311–345. Academic Press, New York.
7. Glasser, S. R., and McCormack, S. A. (1981): Cellular and molecular aspects of decidualization and implantation. In: *Proteins and Steroids in Early Pregnancy,* edited by H. M. Beier and P. Karlson, pp. 245–310. Springer-Verlag, New York.
8. Enders, A. C. (1972): Mechanisms of implantation of the blastocyst. In: *Biology of Reproduction: Basic and Clinical Studies,* edited by J. T. Velardo and B. A. Kasprow, pp. 313–333. Symposium on Reproductive Biology, Sponsored by Third Pan American Congress of Anatomy.
9. Schlafke, S., and Enders, A. C. (1975): Cellular basis of interaction between trophoblast and uterus at implantation. *Biol. Reprod.,* 12:41–65.
10. Wimsatt, W. A. (1975): Some comparative aspects of implantation. *Biol. Reprod.,* 12:1–40.
11. Heap, R. B., Flint, A. P. F., and Gadsby, J. E. (1979): Role of embryonic signals in the establishment of pregnancy. *Br. Med. Bull.,* 35:129–135.
12. Enders, A. C., and Schlafke, S. (1967): A morphological analysis of the early implantation stages in the rat. *Am. J. Anat.,* 120:185–226.
13. Hedlund, K., Nilsson, O., Reinius, S., and Aman, G. (1972): Attachment reaction of the uterine luminal epithelium at implantation: Light and electron microscopy of the hamster, guinea-pig, rabbit and mink. *J. Reprod. Fertil.,* 29:131–132.
14. Nilsson, B. O. (1966): Structural differentiation of luminal membrane in rat uterus during normal and experimental implantations. *Z. Anat.,* 125:152–159.
15. Nilsson, B. O. (1970): Some ultrastructural aspects of ovo-implantation. In: *Ovo-Implantation. Human Gonadotropins and Prolactin,* edited by P. O. Hubinens, F. Lercy, C. Robyn, and P. Leleux, pp. 52–72. S. Karger, New York.
16. Young, M. P., Whicher, J. T., and Potts, D. M. (1968); The ultrastructure of implantation in the golden hamster (*cricetus auratus*). *J. Embryol. Exp. Morphol.,* 19:341–345.
17. Potts, D. M. (1966): The attachment phase of ovoimplantation. *Am. J. Obstet. Gynecol.,* 96:1122–1128.
18. Potts, D. M. (1968): The ultrastructure of implantation in the mouse. *J. Anat.,* 103:77–90.
19. Potts, M. (1969): The ultrastructure of egg-implantation. In: *Advances in Reproductive Physiology,* edited by A. McLaren, pp. 241–267. Logos, London.

20. Psychoyos, A., and Mandon, P. (1971): Scanning electron microscopy of the surface of the rat uterine epithelium during delayed implantation. *J. Reprod. Fertil.*, 26:137–138.
21. Nilsson, O. (1967): Attachment of rat and mouse blastocysts onto uterine epithelium. *Int. J. Fertil.*, 12:5–13.
22. Reinius, S. (1967): Ultrastructure of blastocyst attachment in mouse. *Z. Zellforsch. Mikrosk. Anat.*, 77:257–266.
23. Potts, D. M., and Psychoyos, A. (1967): Evolution de l'ultrastructure des relations ovoendometriales sous l'influence de l'oestrogene, chez la ratte en retard experimental de nidation. *C. R. Acad. Sci. Paris Ser. D*, 264:370–373.
24. Potts, D. M., and Psychoyos, A. (1967): L'ultrastructure des relations ovoendometriales au cours du retard experimental de nidation chez la souris. *C. R. Acad. Sci. Paris Ser. D*, 264:956–958.
25. Mayer, G., Nilsson, O., and Reinius, S. (1967): Cell membrane changes of uterine epithelium and trophoblast during blastocyst attachment in rat. *Z. Anat. Entwick.*, 126:43–48.
26. Tachi, S., Tachi, C., and Lindner, H. R. (1970): Ultrastructural features of blastocyst attachment and trophoblastic invasion in the rat. *J. Reprod. Fertil.*, 21:37–56.
27. Parkening, T. A. (1979): Apposition of uterine luminal epithelium during implantation in senescent golden hamster. *J. Gerontol.*, 34:335–344.
28. Martin, L., Finn, C. A., and Carter, J. (1970): Effects of progesterone and oestradiol on the luminal epithelium of the mouse uterus. *J. Reprod. Fertil.*, 21:461–469.
29. Hedlund, K., and Nilsson, O. (1971): Hormonal requirements for the uterine attachment reaction and blastocyst implantation in the mouse, hamster and guinea-pig. *J. Reprod. Fertil.*, 26:267–269.
30. Pollard, R. M., and Finn, C. A. (1972): Ultrastructure of the uterine epithelium during the hormonal induction of sensitivity and insensitivity to a decidual stimulus in the mouse. *J. Endocrinol.*, 55:293–298.
31. McLaren, A. (1968): A study of blastocysts during delay and subsequent implantation in lactating mice. *J. Endocrinol.*, 42:453–463.
32. Lundkvist, O., Nilsson, B. O., and Bergstrom, S. (1979): Studies on the trophoblast-epithelial complex during decidual induction in rats. *Am. J. Anat.*, 154:211–230.
33. Warren, R., and Enders, A. C. (1964): An electron microscope study of the rat endometrium during delayed implantation. *Anat. Rec.*, 148:177–195.
34. Ljungkvist, I. (1972): Attachment reaction of rat uterine luminal epithelium. IV. The cellular changes in the attachment reaction and its hormonal regulation. *Fertil. Steril.*, 23:847–865.
35. Tachi, S., and Tachi, C. (1979): Ultrastructural studies on maternal-embryonic cell interactions during experimentally induced implantation of rat blastocysts to the endometrium of the mouse. *Dev. Biol.*, 68:203–223.
36. McLaren, A., and Nilsson, O. (1971): Electron microscopy of luminal epithelium separated by beads in the pseudopregnant mouse uterus. *J. Reprod. Fertil.*, 26:379–381.
37. Enders, A. C., and Nelson, D. M. (1973): Pinocytotic activity of the uterus of the rat. *Am. J. Anat.*, 138:277–300.
38. Leroy, F., Van Hoeck, J., and Bogaert, C. (1976): Hormonal control of pinocytosis in the uterine epithelium of the rat. *J. Reprod. Fertil.*, 47:59–62.
39. Parr, M. R., and Parr, E. L. (1974): Uterine luminal epithelium: Protrusions mediate endocytosis, not apocrine secretion, in the rat. *Biol. Reprod.*, 11;:220–233.
40. Lundkvist, O. (1979): Morphometric estimation of stromal edema during delayed implantation in the rat. *Cell Tissue Res.*, 199:339–348.
41. Yochim, J. M., and Saldarini, R. J. (1969): Glucose utilization by the myometrium during early pseudopregnancy in the rat. *J. Reprod. Fertil.*, 20:481–489.
42. Murphy, C. R., Swift, J. G., Mukherjee, T. M., and Rogers, A. W. (1982): Changes in the fine structure of the apical plasma membrane of endometrial epithelial cells during implantation in the rat. *J. Cell Sci.*, 55:1–12.
43. Parr, M. (1982): Apical vesicles in rat uterine epithelium during early pregnancy: A morphometric study. *Biol. Reprod.*, 26:915–924.
44. Pollard, R. M., and Finn, C. A. (1974): Influence of the trophoblast upon differentiation of the uterine epithelium during implantation in the mouse. *J. Endocrinol.*, 62:669–674.
45. Enders, A. C., Hendrickx, A. G., and Schlafke, S. (1983): Implantation in the rhesus monkey: Initial penetration of endometrium. *Am. J. Anat.*, 167:275–298.
46. Parr, M. B., and Parr, E. L. (1982): Relationship of apical domes in the rabbit uterine epithelium during the peri-implantation period to endocytosis, apocrine secretion and fixation. *J. Reprod. Fertil.*, 66:739–744.
47. Bjorkman, N. (1973): Fine structure of the fetal-maternal area of exchange in the epitheliochorial and endotheliochorial types of placentation. *Acta Anat.*, 86(*Suppl.*), 61:1–22.
48. Boshier, D. P. (1969): A histological and histochemical examination of implantation and early placentome formation in sheep. *J. Reprod. Fertil.*, 19:51–61.
49. Wathes, D. C., and Wooding, F. B. P. (1980): An electron microscopic study of implantation in the cow. *Am. J. Anat.*, 159:285–306.
50. Enders, A. C., and Schlafke, S. (1969): Cytological aspects of trophoblast-uterine interaction in early implantation. *Am. J. Anat.*, 125:1–30.
51. Trinkaus, J. P. (1984): Cell adhesion. III. Mechanisms. In: *Cells Into Organs: The Forces That Shape the Embryo*, pp. 120–178. Prentice-Hall, Englewood Cliffs, N.J.
52. Enders, A. C., and Schlafke, S. (1974): Surface coats of the mouse blastocyst and uterus during the preimplantation period. *Anat. Rec.*, 180:31–46.
53. Anderson, T. L., and Hoffman, L. H. (1984): Alterations in epithelial glycocalyx of rabbit uteri during early pseudopregnancy and pregnancy, and following ovariectomy. *Am. J. Anat.*, 171:321–334.
54. Hewitt, K., Beer, A. E., and Grinnell, F. (1979): Disappearance of anionic sites from the surface of the rat endometrial epithelium at the time of blastocyst implantation. *Biol. Reprod.*, 21:691–707.
55. Chavez, D. J., and Anderson, T. L. (1985): The glycocalyx of the mouse uterine luminal epithelium during estrus, early pregnancy, the peri-implantation period and delayed implantation. I. Acquisition of ricinus communis I binding sites during pregnancy. *Biol. Reprod.*, 32:1135–1142.
56. Enders, A. C., and Schlafke, S. (1972): Implantation in the ferret: Epithelial penetration. *Am. J. Anat.*, 133:291–316.
57. Hakansson, S., and Sundkvist, K. G. (1975): Decreased antigenicity of mouse blastocysts after activation for implantation from experimental delay. *Transplantation*, 19:479–484.
58. Hakansson, S., Heyner, S., Sundqvist, K-G., and Bergstrom, S. (1975): The presence of paternal H-2 antigens on hybrid mouse blastocysts during experimental delay of implantation and the disappearance of these antigens after onset of implantation. *Int. J. Fertil.*, 20:137–140.
59. Nilsson, O., Lindqvist, I., and Ronquist, G. (1973): Decreased surface charge of mouse blastocysts at implantation. *Exp. Cell Res.*, 83:421–423.
60. Nilsson, O., Lindqvist, I., and Ronquist, G. (1975): Blastocyst surface charge and implantation in the mouse. *Contraception*, 11:441–450.
61. Jenkinson, E. J., and Searle, R. F. (1977): Cell surface changes on the mouse blastocyst at implantation. *Exp. Cell Res.*, 106:386–390.
62. Clemetson, C. A. B., Moshfeghi, M. M., and Mallikarjuneswara, V. R. (1970): Electrophoretic mobility of the rat blastocyst. *Contraception*, 1:357–360.
63. Nilsson, B. O., and Hjerten, S. (1982): Electrophoretic quantification of the changes in the average net negative charge density of mouse blastocysts implanting *in vivo* and *in vitro*. *Biol. Reprod.*, 27:485–493.
64. Enders, A. C., and Schlafke, S. (1971): Penetration of the uterine epithelium during implantation in the rabbit. *Am. J. Anat.*, 132:219–240.
65. Bergstrom, S., and Nilsson, O. (1976): Blastocyst attachment and early invasion during oestradiol-induced implantation in the mouse. *Anat. Embryol.*, 149:149–154.
66. Konwinski, M., Vorbrodt, A., Solter, D., and Koprowski, H. (1977): Ultrastructural study of concanavalin-A binding to the surface of preimplantation mouse embryos. *J. Exp. Zool.*, 200:311–324.
67. Chavez, D. J., and Enders, A. C. (1981): Temporal changes in lectin binding of peri-implantation mouse blastocysts. *Dev. Biol.*, 87:267–276.
68. Chavez, D. J., and Enders, A. C. (1982): Lectin binding of mouse blastocysts: Appearance of dolichos biflorus binding sites on the

trophoblast during delayed implantation and their subsequent disappearance during implantation. *Biol. Reprod.*, 26:545–552.
69. Sobel, J. S., and Nebel, L. (1976): Concanavalin A agglutinability of the developing mouse trophoblast. *J. Reprod. Fertil.*, 47:399–402.
70. Sobel, J. S., and Nebel, L. (1978): Changes in concanavalin A agglutinability during development of the inner cell mass and trophoblast of mouse blastocysts *in vitro*. *J. Reprod. Fertil.*, 52: 239–248.
71. Nilsson, B. O., Naeslund, G., and Curman, B. (1980): Polar differences of delayed and implanting mouse blastocysts in binding of alcian blue and concanavalin A. *J. Exp. Zool.*, 214:177–180.
72. Carollo, J. R., and Weitlauf, H. M. (1981): Regional changes in the binding of [^{3}H] concanavalin A to mouse blastocysts at implantation: An autoradiographic study. *J. Exp. Zool.*, 218:247–251.
73. Pinsker, M. C., and Mintz, B. (1973): Change in cell-surface glycoproteins of mouse embryos before implantation. *Proc. Natl. Acad. Sci. USA,* 70:1645–1648.
74. Surani, M. A. H. (1979): Glycoprotein synthesis and inhibition of glycosylation by tunicamycin in pre-implantation mouse embryos: Compaction and trophoblast adhesion. *Cell,* 18:217–227.
75. Sherman, M. I., Shalgi, R., Rizzino, A., Sellens, M. H., Gay, S., and Gay, R. (1979): Changes in the surface of the mouse blastocyst at implantation. In: *Maternal Recognition of Pregnancy,* CIBA Foundation Symposium No. 64 (new series), pp. 33–52. Excerpta Medica, New York.
76. Zetter, B. R., and Martin, G. R. (1978): Expression of a high molecular weight cell surface glycoprotein (LETS protein) by preimplantation mouse embryos and teratocarcinoma cells. *Proc. Natl. Acad. Sci. USA,* 75:2324–2328.
77. Gulamhusein, A. P., and Beck, F. (1973): Light and electron microscopic observations at the pre- and early post-implantation stages in the ferret uterus. *J. Anat.*, 115:159–174.
78. Enders, A. C., and Schlafke, S. (1965): The fine structure of the blastocyst: Some comparative studies. In: *Preimplantation Stages of Pregnancy,* CIBA Foundation Symposium, pp. 29–59. Little, Brown, Boston.
79. Parr, E. L. (1973): Shedding of the zona pellucida by guinea pig blastocysts: An ultrastructural study. *Biol. Reprod.*, 8:531–544.
80. Allen, W. R., Hamilton, D. W., and Moor, R. M. (1973): The origin of equine endometrial cups. II. Invasion of the endometrium by trophoblast. *Anat. Rec.*, 177:485–502.
81. Finn, C. A., and Lawn, A. M. (1968): Transfer of cellular material between the uterine epithelium and trophoblast during the early stages of implantation. *J. Reprod. Fertil.*, 15:333–336.
82. Wilson, I. B. (1963): A new factor associated with the implantation of the mouse egg. *J. Reprod. Fertil.*, 5:281–282.
83. Enders, A. C., and Schlafke, S. (1979): Comparative aspects of blastocyst-endometrial interactions at implantation. In: *Maternal Recognition of Pregnancy,* CIBA Foundation Symposium No. 64 (new series), pp. 3–32. Excerpta Medica, New York.
84. Finn, C. A., and Hinchliffe, J. R. (1965): Histological and histochemical analysis of the formation of implantation chambers in the mouse uterus. *J. Reprod. Fertil.*, 9:301–309.
85. Finn, C. A., and Hinchliffe, J. R. (1964): Reaction of the mouse uterus during implantation and deciduoma formation as demonstrated by changes in the distribution of alkaline phosphatase. *J. Reprod. Fertil.*, 8:331–338.
86. Hinchliffe, J. R., and El-Shershaby, A. M. (1975): Epithelial cell death in the oil-induced decidual reaction of the pseudopregnant mouse: An ultrastructural study. *J. Reprod. Fertil.*, 45:463–468.
87. El-Shershaby, A. M., and Hinchliffe, J. R. (1975): Epithelial autolysis during implantation of the mouse blastocyst: An ultrastructural study. *J. Embryol. Exp. Morphol.*, 33:1067–1080.
88. Finn, C. A., and Bredl, J. C. S. (1973): Studies on the development of the implantation reaction in the mouse uterus: influence of actinomycin D. *J. Reprod. Fertil.*, 34:247–253.
89. Moulton, B. C., and Elangovan, S. (1981): Lysosomal mechanisms in blastocyst implantation and early decidualization. In: *Cellular and Molecular Aspects of Implantation,* edited by S. R. Glasser and D. W. Bullock, pp. 335–344. Plenum Press, New York.
90. Roy, S. K., Sengupta, J., and Manchanda, S. K. (1983): Histochemical study of β-glucuronidase in the rat uterus during implantation and pseudopregnancy. *J. Reprod. Fertil.*, 68:161–164.
91. Sengupta, J., Paria, B. C., and Manchanda, S. K. (1981): Effect of an oestrogen antagonist on implantation and uterine leucylnaphthylamidase activity in the ovariectomized hamster. *J. Reprod. Fertil.*, 62:437–440.
92. Van Hoorn, G., and Denker, H. W. (1975): Effect of the blastocyst on a uterine amino acid arylamidase in the rabbit. *J. Reprod. Fertil.*, 45:359–362.
93. Boshier, D. P. (1976): Effects of the rat blastocyst on neutral lipids and nonspecific esterases in the uterine luminal epithelium at the implantation site. *J. Reprod. Fertil.*, 46:245–247.
94. Moulton, B. C. (1974): Ovum implantation and uterine lysosomal enzyme activity. *Biol. Reprod.*, 10:543–548.
95. Finn, C. A. (1982): Cellular changes in the uterus during the establishment of pregnancy in rodents. *J. Reprod. Fertil.* (*Suppl.*), 31:105–111.
96. Cowell, T. P. (1969): Implantation and development of the mouse eggs transferred to the uteri of non-progestational mice. *J. Reprod. Fertil.*, 19:239–245.
97. Steer, H. W. (1970): The trophoblastic knobs of the preimplanted rabbit blastocyst: A light and electron microscopic study. *J. Anat.*, 107:315–325.
98. Steer, H. W. (1971): Implantation of the rabbit blastocyst: The invasive phase. *J. Anat.*, 110:445–462.
99. Larsen, J. F. (1961): Electron microscopy of the implantation site in the rabbit. *Am. J. Anat.*, 109:319–334.
100. Psychoyos, A. (1960): La réaction déciduale est precédée de modifications précoces de la perméabilité capillarie de l'uterus. *C. R. Soc. Biol.*, 154:1384–1387.
101. Psychoyos, A. (1961): Perméabilité capillarie et décidualisation utérine. *C. R. Acad. Sci. Paris,* 252:1515–1517.
102. McLaren, A. (1969): Can mouse blastocysts stimulate a uterine response before losing the zona pellucida? *J. Reprod. Fertil.*, 19:199–201.
103. Loeb, L. (1907): Wounds of the pregnant uterus. *Proc. Soc. Exp. Biol. Med.*, 4:93–96.
104. Loeb, L. (1908): The production of deciduomata and the relation between the ovaries and formation of the decidua. *JAMA,* 50:1897–1901.
105. Loeb, L. (1908): The experimental production of the maternal part of the placenta of the rabbit. *Proc. Soc. Exp. Biol. Med.*, 5:102–105.
106. Deanesly, R. (1971): The differentiation of the decidua at ovo-implantation in the guinea-pig contrasted with that of the traumatic deciduoma. *J. Reprod. Fertil.*, 26:91–97.
107. Lundkvist, O., and Nilsson, B. O. (1982): Endometrial ultrastructure in the early uterine response to blastocysts and artificial deciduogenic stimuli in rats. *Cell Tissue Res.*, 225:355–364.
108. Welch, A. O., and Enders, A. C. (1985): Light and electron microscopic examination of the mature decidual cells of the rat with emphasis on the antimesometrial decidua and its degeneration. *Am. J. Anat.*, 172:1–29.
109. DeFeo, V. J. (1967): Decidualization. In: *Cellular Biology of the Uterus,* edited by R. M. Wynn, pp. 191–290, Appleton-Century-Crofts, New York.
110. Long, J. A., and Evans, H. M. (1922): The oestrus cycle in the rat and its associated phenomena. *Mem. Univ. Calif.*, 6:1–148.
111. Parkes, A. S. (1929): The functions of the corpus luteum. II. The experimental production of placentoma in the mouse. *Proc. R. Soc. Lond.* (*Biol.*), 104:183–188.
112. Kraicer, P. F., and Shelesnyak, M. C. (1959): Détermination de la période de sensibilité maximale de l'endomètre a la décidualisation au moyen de déciduomes provoqués par un traitement empruntant la voie vasculaire. *C. R. Acad. Sci. Paris,* 248:3213–3215.
113. Shelesnyak, M. C., and Kracier, P. F. (1960): Time-limits of uterine sensitivity to decidualization during progestation. *Proc. 1st Int. Congr. Endocrinol.*, (*Copenh.*): 547.
114. DeFeo, V. J. (1963): Determination of the sensitive period for the induction of deciduomata in the rat by different inducing procedures. *Endocrinology,* 73:488–497.
115. DeFeo, V. J. (1963): Temporal aspect of uterine sensitivity in the pseudopregnant or pregnant rat. *Endocrinology,* 72:305–316.
116. Hetherington, C. M. (1968): The development of deciduomata induced by two nontraumatic methods in the mouse. *J. Reprod. Fertil.*, 17:391–393.

117. Harper, M. J. K. (1969): Deciduomal response of the golden hamster uterus. *Anat. Rec.*, 163:563–574.
118. Finn, C. A., and Martin, L. (1972): Endocrine control of the timing of endometrial sensitivity to a decidual stimulus. *Biol. Reprod.*, 7:82–96.
119. McLaren, A., and Michie, D. (1956): Studies on the transfer of fertilized mouse eggs to uterine foster-mothers. I. Factors affecting the implantation and survival of native and transferred eggs. *J. Exp. Biol.*, 33:394–416.
120. Psychoyos, A. (1965): Control de la nidation chez les mammiferes. *Arch. Anat. Micros. Morphol. Exp.*, 54:85–104.
121. Psychoyos, A. (1966): Etude des relations de l'oeuf et de l'endometre au cours du retard de la nidation ou des premieres phases du processes de la nidation chez la ratte. *Compt. Rend. Acad. Sci. Paris Ser. D*, 263:1755–1758.
122. Psychoyos, A. (1966): Recent researches of egg-implantation. In: *Egg Implantation*, CIBA Foundation Study Group 23, pp. 4–28. Churchill, London.
123. Psychoyos, A. (1969): Hormonal factors governing decidualization. *Excerpta Med. Found. Int. Congr. Serv.*, 184:935–938.
124. Psychoyos, A. (1969): Hormonal requirements for egg implantation. In: *Advances in BioSciences. IV. Mechanisms Involved in Conception*, edited by G. Raspe, pp. 275–290. Pergamon Press, London.
125. Noyes, R. W., and Dickmann, Z. (1960): Relationship of ovular age to endometrial development. *J. Reprod. Fertil.*, 1:186–196.
126. Dickmann, Z., and Noyes, R. W. (1960): The fate of ova transferred into the uterus of the rat. *J. Reprod. Fertil.*, 1:197–212.
127. Psychoyos, A. (1967): The hormonal interplay controlling egg-implantation in the rat. In: *Advances in Reproductive Physiology*, edited by A. McLaren, pp. 257–277. Logos Press, London.
128. Humphrey, K. W. (1967): The induction of implantation in the mouse after ovariectomy. *Steroids*, 10:591–600.
129. Shelesnyak, M. C. (1962): Decidualization: The decidua and the deciduoma. *Perspect. Biol. Med.*, 5:503–518.
130. Finn, C. A., and Martin, L. (1967): Patterns of cell division in the mouse uterus during early pregnancy. *J. Endocrinol.*, 39:593–597.
131. Zhinkin, L. N., and Samoshkina, N. A. (1967): DNA synthesis and cell proliferation during formation of deciduomata in mice. *J. Embryol. Exp. Morphol.*, 17:593–605.
132. Hall, K. (1969): Uterine mitosis, alkaline phosphatase and adenosine triphosphatase during development and regression of deciduomata in pseudopregnant mice. *J. Endocrinol.*, 44:91–100.
133. Leroy, F., Galand, P., and Chretien, J. (1969): The mitogenic action of ovarian hormones on the uterine and vaginal epithelium during the oestrus cycle in the rat: An autoradiographic study. *J. Endocrinol.*, 45:441–447.
134. Chaudhury, R. R., and Sethi, A. (1970): Effects of an intra-uterine contraceptive device on mitosis in the rat uterus on different days of pregnancy. *J. Reprod. Fertil.*, 22:33–40.
135. Marcus, G. J. (1974): Mitosis in the rat uterus during the estrous cycle, early pregnancy and early pseudopregnancy. *Biol. Reprod.*, 10:447–452.
136. Tachi, C., Tachi, S., and Lindner, H. R. (1972): Modification by progesterone of oestradiol-induced cell proliferation, RNA synthesis and oestradiol distribution in the rat uterus. *J. Reprod. Fertil.*, 31:59–76.
137. Mehrotra, S. N., and Finn, C. A. (1974): Cell proliferation in the uterus of the guinea-pig. *J. Reprod. Fertil.*, 37:405–409.
138. Marcus, G. J. (1974): Hormonal control of proliferation in the guinea-pig uterus. *J. Endocrinol.*, 63:89–97.
139. Schmidt, I. G. (1943): Proliferation in the genital tract of the normal mature guinea pig treated with colchicine. *Am. J. Anat.*, 73:59–80.
140. Krueger, W. A., and Maibenco, H. C. (1972): DNA replication and cell division in the hamster uterus. *Anat. Rec.*, 173:229–234.
141. Herken, R. (1983): Cell kinetics of early gestation mouse uterus. *Cell Tissue Kinet.*, 16:419–428.
142. Galassi, L. (1968): Autoradiographic study of the decidual cell reaction in the rat. *Dev. Biol.*, 17:75–84.
143. Leroy, F., and Galand, P. (1969): Radioautographic evaluation of mitotic parameters in the endometrium during the uterine sensitivity period in pseudopregnant rat. *Fertil. Steril.*, 20:980–922.
144. O'Grady, J. E., and Heald, P. J. (1976): Uterine nucleic acid and phospholipid metabolism in the early stages of rat pregnancy. *J. Endocrinol.*, 68:33P–34P.
145. Lobel, B.L., Levy, E., and Shelesnyak, M. C. (1967): Studies on the mechanism of nidation. XXXIV. Dynamics of cellular interactions during progestation and implantation in the rat. *Acta Endocrinol. (Suppl.)*, 123:7–109.
146. Clark, B. F. (1973): The effect of oestrogen and progesterone on uterine cell division and epithelial morphology in spayed-hypophysectomized rats. *J. Endocrinol.*, 56:341–342.
147. Allen, E., Smith, G. M., and Gardner, W. U. (1937): Accentuation of the growth effect of Theelin on genital tissues of the ovariectomized mouse by arrest of mitosis with colchicine. *Am. J. Anat.*, 61:321–341.
148. Perrotta, C. A. (1962): Initiation of cell proliferation in the vaginal and uterine epithelia of the mouse. *Am. J. Anat.*, 111:195–204.
149. Epifanova, O. I. (1966): Mitotic cycles in estrogen-treated mice: An autoradiographic study. *Exp. Cell Res.*, 42:562–577.
150. Martin, L., and Finn, C. A. (1968): Hormonal regulation of cell division in epithelial and connective tissues of the mouse uterus. *J. Endocrinol.*, 41:363–371.
151. Finn, C. A., and Martin, L. (1973): Endocrine control of gland proliferation in the mouse uterus. *Biol. Reprod.*, 8:585–588.
152. Martin, L., Finn, C. A., and Trinder, G. (1973): Hypertrophy and hyperplasia in the mouse uterus after oestrogen treatment: An autoradiographic study. *J. Endocrinol.*, 56:133–144.
153. Clark, B. F. (1971): The effects of oestrogen and progesterone on uterine cell division and epithelial morphology in spayed, adrenalectomized rats. *J. Endocrinol.*, 50:527–528.
154. Lee, A., and Dukelow, W. R. (1972): Synthesis of DNA and mitosis in rabbit uteri after oestrogen and progesterone injections and during early pregnancy. *J. Reprod. Fertil.*, 31:473–476.
155. Koseki, Y., and Fujimoto, G. I. (1974): Progesterone effects contrasted with 17-β estradiol on DNA synthesis in epithelial nuclear proliferation in the castrate rabbit uterus. *Biol. Reprod.*, 10:596–604.
156. Nilsson, O. (1958): Ultrastructure of mouse uterine surface epithelium under different estrogenic influences. 1. Spayed animals and oestrus animals. *J. Ultrastruct. Res.*, 1:375–396.
157. Nilsson, O. (1958): Ultrastructure of mouse uterine surface epithelium under different estrogenic influences. 3. Late effect of estrogen administered to spayed animals. *J. Ultrastruct. Res.*, 2:185–199.
158. Nilsson, O. (1958): Ultrastructure of mouse uterine surface epithelium under different estrogenic influences. 2. Early effect of estrogen administered to spayed animals. *J. Ultrastruct. Res.*, 2:73–95.
159. Das, R. M. (1972): The effects of oestrogen on the cell cycle in epithelial and connective tissues of the mouse uterus. *J. Endocrinol.*, 55:21–30.
160. Das, R. M. (1972): The time-course of the mitotic response to oestrogen in the epithelium and stroma of the mouse uterus. *J. Endocrinol.*, 55:203–204.
161. Martin, L., Das, R. M., and Finn, C. A. (1973): The inhibition by progesterone of uterine epithelial proliferation in the mouse. *J. Endocrinol.*, 57:549–554.
162. Das, R. M., and Martin, L. (1973): Progesterone inhibition of mouse uterine epithelial proliferation. *J. Endocrinol.*, 59:205–206.
163. Martin, L., and Finn, C. A. (1969): Duration of progesterone treatment required for a stromal response to oestradiol-17β in the uterus of the mouse. *J. Endocrinol.*, 44:279–280.
164. Finn, C. A., and Martin, L. (1970): The role of the oestrogen secreted before oestrus in the preparation of the uterus for implantation in the mouse. *J. Endocrinol.*, 47:431–438.
165. Finn, C. A., and Martin, L. (1974): The control of implantation. *J. Reprod. Fertil.*, 39:195–206.
166. Finn, C. A., Martin, L., and Carter, J. (1969): A refractory period following oestrogenic stimulation of cell division in the mouse uterus. *J. Endocrinol.*, 44:121–126.
167. Talley, D. J., Tobert, J. A., Armstrong, E. G. Jr., and Villee, C. A. (1977): Changes in estrogen receptor levels during deciduomata development in the pseudopregnant rat. *Endocrinology*, 101:1538–1544.
168. Armstrong, E. G. Jr., Tobert, J. A., Talley, D. J., and Villee, C. A. (1977): Changes in progesterone receptor levels during deciduomata development in the pseudopregnant rat. *Endocrinology*, 101:1545–1551.
169. Logeat, F., Sartor, P., Vu Hai, M. T., and Milgrom, E. (1980): Local effect of the blastocyst on estrogen and progesterone receptors in the rat endometrium. *Science*, 207:1083–1085.

170. Vu Hai, M. T., Logeat, F., and Milgrom, E. (1978): Progesterone receptors in the rat uterus: Variations in cytosol and nuclei during the oestrous cycle and pregnancy. *J. Endocrinol.*, 76:43–48.
171. Martel, D., and Psychoyos, A. (1978): Progesterone-induced oestrogen receptors in the rat uterus. *J. Endocrinol.*, 76:145–154.
172. Clark, J. H., Markaverich, B., Upchurch, S., Eriksson, H., Hardin, J. W., and Peck, E. J. (1980): Heterogeneity of estrogen binding sites: Relationship to estrogen receptors and estrogen response. *Recent Prog. Horm. Res.*, 36:89–134.
173. Do, Y. S., and Leavitt, W. W. (1978): Characterization of a specific progesterone receptor in decidualized hamster uterus. *Endocrinology*, 102:443–451.
174. Martel, D., and Psychoyos, A. (1980): Behavior of uterine steroid receptors at implantation. In: *Progress in Reproductive Biology, Vol. 7*, edited by F. Leroy, C. A. Finn, A. Psychoyos, and P. O. Hubinont, pp. 216–233. Karger, New York.
175. Nilsson, O. (1959): Ultrastructure of mouse uterine surface epithelium under different estrogenic influences. 4. Uterine secretion. *J. Ultrastruct. Res.*, 2:331–341.
176. Nilsson, B. O. (1974): Changes of the luminal surface of the rat uterus at blastocyst implantation: Scanning electron microscopy and ruthenium red staining. *Z. Anat. Entwick.*, 144:337–342.
177. Alden, R. H. (1947): Implantation of the rat egg. II. Alterations in osmiophilic epithelial lipids of the rat uterus under normal and experimental conditions. *Anat. Rec.*, 97:1–19.
178. Elftman, H. (1958): Estrogen control of the phospholipids of the uterus. *Endocrinology*, 62:410–415.
179. Elftman, H. (1963): Estrogen induced changes in the Golgi apparatus and lipid of the uterine epithelium of the rat in the normal cycle. *Anat. Rec.*, 146:139–143.
180. Fuxe, K., and Nilsson, O. (1963): The effect of oestrogen on the histology of the uterine epithelium of the mouse. *Exp. Cell Res.*, 32:109–117.
181. Boshier, D. P., and Holloway, H. (1973): Effects of ovarian steroid hormones on histochemically demonstrable lipids in the rat uterine epithelium. *J. Endocrinol.*, 56:59–67.
182. Hall, K. (1973): Lactic dehydrogenase and other enzymes in the mouse uterus during the peri-implantation period of pregnancy. *J. Reprod. Fertil.*, 34:79–91.
183. Hall, K. (1975): Lipids in the mouse uterus during early pregnancy. *J. Endocrinol.*, 65:233–243.
184. Enders, A. C. (1961): Comparative studies on the endometrium of delayed implantation. *Anat. Rec.*, 139:483–497.
185. Smith, M. S. R., and Wilson, I. B. (1971): Histochemical observations on early implantation in the mouse. *J. Embryol. Exp. Morphol.*, 25:165–174.
186. Wood, C., and Psychoyos, A. (1967): Activité de certaines enzymes hydrolytiques dans l'endomètre et la myomètre au cours de la pseudogestation et de divers états de réceptivité utérine chez la ratte. *C. R. Acad. Sci. Paris, Ser. D*, 265:141–144.
187. Bergstrom, S. (1972): Delay of blastocyst implantation in the mouse by ovariectomy or lactation. A scanning electron microscope study. *Fertil. Steril.*, 23:548–561.
188. Bergstrom, S., and Nilsson, O. (1972): Ultrastructural response of blastocysts and uterine epithelium to progesterone deprivation during delayed implantation in mice. *J. Endocrinol.*, 55:217–218.
189. Christie, G. A. (1966): Implantation of the rat embryo: Glycogen and alkaline phosphatases. *J. Reprod. Fertil.*, 12:279–294.
190. Abraham, R., Hendy, R., Dougherty, W. J., Fulfs, J. C., and Golberg, L. (1970): Participation of lysosomes in early implantation in the rabbit. *Exp. Mol. Pathol.*, 13:329–345.
191. Elangovan, S., and Moulton, B. C. (1980): Blastocyst implantation in the rat and the immunohistochemical distribution and rate of synthesis of uterine lysosomal cathespin D. *Biol. Reprod.*, 23:663–668.
192. Moulton, B. C., and Ingle, C.B. (1981): Uterine lysosomal cathespin D activity, rate of synthesis and immunohistochemical localization following initiation of decidualization in pseudopregnant rats. *Biol. Reprod.*, 25:393–398.
193. Moulton, B. C. (1982): Progesterone and estrogen control of the response of rat uterine lysosomal cathespin D activity to a deciduogenic stimulus. *Endocrinology*, 110:1197–1202.
194. Finn, C. A., and Martin, L. (1971): Endocrine control of the proliferation and secretion of uterine glands in the mouse. *Acta Endocrinol. (Suppl.)*, 155:139.
195. Enders, A. C., and Given, R. L. (1977): The endometrium of delayed and early implantation. In: *Biology of the Uterus*, edited by R. M. Wynn, pp. 203–243. Plenum Press, New York.
196. Given, R. L., and Enders, A. C. (1980): Mouse uterine glands during the peri-implantation period: Fine structure. *Am. J. Anat.*, 157:169–179.
197. Given, R. L., and Enders, A. C. (1978): Mouse uterine glands during the delayed and induced implantation periods. *Anat. Rec.*, 190:271–284.
198. Hooker, C. W., and Forbes, T. R. (1947): A bio-assay for minute amounts of progesterone. *Endocrinology*, 41:158–169.
199. Tachi, C., Tachi, S., and Lindner, H. R. (1974): Effects of ovarian hormones upon nucleolar ultrastructure in endometrial stromal cells of the rat. *Biol. Reprod.*, 10:404–413.
200. Fainstat, T. (1963): Extracellular studies of uterus. I. Disappearance of the discrete collagen bundles in endometrial stroma during various reproductive states in the rat. *Am. J. Anat.*, 112:337–370.
201. Miller, B. G., and Emmens, C. W. (1969): The effects of oestradiol and progesterone on the incorporation of tritiated uridine into the genital tract of the mouse. *J. Endocrinol.*, 43:427–436.
202. Miller, B. G., Owen, W. H., and Emmens, C. W. (1968): The incorporation of tritiated uridine in the uterus and vagina of the mouse during early pregnancy. *J. Endocrinol.*, 41:189–195.
203. Miller, B. G., Owen, W. H., and Emmens, C. W. (1968): Uridine incorporation in the rat genital tract during early pregnancy. *J. Endocrinol.*, 42:351–352.
204. Heald, P. J., and O'Grady, J. E. (1970): The uptake of [^{3}H] uridine into the nucleic acids of the rat uterus during early pregnancy. *Biochem. J.*, 117:65–71.
205. O'Grady, J. E., Heald, P. J. and O'Hare, A. (1970): Incorporation of [^{3}H] uridine into the ribonucleic acid of rat uterus during pseudopregnancy and in the presence of I.C.I. 46474 [*trans*-1-(*p*-β-dimethylaminoethoxyphenyl)-1,2-diphenylbut-1-ene]. *Biochem. J.*, 119:609–613.
206. Heald, P. J., O'Grady, J. E., O'Hare, A., and Vass, M. (1972): Changes in uterine RNA during early pregnancy in the rat. *Biochim. Biophys. Acta*, 262:66–74.
207. Heald, P. J., O'Grady, J. E., and Moffat, G. E. (1972): The incorporation of [^{3}H] uridine into nuclear RNA in the uterus of the rat during early pregnancy. *Biochim. Biophys. Acta*, 281:347–352.
208. O'Grady, J. E., Moffat, G. E., McMinn, L., Vass, M. A., O'Hare, A., and Heald, P. J. (1975): Uterine chromatin template activity during the early stages of pregnancy in the rat. *Biochim. Biophys. Acta*, 407:125–132.
209. Heald, P. J., O'Grady, J. E., O'Hare, A., and Vass, M. (1975): Nucleic acid metabolism of cells of the luminal epithelium and stroma of the rat uterus during early pregnancy. *J. Reprod. Fertil.*, 45:129–138.
210. Kaye, A. M., Icekson, I., and Lindner, H. R. (1971): Stimulation by estrogens of ornitinine and *S*-adenosylmethionine decarboxylases in the immature rat uterus. *Biochim. Biophys. Acta*, 252: 150–159.
211. Saunderson, R., and Heald, P. J. (1974): Ornithine decarboxylase activity in the uterus of the rat during early pregnancy. *J. Reprod. Fertil.*, 39:141–143.
212. Heald, P. J. (1979): Changes in ornithine decarboxylase during early implantation in the rat. *Biol. Reprod.*, 20:1195–1199.
213. Reid, R. J., and Heald, P.J. (1970): Uptake of ^{3}H-leucine into proteins of rat uterus during early pregnancy. *Biochim. Biophys. Acta*, 204:278–279.
214. Reid, R. J., and Heald, P. J. (1971): Protein metabolism of the rat uterus during the oestrous cycle, pregnancy and pseudopregnancy and as affected by an anti-implantation compound, ICI 46,474. *J. Reprod. Fertil.*, 27:73–82.
215. Smith, J. A., Martin, L., King, R. J. B., and Vertes, M. (1970): Effects of oestradiol-17β and progesterone on total and nuclear-protein synthesis in epithelial and stromal tissues of the mouse uterus and of progesterone on the ability of these tissues to bind oestradiol-17β. *Biochem. J.*, 119:773–784.
216. Bell, S. C., Reynolds, S., and Heald, P. J. (1976): Presumptive induced protein synthesis in the rat uterus during early pregnancy. *J. Endocrinol.*, 68:34p–35p.
217. Bell, S. C., Reynolds, S., and Heald, P. J. (1977): Uterine protein synthesis during the early stages of pregnancy in the rat. *J. Reprod. Fertil.*, 49:177–181.

218. Beall, J. R. (1972): Uterine lipid metabolism—A review of the literature. *Comp. Biochem. Physiol.*, 42B:175–195.
219. Goswami, A., Kar, A. B., and Chowdhury, S. R. (1963): Uterine lipid metabolism in mice during the oestrous cycle: Effect of ovariectomy and replacement therapy. *J. Reprod. Fertil.*, 6:287–295.
220. Aizawa, Y., and Mueller, G. C. (1961): The effect *in vivo* and *in vitro* of estrogens on lipid synthesis in the rat uterus. *J. Biol. Chem.*, 236:381–386.
221. Davis, J. S., and Alden, R. H. (1959): Hormonal influence on lipid metabolism of rat uterus. *Anat. Rec.*, 134:725–737.
222. Ray, S. C., and Morin, R. J. (1965): Lipid composition of the nongravid and gravid rabbit endometrium. *Proc. Soc. Exp. Biol. Med.*, 120:849–853.
223. Morin, R. J., and Carrion, M. (1968): *In vitro* incorporation of acetate-1-^{4}C into the phospholipids of rabbit and human endometria. *Lipids*, 3:349–353.
224. Beall, J. R., and Werthessen, N. T. (1971): Lipid metabolism of the rat uterus after mating. *J. Endocrinol.*, 51:637–644.
225. Yochim, J.M. (1971): Intrauterine oxygen tension during the preimplantation period. In: *Biology of the Blastocyst*, edited by R. J. Blandau, pp. 363–382. University of Chicago Press, Chicago.
226. Battellino, L. J., Sabulsky, J., and Blanco, A. (1971): Lactate dehydrogenase isoenzymes in rat uterus: Changes during pregnancy. *J. Reprod. Fertil.*, 25:393–399.
227. Clark, S. W., and Yochim, J. M. (1971): Effect of ovarian steroids on lactic dehydrogenase activity in endometrium and myometrium of the rat uterus. *Endocrinology*, 89:358–365.
228. Clark, S. W., and Yochim, J. M. (1971): Lactic dehydrogenase in the rat uterus during progestation, its relation to intrauterine oxygen tension and the regulation of glycolysis. *Biol. Reprod.*, 5:152–160.
229. Saldarini, R. J., and Yochim, J. M. (1967): Metabolism of the uterus of the rat during early pseudopregnancy and its regulation by estrogen and progesterone. *Endocrinology*, 80:453–466.
230. Surani, M. A. H., and Heald, P. J. (1971): The metabolism of glucose by rat uterus tissue in early pregnancy. *Acta Endocrinol.*, 66:16–24.
231. Yochim, J. M., and Clark, S. W. (1971): Lactic dehydrogenase activity in the uterus of the rat during the estrous cycle and its relation to intrauterine oxygen tension. *Biol. Reprod.*, 5:146–151.
232. Yochim, J.M., and Mitchell, J. A. (1968): Intrauterine oxygen tension in the rat during progestation: Its possible relation to carbohydrate metabolism and the regulation of nidation. *Endocrinology*, 83:706–713.
233. Yochim, J. M., and Pepe, G. J. (1971): Effect of ovarian steroids on nucleic acids, protein, and glucose-6-phosphate dehydrogenase activity in endometrium of the rat; a metabolic role for progesterone in "progestational differentiation." *Biol. Reprod.*, 5:172–182.
234. Mallonee, R. C., and Yochim, J. M. (1980): Uterus of the rat during progestation: Pyridine nucleotide activity and its relation to preimplantation changes in pentose cycle activity. *Biol. Reprod.*, 23: 588–594.
235. Yochim, J. M., and Mallonee, R. C. (1980): Hormonal control of pyridine nucleotide activity in the uterus: A model for progestational differentiation. *Biol. Reprod.*, 23:595–605.
236. Pepe, G. J., and Yochim, J. M. (1971): Pentose cycle activity in endometrium of the rat during progestation: Its regulation by intrauterine oxygen and its relation to the "progestational" action of progesterone. *Endocrinology*, 89:366–377.
237. Cummings, A. M., and Yochim, J. M. (1983): Nicotinamide adenine dinucleotide in rat uterus: Role of progesterone in the regulation of preimplantation differentiation. *Endocrinology*, 112:1407–1411.
238. Cummings, A.M., and Yochim, J. M. (1983): Nicotinamide adenine dinucleotide kinase in the rat uterus: Regulation by progesterone and decidual induction. *Endocrinology*, 112:1412–1419.
239. Yochim, J. M. (1984): Modulation of uterine sensitivity to decidual induction in the rat by nicotinamide: Challenge and extension of a model of progestational differentiation. *Biol. Reprod.*, 30:637–645.
240. Krehbiel, R. H. (1937): Cytological studies of the decidual reaction in the rat during pregnancy and in the production of deciduomata. *Physiol. Zool.*, 10:212–238.
241. Velardo, J. T., Dawson, A. B., Olsen, A. G., and Hisaw, F. L. (1953): Sequence of histological changes in the uterus and vagina of the rat during prolongation of pseudopregnancy associated with the presence of deciduomata. *Am. J. Anat.*, 93:273–305.
242. Lobel, B. L., Tic, L., and Shelesnyak, M. C. (1965): Studies on the mechanisms of nidation. XVII. Histochemical analysis of decidualization in the rat. Part 2. Induction. *Acta Endocrinol.*, 50:469–485.
243. Lobel, B. L., Tic, L., and Shelesnyak, M. C. (1965): Studies on the mechanism of nidation. XVII. Histochemical analysis of decidualization in the rat. Part 3. Formation of the deciduomata. *Acta Endocrinol.*, 50:517–536.
244. Ledford, B. E., Rankin, J. C., Froble, V. L., Serra, M. J., Markwald, R. R., and Baggett, B. (1978): The decidual cell reaction in the mouse uterus: DNA synthesis and autoradiographic analysis of responsive cells. *Biol. Reprod.*, 18:506–509.
245. Finn, C. A., and McLaren, A. (1967): A study of the early stages of implantation in mice. *J. Reprod. Fertil.*, 13:259–267.
246. Sachs, L., and Shelesnyak, M. C. (1955): The development and suppression of polyploidy in the developing and suppressed deciduoma in the rat. *J. Endocrinol.*, 12:146–151.
247. Dupont, H., Duluc, J. A., and Mayer, G. (1971): Evolution cytologique et genese de la polyploidie dans le dèciduome expérimental chez la ratte en gestation unilatérale. *C. R. Acad. Sci. Paris Ser. D*, 272:2360.
248. Ansell, J. D., Barlow, P. W., and McLaren, A. (1974): Binucleate and polyploid cells in the decidua of the mouse. *J. Embryol. Exp. Morphol.*, 31:223–227.
249. Jollie, W., and Benscome, S. A. (1965): Electron microscopic observations on primary decidua formation in the rat. *Am. J. Anat.*, 116:217–236.
250. Lundkvist, O., and Ljungkvist, I. (1977): Morphology of the rat endometrial stroma at the appearance of the pontamine blue reaction during implantation after an experimental delay. *Cell Tissue Res.* 184:453–466.
251. Parkening, T. A. (1976): An ultrastructural study of implantation in the golden hamster. III. Initial formation and differentiation of decidual cells. *J. Anat.*, 122:485–498.
252. O'Shea, J. D., Kleinfeld, R. G., and Morrow, H. A. (1983): Ultrastructure of decidualization in the pseudopregnant rat. *Am. J. Anat.*, 166:271–298.
253. Abrahamsohn, P. (1983): Ultrastructural study of the mouse antimesometrial decidua. *Anat. Embryol.*, 166:263–274.
254. Enders, A. C., Welsh, A. O., and Schlafke, S. (1985): Implantation in the rhesus monkey: Endometrial responses. *Am. J. Anat.*, 173:147–169.
255. Grinnell, F., Head, I. R., and Hoffpauir, J. (1982): Fibronectin and cell shape *in vivo:* Studies on the endometrium during pregnancy. *J. Cell Biol.*, 94:597–606.
256. Finn, C. A., and Lawn, A. M. (1967): Specialized junctions between decidual cells in the uterus of the pregnant mouse. *J. Ultrastruct. Res.*, 20:321–327.
257. Lawn, A. M., Wilson, E. W., and Finn, C. A. (1971): The ultrastructure of human decidual and predecidual cells. *J. Reprod. Fertil.*, 26:85–90.
258. Kleinfeld, R., Morrow, H. A., and DeFeo, V. J. (1976): Intercellular junctions between decidual cells in the growing deciduoma of the pseudopregnant rat uterus. *Biol. Reprod.*, 15:593–603.
259. Abrahamsohn, P., Lundkvist, O., and Nilsson, O. (1983): Ultrastructure of the endometrial blood vessels during implantation of the rat blastocyst. *Cell Tissue Res.*, 229:269–280.
260. Milligan, S. R., and Mirembe, F. M. (1984): Time course of the changes in uterine vascular permeability associated with the development of the decidual cell reaction in ovariectomized steroid-treated rats. *J. Reprod. Fertil.*, 70:1–6.
261. Hoos, P. C., and Hoffman, L. H. (1980): Temporal aspects of rabbit uterine vascular and decidual responses to blastocyst stimulation. *Biol. Reprod.*, 23:453–459.
262. Das, R. M., and Martin, L. (1978): Uterine DNA synthesis and cell proliferation during early decidualization induced by oil in mice. *J. Reprod. Fertil.*, 53:125–128.
263. Ledford, B. E., Rankin, J. C., Markwald, R. R., and Baggett, B. (1976): Biochemical and morphological changes following artificially stimulated decidualization in the mouse uterus. *Biol. Reprod.*, 15:529–535.
264. Shelesnyak, M. C., and Tic, L. (1963): Studies on the mechanism of decidualization. IV. Synthetic processes in the decidualizing uterus. *Acta Endocrinol.*, 42:465–472.

265. Shelesnyak, M. C., and Tic, L. (1963): Studies on the mechanism of decidualization. V. Suppression of synthetic processes of the uterus (DNA, RNA, and protein) following inhibition of decidualization by an antioestrogen, ethanoxytriphetol (MER-25). *Acta Endocrinol.*, 43:462–463.
266. Leroy, F., Bogaert, C., vanHoeck, J., and Delcroix, C. (1974): Cytophotometric and autoradiographic evaluation of cell kinetics in decidual cell growth in rats. *J. Reprod. Fertil.*, 38:441–449.
267. Moulton, B. C., and Blaha, G. C. (1978): Separation of deciduomal cells by velocity sedimentation at unit gravity. *Biol. Reprod.*, 18:141–147.
268. Moulton, B. C. (1979): Effect of progesterone on DNA, RNA and protein synthesis of deciduoma cell fractions separated by velocity sedimentation. *Biol. Reprod.*, 21:667–672.
269. Moulton, B. C., and Koenig, B. B. (1984): Uterine deoxyribonucleic acid synthesis during preimplantation in precursors of stromal cell differentiation during decidualization. *Endocrinology*, 115:1302–1307.
270. Martel, D., and Psychoyos, A. (1981): Estrogen receptors in the nidatory sites of the rat endometrium. *Science*, 211:1454–1455.
271. Ward, W. F., Frost, A. G., and Orsini, M. W. (1978): Estrogen binding by embryonic and interembryonic segments of the rat uterus prior to implantation. *Biol. Reprod.*, 18:598–601.
272. Sartor, P. (1977): Exogenous hormone uptake and retention in the rat uterus at the time of ova-implantation. *Acta Endocrinol.*, 84:804–812.
273. Moulton, B. C., and Koenig, B. B. (1981): Estrogen receptor in deciduoma cells separated by velocity sedimentation. *Endocrinology*, 108:484–488.
274. McConnell, K. N., Sillar, R. G., Young, B. D., and Green, B. (1982): Ploidy and progesterone-receptor distribution in flow-sorted deciduomal nuclei. *Mol. Cell. Endocrinol.*, 25:99–104.
275. Miller, B. G. (1973): Metabolism of RNA and pyrimidine nucleotides in the uterus during the early decidual cell reaction. *J. Endocrinol.*, 59:275–283.
276. Serra, M. J., Ledford, B. E., Rankin, J. C., and Baggett, B. (1978): Changes in RNA polymerase activity in isolated mouse uterine nuclei during the decidual cell reaction. *Biochim. Biophys. Acta*, 521:267–273.
277. Barkai, U., and Kraicer, P. F. (1978): Definition of period of induction of deciduoma in the rat using ornithine decarboxylase as a marker of growth onset. *Int. J. Fertil.*, 23:106–111.
278. Collawn, S. S., Rankin, J., Ledford, B. E., and Baggett, B. (1981): Ornithine decarboxylase activity in the artificially stimulated decidual cell reaction in the mouse uterus. *Biol. Reprod.*, 24:528–533.
279. Tarachand, U., Sivabalan, R., and Eapen, J. (1980): Protein anabolism in endometrium and myometrium during the growth of induced deciduoma in rats. *Experientia*, 36:1154–1156.
280. Yoshinaga, K. (1972): Rabbit antiserum to rat deciduoma. *Biol. Reprod.*, 6:51–57.
281. Yoshinaga, K. (1974): Interspecific cross-reactivity of deciduoma antiserum: Interaction between mouse deciduoma and anti-serum to rat deciduoma. *Biol. Reprod.*, 11:50–55.
282. Joshi, S. G., Szarowski, D. H., and Bank, J. (1981): Decidua-associated antigens in the baboon. *Biol. Reprod.*, 25:591–598.
283. Sacco, A. G., and Mintz, B. (1975): Mouse uterine antigens in the implantation period of pregnancy. *Biol. Reprod.*, 12:498–503.
284. Denari, J. H., and Rosner, J. M. (1978): Studies on biochemical characteristics of an early decidual protein. *Int. J. Fertil.*, 23:123–127.
285. Umapathesivam, K., and Jones, W. R. (1978): An investigation of decidual specific proteins in the rat. *Int. J. Fertil.*, 23:138–142.
286. Denari, J. H., Germino, N. I., and Rosner, J. M. (1976): Early synthesis of uterine proteins after a decidual stimulus in the pseudopregnant rat. *Biol. Reprod.*, 15:1–8.
287. Bell, S. C. (1979): Synthesis of 'decidualization-associated protein' in tissues of the rat uterus and placenta during pregnancy. *J. Reprod. Fertil.*, 56:255–262.
288. Bell, S. C. (1979): Protein synthesis during deciduoma morphogenesis in the rat. *Biol. Reprod.*, 20:811–821.
289. Bell, S. C. (1979): Immunochemical identity of decidualization-associated proteins and α_2 acute-phase macroglobulin in the pregnant rat. *J. Reprod. Immunol.*, 1:193–206.
290. Bell, S. C., Hamer, J., and Heald, P. J. (1980): Induced protein and deciduoma formation in rat uterus. *Biol. Reprod.*, 23:935–940.
291. Notides, A., and Gorski, J. (1966): Estrogen-induced synthesis of a specific uterine protein. *Proc. Natl. Acad. Sci. USA.*, 56:230–235.
292. Manak, R., Wertz, N., Slabaugh, M., Denari, H., Wang, J. T., and Gorski, J. (1980): Purification and characterization of the estrogen-induced protein (IP) of the rat uterus. *Mol. Cell. Endocrinol.*, 17:119–132.
293. Katzenellenbogen, B. S. (1975): Synthesis and inducibility of the uterine estrogen-induced protein, IP, during the rat estrous cycle: Clues to uterine estrogen sensitivity. *Endocrinology*, 96:289–297.
294. Dupont-Mairess, N., and Galand, P. (1975): Estrogen action: Induction of the synthesis of a specific protein (IP) in the myometrium, the stroma and the luminal epithelium of the rat uterus. *Endocrinology*, 96:1587–1591.
295. Lejeune, B. Lecocq, R., Lamy, F., and Leroy, F. (1982): Changes in the pattern of endometrial protein synthesis during decidualization in the rat. *J. Reprod. Fertil.*, 66:519–523.
296. MacDonald, R. G., Morency, K. O., and Leavitt, W. W. (1983): Progesterone modulation of specific protein synthesis in the decidualized hamster uterus. *Biol. Reprod.*, 28:753–766.
297. Leavitt, W. W., MacDonald, R. G., and Shwaery, G. T. (1985): Characterization of deciduoma proteins in hamster uterus: Detection in decidual cell cultures. *Biol. Reprod.*, 32:631–643.
298. Shelesnyak, M. C. (1952): Inhibition of decidual cell formation in the pseudopregnant rat by histamine antagonists. *Am. J. Physiol.*, 170:522–527.
299. Shelesnyak, M. C. (1957): Some experimental studies on the mechanism of ovo-implantation in the rat. *Recent Prog. Horm. Res.*, 13:269–317.
300. Kraicer, P. F., and Shelesnyak, M. C. (1958): The induction of deciduomata in the pseudopregnant rat by systemic administration of histamine and histamine releasers. *J. Endocrinol.*, 17:324–328.
301. Shelesnyak, M. C. (1959): Fall in uterine histamine associated with ovum implantation in pregnant rat. *Proc. Soc. Exp. Biol. Med.*, 100:380–381.
302. Spaziani, E., and Szego, C. M. (1958): The influence of estradiol and cortisol on uterine histamine of the ovariectomized rat. *Endocrinology*, 63:669–678.
303. Spaziani, E., and Szego, C. M. (1959): Further evidence for mediation by histamine of estrogenic stimulation of the rat uterus. *Endocrinology*, 64:713–723.
304. Humphrey, K. W., and Martin, L. (1968): Attempted induction of deciduomata in mice with mast-cell, capillary permeability and tissue inflammatory factors. *J. Endocrinol.*, 42:129–141.
305. Wrenn, T. R., Bitman, J., Cecil, H. C., and Gilliam, D. R. (1964): Uterine deciduomata: Role of histamine. *J. Endocrinol.*, 28:149–152.
306. Finn, C. A., and Keen, P. M. (1962): Influence of systemic antihistamines on formation of deciduoma. *J. Endocrinol.*, 24:381–382.
307. Goldstein, A., and Hazel, M. M. (1955): Failure of an antihistamine drug to prevent pregnancy in the mouse. *Endocrinology*, 56:215–216.
308. Harper, M. J. K. (1965): Failure of various antihistaminic drugs to prevent implantation in rats. *J. Reprod. Fertil.*, 9:359–361.
309. Finn, C. A., and Keen, P. M. (1962): Failure of histamine to induce deciduomata in the rat. *Nature*, 194:602–603.
310. Banik, U. K., and Ketchel, M. M. (1964): Inability of histamine to induce deciduomata in pregnant rats and pseudopregnant rats. *J. Reprod. Fertil.*, 7:259–261.
311. Brandon, J. M., and Wallis, R. M. (1977): Effect of mepyramine, a histamine H_1-, and burinamide, a histamine H_2-receptor antagonist, on ovum implantation in the rat. *J. Reprod. Fertil.*, 50:251–254.
312. Dey, S. K., Villanueva, C., and Abdou, N. I. (1979): Histamine receptors on rabbit blastocyst and endometrial cell membranes. *Nature*, 278:648–649.
313. Brandon, J. M., and Raval, P. J. (1979): Interaction of estrogen and histamine during ovum implantation in the rat. *Eur. J. Pharmacol.*, 57:171–177.
314. Brandon, J. M. (1980): Some recent work on the role of histamine in ovum implantation. In: *Blastocyst-Endometrium Relationships, Progress in Reproductive Biology, Vol 7,* edited by F. Leroy, C. A. Finn, A. Psychoyos, and P. Hubinont, pp. 244–252. S. Karger, New York.

315. Ferrando, G., and Nalbandov, A. V. (1968): Relative importance of histamine and estrogen on implantation in rats. *Endocrinology*, 83:933–937.
316. Dey, S. K., Villanueva, C., Chien, S. M., and Crist, R. D. (1978): The role of histamine in implantation in the rabbit. *J. Reprod. Fertil.*, 53:23–26.
317. Kennedy, T. G. (1983): Embryonic signals and the initiation of blastocyst implantation. *Aust. J. Biol. Sci.*, 36:531–543.
318. Kennedy, T. G., and Armstrong, D. T. (1981): The role of prostaglandins in endometrial vascular changes at implantation. In: *Cellular and Molecular Aspects of Implantation,* edited by S. R. Glasser and D. W. Bullock, pp. 349–363, Plenum Press, New York.
319. Lau, I. F., Saksena, S. K., and Chang, M. C. (1973): Pregnancy blockade by indomethacin, an inhibitor of prostaglandin synthesis: Its reversal by prostaglandins and progesterone in mice. *Prostaglandins,* 4:795–803.
320. Saksena, S. K., Lau, I. F., and Chang, M. C. (1976): Relationship between oestrogen, prostaglandin F_{2a} and histamine in delayed implantation in the mouse. *Acta Endocrinol.*, 81:801–807.
321. Lundkvist, O., and Nilsson, B. O. (1980): Ultrastructural changes of the trophoblast-epithelial complexes in mice subjected to implantation blocking treatment with indomethacin. *Biol. Reprod.*, 22:719–726.
322. Holmes, P. V., and Gordashko, B. J. (1980): Evidence of prostaglandin involvement in blastocyst implantation. *J. Embryol. Exp. Morphol.*, 55:109–122.
323. Gavin, M. A., Dominguez Fernandez-Tejerina, J. C., Montanes de las Heras, M. F., and Vijil Maeso, E. (1974): Efectos de un inhibidor de la biosintesis de las prostaglandinas (indometacina) sobre la implantacion en la rata. *Reproduccion,* 1:177–186.
324. Kennedy, T. G. (1977): Evidence for a role for prostaglandins in the initiation of blastocyst implantation in the rat. *Biol. Reprod.*, 16:286–291.
325. Phillips, C. A., and Poyser, N. L. (1981): Studies on the involvement of prostaglandin in implantation in the rat. *J. Reprod. Fertil.*, 62:73–81.
326. Evans, C. A., and Kennedy, T. G. (1978): The importance of prostaglandin synthesis for the initiation of blastocyst implantation in the hamster. *J. Reprod. Fertil.*, 54:255–261.
327. Hoffman, L. H. (1978): Antifertility effects of indomethacin during early pregnancy in the rabbit. *Biol. Reprod.*, 18:148–153.
328. Kennedy, T. G. (1979): Prostaglandins and increased endometrial vascular permeability resulting from the application of an artificial stimulus to the uterus of the rat sensitized for the decidual cell reaction. *Biol. Reprod.*, 20:560–566.
329. Hoffman, L. H., DiPietro, D.L., and McKenna, T. J. (1978): Effects of indomethacin on uterine capillary permeability and blastocyst development in rabbits. *Prostaglandins,* 15:823–829.
330. Hoos, P. C., and Hoffman, L. H. (1983): The effect of histamine receptor antagonists and indomethacin on implantation in the rabbit. *Biol. Reprod.*, 29:833–840.
331. Castracane, V. D., Saksena, S. K., and Shaikh, A. A. (1974): Effect of IUDs, prostaglandins and indomethacin on decidual cell reaction in the rat. *Prostaglandins,* 6:397–404.
332. Sananes, N., Baulieu, E. E., and le Goascogne, C. (1976): Prostaglandin(s) as inductive factor of decidualization in the rat uterus. *Mol. Cell. Endocrinol.*, 6:153–160.
333. Tobert, J. A. (1976): A study of the possible role for prostaglandins in decidualization using a nonsurgical method for the instillation of fluids into the rat uterine lumen. *J. Reprod. Fertil.*, 47:391–393.
334. Rankin, J. C., Ledford, B. E., Jonsson, H. T., and Baggett, B. (1979): Prostaglandins, indomethacin and the decidual cell reaction in the mouse uterus. *Biol. Reprod.*, 20:399–404.
335. Miller, M. M., and O'Morchoe, C. C. C. (1982): Decidual cell reaction induced by prostaglandin F_{2a} in the mature oophorectomized rat. *Cell Tissue Res.*, 225:189–199.
336. Kennedy, T. G., and Lukash, L. A. (1982): Induction of decidualization in rats by the intrauterine infusion of prostaglandins. *Biol. Reprod.*, 27:253–260.
337. Kennedy, T. G. (1980): Timing of uterine sensitivity for the decidual cell reaction: Role of prostaglandins. *Biol. Reprod.*, 22:519–525.
338. Kennedy, T. G. (1980): Estrogen and uterine sensitization for the decidual cell reaction: Role of prostaglandins. *Biol. Reprod.*, 23:955–962.
339. Kennedy, T. G., and Zamecnik, J. (1978): The concentration of 6-keto-prostaglandin F_{1a} is markedly elevated at the site of blastocyst implantation in the rat. *Prostaglandins,* 16:599–605.
340. Jonsson, H. T., Rankin, J. C., Ledford, B. E., and Baggett, B. (1979): Uterine prostaglandin levels following stimulation of the decidual cell reaction: Effects of indomethacin and tranylcypromine. *Prostaglandins,* 18:847–857.
341. Hoffman, L. H., Davenport, G. R., and Brash, A. R. (1984): Endometrial prostaglandins and phospholipase activity related to implantation in rabbits: Effects of dexamethasone. *Biol. Reprod.*, 30:544–555.
342. Miller, M. M., and O'Morchoe, C. C. C. (1982): Inhibition of artificially induced decidual cell reaction by indomethacin in the mature oopherectomized rat. *Anat. Rec.*, 204:223–230.
343. Hoffman, L. H., Strong, G. B., Davenport, G. R., and Frolich, J. C. (1977): Deciduogenic effect of prostaglandins in the pseudopregnant rabbit. *J. Reprod. Fertil.*, 50:231–237.
344. Kennedy, T. G., Martel, D., and Psychoyos, A. (1983): Endometrial prostaglandin E_2 binding: Characterization in rats sensitized for decidual cell reaction and changes during pseudopregnancy. *Biol. Reprod.*, 29:556–564.
345. Martel, D., Kennedy, T. G., Monier, M. N., and Psychoyos, A. (1985): Failure to detect specific binding sites for prostaglandin F-2_a in membrane preparations from rat endometrium. *J. Reprod. Fertil.*, 75:265–274.
346. Kennedy, T. G., Martel, D., and Psychoyos A. (1983): Endometrial prostaglandin E_2 binding during the estrous cycle and its hormonal control in ovariectomized rats. *Biol. Reprod.*, 29:565–571.
347. Peleg, S., and Lindner, H. R. (1982): The effect of prostaglandins on progestin receptor translocation and on decidual cell reaction *in vivo* and *in vitro*. *Endocrinology,* 110:1647–1652.
348. Leroy, F., Vansande, J., Shetgen, G., and Brasseur, D. (1974): Cyclic AMP and triggering of the decidual reaction. *J. Reprod. Fertil.* 39:207–211.
349. Rankin, J. C., Ledford, B. E., and Baggett, B. (1977): Early involvement of cyclic nucleotides in the artificially stimulated decidual cell reaction in the mouse uterus. *Biol. Reprod.*, 17: 549–554.
350. Kennedy, T. G. (1983): Prostaglandin E_2, adenosine 3′ : 5′-cyclic monophsphate and changes in endometrial vascular permeability in rat uterus sensitized for decidual cell reaction. *Biol. Reprod.*, 29:1069–1076.
351. Johnston, M. E. A., and Kennedy, T. G. (1984): Estrogen and uterine sensitization for the decidual cell reaction in the rat: Role of prostaglandin E_2 and adenosine 3′ : 5′-cyclic monophosphate. *Biol. Reprod.*, 31:959–966.
352. Alleua, J. J., Kenimer, J. G., Jordan, A. W., and Lamanna, C. (1983): Induction of estrogen and progesterone receptors and decidualization in the hamster uterus of cholera toxin. *Endocrinology,* 11:2095–2106.
353. Webb, F. T. G. (1975): The inability of dibutyryl adenosine 3′,-5′-monophosphate to induce the decidual reaction in intact pseudopregnant mice. *J. Reprod. Fertil.*, 42:187–188.
354. Webb, F. T. G. (1975): Implantation in ovariectomized mice treated with dibutyryl adenosine 3′,5′-monophosphate (dibutyryl cyclic AMP). *J. Reprod. Fertil.*, 42:511–517.
355. Holmes, P. V., and Bergstrom, S. (1975): Induction of blastocyst implantation in mice by cyclic AMP. *J. Reprod. Fertil.*, 43:329–332.
356. Heap, R. B., Flint, A. P. F., Gadsby, J. E., and Rice, C. (1979): Hormones, the early embryo and the uterine environment. *J. Reprod. Fertil.*, 55:267–275.
357. Flint, A. P. F., Burton, R. D., Gadsby, J. E., Saunders, P. T. K., and Heap, R. B. (1979): Blastocyst oestrogen synthesis and the maternal recognition of pregnancy. In: *Maternal Recognition of Pregnancy,* CIBA Foundation Symposium No. 64 (new series), pp. 209–238. Excerpta Medica, New York.
358. Atkinson, L. E., Hotchkiss, J., Fritz, G. R., Surve, A. H., Neill, J. D., and Knobil, E. (1975): Circulating levels of steroids and chorionic gonadotropin during pregnancy in the rhesus monkey, with special attention to the rescue of the corpus luteum in early pregnancy. *Biol. Reprod.*, 12:335–345.
359. Blandau, R. J. (1949): Embryo-endometrial interrelationship in the rat and guinea pig. *Anat. Rec.*, 104:331–360.

360. Alden, R. H., and Smith, M. J. (1959): Implantation of the rat egg. IV. Some effects of artificial ova on the uterus. *J. Exp. Zool.*, 142:215–226.
361. McLaren, A. (1968): Can beads stimulate a decidual response in the mouse uterus? *J. Reprod. Fertil.*, 15:313–315.
362. Cole, R. J. (1967): Cinemicrographic observations on the trophoblast and zona pellucida of the mouse blastocyst. *J. Embryol. Exp. Morphol.*, 17:481–490.
363. Bitton-Casimiri, V., Brun, J-L., and Psychoyos, A. (1970): Comportement *in vitro* des blastocysts du 5^{e} jour de la gestation chez la ratte; etude microcinematographique. *C. R. Acad. Sci. Paris Ser. D*, 270:2979–2982.
364. Lejeune, B., Van Hoeck, J., and Leroy, F. (1981): Transmitter role of the luminal uterine epithelium in the induction of decidualization in rats. *J. Reprod. Fertil.*, 61:235–240.
365. Boving, B. G. (1959): Implantation. *Ann. N.Y. Acad. Sci.*, 75:700–725.
366. Boving, B. G. (1963): Implantation mechanisms. In: *Mechanisms Concerned with Conception*, edited by C. G. Hartman, pp. 321–396. Pergamon Press, New York.
367. Hetherington, C. M. (1968): Induction of deciduomata in the mouse by carbon dioxide. *Nature*, 219:863–864.
368. Huff, R. L., and Eik-Nes, K. B. (1966): Metabolism *in vitro* of acetate and certain steroids by six-day-old rabbit blastocysts. *J. Reprod. Fertil*, 11:57–63.
369. Dickmann, Z., and Dey, S. K. (1973): Two theories: The preimplantation embryo is a source of steroid hormones controlling (1) morula-blastocyst transformation, and (2) implantation. *J. Reprod. Fertil.*, 35:615–617.
370. Heap, R. B., Flint, A. P. F., and Gadsby, J. E. (1981): Embryonic signals and maternal recognition. In: *Cellular and Molecular Aspects of Implantation*, edited by S. R. Glasser and D. W. Bullock, pp. 311–325. Plenum Press, New York.
371. Sauer, M. J. (1979): Hormone involvement in the establishment of pregnancy. *J. Reprod. Fertil.*, 56:725–743.
372. Perry, J. S., Heap, R. B., and Amoroso, E. C. (1973): Steroid hormone production by pig blastocysts. *Nature*, 245:45–47.
373. Perry, J. S., Heap, R. B., Burton, R. D., and Gadsby, J. E. (1976): Endocrinology of the blastocyst and its role in the establishment of pregnancy. *J. Reprod. Fertil. (Suppl.)*, 25:85–104.
374. Gadsby, J. E., Heap, R. B., and Burton, R. D. (1980): Oestrogen production by blastocyst and early embryonic tissue of various species. *J. Reprod. Fertil.*, 60:409–417.
375. Gadsby, J. E., Burton, R. D., Heap, R. B., and Perry, J. S. (1976): Steroid metabolism and synthesis in early embryonic tissue of pig, sheep, and cow. *J. Endocrinol.*, 71:45P–46P.
376. Fischer, H. E., Bazer, F. W., and Fields, M. J. (1985): Steroid metabolism by endometrial and conceptus tissues during early pregnancy and pseudopregnancy in gilts. *J. Reprod. Fertil.*, 75:69–78.
377. Flood, D. F. (1974): Steroid-metabolizing enzymes in the early pig conceptus and in the related endometrium. *J. Endocrinol.*, 63:413–414.
378. Heap, R. B., Flint, A. P. F., Hartmann, P. E., Gadsby, J. E., Staples, L. D., Ackland, N., and Hamon, M. (1981): Oestrogen production in early pregnancy. *J. Endocrinol.*, 89:77p–94p.
379. Dhindsa, D. S., and Dziuk, P. J. (1968): Effect of pregnancy in the pig after killing embryos or fetuses in one uterine horn in early gestation. *J. Anim. Sci.*, 27:122–126.
380. Bazer, F. W., and Thatcher, W. W. (1977): Theory of maternal recognition of pregnancy in swine based on estrogen controlled endocrine versus exocrine secretion of prostaglandin F_{2a} by uterine endometrium. *Prostaglandins*, 14:397–401.
381. Frank, M., Bazer, F. W., Thatcher, W. W., and Wilcox, C. J. (1977): A study of prostaglandin F_2 as the leuteolysin in swine. III. Effects of estradiol valerate on prostaglandin F, progestins, estrone, and estradiol concentrations in the utero-ovarian vein of nonpregnant gilts. *Prostaglandins*, 14:1183–1196.
382. Moeljono, M. P. E., Thatcher, W. W., Bazer, F. W., Frank, M., Owens, L. J., and Wilcox, C. J. (1977): A study of prostaglandin F_{2a} as the leuteolysin in swine. II. Characterization and comparison of prostaglandin F, estrogens and progestin concentrations in utero-ovarian vein plasma of nonpregnant and pregnant gilts. *Prostaglandins*, 14:543–555.
383. Zavy, M. T., Bazer, F. W., Thatcher, W. W., and Wilcox, C. J. (1980): A study of prostaglandin F_{2-a} as the leuteolysin in swine. V. Comparison of prostaglandin F, progestins, estrone and estradiol in uterine flushings from pregnant and nonpregnant gilts. *Prostaglandins*, 20:837–851.
384. Heap, R. B., Perry, J. S., Gadsby, J. E., and Burton, K. D. (1975): Endocrine activities of the blastocyst and early embryonic tissue in the pig. *Biochem. Soc. Trans.*, 3:1183–1188.
385. Mondschein, J. S., Hersey, R. M., Dey, S. K., Davis, D. L., and Weisz, J. (1985): Catechol estrogen formation by pig blastocyst during the preimplantation period: Biochemical characterization of estrogen-2/4-dioxylase and correlation with asromatase activity. *Endocrinology*, 117:2339–2346.
386. Hoversland, R. C., Dey, S. K., and Johnson, D. C. (1982): Catechol estradiol induced implantation in the mouse. *Life Sci.*, 30:1801–1804.
387. Pakrasi, P. L., and Dey, S. K. (1983): Catechol estrogens stimulate synthesis of prostaglandin in the preimplantation rabbit blastocyst and endometrium. *Biol. Reprod.*, 29:347–354.
388. Stone, B. A., and Seamark, R. F. (1985): Steroid hormones in uterine washings and in plasma of gilts between days 9 and 15 after oestrus and between days 9 and 15 after coitus. *J. Reprod. Fertil.*, 75:209–221.
389. Dickmann, Z., Dey, S. K., and Sengupta, J. (1975): Steroidogenesis in rabbit preimplantation embryos. *Proc. Natl. Acad. Sci. USA*, 72:298–300.
390. Dickmann, Z., Dey, S. K., and Sen Gupta, J. (1976): A new concept: Control of early pregnancy by steroid hormones originating in the preimplantation embryo. *Vitam. Horm.*, 34:215–242.
391. Bleau, G. (1981): Failure to detect Δ^5-3β-hydroxysteroid oxidoreductase activity in the preimplantation rabbit embryo. *Steroids*, 37:121–132.
392. Seamark, R. F., and Lutwak-Mann, C. (1972): Progestins in rabbit blastocysts. *J. Reprod. Fertil.*, 29:147–148.
393. Fuchs, A. R., and Beling, C. (1974): Evidence for early ovarian recognition of blastocysts in rabbits. *Endocrinology*, 95:1054–1058.
394. Borland, R. M., Erickson, G. F., and Ducibella, T. (1977): Accumulation of steroids in rabbit preimplantation blastocysts. *J. Reprod. Fertil.*, 49:219–224.
395. Singh, M. M., and Booth, W. D. (1978): Studies on the metabolism of neutral steroids by preimplantation rabbit blastocysts *in vitro* and the origin of blastocyst oestrogen. *J. Reprod. Fertil.*, 53:297–304.
396. Fujimoto, S., and Sundaram, K. (1978): The source of progesterone in rabbit blastocysts. *J. Reprod. Fertil.*, 52:231–233.
397. Bullock, D. W. (1977): Steroids from the pre-implantation blastocyst. In: *Development in Mammals, Vol. 2*, edited by M. H. Johnson, pp. 199–208. North-Holland, New York.
398. George, F. W., and Wilson, J. D. (1978): Estrogen formation in the early rabbit embryo. *Science*, 199:200–201.
399. Hoversland, R. C., Dey, S. K., and Johnson, D. C. (1982): Aromatase activity in the rabbit blastocyst. *J. Reprod. Fertil.*, 66:259–263.
400. Wu, J-T., and Lin, G. M. (1982): Effect of aromatase inhibitor on oestrogen production in rabbit blastocysts. *J. Reprod. Fertil.*, 66:655–662.
401. Bhatt, B. M., and Bullock, D. W. (1974): Binding of oestradiol to rabbit blastocysts and its possible role in implantation. *J. Reprod. Fertil.*, 39:65–70.
402. Dey, S. K., Dickmann, Z., and Sen Gupta, J. (1976): Evidence that the maintenance of early pregnancy in the rabbit requires "blastocyst estrogen." *Steroids*, 28:481–485.
403. Sengupta, J., Roy, S. K., and Manchanda, S. K. (1979): Hormonal control of implantation: A possible role of lysosomal function in the embryo-uterus interaction. *J. Steroid Biochem.*, 11:729–744.
404. Wise, T., and Heap, R. B. (1983): Effects of the embryo upon endometrial estrogen synthesis in the rabbit. *Biol. Reprod.*, 28:1097–1106.
405. Dey, S. K., and Dickmann, Z. (1974): Estradiol-17β-hydroxysteroid dehydrogenase activity in preimplantation rat embryos. *Steroids*, 24:57–62.
406. Dey, S. K., and Dickmann, Z. (1974): Δ^5-3β-Hydroxysteroid dehydrogenase activity in rat embryos on days 1 through 7 of pregnancy. *Endocrinology*, 95:321–322.

407. Dickmann, Z., and Dey, S.K. (1974): Steroidogenesis in the preimplantation rat embryo and its possible influence on morula-blastocyst transformation and implantation. *J. Reprod. Fertil.*, 37:91–93.
408. Dickmann, Z., and Dey, S. K. (1974): Evidence that Δ^5-3β-Hydroxysteroid dehydrogenase activity in rat blastocysts is autonomous. *J. Endocrinol.*, 61:513–514.
409. Dickmann, Z., and Sengupta, J. (1974): Δ^5-3β-Hydroxysteroid dehydrogenase activity in preimplantation hamster embryos. *Dev. Biol.*, 40:196–198.
410. Dickmann, Z., Sengupta, J., and Dey, S. S. (1977): Does 'blastocyst estrogen' initiate implantation? *Science*, 195:687–688.
411. Sengupta, J., Dey, S. K., and Dickmann, Z. (1977): Is mouse preimplantation embryogenesis controlled by estrogen originating in the preimplantation embryo? *Anat. Rec.*, 187:709 (abstract).
412. Sengupta, J., Roy, S. K., and Manchanda, S. K. (1981): Effect of an anti-oestrogen on implantation of mouse blastocysts. *J. Reprod. Fertil.*, 62:433–436.
413. Chew, N. J., and Sherman, M. I. (1975): Biochemistry of differentiation of mouse trophoblast: Δ^5,3β-Hydroxysteroid dehydrogenase. *Biol. Reprod.*, 12:351–359.
414. Sherman, M. I., and Atienza, S. B. (1977): Production and metabolism of progesterone and androstenedione by cultured mouse blastocysts. *Biol. Reprod.*, 16:190–199.
415. Marcal, J. M., Chew, N. J., Salomon, D. S., and Sherman, M. I. (1975): Δ^5,β-Hydroxysteroid dehydrogenase activities in rat trophoblast and ovary during pregnancy. *Endocrinology*, 96:1270–1279.
416. Antila, E., Koskinen, J., Niemela, P., and Saure, A. (1977): Steroid metabolism by mouse preimplantation embryos *in vitro*. *Experientia*, 33:1374–1375.
417. Niimura, S., and Ishida, K. (1976): Histochemical studies of Δ^5-3β-, 20α- and 20β-hydroxysteroid dehydrogenases and possible progestagen production in hamster eggs. *J. Reprod. Fertil.*, 48:275–278.
418. Brodie, A. M. H., Wu, J. T., Marsh, D. A., and Brodie, H. J. (1978): Aromatase inhibitors. III. Studies on the antifertility effect of 4-acetoxy-4-androstene-3,17-dione. *Biol. Reprod.*, 18:365–370.
419. Evans, C. A., and Kennedy, T. G. (1980): Blastocyst implantation in ovariectomized, adrenalectomized hamsters treated with inhibitors of steroidogenesis during the pre-implantation period. *Steroids*, 36:41–52.
420. Zavy, M. T., Mayer, R., Vernon, M. W., Bazer, F. W., and Sharp, D. C. (1979): An investigation of the uterine lumenal environment of non-pregnant and pregnant pony mares. *J. Reprod. Fertil.*, (*Suppl.*), 27:403–411.
421. Dey, S. K., Johnson, D. C., and Santos, J. G. (1979): Is histamine production by the blastocyst required for implantation in the rabbit? *Biol. Reprod.*, 21:1169–1173.
422. Dey, S. K., and Johnson, D. C. (1980): Histamine formation by mouse preimplantation embryos. *J. Reprod. Fertil.*, 60:457–460.
423. Dey, S. K. (1981): Role of histamine in implantation: Inhibition of histidine decarboxylase induces delayed implantation in the rabbit. *Biol. Reprod.*, 24:867–869.
424. Johnson, D. C., and Dey, S. K. (1980): Role of histamine in implantation: Dexamethasone inhibits estradiol-induced implantation in the rat. *Biol. Reprod.*, 22:1136–1141.
425. Racowsky, C., and Biggers, J. D. (1983): Are blastocyst prostaglandins produced endogenously? *Biol. Reprod.*, 29:379–388.
426. Dickmann, Z., and Spilman, C. H. (1975): Prostaglandins in rabbit blastocysts. *Science*, 190:997–998.
427. Dey, S. K., Chien, S. M., Cox, C. L., and Crist, R. D. (1980): Prostaglandin synthesis in the rabbit blastocyst. *Prostaglandins*, 19:449–453.
428. Harper, M. J., Norris, C. J., and Rajkumar, K. (1983): Prostaglandin release by zygotes and endometria of pregnant rabbits. *Biol. Reprod.*, 28:350–362.
429. Pakrasi, P. L., and Dey, S. K. (1982): Blastocyst is the source of prostaglandins in the implantation site in the rabbit. *Prostaglandins*, 24:73–77.
430. Shemesh, M., Milaguir, F., Ayalon, N., and Hansel, W. (1979): Steroidogenesis and prostaglandin synthesis by cultured bovine blastocysts. *J. Reprod. Fertil.*, 56:181–185.
431. Lewis, G. S., Thatcher, W. W., Bazer, F. W., and Curl, J. S. (1982): Metabolism of arachidonic acid *in vitro* by bovine blastocysts and endometrium. *Biol. Reprod.*, 27:431–439.
432. Biggers, J. D., Leonov, B. V., Baskar, J. F., and Fried, J. (1978): Inhibition of hatching of mouse blastocysts *in vitro* by prostaglandin antagonists. *Biol. Reprod.*, 19:519–533.
433. Baskar, J. F., Torchiana, D. F., Biggers, J. D., Corey, E. J., Andersen, N. H., and Subramanian, N. (1981): Inhibition of hatching of mouse blastocysts *in vitro* by various prostaglandin antagonists. *J. Reprod. Fertil.*, 63:359–363.
434. Hurst, P. R., and MacFarlane, D. W. (1981): Further effects of nonsteroidal anti-inflammatory compounds on blastocyst hatching *in vitro* and implantation rates in the mouse. *Biol. Reprod.*, 25:777–784.
435. Biggers, J. D., Baskar, J. F., and Torchiana, D. F. (1981): Reduction of fertility of mice by the intrauterine injection of prostaglandin antagonists. *J. Reprod. Fertil.*, 63:365–372.
436. Marcus, G. J. (1981): Prostaglandin formation by the sheep embryo and endometrium as indication of maternal recognition of pregnancy. *Biol. Reprod.*, 25:56–64.
437. Hyland, J. H., Manns, J. G., and Humphrey, W. D. (1982): Prostaglandin production by ovine embryos and endometrium *in vitro*. *J. Reprod. Fertil.*, 65:299–304.
438. Lacroix, M. C., and Kann, G. (1982): Comparative studies of prostaglandins F_{2a} and E_2 in late cyclic and early pregnant sheep: *in vitro* synthesis by endometrium and conceptuses. Effects of *in vivo* indomethacin treatment on establishment of pregnancy. *Prostaglandins*, 23:507–526.
439. Moor, R. M., and Rowson, L. E. A. (1964): Influence of the embryo and uterus on luteal function in the sheep. *Nature* 201:522–523.
440. Moor, R. M., and Rowson, L. E. A. (1966): The corpus luteum of the sheep: Functional relationship between the embryo and the corpus luteum. *J. Endocrinol.*, 34:233–239.
441. Moor, R. M., and Rowson, L. E. A. (1966): The corpus luteum of the sheep: Effect of the removal of embryos on luteal function. *J. Endocrinol.*, 34:497–502.
442. Rowson, L. E. A., and Moor, R. M. (1967): The influence of embryonic tissue homogenate infused into the uterus, on the life span of the corpus luteum in the sheep. *J. Reprod. Fertil.*, 13:511–516.
443. Martal, J., Lacroix, M.-C., Loudes, C., Saunier, M., and Winterberger-Torres, S. (1979): Trophoblastin, an antiluteolytic protein present in early pregnancy in sheep. *J. Reprod. Fertil.*, 56:63–73.
444. Heyman, Y., Camous, S., Fevre, J., Meziou, W., and Martal, J. (1984): Maintenance of the corpus luteum after uterine transfer of trophoblastic vesicles to cyclic cows and ewes. *J. Reprod. Fertil.*, 70:533–540.
445. Godkin, J. D., Bazer, F. W., Moffatt, J., Sessions, F., and Roberts, R. M. (1982): Purification and properties of a major, low molecular weight protein released by the trophoblast of sheep blastocysts at day 13–21. *J. Reprod. Fertil.*, 65:141–150.
446. Godkin, J. D., Bazer, F. W., and Roberts, R. M. (1984): Ovine trophoblast protein 1, an early secreted blastocyst protein, binds specifically to uterine endometrium and affects protein synthesis. *Endocrinology*, 114:120–130.
447. Hansen, P. J., Anthony, R. V., Bazer, F. W., Baumbach, G. A., and Roberts, R. M. (1985): *In vitro* synthesis and secretion of ovine trophoblastic protein-1 during the period of maternal recognition of pregnancy. *Endocrinology*, 117:1424–1430.
448. Godkin, J. D., Bazer, F. W., Thatcher, W. W., and Roberts, R. M. (1984): Proteins released by cultured day 15–16 conceptuses prolong luteal maintenance when introduced into the uterine lumen of cyclic ewes. *J. Reprod. Fertil.*, 71:57–64.
449. Godkin, J. D., Cote, C., and Duby, R. T. (1978): Embryonic stimulation of ovine and bovine corpora lutea. *J. Reprod. Fertil.*, 54:375–378.
450. Ellinwood, W. E., Nett, T. M., and Niswender, G. D. (1979): Maintenance of the corpus luteum of early pregnancy in the ewe. I. Luteotropic properties of embryonic homogenates. *Biol. Reprod.*, 21:281–288.
451. Masters, R. A., Roberts, R. M., Lewis, G. S., Thatcher, W. W., Bazer, F. W., and Godkin, J. D. (1982): High molecular weight glycoproteins released by expanding, pre-attachment sheep, pig and cow blastocysts in culture. *J. Reprod. Fertil.*, 66:571–583.
452. Betteridge, K. J., Eaglesome, M. D., Randall, G. C. B., Mitchell, D., and Sugden, E. A. (1978): Maternal progesterone levels as evidence of luteotrophic or antiluteolytic effects of embryos transferred to heifers 12–17 days after estrus. *Theriogenology*, 9:86.

453. Sreeran, J. M. (1978): Non-surgical embryo transfer in the cow. *Theriogenology,* 9:69–83.
454. Northey, D. L., and French, L. R. (1980): Effect of embryo removal and intrauterine infusion of embryonic homogenates on the lifespan of the bovine corpus luteum. *J. Anim. Sci.,* 50:298–302.
455. Bartol, F. F., Roberts, R. M., Bazer, F. W., Lewis, G. S., Godkin, J. D., and Thatcher, W. W. (1984): Characterization of proteins produced *in vitro* by periattachment bovine conceptus. *Biol. Reprod.,* 32:681–693.
456. Bazer, F. W., Geisert, R. E., Thatcher, W. W., and Roberts, R. M. (1982): The establishment and maintenance of pregnancy. In: *Control of Pig Reproduction,* edited by J. A. Cole and G. R. Foxcroft, pp. 227–252. Butterworths, London.
457. Wyatt, C. (1976): Endometrial components involved in protein synthesis by 16-day pig blastocyst tissue in culture. *J. Physiol. (Lond.),* 260:73P–74P.
458. Saunders, P. T. K., Ziecik, A. J., and Flint, A. P. F. (1980): Gonadotrophin-like substance in pig placenta and embryonic membranes. *J. Endocrinol.,* 85:25P.
459. Rice, C., Ackland, N., and Heap, R. B. (1981): Blastocyst-endometrial interaction and protein synthesis during preimplantation development in the pig studied *in vitro. Placenta,* 2:129–142.
460. Godkin, J. D., Bazer, F. W., Lewis, G. S., Geisert, R. D., and Roberts, R. M. (1982): Synthesis and release of polypeptides by pig conceptuses during the period of blastocyst elongation and attachment. *Biol. Reprod.,* 27:977–987.
461. Fishel, S. B., and Surani, M. A. H. (1980): Evidence for the synthesis and release of a glycoprotein by mouse blastocysts. *J. Reprod. Fertil.,* 59:181–185.
462. Nieder, G. L., Weitlauf, H. M., and Hartman, M. (1986): Synthesis and secretion of stage specific proteins by peri-implantation mouse embryos. *Biol. Reprod.* 36:687–699.
463. Morton, H., Hegh, V., and Clunie, G. J. A. (1974): Immunosuppression detected in pregnant mice by rosette inhibition test. *Nature,* 249:459–460.
464. Morton, H., Hegh, V., and Clunie, G. J. A. (1976): Studies of the rosette inhibition test in pregnant mice: Evidence of immunosuppression? *Proc. R. Soc. Lond. (Biol.)* 193:413–419.
465. Morton, H., Rolfe, B., Clunie, G. J. A., Anderson, M. J., and Morrison, J. (1977): An early pregnancy factor detected in human serum by the rosette inhibition test. *Lancet,* i:394–397.
466. Nancarrow, C. D., Evison, B. M., Scaramuzzi, R. J., and Turnbull, K. E. (1979): Detection of induced death of embryos in sheep by the rosette inhibition test. *J. Reprod. Fertil.,* 57:385–389.
467. Noonan, F. P., Halliday, W. J., Morton, H., and Clunie, G. J. A. (1979): Early pregnancy factor is immunosuppressive. *Nature,* 278:649–650.
468. Clarke, F. M., Morton, H., and Clunie, G. J. A. (1978): Detection and separation of two serum factors responsible for depression of lymphocyte activity in pregnancy. *Clin. Exp. Immunol.,* 32:318–323.
469. Clarke, F. M., Morton, H., Rolfe, B. E., and Clunie, G. J. A. (1980): Partial characterization of early pregnancy factor in the sheep. *J. Reprod. Immunol.,* 2:151–162.
470. Wilson, S., McCarthy, R., and Clarke, F. (1983): In search of early pregnancy factor: Isolation of active polypeptides from pregnant ewe's sera. *J. Reprod. Immunol.,* 5:275–286.
471. Clarke, F. M., and Wilson, S. (1982): Biochemistry of early pregnancy factor. In: *Pregnancy Proteins,* edited by J. G. Grudzinskas, B. Teisner, and M. Seppala, pp. 407–412. Academic Press, New York.
472. Morton, H., Rolfe, B., and Cavanagh, A. (1982): Early pregnancy factor: Biology and clinical significance. In: *Pregnancy Proteins,* edited by J. G. Grudzinskas, B. Teisner, and M. Seppala, pp. 391–405. Academic Press, New York.
473. Morton, H., Rolfe, B. E., McNeill, L., Clarke, P., Clarke, F. M., and Clunie, G. J. A. (1980): Early pregnancy factor: Tissues involved in its production in the mouse. *J. Reprod. Immunol.,* 2: 73–82.
474. Cavanagh, A. C., Morton, H., Rolfe, B. E., and Gidley-Baird, A. (1982): Ovum factor: A first signal of pregnancy? *Am. J. Reprod. Immunol.,* 2:97–101.
475. Nancarrow, C. D., Wallace, A. L. C., and Grewal, A. S. (1981): The early pregnancy factor of sheep and cattle. *J. Reprod. Fertil. (Suppl.),* 30:191–199.
476. Cavanagh, A. C. (1984): Production *in vitro* of mouse early pregnancy factor and purification to homogeneity. *J. Reprod. Fertil.,* 71:581–592.
477. Morton, H., and Clunie, G. J. A. (1979): A test for early pregnancy in sheep. *Res. Vet. Sci.,* 26:261–262.
478. Morton, H., Nancarrow, C. D., Scaramuzzi, R. J., Evison, B. M., and Clunie, G. J. A. (1979): Detection of early pregnancy factor in sheep by rosette inhibition test. *J. Reprod. Fertil.,* 56:75–80.
479. Morton, H., Tinnenberg, H. R., Rolfe, B., Wolf, M., and Mettler, L. (1982): Rosette inhibition test: A multicentre investigation of early pregnancy factor in humans. *J. Reprod. Immunol.,* 4:251–261.
480. Smart, Y. C., Roberts, T. K., Clancy, R. L., and Cripps, A. W. (1981): Early pregnancy factor: Its role in mammalian reproduction research review. *Fertil. Steril.,* 35:397–402.
481. Koh, L. Y., and Jones, W. R. (1982): The rosette inhibition test in early pregnancy diagnosis. *Clin. Reprod. Fertil.,* 1:229–233.
482. Tinnenberg, H. R., Staves, R. P., and Semm, K. (1984): Improvement of the rosette inhibition assay for the detection of early pregnancy factor in humans using the monoclonal antibody, anti-human-lyt-3. *Am. J. Reprod. Immunol.,* 5:151–156.
483. Rolfe, B. E., Morton, H., Cavanagh, A. C., and Gardiner, R. A. (1983): Detection of an early pregnancy factor-like substance in sera of patients with testicular germ cell tumors. *Am. J. Reprod. Immunol.,* 3:97–100.
484. Koch, E., Morton, H., and Ellendorff, F. (1983): Early pregnancy factor: Biology and practical application. *Br. Vet. J.,* 139: 52–58.
485. Morton, H., Morton, D. J., and Ellendorff, F. (1983): The appearance and characteristics of early pregnancy factor in the pig. *J. Reprod. Fertil.,* 69:437–446.
486. Cooper, D. W., and Aitken, R. J. (1981): Failure to detect altered rosette inhibition titres in human pregnancy serum. *J. Reprod. Fertil.,* 61:241–245.
487. Whyte, A., and Heap, R. B. (1983): Early pregnancy factor. *Nature,* 304:121–122.
488. Smart, Y. C., Fraser, I. S., Clancy, R. L., Roberts, T. K., and Crippis, A. W. (1982): Early pregnancy factor as a monitor for fertilization in women wearing intrauterine devices. *Fertil. Steril.,* 37:201–204.
489. Smart, Y. C., Roberts, T. K., Fraser, I. S., Cripps, A. W., and Clancy, R. L. (1982): Validation of rosette inhibition test for detection of early pregnancy in women. *Fertil. Steril.,* 37:779–785.
490. Shaw, F. D., and Morton, H. (1980): The immunological approach to pregnancy diagnosis: A review. *Vet. Rec.,* 106:268–270.
491. Rolfe, B., Cavanagh, A., Forde, C., Bastin, C. C., and Morton, H. (1984): Modified rosette inhibition test with mouse lymphocytes for detection of early pregnancy factor in human pregnancy serum. *J. Immunol. Methods,* 70:1–11.
492. Rolfe, B. E., Morton, H., and Clarke, F. M. (1983): Early pregnancy factor is an immuno-suppressive contaminant of commercial preparations of human chorionic gonadotrophin. *Clin. Exp. Immunol.,* 51:45–52.
493. Rolfe, B. E. (1982): Detection of fetal wastage. *Fertil. Steril.,* 37:655–660.
494. Kent, H. A. Jr. (1973): A polypeptide from oviductal contents which influences ovarian function. *Biol. Reprod.,* 8:38–42.
495. Kent, H. A. Jr. (1975): Contraceptive polypeptide from hamster embryos: Sequence of amino acids in the compound. *Biol. Reprod.,* 12:504–507.
496. Kent, H. A. Jr. (1975): The two to four-cell embryos as source tissue of the tetrapeptide preventing ovulations in the hamster. *Am. J. Anat.,* 144:509–512.
497. Van Niekerk, C. H., and Gerneke, W. H. (1966): Persistence and pathologic cleavage of tubal ova in the mare. *Ondesstepoort J. Vet. Res.,* 31:195–232.
498. Betteridge, K. J., and Mitchell, D. (1972): Retention of ova by the fallopian tube in mares. *J. Reprod. Fertil.,* 31:515.
499. Nieder, G. L., and Corder, C. (1983): Pyruvate and lactate levels in oviducts of cycling, pregnant, and pseudopregnant mice. *Biol. Reprod.,* 28:566–574.
500. O'Neill, C. (1985): Thrombocytopenia is an initial maternal response to fertilization in mice. *J. Reprod. Fertil.,* 73:559–566.

501. Renfree, M. B., and Calaby, J. H. (1981): Background to delayed implantation and embryonic diapause. *J. Reprod. Fertil. (Suppl.)*, 29:1–9.
502. Aitken, R. J. (1977): Embryonic diapause. In: *Development in Mammals, Vol. 1*, edited by M. H. Johnson, pp. 307–359. North-Holland, New York.
503. McLaren, A. (1973): Blastocyst activation. In: *The Regulation of Mammalian Reproduction,* edited by S. J. Segal, R. Crozier, P. A. Corfman, and P. G. Condliffe, pp. 321–328. Charles C Thomas, Springfield, Ill.
504. Brambell, F. W. R. (1937): The influence of lactation on implantation of the mammalian embryo. *Am. J. Obstet. Gynecol.*, 33:942–953.
505. Weitlauf, H. M. (1973): *In vitro* uptake and incorporation of amino acids by blastocysts from intact and ovariectomized mice. *J. Exp. Zool.*, 183:303–308.
506. Weitlauf, H. M. (1974): Effect of actinomycin D on protein synthesis by delayed implanting mouse embryos *in vitro. J. Exp. Zool.*, 189:197–202.
507. Weitlauf, H. M. (1976): Effect of uterine flushings on RNA synthesis by 'implanting' and 'delayed implanting' mouse embryos *in vitro. Biol. Reprod.*, 14:566–571.
508. Weitlauf, H. M. (1978): Factors in mouse uterine fluid that inhibit the incorporation of [3H] uridine by blastocysts *in vitro. J. Reprod. Fertil.*, 52:321–325.
509. Weitlauf, H. M. (1982); A comparison of the rates of accumulation of nonpolyadenylated and polyadenylated RNA in normal and delayed implanting mouse embryos. *Dev. Biol.*, 93:266–271.
510. Weitlauf, H. M. (1985): Changes in the rate of translation with reactivation of delayed implanting mouse embryos. *J. Exp. Zool.*, 236:309–312.
511. Given, R. L., and Weitlauf, H. M. (1982): Resumption of DNA synthesis in delayed implanting mouse blastocysts during activation *in vitro. J. Exp. Zool.*, 224:111–114.
512. Nieder, G. L., and Weitlauf, H. M. (1984): Regulation of glycolysis in the mouse blastocyst during delayed implantation. *J. Exp. Zool.*, 231:121–129.
513. Nieder, G. L., and Weitlauf, H. M. (1985): Effects of metabolic substrates and ionic environment on *in-vitro* activation of delayed implanting mouse blastocysts. *J. Reprod. Fertil.*, 73:151–157.
514. Torbit, C. A., and Weitlauf, H. M. (1975): Production of carbon dioxide *in vitro* by blastocysts from intact and ovariectomized mice. *J. Reprod. Fertil.*, 42:45–50.
515. Weitlauf, H. M., and Kiessling, A. A. (1980): Comparison of overall rates of RNA synthesis in implanting and delayed implanting mouse blastocysts *in vitro. Dev. Biol.*, 77:116–129.
516. Weitlauf, H. M., and Kiessling, A. A. (1981): Activation of 'delayed implanting' mouse embryos *in vitro. J. Reprod. Fertil., (Suppl.)*, 29:191–202.
517. Psychoyos, A., and Bitton-Casimiri, V. (1969): Captation *in vitro* d'un priecurseur d'acide ribonucleique (ARN)-(uridine 5-^{3}H) par le bastocyste de rat: Differences entre blastocysts normaux et blastocysts en diapause. *C. R. Soc. Biol. (Paris)*, 268:188–190.
518. Psychoyos, A., Bitton-Casimiri, V., and Brun, J. L. (1975) Repression and activation of the mammalian blastocyst. In: *Regulation and Differentiated Function in Eukaryote Cells,* edited by G. P. Talwar, pp. 509–514. Raven Press, New York.
519. Mintz, B. (1964): Formation of genetically mosaic mouse embryos and early development of "lethal (t^{12}/t^{12})-normal" mosaics. *J. Exp. Zool.*, 157:273–292.
520. Cole, R. J., and Paul, J. (1965): Properties of cultured preimplantation mouse and rabbit embryos and cell strains derived from them. In: *Preimplantation Stages of Pregnancy,* CIBA Foundation Symposium, pp. 82–111. Little, Brown, Boston.
521. Gwatkin, R. B. L. (1966): Defined media and development of mammalian eggs *in vitro. Ann. N.Y. Acad. Sci.*, 139:79–90.
522. Gwatkin, R. B. L. (1966): Amino acid requirements for attachment and outgrowth of the mouse blastocyst *in vitro. J. Cell Physiol.*, 68:335–344.
523. Naeslund, G. (1979): The effect of glucose-, arginine-, and leucine-deprivation on blastocyst outgrowth *in vitro. Upsala J. Med. Sci.*, 84:9–20.
524. Naeslund, G., Lundkvist, O., and Nilsson, B. O. (1980): Transmission electron microscopy of mouse blastocysts activated and growth arrested *in vivo* and *in vitro. Anat. Embryol.*, 159:33–48.
525. Wordinger, R. J., and Brinster, R.L. (1976): Influence of reduced glucose levels on the *in vitro* hatching, attachment and trophoblast outgrowth of the mouse blastocyst. *Dev. Biol.*, 53:294–296.
526. Van Blerkom, J., Chavez, D. J., and Bell, H. (1979): Molecular and cellular aspects of facultative delayed implantation in the mouse. In: *Maternal Recognition of Pregnancy,* CIBA Foundation Symposium No. 64 (new series), pp. 141–172. Excerpta Medica, New York.
527. Aitken, R. J. (1974): Delayed implantation in roe deer (*Capreolus Capreolus*). *J. Reprod. Fertil.*, 39:225–233.
528. Aitken, R. J. (1974): Calcium and zinc in the endometrium and uterine flushings of the roe deer (*Carreolus Carreolus*) during delayed implantation. *J. Reprod. Fertil.*, 40:333–340.
529. Van Winkle, L. J. (1977): Low Na^+ concentration: A factor contributing to diminished uptake and incorporation of amino acids by diapausing mouse blastocysts? *J. Exp. Zool.*, 202:275–281.
530. Van Winkle, L. J. (1981): Activation of amino acid accumulation in delayed implantation mouse blastocysts. *J. Exp. Zool.*, 218:239–246.
531. Van Winkle, L. J., Campione, A. L., and Webster, D. I. (1983): Sodium ion concentrations in uterine flushings from "implanting" and "delayed implanting" mice. *J. Exp. Zool.*, 226:321–324.
532. Surani, M. A. H. (1977): Cellular and molecular approaches to blastocyst uterine interactions at implantation. In: *Development in Mammals, Vol. 1,* edited by M. H. Johnson, pp. 245–305. North-Holland, New York.
533. Gwatkin, R. B. L. (1969): Nutritional requirements for post-blastocyst development in the mouse. *Int. J. Fertil.*, 14:101–105.
534. Nilsson, B. O., Magnusson, C., Widehn, S., and Hillensjo, T. (1982): Correlation between blastocyst oxygen consumption and trophoblast cytochrome oxidase reaction at initiation of implantation of delayed mouse blastocysts. *J. Embryol. Exp. Morphol.*, 71:75–82.
535. Menke, T. M., and McLaren, A. (1970): Carbon dioxide production by mouse blastocysts during lactational delay of implantation or after ovariectomy. *J. Endocrinol.*, 47:287–294.
536. Aitken, R. J. (1977): The culture of mouse blastocysts in the presence of uterine flushings collected during normal pregnancy, delayed implantation, and pro-oestrus. *J. Embryol. Exp. Morphol.*, 41:295–300.
537. O'Neill, C., and Quinn, P. (1981): Interaction of uterine flushings with mouse blastocysts *in vitro* as assessed by the incorporation of [^{3}H] uridine. *J. Reprod. Fertil.*, 62:257–262.
538. O'Neill, C., and Quinn, P. (1983): Inhibitory influence of uterine secretions on mouse blastocysts decreases at the time of blastocyst activation. *J. Reprod. Fertil.*, 68:269–274.
539. Psychoyos, A., and Casimiri, V. (1981): Uterine blastotoxic factors. In: *Cellular and Molecular Aspects of Implantation,* edited by S. R. Glasser and D. W. Bullock, pp. 327–334. Plenum Press, New York.

THE REPRODUCTIVE SYSTEMS

The Female

The Physiology of Reproduction
edited by E. Knobil and J. Neill *et al.*
Raven Press, Ltd., New York © 1988.

CHAPTER 8

Embryology of Mammalian Gonads and Ducts

Anne Grete Byskov and Poul Erik Høyer

Gonadal formation in mammals takes place early in fetal life. Although the genetic sex is determined at conception, sexual differences between fetuses can first be recognized at the time when the gonads become sex differentiated. The gonads evolve when germ cells and different somatic cells migrate and settle in the gonadal ridges to interact in a finely regulated manner. The following differentiation of the embryonic gonads into an ovary or a testis is crucial for priming the fetus in the female or male direction. Inadequate sexual differentiation of the gonad may alter production of sex hormones and other substances necessary for growth and differentiation of the sex ducts, external genitalia, and other secondary sex characteristics, as well as sex priming of the brain.

EARLY GONADAL FORMATION

The gonads develop along the ventral cranial part of the mesonephros. Two simultaneously occurring events characterize the initial gonadal formation: (a) migration of primordial germ cells (PGC) into the coelomic epithelium and the underlying mesenchymal tissue covering the mesonephros and (b) release and migration of mesonephric cells into the same area.

Primordial Germ Cells

For decades it was believed that the PGC originated in the so-called germinal epithelium, i.e., the coelomic epithelium lining the gonad. However, as early as 1880, Nussbaum (1) proposed an extragonadal origin of the PGC in frog and trout. Subsequently, PGC have also been identified in extragonadal sites in many mammalian species [rat (2,3), mouse (4–6), human (7,8), rabbit (9)].

The migratory pathway and, in particular, the precise origin of the PGC are difficult to establish since they are not easy to distinguish from surrounding cells. Different experiments using cultures of mouse embryonic fragments indicate that the stem cells of the PGC reside in the epiblast of the inner cell mass of the blastocyst (10,11). Studies of X-chromosome inactivation during mouse embryogenesis suggest that somatic cell lines are allocated prior to the germ cell line (12). However, labeling of four- to 16-cell mouse embryos with retroviruses and analyzing the distribution of proviruses in the different tissues developing from such embryos suggest that a germ cell line is set aside very early, maybe in the four- to eight-cell stage, and before allocation of somatic tissues (13).

The sex of migrating primordial germ cells may be recognized by their sex chromatin status. Generally, female cells contain a chromatin body, the Barr body, which represents the inactive X chromosome. Lyon (14) proposed that a dose compensation mechanism is achieved by X-chromosome inactivation in order to avoid the aneuploidy effect by the presence of more than one X chromosome. In somatic cells, inactivation occurs during embryonic life (15–17). In female germ cells, one X chromosome is also inactivated during migration (18), but reactivation has been noticed by the time they reach the ovarian anlage (19–21). In oogonia of human and mouse, only one X chromosome is active (17,22), but reactivation occurs when germ cells enter leptonema (23,24).

The mechanisms by which the PGC are translocated from extragonadal sites to the gonadal ridges are poorly understood. The mobility of PGC suggests that these cells may migrate actively (for review, see ref. 25). The guidance of oriented migration toward the gonads is also uncertain. It appears that fibronectin is present along the migratory pathway (26). The locomotion of PGC *in vitro* is also enhanced by fibronectin in the substrate (27).

A more passive translocation of PGC may occur during the morphogenic rearrangements of the developing tissues (11,28,29). Finally, it is possible that the PGC are attracted by chemotactic substances produced by the gonad (7) as visualized by time-lapse films of chick PGC in culture (30). This attractant does not seem to be class-specific because mouse germ cells settle in chick gonads when mouse hindgut containing germ cells are transplanted into the coelomic cavity of chick embryos (31).

A useful tool for tracing and counting PGC is the cytochemical demonstration of their relatively high activity of alkaline phosphatase (32). Ultrastructural studies have shown that the reaction product is mainly localized to the plasmalemma. It is believed that this enzyme is involved in the transfer of metabolites across the cell surface (4). The alkaline phosphatase-stained PGC have been counted from the time they are seen in the primitive streak until they reach the gonad and then go past the allantois, the hindgut, and the mesentery. In the 8-day-old mouse embryo, about 10 to 100 PGC can be identified (5,6,33). During migration

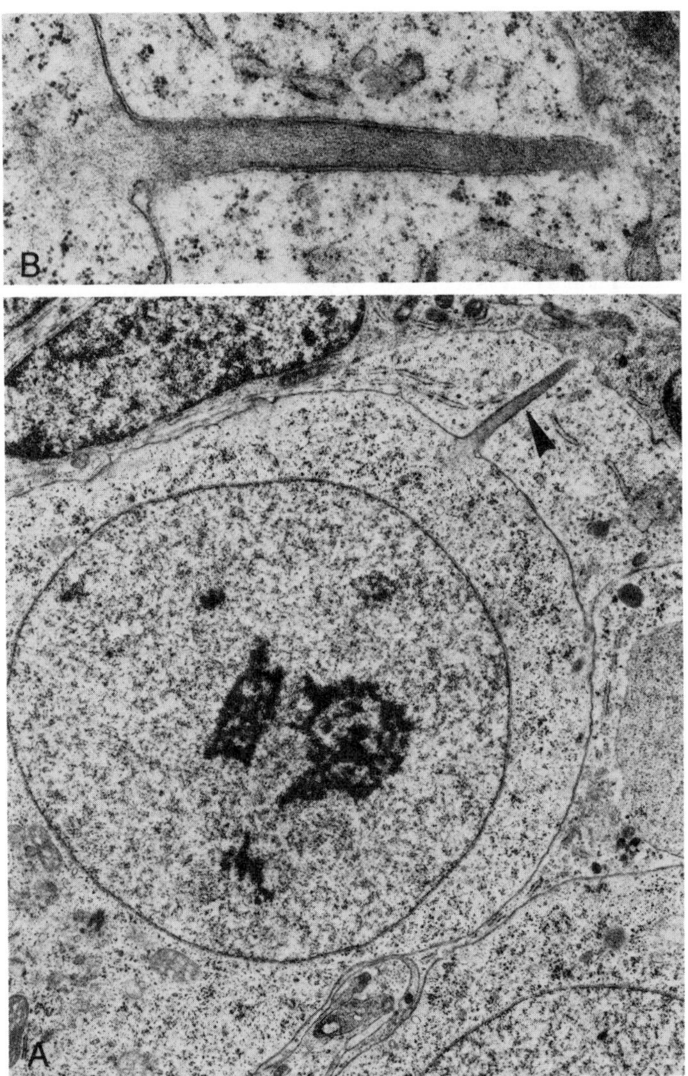

FIG. 1. Oogonium of a 9-week-old fetal human ovary. The plasmalemma forms a finger-like projection (*arrowhead*) with bundles of microfilaments (**B**). (**A**) ×5,800; (**B**) ×30,000.

their number rapidly increases and by day 13 the gonads contain around 10,000 germ cells (34). In the 5-week-old human embryo the number of migrating germ cells is about 700 to 1,300 (7), and by week 8 the germ cell number of the developing gonad is 600,000 (35).

When the PGC arrive at the coelomic epithelium covering the gonadal ridges they seem to be "trapped" by processes from the epithelial cells (36). Soon thereafter, PGC are present in the underlying tissue as well. The PGC of fetal human and pig gonads occasionally exhibit unique straight finger-like projections with closely packed parallel microfilaments (Fig. 1), the function of which is unknown.

Mesonephros

The mesonephros is the second of the three consecutive nephroic structures (pro-, meso-, and metanephros), which develop consecutively during fetal life of all mammals. All three kidneys arise in the nephrogenic cord, which forms from the segmented intermediate mesoderm early in embryonic life. The pronephros develops first from the most cranial segment, the mesonephros develops somewhat later from the intermediate segment, and finally the metanephros, the permanent kidney, arises from the most caudally placed one. The pronephros never functions in mammals, but the pronephric duct serves as an inductor for the formation of the mesonephros and the metanephros (37). The nephrons of mesonephros develop from the nephrogenic cord in a cranial caudal direction and successively form a connection with the pronephric duct, now called the *Wolffian duct*.

In some species, e.g., pig, sheep, rabbit, and human, the mesonephros is a functioning kidney with well-developed glomeruli and tubuli (Fig. 2). However, in other species, e.g., guinea pig and mouse, the mesonephric tissue consists only of tubuli, which in some cases may develop Bowman's capsules but without functional glomeruli (Figs. 3 and 4) (38).

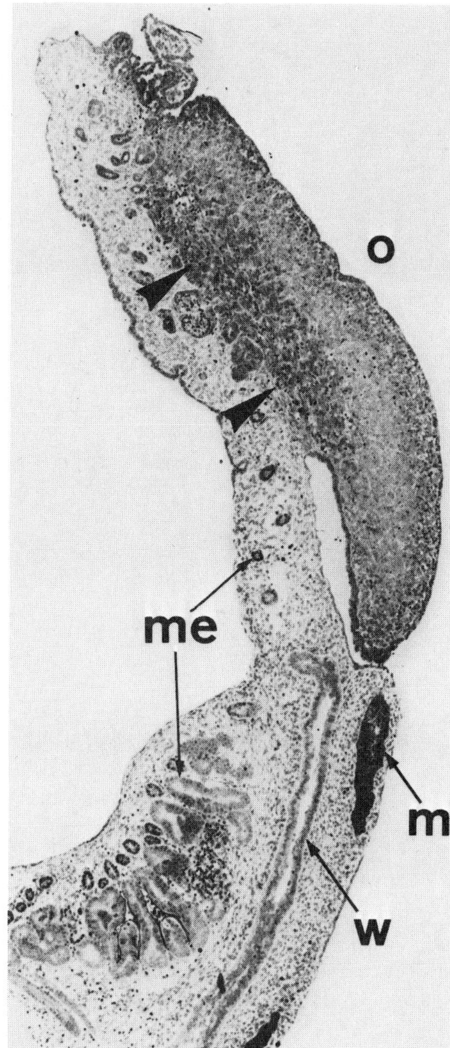

FIG. 2. Ovary-mesonephric complex of an 11-week-old human fetus. The ovary (o) is attached to the cranial part of the mesonephros (*arrowheads*). Caudally, mesonephric tubules (me), the Wolffian duct (w), and the Müllerian duct (m) are seen. ×200.

Although Waldeyer (39) and Balfour (40) proposed more than a century ago that the central cell mass of the gonad originated in the mesonephros (Fig. 5), this idea was virtually neglected until Witschi came to the same conclusion while studying amphibian (41) and mammalian gonads (42). Subsequently, numerous studies have lent support to this idea. For example, in the bovine fetus a broad stream of cells exhibiting strong alkaline phosphatase activity was observed to connect glomerular tuft and the developing gonad (43). Similar cell streams that connect the gonads with the mesonephric tissue have been described in other species, supporting the idea that the mesonephros and the gonads are closely interacting [human (44), sheep (45,46), rabbit (47,48), mouse (49–52)] (Figs. 2, 6, and 7).

Different experiments have shown that the mesonephros influences gonadal development of function. When fetal undifferentiated mouse ovaries are stripped from mesonephric tissues, ovarian differentiation and meiosis are prevented or inhibited when transplanted subcutaneously into nude mice (53). Also, the steroid synthesis by cultured fetal rabbit gonads is influenced by the mesonephros (54,55) (see section entitled "Differentiation of the Testis").

The mesonephros seems to be crucial not only for gonadal development, but also for the formation of the fetal adrenal cortex (56).

Other Cell Types

The future gonadal area consists of a loose mesenchymal tissue covered by the coelomic epithelium and supported by the developing mesonephric tissue.

Mesenchymal cells can be recognized throughout gonadal development of both sexes. At very early stages, the developing gonad is invaded by capillaries (57). A limited

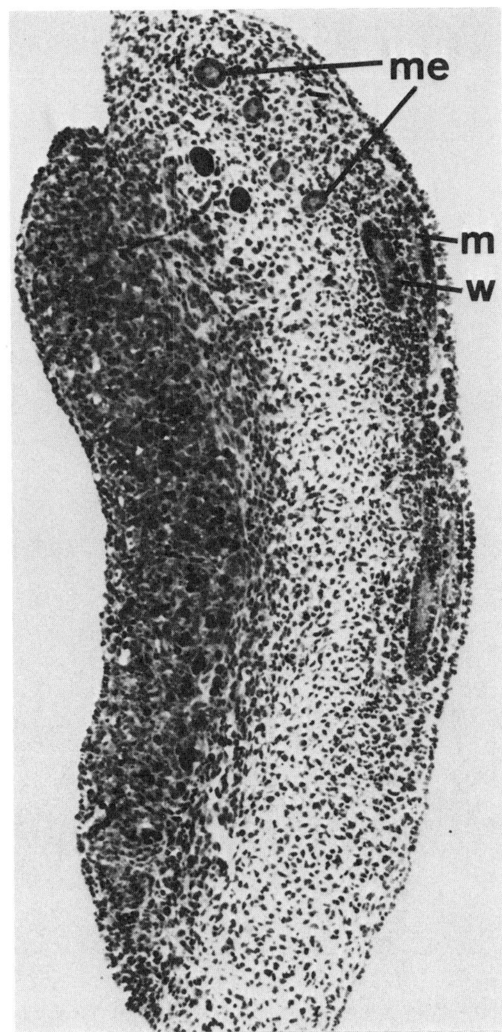

FIG. 3. Ovary-mesonephric complex of a 12½-day-old mouse fetus. The ovary appears as a rather dense homogeneous cell mass. (m) Müllerian duct; (me) mesonephric tubules; (w) Wolffian duct. ×400.

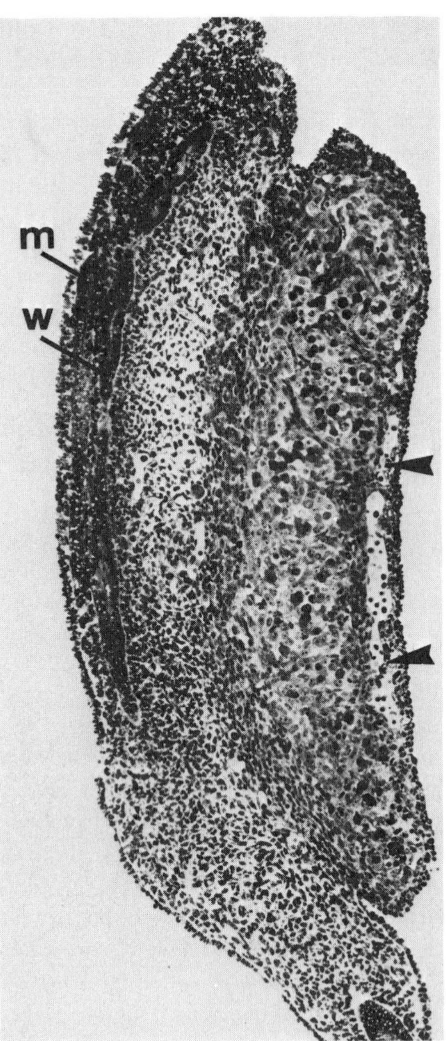

FIG. 4. Testis-mesonephric complex of a 12½-day-old mouse fetus. Beneath the surface epithelium a tunica albuginea (*arrowheads*) is developing. Testicular cords have begun to form in the cranial part of the testis. (m) Müllerian duct; (w) Wolffian duct. ×425.

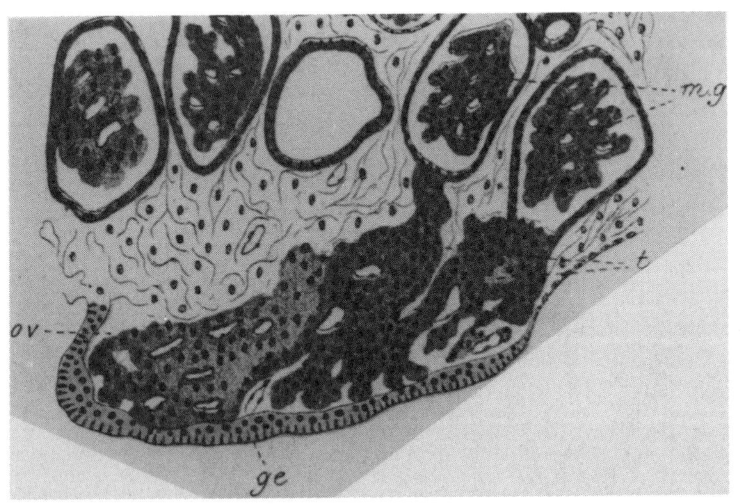

FIG. 5. Drawing showing that cell streams connect the parietal layer of Bowman's capsule with the somatic cells of the developing gonad. This drawing, made by F. M. Balfour in 1878 (see ref. 40), is probably one of the first illustrations indicating that the mesonephros contributes cells to the gonad. (ov) Ovary; (ge) germinal epithelium; (t) tubuliferous tissue, derived from Malpighian bodies; (mg) Malpighian body.

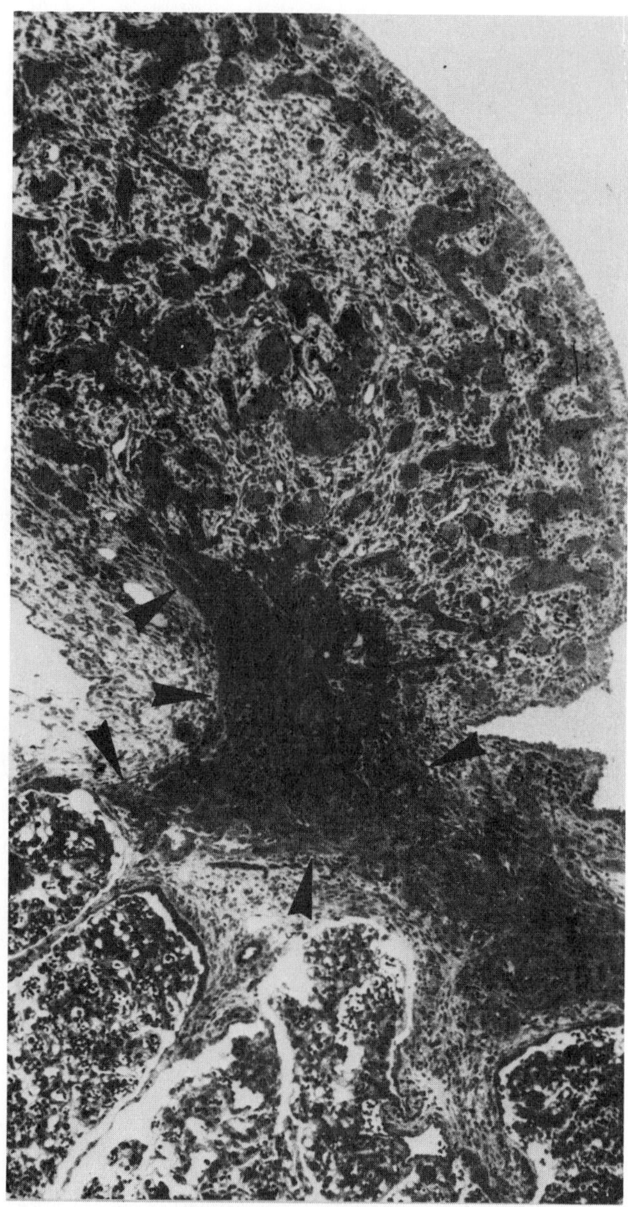

FIG. 6. Part of ovary and mesonephros of a 42-day-old pig fetus. Dense cell masses (*arrowheads*) of mesonephric origin connect the germ cell cords of the ovary with the parietal layers of Bowman's capsules. ×200.

amount of information is available on early innervation of the gonads. However, it is likely that an ingrowth of nerves follows the invasion of blood vessels.

The epithelium that covers the gonad has previously been termed the *germinal epithelium*. This term is very unfortunate because the germ cells do not derive from the epithelium but rather pass through it (see subsection entitled "Primordial Germ Cells"). Before gonadal sex differentiation takes place, no complete separation between the epithelium proper and the underlying tissue exists, since the basal lamina is not yet intact. The epithelial layer consists of pleomorphic proliferating cells, which at places have a cylindrical appearance (58,59). Primordial germ cells, probably in the process of migration, are often contained in the epithelium (60,61).

During gonadal sex differentiation, the coelomic epithelium develops differently in the two sexes. In the male the epithelium is soon delineated by an intact basal lamina, whereby the developing testicular cords become separated from the epithelium. Simultaneously, the epithelium and the outermost testicular cords become separated by a mesenchymal tissue, the developing tunica albuginea. The epithelium initially becomes cuboidal; then later when the testis rapidly increases its volume, it becomes flattened. In some cases, germ cells recognized by their alkaline phosphatase activity are trapped within the epithelium (62) (Fig. 8). In the female, the basal lamina of the coelomic epithelium becomes completed much later in development. As a consequence the epithelium remains, at some locations, in contact with the underlying germ cells (Fig. 9). Germ cells may even be seen within the epithelium a long time after gonadal sex differentiation begins. The morphology of the coelomic epithelium of the ovarian surface varies considerably with age.

A conspicuous cell type with some resemblance to undifferentiated blood cells, particularly lymphocytes, has been found in differentiating gonads of both sexes from different species (A. G. Byskov and P. E. Høyer, *unpublished observations:* human, rabbit, mouse). The cells are rounded and contain many ribosomes, sparse endoplasmic reticulum, and a relatively small, often spherical, nucleus with dense peripheral chromatin. They occur one by one or form aggregates situated close to the germ cells (Fig. 10). In the mouse, such cells disappear after the first week post-birth. The function of these cells remains to be determined.

GONADAL SEX DETERMINATION

Gonadal sex in mammals is normally determined by the genetic sex (63). From experiments with castrated rabbit fetuses, Jost (64,65) concluded that the genital structures basically are "programmed" for femaleness and that development in the male direction opposes the female program. Therefore, the gonadal primordium is considered to develop into an ovary unless a male organizer counteracts this trend and imposes testicular differentiation (66).

In mammals the presence of a Y chromosome is normally associated with development of a testis. Individuals with sex chromosome constitutions XY, XXY, or even XXXXY develop as phenotypical males, and those with XO, XX, or XXX develop as females (67,68). It thus seems that the Y chromosome carries testis-determining sequences (Tds). This gene (or genes) may act by controlling the production of a substance that induces testicular differentiation. Neither testis-determining genes nor substances that induce testicular differentiation have yet been identified.

Testis determination in mammals is effected through the

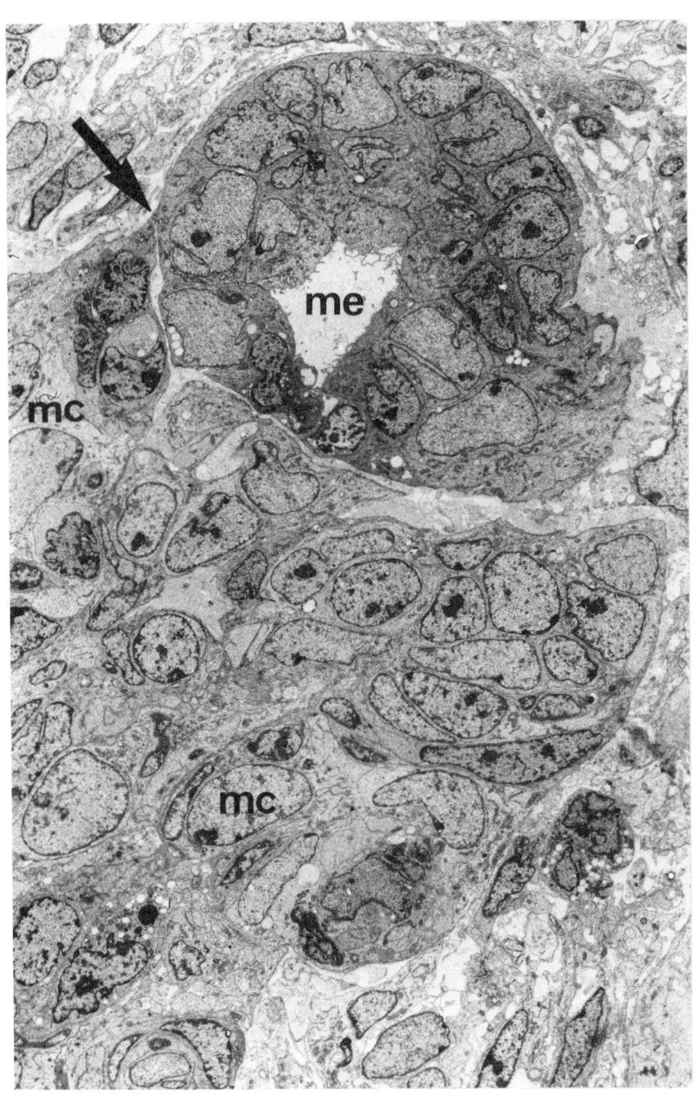

FIG. 7. Cranially placed mesonephric tubule (me) and mesonephric-derived cell mass (mc) of a 9-week-old female human fetus. An opening of the tubule is shown by an arrow. ×1,820.

Y chromosome (69), and the gene sequences in action were visualized in chromosome studies of sex-reversed (Sxr) mice (70), in which XX-Sxr develop as phenotypically normal males (71). The X chromosome of these males contains a body that, during meiosis (72), has been translocated from the Y chromosome (73).

Some years ago it was proposed that a testis-determining substance might be identical to the male-specific H-Y antigen (74), also known as the classical *histocompatible Y antigen* (75). This hypothesis is attractive because, until recently, it was found that almost all mammals possessing a testis were H-Y positive independent of their karyotype (76). The detection of H-Y antigen in these studies is based on serological tests in which it is assumed that antisera raised against male cells will recognize H-Y antigen (serologically detectable male, SDM) (77). However, recently McLaren (78) discovered mice that develop testes but lack H-Y antigenicity, as determined by tests using T-lymphocyte-mediated histocompatibility response as the originally defined H-Y antigen. These specific male mice are variants of Sxr XX mice, which are phenotypical males with testes (70) Previously, phenotypical males with testes, although sterile, have been found to be SDM antigen negative [man (79), mouse (80)]. Although theoretical models may explain why H-Y negative males develop testes (81), it still seems unlikely that the transplantation H-Y antigen is responsible for testicular formation. Since the transplantation H-Y antigen may not be the same as SDM antigen (77,82), it is possible that SDM antigen rather than H-Y antigen might interfere with testicular differentiation.

Results of other experiments lack support with regard to the concept that SDM antigen is the testis inducer, having its primary effect by aggregating fetal male germ cells and Sertoli cells into testicular cords. Epididymal fluid has been reported to be rich in SDM antigen and to exert a reaggregational effect on dispersed rat ovarian cells (83). However, spent culture media from bull and human epididymis (84) or from human testes (85) have the opposite effect on fetal mouse testes, *in vitro,* by preventing testicular cord formation and inducing meiosis. Also, the addition of serum

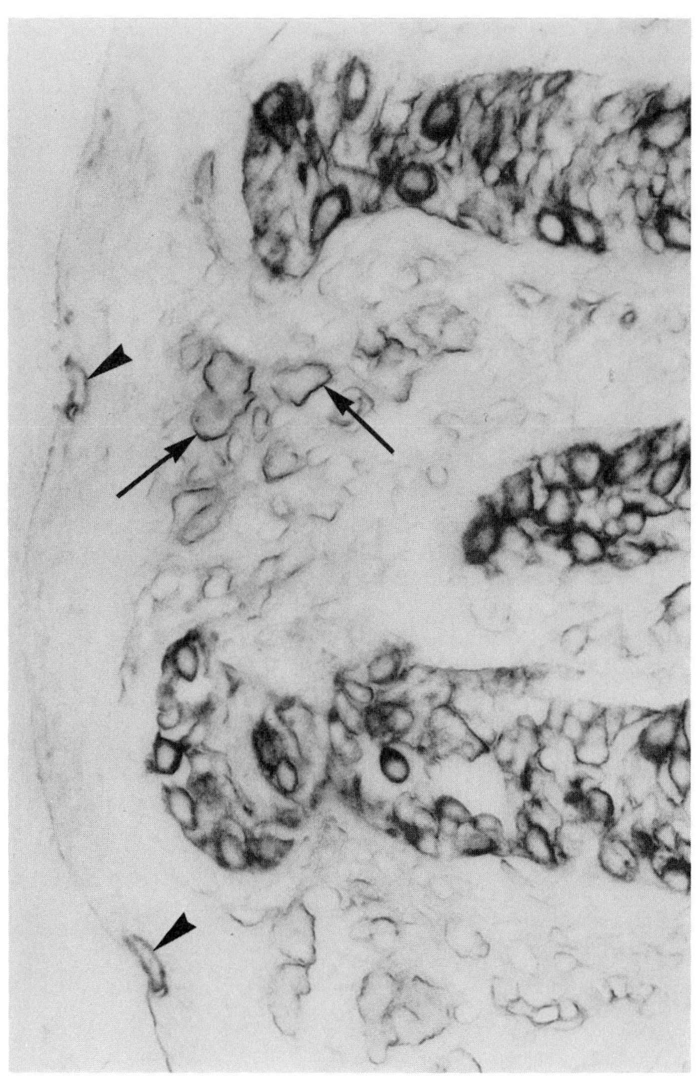

FIG. 8. Alkaline phosphatase activity in a cryosection of a 12-week-old human fetal testis. Germ cells of testicular cords and of the surface epithelium (*arrowheads*) as well as plasmalemma of Leydig cells (*arrows*) exhibit activity. ×311.

to cultures of fetal rat testes prevents testicular cord formation (86).

As indicated above, gonadal sex determination is dependent on the sex chromosome constitution. Chromosomal errors, particularly those affecting the X and Y, which can arise in germ cells during meiosis or in the early mitotic divisions during embryogenesis, may interfere with gonadal differentiation (for review, see ref. 67). However, several chromosomal errors, e.g., XO (Turner's syndrome), XXY (Klinefelter's syndrome), and Tfm (testicular feminization), do not seem to affect the primary sex determination of the gonad, but rather later stages of gonadal differentiation.

An individual in which the gonad develops with both ovarian and testicular tissues is a hermaphrodite, or sex mosaic, and has been described in many species (78), including humans (87). They could develop from fused XX and XY embryos [i.e., chimeras, which have also been made experimentally (88,89)] or as a result of Y-chromosome nondisjunction (90). The gonads of chimeras do not differentiate into an ovary, an ovotestis, or a testis according to the relative proportion of male and female clones (91,92). A male phenotype develops in more than 40% of the cases if the XY cells comprise more than one-third of the cells in the gonads (93). A dominant influence of the male tissue over the female tissue is also demonstrated by the inhibition of growth of the Müllerian duct in fetal mouse hermaphrodites, in which only 15% of testicular tissue caused normal male inhibition of Müllerian duct growth (94).

The gonadal sex of mammals is highly stable, and only in the primitive young marsupials can it be changed experimentally. In the newborn male opossum (95,96) and wallabies (97), the testicular anlage can develop into an ovotestis or an ovary by giving low doses of estradiol propionate. Turner and Asakawa (98) claimed that when embryonic mouse ovaries and testes were grafted closely together under the kidney capsule, the ovary developed testicular tubules. It was proposed that the testis secreted substances that induced differentiation of testicular structures in the ovarian anlage. However, these results could not be reproduced by Ozdzenski et al. (99) or by Burgoyne et al. (100), who suggest instead that the ovarian "testicular cords" are structures of mesonephric origin. Neither in co-cultures between

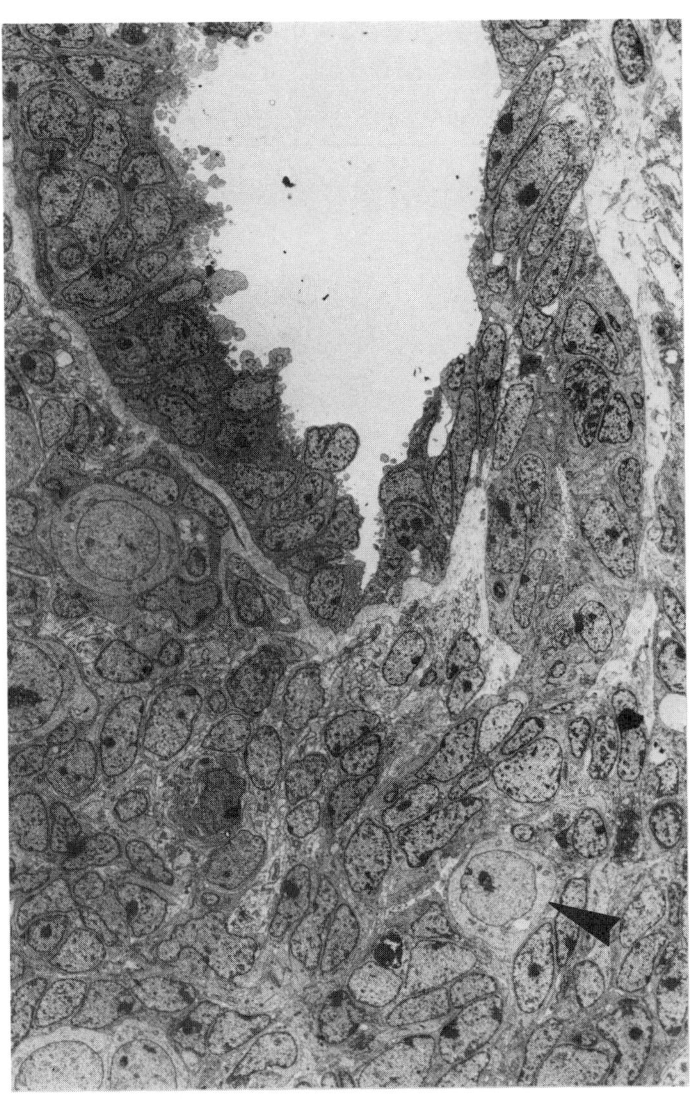

FIG. 9. Part of ovarian cortex of a 9-week-old human fetus showing connections between the down-growing surface epithelium and an oogonium (*arrowhead*). ×1,820.

embryonic mouse ovaries and testis (101) nor between fetal and neonatal rabbit testes and ovaries (102) did any testicular structures develop in the ovaries.

DIFFERENTIATION OF THE OVARY

A functional ovary depends on three major events taking place during early stages of gonadogenesis: the initiation of meiosis, the formation of follicles, and the differentiation of steroid-producing cells.

Different Patterns of Early Ovarian Differentiation

Mesonephric-derived cells populate the gonad a long time before morphological sex differentiation takes place. The ovarian-mesonephric connection is retained during ovarian differentiation, although the mesonephric tissue gradually regresses (Fig. 11). In most species the central part of the differentiating ovary becomes occupied by the invading mesonephric cells (i.e., the intraovarian rete), which push the germ cells toward the periphery. An ovarian cortex richly populated with germ cells and a medulla consisting mainly of mesonephric cells are thereby formed.

Two major patterns of ovarian differentiation can be recognized depending on whether the germ cells of the ovary undergo "immediate" meiosis, without previous steroid production, or "delayed" meiosis (Fig. 12), with steroid secreted before meiosis begins (102). In species with "immediate" meiosis (e.g., mouse, rat, hamster), the germ cells of the ovary enter the first meiotic prophase simultaneously with or shortly after gonadal sex can be recognized morphologically. These ovaries produce little or no steroids *de novo* until follicles are formed. In species with "delayed" meiosis (e.g., pig, sheep, dog, cow), the beginning of meiosis in the female is delayed up to 45 days (cow) with respect to testicular differentiation, i.e., delay period. In contrast to species with immediate meiosis, such ovaries produce

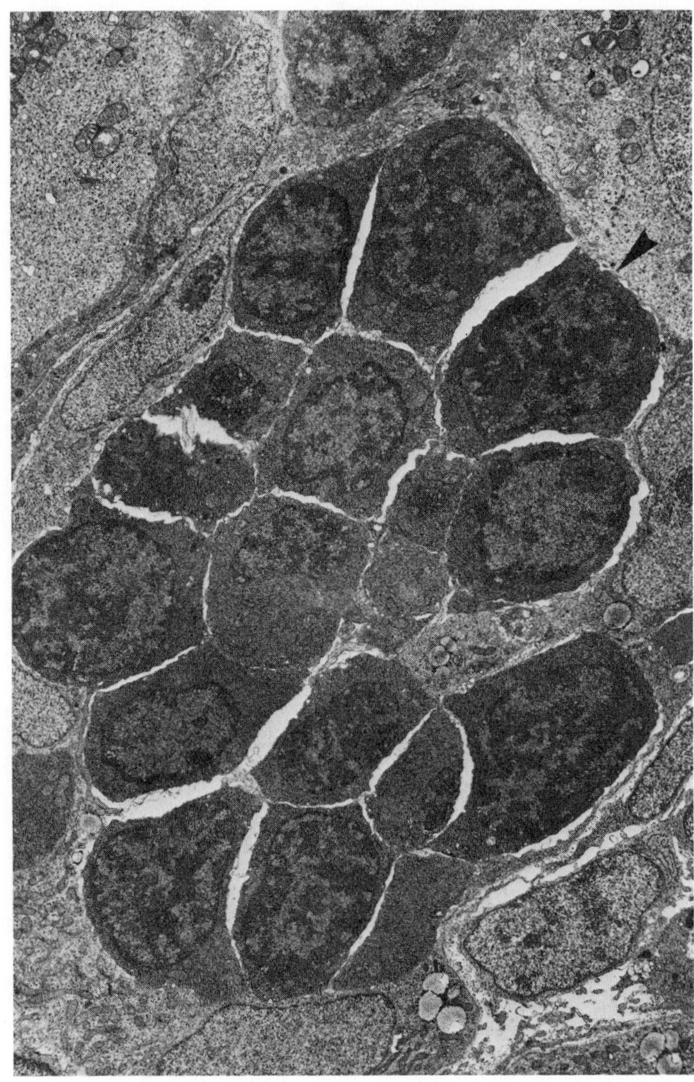

FIG. 10. Aggregate of lymphocyte-like cells in a newborn mouse ovary. At some places, such cells are in contact with oocytes (*arrowhead*). ×4,560.

various amounts of steroids during the delay period (see subsection entitled "Ovary").

In species with immediate meiosis, the ovary appears compact when meiosis begins at an early stage of sex differentiation. The germ cells are distributed uniformly or in clusters throughout the entire ovarian tissue (e.g., mouse, hamster) or in a basically well-defined cortical area (e.g., human).

In ovaries of species with delayed meiosis, the germ cells become enclosed in germ cell cords during the delay period. In some species [pig (103); cat, mink, ferret (104); sheep (43); cow (105)] the germ cell cords are lined with a basal lamina and clearly defined from the surrounding loose mesenchyme (Fig. 13). The cords are irregularly shaped and are tightly packed with somatic cells and germ cells. By the end of the delay period the cell cords begin to break up in the central part of the ovary close to the intraovarian mesonephric cell cords. This process is related to the beginning of meiosis (see subsection entitled "Meiotic Prophase").

In other species (e.g., the rabbit) the germ cell cords are more closely packed in the ovarian cortex and are only clearly recognizable in the inner part, where they connect with the intraovarian mesonephric cell mass.

The development of the human fetal ovary represents a transitory example between immediate and delayed meiosis. Although there is a delay period of 2 to 3 weeks, no or very little steroids are produced *de novo* (see subsection entitled "Ovary"). Intraovarian mesonephric cell cords occupy the medulla before meiosis starts, and the cortically placed germ cells are not confined to cords, but are rather gathered into large clusters (Fig. 14).

Meiotic Prophase

The two meiotic divisions are unique for germ cells. During the first meiotic division, maternal and paternal genes are exchanged before the pairs of chromosomes are divided

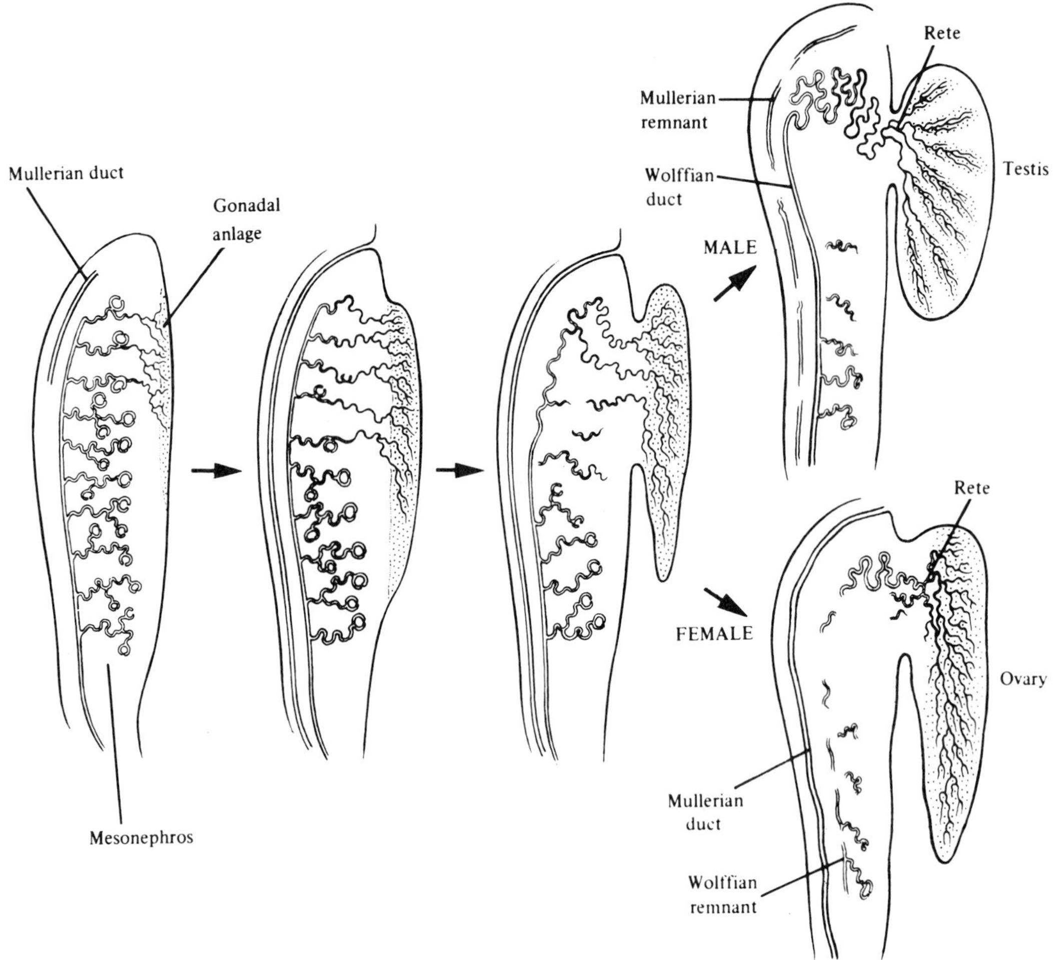

FIG. 11. Transformation of the genital duct system during the period when the gonads pass from the undifferentiated state to recognizable testes and ovaries. [From A. G. Byskov, Chapter 1, in: *Germ Cells and Fertilization,* edited by C. R. Austin and R. V. Short, Cambridge University Press, Cambridge (1982).]

into the two daughter cells, each containing 1n chromosomes and 2c DNA. The second meiotic division occurs without being preceded by DNA synthesis. This division results in formation of the haploid germ cells with a 1n set of chromosomes and 1c DNA (for review see ref. 106).

Although meiosis represents similar events in germ cells of the two sexes, the time schedule and the resulting number of haploid germ cells differ greatly between ovary and testis.

In the female germ cells, meiosis is initiated at early stages of development, often during fetal life. The first germ cells to begin meiosis are always localized at the inner part of the cortex. However, meiosis is arrested in late prophase of the first meiotic phase, and the divisions are delayed and do not take place until much later in the mature animal (around ovulation time). In the male germ cells, meiosis begins at puberty and proceeds without delay (Fig. 15).

Meiosis in each female germ cell results in a single egg and two, or eventually three, abortive cells, the polar bodies, whereas four sperms are produced by each male germ cell (Fig. 15).

Proliferation and Premeiotic DNA Synthesis of Oogonia

The oogonia continue to divide mitotically until they enter meiosis. Fluctuations in the total number of germ cells in fetal and neonatal ovaries of different mammalian species are seen in Fig. 16 (107). The rate of mitosis during the time preceding meiosis varies between species. In species with delayed meiosis, the mitotic activity is low during most of the delay period, but it increases rapidly shortly before meiosis starts [pig (108)]. In species in which meiosis starts shortly after gonadal sex differentiation, the period with low mitotic activity in the oogonial population is nonexistent (mouse) or very short (rat), and meiosis is introduced by a series of mitotic divisions shortly after gonadal sex differentiation (109). Often, groups of germ cells divide synchronously. When meiosis begins, similar groups exhibit synchrony while passing through transitory stages of meiosis (110,111). Germ cells of such groups are often connected by intercellular bridges (112). It has been proposed that a single-stem cell gives rise to such germ cell groups

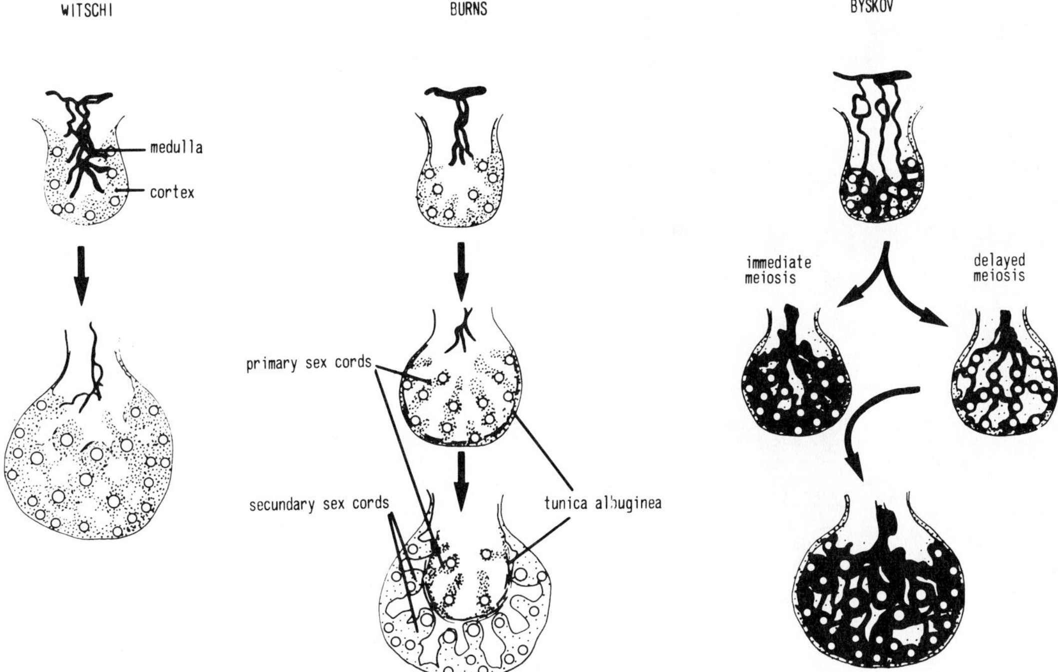

FIG. 12. Schematic drawings of models of ovarian differentiation from Witschi (39,40), Burns (94), and Byskov (197). Witschi and Burns suggest that somatic cells of ovary are mainly derived from surface epithelium, whereas Byskov proposes mesonephric origin. Model by Witschi includes degeneration of medulla and proliferation of cortex. Burns believes that secondary proliferation of surface epithelium forms secondary sex cords, which contribute the bulk of ovarian somatic cells. Byskov's model involves two types of transitory stages of ovarian differentiation, one in which meiosis starts almost simultaneously with gonadal sex differentiation (immediate meiosis) and another in which meiosis is more or less delayed with respect to sex differentiation (delayed meiosis). In both cases, mesonephric-derived cells are main contributors to ovarian cell mass. [Reprinted from A. G. Byskov, Differentiation of mammalian embryonic gonad, *Physiol. Rev.,* 66:71–117 (1986).]

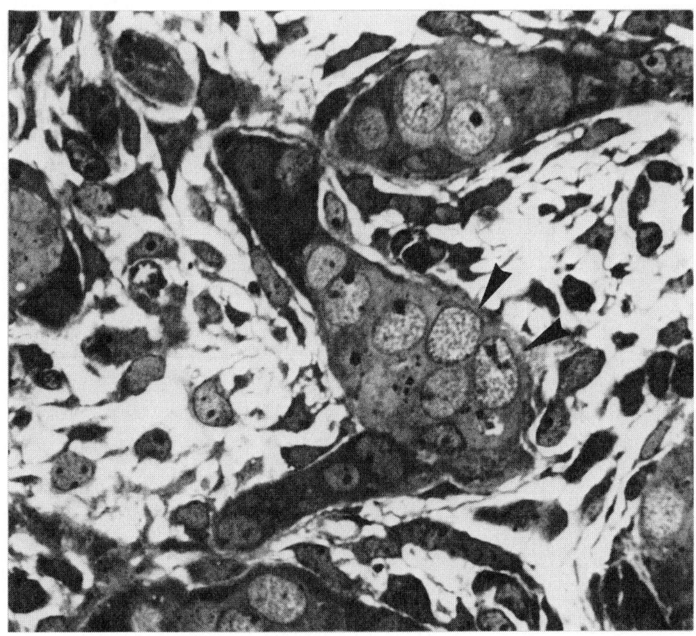

FIG. 13. Germ cell cords of a 42-day-old pig ovary. The cords are tightly packed with somatic cells and germ cells (*arrowheads*). $\times$1,000.

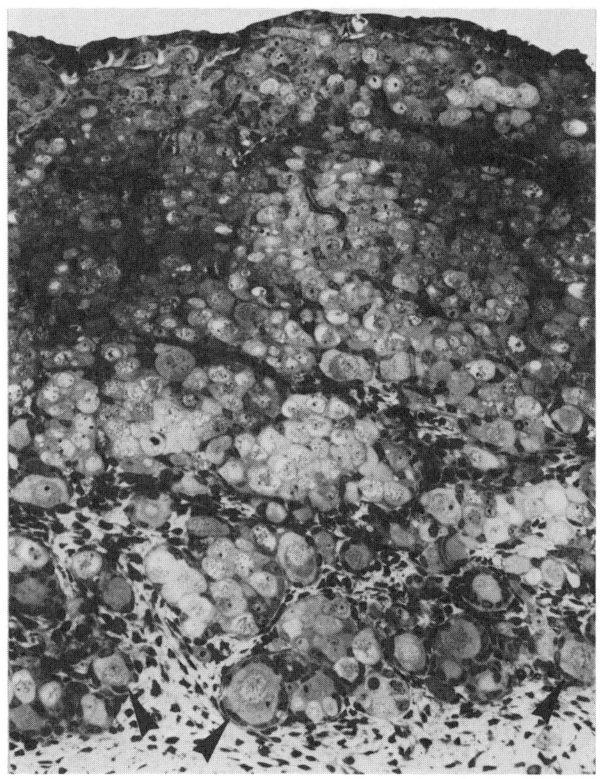

FIG. 14. Part of ovary from a 21-week-old human fetus. Small follicles (*arrowheads*) are present in the inner part of the cortex. The middle part contains oocytes in different stages of meiosis, whereas the peripheral layer still contains oogonia. ×360.

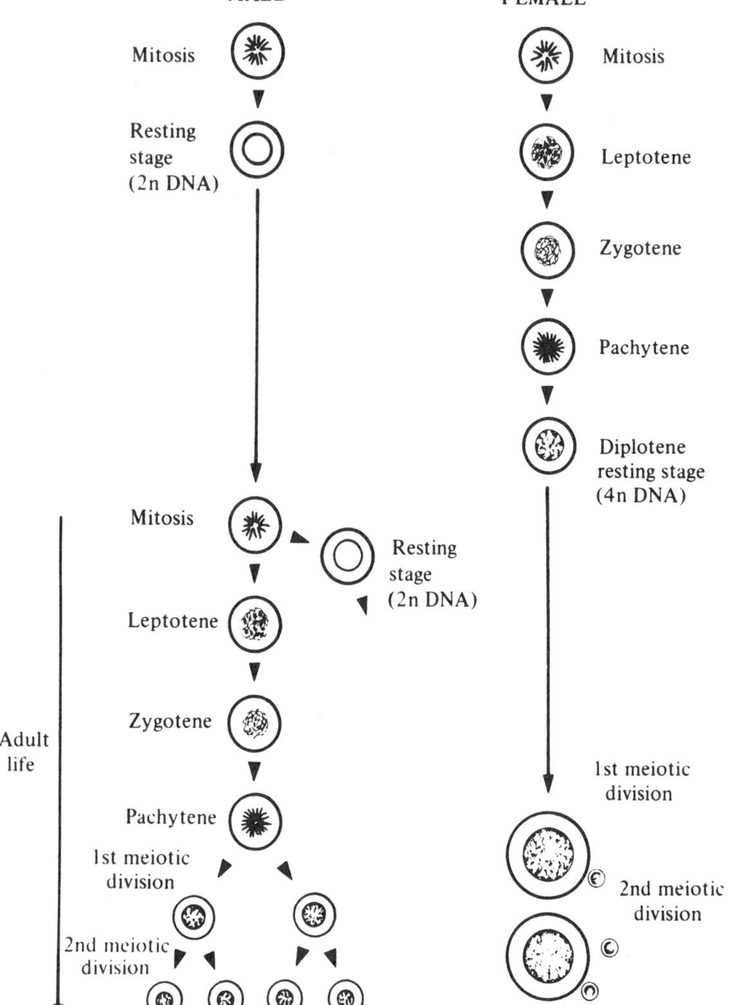

FIG. 15. Life cycles of male and female germ cells. Germ cells of both sexes divide mitotically until, or shortly after, gonadal sex differentiation. The female germ cells all enter meiosis at early stages of development, whereas the male germ cells keep a resting stem cell population which can divide mitotically and from which meiotic cells continue to emerge throughout life. The male germ cells rest with 2c DNA (2c = 2n), whereas the female germ cells rest in the diplotene stage with 4c DNA (4c = 4n). [From A. G. Byskov, Chapter 1, in: *Germ Cells and Fertilization,* edited by C. R. Austin and R. V. Short, Cambridge University Press, Cambridge (1982).]

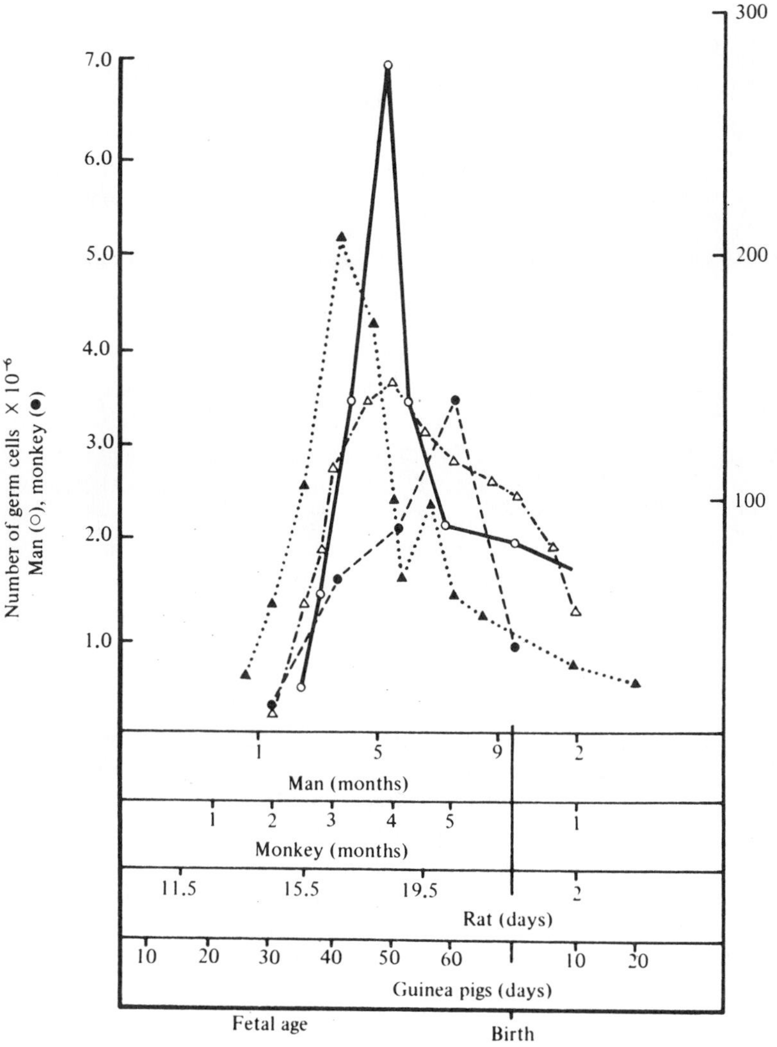

FIG. 16. Graph showing numbers of germ cells in the ovaries of fetuses and neonates in humans, monkeys, rats, and guinea pigs. [From T. G. Baker, Chapter 10, in: *Reproductive Biology,* edited by H. Balin and S. R. Glasser. Excerpta Medica, Amsterdam (1972).]

(113). The bridges may be used to transfer different substances, e.g., gene products in between germ cells (112, 114,115).

The premeiotic DNA synthesis is an important event because this DNA persists throughout the lifetime of the oocyte, lasting until either fertilization or atresia. This DNA synthesis has been studied by means of incorporated isotope-labeled thymidine followed by autoradiography (111,116–118). These studies have shown that no neoformation of oocytes takes place after they enter meiosis. Experiments in which germ cells of fetal ovaries have been eliminated by irradiation confirm that no neoformation takes place (119–121). An exception from this concept occurs in prosimians, in which oogonia-like cells of the adult ovary exhibit DNA synthesis (122,123).

Germ cells of the proliferative phases that precede meiosis are extremely sensitive to irradiation (for review see ref. 124). It seems that the premeiotic division stage is the most sensitive and that sensitivity decreases as meiosis advances (125,126).

Transitory Stages of the Meiotic Prophase in Oocytes

The first meiotic prophase is subdivided into five consecutive stages, namely, leptonema, zygonema, pachynema, diplonema, and diakinesis. ["The adjectives corresponding to the first four stages are leptotene, zygotene, pachytene and diplotene and are often used as nouns" (Goodenough and Levine, ref. 106).]

The leptotene stage is resumed by the end of the premeiotic DNA synthesis. In the immature rabbit, DNA synthesis still seems to take place in leptotene cells (127). In some species a precondensation stage has been recognized [human (128), mouse (129), rabbit (127,130), sheep (131), horse (132)]. During the preleptotene and leptotene stages, the chromosomes begin to condense; they appear in the light microscope as thin, coiled threads with chromomeric periodicity (Fig. 17). Each thread consists of identical sister chromatids.

During the zygotene stage the homologous sister chromatids pair and the synaptonemal complexes are formed

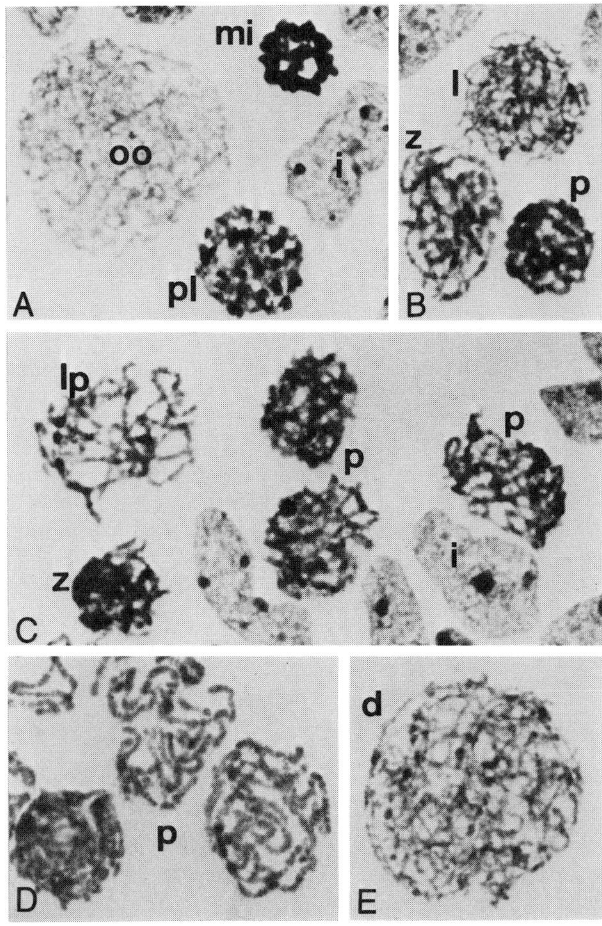

FIG. 17. Feulgen-stained squash preparations of fetal mouse ovaries showing germ cells in different stages of meiosis. ×3,500. (**A**) A 13½-day-old fetus showing an oogonium (oo), preleptotene cells (pl), somatic cells in interphase (i), and one cell in mitosis (mi). (**B**, **C**) A 16½-day-old fetus. Leptotene (l), zygotene (z), pachytene (p), and late pachytene (lp) stage. (**D**, **E**) A 19½-day-old fetus. Diplotene stage (d).

(Fig. 18A and B). The synaptonemal complexes are structures that hold the two homologous chromatids together. Detailed information about the synaptonemal complexes has been provided by three-dimensional reconstructions from serial thin sections of chromosomes (133,134). The process of pairing can also be studied by the surface spreading technique (135). The chromatids coil increasingly during zygonema (Fig. 16). By the end of pachynema, synapsis is completed between homologous chromatids, in which coiling and condensation is maximal (Fig. 16). The maternal and paternal chromatids are now in the position for gene exchange. This important process is called *chiasma* or *crossing over* and takes place between non-sister-chromatid bivalents (set of homologs) in the following stage, i.e., diplonema. In oocytes of the early diplotene stage, the points of crossing over can also be recognized in the light microscope. The amount of chromosomal material that is exchanged between paternal and maternal chromatids can be evaluated by labeling premeiotic oogonia in S-phase with bromodeoxyuridine and studying the oocyte in the metaphase of the second meiotic division (136).

In mammals the diplotene stage (or diplonema) (Fig. 16) lasts for a long time and may (e.g., in the human) take more than 50 years. In general, the chromosomal material becomes very diffuse and is therefore only faintly seen after DNA staining. In some species the chromosomes form lampbrush structures in the diplotene stage, which has been referred to as the *dictyate stage* (137). This condition seems to be related to high radiosensitivity (124).

Germ cells passing through the transitory stages of the meiotic prophase appear to be extremely vulnerable. A large percentage of oocytes that enter meiosis will not reach the diplotene stage but instead will become pyknotic, particularly when entering the zygotene and pachytene stages (138). In the fetal human ovary, only about 5% of the peak number of germ cells reach the diplotene stage (35) (Fig. 18).

It seems that the presence of two active X chromosomes from the beginning of meiosis (see section entitled "Early Gonadal Formation") promotes the survival and function of oocytes. Germ cells of human XO (Turner's syndrome) ovaries begin to degenerate around the third month of fetal life (when meiosis starts), and often these women develop sterile ovaries (139,140). In XO mice, many oocytes degenerate during meiosis (141). It was proposed that germ cells, which during the pachytene stage have unpaired or incompletely paired chromosomes, are selectively destroyed (142,143).

The synthesis of RNA has been studied during the transitory stages of meiosis by autoradiography after uptake of [^{3}H]uridine [rat (109), monkey (144)]. In the rat it was shown that the grain number of oocytes in pachytene stage was 10 times higher than in the previous stages of meiosis (109).

Formation of Follicles

When the oocyte reaches diplonema it must become enclosed in a follicle (Fig. 19). In most species, single oocytes are surrounded by presumptive granulosa cells, which are delineated by an intact basal lamina. In some species, more than one oocyte is enclosed within the same follicle [e.g., primate (145), dog (146)], a phenomenon that is also seen in other species during the immature period (147). If the oocyte in the diplotene stage fails to be enclosed into the follicle, it invariably degenerates.

Follicles begin to form in the inner part of the ovarian cortex, where oocytes first reach diplonema (Fig. 14). Initially the granulosa cells of these developing follicles are connected with the intraovarian mesonephric-derived rete cords (148). That the mesonephric-derived rete cells are in fact the granulosa cell precursors has been supported by *in*

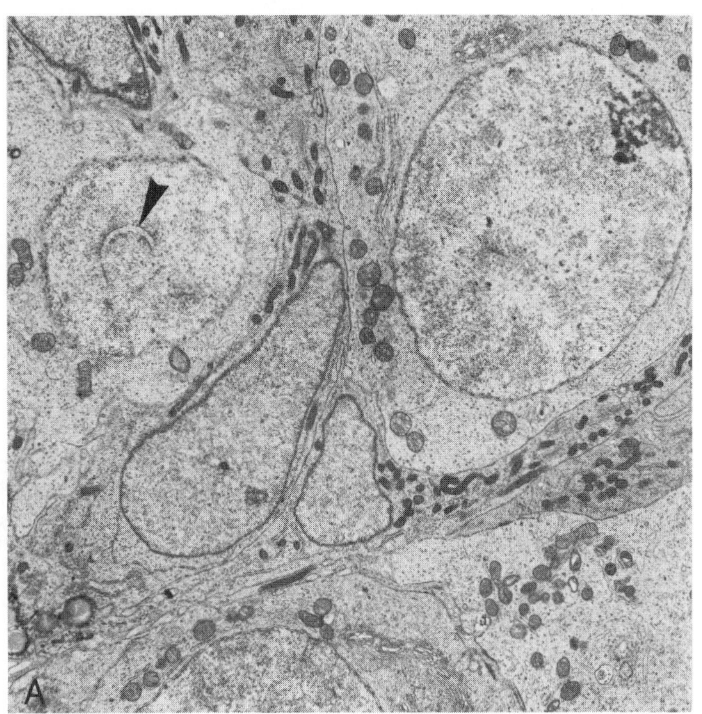

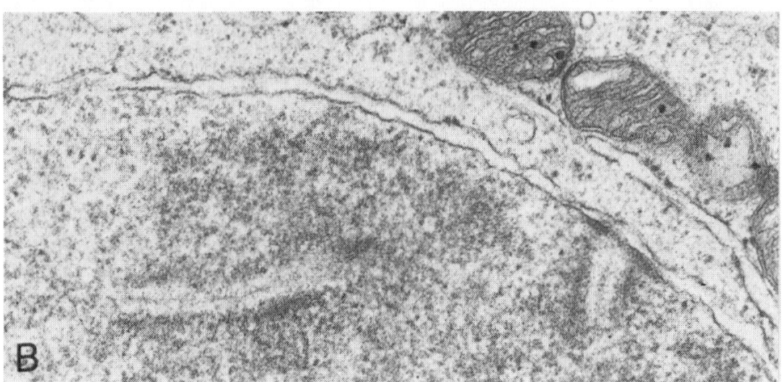

FIG. 18. (**A**) Part of an ovary of a 19-day-old fetal mouse showing oocytes in meiosis (pachytene stage with synaptonemal complex, *arrowhead*). ×6,250. (**B**) Higher magnification of two synaptonemal complexes of an oocyte in the pachytene stage. ×38,000.

vitro experiments which showed that follicle formation depended on whether a sufficient number of mesonephric cells had invaded the developing ovary (149). In addition, these experiments also indicated that the disappearance of the ovarian surface epithelium did not influence folliculogenesis, making it unlikely that this epithelium is an important source of granulosa cells during early formation of follicles. During ovarian maturation, folliculogenesis spreads toward the surface (61).

The first-formed follicles in the center of the fetal or neonatal ovary exhibit a different pattern of formation, growth, and differentiation compared to that of follicles in the mature ovary (150). Early folliculogenesis depends on migration of mitotically dividing extraovarian rete cells into the intraovarian rete (151). Some of these cells surround the diplotene oocytes to become granulosa cells, whereas other intraovarian rete cells become the first interstitial cells (152). Once the rete cells arrive at the ovary, they stop migrating so that they can proliferate, as reported in the rat (151). The accumulation of such granulosa cells is therefore a result of migration and differentiation of rete cells rather than local proliferation. In contrast, the beginning of follicular growth in the mature ovary is a result of proliferation of "preexisting" granulosa cells (153,154). In other respects, early-formed follicles appear to differ from those of the mature ovary. The theory has been advanced that those follicles which remain connected to the intraovarian rete contain an atretic oocyte and are in the process of degeneration (152). Thus, elimination of the connection to the rete may depend on whether the oocyte is healthy or undergoing degeneration.

The mechanisms that trigger initial follicular growth are unknown. Exogenous gonadotrophins have been reported to stimulate the onset of follicular growth in the mouse (155), and gonadotrophins seem to support follicular growth *in vivo* (156) and *in vitro* (157,158). Follicular growth is retarded in hypophysectomized fetal monkeys (156), in anencephalic human fetuses (159), and in infant mice treated with antigonadotrophins (160). The time at which follicles form in different species depends on when the oocytes reach

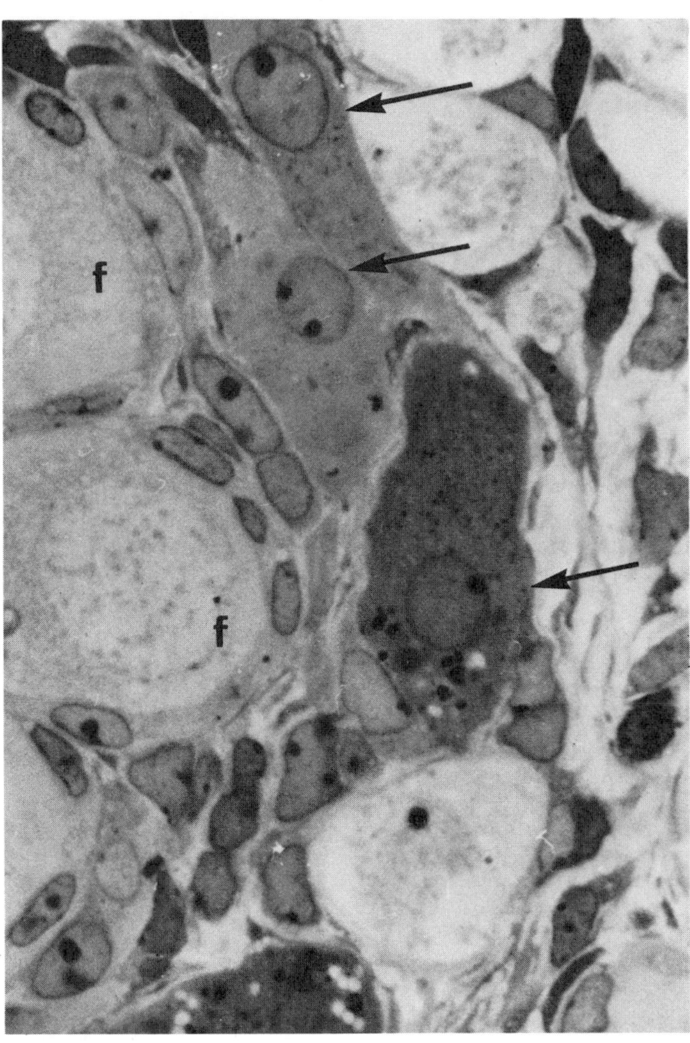

FIG. 19. Part of ovarian cortex of a 23-week-old human fetus showing three interstitial cells (*arrows*) with different content of osmiophilic granules (i.e., various degrees of differentiation), oocytes, and two small follicles (f). ×1,275.

the diplotene stage. This may occur during fetal life (e.g., human, pig, guinea pig) or after birth (e.g., mouse, rat, rabbit, ferret) (for review see refs. 161 and 162).

Early Steroid-Producing Cells

A "typical" steroid-producing cell is traditionally characterized by many mitochondria with tubular cristae, abundant smooth endoplasmic reticulum, and many lipid droplets (163). However, steroid production by the mammalian ovary may occur at times when cells with such characteristics cannot be found, e.g., in the fetal rabbit ovary (103,164). By day 19 the fetal rabbit ovary is able to convert testosterone to estrogen (165) and is also able to secrete steroids *de novo* in cultures (55). The cells, which seem to be responsible for this steroidogenesis, lack the typical ultrastructural characteristics of a steroid-producing cell, except for their content of lipid droplets. However, these cells, which are localized in the mesonephric-derived medulla, do exhibit activity of 3β-hydroxysteroid dehydrogenase shown by quantitative cytochemistry (166).

In species with immediate meiosis, ovarian *de novo* steroidogenesis does not take place until follicles are formed (see section entitled "Early Steroid Hormone Production by the Gonads"). When follicles appear, cells containing mitochondria with tubular cristae, smooth endoplasmic reticulum, and lipid droplets (i.e., the interstitial cells) are recognized in the ovary (166). In the human, these cells are first seen after the 12th week in the inner part of the cortex, close to the follicles (166–168) (Fig. 15). At the 14th week, high NADH diaphorase activity is present in some cells situated in the inner part of the cortex (Fig. 20), but not until the 20th week do a few of these cells show activity of 3β-hydroxysteroid dehydrogenase (166). In the 23-week-old fetus, most of these cells are situated in the inner part of the cortex, but some may also have a more peripheral location.

Different studies indicate that the early steroid-producing cells are derived from cells of mesonephric origin. In particular, the mouse has served as a model to study their ontogeny: A quantitative cytochemical study of 3β-hydroxysteroid dehydrogenase activity in the rete system of

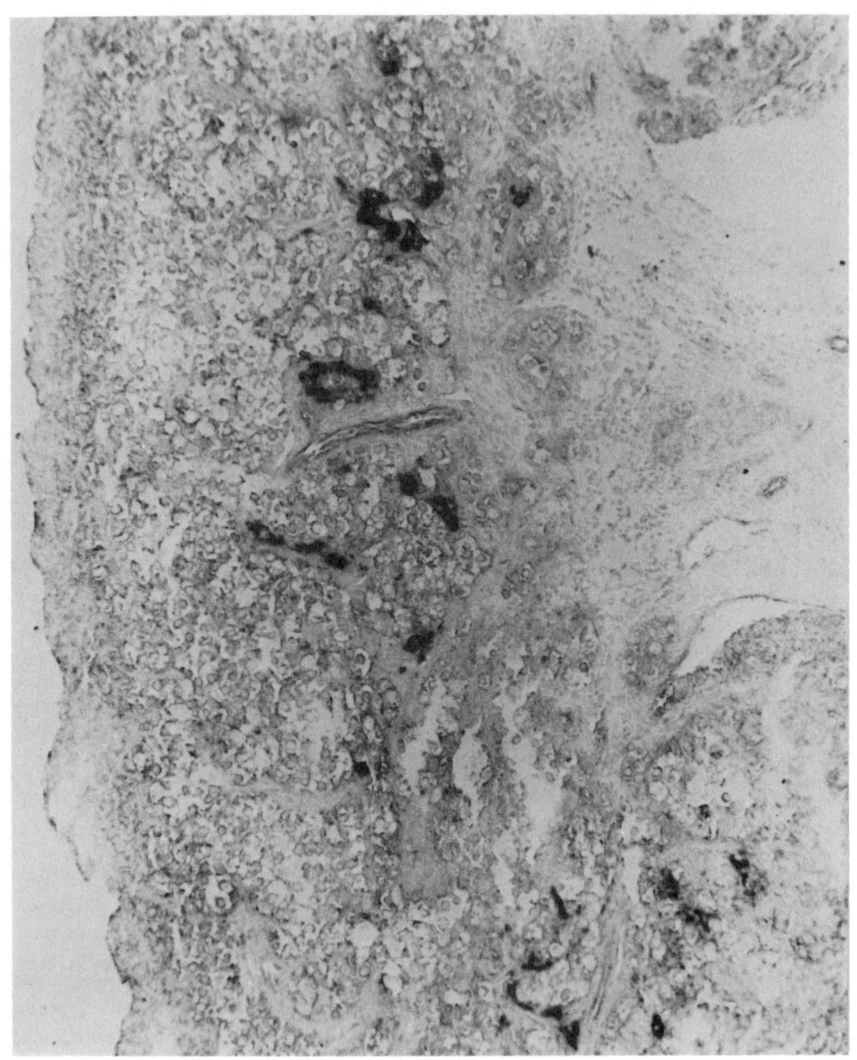

FIG. 20. Part of an ovary of a 20-week-old human fetus. Cells located in the inner part of the cortex exhibit strong NADH diaphorase activity. ×120.

the immature mouse ovary was performed (152). This study showed that by day 7, only those rete cells that position themselves close to the oocytes develop this enzyme activity. During the next 2 weeks the connection between the granulosa cells and the intraovarian rete cells becomes eliminated in some follicles. Only the peripherally situated granulosa cells of these isolated follicles retain some activity of 3β-hydroxysteroid dehydrogenase, whereas the cells closer to the oocytes lose it. However, oocytes, possibly atretic ones, which remain connected to the intraovarian rete, show a uniform enzyme activity in their surrounding granulosa cells (see section entitled "Formation of Follicles"). The activity of these cells, as well as that in cells of the intraovarian rete cords proper, shows a steady increase during the third week of life and represents the first interstitial tissue.

In some species a so-called "hilar rete body," which is formed from the connecting rete (104,169), contains "interstitial hilar gland cells" that exhibit 3β-hydroxysteroid dehydrogenase activity and have a hormone-dependent morphology. In the human fetus, ovarian hilar cells are present from the 13th week onward (168). However, high hCG levels appear to have little effect on the formation of hilar cells, because they are also present in anencephalic fetuses (170).

DIFFERENTIATION OF THE TESTIS

As in the ovary, testicular differentiation and function depend on the enclosure of germ cells into specific compartments, namely the testicular cords (Fig. 21). The subsequent differentiation of the steroid-producing Leydig cells occurs outside these compartments.

Testicular Cords

The first event leading to testicular differentiation seems to be that germ cells gather closely together with some somatic cells, the future Sertoli cells, thereby forming testicular cords. However, different experiments indicate that

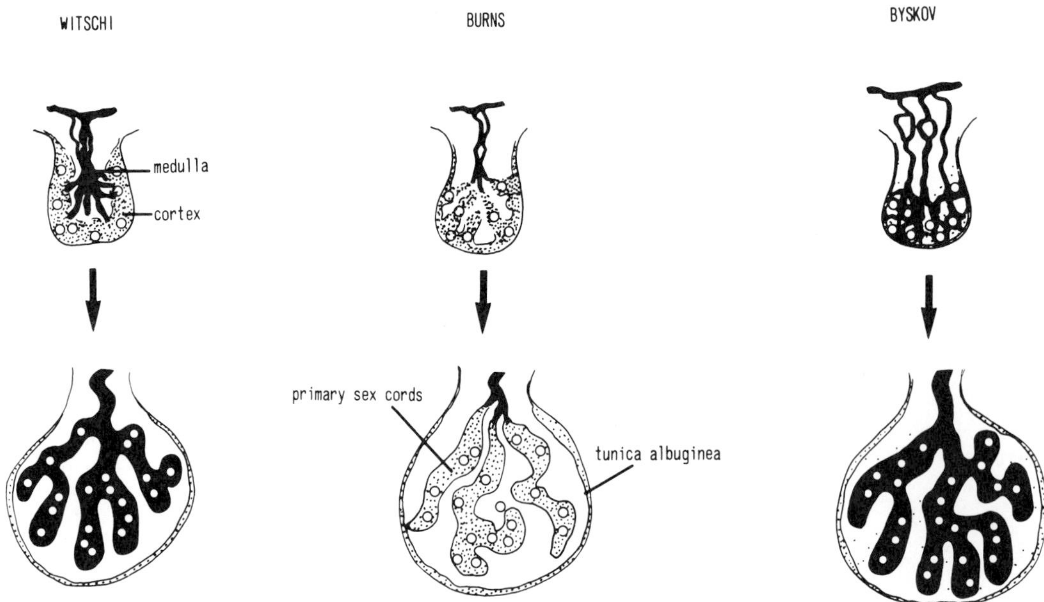

FIG. 21. Schematic drawings of models of testicular differentiation from Witschi (39,40), Burns (94), and Byskov (197). Witschi and Byskov propose that testicular somatic cells originate mainly in the mesonephros. In Witschi's model, epithelial-derived cortex degenerates whereas mesonephric-originated medulla proliferates. In Byskov's model, the epithelium never plays an important role. Burns suggests that surface epithelium proliferates to form primary sex cords, or medullary cords, which develop further into testicular cords. [Reprinted from A. G. Byskov, Differentiation of mammalian embryonic gonad. *Physiol. Rev.,* 66:71–117 (1986).]

germ cells may not be necessary for this process. Testicular cords form in mice in which very few germ cells are present, e.g., in certain mutations (171,172), after irradiation (119), or after treatment with busulphan (173). The trigger mechanism for the gathering of somatic and germ cells remains uncertain. It has been proposed that the male-specific cell surface histocompatibility antigen, H-Y antigen, of the Sertoli cells may play a role (see section entitled "Gonadal Sex Determination"). Clusterin, a glycoprotein (present in the rete testis fluid), which performs a cell-aggregating function and which is possibly secreted by the Sertoli cells, may play a role in the early gathering of germ cells (174). Testicular differentiation appears to be independent of the influence of gonadotrophins (175) and steroid hormones (66).

In the differentiating testis of the human embryo (14-mm crown-rump length), germ cells and presumptive Sertoli cells become tightly packed to form one single plate that, in the 30- to 35-mm embryo, is transformed into a network of anastomosing cords (176). In the newly differentiated fetal rat testis of day 17, the testicular cords are simple arch-formed structures that are arranged more or less perpendicular to the long axis of the testis and connected to the rete testis. During testicular growth, the arches grow in length and become more and more convoluted to form a palisade-like structure without anastomosis (177). Serial sections of the differentiating fetal mouse testis of day 13 indicate that the first aggregations form a few plates or simple arches (Fig. 22) perpendicular to the long axis, thus resembling the rat model.

The precise mechanisms involved in testicular cord formation are not known. However, ultrastructural studies indicate that the formation of an intact basal lamina surrounding the cords is an early and essential event [rat (178), pig (57,179)]. The process of the enclosure of testicular cords occurs fast. In the rat it takes less than 24 hr (178) and often results in cutting off cytoplasm that extends from the Sertoli cells (178,180). Simultaneously, a layer of microfilaments is seen in the Sertoli cells close to the basal surface of the cells. It was suggested that this filamentous layer participates in forming the testicular cords (181). Co-cultures of rat Sertoli cells and peritubular myoid cells indicated that the formation of the basal lamina requires a cooperativity between the two cell types (182). Another important morphogenic element in testicular cord formation may be the deposition of fibronectin in and along the site of the forming basal lamina (183). Throughout testicular differentiation the proximal ends of the testicular cords remain connected to the mesonephric-derived rete testis tissue, which in the human has been called the *rete blastema* (for review see ref. 60). Thus the mesonephric cells have "free access to the intratubular as well as the interstitial space contributing to the Sertoli cell and the Leydig cell precursor" (48). These mesonephric cells exhibit high NADH diaphorase activity in the 9-week-old human male (Fig. 23).

During early stages of testicular differentiation, the coelomic epithelium is connected to the testicular cords for a short period. In the rat the deposition of a continuous layer of fibronectin under the surface epithelium is seen simul-

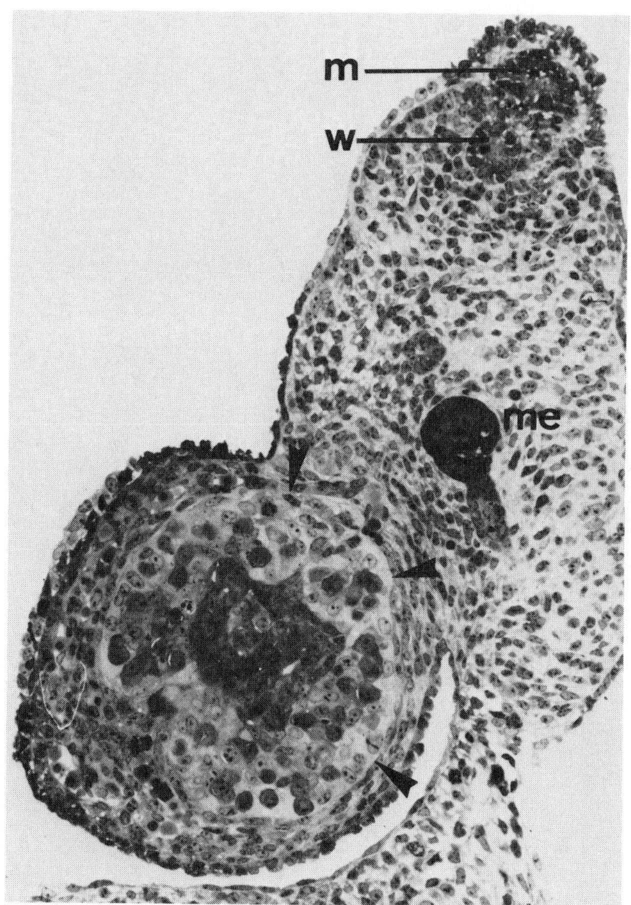

FIG. 22. Cross section of a testicular-mesonephric complex of a 12½-day-old mouse fetus. A newly differentiated testicular cord forms a simple arch (*arrowheads*). (me) Mesonephric tubule; (m) Müllerian duct; (w) Wolffian duct. ×400.

taneously with retraction of the testicular cords from the coelomic epithelium (183). At the same time, an increase in the formation of basal lamina material and other extracellular components is seen beneath the surface epithelium (183). These events represent the formation of the tunica albuginea.

As the testicular anlage grows, the vascularization becomes more prominent. In the fetal pig testis it was proposed that the ingrowing capillaries could stimulate the differentiation of the testicular cords (57). It was described that testicular cords are first differentiated in the periphery; this area is also the first to become vascularized.

The success of testicular cord formation seems to be correlated to an almost complete separation of the testicular tissue from the mesonephric tissue (180). Almost simultaneously with the cord formation the testis becomes rounded, whereby the connection to the mesonephros becomes thin. In the 14-day-old fetal mouse the testis consists only of a few tiny cell cords that connect the testicular cords with the developing tubules of the epididymis. In cultures of fetal undifferentiated mouse testes, testicular cord formation can be more or less prevented by leaving the mesonephros together with the testis. In such cultures, the separation between the testis and the mesonephros is unpaired; also, the testis does not become rounded and it retains a broad connection to the mesonephros (180). The formation of testicular cords *in vitro* can also be prevented in the rat by adding serum from rat and other species (86). Analogs of adenosine cyclic monophosphate also have a preventive effect on testicular cord formation in cultures of fetal mouse testes (184).

Prespermatogonia

When the male germ cells become enclosed in testicular cords they are termed *prespermatogonia* (185) (Fig. 24). If the germ cells are not enclosed in testicular cords, they invariably degenerate (see section entitled "Differentiation of the Testis"). However, enclosure itself does not necessarily ensure normal differentiation. During early testicular development, the prespermatogonia enter waves of mitotic divisions, and simultaneously they undergo morphological differentiation. These events are referred to as *prespermatogenesis* by Hilscher et al. (186), who studied this process in detail in the rat (see also ref. 187). In the fetal rodents [rat (187), mouse (188,189)], many prespermatogonia divide mitotically shortly after testicular differentiation. They are often gathered in clusters in which the cells divide synchronously. Like oogonia, they are connected by intercellular bridges (115,190–192) (Fig. 25). Around day 18 in the rat and day 50 in the pig, prespermatogonia enter the so-called "cap phase" (193), in which the nucleus becomes eccentric and other organelles agglomerate, forming a cap near the nucleus (Fig. 25). This phenomenon is also seen in the fetal pig prespermatogonia (103). The prespermatogonia in the cap phase of the rat are arrested in interphase containing 2c DNA [rat (187), mouse (194)]. Hereafter, virtually no mitoses are seen until the second proliferation wave of mitosis begins, shortly before puberty. The reaction for alkaline phosphatase remains positive in the prespermatogonia, whereas it is lost in diplotene oocytes (see subsection entitled "Transitory Stages of the Meiotic Prophase in Oocytes"). In contrast to oocytes in transitory stages of meiosis, the RNA synthesis remains low in prespermatogonia (109).

The pattern of proliferation of the prespermatogonia of other species (e.g., the rabbit and the pig) differs from that of the rat. In both these species the wave of mitotic divisions is delayed with respect to the time of testicular differentiation [rabbit (195), pig (108)]. This period corresponds to the delay period of the oocytes in these species. Thus, the wave of mitosis in prespermatogonia coincides in time with the onset of meiosis in the female (see section entitled "Control of Meiosis").

In a certain mouse strain (Hi line) it has been shown that in some mice an extended proliferation period of prespermatogonia is correlated to a high incidence of testicular teratomas (188). However, in another group of the same Hi

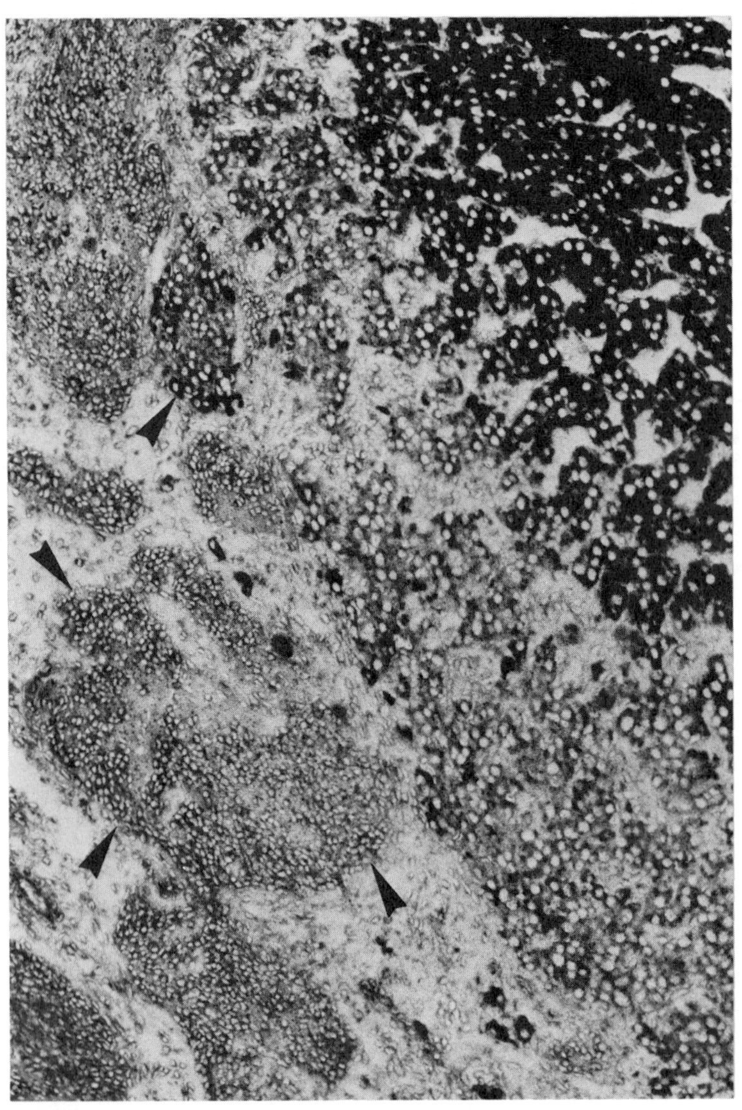

FIG. 23. Cryosection of a 9-week-old human fetal testis showing very strong NADH diaphorase activity in cells of the testicular cords (*upper right corner*). Strong activity is also present in the invading mesonephric cells (*arrowheads*). ×162.

line, about 12% of fetuses at 16 to 18 days of gestation had very few germ cells. All of these had testicular teratomas. It appears that germ cell proliferation must be strictly controlled to ensure their normal differentiation. However, the rate of germ cell degeneration during and shortly after proliferation is normally high [rat (196), rabbit (195)]. Although the reason for this high rate of degeneration is not known, it has been proposed that a certain ratio between germ cells and Sertoli cells is important for germ cell development (195).

Sertoli Cells

Somatic cells that are enclosed in testicular cords are termed *Sertoli cells*.

Like the granulosa cells, the origin of the Sertoli cells is still uncertain. Recent studies indicate that cells derived from the mesonephros contribute to the Sertoli cell population [mouse (52), sheep (46)]. Wartenberg proposed a dual origin of Sertoli cells in the human (44,197) and the rabbit (197), in which a dense dark cell population, the MI cells, could be distinguished from a population of light cells, the MP cells. He proposed that the MI cells (the putative meiosis-inducing cells derived from mesonephros) and the MP cells might be meiosis-preventing cells with origin in the coelomic epithelium. On the other hand, Jost (198) could not find a cellular marker of the dark cells which could trace them as mesonephric cells. However, Witschi (42) and Byskov (199) proposed that testicular somatic cells, including the Sertoli cells, are mainly derived from the mesonephros (for review see ref. 162).

The Sertoli cells proliferate throughout fetal and neonatal development, but when spermatogenesis begins, mitosis in Sertoli cells ceases (200–203). At the initial stages of testicular differentiation the Sertoli cells range from irregular to columnar in shape, with the germ cells embedded between them. Gradually their shape becomes increasingly irregular with cytoplasmic extensions protruding from the apical and lateral borders into neighboring Sertoli cells. This occurs

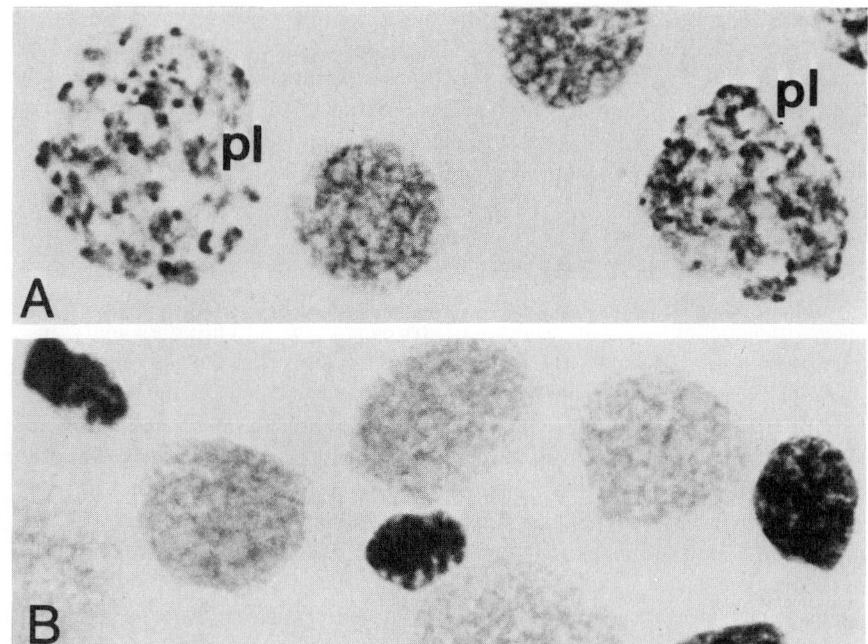

FIG. 24. Feulgen-stained squash preparations of fetal mouse testes showing prespermatogonia. ×5,000. (**A**) A 14½-day-old fetus with two prespermatogonia and two other germ cells in the early preleptotene (pl) stage. (**B**) A 19½-day-old fetus with several lightly stained prespermatogonia and dark somatic cells.

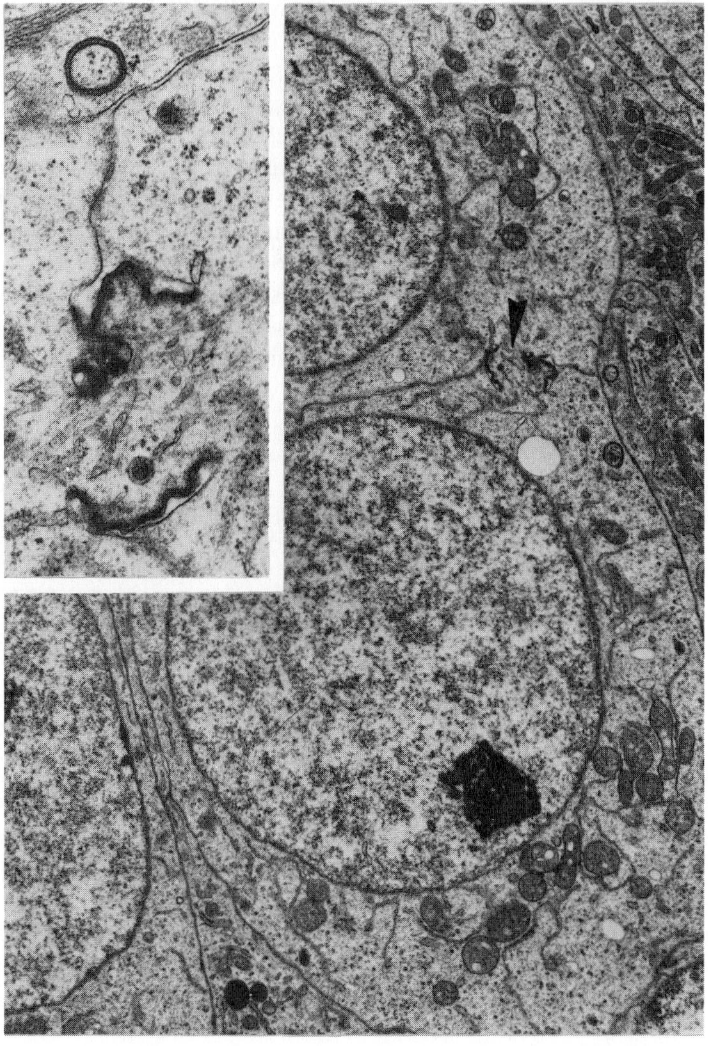

FIG. 25. Part of a testis of a 50-day-old fetal pig showing an intercellular bridge (*arrowhead*) between two prespermatogonia, the lower one having most organelles arranged at one side of its nucleus, thus forming a cap. ×7,640 (**Inset**) Higher magnification of the intercellular bridge. ×30,000.

simultaneously with the changed position of the prespermatogonia from a central to a peripheral location (204). Initially the Sertoli cells are only involved in the formation of desmosomes (205), but gradually the development of incomplete tight junctions and small gap junctions occurs (206). The "tight" junctions lack the parallel and interlacing pattern characteristic of occlusive tight junctions of the fully differentiated Sertoli cells of the adult testis (206). Thus, the fetal Sertoli cells have not yet developed the complex junction attachments, which later form the blood-testis barrier in the adult. It has been proposed that the rearrangement of germ cells from a central to a peripheral position may be caused by a series of formations and disruptions of Sertoli cell junctions (206).

Initially, the ultrastructure of the Sertoli cells resembles that of mesenchymal cells, with a paucity of organelles [rabbit (207), rat (205,208), pig (57,103)]. During later stages, the rough endoplasmic reticulum becomes more prominent, showing a peak in development, which coincides in time with a peak in testosterone production (209,210) and secretion of a protein, the anti-Müllerian hormone (see the subsection entitled "Müllerian Duct" in the section on male differentiation of genital ducts). Simultaneously close approximations between the endoplasmic reticulum and the plasma membrane has been observed in the pig (103) (Fig. 26).

Little information is available concerning steroidogenic capacity of the fetal Sertoli cells. Androgen secretion was found in explanted fetal guinea-pig testes at a stage when no Leydig cells were distinguishable (211). It was suggested that the androgens came from the prospective Leydig cells, although all cell types destined to form testicular cords, including pre-Sertoli cells, were also present. On the other hand, a transitory high activity of 3β-hydroxysteroid dehydrogenase has been detected in the newly formed testicular cord of fetal pig testes before the early differentiation of Leydig cells takes place (212). Moreover, in the early fetal guinea pig, Black and Christensen (213) observed that some Sertoli cells resembled differentiating Leydig cells with regard to some structural features that may be related to steroidogenesis.

Leydig Cells

In contrast to the ovary, the steroid-producing cells of the testis, namely the Leydig cells, develop shortly after gonadal sex differentiation has taken place. They can first be recognized between the testicular cords in the center of the testis as rounded cells with a dense cytoplasm. The origin of the Leydig precursor cells has not yet been clarified. They may arise from mesenchymal cells [human (163,214), pig, (57)] or from mesonephric cells [human, rabbit (197); mouse (49); sheep (46)]. The Leydig cells only proliferate during early stages of differentiation. After birth, mitotic figures in Leydig cells are virtually not seen (204). The differentiating Leydig cells rapidly gain typical morphological appearance of steroid-producing cells, with abundant agranular endoplasmic reticulum, mitochondria with tubular cristae, and lipid droplets (for review see ref. 163) (Fig. 27). Small aggregates of particles as well as gap junctions have been detected on the plasma membrane of differentiating rabbit Leydig cells (112). Gap junctions are also present between differentiated fetal human Leydig cells around the 15th week of fetal life (Figs. 27 and 28). The rise in testosterone secretion by the testis is closely correlated with cytodifferentiation and increase in volume of the Leydig cells (185,215–217) as well as increase in their number (218). Similarly, testosterone secretion declines when the Leydig cells de-differentiate during late fetal life (207,219).

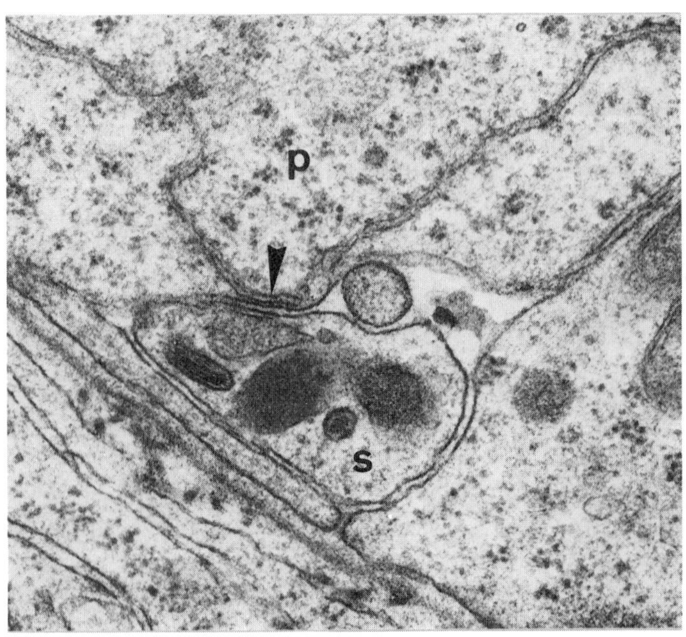

FIG. 26. Peripheral part of a testicular cord from a 50-day-old fetal pig testis. The endoplasmic reticulum of a Sertoli cell (s) and a prespermatogonium (p) are in close proximity to the plasma membranes (*arrowhead*). ×50,000.

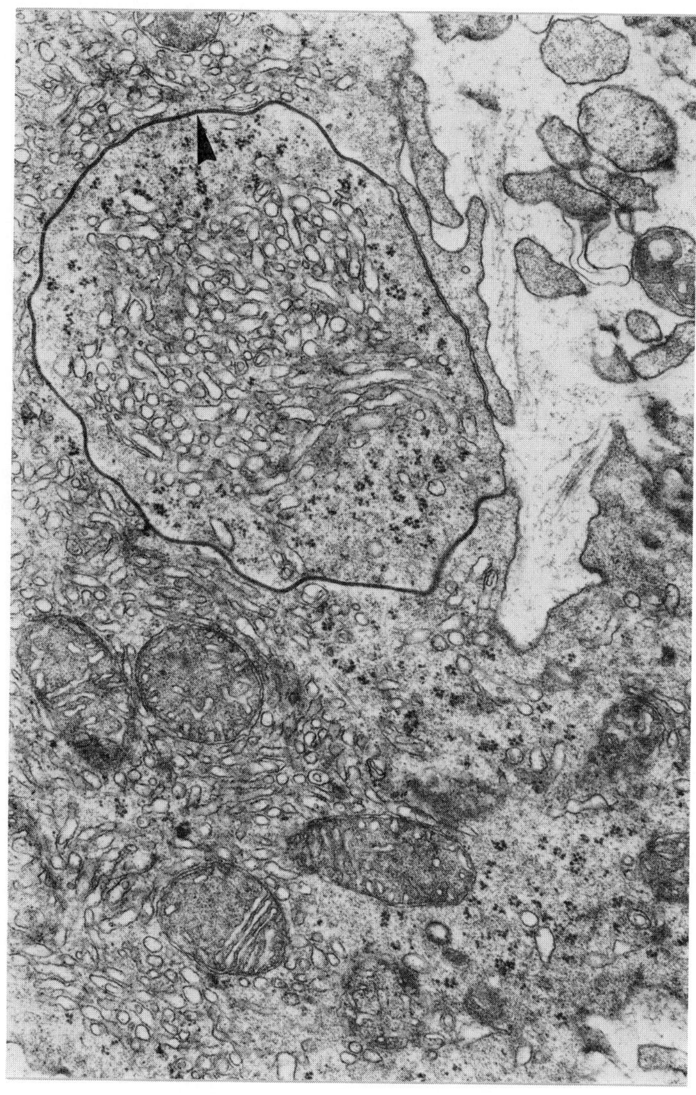

FIG. 27. Leydig cells of a 15-week-old human fetal testis showing abundant agranular endoplasmic reticulum, mitochondria with tubular cristae, and a gap junction between two adjacent cells (*arrowhead*). ×18,400.

The well-differentiated Leydig cells also exhibit high activity of 3β-hydroxysteroid dehydrogenase, NADPH and NADH diaphorases, and glucose-6-phosphate dehydrogenase (220,221) (Figs. 29 and 30). At the same time, high alkaline phosphatase activity is present in the plasma membrane of the Leydig cells (Fig. 8). What triggers the differentiation of the Leydig cells is not known. However, testicular cord formation always precedes the morphological differentiation of Leydig cells. Cultures of minced fetal mouse testes, in which the structure of the testicular cords is disrupted, produce significantly less testosterone, but more progesterone, than do cultures of intact testes (180). The mitochondria of Leydig cells in the minced testes have laminar cristae, and the endoplasmic reticulum is mainly of the granular type, indicating that impaired testicular cord formation influences functional and morphological differentiation of the Leydig cells.

In vitro, testicular cord formation of the fetal mouse testis is also impaired if a low dose of progesterone (2 μg/ml) is added to the culture medium (222), whereas higher doses do not interfere. Thus, with respect to testicular cord formation, it may be crucial that steroidogenesis by the fetal Leydig cells is delayed.

In the fetal rat testis *in vitro,* testicular cord formation can be prevented when the testicular anlage is cultured in a medium containing fetal calf serum (223,224), human serum, or an α-globulin fraction of human serum (184). In such cordless testes, cells exhibiting 3β-hydroxysteroid dehydrogenase activity can be traced, but production of testosterone is considerably lower than in the control cultures (225). It was, however, concluded that cytodifferentiation of the Leydig cells does not depend on normal differentiation of testicular cords.

The influence of gonadotrophins on Leydig cell differentiation and maintenance has been studied in many species (162). The concentration of chorionic gonadotrophin peaks shortly before Leydig cells differentiate (226); by that time, gonadotrophin receptors are present in fetal testicular cells (227,228). Furthermore, *in vitro* studies of hormone production by fetal rabbit testes indicate that some extrinsic

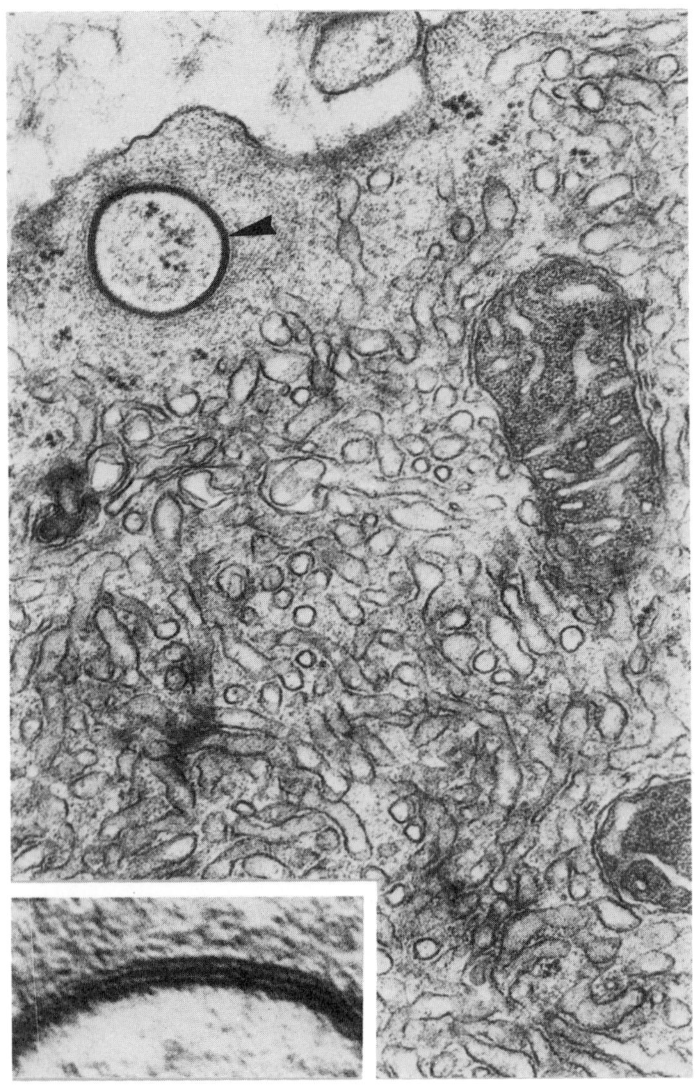

FIG. 28. Peripheral part of the cytoplasm from a Leydig cell of a 15-week-old human fetal testis showing a gap junction between two adjacent cells, one of which forms a finger-like protrusion into the other (*arrowhead*). ×45,600. Inset shows higher magnification of part of the gap junction. ×182,400.

factors initiate steroid synthesis by the fetal testis (54,226). In anencephalic male fetuses, in which the concentration of gonadotrophins is low, few Leydig cells are present (170). Hypophysectomy of fetal monkeys (229) and decapitation of fetal rabbits (175) and fetal monkeys (230) result in depletion of Leydig cells, indicating that the pituitary gland of the fetus is needed for maintenance of Leydig cells. By contrast, in the syndrome of testicular feminization due to lack of androgen receptors, the number of Leydig cells is greatly increased (Fig. 31) and the concentration of gonadotrophins is higher than normal (67). These two conditions also suggest the importance of gonadotrophic stimulation of Leydig cell differentiation and maintenance.

CONTROL OF MEIOSIS

The time at which the first germ cells enter meiosis differs not only between sexes but also between females of different species (see sections entitled "Female Germ Cells" and "Male Germ Cells"). Generally, meiosis begins early in life in the female, whereas in the male, meiosis does not start until puberty. This paradigm has led to the theory that an "internal clock" of the germ cells might regulate meiosis (10). The finding that ectopic mouse germ cells of both sexes, which are localized to the fetal adrenal gland, begin meiosis at the same time that female germ cells enter meiosis in the ovary (231) apparently substantiates the concept that a "meiotic clock" operates autonomously. However, a meiosis-inducing substance has been detected in the fetal human adrenal glands of both sexes at the time when female meiosis starts (L. Westergaard et al., *unpublished results*). It is therefore uncertain whether the germ cells that enter meiosis in the fetal adrenal gland are triggered by a so-called "internal clock" or by substances produced by the somatic cells, as proposed by Tarkowski (232).

The factors that control the different timing of onset of meiosis in female and male germ cells may depend on their genetic constitution. In the female germ cells it seems that both X chromosomes must be active before meiosis begins

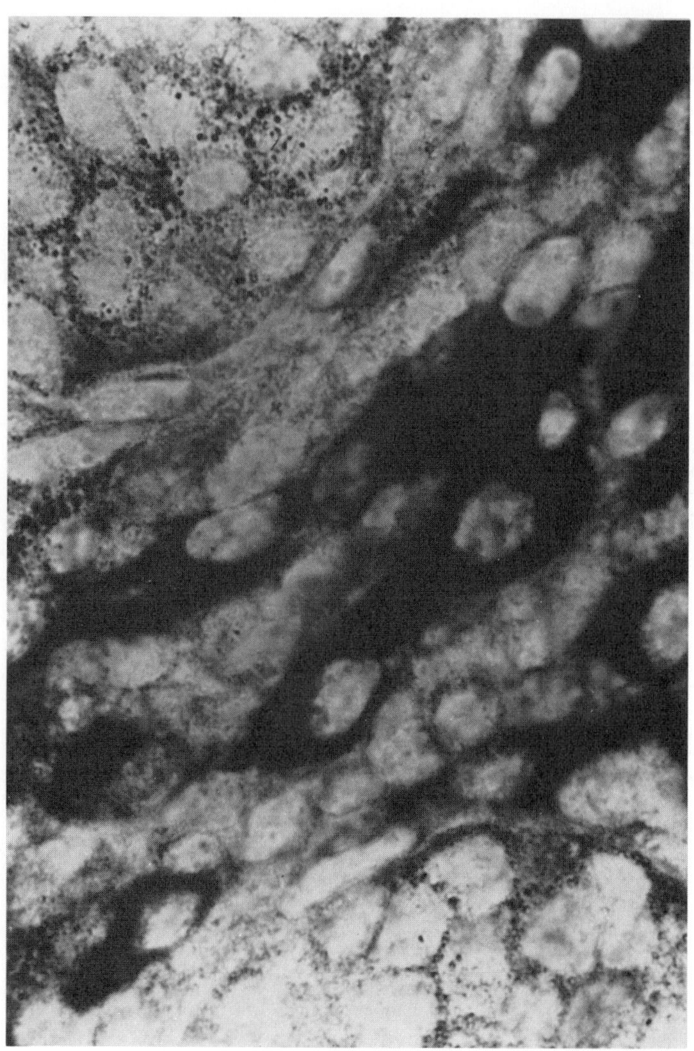

FIG. 29. Cryosection of a 12-week-old human fetal testis showing very strong NADH diaphorase activity in the Leydig cells (*center*). Cells of the testicular cords (*top, bottom*) also show activity. ×1,244.

(14,22,233). However, male germ cells may enter meiosis simultaneously with the female germ cells if they are situated in the vicinity of the mesonephric tissue, outside the testicular cords (234).

It is conceivable that control of meiosis is not controlled by a single parameter but that a series of factors are interacting, such as a "genetic clock," the formation of a specific micromilieu around the germ cells, and the secretion of steroids and specific meiosis-regulating substances. With respect to the latter, meiosis-inducing substances (MIS) can be prepared from media in which ovaries or testes with germ cells undergoing meiosis have been cultured (101). In a similar manner, a meiosis-preventing substance (MPS) is produced by fetal testes in which meiosis is held in abeyance (234). The activity of the two substances is evaluated by their ability to induce or prevent meiosis in cultured fetal mouse testes or ovaries, respectively (86). Although the nature of the two substances is not yet fully understood, different experiments indicate that MIS is a small molecule (less than 2,000 daltons), with hydrophilic as well as hydrophobic characteristics, and that MPS is a small peptide (222). MIS and MPS are apparently not species specific because media containing these substances (obtained from testes of bulls and humans) induce and prevent (respectively) meiosis in fetal mouse testes/ovaries (85).

Female Germ Cells

The first germ cells that enter meiosis in the fetal ovary are always seen in the central basal part of the ovary, close to the mesonephric connection (for review see ref. 162). Gradually more peripherally situated oogonia enter meiosis (Fig. 14). For instance, in the human fetal ovary, the first meiotic germ cells are seen around the third month, whereas peripherally situated germ cells are still entering meiosis during the eighth month (35). Therefore, if an "internal clock" does exist, it must obviously be influenced by factors of the local environment. The old observations that meiosis is initiated close to the mesonephric connection led to the hypothesis that mesonephric-derived cells induce meiosis (104). In support of this theory are the findings that meiosis

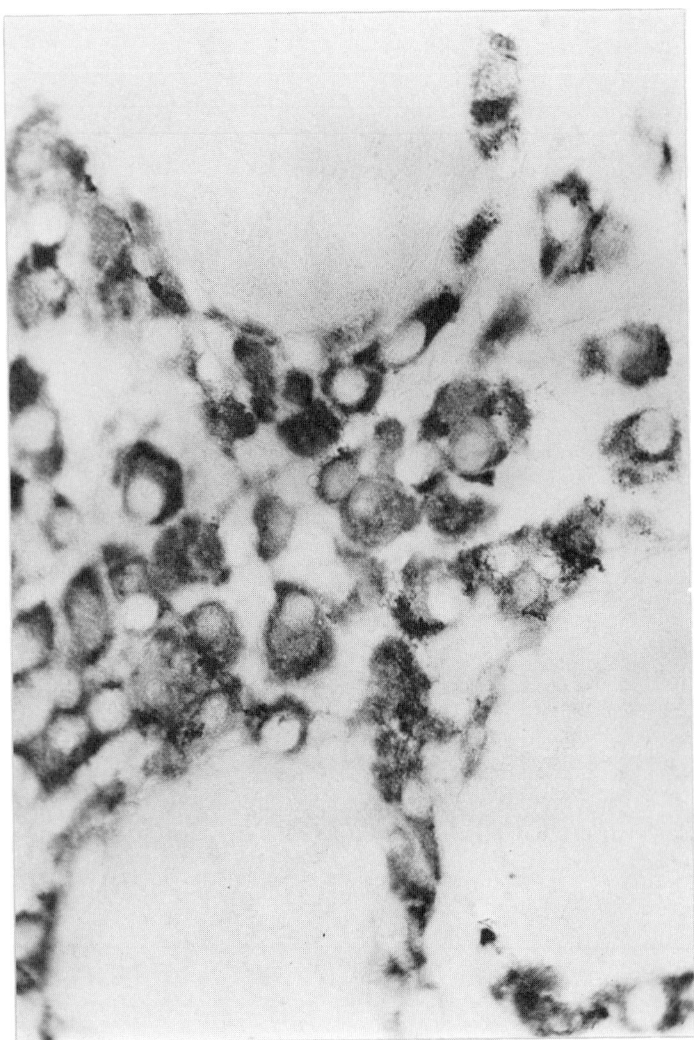

FIG. 30. Cryosection of a 12-week-old human fetal testis showing NADPH diaphorase activity in the Leydig cells, whereas cells of the testicular cords show no or very low activity. ×496.

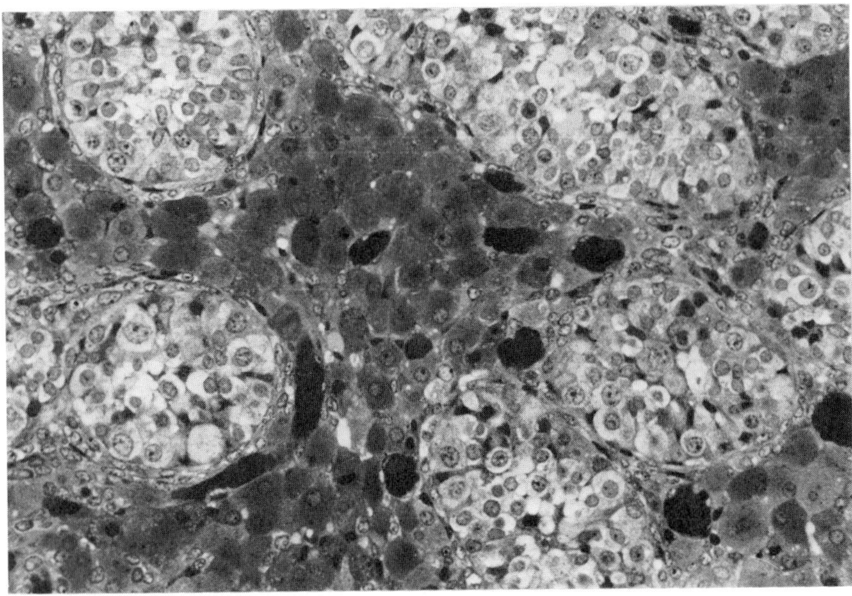

FIG. 31. Part of the testis from a 20-week-old human fetus with testicular feminization. The number and size of the Leydig cells are greatly increased. ×500.

in cultures of fetal ovaries is dependent on the presence of mesonephric tissue in the mouse (53) and hamster (235). However, in other species, meiosis appears not to be influenced by the mesonephros [rat (236), rabbit (102)]. This discrepancy may be related to the pattern of ovarian development in different species, e.g., between species with immediate and delayed meiosis (see section entitled "Different Patterns of Early Ovarian Differentiation"). In the rabbit ovary, which exhibits delayed meiosis, it has not been possible to induce meiosis during the delay period (102). This may be a result of the enclosure of germ cells in cord-like structures, which may create an unfavorable milieu comparable to the conditions in the fetal testicular cords. As mentioned in the sections entitled "Different Patterns of Early Ovarian Differentiation" and "Ovary," steroids are secreted by ovaries during the delay period. Apparently, onset of meiosis does not occur when substantial amounts of steroids are produced by the ovary.

That an MIS is secreted by ovaries at the time when meiosis begins has been shown in co-cultures between fetal mouse ovaries and testes: Ovaries containing germ cells in early stages of meiosis induce meiosis in the male germ cells of co-cultured fetal testes (101). MIS is also present in follicular fluid of preovulatory follicles of human and cow at about 6 hr after the preovulatory gonadotrophic peak (237,238).

The hypothesis has been advanced that meiosis of female germ cells is triggered by MIS and arrested in the diplotene stage by the action of MPS (102) or the so-called *oocyte maturation inhibitor* (OMI), produced by the granulosa cells (239; for review see ref. 240). Thus, meiosis of female germ cells may be controlled by the relative concentration of MIS and MPS (102).

Male Germ Cells

Normally the male germ cells do not enter meiosis until puberty. However, meiotic germ cells are seen in fetal testes of different species at the same time that meiosis begins in the ovary of the coeval female fetus [mouse (129), cat (18), human (241)]. Such meiotic male germ cells are situated outside the testicular cords, in close apposition to the mesonephric tissue (129). As in the female, it seems likely that MIS is produced by the mesonephric-derived tissue and that male germ cells are able to respond to the substance by entering meiosis. The reason that germ cells within testicular cords do not enter meiosis may be due to the presence of MPS within the testicular cords (234). The presence of MPS in testes has been demonstrated in fetal testes co-cultured with fetal ovaries in which meiosis became inhibited (101) and in immature and adult testes that secrete MPS during short-time cultures (86). Since MIS is also produced by the pubertal and adult testes it is possible that also in the testis, meiosis may be regulated by the relative concentration of these two substances.

EARLY STEROID HORMONE PRODUCTION BY THE GONADS

Ovary

For a long time it has been assumed that the fetal ovary was incapable of *de novo* synthesis of steroids. The human fetal ovary, for instance, has been reported to secrete steroids only in the last part of fetal life (242). However, other species, namely those with delayed meiosis, often produce large amounts of estrogen at early stages of ovarian differentiation during the delay period [sheep (243), rabbit (55,165), cow (244), guinea pig (245)]. Obviously the time at which *de novo* steroid synthesis begins varies greatly between species. However, the enclosure of germ cells in specific compartments (either germ cell cords or follicles) seems to play a major role in differentiation of the steroid-producing cells. In primates in which specific germ cell cords are not formed, and in which meiosis begins early, estradiol production *de novo* is not seen until follicles begin to grow late in fetal life (246–248), but the aromatizing system responsible for conversion of androgens to estrogens is already active at the eighth week of fetal life (249). In ovaries of other species, steroid production *de novo* is nil or very low during the period when meiosis occurs [mouse (250), rat (251)].

Early *de novo* steroid production in species with delayed meiosis takes place only during the delay period, when germ cells are enclosed in cord-like structures. By the end of the delay period when meiosis begins, the steroid production decreases or ceases, but it raises again when follicles form (244).

It is not known how steroid synthesis is initiated in the ovary. Thus, it is unclear whether the high level of hCG present before and during early differentiation of the fetal ovary initiates steroid production, but similar to those in the human, the ovaries of these species possess very early the enzymes necessary for conversion of androgens to estrogens [guinea pig (252), rat (253)] (Fig. 32).

Fetal ovarian steroid synthesis by rabbit (209) and rat (251) seems independent of gonadotrophins, whereas gonadotrophins stimulate steroid synthesis by the fetal mouse ovary (250). On the other hand, estradiol production by the fetal bovine ovary is stimulated by luteinizing hormone (LH) during the delay period, but the ovary becomes refractory by the end of the delay period (244). Steroid synthesis by the fetal pig ovary *in vitro* is enhanced by exposure to hCG or LH (254) during the delay period.

It is not known to what extent fetal ovarian cells utilize other steroids, e.g., those that originate in the liver (255) or in the adrenal cortex (256).

Testis

In all the mammalian species that have been studied, the newly sex-differentiated testis is able to synthesize testosterone *de novo* from acetate (for review see ref. 257). Tes-

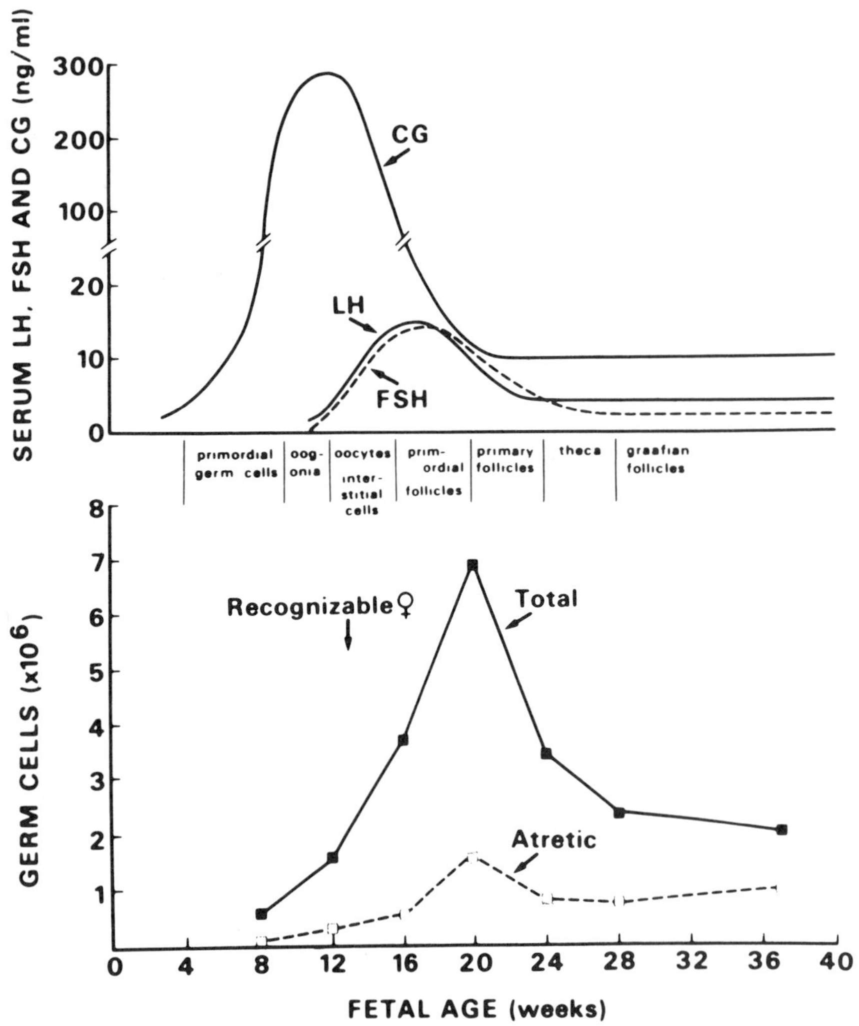

FIG. 32. Schematic summary of the temporal relationship in the female human fetus between mean serum concentrations of: hCG (CG), LH, and FSH; ovarian morphology; and the ovarian content of germ cells. [From J. S. D. Winter, C. Faiman, and F. I. Reyes, Sex steroid production by the human fetus: Its role in morphogenesis and control by gonadotropins. In: *Morphogenesis and Malformation of the Genital System,* edited by R. J. Blandau and D. Bergsma, Alan R. Liss, New York, for The National Foundation–March of Dimes, BD:OAS 13(2):41–58 (1977).]

ticular steroids are responsible for maintenance of growth and differentiation of the internal and external genitalia (64–66,258). Moreover, testicular androgens are necessary for priming the brain in the male direction (259–262). In addition, hormones or substances of testicular origin may control testicular descent from the abdominal position into scrotum (263,264).

As in the ovary, the mechanisms that cause initiation of the steroid synthesis in the fetal testis are not known. *In vitro* experiments have shown that steroid production by sex-differentiated testes can be stimulated by hCG and LH (for review see ref. 265). It is possible that in the human, hCG stimulates fetal androgen production by the testis, because the rise, peak, and fall in hCG content are closely mirrored by testosterone secretion [human (266)] (Fig. 33). In cultures of hCG-treated human fetal testicular tissues, the secretion of testosterone is facilitated by low-density lipoprotein (LDL) cholesterol (267). Since the content of LDL receptors fluctuates with the level of hCG, it is possible that the concentration of LDL cholesterol is regulated by hCG (267). The content of gonadotrophin receptors in fetal testicular tissue rises concomitantly with increasing testosterone secretion. In the human, for example, the number of hCG receptors and the amount of testosterone both reach a peak between the 15th and the 18th week of gestation (268). In the fetal rat the content of LH receptors rises simultaneously with increase in testosterone secretion, but the content of LH receptors continues to increase until after birth, whereas the levels of intratesticular testosterone and hCG decrease (269). The fall in placental hCG during the latter part of fetal life seems to be crucial for the decrease of testosterone production. This may be of particular importance because fetal Leydig cells, at least *in vitro,* remain sensitive to hCG stimulation. In contrast to the adult, cultured fetal Leydig cells of human, monkey, and rat are able to respond to sustained concentration of gonadotrophin by testosterone production without being desensitized (270).

The time at which the peak of testosterone occurs during fetal life also seems to be very important for maturation of the central nervous system. In rat fetuses of stressed mothers, in which the surge of testosterone appears earlier than normal, the male offspring achieves a feminized behavioral pattern (262). Other steroids (e.g., from fetal adrenal gland) may also interfere with testosterone production, since fetal

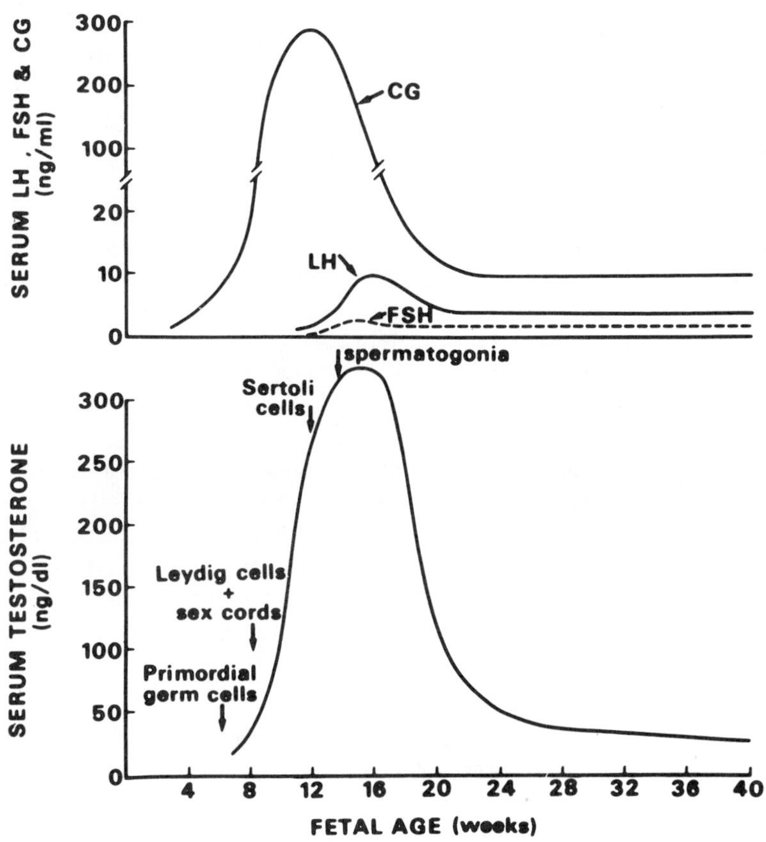

FIG. 33. Schematic summary of the temporal relationship in the male human fetus between mean serum concentrations of hCG (CG), LH, and FSH and of mean serum concentration of testosterone and testicular morphology. [From J. S. D. Winter, C. Faiman, and F. I. Reyes, Sex steroid production by the human fetus: Its role in morphogenesis and control by gonadotropins. In: *Morphogenesis and Malformation of the Genital System,* edited by R. J. Blandau and D. Bergsma, Alan R. Liss, New York, for The National Foundation–March of Dimes, BD:OAS 13(2):41–58 (1977).]

rat testes secrete more testosterone after stimulation with adrenocorticotrophin (271).

FORMATION AND DIFFERENTIATION OF GENITAL DUCTS

Undifferentiated Ducts

The primordia of the genital ducts, namely the Müllerian duct and the Wolffian duct, do not arise simultaneously. The Wolffian duct is the excretory duct of the mesonephros (see subsection entitled "Mesonephros"); it is recognizable before the gonads form. After gonadal sex differentiation, it differentiates into the internal genital tract in the male, whereas in the female the main part degenerates (Fig. 11). The Müllerian duct (i.e., the paramesonephric duct) develops in a cranial-caudal direction along the Wolffian duct around the time when the gonads form. It is likely that the Wolffian duct serves as guidance for this early growth (272). In fact, fusions of plasma membranes of cells from the Wolffian and Müllerian ducts have been observed in the fetal rat in the area where the tip of the Müllerian duct grows caudally (272). The Wolffian duct may even contribute cells to the developing Müllerian duct (273–275). The Müllerian duct serves as anlage of the female genital duct system, whereas in the male it degenerates.

The initial formation of the Müllerian duct appears to start by invagination of the coelomic epithelium lateral to the cranial end of the mesonephric duct. This invagination persists in the female and develops into the abdominal ostium (276). However, in the fetal rabbit, the anlage of the Müllerian duct seems to arise from a cell cord which develops in close contact to the cranial part of the Wolffian duct (A. G. Byskov and P. E. Høyer, *unpublished results*). A similar pattern of development has been described in the chick (277). When the caudal blind tips of the Müllerian ducts reach the pelvic area, they have thus crossed ventrally to the Wolffian ducts to reach and fuse with each other in the midline dorsocranially to the urogenital sinus.

At early stages of differentiation, both mesonephric and paramesonephric ducts are simple, straight tubules lined with a single-layered epithelium consisting of cells ranging from squamous to cylindrical. As they grow, the epithelium becomes taller, with the nuclei situated in the basal part. The epithelial cells of the early Wolffian duct of rat and mouse are rich in glycogen, dense bodies, and lysosomes (278). The rat Müllerian duct has a tiny lumen at the time of sex differentiation. The tightly packed columnar cells are rich in free ribosomes and contain a well-developed supranuclear Golgi apparatus (279). Parallel to the epithelial growth, mesenchymal cells are arranged in concentric layers around the ducts. Further differentiation of the genital ducts is dependent on mesenchymal-epithelial interaction, in which the mesenchyme probably is the target and mediator of morphogenic action by hormones and other substances (for review see ref. 280).

Female Differentiation of Genital Ducts

Female Müllerian Duct (Fig. 2)

In the female the cranial part of the Müllerian duct develops into the oviduct, or the fallopian tubes, the middle part develops into the uterus, and the caudal part may contribute to the cranial part of the vagina. In some species the Müllerian tubes remain separated as paired uteri (e.g., mouse and rat), whereas in others they fuse to form a simplex type of uterus (281). The early differentiating oviduct can be distinguished from the uterus by its coiling and smaller diameter. A muscular layer develops around the oviductal tubules, the epithelium of which invaginates and folds. The epithelial cells may either develop cilia or later become secretory (282). Relatively early in development the oviduct differentiates into three segments: the infundibulum, the ampulla, and the isthmus. In humans and the guinea pig, both of which have an extended gestational period, most of these developmental steps occur during the midgestational period. In species that have a shorter gestation (e.g., the hamster, the mouse, and the rat), differentiation of the oviduct takes place after birth (282).

Differentiation of the uterus starts simultaneously with that of the oviduct. The junction between uterus and oviduct early becomes clearly distinguishable by the abrupt increase in uterine diameter. Demarcation between uterus and vagina takes place later; in the human, this occurs in the latter part of the third month (283), when the vaginal fornices develop. In the human fetus, at about 9½ weeks the uterus begins to differentiate into an upper part (the corpus) and a lower part (the cervix) (284). They are both initially the same length, but the cervix gradually reaches two-thirds of the total length at birth (281). During the second trimester the main components, such as glands and muscular coat, develop. Glands are first seen in the cervical part at 17 weeks, then appear about 2 weeks later in the corpus. At midgestation, mesenchyme surrounding both Wolffian and Müllerian ducts condenses and forms the early muscular layer of the uterus (281). The growing muscular layer of the upper part of the corpus participates in formation of the convex-shaped fundus (284). During the third trimester, mucinous cells appear in the cervix, whereas secretory cells only occasionally are seen in the endometrium at birth. These cytological characteristics may be induced by either estrogens and/or progesterone (285). However, it is not certain how endometrial growth and differentiation are controlled during earlier stages of fetal life.

Early development and growth of the Müllerian duct is generally considered to occur autonomously (286). Apparently, no stimulation is required for differentiation of the female genital tract. Neither decapitation nor castration of fetal female rabbit fetuses prevented growth of the Müllerian duct (64,175). Normal development also takes place in genital tracts of fetal rat cultured in steroid-free culture medium (287). Therefore, neither gonadotrophins nor the ovary are necessary for differentiation of the female genital tract (288). Although the development of paramesonephric ducts is not an estrogen-dependent process (64), estrogen receptors have been detected in Müllerian ducts of fetal rats (286) and guinea pigs (289) during the last part of gestation. However, in a recent *in vitro* study of fetal mouse genital ridges it was shown that growth and differentiation of the oviduct is influenced by the ovary when placed closely together. Newly differentiated fetal mouse ovaries stimulate growth of the stromal tissue of the female duct system, whereas older fetal ovaries suppress growth of both Müllerian duct epithelium and the surrounding stroma (290). Whether an anti-Müllerian hormone (AMH) might be secreted by the ovary in very low concentrations is not known. Anyhow, that the fetal female Müllerian duct can respond to AMH was shown in the classical experiments by Jost (64): Grafts of fetal rabbit testes into fetal rabbit females, close to the genital ducts, induced degeneration of the female Müllerian duct, whereas implants of crystals of testosterone had no effect.

Female Wolffian Duct

During normal female development, the Wolffian duct invariably degenerates because of the lack of androgens. Degeneration begins shortly after gonadal sex differentiation (Fig. 2). In the human it is generally finished in the beginning of the third trimester (278). However, before degeneration is completed, the caudal part of the Wolffian duct gives origin to the ureteric bud and contributes to the bladder and urethra (276). It may also be incorporated in the vaginal plate (291). The Wolffian duct of both sexes of rabbits castrated early in fetal life degenerates unless exposed to implants of testosterone (64). Moreover, in cultures of genital ridges of fetal rats (292,293) and mice, growth and differentiation of the Wolffian duct only occurs when cocultured with testicular tissue or by adding testosterone.

Male Differentiation of Genital Ducts

Male Wolffian Duct

In the male, the cranial part of the Wolffian duct develops into the epididymis, the central portion becomes the vas deferens, and the caudal part forms the ejaculatory duct and the seminal vesicle. Some of the cranial mesonephric tubules, which are connected to the rete testis, are retained as efferent ductules of the epididymis. During differentiation of the epididymis, the Wolffian duct grows in length and becomes heavily convoluted. The epithelium of the duct is columnar and develops numerous microvilli and later develops cilia [rat (294), sheep (295)]. In the human, secretory activity is seen in the third trimester (296). The epididymal duct becomes surrounded by concentrically arranged mesenchymal cells that differentiate into a thin layer of smooth muscle cells. The connection between epididymis and vas deferens becomes clearly marked by the formation of trilaminar smooth muscle layers of the latter duct (297).

The primitive seminal vesicle arises from a distention of the caudal portion of the Wolffian duct, which in the human fetus occurs at the 60-mm stage (62). The seminal vesicle is covered by a tall nonsecretory columnar epithelium with a well-defined basement membrane (298). During differentiation the lumen of the seminal vesicle gradually attains a complicated folded form.

In the human, the caudal part of the Wolffian duct, which becomes the ejaculatory duct, is not clearly demarcated from the seminal vesicle until the third trimester (299). In contrast to the cranial part, no secretory granules are seen during fetal life (299).

Growth and differentiation of the Wolffian duct is controlled by testosterone. This was shown in fetal rabbits (64) and in rats, *in vitro* (292,293) (see section entitled "Female Differentiation of Genital Ducts"). It is testosterone itself and not dihydrotestosterone (DHT) that is responsible for differentiation of the Wolffian duct (300–302). The Wolffian duct becomes dependent on testosterone during the period immediately after sex differentiation, the "critical period," simultaneously with degeneration of the mesonephros (for review see ref. 38). The enzyme that metabolizes testosterone to DHT, namely 5α-reductase, only appears after "stabilization" of the Wolffian duct (297), which occurs during the critical period.

Male Müllerian Duct

In normal males the Müllerian ducts begin regression shortly after testicular differentiation. The regression depends on secretion of a specific Müllerian inhibitor, which is not testosterone (64). This inhibitor is a glycoprotein mentioned earlier in this chapter, namely AMH; it has a molecular weight of about 70,000 daltons (303). It is secreted by the Sertoli cells (304–306) and is interspecies specific, because AMH from one species can induce regression of the Müllerian duct of other species (307,308). These activities of AMH have mainly been assayed *in vitro* using $14\frac{1}{2}$-day-old fetal rat Müllerian ducts (287,305,309).

The Müllerian duct is sensitive to AMH only during a limited period after gonadal sex differentiation. Exposure before or after this critical period is ineffective (310,311). Studies on grafted human embryonic reproductive tracts indicate that the effect of AMH is permanent and irreversible (311).

However, in some species the AMH is produced for an extended period, even when there is no Müllerian duct tissue left (312). It has been proposed that this delayed secretion of AMH might serve other purposes, e.g., inhibition of meiosis (313) and initiation of testicular descent (297,305).

One of the first signs of regression of the Müllerian duct is formation of densely packed fibroblasts around the duct (314,315), indicating that the mesenchyme is an important target in the action of AMH (316). Concomitant with the periductal condensation of mesenchyme, a degradation of the extracellular matrix in this area takes place (317). Biochemical studies indicate that AMH may act by dephosphorylation of membrane proteins (318). In addition, histochemical studies have shown that the membrane-bound enzyme nucleotide pyrophosphatase, which exhibits a broad hydrolytic activity, is localized over the regressing male Müllerian duct of the rat, but absent in the female Müllerian duct (319).

The effect of AMH on male Müllerian duct can be prevented by exogenous estrogens (320). The Müllerian ducts persist in males which have been exposed to diethylstilbestrol (DES), a synthetic estrogen, during fetal life (321,322). Also in mice carrying the testicular feminized mutation gene (Tfm), prenatal exposure to DES inhibits regression of the Müllerian duct (323). Thus, the regression of the Müllerian ducts in males must occur during a critical period of development and depends on a proper hormonal balance.

ACKNOWLEDGMENTS

We wish to thank Hanne Tinggaard and Birgitte Olsen for technical assistance, Keld B. Ottesen for preparing the illustrations, and Karen Grüning and Lotte Nellemann for typing the manuscript.

REFERENCES

1. Nussbaum, M. (1880): Die Differenzierung des Geschlechts im Tierreich. *Arch. Mikrosk. Anat.*, 18:1–121.
2. Rauh, W. (1929): Ursprung des weiblichen Keimzellen und die chromatischen Vorgänge bis zur Entwicklung der Synapsisstadium. Beobachtet an des Ratte (*Mus decum alb.*). *Z. Anat.*, 78:637–668.
3. Eddy, E. M., and Clark, J. M. (1975): Electron microscopic study of migrating germ cells in the rat. In: *Electron Microscopic Concepts of Secretion. Ultrastructure of Endocrine and Reproductive Organs*, edited by M. Hess, pp. 151–167. John Wiley & Sons, New York.
4. Zamboni, L., and Merchant, H. (1973): The fine morphology of mouse primordial germ cells in extragonadal locations. *Am. J. Anat.*, 137:299–335.
5. Chiquoine, A. D. (1954): The identification, origin and migration of the primordial germ cells in the mouse embryo. *Anat. Rec.*, 118:135–145.
6. Mintz, B., and Russell, E. S. (1957): Gene induced embryological modification of primordial germ cells in the mouse. *J. Exp. Zool.*, 134:207–230.
7. Witschi, E. (1948): Migration of the germ cells of human embryos from the yolksac to the primitive gonadal fold. *Contrib. Embryol.*, 32:67–80.
8. McKay, D. C., Hertig, A. T., Adams, E. C., and Danziger, S. (1953): Histochemical observations on the germ cells of human embryos. *Anat. Rec.*, 117:201–219.
9. Chretien, F. C. (1966): Etude de l'origine, de la migration et de la multiplication des cellules germinales chez l'embryon de lapin. *J. Embryol. Exp. Morph.*, 16:591–607.
10. McLaren, A. (1981): *Germ Cells and Soma: A New Look at an Old Problem.* Yale University Press, New Haven.
11. Snow, M. H. L., and Monk, M. (1983): Emergence and migration of mouse primordial germ cells. In: *Current Problems in Germ Cell Differentiation*, edited by A. McLaren and C. C. Wylie, pp. 115–135. Cambridge University Press, Cambridge.

12. McMahon, A., Fosten, M., and Monk, M. (1981): Random X-chromosome inactivation in female primordial germ cells in the mouse. *J. Embryol. Exp. Morph.*, 64:251–258.
13. Soriano, P., and Jaenisch, R. (1986): Retroviruses as probes for mammalian development: Allocation of cells to the somatic and germ cell lineages. *Cell,* 46:19–29.
14. Lyon, M. F. (1961): Gene action in the X-chromosome of the mouse (*Mus musculus*). *Nature,* 190:372–373.
15. Lyon, M. F. (1974): Sex chromosome activity in germ cells. In: *Physiology and Genetics of Reproduction,* edited by F. Fuchs and E. M. Coutinho, pp. 63–71. Plenum Press, New York.
16. Cattanach, B. M. (1975): Control of chromosome inactivation. *Annu. Rev. Genet.*, 9:1–17.
17. Gartler, S. M., Rivewst, M., and Cole, R. E. (1980): Cytological evidence for an inactive X chromosome in murine oogonia. *Cytogenet. Cell Genet.*, 28:203–207.
18. Ohno, S., Klinger, H. P., and Atkin, W. B. (1962): Human oogenesis. *Cytogenetics,* 1:42–51.
19. Teplitz, R., and Ohno, S. (1963): Postnatal induction of oogenesis in the rabbit (*Oryctolagus cuniculus*). *Exp. Cell Res.*, 31:183–189.
20. Ohno, S. (1967): *Sex Chromosomes and Sex Linked Genes*. Springer-Verlag, Berlin.
21. Migeon, B. R., and Jelalian, K. (1977): Evidence for two active X chromosomes in germ cells of female before meiotic entry. *Nature,* 269:242–243.
22. Gartler, S. M., Andina, R., and Gant, N. (1975): Ontogeny of X-chromosome inactivation in the female germ line. *Exp. Cell Res.*, 91:454–457.
23. Andina, R. J. (1978): A study of X chromosome regulation during oogenesis in the mouse. *Exp. Cell Res.*, 111:211–218.
24. West, J. (1982): X chromosome expression during mouse embryogenesis. In: *Genetic Control of Gamete Production and Function,* edited by P. G. Crosignani, B. L. Rubin, and M. Fraccaro, pp. 49–91. Academic Press, London.
25. Eddy, E. M., Clark, J. M., Gong, D., and Fenderson, B. A. (1981): Origin and migration of primordial germ cells in mammals. *Gamete Res.*, 4:333–362.
26. Fujimoto, T., Yoshinaga, K., and Kono, I. (1985): Distribution of fibronectin on the migratory pathway of primordial germ cells in mice. *Anat. Rec.*, 211:271–278.
27. Alvarez-Buylla, A., and Merchant-Larios, H. (1986): Mouse primordial germ cells use fibronectin as a substrate for migration. *Exp. Cell Res.*, 165:362–368.
28. Snow, M. H. L. (1981): Autonomous development of parts isolated from primitive streak stage mouse embryos. Is development clonal? *J. Embryol. Exp. Morphol.*, 65(Suppl.):269–287.
29. Niewkoop, P. D., and Sutasurya, L. A. (1979): *Primordial Germ Cells in the Chordates*. Cambridge University Press, London.
30. Kuwana, T., Maeda-Suga, H., and Fujimoto, T. (1986): Attraction of chick primordial germ cells by gonadal anlage *in vitro*. *Anat. Rec.*, 215:403–406.
31. Rogulska, R., Ozdzenski, W., and Komar, A. (1971): Behaviour of mouse primordial germ cells in the chick embryo. *J. Embryol. Exp. Morphol.*, 25:155–164.
32. Hardisty, M. W. (1978): Primordal germ cells and the vertebrate germ line. In: *The Vertebrate Ovary,* edited by R. E. Jones, pp. 1–45. Plenum Press, New York.
33. Ozdzenski, W. (1967): Observations on the origin of primordial germ cells in the mouse. *Zool. Pol.*, 17:367–379.
34. Tam, P., and Snow, M. H. L. (1981): Proliferation and migration of primordial germ cells during compensatory growth in the mouse embryo. *J. Embryol. Exp. Morphol.* 64:133–147.
35. Baker, T. G. (1963): A quantitative and cytological study of germ cells in the human ovaries. *Proc. R. Soc. Lond. B.*, 158:417–433.
36. Merchant-Larios, H., and Alvarez-Buylla, A. (1986): The role of extracellular matrix and tissue topographic arrangement in mouse and rat primordial germ cell migration. In: *Development and Function of the Reproductive Organs,* edited by A. Eshkol, B. Eckstein, N. Dekel, H. Peters, and A. Tsafriri, *Serono Symposia Review, No. 11*. Raven Press, New York.
37. Du Bois, A. M. (1969): The embryonic kidney. In: *The Kidney, Vol. 1,* edited by C. Rouiller and A. F. Muller, pp. 1–59. Academic Press, New York.
38. Grinsted, J., and Aagesen, L. (1984): Mesonephric excretory function related to its influence on differentiation of fetal gonads. *Anat. Rec.*, 210:551–556.
39. Waldeyer, W. (1870): *Eierstock und Ei*. Engelman, Leipzig.
40. Balfour, F. M. (1878): On the structure and development of the vertebrate ovary. *Q. J. Micr. Sci.*, XVIII:383–445.
41. Witschi, E. (1931): Studies on sex differentiation and sex determination in amphibians. V. Range of the cortex-medulla antagonism in parabiotic twins of Ranidae and Hylidae. *J. Exp. Zool.*, 58:113–145.
42. Witschi, E. (1951): Embryogenesis of the adrenal and the reproductive glands. *Recent Prog. Horm. Res.*, 6:1–23.
43. Gropp, A., and Ohno, S. (1966): Presence of a common embryonic blastema for ovarian and testicular parenchymal (follicular, interstitial and tubular) cells in cattle, Bos taurus. *Z. Zellforsch. Mikrosk. Anat.*, 74:505–528.
44. Wartenberg, H. (1978): Human testicular development and the role of the mesonephros in the origin of a dual Sertoli cell system. *Andrologia,* 10:1–21.
45. Zamboni, L., Bézard, J., and Mauléon P. (1979): The role of the mesonephros in the development of the sheep fetal ovary. *Ann. Biol. Anim. Biochim. Biophys.*, 19(4B):1153–1178.
46. Zamboni, L. Upadhyay, S., Bézard, J., and Mauléon, P. (1981): The role of the mesonephros in the development of the sheep testis and its excurrent pathways. In: *Development and Function of Reproductive Organs,* edited by A. G. Byskov and H. Peters, pp. 31–40. Excerpta Medica, Amsterdam.
47. Kinsky, I. (1979): Bildung des somatischen Gonadenblastems durch die degenerierende Urniereanteile des Kaninchens. *Verh. Anat. Ges.*, 73:403–406.
48. Wartenberg, H. (1979): Der Mesonephros und die gonadenentwicklung. *Verh. Anat. Ges.*, 73:385–401.
49. Byskov, A. G. (1978): The anatomy and ultrastructure of the rete system in the fetal mouse ovary. *Biol. Reprod.*, 19:720–735.
50. Fraedrich, J. (1979): Licht- und elektronmikroskopische Untersuchungen über den Zusammenhang der Mesonephros- und frühen Gonadenentwicklung der weissen Maus. Dissertation. Med. Fak., Bonn, pp. 1–58.
51. Upadhyay, S., Luciani, J. M., and Zamboni, L. (1979): The role of the mesonephros in the development of the indifferent gonads and ovaries of the mouse. *Ann. Biol. Anim. Biochim. Biophys.*, 19(4b):1179–1196.
52. Upadhyay, S., Luciani, J. M., and Zamboni, L. (1981): The role of the mesonephros in the development of the mouse testis and its excurrent pathways. In: *Development and Function of Reproductive Organs,* edited by A. G. Byskov and H. Peters, pp. 18–27. Excerpta Medica, Amsterdam.
53. Byskov, A. G. (1974): Does the rete ovarii act as a trigger for the onset of meiosis? *Nature,* 252:396–397.
54. Grinsted, J., Byskov, A. G., Christensen, I. J. and Jensenius, J. C. (1982): Influence of the mesonephros on fetal and neonatal rabbit gonads. I. Sex-steroid release by the testis *in vitro*. *Acta Endocrinol. (Cophen.)*, 99:272–280.
55. Grinsted, J. (1982): Influence of mesonephros on foetal and neonatal rabbit gonads. II. Sex-steroid release by the ovary *in vitro*. *Acta Endocrinol. (Copenh.)*, 99:281–287.
56. Growder, R. E. (1957): The development of the adrenal gland in man, with special reference to origin and ultimate location of cell types and evidence in favor of the "cell migration" theory. *Contrib. Embryol.*, 251:194–221.
57. Pelliniemi, L. J. (1975): Ultrastructure of gonadal ridge in male and female pig embryos. *Anat. Embryol.*, 147:19–34.
58. Wartenberg, H. (1982): Development of the early human ovary and role of the mesonephros in the differentiation of the cortex. *Anat. Embryol.*, 165:253–280.
59. Wagenen, G. Van, and Simpson, M. E. (1965): *Embryology of the Ovary and Testis. Homo sapiens and Macaca mulatta*. Yale University Press, New Haven.
60. Wartenberg, H. (1981): The influence of the mesonephric blastema on gonadal development and sexual differentiation. In: *Development and Function of Reproductive Organs,* edited by A. G. Byskov and H. Peters, pp. 3–12. Excerpta Medica, Amsterdam.
61. Peters, H., and McNatty, K. P. (1980): *The Ovary. A Correlation of Structure and Function in Mammals*. Granada Publishing, London.

62. Jirasek, J. E. (1971): *Development of the Genital System and Male Pseudohermaphroditism,* John Hopkins Press, Baltimore.
63. Polani, P. E. (1982): Pairing of X and Y chromosomes, non-inactivation of X-linked genes, and the maleness factor. *Hum. Genet.,* 60:207–211.
64. Jost, A. (1947): Recherches sur la différenciation sexuelle de l'embryon de lapin, III. Role des gonades foetales dans la différenciation sexuelle somatique. *Arch. Anat. Micr. Morphol.,* 36:271–315.
65. Jost, A. (1953): Problems in fetal endocrinology. The gonadal and hypophyseal hormones. *Recent Prog. Horm. Res.,* 8:379–418.
66. Jost, A. (1970): General outline about reproductive physiology and its developmental background. In: *Mammalian Reproduction,* edited by H. Gibian and E. J. Plotz, pp. 4–32. Spinger-Verlag, Berlin.
67. Grumbach, M. M., and Conte, F. A. (1985): Disorders of sexual differentiation. In: *Textbook of Endocrinology,* edited by J. D. Wilson and D. W. Foster, pp. 312–401. W. B. Saunders, Philadelphia.
68. Polani, P. E. (1962): Sex chromosome anomalities in man. In: *Chromosomes in Medicine,* edited by J. L. Hamerton. *Little Club Clinics in Developmental Medicine, No. 5,* pp. 74–133. National Spastic Society with William Heinemann Medical Books Ltd., London.
69. Welshons, W. J., and Russell, L. B. (1959): The Y-chromosome as the bearer of male determining factors in the mouse. *Proc. Natl. Acad. Sci. USA,* 45:560–566.
70. Cattanach, B. M., Pollard, C. E., and Hawkes, S. G. (1971): Sex reversed mice: XX and XO males. *Cytogenetics,* 10:318–337.
71. McLaren, A. (1983): Sex reversal in the mouse. *Differentiation,* 23(Suppl.):593–598.
72. Evans, C. W., Robb, D. I., Tuckett, F., and Challoner, S. (1982): Regulation of meiosis in the fetal mouse gonad. *J. Embryol. Exp. Morphol.,* 68:59–67.
73. Singh, L., and Jones, K. W. (1982): Sex reversal in the mouse (*Mus musculus*) is caused by a recurrent nonreciprocal crossover involving the X and an aberrant Y chromosome. *Cell,* 28:205–216.
74. Wachtel, S. S., Ohno, S., Koo, G. L., and Boyse, E. A. (1975): H-Y antigen and male development. In: *Testis in Normal and Infertile Men,* edited by P. Troen and H. R. Nankin, pp. 35–43. Raven Press, New York.
75. Eichwald, E. J., and Silmer, C. R. (1955): Skin. Communication. *Transplant. Bull.,* 2:148–149.
76. Wachtel, S. S., and Koo, G. C. (1981): H-Y antigen in gonadal differentiation. In: *Mechanisms of Sex Differentiation in Animals and Man,* edited by C. R. Austin and R. G. Edwards, pp. 255–299. Academic Press, London.
77. Silvers, W. K., Gasser, D. L., and Eicker, E. M. (1982): H-Y antigen, serologically detectable male antigen and sex determination. *Cell,* 28:439–440.
78. McLaren, A. (1984): Chimeras and sexual differentiation. In: *Chimeras in Developmental Biology,* edited by N. LeDouarin and A. McLaren, pp. 381–399. Academic Press, New York.
79. Teyssier, J. R., Amice-Chambon, U., Bajolle, F., and Pigeon, F. (1983): H-Y antigen negativity associated with a normal male phenotype. *Arch. Androl.,* 11:253–258.
80. Meldvold, R. W., Kohn, H. I., Yerganian, G., and Fawcett, D. W. (1977): Evidence suggesting the existence of two H-Y antigens in the mouse. *Immunogenetics,* 5:33–41.
81. Ohno, S. (1985): The Y-linked testis determining gene and H-Y plasma membrane antigen gene: Are they one and the same? *Endocrine Rev.,* 6:421–431.
82. Simpson, E., McLaren, A., and Chandler, P. (1982): Evidence for two male antigens in mice. *Immunogenetics,* 15:609–614.
83. Müller, U., and Urban, E. (1981): Reaggregation of rat gonadal cells in vitro: Experiments on the function of H-Y antigen. *Cytogenet. Cell Genet.,* 31:104–107.
84. Grinsted, J., Byskov, A. G., and Andreasen, M. P. (1979): Induction of meiosis in fetal mouse testis in vitro by rete testis tissue from pubertal mice and bulls. *J. Reprod. Fertil.,* 56:653–656.
85. Grinsted, J. and Byskov, A. G. (1981): Meiosis inducing and meiosis preventing substances in human male reproductive organs. *Fertil. Steril.,* 35:199–204.
86. Chartrain, I., Magre, S., Maingurd, M., and Jost, A. (1984): Effect of serum on organogenesis of the rat testis in vitro. *In Vitro Cell. Dev. Biol.,* 20:912–922.
87. Niekerk, W. A. Van, and Retief, A. E. (1981): The gonads of human true hermaphrodites. *Hum. Genet.,* 58:117–122.
88. Tarkowski, A. K. (1961): Mouse chimaeras developed from fused eggs. *Nature,* 190:857–860.
89. McLaren, A. (1976): *Mammalian Chimeras.* Cambridge University Press, Cambridge.
90. Eicher, E. M., Beamer, W. G., Washburn, L. L., and Whitten, W. H. (1980): A cytogenetic investigation of inherited true hermaphroditism in BALB/cWt mice. *Cytogenet. Cell Genet.,* 28:104–115.
91. Ford, C. E. (1970): Cytogenetics and sex determination in man and mammals. *J. Biosoc. Sci. (Suppl.),* 2:7–30.
92. Mullen, R. J., and Whitten, W. K. (1971): Relationship of genotype and degree of chimerism in coat color to sex ratios and gametogenesis in chimeric mice. *J. Exp. Zool.,* 178:165–176.
93. Whitten, W. K., Beamer, W. G., and Byskov, A. G. (1979): The morphology of fetal gonads of spontaneous mouse hermaphrodites. *J. Embryol. Exp. Morphol.,* 52:63–78.
94. Yding Andersen, C., Byskov, A. G., and Grinsted, J. (1983): Growth pattern of the sex ducts in foetal mouse hermaphrodites. *J. Embryol. Exp. Morphol.,* 73:59–68.
95. Burns, R. K. (1950): Sex transformation in the opossum: Some new results and a retrospect. *Arch. Anat. Micr.* 39:467–483.
96. Burns, R. K. (1961): Role of hormones in the differentiation of sex. In: *Sex and Internal Secretions,* edited by W. C. Young, pp. 76–160. Williams and Wilkins, Baltimore.
97. Alcorn, G. T. (1975): Ovarian development in the tammar wallaby *Macropus eugenii.* Ph.D. Thesis, MacQuarie University, Australia.
98. Turner, C. D., and Asakawa, H. (1964): Experimental reversal of germ cells in ovaries of fetal mice. *Science,* 143:1344–1345.
99. Ozdzenski, W., Rogulska, T., Batakier, H., Brzozowska, M., Rembiszewska, A., and Stepinska, U. (1976): Influence of embryonic and adult testis on the differentiation of embryonic ovary in the mouse. *Arch. Anat. Microsc. Morphol. Exp.,* 65:285–294.
100. Burgoyne, P. S., Ansell, J.-D., and Tournay, A. (1986): Can the indifferent mammalian XX gonad be sex-reversed by interaction with testicular tissue? In: *Development and Function of the Reproductive Organs,* edited by A. Eshkol, B. Eckstein, N. Dekel, H. Peters, and A. Tsafriri, pp. 23–39. *Serono Symposia Review, No. 11.* Raven Press, New York.
101. Byskov, A. G., and Saxen, L. (1976): Induction of meiosis in foetal mouse testis in vitro. *Dev. Biol.,* 52:193–200.
102. Byskov, A. G. (1979): Regulation of meiosis in mammals. *Ann. Biol. Anim. Biochim. Biophys.,* 19:1251–1261.
103. Byskov, A. G., Høyer, P. E., Björkman, N., Mørk, A. B., Olsen, B., and Grinsted, J. (1986): Ultrastructure of germ cells and adjacent somatic cells correlated to initiation of meiosis in the fetal pig. *Anat. Embryol.,* 175:57–67.
104. Byskov, A. G. (1975): The role of the rete ovarii in meiosis and follicle formation in the cat, mink and ferret. *J. Reprod. Fertil.,* 45:210–219.
105. Hashimoto, Y., and Eguchi, Y. (1955): Histological observations on the gonads in the cattle and the horse fetus. I. The cattle fetus. *Jpn. J. Zootech.,* 26:259–266.
106. Goodenough, V., and Levine, R. P. (1975): *Genetics.* Holt, Rinehart & Winston, London.
107. Baker, T. G. (1972): Oogenesis and ovarian development. In: *Reproductive Biology,* edited by H. Balin and S. Glasser, p. 398–437. Excerpta Medica, Amsterdam.
108. Byskov, A. G., and Grinsted, J. (1981): Production of germ cells and regulation of meiosis. In: *Bioregulators of Reproduction,* edited by G. Jagiello and H. J. Vogel. Academic Press, New York.
109. Hilscher, B., Hilscher, W., Bülthoff-Ohnolz, B., Krämer, U., Birke, A., Pelzer, H., and Gauss, G. (1974): Kinetics of gametogenesis. I. Comparative histological and autoradiographic studies of oocytes and transitional prospermatogonia during oogenesis and prespermatogenesis. *Cell Tissue Res.,* 154:443–470.
110. Borum, K. (1961): Oogenesis in the mouse. A study of meiotic prophase. *Exp. Cell Res.,* 24:495–507.
111. Peters, H., Levy, E., and Crone, M. (1965): Oogenesis in rabbits. *J. Exp. Zool.,* 158:169–180.
112. Gondos, B. (1978): Oogonia and oocytes in mammals. In: *The Vertebrate Ovary,* edited by R. E. Jones, pp. 83–120. Plenum Press, New York.
113. Rüsse, I. (1983): Oogenesis in cattle and sheep. *Bibl. Anat.,* 24:77–92.

114. Beatty, R. A. (1970): Genetic basis for the determination of sex. *Philos. Trans. R. Soc. Lond. (Biol)*, 259:3–13.
115. Gondos, B. (1973): Intercellular bridges and mammalian germ cell differentiation. *Differentiation,* 1:177–182.
116. Kenelly, J. J., Foote, R. H., and Jones, R. C. (1970): Duration of premeiotic deoxyribonucleic acid synthesis and the stages of prophase in rabbit oocytes. *J. Cell Biol.,* 47:477–484.
117. Lima-Di-Faria, A., and Borum, K. (1962): The period of DNA synthesis prior to meiosis in the mouse. *J. Cell Biol.,* 14:381–388.
118. Peters, H., and Crone, M. (1967): DNA synthesis in oocytes of mammals. *Arch. Microsc. Morphol. Exp.,* 56(Suppl. 3–4):160–170.
119. Mintz, B. (1959): Continuity of the female germ cell line from embryo to adult. *Arch. Anat. Microsc. Morphol. Exp.,* 48:155–172.
120. Beaumont, H. M. (1961): Radiosensitivity of oogonia and oocytes in the foetal rat. *Int. J. Radiat. Biol.,* 3:59–72.
121. Mandl, A. M. (1964): The radiosensitivity of germ cells. *Biol. Rev.,* 39:288–371.
122. Ioannou, J. M. (1967): Oogenesis in adult prosimians. *J. Embryol. Exp. Morphol.,* 17:139–145.
123. Anand Kumar, T. C. (1968): Oogenesis in the lorises. *Loris tardigradus lydekkerianus* and *Nucticebris coucang. Proc. R. Soc. Lond. (Biol.),* 169:167–176.
124. Baker, T. G. (1973): The effects of ionizing radiation on the mammalian ovary with particular reference to oogenesis. In: *Handbook of Physiology. Endocrinology, Vol. V,* edited by D. W. Hamilton and R. O. Greep, pp. 349–361. American Physiology Society, Washington, D.C.
125. Beaumont, H. M. (1965): The short term effect of acute X-irradiation on oogonia and oocytes. *Proc. R. Soc. Lond. (Biol.),* 161:550–570.
126. Oakberg, E. F., and Clark, E. (1963): Species comparisons of radiation response of the gonads. In: *Effects of Ionizing Radiation in the Reproductive System,* edited by W. D. Carlson and F. Y. Gassner, pp. 11–24. Pergamon Press, Oxford.
127. Larsen, J., Byskov, A. G., and Christensen, I. J. (1986): Flow cytometry and sorting of meiotic prophase cells of female rabbits. *J. Reprod. Fertil.,* 76:587–596.
128. Stahl, A., and Luciani, J. M. (1971): Individualization d'un stade préleptotene de condensation chromosomique au debut méiose chez l'ovocyte foetal humain. *C. R. Acad. Sci.,* 272:2041–2044.
129. Byskov, A. G. (1978): The meiosis inducing interaction between germ cells and rete cells in the fetal mouse gonad. *Ann. Biol. Anim. Biochim. Biophys.,* 18:327–334.
130. Devictor-Vuillet, M., Luciani, J. M., and Stahl, A. (1973): Etude des stades de début de la méiose chez l'ovocyte de lapin: Comparaison avec l'ovocyte humain. *Ann. Biol. Anim. Biochim. Biophys.,* 13:73–78.
131. Mauléon, P., Devictor-Vuillet, M., and Luciani, J. M. (1976): The preleptotene chromosome condensation and decondensation in the ovary of the sheep embryo. *Ann. Biol. Anim. Biochim. Biophys.,* 16:293–296.
132. Deanesly, R. (1975): Germ cell development and the meiotic prophase in the fetal horse ovary. *J. Reprod. Fertil. (Suppl.),* 23:547–552.
133. Holm, P. B., and Rasmussen, S. W. (1977): Human meiosis I. The human pachytene karyotype analyzed by three dimensional reconstruction of the synaptonemal complex. *Carlsberg Res. Commun.,* 42:283–323.
134. Bojko, M. (1985): Human meiosis IX. Crossing over and chiasma formation in oocytes. *Carlsberg Res. Commun.,* 50:43–72.
135. Speed, R. M. (1982): Meiosis in the foetal mouse ovary. 1. An analysis at the light microscope level using surface spreading. *Chromosoma,* 85:427–437.
136. Polani, P. E., Crolla, J. A., and Seller, M. J. (1981): An experimental approach to female mammalian meiosis: Differential chromosome labeling and an analysis of chiasmata in the female mouse. In: *Bioregulators of Reproduction,* edited by G. Jagiello and H. Vogel, pp. 59–87. Academic Press, New York.
137. Baker, T. G., and Franchi, L. L. (1967): The origin of cytoplasmatic inclusions from the nuclear envelope of mammalian oocytes. *Z. Zellforsch. Mikrosk. Anat.,* 93:45–55.
138. Beaumont, H. M., and Mandl, A. H. (1962): A quantitative and cytological study of oogonia and oocytes in the foetal and neonatal rat. *Proc. R. Soc. Lond. (Biol.),* 155:557–579.
139. Singh, R. P., and Carr, D. H. (1966): The anatomy and histology of XO human embryos and fetuses. *Anat. Rec.,* 155:369–384.
140. Ford, C. E., Jones, K. W., Polani, P. E., De Almeida, J. C. C., and Briggs, J. H. (1959): A sex-chromosome anomaly in a case of gonodal dysgenesis (Turners syndrome). *Lancet,* 1:711–713.
141. Burgoyne, P. S., and Baker, T. G. (1985): Perinatal oocyte loss in XO mice and its implications for the aetiology of gonadal dysgenesis in XO women. *J. Reprod. Fertil.,* 75:633–645.
142. Miklos, G. L. G. (1974): Sex-chromosome pairing and male fertility. *Cytogenet. Cell Genet.,* 13:558–577.
143. Burgoyne, P. S., and Baker, T. G. (1984): Meiotic pairing and gametogenic failure. In: *Controlling Events in Meiosis,* edited by C. W. Evans and H. G. Dickinson, pp. 349–362. Company of Biologists, Cambridge.
144. Baker, T. G., Beaumont, H. M., and Franchi, L. L. (1969): The uptake of tritiated uridine and phenylalanine by the ovaries of rats and monkeys. *J. Cell Sci.,* 4:655–675.
145. Wagenen, G. van, and Simpson, M. E. (1973): Postnatal development of the ovary in *Homo sapiens* and *Macaca mulatta.* Yale University Press, New Haven.
146. Andersen, A. C., and Simpson, M. E. (1973): *The Ovary and the Reproductive Cycle of the Dog (Beagle).* Geron-X, Inc., Los Altos, CA.
147. Brambell, F. W. R. (1956): Ovarian changes. In: *Marshall's Physiology of Reproduction,* edited by A. S. Parkes, pp. 397–542. Longmans, Green, London.
148. Byskov, A. G., and Lintern-Moore, S. (1973): Follicle formation in the immature mouse ovary: The role of the rete ovarii. *J. Anat.,* 116:207–217.
149. Byskov, A. G., Skakkebek, N. E., Stafanger, G., and Peters, H. (1977): Influence of ovarian surface epithelium and rete ovarii on follicle formation. *J. Anat.,* 123:77–86.
150. Mossman, H. W., and Duke, K. L. (1973): *Comparative Morphology of the Mammalian Ovary.* The University of Wisconsin Press, Madison.
151. Stein, L. E., and Anderson, E. H. (1979): A qualitative and quantitative study of rete ovarii development in the fetal rat: Correlation with the onset of meiosis and follicle cell appearance. *Anat. Rec.,* 193:197–211.
152. Høyer, P. E., and Byskov, A. G. (1981): A quantitative cytochemical study of Δ^5, 3β-hydroxysteroid dehydrogenase activity in the rete system of the immature mouse ovary. In: *Development and Function of Reproductive Organs,* edited by A. G. Byskov and H. Peters, pp. 216–224. Excerpta Medica, Amsterdam.
153. Pedersen, T. (1972): Follicle growth in the mouse ovary. In: *Oogenesis,* edited by J. D. Biggers and A. W. Schuetz, pp. 261–276. Butterworths, London.
154. Peters, H. (1978): Folliculogenesis in mammals. In: *The Vertebrate Ovary,* edited by R. E. Jones, pp. 121–144. Plenum Press, New York.
155. Lintern-Moore, S. (1977): Initiation of follicular growth in the infant mouse ovary by exogenous gonadotrophin. *Biol. Reprod.,* 17:635–639.
156. Gulyas, B. J., Hodgen, G. D., Tullner, W. W., and Ross, G. T. (1977): Effects of fetal or maternal hyperphysectomy on endocrine organs and body weight in infant rhesus monkeys (*Macaca mulatta*): With particular emphasis on oogenesis. *Biol. Reprod.,* 16:216–227.
157. Baker, T. G., and Neal, P. (1973): Initiation and control of meiosis and follicular growth in ovaries of the mouse. *Ann. Biol. Anim. Biochim. Biophys.,* 13:137–144.
158. Challoner, S. (1975): Studies of oogenesis and follicular development in the golden hamster. 2. Initiation and control of meiosis *in vitro. J. Anat.,* 119:149–156.
159. Baker, T. G., and Scrimgeour, J. B. (1980): Development of the gonad in normal and anencephalic human fetuses. *J. Reprod. Fertil.,* 60:193–199.
160. Eshkol, A., Lunenfeld, B., and Peters, H. (1970): Ovarian development in infant mice. Dependence on gonadotrophic hormones. In: *Gonadotrophins and Ovarian Development,* edited by W. R. Butt, A. C. Crooke, and M. Ryle, pp. 249–258. Livingstone, Edinburgh.
161. Mauléon, P., and Mariana, J. C. (1976): Oogenesis and folliculogenesis. In: *Reproduction in Domestic Animals,* edited by H. H. Cole and P. T. Cupps, pp. 175–202, Academic Press, New York.

162. Byskov, A. G. (1986): Differentiation of mammalian embryonic gonad. *Phys. Rev.*, 66:71–117.
163. Christensen, A. K. (1975): Leydig cells. In: *Handbook of Physiology, Vol. V*, edited by R. O. Greep and E. B. Astwood, pp. 57–94. Williams and Wilkins, Baltimore.
164. Gondos, B., George, F. W., and Wilson, J. D. (1983): Granulosa cell differentiation and estrogen synthesis in the fetal rabbit ovary. *Biol. Reprod.*, 29:791–798.
165. Milewich, L., George, F. W., and Wilson, J. D. (1977): Estrogen formation by the ovary of the rabbit embryo. *Endocrinology*, 100:187–196.
166. Byskov, A. G., Høyer, P. E., and Westergaard, L. (1985): Origin and differentiation of the endocrine cells of the ovary. *J. Reprod. Fertil.*, 75:299–306.
167. Gondos, B., and Hobel, C. J. (1973): Interstitial cells in the human fetal ovary. *Endocrinology*, 93:736–739.
168. Høyer, P. E. (1980): Histoenzymology of the human ovary: Dehydrogenases directly involved in steroidogenesis. In: *Biology of the Ovary*, edited by P. M. Motta and E. S. Hafez, pp. 52–67. Nijhoff, The Hague.
168. Gougeon, A. (1974): Aspects originaux de la glande interstitielle ovarienne chez le Hérisson: Morphologie, histogenèse, hyperplasie, enzymes de la stéroidogenèse. *Ann. Biol. Anim. Biochim. Biophys.*, 14:53–66.
170. Zondek, L. H., and Zondek, T. (1983): Ovarian hilar cells and testicular Leydig cells in anencephaly. *Biol. Neonate*, 43:211–219.
171. McCoshen, J. A. (1982): In vivo sex differentiation of congeneic germinal cell aplastic gonads. *Am. J. Obstet. Gynecol.*, 142:83–88.
172. Mintz, B., and Russell, E. S. (1955): Developmental modifications of primordial germ cells, induced by W-series genes in the mouse embryo. *Anat. Rec.*, 122:443–449.
173. Merchant, H. (1975): Rat gonadal and ovarian organogenesis with and without germ cells. An ultrastructural study. *Dev. Biol.*, 44:1–21.
174. Blaschuk, O., Burdzy, K., and Fritz, I. B. (1983): Purification and characterization of a cell-aggregating factor (clusterin), the major glycoprotein in ram rete testis fluid. *J. Biol. Chem.*, 258:7714–7720.
175. Jost, A. (1951): Recherches sur la différenciation sexuelle de l'embryon de lapin. IV. Organogénèse sexuelle masculine apres decapitatio du foetus. *Arch. Anat. Micr. Morphol. Exp.*, 40:247–281.
176. Elias, H. (1974): Frühentwicklung der Samenkanälchen beim Menschen. *Verh. Anat. Ges. Versamml.*, 68:123–131.
177. Clermont, Y., and Huckins, C. (1961): Microscopic anatomy of the sex cords and seminiferous tubules in growing and adult albino rats. *Am. J. Anat.*, 180:79–97.
178. Magre, S., and Jost, A. (1980): The initial phases of testicular organogenesis in the rat. An electron microscopy study. *Arch. Anat. Microsc. Morphol.*, 69:297–318.
179. Pelliniemi, L. J. (1976): Ultrastructure of the indifferent gonad in male and female pig embryos. *Tissue Cell*, 8:163–174.
180. Byskov, A. G., Yding Andersen, C., and Westergaard, L. (1983): Dependence of the onset of meiosis on the internal organization of the gonad. In: *Current Problems in Germ Cell Differentiation*, edited by A. McLaren and C. C. Wylie, pp. 215–224. Cambridge University Press, Cambridge.
181. Magre, S., and Jost, A. (1983): Early stages of differentiation of the rat testis: Regulations between Sertoli and germ cells. In: *Current Problems in Germ Cell Differentiation*, edited by A. McLaren and C. C. Wylie, pp. 201–214. Cambridge University Press, Cambridge.
182. Fritz, I. B., Skinner, M. K., and Tung, P. S. (1986): The nature of somatic cell interactions in the seminiferous tubule. In: *Development and Function of Reproductive Organs*, edited by A. Eshkol, B. Eckstein, N. Dekel, H. Peters, and A. Tsafriri, pp. 85–91. *Serono Symposia Review, No. 11*. Raven Press, New York.
183. Paranko, J., Pelliniemi, L. J., Vaheri, A., Foidart, J. M., and Lakkala-Paranko, T. (1983): Morphogenesis and fibronectin in sexual differentiation of rat embryonic gonads. *Differentiation (Suppl.)*, 23:72–81.
184. Taketo, T., Thau, R. B., Adeyemo, O., and Koide, S. S. (1984): Influence of adenosine 3′:5′-cyclic monophosphate analogues on testicular organization of fetal mouse gonads *in vitro*. *Biol. Reprod.*, 30:189–198.
185. Gondos, B. (1980): Development and differentiation of the testis and male reproductive tract. In: *Testicular Development, Structure and Function*, edited by A. Steinberger and E. Steinberger, pp. 3–20. Raven Press, New York.
186. Hilscher, W., Hilscher, B., Gauss, G., Lippers, P., and Bülthoff, B. (1972): Untersuchung zur Kinetik der Gonocyten und Stützzellen der Wistarratte. *Andrologie*, 4:311–325.
187. Hilscher, W. (1981): T1-Prospermatogonia (primodial spermatogonia of Rauh): The "ameiotic" counterpart of early oocytes. *Fortschr. Androl.*, 7:21–32.
188. Nogushi, T., and Stevens, L. C. (1982): Primordial germ cell proliferation in fetal testes in mouse strains with high and low incidences of congenital testicular teratomas. *J. Natl. Cancer Inst.*, 69:907–913.
189. Peters, H. (1970): Migration of gonocytes into the mammalian gonad and their differentiation. *Philos. Trans. R. Soc. Lond. (Biol.)*, 259:91–101.
190. Hilscher, W. (1970): Kinetics of prespermatogenesis and spermatogenesis of the Wistar rat under normal and pathological conditions. *Fortschr. Androl.*, 1:17–20.
191. Huckins, C., and Clermont, Y. (1968): Evolution of gonocytes in the rat testis during late embryonic and early post-natal life. *Arch. Anat. Histol. Embryol.*, 51:343–354.
192. Mauger, A., and Clermont, Y. (1974): Ultrastructure des gonocytes et des spermatogonies de jeune rat. *Arch. Anat. Microsc. Morphol. Exp.*, 63:133–146.
193. Rauh, W. (1929): Das chondriom in der ersten Keimzellen der Ratte. Eine Keimbahnuntersuchung. *Z. Ges. Anat.*, 89:271–309.
194. Larsen, J. K., Byskov, A. G., and Grinsted, J. (1981): Growth and differentiation of foetal mouse gonads in culture studied by flow cytometry on nuclear suspensions. *Acta Pathol. Microbiol. Immunol. Scand. (A) (Suppl.)*, 274:178–182.
195. Gondos, B., and Byskov, A. G. (1981): Germ cell kinetics in the neonatal rabbit testis. *Cell Tissue Res.*, 215:143–151.
196. Beaumont, H. M., and Mandl, A. M. (1963): A quantitative study of primordial germ cells in the male rat. *J. Embryol. Exp. Morphol.*, 11:715–740.
197. Wartenberg, H. (1983): Structural aspects of gonadal differentiation in mammals and birds. In: *Differentiation*, edited by U. Müller and W. W. Franke (Suppl.), pp. 64–71. Springer-Verlag, Berlin.
198. Jost, A. (1985): Initial stages of gonadal development. *Arch. Anat. Micr. Morphol. Exp.*, 74:39–41.
199. Byskov, A. G. (1981): Primordial germ cells and regulation of meiosis. In: *Reproduction in Mammals, Book 1. Germ Cells and Fertilization*, edited by C. R. Austin and R. V. Short, pp. 1–16. Cambridge University Press, Cambridge.
200. Clermont, Y., and Perey, B. (1957): Quantitative study of the cell population of the seminiferous tubules in immature rats. *Am. J. Anat.*, 100:241–268.
201. Nagy, F. (1972): Cell division kinetics and DNA synthesis in the immature Sertoli cells of the rat testis. *J. Reprod. Fertil.*, 28:389–395.
202. Steinberger, A., and Steinberger, E. (1977): The Sertoli cells. In: *The Testis*, edited by A. D. Johnson and W. R. Gomes, pp. 371–399. Academic Press, New York.
203. Sun, E. L., and Gondos, B. (1981): Proliferative activity in the rabbit testis during postnatal development. In: *Development and Function of Reproductive Organs*, edited by A. G. Byskov and H. Peters, pp. 140–148. *International Congress series No. 559*. Excerpta Medica, Amsterdam.
204. Gondos, B. (1977): Testicular development. In: *The Testis, Vol. IV*, edited by A. D. Johnson and W. R. Gomes, pp. 1–37. Academic Press, New York.
205. Jost, A., and Magre, S. (1984): Testicular development phases and dual hormonal control of sexual organogenesis. In: *Sexual Differentiation: Basic and Clinical Aspects*, edited by M. Serio, M. Motta, M. Zanisi, and L. Martini, pp. 1–15. *Serono Symposa Publications, Vol. 11*. Raven Press, New York.
206. Gondos, B., and Sun, E. L. (1981): Cell membrane modifications during human fetal gonadal development. In: *Development and Function of the Reproductive Organs*, edited by A. G. Byskov and H. Peters, pp. 31–40. Excerpta Medica, Amsterdam.

207. Gondos, B., and Conner, L. A. (1973): Ultrastructure of the developing germ cell in the fetal rabbit testis. *Am. J. Anat.*, 136:23–42.
208. Magre, S. (1985): Differentiation des cellules de Sertoli et morphogenese testiculaire chez le foetus de rat. *Arch. Anat. Micr. Morphol. Exp.*, 74:64–68.
209. George, F. W., and Wilson, J. D. (1979): The regulation of androgen and estrogen formation in fetal gonads. *Ann. Biol. Anim. Biochim. Biophys.*, 19(4B):1297–1306.
210. Raeside, J. I., and Sigman, D. M. (1975): Testosterone levels in early fetal testes of domestic pigs. *Biol. Reprod.*, 13:318–321.
211. Ortiz, E., Price, D., and Zaaijer, J. J. P. (1966): Organ culture studies of hormone secretion in endocrine glands of fetal guinea pigs. II. Secretion of androgenic hormone in adrenals and testes during early stages of development. *Koninkl. Nederl. Akademie van Wetenschappen.*, 69:400–408.
212. Moon, Y. S., and Raeside, J. I. (1972): Histochemical studies on hydroxysteroid dehydrogenase activity of fetal pig testis. *Biol. Reprod.*, 7:278–287.
213. Black, V. H., and Christensen, A. K. (1969): Differentiation of interstitial cells and Sertoli cells in fetal guinea pig testes. *Am. J. Anat.*, 124:211–238.
214. Pelliniemi, L. J., and Niemi, M. (1969): Fine structure of the human foetal testis. I. The interstitial tissue. *Z. Zellforsch.*, 99:507–522.
215. Roosen-Runge, E. C., and Anderson, D. (1959): The development of the interstitial cells in the testis of the albino rat. *Acta Anat.*, 37:125–137.
216. Picon, R. (1976): Testosterone secretion by foetal rat testis *in vitro*. *J. Endocrinol.*, 71:231–238.
217. Weisz, J., and Ward, I. L. (1980): Plasma testosterone and progesterone titers of pregnant rats, their male and female fetuses and neonatal offspring. *Endocrinology*, 106:306–316.
218. Tapanainen, J., Kuopio, T., Pelliniemi, L. J., and Huhtaniemi, I. (1984): Rat testicular endogenous steroids and number of Leydig cells between the fetal period and sexual maturity. *Biol. Reprod.*, 31:1027–1035.
219. Pelliniemi, L. J., and Dym, M. (1980): The fetal gonad and sexual differentiation. In: *Maternal-Fetal Endocrinology*, edited by D. Tulchinsky and K. J. Ryan, pp. 252–280. W. B. Saunders, Philadelphia.
220. Niemi, M., Ikonen, M., and Hervonen, A. (1967): Histochemistry and fine structure of interstitial tissue in human foetal testis. In: *Endocrinology of the Testis, Ciba Foundation Colloquium on Endocrinology, Vol. 16*, pp. 31–55.
221. Orth, J., and Weisz, J. (1980): Development of 3β-hydroxysteroid dehydrogenase and glucose-6-phosphatase activity in Leydig cells of the fetal rat testis: A quantitative cytochemical study. *Biol. Reprod.*, 22:1201–1209.
222. Yding Andersen, C., Byskov, A. G., and Grinsted, J. (1981): Partial purification of the meiosis inducing substance (MIS). In: *Development and Function of Reproductive Organs*, edited by A. G. Byskov and H. Peters, pp 73–80. Excerpta Medica, Amsterdam.
223. Magre, S., Agelopoulou, R., and Jost, A. (1981): Action du sérum de foetus de veaun sur la différenciation *in vitro* on le mantien des cordons séminifères du testicule du foetus du rat. *C. R. Acad. Sci. (Paris)*, 292:85–89.
224. Agelopoulou, R., Magre, S., Patsavoudi, E., and Jost, A. (1984): Initial phases of the rat testis differentiation *in vitro*. *J. Embryol. Exp. Morphol.*, 83:15–31.
225. Patsavoudı, E., Magre, S., Castanier, M., Scholler, R., and Jost, A. (1985): Dissociation between testicular morphogenesis and functional differentiation of Leydig cells. *J. Endocrinol.*, 105:235–238.
226. Clements, J. A., Reyes, F. I., Winter, J. S. D., and Faiman, C. (1976): Studies on human sexual development. III. Fetal pituitary and serum, and amniotic fluid concentrations of LH, CG, and FSH. *J. Clin. Endocrinol. Metab.*, 42:9–19.
227. Catt, K. J., Dufau, M. L., Neaves, W. B., Walsh, P. C., and Wilson, J. D. (1975): LH-HCG receptors and testosterone content during differentiation of the testis in the rabbit embryo. *Endocrinology*, 97:1157–1165.
228. George, F. W., Simpson, E. R., Milewich, L., and Wilson, J. D. (1979): Studies on the regulation of the onset of steroid hormone biosynthesis in fetal rabbit gonads. *Endocrinology*, 105:1100–1106.
229. Gulyas, B. J., Tullner, W. W., and Hodgen, G. D. (1977): Fetal and maternal hypophysectomy in Rhesus monkeys (*Macaca mulatta*): Effects on the development of testes and other endocrine organs. *Biol. Reprod.*, 17:650–660.
230. Tseng, M. T., Alexander, N. J., and Kittinger, G. W. (1975): Effects of fetal decapitation on the structure and function of Leydig cells in rhesus monkeys (*Macaca mulatta*). *Am. J. Anat.*, 143:349–362.
231. Zamboni, L., and Upadhyay, S. (1983): Germ cell differentiation in mouse adrenal glands. *J. Exp. Zool.*, 228:173–193.
232. Tarkowski, A. K. (1969): Are genetic factors controlling sexual differentiation of somatic and germinal tissues of a mammalian gonad stable or labile? In: *Environmental Influences on Genetic Expression*, edited by N. Kretchmer and D. N. Walcher, pp. 49–68. National Institutes of Health, Bethesda, MD.
233. Kratzer, P. G., and Chapman, V. M. (1981): X chromosome reactivation in oocytes of *Mus caroli*. *Proc. Natl. Acad. Sci. USA*, 78:3093–3097.
234. Byskov, A. G. (1978): Regulation of initiation of meiosis in fetal gonads. *J. Andrology (Suppl.)*, 2:29–39.
235. Fajer, A. B., Schneider, J., McCall, D., Ances, I. G., and Polakis, S. E. (1979): The induction of meiosis by ovaries of newborn hamsters and its relation to the action of the extraovarian structures in the mesovarium (rete ovarii). *Ann. Biol. Anim. Biochim. Biophys.*, 19(4B): 1273–1278.
236. Stein, L. E., and Anderson, E. (1981): In vitro analysis of ovarian differentiation and the initiation of meiosis in the rat. *Acta Anat.*, 10:189–205.
237. Westergaard, L., Byskov, A. G., VanLook, P. F. A., Angell, R., Aitken, J., Swanston, I. A., and Templeton, A. A. (1985): Meiosis-inducing substances in human preovulatory follicular fluid related to time of follicle aspiration and to the potential of the oocyte to fertilize and cleave *in vitro*. *Fertil. Steril.*, 44:663–667.
238. Westergaard, L., Callesen, H., Hyttel, P., Greve, T., and Byskov, A. G. (1985): Meiosis inducing substance (MIS) in bovine preovulatory follicles. *Zuchthygiene*, 20:217–221.
239. Tsafriri, A., and Channing, C. P. (1975): An inhibitory influence of granulosa cells and follicular fluid upon porcine oocyte meiosis *in vitro*. *Endocrinology*, 96:922–927.
240. Tsafriri, A., Dekel, N., and Bar-Ami, S. (1982): The role of oocyte maturation inhibitor in follicular regulation of oocyte maturation. *J. Reprod. Fertil.*, 64:541–551.
241. Luciani, J. M., Devictor-Vuillet, M., and Stahl, A. (1977): Preleptotene chromosome condensation stage in human foetal and neonatal testes. *J. Embryol. Exp. Morphol.*, 38:175–186.
242. Reyes, F. I., Winter, J. S. D., and Faiman, C. (1973): Studies on human sexual development. I. Fetal gonadal and adrenal sex steroids. *J. Clin. Endocrinol. Metab.*, 37:74–78.
243. Mauléon, P., Bézard, J., and Terqui, M. (1977): Very early and transient secretion of oestradiol-17β by foetal sheep ovary *in vitro*. *Ann. Biol. Anim. Biochim. Biophys.*, 17:399–401.
244. Schemesh, M. (1980): Estradiol-17β biosynthesis by the early bovine fetal ovary during the active and refractory phases. *Biol. Reprod.* 23:577–582.
245. Sholl, S. A., and Goy, R. W. (1978): Androgen and estrogen synthesis in the fetal guinea pig gonad. *Biol. Reprod.*, 18:160–169.
246. Taylor, T., Coutts, J. R. T., and Macnaughton, M. C. (1974): Human foetal synthesis of testosterone from perfused progesterone. *J. Endocrinol.*, 60:321–326.
247. Payne, A. H., and Jaffe, R. B. (1974): Androgen formation from pregnenolene sulfate by the human fetal ovary. *J. Clin. Endocrinol. Metab.*, 39:300–304.
248. Resko, J. A., Ploem, J. G., and Stadelman, H. L. (1975): Estrogens in fetal and maternal plasma of the rhesus monkey. *Endocrinology*, 97:425–430.
249. George, F. W., and Wilson, J. D. (1978): Conversion of androgen to estrogen by the human fetal ovary. *J. Clin. Endocrinol. Metab.*, 47:550–555.
250. Terada, N., Kuroda, H., Namiki, M., Kitamura, Y., and Matsumoto, K. (1984): Augmentation of aromatase activity by FSH in ovaries of fetal and neonatal mice in organ culture. *J. Steroid Biochem.*, 20:741–745.
251. Weniger, J. P., Chouraqui, J., and Zeis, A. (1985): Steroid conversions by the 19-day old foetal rat ovary in organ culture. *Biol. Chem.*, 366:555–559.

252. Rigaudière, N. (1977): Evolution des teneurs en testostérone et dihydrotestostérone dans le plasma le testicule et l'ovaire chez la cobaye au cours de la vie foetale. *C. R. Acad. Sci. (Paris)*, 285:989–992.
253. Picon, R. (1986): Stades initiaux de la stéroidogenèse dans les gonade de mammifères. *Arch. Anat. Micr. Morphol. Exp.*, 74:81–86.
254. Raeside, J. I. (1983): Gonadotrophic stimulation of androgen secretion by the early fetal pig ovary in organ culture. *Biol. Reprod.*, 28:128–133.
255. Carr, B. R., and Simpson, E. R. (1982): Cholesterol synthesis in human fetal tissues. *J. Clin. Endocrinol. Metab.*, 55:447–452.
256. Diczfalusy, E., and Manuso, S. (1969): Oestrogen metabolism in pregnancy. In: *Foetus and Placenta,* edited by A. Klopper and E. Diczfalusy, pp. 191–248. Blackwell Scientific Publications, Oxford.
257. Eik-Nes, K. B (1975): Biosynthesis and secretion of testicular steroids. In: *Handbook of Physiology, Vol. V,* edited by R. O. Greep and E. B. Astwood, pp. 95–115. Williams and Wilkins, Baltimore.
258. Raynard, A., and Frilley, M. (1947): Etat de développement des ébauches mammaires et du cordon vaginal chez les foetus males et femelles de souris, dont le ébauches génitales ont été détruites par une irradiation au moyen des rayons X, a l'age de treize jours. *C. R. Acad. Sci. (Paris)*, 225:1380–1382.
259. Forest, M. G. (1983): Role of androgens in fetal and pubertal development. *Hormone Res.*, 18:69–83.
260. McEwan, B. S. (1980): Gonadal steroids and brain development. *Biol. Reprod.*, 22:43–48.
261. Resko, J. A. (1977): Fetal hormones and development of the central nervous system in primates. *Adv. Sex Horm. Res.*, 3:139–168.
262. Ward, I. L., and Weisz, J. (1980): Maternal stress alters plasma testosterone in fetal males. *Science,* 207:328–329.
263. Habenicht, U.-F. (1983): Hormonal regulation of testicular descent. *Adv. Anat. Embryol. Cell Biol.*, 81:1–54.
264. Hutson, J. M., and Donahoe, P. K. (1986): The hormonal control of testicular descent. *Endocr. Rev.*, 7:270–283.
265. Winter, J. S. D., Faiman, C., and Reyes, F. (1981): Sexual endocrinology of fetal and perinatal life. In: *Mechanisms of sex differentiation in animals and man,* edited by C. R. Austin and R. G. Edwards, pp. 205–253. Academic Press, London.
266. Winter, J. S. D., Faiman, C., and Reyes, F. I. (1977): Sex steroid production by the human fetus: Its role in morphogenesis and control by gonadotrophins. In: *Morphogenesis and Malformation of the Genital System,* edited by R. J. Blandau and D. Bergma, pp. 41–58. Alan R. Liss, New York.
267. Carr, B. R., Parker, C. R., Ohashi, M., MacDonald, P. C., and Simpson, E. R. (1983): Regulation of human fetal testicular secretion of testosterone: Low-density lipoprotein-cholesterol and cholesterol synthesized de novo as steroid precursor. *Am. J. Obstet. Gynecol.*, 146:241–246.
268. Molsberry, R. L., Carr, B. R., and Mendelson, C. R. (1982): Human chorionic gonadotropin binding to human fetal testes as a function of gestational age. *J. Clin. Endocrinol. Metab.*, 55:791–794.
269. Warren, D. W., Huhtaniemi, I. T., Tapanainen, J., Dufau, M. L., and Catt, K. J. (1984): Ontogeny of gonadotropin receptors in the fetal and neonatal rat testis. *Endocrinology,* 114:470–476.
270. Leinonen, P. J., and Jaffe, R. B. (1985): Leydig cell desensitization by human chorionic gonadotropin does not occur in the human fetal testis. *J. Clin. Endocrinol. Metab.*, 61:234–238.
271. Warren, D. W., Schmitt, C. A., and Franzino, S. J. (1984): Adrenocorticotropin stimulates testosterone production by fetal rat testis. *Ann. N.Y. Acad. Sci.*, 438:677–680.
272. Dohr, G., and Tarmann, T. (1984): Contacts between Wollfian and Müllerian cells at the tip of the outgrowing Müllerian duct in rat embryos. *Acta Anat.*, 120:123–128.
273. Grünwald, P. (1941): The relation of the growing Müllerian duct to the Wolffian duct and its importance for the genesis of malformations. *Anat. Rec.*, 81:1–19.
274. Burkl, W., and Pollitzer, G. (1952): Über die genetischen Beziehungen des Müllerschen Ganges zum Wolffschen Gang beim Menschen. *Z. Anat. Entw. Gesch.*, 116:552–572.
275. Frutiger, P. (1969): Zur Frühentwicklung der Ductus paramesonephrici und des Müllerschen Hügels beim Menschen. *Acta Anat.*, 72:233–245.
276. Hamilton, W. J., and Mossman, H. W. (1972): *Human Embryology.* Williams & Wilkins, Baltimore.
277. Didier, E. (1973): Recherches sur la morphogénèse du canal de Müller chez les oiseaux. *Roux Arch. Entw. Mech. Org.*, 172:271–302.
278. Josso, N. (1981): Differentiation of the genital tract: Stimulators and inhibitors. In: *Mechanisms of Sex Differentiation in Animals and Man,* edited by C. R. Austin and R. G. Edwards, pp. 165–203. Academic Press, London.
279. Price, J. M., Donahoe, P. K., Ito, Y., and Hendren, W. H. III (1977): Programmed cell death in the Müllerian duct induced by Müllerian substance. *Am. J. Anat.*, 149:353–376.
280. Cunha, G. R., Shannon, J. M., Neubauer, B. L., Sawayer, L. M., Fujii, H., Taguchi, O., and Chung, L. W. K. (1981): Mesenchymal-epithelial interactions in sex differentiation. *Hum. Genet.*, 58:68–77.
281. O'Rahilly, R. (1973): The embryology and anatomy of the uterus. In: *The Uterus,* edited by H. J. Norris, A. T. Hertig, and M. R. Abell, pp. 17–39. Williams & Wilkins, Baltimore.
282. Price, D., Zaaijer, J. J. P., and Ortiz, E. (1969): Hormonal influences on genetic expression as demonstrated in organ culture studies of reproductive ducts of fetal guinea pigs. *Koninkl. Nederl. Akademie Wetenshappen. Proc. Ser. C,* 72:370–384.
283. Patten, B. M. (1953): *Human Embryology.* McGraw-Hill, New York.
284. Hunter, P. H. (1930): Observations on the development of the human female genital tract. *Contrib. Embryol. Carnegie Inst.*, 22: 91–108.
285. Davies, J., and Kusama, H. (1962): Developmental aspects of the human cervix. *Ann. N.Y. Acad. Sci.*, 97:534–550.
286. Jost, A. (1979): Basic sexual trends in the development of vertebrates. In: *Sex, Hormones and Behaviour,* pp. 5–18. *Ciba Foundation Symposium, No. 62.* Excerpta Medica, Amsterdam.
287. Picon, R. (1969): Action du testicule foetal sur le développement in vitro des canaux de Müller chez le rat. *Arch. Anat. Micr.*, 58:1–9.
288. Somjen, G. J., Kaye, A. M., and Lindner, H. (1976): Demonstration of 8-S-cytoplasmic oestrogen receptor in rat Müllerian duct. *Biochim. Biophys. Acta,* 428:787–791.
289. Pasqualini, J. R., Sumida, C., Gelly, C., and Nguyen, B. L. (1976): Specific 3H-estradiol binding in the fetal uterus and testis of guinea pig. Quantitative evolution of 3H-estradiol receptors in the different fetal tissues (kidney, lung, uterus and testis) during fetal development. *J. Steroid Biochem.*, 7:1031–1038.
290. Byskov, A. G., and Hansen, J. L. (1986): Ovarian influence on the Müllerian duct differentiation. In: *Development and Function of Reproductive Organs,* edited by A. Eshkol, B. Eckstein, N. Deckel, H. Peters, and A. Tsafriri, pp. 85–91. *Serono Symposia Review, No. 11.* Raven Press, New York.
291. Bok, G., and Drews, U. (1983): The role of the Wolffian ducts in the formation of the sinus vagina: An organ culture study. *J. Embryol. Exp. Morphol.*, 73:275–295.
292. Price, D., and Pannabecker, R. (1959): Comparative responsiveness of homologous sex ducts and accessory glands of fetal rats in culture. *Arch. Anat. Micr.*, 48:223–244.
293. Josso, N. (1970): Action de la testostérone sur le canal de Wolff du foetus de rat en culture organotypique. *Arch. Anat. Micr.*, 59:37–50.
294. Flickinger, C. J. (1969): Fine structure of the Wolffian duct and cytodifferentiation of the epididymis in fetal rats. *Z. Zellforsch.*, 96:344–360.
295. Tiedemann, K. (1971): Die Ultrastruktur des Epithels des Wolffschen Ganges und des Ductus Deferens beim Schafembryo. *Z. Zellforsch.*, 113:230–248.
296. Zondek, L. H., and Zondek, T. (1965): The secretory activity of the maturing epididymis compared with maturational changes in other reproductive organs of the foetus, infant and child. *Acta Paediatr. Scand.*, 54:295–305.
297. Wilson, J. D., Griffin, J. E., George, F. W., and Leshim, M. (1983): The endocrine control of male phenotypic development. *Aust. J. Biol. Sci.*, 36:101–128.
298. Flickinger, C. J. (1970): The fine structure and development of the seminal vesicles and prostate in the fetal rat. *Z. Zellforsch.*, 109:1–14.
299. Aumüler, G. (1979): Prostate gland and seminal vesicles. In: *Handbuch der mikroskopischen anatomie des Menschen, 7. Band. Harn- und Geschlechtapparat, 6. Teil.* Springer-Verlag, Berlin.

300. Wilson, J. D., and Siiteri, K. (1973): Developmental pattern of testosterone synthesis in the fetal gonad of the rabbit. *Endocrinology,* 92:1182–1191.
301. Wilson, J. D., and Lasnitski, I. (1971): Dihydrotestosterone formation in fetal tissues of the rabbit and rat. *Endocrinology,* 89:659–668.
302. Siiteri, P. K., and Wilson, J. D. (1974): Testosterone formation and metabolism during male sexual differentiation in the human embryo. *J. Clin. Endocrinol. Metab.,* 38:113–125.
303. Picard, J. Y., Tran, D., and Josso, N. (1978): Biosynthesis of iodinated anti-Müllerian hormone by fetal testes: Evidence for the glycoprotein nature of the hormone and for its disulfide-bonded structure. *Mol. Cell. Endocrinol.,* 12:17–30.
304. Blanchard, M. G., and Josso, N. (1974): Source of the anti-Müllerian hormone synthesized by the fetal testis: Müllerian-inhibiting activity of fetal bovine Sertoli cells in tissue culture. *Pediatr. Res.,* 8:968–971.
305. Donahoe, P. K., Ito, Y., Price, J. M., and Hendren, W. H. III (1977): Müllerian inhibiting substance activity in bovine fetal, newborn and prepuberal testes. *Biol. Reprod.,* 16:238–243.
306. Tran, D., and Josso, N. (1983): Localization of anti Müllerian hormone in the rough endoplasmic reticulum of the developing bovine Sertoli cell using immunocytochemistry with a monoclonal antibody. *Endocrinology,* 111:1562–1567.
307. Josso, N. (1972): Evolution of the Müllerian inhibiting activity of the human testis. Effect of fetal, peri-natal and post-natal human testicular tissue on the Müllerian duct of the fetal rat in organ culture. *Biol. Neonate,* 20:368–379.
308. Tran, D., and Josso, N. (1977): Relationship between ovarian and mammalian anti-Müllerian hormones. *Biol. Reprod.,* 16:267–273.
309. Josso, N., Picard, J.-Y., and Tran, D. (1977): The anti-Müllerian hormone. *Recent Prog. Horm. Res.,* 33:117–163.
310. Josso, N., and Picard, J. -Y. (1986): Anti-Müllerian hormone. *Phys. Rev.,* 66:1038–1090.
311. Taguchi, O., Cunha, G. R., Lawrence, W. D., and Robboy, S. J. (1984): Timing and irreversibility of Müllerian duct inhibition in the embryonic reproductive tract of the human male. *Dev. Biol.,* 106:394–398.
312. Picon, R. (1970): Modifications chez le rat, au cours du developpement du testicule, de son action inhibitrice sur les canaux de Müller in vitro. *C. R. Acad. Sci.,* 271:2370–2372.
313. Jost, A., Vigier, B., and Prépin, J. (1972): Freemartins in cattle: The first steps of sexual organogenesis. *J. Reprod. Fertil.,* 29:349–379.
314. Dyche, W. J. (1979): A comparative study of the differentiation and involution of the Müllerian duct and Wolffian duct in the male and female mouse. *J. Morphol.,* 162:175–210.
315. Wartenberg, H. (1985): Morphological studies on the role of the periductal stroma in the regression of the human male Müllerian duct. *Anat. Embryol.,* 171:311–323.
316. Hayashi, H. H., Shima, H., Hayashi, K., Tvelstaadt, R. L., and Donahoe, P. K. (1984): Immunocytochemical localization of Müllerian inhibiting substance in the rough endoplasmic reticulum and Golgi apparatus in Sertoli cells of the neonatal calf testis using a monoclonal antibody. *J. Histochem. Cytochem.,* 32:649–654.
317. Ikawa, H., Trelstad, R. L., Hutson, J. M., Manganaro, T. F., and Donahoe, P. K. (1984): Changing patterns of fibronectin, laminin, type IV collagen and a basement membrane proteoglycan during rat Müllerian duct regression. *Dev. Biol.,* 102:260–263.
318. Hutson, J. M., Fallat, M. E., Kamagata, S., Donahoe, P. K., and Budzik, G. P. (1984): Phosphorylation events during Müllerian duct regression. *Science,* 233:586–589.
319. Fallat, M. E., Hutson, J. M., Budzik, G. P., and Donahoe, P. K. (1983): The role of nucleotide pyrophosphatase in Müllerian duct regression. *Dev. Biol.,* 100:358–364.
320. Wolff, E. (1939): L'action du diethylstilbestrol sur les organes genitaux de l'embryon de poulet. *C. R. Acad. Sci.,* 208:1532–1535.
321. McLachlan, J. A., Newbold, R. R., and Bullock, B. (1975): Reproductive tract lesions in male mice exposed prenatally to diethylstilbestrol. *Science,* 190:991–992.
322. Newbold, R. R., Suzuki, Y., McLachlan, J. A. (1984): Müllerian duct maintenance in heterotypic organ culture after in vivo exposure to diethylstilbestrol. *Endocrinology,* 115:1863–1868.
323. Kobayashi, S. (1984): Induction of Müllerian duct derivatives in testicular feminized (Tfm) mice by prenatal exposure to diethylstilbestrol. *Anal. Embryol.,* 169:35–39.

The Physiology of Reproduction,
edited by E. Knobil and J. Neill *et al.*
Raven Press, Ltd., New York © 1988.

CHAPTER 9

The Primate Oviduct and Endometrium

Robert M. Brenner and Ila A. Maslar

The cyclic fluctuations in serum estradiol (E_2) and progesterone (P) that occur during the primate menstrual cycle are clearly responsible for the dramatic, cyclic changes that occur throughout the reproductive tract. Although there have been reviews of the primate endometrium (1) and oviduct (2), careful comparisons of the similarities and differences in hormonal responsiveness that exist between these two organs in primates have not been done. We have focused our attention on those similarities and differences in the following review.

CYCLIC CHANGES IN THE PRIMATE OVIDUCT

A number of comprehensive reviews of the biology and cellular ultrastructure of the mammalian oviduct have been published (2–8), and some of these include a considerable amount of information on the oviducts of the common laboratory macaques. The older literature on the comparative gross anatomy of the primate oviduct was summarized by Eckstein (9) in the *Handbook of Primatology*. Most recently, fairly comprehensive studies of the cyclic changes in the oviducts of cynomolgus (10) and pig-tailed macaques (11–13) have been completed. In addition some recent definitive studies (14,15) on the oviducts of women have been reported. What follows is a review of these reports.

Homo sapiens

Novak and Everett (16) provided the first well-documented study of the oviductal cycle in women. These workers showed that in the postmenstrual period the ciliated and secretory cells increased in height to a maximum near midcycle and then diminished in height to a minimum in the premenstrual and menstrual phases. The ciliated cells shrunk more rapidly than the secretory cells, and the apices of the latter projected well beyond the tips of the cilia during the latter part of the cycle. In the older literature, reviewed by Novak and Everett (16), these protruding secretory cells were referred to as "peg" cells and erroneously assumed to be a third cell type of the oviductal epithelium. Verhage et al. (14) reviewed the literature up to 1979 and noted that although there was general agreement that secretory cells varied in cell height in cyclical fashion, there was considerable disagreement on the nature of the changes in the ciliated cells. Some authors (17–20) reported no change in the percentage of ciliation during the cycle, while others (21) observed ciliogenesis with the electron microscope. Verhage et al. (14) studied the oviducts of 24 normally cycling women, 6 each during the early follicular, late follicular, early luteal and late luteal phases of the menstrual cycle. Endometrial biopsies and radioimmunoassay of serum levels of E_2 and P were used to assess the stage of the cycle. Six additional samples were obtained from pregnant women and six from women during the postpartum phase. The cytomorphometrics showed that the epithelial cells attained their maximum height and degree of ciliation during the late follicular phase in both the fimbriae and the ampulla. At the end of the luteal phase some atrophy and deciliation had occurred, especially in the fimbriae. Hypertrophy and reciliation occurred during the early follicular phase. Approximately 10% to 12% of the cells formed new cilia in both the fimbriae and the ampulla during each menstrual cycle. During pregnancy and through the postpartum period, there was further atrophy and deciliation (from 57% ciliation and 30-μm cell height at midcycle to 24% ciliation and 20 μm at parturition). Atrophy and deciliation were associated with elevated serum P levels; hypertrophy and reciliation with low P and moderate E_2 levels. Ultrastructural studies of these tissues showed that the pattern of ciliogenesis was very similar to that described for the rhesus monkey (22). In sum, this careful study indicated that although the ciliation–deciliation cycles that occur in the human oviduct are much less extensive than in the oviducts of nonhuman primates, P antagonizes and E_2 stimulates epithelial cell hypertrophy, secretion, and ciliogenesis in both species. The most recent study of the human oviduct (15) confirmed these conclusions and added that an increase in epithelial mitotic activity occurred during the follicular phase when P was essentially undetectable. Moreover, these workers agreed that deciliation, decrease of epithelial height, and a loss of mitotic activity coincided with elevated levels of P; continuous progestin therapy had the same antiestrogenic effect on the tubal epithelium that was exerted by endogenous P during the luteal phase. The same laboratory had shown previously (23) that estrogens could induce oviductal ciliogenesis in menopausal women. These findings confirm and extend the earlier observations by Andrews (24) that estrogens stimulate oviductal ciliogenesis in postparturient women and that progestins can inhibit this effect.

Jansen (8) has written an interesting review that included an update on the hormonal regulation of oviductal secretions, especially of the human and nonhuman primate oviduct. He notes that around the time of ovulation the secretions of the isthmic region become much more viscous than those of the ampulla. Indeed, the lumen of the isthmus fills with a viscous plug that renders the cilia invisible by scanning electron microscopy. This material was most abundant at midcycle when E_2 levels were highest; P suppressed this secretion. Jansen (8) suggested that this isthmic mucous layer may, like the analogous mucous column in the endocervix, play an important regulatory role in the transport of sperm through the isthmus towards the ampullary–isthmic junction where fertilization normally occurs. Currently, however, there is little biochemical information on the differences in the composition of the fluid secreted by the different regions of the primate oviduct.

Macaca nemestrina

Oviductal cycles have been observed in pig-tailed macaques in a series of studies (11–13). The first of these (11) was a scanning electron microscope study of the oviducts of 23 females. Twelve animals were sampled at midcycle, three during the early follicular, and four in the late luteal phases of the menstrual cycle. Four had been ovariectomized for at least 2 years. One of these four served as an untreated control, and three were treated with estrogen for either 7 or 12 days before the oviducts were sampled.

The results showed that the fimbriae were extensively ciliated during midcycle and sparsely ciliated in the early follicular and late luteal phases. There was evidence of extensive ciliogenesis early in the cycle and signs of ciliary degeneration and shedding late in the cycle. The ampullary epithelium behaved similarly, although the changes were less dramatic. The surface of the isthmus, however, showed little cyclic change. Ovariectomy resulted in almost complete deciliation in the fimbriae and ampulla but not in the isthmus. Treatment with estradiol benzoate restored the epithelium to its heavily ciliated, midcycle appearance.

The second study (12) was an examination of embedded samples of the same tissues that had been examined by scanning microscopy. The percentage of ciliated versus nonciliated cells was determined in 1.5-μm Epon sections by counting through the light microscope. Epithelial ultrastructure was evaluated by transmission electron microscopy. Statistical analysis of the quantitative data confirmed that the number of ciliated cells in the fimbriae and ampullae was significantly higher at midcycle than in the late luteal phase. Considerable variability in the percentage ciliation between animals in the same stage of the cycle and between different blocks of tissue from the same region of the oviduct was noted.

Ultrastructural analysis revealed typical ciliogenic phases in the epithelium during the early follicular phase. In addition, interesting examples were found of internalization of ciliary axonemes into apical protrusions on ciliated cells. The authors suggested that the shedding of such protrusions may be part of the mechanism of deciliation, along with other mechanisms such as the death and extrusion of whole ciliated cells and the apocrine-like shedding of the entire apex of individual ciliated cells.

In the third report on the oviducts of these animals (13), cyclic changes in the oviductal secretory cells were described. In the fimbriae, the secretory cells contained one type of granule that was small and electron dense, whereas in the ampulla and isthmus the secretory cells had two kinds of electron-dense granules and two kinds of electron-lucent vacuoles. The vacuoles had either a fine particulate content or loosely arranged lamellar arrays. The granules either were homogeneous or had tightly packed lamellar arrays. At midcycle the secretory cells were at their tallest, and the various types of granules and vacuoles were most abundant. Early and late in the cycle, the cells were smaller and the granules less abundant, though there was considerable variability from animal to animal and region to region. The authors suggested that the lamellated granules transform into those vacuoles that contain lamellae and that these vacuoles release their contents by exocytosis. They also suggested that a form of apocrine secretion may occur in which electron-dense granules, surrounded by a thin rim of cytoplasm, may be extruded from the cell surface into the lumen. The authors conclude, however, that the exact mode of secretion is impossible to discern from static electron-microscope images and that the presence of the various types of granules and vacuoles is evidence of a very complex process. A more complete understanding of the cytological details of the secretion mechanism awaits studies with tracer molecules.

Cynomolgus and Rhesus Macaques

In the most recent report from our laboratory on cyclic changes in the oviduct (10) we sampled the reproductive tracts of 27 cynomolgus macaques during the menstrual cycle and correlated the cytologic changes in the oviductal epithelium with changes in the serum levels of E_2 and P and with the histology of the ovaries and the endometria.

To provide an adequate sample in the preovulatory, postovulatory, and premenstrual phases of the cycle, we drew blood daily for several days before these periods, performed rapid radioimmunoassays (RIAs) for serum E_2 and P, and then selected the appropriate time for laparotomy.

Ovaries, oviducts, and uteri were fixed (25) and embedded in either Araldite or glycolmethacrylate (GMA) (26). Portions of the oviducts and endometria were assayed for estrogen receptor content (27).

Ciliated cell height and the percentage ciliation were measured in the fimbriae, ampulla, and isthmus as previously described (28). Also, the distance that the tips of the secretory cells extended beyond the basal body row of neighboring ciliated cells was determined with an ocular micrometer at a magnification of 1,000× in 35 to 40 cells per region. This measurement, which we call "secretory tip extension," is a useful index of secretory cell development.

A number of additional cytological features were qualitatively assessed. These included size and roundness of epithelial nuclei, degree of mitotic activity, extent of ciliogenesis as marked by basal body formation, content of glycogen and granules in secretory cells, and degree of pinching-off of ciliated cell tips; the latter is a process similar to apocrine secretion (2).

Two additional criteria were the presence of intraepithelial apoptotic bodies (29,30), an indicator of cell death by apoptosis, and the presence of macrophages filled with nuclear and cellular fragments in subepithelial and intraepithelial locations. These two phenomena have been shown to be hormonally regulated in the uterine luminal epithelium of the hamster (25) and the oviductal epithelium of the cat (31). In an earlier study of the rhesus monkey we reported that the oviduct atrophied and dedifferentiated if P was administered to spayed animals that were being treated with E_2, but we had made no comments about cell death (28). Recently we reviewed the slides from that original study and found that by 2 to 5 days after the initiation of P treatment there were many examples of cell death by apoptosis as well as macrophage invasion. We have also recently reviewed the slides from our earliest report on the oviducts of naturally cycling rhesus monkeys (32). Although the postovulatory samples in the group were not so precisely staged as the current group of cynomolgus macaques, we found examples of oviductal apoptosis and macrophage invasion during the early luteal phase in the oviducts of that group of rhesus as well. Our laboratory had also reported that E_2 withdrawal was a very effective apoptotic stimulus in the uterine luminal epithelium of hamsters (25), and we had concluded that during the natural cycle in the hamster, apoptosis in the uterine luminal epithelium is probably induced by the sharp decline in E_2 combined with the rise in P that occurs during the proestrus–estrus transition. Together, these would induce a sharp estrogen withdrawal in estrogen-dependent cells. A similar pattern of a rapid decline in E_2 after the preovulatory surge and a rise in serum P occurs in the periovulatory period in primates, and this hormonal shift is undoubtedly responsible for the occurrence of cell death, including apoptosis and macrophage invasion, that occurs in the oviducts of cynomolgus and rhesus monkeys. As noted previously, oviductal apoptosis can be induced by P treatment in spayed rhesus receiving continuous injections of E_2. Consequently, in the primate oviduct (as in the luminal epithelium of the hamster uterus) estrogen withdrawal, effective or real, is the stimulus that induces apoptosis.

In our recent work on cynomolgus oviducts (10) we assessed three quantitative and seven qualitative cytologic factors. This led to a more complete analysis of oviductal development than either we or others had previously conducted. Consequently, we were able to define, for cynomolgus macaques, eight specific stages through which the oviduct passes in sequence during the cycle. We have named these stages in order of their appearance during the cycle, as follows: preciliogenic, ciliogenic, ciliogenic-ciliated, ciliated-ciliogenic, ciliated-secretory, early regression, late regression, and full regression. A description of each stage follows, and the stages are illustrated in Figs. 1 to 8. The descriptions were developed through study of the oviducts of cynomolgus macaques, but the same stages occur in rhesus macaques as well.

Preciliogenic (Fig. 1): This phase is marked by the onset of swelling of epithelial cell nuclei, smoothing of the nuclear contours, cellular hypertrophy, and mitotic activity. Light and dark cells are not apparent; generally, no basal bodies are evident.

Ciliogenic (Fig. 2): Mitosis and cellular hypertrophy continue; epithelial nuclei are round and smooth; light and dark cells can now be distinguished, and basal bodies may be apparent in the apical cytoplasm of the light, hypertrophied cells.

Ciliogenic-ciliated (Fig. 3): All the features of the ciliogenic phase persist, but numerous ciliated cells have now developed. Secretory (dark) cells are present but not prominent. The word "ciliogenic" is placed first in the name of this phase to emphasize that ciliogenic cells predominate over ciliated ones.

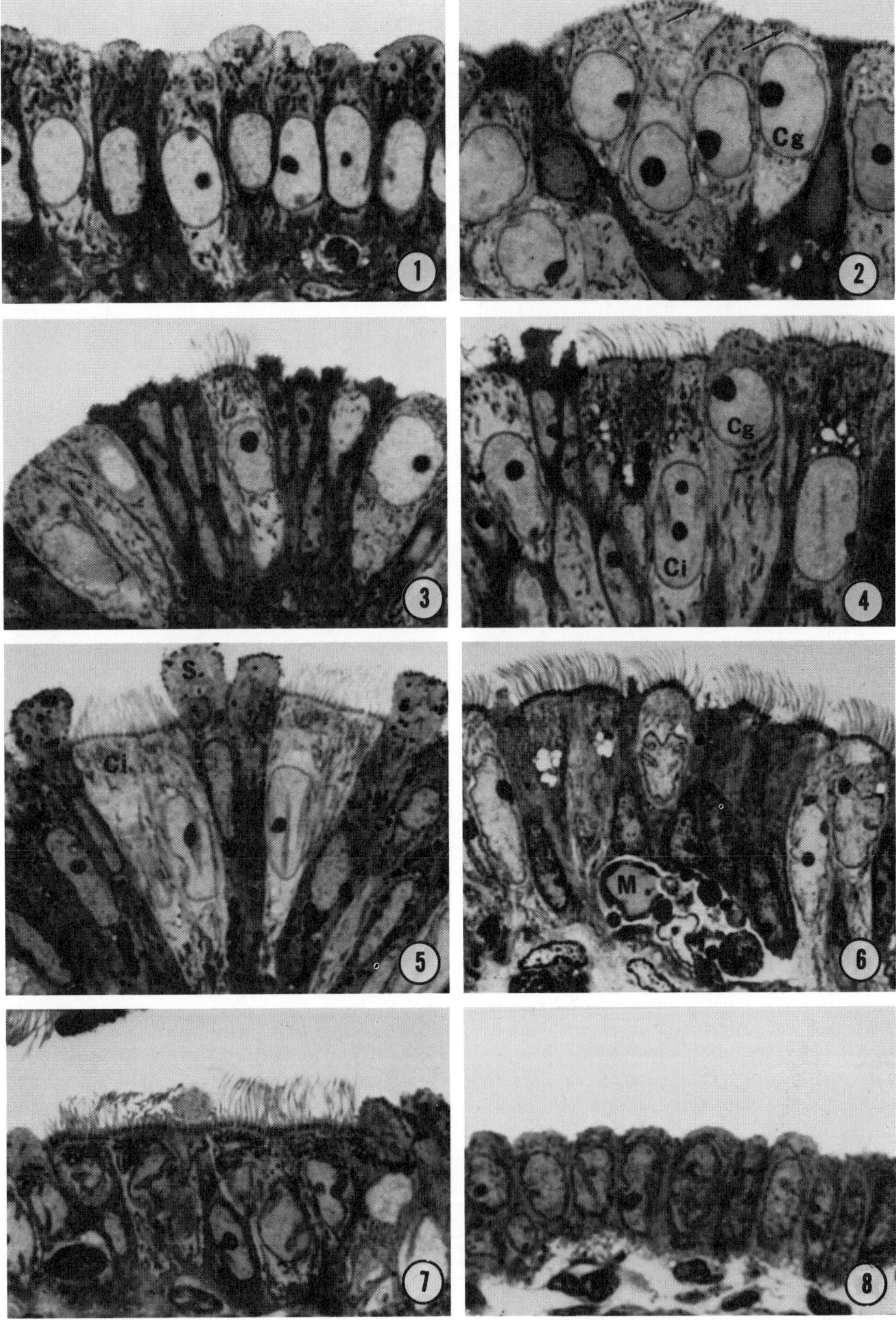

FIGS. 1–8. (*See legends on facing page.*) (From ref. 10.)

Ciliated-ciliogenic (Fig. 4): In this phase, the majority of cells have become ciliated, but a few cells undergoing ciliogenesis can still be found scattered through the epithelium. Moreover, mitotic activity has not yet ceased. Secretory cells have become much more prominent and have developed bulbous tips filled with granules and glycogen. The word "ciliated" is placed first in the name of this phase to emphasize that ciliated cells predominate over ciliogenic ones.

Ciliated-secretory (Fig. 5): In this phase most epithelial cells are either ciliated or secretory, and ciliogenic phases are extremely rare. Secretory cells are fully developed, with bulbous tips rich in granules, glycogen, and some vacuoles. These tips extend well beyond the basal body row in the fimbriae and well past the cilia in the ampulla and isthmus. Epithelial cell nuclear contours are less smooth than during ciliogenesis.

Early regression (Fig. 6): In this phase there are apoptotic and pyknotic epithelial cells scattered throughout the epithelium. Macrophages have invaded the epithelium and are phagocytosing dead cells. There are no other differences from the ciliated-secretory phase.

Late regression (Fig. 7): In this phase, the epithelium is atrophied, secretory activity has diminished, considerable deciliation has occurred, and many ciliated cells appear to be pinching off their tips. Dead cells and macrophages are still present. Epithelial cell nuclei now appear definitely shriveled.

Full regression (Fig. 8): In this phase the epithelium is maximally atrophied and deciliated, epithelial cell nuclei are maximally shriveled, and secretory activity is at a minimum. There are very few dead cells left, and macrophages are less common.

All of the cyclic changes, with one exception, are most evident in the fimbriae, less so in the ampulla, and least in the isthmus. The exception is secretory tip extension, which is least in the fimbriae, larger in the ampulla, and greatest in the isthmus (see Fig. 9).

In Table 1 we list for each animal the predominant ovarian features, the levels of serum E_2 and P, the predominant endometrial features, the mean percentage ciliation in the fimbriae, the oviductal stage, and the days elapsed since the onset of the last menses (cycle day). The animals are presented from the top down in the order of their oviductal (not menstrual) cycles. In five of the six menstruating animals the oviducts were in various phases of the ciliogenic process, so these were ranked first. One menstruating animal (no. 8836) was ranked last because its oviducts were still fully regressed. The ovaries of all menstruating animals had large regressing corpora lutea, serum P levels below 1 ng/ml, and serum E_2 levels that ranged from 35 to 109 pg/ml.

In monkeys with serum E_2 between 88 and 171 pg/ml (medium ovarian follicles) the oviducts were in the ciliogenic-ciliated stage.

In most monkeys with large preovulatory follicles and very high serum E_2 levels (298–583 pg/ml), the oviducts were ciliated-ciliogenic. In one of these (no. 8838), the oviduct had progressed further to the ciliated-secretory state.

Of those animals that we "caught" just after ovulation, one was in the ciliated-secretory state and others showed signs of early regression, namely, scattered epithelial cell death with apoptotic bodies and macrophage invasion.

There were nine monkeys whose oviducts were classified as either late regression or full regression. These were associated either with a large well-developed corpus luteum that was actively secreting progesterone (serum P well above 1 ng/ml) or with a large well-developed one that had early morphological signs of regression and had stopped secreting progesterone (serum P below 1 ng/ml). In eight of these animals the endometrium had become progestational to varied degrees. The other (no. 8836), as previously noted, was menstruating, but its oviduct had not yet come out of the regressed state.

FIG. 1. *Preciliogenic.* Ampulla. All the cells are hypertrophied, and their nuclei are swollen. No basal bodies can be seen by light microscopy. ×1,050.

FIG. 2. *Ciliogenic.* Fimbriae. Ciliogenic (Cg) cells are light, hypertrophied cells with swollen nuclei and enlarged nucleoli; basal bodies (*arrows*) are present in the apical cytoplasm. The dark cells are future secretory cells. ×1,050.

FIG. 3. *Ciliogenic-ciliated.* Ampulla. Most of the light cells are ciliogenic but a few have become ciliated. The dark cells are future secretory cells. ×1,050.

FIG. 4. *Ciliated-ciliogenic.* Ampulla. Most of the light cells have become ciliated (Ci), but some are still ciliogenic (Cg). The dark cells are secretory. ×1,050.

FIG. 5. *Ciliated-secretory.* Ampulla. The light cells are ciliated, the dark cells are secretory. Note the pronounced degree of secretory tip extension. ×1,050.

FIG. 6. *Early regression.* Fimbriae. Large numbers of macrophages (M) filled with nuclear and cellular fragments are present in the epithelium. ×1,050.

FIG. 7. *Late regression.* Ampulla. The epithelium consists of atrophied ciliated and secretory cells with shriveled nuclei. Deciliation is more extensive in some regions than others during this phase. ×1,050. (From ref. 10.)

FIG. 8. *Full regression.* Fimbriae. The epithelial cells are maximally atrophied and dedifferentiated, and their nuclei are maximally shriveled. ×1,050.

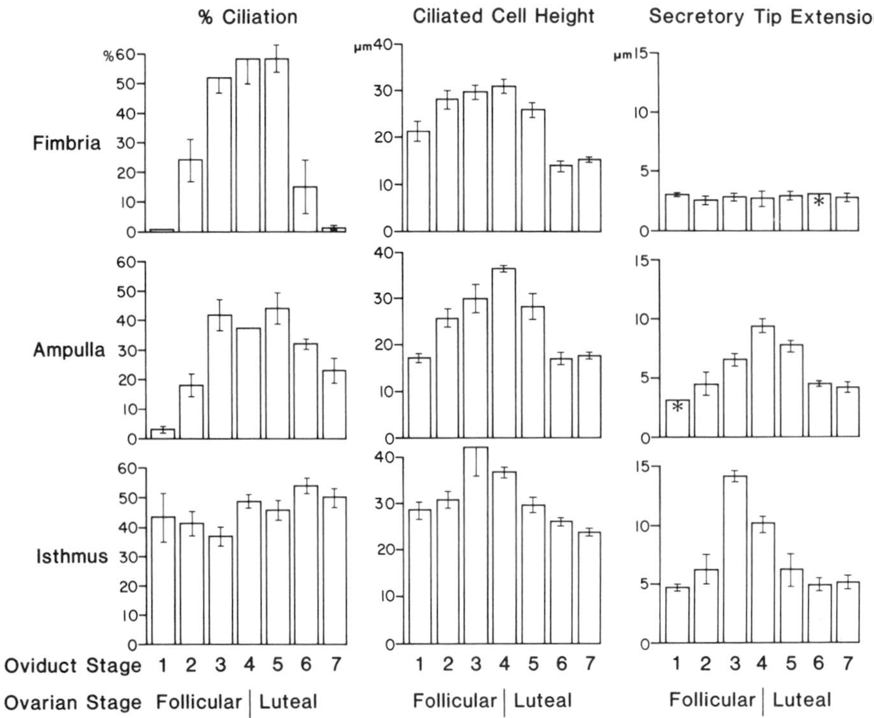

FIG. 9. Comparison of percentage ciliation, cell height, and secretory tip extension in the fimbriae, ampulla and isthmic regions of the oviduct of cynomolgus macaques at different times during the menstrual cycle. The data were grouped according to the oviductal staging sequence described in the text. For convenience of presentation in graphic form, the oviductal stages were given group numbers as follows: *Group 1,* preciliogenic-ciliogenic (n = 3); *Group 2,* ciliogenic-ciliated (n = 6); *Group 3,* ciliated-ciliogenic (n = 3); *Group 4,* ciliated-secretory (n = 2); *Group 5,* early regression (n = 4); *Group 6,* late regression (n = 2); and *Group 7,* full regression (n = 7). Data are presented as means with standard error bars where appropriate. Asterisk indicates sample of one. (From ref. 10.)

TABLE 1. *Oviductal, ovarian, and endometrial features in 27 cycling cynomolgus macaques*

Animal	Cycle day	Mean percentage ciliation in fimbriae	Oviduct stage	E_2 (pg/ml)	P (ng/ml)	Ovarian features	Endometrial stage
9414	1	0	Preciliogenic	93	0.30	Regressing C.L.[a]	Menses
9413	2	0	Ciliogenic	36	0.33	Regressing C.L.	Menses
9449	3	0	Ciliogenic	109	0.54	Regressing C.L.	Menses
9437	2	5.4	Ciliogenic-ciliated	35	0.85	Regressing C.L.	Menses-repair
9420	4	10.5	Ciliogenic-ciliated	76	0.18	Medium follicles	Menses-repair
8819	4	12.0	Ciliogenic-ciliated	152	0.90	Medium follicles	Early proliferative
9425	6	30.0	Ciliogenic-ciliated	88	0.10	Medium follicles	(Tissue lost)
9411	6	50.5	Ciliogenic-ciliated	124	0.10	Large follicle	Early proliferative
9421	6	34.0	Ciliogenic-ciliated	171	0.11	Medium follicle	Early proliferative
9439	13	56.5	Ciliated-ciliogenic	406	0.57	Preovulatory follicle	Midproliferative
9430	11	41.5	Ciliated-ciliogenic	583	0.50	Preovulatory follicle	Midproliferative
9417	10	56.5	Ciliated-ciliogenic	298	0.12	Preovulatory follicle	Midproliferative
8838	40	65.3	Ciliated-secretory	202	0.10	Preovulatory follicle	Late proliferative
8808	14	49.0	Ciliated-secretory	139	2.32	Fresh C.L.	Late proliferative
8817	13	57.0	Early regression	56	0.65	Fresh C.L.	Proliferative-progestational
9436	25	48.5	Early regression	56	2.28	Fresh C.L.	Proliferative-progestational
8833	13	66.8	Early regression	49	2.41	Fresh C.L.	Proliferative-progestational
8821	18	61.0	Early regression	63	4.13	Fresh C.L.	Proliferative-progestational
8828	25	23.5	Late regression	131	5.69	Functional C.L.	Midprogestational
9442	28	5.5	Late regression	62	0.81	Regressing C.L.	Late progestational
8837	25	2.0	Full regression	62	2.90	Functional C.L.	Midprogestational
9416	28	1.0	Full regression	56	0.74	Regressing C.L.	Midprogestational
8815	22	1.0	Full regression	119	12.15	Functional C.L.	Late progestational
8810	32	1.0	Full regression	19	0.20	Regressing C.L.	Late progestational
8825	27	2.0	Full regression	75	7.11	Functional C.L.	Late progestational
8818	30	1.0	Full regression	45	2.66	Functional C.L.	Late progestational
8836	2	2.0	Full regression	60	0.10	Regressing C.L.	Menses

[a]C.L., corpus luteum.
From ref. 10.

The least useful criterion for accurately staging oviducts, as Bartelmez (33) and others have noted for endometria, is the time elapsed since the last menses (the day of the cycle). For example, monkey 8817 was on the 13th day and had a fresh corpus luteum. Monkey 9436 was on day 25 and also had a very fresh corpus luteum. In both these animals the oviductal state (early regression) clearly reflected the hormonal pattern of P elevation with E_2 withdrawal associated with corpus luteum formation. Monkey 9436 had simply had an unusually long follicular phase. Similarly, when monkey 8838 was sampled, 40 days had elapsed since its last recorded menses, but it had a large preovulatory follicle, serum E_2 of 202 pg/ml, late proliferative endometrium, and a ciliated-secretory oviduct. All physiological and morphological data on this animal indicate that it was in a late follicular, preovulatory condition.

Table 1 also indicates that the oviductal stages are roughly equivalent to the typical ovarian stages of the primate menstrual cycle as follows: Preciliogenic and ciliogenic = early follicular; ciliogenic-ciliated = midfollicular; ciliated-ciliogenic = late follicular; ciliated-secretory = periovulatory; early regression = early luteal; late regression = midluteal; and full regression = late luteal.

Fimbrial–Endometrial Relationships

Figures 10 to 16 are micrographs that compare the morphological state of the oviductal fimbriae with that of the endometrium in individual animals at different times in the cycle. Generally when the endometrium is sloughing, the fimbrial epithelium is undergoing ciliogenesis (Figs. 10 and 11); when the endometrium is in the late proliferative stage, the fimbrial epithelium is in the ciliated-secretory state (Figs. 12 and 13); and when the endometrium becomes hypertrophied and progestational, the fimbrial epithelium regresses (Figs. 14–16).

Figure 9 shows that cyclic change in the percentage ciliation is most evident in the fimbriae, less so in the ampulla and absent in the isthmus. The height of the ciliated cells increases to a maximum in the late follicular phase and then decreases to a minimum in the late luteal phase in all three regions. The degree of secretory tip extension does not fluctuate during the cycle in the fimbriae, but in the ampulla and isthmus, secretory tip extension becomes maximal at midcycle.

Odor et al. (12) noted that the oviducts of pig-tailed macaques showed considerable local variability in the degree of ciliated and secretory cell differentiation. In our experience (unpublished), the oviducts of *M. nemestrina* are indeed more variable than those of *M. mulatta* or *M. fascicularis*. However, we do find variability in oviductal responsiveness in the latter two species, and indeed, such variability is the basis of the oviductal staging system that we have described above. For example, we have shown, in a preliminary morphometric study, that nuclear swelling in the oviductal epithelium is one of the earliest responses to E_2 treatment (34). In preciliogenic fimbriae, we have noted that the nuclei of epithelial cells at the bases of mucosal folds may be swollen, while those of cells on the crests of mucosal folds are not. Whether variations in the microenvironment or constitutive differences in E_2 thresholds within the population of epithelial cells are responsible for these differences is not yet known. Our experience suggests that once a cell has responded to E_2 and entered the ciliogenic process, it will ultimately form cilia if E_2 is unopposed by

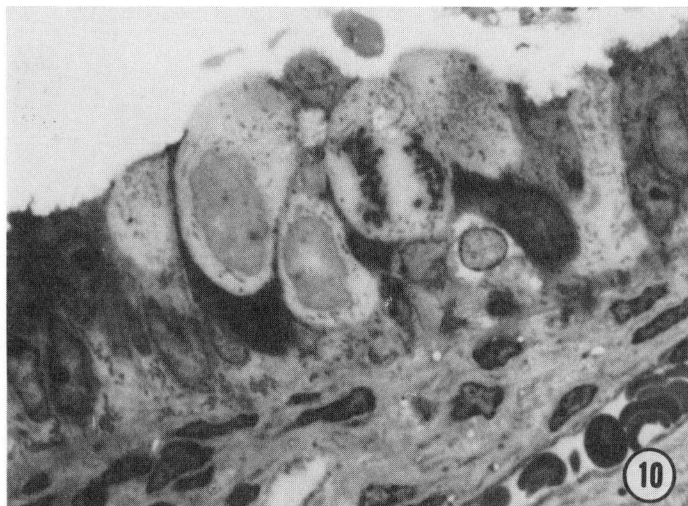

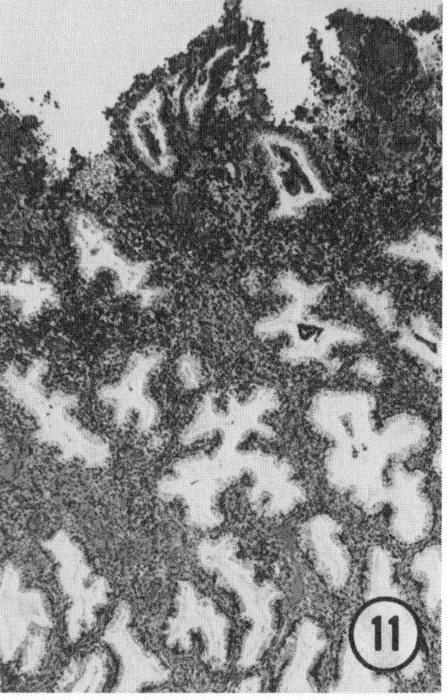

FIGS. 10 and 11. Comparison of fimbriae and endometrium during menses. (From ref. 10.) **FIG. 10.** Fimbriae in the ciliogenic state. A mitotic figure is evident, and there are a number of light, hypertrophied ciliogenic cells. The darker epithelial cells are future secretory cells. ×788. **FIG. 11.** Endometrium during menses. Typical sloughing of the upper zones is evident. ×20.

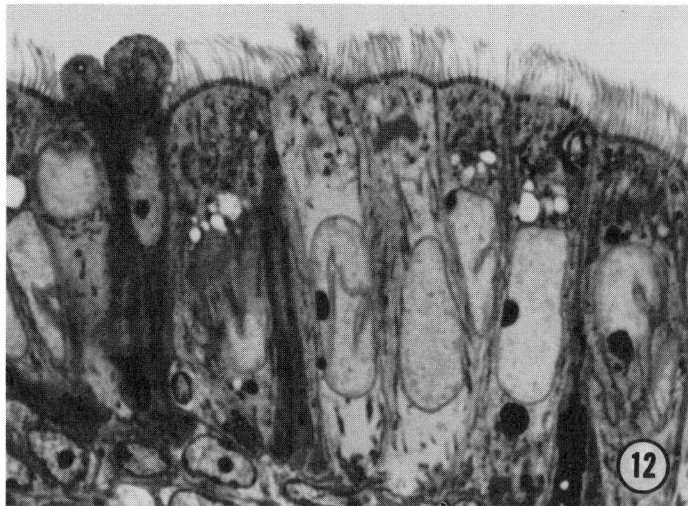

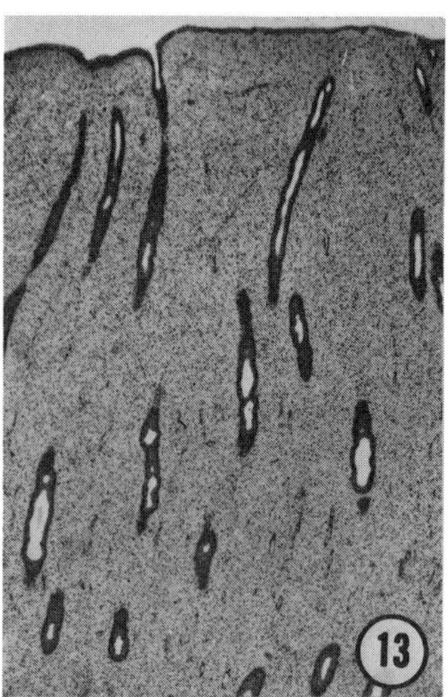

FIGS. 12 and 13. Comparison of fimbriae and endometrium during the preovulatory period. (From ref. 10.). **FIG. 12.** Fimbriae in the ciliated-secretory stage. ×1,575. **FIG. 13.** Endometrium in the late proliferative stage. ×20.

P. But the rate of such differentiation might well differ among individual ciliogenic cells. In the ciliogenic-ciliated stage most cells are ciliogenic but only a few have become ciliated; presumably the latter cells were either the first to enter or the quickest to complete the ciliogenic process. In the ciliated-ciliogenic stage most cells were ciliated but a few were still ciliogenic; presumably the latter cells were either the last to enter or the slowest to complete ciliogenesis. Even in the ciliated-secretory state, when the great majority of cells were either ciliated or secretory, a few ciliogenic cells could still be found; presumably, the latter cells had lagged greatly behind the majority of those cells destined to form cilia.

After ovulation, cell death occurs in some (but not all) of the epithelial cells. Those that die are apparently extremely sensitive to the combination of estrogen withdrawal and progestin increase characteristic of this period; the great majority of the epithelial cells simply atrophy during this

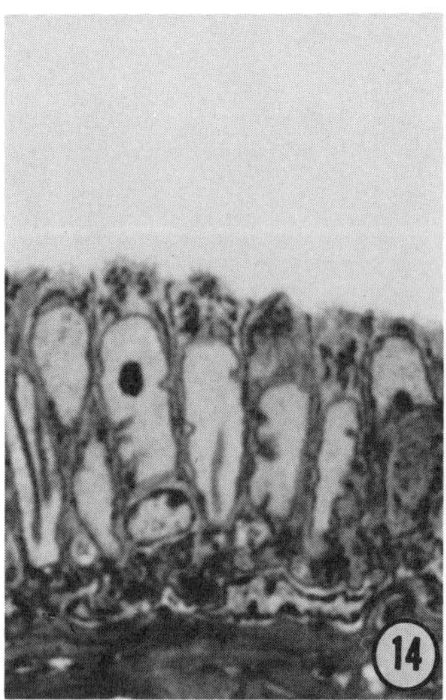

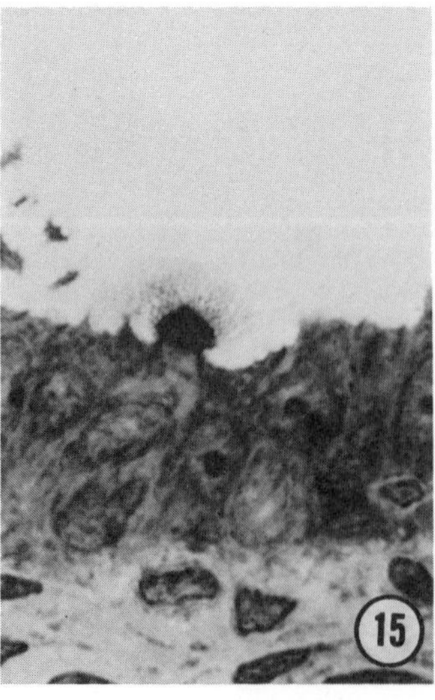

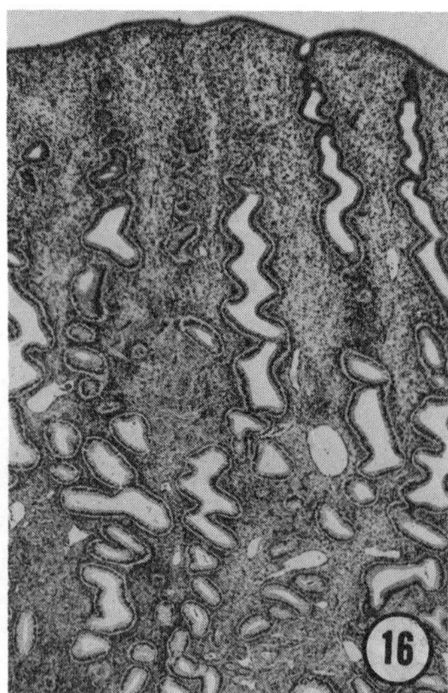

FIGS. 14–16. Comparison of fimbriae and endometrium during the late luteal phase. (From ref. 10.) **FIG. 14.** Fimbriae in the full regression stage. ×1,575. **FIG. 15.** Fimbriae. Another region of the epithelium shown in Fig. 14. An example of the apocrine-like process by which the tips of ciliated cells are pinched off is shown. ×1,575. **FIG. 16.** Endometrium in the late progestational stage. The endometrial glands are highly sacculated. ×20.

time. Differences in the rate of regression during the remainder of the luteal phase also exist. In the fimbriae, many cells lose their cilia quickly, most lose them eventually, but a few never deciliate. Even in long-term ovariectomized animals, a few shrunken and shriveled but fully ciliated cells may persist in the fimbriae. The factors that make some cells so sensitive and others so insensitive to hormonal changes remain to be discovered.

In addition there appear to be cephalocaudal gradients that underlie the regional differences in the hormonal responsiveness of the oviduct. For example, Fig. 9 shows that most of the ciliated cells in the fimbriae lose their cilia by the end of the cycle, while most of those in the isthmus shrink but do not deciliate. The ampulla is somewhat intermediate in this regard. Figure 9 shows that the midcycle bulging of the secretory cell tips is more prominent in the caudal than the cephalad regions of the oviduct. Such cephalocaudal gradients may be remnants of the developmental gradients that exist in the Müllerian duct of the fetus and lead first to the development of the oviduct, the uterus, and the cranial vagina, and then later to development of the fimbriae, ampulla, and isthmus. The biochemical nature of such gradients in either the fetus or the adult remains to be elucidated.

BRIEF OVERVIEW OF ESTROGEN AND PROGESTIN RECEPTORS IN THE PRIMATE OVIDUCT AND UTERUS

The observation that E_2 stimulates the synthesis of E_2 and P receptors in reproductive tract tissues and that sequentially administered P has an opposite, suppressive effect on both receptor systems has been made in several species by several workers (35–38). All published data on E_2 receptor fluctuations during natural menstrual cycles in both human and monkey oviducts and uterus consistently show that nuclear and cytosolic receptor levels are higher during the follicular than during the luteal phase. Figure 17 presents the most recent data from this laboratory on cyclic changes in oviductal and endometrial estrogen receptor (27). These data were obtained from the same 27 cynomolgus macaques represented in Table 1 (10). In the oviduct, the decline in nuclear receptor levels during the luteal phase is associated with cellular atrophy, regression, and loss of differentiated characteristics, whereas in the endometrium, the decline in the estrogen receptor occurs at a time when the endometrium is undergoing extensive progestational development in preparation for implantation. One might expect that, in order to sustain P action, nuclear P receptor levels would be elevated throughout the luteal phase in both organs. However, in both organs, although cytosolic levels of the P receptor are lower during the luteal than the follicular phase, nuclear P receptor levels are reported to be significantly higher only at midcycle or during the first few days of elevated P in the circulation (39–48).

These data are consistent with the view that E_2 treatment increases total P receptor amounts (mostly cytosolic, operationally defined), that sequential P treatment may temporarily increase the amount of P receptor measurable as nuclear, but that eventually there is a reduction of nuclear receptor content during P action. The progestational development of the primate endometrium and the suppression of the differentiated state in the oviduct are both dependent on continuous P action during the cycle, but paradoxically, the action of P tends to decrease the level of its own receptor in both organs. Direct measurements of the endogenous tissue levels of the steroids E_2 and/or P in the reproductive tract by RIA have shown that nuclear and cytosolic E_2 levels in human endometrium and myometrium are higher during the proliferative than during the secretory phase (49) and that P concentrations are greater during the secretory phase in endometrium (50–52) and myometrium (53,54). Recently, West et al. (55) in our laboratory compared endometrial and oviductal nuclear and cytosolic P receptor with P levels measured in aliquots of the same nuclear and cytosolic fractions. Oviducts and endometria were removed from animals after either an artificial follicular phase (14 days E_2) or an artificial luteal phase (E_2, 14 days; then 14 days of E_2 plus P).

In the oviduct, the levels of P receptor in both nuclear and cytosolic fractions in the estrogenized animals were significantly lowered by P treatment. However, in the endometrium, P treatment lowered only the cytosolic, not the nuclear, P receptor levels. In the nuclear fractions prepared from the various tissues, P levels were significantly elevated by P treatment only in the endometrial, not the oviductal, nuclear fractions. In the corresponding cytosolic fractions, P levels were either significantly or substantially increased in all the tissues of the tract. The apparent high level of cytosolic P in tissues from animals treated with P is no doubt due to the inclusion into cytosols of high levels of P from contamination with plasma, lymph, and interstitial fluids. However, nuclei were washed extensively before the measurement of P levels and would have minimal free P.

In sum, the only tissue in which the number of occupied nuclear P receptors was increased after 2 weeks of P treatment was the endometrium. The evidence thus indicates that progestational responses of endometrium are correlated with maintenance of endometrial nuclear P receptor and elevated nuclear P levels. In the oviduct, however, treatment with P results in decreased levels of both nuclear P receptor and P. How P maintains its suppressive effects on the oviduct during the luteal phase is a matter for further research.

THE ENDOMETRIUM OF HIGHER PRIMATES

Anatomical Overview

The endometrium is the mucosa that lines the uterine cavity. Its surface is composed of a simple columnar epi-

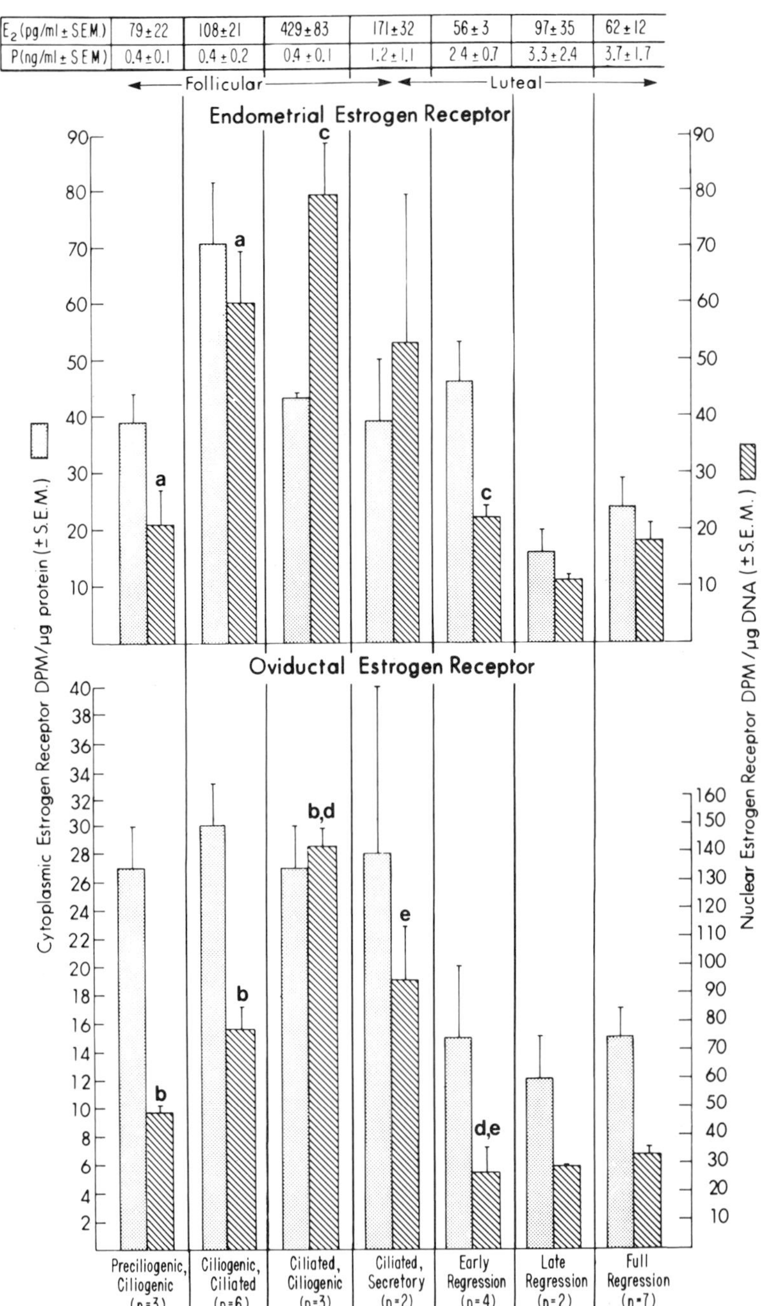

FIG. 17. Nuclear and cytoplasmic estradiol (E_2) receptors in oviducts and endometrium of cynomolgus macaques during the menstrual cycle. The abscissa is a time scale of the cycle from early follicular (left) to late luteal (right). The data are grouped according to the number of animals in each of the oviductal stages. The mean serum levels of E_2 and P in each of these stages are presented in tabular form at the top of the figure. Nuclear receptor levels in groups with the same *lowercase letter* are significantly different from one another (Student's *t*-test, $p < 0.05$). (From ref. 27.)

thelium of secretory and (in women) ciliated cells (56–58) that is continuous with the openings of numerous simple tubular or branched glands that extend to the base of the endometrial–myometrial border. The lamina propria or stroma of the endometrium is a highly cellular connective tissue with an amorphous extracellular matrix containing relatively few connective tissue fibers, similar in appearance to embryonic mesenchyme. The border between the endometrium and the myometrium is irregular and indistinct. There is no intervening submucosal membrane, and pockets of basal endometrium extend into the superficial layer of the myometrium. The morphology of the endometrium depends upon the prevailing hormonal milieu and varies in different regions. On the basis of gross anatomy, the uterus can be divided into three parts: the body or corpus, the top part of which is the fundus (dome), and the isthmus or neck, which leads into the cervix. The endometrium immediately surrounding the openings of the oviducts is often designated as the peritubal-ostium or cornual regions. The isthmus is sometimes referred to as the lower uterine segment. The endometrium of the isthmus is not as thick as that of the corpus and tends to "lag behind" or to fail to develop all of the classic hormone-induced changes in morphology that characterize the endometrium of the corpus. In a fertile cycle, the blastocyst usually implants in the endometrium lining the corpus, most often on the posterior wall of the uterus.

The endometrium can be further subdivided into a series of strata, each with distinct characteristics. Bartelmez described four zones in rhesus (33) and human (59) endometrium (Fig. 18d). Zone I consists of the surface epithelium, a basement membrane, and an underlying band of stromal cells. Zone II contains the straight necks of the glands that run perpendicular to the surface and are surrounded by a relatively dense, cellular stroma. Zone III is composed of a looser or edematous stroma and contains the bodies of the glands, which are "crowded, contorted, and frequently branched." Zone IV is the basal layer adjacent to the myometrium, in which the blind ends of the glands terminate. This basal zone blends into the myometrium without a clear demarcation or connective tissue boundary. An alternate classification, commonly used in medical texts, describes three zones. A thin, superficial, compact layer—the compacta—consists of densely packed stromal cells around the straight necks of the glands. This seems to be equivalent to Bartelmez's zones I and II. Beneath this is a thick, spongy layer—the spongiosa—containing the tortuous bodies of the glands, comparable to zone III, and then a basal layer—the basalis—equivalent to zone IV. The compacta and upper spongiosa (zones I, II, and a portion of III) are also referred to as the functionalis (as opposed to the basalis) because they appear to be more dramatically affected by fluctuations in circulating levels of steroid hormones, derive their blood supply from specialized spiral arterioles rather than the basal arteries that supply the basal endometrium and the myometrium, and are either partially lost or extensively remodeled during parturition or menstruation and the subsequent repair phases of the reproductive cycle.

Development of the Endometrium

In the embryo, the development of the uterus depends upon the caudal extensions of the paramesonephric (Mullerian) ducts, paired structures derived from invaginations of the ceolomic epithelium. The cranial portions of the paramesonephric ducts open into the peritoneal cavity. These develop into the oviducts. The caudal portions grow toward the midline and fuse to form the uterovaginal primordium. The lower part of this structure contributes to the devel-

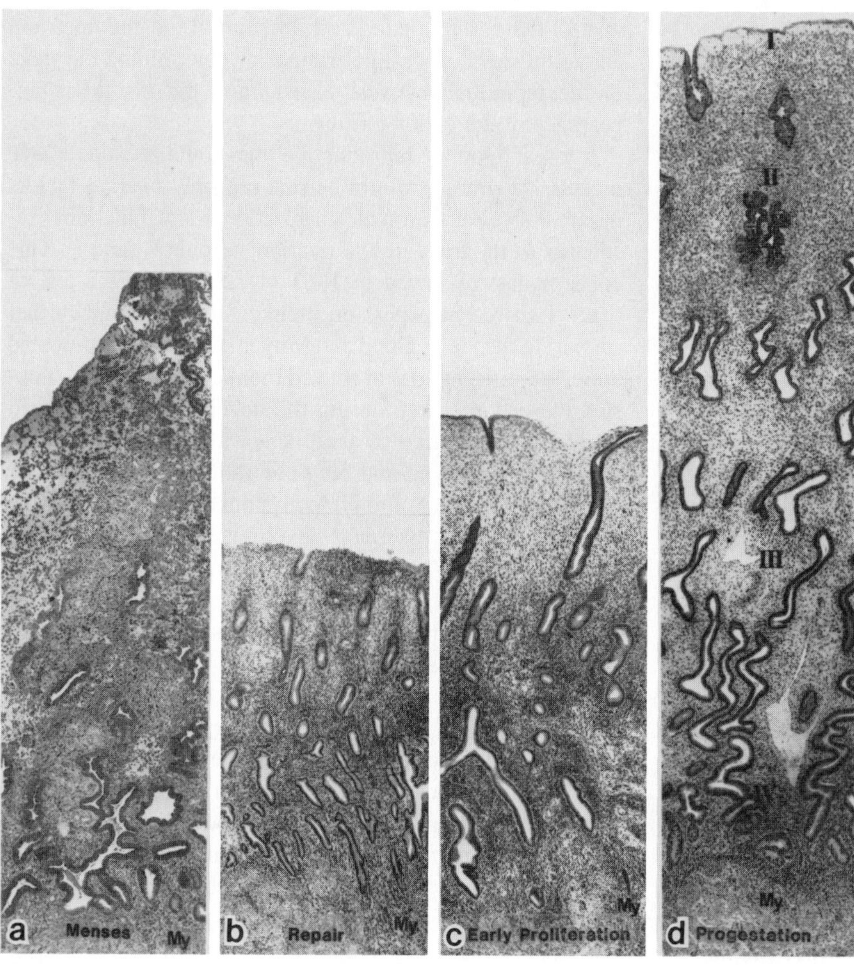

FIG. 18. Composite photomicrograph of endometrium throughout cycle showing zones: (**a**) Menses; (**b**) Repair; (**c**) Early Proliferation; (**d**) Progestation. Myometrium (My). ×20.

opment of the cervix and vagina, the upper portion gives rise to the epithelium and glands of the uterus. The endometrial stroma and myometrium are derived from the adjacent mesenchyme. When the paramesonephric ducts degenerate, as they do in normal male fetuses, the oviducts and uterus do not form. Failure of the paramesonephric ducts to fuse results in a double or bicornuate type of uterus. The persistence of a septum between the two ducts causes a complete or partial partitioning of the uterine cavity. These anomalies in the development of the uterus occur frequently in women; incidence figures of 0.25% have been reported when the analysis included minor abnormalities discovered during postpartum examination (60).

During early fetal development, the uterus is a V-shaped structure located at the anterior end of the fused portion of the paramesonephric ducts. The continuing growth of the uterovaginal primordium caudally, the rostral extension of the fused portion of the paramesonephric ducts, and a proliferation and thickening of the surrounding mesenchyme contribute to the growth of the uterus. By midgestation the caudal two-thirds of the uterus has become a narrow neck or isthmus leading into the cervix, while the cranial portion, the body or corpus of the developing uterus, is short and bulbous. At this time some layering of the mesenchyme is detectable, indicating differentiation of the mucosa, muscularis, and serosa (61). At about this time (approximately 20 weeks in humans), smooth muscle cells begin to appear in the wall of the uterus. The development of this muscular layer during the second half of gestation results in a change in the shape of the fetal uterus. The area between the oviducts bulges upward to form the dome-shaped fundus, and the wall of the corpus becomes thicker than that of the isthmus so that the fetal uterus attains a pear shape similar to that of the adult uterus.

The uterine mucosa also begins to differentiate during the second half of fetal development (61,62). Prior to the fifth month of gestation, the lining of the uterine cavity in human fetuses consists of a single layer of columnar epithelium. There are no glands and the subepithelial stroma is not markedly different in appearance from the deeper mesenchyme that will become the myometrium. As development progresses, the epithelium lining the uterine cavity forms pouches of cells that grow into the underlying mesenchyme. These structures, which will become the endometrial glands, are evident by the seventh month. By this time the endometrium is apparently responding to the high levels of steroid hormones produced by the placenta. The proliferating glandular epithelium resembles that typically found in estrogen-stimulated adult endometrium during the follicular stage of the menstrual cycle. During the eighth month of gestation, the glands begin to coil and the stroma becomes edematous. Witschi (61) described the fetal endometrium at 9 months as "in a hypertrophic, quasi-premenstrual condition. The blood vessels are heavily congested, and the coiled glands are actively secreting." In the newborn human, according to O'Rahilly (63), the endometrium has features of both proliferative and secretory endometrium. "Rarely it resembles progestational endometrium, in which case decidual transformation of the stroma as well as appearances analogous to menstrual changes (such as superficial hemorrhaging and tissue breakdown attributed to estrogen withdrawal) may be found." During infancy and childhood the uterus grows at a rate comparable to overall body growth and the corpus remains smaller than the cervix (61,63). The endometrial glands continue to elongate, eventually reaching the basal portion of the endometrium (62). After puberty, uterine growth is enhanced so that the body of the uterus eventually becomes larger than the cervix. This growth is attributed to the effects of ovarian steroids acting upon both the myometrium and the endometrium.

Cyclic Changes in the Endometrium During the Normal Menstrual Cycle

Hitschmann and Adler (64) described histologic changes in the endometrium in 1908. During the next 30 years, studies on the endometrium of women and of rhesus macaques established that the morphology of the endometrium was directly correlated with coincident changes in the ovary. This finding led to the hypothesis that ovarian hormones control the differentiation and function of the endometrium and to the development of criteria for determining the stage of the reproductive cycle based upon the histologic appearance of the endometrium.

If research on the reproductive tract could be said to have a central dogma, it would be that the only ovarian factors required to elicit complete maturational and functional responses of the tract are the ovarian steroids E_2 and P. This concept, last reviewed in 1961 (1), has stood the test of time. Two recent papers on monkeys (65,66) lend further support to the view. Good and Moyer (65) surgically created uterocutaneous fistulas in spayed monkeys and serially biopsied the endometrium during the development of artificial luteal phases induced by treatment with various E_2–P regimens. They showed that only one ratio of P to E_2 (similar to the physiological ratio typically found during most of the luteal phase) would support development of normal secretory endometria. Abnormal P to E_2 ratios led to imbalances of stromal versus glandular development. Hodgen (66) reported that pregnancy could be established in spayed monkeys treated with Silastic implants of E_2 and P in sequential fashion to recreate the pattern of serum E_2 and P that occurs during the fertile menstrual cycle. The pregnancy was initiated by transfer of an embryo into the fimbrial ostium, so both tubal transport and implantation were supported in these spayed animals. E_2 and P may induce factors that are involved in paracrine interactions within the tissues of the reproductive tract (67), but the evidence seems overwhelming that no other important ovarian factors exist.

In a paper based upon the examination of approximately 8,000 endometrial biopsies, Noyes et al. (68) presented a detailed description of the morphologic features of human endometrium during the normal menstrual cycle and described a scheme for classifying the endometrium relative to an "ideal" 28-day cycle in which the first day of menstruation is day 1. According to this method, ovulation occurs on ideal cycle day 14. Prior to that time, the endometrium can be dated as early, mid-, or late proliferative. During the early proliferative period, days 4 to 7, the surface epithelium is relatively thin and the glands are straight, short, and narrow, with round cross sections. Most of the glandular epithelium is proliferative; however, some of the glands consist of a "cuboidal, ragged, inactive epithelium typical of secretory exhaustion." The stroma is compact; some stromal mitoses are usually found. During the midproliferative period, ideal cycle days 8 to 10, the surface epithelium is columnar, and the glands are longer and have begun to curve so that they tend to be oval or oblong in cross section. The glandular epithelium is proliferative and the stroma is somewhat edematous. The stromal cells appear to be "naked nuclei" with very little cytoplasm. Stromal mitoses are numerous. The late proliferative stage, days 11 to 14, reflects the effects of the increase in circulating estrogen preceding the ovulatory LH surge. The glands, which are growing rapidly, become tortuous. The glandular epithelium appears pseudostratified due to the accelerated proliferation of the elongated cells. The stroma is less edematous than during the midproliferative stage and is also actively growing. The actual duration of the proliferative (follicular) stage depends upon the development of the ovarian follicle and can be highly variable.

When fertilization and implantation do not occur, the luteal phase of a normal cycle usually lasts for 12 to 14 days. During this time the endometrium responds to changes in the circulating levels of progesterone, which, in turn, reflect the differentiation, function, and regression of the corpus luteum. During the first 36 to 48 hr following ovulation (while the new corpus luteum is forming), the morphology of the endometrium is similar to that seen during the late proliferative stage. Then the effects of progesterone begin to become evident. On the basis of these changes, Noyes et al. (68) established precise cycle dates, each corresponding to a distinctive histologic picture. On ideal cycle day 16, the second day after ovulation, glycogen begins to accumulate in the basal portion of the glandular epithelium, and some of the nuclei appear to be displaced or "pushed" into the midportion of the cells, resulting in a pseudostratified configuration. In formalin-fixed material, the glycogen is solubilized, leaving large vacuoles in the base of the cells. This widespread "subnuclear vacuolation" of the glandular epithelium is taken as evidence that a functional, progesterone-producing corpus luteum has been formed. On day 17 the glands become more dilated and tortuous. The nuclei of the glandular epithelial cells form a "more or less orderly row with homogeneous cytoplasm above them and large vacuoles (glycogen deposits) below." By day 18 (4 days postovulation), the vacuoles in the glandular epithelium are smaller and are often located beside the nuclei. At this time the glycogen appears to be moving into the apex of the cells and then into the lumens of the glands. On day 19 very few vacuoles remain in the glandular epithelial cells, and most of the nuclei are once more basal in location. The presence of intraluminal secretion and the absence of both mitotic figures and pseudostratification distinguish day 19 histologic appearance from that of early vacuolation on day 16. Acidophilic secretory material begins to accumulate in the glandular lumens as early as day 17 or 18. These distinctive changes in the appearance of the glandular epithelium have been used to diagnose ovulation (69).

During the first half of the luteal phase of the cycle, progesterone induces significant changes in the glandular epithelium, resulting in extensive glandular secretion at the time when, in a fertile cycle, the blastocyst would arrive in the uterine cavity. In the absence of conception, glandular secretion continues for several days and then diminishes as serum progesterone titers fall. During the final days of the cycle, the glands are dilated and the glandular epithelium is "thrown into tufts," resulting in a "saw-toothed effect." The epithelial cells are cuboidal, with shrunken nuclei and jagged apical surfaces. This appearance, referred to as "secretory exhaustion," is characteristic of the glands at the end of the cycle but is too variable to be useful in dating the endometrium. For this purpose, human endometrium is evaluated by examining the degree to which the stroma has differentiated. On ideal cycle days 21 and 22 (7 to 8 days prior to the onset of menstruation), the endometrial stroma becomes edematous. At this stage the stromal cells are small with dense nuclei and filamentous cytoplasm. On day 23 stromal cells surrounding the spiral arterioles begin to enlarge. This, along with stromal mitoses, "constitute[s] the earliest visible predecidual change." By day 24 predecidual cells are observed "cuffing" the spiral arterioles and stromal mitoses are more numerous. By day 25 hypertrophied stromal cells are also present under the surface epithelium, and by day 27, the upper portion of the endometrial stroma "usually appears as a solid sheet of well-developed decidual-like cells." Differentiation of the decidua is accompanied by a sharp increase in lymphocyte infiltration, beginning on day 24 or 25. Relatively large numbers of polymorphonuclear leukocytes are present on day 26 and are even more numerous by day 27 (68,70).

Similar cyclic changes have been described in the endometrium of non-human primates, e.g., baboon (71–73), and macaque. Of these, the rhesus macaque has been the most extensively studied. The morphology of the endometrium throughout the ovarian cycle (33,59) and early gestation (59,74), as well as during a variety of steroid hormone treatments (75–79), has been described in detail. In comparative studies of uteri removed by hysterectomy, Bartelmez (59) demonstrated that the pattern of cyclic changes in rhesus endometrium is essentially the same as that described for human endometrium. These reports emphasized several points not included in descriptions of the endometrium based predominantly upon the examination of endometrial biopsies: In the early follicular phase of the cycle, there are relatively few mitotic figures present in the endometrium and there is no marked increase in the mitotic activity of the basalis during the "repair" phase of the cycle. The subsequent increase during the midproliferative phase in the number of mitoses found in the surface and glandular epithelium and stroma of the functionalis parallels rising serum estrogen titers. During this period, the glands grow rapidly due to estrogen-stimulated proliferation. This, along with stromal cell proliferation and an increase in edema and ground substance, results in a rapid thickening of the functionalis. During the follicular phase of the cycle, the glandular and surface epithelial cells contain glycogen and produce some secretory material that accumulates in the lumens of the glands, especially in the basal zone of the endometrium. Immediately following ovulation, there is a transitory "regression" of the endometrium characterized by a loss of stromal ground substance and a slight shrinking of the endometrium. Then, under the influence of the new corpus luteum, the glandular secretions become more viscous, richer in mucin and glycogen. This "yields an abundant coagulum on fixation." The glands become coiled, dilated, and sacculated. The development of edema in the superficial layers of the endometrium "not only loosened the stroma but distended the capillary bed." These changes result in the characteristic appearance of the "progestational" or "progravid" endometrium. If implantation and subsequent rescue of the corpus luteum do not occur, progesterone titers fall. A sustained regression of the endometrium follows; this involves a diminution of glandular secretion and an extensive loss of stromal ground substance, causing the upper layers (functionalis) of the endometrium to shrink. This "involution precedes extravasation" (59).

A significant difference in the cyclic changes observed in human and rhesus endometrium is the degree to which the periarteriolar stromal cells differentiate during the final week of the menstrual cycle. In women, a decidual reaction involving increased stromal mitoses and hypertrophy of stromal cells, beginning around the spiral arterioles and then spreading throughout the upper two-thirds of the endometrium, is initiated even when conception and implantation do not occur. The absence of distinct decidual changes, the "cuffing" of the spiral arterioles, in endometrial biopsies obtained during the final 4 to 5 days of the cycle is considered by some clinicians to be diagnostic of a luteal phase defect (80–83) and, if consistently found in consecutive cycles, a significant factor contributing to infertility. A premature decidual reaction, perhaps induced by excessive progesterone production, has also been suggested as a possible contributing factor in failed implantation (84,85). In contrast to the dramatic decidualization of the endometrial stroma in women, the changes that occur in the stroma of the late secretory macaque endometrium appear to be much more subtle. Many of the stromal cells, especially those surrounding the spiral arterioles, enlarge, becoming more rounded and less spindle-shaped in appearance. Figures 19 and 20 illustrate spiral arteries in late luteal macaque endometrium, and Figures 21 and 22 illustrate them in late luteal human endometrium. Exogenous progesterone treatment and pregnancy both result in a marked hypertrophy of the stromal cells in macaque endometrium. Some authors consider this to be a decidual reaction (33,74), while others do not (86). Our view is that the reaction of macaque stromal cells to progesterone is similar in kind but not in degree to that of human stromal cells.

Although it is obvious that a progestational endometrium is essential for a successful pregnancy, very few criteria have been established for determining the competency of the endometrium to maintain a favorable intrauterine environment and to support implantation. The thickness of the endometrium provides a gross indication of the degree to which it has been stimulated during the follicular phase of the cycle by E_2. The number of steroid receptors that can be measured in extracts of endometrium (27,40,87–89) or of isolated cells (90–92) also appears to be correlated with the extent to which the tissue has been "estrogen-primed" and, in some instances, may reflect the capacity of the tissue to respond to progesterone (40,93,94). One effect of progesterone upon the endometrium can be assessed directly, in a qualitative fashion, using morphological end points: Does endogenous or exogenous progesterone induce the specific histologic changes indicative of increased secretion in the glandular epithelium? The development of quantitative criteria for evaluating this response and for determining the hormonal requirements necessary to elicit optimal secretion may follow from the identification of specific proteins produced by the epithelial cells, e.g., progesterone-associated endometrial protein or human α-uterine protein (95–98). Although the physiological significance of these secretory products is not known, it is likely that they are important in supporting the embryo prior to implantation and during the early stages of placental development. This role may be assumed by the epithelial plaque in macaques and then by the glycogen-laden decidualized stromal cells as implantation progresses (74,77). Stromal cells may also protect maternal tissues from the destructive invasion of the trophoblast (99), form a cleavage zone at the time of parturition (99), or contribute to the protection of the allogenic fetoplacental unit from rejection by the maternal immune system (100,101). Recent studies related to this latter possibility have indicated that endometrial granulocytes or "Kornchenzellen" (102,103) cells may be a "functionally distinct population of T cells confined to the highly specialized environment of the decidua" (102). These cells, along with the assortment of lymphocytes, lymphoblasts, and macrophages present in the endometrium, may represent a unique hormone-dependent component of the immune system (102–104). Other studies, most using organ or cell cultures prepared from human endometrium, indicate that decidual cells may synthesize and secrete products that could act within the uterus as paracrine hormones, e.g., prosta-

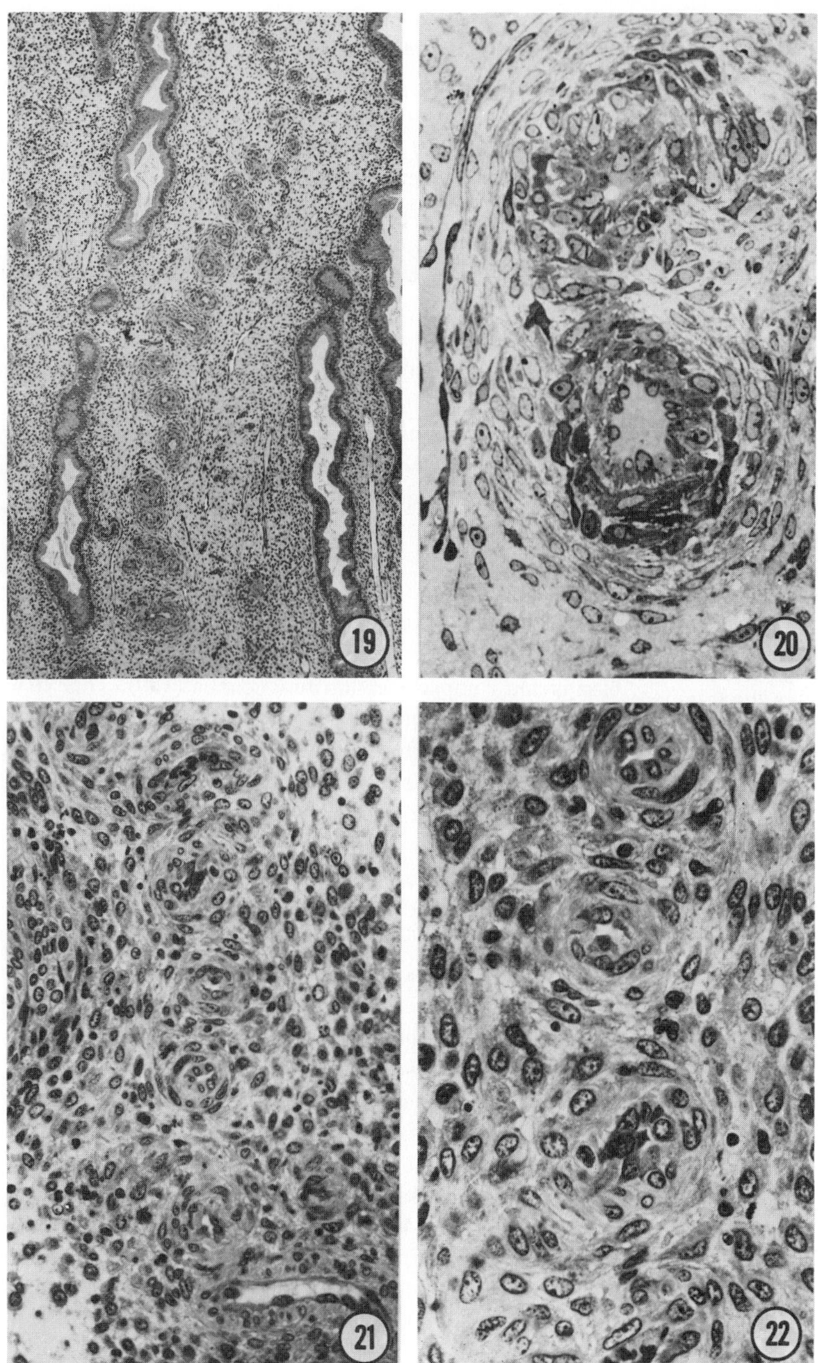

FIGS. 19–22. Comparison of spiral arteries and periarteriolar stromal cells in the macaque and human endometrium during the luteal phase. Enlargement of periarteriolar stromal cells occurs in both species but is more extreme in human endometrium. **FIG. 19.** Macaque. ×140; (From ref. 10.) **FIG. 20.** Macaque. ×480; (From ref. 10.) **FIG. 21.** Human. ×250; **FIG. 22.** Human. X500.

glandins (105,106), relaxin (107,108), vitamin D (109), or prolactin (106,110–113).

Many of the morphological and functional changes that occur in the luteal phase of the cycle and during pregnancy can be induced *in vitro* when explants of proliferative human endometrium are exposed to progesterone. During the first day of culture, basal vacuoles accumulate in the glandular epithelium and, after 1 or 2 days, the glands become secretory (113–116). When these organ cultures are maintained in serum-free nutrient medium containing 50 to 100 ng/ml of progesterone, the stromal cells appear somewhat enlarged and rounded after the first day and, by the end of the first week, resemble the decidual cells of pregnancy endometrium. Decidual prolactin (dPRL), a protein associated with decidualization of the stroma, is released into the medium in detectable quantities by the third or fourth day in culture (113,117). During prolonged incubation in the presence of progesterone, dPRL production increases progressively (Fig. 23). This pattern and the histological appearance of the explants suggest that dPRL production may be a sensitive indicator for progesterone-induced decidualization of the stroma, reflecting a progressive matu-

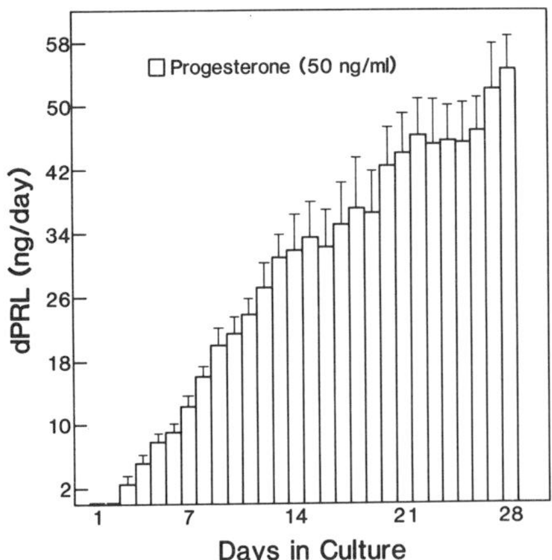

FIG. 23. Prolactin (dPRL) production by proliferative endometrium during organ culture in the presence of progesterone. Explants prepared from four samples of proliferative endometrium were cultured in medium containing 50 ng/ml progesterone for 28 days (two or three cultures from each tissue). The culture medium was replaced daily, and the spent medium was assayed for dPRL. The amounts of dPRL measured in the medium harvested from cultures prepared from the same tissue were averaged, and the values for the four tissues were combined. Each bar represents the mean ± SEM ($n = 4$) amount of dPRL measured in the medium on each day, expressed as nanograms per day/culture. (From ref. 113.)

ration of the hypertrophied stromal cells. This process involves complex ultrastructural changes in the differentiating decidual cells (118–120) and may result in the synthesis and secretion of a variety of decidual proteins. Studies in which radiolabeled amino acids were supplied to organ cultures of human endometrium or decidua have demonstrated that many proteins are synthesized *in vitro* and released into the medium by this tissue (121–125). Only a few of these radiolabeled proteins have been identified, e.g., dPRL (113,125), placental protein 12 (126), pregnancy-associated endometrial α_1- and α_2-globins (122). Additional research will be required to establish which of the various cell populations present in the decidua produces which of these various proteins and to determine their physiological roles during pregnancy.

Menstrual and Repair Phase of the Cycle

Some of the initial descriptions of the histology of the cyclic endometrium suggested that a large amount of tissue, three-quarters of the endometrium, perhaps the entire functionalis, was lost during menstruation (127). From these studies, it was concluded that, during the early follicular stage of each cycle, a new functionalis arose from proliferating stem cells located in the basal or "germinal" layer of the endometrium. That this sort of rapid regeneration was indeed possible was demonstrated by Hartman (128), who removed the entire endometrium from normally cycling macaques by dissecting it out with a scalpel blade and then wiping the uterine cavity clean with a cotton swab. Even after this procedure, the endometrium regenerated completely within 16 to 19 days after surgery. In one such animal, a pregnancy was established 22 days after hysterotomy. This provided convincing evidence that the entire endometrium can regenerate from the deepest portion of zone IV, i.e., from the tiny pockets of endometrium that extend into the myometrium at the endometrial–myometrial junction.

However, the extent of tissue loss during normal menstruation and the subsequent requirement for tissue regeneration from the basal layers during the beginning of the new cycle is certainly less dramatic than that induced by complete surgical "endometriectomy" (Fig. 18a–c). Bartelmez (33,59,129) concluded that very little tissue, only zone I and a portion of zone II, is shed during menstruation and that the marked reduction in the thickness of the endometrium is primarily due to loss of fluid and the resulting collapse of the spongy layer. Thus, postmenstrual endometrium was shown to be not stratum basalis but stratum basalis and compact stratum functionalis (130). This view was partially supported by an extensive study of human endometrium performed by McLennan and Rydell (131), who examined over 500 histologic sections of endometrial–myometrial blocks from 76 uteri removed on days 1 to 6 of the cycle (day 1 = the first day of menses). They found that, although the extent of tissue loss varies widely from one uterus to another, it is "less extensive than many believe it to be." In most cases, an "appreciable fraction of the stratum spongiosum actually disintegrates"; however, "endometrial tissue superficial to the basal layer remains in situ at the end of menstruation." They concluded that "regeneration of the new surface on the fourth day of the cycle, or occasionally as early as the third day, commonly occurs from a residuum of spongiosa rather than from the most basal elements of the endometrium." In a study using scanning electron microscopy, Ferenczy (132) presented yet another interpretation. He found evidence of surface epithelial, stromal, and glandular fragmentation in both the compacta and spongiosa, chiefly in the fundal and corporeal regions. As a result, "large fragments of functionalis were seen to be dissociated from the underlying tissue" and, by day 3, "most of the basal layer appeared to be denuded." Ferenczy concluded that repair of the surface occurred by an epithelial outgrowth from the mouths of the glands and by ingrowth from the surface epithelium of the isthmic and cornual regions that remained intact and that, by the fifth day of the cycle, the endometrial surface is fully re-epithelialized.

The controversy over the extent of tissue loss during menstruation and about the mechanisms involved in repair of the endometrium is made more confusing by a lack of conformity among authors in defining the histologic zones of the endometrium (e.g., the functionalis has been assumed to include all, a portion, or none of zone III by different workers). In addition, there is extensive variability between individual specimens and between regions in the same uterus. This is further complicated by the possible involvement of some pathology in many specimens, especially those of human endometrium, and by the inevitable uncertainty as to whether the cycle preceding hysterectomy was a "normal" one.

Another unresolved problem arises when one attempts to understand how the apparent rapid reorganization of the endometrium during the repair phase of the cycle is accomplished. As Levison (130) points out, "what Bartelmez did not explain was how the long tortuous glands of premenstrual endometrium reverted to the short, straight glands of the early proliferative phase endometrium." The complete loss of the spent secretory glands of the previous cycle and their replacement by new glandular epithelium derived from proliferative basal stem cells provides a simple explanation for the observed phenomenon. As an alternative explanation, Hopwood and Levison (133) have suggested that cellular atrophy and apoptosis play major roles in the remodeling of the endometrium. They report that "electron microscopy of human endometrium indicates that there is considerable loss of glandular epithelial cells with apoptotic bodies (granules containing nuclear fragments) in the late secretory, premenstrual, and menstrual phases." In a subsequent study, Davie et al. (134) described an apparent enlargement of the basal intercellular spaces in the endometrial glands and the movement of cells and cell debris into the endometrial stroma. They proposed that involution of the glands during the perimenstrual portion of the cycle involves the extrusion of cell debris from atrophic and apoptotic epithelial cells into the intercellular space from which components may be recovered following phagocytosis. In this context, it may be significant that, in the regenerating endometrium, stromal fibroblasts and predecidual cells, as well as macrophages, appear to be actively involved in the digestion of residual products (135,136). This model for explaining rapid tissue remodeling without significant cell division is supported by the electron-microscopic study of Flowers and Wilborn (137), who used ruthenium red stain as an indicator for dead or injured cells. Their findings suggested that the secretory spongiosa remains viable during the menstrual period and is converted by autophagocytosis and heterophagocytosis into a replicating endometrium.

Both of the mechanisms described above (extensive tissue loss with menstruation or extensive tissue remodeling with selective cell removal) are consistent with the hypothesis that, for some endometrial cell populations, secretory differentiation results in a prelethal state of terminal differentiation. A major point of disagreement, in addition to the extent of tissue loss during menstruation, centers around the source and location of the stem cells that give rise to a new population of committed endometrial cells. This question seems best approached by examining the available data on cell proliferation patterns in cyclic endometrium. Several of the early studies of endometrial histology included data on the number of mitotic figures observed during various phases of the cycle, all concluding that proliferation, especially in the glandular epithelium, was most pronounced during the late follicular portion of the cycle and was markedly decreased in secretory endometrium. There were few mitotic figures in menstrual endometrium, and no marked increase in mitotic activity could be found in the basal zone (zone IV) during the repair phase immediately following menstruation. The most extensive of these studies was performed by Bensley (138), who evaluated the cyclic fluctuations in the rate of epithelial mitosis in the endometrium from 50 rhesus monkeys for which extensive information about the ovarian status at the time of hysterectomy was available. "A total of 290,812 cells were studied. General surveys covered many thousands more. Records from surface epithelium, superficial glands (Schroder's functionalis), and basal glands were kept separate." Bensley found that the surface epithelium and superficial glands appeared to "respond more promptly to hormonal stimulation" than did the basal glands. In the former, the number of mitotic figures increased rapidly during the follicular phase of the cycle to reach a maximum of 7.7% at the time of ovulation (surface) or 10.5% during the late follicular phase just prior to ovulation (superficial glands). Mitotic activity then declined drastically during the luteal phase of the cycle; no mitoses were found in the late luteal phase. Mitotic activity increased to 2% in the superficial glands in the menstrual and repair phases and to nearly 2% in the surface epithelium during repair. The pattern of mitotic activity in the basal glands was distinctly different: Mitotic activity remained low during the early follicular phase, increased to 4% during the late follicular phase, remained relatively unchanged at 3.5% during the early luteal phase, and was low but detectable, 0.18%, throughout the late luteal phase. No mitoses were observed in the basal glands during the menstrual or repair phase.

More recent studies in which the incorporation of radiolabeled thymidine was used to analyze the proliferation kinetics of the endometrium have largely confirmed Bensley's findings. Ferenczy et al. (135) incubated small slices of human endometrium in Trowell's T8 medium containing [^{3}H]thymidine for 1 hr and then counted radiolabeled nuclei in the outer edges (isotope-accessible portion) of the slices. They detected the highest rates of proliferation in the upper third of the functionalis on cycle days 8 to 10. DNA synthesis in premenstrual endometrium was limited to the surface epithelium, predecidual cells, and the vascular epithelium. In the isthmus and cornual regions and in the basalis the rate of proliferation appeared to be "relatively constant and comparatively lower" than that in the proliferative functionalis. In a second study, Ferenczy et al. (139) focused on endometrial regeneration using the same short-term incubation technique. They concluded that (a) the significant increase in DNA synthesis that was observed in early repair tissues (days 3 and 4) was associated with the gland and surface epithelial cells that were involved in resurfacing the endometrium, (b) that this involved both cellular migration and replication, and (c) that this process was a simple wound-healing reaction that was not dependent upon E_2.

Padykula et al. (140) have also begun to investigate the pattern of proliferation and differentiation in the endometrium of rhesus monkeys. In their studies, endometrial biopsies were taken during the periovulatory period, 1 hr after a single intravascular injection of [^{3}H]thymidine. Autoradiography was performed on seven specimens from four monkeys, and these were classified relative to the preovulatory estrogen surge. Again, epithelial labeling indexes were higher in the functionalis than in the basalis. However, in the most basal layer (zone IV) the percentage of labeled cells increased from 1% at 2 days prior to the estrogen surge to 7% by 3 days after the estrogen surge (approximately 1 day postovulation) (Table 2). Subsequent analysis of two additional biopsies obtained 5 days after the estrogen surge indicated that the labeling index in zone IV continued to increase, reaching 9% during the early luteal phase (141). These data, like those of Bensley (138), indicate "striking zonal differences in mitotic response to the same hormonal milieu" and "point toward the existence of variations in the stimulation of intracellular control mechanisms by estrogen and progesterone." Padykula et al. (140) suggested that the cells produced in zone IV of the basalis during the luteal phase were progenitors for the new endometrium that develops after menstruation. Recently, Press et al. (142) discovered by immunocytochemistry that estrogen receptors persisted in the glands of the deep basalis but not in the upper endometrial zones during the luteal phase. These data support the concept that intrinsic positional differences exist among the cells of the endometrium.

As indicated above, the development of immunocytochemical methods to visualize estrogen receptor with monoclonal antiestrophilins has made it possible to localize estrogen receptor in discrete cell populations (142–145). Through these and other studies (146) a new view of the intracellular localization of the estrogen receptor has developed. In brief, in the absence of E_2 (as in ovariectomized animals) most of the nuclear receptor is located in the nucleus in a loosely bound form, easily extractable into the cytosolic fraction during homogenization. In the presence of E_2, a large portion of the nuclear receptor is transformed into a tightly bound form that resists extraction into the cytosol. In frozen sections of estrogen target tissues processed for immunocytochemistry, all specific estrogen receptor staining has been found within cell nuclei whether E_2 was present *in vivo* or not; any cytoplasmic staining has been found to be nonspecific (142–144,147,148). The micrographs in this review of immunocytochemical preparations (taken from ref. 149) also show only specific nuclear, not cytoplasmic, localization of the estrogen receptor. In the future, improvements in electron-microscopic immunocytochemistry of the estrogen receptor may permit detection of small quantities of the receptor protein in the cytoplasm, where it is synthesized. A recent electron-microscopic study of the progesterone receptor (150) showed that, in the absence of hormone, most of the receptor was present in the nucleus, as has been found for the estrogen receptor, but that small amounts of specific cytoplasmic staining was associated with profiles of the endoplasmic reticulum.

Although it was known that the amount of endometrial estrogen receptor measured in endometrial homogenates during the luteal–follicular transition increased two- to threefold above luteal phase levels (27), it was not known whether such increases occurred at the same rate in each endometrial cell type. To study these relationships. McClellan et al. (149) in this laboratory created artificial menstrual cycles in spayed macaques through the use of E_2- and P-filled Silastic capsules and then sampled the endometrium during the luteal–follicular transition. The spayed animals were treated for 14 days with E_2 followed by 14 days of E_2 plus P. Then the P (but not the E_2) implants were withdrawn and uteri removed 0, 0.5, 1, 2, 3, 4, 5, 7, and 14 days later. Menstruation began 2 to 3 days and repair 4 to 5 days after removal of the P implants. Uterine tissues were assayed biochemically for estrogen receptor content, fixed for histologic examination, and frozen for immunocytochemistry (ICC) of estrogen receptor with monoclonal antiestrophilins (144).

Histological evaluation revealed that on day 0, the endometria were similar to those taken from monkeys in the late luteal phase of the natural cycle. The glands were highly sacculated and the stromal cells were moderately dispersed throughout a light-staining extracellular matrix. After 12 hr of P withdrawal there was a variable increase in stromal edema and a consistent, dramatic increase in cell death by apoptosis, especially in the basalis. By 1 or 2 days after P withdrawal, there was considerable shrinkage and compaction of the stroma due to loss of edema. As a result, there was a greatly increased crowding of the stromal fibroblasts, which led to close associations between the basal lamina of

TABLE 2. *Epithelial labeling index showing zonal distribution of mitotic activity in rhesus macaque endometrium at midcycle*

Day of cycle	Mitotic activity (%)			
	Zone I	II	III	IV
−2	11	10	6	1
−1	10	10	5	2
−1	—	14	7	3
0	11	7	5	4
+1	11	11	5	5
+2	12	13	7	4
+3	9	11	6	7

Endometrial biopsies were taken 1 hr after [^{3}H]thymidine injection. A minimum of 2,000 cells/zone/specimen was used to determine the labeling index. Days of the cycle are normalized (±1 day) to the midcycle LH surge on day 0. (Modified from ref. 140.)

the endometrial glands and the subepithelial stromal cells. The classic, premenstrual invasion of leukocytes into the stroma also occurred during this period. In zones III and IV of the basalis there were numerous dead and dying glandular epithelial cells undergoing apoptosis and pyknosis and an increased number of macrophages filled with cellular debris and nuclear fragments (Fig. 24).

By the third and fourth days of P withdrawal, typical surface hemorrhage and sloughing of surface tissue had occurred and the stroma had become further compacted. By day 5, epithelial cells had migrated from the mouths of the glands and formed a new luminal surface. Epithelial mitoses were abundant except in the basalis. In all animals the surface had healed by day 7 after P withdrawal. Distinct zones I and II were apparent, the glands of the functionalis were straight, and their epithelial cells contained basal deposits of glycogen. In the newly formed zone II, numerous mitotic figures were evident in the glandular epithelium and most stromal fibroblasts had lost the close association with the basal lamina of the glands. By day 14 of P withdrawal there was an increase in overall endometrial thickness, and a further loosening of the stroma in all zones, including the basalis. These histological changes were similar to those described for the natural luteal–follicular transition by Bartelmez in his classic study of the endometrium of the rhesus monkey (33). He used the terms "premenstrual regression" and "regressive phase" to describe the shrinkage and stromal compaction that occur in the endometrium at the beginning of this period, and he mentioned widespread cell death in the glands without specifying the basalis. However, in his study of the menstruating human uterus (129) he presented drawings of dying cells in the basalis (see his figures 35, 36, and 37 in Plate 15) that are excellent illustrations of apoptosis. The withdrawal of P that occurs with the demise of the corpus luteum is no doubt responsible for apoptosis during the natural cycle in the endometrial basalis in macaques and women.

The immunocytochemical studies showed that on day 0 (Fig. 25) nuclear staining for estrogen receptor was absent everywhere except for a few positive glandular epithelial cells in zone IV of the basalis and in some stromal cells associated with the walls of the spiral arteries. All other stromal and glandular epithelial cells were negative. Throughout days 0.5 to 4 of P withdrawal (Figs. 26–28) specific nuclear estrogen receptor immunostaining developed and became intense *only* in stromal fibroblasts, except in the uppermost portions of the functionalis. The glandular epithelial cells of zones I through III remained negative, and the staining of the glands in zone IV decreased. The first indication of epithelial nuclear staining in the glands did not occur until day 5 (Fig. 29). The positive cells were located in the glands of the lower, surviving portions of the functionalis and the upper regions of the basalis. The surface epithelium and the upper portions of the functionalis remained negative. By the seventh day of P withdrawal (Fig. 30), in all three animals sampled, the distribution of glandular estrogen receptor immunostaining was more homogeneous, and many, though not all, epithelial and stromal nuclei were stained. On day 14 there was no apparent change in the number of stained cells, though the intensity of nuclear staining in both glandular epithelial and stromal cells had lessened.

Between days 0 and 3 mitotic activity was nil. No mitoses were recorded in over 15,000 glandular epithelial cells. On day 4 the mitotic index rose to approximately 0.2%; on day 5 (in 2 out of 3 animals sampled) the mitotic activity had

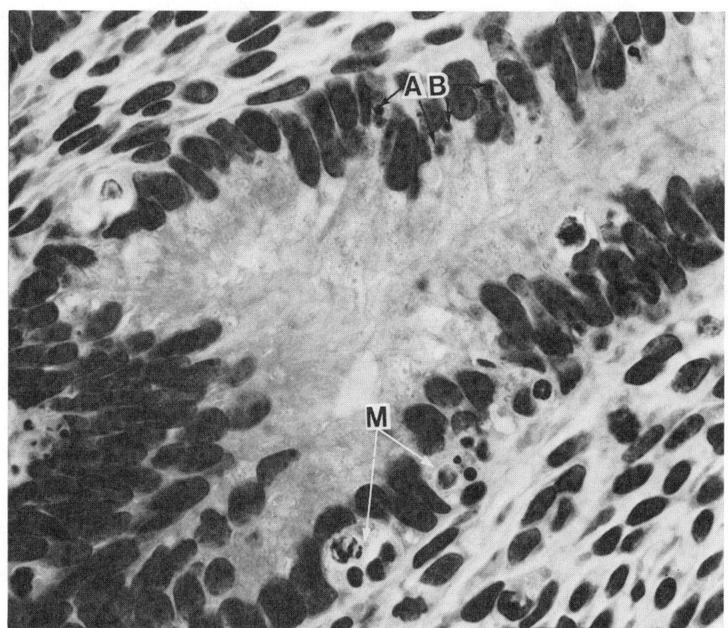

FIG. 24. Photomicrograph of basalis from menstruating macaque. White arrows indicate macrophages (m) and black arrows point to apoptotic bodies (AB). ×640.

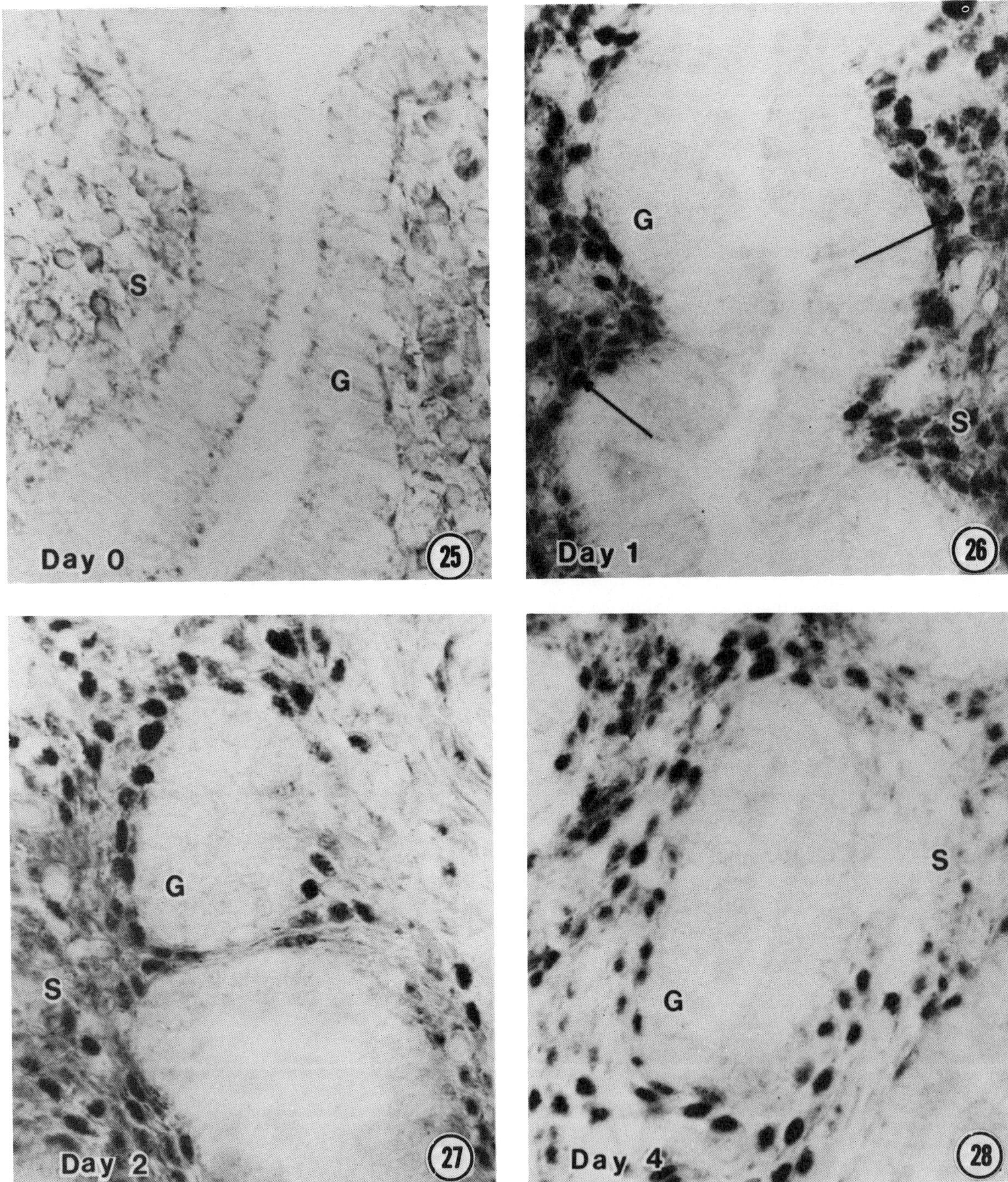

FIGS. 25–30. Spayed macaques were treated sequentially by means of Silastic implants with E_2 (14 days) and then E_2 plus P (14 more days) to create artificial follicular and luteal phases. The P implant (but not the E_2 implant) was removed and uteri were sampled on day 0 (Fig. 25), day 1 (Fig. 26), day 2 (Fig. 27), day 4 (Fig. 28), day 5 (Fig. 29), and day 7 (Fig. 30) of P withdrawal. The sampling period was the equivalent of the natural luteal-follicular transition. Tissues were frozen and processed by immunocytochemistry for estrogen receptors as described in McClellan et al. (144). ×575. (From ref. 149.)

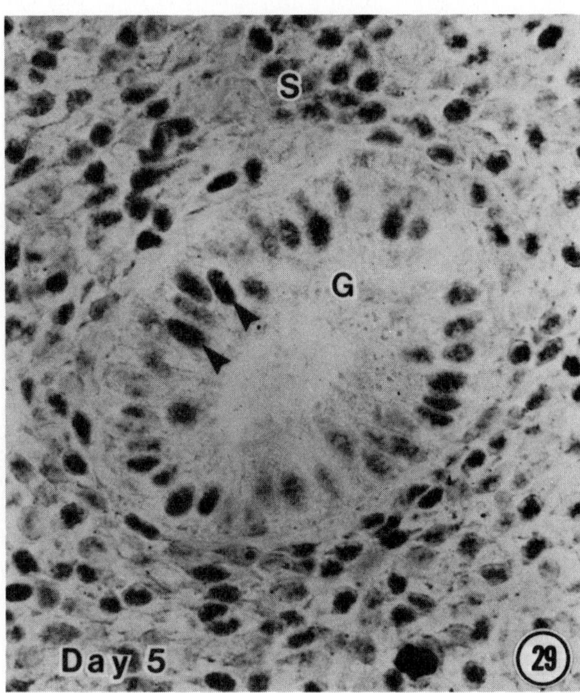

FIG. 29. (*See legend on facing page.*)

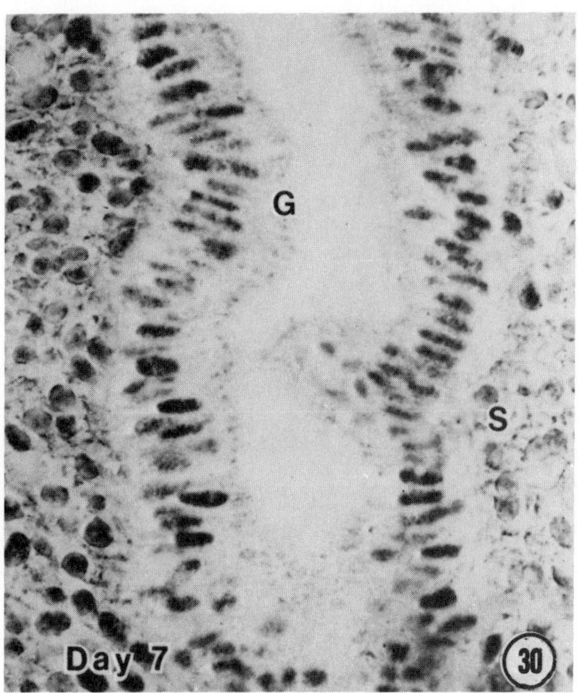

FIG. 30. (*See legend on facing page.*)

risen tenfold to 2%. In all endometria from day 7 and 14 animals the mitotic indices were approximately 2%. Mitoses were not found in the lower basalis except in the 14-day group.

Biochemical assays of estrogen receptor in this study (149) showed that endometrial estrogen receptor concentrations increased linearly during the luteal–follicular transition and roughly paralleled the increase in the number of ICC-positive cells. However, the immunocytochemical results revealed that many epithelial cells were estrogen receptor-negative 5 days after P withdrawal, when the mitotic index in the glands had risen to its maximum level. Compaction of the stroma resulted in close associations between stromal fibroblasts and epithelial cells that would favor interactions between these two cell types during this period. These findings are consistent with a role for stromal cells in mediating the effects of estrogen on those epithelial cells that proliferate during the period of early estrogen action in the primate uterus. Such a stromal–epithelial interaction has been shown to influence the proliferation of normal and neoplastic mammary epithelium (151,152).

However, not all stromal fibroblasts become estrogen receptor-positive during the first few days of P withdrawal. During the sloughing process (days 3–5 of P withdrawal), estrogen receptor staining was negative in the stroma and the glands of the upper regions of the functionalis that disintegrated and were shed during menstruation. The stromal cells that reorganized to form the upper regions of the endometrium (zone I and upper part of zone II) (33,59) after menstrual loss were also negative until days 4 to 5. Estrogen receptor staining was initially negative in the epithelial cells that migrated out from the mouths of the glands to form the new luminal epithelial surface (Fig. 31). These latter observations suggest that the epithelial and stromal cells that participate in early endometrial surface repair do not require estrogen receptors. These data support Ferenczy's suggestion that healing of the surface of the human endometrium is independent of estrogen action (139,153).

We conclude that certain endometrial cells are refractive to P suppression of estrogen receptor (e.g., the glandular epithelium of the basalis and the smooth muscle cells around the spiral arteries), that the suppressed ones renew their estrogen receptor at different rates after P withdrawal, and that the rate of recovery varies with the location of the cell within the endometrial zones. The oviducts were also removed from these same animals and processed by ICC to detect estrogen receptors. Preliminary analysis of these tissues, and of other oviducts taken at intervals from E_2-treated spayed animals (154), indicates that oviductal stromal cells also increase their estrogen receptors at a more rapid rate than the epithelial cells. Whether estrogen receptor-positive stromal cells that are in close apposition to estrogen receptor-negative epithelial cells mediate any of the effects of E_2 on epithelial cell physiology in the macaque reproductive tract remains to be established. There is good evidence for such interaction in other species (67), but unequivocal experimental evidence for stromal–epithelial interactions in macaque endometrium (or oviduct) is not yet at hand.

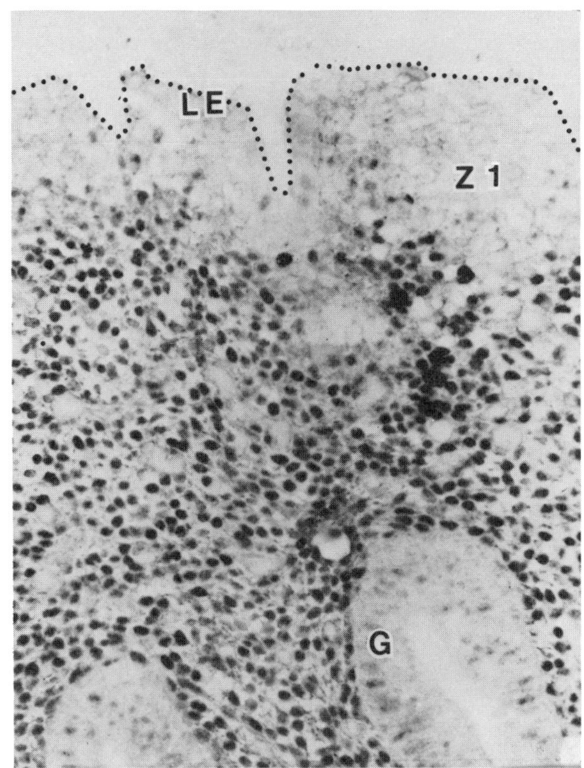

FIG. 31. Frozen section of the upper endometrial functionalis (zone I and upper part of II) on day 5 of P withdrawal. Luminal epithelium (LE) and stromal nuclei of zone I (ZI) were receptor-negative throughout day 5, which included the period of surface healing. The surface is outlined with a dotted line for clarity. ×135. (From ref. 149.)

DISCUSSION

The relationships between the oviduct, the endometrium, and the ovarian steroids in primates can be summarized as follows. Just before the functional corpus luteum begins to regress during the late luteal phase, the oviduct and endometrium are in two entirely different states. Responding to luteal progesterone, the oviductal epithelium has atrophied and regressed, while the endometrium has hypertrophied and become progestational. When the functional corpus luteum regresses, the endometrium responds within a few days by menstruating, and the oviduct responds by entering into the ciliogenic process. The period of transition between two menstrual cycles, from the time of corpus luteum regression through the end of menstruation, can be called the luteal–follicular transition; in rhesus and cynomolgus macaques (35,155) this is a period when serum P levels fall dramatically, while serum E_2 levels change little. In the most recent study from our laboratory of the luteal–follicular transition in macaques there was no difference in the mean serum E_2 levels between nine animals in the late luteal phase (with oviducts undergoing regression) and nine animals in the early follicular phase (with oviducts undergoing ciliogenesis). Only serum P levels were significantly different between these two groups (10). As it is clear that constant levels of E_2 produced by Silastic implants in spayed animals can stimulate oviductal ciliogenesis and secretion and that P can antagonize this effect (28,156,157), it follows that the onset of oviductal ciliogenesis and secretory cell development during the luteal–follicular transition is the result of a decrease in the antagonistic effects of P on estrogen-driven differentiation. The rise in serum E_2 levels that occurs in the midfollicular phase is not necessary for the morphological development of a fully ciliated-secretory oviductal epithelium. Such increases may be important to the rate of secretion of specific oviductal glycoproteins; there is evidence that the rate of transudation of oviductal fluid and the secretion of specific oviductal proteins are stimulated by the rising levels of serum E_2 in the periovulatory period (158,159).

By midcycle the oviduct has completed its differentiation; the endometrium, on the other hand, is far from fully developed. After ovulation, as serum P rises and serum E_2 returns to early follicular phase levels, the endometrium steadily responds by additional stromal cell mitosis and enlargement, gland cell enlargement in all zones, increased glandular sacculation, spiral artery development, increased stromal edema, and (in macaques) increased mitotic activity in zone IV of the basalis (138,140). Under the influence of progesterone, glandular secretory activity in the endometrium is markedly increased, and the composition of that secretion changed (33,59,68). Large amounts of glycogen accumulate in the secretory epithelium (68,136,160) and then in the hypertrophied stromal cells (74,119,136). The activities of specific enzymes are enhanced in both epithelial and stromal components (161–163), and unique progesterone-induced proteins are synthesized (125,164). These biochemical data indicate that progesterone acts upon the estrogen-primed endometrium to induce the expression of an array of steroid-regulated genes. The products of these genes, many of which remain unidentified, are presumably important for supporting the development of the blastocyst, facilitating the process of implantation and maintaining a successful pregnancy.

The oviduct, however, atrophies and dedifferentiates as serum P levels increase. The earliest regressive changes in the oviduct are scattered epithelial cell death, including apoptosis, and an increase in the number of intra- and subepithelial macrophages that phagocytose apoptotic cells and fragments. At the end of the luteal phase the fully regressed oviduct presents a stark contrast to the fully stimulated, hypertrophied endometrium. The finding by West et al. (55) that occupied nuclear P receptor levels are increased during the luteal phase in the endometrium, but not the oviduct, leads to the unexpected conclusion that the stimulatory effects of P as expressed in the development and maintenance of the progestational state in the primate endometrium may require higher levels of occupied nuclear P receptor than do the suppressive effects of P as expressed in oviductal atrophy, diminished ciliation, and reduced secretion. Apparently the antagonistic effects of P action can be sustained in the oviduct throughout the luteal phase without continuous maintenance of elevated levels of occupied nuclear P receptors; the mechanism through which P sustains its antagonistic effects on the oviduct certainly deserves further study. As the luteal phase ends and P levels fall, apoptosis occurs in the deeper zones of the endometrium. Subsequently, estrogen receptor levels increase in both the oviduct and the nonsloughing portions of the endometrium during the luteal–follicular transition. Recent findings (149) suggest that these increases in estrogen receptor occur more rapidly in the stromal than the epithelial cell populations of both organs. It is possible that estrogen receptors in stromal cells mediate some of the effects of estrogen on epithelial proliferation and differentiation in both the oviduct and the endometrium during the early follicular phase. Further research into such cell–cell interactions in the primate female reproductive tract is obviously needed.

We add this final comment on apoptosis. Although the process of apoptosis is the same in all cells that have been examined, the hormonal conditions that induce it in the oviduct and the endometrium are quite different. Wyllie et al. (30) suggested that apoptosis occurs within a particular cell population when the hormone or stimulus that causes mitosis in that population is withdrawn; for example, many adrenocortical cells die by apoptosis when adrenocorticotropin is withdrawn. In the oviductal epithelium, apoptosis occurs after ovulation when serum E_2 falls and serum P rises, a pattern that produces a sharp estrogen withdrawal coupled with loss of estrogen receptors. E_2 is the stimulus that causes mitosis in the oviductal epithelium, and its withdrawal (effective or real) is the appropriate apoptotic signal for oviductal epithelial cells. However, in the endometrial basalis, apoptosis occurs not after ovulation, when serum P rises, but after corpus luteum regression, when serum P falls. All studies, old (138) and new (140), indicate that P is the mitotic signal for the epithelial cells in the endometrial basalis, so withdrawal of P appears to be the stimulus that induces apoptosis in the basalis. Additional research is needed to delineate further the regulatory mechanisms involved in apoptosis, because it is an important process through which cells are deleted from the primate endometrium during the luteal–follicular transition.

Finally, our review of the literature has convinced us that much remains to be learned about the physiology of the endometrial basalis. In macaques, this zone proliferates and hypertrophies dramatically under the influence of luteal P (138,140). Little attention has been paid to this phenomenon, perhaps because so little change is reported to occur in the human endometrial basalis during the cycle. Nevertheless, in macaques, this zone, although very quiescent in the follicular phase, becomes extremely active at the beginning of the luteal phase and reaches its maximal development very near the time of implantation. This does not seem merely coincidental to us. Moreover, unpublished immunocytochemical data from our laboratory show that in rhesus monkeys, as in women (142,148), luteal P suppresses estrogen receptors in all regions of the endometrium except the deeper regions of the basalis. Consequently, we suspect that the glands of the basalis are the only glands in the endometrium that maintain elevated levels of both estrogen and progesterone receptors during the luteal phase. If this is the case, then P and E_2 could have unique, synergistic actions in these cells that could not occur in other endometrial cells. Steroid synergism in the basalis might result in the production of unique proteins, and these might play previously unsuspected roles in implantation and early pregnancy. We realize we end on a rather speculative note, but in our view, studies to explore these various possibilities ought to be intensively pursued.

ACKNOWLEDGMENTS

This review, Publication No. 1523 of the Oregon Regional Primate Research Center, was supported by Grants HD-19182, P30 HD-18185, HD-19917, and RR-00163 from the National Institutes of Health. We would like to thank Drs. Maryanne McClellan and Neal West for their participation in many of the studies and for graciously permitting us to use their findings in this review, Kay Carlisle for help in assembling the figures, and Angela Adler for word-processing assistance. Thanks also to Mr. Ron Severson, science teacher, Lakeridge High School, Lake Oswego, Oregon, for the photomicrograph in Fig. 24, taken during his tenure as a Science Teacher Intern at the Oregon Regional Primate Research Center, Summer 1985.

REFERENCES

1. Hisaw, F. L., and Hisaw, F. L., Jr. (1961): Action of estrogen and progesterone on the reproductive tract of lower primates. In: *Sex and Internal Secretions,* Vol. 1, edited by W. C. Young, p. 556. Williams & Wilkins, Baltimore.
2. Brenner, R. M., and Anderson, R. G. W. (1973): Endocrine control of ciliogenesis in the primate oviduct. In: *Handbook of Physiology, Sect. 7: Endocrinology, The Female Reproductive System,* Vol. 2, edited by R. O. Greep and E. B. Astwood, p. 123. Williams & Wilkins, Baltimore.
3. Hafez, E. S. E., and Blandau, R. J. (eds.) (1969): *The Mammalian Oviduct.* University of Chicago Press, Chicago.
4. Blandau, R. J. (1973): Gamete transport in the female mammal. In: *Handbook of Physiology, Sect. 7: Endocrinology, The Female Reproductive System,* Vol. 2, edited by R. O. Greep and E. B. Astwood, p. 153. Williams & Wilkins, Baltimore.
5. Hafez, E. S. E. (1973): Endocrine control of the structure and function of the mammalian oviduct. In: *Handbook of Physiology, Sect. 7: Endocrinology, The Female Reproductive System,* Vol. 2, edited by R. O. Greep and E. B. Astwood, p. 97. Williams & Wilkins, Baltimore.
6. Hafez, E. S. E. (1973): Anatomy and physiology of the mammalian uterotubal junction. In: *Handbook of Physiology, Sect. 7: Endocrinology, The Female Reproductive System,* Vol. 2, edited by R. O. Greep and E. B. Astwood, p. 87. Williams & Wilkins, Baltimore.
7. Johnson, A. D., and Foley, C. W., eds. (1974): *The Oviduct and Its Functions.* Academic, New York.
8. Jansen, R. P. S. (1984): Endocrine response in the fallopian tube. *Endocrinol. Rev.,* 5:525.
9. Eckstein, P. (1958): Internal reproductive organs. In: *Primatologia,* Vol. 3, edited by H. Hofer, A. H. Schultz, and D. Stark, p. 542. Karger, Basel.

10. Brenner, R. M., Carlisle, K. S., Hess, D. L., Sandow, B. A., and West, N. B. (1983): Morphology of the oviducts and endometria of cynomolgus macaques during the menstrual cycle. *Biol. Reprod.*, 29:1289.
11. Rumery, R. E., Gaddum-Rosse, P., Blandau, R. J., and Odor, D. L. (1978): Cyclic changes in ciliation of the oviductal epithelium in the pig-tailed macaque (*Macaca nemestrina*). *Am. J. Anat.*, 153:345.
12. Odor, D. L., Gaddum-Rosse, P., Rumery, R. E., and Blandau, R. J. (1980): Cyclic variations in the oviductal ciliated cells during the menstrual cycle and after estrogen treatment in the pig-tailed monkey, *Macaca nemestrina*. *Anat. Rec.*, 198:35.
13. Odor, D. L., Gaddum-Rosse, P., and Rumery, R. E. (1983): Secretory cells of the oviduct of the pig-tailed monkey *Macaca nemestrina*, during the menstrual cycle and after estrogen treatment. *Am. J. Anat.*, 166:149.
14. Verhage, H. G., Bareither, M. L., Jaffe, R. C., and Akbar, M. (1979): Cyclic changes in ciliation, secretion and cell height of the oviductal epithelium in women. *Am. J. Anat.*, 156:505.
15. Donnez, J., Casanas-Roux, F., Caprasse, J., Ferin, J., and Thomas, K. (1985): Cyclic changes in ciliation, cell height, and mitotic activity in human tubal epithelium during reproductive life. *Fertil. Steril.*, 43:554.
16. Novak, E., and Everett, H. S. (1928): Cyclical and other variations in the tubal epithelium. *Am. J. Obstet. Gynecol.*, 16:499.
17. Patek, E. (1974): The epithelium of the human fallopian tube. A surface ultrastructural and cytochemical study. *Acta Obstet. Gynecol. Scand. Suppl*, 53:31.
18. Clyman, M. J. (1966): Electron microscopy of the human fallopian tube. *Fertil. Steril.*, 17:281.
19. Brosens, I. A., and Vasquez, G. (1976): Fimbrial microbiopsy. *J. Reprod. Med.*, 16:171.
20. Critoph, F. N., and Dennis, K. J. (1977): The cellular composition of the human oviduct epithelium. *Br. J. Obstet. Gynaecol.*, 84:219.
21. Oberti, C., and Gomez-Rogers, C. (1972): "De novo" ciliogenesis in the human oviduct during the menstrual cycle. In: *Biology of Reproduction: Basic and Clinical Studies, Symposium on Biology of Reproduction, III*, edited by J. T. Velardo and B. A. Kasprow, p. 241. Pan American Congress of Anatomy, New Orleans.
22. Anderson, R. G. W., and Brenner, R. M. (1971): The formation of basal bodies (centrioles) in the rhesus monkey oviduct. *J. Cell Biol.*, 50:10.
23. Donnez, J., Casanas-Rouss, F., Ferin, J., and Thomas, K. (1983): Changes in ciliation and cell height in human tubal epithelium in the fertile and post-fertile years. *Maturitas*, 5:39.
24. Andrews, M. C. (1951): Epithelial changes in the puerperal fallopian tube. *Am. J. Obstet. Gynecol.*, 62:28.
25. Sandow, B. A., West, N. B., Norman, R. L., and Brenner, R. M. (1979): Hormonal control of apoptosis in hamster uterine luminal epithelium. *Am. J. Anat.* 156:15.
26. Bennett, H. S., Wyrick, A. D., Lee, S. W., and McNeil, J. J., Jr. (1976): Science and art in preparing tissues embedded in plastic for light microscopy, with special reference to glycol methacrylate, glass knives and simple stains. *Stain Technol.*, 51:71.
27. West, N. B., and Brenner, R. M. (1983): Estrogen receptor levels in the oviducts and endometria of cynomolgus macaques during the menstrual cycle. *Biol. Reprod.*, 29:1303.
28. Brenner, R. M., Resko, J. A., and West, N. B. (1974): Cyclic changes in oviductal morphology and residual cytoplasmic estradiol binding capacity induced by sequential estradiol-progesterone treatment of spayed rhesus monkeys. *Endocrinology*, 95:1094.
29. Kerr, J. F. R., Wyllie, A. H., and Currie, A. R. (1972): Apoptosis: A basic biological phenomenon with wide ranging implications in tissue kinetics. *Br. J. Cancer*, 26:239.
30. Wyllie, A. H., Kerr, J. F. K., and Currie, A. R. (1980): Cell death: The significance of apoptosis. *Int. Rev. Cytol.*, 68:251–306.
31. Bareither, M. L., and Verhage, H. G. (1981): Control of the secretory cell cycle in cat oviduct by estradiol and progesterone. *Am. J. Anat.*, 162:107.
32. Brenner, R. M. (1969): Renewal of oviduct cilia during the menstrual cycle of the rhesus monkey. *Fertil. Steril.*, 20:599.
33. Bartelmez, G. W. (1951): Cyclic changes in the endometrium of the rhesus monkey (*Macaca mulatta*). *Contrib. Embryol.*, 34:99.
34. Canepa, D. K., and Brenner, R. M. (1983): Hormonal regulation of nuclear shape in macaque oviductal epithelium. *Anat. Rec.*, 205:29A (abstr.).
35. Brenner, R. M., and West, N. B. (1975): Hormonal regulation of the reproductive tract in female mammals. *Annu. Rev. Physiol.*, 37:273.
36. Janne, O., Isomaa, V., Isotalo, H., Kokko, E., and Vierikko, P. (1978): Uterine estrogen and progestin receptors and their regulation. *Ups. J. Med. Sci. (Suppl)*, 22:62.
37. Clark, J. H., and Peck, E. J., Jr. (1979): Female sex steroids: receptors and function. In: *Monographs on Endocrinology*, Vol. 14, edited by F. Gross, M. M. Grumbach, A. Labhart, et al. Springer-Verlag, New York.
38. Leavitt, W. W., MacDonald, R. G., and Okulicz, W. C. (1983): Hormonal regulation of estrogen and progesterone receptor systems. In: *Biochemical Actions of Hormones*, Vol. 10, edited by G. Litwack, p. 323. Academic, New York.
39. Tsibris, J. C. M., Fort, F. L., Cazenave, C. R., et al. (1981): The uneven distribution of estrogen and progesterone receptors in human endometrium. *J. Steroid Biochem.*, 14:997.
40. Levy, C., Robel, P., Gautray, J. P., et al. (1980): Estradiol and progesterone receptors in human endometrium: Normal and abnormal menstrual cycles and early pregnancy. *Am. J. Obstet. Gynecol.*, 136:646.
41. Bayard, F., Damilano, S., Robel, P., and Baulieu, E-E. (1978): Cytoplasmic and nuclear estradiol and progesterone receptors in human endometrium. *J. Clin. Endocrinol. Metab.*, 46:635.
42. Kreitmann-Gimbal, B., Bayard, F., Nixon, W. E., and Hodgen, G. D. (1980): Patterns of estrogen and progesterone receptors in monkey endometrium during the normal menstrual cycle. *Steroids*, 35:471.
43. Pollow, K., Inthraphuvasak, J., Manz, B., Grill, H-J., and Pollow, B. (1981): A comparison of cytoplasmic and nuclear estradiol and progesterone receptors in human fallopian tube and endometrial tissue. *Fertil. Steril.*, 36:615.
44. Robel, P., Mortel, R., and Baulieu, E. E. (1981): Estradiol and progesterone receptors in human endometrium. In: *The Endometrium Hormonal Impacts*, edited by J. De Brux, R. Mortel, and J. P. Gantray, p. 43, Plenum, New York.
45. Ochiai, K. (1980): Cyclic variation and distribution in the concentration of cytosol estrogen and progesterone receptors in the normal human uterus and myoma. *Acta Obstet. Gynecol. Jpn.*, 32:945.
46. Verhage, H. G., Akbar, M., and Jaffe, R. C. (1980): Cyclic changes in cytosol progesterone receptor of human fallopian tube. *J. Clin. Endocrinol. Metab.*, 51:776.
47. Pino, A. M., Devoto, L., Davila, M., and Soto, E. (1984): Changes during the menstrual cycle in cytosolic and nuclear concentrations of progestagen receptor in the human Fallopian tube. *J. Reprod. Fertil.*, 70:481.
48. Lukola, A., and Punnonen, R. (1983): Estrogen and progesterone receptors in human uterus and oviduct. *J. Endocrinol. Invest.*, 6:179.
49. Poortman, J., Thijssen, J. H. H., Landeghem, A. A. J., Wiegerinck, M. A. H. M., and Alsbach, G. P. J. (1983): Subcellular distribution of androgens and estrogens in target tissue. *J. Steroid. Biochem.*, 19:939.
50. Guerrero, R., Landgren, B-M., Montiel, R., Cekan, Z., and Diczfalusy, E. (1975): Unconjugated steroids in the human endometrium. *Contraception*, 11:169.
51. Batra, S., Grundsell, H., and Sjoberg, N-O. (1977): Estradiol-17β and progesterone concentrations in human endometrium during the menstrual cycle. *Contraception*, 16:217.
52. Bayard, F., Rouvet, J. P., Monrozies, M., Boulard, A., and Pontonnier, G. (1975): Endometrial progesterone concentrations during the menstrual cycle. *J. Clin. Endocrinol. Metab.*, 41:412.
53. Schmidt-Gollwitzer, M., Eiletz, J., Genz, T., and Pollow, K. (1979): Determination of estradiol, estrone, and progesterone in serum and myometrium: Correlation with the content of sex steroid receptors and 17β-hydroxysteroid dehydrogenase activity throughout the menstrual cycle. *J. Clin. Endocrinol. Metab.* 49:370.
54. Akerlund, M., Batra, S., and Helm, G. (1981): Comparison of plasma and myometrial tissue concentrations of estradiol-17β and progesterone in nonpregnant women. *Contraception*, 23:447.

55. West, N. B., Hess, D. L., and Brenner, R. M. (1986): Differential suppression of progesterone receptor by progesterone in the reproductive tract of primate macaques. *J. Steroid. Biochem.*, 25:497.
56. White, A. J., and Buchsbaum, H. J. (1973): Scanning electron microscopy of the human endometrium. *Gynecol. Oncol.*, 1:330.
57. Ferenczy, A., and Richart, R. M. (1973): Scanning and transmission electron microscopy of the human endometrial surface epithelium. *J. Clin. Endocrinol. Metab.*, 36:999.
58. Ferenczy, A. (1977): Surface ultrastructural response of the human uterine lining epithelium to hormonal environment. A scanning electron microscopic study. *Acta Cytol.*, 21:566.
59. Bartelmez, G. W. (1957): The phases of the menstrual cycle and their interpretation in terms of the pregnancy cycle. *Am. J. Obstet. Gynecol.*, 74:931.
60. Rock, J. A., and Schlaff, W. D. (1985): The obstetric consequences of uterovaginal anomalies. *Fertil. Steril.*, 43:681.
61. Witschi, E. (1970): Development and differentiation of the uterus. In: *Perinatal Life: Biological and Clinical Perspectives (Proceedings of the 3rd Annual Symposium on the Physiology and Pathology of Human Reproduction)*, p. 11. Wayne State University Press, Detroit.
62. Valdes-Dapena, M. A. (1973): The development of the uterus in late fetal life, infancy, and childhood. In: *The Uterus,* edited by H. J. Norris, A. T. Hertig, and M. R. Abell, p. 40. Williams & Wilkins, Baltimore.
63. O'Rahilly, R. (1973): The embryology and anatomy of the uterus. In: *The Uterus,* edited by H. J. Norris, A. T. Hertig, and M. R. Abell, p. 17. Williams & Wilkins, Baltimore.
64. Hitschmann, F., and Adler, L. (1908): Der Bau der Uterus-schleimhaut des geschlectsreifen Weibes mit besonderer Berucksichtigung der Menstruation. *Monatschr. Geburtsch. Gynakol.*, 27:1.
65. Good, R. G., and Moyer, D. L. (1968): Estrogen-progesterone relationships in the development of secretory endometrium. *Fertil. Steril.*, 19:37.
66. Hodgen, G. D. (1983): Surrogate embryo transfer combined with estrogen-progesterone therapy in monkeys. *JAMA*, 250:2167.
67. Cunha, G. R., Chung, L. W. K., Shannon, J. M., Taguchi, O., and Fujii, H. (1983): Hormone-induced morphogenesis and growth: role of mesenchymal-epithelial interactions. *Recent Prog. Horm. Res.*, 39:559.
68. Noyes, R. W., Hertig, A. T., and Rock, J. (1950): Dating the endometrial biopsy. *Fertil. Steril.*, 1:3.
69. Robertson, W. B. (1984): A reappraisal of the endometrium in infertility. *Clin. Obstet. Gynaecol.*, 11:209.
70. Daly, D. C., Tohan, N., Doney, T. J., Maslar, I. A., and Riddick, D. H. (1982): The significance of lymphocytic-leukocytic infiltrates in interpreting late luteal phase endometrial biopsies. *Fertil. Steril.*, 37:786.
71. MacLennan, A. H., and Wynn, R. M. (1971): Menstrual cycle of the baboon. *Obstet. Gynecol.*, 38:350.
72. Kraemer, D. C., Maqueo, M., Hendrickx, A. G., and Vera Cruz, N. C. (1977): Histology of the baboon endometrium during the menstrual cycle and pregnancy. *Fertil. Steril.*, 28:482.
73. Dollar, J. R., Hand, G. S., Beck, L. R., and Boots, L. R. (1979): The baboon as a primate model for the study of endometrium. *Am. J. Obstet. Gynecol.*, 134:305.
74. Enders, A. C., Welsh, A. O., and Schlafke, S. (1985): Implantation in the rhesus monkey: Endometrial responses. *Am. J. Anat.*, 173:147.
75. Hisaw, F. L., Meyer, R. K., and Fevold, H. L. (1930): Production of a premenstrual endometrium in castrated monkeys by ovarian hormones. *Proc. Soc. Exp. Biol.*, 27:400.
76. Cleveland, R. (1941): Cytologic and histologic observations on the epithelial, connective and vascular tissues of the endometrium of macaques under various experimental conditions. *Endocrinology*, 28:388.
77. Rossman, I. (1940): The deciduomal reaction in the rhesus monkey (*Macaca mulatta*). *Am. J. Anat.*, 66:277.
78. Dallenbach-Hellweg, G., Dawson, A. B., and Hisaw, F. L. (1966): The effect of relaxin on the endometrium of monkeys: Histological and histochemical studies. *Am. J. Anat.*, 119:61.
79. Kelly, W. A., Marston, J. H., and Eckstein, P. (1969): Effect of an intra-uterine device on endometrial morphology and the deciduomal reaction in the rhesus monkey. *J. Reprod. Fertil.*, 19:331.
80. Jones, G. S. (1976): The luteal phase defect. *Fertil. Steril.*, 27:351.
81. DiZerega, G. S., and Hodgen, G. D. (1981): Luteal phases dysfunction infertility: A sequel to aberrant folliculogenesis. *Fertil. Steril.*, 35:489.
82. Shangold, M., Berkeley, A., and Gray, J. (1983): Both midluteal serum progesterone levels and late luteal endometrial histology should be assessed in all infertile woman. *Fertil. Steril.*, 40:627.
83. Witten, B. I., and Martin, S. A. (1985): The endometrial biopsy as a guide to the management of luteal phase defect. *Fertil. Steril.*, 44:460.
84. Noyes, R. W. (1959): The underdeveloped secretory endometrium. *Am. J. Obstet. Gynecol.*, 77:929.
85. Roberts, D. K., Horbelt, D. V., and Powell, L. C., Jr. (1975): The ultrastructural response of human endometrium to medroxyprogesterone acetate. *Am. J. Obstet. Gynecol.*, 123:811.
86. Ramsey, E. M., Houston, M. L., and Harris, J. W. S. (1976): Interactions of the trophoblast and maternal tissues in three closely related primate species. *Am. J. Obstet. Gynecol.* 124:647.
87. Bayard, F., Damilano, S., Robel, P., and Baulieu, E-E. (1978): Cytoplasmic and nuclear estradiol and progesterone receptors in human endometrium. *J. Clin. Endocrinol. Metab.*, 46:635.
88. King, R. J. B., Dyer, G., Collins, W. P., and Whitehead, M. I. (1980): Intracellular estradiol, estrone and estrogen receptor levels in endometria from postmenopausal women receiving estrogens and progestins. *J. Steroid Biochem.*, 13:377.
89. Kreitmann-Gimbal, B., Bayard, F., Nixon, W. E., and Hodgen, G. (1980): Patterns of estrogen and progesterone receptors in monkey endometrium during the normal menstrual cycle. *Steroids*, 35:471.
90. King, R. J. B., Lane, G., Siddle, N., Taylor, R. W., Townsend, P. T., and Whitehead, M. I. (1981): Assessment of oestrogen and progestin effects on epithelium and stroma from pre- and postmenopausal endometria. *J. Steroid Biochem.*, 15:175.
91. King, R. J. B., Townsend, P. T., Siddle, N., Whitehead, M. I., and Taylor, R. W. (1982): Regulation of estrogen and progesterone receptor levels in epithelium and stroma from pre- and postmenopausal endometria. *J. Steroid Biochem.*, 16:21.
92. Fleming, H., Namit, C., and Gurpide, E. (1980): Estrogen receptors in epithelial and stromal cells of human endometrium in culture. *J. Steroid Biochem.*, 12:169.
93. Maynard, P. V., Symonds, E. M., Johnson, J., Baker, P. N., Sant-Cassia, L. J., and Selby, C. (1983): Nuclear progesterone uptake by endometrial tissue in cases of subfertility. *Lancet* 1:310.
94. Laatikainen, T., Andersson, B., Karkkainen, J., and Wahlstrom, T. (1983): Progestin receptor levels in endometria with delayed or incomplete secretory changes. *Obstet. Gynecol.*, 62:592.
95. Joshi, S. G. (1983): A progestagen-associated protein of the human endometrium: basic studies and potential clinical applications. *J. Steroid Biochem.*, 19:751.
96. Joshi, S. G., Henriques, E. S., Smith, R. A., and Szarowski, D. H. (1980): Progestogen-dependent endometrial protein in women: tissue concentration in relation to developmental stage and to serum hormone levels. *Am. J. Obstet. Gynecol.*, 138:1131.
97. Sutcliffe, R. G., Kukulska-Langlands, B. M., Coggins, J. R., Hunter, J. B., and Gore, C. H. (1980): Studies on human pregnancy-associated plasma protein A. *Biochem. J.*, 191:799.
98. Sutcliffe, R. G., Joshi, S. G., Paterson, W. F., and Bank, J. F. (1982): Serological identity between human alpha uterine protein and human progestagen-dependent endometrial protein. *J. Reprod. Fertil.*, 65:207.
99. Mossman, H. W. (1937): Comparative morphogenesis of the fetal membranes and accessory uterine structures. *Contrib. Embryol.*, 158:133.
100. Golander, G., Zakuth, V., Schechter, Y., and Spirer, Z. (1981): Suppression of lymphocyte reactivity in vitro by a soluble factor secreted by explants of human decidua. *Eur. J. Immunol.*, 11:849.
101. Bischof, P., DuBerg, S., Sizonenko, M. T., et al. (1984): In vitro production of pregnancy-associated plasma protein A by human decidua and trophoblast. *Am. J. Obstet. Gynecol.*, 148:13.
102. Bulmer, J. N., and Sunderland, C. A. (1984): Immunohistological characterization of lymphoid cell populations in the early human placental bed. *Immunology*, 52:349.
103. Bulmer, J. N., and Sunderland, C. A. (1983): Bone-marrow origin of endometrial granulocytes in the early human placental bed. *J. Reprod. Immunol.*, 5:383.

104. Laguens, R. M., and Laguens, R. P. (1983): Isolation and characteristics of a macrophage population of human uterine mucosa. *Gynecol. Obstet. Invest.*, 16:136.
105. Korte, K., MacDonald, P. C., Johnston, J. M., Okita, J. R., and Casey, M. L. (1983): Metabolism of arachidonic acid and prostanoids in human endometrial stromal cells in monolayer culture. *Biochim. Biophys. Acta*, 752:423.
106. Hochner-Celnikier, D., Ron, M., Eldor, A., et al. (1984): Growth characteristics of human first trimester decidual cells cultured in serum-free medium: Production of prolactin, prostaglandins and fibronectin. *Biol. Reprod.*, 31:827.
107. Bigazzi, M., Nardi, E., Bruni, P. and Petrucci, F. (1980): Relaxin in human decidua. *J. Clin. Endocrinol. Metab.*, 51:939.
108. Koay, E. S. C., Bagnell, C. A., Bryant-Greenwood, G. D., Lord, S. B., Cruz, A. C., and Larkin, L. H. (1985): Immunocytochemical localization of relaxin in human decidua and placenta. *J. Clin. Endocrinol. Metab.*, 60:859.
109. Weisman, Y., Harell, A., Edelstein, S., David, M., Spirer, Z., and Golander, A. (1979): 1α,25-dihydroxyvitamin D_3 and 24,25-dihydroxyvitamin D_3 *in vitro* synthesis by human decidua and placenta. *Nature*, 281:317.
110. Markoff, E., Zeitler, P., Peleg, S., and Handwerger, S. (1983): Characterization of the synthesis and release of prolactin by an enriched fraction of human decidual cells. *J. Clin. Endocrinol. Metab.*, 56:962.
111. Braverman, M. B., Bagni, A., DeZiegler, D., Den, I., and Gurpide, E. (1984): Isolation of prolactin-producing cells from first and second trimester decidua. *J. Clin. Endocrinol. Metab.*, 58:521.
112. McRae, M. A., Newman, G. R., Walker, S. M., and Jasani, B. (1986): Immunohistochemical identification of prolactin and 24K protein in secretory endometrium. *Fertil. Steril.*, 45:643.
113. Maslar, I. A., and Ansbacher, R. (1986): Effects of progesterone on decidual prolactin production by organ cultures of human endometrium. *Endocrinology*, 118:2102.
114. Kaufman, D. G., Adamec, T. A., Walton, L. A., et al. (1980): Studies of human endometrium in organ culture. *Methods Cell Biol.*, 21B:1.
115. Csermely, T., Demers, L. M., and Hughes, E. C. (1969): Organ culture of human endometrium. *Obstet. Gynecol.*, 34:252.
116. Kohorn, E. I., Rice, S. I., and Gordon, M. (1970): *In vitro* production of nucleolar channel system by progesterone in human endometrium. *Nature*, 228:671.
117. Maslar, I. A., Powers-Craddock, P., and Ansbacher, R. (1986): Decidual prolactin production by organ cultures of human endometrium: Effects of continuous and intermittent progesterone treatment. *Biol. Reprod.*, 34:741.
118. Lawn, A. M., Wilson, E. W., and Finn, C. A. (1971): The ultrastructure of human decidual and predecidual cells. *J. Reprod. Fertil.*, 26:85.
119. Wienke, E., Jr., Cavazos, F., Hall, D. G., and Lucas, F. V. (1968): Ultrastructure of the human endometrial stroma cell during the menstrual cycle. *Am. J. Obstet. Gynecol.*, 102:65.
120. Wewer, U. M., Faber, M., Liotta, L. A., and Albrechtsen, R. (1985): Immunochemical and ultrastructural assessment of the nature of the pericellular basement membrane of human decidual cells. *Lab. Invest.* 53:624.
121. MacLaughlin, D. T., Richardson, G. S., and Sylvan, P. E. (1983): Analysis of human endometrial protein secretions *in vivo* and *in vitro:* Effects of estrogens and progesterone. In: *Steroids and Endometrial Cancer*, edited by V. M. Jasonni et al., p. 93. Raven Press, New York.
122. Bell, S. C., Patel, S., Hales, M. W., Kirwan, P. H., and Drife, J. O. (1985): Immunochemical detection and characterization of pregnancy-associated endometrial α_1- and α_2-globulins secreted by human endometrium and decidua. *J. Reprod. Fertil.*, 74:261.
123. Iacobelli, S., Marchetti, P., Bartoccioni, E., Natoli, V., Scambia, G., and Kaye, A. M. (1981): Steroid-induced proteins in human endometrium. *Mol. Cell Endocrinol.* 23:321.
124. Strinden, S. T., and Shapiro, S. S. (1983): Progesterone-altered secretory proteins from cultured human endometrium. *Endocrinology*, 112:862.
125. Heffner, L. J., Iddenden, D. A., and Lyttle, C. R. (1986): Electrophoretic analyses of secreted human endometrial proteins: Identification and characterization of luteal phase prolactin. *J. Clin. Endocrinol. Metab.*, 62:1288.
126. Rutanen, E-M., Koistinen, R., Wahlstrom, T., Bohn, H., Ranta, T., and Seppala, M. (1985): Synthesis of placental protein 12 by human decidua. *Endocrinology*, 116:1304.
127. Schroder, R. (1915): Anatomische Studien zur normalen und pathologischen Physiologie des Menstruationszyklus. *Arch. Gynaekol.*, 104:27.
128. Hartman, C. G. (1944): Regeneration of the monkey uterus after surgical removal of the endometrium and accidental endometriosis. *Western J. Surg. Obstet. Gynecol.*, 52:87.
129. Bartelmez, G. W. (1933): Histological studies on the menstruating mucous membrane of the human uterus. *Contrib. Embryol.*, 142:142.
130. Levison, D. A. (1985): Lymphoid tissue and cyclical endometrium. *J. Clin. Pathol.*, 38:1316.
131. McLennan, C. E., and Rydell, A. H. (1965): Extent of endometrial shedding during normal menstruation. *J. Obstet. Gynecol.*, 26:605.
132. Ferenczy, A. (1976): Studies on the cytodynamics of human endometrial regeneration. *Am. J. Obstet. Gynecol.*, 124:64.
133. Hopwood, D., and Levison, D. A. (1976): Atrophy and apoptosis in the cyclical human endometrium. *J. Pathol.*, 119:159.
134. Davie, R., Hopwood, D., and Levison, D. A. (1977): Intercellular spaces and cell junctions in endometrial glands: their possible role in menstruation. *Br. J. Obstet. Gynaecol.*, 84:467.
135. Ferenczy, A., Bertrand, G., and Gelfand, M. M. (1979): Proliferation kinetics of human endometrium during the normal menstrual cycle. *Am. J. Obstet. Gynecol.*, 133:859.
136. Cornillie, F. J., Lauweryns, J. M., and Brosens, I. A. (1985): Normal human endometrium. *Gynecol. Obstet. Invest.*, 20:113.
137. Flowers, C. E., Jr., and Wilborn, W. H. (1978): New observations on the physiology of menstruation. *Obstet. Gynecol.*, 51:16.
138. Bensley, C. M. (1951): Cyclic fluctuations in the rate of epithelial mitosis in the endometrium of the rhesus monkey. *Contrib. Embryol.*, 34:87.
139. Ferenczy, A., Bertrand, G., and Gelfand, M. M. (1979): Studies on the cytodynamics of human endometrial regeneration. III. *In vitro* short-term incubation historadioautography. *Am. J. Obstet. Gynecol.*, 134:297.
140. Padykula, H. A., Coles, L. G., McCracken, J. A., King, N. W., Jr., Longcope, C., and Kaiserman-Abramof, I. R. (1984): A zonal pattern of cell proliferation and differentiation in the rhesus endometrium during the estrogen surge. *Biol. Reprod.*, 31:1103.
141. Padykula, H. A., Coles, L. G., McCracken, J. A., Longcope, C., and King, N. W., Jr. (1984): Production of progenitor cells for postmenstrual reconstruction in the cyclic rhesus monkey. *Biol. Reprod. (Suppl.)*, 30:92 (abstr. 123).
142. Press, M. P., Nousek-Goebl, N., King, W. J., Herbst, A. L., and Greene, G. J. (1984): Immunohistochemical assessment of estrogen receptor distribution in the human endometrium throughout the menstrual cycle. *Lab. Invest.*, 51:495.
143. King, W. J., and Greene, G. L. (1984): Monoclonal antibodies localize oestrogen receptor in the nuclei of target cells. *Nature*, 307:745.
144. McClellan, M. C., West, N. B., Tacha, D. E., Greene, G. L., and Brenner, R. M. (1984): Immunocytochemical localization of estrogen receptors in the macaque reproductive tract with monoclonal antiestrophilins. *Endocrinology*, 114:2002.
145. Press, M. F., and Greene, G. L. (1984): An immunocytochemical method for demonstrating estrogen receptor in human uterus using monoclonal antibodies to human estrophilin. *Lab. Invest.*, 50:480.
146. Welshons, W. V., Lieberman, M. E., and Gorski, J. (1984): Nuclear localization of unoccupied oestrogen receptors. *Nature*, 307:747.
147. Brenner, R. M., McClellan, M., and West, N. B. (1986): Immunocytochemistry of the estrogen receptor in the reproductive tract of spayed versus hormone treated macaques. In: *Program of the 68th Annual Meeting of The Endocrine Society*, p. 211 (abstr. 720). Anaheim, California.
148. Press, M. F., Nousek-Goebl, N. A., Bur, M., and Greene, G. L. (1986): Estrogen receptor localization in the female genital tract. *Am. J. Pathol.*, 123:280.
149. McClellan, M., West, N. B., and Brenner, R. M. (1986): Immunocytochemical localization of estrogen receptors in the macaque endometrium during the luteal-follicular transition. *Endocrinology (in press)*.

150. Perrot-Applanat, M., Groyer-Picard, M-T., Logeat, F., and Milgrom, E. (1986): Ultrastructural localization of the progesterone receptor by an immunogold method: Effect of hormone administration. *J. Cell. Biol.,* 102:1191.
151. Enami, J., Enami, S., and Koga, M. (1983): Growth of normal and neoplastic mouse mammary epithelial cells in primary culture: Stimulation by conditioned medium from mouse mammary fibroblasts. *Gann,* 74:845.
152. McGrath, C. M. (1984): Augmentation of the response of normal mammary epithelial cells to estradiol by mammary stroma. *Cancer Res.,* 43:1355.
153. Ferenczy, A. (1977): Studies on the cytodynamics of experimental endometrial regeneration in the rabbit. Historadioautography and ultrastructure. *Am. J. Obstet. Gynecol.,* 128:536.
154. McClellan, M. C., West, N. B., Sternfeld, M. D., Tacha, D. E., and Brenner, R. M. (1983): Immunocytochemistry of estrogen receptors in stroma and epithelium of macaque oviduct during early estrogen action. *Endocrinology,* 112:182 (abstr.).
155. Goodman, A. L., Descalzi, C. D., Johnson, D. K., and Hodgen, G. D. (1977): Composite pattern of circulating LH, FSH, estradiol, and progesterone during the menstrual cycle in cynomolgus monkeys. *Proc. Soc. Exp. Biol. Med.,* 155:479.
156. Verhage, H. G., and Brenner, R. M. (1975): Estradiol-induced differentiation of the oviductal epithelium in ovariectomized cats. *Biol. Reprod.,* 13:104.
157. West, N. B., Verhage, H. G., and Brenner, R. M. (1976): Suppression of the estradiol receptor system by progesterone in the oviduct and uterus of the cat. *Endocrinology,* 99:1010.
158. Hamner, C. E. (1973): Oviductal fluid—composition and physiology. In: *Handbook of Physiology, Sect. 7: Endocrinology, The Female Reproductive System,* Vol. 2, edited by R. O. Greep and E. B. Astwood, p. 123. Williams & Wilkins, Baltimore.
159. Mastroianni, L., Jr., and Stambaugh, R. (1974): Secretory function of the primate oviduct. In: *Physiology and Genetics of Reproduction,* edited by E. M. Coutinho and F. Fuchs, p. 25. Plenum, New York.
160. Gordon, M. (1975): Cyclic changes in the fine structure of the epithelial cells of human endometrium. *Int. Rev. Cytol.,* 42: 127.
161. Sawaragi, I., and Wynn, R. M. (1969): Ultrastructural localization of metabolic enzymes during the human endometrial cycle. *Obstet. Gynecol.,* 34:50.
162. Wilson, E. W. (1969): Alkaline phosphatase in pre-decidual cells of the human endometrium. *J. Reprod. Fert.,* 19:567.
163. Tseng, L. (1980): Hormonal regulation of steroid metabolic enzymes in human endometrium. *Adv. Sex Horm. Res.,* 4:329.
164. Shapiro, S. S., and Forbes, S. H. (1978): Alterations in human endometrial protein synthesis during the menstrual cycle and in progesterone-stimulated organ culture. *Fertil. Steril.,* 30:175.

The Physiology of Reproduction,
edited by E. Knobil and J. Neill *et al.*
Raven Press, Ltd., New York © 1988.

CHAPTER 10

Follicular Steroidogenesis and Its Control

Robert E. Gore-Langton and David T. Armstrong

The follicles are the principal functional units of the mammalian ovary. The function of each follicle is to provide the support system necessary for the female germ cell (oocyte) to attain its maximum potential—that of uniting with a male germ cell (spermatozoan) to produce an embryo capable of development leading to the birth of a normal viable offspring.

The somatic cells of the follicle contribute in several ways to accomplish this function, essential for the reproduction and survival of the species. First, they provide the nutritive requirements of the growing oocyte and, perhaps, the stimulus that initiates its growth. Later they control both the nuclear and cytoplasmic maturation of the oocyte contained in those follicles that are selected for ovulation and contribute to the atresia and oocyte destruction in those that are not. These direct effects of the follicle cells on the development and fate of the enclosed oocyte are mediated via changes they bring about in the microenvironment within the follicle, wrought in large part by products they secrete into the follicular fluid bathing the oocyte. In addition, specialized granulosa cells (cumulus cells) in the innermost layer surrounding the oocyte are coupled, metabolically, to the oocyte by gap junctions through which nutrient substances and regulatory molecules are delivered directly to the ooplasm.

The best-known and best-characterized secretory products of the follicle are the steroid hormones. The follicular steroids fulfill a number of important functions related to reproduction. They function as hormones, in the classical sense, being transported via the circulation to act on a wide variety of "target" tissues and organs comprising not only the reproductive system, but also several other organs and systems, including the central nervous system, musculoskeletal system, cardiovascular system, immune system, liver, and adipose and cutaneous tissues. Steroid actions at many levels contribute to the success of the reproductive process. For example, by action on brain centers that control sexual behavior, they ensure that females are willing and able to mate at the time that mature oocytes are released from the follicle. Actions on the musculature and cilia of the oviduct permit the cumulus–oocyte complex to be picked up by the oviductal fimbria and retained at the site of fertilization, while at the same time assisting with the transport of spermatozoa to that site. Oviductal and uterine smooth muscles, under the influence of steroid hormones, determine the time of entry of the fertilized egg into the uterus, and steroids bring about endometrial changes required for implantation of the developing embryo to occur, for maintenance of pregnancy once it is established, and for delivery of the full-term fetus.

In addition to acting as hormones on structures remote from the ovary, the steroids produced by follicle cells also act locally within the follicles in which they are produced, both as "paracrine" agents, acting on adjacent cells, and as "autocrine" agents, acting on or within the cells in which they are produced. As will be discussed later in this chapter, as well as elsewhere in this volume, steroids produced by the granulosa cells can influence the secretory pattern of the theca cells and the meiotic maturation of the oocyte. They also act on the granulosa cells themselves, influencing both their mitotic rate and their differentiation.

CLASSES OF FOLLICULAR STEROIDS

Chemical Classification

The steroid hormones may be classified on the basis either of their chemical structure or of their principal physiological actions. The hormones of main concern in this chapter are the sex steroids belonging to three major classes: progestins (gestagens, progestagens), androgens, and estrogens. Steroids belonging to all three classes are produced by the ovarian follicles at one or more stage(s) of development.

The chemical classification system relates all steroids to one of several parent, or stem, compounds, all of which comprise a ring complex, made up of three cyclohexane rings (A,B,C) and a cyclopentane ring (D), as illustrated in Fig. 1. To this fully saturated ring complex, referred to as the perhydrocyclopentanophenanthrene nucleus (or, more simply, the steroid nucleus), are attached additional components that vary according to steroid class. The ovarian steroids are all related to, and can be considered as chemical derivatives of, one of the four parent compounds illustrated in Fig. 1.

Cholestane, which comprises the steroid nucleus with methyl groups at the junctions between the A and B rings (at C-10) and the C and D rings (at C-13), and an eight-membered side chain attached to C-17, is the parent compound of cholesterol and other sterols, the biosynthetic precursors of all the steroids to be considered in this chapter. Fission of the side chain between C-20 and C-22 leads to the formation of the C_{21}-steroids (pregnane series), the chemical class to which the progestins belong. Further cleavage of the side chain between C-17 and C-20 produces the C_{19}-steroids (androstane series) to which the androgens belong. Finally, removal of the angular methyl group at C-10 leads to the formation of C_{18}-steroids (estrane series), the class to which the estrogens and related C_{18}-compounds belong.

A systematic method of nomenclature is used to identify each steroid according to which of the above series it belongs, as well as the nature and location of various modifications and chemical substitutions on the parent structure. Modifications of the parent structure include (a) introduction of double bonds between adjacent carbon atoms, either in the ring structure or the side chain; (b) hydroxyl (OH) substituents; and (c) carbonyl groups resulting from oxidation of the hydroxyl substituents. Since the steroid nucleus has a well-defined structure with three-dimensional conformation, the stereochemistry of substitutions must be considered, in order to distinguish between the stereoisomers resulting from substitutions at asymmetric carbons.

Stereoisomers resulting from substituents on the steroid nucleus are distinguished from each other by nomenclature that signifies the side of the plane of the molecule on which the substituent is located. By convention, substituents on the same side of the plane as the angular methyl group at C-10 are considered as having the β-configuration and are signified by a solid valency line (–); those with substituents on the opposite side of the plane have the α-configuration, signified by a broken line (---). For the steroids dealt with here, isomerization at C-3 and C-17 is of particular importance.

The other position of asymmetry of special interest in this chapter is that which occurs at C-5 as a result of orientation of the hydrogen atom there, which can occur on either the α- or β-side of the molecule. This results in *cis–trans* isomerism about the A-B ring junction, the *trans*-isomer resulting

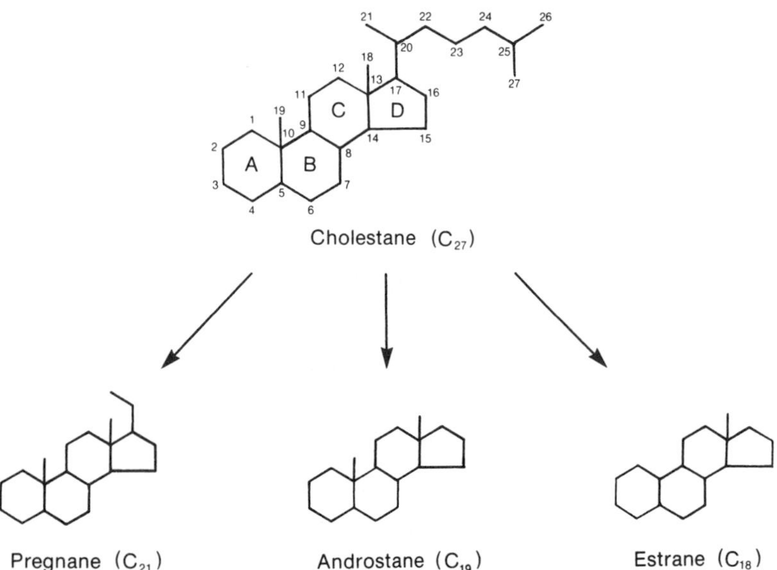

FIG. 1. Chemical classification for the parent structures from which the three main categories of ovarian steroids are derived. All steroid structures are derivatives of cholestane, the parent compound of cholesterol. Decreasing numbers of carbons occur as cholesterol is metabolized to progestins (pregnane series), androgens (androstane series), and estrogens (estrane series).

when the C-5-hydrogen atom is on the α-side of the molecule, i.e., *trans* to the orientation of the angular methyl group at C-10, and the *cis*-isomer resulting when this hydrogen is in the 5β-configuration. The conformation of the steroid nucleus differs markedly, depending on the orientation of the hydrogen at C-5, the A and B rings of 5α-reduced steroids lying in essentially the same plane, whereas those of 5β-reduced steroids are approximately at right angles to each other.

For a more detailed description of steroid structure, including stereochemistry and nomenclature, the reader is referred to the recent concise review by Kellie (1).

Biological Classification

Ovarian steroids are also classified on the basis of their principal biological function into one of the three major classes: progestins, androgens, and estrogens, which for the most part are represented by compounds belonging to the C_{21} (pregnane), C_{19} (androstane), and C_{18} (estrane) series, respectively.

Estrogens

Physiologically, the estrogens, estrone and estradiol-17β, are the most important of the follicular steroids. Their trivial names are reflections of their roles in induction of sexual receptivity (estrus) in female mammals, but they play key roles in many other aspects of female reproductive physiology, as will be considered later. Estrone [3-hydroxy-estra-1,3,5(10)-trien-17-one] was the first sex steroid to be isolated and identified. Doisy et al. (2) crystallized this steroid from human pregnancy urine in 1929, and later from follicular fluid of sows (3). Estradiol-17β [estra-1,3,5(10)-triene-3,17β-diol] is approximately 10 times as potent as estrone in most biological assays and, on a molar basis, is the most active of all steroids produced by the ovary. Several hydroxylated derivatives of these C_{18}-steroids, all of which possess an aromatic A- ring, have been identified recently in follicular fluids and tissues and are therefore assumed to be of follicular origin. These include 2-hydroxyestrone [2,3-dihydroxy-estra-1,3,5(10)-trien-17-one], 2-hydroxyestradiol, and their 2-methylated derivatives, as well as 4-OH-, 6-OH-, and 16-OH-derivatives of estrone and estradiol-17β (4–6).

In addition to the aromatic C_{18}-steroids, other compounds of the estrane series, 19-norandrostenedione (estra-4-ene-3,17-dione) and 19-nortestosterone (17β-hydroxy-estra-4-en-3-one) have been identified in the follicular fluid of the mare (4,7) and sow (8). The physiological function of these nonaromatic C_{18}-steroids remains to be determined.

Androgens

Biological evidence that the ovary produces androgens dates back to observations that ovaries grafted to the ears of male mice were able to reverse castration-induced atrophy of their seminal vesicles and prostate glands (9). The identification of androstenedione and testosterone in follicular fluid (10) followed by the demonstration of formation of these compounds from radiolabeled precursors by follicle cells (11) established the follicle as a significant source of ovarian androgens. As will be considered below, androstenedione and testosterone are the immediate biosynthetic precursors of the estrogenic steroids, estrone and estradiol-17β, respectively, because they are amenable to aromatization.

A number of nonaromatizable C_{19}-steroids, produced by saturation of the A- ring of the steroid nucleus, have also been identified as ovarian androgens of considerable importance (12–14). Ovarian 5α-reduced androgens that have been identified in several species include 5α-dihydrotestosterone (17β-hydroxy-5α-androstan-3-one) (DHT), 5α-androstane-3,17-dione, androsterone and epiandrosterone, and 5α-androstane-3α,17β-diol and its 3β-epimer. There is also recent evidence for ovarian production of 5β-reduced androgens in at least one species, the hamster (15).

Several 16-unsaturated steroids (androsta-4,16-dien-3-one, 5α-androst-16-en-3-one, and 3α-OH-5α-androst-16-ene) have been identified in ovarian tissue following incubation with radiolabeled precursors (16).

Progestins

Pregnenolone (3β-OH-pregn-5-en-20-one) is the most important progestin produced by the follicle because of its key position as the precursor of all the steroid hormones. Its most abundant C_{21} product in the follicle is progesterone (pregn-4-ene-3,20-dione), produced as a biosynthetic intermediate by follicles at all growing stages of development and as a secretory end product in the peri- and postovulatory periods. Other C_{21}-steroids of follicular origin include 17α-OH-progesterone (the immediate precursor of the aromatizable androgens), 20α-dihydroprogesterone (20α-hydroxy-pregn-4-en-3-one) and its 20β-epimer, and 17α,20α- and 17α,20β-pregnenediols. In addition, ring-A-reduced metabolites of each of these pregn-4-ene compounds have been shown to be produced by ovarian tissues of several species (particularly rodents) under certain physiological conditions (13,14,17).

PATHWAYS OF BIOSYNTHESIS AND KEY ENZYMES

Much of our knowledge of steroid biosynthetic processes has been gleaned from investigations on tissues other than the ovary. In particular, studies with adrenal cortex, testis, and human placenta have contributed to most of our current understanding of the steroidogenic enzymes, including their subcellular organization and control mechanisms. The available evidence indicates a high degree of similarity between the processes that are common to the different steroidogenic tissues, including the follicle. We have not attempted to present an exhaustive review of the extensive literature that has led to the present state of knowledge of the subject. The reader is referred to a number of excellent textbooks and reviews (18–20). Our aim in this section, rather, is to provide a summary of the biosynthetic pathways, identifying those individual enzymatic steps and processes that have been shown to be subject to physiological regulation. This brief review will provide a background for the remainder of the chapter, which deals with the control mechanisms as they apply specifically to the steroids of follicular origin. Other chapters will deal with aspects of steroidogenesis that pertain to the corpus luteum and the testis.

Steroid Precursors

The follicular steroids are produced from cholesterol derived from one of three possible sources: (a) preformed cholesterol taken up from the blood, primarily in the form of circulating lipoproteins; (b) preformed cholesterol stored within the ovarian cell, either as free cholesterol, a constituent of cell membranes, or liberated from cholesterol esters stored within cytoplasmic lipid droplets; and (c) cholesterol synthesized *de novo* in the ovarian cell from 2-carbon components derived from metabolism of carbohydrate, fat, or protein within the cell. The extent to which one or another of these sources of cholesterol is utilized for ovarian steroidogenesis varies with animal species and with cell type involved. Utilization of each may be subject to regulation with the quantitative importance of one source or another varying with the physiological state (21).

Most studies of the role of cholesterol from different sources as ovarian steroidogenic precursors have utilized extrafollicular tissues, e.g., corpus luteum (21), interstitial tissue (22), or luteinized granulosa cells in culture (23–25). In these tissues, cholesterol in circulating lipoproteins appears to be the most important source of steroidogenic cholesterol. Considerable evidence has been accumulated supporting a mechanism of uptake that involves binding of extracellular lipoproteins via their apoprotein component to specific receptors located on the cell membrane, followed by internalization of the lipoprotein–receptor complex, uptake of the complexes by lysosomes, degradation of lipoproteins by lysosomal esterases, and release of free cholesterol, which is then able to gain access to the steroidogenic enzymes. Cholesterol from both low-density lipoproteins (LDL) and high-density lipoproteins (HDL) has been implicated as steroidogenic precursor in these tissues (23). Species differences occur in the relative importance of the two classes of lipoproteins; HDL appears to be of greater quantitative importance in rodents, whereas cholesterol associated with LDL is the major circulating form of steroidogenic cholesterol in other species, including humans.

Differences in the vascular anatomy of the various cellular components of the ovary influence the degree to which circulating lipoproteins may serve as steroidogenic precursors. Thus, the corpus luteum, like the adrenal cortex, has an abundant blood supply and a highly permeable capillary endothelium, enabling the large lipoprotein molecules to gain access to lipoprotein receptors on luteal cells *in vivo*. The theca interna of the follicle receives blood from a similarly rich vascular supply and may therefore also be in a position to utilize lipoprotein cholesterol. On the other hand, the granulosa layers of the follicle are isolated from direct contact with the blood supply by a relatively impermeable basement membrane that provides a barrier to large molecules such as LDL (26–28). Only after luteinization has been initiated by the preovulatory luteinizing hormone (LH) surge *in vivo* does penetration of the capillary network occur through the basement membrane, allowing more ready access of lipoproteins to the granulosa cell component of the follicles. Predictions based on these anatomical considerations have been supported by recent experiments with cultured follicles (29) in which steroidogenesis in theca cells was influenced considerably more by the presence or absence of lipoprotein in the culture media than was that in granulosa cells.

Ovarian cells, particularly those in a position to take up extracellular cholesterol from circulating lipoproteins, store substantial amounts of cholesterol in intracellular lipid droplets, primarily as esters of long-chain fatty acids. An equilibrium between the cholesterol–fatty acyl esters in these intracellular depots and free cholesterol is maintained by a balance between two enzymes, acyl coenzyme A:cholesterol-acyl transferase (ACAT) (commonly called cholesterol ester synthetase) and sterol ester hydrolase (cholesterol esterase), the former favoring storage of excess cholesterol in esterified form and the latter catalyzing release of the stored cholesterol. The activities of both these enzymes, as well as of 3-hydroxy-3-methylglutaryl coenzyme A-reductase (HMG CoA reductase), the rate-limiting enzyme in cholesterol biosynthesis (Fig. 2), are under hormonal control, in addition to being regulated by intracellular levels of cholesterol (21). The state of equilibrium between cholesterol esters and free cholesterol and the relative contributions to steroidogenesis of extracellular cholesterol, intracellularly stored cholesterol, and cholesterol synthesized *de novo* from smaller molecular precursors may differ considerably under different prevailing physiological conditions.

FIG. 2. The principal biosynthetic pathways in the ovary for production of the progestins, androgens, and estrogens. Cholesterol may be synthesized *de novo* from acetate or derived from preformed sources. The metabolism of cholesterol to the sex steroids is carried out sequentially by several enzyme systems, each with several catalytic functions. Thus, the conversion of cholesterol to androgens involves three enzyme systems: cholesterol (C_{27}-sterol) side-chain cleavage P-450, C_{21}-steroid side-chain cleavage P-450, and Δ^5-3β-hydroxysteroid dehydrogenase: Δ^{5-4}-isomerase. Subsequent conversion of C_{19}-steroids to estrogens is carried out by aromatase P-450 enzyme(s). The enzyme systems are distributed in different subcellular sites as indicated.

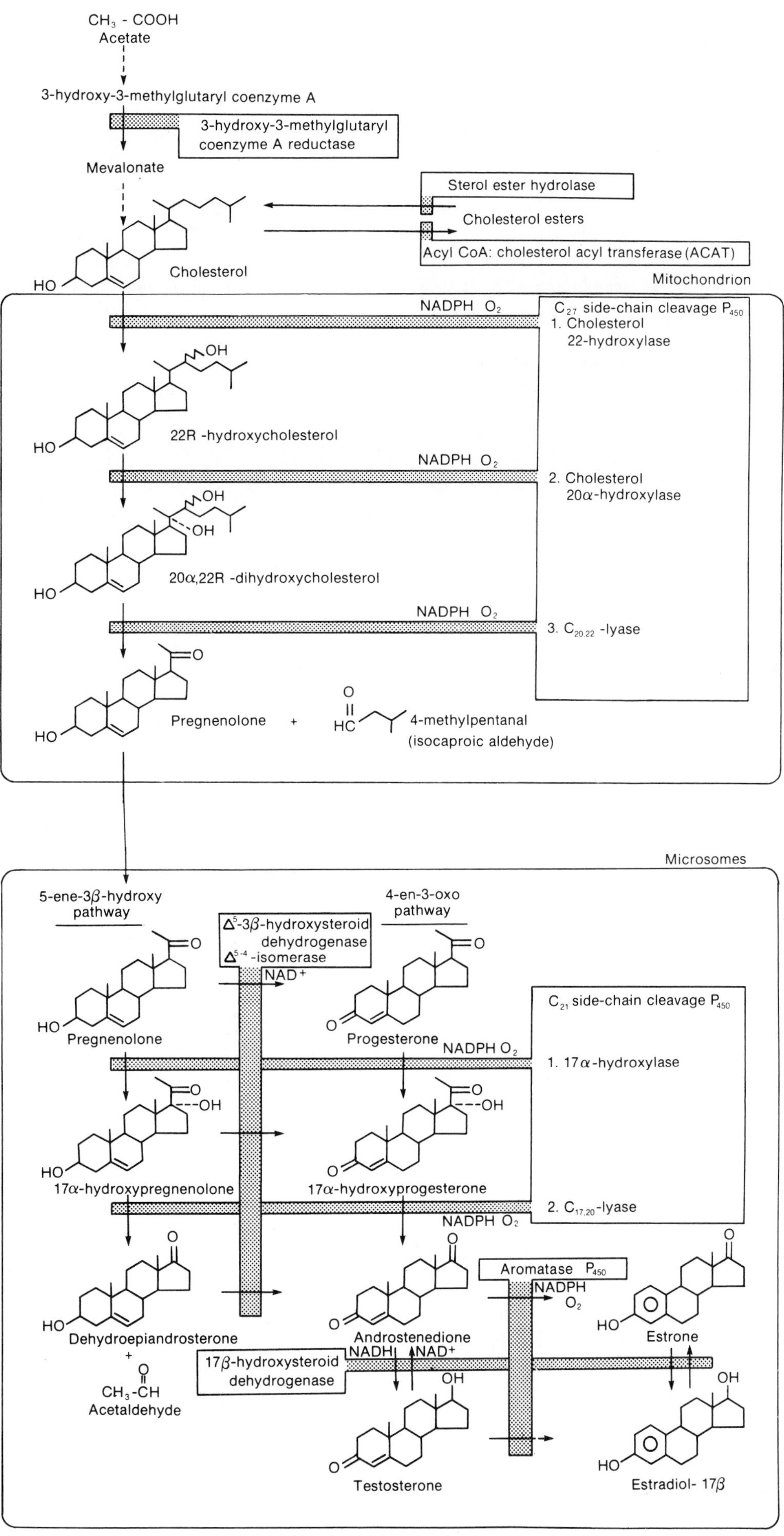

CH_3 - COOH
Acetate
3-hydroxy-3-methylglutaryl coenzyme A
3-hydroxy-3-methylglutaryl coenzyme A reductase
Mevalonate
Sterol ester hydrolase
Cholesterol esters
Acyl CoA: cholesterol acyl transferase (ACAT)
HO
Cholesterol
Mitochondrion
NADPH O_2
C_{27} side-chain cleavage P_{450}
1. Cholesterol 22-hydroxylase
OH
22R -hydroxycholesterol
2. Cholesterol 20α-hydroxylase
20α,22R -dihydroxycholesterol
3. $C_{20,22}$ -lyase
Pregnenolone
+
HC
4-methylpentanal (isocaproic aldehyde)
Microsomes
5-ene-3β-hydroxy pathway
4-en-3-oxo pathway
Δ^5-3β-hydroxysteroid dehydrogenase
Δ^{5-4} -isomerase
NAD^+
Progesterone
C_{21} side-chain cleavage P_{450}
1. 17α-hydroxylase
17α-hydroxypregnenolone
17α-hydroxyprogesterone
2. $C_{17,20}$-lyase
Aromatase P_{450}
NADPH
O_2
Dehydroepiandrosterone
Androstenedione
Estrone
+
CH_3-CH
Acetaldehyde
17β-hydroxysteroid dehydrogenase
NADH
NAD^+
Testosterone
Estradiol- 17β

Cholesterol (C_{27}-Sterol) Side-Chain Cleavage

The first step in the conversion of cholesterol to steroids, and the step generally believed to be rate limiting in steroidogenesis under most conditions, is the cleavage of the C-20,22 bond resulting in the C_{21} compound, pregnenolone, and a 6-carbon fragment, isocaproic aldehyde. The enzyme system that catalyzes this reaction is located on the matrix side of the inner mitochondrial membranes (30). It is a multienzyme complex comprising three components: cytochrome P-450 side-chain cleavage (SCC), which is the terminal (electron-acceptor) oxygenase, a flavin adenine dinucleotide (FAD)-containing flavoprotein, and the sulfur-containing heme protein luteodoxin or adrenodoxin (in luteal and adrenal cells, respectively), which serves to shuttle an electron between the other two components (21). The reaction utilizes nicotinamide adenine dinucleotide phosphate (NADPH) generated within the mitochondria by oxidation of Krebs cycle intermediates or fatty acids. Three moles each of NADPH and of oxygen are utilized per mole of cholesterol undergoing side-chain cleavage.

The generally accepted pathway for biosynthesis of pregnenolone from cholesterol is illustrated in Fig. 2. Evidence summarized by Lieberman et al. (31) suggests that the overall reaction *in vivo* probably does not involve stable, free hydroxylated intermediates as shown here. Instead, it has been proposed that the substrate cholesterol and subsequent transient hydroxylated intermediates remain bound to the P-450_{SCC} until the ultimate product, pregnenolone, is formed and released. The free hydroxylated intermediates that have been isolated from disrupted cell preparations may merely be "inadvertent by-products of the processes which are formed when the cytochrome P-450_{SCC}-substrate complex is denatured" (31).

Metabolism of Pregnenolone

Pregnenolone is the key steroidogenic intermediate common to all classes of steroid hormones produced by the follicles, as well as by other steroidogenic tissues. It is converted to progesterone by a microsomal enzyme, or enzyme complex, Δ^5-3β-hydroxysteroid dehydrogenase:$\Delta^{5\text{-}4}$-isomerase. Although separation of the dehydrogenase from the isomerase activities has been achieved for a bacterial enzyme system, the two enzyme activities in mammalian steroidogenic tissues, including the ovary, have not been separated and appear to function physiologically as a single entity (32). The enzyme utilizes NAD+ as an electron acceptor, and the reaction is essentially irreversible under physiological conditions. Similar, but perhaps not identical enzymes, bring about the conversion of 17α-OH-pregnenolone and dehydroepiandrosterone (DHEA) to 17α-OH-progesterone and androstenedione, respectively (Fig. 2).

C_{21}-Steroid Side-Chain Cleavage

The rate-limiting step in the biosynthesis of androgens in the follicle, as in other androgen-secreting organs, is the 17α-hydroxylase:C-17,20-lyase enzyme complex. A component of the membranes of the agranular endoplasmic reticulum (microsomes), this enzyme system is a cytochrome P-450–containing mixed-function oxidase, requiring NADPH and molecular oxygen. As with the cholesterol side-chain cleavage system, the two reactions (17α-hydroxylation and cleavage of the C-17,20 bond) occur in a concerted fashion in which the 17α-hydroxy intermediate probably remains bound to the enzyme complex without appearing in free form. The reaction can utilize either pregnenolone or progesterone as substrate, resulting in formation of the respective products, DHEA or androstenedione. These two alternative pathways are referred to as the 5-ene-3β-hydroxy (or Δ^5) pathway and the 4-en-3-oxo (or Δ^4) pathway, respectively, although it is uncertain whether the same or separate enzymes are involved (Fig. 2) (33).

This enzymic step is subject to hormonal and feedback regulation, and is one of the key points at which physiological control of follicular steroid secretion occurs.

An alternative mechanism for formation of C_{19}-steroids, involving side-chain cleavage of pregnenolone and progesterone without prior 17-hydroxylation, has been demonstrated in boar testis. The products of the reaction, androst-5,16-dien-3β-ol and androst-4,16-dien-3-one, respectively, have also been identified in porcine and human follicular fluid, suggesting that this minor pathway may function in follicular steroidogenesis under certain conditions (33).

Aromatization of C_{19}-Steroids

The 4-ene-C_{19}-steroids, androstenedione and testosterone, are converted to the estrogens, estrone and estradiol-17β, respectively, by an enzyme complex located in the membranes of the agranular endoplasmic reticulum of several ovarian cell types (to be considered in detail below). This enzyme complex, referred to as "aromatase" because of the aromatic structure of the products, is a cytochrome P-450-containing mixed-function oxidase that catalyzes a multiple-step reaction leading to removal of the methyl group at C-10 as formic acid, followed by rearrangement of ring A to the aromatic structure.

The reaction requires NADPH, and 3 moles of O_2 are consumed. Two of these are involved in two consecutive hydroxylations at C-19, and the overall reaction involves a third hydroxylation, but the exact site of this has not been established with certainty. The overall reaction, illustrating three proposed alternative mechanisms to account for the third mole of oxygen consumed, is depicted as a sequence of steps (Fig. 3). Most evidence supports a concept of enzyme-bound intermediates that do not exist as free compounds, but rather as transition states in which the substrate remains bound to the enzyme complex and undergoes the entire series of reactions before release of the product from the enzyme (31). The final step resulting in the formation of the aromatic A-ring with the loss of the angular methyl group as formic acid may be nonenzymatic and could occur after release from the enzyme complex. Although the mech-

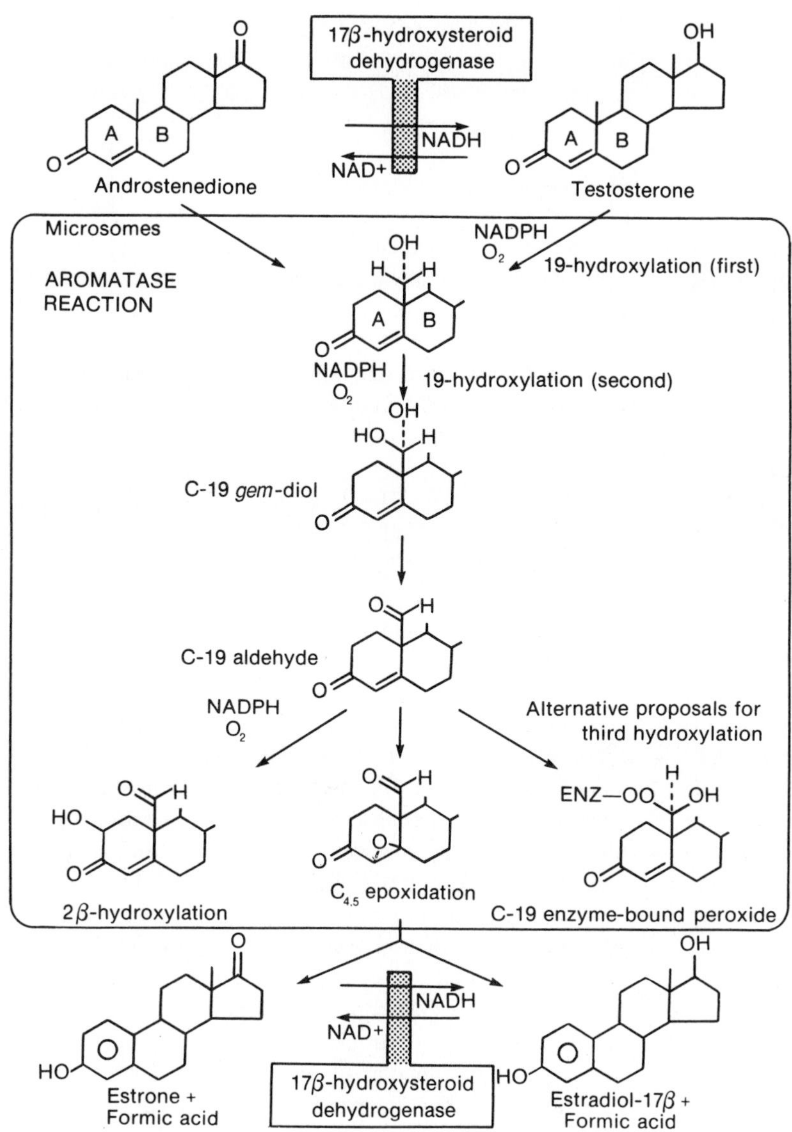

FIG. 3. Proposed sequence of reactions in the aromatization of androstenedione and testosterone. The aromatase enzyme system catalyzes a concerted reaction of enzyme-bound transition states involving three hydroxylations, the first two occurring at C-19, while the site of the third remains controversial: Hydroxylation at C-2β is considered most probable, but alternative mechanisms involving epoxidation or an enzyme-bound peroxide have also been proposed. Note that the C-19 aldehyde form of the enzyme-bound intermediate is more stable than the C-19 *gem* diol and forms spontaneously. Also, the final step resulting in C-10,19 cleavage and rearrangement to the aromatic ring-A may occur by a nonenzymatic mechanism.

anisms of the various steps in the overall reaction have been determined largely from studies of human placental microsome preparations, the available evidence suggests that the reaction in follicle cells proceeds along similar lines (34,35).

Reductive Metabolism of Ovarian Steroids

5α-Reduced Pathways of Progestin and Androgen Metabolism

Enzymatic reduction of 4-en-3-oxo-steroids of both C_{21} and C_{19} classes occurs in ovarian tissues of a variety of species. The enzyme(s) that catalyze this reduction are stereospecific 5α- or 5β-reductase(s) located in the agranular endoplasmic reticulum and utilize(s) NADPH as the source of the reducing protons. In most ovarian systems studied, the reductase is specific for the 5α-configuration (36–38), although 5β-reduced products have been identified from preparations of hamster ovaries (15,39).

In many of the systems studied, 5α-reduction is followed directly by stereospecific reduction of the 3-oxo-group by 3α-hydroxysteroid dehydrogenase leading to formation of 3α-OH-derivatives of the 5α-reduced metabolites. Both the 5α- and 3α-reductions can occur either before or after cleavage of the C-17,20 bond (40), with the result that ring A reduction products of both progestins and androgens are formed by ovarian preparations. Whether these are products of separate enzymes specific for the two classes of steroids or of the same enzymes that do not discriminate between C_{19} and C_{21} steroid substrates has not been established with certainty (see Fig. 4).

3β-Hydroxy derivatives of 5α-reduced progestins and androgens have also been reported following incubation of ovarian homogenates (41,42), suggesting the presence of a 3β-hydroxysteroid dehydrogenase capable of using 5α-reduced steroids as substrates. Because 3β-hydroxy metabolites could not be identified in ovarian vein blood (43) or following incubation of intact ovarian preparations with radiolabeled progesterone (17), the possibility has been raised that 3β-hydroxy products represent artifacts when cell disruption enables the 5α-reduced compounds to gain access to the membrane-bound Δ^5-3β-hydroxysteroid dehydrogenase whose function in conjunction with the Δ^{5-4}-isomerase in the intact cell is conversion of pregnenolone to progesterone (17). On the other hand, high circulating levels of 5α-androstane-3β,17β-diol have been reported in prepubertal rats; these have been found to drop considerably following ovariectomy (44), suggesting that at least a portion of this 3β-reduced androstanediol is of ovarian origin and attesting to the possible physiological significance of the 3β-epimer (45).

20-Hydroxysteroid Dehydrogenases

The C-20-carbonyl group of C_{21} steroids, including progesterone, 17α-hydroxyprogesterone, and ring A-saturated progestins, can undergo enzymic reduction to the corresponding 20-hydroxy derivative(s). The stereospecificity of the 20-hydroxysteroid dehydrogenase enzyme in ovarian cells (corpus luteum, follicles, interstitial cells) of most species is for the 20α configuration, although the bovine corpus luteum, exceptionally, produces the 20β-hydroxy metabolite. The 20-hydroxysteroid dehydrogenases are located in the cytosol portion of those ovarian cells studied, and they preferentially utilize NADPH as the hydrogen donor. The 20α-hydroxysteroid dehydrogenase of rodent corpora lutea undergoes hormonal regulation, thereby providing a means of influencing the biological potency of the C_{21}-steroid product secreted by this organ since the product 20α-hydroxy-pregn-4-en-3-one is considerably less active as a progestational agent than is its precursor, progesterone (46).

Since 20α-reduced steroids are poor substrates for C-17,20-lyase, the activity of the 20α-hydroxysteroid dehydrogenase may play a significant role in determining the amount of C_{21}-substrate available for conversion to androgens in follicular cells (47).

17β-Hydroxysteroid Dehydrogenase

17-Hydroxy- and 17-oxo-steroids are readily interconvertible by a reversible 17β-hydroxysteroid dehydrogenase present in microsomes of several steroidogenic tissues, including the follicle. Enzymes with cofactor requirements for both NAD+ and NADP+ have been described (33). Although both androgens and estrogens serve as substrates for this reaction (Figs. 2,3), it is uncertain whether this is because of a lack of rigorous substrate specificity of the ovarian 17β-hydroxysteroid dehydrogenase or because there are separate enzymes for the C_{18}-steroids and for the C_{19}-steroids, either of the 4-en-3-oxo-, 5-en-3β-hydroxy-, or ring-A-reduced variety.

Hydroxylation of Estrogens

Several hydroxylated estrogens have been reported in follicular fluid of a number of species and are therefore assumed to be of follicular cell origin. These include 2-OH-, 4-OH-, 6-OH-, and 16-OH-estrone and estradiol. Like all hydroxylase reactions, the ovarian enzymes that catalyze these hydroxylations are cytochrome P-450-containing enzymes that require NADPH and molecular oxygen.

The 2-OH- and 4-OH-estrogens are "catechol" estrogens, with 2-OH-estrone and 2-OH-estradiol being of particular interest because of their putative roles in regulation of gonadotropin secretion (48). Once formed, the catechol estrogens are rapidly metabolized to their O-methylated derivatives by the enzyme, catechol-*O*-methyl transferase.

The liver is believed to be the major source of circulating catechol estrogens, but other tissues, particularly various regions of the brain, have received considerable attention as sites of formation of physiological significance. However, the recent demonstration of catechol estrogens and other hydroxylated estrogen metabolites in follicular fluid and tissue (5,6) suggests the follicle may also be a site of formation of this class of compounds. The presence of estrogen-2- and 4-hydroxylase activity in porcine follicular tissues, particularly in membrana granulosa of preovulatory follicles, provides support for follicular production of catechol estrogens and further suggests that production increases during follicular maturation (49). These findings raise questions about the possible physiological significance of these compounds either in follicular regulation or as secretory products of the follicle (50).

STEROIDOGENESIS AND ITS CONTROL BY CELL TYPE

Our intention in this section is to review the individual contributions of the follicular and interstitial cell types to steroidogenesis, with particular regard to the cellular sites of the steroidogenic enzymes and their regulation by gonadotropins, intraovarian steroidal actions, and other known or putative regulatory factors, and to consider the importance of cooperation of the different cell types in the overall

FIG. 4. Reductive pathways of progestin and androgen metabolism in the ovary. *Notes:* 1. The 20α-hydroxysteroid dehydrogenase occurs in ovaries of most species (shown), while in bovines a different enzyme has 20β stereospecificity (not shown). 2. 5α-Reduction occurs similarly for C_{21}- and C_{19}-steroids, but it is not known whether it is the same 4-ene-5α-reductase enzyme acting in each instance. 5β-Reduction, an important reaction in the peripheral metabolism of C_{21}- and C_{19}-steroids, is an additional pathway present in the hamster ovary. 3. Conversion of 5α-reduced steroids via the 3α-hydroxysteroid dehydrogenase (shown) is well documented. An alternative pathway involving a 3β-hydroxysteroid dehydrogenase (not shown) has been demonstrated under limited conditions. The expected 3β-hydroxy products are similar to those shown. The 3β-epimer of androsterone is epiandrosterone.

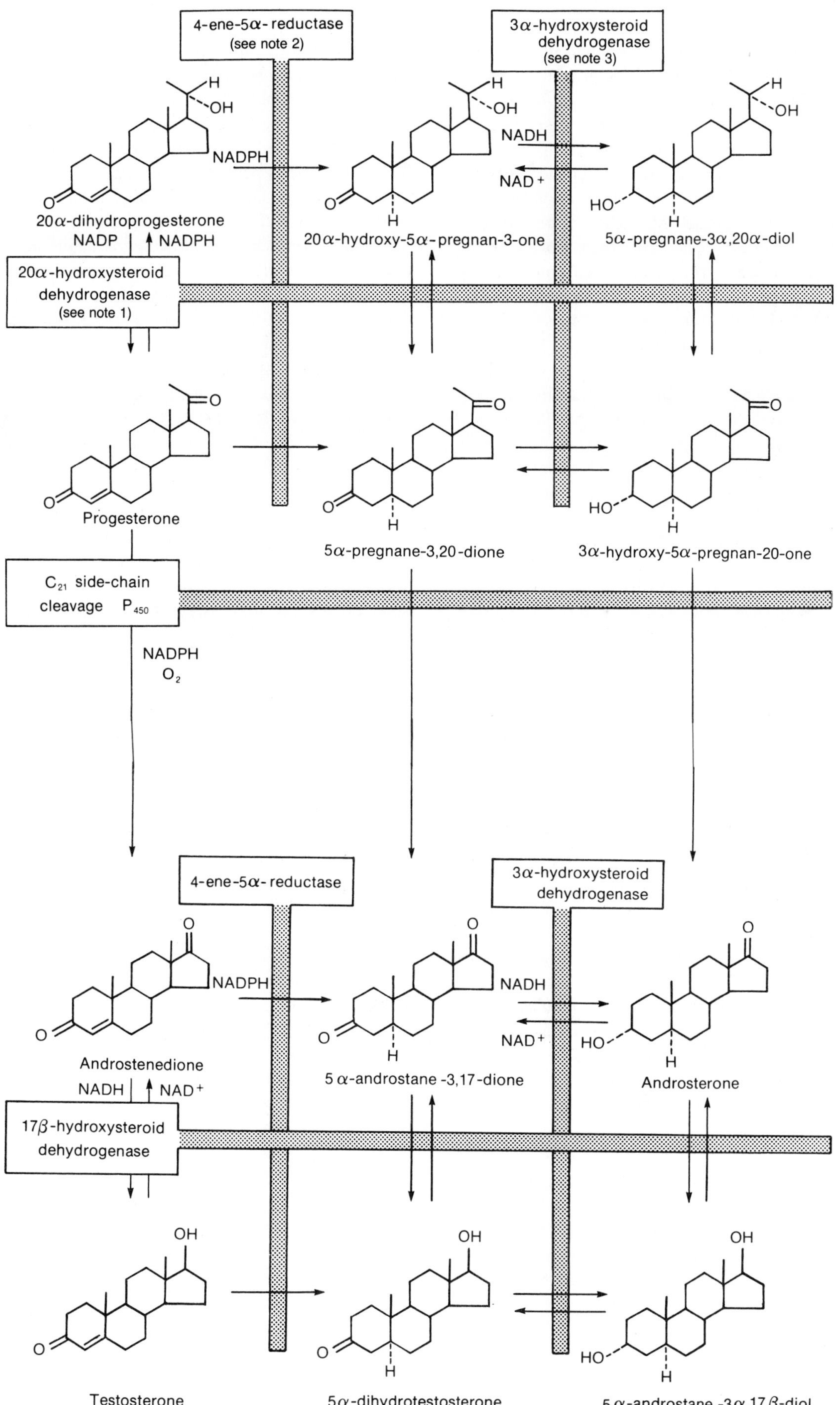

4-ene-5α-reductase
(see note 2)
3α-hydroxysteroid dehydrogenase
(see note 3)
NADPH
NADH
NAD+
20α-dihydroprogesterone
20α-hydroxy-5α-pregnan-3-one
5α-pregnane-3α,20α-diol
NADP
NADPH
20α-hydroxysteroid dehydrogenase
(see note 1)
Progesterone
5α-pregnane-3,20-dione
3α-hydroxy-5α-pregnan-20-one
C21 side-chain cleavage P450
NADPH
O2
4-ene-5α-reductase
3α-hydroxysteroid dehydrogenase
NADPH
NADH
NAD+
Androstenedione
5 α-androstane -3,17-dione
Androsterone
NADH
NAD+
17β-hydroxysteroid dehydrogenase
Testosterone
5α-dihydrotestosterone
5 α-androstane -3α,17β-diol

steroidogenic process in the follicle. We will not consider the molecular mechanisms of gonadotropin action, which are beyond the scope of this chapter, nor will we review the extensive literature that has developed to support the concept that gonadotropins—follicle-stimulating hormone (FSH) and luteinizing hormone (LH)—regulate steroidogenesis and other aspects of follicular maturation by stimulating the production of cyclic AMP (cAMP), the so-called second messenger. These topics have been previously reviewed (51,52). Suffice it to say, cAMP is now well established as the principal, if not the only intracellular mediator of FSH and LH/human chorionic gonadotropin (hCG) actions on the follicular cell types. FSH and LH satisfy virtually all of the criteria orginally set out by Sutherland and colleagues (53) and subsequently extended by Kuo and Greengard (54) to indicate that a hormone mediates its actions via cAMP and cAMP-dependent phosphorylation of proteins. Calcium has a permissive role in the steroidogenic process, as demonstrated for FSH-stimulated steroidogenesis in rat granulosa cells (55).

Steroidogenic Cells and Their Origins

In all mammalian species the principal cell types involved in follicular steroidogenesis are of two basic types: (a) LH-responsive secretory cells, comprising the theca interna cells of the follicular envelope and the interstitial cells of the ovarian stroma, and (b) FSH-responsive cells, consisting exclusively of granulosa cells, which only later in follicular maturation also acquire the ability to respond to LH. These two basic cell types fulfill distinct roles in the steroidogenic process by virtue of their different regulatory hormones and their dissimilar expression of steroidogenic enzymes.

Granulosa and theca/interstitial cells have distinct embryological origins. Granulosa cells appear to be derived mainly, although perhaps not exclusively, from certain cells within the intraovarian rete ovarii which closely resemble granulosa cells in terms of their organelles (56) and microfilaments (57–60). The intraovarian rete ovarii in the prefollicular ovary consists of cell cords and tubules and of mesenchymal cells in the ovarian medulla. Early follicular development occurs centrally in the innermost part of the cortex within the rete cords as rete cells move between and attach to oocytes, differentiate into granulosa cells, and then organize follicles (56,61).

Once follicles form and the granulosa cells become fully enclosed by the follicular basement membrane, it is clear that these cells alone proliferate to produce the membrana granulosa layer. However, this population of granulosa cells does not remain uniform, but as the antral follicle develops, these cells become organized into morphologically distinguishable regions with specialized functions. The granulosa cells in the layer immediately adjacent to the oocyte (i.e., corona radiata cells) establish intimate contact with the oocyte up until the preovulatory stage by means of cellular processes traversing the zona pellucida and forming gap junctional complexes with the oolema. These cells serve as "nurse" cells, providing nutrients for oocyte growth and also presumably exchanging regulatory factors with the oocyte, thereby relaying signals required for the coordinated maturation of the follicle and the oocyte. The cumulus granulosa cells comprise the cellular mass that surrounds the oocyte (i.e., the cumulus oophorus) and attaches the oocyte to the follicle wall. The cumulus cells physically support the oocyte within the follicle and may contribute to its nutritional and regulatory needs. Following ovulation the oocyte–cumulus complex facilitates pick-up by the oviduct and may contribute to the final maturation of the oocyte, as well as the capacitation of spermatozoa that must penetrate through the extracellular material formed by the cumulus cells. The majority of granulosa cells form the so-called mural or parietal granulosa cells lining the follicular cavity. Those mural cells adjacent to the follicular basement membrane are the first to differentiate steroidogenic responsiveness to LH based on the acquisition of LH binding sites (62,63), the expression of Δ^5-3β-hydroxysteroid dehydrogenase activity (64), and the level of cytochrome P-450 (65). In addition, mural granulosa cells at this stage lose the differentiation antigen that is uniformly present on granulosa cells of earlier follicular stages (66). Other *in vitro* evidence suggests that subpopulations of granulosa cells may exist with respect to differential sensitivity to FSH and vasoactive intestinal peptide (VIP) (67).

The theca cells appear to differentiate from mesenchymal cells in the ovarian stroma (68,69). Since the theca layer is not present in primary follicles but differentiates as follicles grow and mature, it is evident that theca cells arise continually throughout reproductive life; the mesenchymal progenitor cells are perhaps pluripotent stem cells that also contribute to cells of loose connective tissue. It has been suggested that in the immature mouse the theca layer might also be formed from certain intraovarian rete cells that are initially contiguous with cells forming the follicular granulosa cells but become separated from association with the oocyte as the follicle is enclosed (70,71). There is similar evidence in the rabbit (72). However, these cells in the mouse appear to give rise principally to the primary interstitial cells (70). Primary interstitial cells in fetal ovaries of the human appear to have distinct steroidogenic activities (see section on the prefollicular ovary, below).

Secondary interstitial cells found in the adult ovary are derived from theca cells of atretic follicles (73–77). Whereas the oocyte and surrounding granulosa cells of an atretic follicle degenerate and are eliminated from the ovary, the theca cells in the follicular envelope survive as small islands of steroidogenic cells in the ovarian stroma. On this basis, certain similarities in function of theca and secondary interstitial cells of adult ovaries might reasonably be expected. However, theca and interstitial cells probably do not have identical biosynthetic properties since the interstitial cells, in contrast with the theca cells, are less likely to be influenced by paracrine regulatory substances secreted by the membrana granulosa; instead, they may receive direct sympathetic innervation. Secondary interstitial cells also differ from theca cells in that their androgen biosynthetic activity not only persists throughout reproductive life (78–80) but continues in aged ovaries (81,82).

In later sections of this chapter we consider the evidence for steroidogenic functions of interstitial cells, theca cells, and granulosa cells in the early stages of ovarian organogenesis and at various stages of follicular development in the adult ovary. However, the characteristic steroidogenic functions of theca and secondary interstitial and granulosa cells in adult ovaries and mature follicles, typical of the follicular phase, are now described.

Pathways and Their Control by Gonadotropins (FSH and LH)

Theca and Interstitial Cells

The most abundant steroid products of mature theca cells of all species are C_{19}-compounds, including the 4-ene-3β-hydroxysteroids and 5α-reduced androgens, which are produced from the catabolism of cholesterol by pathways previously described. As discussed earlier, since the theca interna becomes highly vascularized as the follicle matures, it is reasonable that the internalization of blood-borne lipoprotein provides the major source of cholesterol for steroidogenesis by theca cells *in vivo*. Steroidogenesis in the absence of lipoprotein cholesterol *in vitro* is limited (83).

The preferred enzymatic route for the conversion of cholesterol to androgens in the theca of human (84) and bovine (85) ovary is via the 5-ene-3β-hydroxysteroid pathway. DHEA produced via this pathway is then metabolized to androstenedione. It is apparent that rat ovarian interstitial cell cultures (i.e., consisting of interstitial cells and follicular cell types) produce both 5-ene-3β-hydroxy and 4-en-3-oxo intermediates (86).

LH action via specific receptors present on the theca cells at all follicular stages (87–93), and consequent production of cAMP (81,94–96), provides the principal stimulus for these steroidogenic activities. Studies with cultured ovarian interstitial cells isolated from hypophysectomized rats indicate that the cells constitutively express Δ^5-3β-hydroxysteroid dehydrogenase and have functional LH receptors but are not steroidogenically active unless induced to differentiate with either LH or prostaglandin E_2 (PGE_2) (97). These results with ovarian interstitial cell cultures might reflect similar control mechanisms occurring in thecal tissue, which also responds to LH or PGE_2 with increased androgen secretion (96,98,99).

The steroidogenic action of LH on theca cells apparently increases the activities of 17α-hydroxylase:C-17,20-lyase in ovaries or follicles of rat (100,101,102) and hamster (103). These enzyme activities are rate-limiting and appear to be the site at which LH stimulates C_{19}-steroid production by theca cells, as follicles progress from small antral stages to early preovulatory follicles in the rat (102), and where ovarian androgen production is substantially restricted in late preovulatory follicles (104) (also see the section on preovulatory follicles, below). Recent studies have employed immunoblot analysis to measure the specific contents (i.e., amount of enzyme protein per microgram of tissue protein) of this and other steroidogenic enzymes and their electron donors in follicles dissected from bovine ovaries of mature animals (105). These studies have demonstrated that 17α-hydroxylase P-450 in follicles increased fivefold between medium-sized (9–11 mm) and large (14–18 mm) follicles, indicating that an increase in enzyme protein occurs in the follicular cells (granulosa and theca) as follicles mature. Significantly, this enzyme protein was undetectable in bovine corpora lutea throughout the luteal phase, consistent with the loss of the enzyme activity as follicles luteinize in response to the LH surge. (This aspect is discussed later with respect to late preovulatory follicles after the LH surge.) These changes showed specificity for the 17α-hydroxylase P-450 since its electron donor, NADPH–cytochrome P-450 reductase, has a similar specific content during follicle development and in corpora lutea.

Although progesterone is apparently not limiting as an intermediate for thecal androgen production in small antral follicles, progesterone accumulation in isolated small antral and preovulatory rat follicles is stimulated *in vitro* by hCG, indicating that activation of the LH receptor also stimulates a step in the conversion of cholesterol to progesterone (102). Further studies tended to rule out the possibility that this action was due to decreased progesterone metabolism. Isolated theca cells from small antral and preovulatory rat follicles also produced increased progesterone when stimulated with cAMP, this stimulation being much greater with theca from preovulatory follicles (102). Therefore, it is evident from these studies that progesterone production by theca cells is also hormonally regulated and varies with the stage of follicular development. This effect of LH is probably the result of increased activity of C_{27} side-chain cleavage and is consistent with increased pregnenolone production in LH-stimulated rat ovarian interstitial cell cultures (86). Ultrastructural immunocytochemical visualization of P-450_{SCC} in ovaries of immature rats indicates that this mitochondrial enzyme is initially found in only a few theca cells, but the number of theca cells containing this enzyme increases after pregnant mare serum gonadotropin (PMSG) treatment (30). Significantly, these studies showed a strong reaction for P-450_{SCC} in interstitial cells even before PMSG treatment, with no apparent change as a result of hormonal stimulation.

Androstenedione is the principal aromatizable C_{19}-steroid produced by isolated theca interna tissue or cells, with lesser amounts of testosterone occurring, as described in the rat (94), hamster (103,106), pig (107), sheep (194), cow (85,108,109), and human (110,111). The greater abundance of androstenedione than testosterone is due to a deficiency in 17β-hydroxysteroid dehydrogenase, a fact that has significance in the steroidogenic cooperation of theca and granulosa cells, as discussed later. Rat ovarian interstitial preparations in culture are also active in 5α-reduction of C_{19}-steroids; the major LH-stimulated product is androsterone (86), which may be produced by sequential action of 5α-reductase and 3α-hydroxysteroid dehydrogenase (Fig. 4). The next most abundant 5α-reduced metabolite is 5α-androstane-3α,17β-diol, which can be derived from testosterone according to the same reactions described above for androstenedione or, alternatively, might result from conversion of androsterone to 5α-androstane-3α,17β-diol in a reversible reaction catalyzed by the apparently weak thecal activity of 17β-hydroxysteroid dehydrogenase. It has been demonstrated that 3α-hydroxy-5α-pregnan-20-one is converted to 5α-androstane-3α,17β-diol by supernatants of ovarian homogenates from immature rats, suggesting that this pregnane may be an earlier intermediate in a pathway to the androstanediol (112). Activity of 5α-reductase in thecal tissue from hamster preovulatory follicles may not be regulated by LH (103) but is subject to LH control in thecal/interstitial cells in prepubertal rat ovaries (100,101). There is no change in thecal 5α-reductase activity in the adult rat during pregnancy as follicles develop from small antral to preovulatory stages (113). Activity of ovarian 5α-reductase, which is greatest before the onset of puberty (14,40,45), is greatly decreased in ovaries of adult rats (114–116) and in immature rats in which puberty has been advanced with PMSG (42). The physiological significance of 5α-reduced androgens in the immature rat is indicated by the effect of exogenous 5α-androstane-3β,17β-diol, but not its 3α-epimer, to advance the onset of puberty (117) and by there being sufficient concentrations of the 3β-epimer in blood to account for these changes at puberty (37). FSH has also been shown to induce an epimerization reaction in the immature rat ovary that converts 5α-androstane-3α,17β-diol to the biologically active 3β-epimer (118).

Alternate routes of progesterone catabolism, in addition to those involved in the production of androgens, also occur in theca cells. Transiently increased production of 17α-hydroxyprogesterone in the human at midcycle (119,120) may primarily arise in the theca cells before similar pathways are fully active in the granulosa cells. The corpus luteum becomes the principal source of this steroid in the luteal phase of the human (121). In rat interstitial cells, the principal C_{21} metabolite is 20α-dihydroprogesterone (86). The production of this metabolite is increased by LH treatment, but the amount produced is still less than that of intermediates and products of the 4-en-3-oxosteroid pathway.

Theca cells may also aromatize androgens and contribute directly to ovarian estrogen secretion in varying degrees depending on species and follicular stage, e.g., in human (122–124), monkey (125), mare (126,127), cow (85), hamster (106), sheep (128), and pig (107). However, results of most studies indicate that aromatase activity (i.e., conversion of C_{19}-steroids to estrogens) in the theca cells either is not significantly greater than that in the granulosa cells (e.g., as in pig and sheep) or is considerably less than in the granulosa cells. In studies with cultures of follicular tissue from immature pigs, theca initially has considerably less aromatase activity than granulosa cells expressed on a per follicle basis, but when follicular growth and maturation was induced with PMSG treatment, aromatase activity in theca cells increased substantially while that in granulosa cells declined slightly (107). Studies with sheep follicle cell types also indicate substantially increased estrogen production by theca cells as follicles mature (128). Therefore, in mature follicles of pig and sheep, both theca and granulosa cells appear to have similar abilities *in vitro* to produce estrogens, either from endogenous androgen (theca cells) or supplied substrate (granulosa cells).

Most studies with human theca cells in culture agree that the quantity of estrogen secretion is significant but small (129), regardless of whether the theca is obtained from small or large follicles or at various stages of the menstrual cycle (110). For the preovulatory human follicle it was estimated that 99.9% of the aromatase activity resides in the membrana granulosa (130,131), and there is an excellent positive correlation between granulosa aromatase activity and the concentration of estradiol in follicular fluid (130). These results strongly indicate that thecal cell production of estrogen in the human is relatively minor in comparison to the aromatizing capabilities of granulosa cells from large antral follicles. Results of other studies with human follicle cells in culture (111,124) are difficult to interpret in terms of relative theca and granulosa cell aromatase activities since data are often expressed as estradiol production per culture without corrections for cell number.

There is little direct information to distinguish the steroidogenic functions of secondary interstitial cells from those of the theca interna cells, and the biosynthetic pathways are generally assumed to be similar. However, as already noted, the immunocytochemical staining for $P\text{-}450_{SCC}$ in interstitial cells of immature rat ovary is greater than in theca cells; also, it does not depend on exogenous gonadotropin treatment (30). Whether this difference reflects similar differences in enzymic activity is not known. *In vitro* studies using dispersed ovarian preparations from hypophysectomized rats (designated as ovarian interstitial cells but containing all ovarian cell types) have investigated the regulation of the LH-responsive cell types (86,97). The biosynthetic activities of these mixed cell cultures are similar to those already described for theca cells. Specific isolation of secondary interstitial cells from rat ovarian stroma has not been feasible without significant contamination by theca and follicle cell types but is more readily accomplished in humans and in larger animals. Nevertheless, true interstitial cells (i.e., glandular cells) in the ovarian stroma of the human constitute only about 1% of the ovarian volume during the menstrual cycle, with this value increasing to 4–6% in late pregnancy (132). Human stromal cells obtained on cycle day 18 were incubated with [^{3}H]pregnenolone and [^{14}C]progesterone and were shown to use both 4-en-3-oxo and 5-ene-3β-hydroxy pathways, with the products being androstenedione (the major product), testosterone, progesterone, 17α-hydroxyprogesterone (133), and, under some circumstances, estrone and estradiol (134). Production of these steroids was increased by treatment with hCG. In other studies, cultures of human stromal cells synthesized, androstenedione, 17α-hydroxyprogesterone, progesterone, and estradiol but in lesser amounts than by theca cells (123,135).

Granulosa Cells

Whereas the steroidogenic pathways in the theca and interstitial cells function primarily in the *de novo* production of androgens, the pathways in the granulosa cells are organized principally for the metabolism of C_{19}-steroids (i.e., androgens) to estrogens and for the *de novo* synthesis of progesterone and its C_{21} metabolites. As will be discussed in following sections, cooperation of the theca and granulosa cell compartments appears to be crucial to the control by gonadotropins of follicular steroid hormone secretion in all species studied. This cooperation takes the form of exchange of steroid pathway intermediates, direct steroidal effects on enzyme activities, and paracrine regulation.

Evidence from both *in vivo* and *in vitro* studies indicates that the granulosa cells of large antral and preovulatory follicles are the principal, although not exclusive, site in all species of ovarian aromatase activity and estrogen biosynthesis. Regulation of androgen aromatization in the granulosa cells of all species studied appears to be by the action of FSH (136), which in rat granulosa cell cultures stimulates aromatase enzyme activity as measured in a cell-free assay (137) and requires RNA and protein synthesis for expression of this action (138). Recent studies with rat granulosa cells suggest that aromatase cytochrome P-450, as detected in radiolabeled immunoisolates, is induced by FSH or dibutyryl cAMP (139). In addition, FSH or dibutyryl cAMP has been reported to stimulate two to three times the amount of the NADPH–cytochrome P-450 reductase detected in cultured rat granulosa cells (in immunoisolates and by immunoblot analysis), but this component is apparently in excess of the specific aromatase cytochrome P-450 (140). In addition to this action of FSH to induce aromatase enzyme in granulosa cells, estrogen biosynthesis requires the cooperation of the theca cells in supplying the androgen substrates for the aromatization reaction. This important aspect is discussed in detail in a following section.

The production of progesterone and its metabolites (i.e., progestins) is one of the major biosynthetic activities of granulosa cells in large antral and preovulatory follicles. Progesterone biosynthesis occurs in granulosa cells initially in response to FSH stimulation, but this action is later augmented by LH after its receptors have differentiated. In culture, FSH stimulates progesterone biosynthesis in undifferentiated granulosa cells from immature rats (141–145) and in granulosa cells from various other species, including human (124,129,146), simian (147), porcine (24), and avian (148). A similar effect of FSH on progesterone production has also been shown for cumulus granulosa cells of rat (149). In contrast, LH alone does not stimulate progesterone biosynthesis in cultured granulosa cells from hypophysectomized, estrogen-treated rats but is an effective stimulus *in vitro* following either a 24-hr *in vivo* treatment with FSH to induce LH receptors (142) or after 2 days of FSH priming *in vitro* (150). Many studies in various species substantiate the stimulation of progesterone production by LH in mature granulosa cells from antral follicles. In all species studied the greatest stimulation of progesterone biosynthesis *in vivo* follows the LH surge, often after a transient decrease in production, as granulosa cells undergo differentiation (i.e., luteinization) to form granulosa–lutein cells.

The progesterone biosynthetic pathway (see Fig. 2 and the first three sections on biosynthetic pathways, above) in granulosa cells is typical of all steroidogenic cells, involving conversion of cholesterol to pregnenolone and then to progesterone. In antral and preovulatory follicular stages, intracellular cholesterol is probably almost entirely derived from *de novo* synthesis and perhaps to a small extent from endogenous lipid stores, since cholesterol associated with lipoproteins in blood (28,151) cannot penetrate the avascular granulosa cell layer. Only after ovulation is extracellular lipoprotein likely to be a major source of cholesterol as a precursor for biosynthesis in granulosa–lutein cells (23,152).

The apparent rate-limiting reaction for progesterone biosynthesis, regulated by FSH action on granulosa cells, is cholesterol side-chain cleavage (144,153,154). The effects of hormonal stimulation on this enzyme activity have been suggested to involve an increase in the association of cholesterol with the P-450_{SCC} via a low-molecular-weight activator peptide and to increase the supply of intramitochondrial cholesterol by a cytoskeleton-mediated process, as appears to be the situation in the adrenal cortex (32). There is similar evidence in the ovary for stimulatory effects of LH/hCG on cholesterol transport and activation of the cholesterol side-chain cleavage enzyme (155–157). In rat granulosa cells, FSH stimulates pregnenolone production in the presence of cyanoketone, which inhibits metabolism to progesterone; 25-hydroxycholesterol, which readily enters the mitochondria, further enhances this effect of FSH, suggesting that FSH may also increase cholesterol side-chain cleavage activity in this cell type (153). Concomitant increases in mitochondrial activity of side-chain cleavage enzyme in ovaries of rat (158) and pig (154) further suggest that synthesis of this enzyme may be increased. However, immunoblot analysis of C_{27} side-chain cleavage cytochrome P-450 and its electron donor, adrenodoxin, in dissected bovine follicles has not shown increases in specific contents of either of these enzyme proteins as follicles mature from medium to large sizes (105). These studies report that both P-450_{SCC} and adrenodoxin increase only in corpora lutea at the early-mid luteal phase, which suggests that induction at this stage is primarily the result of earlier LH stimulation.

Additional actions of LH, in luteal tissue of various species, include enhancement of cholesterol availability by (a) stimulating 3-hydroxy-3-methylglutaryl coenzyme A reductase, which is rate-limiting for cholesterol biosynthesis (159); (b) acutely stimulating cholesterol esterase, thereby increasing the availability of free cholesterol from intracellular stores of fatty acid esters (160–162); and (c) increasing the number of lipoprotein receptors (163), thereby enhancing uptake of cholesterol in the form of lipoprotein.

FSH (87), and subsequently LH (164–167), greatly stimulate rat granulosa cell activity of Δ^5-3β-hydroxysteroid dehydrogenase:$\Delta^{5\text{-}4}$-isomerase. It has been suggested that $\Delta^{5\text{-}4}$-isomerase activity may be present in excess in adrenal and testis tissue (168,169), but the issue of whether this enzyme activity and the Δ^5-3β-hydroxysteroid dehydrogenase are separate entities or a single enzyme remains unresolved. Following gonadotropin stimulation, activity of Δ^5-3β-hydroxysteroid dehydrogenase is apparently not limiting for progesterone synthesis in cultured granulosa cells from immature rats, which do not substantially accumulate pregnenolone during FSH-stimulated synthesis of progesterone and 20α-dihydroprogesterone (170). This may not be true in the pig, in which cultured granulosa cells accumulate greater quantities of pregnenolone than progesterone (171).

The metabolism of progesterone to 20α-dihydroprogesterone in granulosa cells (see section on 20-hydroxysteroid dehydrogenase, above) is influenced by FSH stimulation of the 20α-hydroxysteroid dehydrogenase enzyme, as demonstrated by *in vivo* experiments with hypophysectomized, estrogen-treated rats (172) and with cultured rat granulosa cells (173). In contrast, LH is apparently not required for maximal activity of this enzyme in ovaries of proestrous rats (174), and hCG is not an effective stimulus in FSH-primed rat granulosa cells in culture (164). However, various studies in the rat have reported inhibitory or stimulatory actions of LH/hCG on 20α-hydroxysteroid dehydrogenase, concomitant with luteotropic or luteolytic actions, respectively (46,175–177). The conversion of progesterone to 20α-dihydroprogesterone in the rat corpus luteum (178,179) is important in regulating progestational activity during pregnancy (180) and parturition (181,182). The same pathway to 20α-dihydroprogesterone occurs in mouse (183) and human (184); however, in bovine corpus luteum, the principal metabolite is 20β-dihydroprogesterone (184).

Other C_{21} metabolites of progesterone result from the sequential action of 5α-reductase and 3α-hydroxysteroid dehydrogenase, the products being 5α-pregnane-3,20-dione and 3α-hydroxy-5α-pregnan-20-one, respectively (Fig. 4). The extent of formation of these products depends on the 5α-reductase activity, which is greatest in immature rats (115,185). Similar sequential catabolism of 20α-dihydroprogesterone to 20α-hydroxy-5α-pregnan-3-one and then 5α-pregnane-3α,20α-diol is expected (Fig. 4); the latter metabolite has been found to be a significant product in long-term cultures of rat granulosa cells (186). A fully reversible conversion of 5α-pregnane-3,20-dione to 3β-hydroxy-5α-pregnan-20-one is also expected to be catalyzed by the 3β-hydroxysteroid dehydrogenase (see section on 5α-reduced pathways, above), but little is known about the regulation involved.

In contrast with theca cells, granulosa cells of all species studied, with the apparent exception of the bovine (85), do not have significant activities of C_{21} side-chain cleavage enzymes and synthesize little or no C_{19}-steroids from either pregnenolone or progesterone (85,94,99,187–192).

Granulosa cells possess considerable activity of the 17β-hydroxysteroid dehydrogenase enzyme (103,193–196), which acts on both C_{19}-steroids, androstenedione and testosterone, as well as aromatization products, estrone and estradiol (Fig. 2). Although androstenedione is the major ovarian androgen in most species, the 17β-hydroxysteroid dehydrogenase reaction favors the production of estradiol as the major ovarian estrogen. The presence of 5α-reductase and 3α-hydroxysteroid dehydrogenase in granulosa cells also permits theca-derived androgens to be converted to several ring A-reduced metabolites (Fig. 4) according to the same reactions occurring for progesterone metabolism described above. FSH does not influence the production of 5α-reduced metabolites of testosterone (i.e., androsterone and 5α-androstane-3α,17β-diol) in rat granulosa cell cultures (141). Furthermore, FSH was ineffective in maintaining elevated 5α-reductase activity in prepubertal rats after hypophysectomy (197).

From a physiological viewpoint, aromatization of theca-derived androgens is perhaps the most important pathway of androgen metabolism in the granulosa cell. This key concept of cooperation of the follicle cell types in the regulation of estrogen biosynthesis is considered next. Other important actions of theca-derived androgens on estrogen biosynthesis via paracrine mechanisms are considered later (see section on estrogens, below).

Cooperation of Theca and Granulosa Cells

The functional basis of the modern concept of cellular cooperation in follicular estrogen biosynthesis has already been described: Theca cells are stimulated by LH to produce aromatizable androgens, and granulosa cells respond to FSH with increased aromatase activity but without *de novo* production of C_{19}-steroid substrates. We will briefly discuss the historical development of the current "two-cell-type, two-gonadotropin" theory of steroidogenic regulation and then consider the direct *in vitro* experimental evidence in animals and humans that supports this concept and other aspects of cooperation in follicular steroid metabolism.

The early literature implicated the follicle in estrogen biosynthesis (198), with some authors favoring the theca interna cells as the principal site of synthesis (199–201) and others suggesting the follicular epithelium (i.e., membrana granulosa) as the primary source (202). The first substantial evidence of the cooperation of ovarian cell types in estrogen biosynthesis was provided by Falck in 1959 (203) in now-classic experiments in which ovarian cell types in the rat were transplanted either alone or in combination into the anterior eye chamber together with estrogen-sensitive vaginal epithelium as a biological indicator of estrogen production. These studies established that estrogen biosynthesis required the cooperation of granulosa or lutein cells with theca or interstitial cells. Falck mistakenly interpreted these findings as indicating a permissive influence of granulosa or lutein cells (perhaps mediated by progesterone) on estrogen secretion by theca or interstitial cells in the rat. Although this proposal was incorrect for the rat, where thecal biosynthesis does not contribute significantly to estrogen production, in at least certain species C_{21}-steroids from the granulosa cells may indeed be utilized by theca cells for androgen production, thereby contributing to estrogen production by both cell types.

A two-cell theory of the sort suggested by Falck was subsequently proposed for the mare (187), with the additional proposal that granulosa cells have only weak 17α-hydroxylase and little C-17,20-lyase activities. Further studies with isolated ovarian cell types in the pig demonstrated that granulosa cells converted pregnenolone to progestins, but not to androgens, while readily interconverting exogenous testosterone and androstenedione (i.e., by the 17β-hydroxysteroid dehydrogenase) and aromatizing these androgens (193). It was later proposed that C_{19}-steroid precursors in the pig are produced by the theca and are then transferred to the granulosa for conversion to testosterone (188). In this way, estrogen was presumed to be synthesized by granulosa as well as theca cells, although aromatase activity in pig theca was believed to be higher (193).

The next major step in the development of the modern concept of regulation of estrogen biosynthesis was the determination of the cellular sites of FSH and LH action. Much earlier work by Greep and coworkers (204) in hypophysectomized immature rats provided the first hints that FSH and LH act upon different cell types to promote estrogen formation. Subsequently, Hollander and Hollander (205) demonstrated that FSH action *in vivo* or *in vitro* stimulated [^{14}C]testosterone conversion to estradiol by canine ovarian slices. However, up until the 1970s, LH was still considered to be the key, if not the only, steroidogenic hormone in the follicle for a variety of reasons. The action of LH via cAMP was becoming established as an important control mechanism, LH was known to stimulate both androgen and estrogen production by luteal and stromal ovarian preparations (184), and it was later shown to stimulate acute estrogen production by the isolated rabbit follicle (206). Furthermore, use of relatively impure FSH cast doubts on the active hormone in earlier studies. The crucial role of FSH in controlling follicular estrogen biosynthesis in the rat was then established with the findings that explanted ovaries from hypophysectomized immature rats produced estrogen in response to FSH but not to LH and that they required the addition of testosterone as substrate (207). Similar findings with isolated rat granulosa cells in culture determined that FSH acted directly on the granulosa cells to stimulate aromatization (136), thereby extending earlier work demonstrating a similar action of FSH on testicular Sertoli cells (208).

The results of these *in vitro* studies led to the formulation of a modern two cell-type, two gonadotropin theory in which theca interna cells (and perhaps also interstitial cells) are stimulated by LH to produce androgens, which in turn traverse the follicular basement membrane to be utilized for estrogen biosynthesis in an FSH-stimulated reaction within the granulosa cells. Current evidence indicates that this concept is valid for antral and preovulatory follicles in the rat and most other species, despite additional and sometimes significant production of estrogens by theca cells in certain species. Evidence in various species of the exclusive localization of FSH binding sites on granulosa cells and of LH binding sites initially on theca/interstitial and only later on granulosa cells supports the two-cell-type, two-gonadotropin concept described above. The *in vitro* evidence directly supporting the concept of metabolic cooperation in estrogen biosynthesis by the two cell types is of three kinds. First, there is evidence that androgens produced in the theca layer exit from these cells in order to participate in estrogen biosynthesis, the inference being that extracellular androgens diffuse into the granulosa cell layer. Second, the evidence indicates that addition of aromatizable androgens to granulosa cells is essential for significant estrogen production, and addition of pregnenolone or other C_{21} precursors to thecal cells tends to increase androgen production. Third, recombination of isolated theca tissue and granulosa cells by coincubation demonstrates synergism in estrogen synthesis, provided that the two cell types either are stimulated with the appropriate gonadotropins *in vitro* or are derived from mature steroidogenically active follicles. This supporting evidence is discussed below.

First, *in vivo* evidence that FSH and LH act at separate sites and by separate mechanisms in stimulating estrogen secretion has been obtained in studies with hypophysectomized rats. Treatment of hypophysectomized rats with LH has been demonstrated to enhance ovarian androgen (testosterone and dihydrotestosterone) content; however, concomitant administration of FSH was required to elevate estradiol levels. Substitution of LH with aromatizable androgen (testosterone or androstenedione) led to similar increases in estradiol production, provided that the rats had also been treated with FSH (209). Thus, these findings are consistent with a stimulatory action of LH on production of androgens that were then used as substrate for conversion to estradiol in the presence of FSH, thus providing *in vivo* support for the two-cell, two-gonadotrophin mechanism for control of estrogen biosynthesis in the rat.

This cell-cooperation hypothesis requires that androgens of thecal origin must diffuse across the basement membrane separating the granulosa and thecal layers of the follicle in order for androgens to gain access to the aromatase enzyme in the granulosa cells. There is ample evidence that such diffusion does, in fact, occur. Concentrations of aromatizable androgens (i.e., androstenedione and testosterone) in follicular fluid are consistent with their serving as efficient substrates for aromatization by the granulosa cells. Furthermore, even higher concentrations of androgens might be achieved at the level of mural granulosa cells as the result of an androgen gradient, presumed to exist from the theca cells across the follicular basement membrane to the mural cells and finally to the follicular fluid. One study, using an experimental ovarian model in sheep, has provided indirect evidence that extracellular androgen produced in the theca layer must cross into the follicle to allow estrogen biosynthesis by the granulosa cells. In this study, ovaries of ewes were autotransplanted to the carotid–jugular circulation, and endogenous LH pulses were observed to result in episodic secretion of estradiol into the jugular vein (210). Following infusion into the ovarian artery of a high-titer antiserum against androgen, the normally episodic secretion of estradiol was inhibited, suggesting that passage of androgen across the follicular membrane was prevented by binding to antibodies. There is also indirect evidence in the pig that suggests thecal androgen transference to the granulosa cells (107).

Various studies in pig (107), sheep (128), and human (99,124,135,191,211) provide the evidence that granulosa cells must be supplied with an extracellular source of aromatizable androgen substrate in order to synthesize estrogens.

Evidence of substantial theca–granulosa cell synergism in estrogen production *in vitro* has been obtained in coculture studies with follicle cells of sheep (194), hamster (103), and human (122,124,135). Also, evidence of stroma–granulosa synergism in estrogen production in the human was found in one study (124) but not in another (135). Similar studies in sheep have shown that follicle wall preparations (theca and granulosa) were far more effective in the production of estrogen than either cell type alone (128). In the rat, evidence of exclusive production of androgens by theca cells (212) and of aromatization in granulosa cells (141), combined with information that preovulatory estrogen production by the follicle is regulated by LH-stimulated thecal androgen production (102), provides convincing support for the original concept.

Apart from estrogen biosynthesis, there are other forms of follicle cell cooperation in steroid production and metabolism. Theca–granulosa cell synergism has been found for the production of thecal androgen in the sheep (128) and human (124,135). Other studies in the mare (189,213), hamster (103), rat (214), and pig (215) provide evidence that C_{21}-steroid precursors, which may be produced in the granulosa layer, can be metabolized to androgens by the theca cells. In other studies in the rat, comparisons of production of immunoreactive androgen (perhaps DHT) by intact preovulatory follicles or isolated cell types suggest that coordinated activities of both granulosa and theca cells are required for this biosynthetic function (102). Furthermore, theca–granulosa (124,135), as well as stroma–granulosa (135), synergism is also involved in progesterone synthesis in the human.

Intraovarian Regulation by Follicular Steroids

Estrogens

Early experiments demonstrated that estrogens had a stimulatory effect on the ovary (216–223). In experiments in which estrogen was administered to hypophysectomized immature rats, ovarian weight was maintained and ovaries became more responsive to gonadotropic stimulation. Furthermore, the ovarian weight response to gonadotropins was inhibited by antiserum to estradiol (224). Treatment of hypophysectomized rats with gonadotropins increased the number of atretic follicles per ovary, and administration of estrogen partially reversed this effect (225).

Specific uptake and retention of [^{3}H]estradiol *in vivo* by ovaries of immature rats (226,227), incorporation of estradiol into granulosa cells (228), and binding of estradiol to nuclear fractions of rat granulosa (229) and luteal cells (230) indicate the presence of estrogen binding sites in the ovary. Saidudduin and Zassenhaus (231) have characterized estrogen binding components from ovaries of immature rats. Their results suggested that ovarian estrogen binding sites are similar to specific, high-affinity estrogen receptors in uterine tissue.

There is evidence suggesting that estrogen acts within the ovary to inhibit androgen production, the estrogen presumably originating from granulosa cells and androgen from theca. Treatment of intact immature rats with estradiol suppressed ovarian testosterone and 5α-dihydrotestosterone production. Concomitant administration of gonadotropins failed to overcome the inhibition by estrogen, indicating that the effect was not mediated by decreased circulating gonadotropin (232). To provide further evidence for a direct intraovarian action of estrogen, Silastic implants of estradiol were embedded under the ovarian bursa unilaterally. Under these conditions, LH-stimulated androgen content of the ipsilateral ovary was considerably lower than that of the contralateral ovary (232). An inhibitory effect of estradiol on LH-induced androgen content of ovaries from immature hypophysectomized rats was reported as further evidence that a pituitary factor was not involved (232).

Results of *in vitro* experiments have demonstrated similar effects of estrogen on ovarian androgen synthesis. Whole ovaries from estrogen-treated immature, intact, or hypophysectomized rats responded to LH-stimulation *in vitro* with decreased androgen production when compared to that of ovaries obtained from rats that were not treated with estrogen. Dibutyryl cAMP did not increase testosterone production by cultured ovaries of estrogen-pretreated rats (233). Estradiol treatment of immature rats *in vivo* also suppressed androgen secretion by isolated thecal tissue *in vitro* (234). In culture experiments with isolated porcine thecal tissue (234) or dispersed theca cell preparations (235), addition of estrogens directly to the culture medium inhibited LH-stimulated androgen production in a dose-dependent manner, establishing that the inhibitory action of estrogens is directly on theca cells.

All indications are that estrogen inhibits ovarian androgen synthesis at a site distal to cAMP production, probably at an enzymatic step(s) in the steroidogenic pathway between androgens and their C_{21} precursors. In accordance with this hypothesis, estrogen pretreatment of ovaries from intact immature rats *in vivo* has been shown to inhibit conversion of radioactively labeled progesterone to androgens (testosterone, androstenedione, and androsterone) *in vitro*. On the other hand, incorporation into 3α-hydroxy-5α-pregnan-20-one is enhanced, suggesting that estrogen may act by inhibiting the 17α-hydroxylase:C-17,20-lyase enzyme system or by diverting C_{21} substrates into a pathway resulting in the formation of 5α-reduced pregnane compounds (233). In another study, treatment of immature rats with estradiol suppressed the stimulation by hCG of androstenedione, testosterone, 17α-hydroxyprogesterone, and 17α-hydroxypregnenolone production by dispersed ovarian cells in culture. Pregnenolone production was unchanged, while progesterone production was markedly enhanced. Estradiol had no effect on hCG binding capacity, hCG-stimulated cAMP synthesis, or the viability of ovarian steroidogenic cells. It was concluded that exogenous estradiol blocked ovarian androgen formation by reducing the activity of the 17α-hydroxylase enzyme (236). Further *in vitro* evidence with rat ovarian interstitial cell cultures indicates that estradiol directly causes rapid inhibition of 17α-hydroxylase and C-17,20-lyase enzyme activities (237).

There is evidence that estrogens are capable of regulating metabolism of androgens by a direct action on 5α-reductase. Eckstein and Nimrod (238) have shown an inhibitory effect of estradiol on 5α-reductase activity in microsomal preparations from immature rat ovaries. Since the minimal effective concentration of estradiol required to inhibit enzyme activity was in the range measurable in follicular fluid, the authors suggested that estradiol may be physiologically significant in the regulation of androgen metabolism.

Administration of LH to intact immature rats has been shown to affect ovarian progesterone metabolism in a manner identical to that of estrogen. Measured *in vitro,* ovarian androgen production was reduced and 3α-hydroxy-5α-pregnan-20-one secretion stimulated (233). Exposure of ovaries isolated from prepubertal rats to LH alters progesterone metabolism, favoring formation of 5α-reduced pregnane compounds while decreasing androgen and 5α-reduced androgen biosynthesis (239). In cultured preovulatory follicles from PMSG-treated immature rats, LH inhibited C-17,20-lyase activity. Addition of inhibitors of steroid synthesis prevented the inhibitory action of LH on the conversion of 17α-hydroxyprogesterone to androgens but did not affect basal lyase activity. These experiments suggested that the inhibitory action of LH on androgen synthesis may be mediated by the action of another ovarian steroid. That this steroid is estrogen is supported by experiments showing that the aromatase inhibitor, 4-acetoxy-androstane-3,17-dione, blocks the negative effect of LH on androgen synthesis by rat preovulatory follicles *in vitro* (240).

After the ovulatory surge of LH, androgen levels in ovarian tissue, follicular fluid, and ovarian venous blood and serum initially rise and then fall precipitously several hours later (241–243). This apparent inhibitory effect of LH on androgen production raises the possibility that this inhibition represents a physiological role of estrogens in the intrafollicular control of androgen biosynthesis. In support of this possibility, Smith et al. (244) and Kalra and Kalra (245) have measured serum hormone concentrations during the rat estrous cycle and have shown that, shortly after the LH surge on the day of proestrus, estradiol peaks and then rapidly declines. That the rise is dependent on the LH surge has been demonstrated in proestrous hamsters by blocking LH secretion with injections of phenobarbital (246). It may be that the surge of LH initially stimulates theca cells to produce androgens, which are aromatized to estrogens by granulosa cells. The estrogens then inhibit the thecal 17α-hydroxylase:C-17,20-lyase enzyme system, thereby limiting further synthesis of androgens and their subsequent use as substrates for aromatization. The ability of low doses of estradiol to enhance progesterone production by isolated bovine theca cells (247) may be a reflection of precursor accumulation following the inhibitory action of estrogens. This action may contribute to the transition of the follicle from primarily an estrogen-secreting to a progesterone-secreting structure, initiated by the LH surge. The role of estrogens in regulation of the corpus luteum is beyond the scope of this chapter and will be discussed elsewhere in the volume.

Another intrafollicular regulatory action of estrogens that has been clearly established is their ability to enhance ovarian estrogen production through direct actions on granulosa cells. Clomiphene citrate, a weak estrogen, increased estradiol and estrone synthesis from radiolabeled androstenedione by superfused canine ovaries *in vivo* (248). Clomiphene citrate (249), estradiol, estrone, hexestrol, moxestrol, ethinyl estradiol, chlorotrianisene, mestranol (250), and triphenylethylene antiestrogens (251) have also been reported to have similar effects on FSH-induced estrogen synthesis by cultured granulosa cells isolated from ovaries of immature hypophysectomized, DES-primed rats. FSH-induced aromatase activity in rat granulosa cells was enhanced by *in vitro* addition of DES (252). Good correlation was found between receptor binding affinity and biological potency of both natural and synthetic estrogens or antiestrogens, and the stimulatory effect could not be accounted for by increased granulosa cell viability or protein mass (250).

In support of the hypothesis that estrogens are physiological regulators of granulosa cell aromatase activity, the minimal effective dose of estradiol required to elicit a response (3.7×10^{-10} M) is well within the range of estradiol in antral fluid of preovulatory follicles (250). Thus, estrogens may function within the ovary or in individual follicles as end-product amplifiers to enhance FSH-induced aromatase.

Estrogens have been shown to decrease progesterone secretion by porcine (253–256), bovine (247), rat (257), and human (258,259) granulosa cells and by large follicles from bovine ovaries (260). The inhibitory action of estrogens on porcine granulosa cells was both time-and dose-dependent and was demonstrable in short-term, but not long-term, cultures at estradiol concentrations similar to those found *in vivo* (261). Estrogen-inhibition of progesterone production was not dependent on cell density in culture or due to a cytotoxic effect, degree of follicular maturation, or accelerated metabolism of 20α-dihydroprogesterone. Instead, the action of estrogen appeared to limit the conversion of pregnenolone to progesterone, resulting in enhanced pregnenolone accumulation in culture. Increased pregnenolone production in the presence of estrogen was also the result of enhanced cholesterol side-chain cleavage activity (154,261) and mitochondrial content of P-450 (154).

The inhibitory action of estrogen on progesterone production has been corroborated *in vivo*. Administration of estradiol for 3 days decreased LH-induced ovarian progesterone content in hypophysectomized immature rats but not in intact animals. Also, in ovaries of estradiol-treated hypophysectomized rats, dibutyryl cAMP, but not LH, restored *in vitro* progesterone production to values comparable to those of ovaries from control animals. This result suggests that estrogen inhibits progesterone synthesis by acting at a step early in the stimulative cascade, possibly prior to cAMP generation (262).

There are also reports of stimulatory effects of estrogen on progesterone secretion in porcine (24,263) and rat (257,264,265) granulosa cells. Unlike the inhibitory action of estrogen, the stimulatory effect on porcine granulosa cells in culture was only demonstrable in longer-term incubations and was found to be dependent on the density of granulosa cells in culture and the maturational status of the follicle from which cells were isolated (261). Granulosa cells from small, but not larger, follicles responded to estrogen with increased progesterone secretion, an effect that was found to be due to increased activity of Δ^5-3β-hydroxysteroid dehydrogenase:Δ^{5-4}-isomerase. In addition, with estrogen treatment, pregnenolone accumulation was increased, as were cholesterol side-chain cleavage activity and hydrolysis of endogenous cholesterol esters.

Catechol estrogens, which may be synthesized within the follicle (49), have also been shown to stimulate steroidogenesis in rat granulosa cells *in vitro* (266) and corpora lutea (267).

Androgens

With the establishment of the obligatory role of androgens as substrates for estrogen biosynthesis, other possible roles of androgens in follicular function at first received little attention or were dismissed. The antiandrogen, hydroxyflutamide had little or no effect on FSH-induction of enzyme activity or LH receptors in diethylstilbestrol (DES)-primed, hypophysectomized immature rats, suggesting that androgens are not essential for FSH to initiate development of antral follicles (268). In support of this hypothesis, Neumann et al. (269) demonstrated that cyproterone acetate, another antiandrogen, did not disrupt estrous cycles or interfere with ovulation in adult rats. In addition, Lyon and Glenister (270) have reported that Tfm/O mice, a strain in which females carry a gene conferring androgen resistance, have normal reproductive cycles; follicular maturation, conception, and pregnancy occur.

More recently, however, evidence of several sorts has appeared providing convincing evidence of other regulatory functions of androgens in the follicle. Specific androgen binding sites have been identified in ovaries from estrogen-primed, hypophysectomized immature rats (271) and later localized to the granulosa cell compartment (272). Similar androgen-binding proteins are found in sheep granulosa cells (273) and human ovarian cytosol (274).

In healthy, rather than atretic, follicles there is an inverse relationship between intrafollicular concentrations of androgens and estrogens. High ratios of androgens to estrogens in follicular fluid have been associated with nonovular and atretic follicles (229,275,276). However, from these data it is difficult to determine whether the predominance of androgen over estrogen is the cause of atresia or merely a result of the process. Both androgens (221,277) and hCG (278), which stimulate ovarian androgen synthesis, have been shown to promote atresia in rats. Coadministration of antiandrogens or antiserum raised against androgen (278) alleviated this effect of hCG. Further, treatment of immature, hypophysectomized, PMSG-treated rats with DHT induced atresia (279). This latter effect could be at least partially overcome by estradiol. Recently, Opavsky and Armstrong (280) showed an inhibitory effect of LH on the superovulatory response of immature rats to FSH. Although there is considerable circumstantial evidence to implicate androgens in the process of follicular atresia, the mechanisms of this process and the specific role of androgens in controlling the process are poorly understood.

In view of the rather substantial evidence in favoring a negative role for androgens in follicular maturation, it is perhaps surprising to find that androgens have positive effects on follicular growth. Ovarian degeneration occurred in androgen-resistant Tfm/O mice (281), and an antiandrogen accelerated atresia in preovulatory rat follicles (282). Somewhat similarly, treatment of diestrous rats with flutamide resulted in decreased growth and maturation of ovarian follicles (283). Also, an inhibitory action of androgen antisera on hCG-induced ovulation has been reported in hypophysectomized rats (284).

In trying to reconcile the apparent discrepancies between androgen effects within the ovarian follicles, it is worth noting that the antagonistic action of androgen on follicular events, as has been implicated in atresia, is believed to affect only those follicles at the preantral and early antral stages of development. The facilitory effect of androgen may be reserved for those large follicles that have already entered the final stages of development (285).

In culture, androgens have been shown to stimulate progesterone biosynthesis by intact follicles dissected from ovaries of cycling ewes (286) and cows (260) and by granulosa cells isolated from pig (255,256), rat (257,287) and mouse (288) ovaries. In addition, administration of androgens to intact immature rats increased subsequent progesterone accumulation by their isolated ovarian cells *in vitro* (289). Since both aromatizable and nonaromatizable androgens were effective, the response appears to be androgenic rather than dependent on aromatization of androgens to estrogens. This hypothesis is supported by data for the pig, in which implants of antiandrogens (flutamide or hydroxyflutamide) placed in the ovarian interstitium decreased progesterone secretion by isolated granulosa cells *in vitro* (290). Hydroxyflutamide and cyproterone acetate suppressed the stimulatory effect of testosterone on progesterone production by rat granulosa cell incubations (257).

Androgens, in addition to having their own stimulatory effects, enhance FSH-stimulated progestin synthesis (143–145,291). This action was blocked by hydroxyflutamide (292), and the potency of various androgens appeared to be correlated with the extent to which they were converted to testosterone or DHT (195).

Depending on the animal model used, androgens have been shown to act at both pre- and post-cAMP sites. Using granulosa cells isolated from ovaries of immature hypophysectomized, estrogen-treated rats, androstenedione enhanced stimulation of progestin production by the cAMP analog dibutyryl cAMP but had no effect on [^{125}I]FSH binding to the cells, FSH-stimulated cAMP production, or conversion of cAMP to AMP by the phosphodiesterase enzyme (144). On the other hand, in granulosa cells isolated from ovaries of intact immature rats, androgens enhance FSH-responsiveness, as measured by the FSH stimulation of cAMP production (292–294) and [^{125}I]FSH binding (294,295), and suppress cAMP metabolism (292).

Increased C_{21}-steroid production in the presence of androgen is not a reflection of decreased catabolism by 5α-reductase (144), although androgens have been reported to regulate catabolism of progesterone (296,297) through inhibition of 20α-hydroxysteroid dehydrogenase (298). Androgens alone or in combination with FSH have no effect on levels of free or esterified cholesterol in cultured rat granulosa cells (299). However, in these cells, androgen and FSH act synergistically to enhance lipoprotein utilization (300). Both FSH and testosterone independently enhance conversion of cholesterol to pregnenolone, indicating a stimulatory action on cholesterol side-chain cleavage. Combined treatment results in synergism (153,291,299). Transport of cholesterol into mitochondria is unaffected by FSH or androgen (299). Effects of androgens on 3β-hydroxysteroid dehydrogenase are equivocal. Some data suggest that androgens act synergistically with FSH to increase conversion of pregnenolone to progesterone (291), while other data indicate that androgens are ineffective at this site (141).

In contrast to the work using rat tissue, aromatizable androgens have a negative influence on progesterone production by human granulosa cells (124) and on FSH-stimulated progesterone accumulation by granulosa cells isolated from porcine ovaries (171,301). Although estradiol had a similar inhibitory action and nonaromatizable androgens were ineffective, the effect of aromatizable androgens could not be accounted for by conversion to estrogens since 4-acetoxy-4-androstene-3,17-dione, an inhibitor of aromatase, failed to prevent the testosterone-induced decrease in progesterone production (301).

Similar to the action of FSH, dibutyryl cAMP stimulated progesterone production by porcine granulosa cells. Addition of testosterone to cultures suppressed the stimulatory effect of dibutyryl cAMP, indicating that testosterone acts at a site distal to cAMP generation (171). Further studies revealed that androgens had no effect on progesterone metabolism (301); however, they did enhance pregnenolone synthesis in FSH-treated granulosa cell cultures (171). Thus, decreased progesterone production in the presence of androgen appears to be due to restricted conversion of pregnenolone to progesterone through inhibition of Δ^5-3β-hydroxysteroid dehydrogenase:$\Delta^{5\text{-}4}$-isomerase activity. A direct inhibitory action of testosterone on this enzyme has recently been demonstrated (302).

Very little work has been done to investigate intraovarian effects of androgens on thecal steroidogenesis. Androgen has been shown to enhance progesterone secretion by human thecal tissue in culture. The effect on granulosa cell progesterone synthesis was negative, and in combined incubations of theca or stroma plus granulosa cells, no effect of androgen could be discerned (124).

As discussed above, FSH has a regulatory role in ovarian estrogen secretion through induction of aromatase activity in rat granulosa cells. Studies using cultured rat granulosa cells from intact immature rats have demonstrated that, in addition to acting as substrates for FSH-stimulated aromatase, androgens also enhance FSH-induction of enzyme activity (303). Both aromatizable and nonaromatizable androgens were effective, although nonaromatizable androgens (5α-dihydrotestosterone and androsterone) were only 50% as potent as aromatizable androgens (testosterone and androstenedione). Thus, it is clear that this action of androgens is not dependent on their conversion to estrogens. This contention is supported by experiments showing that androgen enhancement of FSH-induced aromatase activity is suppressed by hydroxyflutamide (an androgen receptor blocker) (304,305) and is not affected by 4-acetoxy-4-androstene-3,17-dione (an inhibitor of aromatase) (252) or nafoxidine (an estrogen receptor blocker) (252).

There is evidence to suggest that, in the intact immature rat model, androgens influence granulosa cell aromatase activity by action at a site before cAMP production. Although testosterone enhances FSH-induced aromatase activity, it has no effect on cAMP-induced estrogen synthesis. Androgens enhance the responsiveness of cultured granulosa cells to FSH in the production of cAMP, as well as in stimulating cellular [^{125}I]FSH binding (294).

Aromatization of testosterone to estradiol by granulosa cells, isolated from the largest follicles in ovaries of rats showing diestrous II and proestrous vaginal smears, has been shown to be competitively inhibited by 5α-reduced androgens (306). The same phenomenon was described using human follicles excised at all stages of maturity (307). Apart from alterations in aromatase enzyme activity itself, follicular estrogen biosynthesis may be influenced by the amount of C_{19} substrate available and variation in the ratio of aromatizable to nonaromatizable androgens as the result of changes in 5α-reductase activity. Rat (40) and human (110,308) ovaries have been shown to convert aromatizable androgens actively to 5α-reduced androgens. Since high concentrations of estrogen in follicular fluid have been associated with healthy antral follicles and low estrogen with apparently degenerating follicles (275), alterations in the capacity of granulosa cells to convert androgens to estrogens may be a physiologically important mechanism for regulating concentrations of intrafollicular steroid hormones and development of individual follicles.

Siiteri and Thompson (309) have reported a 2.5-fold increase in 5α-reductase activity and a 5-fold decrease in aromatase activity within a few hours of exposure of ovaries of PMSG-treated rats to hCG. Katz and Armstrong (310) observed a similar decline in aromatase activity following LH treatment. The increased activity of 5α-reductase could contribute to the decreased estradiol secretion, which occurs dramatically following the LH surge, in two ways: (a) by decreasing the intrafollicular levels of aromatizable androgens through increased 5α-reductase activity and (b) by increasing intrafollicular levels of 5α-reduced androgens, which serve as competitive inhibitors of the aromatase enzyme system.

Progestins

It is uncertain whether progestins have any direct role in the intraovarian regulation of ovarian function, and reports are often contradictory. Some investigators have found that administration of exogenous progesterone to estrogen-primed, hypophysectomized immature rats had no effect on ovarian morphology (229,311,312), while others have presented evidence that progesterone has an inhibitory effect on follicular development when given to intact animals (313–316). That the effect of progesterone in these latter experiments might be mediated indirectly by depression of pituitary secretion of gonadotropins, rather than direct inhibition at the follicular level, is suggested by the observation that retardation of follicular growth by progesterone occurs only when plasma concentrations of both FSH and LH are significantly reduced (316). Goodman and Hodgen (317) attempted to avoid this problem by placing progesterone directly in the monkey ovary and suggested that their results supported a direct inhibitory action of progesterone on follicular development.

In prepubertal rats, progesterone implants decrease serum LH concentrations and reduce estradiol accumulation by the isolated follicles but, surprisingly, facilitate the stimulatory effects of low-dose hCG treatment on the growth of small antral follicles and on estrogen synthesis (318). It was suggested that progesterone may facilitate LH action under physiological circumstances when basal LH is low. On the other hand, even in the presence of elevated serum progesterone, preovulatory follicular maturation at the end of pregnancy (i.e., follicles functionally indistinguishable from those at proestrus) is supported by small sustained increases in serum LH, suggesting that progesterone may have no direct inhibitory effect on follicle cell maturation (319).

In support of a direct action of progesterone on ovarian regulation, specific progesterone receptors have been identified in rat ovary (320,321) and subsequently in rat granulosa cells (322,323). Similarly, ovarian progestin binding sites have been reported in rabbit (324), guinea pig (325), cow (326), and human (274,327).

Progesterone has been shown to enhance the ability of cultured rat granulosa cells to respond to FSH in the production of cAMP (293). In another study, synthetic progestin (R5020) increased FSH-stimulation of progesterone and 20α-dihydroprogesterone synthesis in granulosa cells isolated from immature hypophysectomized, estrogen-treated rats. Similarly, R5020 enhanced LH-stimulated progestin production by cells that had previously been primed with FSH to induce LH-receptor formation. Furthermore, in the presence of cyanoketone, an inhibitor of Δ^5-3β-hydroxysteroid dehydrogenase, progesterone augmented the ability of FSH to stimulate pregnenolone synthesis (328). The major criticism of this latter work is that the concentration (1×10^{-6} M) of synthetic progestin required to elicit a response is at the extreme upper limit of physiological progestin concentrations. The possibility that the action of progestin was mediated by nonspecific binding to androgen receptors was considered; however, the apparent autoregulatory actions of progestins were not altered by treatment with antiandrogens, indicating that the effect was not due to binding of progestin to androgen receptors (329).

The effects of several progestins on FSH-stimulated estrogen production by cultured rat granulosa cells isolated from ovaries of immature hypophysectomized, DES-treated rats have been examined (330). FSH-enhanced estrogen secretion was reduced following treatment with progesterone, 20α-dihydroprogesterone, or R5020, a potent synthetic progestin. A study of the relative potencies of the progestins revealed that R5020 was the most effective compound, followed by progesterone and 20α-dihydroprogesterone. This pattern was found to reflect the relative abilities of the progestins to bind to ovarian progestin receptors. Later experiments investigated the mechanism by which R5020 inhibits FSH-induction of aromatase activity. It was concluded that the synthetic progestin acts at a site distal to cAMP production and that it is not a competitive inhibitor of aromatase (331).

In another study of the effect of progesterone on FSH-stimulated estradiol synthesis by cultured rat granulosa cells, it was questioned whether progesterone has the same effect on aromatase activity once activity has been induced *in vivo* (332). In granulosa cells isolated on the morning of proestrus from follicles of immature rats previously treated with PMSG (4 IU), progesterone had a slight suppressive effect on estradiol synthesis. However, it was evident that once aromatizing activity had been induced estradiol synthesis was much less sensitive to inhibition by progesterone.

Likewise, an inhibitory effect of progesterone on estrogen secretion has been demonstrated *in vivo* (246). Progesterone administered to hamsters on the morning of the day of proestrus resulted in a fall in serum estradiol concentration without a concomitant change in blood levels of gonadotropins. The fact that concomitant administration of testosterone did not reverse the effect of progesterone indicated that progesterone acted at the level of the aromatase enzyme system. This study led the authors to speculate that the inhibitory effect of progesterone is one factor in the sharp decline in the serum concentration of estrogen that occurs after the LH surge in normally cycling hamsters (333).

Regulation of androgen production in the ovary by progestins has not been reported; however, both progesterone (334) and 5α-pregnane-3,20-dione (335) are effective inhibitors of the C-17,20-lyase, indicating their potential in intraovarian regulation of androgen biosynthesis.

Other Regulatory Factors and Hormones

Prolactin

Prolactin has long been known as a "luteotrophic" hormone, particularly in rodents but also in several other species. As such, it is involved in initiating luteinization of granulosa cells, in maintaining their level of progesterone synthesis as luteal cells, and in inhibiting the activity of the progesterone catabolizing enzyme, 20α-hydroxysteroid dehydrogenase, the latter particularly in rodents (336). The appearance of specific prolactin receptors in granulosa cells late in follicular development and their induction by FSH in culture (249) indicate the likelihood that prolactin may exert a physiological action on granulosa cells at the stage of terminal differentiation, when they are transformed into luteal cells. In support of this, prolactin has been demonstrated to enhance progesterone production in cultured granulosa cells obtained from preovulatory rat follicles (337) and porcine follicles (338). Striking morphological changes, characteristic of luteinization, were also induced by prolactin in cultured rat granulosa cells (337).

Stimulatory effects of prolactin on steroidogenesis in prepubertal (i.e., nonluteinized) ovaries have also been reported. Thus, prolactin injections (339) or hyperprolactinemia induced by *in vivo* administration of dopaminergic receptor blockers (339,340) have been found to induce precocious puberty, as well as to increase ovarian responsiveness to LH in immature rats. The latter effect appeared to be mediated, in part, by an increase in ovarian LH receptors (339). There is also evidence for a role of prolactin in induction and maintenance of LH receptors on luteal cells at late gestational stages in the rat (341).

In contrast to the stimulatory action of prolactin on progesterone secretion by granulosa cells at a late stage of differentiation, progesterone production by granulosa cells from small immature porcine follicles was markedly inhibited by physiological concentrations of prolactin (338). Exposure of the latter granulosa cells to estradiol reversed this inhibitory effect (342).

Another inhibitory effect of prolactin, on estrogen secretion, was reported for cultured rat granulosa cells obtained from follicles at both preantral and preovulatory stages (343,344). Decreased estrogen secretion *in vitro* appears to be due, at least in part, to an inhibitory action of prolactin on FSH induction of aromatase activity (345,346). The site of this action of prolactin appears to be distal to adenylate cyclase, as prolactin also inhibited the stimulatory action of dibutyryl cAMP. The inhibitory effect of prolactin on rat follicle aromatase activity has also been demonstrated by *in vivo* exposure of intact rats to the hormone (347). In addition, prolactin has been reported to suppress basal and gonadotropin-stimulated estradiol secretion by human ovaries perfused *in vitro* (348).

Evidence for an inhibitory influence of prolactin on androgen secretion, presumably by action on the theca and/or interstitial cells, of rat ovaries has also been reported. Levels of androstenedione in preovulatory follicles of adult rats were significantly decreased by prolactin (347), whereas hypoprolactinemia, induced *in vivo* by bromoergocryptine, was accompanied by markedly increased secretion of 5α-androstane-3α,17β-diol, the major androgen secreted by the prepubertal rat ovary in response to hCG stimulation (349). Addition of prolactin to cultured rat theca–interstitial cell preparations at concentrations within the physiological range for the female rat, and consistent with the binding affinity observed for the specific binding sites (receptors) that have been found on rat theca–interstitial cells, caused a dose-dependent inhibition of LH-stimulated androgen formation (androsterone, 5α-androstandiol) (350). As with granulosa cells, the inhibitory action of prolactin on theca–interstitial cells appears to be exerted at a step after adenylate cyclase, since the stimulatory action of 8-bromo-cAMP, as well as of other activators of adenylate cyclase (PGE_2, choleratoxin), was similarly inhibited by prolactin.

Gonadotropin-releasing Hormone-like Peptides

Evidence that systemic administration of gonadotropin-releasing hormone (GnRH) or its agonists paradoxically inhibit reproductive functions (351) was first attributed exclusively to indirect effects on the hypothalamic–pituitary–gonadal axis. There is indeed evidence showing that continuous or intermittent administration of GnRH or its agonists can cause the pituitary to become refractory to the releasing hormone (352–355) and, through the release of gonadotropins, can induce ovarian receptor loss and desensitization to these hormones (356–359). However, numerous other studies, particularly in the rat, have since established that GnRH binding sites are present in various extrapituitary tissues, including the gonads, and that direct actions of GnRH on somatic cells of ovary and testis occur

(329,360). Furthermore, products with biological activities similar to those of hypothalamic GnRH have been reported in the ovary, testis, placenta, pancreas, other central nervous system (CNS) structures, and in some tumor types (360). We will review only those studies pertinent to possible intraovarian actions of GnRH-like peptides.

Ovarian cell types in the rat that have been demonstrated to have specific high-affinity binding sites for GnRH are granulosa (361,362), luteal (362,363), and theca (364) cells, at all stages of differentiation (364). These binding sites, presumed to be receptors by virtue of the various biological effects reported, are localized in the plasma membrane (365). In granulosa cells, GnRH receptors have been shown to be regulated by GnRH itself (inhibitory and stimulatory effects) and maintained by FSH (362,366). Two binding components have been identified in granulosa cells, of which one is similar to the pituitary GnRH receptor (367,368). Only binding sites of low affinity (369,370) or moderate affinity (371) have been found in human corpus luteum (369,370), consistent with the prolonged treatment required to observe inhibitory effects on progesterone biosynthesis by human granulosa cells *in vitro* (372). One study reports the absence of inhibitory effects of GnRH on progesterone biosynthesis by human granulosa cells (373). Biological effects of GnRH on ovarian cells in rabbit (374), pig (375), and chicken (376,377) also suggest the presence of GnRH-sensitive mechanisms. Lack of ovarian inhibition by GnRH in mice (378) and rhesus monkeys (379) and the absence of specific binding sites in ovine, bovine, and porcine ovaries (380) and in monkey corpora lutea (381) suggest that these species may not share the same GnRH sensitivity found in the rat.

The first evidence for a direct extrapituitary effect of a GnRH agonist on the rat ovary was provided by the study of Rippel and Johnson (382), which showed inhibition of the hCG-stimulated ovarian and uterine weight gains in immature hypophysectomized animals. These findings were substantiated by extrapituitary inhibitory effects of GnRH and its agonists on FSH-stimulated ovarian weight gain and aromatase activity in immature hypophysectomized, estrogen-treated rats and on FSH-stimulated estrogen and progesterone production in cultured rat granulosa cells (383,384). GnRH inhibition of ^3H_2O release from [1β-^{3}H]testosterone, as a measure of aromatase activity, has also been demonstrated in cells from immature estrogen-primed rats (385,386). Other studies in hypophysectomized, PMSG-treated female rats demonstrated that a potent GnRH agonist also inhibited follicular maturation and steroidogenesis (387).

The effect of GnRH in decreasing FSH-stimulated progesterone production appears to be due to actions at several sites, causing inhibition of pregnenolone production (presumed to be an effect on the cholesterol side-chain cleavage enzyme), inhibition of Δ^5-3β-hydroxysteroid dehydrogenase activity (153,386,388), and stimulation of 20α-hydroxysteroid dehydrogenase activity (389), thereby reducing progesterone production and increasing its conversion to 20α-dihydroprogesterone. Inhibitory influences of GnRH on LH/hCG-stimulated estrogen and progesterone production were also demonstrated in cultured rat granulosa cells previously primed with FSH (164,390). Differences in the mechanisms of inhibition of progesterone production were seen with different stimulatory agents. Thus, the inhibitory action on LH/hCG-stimulated progesterone production appeared to involve decreased pregnenolone production (164), whereas the inhibition of prolactin and β-adrenergic agonist-stimulated progesterone production appeared to be the result of an action of GnRH to increase the activity of 20α-hydroxysteroid dehydrogenase, without influencing pregnenolone production (390,391).

Direct effects of GnRH on steroidogenesis in granulosa cells are not limited to inhibition. In the absence of other stimulatory agents, GnRH and its agonists act on granulosa cells from normal or immature hypophysectomized, estrogen-primed rats to increase aromatase activity (386) and the production of pregnenolone, progesterone, and 20α-dihydroprogesterone (153,170,386,388,392). These and other studies indicate that GnRH stimulates the cholesterol side-chain cleavage enzyme (153,170), the Δ^5-3β-hydroxysteroid dehydrogenase (386,388), and 20α-hydroxysteroid dehydrogenase (173). However, GnRH and GnRH agonists do not activate steroidogenesis nearly as well as FSH does. The direct effects of GnRH, either inhibitory or stimulatory, on follicular steroidogenesis *in vivo* appear to depend on the duration of exposure and on the stage of follicular maturation (393,394).

GnRH also has diverse effects on other aspects of granulosa cell cytodifferentiation that may be responsible for some or all of the observed influences on steroidogenesis. FSH-induced formation of LH and prolactin receptors (384,395) and stimulation of receptors for epidermal growth factor (EGF) on rat granulosa cells is inhibited by GnRH and its agonists (396). GnRH also inhibits FSH-stimulated cAMP production in rat (397–399) and porcine (375) granulosa cells. This effect in rat granulosa cells is apparently due to two actions: (a) inhibition of adenylate cyclase (399), which has been attributed to a decrease in the FSH receptor content and to an inhibition of the FSH-regulated increase in its own receptor (400); and (b) stimulation of extracellular phosphodiesterase activity (399), although there are indications that intracellular and total phosphodiesterase activity is decreased by GnRH (401). The inhibition of adenylate cyclase by GnRH is dependent on the type of activating stimulus, since stimulation by isoproterenol or prostaglandin E is not inhibited (400). In contrast, following FSH-stimulation the subsequent increase in cAMP production induced by LH, isoproterenol, or PGE_2 is inhibited by GnRH, in a process requiring calcium (402). Since the inhibitory effects of GnRH can be seen when steroidogenesis is stimulated by cAMP analogs (or by various agents that stimulate cAMP production), it is probable that GnRH causes these effects by actions at site(s) distal to cAMP production. A GnRH agonist partially inhibits dibutyryl cAMP-stimulated aromatase activity in rat granulosa cells in the presence of an inhibitor of phosphodiesterase, indicating that cAMP catabolism is unlikely to fully explain the inhibitory actions (385). Inhibition of the FSH-stimulated increase in cAMP binding sites in rat granulosa cells (170) might be one additional factor in the direct inhibitory effects of GnRH.

Other FSH-stimulated responses that are augmented by GnRH include cellular protein production (403) and prostaglandin synthesis (397). GnRH alone also stimulates cellular protein content (404) and production of lactate (405), plasminogen activator (406), prostaglandins (392), and fibronectin (407). Additional effects of GnRH on phospholipid labeling from ^{32}P and phosphatidylinositol metabolism (408–412) and on arachidonic acid release (413) suggest that pathways involving phosphoinositide metabolism, perhaps related to calcium mobilization and calcium-activated enzymes (414,415), may mediate some of the actions of GnRH at sites distal to cAMP. Neither prostaglandins nor cAMP appears to mediate stimulatory effects of GnRH on progesterone production by granulosa cells from preovulatory rat follicles (416), although a GnRH agonist in the presence of a phosphodiesterase inhibitor has been found to cause very low levels of cAMP to accumulate in the culture medium of granulosa cells from immature estrogen-treated rats (386).

The independent stimulatory actions of GnRH on granulosa cells may activate certain physiological mechanisms since GnRH agonists cause meiotic maturation of follicle-enclosed oocytes *in vitro* (417) and *in vivo* in estrogen- or PMSG-primed, hypophysectomized rats (418,419), as well as ovulation in hypophysectomized rats (420,421). Tertiary atretic follicles seem to be most susceptible to the meiosis-inducing action of GnRH (418). Degenerative changes in oocytes and premature luteinization of granulosa cells, occurring without ovulation (384,400), have been reported as a result of GnRH agonist treatment, suggesting that GnRH both stimulates and disturbs normal regulatory mechanisms. A more recent study indicates that GnRH agonist-induced oocyte maturation in the rat is not abnormal (418), in contrast to earlier reports.

GnRH also has inhibitory effects on ovarian interstitial cells prepared from hypophysectomized immature rats (422). LH-induced differentiation of interstitial cells is blocked by GNRH, and inhibition of androgen production is by selective inhibition of the 17α-hydroxylase:C-17,20-lyase enzyme (423).

The presence of specific receptors for GnRH in ovarian cell types in the rat is reason enough to suspect a physiological role involving locally produced GnRH factors. Yet it is apparent that GnRH decapeptide produced by the hypothalamus is unlikely to have a peripheral action on the ovary by virtue of its extremely low concentrations; the highest concentration in human plasma, collected during the periovulatory period, is on the order of 8×10^{-12} M (424). The first suggestion of a local source of GnRH-like factor(s), so-called gonadocrinins, was the report of an acid-extractable factor in rat follicular fluid and in rat granulosa cell conditioned-medium that was capable of releasing FSH and LH from rat pituitary cells *in vitro* but that was immunologically and chromatographically distinct from GnRH (425). However, the investigators who first reported this factor have been unable to reproduce their findings (426). Other investigators have since found two components in extracts from luteinized rat ovaries that resemble GnRH in a radioreceptor assay using ovarian plasma membranes but that show little immunoassayable activity (427). These ovarian GnRH-like factors are protease sensitive and have molecular weights between 1,000 and 10,000 daltons. They differ from hypothalamic GnRH in that they are more sensitive to heat (inactivated at 50 or 60°C for 5 min), and they are distinct by reverse-phase high-performance liquid chromatography. Since significant quantities of this receptor-active material have also been found in liver and kidney, it would appear that the factors may not be specific ovarian products.

The physiological function(s) of ovarian GnRH-like peptides are unknown. It is conceivable that they are natural GnRH agonists that mediate paracrine or autocrine regulation within the ovary, the biological actions perhaps being similar to those already outlined for GnRH and its synthetic agonists. From this perspective, the direct antigonadotropic actions of GnRH shown in the rat might suggest a role in follicular atresia, perhaps related to selection of the dominant follicle. Alternatively, GnRH-like peptides might be GnRH antagonists. However, evidence obtained in estrogen-primed, hypophysectomized rats indicates that the action of FSH on follicle development is potentiated by a synthetic GnRH antagonist but is inhibited by exogenous GnRH (428). This result suggests that the antagonist was competitive to a GnRH-like factor, presumably of ovarian origin, that inhibits the action of FSH on follicle recruitment to the preovulatory stage.

Glucocorticoids

The influence of the adrenal glands and glucocorticoid treatments on ovarian function has long been recognized from various studies in mice (429) and rats (430–433) and in women (434,435). Although many of the effects of glucocorticoids may be mediated by actions on the hypothalamus and/or pituitary gland (431–433,436), a direct action of these steroids on the ovary cannot be discounted.

Glucocorticoid receptors have been characterized in rat ovaries (437) and localized to granulosa cells (438). Cortisol or dexamethasone have been shown to inhibit FSH-stimulated aromatase activity (439,440) but to enhance FSH-stimulated progesterone production in cultured rat granulosa cells (439,441). The action of glucocorticoids on progesterone production is associated with increased Δ^5-3β-hydroxysteroid dehydrogenase and reduced 20α-hydroxysteroid dehydrogenase activities, resulting in enhanced synthesis and concomitant suppression of metabolism. In porcine granulosa cell incubations, cortisol has no effect on basal progesterone production but is stimulatory in the presence of insulin (442). The physiological significance of these observations is obscure. Concentrations of glucocorticoids required to elicit responses *in vitro* were considered pharmacological. Nevertheless, these observations are interesting from a pathological point of view, and the presence of an ovarian glucocorticoid receptor, as well as of cortisol-binding globulin concentrated in follicular fluid (443,444), suggests that glucocorticoids may be of some physiological significance in the regulation of follicular function.

Growth Factors and Insulin

It is now quite clear that several well-characterized "growth factors" have *in vitro* modulatory effects on granulosa cell differentiation, including effects on steroidogenesis in several species. However, it is uncertain what the concentrations of these factors are within the follicles at different stages, what the cellular sources are either within the ovary or in extraovarian tissues, and what the regulatory or permissive actions are *in vivo*. These factors most likely influence cytodifferentiation in its many facets, rather than specifically affecting the steroidogenic mechanisms. A complete review of this expanding area of investigation is beyond the scope of this chapter, and readers are referred to the reviews available (329,445). We outline below the principal actions of growth factors on steroidogenesis by ovarian cell cultures.

EGF has been shown to bind to high-affinity, low-capacity receptors (446) and to have different influences on the steroidogenic pathways for estrogen and progesterone production in rat granulosa cells. EGF inhibits FSH-stimulated estrogen biosynthesis (i.e., aromatase activity) in granulosa cells from immature hypophysectomized, estrogen-treated rats (446,447), while it augments FSH-stimulated progestin biosynthesis and independently stimulates production of pregnenolone, progesterone, and 20α-dihydroprogesterone (446). EGF has also been reported to impair FSH-stimulated progesterone production in rat granulosa cells by increasing catabolism to 20α-dihydroprogesterone (448). The stimulatory actions of EGF (and perhaps its inhibitory actions as well) may involve sites distal to cAMP production since EGF has been reported to decrease FSH-stimulated cAMP production and to increase cAMP catabolism (448). In studies with pig granulosa cells, EGF inhibited FSH-stimulated estrogen biosynthesis but consistently inhibited FSH or hCG-stimulated progesterone production only after longer periods of treatment in culture (449). In contrast with these actions on rat and pig cells, EGF acts on cultured hen granulosa cells to inhibit LH-stimulated progesterone biosynthesis, apparently by inhibitory actions at the levels of cAMP production, as well as distal to this step but before C_{27} side-chain cleavage (450). Other studies in the rat have shown that the EGF receptor content of granulosa cells is regulated by LH and FSH and is maximum at proestrus of the cycle (396,446), indicating that EGF action may be coordinated with other hormonally regulated events. EGF has also been shown to inhibit androgen production by rat ovarian theca–interstitial cells (451). The only *in vivo* effect of EGF on the follicle so far demonstrated is the retardation of development of early stage follicles when administered to neonatal mice (452). However, there is no evidence to relate this effect to inhibition of estrogen biosynthesis, and it could be due to inhibitory effects on the pituitary.

The source of EGF would appear to be extraovarian, and it has been found in several tissues, as well as in mouse plasma and milk (453). EGF has been purified from submaxillary glands of mice and rats (454,455) and from human urine (456); the structures of the material isolated from these sources are similar but not identical. The fact that androgens greatly stimulate EGF levels in submaxillary glands and plasma (453,457) suggests a possible mechanism for self-regulation of androgen production via EGF action on the theca–interstitial cells. The possibility that EGF-like peptides might be produced locally and have autocrine actions affecting follicular function must also be considered. The EGF-like growth factor, α transforming growth factor (TGF-α), is known to interact with EGF receptors and has been found in several normal tissues (458–460). Also, normal bovine pituitary cells in culture have been reported to produce EGF, EGF-like, and TGF-α-like peptides (461).

Platelet-derived growth factor (PDGF) also increases FSH-stimulated progestin production, which may involve increased sensitivity to FSH and cAMP (448). This *in vitro* action suggests that PDGF release from platelets during follicular rupture may act to stimulate luteal cell production of progesterone.

Several modulatory actions on steroidogenesis have also been shown for insulin and the insulin-like growth factors (IGFs); these latter factors, classically thought to be of hepatic origin, are known as IGF-I [or somatomedin C (Sm-C)] and IGF-II in humans [or rIGF-II/MSA (multiplication stimulating activity) in the rat]. Receptors for SM-C/IGF-I have been reported in granulosa cells of immature pigs (462,463) and of rat (445). Insulin receptors have also been reported on granulosa or luteal cells of rat, pig, and human (464–468). It is not clear whether the effects of insulin on granulosa cells are mediated through insulin receptors or type I IGF receptors (which preferentially bind IGF-I but also bind IGF-II and insulin). However, IGF-I does not appear to interact with insulin receptors.

There is evidence in the rat (445) and pig (469,470) for IGF-I production by granulosa cells in culture and for measurable quantities of IGF-I in follicular fluid from porcine (471,472) and human ovaries (445). Moreover, immunoreactive IGF-I in ovarian extracts increases following treatment of hypophysectomized, estrogen-treated rats with growth hormone (GH) (473), suggesting regulation of ovarian IGF production. Insulin has also been measured in fluid from porcine (472) and human (474) follicles.

The effects of IGF-I on rat granulosa cells cultured under serum-free conditions are to augment the stimulation by FSH of progesterone and 20α-dihydroprogesterone production

(475,476) and of aromatase activity (477). In porcine granulosa cells, IGF-I alone or synergistically with FSH increases progesterone production (462) and also appears to stimulate pregnenolone, progesterone, and 20α-dihydroprogesterone independently, without synergism with FSH (463). Independent stimulatory effects of rIGF-II/MSA have been shown on progesterone production by porcine granulosa cells when cultured in the absence of serum (478), although another study has shown only a synergism with FSH (462). Insulin has also been shown to act synergistically amplifying the stimulatory effect of LDL on progesterone biosynthesis by porcine granulosa cells, the mechanisms involving increased binding, internalization, and degradation of LDL (479).

GH has been shown to augment FSH-stimulated progesterone and 20α-dihydroprogesterone production by cultured granulosa cells from hypophysectomized, estrogen-treated rats by mechanisms involving increased cAMP, as well as stimulation at a site distal to cAMP (480). It has not yet been determined whether this is a direct effect of GH or whether GH-stimulated production of IGF is responsible.

Insulin has steroidogenic effects similar to those of IGF-I, and since effects of insulin and IGF-I are not additive, it is likely that they employ the same mechanism. Progesterone production by rat (464,481) and pig (442,466,467,478, 482,483) granulosa cells is stimulated by insulin, as is FSH-stimulated aromatase activity in rat (481) and human (484) granulosa cells. In contrast, insulin inhibits or is without effect on aromatase activity in porcine granulosa cells (478,485).

Neuroregulatory Substances and Ovarian Innervation

The innervation of the mammalian ovary has been well documented. Although considerable variation exists among species, sympathetic nerves, to a large extent accompanying blood vessels, innervate the ovarian interstitial tissue and perifollicular regions in several species, with follicles at all stages of development having adrenergic nerve terminals in close proximity to the blood vessels of the theca externa. Neither blood vessels nor nerves penetrate the basement membrane to reach the granulosa layers of follicles at any stage of development (486).

Although the physiological significance of the ovarian nerves remains to be established, considerable research has centered around the possible role of adrenergic neurotransmitters in controlling follicular function. Studies by Bahr and Ben-Jonathan (487) have shown that stimulation of the rat ovary with gonadotropin depletes the ovary of the catecholamine. A 40% reduction of ovarian concentrations of noradrenaline occurred 12 hr after PMSG administration to prepubertal rats; this was followed by a further 40% reduction 4 hr after the preovulatory LH surge. FSH, rather than LH or PRL, was found to be the pituitary hormone primarily involved in depletion of noradrenaline from Graafian follicles (488). Noradrenaline levels in porcine follicular fluid have been reported to vary with the stage of the estrous cycle, the highest levels being observed during the follicular phase (days 16–20) (489).

In vivo evidence for possible involvement of ovarian nerves in regulation of steroid secretion has come from ovarian denervation and ovarian nerve stimulation experiments. Decreased activity of Δ^5-3β-hydroxysteroid dehydrogenase was seen in both the interstitial gland cells and corpus luteum of the pregnant rat following ovarian denervation (490). Subsequently, Capps et al. (491) showed that electrical stimulation of the nerves in the ovarian plexus of hypophysectomized rats caused the interstitial cells to hypertrophy and develop ultrastructural features typical of active steroid-secreting cells.

The possible role of catecholamines in the direct regulation of steroid biosynthesis by follicle cells has been examined both *in vivo* and *in vitro*. *In vivo* experiments involved intrafollicular injection of adrenergic agonists and antagonists in rabbits. Beta-adrenergic, but not α-adrenergic, agonists resulted in increased progesterone output by the ovary, without influencing estrogen secretion (492). *In vitro* studies have shown catecholamine stimulation of progesterone production by dispersed luteal or granulosa cells in culture (492–496). These effects could be blocked by the β-adrenergic antagonist propranolol. The steroidogenic response (progesterone synthesis) of cultured rat granulosa cells to noradrenaline and isoproterenol was markedly enhanced by pretreatment of the cells with FSH *in vivo* or *in vitro* (496). Perhaps related to this is the observation of increased levels of high-affinity β_2-adrenergic receptors on granulosa cells during the proestrus associated with puberty in the rat (497). Catecholamine responsiveness of granulosa cells in preovulatory follicles of the rat apparently develops only after the preovulatory LH surge (498).

The interstitial tissue, the most richly innervated component of the ovaries, also contains β_2-adrenergic receptors (497), and addition of the β_2-agonist zinterol to cultured rat interstitial tissue ("residual" tissue, after removal of most granulosa cells) increased output of testosterone and androstenedione from this tissue on the day of proestrus, the peripubertal stage in which the greatest concentration of β_2-receptors were present (497). Addition of epinephrine, norepinephrine and isoproterenol to cultured theca–interstitial cells from hypophysectomized rats also markedly enhanced the secretion of certain androgens in the presence of hCG stimulation. The catecholamines were ineffective in stimulating basal (i.e., in the absence of hCG stimulation) secretion of steroids by the theca–interstitial tissue (despite the fact that they are effective, by themselves, in stimulating cAMP output) (499). Other neurotransmitters that have been detected in the ovary include acetylcholine (based on demonstration of acetylcholinesterase activity) (500), dopamine (487,501), substance P (502,503), VIP (504), and γ-aminobutyric acid (GABA) (329). Although high-affinity binding sites in ovarian tissue have been reported for some of these compounds and certain *in vitro* effects on steroidogenesis occur (505), suggesting possible regulatory roles, information is lacking about the specific effects of these neurotransmitters on steroid biosynthesis in the follicle.

STEROIDOGENESIS AND ITS CONTROL BY FOLLICLE TYPE

Introductory Description of Follicle Types

In the foregoing sections we have described the characteristic steroidogenic functions and control of the separate cell types of the mature ovarian follicle. The purpose of this section is to reexamine the evidence from the perspective of follicular development stage, drawing on related examples from human and animal studies to illustrate principles. It is intended to place the previous discussion of cellular details of steroid formation and regulation into the context of the follicle as a developing biosynthetic structure. We shall consider the dynamic processes of steroid synthesis and secretion occurring within the follicles as follicular maturation proceeds under the control of the pituitary gonadotropic hormones. Although the follicular contribution to ovarian steroid production is at any time the composite secretion of steroids by follicles at various functionally different stages, the most important contribution eventually comes from one or several dominant follicles forming a cohort destined to ovulate.

The stages of follicular development have been described by several classifications that distinguish follicles in terms of oocyte morphology and size, and the number of supporting granulosa cells and their organization. Similar schemes for mouse (506) and human (507) ovaries have defined eight principal types of follicle. The general categories of follicle types are the following: small nongrowing follicles (i.e., primordial follicles classified as types 1–2 in human and 1–3a in mouse); preantral follicles (i.e., single-layered primary and multilaminar secondary follicles classified as types 3–5 in the human and types 3b–5b in the mouse), which are characterized mainly by increases in oocyte size and number of granulosa cells; and antral follicles (i.e., tertiary or Graafian follicles classified as types 6–8 in human and mouse), which feature formation of a fluid-filled antrum and further increases in granulosa cell number. In addition, antral follicles of several species have been referred to previously as either small or large to indicate the extent of their expansion, so this description is also used here. Moreover, large antral follicles are described as either nonovulatory or preovulatory to indicate their maturity according to accepted functional criteria. We shall discuss the differing steroidogenic functions of follicles according to several of these morphological categories.

Initially, a prefollicular phase will be considered. This phase does not represent a follicular stage but, rather, a brief period in ovarian organogenesis before the onset of folliculogenesis, the process whereby germ cells associate with the follicular cells to form primordial follicles. This prefollicular phase can occur in embryonic life, in the neonate, or even in later prepubertal stages depending on the species.

The Prefollicular Ovary

The prefollicular phase of ovarian development would appear to be largely devoid of steroidogenic function in some, but not all, species. However, this view may reflect the great difficulty in assessing steroid production at early stages in certain smaller animals.

Steroid synthesis in rodent ovaries is undetectable or very limited before follicles form (70,508). The rat ovary, which begins forming follicles on postnatal day 1 (509,510), was shown to be unresponsive to gonadotropic stimulation of estrogen production during the fetal period (511). Histochemical activity of Δ^5-3β-hydroxysteroid dehydrogenase has been demonstrated in prefollicular ovaries of rat (512) but only in the interstitial cells, with no activity apparent in granulosa cells. In neonatal mouse ovaries, in which folliculogenesis begins on postpartum day 2 (513–515), significant histochemical activity for Δ^5-3β-hydroxysteroid dehydrogenase first appears in the intraovarian rete cells at 7 days of age (70). However, in all these studies, the presence of histochemical enzyme activity does not establish that the enzyme is functioning as part of a biosynthetic pathway.

In contrast to studies in rodents, prefollicular ovaries of rabbit (516), sheep (517), and cow (518) apparently synthesize or have certain functional enzymes required to synthesize steroids even before initiation of meiosis in the oocytes, which precedes follicle formation. Studies in the rabbit demonstrated conversion of testosterone to estradiol by ovaries at day 18 of gestation, but the presence of endogenous androgen substrate was not determined (516). Other studies showed that gonadotropins were able to stimulate progesterone production by cultured rabbit granulosa cells, isolated from ovaries at the early postnatal period, but only after follicles had formed (519); folliculogenesis begins in this species at 14 days of age (520–522). In bovine ovaries, in which folliculogenesis begins about day 95 of fetal life (523), estradiol production has been detected as early as 45 ± 3 days of fetal age but was biphasic and subsequently declined (518,524). The onset of ovarian estradiol production occurred when the sex of the embryonic gonad was first distinguishable. *De novo* synthesis is believed to occur at this early fetal age since both testosterone and estradiol have been shown to be present in the ovaries. Furthermore, estradiol production *in vitro* is stimulated by LH. Progesterone and prostaglandins are produced even earlier, at day 30 of gestation (518). At much later gestational stages in the bovine, at least a month before term, ovaries *in vitro* convert [^{14}C]progesterone to several hydroxylated metabolites of C_{21}-steroids and to C_{19}-steroids, as well as convert [^{14}C]androstenedione to testosterone and estradiol (525).

These conversions most probably involve enzymes present in both follicular and interstitial cells.

Steroidogenic function in prefollicular human ovaries has not been adequately investigated, but histochemical enzyme activity for Δ^5-3β-hydroxysteroid dehydrogenase has been demonstrated at this stage in the interstitial cells (526–528). Evidence for early steroidogenic function in human fetal ovaries following folliculogenesis is considered later (see section on preantral and early antral follicles, below).

Morphological evidence suggests biosynthetic and secretory activity in granulosa cells in prefollicular ovaries of various species. In general, these cells have numerous ribosomes and branching mitochondria and well-developed Golgi complexes, and they often contain lipid droplets. However, these features are not specific indicators of steroid-synthesizing cells, and they may reflect other biosynthetic functions associated with granulosa cell–oocyte cooperation. In the prefollicular ovary, oocytes and granulosa cells exist together within the irregular cords and nests of the ovarian cortex. The arrangement of oocytes and granulosa cells is closely packed, with extremely close apposition of plasma membranes, since at this time there is no zona pellucida to separate the granulosa cells from the oocyte. At this stage, therefore, granulosa cells may serve primarily to provide nutrients to the oocyte, a function that is certainly continued, in the developing follicles of adults, by the specialized granulosa cells of the corona radiata (60). Granulosa cells in prefollicular ovaries also appear to be active in the phagocytosis of degenerating germ cells.

Oocytes and granulosa cells are entirely interdependent in the formation of follicles, without which neither substantial steroidogenesis nor oocyte growth can occur. Therefore, a most important aspect of the prefollicular phase is the establishment of granulosa cell and oocyte associations leading to folliculogenesis. When the number of oocytes in the fetal ovary is greatly decreased by a genetic defect or destructive treatments, follicles rarely form, and the ovary is deficient in normal steroid production. An example is Turner's syndrome in humans, where the 45,X chromosome constitution results in a failure to differentiate oocytes and follicle organization is disrupted (529–531). The XO condition in mice is far less severe, and females are fertile and appear normal with the exceptions of reduced numbers of oocytes, a shorter reproductive life span (532), and developmental retardation (533). Destruction of oocytes in ovaries of fetal rats by treatment with the antimitotic drug busulphan (534,535) or irradiation (536) leads to a similar conclusion: Without oocytes, follicles do not form, and the resultant ovary consists mainly of stroma containing networks of cords and tubules resembling the intraovarian rete ovarii. Such ovaries lack steroidogenic functions and fail to develop responsiveness to gonadotropins (537).

In summary, the cells of the prefollicular phase in some, but not all, species appear to be steroidogenically inactive and to be unresponsive to gonadotropins in terms of steroid production. However, it is necessary to interpret the significance of these findings cautiously since apparent inactivity may reflect inadequate sensitivity of the assay procedures, while apparent activity of certain enzyme steps need not necessarily indicate biologically important *de novo* production of steroid hormones. Early differentiation of granulosa cells and their organization into follicles would appear to be influenced largely by interactions of these cells with oocytes and gonadotropins, but little is known about other local factors controlling early ovarian differentiation and folliculogenesis, including steroidogenesis.

Preantral and Early Antral Follicles

Preantral follicles develop from primary follicles by enlargement of the oocyte and proliferation of the supporting granulosa cells. The factors responsible for initiation of growth of follicles from the nongrowing pool are unknown but have previously been discussed in terms of regulation by the oocyte or granulosa cells (538). Subsequent development of preantral follicles is not dependent on gonadotropins and continues after hypophysectomy (539). As the follicle enlarges, theca cells differentiate from cells within the ovarian stroma, thereby forming a sheath of flattened cells around the follicular basement membrane. Formation of the theca layer is quite variable among individual follicles in the mouse but becomes distinct at the multilaminar stage. In the hamster, theca appears to differentiate in follicles with seven or eight layers of granulosa cells (540). In the mouse, only later, when the antrum forms, does the theca differentiate further into theca interna and externa (541,542).

Evidence of various types, largely indirect, suggests that in several species limited steroidogenic activity is probably acquired at the preantral stage of follicle development, although it is weakly expressed until the antral stage. FSH receptors are found on rat granulosa cells at all follicular stages, including early preantral follicles (543,544). However, the precise contributions of preantral follicles to ovarian steroid production are not well understood, primarily because of difficulties in studying the relatively low secretory activities of these follicles *in vivo* and because methodology for isolating preantral follicles is not well developed. Only recently has an improved enzymatic and mechanical method been developed for the isolation of various stages of intact preantral follicles in the hamster (540). Research on early follicles has also been neglected in favor of the functionally more important Graafian follicle. Several different approaches for deducing the steroidogenic function of preantral follicles are discussed below.

The formation of preantral follicles in the neonatal period of the rat provides an opportunity to examine gonadotropin responsiveness and steroidogenesis in ovaries containing only small follicles, early preantral follicles, and interstitial cells. Since theca cells from the immature rat produce negligible amounts of estrogens (190) and rat ovarian interstitial cell preparations in culture produce only small quantities of estrogens (86), neonatal ovarian synthesis of estrogens *in vitro* may be an indicator of aromatase activity in the granulosa cells. However, it is also possible that neonatal thecal and interstitial cells at this age differ from those in older rats and are capable of significant estrogen biosynthesis.

Follicle growth in the neonatal rat begins by postpartum day 2, with multilaminar follicles forming by day 6, but it is not until about day 10 that the first follicles containing antra appear in significant numbers. The available data suggest that preantral follicles of the neonatal period may respond to gonadotropins and produce steroids. Quattropani and Weisz (545) have shown that Δ^5-3β-hydroxysteroid dehydrogenase activity is present histochemically in interstitial cells of day 4 rat ovaries and that as early as day 5, ovaries are capable of converting [^{3}H]progesterone to estrogens. These investigators suggested that the interstitial cells were solely responsible for these steroidogenic activities in the neonatal rat. However, FSH binding sites, which are thought to be specific for granulosa cells, have also been demonstrated in the ovary as early as day 5 (546), and FSH has been found to stimulate both cAMP and steroid production by ovaries of 4-day-old rats (547).

Other studies with cultured ovaries from 4-day-old rats have shown that progesterone production is stimulated by $(Bu)_2$cAMP and conversion of testosterone to estradiol is stimulated by $(Bu)_2$cAMP or FSH (548). Furthermore, estrogen production in these studies was not substantially stimulated by FSH alone, but was greatly augmented by FSH in combination with LH (548), which is consistent with a "two-cell type, two-gonadotropin" form of regulation at this early developmental stage.

Recent studies involving similar *in vitro* incubations of rat ovaries have established that purified FSH, LH, or PGE_2 will each stimulate, to a different extent, the production of progesterone, androstenedione, and estradiol by ovaries at day 6 but not earlier (547). In these studies, secondary preantral follicles were the most advanced stages present at this time, suggesting that gonadotropin-regulated *de novo* synthesis of the three major classes of steroids might be produced by the developing preantral follicles in cooperation with the interstitial cells. In these studies, LH was by far the most potent stimulus for androstenedione and estradiol production, but addition of the phosphodiesterase inhibitor 3-isobutyl-1-methylxanthine (MIX) resulted in enhanced responsiveness to both FSH and LH, with FSH then having a potency equal to that of LH. The contention that phosphodiesterase activity limits steroidogenic responsiveness to gonadotropins in early ovaries was confirmed in incubations of 4-day-old ovaries, which only in the presence of MIX allowed increases in androstenedione secretion in response to PGE_2, LH, and FSH and increases in estradiol in response to PGE_2 alone (547). These results indicate that steroidogenic capabilities differentiate in neonatal rat ovaries even before acquisition of full responsiveness to gonadotropins, and certainly well before formation of antral follicles. The responsiveness to LH might also be regulated by local steroid action since other investigators have shown that estrogen treatment of neonatal rats advances the age at which LH-stimulated cAMP can be demonstrated *in vitro* (549).

The extent to which steroidogenic activities seen in neonatal rat ovaries might be influenced by the high circulating levels of FSH (550,551) and other pituitary hormones (552) present during this period is uncertain. It can only be speculated that the steroidogenic pathways seen in neonatal rat ovaries might be similarly expressed as a result of the cooperation of preantral follicles and interstitial cells present in ovaries at later developmental ages, including adults. Steroids secreted by preantral follicles at all developmental ages might influence local concentrations within the ovary, thereby affecting follicular function or maturation. However, the studies described above with whole neonatal ovary incubations do not provide conclusive evidence that significant steroidogenesis occurs within the follicular compartment, as opposed to the interstitial cells.

Similarly, there is no direct information on the steroidogenic function of preantral follicles in the adult human ovary. However, studies have investigated steroidogenic activity of fetal ovarian tissue *in vitro*. Most of the studies have obtained ovarian tissue at fetal ages later than the beginning of folliculogenesis, which occurs at about 8 weeks of gestation in the human (553). Therefore, steroidogenic activities reported might partly reflect functions of early follicles. However, another potentially important steroidogenic cell population is found in the interstitium of ovaries from human fetuses at 12 to 20 weeks gestation (554). These interstitial cells of the embryonic ovary, also called primary interstitial cells (97), are located in the medullary region beneath the cortical cords and are often adjacent to blood vessels. Their fine structure is typical of steroidogenic cells, and they are relatively large (>30 μm greatest diameter).

The evidence for steroidogenesis in human fetal ovaries is based on experiments in which fetal ovarian tissues were incubated in the presence of radioactive steroid precursors. The ability to convert [^{3}H]testosterone or androstenedione into estradiol and estrone was not apparent in undifferentiated gonads of human fetuses at approximately 6 to 8 weeks gestation but was acquired at about 8 to 10 weeks and continued to be present until at least midgestation (555). However, George and Wilson cautioned that their results alone do not give evidence of *de novo* estrogen synthesis from endogenous substrates. Earlier studies with ovaries from more advanced fetuses (16–22 weeks gestation) did not find evidence of C_{19}-steroid synthesis from [^{14}C]progesterone (556) or from [1-^{14}C]acetate (557), but in the latter study acetate was converted to lanosterol, cholesterol, and smaller quantities of pregnenolone and progesterone. A further study in which fetal ovarian tissue was incubated with [^{14}C]pregnenolone found progesterone to be the main product, but products of the 5-ene-3β-hydroxysteroid pathway, 17α-hydroxypregnenolone and dehydroepiandrosterone, were also identified (558). An earlier study demonstrated the active conversion of [^{14}C]progesterone to

20α-dihydroprogesterone in fetal ovaries at 19 weeks but not at 12 to 15 weeks of gestation (559). More recently, in organ cultures of ovaries from three fetuses (12, 20, and 22 weeks gestation), release of progesterone, dehydroepiandrosterone, androstenedione, estrone, and estradiol (560) was reported. It was also found that progesterone production *in vitro* was stimulated by $(Bu)_2cAMP$ and, to a lesser extent, by LH/FSH.

A most interesting finding is the substantial conversion by fetal human ovaries (at approximately 12.5–17.5 weeks gestation) of $[^3H]$pregnenolone sulfate into pregnenolone, 17α-hydroxypregnenolone, dehydroepiandrosterone, and androstenedione but without formation of progesterone, testosterone, or estrogens (561). This indicates the presence of steroid sulfatase activity in the fetal ovary and the ability to convert C_{21}-steroids to C_{19}-steroids via the 5-ene-3β-hydroxysteroid pathway, similar to the preferred pathway to androstenedione in the adult ovary (84). The presence of a high concentration of pregnenolone sulfate in fetal blood (562) suggests there is a natural substrate available. These studies indicate that the human fetal ovary is steroidogenically active at developmental stages after initiation of folliculogenesis but when embryonic interstitial cells are also present. It is possible that both early follicular cells and interstitial cells contribute to the conversions observed. However, the presence of the interstitial cells precludes deductions regarding the steroidogenic functions of early stages of human follicles. As mentioned previously, interstitial cells in the human ovary are histochemically reactive for Δ^5-3β-hydroxysteroid dehydrogenase even in prefollicular stages.

One study with fetal ovaries of rhesus monkeys indicates that the capacity for *de novo* production of estradiol is acquired only in late gestation, when multilayered and antral follicles have already developed (563); this suggests that preantral follicles may not contribute significantly to estrogen production in this species, at least during fetal life.

A more direct, but little used approach to assess steroidogenesis in preantral follicles at various stages of development has been to obtain dispersed follicles by enzymatic and/or mechanical procedures. In one study, dispersed ovarian tissues from immature mice were cultured *in vivo* as transplants, either implanted subcutaneously in gelfoam sponges or diffusion chambers or as cells implanted into intraocular sites (564). Intraocular transplants were accompanied by a fragment of vaginal epithelium as a biological indicator of estrogen production. These studies demonstrated that subcutaneous transplants into ovariectomized mice caused vaginal opening and onset of estrous cycles similar to that seen in nonovariectomized controls, and intraocular transplants promoted cornification of the vaginal fragment. In the latter situation, follicles transplanted together with dispersed ovarian cells, presumably containing androgen-secreting interstitial cells, were far more effective in causing vaginal cornification. Most importantly, it was noted that vaginal cornification, taken as a measure of estrogen production, was apparent only when growth of follicles and concomitant maturation of antra were observed. Therefore, while preantral follicles might have contributed to estrogen production by transplants of dispersed ovarian tissues, these studies suggest that substantial secretion of estrogens requires antral follicles.

Enzymatic dispersion of the ovarian compartments has also been used successfully to harvest all but the most mature antral follicles from rabbit ovaries (565). Measurements of follicular steroid content, which undoubtedly reflect steroid uptake from other compartments and follicles at different stages, as well as biosynthesis, suggest a progressive increase in levels of progesterone and estrogen as follicles develop from small primary to large antral stages. However, since *de novo* synthesis was not conclusively demonstrated, these results do not necessarily establish the steroidogenic abilities of early rabbit follicles.

Preantral follicles have been isolated from ovaries of cyclic hamsters and incubated *in vitro* to assess LH-stimulated steroid production (566). These studies indicate that isolated preantral follicles show a shift in LH-stimulated steroid products, depending on the time of follicle isolation relative to the endogenous LH surge. Before the LH surge during proestrus, androstenedione production predominated; immediately following the endogenous LH surge, the isolated preantral follicles produced only progesterone. The ability to produce androstenedione, and additionally estradiol, reappeared in follicles isolated on the afternoon of estrus. Subsequently, isolated small antral follicles, which had developed from preantral follicles present at estrus, produced mainly estradiol and androstenedione, with only smaller amounts of progesterone. It is apparent that steroidogenesis can occur in isolated preantral hamster follicles and that *in vivo* the LH surge may act to synchronize steroidogenesis by these follicles (566).

Many *in vivo* studies with immature normal or hypophysectomized rats indicate that ovaries consisting primarily of larger preantral follicles are steroidogenically responsive to gonadotropins (FSH and/or LH). However, these animal models do not allow the action of FSH in inducing steroidogenic activity to be distinguished from the concurrent effect of FSH on formation of follicular antra. Large preantral follicles that form in hypophysectomized rats do not show autonomous synthesis of estrogens but require stimulation with FSH and either LH or aromatizable androgen (209). It would appear that significant aromatase activity occurs only as antral follicles form in response to FSH stimulation.

Several models exist for the culture of granulosa cells from ovaries containing primarily small and preantral follicles. Granulosa cells can be obtained either from normal immature rats before large antral follicles have formed or from immature hypophysectomized rats, in which very few small tertiary follicles will form in the absence of gonadotropin stimulation. In both models, treatment with estrogen is often used to stimulate the numbers of relatively uniform preantral follicles; in addition, this treatment greatly increases the responsiveness of the cells to FSH. Regardless of the model employed, granulosa cells isolated from ovaries of these animals show minimal production of progestins or estrogens when cultured without gonadotropins, even in the presence of aromatizable substrates. Other features of granulosa cytodifferentiation, such as LH receptor formation, are also absent in cells cultured without gonadotropins, indicating that these cells are minimally differentiated. Therefore, it is apparent that key steroidogenic enzymes are lacking or weakly expressed in granulosa cells of preantral follicles in hypophysectomized or normal immature rats. Since preantral follicles can, and probably do, develop without gonadotropin support, it is likely that the granulosa cells of at least early preantral stages are not very active steroid producers. However, it is probable that cyclical increases in circulating gonadotropins act in a coordinate fashion to stimulate cytodifferentiation and steroidogenesis in granulosa cells of late preantral follicles. Granulosa cells from preantral follicles of rats respond in culture to FSH with increased secretion of C_{21}-steroids and increased aromatase activity. These steroidogenic effects *in vitro* usually appear after a delay of about 24 hr, suggesting the need for induction of steroidogenic enzymes.

Certain steroidogenic enzymes are present (although perhaps not maximally expressed) in preantral follicles that have not been stimulated with gonadotropins. Granulosa cells isolated from immature rats and placed in culture are able to convert exogenous pregnenolone to progesterone, 20α-dihydroprogesterone, and, probably in lesser amounts, 5α-reduced C_{21}-steroid metabolites (47). They also convert testosterone rapidly to its 5α-reduced metabolites, including 5α-androstane-3α,17β-diol and androsterone (141). Histochemical demonstration of Δ^5-3β-hydroxysteroid dehydrogenase activity in the rat ovary indicates that this enzyme is strongly expressed in granulosa cells of preovulatory follicles but is only weakly expressed in earlier antral stages (567). This is consistent with the biochemical evidence that induction of this enzyme requires FSH stimulation of the granulosa cells (141).

A variety of factors might be responsible for limiting the steroidogenic competency of preantral follicles. Although the granulosa cells have FSH receptors that, at least in late preantral follicles, are functionally coupled to adenylate cyclase, these receptors do not function optimally since estrogen is required to augment FSH-stimulated cAMP production. This increased cAMP response in turn allows FSH to increase aromatase activity and estrogen synthesis and to increase the number of gonadotropin receptors and cAMP binding sites (568). These changes are associated with development of the antral follicle. Further, although it is generally assumed that circulating FSH and LH are similarly available to the granulosa cells of preantral and later-stage follicles by diffusion from capillaries of the theca layer through the follicular wall and into the granulosa cell layers, this assumption has not been critically tested. However, molecular size per se is not a limiting factor for gonadotropin penetration of the follicular membrane (569). The ability of healthy and steroidogenically active follicles to concentrate gonadotropins in follicular fluid suggests the probable importance of the availability of FSH to steroid production. Thus, while it is clear that follicle cells isolated from large preantral follicles respond to gonadotropins and require them for steroid production, it is uncertain to what extent preantral follicles from various species secrete steroids *in vivo* in response to normal cyclical fluctuations in circulating gonadotropin levels.

Antral to Early Preovulatory Follicles

There is general agreement that the antral stages of follicular development, and especially the early preovulatory follicles, are by far the most important source of ovarian steroids during the female cycle. This changing pattern of steroid secretion is associated with increased follicle cell growth and cytodifferentiation and considerable expansion of the antrum, which occur in response to changing levels of FSH and LH. The ability to secrete significant quantities of estrogens, a function acquired as antral follicles form, is of key importance in increasing the responsiveness of the granulosa cells to FSH and subsequently to LH (570–572). The direct action of estrogen at the follicular level and the additional indirect effect of feedback inhibition of gonadotropin secretion are important contributing factors in follicular selection.

The formation of the fluid-filled antrum provides a convenient morphological marker of the stage in follicle development when gonadotropin-dependent growth of the follicle approximately begins and steroid secretion greatly increases. Antrum formation is induced by the action of FSH, but not LH alone, and presumably reflects changes in the FSH-dependent secretory function of the granulosa cells, as well as influx of interstitial fluid (569,573). Increased follicular vascularization and steroidal effects on follicular vascular permeability could also be factors in antral fluid accumulation (569). However, antrum formation is apparently not a necessary feature of preovulatory follicular maturation in all species, since in several exceptional families (i.e., *Tenrecidae* and *Erinaceidae*), ovaries do not form antral follicles (574).

Granulosa cells of early antral follicles do not generally have ultrastructural features characteristic of steroid-secreting cells. This was originally taken as evidence of their nonsteroidogenic function until later histochemical and biochemical evidence changed that view. Only after the LH surge are substantial ultrastructural changes seen in organelles associated with steroidogenesis in the granulosa cells. These changes, which are considered the earliest signs of morphological luteinization and may occur prior to ovulation in certain species (575), are discussed in the next section.

We have already reviewed the evidence for steroid pathways present in mature granulosa and theca cells of antral follicles and considered the types of cellular cooperation involved in regulating steroid production at this stage. In this section, we consider only the additional evidence indicating that the major sources of ovarian estrogens and progesterone during the follicular phase are the large antral and preovulatory follicles, and that both small and large antral follicles are significant sources of androgens prior to the LH surge. This evidence comes mainly from measurements comparing steroid levels in ovarian venous plasma or in follicular fluid with those in peripheral plasma.

Steroid measurements in ovarian venous plasma reflect rates of ovarian secretion into the circulation. For example, a close relationship between follicular production of certain steroids and secretion into blood is apparent, since pulsatile release of LH in sheep is followed rapidly by steroid secretion into the ovarian vein, with peak levels of estradiol and androstenedione occurring 30 min after each pulse (576). In comparison, steroid measurements in follicular fluid provide a static profile of the pool of steroids secreted primarily by the granulosa and theca cells of one follicle. However, the concentrations of steroids in follicular fluid reflect not only secretion into the fluid, but also changes due to metabolism and dilution as fluid accumulates. Transfer of steroids from follicular fluid to venous plasma occurs only slowly. As demonstrated in the mare, the hourly transfer of radiolabeled pregnenolone and androstenedione from follicular fluid to ovarian vein was approximately 3% to 9% (189). The export of free and conjugated steroids from follicular fluid might also be impaired by binding globulins in the fluid (577,578). In this regard, species differences occur since sex hormone-binding globulin is present in blood plasma and follicular fluid of the cow and sheep but not the pig (579).

Estrogens

Estrogen secretion in women is highest during the late follicular phase of the menstrual cycle (580). At this time, estrogen levels are significantly higher in ovarian venous plasma from ovaries containing a large antral follicle (>8 mm diameter) compared with contralateral ovaries containing small antral follicles (<8 mm diameter) (581). This difference is about 15-fold for estradiol and 7-fold for estrone. Furthermore, venous plasma levels of estrogens from ovaries containing small follicles are only about 1.6-fold greater than levels in peripheral plasma, indicating the relatively low rate of estrogen secretion by small antral follicles. At other times in the cycle, from menstruation to the early follicular phase, when peripheral estrogen levels are low, there are no differences in venous plasma levels between right and left ovaries (581).

Follicular fluid levels of estrogens measured in small and large antral follicles (according to the sizes described above) throughout the human menstrual cycle provide additional evidence that it is the large antral follicles of the middle and late follicular phase that secrete the greatest quantities of estrogens (581,582). In several different studies, fluids from large follicles at late follicular phase have been reported to have mean estradiol concentrations in the range of 1,500 to 2,400 ng/ml (581–585). In contrast with these types of follicles, fluid obtained from large antral follicles at early follicular or luteal phases of the cycle had low estrogen concentrations that did not differ from those in small antral follicles (581). Furthermore, small antral follicles (<8 mm diameter) showed only small fluctuations in concentrations of estrogens throughout the follicular and luteal phases. However, a more recent study in the human indicates that relatively high intrafollicular concentrations of estradiol (>200 ng/ml) are also found in certain small antral follicles (4–7 mm in diameter) from follicular and luteal phases of the cycle (586), when these follicles are judged to be healthy. In this study, a healthy follicle was defined as having a nondegenerative oocyte and at least 50% of the maximum number of granulosa cells present for a given follicular diameter. Therefore, estrogen concentrations in human follicular fluid are substantially elevated only in healthy antral follicles and are greatest in healthy large antral follicles that have developed at the appropriate stage of the cycle, i.e., preovulatory follicles.

Consistent with the observations on follicular fluid levels of estrogens, much higher levels of aromatase activity, determined *in vitro,* are present in large preovulatory follicles compared with nonovulatory antral follicles taken during the late follicular phase in women (131,587). Furthermore, aromatase activity in granulosa cells of the dominant follicle in humans becomes maximal during the midfollicular phase and cannot be further stimulated by FSH *in vitro* (131,586). In comparison, when FSH and LH levels are suppressed by steroid negative feedback from the corpus luteum during the human luteal phase, follicles are not recruited for preovulatory estrogen biosynthesis; hence, follicular fluid concentrations of estrogens remain low.

Estrogenic follicles in the human are distinguished by two other important features. First, elevated estradiol concentrations in these follicles occur only when intrafollicular FSH is also elevated (>1.3 mU/ml), indicating the key regulatory role of FSH (582). Second, the importance of granulosa cells in estrogen production is further indicated by the positive relation between the number of granulosa cells and the intrafollicular estradiol concentration for a given size of antral follicle (588). Thus, it appears that preovulatory follicles prior to the midcycle LH surge are characterized by much higher estrogen biosynthetic activity and estrogen content, higher FSH concentrations, and more granulosa cells than in nonovulatory or atretic follicles (131,584,589,590).

Studies of numerous other species—including sheep (591), cows (109), pigs (592), rabbits (593), and rats (594)—report similarly high levels of estrogens in follicular fluid from large antral follicles, with maximal concentrations occurring in the preovulatory period, before or immediately after the LH surge. On the other hand, fluid from atretic follicles of various species, like the human, characteristically exhibits substantially lower estradiol concentrations (109,276, 588,595,596).

Over 90% of the circulating estradiol secreted during the late follicular phase of monotocous species originates from the dominant follicle (597,598). In women, normally only one antral follicle matures to preovulatory eminence. Estradiol levels in the fluid of the dominant follicle before the midcycle LH surge is on the order of 1 to 2 μg/ml (131,569,597), and similar estrogen levels have been found in fluids from ovaries of cyclic (597,599–602) and gonadotropin-stimulated (603,604) women. Results from various other monotocous species are comparable (187,213,603,605–607). Therefore, this evidence indicates that the dominant follicle is the principal source of the preovulatory estrogen surge that appears in plasma. This conclusion has been directly supported by studies in women that measured the large decrease in ovarian venous plasma levels of estradiol and estrone following surgical enucleation (i.e., intact removal) of the largest follicle (608). This preovulatory estrogen production is apparently regulated by LH-stimulated production of aromatizable androgens in the theca cells (discussed below; see also the section on post-LH surge preovulatory follicles), in agreement with evidence that granulosa aromatase activity is already maximally stimulated in early preovulatory follicles and cannot be further stimulated by FSH in cells from follicles >12 mm in diameter at midfollicular phase (586).

Some insight into the physiological factors regulating follicular estrogen biosynthesis during the preovulatory period has been provided from *in vitro* incubations of follicles at different stages of the estrous cycle. In the rat, regulation of estradiol production by isolated preovulatory follicles appears to be principally at the level of production of aromatizable androgens. When follicles from ovaries of 5-day cycling rats were incubated individually, accumulation of estradiol in the culture medium increased from low levels at diestrus I to high levels at proestrus (609). Estradiol accumulation by follicles obtained at either diestrus or proestrus was increased by addition of androstenedione or testosterone (indicating the presence of aromatase activity) or by addition of 17α-hydroxyprogesterone or progesterone (indicating the presence of 17α-hydroxylase:C-17,20-lyase enzyme required for conversion of progesterone to androgens). In these studies measurements of follicular enzyme activities at diestrus and proestrus demonstrated little change in lyase activity and a small increase in aromatase activity at proestrus. Since C-17,20-lyase activity was always more limiting than aromatase activity, it was concluded that increased estradiol production at proestrus might be due to an increase in endogenous production of progesterone, with greater conversion to androgens. This was supported by the finding that pregnenolone accumulation in medium from follicle incubations, carried out in the presence of cyanoketone to inhibit metabolism to progesterone, increased between diestrus and proestrus (609). Other studies (as already discussed in the section on the theca) have indicated that increased thecal cell activities of 17α-hydroxylase:C-17,20-lyase are principally responsible for the increases in androgen production that occur as small antral follicles become preovulatory (102). Therefore, together, these results are consistent with the idea that LH-stimulated production of thecal androgens (via affects on C_{21} and C_{27} side-chain cleavage) is the controlling factor in estrogen secretion at proestrus in the rat. In this respect, the regulation of preovulatory estrogen secretion in the rat and human appears to be similar.

The regulation of follicular estrogen biosynthesis in developing follicles might in part be accomplished by secreted regulatory protein(s) that have been identified in fluids of preovulatory follicles in the human (610,611) and pig (612) and that have been shown to inhibit granulosa cell aromatase activity and reduce responsiveness to gonadotropins (611–613). The regulatory protein(s) might be one means by which the "selected" or dominant follicle in monotocous species causes neighboring follicles to become atretic. The positive relationship in preovulatory follicles between estrogen concentrations in follicular fluid and levels of aromatase-inhibiting activity suggests that the dominant follicle is insensitive to this inhibitor (613). Evidence in women that this factor is secreted into the venous blood of ovaries containing a preovulatory follicle but not of contralateral ovaries suggests that interovarian, as well as intraovarian, regulation may be involved (614).

Androgens

Follicular fluid measurements demonstrate that antral follicles at all stages of the menstrual cycle in women are significant sources of C_{19}-steroids including androstenedione, testosterone, and their 5α-reduced metabolites. Since androstenedione and testosterone are not synthesized *de novo* in significant quantities by granulosa cells, they must be secreted into the follicular fluid by the theca cells of the follicle and perhaps also by the interstitial cells. However, granulosa and theca cells are capable of 5α-reduction of testosterone to 5α-dihydrotestosterone and further metabolism to 5α-androstane-3α,17β-diol and androsterone, so these metabolites might arise partly by conversion in the granulosa cells. Follicular fluid of women (275,615) and pigs (616) and extracts of rat ovary (79) contain 5α-dihydrotestosterone. The relative levels of androstenedione and testosterone in follicular fluid are probably also influenced by interconversion via 17β-hydroxysteroid dehydrogenase in the granulosa cells, as discussed earlier.

In women, the dominant androgen, androstenedione, has been measured in small and large antral follicles throughout the menstrual cycle (581). Concentrations of androstenedione in follicular fluid are between 100 and 500 times that in peripheral plasma (569). The highest concentrations of androstenedione in follicular fluid are found at midfollicular phase (745 ng/ml), with a substantial decrease occurring by the late follicular phase (120 ng/ml) (584). At the late follicular phase there is a significantly greater concentration of androstenedione in small antral follicles (726 ng/ml) than in large antral follicles (266 ng/ml) (581). At all other phases of the menstrual cycle, the differences between androgen concentrations in large and small antral follicles are not significant. Concentrations of testosterone, although considerably lower than androstenedione, show a similar pattern of change, with the highest levels occurring in small antral follicles at midcycle (104 ng/ml) but with lower concentrations in large antral follicles throughout the follicular phase (25–38 ng/ml) (581).

Androgen concentrations might be less in large antral follicles at the late follicular phase partly because of substantially greater conversion to estrogens and partly because of greater secretion into the blood due to the increased vascularization of the theca (581,617). Another contributing factor in the declining level of androgens observed in follicular fluid during the later stages of preovulatory follicle growth may be the inhibitory influence of the increasing estradiol concentrations on androgen biosynthesis in the theca cells (618,619). This possibility is supported by observations that the decline in androstenedione concentration occurring between the middle and late follicular phases is seen only in normal healthy follicles characterized by detectable levels of FSH in follicular fluid, while increased androstenedione concentrations are observed in follicles with undetectable FSH (584). Therefore, the role of FSH in inducing aromatase activity in granulosa cells appears to be an important factor in regulating follicular androgen concentrations. Estradiol, produced as a result of FSH-induced aromatase activity in granulosa cells, may feed back on the theca cells to inhibit production of its precursors, the aromatizable androgens. Such an intrafollicular negative-feedback system could be significant in limiting the rate of increase of estrogen secretion during the final stages of follicular growth; this would provide adequate time for completion of the process of cytoplasmic maturation of the oocyte before ovulation. An intrafollicular negative-feedback mechanism such as this could be particularly significant in polytocous species as a means of holding in check the most mature follicles in the selected ovulatory population: The less mature of the selected follicles could thereby continue to develop, thus resulting in a synchronous population by the time of the LH surge.

In bovine antral follicles, as in the human, changes in androgen and estrogen concentrations in follicular fluid are inversely related as follicles mature. Estradiol concentrations increase greatly as bovine follicles progress from small to large sizes, while androstenedione and testosterone concentrations decrease (620). A sharper decline in testosterone than androstenedione suggests that, as previously demonstrated (621,622), testosterone is the preferred substrate for aromatization in bovines, in contrast to the situation in the human. Another apparent difference from humans is that the concentration of FSH in bovine follicular fluid is not related to the high ratio of estradiol to androgen found in large follicles (620). This suggests that intrafollicular FSH is less likely to be a limiting factor for aromatization in bovine follicles than in human follicles. The bovine follicle may be exceptional also in another respect, since granulosa cells in this species have been reported to convert pregnenolone to 17α-hydroxprogesterone, and 17α-hydroxypregnenolone to androstenedione, indicating a possible role for these cells in C_{19}-steroid formation (85).

In the hamster, a different relationship of whole follicular concentrations of androgens and estrogens was seen in antral follicles stimulated with PMSG (623). After treatment with PMSG, testosterone and estrogen levels initially increased, the greatest concentrations occurring in middle-sized follicles; at longer intervals, however, testosterone concentrations decreased sharply in medium and large follicles, while estradiol and estrone concentrations declined less abruptly. Therefore, according to this model system in the hamster, a possible difference from other species is that androgen availability might become limiting to estrogen biosynthesis even before large antral follicles have formed.

Nonaromatic C_{18}-steroids are present in the follicular fluid of the mare and sow and are presumed to be products of follicular steroidogenesis. Equine follicular fluid was first shown to contain high levels of 19-norandrostenedione, with concentrations of this steroid at estrus being 30 to 160 ng/ml (4). More recently, 19-nortestosterone was also identified as a minor component in equine follicular fluid (6). Equine granulosa cells convert testosterone primarily to estrogens but also produce 19-nortestosterone and, apparently, lower amounts of 19-norandrostenedione (126), indicating an intrafollicular site of 19-norsteroid biosynthesis. Limited studies on follicular stages in the mare report that the highest concentrations of 19-norandrostenedione are present in fluids from large and preovulatory follicles, with lower levels present in less mature and atretic follicles (7). Porcine follicular fluid from preovulatory follicles obtained on days 19 and 20 of the estrous cycle also contains high concentrations of 19-norandrostenedione (21–25 μmol/liter, 5720–6810 ng/ml), with 19-nortestosterone being tentatively identified as a minor component (8). Follicular fluid concentrations of 19-norandrostenedione were increased after treatment of immature pigs with PMSG and decreased following subsequent hCG treatment (624). The physiological significance of 19-norsteroids in the follicle is not known, but they have been proposed as possible intermediates in estrogen biosynthesis in the mare (7) and as competitive inhibitors of aromatization in the pig (8). Furthermore, 19-norandrostenedione (0.5 μmol/liter) acts synergistically with cAMP to inhibit porcine oocyte maturation *in vitro,* suggesting another possible regulatory role in this species (625). Human ovarian tissue *in vitro* has been reported to convert testosterone to 19-norsteroids (626), but it has not been established that these steroids are present in human ovaries.

Progestins

Progesterone concentrations in follicular fluid of human follicles are much lower than in tissue of corpora lutea (627), but they vary substantially during the menstrual cycle and in small and large antral follicles. During the late follicular phase, concentrations are significantly higher in large antral follicles (~1300 ng/ml) than in small ones (~270 ng/ml) (582). Furthermore, the increase in follicular fluid progesterone concentration in large antral follicles occurs during the transition from midfollicular (760 ng/ml) to late follicular phases (1720 ng/ml), and this increase is associated with the presence of detectable levels of LH in the fluid (582). These increases in progesterone in the late follicular phase presumably reflect the increased secretion by granulosa cells; increased granulosa stimulation by LH would be expected as LH levels progressively rise in the second half of the follicular phase, at a time when FSH levels decline (628). LH has been shown to stimulate progesterone secretion by human granulosa cells from large antral follicles treated with FSH and estrogen (629). This effect of LH on human granulosa cells is presumably as a consequence of LH receptor induction, similar to that demonstrated in rat granulosa cells *in vivo* (87) and in culture (329). Luteinization of human granulosa cells appears to begin before ovulation since cells isolated in the preovulatory period produce large amounts of progesterone (630).

Pregnenolone, the immediate precursor of progesterone, is also substantially increased in fluid from large antral follicles at middle and late follicular phases in women (582). Levels on the order of 10 μg/ml are reported. Pregnenolone concentrations are also elevated in fluid from human preovulatory follicles aspirated 32 to 33 hr after treatment with hCG at midcycle, before the LH surge (631). Pregnenolone has been measured in bovine follicular fluid, with concentrations exceeding those of progesterone in the large preovulatory follicles present at proestrus (109).

Although the cellular origin of follicular fluid pregnenolone is uncertain, the likelihood that the granulosa cells are the source is supported by observations of high rates of pregnenolone secretion by cultured porcine granulosa cells (215). Evidence has been presented to suggest that pregnenolone in follicular fluid, secreted by granulosa cells, may undergo metabolism to progesterone by bovine theca cells (632) and to aromatizable androgens by porcine theca cells (215).

Preovulatory Follicles After the LH Surge

The ovulation-inducing LH surge causes concomitant changes in follicle cell structure, proliferative activity, and steroidogenesis of the preovulatory follicles. These changes occur in the interval between the LH peak and ovulation, this interval being relatively constant for each species; for example, 12 to 15 hr in mouse or rat and approximately 28 to 36 hr in human (633).

Ultrastructural changes occurring in granulosa cells of women prior to ovulation include a continuous change from granular to smooth endoplasmic reticulum (634,635) and a change to a more homogeneous chromatin structure (636). Typical characteristics of luteinization, such as an increase in smooth endoplasmic reticulum and the appearance of mitochondria with tubular cristae, begin to appear even before ovulation in many species (575). The ovulatory stimulus is also associated with changes in the quantities and types of gap junctions present between granulosa cells, as in the rabbit (637,638).

Mitoses are abundant in granulosa cells of large preovulatory follicles of certain species, including human (639), hamster (640), and guinea pig (641), but mitotic activity declines sharply between the LH surge and ovulation. In women the high mitotic index and nucleocytoplasmic ratio of granulosa cells in preovulatory follicles are apparently lowered even before the beginning of the LH surge (639). In the estrous rabbit, mitotic activity is greatest in cells of nonvesicular follicles but similarly declines following the mating-induced LH surge (642). These observations suggest that either the LH surge or perhaps related events preceding it are involved in suppressing granulosa cell proliferative activity as cells begin to luteinize. It is unknown whether these proliferative and steroidogenic changes are causally related. However, *in vivo* studies of PMSG/hCG superovulated rats indicate that increased steroidogenic activity develops only after DNA synthesis arrests (158,643), and recent *in vitro* studies with rat granulosa cells suggest that cell proliferation in culture and steroidogenic expression are inversely related (186).

Histochemical evidence of increased steroidogenic activity is also apparent as ovulation approaches. Activity of Δ^5-3β-hydroxysteroid dehydrogenase is weak in granulosa cells of developing antral follicles but increases about the time of the estrogen surge (644,645). Similarly in the hamster, activity of this enzyme increases towards the time of ovulation (640,646,647), when follicular progesterone synthesis increases (648). This enzyme is also active in granulosa cells of preovulatory human follicles, whereas it is limited to thecal cells in smaller antral follicles (585,649). In contrast with these changes in the granulosa cells, theca interna cells show high activity of Δ^5-3β-hydroxysteroid dehydrogenase throughout the maturation of the follicle.

Steroid production is substantially altered in the preovulatory period following the LH surge. Within minutes of the LH surge there is a transient increase in progesterone and estrogen secretion in several animal species, including rat, monkey, and rabbit, followed by a marked decline to basal levels within several hours (241,310,593,650–653). This inhibitory phase following the LH surge or after hCG treatment is marked by decreased concentrations of aromatizable androgens and estrogens in follicular fluid or ovaries of all species studied, including rat (243), hamster (654), sheep (655), bovine (656), and human (657,658).

In the rat, a large preovulatory peak of progesterone and 20α-dihydroprogesterone occurs close to the time of the LH peak. These extremely high levels of progestins (i.e., greater than in the short luteal phase at diestrus) are probably derived from the granulosa cells as they begin the process of luteinization, although the extent of contributions from theca–interstitial cells is uncertain. LH stimulates progesterone secretion *in vitro* by mature granulosa cells of the rat (293,571), and *in vivo* pretreatment with testosterone significantly enhances this secretion (289). Measurements of steroids in follicular fluid of preovulatory follicles have been made in rats first given low-dose PMSG treatment to induce follicle maturation and then LH to induce ovulation (243). In these studies, the progesterone concentration in follicular fluid increased sevenfold within 1 hr of LH treatment and remained elevated throughout the 10-hr study. Androstenedione and estradiol concentrations in fluid were elevated before LH treatment, increased slightly 1 to 2 hr after LH, and then fell to extremely low levels by 6 hr. In other studies, inhibition of steroidogenesis, and in particular of estradiol production, occurs during the latter half of the preovulatory period in rat (104,310,650,653), sheep (659), and pig (660). In the rabbit, where the LH surge is a reflex response induced by mating, follicles isolated at 2 and 12 hours after mating showed, respectively, a rapid rise then a fall in progesterone and estradiol synthesis from [^{14}C]acetate (651).

A similar type of steroidogenic regulation occurs in the human ovary following the LH surge. Human ovarian slices initially showed increased conversion of [^{14}C]acetate into pregnenolone, progesterone, 17α-hydroxyprogesterone, androstenedione (principal androgen), and estrogens (661). Subsequently, there was substantial reduction in the synthesis of pregnenolone and 17α-hydroxyprogesterone and, at the same time, almost complete inhibition of androgen and estrogen production (661). Fluid from human follicles after the LH surge also shows a progressive decrease over 38 hr in concentrations of estradiol and androstenedione, testosterone, and dehydroepiandrosterone (657). Similar results have been obtained in other studies (588,615,631). Despite the decrease in estradiol concentrations in human follicular fluid following the LH surge, preovulatory follicles still have the ability to aromatize androgens *in vivo* (583) and *in vitro* (662). Progesterone production decreases only slightly in the preovulatory period and then rises steadily towards ovulation (630,663), while estradiol synthesis remains low (651). Luteinization is well advanced 15 to 20 hr after the beginning of the LH surge, as indicated by high progesterone concentrations in follicular fluid (~13 μg/ml), with a further increase occurring (~18 μg/ml) after more than 27 hr (662). Progesterone concentrations in follicular fluid have been observed to peak between 5 and 25 hr after the onset of the LH surge, while the concentrations of 17α-hydroxyprogesterone change little (657). Measurements of steroids in blood during the preovulatory period in women provide similar evidence of changes in ovarian steroid secretion (630).

Regulation of the transient inhibition of steroid production in the preovulatory period of all species probably occurs at several levels. Evidence from luteal cells (356,357,664) and granulosa cells (358,359) indicates that relatively high concentrations of LH cause a transient desensitization at the gonadotropin receptor level such that target cells become refractory to gonadotropin stimulation of adenylate cyclase and steroid production. Desensitization in granulosa cells is followed by a down-regulation of receptors for LH, FSH, and estrogen (665,666). Normally during the luteal phase new receptors form and cells regain their sensitivity to LH at a time when progesterone production greatly increases. Pulsatile release of tonic levels of LH during the follicular phase may be important in preventing desensitization and down-regulation, which naturally occur in response to high concentrations and prolonged exposure to LH at midcycle.

Inhibition of estradiol production following the preovulatory LH surge is primarily the result of decreased androgen production in theca and interstitial cells. In an *in vitro* study with rat Graafian follicles in culture, inhibition of androgen secretion appeared to result from reduced 17α-hydroxylase and/or C-17,20-lyase activity since there was a concomitant inhibition of estradiol, androstenedione, and testosterone accumulation 4 to 6 hr after LH treatment (104). The authors of this study suggested that an LH-stimulated protein factor might inhibit enzymes required for cleavage of the C-17 side chain of progesterone. A subsequent study with PMSG-primed immature rats showed that a maximal ovulatory dose of LH *in vivo* caused an initial increase in ovarian androgen after 2 hr and then a reduction in androgens and estradiol 4 to 8 hr after LH injection, with serum concentrations declining after 6 hr (310). Aromatase activity in the ovarian microsomal fraction was also inhibited in a noncompetitive manner between 4 and 8 hr after LH treatment *in vivo*, consistent with either inactivation of the aromatase complex or reduced biosynthesis and rapid turnover of this enzyme. These results led to the suggestion that LH-induced inhibition of estrogen production in the rat occurred mainly at the level of 17α-hydroxylase:C-17,20-lyase, followed by a secondary decrease in aromatase activity (310). Other *in vivo* and *in vitro* studies in rats provide clear evidence that the major cause of the rapid decline in estrogen secretion after the LH surge is limited availability of aromatizable androgens, due to the decreased rate of C_{21} side-chain cleavage. The decreased ovarian content of estradiol following injection of hCG could be completely prevented by *in vivo* administration of testosterone (667) or by *in vitro* incubation of isolated follicles with aromatizable substrate (668). The decreased levels of 17α-hydroxylase:C-17,20-lyase responsible for the declining androgen production have been found to be associated with a marked reduction in the microsomal cytochrome P-450 levels in the preovulatory ovary. These experiments involving inhibitors of RNA and protein synthesis provided evidence that the LH-induced decline in activity of these rate-limiting enzymes was dependent on continuing synthesis of RNA and protein (669).

Recent studies indicate that the inhibition of the C_{21} side-chain cleavage reaction following treatment of proestrous rats with an ovulatory dose of hCG is at the levels of NADPH- and NADH-linked lyase reactions and selectively at the NADH-linked 17α-hydroxylase (670). It is possible that these apparently distinct lyase and hydroxylase activities detected after cell disruption do not reflect the true nature of the C_{21} side-chain cleavage system. As mentioned previously, direct immunoblot measurements of cytochrome P-450 for this enzyme in bovine follicles established that the enzyme protein decreases to undetectable levels at the earliest stage of corpora lutea formation (105). Inhibition of aromatase cannot be ruled out as a minor regulatory mechanism following LH treatment. Preovulatory estrogen secretion, which peaks slightly before the LH surge, has been suggested to mediate the inhibitory action on androgen production by a direct intraovarian action on the ovary (233). Support for this idea has been provided by results of *in vitro* studies indicating that estradiol inhibits androgen production by rat ovarian interstitial cell preparations (86). Evidence for a similar inhibitory effect of estradiol on androgen production by isolated porcine theca cells has also been reported (619) and recently confirmed (235).

Morphological signs of theca cell regression suggest that the activity of this cell type is reduced in the late preovulatory period in sheep (671) and human (672). Other studies of advanced human preovulatory follicles show that there are fewer theca cells and that they are associated with hemorrhagic lesions when androgen synthesis is minimal (661). However, in the rat, estrogen-priming *in vivo* actually increases the *in vitro* LH-stimulated progesterone response of theca cell preparations, suggesting that viability of theca cells is maintained despite reduced androgen production (234).

Prostaglandins may also be involved in steroidogenic regulation during the preovulatory period. High levels of prostaglandins (F and E series) are found in follicular fluid of the late preovulatory follicles of many species, including the rabbit (673,674), rat (675–677), pig (678,679), and human (680). Prostaglandin synthesis is presumably stimulated via the action of LH in increasing cAMP. PGF is undetectable in human follicular fluid prior to the LH peak but is high in ovulatory follicles and at ovulation (569,678). Prostaglandins may be involved in desensitization to gonadotropins. However, PGE_2, which stimulates progesterone production by human granulosa cells *in vitro* (681), may also maintain or increase progesterone secretion in the late preovulatory period. Furthermore, PGE_2 stimulates androgen production by thecal cells (99,682). Adenylate cyclase is desensitized to LH and FSH at this time, but granulosa cells remain responsive to PGE_2 (665). Prostaglandins might also mediate effects of LH on increased blood flow and intraovarian distribution of blood (683), thereby influencing steroid secretion into the circulation. A further important role of prostaglandins at ovulation is probably in follicular rupture since this process is blocked by inhibitors of prostaglandin synthetase (684,685) and by systemic (686) or intrafollicular injection of antiserum against prostaglandins (675).

SUMMARY AND CONCLUDING COMMENTS

As reviewed in this chapter, the follicle is the principal steroidogenic unit of the ovary. Its biosynthetic activities, and the factors that regulate them, change greatly as it emerges from the pool of resting follicles and undergoes progressive stages of differentiation. This progression leads ultimately to ovulation and luteinization of a small minority of those follicles that leave the resting pool, with the vast majority being aborted in atresia.

The steroidogenic output of the follicle at essentially all stages is a function of the concerted actions of its two types of somatic cells, the theca and granulosa cells, whose steroidogenic profiles differ in some significant ways. These differences are the result of differences in hormone receptors on their cell membranes, in specific steroidogenic enzyme activities, and in compartmentalization within the follicle, which restricts vascularization to the thecal layers and thus creates substantially different microenvironments for the two cell types.

The steroidogenic cells of the follicle are under primary control by the pituitary gonadotropic hormones, FSH and LH, with many of the actions of these hormones being influenced or modulated by a number of intraovarian factors, principally the steroid products of these cells. The gonadotropins initiate the chain of responses in their respective target cells through interaction with specific high-affinity binding sites (receptors) on the cell surfaces. Variation in the cellular concentrations of these receptors appears to dictate the fate of a given follicle, including its level of steroid output at a given stage of development.

The actions of FSH are restricted to the granulosa cells, as all other ovarian cell types appear to lack FSH receptors. In contrast, LH actions are exerted on both follicle cell types, as well as on cells of the interstitial gland and corpus luteum. Granulosa cells at all stages of follicular development appear to possess FSH receptors, whereas they acquire LH receptors and responsiveness only at later developmental stages. Theca cells acquire LH receptors and responsiveness at considerably earlier stages of follicular development than do granulosa cells.

FSH and LH exert major effects on steroidogenesis in their respective follicle target cells at least in part through activation of membrane-bound adenylate cyclase, thereby increasing the rate of synthesis of cAMP from ATP. The resulting increased intracellular cAMP levels bring about a variety of physiological responses of the cells through coupling mechanisms that generally involve phosphorylation and activation of protein kinases. Steroidogenic responses depend upon the identity and levels of rate-limiting enzymes that the particular target cells possess at the time of stimulation or acquire subsequently.

The earliest steroidogenic response of undifferentiated granulosa cells (those present at early preantral stages of follicle development) to FSH is increased activity of the aromatase enzyme complex. Given an adequate supply of aromatizable androgens (testosterone or androstenedione), the granulosa cells, thus stimulated, are able to increase their rate of synthesis and secretion of estrogens. However, because of an essential absence of the androgen biosynthetic enzymes (17α-hydroxylase:C-17,20-lyase complex) in granulosa cells, estrogen secretion following FSH stimulation depends on an exogenous supply of androgen, and substrate supply becomes the rate-limiting factor *in vivo* and *in vitro* for estrogen biosynthesis by granulosa cells at early developmental stages.

FSH also increases the ability of the granulosa cells to secrete progestins through induction of two other rate-limiting steps in the steroidogenic pathway, cholesterol side-chain cleavage P-450$_{SCC}$ and the Δ^5-3β-hydroxysteroid dehydrogenase:$\Delta^{5\text{-}4}$-isomerase enzyme complex. The cholesterol substrate required by the granulosa cells for progestin production *in vivo* (over and above that provided by low rates of constitutive synthesis in the granulosa cells themselves) is provided in the form of lipoprotein-bound cholesterol reaching the follicle via the blood supply. Lack of vascularization of the granulosa cell layer and essential impermeability of the basement membrane surrounding the granulosa layer to the large lipoprotein molecules limit progesterone production by granulosa cells until later preovulatory stages.

As the follicle matures, plasma membrane receptors for LH and prolactin are acquired by the granulosa cells. FSH appears to be the primary inducer of these receptors, but the induction is enhanced by autocrine and/or paracrine actions of the estrogen produced intracellularly in response to FSH stimulation and acting synergistically with FSH. Once the granulosa cells acquire receptors for LH, this gonadotropin becomes an additional stimulus to cAMP-regulated processes, particularly the further stimulation of the progesterone-synthesizing enzymes.

Androgen production appears to be the principal steroidogenic function of the theca cells. These cells therefore play a major role in enabling production of estrogen by the follicle, as they supply the substrate that is the rate-limiting factor in estrogen biosynthesis by the aromatase enzyme complex in granulosa cells. Since LH is required for significant rates of androgen production by the theca cells, this gonadotropin may be regarded as the primary regulatory factor in controlling estrogen secretion by all but the most immature of follicles. It is this action of LH on theca cells, together with the action of FSH in induction of aromatase activity in granulosa cells, that forms the basis of the "two-cell, two-gonadotropin" theory for control of estrogen secretion in the follicle.

The increased androgen secretion by theca cells, under LH stimulation, appears to be the result of increased activities of two sets of steroidogenic enzymes—the cholesterol side-chain cleavage system and the 17α-hydroxylase:C-17,20-lyase complex. Under certain physiological conditions, when the latter enzyme complex is rate-limiting, the products of the former may accumulate with the result that the theca cells become a significant source of C_{21}-steroid (progestin) secretion. Under other conditions, C_{21}-steroid synthesis may not keep pace with the activity of the 17α-hydroxylase:C-17,20-lyase complex, in which case exogenous progestin of granulosa cell origin may provide significant amounts of the C_{21}-substrate for theca cell androgen output. This then, forms the basis of a second two-cell theory, for follicular steroidogenesis, in which granulosa and theca cells cooperate in the production of androgens by the follicle.

Under certain conditions, in some species more than others, the theca cells appear to possess a sufficient aromatase enzyme system to become a significant source of estrogen secretion as well.

Various steroidal influences on the activities of the steroidogenic enzymes in both granulosa and theca cells come into play as the follicles become more steroidogenically active under the influence of FSH and LH, as summarized in Fig. 5. At least some of the modulating effects of steroids appear to be mediated via intracellular steroid receptor, i.e., the demonstrated existence of estrogen receptors in granulosa cells, and the intraovarian actions of estrogens mentioned above. Other steroid effects appear to occur through direct action on steroidogenic enzymes.

In granulosa cells, the action of FSH in induction of aromatase is enhanced by androgens, as well as by estrogens, and inhibited, under certain circumstances, by 5α-reduced androgens and perhaps by progesterone. The 5α-reduced androgens also act as competitive inhibitors of the aromatase system. Both stimulatory and inhibitory actions of androgens have been reported on FSH-induced progesterone biosynthesis in granulosa cells. The stimulatory action, studied extensively in rat granulosa cells, appears to involve enhancement of FSH induction of the cytochrome P-450$_{SCC}$ and the Δ^5-3β-hydroxysteroid dehydrogenase:$\Delta^{5\text{-}4}$-isomerase enzymes. The inhibitory action, demonstrated with porcine granulosa cells, appears to be primarily at the level of the Δ^5-3β-hydroxysteroid dehydrogenase:$\Delta^{5\text{-}4}$-isomerase complex.

Estrogens have been shown to influence androgen biosynthesis by theca cells, through inhibition at the level of the 17α-hydroxylase:C-17,20-lyase system. This paracrine action of estrogen may function as an intrafollicular negative-feedback system to limit its own production in granulosa cells through regulation of substrate availability.

Prolactin appears to exert inhibitory influences on estrogen biosynthesis, by inhibiting both FSH-induced aromatase activity in granulosa cells and LH-induced androgen production by theca/interstitial cells. A further well-established action of prolactin is its role in stimulating progesterone

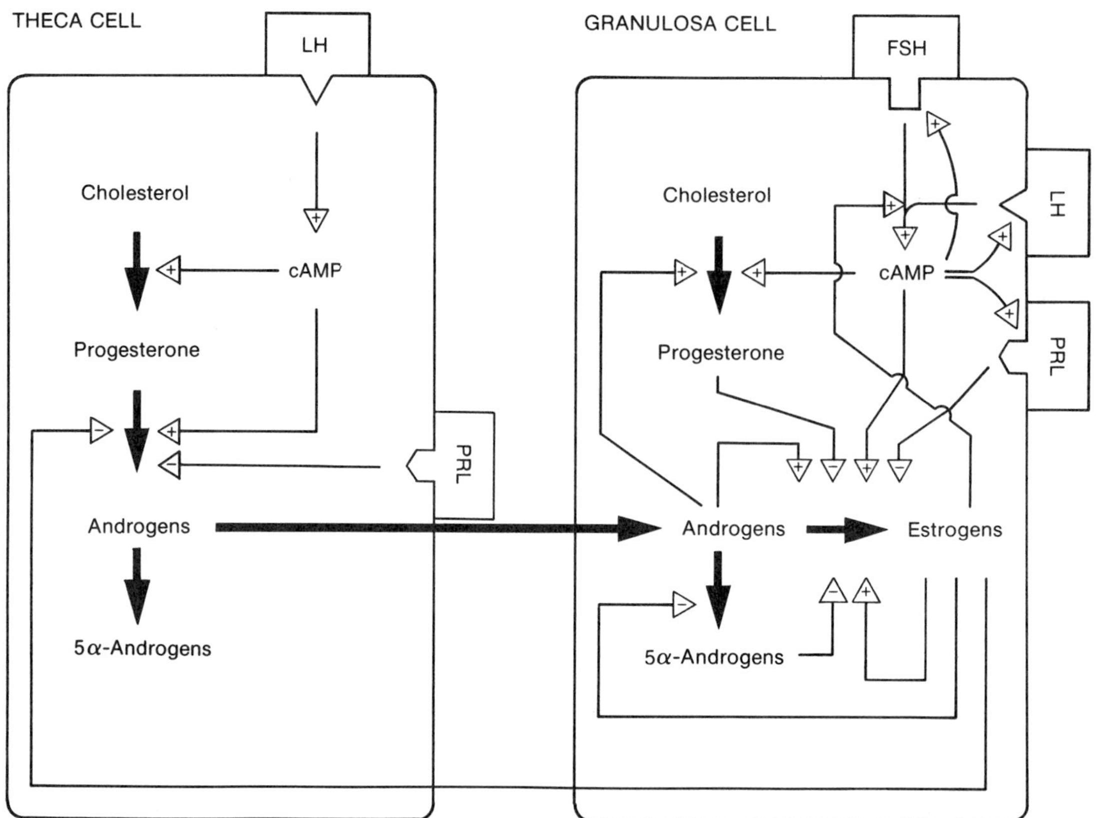

FIG. 5. Principal sites of regulation of follicular steroidogenesis in the rat. The scheme compresses into one diagram the principal regulatory sites of action of gonadotropins and steroids that have been demonstrated either at various stages of follicular maturation *in vivo* or with isolated cell types. (See section on steroidogenesis and its control by cell type for details.) The proposed sequence of events is as follows. Undifferentiated granulosa cells initially respond exclusively to FSH, by a cAMP-dependent mechanism, thereby stimulating activities of enzymes required for the metabolism of cholesterol to progesterone and for the conversion of theca-derived androgens to estrogens. Steroid biosynthesis in the theca cells is stimulated exclusively by LH. As the follicle matures, plasma membrane receptors for LH and prolactin (PRL) are acquired by the granulosa cells as a result of both FSH action and stimulation by estrogen on this process. LH may initially contribute to granulosa cell differentiation by augmenting the various cAMP-dependent processes. A variety of steroidal influences on the activities of steroidogenic enzymes may come into play as the follicles become more biosynthetically active. These effects may occur as the result of receptor-mediated actions of estrogens, androgens, and progesterone, thereby influencing responsiveness to FSH and LH, or steroids may directly alter enzymatic activities; these different actions of steroids are not distinguished in the above scheme. The apparent induction of aromatase activity is augmented by androgenic and estrogenic actions but is inhibited by progestins under certain circumstances. 5α-Reduced metabolites of androgens may competitively inhibit the aromatase enzyme, and estrogens may inhibit 5α-reductase. Prolactin has been shown to inhibit the induction of aromatase activity *in vitro* and also does so *in vivo* under certain physiological conditions, but its role in regulating estrogen synthesis during the ovarian cycle is still uncertain. Androgens may also facilitate the synthesis of progesterone. Following the LH surge, steroid production is briefly stimulated and then suppressed as granulosa and theca cells become desensitized to gonadotropin stimulation. Transiently increased estrogen secretion by granulosa cells causes inhibition of follicular estrogen biosynthesis by inhibiting androgen biosynthesis in the theca cells. Progesterone biosynthetic activity is restored subsequently and increases greatly as follicle cells luteinize.

production by granulosa cells undergoing luteinization during the periovulatory period. The resulting high levels of progesterone may further contribute to the inhibition of estrogen synthesis in the follicle by prolactin.

The cyclic changes in follicular steroid biosynthesis during the estrous or menstrual cycle—as well as the more basal secretion rates of follicular activity during other physiological states such as pregnancy, seasonal and lactational anestrus (or amenorrhea), and prepuberty—can probably be explained on the bases of the coordinated actions of those cellular mechanisms and regulatory agents discussed in this chapter. The physiological importance of the pituitary gonadotropins and prolactin, as well as of the steroidal products of the follicular cells, is widely accepted. There are a number of other regulatory molecules whose specific roles in ovarian regulation are less well established but for which there is mounting evidence, largely from *in vitro* studies with isolated ovarian cells, of at least a supporting or permissive role in follicular regulation. Those we have included in this review are GnRH-like peptides, corticosteroids, insulin and other growth factors, and various neurotransmitters. We have undoubtedly overlooked others of emerging importance. Whether the demonstrated effects of these substances represent physiologically important actions or merely modulations peculiar to the *in vitro* systems remains uncertain. Nevertheless, it is abundantly clear that the follicular microenvironment, as embodied in the fluid of antral follicles, contains a wide array of varied substances (including steroids, eicosanoids, peptides, proteins, glycoproteins, and proteoglycans), some of which have hormonal or other biological activities *in vitro* and which could have significant regulatory effects on gonadotropin action and/or follicular steroidogenesis.

ACKNOWLEDGMENTS

We wish to thank Dr. S.A.J. Daniel for expert assistance in preparing material for portions of this chapter and Dr. M. W. Khalil for valuable discussions. We are also indebted to Mr. G. Barbe, Mrs. H. E. Ross, and Ms. U. Williams for diligent assistance in the preparation of the manuscript. The authors' research is supported by a group grant from the Medical Research Council (MRC) of Canada; D.T.A. is a Career Investigator of the MRC, and R.E.G.-L. is the recipient of a Career Scientist Award from the Ontario Ministry of Health, Health Research Personnel Development Program.

REFERENCES

1. Kellie, A. E. (1984) Structure and nomenclature. In: *Biochemistry of Steroid Hormones,* edited by H. L. J. Makin, pp. 1–19. Blackwell Scientific, Oxford, UK.
2. Doisy, E. A., Veler, C. D., and Thayer, S. (1929): Folliculin from urine of pregnant women. *Am. J. Physiol.,* 90:329–330.
3. MacCorquodale, D. W., Thayer, S. A., and Doisy, E. A. (1936): The isolation of the principal estrogenic substance of liquor folliculi. *J. Biol. Chem.,* 115:435–448.
4. Short, R. V. (1961): Steroid concentrations in the follicular fluid of mares at various stages of the reproductive cycle. *J. Endocrinol.,* 22:153–163.
5. Dehennin, L., Blacker, C., Reiffsteck, A., and Scholler, R. (1984): Estrogen 2-, 4-, 6- or 16-hydroxylation by human follicles shown by gas chromatography-mass spectrometry associated with stable isotope dilution. *J. Steroid Biochem.,* 20:465–471.
6. Silberzahn, P., Almahbobi, G., Dehennin, L., and Merouane, A. (1985): Estrogen metabolite in equine ovarian follicles; gas chromatographic-mass spectrometric determinations in relation to follicular ultrastructure and progestin content. *J. Steroid Biochem.,* 22:501–505.
7. Silberzahn, P., Dehennin, L., Zwain, I., and Reiffsteck, A. (1985): Gas chromatography-mass spectrometry of androgens in equine ovarian follicles at ultrastructurally defined stages of development. Identification of 19-nortestosterone in follicular fluid. *Endocrinology,* 117:2176–2181.
8. Khalil, M. W., and Walton, J. S. (1985): Identification and measurement of 4-oestren-3,17-dione (19-norandrostenedione) in porcine ovarian follicular fluid using high performance liquid chromatography and capillary gas chromatography-mass spectrometry. *J. Endocrinol.,* 107:375–381.
9. Hill, R. T. (1937): Ovaries secrete male hormone. I. Restoration of the castrate type of seminal vesicle and prostate glands to normal by grafts of ovaries in mice. *Endocrinology,* 21:495–502.
10. Short, R. V. (1960): Steroids present in the follicular fluid of the mare. *J. Endocrinol.,* 20:147–156.
11. Ryan, K. J., and Petro, Z. (1966): Steroid biosynthesis by human ovarian granulosa and thecal cells. *J. Clin. Endocrinol. Metab.,* 26:46–52.
12. Springer, C., and Eckstein, B. (1971): Regulation of production in vitro of 5α-androstane-3α,17β-diol in the immature rat ovary. *J. Endocrinol.,* 50:431–439.
13. Zmigrod, A., Lindner, H. R., and Lamprecht, S. A. (1972): Reductase pathways of progesterone metabolism in the rat ovary. *Acta Endocrinol. (Copenh.),* 69:141–152.
14. Karakawa, T., Karachi, K., Aono, T., and Matsumoto, K. (1976): Formation of 5α-reduced C_{19}-steroids from progesterone in vitro by a pathway through 5α-reduced C_{21}-steroids in ovaries of late prepubertal rats. *Endocrinology,* 98:571–579.
15. Tsuji, M., Terada, N., Sato, B., and Matsumoto, K. (1982): 5β- and 5α-reductases for 4-ene-3-ketosteroids in golden hamster ovaries at different stages of development. *J. Steroid Biochem.,* 16:207–213.
16. Gower, D. B. (1972): 16-Unsaturated C_{19}-steroids. A review of their chemistry, biochemistry and possible physiological role. *J. Steroid Biochem.,* 3:45–103.
17. Armstrong, D. T. (1979): Alterations of progesterone metabolism in immature rat ovaries by luteinizing hormone. *Biol. Reprod.,* 21:1025–1033.
18. Fieser, L. F., and Fieser, M. (1959): *Steroids.* Reinhold, New York.
19. Dorfman, R. T., and Ungar, F. (1965): *Metabolism of Steroid Hormones.* Academic, New York.
20. Makin, H. L. J. (ed.) (1984): *Biochemistry of Steroid Hormones.* Blackwell, Oxford, UK.
21. Strauss III, J. F., Schuler, L. A., Rosenblum, M. F., and Tanaka, T. (1981): Cholesterol metabolism by ovarian tissue. *Adv. Lipid Res.,* 18:99–157.
22. Solod, E. A., Armstrong, D. T., and Greep, R. O. (1966): Action of luteinizing hormone on conversion of ovarian cholesterol stores to steroid secreted in vivo and synthesized in vitro by the pseudopregnant rabbit ovary. *Steroids,* 7:607–620.
23. Gwynne, J. T., and Strauss III, J. F. (1982): The role of lipoproteins in steroidogenesis and cholesterol metabolism in steroidogenic glands. *Endocr. Rev.,* 3:299–329.
24. Veldhuis, J. D., Klase, P. A., Strauss III, J. F., and Hammond, J. M. (1982): Facilitative interactions between estradiol and luteinizing hormone in the regulation of progesterone production by cultured swine granulosa cells: relation to cholesterol metabolics. *Endocrinology,* 111:441–447.
25. Rajendran, K. C., Hwang, J., and Menoir, K. M. J. (1983): Binding, degradation and utilization of plasma high density and low density lipoproteins for progesterone production in cultured rat luteal cells. *Endocrinology,* 112:1746–1753.
26. Shalgi, R., Kraicer, P., Renoir, A., Pinto, M., and Soferman, N. (1973): Proteins of human follicular fluid: the blood–follicle barrier. *Fertil. Steril.,* 24:429–434.
27. Chang, S. C. S., Jones, J. D., Ellefson, R. D., and Ryan, R. J. (1976): The porcine ovarian follicle: I. Selected chemical analysis of follicular fluid at different developmental stages. *Biol. Reprod.,* 15:321–328.
28. Simpson, E. R., Rochelle, D. B., Carr, B. R., and MacDonald, P. C. (1980): Plasma lipoproteins in follicular fluid of human ovaries. *J. Clin. Endocrinol. Metab.,* 51:1469–1471.
29. Wang, S. C., and Greenwald, G. S. (1984): Effect of lipoproteins, 25-hydroxycholesterol and luteinizing hormone on in vitro follicular steroidogenesis in the hamster and rat. *Biol. Reprod.,* 31:271–279.
30. Farkash, Y., Timberg, R., and Orly, J. (1986): Preparation of antiserum to rat cytochrome P-450 cholesterol side chain cleavage, and its use for ultrastructural localization of the immunoreactive enzyme by protein A–gold technique. *Endocrinology,* 118:1353–1365.
31. Lieberman, S., Greenfield, N. J., and Wolfson, A. (1984): A heuristic proposal for understanding steroidogeneic processes. *Endocr. Rev.,* 5:128–148.
32. Hall, P. F. (1984): Cellular organization for steroidogenesis. *Int. Rev. Cytol.,* 86:53–95.

33. Gower, D. B. (1984): The role of cytochrome P-450 in steroidogenesis and properties of some of the steroid-transforming enzymes. In: *Biochemistry of Steroid Hormones,* edited by H. L. J. Makin, pp. 230–292. Blackwell Scientific, Oxford, UK.
34. Kautsky, M. P., and Hagerman, D. D. (1980): Kinetic properties of steroid 19-hydroxylase and estrogen synthetase from porcine ovary microsomes. *J. Steroid Biochem.,* 13:1283–1290.
35. Brodie, A. M., Schwarzel, W. C., and Brodie, H. J. (1976): Studies on the mechanism of estrogen biosynthesis in the rat ovary. *J. Steroid Biochem.,* 7:787–793.
36. Mason, N. R. (1970): Steroid A-ring reduction by rat ovaries. *Endocrinology,* 87:350–355.
37. Eckstein, B., and Ravid, R. (1974): On the mechanism of the onset of puberty: identification and pattern of 5α-androstane-3β,17β-diol and its 3α-epimer in peripheral blood of immature female rats. *Endocrinology,* 94:224–229.
38. Mizutani, S., Akashi, S., Terada, N., and Matsumoto, K. (1979): A comparison of metabolism of progesterone to 5α-steroids in monkey, mouse and rat ovaries. *J. Steroid Biochem.,* 10:549–552.
39. Furubayashi, Y., Terada, N., Sato, B., and Matsumoto, K. (1982): Localization of Δ^4-5β- and 5α-reductases and 17β-ol-dehydrogenase in immature golden hamster testis. *Endocrinology,* 111:269–272.
40. Inaba, T., Imori, T., and Matsumoto, K. (1978): Formation of 5α-reduced C_{19}-steroids from progesterone in vivo by 5α-reduced pathway in immature rat ovaries. *J. Steroid Biochem.,* 9:1105–1110.
41. Zmigrod, A., and Lindner, H. R. (1969): Metabolism of progesterone by the rat ovary: formation of 3β-hydroxy-5α-pregnan-20-one by ovarian microsomes. *Acta Endocrinol. (Copenh.),* 61:618–628.
42. Armstrong, D. T., Kraemer, M. A., and Hixon, J. E. (1975): Metabolism of progesterone by rat ovarian tissue: influence of pregnant mare serum gonadotrophin and prolactin. *Biol. Reprod.,* 12:599–608.
43. Ichikawa, S., Morioka, H., and Sawada, T. (1971): Identification of the neutral steroids in the ovarian venous plasma of LH-stimulated rats. *Endocrinology,* 88:372–383.
44. Eckstein, B. (1974): The origin of 5α-androstane-3α,17β-diol and its 3β epimer in peripheral blood of immature female rats. *J. Steroid Biochem.,* 5:577–580.
45. Eckstein, B. (1983): Blood concentrations and biological effects of androstanediols at the onset of puberty in the female rat. *J. Steroid Biochem.,* 19:883–886.
46. Hashimoto, I., and Wiest, W. G. (1969): Luteotrophic and luteolytic mechanisms in rat corpora lutea. *Endocrinology,* 80:886–892.
47. Goldring, N. B., and Orly, J. (1985): Concerted metabolism of steroid hormones produced by cocultured ovarian cell types. *J. Biol. Chem.,* 260:913–920.
48. MacLusky, N. J., Naftolin, F., Krey, L. C., and Franks, S. (1981): The catechol estrogens. *J. Steroid Biochem.,* 15:111–124.
49. Hammond, J. M., Hershey, R. M., Walega, M. A., and Weisz, J. (1986): Catecholestrogen production by porcine ovarian cells. *Endocrinology,* 118:2292–2299.
50. Ball, R., and Knuppen, R. (1980): Catechol oestrogens (2- and 4-hydroxyoestrogen): chemistry, biogenesis, metabolism, occurrence and physiological significance. *Acta Endocrinol. (Copenh.),* 93 (Suppl. 232):1–27.
51. Richards, J. S. (1979): Hormonal control of ovarian follicular development. *Rec. Prog. Horm. Res.,* 35:343–368.
52. Richards, J. S. (1980): Maturation of ovarian follicles: actions and interactions of pituitary and ovarian hormones on follicular cell differentiation. *Physiol. Rev.,* 60:51–89.
53. Robison, G. A., Butcher, R. W., and Sutherland, E. W. (1971): *Cyclic AMP.* Academic, New York.
54. Kuo, J. F., and Greengard, P. (1969): Cyclic nucleotide-dependent protein kinases. IV. Widespread occurrence of adenosine 3′,5′-monophosphate-dependent protein kinase in various tissues and phyla of the animal kingdom. *Proc. Natl. Acad. Sci. USA,* 64:1349–1355.
55. Carnegie, J., and Tsang, B. K. (1983): Follicle-stimulating hormone-regulated granulosa cell steroidogenesis: involvement of the calcium-calmodulin system. *Am. J. Obstet. Gynecol.,* 145:223–228.
56. Byskov, A. G. (1978): The anatomy and ultrastructure of the rete system in the fetal mouse ovary. *Biol. Reprod.,* 19:720–735.
57. Byskov, A. G., and Rasmussen, G. (1973): Ultrastructural studies of the developing follicle. In: *The Development and Maturation of the Ovary and Its Function, International Congress Series No. 267* edited by H. Peters, pp. 55–62. Excerpta Medica, Amsterdam.
58. Bjersing, L. (1967): On the ultrastructure of follicles and isolated follicular granulosa cells of porcine ovary. *Z. Zellforsch. Mikrosk. Anat.,* 82:173–186.
59. Motta, P., and Didio, L. J. A. (1974): Microfilaments in granulosa cells during the follicular development and transformation in corpus luteum in the rabbit ovary. *J. Submicrosc. Cytol.,* 6:15–27.
60. Zamboni, L. (1974): Fine morphology of the follicle wall and follicle cell–oocyte association. *Biol. Reprod.,* 10:125–149.
61. Byskov, A. G. (1975): The role of rete ovarii in meiosis and follicle formation in the cat, mink and ferret. *J. Reprod. Fertil.,* 45:201–289.
62. Amsterdam, A., Koch, Y., Lieberman, M. E., and Lindner, H. R. (1975): Distribution of binding sites for human chorionic gonadotropin in the preovulatory follicle of the rat. *J. Cell Biol.,* 67:894–900.
63. Midgley, Jr., A. R. (1972): Gonadotropin binding to frozen sections of ovarian tissue. In: *Gonadotropins,* edited by B. B. Saxena, C. G. Beling, and H. M. Gandy, pp. 248–260. Wiley-Interscience, New York.
64. Zoller, L. C., and Weisz, J. (1979): A quantitative cytochemical study of glucose-6-phosphate dehydrogenase and Δ^5-3β-hydroxysteroid dehydrogenase activity in membrana granulosa of the ovulable type of follicle of the rat. *Histochemistry,* 62:125–135.
65. Zoller, L. C., and Weisz, J. (1978): Identification of cytochrome P-450 and its distribution in the membrana granulosa of the preovulatory follicle using quantitative cytochemistry. *Endocrinology,* 103:310–313.
66. Erickson, G. F., Hofeditz, C., Unger, M., Allen, W. R., and Dulbecco, R. (1985): A monoclonal antibody to a mammary cell line recognizes two distinct subtypes of ovarian granulosa cells. *Endocrinology,* 117:1490–1499.
67. Kasson, B. G., Median, R., Davoren, J. B., and Hsueh, A. J. W. (1985): Identification of subpopulations of rat granulosa cells: sedimentation properties and hormonal responsiveness. *Endocrinology,* 117:1027–1034.
68. Weakly, B. S. (1966): Electron microscopy of the oocyte and granulosa cells in the developing ovarian follicles of the golden hamster. *J. Anat.,* 100:503–534.
69. Hoage, T. R., and Cameron, I. L. (1976): Folliculogenesis in the ovary of the mature mouse: an autoradiographic study. *Anat. Rec.,* 184:699–710.
70. Høyer, P. E., and Byskov, A. G. (1981): A quantitative cytochemical study of Δ^5, 3β-hydroxysteroid dehydrogenase activity in the rete system of the immature mouse ovary. In: *Development and Function of Reproductive Organs,* edited by A. G. Byskov and H. Peters, pp. 216–224. Excerpta Medica, Amsterdam.
71. Quattropani, S. L. (1973): Morphogenesis of the ovarian interstitial tissue in the neonatal mouse. *Anat. Rec.,* 177:569–584.
72. Mori, H., and Matsumoto, K. (1970): On the histogenesis of the ovarian interstitial gland in rabbits. I. Primary interstitial gland. *Am. J. Anat.,* 129:289–306.
73. Kingsbury, B. F. (1939): Atresia and the interstitial cells of the ovary. *Am. J. Anat.,* 65:309–331.
74. Dawson, A. B., and McCabe, M. (1951): The interstitial tissue of the ovary in infantile and juvenile rat. *J. Morphol.,* 88:543–571.
75. Rennels, E. G. (1951): Influence of hormones on the histochemistry of ovarian interstitial tissue in the immature rat. *Am. J. Anat.,* 88:63–108.
76. Deanesly, R. (1972): Origins and development of interstitial tissue in ovaries in rabbit and guinea-pig. *J. Anat.,* 113:251–260.
77. Guraya, S. S., and Greenwald, G. S. (1968): A comparative histochemical study of interstitial tissue and follicular atresia in the mammalian ovary. *Anat. Rec.,* 149:411–434.
78. McNatty, K. P. (1981): Hormonal correlates of follicular development in the human ovary. *Aust. J. Biol. Sci.,* 34:249–268.
79. Bélanger, A., Cusan, L., Caron, S., Barden, N., and Dupont, A. (1981): Ovarian progestins, androgens and estrogen throughout the 4-day estrous cycle in the rat. *Biol. Reprod.,* 24:591–596.
80. Sridaran, R., and Gibori, G. (1983): Intraovarian localization of luteinizing hormone/human chorionic gonadotropin stimulation of testosterone and estradiol synthesis in the pregnant rat. *Endocrinology,* 112:1770–1776.

81. Dennefors, B. L., Janson, P., Knutson, F., and Hamberger, L. (1980): Steroid production and responsiveness to gonadotrophin in isolated stromal tissue of human menopausal ovaries. *Am. J. Obstet. Gynecol.*, 136:997–1002.
82. Longcope, C., Hunter, R., and Franz, C. (1980): Steroid secretion by the postmenopausal ovary. *Am. J. Obstet. Gynecol.*, 138:564–568.
83. Dyer, C. A., Erickson, G. F., and Curtiss, L. K. (1985): Functional heterogeneity in the ability of high density lipoproteins to enhance gonadotropin-induced androgen production in cultured rat theca-interstitial cells. In: *Lipoprotein and Cholesterol Metabolism in Steroidogenic Tissues*, edited by J. F. Strauss III and K. M. J. Menon, pp. 141–146. Strickley, Philadelphia.
84. Aakvaag, A. (1969): Pathways in the biosynthesis of androstenedione in the human ovary in vitro. *Acta Endocrinol. (Copenh.)*, 60:517–526.
85. Lacroix, E., Eechaute, W., and Leusen, I. (1974): The biosynthesis of oestrogens by cow follicles. *Steroids*, 23:337–356.
86. Magoffin, D. A., and Erickson, G. F. (1982): Primary culture of differentiating ovarian androgen-producing cells in defined medium. *J. Biol. Chem.*, 257:4507–4513.
87. Zeleznik, A. J., Midgley Jr., A. R., and Reichert Jr., L. E. (1974): Granulosa cell maturation in the rat: increased binding of human chorionic gonadotropin following treatment with follicle-stimulating hormone in vivo. *Endocrinology*, 95:818–825.
88. Lindner, H. R., Amsterdam, A., Salomon, Y., Tsafriri, A., Nimrod, A., Lamprecht, S. A., Zor, U., and Koch, Y. (1977): Intraovarian factors in ovulation: determinants of follicular response to gonadotropins. *J. Reprod. Fertil.*, 51:215–235.
89. Zeleznik, A. J., Schuler, H. M., and Reichert Jr., L. E. (1981): Gonadotropin-binding sites in the rhesus monkey ovary: role of the vasculature in the selective distribution of human chorionic gonadotropin in the preovulatory follicle. *Endocrinology*, 109:356–362.
90. Oxberry, B. A., and Greenwald, G. S. (1982): An autoradiographic study of the binding of ^{125}I-labelled follicle-stimulating hormone, human chorionic gonadotrophin and prolactin to the hamster ovary throughout the estrous cycle. *Biol. Reprod.*, 27:505–516.
91. Shaha, C., and Greenwald, G. S. (1983): Development of steroidogenic activity in the ovary of the prepubertal hamster. I. Response to in vivo or in vitro exposure to gonadotropins. *Biol. Reprod.*, 28:1231–1241.
92. Uilenbroek, J. T. J., and van der Linden, R. (1983): Changes in gonadotrophin binding to rat ovaries during sexual maturation. *Acta Endocrinol. (Copenh.)*, 104:413–419.
93. Henderson, K. M., Kieboom, L. E., McNatty, K. P., Lun, S., and Heath, D. A. (1984): ^{125}I-HCG binding to bovine thecal tissue from healthy and atretic antral follicles. *Mol. Cell. Endocrinol.*, 34:91–98.
94. Hamberger, L., Hillensjö, T., and Ahren, K. (1978): Steroidogenesis in isolated cells of preovulatory rat follicles. *Endocrinology*, 103:771–777.
95. Weiss, T. J., Armstrong, D. T., McIntosh, J. E. A., and Seamark, R. F. (1978): Maturational changes in sheep ovarian follicles: gonadotrophic stimulation of cyclic AMP production by isolated theca and granulosa cells. *Acta Endocrinol. (Copenh.)*, 89:158–165.
96. Tsang, B. K., Moon, Y. S., Simpson, C. W., and Armstrong, D. T. (1979): Androgen biosynthesis in human ovarian follicles: cellular source, gonadotropic control, and andenosine 3′,5′-monophosphate mediation. *J. Clin. Endocrinol. Metab.*, 48:153–158.
97. Erickson, G. F., Magoffin, D. A., Dyer, C. A., and Hofeditz, C. (1985): The ovarian androgen producing cells: a review of structure/function relationships. *Endocr. Rev.*, 6:371–399.
98. Erickson, G. F., and Ryan, K. J. (1976): Stimulation of testosterone production in isolated rabbit thecal tissue by LH/FSH, dibutyryl cyclic AMP, $PGF_{2\alpha}$, and PGE_2. *Endocrinology*, 99:452–458.
99. Tsang, B. K., Armstrong, D. T., and Whitfield, J. F. (1980): Steroid biosynthesis by isolated human ovarian follicular cells in vitro. *J. Clin. Endocrinol. Metab.*, 51:1407–1411.
100. Fukuda, S., Terakawa, N., Sato, B., Imori, T., and Matsumoto, K. (1979): Hormonal regulation of activities of 17β-ol-dehydrogenases, aromatase and 4-ene-5α-reductase in immature ovaries. *J. Steroid Biochem.*, 11:1421–1427.
101. Aono, T., Kitamura, Y., Fukuda, S., and Matsumoto, K. (1981): Localization of 4-ene-5α-reductase, 17β-ol-dehydrogenase and aromatase in immature rat ovary. *J. Steroid Biochem.*, 14:1369–1377.
102. Bogovich, K., and Richards, J. S. (1982): Androgen biosynthesis in developing ovarian follicles: evidence that luteinizing hormone regulates thecal 17α-hydroxylase and C_{17-20}-lyase activities. *Endocrinology*, 111:1201–1208.
103. Makris, A., and Ryan, K. J. (1980): The source of follicular androgen in the hamster follicle. *Steroids*, 35:53–64.
104. Lieberman, M. E., Barnea, A., Bauminger, S., Tsafriri, A., Collins, W. P., and Lindner, H. R. (1975): LH effect on the pattern of steroidogenesis in cultured Graafian follicles of the rat: dependence on macromolecular synthesis. *Endocrinology*, 96:1533–1542.
105. Rodgers, R. J., Waterman, M. R., and Simpson, E. R. (1986): Cytochromes $P\text{-}450_{scc}$, $P\text{-}450_{17\alpha}$, adrenodoxin, and reduced nicotinamide adenine dinucleotide phosphate-cytochrome P-450 reductase in bovine follicles and corpora lutea. Changes in specific contents during the ovarian cycle. *Endocrinology*, 118:1366–1374.
106. Makris, A., and Ryan, K. J. (1975): Progesterone, androstenedione, testosterone, estrone, and estradiol synthesis in hamster ovarian follicle cells. *Endocrinology*, 96:694–701.
107. Evans, G., Dobias, M., King, G. J., and Armstrong, D. T. (1981): Estrogen, androgen, and progesterone biosynthesis by theca and granulosa of preovulatory follicles in the pig. *Biol. Reprod.*, 25:673–682.
108. McNatty, K. P., Heath, D. A., Lun, S., Fanin, J. M., McDiarmid, J. M., and Henderson, K. M. (1984): Steroidogenesis by bovine theca interna in an in vitro perfusion system. *Biol. Reprod.*, 30:159–170.
109. Fortune, J. E., and Hansel, W. (1985): Concentrations of steroids and gonadotropins in follicular fluid from normal heifers and heifers primed for superovulation. *Biol. Reprod.*, 32:1069–1079.
110. McNatty, K. P., Makris, A., Reinhold, V. N., DeGrazia, C., Osathanondh, R., and Ryan, K. J. (1979): Metabolism of androstenedione by human ovarian tissues in vitro with particular references to reductase and aromatase activity. *Steroids*, 34:429–443.
111. McNatty, K. P., Makris, A., Osathanondh, R., and Ryan, K. J. (1980): Effects of luteinizing hormone on steroidogenesis by thecal tissue from human ovarian follicles in vitro. *Steroids*, 36:53–63.
112. Lerner, N., and Eckstein, B. (1976): Identification of two 5α-reduced pregnanes as major metabolites of progesterone in immature rat ovaries (1000 × g supernatant) in vitro. *Endocrinology*, 98:179–188.
113. Bogovich, K., Scales, L. M., Higginbottom, E., Ewing, L. L., and Richards, J. S. (1986): Short term androgen production by rat ovarian follicles and long term steroidogenesis by thecal explants in culture. *Endocrinology*, 118:1379–1386.
114. Eckstein, B., Mechoulam, R., and Burstein, S. H. (1970): The identification of 5α-androstane-3α,17β-diol as a principal metabolite of pregnenolone in rat ovary at the onset of puberty. *Nature*, 228:866–868.
115. Suzuki, K., Kawakura, K., and Tamaoki, B. I. (1978): Effect of pregnant mare's serum gonadotrophin on the activities of 5α-reductase, aromatase, and other enzymes in the ovaries of immature rats. *Endocrinology*, 102:1595–1605.
116. Eckstein, B., and Ravid, R. (1979): Changes in pathways of steroid production taking place in the rat ovary around the time of the first ovulation. *J. Steroid Biochem.*, 11:593–597.
117. Eckstein, B., Golan, R., and Mishinsky, J. S. (1973): Onset of puberty in the immature female rat induced by 5α-androstane-3β,17β-diol. *Endocrinology*, 92:941–945.
118. Eckstein, B., and Springer, C. (1971): Induction of an ovarian epimerase system catalyzing the transformation of 5α-androstane-3α,17β-diol to 5α-androstane-3β,17β-diol after treatment of immature rats with gonadotropins exhibiting FSH-like activity. *Endocrinology*, 89:347–352.
119. Florensa, E., Sommerville, I. F., Harrison, R. F., Johnson, M. W., and Youssefnejadian, E. (1976): Plasma 20α-dihydroprogesterone, progesterone and 17-hydroxyprogesterone: daily and four-hourly variations during the menstrual cycle. *J. Steroid Biochem.*, 7:769–777.
120. Holmdahl, T. H., and Johansson, E. D. B. (1972): Peripheral plasma levels of 17α-hydroxyprogesterone, progesterone and oestradiol during normal menstrual cycles in women. *Acta Endocrinol. (Copenh.)*, 71:743–754.
121. Aedo, A. R., Langren, B. M., Cekan, Z., and Diczfalusy, E. (1976): Studies on the pattern of circulating steroids in the normal menstrual cycle. *Acta Endocrinol. (Copenh.)*, 82:600–616.

122. Ryan, K. J., Petro, Z., and Kaiser, J. (1968): Steroid formation by isolated and recombined ovarian granulosa and theca cells. *J. Clin. Endocrinol. Metab.*, 28:355–358.
123. Channing, C. P. (1969): Steroidogenesis and morphology of human ovarian cell types in tissue culture. *J. Endocrinol.*, 45:297–308.
124. Batta, S. K., Wentz, A. C., and Channing, C. P. (1980): Steroidogenesis by human ovarian cell types in culture: influence of mixing of cell types and effect of added testosterone. *J. Clin. Endocrinol. Metab*, 50:274–279.
125. Channing, C. P., Wentz, A. C., and Jones, G. (1978): Steroid secretion by monkey and human ovarian cell types in vivo and in vitro. In: *Symposium on the Ovary held in Fresnes, France,* edited by R. Scholler, pp. 71–86. Editions Sepe, Paris.
126. Ryan, K. J., and Short, R. V. (1965): Formation of estradiol by granulosa and thecal cells of the equine ovarian follicle. *Endocrinology,* 76:108–114.
127. Channing, C. P., and Grieves, S. A. (1969): Studies on tissue culture of equine ovarian cell types: steroidogenesis. *J. Endocrinol.*, 43:391–402.
128. Armstrong, D. T., Weiss, T. J., Selstam, G., and Seamark, R. F. (1981): Hormonal and cellular interactions in follicular steroid biosynthesis by the sheep ovary. *J. Reprod. Fertil. (Suppl. 30)*, 30:143–154.
129. Moon, Y. S., Tsang, B. K., Simpson, C., and Armstrong, D. T. (1978): 17β-Estradiol biosynthesis in cultured granulosa and thecal cells of human ovarian follicles: stimulation by follicle-stimulating hormone. *J. Clin. Endocrinol. Metab.*, 47:263–267.
130. Hillier, S. G. (1981): Regulation of follicular oestrogen biosynthesis: a survey of current concepts. *J. Endocrinol.*, 89:3P–18P.
131. Hillier, S. G., van den Boogaard, A. J. M., Reichert Jr., L. E., and van Hall, E. V. (1981): Control of preovulatory follicular estrogen biosynthesis in the human ovary. *J. Clin. Endocrinol. Metab.*, 52:847–856.
132. Mossman, H. W., Koering, M. J., and Ferry Jr., D. (1964): Cyclic changes of interstitial gland tissue of the human ovary. *Am. J. Anat.*, 115:235–256.
133. Leymarie, P., and Savard, K. (1968): Steroid hormone formation in the human ovary. VI. Evidence for two pathways of synthesis of androgens in the stromal compartment. *J. Clin. Endocrinol. Metab.*, 28:1547–1554.
134. Marsh, J. M., Savard, K., and LeMaire, W. J. (1976): Steroidogenic capacities of the different compartments of the human ovary. In: *The Endocrine Function of The Human Ovary,* edited by V. H. T. James, M. Serio, and G. Giusti, pp. 37–45. Academic, London.
135. McNatty, K. P., Makris, A., De Grazia, C., Osathanondh, R., and Ryan, K. J. (1980): Steroidogenesis by recombined follicular cells from the human ovary in vitro. *J. Clin. Endocrinol. Metab.*, 51:1286–1292.
136. Dorrington, J. H., Moon, Y. S., and Armstrong, D. T. (1975): Estradiol-17β biosynthesis in cultured granulosa cells from hypophysectomized immature rats; stimulation by follicle-stimulating hormone. *Endocrinology,* 97:1328–1331.
137. Gore-Langton, R. E., and Dorrington, J. H. (1981): FSH induction of aromatase in cultured rat granulosa cells measured by a radiometric assay. *Mol. Cell. Endocrinol.*, 22:135–151.
138. Wang, C., Hsueh, A. J. W., and Erickson, G. F. (1982): The role of cyclic AMP in the induction of estrogen and progestin synthesis in cultured granulosa cells. *Mol. Cell. Endocrinol.*, 25:73–83.
139. Mendelson, C. R., Durham, C., Evans, C., and Simpson, E. R. (1985): The induction of aromatase activity in estrogen-producing cells is mediated by the increased synthesis of aromatase cytochrome P-450. *67th Annual Meeting of The Endocrine Society,* p. 77 (Abstr. 307).
140. Durham, C. R., Zhu, H., Masters, B. S. S., Simpson, E. R., and Mendelson, C. R. (1985): Regulation of aromatase activity of rat granulosa cells: induction of synthesis of NADPH-cytochrome P-450 reductase by FSH and dibutyryl cyclic AMP. *Mol. Cell. Endocrinol.*, 40:211–219.
141. Dorrington, J. H., and Armstrong, D. T. (1979): Effect of FSH on gonadal functions. *Rec. Prog. Horm. Res.*, 35:301–342.
142. Hillier, S. G., Zeleznik, A. J., and Ross, G. T. (1978): Independence of steroidogenic capacity and luteinizing hormone receptor induction in developing granulosa cells. *Endocrinology,* 102:937–946.
143. Armstrong, D. T., and Dorrington, J. H. (1976): Androgens augment FSH-induced progesterone secretion by cultured rat granulosa cells. *Endocrinology,* 99:1411–1414.
144. Nimrod, A. (1977): Studies on the synergistic effect of androgen on the stimulation of progestin secretion by FSH in cultured rat granulosa cells: a search for the mechanism of action. *Mol. Cell. Endocrinol.*, 8:201–211.
145. Nimrod, A., and Lindner, H. R. (1976): A synergistic effect of androgen on the stimulation of progesterone secretion by FSH in cultured rat granulosa cells. *Mol. Cell. Endocrinol.*, 5:315–320.
146. McNatty, K. P., Makris, A., De Grazia, C., Osathanondh, R., and Ryan, K. J. (1979): The production of progesterone, androgens and oestrogens by human granulosa cells in vitro and in vivo. *J. Steroid Biochem.*, 11:775–779.
147. Channing, C. P. (1974): Temporal effects of LH, hCG, FSH and dibutyryl cyclic 3′,5′-AMP upon luteinization of rhesus monkey granulosa cells in culture. *Endocrinology,* 94:1215–1223.
148. Hammond, R. W., Burke, W. H., and Hertelendy, F. (1981): Influence of follicular maturation of progesterone release in chicken granulosa cells in response to turkey and ovine gonadotropins. *Biol. Reprod.*, 24:1048–1055.
149. Hillensjö, T., Magnusson, C., Svensson, U., and Thelander, H. (1981): Effects of luteinizing hormone and follicle-stimulating hormone on progesterone synthesis by cultured rat cumulus cells. *Endocrinology,* 108:1920–1924.
150. Wang, C., Hsueh, A. J. W., and Erickson, G. F. (1981): LH stimulation of estrogen secretion in cultured granulosa cells. *Mol. Cell. Endocrinol.*, 24:17–28.
151. Chang, S. C. S., Jones, J. D., Ellefson, R. D., and Ryan, R. J. (1976): The porcine ovarian follicle. I. Selected chemical analysis of follicular fluid at different developmental stages. *Biol. Reprod.*, 15:321–328.
152. Carr, B. R., MacDonald, P. C., and Simpson, E. R. (1982): The role of lipoproteins in the regulation of progesterone secretion by the human corpus luteum. *Fertil. Steril.*, 38:303–311.
153. Jones, P. B. C., and Hsueh, A. J. W. (1982): Pregnenolone biosynthesis by cultured granulosa cells: modulation by follicle-stimulating hormone and gonadotropin-releasing hormone. *Endocrinology,* 111:713–721.
154. Toaff, M.E ., Strauss III, J. F., and Hammond, J. M. (1983): Regulation of cytochrome $P\text{-}450_{SCC}$ in immature porcine granulosa cells by FSH and estradiol. *Endocrinology,* 112:1156–1158.
155. Boyd, G. S., Arthur, J. R., Beckett, G. J., Mason, J. I., and Trzeciak, W. H. (1975): The role of cholesterol and cytochrome P-450 in the cholesterol side-chain cleavage reaction in adrenal cortex and corpora lutea. *J. Steroid Biochem.*, 6:427–436.
156. Robinson, J., Stevenson, P. M., Boyd, G. S., and Armstrong, D. T. (1975): Acute in vivo effects of hCG and LH on ovarian mitochondrial cholesterol utilization. *Mol. Cell. Endocrinol.*, 2:149–155.
157. Mori, M., and Marsh, J. M. (1982): The site of luteinizing hormone stimulation of steroidogenesis in mitochondria of the rat corpus luteum. *J. Biol. Chem.*, 257:6178–6183.
158. Naumoff, P. A., and Stevenson, P. M. (1981): The differential development of mitochondrial cytochrome P-450 and the respiratory cytochromes in rat ovary. *Biochim. Biophys. Acta,* 673:359–365.
159. Schuler, L. A., Toaff, M. E., and Strauss III, J. F. (1981): Regulation of ovarian cholesterol metabolism: control of 3-hydroxy-3-methylglutaryl coenzyme A reductase and acyl coenzyme A:cholesterol acyltransferase. *Endocrinology,* 108:1476–1486.
160. Behrman, H. R., and Armstrong, D. T. (1969): Cholesterol esterase stimulation by luteinizing hormone in luteinized rat ovaries. *Endocrinology,* 85:474–480.
161. Caffrey, J. L., Fletcher, P. W., Diekman, M. A., O'Callaghan, P. L., and Niswender, G. D. (1979): The activity of ovine luteal cholesterol esterase during several experimental conditions. *Biol. Reprod.*, 21:601–608.
162. Henderson, K. M., Gorban, A. M. S., and Boyd, G. S. (1981): Effect of LH factors regulating ovarian cholesterol metabolism and progesterone synthesis in PMSG-primed immature rats. *J. Reprod. Fertil.*, 61:373–380.
163. Hwang, J., and Menon, J. M. J. (1983): Characterization of low density and high density lipoprotein receptors in the rat corpus luteum and regulation by gonadotropin. *J. Biol. Chem.*, 258:8020–8027.

164. Jones, P. B. C., Valk, C. A., and Hsueh, A. J. W. (1983): Regulation of progestin biosynthetic enzymes in cultured rat granulosa cells: Effects of prolactin, β_2-adrenergic agonist, human chorionic gonadotropin and gonadotropin-releasing hormone. *Biol. Reprod.*, 29:572–585.
165. Rubin, B. L., Deane, H. W., Hamilton, J. A., and Driks, E. C. (1963): Changes in Δ^5-3β-hydroxysteroid dehydrogenase activity in the ovaries of maturing rats. *Endocrinology*, 72:924–930.
166. Koritz, S. B. (1967): On the regulation of pregnenolone synthesis. In: *Functions of the Adrenal Cortex*, edited by K. McKerns, pp. 27–48. Appleton-Century-Crofts, New York.
167. Madej, E. (1980): Effect of exogenous hormones on the activity of Δ^5-3β-hydroxysteroid dehydrogenase in cultured granulosa cells from proestrous and preovulatory rat ovarian follicles. *Acta Histochem.*, 67:253–260.
168. Neville, A. M., and Engel, L. L. (1968): Steroid Δ-isomerase of the bovine adrenal gland: kinetics, activation by NAD and attempted solubilization. *Endocrinology*, 83:864–872.
169. Philpott, J. E., and Peron, F. G. (1971): A microassay procedure for Δ^5-3β-hydroxysteroid dehydrogenase based on substrate depletion. *Endocrinology*, 88:1082–1085.
170. Dorrington, J. H., McKeracher, H. L., Chan, A., and Gore-Langton, R. E. (1984): Luteinizing hormone-releasing hormone independently stimulates cytodifferentiation of granulosa cells. In: *Hormonal Control of The Hypothalamo-pituitary-gonadal Axis. Biochemical Endocrinology Series*, edited by K. W. McKerns and Z. Naor, pp. 467–478. Plenum, New York.
171. Lischinsky, A., Evans, G., and Armstrong, D. T. (1983): Site of androgen inhibition of FSH-stimulated progesterone production in porcine granulosa cells. *Endocrinology*, 113:1999–2003.
172. Eckstein, B., and Nimrod, A. (1979): Effect of human chorionic gonadotropin and prolactin on 20α-hydroxysteroid dehydrogenase activity in granulosa cells of immature rat ovary. *Endocrinology*, 104:711–714.
173. Jones, P. B. C., and Hsueh, A. J. W. (1981): Direct stimulation of ovarian progesterone metabolizing enzyme by gonadotropin-releasing hormone in cultured granulosa cells. *J. Biol. Chem.*, 256:1248–1254.
174. Eckstein, B., Raanan, M., Lerner, N., Cohen, S., and Nimrod, A. (1977): The appearance of 20α-hydroxysteroid dehydrogenase activity in preovulatory follicles of immature rats treated with pregnant mare serum gonadotropin. *J. Steroid Biochem.*, 8:213–216.
175. Hickman-Smith, D., and Kuhn, N. J. (1976): A proposed sequence of hormones controlling the induction of luteal 20α-hydroxysteroid dehydrogenase and progesterone withdrawal in the late-pregnant rat. *Biochem. J.*, 160:663–670.
176. Loewit, K., and Zambelis, N. (1979): Progesterone and 20α-hydroxysteroid dehydrogenase regulation in the corpus luteum of the pregnant rat. *Acta Endocrinol. (Copenh.)*, 90:176–184.
177. Suzuki, K., and Tamaoki, B. I. (1979): Enzymological studies of rat luteinized ovaries in relation to acute reduction of aromatizable androgen formation and stimulated production of progestins. *Endocrinology*, 104:1317–1323.
178. Wiest, W. G. (1959): Conversion of progesterone to 4-pregn-20α-ol-3-one by rat ovarian tissue in vitro. *J. Biol. Chem.*, 234:3115–3121.
179. Wiest, W. G., Kidwell, W. R., and Kirschbaum, T. H. (1963): Induction of rat ovarian 20α-hydroxysteroid dehydrogenase activity by gonadotrophic hormone administration. *Steroids*, 2:617–630.
180. Csapo, A. I., and Wiest, W. G. (1969): An examination of the quantitative relationship between progesterone and the maintenance of pregnancy. *Endocrinology*, 85:735–746.
181. Wiest, W. G. (1968): On the function of 20α-hydroxypregn-4-en-3-one during parturition in the rat. *Endocrinology*, 83:1181–1184.
182. Diaz-Zagoya, J. C., Wiest, W. G., and Arias, F. (1979): 20α-Hydroxysteroid oxidoreductase activity and 20α-dihydroprogesterone concentration in human placenta before and after parturition. *Am. J. Obstet. Gynecol.*, 133:673–676.
183. Loutfi, G., Peron, F., and Dorfman, R. I. (1962): Formation of 20α-hydroxy-Δ^4-pregnen-3-one and Δ^4-androsten-3,17-dione in rodent ovaries. *Endocrinology*, 71:983–985.
184. Savard, K., Marsh, J. M., and Rice, B. F. (1965): Gonadotropins and ovarian steroidogenesis. *Rec. Prog. Horm. Res.*, 21:285–356.
185. Eckstein, B., and Lerner, N. (1977): Changes in ovarian 5α-steroid reductase and 20α-hydroxysteroid dehydrogenase activity produced by induction of first ovulation with gonadotropin. *Biochim. Biophys. Acta*, 489:143–149.
186. Epstein-Almog, R., and Orly, J. (1985): Inhibition of hormone-induced steroidogenesis during cell proliferation in serum-free cultures of rat granulosa cells. *Endocrinology*, 116:2103–2112.
187. Short, R. V. (1962): Steroids in the follicular fluid and the corpus luteum of the mare: A "two-cell type" theory of ovarian steroid synthesis. *J. Endocrinol.*, 24:59–63.
188. Bjersing, L., and Carstensen, H. (1967): Biosynthesis of steroids by granulosa cells of the porcine ovary in vitro. *J. Reprod. Fertil.*, 14:101–111.
189. Younglai, E. V., and Short, R. V. (1970): Pathways of steroid biosynthesis in the intact Graafian follicle of mares in oestrus. *J. Endocrinol.*, 47:321–331.
190. Fortune, J. E., and Armstrong, D. T. (1978): Hormonal control of 17β-estradiol biosynthesis in proestrous rat follicles: estradiol production by isolated theca versus granulosa cells. *Endocrinology*, 102:227–235.
191. Fowler, R. E., Fox, N. L., Edwards, R. G., Walters, D. E., and Steptoe, P. C. (1978): Steroidogenesis by cultured granulosa cells aspirated from human follicles using pregnenolone and androgen as precursors. *J. Endocrinol.*, 77:171–183.
192. Johnson, D. C., and Hoversland, R. C. (1983): Oestradiol synthesis by granulosa cells from immature rats treated with pregnant mare's serum gonadotrophin. *Acta Endocrinol. (Copenh.)*, 104:74–79.
193. Bjersing, L., and Carstensen, H. (1964): The role of the granulosa in the biosynthesis of ovarian steroids. *Biochim. Biophys. Acta*, 86:637–639.
194. Moor, R. M. (1977): Sites of steroid production in ovine Graafian follicles in culture. *J. Endocrinol.*, 73:143–150.
195. Nimrod, A., Rosenfield, R. L., and Otto, P. (1980): Relationship of androgen action to androgen metabolism in isolated rat granulosa cells. *J. Steroid Biochem.*, 13:1015–1019.
196. Moon, Y. S., and Duleba, A. J. (1982): Comparative studies of androgen metabolism in theca and granulosa cells of human follicles in vitro. *Steroids*, 39:419–430.
197. Terakawa, N., Kondo, K., Aono, T., Kurachi, K., and Matsumoto, K. (1978): Hormonal regulation of 4-ene-5α-reductase activity in prepubertal rat ovaries. *J. Steroid Biochem.*, 9:307–311.
198. Allen, E., and Doisy, E. A. (1927): Ovarian and placental hormones. *Physiol. Rev.*, 7:600–650.
199. Mossman, H. W. (1937): The thecal gland and its relation to the reproductive cycle. A study of the cyclic changes in the ovary of the pocket gopher, *Geomys Bursarius* (Shaw). *Am. J. Anat.*, 61:289–319.
200. Corner, G. W. (1983): The sites of formation of estrogenic substances in the animal body. *Physiol. Rev.*, 18:154–172.
201. Hisaw, F. L. (1947): Development of the Graafian follicle and ovulation. *Physiol. Rev.*, 27:95–119.
202. Allen, E. (1941): Glandular physiology and therapy. *JAMA*, 116:405–413.
203. Falck, B. (1959): Site of production of oestrogen in rat ovary as studied in micro-transplants. *Acta Physiol. Scand. Suppl. 47*, 163:1–101.
204. Greep, R. O., van Dyke, H. B., and Chow, B. F. (1942): Gonadotropins of the swine pituitary. I. Various biological effects of purified thylakentrin (FSH) and pure metakentrin (ICSH). *Endocrinology*, 30:635–649.
205. Hollander, N., and Hollander, V. (1958): The effect of follicle-stimulating hormone on the biosynthesis in vitro of estradiol-17β from acetate-1-C^{14} and testosterone-4-C^{14}. *J. Biol. Chem.*, 233:1097–1099.
206. Mills, T. M., Davies, P. J. A., and Savard, K. (1971): Stimulation of estrogen synthesis in rabbit follicles by luteinizing hormone. *Endocrinology*, 88:857–862.
207. Moon, Y. S., Dorrington, J. H., and Armstrong, D. T. (1975): Stimulatory action of follicle-stimulating hormone on estradiol-17β secretion by hypophysectomized rat ovaries in organ culture. *Endocrinology*, 97:244–247.
208. Dorrington, J. H., and Armstrong, D. T. (1975): Follicle-stimulating hormone stimulates estradiol-17β synthesis in cultured Sertoli cells. *Proc. Natl. Acad. Sci. USA*, 72:2677–2681.

209. Armstrong, D. T., and Papkoff, H. (1976): Stimulation of aromatization of exogenous and endogenous androgens in ovaries of hypophysectomized rats in vivo by follicle-stimulating hormone. *Endocrinology,* 99:1144–1151.
210. Baird, D. T. (1977): Evidence in vivo for the two-cell hypothesis of ovarian estrogen synthesis by the sheep Graafian follicle. *J. Reprod. Fertil.,* 50:183–185.
211. Fowler, R. E., Fox, N. L., Edwards, R. G., and Steptoe, P. C. (1978): Steroid production from 17α-hydroxypregnenolone and dehydroepiandrosterone by human granulosa cells in vitro. *J. Reprod. Fertil.,* 54:109–117.
212. Fortune, J. E., and Armstrong, D. T. (1977): Androgen production by theca and granulosa isolated from proestrous rat follicles. *Endocrinology,* 100:1341–1347.
213. Short, R. V. (1962): Steroids present in the follicular fluid of the cow. *J. Endocrinol.,* 23:401–411.
214. Fortune, J. E. (1981): Bovine theca and granulosa cells interact to promote androgen and progestin production. *Biol. Reprod. (Suppl. 1),* 24:39A (abstr. 33).
215. Lischinsky, A., and Armstrong, D. T. (1983): Granulosa cell stimulation of thecal androgen synthesis. *Can. J. Physiol. Pharmacol.,* 61:472–477.
216. Pencharz, R. I. (1940): Effect of estrogens and androgens alone and in combination with chorionic gonadotropin on the ovary of the hypophysectomized rat. *Science,* 91:554–555.
217. Williams, P. C. (1940): Effect of stilbestrol on the ovaries of hypophysectomized rats. *Nature,* 145:388–389.
218. Simpson, M. E., Evans, H. M., Fraenkel-Conrat, H. L., and Li, C. H. (1941): Synergism of estrogens with pituitary gonadotropins in hypophysectomized rats. *Endocrinology,* 28:37–41.
219. Williams, P. C. (1944): Ovarian stimulation by oestrogens: effects in immature hypophysectomized rats. *Proc. R. Soc. London [Biol.],* 132:189–199.
220. Payne, R. W., and Hellbaum, A. A. (1955): The effect of estrogens on the ovary of the hypophysectomized rat. *Endocrinology,* 57:193–199.
221. Payne, R. W., and Runser, R. H. (1958): The influence of estrogen and androgen on the ovarian response of hypophysectomized immature rats to gonadotropins. *Endocrinology,* 62:313–321.
222. Bradbury, J. T. (1961): Direct action of estrogen on the ovary of the immature rat. *Endocrinology,* 68:112–120.
223. Smith, B. D. (1961): The effect of diethylstilbestrol on the immature rat ovary. *Endocrinology,* 69:238–245.
224. Reiter, E. O., Goldenberg, R. L., Vaitukaitis, J. L., and Ross, G. T. (1972): Evidence for a role of estrogen in ovarian augmentation reaction. *Endocrinology,* 91:1518–1522.
225. Harman, S. M., Louvet, J. P., and Ross, G. T. (1975): Interaction of estrogen and gonadotrophins on follicular atresia. *Endocrinology,* 96:1145–1152.
226. Saiduddui, S. (1971): ^{3}H-estradiol uptake by the rat ovary. *Proc. Soc. Exp. Biol. Med.,* 138:651–660.
227. Saiduddui, S., and Milo Jr., G. E. (1974): Effect of hypophysectomy and pretreatment on uptake and retention of estradiol by the ovary. *Proc. Soc. Exp. Biol. Med.,* 146:513–517.
228. Stumpf, W. E. (1969): Nuclear concentration of ^{3}H-estradiol in target issues. Dry-mount autoradiography of vagina, oviduct, ovary, testis, mammary tumor, liver and adrenal. *Endocrinology,* 85:31–37.
229. Richards, J. S. (1975): Estradiol receptor content of rat granulosa cells during follicular development: modification by estradiol and gonadotropins. *Endocrinology,* 97:1174–1184.
230. Richards, J. S. (1974): Estradiol binding to rat corpora lutea during pregnancy. *Endocrinology,* 95:1046–1053.
231. Saidudduin, S., and Zassenhaus, H. P. (1977): Estradiol-17β receptors in the immature rat ovary. *Steroids,* 29:197–213.
232. Leung, P. C. K., Goff, A. K., Kennedy, T. G., and Armstrong, D. T. (1978): An intraovarian inhibitory action of estrogen and androgen production in vivo. *Biol. Reprod.,* 19:641–647.
233. Leung, P. C. K., and Armstrong, D. T. (1979): Estrogen treatment of immature rats inhibits ovarian androgen production in vitro. *Endocrinology,* 104:1411–1417.
234. Leung, P. C. K., and Armstrong, D. T. (1980): Further evidence in support of a short-loop feedback action of estrogen on ovarian androgen production. *Life Sci.,* 27:415–420.
235. Hunter, M. G., and Armstrong, D. T. (1986): Estrogens inhibit steroid production by dispersed porcine thecal cells. *Biol. Reprod. (Suppl. 1),* 34:196 (abstr. 293).
236. Magoffin, D. A., and Erickson, G. F. (1981): Mechanism by which 17β-estradiol inhibits ovarian androgen production in the rat. *Endocrinology,* 108:962–969.
237. Magoffin, D. A., and Erickson, G. F. (1982): Direct inhibitory effects of estrogen on LH-stimulated androgen synthesis by ovarian cells cultured in defined medium. *Mol. Cell. Endocrinol.,* 28:81–89.
238. Eckstein, B., and Nimrod, A. (1977): Properties of microsomal Δ^4-3-ketosteroid 5α-reductase in immature rat ovary. *Biochim. Biophys. Acta,* 499:1–9.
239. Armstrong, D. T. (1979): Alterations of progesterone metabolism in immature rat ovaries by luteinizing hormone. *Biol. Reprod.,* 21:1025–1033.
240. Evans, G., Leung, P. C. K., Brodie, A. M. H., and Armstrong, D. T. (1981): Effect of an aromatase inhibitor (4-acetoxy-4-androstene-3,17-dione) on the stimulatory action of luteinizing hormone on estradiol-17β synthesis by rat preovulatory follicles in vitro. *Biol. Reprod.,* 25:290–294.
241. Armstrong, D. T., Dorrington, J. H., and Robinson, J. (1976): Effects of indomethacin and aminoglutethimide phosphate in vivo on luteinizing-hormone-induced alterations on cyclic adenosine monophosphate, prostaglandin F, and steroid levels in preovulatory rat ovaries. *Can. J. Biochem.,* 54:796–802.
242. Bahr, J. M. (1978): Simultaneous measurement of steroids in follicular fluid and ovarian venous blood in the rabbit. *Biol. Reprod.,* 18:193–197.
243. Goff, A. K., and Henderson, K. M. (1979): Changes in follicular fluid and serum concentrations of steroids in PMS-treated immature rats following LH administration. *Biol. Reprod.,* 20:1153–1157.
244. Smith, M. S., Freeman, M. E., and Neill, J. D. (1975): The control of progesterone secretion during the estrous cycle and early pseudopregnancy in the rat: prolactin gonadotropin and steroid levels associated with rescue of the corpus luteum of pseudopregnancy. *Endocrinology,* 96:219–226.
245. Kalra, S. P., and Kalra, P. S. (1974): Temporal interrelationships among circulating levels of estradiol, progesterone and LH during the rat estrous cycle: effects of exogenous progesterone. *Endocrinology,* 95:1711–1718.
246. Saidapur, S. K., and Greenwald, G. S. (1979): Regulation of 17β-estradiol synthesis in the proestrous hamster: role of progesterone and luteinizing hormone. *Endocrinology,* 105:1432–1439.
247. Fortune, J. E., and Hansel, W. (1979): The effects of 17β-estradiol on progesterone secretion by bovine theca and granulosa cells. *Endocrinology,* 104:1834–1838.
248. Engels, J. A., Friedlander, R. L., and Eik-Nes, K. B. (1968): An effect in vivo of clomiphene on the rate of conversion of androstenedione-C^{14} to estrone-C^{14} and estradiol-C^{14} by the canine ovary. *Metabolism,* 17:189–198.
249. Zhuang, L.-Z., Adashi, E. Y., and Hsueh, A. J. W. (1982): Direct enhancement of gonadotropin-stimulated ovarian estrogen biosynthesis by estrogen and clomiphene citrate. *Endocrinology,* 110:2219–2221.
250. Adashi, E. Y., and Hsueh, A. J. W. (1982): Estrogens augment the stimulation of ovarian aromatase activity by follicle-stimulating hormone in cultured rat granulosa cells. *J. Biol. Chem.,* 257:6077–6083.
251. Welsh Jr., T. H., Jia, X.-C., Jones, P. B. C., Zhuang, L.-Z., and Hsueh, A. J. W. (1984): Disparate effects of triphenylethylene antiestrogens on estrogen and progestin biosyntheses by cultured rat granulosa cells. *Endocrinology,* 115:1275–1282.
252. Daniel, S. A. J., and Armstrong, D. T. (1983): Involvement of estrogens in the regulation of granulosa cell aromatase activity. *Can. J. Physiol. Pharmacol.,* 61:507–511.
253. Thanki, K. H., and Channing, C. P. (1976): Influence of serum, estrogen, and gonadotropins upon growth and progesterone secretion by cultures of granulosa cells from small porcine follicles. *Endocr. Res. Commun.,* 3:319–333.
254. Thanki, K. H., and Channing, C. P. (1978): Effects of follicle-stimulating hormone and estradiol upon progesterone secretion by porcine granulosa cells in tissue culture. *Endocrinology,* 103:74–80.

255. Schomberg, D. W., Stouffer, R. L., and Tyrey, L. (1976): Modulation of progestin secretion in ovarian cells by 17β-hydroxy-5-androstan-3-one (dihydrotestosterone): a direct demonstration in monolayer culture. *Biochem. Biophys. Res. Commun.*, 68:77–81.
256. Haney, A. F., and Schomberg, D. W. (1978): Steroidal modulation of progesterone secretion by granulosa cells from large porcine follicles: a role for androgens and estrogens in controlling steroidogenesis. *Biol. Reprod.*, 19:242–248.
257. Hillier, S. G., Knazek, R. A., and Ross, G. T. (1977): Androgenic stimulation of progesterone production by granulosa cells from preantral ovarian follicles: further in vitro studies using replicate cell cultures. *Endocrinology*, 100:1539–1549.
258. Bieszczad, R. R., McClintock, J. S., Pepe, G. J., and Dimino, M. J. (1982): Progesterone secretion by granulosa cells from different sized follicles of human ovaries after short term incubation. *J. Clin. Endocrinol. Metab.*, 55:181–184.
259. Veldhuis, J. D., Klase, P. A., Sandon, B. A., and Kolp, L. A. (1983): Progesterone secretion by highly differentiated human granulosa cells isolated from preovulatory Graafian follicles, induced by endogenous gonadotropins and human chorionic gonadotropin. *J. Clin. Endocrinol. Metab.*, 57:287–291.
260. Shemesh, M., and Ailenberg, M. (1977): The effect of androstenedione on progesterone accumulation in cultures of bovine ovarian follicles. *Biol. Reprod.*, 17:499–505.
261. Veldhuis, J. D. (1985): Bipotential actions of estrogens on progesterone biosynthesis by ovarian cells. II. Relation of estradiol's stimulatory actions to cholesterol and progestin metabolism in cultured swine granulosa cells. *Endocrinology*, 117:1076–1083.
262. Leung, P. C. K., and Armstrong, D. T. (1979): A mechanism for the intraovarian inhibitory action of estrogen on androgen production. *Biol. Reprod.*, 21:1035–1042.
263. Goldenberg, R. L., Bridson, W. E., and Kohler, P. O. (1972): Estrogen stimulation of progesterone synthesis by porcine granulosa cells in culture. *Biochem. Biophys. Res. Commun.*, 48:101–107.
264. Bernard, J. (1975): Effect of follicular fluid and oestradiol on the luteinization of rat granulosa cells in vitro. *J. Reprod. Fertil.*, 45:453–460.
265. Welsh Jr., T. H., Zhuang, L.-Z., and Hsueh, A. J. W. (1983): Estrogen augmentation of gonadotropin-stimulated progestin biosynthesis in cultured rat granulosa cells. *Endocrinology*, 112:1916–1924.
266. Hudson, K. E., and Hillier, S. G. (1985): Catechol estradiol control of FSH-stimulated granulosa cell steroidogenesis. *J. Endocrinol.*, 106:R1–R4.
267. Khan, M. I., and Gibori, G. (1984): Catechol estrogens and their role in luteal steroidogenesis. *Biol. Reprod.*, 30 (Suppl. 1):127 (abstr. 194).
268. Zeleznik, A. J., Hillier, S. G., and Ross, G. T. (1979): Follicle-stimulating hormone-induced follicular development: an examination of the role of androgens. *Biol. Reprod.*, 21:673–681.
269. Neumann, F., von Berswordt-Wallrabe, R., Elger, W., Steinbeck, K., Hann, J. D., and Kramer, M. (1970): Aspects of androgen-dependent events as studied by antiandrogens. *Recent Prog. Horm. Res.*, 26:337–410.
270. Lyon, M. F., and Glenister, P. H. (1974): Evidence from Tfm/O that androgen is inessential for reproduction in female mice. *Nature*, 247:366–367.
271. Schreiber, J. R., Reid, R., and Ross, G. T. (1976): A receptor-like testosterone binding protein in ovaries from estrogen-stimulated hypophysectomized immature female rats. *Endocrinology*, 98:1206–1213.
272. Schreiber, J. R., and Ross, G. T. (1976): Further characterization of rat ovarian testosterone receptor with evidence for nuclear translocation. *Endocrinology*, 99:590–596.
273. Campo, S. M., Carson, R. S., and Findlay, J. K. (1984): Distribution and characterisation of specific androgen-binding sites within the ovine follicle. *15th Annual Conference of the Australian Society for Reproductive Biology, Canberra*, p. 27 (abstr.).
274. Milwidsky, A., Younes, M. A., Besch, N. F., Besch, P. K., and Kaufman, R. H. (1980): Receptor-like binding proteins for testosterone and progesterone in the human ovary. *Am. J. Obstet. Gynecol.*, 138:93–98.
275. McNatty, K. P., Moore Smith, D., Makris, A., Osathanondh, R., and Ryan, K. J. (1979): The microenvironment of the human antral follicle: interrelationships among the steroid levels in antral fluid, the population of granulosa cells, and the status of the oocyte in vivo and in vitro. *J. Clin. Endocrinol. Metab.*, 49:851–860.
276. Carson, R. S., Findlay, J. K., Clarke, I. J., and Burger, H. G. (1981): Estradiol, testosterone, and androstenedione in ovine follicular fluid during growth and atresia of ovarian follicles. *Biol. Reprod.*, 24:105–113.
277. Hillier, S. G., and Ross, G. T. (1979): Effects of exogenous testosterone on ovarian weight, follicular morphology and intraovarian progesterone concentration in estrogen-primed hypophysectomized immature female rats. *Biol. Reprod.*, 20:261–268.
278. Louvet, J. P., Harman, S. M., Schreiber, J. R., and Ross, G. T. (1975): Evidence for a role of androgens in follicular maturation. *Endocrinology*, 97:366–372.
279. Bagnell, C. A., Mills, T. M., Costoff, A., and Mahesh, V. B. (1982): A model for the study of androgen effects of follicular atresia and ovulation. *Biol. Reprod.*, 27:903–914.
280. Opavsky, M. A., and Armstrong, D. T. (1985): The effectiveness of FSH in inducing superovulation is influenced by LH. *Biol. Reprod.*, 32 (Suppl. 1):71 (abstr. 67).
281. Ohno, S., Christian, L., and Attardi, B. (1973): Role of testosterone in normal female function. *Nature*, 243:119–120.
282. Peluso, J. J., Brown, I., and Steger, R. W. (1979): Effects of cyproterone acetate, a potent antiandrogen, on the preovulatory follicle. *Biol. Reprod.*, 21:929–936.
283. Kumari, G. L., Datta, J. K., Das, R. P., and Roy, S. (1978): Evidence for a role of androgens in the growth and maturation of ovarian follicles in rats. *Horm. Res.*, 9:112–120.
284. Mori, T., Suzuki, A., Nishimura, T., and Kambegawa, A. (1977): Evidence for androgen participation in induced ovulation in immature rats. *Endocrinology*, 101:623–626.
285. Tsafriri, A., and Braw, R. H. (1984): Experimental approaches to atresia in mammals. In: *Oxford Reviews of Reproductive Biology*, Vol. 6, edited by R. E. Clarke, pp. 226–265. Clarendon Press, Oxford.
286. Moor, R. M., Hay, M. F., and Seamark, R. F. (1975): The sheep ovary: regulation of steoidogenic, haemodynamic and structural changes in the largest follicle and adjacent tissue before ovulation. *J. Reprod. Fertil.*, 45:595–604.
287. Lucky, A. W., Schreiber, J. R., Hillier, S. G., Schulman, J. D., and Ross, G. T. (1977): Progesterone production by cultured preantral rat granulosa cells: stimulation by androgens. *Endocrinology*, 100:128–133.
288. Corredor, A., and Flickinger, G. L. (1983): Hormonal regulation of progesterone secretion by cultured mouse granulosa cells. *Biol. Reprod.*, 29:1142–1146.
289. Leung, P. C. K., Goff, A. K., and Armstrong, D. T. (1979): Stimulatory action of androgen administration in vivo on ovarian responsiveness to gonadotropins. *Endocrinology*, 104:1119–1123.
290. Schomberg, D. W., Williams, R. F., Tyrey, L., and Ulberg, L. C. (1978): Reduction of granulosa cell progesterone secretion in vitro by intraovarian implants of antiandrogen. *Endocrinology*, 102:984–987.
291. Welsh Jr., J. H., Jones, P. B. C., Ruiz de Galaretta, C. M., Fanjul, L. F., and Hsueh, A. J. W. (1982): Androgen regulation of progestin biosynthetic enzymes in FSH-treated rat granulosa cells in vitro. *Steroids*, 40:691–700.
292. Hillier, S. G., and deZwart, F. A. (1982): Androgen/antiandrogen modulation of cyclic AMP-induced steroidogenesis during granulosa cell differentiation in tissue culture. *Mol. Cell. Endocrinol.*, 28:347–361.
293. Goff, A. K., Leung, P. C. K., and Armstrong, D. T. (1979): Stimulatory action of follicle-stimulating hormone and androgens on the responsiveness of rat granulosa cells to gonadotropins in vitro. *Endocrinology*, 104:1124–1129.
294. Daniel, S. A. J., and Armstrong, D. T. (1984): Site of action of androgens on follicle-stimulating hormone-induced aromatase activity in cultured rat granulosa cells. *Endocrinology*, 114:1975–1982.
295. Knecht, M., Darbon, J. M., Ranta, T., Baukal, A. J., and Catt, K. J. (1984): Estrogens enhance the adenosine 3′,5′-monophosphate-mediated induction of follicle-stimulating hormone and luteinizing hormone receptors in rat granulosa cells. *Endocrinology*, 115:41–49.

296. Duleba, A. J., Takahashi, H., and Moon, Y. S. (1983): Androgenic modulation of progesterone metabolism by rat granulosa cells in culture. *Steroids,* 42:321–330.
297. Moon, Y. S., Duleba, A. J., and Takahashi, H. (1984): Differential actions of LH and androgens on progesterone catabolism by rat granulosa cells. *Biochem. Biophys. Res. Commun.,* 119:694–699.
298. Moon, Y. S., Duleba, A. J., Kuir, K. S., and Yuen, B. H. (1985): Alterations of 20α-hydroxysteroid dehydrogenase activity in cultured rat granulosa cells by follicle-stimulating hormone and testosterone. *Biol. Reprod.,* 32:998–1009.
299. Nimrod, A. (1981): On the synergistic action of androgen and FSH on progestin secretion by cultured rat granulosa cells. Cellular and mitochondrial cholesterol metabolism. *Mol. Cell. Endocrinol.,* 21:51–62.
300. Schrieber, J. R., Nakamura, K., and Weinstein, D. B. (1983): Androgen and FSH synergistically stimulate rat ovary granulosa cell utilization of rat and human lipoproteins. In: *Factors Regulating Ovarian Function,* edited by G. Greenwald and P. F. Terranova, pp. 311–315. Raven Press, New York.
301. Evans, G., Lischinsky, A., Daniel, S. A. J., and Armstrong, D. T. (1984): Androgen-inhibition of FSH-stimulated progesterone production by granulosa cells of pre-pubertal pig. *Can. J. Physiol. Pharmacol.,* 62:840–845.
302. Tan, C. H., and Armstrong, D. T. (1984): FSH-stimulated 3β-HSD activity of porcine granulosa cells: inhibition by androgens. *Proceedings of the 3rd Joint Meeting of the British Endocrine Societies, Edinburgh,* Abstr. 12.
303. Daniel, S. A. J., and Armstrong, D. T. (1980): Enhancement of follicle-stimulating hormone-induced aromatase by androgens in cultured rat granulosa cells. *Endocrinology,* 107:1027–1033.
304. Armstrong, D. T., Daniel, S. A. J., Salhanick, A. R., and Sheela Rani, C. S. (1980): Hormonal interactions in regulation of steroid biosynthesis by the ovarian follicle. In: *Functional Correlates of Hormone Receptors in Reproduction,* edited by V. B. Makesh, T. G. Muldoon, B. B. Saxena, and W. A. Sadler, pp. 245–260. Elsevier/North-Holland, New York.
305. Hillier, S. G., and deZwart, F. A. (1981): Evidence that granulosa cell induction/activation by follicle-stimulating hormone is an androgen receptor-regulated process in vitro. *Endocrinology,* 109:1303–1305.
306. Hillier, S. G., van den Boogaard, A. M. J., Reichert Jr., L. E., and van Hall, E. V. (1980): Alterations in granulosa cell aromatase activity accompanying preovulatory follicular development in the rat ovary with evidence that 5α-reduced C_{19} steroids inhibit the aromatase reaction in vitro. *J. Endocrinol.,* 84:409–419.
307. Hillier, S. G., van den Boogaard, A. M. J., Reichert Jr., L. E., and van Hall, E. V. (1980): Intraovarian sex steroid hormone interactions and the regulation of follicular maturation: aromatization of androgens by human granulosa cells in vitro. *J. Clin. Endocrinol. Metab.,* 50:640–647.
308. Smith, O. W., Ofner, P., and Vena, R. L. (1974): In vitro conversion of testosterone-4-^{14}C to androgens of the 5α-androstane series by normal human ovary. *Steroids,* 24:311–315.
309. Siiteri, P. K., and Thompson, E. A. (1975): Studies of human placental aromatase. *J. Steroid Biochem.,* 6:317–322.
310. Katz, Y., and Armstrong, D. T. (1976): Inhibition of ovarian estradiol-17β secretion by luteinizing hormone in prepubertal, pregnant mare serum-treated rats. *Endocrinology,* 99:1442–1447.
311. Saidudduin, S., and Zassenhaus, H. P. (1978): Effect of testosterone and progesterone on the estradiol receptor in the immature rat ovary. *Endocrinology,* 102:1069–1076.
312. Smith, B. D., and Bradbury, J. T. (1966): Influence of progestins on ovarian responses to estrogen and gonadotrophins in immature rats. *Endocrinology,* 78:297–301.
313. Jesel, L. (1970): Données nouvelles sur le contrôle exercé par le corps jaune sur la croissance folliculaire au début du cycle oestral chez le Cobaye. *C. R. Acad. Sci., Ser D,* 271:1693–1696.
314. Hori, T., Kato, G., and Miyake, T. (1973): Acute effects of ovarian steroids upon follicular growth in the cycling rat. *Endocrinol. Jpn.,* 20:475–482.
315. Buffler, G., and Roser, S. (1974): New data concerning the role played by progesterone in the control of follicular growth in the rat. *Acta Endocrinol.,* 75:569–578.
316. Beattie, C. W., and Corbin, A. (1975): The differential effects of diestrous progesterone administration on proestrous gonadotrophin levels. *Endocrinology,* 97:885–890.
317. Goodman, A. L., and Hodgen, G. D. (1977): Systemic versus intraovarian progesterone replacement after luteectomy in rhesus monkeys: differential patterns of gonadotropins and follicle growth. *J. Clin. Endocrinol. Metab.,* 45:837–840.
318. Richards, J. S., and Bogovich, K. (1982): Effect of human chorionic gonadotropin and progesterone on follicular development in the immature rat. *Endocrinology,* 111:1429–1438.
319. Bogovich, K., Richards, J. S., and Reichert Jr., L. E. (1981): Obligatory role of LH in the initiation of preovulatory follicular growth in the pregnant rat: specific effects of human chorionic gonadotropin and follicle-stimulating hormone on LH receptors and steroidogenesis in theca, granulosa and luteal cells. *Endocrinology,* 109:860–867.
320. Schrieber, J. R., and Hsueh, A. J. W. (1979): Progesterone "receptor" in rat ovary. *Endocrinology,* 105:915–919.
321. Schreiber, J. R., Hsueh, A. J. W., and Baulieu, E. E. (1983): Binding of the anti-progestin RU-486 to rat ovary steroid receptors. *Contraception,* 28:77–85.
322. Schreiber, J. R., and Erickson, G. F. (1979): Progesterone receptor in the rat ovary: further characterization and localization in the granulosa cell. *Steroids,* 34:459–469.
323. Naess, O. (1981): Characterization of cytoplasmic progesterone receptors in rat granulosa cells: evidence for nuclear translocation. *Acta Endocrinol.,* 98:288–294.
324. Philibert, D., Ojasoo, T., and Raynaud, J. P. (1977): Properties of the cytoplasmic progestin-binding protein in the rabbit uterus. *Endocrinology,* 101:1850–1861.
325. Pasqualini, J. R., and Nguyen, B. J. (1980): Progesterone receptors in fetal uterus and ovary of the guinea pig. Evolution during fetal development and induction and stimulation in estradiol-primed animals. *Endocrinology,* 106:1160–1165.
326. Jacobs, B. R., and Smith, R. G. (1980): Evidence for a receptor-like protein for progesterone in bovine ovarian cytosol. *Endocrinology,* 106:1276–1282.
327. Jacobs, B. R., Suchocki, S., and Smith, R. G. (1980): Evidence for human ovarian progesterone receptor. *Am. J. Obstet. Gynecol.,* 138:332–336.
328. Fanjul, L. F., de Galarreta, R., and Hsueh, A. J. W. (1983): Progestin augmentation of gonadotrophin-stimulated progesterone production by cultured rat granulosa cells. *Endocrinology,* 112:405–407.
329. Hsueh, A. J. W., Adashi, E. Y., Jones, P. B. C., and Welsh, T. H. (1984): Hormonal regulation of the differentiation of cultured ovarian granulosa cells. *Endocr. Rev.,* 5:76–127.
330. Schreiber, J. R., Nakamura, K., and Erickson, G. F. (1980): Progestins inhibit FSH-stimulated steroidogenesis in cultured rat granulosa cells. *Mol. Cell. Endocrinol.,* 19:165–173.
331. Schreiber, J. R., Nakamura, K., and Erickson, G. F. (1981): Progestins inhibit FSH-stimulated granulosa estrogen production at a post-cAMP site. *Mol. Cell. Endocrinol.,* 21:161–170.
332. Fortune, J. E., and Vincent, S. E. (1983): Progesterone inhibits the induction of aromatase activity in rat granulosa cells in vitro. *Biol. Reprod.,* 28:1078–1089.
333. Greenwald, G. S. (1974): Gonadotropin regulation of follicular development. In: *Gonadotropins and Gonadal Function,* edited by N. R. Moudgal, pp. 205–212. Academic, New York.
334. Mahajan, D. K., and Samuels, L. T. (1975): Inhibition of 17,20(17-hydroxyprogesterone)-lyase by progesterone. *Steroids,* 25:217–228.
335. Brophy, P. J., and Gower, D. B. (1974): Studies on the inhibition by 5α-pregnane-3,20-dione of the biosynthesis of 16-androstenes and dehydroepiandrosterone in boar testis preparations. *Biochim. Biophys. Acta,* 360:252–259.
336. Rothchild, I. (1981): The regulation of the mammalian corpus luteum. *Rec. Prog. Horm. Res.,* 37:183–298.
337. Crisp, T. M. (1977): Hormone requirements for early maintenance of rat granulosa cell cultures. *Endocrinology,* 101:1286–1297.
338. Veldhuis, J. D., Klase, P., and Hammond, J. M. (1980): Divergent effects of prolactin upon steroidogenesis by porcine granulosa cells in vitro: influence of cytodifferentiation. *Endocrinology,* 107:42–46.
339. Advis, J. P., Richards, J. S., and Ojeda, S. R. (1981): Hyperprolactinemia-induced precocious puberty: studies on the mechanism(s)

by which prolactin enhances ovarian progesterone responsiveness to gonadotropins in prepubertal rats. *Endocrinology,* 108:1333–1342.

340. Advis, J. P., and Ojeda, S. R. (1978): Hyperprolactinemia-induced precocious puberty in the female rat: ovarian site of action. *Endocrinology,* 103:924–935.
341. Gibori, G., and Richards, J. S. (1978): Dissociation of two distinct luteotropic effects of prolactin: regulation of luteinizing hormone-receptor content and progesterone secretion during pregnancy. *Endocrinology,* 102:767–774.
342. Veldhuis, J. D., and Hammond, J. M. (1980): Oestrogens regulate divergent effects of prolactin in the ovary. *Nature,* 284:262–264.
343. Wang, C., Hsueh, A. J. W., and Erickson, G. F. (1980): Prolactin inhibition of estrogen production by cultured rat granulosa cells. *Mol. Cell. Endocrinol.,* 20:135–144.
344. Wang, C., and Chan, V. (1982): Divergent effects of prolactin on estrogen and progesterone production by granulosa cells of rat Graafian follicles. *Endocrinology,* 110:1085–1093.
345. Dorrington, J., and Gore-Langton, R. E. (1981): Prolactin inhibits oestrogen synthesis in the ovary. *Nature,* 290:600–602.
346. Dorrington, J. H., and Gore-Langton, R. E. (1982): Antigonadal action of prolactin: further studies on the mechanism of inhibition of follicle-stimulatory hormone-induced aromatase activity in rat granulosa cell cultures. *Endocrinology,* 110:1701–1707.
347. Tsai-Morris, C. H., Ghosh, M., Hirshfield, A. N., Wise, P. M., and Brodie, A. M. H. (1983): Inhibition of ovarian aromatase by prolactin in vivo. *Biol. Reprod.,* 29:342–346.
348. Demura, R., Ono, M., Demura, H., Shizume, K., and Oouchi, H. (1982): Prolactin directly inhibits basal as well as gonadotropin-stimulated secretion of progesterone and 17β-estradiol in the human ovary. *J. Clin. Endocrinol. Metab.,* 54:1246–1250.
349. Advis, J. P., Wiener, S. L., and Ojeda, S. R. (1981): Changes in ovarian 3α-androstanediol response to human chorionic gonadotropin during puberty in the rat: modulatory role of prolactin. *Endocrinology,* 109:223–228.
350. Magoffin, D. A., and Erickson, G. P. (1982): Prolactin inhibition of luteinizing hormone-stimulated androgen synthesis in ovarian interstitial cells cultured in defined medium: mechanism of actions. *Endocrinology,* 111:2001–2007.
351. Fraser, H. M. (1982): Antifertility effects of GnRH. *J. Reprod. Fertil.,* 64:503–515.
352. de Koning, J., van Dieten, J. A. M. J., and van Rees, G. P. (1978): Refractoriness of the pituitary gland after continuous exposure to luteinizing hormone releasing hormone. *J. Endocrinol.,* 79:311–318.
353. Rippel, R. H., Johnson, E. S., and White, W. F. (1974): Effect of consecutive injections of synthetic gonadotropin-releasing hormone on LH release in anestrous and ovariectomized ewes. *J. Anim. Sci.,* 39:907–914.
354. Sandow, J., van Rechenberg, W., Kuhl, H., Baumann, R., Krauss, B., Jerzabek, G., and Killie, S. (1979): Inhibitory control of the pituitary LH secretion by LHRH in male rats. *Horm. Res.,* 11:303–317.
355. Fraser, H. M., Laird, N. C., and Blakeley, D. M. (1980): Decreased pituitary responsiveness and inhibition of the luteinizing hormone surge and ovulation in the stump-tailed monkey (*Macaca arctoides*) by chronic treatment with an agonist of luteinizing hormone-releasing hormone. *Endocrinology,* 106:452–457.
356. Conti, M., Harwood, J. P., Hsueh, A. J. W., Dufau, M. L., and Catt, K. J. (1976): Gonadotropin-induced loss of hormone receptors and desensitization of luteal adenylate cyclase in the ovary. *J. Biol. Chem.,* 251:7729–7731.
357. Hunzicker-Dunn, M., and Birnbaumer, L. (1976): Adenylate cyclase activities in ovarian tissues. IV. Gonadotropin-induced desensitization of luteal adenylyl cyclase throughout pregnancy and pseudopregnancy in the rabbit and rat. *Endocrinology,* 99:211–222.
358. Jonassen, J. A., and Richards, J. S. (1980): Granulosa cell desensitization: effects of gonadotropins on antral and preantral follicles. *Endocrinology,* 106:1786–1794.
359. Jonassen, J. A., Bose, K., and Richards, J. S. (1982): Enhancement and desensitization of hormone-responsive adenylate cyclase in granulosa cells of preantral and antral ovarian follicles: effects of estradiol and follicle-stimulating hormone. *Endocrinology,* 111:74–79.
360. Hseuh, A. J. W., and Jones, P. B. C. (1981): Extrapituitary actions of gonadotropin-releasing hormone. *Endocr. Rev.,* 2:437–461.
361. Jones, P. B. C., Conn, P. M., Marian, J., and Hsueh, A. J. W. (1980): Binding of gonadotropin-releasing hormone agonist to rat ovarian granulosa cells. *Life Sci.,* 27:2125–2132.
362. Pieper, D. R., Richards, J. S., and Marshall, J. C. (1981): Ovarian gonadotropin-releasing hormone (GnRH) receptors: characterization, distribution, and induction by GnRH. *Endocrinology,* 108:1148–1155.
363. Clayton, R. N., Harwood, J. P., and Catt, K. J. (1979): Gonadotropin-releasing hormone analogue binds to luteal cells and inhibits progesterone production. *Nature,* 282:90–92.
364. Pelletier, G., Sequin, C., Dube, D., and St.-Arnaud, R. (1982): Distribution of LHRH receptors in the rat ovary. *Biol. Reprod.,* 26 (Suppl. 1):151 (abstr. 230).
365. Marian, J., and Conn, P. M. (1983): Subcellular localization of the receptor for gonadotropin-releasing hormone in pituitary and ovarian tissue. *Endocrinology,* 112:104–112.
366. Ranta, T., Knecht, M., Kody, M., and Catt, K. J. (1983): GnRH receptors in cultured rat granulosa cells: mediation of the inhibitory and stimulatory actions of GnRH. *Mol. Cell. Endocrinol.,* 27:233–240.
367. Hazum, E., and Nimrod, A. (1982): Photoaffinity-labeling and fluorescence-distribution studies of gonadotropin-releasing hormone receptors in ovarian granulosa cells. *Proc. Natl. Acad. Sci. USA,* 79:1747–1750.
368. Hazum, E. (1981): Photoaffinity labeling of luteinizing hormone releasing hormone receptor of rat pituitary membrane preparations. *Endocrinology,* 109:1281–1283.
369. Clayton, R. N., and Huhtaniemi, I. T. (1982): Absence of gonadotropin-releasing hormone receptors in human gonadal tissue. *Nature,* 299:56–59.
370. Popkin, R., Bramley, T. A., Currie, A., Shaw, R. W., Baird, D. T., and Fraser, H. M. (1983): Specific binding of luteinizing-hormone releasing hormone to human luteal tissue. *Biochem. Biophys. Res. Commun.,* 114:750–756.
371. Bramley, T. A., Menzies, G. S., and Baird, D. T. (1985): Specific binding of gonadotropin-releasing hormone and an agonist to human corpus-luteum homogenates—characterization, properties, and luteal phase levels. *J. Clin. Endocrinol. Metab.,* 61:834–841.
372. Tureck, R. W., Mastroianni Jr., L., Blasco, L., and Strauss III, J. F. (1982): Inhibition of human granulosa cell progesterone secretion by a gonadotropin-releasing hormone agonist. *J. Clin. Endocrinol. Metab.,* 54:1078–1080.
373. Casper, R. F., Erickson, G. F., Rebar, R. W., and Yen, S. S. C. (1982): The effect of luteinizing hormone releasing factor and its agonist on cultured human granulosa cells. *Fertil. Steril.,* 37:406–409.
374. Koos, R. D., Ahren, K. E. B., Janson, P. O., and LeMaire, W. J. (1982): Effect of a GnRH agonist on the rabbit ovary perfused in vitro. *64th Annual Meeting of the Endocrine Society,* p. 178 (abstr. 395).
375. Massicotte, J., Veilleux, R., Lavoie, M., and Labrie, F. (1980): An LHRH agonist inhibits FSH-induced cyclic AMP accumulation and steroidogenesis in porcine granulosa cells in culture. *Biochem. Biophys. Res. Commun.,* 94:1362–1366.
376. Takats, A., and Hertelendy, F. (1982): Adenylate cyclase activity of avian granulosa: effect of gonadotropin-releasing hormone. *Gen. Comp. Endocrinol.,* 48:515–524.
377. Hertelendy, F., Linker, F., Asem, E. K., and Raab, B. (1982): Synergistic effect of gonadotropin releasing hormone on LH-stimulated progesterone production in granulosa cells of the domestic fowl (*Gallus domesticus*). *Gen. Comp. Endocrinol.,* 48: 117–122.
378. Bex, F. J., Corbin, A., and France, E. (1982): Resistance of the mouse to the antifertility effects of LHRH agonists. *Life Sci.,* 30:1263–1269.
379. Asch, R. H., Eddy, C. A., and Schally, A. V. (1981): Lack of luteolytic effect of D-Trp-6-LH-RH in hypophysectomized rhesus monkeys (*Macaca mulatta*). *Biol. Reprod.,* 25:963–968.
380. Brown, J. L., and Reeves, J. J. (1983): Absence of specific luteinizing hormone releasing hormone receptors in ovine, bovine and porcine ovaries. *Biol. Reprod.,* 29:1179–1182.
381. Asch, R. H., VanSickle, M., Rettori, V., Balmaceda, J. P., Eddy, C. A., Coy, D. H., and Schally, A. V. (1981): Absence of LHRH

binding sites in corpora lutea from rhesus monkeys (*Macacca mulatta*). *J. Clin. Endocrinol. Metab.*, 53:215–217.

382. Rippel, R. H., and Johnson, E. S. (1976): Inhibition of hCG-induced ovarian and uterine weight augmentation in the immature rat by analogs of GnRH. *Proc. Soc. Exp. Biol. Med.*, 152:432–436.
383. Hsueh, A. J. W., and Erickson, G. F. (1979): Extrapituitary action of gonadotropin-releasing hormone: direct inhibition of ovarian steroidogenesis. *Science*, 204:845–855.
384. Hsueh, A. J. W., Wang, C., and Erickson, G. F. (1980): Direct inhibitory effect of gonadotropin-releasing hormone upon follicle-stimulating hormone induction of luteinizing hormone receptor and aromatase activity in rat granulosa cells. *Endocrinology*, 106:1697–1705.
385. Gore-Langton, R. E., Lacroix, M., and Dorrington, J. H. (1981): Differential effects of luteinizing hormone-releasing hormone on follicle-stimulating hormone-dependent responses in rat granulosa cells and Sertoli cells in vitro. *Endocrinology*, 108:812–819.
386. Dorrington, J. H., McKeracher, H. L., Chan, A. K., and Gore-Langton, R. E. (1983): Hormonal interactions in the control of granulosa cell differentiation. *J. Steroid Biochem.*, 19:17–32.
387. Ying, S.-Y., and Guilleman, R. (1979): (DTrp^6-Pro^9-NEt)-luteinising hormone-releasing factor inhibits follicular development in hypophysectomised rats. *Nature*, 280:593–595.
388. Jones, P. B. C., and Hsueh, A. J. W. (1982): Regulation of 3β-hydroxysteroid dehydrogenase by gonadotropin-releasing hormone and follicle-stimulating hormone in cultured rat granulosa cells. *Endocrinology*, 110:1663–1671.
389. Jones, P. B. C., and Hsueh, A. J. W. (1981): Regulation of ovarian 20α-hydroxysteroid dehydrogenase by gonadotropin-releasing hormone and its antagonist in vitro and in vivo. *J. Steroid Biochem.*, 14:1169–1175.
390. Jones, P. B. C., and Hsueh, A. J. W. (1981): Direct effects of gonadotropin-releasing hormone and its antagonist upon ovarian functions stimulated by FSH, prolactin and LH. *Biol. Reprod.*, 24:747–759.
391. Jones, P. B. C., and Hsueh, A. J. W. (1981): Regulation of progesterone metabolizing enzyme by adrenergic agents, prolactin and prostaglandins in cultured rat ovarian granulosa cells. *Endocrinology*, 109:1347–1354.
392. Clark, M. R. (1982): Stimulation of progesterone and prostaglandin E accumulation by luteinizing hormone-releasing hormone (LHRH) and LHRH analogs in rat granulosa cells. *Endocrinology*, 110:146–152.
393. Sheela Rani, C. S., Ekholm, C., Billig, H., Magnusson, C., and Hillensjö, T. (1983): Biphasic effect of gonadotropin releasing hormone on progestin secretion by rat granulosa cells. *Biol. Reprod.*, 28:591–597.
394. Popkin, R., Fraser, H. M., and Jonassen, J. (1983): Stimulation of androstenedione and progesterone release by LHRH and LHRH agonist from isolated rat preovulatory follicles. *Mol. Cell. Endocrinol.*, 29:169–179.
395. Hsueh, A. J. W., and Ling, N. C. (1979): Effect of an antagonistic analog of gonadotropin-releasing hormone upon ovarian granulosa cell function. *Life Sci.*, 25:1223–1230.
396. St.-Arnaud, R., Walker, P., Kelly, P. A., and Labrie, F. (1983): Rat ovarian epidermal growth factor receptors: characterization and hormonal regulation. *Mol. Cell. Endocrinol.*, 31:43–52.
397. Clark, M. R., Thibier, C., Marsh, J. M., and LeMaire, W. J. (1980): Stimulation of prostaglandin accumulation by luteinizing hormone-releasing hormone (LHRH) and LHRH analogs in rat granulosa cells in vitro. *Endocrinology*, 107:17–23.
398. Knecht, M., Katz, M. S., and Catt, K. J. (1981): Gonadotropin-releasing hormone inhibits cyclic nucleotide accumulation in cultured rat granulosa cells. *J. Biol. Chem.*, 256:34–36.
399. Knecht, M., and Catt, K. J. (1981): Gonadotropin-releasing hormone: regulation of adenosine 3′,5′-monophosphate in ovarian granulosa cells. *Science*, 214:1346–1348.
400. Ranta, T., Baukal, A., Knecht, M., Korhonen, M., and Catt, K. J. (1983): Inhibitory actions of a gonadotropin-releasing hormone agonist on ovarian follicle-stimulating hormone receptors and adenylate cyclase in vitro. *Endocrinology*, 112:956–964.
401. Jones. P. B. C., and Hsueh, A. J. W. (1983): Modulation of steroidogenic enzymes by gonadotropin-releasing hormone in cultured granulosa cells. In: *Factors Regulating Ovarian Function*, edited by G. S. Greenwald and P. F. Terranova, pp. 275–279. Raven Press, New York.
402. Ranta, T., Knecht, M., Darbon, J.-M., Baukal, A. J., and Catt, K. J. (1983): Calcium dependence of the inhibitory effect of gonadotropin-releasing hormone on luteinizing hormone-induced cyclic AMP production in rat granulosa cells. *Endocrinology*, 113:427–429.
403. Hsueh, A. J. W., and Jones, P. B. C. (1982): Direct hormonal modulation of ovarian granulosa cell maturation: effects of gonadotropin-releasing hormone. In: *Proceedings IVth Regnier de Graaf Symposium: Follicular Maturation and Ovulation*, edited by R. Rolland, E. V. Van Hall, S. G. Hillier, K. P. McNatty, and J. Schoemaker, pp. 19–33. Excerpta Medica, Amsterdam.
404. Hsueh, A. J. W., and Jones, P. B. C. (1982): Regulation of ovarian granulosa and luteal cell functions by gonadotropin-releasing hormone and its antagonist. *Adv. Exp. Med. Biol.*, 147:223–262.
405. Billig, H., Magnusson, C., Ekholm, C., and Hillensjö, T. (1982): Biphasic effect of a GnRH agonist on glycolysis in cultured rat granulosa cells. *Biol. Reprod.*, 26 (Suppl 1): 152A (abstr. 231).
406. Wang, C. (1983): Luteinizing hormone-releasing hormone stimulates plasminogen activator production by rat granulosa cells. *Endocrinology*, 112:1130–1132.
407. Dorrington, J. H., and Skinner, M. K. (1986): Cytodifferentiation of granulosa cells induced by gonadotropin-releasing hormone promotes fibronectin secretion. *Endocrinology*, 118:2065–2071.
408. Naor, Z., and Yavin, E. (1982): Gonadotropin releasing hormone stimulates phospholipid labeling in cultured granulosa cells. *Endocrinology*, 111:1615–1619.
409. Leung, P. C. K., Raymond, V., and Labrie, F. (1983): Stimulation of phosphatidic acid and phosphatidylinositol labeling in luteal cells by luteinizing hormone-releasing hormone. *Endocrinology*, 112: 1138–1140.
410. Davis, J. S., Farese, R. V., and Clark, M. R. (1983): Gonadotropin-releasing hormone (GnRH) stimulates phosphatidylinositol metabolism in rat granulosa cells: mechanism of action of GnRH. *Proc. Natl. Acad. Sci. USA*, 80:2049–2053.
411. Davis, J. S., West, L. A., and Farese, R. V. (1986): Gonadotropin-releasing hormone (GnRH) rapidly stimulates the formation of inositol phosphates and diacylglycerol in rat granulosa cells: further evidence for the involvement of Ca^{2+} and protein kinase C in the action of GnRH. *Endocrinology*, 118:2561–2571.
412. Minegishi, T., and Leung, P. C. K. (1985): Effects of prostaglandins and luteinizing hormone-releasing hormone on phosphatidic acid-phosphatidylinositol labelling in rat granulosa cells. *Can. J. Physiol. Pharmacol.*, 63:320–324.
413. Minegishi, T., and Leung, P. C. K. (1985): Luteinizing hormone-releasing hormone stimulates arachidonic acid release in rat granulosa cells. *Endocrinology*, 117:2001–2007.
414. Berridge, M. J. (1981): Phosphatidylinositol hydrolysis: a multifunctioned transducing mechanism. *Mol. Cell. Endocrinol.*, 24:115–140.
415. Nishizuka, Y. (1984): The role of protein kinase C in cell surface signal transduction and tumour promotion. *Nature*, 308:693–698.
416. Zilberstein, M., Sakut, H., Eli, Y., and Naor, Z. (1984): Regulation of prostaglandin E, progesterone, and cyclic adenosine monophosphate production in ovarian granulosa cells by luteinizing hormone and gonadotropin-releasing hormone and gonadotropin-releasing hormone agonist: comparative studies. *Endocrinology*, 114:2374–2381.
417. Hillensjö, T., and LeMaire, W. J. (1980): Gonadotropin-releasing hormone agonists stimulate meiotic maturation of follicle-enclosed rat oocytes in vitro. *Nature*, 287:145–146.
418. Banka, C. L., and Erickson, G. F. (1985): Gonadotropin-releasing hormone induces classical meiotic maturation in subpopulations of atretic preantral follicles. *Endocrinology*, 117:1500–1507.
419. Dekel, N., Sherizly, I., Phillips, D. M., Nimrod, A., Zilberstein, M., and Naor, Z. (1985): Characterization of the maturational changes induced by a GnRH analogue in the rat ovarian follicle. *J. Reprod. Fertil.*, 75:461–466.
420. Corbin, A., and Bex, F. J. (1981): Luteinizing hormone releasing hormone agonists induce ovulation in hypophysectomized proestrous rats: direct ovarian effect. *Life Sci.*, 29:185–192.
421. Ekholm, C., Hillensjö, T., and Isaksson, O. (1981): Gonadotropin-releasing hormone agonists stimulate oocyte meiosis and ovulation in hypophysectomized rats. *Endocrinology*, 108:2022–2024.

422. Magoffin, D. A., Reynolds, D. S., and Erickson, G. F. (1981): Direct inhibitory effect of GnRH on androgen secretion by ovarian interstitial cells. *Endocrinology,* 109:661–663.
423. Magoffin, D. A., and Erickson, G. F. (1982): Mechanism by which GnRH inhibits androgen synthesis directly in ovarian interstitial cells. *Mol. Cell. Endocrinol.,* 27:191–198.
424. Elkind-Hirsch, K., Ravnikar, V., Schift, I., Tulchinsky, D., and Ryan, K. J. (1982): Determinations of endogenous immunoreactive luteinizing hormone-releasing hormone in human plasma. *J. Clin. Endocrinol. Metab.,* 54:602–607.
425. Ying, S.-Y., Ling, N., Bohlen, P., and Guillemin, R. (1981): Gonadocrinins: peptides in ovarian follicular fluid stimulating the secretion of pituitary gonadotropins. *Endocrinology,* 108:1206–1215.
426. Esch, F., Ling, N., Ying, S.-Y., and Guillemin, R. (1982): Peptides of gonadal origin involved in reproductive biology. In: *Role of Peptides and Proteins in Control of Reproduction,* edited by S. M. McCann and D. S. Dhindsa, Proceedings of National Institute of Health Workshop, Bethesda, MD.
427. Aten, R. F., Williams, T., and Behrman, H. R. (1986): Ovarian gonadotropin-releasing hormone-like protein(s): demonstration and characterization. *Endocrinology,* 118:961–967.
428. Birnbaumer, L., Shahabi, N., Rivier, J., and Vale, W. (1985): Evidence for a physiological role of gonadotropin-releasing hormone (GnRH) or GnRH-like material in the ovary. *Endocrinology,* 116:1367–1370.
429. Jarrett, R. J. (1965): Effect and mode of action of adrenocorticotrophic hormone upon the reproductive tract of the female mouse. *Endocrinology,* 76:434–440.
430. Ramaley, J. A. (1973): Role of the adrenal in PMSG-induced ovulation before puberty: effect of adrenalectomy. *Endocrinology,* 92:881–887.
431. Baldwin, D. M., and Sawyer, C. H. (1974): Effect of dexamethasone on LH release and ovulation in the cyclic rat. *Endocrinology,* 94:1397–1403.
432. Yaginuma, T., and Kobayashi, T. (1977): Effect of stress, metyrapone and adrenalectomy on compensatory ovarian hypertrophy. *Endocrinol. Jpn.,* 24:403–407.
433. Baldwin, D. M. (1979): The effect of glucocorticoids on estrogen-dependent luteinizing hormone release in the ovariectomized rat and on gonadotropin secretion in the intact female. *Endocrinology,* 105:120–128.
434. Cortes-Gallegos, V., Gallegos, A. J., Bedolla Tovar, N., Cervantes, C., and Parra, A. (1975): Effect of paramethasone acetate on ovarian steroids and gonadotropins. I. Normal menstrual cycle. *J. Clin. Endocrinol. Metab.,* 41:215–220.
435. Cunningham, G. R., Goldzieher, J. W., de la Pena, A., and Oliver, M. (1978): The mechanism of ovulation inhibition by triamcinolone acetonide. *J. Clin. Endocrinol. Metab.,* 46:8–14.
436. Hagino, N., Watanabe, M., and Goldzieher, J. W. (1969): Inhibition by adrenocorticotrophin of gonadotrophin-induced ovulation in immature female rats. *Endocrinology,* 84:308–314.
437. Schreiber, J. R., Nakamura, K., and Erickson, G. F. (1982): Rat ovary glucocorticoid receptor: identification and characterization. *Steroids,* 39:569–584.
438. Louvet, J. P., Baislic, M., Bayard, F., and Boulard, C. (1977): Glucocorticoid receptors in rat ovarian granulosa cell cytosol. *59th Annual Meeting of the Endocrine Society,* p. 363 (abstr. 601).
439. Hsueh, A. J. W., and Erickson, G. F. (1978): Glucocorticoid inhibition of FSH-induced estrogen production in cultured rat granulosa cells. *Steroids,* 32:639–648.
440. Schoonmaker, J. N., and Erickson, G. F. (1983): Glucocorticoid modulation of follicle-stimulating hormone-mediated granulosa cell differentiation. *Endocrinology,* 113:1356–1363.
441. Adashi, E. Y., Jones, P. B. C., and Hsueh, A. J. W. (1981): Synergistic effect of glucocorticoids on the stimulation of progesterone production by follicle-stimulating hormone in cultured rat granulosa cells. *Endocrinology,* 109:1888–1894.
442. Channing, C. P., Tsai, V., and Sachs, D. (1976): Role of insulin, thyroxin and cortisol in luteinization of porcine granulosa cells grown in chemically defined media. *Biol. Reprod.,* 15:235–247.
443. Mahajan, D. K., and Little, A. B. (1978): Specific cortisol binding protein in porcine follicular fluid. *Biol. Reprod.,* 17:834–842.
444. Mahajan, D. K., Billiar, R. B., and Little, A. B. (1980): Isolation of cortisol binding globulin (CBG) from porcine follicular fluid by affinity chromatography. *J. Steroid Biochem.,* 13:67–71.
445. Adashi, E. Y., Resnick, C. E., D'ercole, A. J., Svoboda, M. E., and Van Wyk, J. J. (1985): Insulin-like growth factors as intraovarian regulators of granulosa cell growth and function. *Endocr. Rev.,* 6:400–420.
446. Jones, P. B. C., Welsh Jr., T. H., and Hsueh, A. J. W. (1982): Regulation of ovarian progestin production by epidermal growth factor in cultured rat granulosa cells. *J. Biol. Chem.,* 257:11268–11273.
447. Hsueh, A. J. W., Welsh Jr., T. H., and Jones, P. B. C. (1981): Inhibition of ovarian and testicular steroidogenesis by epidermal growth factor. *Endocrinology,* 108:2002–2004.
448. Knecht, M., and Catt, K. J. (1983): Modulation of cAMP-mediated differentiation in ovarian granulosa cells by epidermal growth factor and platelet-derived growth factor. *J. Biol. Chem.,* 258: 2789–2794.
449. Schomberg, D. W., May, J. V., and Mondschein, J. S. (1983): Interactions between hormones and growth factors in the regulation of granulosa cell differentiation in vitro. *J. Steroid Biochem.,* 19:291–295.
450. Pulley, D. D., and Marrone, B. L. (1986): Inhibitory action of epidermal growth factor on progesterone biosynthesis in hen granulosa cells during short term culture: two sites of action. *Endocrinology,* 118:2284–2291.
451. Erickson, G. F., and Case, E. (1983): Epidermal growth factor antagonizes ovarian theca–interstitial cytodifferentiation. *Mol. Cell. Endocrinol.,* 31:71–76.
452. Lintern-Moore, S., Moore, G. P. M., Panaretto, B. A., and Robertson, D. (1981): Follicular development in the neonatal mouse ovary; effect of epidermal growth factor. *Acta Endocrinol. (Copenh.),* 96:123–126.
453. Byyny, R. L., Orth, D. N., Cohen, S., and Doyne, E. S. (1974): Epidermal growth factor: effects of androgens and adrenergic agents. *Endocrinology,* 95:776–782.
454. Savage, C. R., and Cohen, S. (1972): Epidermal growth factor and a new derivative: rapid isolation procedures and biological and chemical characterization. *J. Biol. Chem.,* 247:7609–7611.
455. Moore Jr., J. B. (1978): Purification and partial characterization of epidermal growth factor isolated from the male rat submaxillary gland. *Arch. Biochem. Biophys.,* 189:1–7.
456. Cohen, S., and Carpenter, G. (1975): Human epidermal growth factor: isolation and chemical and biological properties. *Proc. Natl. Acad. Sci. USA,* 72:1317–1321.
457. Byyny, R. L., Orth, D. N., Cohen, S., and Island, D. P. (1971): Epidermal growth factor radioimmunoassay: effects of age, androgen and adrenergic agents on EGF storage and release. *53rd Annual Meeting of the Endocrine Society,* p. A45 (abstr. 6).
458. Nexo, E., Hollenberg, M. D., Figueroa, A., and Pratt, R. M. (1980): Detection of epidermal growth factor-urogastrone and its receptor during fetal mouse development. *Proc. Natl. Acad. Sci. USA,* 77:2782–2785.
459. Sporn, M. B., Roberts, A. B., Shull, J. H., Smith, J. M., Ward, J. M., and Sodek, J. (1983): Polypeptide transforming growth factors isolated from bovine sources and used for wound healing in vivo. *Science,* 219:1329–1331.
460. Twardzik, D. R., Ranchalis, J. E., and Todaro, G. J. (1982): Mouse embryonic transforming growth factors related to those isolated from tumour cells. *Cancer Res.,* 42:590–593.
461. Kudlow, J. E., and Korbin, M. S. (1984): Secretion of epidermal growth factor-like mitogens by cultured cells from bovine anterior pituitary glands. *Endocrinology,* 115:911–917.
462. Baranao, J. L. S., and Hammond, J. M. (1984): Comparative effects of insulin and insulin-like growth factors on DNA synthesis and differentiation of porcine granulosa cells. *Biochem. Biophys. Res. Commun.,* 124:484–490.
463. Veldhuis, J. D., and Furlanetto, R. W. (1985): Trophic actions of human somatomedin C/insulin-like growth factor I on ovarian cells: in vitro studies with swine granulosa cells. *Endocrinology,* 116:1235–1242.
464. Ladenheim, R. G., Tesone, M., and Charreau, E. H. (1984): Insulin action and characterization of insulin receptors in rat luteal cells. *Endocrinology,* 115:752–756.

465. Rein, M. S., and Schomberg, D. W. (1982): Characterization of insulin receptors on porcine granulosa cells. *Biol. Reprod.*, 26 (Suppl. 1):113A (abstr. 154).
466. Otani, T., Mauro, T., Yukimur, N., and Mochizuki, M. (1985): Effect of insulin on porcine granulosa cells: implications of a possible receptor mediated action. *Acta Endocrinol. (Copenh.)*, 108:104–110.
467. Veldhuis, J. D., Tamura, S., Kolp, L., Furlanetto, R. W., and Larner, J. (1984): Mechanisms subserving insulin action in the gonad: evidence that insulin induces specific phosphorylation of its immunoprecipitable receptor on ovarian cells. *Biochem. Biophys. Res. Commun.*, 120:144–149.
468. Poretsky, L., Grigorescu, F., and Flier, J. S. (1985): Insulin but not IGF-I receptors are widely distributed in normal human ovary. *67th Annual Meeting of the Endocrine Society*, p. 204 (abstr. 814).
469. Hammond, J. M., Knight, A. P., and Rechler, M. M. (1984): Somatomedin secretion by porcine granulosa cells: a potential mechanism for regulating ovarian follicular growth. *Clin. Res.*, 32:485A (abstr.).
470. Hammond, J. M., Baranao, J. L. F., Skaleris, D. A., Rechler, M. M., and Knight, A. P. (1984): Somatomedin (Sm) production by cultured porcine granulosa cells (GC). *J. Steroid Biochem.*, 20:1597 (abstr. 128).
471. Hammond, J. M. (1981): Peptide regulators in the ovarian follicle. *Aust. J. Biol. Sci.*, 34:491–504.
472. Hammond, J. M., Yoshida, K., Veldhuis, J. D., Rechler, M. M., and Knight, A. P. (1983): Intrafollicular role of somatomedins: comparison with effect of insulin. In: *Factors Regulating Ovarian Function*, edited by G. S. Greenwald and P. F. Terranova, pp. 197–201. Raven Press, New York.
473. Davoren, J. B., and Hsueh, A. J. W. (1986): Growth hormone increases ovarian levels of immunoreactive somatomedin C/insulin-like growth factor I in vivo. *Endocrinology*, 118:888–898.
474. Diamond, M. P., Webster, B. W., Carr, R. K., Wentz, A. C., and Osteen, K. G. (1985): Human follicular-fluid insulin concentrations. *J. Clin. Endocrinol. Metab.*, 61:990–992.
475. Adashi, E. Y., Resnick, C. E., Svoboda, M. E., and Van Wyk, J. J. (1984): A novel role for somatomedin-C in the cytodifferentiation of the ovarian granulosa cell. *Endocrinology*, 115:1227–1229.
476. Adashi, E. Y., Resnick, C. E., Svoboda, M. E., and Van Wyk, J. J. (1985): Somatomedin-C synergizes with follicle-stimulating hormone in the acquisition of progesterone biosynthetic capacity by cultured rat granulosa cells. *Endocrinology*, 116:2135–2142.
477. Adashi, E. Y., Resnick, C. E., Brodie, A. M. H., Svoboda, M. E., and Van Wyk, J. J. (1985): Somatomedin-C-mediated potentiation of follicle-stimulating hormone-induced aromatase activity of cultured rat granulosa cells. *Endocrinology*, 117:2313–2320.
478. Veldhuis, J. D., Kolp, L. A., Toaff, M. E., Strauss III, J. F., and Demers, L. M. (1983): Mechanisms subserving the trophic actions of insulin on ovarian cells: in vitro studies using swine granulosa cells. *J. Clin. Invest.*, 72:1046–1057.
479. Veldhuis, J. D., Nestler, J. E., Strauss III, J. F., and Gwynne, J. T. (1986): Insulin regulates low density lipoprotein metabolism by swine granulosa cells. *Endocrinology*, 118:2242–2253.
480. Jia, X.-C., Kalmijn, J., and Hsueh, A. J. W. (1986): Growth hormone enhances follicle-stimulating hormone-induced differentiation of cultured rat granulosa cells. *Endocrinology*, 118:1401–1409.
481. Davoren, J. B., and Hsueh, A. J. W. (1984): Insulin enhances FSH-stimulated steroidogenesis by cultured rat granulosa cells. *Mol. Cell. Endocrinol.*, 35:97–105.
482. Veldhuis, J. D., and Kolp, L. A. (1985): Mechanisms subserving insulin's differentiating actions on progestin biosynthesis by ovarian cells: studies with cultured swine granulosa cells. *Endocrinology*, 116:651–659.
483. Ciancio, M. J., and LaBarbera, A. R. (1984): Insulin stimulates granulosa cells: increased progesterone and cAMP production in vitro. *Am. J. Physiol.*, 10:E468–E474.
484. Garzo, V. G., and Dorrington, J. H. (1984): Aromatase activity in human granulosa cells during follicular development and the modulation by follicle-stimulating hormone and insulin. *Am. J. Obstet. Gynecol.*, 148:657–662.
485. May, J. V., and Schomberg, D. W. (1981): Granulosa cell differentiation in vitro: effect of insulin on growth and functional integrity. *Biol. Reprod.*, 25:421–431.
486. Burden, H. W. (1972): Adrenergic innervation in ovaries of the rat and guinea pig. *Am. J. Anat.*, 133:455–462.
487. Bahr, J. M., and Ben-Jonathan, N. (1981): Pre-ovulatory depletion of ovarian catecholamine. *Endocrinology*, 108:1815–1820.
488. Ben-Jonathan, N., Brown, R. H., Laufer, N., Reich, R., and Bahr, J. M. (1982): Norepinephrine in Graafian follicles is depleted by follicle-stimulating hormone. *Endocrinology*, 110:457–461.
489. Bahr, J. M., and Ben-Jonathan, N. (1985): Elevated catecholamine in porcine follicular fluid before ovulation. *Endocrinology*, 117:620–623.
490. Burden, H. W., and Lawrence, I. E. (1977): The effects of denervation on the localization of Δ^5-3β-hydroxysteroid dehydrogenase activity in the rat ovary during pregnancy. *Acta Anat.*, 97:286–290.
491. Capps, M. L., Lawrence, I. E., and Burden, H. W. (1978): Ultrastructure of the cells of the ovarian interstitial gland in hypophysectomized rats. The effects of stimulation of the ovarian plexus and of denervation. *Cell Tissue Res.*, 193:433–442.
492. Bahr, J., Kao, L., and Nalbandov, A. V. (1974): The role of catecholamine and nerves in ovulation. *Biol. Reprod.*, 10:273–290.
493. Condon, W. A., and Black, D. L. (1976): Catecholamine-induced stimulation of progesterone by the bovine corpus luteum in vitro. *Biol. Reprod.*, 15:573–578.
494. Jordan III, A. W., Caffrey, J. L., and Niswender, G. D. (1978): Catecholamine-induced stimulation of progesterone and adenosine 3′,5′-monophosphate production by dispersed ovine luteal cells. *Endocrinology*, 103:385–392.
495. Kliachko, S., and Zor, U. (1981): Increase in catecholamine-stimulated cyclic AMP and progesterone synthesis in rat granulosa cells during culture. *Mol. Cell Endocrinol.*, 23:23–32.
496. Adashi, E. Y., and Hsueh, A. J. W. (1981): Stimulation of β-adrenergic responsiveness by follicle-stimulating hormone in rat granulosa cells in vitro and in vivo. *Endocrinology*, 108:2170–2178.
497. Aguado, L. I., Petrovic, S. L., and Ojeda, S. R. (1982): Ovarian β-adrenergic receptors during the onset of puberty: characterization, distribution and coupling to steroidogenic responses. *Endocrinology*, 110:1124–1132.
498. Sheela Rani, C. S., Nordenström, K. Norjavaara, E., and Ahren, K. (1983): Development of catecholamine responsiveness in granulosa cells from preovulatory rat follicles—dependence on preovulatory luteinizing hormone surge. *Biol. Reprod.*, 28:1021–1031.
499. Dyer, C. A., and Erickson, G. F. (1985): Norepinephrine amplifies human chorionic gonadotropin-stimulated androgen biosynthesis by ovarian theca-interstitial cells. *Endocrinology*, 116:1645–1652.
500. Burden, H. W., and Lawrence Jr., I. E. (1978): Experimental studies on the acetylcholinesterase-positive nerves in the ovary of the rat. *Anat. Rec.*, 190:233–242.
501. Farrar, J. A., Handeberg, G. M., Hartley, M. L., and Pennefather, J. N. (1980): Catecholamine levels in the guinea pig ovary, myometrium and costo-uterine muscle during the estrous cycle and in the ovary remaining after unilateral ovariectomy. *Biol. Reprod.*, 22:473–479.
502. Ojeda, S. R., Costa, M. E., Katz, K. H., and Hersh, L. B. (1985): Evidence for the existence of substance P in the prepubertal rat ovary. I. Biochemical and physiological studies. *Biol. Reprod.*, 33:286–295.
503. Dees, W. L., Kozlowski, G. P., Dey, R., and Ojeda, S. R. (1985): Evidence for the existence of substance P in the prepubertal rat ovary. II. Immunocytochemical localization. *Biol. Reprod.*, 33:471–476.
504. Larson, L. I., Fahrenkrug, J., and Schaffalitsky de Misckadell, O. B. (1977): Vasoactive intestinal polypeptide occurs in nerves of the female genitourinary tract. *Science*, 197:1374–1375.
505. Davoren, J. B., and Hsueh, A. J. W. (1985): Vasoactive intestinal peptide: a novel stimulator of steroidogenesis by cultured rat granulosa cells. *Biol. Reprod.*, 33:37–52.
506. Pedersen, T., and Peters, H. (1968): Proposal for a classification of oocytes and follicles in the mouse ovary. *J. Reprod. Fertil.*, 17:555–557.
507. Peters, H., Byskov, A. G., and Grinsted, J. (1978): Follicular growth in fetal and prepubertal ovaries in humans and other primates. In: *Clinics in Endocrinology and Metabolism. Reproductive Endocrinology*, edited by G. T. Ross and M. B. Lipsett, pp. 469–485. Saunders, London.
508. Noumura, T., Weisz, J., and Lloyd, C. W. (1966): In vitro conversion of 7-H^3 progesterone to androgens by the rat testis during the second half of fetal life. *Endocrinology*, 78:245–253.

509. Arai, H. (1920): On the postnatal development of the ovary (albino rat) with special reference to the number of ova. *Am. J. Anat.*, 27:405–462.
510. Beaumont, H., and Mandl, A. M. (1962): A quantitative and cytological study of oogonia and oocytes in the foetal and neonatal rat. *Proc. R. Soc. London [Biol.]* 155:557–579.
511. Levina, S. E., Gyevai, A., and Horvath, E. (1975): Responsiveness of the ovary to gonadotrophins in pre- and perinatal life: estrogen secretion in tissue and organ cultures. *J. Endocrinol.*, 65: 219–223.
512. Schlegel, R. J., Farias, E., Russo, N. C., Moore, J. R., and Gardner, L. I. (1967): Structural changes in the fetal gonads and gonaducts during maturation of an enzyme, steroid 3β-ol-dehydrogenase, in the gonads, adrenal cortex and placenta of fetal rats. *Endocrinology*, 81:565–572.
513. Brambell, F. W. R. (1927): The development and morphology of the gonads of the mouse. 1. The morphogenesis of the indifferent gonad and of the ovary. *Proc. R. Soc. London [Biol.]*, 101:391–408.
514. Borum, K. (1961): Oogenesis in the mouse. A study of the meiotic prophase. *Exp. Cell Res.*, 24:495–507.
515. Peters, H. (1969): The development of the mouse ovary from birth to maturity. *Acta Endocrinol. (Copenh.)*, 62:98–116.
516. Milewich, L., George, F. W., and Wilson, J. D. (1977): Estrogen formation by the ovary of the rabbit embryo. *Endocrinology*, 100:187–196.
517. Mauléon, P., Bezard, J., and Terqui, M. (1977): Very early and transient 17β-estradiol secretion by fetal sheep ovary—in vitro study. *Ann. Biol. Anim. Biochim. Biophys.*, 17:339–401.
518. Shemesh, M., Ailenberg, M., Milaguir, F. Ayalon, N., and Hansel, W. (1978): Hormone secretion by cultured bovine pre- and postimplantation gonads. *Biol. Reprod.*, 19:761–767.
519. Erickson, G. F., Challis, J. R. G., and Ryan, K. J. (1974): A developmental study on the capacity of rabbit granulosa cells to respond to trophic hormones and secrete progesterone in vitro. *Dev. Biol.*, 40:208–224.
520. Mauléon, P. (1961): Utilization de la colchicine dans l'étude des divisions goniales de l'ovaire d'embryons de brebis et analyse de quelques résultats. *Ann. Biol. Anim. Biochem. Biophys.*, 1:70–73.
521. Teplitz, R., and Ohno, S. (1963): Postnatal induction of ovogenesis in the rabbit (*Oryctolagus cuniculus*). *Exp. Cell Res.*, 31:183–189.
522. Peters, H., Levy, E., and Crone, M. (1965): Oogenesis in rabbits. *J. Exp. Zool.*, 158:169–180.
523. Mauléon, P. (1967): Cinétique de l'ovogenèse chez les mammifères. *Arch. Anat. Microsc. Morphol. Exp.* (Suppl).3/4:125–150.
524. Shemesh, M. (1980): Estradiol-17β biosynthesis by the early bovine fetal ovary during the active and refractory phases. *Biol. Reprod.*, 23:577–582.
525. Roberts, J. D., and Warren, J. C. (1964): Steroid biosynthesis in the fetal ovary. *Endocrinology*, 74:846–852.
526. Goldman, A. A., Yakovac, W. C., and Bongiovanni, A. M. (1966): Development of activity of 3β-hydroxysteroid dehydrogenase in human fetal tissues and in two anencephalic newborns. *J. Clin. Endocrinol. Metab.*, 26:14–22.
527. Cavallero, C., and Magrini, U. (1966) Histochemical studies on 3β-hydroxysteroid dehydrogenase and other enzymes in the steroid-secreting structures of human foetus. In: *Second International Congress on Hormonal Steroids, International Congress Ser. 132,* edited by L. Martini, F. Fraschini, and M. Motta, pp. 667–674. Excerpta Medica, Amsterdam.
528. Brandau, H., and Lehmann, V. (1970): Histoenzymatische untersuchungen an menschlichen gonaden wahrend der intrauterinen entwicklung. *Z. Geburtshilfe Gynaekol.*, 173:233–249.
529. Singh, R. F., and Carr, D. H. (1966): The anatomy and histology of XO human embryos and fetuses. *Anat. Rec.*, 155:369–383.
530. Morishima, A., and Grumbach, M. M. (1968): The interrelationship of sex chromosome constitution and phenotype in the syndrome of gonadal dysgenesis and its variants. *Ann NY Acad. Sci.*, 155:695–715.
531. Weiss, L. (1971): Additional evidence of gradual loss of germ cells in the pathogenesis of streak ovaries in Turner's syndrome. *J. Med. Genet.*, 8:540–544.
532. Lyon, M. F., and Hawker, S. G. (1973): Reproductive lifespan in irradiated and unirradiated chromosomally XO mice. *Genet. Res.*, 21:185–194.
533. Burgoyne, P. S., and Baker, T. G. (1981): The XO ovary—development and function. In: *Development and Function of Reproductive Organs, International Congress Series No. 559,* edited by A. G. Byskov and H. Peters, pp. 122–128. Excerpta Medica, Amsterdam.
534. Vanhems, E., and Bousquet, J. (1971): Influence du misulban sur le développement de l'ovaire du rat. *Ann. Endocrinol. (Paris)*, 33:119–128.
535. Merchant Larios, H. (1976): The role of germ cells in the morphogenesis and cytodifferentiation of the rat ovary. In: *Progress in Differentiation Research,* edited by N. Müller-Bérat, pp. 453–462. North-Holland, Amsterdam.
536. Beaumont, H. M. (1961): Radiosensitivity of oogonia and oocytes in the foetal rat. *Int. J. Rad. Biol.*, 3:59–72.
537. Reddoch, R. B., Pelletier, R. M., Barbe, G. J., and Armstrong, D. T. (1986): Lack of ovarian responsiveness to gonadotropic hormones in infantile rats sterilized with Busulfan. *Endocrinology*, 119:879–886.
538. Edwards, R. G., Fowler, R. E., Gore-Langton, R. E., et al. (1977): Normal and abnormal follicular growth in mouse, rat and human ovaries. *J. Reprod. Fertil.*, 51:237–263.
539. Nakano, R., Mizuno, T., Katayama, K., and Tojo, S. (1975): Growth of ovarian follicles in the absence of gonadotrophins. *J. Reprod. Fertil.*, 45:545–546.
540. Roy, S. K., and Greenwald, G. S. (1985): An enzymatic method for dissociation of intact follicles from the hamster ovary: histological and quantitative aspects. *Biol. Reprod.*, 32:203–215.
541. Brambell, F. W. R. (1928): The development and morphology of the gonads of the mouse. 3. The growth of the follicles. *Proc. R. Soc. London [Biol.]*, 102:258–272.
542. Harrison, R. J., and Weir, B. J. (1977): Structure of the mammalian ovary. In: *The Ovary,* Vol. 1, edited by S. Zuckerman and B. J. Weir, pp. 113–217, Academic, New York.
543. Presl, J., Pospisil, J., Figarova, V., and Krabec, Z. (1974): Stage dependent changes in binding of iodinated FSH during ovarian follicle maturation in rats. *Endocrinol. Exp. (Bratisl.)*, 8:291–298.
544. Nimrod, A., Erickson, G. F., and Ryan, K. J. (1976): A specific FSH receptor in rat granulosa cells: properties of binding in vitro. *Endocrinology*, 98:56–64.
545. Quattropani, S. L., and Weisz, J. (1973): Conversion of progesterone to estrone and estradiol in vitro by the ovary of the infantile rat in relation to the development of its interstitial tissue. *Endocrinology*, 53:1269–1276.
546. Peluso, J. J., Steger, R. W., and Hafez, E. S. E. (1976): Development of gonadotropin-binding sites in the immature rat ovary. *J. Reprod. Fertil.*, 47:55–58.
547. Reddoch, R. B., and Armstrong, D. T. (1984): Interactions of a phosphodiesterase inhibitor, 3-isobutyl-1-methyl xanthine, with prostaglandin E_2, follicle-stimulating hormone, luteinizing hormone, and dibutyryl cyclic 3′,5′-adenosine monophosphate (cAMP) in cAMP and steroid production by neonatal rat ovaries in vitro. *Endocrinology*, 115:11–18.
548. Funkenstein, B., Nimrod, A., and Lindner, H. R. (1980): The development of steroidogenic capability and responsiveness to gonadotropins in cultured neonatal rat ovaries. *Endocrinology*, 106:98–106.
549. Kolena, J. (1976): Reversal of the unresponsiveness of neonatal rat ovary to LH in cAMP synthesis by estrogen. *Horm. Res.*, 7:152–157.
550. Dohler, K. D., and Wuttke, W. (1975): Changes with age in levels of serum gonadotropins, prolactin and gonadal steroids in prepubertal male and female rats. *Endocrinology*, 97:898–907.
551. Meijs-Roelofs, H. M. A., deGreef, W. J., and Uilenbroek, J. T. J. (1975): Plasma progesterone and its relationship to serum goadotropins in immature female rats. *J. Endocrinol.*, 64:329–334.
552. Ramaley, J. A. (1979): Development of gonadotropin regulation in the prepubertal mammal. *Biol. Reprod.*, 20:1–31.
553. van Wagenen, G., and Simpson, M. E. (1965): *Embryology of The Ovary and Testis. Homo Sapiens and Macaca Mulatta.* Yale University Press, New Haven, CT.
554. Gondos, B., and Hobel, C. J. (1973): Interstitial cells in the human fetal ovary. *Endocrinology*, 93:736–739.
555. George, F. W., and Wilson, J. D. (1978): Conversion of androgen to estrogen by the human fetal ovary. *J. Clin. Endocrinol. Metab.*, 47:550–555.

556. Taylor, T., Coutles, J. R. T., and MacNaughton, M. C. (1974): Human foetal synthesis of testosterone from perfused progesterone. *J. Endocrinol,* 60:321–326.
557. Jungmann, R. A., and Schweppe, J. S. (1968): Biosynthesis of sterols and steroids from acetate ^{14}C by human fetal ovaries. *J. Clin. Endocrinol. Metab.,* 28:1599–1604.
558. Schindler, A. E., and Friedrich, E. (1975): Steroid metabolism of foetal tissues. I. Metabolism of pregnenolone-4-^{14}C by human foetal ovaries. *Endokrinologie,* 65:72–79.
559. Bloch, E. (1964): Metabolism of [4-^{14}C]-progesterone by human fetal testis and ovaries. *Endocrinology,* 74:833–845.
560. Wilson, E. A., and Jawad, M. J. (1979): The effects of trophic agents on fetal ovarian steroidogenesis in organ culture. *Fertil. Steril.,* 32:73–79.
561. Payne, A. H., and Jaffe, R. B. (1974): Androgen formation from pregnenolone sulfate by the human fetal ovary. *J. Clin. Endocrinol. Metab.,* 39:300–304.
562. Huhtaniemi, I., and Vihko, R. (1970): Determination of unconjugated and sulfated neutral steroids in fetal blood of early and mid-pregnancy. *Steroids,* 16:197–206.
563. Ellinwood, W. M., McClellan, M. C., Brenner, R. M., and Resko, J. A. (1983): Estradiol synthesis by fetal monkey ovaries correlates with antral follicle formation. *Biol. Reprod.,* 28:505–516.
564. Grob, H. S. (1969): Growth and endocrine function of isolated ovarian follicles cultivated in vivo. *Biol. Reprod.,* 1:320–323.
565. Nicosia, S. V., Evangelista, I., and Batta, S. K. (1975): Rabbit ovarian follicles. I. Isolation technique and characterization at different stages of development. *Biol. Reprod.,* 13:423–447.
566. Terranova, P. F., and Garza, F. (1983): Relationship between the preovulatory luteinizing hormone (LH) surge and androstenedione synthesis of preantral follicles in the cyclic hamster: Detection by in vitro responses to LH. *Biol. Reprod.,* 29:630–636.
567. Høyer, P. E., and Anderson, H. (1977): Histochemistry of 3β-hydroxysteroid dehydrogenase in rat ovary. *Histochemistry,* 51:167–193.
568. Richards, J. S. (1980): Maturation of ovarian follicles: actions and interactions of pituitary and ovarian hormones on follicular cell differentiation. *Physiol. Rev.,* 60:51–89.
569. McNatty, K. P. (1978): Follicular fluid. In: *The Vertebrate Ovary,* edited by R. E. Jones, pp. 215–259. Plenum Press, New York.
570. Richards, J. S., Jonasson, J. A., Rolfes, A. I., Kersey, K., and Reichert Jr., L. E. (1979): Adenosine 3′,5′-monophosphate, luteinizing hormone receptor, and progesterone during granulosa cell differentiation: effects of estradiol and follicle-stimulating hormone. *Endocrinology,* 104:765–773.
571. Sheela Rani, C. S., Salhanick, A. R., and Armstrong, D. T. (1981): Follicle-stimulating hormone induction of luteinizing hormone receptor in cultured rat granulosa cells: an examination of the need for steroids in the induction process. *Endocrinology,* 108:1379–1385.
572. Wang, C., Hsueh, A. J. W., and Erickson, G. F. (1979): Induction of functional prolactin receptors by follicle-stimulating hormone in rat granulosa cells in vivo and in vitro. *J. Biol. Chem.,* 254:11330–11336.
573. Edwards, R. G. (1974): Follicular fluid. *J. Reprod. Fertil.,* 37:189–219.
574. Mossman, H. W., and Duke, K. L. (1973): *Comparative Morphology of the Mammalian Ovary.* University of Wisconsin Press, Madison.
575. Bjersing, L. (1978): Maturation, morphology, and endocrine function of the follicular wall in mammals. In: *The Vertebrate Ovary,* edited by R. E. Jones, pp. 181–214. Plenum, New York.
576. Baird, D. T., Swanston, I., and Scaramuzzi, R. J. (1976): Pulsatile release of LH and secretion of ovarian steroids in sheep during the luteal phase of the estrous cycle. *Endocrinology,* 98:1490–1496.
577. Giorgi, E. P., Addis, M., and Columbo, G. (1969): The fate of free and conjugated oestrogens injected into the Graafian follicles of equines. *J. Endocrinol.,* 43:37–50.
578. Martin, B., Rotten, D., Jolivet, A., and Gautray, J. P. (1981): Binding of steroids by proteins in follicular fluid of the human ovary. *J. Clin. Endocrinol. Metab.,* 53:443–447.
579. Cook, B., Hunter, R. H. F., and Kelly, A. S. L. (1977): Steroid-binding proteins in follicular fluid and peripheral plasma from pigs, cows and sheep. *J. Reprod. Fertil.,* 51:65–71.
580. Baird, D. T. (1976): Ovarian steroid secretion and metabolism in women. In: *The Endocrine Function of the Human Ovary,* edited by V. H. T. James, M. Seiro, and G. Giusti, pp. 125–133. Academic, London.
581. McNatty, K. P., Baird, D. T., Bolton, A., Chambers, P., Corker, C. S., and McLean, H. (1976): Concentration of oestrogens and androgens in human ovarian venous plasma and follicular fluid throughout the menstrual cycle. *J. Endocrinol.,* 71:77–85.
582. McNatty, K. P., Hunter, W. M., McNeilly, A. S., and Sawers, R. S. (1975): Changes in the concentration of pituitary and steroid hormones in the follicular fluid of human Graafian follicles throughout the menstrual cycle. *J. Endocrinol.,* 64:555–571.
583. Kemeter, P., Salzer, H., Breitenecker, G., and Friedrich, F. (1975): Progesterone, oestradiol-17β, and testosterone levels in the follicular fluid of tertiary follicles and Graafian follicles of human ovaries. *Acta Endocrinol. (Copenh.),* 80:686–704.
584. McNatty, K. P., and Baird, D. T. (1978): Relationship between follicle-stimulating hormone, androstenedione and oestradiol in human follicular fluid. *J. Endocrinol.,* 76:527–531.
585. Breitenecker, G., Friedrich, F., and Kemeter, P. (1978): Further investigations on the maturation and degeneration of human ovarian follicles and their oocytes. *Fertil. Steril.,* 29:336–341.
586. McNatty, K. P. (1982): Ovarian follicular development from the onset of luteal regression in humans and sheep. In: *Proceedings IVth Regnier de Graaf Symposium: Follicular Maturation and Ovulation,* edited by R. Rolland, E. V. van Hall, S. G. Hillier, K. P. McNatty, and J. Schoemaker, pp. 1–18. Excerpta Medica, Amsterdam.
587. Hillier, S. G., van Hall, E. V., van den Boogaard, A. J. M., de Zwart, F. A., and Keyzer, R. (1982): Activation and modulation of the granulosa cell aromatase system: experimental studies with rat and human ovaries. In: *Proceedings IVth Regnier de Graaf Symposium: Follicular Maturation and Ovulation,* edited by R. Rolland, E. V. van Hall, S. G. Hillier, K. P. McNatty, and J. Schoemaker, pp. 51–70. Excerpta Medica, Amsterdam.
588. Bomsel-Helmreich, O., Gougeon, A., Thebault, A., et al. (1979): Healthy and atretic human follicles in the preovulatory phase: differences in evolution of follicular morphology and steroid content of follicular fluid. *J. Clin. Endocrinol. Metab.,* 48:686–694.
589. Westergaard, L., McNatty, K. P., Christensen, I., Larsen, J. K., and Byskov, A. G. (1982): Flow cytometric deoxyribonucleic acid analysis of granulosa cells aspirated from human ovarian follicles. A new method to distinguish healthy and atretic ovarian follicles. *J. Clin. Endocrinol. Metab.,* 55:693–698.
590. McNatty, K. P., Hillier, S. G., van den Boogaard, A. M. J., Trimbos-Kemper, T. C. M., Reichert Jr., L. E., and van Hall, E. V. (1983): Follicular development during the luteal phase of the human menstrual cycle. *J. Clin. Endocrinol. Metab.,* 56:1022–1031.
591. McNatty, K. M., Gibb, M., Dobson, C., Thurley, D. C., and Findlay, J. K. (1981): Changes in the concentration of gonadotrophic and steroidal hormones in the antral fluid of ovarian follicles throughout the estrous cycle of the sheep. *Aust. J. Biol. Sci.,* 34:67–80.
592. Eiler, H., and Nalbandov, A. V. (1977): Sex steroids in follicular fluid and blood plasma during the estrous cycle of pigs. *Endocrinology,* 100:331–338.
593. Patwardhan, V. V., and Lanthier, A. (1976): Effect of an ovulatory dose of luteinizing hormone on the concentration of oestrone, oestradiol and progesterone in the rabbit ovarian follicles. *Acta Endocrinol. (Copenh.),* 82:792–800.
594. Fujii, T., Hoover, D. J., and Channing, C. P. (1983): Changes in inhibin activity, and progesterone, oestrogen and androstenedione concentrations in rat follicular fluid throughout the oestrous cycle. *J. Reprod. Fertil.,* 69:307–314.
595. Moor, R. M., Hay, M. F., Dott, H. M., and Cran, D. G. (1978): Macroscopic identification and steroidogenic function of atretic follicles in sheep. *J. Endocrinol.,* 77:309–318.
596. Tsuji, K., Sowa, M., and Nakano, R. (1983): Relationship among the status of the human oocyte, the 17β-estradiol concentration in the antral fluid and the follicular size. *Endocrinol. Jpn.,* 30:251–254.
597. Baird, D. T., and Fraser, I. S. (1975): Concentration of oestrone and oestradiol-17β in follicular fluid and ovarian venous blood of women. *Clin. Endocrinol.,* 4:259–266.
598. Baird, D. T. (1983): Factors regulating the growth of the preovulatory follicle in the sheep and human. *J. Reprod. Fertil.,* 69:343–352.
599. Smith, O. W. (1960): Estrogens in the ovarian fluids of normally menstruating women. *Endocrinology,* 67:698–707.

600. Short, R. V., and London, D. R. (1961): Defective biosynthesis of ovarian steroids in the Stein-Leventhal syndrome. *Br. Med. J.*, 1:1764–1727.
601. deJong, F. H., Baird, D. T., and van der Molen, H. J. (1974): Ovarian secretion rates of oestrogens, androgens and progesterone in normal women and in women with persistent ovarian follicles. *Acta Endocrinol. (Copenh.)*, 77:575–587.
602. Sanyal, M. K., Berger, M. J., Thompson, I. E., Taymor, M. L., and Horne Jr., H. W. (1974): Development of Graafian follicles in adult human ovary. I. Correlation of estrogen and progesterone concentration in antral fluid with growth of follicles. *J. Clin. Endocrinol. Metab.*, 38:828–835.
603. Short, R. V. (1964): Steroid concentrations in the fluid from normal and polycystic (Stein-Leventhal) ovaries. In: *Proceedings of the Second International Congress of Endocrinology. International Congress Ser. No. 83,* pp. 940–943. Excerpta Medica, Amsterdam.
604. Edwards, R. G., Steptoe, P. C., Abraham, G. E., Walters, E., Purdy, J. M., and Fotherby, K. (1972): Steroid assays and preovulatory follicular development in human ovaries primed with gonadotrophins. *Lancet,* 2:611–615.
605. Knudsen, O., and Velle, W. (1961): Ovarian oestrogen levels in the nonpregnant mare: relationship to histological appearance of the uterus and to clinical status. *J. Reprod. Fertil.*, 2:130–137.
606. Short, R. V. (1962): Steroid concentrations in normal follicular fluid and ovarian cyst fluid from cows. *J. Reprod. Fertil.*, 4:27–45.
607. Channing, C. P., and Coudert, S. P. (1976): Contribution of granulosa cells and follicular fluid to ovarian estrogen secretion in the rhesus monkey in vivo. *Endocrinology,* 98:590–597.
608. Aedo, A. R., Pedersen, P. H., Pedersen, S. C., and Diczfalusy, E. (1980): Ovarian steroid secretion in normally menstruating women. I. The contribution of the developing follicle. *Acta Endocrinol. (Copenh.)*, 95:212–221.
609. Uilenbroek, J. T. J., van der Schoot, P., den Besten, D., and Woutersen, P. J. A. (1982): Control of steroidogenesis during growth and early atresia of preovulatory rat follicles. In: *Proceedings of the IVth Regnier De Graaf Symposium. Follicular Maturation and Ovulation,* edited by R. Rolland, E. V. van Hall, S. G. Hillier, K. P. McNatty, and J. Schoemaker, pp. 71–82. Excerpta Medica, Amsterdam.
610. diZerega, G. S., Marrs, R. P., Roche, P. C., Campeau, J. D., and Kling, O. R. (1983): Identification of proteins in pooled human follicular fluid which suppress follicular response to gonadotropins. *J. Clin. Endocrinol. Metab.*, 56:35–41.
611. diZerega, G. S., Marrs, R. P., Campeau, J. D., and Kling, O. R. (1983): Human granulosa cell secretion of protein(s) which suppress follicular response to gonadotropins. *J. Clin. Endocrinol. Metab.*, 56:147–155.
612. Kling, O. R., Roche, P. C., Campeau, J. D., Nishimura, K., Nakamura, R. M., and diZerega, G. S. (1984): Identification of protein(s) in porcine follicular fluid which suppress follicular response to gonadotropins. *Biol. Reprod.*, 30:564–572.
613. diZerega, G. S., Campeau, J. D., Nakamura, R. M., Ujita, E. L., Lobo, R., and Marrs, R. P. (1983): Activity of a human follicular fluid protein(s) from spontaneous and induced ovarian cycles. *J. Clin. Endocrinol. Metab.*, 57:838–846.
614. diZerega, G. S., Goebelsman, U., and Nakamura, R. M. (1982): Identification of protein(s) secreted by the preovulatory ovary which suppresses the follicle response to gonadotropins. *J. Clin. Endocrinol. Metab.*, 54:1091–1096.
615. Brailly, D., Gougeon, A., Milgrom, E., Bomsel-Helmreich, O., and Papiernik, E. (1981): Androgen and progestins in the human ovarian follicle: differences in the evolution of preovulatory, healthy nonovulatory and atretic follicles. *J. Clin. Endocrinol. Metab.*, 53:128–134.
616. Veldhuis, J. D., Klase, P. A., and Hammond, J. M. (1981): Sex steroids modulate prolactin action in spontaneously luteinizing porcine granulosa cells in vitro. *Endocrinology,* 108:1463–1468.
617. Schaar, H. (1976): Funktionelle morphologie der theca interna im blaschenfollikel des menschlichen ovars. *Acta Anat.*, 94:283–298.
618. Leung, P. C. K., and Armstrong, D. T. (1980): Interactions of steroids and gonadotropins in the control of steroidogenesis in the ovarian follicle. *Annu. Rev. Physiol.*, 42:71–82.
619. Tsang, B. K., Leung, P. C. K., and Armstrong, D. T. (1979): Inhibition by estradiol-17β of porcine thecal androgen production in vitro. *Mol. Cell. Endocrinol.*, 14:131–139.
620. Henderson, K. M., McNeilly, A. S., and Swanston, I. A. (1982): Gonadotrophin and steroid concentrations in bovine follicular fluid and their relationship to follicle size. *J. Reprod. Fertil.*, 65:467–473.
621. Henderson, K. M., and Swanston, I. A. (1978): Androgen aromatization by luteinized bovine granulosa cells in tissue culture. *J. Reprod. Fertil.*, 52:131–134.
622. Henderson, K. M., and Moon, Y. S. (1979): Luteinization of bovine granulosa cells and corpus luteum formation associated with loss of androgen aromatizing ability. *J. Reprod. Fertil.*, 56:89–97.
623. Matson, P. L., Tyler, J. P. P., and Collins, W. P. (1981): Follicular steroid content and oocyte meiotic status after PMSG stimulation of immature hamsters. *J. Reprod. Fertil.*, 61:443–452.
624. Khalil, M. W., and Snow, K. (1985): 19-norandrostenedione (4-estren-3,17-dione) levels in follicular fluid during ovarian follicular development in gilts. *Biol. Reprod.*, 32 (Suppl. 1): 122 (abstr. 170).
625. Daniel, S. A. J., Khalil, M. W., and Armstrong, D. T. (1986): 19-Norandrostenedione (4-estrene-3,17-dione) inhibits porcine oocyte maturation in vitro. *Gamete Res.*, 13:173–184.
626. Axelrod, L. R., and Goldzieher, J. W. (1970): The effect of cofactors on steroid biosynthesis in normal ovarian tissue. *Biochim. Biophys. Acta,* 202:349–353.
627. Swanston, I., McNatty, K. P., and Baird, D. T. (1977): The concentration of prostaglandin $F_{2\alpha}$ and steroids in the human corpus luteum. *J. Endocrinol.*, 73:115–122.
628. Yen, S. S. C. (1978): The human menstrual cycle (integrative function of the hypothalamic–pituitary–ovarian–endometrial axis). In: *Reproductive Endocrinology,* edited by S. S. C. Yen and R. B. Jaffe, pp. 126–151. Saunders, Philadelphia.
629. McNatty, K. P., and Sawers, R. S. (1975): Relationship between the endocrine environment within the Graafian follicle and the subsequent rate of progesterone secretion by human granulosa cells in vitro. *J. Endocrinol.*, 66:391–400.
630. Laborde, N., Carril, M., Cheviakoff, S., Croxatto, H. D., Pedroza, E., and Rosner, J. M. (1976): The secretion of progesterone during the periovulatory period in women with certified ovulation. *J. Clin. Endocrinol. Metab.*, 43:1157–1163.
631. Fowler, R. E., Chan, S. T. H., Walters, D. E., Edwards, R. G., and Steptoe, P. C. (1977): Steroidogenesis in human follicles approaching ovulation as judged from assays of follicular fluid. *J. Endocrinol.*, 72:259–271.
632. Fortune, J. E. (1981): Bovine theca and granulosa cells interact to promote androgen and progestin production. *Biol. Reprod.*, 24 (Suppl. 1): 39A (abstr.).
633. Peters, H., and McNatty, K. P. (1980): *The Ovary*. Granada, London.
634. Mestwerdt, W. (1977): Die follikel-granulosazellen in beziehung zur steroid-biosynthese in der periovulationsphase. *Fortschr. Med.*, 95:361–365.
635. Mestwerdt, W., Müller, O., and Brandau, H. (1977): Die differenzierte struktur und funktion der granulosa und theka in verschiedenen follikelstadien menschlicher ovarien. 2. Mittleilung: der reifende, reife, sprungreife und frisch geplatzte follikel. *Arch. Gynaekol.*, 222:115–136.
636. Mestwerdt, W., Müller, O., and Brandau, H. (1977): Die differenzierte struktur und funktion der granulosa und theka in verschiedenen follikelstadien menschlicher ovarien. 1. mitteilung: der primordial-, primar-, sekundar- und ruhende tertiarfollikel. *Arch. Gynakol.*, 222:45–71.
637. Albertini, D. F., and Anderson, E. (1974): The appearance and structure of intercellular connections during the ontogeny of the rabbit ovarian follicle with particular reference to gap junctions. *J. Cell Biol.*, 63:234–250.
638. Bjersing, L., and Cajander, S. (1974): Ovulation and the mechanism of follicle rupture. VI. Ultrastructure of theca interna and the inner vascular network surrounding rabbit Graafian follicles prior to induced ovulation. *Cell Tissue Res.*, 153:31–44.
639. Delforge, J. P., Thomas, K., Roux, F. Carneiro de Siqueira, J., and Ferin, J. (1972): Time relationships between granulosa cell growth and luteinization, and plasma luteinizing hormone discharge in human. I. A morphometric analysis. *Fertil. Steril.*, 23:1–11.

640. Norman, R. L., and Greenwald, G. S. (1972): Follicular histology and physiological correlates in the preovulatory hamster. *Anat. Rec.*, 173:95–108.
641. Hermreck, A. S., and Greenwald, G. S. (1964): The effects of unilateral ovariectomy on follicular maturation in the guinea pig. *Anat. Rec.*, 148:171–176.
642. Boucek, R. J., Telegdy, G., and Savard, K. (1967): Influence of gonadotropin on histochemical properties of the rabbit ovary. *Acta Endocrinol. (Copenh.)*, 54:295–310.
643. Klinken, S. P., and Stevenson, P. M. (1977): Changes in enzymatic activities during the artificially stimulated transition from follicular to luteal cell types in rat ovary. *Eur. J. Biochem.*, 81:327–332.
644. Pupkin, M., Bratt, H., Weisz, J., Lloyd, C. W., and Balogh Jr., K. (1966): Dehydrogenases in the rat ovary. I. A histochemical study of Δ^5-3β- and 20α-hydroxysteroid dehydrogenases and enzymes of carbohydrate oxidation during the estrous cycle. *Endocrinology*, 79:316–327.
645. Bjersing, L. (1977): Ovarian histochemistry. In: *The Ovary*, Vol. 1, edited by S. Zuckerman and B. J. Wier, pp. 303–391. Academic, New York.
646. Wingate, A. L. (1970): A histochemical study of the hamster ovary. *Anat. Rec.*, 166:399 (abstr.).
647. Blaha, G. C., and Leavitt, W. W. (1970): The distribution of Δ^5-3β-hydroxysteroid activity in the golden hamster during the estrous cycle, pregnancy, and lactation. *Biol. Reprod.*, 3:362–368.
648. Norman, R. L., and Greenwald, G. S. (1971): Effect of phenobarbital, hypophysectomy, and X-irradiation on preovulatory progesterone levels in the cyclic hamster. *Endocrinology*, 89:598–605.
649. Friedrich, F., Breitenecker, G., Salzer, H., and Holzner, J. H. (1974): The progesterone content of the fluid and the activity of the steroid-3β-ol-dehydrogenase within the wall of the ovarian follicles. *Acta Endocrinol. (Copenh.)*, 76:343–352.
650. Hillensjö, T., Bauminger, S., and Ahrén, K. (1976): Effect of luteinizing hormone on the pattern of steroid production by preovulatory follicles of pregnant mare's serum gonadotropin-injected immature rats. *Endocrinology*, 99:996–1002.
651. LeMaire, W. J., and Marsh, J. M. (1975): Interrelationships between prostaglandins, cyclic AMP and steroids in ovulation. *J. Reprod. Fertil.*, 22 (Suppl.):53–74.
652. Younglai, E. V. (1977): Steroid production by isolated rabbit ovarian follicles: effects of luteinizing hormone from mating to implantation. *J. Endocrinol.*, 73:59–65.
653. Hori, T., Ide, M., and Miyake, T. (1969): Pituitary regulation of preovulatory oestrogen secretion in the rat. *Endocrinol. Jpn.*, 16:351–360.
654. Hubbard, C. J., and Greenwald, G. S. (1982): Cyclic nucleotides, DNA, and steroid levels in ovarian follicles and corpora lutea of the cyclic hamster. *Biol. Reprod.*, 26:230–240.
655. Murdoch, W. J., and Dunn, T. G. (1982): Alterations in follicular steroid hormones during the preovulatory period in the ewe. *Biol. Reprod.*, 24:1171–1181.
656. Dieleman, S. J., Bevers, M. M., Poortman, J., and van Tol, H. T. M. (1983): Steroid and pituitary hormone concentrations in the fluid of preovulatory bovine follicles relative to the peak of LH in the peripheral blood. *J. Reprod. Fertil.*, 69:641–649.
657. Testart, J. Castanier, M., Feinstein, M.-C., and Frydman, R. (1982): Pituitary and steroid hormones in the preovulatory follicle during spontaneous or stimulated cycles. In: *Follicular Maturation and Ovulation*, edited by R. Rolland, E. V. van Hall, S. G. Hillier, K. P. McNatty, and J. Schoemaker, pp. 193–201. Excerpta Medica, Amsterdam.
658. Van Look, P. F. A., Templeton, A. A., Swantson, I. A., et al. (1984). The effect of hCG on steroid levels in human Graafian follicles. *Proceedings of the 3rd Joint Meeting of the British Endocrine Societies, Edinburgh*, Abstract.
659. Moor, R. M. (1974): The ovarian follicle of the sheep: inhibition of oestrogen secretion by luteinizing hormone. *J. Endocrinol.*, 61:455–463.
660. Bockaert, J., Hunzicker-Dunn, M., and Birnbaumer, L. (1976): Hormone-stimulated desensitization of hormone-dependent adenylyl cyclase: dual action of luteinizing hormone on pig Graafian follicle membranes. *J. Biol. Chem.*, 251:2653–2663.
661. Mori, T., Fujita, Y., Suzuki, A., Kinoshita, Y., Nishimura, T., and Kambegawa, A. (1978): Functional and structural relationships in steroidogenesis in vitro by human ovarian follicles during maturation and ovulation. *J. Clin. Endocrinol. Metab.*, 47:955–966.
662. Edwards, R. G., Steptoe, P. C., Fowler, R. E., and Baille, J. (1980): Observations on preovulatory human ovarian follicles and their aspirates. *Br. J. Obstet. Gynaecol.*, 87:769–779.
663. Landgren, B.-M., Aedo, A.-R., Nunez, M., Cekan, S. Z., and Diczfalusy, E. (1977): Studies on the pattern of circulating steroids in the normal menstrual cycle. *Acta Endocrinol. (Copenh.)*, 84:620–632.
664. Kirchick, H. J., and Birnbaumer, L. (1983): Luteal adenylyl cyclase does not develop sensitivity to desensitization by human chorionic gonadotropin in the absence of nonluteal ovarian tissue. *Endocrinology*, 113:2052–2058.
665. Richards, J. S., Ireland, J. J., Rao, M. C., Bernath, G. A., Midgley Jr., A. R., and Reichert Jr., L. E. (1976): Ovarian follicular development in the rat: hormone receptor regulation by estradiol, follicle-stimulating hormone and luteinizing hormone. *Endocrinology*, 99:1562–1570.
666. Rao, M. C., Richards, J. S., Midgley Jr., A. R., and Reichert Jr., L. E. (1977): Regulation of gonadotropin receptors by luteinizing hormone in granulosa cells. *Endocrinology*, 101:512–523.
667. Suzuki, K., and Tamaoki, B. I. (1980): Postovulatory decrease in estrogen production is caused by the diminished supply of aromatizable androgen to ovarian aromatase. *Endocrinology*, 107:2115–2116.
668. Hillensjö, T., Hamberger, L., and Ahrén, K. (1977): Effect of androgens on the biosynthesis of estradiol-17β by isolated preovulatory follicles. *Mol. Cell. Endocrinol.*, 9:183–193.
669. Suzuki, K., and Tamaoki, B. I. (1983): Acute decrease by human chorionic gonadotropin of the activity of preovulatory ovarian 17α-hydroxylase and C-17-20-lyase is due to decrease of microsomal cytochrome P-450 through de novo synthesis of ribonucleic acid and protein. *Endocrinology*, 113:1985–1991.
670. Eckstein, B., and Tsafriri, A. (1986): The steroid C-17,20-lyase complex in isolated Graafian follicles: effects of human chorionic gonadotropin. *Endocrinology*, 118:1266–1270.
671. Bjersing, L., Hay, M. F., Kann, G., et al. (1972): Changes in gonadotrophins, ovarian steroids and follicular morphology in sheep at oestrus. *J. Endocrinol.*, 52:465–479.
672. Watzka, M. (1957): Weibliche genitalorgane. Das ovarium. In: *Handbuch der Mikroskopischen Anatomies des Menschen*, Vol. 7, edited by M. V. Mollendorf and W. Bargmann, pp. 1–178. Springer, Berlin.
673. LeMaire, W. J., Yang, N. S. T., Behrman, H. H., and Marsh, J. M. (1973): Preovulatory changes in the concentration of prostaglandins in rabbit Graafian follicles. *Prostaglandins*, 3:367–376.
674. Yang, N. S. T., Marsh, J. M., and LeMaire, W. J. (1974): Postovulatory changes in the concentrations of prostaglandins in rabbit Graafian follicles. *Prostaglandins*, 6:37–44.
675. Armstrong, D. T., Moon, Y. S., and Zamecnik, J. (1974): Evidence for a role of prostaglandins in ovulation. In: *Gonadotropins and Gonadal Function*, edited by N. R. Moudgal, pp. 345–356. Academic, New York.
676. Armstrong, D. T., and Zamecnik, J. (1975): Pre-ovulatory elevation of rat ovarian prostaglandin F, and its blockade by indomethacin. *Mol. Cell. Endocrinol.*, 2:125–131.
677. Bauminger, S., and Lindner, H. R. (1975): Periovulatory changes in ovarian prostaglandin formation and their hormonal control in the rat. *Prostaglandins*, 9:737–751.
678. Ainsworth, L. Baker, R. D., and Armstrong, D. T. (1975): Preovulatory changes in follicular fluid prostaglandin F levels in swine. *Prostaglandins*, 9:915–925.
679. Tsang, B. K., Ainsworth, L., Downey, B. R., and Armstrong, D. T. (1979): Pre-ovulatory changes in cyclic AMP and prostaglandin concentrations in follicular fluid of gilts. *Prostaglandins*, 17:141–148.
680. Plunkett, E. R., Moon, Y. S., Zamecnik, J., and Armstrong, D. T. (1975): Preliminary evidence of a role for prostaglandin F in human follicular function. *Am. J. Obstet. Gynecol.*, 123:391–397.
681. Henderson, K. M., and McNatty, K. P. (1975): A biochemical hypothesis to explain the mechanism of luteal regression. *Prostaglandins*, 9:779–798.
682. Armstrong, D. T. (1981): Prostaglandins and follicular functions. *J. Reprod. Fertil.*, 62:283–291.

683. Janson, P. O. (1975): Effects of luteinizing hormone on blood flow in the follicular rabbit ovary as measured by radioactive microspheres. *Acta Endocrinol. (Copenh.),* 79:122–133.
684. Armstrong, D. T., and Grinwich, D. L. (1972): Blockade of spontaneous and LH-induced ovulation in rats by indomethacin, an inhibitor of prostaglandin biosynthesis. *Prostaglandins,* 1:21–28.
685. Grinwich, D. L., Kennedy, T. G., and Armstrong, D. T. (1972): Dissociation of ovulatory and steroidogenic actions of luteinizing hormone in rabbits with indomethacin, an inhibitor of prostaglandin synthesis. *Prostaglandins,* 1:89–95.
686. Lau, I. F., Saksena, S. K., and Chang, M. C. (1974): Prostaglandins F and ovulation in mice. *J. Reprod. Fertil.,* 40:467–469.

The Physiology of Reproduction, edited by E. Knobil and J. Neill *et al.* Raven Press, Ltd., New York © 1988.

CHAPTER 11

Follicular Selection and Its Control

Gilbert S. Greenwald and Paul F. Terranova

"One of the most intriguing mysteries in ovarian physiology is what factors determine whether one follicle remains quiescent, another begins to develop but later becomes atretic, while still a third matures and ovulates" (1).

The above description of the fate of three primordial follicles sets the theme for this chapter. In view of the paucity of information about primordial follicles, emphasis is upon follicles once they have entered into the growing pool. We hope to provide a balanced account of follicular development in the cyclic, pregnant, and lactating animal. A comparative approach that will point out significant species similarities and differences is stressed. Moreover, an attempt will be made to cover all aspects of folliculogenesis.

Folliculogenesis has attracted a great deal of attention and, where feasible, this chapter focuses on recent findings. Table 1 lists a series of relevant reviews and chapters—which is by no means complete. Further entree to the literature on follicular development can be gained by consulting the volumes published during the past 10 years (Table 2).

EARLY STAGES OF FOLLICULAR DEVELOPMENT

The majority of mammals restrict oogonial proliferation to prenatal development or to the early postnatal period (29); the rare exceptions are lemurs, in which mitotic activity of germ cells is demonstrable even in the adult (30). Thus, in most mammals oogonia are transformed before or soon after birth into primary oocytes that are characterized by a prolonged meiotic prophase and surrounded by a squamous layer of pregranulosa cells. These *primordial follicles* constitute the resting stockpile of nongrowing follicles that are progressively depleted during the reproductive life span. Primordial follicles continuously (presumably) leave the nongrowing pool by being converted into *primary follicles* in which the oocyte is surrounded by a unilaminar layer of cuboidal granulosa cells—the descendents of the pregranulosa cells. The follicle is then launched on its career as a growing or developing follicle, culminating in either ovulation or, more likely, atresia at some stage in its subsequent development. According to Peters (31), the initiation of

TABLE 1. *Reviews and chapters relevant to follicular selection*

Year	Author
1947	Hisaw (2)
1956	Brambell (3)
1959	Falck (4)
1974	Greenwald (5)
1977	Channing and Tsafriri (6)
1977	Lindner et al. (7)
1977	Armstrong and Dorrington (8)
1980	Richards (9)
1981	diZerega and Hodgen (10)
1983	Erickson (11)
1984	Hsueh et al. (12)
1984	Tsafriri and Braw (13)
1985	Hillier (14)

follicle growth is not dependent on gonadotropins since unilateral ovariectomy of 2-day-old mice does not change the number of normal developing follicles present 12 days later. On the other hand, continuous daily injection from birth of an antiserum to gonadotropins leads to signs of altered follicular development by 5 days of age and definite effects from 7 days onwards (32). Follicular development in gonadotropin-deprived mice rarely progresses beyond the 40-cell stage, corresponding to a type 3b follicle: the smallest medium-sized follicle with an oocyte slightly larger than 20 μm in diameter (33). Transplantation of ovaries of 1-day-old rats to ovariectomized or ovariectomized-hypophysectomized adult female rats results 15 days later in the same number of small and medium follicles (up to two layers of granulosa cells), but the transplants in the gonadotropin-rich environment contain many more secondary follicles (multilaminar granulosa layers) and large follicles with incipient formation of an antral cavity. The oocytes are also considerably larger in the transplants in the ovariectomized hosts (34). The conclusion is that gonadotropins, especially follicle-stimulating hormone (FSH), enhance early follicle cell development and early oocyte growth. In the immature mouse (33) and rat (35), more follicles start to grow per day in young animals (7-day-old mice, 16-day-old rats) than in older ones. This perhaps can be explained on the basis of high levels of gonadotropins in the prepubertal rodent (rat: 36; hamster: 37). The reduced number of growing follicles recruited per day in 3-week-old mice has been attributed to a factor produced by atretic follicles that reduces growth initiation (31). The fact that large follicles have already differentiated by 21 days of age (33) raises the possibility that production of steroids and/or inhibin by the enlarging follicles can act via the hypothalamic–pituitary axis to account for fewer follicles entering into the growing pool.

With age the number of primordial follicles declines in parallel with the number of growing follicles (mouse: 38,39; rat: 40; human: 41,42). The size of the pool of primordial follicles determines the fraction that is stimulated to grow. A reduction in the size of the pool reduces the number recruited into the growing pool. In the mouse, this relationship holds true whether the nongrowing pool is reduced by age or artificially by injection of dimethyl-benzanthracene (38) or by early androgenization (31). There is considerable individual variation in the number of primordial follicles in man (41) and rhesus monkey (43). The number of primordial follicles shows significant differences among three strains of rats (44). Interestingly, the strain with the greatest number of primordial follicles also has the greatest number of growing follicles and is most responsive to exogenous FSH. It is disconcerting, however, that this strain is the less fecund, as judged by a higher incidence of sterile matings and smaller litter sizes; whether there are differences in ovulation rate between the strains is unknown (45).

TABLE 2. *Relevant books on the ovarian follicle, 1977–1985*

Year	Title	Author(s)
1977	*The Ovary*, 2nd ed.	Zuckerman and Weir (15)
1978	*The Vertebrate Ovary*	Jones (16)
1978	*Control of Ovulation*	Crighton et al. (17)
1979	*Ovarian Follicular Development and Function*	Midgley and Sadler (18)
1979	*Ovarian Follicular and Corpus Luteum Function*	Channing et al. (19)
1980	*Conception in the Human Female*	Edwards (20)
1980	*Biology of the Ovary*	Motta and Hafez (21)
1981	*Dynamics of Ovarian Function*	Schwartz and Hunzicker-Dunn (22)
1982	*Intraovarian Control Mechanisms*	Channing and Segal (23)
1983	*Factors Regulating Ovarian Function*	Greenwald and Terranova (24)
1982–84	*Reproduction in Mammals*, 2nd ed.	Austin and Short (25)
1984	*Marshall's Physiology of Reproduction/Reproductive Cycles of Vertebrates*, 4th ed.	Lamming (26)
1985	*Biology of Ovarian Follicles in Mammals*	Guraya (27)
1985	*Proceedings of the Fifth Ovarian Workshop*	Toft and Ryan (28)

One of the most critical steps in folliculogenesis is the transformation of primordial into primary follicles. Intuitively, it seems likely that the conversion of the flattened pregranulosa cells into a cuboidal epithelium depends on cues provided by the oocytes, but the nature of the signal is unclear. Several lines of evidence indicate that the pregranulosa cells are unable to form follicles in the absence of the oocyte. Injection of busulfan (an alkylating agent) into pregnant rats destroys all primordial germ cells, and consequently, a sterile gonad devoid of steroidogenic tissue is formed (46). Similarly, a mutant mouse strain may have 2 to 20 oocytes at birth, but their disappearance by 3 months prevents any further follicular development (47).

By a series of mitotic divisions, the unilaminar primary follicle is converted into a multilaminated preantral stage designated a *secondary follicle;* at various times in its life history the secondary follicle becomes invested with thecal cells. Finally, with the appearance of an antral cavity, the secondary follicle is converted into a *tertiary follicle*. The morphological and biochemical changes associated with these changes will be discussed later. At this point, we are concerned with a very basic issue: Is the growth and differentiation of primary and secondary follicles under the influence of gonadotropins, or is it only with the development of an antral cavity that the tertiary follicle becomes dependent on FSH and luteinizing hormone (LH)?

The relatively constant number of preantral follicles throughout the estrous cycle has often been cited as evidence that they are unaffected—or at most slightly affected—by changes in gonadotropins. Thus, throughout the cycle of the mouse, no cyclic changes in numbers exist for follicles of types 3a to 6 [type 6 = incipient formation of antral cavity (48)]. Based on large sample sizes (11–18 rats/day of cycle), at least 21 follicles/ovary are recruited from less than 260 μm into greater than 260 μm between proestrus and estrus (49). Moreover, the number of smaller follicles (70–110 μm) significantly increases at diestrus; a definite antrum (i.e., a tertiary follicle) is present in follicles 120 to 130 μm in diameter. Hence, the number of preantral follicles *does* change during the estrous cycle of the rat. It is noteworthy that rat follicles less than 70 μm in diameter are never atretic (49). Similarly, in the periovulatory period of the rhesus monkey, there is a significant increase in the percentage of small preantral follicles ranging from 100 to 200 μm in diameter; the transition to an antral follicle occurs between 200 and 250 μm (43). Based on the terminology of Pedersen and Peters (50), there are significantly more type 3b and 4 rat follicles at estrus and metestrus than on other days of the cycle (51). Of perhaps greater significance, the duration of the DNA synthesis phase is shorter for all primary and secondary follicles at estrus than at other stages of the cycle (51), and this is also true for the cyclic mouse (48). The number of preantral follicles with two to five layers of granulosa cells does not vary during the hamster cycle (52). However, preantral hamster follicles, with one to five layers of granulosa cells show significant increases in [^{3}H]thymidine incorporation on proestrus and estrus as evaluated by autoradiography (53) or after in vitro incubation with [^{3}H]thymidine (54). Thus, the dogma of the unchanging number and responsiveness of preantral follicles is refuted in a number of species.

Still another way of demonstrating that preantral follicles *can* be stimulated in intact animals by gonadotropins is by evaluation of the effects of superovulation induced by pregnant mare serum (PMS). For example, 26- to-28-day-old mice ovulate 60 ova in response to 10 IU PMS followed 56 hr later by 5 IU human chorionic gonadotropin (hCG): rats 24 to 30 days old ovulate 50 eggs after 30 IU PMS and an ovulating dose of 10 IU hCG (55). Adult rats injected with 50 IU PMS and then with 15 IU hCG 3 days later ovulate 43 ova per animal (56). The number of ova ovulated hardly makes it feasible that reduced atresia of tertiary follicles can solely account for these results; rather, recruitment of preantral follicles seems to be an essential component. Unequivocal evidence that preantral follicles are recruited by PMS treatment is provided by the cyclic hamster. Injection of 30 IU PMS on estrus (day 1 of cycle) results in the ovulation of 54 ova by the next cycle, and this is associated by day 2 with a doubling in the number of follicles greater than 267 μm in diameter (57). Within 4 hr after the injection of 30 IU PMS on estrus, hamster follicles with four to five layers of granulosa cells respond by a significant reduction in their numbers and a concomitant increase in follicles with incipient formation of an antral cavity (58). Collectively, these results point to significant effects of gonadotropins on secondary (and even primary) follicles in intact animals.

It is frequently stated that gonadotropic hormones are unessential for early growth of follicles and that FSH and LH become indispensable for further development only at the transformation of the secondary to a tertiary follicle. Although species differences may exist, a careful perusal of the literature indicates that early follicular development *is* influenced by gonadotropins, but the picture is confusing because of the frequent subjective, anecdotal evaluations and the way even quantitative data have been presented. What follows, then, is a species-by-species account of the effects of hypophysectomy on follicular development that attempts to provide a balanced view on this important subject.

Rat

Rats hypophysectomized at 28 days of age were killed at various postoperative intervals, and healthy follicles were classified as primary or vesicular; the former category includes preantral follicles with two or more layers of granulosa cells (59). By 10 and 38 days after hypophysectomy, the average number of primary follicles was 102 and 20, respectively, compared with 213 on the day after operation; similarly the number of vesicular follicles at the same time intervals were 99 and 3 compared with 160 on day 1. The maximal diameter of follicles maintained posthypophysectomy was 250 μm, but the number obviously falls sharply with time. An often-cited, but somewhat confusing study by Paesi (60) dealt with hypophysectomy of young rats weighing 61 to 72 g. A week after operation, there was a 71% increase in the smallest follicles (23–32 μm in diameter). Since primordial follicles were not counted, presumably these were primary follicles with one layer of cuboidal granulosa cells. Approximately 20% of the small follicles showed signs of beginning atresia. One week after hypophysectomy, the largest follicles present were 360 μm compared preoperatively to 576 μm. The accumulation of small follicles might represent a decrease in the number of follicles developing into larger stages per unit of time (60). An excellent, thorough study by De Reviers (61) dealt with follicular development in the immature rat, with follicles classified by the volume of granulosa cells. Volume ranged from 1,259 μm^2 for primary follicles to 25,200 μm^2 for large tertiary follicles. Ten days after hypophysectomy at 27 days of age, there is a 43% reduction in the number of smallest follicles (types 3b and 4) and a 37% reduction in intermediate follicles (type 5a and 6) and no larger stages (type 6–8) present compared to intact 28-day-old rats. In hypophysectomized rats killed 105 or 135 days later, the total number of small follicles varied from 8 to 48, and only sporadic numbers of intermediate follicles were present. De Reviers pointed out that long-term hypophysectomy of male rats leads to the development of gonadotropin-like cells in the pars tuberalis as evidenced by immunocytology (cited in 61). Even the long-term hypophysectomized rat may therefore not be completely devoid of some gonadotropin reserve. Ovine FSH is capable of stimulating follicular growth in rats hypophysectomized for as long as 25 days, and this effect is manifested on all stages of folliculogenesis. The action of FSH—depending on dose—involves diminished atresia but also increased recruitment. The recruitment may even affect primordial follicles, as demonstrated by injecting [^{3}H]thymidine 1 hr before hypophysectomy with the rats killed 72 hr later. There was approximately a threefold greater labeling index in type 3b follicles after FSH treatment (61).

An unpublished study has considered follicular development in adult hypophysectomized rats with the endpoint—21 days later—expressed as numerical density of follicles based on their diameter (cited in 62). Follicles smaller than 60 μm were not measured. The results indicate a significant decline in follicles larger than 175 μm by 3 weeks after hypophysectomy. A single injection of Armour FSH (4 mg) resulted in a significant increase in the number of follicles 75 to 125 μm in diameter 24 hr later. A recent study reconfirms a number of the above findings: Rats hypophysectomized at 26 days of age showed significant declines in secondary and tertiary follicles 3 days later; e.g., the number of follicles with two to three layers of granulosa cells were reduced to 107 ± 12 per ovary from the normal value of 175 ± 22 (63). The number of healthy tertiary follicles was even more affected by 3 days: 4.5 ± 1.2 versus 39 ± 3 in intact controls.

The above results are so striking that one wonders why there is any question about the dependency of preantral rat follicles on gonadotropin support. In part, this is because some investigators have been more impressed by the ability of at least *some* follicles in the hypophysectomized rat to maintain some semblance of normal function. Thus, rats hypophysectomized on day 22 and injected 10 days later with [^{3}H]thymidine show a degree of labeling of granulosa cells in small follicles similar to that in intact animals (64). The authors state that "although many follicles were atretic, a few follicles with more than one layer of granulosa cells persisted." In another study, hypophysectomized rats were implanted 5 days postsurgery with pumps containing [^{3}H]thymidine and were then killed 8 days later (65). Follicles were heavily labeled over the granulosa cells: "Some of the labeled follicles were healthy," but "many labeled follicles were atretic." Again, the author was more impressed with the qualitative aspects—not quantitative—of follicular growth after hypophysectomy.

Mouse

Hypophysectomy of 12 postpubertal mice resulted in few follicles developing beyond the two-layered granulosa stage, but the authors recognized the tentativeness of the conclusion because of the heterogeneous ages of the mice and different survival times (66). It is interesting, however, that in intact cyclic mice follicles are committed to either normal development or atresia by the time the third layer of granulosa cells has differentiated; a clearly established thecal layer is evident at this stage (67).

Hamster

In hamsters hypophysectomized on estrus, 1 to 28 days postsurgery, 99% of the follicles have five or fewer layers of granulosa cells, which is considerably below the size of the largest preantral follicle (68). With time, a greater percentage of follicles than normal accumulates in the group with two to three layers of granulosa cells. After a hiatus of a week, daily injection of 200 μg ovine FSH (NIH-S7) for 4 days, followed by hCG, resulted in the ovulation of an average of 32 ova. Interestingly, 200 μg FSH on the first day of treatment followed by 50 μg/day thereafter led to ovulation of 9 ova—a regimen and number of ovulations simulating the pattern in the intact cyclic hamster. Three days after immature hamsters were hypophysectomized, the number of healthy secondary and tertiary follicles was reduced from 405 to 251 per ovary and there was already a significant reduction in follicles with two to eight layers of granulosa cells and larger follicles had vanished (63). Similar results have also been observed in the adult hypophysectomized hamster (69). Four days after hypophysectomy of adult hamsters, considerable amounts of FSH can still be eluted from the nonluteal ovary and with significantly greater FSH receptor affinity than from follicles of intact hamsters (70). This finding has two important implications: Small preantral follicles have a greater affinity for FSH than large ones (there is no appreciable FSH binding by the interstitium), and it may take considerable time, depending on the species, before FSH completely disappears from the ovary of the hypophysectomized animal and a truly anhormonal environment is established.

Guinea Pig

An often-cited paper (71) reported on three hypophysectomized animals that were killed 12 days after surgery: "There was no reduction in the number of nonvesicular follicles." This is strictly an anecdotal account. Subsequently, 3- to 4-week-old guinea pigs were hypophysectomized and groups of three or four animals killed over the next 4 days (72). Follicles in the range of 140 to 800 μm in diameter were counted. The percentage of normal follicles from 140 to 356 μm did not appreciably differ between controls and hypophysectomized guinea pigs over the next 14 days. Only one of three animals killed on day 4 had any normal vesicular follicles, and in the other animals, all follicles beyond the primordial stage were atretic. Paradoxically, by 6 and 14 days all ovaries contained vesicular follicles and a greater percentage were healthy: 63% versus 14% on day 4. No explanation was offered for these unusual results. Is it a matter of small sample size or with time does another source of gonadotropins develop in the hypophysectomized guinea pig (pars tuberalis)?

Sheep

Ewes were hypophysectomized at estrus, with one ovary removed 4 days later and the other removed 70 days after treatment (73). All follicles with three or more layers of granulosa cells were counted. Four days after hypophysectomy the number of preantral follicles (<0.06–0.2 mm) did not differ from controls, but by 70 days posthypophysectomy there were fewer follicles 0.06 to 0.2 mm compared to the day 4 control group (approximately 50% less in each size range). In hypophysectomized ewes, even in the short-term group, all follicles larger than 2.0 mm were atretic. The long-term hypophysectomized ewes had about 30 healthy small vesicular follicles (0.23 mm in diameter). Thus, the ewe seems to be relatively impervious to the absence of gonadotropic hormones in developing small tertiary follicles. One wonders how *soon* after hypophysectomy do changes become apparent in the follicular population of the ewe.

Human

The effects of hypophysectomy on follicular development in the ovary have not been considered. However, two interesting clinical syndromes are pertinent. Follicular development past the primordial stage is rarely observed in women with hypogonadotropic hypogonadism and anosmia (olfactogenital dysplasia) (74). Total urinary gonadotropins are below the limits of detection in a mouse uterine bioassay, but exogenous gonadotropins can induce ovulation. In contrast, in the gonadotropin-resistant ovary syndrome, serum FSH and LH levels are elevated and can be further increased by luteinizing hormone releasing hormone (LHRH) (75), and the ovaries are not responsive to human menopausal gonadotropin (76). Follicular development is limited to primordial and a few primary follicles. It is assumed that there is a deficiency in gonadotropin receptors or a postreceptor defect. Hence, long-term follicular development is severely impaired in the human ovary in the absence of physiologically effective actions of gonadotropins.

From the above account, it seems that a strong case can be made for several species that folliculogenesis—even in its early stages—is influenced by gonadotropins; following hypophysectomy some follicles can progress to the secondary stage, but, quantitatively, follicular growth is severely curtailed. Obviously, more research involving quantitative evaluation of follicular development, in a number of species, is required to establish definitely the precise effects of gonadotropins on the early stages of folliculogenesis.

STRUCTURE AND FUNCTION OF THE ANTRAL FOLLICLE

A biphasic pattern of oocyte and follicle growth in eutherian mammals was clearly established in studies performed 50 to 60 years ago (3). During the first phase, oocyte and follicle growth are linearly and positively correlated. Once the follicle is close to its maximal size, shortly before formation of the antral cavity, a second phase ensues in which follicle growth, consisting of mitotic activity of the granulosa and thecal cells and accumulation of follicular fluid, becomes the dominant element. This same relationship exists in monotremes and marsupials (77).

A very intimate relationship exists between the oocyte and surrounding granulosa cells. Oocytes of the nongrowing pool in the mouse ovary are surrounded by two to eight squamous follicle cells but exhibit active RNA synthesis and low, but significant, levels of RNA polymerase (78). When nine follicle cells surround the oocyte, 96% of the follicular epithelium is cuboidal and oocyte growth is initiated, as detected by an increase in nucleolar RNA polymerase. Of the total oocyte population in 30-day-old mouse ovaries, 81% were in the nongrowing pool and only 2% of the total population were surrounded by nine or more granulosa cells. It is well established that RNA synthesis in mammalian oocytes increases during follicle growth and reaches a peak before an antral cavity is formed (for literature, see ref. 79). Thereafter, [^{3}H]uridine uptake declines rapidly and is low in the oocytes of mature follicles. Protein synthesis by mouse oocytes increases linearly and is greatest in medium (60–70 μm in vitellus diameter) and large (75–90 μm in diameter) oocytes; the latter were collected from large antral follicles (80). That the oocyte in turn influences granulosa development has been illustrated by several experiments. An oocyte-specific antigen from Lewis rats was collected and an antiserum raised in male rats; only oocytes reacted with the antiserum (81). When dissociated ovarian cells were incubated in the presence of normal rat serum, 40% to 50% reaggregated in a folliclelike structure, whereas when anti-oocyte serum was used, the percentage of granulosa cells forming "follicles" was reduced to 20% to 30%. A specific oocyte antigen—which is trypsin labile—may therefore induce follicular differentiation.

In preantral rat follicles with oocyte diameter greater than 80 μm, the granulosa cells nearest the oocyte have a much higher labeling index than more distant cells, and after antral formation, labeling and mitotic indices in cumulus cells are three times as great as in the mural granulosa (82). A gradient in labeling index also is demonstrable in the mural granulosa, the layer adjacent to the antrum having a much higher labeling index than the deeper layers. Similarly, proestrous rats exposed to continuous infusion of [^{3}H]thymidine for 24 hr show a centripetal labeling pattern with intensive marking of granulosa cells bordering on the antral cavity and in the cumulus oophorus (83). In contrast, in 27-day-old rats, similarly sized follicles do not show this regional distribution.

Morphometric analysis of sheep oocytes reveals that in the smallest follicles (0.2–0.4 mm in diameter), the Golgi apparatus is located at the periphery and the cell membrane is folded and consists of numerous slender villi; thus, the surface area is about five times greater than a sphere of similar dimensions (84). As the follicle grows to about 2 mm, the mitochondria align along the periphery of the oocyte and the microvilli now only increase the surface area of the oocyte twofold.

The most intimate relationship of the oocyte and cumulus cells obviously involves the granulosa cells that ultimately form the corona radiata, and this relationship is established by the primary follicle (for literature, see ref. 85). A series of follicular villi abut as gap junctions on the plasmalemma of the oocyte, before the zona pellucida develops, and more than 85% of the nutrients are first taken up by the neighboring granulosa cells before being transferred to the oocyte (for literature, see ref. 86). However, nonpolar amino acids such as leucine and valine may be able to bypass granulosa cells and interact directly with the mouse oocyte, whereas most amino acids enter mouse oocytes cooperatively (87). The origin of the zona pellucida has long been controversial, and species differences may very well account for the uncertainty concerning whether it is derived from the oocyte, follicle cells, or both (85). Recent biochemical evidence indicates that denuded mouse oocytes synthesize and secrete zona pellucida proteins (88,89). In the rabbit, the zona pellucida proteins are first observed immunocytochemically in the oocyte when it is still surrounded by squamous follicle cells. The extracellular assemblage of the glycoproteins forming the zona pellucida intensifies when two or more layers of follicular cells have formed, and the antigens are then apparent not only in the oocyte but in the inner layer of granulosa cells as well (90). This suggests a joint derivation of the zona pellucida. Rabbits immunized with porcine zonae pellucidae ultimately show impeded follicular growth, with no normal follicles having two or more layers of differentiating granulosa cells (91). The stage of follicular development affected by the increasing titer of zona pellucida antibodies occurs when the extracellular matrix first appears between the oocyte and follicle cells. There is a reduction in the number of primordial and primary follicles. In this connection, it is intriguing that after neonatal thymectomy or in naturally athymic "nude" mice, a similar type of ovarian dysgenesis develops with age (see ref. 92). One wonders whether a common thread runs through both situations.

With the onset of formation of the antral cavity, follicular growth accelerates as a result of increased mitotic activity and accumulation of follicular fluid. Throughout the estrous cycle of the rat, 90% of the follicles are less than 300 μm and the volume of follicular fluid first increases in amount when a diameter of 300 μm is reached (93). Mitotic activity in granulosa and theca is maximal in follicles 200 to 300 μm in diameter and is approximately three times higher in granulosa cells (93). The mitotic index then falls in a linear fashion, the nadir for both compartments being reached in follicles 600 to 700 μm in diameter. There is a metestrous peak in mitotic activity in both granulosa and theca in follicles 401 to 500 μm, which presumably results in their ovulation at the next estrus. The volume of the antral cavity in the rat shows three distinct growth phases: a low plateau in follicles 200 to 300 μm, accelerated growth between 300 to 600 μm, and a final preovulatory spurt in follicles 700 μm. In follicles 600 μm in diameter, the volumes of granulosa, theca, and antrum are about 6:2:1, respectively.

Three peaks of mucopolysaccharides are present in porcine follicular fluid, representing chondroitin-like material, heparan sulfate, and an unidentified compound. All three fractions are maximal (expressed as μg/follicle) in follicles 6 to 12 mm in diameter (94). A more detailed biochemical analysis of proteoglycans in porcine follicular fluid was provided by Yanagishita et al. (95). Porcine FSH stimulates the incorporation of [^{3}H]glucosamine into mucopolysaccharides by granulosa cells from small porcine follicles (<2 mm), and the stimulating effects are mimicked by dibutyryl cyclic AMP (cAMP) and prostaglandin (PG) E_2 (96). The function of proteoglycans in follicular fluid is still unknown.

Both the granulosa and thecal compartments act as functional syncitia through the presence of homocellular gap junctions, which persist in rat preantral follicles even after 90 days of hypophysectomy (97). However, within 48 hr of injection of estradiol the gap junction surface area is increased in granulosa cells (fivefold greater than control values in intact rats); hCG has a similar effect on theca. Neither hormone is effective on the other compartment. A quantitative ultrastructural study of granulosa cell gap junctions in rat and rabbit follicles confirmed previous observations that an ovulatory dose of hCG within 5 to 12 hr leads to rapid loss of gap junctions; in the rabbit, granulosa cells of ruptured follicles have only 15% of the amount of junctional membrane found in unstimulated large follicles (98). The importance of granulosa gap junctions in cell-to-cell communication is reinforced by a recent study (99). Granulosa cells were aspirated from preovulatory follicles of mature sows at days 18 to 20 of the cycle (when they have already been exposed to increasing levels of LH). Only 20% to 35% of the granulosa cells bound FSH or hCG, and yet at 70% to 80% confluency nearly all granulosa cells contained dissociated cAMP-dependent protein kinase; at less than 20% confluency, only one third or fewer cells had dissociated protein kinase. The results show the importance of gap junctions in spreading a hormonal signal among granulosa cells.

There are considerable species differences in the ability of granulosa cells to convert pregnenolone to progesterone. In most species, it is not until shortly before the onset of the preovulatory surge in gonadotropins that significant 3β-hydroxysteroid dehydrogenase (3β-HSD) activity is evident in granulosa cells. For example, in the sheep the dominant follicle shows significant 3β-HSD activity (histochemically detectable) in the theca, whereas the enzyme is not present in the membrana granulosa until a few hours before ovulation (100).The ultrastructural characteristics of the granulosa from large preovulatory follicles from sheep show few of the features associated with steroidogenesis, and even in the immediate period prior to ovulation there is no evidence of structural changes indicative of luteinization (101). Human granulosa cells show ultrastructural characteristics of protein synthesis until the periovulatory increase in LH, when morphometric analysis reveals a striking increase in smooth endoplasmic reticulum and other features indicative of increased steroidogenesis (102). Histochemical detection of 3β-HSD is also low in the preovulatory human follicle compared with the thecal reaction (103). Similarly, the ultrastructural organization of granulosa cells from preovulatory rhesus follicles shows features not associated with steroidogenesis, whereas atretic follicles have extensive smooth endoplasmic reticulum and large mitochondria with tubular cristae (104). These electron-microscopic features are more indicative of 3β-HSD than of other enzymes since in both species granulosa cells can convert androgens to estrogens. Does the buildup of progesterone in follicular fluid in the immediate preovulatory period in humans represent a granulosa or thecal derivative? An enlightening histochemical comparison showed a much more intense reaction for 3β-HSD in the granulosa and theca of preovulatory follicles of the rat than hamster—both qualitatively and quantitatively (105). The activity in both species was much greater in the peripheral granulosa cells bordering on the basal lamina. Could this difference partly account for the premature histological and biochemical signs of luteinization of granulosa cells observed in the preovulatory rat follicle compared with most other species? In summary, 3β-HSD activity is sparse in granulosa cells of most species until rising titers of LH enhance its ability to synthesize progesterone (see ref. 106). In the cow follicle, the major steroid product of the granulosa cells is pregnenolone, which is apparently then exported to the thecal layer for ultimate conversion to androgens (107). Hence, there is traffic in both directions between theca and granulosa. In the proestrous hamster follicle neither pregnenolone or progesterone is synthesized by granulosa cells incubated for 2 hr with or without LH, whereas isolated theca produces considerable amounts of pregnenolone in response to LH (108).

It has become evident in recent years that granulosa cells do not constitute a homogeneous tissue but rather show interesting regional specializations. This has been especially well demonstrated by quantitative cytochemistry. In the rat, there are distinctive differences between the peripheral portion of the membrana granulosa, the periantral granulosa cells and the cumulus region. At proestrus, cells of the peripheral one half to two thirds of the membrana granulosa are pseudostratified, with cell processes extending to the basal lamina; these follicles are the ones destined to ovulate (109). In contrast, the rest of the membrana granulosa consists of stratified, rounded cells with rounded nuclei. On proestrus, growing follicles with a diameter of 400 μm first show signs of pseudostratification, and there are about three times as many showing this reaction as the number expected to ovulate. Elimination of the excess number of pseudostratified follicles proceeds rapidly after diestrus 1 and is completed by the evening of diestrus 2. Thus, the ovulable type of follicle is distinguished on the basis of the organization of the peripheral granulosa cells. On estrus and diestrus 1, there is little appreciable difference in 3β-HSD activity among peripheral, antral, and cumulus granulosa cells (110). However, by diestrus 2 and proestrus, 3β-HSD is two- to threefold higher in peripheral granulosa. A similar regional difference is demonstrable for glucose-6-phosphate dehydrogenase of the type associated with hydroxylation reactions involved in steroid biosynthesis (110). Other evidence of granulosa heterogeneity is provided by a difference in lysosomal membrane permeability, which is greatest in peripheral granulosa cells, followed by periantral and then cumulus cells (111); presumably the former is the most active steroidogenic region of the granulosa. Lipid droplets are also concentrated in the peripheral granulosa cells but much less than in the theca interna (105). The one characteristic feature of the cumulus cells of ovulable rat follicles is that periodic acid-Schiff-positive granules are restricted to this region. A morphometric ultrastructural study of rat preovulatory follicles also confirms regional differences in the granulosa (105). The peripheral region contains the greatest volume of mitochondria, smooth endoplasmic reticulum, and lipid droplets. In contrast, the cumulus oophorus has the highest volume of rough endoplasmic reticulum—indicative of protein synthesis—and no lipid droplets. The oocyte–cumulus complex of rats collected before the LH surge secrete low amounts of progesterone throughout 2 days of culture (<10 pg/cumulus/day), whereas cumulus cells harvested after the LH surge accumulate 300 to 400 pg progesterone/day (112). A mouse monoclonal antibody generated against a mammary tumor cell line recognizes a surface antigen in rat granulosa cells (113). Throughout the development of the preantral follicle, the plasma membrane of all granulosa cells gives a strong positive response for the antibody. However, once the antral cavity appears, 75% of the granulosa cells in the mural granulosa lack the antibody, and its disappearance is initiated by FSH treatment within 12 hr. A dramatic demonstration of the symbiosis between cumulus cells and oocyte is provided by culturing denuded, corona-enclosed and cumulus-enclosed ovine oocytes for 24 hr before transferring them to suitable inseminated recipients (114). For the three classes, the percentages of transferred ova developing into blastocysts were 1.9%, 1.8%, and 42.6%, respectively. However, when corona oocytes were supplemented with 5×10^6 granulosa cells (presumably mural cells), 37.2% developed into blastocysts.

Regional differences in FSH, hCG, and prolactin (PRL) receptors have also been demonstrated in granulosa cells. In the preantral follicle, FSH binding sites are limited to granulosa cells and LH (hCG) binding sites are restricted to the theca. With time, LH binding sites appear in granulosa cells and the mature ovulable follicle therefore can be distinguished by LH and FSH binding sites in granulosa and LH binding in theca (for literature, see refs. 7, 9, 11, 12).

Hypogonadal mice, injected intravenously with labeled hormones, bind hCG only to thecal and interstitial cells and FSH to granulosa cells. When treated with LHRH for 5 days, mature follicles differentiate, with some showing hCG binding now encompassing both theca and granulosa (115). In small sheep follicles (1–3 mm in diameter), cAMP production by granulosa cells is stimulated by FSH but not hCG (116) and similar observations have been made for porcine granulosa cells (see ref. 117). Topical autoradiography using slices of porcine ovaries reveals that granulosa cells from small follicles (1–2 mm) bind much more FSH than medium (3–5 mm) or large (6–10 mm) follicles, and hCG binding is slight in granulosa cells until large follicles are developed (118). When the largest antral follicles are collected on each day of the rat estrous cycle, the binding of FSH to granulosa cells is constant throughout the cycle at about 3,000 cpm/μg DNA, whereas hCG binding does not begin to increase until diestrus 2, with maximal values obtained on proestrus and dramatic increases even before the preovulatory surges of gonadotropins (119). Maximal hCG binding to theca also occurs on proestrus. Intravenous injection of rats with labeled hCG, followed by autoradiography, showed that mural granulosa cells adjacent to the basement membrane demonstrated maximal grain counts, 10-fold greater than the periantral layer (120). It is noteworthy that hCG binding to cumulus and oocyte is no greater than background (120). A quantitative study showed no binding of hCG to the rat oocyte; the affinity to cumulus and mural granulosa cells was the same, but the number of binding sites was very different: 223 sites/cumulus cell versus 2000/mural cell (121). Using topical autoradiography, and determining grain densities, there is no hCG binding to granulosa cells of rat follicles 400 to 500 μm in diameter—which are small antral follicles (122). The first noticeable binding of hCG was in the outermost granulosa layers of 500- to 600-μm follicles, and with increased size, hCG binding spread to finally encompass the entire mural granulosa in follicles >600 μm. Throughout the estrous cycle, hCG binding to cumulus and oocyte was no greater than background. An autoradiographic study of the hamster ovary revealed that FSH binding to granulosa cells was present in the smallest preantral to large antral follicle and also to the *oocyte* with increasing intensity as the oocyte enlarged; hCG or PRL did not bind to the granulosa of preantral follicles, but newly formed antral follicles on day 2 showed a light activity in peripheral granulosa cells that gradually spread to engulf all of the mural granulosa (123). Neither hCG nor PRL binding was detected on the mural granulosa or oocyte of preantral follicles. Hamster oocytes from which the zona pellucida has been removed still show specific FSH binding sites (124). Hydroxysteroid dehydrogenases have been demonstrated histochemically in the oocytes of several species (125), and one wonders whether mammalian oocytes are capable of producing steroids in response to gonadotropins, a well-established phenomenon in amphibians. Thus, regional differences in receptor distribution in mural and cumulus granulosa cells parallel morphological and biochemical localizations.

THECAL STRUCTURE AND FUNCTION

Primordial follicles in the mouse ovary 4 to 6 days after birth are surrounded by a unilaminar layer of connective tissue; on the transformation of primordial to primary follicles (i.e., a single layer of cuboidal granulosa cells), a theca folliculi, consisting of fibroblasts and epithelial cells and possibly transitional cells, begins to differentiate (126). Even after the administration of PMS and hCG, the same cell types are present in the differentiated theca of Graafian follicles (126). In the rat, a theca externa is first apparent around small antral follicles, 0.1 to 0.25 mm in diameter, consisting of fibroblasts, smooth muscle cells, and an intermediate variety (127). Some of the cells definitely show the ultrastructural characteristics of smooth muscle cells, and this is reinforced by the immunofluorescent demonstration of actin and myosin in several cell layers of the theca externa surrounding large Graafian follicles (128). In "smaller" rat follicles, the fluorescent band is only one to four layers thick and often incomplete; follicles surrounded by one or two layers of granulosa cells already show a weak, but definite fluorescence indicative of actin and myosin. Homocellular gap junctions link thecal cells in multilaminar follicles in the hypophysectomized rat and hCG treatment increases the size and frequency of gap junctions and leads to thecal hypertrophy (97). Based on the definite presence of smooth muscles in the theca externa, the possibility has been raised for a number of species of a contractile component involved in ovulation (see citations in ref. 129). This is consistent with the distribution of cholinergic and adrenergic nerves in the theca externa of numerous species and the ability to stimulate contractility of the bovine follicle *in vitro* and induce ovulation in the *in vitro* perfused rabbit ovary (130,131). However, when ovarian denervation is performed by freezing the ovarian pedicle (thus eliminating ovarian sympathetic innervation for 10 days), normal ovulation rates continue (132).

The aggregation and ultimate differentiation of the theca folliculi is assumed to occur under the influence of growth factors emanating from the oocyte–granulosa complex, but there is no direct evidence to substantiate a causal relationship. In combined cultures of porcine thecal and granulosa cells, the reaggregated "follicle" tends to have the thecal cells arranged as the peripheral tissue (133). A causal relationship between the number of granulosa cell gap junctions and thecal development has been suggested for growing rat follicles (134). After the induction of ovulation by hCG in the rabbit, the temporal sequence in growing follicles is an increase in the labeling index of granulosa cells by 20 to 28 hr and a lag until 40 hr for an increase in the labeling index of endothelial thecal cells (135). On the other hand, a cytosol thecal extract (porcine) enhances the *in vitro* proliferation of granulosa cells and BALB/3T3 cells (136). Reciprocal interactions undoubtedly exist between theca and granulosa which must be constantly kept in mind when the morphological, biochemical and steroidogenic properties of the isolated compartments are considered.

The theca interna of sheep follicles, <3.0 mm in diameter, already consists of 8 to 12 layers of flattened cells and capillaries. Some 20% of the cells have the ultrastructural features of steroidogenically active cells, and others are fibroblasts; the majority are undifferentiated (137). In follicles 3 to 5.9 mm, approximately 40% of the theca interna cells possess tubular endoplasmic reticulum, and the largest follicles on day 15 contain about 50% steroidogenically active cells. In all species, the theca interna is separated from the granulosa cells by a distinct PAS-positive band, the basal lamina [e.g., in the cow (138)]. In the mouse, the basal layer consists of laminin-a noncollagenous glycoprotein (139), which is believed to be synthesized by basal epithelial or endothelial cells rather than fibroblasts. The basal lamina is intact until shortly before ovulation. The time of appearance of a well-differentiated theca interna relative to the development of granulosa cells varies from species to species: mouse, three layers of granulosa cells (67); hamster, six layers of granulosa cells (140); sheep, follicles 2 to 3 mm (137); rhesus, three layers of granulosa cells, 100 to 125 μm in diameter (Koering, personal communication); human, preantral 180 to 240 μm in diameter (42). It is intriguing that in the first three species normal development of granulosa cells can proceed posthypophysectomy to the stage before a differentiated theca interna is found, albeit with a greatly reduced number of healthy follicles.

In the sheep follicle, maximal differentiation of the theca interna occurs in late estrus, but even then, not all cells contain smooth endoplasmic reticulum (137). It is not until late estrus that numerous lipid droplets accumulate in the ovine theca interna—a usual sign of reduction in steroidogenesis. The first signs of discontinuity in the basal lamina also then appear (137). In the bovine theca interna, 3 to 4 days before ovulation, two cell populations emerge consisting of large epithelial cells with round nuclei increasing in area and another group of fibroblastlike cells in which nuclear profile area does not increase; ultimately the fibroblastic thecal cells contribute to the small luteal cells at the periphery of the corpus luteum and the epithelial variety disperse into the stroma (138). It is possible with large porcine follicles (1.0–1.2 cm in diameter) to separate the theca interna as a discrete layer and mince it with scissors and then with gentle trypsinization disperse the thecal cells (141). The thecal cells from these large preovulatory follicles differ in several respects from porcine granulosa cells in that the former contain many more lipid droplets, histochemically show very intense 3β-HSD activity, and in the first 2 days of culture produce 13 times more estrogen than granulosa cells. Similar substantial thecal production of estrogens has been observed in mature pig follicles obtained after injection of PMS and hCG (142). Cultured human thecal cells, similarly isolated by collagenase–hyaluronidase digestion, *in vitro* produce high levels of androstenedione for 8 days (30 ng $\times$ 10^5 cells), moderate levels of estradiol (2 ng $\times$ 10^5 cells) and, beyond day 4, undetectable levels of either. On the other hand, progesterone is produced at high levels (20 ng $\times$ 10^5 cells) throughout the 10 days of culture (143).

An abundant literature on rodents and many other species points to the theca as the major source of androgen precursors, which are then transported to the granulosa compartment for conversion to estrogens (see Chapter 10). In the rat, theca from small antral follicles do not accumulate testosterone, dihydrotestosterone (DHT), or androstenedione in response to 8-bromo-cAMP, in contrast to large preovulatory follicles (144). Similarly, thecal cells from rat follicles increase progesterone synthesis in response to dibutyryl-cAMP or hCG, with comparable values in interstitial gland cells (145). Stromal cells (theca and interstitium) have considerably more 5α-reductase activity than granulosa cells from both small and large rat follicles, consistent with a much greater production of 5α-pregnane-3,20-dione and 5α-androstene-3,17-dione. These findings agree with a topical autoradiographic study of the rat ovary, which showed that hCG binding to theca interna was detectable in follicles 100 to 200 μm in diameter and that grain density doubled again in follicles >600 μm (122).

It seems quite likely that LH receptors must develop in the theca folliculi before it can differentiate into theca externa and interna, but this critical stage has not yet been studied. A fluorescein–hCG conjugate, injected intravenously, is localized in scattered patches of interstitial cells during the early follicular phase of cynomolgus monkeys; although at this stage numerous antral follicles are present, no concentrated band of hCG is evident, and none is demonstrable on preantral follicles (146). On day 7, a single follicle in both ovaries was surrounded by a fluorescent ring of hCG, although there were as many as four to eight follicles 1 to 3 mm in diameter per ovary. The fluorescent follicle—the putative dominant follicle—was not the largest. However, on day 9 the dominant follicle was surrounded by 8 to 14 layers of thecal cells, was more intensively fluorescent than on day 7, and was the largest follicle present.

In addition to its differentiation as a steroidogenic tissue, the theca interna *pari passu* develops a vascular supply, and the two events may very well be related. Primordial rat follicles do not have an independent blood supply; it is not until a multilaminar granulosa and theca have formed (follicular diameter 80–160 μm) that a vascular wreath develops in the inner portion of the theca interna adjacent to the membrana granulosa (147). The theca interna vasculature, in turn, is linked to an outer series of arterioles and venules in the theca externa. This pattern is unchanged throughout development except for expansion of blood vessels to keep pace with follicular growth. The pattern described for the vasculature of the rat follicle is essentially duplicated in all mammals. In ovaries removed from rhesus monkeys on day 9 or 10 of the cycle, morphometric analysis of the dominant follicle showed that 48% of the theca was vascularized compared to 25% vascularity in smaller antral follicles (148). When iodinated hCG was injected intravenously, the theca of the dominant follicle was heavily labeled, whereas smaller follicles showed little if any activity. Thus, selective vascularization of one follicle was associated with its greater ability to extract and concentrate hCG from the peripheral circulation. The steroidogenic output of androstenedione by perfused bovine theca correlates with the flow rate of the medium in the presence or absence of LH; the theca were from large (≥10 mm in diameter) preovulatory follicles (149).

The blood supply of the ovary can be increased by several mechanisms: (a) intraovarian growth of new blood vessels (angiogenesis); (b) growth of larger blood vessels; (c) vasodilation of existing capillaries; and (d) an increase in the delivery of blood to the ovary. We will concentrate on angiogenesis. On the basis of earlier studies (147,148), we propose that follicular growth is angiogenic dependent, i.e., the increase in granulosal and thecal cells must be accompanied and/or preceded by an increase in new capillaries that grow towards and within the theca of growing follicles. Ovaries excised from PMS-treated rats exhibit considerable vascularity 3 days after being placed on the chorioallantoic membrane of chicken eggs (150). Ovaries from untreated rats showed moderate to no vascularization. In the PMS-treated rat, vascularity was most intense around follicles, and the theca was filled with nucleated chicken erythrocytes; however, these vessels did not penetrate the basal lamina. It is hypothesized that the granulosa cell may be the likely source of angiogenic factor because the new capillaries grow into the theca towards the granulosa cells (150).

Consistent with this concept, follicular fluid from porcine and human ovaries contains an angiogenic product (151,152), and the corpus luteum is also a source of an angiogenic factor (153). Using gel filtration with ammonium sulfate precipitation, two fractions of angiogenic activity were found in follicular fluid using as an endpoint aortic endothelial cell movement and proliferation in vitro and corneal angiogenesis in vivo (152). One factor with a molecular weight of 45,000 to 65,000 daltons and another fraction of less than 1,500 daltons exhibited angiogenic activity. On the other hand, proliferation of cultured bovine capillary endothelial cells is enhanced by extracts of porcine luteal and thecal cells but *not* by granulosa cells or follicular fluid (154). Hence, the normally vascularized follicular compartment may have intrinsic ability to increase local angiogenesis. Whether the bovine thecal cells per se or the contained endothelial component is the source of the angiogenic factor remains to be established.

FOLLICULAR ATRESIA

Follicular atresia is a universal phenomenon, characteristic of both mammalian and nonmammalian vertebrates (155). In the latter group, follicles are obliterated by massive phagocytic activity by granulosa cells, which in turn degenerate; morphological changes are usually more subtle in the case of atresia in the mammalian ovary. It is estimated that greater than 99% of follicles become atretic in the human ovary and about 77% in the mouse (156). The number of follicles developing to the preovulatory stage are thus far fewer than the number undergoing atresia. Follicles can become atretic at any stage of development. Once a follicle enters the growing pool, it either goes on to ovulate or becomes atretic; the chances are that it will become atretic since more follicles are recruited during a cycle than usually ovulate. However, follicles in the nongrowing pool may also degenerate (157). The factors initiating atresia have intrigued scientists for many years, and the factors regulating such a finely controlled mechanism are obviously worthy of investigation. Another intriguing question is whether one can predict when a follicle will become atretic, i.e., what biochemical markers indicate that a follicle is destined for atresia (assessed morphologically). In the search for these markers, several models of atresia have been developed, and they will be discussed later. First, a description of the process of natural atresia is given.

The Normal Process of Atresia: Membrana Granulosa

Two patterns of atresia are discernible in canine follicles. Type A involves prominent necrotic changes in oocyte and zona pellucida, whereas alterations of the granulosa cells are secondary; Type B atresia is typified by distinctive degenerative changes in the granulosa with an almost unchanged oocyte and zona pellucida (158). Type A atresia predominates in secondary follicles (i.e., preantral), whereas Type B atresia is the only variety encountered in tertiary follicles.

It is difficult to discern when follicular atresia begins. Some investigators have used the presence of one or two pyknotic granulosa nuclei in the largest cross section of the follicle as the major criterion. This definition seems somewhat arbitrary since even in the rodent tertiary follicle there are thousands of cells. A much more reliable number for early atresia was set up by Byskov (159), who used 5% pyknotic granulosa cells (in the largest cross section) as a sign of definite but early atresia. Healthy nonovulatory human follicles have a low pyknotic index (mean ± SE = 1.2%) and a high mitotic index (11.5%), whereas atretic follicles contain 10.9% pyknotic nuclei (160). Correlating flow cytometry of granulosa cells and follicular fluid estradiol in human follicles reveals that a DNA-S phase of ≥16% correlates with follicular health (86%), whereas an S-fraction <16% includes 95% atretic follicles (161). Morphological analysis of the largest follicle in ovaries from eight monkeys revealed that pyknosis normally occurs to some degree even in the dominant viable follicle. Moreover, the pyknotic index may vary considerably from one histologic section to another (162). This reinforces the difficulty of assessing the onset of spontaneous follicular atresia.

It has been proposed by Byskov (159) that atresia in the granulosa cell layer in the mouse occurs in three progressive phases. In *stage I,* up to 20% of the granulosa cells of the earliest atretic follicles exhibit pyknosis and fragmentation, and these cells usually are adjacent to the antral cavity. This coincides with a reduction in [^{3}H]thymidine incorporation by the granulosa cells—expressed as labeling index (LI), the number of labeled cells expressed as a percentage of the total granulosa cells counted. Others have also reported a decreased uptake of [^{3}H]thymidine in atretic mouse follicles (48) and dog follicles (158), as well as decreased ^{32}P uptake (163), both of which relate to the reduction in mitosis. An early study by Deane (164) revealed the presence of Feulgen-positive globules that were probably the fragmented nuclei of pyknotic cells observed by Byskov (159). In stage I atresia and in normal follicles the basement membrane is intact. Two days after pulse labeling, mouse follicles in stage I show a marked increase in LI compared with the index at time zero, presumably because of a reutilization of DNA released from dying cells by granulosa cells that are still viable (159). In addition, normal follicles exhibit essentially no pyknotic granulosa cells. *Stage II* is a step further into atresia; the granulosa cells incorporate little, if any, [^{3}H]thymidine, and pyknotic granulosa cells are abundant (5–20%). Leukocytes begin to invade the membrana granulosa, correlating with a breakdown of the basement membrane. Lymphoid cells migrate into rat follicles on the evening of late diestrus as an antecedent to irreversible atresia (165). Subsequent studies involving immunoperoxidase staining have shown that stage II atretic rat follicles are occasionally invaded by cytotoxic T-lymphocytes, suggesting a role of the immune system in follicular differentiation and degeneration (166). In *stage III* atresia the follicles are shrunken. Most of the parameters are similar to stage II atresia, except that the percentage of pyknotic cells is only 5%, probably due to a clearing of pyknotic granulosa cells from the follicles by macrophages and other scavenger-type cells.

In adult cyclic rats, the number of midsized follicles (350–550 μm) increases from estrus to diestrus. A positive correlation is apparent when the percentage of viable granulosa cells is measured by trypan blue exclusion and compared with the viability of the oocyte, as judged by fluorescence on exposure to fluorescein diacetate (167). At diestrus and proestrus, follicles >550 mm with ≥60% granulosa viability were associated with healthy oocytes; e.g., at proestrus, of 7.3 large antral follicles per ovary, only 4 were normal. As rat follicles become atretic, ultrastructurally, intercellular spaces between granulosa cells increase (168); this most likely represents a loss of gap junctions, which are reduced in atretic follicles (134). In medium-sized preantral follicles in the rat, incipient atretic changes in granulosa cells have a patchy distribution in that some cells show nuclear condensation (pyknosis) and marked dilatation of cytoplasmic organelles, with the cytoplasm and microvilli of the oocyte still well preserved (169). Adjacent normal granulosa cells are found to undergo mitosis. The granulosa cells also become flattened and lose cytoplasmic evaginations during atresia, whereas normal granulosa cells are spherical and have irregular cytoplasmic projections. These cytoplasmic projections normally correlate with the development of LH binding to granulosa cells (170). Thus, the loss of microvilli corresponds to loss of LH binding and the onset of atresia (171). With the loss of gap junctions and the loss of LH binding to granulosa cells, it is highly probable that the intercellular communication and trophic actions of LH needed to maintain an intact, well-structured membrana granulosa are lost.

An unusual variant of granulosa degeneration is present in the sheep follicle (172). The process again begins in granulosa cells bordering on the antral cavity. Phagocytic cells representing transformed granulosa cells increase in number as atresia progresses, akin to the process in nonmammalian vertebrates (155). During secondary atresia, atretic bodies develop from the fusion of many nuclei; these multinucleated structures vary in diameter from 15 to 400 μm. Atretic sheep follicles (2–6 mm in diameter) have been reported to "regenerate" *in vitro* within 3 days by a two- to fourfold increase in the thickness of the granulosa layer (173). However, no mitotic figures are observed and histologically the cells are definitely not normal granulosa cells.

It is possible to make a gross identification of atretic and healthy follicles in sheep (174), pig (175), and cow (176) based primarily on the vascularization of the theca, integrity of the membrana granulosa, and translucency of the follicle. In fact, in the ewe, normal and advanced atretic follicles can be correctly identified by histological criteria in over 95% of the cases (174).

During atresia the granulosa cells from atretic follicles of the rabbit take up less ^{35}S (177), suggesting a decrease in the synthesis of sulfate-containing mucopolysaccharides. In contrast, atretic bovine follicles have low levels of estrogen but high levels of progesterone and chondroitin sulfate in follicular fluid (178). This relationship is significant when chondroitin sulfate concentration is plotted against estrogen or the estrogen:progesterone ratio but not when histology is used as the variable.

Histochemical and biochemical alterations in granulosa cells often precede definite morphologic changes in atretic granulosa cells (for citations, see ref. 179). These include an increase in lysosomal enzymes such as acid phosphatase and aminopeptidase (180), and their role in the induction of atresia has been recently evaluated (181). Using recombinant DNA technology it should be possible to determine the gene regulating these granulosa cell enzymes and then, by turning on the gene, induce widespread atresia. In atretic follicles of a number of species (e.g., humans), the histochemical appearance of 3β-HSD and lipid droplets in granulosa cells is characteristic of atresia (182).

Granulosa cells from healthy human follicles maintained *in vitro* for 48 hr produced large amounts of estradiol and progesterone and small amounts of androstenedione without added steroid precursors (183). The follicles were judged to be normal, based on their possessing at least 75% of the maximal number of granulosa cells for their diameters. Follicles with <50% of optimal cell numbers of granulosa cells were judged atretic, and they frequently had a degenerating oocyte, low levels of estradiol, and undetectable levels of FSH in follicular fluid. Incubation of these granulosa cells produced elevated levels of androstenedione, testosterone, and DHT but negligible amounts of progesterone and estradiol. Thus, atresia of human follicles was associated with differentiation of granulosa cells into androgen-producing cells.

Oocyte

The common characteristic of atresia in the oocyte from the large follicles of many species is the meioses-like alterations called pseudomaturation or pseudocleavage. This includes breakdown of the germinal vesicle, alignment of the chromosomes in metaphase, and possibly expulsion of a polar body (184). One of the first signs of atresia in some follicles is the shrinkage of the oocyte (157,185). This is then either accompanied or followed by pseudomaturation. An increase in argyrophilic substances is observed in the oocytes of atretic rat follicles prior to the degenerative changes in the granulosa cells (186). This correlates ultrastructurally with an increase in granules in oocytes from atretic rat follicles (187). In nonpregnant women, synchronous degeneration of oocyte and granulosa occurs even in small antral follicles (188).

Previous studies have shown that the organelles of the oocyte from atretic follicles tend to aggregate (187,189). The nuclear envelope loses its bilaminar appearance, increases its width, and becomes uneven (187) or ruptures (190); thus, the plasmalemma of the oocyte becomes less distinct compared to that of healthy follicles.

A change in the histochemical staining properties of the porcine zona pellucida of atretic follicles is quite striking. In healthy follicles the zona pellucida stains uniformly green with Shorr's S3 and hematoxylin (191); in obviously atretic follicles, it stains a bright orange. In some follicles (presumably healthy and with no morphological signs of atresia), the zona pellucida is partially stained orange and green. These results indicate that Shorr's S3 stain may reveal a very early sign of atresia, that is, prior to observable changes in the follicular wall. Apparently, there are biochemical alterations in the mucopolysaccharides that reflect these changes in staining of the zona pellucida (191). Based on the altered staining properties of the atretic zona pellucida, it was estimated that 56% of preantral pig follicles were atretic compared to 73% and 84%, respectively, of medium (3–5 mm) and large follicles (6–12 mm). Shorr's stain is frequently used in exfoliative cytology to identify cornified vaginal cells, which biochemically represent a stage involving the formation of disulfide bonds in the epithelium. It is possible that physicochemical changes in the mucoproteins of the porcine zona pellucida may lead to similar changes during atresia.

Follicles of most species in late stages of atresia exhibit germinal vesicle breakdown (GVB). When the oocytes from atretic rat follicles are cultured, GVB increased; however, 23% of the oocytes fragmented (187). Addition of pyruvate, which facilitates GVB (192), did not increase GVB in atretic follicles (187). In the rat cumulus cells lose contact with the oocyte during atresia (157). Ultrastructurally, small gap junctions exist between the oocyte and the cumulus, and these are reduced in atretic follicles (193).

In atretic rat follicles, the time from the degeneration of the entire granulosa wall until observable changes begin in the oocyte is estimated to take 24 hr and another 24 hr elapses before the oocyte is completely denuded of cumulus cells (194). The ultimate death of the oocyte is typical in most mammals. However, the oocyte of the atretic sheep follicle (3–5 mm) is extremely resistant to degenerative changes: Oocytes that are cultured in atretic follicles for 24 hr with FSH, LH, and estradiol and are then transferred to the oviducts of inseminated ewes developed into blastocysts in 46% of the transfers (195).

Theca

In a number of species, including rodents (196) and primates (197), thecal hypertrophy is a characteristic of follicles undergoing atresia. Ultrastructural examination of the thecal cells in atretic rat follicles reveals lipid droplets, an agranular endoplasmic reticulum and mitochondria with tubular cristae typical of steroid-secreting cells (198). The thecal cells of atretic follicles are cuboidal with a large nucleus-to-cytoplasm ratio and excessively folded plasma membranes. This transformation of rat thecal cells during atresia is similar to the morphology of the secondary interstitium; thus, in many species the theca cells of atretic follicles are progenitors of the secondary interstitium. The fact that these cells are functionally similar to interstitial cells is shown by the large amounts of progesterone secreted *in vitro* in response to hCG (198) and the presence of 3β-HSD activity (196,198). In hamster models of atresia, isolated theca respond to LH in vitro with an increase of progesterone, whereas theca from healthy antral follicles produce only small amounts of progesterone (199,200).

In several species, the ultimate fate of the theca is complete regression without any contribution to the interstitium. This is exemplified by the pig (191), cow (138), and sheep (201). This has been especially well studied in sheep (201), in which during secondary atresia, thecal cells undergo condensation, fragmentation, and ultimate phagocytosis by still-healthy thecal cells. Thecal deletion in sheep therefore arises from the phenomenon of apoptosis, a basic process in kinetics of normal and abnormal tissue growth.

Degenerating cellular material accumulates and blocks the thecal capillaries of the atretic ovine follicle. This is an occasional finding in primary atresia, which becomes more marked as atresia progresses (201). Similarly, in tertiary atresia, the number of red blood cells per unit area and capillary area are significantly reduced in the ovine follicle (172). Estimates of follicular blood flow by radiolabeled microspheres fail to show any difference between normal and early atretic ovine follicles (202). The results may be confounded by the use of halothane to induce anesthesia. However, a similar study with conscious sheep also failed to distinguish between normal and early atretic follicles by thecal capillary blood flow. It was only in more advanced stages of atresia that thecal blood flow was reduced compared to normal follicles (cited in ref. 203). Thus, the evidence accumulated so far indicates that altered blood flow is a secondary, rather than controlling, factor in the onset of atresia. However, subtle changes in redistribution of blood between the inner and outer capillary wreathes of the theca would be difficult to evaluate with present methodology.

One of the last steps in atresia is complete collapse of the follicle. Shortening of smooth muscle cells in the theca externa of atretic follicles has been reported in mice (204), and this may be the cause of the final shrinkage.

After considering atretic changes in granulosa and theca, it is appropriate to review altered steroidogenesis during spontaneous follicular atresia. Slices of human antral follicles, classified into stages of atresia histologically, were incubated with [^{14}C]acetate (205). Stage I atresia was defined as the appearance of crumbling, regressing granulosa cells; stage II as the virtual complete disappearance of granulosa cells and hypertrophy and hyperplasia of thecal cells; and stage III the regression of the theca. In all three stages, androstenedione was the principal steroid product, without any incorporation of acetate into progesterone. During the third stage of atresia, 17-hydroxyprogesterone was the only other steroid formed. As previously mentioned, granulosa cells from atretic human follicles lose their capacity to produce estradiol, estrone, and progesterone in association with the absence of FSH in follicular fluid (206). Theca from human healthy and atretic follicles incubated for 15 hr show significantly greater production of progesterone and testosterone by the atretic theca (207). Addition of 5 or 10 ng LH/ml enhanced the production of androstenedione, testosterone, and DHT to the same extent, whereas the theca of atretic follicles showed no increases in estrone or estradiol but a greatly enhanced ability to accumulate progesterone (with 10 ng of LH).

Incubation of healthy and atretic porcine follicles for 24 hr has shown that atretic follicles produce less estradiol but considerably more androstenedione, testosterone, and DHT (175). Progesterone secretion by atretic follicles is not increased in response to hCG. Follicular fluid concentrations of estrogen, testosterone, and androstenedione are significantly less in atretic porcine follicles (208). Estrogen production by pig granulosa cells in the presence or absence of equimolar amounts of testosterone or androstenedione was highly elevated in granulosa from healthy follicles, as was also true for progesterone production after the addition of FSH. Conversely, production of estradiol was much less by the theca of atretic follicles, but the production rates of testosterone and androstenedione were virtually identical in normal and healthy theca. The conclusion is that the loss of aromatase activity by porcine granulosa cells is the first step affected by atresia, in agreement with a similar sequence in the human follicle (206).

Steroid concentrations in pools of ovine antral fluid show

that in normal follicles the molar ratio of estrogen to testosterone plus androstenedione is always >1 (209). As atresia progresses the ratio shifts in favor of androgen primarily because of a fall in estradiol. In large (⩾3.5 mm) atretic follicles, as judged by morphological criteria, follicles with signs of early degeneration have reduced aromatase activity, consistent with the idea that, in the ewe, lack of androgen substrate is not the limiting factor (210). In atretic ovine follicles (>4 mm), binding of [^{125}I]FSH and LH does not differ from that in healthy follicles until the most advanced stage of atresia (211). However, for intermediate-sized antral follicles (2–4 mm), the loss of FSH binding by granulosa cells precedes the decline in hCG binding. It was concluded that the decline in binding of the labeled gonadotropins as atresia progresses is more likely a consequence than a cause of follicular regression.

Bovine follicles from days 3 to 13 of the estrous cycle were assigned to healthy or atretic status based on follicular concentration of estradiol (estrogen active or inactive) and histology (212). From days 3 to 7, a single large estrogen active follicle is present. During this time span the estrogen-inactive follicles exhibit significantly less binding of hCG to theca and granulosa and reduced FSH binding to granulosa. Analysis of the data is complicated by the few estrogen-inactive follicles, their significantly fewer granulosa cells on days 5 and 7, and a lack of agreement between histological classification and follicular fluid ratios of estrogen to progesterone. There is no difference in [^{125}I]hCG binding to bovine theca interna from healthy and atretic antral follicles (176). When perfused *in vitro,* the output of androstenedione by theca interna of normal bovine follicles is considerably enhanced by equimolar concentrations of LH or hCG, but theca of atretic follicles are unresponsive. Lack of available receptors, therefore, does not seem to account for the failure of androgen production by large atretic bovine follicles. Rather, distal events seem to be affected. A subsequent study (213) classified the theca of large bovine follicles (>8 mm) into three types based on the number and steroidogenic capacities of the associated granulosa cells. Type I theca (normal follicles) perfused *in vitro* with LH respond by secreting increased cAMP, androstenedione, and testosterone; Type II theca (from possibly early atretic follicles) secrete increased cAMP and progesterone but not androgens; and Type III theca (definitely atretic) do not increase cAMP or steroids in response to LH. The theca of all three types contain LH receptors. These results are strikingly similar to findings with some of the rodent models (see below).

Experimental Induction of Follicular Atresia

During the past 15 years several models involving rodents have been developed to study atresia, with a number of the experimental designs based on previously described procedures (Table 3). Despite disparities in species and experimental design, the models have yielded remarkably similar conclusions but differ in key aspects from spontaneous atresia in sheep and human (see above). With one exception (198), the models focus on tertiary follicles, but they could just as well be utilized to study atresia of preantral follicles. As expected, the models using hypophysectomized animals show more rapid onset of morphological and steroidogenic

TABLE 3. *Rodent models of follicular atresia*

Model	Reference(s)
1. Hypophysectomy of proestrous rat	Braw et al., 1981 (214)
2. Hypophysectomy + PMS followed by anti-PMS (hamster)	Bill and Greenwald, 1981 (215)
3. Pentobarbital delay of ovulation in rat	Braw and Tsafriri, 1980 (216) Uilenbroek et al., 1980 (217)
4. Phenobarbital delay of ovulation in hamster	Terranova, 1980 (218)
5. PMS to immature mouse	Peters et al., 1975 (219)
6. PMS to immature rat	Peluso and Steger, 1978 (220) Braw and Tsafriri, 1980b (221)
7. PMS to immature hamster	Matson et al., 1984 (222)
8. Hypophysectomy of prepubertal rat, treatment with E_2 or DES, then hormone withdrawal	Schwall and Erickson, 1981 (198)
9. Androgen treatment of hypophysectomized rat	Bagnell et al., 1982 (223)

TABLE 4. *Methods of inducing superovulation*

1. Administration of pregnant mare serum (domestic species and laboratory rodents)
2. Effects of FSH and LH
3. Active immunization with steroids (sheep)
4. Passive immunization with steroid antisera (sheep)
5. Bovine follicular fluid (sheep)
6. Pulsatile administration of GNRH
7. Clomiphene citrate, human menopausal gonadotropin (human)
8. Effect of anti-LH

changes indicative of atresia than those using intact animals. Thus, within 12 hr after hypophysectomy of proestrous rats *in vitro* accumulation of progesterone is significantly increased by explanted follicles; conversely, estradiol is approximately halved (214). Morphological signs of early atresia are evident by 24 hr, with about 10% of the granulosa cells pyknotic; mitotic figures are still present, however. By 2 days after hypophysectomy, germinal vesicle breakdown and polar body exclusion occur in most oocytes and the resumption of meiosis is associated with a 95% increase in oxygen consumption by the oocyte (224).

The onset of atresia is even more dramatic when PMS is neutralized by anti-PMS in the hypophysectomized hamster: Within 1 hr, serum estradiol is reduced 55% (215), and the earliest histological signs of atresia are discernible within 4 hr by a significant increase in pyknotic cells in the cumulus oophorus, from 0.3% to 23.4% (225). At 2 hr after anti-PMS, cAMP increases 108% above control levels, while cGMP rises 117% at 4 hr; beginning at 12 hr, cAMP steadily declines (226). Pyknotic cells begin to appear in the mural granulosa by 8 hr, when there are still 65 mitotic figures in the largest cross section of the follicle. By 48 hr, the number of pyknotic granulosa nuclei is maximal and mitoses are absent. By 72 hr, the granulosa layer is virtually eliminated, and DNA values indicate that only 20% of the original number of cells is left in the follicle (226). The thickness of the theca shows a transitory increase at 12 hr (225), which does not persist, unlike the situation observed during spontaneous atresia in the hamster. Steroid production by isolated hamster granulosa and theca parallels the structural demise of the follicle. Necrotic changes in the granulosa cells are too widespread beyond 24 hr to warrant further steroid determinations (200). The salient observations are that thecal shells exposed to LH produce large amounts of androstenedione and 17-hydroxyprogesterone for the first 24 hr after anti-PMS but continue to produce appreciable quantities of progesterone for at least 72 hr. This confirms previous observations with this model. When intact follicles are incubated with 200 ng LH, cAMP also increases for up to 72 hr, presumably a response of the theca (227). Thus, the loss of C-17,20 lyase in theca of the atretic hamster follicle is a critical event in atresia, an observation consistent with several other rodent models (see below). Twenty-four hours after administration of anti-PMS, grain counts of ^{125}I-labeled FSH and LH on granulosa cells are reduced by 69% and 53%, respectively, of control values and receptor binding declines to 5% and 24%, respectively, at 72 hr (228). It is noteworthy that hCG binding to thecal cells and the interstitium is maintained at the same levels throughout the 72 hr after the induction of atresia, which points to the extreme resistance of these tissues to hormone withdrawal.

Another series of models deal with the administration of barbiturates at proestrus to block preovulatory surges of LH and FSH and hence extend the life span of antral follicles beyond their normal 2 to 3 days duration (Table 3; models 3–4). With these models, atresia unfolds at a slower pace. After 3 days of ovulatory delay by repeated injections of phenobarbital, early signs of atresia in the cyclic hamster are manifested by pyknotic nuclei in the membrana granulosa cells bordering on the antral cavity and in granulosa cells of the cumulus oophorus plus oocyte changes (218). During the period of ovulatory delay, the tertiary follicles continue to enlarge, expanding from 561 μm in diameter at proestrus to 680 μm on the next day. A new set of follicles is recruited by 3 days of ovulatory delay, possibly in response to elevated serum levels of FSH. After 2 days of phenobarbital treatment, spontaneous ovulation results in about 18 ova being shed, most likely representing a composite of both delayed and new follicles. On days 2 and 3 of delay, follicles incubated in the presence of LH produce more progesterone and less androstenedione and estradiol than proestrous follicles (229). However, when explanted follicles were provided with androstenedione as a precursor, estrogen accumulation was maintained at high levels, indicating that impaired estrogen secretion by the follicle is

TABLE 5. *Actions of FSH on follicular steroids and receptors during the early stages of development*

Action	Reference(s)
Increase in 3β-hydroxysteroid dehydrogenase, induction of LH (hCG) receptors	Zeleznik et al. 1974 (351)
Stimulates estradiol secretion by granulosa cells when incubated with testosterone	Dorrington et al. 1975 (369)
Adenyl cyclase stimulation and progesterone secretion	Hillier et al. 1978, 1980 (370,371)
Stimulates aromatase activity	Erickson and Hsueh, 1978 (347)
Stimulates prolactin receptor formation	Wang et al., 1979 (372)
Stimulates epidermal growth factor (EGF) and FSH receptor formation	EGF: Jones et al., 1982 (373) FSH: Richards et al., 1976 (335), Ireland and Richards, 1978 (374)

TABLE 6. *Follicular development in the human ovary*[a]

Class of follicle	Description and time of entry into class	Diameter and number of granulosa cells	Mitotic index of granulosa cells	Time in each class (days)	Atretic follicles[b] (%)
1	Preantral with theca: Cycle 1 Luteal	190–240 μm $3–5 \times 10^3$	3.8	25	23.6
2	Beginning antrum: Cycle 2 End follicular phase	400 μm 15×10^3	4.1	20	35.4
3	Antral: Cycle 3 Follicular phase	1 mm 75×10^3	5.3	15	15.3
4	Antrum: Cycle 3 Midcycle phase	2 mm 375×10^3	8.5	10	24.2
5	Antrum: Cycle 3 Late luteal phase	5 mm 1.9×10^6	10.1	5	58.0
6	Antrum: Cycle 4 Early follicular phase	10 mm 9.4×10^6	10.6	5	76.8
7	Antrum: Cycle 4 Midfollicular phase	16 mm 47×10^6	10.7	5	50
8	Preovulatory: Cycle 4 Late follicular phase	20 mm 60×10^6	5.2[c] 0.5[d]	5	0

[a]After refs. 42, 493.
[b]Throughout cycle.
[c]Before LH surge.
[d]After LH surge.

not attributable to loss of aromatase activity but rather to a deficiency of androgen precursor. The *in vitro* ability of the hamster theca to respond to LH by producing androstenedione decreased, but with a concomitant increase in progesterone accumulation, as ovulatory delay was lengthened (199).

Determination of FSH and LH (hCG) receptors in delayed follicles revealed that LH binding increased slightly or remained essentially unchanged during 3 days of delay (230); FSH binding decreased steadily throughout delay. Binding favored LH, and therefore, an increase in receptors may account for the increase in progesterone secretion in delayed follicles.

Similar results were obtained in the proestrous rat injected with pentobarbital (model 3). After 3 or 4 days of Nembutal treatment, most of the oocytes were in the dictyate stage, but pyknotic nuclei, as well as mitotic figures, characterized the membrana granulosa. Meiosis-like changes in the oocyte were observed by 4 days of ovulatory delay (216). Stage I atresia existed by day 3 and stages I and II by day 4. By day 4 of treatment, injection of hCG resulted in the ovulation of 3.4 ova per animal compared with 11.0 on proestrus. A more drastic regimen involved Nembutal injected at proestrus (day 0) along with 4 mg progesterone (231). Preovulatory follicles regressed 2 days later and were being replaced by a new set of follicles, capable of a full ovulatory response to hCG (10.8 ova) by the next day. The reason for the rapidity of replacement of the preovulatory follicles was a drastic curtailment in LH secretion and a second surge of FSH on day 2.

Before morphological signs of atresia are apparent in the pentobarbital-treated rat, steroid secretion is modified within a day, as evidenced by estradiol and androgen accumulations of about 20% to 25% of proestrous values (216,217). On the other hand, progesterone accumulation over a 4-hr period is unaffected (217). One day after ovulation is blocked, specific binding of hCG to follicles is significantly increased and FSH binding is comparable to proestrous values. Changes in receptor numbers therefore occur as a secondary event in this model of atresia as well as in others. *In vitro* steroidogenic activity of the delayed ovulating rat follicles duplicates the pattern in the hamster: Accumulation of androgen and estradiol is drastically decreased by 1 day of Nembutal treatment, and addition of testosterone to the medium leads to a fivefold increase in estradiol (217). Measurement of steroidogenic enzymes by ^{3}H-exchange assays showed that 1 day of Nembutal treatment significantly reduced C-17,20 lyase and 17α-hydroxylase, with a fall in aromatase activity by day 2 (232). Again, the unavailability of androgen substrate, presumably thecal in origin, was one of the first biochemical markers of atresia. When bromocryptine—a dopaminergic agonist—is injected daily along with pentobarbital, the ability to ovulate in response to hCG is prolonged for as long as 3 days, but normal follicular structure and the *in vitro* ability to secrete high levels of estrogen are maintained (233). It is presumed that bromocryptine acts by decreasing PRL secretion, which may have direct inhibitory effects on follicular secretion of estrogen. As enumerated several times in this chapter, the secretion of high levels of estrogen is *sine qua non* for normal tertiary follicles. The pattern of atresia in rat follicles after pentobarbital administration parallels the sequence observed in spontaneous atresia with a delay of about 2 days in all events (234). During the cycle the life span of antral follicles in the rat can be extended to a total of only 5 to 6 days before regressive changes become evident.

Another group of models of induced follicular atresia involves the injection of immature animals with PMS, which leads to the waxing and waning of preovulatory antral follicles (Table 3; models 5–7). For example, 24 hr after injection of 22-day-old mice with 5 IU PMS there is no change in the total number of "large" follicles, but the balance between healthy and atretic follicles is shifted so that only 33% of the population is atretic compared to 76% in controls (219). Similarly, administration of 15 IU PMS to 26-day-old rats does not alter the total number of preantral and antral follicles present 24 hr later but decreases the proportion between nonatretic and atretic follicles (221). Both of these studies emphasize that PMS "rescues" follicles from atresia in mice and rats, but species differences and the dose of PMS administered suggest recruitment of follicles as another important role for the hormone in inducing superovulation (see below).

In 26-day-old rats, follicles capable of ovulating to hCG are present 48 hr after IP injection of 5 IU PMS, and they then rapidly degenerate by 60 to 72 hr (235). The follicles can no longer ovulate 72 hr after a challenging dose of hCG; by 60 hr, acid phosphatase begins to build up in the membrana granulosa. By 60 hr after PMS, LH binding is reduced by 46% (235), whereas FSH binding is unaffected until 56 hr (220). Incorporation of [^{3}H]thymidine into the total ovary did not vary between 48 and 96 hr after PMS, but the labeling index of antral follicles fell significantly at 96 hr; this marked the onset of early atresia as judged by the appearance of pyknotic granulosa cells (220). The critical role of FSH in maintaining an optimal environment for the granulosa cells is evident. Ultrastructurally, the earliest signs of atresia are evident by 72 hr; 28% of tertiary follicles are atretic, as evidenced by focal areas of degeneration in granulosa cells, while others are normal (168). By 96 hr all antral follicles contained at least two pyknotic nuclei and microvilli were diminishing. Thus, cell-to-cell communication is disrupted. Ovarian concentrations of testosterone and estradiol are significantly lower by 72 and 96 hr compared to 48 hr after PMS (168).

By 72 to 78 hr, immature hamsters (25 days old) injected with 40 IU PMS—a superovulatory dose—show normal *in vitro* follicular outputs of progesterone, 17-hydroxyprogesterone, and estradiol in response to LH (222). After 96 to 102 hr, advanced atresia (established histologically) had affected antral follicles in some ovaries, correlating with significantly higher accumulations of progesterone and greatly elevated plasma levels of the hormone or use *in vivo*. An estrogen–progesterone shift is thus demonstrable comparable to the changes observed in healthy tertiary follicles on proestrus after the preovulatory release of gonadotropins.

The above models concentrated on atresia induced in antral follicles. Another one deals with preantral follicles and emphasizes thecal changes. The model involves hypophysectomized 21-day-old rats with Silastic implants of diethylstilbestrol (DES), which are removed from half the animals on day 24; necropsy is performed 2 and 4 days later (198). In the animals in which estrogen levels are maintained, numerous preantral follicles with fibroblastic thecal cells are present. In contrast, after DES withdrawal the thecal cells hypertrophy and develop the ultrastructural features of steroidogenic tissues. It is fascinating that these thecal changes occur in a presumably anhormonal environment. After DES withdrawal, hCG binding and the number of 3β-hydroxysteroid-reactive cells increase, presumably reflecting thecal and interstitial cells. Four days after estrogen withdrawal, when follicular activity is maximal, in vitro steroidogenesis in the presence of hCG is greatly enhanced for progesterone, 20-dihydroprogesterone, and androstenedione. In both control and estrogen-withdrawn cells, testosterone, DHT, and estrogen are undetectable. The increase in androgen production by the theca–interstitium is therefore apparently a secondary event in atresia of preantral follicles. Considerable attention has been devoted to a possible atretogenic role of androgens, as opposed to the antiatretic effects of estrogens (236–238). For example, in PMS-hCG-treated immature rats, pretreatment with the antiandrogens cyproterone acetate or flutamide reduces the ovulation rate to hCG by 50% (239). Ovarian concentrations of estradiol, testosterone, and progesterone, however, are unaffected by flutamide; a better endpoint would be *in vitro* accumulation of steroids by the antral follicles. In control rats, 76% of the follicles >500 μm were healthy 48 hr after PMS; injection of either flutamide or CI 628 (an anti-estrogen) decreases the number of nonatretic follicles to 14% and 9%, respectively (239). Granulosa cell viability, assessed by trypan blue exclusion, is reduced and is 20 times more sensitive to the anti-estrogen than the anti-androgen.

Since granulosa cells have specific androgen receptors (240,241), it is likely that the atretogenic actions of androgens are exerted directly on these cells. Interestingly, testosterone reduces the availability of estrogen receptors (242). A role for DHT in inducing atresia has been the subject of several studies. Thus, DHT administered to hypophysectomized PMS treated rats causes a significant reduction in primary, secondary, and tertiary follicles, and coadministration of estrogen reverses this effect (223). However, using the same animal model and the same protocol a recent study failed to demonstrate a direct atretogenic effect of DHT (243). In the immature rat DHT reduces the formation of LH receptors induced by FSH (244,245). Since DHT does not alter FSH-stimulable adenylate cyclase and estradiol production, it is postulated that it acts as an anti-estrogen by blocking the action of estradiol on the estradiol receptor, thus promoting atresia. Estradiol is required for FSH action in rat granulosa cells (246). Another possible mechanism of action of DHT is to block aromatase activity in rat granulosa cells (247). It has been suggested that if androgen production exceeds the ability of granulosa cells to aromatize it to estrogen, then DHT will be formed and perhaps lead to atresia (8). Excessive LH stimulation of the theca of small rat follicles increases DHT significantly, whereas the granulosa cell population is great enough in large follicles to convert most of the androgen to estrogen (247). At least for the rat, a proper balance between LH stimulation, androgen production, and aromatization are necessary to promote estrogen formation and the prevention of atresia. In other species, such as human and sheep, the presence of high levels of androgens in follicular fluid of atretic follicles may not be causative but merely represent the accumulation of large amounts of precursors because of insufficient aromatase activity.

Collectively, the rodent models of atresia show a consistent pattern. The morphological changes duplicate those observed during spontaneous atresia. The steroid profiles demonstrate a fall in estrogen as the primary steroidogenic effect, attributable to a shut-down in thecal androgen secretion. The same changes prevail in the normal preovulatory period of rat and hamster (for literature, see ref. 248). In contrast, comparable to the changes during atresia, in the proestrous ewe the abrupt fall in serum levels of estradiol is not associated with a concomitant decline in androgens (249). Species differences may therefore exist regarding the hormonal basis of estrogen withdrawal.

A charge frequently leveled against models of atresia is that they may not accurately reflect events in normal, spontaneous atresia. However, an unpublished study by Greenwald involving the hamster indicates excellent agreement between the morphological and hormonal changes encountered during induced and spontaneous atresia. The experimental design consisted of dissecting the 10 largest follicles from one ovary of intact cyclic hamsters for each day of the cycle. The follicles were incubated for a baseline 1-hr period followed by the addition of LH for another hour. The media were saved for determinations of steroids and the follicles then prepared for histological examination to assess whether they were healthy or atretic. Follicles with the earliest signs of atresia have steroid profiles comparable to healthy follicles and normal vascularity, as judged by the number of red blood cells present in thecal capillaries. When approximately a third to a half of the membrana granulosa cells are pyknotic and degenerating, a concurrent fall in *both* androstenedione and estradiol accumulation is apparent in the baseline and LH-stimulated incubations. Thecal vascularity is then also drastically reduced.

All of the aforementioned models of atresia have dealt with polytocous species. A model for inducing atresia in rhesus monkeys is based on exposure to elevated levels of estradiol-17β in Silastic implants for 24 hr (250). After-treatment at day 5, the contents of the single dominant follicle are aspirated on day 10. Follicular fluid concentrations of estrogen and progesterone were reduced three- and sevenfold, respectively, from control follicles. In light of the previous discussion on spontaneous atresia in the human, it would have been worthwhile to also measure androgens. The viability of granulosa cells had already diminished in the estrogen-treated follicles, but treatment with human FSH restored progesterone to control levels. At the end of 3 days of culture, the percentage of granulosa cells binding [^{125}I]hFSH did not differ in control and treated animals.

FOLLICULAR DEVELOPMENT AND SUPEROVULATION

An experimental increase in ovulation rate is an important procedure for analyzing follicular regulation in laboratory species, farm animals, and humans for in vitro fertilization programs. For our purposes, superovulation is defined as an approximate doubling in the normal ovulation rate. Table 4 (p. 401) lists various methods that have been used, all of which act by affecting either exogenous or endogenous levels of gonadotropins. Three mechanisms of action have been suggested for the effects of gonadotropins on follicular development: (a) Follicles already undergoing early atresia are presumably "rescued" as a result of vigorous mitotic activity in granulosa and/or thecal compartments; (b) smaller healthy follicles are recruited into a more active growth phase; and (c) the rate of follicular atresia is reduced. The last two mechanisms are not mutually exclusive and, indeed, are the most likely combination accounting for superovulation.

Since its isolation some 50 years ago, PMS has been the most extensively utilized gonadotropin for inducing superovulation in laboratory animals and large domestic species (251). This unique molecule is structurally akin to hCG (252) and functions almost exclusively as an LH-like hormone in the mare and stallion (253,254). In other species, however, PMS serves in a dual capacity as an FSH and LH molecule (253–256). In one study using radioreceptor assays for FSH and LH, the molar ratio of FSH:LH was 0.20 in pig, 0.25 in rat tissue, and 0.0 in the horse (256). Rat, cow, and pig gonadal tissues bind as much labeled PMS as LH on a molar basis, whereas equine tissues bind only 4% as much PMS as LH, or less (253). For this reason, several investigators have substituted "equine chorionic gonadotropin" for PMS, but the latter designation may be too firmly entrenched to be displaced.

The FSH:LH bioactivity ratio of PMS is almost impossible to evaluate because of the various endpoints that have been used in various studies. Equine pituitary LH also has significant FSH activity in rat and pig (254,256). Two other features of PMS contribute to its efficacy in stimulating follicular growth: its long half-life, attributable to its high sialic acid content (252), and its ability to increase cholesterol side-chain cleavage, cholesterol esterase activity, and cytochrome P-450 when injected into immature rats (257), and therefore overall increased steroidogenesis in rabbits (258), hamsters (259), and other species. At the same time, in large domestic species, increased steroid levels in response to PMS can be detrimental because of disturbances to the hypothalamic–pituitary axis.

The effects of PMS on follicular development have been established for several species. Administration of PMS on day 2 or 3 of the ovine cycle results in the formation of numerous large follicular cysts (≥20 mm), which ultimately become luteinized without ovulating (260). If, however, PMS is injected on days 5 to 7, an average of 7.3 luteinized follicles with stigmata (indicative of ovulation) are present 9 to 10 days later and, concomitantly, the number of cystic follicles is reduced. For a number of species, including sheep, the follicular population of the two ovaries of one animal show considerably less variation than between-animal variation (sheep: 261; hamster: 262; heifer: 263), and a number of studies have taken advantage of this feature in their experimental design. In one investigation, sheep were either unilaterally ovariectomized on day 12 of the cycle (controls) or were injected with PMS and the other ovary removed 24 or 40 hr later (264). In the control group, 74% of the follicles were between 2 and 2.9 mm in diameter and 7% were between 3 and 3.9 mm. Twenty-four hours after PMS, only 50% of the follicles were in the smallest size category, and 24% were in the 3- to 3.9-mm range. Moreover, between 24 and 48 hr after PMS, the number of healthy follicles >2 mm was substantially increased, but the number of atretic follicles was unchanged. It was concluded that either recruitment and/or reduced atresia account for the increased number of large follicles after PMS.

Similar conclusions were reached for heifers that were unilaterally ovariectomized on day 7, were immediately injected with PMS, and then had the remaining ovary removed 148 ± 23 hr later—after the onset of the preovulatory surge of LH (263). Follicles >70 μm were counted and assessed for normality or early to late atresia. An antral cavity began to form between 115 to 280 μm. Unilateral ovariectomy alone did not affect the number of normal preantral or antral follicles or the number of atretic follicles. After PMS, the remaining ovary significantly increased the number of preantral follicles and follicles with incipient formation of an antral cavity; the number of antral follicles was not affected. For the first two categories of follicles, PMS approximately doubled the mitotic index without changing that for normal or early atretic antral follicles. PMS treatment delayed antrum formation in follicles <0.5 mm. After PMS, follicles >5 mm contained significantly fewer granulosa cells than control ovaries, suggesting that the antrum was correspondingly larger in the former group. The investigators believed that some follicles were "rescued" from early atresia because abundant pyknotic cells were sometimes present in fresh corpora lutea and especially in luteinized follicles. The above findings on increased numbers of preantral and early antral follicles after PMS lend more credence to recruitment and reduced atresia as the factors responsible for increased numbers of healthy follicles. Similar conclusions were reached in another study in which four cows were injected with PMS and the entire antral population of follicles (>3 mm) analyzed 48 hr later (265). In the treated animals, 70% of the follicles were healthy or very early atretic compared to 35% in the untreated controls; counting only healthy follicles, the percentages were 38.4% and 16.2%, respectively. Repeated PMS-induced superovulations in cows did not affect the ovulation rate or viable embryos recovered (265), and similar results have been obtained in the hamster (266). Hence, antibody formation to repeated exposure to PMS is not a problem. The ovulatory response in PMS-treated cows is enhanced by injection of PMS antiserum on the day of standing heat (267). The number of corpora lutea increased to 15.7 compared to 9.4 in PMS-treated controls, and the number of large unruptured follicles decreased from 6.5 to 2.8.

The hamster is the rodent species par excellence for evaluating the effects of PMS on ovulation and follicular development (268). This stems from the precision of its 4-day cycle and the ease with which spontaneous superovulation can be induced, in contrast to the rat (see below). On day 1 of the cycle (estrus), each ovary of the hamster has normally recruited 10 *developing follicles* that are large preantral stages. In the ensuing days, the preantral follicles mature into antral stages, and the number per ovary is reduced between days 3 and 4 (morning of proestrus) to approximately 5, thus accounting for the normal ovulation of about 10 ova. When a small dose of PMS (5 IU) is injected on day 1, the hamsters ovulate 20 eggs by preventing atresia of the developing follicles, normally eliminated between days 3 and 4. In the light of recent findings on the dual FSH and LH actions of PMS on the rodent ovary, the question arises of whether one or both of these gonadotropin activities save the developing follicles. With administration of increasing doses of PMS on day 1, a plateau of 70 ovulations is reached with 30 or 60 IU PMS. This results from the recruitment of smaller *reserve follicles* that would normally have taken several cycles to reach large preovulatory stages. Within 24 hr of the injection of 30 IU PMS, the hamster ovary contains 27 ± 4 follicles >267 μm, as compared with 14 ± 3 follicles in controls, and the combined developing and reserve follicles are maintained for the rest of the cycle (57). In the hamster, clear-cut recruitment and subsequent reduced atresia represents the follicular responses to PMS. This has been further substantiated: As early as 4 hr after PMS, preantral follicles with four or more layers of granulosa cells (these are the reserve follicles) are mobilized and begin to develop antral cavities (58). This also illustrates the rapidity with which follicles in the rodent ovary can be recruited by various perturbations, in contrast to the large domestic species in which follicular kinetics operate at a much slower pace. The combined effect of the developing and reserve follicles ultimately results in a three- to fourfold increase in the number of antral follicles and, concomitantly, in enormous increases in estrogen. For example, after 30 IU PMS on day 1 of the hamster cycle, serum estradiol on the afternoon of day 3 is 929 pg/ml, which, however, does not interfere with the normal operation of the hypothalamic–pituitary axis and ovulation of an average of 63 ova at the end of a normal 4-day cycle (269).

The effects of PMS administration to the cyclic rat are quite different. After the injection of 5 IU PMS during estrus, follicular development is accelerated, and there is a prompt appearance on the same day of approximately three times as many follicles larger than 55×10^6 μm^3 than in untreated animals; however, only the normal number of ova are spontaneously ovulated (56). Higher doses of PMS (10–50 IU) recruit an even greater number of healthy follicles; even so, there is no spontaneous ovulation, although hCG treatment on day 3 causes the ovulation of 29 to 43 ova. It is presumed that rising and excessive titers of estrogens impair the proestrous release of LH and, consequently, prevent ovulation. The salient point of this study (56) is that higher doses of PMS *can* increase the rate of recruitment of follicles and reduce atresia in the cyclic rat. Injection of 7.5 IU PMS on day 24 to immature rats results 24 hr later in high mitotic indices in granulosa cells of all sizes of follicles, and this is already manifested in the smallest follicles studied, those with 90 cells in the largest cross section (65). This corresponds to follicles that are about 120 μm in diameter (270), and they are therefore very small preantral stages.

In addition to PMS, superovulation has been induced in several species with "purified" preparations of FSH. The most provocative finding, though, is the ability of LH to induce superovulation in cyclic hamsters and guinea pigs (69). High tonic levels of the hormone are maintained in hamsters by implanting an osmotic minipump on day 1 of the cycle. When 400 μg of ovine LH was infused, approximately 32 ova were shed at the next estrus. Several experiments eliminated the possibility that FSH contamination accounted for these results. Even more striking, hamsters hypophysectomized on day 1 and implanted with LH maintained large antral follicles through day 4. Infusion of LH into guinea pigs doubled the ovulation rate, whereas similar treatment of cyclic mice and rats was ineffective. Possibly excessive levels of estrogen may be acting as a negative-feedback influence in the mouse and rat.

Continuous infusion of LH increases blood flow to the hamster ovary on day 3 and induces a depletion of ovarian histamine (271). Injection of an antihistamine reduces the number of ova shed in LH-implanted hamsters but not in controls. It is possible that increased ovarian blood flow may enhance delivery of FSH to the ovary, which seems to be necessary as a synergist for LH-induced superovulation. In the hamster, thousands of mast cells are located in the hilum of the ovary surrounding the blood vessels that enter and exit from the ovary (272). Since the LH surge on proestrus causes mast cell degranulation in the hamster (272) and LH causes ovarian histamine discharge (271,273,274), it seems plausible that mast cells and histamine are mediators in part of LH-induced superovulation in the hamster. Indeed, antihistamines block ovulation in several species by preventing follicular rupture (275–277). Several questions arise at this point: What factors are involved in the LH-induced increase in ovarian blood flow? Do PMS and FSH induce ovulation by the same mechanism(s)? Are mast cells essential for LH-induced superovulation?

Other methods to induce superovulation rely upon the experimental manipulation of endogenous gonadotropin levels (Table 4). Active immunization of female sheep against estrogens increases basal levels of LH and FSH and increases pulsatile LH release to levels encountered in ovariectomized animals (for literature, see ref. 278). The ovulation rate is increased from 1.5 to 3 by this treatment. Active immunization against androstenedione increases the ovulation rate from 1.50 ± 0.25 to 2.00 ± 0 and the number of surface follicles >3 mm in diameter from 1 to 3, respectively (279). It has been proposed that active immunization against steroids increases the ovulation rate by disrupting the normal negative-feedback effects of estradiol and/or by a reduction in follicular atresia. A variation of this technique involves passive immunization with antisera to steroids given as a single intravenous injection on the first day of estrus (280). Controls ovulated 1.3 ova compared to 2.1 ova after administration of the estradiol antisera, and the mean number of lambs born alive was 1.3 versus 1. This was attributable to a higher incidence of twinning in the group treated with the antisera. A mixture of antisera to estradiol, estrone, androstenedione, and testosterone was the most efficacious, increasing the ovulation rate to 2.1 and the lambing rate to 1.5.

Intravenous injection of bovine follicular fluid to ewes on days 1 to 11 of the cycle increased the ovulation rate to 3.4 ± 0.3, as compared with 2.3 ± 0.3 in controls (281). The treatment significantly lowered FSH levels over the first 7 days, the levels returning to control values thereafter. Throughout the luteal phase, daily LH concentrations and pulse frequency and amplitude were significantly increased in the treated group. With the onset of induced luteolysis, the ewes injected with follicular fluid showed fourfold greater levels of FSH and about a twofold increase in LH compared with controls. It was pointed out that the treatment prevented the postestrous surge of FSH and that the hypersecretion of FSH at the onset of the follicular phase presumably accounts for the increased ovulation rate. However, since the onset of estrus was significantly delayed (89 vs. 41 hr), the return to control levels of FSH on day 8 and thereafter may constitute the time when "privileged follicles" may have been exposed to the amounts of FSH required for their ultimate selection after luteal regression.

The pulsatile infusion of gonadotropin releasing hormone (GNRH) using Alza osmotic minipumps has been used to increase ovulation rate and estrus in zoo-maintained animals (282). The advantages are that synthetic GNRH seems to be universally capable of stimulating the species' own FSH and LH; consequently, physiological stimulation of the ovaries is simulated and "natural" mating behavior is elicited.

Various regimens have been used to induce superovulation in humans (283), including clomiphene citrate followed by hCG, clomiphene plus human menopausal gonadotropin (hMG) followed by hCG and hMG followed by hCG. There is still room for improvement in the methodology. A new approach involves intravenous infusion of pulsatile LHRH or FSH with a controlled LH surge, similar to the system described for zoo-maintained species. A detailed consideration of superovulation in the human is beyond the scope of this chapter.

A chance discovery led to the surprising finding that a potent equine antiserum to bovine LH (anti-LH) is able to induce superovulation in several species. A single injection of anti-LH interrupted pregnancy in hamsters and rats, and at subsequent estrus, the hamster superovulated 29 ova, whereas the rat ovulated the normal number of 13 eggs (284). Cyclic hamsters injected subcutaneously with 100 μl anti-LH at estrus (day 1) spontaneously ovulated 31.5 eggs after a cycle lengthened to 5 days from the normal 4 days (285). The major effect of the anti-LH was to induce atresia of the larger preantral follicles by day 2 followed by a rebound in follicular recruitment by the next day, so that a greater than normal number of antral and intermediate follicles repopulated the ovaries. Quite distinct from the superovulatory effects of PMS, with anti-LH, serum levels of estradiol throughout the cycle are within the normal limits of control animals; hence aromatase activity is not increased. The anti-LH was only effective in inducing superovulation in the cyclic hamster when it was administered on estrus or proestrus, i.e., at times when serum levels of FSH are normally elevated. After removal of the interfering LH antibodies from serum by Sephadex G-200 chromatography, radioimmunoassays for FSH and LH revealed normal levels of FSH throughout the cycle, but LH levels were nondetectable on day 2 and in most hamsters on day 3 (286). We had anticipated that anti-LH treatment would elicit a castration response and consequent hypersecretion of FSH and LH; indeed, the possibility cannot be discounted that more frequent samples between days 2 and 3 might detect a rebound release of elevated levels of FSH and/or LH. However, if the results are taken at face value, the sustained secretion of progesterone for 2 days by the autonomous corpora lutea might act as a sufficient negative-feedback influence to prevent hypersecretion of gonadotropins. Our hypothesis concerning the mechanism of anti-LH's ability to induce superovulation in the hamster is that by temporarily eliminating LH action on the ovary, a "pure" FSH effect is manifested, thus increasing its mitogenic effects on granulosa cells (see ref. 286 for pertinent references on FSH:LH ratios). Several recent papers also point to altered FSH:LH ratios affecting follicular development, with higher amounts of LH reducing the mitogenic action of FSH. Thus, administration to immature rats of PMS with different FSH:LH ratios, followed by an ovulating dose of hCG, causes reduced ovulation rates at lower ratios (255). Similarly, immature rats with mini-osmotic pumps delivering 240 μg porcine FSH/day ovulated 69 ± 10 eggs. When FSH was held constant and increasing amounts of LH concurrently infused, the ovulation rate progressively declined (287). On the other hand, in *hypophysectomized* proestrous hamsters injected daily with 5 μg/day ovine FSH plus 5, 10, or 20 μg LH, the number of follicles that matured or ovulated in response to hCG did not decline (288).

The ability of anti-LH to induce superovulation in the cyclic hamster is restricted to its first administration; a second injection—even 3 months later—results in the ovulation of only 6 ova at the end of a 4-day cycle (266). Injection of normal horse serum at estrus followed 14 days later by anti-LH results in the ovulation of only 18 ova. Evidently, after the initial exposure the hamster rapidly forms antibodies to equine immunoglobulins. Injection of guinea pigs on day 12 of the cycle with 0.8 ml anti-LH prolonged the estrous cycle by 3 days and increased the ovulation rate from 2.9 to 5.6 ova (289). To our knowledge this is the only treatment, other than the continuous infusion of LH, that has increased ovulation rate in the guinea pig (69). Equine anti-bovine LH injected on day 10 of the cycle also increases the number of ova shed in cyclic ewes from 2.1 ± 0.1 in control animals to 2.7 ± 0.2, with estrus being delayed by 0.6 days (290). It has likewise been successful in increasing the ovulation rate in pregnant mice, injected with anti-LH on day 4; on day 8 the animals (from a control line) ovulated 16 eggs compared with the normal number of 8.8 at estrus. A high ovulating strain that normally ovulates 16 eggs ovulated 30 eggs when similarly treated (Barkley and Greenwald, unpublished data). However, anti-LH does not increase the ovulation rate of pregnant (284) or cyclic rats (Terranova and Greenwald, unpublished data). This intriguing model deserves further study.

EFFECTS OF UNILATERAL OVARIECTOMY ON FOLLICULAR DEVELOPMENT

Unilateral ovariectomy (ULO) is a time-honored procedure that has been useful in elucidating follicular kinetics in species as disparate as pigs, chickens, Drosophila (for literature, see ref. 291), geckos (292), and the California leaf-nosed bat (293). The latter species normally always ovulates from the right ovary, but following its removal the left ovary becomes active.

The effects of ULO in mammals can be analyzed in terms of compensatory hypertrophy of the contralateral ovary (i.e., increased weight), representing persistence of increased numbers of corpora lutea (e.g., the rat) and enhanced follicular activity. For our purposes, the effects of ULO on follicular development within the cycle in which the procedure was performed is a more meaningful endpoint, providing information on how late in the cycle successful follicular recruitment and hence increased ovulation rate can be elicited. This can be contrasted with the long-term effects of ULO on follicular compensation, which involves different adjustments in pituitary–ovarian function.

The first experiment involving ULO dates back to an often-quoted study of Hunter (294), who followed the farrowing records of two sows, one of which had been semispayed. Over the first eight litters, the intact sow produced 87 young and the semispayed sow 76; thereafter, however, the control animal delivered 5 more litters consisting of 75 young. A pioneering study of Arai (295) established ovarian compensation in the rat after ULO and demonstrated that the surviving ovary had about twice as many corpora lutea and a greater number of mature follicles than the intact animal. Working with the rabbit, Lipschutz (296) proposed that ovarian hypertrophy following ULO was caused by an increased follicular development that depended on some "general body factor." He proposed one of the basic tenets of follicular selection, the law of follicular constancy: "The number of ova entering into follicular development, the rhythm of follicular development and the degree which is attained by follicular development are constant and are controlled by somatic factors outside the ovary. Ovarian hypertrophy means those integrative processes which take place in the ovarian fragment after partial castration which are not to be characterized by the increase in weight, but only by those processes which are dictated by the Law of Follicular Constancy" (296).

Short-Term Effects of ULO

The first species in which the immediate effects of ULO on compensatory ovulation were established was the hamster (262). Removal of one ovary at 9:00 a.m. for the first 3 days of the 4-day estrous cycle was followed by a doubling in the number of ovulations from the remaining ovary. It was initially believed that a reduction in atresia of larger follicles between days 3 and 4 spared follicles and therefore resulted in compensatory ovulation (262). Recently, however, it was shown that ULO on day 3 within 4 hr mobilizes preantral follicles with six to seven layers of granulosa cells and converts them into small antral follicles (297). This puts the hamster in line with other species (see below) and also points to the rapidity with which follicles can respond in species with short estrous cycles.

Compensatory ovulation in cyclic rats after ULO depends on the length of the estrous cycle: in rats with 4-day cycles, ULO as late as day 3 results in a doubling of the number of ovulations from the remaining ovary. Slightly more leeway exists in rats with 5-day cycles, in which removal of one ovary as late as 2 a.m. of diestrus 2 results in follicular compensation (298). Increased proliferation of smaller follicles results in a doubling of the number of large follicles following ULO and consequently maintains the normal ovulation rate characteristic of the rat (299). Compensatory ovulation does not occur after ULO of 4-day cyclic rats at 1700 or 2000 hr of diestrus, although a surge in FSH begins 6 hr later (300). However, if a day is added to the cycle by treatment with pentobarbital on proestrus, the animals *do* compensate by reduced follicular atresia, as well as by recruitment of smaller follicles. Mice unilaterally ovariectomized at random times during the cycle invariably double the number of ova shed within 3 days after the procedure (301). As an induced ovulator, the rabbit's response to ULO is of interest. Within 48 hr of ULO, the number of follicles $\geq$1 mm increases two- to threefold in the remaining ovary, and injection of hCG 4 days later results in ovulation of 11.4 ova (302).

What are the effects of ULO in species with long estrous cycles? The guinea pig can compensate as late as day 10 of the cycle by doubling the ovulation rate from the remaining ovary; an increased rate of transformation of smaller-sized follicles into larger ones accounts for the results (303). In contrast, ULO of Finn-Dorset sheep on day 2, 8, or 14 does not affect the number of ova shed (measured by number of corpora lutea) at the very next estrus (304). On the other hand, unilateral ovariectomy of Leicester-Merino ewes at day 14 results in compensatory ovulation by the next cycle (ULO, 2 corpora lutea; intact, 1.70) but is only partially effective when hemicastration is deferred to day 16 (305). In a breed of sheep with high ovulation rate (2.4 corpora lutea), ULO on day 10 of the cycle results in an overall ovulation of 2.2 from the remaining ovary (73). Four days after ULO there is no significant increase in any size range of preantral follicles and antral follicles (73). Unilateral ovariectomy on day 2 of the porcine estrous cycle results by day 13 in a compensatory increase in the number of large follicles (5–12.9 mm in diameter) (306). Sows unilaterally ovariectomized on day 2 of the estrous cycle ovulate as many ova at the next estrus as intact animals: 18.1 and 16.0 corpora lutea, respectively (307). There are obvious species differences between the sow and the ewe. The ewe after ULO ultimately does increase its ovulation rate per ovary, but the 2-year lamb production is significantly lower than that of intact ewe: 1.35 versus 1.61 (308). Evidently, follicles cannot be recruited as readily in the ewe as in other species. In contrast, within 6 hr after ULO on day 3 of the hamster cycle, there is already a 66% depletion of stage 4 follicles (with four layers of granulosa cells) into stage 5 (five-layered follicles) (141). Moreover, by 6 hr after ULO, incubation of follicles with [^{3}H]thymidine shows a significantly lower rate of incorporation than comparable follicles from intact animals (309). This points to the rapidity with which follicles can be mobilized in animals with short estrous cycles.

What are the effects of ULO on species that are normally monovular? In the cow, ULO on day 8 of the cycle results, by the next estrus, in a redistribution of follicular size, there being a greater representation of the 9- to 16-mm class than in controls. However, in the one-ovary group, the largest follicle is smaller than in the control, although the next largest follicle is consistently larger in the ULO group (310). The authors raise the interesting question of whether the potential for twin ovulation is enhanced in the ULO group, but to our knowledge this possibility has never been tested. Seven days after ULO of the heifer there is a significant increase in the number of follicles 5 to 6 mm and >9 mm in diameter; this increase can be blocked by daily injection of bovine follicular fluid (311).

Rhesus monkeys hemicastrated for 3 months show ovarian hypertrophy of the remaining ovary and, histologically, numerous "large follicles and corpora lutea in various stages of development" (312). Hemiovariectomized cynomolgus monkeys have more ovulatory cycles per 13 months than intact animals: 9.8 versus 5.8. Also, in 49% of the cycles, serum progesterone was >9 ng/ml, compared with 26% in the intact group (313). Ovulation was verified by laparoscopy on days 11 and 21 of each cycle, and there evidently was no increase in ovulation rate, which would surely have been noted. As expected, there is even more of a dearth of information about the effects of ULO in the human female. The only concrete evidence, albeit incomplete, is provided in a study by Speert and colleagues of a series of 16 patients who required a second laparotomy within 2 years after removal of one ovary for complications of tubal pregnancy (314). In 6 patients the ovary was enlarged because of luteal or follicular cysts, but the remaining ovary appeared normal in the other patients. A long-term unilaterally ovariectomized woman had only one corpus luteum in the remaining ovary (315). The availability of sonographic techniques to visualize temporal changes in large follicles now makes it feasible to explore the long-term effects of ULO in primates.

It is apparent from the literature discussed so far that compensatory follicular development (and therefore ultimately maintenance of the number of ovulations characteristic of the species) depends on rapid recruitment of small follicles as an acute response to ULO. What hormonal changes account for such a prompt response? Before the advent of radioimmunoassays, it was proposed that ULO did not result in an increase in pituitary gonadotropins, but rather had a "sparing effect," so that the amount of hormone normally available to two ovaries now exerted its actions on the remaining ovary. What is now established beyond doubt is that the acute effect of ULO or ablation of the dominant follicle is manifested in a sharp transient increase in serum levels of FSH, with variable and less striking changes in LH. This has now been observed in hamster (316), rat (for literature, see ref. 317), rabbit (302), gilt (318), cow (311), ewe (305), and human (319). The increase in FSH after ULO is analogous to the periovulatory increase that occurs in most mammals and that is believed to recruit the next cohort of follicles. In the immediate period following ULO there is no change in serum levels of estradiol in the hamster (320) or rat (317). Hence, removal of negative steroid feedback does not seem to be the major factor accounting for the transient increase in FSH. The effects of ULO on rats hemicastrated on diestrus 2 (when antral follicles are present) are reversed by administration of inhibin, suggesting that this may be the key ingredient removed by semispaying (317). Similarly, compensatory ovarian hypertrophy is prevented in unilaterally ovariectomized gilts by daily treatment with porcine follicular fluid (318). The authors caution that their results do not rule out a direct inhibitory effect on follicular growth, although serum FSH was significantly increased in semispayed gilts injected with porcine serum.

At various times it has been suggested that ovarian nerves play a role in compensatory follicular development, but ovarian sympathectomy by injecting 6-hydroxydopamine into an artificially closed ovarian bursa fails to prevent the increase in follicular number after ULO of the contralateral ovary (reviewed in ref. 321).

Long-Term Effects of ULO

Following ULO of the cyclic hamster, compensatory ovulation occurs in the next 14 cycles without deviating from the normally rigid 4-day cycle (322). The hemicastrated rat, on the other hand, compensates completely for only 10 cycles and thereafter ovulates 7 to 9 ova from the remaining ovary. Comparable results for the rat were obtained by Peppler (323), who observed that rats hemiovariectomized for 3 months shed 10.9 ova from the remaining ovary, whereas by 6 months only 4.9 ova were shed. In long-term hemicastrated rats (3 months), the remaining ovary when examined at metestrus contained a similar number of follicles (>357 μm) as intact animals (323), suggesting that follicular selection took place later in the cycle. In rats hemicastrated for 20 to 30 days the total number of large antral follicles (>400 μm) by metestrus was the same in ULO and intact rats, and it appears that this was accomplished by a significant reduction in atresia of follicles in the 350- to 399-μm category (324). A subsequent paper by Hirshfield explored the problem in greater detail (325). Semispayed rats had twice as many follicles >450 μm at proestrus than did intact rats, thus accounting for compensatory ovulation. By metestrus and diestrus there were already twice as many follicles in the semispayed group, and this was associated with decreased atresia. Seventy days after ULO of sheep, there is a significant increase in the number of small preantral follicles (<0.06 to 0.07 mm in diameter) and antral follicles, especially in the range of 2.0 to 3.6 mm (73). Again, this indicates the sluggish responsiveness of sheep follicles to ULO, but it must be realized that the increase in number of follicles may occur considerably earlier than the third or fourth cycle.

What hormonal patterns can account for follicular compensation in the long-term hemicastrate? For both the rat (326) and hamster (316), the second surge of FSH that is normally restricted to estrus is extended into the second day of the cycle, and this appears to be the signal that recruits additional follicles (300–450 μm in the rat) into the ovulatory range.

It is beyond the scope of this chapter to consider the effects of ULO on truly long-term reproductive performance. The primary studies were carried out by Zuckerman and his associates in rats (reviewed in ref. 327). A recent study shows that stage I follicles (one layer of flattened granulosa cells), which constitute the "follicular pool," are significantly reduced by 4 weeks in hemicastrated mice but that the number of growing follicles is maintained or even increased (327). There is no difference in the percentage of oocytes undergoing atresia between semispayed and control mice for any stage of follicular development, but the stage of the estrous cycle when the animals were killed was not taken into account.

The overall impression from both the short- and long-term effects of ULO is that FSH is essential for either increased follicular recruitment and/or reduced atresia. Whether FSH is acting through the now classical cyclic nucleotide pathways has not been established for any of the experimental models for ULO.

FOLLICULAR DEVELOPMENT DURING THE ESTROUS CYCLE OF RAT AND HAMSTER

The rat and hamster have been selected as representative rodent species with short cycles in which follicular events occur at a much different rate than in mammals with long cycles such as sheep and humans. Schwartz (328) was one of the first to propose that the secondary surge of FSH on estrus initiates recruitment of growing follicles in the rat and that these follicles are ovulated at the next estrus (4 or 5 days later). However, other factors preceding the (secondary) FSH surge of the immediate cycle are apparently also involved in the regulation of follicle development. Kinetic studies using the mouse, hamster, and rat have shown that the large preovulatory follicles that ovulate in response to the LH surge actually enter the growing pool of follicles some 20 days earlier. These follicles may have been recruited by a gonadotropin surge and were then exposed to three to four consecutive surges of gonadotropins before ovulating.

It appears that primordial follicles enter the growing pool at a constant rate regardless of the day of the mouse estrous cycle, as evidenced by a similar rate of incorporation of tritiated thymidine by granulosa cells of small follicles on each day of the cycle (48). Follicles entering the growing pool on day 1 (estrus), when FSH levels are elevated, may be stimulated by the gonadotropic stimulus to move into more advanced stages of development. For example, in the hamster, stage I follicles (2–3 layers of granulosa cells) that are present on estrus progress to stage II (4–5 layers of granulosa cells) after 8 days (329). At the next estrus (when FSH levels are elevated) these follicles migrate after an additional 8 days to the next stage of development (stage III, 6–7 layers of granulosa cells). However, stage III and IV follicles (8 or more layers of granulosa cells but no antrum) present on estrus may either move into the preovulatory stages within 4 days or become atretic. Thus, from stage I to the preovulatory phase takes approximately 20 days. It is unknown how long it takes for primary follicles to be transformed into stage I follicles in the hamster. Based on [^{3}H]thymidine studies in the cyclic rat, follicles with one to two layers of granulosa cells (type 3b) take approximately 22 days to develop to stage 6 (antral follicle: 200 μm in diameter) (51). If 4 days is included for the transit time through types 7 and 8 (330,331), then a total of approximately 27 days elapses between type 3b to 8.

During the 20 to 30 days of growth, the follicles are exposed to four or five consecutive LH/FSH surges at recurring intervals. These surges have been shown to affect small developing follicles in the rat and hamster (332,333). In the hypophysectomized, estradiol-treated immature rat, treatment with 5 IU hCG followed by 2 μg human FSH resulted in a 15-fold increase in granulosal cell LH receptors by 36 hr; FSH receptor increased 3-fold by 48 hr, and antral follicular development was markedly enhanced (332). Neither FSH nor hCG alone increased the FSH and LH receptors to maximal levels. In fact, FSH followed by hCG 12 hr later was unable to increase the granulosa cell FSH and LH receptors to the same magnitude as hCG followed by FSH. The major point is that hCG (in synergy with FSH) increased its own receptor in the developing antral follicles. This action of hCG is similar to that of FSH on small antral follicles. The mechanism by which hCG increases the action of FSH is unknown. Very low levels of hCG binding sites are present in the theca and granulosa cells of estradiol-primed rats (334–336), and hCG can stimulate theca cell hypertrophy. Therefore, hCG may synergize with FSH using a thecal cell intermediary product (332). Neither testosterone nor estradiol mimicked the concerted effect of hCG and FSH to increase hCG receptor sites (332).

The LH surge in the hamster enhances progesterone production and inhibits androstenedione production in theca of preantral follicles (333). Large preantral follicles (stages III and IV) isolated immediately before, during, and after the LH surge on proestrus were incubated in vitro with LH to stimulate steroidogenesis. Before the LH surge, follicles produced 2.4 ± 0.3 ng androstenedione (A) per follicle and very low amounts of progesterone (P) (<250 pg) and estradiol (E_2, <100 pg). During the peak of the LH surge, preantral follicles produced 1.8 ± 0.2 ng P and 1.9 ± 0.1 ng A and less than 100 pg E_2. Immediately after the LH surge, preantral follicles were unable to produce A and E_2 but produced 8.1 ± 3.1 ng P at 1500 hr on estrus; A secretion was also restored. Thereafter, steroid secretion returned to levels similar to that observed prior to the surge. These results have their exact counterpart in the altered steroidogenic profile of large preovulatory follicles after exposure to the ovulatory surges of gonadotropins. The LH surge may therefore synchronize the onset of androstenedione and estradiol synthesis during follicular development. LH appears to inhibit FSH action on steroidogenesis immediately after the surge but acts in synergy with FSH at later stages of development. FSH then acts on steroidogenically synchronized follicles after recruitment into the growing population.

Clear-cut evidence that small growing follicles are influenced by periovulatory changes in gonadotropins is provided in a series of recent studies based on the ability to dissect intact follicles from the hamster ovary enzymatically (140). Small preantral follicles with one to five layers of granulosa cells lack any thecal investment. When such follicles are incubated with [^{3}H]thymidine for 4 hr, a significant increase in incorporation occurs between the morning of proestrus and 1500 hr—when the preovulatory surges of FSH and LH are in progress (54). A second increase in DNA synthesis is evident on the morning of estrus that not only involves the smallest preantral follicles but also includes all larger healthy stages as well. These results are consistent with a previous autoradiographic study (53). Phenobarbital injected at 1300 hr proestrus blocks the normal rise in FSH and LH and prevents the increase in [^{3}H]thymidine incorporation in all follicular stages; however, the effects can be reversed in the small preantral follicles by injection of FSH but not LH (309). The ability of FSH to enhance DNA synthesis of small preantral follicles can also be demonstrated *in vitro,* where it is associated with increased cAMP activity (Roy and Greenwald, *unpublished data*).

Follicular Development During the Cycle: Estrus

On the first day of the hamster's cycle (estrus), serum FSH is elevated, being two- to sixfold higher than on day 2 (337–339). There is a biphasic pattern on day 4 (proestrus), with peak FSH levels attained at 1600 hr on day 4; a decline to low levels by 2100 hr is then followed by a steady increase to the high levels observed on day 1. The secondary FSH surge in the rat is not as discrete as in the hamster (340,341). A single increase of serum FSH in the rat lasts for about 24 hr (afternoon of proestrus until just before noon estrus). The reason for the increase in estrous levels of FSH in the rat is the decline late on proestrus and early on estrus in ovarian venous blood levels of inhibin-like activity (342), coinciding with a decrease in follicular fluid levels of inhibin (343) and in secretion of inhibin by granulosa cells in culture (344). A negative correlation also exists between the decrease in the number of antral follicles (due to ovulation) and rising FSH levels (345). In the hamster, charcoal-treated extracts of ovaries collected on proestrus reduce the serum levels of FSH but not ovaries gathered on other days of the cycle (346). It thus appears that the proestrous follicles produce substantial amounts of inhibin, granulosa cells being the principal source (347).

A strong inverse relationship exists between peripheral serum levels of FSH and inhibin levels in ovarian venous plasma in the rat (342). Inhibin activity was determined by its ability to reduce the 24 hr secretion of FSH in a dispersed rat pituitary cell culture system. On proestrus, in association with the LH surge, ovarian venous inhibin levels decreased, indicating that early luteinization altered the ability of the granulosa cells from mature follicles to produce inhibin (342,348). Thus, the pituitary was released of its FSH feedback regulation by a decrease in inhibin levels, and the subsequent secondary FSH surge ensued (349).

In the hamster, the major targets of FSH on estrus are large preantral follicles (with 8 or more layers of granulosa cells) (52,350) and in the rat, antral follicles 350 to 550 μm in diameter (167,299,331). Histological methods used to assess these changes in follicle development include quantitative analysis of the number and size of follicles on each day of the cycle and quantitative autoradiography of the extent of incorporation of [^{3}H]thymidine into granulosa cells of the various sized follicles. Using autoradiography, these classes of follicles possess FSH and LH receptors in both species (119,123). In rat and hamster, FSH receptors are located on granulosa cells (123,351). LH receptors are located on the theca of large preantral follicles and on the granulosa of antral follicles. Evidently, FSH induces granulosa cell steroidogenesis and increased numbers of LH receptors associated with preovulatory follicular development. In the immature rat (either intact or hypophysectomized), local ovarian effects of exogenous estrogen enhance the responsiveness of the ovary to FSH (352–354). Two types of estrogen receptors have been characterized in rat granulosa cells: one is present only in the cytosol and does not appear to be involved in genomic responses; the other has the K_a and steroid specificity typical of estrogen-binding systems (355). In the intact and hypophysectomized immature hamster, however, estrogens do not increase the number of large preantral follicles (63). Either 1 or 2 mg of estradiol cyclopentylpropionate (ECP) or DES given daily on days 23 to 25 to intact or hypophysectomized immature hamsters and rats led to drastic differences in ovarian follicular development (hamster, reduced; rat, enhanced), whereas increases in uterine weights were similar in both species.

Several lines of evidence indicate that *both* FSH and LH control follicular development in the hamster and rat. The release of FSH on estrus after (or coincidental with) the decline in inhibin secretion stimulates follicular development. In the hamster, injection of ECP, a long-acting estrogen, on estrus prevents the secondary FSH surge at the next cycle; thus, mature follicles fail to develop (356). When FSH secretion on estrus is reduced by injections of bovine follicular fluid, the number of ovulations in hamsters is proportional to the release of FSH during estrus (357). Complete inhibition of estradiol secretion and ovulation in the next cycle occurs only after abolishment of the preceding proestrous and estrous surges of FSH (357), whereas another study reported complete inhibition of the secondary FSH surge and of ovulation with ECP given as a single injection on estrus (356). The differences in the two studies may be due to the degree of suppression of FSH secretion.

A significant correlation exists between the estrous release of FSH and the recruitment of large preantral follicles (stage IV)—the pool from which the ovulatory follicles are selected 4 days later (358). The preovulatory secretion of FSH on proestrus may also be important in recruiting follicles because neutralization of circulating FSH with appropriate antisera decreased the secretion of estradiol and the number of ova shed at the next cycle in the hamster (359). Immature hamsters injected with PMS show maximal in vitro incorporation of [^{3}H]thymidine into the ovaries by 18 hr; intraperitoneal injection of FSH antiserum in the initial 8 hr, but not later, inhibits the response (359). Hence, the continued presence of PMS is not necessary. The same methodology nicely demonstrates the synergistic interaction of estrogens alone or with FSH in the immature rat. Unfortunately, the effects of estrogen were not tested in the hamster model.

As previously mentioned, hamster follicles that will ovulate at the subsequent cycle can be identified on the morning of estrus (day 1) as preantral follicles with 8 to 12 layers of granulosa cells (52). In chronically hypophysectomized hamsters, follicles do not grow beyond stages 2 or 3 (68). In order to stimulate growth of preovulatory follicles, either a single large dose of FSH (200 μg) is required initially or the normal endogenous secondary surge of FSH is required (69,288). This must be followed by LH (69,288) or LH and FSH (288). A normal or exogenous surge of FSH is therefore essential to initiate development of preantral follicles that will ovulate 4 days later.

There are many actions of FSH that ensure proper development of the follicle to the preovulatory stage (Table 5, p. 401). FSH-stimulated secretion of estradiol by rat granulosa cells has a lag period of about 1 day *in vitro* (347) coinciding with antrum formation (in the hamster) and the onset of estradiol secretion (in the hamster and rat) on diestrus 1 or 2 (day 2–3) of the cycle (52,341,360). It has long been known that both FSH and LH are necessary to maintain the secretion of estradiol by growing follicles (361–363). Even though FSH is capable of stimulating estradiol and aromatase, *in vitro* studies with FSH-primed rat granulosa cells have shown that LH also maintains estrogen production (364,365). Supporting *in vivo* evidence of this concept comes from the hamster hypophysectomized on estrus (when FSH levels in sera are elevated) and given constant infusion of LH using Alzet osmotic minipumps (69) or daily injections of hCG (288). Treatment with LH induces the development of normal estrogen-secreting preovulatory follicles 3 days later. The ability of LH alone to maintain follicle development depends on the time of prior FSH priming, i.e., LH pumps inserted immediately and 6 hr (but not 12 hr) after FSH priming induced normal follicular growth (366).

Does this mean that after estrus only LH or hCG is required for normal follicular development? In hypophysectomized hamsters treated with 5 μg ovine FSH on day 1 and 20 μg LH in polyvinylpyrrolodinone from days 1 to 4, serum levels of FSH are undetectable beyond day 2, but on day 4 the number of occupied FSH receptors in large antral follicles is two thirds the value in follicles from intact hamsters (70). This is consistent with the observation that the hamster anterior pituitary on estrus (when the second serum peak of FSH is in progress) contains >80% of FSH which migrates after electrofocusing at P.I. values of 4.5 or less (367). The high glycoprotein content of FSH on estrus, therefore, may affect its plasma half-life and postreceptor biologic activity. In the intact hamster, a potent FSH antiserum blocks ovulation when injected on every day of the cycle except for the morning of proestrus (368). Hence, the antral follicle is dependent for FSH throughout most of its existence. The point is that both FSH and LH are needed for normal follicular maturation, but their ratios and importance may vary at different stages of the cycle. This is most impressively demonstrated in studies involving perfusion of rat ovaries for 4 days with changing FSH:LH ratios comparable to the *in vivo* profiles found during the normal 4-day estrous cycle (375). Follicular growth culminates 4 days later in ovulation of an average of 4.3 oocytes/ovary.

Diestrus

During early diestrus, serum levels of progesterone are elevated in the hamster and rat (341,360,376), coinciding with luteal secretion of progesterone (377–380). Follicles continue to grow during diestrus in the rat, and LH levels begin to increase (381,382). Measurement of the steroid content of the largest follicles excised from 4-day cyclic rats showed that follicular estrogen first increased significantly on diestrus (e.g., at 1100 hr to 78 pg/follicle); in contrast, measurable levels of progestogens were first detected at 1100 hr of proestrus—about 1 ng/follicle (383). In granulosa cells from small- to medium-sized rat follicles, 1 μg FSH/ml, but not LH (10–100 μg/ml), stimulated cAMP formation, whereas both gonadotropins enhanced cAMP synthesis by granulosa cells from preovulatory follicles (384). These results are similar to experiments on isolated granulosa cells from porcine follicles of different sizes. The elevated LH may cause the enhancement of follicular development in the rat. On diestrus 1, circulating levels of LH are higher than on other days of the cycle except for the afternoon of proestrus. The elevation in peripheral LH is due to an increase in LH pulse amplitude and a shortening of the LH pulse interval (381). This confirms previous reports that LH levels are elevated on diestrus 1 in the rat (382,385–387) but, importantly, establishes that LH levels are then pulsatile. Although it is not definitely known why LH levels increase on diestrus 1, it has been hypothesized that the low serum levels of progesterone and estradiol are causal factors (381,388). Injection of an LHRH antagonist on diestrus 1 reduces mean LH by changing amplitude but not frequency and leads within 8 hr to an increased percentage of early atretic follicles from 351 to 450 μm in diameter (389). In rats, pentobarbital administered on diestrus 1 delays vaginal cornification and uterine ballooning, presumably by decreasing circulating LH levels and therefore estradiol secretion (390,391); hCG given concurrently with pentobarbital restores vaginal cornification and uterine ballooning to normal levels. It has also been shown that injection of LH antisera on various days of the cycle in the hamster and rat prolongs the cycle by 1 to 2 days (285,392,393), indicating that during this phase of the cycle LH is crucial in follicular development.

Additional evidence for the necessity of LH in follicle

development in the hamster and rat comes from studies using subcutaneous injection of progesterone on various days of the cycle. Injection of progesterone (2.5–5 mg on day 1 of the cycle) delays ovulation 1 to 5 days in the hamster (394,395). If the day of progesterone administration is shifted to day 3 of the hamster cycle, then 25 to 50 μg progesterone consistently reduces serum LH and delays ovulation by a day (396); in contrast, 250 μg progesterone on diestrus 2 of the rat postpones ovulation (397). In the hamster, progesterone injected on day 3 reduces serum levels of LH and estradiol, and thecal androstenedione production by antral follicles *in vitro*; follicular aromatizing ability is unaffected (398). Exogenous LH (combined with progesterone) restored estradiol secretion on day 3 by the antral follicles. Thus, exogenous progesterone induces a decline in LH, causing reduced thecal secretion of androstenedione by antral follicles; in turn, this reduces the amount of precursor available for aromatization to estradiol. Ovulation is delayed a day presumably because of the lack of the positive feedback action of estradiol at the hypothalamic–pituitary axis, thus postponing the surge of gonadotropins until estradiol levels return to normal. It is also possible that at this phase of the cycle progesterone has a direct inhibitory action on the secretion of GnRH. Paradoxically, in the adult rat the LH pulse height and the mean serum LH are lower on diestrus 2 (day 3) than on day 2, when progesterone levels in the sera are basal (382). Thus, the decline in progesterone associated with luteal regression is accompanied by a decline in LH levels even though follicular development and estradiol secretion are increasing. Within 1 hr of a single subcutaneous injection of 800 μg progesterone at 0900 hr on rat diestrus 2, a precipitous decline in serum estradiol occurs in association with a fall in LH lasting for 48 hr and a temporary decline in FSH; but serum testosterone does not change (399). Follicular LH (hCG) receptors increase during the early antral phase of development (9), and the sensitivity of the follicle to LH may therefore increase dramatically. In hamsters and rats with 4 day cycles, functional luteolysis on day 3 is not associated with any increase in ovarian venous blood flow (400,401), although this may not necessarily reflect the picture at the level of thecal blood supply.

Hourly LH pulses *in vitro* plus tonic FSH or tonic LH alone induce follicular growth within 3 hr in ovaries of diestrous (1) adult rats (402). It was estimated that in the larger size classes of follicles, tonic LH increased the number of cells by 5×10^4, attesting to the rapidity of response of the rodent ovary. During early diestrus small antral follicles arising from the large preantral follicles present the day before have differentiated in the hamster (53,403). In the rat, the range in size of small antral follicles observed on estrus (352–517 μm in diameter) decreases on diestrus to 448 to 517 μm; thereafter, the follicles grow about 50 to 60 μm per day until proestrus (299). Immature 26-day-old rats primed with 10 IU PMS and killed at intervals corresponding to mid-diestrus and later show a striking *in vitro* increase in testosterone accumulation by granulosa cells at late diestrus, with levels then reverting to low values (404). Follicles at late diestrus were at small- and medium-sized stages. A caveat to this study and others is that priming with PMS may alter the steroidogenic pathways and may not represent the status of adult cyclic animals.

It is postulated for the cyclic rat that the largest follicles on day 1 (estrus) may become atretic the next day and that the follicles destined to ovulate 4 days later are derived from a smaller group of follicles present on day 1 (270). This hypothesis is based on the observation that the number of granulosa cells (in the largest cross section) of the largest healthy follicles on day 2 have 1,200 cells rather than the expected 1,700 cells. Proliferation rates of granulosa cells determined on day 1 indicate that the follicles with 1,200 cells on day 2 would have been derived from follicles with 750 cells in the largest cross section. The largest healthy follicles on day 1 may therefore not necessarily give rise to the follicles ovulating 3 to 4 days later.

On days 3 and 4 of the cycle, follicles in both species continue to grow presumably (and primarily) under the influence of LH. During this period of time, subtle LH pulses continue (381,382). In progesterone-delayed ovulation of immature rats, slight but sustained increases in circulating LH occur after removal of the progesterone implants (405). The small increases in LH are presumably required for continued follicular maturation, production of estradiol, and increased LH binding to the follicle. The synchrony in the timing of ovulation following removal of the progesterone implants was similar to the effects of the normal decline in serum progesterone associated with luteal regression. Studies by Schwartz (379) and Greenwald (403) suggested that the decline in luteal production of progesterone regulated the time of onset of the next ovulation. For example 5-day cyclic rats exhibit an extra day of luteal progesterone secretion (406–408). Conversely, injection of rats with bromocryptine (BRC), which decreases PRL secretion, shortens the estrous cycle from 5 to 4 days by prematurely withdrawing luteal support (409,410).

Interestingly, no significant differences in the number or size of the larger (preovulatory) follicles on diestrus 2 are observed between BRC-treated (4-day cycle) and 5-day cyclic rats (409). The failure of BRC to affect follicular diameter was later reconfirmed, although follicular size was significantly larger in 4-day than in 5-day cyclic rats irrespective of whether they had received BRC (410). Shortening of the cycle to 4 days with BRC did not alter the ovulation rate (approximately 10 ova/rat), as assessed by the number of fresh corpora lutea at the end of the next cycle. Follicular estradiol accumulation *in vitro* (4-hr incubation) by large antral follicles taken on diestrus 2 is greater from rats treated with BRC than control animals (9.0 ± 0.8 and 7.0 ± 0.4 pmol/follicle/4 hr, respectively) (409), indicating that prolactin and/or progesterone may suppress follicular production of estradiol.

The change after luteolysis has been termed the "luteal-follicular" shift because of the coincident demise of the corpus luteum and the rise of follicular dominance (403). In 4-day cyclic rats, follicular progesterone, testosterone, and estrogen significantly increase at diestrus when serum progesterone declines (343). Steroid levels in the serum, corpora lutea, and nonluteal portion of the ovary of the cyclic hamster during this period reveal an inverse relationship between progesterone and estradiol (378) and the ratio of FSH to LH changes in favor of LH, which agrees with the hypothesis that LH is a major factor regulating follicular secretion of estrogen (405).

It has been proposed that during the luteal phase of the cycle, progesterone might be inhibitory by either a direct or indirect action on the follicle since secretion of estrogen is impaired. However, for intact animals there is no evidence supporting a direct inhibitory action of progesterone on the ovary; in fact, progesterone stimulates ovarian responsiveness of hCG in the immature rat (411). A long-term inhibitory effect of progesterone on production of estradiol by proestrous rat follicles has been demonstrated but the amounts of progesterone required are probably pharmacological (412).

Evidence for an inhibitory action of prolactin on follicular estradiol synthesis is derived from a model using PRL-treated cyclic rats (413). Injection of 100 μg PRL at 1500 hr diestrus 1 and 0900 and 1700 hr of diestrus 2 reduces follicular estradiol production from control values. Of seven animals injected with PRL, three exhibited activated corpora lutea, as evidenced by elevated serum levels of progesterone; this group also had lower serum levels of LH and estradiol. (This mechanism of inhibition of follicular estradiol has been attributed earlier to progesterone's ability to suppress LH secretion.) In the other PRL-treated animals, serum progesterone, LH, and estradiol levels were the same as in saline-injected rats; however, follicular estradiol production was suppressed *in vitro*.

The mechanism by which PRL inhibits follicular estradiol production may involve effects on the aromatase or hydroxyl-lyase enzyme systems. Since prolactin receptors are present on the granulosa cells of Graafian follicles (334) and on theca-interstitial cells (336), both of these sites may be potential targets for PRL-induced suppression of estradiol secretion.

Prolactin also has been shown to inhibit estradiol synthesis *in vitro*. Granulosa cells taken from DES–FSH-treated immature hypophysectomized rats were cultured for 2 to 4 days in the presence of 10^{-7} M androstenedione and 100 ng/ml of either FSH or LH (365). Addition of increasing quantities of PRL to the culture media suppressed, in a dose-dependent manner, the secretion of estradiol but not of progesterone. These results indicate that PRL may have a specific inhibitory effect on granulosal cell aromatase. However, long-term culture of ovarian (theca-interstitial) cells from hypophysectomized immature rats reveals that PRL inhibits LH-induced androgen synthesis (414). Progesterone was not produced in large quantities even when androgen secretion was maximal.

FOLLICULAR DEVELOPMENT DURING THE ESTROUS CYCLES OF SHEEP, COW, AND SOW

These species are singled out for consideration because of the considerable research attention they have received and their different mode(s) of coping with the problem of follicular selection as compared with species with short cycles. Strain differences exist, especially in sheep, but for the sake of convenience the generic designations will be used when feasible. The length of the estrous cycle is usually about 17 days in the sheep and 21 days in both the cow and the sow. The first day of estrus is designated as day 0 of the cycle.

Before considering follicular kinetics in the ewe, it is worthwhile considering peripheral levels of gonadotropins and steroids throughout the estrous cycle. Following the proestrous surge of FSH, a second elevation of FSH occurs 1 to 2 days later (249,415) although this has not been observed consistently in all studies even with blood samples taken at frequent intervals (416,417). Occasional sporadic peaks of FSH are detectable during the luteal phase but with no definite rhythms recurring at intervals of several days. Pulses of FSH occur about every 2 hr during the luteal and follicular phases of the cycle (249). In contrast, episodic pulses of LH recur about every 2.5 hr during the luteal phase, accelerating to about one per hour during the follicular phase. Peripheral serum levels of estradiol are at peak levels (10–25 pg/ml) on days 4 to 6 of the cycle (417,418), with a second increase apparent at the onset of luteolysis. The first peak occurs when circulating levels of both FSH and LH are high. Pulsatile release of estradiol is linked to LH, and the relationship is especially apparent when estradiol is measured in ovarian venous blood (for literature, see ref. 249). The secretion of androstenedione and testosterone are correlated with that of estradiol. The corpus luteum has a life span of 14 to 15 days, and at its peak progesterone secretion in the midluteal phase, serum LH and FSH are at their nadir. During the luteal phase, the peripheral concentration and secretion rate of progesterone are not influenced by the pulsatile release of LH (419). With the demise of the corpus luteum, a progressive 5-fold increase in serum LH is elicited; there seems little doubt that negative-feedback action of progesterone is the major regulatory steroid affecting LH secretion (418) and hence the selection of the ovulable follicle(s). In ovariectomized ewes, Silastic implants of estradiol plus progesterone, which duplicate the hormone profiles of intact animals, restore tonic LH levels to normal values but do not depress the postcastrational hypersecretion of FSH (416). Inhibin is the most likely choice for the putative hormone.

In cyclic Texel ewes, an antral cavity begins to form in follicles about 0.5 mm in diameter, and a pair of ovaries contains on average about 32% healthy tertiary follicles (420). Of the normal tertiary follicles, 83% are <2 mm in diameter, and for follicles >2 mm, there is an average of 3.6 normal and 8.7 atretic. Based on follicular volumes, two "waves" of follicular development are discernible. The first, from day 1 to 12, culminates in a large tertiary follicle on days 7 to 9 that ultimately becomes atretic. The second wave, from day 12 to 0, usually recruits two large follicles; these grow rapidly in size on day 15 following luteolysis on day 14. Although Brand and deJong referred to waves of follicular development, they were well aware of the constant presence of small follicles (up to 2 mm in diameter) throughout the cycle, and they emphasized "that during the oestrous cycle the tertiary follicle population is constant and that an equilibrium exists between the production of follicles in a certain size class and their disappearance from that class, either by passing to a higher size class or by atresia." The fate of the two largest follicles (F_1 and F_2) on day 10 or 14 has been monitored by marking them with india ink and then intravenously injecting gonadotropins within 1 hr (421). In uninjected ewes, the follicles marked on day 10 never ovulated, whereas on day 14, the F_1 as well as some unmarked follicles ovulated but none of the F_2 group did. In the absence of the corpus luteum, cauterization of the largest follicle on day 0, 3.5, or 7 is followed by a surge of FSH and ovulation occurs approximately 4 days later (see ref. 420). After luteolysis induced by a prostaglandin analog (cloprostenol), follicles 2 to 4 mm or >4 mm in diameter have the ability to trigger an LH surge within the normal time span: 55 to 60 hr (422). If, however, the largest follicles are 2 mm (after cauterization of the larger ones), the LH surge is delayed by 24 hr. Thus, considerable flexibility exists in the size range of follicles in the final selection process. The corpus luteum exerts a local effect on follicular development in the ewe; during the luteal phase there are more follicles ≥4 mm on the ovary bearing the corpus luteum than on the contralateral ovary (423). A very thorough paper (424) documents changes in follicular dynamics in Merino ewes by estimating the doubling time of granulosa cells utilizing mitotic index and an estimate of 0.43 hr for mitotic time (obtained by using colchicine). The growth rate of follicles up to 0.7 mm was slow (estimated times in classes 1 to 6, 37 days) and accelerated in larger stages: approximately 8 days to reach 5 mm. An important point is that a follicle ovulating at the end of any cycle would have been about 0.5 mm in diameter on day 6 or 7 of the cycle. Early atresia was rare in follicles <1 mm in diameter. Following subcutaneous injection of PMS, there were twice as many follicles (>0.5 mm) 48 hr later as in untreated ewes, with the greatest increase in follicles >2.5 mm. This was associated with significantly higher mitotic indices and a concomitant reduction in atresia in the larger classes of follicles.

A similar study compared follicular kinetics for two strains of ewes with different ovulation rates: Romanov and Ile-De-France (average ovulations 3.0 and 1.6, respectively) (425). Only follicles with three or more layers of granulosa cells were counted, and antrum formation began at a follicular diameter of about 0.2 mm in both strains. There was no difference between breeds in follicular growth rates, although there are 1.5 to 2.0 times as many follicles (>0.09 mm) in the Romanov than in Ile-De-France ewes (261). After pooling the data from the two breeds, it was estimated that the mean time for a follicle to pass from three layers of granulosa cells (~200 cells) to the start of antrum formation (5,000 cells) was 130 days and to the preovulatory stage another 45 days, for a total of about 6 months.

Another study (426) compared follicular growth in a high ovulating breed, D'Man (mean ovulation rate, 2.9), and a low ovulating breed, Timahite (rate, 1.1). The major differences between the two are that the D'Man ewes have a greater number of follicles >1,285 μm (large follicles with an antrum) and a lower rate of atresia (54.9% vs. 66.7%) for follicles 1,084 to 2,141 μm in diameter. In addition, there are significantly more follicles 118 to 462 μm (follicles beginning to develop an antrum)—a critical phase in follicular growth—in the D'Man ewe.

A breed that has attracted considerable and justifiable attention is the Booroola ewe: Some animals ovulate as many as 10 or 11 eggs. There is a genetic basis for this high spontaneous ovulation rate (for literature, see ref. 427). One possible factor accounting for the prolificacy of the breed is that on day 3 of the cycle, pituitary content of FSH is approximately twice that in control ewes; however, electrofocusing reveals no qualitative difference in FSH (428). There are obvious problems in extrapolating pituitary content to peripheral levels of FSH. However, the inhibin content of ovaries of Booroola ewes collected at the midluteal phase is only a third the value of control animals (427), which is consistent with the possibility of higher circulating levels of FSH. The latter, however, is still to be demonstrated. Alternatively, the increased ovulation rate may be attributable to increased sensitivity to normal levels of gonadotropins. This possibility has been explored by comparing Booroola × Romney ewes ovulating 3.3 ova (F+) to animals ovulating 1.1 (+ +) (429). The animals were injected with cloprostenol on day 10, blood samples collected 0 to 48 hr later, and all follicles ≥2 mm in diameter were dissected. The main finding was that in F+ ewes, follicles mature at a smaller diameter (3.5 vs. 5 mm), as evidenced by their ability to synthesize estradiol. The fact that there is no difference in androstenedione output in response to LH between the two strains points to differences in aromatase activity by the granulosa cells as the controlling factor. Two interesting correlations were evident: Nonatretic follicles from F+ ewes had about one third as many granulosa cells as the + + ewes, and corpora lutea of the F+ ewes weighed 0.39 times as much as those of + + ewes. From this observation, the logical conclusion is reached that a granulosa mass from 3F+ follicles equals the estrogen production rate of one follicle from the + + group. In comparing highly fecund F+ and Booroola ewes to control flocks with ovulation rates of ~1.4, the Booroolas ovulate significantly earlier (7.5 hr) but usually with no differences in peak LH concentrations or the interval between the onset of estrus and LH discharge (430). This again points to differences in follicular responsiveness established in the late luteal phase as the principal factor leading to increased ovulation rate in the Booroola.

On day 13 of the cycle, the corpus luteum is still functional in Welsh mountain sheep, and the concentration of progesterone in ovarian venous plasma is about a 1,000-fold higher than peripheral levels (431). Even at this stage, however, the largest nonatretic follicle secretes appreciable quantities of estrogen: from 145 to 390 pg/ml in ovarian venous plasma. This trend is accentuated on day 15, when, in most instances, the corpus luteum is regressing.

From days 2 to 5, the largest follicle secreting estrogen has the enzyme 3β-HSD restricted to the theca interna; after a hiatus on days 8 to 11, beginning on day 13 to 0, a presumably new set of follicles show enzymatic activity limited to the theca (100). Within 24 to 48 hr after injection of PMS on day 13, the number of 5-mm follicles increases, and concomitantly strong 3β-HSD activity is demonstrable in the theca—but not in the granulosa—of all these follicles.

A subsequent investigation revealed that *in vivo* exposure to PMS for only 5 min enables about 25% of follicles >2 mm in diameter to secrete estrogen *in vitro* (432). Lengthening the time of exposure to PMS to 12 hr fails to increase the proportion of estrogen-secreting follicles, consistent with the finding that for any follicular class, about a third of the follicles are nonatretic (e.g., ref. 420). Thus, for the ewe the concept of estrogen "activated" versus "nonactivated" follicles is extremely important, as only one or two of the largest follicles fall into the former category. The notable exception is between days 2 and 4 of the cycle, for example, many explanted follicles are steroidogenically active (432) at a time approximating the second surge of FSH. Secretion rates of androstenedione and estradiol are increased (but not significantly) on day 3 of the cycle (433). The concentration of FSH in follicular fluid is about threefold higher in follicles in which the estradiol:androstenedione ratio is >1, and the FSH values are comparable to peripheral levels (433). In experiments involving ewes with ovary and adnexa autotransplanted to the neck, the secretion rate between days 12 and 15 of estradiol, but not progesterone, increased within 5 min of each LH pulse; everything points to a causal relationship between the two events (419). Addition of 0.25 to 10.0 μg LH to explanted follicles of PMS-treated ewes results in drastic curtailment of estrogen production 48 hr later, whereas progesterone production increases dramatically by 24 hr (434). However, within 4 hr of the addition of LH, a transitory increase in estrogen accumulation occurs, and this is followed by inhibition. It must be kept in mind that the amounts of LH added *in vitro* were comparable to estrous surge levels and not to the pulsatile pattern encountered on days 12 to 14.

An interesting approach combined topical autoradiography of [^{125}I]hCG binding sites with determinations of follicular fluid concentrations of steroids (435). During the luteal phase of the ewe, all follicles >2 mm were dissected, antral fluid aspirated, and the follicle prepared for autoradiography. Follicles fell into three categories of hCG binding: to theca and granulosa (type I); LH receptors restricted to theca (type II); and no LH receptors in either cell type (type III). During the luteal phase, the type I follicles contained the highest values of progesterone in follicular fluid (ca. 120 ng/ml), which were 10-fold higher than the concentrations of testosterone and estradiol. During the follicular phase, these follicles had the highest concentration of estradiol (120 ng/ml), and the type II follicles contained high levels of testosterone (55 ng/ml) and very low levels of estradiol (2.5 ng/ml). LH was detectable (>2.5 ng/ml) in 86% of follicles examined, there being no significant differences between small (<5 mm) and large follicles (>5 mm), except during behavioral estrus (433).

As is already evident, the follicles destined to ovulate in the ewe do not differentiate until about the time of luteolysis (436). This has been demonstrated during the normal estrous cycle (e.g., see ref. 431) and following induced luteolysis and other experimental manipulations. Utilizing ovarian or utero-ovarian autotransplants, with luteolysis induced on day 10, there is an abrupt two- to threefold increase in the episodic rate of release of LH, with no change in pulse amplitude; concomitantly, the pulse rate of plasma FSH was unchanged, with the pulse amplitude reduced by 60% (249). The episodic release of LH was mirrored within a few minutes by a rise in estradiol and androgens. As luteolysis progressed, plasma FSH dropped because of the reduced amplitude of the pulses. A surge of FSH accompanied the LH peak, followed by a second FSH peak about 22 hr later. Very similar results are obtained in ewes with ovaries *in situ* and with prostaglandin-induced luteolysis (with or without PMS) on days 9 and 10 (437). The ewes were ovariectomized from 0 to 48 hr after the onset of luteolysis and all follicles ≥1.0 mm in diameter dissected; the follicles were classified as healthy or atretic based on whether they contained ≥50% or ≤50% of the maximal number of granulosa cells for a given follicular diameter. It was not until 10 hr after the induction of luteolysis that a large estrogen-activated follicle (≥5 mm in diameter) was consistently present. Analysis of the percentage of healthy follicles by diameters suggests that the dominant follicle is capable of doubling the number of granulosa cells in 6 to 10 hr. As the dominant follicles rise to prominence, there is a steady fall in the number of healthy follicles (≥1 mm) from 50% at time 0 to less than 20% by 24 hr; this decline is possibly related to the decrease in FSH levels. Injection of PMS temporarily delays at 10 hr the fall in follicular numbers, apparently by recruiting smaller stages; by 24 hr, however, the percentage of healthy follicles reverts to control levels. Another approach to identifying the ovulatory follicle is to synchronize estrus by using progesterone implants; removal of the implants sets in motion the same set of changes already described following spontaneous or induced regression of the corpus luteum (438). As the preovulatory period progressed, the dominant follicles were larger and had greater concentrations of estradiol in follicular fluid and increased numbers of LH/hCG receptors in theca and granulosa cells than did nonovulatory follicles. Suffolk sheep have an ovulation rate of 1.3, whereas Finnish Landrace ovulate 2.7 ova. Correlated with these rates, Suffolk ewes have 1.2 follicles with hCG binding to both theca and granulosa cells compared with 2.9 follicles in Finnish Landrace (438).

It is apparent from these studies that the differentiation of the dominant follicles is associated with increased LH levels but with FSH unaffected or, if anything, reduced. In support of this contention, intravenous administration of LHRH antiserum in the preovulatory period promptly eliminates the pulsatile release of LH without affecting basal levels; the pulsatile release of estradiol is abolished with no change in secretion rate of testosterone or plasma levels of FSH (439). Anestrous ewes have 35 follicles ≥1 mm diameter, whereas there are 24 follicles on days 9 to 10 of the estrous cycle (440). The anestrous pattern is associated with elevated levels of FSH and progesterone and, conversely, a reduction in the number of high-amplitude LH peaks (2.4/9 hr vs. 5.3/9 hr on day 10 of the cycle). Continuous infusion of low doses of GNRH in anestrous ewes resulted in 23 of 24 ovulating, with estrus detected 37 hr, on average, after the start of infusion (441). LH concentration in sera significantly increased; FSH values were not reported. The corpora lutea induced by GNRH were functional for at least 9 days. Intravenous pulse administration of LH (10 μg every 1 or 2 hr for 29–91 days) to anestrous ewes simulates pulse rates comparable to those in the luteal and follicular phases (440). This regimen is sufficient to induce normal cyclic progestational activity for at most two cycles; the period of subsequent acyclicity is associated with reduced FSH concentrations. Injection of anestrous ewes with bovine follicular fluid lowered plasma FSH concentrations by 70% and reduced the number of healthy follicles ≥2 mm in diameter. Hourly intravenous injections of 50 μg FSH plus follicular fluid reversed the effects and significantly increased the number of large nonatretic follicles (≥3 mm) (442).

Collectively, these results suggest that following the onset of luteolysis, pulsatile release of LH is the controlling factor in the emergence of the dominant follicles, with FSH playing a strictly subordinate role. This does not rule out a possible primary role of FSH at earlier critical stages of follicular maturation. Indeed, injection of 500 IU PMS along with prostaglandins increases the ovulation rate in Romney ewes (437). Moreover, infusion of FSH from 24 hr before until 60 hr after induced luteolysis in the ewe results in a mean ovulation rate of 8, as compared with a rate of 3 for animals in which infusion was started concurrently with the induction of luteolysis (Baird and Webb, *personal communication,* cited in ref. 436). Similarly, after prostaglandin-induced luteal regression, intravenous injection of bovine follicular fluid significantly decreases FSH levels without affecting the number of ovulations (443). Infusion of ovine FSH for 48 hr plus injection of follicular fluid resulted in an ovulation rate of 14.6 ova.

FOLLICULAR DEVELOPMENT IN THE COW

Following the estrous surge there is a very definite second peak of circulating FSH, lasting for 2 to 3 days (212,444). FSH levels have been reported to peak on days 4, 8, 12 or 13, 17, and 18, but these results are based on relative percentage changes (444). Schams et al. believe these peaks are temporally related to periods of enhanced follicular growth, but this is pure conjecture. During the early luteal phase (day 4), 8.5 pulses of FSH are recorded per 12 hr compared with 6.3 on day 11; pulse amplitude is also unchanged: 18.5 vs. 16.6 ng/ml (445). Separate FSH pulses (with minimal LH increases) are encountered about 41% of the time in the midluteal phase; these are concomitant with or soon followed by pulses of progesterone (445). With the onset of luteolysis, no change in plasma FSH is observed for as long as 12 hr (446,447), but the levels fall significantly by 24 to 36 hr (446). The second postestrous peak in FSH on day 4 is not associated with an increase in LH. On day 4, there are 8 LH peaks per 12 hr, the number falling to 3.6 on day 11 when progesterone levels are maximal (445). Ninety-six percent of all LH/FSH pulses are followed within 60 min by a peak in estradiol (445). With the onset of induced luteolysis, a significant increase of mean plasma LH occurs within 1 to 3 hr; this is related to a 4-fold increase in pulse frequency and amplitude (445,447). During the luteal phase, plasma estradiol rises to a peak of 6 pg/ml on day 6 (448), and there are 7 pulses of estradiol per 12 hr; by the midluteal phase, this value has fallen by half, in conjunction with the change in LH pulse frequency (445). Following induced luteolysis, the pulse frequency for estradiol increases within 4 to 6 hr but without changes in pulse amplitude (446). In healthy preantral follicles, the principal thecal androgen produced in vitro is androstenedione, with about a fifth as much testosterone present (149). During the early follicular phase, the average width of the theca interna is considerably thinner than in the preovulatory follicle (72.8 vs. 237 μm) (449). Before the LH surge, 3β-hydroxysteroid dehydrogenase is presumably deficient in cow granulosa cells, as is the case in sheep and numerous other species. A slow increase in peripheral estradiol levels begins before progesterone falls (448).

Progesterone levels in the cyclic cow begin to increase from about day 4, reach a plateau around day 10, and decline to basal levels by day 17 or 18 (444). Luteal phase levels of progesterone average about 4 ng/ml (445,447), with pulse amplitude and mean concentrations peaking at about day 11. Progesterone drops very rapidly after induced luteolysis, falling 67% by 20 min (446). An inverse relationship exists between progesterone and LH levels in the cow (450), as in the ewe. Insertion of vaginal coils loaded with progesterone into cattle during the luteal or follicular phases usually lowers serum LH, but FSH is unaffected. On removal of the coils and injection of $PGF_{2\alpha}$, serum LH increases but not FSH. Hence, a case can be made for FSH being controlled by a separate releasing hormone or, more likely, by the secretion of inhibin (450).

How do these cyclic changes in hormone levels relate to follicular development in the cow? When the largest follicle was marked between days 9 and 17, none ovulated; the likelihood of the largest follicle ovulating increased abruptly at day 18 and in 5 of 6 animals, the largest or next-to-largest follicle was selected by day 18 (451). When the largest follicle (F_1) and second largest follicle (F_2) are marked on different days of the cycle and examined 5 days later, the follicles are still present on days 8 and 13 but have regressed considerably by day 18 (452). Thus, between days 13 and 18, there is an increase in the rate of replacement and turnover of large follicles. This is further accentuated by day 18 in that the F_1 follicle only ovulated when ovulation occurred within 3 days. The greatest number of small follicles (1–3 mm) is observed on day 3, presumably in response to the second FSH surge (452). Medium-sized follicles (3–6 mm) are most numerous on day 13. In contrast, the number of large follicles (>6 mm) does not vary throughout the cycle. When all follicles >5 mm in diameter are destroyed on day 13, it takes 5 days for F_1 and F_2 follicles to emerge from the medium-sized group. Similarly, if the ovary bearing the F_1 follicle is removed between days 4 and 12, the remaining ovary compensates within 4 days, but if the ovary contralateral to the F_1 follicle is removed, follicular development is unchanged (453). The dominant follicle may therefore inhibit smaller follicles by an intraovarian mechanism. When all grossly visible follicles are eliminated from both ovaries on day 10 by electrocautery and x-irradiation of the ovaries, luteal life span is significantly extended (454). This indicates that the normal presence of follicles during mid- to late diestrus is essential for luteolysis in the cow. The above results are consistent with earlier histological studies, which showed that 23.7% normal and 76.3% atretic follicles were present per pair of ovaries during the cycle (455). Follicles undergoing early atresia (defined in ref. 455) constituted 20.3% of the atretic population. Normal follicles >5 mm were not found during the luteal phase, whereas follicles 8 to 18 mm developed during the follicular phase. Using the mitotic time of sheep granulosa cells, the time required for bovine follicles to pass from one class to another has been analyzed (456). The time required for Graafian follicles to grow from 0.4 to 10 mm is about 22 days, the approximate length of the estrous cycle. It is therefore tempting to speculate that the postestrous FSH surge stimulates the follicles that will ultimately ovulate 20 to 22 days later. Histological signs of atresia were first observed in follicles at least 1.7 mm in diameter (456). The maximum growth rate of granulosa cells in cow follicles is reached in larger follicles (1.5 mm diameter) than in the sheep (0.10 mm), suggesting that bovine Graafian follicles need to persist longer and grow to a greater size before they can respond to an ovulatory amount of LH. There is an excellent correlation between macroscopic and histological criteria for follicular normality (93.3%) and atresia (95.5%) in bovine follicles ranging from 2 to 22 mm in diameter (457). As to be expected, for follicles from 2 to 5 mm in diameter, there is a progressive decline in follicular fluid estradiol as atresia proceeds from early to advanced stages (457).

The number of large follicles (≥8 mm) increases from day 6 (1.3) to day 12 (1.8) and day 18 (2.1), and healthy follicles with FSH binding to granulosa cells and hCG binding to granulosa and thecal cells are already present at day 6 (458). Thus, even at day 6, follicles that could be thought of as preovulatory have differentiated, since removal of the corpus luteum or treatment with prostaglandins results in ovulation 2 or 3 days later. However, the ultimate normal fate of these follicles is atresia. On day 18, two large follicles are invariably present, one with considerably more estradiol than the other, the latter evidently destined to degenerate (458).

Ovaries collected from cows (with no information available about their reproductive history) had follicular fluid aspirated from all surface follicles, and the follicles were classified into three size ranges based on antral fluid volume (459). As follicle size increased, FSH concentration in follicular fluid was unchanged, LH decreased significantly by 27%, and prolactin increased 2-fold. These changes were associated with a shift in the estradiol:androgen ratio, such that 83% of the large follicles were predominantly estrogenic, as compared with only 7% of the small follicles. From days 3 to 7 of the cycle, the number of estrogen-active follicles (based on steroid determinations from follicular fluid) decreased from 2 to 1 per heifer, with a gradual increase to day 7 in follicular diameter (14 mm) and number of granulosa cells (12×10^6) (212). Through day 7, an average of one large estrogen-inactive follicle was present per heifer, which was usually judged to be atretic on histological grounds. On day 9, all follicles were estrogen inactive; by day 13, however, small active follicles (10 mm) reappeared. The estrogen-active follicle is distinguishable by specific hCG binding to both theca and granulosa cells and FSH binding to granulosa cells. This was especially evident on day 17, when receptor levels were about twice as high in both compartments compared with the inactive follicle (212).

The proestrous follicle (24 hr after progesterone declined to <1 ng/ml) averages 16 mm in diameter, with follicular fluid LH and FSH concentrations of 1.48 and 0.42 ng/ml, respectively. Estrogen concentration in the follicle (estradiol plus estrone, with the latter about 20-fold less) was 39 times the combined concentration of testosterone and androstenedione (460). This correlates with increased serum levels of LH but unchanged FSH levels (447). The estrogen-activated follicle has significantly greater FSH binding to granulosa cells and hCG binding to granulosa and thecal cells than the large estrogen-inactive follicles, which are usually atretic by histological criteria. Large atretic follicles (>1 cm) have estradiol concentrations 150-fold lower than normal preovulatory follicles (460). Thus, in the cow, as in the ewe, regression of the corpus luteum leads to the final selection of the ovulatory follicle, principally as a result of increased LH activity, after FSH and LH priming actions.

Ovaries were removed from cows 2 hr after behavioral estrus and the nine largest follicles from each pair were dissected. The dominant follicle was 15 mm in diameter; others were as small as 2 to 3 mm (461). Estradiol secretion by the largest follicle in vitro was at a rate of 2 to 3 orders of magnitude greater than the smaller follicles, but small follicles ipsilateral to the dominant follicle secreted 3 times as much estradiol as the population on the contralateral ovary. Injection of porcine FSH for 4 days beginning on day 9 of the bovine cycle results in superovulation of 11 eggs per animal after induced luteolysis (462). Twelve hours after the onset of estrus, estrogen concentrations in follicular fluid were similar to those observed in normal preovulatory follicles except for much lower amounts of estradiol.

FOLLICULAR DEVELOPMENT DURING THE PORCINE ESTROUS CYCLE

Serum FSH shows a minor rise, concomitant with the proestrous LH surge, and a second rise in FSH about 27 hr later, paralleling an increase in progesterone (463). Mean values of FSH are maximal on day 3, when estradiol is minimal. Contrary to the ewe and cow, the gilt shows greater pulsatile activity for FSH and LH during the luteal than the follicular phase of the cycle. On day 12 of the cycle, pulsatile release of LH was usually followed within about an hour by pulses of estradiol. Two separate surges of prolactin are observed during the cycle, one during the proestrous increase of estradiol and one during estrus. Maximal values of serum progesterone are reached between days 9 and 14 of the cycle, before drastically falling on day 15 (463,464). The hormonal pattern in the pig has not been studied as closely as other domestic species, but the available evidence indicates that the demise of luteal function does not increase basal or pulsatile levels of LH (463). Plasma concentrations of estrone and estradiol do not begin to increase during proestrus until plasma progesterone falls between days 15 and 18, and other than the proestrous surge, levels range from 8 to 12 pg/ml throughout the rest of the cycle (464).

The selection of follicles for ovulation occurs before day 17, as evidenced by the lack of compensatory ovulation when unilateral ovariectomy is performed on day 15 or 17 (465). On day 3 of the cycle no follicles >4 mm are present in the ovaries, but by day 9 follicles between 4 and 8 mm begin to repopulate the ovary (466). On day 13, the largest follicles range from 3 to 6 mm, with an average diameter of 4 mm (467). By day 16, average diameter is 4.8 mm, and only one of six gilts possessed large follicles (6–9 mm). Injection of 1,000 IU hCG on day 12 results in the presence on day 16 of both medium and large follicles in all animals with follicular estrogen and progesterone concentrations 2- and 40-fold greater than the levels in control follicles, respectively. In randomly selected gilts, the right ovary on day 13 contained 48 follicles 1 to 6 mm; by day 19, there were 29 follicles in this size range and there was an average of only 1.5 large follicles (7–10 mm) per ovary (465). Follicular selection is evidently completed by day 17 since 91% of 5- to 6-mm follicles marked between days 17 and 21 are represented 6 days later by corpora lutea (468).

When all grossly visible follicles (>1 mm) of Poland China gilts are destroyed by electrosurgical cauterization on day 14 (late luteal phase), the largest clear follicles present 6 days later were 8 mm in diameter (469). Thus, the follicles grew 7 mm or 0.4515 log mm^3/day. Based on this figure, it is estimated that the ultimate ovulatory follicles, which are 7 to 11 mm at estrus, begin to develop around day 5 or 6 and that they require 15.6 days to complete development. Again, the second postestrous FSH increase may be an important selective factor.

As in the case of the other barnyard species, the largest follicles present at metestrus (>8 mm) have significantly greater follicular fluid levels of estrogens than androgens, and this relationship persists through diestrus and proestrus (470). Similarly, prepubertal gilts treated with PMS show a daily follicular increase of 1 to 2 mm in diameter; this is associated with increasing follicular fluid concentrations of estrone, estradiol, and progesterone, comparable to the levels in the cyclic sow before and at the onset of estrus (471).

FOLLICULAR DEVELOPMENT DURING THE MENSTRUAL CYCLE OF *MACACA* AND HUMAN

Follicles from *Macaca mulatta* pass from preantral to antral stages between 200 and 250 μm (43). A significant increase in the mean percentage of follicles 100 to 200 μm is evident in the periovulatory period, evidently influenced by the midcycle increases in steroids (estrogens?) and gonadotropins (FSH?). Atresia is very limited in preantral follicles from 40 to 159 μm in diameter, varying from less than 1% to a maximum of about 3%. Primordial follicles constitute 80 to 95% of the preantral follicles and range from 26,000 to 242,000 per pair of ovaries. In general, the mean number of preantral follicles varies directly with the size of the primordial follicle pool; similar numbers of primordial and preantral follicles are present in the right and left ovaries (43).

Very few antral follicles >1 mm are present during the luteal phase until the corpus luteum shows histological signs of regression in the premenstrual period (472). This coincides with a significant increase in serum FSH without a change in LH levels (e.g., 473,474). The greatest number of atretic follicles throughout the cycle are 0.5 to 1.0 mm in diameter, medium-sized follicles (472). During the midluteal phase, preantral follicles (≤257 μm in diameter) incorporate [^{3}H]thymidine with a labeling frequency from 10% in follicles with one layer of granulosa cells to 60% in follicles with 6 or more layers (475). Hence, the failure of advanced follicular development during the luteal phase is not attributable to a deficiency in growing preantral follicles. The limited follicular development during the luteal phase is most likely due to changes in pulse frequency and amplitude of gonadotropins as GNRH pulses are modulated. Thus, in measuring bioactive LH, an average of about one pulse per 90 min occurs during the early luteal phase; the frequency changes to one pulse per 7 to 8 hr during the late luteal phase (476). During the early follicular phase (days 2–5), the largest healthy follicles are 2 mm or less and there are usually two follicles about the same size. However, by days 7 to 9, one follicle was considerably larger than the other in 3 of 4 sets of ovaries, and this was further accentuated by days 11–13 (preovulatory stage), when the largest follicle was usually about 6 mm. Based on *in vivo* observations, the largest follicle grows from 1.7 to 9.4 mm during the 11 days before the LH surge, and the dominant follicle, destined to ovulate, can be confidently identified in 75% of repeated laparoscopies 7 days before the LH peak and in 100% of cases by 5 days before the peak (477). As the day of the LH peak approaches, the follicle grows about 1 mm/day, as compared with 0.5 mm daily 10 days before the LH peak. Peripheral levels of estradiol increase rapidly from day 3 to 0 (the day of the LH surge), presumably reflecting the activity of the dominant follicle.

As follicle diameter increases from 1 to 7 mm, serum FSH decreases; thereafter, however, increased diameter correlates with rising levels of FSH. Ovulation occurs with equal frequency in each ovary, regardless of the location of the previous corpus luteum (478). By day 8 of the cycle, the ovarian venous effluent on the side of the dominant follicle already contains significantly more estradiol than the contralateral drainage (473). Even on day 8 or 12 of the cycle, the dominant follicle may contain as many as 1.2% pyknotic granulosa cells and still be normal. Thus, the presence of one or two pyknotic nuclei is hardly grounds for classifying any follicle as atretic.

As already mentioned, a technique that has yielded a great deal of useful information about follicular development in large domestic species is extirpation of follicles and corpora lutea, and it has been equally successful in primates. Cautery of the largest follicle present on days 10 to 12 of the rhesus cycle blocks ovulation, and surges of LH and FSH occur 12.4 days later (479). Hence, the follicle destined to ovulate was already selected, and no others were able to immediately substitute for its loss. Following follicle cautery, basal levels of LH and FSH (measured daily in ketamine-injected monkeys) were relatively stable, although a few animals showed slightly elevated levels the next day. Following luteectomy 4 to 6 days after the LH surge, preoperative levels of LH and FSH were maintained until 12.8 days later, when typical midcycle surges of the gonadotropins were observed (479). Ovulation invariably occurred in the contralateral ovary (for literature, see ref. 480), and within 4 days after luteectomy, the contralateral ovary in monkeys with both ovaries present already had more medium-sized (0.5–1.0 mm) and large (1.1–1.5 mm) follicles (473). Another study involving luteectomy revealed that on days 17 to 19 of the cycle, the new dominant follicle always originated on the side opposite the ovarian vein with the highest concentration of progesterone (481).

The fact that ovulation in about 90% of cases occurred in the contralateral ovary raised the possibility that trauma following follicular ablation or luteectomy might have temporarily affected the ipsilateral ovary, and the above experiments were therefore repeated in hemiovariectomized rhesus monkeys (480). After luteal extirpation in these animals a sustained and large increase in serum FSH was always observed, suggesting that when two ovaries are present, the contralateral ovary is responsible for the negative feedback on tonic FSH release, now thought to be due to its production of inhibin. Collectively, these experiments led to the concept of recruitment of follicles at the end of the luteal phase and selection of the dominant follicle by days 5 to 7 of the follicular phase (for references, see ref. 482).

Presumably the higher levels of FSH in the early follicular phase aid in the selection of the dominant follicle. When charcoal treated porcine follicular fluid was injected IP every 8 hr from days 1 to 4, serum FSH decreased 50% to 80% with no change in LH (483). Following this treatment, on days 10 to 14, the dominant follicle was much smaller than usual and contained very few granulosa cells; in vitro these cells secreted negligible amounts of progesterone and did not luteinize. Moreover, within 4 days the cells became necrotic. When porcine follicular fluid was administered daily from days 1 to 3, serum FSH was depressed from days 2 to 4, followed by a rebound to elevated levels on day 6 (474). Nevertheless, the animals ovulated with a follicular phase comparable in duration to control cycles. The resultant corpus luteum, secreted significantly less progesterone during the first half of the luteal phase.

Porcine follicular fluid (PFF) administered from days 1 to 5 or days 6 to 12 significantly reduced serum FSH concentrations and estradiol without affecting LH (484). After cessation of PFF there was a rebound in FSH levels. Treatment during menses led to a delay in midcycle FSH and LH peaks until day 17, with formation of a normal, functional corpus luteum. On the other hand, when PFF was deferred until days 6 to 12, midcycle gonadotropin surges were delayed until day 26. It appears that the early treatment deferred the appearance of the dominant follicle, whereas later treatment resulted in atresia. The dominant follicle therefore requires the continued presence of FSH throughout its development.

The clear opposite of reducing serum FSH levels by PFF is to increase circulating levels by treatment with hMG (484). When hMG was administered from days 1 to 3 or 4 to 6, estradiol secretion increased immediately as more follicles were recruited. However, when hMG was administered after day 7 (when the dominant follicle has emerged), the other follicles were now unable to respond with increased estradiol secretion; presumably most of them were now atretic. Thus, after the selection of the dominant follicle, the other follicles, members of the same cohort, are unresponsive. Evidence has been presented that a follicular regulatory protein (FRP) produced by the dominant follicle suppresses estrogen production by other developing antral follicles without affecting FSH levels; it is therefore distinct from inhibin (reviewed in ref. 482; also see section below on human folliculogenesis). The maturing follicle in cynomolgus monkeys is the source of increasing titers of estradiol. When, after unilateral ovariectomy (ULO on day 0), estradiol antibodies are infused from days 5 to 10, serum FSH and LH increase, and 10 days after hemispaying the remaining ovary of two animals contained two large follicles and the third contained four (485). Accordingly, it appears that the dominant follicle's production of estrogen acts as the principal modulator of development of other follicles by its ability to suppress gonadotropin levels. This is contrary to the notion that a follicular regulatory protein produced by the dominant follicle accounts for its outstripping the other members of the cohort.

Another approach to analyzing follicular development in the rhesus is to induce follicular atresia by Silastic implants of estradiol on days 5 to 7 of the rhesus cycle (for literature, see ref. 486). The resultant serum concentrations of estradiol, 100 to 400 pg/ml/24 hr, led to transient declines in FSH and LH, followed by a rebound and unusually high levels of both hormones on day 8. Dierschke et al. (486) believe that exogenous estrogen acts directly at the ovary or indirectly by the transitory depression of FSH to induce follicular atresia. It seems equally plausible that the rebound in LH is responsible for atresia: Injection of hCG (1,000 IU) on day 9 or 11, prior to the spontaneous midcycle surges of LH and FSH, leads to apparent atresia of the dominant follicle, as evidenced by the absence of midcycle increases in peripheral estrogen and gonadotropins (487). Progesterone administration by injection or Silastic implants on day 6 of the rhesus cycle similarly affects the dominant follicle, resulting in very low levels of serum estradiol (30–50 pg/ml) throughout the course of treatment (for literature, see ref. 488).

During the follicular phase of the rhesus cycle, as follicles increase in size from 3 to 6 mm to 6 to 8 mm, follicular fluid estrogen increases from 100 to 2,200 ng/ml (489), in agreement with the estrogen-activated follicles already described for other species. Before the LH surge *in vitro* progesterone secretion and morphological luteinization of granulosa cells from follicles less than or greater than 6 mm are minimal in 2- to 8-day cultures (489). On the other hand, follicles removed during the early LH surge (when they are 6–8 mm) or mid-LH surge (10–11 mm) show *in vitro* morphological luteinization of granulosa cells and significant progesterone secretion by granulosa and thecal cells. Moreover, the theca (without the addition of an androgen precursor) produces considerable amounts of estrogen, whereas the granulosa cells are inactive.

These results have been confirmed in short-term (3 hr) incubations of granulosa and thecal cells from dominant follicles removed on day 12 of the rhesus cycle—2 days before the normal LH surge (490). The follicles were 5.2 mm in diameter and contained 3.32×10^6 granulosa cells. A tritiated exchange assay with [1,2^{3}H]androstenedione (a measure of aromatase activity) showed that granulosa cells produced 341 fmol ^3H_2O, compared with 89 fmol by thecal cells. In this connection, when peripheral estradiol was >150 pg/ml, aspiration of as many granulosa cells as possible from the dominant follicle results 15 min later in a fall of about 70% in the concentrations of progesterone, estradiol, and androstenedione from preaspiration levels (491).

FOLLICULAR DEVELOPMENT IN THE HUMAN

Until recently, quantitative histological analyses of the human ovary were extremely limited—for obvious reasons. It is well established that the number of primordial and growing (≥100 μm) follicles diminishes with age: *primordial* ages 6 to 9, 484,000 vs. 8,236 at age 40 to 44; *growing* ages 6 to 9, 15,220 vs. 6,190 at age 40 to 44 (41). The number of Graafian follicles (>1 mm) averaged 63 per pair of ovaries over the same time span, with only three of seven women having follicles in this size range at ages 40 to 44. Another frequently cited study dealt with follicular development during the menstrual cycle, with histological evaluation of the endometrium used to date the ovaries (492). The heart of that paper is Table 21. Presenting the data on 17 ovaries from women aged 18 to 33 years, the table shows the gradual emergence during the late follicular phase (days 11–14) of a large viable follicle, 10 to 13 mm in diameter, whereas on day 1 of the cycle, the largest follicles are 3 to 4 mm. There are more small antral follicles 1 to 2 mm in diameter present from day 12 to 14 (15.2/ovary) than in the earlier follicular phase; the number of healthy small follicles declines in the earlier luteal phase (days 16–18) to an average of 8.5/ovary, with the maximal number present on days 20 to 27 (28/ovary). Although a heroic amount of effort went into Block's studies, the knowledge gained was rather limited.

The situation was dramatically changed by a series of interesting and provocative findings by Gougeon (42,493). The studies involved histological analyses of ovaries of 33 women with regular menstrual cycles (28 ± 2 days) who had been ovariectomized for extraovarian pathology. Days of the cycle were judged by plasma levels of estradiol, progesterone, LH, FSH, and, in some instances, endometrial biopsy. Serial sections (10 μm) of each ovary were cut, both ovaries being available for sectioning from 22 patients.

Some salient findings are outlined in Table 6 (p. 402). The follicles are classified in eight stages, based primarily on diameter and number of granulosa cells. Estimates of the doubling time of granulosa cells are calculated from *in vitro* determinations of the mitotic time [1.36 hr, the same time as in the sheep (424)] and mitotic index (494). Based on these estimates, the length of time spent in each class of follicular development is listed in Table 6. The mean time for a preantral follicle (stage 1) to ovulation is about 85 to 90 days, about $3\frac{1}{2}$ cycles. Note that the most active stages in granulosa proliferation occur in classes 4 through 7. The overall rates of atresia are also shown in Table 6. Atresia of follicles 1 to 2 mm—classes 1 through 4—is relatively constant throughout the menstrual cycle and is unaffected by cyclic hormonal changes (495). In contrast, the atretic rate for classes 5 and 6 is higher and inversely proportional to circulating gonadotropin levels; it is highest during the early and midluteal phase, when almost all class 8 follicles are atretic. Table 6 lists the overall mitotic indices throughout the cycle (494). These rates, however, are not constant, and there is an especially brisk increase for class 5 and 6 follicles at the end of the cycle (day 28) (495). Analysis of the largest healthy and atretic follicles throughout the cycle revealed that the dominant follicle could be identified by size during the early follicular phase, days 1 through 5, although it did not differ in vascularization or thecal or granulosa development from other healthy follicles. By days 6 and 10, the dominant follicle (now 13.3 mm) did differ in these features from other healthy follicles (315). Excluding the dominant follicle, the next healthiest follicle never exceeded 6 mm in the follicular phase or 4 mm in the luteal phase. Based on the mitotic index, follicles 2 to 5 mm in diameter (classes 4 and 5 in Table 6) are very active in the late luteal phase and represent the population from which the dominant follicle may already be selected. It is interesting that the largest healthy follicle was invariably located on the ovary contralateral to the previous ovulation (315). A subsequent study (496) showed that this phenomenon occurred in 87.6% of cases. This conclusion was based on the ability to make a histological identification of the age of the corpus luteum over five cycles. If the histological criteria are valid, this would be quite contrary to previous assertions that ovulation in the human is random, uninfluenced by the side of the last corpus luteum. The pattern of alternating ovulations is explained on the basis of differences in the intraovarian hormonal milieu, such that a 5-day asynchrony exists in the population of follicles developing in the "ovulating" ovary and the contralateral one (497). It is proposed that this local effect comes into play when the follicles begin to develop an antral cavity (class 2). The follicles on the side of the corpus luteum, i.e., the ovulating ovary, have a significantly higher mitotic index but are smaller than in the contralateral side; in the next cycle, class 3 and 4 follicles now develop earlier in the ipsilateral, nonovulating ovary. Alternation of ovulation is an interesting and unsettling phenomenon if true: Ultrasonography should be able to show whether, in fact, it is occurring. Table 6 also shows when follicles pass from one stage to another during the menstrual cycle, illustrating how a class 1 follicle that will ovulate approximately 3 months later is selected. It is postulated that follicles move continuously out of the resting pool into class 1 and that the growth of follicles <2 mm requires only small amounts of gonadotropins, whereas larger sizes are influenced by cyclic changes in gonadotropin levels (498). The critical factor for class 1 follicles is whether their development is initiated in the periovulatory period. These "privileged" follicles develop a theca under the influence of high levels of LH at the midcycle surge; consequently, they may have a greater ability to produce androgens, which, transported to the granulosa compartment, enhance estrogen secretion (the last speculation is by G. S. Greenwald). Class 1 follicles developing at other times during the cycle are destined to become atretic at some stage. Thus, a class 1 follicle fortuitously emerging in the proper hormonal milieu is the one selected to ovulate. This scheme proposes a very early stage for follicular selection and is probably too rigid. There is more leeway in the system, as evidenced by the effects of administering human menopausal gonadotropin (hMG), which acts on much more advanced classes of follicles (see below).

The point remains that the overwhelming number of follicles leaving the resting pool undergo atresia. It must be kept in mind, however, that even large preovulatory follicles (12–27 mm in diameter) contain pyknotic nuclei (1 ± 0.2%), but this is balanced by a moderate mitotic index (4.6 ± 0.8%) (160). In contrast, frankly atretic large follicles (>6 mm) have a high pyknotic index (10.9 ± 2.1%) 2 days before the LH surge. Healthy dominant human follicles show a strong reaction for 3β-HSD in the theca and limited activity in the granulosa; it is not until after the LH surge that an intense reaction develops in the granulosa cells. Follicles in advanced atresia show low or moderate 3β-HSD activity in the theca and almost none in the granulosa.

Criteria proposed for determining a follicle's potential for further development are whether it contains (a) more than 50% of the maximal complement of granulosa cells for its size and (b) a normal oocyte (206). Thus, a 4-mm follicle has about 1×10^6 granulosa cells and a 12-mm normal follicle has 10×10^6 granulosa cells. Based on these criteria and the concentration of steroids in follicular fluid, 90% of follicles ≥1 mm in diameter were undergoing degenerative changes. After reaching a diameter of ~4 mm, only one or at most two follicles per follicular phase of the cycle are capable of continued mitotic activity to reach the 50 to 100 million granulosa cells characteristic of the preovulatory follicle. According to the aforementioned histologic studies of Gougeon and hormonal correlates from antral fluid (499), it is evident that the follicle destined to ovulate has normally emerged by days 1 to 5 as a healthy 4-mm follicle. On day 1 of the cycle, although the dominant follicle cannot be grossly identified, ovarian venous plasma collected from both ovaries already shows unilaterally high concentrations of progesterone, estradiol, and estrone, and this is even more apparent by days 4 to 9 and thereafter, when a large follicle can be identified (e.g., refs. 500–502). Moreover, by the midfollicular phase, high unilateral concentrations of the above steroids in ovarian effluent are also associated with asymmetry in levels of androstenedione and testosterone.

Granulosa cells harvested from 6- to 9-mm follicles on day 9 produce small amounts of estradiol (2 ng/10^6 cells) for 3 hr with 10^{-7} M testosterone or androstenedione but show an eightfold increase when FSH is combined with either of the androgens (247). In contrast, granulosa cells collected from a large dominant follicle (20 mm) accumulate ~60 ng estradiol/10^6 cells/3 hr in the presence of testosterone, and FSH has no synergistic action. Thus, the early developing follicle depends on FSH for regulation of aromatase enzymes in granulosa cells. It is interesting that 5α-reduced androgens at physiological concentrations can inhibit aromatization of testosterone in FSH-stimulated granulosa cells of small (5–9 mm) follicles (247).

For follicles <8 mm in diameter, the follicular fluid concentration of FSH is maximal at the early follicular, early luteal, and late luteal phases, during or just after peak levels of FSH in peripheral plasma (503). Large follicles appear during the midfollicular phase, with 38% having detectable levels of FSH in follicular fluid; 11% of these follicles contain measurable amounts of LH. By the late follicular phase, 83% of large follicles have detectable FSH in follicular fluid and 70% similarly have LH present. Follicles with high concentrations of FSH in follicular fluid also have a high ratio of estradiol to androstenedione in antral fluid (504). Judged by ultrasound scanning, the volume and diameter of the dominant follicle averaged 9.8 mm (range: 6–13 mm) 5 days before ovulation; thereafter, an exponential growth phase ensued, culminating in a maximal diameter of 21 ± 3.5 mm (SD) with a range from 14 to 28 mm (505). During the 9 days after the LH peak, all follicles from 4 to 10 mm are usually atretic, based on histological criteria (103). Such follicles invariably have an androstenedione:estradiol ratio greater than unity (506). Progesterone concentrations in follicular fluid are maximal in the late follicular phase, which correlates with detectable antral fluid levels of LH and FSH (506). Progesterone secretion by granulosa cells increases from 6 to 30 μg/24 hr/10^6 cells as follicles enlarge from 5 to 25 mm (507). Addition of LH to granulosa cells from follicles 5 to 15 mm enhances progesterone secretion by 2.5-fold but does not stimulate further increases in larger follicles. For 5- to 18-mm follicles, 5 μg estradiol/ml significantly decreases progesterone secretion, with almost 60% inhibition of progesterone by granulosa cells from 18-mm follicles (507).

Prolactin in follicular fluid is maximal in the early follicular phase and falls to its lowest levels during the late follicular phase for all follicles, irrespective of size; a second peak occurs in the midluteal stage (503). In situations in which peripheral levels of prolactin are >100 ng/ml, 96% of the follicles lack detectable amounts of FSH and antral fluid concentration of estradiol is depressed (506). In addition, accompanying hyperprolactinemia, follicles >4 mm were apparently undergoing atresia, based on the reduced number of granulosa cells for their diameter.

In large preovulatory follicles, both diced theca and granulosa cells appear capable of producing progesterone, androstenedione, and estradiol, with progesterone the dominant steroid secreted by granulosa cells and androstenedione the major steroid produced by theca (for literature, see ref. 508). When expressed as ng steroid/mg protein × 2 hr, thecal and granulosa cells released estradiol at approximately the same rate in the absence or presence of hCG (508). In contrast, collagenase-dispersed preparations, incubated with a fixed amount of testosterone, show that granulosa cells have at least 700 times the aromatase activity of the theca when expressed as steroid/10^5 cells/24 hr (247). Considerable differences in experimental design make it difficult to compare the two studies.

Based on these findings and others, McNatty (499,506) proposed that a preantral follicle destined for further development is transformed to an antral stage concurrent with high levels of FSH in plasma and its antral fluid. The latter minimizes atresia by increasing mitotic activity of granulosa cells and increasing aromatase activity in the cells, thus enhancing estrogen secretion. The combined interactions of FSH and estrogen act as a positive feedback to further enhance granulosa cell mitosis and estrogen accumulation in the follicle. The action of LH on the theca stimulates androstenedione, which in the favored follicle is converted to estrogens and thus further shifts the estrogen:androgen ratio. Preantral follicles not emerging when the concentration of follicular fluid FSH can be increased are therefore much more likely to be androgenic follicles and hence prone to atresia.

The potential to recruit follicles for ovulation obviously encompasses larger follicles—presumably ~4 mm at the onset of the follicular phase—as demonstrated by the ability of human menopausal gonadotropin or FSH administered on days 3 and 4 to increase the number of oocytes induced by hCG administered on day 8 (for literature, see ref. 509). Injection of hMG at the late luteal phase instead of the early follicular phase is even more successful in increasing the mitotic index of granulosa cells and increasing the induced ovulation rate to 3.7 ova (510).

The human—like the rhesus—responds to removal of the dominant follicle or corpus luteum by ovulating 12.7 and 14.6 days later, respectively (511). Following either procedure, ovulation invariably occurs in the ipsilateral ovary, contrary to the situation in the rhesus. Unlike the rhesus, there is a clear-cut, transient increase in FSH and LH after follicular ablation in the human (319,512). Whether a true species difference exists or whether effects of anesthesia are responsible remains to be established. It would indeed be unusual if recruitment of the next follicle in the rhesus is not associated with transient increases in gonadotropins. The restraining influence of the human corpus luteum on gonadotropin levels is evident.

A protein aspirated and pooled from human follicular fluid of hyperstimulated ovaries inhibits ovarian weight increase and serum estradiol in suitably primed hypophysectomized immature rats (513). The putative FRP is heat and trypsin labile and has also been recovered from the ovarian venous drainage on the side of the dominant follicle. FRP is produced by granulosa cells (recoverable from spent medium during the first 48 hr of incubation) and does not affect FSH binding to rat granulosa cells but does decrease their aromatase activity (514). It is speculated that FRP may be an important intraovarian regulator of folliculogenesis and may account for the selection of the dominant follicle in primates and other species (for review, see ref. 482). The substance appears to be distinctly different from inhibin based on its biophysical properties (515).

Considerably more work is needed before a physiological role of FRP can be established. At present, activity is based on pooled antral fluid from hyperstimulated ovaries and sampling from *individual* follicles (preferably from nonstimulated ovaries) is needed to establish whether a hierarchical relationship exists between FRP in the dominant follicle and other members of the cohort.

FOLLICULAR DEVELOPMENT DURING PREGNANCY

This topic is of interest for several reasons: (a) Is there any "wavelike" development of follicles during pregnancy comparable to the length of the estrous cycle and therefore recurring every *n* days? (b) How does the negative-feedback effect of high steroid levels affect the hypothalamic-pituitary axis and hence follicular growth? (c) In species in which corpora lutea are essential throughout pregnancy and produce progesterone as the main hormone, the follicles obviously are the principal source of ovarian estrogens. (d) Are follicles developing during pregnancy "mature" enough to ovulate in response to hCG?

Follicular development in the pregnant mouse can be divided into three stages: (a) From day 1 to 8 (day 1 = morning after mating), the largest follicles present are up to 473 μm in diameter and atresia of large follicles is minimal; (b) from day 10 to 14, follicular atresia is maximal and the largest follicles are usually 373 μm or less; (c) from day 16 to 19, follicular atresia is again minimal and from day 18 and on, large follicles reappear in preparation for postpartum ovulation (516). This profile correlates with the ability to induce ovulation with 5 IU hCG. Thus, between days 12 and 14, only 37% of injected animals ovulate; the nadir is reached at day 12, when the mean number of ovulations is 5.2—only half the normal number. Subcutaneous injection of 5 IU PMS on day 10 followed by hCG on day 12 results in 91% of the mice ovulating an average of 11.2 ova (516).

When pregnant mice were pulse-labeled by injecting [^{3}H]thymidine, small to large follicles were labeled on every day, showing that there is continuous growth of follicles (50). At any time during pregnancy about 14 small follicles begin to grow compared with 19 per day during the estrous cycle, but there is no difference in the transit time. It is interesting that the labeling index of type 6 and 7 follicles (incipient formation of antral cavity and coalesced cavity, respectively) tend to decrease during midpregnancy (*cf.* above results on induced ovulation with hCG). It was estimated that type 3b follicles (with 21–60 granulosa cells) moving out of the resting pool on day 1 of pregnancy are the ones that ultimately ovulate at postpartum estrus.

These morphological findings show interesting correlations with the gonadotropin pattern during mouse pregnancy. Using 50 μl of plasma, there are LH peaks on days 4 and 11 of gestation with no significant changes in FSH throughout this period (517). However, from days 12 to 15, LH is frequently undetectable in the amount of plasma assayed, whereas plasma FSH does not differ from earlier values. On the day of parturition, there is a sharp increase in both FSH and LH (517) coincident with restoration of follicular kinetics to the pattern characteristic of the estrous cycle (50).

Follicular growth and gonadotropin profiles are quite different between the pregnant mouse and rat. Until day 14 of pregnancy in the rat, healthy follicles up to 600 μm are present, but this is followed by a hiatus on days 16 and 18, when the largest antral follicles are only 400 to 500 μm. Differentiation of larger follicles begins on day 20, culminating in follicles >600 μm on day 22 and at delivery on day 23 (518). Follicles 300 to 400 μm in diameter are present on every day of pregnancy and are especially abundant on the first 4 days of gestation. Ovulation with 20 IU hCG (sc) could not be induced before day 21, but priming with 25 IU PMS on day 15, 72 hr before hCG treatment, resulted in ovulation. It was concluded that even though medium and large antral follicles are present throughout most of gestation, the follicles were "physiologically immature." Subsequently, several other investigators who injected pregnant rats with hCG reported different results, depending possibly on differences in strain, colony, and route of administration (519). However, the consensus was that days 15 and 16 represented the nadir in follicular responsiveness to hCG.

In this connection, it is interesting that serum levels of FSH and LH are at their lowest values on day 16, with serum LH abruptly increasing on days 20 and 22 and with FSH recovering on day 18 (520). Furthermore, on day 16 the corpora lutea of pregnancy have the highest concentrations of estradiol with the lowest levels in the nonluteal ovary, suggesting that between days 14 and 18 secretion of testosterone and estradiol represents proportionately more luteal than follicular activity. Ovarian venous plasma on day 15 of pregnancy also does not contain detectable amounts of inhibin, a further indication of the nonfunctional status of the follicles (521).

Richards and colleagues have recently explored this problem in depth, focusing on follicular development on day 16 of pregnancy. Between days 14 and 19, FSH and hCG binding reach their nadir in granulosa cells, and hCG receptors in thecal shells are also minimal (522). This was associated with minimal accumulation of estradiol *in vitro*, although providing testosterone as a substrate increased estrogen levels to values observed on days 4 to 12. Hence, on day 15 the aromatizing system is still intact in the granulosa compartment. Follicular morphology on day 16 revealed that the follicles lacked the features typical of steroidogenically active tissue (523). Following daily injection on days 14 and 15 of 1.5 IU hCG, however, the theca hypertrophied and the orientation of granulosa cells was altered with extensive lipid deposition in both tissues. The most salient finding was that isolated thecal shells produced considerable testosterone *in vitro* after exposure to hCG: from 17 to 175 pg/thecae/5 hr (523). The action of hCG is specific in that twice-daily injections of FSH on days 14 and 15 fails to increase thecal LH receptor content or intrinsic ability of follicles to accumulate estradiol (524). The small antral follicles normally present on day 16, when incubated with [^{3}H]progesterone, fail to convert it appreciably to labeled 17α-OH progesterone or androgens, in contrast to normal preovulatory follicles on day 23 (525). Collectively, these experiments demonstrate that the relative paucity of serum LH on day 16 accounts for inadequate biochemical development of the theca with a consequent deficit in 17α-hydroxylase and C-17,20 lyase. This condition is then reversed by rising titers of LH commencing on day 20 of gestation.

Follicular development in the pregnant hamster is diametrically opposed to the pattern described for the rat. Large healthy antral follicles >415 μm in diameter are always present in the hamster ovary, with about 10 per pair of ovaries from day 4 to 10; this number reaches a peak of 35 to 40 on day 12 (526). This is paralleled by the ability of hCG to induce ovulation at any time during gestation: The mean of 10 to 13 ovulations from days 4 to 8 culminated in a peak of 35 ovulations on day 12 (526). Hence, at midpregnancy, the hamster matures sufficient follicles to result in superovulation. Healthy follicles 277 to 322 μm in diameter (the smallest ones measured) were continuously present throughout gestation, indicating constant recruitment of preantral stages. The concentration of FSH on day 1 of the 16-day pregnancy was about fivefold greater than the levels on subsequent days (527). When sampled at 0900 hr at 2-day intervals throughout pregnancy, serum FSH was approximately twice as great as 0900 hr proestrous values (~180 versus 93 ng/ml), and serum LH was 20 ng/ml, which was comparable to 0900 hr proestrous values (528). In contrast, in the pregnant rat, serum FSH is comparable to proestrous values, but LH ranges from 4 to 8 ng/ml from day 4 to 18, whereas serum LH is approximately 30 ng on the morning of proestrus (399). Thus, the relative deficiency of LH may account for the differences in follicular development between the pregnant rat and hamster. Hamster follicles *in vitro* can be stimulated by 10 ng LH at any time during gestation to accumulate estradiol, although the response is drastically curtailed by day 16—the day of delivery (528). Again, this is a striking difference from the rat.

Follicular development in the pregnant rabbit resembles the pattern found in the hamster. The intravenous injection of 25 IU hCG up to 12 days of pregnancy results in the ovulation of 11 ova, but similar treatment on day 21 leads to the ovulation of an average of 21 eggs (529). The enhanced ovulatory response to hCG is associated with increasing numbers of antral follicles 1 mm in diameter or greater: on days 8 to 11 a mean number of 14 follicles compared to day 17, when the ovaries average 23 follicles (529). Serum levels of FSH and LH measured at 3-day intervals throughout rabbit pregnancy do not correlate with the midgestational change in follicular number (530), but the sampling intervals tested in the hamster and other species are also not frequent enough for any valid comparisons. In estrous does, approximately 50% of the follicles are <1.6 mm in diameter and the remainder are >1.6 mm (531). Some of these large follicles contain elevated levels of testosterone and progesterone but low estradiol; presumably these follicles are atretic. After inducing ovulation with hCG, only 15% of the remaining follicles are large; by day 6 of pseudopregnancy, however, there is a redistribution, with 75% of the follicles being classified as large. Correlated with the recruitment of large follicles, on day 6, the follicles now contain high levels of estradiol, testosterone, and progesterone. Rabbit corpora lutea first become dependent on estrogen on day 6, and the large follicles recruited by the periovulatory surge of FSH on days 1 and 2, with tonic levels of LH (530), evidently fulfill this need.

The pregnant guinea pig resembles the hamster and rabbit in that large preovulatory follicles (500–700 μm) are present throughout gestation, with the peak number attained on day 66 in preparation for postpartum estrus (532,533). Ovulation can be induced at any time in pregnant guinea pigs by intravenous injection of 50 IU hCG (534); the follicles are less sensitive on days 8 through 20 than on days 41 through 62, and the average ovulation rate is about twice as great in the last trimester (2.0 versus 3.9, respectively).

There is very little information available about follicular development during pregnancy in large domestic species. In cross-bred pigs, the total number of follicles up to 8 mm in diameter is greater up to 40 days of gestation, and by 110 days (shortly before delivery) there are no 7- to 8-mm follicles and few in the 4- to 6-mm class (535). Small follicles (1–2 mm) were relatively constant from days 23 to 63 in three breeds of sow (127); over the same time span, medium follicles (3–5 mm) were also fairly constant (61), with large follicles (6–10 mm) averaging 4.8 per pregnant sow (536).

In the pregnant cow, 32.6% of the follicles are normal and 67.4% are atretic (455). Follicles larger than 5 mm in diameter are absent throughout pregnancy, and in late pregnancy (243 days) the largest follicles are only 2 mm. Small follicles <1 mm in diameter are present throughout pregnancy and in fact constitute the dominant group. Despite the paucity of follicular development, plasma estradiol and estrone rise progressively throughout gestation, peaking in the last trimester (537). At term, estrone levels are eight times as high as estradiol; evidently, a nonfollicular source of estrogens exists if the two cited studies are comparable. During bovine gestation, FSH pulses average five or six per 12 hr throughout pregnancy, whereas LH pulses average between one and two in the first and third trimesters and are almost wholly abolished in midgestation (537). The relationship between these peripheral hormone values and follicular quiescence during pregnancy is most likely related to differences from the bovine estrous cycle, in which basal levels of progesterone, estradiol, and FSH are considerably less than during gestation and LH pulses per 12 hr are three- to sevenfold greater during the cycle (538). Hence, reduced steroid feedback characterizes the estrous cycle, with resultant modifications in pulsatile FSH and LH patterns.

There are no quantitative accounts available for the human ovary during pregnancy. Up to 10 weeks, the ovary is populated by large Graafian follicles (averaging 10 mm in diameter) that are atretic based on the usual degenerative status of the ovum, a granulosa layer only three cells thick and an undeveloped thecal layer (539). This is very similar to the condition of the ovary shortly after ovulation. After 10 weeks, many new Graafian follicles differentiate but rarely grow much larger than 4 mm, and ultimately all show signs of atresia; degeneration of the granulosa cells is accompanied by excessive development of the theca. A later paper of Govan (540) dealt with ovarian activity from 26 to 40 weeks. During the first 7 weeks, there was little follicular activity, but beginning at 33 weeks and continuing until term, Graafian follicles 2 to 4 mm reappeared with considerable mitotic activity in the granulosa cells. Usually, however, most of these follicles were atretic. When the follicles were approximately 3 mm, mitoses appear in the theca layer and the theca persists after the complete disappearance of granulosa cells but lacks 3β-ol-dehydrogenase. A characteristic finding during pregnancy is the proliferation and luteinization of thecal cells surrounding both normal and atretic follicles (541), presumably in response to the elevated hCG levels. In another study, involving samples collected at cesarian section, 298 follicles were available for analysis (542). The average diameter (extrapolated from follicular fluid measurements) was 2.75 mm, and degenerative changes were apparent in the failure to recover oocytes from 50% of the follicles; 79% of oocytes recovered from the remaining follicles were undergoing lysis. At term no follicles larger than 6 mm were present. After 2 hr of incubation, the predominant steroid released was androstenedione, about eightfold more than progesterone and estradiol (543). High concentrations of PGE_2 or PGF_2 (10 μg/ml) significantly increased cAMP formation by the follicles, whereas hCG was ineffective. The still functioning theca was presumably the source of the androgen and also was the tissue responsive to the prostaglandins. During the third trimester of human pregnancy, follicles normally develop to about 6 mm in diameter, and based on flow cytometry, only 7% are judged to be healthy (544). The steroid profiles in follicular fluid differed from aspirates from cycling women in having higher concentrations of progesterone and lower levels of androstenedione.

These scattered observations indicate that the human ovary is not quiescent during pregnancy, but follicles grow only to about 4 to 6 mm before degenerative changes intervene. The puzzling question is what gonadotropins account for even this limited proliferation of follicles in view of the very low and frequently undetectable levels of FSH during human gestation (545,546). Human chorionic gonadotropin is obviously the principal circulating gonadotropin, and at various times it has been proposed that hCG has intrinsic but variable FSH activity. It is interesting that deglycosylated hCG acts as a partial agonist at the FSH receptor in rat granulosa cells, whereas native hCG shows only negligible cross-reactivity (547). Moreover, the relative binding affinity of deglycosylated hCG for LH receptors is twice that of native hCG. It is therefore possible that modified hCG may be able to substitute, in part, for FSH in stimulating follicular recruitment.

EFFECTS OF LACTATION ON FOLLICULAR DEVELOPMENT

In all mammals studied lactation impairs follicular development. Among laboratory species, this has been most clearly demonstrated in the rat, in which the suckling stimulus of small versus large litters influences the degree of follicular inhibition (reviewed in ref. 548). Thus, mothers nursing eight pups show a decrease in follicular number, with the nadir reached at day 8 of lactation; between days 4 and 12, follicles >400 μm are absent. In contrast, a few follicles in this range are always present in dams nursing two pups (548). Follicular immaturity in rats with eight pups was reflected in very low levels of estradiol, both *in vivo* and *in vitro*. On removal of the litter on day 3 of lactation, a significant increase is evident by 30 hr in the number of follicles 201 to 600 μm in diameter, and the animals ovulate by 96 hr (549). The hormone profiles found in rats nursing eight pups exemplify a rather universal pattern during lactation: normal cyclic serum levels of FSH, elevated PRL, and extremely reduced LH. Daily injection of 0.5 to 1.0 IU hCG or 50 μg ovine LH from day 2 to 5, followed by an ovulatory injection of hCG, results in ovulation of the normal complement of ova by the next morning (548). After the removal of the litter on day 3 of lactation at 1100 hr, significant increases occur 24 hr later in serum LH and FSH with a concurrent fall in PRL (549). The missing ingredient during intense suckling stimulus therefore appears to be LH. *In vitro* production rates of testosterone and estradiol by the nonluteal ovary are drastically reduced in rats nursing two or eight pups on day 2 of lactation, but a positive staircase increase occurs in the former group over the next 8 days. It thus appears likely that the deficiency in LH leads to decreased androgen production by the theca and presumably reduced estrogen production by the granulosa compartment. Reduced estrogen secretion may also reflect lower aromatase activity. This does not negate the role of high levels of PRL during lactation, which may act directly or indirectly on the ovary. For example, high levels of PRL inhibit follicular estrogen production in the rat (413,550). The respective roles of LH and PRL in affecting follicular function during lactation is a theme recurring throughout this section. In addition to the high baseline levels of PRL during lactation, the suckling-induced response must also be considered. In rats suckling eight pups, the magnitude of PRL release in 20-day postpartum mothers is considerably reduced and the return to baseline levels accelerated (551). Substituting 10-day-old pups with the 20-day postpartum mother does not enhance PRL release, indicating that the intensity of the suckling stimulus is not a factor. As will be seen for other species, the hypothalamic–pituitary mechanism mediating suckling release of prolactin becomes refractory with time. Rats with prolonged lactation for 72 to 105 days (produced by substituting litters at approximately 2-week intervals) and then mated usually deliver at 22 days (552). This suggests that FSH and especially LH are of greater significance in the rat than suckling release of PRL in regulating follicular development.

Bromocriptine treatment of suckling rats mated at postpartum estrus suppresses serum PRL and progesterone levels, and the uterus contains unimplanted embryos even if progesterone is injected concurrently with bromocriptine (553). Removal of PRL evidently fails to increase secretion of follicular estrogen, which is the key to triggering ovulation in the rat. This also suggests that the primary role of PRL is at the hypothalamic–pituitary axis, not at the follicular level. In postpartum rats nursing seven pups, diestrus lasts for 3 weeks and is associated with reduced LH secretion, hyperprolactinemia, and increased serum progesterone (554). Daily administration of bromocriptine to lactating rats shortens the duration of diestrus to 11 days by depressing the secretion of both PRL and progesterone to baseline levels.

It is well established that lactation prevents the postcastration rise in gonadotropins in the rat (reviewed in ref. 555), and with the increase in understanding of neuroendocrine mechanisms, it was logical to infer that the hypothalamic–pituitary axis is a controlling factor. Indeed, there is a significant fall during lactation in pituitary LHRH receptor concentration (556). There is no change in pituitary affinity for GNRH receptors, but there are about 50% fewer binding sites than at estrus (557). Moreover, removal of an eight-pup litter from ovariectomized mothers results in a sharp increase in GNRH pituitary receptors 24 hr later. Rats ovariectomized on day 10 show a significant increase in LH secretion by the next day; this can be blocked by exogenous PRL without, however, affecting the LH response to LHRH (555). The action of PRL is therefore presumably exerted in part at the hypothalamic level. On the other hand, pituitaries of lactating rats nursing eight pups exposed *in vitro* to pulsatile GNRH release as much FSH but considerably less LH than pituitaries of animals nursing two pups (558). This points to an action of the suckling stimulus (PRL?) directly modifying pituitary response to GHRH. As will become apparent, changes in the frequency and magnitude of GNRH release most likely account for the low serum levels of LH during lactation.

Swiss mice nursing six young show a pattern very similar to the rat. During the first 11 days postpartum the largest vesicular follicles are 350 μm in diameter; thereafter, the follicles enlarge to 450 μm, the corpora lutea of pregnancy regress, and the vagina becomes mucified, indications of estrogen–progesterone interaction (559).

The most extreme effect of lactation on follicular development has been observed in the hamster. Unlike the rat and mouse, there is no postpartum ovulation in the hamster; instead, the large number of vesicular follicles developed during pregnancy quickly regress and consequently the thecal cells are incorporated into the interstitium (560). The net result is an ovary characterized by interstitial hypertrophy, with follicular development limited to preantral follicles with seven to eight layers of granulosa cells. This unusual ovary is maintained by as few as one or two suckling young. Removal of all young on day 2 or 14 of lactation results in ovulation exactly 4 days later (560). The hormonal basis for the acyclic ovary is a daily massive release at 1600 hr of FSH and LH (561), evidently in a ratio incompatible with the differentiation of antral follicles. Concomitant with the daily gonadotropin surge, serum progesterone increases as lactation progresses. The progesterone is secreted by the interstitium, and several lines of evidence indicate its release is in response to the LH surge (561).

Because of the species' economic importance, considerable attention has been devoted to follicular development in the postpartum cow. The degree of follicular inhibition is influenced by two factors: Suckling and its intensity delay the return to estrus. For example, beef cows that were nonsuckled, suckled once daily for 30 min, or suckled *ad libitum* by two calves ovulated, on average, 31, 41, and 76 days after parturition, respectively (562). Another factor complicating follicular development in the cow is the well-documented inhibitory effect of the corpus luteum of pregnancy or the ipsilateral uterine horn (563). In nonsuckling dairy cows, nonatretic follicles begin to form an antral cavity at 0.16 mm in diameter (564). On day 15 postpartum, 77% of the largest healthy antral follicles present are 0.16 to 1.6 mm, and by day 35, only 1.5% of the smallest class are represented. Thus, during the early postpartum period, there is no constant replenishment of small antral follicles by preantral stages. On day 15 the percentage of follicles from 0.29 to 1.6 mm increased, presumably at the expense of the smallest antral follicles. At all times the ovary containing the corpus luteum had more nonatretic follicles than the contralateral ovary. In another study, follicles >3 mm were removed from the ovaries of suckling and nonsuckling beef cows on day 5 postpartum, and the number of healthy and atretic follicles was estimated based on estrogen content in follicular fluid and histology (563). Follicles from the nonsuckled cows were already considerably larger: 50% were >6 mm compared with 33% for suckled cows. Moreover, individual follicles from suckled cows had half the concentration of estrogen compared to follicles from the nonsuckled group. The "carry-over" effect of the corpus luteum was also evident in that the percentage of follicles containing estrogen in the ovary with the corpus luteum was about a third the value of the contralateral ovary (563). Another study evaluated follicular parameters in beef cows that were suckled or weaned on day 21 postpartum with the endpoint on day 25 (565). For combined follicles from 1 to >6 mm in the weaned group, there was a 68% increase in LH receptors but no difference in FSH binding sites. The only hormone that differed in follicular fluid concentration was PRL, which was 53% higher in follicles from the weaned cows. Subsequently, the same authors (566) measured changes at 24-hr intervals after weaning on day 21 postpartum. Utilizing the largest follicle in the ovary, an increase in FSH receptors was observed 48 hr after weaning, whereas the increase in hCG receptors did not occur until 96 hr.

In the suckling cow, serum levels of FSH and LH are depressed compared to weaned animals (567), and this is associated with an altered pattern of gonadotropin release. In cows nursing two young *ad libitum,* the LH pulse rate is about one every 6 hr, contrasted to three per 6 hr in weaned animals (562). After weaning on day 21, the number of LH pulses is approximately threefold greater in the weaned animals (565). In milked cows, FSH is secreted in the early postpartum period in discrete pulses comparable in frequency and magnitude to the profiles during pregnancy; there is a gradual increase in pulsatile release of LH in the first 1 to 2 weeks postpartum (see ref. 568). Again, LH levels are more affected than FSH levels by lactation in the cow. When pituitary explants of weaned and suckled cows are exposed to GNRH, LH secretion is doubled in the former group (566). Following weaning, over the next 4 days, basal levels of serum LH increase in linear fashion, whereas FSH is unaffected (566). It has frequently been noted that the first cycle after parturition in the cow is significantly shorter than subsequent ones judged both by serum progesterone levels and behavioral estrus. This inadequate luteal phase is similar to a disorder of the human female, and in both cases inadequate gonadotropin priming of follicles may be responsible. On day 7 postpartum, suckled beef cows have lower serum concentrations and pulse frequencies of LH and FSH than nonsuckled animals (567). The FSH was measured by a homologous radioimmunoassay, but in another study in which a heterologous FSH assay was used, serum levels of the hormone were within the normal estrous range (569).

In summary, the suckling stimulus in the bovine alters the frequency of LH (and FSH?) pulses; consequently, follicular development is impaired. As one might anticipate, pulsatile injection of GNRH has been used to reverse this situation and to induce ovulation within 4 days of treatment of suckling cows (570).

Lactational anestrus in the sow usually lasts 6 weeks or longer and is, as usual, associated with altered follicular development. During the first 4 weeks of lactation, only 47% of the follicles >1 mm in diameter are normal, and the largest healthy follicles are <4 mm (571). Beginning at the sixth week, normal follicles comprise 64% of the population, and a few follicles begin to emerge that are ≥4 mm. On the day after weaning, there are numerous follicles <5 mm in diameter; by 4.8 days, the ovaries contain an average of 7 follicles >10 mm and 15 follicles 5 to 10 mm in diameter (572). Follicular development in the sow is therefore held in abeyance until the suckling stimulus is removed. Before weaning, serum FSH values are similar to those observed during the estrous cycle, whereas LH values are depressed (573). Serum PRL is elevated compared to cyclic values. Pigs ovariectomized 2 to 4 days after farrowing show a prompt increase in FSH throughout a 30-day period of lactation, while serum LH does not differ between ovariectomized and intact animals over this period (574). The divergent profiles evidently result from two different control mechanisms, with FSH being normally restrained in the intact sow by inhibin produced by the numerous 1- to 5-mm follicles present throughout the postpartum period. After weaning, significant increases in serum FSH and LH presumably are responsible for the rapid maturation of follicles (572). Weaning to estrous intervals range from 3 to 10 days, and PRL levels decline to basal concentration 1 to 2 hr after weaning (575). Both LH and FSH concentrations rose in the 12-hr postweaning period and an increase in pulse frequency per 12 hr was especially pronounced for LH. As a corollary to these results, pulsatile administration of GNRH to lactating sows 25 days postpartum is as effective as weaning in leading to fertile estrus within 4 days (576).

Although there is no morphological evidence on follicular growth during lactation in the primate, indirect monitoring of gonadotropins and steroid hormones indicates that suckling inhibits follicular development. For example, in lactating rhesus monkeys, weaning normally occurs 9 to 12 months postpartum. Under these circumstances, serum LH is low during the first 9 months and values typical of the follicular phase of the cycle are not attained until about 1 year (577). In the absence of a suckling stimulus, basal LH levels begin to rise after the first month. Serum FSH is also reduced during the first 6 months postpartum in lactating rhesus, and normal follicular levels are not attained until 10 months. LH surges cannot be consistently elicited by injection of estradiol benzoate until 10 months in lactating monkeys, whereas in nonsuckling females, they can be elicited within the first month postpartum. This included a group of cycling monkeys who served as foster mothers after being primed twice daily with thyrotropin-releasing hormone to become hyperprolactinemic. They responded to estradiol benzoate exactly like the normal postpartum suckling monkeys, ruling out pregnancy per se as the factor responsible for ovarian refractoriness in lactating animals.

In suckling or nonsuckling rhesus monkeys ovariectomized on day 24 or 25 postpartum, serum LH and FSH are suppressed by lactation (578). (Compare with results in the sow.) It is also noteworthy that pituitaries of lactating females contain only about 8% as much LH compared to a pool of pituitaries from cycling rhesus; FSH concentrations were similar between the two groups.

Basal serum PRL gradually falls in lactating rhesus but still runs at about 150 ng/ml from 60 to 180 days, whereas it declines drastically within 48 hr in nonsuckled monkeys (577). The diurnal rhythm of PRL secretion, which is absent during pregnancy, is resumed within the first week postpartum (579). These altered patterns of gonadotropin secretion associated with lactation are also reflected in low serum levels of estradiol and progesterone (577,579). In the former study, serum progesterone averaged 0.4 ± 0.1 ng/ml for up to 80 days postpartum, confirmatory evidence that suckling can partially "rejuvenate" the corpus luteum of pregnancy and restore some modicum of secretory activity, albeit at a low level. This is consistent with recent observations that bromocriptine administered to suckling monkeys curtails serum PRL and progesterone (580).

In women, lactation delays the onset of first ovulation but the duration and patterns of suckling stimulus are variables that confound the results (reviewed in refs. 581,582). No morphological studies are available, so that the extent to which follicular maturation is impaired is unknown. By 3 weeks after delivery, FSH levels are within the range of normal follicular values (583,584) and LH is reported to be within the normal range by 4 to 5 weeks (583). However, the pulsatile secretion of LH appears to be too low to induce estradiol secretion (584). Urinary estrogen is low in breast-feeding women until 40 weeks after delivery (582). The first ovulation in nonlactating women occurred between 43 and 87 days after delivery and was associated with increases in urinary pregnanediol or plasma progesterone (584). In the lactating group, there was no evidence of ovarian cyclicity until after weaning or after at least 150 days of lactation. After injection of 1 mg estradiol benzoate, a positive-feedback increase in LH, was still absent in 7 lactating women at 100 days postpartum. For the first 2 weeks after delivery, the response of non-nursing mothers, to GNRH is negative; this is followed by gradually increasing responsiveness, with FSH responding before LH (585). Similar results have been reported for lactating and nonlactating women, both showing similar normal profiles of FSH and LH in response to GNRH by 4 to 5 weeks postpartum (583).

Prolactin levels decline rapidly after delivery but are maintained by suckling in lactating women for long periods (see ref. 586). The question then is, With fairly early resumption of basal levels of FSH and LH and response to GNRH, why is follicular maturation delayed so long in lactating women? More data is needed before it can be resolved whether PRL, directly or indirectly, plays a role or whether changes in GNRH pulsatile release is the controlling factor in lactational amenorrhea (see ref. 587).

SUMMARY AND CONCLUSIONS

1. Knowledge of the nongrowing pool of follicles—the primordial stages—is still woefully lacking. The fact that primary follicles, the first step in follicular differentiation, are always present in rather constant numbers, and regardless of reproductive status, suggests that primordial follicles are recruited continuously on a daily basis. It is possible that their mobilization is random. On the other hand, proximity to nerve endings, blood vessels, larger follicles, or corpora lutea might conceivably influence their exit from the resting pool. There are even a few hints in the literature (e.g., ref. 61) that primordial follicles in the rat can be affected by gonadotropins. Whether primordial follicles enter the growing pool by chance or design, their time of transformation into primary follicles may be the decisive factor in deciding their ultimate fate. Gougeon has referred to "privileged follicles," which emerge at a time when critical changes in gonadotropin levels, e.g., the periovulatory period, may endow them with selective advantages for further normal differentiation. Gougeon believes that in the human, privileged status is bestowed on preantral follicles with 3 to 5 $\times$ 10^3 granulosa cells (class 1 follicles), whose development is initiated in the periovulatory window; these follicles develop a theca under the influence of high midcycle levels of LH. In the hamster, and other species as well, privileged follicles may involve still earlier stages in folliculogenesis: Primary follicles present on the morning of proestrus show dramatic increases in *in vitro* incorporation of [^{3}H]thymidine in response to the periovulatory increases in gonadotropins. It is therefore possible that hamster follicles developing in synchrony with surges of FSH and LH recurring every 4 days constitute the group selected to ovulate after 4 or 5 cycles of development.

2. It is often stated that primary and secondary follicles, i.e., preantral stages, are largely independent of gonadotropic support. Although species differences may well exist, a strong case can be made that laboratory rodents *are* dependent on gonadotropins—especially FSH—at early stages of folliculogenesis. The literature on this subject is difficult to interpret because so much is based on subjective evaluations. Some investigators have been more impressed by the qualitative ability of some preantral follicles to develop following hypophysectomy than the fact that the number is drastically reduced from intact animals. Careful quantitative studies are needed for a number of species focusing on follicular development (healthy and atretic) in the posthypophysectomy period and the recrudescence in response to FSH preparations. *In vitro* steroidogenesis by preantral fol-

licles from hypophysectomized versus that of intact animals would be another useful endpoint. However, there may very well be species differences in how far follicular development proceeds in the absence of gonadotropins.

3. An interesting finding of the past decade is the observation that regional differences exist in the granulosal compartment of antral follicles. This is reflected in distinct localization of peptide receptors, enzymes, steroidogenic potential, and presumably metabolic processes as well between the membrana granulosa and the cumulus oophorus. These structural and functional distinctions originate from the intimate relationship between the oocyte and its surrounding investment of granulosa cells. One wonders how early in the history of the preantral follicle can the future differences between cumulus and membrana granulosa be discerned. The different roles of the membrana granulosa and the cumulus-oocyte complex in the postovulatory period are obviously related to their different topographic and functional organizations in the maturing follicle.

4. Several lines of evidence show that in the rat and hamster the second periovulatory surge of FSH is responsible for the final recruitment of the large growing follicles that will ovulate 4 to 5 days later. This does not rule out the necessity of low tonic levels of LH since its neutralization in the hamster by anti-LH precipitates atresia in the face of normal serum levels of FSH. The role of the second FSH increase during the first few postovulatory days is less clear in species with long cycles. Is it also essential for the selection of the follicles that ultimately ovulate? Early in the cycle, follicles in the ewe and cow are 0.4 and 0.5 mm, respectively, and kinetic studies indicate that follicles in this size range grow in the course of the current cycle to become the ovulatory follicles. Is it possible that further differentiation of these follicles is influenced by the postestrous FSH peak? This is a difficult question to resolve experimentally; for example, in sheep, suppression of the second FSH peak by inhibin is usually followed by a rebound in FSH levels.

5. A wide variety of stimuli induce superovulation, including pituitary and placental gonadotropins, antisera to some steroids, antisera to inhibin, and clomiphene—an estrogen antagonist. It appears that highly pure FSH-like compounds (with high FSH:LH ratios) stimulate development of supernumerary follicles better than gonadotropins containing low FSH:LH ratios. However, in the hamster and guinea pig, continuous LH stimulation can induce spontaneous superovulation. Superovulation may result from a combination of recruitment of new follicles into the population and prevention of atresia of larger follicles; this may depend on the stage of the cycle that gonadotropic stimulus is provided. The mechanism of superovulation may also involve an increase in ovarian blood flow, and thus the delivery rate of essential nutrients for the sudden increase in follicular growth. The temporal changes in ovarian blood flow after a superovulatory stimulus are largely unknown. It is tempting to speculate that increases in ovarian blood flow parallel (or precede) increases in the number of follicles. Superovulation also involves stimulation of ovarian FSH and LH receptors. FSH's ability to increase granulosa cell division, aromatase activity, and LH receptor formation and LH's ability to stimulate thecal androgen production are instrumental in causing superovulation. Excessive LH stimulation (in the case of gonadotropins with low FSH:LH ratios) may in some species down-regulate LH receptors, reduce androgen secretion, and induce atresia of developing follicles. A better understanding of the mechanism(s) of superovulation ultimately will provide insight into the nature of superovulatory compounds, the appropriate timing of the stimuli, and the factors reducing the variability of the number of ova shed and increasing the quality of the ova.

6. Whether species have short or long cycles, the demise of luteal function accelerates follicular development and estrogen secretion. Thus, the main variable in determining the duration of the estrous cycle in the rat is whether the corpora lutea secrete progesterone for 2 or 3 days. The precision of the 4-day cycle of the hamster correlates with the rigid life span of the corpora lutea. The final impetus for follicular selection in the human is geared to luteolysis, which triggers a small, short-lived spurt of FSH. In the sheep and cow, the follicular phase is especially clearly demarcated by the spontaneous or induced regression of the corpus luteum. The luteal–follicular shift, therefore, is of paramount importance in the final selection of the ovulatory follicle(s) and is associated with progesterone withdrawal. In most cases, after luteolysis, baseline levels of FSH are unaffected, but LH increases as a consequence of an increased pulsatile release pattern. Although, I (G. S. Greenwald) have previously speculated that progesterone may directly affect follicular responsiveness, the overwhelming mass of evidence points to a classical inhibitory action on the hypothalamic–pituitary axis and, with the withdrawal of progesterone, increased secretion of LH. Presumably, the presence of higher titers of LH leads to increased secretion of androgens by the theca and concomitantly increases levels of estrogen and the development of a positive-feedback circuit in the now dominant follicles. According to this concept, although FSH is essential for the recruitment of the developing follicles (the cohort leading to the selection of the dominant follicles), the final maturation becomes more and more dependent on LH. This is also clearly shown in the pregnant rat, in which the maturation of the follicles destined to ovulate at postpartum estrus is brought about by rising titers of LH, beginning on day 20.

7. The estrous cycles of hamster, rat, and mouse usually recur at 4- to 5-day intervals, as compared with 18 to 22 days for sheep, pigs, and cows. One would intuitively assume that folliculogenesis proceeds at different rates depending on cycle length and indeed this is the case. For the laboratory rodents, it is estimated that about 3 weeks are required between the time a follicle enters the growing pool and ovulates. In contrast, similar estimates for the ewe are 6 months, and for the human, 85 days. Consequently, perturbations are quickly sensed and promptly responded to by

rodent follicular populations, as exemplified by their rapid mobilization after unilateral ovariectomy or administration of PMS—and their possible rapid onset of regression after hypophysectomy.

8. There is no evidence to support the concept of "waves" of follicular activity during cycles of long duration or pregnancy. In both situations, the population of primary follicles is continually replenished from the resting pool, and all stages of follicular growth are represented—from primary to tertiary. For example, in sheep and cow, estrogen-secreting antral follicles are present during the luteal phase, but their full development is held in check by progesterone, and the follicles wax and wane as their physiological life span is exceeded. A critical unanswered question is whether the follicles ultimately selected to ovulate at the end of pregnancy (rat) or the cycle (ewe) are ever exposed to elevated levels of FSH or whether they can mature after exposure to tonic levels of FSH but with increased levels of LH superimposed as the controlling factor. As previously mentioned, the concept of follicles emerging from the resting pool when FSH levels are high (in the immediate postovulatory period) may be the signal. For example, it takes about 21 days in the cyclic rat for a primary follicle to grow into a large preovulatory follicle. Is it merely coincidental that postpartum ovulation routinely occurs on day 23. Obviously, this line of reasoning does not apply to species with long gestation lengths.

9. Recent years have witnessed renewed interest in follicular degeneration based on models to induce atresia or investigations of the spontaneous event. Species seem to be divided into two categories in terms of the hormonal withdrawal pattern by antral follicles: in rodents, the loss of thecal androgen seems to precede the loss of granulosal aromatase activity, whereas in the ewe and human the reverse sequence exists. In both groups, the loss of estrogen secretion by the atretic follicle is the common denominator. The deficit in estrogen secretion in a young antral follicle presumably curtails mitoses in the granulosa cells, and the follicle therefore lags further and further behind. The question remains, however, whether the loss of estrogen (or androgen) production is a primary or secondary event in atresia of tertiary follicles. It is virtually impossible to answer this question by examining follicles undergoing spontaneous atresia because of the difficulty in pinpointing the moment when degeneration begins and determining the criteria for this early step. The histologic presence of a few pyknotic nuclei may be normal and of no consequence to a granulosa population of several thousand to million cells (depending on the species). By the time the follicle can definitely be classified as atretic, it is too late to establish causal relationships. Hence, it is our prejudice that experimental models in which atresia occurs as a timed, predictable event will be the only way to determine the prime mover. Although emphasis on atresia has focused on tertiary follicles, certainly the process is even more widespread in younger follicles, and entirely different mechanisms may be involved in their regression. A few studies have looked at FSH and LH receptors at the onset of atresia and found no differences in total numbers from normal follicles. A more meaningful endpoint may be the number of occupied receptors that are coupled to adenylate cyclase. We believe that a change distal to the peptide receptor may be the earliest signal of atresia.

The most dramatic histological signs of atresia occur in the granulosa cells, and consequently this compartment has received the most attention. The theca is the most resistant portion of the atretic follicle, and morphological alterations may not occur until several days after granulosa cells are affected. It is possible though—at least for rodents—that the theca may be the key to antral follicular development and atresia. Hisaw originally postulated that an "undeveloped" theca might be responsible for atresia. Although the morphological development of the theca in rodents may be normal, we suggest that biochemical "immaturity" may lead to atresia by impaired production of androgens, which in turn deprives the granulosa cells of substrate for conversion to estrogens. We base this belief on the pattern of steroidogenesis in induced and spontaneous atresia and the ability of exogenous LH to salvage the developing follicles that normally become atretic between days 3 and 4 of the hamster estrous cycle. This does not exclude an additional role for LH in recruiting more than the normal number of 20 developing follicles in the hamster. The critical factor in the final maturation of developing follicles may be the LH receptor level in theca interna cells. This may determine the ability of the cells to produce androstenedione and the vascularity of the theca. These two properties of the theca are so inextricably bound that it may be impossible to dissociate them. At present, however, it appears that the inception of atresia is not associated with decreases in vascularity, which may be a secondary event comparable to the sequence in luteolysis. Although the theca may be the pivotal tissue in rodent atresia, in other species the receptor deficiency may reside in the granulosa compartment involving LH and/or FSH receptors. Reasons for this possibility have been cited.

10. In this account, the follicle has largely been considered as an isolated component, uninfluenced by other ovarian compartments. The interrelationships between follicles and corpora lutea, follicles and interstitium have been barely touched. Moreover, do tertiary follicles affect preantral stages if they share a common vascular supply? Coculture of these various tissues might be a rewarding approach.

11. Follicular development during lactation is impaired because of altered pulsatile release of LH and elevated levels of PRL. The problem of hormonal control during lactation is also complicated by species differences. What remains to be established are the relative roles of GNRH and PRL and how much of their effects are exerted indirectly or directly at the ovarian level.

12. Fifteen years ago, one could confidently predict that *in vitro* studies of antral follicles, granulosa, and thecal cells and peptide receptor distribution and follicular kinetics would

be profitable areas of investigation. It is also equally obvious that molecular biology—an area untouched in this review—will have significant impact on the problems of folliculogenesis, as will the *in vitro* effects of growth factors interacting with peptide and steroid hormones. It is worth reiterating, however, that more classical techniques still have a great deal to offer in this field and should not be neglected or discarded.

ACKNOWLEDGMENTS

The original work of the authors included in this chapter was supported by NIH Grants HD00596-25 (G.S.G.) and HDK00478 and HD20389 (P.F.T.). We thank Mrs. Darlene Limback for help in assembling the bibliography and Mrs. Linda Carr for typing the manuscript.

REFERENCES

1. Greenwald, G. S. (1972): Editorial. Of eggs and follicles. *Am. J. Anat.*, 135:1–4.
2. Hisaw, F. L. (1947): Development of the graafian follicle and ovulation. *Physiol. Rev.*, 27:95–119.
3. Brambell, F. W. R. (1956): Ovarian changes. In: *Marshall's Physiology of Reproduction* edited by A. S. Parkes, pp. 397–542. Longmans, Green, New York.
4. Falck, B. (1959): Site of production of oestrogen in rat ovary as studied in micro-transplants. *Acta Physiol. Scand. Suppl. 163*, 47:5–101.
5. Greenwald, G. S. (1974): Role of follicle-stimulating hormone and luteinizing hormone in follicular development and ovulation. In: *Handbook of Physiology/Endocrinology, Vol. 4: Part 2,* edited by E. Knobil and W. H. Sawyer, pp. 293–323. American Physiological Society, Washington, D.C.
6. Channing, C. P., and Tsafriri, A. (1977): Mechanism of action of luteinizing hormone and follicle-stimulating hormone on the ovary in vitro. *Metabolism,* 26:413–468.
7. Lindner, H. R., Amsterdam, A., Salomon, Y., et al. (1977): Intraovarian factors in ovulation: determinants of follicular response to gonadotrophins. *J. Reprod. Fertil.*, 51:215–235.
8. Armstrong, D. T., and Dorrington, J. H. (1977): Estrogen biosynthesis in the ovaries and testes. In: *Regulatory Mechanisms Affecting Gonadal Hormone Action,* edited by J. A. Thomas and R. H. Singhal, pp. 215–258. University Park Press, Baltimore.
9. Richards, J. S. (1980): Maturation of ovarian follicles: actions and interactions of pituitary and ovarian hormones on follicular cell differentiation. *Physiol. Rev.*, 60:51–89.
10. diZerega, G. S., and Hodgen, G. D. (1981): Folliculogenesis in the primate ovarian cycle. *Endocrine Rev.*, 2:27–49.
11. Erickson, G. F. (1983): Primary cultures of ovarian cells in serum-free medium as models of hormone-dependent differentiation. *Mol. Cell. Endocrinol.*, 29:21–49.
12. Hsueh, A. J. W., Adashi, E. Y., Jones, P. B. C., and Welsh, T. H., Jr. (1984): Hormonal regulation of the differentiation of cultured ovarian granulosa cells. *Endocrine Rev.*, 5:76–127.
13. Tsafriri, A., and Braw, R. H. (1984): Experimental approaches to atresia in mammals. *Oxford Rev. Reprod. Biol.*, 6:226–265.
14. Hillier, S. G. (1985): Sex steroid metabolism and follicular development in the ovary. *Oxford Rev. Reprod. Biol.*, 7:168–222.
15. Zuckerman, S. S., and Weir, B. J., eds. (1977): *The Ovary, 2nd ed.* Academic, New York.
16. Jones, R. E., ed. (1978): *The Vertebrate Ovary. Comparative Biology and Evolution.* Plenum, New York.
17. Crighton, D. B., Foxcroft, G. R., Haynes, N. B., and Lamming, G. E. (1978): *Control of Ovulation.* Butterworths, Boston.
18. Midgley, A. R., Jr., and Sadler, W. A., eds. (1979): *Ovarian Follicular Development and Function.* Raven Press, New York.
19. Channing, C. P., Marsh, J. M., and Sadler, W. A., eds. (1979): *Ovarian Follicular and Corpus Luteum Function.* Plenum, New York.
20. Edwards, R. G. (1980): *Conception in the Human Female.* Academic, New York.
21. Motta, P. M., and Hafez, E. S. E., eds. (1980): *Biology of the Ovary.* Martinus Nijhoff Publishers, The Hague.
22. Schwartz, N. B., and Hunzicker-Dunn, M., eds. (1981): *Dynamics of Ovarian Function.* Raven Press, New York.
23. Channing, C. P., and Segal, S. J., eds. (1982): *Intraovarian Control Mechanisms.* Plenum, New York.
24. Greenwald, G. S., and Terranova, P. F., eds. (1983): *Factors Regulating Ovarian Function.* Raven Press, New York.
25. Austin, C. R., and Short, R. V., eds. (1982–84): *Reproduction in Mammals, 2nd ed.* Cambridge University Press, New York.
26. Lamming, G. E., ed. (1984): *Marshall's Physiology of Reproduction. Vol. 1, 4th Ed., Reproductive Cycles of Vertebrates.* Churchill Livingstone, New York.
27. Guraya, S. S. (1985): *Biology of Ovarian Follicles in Mammals.* Springer-Verlag, New York.
28. Toft, D. O., and Ryan, R. J., eds. (1985): *Proceedings of the Fifth Ovarian Workshop.* Ovarian Workshops, Champaign, IL.
29. Mauleon, P. (1967): Cinetique de l'ovogenese chez les mammiferes. *Arch. Anat. Microsc. Morphol. Exp.*, 56:125–150.
30. Gerard, P., and Herlant, M. (1953): Sur la persistance de phenomenes d'oogenese chez les lemuriens adultes. *Arch. Biol.*, 64:97–111.
31. Peters, H., Byskov, A. G., and Faber, M. (1973): Intraovarian regulation of follicle growth in the immature mouse. In: *The Development and Maturation of the Ovary and its Functions,* edited by H. Peters, pp. 20–23. Excerpta Medica, Amsterdam.
32. Lunenfeld, B., Kraiem, Z., and Eshkol, A. (1975): The function of the growing follicle. *J. Reprod. Fertil.*, 45:567–574.
33. Peters, H. (1969): The development of the mouse ovary from birth to maturity. *Acta Endocrinol.*, 62:98–116.
34. de Wolff-Exalto, E. A. (1982): Influence of gonadotrophins on early follicle cell development and early oocyte growth in the immature rat. *J. Reprod. Fertil.*, 66:537–542.
35. Hage, A. J., Groen-Klevant, A. C., and Welschen, R. (1978): Follicle growth in the immature rat ovary. *Acta Endocrinol.*, 88:375–382.
36. Uilenbroek, J. T. J., de Wolff-Exalto, E. A., and Blankenstein, M. A. (1976): Serum gonadotrophins and follicular development in immature rats after early androgen administration. *J. Endocrinol.*, 68: 461–468.
37. Vomachka, A. J., and Greenwald, G. S. (1979): The development of gonadotropin and steroid hormone patterns in male and female hamsters from birth to puberty. *Endocrinology,* 105:960–966.
38. Krarup, T., Pedersen, T., and Faber, M. (1969): Regulation of oocyte growth in the mouse ovary. *Nature,* 224:187–188.
39. Gosden, R. G., Laing, S. C., Felicio, L. S., Nelson, J. F., and Finch, C. E. (1983): Imminent oocyte exhaustion and reduced follicular recruitment mark the transition to acyclicity in aging C57BL/6J mice. *Biol. Reprod.*, 28:255–260.
40. Mandl, A. M., and Shelton, M. (1959): A quantitative study of oocytes in young and old nulliparous laboratory rats. *J. Endocrinol.*, 18:444–450.
41. Block, E. (1952): Quantitative morphological investigations of the follicular system in women. Variations at different ages. *Acta Anat.*, 14:108–123.
42. Gougeon, A. (1981): Cinetique de la croissance et de l'involution des follicules ovariens pendant le cycle menstruel chez la femme. Thesis, Université Pierre and Marie Curie.
43. Koering, M. J. (1983): Preantral follicle development during the menstrual cycle in the *Macaca mulatta* ovary. *Am. J. Anat.*, 166:429–433.
44. Mauleon, P., and Rao, K. H. (1963): Variations genetiques des populations foliculaires dans les ovaires de rates impuberes. *Ann. Biol. Anim. Bioch. Biophys.*, 3:21–31.
45. Mauleon, P., and Pelletier, J. (1964): Variations genetiques du fonctionnement hypophysaire de trois souches de rattes immatures, relations avec la fertilite. *Ann. Biol. Anim. Bioch. Biophys.*, 4:105–112.
46. Merchant, H. (1975): Rat gonadal and ovarian organogenesis with and without germ cells. An ultrastructural study. *Dev. Biol.*, 44:1–21.

47. Merchant-Larios, H., and Centeno, B. (1981): Morphogenesis of the ovary from the sterile W/Wv mouse. In: *Eleventh International Congress of Anatomy: Advances in the Morphology of Cells and Tissues,* pp. 383–392. Liss, New York.
48. Pedersen, T. (1970): Follicle kinetics in the ovary of the cyclic mouse. *Acta Endocrinol.,* 64:304–323.
49. Butcher, R. L., and Kirkpatrick-Keller, D. (1984): Patterns of follicular growth during the four-day estrous cycle of the rat. *Biol. Reprod.,* 31:280–286.
50. Pedersen, T., and Peters, H. (1971): Follicle growth and cell dynamics in the mouse ovary during pregnancy. *Fertil. Steril.,* 22:42–52.
51. Groen-Klevant, A. C. (1981): An autoradiographic study of follicle growth in the ovaries of cyclic rats. *Acta Endocrinol.,* 96:377–381.
52. Greenwald, G. S. (1974): Quantitative aspects of follicular development in the untreated and PMS-treated cyclic hamster. *Anat. Rec.,* 178:139–143.
53. Chiras, D. D., and Greenwald, G. S. (1980): Analysis of ovarian follicular development and thymidine incorporation in the cyclic golden hamster. *Am. J. Anat.,* 157:309–317.
54. Roy, S. K., and Greenwald, G. S. (1986): Quantitative analysis of in vitro incorporation of [^{3}H] thymidine into hamster follicles during the oestrous cycle. *J. Reprod. Fertil.,* 77:143–152.
55. Zarrow, M. X., and Wilson, E. D. (1961): The influence of age on superovulation in the immature rat and mouse. *Endocrinology,* 69:851–855.
56. Welschen, R., and Rutte, M. (1971): Ovulation in adult rats after treatment with pregnant mare serum gonadotrophin during oestrus. *Acta Endocrinol.,* 68:41–49.
57. Greenwald, G. S. (1962): Analysis of superovulation in the adult hamster. *Endocrinology,* 71:378–389.
58. Chiras, D. D., and Greenwald, G. S. (1978): Ovarian follicular development in cyclic hamsters treated with a superovulatory dose of pregnant mare's serum. *Biol. Reprod.,* 19:895–901.
59. Lane, C. E., and Greep, R. O. (1935): The follicular apparatus of the ovary of the hypophysectomized immature rat and the effects of hypophyseal gonadotropic hormones on it. *Anat. Rec.,* 63:139–146.
60. Paesi, F. J. A. (1949): The influence of hypophysectomy and of subsequent treatment with chorionic gonadotrophin on follicles of different size in the ovary of the rat. *Acta Endocrinol.,* 3:89–104.
61. De Reviers, M. M. (1974): Étude quantitative de l'action des hormones gonadotropes hypophysaires sur la population folliculaire de l'ovaire de ratte immature—signification biologique du dosage de l'hormone folliculo-stimulante par le test de Steelman et Pohley. Thesis, L'Université de Tours.
62. Edwards, R. G., Fowler, R. E., Gore-Langton, R. E., Gosden, R. G., Jones, E. C., Readhead, C., and Steptoe, P. C. (1977): Normal and abnormal follicular growth in mouse, rat and human ovaries. *J. Reprod. Fertil.,* 51:237–263.
63. Kim, I., Shaha, C., and Greenwald, G. S. (1984): A species difference between hamster and rat in the effect of oestrogens on growth of large preantral follicles. *J. Reprod. Fertil.,* 72:179–185.
64. Nakano, R., Mizuno, T., Katayama, K., and Tojo, S. (1975): Growth of ovarian follicles in rats in the absence of gonadotrophins. *J. Reprod. Fertil.,* 45:545–546.
65. Hirshfield, A. N. (1985): Comparison of granulosa cell proliferation in small follicles of hypophysectomized, prepubertal, and mature rats. *Biol. Reprod.,* 32:979–987.
66. Faddy, M. J. E., Jones, E. C., and Edwards, R. G. (1976): An analytical model for ovarian follicle dynamics. *J. Exp. Zool.,* 197:173–185.
67. Oakberg, E. F. (1979): Follicular growth and atresia in the mouse. *In Vitro,* 15:41–49.
68. Moore, P. J., and Greenwald, G. S. (1974): Effect of hypophysectomy and gonadotropin treatment on follicular development and ovulation in the hamster. *Am J. Anat.,* 139:37–48.
69. Garza, F., Shaban, M. A., and Terranova, P. F. (1984): Luteinizing hormone increases the number of ova shed in the cyclic hamster and guinea-pig. *J. Endocrinol.,* 101:289–298.
70. Kim, I., and Greenwald, G. S. (1986): Occupied and unoccupied FSH receptors in follicles of cyclic, hypophysectomized or hypophysectomized/gonadotropin-treated hamsters. *Mol. Cell. Endocrinol.,* 44:141–145.
71. Dempsey, E. W. (1937): Follicular growth rate and ovulation after various experimental procedures in the guinea pig. *Am. J. Physiol.,* 120:126–132.
72. Perry, J. S., and Rowlands, I. W. (1963): Hypophysectomy of the immature guinea-pig and the ovarian response to gonadotrophins. *J. Reprod. Fertil.,* 6:393–404.
73. Dufour, J., Cahill, L. P. and Mauleon, P. (1979): Short- and long-term effects of hypophysectomy and unilateral ovariectomy on ovarian follicular populations in sheep. *J. Reprod. Fertil.,* 57:301–309.
74. Goldenberg, R. L., Powell, R. D., Rosen, S. W., Marshall, J. R., and Ross, G. T. (1976): Ovarian morphology in women with anosmia and hypogonadotropic hypogonadism. *Am. J. Obstet. Gynecol.,* 126:91–94.
75. Lim, H. T., Meinders, A. E., deHaan, L. D., and Bronkhorst, F. B. (1984): Anovulation presumably due to the gonadotrophin-resistant ovary syndrome. *Eur. J. Obstet. Gynecol. Reprod. Biol.,* 16:327–337.
76. Talbert, L. M., Raj, M. H. G., Hammond, M. G., and Greer, T. (1984): Endocrine and immunologic studies in a patient with resistant ovary syndrome. *Fert. Steril.,* 42:741–744.
77. Lintern-Moore, S., and Moore, G. P. M. (1977): Comparative aspects of oocyte growth in mammals. In: *Reproduction and Evolution. Proceedings of the Fourth Symposium on Comparative Biology of Reproduction, Canberra, December 1976,* edited by J. H. Calaby and C. H. Tyndale-Biscoe, pp. 215–219. Australian Academy of Science, Canberra City.
78. Lintern-Moore, S., and Moore, G. P. M. (1979): The initiation of follicle and oocyte growth in the mouse ovary. *Biol. Reprod.,* 20:773–778.
79. Moore, G. P. M., Lintern-Moore, S., Peters, H., and Faber, M. (1974): RNA synthesis in the mouse oocyte. *J. Cell Biol.,* 60:416–422.
80. Canipari, R., Pietrolucci, A., and Mangia, F. (1979): Increase of total protein synthesis during mouse oocyte growth. *J. Reprod. Fertil.,* 57:405–413.
81. Muller, U., and Urban, E. (1981): An oocyte-specific antigen and its possible role in the organization of the ovarian follicle of the rat. *Differentiation,* 20:274–277.
82. Takaoka, H., Satoh, H., Makinoda, S., Moriya, S., and Ichinoe, K. (1985): Granulosa-cell growth factor in oocyte and its transport systems. *Acta Obstet. Gynaecol. Jpn.,* 37:92–98.
83. Hirshfield, A. N. (1986): Patterns of [^{3}H] thymidine incorporation differ in immature rats and mature, cycling rats. *Biol. Reprod.,* 34:229–235.
84. Cran, D. G., Moor, R. M., and Hay, M. F. (1980): Fine structure of the sheep oocyte during antral follicle development. *J. Reprod. Fertil.,* 59:125–132.
85. Tesoriero, J. V. (1984): Comparative cytochemistry of the developing ovarian follicles of the dog, rabbit, and mouse: origin of the zona pellucida. *Gamete Res.,* 10:301–318.
86. Shimizu, S., Tsuji, M., and Dean, J. (1983): In vitro biosynthesis of three sulfated glycoproteins of murine zonae pellucidae by oocytes grown in follicle culture. *J. Biol. Chem.,* 258:5858–5863.
87. Colonna, R., and Mangia, R. (1983): Mechanisms of amino acid uptake in cumulus-enclosed mouse oocytes. *Biol. Reprod.,* 28:797–803.
88. Wassarman, P. M., Bleil, J. D., Cascio, S. M., LaMarca, M. J., Letourneau, G. E., Mrozak, S. C., and Schultz, R. M. (1981): Programming of gene expression during mammalian oogenesis. In: *Bioregulators of Reproduction,* edited by G. Jagiello and H. J. Vogel, pp. 119–150. Academic, New York.
89. Dunbar, B. S. (1983): Morphological, biochemical, and immunochemical characterization of the mammalian zona pellucida. In: *Mechanism and Control of Animal Fertilization,* pp. 139–175. Academic, New York.
90. Wolgemuth, D. J., Celenza, J., Bundman, D. S., and Dunbar, B. S. (1984): Formation of the rabbit zona pellucida and its relatioship to ovarian follicular development. *Dev. Biol.,* 106: 1–14.
91. Skinner, S. M., Mills, T., Kirchick, H. J., and Dunbar, B. S. (1984): Immunization with zona pellucida proteins results in abnormal ovarian follicular differentiation and inhibition of gonadotropin-induced steroid secretion. *Endocrinology,* 115:2418–2432.

92. Michael, S. D. (1983): Interactions of the thymus and the ovary. In: *Factors Regulating Ovarian Function,* edited by G. S. Greenwald and P. F. Terranova, pp. 445–464. Raven, New York.
93. Lane, C. E., and Davis, F. R. (1939): The ovary of the adult rat. I. Changes in growth of the follicle and in volume and mitotic activity of the granulosa and theca during the estrous cycle. *Anat. Rec.,* 73:429–442.
94. Ax, R. L., and Ryan, R. J. (1979): The porcine ovarian follicle. IV. Mucopolysaccharides at different stages of development. *Biol. Reprod.,* 20:1123–1132.
95. Yanagishita, M., Rodbard, D., and Hascall, V. C. (1979): Isolation and characterization of proteoglycans from porcine ovarian follicular fluid. *J. Biol. Chem.,* 254:911–920.
96. Schweitzer, M., Jackson, J. C., and Ryan, R. J. (1981): The porcine ovarian follicle. VII. FSH stimulation of in vitro [^{3}H]-glucosamine incorporation into mucopolysaccharides. *Biol. Reprod.,* 24:332–340.
97. Burghardt, R. C., and Anderson, E. (1981): Hormonal modulation of gap junctions in rat ovarian follicles. *Cell Tissue Res.,* 214:181–193.
98. Larsen, W. J., Tung, H. N., and Polking, C. (1981): Response of granulosa cell gap junctions to human chorionic gonadotropin (hCG) at ovulation. *Biol. Reprod.,* 25:1119–1134.
99. Fletcher, W. H., and Greenan, J. R. T. (1985): Receptor mediated action without receptor occupancy. *Endocrinology,* 116:1660–1662.
100. Hay, M. F., and Moor, R. M. (1975): Distribution of Δ5-3β-hydroxysteroid dehydrogenase activity in the graafian follicle of the sheep. *J. Reprod. Fertil.,* 43:313–322.
101. Cran, D. G., Hay, M. F., and Moor, R. M. (1979): The fine structure of the cumulus oophorus during follicular development in sheep. *Cell Tissue Res.,* 202:439–451.
102. Mestwerdt, W., and Muller, O. (1978): Elektronenoptisch-morphometrische Untersuchungen zum Luteinisierungsprozess der Follikelgranulosazelle menschlicher Ovarien. *Arch. Gynaekol.,* 225: 51–65.
103. Bomsel-Helmreich, O., Gougeon, A., Thebault, A., Saltarelli, D., Milgrom, E., Frydman, R., and Papiernik, E. (1979): Healthy and atretic human follicles in the preovulatory phase: differences in evolution of follicular morphology and steroid content of follicular fluid. *J. Clin. Endocrinol. Metabol.,* 48:686–694.
104. Amin, H., Richart, R. M., and Brinson, A. O. (1976): Preovulatory granulosa cells and steroidogenesis. An ultrastructural study in the rhesus monkey. *Obstet. Gynecol.,* 47:562–568.
105. Zoller, L. C. (1984): A comparison of rat and hamster preovulatory follicles: an examination of differences in morphology and enzyme activity using qualitative and quantitative analyses. *Anat. Rec.,* 210:279–291.
106. Bjersing, L. (1978): Maturation, morphology, and endocrine function of the follicular wall in mammals. In: *The Vertebrate Ovary. Comparative Biology and Evolution,* edited by R. E. Jones, pp. 181–214. Plenum, New York.
107. Fortune, J. E. (1986): Bovine theca and granulosa cells interact to promote androgen production. *Biol. Reprod.,* 35:292–299.
108. Makris, A., Olsen, D., and Ryan, K. J. (1983): Significance of the Δ5 and Δ4 steroidogenic pathways in the hamster preovulatory follicle. *Steroids,* 42:641–651.
109. Weisz, J., and Zoller, L. C. (1979): Quantitative cytochemistry in the study of regional specialization in the membrana granulosa of the ovulable type of follicle. In: *Quantitative Cytochemistry and Its Applications,* edited by J. R. Pattison, L. Bitensky, and J. Chayen, pp. 269–283. Academic, New York.
110. Zoller, L. C., and Weisz, J. (1979): A quantitative cytochemical study of glucose-6-phosphate dehydrogenase and Δ5-3β-hydroxysteroid dehydrogenase activity in the membrana granulosa of the ovulable type of follicle of the rat. *Histochemistry,* 62:125–135.
111. Zoller, L. C., and Enelow, R. (1983): A quantitative histochemical study of lactate dehydrogenase and succinate dehydrogenase activities in the membrana granulosa of the ovulatory follicle of the rat. *Histochem. J.,* 15:1055–1064.
112. Hillensjo, T., Magnusson, C., Svensson, U., and Thelander, H. (1981): Effect of luteinizing hormone and follicle-stimulating hormone on progesterone synthesis by cultured rat cumulus cells. *Endocrinology,* 108:1920–1924.
113. Erickson, G. F., Hofeditz, C., Unger, M., Allen, W. R., and Dulbecco, R. (1985): A monoclonal antibody to a mammary cell line recognizes two distinct subtypes of ovarian granulosa cells. *Endocrinology,* 117:1490–1499.
114. Staigmiller, R. B., and Moor, R. M. (1984): Effect of follicle cells on the maturation and developmental competence of ovine oocytes matured outside the follicle. *Gamete Res.,* 9:221–229.
115. Charlton, H. M., Parry, D., Halpin, D. M. G., and Webb, R. (1982): Distribution of ^{125}I-labelled follicle-stimulating hormone and human chorionic gonadotrophin in the gonads of hypogonadal (hpg) mice. *J. Endocrinol.,* 93:247–252.
116. Armstrong, D. T., Weiss, T. J., Selstam, G., and Seamark, R. F. (1981): Hormonal and cellular interactions in follicular steroid biosynthesis by the sheep ovary. *J. Reprod. Fertil. Suppl.,* 30:143–154.
117. Channing, C. P., Schaerf, F. W., Anderson, L. D., and Tsafriri, A. (1980): Ovarian follicular and luteal physiology. In: *Reproductive Physiology. III. International Review of Physiology,* edited by R. O. Greep, pp. 117–201. University Park Press, Baltimore.
118. Nakano, R., Sasaki, K., Shima, K., and Kitayama, S. (1983): Follicle-stimulating hormone and luteinizing hormone receptors on porcine granulosa cells during follicular maturation: an autoradiographic study. *Exp. Clin. Endocrinol.,* 81:17–23.
119. Uilenbroek J. T. J., and Richards, J. S. (1979): Ovarian follicular development during the rat estrous cycle: gonadotropin receptors and follicular responsiveness. *Biol. Reprod.,* 20:1159–1165.
120. Amsterdam, A., Koch, Y., Lieberman, M. E., and Lindner, H. R. (1975): Distribution of binding sites for human chorionic gonadotropin in the preovulatory follicle of the rat. *J. Cell. Biol.,* 67:894–900.
121. Lawrence, T. S., Dekel, N., and Beers, W. H. (1980): Binding of human chorionic gonadotropin by rat cumuli oophori and granulosa cells: a comparative study. *Endocrinology,* 106:1114–1118.
122. Bortolussi, M., Marini, G., and Reolon, M. L. (1979): A histochemical study of the binding of ^{125}I-HCG to the rat ovary throughout the estrous cycle. *Cell Tissue Res.,* 197:213–226.
123. Oxberry, B. A., and Greenwald, G. S. (1982): An autoradiographic study of the binding of ^{125}I-labeled follicle-stimulating hormone, human chorionic gonadotropin and prolactin to the hamster ovary throughout the estrous cycle. *Biol. Reprod.,* 27:505–516.
124. Roy, S. K., and Greenwald, G. S. (1985): Evidence for binding sites for FSH and hCG in mammalian oocytes. In: *Proceedings of the Fifth Ovarian Workshop,* edited by D. O. Toft and R. J. Ryan, pp. 143–147. Ovarian Workshops, Champaign, IL.
125. Niimura, S., and Ishida, K. (1983): Histochemical demonstration of hydroxysteroid dehydrogenases in the oocytes in antral follicles of pigs, cattle and horses. *Jpn. J. Anim. Reprod.,* 29:150–153.
126. Hiura, M., and Fujita, H. (1977): Electron microscopy of the cytodifferentiation of the theca cell in the mouse ovary. *Arch. Histol. Jpn.,* 40:95–105.
127. O'Shea, J. D. (1970): An ultrastructural study of smooth muscle-like cells in the theca externa of ovarian follicles in the rat. *Anat. Rec.,* 167:127–140.
128. Amsterdam, A., Lindner, H. R., and Stewart, U. G. (1977): Localization of actin and myosin in the rat oocyte and follicular wall by immunofluorescence. *Anat. Rec.,* 187:311–328.
129. Capps, M. L., Lawrence, I. E., Jr., and Burden, H. W. (1981): Cellular junctions in perifollicular contractile tissue of the rat ovary during the preovulatory period. *Cell Tissue Res.,* 219:133–141.
130. Walles, B., Edvinsson, L., Owman, C., Sjoberg, N. O., and Sporrong, B. (1976): Cholinergic nerves and receptors mediating contraction of the graafian follicle. *Biol. Reprod.,* 15:565–572.
131. Kobayashi, Y., Sjoberg, N. O., Walles, B., Owman, C., Wright, K. H., Santulli, R., and Wallach, E. E. (1983): The effect of adrenergic agents on the ovulatory process in the in vitro perfused rabbit ovary. *Am. J. Obstet. Gynecol.,* 145:857–864.
132. Wylie, S. N., Roche, P. J., and Gibson, W. R. (1985): Ovulation after sympathetic denervation of the rat ovary produced by freezing its nerve supply. *J. Reprod. Fertil.,* 75:369–373.
133. Stoklosowa, S., Gregoraszczuk, E., and Channing, C. P. (1982): Estrogen and progesterone secretion by isolated cultured porcine thecal and granulosa cells. *Biol. Reprod.,* 26:943–952.
134. Merk, F. B., Albright, J. T., and Botticelli, C. R. (1973): The fine structure of granulosa cell nexuses in rat ovarian follicles. *Anat. Rec.,* 175:107–126.
135. Kranzfelder, D., Korr, H., Mestwerdt, W., and Maurer-Schultze, B. (1984): Follicle growth in the ovary of the rabbit after ovulation-

inducing application of human chorionic gonadotropin. *Cell. Tissue Res.*, 238:611–620.

136. Makris, A., Klagsbrun, M. A., Yasumizu, T., and Ryan, K. J. (1983): An endogenous ovarian growth factor which stimulates BALB/3T3 and granulosa cell proliferation. *Biol. Reprod.*, 29:1135–1141.
137. O'Shea, J. D., Cran, D. G., Hay, M. F., and Moor, R. M. (1978): Ultrastructure of the theca interna of ovarian follicles in sheep. *Cell Tissue Res.*, 187:457–472.
138. Priedkalns, J., Weber, A. F., and Zemjanis, R. (1968): Qualitative and quantitative morphological studies of the cells of the membrana granulosa, theca interna and corpus luteum of the bovine ovary. *Z. Zellforsch.*, 85:501–520.
139. Wordinger, R. J., Rudick, V. L., and Rudick, M. J. (1983): Immunohistochemical localization of laminin within the mouse ovary. *J. Exp. Zool.*, 228:141–143.
140. Roy, S. K., and Greenwald, G. S. (1985): An enzymatic method for dissociation of intact follicles from the hamster ovary: histological and quantitative aspects. *Biol. Reprod.*, 32:203–215.
141. Stoklosowa, S., Bahr, J., and Gregoraszczuk, E. (1978): Some morphological and functional characteristics of cells of the porcine theca interna in tissue culture. *Biol. Reprod.*, 19:712–719.
142. Tsang, B. K., Ainsworth, L., Downey, B. R., and Marcus, G. J. (1985): Differential production of steroids by dispersed granulosa and theca interna cells from developing preovulatory follicles of pigs. *J. Reprod. Fertil.*, 74:459–471.
143. Katayama, E. (1984): Monolayer culture of human ovarian thecal cells—A study on morphological and functional characteristics. *Acta Obstet. Gynaecol. Jpn.*, 36:927–936.
144. Bogovich, K., and Richards, J. S. (1984): Androgen synthesis during follicular development: evidence that rat granulosa cell 17-ketosteroid reductase is independent of hormonal regulation. *Biol. Reprod.*, 31:122–131.
145. Koninckx, P. R. (1981): New aspects of ovarian function in man and in rat. Thesis, Katholieke Universiteit Leuven, Leuven.
146. diZerega, G. S., and Hodgen, G. D. (1980): Fluorescence localization of luteinizing hormone/human chorionic gonadotropin uptake in the primate ovary. II. Changing distribution during selection of the dominant follicle. *J. Clin. Endocrinol. Metab.*, 51:903–907.
147. Bassett, D. L. (1943): The changes in the vascular pattern of the ovary of the albino rat during the estrous cycle. *Am. J. Anat.*, 73:251–291.
148. Zeleznik, A. J., Schuler, H. M., and Reichert, L. E., Jr. (1981): Gonadotropin-binding sites in the rhesus monkey ovary: role of the vasculature in the selective distribution of human chorionic gonadotropin to the preovulatory follicle. *Endocrinology,* 109:356–362.
149. McNatty, K. P., Heath, D. A., Lun, S., Fannin, J. M., McDiarmid, J. M., and Henderson, K. M. (1984): Steroidogenesis by bovine theca interna in an in vitro perifusion system. *Biol. Reprod.*, 30:159–170.
150. Koos, R. D., and LeMaire, W. J. (1983): Factors that may regulate the growth and regression of blood vessels in the ovary. *Semin. Reprod. Endocrinol.*, 1:295–307.
151. Frederick, J. L., Shimanuki, T., and diZerega, G. S. (1984): Initiation of angiogenesis by human follicular fluid. *Science,* 224:389–390.
152. Frederick, J. L., Nuguyen, H., Preston, D. S., Frederick, J. J., Campeau, J. D., Ono, T., and diZerega, G. S. (1985): Initiation of angiogenesis by porcine follicular fluid. *Am. J. Obstet. Gynecol.*, 152:1073–1078.
153. Gospodarowicz, D., Cheng, J., Lui, G. M., Baird, A., Esch, F., and Bohlen, P. (1985): Corpus luteum angiogenic factor is related to fibroblast growth factor. *Endocrinology,* 117:2283–2391.
154. Makris, A., Ryan, K. J., Takehiko, Y., Hill, C. L., and Zetter, B. R. (1984): The nonluteal porcine ovary as a source of angiogenic activity. *Endocrinology,* 15:1672–1677.
155. Saidapur, S. K. (1978): Follicular atresia in the ovaries of nonmammalian vertebrates. *Int. Rev. Cytol.*, 54:225–244.
156. Byskov, A. G. (1978): Follicular atresia. In: *The Vertebrate Ovary. Comparative Biology and Evolution,* edited by R. E. Jones, pp. 533–562. Plenum, New York.
157. Ingram, D. L. (1962): Atresia. In: *The Ovary,* edited by S. S. Zuckerman, A. M. Mandl, and P. Eckstein, pp. 247–273. Academic, New York.
158. Spanel-Borowski, K. (1981): Morphological investigations on follicular atresia in canine ovaries. *Cell Tisue Res.*, 214:155–168.
159. Byskov, A. G. S. (1974): Cell kinetic studies of follicular atresia in the mouse ovary. *J. Reprod. Fertil.*, 37:277–285.
160. Brailly, S., Gougeon, A., Milgrom, E., Bomsel-Helmreich, O., and Papiernik, E. (1981): Androgens and progestins in the human ovarian follicle: differences in the evolution of preovulatory, healthy nonovulatory, and atretic follicles. *J. Clin. Endocrinol. Metab.*, 53: 128–133.
161. Westergaard, L., McNatty, K. P., Christensen, I., Larsen, J. K., and Byskov, A. G. (1982): Flow cytometric deoxyribonucleic acid analysis of granulosa cells aspirated from human ovarian follicles. A new method to distinguish healthy and atretic ovarian follicles. *J. Clin. Endocrinol. Metab.*, 55:693–698.
162. Koering, M. J., Goodman, A. L., Williams, R. F., and Hodgen, G. D. (1982): Granulosa cell pyknosis in the dominant follicle of monkeys. *Fert. Steril.*, 37:837–844.
163. Odeblad, E. (1952): Contributions to the theory and technique of quantitative autoradiography with ^{32}P with special reference to the granulosa tissue of the graafian follicles in the rabbit. *Acta Radiol. (Stockh.) Suppl.*, 93:1–123.
164. Deane, H. W. (1952): Histochemical observations on the ovary and oviduct of the albino rat during the estrous cycle. *Am. J. Anat.*, 91:363–414.
165. Bukovsky, A., Presl, J., and Zidovsky, J. (1979): Migration of lymphoid cells into the granulosa of rat ovarian follicles. *IRCS Med. Sci.*, 7:603–604.
166. Bukovsky, A., Presl, J., and Holub, M. (1984): The ovarian follicle as a model for the cell-mediated control of tissue growth. *Cell Tissue Res.*, 236:717–724.
167. Peluso, J. J., and England-Charlesworth, C. (1982): Development of preovulatory follicles and oocytes during the oestrous cycle of mature and aged rats. *Acta Endocrinol.*, 100:434–443.
168. Peluso, J. J., England-Charlesworth, C., Bolender, D. L., and Steger, R. W. (1980): Ultrastructural alterations associated with the initiation of follicular atresia. *Cell Tissue Res.*, 211:105–115.
169. Gondos, B. (1982): Ultrastructure of follicular atresia in the rat. *Gamete Res.*, 5:199–206.
170. Ryan, R. J., and Lee, C. Y. (1976): The role of membrane bound receptors. *Biol. Reprod.*, 14:16–29.
171. Peluso, J. J., Steger, R. W., and Hafez, E. S. E. (1977): Surface ultrastructural changes in granulosa cells of atretic follicles. *Biol. Reprod.*, 16:600–604.
172. Hay, M. F., Cran, D. G., and Moor, R. M. (1976): Structural changes occurring during atresia in sheep ovarian follicles. *Cell Tissue Res.*, 169:515–529.
173. Hay, M. F., Moor, R. M., Cran, D. G., and Dott, H. M. (1979): Regeneration of atretic sheep ovarian follicles in vitro. *J. Reprod. Fertil.*, 55:195–207.
174. Moor, R. M., Hay, M. F., Dot, H. M., and Cran, D. G. (1978): Macroscopic identification and steroidogenic function of atretic follicles in sheep. *J. Endocrinol.*, 77:309–318.
175. Meinecke, B., Meinecke-Tillmann, S., and Gips, H. (1982): Experimentelle Untersuchungen zur Steroidsekretion intakter und atretischer Follikel in vitro. *Berl. Munch. Tierarztl. Wochenschr.*, 95:107–111.
176. Henderson, K. M., Kieboom, L. E., McNatty, K. P., Lun, S., and Heath, D. A. (1984): [^{125}I]hCG binding to bovine thecal tissue from healthy and atretic antral follicles. *Mol. Cell. Endocrinol.*, 34:91–98.
177. Zachariae, F. (1957): Studies in the mechanism of ovulation. Autoradiographic investigations on the uptake of radioactive sulphate (^{35}S) into the ovarian follicular mucopolysaccharides. *Acta Endocrinol.*, 26:215–224.
178. Bellin, M. E., and Ax, R. L. (1984): Chondroitin sulfate: an indicator of atresia in bovine follicles. *Endocrinology,* 114:428–434.
179. Guraya, S. S. (1973): Follicular atresia. *Proc. Indian Natl. Sci. Acad.*, 39:311–332.
180. Lobel, B. L., Rosenbaum, R. M., and Deane, H. W. (1961): Enzymic correlates of physiological regression of follicles and corpora lutea in ovaries of normal rats. *Endocrinology,* 68:232–247.
181. Ryan, R. J. (1981): Follicular atresia: some speculations on biochemical markers and mechanisms. In: *Dynamics of Ovarian Func-*

tion, edited by N. B. Schwartz and M. Hunzicker-Dunn. Raven Press, New York.
182. Breitenecker, G., Friedrich, F., and Kemeter, P. (1978): Further investigations on the maturation and degeneration of human ovarian follicles and their oocytes. *Fertil. Steril.,* 29:336–341.
183. McNatty, K. P., Makris, A., De Grazia, C., Osathanondh, R., and Ryan, K. J. (1979): Steroidogenesis in granulosa cells and corpus luteum. The production of progesterone, androgens and oestrogens by human granulosa cells in vitro and in vivo. *J. Steroid Biochem.,* 11:775–779.
184. Austin, C. R. (1961): *The Mammalian Egg.* Blackwell, Oxford, UK.
185. Byskov, A. G. (1979): Atresia. In: *Ovarian Follicular Development and Function,* edited by A. R. Midgley and W. A. Sadler, pp. 41–57. Raven Press, New York.
186. Dawson, A. B. (1952): Argyrophilic inclusions in the cytoplasm of the ova of the rat in normal and atretic follicles. *Anat. Rec.,* 112:37–59.
187. Peluso, J. J., Bolender, D. L., and Perri, A. (1979): Temporal changes associated with the degeneration of the rat oocyte. *Biol. Reprod.,* 20:423–430.
188. Westergaard, L. (1985): Follicular atresia in relation to oocyte morphology in non-pregnant and pregant women. *J. Reprod. Fertil.,* 74:113–118.
189. Vasques-Nin, G. H., and Sotelo, J. R. (1967): Electron microscope study of the atretic oocytes of the rat. *Z. Zelforsch. Abt. Histochem.,* 80:518–533.
190. Baker, T. G., and Franchi, L. L. (1967): The fine structure of oogonia and oocytes in human ovaries. *J. Cell. Sci.,* 2:213–234.
191. Centola, G. M. (1982): Light microscopic observations of alterations in staining of the zona pellucida of porcine follicular oocytes: possible early indications of atresia. *Gamete Res.,* 6:293–304.
192. Donahue, R. P., and Stern, S. (1968): Follicular cell support of oocyte maturation: production of pyruvate in vitro. *J. Reprod. Fertil.,* 17:395–398.
193. Albertini, D. F., and Anderson, E. (1974): The appearance and structure of intercellular connections during the ontogeny of the rabbit ovarian follicle with particular reference to gap junctions. *J. Cell. Biol.,* 63:234–250.
194. Osman, P. (1985): Rate and course of atresia during follicular development in the adult cyclic rat. *J. Reprod. Fertil.,* 73:261–270.
195. Moor, R. M., and Trounson, A. O. (1977): Hormonal and follicular factors affecting maturation of sheep oocytes in vitro and their subsequent developmental capacity. *J. Reprod. Fertil.,* 49:101–109.
196. Guraya, S. S., and Greenwald, G. S. (1964): A comparative histochemical study of interstitial tissue and follicular atresia in the mammalian ovary. *Anat. Rec.,* 149:411–434.
197. Mossman, H. W., Koering, M. J., and Ferry, D., Jr. (1964): Cyclic changes of interstitial gland tissue of the human ovary. *Am. J. Anat.,* 115:235–256.
198. Schwall, R., and Erickson, G. F. (1981): Functional and morphological changes in rat theca cells during atresia. In: *Dynamics of Ovarian Function,* edited by N. B. Schwartz and M. Hunzicker-Dunn, pp. 29–34. Raven Press, New York.
199. Terranova, P. F., Martin, N. C., and Chien, S. (1982): Theca is the source of progesterone in experimentally induced atretic follicles of the hamster. *Biol. Reprod.,* 26:721–727.
200. Silavin, S. L., and Greenwald, G. S. (1984): Steroid production by isolated theca and granulosa cells after initiation of atresia in the hamster. *J. Reprod. Fertil.,* 71:387–392.
201. O'Shea, J. D., Hay, M. F., and Cran, D. G. (1978): Ultrastructural changes in the theca interna during follicular atresia in sheep. *J. Reprod. Fertil.,* 54:183–187.
202. Bruce, N. W., and Moor, R. M. (1976): Capillary blood flow to ovarian follicles, stroma and corpora lutea of anaesthetized sheep. *J. Reprod. Fertil.,* 46:299–304.
203. Findlay, J. K., and Carson, R. S. (1980): Selective binding of gonadotrophins and the control of follicular growth and atresia. In: *Advances in Physiological Science, Vol. 15: Reproduction and Development,* edited by B. Flerko, G. Setalo, and L. Tima, pp. 79–89. Pergamon, Budapest.
204. Motta, P. M., and Familiari, G. (1981): Occurrence of contractile tissue in the theca externa of atretic follicles in the mouse ovary. *Acta Anat.,* 109:103–114.
205. Mori, T., Fujita, Y., Nihnobu, K., Ezaki, Y., Kubo, K., and Nishimura, T. (1982): Steroidogenesis in vitro by human ovarian follicles during the process of atresia. *Clin. Endocrinol.,* 16:391–400.
206. McNatty, K. P., Smith, D. M., Makris, A., Osathanondh, R., and Ryan, K. J. (1979): The microenvironment of the human antral follicle: interrelationships among the steroid levels in antral fluid, the population of granulosa cells, and the status of the oocyte in vivo and in vitro. *J. Clin. Endocrinol. Metab.,* 49:851–860.
207. McNatty, K. P., Makris, A., Osathanondh, R., and Ryan, K. J. (1980): Effects of luteinizing hormone on steroidogenesis by thecal tissue from human ovarian follicles in vitro. *Steroids,* 36:53–63.
208. Maxson, W. S., Haney, A. F., and Schomberg, D. W. (1985): Steroidogenesis in porcine atretic follicles: loss of aromatase activity in isolated granulosa and theca. *Biol. Reprod.,* 33:495–501.
209. Carson, R. S., Findlay, J. K., Clarke, I. J., and Burger, H. G. (1981): Estradiol, testosterone, and androstenedione in ovine follicular fluid during growth and atresia of ovarian follicles. *Biol. Reprod.,* 24:105–113.
210. Tsonis, C. G., Carson, R. S., and Findlay, J. K. (1984): Relationships between aromatase activity, follicular fluid oestradiol-17β and testosterone concentrations, and diameter and atresia of individual ovine follicles. *J. Reprod. Fertil.,* 72:153–163.
211. Carson, R. S., Findlay, J. K., Burger, H. G., and Trounson, A. O. (1979): Gonadotropin receptors of the ovine ovarian follicle during follicular growth and atresia. *Biol. Reprod.,* 21:75–87.
212. Ireland, J. J., and Roche, J. F. (1983): Development of nonovulatory antral follicles in heifers: changes in steroids in follicular fluid and receptors for gonadotropins. *Endocrinology,* 112:150–156.
213. McNatty, K. P., Lun, S., Heath, D. A., Kieboom, L. E., and Henderson, K. M. (1985): Influence of follicular atresia on LH-induced cAMP and steroid synthesis by bovine thecae interna. *Mol. Cell Endocrinol.,* 39:209–215.
214. Braw, R. H., Bar-Ami, S., and Tsafriri, A. (1981): Effect of hypophysectomy on atresia of rat preovulatory follicles. *Biol. Reprod.,* 25:989–996.
215. Bill, C. H., II, and Greenwald, G. S. (1981): Acute gonadotropin deprivation. I. A model for the study of follicular atresia. *Biol. Reprod.,* 24:913–921.
216. Braw, R. H., and Tsafriri, A. (1980): Follicles explanted from pentobarbitone-treated rats provide a model for atresia. *J. Reprod. Fertil.,* 59:259–265.
217. Uilenbroek, J. T. J., Woutersen, P. J. A., and van der Schoot, P. (1980): Atresia of preovulatory follicles: gonadotropin binding and steroidogenic activity. *Biol. Reprod.,* 23:219–229.
218. Terranova, P. F. (1980): Effects of phenobarbital-induced ovulatory delay on the follicular population and serum levels of steroids and gonadotropins in the hamster: a model for atresia. *Biol. Reprod.,* 23:92–99.
219. Peters, H., Byskov, A. G., Himelstein-Braw, R., and Faber, M. (1975): Follicular growth: the basic event in the mouse and human ovary. *J. Reprod. Fertil.,* 45:559–566.
220. Peluso, J. J., and Steger, R. W. (1978): Role of FSH in regulating granulosa cell division and follicular atresia in rats. *J. Reprod. Fertil.,* 54:275–278.
221. Braw, R. H., and Tsafriri, A. (1980): Effect of PMSG on follicular atresia in the immature rat ovary. *J. Reprod. Fertil.,* 59:267–272.
222. Matson, P. L., Gledhill, B., and Collins, W. P. (1984): Effect of LH on steroidogenesis by hamster follicles isolated at defined stages of development. *J. Reprod. Fertil.,* 70:675–681.
223. Bagnell, C. A., Mills, T. M., Costoff, A., and Mahesh, V. B. (1982): A model for the study of androgen effects on follicular atresia and ovulation. *Biol. Reprod.,* 27:903–914.
224. Magnusson, C., Bar Ami, S., Braw, R., and Tsafriri, A. (1983): Oxygen consumption by rat oocytes and cumulus cells during induced atresia. *J. Reprod. Fertil.,* 68:97–103.
225. Hubbard, C. J., and Greenwald, G. S. (1985): Morphological changes in atretic graafian follicles during induced atresia in the hamster. *Anat. Rec.,* 212:353–357.
226. Hubbard, C. J., and Greenwald, G. S. (1981): Changes in DNA, cyclic nucleotides and steroids during induced follicular atresia in the hamster. *J. Reprod. Fertil.,* 63:455–461.
227. Hubbard, C. J., and Greenwald, G. S. (1983): In vitro effects of luteinizing hormone on induced atretic graafian follicles in the hamster. *Biol. Reprod.,* 28:849–859.

228. Shaha, C., and Greenwald, G. S. (1982): Autoradiographic analysis of changes in ovarian binding of FSH and hCG during induced follicular atresia in the hamster. *J. Reprod. Fertil.*, 66:197–201.
229. Terranova, P. F. (1981): Steroidogenesis in experimentally induced atretic follicles of the hamster: a shift from estradiol to progesterone synthesis. *Endocrinology,* 108:1885–1890.
230. Na, J. Y., Garza, F., and Terranova, P. F. (1985): Alterations in follicular fluid steroids and follicular hCG and FSH binding during atresia in hamster. *Proc. Soc. Exp. Biol. Med.*, 179:123–127.
231. Mizuno, O., Otani, T., Shirota, M., and Sasamoto, S. (1983): Maturation of ovarian follicles after inhibition of ovulation in rats. *J. Endocrinol.*, 97:113–119.
232. Uilenbroek, J. T. J., van der Linden, R., and Woutersen, P. J. A. (1984): Changes in oestrogen biosynthesis in preovulatory rat follicles after blockage of ovulation with pentobarbitone sodium. *J. Reprod. Fertil.*, 70:549–555.
233. van der Schoot, P., den Besten, D., and Uilenbroek, J. T. J. (1982): Atresia of preovulatory follicles in rats treated with sodium pentobarbital: effects of bromocriptine. *Biol. Reprod.*, 27:189–199.
234. Freeman, M. E., Butcher, R. L., and Fugo, N. W. (1970): Alteration of oocytes and follicles by delayed ovulation. *Biol. Reprod.*, 2:209–215.
235. Peluso, J. J., Steger, R. W., and Hafez, E. S. E. (1977): Sequential changes associated with the degeneration of preovulatory rat follicles. *J. Reprod. Fertil.*, 49:215–218.
236. Louvet, J. P., Harman, S. M., Schreiber, J. R., and Ross, G. T. (1975): Evidence for a role of androgens in follicular maturation. *Endocrinology,* 97:366–372.
237. Hillier, S. G., and Ross, G. T. (1979): Effects of exogenous testosterone on ovarian weight, follicular morphology and intraovarian progesterone concentration in estrogen-primed hypophysectomized immature female rats. *Biol. Reprod.*, 20:261–268.
238. Harmon, S. M., Louvet, J. P., and Ross, G. T. (1975): Interaction of estrogen and gonadotrophins on follicular atresia. *Endocrinology,* 96:1145–1152.
239. Peluso, J. J., Charlesworth, J., and England-Charlesworth, C. (1981): Role of estrogen and androgen in maintaining the preovulatory follicle. *Cell Tisue Res.*, 216:615–624.
240. Schreiber, J. R., Reid, R., and Ross, G. T. (1976): A receptor-like testosterone-binding protein in ovaries from estrogen-stimulated hypophysectomized immature female rats. *Endocrinology,* 98:1206–1213.
241. Schreiber, J. R., and Ross, G. T. (1976): Further characterization of a rat ovarian testosterone receptor with evidence for nuclear translocation. *Endocrinology,* 99:590–596.
242. Saiduddin, S., and Zassenhaus, H. P. (1978): Effect of testosterone and progesterone on the estradiol receptor in the immature rat ovary. *Endocrinology,* 102:1069–1076.
243. Kohut, J. K., Jarrell, J. F., and Younglai, E. V. (1985): Does dihydrotestosterone induce atresia in the hypophysectomized immature female rat treated with pregnant mare's serum gonadotropin? *Am. J. Obstet. Gynecol.*, 151:250–255.
244. Farookhi, R. (1980): Effects of androgen on induction of gonadotropin receptors and gonadotropin-stimulated adenosine 3′-5′-monophosphate production in rat ovarian granulosa cells. *Endocrinology,* 106:1216–1223.
245. Farookhi, R. (1981): Atresia: A hypothesis. In: *Dynamics of Ovarian Function,* edited by N. B. Schwartz and M. Hunzicker-Dunn, pp. 13–23. Raven Press, New York.
246. Tonetta, S. A., Spicer, L. J., and Ireland, J. J. (1985): CI628 inhibits follicle-stimulating hormone (FSH)-induced increases in FSH receptors of the rat ovary: requirement of estradiol for FSH action. *Endocrinology,* 116:715–722.
247. Hillier, S. G., van den Boogaard, A. M. J., Reichert, L. E., Jr., and van Hall, E. V. (1980): Intraovarian sex steroid hormone interactions and the regulation of follicular maturation: aromatization of androgens by human granulosa cells in vitro. *J. Clin. Endocrinol. Metab.*, 50:640–647.
248. Greenwald, G. S., and Limback, D. L. (1984): Effects of treatment with cycloheximide at proestrus on subsequent in vitro follicular steroidogenesis in the hamster. *Biol. Reprod.*, 30:1105–1116.
249. Baird, D. T., Swanston, I. A., and McNeilly, A. S. (1981): Relationship between LH, FSH, and prolactin concentration and the secretion of androgens and estrogens by the preovulatory follicle in the ewe. *Biol. Reprod.*, 24:1013–1025.
250. Hutz, R. J., Dierschke, D. J., and Wolf, R. C. (1986): Markers of atresia in ovarian follicular components from rhesus monkeys treated with estradiol-17β. *Biol. Reprod.*, 34:65–70.
251. Cole, H. H. (1975): Studies on reproduction with emphasis on gonadotropins, antigonadotropins and progonadotropins. *Biol. Reprod.*, 12:194–211.
252. Moore, W. T., Jr., Burleigh, B. D., and Ward, D. N. (1980): Chorionic gonadotropins: comparative studies and comments on relationships to other glycoprotein hormones. In: *Chorionic Gonadotropin* edited by S. J. Segal, pp. 89–126. Plenum, New York.
253. Stewart, F., and Allen, W. R. (1979): The binding of FSH, LH and PMSG to equine gonadal tissues. *J. Reprod. Fertil. Suppl.*, 27:431–440.
254. Licht, P., Gallo, A. B., Aggarwal, B. B., Farmer, S. W., Castelino, J. B., and Papkoff, H. (1979): Biological and binding activities of equine pituitary gonadotrophins and pregnant mare serum gonadotrophin. *J. Endocrinol.*, 83:311–322.
255. Murphy, B. D., Mapletoft, R. J., Manns, J., and Humphrey, W. D. (1984): Variability in gonadotrophin preparations as a factor in the superovulatory response. *Theriogenology,* 21:117–125.
256. Combarnous, Y., Guillou, F., Martinat, N., and Cahoreau, C. (1984): Origine de la double activite FSH + LH de la choriogonadotropine equine (eCG/PMSG). *Ann. Endocrinol. (Paris),* 45:261–268.
257. Leaver, H. A., and Boyd, G. S. (1981): Action of gonadotrophic hormones on cholesterol side-chain cleavage and cholesterol ester hydrolase in the ovary of the immature rat. *J. Reprod. Fertil.*, 63:101–108.
258. Younglai, E. V. (1984): Effects of pregnant mare's serum gonadotrophin administered in vivo on steroid accumulation by isolated rabbit ovarian follicles. *Acta Endocrinol.*, 107:531–537.
259. Matson, P. L., Tyler, J. P. P., and Collins, W. P. (1981): Follicular steroid content and oocyte meiotic status after PMSG stimulation of immature hamsters. *J. Reprod. Fertil.*, 61:443–452.
260. Cran, D. G. (1983): Follicular development in the sheep after priming with PMSG. *J. Reprod. Fertil.*, 67:415–423.
261. Cahill, L. P., Mariana, J. C., and Mauleon, P. (1979): Total follicular populations in ewes of high and low ovulation rates. *J. Reprod. Fertil.*, 5:27–36.
262. Greenwald, G. S. (1961): Quantitative study of follicular development in the ovary of the intact or unilaterally ovariectomized hamster. *J. Reprod. Fertil.*, 2:351–361.
263. Monniaux, D., Mariana, J. C., and Gibson, W. R. (1984): Action of PMSG on follicular populations in the heifer. *J. Reprod. Fertil.*, 70:243–253.
264. Dott, H. M., Hay, M. F., Cran, D. G., and Moor, R. M. (1979): Effect of exogenous gonadotrophin (PMSG) on the antral follicle population in the sheep. *J. Reprod. Fertil.*, 56:683–689.
265. Moor, R. M., Kruip, T. A. M., and Green, D. (1984): Intraovarian control of folliculogenesis: limits to superovulation? *Theriogenology,* 21:103–116.
266. Greenwald, G. S., and Terranova, P. F. (1983): Development in the cyclic hamster of refractoriness to the superovulatory action of anti-LH serum. *J. Reprod. Fertil.*, 69:297–301.
267. Dhondt, D., Bouters, R., Spincemaille, J., Coryn, M., and Vandeplassche, M. (1978): The control of superovulation in the bovine with a PMSG-antiserum. *Theriogenology,* 9:529–534.
268. Greenwald, G. S. (1979): Analysis of superovulation in the hamster: 1962–1978. *Ann. Biol. Anim. Bioch. Biophys.*, 19:1483–1487.
269. Greenwald, G. S. (1973): Effect of an anti-PMS serum on ovulation and estrogen secretion in the PMS-treated hamster. *Biol. Reprod.*, 9:437–446.
270. Hirshfield, A. N. (1984): Stathmokinetic analysis of granulosa cell proliferation in antral follicles of cyclic rats. *Biol. Reprod.*, 31:52–58.
271. Krishna, A., Terranova, P. F., Matteri, R. L., and Papkoff, H. (1986): Histamine and increased ovarian blood flow mediate LH-induced superovulation in the cyclic hamster. *J. Reprod. Fertil.*, 76:23–29.
272. Krishna, A., and Terranova, P. F. (1985): Alterations in mast cell degranulation and ovarian histamine in the proestrous hamster. *Biol. Reprod.*, 32:1211–1217.

273. Szego, C. M., and Gitin, E. S. (1964): Ovarian histamine depletion during acute hyperaemic response to luteinizing hormone. *Nature,* 201:682–684.
274. Lipner, H. (1971): Ovulation from histamine depleted ovaries. *Proc. Soc. Exp. Biol. Med.,* 136:111–114.
275. Wallach, E. E., Wright, K. H., and Hamada, Y. (1978): Investigation of mammalian ovulation with an in vitro perfused rabbit ovary preparation. *Am. J. Obstet. Gynecol.,* 132:728–738.
276. Knox, E., Lowry, S., and Beck, L. (1979): Prevention of ovulation in rabbits by antihistamine. In: *Ovarian Follicular Development and Function,* edited by A. R. Midgley and W. A. Sadler, pp. 159–163. Raven Press, New York.
277. Kobayashi, Y., Wright, K. H., Santulli, R., Kitai, H., and Wallach, E. E. (1983): Effect of histamine and histamine blockers on the ovulatory process in the in vitro perfused rabbit ovary. *Biol. Reprod.,* 28:385–392.
278. Scaramuzzi, R. J., Martensz, N. D., and Van Look, P. F. A. (1980): Ovarian morphology and the concentration of steroids, and of gonadotrophins during the breeding season in ewes actively immunized against oestradiol-17β or oestrone. *J. Reprod. Fertil.,* 59:303–310.
279. Scaramuzzi, R. J., Baird, D. T., Clarke, I. J., Martensz, N. D., and Van Look, P. F. A. (1980): Ovarian morphology and the concentration of steroids during the oestrous cycle of sheep actively immunized against androstenedione. *J. Reprod. Fertil.,* 58:27–35.
280. Land, R. B., Morris, B. A., Baxter, G., Fordyce, M., and Forster, J. (1982): Improvement of sheep fecundity by treatment with antisera to gonadal steroids. *J. Reprod. Fertil.,* 66:625–634.
281. Wallace, J. M., and McNeilly, A. S. (1985): Increase in ovulation rate after treatment of ewes with bovine follicular fluid in the luteal phase of the oestrous cycle. *J. Reprod. Fertil.,* 73:505–515.
282. Lasley, B. L. (1984): Treating infertility: CRES employs innovative method. *CRES Rep.,* 2:No. 2.
283. Jones, G. S. (1984): Update on in vitro fertilization. *Endocrine Rev.,* 5:62–75.
284. Terranova, P. F., and Greenwald, G. S. (1979): Antiluteinizing hormone: chronic influence on steroid and gonadotropin levels and superovulation in the pregnant hamster. *Endocrinology,* 104:1013–1019.
285. Greenwald, G. S., and Terranova, P. F. (1981): Induction of superovulation in the cyclic hamster by a single injection of antiluteinizing hormone serum. *Endocrinology,* 108:1903–1908.
286. Terranova, P. F., and Greenwald, G. S. (1981): Alteration of the serum follicle-stimulating hormone to luteinizing hormone ratio in the cyclic hamster treated with antiluteinizing hormone: relationship to serum estradiol, free antiluteinizing hormone, and superovulation. *Endocrinology,* 108:1909–1914.
287. Opavsky, M. A., and Armstrong, D. T. (1985): The effectiveness of FSH in inducing superovulation is influenced by LH. *Biol. Reprod. Suppl. 1,* 32:71.
288. Kim, I., and Greenwald, G. S. (1984): Hormonal requirements for maintenance of follicular and luteal function in the hypophysectomized cyclic hamster. *Biol. Reprod.,* 30:1063–1072.
289. Terranova, P. F., and Greenwald, G. S. (1981): Increased ovulation rate in the cyclic guinea pig after a single injection of antiserum to LH. *J. Reprod. Fertil.,* 61:37–42.
290. Fitzgerald, J. A., Ruggles, A. J., and Hansel, W. (1985): Increased ovulation rate of adult ewes treated with anti-bovine LH antiserum during the normal breeding season. *J. Anim. Sci.,* 60:749–754.
291. Peppler, R. D. (1968): Method and mechanism of ovulatory compensation following unilateral ovariectomy in the rat. Thesis, University of Kansas.
292. Jones, R. E., and Summers, C. H. (1984): Compensatory follicular hypertrophy during the ovarian cycle of the house gecko, *Hemidactylus frenatus. Anat. Rec.,* 209:59–65.
293. Bleier, W. J., and Ehteshami, M. (1981): Ovulation following unilateral ovariectomy in the California leaf-nosed bat (*Macrotus californicus*). *J. Reprod. Fertil.,* 63:181–183.
294. Hunter, J. (1787): An experiment to determine the effect of extirpating one ovarium upon the number of young produced. *Phil. Trans.,* 17:233–239.
295. Arai, H. (1920): On the cause of the hypertrophy of the surviving ovary after semispaying (albino rat) and on the number of ova in it. *Am. J. Anat.,* 28:59–79.
296. Lipschutz, A. (1928): New developments in ovarian dynamics and the law of follicular constancy. *Br. J. Exp. Biol.,* 5:283–291.
297. Chiras, D. D., and Greenwald, G. S. (1978): Acute effects of unilateral ovariectomy on follicular development in the cylic hamster. *J. Reprod. Fertil.,* 52:221–225.
298. Peppler, R. D., and Greenwald, G. S. (1970): Effects of unilateral ovariectomy on ovulation and cycle length in 4- and 5-day cycling rats. *Am. J. Anat.,* 127:1–8.
299. Peppler, R. D., and Greenwald, G. S. (1970): Influence of unilateral ovariectomy on follicular development in cycling rats. *Am. J. Anat.,* 127:9–14.
300. Otani, T., and Sasamoto, S. (1982): Plasma and pituitary hormone changes and follicular development after unilateral ovariectomy in cyclic rats. *J. Reprod. Fertil.,* 65:347–353.
301. McLaren, A. (1966): Regulation of ovulation rate after removal of one ovary in mice. *Proc. R. Soc. London [Biol.],* 166:316–340.
302. Fleming, M. W., Rhodes, R. C., III, and Dailey, R. A. (1984): Compensatory responses after unilateral ovariectomy in rabbits. *Biol. Reprod.,* 30:82–86.
303. Hermreck, A. S., and Greenwald, G. S. (1964): The effects of unilateral ovariectomy on follicular maturation in the guinea pig. *Anat. Rec.,* 148:171–176.
304. Land, R. B. (1973): Ovulation rate of Finn-Dorset sheep following unilateral ovariectomy or chlorpromazine treatment at different stages of the oestrous cycle. *J. Reprod. Fertil.,* 33:99–105.
305. Findlay, J. K., and Cumming, I. A. (1977): The effect of unilateral ovariectomy on plasma gonadotropin levels, estrus and ovulation rate in sheep. *Biol. Reprod.,* 17:178–183.
306. Brinkley, H. J., and Young, E. P. (1969): Effects of unilateral ovariectomy or the unilateral destruction of ovarian components on the follicles and corpora lutea of the nonpregnant pig. *Endocrinology,* 84:1250–1256.
307. Brinkley, H. J., Wickersham, E. W., First, N. L., and Casida, L. E. (1964): Effect of unilateral ovariectomy on the structure and function of the corpora lutea of the pig. *Endocrinology,* 74:462–467.
308. Sundaram, S. K., and Stob, M. (1967): Effect of unilateral ovariectomy on reproduction and induced ovulation in ewes. *J. Anim. Sci.,* 26:374–376.
309. Roy, S. K., and Greenwald, G. S. (1986): Effects of FSH and LH on incorporation of [^{3}H] thymidine into follicular DNA. *J. Reprod. Fertil.* 78:201–209.
310. Saiduddin, S., Rowe, R. F., and Casida, L. E. (1970): Ovarian follicular changes following unilateral ovariectomy in the cow. *Biol. Reprod.,* 2:408–412.
311. Johnson, S. K., Smith, M. F., and Elmore, R. G. (1985): Effect of unilateral ovariectomy and injection of bovine follicular fluid on gonadotropin secretion and compensatory ovarian hypertrophy in prepuberal heifers. *J. Anim. Sci.,* 60:1055–1060.
312. Cochrane, R. L., and Holmes, R. L. (1966): Unilateral ovariectomy and hypophysectomy in the rhesus monkey. *J. Endocrinol.,* 35:427–428.
313. Sopelak, V. M., and Hodgen, G. D. (1984): Contralateral tubal-ovarian apposition and fertility in hemiovariectomized primates. *Fertil. Steril.,* 42:633–637.
314. Speert, H., Na Sh, W., and Kaplan, A. L. (1956): Tubal pregnancy. Some observations on external migration of the ovum and compensatory hypertrophy of the residual ovary. *Obstet. Gynecol.,* 7:322–324.
315. Gougeon, A., and Lefevre, B. (1983): Evolution of the diameters of the largest healthy and atretic follicles during the human menstrual cycle. *J. Reprod. Fertil.,* 69:497–502.
316. Bast, J. D., and Greenwald, G. S. (1977): Acute and chronic elevations in serum levels of FSH after unilateral ovariectomy in the cyclic hamster. *Endocrinology,* 100:955–966.
317. Welschen, R., Dullaart, J., and deJong, F. H. (1978): Interrelationships between circulating levels of estradiol-17β, progesterone, FSH and LH immediately after unilateral ovariectomy in the cyclic rat. *Biol. Reprod.,* 18:421–427.
318. Redmer, D. A., Christenson, R. K., Ford, J. J., and Day, B. N. (1985): Effect of follicular fluid treatment on follicle-stimulating hormone, luteinizing hormone and compensatory ovarian hypertrophy in prepuberal gilts. *Biol. Reprod.,* 32:111–119.

319. Baird, D. T., Backstrom, T., McNeilly, A. S., Smith, S. K., and Wathen, C. G. (1984): Effect of enucleation of the corpus luteum at different stages of the luteal phase of the human menstrual cycle on subsequent follicular development. *J. Reprod. Fertil.*, 70:615–624.
320. Baranczuk, R., and Greenwald, G. S. (1973): Peripheral levels of estrogen in the cycling hamster. *Endocrinology,* 92:805–812.
321. Curry, T. E., Jr., Lawrence, I. E., Jr., and Burden, H. W. (1984): Effect of ovarian sympathectomy on follicular development during compensatory ovarian hypertrophy in the guinea-pig. *J. Reprod. Fertil.*, 71:39–44.
322. Chatterjee, A., and Greenwald, G. S. (1972): The long-term effects of unilateral ovariectomy of the cycling hamster and rat. *Biol. Reprod.*, 7:238–246.
323. Peppler, R. D. (1971): Effects of unilateral ovariectomy on follicular development and ovulation in cycling, aged rats. *Am. J. Anat.*, 132:423–428.
324. Hirshfield, A. N. (1982): Follicular recruitment in long-term hemicastrate rats. *Biol. Reprod.*, 27:48–53.
325. Hirshfield, A. N. (1983): Compensatory ovarian hypertrophy in the long-term hemicastrate rat: size distribution of growing and atretic follicles. *Biol. Reprod.*, 28:271–278.
326. Butcher, R. L. (1977): Changes in gonadotropins and steroids associated with unilateral ovariectomy of the rat. *Endocrinology,* 101:830–839.
327. Baker, T. G., Challoner, S., and Burgoyne, P. S. (1980): The number of oocytes and the rate of atresia in unilaterally ovariectomized mice up to 8 months after surgery. *J. Reprod. Fertil.*, 60:449–456.
328. Schwartz, N. B., Cobbs, S. B., and Ely, C. A. (1972): What is the function(s) of the proestrous FSH surge in the rat. In: *Endocrinology, Proceedings of the 4th International Congress of Endocrinology, Washington (June 1972), Excerpta Med. Int. Cong. Ser. No. 273,* pp. 897–902. Excerpta Medica, Amsterdam.
329. Chiras, D. D., and Greenwald, G. S. (1977): An autoradiographic study of long-term follicular development in the cylic hamster. *Anat. Rec.*, 188:331–337.
330. Welschen, R. (1973): Amounts of gonadotropins required for normal follicular growth in hypophysectomized adult rats. *Acta Endocrinol. (Copenh.)*, 72:137–155.
331. Hirshfield, A. N., and Midgley, A. R., Jr. (1978): Morphometric analysis of follicular development in the rat. *Biol. Reprod.*, 19:597–605.
332. Ireland, J. J., and Richards, J. S. (1978): A previously undescribed role for luteinizing hormone (LH:hCG) on follicular cell differentiation. *Endocrinology,* 102:1458–1465.
333. Terranova, P. F., and Garza, F. (1983): Relationship between the preovulatory luteinizing hormone (LH) surge and androstenedione systhesis of preantral follicles in the cyclic hamster: detection by in vitro responses to LH. *Biol. Reprod.*, 29:630–636.
334. Richards, J. S., and Midgley, A. R., Jr. (1976): Protein hormone action: a key to understanding follicular and luteal cell development. *Biol. Reprod.*, 14:82–94.
335. Richards, J. S., Ireland, J. J., Rao, M. C., Bernath, G. A., Midgley, A. R., Jr., and Reichert, L. E., Jr. (1976): Ovarian follicular development in the rat: hormone receptor regulation by estradiol, follicle stimulating hormone and luteinizing hormone. *Endocrinology,* 99:1562–1570.
336. Midgley, A. R., Jr. (1973): Autoradiographic analysis of gonadotropin binding to rat ovarian tissue sections. *Adv. Exp. Med. Biol.*, 36:365–378.
337. Bast, J. D., and Greenwald, G. S. (1974): Serum profiles of follicle-stimulating hormone, luteinizing hormone and prolactin during the estrous cycle of the hamster. *Endocrinology,* 94:1295–1299.
338. Bex, F. J., and Goldman, B. D. (1975): Serum gonadotropins and follicular development in the Syrian hamster. *Endocrinology,* 96:928–933.
339. Siegel, H. I., Bast, J. D., and Greenwald, G. S. (1976): The effects of phenobarbital and gonadal steroids on periovulatory serum levels of luteinizing hormone and follicle stimulating hormone in the hamster. *Endocrinology,* 98:48–55.
340. Gay, V. L., Midgley, A. R., Jr., and Niswender, G. D. (1970): Patterns of gonadotropin secretion associated with ovulation. *Fed. Proc.*, 29:1880–1887.
341. Butcher, R. L., Collins, W. E., and Fugo, N. W. (1974): Plasma concentrations of LH, FSH, prolactin, progesterone and estradiol-17β throughout the 4-day estrous cycle of the rat. *Endocrinology,* 94:1704–1708.
342. DePaolo, L. U., Shander, D., Wise, P. M., Barraclough, C. A., and Channing, C. P. (1979): Identification of inhibin-like activity in ovarian venous plasma of rats during the estrous cycle. *Endocrinology,* 105:647–654.
343. Fujii, T., Hoover, D. J., and Channing, C. P. (1983): Changes in inhibin activity, and progesterone, oestrogen and androstenedione concentrations, in rat follicular fluid throughout the oestrous cycle. *J. Reprod. Fertil.*, 69:307–314.
344. Sander, H. J., van Leeuwen, E. C. M., and deJong, F. H. (1984): Inhibin-like activity in media from cultured rat granulosa cells collected throughout the oestrous cycle. *J. Endocrinol.*, 103:77–84.
345. Welschen, R., Hermans, W. P., and deJong, F. H. (1980): Possible involvement of inhibin in the interrelationship between numbers of antral follicles and peripheral FSH concentrations in female rats. *J. Reprod. Fertil.*, 60:485–493.
346. Chappel, S. C. (1979): Cyclic fluctuations in ovarian FSH-inhibiting material in golden hamsters. *Biol. Reprod.*, 21:447–453.
347. Erickson, G. F., and Hsueh, A. J. W. (1978): Secretion of inhibin by rat granulosa cells in vitro. *Endocrinology,* 103:1960–1963.
348. Lee, V. W. K. (1983): PMSG treated immature female rat—a model system for studying control of inhibin secretion. In: *Factors Regulating Ovarian Function,* edited by G. S. Greenwald and P. F. Terranova, pp. 157–161. Raven Press, New York.
349. Schwartz, N. B., and Channing, C. P. (1977): Evidence for ovarian "inhibin": suppression of the secondary rise in serum follicle stimulating hormone levels in proestrous rats by injection of porcine follicular fluid. *Proc. Natl. Acad. Sci. USA,* 74:5721–5724.
350. Chiras, D. D., and Greenwald, G. S. (1978): Effects of steroids and gonadotropins on follicular development in the hypophysectomized hamster. *Am. J. Anat.*, 152:307–320.
351. Zeleznik, A. J., Midgley, A. R., Jr., and Reichert, L. E., Jr. (1974): Granulosa cell maturation in the rat: increased binding of human chorionic gonadotropin following treatment with follicle stimulating hormone in vivo. *Endocrinology,* 95:818–825.
352. Pencharz, R. I. (1940): Effect of estrogens and androgens alone and in combination with chorionic gonadotropin on the ovary of the hypophysectomized rat. *Science,* 91:554–555.
353. Williams, P. C. (1940): Effect of stilbestrol on the ovaries of hypophysectomized rats. *Nature,* 145:388–389.
354. Smith, B. D., and Bradbury, J. T. (1963): Ovarian response to gonadotropins after pre-treatment with diethylstilbestrol. *Am. J. Physiol.*, 204:1023–1027.
355. Kudolo, G. B., Elder, M. G., and Myatt, L. (1984): A novel oestrogen-binding species in rat granulosa cells. *J. Endocrinol.*, 102:83–91.
356. Greenwald, G. S. (1975): Proestrous hormone surges dissociated from ovulation in the estrogen treated hamster. *Endocrinology,* 97:878–884.
357. Chappel, S. C., and Selker, F. (1979): Relation between the secretion of FSH during the periovulatory period and ovulation during the next cycle. *Biol. Reprod.*, 21:347–352.
358. Greenwald, G. S., and Siegel, H. I. (1982): Is the first or second periovulatory surge of FSH responsible for follicular recruitment in the hamster? *Proc. Soc. Exp. Biol. Med.*, 170:225–230.
359. Sheela Rani, C. S., and Moudgal, N. R. (1977): Role of the proestrous surge of gonadotropins in the initiation of follicular maturation in the cyclic hamster: a study using antisera to follicle stimulating hormone and luteinizing hormone. *Endocrinology,* 101: 1484–1494.
360. Page, R. D., and Butcher, R. L. (1982): Follicular and plasma patterns of steroids in young and old rats during normal and prolonged estrous cycles. *Biol. Reprod.*, 27:383–392.
361. Fevold, H. L. (1941): Synergism of follicle stimulating hormone and luteinizing hormone in producing estrogen secretion. *Endocrinology,* 28:33–36.
362. Greep, R. O., Van Dyke, H. B., and Chow, B. F. (1942): Gonadotropins of the swine pituitary. I. Various biological effects of purified thylakentrin (FSH) and pure metakentrin (ICSH). *Endocrinology,* 30:635–649.

363. Lostroh, A., and Johnson, R. E. (1966): Amounts of interstitial cell stimulating hormone and follicle stimulating hormone required for development, uterine growth and ovulation in the hypophysectomized rat. *Endocrinology*, 79:991–996.
364. Erickson, G. F., Wang, C., and Hsueh, A. J. W. (1979): FSH induction of functional LH receptors in granulosa cells cultured in a chemically defined medium. *Nature*, 279:336–337.
365. Wang, C., Hsueh, A. J. W., and Erickson, G. F. (1981): LH stimulation of estrogen secretion in cultured granulosa cells. *Mol. Cell. Endocrinol.*, 24:17–28.
366. Goodwin, J. A., and Terranova, P. F. (1985): Relationship between LH dependency of preantral follicles and the secondary FSH surge: effects of hypophysectomy and correlation with hCG and FSH binding and follicular steroids. In: *Proceedings of the 5th Ovarian Workshop*, edited by D. O. Toft and R. J. Ryan, pp. 243–248. Raven Press, New York.
367. Cameron, J. L., and Chappel, S. C. (1985): Follicle-stimulating hormone within and secreted from anterior pituitaries of female golden hamsters during the estrous cycle and after ovariectomy. *Biol. Reprod.*, 33:132–139.
368. Sheela Rani, C. S., and Moudgal, N. R. (1977): Examination of the role of FSH in periovulatory events in the hamster. *J. Reprod. Fertil.*, 50:37–45.
369. Dorrington, J. H., Moon, Y. S., and Armstrong, D. T. (1975): Estradiol biosynthesis in cultured granulosa cells from hypophysectomized immature rats: stimulation by follicle stimulating hormone. *Endocrinology*, 97:1328–1331.
370. Hillier, S. G., Zeleznik, A. J., and Ross, G. T. (1978): Independence of steroidogenic capacity and luteinizing hormone receptor induction in developing granulosa cells. *Endocrinology*, 102:937–946.
371. Hillier, S. G., Zeleznik, A. J., Knazek, R. A., and Ross, G. T. (1980): Hormonal regulation of preovulatory follicle maturation in the rat. *J. Reprod. Fertil.*, 60:219–229.
372. Wang, C., Hsueh, A. J. W., and Erickson, G. F. (1979): Induction of functional prolactin receptors by follicle stimulating hormone in rat granulosa cells in vivo and in vitro. *J. Biol. Chem.*, 254:11330–11336.
373. Jones, P. B. C., Welsh, T. H., Jr., and Hsueh, A. J. W. (1982): Regulation of ovarian progestin production by epidermal growth factor in cultured rat granulosa cells. *J. Biol. Chem.*, 257:11268–11273.
374. Ireland, J. J., and Richards, J. S. (1978): Acute effects of estradiol and FSH on specific binding of human [I^{125}] iodo FSH to rat ovarian granulosa cells in vivo and in vitro. *Endocrinology*, 102:876–883.
375. Gruenberg, M. L., Steger, R. W., and Peluso, J. J. (1983): Follicular development, steroidogenesis and ovulation within ovaries exposed in vitro to hormone levels which mimic those of the rat estrous cycle. *Biol. Reprod.*, 29:1265–1275.
376. Saidapur, S., and Greenwald, G. S. (1978): Peripheral blood and ovarian levels of sex steroids in the cyclic hamster. *Biol. Reprod.*, 18:401–408.
377. Leavitt, N. N., Barcom, C. R., Bagwell, J. N., and Blaha, C. C. (1973): Structure and function of the hamster corpus luteum during the estrous cycle. *Am. J. Anat.*, 136:235–250.
378. Terranova, P. F., and Greenwald, G. S. (1978): Steroid and gonadotropin levels during the luteal-follicular shift of the cylic hamster. *Biol. Reprod.*, 18:170–175.
379. Schwartz, N. B. (1969): A model for the regulation of ovulation in the rat. *Recent Prog. Horm. Res.*, 25:1–55.
380. Smith, M. S., Freeman, M. E., and Neill, J. D. (1973): The control of progesterone secretion during the estrous cycle and early pseudopregnancy in the rat: prolactin, gonadotropin and steroid levels associated with rescue of the corpus luteum of pseudopregnancy. *Endocrinology*, 96:219–226.
381. Gallo, R. V. (1981): Pulsatile LH release during periods of low level LH secretion in the rat estrous cycle. *Biol. Reprod.*, 24:771–777.
382. Fox, S. R., and Smith, M. S. (1985): Changes in the pulsatile pattern of luteinizing hormone secretion during the rat estrous cycle. *Endocrinology*, 116:1485–1492.
383. Szoltys, M. (1981): Oestrogens and progestagens in rat ovarian follicles during the oestrous cycle. *J. Reprod. Fertil.*, 63:221–224.
384. Hamberger, L., Nordenstrom, K., Rosberg, S., and Sjogren, A. (1978): Acute influence of LH and FSH on cyclic AMP formation in isolated granulosa cells of the rat. *Acta Endocrinol.*, 88:567–579.
385. Naftolin, F., Brown-Grant, K., and Corker, C. S. (1972): Plasma and pituitary luteinizing hormone and peripheral plasma oestradiol concentrations in the normal oestrous cycle of the rat and after experimental manipulation of the cycle. *J. Endocrinol.*, 53:17–30.
386. Kalra, S. P., and Kalra, P. S. (1974): Temporal interrelationships among circulating levels of estradiol, progesterone and LH during the rat estrous cycle. *Endocrinology*, 95:1711–1718.
387. Goodman, R. L. (1978): A quantitative analysis of the physiological role of estradiol and progesterone in the control of tonic and surge secretion of luteinizing hormone in the rat. *Endocrinology*, 102:142–150.
388. Goodman, R. L., and Daniel, K. (1985): Modulation of pulsatile luteinizing hormone secretion by ovarian steroids in the rat. *Biol. Reprod.*, 32:217–225.
389. Devorshak-Harvey, E., Peluso, J. J., Bona-Gallo, A., and Gallo, R. V. (1985): Effect of alterations in pulsatile luteinizing hormone release on ovarian follicular atresia and steroid secretion on diestrus 1 in the rat estrous cycle. *Biol. Reprod.*, 33:103–111.
390. Okamoto, M. T., Nobunaga, T., and Suzuki, Y. (1972): Delay in ovulation with pentobarbital anesthesia applied at various stages of the 4-day cyclic rat. *Endocrinol. Jpn.*, 19:11–17.
391. Dominquez, R., and Smith, E. R. (1974): Barbiturate blockade of ovulation on days other than proestrus in the rat. *Neuroendocrinology*, 14:212–223.
392. Schwartz, N. B., and Gold, J. J. (1967): Effect of a single dose of anti-LH serum at proestrus on the rat estrous cycle. *Anat. Rec.*, 157:137–150.
393. Laurence, K. A., and Ichikawa, S. (1969): Effects of antiserum to bovine LH on the estrous cycle and early pregnancy in the female rat. *Int. J. Fertil.*, 14:8–15.
394. Greenwald, G. S. (1965): Effect of a single injection of diethylstilbestrol or progesterone on the hamster ovary. *J. Endocrinol.*, 33:13–23.
395. Greenwald, G. S. (1977): Exogenous progesterone: influence on ovulation and hormone levels in the cyclic hamster. *J. Endocrinol.*, 73:151–155.
396. Greenwald, G. S. (1978): Modification by exogenous progesterone of estrogen and gonadotropin secretion in the cyclic hamster. *Endocrinology*, 103:2315–2322.
397. Beattie, C. W., and Corbin, C. W. (1975): The differential effects of diestrous progestogen administration on proestrous gonadotropin levels. *Endocrinology*, 97:885–890.
398. Garza, F., and Terranova, P. F. (1984): Inhibition of thecal androstenedione production by exogenous progesterone in the cyclic hamster. *J. Reprod. Fertil.*, 70:493–498.
399. Taya, K., Terranova, P. F., and Greenwald, G. S. (1981): Acute effects of exogenous progesterone on follicular steroidogenesis in the cyclic rat. *Endocrinology*, 108:2324–2330.
400. Varga, B., and Greenwald, G. S. (1979): Cyclic changes in utero-ovarian blood flow and ovarian hormone secretion in the hamster: effects of adrenocorticotropin, luteinizing hormone, and follicle-stimulating hormone. *Endocrinology*, 104:1525–1531.
401. Varga, B., Horvath, E., Folly, G., and Stark, E. (1985): Study of the luteinizing hormone-induced increase of ovarian blood flow during the estrous cycle in the rat. *Biol. Reprod.*, 32:480–488.
402. Peluso, J. J., Luttmer, S., and Gruenberg, M. L. (1984): Modulatory action of FSH on LH-induced follicular growth in rats. *J. Reprod. Fertil.*, 72:173–177.
403. Greenwald, G. S. (1978): Follicular activity in the mammalian ovary. In: *The Vertebrate Ovary*, edited by R. E. Jones, pp. 639–689. Plenum, New York.
404. Nordenstrom, K., and Johanson, C. (1985): Steroidogenesis in isolated rat granulosa cells—changes during follicular maturation. *Acta Endocrinol.*, 108:550–556.
405. Richards, J. S., Jonassen, J. A., and Kersey, K. A. (1980): Evidence that changes in tonic luteinizing hormone secretion determine the growth of preovulatory follicles in the rat. *Endocrinology*, 107:641–647.
406. Roser, S., and Block (1971): Étude comparative des variations de la progestérone plasmatique ovarienne au cours de cycles de respectivement 4 et 5 jour, chez la ratte. *C. R. Soc. Biol.*, 165:1995–1998.
407. van der Schoot, P., and de Greef, W. J. (1976): Dioestrous progesterone and pro-estrous luteinizing hormone in 4- and 5-day cycles of female rats. *J. Endocrinol.*, 70:61–68.

408. Nequin, L. G., Alvarez, J., and Shwartz, N. B. (1979): Measurement of serum steroid and gonadotropin levels and uterine and ovarian variables throughout 4 day and 5 day estrous cycles in the rat. *Biol. Reprod.*, 20:659–670.
409. van der Schoot, P., and Uilenbroek, J. T. J. (1983): Reduction of 5-day cycle length of female rats by treatment with bromocriptine. *J. Endocrinol.*, 97:83–89.
410. Boehm, N., Plas-Roser, S., and Aron, C. (1984): Prolactin and the control of cycle length in the female rat. *Acta Endocrinol.*, 106:188–192.
411. Richards, J. S., and Bogovich, K. (1982): Effects of human chorionic gonadotropin and progesterone on follicular development in the immature rat. *Endocrinology*, 111:1429–1438.
412. Fortune, J. E., and Vincent, S. E. (1983): Progesterone inhibits the induction of aromatase activity in rat granulosa cells in vitro. *Biol. Reprod.*, 28:1078–1089.
413. Uilenbroek, J. T. J., van der Schoot, P., den Besten, D., and Lankhorst, R. R. (1982): A possible direct effect of prolactin on follicular activity. *Biol. Reprod.*, 27:1119–1125.
414. Magoffin, D. A., and Erickson, G. F. (1981): LH induction of androgen biosynthesis in cultured ovarian cells: inhibitory effect on prolactin. In: *Dynamics of Ovarian Function*, edited by N. B. Schwartz and M. Hunzicker-Dunn, pp. 55–60. Raven Press, New York.
415. L'Hermite, M., Niswender, G. D., Reichert, L. E., Jr., and Midgley, A. R., Jr. (1972): Serum follicle-stimulating hormone in sheep as measured by radioimmunoassay. *Biol. Reprod.*, 6:325–332.
416. Goodman, R. L., Pickover, S. M., and Karasch, F. J. (1981): Ovarian feedback control of follicle-stimulating hormone in the ewe: evidence for selective suppression. *Endocrinology*, 108:772–777.
417. McNatty, K. P., Dobson, C., Gibb, M., Kieboom, L., and Thurley, D. C. (1981): Accumulation of luteinizing hormone, oestradiol and androstenedione by sheep ovarian follicles in vivo. *J. Endocrinol.*, 91:99–109.
418. Hauger, R. L., Karsch, F. J., and Foster, D. L.(1977): A new concept for control of the estrous cycle of the ewe based on the temporal relationships between luteinizing hormone, estradiol and progesterone in peripheral serum and evidence that progesterone inhibits tonic LH secretion. *Endocrinology*, 101:807–817.
419. Baird, D. T., Swanston, I., and Scaramuzzi, R. J. (1976): Pulsatile release of LH and secretion of ovarian steroids in sheep during the luteal phase of the estrous cycle. *Endocrinology*, 98:1490–1495.
420. Brand, A., and deJong, W. H. R. (1973): Qualitative and quantitative micromorphological investigations of the tertiary follicle population during the oestrous cycle in sheep. *J. Reprod. Fertil.*, 33:431–439.
421. Bherer, J., Matton, P., and Dufour, J. J. (1977): Fate of the two largest follicles in the ewe after injection of gonadotrophins at two stages of the estrus cycle. *Proc. Soc. Exp. Biol. Med.*, 154:412–414.
422. Tsonis, C. G., Cahill, L. P., Carson, R. S., and Findlay, J. K. (1984): Identification at the onset of luteolysis of follicles capable of ovulation in the ewe. *J. Reprod. Fertil.*, 70:609–614.
423. Dailey, R. A., Fogwell, R. L., and Thayne, W. V. (1982): Distribution of visible follicles on the ovarian surface in ewes. *J. Anim. Sci.*, 54:1196–1204.
424. Turnbull, K. E., Braden, A. W. H., and Mattner, P. E. (1977): The pattern of follicular growth and atresia in the ovine ovary. *Aust. J. Biol. Sci.*, 30:229–241.
425. Cahill, L. P., and Mauleon, P. (1980): Influences of season, cycle and breed on follicular growth rates in sheep. *J. Reprod. Fertil.*, 58:321–328.
426. Lahlou-Kassi, A., and Mariana, J. C. (1984): Ovarian follicular growth during the oestrous cycle in two breeds of ewes of different ovulation rate, the D'man and the Timahdite. *J. Reprod. Fertil.*, 72:301–310.
427. Cummins, L. J., O'Shea, T., Bindon, B. M., Lee, V. W. K., and Findlay, J. K. (1983): Ovarian inhibin content and sensitivity to inhibin in Booroola and control strain Merino ewes. *J. Reprod. Fertil.*, 67:1–7.
428. Robertson, D. M., Ellis, S., Foulds, L. M., Findlay, J. K., and Bindon, B. M. (1984): Pituitary gonadotrophins in Booroola and control Merino sheep. *J. Reprod. Fertil.*, 71:189–197.
429. McNatty, K. P., Henderson, K. M., Lun, S., et al. (1985): Ovarian activity in Booroola × Romney ewes which have a major gene influencing their ovulation rate. *J. Reprod. Fertil.*, 73;109–120.
430. Bindon, B. M., Piper, L. R., and Thimonier, J. (1984): Preovulatory LH characteristics and time of ovulation in the prolific Booroola Merino ewe. *J. Reprod. Fertil.*, 71:519–523.
431. Bjersing, L., Hay, M. F., Kan, G., et al. (1972): Changes in gonadotrophins, ovarian steroids and follicular morphology in sheep at oestrus. *J. Endocrinol.*, 52:465–479.
432. Hay, M. F., and Moor, R. M. (1975): Functional and structural relationships in the graafian follicle population of the sheep ovary. *J. Reprod. Fertil.*, 45:583–593.
433. McNatty, K. P., Gibb, M., Dobson, C., Thurley, D. C., and Findlay, J. K. (1981): Changes in the concentration of gonadotrophic and steroidal hormones in the antral fluid of ovarian follicles throughout the oestrous cycle of the sheep. *Aust. J. Biol. Sci.*, 34:67–80.
434. Moor, R. M. (1974): The ovarian follicle of the sheep: inhibition of oestrogen secretion by luteinizing hormone. *J. Endocrinol.*, 61:455–463.
435. England, B. G., Webb, R., and Dahmer, M. K. (1981): Follicular steroidogenesis and gonadotropin binding to ovine follicles during the estrous cycle. *Endocrinology*, 109:881–887.
436. Driancourt, M. A., Gibson, W. R., and Cahill, L. P. (1985): Follicular dynamics throughout the oestrous cycle in sheep. A review. *Reprod. Nutr. Dev.*, 25:1–15.
437. McNatty, K. P., Gibb, M., Dobson, C., et al. (1982): Preovulatory follicular development in sheep treated with PMSG and/or prostaglandin. *J. Reprod. Fertil.*, 65:111–123.
438. Webb, R., and England, B. G. (1982): Identification of the ovulatory follicle in the ewe: associated changes in follicular size, thecal and granulosa cell luteinizing hormone receptors, antral fluid steroids, and circulating hormones during the preovulatory period. *Endocrinology*, 110:873–881.
439. McNeilly, A. S., Fraser, H. M., and Baird, D. T. (1984): Effect of immunoneutralization of LH releasing hormone on LH, FSH and ovarian steroid secretion in the preovulatory phase of the oestrous cycle in the ewe. *J. Endocrinol.*, 101:213–219.
440. McNatty, K. P., Hudson, N. L., Henderson, K. M., et al. (1984): Changes in gonadotropin secretion and ovarian antral follicular activity in seasonally breeding sheep throughout the year. *J. Reprod. Fertil.*, 70:309–321.
441. McLeod, B. J., Haresign, W., and Lamming, G. E. (1983): Induction of ovulation in seasonally anoestrous ewes by continuous infusion of low doses of Gn-RH. *J. Reprod. Fertil.*, 68:489–495.
442. McNatty, K. P., Hudson, N., Gibb, M., et al. (1985): FSH influences follicle viability, oestradiol biosynthesis and ovulation rate in Romney ewes. *J. Reprod. Fertil.*, 75:121–131.
443. McNeilly, A. S. (1985): Effect of changes in FSH induced by bovine follicular fluid and FSH infusion in the preovulatory phase on subsequent ovulation rate and corpus luteum function in the ewe. *J. Reprod. Fertil.*, 74:661–668.
444. Schams, D., Schallenberger, E., Hoffman, B., and Karg, H. (1977): The oestrous cycle of the cow: hormonal parameters and time relationships concerning oestrus, ovulation, and electrical resistance of the vaginal mucus. *Acta Endocrinol.*, 86:180–182.
445. Walters, D. L., Schams, D., and Schallenberger, E. (1984): Pulsatile secretion of gonadotrophins, ovarian steroids and ovarian oxytocin during the luteal phase of the oestrous cycle in the cow. *J. Reprod. Fertil.*, 71:479–491.
446. Schallenberger, E., Schams, D., Bullermann, B., and Walters, D. L. (1984): Pulsatile secretion of gonadotrophins, ovarian steroids and ovarian oxytocin during prostaglandin-induced regression of the corpus luteum in the cow. *J. Reprod. Fertil.*, 71:493–501.
447. Ireland, J. J., and Roche, J. F. (1982): Development of antral follicles in cattle after prostaglandin-induced luteolysis: changes in serum hormones, steroids in follicular fluid, and gonadotropin receptors. *Endocrinology*, 111:2077–2086.
448. Glencross, R. G., Munro, I. B., Senior, B. E., and Pope, G. S. (1973): Concentrations of oestradiol-17β, oestrone and progesterone in jugular venous plasma of cows during the oestrous cycle and in early pregnancy. *Acta Endocrinol.*, 73:374–384.
449. Dieleman, S. J., Kruip, T. A. M., Fontijne, P., de Jong, W. H. R., and van der Weyden, G. C. (1983): Changes in oestradiol, progesterone and testosterone concentrations in follicular fluid and in the micromorphology of preovulatory bovine follicles relative to the peak of luteinizing hormone. *J. Endocrinol.*, 97:31–42.

450. Roche, J. F., and Ireland, J. J. (1981): The differential effect of progesterone on concentrations of luteinizing hormone and follicle-stimulating hormone in heifers. *Endocrinology,* 108:568–572.
451. Dufour, J., Whitmore, H. L., Ginther, O. J., and Casida, L. E. (1972): Identification of the ovulating follicle by its size on different days of the estrous cycle in heifers. *J. Anim. Sci.,* 34:85–87.
452. Matton, P., Adelakoun, V., Couture, Y., and Dufour, J. J. (1981): Growth and replacement of the bovine ovarian follicles during the estrous cycle. *J. Anim. Sci.,* 52:813–820.
453. Staigmiller, R. B., and England, B. G. (1982): Folliculogenesis in the bovine. *Theriogenology,* 17:43–52.
454. Fogwell, R. L., Cowley, J. L., Wortman, J. A., Ames, N. K., and Ireland, J. J. (1985): Luteal function in cows following destruction of ovarian follicles at midcycle. *Theriogenology,* 23:389–398.
455. Choudary, J. B., Gier, H. T., and Marion, G. B. (1968): Cyclic changes in bovine vesicular follicles. *J. Anim. Sci.,* 27:468–471.
456. Scaramuzzi, R. J., Turnbull, K. E., and Nancarrow, C. D. (1980): Growth of graafian follicles in cows following luteolysis induced by the prostaglandin $F_{2\alpha}$ analogue, cloprostenol. *Aust. J. Biol. Sci.,* 33:63–69.
457. Kruip, T. A. M., and Dieleman, S. J. (1982): Macroscopic classification of bovine follicles and its validation by micromorphological and steroid biochemical procedures. *Reprod. Nutr. Dev.,* 22:465–473.
458. Merz, E. A., Hauser, E. R., and England, B. G. (1981): Ovarian function in the cycling cow: relationship between gonadotropin binding to theca and granulosa and steroidogenesis in individual follicles. *J. Anim. Sci.,* 52:1457–1468.
459. Henderson, K. M., McNeilly, A. S., and Swanston, I. A. (1982): Gonadotrophin and steroid concentrations in bovine follicular fluid and their relationship to follicle size. *J. Reprod. Fertil.,* 65:467–473.
460. Fortune, J. E., and Hansel, W. (1985): Concentrations of steroids and gonadotropins in follicular fluid from normal heifers and heifers primed for superovulation. *Biol. Reprod.,* 32:1069–1079.
461. Staigmiller, R. B., England, B. G., Webb, R., Short, R. E., and Bellows, R. A. (1982): Estrogen secretion and gonadotropin binding by individual bovine follicles during estrus. *J. Anim. Sci.,* 55:1473–1482.
462. Thayer, K. M., Forrest, D. W., and Welsh, T. H., Jr. (1985): Real-time ultrasound evaluation of follicular development in superovulated cows. *Theriogenology,* 23:233.
463. van de Wiel, D. F. M., Erkens, J., Koops, W., Vos, E., and van Landeghem, A. A. J. (1981): Periestrous and midluteal time courses of circulating LH, FSH, prolactin, estradiol-17β and progesterone in the domestic pig. *Biol. Reprod.,* 24:223–233.
464. Magness, R. R., Christenson, R. K., and Ford, S. P. (1983): Ovarian blood flow throughout the estrous cycle and early pregnancy in sows. *Biol. Reprod.,* 28:1090–1096.
465. Clark, J. R., Brazier, S. G., Wiginton, L. M., Stevenson, G. R., and Tribble, L. F. (1982): Time of ovarian follicle selection during the porcine estrous cycle. *Theriogenology,* 18:697–709.
466. Parlow, A. F., Anderson, L. L., and Melampy, R. M. (1964): Pituitary follicle-stimulating hormone and luteinizing hormone concentrations in relation to reproductive stages of the pig. *Endocrinology,* 75:365–376.
467. Guthrie, H. D., and Knudsen, J. F. (1984): Follicular growth and production of estrogen and progesterone after injection of gilts with human chorionic gonadotropin on day 12 of the estrous cycle. *J. Anim. Sci.,* 59:1295–1302.
468. Hunter, R. H. F., and Baker, T. G. (1975): Development and fate of porcine graafian follicles identified at different stages of the oestrous cycle. *J. Reprod. Fertil.,* 43:193–196.
469. Dailey, R. A., Clark, J. R., Staigmiller, R. B., First, N. L., Chapman, A. B., and Casida, L. E. (1976): Growth of new follicles following electrocautery in four genetic groups of swine. *J. Anim. Sci.,* 43:175–183.
470. Bamberg, E., Choi, H. S., Hassaan, N. K., Klaring, W. J., Mostl, E., and Stockl, W. (1980): Steroidhormongehalt in Blut und Ovarfollikeln des Rindes wahrend des Zyklus. *Zbl. Vet. Med.,* 27:186–194.
471. Ainsworth, L., Tsang, B. K., Downey, B. R., Marcus, G. J., and Armstrong, D. T. (1980): Interrelationships between follicular fluid steroid levels, gonadotropic stimuli, and oocyte maturation during preovulatory development of porcine follicles. *Biol. Reprod.,* 23:621–627.
472. Koering, M. J. (1969): Cyclic changes in ovarian morphology during the menstrual cycle in *Macaca mulatta. Am. J. Anat.,* 126:73–101.
473. Koering, M. J., Baehler, E. A., Goodman, A. L., and Hodgen, G. D. (1982): Developing morphological asymmetry of ovarian follicular maturation in monkeys. *Biol. Reprod.,* 27:989–997.
474. Stouffer, R. L., Hodgen, G. D., Ottobre, A. C., and Christian, C. D. (1984): Follicular fluid treatment during the follicular versus luteal phase of the menstrual cycle: effects on corpus luteum function. *J. Clin. Endocrinol. Metab.,* 48:1027–1033.
475. Zeleznik, A. J., Wildt, L., and Schuler, H. M. (1980): Characterization of ovarian folliculogenesis during the luteal phase of the menstrual cycle in rhesus monkeys using [^{3}H]thymidine autoradiography. *Endocrinology,* 107:982–988.
476. Ellinwood, W. E., Norman, R. L., and Spies, H. G. (1984): Changing frequency of pulsatile luteinizing hormone and progesterone secretion during the luteal phase of the menstrual cycle of rhesus monkeys. *Biol. Reprod.,* 31:714–722.
477. Clark, J. R., Dierschke, D. J., Meller, P. A., and Wolf, R. C. (1979): Hormonal regulation of ovarian folliculogenesis in rhesus monkeys. II. Serum concentrations of estradiol-17β and follicle stimulating hormone associated with growth and identification of the preovulatory follicle. *Biol. Reprod.,* 21:497–503.
478. Clark, J. R., Dierschke, D. J., and Wolf, R. C. (1978): Hormonal regulation of ovarian folliculogenesis in rhesus monkeys: I. Concentrations of serum luteinizing hormone and progesterone during laparoscopy and patterns of follicular development during successive menstrual cycles. *Biol. Reprod.,* 17:779–783.
479. Goodman, A. L., Nixon, W. E., Johnson, D. K., and Hodgen, G. D. (1977): Regulation of folliculogenesis in the cycling rhesus monkey: selection of the dominant follicle. *Endocrinology,* 100: 155–161.
480. Goodman, A. L., Nixon, W. E., and Hodgen, G. D. (1979): Between-ovary interaction in the regulation of follicle growth, corpus luteum function, and gonadotropin secretion in the primate ovarian cycle. III. Temporal and spatial dissociation of folliculogenesis and negative feedback regulation of tonic gonadotropin release after lutectomy in rhesus monkeys. *Endocrinology,* 105:69–73.
481. diZerega, G. S., and Hodgen, G. D. (1982): The interovarian progesterone gradient: a spatial and temporal regulator of folliculogenesis in the primate ovarian cycle. *J. Clin. Endocrinol. Metab.,* 54:495–499.
482. diZerega, G. S., Campeau, J. D., Ujita, E. L., et al. (1983): The possible role for a follicular protein in the intraovarian regulation of folliculogenesis. *Sem. Reprod. Endocrinol.,* 1:309–320.
483. Channing, C. P., Anderson, L. D., Hoover, D. J., Gagliano, P., and Hodgen, G. (1981): Inhibitory effects of porcine follicular fluid on monkey serum FSH levels and follicular maturation. *Biol. Reprod.,* 25:885–903.
484. diZerega, G. S., Turner, C. K., Stouffer, R. L., Anderson, L. D., Channing, C. P., and Hodgen, G. D. (1981): Suppression of follicle-stimulating hormone-dependent folliculogenesis during the primate ovarian cycle. *J. Clin. Endocrinol. Metab.,* 52:451–456.
485. Zeleznik, A. J., Hutchison, J. S., and Schuler, H. M. (1985): Interference with the gonadotropin-suppressing actions of estradiol in macaques overrides the selection of a single preovulatory follicle. *Endocrinology,* 117:991–999.
486. Dierschke, D. J., Hutz, R. J., and Wolf, R. C. (1985): Induced follicular atresia in rhesus monkeys: strength–duration relationships of the estrogen stimulus. *Endocrinology,* 117:1397–1403.
487. Williams, R. F., and Hodgen, G. D. (1980): Disparate effects of human chorionic gonadotropin during the late follicular phase in monkeys: normal ovulation, follicular atresia, ovarian acyclicity, and hypersecretion of follicle-stimulating hormone. *Fertil. Steril.,* 33:64–68.
488. Wilks, J. W., Spilman, C. H., and Campbell, J. A. (1983): Arrest of folliculogenesis and inhibition of ovulation in the monkey following weekly administration of progestins. *Fertil. Steril.,* 40:688–692.
489. Channing, C. P. (1980): Progesterone and estrogen secretion by cultured monkey ovarian cell types: influences of follicular size, serum luteinizing hormone levels, and follicular fluid estrogen levels. *Endocrinology,* 107:342–352.

490. Vernon, M. W., Dierschke, D. J., Sholl, S. A., and Wolf, R. C. (1983): Ovarian aromatase activity in granulosa and theca cells of rhesus monkeys. *Biol. Reprod.*, 28:342–349.
491. Marut, E. L., Huang, S. C., and Hodgen, G. D. (1983): Distinguishing the steroidogenic roles of granulosa and theca cells of the dominant ovarian follicle and corpus luteum. *J. Clin. Endocrinol. Metab.*, 57:925–930.
492. Block, E. (1951): Quantitative morphological investigations of the follicular system in women. Variations in the different phases of the sexual cycle. *Acta Endocrinol.*, 8:33–54.
493. Gougeon, A. (1981): Rate of follicular growth in the human ovary. In: *Follicular Maturation and Ovulation—Proceedings of the IVth Reinier de Graaf Symposium, International Congress Ser. No. 560*, edited by R. Rolland, E. V. van Hall, S. G. Hillier, K. P. McNatty, and J. Schoemaker, pp. 155–163. Excerpta Medica, Princeton, NJ.
494. Gougeon, A. (1984): Vitesse de croissance des follicules dans l'ovaire humain. *Contraception-Fertilite-Sexualite*, 12:839–845.
495. Gougeon, A. (1984): Influence des variations hormonales cycliques (steroides et gonadotropines) sur la croissance folliculaire dans l'ovaire humain. *Contraception-Fertilite-Sexualite*, 12:615–620.
496. Gougeon, A., and Lefevre, B. (1984): Histological evidence of alternating ovulation in women. *J. Reprod. Fertil.*, 70:7–13.
497. Gougeon, A. (1984): Croissance folliculaire dans l'ovaire humain pendant le cycle menstruel: mise en evidence de regulations intraovariennes. *Contraception-Fertilite-Sexualite*, 12:733–738.
498. Gougeon, A. (1984): Le follicule ovulatoire humain. A quel moment du cycle est-il selectionne et par quels mecanismes? Une tentative de reponse. *Contraception-Fertilite-Sexualite*, 12:1397–1405.
499. McNatty, K. P. (1981): Hormonal correlates of follicular development in the human ovary. *Aust. J. Biol. Sci.*, 34:249–268.
500. Lloyd, C. W., Lobotsky, J., Baird, D. T., et al. (1971): Concentration of unconjugated estrogens, androgens and gestagens in ovarian and peripheral venous plasma of women: The normal menstrual cycle. *J. Clin. Endocrinol.*, 32:155–166.
501. deJong, F. H., Baird, D. T., and van der Molen, H. J. (1974): Ovarian secretion rates of oestrogens, androgens and progesterone in normal women and in women with persistent ovarian follicles. *Acta Endocrinol.*, 77:575–587.
502. Baird, D. T., and Fraser, I. S. (1974): Blood production and ovarian secretion rates of estradiol-17β and estrone in women throughout the menstrual cycle. *J. Clin. Endocrinol. Metab.*, 38:1009–1017.
503. McNatty, K. P., Hunter, W. M., McNeilly, A. S., and Sawers, R. S. (1975): Changes in the concentration of pituitary and steroid hormones in the follicular fluid of human graafian follicles throughout the menstrual cycle. *J. Endocrinol.*, 64:555–571.
504. McNatty, K. P., and Baird, D. T. (1978): Relationship between follicle-stimulating hormone, androstenedione and oestradiol in human follicular fluid. *J. Endocrinol.*, 76:527–531.
505. Queenan, J. T., O'Brien, K. G. D., Bains, L. M., Simpson, J., Collins, W. P., and Campbell, S. (1980): Ultrasound scanning of ovaries to detect ovulation in women. *Fertil. Steril.*, 34:99–105.
506. McNatty, K. P. (1978): Cyclic changes in antral fluid hormone concentrations in humans. *Clin. Endocrinol. Metab.*, 7:577–600.
507. Bieszczad, R. R., McClintock, J. S., Pepe, G. J., and Dimino, M. J. (1982): Progesterone secretion by granulosa cells from different sized follicles of human ovaries after short term incubation. *J. Clin. Endocrinol. Metab.*, 55:181–184.
508. Dennefors, B. L., Nilsson, L., and Hamberger, L. (1982): Steroid and adenosine 3′, 5′-monophosphate formation in granulosa and thecal cells from human preovulatory follicles in response to human chorionic gonadotropin. *J. Clin. Endocrinol. Metab.*, 54:436–441.
509. Bernardus, R. E., Jones, G. S., Acosta, A. A., et al. (1985): The significance of the ratio in follicle-stimulating hormone and luteinizing hormone in induction of multiple follicular growth. *Fertil. Steril.*, 43:373–378.
510. Gougeon, A., Lefevre, B., and Testart, J. (1984): Recrutement et selection du follicule dominant pendant le cycle menstruel spontane ou stimule chez la femme. In: *Periode Peri-ovulatoire. Colloque de la societe francaise pour l'etude de la fertilite*, pp. 1–11.
511. Nilsson, L., Wikland, M., and Hamberger, L. (1982): Recruitment of an ovulatory follicle in the human following follicle-ectomy and luteectomy. *Fertil. Steril.*, 37:30–34.
512. Araki, S., Chikazawa, K., Akabori, A., Ijima, K., and Tamada, T. (1983): Hormonal profile after removal of the dominant follicle and corpus luteum in women. *Endocrinol. Jpn.*, 30:55–70.
513. diZerega, G. S., Marrs, R. P., Roche, P. C., Campeau, J. D., and Kling, O. R. (1983): Identification of proteins in pooled human follicular fluid which suppress follicular response to gonadotropins. *J. Clin. Endocrinol. Metab.*, 56:35–41.
514. diZerega, G. S., Marrs, R. P., Campeau, J. D., and Kling, O. R. (1983): Human granulosa cell secretion of protein(s) which suppress follicular response to gonadotropins. *J. Clin. Endocrinol. Metab.*, 56:147–155.
515. Chari, S., Daume, E., Sturm, G., Vaupel, H., and Schuler, I. (1985): Regulators of steroid secretion and inhibin activity in human ovarian follicular fluid. *Mol. Cell. Endocrinol.*, 41:137–145.
516. Greenwald, G. S., and Choudary, J. B. (1969): Follicular development and induction of ovulation in the pregnant mouse. *Endocrinology*, 84:1512–1516.
517. Murr, S. M., Bradford, G. E., and Geschwind, I. I. (1974): Plasma luteinizing hormone, follicle-stimulating hormone and prolactin during pregnancy in the mouse. *Endocrinology*, 94:112–116.
518. Greenwald, G. S. (1966): Ovarian follicular development and pituitary FSH and LH content in the pregnant rat. *Endocrinology*, 79:572–578.
519. Taya, K., and Sasamoto, S. (1977): Induction of ovulation by exogenous gonadotrophin during pseudopregnancy, pregnancy or lactation in rats. *J. Reprod. Fertil.*, 51:467–468.
520. Taya, K., and Greenwald, G. S. (1981): In vivo and in vitro ovarian steroidogenesis in the pregnant rat. *Biol. Reprod.*, 25:683–691.
521. Taya, K., Kimura, J., and Sasamoto, S. (1984): Inhibin activity in ovarian venous plasma during pregnancy, pseudopregnancy and lactation in the rat. *Endocrinol. Jpn.*, 31:427–433.
522. Richards, J. S., and Kersey, K. A. (1979): Changes in theca and granulosa cell function in antral follicles developing during pregnancy in the rat: gonadotropin receptors, cyclic AMP and estradiol-17β. *Biol. Reprod.*, 21:1185–1201.
523. Carson, R. S., Richards, J. S., and Kahn, L. E. (1981): Functional and morphological differentiation of theca and granulosa cells during pregnancy in the rat: dependence on increased basal luteinizing hormone activity. *Endocrinology*, 109:1433–1441.
524. Bogovich, K., Richards, J. S., and Reichert, L. E., Jr. (1981): Obligatory role of luteinizing hormone (LH) in the initiation of preovulatory follicular growth in the pregnant rat: specific effects of human chorionic gonadotropin and follicle-stimulating hormone on LH receptors and steroidogenesis in theca, granulosa and luteal cells. *Endocrinology*, 109:860–867.
525. Bogovich, K., and Richards, J. S. (1982): Androgen biosynthesis in developing ovarian follicles: evidence that luteinizing hormone regulates thecal 17α-hydroxylase and C17-20-lyase activities. *Endocrinology*, 111:1201–1208.
526. Greenwald, G. S. (1967): Induction of ovulation in the pregnant hamster. *Am. J. Anat.*, 121:249–258.
527. Bast, J. D., and Greenwald, G. S. (1974): Daily concentrations of gonadotrophins and prolactin in the serum of pregnant or lactating hamsters. *J. Endocrinol.*, 63:527–532.
528. Greenwald, G. S., Voogt, J. L., and Limback, D. (1984): In vitro follicular and luteal steroidogenesis in the pregnant hamster with preliminary studies in the rat. *Biol. Reprod.*, 30:93–104.
529. Adams, C. E. (1968): Ovarian response to human chorionic gonadotrophin and egg transport in the pregnant and post-parturient rabbit. *J. Endocrinol.*, 40:101–105.
530. Osteen, K. G., and Mills, T. M. (1979): Serum LH and FSH levels in the pregnant rabbit. *Proc. Soc. Exp. Biol. Med.*, 162:454–457.
531. Osteen, K. G., and Mills, T. M. (1980): Changes in the size, distribution and steroid content of rabbit ovarian follicles during early pseudopregnancy. *Biol. Reprod.*, 22:1040–1046.
532. Labhsetwar, A. P., and Diamond, M. (1970): Ovarian changes in the guinea pig during various reproductive stages and steroid treatments. *Biol. Reprod.*, 2:53–57.
533. Bujard, E. (1953): L'ovaire de cobaye (etudes statistiques des follicules ovariques) I. L'ovaire gravide. *Rev. Suisse Zool.*, 60:615–652.
534. Rowlands, I. W. (1956): The corpus luteum of the guinea pig. In: *CIBA Foundation Colloquia on Ageing*, Vol. 2, edited by G. Wolstenholme and E. Millar, pp. 69–85. Little, Brown, Boston.

535. Melampy, R. M., Henricks, D. M., Anderson, L. L., Chen, C. L., and Schultz, J. R. (1966): Pituitary follicle-stimulating hormone and luteinizing hormone concentrations in pregnant and lactating pigs. *Endocrinology,* 78:801–804.
536. Dufour, J. J., and Fahmy, M. H. (1974): Follicular and luteal changes during early pregnancy in three breeds of swine. *Can. J. Anim. Sci.,* 54:29–33.
537. Schallenberger, E., Rampp, J., and Walters, D. L. (1985): Gonadotrophins and ovarian steroids in cattle. II. Pulsatile changes of concentrations in the jugular vein throughout pregnancy. *Acta Endocrinol.,* 108:322–330.
538. Schallenberger, E., Schondorfer, A. M., and Walters, D. L. (1985): Gonadotrophins and ovarian steroids in cattle. I. Pulsatile changes of concentrations in the jugular vein throughout the oestrous cycle. *Acta Endocrinol.,* 108:312–321.
539. Govan, A. D. T. (1968): The human ovary in early pregnancy. *J. Endocrinol.,* 40:421–428.
540. Govan, A. D. T. (1970): Ovarian follicular activity in late pregnancy. *J. Endocrinol.,* 48:235–241.
541. Starup, J., and Visfeldt, J. (1974): Ovarian morphology in early and late human pregnancy. *Acta Obstet. Gynecol. Scand.,* 53:211–218.
542. Dekel, N., David, M. P., Yedwab, G. A., and Kraicer, P. F. (1977): Follicular development during late human pregnancy. *Int. J. Fertil.,* 22:24–29.
543. Dennefors, B. L., and Nilsson, L. (1981): Steroid production and responsiveness to gonadotropin and prostaglandins of human ovarian follicles at term pregnancy. *Fertil. Steril.,* 35:232–233.
544. Westergaard, L., McNatty, K. P., and Christensen, I. J. (1985): Steroid concentrations in fluid from human ovarian antral follicles during pregnancy. *J. Endocrinol.,* 107:133–136.
545. Parlow, A. F., Daane, T. A., and Dignam, W. J. (1970): On the concentration of radioimmunoassayable FSH circulating in blood throughout human pregnancy. *J. Clin. Endocrinol.,* 31:213–214.
546. Mishell, D. R., Jr., Thorneycroft, I. H., Nagata, Y., and Nakamura, R. M. (1973): Steroid and gonadotropin levels in normal pregnancies and pregnancies following HMG therapy. In: *Gonadotropin in Female Infertility,* edited by E. Rosemberg, pp. 201–207. Excerpta Medica, Amsterdam.
547. Ranta, T., Chen, H. C., Shimohigashi, Y., Baukal, A. J., Knecht, M., and Catt, K. (1985): Enhanced follicle-stimulating hormone activity of deglycosylated human chorionic gonadotropin in ovarian granulosa cells. *Endocrinology,* 116:59–64.
548. Taya, K., and Greenwald, G. S. (1982): Mechanisms of suppression of ovarian follicular development during lactation in the rat. *Biol. Reprod.,* 27:1090–1101.
549. Taya, K., and Sasamoto, S. (1980): Initiation of follicular maturation and ovulation after removal of the litter from the lactating rat. *J. Endocrinol.,* 87:393–400.
550. Tsai-Morris, C. H., Ghosh, M., Hirshfield, A. N., Wise, P. M., and Brodie, A. M. H. (1983): Inhibition of ovarian aromatase by prolactin in vivo. *Biol. Reprod.,* 29:342–346.
551. Selmanoff, M., and Selmanoff, C. (1983): Role of pup age, estradiol 17-β and pituitary responsiveness in the differences in the suckling-induced prolactin response during early and late lactation. *Biol. Reprod.,* 29:400–411.
552. Bruce, H. M. (1961): Observations on the suckling stimulus and lactation in the rat. *J. Reprod. Fertil.,* 2:17–34.
553. Gosden, R. G., Russell, J. A., Clarke, J., and Piper, I. (1981): Effects of inhibiting prolactin secretion on the maintenance of embryonic diapause in the suckling rat. *J. Endocrinol.,* 88:197–203.
554. Hansen, S., Sodersten, P., and Eneroth, P. (1983): Mechanisms regulating hormone release and the duration of dioestrus in the lactating rat. *J. Endocrinol.,* 99:173–180.
555. Smith, M. S. (1981): Site of action of prolactin in the suppression of gonadotropin secretion during lactation in the rat: effect on pituitary responsiveness to LHRH. *Biol. Reprod.,* 24:967–976.
556. Reeves, J. J., Tarnavsky, G. K., and Platt, T. (1982): Pituitary and ovarian luteinizing hormone releasing hormone receptors during the estrous cycle, pregnancy and lactation in the rat. *Biol. Reprod.,* 27:316–319.
557. Smith, M. S. (1984): Effects of the intensity of the suckling stimulus and ovarian steroids on pituitary gonadotropin-releasing hormone receptors during lactation. *Biol. Reprod.,* 31:548–555.
558. Smith, M. S. (1982): Effect of pulsatile gonadotropin-releasing hormone on the release of luteinizing hormone and follicle-stimulating hormone in vitro by anterior pituitaries from lactating and cycling rats. *Endocrinology,* 110:882–890.
559. Greenwald, G. S. (1958): A histological study of the reproductive tract of the lactating mouse. *J. Endocrinol.,* 17:17–23.
560. Greenwald, G. S. (1965): Histologic transformation of the ovary of the lactating hamster. *Endocrinology,* 77:641–650.
561. Bridges, R. S., and Goldman, B. D. (1975): Diurnal rhythms in gonadotropins and progesterone in lactating and photoperiod induced acyclic hamsters. *Biol. Reprod.,* 13:617–622.
562. Garcia-Winder, M., Imakawa, K., Day, M. L., Zalesky, D. D., Kittok, R. J., and Kinder, J. E. (1984): Effect of suckling and ovariectomy on the control of luteinizing hormone secretion during the postpartum period in beef cows. *Biol. Reprod.,* 31:771–778.
563. Bellin, M. E., Hinshelwood, M. M., Hauser, E. R., and Ax, R. L. (1984): Influence of suckling and side of corpus luteum or pregnancy on folliculogenesis in postpartum cows. *Biol. Reprod.,* 31:849–855.
564. Dufour, J. J., and Roy, G. L. (1985): Distribution of ovarian follicular populations in the dairy cow within 35 days after parturition. *J. Reprod. Fertil.,* 73:229–235.
565. Walters, D. L., Kaltenbach, C. C., Dunn, T. G., and Short, R. E. (1982): Pituitary and ovarian function in postpartum beef cows. I. Effect of suckling on serum and follicular fluid hormones and follicular gonadotropin receptors. *Biol. Reprod.,* 26:640–646.
566. Walters, D. L., Short, R. E., Convey, E. M., Staigmiller, R. B., Dunn, T. G., and Kaltenbach, C. C. (1982): Pituitary and ovarian function in postpartum beef cows. II. Endocrine changes prior to ovulation in suckled and nonsuckled postpartum cows compared to cycling cows. *Biol. Reprod.,* 26:647–654.
567. Williams, G. L., Talavera, F., Petersen, B. J., Kirsch, J. D., and Tilton, J. E. (1983): Coincident secretion of follicle-stimulating hormone and luteinizing hormone in early postpartum beef cows: effects of suckling and low-level increases of systemic progesterone. *Biol. Reprod.,* 29:362–373.
568. Peters, A. R., Pimentel, M. G., and Lamming, G. E. (1985): Hormone responses to exogenous GnRH pulses in post-partum dairy cows. *J. Reprod. Fertil.,* 75:557–565.
569. Webb, R., Lamming, G. E., Haynes, N. B., and Foxcroft, G. R. (1980): Plasma progesterone and gonadotrophin concentrations and ovarian activity in post-partum dairy cows. *J. Reprod. Fertil.,* 59:133–143.
570. Walters, D. L., Short, R. E., Convey, E. M., Staigmiller, R. B., Dunn, T. G., and Kaltenbach, C. C. (1982): Pituitary and ovarian function in postpartum beef cows. III. Induction of estrus, ovulation and luteal function with intermittent small-dose injections of GnRH. *Biol. Reprod.,* 26:655–662.
571. Kunavongkrit, A., Einarsson, S., and Settergren, I. (1982): Follicular development in primiparous lactating sows. *Anim. Reprod. Sci.,* 5:47–56.
572. Cox, N. M., and Britt, J. H. (1982): Relationships between endogenous gonadotropin-releasing hormone, gonadotropins, and follicular development after weaning in sows. *Biol. Reprod.,* 27:70–78.
573. Edwards, S., and Foxcroft, G. R. (1983): Endocrine changes in sows weaned at two stages of lactation. *J. Reprod. Fertil.,* 67:161–172.
574. Stevenson, J. S., Cox, N. M., and Britt, J. H. (1981): Role of the ovary in controlling luteinizing hormone, follicle-stimulating hormone, and prolactin secretion during and after lactation in pigs. *Biol. Reprod.,* 24:341–353.
575. Shaw, H. J., and Foxcroft, G. R. (1985): Relationships between LH, FSH and prolactin secretion and reproductive activity in the weaned sow. *J. Reprod. Fertil.,* 75:17–28.
576. Cox, N. M., and Britt, J. H. (1982): Pulsatile administration of gonadotropin releasing hormone to lactating sows: endocrine changes associated with induction of fertile estrus. *Biol. Reprod.,* 27:1126–1137.
577. Plant, T. M., Schallenberger, E., Hess, D. L., McCormack, J. T., Dufy-Barbe, L., and Knobil, E. (1980): Influence of suckling on gonadotropin secretion in the female rhesus monkey (*Macaca mulatta*). *Biol. Reprod.,* 23:760–766.
578. Weiss, G., Butler, W. R., Dierschke, D. J., and Knobil, E. (1976): Influence of suckling on gonadotropin secretion in the postpartum rhesus monkey. *Proc. Soc. Exp. Biol. Med.,* 153:330–331.

579. Williams, R. F., and Hodgen, G. D. (1980): Reinitiation of the diurnal rhythm of prolactin secretion in postpartum rhesus monkeys. *Biol. Reprod.*, 23:276–280.
580. Richardson, D. W., Goldsmith, L. T., Pohl, C. R., Schallenberger, E., and Knobil, E. (1985): The role of prolactin in the regulation of the primate corpus luteum. *J. Clin. Endocrinol. Metab.*, 60:501–504.
581. Thomson, A. M., Hytten, F. E., and Black, A. E. (1975): Lactation and reproduction. *Bull. WHO*, 52:337–349.
582. Howie, P. W., and McNeilly, A. S. (1982): Effect of breast-feeding patterns on human birth intervals. *J. Reprod. Fertil.*, 65:545–557.
583. Jeppsson, S., Rannevik, G., Thorell, J. I., and Wide, L. (1977): Influence of LH/FSH releasing hormone (LRH) on the basal secretion of gonadotrophins in relation to plasma levels of oestradiol, progesterone and prolactin during the post-partum period in lactating and in non-lactating women. *Acta Endocrinol.*, 84:713–728.
584. Baird, D. T., McNeilly, A. S., Sawers, R. S., and Sharpe, R. M. (1979): Failure of estrogen-induced discharge of luteinizing hormone in lactating women. *J. Clin. Endocrinol. Metab.*, 49:500–506.
585. Keye, W. R., Jr., and Jaffe, R. B. (1976): Changing patterns of FSH and LH response to gonadotropin-releasing hormone in the puerperium. *J. Clin. Endocrinol. Metab.*, 42:1133–1138.
586. McNeilly, A. S. (1980): Prolactin and the control of gonadotrophin secretion in the female. *J. Reprod. Fertil.*, 58:537–549.
587. McNeilly, A. S., Glasier, A., Jonassen, J., and Howie, P. W. (1982): Evidence for direct inhibition of ovarian function by prolactin. *J. Reprod. Fertil.*, 65:559–569.

The Physiology of Reproduction,
edited by E. Knobil and J. Neill *et al.*
Raven Press, Ltd., New York © 1988.

CHAPTER 12

Mechanism of Mammalian Ovulation

Harry Lipner

Ovulation marks the culmination of a series of events initiated by the surge of luteinizing hormone (LH) and characterized by resumption of meiosis and germinal vesicle breakdown, initiation of luteinization of the granulosa cells, and restructuring of the follicle wall, with resultant follicular rupture and release of a mature fertilizable ovum. Study of the control of ovulation has spawned a large literature, including that on hormonal controls and detailed morphological and biochemical analyses of the preovulatory follicle. These contributions have extended our understanding of the cellular mechanisms associated with steroidal and nonsteroidal biosynthesis, collagenolysis, and vascular changes associated with ovulation but have not yet fully explained the intimate details of follicular rupture. There are a number of reviews that offer interesting insights into the phenomenon of ovulation (34,48,103,144,151–153,155,201,292,310 317,350,386,422).

HISTORICAL BACKGROUND

The study of ovulation began with the discovery of the follicle (227) and that it contained an ovum (118). The cellular composition of the ovary and the follicle wall then occupied workers for the next 170 years in an attempt to settle a raging argument over whether there is smooth muscle in the follicle wall. When the question was resolved in the affirmative, the role of smooth muscle in ovulation was disputed and finally characterized as probably conducive but not essential. Beginning 70 years ago, the suggestion of a role for proteolytic enzymes initiated a new and continuing study of their presence, substrate(s), and controls. A role for the nerve supply to the ovary was bitterly disputed, the answer depending on whether one accepted that nerves penetrated only to the follicle, supplied only the outer two layers, or reached all the layers of the follicle. Not to be excluded in the study of ovulation is the control of the vascular supply to both ovary and follicle, as changes in blood flow manifested by the follicle "blush" have been a subject of intense examination almost from the suggestion 130 years ago that the ovary is an erectile organ (425).

Smooth Muscle

Regnier de Graaf (227) described the ovary as differing from the testis because it lacked tubules and instead had vesicles on its surface, which he mistakenly called eggs or ova. One hundred twenty-five years later, Cruikshank (118) demonstrated ova in rabbit fallopian tubes. This observation initiated the search for an explanation of follicle rupture. Von Kolliker (258) was the first to note smooth muscle in the ovary, and Aeby (4,5) described smooth muscle in the frog ovary, suggested it was involved in the discharge of ova, and explained the observations by Pfluger (399) that frog ovaries showed spontaneous movements. Rouget (425) assumed that smooth muscle around the blood vessels in the ovary and mesovarium allowed the ovary to behave as an erectile organ, discharging ova as the erect penis discharged semen. This concept was accepted as late as 1905 by Heape (209). Grohe (200) described smooth muscle in pig ovaries in the hilus, extending to and encircling the follicle and in close association with blood vessels. Heape (209) noted that rabbits ovulate approximately 10 hr after mating and that only estrus does permit coition. Mature follicles in unmated rabbits fail to release their ova, and the ova and follicles degenerate and regress. He further demonstrated that an intact blood supply to the ovary was essential for follicle rupture but that the presence of sperm was unnecessary. He described growth of the follicles, the appearance of liquor folliculi, and the thinning of the wall to the point at which the contained ovum became visible, the blood vessels around the maturing follicle increased in number, enlarged, and became congested, and the follicle projected above the ovarian surface. After mating, the swollen Graafian follicle underwent changes involving the relationship of the cells of the corona radiatum to the ovum, and approximately 10 hr after mating, follicle rupture occurred. Heape noted that pressure in the follicle was not an adequate explanation because unmated rabbits also had enlarged, projecting follicles. He thought that the innervation of the ovary and the possible behavior of the ovary as an erectile tissue made for a plausible explanation. Despite the earlier histological evidence of smooth muscle in the ovary and follicle, von Winiwarter and Sainmont (506) failed to demonstrate that either electrical or chemical stimuli caused follicle rupture, but they proceeded to demonstrate what they interpreted as smooth muscle in the cat ovarian follicle wall and subsequently in the human follicle (505).

Thomson (466) introduced what should be called the "multifactor hypothesis of ovulation." He suggested that the distribution of smooth muscle in the follicle wall, for whose presence he largely depended on the reports of earlier workers and his own observations based on tinctorial characteristics of tissues, conformed closely to the distribution of blood vessels and the capillary wreath previously described by Clark (108). Thomson (466) found smooth muscle in the human ovary to be less abundant than in other species but present in sufficient quantity to act as he thought it did in those species. He suggested that the increase in follicle size was caused by the increase in volume of the liquor folliculi and a consequent increase in intrafollicular pressure and that enzymes in the liquor folliculi, whose presence was demonstrated by Schochet (428), caused digestion of the theca, leading to ovulation. Thomson (466), as had Heape (209) and von Winiwarter (505) before him, accepted that there was an intimate association between ovulation and menstruation and that the vascular changes associated with the latter induced the vascular changes involved in the former. He therefore assumed that the increase in follicular volume must be caused by an increase in transudation resulting from vascular engorgement and that the combination of increased fluid, proteolysis of the theca, and smooth muscle contraction would lead to the increase in intrafollicular pressure, resulting in ovulation.

Corner (114,115) described smooth muscle in sow ovarian follicles, and Guttmacher and Guttmacher (202) confirmed these observations and suggested that the smooth muscle was responsible for ovulation under the stimulation of the nerve fibers that they traced into the follicle wall. The significance of their study is that they caused contraction of sow follicle wall strips *in vitro* with low pH, barium chloride, and physostigmine sulfate, but caused relaxation with high pH, epinephrine, and atropine. They concluded that ovulation was contributed to by contraction of smooth muscle under autonomic control and that increased intrafollicular pressure resulting from increased arterial pressure was not sufficient to cause ovulation.

Kraus (263) evaluated the roles of increased intrafollicular pressure, proteolytic enzymes and the presence of smooth muscle as factors in the mechanism of ovulation in the frog, hen, and rabbit. In the frog, pressure applied at the base induced rupture in the stigma area, but introduction of saline into the follicle was without effect. In the hen, application of external pressure induced rupture at unpredictable sites; however, late in follicular development, such pressure produced rupture at the stigma even though the hens were dead. Saline injections into the follicles were ineffectual. In the rabbit, pressure induced rupture, whether it was applied externally or by intrafollicular injection of saline. Kraus (263) noted that, in the frog and hen, increased intrafollicular pressure may be an adequate explanation if combined with proteolytic changes in the follicle wall. In the rabbit, however, the pattern of discharge of follicular fluid argued against a sharp increase in intrafollicular pressure, but for an orderly progression of morphological change.

Although smooth muscle had been reported in ovarian follicles by a number of workers, subsequent workers failed to confirm its presence in humans (429), swine (20), or rabbits (206). Claesson (107) attempted to resolve the divergent results obtained by histologists by utilizing polarization microscopy. He found perifollicular spindle-shaped cells resembling smooth muscle in the ovaries of cow, swine, rabbit, guinea pig, and rat. However, by using polarization microscopy he failed to find the high intrinsic birefringence characteristic of muscle, but did find the high form birefringence characteristic of connective tissue. The absolute objectivity of polarization microscopy completely negated all previous histological evidence, including Claesson's own, of smooth muscle in the follicle wall and threw doubt on the reliability of any physiological data.

The Vascular System

Direct microscopic observation of ovulation in rabbits was achieved by Walton and Hammond (495), who timed the process from coitus to rupture and confirmed the time reported earlier by Heape (209). They described the follicle as a broad-based convex structure, covered with a fine capillary network, protruding above the surface of the ovary. The first sign of impending ovulation was the appearance of the macula pellucida, which implied an obliteration of the blood flow to the apex, followed by further protrusion of the follicle. The macula pellucida became a pimple and ruptured, and the capillaries at the base of the pimple ruptured before the pimple did. The rupture of the capillaries was interpreted to mean that thecal rupture preceded rupture of the surface. "The whole process of ovulation, the congestion and swelling of the follicle, the formation of a pimple at the surface and the gradual rupture and extrusion of contents strongly resembles the formation and rupture of a boil and, not unlikely, somewhat similar mechanisms are involved" (495). The investigators further noted that the liquor folliculi did not squirt from the follicle but flowed as the walls gradually collapsed. Kelly (248) confirmed with little variation the observations made by Walton and Hammond (495). Markee and Hinsey (310) confirmed the earlier observations by Walton and Hammond (495) and Kelly (248) but noted that the mature follicle developed an avascular area surrounded by dilated vessels before there was any sign of a papilla. They also examined the rupture points and noted that they were uniformally oval shaped, with no appearance of the tearing they assumed would be present if there had been an increase in intrafollicular pressure resulting either from smooth muscle contraction or from a rise in ovarian blood pressure. They thus concurred with Guttmacher and Guttmacher (202), who had failed to induce follicle rupture in Graafian follicles by injecting saline into ovarian arteries and raising the intraarterial pressure to 300 mm Hg.

Despite suggestions that ovulation occurred with minimal intrafollicular pressure changes, contrary observations continued to appear. Smith (444,445) noted that follicular fluid rose to 1 cm or less into a fine-tipped tube inserted into a Graafian follicle of an uninjected mature rabbit, but it rose to a height of 5 or 6 cm from the Graafian follicle of a pregnancy-urine-injected rabbit, suggesting that the latter fluid was under greater pressure. Hill et al. (214) applied the newly introduced cinemicrographic technique to the study of ovulation in the rabbit. These workers interpreted their observations as indicating that "follicular rupture is truly explosive in nature." These observations supported the idea that a tension was exerted on the intrafollicular contents and that rupture was a result of the pressure generated by the follicle wall.

Although Schochet (428) had suggested that ovulation might be a result of enzymatic degradation of the follicle wall, and Thomson (466) had included this idea in what I call the multifactor hypothesis, little work was done on the enzymatic degradation of the follicle until Espey and Lipner (157) noted the effect of enzymes injected into the follicle.

Depolymerization of Mucopolysaccharide

Because after 1947 it was generally accepted that smooth muscle was absent from the follicle wall or present in insufficient amounts to affect intrafollicular pressure (107), and Guttmacher and Guttmacher (202) had discounted the increase in intravascular pressure as a source of intrafollicular pressure, an alternative mechanism was needed to explain the assumed increase in intrafollicular pressure. Zachariae (106,226,518–520) suggested that the mucopolysaccharides synthesized by the granulosa cells and secreted into the follicle antrum were subjected to depolymerization to smaller molecular species, inducing an increase in the number of osmotically active molecules, and thus increased the volume of fluid in the follicle and the intrafollicular pressure. Nine hours after mating, rabbits were laparotomized, the ovaries were located, and Evans blue was administered. Graafian follicles of unmated rabbits showed little accumulation of Evans blue at 20 min and slightly more at 30 min. The Graafian follicles of mated rabbits began to accumulate the dye within 5 min and were intensely stained by 20 min. The permeability of the follicle wall had increased, and, because Evans blue is bound to plasma proteins, it was unlikely that the mucopolysaccharide depolymerization hypothesis could explain the increase in follicle volume or rupture as being caused by increased pressure. That ovulation might be a result of smooth muscle contraction was again suggested by Lipner and Maxwell (295), who found that rabbit Graafian follicles autotransplanted to the anterior chamber of the eye underwent changes in shape within minutes after administration of pregnancy urine.

Neural Control of Ovulation

A role for neural control of ovulation has periodically been suggested, beginning with the recognition that sympathetic nerves entered the ovary at the hilus along with the vacular supply (177,218,487). The nerves entering the ovary either accompanied blood vessels or went directly to the follicles (417). Opinions on the subsequent distribution of the nerves divided anatomists into three schools of thought: (a) those believing the nerves penetrated all layers of the follicle wall (63,182,210,417,507); (b) those believing only the two outermost layers of the follicle wall received neural innervation (1,202); and (c) those believing only the vessels in the follicle wall were innervated (129,308,415).

Physiological studies initiated by von Winiwarter and Sainmont (506), who stimulated follicles *in situ* either chemically or electrically, were extended by Thomson (466), who noted that epinephrine was stimulatory *in vitro,* continued by Guttmacher and Guttmacher (202), who found that epinephrine was inhibitory and that acetylcholine was excitatory and supported by the demonstration of norepinephrine in ovarian tissue (164). The whole significance of the neural innervation was challenged by the demonstration by Hinsey and Markee (217) that rabbits in which the vagal, thoracolumbar, and sacral innervations to the ovary were destroyed could still ovulate in response to stimulation with pregnancy urine. Modern study of ovulation has made use of all the tools of anatomy, physiology, pharmacology, and biochemistry to analyze the mechanism. Although there are still some questions to be resolved, a more coherent description of ovulation has now become possible.

THE STRUCTURE OF THE OVARIAN FOLLICLE

General Features of Follicular Morphology

The structure of the ovarian follicle has been extensively reviewed by Nagel (344), Klebs (250), and most recently Mossman and Duke (334). Both structure and function have been reviewed by Bjersing (48), Erickson et al. (147), and Guraya (201).

The adult ovary of mammals is invested with an epithelial membrane, the germinal epithelium, overlying a tough connective membrane, the tunica albuginea. Immediately beneath the tunica albuginea is the ovarian cortex, in which are located the follicles in various stages of maturation or degeneration.

The primordial follicles are surrounded by a single layer of granulosa cells; with maturation, the granulosa cells increase in number and begin to form layers, which appear stratified or pseudostratified (49,293). As the granulosa cells increase in number, an encapsulating sheath, the theca, composed of the surrounding stroma, delineates the developing follicle, separating it from adjacent primordial follicles. The theca becomes differentiated, as antrum formation begins, into a well-vascularized theca interna consisting of several layers of rounded steroid-secreting cells and an equally well-vascularized theca externa composed of spindle-shaped cells (371,372).

The outer wall of the preovulatory follicle is generally described as being composed of six layers. The most superficial is the surface germinal epithelium, which rests on a basal lamina, which in turn merges with the tunica albuginea; these three elements constitute the serosa of the ovary, which is comparable to the serosae of other organs suspended in the abdominal cavity. The wall of the follicle abutting the tunica albuginea is composed of the theca externa, then the theca interna, which rests on the lamina propria, which excludes all direct vascular supply to the innermost layer, the membrana granulosa.

Detailed Features of Follicular Morphology

Germinal Epithelium

The comparative aspects of the structure of the ovary have been examined by Mossman and Duke (334), and the following discussion is largely based on their evaluation of the literature.

The ovary is attached to the body wall by the mesovarium and, except for the line of junction of the peritoneum, is completely enveloped. It is at this junction, the hilus, that blood vessels and nerves enter the ovary. The serosal layer enveloping the ovary consists, as it does for most mammalian organs, of a simple squamous epithelium overlying a fibrous connective tissue layer. In the course of embryogenesis, the epithelial cells overlying the ovary undergo a transformation from squamous to low columnar epithelium lying upon a basement membrane, which separates the epithelium from the connective tissue layer. The columnar nature of the epithelium persists especially in the region of the hilus, but ranges from squamous to low columnar in other areas of the ovary. In some species of small mammals, the basement membrane is absent, and there may not be a clear distinction between the underlying cells and the surface epithelium. Mossman and Duke (334) conclude that the serosa of the mammalian ovary is relatively embryonic, but that "it actually bears a much more intimate morphological and physiological relation to the organ as a whole than does that of other organs. . . . Even the adult ovary retains much of its embryonic character, its epithelium having a more or less continuous and formative relationship with it. For this reason, the epithelial covering of the ovary is regarded as different from the rest of the coelom, and in view of its function in gonadal development should be called surface germinal epithelium (epithelium germinale superficiale)."

The relationship of the superficial germinal epithelium to cortical development of the ovary was first described by Pfluger (400) and in ovaries of fetal and neonatal dogs and humans (337). The superficial epithelium was termed germinal epithelium by Waldeyer (487). Ultrastructural examination of germinal epithelium of the mouse ovarian surface by Wischnitzer (508) revealed an epithelium similar to that described by light microscopy, with the addition of microvillus projections and the usual cell organelles. Espey (148,150) described the germinal epithelium of the rabbit ovary but was more concerned with the underlying structures. A later study noted the presence of electron-dense particles in the germinal epithelium (410). Byskov (86) also studied the surface germinal epithelium in the mouse ovary but only confirmed the description by Wischnitzer (508).

In 1971, Motta et al. (335) examined the ovarian surface epithelium of guinea pigs, mice, rats, rabbits, and humans and correlated the changes in the epithelium with the follicular events preceding ovulation. The observations were similar in all the species examined. The cells were hemispheric, with the convexity directed outward and the surface covered with microvilli. The cells tended to flatten and become squamous only on the apices of enlarging preovulatory follicles, with short evaginations appearing on their surfaces, suggesting increased cellular activity. The surface epithelium disappears shortly before follicular rupture. The proliferative activity of the surface epithelium is minimal prior to ovulation and shows a resurgence adjacent to the stigma immediately after ovulation (375).

The role of the surface germinal epithelium in rupture of the follicle was again evaluated in a series of studies by Bjersing and Cajander (49–51), Cajander (87), and Cajander and Bjersing (88,89). They hypothesized that, with time, the surface germinal epithelium undergoes a series of transformations that provide the enzyme(s) that digest the surface layers of the follicle and induce rupture. The release of LH was the assumed initiator; however, this hypothesis fails to explain the changes in vascularity and neural activity or the series of biochemical changes (steroidal and nonsteroidal) that occur during the periovulatory period.

Tunica Albuginea

The serosal cover of the ovary consists of the surface germinal epithelium, a thin, almost cell-free layer of amorphous translucent material in which are embedded collagen bundles, and a relatively thin layer of fibroblasts surrounded by interwoven compact collagen fibers. It is this last area that is usually referred to as the *tunica albuginea*. Mossman and Duke (334) note that in small mammals (shrews and mice) the tunica albuginea is absent. In rats it appears as an indistinct subepithelial fibrous layer, but in the porcupine it is a distinct subepithelial fibrous capsule and should be considered the analog of the testicular tunica albuginea. The surface epithelium of the ovary in young women is underlayered by a thin subepithelial fibrous capsule with little transition into the ovarian cortex.

Theca Externa

The outermost coat of the preovulatory follicle subjacent to the tunica albuginea is composed of several layers (two to five or seven) of fusiform cells and an extensive capillary network. The fusiform cells are of two types. One of these is designated as stromal or fibroblast cells and is characterized by an endoplasmic reticulum with cisternae ramifying through the cytoplasm, which contains occasional mitochondria and free ribosomal particles. The second type of fusiform cell is ultrastructurally similar to smooth muscle. In these cells are bundles of thin filaments, numerous free ribosomes, lipid droplets, glycogen granules, mitochondria with long cristae, and a Golgi vesicular complex. The plasma membrane contains caveolae intracellulares (invaginations) and occasionally myoneural junctions. The muscle cells are present in fascicles, in small groups, or as isolated cells. They are interspersed among the fibroblasts and form incomplete layers in the thecae externae of developing, mature, and atretic follicles and are present around corpora lutea and interstitial cells.

Smooth muscle. Smooth muscle has been described in the theca externa in most mammals: rat (18,181,369,377), sheep (370), monkey (360,377), mouse (18,181,336), cat (18,68,181,360), guinea pig (68), rabbit (18,53,68,360), human (360), hamster (318,389,391), gerbil (318), and cow (490). Although the smooth muscle cells may be under neural control, cellular junctions among the perifollicular smooth-muscle cells may allow direct communication and sequential response (93).

Collagen. The theca externa invariably contains collagen fibers occurring in bands and interspersed among the fibroblasts and smooth muscle cells. The mechanisms determining the rupture of the Graafian follicle primarily involve the degradation of the follicle wall (152,292). The primary component responsible for the wall's tensile strength is its collagen content (149). It is therefore essential that some discussion of collagen precede any review of the studies regulating its degradation. The following discussion is based on the reviews by Miller (320), Eyre (167), Jackson (222), and Fessler and Fessler (170).

The word *collagen* is now used as a generic term describing a population of distinct, but chemically related, macromolecular species (320). Table 1 lists the known vertebrate collagens and divides them into types based on their physicochemical properties. The properties shared by the 11 currently recognized collagens are that they (a) contain sizable domains in which the collagen helical fold is present and (b) contribute structurally to the formation of extracellular supramolecular aggregates. Miller (320) has divided the collagens into three molecular groups. Group 1 molecules are those collagens that give rise to fibers; Group 2 molecules are those composed of very large aggregates that give rise to the open mesh-like arrangements of basement membranes. The organization of the Group 3 molecules is currently undescribed and not of interest in the context of collagens found in the ovarian follicle wall.

Collagen is a ubiquitous protein component of connective tissues. A generalized view of such tissues reveals them to be composed of a fibrous meshwork of collagen and elastin embedded in an amorphous polyionic matrix of proteoglycans and glycoproteins. Interspersed among the fibers are the cells giving origin to these fibrous proteins. The array of connective tissues in vertebrates is large, and the amounts of collagen in these tissues are variable.

Final collagen as it appears in tissues consists of three alpha polypeptide chains. Each chain consists of a central collagen fold with a short telopeptide chain at each end.

TABLE 1. *Properties of selected group I and group II collagen molecules*[a]

Collagen	Chain molecular weight	Molecular species	Form of aggregates
Type I	95,000	$[\alpha_1(I)]_2[\alpha_2(I)]$ $[\alpha_1(I)]_3$	Fibers
Type II	95,000	$[\alpha_1(II)]_3$	Fibers-fibrils
Type III	95,000–100,000	$[\alpha_1(III)]_3$	Reticular networks
Type IV	170,000–185,000	$[\alpha_1(IV)]_2[\alpha_2(IV)]$ $[\alpha_1(IV)]_3$ $[\alpha_2(IV)]_3$	Open mesh-like aggregates of basement membranes
Type V	130,000–200,000	$[\alpha_1(V)]_2[\alpha_2(V)]$ $[\alpha_1(V)]_3$ $[\alpha_1(V)][\alpha_2(V)][\alpha_3(V)]$	Aggregates of unknown structure in pericellular and perifibrillar genes

[a]Modified from Miller (320).

Roman numerals indicate the genetic types of collagen chain within a species. Types II, III, and probably IV are composed of three identical chains. Type I is a heterotrimer composed of two alpha-1 and one alpha-2 $[(\alpha_1(I))_2(\alpha_2(I))]$ chains. Type IV is found in basement membranes and is the best-characterized collagen type. It is the largest and has many 3-α hydroxyproline residues. The different collagen types tend to be distributed in particular tissues. Thus chondrocytes are a primary source of Type II, which is largely present in hyaline cartilage. Type I is formed by osteocytes and corneal and tendon fibroblasts. Smooth-muscle cells are capable of synthesizing all of the types of collagen. Blood-vessel smooth-muscle cells in culture express both Type I and Type III collagens in variable amounts. Structures that resist deformation, such as bone, generally contain Type I collagen. Elastic connective tissues contain Types I and III, whereas Type IV is the collagen found between the underlying stroma and epithelium. Type II is restricted to structures that resist deformation, such as the cartilagenous tissues and vitreous humor of the eye.

Type I and III collagens have been identified by immunohistochemical methods in the theca of the Graafian follicle (382) and appear as bundles of fibers distributed among the smooth-muscle cells and fibroblasts, whereas the lamina propria between the theca interna and the granulosa cells contains Type IV collagen (31,382).

Martin and Miller-Walker (312) used a solution of sodium dodecyl sulfate incubated with hamster ovaries to strip away the overlying germinal epithelium and examine the distribution of collagen fibers in the follicle wall. They observed bands of parallel fibers arranged in layers beginning at the base of the follicle and extending into its apex, where they fan out into a meshwork covering the apex. Although similar studies have not been performed on the follicles of other species, ultrastructural study has indicated the presence of collagen fibers. Continued presence of collagen at ovulation is described in hamsters (312) and in rats (477), but dissolution of collagen has been reported in rat (120,328, 362,385,412), human (179,359), and rabbit (148).

Collagen degradation can follow two pathways. Its triple helical configuration is resistant to proteolysis. Collagenase, a specific metalloprotease, completely splits the molecule, producing fragments that are three-fourths and one-fourth of the molecule. At 37°C, these fragments unwind, giving rise to three separate gelatin chains, which are rapidly attacked by proteases. Extracellular serine proteases may attack the residual collagen molecule at the telopeptide portion, splitting the cross-linking and at 37°C denaturing the soluble telopeptide-free collagen to gelatin chains. A second pathway involves granulocytic or fibroblastic phagocytosis and intracellular degradation (510). The proteoglycan ground substance surrounding the collagen fibrils is degraded by serine proteases and elastase and these probably contribute to the complete proteolysis of collagenase-degraded collagen (343).

The sources of collagenase. Granulocytic proteases. The human polymorphonuclear leukocyte (granulocyte) contains in its granules (a) neutral proteases that exhibit collagenase activity associated with a metalloprotease, (b) serine proteases having elastase and low-level collagenase activity, and (c) cathepsin G (chymotrypsin-like cationic protein). The collagenase is strongly bound to plasma α_2-macroglobulin and less well bound to plasma β_1-anticollagenase. The elastase is strongly bound to plasma α_1-antitrypsin and mucus inhibitor I and weakly bound to α_2-macroglobulin. The secretion of neutral proteases is low except during phagocytosis, and endogenous protease inhibitors normally keep the low levels in check, but local high concentrations of the enzymes may be achieved when the excess saturates the local inhibitory concentrations (354) during inflammatory reactions.

Tissue collagenase. In addition to granulocytes, a wide variety of cells are capable of producing collagenase; however, with the exception of the granulocyte, there is little evidence of intracellular storage of active collagenase. Collagenase production is dependent on induction of DNA-mediated synthesis rather than on cellular release of preformed enzyme. Collagenase may be synthesized and stored in an inactive form, or both the enzyme and an inhibitor may be present simultaneously; their concurrent release would prevent the appearance of an active enzyme (511).

Murphy and Sellers (343) hypothesize that all connective tissues synthesize collagenase inhibitors that complex with collagenase and that the resulting latent enzyme complex is, in turn, bound to collagen. In its latent form, collagenase is not subject to α_2-macroglobulin inactivation. Latent collagenase may be a proenzyme requiring enzymatic activation. A number of endogenous proteinases have been demonstrated to activate the latent collagenase by cleavage of a small peptide. The endogenous activator may also be present in a latent form requiring plasmin, kallikrein, or lysosomal proteinases such as cathepsin B and trypsin for activation (343). Plasmin is a very effective activator of latent collagenase; however, it is present in body fluids in the inactive plasminogen form and requires activation by plasminogen activator or streptokinase. Rheumatoid synovial cells secrete both latent collagenase and plasminogen activator and, in the presence of the local inflammation and large amounts of plasminogen, a situation adequate for activation of collagenase is created (501). Latent collagenase can also be activated by thiol-binding reagents such as α-aminophenylmercuric acetate, *N*-ethylmaleimide, and *p*-chloromercuribenzoate. The collagenase activity is as great with these compounds as with trypsin, and no synergism between trypsin and thiol-binding reagents is found (343).

Theca Interna

Erickson et al. (147) elegantly summarized the literature on the structure and function of the interstitial cells of the ovary, and detailed references can be found in their review. They note that there are four varieties of interstitial cells. Primary interstitial cells constitute a transient population of endocrine cells contained in the medullary compartment of the developing ovary. These cells lack the ability to synthesize steroids *de novo,* but they convert pregnenolone sulfate to dehydroepiandrosterone and androstenedione (in humans). Theca interstitial cells are perhaps the most important group of interstitial cells. These cells are found in the theca interna of the developing follicle. They are derived from stromal cells; cytodifferentiation occurs concurrent with their invasion by arterioles and the formation of a capillary wreath. The cells acquire 3β-hydroxysteroid dehydrogenase and undergo the subsequent cytodifferentiation that characterizes the true theca interstitial cell. On the ultramicroscopic level, there appear to be at least two types of theca-interna cells, light and dark cells; both have the ultrastructure of steroidogenic cells. The third variety of interstitial cells are those found around atretic follicles. These cells are innervated by adrenergic nerves and, in culture, respond to catecholamine stimulation by increasing their production of androgen. Finally, the fourth variety of interstitial cells are those found in the hilus. These cells resemble the Leydig cells of the testis and respond to LH stimulation by increasing their testosterone synthesis and secretion (265).

Lamina Propria

The theca interna and its vascular supply are separated from the membrana granulosa by the lamina propria. This amorphous boundary is composed of laminin, Type IV collagen, fibronectin, and heparan sulfate proteoglycan. Induction of ovulation with human chorionic gonadotropin (hCG) causes fragmentation of the lamina and invasion by thecal cells and capillaries (31,382), probably under the influence of induced angiogenic factor (260,306).

Membrana Granulosa

The parietal membrana granulosa of the preovulatory follicle in the rabbit is described as a stratified epithelium or a pseudostratified epithelium four to five cells thick (49,293). The cells close to the lamina propria appear columnar, whereas those lining the antrum appear polyhedral. Many of the luminal cells have long slender projections extending to the lamina propria (49,293).

The membrana granulosa in the human preovulatory follicle is six to 12 cells thick but appears similar to that in the rabbit. The cells of the basal layer are columnar, and those of the other layers are polyhedral. After the LH surge, the antral cells become disorganized, and the cells and their nuclei increase in size (60). The ultrastructural appearance of the cells of the membrana granulosa is consistent with a steroid secretory function. They contain a granular endoplasmic reticulum, and at estrus 3β and 17β-hydroxysteroid dehydrogenase activity is high, at the time that estrogen secretion by the follicle is maximal (48,326).

Steroid biosynthesis is generally associated with secretory function of the cells of the membrana granulosa; however, other nonsteroidal factors are synthesized and secreted by these cells. Among these are the prostaglandins, inhibin, a 32K molecular weight protein that inhibits basal secretion of FSH (102,146) plasminogen activator (90,351) and peptide growth regulators (207,208).

The granulosa cells also secrete the components of the extracellular matrix. Fibronectin is secreted by the granulosa cells before FSH induces the cytodifferentiation that inhibits its further production (443). The guinea pig ovarian follicle incorporates $^{35}SO_4$ into glycosaminoglycans, which also contribute to the extracellular matrix composing the early follicular fluid (110).

Three varieties of granulosa cells occupy the area beneath the lamina propria in rat preovulatory follicles. Lying on the lamina propria is a parietal layer of columnar cells joined at their lateral margins by gap junctions (Type I). Adjacent to this basal layer and extending to the antrum are polygonal cells joined to each other as well as to the apices of the parietal cells by gap junctions (Type II). Antral cells floating in follicular fluid free of contact with subjacent cells or with each other appear shortly before follicular rupture (Type III) (175). The Type I and Type II cells on the morning of proestrus contain small mitochondria with lamellar cristae, moderately developed Golgi apparatus, inconspicuous lysosomes, and only small amounts of lipid inclusions. Late in proestrus, Type I cells have only short segments of rough endoplasmic reticulum (RER), but the smooth endoplasmic reticulum (SER) shows profuse cisternal dilations. Mitochondria are increased in size and number and appear spherical; the cristae are tubular. Lipid inclusions are plentiful, and Golgi cisternae are enlarged. The ultrastructural appearance of the membrana granulosa has been similarly described in several species, including the rat (55,175), mouse (86), rabbit (148), cow (309,406), and human (180).

Existence of cell-cell contacts was reported by Bjorkman (55) and Byskov (86); however, their significance was unappreciated until Espey and Stutts (160) and Merk et al. (319) identified them as gap junctions between the granulosa cells and annular gap junctions contained within the cytoplasm. Espey and Stutts (160) suggested the latter might be a mechanism for exchange of cytoplasm between the cells; their internalization might be a mechanism for decreased intercellular adhesion. The structure of the gap junction in different organisms and tissues has been reviewed by Larsen (271); Peracchia (393,394) and Loewenstein (299) have reviewed structure, mechanism of formation, control of permeability, number of particles, and adhesion. Uncoupling and decreased numbers of gap junction particles may result from decreased intracellular Ca^{2+} concentration, intracellular acidification (394), or decreased intracellular concentrations of cAMP (299). Both follicle stimulating hormones (FSHs) and LH increase intracellular concentrations of cAMP; therefore the effects of these hormones should be to increase the numbers of gap junctions among the granulosa cells.

Albertini and Anderson (14) reported that gap junctions appear among granulosa cells concurrently with the appearance of the antrum (23). However, Fletcher (172,173) noted them among granulosa cells in 3-day-old rats, and Burghardt and Matheson (78) found them present in preantral follicles and probably present from the earliest appearance of granulosa cells. Albertini and Anderson (14) found that gap junctions of the granulosa cells increase in size as the follicles grow. Using tracers, Albertini et al. (15) demonstrated that annular gap junctions arise by invagination of the cell surface. Larsen and Tung (272) and Larsen et al. (273,274) described the probable mechanism for internalization of gap junctions through an endocytotic process.

The cAMP formed in rat granulosa cells in response to FSH exposure is transferred across heterologous gap junctions to co-cultured mouse myocardial cells, which manifest the effect by an increased beat (277). Furthermore, addition of FSH to the medium of cultures of rat granulosa cells causes the cells to change from a flattened epithelioid shape to a semispherical form but with retention of cytoplasmic processes in contact with adjacent cells and with the substrate (278). In *in vivo* studies, Burghardt and Matheson (78) found that FSH amplifies the sequence of gap junction growth and turnover in young follicles and increases internalization in mature follicles. Prolonged exposure of cultured granulosa cells to FSH increases membrane microviscosity (454) and probably reduces the lateral mobility of granules in the cell surface, thus contributing to the internalization of gap junctions.

Although Bjersing and Cajander (52) and Coons and Espey (113) had noted a decrease in the number of gap junctions after hCG and as the time of ovulation approaches, Larsen et al. (274), in a quantitative analysis of the gap junction, found that hCG induces an increase in the proportion of small surface gap junctions in the granulosa cells and a marked decrease in the proportion of large surface gap junctions. They also found a decrease in the amount of gap junction membranes in the granulosa cells. Burghardt and Matheson (78) hypothesize that synthesis and turnover of gap junctions are amplified by mechanisms that increase intracellular cAMP and that the ratio of surface to internalized gap junctions is dependent on the state of maturation of the follicle. FSH promotes formation of surface gap junctions in early stages of follicle growth and turnover of gap junctions in later stages of follicle growth, and LH takes over this role in the later stages (76–78).

The significance of the ultrastructural organization of the membrane granulosa resides in the observation that the cells composing it are heterogeneous; those located near the basal lamina possess larger numbers of LH receptors than those closer to the antrum (21,241) and, by cell-cell communication, permit uniform responses by cells separated from the vascular system (186). Prolactin receptors are more prevalent in the antral than in the mural (parietal) granulosa cells (140), and the enzyme populations are a function of location in the membrane granulosa (521,522).

THE NEURAL INNERVATION OF THE OVARY

Neural Innervation of Ovary and Follicles

The gross anatomy of the nerve supply to the ovary was described in 1867 by Frankenhauser (177). The nerves originate at spinal segments T_{10} and T_{11} (268,502), give rise to an aortorenal plexus, and follow the ovarian artery as a nerve plexus into the ovary at the hilus (345). Sensory fibers originate at spinal segment T_{10} and accompany the sympathetic fibers. The parasympathetic innervation is derived from the vagus (212,213,286). Spinal segments S-2 to S-4 may also contribute to the parasympathetic innervation (323); however, denervation studies suggest that these, if they exist, are inconsequential. In the rat the parasympathetic innervation is primarily vagal in origin (19,71,73,74,171,212). Furthermore, much of the innervation is probably composed of visceral afferent fibers, since in the rabbit only 10% of the abdominal vagal fibers are motor neurons (165).

Early studies of the microscopic distribution of the autonomic nerve distribution utilized silver impregnation techniques, which were subject to artifact because of the tendency of the method to stain reticular and elastic fibers as

TABLE 2. *Comparison of adrenergic innervation by fluorescence microscopy with concentration of norepinephrine in mammalian ovaries*[a]

Innervation	Concentrations (μg/g)	Reference
Rich		
Cow	1.96 ± 0.19	444
Sheep		
Cat	4.93 ± 1.30	424
Guinea pig	2.29 ± 0.35	449
Left	2.32 ± 0.30	267
Right	2.16 ± 0.20	267
Intermediary		
Human	0.86 ± 0.30	378
	0.57	224
Pig	0.25 ± 0.04	449
Dog[b]		449
Rat	0.50 ± 0.03	449
Opossum[b]		449
		449
Sparse		
Rabbit	0.20 ± 0.02	442
	0.22 ± 0.02	58
Mouse	0.63 ± 0.11	449
Hedgehog	0.71 ± 0.12	449
Syrian hamster	0.41 ± 0.09	449
Squirrel monkey	0.17	224
Rhesus monkey	0.35 ± 0.06	380

[a]Modified from Stefenson et al. (449).
[b]Qualitative evaluation.

well as nerve fibers (32,71). Development of the histochemical fluorescence method for biogenic amines (168,169) marks the beginning of the new era in the study of the adrenergic innervation of the ovary. Concurrently, refinements in the histochemical methods for demonstrating acetylcholinesterase and distinguishing it from nonspecific cholinesterases have led to more precise descriptions of the parasympathetic innervation of the ovary (67,239).

Autonomic innervation of the ovary has been studied extensively in a number of species for the development of innervation (234) and for the distribution of nerve fibers in the cortex and in and around the follicles (69,70,378,379,424). The fluorescence has been identified as being primarily norepinephrine (378). Innervation of the cortical stroma and the follicles, as well as the nerve distribution in the theca externa and theca interna, has been found in all species examined. A distinguishing characteristic is the density of innervation, which varies from slight to intense. The adrenergic innervation based on qualitative histochemical evaluation is compared with concentrations of norepinephrine in Table 2 (in the case of sheep, dog, and opossum, only the qualitative histochemical evaluation is indicated) (449).

The presence of specific acetylcholinesterase has been demonstrated histochemically, with concentration arrived at on the basis of qualitative evaluation. In human, dog, rat, and hamster, the appearance of the cholinergic fibers is similar, with a dense network of these fibers associated with blood vessels and follicles. The follicles of the human ovary have an especially dense innervation. The incidence of cholinergic fibers is less than that of adrenergic fibers. The rabbit ovary has a sparse and random distribution of cholinergic fibers (449).

In strips prepared from bovine ovarian follicles, the smooth muscle cells lie in the theca externa in groups parallel to the surface, with distances of 30 to 100 nm between them. Bundles of nonmyelinated nerves in the stroma send branches to the smooth muscle cells as well as to the smooth muscle of the blood vessels. The naked nerve terminals lie in close proximity to the smooth-muscle cells, as close as 50 nm. In the absence of specialized junctions, this is a distance short enough for diffusion to provide innervation. These nerve terminals contain dense-cored synaptic vesicles and are presumed to be adrenergic nerves. Also present are nerve terminals containing empty synaptic vesicles, and because these tend to correspond to the nerve distribution of cholinesterase-containing nerves, they are presumed to be cholinergic nerves (492). Similarly, the presence of both adrenergic and cholinergic nerves in the ovarian follicle wall has been noted in humans (378,379,433), rats, guinea pigs, and rabbits (60,74,232), and cats (424). The concentration of norepinephrine in the ovary is a function of its innervation by the ovarian plexus, because crushing of the nerves on the guinea pig ovarian artery results, after 8 days, in a decrease in the concentration of norepinephrine in the treated ovary, whereas sectioning the hypogastric nerve has no effect on the norepinephrine concentration (267).

Physiological Studies

Noncontractile Effects of Autonomic Innervation

Adrenergic innervation of the ovary has been associated with follicular growth (64,119), cyclicity (286,459), puberty (6,7,333), innervation of the guinea-pig ovarian interstitial gland (457), progesterone synthesis (3,105,240, 348,409,525), compensatory ovarian hypertrophy (73, 193), and ovulation (96,124,176,217,223,228,235,302, 497–500) (Table 3).

Prostaglandins, Oxytocin, and Ovarian Contractility

In addition to the autonomic transmitters, a number of substances also induce contractions of the ovary *in vivo* and *in vitro* or of follicle strips *in vitro*. Prostaglandin $F_{2\alpha}$ induces contractions and prostaglandin E_2 (PGE_2) relaxation (116,117,130,187–189,303,450,483). Oxytocin induces ovarian contractions throughout the estrous cycle (419); however, Sterin-Borda et al. (450) observed more marked contractions during the periovulatory period (late proestrus), with a greater activity in the left ovary than in the right. Serotonin (5-hydroxytryptamine) causes contractions of the preovulatory hamster ovary (464). The complexity of neurohumoral-induced effects is further exaggerated by demonstrations of several [enkephalin, substance P, vasoactive intestinal peptide, neurotensin, somatostatin, gastric-releas-

TABLE 3. *Neural regulation of noncontractile mechanisms in the ovary*

Species	Treatment	Response	Reference
Rat	Surgical sympathectomy	Normal estrous cyclicity	459
Rat	Ovarian autografts	Ovulation	124
Mouse	Denervation of ovary	Delayed vaginal opening, failure of normal estrous cyclicity, failure of follicle maturation, failure of corpus luteal formation	197
Rat	Reserpine to immature rats treated with PMSG/hCG	Inhibition of ovulation effect partially reversed with pargyline	176
Rat	Ovarian autografts	Normal ovulation	133
Mouse	Denervation of ovary	Delayed vaginal opening, decreased ovarian weight, erratic estrous cycles, decreased follicle maturation, failure of corpus luteal formation	198
Mouse	Norepinephrine to hypophysectomized mice	Slight regression of interstitial elements, increased numbers of type 3b and 4 follicles, decreased numbers of atretic follicles	199
Mouse	Unilateral denervation of PMSG/hCG	Devervated ovary had reduced numbers of maturing follicles; after gonadotropins effects were exacerbated	64
Mouse	6-Hydroxydopamine	Decreased litter size	96
Mouse	6-Hydroxydopamine	No effect on fertility	228
Guinea pig	None	Interstitial gland of ovary innervated by adrenergic nerves	457
Rat	Ovarian autografts	No correlation between density of innervation and plasma levels of progesterone and estradiol	105
Rat	None	Interstitial gland of ovary innervated by autonomic nerves	276
Rat	Denervation	Decreased 3β-hydroxysteroid dehydrogenase activity during pregnancy only	72
Rat	Vagotomy and 6-hydroxydopamine	Disrupts estrous cycles, interrupts estrous cycles, decreases compensatory ovary hypertrophy	73
Rat	Adrenalectomized hyphophysectomized electrical stimulation of areas of brain	Increased secretion of progesterone and estradiol	244 245
Rat	β-adrenergic stimulation	Secretion of progesterone	525
Rat	Ovarian denervation	Acute decreased secretion of progesterone	6,7,356
Rat	Ovarian denervation in pubescent rats	Depletion of ovarian norepinephrine, no effect on puberty or first ovulation	7
Rat	Catecholamines in ovarian bursa	Increased numbers of ovulation	427

ing peptide, bombesin, neuropeptide Y (451)] different peptides and indolamine (serotonin) associated with autonomic nerves (83).

Neural Innervation and Ovulation

A frequently examined issue has been the role of the neural innervation in ovulation. In acute experiments, in which hormonal treatment to the animal is followed by *in vitro* perfusion of the ovary, ovulation occurs. Examples of such experiments are those by Wallach et al. (488). In such studies the nerve terminals may still provide the control of smooth-muscle contractility necessary for ovulation. This criticism has led to various attempts to demonstrate the independence of the ovulatory mechanism from the neural innervation demonstrated anatomically.

Autotransplantation of the rat ovary into subcutaneous sites has no effect on the incidence of ovulation (124); however, Jacobowitz and Laties (223) noted that ovarian autotransplants into the anterior chamber of the cat eye were reinnervated by adrenergic fibers with the revascularization. Because Deanesley did not examine the transplants for a neural reinnervation, it is possible that the functional ovarian tissue ovulated because it was reinnervated. Spinal cord transection in the absence of abdominal vagotomy is an inadequate experimental determination of the role of neural innervation in follicular maturation and ovulation (184).

Weiner et al. (497) utilized the technique of stripping the neural plexus around the rabbit ovarian artery to denervate the ovary. The ovaries lost all evidence of histofluorescence, but ovarian size and follicle number were unaffected. Rabbits with one denervated ovary ovulate equally frequently on the denervated and control sides in response to hCG and with coital stimulation (498,499). The denervated ovary shows spontaneous contractile activity and responds to norepinephrine with a sharp increase in tone and rapid small contractions; exposure to the α-adrenergic blocking drug phenoxybenzamine totally inhibited the contractile activity, as did exposure to isoproterenol, a β-adrenergic agonist, but propranolol, a β-adrenergic blocking drug, enhanced the activity (500). Retention of, and even increased, sensitivity to agonists is a common characteristic of denervated smooth muscle (203), and because most receptor structures are retained in the membrane, inhibition of contractility by α-receptor antagonists is demonstrable (500).

Demonstration that 6-hydroxydopamine causes selective degeneration of adrenergic terminals, i.e., a chemical sympathectomy (471), resulted in its application to ovarian function. Administered to mice, 6-hydroxydopamine had no effect on the estrous cycle or ovulation (96,228), nor did it affect these parameters of ovarian function when administered in rats (302).

Autonomic Innervation and Ovarian Contractility

Another approach to studying the role of autonomic innervation to the ovary has been the utilization of cholinomimetic and sympathomimetic agonists and antagonists applied in *in vitro* organ bath systems. This technique, with many modifications and refinements (427), has become standard for studying the effects of various reagents on contractility of the follicle wall. Contractions of ovarian follicles were first reported in autotransplanted follicles in the anterior chamber of the rabbit eye (295) in response to hCG stimulation. Guttmacher and Guttmacher (202) had demonstrated that ovarian strips could be induced to contract, but spontaneous contractions of ovaries of cats suspended in an organ bath were observed by Rocerto et al. (420). They also noted the enhanced contractile activity caused by norepinephrine and epinephrine, as well as the inhibition of norepinephrine-induced increased frequency of contractions caused by phenoxybenzamine. These observations have been confirmed *in vivo* in rabbits (482,483) and in monkeys (254,484).

The *in vitro* method has been used to demonstrate the presence of spontaneous contractions in whole human ovaries (116,383) and in human and canine ovarian strips (188,357,358,489). The human ovarian strips showed minimal spontaneous contractility, which, however, could be induced with cholinergic and adrenergic compounds (357,489). In general, some cholinergic drugs (acetylcholine, bethanechol, and neostigmine) enhanced contractility, some (methacholine and pilocarpine) exerted variable effects, and atropine depressed response (126).

Effects of cholinomimetic and sympathomimetic drugs on ovarian and follicle strip contractility have been studied most elegantly and systematically by the Swedish group (235,379,427,446,489–494). Both the cat and the guinea-pig ovary show an increase in tone and contractility when exposed *in vitro* to norepinephrine; however, the guinea-pig response appears only in the presence of a β-receptor antagonist. The contractility induced with norepinephrine is abolished with α-receptor blockade. These effects were also examined in strips prepared from the protruding part of bovine or human follicles. The bovine follicle strip contracted in response to norepinephrine; contraction was blocked irreversibly by phenoxybenzamine and reversibly by piperoxan, both α-adrenergic receptor antagonists; however, the piperoxan is an α_2-receptor antagonist and therefore contraction is caused by competitive inhibition of norepinephrine-induced contractions (490). The human follicle strip also contracted in response to norepinephrine; however, the addition of a β-receptor antagonist intensified the contraction (489). The order of potency for the catecholamines in the bovine follicle strip is norepinephrine > epinephrine > phenylephrine > isoproterenol (490).

The contractile potency relationship of catecholamines, when tested on human follicle strips, is norepinephrine > epinephrine > phenylephrine > isoproterenol, indicating that an α-adrenergic receptor is involved in generating the response. Relaxation induced by the catecholamines was evaluated by induction of a tonic contraction with carbamylcholine in α-receptor-antagonized strips. The potency

TABLE 4. *Studies of spontaneous and stimulated contractility of the ovary or follicle*

Species	Procedure	Treatment	Reference
Rabbit	*In vitro*	Pharmacologic agents	202
Rabbit	*In vivo*	Transplanted/hCG	295
Rabbit	*In vivo*	Spontaneous	157
Cat	*In vitro*	Spontaneous	420
Human	*In vivo*	Prostaglandins $F_{2\alpha}$ and E_2	116
Human	*In vitro*	Spontaneous	383
Rabbit	*In vitro*	Prostaglandins $F_{2\alpha}$ and E_2	482
Monkey	*In vivo*	Spontaneous	484
	In vitro	Prostaglandins	
		α-Adrenergic blockers	
		β-Adrenergic blockers	
Rabbit	*In vivo*	Prostaglandins	130
Human	*In vitro*	Electrical stimulation	360
	In vitro	Neurotransmitters	358
		Prostaglandins	357
Sheep	*In vitro*	Spontaneous contractions	373
		Catecholamines	
		Prostaglandin $F_{2\alpha}$	
Cat	*In vitro*	Spontaneous	489
Guinea pig	*In vitro*	Cholinergic agonists	
Cow	*In vitro*	Adrenergic agonists	
Human	*In vitro*	Adrenergic agonists	
		Cholinergic agonists	
Guinea pig	*In vitro*	Spontaneous contractions	188
		Oxytocin	
		Prostaglandin $F_{2\alpha}$	
Human	*In vitro*	Neurotransmitter	188
		Prostaglandins	189
Human	*In vitro*	Adrenergic agonists	379
		Electrical stimulation	
Cow	*In vitro*	Adrenergic agonists	490
Rabbit	*In vivo*	Cholinergic agonists	126
	In vitro		
Human	*In vitro*	Neurotransmitters	303
Guinea pig	*In vitro*	Prostaglandins	303
Rat	*In vitro*	Oxytocin	419
Rat	*In vitro*	Spontaneous	450
		Prostaglandins	
		Oxytocin	
Rabbit	*In vivo*	Spontaneous	480–482, 512
Rabbit	*In vivo*	Denervated	500
		Spontaneous	
		α-Adrenergic agonists	
	In vitro	Electrical stimulation	
		Inhibitors	
Cow	*In vitro*	Electrical stimulation	494

rank of the test compounds was isoproterenol > norepinephrine > terbutaline > epinephrine. Relaxation of the follicle wall is mediated through β-receptors. The relaxation is antagonized by propranolol but not by practolol (β_1-antagonist), indicating the relaxation effect is probably caused by a β_2-receptor (493).

Both acetylcholine and carbamylcholine induce contractions of the follicle strips, and after addition of atropine, contraction is elicited only at higher concentrations of the agonists. These observations suggest that both the parasympathetic and the sympathetic divisions of the autonomic nervous system can induce a contractile response in the follicle (379). Dose-response curves generated in the presence of acetylcholine and carbamylcholine alone or in the presence of atropine indicate that muscarinic receptors are probably on the smooth-muscle cells (492).

Electrical stimulation of bovine follicle wall strips induces a frequency-dependent contraction that is abolished in the presence of bretylium, phentolamine, and reserpine, indicating that adrenergic nerves and α-receptors are involved in the response (494) (Table 4).

A possible role for the adrenoreceptor agonists in ovulation has been examined in an *in vitro* perfusion system utilizing rabbit ovaries (427). Terbutaline, a β_2-adrenoreceptor agonist, increased the incidence of ovulations in ovaries from hCG-treated rabbits. The mechanism for this effect may be dependent on β_2-receptor activation of cAMP formation, with the latter, in turn, increasing progesterone secretion (*vide supra*). Blockade of α-receptors with phentolamine and phenoxybenzamine (α_1-receptor antagonists) reduced the incidence of follicular rupture induced with hCG. Clonidine, an α-agonist, somewhat stimulated the ovulatory process, and piperoxan, an α_2-antagonist, blocks follicular contractility. It thus appears that both α- and β-adrenoreceptor agonists enhance the response to gonadotropin-induced ovulation. The sites of their actions probably involve the follicular wall (α-adrenergic response) and an enhancement of hormonal action in the theca interna and membrana granulosa (427).

Introduction of norepinephrine, terbutaline, and 4-aminopyridine into the bursa around the ovary increased the number of ovulations in pregnant-mare-serum-gonadotropin (PMSG)-primed LH-triggered immature rats (235). In this study, phentolamine partially blocked the norepinephrine-enhanced response and decreased the number of ovulations when administered alone. Terbutaline enhanced the number of ovulations, and propranolol counteracted the effect, whereas the nonspecific β-receptor agonist isoproterenol was ineffective. These data further support the argument that activation of the α-receptors exerts a follicle-wall effect and that β-receptors exert an effect via a hormonal mechanism (235).

The specific role of the cholinergic receptors is undefined, but Ojeda et al. (356) note that, in the rat, abdominal vagotomy delays onset of puberty and disturbs ovarian function. Abdominal vagotomy also depresses LH and FSH secretion in unilaterally ovariectomized rats (73). In rats, section of the ovarian artery has no effect on the integrity of the ovary because of an extensive anastomosis of the utero-ovarian and ovarian blood vessels. Section of the ovarian artery resulted, however, in the disappearance of histofluorescence and specific acetylcholinesterase-positive nerves. Chemical sympathectomy with 6-hydroxydopamine caused loss of histofluorescence but some retention of acetylcholinesterase-positive nerves in the hilar and medullary regions. Pelvic neurectomy or abdominal vagotomy had no effect on ovarian adrenergic or acetycholinesterase-positive nerves. Combined pelvic neurectomy, abdominal vagotomy, and chemical sympathectomy resulted in loss of adrenergic nerves but persistence of acetycholinesterase-positive nerves in the hilar and medullary areas. These observations result in the suggestion that the small incidence of acetycholinesterase-positive fibers is derived from the vagus but that most of the acetylcholinesterase is in the adrenergic nerves (74) (Table 3).

The discharge of norepinephrine at adrenergic terminals is accompanied by other substances, which may modulate further norepinephrine release. These include adenosine, prostaglandins, histamine, 5-hydroxytryptamine, acetylcholine (83), and perhaps β-endorphin (288). The concept that acetylcholine enhances the secretion of norepinephrine was initially introduced by Burn (80–82,256,408). The ability of atropine to block contractile activity in the ovarian strip (489) may be a result of mechanisms other than blockade of a muscarinic receptor on the smooth-muscle cell because ". . . with few exceptions sympathetic neurons are endowed with two presynaptic receptor systems for cholinergic drugs. Nicotinic agonists depolarize the nerve endings and evoke a calcium-dependent release of noradrenaline, whereas muscarinic agonists inhibit calcium-dependent release processes such as release evoked by electrical pulses, high potassium concentrations and nicotinic drugs" (448).

The consensus is that the neural innervation of the follicle probably modulates the mechanism of ovulation and that the smooth muscle in the follicle wall plays no critical role in ovulation (75,131), but a contrary opinion implies a major role (380).

THE OVARIAN BLOOD SUPPLY

Morphology

The blood supply to the ovary was first studied in detail by Clark (108) and was reviewed by Reynolds (416), who described the embryogenesis and the adult vasculature of the ovary, and by Ellinwood et al. (143), who reviewed the various methods available for measuring blood flow through the ovary and paid particular attention to the probable role of the uteroovarian veins in control of corpus luteal function. The blood and lymph supply of the ovary has also been extensively reviewed by Gillet et al. (185).

In most mammals the ovarian arteries arise from the abdominal aorta inferior to the renal arteries and reach the ovaries through the mesovarium. The ovarian artery at the hilus gives rise to many primary and secondary spiral arteries. The latter give origin to a rich capillary plexus (237,416), which surrounds the follicle with a dense basketwork of capillaries. In rabbits the venules draining the capillary plexus are more numerous and have a larger diameter and thinner wall than the arterioles (237). The post-capillary venules merge into secondary and primary veins and take a direct route to emerge from the ovary at the hilus (84).

Growth of the capillary plexus in the rabbit ovarian follicle has been examined by determining the incidence of labeled cells in the membrana granulosa and in the endothelial cells of the theca interna after stimulation with hCG. The labeling index for both sets of cells is correlated with follicle size and increases in parallel with it. Because the relative number of capillaries constituting the capillary plexus remains constant as the cohort of tertiary follicles (250–900 μm in diameter) grows in response to hCG stimulation, the size of the plexus must increase to keep pace with the growth of the follicle (262). Growth of the capillary plexus in the preovulatory follicle may be under the control of an angiogenic factor, whose presence has been demonstrated in extracts of nonluteal porcine ovarian tissue (306) and in extracts of rat follicles (260).

At the level of the preovulatory follicle, the initiation of ovulation may be said to be presaged by a hyperemia (523), later followed by an edema (49,84,86) involving the theca externa and interna. Espey (153) has hypothesized that ovulation may be an inflammatory process. Consequently a number of workers have examined the morphology of the microvasculature of the rabbit preovulatory follicle and the changes in its permeability (236,237,363–368) and that of the capillary plexus of the human follicle (361).

The vascular supply to primary follicles is represented by a simple capillary network whose complexity grows with growth of the follicle, assuming the appearance of a multilayered capillary plexus. The capillaries take origin directly from, and frequently at right angles to, the arterioles and drain abruptly into venules. This pattern makes possible a high arterial pressure throughout the microvasculature. The venules are readily distinguishable from the arterioles by their larger diameter and by the larger number of capillaries entering into them (361).

After treatment with hCG, preovulatory follicles enlarge without apparent change in the capillaries. Prior to rupture of the apex, the capillaries become dilated and the injection resin leaks into the interstitial space (236,237). Increase in capillary permeability is manifested by increased numbers of pinocytotic vesicles, endothelial fenestrations, and interendothelial gaps (49,366). The pinocytotic vesicles are present without change in number, size, or distribution throughout the preovulatory phase. Fenestrations increase in number, reaching maximum at 4 hr, and interendothelial gaps large enough to allow carbon particles to pass through appear late, at 10 and 12 hr after administration of hCG (365). That the interendothelial gaps were large enough to allow carbon particles to pass through implies that at a much earlier stage they were large enough to allow macromolecules to pass through; this is especially likely because increase in the accumulation of iodinated serum albumin by PMSG-stimulated hCG-triggered immature rat ovarian follicles is linear from the time of the initial bolus of hCG to ovulation (296).

Quantitation of the Preovulatory Blood Flow

That hyperemia is a prelude to ovulation has long been appreciated. Its presence was noted by Zondek et al. (523), although Heape (209) had noted the congested state of the blood vessels of the Graafian follicle. In rabbit follicles autotransplanted to the anterior chamber of the eye, the onset of the hyperemia was described as occurring within minutes after administration of hCG (295). This observation has been quantitated both in the whole ovary and in follicles in a number of studies with several different techniques. Ellis (144), Lipner and Smith (296), and Wada (486) measured radioiodinated serum albumin content of rat ovaries; Wurtman (513) employed a ^{42}K indicator fractionation technique. The thermocouple technique for blood flow measurements (143) was used by Makinada (305) for hemodynamic study of blood flow through the ovarian cortex. Direct outflow of blood was measured in rats (401), in sheep (112,219,315), and in pigs (112). The method of choice for quantitating blood flow through the ovary and follicles with the least number of artifacts, and the method most frequently employed, is the radioactive microsphere technique (RMS) introduced by Janson (225) for ovarian studies (143).

Physiological Changes in Blood Flow

Wurtman (513), using the indicator method, measured an increased ovarian blood flow within 6 sec after administration of LH, whereas Janson (225) recorded, using the RMS technique, an increased blood flow within 2 min. The increased blood flow occurs in the absence of any change in arterial pressure and is therefore attributable to a decrease in vascular resistance, most probably as a result of arteriolar vasodilation (225). Blasco et al. (57), also using the RMS technique in the rabbit, observed that blood flow through the ovary during the preovulatory phase increased fourfold by 4 hr after hCG administration, whereas blood flow (expressed as percent of cardiac output) to other organs (oviduct, uterus, brain, kidney) did not change. Lee and Novy (280), using the RMS technique, confirmed that blood flow in the rabbit ovary increased after administration of either 10 μg or 100 μg of LH and that the increase was independent of the dose of LH. The increase in absolute blood flow through the ovaries was at peak at 10 min (the earliest time measured after the control measurement) and had begun to decline by 60 min. To measure the blood flow to the dominant preovulatory follicle by the RMS technique, Murdoch et al. (342) excised the follicle and divided it into apical and basal portions and follicular fluid, then correlated the radioactivity with change in serum LH. Blood flow to the follicle (apex + base) was elevated after the rise in LH began during the 0-to-12-hr period, declined during the 12-to-16-hr period, and continued to decline at 20 hr and until after ovulation at 24 hr or later. No preferential blood flow to apex or base was observed, and no leakage of labeled microspheres into the follicular fluid was noted (342). The hyperemia initiated by LH is rapid in onset and persists for the rest of the rising limb of the LH surge, after which it either reaches a plateau or declines, suggesting that the blood flow, having reached a maximum, becomes constant for that period of the life of the follicle. Although blood flow is constant, the amount of protein passing through the walls of the capillary plexus increases (296) commensurate with the increasing edema and increasing follicular fluid volume (292).

Vasodilatory Substances and Ovarian Blood Flow

Histamine

The earliest response of the capillary plexus of the preovulatory follicle, occurring within seconds of the onset of the LH surge or administration of a bolus of LH or hCG, is a hyperemia (523), which persists and develops into an edematous reaction (153). The mechanism for the rapid response is undefined but may be caused by a rapid release of histamine (229,291,331,461,462,513) by mast cells located around the blood vessels in the hilus (230,264,491). The effect is most apparent in the preovulatory follicles, probably because of their extensive vascularization. The capillary and venule endothelia are the most likely sites for the changed permeability leading to edema. The formation of edema is primarily a result of increased macromolecular (protein) efflux, with consequent decrease in the lymph/plasma total-protein ratio thus decreasing the transmural colloid osmotic pressure gradient (192). Contractile elements in the endothelial cell and the pericytes activated by Ca^{2+} are hypothesized to enlarge the intercellular junctions, enlarging pores through which the protein can pass. Activation of the contractile elements requires the interaction of vasodilator substances with cellular receptors and an augmentation of Ca^{2+} influx, which also induces formation of prostaglandins. The latter facilitate influx of more Ca^{2+} and contraction of the pericyte (321). The major site of action of most substances that increase macromolecular permeability is the postcapillary venule. The permeability of the postcapillary venule is increased by the mediators listed in Table 5.

A number of inhibitors of postcapillary venule permeability have been described that also antagonize effects induced by histamine (Table 6). Among the early attempts to manipulate the level of histamine in the rat ovary and to block its action was that by Lipner (291). He used an H_1 blocker and also attempted to deplete the histamine levels; however, the rats ovulated, indicating either inadequate de-

TABLE 5. *Mediators of postcapillary venule permeability*[a]

Histamine, 5-hydroxytryptamine
Bradykinin, substance P
ADP, adenosine, inosine
Prostaglandins E_1, E_2, F_2
Leukotrienes C_4, D_4, E_4, B_4

[a]Modified from Svensjo and Grega (456).

TABLE 6. *Inhibitors of histamine-induced permeability*[a]

β_2-Receptor agonists (isoprenaline, terbutaline, salbutamol)
Calcium antagonist (Verapamil)
Glucocorticoids (budesonide, dexamethasone, methylprednesoline)
H_1-blocker antihistamine (pyrilamine)
Phosphodiesterase inhibitors (theophylline, xanthines)
Arginine vasopressin

[a]Modified from Svensjo and Grega (456).

pletion of histamine and blockade or that hCG could drive the ovulation cascade independently of histamine. Blockade of ovulation with H_1 antihistamines has been observed *in vivo* in rabbits (253) and *in vitro* in a perfused rabbit ovary (488); however, histamine may not be essential for ovulation, because other vasodilatory substances are probably also involved. In a study using the *in vitro* perfused rabbit ovary preparation, neither H_1 blockade with chlorpheniramine nor H_2 blockade with cimetidine, nor combination of the two, could block hCG-induced ovulation (255), even though in this preparation histamine alone could induce a low incidence of follicle rupture. Questions about the role of histamine in the cascade of events leading to ovulation are raised that still require resolution. Especially pertinent is the observation that the hCG-stimulated ovaries, even with exposure to H_1 and/or H_2 blockade, still show the edema so well summarized by Espey (153).

Estrogens are capable of inducing a vasodilation in reproductive tissues (of most mammals) (423,461). The factor usually associated with the estrogenic response is histamine, although other vasodilatory substances are unexplored. Because the estrogenic effect has a 30-min latency period and the response to LH or hCG is almost instantaneous (513), estrogen is probably not an immediate intermediate but may be involved in later maintenance of the hyperemia.

Bradykinin

Plasmin acting on prekallikrein generates the protease kallikrein, which releases from a high-molecular-weight plasma kininogen the nonapeptide bradykinin; low-molecular-weight plasma kininogen is converted by a tissue protease, kallikrein, to the decapeptide kallidin, which by the action of an aminopeptidase is converted to bradykinin. The kinins act on the arterioles to induce vasodilation and on the small venules to increase the permeability of the microcirculation, leading to edema. Kinins also release histamine from mast cells, which then augment the kinin vascular effect (134).

Bradykinin is present in follicular fluid (407); its concentrations in the follicle increase as the preovulatory follicle approaches the time of ovulation, and the levels reached are depressed by large doses of indomethacin, which block ovulation (161). The importance of this observation is obscure because the experiment does not distinguish between the actions of prostaglandins and bradykinin. Bradykinin releases arachidonic acid from cell membranes (266), and it is probable that in this study (161) the indomethacin exerted a dual effect. *In vitro,* neither bradykinin, histamine, nor angiotensin II had any effect on the rate of prostaglandin synthesis (259). Therefore, although increased synthesis of bradykinin parallels the increased synthesis of the prostaglandins, it has a minimal relationship to the early hyperemic reaction and to the induction of ovulation. Bradykinin may, however, contribute to the edema subsequent to the LH surge. Because plasmin synthesis is blocked by indomethacin (92), the postindomethacin increase in follicle volume is probably not caused by bradykinin, but other vasoactive substances that may still be active.

Prostaglandins

Although the prostaglandins studied in follicular function are generally limited to $PGF_{2\alpha}$ and PGE_2, the use of the nonsteroidal anti-inflammatory drugs (NSAIDs) results in the inhibition of the synthesis of prostacyclin (PGI_2), a vasodilator; PGE_2, an inducer of erythema and edema; $PGE_{2\alpha}$, in many tissues a vasodilator; and thromboxane (TXA_2), a vasoconstrictor. Furthermore, NSAIDs may inhibit chemotaxis of cells involved in the inflammatory process, inhibit labilization of membrane by lysosomes, antagonize the action of histamine and bradykinin, inhibit biosynthesis of mucopolysaccharides, uncouple oxidative phosphorylation, activate fibrinolytic activity, stabilize and block sulfhydryldisulfide reaction, inhibit production of collagenase, and suppress lymphocyte function (346).

The effect of indomethacin on ovarian and follicular blood flow has been studied because the mechanism for the essential role of the prostaglandin in ovulation is still considered to be in doubt in some laboratories. At dose levels that block ovulation, Lee and Novy (280) observed a reduction in absolute blood flow to 1.03 ml/min/g of ovary from an unstimulated control level of 1.68, a decrease of 40%. The increase of blood flow in indomethacin-treated rabbits after administration of LH at 10 min was 2.4-fold; at 30 min it was 3.0-fold, and by 60 min it was 3.4-fold. In the group treated with LH only, the comparable increases were 3.4-, 3.5-, and 2.5-fold for similar intervals. Systemic treatment with indomethacin causes a reduction in prostaglandin levels in most vascular beds, a reduction in blood flow, and an enhanced vasoconstrictor response; by analogy, it probably attenuates the ovarian response to vasodilator stimuli, and $PGF_{2\alpha}$ induces an increase in ovarian blood flow (349). The importance of the prostaglandin vasodilator mechanism in the generation of the early hyperemic response is questionable in any case, because the peak of prostaglandin synthesis occurs hours after the initiation of the maximum vascular response to LH. Since LH exerts its cellular effects by activating adenylate cyclase in its target cells, it is possible that either cAMP or progesterone might effect the vascular response (339); however, there is no latency between the onset of progesterone secretion and augmented ovarian blood flow in ewes during the estrous cycle, as determined with Doppler ultrasonic transducers (347). That the effect of prostaglandins on the vascular supply to the follicle is not related to ovulation was further demonstrated in ewes by Murdoch and Myers (340). They found, after administration of indomethacin, that the amount of blood in the follicles was greatly increased, that the follicles were increased in diameter (an observation also made by others; see ref. 243) because of an increased volume of follicular fluid, and that the amount of $PGE_{2\alpha}$ in the follicle wall was reduced, but that the amount of blood in the vessels of the wall was very noticeable. In order for fluid to accumulate in the follicle, blood flow must persist (292), and it becomes questionable that inhibition of ovulation by blockade of prostaglandin synthesis is mediated by controlling follicle blood flow.

THE ROLE OF SMOOTH MUSCLE IN OVULATION

Presence of smooth muscle in both the stroma of the ovary and the follicle wall (Table 7) has generated a search for its role in ovulation. The presence of smooth muscle in ovarian stroma and preovulatory follicle, coupled with its contractility, initiated the suggestion, first introduced by Rouget (425), that ovulation is either induced or facilitated by the contractions. Because no increase in pressure in the preovulatory follicle has been demonstrated, it is unlikely that the smooth muscle contributes to an increase in pressure (56,65,156,292). However, it is still possible that the contraction of the smooth muscle causes the wall of the follicle to collapse, facilitating the evacuation of the contents of the follicle (313,481) at the rupture point. The hamster rupture point tends to be small and may require contraction of the smooth muscle to facilitate discharge of the ovum (390,463); however, this mechanism is not generally observed. Despite the many efforts to demonstrate a role of smooth muscle in ovulation (313,430,464), no cause-and-effect data have been presented. The conclusion at present is that smooth-muscle contractions play no role in follicular rupture, but perhaps facilitate evacuation of follicle contents.

TABLE 7. *Distribution of smooth muscle in ovaries*

Species	Location	Reference
Rat	Theca externa	369
	Corpora lutea	
Rat	Theca externa	377
	Interstitial tissue	
	Atretic follicles	
Monkey	Atretic follicles	377
Sheep	Theca externa	370
Human	Theca externa	360
Rabbit	Theca externa	360
	Corpora lutea	53
	Cortical stroma	18
Cat	Cortical stroma	181
	Theca externa	68
Monkey	Theca externa	
Cat	Cortical stroma	
Rabbit	Theca externa	68
Guinea pig	Theca externa	
Hamster	Theca externa	318
	Corpora lutea	
	Interstitial tissue	
Gerbil	Theca externa	318
	Corpora lutea	
	Interstitial tissue	
Hamster	Theca externa	391
Cow	Theca externa	490

FOLLICULAR FLUID

The growing follicle undergoes a transformation from a solid mass of cells enclosing the ovum to a fluid-filled follicle containing a centrally located antrum into which projects a column of cells, the cumulus oophorus, continuous with the membrana granulosa. The ovum, surrounded by the corona radiata, sits attached to the cumulus oophorus and is positioned eccentrically within the antrum (397). Initially there appear, among the multiplying granulosa cells, small fluid-filled areas, which become confluent and give rise to a single fluid-filled antrum. This follicular configuration is characteristic of many, but not all, mammals (334).

The composition of the follicular fluid (liquor folliculi) changes as the follicle matures and the antral volume increases. Young antral follicles contain a primary fluid largely composed of proteoglycans. The proteoglycans become diluted by a gradual influx of fluid derived from the plasma enriched by the steroids and minute amounts of proteins synthesized by the theca interna and granulosa cells.

Except in the case of large mammal follicles (human, cow, and pig), data on the composition of the fluid are frequently based on analyses of pools of fluid collected from small, medium, and large follicles. However, by the definition developed by Peters (397), all the antral follicles belong to the category of large follicles because their oocytes are large, and only the membrana granulosa and theca interna increase in cell number while the antrum increases in volume.

Physical Characteristics

The follicular fluid in the preovulatory follicle is very similar to plasma. It is straw-colored, although it may at times appear yellow, and has a variable viscosity, an osmolality equal to that of plasma, and an electrolyte content, with minor variations, almost equal to that of plasma [rabbit (79,122,436)]. The gas content of human follicular fluid has been compared to that of plasma with differing results; the Po_2 is highly variable and not correlated with follicular histology, but the Pco_2 is correlated approximately with pH 7.3 (435). Fraser et al. (178) note that the Po_2 is higher in ovarian venous blood than in peripheral blood in women and suggest that arteriovenous shunts may account for the higher Po_2 levels and that therefore the follicular fluid Po_2 should be lower than the Po_2 of ovarian and peripheral venous blood. Unfortunately these studies are not comparable because Shalgi et al. (435) examined the follicular fluid, whereas Fraser et al. (178), studied only ovarian venous blood and peripheral venous blood. In the rabbit ovary, no evidence of arteriovenous shunts was found in studies based on *in situ* perfusion with microspheres (8).

Although we could not record a potential difference across the follicle wall in rats or rabbits (292), a small positive potential ($+1.2 \pm 0.3$ mV) has been reported across the wall of the mouse follicle in cycling mice, with an increase of $+3.8 \pm 0.8$ mV immediately before ovulation. These effects are modulated by sodium pentobarbital, sodium cyanide, and ouabain, inducing a positive potential, whereas PGE_1 and $PGF_{2\alpha}$ caused negative potentials; the changes involved are extremely small, and their meanings are difficult to interpret (526).

Proteins

The protein content and composition of follicular fluid have been examined in cows (22,94,128,301,485,520), pigs (316,440), rabbits (122), rats (434), and women (249,307,396,437). The total protein content of the follicular fluid is equal to or lower than that of serum (Table 8). It may vary with stage of the estrous cycle (387), but the protein content in all the follicles is similar regardless of size (22). The specific proteins show some variability; fibrinogen is present in lowest concentration, or absent, in pigs (440), cows (128), and women (307) and only 60% excluded (437). Rat follicles contain all the protein present in plasma (41) (Table 9).

TABLE 8. *Comparison of protein concentrations in plasma and ovarian follicular fluid in several species*

	Serum (g/100 ml)	Follicular fluid (g/100 ml)	Fluid/serum ratio	Reference
Cow		4.7–5.6		301
Cow	5.6	4.5	0.80	94
Cow	6.6	5.6	0.85	520
Cow	9.1	7.0	0.77	128
Cow		6.57	0.86	22
Pig			0.76	440
Pig	8.35	7.19[a]	0.86	316
Rabbit	6.94	7.0[b]	0.99	122
		6.8[b]	1.02	
Woman	7.4	5.5		396
Woman	7.4[c]	5.5	0.74	249
Woman	7.6	3.6	0.47	307
	6.8	3.6	0.53	307
Woman	5.8	5.8	1.0	436

[a]Mean of small and large follicles.
[b]Arterial and venous plasma, respectively.
[c]Plasma value.

Attempts to demonstrate the presence of proteins specific to the follicular fluid of pigs (440), cows (128), rats (41), and humans (307,436,437) by immunizing rabbits with follicular fluid have been uniformly unsuccessful, but immunoglobulin has been observed in the female rabbit reproductive tract (460). The failure to demonstrate the presence of antigenic components in follicular fluid foreign to plasma, however, indicates that the immunologic technique is insufficiently sensitive to detect such substances, because rat granulosa cells secrete inhibin (146), and inhibin has been demonstrated to occur in the follicular fluids of cows, pigs, horses, and humans (121,231,322,432). Various factors suspected to be present in follicular fluid have been noted (132,174,251,279,325) and summarized (101,201,207, 208,418).

The control of the permeability of the capillaries of all antral follicles, small or large, must be subject to the same factors because the protein contents of the fluid collected from small and large follicles are, with minor variation, similar (22). Furthermore, the permeability of the capillary wall must be high, because the protein content of the follicular fluid is very similar to that of serum (Table 8), and only the distributions of specific proteins differ (Table 9). Although a blood-follicle wall barrier has been suggested (437), the exclusion of molecules with molecular weights greater than 1,300,000 and partial exclusion of fibrinogen, with a molecular weight of 340,000, suggests a passive phenomenon of molecular sieving; however, even the largest molecules are found in the follicular fluid (441).

Hormones

The concentrations of hormones in the follicular fluid have been summarized by McNatty (317) and more recently by Guraya (201). The largest body of information on the gonadotropin content is based on studies of women. In general the levels of FSH and LH reflect the circulating blood levels, but prolactin levels are more closely and inversely related to follicular fluid volumes. The steroid concentrations reflect the stimulation of biosynthesis and are dependent on the rate of synthesis and diffusion from the theca interna and membrana granulosa and on the presence of steroid-binding proteins that cause enrichment of the steroid concentration in the follicular fluid (317).

The integrity of the follicle is dependent on the sequential exposure of its constituent cell population to FSH and LH, with prolactin serving to modulate the synthesis of steroids and the response to FSH and to affect follicle growth and development (147).

Enzymes

Schochet (428) initiated the search for the enzymatic mechanism of ovulation by demonstrating that follicular fluid could attack fibrin, boiled connective tissue, muscle, and ovarian tissue. The spectrum of enzymes identified in

TABLE 9. *Distribution of plasma proteins in serum and follicular fluid (F.F.)*[a]

Protein	Molecular weight	Women (396)		Women (249)		Women (437)		Cow (22,520)	
		Serum	F.F.	Serum	F.F.	Serum	F.F.	Serum	F.F.
Total protein		7.17	5.66	7.4	5.5	5.8	5.8	6.6	5.6
				% of Protein in serum or follicular fluid					
Albumin	69,000		45.1	56.5	63.5	52	69	61.4	64.8
α_1-Glycoprotein			6.6	3.5	2.8				
α-Globulin								12.2	7.7
α_1-Globulin									
α_2-Globulin			6.8	9.7	6.1				
β-Globulin			13.8	11.4	10.6				
β_1-Globulin								10.3	9.8
β_2-Globulin								8.8	10.5
IgG	150,000		27.8	19.2	15.2			7.3	8.4
Transferrin									
Fibrinogen	340,000					3.7	1.1		
Haptoglobulin									
IgA									
α_2-Macroglobulin									
IgM	900,000								
β_1-Lipoprotein	1,300,000		Present (441)				Undetectable		

[a]Andersen et al. (22) identified 37 individual proteins common to plasma and bovine follicular fluid by precipitate and 40 by crossed immunoelectrophoresis, including fibrinogen and its split products.

the follicular fluid from women, cows, and sows is listed in Table 10. Except for plasmin and collagenase, it is doubtful that these enzymes play a direct role in ovulation. It is also questionable that the enzyme in rabbit and sow follicular fluid that attacked the synthetic collagenase substrate carbobenzoxy-Gly-Pro-Gly-Gly-Pro-Ala (158,159,362) is a true mammalian collagenase, because this synthetic substrate is not attacked by animal collagenase, and enzymes that cleave this substrate have no action on collagen (327). Plasminogen activator in the follicular fluid (43,44,452) may be the significant enzyme that initiates the proteolytic cascade that ultimately degrades the collagen and leads to rupture of the follicle (*vide infra*) (Table 10).

Proteoglycans

Metachromasia in tissues is a well-established phenomenon, as are its association with the follicular fluid of young

TABLE 10. *Enzymes in follicular fluid*

Enzyme	Rat (42)	Porcine (238,292)	Bovine (317)	Human (97–99)	Rabbit (161)
Endopeptidase		+		+	
Aminopeptidase		+		+	
Proteinase		+			
Plasminogen activator	+		+		
Plasmin	+				
Dipeptidase				+	
Acid phosphatase				+	
Alkaline phosphatase		+		+	
Adenosine triphosphatase		+		+	
Fructose diphosphate aldolase					
Lactate dehydrogenase		+		+	
Hyaluronidase				+	
Amino transferase-aspartate		+			
Amino transferase-alanine		+			
Pyrophosphatase				+	
Kallikrein			+	+	+
Nucleotidase				+	
Thromboplasmin				+	
Collagenase (151)		+		+	
Adenosine triphosphatase				+	

follicles, its decreasing intensity of staining with maturation of the follicle, and its digestibility with hyaluronidase (509). These properties led to the suggestion that the substance was composed of mucopolysaccharides (509). Administration of $^{35}SO_4$ results in autoradiographic labeling of the follicular fluid because of secretion by the granulosa cells, during antrum formation (191,518,520), of a material identified as acid mucopolysaccharides (now called proteoglycans) (467).

The follicular fluid in follicles with newly formed antra is jelly-like (61,204,352,518) and becomes more fluid but remains viscous (141,142) as the follicles mature. The antra of mature follicles, prepared from rat ovaries fixed in aldehyde and stained with chromic acid and phosphotungstic acid, contain a complex network of fine reticular configuration (233); however, at lower magnification, the follicular fluid appears as a homogeneous granular precipitate (24).

Proteoglycans are composed of a core of protein, to which is attached polysaccharide chains called *glycosaminoglycans* (GAGs). Seven classes of GAGs with common characteristics have been identified. They contain long heteropolysaccharide chains composed of largely repeating units of disaccharides, in which one sugar is a hexosamine and the other is a uronic acid with sulfate groups. The carboxyl and sulfate groups are among the factors that make the GAGs highly charged polyanions. Because they hold cations and water within their domains, the proteoglycans give tissues their resiliency, form solutions of high elasticity and viscosity, and stabilize the fibrous and cellular elements of tissues.

Antrum formation in estrogen-primed hypophysectomized immature female rats occurs in response to administration of FSH (190). In a similar model, labeled sulfate is incorporated into proteoglycans linearly with the log of the dose of FSH (338). The predominant glycosaminoglycans of the follicular fluid are chondroitin sulfate and heparan sulfate (29,30,46,183,338,514,515), with chondroitin sulfate the major glycosaminoglycan of the proteoglycan found in the rat (514), pig (29,515), and cow (35,194,195). The predominant glycosaminoglycan secreted *in vitro* by rat granulosa cells (514,516) and bovine granulosa cells (46,47,285) is chondroitin sulfate. Healthy follicles have elevated concentrations of estrogen and low concentrations of progesterone and chondroitin sulfate, whereas atretic follicles have low amounts of estrogen and elevated concentrations of progesterone and chondroitin sulfate (45). The accompaniments of follicular maturation are rising concentrations of estrogen and declining concentrations of chondroitin sulfate and heparan sulfate (85). Elevated levels of cAMP increase the synthesis of proteoglycans by rat ovarian granulosa cells, because incorporation of $^{35}SO_4$ into proteoglycans is stimulated by ovine FSH and LH, human chorionic gonadotropin, PGE_1, PGE_2, *N,O′*-dibutyryl cAMP, theophylline, and testosterone (516). Treatment of bovine granulosa cells by using phenothiazine drugs such as trifluoroperazine, chlorpromazine, and chlorpromazine sulfate to inhibit calmodulin or by decreasing the concentration of calcium in the medium with EGTA inhibits the synthesis of proteoglycans in response to stimulation with either ovine or rat FSH. The synthesis of proteoglycans in response to stimulation by FSH requires activation of adenylate cyclase and the presence of calcium ions (285).

The formation of the secondary follicular fluid in the preovulatory follicle occurs with the onset of the LH surge and reflects the series of events associated with changes in the follicle wall. There is an almost instantaneous increase in follicular blood flow manifested by the vasodilation. Somewhat later (6 hr after the LH surge) the increase in capillary and venule permeability is accompanied by increased volumes of interstitial fluid containing high concentrations of plasma proteins. The gradually rising concentrations of the prostaglandins and leukotrienes induce contraction of the smooth muscle in the postcapillary venules (456), thus increasing the intracapillary pressure further and enhancing the rate of transudation of plasma (321). There is an increase in tone of the smooth muscle of the follicle wall in response to sympathetic nerve terminal secretion of norepinephrine and co-transmitter substances. Later the β_2-adrenergic effects are exerted on the membrana granulosa, causing further increase of prostaglandin secretion and thus maintaining the increased smooth muscle tone and venule permeability (456). The consequence of these processes is to raise the free fluid pressure (as measured in the antrum) to a positive value, indicating that the factors that prevent accumulation of fluid (low interstitial-fluid protein concentration, lymphatic protein removal, and low venule resistance) are no longer effective and that conditions for accumulation of increased extracellular fluid volumes now exist (192).

The importance of the proteoglycans in the follicle is probably dependent on the negative charges of the glycosaminoglycans, which create Donnan osmotic and hydromechanical forces (62). These act as a sink and probably are responsible for the slow initial influx of fluid and gradual expansion of the antral space.

PREOVULATORY MORPHOLOGICAL CHANGES ASSOCIATED WITH OVULATION

Heape (209) thought that the cause of follicular rupture was obscure. Eighty years later the cause still under investigation is less obscure, but is still far from being revealed in its totality. The morphological changes have been examined in much detail, but only in a relatively small number of species, and though there appears to be much similarity in these changes, many more species need to be examined.

In the rabbit and rat the volume of the preovulatory follicle after a coital stimulus or hCG increases linearly (296,495). Concurrent with the increase in follicular volume, there is an increase in collagen synthesis indicated by a threefold increase in the content of hydroxyproline in ovaries of PMSG-primed immature rats. After the endogenous surge of LH, there is a further twofold increase in ovarian hydroxyproline and a subsequent abrupt decline (328). Preovulatory follicles therefore undergo a period of enhanced collagen synthesis followed by a degradation of collagen.

The appearance of the preovulatory follicle as it approaches rupture has been described in great detail. In mice (86) and rabbits (104) the follicle protrudes above the surface of the ovary as its volume increases, the capillaries in the theca appear packed with erythrocytes, and the endothelium is flattened; with time, perforations appear in the capillary walls. As time of rupture approaches, the thecal cells at the base of the follicle break through the lamina propria and begin to intermingle with the parietal granulosa cells, which show a marked increase in smooth endoplasmic reticulum, signaling their transformation to lutein cells. At the apex, the germinal epithelium lies on (a) a basement membrane containing fibroblasts (the theca) and (b) a basement membrane, the lamina propria, of the membrana granulosa. The germinal cells flatten as the follicle protrudes and gives rise to the stigma and then disappear as rupture becomes imminent. The underlying fibroblasts are no longer present, but collagen fibers are seen. The theca cells beneath the fragmented epithelial layer appear necrotic. At rupture, the theca cells are lost, as is the lamina propria of the membrana granulosa. The latter cells protrude through the developing rupture point and appear intact. Similar changes have been described in the rabbit and human, with the added observation that the collagen in the apex becomes sparse (49–54,148,359).

As the time of ovulation approaches, the preovulatory follicle develops a protrusion called the *stigma*. In the rat the stigma assumes one of two different configurations. Stigmas may appear as extensively bulging vesicles, called *bleb-type,* or as small flat avascular areas, called *flat-type*. The bleb-type stigmas lose their epithelial cover, exposing densely arranged fibroblasts, with multivesicular bodies (150) protruding but without collagen fibers present, surrounding a pore. The surface epithelium sloughs off the avascular area of the flat-type stigmas, revealing an underlying stroma composed of coarse longitudinal and smaller circular fibers. Beneath these are fibroblasts surrounding a small opening in the stroma, through which granulosa cells protrude (477).

Throughout the estrous cycle, cell replication does not occur in the theca externa of mature rat follicles, but the granulosa cells and theca interna incorporate [^{3}H]thymidine into nuclear DNA during diestrus and stop taking up [^{3}H]thymidine during estrus (478). Thus, although follicle-wall synthetic activities are present, they derive from a constant cell population.

Increased extravasation of fluid in the follicle wall is frequently described (49–54,86,148,209,495) and is summarized by Espey (153). Edema and follicle enlargement occur even when ovulation is blocked with indomethacin (25,162,517). The determinants of ovulation therefore are neither edema nor inflammation per se but, instead, synthetic mechanisms inherent to the preovulatory follicle and initiated by LH.

PREOVULATORY CHEMICAL CHANGES ASSOCIATED WITH OVULATION

The surge of LH that occurs at midcycle in women and subhuman primates, in proestrus in spontaneously cycling mammals, or subsequent to coitus in reflex ovulators is followed by a series of changes in the follicle wall that lead to its disruption and the discharge of the ovum (431). These changes are initiated with the rising concentration of LH and, after 1 hr of exposure to LH, become independent of subsequent hormonal stimulation (292). The cascade of changes may be interrupted by blockade of protein synthesis with cycloheximide or actinomycin D (17,38,403,404), by blockade of steroid synthesis with cyanoketone or aminoglutethimide (294,297), with antiprogesterone antiserum (329,458), or with antitestosterone antiserum (330), by blockade of prostaglandin synthesis with indomethacin (25), or by interruption of the plasminogen activator-plasminogen cascade (92).

Protein Synthesis

The rabbit, because it is a reflex ovulator, is an interesting model for the study of ovulation. The interval from the stimulus, either coital or hormonal (LH or hCG), to the time of ovulation is 10 to 12 hr (209). During this 10- to 12-hour interval, all the important changes initiated by LH must occur. A role for protein synthesis in ovulation was first explored by means of the intrafollicular injection of actinomycin D (an inhibitor of transcription, blocking synthesis of mRNA) and cycloheximide (an inhibitor of translation, blocking peptide-chain initiation and chain elongation) (403,404). Both compounds block ovulation when introduced into the follicle up to 5 hr post-coitally. This observation made with actinomycin D was confirmed in both mature and immature hamsters (38). Diphtheria toxin and cycloheximide, both of which block translation by inhibiting peptide chain elongation, inhibited ovulation in hamsters (17). Increasing the dose of either inhibitor extended the duration of inhibition, probably indicating that protein synthesis is an ongoing process throughout the crucial period. Alleva et al. (17) note that, even though ovulation is blocked by diphtheria toxin or cycloheximide, behavioral estrus that is progesterone dependent is unaffected. They conclude that either the blocked protein synthesis is most probably associated with enzymes involved in follicle-wall degradation (and not with steroid synthesis) or behavioral estrus is controlled by smaller amounts of progesterone than is ovulation.

Steroidogenesis

The biosynthesis of steroids by the theca interna and granulosa cells has been reviewed by Erickson et al. (147), with special emphasis on the ovarian production of androgen. The best explanation for estrogen production in the follicle is based on the two-cell two-hormone hypothesis.

FSH serves to induce LH receptors, and the LH causes the theca interna to shift from a progesterone- to an androgen-secreting tissue. In the presence of granulosa cells, the androgen is converted to estrogen, and follicular growth and development ensue. The preovulatory surge of LH terminates estrogen synthesis by the preovulatory follicle, and the theca cells change from an androgen- to a progesterone-secreting tissue (147).

Blockade of ovulation occurs when immature rats treated with PMSG/hCG or PMSG/LH are pretreated with cyanoketone (2α-cyano-4,4,17α-trimethylandrost-5-en-17β-ol-3-one), a 3β-hydroxysteroid dehydrogenase inhibitor (297); aminoglutethimide, a 20α-hydroxycholesterol dehydrogenase inhibitor; or Su 10603, a 17α-hydroxylase inhibitor (294). The authors suggested that progesterone was a precursor molecule essential for ovulation. Bullock and Kappauf (66), using immature rats primed with PMSG/hCG and treated with aminoglutethimide or cyanoketone, found that ovulation was unaffected by aminoglutethimide, even though serum progesterone was depressed, and that with cyanoketone at the largest dose, both depression of serum progesterone and blockade of ovulation occurred. They concluded that neither progesterone nor steroids were involved in the ovulatory mechanism. This conclusion was seemingly reinforced by Hamada et al. (205), who noted that a slightly higher number of perfused rabbit ovaries ovulated when exposed to hCG and progesterone than when perfused with hCG alone. More recently, apparent dissociation of steroid biosynthesis and ovulation was again observed. Perfusion of immature rat ovaries with LH 48 hr after they were primed with PMSG resulted in follicular rupture and an increase in the concentration of estradiol in the medium and in the follicular fluid. Addition of 4-hydroxyandrostene-3,17-dione prevents the increase in estradiol but does not prevent ovulation (261). Although the concentrations of both progesterone and estrogen were reduced, the continued synthesis of neither steroid was completely blocked, and it is not known what levels of steroid, if any, are necessary to allow ovulation.

There is, however, an interesting body of literature supporting the observation that progesterone, testosterone, and, by implication, estradiol are involved in ovulation. Intrafollicular injection of normal rabbit serum (Fig. 1) does not affect the incidence of ovulation (Fig. 2), but ovine progesterone antiserum reduces the incidence of ovulation to 20% (Fig. 3), whereas rabbit estrogen antiserum or progesterone antiserum adsorbed with progesterone are ineffective in blocking or even reducing the incidence of ovulation (Fig. 4). Furthermore, hamster ovaries explanted into progesterone-containing media have multiple ovulations (36,37). Rondell (421) noted that estradiol and progesterone increase the distensibility of follicle-wall strips; however, there is no direct link between this phenomenon and ovulation.

A relationship between steroids and ovulation has been established by the use of antitestosterone antiserum and antiprogesterone antiserum in rats (329,330) and in humans and ewes (33). In these studies (329,330), ovulation was blocked in PMSG/hCG-treated immature rats with antiserum against either progesterone or testosterone, and the effect of the antiprogesterone antiserum was reversed by administration of progesterone within 6 hr after the hCG treatment. Antiprogesterone antiserum was ineffective if administered more than 6 hr after the hCG treatment (257). This observation in the rat parallels that by Swanson and Lipner (458) (Fig. 3) and supports that concept that steroids may be involved in ovulation.

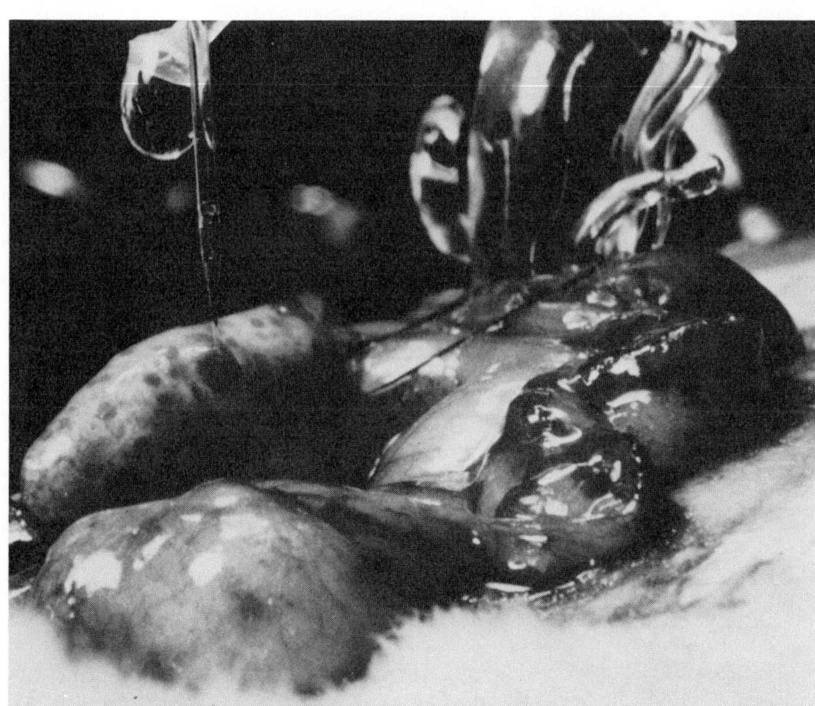

FIG. 1. Appearance of the operative field with preovulatory follicle receiving an injection in an exteriorized ovary. The tissue is kept warm and moist with a continuous 37°C drip of mammalian Ringer's solution. In the foreground are a fat body and the oviduct. [From Swanson and Lipner (1977), *unpublished report.*]

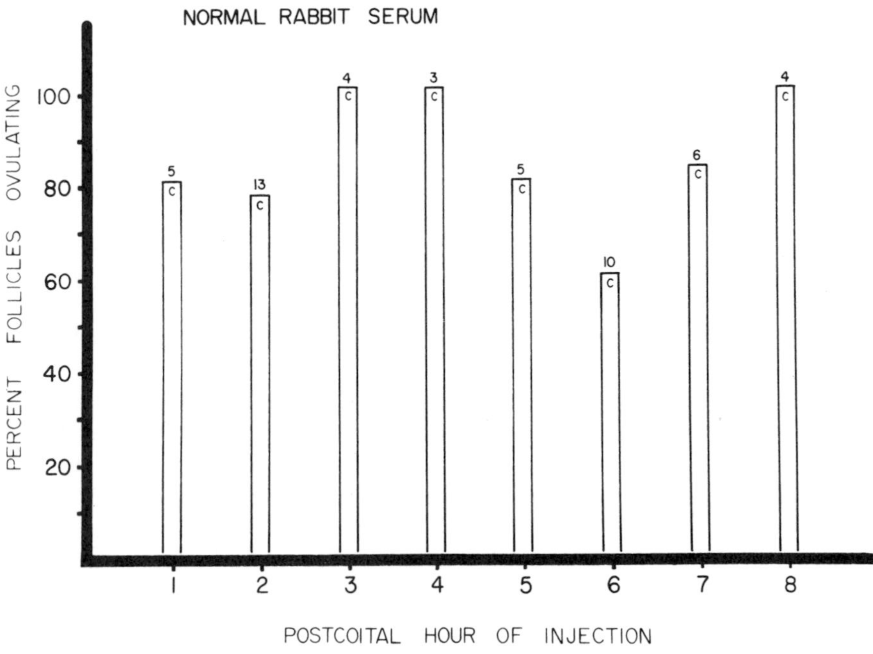

FIG. 2. Follicles (numbers above columns) injected with 0.1 μl of normal rabbit serum at various intervals post-coitus. No significant difference is noted between the columns, and the range of ovulations was from 60 to 100%. On average, only 80% of follicles ovulate. [From Swanson and Lipner (1977), *unpublished report.*]

Bellin and Ax (45) noted that healthy follicles have elevated levels of estradiol. The path to estradiol synthesis includes testosterone from sources extrinsic to the estrogen-secreting cell; therefore, the most probable sites for inhibition of the ovulatory mechanism are at stages preceding the synthesis of estrogen (294,297,329,330). This finding explains the failure of MER-25 (297) and of antiestrogen antiserum introduced directly into the follicle to inhibit ovulation (Fig. 4). In immature rats primed with PMSG/hCG, both indomethacin and cycloheximide reduce the levels of estradiol and progesterone in the ovaries. In the ovaries of rats not treated with the inhibitors, the concentrations of estradiol and progesterone are inversely related, and the steroid changes precede the rise in prostaglandins. Thus one may postulate that the steroids contribute to the regulation of prostaglandin production, which in turn may regulate enzyme production (154).

Prostaglandins

Arachidonic acid is converted by prostaglandin cyclooxygenase to the endoperoxide intermediate PGH_2, which is then converted by the action of isomerases to a number of biologically active molecules, among which prostaglandin E_2 (PGE_2), prostaglandin F_2 alpha ($PGF_{2\alpha}$), and prostacyclin ($PGI_{2\alpha}$) are the most abundant (455). $PGI_{2\alpha}$ is unstable, and

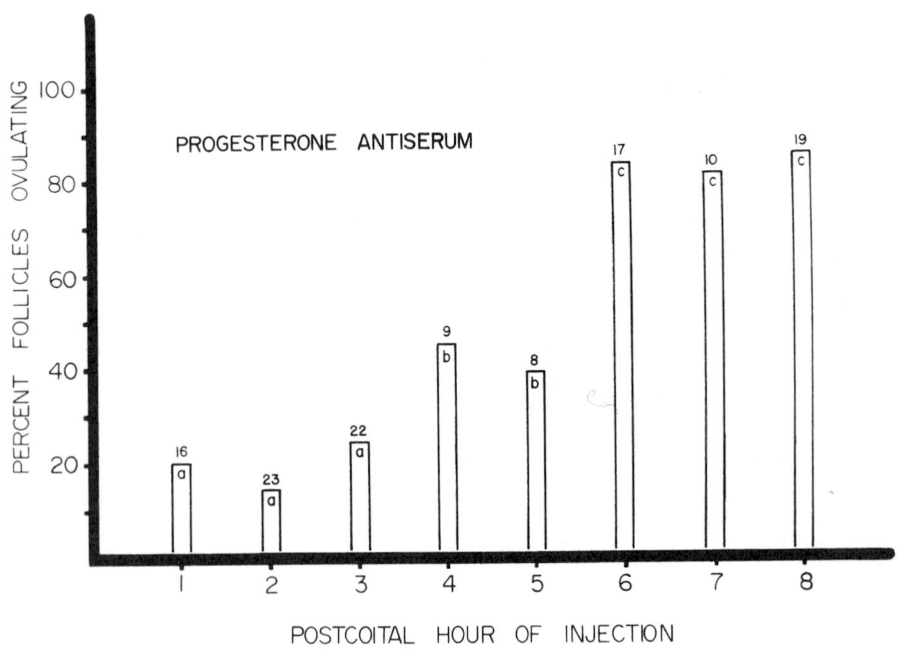

FIG. 3. Follicles (numbers above columns) were injected with 0.1 μl of ovine progesterone antiserum (produced in sheep against progesterone-BSA conjugate, with a low cross-reactivity against estrogens and progestagens, other than progesterone; a gift from Dr. J. D. Neill and Dr. M. Freeman). There is no significant difference between the columns that have the same letters. Columns with different letters were significantly different at $p < 0.01$. [From Swanson and Lipner (1977), *unpublished report.*]

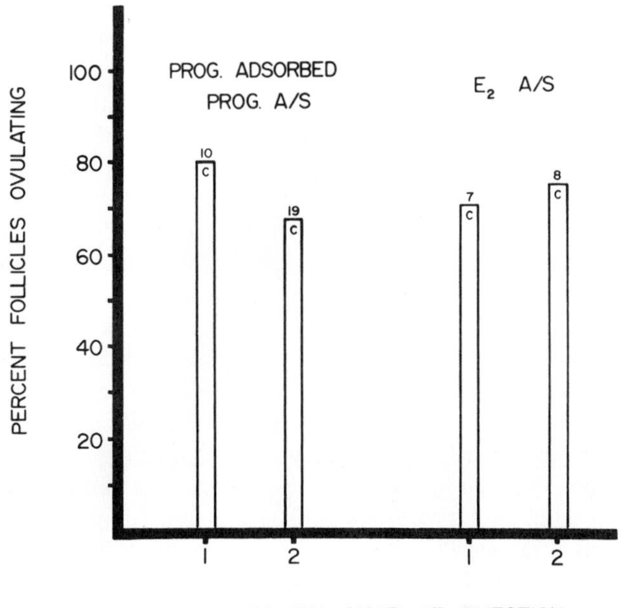

FIG. 4. Follicles (numbers above columns) injected with ovine progesterone antiserum and adsorbed with progesterone (*left side*) or injected with rabbit estrogen antiserum (batch E_2-7α-H was a gift from Dr. K. Wright and Dr. D. C. Collins, prepared in rabbits with estradiol-17β-carboxymethoxine thyroglobulin). No significant difference was found from the expected incidence of ovulation with either treatment. [From Swanson and Lipner (1977), *unpublished report.*]

its presence is manifested by that of the stable molecule 6-keto-$PGF_{1\alpha}$. Prostaglandin cyclooxygenase is subject to inhibition by NSAIDs such as aspirin, ibuprofen, piroxicam, and indomethacin. Inhibition of prostaglandin cyclooxygenase effectively blocks the synthesis of all the prostaglandins of the PGH_2 series. An alternative pathway for the oxygenation of arachidonic acid is provided by lipoxygenase enzymes, which are insensitive to NSAIDs. The products of the lipoxygenase enzymes are hydroperoxyeicosatetranoic acids (HPETEs). Among the latters' degradation products are 5-hydroperoxyeicosatetranoic acid, which can, by epoxide formation, give rise to the leukotrienes (266). The prostaglandins have numerous and varied actions, among which are smooth-muscle contractile ($PGF_{2\alpha}$) or relaxant (PGE_2) activity, activation of adenylate cyclase, participation in the inflammatory reaction, and activation of proteolytic enzymes. One of the important actions of the leukotrienes is in their chemotactic effect on polymorphoneutrophils and their involvement in the inflammatory reaction.

Inhibition of cyclooxygenase with indomethacin blocks ovulation (25), and blockade of lipoxygenase activity with nordihydroguaiaretic acid (a nonspecific inhibitor of both prostaglandin cyclooxygenase and lipoxygenase; see ref. 384), 3-amino-1-(3-trifluoromethylphenyl)-2-pyrazoline hydrochloride (BW 755C), and FPL-55712 (lipoxygenase inhibitors; see ref. 95) results in partial blockade of ovulation (413). Furthermore, rat ovarian and follicular homogenates both possess lipoxygenase activity that increases after *in vivo* administration of hCG (414). These observations implicate the leukotrienes as well as the prostaglandins in follicular rupture.

Rat granulosa cells obtained from PMSG-treated immature rats form 6-keto-$PGF_{1\alpha}$ and PGE_2, with maximum stimulation occurring in the presence of arachidonic acid and LH. Although arachidonic acid, LH, and lueteinizing hormone releasing hormone (LHRH)-ethylamide (a potent LHRH agonist) stimulate prostaglandin formation, it has been found that histamine, bradykinin, and angiotensin II have no effects on the rate of prostaglandin synthesis (259). The significance of the ability of the granulosa cells to synthesize 6-keto-$PGF_{1\alpha}$ resides in the observation that prostacyclin ($PGI_{2\alpha}$, a major arachidonic acid metabolite; see ref. 405) and the 6-keto-$PGF_{1\alpha}$ that appears as a stable oxidative product of the $PGI_{2\alpha}$ decrease the incorporation of [^{3}H]proline into human cervical tissue during the follicular phase and increase the incorporation of the labeled amino acid during the luteal phase of the menstrual cycle (503). The steroid milieu of the tissue apparently influences the action of the prostaglandin. A similar control of collagen synthesis probably holds in the Graafian follicle, because incorporation of [^{3}H]proline into the tunica albuginea of human preovulatory follicles is depressed by PGE_2 (127).

Prostaglandins acting on cultured follicles mimic the effects exerted by LH. PGE_2 can induce adenylate cyclase activity, activate protein kinase (269,270) and ornithine decarboxylase (270,376), increase glucose oxidation (395), and induce luteinization and resumption of meiotic division of the oocyte (289,474). $PGF_{2\alpha}$ is less effective than PGE_2 in increasing cAMP accumulation and in inducing the first meiotic division of the oocyte (290). Any substance capable of increasing cAMP accumulation is effective at inducing maturation of follicle-enclosed ova. Among these compounds are LH, FSH, PGE_2, and $PGF_{2\alpha}$. Whereas FSH induces secretion of progesterone, LH and PGE_2 induce the secretion of progesterone, androstenedione, and estradiol (289).

The action of LH on the biosynthetic activities of cultured follicles is independent of concurrent synthesis of prostaglandins. In the presence of flufenamic acid [*N*-(α,α,α-trifluoro-*m*-tolyl) anthranilic acid], indomethacin, or aspirin (prostaglandin cyclooxygenase inhibitors), LH stimulates cAMP accumulation and progesterone release from the follicles (289). Furthermore, after prolonged exposure to LH, a subsequent stimulation with LH elicits no further activation of adenylate cyclase (282), but PGE_2 provokes additional adenylate cyclase activation (289). The actions of LH and PGE_2 are independent and parallel, and PGE_2 mimics the LH effects (290).

Although whole rabbit or rat follicles respond to exposure to LH with increased prostaglandin synthesis (40,281), demonstration that isolated follicle components secrete prostaglandins under gonadotropic stimulation has been achieved only occasionally. Rabbit granulosa cells secrete $PGF_{2\alpha}$ but are unstimulated by human menopausal gonadotropin (hMG with LH/FSH activity) (100). Rabbit follicles dissected into thecal wall and granulosa components secrete prostaglandins, but neither follicle component is stimulated by LH (474). The granulosa cells from PMSG-treated immature rats do, however, show a response to LH with an increase in PGE synthesis (109). There is an increase in PGF in pieces of follicles of human ovarian tissue after incubation for 72 hr and continuous exposure to hCG and hMG (402); in human granulosa cells, hCG or hCG and hMG stimulate PGE production (388). Rat ovarian theca incubated with FSH increases PGE formation 15-fold over basal levels and threefold over the stimulated rate in granulosa from the same follicle (524). Theca and granulosa from gilts treated with PMSG and hCG and then cultured with LH or FSH are differently affected. FSH exerts no additional stimulation, but LH stimulates the granulosa to increase production of PGE_2 (166). In a study of dispersed granulosa cells and theca interna cells obtained from prepubertal gilts treated with PMSG and hCG, both cell types produce $PGF_{2\alpha}$ and PGE_2; the latter was the major product produced. Neither FSH nor LH induced responses in these cell types (11). Either the appropriate *in vitro* conditions have yet to be achieved, there is a step (or steps) yet to be elucidated, or the interaction of the theca interna and granulosa is required for the gonadotropin stimulus to be effective. Furthermore, the greatest success with LH stimulation occurs after previous exposure to PMSG. These observations are very similar to those describing the control of the production of plasminogen activator and suggest that maturation of the follicle subsequent to exposure to FSH must precede the response to LH (see subsection entitled "Plasminogen").

In the absence of prostaglandins the final phase of ovulation—the follicular rupture—does not occur (281). Thus, although LH induces the process of ovulation, prostaglandins must be present for the final phase. Inhibition of prostaglandin synthesis by administration of indomethacin blocks ovulation in rats (25,324,475), rabbits (26,196,353), marmoset monkeys (304), and gilts (10).

The concentrations of PGE and PGF in the ovaries, follicles, and follicular fluid are indicated in Table 11. In rats, rabbits, humans, and swine the prostaglandin levels rise as time of ovulation approaches. In rabbits, $PGF_{2\alpha}$ increases 10-fold and PGE_2 increases fivefold 5 hr after an ovulatory dose of hCG, and by 10 hr these prostaglandin concentrations have increased 60-fold and 15-fold, respectively (284). PGE_2 is present in higher concentrations initially than is $PGF_{2\alpha}$, and only by 9 hr does the ratio of PGE_2 to PGF_2 approach unity. In rats and sheep the increase in follicular prostaglandin is initiated by the LH surge and reaches maximum concentration as time of ovulation approaches (39,289,341). Prepubertal pigs treated with PMSG and hCG ovulate approximately 116 hr after the administration of the hCG. PGF in the follicular fluid of preovulatory follicles increases to a maximum by 90 to 92 hr (9). That prostaglandins are probably involved in ovulation in humans is indicated by the increased synthesis of prostaglandins by human ovaries exposed to human menopausal gonadotropin (402) (Table 11).

Prostaglandins have been implicated in a number of diverse effects on the ovarian follicle. $PGF_{2\alpha}$ may be involved in maturation of guinea-pig (465), and prostaglandins in maturation of mouse (137), ovarian follicles. PGE_2 inhibits the synthesis of collagen within the tunica albuginea of preovulatory human follicles (127) but stimulates the synthesis of proteoglycans in this tissue (468). In mice, PGE_2 induces cumulus expansion associated with synthesis of hyaluronic acid (145). In rabbits, blockade of prostaglandin synthesis with indomethacin prevents the appearance of proteolytic enzymes (collagenases) specifically associated with collagen degradation (215,216,246). $PGF_{2\alpha}$ injected into rabbit Graafian follicles induces the expulsion of the ovum along the path through the follicle wall created by the cannula (27), and $PGF_{2\alpha}$ injected intraaortically in indomethacin-treated rabbits increases ovarian contractility (130).

Follicle walls prepared from human ovarian follicles are spontaneously contractile and manifest a significant increase in tone when exposed to $PGF_{2\alpha}$, but a small decrease in tone when exposed to PGE_2 (357,358). In a similar study performed on sow ovarian follicles, $PGF_{2\alpha}$ decreased the tension generated in early and late preovulatory strips, whereas PGE_2 increased the basal tension (187,188). Guinea-pig ovaries develop a marked increase in isometric tension when exposed to either oxytocin or $PGF_{2\alpha}$ during late proestrus (189).

The effect of the prostaglandins on contractility of whole rabbit ovaries has also been examined both *in vivo* and *in vitro*. $PGF_{2\alpha}$ causes an increase in intraovarian pressure and contractions of human ovarian stroma *in situ*, whereas PGE_2 has no effect on the intraovarian pressure, but the combination of the two prostaglandins in equal quantities is stimulatory (116). *In vitro* study of human ovarian tissue prepared from proliferative-phase follicles indicates that PGE_2 causes a decrease, and $PGF_{2\alpha}$ an increase, in tonic contractions (117). *In situ* ovaries are spontaneously contractile even without prior exposure to hCG. $PGF_{2\alpha}$ administered via the aorta increases tone and amplitude of contractions, and PGE_2 similarly administered induces a reduction in tone and contractile activity. *In vitro* measurements yield similar responses to the two prostaglandins. In hCG-treated rabbits the ovaries both *in vivo* and *in vitro* were spontaneously active, and $PGF_{2\alpha}$ stimulates increases in tone and amplitude of contraction (483). Although the prostaglandins affect the smooth muscle of the ovary and probably the follicle, a relationship to ovulation is still not established. The effect of $PGF_{2\alpha}$ on ovaries of most animals examined is to increase tone and contractility of the smooth muscle in the follicle wall. PGE_2, on the other hand, causes a reduction in the tonic contraction and obliterates contractile activity.

The number of actions elicited by the prostaglandins on tissues are numerous and diverse, but the mechanism by which they act on the ovary to elicit ovulation is now be-

TABLE 11. *Prostaglandin levels in ovaries, follicles, or follicular fluid*

			Prostaglandin (pg/mg)		Prostaglandin (pg/follicle or pg/ml)		
Species	Treatment	Tissue	PGE	PGF	PGE	PGF	Reference
Rat	Estrous cycle	Graafian follicle					283
	Proestrus						
	8:00 a.m.		11 + 1.0	18 + 2.5			
	12:00 p.m.		10 + 1.0	19 + 3.0	37	77	
	4:00 p.m.		14 + 3.0	22 + 6.0	37	77	
	8:00 p.m.		370 + 210	247 + 102	1,050 + 51	746 + 2,701	
	12:00 a.m.		746 + 275	369 + 63	2,570 + 509	1,380 + 263	
	Estrus						
	4:00 a.m.		49 + 43	69 + 50	118 + 100	161 + 132	
	8:00 a.m.		25 + 7.0	27 + 6.0	66 + 21	70 + 17	
Rabbit	None	Graafian follicle				20	26
	50 g NIH-LH-B7 (9½ hr post-LH)					742 + 174	
Rabbit		Graafian follicle					284
	None	(5)[a]	70.0 + 27.9	15.2 + 5.9			
	hCG (100 IU)						
	after 1 hr	(4)	107 + 45	19 + 4.3			
	after 5 hr	(4)	335 + 191	296 + 321			
	after 9 hr	(5)	816 + 246	763 + 247			
Human		Whole follicle, preovulatory			3,160	840	388
		Late proliferative follicle					
		Theca			70.6	87	
		granulosa			n.d.[b]	n.d	
Swine (prepubertal)	PMSG, hCG	Pooled follicular fluid					476
	Time after hCG (hr)						
	0	(4)			1,200 + 200	160 + 20	
	4	(4)			1,100 + 100	140 + 30	
	30	(5)			6,300 + 800	6,100 + 1,100	
	35	(6)			37,600 + 26,300	38,600 + 1,800	
	38	(4)			176,000 + 26,000	231,000 + 55,000	
	40	(4)			196,000 +	192,000 + 161,000	
Sheep[c]	Estrous cycle	Follicle wall					341
	Pre LH rise				2,300	5,700	
	Hours after LH rise						
	0				2,600	6,600	
	4				2,600	6,600	
	8				13,000	11,000	
	12				15,000	12,600	
	16–20				5,000	10,600	

[a]Numbers in parentheses indicate the number of animals.
[b]n.d., not detected.
[c]Values are approximate, based on Fig. 5 [Murdoch et al. (341)].

coming more apparent (92,412). NSAIDs block the synthesis of prostaglandins and inhibit ovulation, but dexamethasone, a very effective steroidal anti-inflammatory drug, has little or no effect on ovulatory rate (161). NSAIDs also inhibit the activation of neutrophils and inhibit calcium ion (Ca^{2+}) movement into them; they therefore prevent the release of other inflammation-provoking substances (2). These observations can be extended to the ovarian follicle; NSAIDs may prevent the release of enzymes from polymorphoneutrophils as well as from other cells that participate in ovulation. However, it should be noted that PGE_2 affects ovulation in indomethacin-blocked animals (25,473) and thus plays a major role in ovulation. PGE_2 causes vasodilation and smooth-muscle relaxation, and PGF_2 causes venomotor smooth muscle contraction and elicits this effect on ovarian follicle smooth muscle (358). PGE_2 is the predominant prostaglandin in the follicle, but the $PGF_{2\alpha}$ may exert an effect on the smooth-muscle elements of the follicle wall (130). Furthermore, antiserum to $PGF_{2\alpha}$ injected into preovulatory follicles of LH-primed rabbits blocks ovulation of the antiserum-treated follicles only (26); in indomethacin-blocked rats, ovulation can be induced by administration of PGE_2 (473,475). These diverse observations have now become interpretable as a result of more recent studies (see subsections entitled "Plasminogen" and "Collagenolysis").

Plasminogen

Enzymatic degradation of the follicle wall is probably the best hypothesis explaining follicular rupture (42,44, 151,152,292). Espey (152) is a proponent of the concept that activation of the fibroblast and its release of an activator (Fig. 5, step 3) to convert latent collagenase is the mechanism controlling ovulation. The plasminogen-activator–plasminogen hypothesis (Fig. 5) is the most recent and most likely explanation of the mechanism initiating the cascade that leads to follicular rupture. The study of this system has resulted in an intensive evaluation of the various steps in the postulated cascade.

The plasminogen-activator–plasminogen system may be important in situations where controlled proteolysis and tissue degradation are necessary, as in involution of the mammary gland at termination of lactation (374), rupture of the ovarian follicle at the time of ovulation (42,44,452), and embryonic reorganization (311,453). The advantages of this system are based on the ability of the cell to secrete small amounts of a specific protease (plasminogen activator) to generate a second protease (plasmin) with a broad range of substrates. The second protease (plasmin) has its pH optimum at the pH of extracellular fluid. The proenzyme (plasminogen) is present in plasma in high concentrations (0.5

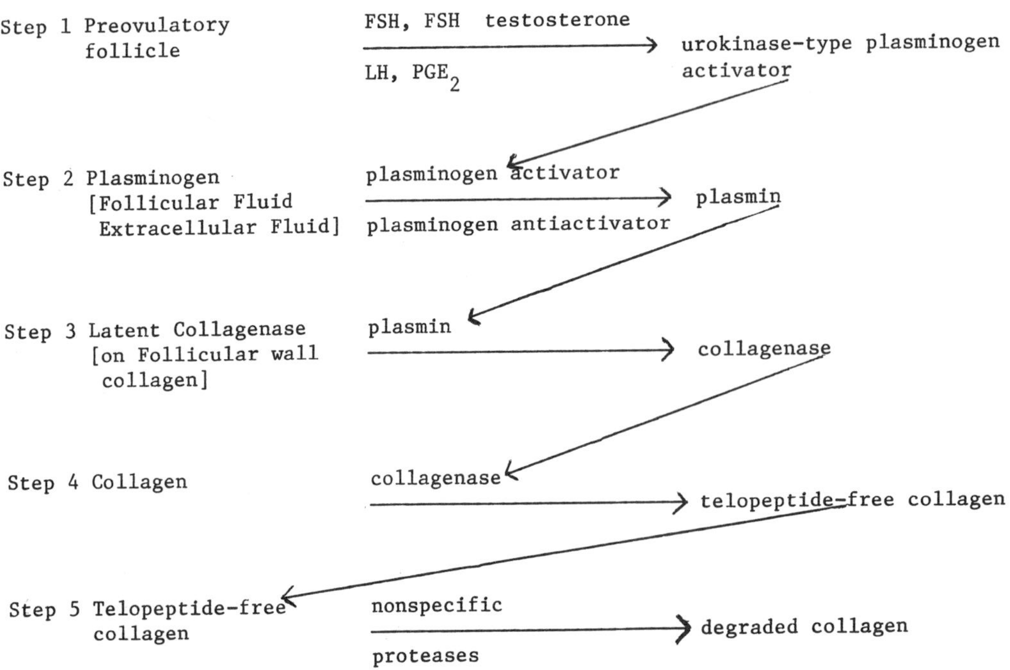

FIG. 5. A hypothesis describing the proteolytic cascade involved in degradation of the collagen in the preovulatory follicle wall. Step 1: The preovulatory follicle stimulated by gonadotropins secretes urokinase-type plasminogen activator. Step 2: Urokinase-type plasminogen activator converts plasminogen to plasmin, and the production of plasminogen antiactivator is decreased under the influence of the gonadotropins. Step 3: Latent collagenase is activated by the plasmin, and active collagenase is generated. Step 4: The collagenase attacks the collagen, giving rise to telopeptide-free collagen. Step 5: Telopeptide-free collagen is degraded by nonspecific proteases.

mg/ml), and the space of action of plasmin is limited by the presence of plasma protease inhibitors (311). Secretion of plasminogen activator produced by bovine aortic endothelial cells (438) and macrophages (479) is subject to inhibition by similar compounds (Table 12). Plasminogen activator production by granulosa cells is subject to stimulation by a number of substances (Table 13).

Plasminogen is a glycoprotein contained in the plasma and is converted to a serine protease by proteolytic modification. Circulating plasminogen is present as two noninterconvertible isozymic forms differing only in their state of glycosylation. In adult animals, they are principally synthesized in the liver and are continuously secreted (59). Plasminogen is converted to the active serine protease by two different plasminogen activators (PAs): urokinase (uPA), found in urine (504); and tissue-type activator (tPA), found in animal tissue homogenates (28) and human tissue extracts (16). The two PAs are immunologically unrelated, and each is immunoprecipitated by a specific antiserum. Urokinase (MW 40,000–52,000) is secreted by endothelial cells; tPA (MW 74,000) is contained in endothelial cells (287) and is probably the vascular PA that is released upon adequate stimulation and that binds to and requires fibrin for its activity (111). Cultured granulosa cells produce both uPA and tPA (91,92,252,351,412).

Plasminogen activators are present in human ovarian tissue extracts (16), in bovine follicular fluid, and in the supernatant fluid of follicle-wall homogenates (42). The follicular fluid also contains plasma protease inhibitors that are destroyed in acid media (42) and which may be derived from the plasma and anti-plasminogen activator whose secretion by granulosa cells is inhibited by gonadotropins (351). Granulosa cell lysates, prepared from ovarian preovulatory follicles of immature rats treated with PMSG/LH or from

TABLE 12. *Inhibitors of the secretion of plasminogen activator activity*

Compound	Test tissue	Reference
Cycloheximide Colchicine Hydrocortisone Dibutyryl cAMP Theophylline	Bovine endothelial cells	438
Cholera toxin Colchicine Dibutyryl cAMP Epinephrine Isoproterenol Prostaglandin E_1 Prostaglandin E_2 Steroid hormones (dexamethasone) Vinblastine	Peritoneal macrophages	479

TABLE 13. *Substances increasing granulosa cell production of plasminogen activator*

Substance	Reference
Dibutyryl cAMP	44
Dibutyryl cAMP + theophylline	44
LH	44
Prostaglandin E_1	44
Prostaglandin E_2	44
FSH	452
FSH + testosterone	298
Cholera toxin	496

mature proestrous rats, contain PA, which increases in concentration as time of ovulation approaches (44).

Granulosa cells cultured with FSH or LH *in vitro* produce PA, but FSH in this system is more effective than LH. Cyclic AMP and its analogs also stimulate production of PA, and theophylline potentiates the response of the granulosa cells to LH. PGE_1 and PGE_2 stimulate production of granulosa-cell PA; the largest responses are obtained in the range between 10^{-8} and 10^{-6} M. Because the gonadotropins and the prostaglandins stimulate the adenylate cyclase pathway of the cell, cAMP probably activates the protein synthetic system, leading to increased production of PA (452). Peak levels of PA activity in PMSG-stimulated immature-rat granulosa cells in culture are obtained at concentrations of 30 ng FSH/ml, with the response beginning after 2 hr of exposure to the gonadotropin (43,92). An extensive analysis of the hormones stimulating PA activity of immature-rat granulosa cells found rat, equine, human, porcine, ovine, bovine, and rabbit FSH to be effective (314) at culture concentrations of less than 10 ng/ml. This study is noteworthy because 32 hormones were examined, and only FSH from mammalian species was effective at stimulating PA activity. In contrast, Too et al. (469,470), in a similar system, i.e., PMSG-primed immature-rat ovarian granulosa cells in culture, found that 5 μg/ml FSH and 5 μg/ml relaxin stimulated PA activity after 20 hr of incubation. These workers also found that relaxin had no effect on cAMP levels of the granulosa cells but that FSH did, confirming the findings of Strickland and Beers (452). They also noted that, in response to relaxin, the granulosa cells released both latent and active collagenase as well as proteoglycanase. Although the latter enzyme may be released, collagenase has been identified in follicular fluid only by Espey and Rondell (158,159) and Okazaki et al. (362) (*vide supra*).

The hormonal treatment of rats prior to collection of their ovaries and culture of the granulosa cells determines the effectiveness with which LH can elicit a PA response. The granulosa cells of hypophysectomized or intact immature rats treated with diethylstilbestrol (DES) are unaffected by LH but are highly responsive to FSH (252,298,351,496). Subsequent to incubation with FSH, the undifferentiated granulosa cells become responsive to LH (351,496). The granulosa cells obtained from PMSG-primed immature rats produce PA in response to addition of FSH to the culture medium after a 2-hr induction period, but in response to LH only after a longer lag period (92). However, whole proestrous preovulatory follicles cultured for 6 hr in the presence of LH, FSH, or prolactin (PRL) are fivefold more responsive to LH than to FSH, and PRL is ineffective in inducing PA production (411).

Because an early response of the preovulatory follicle to LH is increased steroid synthesis, and blockade of steroid synthesis prevents ovulation, a relationship between steroids and PA production has been examined. Cyanoketone induces suppression of plasminogen production in the preovulatory ovaries of immature rats primed with PMSG/hCG, and progesterone reverses this effect (355). Granulosa cell cultures, however, fail to show enhanced PA production when exposed to steroids (298,452), but, although proestrous preovulatory follicles incubated with steroids (pregnenolone, progesterone, testosterone, estradiol) fail to show enhanced follicular PA, addition of estradiol to culture medium containing LH-stimulated follicles further enhances PA production. In this same model, aminoglutethimide phosphate inhibits LH-stimulated PA production, and the inhibition is reversed by addition of progesterone, testosterone, or estradiol but not by dihydrotestosterone (411). An explanation for these effects, though tentative, is that the steroid cascade is involved in the production of PA.

Hypotheses on the production of two types of plasminogen activator by the follicle and their relationship to ovulation have arisen as extensions of the early observation of the presence of PA in the follicle (42). Criticisms of the plasminogen-activator–plasminogen hypothesis (152) are that tissue-type plasminogen activator requires fibrin to be activated, that fibrinogen is present in follicular fluid in lower concentrations than in plasma, and that anticoagulant activity is present in follicular fluid (242,381,447). However, urokinase-type plasminogen activator does not have these limitations. Analysis of the two types of plasminogen activator produced by the major component of the preovulatory follicle, the granulosa cells, by means of antibodies specific for each, indicates that the tissue-type enzyme is produced predominantly; however, whole follicles produce primarily the urokinase-type plasminogen activator (91).

Unstimulated, undifferentiated granulosa cells secrete the urokinase-type plasminogen activator, and addition of FSH induces the secretion of tissue-type enzyme as indicated by sodium dodecyl sulfate polyacrylamide gel electrophoresis (351). After 2 days of priming with low concentrations of FSH, either FSH or LH induces the secretion of the tissue-type plasminogen activator. Thus, either gonadotropin induces the formation of tissue-type plasminogen activator in differentiated granulosa cells.

That the production of plasminogen activator represents induction of protein synthesis in granulosa cells is indicated by the response to the presence of protein-synthesis inhibitors in the culture medium. FSH induces cellular plasminogen activator, as measured by lysis of a chromogenic substrate, within 2 hr in undifferentiated granulosa cells; within 6 hr, 80% of maximal enzyme activity is contained in the cells; negligible plasminogen activator activity is released into the culture medium. Both actinomycin D and cycloheximide suppress cellular plasminogen-activator production when added to the culture medium early in the incubation period, and reduced secretion occurs when they are added at 44 to 48 hr of the incubation (252).

The formation of plasmin or other proteases in the preovulatory follicle has also been evaluated. Fibrinolytic activity in the external area of the preovulatory follicle reaches a maximum about 2 hr before ovulation in the rat (12), and *trans*-aminomethyl cyclohexane carboxylic acid (t-AMCHA), an inhibitor of fibrinolysis, suppresses the appearance of fibrinolytic activity, decreases the appearance of ova, and postpones the time of ovulation. t-AMCHA administered to PMSG/hCG-treated immature rats or to proestrous rats suppresses ovulation almost completely (12,13). Treatment with protease inhibitor also reduces the incidence of ovulation, suggesting that nonspecific proteolytic enzymes may also be involved (220,392,413).

Serine protease inhibitors or indomethacin block ovulation without inhibition of ovarian plasminogen activator, and only at high doses of indomethacin is blockade of both ovarian plasminogen-activator production and ovulation achieved (163,439); however, Reich et al. (411) found that indomethacin had no effect on production of plasminogen activators. The type of plasminogen activator is probably the key determinant with regard to plasminogen-activator production and ovulation. Indomethacin added to follicles *in vitro* prevents the LH-stimulated increase in plasminogen activator; however, when indomethacin is administered *in vivo* to PMSG/hCG-primed rats and the preovulatory follicles and granulosa cells are cultured, the situation is strikingly changed. At doses of indomethacin that induce blockade of ovulation, the granulosa cells still produce and secrete tissue-type plasminogen activator, but whole-follicle production of urokinase-type plasminogen activator is reduced to basal levels (Table 14) (92).

Correlated with this last observation are the reports that prostaglandins reverse the effect of indomethacin, that PGE_2 is more involved in reversal of ovum maturation and cumulus mucification (138), and that $PGF_{2\alpha}$ is more involved in the reversal of the indomethacin-imposed blockade of ovulation (135,136,426). Antiserum to PGE_2 is a less effective inhibitor of ovulation than is antiserum to $PGF_{2\alpha}$ (26,275). Fibroblast proliferation is stimulated by $PGF_{2\alpha}$ (125,211), and both prostaglandins stimulate fibroblasts to produce latent collagenase (123,139,300,398). Latent collagenase thus may be activated by urokinase, by plasminogen activator, by the plasmin generated by the PA, or by fibrobasts.

TABLE 14. *Effect of indomethacin or ovarian PA production and ovulation in rats treated with hCG*[a]

Indomethacin (mg)	Granulosa tPA	Follicular fluid tPA	Follicular uPA	No. ovulating/No. treated
0	37.2 ± 26.2	2.4 ± 1.4	5.0 ± 3.7	15/20
1	57.4 ± 11.4	4.0 ± 0.6	2.4 ± 3.4	6/19
2	19.2 ± 24.3	2.3 ± 3.8	1.0 ± 1.0	3/20
5	17.6 ± 11.4	1.9 ± 0.8	0.6 ± 0.3	1/15

[a]PMSG-primed 26-day-old rats treated with hCG and indomethacin solvent or hCG and indomethacin. The data are expressed as a percentage of solubilized substrate. For experimental details, see original report. Modified from Canipari and Strickland (92).

Collagenolysis

Injection of collagenolytic enzyme (bacterial collagenase) into preovulatory follicles initiates the preovulatory changes leading to rupture of the follicle but at an accelerated pace (157). Early observations of collagenolytic activity in ovaries (158,159,362) using the synthetic collagen substrate *N*-carbobenzoxy-Gly-Pro-Gly-Gly-Pro-Ala were invalidated when it was noted that this substrate is not attacked by true mammalian collagenase (327). Collagenolytic activity in rat preovulatory follicles was demonstrated with a microassay; its presence in a latent form was noted, as was its increase in activity on treatment of immature rats with PMSG/hCG (327).

Collagenolytic activity in the rabbit ovary (246,247) and in the human ovary was studied with a collagenase-specific peptide, and three other noncollagenolytic peptidases were studied with other synthetic peptides (179). All the peptidases had a marked preovulatory decrease in activity at the apex of the follicle. The activity in the granulosa cell layer increased near the time of ovulation (179), suggesting a role for collagenase in ovulation. In a study of rat-follicle collagenolytic activity, in which Type I collagen was used as the substrate and disappearance of collagen was determined by disappearance of hydroxyproline, collagen disappeared from the follicle and collagenase activity, activated with trypsin or aminophenylmercuric acetate, was present up to the time of ovulation. The presence of collagenolytic activity at the apex of the follicle (and that it is responsible for breakdown of the follicular collagen) was not, however, demonstrated (328).

Collagenolytic activity in the ovaries of immature rats primed with PMSG/hCG rises to a peak at 8 hr after the injection of the hCG and remains high at 12 hr, correlating with maximal release of ova (120). Collagenolysis was also demonstrated with two different methods by Reich et al. (412). These workers labeled ovaries with L[^{3}H]proline, introduced into the ovarian bursa, and observed the disappearance of [^{3}H]hydroxyproline from ovaries of adult rats through the estrous cycle, after nembutal was administered at proestrus (blocking the LH surge) or in response to ad ministered hCG; this effect was also observed in immature rats treated with PMSG/hCG. Excellent correlation was obtained between increased disappearance of labeled amino acid and either endogenous LH surge or exogenous hCG. That collagenase was the probable enzyme involved was also demonstrated by blockade of ovulation by introduction of cysteine (blockade of metalloprotease) into the ovarian bursa of immature rats treated with PMSG/hCG. The investigators also demonstrated that the addition of *p*-aminophenylmercuric acetate or plasmin to [^{3}H]proline-labeled collagen extracts of preovulatory ovaries from adult rats, or from PMSG/hCG, induced high levels of collagenolytic activity, as demonstrated by solubilization of [^{3}H]hydroxyproline. These data further support the hypotheses that ovulation is dependent on activation of latent collagenase and that plasmin is probably the enzyme involved in its activation. Utilizing a variety of proteinase inhibitors, Ichikawa et al. (220) found that two different proteolytic enzymes are involved in the blockade of ovulation in explanted hamster preovulatory follicles. Talopeptin, a metalloproteinase inhibitor, inhibits mammalian collagenase and blocks ovulation (221), and microbial alkaline proteinase inhibitor blocks ovulation at the late stage of the ovulatory process, indicating that other proteinases are probably involved in further degradation of the telopeptide-free collagen formed by collagenase. These observations are summarized in a five-step cascade leading to the degradation of the collagen in the follicle wall and its rupture (Fig. 5). The smooth muscle in the wall may contribute to the expulsion of the antral contents subsequent to the degradative changes.

SUMMARY

Ovulation is initiated by the surge of LH (431). Almost immediately the preovulatory follicle becomes hyperemic and subsequently edematous, even in the presence of indomethacin, while progesterone and other steroid syntheses persist unaffected. Protein synthesis (17,32,403,404) initiated by LH is responsible for cellular differentiation of the membrana granulosa to lutein cells and secretion of steroids and plasminogen activator (42,298,349,351). Activation of adenylate cyclase initiates many of these responses, including prostaglandin secretion (109,269,270,281,476). The theca interna also responds to LH stimulation by increased secretion of progesterone (257) and androgens (147) as well as prostaglandins (11,40,388) and plasminogen activator (252). The secretion of other substances by the follicle probably also occurs, but these are as yet uncharacterized. The adrenergic neurons in the follicle wall are activated either by the LH or neurogenically and secrete norepinephrine. Histamine released from mast cells (264,291,461) and the α-adrenergic agonist effects may be to enhance the hyperemia (513,523) by affecting the contractility of the endothelial cells, the pericytes, and the postcapillary venules (192,321,349,364). The β-adrenergic agonist effect may be to enhance secretion of progesterone (245,525). The prostaglandins (42,92,411) increase plasminogen-activator production, as does progesterone. The enhanced secretion of plasminogen activator (13) then converts the plasminogen in the follicular fluid and extracellular edema fluid to plasmin (43); the latter acts on latent collagen attached to the collagen fibers (343). Induced collagenolysis (221) and serine proteases (220) then complete the proteolysis of the collagen (120,327,328,362,412). The net effect is to decrease the tensile strength of the follicle wall to the point at which rupture occurs under the existing intrafollicular pressure of 15 to 20 mm Hg (56,65) (Fig. 6).

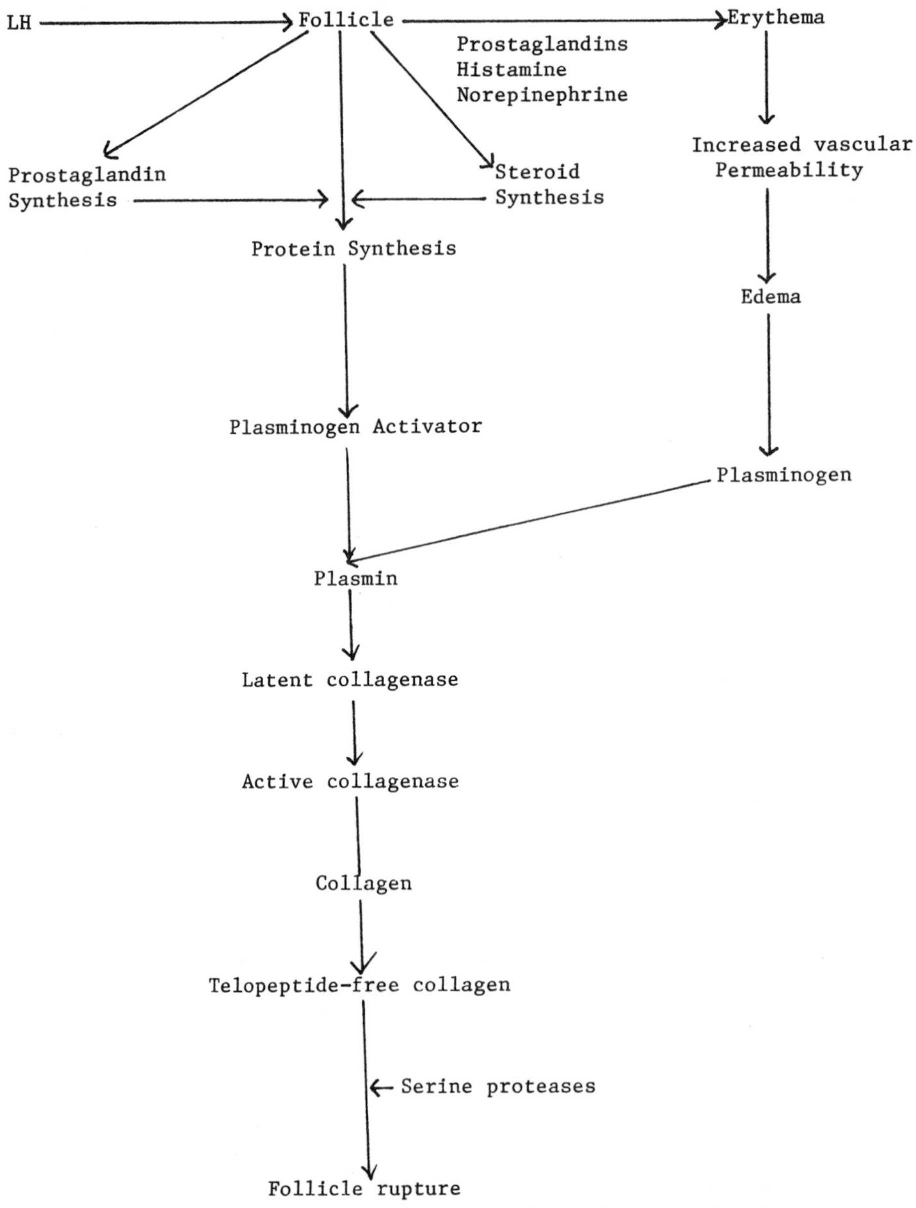

FIG. 6. Multifactor hypothesis of ovulation (see text of "Summary").

ACKNOWLEDGMENTS

The references contained in this review extend only to early 1986 and are far from inclusive. There are many reports omitted largely because I am unaware of them or because they were peripheral to the areas reviewed. To those omitted, I apologize.

I wish to thank my wife Janet for her forebearance. Special notes of appreciation go to Linda Mathews, who plowed through my rough drafts and made the writing and completion possible, and to Dr. Anne Thistle for her editorial efforts.

REFERENCES

1. Abel, W., and McIlroy, A. L. (1912): The arrangement and distribution of nerves in certain mammalian ovaries. *Proc. R. Soc. Med. Obstet. Gynecol.*, 6:240–247.
2. Abramson, S., Korchak, H., Ludewig, R., Edelson, H., Haines, K., Levin, R. I., Herman, R., Rider, L., Kimmel, S., and Weissmann, G. (1985): Modes of action of aspirin-like drugs. *Proc. Natl. Acad. Sci. USA*, 82:7227–7231.
3. Adashi, E. Y., and Hsueh, A. J. W. (1981): Stimulation of beta-2-adrenergic responsiveness by follicle stimulating hormone in rat granulosa cells *in-vitro* and *in-vivo*. *Endocrinology*, 108:2170–2178.
4. Aeby, C. (1859): Uber glatten Muskelfassen in Ovarium und Mesovarium von Wirbelthieren. *Arch. Anat. Physiol. Wissensch. Med.*, 675–676.
5. Aeby, C. (1861): Die glatten Muskelfassen in den Eierstocken der Wirbelthiere. *Arch. Anat. Physiol. Wissensch. Med.*, 1:635–645.
6. Aguado, L. I., and Ojeda, S. R. (1984): Pre-pubertal ovarian function is finely regulated by direct adrenergic influences: Role of noradrenergic innervation. *Endocrinology*, 114:1845–1853.
7. Aguado, L. I., and Ojeda, S. R. (1984): Ovarian adrenergic nerves play a role in maintaining preovulatory steroid secretion. *Endocrinology*, 114:1944–1946.
8. Ahren, K., Janson, P. O., and Selstam, G. (1974): Search for arteriovenous shunts in the rabbit ovary in situ using perfusion of microspheres. *J. Reprod. Fertil.*, 41:133–142.
9. Ainsworth, L., Baker, R. D., and Armstrong, D. T. (1975): Preovulatory changes in follicular fluid prostaglandin F levels in swine. *Prostaglandins*, 9:915–925.
10. Ainsworth, L., Tsang, B. K., Downey, B. R., Baker, R. D., Marcus, T. J., and Armstrong, D. T. (1979): Effects of indomethacin on ovulation and luteal function in gilts. *Biol. Reprod.*, 21:401–412.
11. Ainsworth, L., Tsang, B. H., Marcus, G. J., Downey, B. R. (1984): Prostaglandin production by dispersed granulosa and theca interna cells from porcine preovulatory follicles. *Biop. Reprod.*, 31:115–121.
12. Akazawa, K., Matsuo, O., Kosugi, T., Mihara, H., and Mori, N. (1983): The role of plasminogen activator in ovulation. *Acta Physiol. Lat. Am.*, 33:105–110.
13. Akazawa, K., Mori, N., Kosugi, T., Matuso, O., and Mihara, H. (1983): Localization of fibrinolytic activity in ovulation of the rat follicle as determined by the fibrin slide method. *Jpn. J. Physiol.*, 33:1011–1018.
14. Albertini, D. F., and Anderson, E. (1974): The appearance and structure of intercellular connections during the ontogeny of the rabbit ovarian follicle with particular reference to gap junctions. *J. Cell Biol.*, 63:234–250.
15. Albertini, D. F., Fawcett, D. W., and Olds, P. J. (1975): Morphological variation in gap junctions of ovarian granulosa cells. *Tissue Cell*, 7:389–405.
16. Albrechtsen, O. K. (1957): The fibrinolytic activity of human tissues. *Br. J. Haematol.*, 3:284–291.
17. Alleva, J. J., Bonventre, P. F., and Lamanna, C. (1979): Inhibition of ovulation in hamsters by the protein synthesis inhibitors diphtheria toxin and cycloheximide. *Proc. Soc. Exp. Biol. Med.*, 162:170–174.
18. Amenta, F., Allen, D. J., Didio, L. J. A., and Motta, P. (1979): A transmission electronmicroscopic study of smooth muscle cells in the ovary of rabbits, cats, rats, and mice. *J. Submicrosc. Cytol.*, 11:39–52.
19. Amenta, F., Cavallotti, C., De Rossi, M., and Evangelisti, F. (1981): Acetylcholinesterase containing nerve fibers in guinea-pig ovary. *J. Neural Transm.*, 52:295–302.
20. Amman, K. (1936): *Histologie des Schweine-Eierstockes unter besonderer Beruksichtigung des Ovarialzylus.* Druck von Humber & Co. Aktiengesellschaft, Fravenfeld.
21. Amsterdam, A., Koch, Y., Lieberman, M. E., and Lindner, H. L. (1975): Distribution of binding sites for human chorionic gonadotropin in the preovulatory follicle of the rat. *J. Cell. Biol.*, 67:894–902.
22. Andersen, M. M., Kroll, J., Byskov, A. G., and Faber, M. (1976): Protein composition in the fluid of individual bovine follicles. *J. Reprod. Fertil.*, 48:109–118.
23. Anderson, E. (1979): Follicular morphology. In: *Ovarian Follicular Development*, edited by A. R. Midgley, Jr., and W. A. Sadler, pp. 91–105. Raven Press, New York.
24. Apkarian, R., and Curtis, J. C. (1981): SEM cryofracture study of ovarian follicles of immature rats. *Scan. Electron. Miscrosc.*, 4:165–172.
25. Armstrong, D. T., and Grinwich, D. L. (1972): Blockade of spontaneous and LH-induced ovulation in rats by indomethacin, an inhibitor of prostaglandin biosynthesis. *Prostaglandins*, 1:21–28.
26. Armstrong, D. T., Grinwich, D. L., Moon, Y. S., and Zanecnik, J. (1974): Inhibition of ovulation in rabbits by intrafollicular injection of indomethacin and PGF_2 anti-serum. *Life Sci.*, 14:129–140.
27. Armstrong, D. T., Moon, Y. S., and Zanecnik, J. (1974): Evidence for a role of ovarian prostaglandins in ovulation. In: *Gonadotropins and Gonadal Function*, edited by N. R. Moudgal, pp. 345–356. Academic Press, New York.
28. Astrup, T., and Permin, P. M. (1947): Fibrinolysis in the animal organism. *Nature*, 159:681–682.
29. Ax, R. L., and Ryan, R. J. (1978): The porcine ovarian follicle. IV. Mucopolysaccharides at different stages of development. *Biol. Reprod.*, 20:1123–1132.
30. Ax, R. L., and Ryan, R. J. (1979): FSH stimulation of ^{3}H-glucosamine-incorporation into proteoglycans by porcine cells in vitro. *J. Clin. Endocrinol. Metab.*, 49:646–648.
31. Bagavandoss, P., Midgley, A. R., Jr., and Wicha, M. (1983): Developmental changes in the ovarian follicular basal lamina detected by immunofluorescence and electron microscopy. *J. Histochem. Cytochem.*, 31:633–640.
32. Bahr, J., Kao, L., and Nalbandov, A. V. (1974): The role of catecholamines and nerves in ovulation. *Biol. Reprod.*, 10:273–290.
33. Baird, D. T. (1983): Factors regulating the growth of the preovulatory follicle in the sheep and human. *J. Reprod. Fertil.*, 69:343–352.
34. Balboni, G. C. (1983): Structural changes: Ovulation and luteal phase. In: *The Ovary*, edited by G. B. Serra, pp. 123–141. Raven Press, New York.
35. Ball, G. D., Bellin, M. E., Ax, R. L., and First, N. L. (1982): Glycosaminoglycans in bovine cumulus-oocyte complexes: Morphology and chemistry. *Mol. Cell. Endocrinol.*, 28:113–122.
36. Baranczuk, R. J., and Fainstat, T. (1976): Progesterone-induced ovulation of the hamster ovary *in vitro*. *J. Endocrinol.*, 70:317–318.
37. Baranczuk, R. J., and Fainstat, T. (1976): In vitro ovulation from adult hamster ovary. *Am. J. Obstet. Gynecol.*, 124:517–522.
38. Barros, C., and Austin, C. R. (1968): Inhibition of ovulation by systemically administered actinomycin D in the hamster. *Endocrinology*, 83:177–179.
39. Bauminger, S., Lieberman, M. E., and Lindner, H. R. (1975): Steroid-independent effect of gonadotropins on prostaglandin synthesis in rat graafian follicles *in vitro*. *Prostaglandins*, 9:753–764.
40. Bauminger, S., and Lindner, H. R. (1975): Periovulatory changes in ovarian prostaglandin formation and their hormonal control in the rat. *Prostaglandins*, 9:737–751.
41. Beck, L. R., and Shelden, R. M. (1972): Antigenicity of rat follicular fluid. *Fertil. Steril.*, 23:910–914.
42. Beers, W. H. (1975): Follicular plasminogen and plasminogen activator and the effect of plasmin on ovarian follicle wall. *Cell*, 6:379–386.

43. Beers, W. H., Strickland, S., and Reich, E. (1975): Ovarian plasminogen activator: Relationship to ovulation and hormonal regulation. *Cell,* 6:387–394.
44. Beers, W. H., and Strickland, S. (1978): A cell culture assay for follicle-stimulating hormone. *J. Biol. Chem.,* 253:3877–3881.
45. Bellin, M. E., and Ax, R. L. (1984): Chondroitin sulfate: An indicator of atresia in bovine follicles. *Endocrinology,* 114:428–434.
46. Bellin, M. E., Hinshelwood, M. M., Robinson, G. M., Ax, R. L., and Hauser, E. R. (1983): Estrogen, heparan sulfate, and chondroitin sulfate in relation to morphology of individual bovine follicles. In: *Factors Regulating Ovarian Function,* edited by G. S. Greenwald and P. F. Terranova, pp. 45–48. Raven Press, New York.
47. Bellin, M. E., Lenz, R. W., Steadman, L. E., and Ax, R. L. (1983): Proteoglycan production by bovine granulosa cells *in vitro* occurs in response to FSH. *Mol. Cell. Endocrinol.,* 29:51–65.
48. Bjersing, L. (1978): Maturation, morphology, and endocrine function of the follicular wall in mammals. In: *The Vertebrate Ovary,* edited by R. E. Jones, pp. 181–214. Plenum Press, New York.
49. Bjersing, L., and Cajander, S. (1974): Ovulation and the mechanism of follicle rupture. I. Light microscopic changes in rabbit ovarian follicles prior to induced ovulation. *Cell Tissue Res.,* 149:287–300.
50. Bjersing, L., and Cajander, S. (1974): Ovulation and the mechanism of follicle rupture. II. Scanning electron microscopy of rabbit germinal epithelium prior to induced ovulation. *Cell Tissue Res.,* 149:301–312.
51. Bjersing, L., and Cajander, S. (1974): Ovulation and the mechanism of follicle rupture. III. Transmission electron microscopy of rabbit germinal epithelium prior to induced ovulation. *Cell Tissue Res.,* 149:313–327.
52. Bjersing, L., and Cajander, S. (1974): Ovulation and the mechanism of follicle rupture IV. Ultrastructure of membrana granulosa of rabbit graafian follicles prior to induced ovulation. *Cell Tissue Res.,* 153:1–14.
53. Bjersing, L., and Cajander, S. (1974): Ovulation and the mechanism of follicle rupture. V. Ultrastructure of tunica albuginea and theca externa of rabbit graafian follicles prior to induced ovulation. *Cell Tissue Res.,* 153:15–30.
54. Bjersing, L., and Cajander, S. (1974): Ovulation and the mechanism of follicle rupture. VI. Ultrastructure of theca interna and the inner vascular network surrounding rabbit graafian follicles prior to induced ovulation. *Cell Tissue Res.,* 153:31–44.
55. Bjorkman, N. (1962): A study of the ultrastructure of the granulosa cells of the ovary. *Acta Anat.,* 51:125–147.
56. Blandau, R. J., and Rumery, R. E. (1963): Measurements of intrafollicular pressure in the ovulatory and preovulatory follicles of the rat. *Fertil. Steril.,* 14:330–341.
57. Blasco, L., Wu, C. H., Flickinger, G. L., Pearlmutter, D., and Mikhail, G. (1975): Cardiac output and genital blood flow distribution during the preovulatory period in rabbits. *Biol. Reprod.,* 13:581–586.
58. Bodkhe, R. R., and Harper, M. J. K. (1972): Changes in the amount of adrenergic neurotransmitter in the genital tract of untreated rabbits and rabbits given reserpine or ipronizid during the time of egg transport. *Biol. Reprod.,* 6:288–299.
59. Bohmfalk, J. F., and Fuller, G. M. (1980): Plasminogen is synthesized by primary cultures of rat hepatocytes. *Science,* 209:408–410.
60. Bomsel-Helmrich, O., Gougeon, A., Thebault, A., Saltarelli, D., Milgron, E., Frydman, R., and Papiernik, E. (1979): Healthy and artretic human follicles in the preovulatory phase: Differences in evolution of follicular morphology and steroid content of follicular fluid. *J. Clin. Endocrinol. Metab.,* 48:686–694.
61. Bostrom, H., and Odeblad, O. (1952): Autoradiographic observation on the uptake of S^{35} in the genital organs of the female rat and rabbit after injection of labelled sodium sulphate. *Acta Endocrinol. (Copenh.),* 10:89–96.
62. Brace, R. A. (1981): Progress toward resolving the controversy of positive vs negative interstitial fluid pressure. *Circ. Res.,* 49:281–297.
63. Brill, W. (1915): Untersuchungen uber die Nerven des Ovariums. *Arch. Mikr. Anat.,* 86(Sect. 1):338–376.
64. Brink, C. E., and Grob, H. S. (1973): Response of the denervated mouse ovary to exogenous gonadotropins. *Biol. Reprod.,* 9:108 (abstract No. 120).
65. Bronson, R. A., Bryant, G., Balk, M., Emanuels, N. (1979): Intrafollicular pressure within preovulatory follicles of the pig. *Fertil. Steril.,* 31:205–213.
66. Bullock, D. W., and Kappauf, B. H. (1973): Dissociation of gonadotropin-induced ovulation and steroidogenesis in immature rats. *Endocrinology,* 92:1625–1628.
67. Bulmer, D. (1965): A histochemical study of ovarian cholinesterases. *Acta Anat.,* 62:254–265.
68. Burden, H. W. (1972): Ultrastructural observations on ovarian perifollicular smooth muscle in the cat, guinea pig, and rabbit. *Am. J. Anat.,* 133:125–142.
69. Burden, H. W. (1972): Adrenergic innervation in ovaries of the rat and guinea pig. *Am. J. Anat.,* 133:455–462.
70. Burden, H. W. (1973): The distribution of smooth muscle in the cat ovary with a note on its adrenergic innervation. *J. Morphol.,* 140:467–476.
71. Burden, H. W. (1978): Ovarian innervation. In: *The Vertebrate Ovary,* edited by R. E. Jones, pp. 615–638. Plenum Press, New York.
72. Burden, H. W., and Lawrence, I. E. (1977): The effects of denervation on the localization of Δ^5-3β-hydroxysteroid dehydrogenase activity in the rat ovary during pregnancy. *Acta Anat.,* 97: 286–290.
73. Burden, H. W., and Lawrence, I. E., Jr. (1977): The effect of denervation on compensatory ovarian hypertrophy. *Neuroendocrinology,* 23:368–378.
74. Burden, H. W., and Lawrence, I. E., Jr. (1978): Experimental studies on the acetylcholinesterase positive nerves in the ovary of the rat. *Anat. Rec.,* 190:233–242.
75. Burden, H. W., and Lawrence, I. E. (1980): Nerve supply of the ovary. In: *Biology of the Ovary,* edited by P. M. Motta and E. S. E. Hafez, pp. 99–105. Martinus Nijhoff, The Hague.
76. Burghardt, R. C., and Anderson, E. (1979): Hormonal modulation of ovarian interstitial cells with particular reference to gap junctions. *J. Cell Biol.,* 81:104–114.
77. Burghardt, R. C., and Anderson, E. (1981): Hormonal modulation of gap junctions in rat ovarian follicles. *Cell Tissue Res.,* 214:181–194.
78. Burghardt, R. C., and Matheson, R. L. (1982): Gap junction amplification in rat ovarian granulosa cells. *Dev. Biol.,* 94:206–215.
79. Burgoyne, P. S., Borland, R. M., Biggers, J. D., and Lechene, C. P. (1979): Elemental composition of rabbit control fluid during preovulatory follicular swelling. *J. Reprod. Fertil.,* 57:515–523.
80. Burn, J. H. (1961): A new view of adrenergic nerve fibers explaining the action of reserpine, bretylium and guanethidine. *Br. Med. J.,* 1:1623–1627.
81. Burn, J. H. (1966): Adrenergic transmission introductory remarks. *Pharmacol. Rev.,* 18:459–470.
82. Burn, J. H., and Rand, M. J. (1965): Acetylcholine in adrenergic transmission. *Annu. Rev. Pharmacol.,* 5:163–182.
83. Burnstock, G. (1986): The changing face of autonomic neurotransmission. *Acta Physiol. Scand.,* 126:67–92.
84. Burr, J. H., and Davis, J. R. (1951): The vascular system of the rabbit ovary and its relationship to ovulation. *Anat. Rec.,* 111:273–297.
85. Bushmeyer, S. M., Bellin, M. E., Brantmeier, S. A., Boehm, S. K., Kubajak, C. L., and Ax, R. L. (1985): Relationships between bovine follicular fluid glycosaminoglycans and steroids. *Endocrinology,* 117:879–885.
86. Byskov, A. G. S. (1969): Ultrastructural studies on the preovulatory follicle in the mouse ovary. *Z. Zell Forsch. Mikroskop. Anat.,* 100:285–299.
87. Cajander, S. (1976): Structural alterations of rabbit ovarian follicles after mating with special reference to the overlying surface epithelium. *Cell Tissue Res.,* 173:437–449.
88. Cajander, S., and Bjersing, L. (1975): Fine structural demonstration of acid phosphatase in rabbit germinal epithelium prior to induced ovulation. *Cell Tissue Res.,* 164:279–289.
89. Cajander, S., and Bjersing, L. (1976): Further studies of the epithelium covering preovulatory rabbit follicles with special reference to lysosomal alterations. *Cell Tissue Res.,* 169:129–141.
90. Canipari, R., and Strickland, S. (1985): Hormonal regulation of plasminogen activator in the rat ovary. *Biol. Reprod.,* 32(Suppl. 1):183 (abstract No. 292).

91. Canipari, R., and Strickland, S. (1985): Plasminogen activator in the rat ovary. Production and gonadotropin regulation of the enzyme in granulosa and thecal cells. *J. Biol. Chem.*, 260:5121–5125.
92. Canipari, R., and Strickland, S. (1986): Studies on the hormonal regulation of plasminogen activator production in the rat ovary. *Endocrinology*, 118:1652–1659.
93. Capps, M. L., Lawrence, I. E., Jr., and Burden, H. W. (1981): Cellular functions in perifollicular contractile tissue of the rat ovary during the preovulatory period. *Cell Tissue Res.*, 219:133–141.
94. Caravaglios, R., and Cilotti, R. (1957): A study of the proteins in the follicular fluid of the cow. *J. Endocrinol.*, 15:273–278.
95. Casey, F. B., Appleby, B. J., and Buck, D. C. (1983): Selective inhibition of lipoxygenase metabolic pathway of arachodonic acid by the SRS-A antagonist, FPL 55712. *Prostaglandins*, 25:1–11.
96. Castren, O., Airaksinen, M. M., Fristrom, S., and Saarikoski, S. (1973): Decrease of litter size and fetal monoamines by 6-hydroxydopamine in mice. *Experientia*, 29:576–578.
97. Caucig, H., Friedrich, F., Breitenecker, G., and Golob, E. (1972): Enzyme activity in the fluid of the human ovarian follicle. *Gynecol. Obstet. Invest.*, 3:215–220.
98. Caucig, H., Friedrich, F., Hager, R., and Golob, E. (1971): Enzym untersuchungen in Follikel- und Zystenflussigkeit des Menchlichen Ovars. *Acta Endocrinol.* (*Copenh.*) (*Suppl.*), 152:52 (abstract No. 52).
99. Cerletti, P., and Zichella, L. (1961): Nucleotidases, nucleotides, vitamins and coenzymes in the follicular fluid of human ovary. *Clin. Chim. Acta*, 6:581–582.
100. Challis, J. R. G., Erickson, G. F., and Ryan, K. J. (1974): Prostaglandin F production in vitro by granulosa cells from rabbit preovulatory follicles. *Prostaglandins*, 7:183–193.
101. Channing, C. P., Schaerf, F. W., Anderson, L. D., and Tsafriri, A. (1980): Ovarian follicular and luteal physiology. In: *Reproductive Physiology III, International Review of Physiology, Vol. 22*, edited by R. O. Greep, pp. 117–201. University Park Press, Baltimore.
102. Channing, C. P., Tanabe, K., Chacon, M., and Tildon, J. T. (1984): Stimulatory effects of FSH and luteinizing hormone upon secretion of progesterone and inhibin activity by cultured infant human ovarian granulosa cells. *Fertil. Steril.*, 42:598–605.
103. Channing, C. P., and Tsafriri, A. (1977): Mechanism of action of luteinizing hormone and follicle-stimulating hormone on the ovary in vitro. *Metabolism*, 26:413–468.
104. Cherney, D. D., Didio, L. J. A., and Motta, P. (1975): The development of rabbit ovarian follicles following copulation. *Fertil. Steril.*, 26:257–271.
105. Chihal, H. J. W., Weitsen, H. A., Stone, S. C., and Peppler, R. D. (1976): Autonomic innervation and plasma estradiol-17 and progesterone levels in rats with subcutaneous ovarian autografts. *Cell Tissue Res.*, 175:113–121.
106. Christiansen, J. A., Jensen, C. E., and Zachariae, F. (1958): Studies on the mechanism of ovulation. Some remarks on the effect of depolymerization of high-polymers on the preovulatory growth of follicles. *Acta Endocrinol.*, 29:115–117.
107. Claesson, L. (1947): Is there any smooth musculature in the wall of the Graafian follicle? *Acta Anat.*, 3:295–311.
108. Clark, J. G. (1899): Origin, development and degeneration of the blood vessels of the ovary. *Bull. J. Hopkins Hosp.*, 94, 95, 96:40–44.
109. Clark, M. R., Marsh, J. M., and Lemaire, W. J. (1978): Stimulation of prostaglandin accumulation in preovulatory rat follicles by adenosine 3′-5′ monophosphate. *Endocrinology*, 102:39–44.
110. Clinton, M., Long, W. F., Williamson, F. B., Hutchinson, J. S., and Seddon, B. (1983): Incorporation of ^{35}S into glycosaminoglycans of ovarian follicular and luteal tissue isolated during the guinea pig estrous cycle. *Biochem. Biophys. Res. Commun.*, 111:574–580.
111. Collen, D. (1980): On the regulation and control of fibrinolysis. *Thromb. Haemost.*, 43:77–85.
112. Cook, B., Kaltenback, C. C., Niswender, G. D., Norton, H. W., and Nalbandov, A. V. (1969): Short-term ovarian responses to some pituitary hormones infused *in vivo* in pigs and sheep. *J. Animal Sci.*, 29:711–718.
113. Coons, L. W., and Espey, L. L. (1977): Quantitation of nexus junctions in the granulosa cell layer of rabbit ovarian follicles during ovulation. *J. Cell Biol.*, 74:321–325.
114. Corner, G. W. (1919): On the origin of the corpus luteum of the sow from both granulosa and theca interna. *Am. J. Anat.*, 26:117–183.
115. Corner, G. W. (1919): Cyclic changes in the ovaries and uterus of the sow, and their relation to the mechanism of implantation. In: *Publications of the Carnegie Institute, No. 276* (contribution to *Embryology*, No. 64), pp. 119–145.
116. Coutinho, E. M., and Maia, H. (1971): The contractile response of the human uterus, fallopian tubes and ovary to prostaglandins in vivo. *Fertil. Steril.*, 22:539–542.
117. Coutinho, E. M., Maia, H., and Maia, H., Jr. (1974): Ovarian contractility. *Basic Life Sci.*, 4:127–137.
118. Cruikshank, W. C. (1797): Experiments in which on the third day after impregnation the ova of rabbits were found in the fallopian tubes, on the fourth after, in the uterus with the first appearances of the fetus. *Philos. Trans. R. Soc. Lond.*, (Biol.), 87:197–214.
119. Curry, T. E., Jr., Lawrence, I. E., Jr., and Burden, H. W. (1984): Ovarian sympathectomy in the guinea-pig. 2. Effects on follicular development during the prepubertal period and following exogenous gonadotropin stimulation. *Cell Tissue Res.*, 236:593–596.
120. Curry, T. E., Dean, D. D., Woessner, J. F., Jr., and LeMaire, W. J. (1985): The extraction of a tissue collagenase associated with ovulation in the rat. *Biol. Reprod.*, 33:981–991.
121. Daume, E., Chari, S., Hopkinson, C. R. N., Sturm, G., and Hirschhauser, C. (1978): Nachweis von Inhibin-aktivitat in der Follikelflussigkeit menschlicher Ovarien. *Klin. Wochenschr.*, 56:369–370.
122. David, A., Frenkel, G., and Kraicer, P. F. (1973): Chemical composition of rabbit follicular fluid. *Fertil. Steril.*, 24:227–229.
123. Dayer, J. M., Krane, S. M., Russel, R. G. G., and Robinson, D. R. (1976): Production of collagenase and prostaglandins by isolated adherent rheumatoid synovial cells. *Proc. Natl. Acad. Sci. USA*, 73:945–949.
124. Deanesly, R. (1956): Cyclic function in ovarian grafts. *J. Endocrinol.*, 13:211–220.
125. DeAsua, L. J., Clingan, D., and Rudland, P. S. (1975): Initiation of cell proliferation in cultured mouse fibroblasts by prostaglandin $F_{2\alpha}$. *Proc. Natl. Acad. Sci. USA*, 72:2724–2728.
126. De La Cruz, A., Wright, K. H., and Wallach, E. E. (1976): The effects of cholinergic agents on ovarian contractility in the rabbit. *Obstet. Gynecol.*, 47:272–278.
127. Dennefers, B., Tjugum, J., Norstrom, A., Janson, P. O., Nilsson, L., Hamberger, L., and Wilhelmsson, L. (1982): Collagen synthesis inhibition by PGE_2 within the human follicular wall—One possible mechanism underlying ovulation. *Prostaglandins*, 24:295–302.
128. Desjardins, C., Kirton, K. T., and Hafs, H. D. (1966): Some chemical, immunochemical and electrophoretic properties of bovine follicular fluid. *J. Reprod. Fertil.*, 11:237–244.
129. deVos, J. (1894): Etude sur l'innervation de l'ovaire. *Bull Acad. Med. Belge Ser. 4*, 8:552–558.
130. Diaz-Infante, A., Jr., Wright, K. H., and Wallach, E. E. (1974): Effects of indomethacin and prostaglandin $F_{2\alpha}$ on ovulation and ovarian contractility in the rabbit. *Prostaglandins*, 5:567–579.
131. Didio, L. J. A., Allen, D. J., Correr, S., and Motta, P. M. (1980): Smooth muscle in the ovary. In: *Biology of the Ovary*, edited by P. M. Motta and E. S. E. Hafez, pp. 107–118. Martinus Nijhoff, The Hague.
132. di Zerega, G. S., Goembelsmann, U., and Nakamura, R. M. (1982): Identification of protein(s) secreted by the preovulatory ovary which suppresses the follicle response to gonadotropins. *J. Clin. Endocrinol. Metab.*, 54:1091–1096.
133. Dominques, R., and Riboni, L. (1971): Failure of ovulation in autografted ovary of hemispayed rat. *Neuroendocrinology*, 7:164–170.
134. Douglas, W. W. (1980): Polypeptides—Angiotensin, plasma kinins, and others. In: *The Pharmacological Basis of Therapeutics, 6th ed.*, edited by A. G. Gilman, L. S. Goodman, and A. Gilman, pp. 659–663. Macmillan, New York.
135. Downey, B. R., and Ainsworth L. (1980): Reversal of indomethacin blockade of ovulation in gilts by prostaglandins. *Prostaglandins*, 19:17–22.
136. Downs, S. M., and Longo, F. J. (1982): Effects of indomethacin on preovulatory follicles in immature superovulated mice. *Am. J. Anat.*, 164:265–274.

137. Downs, S. M., and Longo, F. J. (1983): Prostaglandins and preovulatory follicular maturation in mice. *J. Exp. Zool.*, 228:99–108.
138. Downs, S. M., and Longo, F. J. (1983): An ultrastructural study of preovulatory apical development in mouse ovarian follicles: Effects of indomethacin. *Anat. Rec.* 205:159–168.
139. Dowsett, M., Eastman, A. R., Easty, D. M., Easty, G. C., Powles, T. J., and Neville, A. M. (1976): Prostaglandin mediation of collagenase-induced bone resorption. *Nature,* 263:72–74.
140. Dunaif, A. E., Zimmerman, E. A., Friesen, H. G., and Frantz, A. G. (1982): Intracellular localization of prolactin receptors and prolactin in the rat ovary by immunocytochemistry. *Endocrinology,* 110:1465–1471.
141. Edwards, R. G. (1974): Follicular fluid. *J. Reprod. Fertil.*, 37:189–219.
142. Edwards, R. G., Steptoe, P. C., Fowler, R. E., and Baillie, J. (1980): Observations on preovulatory human ovarian follicles and their aspirates. *Br. J. Obstet. Gynaecol.*, 87:769–779.
143. Ellinwood, W. E., Nett, T. M., and Niswender, G. D. (1978): Ovarian vasculature: Structure and function. In: *The Vertebrate Ovary: Comparative Biology and Evolution,* edited by R. E. Jones, pp. 583–416. Plenum Press, New York.
144. Ellis, S. (1961): Bioassay of luteinizing hormone. *Endocrinology,* 68:334–340.
145. Eppig, J. J. (1981): Prostaglandin E_2 stimulates cumulus expansion and hyaluronic acid synthesis by cumuli oophori isolated from mice. *Biol. Reprod.*, 25:191–195.
146. Erickson, G. F., and Hsueh, A. J. W. (1978): Secretion of "inhibin" by rat granulosa cells *in vitro*. *Endocrinology,* 103:1960–1963.
147. Erickson, G. F., Magoffin, D. A., Dyer, C. A., and Hofeditz, C. (1985): The ovarian androgen producing cells: A review of structure/function relationships. *Endocr. Rev.*, 6:371–399.
148. Espey, L. L. (1967): Ultrastructure of the apex of the rabbit Graafian follicle during the ovulatory process. *Endocrinology,* 81:267–276.
149. Espey, L. L. (1967): Tenacity of porcine Graafian follicle as it approaches ovulation. *Am. J. Physiol.*, 212:1397–1401.
150. Espey, L. L. (1971): Decomposition of connective tissue in rabbit ovarian follicles by multivesicular structures of thecal fibroblasts. *Endocrinology,* 88:437–444.
151. Espey, L. L. (1974): Ovarian proteolytic enzymes and ovulation. *Biol. Reprod.*, 10:216–235.
152. Espey, L. L. (1978): Ovulation. In: *The Vertebrate Ovary,* edited by R. E. Jones, pp. 503–532. Plenum Press, New York.
153. Espey, L. L. (1980): Ovulation as an inflammatory reaction: a hypothesis. *Biol. Reprod.*, 22:73–106.
154. Espey, L. L. (1986): Simultaneous determination of ovarian prostaglandin E_2, prostaglandin $F_{2\alpha}$, 6-keto-prostaglandin $F_{1\alpha}$, β-estradiol and progesterone during ovulation in the PMSG/hCG-primed immature rat. *Biol. Reprod.*, 34 (Suppl. 1), 151 (abstract).
155. Espey, L. L., and Coons, P. J. (1976): Factors which influence ovulatory degradation of rabbit ovarian follicles. *Biol. Reprod.*, 14:233–245.
156. Espey, L. L., and Lipner, H. (1963): Measurement of intrafollicular pressures in the rabbit ovary. *Am. J. Physiol.*, 205:1067.
157. Espey, L. L., and Lipner, H. (1965): Enzyme-induced rupture of rabbit Graafian follicle. *Am. J. Physiol.*, 208:208–213.
158. Espey, L. L., and Rondell, P. (1967): Estimation of mammalian collagenolytic activity with a synthetic substrate. *J. Appl. Physiol.*, 23:757–761.
159. Espey, L. L., and Rondell, P. (1968): Collagenolytic activity in the rabbit and sow Graafian follicle during ovulation. *Am. J. Physiol.*, 214:326–329.
160. Espey, L. L., and Stutts, R. H. (1972): Exchange of cytoplasm between two cells of the membrana granulosa in rabbit ovarian follicles. *Biol. Reprod.*, 6:168–175.
161. Espey, L., Miller, D., and Margolius, H. S. (1985): Indomethacin and cycloheximide inhibition of ovarian kinin-generating activity during ovulation in the PMSG/hCG-primed immature rat. *Biol. Reprod.*, 32(Suppl. 1) (abstract No. 291).
162. Espey, L. L., Coons, P. J., Marsh, J. M., and LeMaire, W. J. (1981): Effect of indomethacin on preovulatory changes in the ultrastructure of rabbit Graafian follicles. *Endocrinology,* 108:1040–1048.
163. Espey, L., Shimada, H., Okamura, H., and Mori, T. (1985): Effect of various agents on ovarian plasminogen activator activity during ovulation in pregnant mare's serum gonadotropin-primed immature rats. *Biol. Reprod.*, 32:1087–1094.
164. von Euler, U. S., and Hammarstrom, S. (1937): Ueber Vorkommen und Wirkung von Adrenalin in Ovarien. *Scand. Arch. Physiol.*, 77:163–178.
165. Evans, D. H. L., and Murray, J. G. (1954): Histological and functional studies on the fibre composition of the vagus nerve of the rabbit. *J. Anat.*, 88:320–337.
166. Evans, G., Dobias, M., King, C. J., and Armstrong, D. T. (1983): Production of prostaglandins by porcine preovulatory follicular tissue and their roles in intrafollicular function. *Biol. Reprod.*, 28:322–328.
167. Eyre, D. R. (1980): Collagen: Molecular diversity in the body's protein scaffold. *Science,* 207:1315–1322.
168. Falck, B. (1962): Observations on the possibilities of the cellular localization of monoamines by a fluorescence method. *Acta Physiol. Scand.*, 56:1–25.
169. Falck, B., and Owman, C. (1965): A detailed methodological description of the fluorescence method for the cellular demonstration of biogenic monoamines. *Acta Univ. Lundensis Sect. II,* 7:5–23.
170. Fessler, J. H., and Fessler, L. I. (1978): Biosynthesis of procollagen. *Annu. Rev. Biochem.*, 47:129–162.
171. Fink, G., and Schofield, G. C. (1971): Experimental studies on the innervation of the ovary in cats. *J. Anat.*, 109:115–126.
172. Fletcher, W. H. (1975): Assembly of an "enclosed gap junction" by the granulosa cells of developing ovarian follicles in sexually immature rats. *J. Cell Biol.*, 67:116a(abstract no. 232).
173. Fletcher, W. H. (1979): Intercellular junctions in ovarian follicles: A possible functional role in follicle development. In: *Ovarian Follicular Development and Function,* edited by A. R. Midgley and W. A. Sadler, pp. 113–120. Raven Press, New York.
174. Fletcher, P. W., Dias, J. A., Sanzo, M. A., and Reichert, L. E., Jr. (1982): Inhibition of FSH action on granulosa cells by low molecular weight components of follicular fluid. *Mol. Cell. Endocrinol.*, 25:303–316.
175. Fletcher, W. H., and Everett, J. W. (1973): Ultrastructural reorganization of rat granulosa cells on the day of proestrus. *Anat. Rec.*, 175:320a.
176. France, E. S. (1969): Reversal by pargyline of reserpine block of induced ovulation—Direct ovarian effects. *Neuroendocrinology,* 6:77–89.
177. Frankenhauser. R. (1867): *Die Nerven der Gebarmuter und ihre Endegigungen in den glatten Muskelfasern*. F. von Mauke, Jena.
178. Fraser, I., Baird, D. T., and Cockburn, F. (1973): Ovarian venous blood PO_2, PCO_2 and pH in women. *J. Reprod. Fertil.*, 33:11–17.
179. Fukumoto, M., Yajima, Y., Okamura, H. and Midorikawa, O. (1981): Collagenolytic enzyme activity in human ovary: An ovulatory enzyme system. *Fertil. Steril.*, 36:746–750.
180. Fukushimo, M. (1977): Intercellular junctions in the human developing preovulatory follicle and corpus luteum. *Int. J. Fertil.*, 22:206–216.
181. Fumagalli, Z., Motta, P., and Calvieri, S. (1971): The presence of smooth muscular cells in the ovary of several mammals as seen under the electron microscope. *Experientia,* 27:682–683.
182. von Gawronsky, N. (1894): Ueber verbreitung und Endigung der Nerven in den weiblichen Genitalien. *Arch. Gynecol.*, 47:271–283.
183. Gebauer, H., Lindner, H. R., and Amsterdam, A. (1978): Synthesis of heparin-like glycosamine-glycans in rat ovarian slices. *Biol. Reprod.*, 18:350–358.
184. Gelderd, J. G., and Peppler, R. D. (1979): Effect of spinal cord transection on the reproductive system in the female rat. *Neuroendocrinology,* 29:293–299.
185. Gillet, J. Y., Maillet, R., and Gautier, C. (1980): Blood and lymph supply of the ovary. In: *Biology of the Ovary,* edited by P. M. Motta and E. S. E. Hafez, pp. 86–98. Martinus Nijhoff, The Hague.
186. Gilula, N. B., Epstein, M. L., and Beers, W. H. (1978): Cell-to-cell communication and ovulation. A study of the cumulus-oocyte complex. *J. Cell Biol.*, 78:58–75.
187. Gimeno, M. F., Borda, E., Sterin-Borda, L., Vidal, J. H., and Gimeno, A. L. (1976): Pharmacologic influences on human ovarian contractions. *Obstet. Gynecol.*, 47:218–222.
188. Gimeno, M. F., Gimeno, A. L., and Rettori, V. B. (1975): Physiologic and pharmacologic studies on the motility of isolated guinea pig ovaries. *Fertil. Steril.*, 26:422–426.

189. Gimeno, M. F., Sterin-Speziale, N., Landa, A., Bonacossa, A., and Gimeno, A. L. (1977): Drug-induced motility of sow (*Sus scrofa*) Graafian follicles isolated during pre- and postovulatory periods of the sex cycle. *Act Physiol. Lat. Am.*, 27:321–331.
190. Goldenberg, R. L., Vaitukaitis, J. L., and Ross, G. T. (1972): Estrogen and follicle stimulating hormone interactions on follicle growth in rats. *Endocrinology,* 90:1492–1498.
191. Gothie, S. (1954): Etude comparee de la repartition du P^{32} et du ^{35}S dans l'organisme de lapire, specialement dans l'ovaire. *C. R. Soc. Biol.*, 148:1210–1213.
192. Grega, G. J., Adamski, S. W., and Dobbins, D. E. (1986): Physiological and pharmacological evidence for the regulation of permeability. *Fed. Proc.*, 45:96–100.
193. Grenedai, I., Marchetti, B., Maugeri, S., Roxas, M. A., and Scapagnini, V. (1978): Prevention of compensatory ovarian hypertrophy by local treatment of the ovaries with 6-OHDA. *Neuroendocrinology,* 27:272–278.
194. Grimek, H. J., and Ax, R. L. (1982): Chromatographic comparisons of chondroitin-containing proteoglycans from small and large bovine ovarian follicles. *Biochem. Biophys. Res. Commun.*, 104: 1401–1406.
195. Grimek, H. J., Bellin, M. E., and Ax, R. L. (1984): Characteristics of proteoglycans isolated from small and large bovine ovarian follicles. *Biol. Reprod.*, 30:397–409.
196. Grinwich, D. L., Kennedy, T. G., and Armstrong, D. T. (1972): Dissociation of ovulatory and steroidogenic actions of luteinizing hormone in rabbits with indomethacin, an inhibitor of prostaglandin biosynthesis. *Prostaglandins,* 1:89–96.
197. Grob, H. S. (1969): Effects of denervation of mouse ovary. *Am. Zool,* 9:1086 (abstract No. 141).
198. Grob, H. S. (1972): Effects of abdominal ovarian denervation on vaginal opening, estrus and ovarian histology. *Fed. Proc.*, 31:265 (abstract No. 296).
199. Grob, H. S., and Brink, C. E. (1973): Effects of exogenous norepineprine on the ovaries of hypophysectemized mice. *Fed Proc.*, 32:213 (abstract No. 10).
200. Grohe, F. (1863): Uber den Bau und das Wachstum des menschlichen Eierstocks. *Arch. Pathol. Anat. Physiol.* 26:271–306.
201. Guraya, S. S. (1985): *Biology of Ovarian Follicles in Mammals.* Springer-Verlag, Berlin.
202. Guttmacher, M. S., and Guttmacher, A. F. (1921): Morphological and physiological studies on the musculature of the mature Graafian follicle of the sow. *Bull. J. Hopkins Hosp.*, 32:394–399.
203. Guyton, A. C. (1986): *Textbook of Medical Physiology,* 7th ed., p. 693. W. B. Saunders, Philadelphia.
204. Hadek, R. (1963): Electron microscope study on primary liquor folliculi secretion in the mouse ovary. *J. Ultrastruct. Res.*, 9:445–458.
205. Hamada, Y., Bronson, R. A., Wright, K. H., and Wallach, E. E. (1977): Ovulation in the perfused rabbit ovary: The influence of prostaglandins and prostaglandin inhibitors. *Biol. Reprod.*, 17:58–63.
206. Hammond, J., and Marshall, F. H. A. (1925): *Reproduction in the Rabbit.* Oliver and Boyd, London.
207. Hammond, J. M. (1981): Peptide regulators in the ovarian follicle. *Aust. J. Biol. Sci.*, 34:391–504.
208. Hammond, J. M., Barrando, L. S., Skaleris, D., Knight, A. B., Romanus, J. A., and Rechler, M. M. (1985): Production of insulin-like growth factors by ovarian granulosa cells. *Endocrinology,* 117:2553–2555.
209. Heape, W. (1905): Ovulation and degeneration of the ova in the rabbit. *Proc. R. Soc. Lond. (Biol.),* 76B:260–268.
210. von Herff, O. (1892): Ueber den fienesen Verlauf der Nerven im Eierstock des Menschen. *Z. Geburtschilfe Gynakol.*, 24:289–308.
211. Hial, V., DeMello, M. C. F., Horakova, Z., and Beaven, M. A. (1977): Antiproliferative activity of antiinflammatory drugs in two mammalian cell culture lines. *J. Pharmacol. Exp. Ther.*, 202:446–454.
212. Hill, R. T. (1949): Adrenal cortical physiology of spleen grafted and denervated ovaries in the mouse. *Exp. Med. Surg.*, 7:86–98.
213. Hill, R. T. (1962): Paradoxical effects of ovarian secretions. In: *The Ovary, Vol. II,* edited by S. Zuckerman, pp. 231–261. Academic Press, New York.
214. Hill, R. T., Allen, E., and Kramer, T. C. (1935): Cinemicrographic studies of rabbit ovulation. *Anat. Rec.*, 63:239–245.
215. Himeno, N., Kawamura, N., Okamura, H., Mori, T., Fukumoto, M., and Midorikawa, O. (1984): Collagen synthetic activity in rabbit ovary during ovulation and its blockage by indomethecin. *Acta Obstet. Gynaecol. Jpn.*, 36:1930–1934.
216. Himeno, N., Kawamura, N., Okamura, H., Mori, T., Fukumoto, M., and Midorikawa, O. (1984): The effect of prostaglandin F-2-alpha on collagen synthesis in rabbit ovary during the ovulatory process. *Acta Obstet. Gynaecol. Jpn.* 36:2494–2495 (in Japanese).
217. Hinsey, J. C., and J. E. Markee. (1932): A search for neurological mechanisms in ovulation. *Proc. Soc. Exp. Biol. Med.*, 30:136–138.
218. His, W. (1865): Beobachtungen ueber den Bau des Saugethiereierstockes. *Arch. Mikr. Anat.*, 1:97–105.
219. Hixon, J. E., and Clegg, M. T. (1969): Influence of the pituitary on ovarian progesterone output in the eye: Effects of hypophysectomy and gonadotropic hormones. *Endocrinology,* 84:828–834.
220. Ichikawa, S., Morioka, H., Oda, M., Oda, K., and Murao, S. (1983): Effects of various proteinase inhibitors on ovulation of explanted hamster ovaries. *J. Reprod. Fertil.*, 68:407–412.
221. Ichikawa, S., Ohta, M., Morioka, H., and Murao, S. (1983): Blockage of ovulation in the explanted hamster ovary by a collagenase inhibitor. *J. Reprod. Fertil.*, 68:17–19.
222. Jackson, D. S. (1980): The substrate collagen. In: *Collagenase in Normal and Pathological Connective Tissues,* edited by D. E. Woolley and J. M. Evanson, pp. 1–10. John Wiley & Sons, New York.
223. Jacobowitz, D., and Laties, A. M. (1970): Adrenergic reinnervation of the cat ovary transplanted to the anterior chamber of the eye. *Endocrinology,* 86:921–924.
224. Jacobowitz, D., and Wallach, E. E. (1967): Histochemical and chemical studies of the autonomic innervation of the ovary. *Endocrinology,* 81:1132–1139.
225. Janson, P. O. (1975): Effects of luteinizing hormone on blood in the follicular rabbit ovary as measured by radioactive microspheres. *Acta Endocrinol.*, 79:122–123.
226. Jensen, C. E., and Zachariae, F. (1958): Studies on the mechanism of ovulation. Isolation and analysis of acid mucopolysaccharides in bovine follicular fluid. *Acta Endocrinol.*, 27:356–368.
227. Jocelyn, H. D., and Setchell, B. P. (1972): Translation of Regnier de Graaf. On Human Reproductive Organs from the Latin Text *Tractus de Vivorum Organis Generationi Inservientibus* (1668) and *DeMulierum Organis Generationi Inservientibus Tractatus Novus* (1672), Chapter XII, pp. 131–135. *Reprod. Fertil.*, (*Suppl.*), 17:131–135.
228. Johns, A., Chlumecky, J., Cottle, M., and Paton, D. M. (1975): Effect of chemical sympathectomy and adrenergic agonists on the fertility of mice. *Contraception,* 11:563–570.
229. Jonassen, F., Granerus, G., and Wetterquist, H. (1976): Histamine metabolism during the menstrual cycle. *Acta Obstet. Gynecol. Scand.*, 55:297–304.
230. Jones, R. E., Duvall, D., and Guillette, L. J., Jr. (1980): Rat ovarian mast cells: Distribution and cyclic changes. *Anat. Rec.*, 197:489–493.
231. deJong, F. H., and Sharpe, R. M. (1976): Evidence for inhibin-like activity in bovine follicular fluid. *Nature,* 263:71–72.
232. Jordan, S. M. (1970): Adrenergic and cholinergic innervation of the reproductive tract and ovary in the guinea pig and rabbit. *J. Physiol. (Lond.),* 210:115–117.
233. Kang, H. H., Anderson, W. A., Chang, S. C., and Ryan, R. J. (1979): Studies on the structure of the extracellular matrices of the mammalian follicles as revealed by high-voltage electromicroscopy and cytochemistry. In: *Ovarian Follicular Development and Function,* edited by A. R. Midgley and W. A. Sadler, pp. 121–135. Raven Press, New York.
234. Kannisto, P., Owman, C., Rosengren, E., and Walles, B. (1984): Intraovarian adrenergic nerves in the guinea pig: Development from fetal life to sexual maturity. *Cell Tissue Res.*, 238:235–240.
235. Kannisto, P., Owman, C., and Walles, B. (1985): Involvement of local adrenergic receptors in the process of ovulation in gonadotrophin-primed immature rats. *J. Reprod. Fertil.*, 75:357–362.
236. Kanzaki, H. (1981): Scanning electronmicroscopic study on corrosive casts for rabbit ovarian follicle microvasculature during the ovulatory and luteinizing process. *Acta Obstet. Gynecol. Jpn.*, 33:1925–1933.
237. Kanzaki, H., Okamura, H., Okuda, Y., Takenaka, A., Morimoto, K., and Nishimura, T. (1982): Scanning electron microscopic study

of rabbit ovarian follicle microvasculature using resin injection-corrosion casts. *J. Anat.*, 134:697–704.
238. Kapri, A., and Aratei, H. (1965): The biochemistry of the follicular fluid. *Rev. Roum. Biochim.*, 2,3:243–248.
239. Karnovsky, M. J., and Roots, L. (1964): A "direct-coloring" thicoholine method for cholinesterases. *J. Histochem. Cytochem.*, 12:219–221.
240. Kasson, B. G., and Hsueh, A. J. (1985): Cholinergic inhibition of follicle-stimulating hormone-induced progesterone production by cultured rat granulosa cells. *Biol. Reprod.*, 33:1158–1167.
241. Kasson, B. G., Meidan, R., Davoren, J. B., and Hseuh, A. J. (1985): Identification of subpopulations of rat granulosa cells: Sedimentation properties and hormonal responsiveness. *Endocrinology*, 117: 1027–1034.
242. von Kaulla, K. N., and Shettles, L. B. (1956): Thromboplastic activity of human cervical mucus and ovarian follicular and seminal fluids. *Fertil. Steril.*, 7:166–169.
243. Kawai, Y., Satoh, K., Mitsuhashi, N., Hasumi, K., Sakakibara, K., Kinoshita, K., Wu, T., and Sakamoto, S. (1981): Prostaglandin and luteinized unruptured follicles: The follicles of gilts treated with the inhibitors of prostaglandin production. *Folia Endocrinol. Jpn.*, 57:1475–1488.
244. Kawakami, M., Kubo, K., Uemura, T., and Nagase, M. (1979): Evidence for the existence of extra-hypophyseal neural mechanisms controlling ovarian steroid secretion. *J. Steroid Biochem.*, 11:1001–1005.
245. Kawakami, M., Kubo, K., Uemura, T., Nagase, M., and Hayashi, R. (1981): Involvement of ovarian innervation in steroid secretion. *Endocrinology*, 109:136–145.
246. Kawamura, N., Himeno, N., Okamura, H., Mori, T., Fukumoto, M., and Midorikawa, O. (1984): Effect of indomethacin on collagenolytic enzyme activities in rabbit ovary. *Acta Obstet. Gynaecol. Jpn.*, 36:2099–2105.
247. Kawamura, N., Yajema, Y., Huang, C. H., Okuda, Y., Fukumoto, M., Okamura, H., and Nishimura, T. (1981): DNP-peptidase activity in the rabbit ovary. *Acta Obstet. Gynecol. Jpn.* 33:1684–1688.
248. Kelly, G. L. (1931): Direct observation of rupture of the Graafian follicle in a mammal. *J. Fla. Med. Assoc.*, 17:422–423.
249. Kiekhofer, W., Holmen, G. J., and Peckham, B. (1962): Some chemical characteristics of ovarian and parovarian cystic fluids. *Obstet. Gynecol.*, 20:471–483.
250. Klebs, E. (1861): Die Eierstockseier der Wirbelthiere. *Arch. Pathol. Anat. Physiol.*, 21 and 28:362–366. (quoted from Nagel).
251. Kling, O. R., Roche, P. C., Campeau, J. D., Nishimura, K., Nakamura, R. M., and di Zerega, G. S. (1984): Identification of a porcine fluid fraction which suppressed follicular response to gonadotropins. *Biol. Reprod.*, 30:564–572.
252. Knecht, M. (1986): Production of a cell-associated and secreted plasminogen activator by cultured rat granulosa cells. *Endocrinology*, 118:348–353.
253. Knox, E., Lowry, S., and Beck, L. (1979): Prevention of ovulation in rabbits by antihistamines. In: *Ovarian Follicular Development and Function*, edited by A. R. Midgley and W. A. Sadler, pp. 159–161. Raven Press, New York.
254. Kobayashi, Y., Sjoberg, N. O., Walles, B., Owman, C., Wright, K. H., Santulli, R., and Wallach, E. E. (1983): Effect of adrenergic agents on the ovulatory process in the *in-vitro* perfused rabbit ovary. *Am. J. Obstet Gynecol.*, 145:857–864.
255. Kobayashi, Y., Wright, K. H., Santulli, K., Kitai, H., and Wallach, E. G. (1983): Effect of histamine and histamine blockers on the ovulatory process in vitro perfused rabbit ovary. *Biol. Reprod.*, 28:385–392.
256. Koelle, G. B. (1962): A new general concept of the neurohumoral functions of acetylcholine and acetylcholinesterase. *J. Pharm. Pharmacol.*, 14:65.
257. Kohda, H., Mori, T., Ezaki, Y., Nishimura, T., and Kambegawa, A. (1980): A progesterone-dependent step in ovulation induced by human chorionic gonadotrophin in immature rats primed with pregnant mare serum gonadotrophin. *J. Endocrinol.*, 87:105–107.
258. von Kolliker, A. (1849): Beitrage zur kenntniss der glatten Muskeln. *Abhandl. Wiss. Zool.*, 1:48–87.
259. Koos, R. D., and Clark, M. R. (1982): Production of 6-keto-prostaglandin F-1-alpha by rat granulosa cells *in vitro*. *Endocrinology*, 11:1513–1518.
260. Koos, R. D., and LeMaire, W. J. (1983): Evidence for an angiogenic factor from rat follicles. In: *Factors Regulating Ovarian Functions*, edited by G. S. Greenwald and P. F. Terranova, pp. 191–196. Raven Press, New York.
261. Koos, R. D., Feiertag, M. A., Brodie, A. M. H., and LeMaire, W. J. (1984): Inhibition of estrogen synthesis does not inhibit luteinizing hormone-induced ovulation. *Am. J. Obstet. Gynecol.*, 148:939–945.
262. Kranzfelder, D., Korr, H., Mestwerdt, W., and Maurer-Schultze, B. (1984): Follicle growth in the ovary of the rabbit after ovulation-inducing application of human chorionic gonadotropin. *Cell Tissue Res.*, 238:611–620.
263. Kraus, S. D. (1947): Observations on the mechanism of ovulation in the frog, hen and rabbit. *West J. Surg. Obstet. Gynecol.*, 55:424–437.
264. Krishna, A., and Terranova, P. F. (1985): Alterations in mast cell degranulation and ovarian histamine in the proestrous hamster. *Biol. Reprod.*, 32:1211–1217.
265. Kristek, F., Tesarik, J., and Unzeiting, V. (1984): Ultrastructure of the human theca. *Folia Morphol.*, 32:5–8.
266. Kuehl, F. A., Jr., and Egan, R. W. (1980): Prostaglandins, arachidonic acid and inflammation. *Science*, 210:978–984.
267. Kulkarni, P. S., Wakade, A. R., and Kirpekar, S. M. (1976): Sympathetic innervation of guinea pig uterus and ovary. *Am. J. Physiol.*, 230:1400–1405.
268. Kuntz, A. (1945): *The Autonomic Nervous System, 3rd ed.* Lea and Febiger, Philadelphia.
269. Lamprecht, S. A., Zor, U., Tsafriri, A., and Lindner, H. R. (1971): Action of prostaglandin E_2 and luteinizing hormone on cyclic adenosine 3′-5′-monophosphate production and protein kinase activity in fetal, early postnatal and adult rat ovaries. *Isr. J. Med. Sci.*, 7:704–705.
270. Lamprecht, S. A., Zor, U., Tsafriri, A., and Lindner, H. R. (1973): Action of prostaglandin E_2 and of luteinizing hormone on ovarian adenylate cyclase, protein kinase, and ornithine decarboxylase activity during postnatal development and maturity in the rat. *J. Endocrinol.*, 57:217–233.
271. Larsen, W. J. (1977): Structural diversity of gap junctions: A review. *Tissue Cell*, 9:373–394.
272. Larsen, W. J., and Tung, H. N. (1978): Origin and fate of cytoplasmic gap junctional vesicles in rabbit granulosa cells. *Tissue Cell*, 10:585–598.
273. Larsen, W. J., Tung, H. N., Murray, S. A., and Swenson, C. A. (1979): Evidence for the participation of actin microfilaments and bristle coats in the internalization of gap junction membrane. *J. Cell Biol.*, 83:576–583.
274. Larsen, W. J., Tung, H. N., and Polking, C. (1981): Response of granulosa cell gap junctions to human chorionic gonadotropin (hCG) at ovulation. *Biol. Reprod.*, 25:1119–1134.
275. Lau, I. F., Saksena, S. K., and Chang, M. C. (1974): Prostaglandins F and ovulation in mice. *J. Reprod. Fertil.*, 40:467–469.
276. Lawrence, I. E., and Burden, H. W. (1976): The autonomic innervation of the interstitial gland of the rat ovary during pregnancy. *Am. J. Anat.*, 147:81–94.
277. Lawrence, T. S., Beers, W. H., and N. B. Gilula. (1978): Transmission of hormonal stimulation by cell-to-cell communication. *Nature*, 272:501–506.
278. Lawrence, T. S., Ginzberg, R. D., Gilula, N. B., and W. H. Beers. (1979): Hormonally induced cell shape changes in cultured rat ovarian granulosa cells. *J. Cell Biol.*, 80:21–36.
279. Ledwitz-Rigby, F., and Ribgy, B. W. (1983): The actions of follicular fluid factors on steroidogenesis by cultured ovarian granulosa cells. *J. Steroid Biochem.*, 19:127–131.
280. Lee, W., and Novy, M. J. (1978): Effects of luteinizing hormone and indomethacin on blood flow and steroidogenesis in the rabbit ovary. *Biol. Reprod.*, 18:799–807.
281. LeMaire, W. J., and Marsh, J. M. (1975): Interrelationships between prostaglandins, cyclic AMP and steroids in ovulation. *J. Reprod. Fertil. (Suppl.)*, 22:53–74.
282. LeMaire, W. J., Davies, P. J., and Marsh, J. M. (1976): The role of prostaglandins in the development of refractoriness to LH stimulation by Graafian follicles. *Prostaglandins*, 12:271–279.
283. LeMaire, W. J., Leidner, R., and Marsh, J. M. (1975): Pre- and postovulatory changes in the concentration of prostaglandins in rat Graafian follicles. *Prostaglandins*, 9:221–229.

284. LeMaire, W. J., Yang, N. S. T., Behrman, H. R., and Marsh, J. M. (1973): Preovulatory changes in the concentration of prostaglandins in rabbit Graafian follicles. *Prostaglandins,* 3:367.

285. Lenz, R. W., Ax, R. L., and First, N. L. (1982): Proteoglycan production by bovine granulosa cells *in vivo* is regulated by calmodulin and calcium. *Endocrinology,* 110:1052–1054.

286. LePere, R. H., Benoit, P. E., Hardy, R. C., and Goldzieher, J. W. (1966): The origin and function of the ovarian nerve supply in the baboon. *Fertil. Steril.,* 17:68–75.

287. Levin, E. G., and Loskutoff, D. J. (1982): Cultured bovine endothelial cells produce both urokinase and tissue-type plasminogen activators. *J. Cell Biol.* 94:631–636.

288. Lim, A. T., Lolait, S., Barlow, J. W., Wai Sum, O., Zois, I., Toh, B. H., and Funder, J. W. (1983): Immunoreactive beta-endorphin in sheep. *Nature,* 303:709–711.

289. Lindner, H. R., Tsafriri, A., Lieberman, M. E., Zor, U., Koch, Y., Bauminger, S., and Barne, A. (1974): Gonadotropin action on cultured Graafian follicles: Induction of maturation division of the mammalian oocyte and differentiation of the luteal cell. *Rec. Prog. Hormone Res.,* 30:79–138.

290. Lindner, H. R., Zor, U., Kohen, F., Bauminger, S., Armsterdam, A., Lahar, M., and Salomon, Y. (1980): Significance of prostaglandins in the regulation of cyclic events in the ovary and uterus. *Adv. Prostaglandin Thromboxane Leukotriene Res.,* 8:1371–1390.

291. Lipner, H. (1971): Ovulation from histamine depleted ovaries. *Proc. Soc. Exp. Biol. Med.,* 136:111–114.

292. Lipner, H. (1973): Mechanism of mammalian ovulation. In: *Handbook of Physiology—Endocrinology II, Part 1,* Chapter 18, pp. 409–437.

293. Lipner, H., and Cross, N. L. (1968): Morphology of the membrana granulosa of the ovarian follicle. *Endocrinology,* 82:638–641.

294. Lipner, H., and Greep, R. O. (1971): Inhibition of steroidogenesis at various sites in the biosynthetic pathway and the relationship to induced ovulation. *Endocrinology,* 88:602–607.

295. Lipner, H., and Maxwell, B. A. (1960): Hypothesis concerning the role of follicular contractions in ovulation. *Science,* 131:1737–1738.

296. Lipner, H., and Smith, M. S. (1971): A method for determining the distribution and source of protein in preovulatory rat ovaries. *J. Endocrinol.,* 50:1–14.

297. Lipner, H., and Wendelkin, L. (1971): Inhibition of ovulation by inhibition of steroidogenesis in immature rats. *Proc. Soc. Exp. Biol. Med.,* 136:1141–1145.

298. Liu, W. K., Burleigh, B. D., and Ward, D. N. (1981): Steroid and plasminogen activator production by cultured rat granulosa cells in response to hormone treatment. *Mol. Cell. Endocrinol.* 21:63–73.

299. Loewenstein, W. R. (1981): Junctional intercellular communication: The cell-to-cell membrane channel. *Physiol. Rev.,* 61:829–913.

300. Lupulescu, A. P. (1977): Cytologic and metabolic effects of prostaglandins on rat skin. *J. Invest. Dermatol.,* 68:138–145.

301. Lutwak-Mann, C. (1954): Note on the chemical composition of bovine follicular fluid. *J. Agr. Sci.,* 44:477–480.

302. Macdonald, E. J., and Airaksinen, M. M. (1974): The effect of 6-hydroxydopamine on the oestrus cycle and fertility of rats. *J. Pharm. Pharmacol.,* 26:518–521.

303. Mai, H., Jr., Barbosa, I., and Coutinho, E. M. (1975): Effects of aminophylline, imidazole and indomethacin on spontaneous and prostaglandin induced ovarian contractions *in vitro. Int. J. Fertil.,* 20:82–86.

304. Mai, H., Jr., Barbosa, I., and Coutinho, E. M. (1978): Inhibition of ovulation in marmoset monkeys by indomethacin. *Fertil. Steril.,* 29:565–570.

305. Makinada, S. (1980): Hemodynamics and histological studies on ovarian blood flow during ovulation. *Hokkaido J. Med. Sci.,* 55:521–526.

306. Makris, A., Ryan, K. H., Hasumizu, T., Hill, C. L., and Zetter, B. R. (1984): The nonluteal porcine ovary as a source of angiogenic activity. *Endocrinology,* 115:1672–1677.

307. Manarang-Pangan, S., and Menge, A. C. (1971): Immunologic studies on human follicular fluid. *Fertil. Steril.,* 22:367–372.

308. Mandl, L. (1895): Ueber Anordnung und Endigungsweise der Nerven im Ovarium. *Arch. Gynecol.,* 48:376.

309. Marion, G. B., Gier, H. T., and Choudary, J. B. (1968): Micromorphology of the bovine ovarian follicular system. *J. Anim. Sci.,* 27:451–465.

310. Markee, J. E., and Hinsey, J. C. (1936): Observations on ovulation in the rabbit. *Anat. Rec.,* 64:309–319.

311. Marotti, K. R., Belin, D., and Strickland, S. (1982): The production of distinct forms of plasminogen activator by mouse embryonic cells. *Dev. Biol.* 90:154–159.

312. Martin, G. G., and Miller-Walker, W. C. (1983): Visualization of the 3-dimensional distribution of collagen fibrils over pre-ovulatory follicles in the hamster *Mesocricetus auratus. J. Exp. Zool.,* 225:311–320.

313. Martin, G. G., and Talbot, P. (1981): The role of follicular smooth muscle cells in hamster ovulation. *J. Exp. Zool.,* 216:469–482.

314. Martinat, N., and Combarnous, Y. (1983): The release of plasminogen activator by rat granulosa cells is highly specific for FSH activity. *Endocrinology,* 119:433–435.

315. McCracken, J. A., Baird, D. T., and Goding, J. R. (1971): Factors affecting the secretion of steroids from autotransplanted ovary in the sheep. *Recent Prog. Hormone Res.,* 27:537–582.

316. McGaughey, R. W. (1975): A comparison of the fluids from small and large ovarian follicles of the pig. *Biol. Reprod.,* 13:147–153.

317. McNatty, K. P. (1978): Follicular fluid. In: *The Vertebrate Ovary,* edited by R. E. Jones, pp. 215–259. Plenum Press, New York.

318. McReynolds, H. D., Siraki, C. M., Bramson, P. H., and Pollock, R. J., Jr. (1973): Smooth muscle-like cells in ovaries of the hamster and gerbil. *Z. Zellforsch.,* 140:1–8.

319. Merk, F. B., Albright, J. T., and Botticelli, C. R. (1973): The fine structure of granulosa cell nexuses in rat ovarian follicles. *Anat. Rec.,* 175:107–125.

320. Miller, E. J. (1985): Recent information on the chemistry of the collagens. In: *The Chemistry and Biology of Mineralized Tissues,* edited by W. T. Butler, pp. 80–93. EBSCO Media, Birmingham, AL.

321. Miller, F. N., and Sims, D. E. (1986): Contractile elements in the regulation of macromolecular permeability. *Fed. Proc.,* 45: 84–88.

322. Miller, K. F., Wesson, J. A., and Ginther, O. J. (1979): Changes in concentration of circulating gonadotrophins following administration of equine follicular fluid to ovariectomized mares. *Biol. Reprod.,* 21:867–872.

323. Mitchell, G. A. G. (1938): Innervation of ovary, uterine tube, testis and epididymis. *J. Anat.,* 72:508–517.

324. Mitsuhashi, N. (1981): Studies on the mechanism and the significance of prostaglandin biosynthesis by the ovary, ovulation block by the indomethacin and incubation of the follicle. *Acta Obstet. Gynaecol. Jpn.,* 33:479–488.

325. Montz, F. J., Ujita, E. L., Campeau, J. D., and diZerega, G. S. (1984): Inhibition of luteinizing hormone, human chorionic gonadotropin binding to porcine granulosa cells by a follicular fluid protein. *Am. J. Obstet. Gynecol.,* 148:436–441.

326. Moor, R. M., Hay, M. F., and Seamark, R. F. (1975): The sheep ovary: Regulation of steroidogenic, haemodynamic and structural changes in the largest follicle and adjacent tissue before ovulation. *J. Reprod. Fertil.,* 45:595–604.

327. Morales, T. I., Woessner, J. F., Howell, D. S., Marsh, J. M., and LeMaire, W. J. (1978): A microassay for the direct demonstration of collagenolytic activity in Graafian follicles of the rat. *Biochim. Biophys. Acta,* 524:428–434.

328. Morales, T. I., Woessner, J. F., Jr., Marsh, J. M., and LeMaire, W. J. (1983): Collagen, collagenase and collagenolytic activity in rat Graafian follicles during follicular growth and ovulation. *Biochim. Biophys. Acta,* 756:119–122.

329. Mori, T., Suzuki, A., Nishimura, T., and Kambegawa, A. (1977): Inhibition of ovulation in immature rats by antiprogesterone antiserum. *J. Endocrinol.,* 73:185–186.

330. Mori, T., Suzuki, A., Nishimura, T., and Kambegawa, A. (1977): Evidence for androgen participation in induced ovulation in immature rats. *Endocrinology,* 101:623–626.

331. Morikawa, H., Okamura, H., Takenaka, A., Morimoto, K., and Nishimura, T. (1981): Histamine concentration and its effect on ovarian contractility in humans. *Int. J. Fertil.,* 26:283–286.

332. Morimoto, K., Okamura, H., Kanzaki, H., Okuda, Y., Takenaka, A., and Nishimura, T. (1981): Adrenergic nerve supply to bovine ovarian follicles. *Int. J. Fertil.,* 26:14–19.

333. Morimoto, K., Okamura, H., and Tanaka, C. (1982): Development and periovulatory changes of ovarian norepinephrine in the rat. *Am. J. Obstet. Gynecol.,* 143:389–392.

334. Mossman, H. W., and Duke, K. L. (1973): *Comparative Morphology of the Mammalian Ovary*. University of Wisconsin Press, Madison, Wis.
335. Motta, P.; Cherney, D. D., and Didio, L. J. A. (1971): Scanning and transmission electromicroscopy of the ovarian surface in mammals with special reference to ovulation. *J. Submicr. Cytol.* 3:85–100.
336. Motta, P. M., and Familiari, G. (1981): Occurrence of a contractile tissue in the theca externa of atretic follicles in the mouse ovary. *Acta Anat. (Basal),* 109:103–114.
337. Motta, P. M., and Makabe, S. (1982): Development of the ovarian surface and associated germ cells in the human fetus: a correlated study by scanning electron microscopy and transmission electron microscopy. *Cell Tissue Res.*, 226:493–510.
338. Mueller, P. L., Schreiber, J. R., Lucky, A. W., Schulman, J. D., Rodbard, D., and Ross, G. T. (1978): Follicle-stimulating hormone stimulates ovarian synthesis of proteoglycans in estrogen-stimulated hypopohysectomized immature female rats. *Endocrinology,* 102:824–831.
339. Murdoch, W. J., and Dunn, T. G. (1982): Alterations in follicular steroid hormones during the preovulatory period in the ewe. *Biol. Reprod.*, 27:300–307.
340. Murdoch, W. J., and Myers, D. A. (1983): Effect of treatment of estrous ewes with indomethacin on the distribution of ovarian blood to the periovulatory follicle. *Biol. Reprod.*, 29:1229–1232.
341. Murdoch, W. J., Dailey, R. A., and Inskeep, E. K. (1981): Preovulatory changes in prostaglandins E_2 and F_2 in ovine follicles. *J. Animal Sci.*, 53:192—205.
342. Murdoch, W. J., Nix, K. J., and Dunn, T. G. (1983): Dynamics of ovarian blood supply to periovulatory follicles of the ewe. *Biol. Reprod.*, 28:1001–1006.
343. Murphy, G., and Sellers, A. (1980): The extracellular regulation of collagenase activity. In: *Collagenase in Normal and Pathological Connective Tissues,* edited by D. E. Woolley and J. M. Evanson, pp. 65–81. John Wiley & Sons, New York.
344. Nagel, W. (1896): Harn und Geschlechtsorgane. In: *Handbuck der Anatomie des Menschen. Bd. VII,* edited by K. von Bardeleben, pp. 42–64. Verlag G. Fischer, Jena.
345. Neilson, D., Jones, G. S., Woodruff, J. D., and Goldberg, B. (1970): The innervation of the ovary. *Obstet. Gynecol. Surv.*, 25:889–904.
346. Nickander, R., McMahon, F. G., and Ridolfo, A. S. (1979): Nonsteroidal antiinflammatory agents. *Annu. Rev. Pharmacol. Toxicol.*, 19:469–490.
347. Niswender, G. D., Reimers, T. J., Diekman, M. A., and Nett, T. M. (1976): Blood flow: A mediator of ovarian function. *Biol. Reprod.*, 14:64–81.
348. Norjavaara, E., Selstam, G., and Ahren, K. (1982): Catecholamine stimulation of cyclic AMP and progesterone production in the rat corpora lutea of different ages. *Acta Endocrinol. (Copenh.),* 100:613–622.
349. Novy, M. J., and Cook, M. J. (1973): Redistribution of blood flow by prostaglandin F_2 in the rabbit ovary. *Am. J. Obstet. Gynecol.*, 117:381–385.
350. Nowacki, R. (1977): Das zeitgenossische Bild desreifen ovarialfollikels der Saugetiere. *Zbl. Vet. Med. C Anat. Hist. Embryol.*, 6:217–239.
351. Ny, T., Bjersing, L., Hsueh, A. J. W., and Loskutoff, D. J. (1985): Cultured granulosa cells produce two plasminogen activators, each regulated by gonadotropins. *Endocrinology,* 116:1666–1668.
352. Odin, L. (1959): Studies on the chemistry of ovarian cyst contents. *Acta Soc. Med. Upsala,* 64:25–91.
353. O'Grady, J. P., Caldwell, B. V., Auletta, F. J., and Speroff, L. (1972): The effects of an inhibitor of prostaglandin synthesis (indomethacin) on ovulation, pregnancy and pseudopregnancy in the rabbit. *Prostaglandins,* 1:97–106.
354. Ohlsson, K. (1980): Polymorphonuclear leucocyte collagenase. In: *Collagenase in Normal and Pathological Connective Tissues,* edited by D. E. Woolley and J. M. Evanson, pp. 209–222. John Wiley & Sons, New York.
355. Ohno, Y., and Mori, T. (1985): Correlation between progesterone and plasminogen activator in rat ovaries during the ovulatory process. *Acta Obstet. Gynaecol. Jpn.*, 37:247–256.
356. Ojeda, S. R., White, S. S., Aguado, L. I., and Andersen, J. M. (1983): Abdominal vagotomy delays the onset of puberty and inhibits ovarian function in the female rat. *Neuroendocrinology,* 36:261–267.
357. Okamura, H., Okazaki, T., and Nakajima, A. (1974): Human ovarian contractility in vitro. *Acta Obstet. Gynecol. Jpn.*, 21:89–96.
358. Okamura, H., Okazaki, T., and Nakajima, A. (1974): Effects of neurotransmitters and prostaglandins on human ovarian contractility. *Obstet. Gynecol.*, 44:720–726.
359. Okamura, H., Takenaka, A., Yajima, Y., and Nishimura, T. (1980): Ovulatory changes in the wall at the apex of the human Graafian follicle. *J. Reprod. Fertil.*, 58:153–155.
360. Okamura, H., Virutamasen, P., Wright, K. H., and Wallach, E. E. (1972): Ovarian smooth muscle in the human being, rabbit, and cat. *Am. J. Obstet. Gynecol.*, 112:183–191.
361. Okamura, H., Okuda, Y., Kanzaki, H., Takenaka, A., Morimoto, K., and Nishimura, T. (1981): Ultrastructural observation of the ovulatory changes in the capillary of the human follicular apex. *Acta Obstet. Gynecol. Jpn.*, 33:215–221.
362. Okazaki, T., Okamura, H., and Nishimura, T. (1973): Collagenolytic activity in rat ovary during ovulation. *Acta Obstet. Gynecol. Jpn.*, 20:112–117.
363. Okuda, Y. (1983): An ultrastructural study on capillary permeability of the rabbit ovarian follicles during ovulation. *J. Clin. Electron Microsc.*, 16:117–134.
364. Okuda, Y., Okamura, H., Kanzaki, H., and Takenaka, A. (1983): Capillary permeability of rabbit ovarian follicles prior to ovulation. *J. Anat.*, 137:263–269.
365. Okuda, Y., Okamura, H., Kanzaki, H., Takenaka, A., Morimoto, K., and Nishimura, T. (1980): An ultrastructural study of capillaries of rabbit follicles during ovulatory process. *Acta Obstet. Gynecol. Jpn.*, 32:739–748.
366. Okuda, Y., Okamura, H., Kanzaki, H., Takenaka, A., Morimoto, K., and Nishimura, T. (1980): An ultrastructural study of capillary permeability of rabbit follicles during ovulation using carbon traces. *Acta Obstet. Gynecol. Jpn.*, 32:859–867.
367. Okuda, Y., Okamura, H., Kanzaki, H., Takenaka, H., Morimoto, K., and Nishimura, T. (1982): An ultrastructural study of capillary permeability of rabbit ovarian follicles using horse radish peroxidase as a tracer. *Acta Obstet. Gynecol. Jpn.*, 34:181–186.
368. Okuda, Y., Okamura, H., Kanzaki, H., Fujii, S., Takenaka, A., and Wallach, E. E. (1983): An ultrastructural study of ovarian perifollicular capillaries in the indomethacin-treated rabbit. *Fertil. Steril.*, 39:85–92.
369. O'Shea, J. D. (1970): An ultrastructural study of smooth muscle-like cells in the theca externa of ovarian follicles in the rat. *Anat. Rec.*, 167:127–140.
370. O'Shea, J. D. (1971): Smooth muscle-like cells in the theca externa of ovarian follicles in the sheep. *J. Reprod. Fertil.*, 24:283–285.
371. O'Shea, J. D. (1981): Structure-function relationships in the wall of the ovarian follicle. *Aust. J. Biol. Sci.*, 34:379–394.
372. O'Shea, J. D., Cran, D. G., Hay, M. F., and Moor, R. M. (1978): Ultrastructure of the theca interna of ovarian follicles in sheep. *Cell Tissue Res.*, 187:457–472.
373. O'Shea, J. D., and Phillips, R. E. (1974): Contractility in vitro of ovarian follicles from sheep, and the effects of drugs. *Biol. Reprod.*, 10:370–379.
374. Ossowski, L., Biegel, O., and Reich, E. (1979): Mammary plasminogen activator: Correlation with involution, hormonal modulation and comparison between normal and neoplastic tissues. *Cell,* 16:929–940.
375. Osterholzer, H. O., Johnson, J. H., and Nicosia, S. V. (1985): An autoradiographic study of rabbit ovarian surface epithelium before and after ovulation. *Biol. Reprod.*, 53:729–738.
376. Osterman, J., and Hammond, J. M. (1978): Prostaglandin stimulation of ovarian ornithine decarboxylase EC-4.1.1.17 *in vitro. Biochem. Biophys Res. Commun.*, 83:794–799.
377. Osvaldo-Decima, L. (1970): Smooth muscle in the ovary of the rat and monkey. *J. Ultrastruct. Res.*, 29:218–237.
378. Owman, C., Rosengren, E., and Sjoberg, N. O. (1967): Adrenergic innervation of the human female reproductive organs: A histochemical and chemical investigation. *Obstet. Gynecol.*, 30:763–773.
379. Owman, C., Sjoberg, N. O., Svensson, K. G., and Walles, B. (1975): Autonomic nerves mediating contractility in the human graafian follicle. *J. Reprod. Fertil.*, 45:553–556.

380. Owman, C., Sjoberg, N. O., Wallach, E. E., Walles, B., and Wright, K. H. (1979): Neuromuscular mechanisms of ovulation. In: *Human Ovulation: Mechanisms, Prediction, Detection and Regulation*, edited by E. S. E. Hafez, pp. 57–100. Elsevier/North Holland, Amsterdam.
381. Palla, V. (1952): Azione del solfata di protamina sulla sostanza eparinosimile del liquor folliculi. *Minerva Ginecol.*, 4:164–174.
382. Palotie, A., Peltenen, L., Foidart, J. M., and Rajaniemi, H. (1984): Immunohistochemical localization of basement membrane components and interstitial collagen types in preovulatory rat ovarian follicles. *Coll. Relat. Res.*, 4:279–287.
383. Palti, Z., and Freund, M. (1972): Spontaneous contractions of the human ovary in vitro. *J. Reprod. Fertil.*, 28:113–115.
384. Panganamala, R. V., Miller, J. S., Gwebu, E. T., Sharma, H. M., and Cornwell, D. G. (1977): Differential inhibitory effects of vitamin E and other antioxidants on prostaglandin synthetase, platelet aggregation and lipoxidase. *Prostaglandins*, 14:261–271.
385. Parr, E. L. (1974): Histological examination of the rat ovarian follicle wall prior to ovulation. *Biol. Reprod.*, 11:483–503.
386. Parr, E. L. (1975): Rupture of ovarian follicles at ovulation. *J. Reprod. Fertil. (Suppl.)*, 22:1–22.
387. Pascu, T., Tudorascu, R., Stancioiu, N., and Lunca, H. (1971): Concentration des proteines totales et des fractions proteiques dans le liquide folliculaire normal, pendant les differentes phases due cycle oestral, et dans le liquide des kystes folicularies ovariens, ainse que dans le sang des mimes vaches. *Recl. Med. Vet.*, 147:979–991.
388. Patwardhan, V. V., and Lanthier, A. (1981): Prostaglandin E and prostaglandin F in human ovarian follicles: Endogenous contents and *in-vitro* formation by theca and granulosa cells. *Acta Endocrinol.*, 97:543–550.
389. Pendergrass, P. B. (1980): Ultrastructural comparison of smooth muscle from ovarian follicle and oviduct of the golden hamster. *Cell Tissue Res.*, 209:43–48.
390. Pendergrass, P. B., and Reber, M. (1980): Scanning electron microscopy of the Graafian follicle during ovulation in the golden hamster. *J. Reprod. Fertil.*, 59:21–24.
391. Pendergrass, P. B., and Talbot, P. (1979): The distribution of contractile cells in the apex of the preovulatory hamster follicle. *Biol. Reprod.*, 20:205–213.
392. Penkala, J. E., and Talbot, P. (1984): Inhibitors of proteinase activity block in vivo ovulation in the golden hamster. *J. Cell Biol.*, 99:391 (abstract).
393. Peracchia, C. (1980): Structural correlates of gap junction permeation. *Int. Rev. Cytol.*, 66:81–146.
394. Peracchia, C. (1984): Communicating junctions and calmodulin: Inhibition of electrical uncoupling in Xenopus embryo by calmidazolium. *Membr. Biol.*, 81:49–58.
395. Perklev, T., and Ahren, K. (1971): Effects of prostaglandins, LH and polyphloretin phosphate on the lactic acid production of the prepubertal rat ovary. *Life Sci.*, 10:1387–1393.
396. Perloff, W. H., Schultz, J., Farris, E., and Balin, H. (1955): Some aspects of the chemical nature of human ovarian follicular fluid. *Fertil. Steril.*, 6:11–17.
397. Peters, H. (1969): The development of the ovary from birth to maturity. *Acta Endocrinol. (Copenh.).*, 62:98–116.
398. Pettigrew, D. V., Ho, G. H., Sodek, J., Brunette, D. M., and Wang, H. M. (1978): Effect of oxygen tension and indomethacin on production of collagenase and neutral proteinase enzymes and their latent forms by porcine gingival explants in culture. *Arch. Oral Biol.*, 23:767–777.
399. Pfluger, E. (1857): Ueber die Bewegungen der Ovarien. *Arch. Anat. Physiol. Wissensch. Med.*, 1:30–32.
400. Pfluger, E. F. W. (1863): *Ueber die Eierstocke der Saugethiere und des Menschen*. W. Englemann, Leipzig.
401. Piacsek, B. E., and Huth, J. F. (1971): Changes in ovarian venous blood flow following cannulation: Effect of luteinizing hormone (LH) and antihistamine. *Proc. Soc. Exp. Biol. Med.*, 138:1022–1024.
402. Plunkett, E. R., Moon, Y. S., Zamecnik, J., and Armstrong, D. (1975): Preliminary evidence of a role for prostaglandin F in human follicular function. *Am. J. Obstet. Gynecol.*, 123:391–397.
403. Pool, W. R., and Lipner, H. (1965): Inhibition of ovulation in the rabbit by actinomycin D. *Nature*, 203:1385–1387.
404. Pool, W. R., and Lipner, H. (1966): Inhibition of ovulation by antibiotics. *Endocrinology*, 79:858–864.
405. Poyser, N. L., and Scott, F. M. (1980): Prostaglandin and thromboxyane production by the rat uterus and ovary in vitro during the estrous cycle. *J. Reprod. Fertil.*, 60:33–40.
406. Priedkalns, J., Weber, A. F., and Zemjanis, R. (1968): Qualitative and quantitative morphological studies of the cells of the membranosa, theca interna and corpus luteum of the bovine ovary. *Z. Zellforsch.*, 85:501–520.
407. Ramwell, P. W., Shaw, J. E., and Jessup, S. J. (1969): Follicular fluid kinin and its action on fallopian tube. *Endocrinology*, 84:931–936.
408. Rand, M. J., and Trinker, F. R. (1966): Pharmacological agents affecting the release and activity of catecholamines. *Br. J. Anaesth.*, 38:666–689.
409. Ratner, A., Weiss, G. R., and Sanborn, C. R. (1980): Stimulation by B_2-adrenergic receptors of the production of cyclic AMP and progesterone in rat ovarian tissue. *J. Endocrinol.*, 87:123–129.
410. Rawson, J. M., and Espey, L. L. (1977): Concentration of electron dense granules in the rabbit ovarian surface epithelium during ovulation. *Biol. Reprod.*, 17:561–566.
411. Reich, R., Miskin, R., and Tsafriri, A. (1985): Follicular plasminogen activator: Involvement in ovulation. *Endocrinology*, 116:516–521.
412. Reich, R., Tsafriri, A., and Mechanic, G. L. (1985): The involvement of collagenolysis in ovulation in the rat. *Endocrinology*, 116:522–527.
413. Reich, R., Kohen, F., Naor, Z., and Tsafriri, A. (1983): Possible involvement of lipoxygenase products of arachidonic acid pathway in ovulation. *Prostaglandins*, 26:1011–1020.
414. Reich, R., Kohen, F., Slager, R., and Tsafriri, A. (1985): Ovarian lipoxygenase activity and its regulation by gonadotropin in the rat. *Prostaglandins*, 30:581–590.
415. Retzius, G. (1893): Ueber die Nerven der Ovarium und Hoden. *Biol. Untersuch.*, 5:31–34.
416. Reynolds, S. R. M. (1973): Blood and lymph vascular systems of the ovary. In: *Handbook of Physiology, Vol. II*, Section 7, pp. 261–316, American Physiological Society, Washington, D.C.
417. Riese, H. (1891): Die feinsten Nervenfasern und ihre Endigungen in Ovarium der Saugethiere und des Menschen. *Anat. Anz.*, 6:400–420.
418. Rigby, B. W., Ling, S. Y., and Ledwitz-Rigby, F. L. (1983): In search of the elusive follicular fluid factors. In: *Factors Regulating Ovarian Function*, edited by G. S. Greenwald and P. F. Terranova, pp. 179–183. Raven Press, New York.
419. Roca, R., Garofalo, E., Piriz, H., Martino, I., Rieppi, G., and Sala, M. (1976): Effects of oxytocin on *in vitro* ovarian contractility during the estrous cycle of the rat. *Biol. Reprod.*, 15:464–466.
420. Rocerto, T., Jacobowitz, D. and Wallach, E. (1969): Observations of spontaneous contractions of the cat ovary *in vitro*. *Endocrinology*, 84:1336–1341.
421. Rondell, P. (1964): Follicular pressure and distensibility. *Am. J. Physiol.*, 207:590–594.
422. Rondell, P. (1970): Biophysical aspects of ovulation. *Biol. Reprod. Suppl.*, 2:64–89.
423. Rosenfeld, C. R., Morriss, F. H., Jr., Battaglia, F. C., Mokowski, E. L., and Mescha, G. (1976): Effect of estradiol-17β on blood flow to reproductive and nonreproductive tissues in pregnant ewes. *Am. J. Obstet. Gynecol.*, 124:618–629.
424. Rosengren, E., and Sjoberg, M. O. (1967): The adrenergic nerve supply to the female reproductive tract of the cat. *Am. J. Anat.*, 121:271–284.
425. Rouget, C. (1858): Recherches sur les organes erectiles de la femme et sur l'appareil musculataire tubo ovarien dans luvs rapports avec l'ovulation et la menstruation. *J. Physiol. (Paris)*, 1:320–343.
426. Sato, T., Taya, K., Jyiyo, T., and Igarashi, M. (1974): Ovulation block by indomethacin, an inhibitor of prostaglandin synthesis: A study of its site of action in rats. *J. Reprod. Fertil.*, 39: 33–40.
427. Schmidt, G., Owman, C., Sjoberg, N. O., and Walles, B. (1985): Influence of adrenoreceptor agonists and antagonists on ovulation in the rabbit ovary perfused in vitro. *J. Auton. Pharmacol.*, 5:241–250.
428. Schochet, S. S. (1916): A suggestion as to the process of ovulation and ovarian cyst formation. *Anat. Rec.* 10:447–457.
429. Schröder, R. (1930): Weibliche Genitalorgane. In: *Handbuch mikroanatomische des Menschen. Vol. II*, edited by W. von Mollendorff, pp. 1–329. Springer-Verlag, Berlin.

430. Schroeder, P. C., and Talbot, P. (1982): Intrafollicular pressure decreases in hamster preovulatory follicles during smooth muscle cell contraction *in vitro*. *J. Exp. Zool.*, 224:417–426.
431. Schwartz, N. B., and Channing, C. P. (1977): Evidence for ovarian inhibin: Suppression of the secondary rise in serum follicle stimulating hormone levels in proestrous rats by injection of porcine follicular fluid. *Proc. Natl. Acad. Sci. USA*, 74:5721–5724.
432. Schwartz, N. B., and McCormack, C. E. (1972): Reproduction: Gonadal function and its regulation. *Annu. Rev. Physiol.*, 34:425–472.
433. Semenova, I. I. (1969): Adrenergic innervation and distribution of cholinesterases in the human ovary. *Bull. Eksp. Biol. Med.*, 68:103–106.
434. Shalgi, R., Kaplan, R., and Kraicer, P. F. (1977): Proteins of follicular, bursal and ampullar fluids of rats. *Biol. Reprod.*, 17:333–338.
435. Shalgi, R., Kraicer, P. F., and Soferman, N. (1972): Gases and electrolytes of human follicular fluid. *J. Reprod. Fertil.*, 28:335–340.
436. Shalgi, R., Kraicer, P. G., and Soferman, N. (1972): Human follicular fluid. *J. Reprod. Fertil.*, 31:515–516.
437. Shalgi, R., Kraicer, P., Rimon, A., Pinto, M., and Soferman, N. (1973): Proteins of human follicular fluid: The blood-follicle barrier. *Fertil. Steril.*, 24:429–434.
438. Shepro, D., Schleef, R., and Hecktman, H. B. (1980): Plasminogen activator activity by cultured bovine aortic endothelial cells. *Life Sci.* 26:415–422.
439. Shimada, H., Okamura, H., Nada, Y., Suzuki, A., Tojo, S., and Takada, A. (1983): Plasminogen activator in rat ovary during the ovulatory process: Independence of prostaglandin mediation. *J. Endocrinol.*, 97:201–205.
440. Shivers, C. A., Metz, C. B., and Lutwak-Mann, C. (1964): Some properties of pig follicular fluid. *J. Reprod. Fertil.*, 8:115–120.
441. Simpson, E. R., Rochelle, D. B., Carr, B. R., Macdonald, P. C., Cecil, H., and Green, J. (1980): Plasma lipoproteins in follicular fluid of human ovaries. *J. Clin. Endocrinol. Metab.*, 51:1469–1471.
442. Sjoberg, N. O. (1968): Increase in transmitter content of adrenergic nerves in the reproductive tract of female rabbits after oestrogen treatment. *Acta Endocrinol.*, 57:405–413.
443. Skinner, M. K., McKeracher, H. L., and Dorrington, J. H. (1985): Fibronectin as a marker of granulosa cell cytodifferentiation. *Endocrinology*, 117:886–892.
444. Smith, J. T. (1934): Some observations on the rupture of the Graafian follicles in rabbits. *Am. J. Obstet. Gynecol.*, 27:728–730.
445. Smith, J. T. (1937): Rupture of Graafian follicles. *Am. J. Obstet. Gynecol.*, 33:820–827.
446. Sporrong, B., Kannisto, P., Owman, C., Sjoberg, N. O., and Walles, B. (1985): Histochemistry and ultrastructure of adrenergic and acetylcholinesterase-containing nerves supplying follicles and endocrine cells in the guinea pig ovary. *Cell Tissue Res.*, 240: 505–511.
447. Stangroom, J. E., and Weevers, R. deG. (1962): Anticoagulant activity of equine follicular fluid. *J. Reprod. Fertil.*, 3:269–282.
448. Starke, K. (1979): Presynaptic regulation of release in the central nervous system. In: *The Release of Catecholamines from Adrenergic Neurons*, edited by D. M. Paton, pp. 143–184. Pergamon Press, New York.
449. Stefenson, A., Owman, C. M., Sjoberg, N. O., Sporrong, B., and Walles, B. (1981): Comparative study of the autonomic innervation of the mammalian ovary with particular regard to the follicular system. *Cell Tissue Res.*, 215:47–62.
450. Sterin-Borda, L., Borda, E., Gimeno, M. F., and Gimeno, A. L. (1976): Spontaneous and prostaglandin or oxytocin induced motility of rat ovaries isolated during different stages of the estrous cycle: Effects of norepinephrine. *Fertil. Steril.*, 27:319–327.
451. Stjernquist, M., Emson, P., Owman, C., Sjoberg, N. O., Sundler, F., and Tatemoto, K. (1983): Neuropeptide Y in the female reproductive tract of the rat. Distribution of nerve fibers and motor effects. *Neurosci. Lett.*, 39:279–284.
452. Strickland, S., and Beers, W. H. (1976): Studies on the role of plasminogen activator in ovulation. *In vitro* response of granulosa cells to gonadotropins, cyclic nucleotides and prostaglandins. *J. Biol. Chem.*, 251:5694–5702.
453. Strickland, S., Reich, E., and Sherman, M. I. (1976): Plasminogen activator in early embryogenesis. Enzyme production by trophoblast and parietal endoderm. *Cell*, 9:231–240.
454. Strulovici, B., Lindner, H. R., Shinitzky, M., and Zor, U. (1981): Elevation of apparent membrane viscosity in ovarian cells by follicle stimulating hormone. *Biochim. Biophys. Acta*, 640: 159–168.
455. Sun, F. F., Chapman, J. P., and McGuire, J. C. (1977): Metabolism of prostaglandin endoperoxide in animal tissues. *Prostaglandins*, 14:1055–1074.
456. Svensjo, E., and Grega, G. J. (1986): Evidence for endothelial cell-mediated regulation of macromolecular permeability by post-capillary venules. *Fed. Proc.*, 45:89–95.
457. Svensson, K. G., Owman, C., Sjoberg, N.-O., Sporrong, B., and Walles, B. (1975): Ultrastructural evidence for adrenergic innervation of the interstitial gland in the guinea pig ovary. *Neuroendocrinology*, 17:40–47.
458. Swanson, R. J., and Lipner, H. (1977): Mechanism of ovulation: Effect of intrafollicular progesterone antiserum. *Fed. Proc.*, 36:390 (abstract).
459. Sweet, L. K., and Thorp, E. G. (1929): The effect of lower abdominal sympathectomy on the estrous cycle. *Am. J. Physiol.*, 89:50–53.
460. Symons, D. B. A., and Herbert, J. (1971): Incidence of immunoglobulins in fluids of the rabbit tracts and the distribution of IgG-globulin in the tissues of the female tract. *J. Reprod. Fertil.*, 24:55–62.
461. Szego, C. M. (1965): Role of histamine in mediation of hormone action. *Fed. Proc.*, 24:1343–1352.
462. Szego, C. M., and Giten, E. S. (1964): Ovarian histamine depletion during acute hyperaemic response to luteinizing hormone. *Nature*, 201:682–684.
463. Talbot, P., and Chacon, R. S. (1982): *In vitro* ovulation of hamster oocytes depends on contraction of follicular smooth muscle cells. *J. Exp. Zool.*, 224:409–415.
464. Talbot, P., and Schroeder, P. C. (1982): 5-Hydroxytryptamine causes contraction of smooth muscle cells in preovulatory hamster follicles. *J. Exp. Zool.*, 224:427–436.
465. Tam, W. H., and Roy, R. J. (1982): A possible role of prostaglandin F-2-α in the development of ovarian follicle in guinea pigs. *J. Reprod. Fertil.*, 66:277–282.
466. Thomson, A. (1919): The ripe human Graafian follicle, together with some suggestions as to its mode of rupture. *J. Anat.*, 54:1–40.
467. Thorsoe, H. (1962): Hexuronic acid, hexosamine and radiosulphate uptake in ovaries of myxoedematous rabbits. *Acta Endocrinol. (Copenh.)*, 41:613–618.
468. Tjugum, J., Norstrom, A., and Dennefors, B. (1983): Influence of prostaglandin E_2 on proteoglycan synthesis in the human ovarian follicle wall. *Prostaglandins*, 25:71–77.
469. Too, C. K. L., Weiss, T. J., and Bryant-Greenwood, G. D. (1982): Relaxin stimulates plasminogen activator secretion by rat granulosa cells *in vitro*. *Endocrinology*, 111:1424–1426.
470. Too, C. K. L., Bryant-Greenwood, G. D., and Greenwood, F. C. (1984): Relaxin increases the release of plasminogen activator, collagenase and proteoglycanase from rat granulosa cells *in vitro*. *Endocrinology*, 115:1043–1050.
471. Tranzer, J. P., and Thoenen, H. (1968): An electron microscopic study of selective acute degeneration of sympathetic nerve terminals after administration of 6-hydroxydopamine. *Experientia*, 24:155–156.
472. Triebwasser, W. F., Clark, M. R., LeMaire, W. J., and Marsh, J. M. (1978): Localization and *in vitro* synthesis of prostaglandins in components of rabbit preovulatory Graafian follicles. *Prostaglandins*, 16:621–632.
473. Tsafriri, A., Lindner, H. R., Zor, U., and Lamprecht, S. A. (1972): Physiological role of prostaglandins in the induction of ovulation. *Prostaglandins*, 2:1–10.
474. Tsafriri, A., Lindner, H. R., Zor, U., and Lamprecht, S. A. (1972): *In vitro* induction of meiotic division in follicle-enclosed rat oocytes by LH, cyclic AMP and prostaglandin E_2. *J. Reprod. Fertil.*, 31:39–50.
475. Tsafriri, A., Koch, Y., and Lindner, H. R. (1973): Ovulation rate and serum LH levels in rats treated with indomethacin or PGE_2. *Prostaglandins*, 3:461–467.

476. Tsang, B. K., Ainsworth, L., Downey, B. R., and Armstrong, D. T. (1979): Preovulatory changes in cyclic AMP and prostaglandin concentrations in follicular fluid of gilts. *Prostaglandins,* 17:141–148.
477. Tsujimoto, D., Katayama, K., Tojo, S., and Mizoguti, H. (1982): Scanning electron microscopic studies on stigmas in rat ovaries. *Acta Obstet. Gynecol. Scand.,* 61:269–273.
478. Tuohimaa, P., and Niemi, M. (1969): Cell renewal in the ovarian follicles of the rat during the oestrous cycle and in persistent estrus. *Acta Endocrinol.,* 62:306–314.
479. Vassalli, J-D., Hamilton, J., and Reich, E. (1976): Macrophage plasminogen activator: Modulation of enzyme production by anti-inflammatory steroids, mitotic inhibitors and cyclic nucleotides. *Cell,* 8:271–281.
480. Virutamasen, P., Hickok, R. L., and Wallach, E. E. (1971): Local ovarian effects of catecholamines on human chorionic gonadotrophin-induced ovulation in the rabbit. *Fertil. Steril.,* 22:235–243.
481. Virutamasen, P., Smitarsiri, Y., and Fuchs, A. R. (1976): Intraovarian pressure changes during ovulation in rabbits. *Fertil. Steril.,* 27:188–196.
482. Virutamasen, P., Wright, K. H., and Wallach, E. E. (1972): Effects of catecholamines on ovarian contractility in the rabbit. *Obstet. Gynecol.,* 39:225–236.
483. Virutamasen, P., Wright, K. H., and Wallach, E. E. (1972): Effects of prostaglandins E_2 and $F_{2\alpha}$ on ovarian contractility in the rabbit. *Fertil. Steril.,* 23:675–682.
484. Virutamasen, P., Wright, K. H., and Wallach, E. E. (1973): Monkey ovarian contractility: Its relationship to ovulation. *Fertil. Steril.,* 24:763–771.
485. Wada, H. (1978): The biochemical and biological properties of bovine follicular fluid compared with blood serum. *Bull. Azabu Vet. Coll.,* 3:313–331.
486. Wada, H. (1981): Effects of gonadotropins steroid hormones and histamine on the blood follicle barrier of the ovary. *Med. J. Kobe Univ.,* 42:57–66.
487. Waldeyer, W. (1870): *Eierstock and Ei.* von Wilhelm Englemann, Leipzig.
488. Wallach, E. E., Wright, K. H., and Hamada, Y. (1978): Investigation of mammalian ovulation with an *in vitro* perfused rabbit ovary preparation. *Am. J. Obstet. Gynecol.,* 132:728–738.
489. Walles, B., Edvinsson, L., Falck, B., Nybell, G., Owman, C., Sjoberg, N. O., and Svensson, K. G. (1974): Modifications of ovarian and follicular contractility by amines. A mechanism involved in ovulation. *Eur. J. Obstet. Gynecol. Reprod. Bio.,* 4/1 (Suppl.): S103–S107.
490. Walles, B., Edvinsson, L., Owman, C., Sjoberg, N. O., and Svensson, K. G. (1975): Mechanical response in the wall of ovarian follicles mediated by adrenergic receptors. *J. Pharmacol. Exp. Ther.,* 193:460–473.
491. Walles, B., Edvinsson, L., Falck, B., Owman, C., Sjoberg, N. O., and Svensson, K. G. (1975): Evidence for a neuromuscular mechanism involved in the contractility of the ovarian follicular wall. Fluorescence and electron microscopy and effects of tyramine on follicle strips. *Biol. Reprod.,* 12:239–248.
492. Walles, B., Edvinsson, L., Owman, C., Sjoberg, N. O., and Sporrong, B. (1976): Cholinergic nerves and receptors mediating contraction of the graafian follicle. *Biol. Reprod.,* 15:565–572.
493. Walles, B., Falck, B., Owman, C., and Sjoberg, N. O. (1977): Characterization of autonomic receptors in the smooth musculature of human Graafian follicle. *Biol. Reprod.,* 17:423–431.
494. Walles, B., Owman, C., and Sjoberg, N. O. (1982): Contraction of the ovarian follicle induced by local stimulation of its sympathetic nerves. *Brain Res. Bull.,* 9:757–760.
495. Walton, A., and Hammond, J. (1928): Observations on ovulation in the rabbit. *J. Exp. Biol.,* 6:190–204.
496. Wang, C., and Leung, A. (1983): Gonadotropins regulate plasminogen activator production by rat granulosa cells. *Endocrinology,* 112:1201–1207.
497. Weiner, S., Wright, K. H., and Wallach, E. E. (1975): Selective ovarian sympathectomy in the rabbit. *Fertil. Steril.,* 26:353–362.
498. Weiner, S., Wright, K. H., and Wallach, E. E. (1975): Studies on the function of the denervated rabbit ovary: Human chorionic gonadotrophin-induced ovulation. *Fertil. Steril.,* 26:363–368.
499. Weiner, S., Wright, K. H., and Wallach, E. E. (1975): Lack of effect of ovarian denervation on ovulation and pregnancy in the rabbit. *Fertil. Steril.,* 26:1083–1089.
500. Weiner, S., Wright, K. H., and Wallach, E. E. (1977): The influence of ovarian denervation and nerve stimulation on ovarian contractions. *Am. J. Obstet. Gynecol.,* 128:154–160.
501. Werb, Z., Mainardi, C. L., Vater, C. A., and Harris, E. O., Jr. (1977): Endogenous activation of latent collagenase by rheumatoid synovial cells. *N. Engl. J. Med.,* 296:1017–1023.
502. White, J. C. (1943): Sensory innervation of the viscera. Studies on visceral afferent neurones in man based on neurosurgical procedures for the relief of intractable pain. *Res. Publ. Assoc. Res. Nerv. Ment. Dis.,* 23:373–390.
503. Wilhelmsson, L., Norstrom, A., and Hamberger, L. (1981): Influence of 6-keto-$PGF_{1\alpha}$ on collagen synthesis in the human cervix during various phases of the menstrual cycle. *Prostaglandins,* 22:125–130.
504. Williams, J. R. B. (1951): The fibrinolytic activity of urine. *Br. J. Exp. Pathol.,* 32:530–537.
505. von Winiwarter, H. (1910): Contribution a l'etude de l'ovarire humain. *Arch. Biol..* 25:683–755.
506. von Winiwarter, H., and Sainmont, G. (1909): Nouvelles recherches sur l'ovogenese et l'organogenese de l'ovaire des Mammiferes Chat. *Arch. Biol. (Liege),* 24:627–651.
507. Winterhalter, E. H. (1896): Ein sympathisches Ganglion in menschichen Ovarian. *Arch. Gynecol.,* 51:49–55.
508. Wischnitzer, S. (1965): The ultrastructure of the germinal epithelium of the mouse ovary. *J. Morphol.,* 117:387–400.
509. Wislocki, G. B., Bunting, H., and Dempsey, E. W. (1947): Metachromasia in mammalian tissues and its relationship to mucopolysaccharides. *Am. J. Anat.,* 81:1–37.
510. Woessner, J. F., Jr. (1982): Enzymatic mechanisms for the degradation of connective tissue matrix. In: *Symposium on Idiopathic Low Back Pain,* edited by A. White and S. L. Gordon, pp. 391–400. Mosby, St. Louis.
511. Woolley, D. E., and Evanson, J. M. (1980): Present status and future prospects in collagenase research. In: *Collagenase in Normal and Pathobiological Connective Tissues,* edited by D. E. Woolley and J. M. Evanson, pp. 241–250. John Wiley & Sons, New York.
512. Wright, K. H., Wallach, E. E., Fromm, E., and Jeutter, D. C. (1976): Studies of rabbit ovarian contractility using chronically implanted transducers. *Fertil. Steril.* 27:310–318.
513. Wurtman, R. J. (1964): An effect of luteinizing hormone on the fractional perfusion of the rat ovary. *Endocrinology,* 75:927–933.
514. Yanagishita, M., and Hascal, V. C. (1979): Biosynthesis of proteoglycans by rat granulosa cells cultured *in vitro. J. Biol. Chem.,* 254:12355–12364.
515. Yanagishita, M., Rodbard, D., and Hascal, V. C. (1979): Isolation and characterization of proteoglycans from porcine ovarian follicular fluid. *J. Biol. Chem.,* 254:911–920.
516. Yanagishita, M., Hascal, V. C., and Rodbard, D. (1981): Biosynthesis of proteoglycans by rat granulosa cells cultured *in vitro*: Modulation by gonadotropins, steroid hormones prostaglandins, steroid hormones, and prostaglandins and a cyclic nucleotide. *Endocrinology,* 109:1641–1649.
517. Yang, N. S. T., Marsh, J. M., and LeMaire, W. J. (1973): Prostaglandin changes induced by ovulatory stimuli in rabbit Graafian follicles. The effect of indomethacin. *Prostaglandins,* 4:395–404.
518. Zachariae, F. (1957): Studies on the mechanism of ovulation: Autoradiographic investigations on the uptake of radioactive sulphate (^{35}S) into the ovarian mucopolysaccharides. *Acta Endocrinol. (Copenh.),* 26:215–223.
519. Zachariae, F. (1958): Studies on the mechanism of ovulation. Permeability of the blood-liquor barrier. *Acta Endocrinol.,* 27:339–342.
520. Zachariae, F., and Jensen, C. E. (1958): Studies on the mechanism of ovulation. Histochemical and physico-chemical investigations on genuine follicular fluids. *Acta Endocrinol.,* 27:343–355.
521. Zoller, L. C., and Weisz, J. (1979): A quantitative cytochemical study of glucose-6-phosphate dehydrogenase and Δ^5-3β-hydroxysteroid dehydrogenase activity in membrana granulosa of the ovulable type of follicle of the rat. *Histochemistry,* 62:125–132.

522. Zoller, L. C., and Weisz, J. (1980): A demonstration of regional differences in lysosome membrane permeability in the membrana granulosa of Graafian follicles in cryostat sections of the rat ovary: A quantitative cytochemical study. *Endocrinology,* 106:871–877.
523. Zondek, B., Sulman, F., and Black, R. (1945): The hyperemia effect of gonadotropins on the ovary. *J. Am. Med. Assoc.,* 128: 939–944.
524. Zor, U., Strulovici, B., Braw, R., Lindner, H. R., and Tsafriri, A. (1983): FSH induced prostaglandin E formation in isolated rat ovarian theca. *J. Endocrinol.,* 97:43–50.
525. Zsolmar, B., Varga, B., and Horvath, E. (1982): Increase of ovarian progesterone secretion by B_2-adrenergic stimulation in oestrous rats. *Acta Endocrinol. (Copenh.),* 101:268–272.
526. McCaig, C. D. (1985): A potential difference across mouse ovarian follicle. *Experientia* 41:609–611.

The Physiology of Reproduction, edited by E. Knobil and J. Neill *et al.* Raven Press, Ltd., New York © 1988.

CHAPTER 13

The Corpus Luteum and Its Control

Gordon D. Niswender and Terry M. Nett

The corpus luteum is a transient endocrine organ formed from cells of the follicle following ovulation (Fig. 1). That the corpus luteum is required for a successful pregnancy was first discovered early in the twentieth century by Frankel (1), who found that pregnancy in rabbits was terminated following removal of corpora lutea. Similar findings have since been reported in many different species of mammals. Even though the requirement for the corpus luteum during normal pregnancy was documented in 1903, the nature of the substance that the corpus luteum produced to maintain pregnancy remained unknown for some two decades. In 1929, Allen and Corner (2) showed that a lipoidal extract of the corpus luteum could maintain pregnancy in rabbits ovariectomized a few days after mating. The component in the extract responsible for the maintenance of pregnancy was subsequently called progesterone. Its purification and crystallization was first achieved in the laboratory of Allen and Wintersteiner in 1934 (3). Since that time, there has been a major interest in understanding the factors that regulate the life span and function of the corpus luteum. Development of methods to limit the function of this gland should have a major effect on limiting reproduction in humans, rodents and pet animals. In addition, 25% to 55% of all mammalian embryos are lost during early gestation and much of this loss appears to be due to inadequate luteal function. Development of procedures to prevent this loss would have a dramatic impact on increasing the production of food animals.

The authors thank Dr. Heywood Sawyer for the electron micrographs and Ms. Kathy Miller for typing this manuscript.

BIOLOGICAL FUNCTIONS OF PROGESTERONE

The primary function of the corpus luteum is to secrete progesterone. Progesterone has several biological effects on target tissues in the reproductive system to prepare them for support of pregnancy or to provide nourishment to the conceptus. The following is a brief description of the general effects of progesterone on the reproductive organs of the female during the estrous cycle and in early pregnancy. It is not intended to provide a comparative description of the actions of progesterone in a variety of species.

Reproductive Tract

A primary target for progesterone is the mucosal lining of the genital tract. For progesterone to affect the genital tract, the cells must first have been exposed to estradiol, which induces the formation of receptors for progesterone (4). Estrogens act on the oviductal epithelium to promote growth and proliferation of the cells and to induce ciliogenesis. Following ovulation, cilitated cells in the fimbriated end of the oviduct appear to direct the ovum and associated cumulus cells into the infundibulum and then downward toward the ampulla. Together, estrogen and progesterone also regulate contractions of the oviduct that influence the rate of transport of the ovum to the uterus (5). These con-

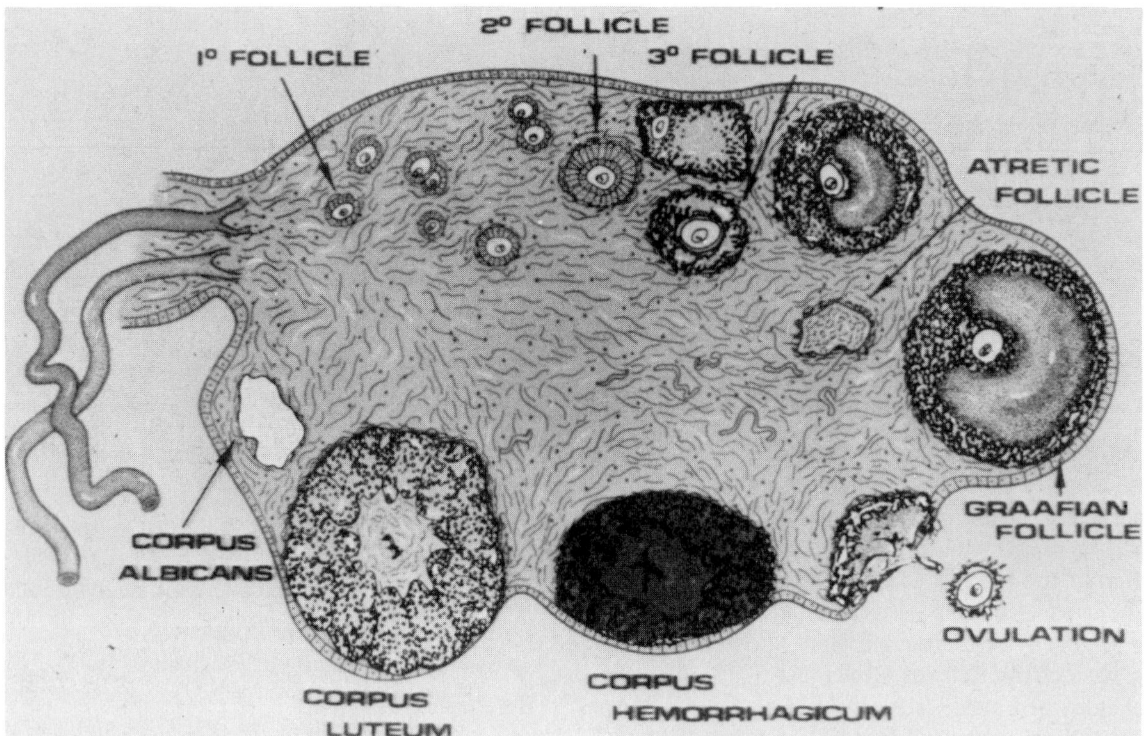

FIG. 1. Composite diagram of the mammalian ovary. Progressive stages in follicular growth and development are depicted. The primary (1°) follicle has a single layer of granulosal cells surrounding the ovum. The secondary (2°) follicle has multiple layers of granulosal cells, and the theca layers begin to differentiate. The tertiary (3°) follicle has fully developed granulosal, theca interna, and theca externa layers, and an antrum has formed and filled with follicular fluid. The Graafian, or ovulatory, follicle continues to grow until ovulation occurs. The cavity of the ovulated follicle fills with blood (the corpus hemorrhagicum) and the corpus luteum develops after a number of morphological and biochemical changes that are described in the text.

tractions are coordinated in a manner that results in the delivery of the conceptus to the uterus at an appropriate time. Progesterone contributes to the secretory activity of the oviductal epithelium to induce the secretion of a fluid that supports the early development of the conceptus. Progesterone also appears to induce regression of the oviductal epithelium, which is characterized by a sloughing of the apical portion of the epithelial cells (6).

One of the most significant actions of progesterone is to prepare the uterus for pregnancy. The uterine mucosa is composed of a surface layer of columnar epithelial cells overlying a stroma composed of spindle-shaped cells permeated by blood vessels. Numerous glands permeate the surface layer and dip into the stroma. These glands are lined by columnar epithelial cells, some of which are ciliated, whereas others are nonciliated and appear to be secretory. Under the influence of estradiol, the uterine mucosa thickens due to mitotic proliferation of the epithelium and stroma, and the tubular glands lengthen but remain straight. Nuclei in the epithelial cells tend to be located near the center of the cells. Progesterone, secreted by the developing corpus luteum, inhibits cell division, induces a marked coiling of the glands, and increases the vascularity of the stroma substantially (7). There is a dramatic reduction in cell proliferation and an increase in glycogen content of the epithelial cells. The nuclei of the epithelial cells become more basally oriented and their cytoplasm becomes vacuolar. These changes prepare the endometrial cells to provide nourishment and support to the conceptus until attachment (or implantation) and placentation occurs. In many species, progesterone also acts on the cells of the myometrium to block organized contractions.

During nonfertile cycles, the progestational endometrium undergoes deterioration when serum levels of progesterone decrease as the corpus luteum ceases to function. Although the uteri of all species undergo regressive changes as serum levels of progesterone fall, it is most dramatic in primates, in which the lining of the uterus actually is sloughed and results in menstruation.

Under the influence of estrogen, the cervix secretes a mucus rich in glycoprotein that appears to align in filaments, facilitating passage of sperm through the cervical canal. Under the influence of progesterone, the consistency of the cervical mucus changes and becomes highly viscous. The glycoprotein filaments form networks that impede passage of materials either into or out of the uterus. Thus, when circulating levels of progesterone are high, the cervix provides an effective barrier between the uterus and the external environment (7).

Estrogens promote proliferation and cornification of the

vaginal epithelium. As the vaginal epithelium thickens, the superficial layers are not close to blood vessels; this leads to keratinization and loss of nuclei. These cells are then sloughed off. This trend is reversed by progesterone. Under the influence of progesterone, the vaginal epithelium thins and is characterized by small nucleated cells. The thinness of the vaginal epithelium allows escape of leukocytes, which may appear in vaginal smears from animals under the influence of progesterone. These changes have been most completely characterized in rodents (8) and dogs (9) but occur to a lesser extent in other species as well.

Mammary Gland

Besides its effects on the female reproductive tract, progesterone also acts to promote lobuloalveolar development of the mammary glands. In order for progesterone to be effective in this regard, the mammary gland must have been exposed to estrogen, and anterior pituitary hormones must also be present, i.e., progesterone alone has little, if any, effect on mammary tissue (10). Progesterone receptors are present in the mammary gland, but little is known concerning their role in the regulation of mammary gland growth or lactogenesis. During estrous (or menstrual) cycles, progesterone appears to have little effect on mammary gland growth. However, during the prolonged secretion of progesterone that occurs during pregnancy, there is considerable development of the lobuloalveolar system. The extent to which this development can be credited to progesterone versus that which is due to stimulation by placental lactogen and prolactin has not been resolved.

Hypothalamus and Anterior Pituitary Gland

Under the influence of estradiol during the follicular phase of the cycle, gonadotropin secretion is characterized by decreasing serum concentrations of follicle-stimulating hormone (FSH) and increasing concentrations of luteinizing hormone (LH) in most species. The increasing baseline concentrations of LH result from secretion of low-amplitude, high-frequency pulses of LH during the follicular phase of the cycle (11–14). During the luteal phase of the cycle, when serum levels of progesterone are elevated, the pattern of gonadotropin secretion changes dramatically. Pulses of LH are infrequent and are of higher amplitude than those observed during the follicular phase of the cycle. This appears to be due to a direct influence of progesterone on the "gonadotropin-releasing hormone pulse generator" in the hypothalamus. Secretion of FSH is not greatly affected by progesterone. As a result, in those species in which the corpus luteum does not secrete estradiol the secretion of FSH is rather stable at a relatively high baseline during the luteal phase of the cycle. In primates the corpus luteum secretes estradiol, and basal concentrations of FSH remain suppressed during the luteal phase and do not increase until after regression of the corpus luteum (13,15).

Other Hormones Produced by the Corpus Luteum

In addition to progesterone, the corpus luteum also secretes a variety of other hormones. In primates, the corpus luteum is a source of estrogens, but this does not appear to be the case in most other species. In several species, including human (16), pig (17), and rat (18), the corpus luteum produces relaxin. The function of ovarian relaxin is unclear. It may act synergistically with estrogen and progesterone to prepare the endometrium for implantation and development of the blood supply to the conceptus in primates. Near term, several changes in the birth canal that are required for parturition are induced by relaxin; however, in most species the fetoplacental unit appears to be the major source of relaxin in late gestation. Corpora lutea from a variety of species also contain oxytocin (19,20). The biological function of luteal oxytocin is unknown, but an involvement in luteolysis has been suggested (21). There is also evidence that the corpus luteum from some species, particularly primates, can secrete the prostaglandin $PGF_{2\alpha}$ (22,23).

FORMATION OF THE CORPUS LUTEUM

Morphological Changes Associated with Luteinization

Formation of the corpus luteum is initiated by a series of morphological and biochemical changes in the cells of the theca interna and membrana granulosa of the preovulatory follicle. This is termed luteinization. These changes occur as a result of the dramatic increases in serum levels of LH associated with the preovulatory surge of this hormone.

The most complete description of the morphological changes associated with luteinization in the rat is that of Anderson and Little (24). Following the ovulatory stimulus, but prior to ovulation, there is hypertrophy of granulosal cells and nuclear activation. After ovulation, the basement membrane breaks down, and blood vessels from the theca interna invade the cavity of the ruptured follicle. The growth of these new vessels appears to be due to an angiogenic factor that must be secreted soon after rupture of the follicle. In rats, the number and size of gap junctions between granulosal cells increases as the follicle matures but then decreases just prior to ovulation. During luteinization, many gap junctions reappear between the developing luteal cells in rats. As will be discussed later, the presence of gap junctions between luteal cells during the reproductive cycle is not a universal phenomenon. Gonadotropic hormones appear to amplify and modulate, rather than to induce, the formation of gap junctions. The appearance of gap junctions may be dependent upon intracellular levels of cAMP (25).

Cytoplasmic projections, which are characteristic of rat

granulosal cells, are also found on luteal cells. However, the rather thin microvilli frequently seen on granulosal cells are not seen on luteal cells. These cytoplasmic projections contain receptors for LH (26,27) and have septate-like junctions between them (28). All of the cells of the follicle do not differentiate synchronously following ovulation. The amount of smooth endoplasmic reticulum and the number of mitochondria both increase during luteinization. Mitochondria in granulosal cells have lamellar cristae, while those in luteal cells have primarily tubular cristae. Luteal cells during early and midpregnancy in rats also contain lipid droplets and well-developed Golgi complexes.

In the ewe, the first signs of luteinization occur prior to ovulation. Dispersion of nuclear chromatin and formation of a nucleolus occurs with a concomitant increase in the number of polyribosomes. This suggests that RNA and protein synthesis are important at this stage. There are numerous gap junctions between adjacent granulosal cells in the preovulatory follicle, along with desmosome-like structures (29). The formation of smooth endoplasmic reticulum and alterations in mitochondria occur 30 to 40 hr after the ovulatory surge of LH. The elaboration of smooth endoplasmic reticulum is necessary for normal biosynthesis of steroids and is the site of localization of 3β-hydroxysteroid dehydrogenase, which is acquired by the granulosal cells within a few hours following ovulation (30). This is the first time that these cells are capable of synthesizing progesterone. In addition, after ovulation the mitochondria become rounded and develop villiform cristae. The development of the smooth endoplasmic reticulum and mitochondria in granulosal-luteal cells is correlated with the initial rise in serum levels of progesterone. Gap junctions are no longer apparent in the ovine corpus luteum by 48 hr after ovulation. Based on detailed morphological studies of the ovulatory follicle and developing corpus luteum, it has been concluded that granulosal cells differentiate into the large steroidogenic luteal cells found in the mature corpus luteum in ewes (29,31) and cows (32).

In the ewe, the cells of theca interna in the preovulatory follicle possess abundant lipid droplets. Alkaline phosphatase and 3β-hydroxysteroid dehydrogenase are restricted to this cell type prior to ovulation (31). In contrast to granulosal cells, only occasional mitotic figures are seen in the cells of the theca interna. Within 24 hr of ovulation, cells derived from the theca interna begin migrating from their original sites into the deeper, granulosal-derived areas of luteal tissue (33). At later stages, cells derived from the theca interna remain concentrated in the septa derived from follicular infoldings but are also widely distributed throughout the luteal tissue.

Ontogeny of Luteal Receptors for Hormones

Since luteinization and formation of the corpus luteum is simply a natural extension of follicular growth and ovulation, this section will begin with a discussion of the changes that occur in receptors during follicular development. The induction and first appearance of receptors for LH during the course of follicular development has been intensely studied, particularly in granulosal cells. Granulosal cells obtained from immature rat or pig follicles possess few, if any, receptors for LH (34,35). However, as follicles mature and increase in size, the number of receptors for LH increases dramatically (36–40). On the basis of studies that have employed estradiol–FSH-primed, hypophysectomized rats, it appears that the initial appearance and subsequent increase in the number of receptors for LH in granulosal cells is a result of the synergistic action of estrogen and FSH (39,41). According to Richards et al. (39): (a) Estradiol-17β acts on granulosal cells to increase the concentration of its own receptor and induces receptors for FSH; (b) FSH acts on estrogen-primed granulosal cells to increase receptors for both FSH and LH; and (c) LH acts on estrogen–FSH-primed cells to effect a decrease in receptors for estradiol, FSH, and LH and at the same time promote an increase in the number of receptors for prolactin. Data from studies that have employed intact, normally cycling rats also indicate that the appearance of an increased number of receptors for LH is a result of the combined action of estrogen and FSH (42). Once granulosal cells acquire receptors for LH, they are rendered sensitive to LH and are capable of undergoing luteinization. As demonstrated by Richards et al. (43), the ability of LH to induce luteinization is related to its ability to increase the intracellular concentrations of cAMP. In hypophysectomized rats administration of LH or human chorionic gonadotropin (hCG) to cause ovulation and luteinization of follicular cells is followed by a decrease ("down-regulation") in the number of LH receptors on granulosal cells. However, since Nimrod et al. (42) were unable to detect any significant loss of receptors for LH under physiological conditions, the reason for down-regulation of LH receptors observed during LH-induced luteinization in hypophysectomized animals (39,43,44) is uncertain.

The pattern of development of receptors for LH in follicular granulosal cells in pigs (37) and sheep (45) appears to be similar to that described for rats. There is little information regarding receptors for LH in follicular thecal cells. In sheep it appears that receptors for LH appear first in the thecal cells in small follicles and that as the follicle enlarges there is a slight decline in the capacity of thecal cells to bind LH concomitant with a dramatic increase in LH binding to granulosal cells (45).

In rats, prolactin is necessary to maintain normal numbers of receptors for LH in the developing corpus luteum (41). This role is consistent with the known biological effects of prolactin on luteal function in this species. However, the situation in other species is not so clear, since prolactin does not appear to influence luteal function in cattle (46–49) or sheep (48,49). Although receptors for prolactin have been reported in porcine luteal tissue (50), the exact role of this hormone in regulating luteal receptors for LH in species other than rodents will require additional experimentation. In porcine luteal cells, prolactin appears to influence the number of receptors for low-density lipoprotein (51), and it may therefore play a role in regulating substrate availability for steroidogenesis.

LUTEAL PHASE OF THE ESTROUS CYCLE

Morphology of Luteal Cells

In the late 1800s and early 1900s there were two hypotheses concerning the follicular cell type responsible for formation of the corpus luteum. The first held that the corpus luteum was derived exclusively from granulosal cells of the follicle while the cells from the theca interna degenerated shortly after ovulation. The second hypothesis held exactly the opposite view. In 1906, Loeb (52) performed a detailed morphological analysis of the ovary in the guinea pig during the period of luteinization and concluded that cells from both the theca interna and granulosal layers of the ovarian follicle were involved in formation of the corpus luteum. Corner (53) came to the same conclusion concerning the corpus luteum of the sow, as have subsequent investigators examining corpora lutea in cows (32,54–56), ewes (31), rats (57), and women (58).

Since the cells of the corpus luteum appear to be derived from at least two different types of follicular steroid-secreting cells (thecal and granulosal cells), it is not surprising that the corpus luteum consists of at least two distinct types of steroidogenic luteal cells in several species (53,59–61). The two types of steroidogenic cells are morphologically distinct. The so-called large luteal cells (32,33,56,62–66)—also referred to as granulosa-lutein (60,67), Type II (68), and D cells (69)—are the most readily distinguished cells in the corpus luteum (Fig. 2). They are the largest, strictly endocrine cells in the body and range from approximately 20 μm in diameter in rodents to 40 μm or more in humans (70). Under the light microscope, large luteal cells appear polyhedral, with a lightly staining cytoplasm and a large, centrally located nucleus with a distinct nucleolus. In contrast, small luteal cells have a diameter of 22 μm or less and appear spindle-shaped with darkly staining cytoplasm, large lipid droplets, and an irregularly shaped nucleus that often contains what has been described as cytoplasmic inclusion. Alternative terms for small luteal cells include theca-lutein (60,67), Type I (68), and I cells (69). On a volume basis, large luteal cells comprise about 25% to 35% of the corpus luteum in sheep, whereas small luteal cells represent approximately 12% to 18% of the luteal volume (71,72). The corpus luteum also contains vascular elements and connective tissue. During the period of maximum secretion of progesterone, vascular elements account for approximately 11% of luteal volume (71). The remainder of the corpus luteum is composed of connective tissue (22–29%) and fibroblasts (7–11%) (71,72).

Ultrastructurally, large luteal cells contain all of the elements of steroid-secreting cells, that is, numerous mitochondria and an abundance of smooth endoplasmic reticulum (Fig. 3) (73). Mitochondria in large luteal cells can take on a variety of shapes: spherical, cup-shaped, or elongated (70); in fact, it is not uncommon to find each of these shapes of mitochondria within a single cell. There is also considerable variation in the size of mitochondria in large luteal cells. In most species, mitochondria with tubular cristae predominate, but some with lamelliform cristae may also be observed. Clustering and regional exclusion of mitochondria are also common features noted in large luteal cells (70).

Large luteal cells have an abundance of smooth endoplasmic reticulum, which is characteristically most prevalent in the peripheral region of the cell. In fact, it is often the most abundant cytoplasmic component found at the cell's periphery. The smooth endoplasmic reticulum is in the form of branched tubules, tubular sheets, and fenestrated cisternae. Often the fenestrated cisternae are centered around a mitochondrion or lipid droplet. The branched tubules may form an anastomotic network that traverses the entire cell.

The Golgi complex is quite extensive in large luteal cells and is usually located at one side of the nucleus and occupies

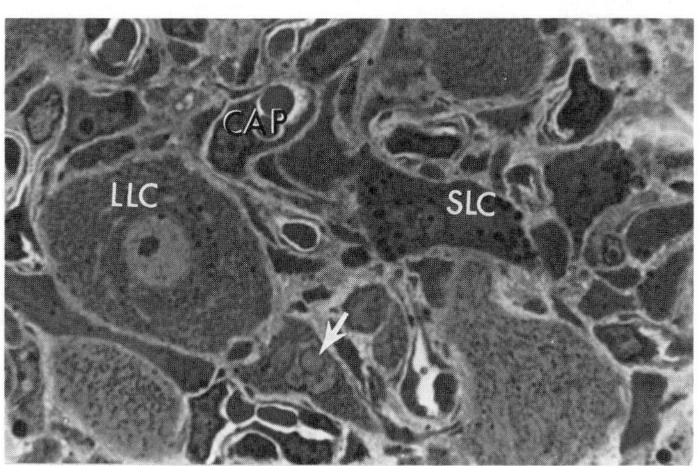

FIG. 2. Large luteal cells (LLC) can be easily distinguished from small luteal cells (SLC) in 1-μm-thick sections stained with toluidine blue. Small luteal cells are usually spindle-shaped, whereas LLC are typically spherical or polyhedral. In addition, the dark-staining cytoplasm of SLC contains large lipid droplets. The nuclei of SLC sometimes possess cytoplasmic inclusions (*arrow*). Both cell types are in close apposition to capillaries (CAP). ×800. (From ref. 61.)

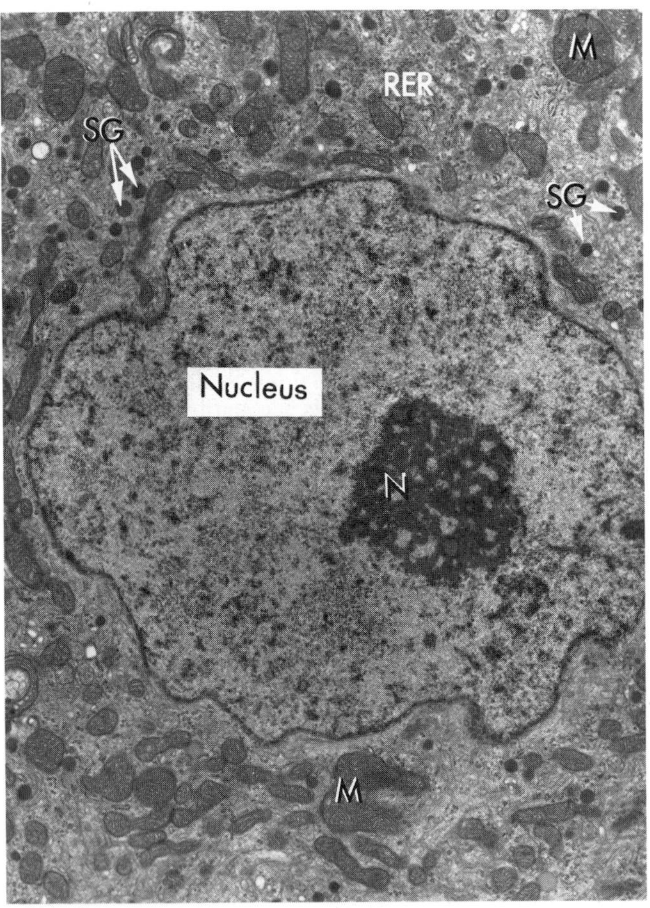

FIG. 3. Electron micrograph showing a portion of a large luteal cell (LLC). The presence of numerous electron-dense, membrane-bound secretory granules (SG) in the cytoplasm of LLC distinguishes these cells from small luteal cells (SLC) (see Fig. 5). Note the absence of lipid droplets comparable to those found in SLC. Mitochondria (M), nucleolus (N), rough endoplasmic reticulum (RER). ×7,200. (From ref. 61.)

a comparable volume. There is a paucity of tubular smooth endoplasmic reticulum and mitochondria in the area of the Golgi complex. Unlike other cell types, there is an indication that the smooth endoplasmic reticulum is in direct communication with the Golgi cisternae (74).

There are abundant electron-dense, membrane-bound secretory granules in the cytoplasm of large luteal cells (Fig. 3). These granules are similar in size to lysosomes and peroxisomes, but they are a distinct form of granule (75) and their contents do not include acid phosphatase or catalase activity (75–77). Contents of the granules are released at the surface of the cell by exocytosis (Fig. 4) (78–80). The exocytotic release of granular contents is correlated with the secretion of progesterone both *in vivo* (76) and *in vitro* (80). Based on these observations, several investigators proposed that these granules contain progesterone (and a protein that binds progesterone) and provide a mechanism for the active secretion of progesterone from the luteal cell (76–82). However, at the current time this hypothesis seems unlikely since small steroidogenic luteal cells have few, if any, secretory granules. Thus, the mechanisms for secretion of progesterone would have to be different in the two cell types. In contrast, others argue that progesterone exits the cell by simple diffusion due to a concentration gradient between intracellular concentrations and those in the blood (70,83). At least one of the components in secretory granules in large luteal cells in cattle (84) and sheep (20,85) is oxytocin. Relaxin has also been identified in similar granules in rats (86,87), pigs (88–90), and cows (91). It is possible that the granules may contain more than one secretory product or that there are different types of granules within the same cell.

The ultrastructural appearance of small luteal cells is distinct from that of large luteal cells (Fig. 5). The nucleus is irregular in shape, and in approximately 10% of the cells it

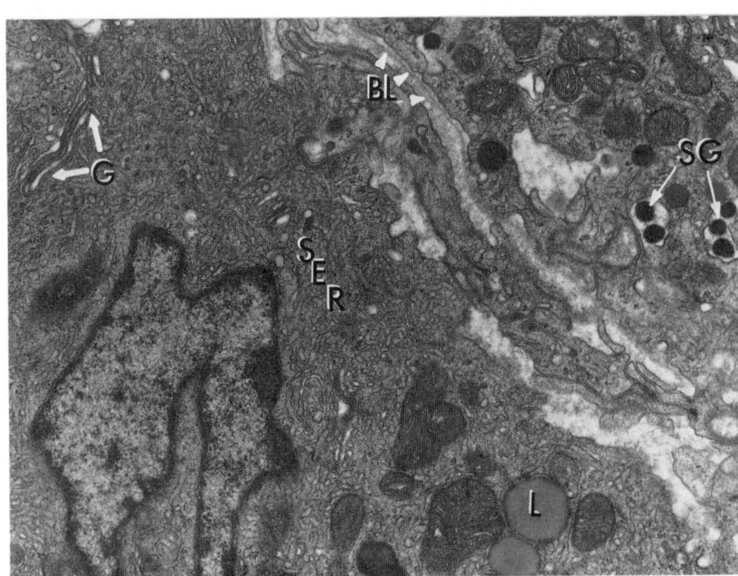

FIG. 4. Both small (lower left) and large (upper right) luteal cells possess fine structural characteristics consistent with a steroid-secreting function, i.e., extensive smooth endoplasmic reticulum (SER), lipid droplets (L), and Golgi apparatus (G). However, LLC also have characteristics typical of protein-secreting cells, including secretory granules (SG), some of which have been exocytosed. Large luteal cells possess a more conspicuous basal lamina (BL) than do small luteal cells. ×14,800. (From ref. 61.)

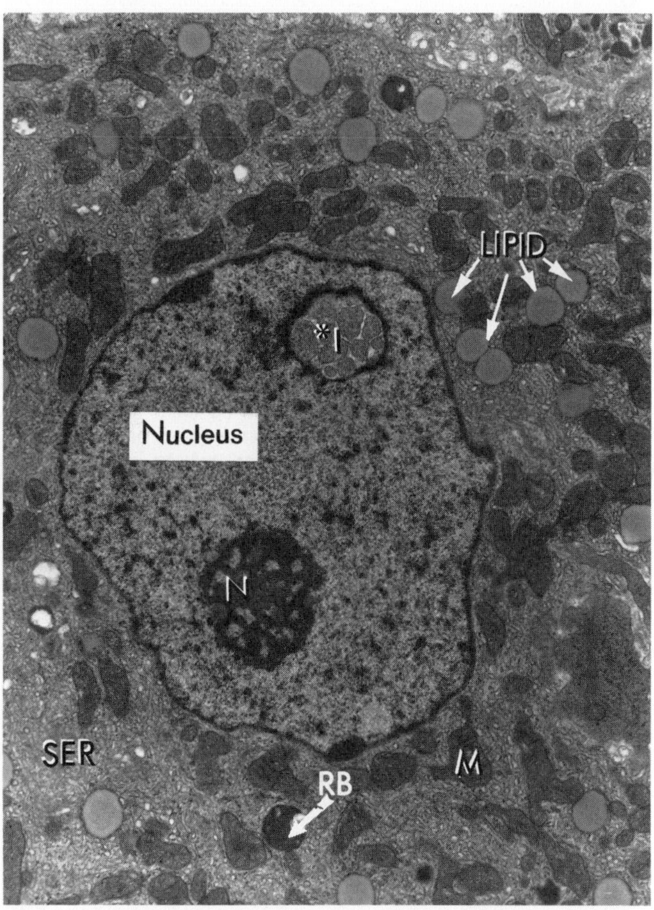

FIG. 5. Electron micrograph showing a portion of a small luteal cell. The cytoplasm is characterized by an abundance of smooth endoplasmic reticulum (SER), numerous mitochondria (M), and lipid droplets. Residual bodies (RB) are often observed in these cells. Besides the nucleolus (N), the nucleus contains what appears to be a cytoplasmic inclusion (I). ×7,200. (From ref. 61.)

appears to contain areas of cytoplasm bounded by a completely inverted nuclear envelope (Fig. 5) (33). However, to date no one has serially sectioned the nucleus of the small luteal cell to establish whether these structures represent true cytoplasmic inclusions, or rather, if they are simply cytoplasmic invaginations into the nucleus (Fig. 4). The characteristic small luteal cell contains a moderate number of mitochondria of variable size. Their profile may appear as round, elongated, or branching. Both tubular and lamelliform cristae have been observed. Large amounts of endoplasmic reticulum are present in small luteal cells. The endoplasmic reticulum is predominantly of the smooth, tubular type, but scattered clusters of attached ribosomes are also present. The Golgi complex is less pronounced in the small luteal cell than in large luteal cells, is located perinuclearly, and is associated with numerous small coated or uncoated vesicles (33). A characteristic feature of the small luteal cell is the absence of the secretory granules that are present in the large luteal cell. Small luteal cells also contain numerous lipid droplets, which are virtually absent in large luteal cells.

Hypophyseal Regulation of Luteal Function

In most species three organ systems regulate the function of the corpus luteum. The anterior pituitary gland secretes LH, which is the primary hormone responsible for regulating the secretion of progesterone. In several rodent species, hypophyseal prolactin is also an important regulator of luteal function. In most nonprimate species the uterus has a luteolytic effect during the late luteal phase of the estrous cycle. Finally, the conceptus has either direct or indirect luteotropic effects in most mammalian species.

Rats

Rothchild (92) has recently reviewed the factors that regulate the function of the corpus luteum in most species, with particular attention to the rat. In rats, the secretion of progesterone during the estrous cycle is short-lived and appears to be autonomous the first day of diestrus but requires prolactin during the second day (93). Postovulatory secretion of progesterone in rats has a pattern similar to the responsiveness of adenylate cyclase to LH (94). Although some minor differences may be present, it appears that the endocrine events controlling the life span and function of the corpus luteum during the estrous cycle in other rodents such as mice, hamsters, and gerbils are similar to those described here for the rat. The one exception appears to be that prolactin, LH, and FSH are required for normal secretion of progesterone in hamsters (59).

Rabbits

Hormonal regulation of luteal function in the rabbit has been reviewed by Hilliard (96) and by Keyes et al. (97). In rabbits, ovulation is induced by cervical stimulation, which causes the preovulatory surge of LH that results in ovulation. Maintenance of the structure and function of the corpus luteum requires estradiol (97). Despite a dependence on estradiol for maintenance of the corpus luteum, rabbit luteal tissue exhibits an acute steroidogenic response to LH (98), contains high-affinity receptors for LH (99), and possesses LH-sensitive adenylate cyclase (94). The corpus luteum of the rabbit contains two cell types: with small luteal cells that are responsive to LH and large cells that do not respond to LH with enhanced secretion of progesterone (100). There is no direct steroidogenic response to estradiol. Thus, the mechanisms whereby estradiol maintains the corpus luteum are not clear.

Domestic Ruminants

There has been considerable controversy regarding the requirement of the anterior pituitary gland for the regulation of luteal function in ewes and cows. In 1963, Denamur and Mauleon (101) reported that formation and maintenance of the corpus luteum in prepubertal ewes was not influenced by hypophysectomy. However, Kaltenbach et al. (102) found that hypophysectomy on day 1 after a normal or induced ovulation resulted in failure of the corpus luteum to form, while hypophysectomy on day 5 resulted in regression of the partially formed corpus luteum. In subsequent studies, Denamur et al. (103) demonstrated that hypophysectomy of hysterectomized ewes also resulted in regression of the corpus luteum. Thus, there is agreement that hypophysectomy will prevent further luteal development and/or cause at least partial regression of existing luteal tissue.

Even more controversial than the effects of hypophysectomy on luteal function are the results of studies designed to determine which hypophyseal hormone(s) are responsible for maintenance of luteal function. Injections of prolactin resulted in maintenance of luteal weight in hypophysectomized, hysterectomized ewes (103,104), but this hormone was without effect when infused into hypophysectomized ewes with an intact uterus (105).

Injections of LH would not maintain luteal weight in hypophysectomized, hysterectomized ewes (103). On the other hand, infusion of LH, but not prolactin or estradiol was followed by maintenance of the corpus luteum in hypophysectomized ewes with an intact uterus (105). Based on these studies, it was suggested that LH was the primary luteotropic hormone in ewes. However, data from subsequent studies (106,107) suggest it is likely that prolactin also plays a role in regulating luteal function in hypophysectomized, nonhysterectomized ewes. Interpretation of the data from these studies is complicated by the fact that the preparations of hormones used for replacement therapy were only partially purified. In addition, it is very difficult to completely remove the anterior pituitary gland from ewes without leaving a few cells adhered to the sella turcica or in the pars tuberalis. Since there would be no hypothalamic control of prolactin secretion in these animals, these cells could begin to hypersecrete prolactin, resulting in normal circulating concentrations of this hormone within a relatively short time (107). In fact, Schroff et al. (107) reported that hypophysectomized ewes in which LH maintained luteal weight invariably had normal serum concentrations of prolactin. Thus, there are data that following hypophysectomy both LH and prolactin may be required for maintenance of normal luteal function in ewes.

The results of a number of additional studies are relevant regarding the roles of LH and prolactin in the regulation of luteal function. Constant infusions of LH prolonged the life span and function of corpora lutea in cyclic ewes (108), LH enhanced secretion of progesterone from the ovary *in situ* (109) or from luteal tissue *in vitro* (110,111), and daily injections of antiserum to LH caused luteal regression in cycling ewes (112). Similar data for cattle led Hansel et al. (46) to conclude that LH was the primary luteotropin in this species.

Although there is evidence that prolactin is important for maintenance of the corpus luteum in hypophysectomized ewes, confirming data in intact animals are not available. When serum concentrations of prolactin were reduced in ewes by >95% for an entire estrous cycle by injections of 2-bromo-α-ergocryptine there was no effect on serum concentration of progesterone or length of the estrous cycle (49). Similar data are available for cows (47). Infusion of prolactin into intact ewes did not extend the life span of the corpus luteum (48), nor did infusion of prolactin into the ovarian artery result in enhanced secretion of progesterone (113). Finally, P. O'Callaghan and G. Niswender (*unpublished data*) have been unable to demonstrate luteal receptors for prolactin in cycling ewes under a variety of conditions. However, others (114) have reported that radioiodinated human growth hormone will bind to luteal membranes to a greater extent than will radioiodinated ovine prolactin and that this binding can be inhibited by ovine prolactin. These authors concluded that luteal receptors for prolactin are present and that their numbers change during pregnancy. Thus, controversy persists regarding the role of prolactin in the regulation of luteal function in domestic ruminants.

Pigs

Removal of the pituitary gland during the first 2 days of the estrous cycle did not affect corpora lutea of the estrous cycle in pigs (115). Based on these data it was concluded that corpora lutea in cyclic pigs were capable of normal function without gonadotropic support after the initial stimulation of ovulation. Duncan et al. (116) were first to study progesterone synthesis by porcine luteal tissue *in vitro* and Cook et al. (117) demonstrated that LH stimulated the synthesis of progesterone.

Horses

Because of the unique structure of the equine ovary, ovulation can occur at only one site on the ovary, the ovulation fossa (60). As a result of this anatomical feature, essentially the entire structure of the corpus luteum is contained within the ovarian stroma (Fig. 6). Anatomically, the corpus luteum of the mare reaches its maximum diameter within approximately 3 days of ovulation (118), but maximum secretion of progesterone does not occur until about 9 days after ovulation (119).

Based on histological studies (120,121), it appears that the secretory elements of the equine corpus luteum are derived primarily, if not exclusively, from granulosal cells. The thecal cells begin degenerating just prior to ovulation, and their degeneration is nearly complete by 24 hr after ovulation. In contrast, granulosal cells, which are approximately 10 μm in diameter at ovulation, have enlarged to

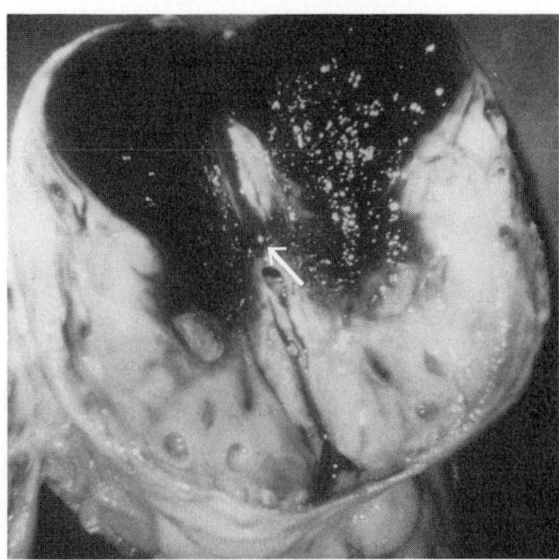

FIG. 6. Ovary from a mare cut midsagittally. The dark area is a developing corpus luteum. Note the constricted portion of the corpus luteum near the center of the ovary. This represents the tract in which the follicle grew from the periphery of the ovary to the ovulation fossa (*arrow*).

15 μm by 24 hr following ovulation and undergo cytological changes characteristic of luteinization. Luteinization of the granulosal cells appears to be complete by 3 days post-ovulation, but they continue to hypertrophy until day 9 (average diameter, 37.5 μm), when maximal secretory activity is achieved. On day 9, in addition to the large, light-staining luteal cells, approximately 15% of the luteal cells are small cells. These small cells are eosinophilic and are thought to represent a resting stage that can be converted to the large, light-staining luteal cells. By 12 days postovulation the large luteal cells begin to decrease in diameter, and by day 16 their diameter averages 20 μm. The reduction in their size is correlated with a decrease in circulating concentrations of progesterone.

Endocrinologically, the corpus luteum of the mare appears to be primarily dependent upon luteinizing hormone. Antisera raised against the gondotropin fraction of equine pituitary extracts will induce luteal regression (122). Likewise, administration of hCG or equine pituitary extract can extend the life span of the corpus luteum in mares (118). The concentration of receptors for LH in the corpus luteum of the mare parallels the circulating concentrations of progesterone (123). Interestingly, the affinity of these receptors for LH also appears to increase when the secretion of progesterone is maximal. This phenomenon appears to be unique to the equine corpus luteum.

Dogs

In the bitch, ovulation does not occur until 24 to 72 hr after the preovulatory LH surge. Luteinization of ovarian follicles (and secretion of progesterone) begins prior to ovulation (124,125), possibly due to the extended interval between the LH surge and ovulation. There is a slight increase in secretion of progesterone concomitant with the onset of the LH surge. This increase is important for the display of sexual receptivity by the bitch (124). Luteal growth continues for 10 to 20 days after ovulation, at which time secretion of progesterone is maximal. This is followed by decreasing luteal activity, with circulating concentrations of progesterone returning to basal levels by 55 to 90 days after ovulation in the pseudopregnant bitch. Concentrations of progesterone in the pregnant bitch appear to be similar to (126–128) or greater than those in the pseudopregnant bitch (129,130). Cessation of progesterone secretion is much more synchronous at the end of pregnancy, with a decrease to less than 1 ng/ml of blood occurring about 63 to 65 days after the LH surge.

Luteal function in the bitch requires the presence of pituitary hormones throughout pregnancy or pseudopregnancy since secretion of progesterone ceases following hypophysectomy (131). Two hypophyseal hormones, LH and prolactin, appear to be necessary for maintenance of the corpus luteum. Apparently, both hormones must be present continuously for normal luteal function. Administration of an antiserum to LH results in a dramatic decline in secretion of progesterone (132). Likewise, administration of ergocryptine to reduce circulating levels of prolactin also results in a drastic reduction in circulating concentrations of progesterone.

Receptors for both LH and prolactin have been quantified in canine corpora lutea throughout the estrous cycle (Fernandes et al., *unpublished observations*). The concentration of receptors for LH remains unchanged throughout the cycle; however, concentrations of receptors for prolactin are high through day 40 but appear to decline at days 50 and 60. The physiological significance of these observations remains to be established.

Primates

Continued low levels of LH are necessary for normal luteal function in hypophysectomized women (133). Treatment of normally cycling women during the luteal phase of the estrous cycle with LH or hCG increased the circulating levels of progestin and extended the life of the corpus luteum (134). LH also enhances the secretion of progesterone from human (135) or monkey (136) luteal tissue *in vitro*. Treatment of monkeys with antiserum to LH during the luteal phase of the menstrual cycle resulted in menstruation 2 to 4 days later (137). Thus, it appears that in primates LH is the hormone responsible for maintenance of the life span and function of the corpus luteum.

Regulation of Progesterone Secretion

The mechanisms involved in the synthesis and secretion of progesterone are complex, although this hormone is the first biologically active compound produced in the steroid biosynthetic pathway (Fig. 7). Cholesterol bound to low-

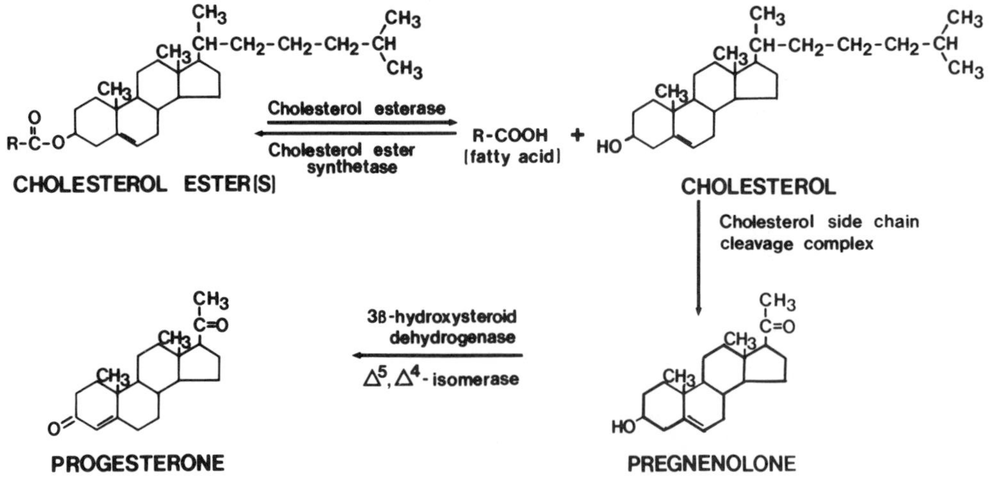

FIG. 7. Biosynthetic pathway for synthesis of progesterone from cholesterol ester. The conversion of cholesterol ester to cholesterol is a reversible reaction. Cholesterol side-chain cleavage complex within the mitochondrion converts cholesterol to pregnenolone, which is converted to progesterone in the smooth endoplasmic reticulum by 3β-hydroxysteroid dehydrogenase/Δ^5,Δ^4-isomerase.

density lipoprotein (LDL) or, in some species, high-density lipoprotein (HDL) produced by the liver is the primary substrate for progesterone synthesis. However, under some conditions, luteal cells also synthesize cholesterol from acetate for use in the steroidogenic pathway. The steroidogenic luteal cell contains LDL (or HDL) receptors that are involved in the transport of lipoprotein from outside to inside the cell. The LDL–LDL receptor complex is internalized by endocytosis. The endocytotic vesicles combine with lysosomes and the cholesterol is liberated. The free cholesterol leaves the lysosome and is either esterified and stored as lipid droplets or is used for steroid biosynthesis or in the membrane constitutents of the cell. For biosynthesis of progesterone, cholesterol is transported to the mitochondria, where it is converted to pregnenolone by side-chain cleavage. The pregnenolone is converted to progesterone by 3β-hydroxysteroid dehydrogenase/Δ^5,Δ^4-isomerase in the smooth endoplasmic reticulum, and the progesterone is secreted. The luteal cell has a limited capacity to store progesterone.

The single most important endocrine factor involved in regulating the synthesis and secretion of progesterone in the corpus luteum, irrespective of species, is LH. LH increases the synthesis and secretion of progesterone *in vivo* (138,139) or when incubated with luteal slices or cells *in vitro* (110,111,117,140,141).

Receptors for LH

The presence of specific receptors for LH in the ovary and testis was first demonstrated by the ability of these tissues to preferentially bind and concentrate radioactively labeled LH or hCG *in vivo* (34). Subsequent studies designed to determine the subcellular distribution of binding sites, the kinetics of hormone–receptor binding, and the physiochemical properties of the receptor molecule have employed tissue slices (142), dispersed cells (143–145), homogenates or particulate fractions (146–149), and isolated membranes (150–152) prepared from target tissues. To date it has not been possible to isolate and purify receptors for LH in quantities sufficient for a complete chemical characterization; however, several lines of evidence suggest that the receptor molecule is a glycolipoprotein (149,150,153).

Since it has not been feasible to label receptors for protein hormones directly, these molecules have been labeled indirectly using LH or hCG coupled to various markers, such as ferritin (154), fluorescein (155), or radioiodine (156). It has been demonstrated repeatedly that hCG and LH compete for the same specific receptor, and hCG has been labeled most frequently. However, it has recently become clear that the steroidogenic response, the time required for internalization of the hormone–receptor complex, and the lateral mobility in the membrane of the occupied LH receptor are different for LH and hCG (61).

Results from studies that have employed LH covalently linked to ferritin (154) or agarose beads (157), as well as data from autoradiographic (27,158–160), immunocytochemical (160,161), and immunofluorescent studies (155,162) and cell fractionation (151,152,163) have clearly demonstrated that receptors for LH are localized in the plasma membrane of target cells. In rat luteal cells the majority of hCG binding sites are localized along regions of the cell surface facing capillaries, which is characterized by microvillus folds, whereas the basolateral surfaces of the luteal cells are characterized by junctional complexes and contain very few binding sites (27). Thus, not only are receptors for LH localized in the plasma membrane, they also appear to be concentrated in specific regions of the membrane and not distributed uniformly over the entire cell surface.

Once the corpus luteum begins to develop, the secretion

of progesterone by this gland in women (164), rats (165), and cows (166) appears to be highly correlated with the number of receptors for LH. One of the most complete studies to date regarding the relationship between the total number of receptors, the number occupied by endogenous hormone, and secretion of progesterone by the corpus luteum is that of Diekman et al. (167). The total number of receptors for LH increased 40-fold between days 2 and 14 of the cycle in ewes (Fig. 8). There was a 6-fold increase in both the number of receptors occupied by endogenous hormone and the weight of the corpus luteum and a 10-fold increase in serum concentrations of progesterone during this same period. However, less than 0.5% of the total number of receptors was occupied by endogenous hormone. By day 16 (late luteal phase), both the total number of receptors and the number occupied by endogenous LH had decreased by 75%. During early pregnancy, the numbers of total and occupied receptors were very similar to those observed during the midluteal phase of the cycle (167). There was a high

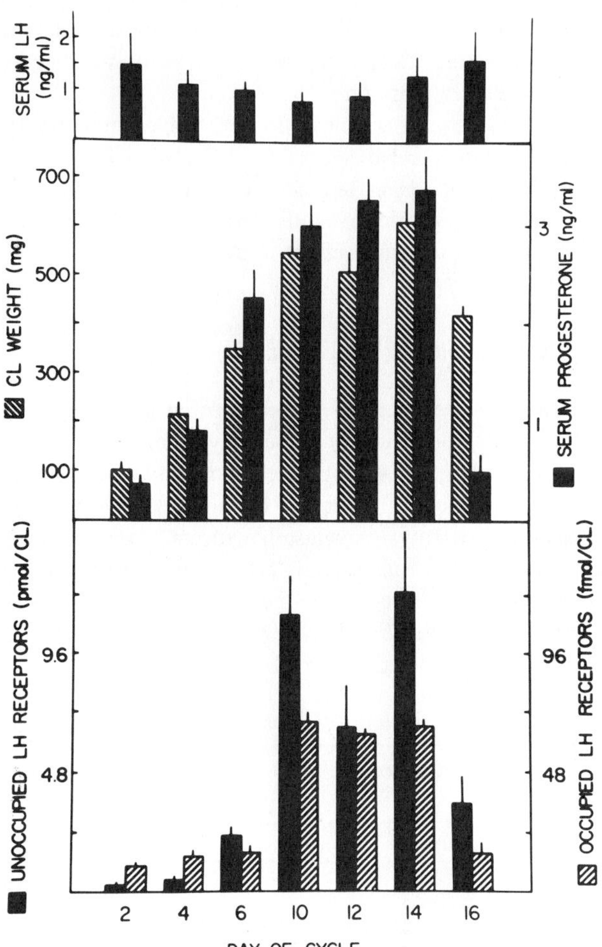

FIG. 8. Serum levels of LH (top panel) and progesterone (middle panel), weight of corpora lutea (middle panel), and number of occupied and unoccupied receptors for LH in ovine corpora lutea (bottom panel) collected throughout the estrous cycle from ewes ($n = 6$). (From ref. 167.)

degree of correlation between the total number of LH receptors, the number occupied by endogenous LH, and serum concentrations of progesterone. However, the biological significance of this finding has recently been questioned. There is little correlation between episodic peaks of LH in serum and systemic levels of progesterone during the midluteal phase of the estrous cycle in ewes (168). In addition, when serum levels of LH were increased approximately 1,000-fold during the midluteal phase of the estrous cycle, the increase in serum levels of progesterone was less than 2-fold and lasted less than 6 hr (169). These findings can apparently be explained by the recent observation that in ewes >80% of the progesterone secreted by the corpus luteum is derived from the large steroidogenic luteal cells, which have few, if any, LH receptors (61). However, it should not be inferred from these data that LH is not important for normal secretion of progesterone. Injections of hCG or LH will increase the numbers of large luteal cells; concomitantly the numbers of small luteal cells will decrease (61). Thus, LH may regulate the differentiation of small to large luteal cells, a suggestion originally presented by Donaldson and Hansel (32) for cattle. Therefore, although the secretion of progesterone by large luteal cells is not regulated directly by LH, the number of large luteal cells may depend, at least in part, on this hormone.

The observation that <1% of the receptors for LH in the ovary (167) are occupied under conditions of maximal steroid secretion has led to the concept of "spare" receptors for this tropic hormone. However, it seems unlikely that these receptors are really spare, since circulating levels of LH are so low (0.5–1.5 ng/ml) that the large number of receptors is required to insure that sufficient numbers are occupied by endogenous hormone to stimulate steroidogenesis. In addition, intracellular levels of cAMP continue to increase with increased occupancy of LH receptors, even after steroidogenesis is maximal (170,171). This observation suggests that the receptors are coupled to adenylate cyclase and biologically functional. It may well be that cAMP is important for aspects of luteal cell function not acutely related to secretion of progesterone. For example, cAMP seems to be necessary for luteinization of granulosal cells (43) and maintenance of the characteristic morphology of luteal cells grown in culture (172). It is also possible that cAMP may be the intracellular agent involved in differentiation of small luteal cells into large ones if such differentiation can be unequivocally demonstrated (61).

A variety of factors may influence the concentration of LH receptors in the ovary (35), but the primary factor appears to be LH itself. Exposure of luteal tissue to high concentrations of LH or hCG invariably results in a dramatic loss (up to 90% in some cases) of LH receptors known as "down-regulation" (144,156,169,173,174). The loss induced by homologous hormone is time and dose dependent, and it is accompanied by a concomitant loss in hCG-stimulated adenylate cyclase activity and/or steroid production (174,175). However, at present sufficient information is not available for a meaningful evaluation of the physiological significance of down-regulation of LH receptors. Although it is tempting to conclude that the loss of adenylate cyclase activity and tissue responsiveness is related to receptor loss, there may also be a secondary lesion involved, since the administration of dibutyryl cAMP does not stimulate steroidogenesis in desensitized tissues (173).

Two mechanisms have been proposed to explain the loss of LH receptors following administration of a large dose of LH or hCG. Receptors for LH could be inactivated or sequestered within the plasma membrane and thus become inaccessible for binding (145,174) or the hormone receptor complex may be internalized (160). The latter possibility seems most likely since there is good evidence that the LH-receptor complex enters the cell via small endocytotic vesicles (27,145,160,162) and the hormone is subsequently degraded by lysosomal enzymes (176–179). That internalization of the hormone is a degradatory process rather than a mechanism for action by the hormone is suggested by the fact that chloroquine, a lysosomal enzyme inhibitor, blocks degradation of the hormone by the target cell but does not reduce steroid secretion (177). In addition, ovine luteal cells exposed to a 15-min pulse of LH secrete enhanced quantities of progesterone for 3 to 4 hr, whereas exposure to a 15-min pulse of hCG results in enhanced secretion of progesterone for more than 6 hr (180). Since the hCG–LH receptor complex is internalized approximately 50 times more slowly than the oLH–LH receptor complex, these data suggest that internalization of the hormone–receptor complex is the mechanism whereby the cell deactivates itself after stimulation (61).

Our current working hypothesis is that the functional life of the receptor for LH in ovine luteal cells is a single binding of hormone followed by internalization and degradation of the hormone. The receptor appears to be recycled to the plasma membrane (181), probably in a manner similar to that proposed for other peptide hormones (182). This suggests that regulation of the biological effects of LH on luteal cells is a very precise phenomenon and may also explain how the hormone-stimulated cell returns to basal activity.

Data obtained *in vivo* by Suter et al. (1969) provide additional insight into the mechanisms involved in loss and renewal of receptors for LH in ewes administered a pharmacological dose of LH during the midluteal phase of the estrous cycle. There was a dramatic increase in receptors occupied by LH within 10 min after the injection, after which the number of receptors occupied by LH decreased rapidly and returned to basal levels within 6 hr (Table 1). In contrast, the number of unoccupied receptors had decreased dramatically within 12 hr but had returned to preinjection levels within 48 hr. There were three interesting observations from this study. First, the total number of receptors (occupied plus unoccupied) for LH in the crude membrane fraction increased significantly within 10 min of the LH injection ("up-regulation"). Second, although the total number of receptors for LH was decreased within 12 to 24 hr after the injection of LH, at no time during the study did serum concentrations of progesterone fall below preinjection levels. Thus, the biological significance of "down-regulation" of ovine luteal receptors is unclear. Finally, the number of receptors occupied at 10 min after injection of LH was almost perfectly correlated with the number of receptors lost by 24 hr. This finding certainly suggests that loss of receptors for LH in ovine luteal cells is a function of occupancy by hormone.

In rats, $PGF_{2\alpha}$ also appears to be involved in regulating the number of luteal receptors for LH (183). The number of receptors for LH in rats administered a luteolytic dose of $PGF_{2\alpha}$ decreases dramatically. However, $PGF_{2\alpha}$ does not appear to have the same effect in ewes (184).

Effects of LH on Steroidogenesis

There has been general agreement that the receptor for LH is linked biochemically to the enzyme adenylate cyclase and that binding of LH to this receptor results in activation of adenylate cyclase in corpora lutea (185). The hormonal regulation of adenylate cyclase has recently been reviewed in detail by Birnbaumer et al. (186). The critical steps in the activation of intracellular mechanisms via this process are outlined in Fig. 9. Most cell types have receptors for

TABLE 1. *Number of receptors for LH and content of progesterone in the corpus luteum (CL) after injection of 1 mg LH*

Time after LH (hr)	Unoccupied receptors (mol/CL × 10^{12})	Occupied receptors (mol/CL × 10^{12})	Total receptors (mol/CL × 10^{12})
0	2.63 ± 0.48	0.41 ± 0.66	3.04 ± 0.88
0.17	2.48 ± 0.48	5.43 ± 0.73[a]	7.91 ± 0.99[a]
2	1.45 ± 0.48	1.51 ± 0.73	2.96 ± 0.99
6	1.54 ± 0.48	0.52 ± 0.66	2.06 ± 0.88
12	0.90 ± 0.48[a]	0.98 ± 0.66	1.88 ± 0.88
24	0.95 ± 0.48[a]	0.21 ± 0.72	1.16 ± 0.98[a]
48	3.32 ± 0.54	0.41 ± 0.73	3.73 ± 0.99
72	3.29 ± 0.48	0.46 ± 0.73	3.75 ± 0.99

Each value represents the least-squares mean ± SEM of 7 determinations.
[a]Values significantly different from control ($t = 0$, $p < 0.05$).

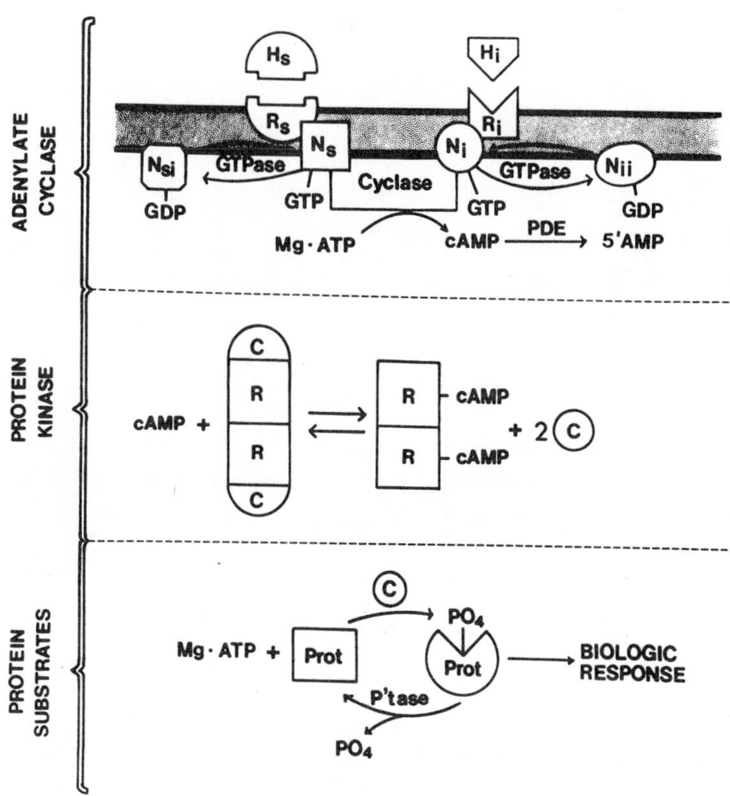

FIG. 9. Schematic representation of the molecular events that occur as part of hormonal regulation of the biologic responses of target cells. *Adenylate cyclase*: Hormone, either stimulatory (Hs) or inhibitory (Hi), interacts with its cell membrane bound receptor (Rs or Ri), which results in activation of the appropriate regulatory component(s) of adenylate cyclase (Ns or Ni). The dissociation of GDP from the inactive Nsi or Nii and binding of GTP activates Ns or Ni. This results in activation of the catalytic subunit (cyclase), which converts ATP to cAMP. *Protein kinase*: The cAMP binds to the receptor (R) subunit of cAMP-dependent protein kinase, causing dissociation and activation of the catalytic subunit (C). *Protein substrate*: The catalytic subunit of protein kinase alters the activity of various protein substrates (Prot) via phosphorylation, leading to activation of these proteins and modification of the biologic response (see Fig. 10). Points for negative regulation of this system include activation of Ni, GTPase inactivation of Ns, phosphodiesterase (PDE) conversion of cAMP to 5'-AMP, dissociation of cAMP from R, and dephosphorylation of phosphorylated protein substrate by phosphatase (Ptase).

multiple regulatory agents, some of which stimulate (Rs) adenylate cyclase, while others are inhibitory (Ri). The stimulatory or inhibitory actions of the hormone receptor complexes are mediated via two transducing or coupling proteins. The protein complex involved in activating adenylate cyclase has been called the Gs- (187) or Ns-protein (186), while the protein that inhibits adenylate cyclase has been termed Gi (187) or Ni (186). These proteins will be referred to as Ns or Ni in this discussion. The activity of Ns is regulated by guanine nucleotide binding. The stimulatory, occupied hormone receptor interacts with Ns-promoting GTP binding through a Mg-dependent process that results in activation of Ns. Dissociation of GDP from Ns is also a normal regulated component of the system. The activated Ns then stimulates the catalytic component of adenylate cyclase, resulting in the conversion of Mg · ATP to cAMP. Ns has inherent GTPase activity, which converts the bound GTP to GDP, resulting in inactivation of Ns unless dissociation of the GDP and further GTP binding occurs. Stimulatory hormones have been demonstrated to enhance the rate of exchange of GDP for GTP on Ns. Inhibitory hormones bind to their receptor, which activates Ni and results in an inhibition of the activity of adenylate cyclase. Oxytocin and vasopressin have been shown to activate Ni in rat Leydig cells and to prevent LH-stimulated increases in testosterone secretion. However, this phenomenon cannot be demonstrated in ovine luteal tissue.

In the bovine and ovine corpus luteum, LH and epinephrine are capable of activating adenylate cyclase (171,185,188), but it is not clear whether LH and epinephrine influence the activity of the same or different pools of the enzyme (171,188). Intracellular mediation of biological responses by cAMP involves several points of regulation (Fig. 9). Intracellular cAMP that is produced binds to the regulatory subunit of the cAMP-dependent protein kinase (189,190) or is degraded to 5'-AMP by a cAMP-phosphodiesterase (185). The binding of cAMP to the protein kinase promotes dissociation (activation) of the catalytic subunit of this enzyme. The activated catalytic subunit utilizes Mg · ATP to phosphorylate endogenous protein substrates, which results in altered activity (stimulated or inhibited) of these biological regulators. Consequently, a biologic response ensues. These responses may be reversed by dephosphorylation of the protein substrate by a phosphoprotein phosphatase (191). It is generally accepted that all of the intracellular effects of cAMP are mediated via the cAMP-dependent protein kinase (192).

The activity of protein kinase is enhanced in steroidogenic tissue at concentrations of LH that do not result in measurable increases in cAMP (156,193). The increase in protein kinase activity and steroid secretion are highly correlated. Thus, it seems reasonable to assume that increased activity of protein kinase due to elevated intracellular levels of cAMP in some compartments is involved in the stimulation of steroidogenesis by LH. Increased protein kinase activity can influence the function of the luteal cell via several mechanisms (Fig. 10). (1) Protein kinases may influence nuclear events, gene expression, and protein syn-

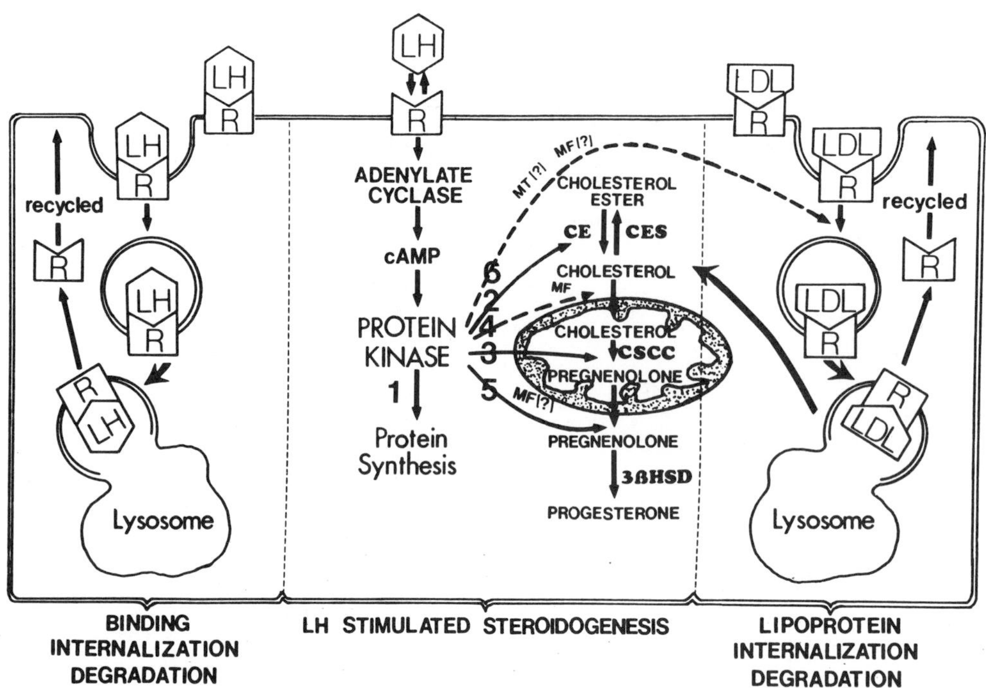

FIG. 10. Schematic representation of the intracellular events involved in LH-stimulated steroidogenesis. LH binds to its receptor in the cell membrane and activates adenylate cyclase, resulting in increased intracellular levels of cAMP and activation of protein kinase (Fig. 9). The active protein kinase (1) stimulates protein synthesis; (2) activates cholesterol esterase (CE); (3) activates cholesterol side-chain cleavage complex; (4) stimulates transport of cholesterol into the mitochondrion; (5) may stimulate transport of pregnenolone out of the mitochondrion and/or; (6) may stimulate the uptake of low-density lipoprotein (LDL), thus increasing cholesterol for substrate. In some species high-density lipoprotein is the preferred moiety for cholesterol uptake. See text for details of the various actions of protein kinase. The LDL is degraded in the lysosome, providing cholesterol for steroidogenesis. The LH and its receptor (R) is internalized, and the LH is degraded in lysosomes. The receptors for LH and LDL are probably recycled to the plasma membrane.

thesis (194), including a cholesterol-binding protein (195), or they may enhance protein synthesis by phosphorylation of ribosomes (196). The exact sites in the steroidogenic pathway where protein synthesis is required have not been elucidated, but several have been suggested. (2) Phosphorylation of cholesterol esterase activates this steroidogenic enzyme (197,198). (3) It also appears that phosphorylation of a component (cytochrome P-450) of the cholesterol side-chain cleavage enzyme complex (199–201) is required for activation of this enzyme complex. (4) Transport of cholesterol into the mitochondria has been shown to involve microfilaments (202). (5) Microfilaments may also play a role in the transport of pregnenolone out of the mitochondria and/or (6) the internalization and transport of LDL receptors to lysosomes. The polymerization and activity of microfilaments is thought to be modified by protein kinase and phosphorylation. More recently, alterations in phospholipid turnover have been demonstrated following stimulation of steroidogenic tissues with 8-bromo-cAMP or LH (203). Each of these sites of regulation of steroidogenesis will be discussed in more detail below.

The steroids and sterols involved in steroidogenesis are only slightly soluble in aqueous media; therefore, diffusion alone does not seem sufficient to shuttle substrates from one enzymatic site to another. This problem is partially alleviated by the close association of several of the steroidogenic enzymes in linked complexes (e.g., the cholesterol side-chain cleavage complex), although transport may be further assisted by close proximity of steroidogenically related organelles (204). Hepatocytes alleviate the problem of substrate transport by synthesizing sterol binding proteins, which render the otherwise insoluble sterols soluble in the aqueous cytoplasm (205). The hepatic enzymes involved in the synthesis of cholesterol appear to be dependent on these proteins to facilitate substrate transport and transfer to successive enzymes in the pathway. A similar process appears to occur in luteal tissue since binding proteins for cholesterol (206,207) and pregnenolone (208) have been identified. Since ongoing protein synthesis is essential for the steroidogenic response (170,209–211), and the protein(s) synthesized has a very short half-life (211), it is possible that the protein(s) is a steroid carrier protein. In the case of luteal cells, the synthesis and/or activation of this carrier protein may be sensitive to stimulation by tropic hormones. It appears that ongoing protein synthesis is necessary for transport of cholesterol to the cytochrome P-450 component of the side-chain cleavage enzyme complex, and this appears to be one mechanism involved in stimulation of progesterone secretion in luteal tissue by LH (212).

All of the enzymes involved in steroidogenesis in luteal tissue (cholesterol esterase, cholesterol side-chain cleaveage complex, and 3β-hydroxysteroid dehydrogenase:Δ^5,Δ^4-isomerase complex) are sensitive to end-product inhibition (213). This end-product inhibition is of such magnitude that it makes reliable measurement of 3β-hydroxysteroid dehydrogenase-isomerase activity very difficult (214). In fact, the affinity of this enzyme complex for the end product, progesterone, is six times greater than for the precursor, pregnenolone (214). Reduced end-product inhibition of this enzyme would also be expected to decrease the inhibitory effects exerted by other products synthesized previously in the steroidogenic pathway. Steroid binding proteins could provide a mechanism for reducing end-product inhibition of the key steroidogenic enzymes.

Steroidogenesis in luteal tissue is less complex than in other steroidogenic tissues, since the major product, progesterone, is formed early in the steroidogenic pathway. Cholesterol is the initial substrate for luteal steroidogenesis. It may be extracted from the circulation, released from intracellular stores of cholesterol esters, or synthesized *de novo* from acetate. Although all three sources of cholesterol have been implicated in the steroidogenic response of luteal cells to LH (215–220), there are substantial quantities of cholesterol (both free and esterified) already present within luteal cells. Regulation of cholesterol uptake via the LDL-receptor pathway is likely to involve microfilaments and may be regulated, at least to a degree, by LH. The release of cholesterol from pools of fatty acid esters is a possible target for the acute action of LH (220). It is clear that cholesterol esterase is activated by a cAMP-dependent protein kinase (197,198). Therefore, this enzyme appears to be one important point for the regulation of steroidogenesis by LH.

Activation of cholesterol side-chain cleavage complex by a cAMP-dependent protein kinase has also been reported, and it was suggested that the phosphorylated moiety was cytochrome P-450 (199). This enzyme is a key one in the steroidogenic pathway and is thought by many to be the rate-limiting factor in steroidogenesis. Thus, its regulation by cAMP-dependent protein kinase may be the most important step in LH regulation of steroidogenesis. There is no evidence for acute hormonal regulation of 3β-hydroxysteroid dehydrogenase:Δ^5,Δ^4-isomerase complex, and this enzyme appears to be present in considerable excess in luteal tissue (214). The synthesis of new enzyme seems unlikely in the case of cholesterol side-chain cleavage complex (mitochondria) or 3β-hydroxysteroid dehydrogenase-isomerase complex (smooth endoplasmic reticulum), since both of these enzyme complexes are integral components of intracellular membranes (214,221). The turnover of these organelles is much too slow to account for the rapid, acute steroidogenic response that follows LH stimulation. However, synthesis of new enzyme might be expected as part of the chronic response to LH. Since cholesterol esterase is thought to be a cytoplasmic or soluble enzyme (214,220), its activity could be modified more easily as a result of increased synthesis or a decline in its degradation rate.

As a final consideration, cAMP may be involved directly in the chronic response of luteal cells to LH. Gospodarowicz and Gospodarowicz (172) have indicated that bovine luteal cells grown in culture tend to dedifferentiate with time but reform into luteal cells on addition of LH or cAMP, apparently as a result of the effects of cAMP on microtubules. Thus, it appears that cAMP may be important for the maintenance of the normal morphology of luteal cells *in vivo* and for the maintenance of the intracellular components necessary for steroid synthesis and secretion. It has also been suggested that LH-stimulated cAMP may be important for the differentiation of small to large luteal cells in ewes (61) and cows (32).

The data presented above suggest that LH may stimulate the synthesis of progesterone via a number of mechanisms, including protein kinase activation of cholesterol esterase and a component of side-chain cleavage enzyme complex, and synthesis and/or activation of transport mechanisms responsible for enhancing substrate availability and/or relief of end-product inhibition. It is not necessary that the effects of LH be limited to one of these mechanisms. In fact, it seems likely that LH stimulates secretion of progesterone via several mechanisms.

The above discussion has dealt primarily with the effects of LH on progesterone secretion from small luteal cells, which contain the majority of the LH receptors. However, in sheep—and probably in many other species—most of the progesterone is secreted by large luteal cells (61). Secretion of progesterone from large cells does not appear to be regulated by the cAMP second messenger system, although these cells contain adenylate cyclase (222). Treatment of large luteal cells with cholera toxin or forskolin to activate adenylate cyclase nonspecifically results in a dramatic increase in intracellular cAMP, but there is no concomitant increase in progesterone production (222). This was true even though an enhanced occupancy of cAMP-dependent protein kinase was demonstrated. In contrast, secretion of progesterone from large luteal cells is enhanced by PGE_2, although this response is not mediated via adenylate cyclase (223). Further studies are required to elucidate the mechanisms regulating synthesis of progesterone in large cells. It is possible that during differentiation these cells lose the ability to inhibit the cAMP-dependent processes (i.e., they have reduced levels of phosphodiesterase or protein phosphatases). Since the conversion of cAMP to 5′-AMP and the dephosphorylation of proteins by phosphatase are thought to be key mechanisms involved in limiting the stimulatory effect of increased intracellular levels of cAMP, reduced levels or a total lack of these enzymes would be expected to result in a permanent stimulation of steroidogenesis. Further research is needed to unravel the mechanisms controlling secretion of progesterone by large cells.

LUTEOLYSIS

Uterine Involvement in Luteal Regression

The first evidence of uterine involvement in the luteolytic process was presented in 1923 (224), when Loeb reported that removal of the uterus (hysterectomy) lengthened the life span of the corpus luteum in guinea pigs. Extension of the life span of the corpus luteum following hysterectomy was later demonstrated in pseudopregnant rats (225,226), mice (227,228), hamsters (229–231) and rabbits (232–234). Maintenance of the corpus luteum also occurs following hysterectomy in cattle, sheep (235), swine (236), and horses (237,238).

In other species, the presence of the uterus is not required for luteolysis. Most notably, in several species of primates—including rhesus monkeys (239), cynomologus monkeys (240), and humans (241,242)—removal of the uterus has no effect on normal cyclic activity. In addition, hysterectomy has no effect on the life span of the corpus luteum in the opossum (243), dog (128,244), or ferret (245). In contrast to pseudopregnant animals, the normal estrous cycle of the rat (246), mouse (247), and hamster (229,230) is not prolonged by hysterectomy.

Although there is variation among species in the length of time that corpora lutea survive in hysterectomized animals, corpora lutea generally retain both structural and functional integrity for at least the duration of a normal pregnancy in guinea pigs (248–250), sheep (251–253), cattle (254,255), pigs (236,256–258), and rats (259). Following hysterectomy of rabbits or horses, luteal function is maintained at levels lower than those established during the luteal phase (238,260–262).

In many species, the effects of the uterus on luteal function are exerted locally. Unilateral hysterectomy (removal of one uterine horn) in sheep (263,264), cattle (265), swine (266), guinea pigs (267,268), pseudopregnant hamsters (269), and pseudopregnant rats (270) results in luteal regression in the ovary adjacent to the intact horn but prevents regression in the opposite ovary. The rabbit and horse are exceptions in that corpora lutea will undergo regression despite unilateral removal of the adjacent uterine horn (237,271). Thus, it is apparent that the luteolytic factor emanating from the uterus in most species exerts its effect only on the adjacent ovary. Therefore, it is unlikely that it is transported from uterus to ovary through the systemic circulation.

The mechanism of this transport is not clear. The corpora lutea are maintained when the connections (vascular and otherwise) between the ovary and uterus are severed in ewes (263), cows (272), guinea pigs (273–275), and pseudopregnant rats (268,270,276). Autotransplantation of either the uterus or ovary, while leaving the other organ *in situ*, results in extended luteal function in ewes (277,278) and guinea pigs (279–281). However, when the uterus and ovaries are transplanted to the neck as as unit, normal cyclic ovarian behavior continues in ewes (282). On the contrary, luteolysis is merely delayed following autotransplantation of the uterus or endometrial tissue in hamsters (229).

The uterine luteolytic factor appears to pass directly from the uterine vein to the ovarian artery in the ewe. This conclusion is based primarily on the results of the elegant anatomical and vascular anastomoses studies of Ginther and his colleagues (for a review, see ref. 283). If the uterine vein draining the intact horn of unilaterally hysterectomized ewes is anastomosed to the uterine vein from the hysterectomized side, only the corpora lutea on the hysterectomized side will regress (284,285) (Fig. 11). Reversal of the normal pattern of luteal regression in unilaterally hysterectomized ewes also occurs if the ovarian artery supplying the ovary on the uterine intact side is anastomosed to the artery on the hysterectomized side (284,285) (Fig. 12). A similar effect of uterine venous and ovarian arterial anastomoses has been described for cattle (286).

Although there do not appear to be vascular connections between the uterine vein and ovarian artery, there are regions of extensive contact between these 2 vessels throughout the broad ligament and up to their respective junctions with the vena cava and aorta (287,288). The ovarian artery is extremely tortuous, and collateral channels and venules separate from the uterine vein, wrapping around the artery and

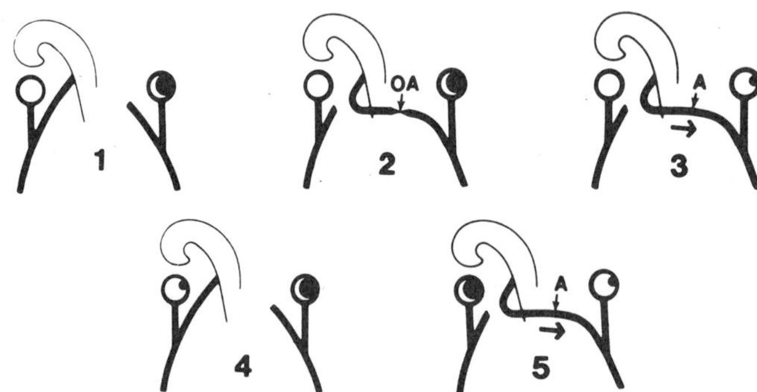

FIG. 11. Effects of unilateral hysterectomy and uterine venous anastomosis on luteolysis in sheep. Arrows indicate the direction of blood flow. A large or small black dot in an ovary indicates the corpus luteum was maintained or regressed, respectively, 20 days after ovulation. Unilateral hysterectomy (1, 4) resulted in luteal maintenance on the hysterectomized side and luteal regression on the uterine-intact side (4). Anastomosis of the uterine vein from the intact to the hysterectomized side resulted in luteal regression on the hysterectomized side if the anastomosis was patent (3), but the corpus luteum was maintained when the anastomosis was occluded (OA) (2). When corpora lutea were present on both ovaries, diversion of the uterine drainage from the uterine-intact side to the hysterectomized side resulted in luteal maintenance on the uterine-intact side and luteal regression on the hysterectomized side (5). (From ref. 284.)

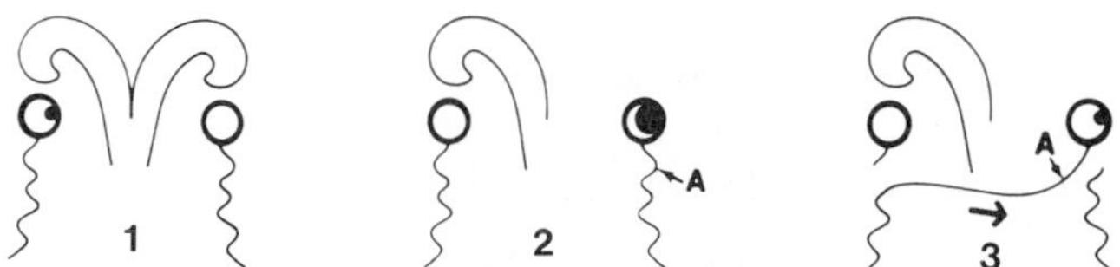

FIG. 12. Effects of unilateral hysterectomy and ovarian arterial anastomosis (A) on luteal regression in sheep. A large or small black dot in an ovary indicates the corpus luteum was maintained or regressed, respectively, 20 days after ovulation. In control ewes, luteal regression occurred at the appropriate time (1). Unilateral hysterectomy resulted in luteal maintenance on the hysterectomized side (2). Anastomosis of the ovarian artery from the uterine-intact side to the ovarian artery on the hysterectomized side resulted in luteal regression on the hysterectomized side (3). The arrow indicates the direction of blood flow. (From ref. 284.)

thus increases the area of contact between the two vessels (289). The vessels share a common tunica adventitia and have thinner walls in regions where they make contact (290). Similar gross morphological venoarterial relationships have been observed in guinea pigs, rats, hamsters (291), pigs (288), and cows (292). Interestingly, there is a very little contact between the uterine vein and ovarian artery in the rabbit and horse, two species in which the uterine luteolytic effect is not exerted locally (288,291,293).

Identification of $PGF_{2\alpha}$ as the Uterine Luteolytic Factor

Although the luteolytic effect of the uterus was recognized more than 60 years ago, the mechanisms involved in this effect were difficult to elucidate. A major breakthrough in this area occurred when the luteolytic actions of $PGF_{2\alpha}$ were demonstrated in pseudopregnant rats (294). This initial observation was rapidly extended to other species, and $PGF_{2\alpha}$ has been shown to exert a luteolytic effect in cattle (295–298), sheep (299–301), guinea pigs (302), goats (303), horses (304–306), pseudopregnant rodents—i.e., mice (307), hamsters (308), and rabbits (309,310)—and to a limited extent in swine (311–314).

Interestingly, in rhesus monkeys (315,316), humans (317,318), and dogs (319), species in which the uterus has no clear luteolytic effect, there is a transitory suppression in the secretion of progesterone following short-term infusions (up to 12 hr) with $PGF_{2\alpha}$ during the luteal phase of the cycle. In fact, premature luteal regression can be induced in rhesus monkeys (320) and dogs (321) by more prolonged treatment regimens with high levels of $PGF_{2\alpha}$. Extremely high doses of $PGF_{2\alpha}$ are ineffective in causing luteal regression in the cat (322). If endogenous $PGF_{2\alpha}$ is involved in the normal luteolytic process in these species, it is probably not of uterine origin.

Although treatment of animals with $PGF_{2\alpha}$ caused premature luteolysis, this did not prove that it was the uterine factor involved in this process normally. However, considerable evidence has accumulated to suggest that $PGF_{2\alpha}$ is the factor of uterine origin responsible for luteolysis in both large domestic species and rodents. Treatment of intact animals with inhibitors of prostaglandin synthesis, such as indomethacin, will block spontaneous luteolysis in cattle, sheep, and guinea pigs. The length of pseudopregnancy can be prolonged in rabbits (323), rats, hamsters (324), and mice (325) by treatment with indomethacin. Thus, synthesis of prostaglandins (presumably $PGF_{2\alpha}$) appears to be required for normal luteolysis. Perhaps the best evidence that $PGF_{2\alpha}$ is the uterine luteolytic factor is the fact that spontaneous luteal regression can be prevented by active or passive immunization of sheep (326,327), cattle (328), and guinea pigs (250) to $PGF_{2\alpha}$.

Prostaglandin $F_{2\alpha}$ has been isolated from endometrial tissue of several species, and its concentration is maximal during the period of luteal regression in cattle (329), sheep (330), guinea pig (331), horses (332), swine (333), pseudopregnant rats (334), and pseudopregnant rabbits (335). In addition, secretion of $PGF_{2\alpha}$ into the uterine vein is temporally associated with both spontaneous and hormonally induced luteal regression in several species. The concentrations of $PGF_{2\alpha}$ in uterine venous blood increases as spontaneous luteolysis commences in swine (336,337), horses (338), and pseudopregnant rabbits (335) and rats (339).

Based on the available data, it seems reasonable to conclude that $PGF_{2\alpha}$ is the factor, of uterine origin, responsible for luteolysis in the large domestic species and pseudopregnant rodents.

Mechanism of Action of $PGF_{2\alpha}$

A number of different mechanisms have been proposed to explain the luteolytic effects of $PGF_{2\alpha}$: (a) a rapid and dramatic decrease in luteal blood flow (71,139); (b) a reduction in the number of receptors for LH (340); (c) an uncoupling of the LH receptor from adenylate cyclase (341); and (d) a cytotoxic effect (342). Although there is good evidence for all of these actions, the effects of $PGF_{2\alpha}$ appear to differ among species, and the actions demonstrable *in vivo* often differ from those observed *in vitro*.

Injections of a luteolytic dose of $PGF_{2\alpha}$ into rats does not appear to decrease ovarian blood flow (183). However, it does dramatically decrease the binding of LH to luteal cells *in vivo* by an unexplained mechanism. There is a direct block of adenylate cyclase activation by LH in isolated rat luteal cells. Finally, there is an eventual loss of LH receptors due to inhibition of the actions of prolactin.

In ewes, the first effect of $PGF_{2\alpha}$ appears to be a rapid decrease in luteal blood flow (139) (Fig. 13). The decrease in blood flow is highly correlated with decreased levels of progesterone in serum. There is no decrease in the number of receptors for LH in ewes administered a luteolytic dose of $PGF_{2\alpha}$ until well after a dramatic decrease in serum levels

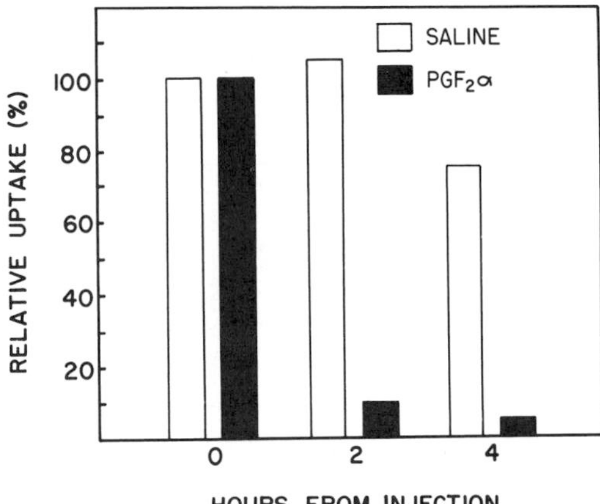

FIG. 13. Relative blood flow to the corpus luteum before and after administration of $PGF_{2\alpha}$ or saline to ewes on day 9 of the estrous cycle. Data are expressed as percentage of the uptake of radioactive microspheres prior to treatment. (From ref. 71.)

of progesterone has occurred (184). A number of effects of $PGF_{2\alpha}$ have also been demonstrated *in vitro*. There is a total block of LH-induced increases in the production of cAMP and progesterone secretion (Fig. 14). This observation is particularly interesting since the majority of receptors for LH are on small steroidogenic cells, whereas receptors for $PGF_{2\alpha}$ are on large luteal cells (66). This suggests that there must be large cell–small cell communication in the corpus luteum. This concept is further substantiated by the observation that the number of large luteal cells and the levels of serum progesterone are reduced significantly within 12 hr of a luteolytic dose of $PGF_{2\alpha}$ but that the number of small cells does not decrease until 24 hr (343). $PGF_{2\alpha}$ has been shown to be cytotoxic to large luteal cells *in vitro*, an effect that was reversed by coincubation in the presence of PGE_2 (342).

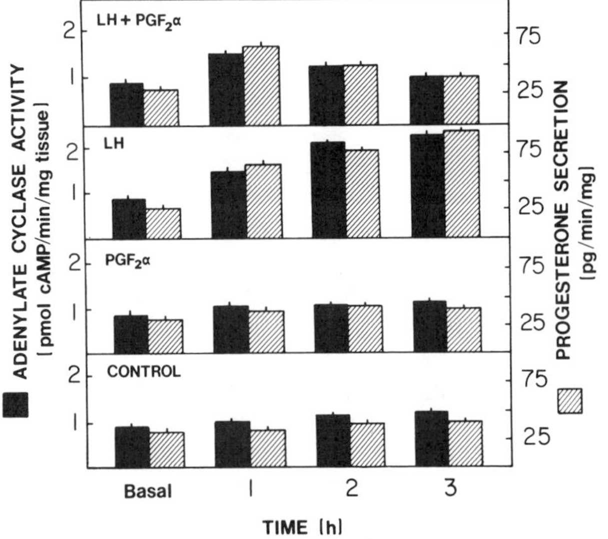

FIG. 14. Adenylate cyclase activity and rate of progesterone accumulation from ovine luteal tissue following stimulation with Medium 199 alone (control), $PGF_{2\alpha}$ (250 ng/ml), LH (100 ng/ml), or LH plus $PGF_{2\alpha}$. The values represent means ± SEM from triplicate determinations at each time point. (From ref. 341).

The biological significance of the data obtained *in vitro* is questionable since LH stimulation of progesterone secretion from luteal tissue obtained at various times after a luteolytic dose of $PGF_{2\alpha}$ does not decrease even at times where serum levels of progesterone have declined (344). Weston and Hixon (344) suggested that the most important action of $PGF_{2\alpha}$ *in vivo* was its dramatic effect on luteal blood flow.

Morphological Changes during Luteal Regression

During regression of the corpus luteum following pregnancy in rats a number of distinct morphological changes occur (24). The plasma membrane of cells from the regressing corpus luteum contain membrane specializations, including gap junctions, maculae adherentes, coated invaginations, and microvilli similar to those of the corpus luteum of pregnancy. Many lipid droplets were found in the cytoplasm during early luteolysis, a time when luteal triglycerides have been shown to increase 10-fold (24). There is a decrease in the quantity of smooth endoplasmic reticulum and an increase in the number of autophagic vacuoles and heterolysosomes. As regression progresses, many of the cells show an increased number of cytoplasmic vacuoles. The degenerating cells appear to be removed by macrophages (345).

A number of morphological changes appear to be common among several species during luteolysis. The increase in the number of lipid droplets and cytoplasmic vacuoles has also been observed in rabbits (346), pigs (345), humans (347), and sheep (348). Other morphological characteristics of the degenerating cells also appear to be similar in several species. However, macrophages do not appear to be involved in removing the cell debris in regressing rabbit corpora lutea (346).

The degenerative changes in the ovine corpus luteum noted near the end of the estrous cycle and observed following treatment with $PGF_{2\alpha}$ have been studied extensively. The densely staining secretory granules observed during periods of maximal secretion of progesterone decrease in number throughout the period of luteal regression. Concurrent with the decrease in numbers of secretory granules is the appearance of autophagosomes (71). Autophagosomes appear to be sites of cytoplasmic involution, and their numbers increase as regression of the corpus luteum proceeds.

Another early change that occurs during regression of the corpus luteum is in the vascular component. The percentage volume of the corpus luteum occupied by vascular elements decreases linearly during the last few days of the estrous cycle (139). Likewise, in sheep there is a rapid decrease in the number of red blood cells and luminal volume of capillaries in the corpus luteum after treatment with $PGF_{2\alpha}$ (71). A swelling of the endothelial cells appears to be responsible for the initial reduction in luminal volume. The decreased luminal volume most likely results in a decreased perfusion of luteal tissue and probably causes blood to be shunted away from the corpus luteum (139,349,350).

As luteal regression continues, there is an accumulation of lipid droplets in the cells and the steroidogenic cells decrease in size. The shrinkage of the cells results in a clumping of subcellular components. This is particularly noticeable in the case of mitochondria. Normally, there is little, if any, evidence of lipid accumulation in the cells of ovine corpus luteum; however, during regression there is a striking increase in intracellular lipid, with the lipid droplet becoming the most prominent organelle near the end of the estrous cycle.

Lysosomes are present in luteal cells throughout the estrous cycle; however, they appear to increase in number as regression of the corpus luteum progresses (77). During the midluteal phase of the cycle, acid phosphatase activity is restricted to lysosomes and the inner cisternae of the Golgi apparatus. During regression an increase in number of primary lysosomes appears to occur as a result of pinching off from the lateral margins of the inner Golgi cisternae. As regression progresses, the intracellular organelles become increasingly disorganized, and acid phosphatase activity is found with the degenerating organelles. The cellular disorganization during luteal regression is not restricted to steroidogenic cells but involves essentially all cells comprising the corpus luteum.

LUTEAL FUNCTION DURING PREGNANCY

Maternal Recognition of Pregnancy

In most mammalian species, progesterone must be secreted throughout gestation to maintain a uterine environment conducive to pregnancy. In some species, carnivores and marsupials, for example, gestation lasts no longer than a normal luteal phase. Therefore, there is no need for the conceptus to alter luteal function since the corpus luteum provides adequate progestational support. Most other mammalian species have developed a means of shortening the life span of the corpus luteum in the event of a nonfertile cycle so as to increase reproductive efficiency. The luteolytic mechanism discussed in the preceding section provides such a means. Along with the development of a uterine luteolytic mechanism, some means of maintaining the uterus in a progestational state during pregnancy must also be developed if successful reproduction is to occur. The simplest solution would be for the conceptus itself to secrete progesterone and ensure its own survival. In many species, the placenta is a very active endocrine tissue, secreting several hormones, including progesterone. However, in most species, the ability of the conceptus to secrete progesterone is not developed until after the corpus luteum of the estrous cycle would have normally regressed, e.g., sheep (351). Thus, in order to maintain adequate progestational support for a developing pregnancy it is necessary to prevent luteal regression. The process by which the conceptus acts to maintain luteal secretion of progesterone has been termed maternal recognition of pregnancy. The mechanism by which this process is accomplished differs from species to species, and a few examples will be considered in the following discussion.

Rat

The estrous cycle of the rat lasts only 4 to 5 days. The corpus luteum of the estrous cycle secretes progesterone for just 24 to 48 hr and never becomes fully functional (352, 353). Sterile mating or cervical stimulation results in pseudopregnancy. During pseudopregnancy the corpus luteum continues to secrete progesterone for up to 12 days (253,259). Maintenance of the corpus luteum of gestation or pseudopregnancy appears to involve two separate endocrine effects. First, fertile mating (or cervical stimulation leading to pseudopregnancy) results in activation of a neural reflex arc leading to a dramatic increase in serum concentrations of prolactin within 2 hr that persists as long as 48 hr (354). The increased serum levels of prolactin are dependent upon stimulation of the pelvic nerve since bilateral resection of the pelvic nerve prevents the enhanced secretion of prolactin in mated rats. Freeman et al. (355) subsequently showed that cervical stimulation results in both diurnal and nocturnal surges of prolactin that last throughout pseudopregnancy. A similar phenomenon appears to exist during pregnancy since Butcher et al. (356) reported two surges of prolactin per day during early pregnancy. Thus, it seems clear that in rats cervical stimulation on the morning of estrus leads to increased secretion of prolactin and enhanced concentrations of progesterone in serum. The increase in prolactin secretion appears to be responsible for prolongation of luteal function since daily injections of prolactin will maintain the corpus luteum in cycling rats (357) and since a single injection of ergocornine (an inhibitor of prolactin secretion) on days 6, 7, 8, or 9 terminates pseudopregnancy (358). The enhanced secretion of prolactin during pregnancy or pseudopregnancy is responsible for increasing the number of luteal LH receptors and thus enhancing the steroidogenic responsiveness of this tissue to the hormone (41). These events appear sufficient to ensure that a proper endocrine environment is provided for implantation and normal development of the embryo during early pregnancy.

In the rat, gestation lasts about 22 days, and corpora lutea are required through day 17 to maintain pregnancy (359). The ovary is the primary source of progesterone throughout gestation, and replacement therapy with progesterone is all that is required to maintain pregnancy in ovariectomized rats (359). The process of maternal recognition of pregnancy in the rat involves prolonging the life span of the corpus luteum of pseudopregnancy.

The corpus luteum of early pregnancy is dependent on prolactin only through day 7 (360). Serum concentrations of progesterone during early pregnancy are very similar to those in pseudopregnancy; however, instead of decreasing on day 11, as in pseudopregnant rats, the concentration of progesterone in serum increases to about twice that seen in pseudopregnancy and is maintained at this higher level through day 20 (259). The corpora lutea of pseudopregnant rats are maintained following hysterectomy (225) or after induction of decidual tissue in the uterus (361,362); however, the concentration of progesterone in serum remains at the same lower level established early in pseudopregnancy in both of these situations (259).

A complete picture of uterine secretion of $PGF_{2\alpha}$ in pregnant and pseudopregnant rats is not available. Uterine content and uterine venous concentrations of $PGF_{2\alpha}$ are maximal on days 10 through 12 of pseudopregnancy (334,339), and this increase may initiate luteolysis. However, a similar increase in uterine venous concentrations of $PGF_{2\alpha}$ was observed on day 10 in pregnant rats (363). The ability of placental tissue from rats to synthesize $PGF_{2\alpha}$ is maximal on day 11 (364). Despite the increase in synthesis and secretion of $PGF_{2\alpha}$ from the uterus during pregnancy, the corpora lutea do not regress.

Maintenance of the corpus luteum during the second half of gestation in rats depends upon the secretion of placental luteotropin (365,366). Luteotropic activity was first demonstrable by bioassay in serum on day 11 of pregnancy, reached peak levels on day 12, and had begun to decrease on day 13 (366). A substance with prolactin-like activity, rat placental lactogen (rPL) has been isolated and purified from placental tissue of rats (367,368). It is detectable in the serum of pregnant rats on days 8 through 15 (367,369). A similar lactogenic substance exists in decidual tissue of pseudopregnant rats (358). Placental tissue also secretes a substance with LH-like properties, a rat chorionic gonadotropin (rCG), whereas decidual tissue does not (370,371).

These substances, secreted by the placenta and decidual endometrium, can account for all of the endocrine changes associated with maternal recognition of pregnancy. The rPL, of placental or decidual origin, may provide adequate lactogenic support by day 8 such that prolactin is no longer necessary. Rat PL may also reduce the sensitivity of the corpus luteum to $PGF_{2\alpha}$. Behrman et al. (340) have shown that treatment of pseudopregnant rats with prolactin reduces the ability of exogenous $PGF_{2\alpha}$ to induce luteal regression. The rCG, secreted by the placenta, may be responsible for the increased secretion of progesterone observed during the second half of pregnancy. This substance is not present in hysterectomized or decidualized pseudopregnant rats, which maintain luteal function at a lower level than in pregnant rats.

Based on these observations, it appears that the conceptus alters luteal function in at least three ways: (a) It shortens the period over which the corpus luteum requires prolactin to maintain normal function; (b) it exerts a direct stimulatory effect on the corpus luteum not observed in hysterectomized pseudopregnant rats; and (c) it reduces the sensitivity of the corpus luteum to the luteolytic effect of $PGF_{2\alpha}$.

Rabbit

The rabbit is a reflex-ovulator; therefore, corpora lutea are found only after mating, cervical stimulation, or hormonal induction of ovulation. If the ovulatory stimulus is not a fertile mating, a pseudopregnancy results, and corpora lutea secrete progesterone for about 16 to 17 days (372). Follicular secretion of estrogens, stimulated by LH, is required to maintain normal luteal function throughout pseudopregnancy (373).

Chronic treatment of intact pseudopregnant rabbits with estradiol-17β stimulates luteal secretion of progesterone but has no effect on the life span of the corpus luteum (261,373). Hysterectomy has just the opposite effect. It lengthens the life span of the corpus luteum but only slows the reduction in luteal function, which begins about day 12. Luteal function is then maintained at a much lower level for several days (261,262,372). Maximal luteal function is maintained if hysterectomized, pseudopregnant rabbits are treated with estradiol-17β (261). These data may indicate that the corpus luteum has some intrinsic control over its own sensitivity to the luteotropic action of estrogens. Perhaps sensitivity to estradiol-17β decreases after day 10.

A significant increase in the concentration of $PGF_{2\alpha}$ in uterine tissue and uterine venous plasma occurs on day 17 of pseudopregnancy (262,335). Uterine production of $PGF_{2\alpha}$ may be stimulated by the decrease in concentrations of progesterone and/or increase in concentrations of estradiol-17β in serum that occurs during the last few days of pseudopregnancy (374). The increase in uterine secretion of $PGF_{2\alpha}$ is responsible for regression of the corpus luteum.

In the pregnant rabbit, corpora lutea continue to secrete progesterone for 31 days, the duration of gestation (374). Corpora lutea are required throughout gestation to maintain pregnancy in the rabbit, and replacement with progesterone is an adequate substitute in ovariectomized pregnant does (375,376). The placenta of the rabbit does not produce progesterone (377).

Corpora lutea develop a dependence on some placental product around day 12. Removal of the conceptus before day 12 results in a temporal pattern in the concentration of progesterone very similar to that seen during pseudopregnancy (378,379). However, removal of the conceptus on day 12 or thereafter results in a very precipitous decline in the concentration of progesterone in serum. Removal of fetuses alone has very little effect (380,381). Unlike embryonic tissue from rats, the rabbit conceptus is devoid of LH-like activity throughout pregnancy (382,383).

The corpus luteum is dependent on follicular estrogens throughout pregnancy (384). Treatment of pregnant rabbits with very high doses of estradiol-17β following removal of the conceptus on day 18 results in maintenance of luteal function (381). However, physiological doses of estradiol-17β are ineffective in maintaining the corpus luteum following hysterectomy on day 21 of pregnancy (384). These data imply that the presence of the embryo reduces the amount of estrogen required to maintain luteal function, i.e., it increases luteal sensitivity to estrogen.

There are dramatic changes in uterine secretion of prostaglandins in pregnant rabbits (262,335). The increase in secretion of $PGF_{2\alpha}$ on day 17 of pseudopregnancy is absent in pregnancy, perhaps because secretion of progesterone is maintained at a very high level throughout pregnancy. Beginning on day 11 of pregnancy, there is an increase in uterine secretion of PGE_2, the amount secreted being proportional to the number of embryos in the uterus. The luteotropic properties of PGE_2 in rabbits have not been examined, but PGE_1 does stimulate luteal adenylate cyclase activity (385). The concentration of PGE_2 is extremely high in the fetal portion of the placenta (335), and rabbit blastocysts secrete PGE_2 during incubation *in vitro* (386). It is possible that PGE_2 is the placental factor that enhances luteal sensitivity to follicular estrogens.

Guinea Pig

As for all of the remaining species to be discussed, the guinea pig is a spontaneous ovulator. It has recurrent estrous cycles about 16 days long. During the cycle, the concentration of progesterone in serum reaches a maximum on day 6 and is maintained at this level through day 11, after which levels fall as the corpora lutea regress (387,388). As noted previously, uterine secretion of $PGF_{2\alpha}$ increases during the period of luteolysis (389,390).

Corpora lutea must continue to secrete progesterone through the first 30 days of gestation. Replacement therapy with progesterone will maintain pregnancy in ovariectomized guinea pigs (391,392). The placenta begins to synthesize some progesterone as early as day 15 and becomes the primary source from day 40 through the remainder of gestation (393).

The concentrations of progesterone in serum through the first 10 days of gestation are very similar to those observed during the estrous cycle; however, by day 20 the concentration of progesterone has increased nearly 100-fold (394). The progesterone is primarily of luteal origin (393), and the levels reached are much higher than in animals in which the corpora lutea can be maintained by either hysterectomy or treatment with indomethacin (250). The corpora lutea also increase in size during this period (395,396). One factor that contributes to the increase in the circulating concentrations of progesterone is a reduction in the metabolic clearance rate for progesterone (397,398). This reduction may be due to an increase in the concentration of circulating proteins capable of binding progesterone. However, this change in clearance rate cannot completely account for the increase in the concentration of progesterone observed. The production of progesterone by the corpora lutea must increase during this period as well (394). Thus, the conceptus appears to exert at least three effects: (a) it prevents luteal regression, (b) stimulates luteal growth and secretion of progesterone, and (c) reduces the metabolic clearance rate of progesterone.

The concentrations of $PGF_{2\alpha}$ in uterine venous plasma of pregnant guinea pigs on days 12 through 16 postestrus are lower than those in nonpregnant guinea pigs over the same period (399,400). Homogenates of uteri collected from pregnant guinea pigs on day 15 produced less $PGF_{2\alpha}$ *in vitro* than did similar homogenates from nonpregnant guinea pigs (396). Thus, the failure of the corpus luteum of early pregnancy to undergo luteal regression may be due to the lack of synthesis and secretion of $PGF_{2\alpha}$ from the uterus. It is equally possible that maintenance of the corpus luteum keeps the hormonal environment in a state not conducive to maximal secretion of $PGF_{2\alpha}$.

As in the rat, an LH-like substance, a guinea pig CG, has been identified in placental tissue (401). The concentrations of the substance in placental tissue are maximal on day 18 postestrus, coinciding with the period of luteal growth and increased secretion of progesterone. Babra et al. (402) have purified the substance and found it to be structurally similar and of comparable biological potency to hCG.

Domestic Ruminants

In the ewe, the corpus luteum must be present through the first 50 days of gestation to maintain pregnancy (403,404). Pregnancy can be maintained in ovariectomized ewes by treatment with progesterone (405,406). The placenta begins to secrete progesterone around day 50 of gestation (351) and provides adequate progestational support for the remainder of gestation. Following removal of embryos on day 13 or thereafter, the life span of the corpus luteum is extended (407), indicating that the embryo has a luteotropic effect by this time. However, embryos can be successfully transferred to synchronized recipients as late as day 12 postestrus and the corpus luteum will be maintained (408). Thus, the critical period for maternal recognition of pregnancy in the ewe is days 12 to 13.

The concentrations of progesterone in serum of pregnant and nonpregnant ewes are similar through the first 14 days postestrus (409) and are maintained at this level through the first 50 days of gestation (410). Thus, it appears that the only effect of the conceptus on the corpus luteum is to prevent luteal regression. Investigations into the mechanism by which the conceptus maintains luteal function have centered around two possibilities. The first is that the conceptus suppresses uterine secretion of $PGF_{2\alpha}$. The second is that the conceptus reduces the sensitivity of the corpus luteum to the luteolytic effects of $PGF_{2\alpha}$. With respect to the first possibility, concentrations of $PGF_{2\alpha}$ in uterine venous plasma of pregnant and nonpregnant ewes have been examined in numerous studies. It seems clear, from measurements of both $PGF_{2\alpha}$ and its major metabolite 13,14-dihydro-15-keto-$PGF_{2\alpha}$ (PGFM), that the high-amplitude surges in secretion, which occur during and after luteolysis in nonpregnant ewes, are absent in pregnant ewes (411–414). However, basal levels of $PGF_{2\alpha}$ in uterine venous plasma collected at frequent intervals are higher in pregnant than in cycling ewes. Basal concentrations of PGFM in peripheral plasma are greater in pregnant animals, reaching a maximum value on day 14 or 15 (414,415). Prior to luteal regression, the concentrations of $PGF_{2\alpha}$ in the serum of pregnant ewes are similar to or greater than those in nonpregnant ewes (411,412,416–420).

The concentrations of $PGF_{2\alpha}$ in uterine tissue and uterine luminal flushings are greater in pregnant than in nonpregnant ewes (417,418,421,422). The ability of uterine tissue to secrete $PGF_{2\alpha}$ *in vitro* is also greater in pregnant ewes (418,423). Thus, the gravid uterus retains the ability to synthesize $PGF_{2\alpha}$; however, the pattern of secretion appears to be altered. It is impossible to determine if the change in the pattern of secretion of $PGF_{2\alpha}$ is a cause or an effect of luteal maintenance given the current lack of knowledge concerning steroidal regulation of uterine secretion of $PGF_{2\alpha}$.

Homogenates of day 14 to 16 conceptuses maintain the corpus luteum when infused into the uterine lumen (424–426). The active component within the homogenate is heat labile and susceptible to proteolytic digestion. There is no LH- or prolactin-like bioactivity associated with these homogenates (425). Homogenates of 22-day-old embryos lack the ability to maintain the corpus luteum.

Infusion into the uterine horn of a mixture of large-molecular-weight substances secreted *in vitro* by the ovine conceptus collected on day 15 or 16 maintains luteal function in nonpregnant ewes (427) and reduces uterine secretion of $PGF_{2\alpha}$ in response to treatment with estradiol-17β (415). Godkin et al. (427,428) have isolated a protein from this mixture that is able to maintain the corpus luteum. It binds specifically to the uterine endometrium (429) and probably exerts its effects through an alteration in uterine function.

In addition to proteins, the ovine conceptus secretes $PGF_{2\alpha}$ and PGE_2 (430,431). The ovine conceptus lacks the ability to form estrogens (432). Embryonic secretion of $PGF_{2\alpha}$ may account for the very high concentrations of $PGF_{2\alpha}$ in uterine flushings and for the increase in basal secretion of $PGF_{2\alpha}$ observed in early pregnancy.

Secretion of PGE_2 by endometrial tissue *in vitro* is also greater in pregnant than in nonpregnant ewes (418, 431,433,434). Therefore, both the uterus and conceptus may contribute to the increased concentrations of PGE_2 observed in pregnant ewes during the critical period for maternal recognition of pregnancy (418,420,435). Infusion of PGE_2 into the uterine lumen of nonpregnant ewes delays luteal regression (436,437). It also suppresses the luteolytic action of exogenously administered estradiol-17β (438) and $PGF_{2\alpha}$ (439–441).

The luteotropic effect of the embryo is exerted locally (442). Anastomosis of the uterine vein draining the gravid horn to the opposite uterine vein results in luteal maintenance on the ovary opposite the embryo (443) (Fig. 15). Similar cross anastomosis of the ovarian arteries produces similar results, indicating that the embryonic signal is passed from the uterine vein to the ovarian artery (444) (Fig. 16). The sensitivity of the corpus luteum to the luteolytic action of $PGF_{2\alpha}$ appears to be altered in early pregnancy. Intrafollicular or periarterial injections of $PGF_{2\alpha}$ were less effective in inducing luteal regression in pregnant than in nonpregnant ewes on day 12 or 13 (436,444,445). In addition, the dose of $PGF_{2\alpha}$ required to induce continued luteolysis when given intramuscularly was less in cycling ewes than in pregnant ewes (446). Luteal resistance to $PGF_{2\alpha}$ was absent on day 10 after mating, was greatest from days 13 to 16, and was again absent by day 20 (Fig. 17). Thus, the resistance to $PGF_{2\alpha}$ was transient and coincided with the known time for maternal recognition of pregnancy. The factor responsible for this resistance to $PGF_{2\alpha}$ appeared to be of conceptal origin since corpora lutea from ewes with two embryos were more resistant to $PGF_{2\alpha}$ then corpora lutea from ewes with a single embryo.

Based on these data, a model has been developed to describe how the conceptus might act to maintain the corpus luteum of early pregnancy (Fig. 18). In both pregnant and nonpregnant ewes, $PGF_{2\alpha}$ is secreted from the uterus beginning on days 12 to 13. In the nonpregnant ewe, luteolysis is initiated and secretion of progesterone declines. This al-

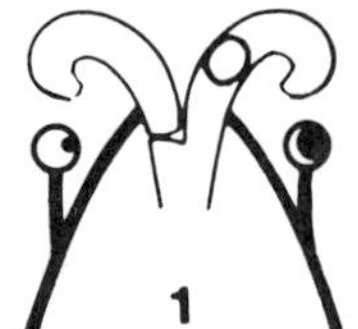

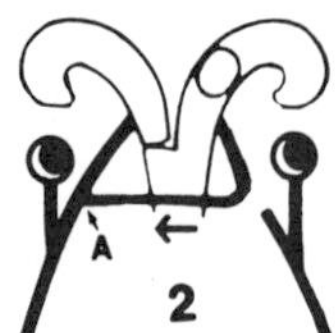

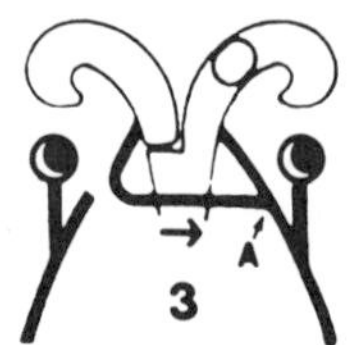

FIG. 15. Effects of unilateral pregnancy and uterine venous anastomosis (A) on luteal regression in sheep. Arrows indicate the direction of venous blood flow. A large or small black dot in an ovary indicates the corpus luteum was maintained or regressed, respectively, 20 days after ovulation and breeding. Unilateral pregnancy resulted in luteal maintenance when the corpus luteum and gravid horn were on the same side and luteal regression when on opposite sides (1). Anastomosis of uterine vein from the gravid side to the nongravid side resulted in luteal maintenance on the nongravid side as well (2). Luteal regression did not occur when the venous drainage from the nongravid side was anastomosed with the uterine vein on the gravid side (3). This indicates that the conceptus produces a substance(s) that overrides the luteolytic effect of $PGF_{2\alpha}$ from a nongravid uterus. (From ref. 443.)

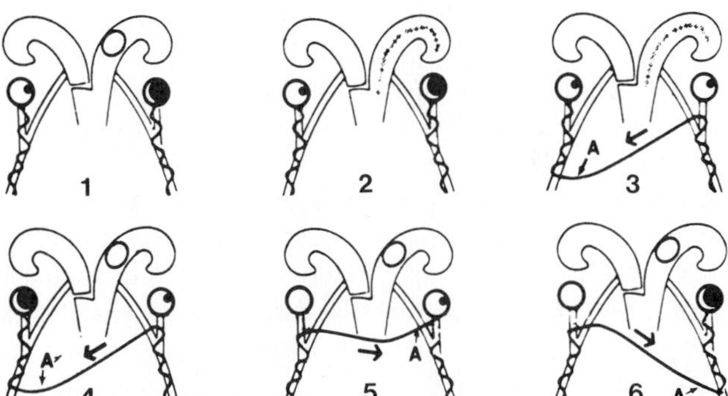

FIG. 16. Effects of unilateral pregnancy and ovarian arterial anastomosis on luteal regression in sheep. Arrows indicate the direction of arterial blood flow. A large or small black dot in an ovary indicates the corpus luteum was maintained or regressed, respectively, 20 days after ovulation and breeding. Unilateral pregnancy resulted in luteal maintenance when the corpus luteum and gravid horn were on the same side and luteal regression when on opposite sides (1). Unilateral destruction of the endometrium with phenol had an effect similar to pregnancy on luteal function when the ovarian arteries were left intact (2). Luteal regression occurred when the artery ipsilateral to the uterine horn treated with phenol was anastomosed to the ovarian artery on the contralateral side (3). This indicates the lack of an effect of the surgical anastomosis on luteal maintenance. Arterial anastomosis from the gravid side to the nongravid side resulted in luteal maintenance on the nongravid side (4). Arterial anastomosis from the nongravid side to the gravid side resulted in luteal regression when the anastomosis was done close to the gravid ovary (5) but not when done a few centimeters from the gravid ovary. This indicates that the luteolytic effect from the nongravid uterine horn was transferred into the ovarian artery, but its effect could be overridden by a substance(s) transferred from the uterine vein of the gravid uterine horn to the ovarian artery (6). (From ref. 444.)

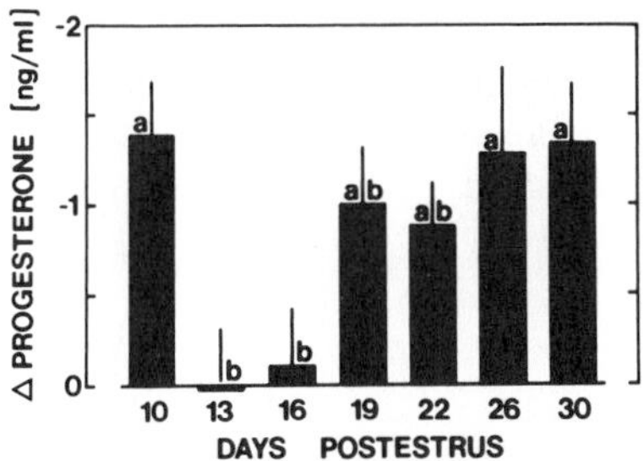

FIG. 17. Effect of treatment with $PGF_{2\alpha}$ (4 mg/58 kg body weight) on the decrease in the concentration of progesterone in serum (progesterone) of pregnant ewes treated on various days postbreeding. The corpus luteum was resistant to the luteolytic effects of $PGF_{2\alpha}$ on days 13 and 16, as indicated by absence of a decrease in serum levels of progesterone on these days. Groups with different superscripts are different ($p<0.05$). (From ref. 446.)

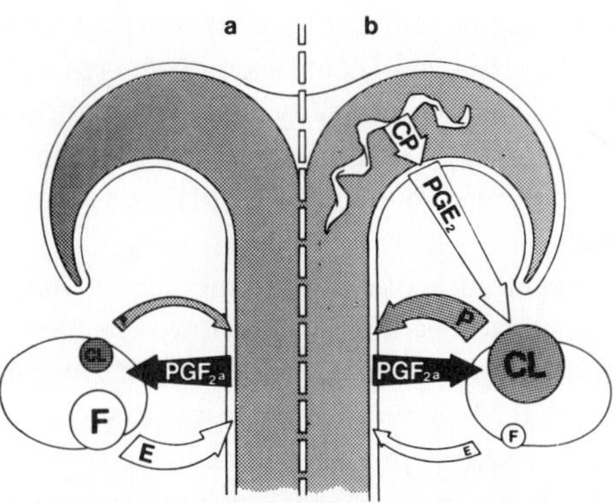

FIG. 18. Model depicting the major hormonal interactions among the conceptus, uterus, and ovary during luteolysis (a) and early pregnancy (b). During luteolysis, major episodic release of $PGF_{2\alpha}$ from the nonpregnant uterus induces luteolysis via mechanisms discussed in the text. As serum levels of progesterone (P) decrease, follicular (F) growth and estradiol (E) production increase, leading to further secretion of $PGF_{2\alpha}$. During early pregnancy, secretion of a conceptus protein (CP) enhances the secretion of PGE_2 from the uterus, antagonizing the luteolytic actions of $PGF_{2\alpha}$. The corpus luteum (CL) is maintained and serum levels of progesterone remain high, suppressing follicular growth and estradiol secretion. This results in an altered pattern of $PGF_{2\alpha}$ secretion, with a reduction in the estradiol-induced episodic release of $PGF_{2\alpha}$ but an elevated basal release.

lows increased follicular development and, as a result, increased secretion of estradiol-17β. The combination of falling progesterone and increasing estradiol-17β results in the very high amplitude surges of $PGF_{2\alpha}$ typically found during late luteolysis and the follicular phase. In the pregnant ewe, the conceptus secretes a protein that stimulates uterine secretion of PGE_2, which protects the corpus luteum from the luteolytic effect of $PGF_{2\alpha}$. As a consequence, the concentration of progesterone in serum is maintained at a normal level, follicular development is suppressed, and the concentration of estradiol-17β remains low. The luteal phase steroid environment is maintained, and a different pattern of $PGF_{2\alpha}$ secretion is the result.

In the pregnant cow, the corpus luteum must be present for the first 200 days of gestation (447). Pregnancy can be maintained in ovariectomized cows by treatment with progesterone (448). The adrenal gland appears to secrete enough progesterone to maintain pregnancy after day 200 (449). The placental contribution to circulating concentrations of progesterone, even after day 200, appears to be negligible.

Embryos can be successfully transferred as late as day 16 postestrus (450). The corpus luteum is maintained despite removal of embryos on day 17 or thereafter (451,452). Thus, the critical period for maternal recognition of pregnancy in the cow are days 16 to 17.

Some researchers have found that the concentrations of progesterone in serum are similar in pregnant and nonpregnant cows through days 17 to 18 postestrus (453,454). Others, using more frequent sampling protocols, have found significantly higher concentrations of progesterone in serum or milk of pregnant cows compared to both bred and nonbred, nonpregnant animals, as early as day 6 postestrus (455–458). Based on these reports, the existence of an embryonic luteotropin secreted by the bovine blastocyst has been proposed (459).

The concentration of $PGF_{2\alpha}$ in uterine venous plasma on day 18 postestrus is significantly lower in pregnant cows compared to nonpregnant cows (458). The high-amplitude surges of PGFM in peripheral plasma associated with luteolysis are absent in pregnant animals (460). However, the basal concentration of PGFM appears to increase during early pregnancy (461,462).

Homogenates of 17- or 18-day-old embryos have been infused into the uterine lumen, resulting in prolonged luteal function (451,452). Knickerbocker et al. (463) have incubated 16- to 18-day-old conceptuses and infused the incubation medium (after dialysis) into the uterus to achieve similar results. Infusion of this mixture of large-molecular-weight, conceptus secretory products mimicked the suppressive effect of the embryo on secretion of PGF_2 from the uterus in response to treatment with estradiol-17β (464). The active factor(s) within this mixture appears to be a protein similar to that identified in sheep.

Bovine conceptuses secrete $PGF_{2\alpha}$, PGE_2, progesterone, estradiol-17β, and 5-α-reduced steroids *in vitro* (432,465–468). Infusion of PGE_2 into the uterine lumen prolongs luteal life span for the duration of the infusion (452,469). Reynolds et al. (470) suggested that there may be some interaction between estradiol and PGE_2 in regulating luteal function in cows.

The conceptus prevents luteal regression through a local pathway similar to that used to transport the uterine luteolysin. If the uterine horns are surgically isolated from each other, only corpora lutea on the ovary adjacent to the gravid uterine horn are maintained (471). If the uterine vein draining the gravid uterine horn is anastomosed to the uterine vein draining the opposite horn, the corpus luteum on the ovary opposite the gravid horn is maintained (472). This type of preparation combines the uterine venous effluent from both the gravid and nongravid uterine horns. If the embryo acts primarily by reducing uterine secretion of $PGF_{2\alpha}$, then maintenance of the corpus luteum must be due to a dilution of the $PGF_{2\alpha}$ coming from the nongravid horn. Alternatively, the gravid uterine horn may be actively secreting a substance that acts in a local fashion to reduce the luteolytic effectiveness of $PGF_{2\alpha}$. As with $PGF_{2\alpha}$, the physical properties and rapid metabolism of PGE_2 are compatible with the local nature of this effect. The ability of large-molecular-weight conceptus secretory products to prolong luteal function may be due to a direct inhibition of uterine secretion of $PGF_{2\alpha}$ or a stimulation of uterine secretion of an antiluteolytic factor such as PGE_2. Prostaglandin E_2 stimulates secretion of progesterone by bovine luteal tissue *in vitro* (473,474).

Pigs

The corpus luteum of the sow must continue to secrete progesterone throughout gestation (115 days) to maintain pregnancy (475) and progesterone replacement therapy is sufficient to maintain pregnancy in ovariectomized sows (476). The increase in uterine secretion of $PGF_{2\alpha}$ associated with luteolysis in cycling pigs does not occur in pregnant pigs (337,477,478). Endometrial tissue from pregnant sows secretes less $PGF_{2\alpha}$ *in vitro* than similar tissue from nonpregnant sows (477,479). However, there is a very significant increase in the concentration of $PGF_{2\alpha}$ in flushings of the uterine lumen (480).

Treatment with estrogens, for as little as five days (days 11–15) will maintain normal luteal function in nonpregnant sows for up to 300 days (481–483). Uterine secretion of $PGF_{2\alpha}$ both *in vivo* and *in vitro,* is reduced by treatment of nonpregnant sows with estrogen *in vivo* (477,483,484). This treatment is also associated with an accumulation of $PGF_{2\alpha}$ in the uterine lumen (483,485). In these respects, treatment with estrogen mimics the effects of the conceptus.

The porcine conceptus synthesizes and secretes estrogens as early as day 12 (432,486,487). On the basis of these data, it has been proposed that the corpus luteum of early pregnancy in the pig is maintained by the secretion of estrogens from the conceptus. In addition to the inhibitory effect that estrogens have on uterine synthesis of prostaglandins, Bazer and Thatcher (488) have proposed that estrogens alter the direction of secretion of $PGF_{2\alpha}$, so that $PGF_{2\alpha}$ moves into the uterine lumen rather than into the uterine vein. An essential role for embryonic synthesis of estrogens in the maintenance of corpora lutea of pregnancy remains to be demonstrated. No attempt has been made to prevent luteal maintenance by administering either inhibitors of estrogen synthesis or estrogen antagonists.

In addition to estrogens, porcine embryos synthesize PGE_2 and $PGF_{2\alpha}$ (484,489) and concentrations of PGE_2 in the uterine lumen increase during early pregnancy (490). The role of PGE_2 in the process of maternal recognition of pregnancy in the sow has not been examined. Secretion of $PGF_{2\alpha}$ by the conceptus may contribute more to the accumulation of $PGF_{2\alpha}$ in the uterine lumen during early pregnancy than the proposed redirection of secretion of the limited amount of $PGF_{2\alpha}$ synthesized by the pregnant uterus.

Horse

The mechanism(s) responsible for maintenance of the primary corpus luteum during early pregnancy in the mare are not well understood. As in other species, $PGF_{2\alpha}$ appears to be responsible for regression of the corpus luteum at the end of the estrous cycle of the mare (313). On days 10 and 14 of pregnancy, the concentration of PGF in the uterine venous blood is lower than in nonpregnant mares (338).

There does not appear to be a redirecting of the secretion of $PGF_{2\alpha}$ into the uterine lumen. Further, there does not appear to be a reduction in the sensitivity of the corpus luteum to $PGF_{2\alpha}$ during early pregnancy. On the contrary, the ability of the corpus luteum to bind $PGF_{2\alpha}$ increases rather than decreases during early pregnancy (332).

The corpus luteum must continue to secrete progesterone through the first 50 to 70 days of gestation (491). During this period, pregnancy can be maintained in mares after ovariectomy by treatment with progesterone (491). The corpus luteum is maintained following removal of the embryo on day 16 or thereafter (492). The concentration of progesterone in serum of pregnant mares follows a temporal pattern similar to that of the nonpregnant mare through the first 12 days postestrus (260,493). From this point, the concentration of progesterone declines gradually, establishing a lower basal level between days 20 and 35 (494). About days 35 to 40, the concentration increases again, with maximal levels being achieved on day 100. This is in contrast to the pattern observed in hysterectomized mares (238,260). In that case, the gradual decline initiated on day 12 continues until luteal function is lost completely sometime between days 100 and 200.

Certainly, the conceptus is involved in recognition of pregnancy and the subsequent maintenance of the primary corpus luteum. At least two different mechanisms seem to be involved. First, unfertilized ova are trapped in the oviduct of mares, where they degenerate over a period of months (495). In contrast, the fertilized ovum produces a substance that insures its selective passage through the oviduct and into the uterus. Once in the uterus, the conceptus must come into contact with essentially the entire endometrial surface to prevent luteal regression. Since the equine conceptus does not elongate, but rather remains spherical until well into the second month of gestation, endometrial contact is achieved by migration of the conceptus throughout the uterus. In fact, the equine conceptus appears to traverse the entire uterus about every 2 hr during the critical period for recognition of pregnancy (496).

The interaction of the conceptus with the endometrium is speculated to prevent production and secretion of $PGF_{2\alpha}$ (496). The nature of the substance produced by the conceptus to inhibit production of $PGF_{2\alpha}$ has not been identified, but it is believed it may be estrogen. The equine conceptus is capable of synthesizing estradiol *in vitro* (497), and small quantities of estrogen induce a uterine tone characteristic of pseudopregnancy. Once the corpus luteum of pregnancy is established, the secretion of progesterone gradually decreases until secretion of equine chorionic gonadotropin begins on about day 35 (494).

In the mare, increases in secretion of FSH occur at approximately 10-day intervals throughout early pregnancy (498), and this results in surges of follicular activity (499). Secretion of massive quantities of equine chorionic gonadotropin beginning around day 35 of gestation induces ovulation of these follicles and the formation of secondary corpora lutea (500). Function of the primary corpus luteum is also stimulated by equine chorionic gonadotropin (501). The secondary corpora lutea appear similar to the primary corpus luteum in structure and function. They secrete progesterone until their trophic support (equine chorionic gonadotropin) disappears from the circulation at approximately day 150 of gestation, at which time they regress along with the primary corpus luteum. Progestational support for the remainder of pregnancy in the mare is provided by the feto-placental unit (502).

Primates

The most simplistic mechanisms for maternal recognition of pregnancy appear to exist in women and other nonhuman primates. In these species the placenta begins to secrete a chorionic gonadotropin as early as 8 to 12 days postconception. This chorionic gonadotropin is responsible for extension of the life span and function of the corpus luteum.

Human chorionic gonadotropin has been studied extensively. It is a glycoprotein with a structure similar to that of hLH. The α-subunits of the two hormones are essentially identical, but there are an additional 32 amino acids with associated carbohydrate moieties on the β-subunit of hCG. In addition, hCG has considerably more total carbohydrate than does hLH. Human CG and hLH have been shown to bind to the same receptor and to stimulate adenylate cyclase and progesterone secretion. However, recent data suggest that there are some differences in the receptor-mediated actions of the two hormones. *In vitro* studies with ovine luteal cells have indicated that hCG induces a more prolonged steroidogenic response compared with ovine LH (180). Similar data have been obtained with Leydig tumor cells (503). The apparent reason for this is that the hCG–LH receptor complex is internalized at a much slower rate than in the LH–LH receptor complex. This reduced rate of internalization is apparently due to a dramatically reduced lateral mobility of hCG–LH receptor complexes in the ovine luteal cell membrane compared with oLH–LH receptor complexes (504). Binding of hCG to the LH receptor results in immobilization of the receptor via a reaction apparently involving microfilaments (505). The high content of carbohydrate in hCG is also responsible for a much reduced rate of clearance of this hormone from the blood. Thus, the unique chemical composition of hCG results in dramatic increases in its circulatory life in blood and enhanced hCG-receptor life on the plasma membrane of the luteal cell. Both of these actions result in a prolonged biological effect and enhanced secretion of progesterone.

Human CG is secreted by the syncytiotrophoblastic cell in the placenta. Levels of hCG in serum begin to rise by day 8 postconception and reach peak levels around the 14th week of pregnancy. Serum hCG levels then begin to decline.

The placenta can secrete sufficient quantities of progesterone by the 20th week so that continued maintenance of the corpus luteum is not required.

That hCG is the primary luteotropin in primates has been substantiated by the fact that treatment with this hormone extended the life span and function of the corpus luteum in normally cycling woman (134). In addition, administration of an hCG antiserum to monkeys will cause premature luteolysis (137). Thus, it appears that chorionic gonadotropin is the only factor required for maternal recognition of pregnancy in most primates, including humans.

REFERENCES

1. Frankel, L. (1903): Die function des corpus luteum. *Arch Gynaekol.*, 68:438–443.
2. Allen, W. M., and Corner, G. W. (1929): Physiology of the corpus luteum: Production of special uterine reaction (progestational proliferation) by extracts of corpus luteum. *Am. J. Physiol.*, 88:326–334.
3. Allen, W. M., and Wintersteiner, O. (1934): Crystalline progestin. *Science*, 80:190–191.
4. Muldoon, T. G. (1980): Regulation of steroid hormone receptor activity. *Endocrine Rev.*, 1:339–364.
5. Blandau, R. J., Brackett, B., Brenner, R. M., et al. (1977): The oviduct. In: *Frontiers in Reproduction and Fertility Control*, edited by R. O. Greep and M. A. Koblinsky, pp. 132–145. MIT Press, Cambridge, MA.
6. Brenner, R. M., and Anderson, R. G. W. (1973): Endocrine control of ciliogenesis in the primate oviduct. In: *Handbook of Physiology*, edited by R. O. Greep and E. B. Astwood, pp. 123–139. Williams & Wilkins, Baltimore.
7. Porter, D. G., and Finn, C. A. (1977): The biology of the uterus. In: *Frontiers in Reproduction and Fertility Control*, edited by R. O. Greep and M. A. Kolinsky, pp. 146–156. MIT Press, Cambridge, MA.
8. Zarrow, M. X., Yochim, J. M., and McCarthy, J. L. (1964): *Experimental Endocrinology*. Academic, New York.
9. Gier, H. T. (1960): Estrous cycle in the bitch; vaginal fluids. *Vet. Scope*, 5:2–9.
10. Topper, Y. J., and Freeman, C. S. (1980): Multiple hormone interactions in the developmental biology of the mammary gland. *Physiol. Rev.*, 60:1049–1106.
11. Baird, D. T., and Scaramuzzi, R. J. (1976): Changes in the secretion of ovarian steroids and pituitary luteinizing hormone in the periovulatory period in the ewe: The effect of progesterone. *J. Endocrinol.*, 70:237–245.
12. Karsch, F. J., Foster, D. L., Legan, S. J., Ryan, K. D. and Peter, G. K. (1979): Control of the preovulatory endocrine events in the ewe: interrelationship of estradiol, progesterone and luteinizing hormone. *Endocrinology*, 105:421–426.
13. Knobil, E. (1980): The neuroendocrine control of the menstrual cycle. *Rec. Prog. Horm. Res.*, 36:53–88.
14. Rahe, C. H., Owens, R. E., Fleeger, J. L., Newton, H. J., and Harms, P. G. (1980): Patterns of plasma luteinizing hormone in the cyclic cow: Dependence upon period of the cycle. *Endocrinology*, 107:498–503.
15. Midgley, A. R., Jr., and Jaffe, R. B. (1968): Regulation of human gonadotropins: IV. Correlation of serum follicle-stimulating hormone and luteinizing hormone during the menstrual cycle. *J. Clin. Endocrinol. Metab.*, 28:1699–1703.
16. Weiss, G. (1981): Human relaxin: Source and stimulus. In: *Relaxin*, edited by H. D. Neill and G. D. Bryant-Greenwood, pp. 167–168. Elsevier North-Holland, New York.
17. Sherwood, O. D., and O'Byrne, E. M. (1974): Purification and characterization of porcine relaxin. *Arch Biochem. Biophys.*, 160:185–196.
18. Goldsmith, L. T., Grob, H. S., Scherer, K., Surve, A., Steinmetz, G. B., and Weiss, G. (1981): Placental control of ovarian immunoreactive relaxin secretion in the pregnant rat. *Endocrinology*, 109:548–552.
19. Wathes, D. C., and Swann, R. W. (1982): Is oxytocin an ovarian hormone? *Nature*, 297:225–227.
20. Sawyer, H. R., Moeller, C. L., and Kozlowski, G. P. (1986): Immunocytochemical localization of neurophysin and oxytocin in ovine corpora lutea. *Biol. Reprod.*, 34:543–548.
21. Flint, A. P. F., and Sheldrick, E. L. (1985): Ovarian peptides and luteolysis. In: *Implantation of the Human Embryo*, edited by R. G. Edwards, J. M. Purdy, and P. C. Steptoe, pp. 235–242. Academic, London.
22. Balmaceda, J., Asch, R. M., Fernandez, E. D., Valenzuela, G., Eddy, C. A., and Pauerstein, C. J. (1979): Prostaglandin production by rhesus monkey corpora lutea *in vitro*. *Fertil. Steril.*, 31:214–216.
23. Shutt, D. A., Shearman, R. P., Lyneham, R. C., Clark, A. H., McMahon, A. H., and Goh, P. (1975): Radioimmunoassay of progesterone, 17-hydroxyprogesterone, estradiol-17β and prostaglandin F in human corpus luteum. *Steroids*, 26:299–310.
24. Anderson, E., and Little, B. (1985): The ontogeny of the rat granulosa cell. In: *Proceedings of the Fifth Ovarian Workshop*, edited by D. O. Toft and R. J. Ryan, pp. 203–225. Ovarian Workshops, Champaign, IL.
25. Azarnia, R., Dahl, G., and Lowenstein, W. R. (1981): Cell junction and cyclic AMP: III. Promotion of junctional membrane permeability and junction membrane particles in a junction-deficient cell type. *J. Membrane Biol.*, 63:133–146.
26. Amsterdam, A., and Tsafriri, A. (1979): *In vitro* binding of ^{125}I-human chorionic gonadotropin (hCG) in the preovulatory follicle: absence of receptor sites on oocyte. *J. Cell Biol.*, 83:255.
27. Anderson, W., Kang, Y., Perotti, M. E., Bramley, T. A., and Ryan, R. J. (1979): Interactions of gonadotropins with corpus luteum membranes. III. Electron microscopic localization of [^{125}I]-hCG binding to sensitive and desensitized ovaries seven days after PMSG-hCG. *Biol. Reprod.*, 20:362–376.
28. Albertini, D., and Anderson, E. (1975): Structural modifications of lutein cell gap junctions during pregnancy in the rat and the mouse. *Anat. Rec.*, 181:171–194.
29. McClellan, M. C., Diekman, M. A., Abel, J. H., Jr., and Niswender, G. D. (1975): Luteinizing hormone, progesterone and the morphological development of normal and superovulated corpora lutea in sheep. *Cell Tissue Res.*, 164:291–307.
30. Hay, M. F., and Moor, R. M. (1975): Distribution of Δ^5-3β-hydroxysteroid dehydrogenase activity in the Graafian follicle of the sheep. *J. Reprod. Fertil.*, 43:313–322.
31. O'Shea, J. D., Cran, D. G., and Hay, M. F. (1980): Fate of the theca interna following ovulation in the ewe. *Cell Tissue Res.* 210:305–319.
32. Donaldson, L., and Hansel, W. (1965): Histological study of bovine corpora lutea. *J. Dairy Sci.*, 48:905–909.
33. O'Shea, J. D., Cran, D. G., and Hay, M. F. (1979): The small luteal cell of the sheep. *J. Anat.*, 128:239–251.
34. Channing, C., and Kammerman, S. (1974): Binding of gonadotropins to ovarian cells. *Biol. Reprod.*, 10:179–198.
35. Richards, J. S. (1979): Hormone regulation of hormone receptors in ovarian follicular development. In: *Ovarian Follicular Development*, edited by A. R. Midgley and W. A. Sadler, pp. 225–242. Raven, New York.
36. Zeleznik, A. J., Midgley, A. R., Jr., and Reichert, L. E., Jr. (1974): Granulosa cell maturation in the rat: Increased binding of human chorionic gonadotropin following treatment with follicle-stimulating hormone *in vivo*. *Endocrinology*, 95:818–825.
37. Kammerman, S., and Ross, J. (1975): Increase in numbers of gonadotropin receptors on granulosa cells during follicle maturation. *J. Clin. Endocrinol. Metab.*, 41:546–550.
38. Lee, C. Y. (1976): The porcine ovarian follicle: III. Development of chorionic gonadotropin receptors associated with increase in adenyl cyclase activity during follicle maturation. *Endocrinology*, 99:42–48.
39. Richards, J. S., Ireland, J. J., Rao, M. C., Bernath, G. A., Midgley, A. R., Jr., and Reichert, L. E., Jr. (1976): Ovarian follicular development in the rat: Hormone receptor regulation by estradiol, follicle stimulating hormone and luteinizing hormone. *Endocrinology*, 99:1562–1570.

40. Chang, S. C. S., Anderson, W., Lewis, J. C., Ryan, R. J., and Kang, Y. H. (1977): The porcine ovarian follicle. II. Electron microscopic study of surface features of granulosa cells at different stages of development. *Biol Reprod.,* 16:349–357.
41. Richards, J. S., and Williams, J. L. (1976): Luteal cell receptor content for prolactin (PRL) and luteinizing hormone (LH). Regulation by LH and PRL. *Endocrinology,* 99:1571–1581.
42. Nimrod, A., Bedrak, E., and Lamprecht, S. A. (1977): Appearance of LH-receptors and LH-stimulable cyclic AMP accumulation in granulosa cells during follicular maturation in the rat ovary. *Biochem. Biophys. Res. Commun.,* 78:977–984.
43. Richards, J. S., Jonassen, J. A., Rolfes, A. I., Kersey, K., and Reichert, L. E., Jr. (1979): Adenosine 3′,5′-monophosphate, luteinizing hormone receptor, and progesterone during granulosa cell differentiation: Effects of estradiol and follicle-stimulating hormone. *Endocrinology,* 104:765–773.
44. Rao, M. C., Richards, J. S., Midgley, A. R., Jr., and Reichert, L. E., Jr. (1977): Regulation of gondotropin receptors by luteinizing hormone in granulosa cells. *Endocrinology,* 101:512–523.
45. Carson, R. S., Findlay, J. K., and Burger, H. G. (1979): Receptors for gonadotrophins in the ovine follicle during growth and atresia. In: *Advances in Experimental Medicine and Biology, Vol. 112: Ovarian Follicular and Corpus Luteum Function,* edited by C. P. Channing, J. Marsh, and W. A. Sadler, pp. 89–94. Plenum, New York.
46. Hansel, W., Concannon, P. W., and Lukaszewska, J. H. (1973): Corpora lutea of the large domestic animals. *Biol. Reprod.,* 8:222–245.
47. Hoffman, B., Schams, D., Bopp, R., Ender, M. L., Giminez, T., and Karg, H. (1974): Luteotrophic factors in the cow: evidence for LH rather than prolactin. *J. Reprod. Fertil.,* 40:77–85.
48. Karsh, F. J., Cook, B., Ellicott, A. R., Foster, D. L., Jackson, G. L., and Nalbandov, A. V. (1971): Failure of infused prolactin to prolong the lifespan of the corpus luteum of the ewe. *Endocrinology,* 89:272–275.
49. Niswender, G. D. (1974): Influence of 2-Br-α-ergocryptine on the serum levels of prolactin and the estrous cycle in sheep. *Endocrinology,* 94:612–615.
50. Rolland, R., Hammond, J. M., Schellekens, L. A., Lequin, R. M., and deJong, F. H. (1976): Prolactin and ovarian function. In: *Endocrine Function of the Human Ovary,* edited by V. H. T. James, M. Serio, and G. Giusti, pp. 305–321. Academic, New York.
51. Murphy, B. D., and Rajkuman, K. (1985): Prolactin as a luteotropin. *Can. J. Physiol. Pharmacol.,* 63:257–264.
52. Loeb, L. (1906): The formation of the corpus luteum of the guinea pig. *JAMA,* 46:416–423.
53. Corner, G. W. (1919): On the origin of the corpus luteum of the sow from both granulosa and theca interna. *Am. J. Anat.,* 26:117–183.
54. McNutt, G. W. (1924): The corpus luteum of the ox ovary in relation to the estrous cycle. *J. Am. Vet. Med. Assoc.,* 65:556–597.
55. Lobel, B. L., and Levy, E. (1968): Enzymatic correlates of development, secretory function and regression of follicles and corpora lutea in the bovine ovary. *Acta Endocrinol. Suppl.,* 132:7–63.
56. Priedkalns, J., Weber, A. F., and Zemjanis, R. (1968): Qualitative and quantitative morphological studies of the cells of the membrane granulosa, theca interna and corpus luteum of the bovine ovary. *Z. Zellforsch.,* 85:501–520.
57. Pederson, E. S. (1951): Histogenesis of lutein tissue of the albino rat. *Am. J. Anat.,* 88:397–416.
58. Guraya, S. (1971): Morphology, histochemistry and biochemistry of human ovarian compartments and steroid hormone synthesis. *Physiol. Rev.,* 51:785–897.
59. Warbritton, V. (1934): The cytology of the corpora lutea of the ewe. *J. Morphol.,* 56:186–202.
60. Mossman, H. W., and Duke, K. L. (1973): Some comparative aspects of the mammalian ovary. In: *Handbook of Physiology,* Sect. 7, Vol. 2, Pt. I, pp. 389–402. American Physiological Society, Bethesda, MD.
61. Niswender, G. D., Schwall, R. H., Fitz, T. A., Farin, C. E., and Sawyer, H. R. (1985): Regulation of luteal function in domestic ruminants: new concepts. *Rec. Prog. Horm. Res.,* 41:101–142.
62. Deane, H. W., Hay, M. F., Moor, R. M., Rowson, L. E. A., and Short, R. V. (1966): The corpus luteum of the sheep: relationships between morphology and function during the oestrous cycle. *Acta Endocrinol.,* 51:245–263.
63. Lemon, M., and Loir, M. (1977): Steroid release *in vitro* by two luteal cell types in the corpus luteum of the pregnant sow. *J. Endocrinol.,* 72:351–359.
64. Ursely, J., and Leymarie, P. (1979): Varying response to luteinizing hormone of two luteal cell types isolated from bovine corpus luteum. *Endocrinology,* 83:303–310.
65. Koos, R. D., and Hansel, W. (1981): The large and small cells of the bovine corpus luteum: ultrastructural and functional differences. In: *Dynamics of Ovarian Function,* edited by N. B. Schwartz and M. Hunzicker-Dunn, pp. 197–203. Raven Press, New York.
66. Fitz, T. A., Mayan, M. H., Sawyer, H. R., and Niswender, G. D. (1982): Characterization of two steroidogenic cell types in the ovine corpus luteum. *Biol. Reprod.,* 27:703–711.
67. Sinha, A. A., Seal, J. S., and Doe, R. P. (1971): Ultrastructure of the corpus luteum of the white-tailed deer during pregnancy. *Am. J. Anat.,* 132:189–206.
68. Foley, R. C., and Greenstein, J. S. (1958): Cytological changes in the bovine corpus luteum during early pregnancy. In: *Reproduction and Infertility,* edited by F. X. Gassner, pp. 88–96. Pergamon, New York.
69. Wilkinson, R. F., Anderson, E., and Aalberg, J. (1976): Cytological observations of dissociated rat corpus luteum. *J. Ultrastruct. Res.,* 57:168–184.
70. Enders, A. C. (1973): Cytology of the corpus luteum. *Biol. Reprod.,* 8:158–182.
71. Nett, T. M., McClellan, M. C., and Niswender, G. D. (1976): Effects of prostaglandins on the ovine corpus luteum: Blood flow, secretion of progesterone and morphology. *Biol. Reprod.,* 15:66–78.
72. Rodgers, R. J., O'Shea, J. D., and Bruce, N. W. (1984): Morphometric analysis of the cellular composition of the ovine corpus luteum. *J. Anat.,* 138:757–769.
73. Christensen, A. K., and Gillim, S. W. (1969): The correlation of fine structure and function in steroid-secreting cells, with emphasis on those in the gonads. In: *The Gonads,* edited by K. W. McKerns, pp. 415–488. Appleton-Century-Crofts, New York.
74. Fawcett, D. T., Long, J. A., and Jones, A. L. (1969): The ultrastructure of endocrine glands. *Rec. Prog. Horm. Res.,* 25:15–380.
75. Paavola, L. G., and Christensen, A. K. (1981): Characterization of granule types in luteal cells of sheep at the time of maximum progesterone secretion. *Biol. Reprod.,* 25:203–215.
76. Gemmell, R. T., Stacy, B. D., and Thorburn, G. D. (1974): Ultrastructural study of secretory granules in the corpus luteum of sheep during the estrous cycle. *Biol. Reprod.,* 16:499–512.
77. McClellan, M. C., Abel, J. H., Jr., and Niswender, G. D. (1977): Functions of lysosomes during luteal regression in normally cycling and $PGF_{2\alpha}$-treated ewes. *Biol. Reprod.,* 16:499–512.
78. Corteel, M. (1973): Etude histologique de la transformation du follicle pre-ovulatoire en corps jaune cyclique chez la brebis. *Annu. Biol. Anim. Biochim. Biophys. Suppl.,* 13:249–258.
79. Gemmell, R. T., and Stacy, B. D. (1979): Granule secretion by the luteal cell of the sheep: the fate of the granule membrane. *Cell Tissue Res.,* 197:413–419.
80. Sawyer, H. R., Abel, J. H., Jr., McClellan, M. C., Schmitz, M., and Niswender, G. D. (1979): Secretory granules and progesterone secretion by ovine corpora lutea *in vitro*. *Endocrinology,* 104:476–586.
81. Quirk, S. J., Wilcox, D. L., Parry, D. M., and Thorburn, G. D. (1979): Subcellular location of progesterone in the bovine corpus luteum: A biochemical, morphological and cytochemical investigation. *Biol. Reprod.,* 20:1133–1145.
82. Parry, D. M., Wilcox, D. L., and Thorburn, G. D. (1980): Ultrastructural and cytochemical study of the bovine corpus luteum. *J. Reprod. Fertil.,* 60:349–457.
83. Carlson, J. C., Gruber, M. Y., and Thompson, J. E. (1983): A study of the interaction between progesterone and membrane lipids. *Endocrinology,* 113:190–194.
84. Wathes, D. C., Swann, R. W., Birkett, S. D., Porter, D. G., and Pickering, B. T. (1983): Characterization of oxytocin, vasopressin and neurophysin from the bovine corpus luteum. *Endocrinology,* 113:693–698.
85. Rodgers, R. J., O'Shea, J. D., Findlay, J. K., Flint, A. P. F., and Sheldrick, E. L. (1983): Large luteal cells the source of oxytocin in sheep. *Endocrinology,* 113:2302–2304.

86. Anderson, M. L., and Long, J. A. (1978): Localization of relaxin in the pregnant rat. Bioassay of tissue extracts and cell fractionation studies. *Biol. Reprod.*, 18:110–117.
87. Anderson, M. B., and Sherwood, O. D. (1984): Ultrastructural localization of relaxin immunoreactivity in corpora lutea of pregnant rats. *Endocrinology*, 114:1124–1127.
88. Belt, W. D., Anderson, L. L., Cavazos, L. A., and Melampy, R. M. (1971): Cytoplasmic granules and relaxin levels in porcine corpora lutea. *Endocrinology*, 89:1–10.
89. Kendall, J. Z., Plopper, C. G., and Bryant-Greenwood, G. D. (1978): Ultrastructural immunoperoxidase demonstration of relaxin in corpora lutea from a pregnant sow. *Biol. Reprod.*, 18:94–98.
90. Fields, P. A. (1984): Ultrastructural localization of relaxin in corpora lutea of pregnant, pseudopregnant and cycling gilts using porcine relaxin antiserum and goat anti-rabbit IgG-colloidal gold. *Biol. Reprod.*, 30 (Suppl. 1):116A.
91. Fields, M. J., Fields, P. A., Castro-Hernandez, A., and Larkin, L. H. (1980): Evidence for relaxin in corpora lutea of late pregnant cows. *Endocrinology*, 107:869–876.
92. Rothchild, I. (1981): The regulation of the mammalian corpus luteum. *Rec. Prog. Horm. Res.*, 37:183–283.
93. Rothchild, I. (1965): Interrelations between progesterone and the ovary, pituitary, and central nervous system in the control of ovulation and the regulation of progesterone secretion. *Vitam. Horm.*, 23:209–327.
94. Hunzicker-Dunn, M., and Birnbaumer, L. (1976): Adenylyl cyclase activities in ovarian tissues. IV. Gonadotropin-induced desensitization of the luteal adenylyl cyclase throughout pregnancy and pseudopregnancy in the rabbit and the rat. *Endocrinology*, 99:211–222.
95. Greenwald, G. S. (1967): Further observations on the luteotropic complex of the hamster. *Arch. Anat. M.*, 56:281–291.
96. Hilliard J. (1973): Corpus luteum function in guinea pigs, hamsters, rats, mice and rabbits. *Biol. Reprod.*, 8:203–211.
97. Keyes, P. L., Gadsby, J. E., Yuh, K.-C. M., and Bill, C. H., II (1983): The corpus luteum. In: *International Review of Physiology, Reproductive Physiology*, Vol. 4, edited by R. O. Greep, pp. 57–97. University Park Press, Baltimore, MD.
98. Damle, S., LaBarbera, A. R., and Hunzicker-Dunn, M. (1984): Progesterone production by rabbit corpora lutea *in vitro*: Regulation by LH and epinephrine. *Program of the 17th Annual Meeting of the Society for the Study of Reproduction*. Laramie, WY. p. 115.
99. Yuh, K-C. M., Bill, C., II, and Keyes, P. L. (1984): Transient development and function of rabbit corpora lutea after hypophysectomy. *Am. J. Physiol.*, 247:E808–814.
100. Hoyer, P. B., Keyes, P. L., and Niswender, G. D. (1986): Size distribution and hormonal responsiveness of dispersed rabbit luteal cells during pseudopregnancy. *Biol. Reprod. (in press)*.
101. Denamur, R., and Mauleon, P. (1963): Effets de l'hypophysectomie sur la morphologie et l'histologie du corps jaune des ovins. *C. R. Acad. Sci.*, 257:264–267.
102. Kaltenbach, C. C., Graber, J. W., Niswender, G. D., and Nalbandov, A. V. (1968): Effect of hypophysectomy on the formation and maintenance of corpora lutea in the ewe. *Endocrinology*, 82:753–759.
103. Denamur, R., Martinet, J., and Short, R. V. (1973): Pituitary control of the ovine corpus luteum. *J. Reprod. Fertil.*, 32:207–220.
104. Thibault, C. (1966): Luteal maintenance of hypophysectomized and hysterectomized sheep. *J. Reprod. Fertil.*, (Suppl. 1):63.
105. Kaltenbach, C. C., Graber, J. W., Niswender, G. D., and Nalbandov, A. V. (1968): Luteotrophic properties of some pituitary hormones in nonpregnant or pregnant hypophysectomized ewes. *Endocrinology*, 82:818–824.
106. Hixon, J. E., and Clegg, M. T. (1969): Influence of the pituitary on ovarian progesterone output in the ewe: Influence of hypophysectomy and gonadotropic hormones. *Endocrinology*, 84:828–834.
107. Schroff, C., Klindt, F. M., Kaltenbach, C. C., Graber, J. W., and Niswender, G. D. (1971): Maintenance of corpora lutea in hypophysectomized ewes. *J. Anim. Sci.*, 33:268.
108. Karsch, F. J., Roche, J. F., Noveroske, J. W., Foster, D. L., Norton, H. W., and Nalbandov, A. V. (1971): Prolonged maintenance of the corpus luteum of the ewe by continuous infusion of luteinizing hormone. *Biol. Reprod.*, 4:129–136.
109. Domanski, E., Skrezczkowski, L., Stupnicka, E., Fitko, R., and Dobrowlski, W. (1967): Effect of gonadotropins on the secretion of progesterone and oestrogens by the sheep ovary perfused *in situ*. *J. Reprod. Fertil.*, 14:365–372.
110. Kaltenbach, C. C., Cook, B., Niswender, G. D., and Nalbandov, A. V. (1967): Effect of pituitary hormones on progesterone synthesis by ovine luteal tissue *in vitro*. *Endocrinology*, 81:1407–1409.
111. Simmons, K. R., Caffrey, J. L., Phillips, J. L., Abel, J. H., Jr., and Niswender, G. D. (1976): A simple method for preparing suspensions of luteal cells. *Proc. Soc. Exp. Biol. Med.*, 152:366–371.
112. Fuller, G. B., and Hansel, W. (1970): Regression of sheep corpora lutea after treatment with antibovine luteinizing hormone. *J. Anim. Sci.*, 31:99–103.
113. McCracken, J. A., Baird, D. T., and Goding, J. R. (1971): Factors affecting the secretion of steroids from the transplanted ovary of the sheep. *Rec. Prog. Horm. Res.*, 27:537–582.
114. Jammes, H., Schirar, A., and Djiane, J. (1985): Differential patterns in luteal prolactin and LH receptors during pregnancy in sows and ewes. *J. Reprod. Fertil.*, 73:27–35.
115. du Mesnil du Buisson, F., and Leglise, P. C. (1963): Effet de l'hypophysectomie sur les corps jaunes de la truie. Resultats preliminaires. *C. R. Acad. Sci.*, 257:261–263.
116. Duncan, G. W., Bowerman, A. M., Anderson, L. L., Hearn, W. R., and Melampy, R. M. (1961): Factors influencing *in vitro* synthesis of progesterone. *Endocrinology*, 68:199–207.
117. Cook, B., Kaltenbach, C. C., Norton, H. W., and Nalbandov, A. V. (1967): Synthesis of progesterone *in vitro* by porcine corpora lutea. *Endocrinology*, 81:573–584.
118. Ginther, O. J. (1979): *Reproductive Biology of the Mare. Basic and Applied Aspects*. McNaughton and Gunn, Ann Arbor, MI.
119. Nett, T. M., Pickett, B. W., Seidel, G. E., Jr., and Voss, J. L. (1976): Levels of luteinizing hormone and progesterone during the estrous cycle and early pregnancy in mares. *Biol. Reprod.*, 14:412–415.
120. Harrison, R. J. (1946): The early development of the corpus luteum in the mare. *J. Anat.*, 80:160–166.
121. Van Niekerk, C. H., Morgenthal, J. C., and Gerneke, W. H. (1975): Relationship between the morphology of and progesterone production by the corpus luteum of the mare. *J. Reprod. Fertil. Suppl.*, 23:171–175.
122. Pineda, M. H., Ginther, O. J., and McShan, W. H. (1972): Regression of corpus luteum in mares treated with an antiserum against an equine pituitary fraction. *Am. J. Vet. Res.*, 33:1767–1773.
123. Roser, J. F., and Evans, J. W. (1983): Luteal luteinizing hormone receptors during the postovulatory period in the mare. *Biol. Reprod.*, 29:499–510.
124. Concannon, P. W., Hansel, W., and McEntee, K. (1977): Changes in LH, progesterone and sexual behavior associated with preovulatory luteinization in the bitch. *Biol. Reprod.*, 17:604–613.
125. Wildt, D. E., Panko, W. B., Chakraborty, P., and Seager, S. W. (1979): Relationship of serum estrone, estradiol-17β and progesterone to LH, sexual behavior and time of ovulation in the bitch. *Biol. Reprod.*, 20:648–658.
126. Nett, T. M., Akbar, A. M., Phemister, R. D., Holst, P. A., Reichert, L. E., Jr., and Niswender, G. D. (1975): Levels of luteinizing hormone, estradiol and progesterone in serum during the estrous cycle and pregnancy in the beagle bitch. *Proc. Soc. Exp. Biol. Med.*, 148:134–139.
127. Reimers, R. J., Phemister, R. D., and Niswender, G. D. (1978): Radioimmunological measurement of follicle-stimulating hormone and prolactin in the dog. *Biol. Reprod.*, 19:673–679.
128. Olson, P. N., Bowen, R. A., Behrendt, M. D., Olson, J. D., and Nett, T. M. (1984): Concentrations of progesterone and luteinizing hormone in the serum of diestrous bitches before and after hysterectomy. *Am. J. Vet. Res.*, 45:149–153.
129. Smith, M. S., and McDonald, L. E. (1974): Serum levels of luteinizing hormone and progesterone during the estrous cycle, pseudopregnancy and pregnancy in the dog. *Endocrinology*, 94:404–412.
130. Concannon, P. W., Hansel, W., and Visek, W. V. (1975): The ovarian cycle of the bitch: plasma estrogen, LH and progesterone. *Biol. Reprod.*, 13:112–121.
131. Concannon, P. W. (1980): Effects of hypophysectomy and of LH administration on luteal phase plasma progesterone levels in the beagle bitch. *J. Reprod. Fertil.*, 58:407–410.
132. Concannon, P. W. (1983): Reproductive physiology and endocrine patterns of the bitch. In: *Current Veterinary Therapy VIII*

Small Animal Practice, edited by Robert W. Kirk, pp. 886–901. Saunders, Philadelphia.

133. VandeWiele, R. L., Bogumil, J., Dyrenfurther, I., et al. (1970): Mechanisms regulating the menstrual cycle in women. *Rec. Prog. Horm. Res.,* 26:63–90.

134. Hanson, F. W., Powell, J. E., and Stevens, V. C. (1971): Effects of hCG and human pituitary LH on steroid secretion and functional life of the human corpus luteum. *J. Clin. Endocrinol. Metab.,* 32:211–215.

135. Rice, B. F., Hammerstein, J., and Savard, K. (1964): Steroid hormone formation in the human ovary. II. Action of gonadotropins *in vitro* in the corpus luteum. *J. Clin. Endocrinol. Metab.,* 24:606–615.

136. Stouffer, P. L., Nixon, W. E., Gulyas, B. J., and Hodgen, G. D. (1977): Gonadotropin sensitive progesterone production by rhesus monkey luteal cells *in vitro*: A function of age of the corpus luteum during the menstrual cycle. *Endocrinology,* 100:506–512.

137. McDonald, G. J. (1971): Effect of hCG antiserum (A/S) on ovulation and corpus luteum function in the monkey, *Macaca fascicularis. Proceedings of the IV Annual Meeting of the Society for the Study of Reproduction, Abstr. 16.*

138. Schomberg, D. W., Coudert, S. P., and Short, R. V. (1967): Effects of bovine luteinizing hormone and human chorionic gonadotrophin on the bovine corpus luteum *in vivo. J. Reprod. Fertil.,* 14:277–285.

139. Niswender, G. D., Reimers, T. J., Diekman, M. A., and Nett, T. M. (1976): Blood flow: A mediator of ovarian function. *Biol. Reprod.,* 14:64–81.

140. Armstrong, D. T., and Black, D. L. (1966): Influence of luteinizing hormone on corpus luteum metabolism and progesterone biosynthesis throughout the bovine estrous cycle. *Endocrinology,* 78:937–944.

141. Williams, M. T., and Marsh, J. M. (1978): Estradiol inhibition of luteinizing hormone-stimulated progesterone synthesis in isolated bovine luteal cells. *Endocrinology,* 103:1611–1618.

142. Lee, C. Y., and Ryan, R. J. (1971): The uptake of human luteinizing hormone (hLH) by slices of luteinized rat ovaries. *Endocrinology,* 89:1515–1523.

143. Papaionannou, S., and Gospodarowicz, D. (1975): Comparison of the binding of human chorionic gonadotropin to isolated bovine luteal cells and bovine luteal plasma membranes. *Endocrinology,* 97:114–124.

144. Conti, M., Harwood, J. P., Dufau, M. L., and Catt, K. J. (1976): Effect of gonadotropin-induced receptor regulation on biological responses of isolated rat luteal cells. *J. Biol. Chem.,* 252:8867–8874.

145. Conn, P. M., Conti, M., Harwood, J. P., Dufau, M. L., and Catt, K. J. (1978): Internalisation of gonadotrophin-receptor complex in ovarian luteal slices. *Nature,* 274:598–600.

146. DeKrester, D. M., Catt, K. J., and Paulsen, C. A. (1971): Studies on the *in vitro* testicular binding of iodinated luteinizing hormone in rats. *Endocrinology,* 88:332–337.

147. Catt, K. J., Dufau, M. L., and Tsuruhara, T. (1971): Studies of a radioligand-receptor assay system for luteinizing hormone and chorionic gonadotropin. *J. Clin. Endocrinol. Metab.,* 32:860–863.

148. Lee, C. Y., and Ryan, R. J. (1972): Luteinizing hormone receptors. Specific binding of human luteinizing hormone to homogenates of luteinized rat ovaries. *Proc. Natl. Acad. Sci. USA,* 69:3520–3523.

149. Lee, C. Y., and Ryan, R. J. (1973): Interaction of ovarian receptors with human luteinizing hormone and human chorionic gonadotropin. *Biochemistry,* 12:4609–4620.

150. Gospodarowicz, D. (1973): Properties of the luteinizing hormone receptor of the isolated bovine corpus luteum plasma membrane. *J. Biol. Chem.,* 248:5042–5049.

151. Bramley, T. A., and Ryan, R. J. (1978): Interactions of gonadotropins with corpus luteum membranes. I. Properties and distributions of some marker enzyme activities after subcellular fractionation of the superovulated rat ovary. *Endocrinology,* 103:778–795.

152. Bramley, T. A., and Ryan, R. J. (1978): Interactions of gonadotropins with corpus luteum membranes. II. The identification of two distinct surface membrane fractions from superovulated rat ovaries. *Endocrinology,* 103:796–804.

153. Dufau, M. L., and Catt, K. J. (1976): Gonadal receptors for luteinizing hormone and human chorionic gonadotropin. In: *Cell Membrane Receptors for Viruses, Antigens and Antibodies, Polypeptide Hormones and Small Molecules,* edited by R. F. Beers and E. G. Bassett, pp. 135–152. Raven Press, New York.

154. Luborsky, J. L., Slater, W. R. and Behrman, H. R. (1984): Luteinizing hormone (LH) receptor aggregation: Modification of ferritin-LH binding and aggregation by prostaglandin $F_{2\alpha}$ and ferritin-LH. *Endocrinology,* 115:2217–2226.

155. Hsueh, A. J., Dufau, M. L., Katz, S. J., and Catt, K. J. (1976): Immunofluorescence labeling of gonadotropin receptors in enzyme-dispersed interstitial cells. *Nature,* 261:710–711.

156. Dufau, M. L., and Catt, K. J. (1978): Gonadotropin receptors and regulation of steroidogenesis in the testis and ovary. *Vitam. Horm.,* 36:462–592.

157. Dufau, M. L., Catt, K. J., and Tsuruhara, T. (1971): Gonadotropin stimulation of testosterone production by the rat testis *in vitro. Biochem. Biophys. Acta,* 252:574–579.

158. Rajaniemi, H., and Vanha-Perttula, T. (1972): Specific receptor for LH in the ovary: Evidence by autoradiography and tissue fractionation. *Endocrinology,* 90:1–9.

159. Han, S. S., Rajaniemi, H., Cho, M. I., Hirshfield, A. N., and Midgley, A. R., Jr. (1974): Gonadotropin receptors in rat ovarian tissue. II. Subcellular localization of LH binding sites by electron microscopic radioautography. *Endocrinology,* 95:589–598.

160. Chen, T. T., Abel, J. H., McClellan, M. C., Sawyer, H. R., and Niswender, G. D. (1977): Localization of gonadotropic hormones in lysosomes of ovine luteal cells. *Cytobiologie,* 14:412–420.

161. Petrusz, P., and Sar, M. (1978): Light microscopic localization of gonadotropin bindings sites in ovarian target cells. In: *Cell Membrane Receptors for Drugs and Hormones,* edited R. W. Straub and L. Boles, pp. 167–182. Raven Press, New York.

162. Amsterdam, S., Kohen, F., Nimrod, A., and Lindner, H. R. (1979): Lateral mobility and internalization of hormone receptors to human chorionic gonadotropin in cultured rat granulosa cells. In: *Advances in Experimental Medicine and Biology, Vol. 112: Ovarian Follicular and Corpus Luteum Function,* edited by C. P. Channing, J. Marsh, and W. A. Sadler, pp. 69–75. Plenum, New York.

163. Rajaniemi, H. J., Hirshfield, A. N., and Midgley, A. R., Jr. (1974): Gonadotropin receptors in rat ovarian tissue. I. Localization of LH binding sites by fractionation of subcellular organelles. *Endocrinology,* 95:579–587.

164. Lee, C. Y ., Coulan, C. B., Jiang, N. S., and Ryan, R. J. (1973): Receptors for human luteinizing hormone in human corpora luteal tissue. *J. Clin. Endocrinol. Metab.,* 36:148–152.

165. Hacik, T., and Kolena, J. (1975): Production of oestradiol, cAMP and ^{125}I-hCG binding by rat ovaries during the reproductive cycle. *Endokrinologie,* 66:15–23.

166. Rao, C. V., Estergreen, V. L., Carman, F. R., Moss, G. E., and Frandle, K. A. (1976): Receptors for prostaglandin $(PG)F_{2\alpha}$ and human choriogonadotropin (hCG) in cell membranes of ovine corpora lutea (CL) throughout estrous cycle. *Vth International Congress of Endocrinology, (abstr.).*

167. Diekman, M. A., O'Callaghan, P., Nett, T. M., and Niswender, G. D. (1978): Validation of methods and quantification of luteal receptors for LH throughout the estrous cycle and early pregnancy in ewes. *Biol. Reprod.,* 19:999–1009.

168. Baird, D. T., Swanston, I., and Scaramuzzi, R. J. (1976): Pulsatile release of LH and secretion of ovarian steroids in sheep during the late luteal phase of the estrous cycle. *Endocrinology,* 98:1490–1496.

169. Suter, D. E., Fletcher, P. W., Sluss, P. M., Reichert, L. E., Jr., and Niswender, G. D. (1980): Alterations in the number of ovine luteal receptors for LH and progesterone secretion induced by homologous hormone. *Biol. Reprod.,* 22:205–210.

170. Mendelson, C., Dufau, M., and Catt, K. (1975): Gonadotropin binding and stimulation of cyclic adenosine 3′:5′ monophosphate and testosterone production in isolated Leydig cells. *J. Biol. Chem.,* 250:8818–8823.

171. Jordan, A. W., III, Caffrey, J. L., and Niswender, G. D. (1978): Catecholamine-induced stimulation of progesterone and adenosine 3′,5′-monophosphate production by dispersed ovine luteal cells. *Endocrinology,* 103:385–392.

172. Gospodarowicz, D., and Gospodarowicz, F. (1975): The morphological transformation and inhibition of growth of bovine luteal cells in tissue culture induced by luteinizing hormone and dibutyryl cyclic AMP. *Endocrinology,* 96:458–467.

173. Conti, M., Harwood, J. P., Dufau, M. L., and Catt, K. J. (1977): Regulation of luteinizing hormone receptors and adenylate cyclase activity by gonadotrophin in the rat ovary. *Mol. Pharmacol.* 13:1024–1032.

174. Harwood, J. P., Conti, M., Conn, P. M., Dufau, M. L., and Catt, K. J. (1978): Receptor regulation and target cell responses: Studies in the ovarian luteal cells. *Mol. Cell. Endocrinol.*, 11:121–135.
175. Catt, K. J., Harwood, J. P., Richert, N. P., Conn, P. M., Conti, M., and Dufau, M. L. (1978): Luteal desensitization: Hormone regulation of LH receptors, adenylate cyclase and responses in the luteal cell. In: *Ovarian Follicular and Corpus Luteum Function,* edited by C. P. Channing, J. Marsh, and W. A. Sadler, pp. 647–662. Plenum, New York.
176. Abel, J. H., Chen, T. T., Endres, D. B., et al. (1978): Sites of binding and metabolism of gonadotropic hormones in the mammalian ovary. In: *Cell Membrane Receptors for Drugs and Hormones,* edited by R. W. Straub and L. Bolis, pp. 183–202. Raven Press, New York.
177. Ascoli, M., and Puett, D. (1978): Inhibition of the degradation of receptor-bound human choriogonadotropin by lysosomotropic agents, protease inhibitors, and metabolic inhibitors. *J. Biol. Chem.*, 253:7839–7843.
178. Chen, T. T., McClellan, M. C., Diekman, M. A., Abel, J. H., and Niswender, G. D. (1981): Localization of human chorionic gonadotropin in the lysosomes of ovine luteal cells. In: *Structure and Function of the Gonadotropins,* edited by K. W. McKerns, pp. 591–612. Plenum, New York.
179. Ahmed, C. E., Sawyer, H. R., and Niswender, G. D. (1981): Internalization and degradation of human chorionic gonadotropin in ovine luteal cells: Kinetic studies. *Endocrinology,* 109:1380–1387.
180. Bourdage, R. J., Fitz, T. A., and Niswender, G. D. (1984): Differential steroidogenic response of ovine luteal cells to ovine luteinizing hormone and human chorionic gonadotropin. *Proc. Soc. Exp. Biol. Med.*, 175:483–486.
181. Suter, D. E., and Niswender, G. D. (1983): Internalization and degradation of human chorionic gonadotropin in ovine luteal cells: Effects of inhibition of protein synthesis. *Endocrinology,* 112:838–845.
182. Willingham, M. C., and Pastan, I. (1984): Endocytosis and membrane traffic in cultured cells. *Recent Prog. Horm. Res.*, 40:569–587.
183. Behrman, H. R., Luborsky-Moore, J. L., Pang, C. Y., Wright, K., and Dorflinger, L. J. (1979): Mechanisms of $PGF_{2\alpha}$ action in functional luteolysis. In: *Ovarian Follicular and Corpus Luteum Function, Advances in Experimental Medicine and Biology,* Vol. 112: edited by C. P. Channing, J. Marsh, and W. A. Sadler pp. 557–571. Plenum, New York.
184. Diekman, M. A., O'Callaghan, P., Nett, T. M., and Niswender, G. D. (1978): Effect of prostaglandin $F_{2\alpha}$ on the number of LH receptors in ovine corpora lutea. *Biol. Reprod.*, 19:1010–1013.
185. Marsh, J. (1975): The role of cAMP in gonadal function. *Adv. Cyclic Nucleotide Res.*, 6:137–199.
186. Birnbaumer, L., Codina, J., Mattera, R., et al. (1985): Regulation of hormone receptors and adenylyl cyclases by guanine nucleotide binding N proteins. *Recent Prog. Horm. Res.*, 41:41–94.
187. Gilman, A. G. (1984): G. proteins and dual control of adenylate cyclase. *Cell,* 36:577–579.
188. Condon, W. A., and Black, D. L. (1976): Catecholamine-induced stimulation of progesterone by the bovine corpus luteum *in vitro. Biol. Reprod.*, 15:573–578.
189. Flockhart, D. A., and Corbin, J. D. (1982): Regulatory mechanisms in the control of protein kinases. *CRC Crit. Rev. Biochem.*, 12:133–186.
190. Nimmo, H. G., and Cohen, P. (1977): Hormonal control of protein phosphorylation. *Adv. Cyclic Nucleotide Res.*, 8:145–266.
191. Krebs, E. G., and Beavo, J. A. (1979): Phosphorylation-dephosphorylation of enzymes. *Annu. Rev. Biochem.*, 48:923–959.
192. Kuo, J. F., and Greengard, P. (1969): Cyclic nucleotide-dependent protein kinase. IV. Widespread occurrence of adenosine 3′,5′-monophosphate-dependent protein kinase in various tissues and phyla of the animal kingdom. *Proc. Natl. Acad. Sci. USA,* 64: 1349–1353.
193. Ling, W. Y., and Marsh, J. M. (1977): Reevaluation of the role of cyclic adenosine 3′,5′ monophosphate and protein kinase in the stimulation of steroidogenesis by luteinizing hormone in bovine corpus luteum slices. *Endocrinology,* 100:1571–1578.
194. Jungmann, R. A., and Hunzicker-Dunn, M. (1978): Mechanism of action of gonadotropins and the regulation of gene expression. In: *Structure and Function of the Gonadotropins,* edited by K. W. McKerns, pp. 1–29. Plenum, New York.
195. Simpson, E. R., McCarthy, J. L., and Peterson, F. A. (1978): Evidence that the cycloheximide sensitive site of adrenocorticotropic hormone action is in the mitochondrion. Changes in pregnenolone formation, cholesterol content, and the electron paramagnetic resonance spectra of cytochrome P-450. *J. Biol. Chem.*, 253:3135–3139.
196. Azhar, S., and Menon, K. M. J. (1975): Adenosine 3′,5′-monophosphate dependent phosphorylation of ribosomes and ribosomal subunits from bovine corpus luteum. *Biochem. Biophys. Acta,* 392:64–74.
197. Trzeciak, W. H., and Boyd, G. S. (1974): Activation of cholesteryl esterase in bovine adrenal cortex. *Eur. J. Biochem.*, 46:201–207.
198. Caffrey, J. L., Fletcher, P. W., Diekman, M. A., O'Callaghan, P. L., and Niswender, G. D. (1979): The activity of ovine luteal cholesterol esterase during several experimental conditions. *Biol. Reprod.*, 21:601–608.
199. Caron, M. G., Goldstein, S., Savard, K., and Marsh, J. (1975): Protein kinase stimulation of a reconstituted cholesterol side chain cleavage enzyme system in the bovine corpus luteum. *J. Biol. Chem.*, 250:5137–5143.
200. Downing, J. R., and Dimino, M. J. (1979): Studies on mitochondrial protein kinase activity of porcine corpora lutea. *Endocrinology,* 105:570–573.
201. Neymark, M. A., Biersyezad, R. R., and Dimino, M. J. (1984): Phosphorylation of mitochondrial proteins in isolated porcine ovarian follicles after treatment with luteinizing hormone. *Endocrinology,* 114:588–593.
202. Hall, P. F. (1985): Trophic stimulation of steroidogenesis: In search of the elusive trigger. *Recent Prog. Horm. Res.* 41:1–31.
203. Lowitt, S., Farese, R. V., Sabor, M. A., and Root, A. W. (1982): Rat leydig cell phospholipid content is increased by luteinizing hormone and 8-bromo-cyclic AMP. *Endocrinology,* 111:1415–1417.
204. Ogle, T. F. (1974): Effects of ACTH on organelle interrelationships in the corpus luteum of the pregnant deermouse. *Cell Tissue Res.*, 153:195–209.
205. Scallen, T. J., Srikantaiah, M. V., Seetharam, B., Hansbury, E., and Gavey, K. L. (1974): Sterol carrier protein hypothesis. *Fed. Proc.*, 33:1733–1746.
206. Erickson, S. K., Meyer, D. J., and Gould, F. T. (1978): Purification and characterization of a new cholesterol binding protein from rat liver cytosol. *J. Biol. Chem.*, 253:1817–1826.
207. Strott, C. A., and Lyons, C. D. (1978): Studies of cholesterol binding in the soluble fraction of the adrenal cortex of the guinea pig. *J. Steroid Biochem.*, 9:721–730.
208. Strott, C. A. (1977): A prenenolone-binding protein in soluble fraction of guinea pig adrenal cortex. *J. Biol. Chem.*, 252:464–470.
209. Ferguson, J. J., Jr. (1962): Puromycin and adrenal responsiveness to adrenocorticotropic hormone. *Biochem. Biophys. Acta,* 57:616–617.
210. Garren, L. D. (1968): The mechanism of action of adrenocorticotropic hormone. *Vitam. Horm.*, 26:119–145.
211. Schulster, D., Richardson, M. C., and Palfreyman, J. W. (1974): The role of protein synthesis in adrenocorticotropin action: Effects of cycloheximide and puromycin on the steroidogenic response of isolated adrenocortical cells. *Mol. Cell. Endocrinol.*, 2:17–29.
212. Hermier, C., Combarnous, Y., and Jutisz, M. (1971): Role of a regulating protein and molecular oxygen in the mechanism of action of luteinizing hormone. *Biochem. Biophys. Acta,* 244:625–633.
213. Hochberg, R. B., vader Hoeven, T. A., Welch, S., and Lieberman, S. (1974): A simple and precise assay of the enzymatic conversion of cholesterol into pregnenolone. *Biochemistry,* 13:603–609.
214. Caffrey, J. L., Nett, T. M., Abel, J. H., Jr., and Niswender, G. D. (1979): Activity of 3β-hydroxy-Δ^5 steroid dehydrogenase/Δ^5,Δ^4-isomerase in the ovine corpus luteum. *Biol. Reprod.*, 20:279–287.
215. Werbin, H., and Charkoff, I. L. (1961): Utilization of adrenal gland cholesterol for synthesis of cortisol by the intact normal and the ACTH-treated guinea pig. *Arch. Biochem. Biophys.*, 93:474–482.
216. Armstrong, D. T., O'Brien, J., and Greep, R. O. (1964): Effects of luteinizing hormone on progestin biosynthesis in the luteinizing rat ovary. *Endocrinology,* 75:488–500.
217. Krum, A. A., Morris, M. D., and Bennett, L. J. (1964): Role of cholesterol in the *in vivo* biosynthesis of adrenal steroids by the dog. *Endocrinology,* 74:543–547.

218. Ichii, S., Forchielli, E., and Dorfman, R. I. (1963): *In vitro* effect of gonadotropins on the soluble cholesterol side-cleaving enzyme of bovine corpus luteum. *Steroids,* 2:631–656.
219. Melby, J. C., Egdahl, R. H., and Dale, S. L. (1967): Role of circulating free cholesterol of plasma in adrenal steroidogenesis. *Clin. Res.,* 15:263.
220. Behrman, H. R., and Armstrong, D. T. (1969): Cholesterol esterase stimulation by luteinizing hormone in luteinized rat ovaries. *Endocrinology,* 85:474–480.
221. Koritz, S. B. (1967): On the regulation of pregnenolone synthesis. In: *Functions of the Adrenal Cortex,* Vol. 1, edited by K. M. McKerns, pp. 27–48. Appleton-Century-Crofts, New York.
222. Hoyer, P. B., Fitz, T. A., and Niswender, G. D. (1984): Hormone-independent activation of adenylate cyclase in large steroidogenic ovine luteal cells does not result in increased progesterone secretion. *Endocrinology,* 114:604–608.
223. Fitz, T. A., Hoyer, P. B., and Niswender, G. D. (1984): Interactions of prostaglandins with subpopulations of ovine luteal cells. I. Stimulatory effects of prostaglandins E_1, E_2, and I_2. *Prostaglandins,* 28:119–126.
224. Loeb, L. (1923): The effect of extirpation of the uterus on the life and function of the corpus luteum in the guinea pig. *Proc. Soc. Exp. Biol. Med.,* 20:441–464.
225. Bradbury, J. T. (1937): Prolongation of the life of the corpus luteum by hysterectomy in the rat. *Anat. Rec.,* 70(Suppl. 1):51 (abstr.).
226. Bradbury, J. T., Brown, W. E., and Gray, L. A. (1950): Maintenance of the corpus luteum and physiologic actions of progesterone. *Recent Prog. Horm. Res.* 5:151–194.
227. Bartke, A. (1970): Influences of an IUD on the leucocytic content of the uterus and on the duration of pseudopregnancy in mice. *J. Reprod. Fertil.,* 23:243–247.
228. Critser, E. S., Rutledge, J. J., and French, R. L. (1980): Role of the uterus and the conceptus in regulating luteal lifespan in the mouse. *Biol. Reprod.,* 23:558–563.
229. Caldwell, B. V., Mazer, R. S, and Wright, P. A. (1967): Luteolysis as affected by uterine transplantation in the Syrian hamster. *Endocrinology,* 80:477–482.
230. Duby, R. T., McDaniel, J. W., Spilman, C. H., and Black, D. L. (1969): Utero-ovarian relationships in the golden hamster. I. Ovarian periodicity following hysterectomy. *Acta Endocrinol.,* 60: 595–602.
231. Lukaszewska, J. H., and Greenwald, G. S. (1969): Comparison of luteal function in pseudopregnant and pregnant hamsters. *J. Reprod. Fertil.,* 20:185–187.
232. Asdell, S. A., and Hammond, J. (1933): The effect of prolonging the life of the corpus luteum in the rabbit by hysterectomy. *Am. J. Physiol.,* 103:600–605.
233. Gillard, J. L. (1937): The effects of hysterectomy on mammary development in the rabbit. *Am. J. Physiol.,* 120:300–303.
234. Chu, J. P., Lee, C. C., and You, S. S. (1946): Functional relation between the uterus and the corpus luteum. *J. Endocrinol.,* 4:392–398.
235. Wiltbank, J. N., and Casida, L. E. (1956): Alteration of ovarian activity by hysterectomy. *J. Anim. Sci.,* 15:134–140.
236. Spies, H. G., Zimmerman, D. R., Self, H. L., and Casida, L. E. (1960): Effect of exogenous progesterone on the corpora lutea of hysterectomized gilts. *J. Anim. Sci.,* 19:101–108.
237. Ginther, O. J., and First, N. L. (1971): Maintenance of the corpus luteum in hysterectomized mares. *Am. J. Vet. Res.,* 32:1687–1691.
238. Stabenfeldt., G. H., Hughes, J. P., Wheat, J. D., Evans, J. W., Kennedy, P. C., and Cupps, P. T. (1974): The role of the uterus in ovarian control in the mare. *J. Reprod. Fertil.,* 37:343–351.
239. Neill, J. D., Johansson, E. D. B., and Knobil, E. (1969): Failure of hysterectomy to influence the normal pattern of cyclic progesterone secretion in the rhesus monkey. *Endocrinology,* 84:464–465.
240. Castracane, V. D., Moore, G. T., and Shaikh, A. A. (1979): Ovarian function in hysterectomized *Macaca fascicularis. Biol. Reprod.,* 20:462–472.
241. Beling, C. G., Marcus, S. L., and Markam, S. M. (1970): Functional activity of the corpus luteum following hysterectomy. *J. Clin. Endocrinol. Metab.,* 30:30–39.
242. Doyle, L. L., Barclay, D. L., Duncan, G. W., Kirton, K. T. (1971): Human luteal function following hysterectomy as assessed by plasma progestin. *Am. J. Obstet. Gynecol.,* 110:92–97.
243. Hartman, C. G. (1925): Hysterectomy and the oestrous cycle in the opossum. *Am. J. Anat.,* 35:25–29.
244. Hadley, J. C. (1975): The effect of serial uterine biopsies and hysterectomy on peripheral blood levels of total unconjugated oestrogen and progesterone in the bitch. *J. Reprod. Fertil.,* 45:389–393.
245. Deanesly, R. and Parkes, A. S. (1933): The effect of hysterectomy on the oestrous cycle of the ferret. *J. Physiol. (Lond.),* 78:80–84.
246. Durrant, E. P. (1927): Studies on vigor. XI. Relationship of hysterectomy to voluntary activity in the white rat. *Am. J. Physiol.,* 82:14–18.
247. Dewar, A. D. (1973): Effects of hysterectomy on corpus luteum activity in the cyclic, pseudopregnant and pregnant mouse. *J. Reprod. Fertil.,* 33:77–89.
248. Rowlands, I. W., and Short, R. V. (1959): The progesterone content of the guinea-pig corpus luteum during the reproductive cycle and after hysterectomy. *J. Endocrinol.,* 19:81–86.
249. Heap, R. B., Perry, J. S., and Rowlands, I. W., (1967): Corpus luteum function in the guinea-pig; arterial and luteal progesterone levels, and the effects of hysterectomy and hypophysectomy. *J. Reprod. Fertil.,* 13:537–553.
250. Poser, N. L., and Horton, E. N. (1975): Plasma progesterone levels in guinea-pigs actively immunized against prostaglandin $F_{2\alpha}$, hysterectomized or treated with intra-uterine indomethacin. *J. Endocrinol.,* 67:81–88.
251. Kiracofe, G. H., and Spies, H. G. (1966): Length of maintenance of naturally formed and experimentally induced corpora lutea in hysterectomized ewes. *J. Reprod. Fertil.,* 11:275–279.
252. Moor, R. M., Hay, M. F., Short, R. V., and Rowson, L. E. A. (1970): The corpus luteum of the sheep: effect of uterine removal during luteal regression. *J. Reprod. Fertil.,* 21:319–326.
253. Sheldrick, E. L., and Flint, A. P. F. (1983): Regression of the corpora lutea in sheep in response to cloprostenol is not affected by loss of luteal oxytocin after hysterectomy. *J. Reprod. Fertil.,* 68:155–160.
254. Malven, P. V., and Hansel, W. (1964): Ovarian function in dairy heifers following hysterectomy. *J. Dairy Sci.,* 47:1388–1393.
255. Anderson, L. L., Bowerman, A. M., and Melampy, R. M. (1965): Oxytocin on ovarian function in cycling and hysterectomized heifers. *J. Anim. Sci.,* 24:864–868.
256. Anderson, L. L., Butcher, R. L., and Melampy, R. M. (1961): Subtotal hysterectomy and ovarian function in gilts. *Endocrinology,* 68:571–580.
257. Masuda, H., Anderson, L. L., Henricks, D. M., and Melampy, R. M. (1967): Progesterone in ovarian venous plasma and corpora lutea of the pig. *Endocrinology,* 80:240–246.
258. Moeljono, M. P. E., Bazer, F. W., and Thatcher, W. W. (1976): A study of prostaglandin $F_{2\alpha}$ as the luteolysin in swine. I. Effect of prostaglandin $F_{2\alpha}$ in hysterectomized gilts. *Prostaglandins,* 11:737–743.
259. Pepe, G. J., and Rothchild, I. (1974): A comparative study of serum progesterone levels in pregnancy and in various types of pseudopregnancy in the rat. *Endocrinology,* 95:275–279.
260. Squires, E. L., Wentworth, B. C., and Ginther, O. J. (1975): Progesterone concentration in blood of mares during the estrous cycle, pregnancy and after hysterectomy. *J. Anim. Sci.,* 39:759–767.
261. Miller, J. B., and Keyes, P. L. (1976): A mechanism for regression of the rabbit corpus luteum: uterine induced loss of luteal responsiveness to 17β-estradiol. *Biol. Reprod.,* 15:511–518.
262. Lytton, F. D. C., and Poyser, N. L. (1982): Concentrations of $PGF_{2\alpha}$ and PGE_2 in the uterine venous blood of rabbits during pseudopregnancy and pregnancy. *J. Reprod. Fertil.,* 64:421–429.
263. Inskeep, E. K., and Butcher, R. L. (1966): Local component of utero-ovarian relationships in the ewe. *J. Anim. Sci.,* 25:1164–1168.
264. Moor, R. M., and Rowson, L. E. A. (1966): Local uterine mechanisms affecting luteal function in sheep. *J. Reprod. Fertil.,* 11:307–310.
265. Ginther, O. J., Woody, C. O., Mahajan, S. Janakiraman, K., and Casida, L. E. (1967): Effect of oxytocin administration on the oestrous cycle of unilaterally hysterectomized heifers. *J. Reprod. Fertil.,* 14:225–229.
266. du Mesnil du Buisson, F. (1961): Regression unilaterale des corpes jaunes apres hysterectomie partielle chez la truie. *Ann. Biol. Anim. Biochim. Biophys.,* 1:105–112.
267. Fisher, T. V. (1965): Local uterine inhibition of the corpus luteum in the guinea pig. *Anat. Rec.,* 151:350 (abstr.).

268. Butcher, R. L., Barley, D. A., and Inskeep, E. K. (1969): Local relationship between the ovary and uterus of rats and guinea pigs. *Endocrinology,* 4:476–481.
269. Duby, R. T., McDaniel, J. W., Spilman, C. H., and Black, D. L., (1969): Utero-ovarian relationships in the golden hamster. II. Quantitative and local influences of the uterus on ovarian function. *Acta Endocrinol.,* 60:603–610.
270. Barley, D. A., Butcher, R. L., and Inskeep, E. K. (1966): Local nature of utero-ovarian relationships in the pseudopregnant rat. *Endocrinology,* 79:119–124.
271. Hunter, G. L., and Casida, L. E. (1967): Absence of local effects of the rabbit uterus on weight of corpus luteum. *J. Reprod. Fertil.,* 13:179–181.
272. Hixon, J. E., and Hansel, W. (1974): Evidence for preferential transfer of prostaglandin $F_{2\alpha}$ to the ovarian artery following intrauterine administration in cattle. *Biol. Reprod.,* 11:543–552.
273. Bland, K. P., and Donovan, B. T. (1969): Observations on the time of action and the pathway of the uterine luteolytic effect of the guinea pig. *J. Endocrinol.,* 43:259–264.
274. Ginther, O. J. (1969): Utero-ovarian relationships in progesterone-treated guinea pig. *Am. J. Vet. Res.,* 30:261–267.
275. Fisher, T. V. (1971): Local pathway controlling luteal function in the guinea pig. *Biol. Reprod.,* 4:126–128.
276. O'Shea, J. D., and Lee, C. S. (1972): Local uterine luteolysis in the rat. *J. Reprod. Fertil.,* 28:155–156.
277. Goding, J. R., Harrison, F. A., Heap, R. B., and Linzell, J. L. (1967): Ovarian activity in the ewe after autotransplantation of the ovary or uterus to the neck. *J. Physiol. (Lond.),* 191:129–130.
278. Baird, D. T., Goding, J. R., Ichikawa, Y., and McCracken, J. A. (1968): The secretion of steroids from the autotransplanted ovary in the ewe spontaneously and in response to systemic gonadotrophin. *J. Endocrinol.,* 42:283–299.
279. Butcher, R. L., Chow, K. Y., and Melampy, R. M. (1962): Effect of uterine auto-transplants on the estrous cycle in the guinea pig. *Endocrinology,* 70:442–443.
280. Bland, K. P., and Donovan, B. T. (1968): The effect of autotransplantation of the ovaries to the kidneys or the uterus on the oestrous cycle of the guinea pig. *J. Endocrinol.,* 41:95–103.
281. Bland, K. P., and Donovan, B. T. (1970): Oestrogen and progesterone and the function of the corpora lutea in the guinea pig. *J. Endocrinol.,* 47:225–230.
282. Harrison, F. A., Heap, R. B., and Linzell, J. L. (1968): Ovarian function in the sheep after autotransplantation of the ovary and the uterus to the neck. *J. Endocrinol.,* 40:viii.
283. Ginther, O. J. (1974): Internal regulation of physiological processes through venoarterial pathways: a review. *J. Anim. Sci.,* 39:550–564.
284. Ginther, O. J., Del Campo, C. H., and Rawlings, C. A. (1973): Vascular anatomy of the uterus and ovaries and the unilateral luteolytic effect of the uterus: a local venoarterial pathway between uterus and ovaries in sheep. *Am. J. Vet. Res.,* 34:723–728.
285. Mapletoft, R., and Ginther, O. J. (1975): Adequacy of main uterine vein and the ovarian artery in the local venoarterial pathway for uterine-induced luteolysis in ewes. *Am. J. Vet. Res.,* 36:957–963.
286. Mapletoft, R. J., Del Campo, M. R., and Ginther, O. J. (1976): Local venoarterial pathway for uterine-induced luteolysis in cows. *Proc. Soc. Exp. Biol. Med.,* 153:289–294.
287. Del Campo, C. H., and Ginther, O. J. (1973): Vascular anatomy of the uterus and ovaries and the unilateral luteolytic effect of the uterus: horses, sheep and swine. *Am. J. Vet. Res.,* 34:305–316.
288. Del Campo, C. H., and Ginther, O. J. (1973): Vascular anatomy of the uterus and ovaries and the unilateral luteolytic effect of the uterus: angioarchitecture in sheep. *Am. J. Vet. Res.,* 34:1377–1386.
289. Ginther, O. J., and Del Campo, C. H. (1973): Vascular anatomy of the uterus and ovaries and the unilateral luteolytic effect of the uterus: Areas of close apposition between the ovarian artery and vessels which contain uterine venous blood in sheep. *Am. J. Vet. Res.,* 34:1387–1393.
290. Del Campo, C. H., and Ginther, O. J. (1974): Vascular anatomy of the uterus and ovaries and the unilateral luteolytic effect of the uterus: Histologic structure of uteroovarian vein and ovarian artery in sheep. *Am. J. Vet. Res.,* 35:397–399.
291. Del Campo, C. H., and Ginther, O. J. (1973): Vascular anatomy of the uterus and ovaries and the unilateral luteolytic effect of the uterus: guinea pigs, rats, hamsters and rabbits. *Am. J. Vet. Res.,* 33:2561–2578.
292. Ginther, O. J., and Del Campo, C. H. (1974): Vascular anatomy of the uterus and ovaries and the unilateral luteolytic effect of the uterus: Cattle. *Am. J. Vet. Res.,* 35:193–203.
293. Ginther, O. J., Garcia, M. C., Squires, E. L., and Steffenhagen, W. P. (1972): Anatomy of uterus and ovaries in mares. *Am. J. Vet. Res.,* 33:1687–1691.
294. Pharriss, B. B., and Wyngarden, L. (1969): The effect of prostaglandin $F_{2\alpha}$ on the progestogen content of ovaries from pseudopregnant rats. *Proc. Soc. Exp. Biol. Med.,* 130:92–94.
295. Lauderdale, J. W. (1972): Effects of $PGF_{2\alpha}$ on pregnancy and estrous cycle of cattle. *J. Anim. Sci.,* 35:246.
296. Liehr, R. A., Marion, G. B., and Olson, H. H. (1972): Effects of prostaglandin on cattle estrous cycles. *J. Anim. Sci.,* 35:247.
297. Louis, T. M., Hafs, H. D., and Morrow, D. A. (1972): Estrus and ovulation after uterine prostaglandin $F_{2\alpha}$ in cows. *J. Anim. Sci.,* 35:247.
298. Rowson, L. E. A., Tervit, H. R., and Brand, A. (1972): The use of prostaglandins for synchronization of oestrus in cattle. *J. Reprod. Fertil.,* 29:145.
299. McCracken, J. A., Glew, M. E., and Scaramuzzi, R. (1970): Corpus luteum regression induced by prostaglandin $F_{2\alpha}$. *J. Clin. Endocrinol. Metab.,* 30:544–546.
300. Barrett, S., DeB. Blockey, M. A., Brown, J. M., Cumming, J. A., Goding, J. R., Mole, B. J., and Obst., J. M. (1971): Initiation of the oestrous cycle in the ewe by infusions of $PGF_{2\alpha}$ to the autotransplanted ovary. *J. Reprod. Fertil.,* 24:136–137.
301. Thorburn, G. D., and Nicol, D. H. (1971): Regression of the ovine corpus luteum after infusion of prostaglandin $F_{2\alpha}$ into the ovarian artery and uterine vein. *J. Endocrinol.* 51:785.
302. Chaichareon, D. P., Mickley, P. E., and Ginther, O. J. (1974): Effect of prostaglandin $F_{2\alpha}$ on corpora lutea in guinea pigs and Mongolian gerbils. *Am. J. Vet. Res.,* 35:685–687.
303. Ott, R. S., Nelson, D. R., and Hixon, J. E. (1980): Peripheral serum progesterone and luteinizing hormone concentrations of goats during synchronization of estrus and ovulation with prostaglandin $F_{2\alpha}$. *Am. J. Vet. Res.,* 41:1432–1434.
304. Douglas, R. H., and Ginther, O. J. (1972): Effect of prostaglandin $F_{2\alpha}$ on the length of diestrus in mares. *Prostaglandins,* 2:265–268.
305. Allen, W. R., and Rowson, L. E. A. (1973): Control of the mare's oestrous cycle by prostaglandins. *J. Reprod. Fertil.,* 33:539–543.
306. Noden, P. A., Hafs, H. D., and Oxender, W. D. (1974): Estrus, ovulation, progesterone and luteinizing hormone after prostaglandin $F_{2\alpha}$ in mares. *Proc. Soc. Exp. Biol. Med.,* 145:145–150.
307. Bartke, A., Merrill, A. P., and Baker, C. F. (1972): Effects of prostaglandin $F_{2\alpha}$ on pseudopregnancy and pregnancy in mice. *Fertil. Steril.,* 23:543–547.
308. Harris, K. H., and Murphy, B. D. (1981): Luteolysis in the hamster: Abrogation by gonadotropin and prolactin pretreatment. *Prostaglandins,* 21:177–187.
309. Scott, R. S., and Rennie, P. I. C. (1970): Factors controlling the lifespan of the corpora lutea in the pseudopregnant rabbit. *J. Reprod. Fertil.,* 23:415–422.
310. Gutknecht, G. D., Duncan, G. W., and Wyngarden, L. J. (1972): Inhibition of prostaglandin $F_{2\alpha}$ or LH induced luteolysis in the pseudopregnant rabbit by 17β-estradiol. *Proc. Soc. Exp. Biol. Med.,* 139:406–410.
311. Diehl, J. R., and Day, B. N. (1973): Effect of prostaglandin $F_{2\alpha}$ on luteal function in swine. *J. Anim. Sci.* 37:307.
312. Gleeson, A. R. (1974): Luteal function of the cyclic sow after infusion of prostaglandin $F_{2\alpha}$ through a uterine vein. *J. Reprod. Fertil.,* 36:518–522.
313. Douglas, R. H., and Ginther, O. J. (1975): Effect of prostaglandin $F_{2\alpha}$ on estrous cycles or corpus luteum in mares and gilts. *J. Anim. Sci.,* 40:518–522.
314. Hallford, D. M., Wetteman, R. P., Turman, E. J., and Omtvedt., I. T. (1975): Luteal function in gilts after prostaglandin $F_{2\alpha}$. *J. Anim. Sci.,* 41:1706–1710.
315. Kirton, K. T., Pharriss, B. B., and Forbes, A. D. (1970): Luteolytic effect of prostaglandin $F_{2\alpha}$ in primates. *Proc. Soc. Exp. Biol. Med.,* 133:314–316.
316. Auletta, F. J., Caldwell, B. V., and Speroff, L. (1973): Prostaglandin $F_{2\alpha}$ induced steroidogenesis and luteolysis in the primate corpus luteum. *J. Clin. Endocrinol. Metab.,* 36:405–407.
317. Lehmann, F., Peters, F., Breckholdt, M., and Bettendorf, G. (1972): Plasma progesterone levels during infusion of prostaglandin $F_{2\alpha}$ in the human. *Prostaglandins,* 1:269–277.

318. Wentz, A. C., and Jones, G. E. S. (1973): Transient luteolytic effect of prostaglandin $F_{2\alpha}$ in the human. *Obstet. Gynecol.*, 42:172–181.
319. Jochle, W., Tomlinson, R. V., and Andersen, A. C. (1973): Prostaglandin effects on plasma progesterone levels in the pregnant and cycling dog (beagle). *Prostaglandins*, 3:209–217.
320. Auletta, F. J., Kamps, D. L., Pories, S., Bisset, J., and Gibson, M. (1984): An intra-corpus luteum site for the luteolytic action of prostaglandin $F_{2\alpha}$ in the rhesus monkey. *Prostaglandins*, 27:285–298.
321. Concannon, P. W., and Hansel, W. (1977): Prostaglandin $F_{2\alpha}$ induced luteolysis hypothermia and abortions in beagle bitches. *Prostaglandins*, 13:533–542.
322. Wildt, D. E., Panko, W. B., and Seager, S. W. J. (1979): Effect of prostaglandin $F_{2\alpha}$ on endocrine-ovarian function in the domestic cat. *Prostaglandins*, 18:883–892.
323. O'Grady, J. P., Caldwell, B. V., Auletta, F. J., and Speroff, L. (1972): The effects of an inhibitor of prostaglandin synthesis (indomethacin) on ovulation, pregnancy and pseudopregnancy in the rabbit. *Prostaglandins*, 1:98–106.
324. Lau, I. F., Saksena, S. K., and Chang, M. C. (1975): Effects of indomethacin, an inhibitor of prostaglandin biosynthesis, on the length of pseudopregnancy in rats and hamsters. *Acta. Endocrinol.*, 78:343–348.
325. Critser, E. S., Rutledge, J. J., and French, L. R. (1981): Effect of indomethacin on the interestrous interval of intact and hysterectomized pseudopregnant mice. *Biol. Reprod.*, 24:1000–1005.
326. Scaramuzzi, R. J., and Baird, D. T. (1976): The oestrous cycle of the ewe after active immunization against prostaglandin $F_{2\alpha}$. *J. Reprod. Fertil.*, 46:39–47.
327. Fairclough, R. J., Smith, J. F., Peterson, A. J., and McGowan, L. (1976): Effect of oestradiol-17β, progesterone and prostaglandin $F_{2\alpha}$ antiplasma on luteal function in the ewe. *J. Reprod. Fertil.*, 46:523–524.
328. Fairclough, R. J., Smith, J. F., and McGowan, L. T. (1981): Prolongation of the oestrous cycle in cows and ewes after passive imunization with PGF antibodies. *J. Reprod. Fertil.*, 62:213–219.
329. Shemesh, M., and Hansel, W. (1975): Levels of prostaglandin F in bovine endometrium, uterine venous, ovarian arterial and jugular plasma during the estrous cycle. *Proc. Soc. Exp. Biol. Med.*, 148:123–126.
330. Wilson, L. Jr., Cenedella, R. J., Butcher, R. L., and Inskeep, E. K. (1972): Levels of prostaglandins in the uterine endometrium during the ovine estrous cycle. *J. Anim. Sci.*, 34:93–99.
331. Poyser, N. L. (1972): Production of prostaglandins by the guinea-pig uterus. *J. Endocrinol.*, 54:147–159.
332. Vernon, M. W., Zavy, M. T., Aisquith, R. L., and Sharp, D. C. (1981): Prostaglandin $F_{2\alpha}$ in the equine endometrium: Steroid production and production capacities during the estrous cycle and early pregnancy. *Biol. Reprod.*, 25:581–589.
333. Guthrie, H. D., and Rexroad, C. E., Jr. (1980): Progesterone secretion and prostaglandin F release *in vitro* by endometrial and luteal tissue of cyclic pigs. *J. Reprod. Fertil.*, 60:157–163.
334. Doebler, J. A., Wickersham, E. W., and Anthony, A. (1981): Uterine prostaglandin $F_{2\alpha}$ content and 20-α-hydroxy-steroid dehydrogenase activity in individual ovarian compartments during pseudopregnancy in the rat. *Biol. Reprod.*, 24:871–878.
335. Lytton, F. D. C., and Poyser, N. L. (1982): Prostaglandin production by the rabbit uterus and placenta *in vitro*. *J. Reprod. Fertil.*, 66:591–599.
336. Gleeson, A. R., Thorburn, G. D., and Cox, R. I. (1974): Prostaglandin F concentrations in the utero-ovarian vein plasma of the sow during the late luteal phase of the oestrous cycle. *Prostaglandins*, 5:521–529.
337. Moeljono, M. P. E., Thatcher, W. W., Bazer, F. W., Frank, M., Owens, L. J., and Wilcox, C. J. (1977): A study of prostaglandin $F_{2\alpha}$ as the luteolysin in swine: II. Characterization and comparison of prostaglandin F, estrogens and progestin concentrations in utero-ovarian vein plasma of nonpregnant and pregnant gilts. *Prostaglandins*, 14:543–555.
338. Douglas, R. H., and Ginther, O. J. (1976): Concentrations of prostaglandin F in uterine venous plasma of anesthetized mares during the estrous cycle and early pregnancy. *Prostaglandins*, 11:251–260.
339. Castracane, V. D., and Shaikh, A. A. (1976): Effect of decidual tissue on the uterine production of prostaglandins in pseudopregnant rats. *J. Reprod. Fertil.*, 46:101–104.
340. Behrman, H., Grinwich, D. H., Hichens, M., and MacDonald, G. J. (1978): Effect of hypophysectomy, prolactin and prostaglandin $F_{2\alpha}$ on gonadotropin binding *in vivo* and *in vitro* in the corpus luteum. *Endocrinology*, 103:349–357.
341. Fletcher, P. W., and Niswender, G. D. (1982): Effect of $PGF_{2\alpha}$ on progesterone secretion and adenylate cyclase activity in ovine luteal tissue. *Prostaglandins*, 20:803–818.
342. Silvia, W. J., Fitz, T. A., Mayan, M. H., and Niswender, G. D. (1984): Cellular and molecular mechanisms involved in luteolysis and maternal recognition of pregnancy in the ewe. *Anim. Reprod. Sci.*, 7:57–74.
343. Braden, T. D., and Niswender, G. D. (1985): Differential loss of the two steroidogenic cell types in the ovine corpus luteum following prostaglandins $(PG)F_{2\alpha}$. *Biol. Reprod.*, 30 (Suppl. 1):14.
344. Weston, P. G., and Hixon, J. E. (1980): Effects of *in vivo* prostaglandin $F_{2\alpha}$ administration on *in vitro* progesterone synthesis by bovine corpora lutea. *Biol. Reprod.*, 22:259–268.
345. Paavola, L. G. (1979): The corpus luteum of the guinea pig. IV. Fine structure of macrophages during pregnancy and postpartum luteolysis and the phagocytosis of luteal cells. *Am. J. Anat.*, 154:337–364.
346. Koering, M. J., and Thor, M. J. (1978): Structural changes in the regressing corpus luteum of the rabbit. *Biol. Reprod.*, 17:719–733.
347. VanLennys, E. W., and Madden, L. M. (1965): Electron microscopic observations of the involution of the human corpus luteum of menstruation. *A. Zellforsch. Mikrosk. Anat.*, 66:365–380.
348. Corteel, M. (1975): Luteolysis induced by prostaglandin $F_{2\alpha}$ compared with natural luteolysin in the ewe. *Ann. Biol. Anim. Biochem. Biophys.*, 15:175–180.
349. Thorburn, G. D., and Hales, J. R. S. (1972): Selective reduction in blood flow to the ovine corpus luteum after infusion of prostaglandins $F_{2\alpha}$ into a uterine vein. *Proc. Aust. Physiol. Pharmacol. Soc.*, 3:145.
350. Novy, M. J., and Cook, M. J. (1973): Redistribution of blood flow by prostaglandin $F_{2\alpha}$ in the rabbit ovary. *Am. J. Obstet. Gynecol.*, 117:381–385.
351. Ricketts, A. P., and Flint, A. P. F. (1980): Onset of synthesis of progesterone by ovine placenta. *J. Endocrinol.*, 86:337–347.
352. Butcher, R. L., Collins, W. E., and Fugo, N. W. (1974): Plasma concentration of LH, FSH, prolactin, progesterone and estradiol-17β throughout the 4-day estrous cycle of the rat. *Endocrinology*, 94:1704–1708.
353. Smith, M. S., Freeman, M. E., and Neill, J. D. (1975): The control of progesterone secretion during the estrous cycle and early pseudopregnancy in the rat: prolactin, gonadotropin and steroid levels associated with rescue of the corpus luteum of pseudopregnancy. *Endocrinology*, 96:219–226.
354. Spies, H. G., and Niswender, G. D. (1971): Levels of prolactin, LH and FSH in the serum of intact and pelvic-neuroectomized rats. *Endocrinology*, 88:937–943.
355. Freeman, M. E., Smith, M. S., Nazian, S. J., and Neill, J. D. (1974): Ovarian and hypothalamic control of the daily surges of prolactin secretion during pseudopregnancy. *Endocrinology*, 94:875–882.
356. Butcher, R. L., Fugo, N. W., and Collins, W. E. (1972): Semicircadian rhythm in plasma levels of prolactin during early gestation in the rat. *Endocrinology*, 90:1125–1127.
357. von Berswoldt-Wallabre, I., Geller, H. F., and Herlyn, U. (1964): Temporal aspects of decidual cell reaction. I. Induction of decidual cell reaction in lactogenic hormone treated and in pseudopregnant rats. *Acta Endocrinol.*, 45:349–352.
358. Gibori, G., Rothchild, I., Pepe, G. J., Morishige, W. K., and Lam, P. (1974): Luteotropic action of decidual tissue in the rat. *Endocrinology*, 95:1113–1118.
359. Csapo, A. I., and Wiest, W. G. (1969): An examination of the quantitative relationship between progesterone and the maintenance of pregnancy. *Endocrinology*, 85:735–746.
360. Morishige, W. K., and Rothchild, I. (1974): Temporal aspects of the regulation of corpus luteum function by luteinizing hormone, prolactin and placental luteotrophin during the first half of pregnancy in the rat. *Endocrinology*, 95:260–274.
361. Ershoff, B. H., and Devel, H. I., Jr. (1943): Prolongation of pseudopregnancy by induction of deciduomata. *Proc. Soc. Exp. Biol. Med.*, 54:167–168.

362. Peckham, B. M., and Greene, R. R. (1948): Prolongation of pseudopregnancy by induction of deciduomata. *Proc. Soc. Exp. Biol. Med.*, 69:417–418.
363. Shaikh, A. A., Naqvi, R. H., and Saksena, S. K. (1977): Prostaglandins E and F in uterine venous plasma in relation to peripheral plasma levels of progesterone and 20α-hydroxyprogesterone in the rat throughout pregnancy and parturition. *Prostaglandins*, 13:311–320.
364. Carminati, P., Luzzani, F., Soffientini, A., and Lerner, L. (1975): Influence of day of pregnancy on rat placental, uterine and ovarian prostaglandin synthesis and metabolism. *Endocrinology*, 97:1071–1079.
365. Astwood, E. B., and Greep, R. O. (1938): A corpus luteum-stimulating substance in the rat placenta. *Proc. Soc. Exp. Biol. Med.*, 38:713–716.
366. Linkie, D. M., and Niswender, G. D. (1972): Characterization of rat placental luteotropin: Physiology and biochemical properties. *Biol. Reprod.*, 8:48–57.
367. Kelly, P. A., Shiu, R. P. C., Robertson, M. C., and Friesen, H. G. (1975): Characterization of rat chorionic mammotropin. *Endocrinology*, 96:1187–1195.
368. Robertson, M. C., and Friesen, H. G. (1975): The purification and characterization of rat placental lactogen. *Endocrinology*, 97:621–629.
369. Robertson, M. C., Gillespie, B. and Friesen, H. G. (1982): Characterization of the two forms of rat placental lactogen (rPL): rPL-I and rPL-II. *Endocrinology*, 111:1862–1866.
370. Haour, F., Tell, G., Sanchez, P., and Debre, R. (1976): Mise en evidence et dosage d'une gonadotrophine chorionique chez le rat (rCG). *C. R. Acad. Sci., Ser. D*, 282:1183–1186.
371. Jayatilak, P. G., Glasser, L. A., Warshaw, M. L., Herz, Z., Gruber, J. R., and Gibori, G. (1984): Relationship between luteinizing hormone and decidual luteotropin in the maintenance of luteal steroidogenesis. *Biol. Reprod.*, 31:556–564.
372. Hilliard, J., Scaramuzzi, R. J., Penardi, R. and Sawyer, C. H. (1974): Serum progesterone levels in hysterectomized pseudopregnant rabbits. *Proc. Soc. Exp. Biol. Med.*, 145:151–153.
373. Bill, II, C. H., and Keyes, P. L. (1983): 17β-estradiol maintains normal function of corpora lutea throughout pseudopregnancy in hypophysectomized rabbits. *Biol. Reprod.*, 28:608–617.
374. Browning, J. Y., Keyes, P. L., and Wolf, R. C. (1980): Comparison of serum progesterone, 20α-dihydroprogesterone and estradiol-17β in pregnant and pseudopregnant rabbits: evidence for postimplantation recognition of pregnancy. *Biol. Reprod.*, 23:1014–1019.
375. Wu, D. H., and Allen, W. M.: Maintenance of pregnancy in castrated rabbits by 17-α-hydroxy-progesterone caproate and by progesterone. *Fertil. Steril.*, 10:439–460.
376. Kwun, J. K., and Emmens, C. W. (1974): Hormonal requirements for implantation and pregnancy in the ovariectomized rabbit. *Aust. J. Biol. Sci.*, 27:275–283.
377. Thau, R., and Lanman, J. T. (1974): Evaluation of progesterone synthesis in rabbit placentas. *Endocrinology*, 94:925–926.
378. Browning, J. Y., and Wolf, R. C. (1981): Maternal recognition of pregnancy in the rabbit: effect of conceptus removal. *Biol. Reprod.*, 24:293–297.
379. Nowak, R. A., and Bahr, J. (1983): Maternal recognition of pregnancy in the rabbit. *J. Reprod. Fertil.*, 69:623–627.
380. Klein, M. (1933): Sur l'ablation des embryons chez la lapine gravid et sur les facteurs qui determinent le maintien du corps jaune pendant la deuxieme partie de la grosesse. *C. R. Soc. Biol.*, 113:441–443.
381. Lanman, J. T., and Thau, R. (1979): Effect of the fetal placenta and of a rabbit pituitary extract on plasma progesterone in fetectomized rabbits. *J. Reprod. Fertil.*, 57:341–344.
382. Ellinwood, W. E., Seidel, G. E., and Niswender, G. D. (1979): Secretion of gonadotropic factors by the preimplantation rabbit blastocyst. *Proc. Soc. Exp. Biol. Med.*, 161:136–141.
383. Browning, J. Y., Amis, M. A., Meller, P. A., Bridson, W. E., and Wolf, R. C. (1982): Luteotropic and antiluteolytic activities of the rabbit conceptus. *Biol. Reprod.*, 27:665–672.
384. Gadsby, J. E., Keyes, P. L., and Bill, II, C. H. (1983): Control of corpus luteum function in the pregnant rabbit: Role of estrogen and lack of a direct luteotropic role of the placenta. *Endocrinology*, 113:2255–2262.
385. Abramowitz, J. A., and Birnbaumer, L. (1979): Prostacyclin activation of adenylyl cyclase in rabbit corpus luteum membranes: Comparison with 6-keto-prostaglandin $F_{1\alpha}$ and prostaglandin E_1. *Biol. Reprod.*, 21:609–616.
386. Harper, M. J. K., Norris, C. J., and Rajkumar, K. (1983): Prostaglandin release by zygotes and endometria of pregnant rabbits. *Biol. Reprod.*, 28:350–362.
387. Croix, D., and Franchimont, P. (1975): Changes in serum levels of gonadotropins, progesterone and estradiol during the estrous cycle of the guinea pig. *Neuroendocrinology*, 19:1–11.
388. Blatchley, F. R., Donovan, B. T., and Ter Haar, M. B. (1976): Plasma progesterone and gonadotrophin levels during the estrous cycle of the guinea pig. *Biol. Reprod.*, 15:29–38.
389. Blatchley, F. R., Donovan, B. T., Horton, E. W., and Poyser, N. L. (1972): The release of prostaglandins and progesterone into the utero-ovarian venous blood of guinea-pigs during the oestrous cycle and following oestrogen treatment. *J. Physiol. (Lond.)*, 223: 69–88.
390. Granstrom, E., and Kindahl, H. (1976): Radioimmunoassay for urinary metabolites of prostaglandin $F_{2\alpha}$. *Prostaglandins*, 12: 759–783.
391. Artunkal, T., and Colonge, R. A. (1949): Action de l'ovariectomie sur la gestation du cobaye. *C. R. Soc. Biol.*, 143:1590–1592.
392. Csapo, A. L., Puri, C. P., and Tano, S. (1981): Relationship between timing of ovariectomy and maintenance of pregnancy in the guinea-pig. *Prostaglandins*, 22:131–140.
393. Illingworth, D. V., and Challis, J. R. G. (1973): Concentrations of oestrogens and progesterone in the plasma of ovariectomized and ovariectomized norgestrel-treated pregnant guinea-pigs. *J. Reprod. Fertil.*, 34:289–296.
394. Challis, J. R. G., Heap, R. B., and Willingworth, D. V. (1971): Concentrations of estrogen and progesterone in the plasma of non-pregnant, pregnant and lactating guinea-pigs. *J. Endocrinol.*, 51:333–345.
395. Moor, R. M. (1968): Effect of embryo on corpus luteum function. *J. Anim. Sci.*, 27(Suppl. 1):97–118.
396. Maule-Walker, F. M., and Poyser, N. L. (1974): Production of prostaglandins by the early pregnant guinea-pig uterus *in vitro*. *J. Endocrinol.* 61:265–271.
397. Heap, R. B., and Deanesly, R. (1967): The increase in plasma progesterone levels in the pregnant guinea-pig and its possible significance. *J. Reprod. Fertil.*, 14:339–341.
398. Illingworth, D. V., Heap, R. B., and Perry, J. S. (1970): Changes in the metabolic clearance rate of progesterone in the guinea pig. *J. Endocrinol.*, 48:409–417.
399. Blatchley, F. R., Maule-Walker, F. M., and Poyser, N. L. (1975): Progesterone, prostaglandin $F_{2\alpha}$ and oestradiol in the utero-ovarian venous plasma of nonpregnant and early, unilaterally pregnant guinea-pigs. *J. Endocrinol.*, 67:225–229.
400. Antonini, R., Turner, T. T., and Pauerstein, C. J. (1976): The hormonal control of the guinea-pig corpus luteum during early pregnancy. *Fertil. Steril.*, 27:1322–1325.
401. Hymphreys, E. M., Hobson, B. M., and Wide, L. (1981): Gonadotrophic activity of the guinea-pig placenta during pregnancy. *J. Reprod. Fertil.*, 65:231–238.
402. Babra, C.S., Lynch, S. S., Foxcroft, G. R., Robinson, G., and Amoroso, E. C. (1984): Purification and characterization of guinea-pig chorionic gonadotrophin. *J. Reprod. Fertil.*, 71:227–233.
403. Casida, L. E., and Warwick, E. J. (1945): The necessity of the corpus luteum for maintenance of pregnancy in the ewe. *J. Anim. Sci.*, 4:34–36.
404. Denamur, R., and Martinet, J. (1955): Effets de l'ovariectomie chez la brebis pendant la gestation. *C. R. Seanc. Soc. Biol.*, 149:2105–2107.
405. Moore, N. W., and Rowson, L. E. A. (1959): Maintenance of pregnancy in ovariectomized ewes by means of progesterone. *Nature*, 184:1410.
406. Bindon, B. M. (1971): The role of progesterone in implantation in the sheep. *Aust. J. Biol Sci.*, 24:149–158.
407. Moor, R. M., and Rowson, L. E. A. (1966): The corpus luteum of the sheep: Effect of the removal of embryos on luteal function. *J. Endocrinol.*, 34:497–502.
408. Moor, R. M., and Rowson, L. E. A. (1966): The corpus luteum of the sheep: Functional relationship between the embryo and corpus luteum. *J. Endocrinol.*, 34:233–239.
409. Bindon, B. M. (1971): Systematic study of preimplantation stages of pregnancy in the sheep. *Aust. J. Biol Sci.*, 24:131–147.

410. Bassett, J. M., Oxborrow, T. J., Smith, I. D., and Thorburn, G. D. (1969): The concentration of progesterone in the peripheral plasma of the pregnant ewe. *J. Endocrinol.*, 45:449–457.
411. Thorburn, G. D., Cox, R. I., Currie, W. B., Restall, B. J., and Schneider, W. (1973): Prostaglandin F concentration in the utero-ovarian venous plasm of the ewe during the estrous cycle. *J. Reprod. Fertil. (Suppl.)* 18:151–158.
412. Barcikowski, B., Carlson, J. C., Wilson, L., and McCracken, J. A. (1974): The effect of endogenous and exogenous estradiol-17β on the release of prostaglandin $F_{2\alpha}$ from the ovine uterus. *Endocrinology*, 95:1340–1349.
413. Peterson, A. J., Tervit, H. R., Fairclough, R. J., Havik, P. G., and Smith, J. F. (1976): Jugular levels of 13,14-dihydro-15-keto-prostaglandin F and progesterone around luteolysis and early pregnancy in the ewe. *Prostaglandins*, 12:551–558.
414. Zarco, L., Stabenfeldt, G. H., Kindahl, H., Bradford, G. E., and Basu, S. (1984): A detailed study of prostaglandin $F_{2\alpha}$ release during luteolysis and establishment of pregnancy in the ewe. *Biol. Reprod. (Suppl. 1)* 30:153.
415. Fincher, K. B., Hanson, P. J., Thatcher, W. W., Roberts, R. M., and Bazer, F. W. (1984): Ovine conceptus secretory proteins suppress induction of prostaglandins $F_{2\alpha}$ release by estradiol and oxytocin. *J. Anim. Sci. (Suppl. 1)*, 59:369.
416. Nett, T. M., Staigmiller, R. B., Akbar, A. M., Diekman, M. A., Ellinwood, W. E., and Niswender, G. D. (1976): Secretion of prostaglandin $F_{2\alpha}$ in cycling and pregnant ewes. *J. Anim. Sci.*, 42:876–880.
417. Lewis, G. S., Wilson, L., Jr., Wilks, J. W., et al. (1977): Prostaglandin $F_{2\alpha}$ and its metabolites in uterine and jugular venous plasma and endometrium of ewes during early pregnancy. *J. Anim. Sci.*, 45:320–327.
418. Ellinwood, W. E., Nett, T. M., and Niswender, G. D. (1979): Maintenance of the corpus luteum of early pregnancy in the ewe. II. Prostaglandin secretion by the endometrium *in vitro* and *in vivo*. *Biol. Reprod.*, 21:845–856.
419. Ottobre, J. S., Vincent, D. L., Silvia, W. J., and Inskeep, E. K. (1984): Aspects of regulation of uterine secretion of prostaglandins during the oestrous cycle and early pregnancy. *Anim. Reprod. Sci.*, 7:75–100.
420. Silvia, W. J., Ottobre, J. S., and Inskeep, E. K. (1984): Concentrations of prostaglandins E_2, $F_{2\alpha}$ and 6-keto-prostaglandin $F_{1\alpha}$ in the utero-ovarian venous plasma of nonpregnant and early pregnant ewes. *Biol. Reprod.*, 30:936–944.
421. Wilson, L., Jr., Butcher, R. L., and Inskeep, E. K. (1972): Prostaglandin $F_{2\alpha}$ in the uterus of ewes during early pregnancy. *Prostaglandins*, 1:479–482.
422. Findlay, J. K., Colvin, N., Swaney, J., and Doughton, B. (1983): Prostaglandin F and 13-14-dihydro-15-keto prostaglandin F in the endometrium and uterine flushings of sheep before implantation. *J. Reprod. Fertil.*, 68:343–349.
423. Findlay, J. K., Ackland, N., Burton, R. D., et al. (1981): Protein, prostaglandin and steroid synthesis in caruncular endometrium of sheep before implantation. *J. Reprod. Fertil.*, 62:361–377.
424. Rowson, L. E. A., and Moor, R. M. (1967): The influence of embryonic tissue homogenate infused into the uterus, on the lifespan of the corpus luteum in sheep. *J. Reprod. Fertil.*, 13:511–516.
425. Ellinwood, W. E., Nett, T. M., and Niswender, G. D. (1979): Maintenance of the corpus luteum of early pregnancy in the ewe. I. Luteotropic properties of embryonic homogenates. *Biol. Reprod.*, 21:281–288.
426. Martal, J., LaCroix, M. C., Loudes, C., Saunier, M., and Wintenberger-Torres, S. (1979): Trophoblastin, an antiluteolytic protein present in early pregnancy in sheep. *J. Reprod. Fertil.*, 56:63–73.
427. Godkin, J. D., Bazer, F. W., Thatcher, W. W., and Roberts, R. M. (1984): Proteins released by cultured day 15–16 conceptuses prolong luteal maintenance when introduced into the uterine lumen of cyclic ewes. *J. Reprod. Fertil.*, 71:57–64.
428. Godkin, J. D., Bazer, F. W., Moffatt, J., Sessions, F., and Roberts, R. M. (1982): Purification and properties of a major, low molecular weight protein released by the trophoblast of sheep blastocysts at day 13–21. *J. Reprod. Fertil.*, 65:141–150.
429. Godkin, J. D., Bazer, F. W., and Roberts, R. M. (1984): Ovine trophoblast protein I, an early secreted blastocyst protein, binds specifically to uterine endometrium and affects protein synthesis. *Endocrinology*, 114:120–130.
430. Hyland, J. H., Manns, J. G., and Humphrey, W. D. (1982): Prostaglandin production by ovine endometrim *in vitro*. *J. Reprod. Fertil.*, 65:299–304.
431. LaCroix, M. C., and Kann, G. (1982): Comparative studies of prostaglandins $F_{2\alpha}$ and E_2 in late cyclic and early pregnant sheep: *In vitro* synthesis by endometrium and conceptus; effect of *in vivo* indomethacin treatment on establishment of pregnancy. *Prostaglandins*, 23:507–526.
432. Gadsby, J. E., Heap, R. B., and Burton, R. D. (1980): Oestrogen production by blastocyst and early embryonic tissue of various species. *J. Reprod. Fertil.*, 60:409–417.
433. Marcus, G. J. (1981): Prostaglandin formation by the sheep embryo and endometrium as an indication of maternal recognition of pregnancy. *Biol. Reprod.*, 25:56–64.
434. LaCroix, M. C., and Kann, G. (1983): Discriminating analysis of "in vitro" prostaglandin release by myometrial and luminal sides of the ewe endometrium. *Prostaglandins*, 25:853–869.
435. Vincent, D. L., and Inskeep, E. K. (1984): Effects of ovariectomy and progesterone replacement on uteroovarian venous prostaglandins (PG). *J. Anim. Sci. (Suppl. 1)*, 59:368.
436. Pratt, B. R., Butcher, R. L., and Inskeep, E. K. (1977): Antiluteolyic effect of the conceptus and of PGE_2 in ewes. *J. Anim. Sci.*, 45:784–791.
437. Magness, R. R., Huie, J. M., and Weems, C. W. (1981): Effect of chronic ipsilateral or contralateral intrauterine infusion of prostaglandin E_2 (PGE_2) on luteal function of unilaterally ovariectomized ewes. *Prostagland. Med.*, 6:389–401.
438. Colcord, M. L., Hoyer, G. L., and Weems, C. W. (1978): Effect of prostaglandin E_2 (PGE_2) as an anti-luteolysin in estrogen-induced luteolysis in ewes. *J. Anim. Sci. (Suppl 1)*, 47:352.
439. Henderson, K. M., Scaramuzzi, R. J., and Baird, D. T. (1977): Simultaneous infusion of prostaglandin E_2 antagonizes the luteolytic action of prostaglandin $F_{2\alpha}$ *in vitro*. *J. Endocrinol.*, 72:379–383.
440. Mapletoft, R. J., Miller, K. F., and Ginther, O. J. (1977): Effects of $PGF_{2\alpha}$ and PGE_2 on corpora lutea in ewes. *J. Anim. Sci. (Suppl 1)*, 45:185.
441. Reynolds, L. P., Stigler, J., Hoyer, W. L., et al. (1981): Effect of PGE_1 or PGE_2 of $PGF_{2\alpha}$-induced luteolysis in nonbred ewes. *Prostaglandins*, 21:957–972.
442. Moor, R. M., and Rowson, L. E. A. (1966): Local maintenance of the corpus luteum in sheep in embryos transferred to various isolated portions of the uterus. *J. Reprod. Fertil.*, 12:539–550.
443. Mapletoft, R. J., Del Campo, M. R., and Ginther, O. J. (1975): Unilateral luteotropic effect of uterine venous effluent of a gravid uterine horn in sheep. *Proc. Soc. Exp. Biol. Med.*, 150:129–133.
444. Mapletoft, R. J., Lapin, D. R., and Ginther, O. J. (1976): The ovarian artery as the final component of the local pathway between a gravid uterine horn and ovary in ewes. *Biol. Reprod.*, 15:414–421.
445. Inskeep, E. K., Smutny, W. J., Butcher, R. L., and Pexton, J. E. (1975): Effects of intrafollicular injections of prostaglandins in nonpregnant and pregnant ewes. *J. Anim. Sci.*, 41:1098–1104.
446. Silvia, W. J., and Niswender, G. D. (1986): Maintenance of the corpus luteum of early pregnancy in the ewe. IV. Changes in luteal sensitivity to prostaglandin $F_{2\alpha}$ throughout early pregnancy. *J. Anim. Sci.*, 63:1201–1207.
447. Estergreen, V. L., Frost, O. L., Gomes, W. R., Erb, R. E., and Bullard, J. F. (1967): Effect of ovariectomy on pregnancy maintenance and parturition in dairy cows. *J. Dairy Sci.*, 50:1293–1295.
448. Tanabe, T. Y., Hokanson, J. F., and Griel, L. C. (1968): Minimal exogenous progesterone requirements for maintenance of pregnancy in dairy cows after corpus luteum removal via laparotomy. *Proceedings of the 2nd World Conference on Animal Productivity*, p. 370.
449. Wendorf, G. L., Lawyer, M. S., and First, N. L. (1983): Role of the adrenals in maintenance of pregnancy in cows. *J. Reprod. Fertil.*, 68:281–287.
450. Betteridge, K. G., Egglesome, M. D., Randall, G. C. B., and Mitchell, D. (1980): Collection, description and transfer of embryos from cattle 10–16 days after oestrus. *J. Reprod. Fertil.*, 59:205–216.
451. Northey, D. L., and French, L. R. (1980): Effect of embryo removal and intrauterine infusion of embryonic homogenates on the lifespan of the bovine corpus luteum. *J. Anim. Sci.*, 50:298–302.
452. Dalla Porta, M. A., and Humblot, P. (1983): Effect of embryo removal and embryonic extracts or PGE_2 infusions on luteal function in the bovine. *Theriogenology*, 19:122.

453. Shemesh, M., Ayalon, N., and Lindner, H. R. (1968): Early effect of conceptus on plasma progesterone level in the cow. *J. Reprod. Fertil.*, 15:161–164.
454. Pope, G. S., Gupta, S. K., and Numro, I. B. (1969): Progesterone levels in systemic plasma of pregnant, cycling and ovariectomized cows. *J. Reprod. Fertil.*, 20:369–381.
455. Henricks, D. M., Lamond, D. R., Hill, J. R., and Dickey, J. F. (1971): Plasma progesterone concentrations before mating and in early pregnancy in the beef heifer. *J. Anim. Sci.*, 33:450–454.
456. Erb, R. E., Garverick, H. A., Randel, R. D., Brown, B. L., and Callahan, C. J. (1976): Profiles of reproductive hormones associated with fertile and nonfertile inseminations of dairy cows. *Theriogenology*, 5:227–242.
457. Bulman, D. C., and Lamming, G. E. (1978): Milk progesterone levels in relation to conception, repeat breeding and factors influencing acyclicity in dairy cows. *J. Reprod. Fertil.*, 54:447–458.
458. Lukaszewska, J. H., and Hansel, W. (1980): Corpus luteum maintenance during early pregnancy in the cow. *J. Reprod. Fertil.*, 59:485–493.
459. Hansel, W. (1981): Plasma hormone concentrations associated with early embryo mortality in heifers. *J. Reprod. Fertil. (Suppl.)*, 30:231–239.
460. Kindahl, H., Edqvist, L. E., Bane, A., and Granstom, E. (1976): Blood levels of progesterone and 15-keto-13,14-dihydro-prostaglandin $F_{2\alpha}$ during the normal estrous cycle and early pregnancy in heifers. *Acta Endocrinol.*, 82:134–149.
461. Williams, W. F., Lewis, G. S., Thatcher, W. W., and Underwood, C. S. (1983): Plasma 13,14-dihydro-15-keto-$PGF_{2\alpha}$ (PGFM) in pregnant and open heifers prior to and during laparotomy and following intrauterine injection of $PGF_{2\alpha}$. *Prostaglandins*, 25:891–899.
462. Thatcher, W. W., Wolfenson, D., Curl, J. S., et al. (1984): Prostaglandin dynamics associated with development of the bovine conceptus. *Anim. Reprod. Sci.*, 7:149–176.
463. Knickerbocker, J. J., Thatcher, W. W., Bazer, F. W., et al. (1984): Proteins secreted by cultured day 17 bovine conceptuses extend luteal function in cattle. *Proceedings of the 10th International Congress on Animal Reproduction and Artificial Insemination*, p. 88 (abstr.).
464. Knickerbocker, J. J., Thatcher, W. W., Bazer, F. W., Barron, D. H., and Roberts, R. M. (1984): Inhibition of estradiol-17β(E) induced uterine prostaglandin $F_{2\alpha}$ ($PGF_{2\alpha}$) production by bovine conceptus secretory proteins (CSP). *J. Anim. Sci. (Suppl 1)*, 59:368 (abstr.).
465. Shemesh, M. F., Milaguir, F., Ayalon, N., and Hansel, W. (1979): Steroidogenesis and prostaglandin synthesis by cultured bovine blastocysts. *J. Reprod. Fertil.*, 56:181–185.
466. Chenault, J. R. (1980): Steroid metabolism by the early bovine conceptus. 1. 5α-reduction of neutral C_{19}-steroids. *J. Steroid Biochem.*, 13:499–506.
467. Lewis, G. S., Thatcher, W. W., Bazer, F. W., and Curl, J. S. (1982): Metabolism of arachidonic acid *in vitro* by bovine blastocysts and endometrium. *Biol. Reprod.*, 27:431–439.
468. Ely, R. M., Thatcher, F. W., Bazer, F. W., and Fields, M. J. (1983): Steroid metabolism by the bovine uterine endometrium and conceptus. *Biol. Reprod.*, 28:804–816.
469. Chenault, J. R. (1983): Response of bovine corpora lutea to intrauterine prostaglandin E_2 infusion *J. Anim. Sci. (Suppl 1)*, 57:323–324 (abstr.).
470. Reynolds, L. P., Robertson, D. A., and Ford, S. P. (1983): Effects of intrauterine infusion of oestradiol-17β and prostaglandin E_2 on luteal function in nonpregnant heifers. *J. Reprod. Fertil.*, 69:703–709.
471. Del Campo, M. R., Rowe, R. F., French, L. R., and Ginther, O. J. (1977): Unilateral relationship of embryos and the corpus luteum in cattle. *Biol. Reprod.*, 16:580–585.
472. Del Campo, M. R., Mapletoft, R. J., Rowe, R. F., Critser, J. K., and Ginther, O. J. (1980): Unilateral utero-ovarian relationship in pregnant cattle and role of uterine vein. *Theriogenology*, 14:185–193.
473. Marsh, J. M. (1970): The stimulatory effect of PGE_2 on adenyl cyclase in the bovine corpus luteum. *FEBS Lett.*, 7:283–286.
474. Speroff, L., and Ramwell, P. W. (1970): Prostaglandin stimulation of *in vitro* progesterone synthesis. *J. Clin. Endocrinol Metab.*, 30:345–350.
475. du Mesnil du Buisson, F., and Dauzier, L. (1957): Influence de l'ovariectomie chez la truie pendant la gestation. *C. R. Soc. Biol.*, 151:311–313.
476. Ellicott, A. R., and Dzuik, P. J. (1973): Minimum daily dose of progesterone and plasma concentration for maintenance of pregnancy in ovariectomized gilts. *Biol. Reprod.*, 9:300–304.
477. Guthrie, H. D., and Rexroad, C. E., Jr. (1981): Endometrial prostaglandin F release in vitro and plasma 13,14-dihydro-15-keto-prostaglandin F_2 in pigs with luteolysis blocked by pregnancy, estradiol benzoate or human chorionic gonadotropin. *J. Anim. Sci.*, 52:330–339.
478. Schille, W. M., Karlbom, I., Einarsson, S., Larsson, K., Kindahl, H., and Edqvist, L. E. (1979): Concentration of progesterone and 15-keto-13,14-dihydro-prostaglandin $F_{2\alpha}$ in peripheral plasma during the estrous cycle and early pregnancy in gilts. *Zentralbl. Veterinaermed., Reihe A*, 26:169–181.
479. Watson, J., and Pack, C. E. (1979): Steroid and prostaglandin secretion by the corpus luteum, endometrium and embryo of cyclic and pregnant gilts. *J. Endocrinol.*, 82:425–428.
480. Zavy, M. T., Bazer, F. W., Thatcher, W. W., and Wilcox, C. J. (1980): A study of prostaglandin $F_{2\alpha}$ as the luteolysis in swine. V. Comparison of prostaglandin F, progestins, estrone and estradiol in uterine flushings from pregnant and nonpregnant gilts. *Prostaglandins*, 20:837–851.
481. Kidder, H. E., Casida, L. E., and Grummer, R. H. (1955): Some effects of estrogen injections on the estrual cycle of gilts. *J. Anim. Sci.*, 14:470–474.
482. Gardner, M. L., First, N. L., and Casida, L. E. (1963): Effect of exogenous estrogens on corpus luteum maintenance in gilts. *J. Anim. Sci.*, 22:132–134.
483. Frank, M., Bazer, F. W., Thatcher, W. W., and Wilcox, C. J. (1977): A study of prostaglandin $F_{2\alpha}$ as the luteolysin in swine. III. Effects of estradiol valerate on prostaglandin F, progestin, estrone and estradiol concentration in the utero-ovarian veins of nonpregnant gilts. *Prostaglandins*, 14:1183–1196.
484. Guthrie, H. D., and Lewis, G. S. (1984): Hormone production and $[^3H]$-$PGF_{2\alpha}$ metabolism by endometrium, lung and embryonal membranes of cyclic and pregnant gilts. *J. Anim. Sci. (Suppl 1)*, 59:351.
485. Geisert, R. D., Thatcher, W. W., Roberts, R. M., and Bazer, F. W. (1982): Establishment of pregnancy in the pig: III. Endometrial secretory response to estradiol valerate administered on day 11 of the estrous cycle. *Biol. Reprod.*, 27:957–965.
486. Perry, J. S., Heap, R. B., and Amoroso, E. C. (1973): Steroid hormone production by pig blastocysts. *Nature*, 245:45–47.
487. Heap, R. B., Flint, A. P. F., Hartman, P. E., et al. (1981): Oestrogen production in early pregnancy. *J. Endocrinol.* 89:77–94.
488. Bazer, F. W., and Thatcher, W. W. (1977): Theory of maternal recognition of pregnancy in swine based on estrogen controlled endocrine versus exocrine secretion of prostaglandin $F_{2\alpha}$ by the uterine endometrium. *Prostaglandins*, 14:397–399.
489. Lewis, G. S., and Waterman, R. A. (1983): Metabolism of arachidonic acid *in vitro* by porcine blastocysts and endometrium. *Prostaglandins*, 25:871–880.
490. Geisert, R. D., Renegar, R. H., Thatcher, W. W., Roberts, R. M., and Bazer, F. W. (1982): Establishment of pregnancy in the pig: I. Interrelationships between preimplantation development of the pig blastocyst and uterine endometrial secretions. *Biol. Reprod.*, 27:925–939.
491. Holtan, D. W., Squires, D. L., Lapin, D. R., and Ginther, O. J. (1979): Effect of ovariectomy on pregnancy in mares. *J. Reprod. Fertil. (Suppl.)*, 27:395–401.
492. Hershman, L., and Douglas, R. H. (1979): The critical period for the maternal recognition of pregnancy in pony mares. *J. Reprod. Fertil. (Suppl.)*, 27:395–401.
493. Holtan, D. W., Nett, T. M., and Estergreen, V. L. (1975): Plasma progestins in pregnant, postpartum and cycling mares. *J. Anim. Sci.*, 40:251–260.
494. Nett, T. M., and Pickett, B. W. (1979): Effect of diethylstilbestrol on the relationship between LH, PMSG and progesterone during pregnancy in the mare. *J. Reprod. Fertil. (Suppl.)*, 27:465–470.
495. van Niekerk, C. H., and Gerneke, W. H. (1966): Persistence and parthogenetic cleavage of tubal ova in the mare. *Onderspoort J. Vet Res.*, 31:195–232.
496. Leith, G. S., and Ginther, O. J. (1984): Characterization of intrauterine mobility of the early equine conceptus. *Theriogeneology*, 22:401–408.
497. Mayer, R. E., Vernon, M. W., Zavy, M. T., Bazer, F. W., and Sharp, D. C. (1977): Estrogen production by the early equine con-

ceptus. *Proceedings of the 69th Annual Meeting of the American Society of Animal Science,* p. 186.
498. Evans, M. J., and Irvine, C. H. G. (1975): Serum concentrations of FSH, LH and progesterone during the estrous cycle and early pregnancy in the mare. *J. Reprod. Fertil. (Suppl.),* 23:193–200.
499. Allen, W. E. (1974): Ovarian changes during gestation in pony mares. *Equine Vet. J.,* 6:135–138.
500. Cole, H. H., Howell, C. E., and Hart, G. H. (1931): Changes occurring in the ovary of the mare during pregnancy. *Anat. Rec.,* 49:199–210.
501. Squires, E. L., Stevens, W. B., Pickett, B. W., and Nett, T. M. (1979): Role of pregnant mare serum gonadotropin in luteal function of pregnant mares. *Am. J. Vet. Res.,* 40:889–891.
502. Moss, G. E., Estergreen, V. L., Becker, S. R., and Grant, B. D. (1979): The source of 5α-pregnanes that occur during gestation in the mare. *J. Reprod. Fertil.,* 27:511–519.
503. Ascoli, M. (1981): Receptor mediated uptake and degradation of human choriogonadotropin: fate of hormone subunits. *Ann. NY Acad. Sci.,* 383:151–173.
504. Niswender, G. D., Roess, D. A., Sawyer, H. R., Silvia, W. J., and Barisas, B. G. (1985): Differences in lateral mobility of receptors for LH in the luteal cell plasma membrane when occupied by oLH vs. hCG. *Endocrinology,* 116:164–169.
505. Roess, D. A., Niswender, G. D., and Barisas, B. G. (1985): Cytoskeletal modulation of hCG-LH receptor complex mobility on ovine luteal cells. *Proceedings of the 67th Annual Meeting of the Endocrine Society,* p. 71 (abstr. 281).

The Physiology of Reproduction,
edited by E. Knobil and J. Neill *et al.*.
Raven Press, Ltd., New York © 1988.

CHAPTER 14

Local Nonsteroidal Regulators of Ovarian Function

Alex Tsafriri

> "There should be no other motive for study except gaining knowledge, and there is no other purpose in truth than knowing it is the truth. . . . Only man's ignorance makes him seek another aim for this ultimate aim."
>
> RABBI MOSHE BEN MAIMON (MAIMONIDES, 1138–1204)
> Introduction to Commentary to Chapter X of *Sanhedrin*

This thesis of Rabbi Moshe ben Maimon (Maimonides), a most prominent medieval referee of Jewish law, theologian, philosopher, and practicing physician, was originally formulated regarding theology, but can be equally well adapted to any scientific endeavor. I believe that the quest for knowledge is, and should remain, the prime motivation of any scientific activity. It was argued that since complete understanding of any aspect of nature may be an unrealistic goal never to be attained, perhaps the best that we can hope for is to derive practical applications leading to the betterment of our society. Although the limitations of science and its asymptotic nature cannot be denied, overemphasis of the applied value of scientific inquiry may adversely affect both the advancement of our understanding and, in the long run, the utilization of this knowledge for human benefit.

The issue of local ovarian regulation, to be overviewed here, is in its formative stage. This is evidenced by the rapid accumulation of new data and suggestions of additional local mechanisms, which makes it nearly impossible to avoid deletions and to overlook pertinent studies. Hence, this review should be considered an interim account of intraovarian control mechanisms. As such, the emphasis is put on its comprehensiveness, rather than on selectiveness. Furthermore, in most of the cases, the studies cited are presented at face value. It is hoped that this may serve as an introduction to young researchers of this field and promote further inquiry into ovarian regulation. Several reviews (1,2) and multiauthor books (3–7) have been recently published on paracrine regulation of gonadal function.

BACKGROUND

The concept of local gonadal regulators and regulation can be traced to the early days of ovarian research. Thus, differentiation of the gonads was hypothesized by Witschi (8) to result from the interaction of two morphogenetic substances termed cortexine and medullarine. Cortexine, which was later renamed cortecin (9), was postulated as the inducer of ovarian tissue and medullarine as inducer of testicular tissue.

The rapid and impressive progress in the understanding of ovarian endocrine function, including production and secretion of steroids (10,11) and the regulation of ovarian activity by gonadotropins (12), led to the widely accepted view that the ovary is the source of ova and of steroid hormones and that it is controlled by hypophyseal hormones. Relaxin remained for some time a disturbing and largely neglected exception in this outlook.

Development and application of more refined and sophisticated approaches to the study of reproductive processes and organs, such as radioimmunoassays, the vast array of chromatographic techniques and culture *in vitro* of ovarian follicles, corpora lutea, and isolated cells, led to an increase in resolution and hence to a realization of a higher level of complexity in the control of ovarian activity. Studies revealed ovarian nonsteroidal substances exerting biological effects on the ovary or ovarian cells and other organs. In addition, it became increasingly difficult to explain all the details of ovarian function by the action of hypophyseal hormones alone. Thus the initiation of meiosis in fetal ovaries, recruitment of primordial follicles, selection of ovulatory and atretic follicles, and follicular inhibition of precocious oocyte maturation cannot be attributed solely to changes in gonadotropin levels. Therefore, local factors were suggested to be superimposed and to modulate gonadotropin actions on these processes. Furthermore, analysis of ovarian activity revealed yet another type of local regulation: the coordinated production of steroids by granulosa and theca cells, known as the two-cell hypothesis (13) (R. E. Gore-Langton and D. T. Armstrong, *this volume*), and the regulatory functions of steroids within the ovary, probably exerted through variation in their local concentration (13) (G. S. Greenwald and P. F. Terranova, *this volume*).

ENDOCRINE, PARACRINE, AND AUTOCRINE REGULATION

The classical definition of endocrinology maintained that a group of cells located in endocrine glands releases chemical messengers, or hormones, which reach their target through the blood stream and thereby affect other tissues, organs, or body functions (14). This system of communication was in contradistinction to the previously known nervous system. The line of demarcation between these two systems became obscured very early when neurotransmitters were first identified. Recent work revealed a wealth of intercellular communication systems that do not conform with the classical definitions set for either the endocrine or the nervous system (Fig. 1). Thus, for example, hormones were found in organs that were not considered endocrine glands or primary sources of the hormones. Conversely, many messenger molecules that cannot be considered hormones, since they reach their target cells without passing through the circulatory system, are indistinguishable from hormones in their structure, interaction with their target cells, and biological actions. Furthermore, many bona fide hormones were also found to act locally without being first transported through the circulation. These and other considerations, including the finding of substances resembling vertebrate hormonal peptides in more primitive multicellular or even unicellular organisms, led to the evolutionary approach unifying all modes of intercellular communication (15,16). According to this approach, intercellular communication by soluble messenger molecules was devised even before the appearance of multicellular organisms. The development of highly specialized cells devoted largely or exclusively to intercellular communication (i.e., nerves and endocrine glands) is the result of extreme cellular differentiation. Thus, the classical endocrine systems inherited their key molecular components (messenger and receptor mechanisms) from simpler unicellular ancestors.

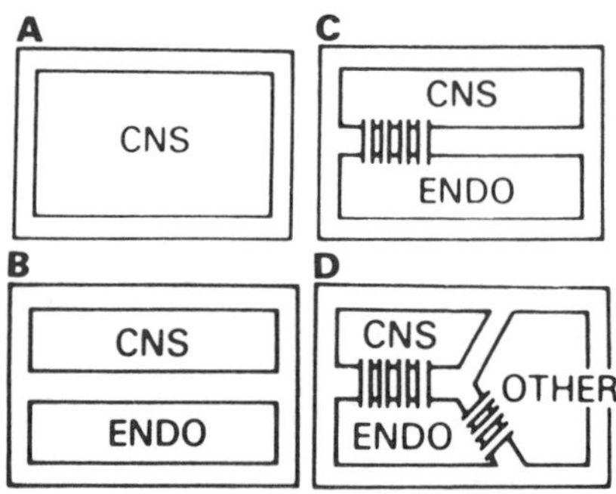

FIG. 1. Evolution of concepts about intercellular communication. **A**: The central nervous system (CNS) was considered to be the unique coordinator among cells of multicellular animals; **B**: integration and coordination were performed by two separate but equal systems, the CNS and the endocrine system (ENDO); **C**: penetrations in the boundaries that separate the two systems became apparent, especially in recent years; and **D**: there are a large number of examples of intercellular communication that we now recognize which do not fit either system, designated OTHER. From Roth et al. (16), by permission of Clinical Research.

These molecules, whether remaining conserved or undergoing substantial evolution, very often assumed new functions (17,18). Such a comprehensive view encompassing any intercellular chemical messenger molecules as hormones (Fig. 2) discerns three variations of endocrine regulation (Fig. 3):

1. The classical endocrine system—endocrine glands secreting their hormones into the circulation (including blood or lymph) through which they are transported to their target

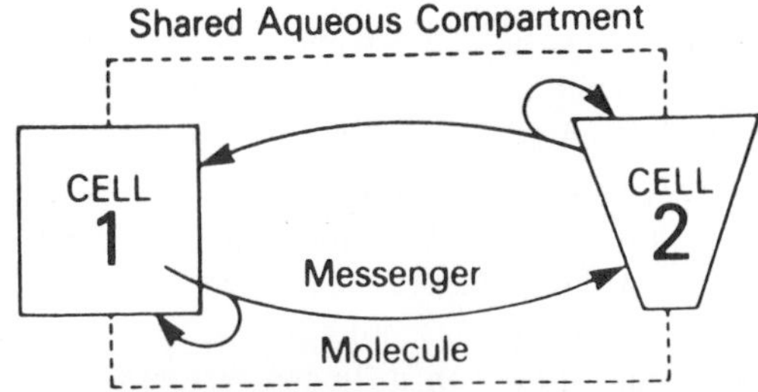

FIG. 2. Features of an intercellular communication system. The secretory cell (cell 1) synthesizes and releases a soluble messenger (signal) into a shared aqueous compartment and acts on the target cell (cell 2). In the classical endocrine system, cell 1 is a glandular cell, the signal molecule is a hormone, and the shared aqueous compartment is blood, whereas in the nervous system cell 1 is a neuron, the signal molecule a neurotransmitter and the shared aqueous compartment a synapse. Applying the term hormone to any intercellular messenger molecule extends endocrine interactions to include paracrine and endocrine regulation (see Fig. 3). From Roth et al. (16), by permission of Clinical Research.

organs or cells. The specialized endocrine glands differ from other hormone secreting cells in their ability to produce large quantities of the hormone, store it, and release it into the circulation upon the appropriate trigger.

2. Paracrine control mechanisms involve local diffusion of hormone to their target cells (19,20). In primitive organisms lacking circulatory system or endocrine glands, this is the principal mode of humoral regulation. Paracrine regulation is probably important in vertebrates during early embryonic development prior to the establishment of circulation and endocrine glands.

3. Autocrine regulation, originally suggested by Sporn and Todaro on the basis of studies with transformed cells, "whereby a cell secretes a hormone-like substance for which the cell has functional external receptors" (21). This definition warrants extension to include not only peptides interacting with external membranal receptors, but to any regulatory molecule that interacts with cellular receptors. Thus, regulatory functions of steroid hormones in the gonads should be included in autocrine regulation, according to my view, provided that cellular production, interaction with receptors, and typical postreceptor responses can be discerned within the same cell type.

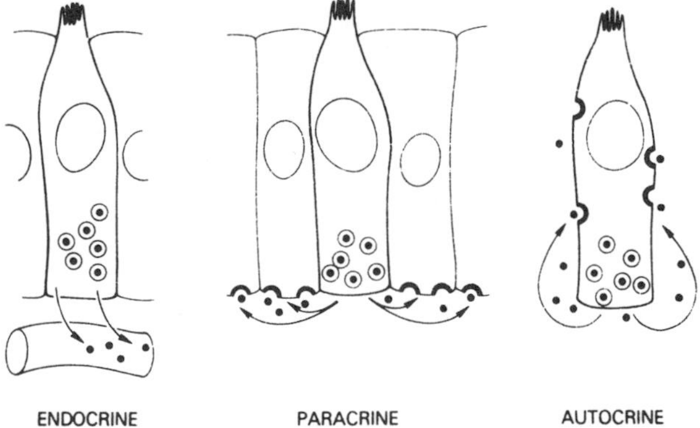

FIG. 3. Diagrammatic representation of the variants of communication employed by the hormonal system. Regulatory chemical messengers are shown in latent form within the cell. The thickened, semicircular regions of the cell membrane represent receptor sites, but receptors to some hormones may be intracellular. From Sporn and Todaro (21), by permission of The New England Journal of Medicine.

Several terms were suggested for intercellular messenger molecules which do not conform to the classical definition of hormone: regulatory or growth factors, regulins and chemitters (22), and cybernins (23). Except for the general term factor, none of the specific terms are in common usage. It is most proper to extend the definition of hormone to all intercellular regulatory messenger molecules and adopt the radical suggestion of O'Malley (24) to concentrate on hormones and their functions, rather than glands and hormones. Hence, throughout this review the term hormone will be applied to any regulatory messenger molecules.

OVARIAN PARACRINE AND AUTOCRINE REGULATION

Sharpe (2) suggested the following criteria for intragonadal hormones: (a) evidence that the hormone is produced within the gonad; (b) receptors for this hormone are present within the gonad; and (c) demonstrated biological actions within the gonad. Ideally, only hormones that fulfill all these criteria should be considered intragonadal hormones. Nevertheless, in the present state most of the nonsteroidal hormones to be included in paracrine or autocrine regulation of ovarian function cannot withstand rigorous examination by these three criteria. In most of the cases, the hormone has not been chemically characterized, and hence no receptor binding studies could be performed and no unequivocal evidence for local production could be obtained. Furthermore, the intragonadal function is deduced in few cases from *in vivo* and in most cases from *in vitro* model systems which do not necessarily represent the physiological situation. Therefore, included here as intraovarian hormones are these fulfilling two more lenient criteria: (a) they are found in the ovary and there is no evidence of extraovarian origin; and (b) a biological effect of the hormone can be demonstrated on the ovary *in situ* or *in vitro* or on ovarian cell preparations *in vitro*.

Adoption of these two criteria mentioned above results in a chemically mixed group of substances: amines, peptides, steroids and eicosanoids (Table 1). Some of them are chemically characterized and have, in addition, extraovarian source(s) and targets. This group includes, for example, steroids, eicosanoids (prostaglandins and hydroperoxides), oxytocin, vasopressin, and proopiomelanocortin-derived peptides. A more difficult group to deal with is that of ovarian factors eliciting biological responses in ovarian tissue and that are still in the process of their chemical characterization and purification (Table 2), such as follicular

TABLE 1. *Putative paracrine/autocrine regulators of ovarian function*

Hormone	Section[a]
Adenosine	Adenosine and Other Purines
Angiogenic factors	Ovarian Angiogenic Factors
Catecholamines	Neurotransmitters
Epidermal growth factor (EGF) and fibroblast growth factor (FGF)	EFG and FGF Actions on Ovarian Cells
Eicosanoids	Eicosanoids
Follicular regulatory protein(s) (FRP)	Follicular Regulatory Proteins
FSH-binding inhibitor (FSH-BI)	FSH-binding Inhibitor
γ-Aminobutyric acid (GABA)	γ-Aminobutyric Acid (GABA)
GnRH-like peptide(s)	GnRH-like Peptides
Insulin-like growth factors (IGFs)	Role of Insulin and IGFs
LH-binding inhibitor (LH-BI)	LH-binding Inhibitor
Luteinization inhibitor (LI) or atretogenic factor	Luteinization Inhibitor
Luteinization stimulator (LS) or maturation stimulator	Luteinization Stimulator
Oocyte maturation inhibitor (OMI)	Oocyte Maturation Inhibitor (OMI)
Ovarian growth stimulator(s)	Ovarian Growth-stimulating Actions
Oxytocin	Neurohypophyseal Hormones
Platelet-derived growth factor (PDGF)	Effect of PDGF and Copurifying Factors
Proopiomelanocortin-derived hormones	GnRH Binding and Mechanism of Action in the Ovary
Relaxin	O.D. Sherwood (*this volume*)
Steroids	R.E. Gore-Langton and D.T. Armstrong (*this volume*); G.S. Greenwald and P.F. Terranova (*this volume*)
Substance P	Other Neurotransmitters
Vasoactive intestinal peptide (VIP)	Vasoactive Intestinal Peptide (VIP)
Vasopressin	Neurohypophyseal Hormones

[a]In parentheses reference is given to other chapters in this volume; otherwise the section of this review is indicated.

regulatory proteins (FRP); oocyte maturation inhibitor (OMI), LH-binding inhibitors (LH-BI), FSH-binding inhibitors (FSH-BI), luteinization stimulator (LS), and luteinization inhibitor (LI). Since their chemical nature has not as yet been elucidated, some of them may actually be similar or identical to other hormones or some of their disparate activities may be assigned to the same molecule. The purification of these factors is proceeding very slowly partly because of the very nature of these factors and partly because of inadequacies in assay and purification procedures. Acting locally, they are produced in minuscule quantities and act within discrete areas, some of them seemingly unstable and possibly subject to very rapid degradation. They appear to act in conjunction with other hormones, such as gonadotropins and steroids, and to assume a modulatory role. Therefore, their action may differ substantially according to the physiological or endocrine status of the gonad. In comparison with the classical endocrine hormones, which can be considered "macro regulators," the autocrine and paracrine hormones seem to be involved mainly in fine tuning. These biological characteristics pose major practical difficulties for the purification, particularly in two areas: the assay systems used to monitor purification and insufficient resolution of the purification procedures. Most of the *in vitro* assays are slow and cumbersome, and their relevance to physiological regulation is questionable. Moreover, the lack of standard preparations and assay procedures makes comparison of different research groups' results very difficult. The sources of putative intraovarian regulators, follicular fluid (FFl), ovarian extracts, and conditioned tissue culture media are extremely complex and variable according to subtle physiological and endocrine conditions and impose high demands on the purification procedure. Finally, the factor isolated from follicular fluid or other biological sources may not be the potent native hormone but a chemically modified product retaining some of the original activity or mimicking the action of an unrelated hormone.

The present state of our knowledge does not permit a consistent classification of ovarian hormones according to either their precise chemical nature or ovarian function. Hence, they will be grouped as convenient, according to any of these criteria. Steroids are synthesized in the ovary, and their intraovarian receptors and actions, in addition to their extragonadal effects, have been convincingly demonstrated. Steroids belong, therefore, to intraovarian hormones but will be dealt with elsewhere in R. E. Gore-Langton and D. T. Armstrong (*this volume*) and G. S. Greenwald and P. F. Terranova (*this volume*). Likewise, eicosanoids (prostaglandins and hydroperoxides) will be discussed by H. Lipner (*this volume*) and relaxin by O. D. Sherwood (*this volume*), and hence their intragonadal actions will be described here only briefly.

OOCYTE MATURATION INHIBITOR (OMI)

Life History of the Mammalian Ovum

Meiotic maturation in the mammalian female is a protracted process, subject to multiple stop–go controls. Meiotic maturation in mammalian oocytes is initiated during prenatal life or shortly after birth, but the process is arrested (*first meiotic arrest*) at the diplotene stage, usually referred to as the dictyate stage of the prophase of first meiotic division (Fig. 4). The meiotic arrest is maintained throughout oocyte

TABLE 2. *Ovarian local regulators not identified with other known hormones*

Hormone	Ovarian source	Species	Chemical nature	Actions	References
Follicular regulatory proteins(s)	granulosa cells, identified in FF1 and venous drainage of preovulatory follicles	human, sow, ewe, and rat	heat and trypsin labile; 12,000–15,000 MW	inhibition of FSH stimulated actions on the follicle, including aromatase and follicular development	258–260, 268
FSH-binding inhibitor	follicular fluid, increased concentration in atretic follicles	human, sow, and cow	peptide (?) ~1,000 MW	inhibits binding of FSH to receptor	121, 132, 133
LH-binding inhibitor	corpora lutea	human, sow, ewe, goat, cat, dog, and rat	~20,000 MW	inhibits binding of LH to receptor	122–124
Luteinization inhibitor (atretogenic factor)	fluid from small follicles; granulosa cell-conditioned medium	human, sow, cow, and mare	130,000–500,000 MW	inhibition of progesterone synthesis and morphological luteinization	278, 279, 293
Luteinization stimulator (maturation)	fluid from large follicles; granulosa cell-conditioned medium	sow	~60,000 MW	stimulation of steroid production and morphological luteinization	278, 279, 296, 307
Oocyte maturation inhibitor	follicular fluid, granulosa cell-conditioned medium	human, sow, cow, ewe, rat, hamster, and rabbit	~1,000 peptide (?), hypoxanthine, or other purine base (?)	inhibition of spontaneous resumption of meiosis *in vitro*	53, 54, 79, 80

and follicular development to the Graafian follicle stage. *In vivo* the meiotic process is resumed only in fully grown oocytes in follicles responding to the preovulatory surge of gonadotropins (25) and in follicles undergoing atresia (26). At ovulation, in most mammalian species, a secondary oocyte arrested at the metaphase of the second meiotic division (*second meiotic arrest*) is released. The second meiotic division is completed only after fertilization or a parthenogenetic stimulus by abstriction of the second polar body.

The mechanism(s) involved in the regulation of meiosis in the fetus remain obscure. It has been proposed that meiosis in mammals is regulated by products of the somatic cells of the gonad: a meiosis-inducing substance (MIS) and a meiosis-preventing substance (MPS) (27). This suggestion is based on experiments in which MIS activity was demonstrated by the ability to promote meiosis in fetal mouse testis *in vitro,* whereas MPS retarded the initiation of meiosis in fetal mouse ovaries *in vitro* (27). That the somatic compartment of the ovary influences the meiotic behavior of germ cells is further supported by the observation that the first meiotic arrest coincides with folliculogenesis, that is, enclosure of the germ cells with somatic cells, and that oocytes which do not become enclosed with follicle cells usually undergo further abortive meiotic changes and degenerate (28).

Here the paracrine regulation of the progress of the dictyate oocyte to the metaphase of the second meiotic division will be reviewed. These changes will be regarded as *resumption of meiosis* (or of *maturation*) or *ovum maturation* even though they do encompass only a limited aspect of the meiotic process. The first change associated with preovulatory resumption of meiosis, that is, the breakdown of the germinal vesicle (GVBD), is most easily observed by microscopic observation of the ovum and hence frequently used as an experimental criterion for ovum maturation (Figs. 4 and 5). This seems to be a proper criterion when the study is aimed at the identification of mechanisms controlling the resumption of meiosis. However, GVBD should not be considered indicative of fertilizability of the ovum or of its competence to give a viable embryo (29–31).

The resumption of meiosis in nonatretic follicles *in vivo* is critically dependent upon the preovulatory surge of gonadotropins. Blocking the surge by pentobarbitone or similar drugs prevents ovum maturation as well as other ovulatory changes (25) and administration of exogenous luteinizing hormone (LH) to pentobarbitone-treated rats results in GVBD within 2.5 to 3.5 hr (32,33).

Three *in vitro* models have been employed for investigating hormonal and follicular control of meiotic maturation in mammalian oocytes (Fig. 5). The simplest is that established by Pincus and Enzmann (34), who demonstrated that rabbit oocytes liberated from their follicles undergo spontaneous maturation in culture without any need for hormonal stimulation. Such spontaneous maturation of cultured oo-

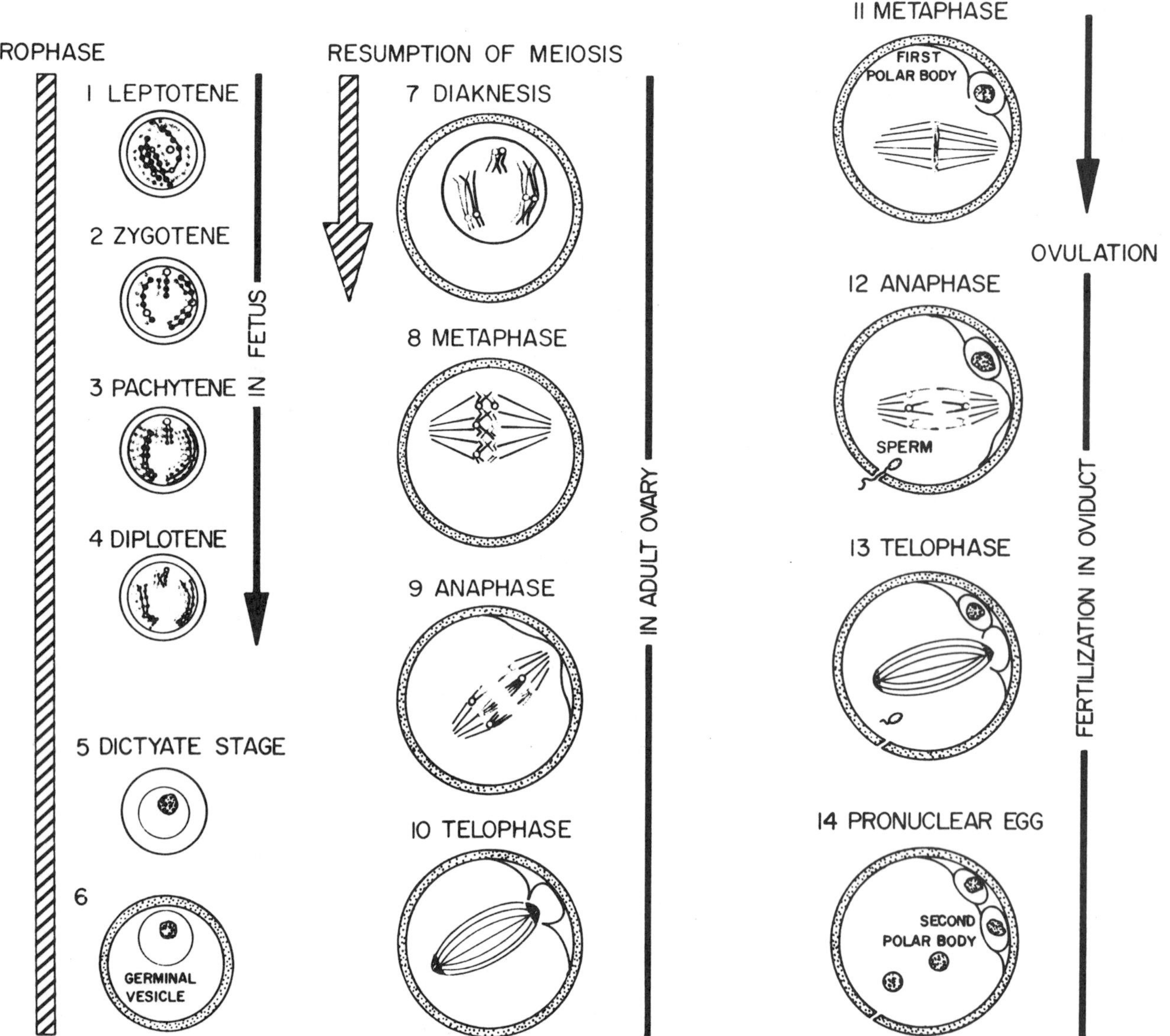

FIG. 4. Oocyte meiosis. For simplicity, only three pairs of chromosomes are depicted. (1–4) Prophase stages of the first meiotic division that occur in most mammals during fetal life. At zygotene (2) the homologous maternal and paternal chromosomes begin to pair. At pachytene (3) they are paired along their entire length, thus forming bivalents. During pachytene, each homolog cleaves longitudinally to form two sister chromatids, so that each bivalent forms a tetrad. During this stage, interchange of genetic material between maternal and paternal chromatids may occur by crossing over. At diplotene (4), the chromosomes begin to separate, remaining united at the chiasmata. The meiotic process is arrested at this stage (first meiotic arrest), and the oocyte enters the dictyate stage. When meiosis is resumed, the first maturation division is completed (7–11). Ovulation usually occurs at the metaphase II stage (11) (second meiotic arrest), and the second meiotic division (12–14) is completed in the oviduct following sperm penetration. From Tsafriri (36), by permission of Plenum, New York.

cytes either denuded of their cumulus cells or within their cumulus complex was confirmed in all mammalian species examined (35,36) and has been widely employed for studying some physiological aspects of oocyte maturation. It should be noted, however, that oocytes isolated from preantral follicles do not resume meiosis spontaneously in culture. The ability to mature spontaneously *in vitro* (meiotic competence) is acquired only when the oocyte enters its final stage of growth. Meiotic competence is gradually acquired at the age of 15 to 21 days in mice (37,38) and 20 to 26 days in rats (39). The development of meiotic competence appears to be regulated by follicle-stimulating hormone (FSH), an action which is, at least partially, mediated by follicular estrogen production (40). In the second model, consisting of explanted preovulatory follicles, resumption of meiosis is dependent upon hormonal stimulation *in vivo* or *in vitro*

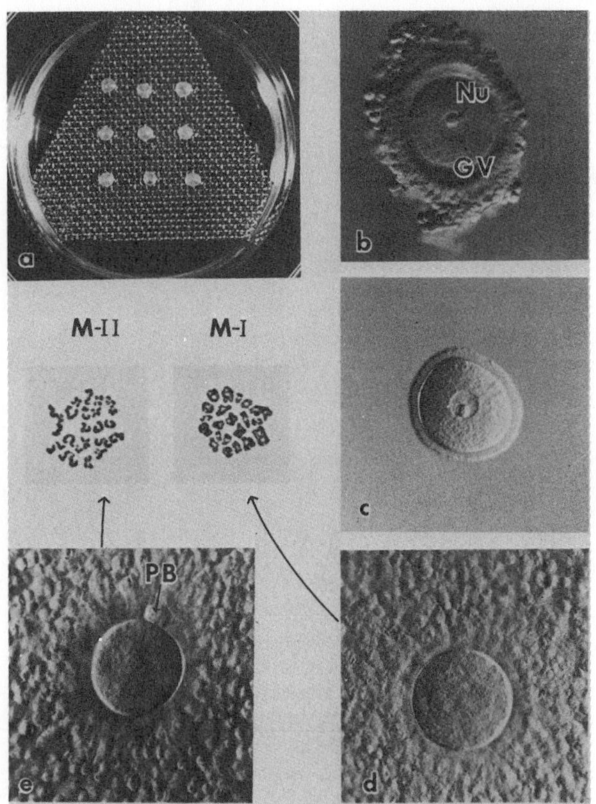

FIG. 5. Oocyte maturation in the rat. **a**: Explanted preovulatory follicles. **b–e**: Oocytes viewed with Nomarski interference optics: isolated oocyte cultured with its intact cumulus mass (**b**). GV, germinal vesicle; Nu, nucleolus. **c**: Denuded oocyte. **d**: GVBD; M-I (*inset*), bivalents in metaphase I. **e**: Secondary oocyte. PB, polar body; M-II (*inset*), chromosomes (dyads) seen at metaphase II. Chromosomes were prepared according to the method of Tarkowski (1966) and photographed under phase contrast. From Tsafriri (53), by permission of Academic Press, New York.

(41). This model has been employed extensively for studying the hormonal control of resumption of meiosis in a variety of mammalian species (29,36,41–46).

The finding that oocytes removed from their follicle mature spontaneously in culture, whereas maturation in follicle-enclosed oocytes is dependent upon hormonal stimulation, led to the suggestion that within the follicle meiosis is prevented through follicular inhibitory action. In order to test this hypothesis a third *in vitro* model was adopted: coculture of oocytes with various follicular components (47–52). Such studies corroborated the concept of follicular inhibitory action and led to partial characterization and purification of a factor, oocyte maturation inhibitor (OMI) (53–55). It should be remembered, however, that the coculture of oocytes with follicular components can hardly restore the precise follicular interactions between the ovum and its micromilieu. Furthermore, OMI purified from the follicular fluid may not necessarily be the native molecule regulating meiosis upon direct transfer from follicle cells to the ovum through the gap junctions connecting these two follicular compartments. At the most, we can hope for an approximation and the gaining of some insight into the paracrine mechanisms participating in follicular control of meiosis *in situ*. Here an overview of the present status of paracrine regulation of ovum maturation will be presented.

Paracrine Regulation of Ovum Maturation

The spontaneous maturation of isolated oocytes in culture led Pincus and Enzmann (34) to suggest that follicle cells in mammals "supply to the ovum a substance or substances which directly inhibit nuclear maturation." This suggestion was supported by the inhibition of the resumption of meiosis of porcine oocytes cocultured with segments of follicle wall, but not with its theca layer (48,49) or ovarian bursa (50). Similarly, when porcine oocytes (up to 12) were transferred to host follicles and cultured in hormone free-medium maturation was prevented (46,56) and maturation of rat oocytes injected into porcine follicles was markedly delayed (56). Further, coculture of porcine oocytes with porcine granulosa cells inhibited the spontaneous resumption of meiosis (49,57). The inhibitory effect of granulosa cells depended upon their concentration in culture. Granulosa cells collected from small follicles inhibited meiosis more effectively than cells from medium or large follicles (49,58). Similarly, when rat oocytes were added to rat granulosa cells previously cultured for 24 or 48 hr, resumption of meiosis was suppressed and the degree of inhibition depended upon the number of granulosa cells in the culture. This inhibitory effect of rat granulosa cells was reversed by the addition of LH to the cocultures (59,60).

Extracts of granulosa cells, as well as granulosa cell-conditioned medium (i.e., a medium in which granulosa cells were cultured previously), inhibited the resumption of meiosis (58,60–65). Collectively these results suggest that within the follicle meiosis is kept in abeyance by an OMI produced by granulosa cells. It was found that addition of FSH or prolactin to suspension cultures of porcine granulosa cells facilitates the accumulation of OMI in the medium, whereas testosterone or dihydrotestosterone reduced it (1,64). These studies led to a hypothesis linking porcine follicular development, steroid synthesis, and OMI production (Fig. 6).

FFl from ovaries of rabbit, ovine, bovine, porcine, hamster, and human origin exerted an inhibitory effect upon the spontaneous maturation of isolated oocytes (47,49,59,66–72). This inhibitory effect is not species-specific (59,66, 71,72). The OMI activity in porcine FFl appears to decline in the course of follicular growth. This was demonstrated by assaying FFl freshly collected from small, medium, and large follicles (71) or fluid collected from pigs on specified days of their reproductive cycle (68). Similarly, in FFl collected from women participating in *in vitro* fertilization-

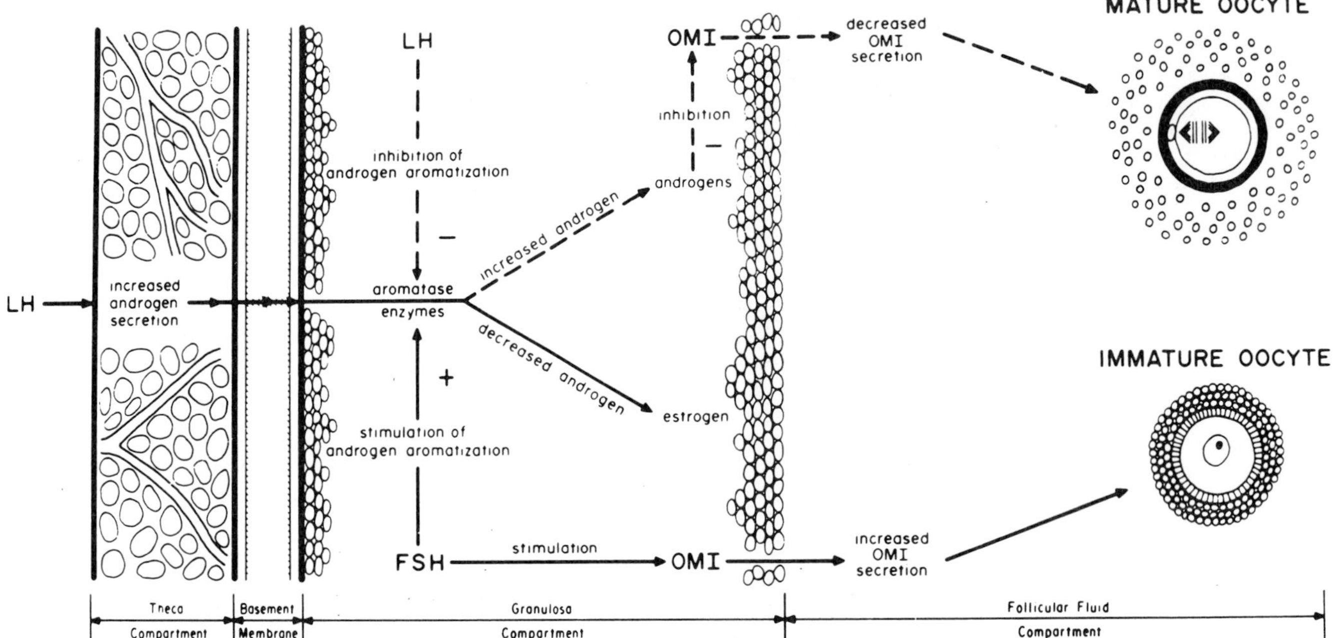

FIG. 6. A hypothesis of the control of OMI secretion by hormones within the porcine follicle. Prior to ovulation luteinizing hormone interacts with the theca interna cells of the ovarian follicle (*left*) to maintain increased androgen biosynthesis. In addition to aromatization by the theca cells, the androgen transverses the basement membrane to interact with the granulosa cells (*center*). Androgen is converted in part in granulosa cells to estrogen by the aromatase enzyme complex which is stimulated by FSH. Furthermore, FSH directly stimulates the secretion of OMI from granulosa cells and maintains the oocyte in an immature state (*lower right*). At any time during follicular development, the loss of FSH responsiveness or receptors, the aromatase enzymes, and/or an increase in androgen would result in atresia and the attenuation of OMI secretion; thereby the oocyte is allowed to undergo maturation (*upper right*) and degeneration in the unruptured follicle. An analogous situation may occur during the LH surge; that is, LH stimulates theca cell androgen secretion while inhibiting its conversion to estrogen in granulosa cells. As a result, the increased androgen would also attenuate OMI secretion allowing the oocyte to resume meiosis. From Anderson et al. (64), by the permission of Gamete Research.

embryo transfer program, the OMI activity was significantly lower in follicles yielding mature and fertilizable oocytes than follicles yielding immature or atretic oocytes (69,70).

Characterization of OMI

Assays of OMI

Pig oocytes from either medium or large follicles were frequently employed for bioassay of OMI (49,66,72). This assay requires a steady source of a large number of porcine ovaries, a long incubation period (42–44 hr), and fixation and staining of the ova after the incubation. Rat (59,73) and mouse (52,74) oocytes were also used for assaying OMI. Murine oocytes are widely available and the culture period is much shorter (up to 4–6 hr). Nevertheless, OMI assays involving mammalian ova are cumbersome and tedious, require experienced personnel, and can be applied only to a limited number of samples.

Recently inhibitory effects of human follicular fluid on maturation of amphibian oocytes was demonstrated (75,76). It is postulated that the inhibition resulted from the presence of OMI in this fluid (69,73).

S. H. Pomerantz and P. Bilello (562a) developed an assay for OMI using inhibition of the progesterone-mediated maturation of *Xenopus* oocytes as the test system. The attractive features of this assay are its speed (about 10–12 hr for a complete assay) and economy (it can be done by one person and a large number of fractions can be assayed at one time because one toad can furnish 600–1,000 oocytes from each ovary).

The results of the *Xenopus* assay were compared with those of pig oocyte assays. Both assays gave essentially the same results for the fractionation of relatively pure preparations obtained by reverse-phase high performance liquid chromatography (HPLC) (see Characterization and Purification of OMI, *this chapter*).

Characterization and Purification of OMI

Tsafriri et al. (77) reported that OMI passed through an Amicon PM-10 filter which has a molecular weight cut off of 10,000. Chromatography of the concentrated filtrate on Sephadex G-25 (71,77) revealed that OMI had a molecular weight <2,000 and that two peaks of activity were present. Tsafriri et al. (77) found that FFl lost OMI activity when it was treated with trypsin but retained its activity on freezing and thawing treatment with charcoal and when it was heated to 60°C for 20 min. S. H. Pomerantz (*unpublished experiments*) showed that bacterial protease from *Streptomyces griseus* (Sigma) destroyed all of the OMI activity of a partially purified Biogel P2 fraction. Treatment of the same fraction with trypsin left no significant activity. These results are all consistent with OMI being a peptide of low molecular weight. OMI from bovine FFl appears to have similar properties (65).

After lyophilization to dryness of the PM-10 filtrate, OMI could be extracted with acetic acid dissolved in methanol (1). This step was then followed by gel filtration chromatography on Sephadex G-25 or Biogel P2 (S. H. Pomerantz and Bilello, *unpublished experiments*). After gel filtration ion exchange chromatography on CM-Sephadex and DEAE-Sephadex was applied (1,72). These steps showed OMI to be an acidic compound since it was bound to DEAE, but not CM-Sephadex. However, these procedures resulted in a modest purification and a poor yield, and a lengthy period of time was required.

The current procedure used by Pomerantz exploits the acidic nature of OMI. First, pig FFl is filtered through an Amicon PM-10 filter as in the earlier procedures and the filtrate is diluted with an equal volume of water and passed onto a column of QAE-Sephadex. This strongly basic ion exchange resin binds OMI; the latter is eluted from the column with a steep gradient of NH_4HCO_3. Two (or sometimes three) peaks of OMI activity are detected by assays with pig oocytes. Each peak is then treated separately by chromatography on reverse-phase HPLC. Two main and one minor fraction were obtained from the two principal OMI fractions from QAE-Sephadex. The purification from FFl is about 150,000 fold for one main peak and 80,000 for the other, with a combined recovery of about 34%. Anion exchange HPLC and gel filtration HPLC are two additional procedures that will be exploited in the continuation of the purification to obtain homogeneous samples of OMI.

By the use of mouse oocytes as an assay system, an inhibitory effect of porcine FFl was demonstrated and this inhibition was potentiated by cyclic AMP (52,74). By monitoring purification of OMI from porcine FFl, Downs and his colleagues (79) reached the conclusion that hypoxanthine is the predominant low molecular weight component of porcine FFl that inhibits mouse oocyte maturation. This conclusion is based on the findings that the potent inhibitory fraction of porcine FFl had an absorption maximum (250 nm) identical to that of hypoxanthine; had a retention time on HPLC of pure hypoxanthine; exerted inhibition of oocyte maturation identical to that exhibited by a commercial preparation of hypoxanthine; had a hypoxanthine concentration of about 1.41 mM in porcine FFl which could account for the majority of the inhibitory activity of porcine FFl on mouse oocytes. Similarly, Chari et al. (73), using human FFl, did not find reduction in OMI activity by proteolytic treatment, thus supporting the notion that it is not a peptide. The concentrations of hypoxanthine (2–4 mM) and of adenosine (0.35–0.70 mM) in mouse FFl could account for inhibition of oocyte maturation, since even the lower concentration of these two purines combined inhibited the spontaneous maturation of mouse oocytes during a 24-hr incubation period *in vitro* (80). Nevertheless, the same authors were unable to detect a reduction in FFl hypoxanthine and adenosine concentration 2 hr after hCG administration, that is, just before GVBD. It is possible that the concentration of these purines in FFl does not necessarily reflect their levels within the oocyte, which are probably more relevant for maintenance of meiotic arrest. Hypoxanthine or adenosine were not detected in bovine FFl, in spite of the presence of low molecular weight component which was inhibitory for ovum maturation (J. J. Eppig, *personal communication*). Guanosine and hypoxanthine dose-dependently inhibited the spontaneous maturation of rat oocytes. Guanosine was more effective, 50 μM inhibiting resumption of meiosis to the same extent as 2 mM hypoxanthine. FSH potentiated the inhibitory action of both purines (81). By contrast, in another study, adenosine, but not inosine hypoxanthine or guanosine, synergized with FSH in inhibiting maturation of rat oocytes (82). The identification of hypoxanthine or other purines as inhibitors of oocyte maturation is most interesting and should be carefully examined using follicular fluids and oocytes of additional species for bioassay. It should be noted, however, that Downs and his colleagues (79) observed an additional inhibitory fraction which was not removed by charcoal extraction. The resistance of OMI activity to proteolytic activity cannot be taken as conclusive evidence that OMI is not a peptide. A small peptide may be a very poor substrate for proteases and the appropriate sensitive peptide bonds may not be present. Hence the final identification of OMI as a purine base or a peptide of a combination of both must await confirmation in several mammalian test systems.

OMI as a Physiological Regulator of Ovum Maturation

Reversibility of Inhibition by Follicular Factor(s)

In order to serve as a physiological regulator of meiosis, a substance has to fulfill the following criteria: It should be present in a compartment relevant to regulation of meiosis at the proper timing; its action should be reversible with no adverse effects on further stages of ovum maturation, fertilization, and embryonic development; and the physiological trigger of resumption of meiosis, gonadotropin, should be able to either bypass its inhibitory action or cause its degradation or removal from the relevant compartment. The inhibitory action of porcine FFl and of its partially purified fractions could be reversed by either transferring the oocytes after an initial 24 hr incubation with the inhibitor to a medium without OMI (71,83,84) or by the addition of an antibody prepared against the low molecular weight fraction of porcine FFl (60). Similarly, the inhibition of maturation of mouse oocytes by hypoxanthine and adenosine was completely reversible by withdrawal of the purines, 47% of the ova were competent of fertilization, and 30% of these developed to the expanded blastocyst stage (78,80). Thus the inhibition of meiosis, by both the apparently peptide OMI from porcine FFl and of hypoxanthine and adenosine, appears not to be due to a toxic and irreversible action.

In vivo or in follicle-enclosed oocytes *in vitro,* resumption of meiosis is induced by LH. Hence the ability of LH to overcome the inhibition of meiosis by FFl or by coculture with granulosa cells lends support for the physiological role of OMI in the regulation of meiosis. It was found that the addition of LH to cultures of porcine oocytes with porcine FFl or its purified fractions overcame their inhibition of meiosis (49). Also, the inhibitory action of bovine or hamster FFl (65), of porcine FFl, rat granulosa cell "conditioned" medium, as well as coculture with rat granulosa cells (59,60) were all alleviated by the addition of LH, closely resembling the regulation *in vivo* of oocyte maturation.

By contrast, the charcoal extracted inhibitor from porcine FFl [later identified as hypoxanthine (79)] prevented the gonadotropin reversal of cAMP-dependent meiotic arrest of mouse oocytes. This finding is difficult to reconcile with the suggested role of hypoxanthine as a physiological regulator of meiosis in the follicle.

Role of cAMP in Regulation of Meiosis

Many of the agents inducing the maturation of follicle-enclosed oocytes *in vitro* also stimulate production of cAMP (41,85). Injection of the cAMP derivative dibutyryl cAMP (dbcAMP) into the follicular antrum (41) or short-term exposure of follicles to 8-bromo-cAMP (86), dbcAMP, or isobutyl methyl xanthine (IBMX) (87) triggered the resumption of meiosis. By contrast, the continuous presence of cAMP derivatives or several inhibitors of phosphodiesterase prevented the induction of meiosis by LH (85,86,88). The spontaneous maturation of isolated oocytes from mice and rats was prevented in the presence of cAMP derivatives or phosphodiesterase inhibitors (43,86,89–91).

It seems, therefore, that enhanced production of cAMP in the somatic cell compartment of the follicle is involved in the mediation of the meiosis-inducing action of LH, while elevated cAMP in the oocyte inhibits the resumption of meiosis. It has been suggested that cAMP serves as a physiological regulator of meiosis in mammalian oocytes (85,88,91,92). Indeed, a decrease in oocyte cAMP precedes resumption of meiosis, and when this decrease is prevented resumption of meiosis is blocked or substantially delayed (93–95). Similarly, incubation of rat oocytes with an invasive adenylate cyclase from bacteria of the genus Bordetella elevated oocyte cAMP levels and inhibited resumption of meiosis; removal of the enzyme resulted in a drop of oocyte cAMP levels and meiosis (96). These results support the notion that elevated levels of oocyte cAMP maintain meiotic arrest and that an intraoocyte drop in cAMP allows the resumption of meiosis.

Studies employing forskolin, a potent and reversible activator of adenylate cyclase, provide further support for this hypothesis. Addition of forskolin to the medium induced resumption of meiosis in rat follicle-enclosed oocytes (97). By contrast, forskolin inhibited the spontaneous maturation of cumulus-enclosed oocytes and had no effect on the maturation of denuded oocytes (98,99). Similar results were obtained when cholera toxin was used (87). These results seem to indicate that activation of adenylate cyclase in the whole follicle induces resumption of meiosis; activation of adenylate cyclase in the cumulus–oocyte complex results in inhibition of meiosis; and the oocyte is devoid of adenylate cyclase or the level of cAMP produced by the oocyte is not sufficient to maintain meiotic arrest. Indeed, evidence for transfer of cAMP from the cumulus cells to the ovum has been obtained in rat, mouse, hamster, and porcine oocytes (98–102). These studies leave little doubt regarding the important role of oocyte cAMP in the resumption of meiosis in mammals. However, the question of whether the oocyte synthesizes a sufficient amount of cAMP to inhibit meiosis, and whether cAMP is transferred from the cumulus to the oocyte, was answered by contrasting experimental results. Thus, while forskolin did not affect the resumption of meiosis in denuded oocytes of the rat (98,99) and hamster (100), in other studies it was inhibitory in mouse (103,104), rat (105), and pig (101) denuded oocytes. The varying results may be related, at least in part, to species and strain differences, as well as to the experimental procedures employed. Quantitative differences among species or even strains in oocyte adenylate cyclase, coupled with differences in cumulus cell-oocyte transport of cAMP, can easily be envisioned. Examination of these parameters in several species supports this notion (*see above*). Nevertheless, the essential role of oocyte cAMP in the regulation of mammalian meiosis seems well established. The observed synergism of cAMP and OMI in inhibiting spontaneous maturation *in vitro* of isolated oocytes (54,93,94,106,107) is suggestive of interaction of cAMP and follicular OMI in the control of oocyte maturation. This concept further emphasizes the multifactorial control of resumption of meiosis.

Role of Cumulus Cells

The cumulus cells appear to have an important role in the regulation of meiosis. Whereas OMI from porcine follicular fluid inhibited the resumption of meiosis by oocytes cultured within their intact cumuli, it did not interfere with the maturation of denuded oocytes of the pig (84) or rat (108). By contrast, porcine FFl attenuated maturation of mouse denuded oocytes. Nevertheless, in this study too, the suppression of meiosis resumption in mouse denuded oocytes was consistently less than in cumulus-enclosed oocytes (52). It appears, therefore, that the inhibitory action of OMI upon meiosis is exerted, at least partially, through the mediation of cumulus cells.

The cumulus cells are apparently involved also in the mediation of the meiosis-inducing action of LH. Whereas it was not possible to demonstrate specific receptors of LH on the oocyte, specific LH/hCG receptors were demonstrated on cumulus cells (109,110). This finding was further supported by the response of the whole oocyte–cumulus complex to gonadotropins, involving enhanced steroidogenesis (111,112), lactate production (113) cumulus mucification (114), and activation of adenylate cyclase (104). LH accelerated resumption of meiosis in mouse oocytes pretreated with dbcAMP and IBMX, and LH was effective only in oocytes cultured within their cumulus complex but not in denuded oocytes (115). It was suggested that acceleration of meiosis by LH is mediated by an increase in cumulus cell cAMP levels which promotes a decrease in maturation inhibitors. The finding that the prevention of the LH-induced increase in cAMP with *N*α-*p*-tosyl-L-lysine chloromethyl ketone (TLCK), inhibiting also the LH-induced acceleration of oocyte maturation, lends support to this notion (115). Germinal vesicle breakdown in rat (60) and rabbit (116) isolated oocytes maturing spontaneously occurs 1 to 2 hr earlier than GVB in follicle-enclosed oocytes stimulated by LH. This suggests that by isolating an oocyte from its follicle, some regulatory step(s) essential for triggering meiosis *in vivo* is bypassed. This may include merely the removal of the inhibitory signal (OMI) by decreased synthesis, increased degradation, or a combination of both, or alternatively the generation of a positive signal which triggers the resumption of meiosis. Some of these alternative regulatory mechanisms of meiosis are reviewed and compared in mammalian, amphibian, and echinoderm oocytes (117). The putative role of steroids in the control of resumption of meiosis is dealt with elsewhere (53,54,106,117).

Some investigators were unable to demonstrate OMI activity of follicular preparations. Granulosa cells did not inhibit maturation of cow, sow, or ewe oocytes, whereas FFl showed such activity (67); porcine follicular fluid was inactive whereas coculture with granulosa cells inhibited resumption of meiosis (57,62); and bovine and porcine FFl as well as granulosa cells were inactive (51), but coculture with follicle hemisection prevented meiosis and this was overcome by addition of LH (50). These varying findings may be related, at least in part, to the low OMI activity of follicular fluid and of granulosa cell cultures, the finding that fluid and granulosa cells from large follicles are devoid of OMI activity, the instability of OMI, and differences in methods of oocyte collection and culture. The multitude of studies from numerous other laboratories demonstrating OMI activity attest to the paracrine regulation of the resumption of meiosis. Nevertheless, purification and chemical characterization of OMI are needed to further our understanding of the exact biochemical and cellular mechanisms controlling the preovulatory resumption of meiosis.

GONADOTROPIN-BINDING INHIBITORS

A plausible mechanism for paracrine modulation of gonadotropin action could be interference with signal reception at the level of the receptor. Indeed, inhibitors of FSH- and LH-binding have been isolated from ovarian [and also from testicular (118–120)] tissues. Since these studies have been reviewed recently by the leaders of this field (121–125), only a brief overview of these studies are presented here. It has already been indicated (121) that many factors may interfere with radioligand binding *in vitro,* hence it is very difficult (especially when working on crude extracts) to distinguish between regulatory significant gonadotropin-binding inhibitor and perturbance of the assay conditions. The alternative assays, measuring biological responses to gonadotropic challenge, may be misleading as far as binding is concerned, especially when tested *in vivo*.

FSH-Binding Inhibitor

Follicle-stimulating hormone-binding inhibitors (FSH-BI) were first described in buffer or water extracts of rat testis (126). Later studies described similar factors in bovine follicular fluid (127), human serum (128), and seminal plasma (129). This chapter only discusses studies on ovarian FSH-BI.

Bovine and porcine follicular fluid contain FSH-BI, separable by diafiltration through membranes with calibrated pore sizes, with molecular weights (MW) of less than 500, between 500 to 5,000, and greater than 5,000 (121,130–133) (Fig. 7).

Approximately 50% of the FSH-BI activity of follicular fluid is present in the very small MW subfraction. However, this activity most probably results from the *in vitro* effect of concentrated salts (134,135). The electrolyte concentration of porcine follicular fluid does not vary significantly with follicular development; hence it is unlikely that differences in FSH-BI potency from follicles varying in their size result from their electrolyte concentration (121).

The large molecular weight subfraction of follicular fluid was estimated to represent approximately 30% of total FSH-BI activity. Nevertheless, this fraction contains several substances, such as FSH, proteoglycans, and proteases, which may interfere with FSH binding *in vitro*. In addition, an enteric bacterium, *Serratia liquifaciens,* can contaminate porcine follicular fluid and secretes a large MW FSH-BI (136,137). Therefore, Reichert and his colleagues studied

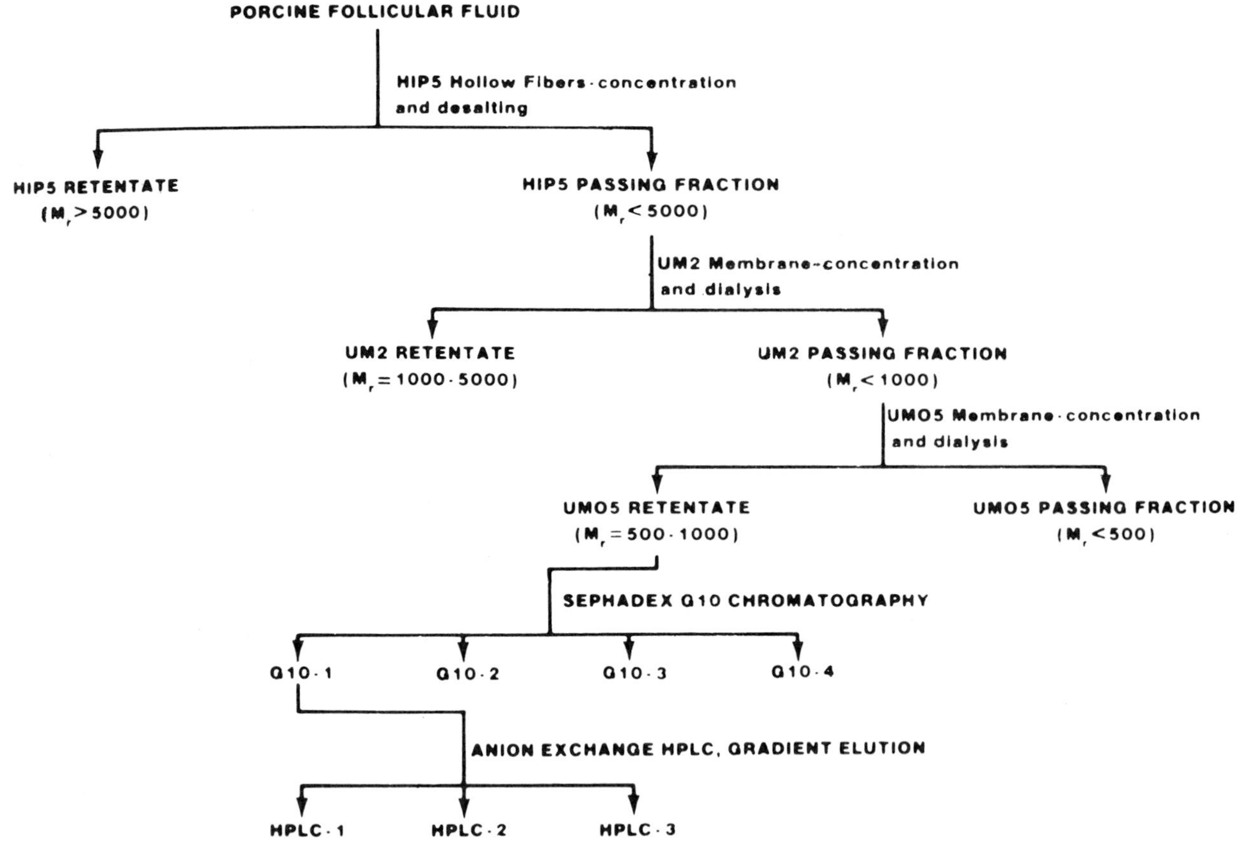

FIG. 7. Flow diagram for the isolation of low M_r FSH-binding inhibitors from porcine FFl: a total of 2.5 l of FFl in 500-ml aliquots was fractionated according to this procedure. M_r is the apparent molecular weight based on pore sizes of the fibers or membranes employed. Sephadex G10 fractions from separate runs were pooled and then further purified by HPLC. UM2 retentates were also subjected to further purification as shown for UM05 retentate. G10-2 and G10-3 fractions were also subjected to anion-exchange HPLC. From Sluss and Reichert (133), by the permission of the Society for the Study of Reproduction.

in detail the intermediate-sized (500–5,000 MW) subfractions, which account for only approximately 15% of the FSH-BI activity of follicular fluid (Fig. 7). Sephadex G10 chromatography of the intermediate-sized subfraction, followed by anion-exchange HPLC demonstrated several low molecular weight (approx. 1,000) FSH-BI components (133). One component was identified as putrescine and another was suggested to be a peptide of 10 to 11 amino acids, but additional components have not been characterized as yet (121,138).

Several lines of reasoning led Reichert and his co-workers (121) to suggest that the intermediate-sized (i.e., 500–5,000 MW) subfraction is the physiologically relevant FSH-BI: (a) This was the only fraction, besides unfractionated follicular fluid, to also exhibit post-binding responses such as FSH-stimulated adenylate cyclase in intact granulosa cells and homogenates (131); and (b) the FSH-BI activity of this fraction was related to the physiological state of follicular fluid pools. Thus the concentration of FSH-BI was higher in pools of bovine follicle fluid obtained from animals in the luteal phase of their cycle, as compared to that of pregnant animals (132). Furthermore, concentration of FSH-BI was correlated with the degree of follicular atresia as defined by biochemical parameters (132) (Fig. 8). This finding suggests that FSH-BI may play a role in the induction or propagation of follicular atresia by attenuating the responsiveness of granulosa cells to FSH. Examination of FSH-BI in individual follicles at various stages of atresia as well as the ability of native or synthetic FSH-BI to induce atresia is required in order to confirm such a role of FSH-BI in the processes leading to atresia.

LH-Binding Inhibitor

Inhibitors of luteinizing hormone binding (LH-BI) have been demonstrated in extracts of rat (139,140), pig (141,142), cat, dog, sheep, goat (143), and human (144,145) corpora lutea. This inhibition of LH binding could result from competition of tissue LH or of LH destruction by a protease present in the extract. Both of these possibilities seem unlikely, since boiling of rat corpora lutea extracts destroys only a small fraction (<20%) of LH-BI activity and exposure of LH to these extracts does not alter the physical and chemical properties of LH (125). Furthermore, several

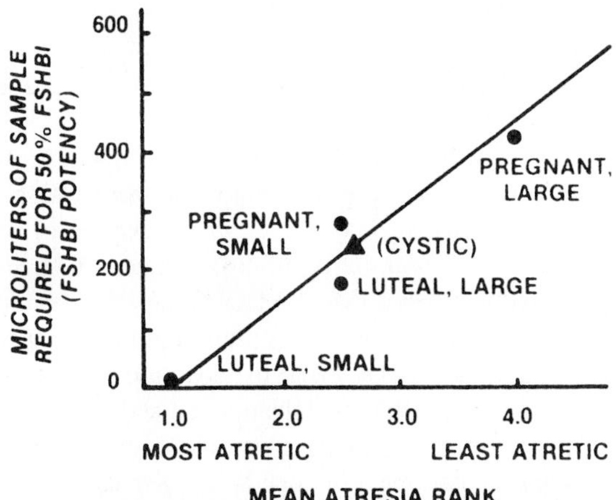

FIG. 8. Correlation between FSH-BI potency of low M_r fraction of FFI and atresia rank of pooled FFI of various-sized follicles from pregnant and luteal phase cows. Data were compared by least squares linear regression analysis. The correlation coefficient (r) was 0.967 for the 4 pools of FFI (identified in parentheses in the figure) which represents a significant (P = 0.02) linear relationship between the two parameters. FSH-BI_{50} of FF from cystic follicles (▲) is plotted on the regression line for comparison but was not included in the regression analysis. Note that the greater the concentration of inhibitor in the sample, the less volume (μl) required to obtain 50% inhibition of FSH binding to receptor (FSH-BI potency). From Sluss et al. (132), by the permission of the Society for the Study of Reproduction.

experimental approaches did not show appreciable binding of LH to LH-BI, thus supporting the notion that LH-BI activity is not due to solubilized LH receptors in the extracts (125).

LH-BI activity is present in freshly collected corpora lutea of pregnant rat, dog, sheep, goat (146), and rat (125) but not from fresh pseudopregnant rat and porcine corpora lutea (141,146). In all cases, storage at −20°C increased the LH-BI activity extractable from corpora lutea, but not in tissues other than luteinized ovary (125). This increase in LH-BI activity is thought to be related to the association of LH-BI with some cellular fraction. Storage appears to release (or to make readily extractable) LH-BI from these cellular sites. The finding that LH-BI could be extracted from fresh pseudopregnant rat ovaries with a nonionic detergent, Triton X-100, supports this notion (143).

In addition to direct demonstration of inhibition of LH binding by LH-BI, studies were conducted to examine post-binding responses. Thus, LH-BI inhibited LH/hCG-stimulated, but not basal, progesterone synthesis by ovary slices of pseudopregnant rats (143,146). Similarly, Kumari and her colleagues (147) demonstrated inhibition of progesterone synthesis by LH-BI preparations whether treated or not by charcoal. *In vivo* effects of LH-BI preparations on ovulation were reported in rabbits (148), rats, and mice (149). However, since crude preparations were used, activities other than LH-BI cannot be excluded at the present.

Aqueous extracts of rat luteinized ovaries contained LH-BI activity in both dialysate and the nondialyzable fraction (139), whereas in the pig luteal extracts only the nondialyzable activity was observed (122,125). The nondialyzable LH-BI from both rat and porcine extracts exhibited similar properties upon gel filtration and ion-exchange chromatography. It seemed that LH-BI exists in more than one molecular form, the major components with MW of around 20,000 (125).

The finding that $PGF_{2\alpha}$, the physiological regulator of corpus luteum function, inhibited hCG binding to corpora lutea receptors *in vivo* (150) may probably be interpreted to involve activation of LH-BI related mechanism, but experimental evidence linking this LH-BI action to $PGF_{2\alpha}$ is lacking at the present. Hence, the physiological role of LH-BI remains obscure at present and should be the subject of physiological studies employing pure LH-BI fractions.

MITOGENIC AND GROWTH FACTORS

The ovarian follicle undergoes most impressive cell proliferation during its growth. Thus, it is estimated that a primordial follicle with approximately 50 granulosa cells (151) reaches more than 5×10^7 granulosa cells in preovulatory follicles in the human (152). Of course, these estimates may vary among species, different ovarian cell populations, and even researchers, but there is no question that cell replication is a major feature of ovarian activity.

The earliest stages of follicular growth seem to be independent of circulating gonadotropins (153,154). Therefore, it is generally assumed that the initiation of follicular growth is regulated by ovarian autocrine and paracrine hormones. Furthermore, even after antrum formation, when follicular development is dependent upon gonadotropins and estrogen, it is difficult to assign all aspects of follicular growth and selection solely to these hormones. The experiments demonstrating the ability of granulosa cells to reverse serum-attenuated cell differentiation *in vitro* and the dependence of this reversal on the density of the cultured granulosa cells (155) support this notion.

After antrum formation there is a further 100- to 1,000-fold increase in follicular granulosa cell number (152). It has been demonstrated that FSH and estradiol enhance synergistically granulosa cell proliferation *in vivo* (156) and *in vitro* (157–159). In recent years much work has been directed toward discovery of nongonadotropin and nonsteroidal growth-stimulating ovarian actions. This approach was complemented by testing the actions of known polypeptide growth factors on ovarian cells *in vivo* or *in vitro*. The studies involving ovarian tissues were reviewed recently (13,160–164). Much of the research on growth factors is centered on their growth-promoting actions. It should be noted, however, that these factors may also modulate differentiation and this action may be uncoupled from their effects on cellular proliferation (165–172). The following growth factors or growth factor families have been mostly considered regarding their putative involvement in ovarian physiology.

Epidermal growth factor (EGF). EGF was originally extracted from mouse submaxillary glands (173). It is mitogenic in ectodermal- and endodermal-derived cells *in vitro* (174–176).

Fibroblast growth factor (FGF). FGF has been originally purified from bovine pituitary (177) and is similar to EGF in its physiological actions, but exhibits somewhat different cell specificity (175). FGF was recently purified to homogeneity and characterized (178,179).

Platelet-derived growth factor (PDGF). PDGF is stored in alpha granules of blood platelets and released during clot formation and may be involved in tissue repair processes (180–182).

Insulin and insulin-like growth factors (IGFs). This is a family of serum-derived factors closely related to insulin. A gene duplication approximately 600 million years ago led to the diversion of a common precursor molecule into insulin and IGF as distinct hormones (183). The IGF family consists of several homologous, low molecular weight, single chain polypeptide growth factors named after their remarkable similarity to insulin. These were originally isolated on the basis of their two different metabolic actions: (a) the ability to stimulate sulfate incorporation into cartilage (sulfation factor activity); and (b) nonsuppressible insulinlike activity (NSILA), demonstrating insulinomimetic actions originally tested in adipocytes (184,185). On the basis of net charge, the IGFs can be classed into two distinct groups: (a) basic IGFs (isoelectric points 8.1–8.5) which include human IGF-I (hIGF-I), identified with somatomedin C (SmC) (186–188) and its suggested murine equivalent, basic rat somatomedin, labeled rat IGF-I (rIGF-I) (189); and (b) neutral IGFs, including human IGF-II (hIGF-II) and its probable murine counterpart, multiplication stimulating activity (MSA), also referred to as rat IGF-II (rIGF-II).

Angiogenic factors. In view of the rapid changes in ovarian vasculature associated with follicular growth, atresia, periovulatory changes, corpus luteum formation, and regression, it is reasonable to search for angiogenic factor(s) in the ovary (164). Angiogenic factors have been isolated from both tumor and nontumor sources. They vary in their apparent molecular weight from 200 to 100,000 and have not yet been fully characterized and purified to homogeneity (164). The recent purification and characterization of angiogenin, an angiogenic protein from human carcinoma cells (190–192) and the demonstration of angiogenic activity of FGF (178,179,193) may soon result in elucidation of ovarian angiogenic hormone(s) and its relationship to other growth factors (194).

Ovarian Growth-Stimulating Actions

Under this subheading a short review of unidentified ovarian growth activites will be presented. Of course, this separation does not imply that they differ from the growth factors to be dealt with in the following sections. Also, not all the factors dealt with in these sections have been proven to be produced in the ovary.

Evidence suggesting that follicular theca components secrete substances that enhance granulosa cell proliferation *in vitro* was obtained by recombining *in vitro* thecal tissue and granulosa cells (195). Similarly, Makris and her colleagues (196,197) have isolated a thecal factor stimulating porcine granulosa cell and BALB/3T3 cell proliferation. Using ornithine decarboxylase (ODC) activity as an indirect marker of mitogenic activity (198–200). Hammond and co-workers (201,202) found ODC-stimulating activity in two molecular weight ranges in porcine FFl: one $<$ 10,000 daltons and another $>$30,000 daltons. Since FFl was shown to exert substantial somatomedin activity in the $<$10,000 fraction (161,202), it may account for the low molecular weight activity (*see* Role of Insulin and IGFs *below*).

EGF and FGF Actions on Ovarian Cells

The initial studies of Gospodarowicz and his colleagues (203–205) demonstrated the mitogenic activity of EGF and FGF on bovine, porcine, rabbit, guinea pig, and human granulosa cells *in vitro*. By contrast, granulosa cells of intact or hypophysectomized-estrogen treated rats or bovine luteal cells *in vitro* did not proliferate in response to EGF or FGF (205–207), but follicle growth in the rat was promoted by EGF administration *in vivo* (175). This disparate sensitivity of ovarian cells cannot be interpreted at the present; both rat granulosa cells (208,209) and bovine granulosa cells (206) possess EGF receptors. Neutral extracts of nonluteinized rat ovaries revealed the presence of immunoreactive FGF, and only a small increase was observed following luteinization (194).

These growth factors, in addition to their mitogenic action, affected granulosa cell LH receptor development and steroidogenesis. FGF was a potent inhibitor of FSH-stimulated aromatase activity in rat granulosa cells (194). Similarly, Mondschein and Schomberg demonstrated that EGF and FGF suppress FSH-induced LH receptors in serum-free cultures (210). This effect is probably exerted mainly distal to cAMP formation, since EGF also attenuated 8-Br-cAMP- or cholera-toxin-induced action on LH receptors (211,212). Using different experimental protocols, varying results were obtained regarding EGF action on granulosa cell cAMP. Thus, EGF reduced adenylate cyclase and enhanced phosphodiesterase activity and hence lowered cAMP in granulosa cell cultures (213), but no such EGF action was observed in response to short-term FSH stimulation of rat and porcine granulosa cell cultures (214).

EGF, but not FGF, inhibits FSH-stimulated estrogen production by rat granulosa cells *in vitro*. This effect is exerted, at least partially, distal to cAMP formation, as EGF suppressess cholera toxin-, diBu-cAMP-, and PGE_2-induced estrogen biosynthesis (207,208). Similarly, EGF depresses aromatase activity in porcine unstimulated granulosa cell cultures (211,212). By contrast, EGF seems to exert stimulatory effects on basal and FSH-stimulated progestin synthesis by an increase in pregnenolone production and the activities of 3β-HSD and 20α-HSD (208,213).

In another study, when only 20α-hydroxy progesterone was measured in 3-day cultures of rat granulosa cells, EGF exerted only marginal effects which were inhibitory or stimulatory depending on the dose of EGF (163). In porcine granulosa cells, EGF depressed basal and hormone-stimulated progesterone secretion (211,212,215). These disparate effects of EGF may be related to the differences in the experimental design employed.

EGF acts on additional ovarian compartments. It inhibits androgen production by a theca-interstitial cell preparation *in vitro* (216) and suppresses follicular development in neonatal mice *in vivo* (217). Finally, EGF induces the resumption of meiosis in explanted preovulatory rat follicles (218).

Specific high affinity, low capacity EGF-binding sites have been demonstrated in rat granulosa cells (208,209) suggesting a receptor mediated mechanism of action. After occupancy the EGF receptors of granulosa and luteal cells are internalized, and the label is associated with cell nuclei (206,219–221). Administration of LH and FSH, but not prolactin, increased total ovarian EGF receptors (208,209). Furthermore, ovarian EGF receptor number changes throughout the rat reproductive cycle, being higher on proestrus and lower during diestrus (208).

The general pattern of the differentiative actions of EGF and FGF on the ovary is somewhat reminiscent of the actions of GnRH (*see* GnRH-like Peptides *below*). In terms of physiological function the common denominator may be atretogenic activity. Their proliferative actions are, however, incompatible with atretogenic function. Further studies are therefore needed in order to define the role of EGF and FGF in ovarian physiology.

Effect of PDGF and Copurifying Factors

PDGF was reported to enhance FSH stimulation of granulosa cell LH receptors *in vitro* both in the absence and in the presence of serum (210,213,214,222). PDGF also enhanced cholera-toxin induction of LH receptors, but this action was exerted only when serum was present in the culture medium (214). Recent studies utilizing CM Sephadex, Blue Sepharose, and Biogel P-60 chromatography yielded a PDGF component that was mitogenic in BALB/3T3 cells but had no effect on FSH-induced granulosa cell LH receptors. In contrast, a smaller molecular weight component (~ 21,000) markedly enhanced FSH induction of LH receptors (163). These results suggest that the above reviewed effects of PDGF on granulosa cells are due to a platelet product other than PDGF itself. The varying findings of the two groups working on PDGF effects on granulosa may therefore be due to the different preparation of PDGF used. It will be most interesting to follow the nature of the PDGF component acting on granulosa cells and to examine its physiological role.

Role of Insulin and IGFs

The use of insulin to supplement culture media for ovarian cells, the presence of ovarian insulin receptors, and insulin action on granulosa cell metabolism and steroidogenesis have been recently reviewed (13,223,224). Since apparently no claim was made of local production of insulin, only the actions of IGFs on ovarian tissues and their possible role as local regulators of ovarian function will be addressed. This topic was recently reviewed by Adashi and his colleagues (162).

Addition of SmC/IGF-I to granulosa cells from small (4–6 mm) bovine follicles caused mitogenic response in serum-free cultures (220). Likewise, both IGF-I and IGF-II or insulin enhanced [^{3}H]-thymidine incorporation into DNA of porcine granulosa cells (225). Addition of SmC/IGF-I to rat granulosa cells augmented FSH-stimulated progesterone accumulation and had only limited effect on their basal production (226,227). Similarly SmC/IGF-I stimulated progesterone synthesis by porcine granulosa cells *in vitro* (225,228). In porcine granulosa cell cultures MSA/IGF-II synergized with FSH in stimulating progesterone secretion (223,225). Similarly, SmC/IGF-I synergized with estradiol-17β in enhancing porcine granulosa cell progesterone and pregnenolone biosynthesis (229).

SmC/IGF-I synergized with FSH in enhancing aromatase activity of rat granulosa cells, but had no effect on basal aromatase activity (230). By contrast, SmC/IGF-I stimulated sulfate incorporation into extracellular proteoglycans in both FSH-treated and untreated rat granulosa cells (231). Finally, SmC/IGF-I synergized with FSH in inducing LH receptors (232).

This short review of some of the recently published effects of IGFs clearly supports the notion that they may be involved in regulation of follicular growth and differentiation. This conclusion is reinforced by the demonstration of IGFs specific binding by porcine (225) and rat (162,233) granulosa cells.

Porcine follicular fluid was found to contain MSA-like somatomedin (234–236). IGF-I levels were higher in fluid of preovulatory follicles than in serum of immature follicles (236). Studies with granulosa cells *in vitro* lend further support to local production of IGFs in the ovary. Thus, rat granulosa cells produced *in vitro* measurable SmC/IGF-I whether stimulated with FSH or not (162). In contrast, porcine granulosa cells responded to the addition of FSH and estradiol-17β with increased release of IGF-I as measured by a radioreceptor assay and by RIA (234–236), and IGF production continued for 6 to 10 days. Using immunohistochemical technique employing different antibodies, SmC/IGF-I was localized in oocytes, theca, and granulosa cells of primordial follicles, and the reaction diminished with follicular development (237). Conclusive proof for IGF formation in the ovaries and precise determination of their types must await the availability of proper cDNA clones.

In summary, the present data support the notion that ovarian granulosa cells produce and respond to IGFs. Unpublished studies quoted by Adashi et al. (162) suggest the presence of IGF receptors also in nongranulosa ovarian compartments. Therefore it is possible that IGFs play both an autocrine and paracrine regulatory role in ovarian function.

Ovarian Angiogenic Factors

Here the evidence for the presence of angiogenic factor(s) in ovarian tissues will be summarized, and their nature and the relation of angiogenic activity to ovarian function will be discussed in brief. A broader review, including description of vascular changes in the ovary throughout the reproductive cycle, their comparison to such changes during wound healing, inflammation, tumor growth, and other derangements, and a brief description of the assay systems utilized in the search for angiogenic factors, has been published recently (164).

Ovarian angiogenic activity was first demonstrated in bovine corpus luteum (238). This was followed by similar results using rabbit (239), pig (240), and rat (164,241) corpora lutea. Noteworthy is the finding that 1- or 2-day-old rat corpora lutea had high angiogenic activity, whereas 6-day-old corpora lutea of pseudopregnancy exerted a lesser degree of activity, and those of 10 days were devoid of such activity (164,241). These studies utilized several of the *in vivo* and *in vitro* assays available for studying angiogenic activity and testing endothelial cell proliferation and migration. Further support for the involvement of angiogenic activity in corpus luteum formation was obtained recently by *in situ* radioautography of newly formed rat corpora lutea and demonstration of an increase in ^{3}H-thymidine incorporation into endothelial cells (242).

These studies were extended also to nonluteinized ovarian tissue by testing angiogenic activity of ovarian extracts or fragments of PMSG-treated immature mice or rats (241,243). Both studies demonstrated PMSG-stimulated angiogenic activity and vascularization was most intense around follicles (241). Further studies demonstrated angiogenic activity in extracts of porcine nonluteal ovaries (244), rabbit (245), and primate (246) follicles, and follicular fluid of pigs (247) and of hormone-stimulated women (248). Ovarian origin of this angiogenic activity is suggested by the accumulation of such activity in media in which intact follicles (241), thecal tissues (243,246), granulosa cells (245,249), and luteal cells (250) were cultured previously. The studies demonstrate the presence of angiogenic activity in ovarian tissues of several mammalian species and in both early luteal and hormone-stimulated follicular tissues. Considering the ample morphological evidence (164,251,252) suggesting massive changes in vascularization associated with follicular and corpus luteum development and their demise at atresia and luteolysis, the role of angiogenic hormones cannot be overemphasized. Thus, increase in angiogenic activity was associated with PMSG treatment, which enhances follicular development, and with early stages of corpus luteum development. Conversely, in aging corpora lutea, angiogenic activity decreases. These findings give credence to the important regulatory role of an angiogenic factor in follicle selection and corpus luteum function. Indeed, the importance of follicular vasculature for supply of gonadotropins to monkey follicles has been suggested (253), and a decrease in follicular vasculature was associated with atresia (254–256). It remains to be determined whether these angiogenic changes have a regulatory role in ovarian activity or are merely an expression of other regulatory signals. Therefore, purification of the ovarian angiogenic hormone(s) is of major importance for further studies.

The angiogenic factor from porcine nonluteinized ovaries has been preliminarily characterized as a heat-labile, nondialyzable, protease-sensitive, cationic peptide that was soluble in 40%, but not 60%, ammonium sulfate (244). The bovine corpus luteum angiogenic factor has been purified to apparent homogeneity and found to be related to FGF (257). If these results extend to other mammalian species and also prove true for nonluteinized follicular angiogenic factor(s), current concepts regarding ovarian angiogenesis and ovarian cell proliferation must be altered. Further studies are definitely required in order to elucidate the role of ovarian autocrine and paracrine hormones in regulating ovarian cell proliferation and angiogenesis. The purification of corpus luteum angiogenic factor should lead to the localization of its cellular origin and of the mechanisms controlling its production.

FOLLICULAR REGULATORY PROTEINS

Proteins from the venous drainage of human preovulatory follicles or pooled follicular fluid that can suppress follicular responses to gonadotropins have been described and referred to as follicle regulatory proteins (FRP). A detailed account of these studies can be found in recent reviews by diZerega and his colleagues (258–260). It was suggested that these proteins are produced by the dominant follicle and suppress the responsiveness of follicles lower in the hierarchy.

Recently, FRPs were defined as the fraction remaining after precipitation with 20% to 30% saturated ammonium sulfate, dialysis and elution from an Orange-A-sepharose column with 0.5 M KCl, and molecular sieving (12,500–15,000 daltons). It is heat and trypsin labile (259). FRP activities were described, in addition to human ovaries, also in porcine (261), ovine (262), and bovine (263) follicular fluid. Furthermore, FRP activity could be demonstrated in media in which human granulosa cells have been cultured, thus suggesting its granulosa cell origin (264).

The initial studies on FRP activity included administration of FFl or its enriched FRP fraction to hypophysectomized, diethylstilbestrol-treated immature rats and assessed by the inhibition of ovarian weight and serum estradiol increase in response to human menopausal gonadotropin challenge (265,266). Further demonstration of FRP activity entailed its administration to normally cycling monkeys, leading to reduced peripheral serum estradiol, without markedly affecting serum FSH concentration, and resulted in either apparent anovulation or inadequate luteal phase (267). Ovine FRP activity was demonstrated by the inhibition of follicular growth and the rise in serum estradiol in response to exogenous PMSG challenge of hypophysectomized ewes (262). In these studies a reduction in the mitotic index of granulosa cells in <2 mm follicles was observed, thus suggesting an antiproliferative activity (262). These studies were extended to unilaterally ovariectomized ewes in which visible follicles were ablated by electrocautery. Ovine FFl inhibited PMSG sustained follicular growth by decreasing mitosis in follicles < 2 mm. This resulted in an increase in the number of < 2-mm and decrease in > 4-mm follicles (268).

The mechanism(s) involved in FRP action were examined using *in vitro* cultures of granulosa cells. Thus, FSH-induced adenylate cyclase activity was decreased by FRP when porcine granulosa cells were challenged by forskolin or Gpp(NH)p and this was not changed in the presence of IBMX (269). Likewise, FRP inhibited FSH-induced LH/hCG receptors in cultured porcine granulosa cells (269). The actions of FRP on granulosa cell steroidogenesis were very complex. FRP from porcine or human follicular fluid inhibits aromatase activity in porcine (264,270) and rat preantral (271) granulosa cells, and this effect in rat cells can be counteracted with higher FSH doses. FRP exerted biphasic effects on FSH-enhanced rat and porcine granulosa cell progestin synthesis, low doses being stimulatory and highly inhibitory (271,272). The effect on porcine granulosa cells was limited to those from small and medium size follicles, but had no effect on granulosa cells from large follicles (272). Likewise, in our preliminary studies FRP had no clear-cut inhibitory actions on explanted intact preovulatory rat follicles (Abisogun et al., *unpublished information*). Undoubtedly, the complex nature of FRP action on steroidogenesis warrants further studies in order to enable us to understand its physiological role. One possibility is that FRP preparations contain several, and probably counteracting, biological activities that are differentially expressed in various model test systems.

As is the case with other putative ovarian regulators, the need for purification and chemical characterization of FRP(s) cannot be overemphasized. In its biological actions FRP bears some resemblance to luteinization regulators and, at least the FRP of ovine origin, has mitogenic activity. It does not inhibit FSH binding and hence apparently is not FSH-BI.

The finding that FSH can override FRP inhibitory action on estrogen production is compatible with the positive correlation between estrogen levels and FRP in the human follicle (273,274) and the finding that follicles with the highest concentration of estradiol in their follicular fluid also have the highest concentrations of FSH (275). As reduction in follicular estrogen production is associated with early stages of atresia (26,276), FRP may induce atresia in other follicles by blocking aromatase activity whereas the dominant follicle is protected by the local high FSH levels. Thus production of FRP by a follicle may regulate differentially its own steroid synthesis and that of other follicles. The physiological action of an FRP-like paracrine hormone probably underlies the recently described ability of exogenous PMSG to recruit follicles only during a narrowly delimited portion of the estrous cycle, when preovulatory follicles are not present in the ovary (277).

REGULATORS OF LUTEINIZATION

The findings that follicular fluid alters the *in vitro* responses of cultured granulosa cells to gonadotropins suggest that paracrine factors are involved in the differentiation of granulosa cells. Thus, responsiveness of granulosa cells to gonadotropins, according to this view, is not entirely dependent upon gonadotropin receptors but modified also by locally produced hormonal regulators. One such activity was stimulation of the secretion of both progesterone and estrogens, enhancement of morphological differentiation, and potentiation of FSH and LH action on granulosa cells from immature antral follicles. This activity is referred to as luteinization (and in later studies as maturation) stimulator (LS) (278,279). The other activity is consistently observed in fluid from small follicles and referred to as luteinization inhibitor (LI) and more recently as atretogenic factor (278,279).

Most of the studies on LS and LI were performed using follicular fluid and conditioned media of granulosa cells obtained from pigs (142,278–280). But similar effects were reported using human (281,282), cow (283–285), and mare (286,287) follicular fluid.

The preponderance of LI activity in pools of fluid from small follicles and of LS in that from large follicles, led Channing and her colleagues (1) to suggest that the ratio between the stimulatory and inhibitory activity in the follicle plays an essential role in follicle selection. In accordance, it was found that fluid from midcycle bovine follicles decreased granulosa cell secretion of progesterone and prostaglandin *in vitro,* but fluid from preovulatory follicles was devoid of such inhibitory activity (283). Likewise, fluid from viable mare follicles enhanced FSH-stimulated steroidogenesis, but fluid from atretic follicles was inhibitory (287).

The most commonly applied approach to test for LS was to use fluid from large follicles and test its action on granulosa cells from small follicles, whereas LI activity was tested on the behavior of cells from large follicles.

Luteinization Stimulator

Porcine granulosa cells from either small or large follicles, cultured for 2 days with fluid from large follicles, exhibited higher lipid content than cells cultured in serum (288,289). This morphologic observation was coupled with stimulatory action of porcine follicular fluid from large follicles on granulosa cell steroidogenesis *in vitro*. Incubation of granulosa cells from small follicles with fluid from large ones significantly enhanced progesterone accumulation within 2 to 5 min of the addition of the fluid and reached 10- to 12-fold stimulation within 24 to 48 hr with follicular fluid from large follicles, as compared to cells incubated with serum. Since the granulosa cell content of progesterone was very low (<0.15 ng/5 $\times$ 10^5 cell) prior to incubation, it appears that the fluid from large follicles stimulated progesterone synthesis and not merely its release (290,291). Fluid from small follicles often failed to stimulate progesterone secretion during the first 2 days of incubation, but after 4 to 6 days of culture it enhanced progesterone accumulation by two- to fivefold (291).

In addition to its stimulation of basal progesterone accumulation by granulosa cells from small follicles, fluid from large follicles also enhanced FSH action, suggesting that it increases responsiveness to FSH. Evidence that this action of FFl is not solely due to its FSH content includes the inability of added FSH to elicit similar response to serum and the fact that addition of antiserum to FSH did not abolish this activity of follicular fluid (292,293). Likewise, FFl also enabled LH to stimulate progesterone accumulation by granulosa from small follicles, whereas LH was inactive when incubated with the same cells in the presence of serum (291). This concurs with studies demonstrating the stimulation of LH receptor development by treatment with FFl (294–296).

Follicular fluid from large follicles also enhanced the conversion of added testosterone to estrogen by cultures of granulosa cells explanted from small and large follicles. But the time course of stimulation was entirely different in these two cell types; a 24-hr incubation was sufficient for enhanced estrogen accumulation by cells from large follicles, whereas 72 hr were necessary before cells from small follicles exhibited an increase in estrogen formation (279,297).

The LS activity survives charcoal extraction and long-term storage but is lost by successive freeze-thawing. Partial purification was achieved by ethanol precipitation and Sephacryl S-300 fractionation. The LS activity eluted in the 60,000-dalton range (298).

Luteinization Inhibitor

Granulosa cells explanted from porcine large follicles undergo *in vitro* a series of morphological and endocrine changes commonly referred to as luteinization (299). Addition of follicular fluid from small and medium-sized porcine follicles prevents these luteinizationlike changes (300) as well as FSH induction of LH/hCG receptors and progesterone synthesis from cells explanted from small follicles (1,294,295). Similar inhibitory activities were demonstrated in follicular fluid of other species. Thus, bovine follicular fluid exhibited inhibition of morphological luteinization (284,301) and RNA synthesis (285) in cultured rat granulosa cells *in vitro*. Likewise, human FFl prevented gonadotropin stimulation of cAMP (281) and progesterone accumulation (282). Since most of the studies on LI were performed using porcine FFl, these will be reviewed here in more detail.

Morphometric analysis of granulosa cells from large follicles cultured for 2 days with FFl from small follicles revealed significantly fewer lipid droplets, mitochondria, smooth endoplasmic reticulum, and lysosomes than either of the control groups cultured with FFl from large follicles or with porcine serum (289).

Conversely, in cultures of granulosa cells from large follicles with FFl from small ones basal as well as FSH-, LH- and prostaglandin-stimulated progesterone, secretion was reduced to 10% to 20% of the levels attained by cells cultured in serum controls (279,300). Increasing the dose of gonadotropins above the maximally stimulating dose did not overcome the inhibition of porcine FFl (278,302). The inhibition of progesterone synthesis by FFl was dose-dependent, and a minimum exposure of 24 hr to the fluid was required for demonstrating the inhibitory effect (279,300).

Incubation of porcine granulosa cells from large follicles with fluid from porcine small follicles decreased both basal and NaF-, LH-, and epinephrine-stimulated adenylate cyclase activity. A minimal incubation with FFl for 24 hr was required to exhibit this effect (303). Further increase of the LH dose added to the medium did not overcome the effect of FFl on adenylate cyclase, but addition of 8-Br-cAMP, dibutyryl-cAMP, or IBMX partially reversed the inhibitory action of FFl from small follicles on progesterone accumulation. Furthermore, a combination of LH and IBMX or 8-bromo-cAMP and IBMX fully restored progesterone secretion in the presence of FFl. Thus the inhibitory effect of FFl is exerted distal to hormone binding. Accordingly, porcine fluid (303) did not inhibit LH binding, and bovine fluid depressed binding to a minor degree (304,305). Nevertheless, the precise mode of action of the porcine and bovine inhibitors may differ. Porcine fluid inhibited adenylate cyclase activity generally (i.e., basal and LH-, epinephrine-, and NaF-stimulated), arguing for an action on the catalytic subunit of the enzyme, whereas fluid from bovine follicles had minimal effect on fluoride-stimulated adenylate cyclase, consistent with interruption of LH receptor–adenylate cyclase coupling. It should be noted, however, that the studies with porcine fluid have utilized granulosa cells, whereas those with bovine fluid were performed on granulosa cell membrane preparations and could not be extended to intact cells (A. Amsterdam, *personal communication*).

Partial purification of LI and its separation from porcine

FFl inhibin was achieved by 75% ethanol precipitation and Matrix gel Red A column chromatography or 36% ethanol precipitation and DEAE-trisacryl chromatography (306,307). Further purification of the LI activity obtained by the latter procedure by TSK-3000SW high performance liquid chromatography (HPLC) yielded a principal LI activity of 130,000 and another of 500,000 dalton (306,307). Interestingly, it was noted that treating follicular fluid with a chaotropic agent, 5 M guanidine, increased apparent LI activity of FFl. This finding raised the hypothesis that LI activity may be regulated by its aggregation with FFl proteins (306–308).

It now appears that both LS and LI activities are present in follicles at various stages of follicular development (1,279,308). Therefore a hypothetical model was suggested, ascribing to the changing ratio of LS/LI the modulation of follicular response to circulating gonadotropins. According to this model, only growing follicles containing sufficient LS activity will grow and reach ovulation, while most of the follicles, with excess LI activity, will become unresponsive to gonadotropin and be doomed to atresia (308). Indeed, fluid from mare atretic follicles inhibited steroidogenic activity of porcine granulosa cells, but fluid from large follicles of estrous mares synergized with FSH in enhancing granulosa cell steroidogenesis (287). It remains to be determined whether this atretogenic factor has a role in causing atresia or is merely a product of atretic follicles. Furthermore, it is not known at this stage whether this atretogenic factor is identical or similar to LI. Only purification of LI and LS to homogeneity will enable examination of the mechanisms controlling their production and action. This will allow us to assess the physiological role of these putative hormones in follicular development and selection.

GnRH-LIKE PEPTIDES

The direct effects of GnRH and its synthetic analogs on the ovary are numerous, and the literature on its intragonadal actions exceeds that of any other gonadal peptides. Various aspects of these studies have been reviewed extensively (13,309–316). Evidence for a GnRH-like peptide being a gonadal hormone is based on the following findings: (a) GnRH exerts both inhibitory and stimulatory actions on the ovary and ovarian cells; (b) receptors for GnRH were demonstrated within the ovary; (c) several reports suggest the presence of a GnRH-like peptide in the ovary. The physiological role of GnRH in regulating ovarian function was recently substantiated by the ability of GnRH antagonists to potentiate the action of FSH and enhance follicular development (317). It should be emphasized that it is unlikely that hypothalamic GnRH reaches the ovary in physiologically active concentrations because of its dilution in the circulation (318) and its rapid degradation in the pituitary, brain, kidney, liver, and serum (319,320). The rapid degradation of GnRH is the major reason for using GnRH agonistic analogs exhibiting higher resistance to degrading enzymes (321). Here an overview of the direct actions of GnRH and its analogs on the ovary, their binding, and suggested mechanism of action will be presented. In addition, the evidence for the suggested role of an ovarian GnRH-like peptide in regulating ovarian function will be discussed.

Inhibitory Actions of GnRH on the Ovary

A direct ovarian effect of GnRH was demonstrated by Rippel and Johnson (322) who observed a decrease in hCG-augmented ovarian weight in immature hypophysectomized rats treated with GnRH. These findings were confirmed in hypophysectomized rats stimulated with PMSG (323) or FSH (324) and shown to be associated with inhibition of ovarian steroidogenesis (324).

In vitro studies demonstrated direct effects of GnRH on primary cultures of granulosa cells. These major effects are suppression of FSH-stimulated steroidogenesis, LH, and Prl receptors (309). The action on granulosa cell steroidogenesis is exerted at multiple sites: inhibition of FSH-stimulated cAMP production (325,326); protein kinase activation and labeling of type II cAMP-binding subunits of protein kinase (327); progesterone and estrogen production (324,328); inhibition of aromatase (329–331), 3β-hydroxysteroid dehydrogenase (332) and possibly the cholesterol side-chain cleavage enzyme (332); and stimulation of 20α-steroid dehydrogenase (333). The GnRH inhibition of FSH-enhanced steroidogenesis and LH and Prl receptor formation is blocked by concomitant treatment with GnRH antagonists (329,333–335). Likewise, the prostaglandin E_2-, cholera toxin-, and cAMP derivatives-stimulated estrogen production were all inhibited by GnRH (326,329,333,336,337).

The inhibitory action of GnRH on the ovary is exerted on other ovarian compartments in addition to the granulosa cells. Thus GnRH inhibits basal and LH-stimulated androgen synthesis by rat ovarian interstitial cells (338,339). Likewise, GnRH inhibits LH/hCG-stimulated progesterone secretion by rat luteal cells *in vitro* (328,340–342) or *in vivo* (342) and desensitizes the luteal LH receptors of cultured luteal cells within 24 hr (343). It seems that as in granulosa cells, GnRH does not interfere with LH binding in luteal cells but prevents the activation of adenylate cyclase. In intact luteal cells, unlike the granulosa cells, the inhibition of progesterone secretion by GnRH is reversed by dibutyryl cAMP (340,344).

Stimulatory Effects of GnRH on the Ovary

GnRH, given alone, stimulates some ovarian activities (13). Thus, GnRH stimulates granulosa cell production of estrogen, progesterone, 20α-hydroxyprogesterone, and prostaglandin and lactate (330–332,345–348). Nevertheless, the most consistent stimulatory action of GnRH on ovarian function is exerted on mature preovulatory follicles. GnRH induces ovulation in hypophysectomized rats

(349,350). This action of GnRH, but not of LH, was blocked by GnRH antagonists (351,352). Hence, GnRH or ovarian GnRH-like peptide is capable of mimicking LH action on ovulation, but does not seem to be involved in the mediation of LH action on ovulation. The action of GnRH on follicular rupture at ovulation seems to be related to its ability to stimulate *in vitro* granulosa cell and follicular prostaglandin (345,346,353), and plasminogen activator (354,355) synthesis, both involved in follicular rupture at ovulation (see H. Lipner, *this volume*). Thus, inhibitors of prostaglandins prevented the induction of ovulation by GnRH (351,352,356). Likewise, GnRH induced ovulation and stimulated progesterone secretion in perfused rat and rabbit ovaries, but it was much more effective in this respect in rat ovaries (357).

Explantation of preovulatory rat follicles *in vitro* allowed detailed analysis of GnRH effects. It induced resumption of ovum maturation, cumulus cell dispersion, and mucification and stimulated oocyte respiration (352,358,359). Unlike its effect on follicular rupture, the action of GnRH on the ovum is not prevented by indomethacin and hence does not seem to be mediated by follicular prostaglandin production (351). Recent studies indicate that the action of GnRH on ovum maturation involves protein kinase C. Thus, phospholipase C, phorbol ester, and diacylglycerol induced resumption of meiosis in follicle-enclosed oocytes and synergized with GnRH in this action (360). Furthermore, inhibitors of the lipoxygenase pathway of arachidonic acid inhibited the resumption of meiosis induced by GnRH, but not by LH, suggesting the involvement of this pathway in mediating GnRH action on ovum maturation (361). GnRH stimulated the accumulation in the medium of pregnenolone, progesterone, 20α-OH-progesterone, androstenedione, testosterone, and estradiol 17-β upon short incubation (up to 6–8 hr) of rat preovulatory follicles (362,363). While GnRH-induced accumulation of progestins continued beyond the initial 6 hr of incubation, androgen accumulation was reduced, in a similar pattern to that following stimulation with LH (363). GnRH mimicked several actions of LH on the rat preovulatory follicle, but not in all respects. Thus, the stimulatory effects of LH on steroidogenesis were expressed earlier and reached higher maximal response than with GnRH (363).

GnRH Binding and Mechanism of Action in the Ovary

Evidence for ovarian GnRH-binding sites was obtained by ovarian uptake of ^{125}I-GnRH analog *in vivo* in intact and hypophysectomized rats (364). Detailed *in vitro* studies led to the conclusion that GnRH exerts its gonadal actions via membrane receptors showing similar specificity and affinity for GnRH and its analogs as GnRH receptors in the anterior pituitary (310,365). Conclusive evidence for specific high affinity GnRH receptors has been obtained in granulosa and luteal cells (341,343,366–369). The number and affinity of GnRH receptors did not show conspicuous changes during the day, stage of the estrous cycle, or hypophysectomy, but the number of GnRH receptors in luteal membranes of cycling rats was half that of granulosa cells (368). Ovarian GnRH-binding sites are present already at the age of 10 days to reach a maximum on day 20 (370), and decline during early proestrous phase of puberty (371). Binding studies utilizing fluorescent derivative of GnRH revealed initial uniform distribution on granulosa cell surface followed by formation of patches and internalization (372). Photoaffinity labeling of ovarian GnRH receptors results in identification of two specific components with apparent MW of 60,000 and 54,000 daltons (315,372); since only the former component is present in the pituitary (373), the latter component of the ovarian receptors may be related to different and specific functions of GnRH in the ovary.

GnRH-binding sites decreased in PMSG- or FSH-treated rats after induction of ovulation by LH/hCG (366–368). By contrast, FSH maintains GnRH receptor content of granulosa cells *in vitro* (374) and GnRH *in vivo* may increase or decrease its own receptors, depending on the dose and time of treatment (367,368,374). Ovarian GnRH receptors do not seem to alter during the estrous cycle (341,375).

The earliest cellular response subsequent to GnRH binding to its ovarian receptor reported to date is an increase in phospholipid (phosphatidylinositol-PI and phosphatidic acid-PA) labeling in cultured granulosa and luteal cells (376–380). The effect could be demonstrated as early as 2 to 5 minutes after the addition of the agonist. The antigonadotropic action of GnRH in rat ovarian cells appears to be dependent and mediated by calcium (312,381,382). GnRH stimulated arachidonic acid release from prelabeled granulosa cells in culture (383). Thus, GnRH action on the ovary (as in the pituitary) may involve the recently described (384–386) mechanism integrating inositol phospholipid turnover, calcium mobilization, protein phosphorylation, and arachidonic acid metabolism in signal transduction (313,314). This is considered a major alternative pathway for peptide hormones which do not exert their action through cyclic nucleotide mediation (387). LH action on the ovary is exerted through the mediation of cAMP (388,389). By contrast, no clear-cut stimulatory effects of GnRH on ovarian cAMP production could be detected (345,353,390). It seems, therefore, that in spite of the fact that GnRH mimics the ovulation triggering action of LH, its action is mediated through different mechanism(s). In explanted rat preovulatory follicles, inhibitors of cyclooxygenase and lipoxygenase attenuated GnRH-induced progesterone synthesis and activity of plasminogen activator, but had no effect on these parameters when LH was added to the medium (355). Thus, it is possible that at least part of the actions of GnRH on the follicle are exerted through changes in arachidonic acid metabolism and its active metabolites. Further studies are required in order to define the precise molecular mechanisms involved in the stimulatory as well as the inhibitory actions of GnRH in ovarian cells.

Possible Role of GnRH in Ovarian Physiology

Ovarian GnRH-like Peptides

The evidence reviewed in the previous sections of GnRH reception and action in the ovary needs complementary evidence for local production in order to qualify as a paracrine/autocrine regulator of ovarian function. However, the evidence for ovarian production of GnRH or GnRH-like peptide is scanty at the present. The original report of ovarian GnRH-like peptide (391) could not be confirmed and was probably the result of contamination during purification (392). However, several studies reported the presence of a GnRH-like substance in porcine follicular fluid (393), ovaries (394), and rat ovaries (395). While these studies are suggestive of GnRH production in the ovary, more detailed reports and studies are needed for establishing this. Noteworthy are the more conclusive reports on GnRH-like peptide(s) in the male gonad (2) which may be indicative also for ovarian synthesis of a GnRH-like peptide.

GnRH Action and Reception in Different Species

Most of the studies on ovarian GnRH reception and action were performed in the rat. Hence, if GnRH plays a regulatory role in ovarian physiology, it is important to see whether these findings can be confirmed in other species too. Attempts to demonstrate high affinity ovarian GnRH receptors yielded, thus far, negative results in sheep, cow, and pig (396), monkey (397), and human (398), but low affinity receptors were demonstrated in human corpus luteum (399). Nevertheless, other studies have demonstrated direct effects of GnRH on the ovary of rabbit (357), pig (325), cow (400), monkey (312), and human (401) ovaries. In the two latter species, other authors under different experimental conditions did not observe any effects of GnRH agonists *in vitro* (402–405). Collectively, these studies attest to the fact that the rat is not the only species in which ovarian effects of GnRH could be demonstrated, but, at the same time, suggest that rat ovaries are by far more responsive to the agonists tested than other species. The failure to demonstrate high affinity binding sites in other species may be due to the poor ability of the labeled GnRH analogs used to interact with the gonadal GnRH-like peptide receptors in these species. In addition, even in the rat ovaries, the number of GnRH receptors is low and their demonstration posed many technical and methodological difficulties.

Physiological Attributes of GnRH Action on the Ovary

In general, the inhibitory effects of GnRH on nonluteal ovarian tissue make it likely that ovarian GnRH-like peptide may have a role in the regulation of follicular atresia. Furthermore, even some of GnRH stimulatory actions are compatible with such an atretogenic function. Thus, elevation of progestin secretion (prostesterone and 20α-hydroxyprogesterone) (*see above*) (406) and precocious maturation of the oocyte in preantral follicles (407) by GnRH may be indicative and associated with early atretic changes (26). In fact, the meiosis-inducing action of GnRH in immature, estrogen-primed hypophysectomized rats was limited to a subpopulation of atretic preantral follicles (408). The recent finding that antagonists of GnRH given concomitantly with FSH enhance its stimulatory action on follicular development and maturation of follicles to an ovulable stage (317) strongly supports the notion that an ovarian GnRH-like peptide is involved in the regulation of follicular development and follicle selection as a physiological atretic signal.

The inhibitory actions of GnRH on luteal cells are very similar to that of $PGF_{2\alpha}$, which serves as a natural luteolysin (405). Both GnRH and $PGF_{2\alpha}$ cause a rapid and marked increase in labelling of PA and PI of rat luteal cells in culture (379,380). Thus, it is possible that a GnRH-like peptide plays a physiological role in regulating corpus luteum function.

In terms of physiological function of an ovarian GnRH-like peptide, the ovulation-inducing actions of GnRH seem difficult to interpret. One possible interpretation is that GnRH-like peptides mediate LH action on the preovulatory follicle. Inasmuch as LH action on the ovary could not be blocked by antagonistic analogs of GnRH, whereas the action of GnRH was blocked by such drugs (351,352), makes this interpretation unlikely. Alternatively, it is possible that the vital role of ovulation in reproduction resulted in the development of several parallel triggering or amplifying mechanisms. The findings that GnRH acts through cAMP-independent pathways, whereas LH acts through cAMP, may be related to such a role, but at the present time there is no hard experimental evidence to support this notion. Nevertheless, it is possible that the action of GnRH on the preovulatory follicle is not physiological and is related to the ability of GnRH to activate arachidonic acid metabolism, which is also activated by LH and is involved in ovulation (H. Lipner, *this volume* and the section on GnRH binding and mechanism of action in the ovary). Further studies are required in order to distinguish between these alternative possibilities. In any case, GnRH has proved to be a powerful tool to probe into some of the normally obscured mechanisms of ovarian function.

OTHER PUTATIVE LOCAL REGULATORS OF OVARIAN FUNCTION

In this section the local regulatory actions in the ovary of hormones, neutrotransmitters, and factors known from nonreproductive organs and tissues will be described. The list of such factors implicated in ovarian function by their action *in vivo* or *in vitro* is growing rapidly. Nevertheless, the scarcity of data supporting these claims by demonstrating their ovarian production and reception made it very difficult to decide which hormones or factors to include as ovarian regulators. Hence it seems very likely that future research will extend the list of hormones included here, whereas some of these included will not withstand rigorous examination by the criteria set for local ovarian regulators. Also, enzymes or constitutive molecules were not included in this review, even if they may assume important functions in ovarian physiology. Thus, for example, plasminogen activator which plays a central role in follicular rupture at ovulation (see H. Lipner, *this volume*) (409) or proteoglycans with their putative regulatory functions (410,411) and similar substances were not included. The role of relaxin as ovarian regulator is discussed elsewhere by H. Lipner (*this volume*) and O.D. Sherwood (*this volume*).

Neurotransmitters

Role of Catecholamines

The recent studies demonstrating biosynthesis of norepinephrine (NE) from its precursor tyrosine by ovarian slices (412) and explanted follicles (413), coupled with previous demonstration of its ovarian receptors (414–421) and actions (414–416,418,422–435) in the ovary, justify inclusion of catecholamines among ovarian regulators.

Most of the initial studies regarding the ovarian role of adrenergic agents were concerned with their involvement in ovulation and compensatory ovarian hypertrophy (436). Such studies did not bring forward convincing evidence for the role of catecholamines in ovulation (437–440). However, these studies may be complicated by possible ingrowth of adrenergic nerves accompanying revascularization (441–443) and by local production of catecholamines. Furthermore, recently an increase in sensitivity of ovarian cells to adrenergic agents was associated with ovarian denervation (444). Likewise, culture of granulosa cells in the absence of catecholamines increased very much their sensitivity to adrenergic stimuli, whereas addition of catecholamines down-regulated adrenergic receptors. It was suggested, therefore, that the adrenergic tone *in vivo* and *in vitro* may modulate ovarian cell responsiveness to adrenergic stimuli (444).

Local treatment of rat ovary with 6-hydroxydopamine (chemical sympathectomy) increased contralateral ovarian weight, and after unilateral ovariectomy the treatment of the remaining ovary prevented compensatory changes in that ovary (445,446). As unilateral ovariectomy and the resulting compensatory ovarian hypertrophy were associated with increased uptake of ^{3}H-lysine and ^{3}H-uridine into the contralateral hypothalamic arcuate nucleus (447), the existence of a gonadal-hypothalamic neural axis or neural reflex mechanism necessary for the development of the hypotrophy was postulated (447). Nevertheless, in guinea pigs, a species with dense ovarian adrenergic innervation, chemical sympathectomy did not cause hypertrophy in the contralateral ovary, nor did 6-hydroxydopamine prevent hypertrophy of the remaining ovary (448). These species differences may be related to the varying density of ovarian adrenergic nerves. Sympathectomy somewhat impaired follicular development in mice (449) and guinea pigs (448,450). It is likely that ovarian catecholamines modulate follicular growth and response to gonadotropins, but the precise nature of its actions remains obscure.

The presence of β-adrenergic receptors in the ovary of immature rats, in both granulosa cells and residual tissue compartments, has been demonstrated (418). The concentration of these receptors increases between the late juvenile period and the morning of first proestrus and then decreases markedly at the first preovulatory surge of gonadotropins. Furthermore, adrenergic agonists elicit only a small increase in progesterone and marked increase in aromatizable androgens prior to ovulation. After ovulation, the action of the adrenergic agonist on progesterone release was enhanced and on adrogens was reduced (418). Both, ovarian content and biosynthesis of norepinephrine increased remarkably during the juvenile period (days 25–30) of rats (412). These data prompted Ojeda and Aguado (444) to suggest a modulatory action of catecholamines in prepubertal ovarian function. Nevertheless, bilateral section of the superior ovarian nerve 24 days of age did not alter the time of vaginal opening or of first ovulation (444). The superior ovarian nerve travels along the suspensory ligament and is one source of rat ovarian innervation, the other being the plexus nerve accompanying the ovarian artery.

By the use of double isotope radioenzymatic assay, a significant depletion of ovarian catecholamines following PMSG-treatment of immature rats was observed (451). The norepinephrine content of Graafian follicles is markedly reduced within 4 hr after the preovulatory surge of gonadotropins. FSH, rather than LH or prolactin, seems to be responsible for follicular norepinephrine depletion (452,453). Catecholamines have been identified in porcine (454) and human (455) follicular fluid. Recently, follicular fluid catecholamine content was assayed throughout porcine estrous cycle; NE concentrations remained constant during the luteal phase (days 1–15; 1.7 ± 0.2 ng/ml FF1), but were elevated significantly during the follicular phase (days 16–20; 2.9 ± 0.4 ng/ml); epinephrine had a similar pattern, but at much lower concentrations. In contrast, serum NE and epinephrine concentrations did not change during the luteal and follicular stages of the cycle (456).

Ovarian adenylate cyclase activation by catecholamines has been demonstrated. Studies in the pig (423), rabbit (432,457), and rat (434,458–461) agree that follicular tissues are relatively insensitive to catecholamines, whereas corpora lutea or its cells respond readily with enhanced adenylate cyclase activity.

In granulosa cells isolated from immature hypophysectomized-estrogen-treated rats addition of FSH stimulates the acquisition of responsiveness to catecholamines in terms of progesterone production within 2 days (430). In PMSG-treated rats, LH rather than FSH seems to induce responsiveness more effectively to catecholamines in terms of adenylate cyclase activation and progesterone secretion (434,462). That the development of rat granulosa cell responsiveness to catecholamines *in vivo* is dependent upon hormonal stimulation (FSH, LH, and prostaglandins) is commonly accepted; thus hypophysectomy or administration of indomethacin prevented the development of responsiveness to catecholamines by granulosa cells (460). By contrast, spontaneous development of catecholamine receptors and responsiveness in granulosa cells cultured *in vitro* for 2 days in serum containing or serum devoid media was observed (416,460). Likewise, Orly et al. (462) noted an increase in responsiveness of rat granulosa cells to catecholamines in serum- and hormone-free media. Conversely, other studies demonstrated that *in vitro* too, responsiveness to catecholamines is hormone dependent (430,434). It is very difficult to explain these disparate results, since no obvious differences in the experimental protocol or culture conditions can be pointed out. Therefore, understanding the role of gonadotropins and the biochemical mechanisms mediating their action in inducing responsiveness to catecholamines must await additional studies.

Catecholamine stimulation of corpus luteum progesterone secretion has been demonstrated in the rat (428,429, 433,458,460), rabbit (427,432,455,463,464), ewe (426), and cow (422,425). The action of catecholamines to enhance progesterone accumulation is attributed, in part, to their reduction of 20α-SDH activity (431) and, in part, to enhanced pregnenolone production and stimulation of 3β-SDH activity (465).

The luteotrophic action of catecholamines on the corpus luteum was found to be enhanced between day 2 and 4 and thereafter luteal response declines (461), which seems to be associated with changes in the content of adrenergic receptors (421). $PGF_{2\alpha}$, which exerts a luteolytic action in aging corpora lutea (466–469), inhibited the leuteotrophic effect of epinephrine. This action, too, was dependent on the age of the corpus luteum: 1-day-old corpora lutea were not affected by $PGF_{2\alpha}$, whereas in 3-day-old ones $PGF_{2\alpha}$ inhibited the stimulatory action of epinephrine on tissue levels of cAMP and production of progesterone (470).

In addition to the steroidogenic effects of adrenergic agents on luteinized granulosa cells and corpora lutea, stimulatory actions were also observed in interfollicular tissues of the rat. Thus, stimulation of the neural plexus in hypophysectomized rats caused interstitial cells to develop morphological features of steroidogenically active cells (471). Likewise, adrenergic agents enhance hCG-induced rise in androgen secretion by ovarian theca-interstitial cells (435).

The studies reviewed seem to suggest a modulatory role of adrenergic agents in follicular development and corpus luteum function. However, conflicting data and several paradoxical observations make it very difficult at this time to draw a comprehensive mechanistic outline of the physiological role of adrenergic agents in ovarian function. This will probably be achieved by additional studies in the future.

γ-Aminobutyric Acid

γ-Aminobutyric acid (GABA) is known as the major inhibitory neurotransmitter in the mammalian central nervous system (472). High GABA levels, comparable to those in the brain, have recently been demonstrated in the ovary (473–475). Ovarian GABA concentration and content increased during days 3 to 14 of pregnancy and were diminished on day 21 (476). Furthermore, the ovarian levels of glutamic acid decarboxylase, the primary enzyme responsible for GABA biosynthesis in the brain, correlate well with endogenous GABA concentrations (475,477,478). But in contrast to the high levels of GABA and its synthesizing enzyme in the whole ovary, both GABA and the enzyme are undetectable in granulosa cell preparations (475). Furthermore, ovarian glutamic acid decarboxylase was not precipitated by an antibody directed against the rat neuronal enzyme (479). It was concluded, therefore, that ovarian GABA should not be taken as evidence for GABAergic innervation. In addition, the relatively low enzyme activity measured in the ovary may be artefactual and be formed indirectly from glutamate (479).

GABA-binding sites were described in ovarian tissue (477,478,480–482) and granulosa cells (475). Thus, granulosa cells have specific high affinity binding sites but do not contain GABA or GABA-biosynthesizing enzyme. The demonstrations of ovarian production and specific binding of GABA suggest a modulatory action of GABA in the ovary. Intrabursal administration of GABA to pseudopregnant rats increased ovarian blood flow, enhanced estradiol 17β release, and decreased progesterone secretion (483). Additional studies are needed for evaluating the physiological role of GABA in ovarian function.

Vasoactive Intestinal Peptide (VIP)

VIP and VIPergic nerve fibers were described in the ovarian stroma of laboratory animals and human ovaries (484–486), and even occasional association with antral follicles was noted in immature rat ovaries (487). Furthermore, in our unpublished studies using very high specific activity labeled VIP gene fragments (488) as hybridization probes on ovarian RNA (489), we have located VIP encoding mRNA in ovarian tissues (I. Gozes and A. Tsafriri, *unpublished data*) which may suggest the presence of VIP-synthesizing cells within the ovary.

VIP actions on immature rat granulosa cells have been reported. VIP enhanced both progestin and estrogen production *in vitro* by granulosa cells of hypophysectomized estrogen-treated rats. This effect was, at least partially, exerted through cAMP-mediated mechanisms and entailed increased availability of pregnenolone, stimulation of 3β-HSD, and decrease in 20α-HSD activities and stimulation of aromatase (490). Upon separation of granulosa cells on Metrizamide density gradient, VIP preferentially stimulated steroid production in cells with lower density as compared with FSH which stimulated steroidogenesis in cells with the highest density (491). Similar results were obtained in granulosa cells of intact immature rats, VIP enhanced progesterone release from cells explanted from infantile (12 day old), juvenile (30 day old), and peripubertal rats, whereas estradiol release was stimulated by VIP during the two latter developmental stages and reached maximum during proestrus phases of puberty (487).

These initial studies, indicating VIP production and action in ovarian tissues, should be complemented with more studies in order to assess the possible modulatory role of VIP or VIPergic nerves in ovarian function.

Other Neurotransmitters

Studies using retrograde transport of horseradish peroxidase demonstrated vagal ovarian innervation (492). Abdominal vagotomy, which does not affect adrenergic innervation, decreases steroid secretion (493) and delays onset of puberty (494). These studies make it reasonable to assume that additional neurotransmitters may be involved in modulating ovarian activity.

Recently, substance P-containing fibers have been observed by immunohistofluorescence in juvenile and prepubertal rat ovaries. These fibers were closely associated with the theca externa of antral follicles, interstitial tissue, and tunica adventitia of small blood vessels (495). Substance P was found in ovaries of mature hamsters (496) and in prepubertal rats (497). Nevertheless, addition of substance P to cultured granulosa cells had no effect on their steroidogenic activity, and hence involvement in the regulation of ovarian blood flow was suggested (487,497).

Neurohypophyseal Hormones

The role of oxytocin in luteal regression in ruminants through its action of the uterus has recently been reviewed (498) (G.D. Niswender and T.M. Nett, *this volume*) and as such is not a local ovarian regulator. Nevertheless, recently follicular production of oxytocin in human (499) and bovine (500,501) follicular tissues was demonstrated. In the human and rat, luteal oxytocin levels are considered as too low to allow for extragonadal actions (502,503). Evidence has been presented to suggest that oxytocin affects follicular development in the mouse (504). In ovine corpora lutea only the large cells contain oxytocin (505). Conversely, oxytocin inhibits LH-stimulated progesterone secretion from small cells of ovine corpus luteum (506), thus suggesting the presence of oxytocin receptors in small cells and supporting a paracrine role for oxytocin in ovine corpus luteum. Oxytocin at high concentration inhibited basal and hCG-stimulated steroidogenesis in bovine and human luteal cells, while at low concentration it stimulated basal steroidogenesis (507,508). By contrast, oxytocin had no effect on progesterone and cAMP production of rat luteal cells in culture (509).

Arginine vasopressin was found in human ovaries and follicular fluid at concentrations significantly higher than in serum (499,510–513), suggesting local production. Arginine vasopressin was also demonstrated in rat and sheep ovaries (514,515), including demonstration of vasopressin-neurophysin II gene expression in the ovary (516). However, at the present, it is very difficult to base any conclusions regarding the local regulatory role of neurohypophyseal hormones in ovarian function on this evidence.

Proopiomelanocortin-Derived Hormones

Proopiomelanocortin (POMC) is a known precursor for a variety of peptide hormones including ACTH, MSHs, lipotropins, and β-endorphin. Immunostainable β-endorphin was demonstrated in rat corpora lutea (517) and in porcine follicular fluid (518). Immunostaining of POMC-derived peptides was predominantly associated with corpora lutea of cycling and pregnant mouse ovaries; weak staining was present also in the ovarian interstitium of 15- and 24-day-old mice but not in follicles and ovaries of mouse embryos (519). Likewise, ovine granulosa cells luteinizing in culture secreted POMC-derived peptides (520). Administration of PMSG to immature mice markedly increases immunostainable β-endorphin in both the follicles and interstitium. By contrast, treatment with hCG/LH stimulated β-endorphin-like staining only in the ovarian interstitium (521,522). Immunoreactive β-endorphin was located also in adult rat ovaries in luteal, granulosa, and interstitial cells. Furthermore, ovarian immunoreactive β-endorphin levels were the lowest at estrus and significantly raised in stepwise manner over metestrus and diestrus to a peak at proestrus (523). Using rat pituitary POMC cDNA as a hybridization probe, POMC-like mRNA was identified in ovaries of the rat, mouse, and monkey. Furthermore, expression of ovarian POMC gene, as revealed by hybridization with POMC cDNA, was increased following PMSG treatment of immature rats or by pregnancy (524).

Thus, the ovaries like other steroidogenic organs, such as the adrenal and the testis, contain POMC, and its ovarian production is regulated by gonadotropins. At present we do not have any clues regarding the physiological role of POMC-derived peptides in ovarian physiology.

Adenosine and Other Purines

In the above sections on ovum maturation, the putative role of purine and pyrimidine bases in the regulation of meiosis has been discussed.

Adenosine and other purines have been shown to enhance gonadotropin-stimulated cAMP accumulation in rat granulosa and luteal cells (525–528) and in periovulatory human granulosa cells (527). Adenosine exerted both stimulatory and inhibitory effects. Thus, acute stimulation with adenosine resulted in amplification of FSH-stimulated cAMP production during the first 6 to 20 hr of culture. During the second 24 hr of culture adenosine inhibited FSH-induced responses such as cAMP and progesterone production and expression of FSH and LH receptors (529). In rat luteal cells adenosine also enhances LH-stimulated progesterone synthesis. Adenosine amplification of cAMP and progesterone is a function of corpus luteum age, decreasing from days 4 to 11. Furthermore, adenosine antagonizes the luteolytic actions of $PGF_{2\alpha}$ (530). These effects of adenosine led to the suggestion that adenosine may play a modulatory role in the ovary (531).

Granulosa cell ATP levels were rapidly and markedly increased by adenosine (528,531–533). This effect of adenosine occurred in the absence and presence of gonadotropins (533). By contrast, gonadotropins suppressed granulosa cell ATP levels both in cultures containing and devoid of adenosine (528,534). The finding that adenosine enhanced LH-dependent cAMP to a greater extent than that stimulated by FSH led to the suggestion that adenosine may function as a promoter of follicular atresia (534).

Adenosine may be involved in adenylate cyclase activity in two principal ways: direct regulation of enzyme activity via membranal adenosine receptors (535) and as a substrate to the enzyme by conversion to ATP (536). Adenosine receptors have been demonstrated in testicular cells (537–539), and evidence for granulosa cell adenosine receptors has been presented (540). The suggested role of adenosine as local ovarian regulator should be confirmed by demonstration of specific receptors on ovarian cells and by clarification of the physiological role of adenosine in ovarian activity. The putative actions of adenosine include mediation of atresia, promotion and maintenance of corpora lutea, and regulation of oocyte maturation (534).

Eicosanoids

The role of arachidonic acid metabolites in ovarian physiology, and especially in follicular rupture at ovulation and in corpus luteum development and demise, is detailed in H. Lipner (*this volume*) and G. D. Niswender and T. M. Nett (*this volume*).

Here the role of eicosanoids, products of C_{20} fatty acids (541), as local ovarian regulators will be outlined in brief. Ample evidence for ovarian production and action of products of the cyclooxygenase has been presented (542–545). Recently, the activity of ovarian lipoxygenase has been demonstrated. Ovarian and follicular lipoxygenase activity was enhanced by LH/hCG stimulation *in vivo* or *in vitro* (546,547). Furthermore, inhibitors of lipoxygenase prevented follicular rupture dose-dependently (546,547). Inhibitors of both pathways of arachidonic acid metabolism, namely of cyclooxygenase and lipoxygenase, did not affect follicular plasminogen activator, but prevented LH-induced increase in ovarian collagenolytic activity (548). Prostaglandins have been implicated in paracrine regulation of cumulus expansion (549,550). Thus, cumulus cells cocultured with granulosa cells or in a granulosa cell conditioned medium underwent cumulus expansion. Addition of cyclooxygenase inhibitors to the granulosa cell cultures prevented the action of conditioned media on cumulus expansion, whereas they did not prevent expansion of cumuli in response to hormonal stimuli (551). The evidence for arachidonic acid metabolite receptors in ovarian tissue is much more limited. Nevertheless, the clear effects of these metabolites on ovarian function and their production in the ovary justify considering eicosanoids as local ovarian hormones. Further studies aimed at localization of ovarian receptors of eicosanoids and elucidation of cellular and molecular mechanisms underlying their involvement in follicular rupture and corpus luteum function are definitely required.

CONCLUSIONS

Throughout this review we have considered a multitude of ovarian paracrine/autocrine hormones. Nevertheless, the story of local ovarian regulation is probably, to a large measure, unknown as yet. This underlies the steadily increasing number of reports on new putative ovarian regulators and the additional data on previously described ones. This is one of the reasons why a comprehensive overview of local regulation of ovarian function was presented here, rather than a critical evaluation of each system. The data available at the present do not allow, in too many instances, a profound assessment. Another reason for the approach adopted is the implication of local regulators in a broad spectrum of ovarian activities, far beyond the area of the author's own research interests. In spite of the intent to include any local regulators, some have been overlooked due to the author's unawareness, the scarcity of information, and difficulty of fitting them into proper perspective. Thus, for example, a nonidentified low-molecular ovarian substance was demonstrated to induce steroidogenesis in cultured granulosa cells (552); melatonin was found to directly stimulate progesterone secretion in cultured granulosa cells (553); somatostatin-like immunoreactivity was detected in porcine ovaries (554); and synthetic somatostatin inhibited the spontaneous maturation of porcine oocytes in culture (556).

Most of the cell types considered regarding their ovarian regulatory function were those also having clear endocrine functions, granulosa, theca, and interstitial cells. The close proximity of additional cells in the ovary, such as fibroblasts, macrophages, and mast cells, suggests that they also participate in paracrine regulation of ovarian activity. Indeed, alterations in ovarian histamine concentration (555,557) and mast cell degranulation (558) were observed after the preovulatory surge of gonadotropins. Likewise, peritoneal macrophages (559) or their extract (560) increased progesterone secretion by mice granulosa cells in culture, and pelvic macrophages stimulated progesterone secretion by human granulosa cells *in vitro* (561). These studies provide a basis for further search for the participation of additional cell types in ovarian paracrine control.

Finally, the very wide spectrum of agents modulating ovarian activity warrants special notice. Ovarian cells have both intracellular and plasma membrane receptors. On the basis of the mode of signal transduction, membranal receptors are classified into four subtypes: (a) receptors regulating cyclic AMP formation; (b) receptors modulating intracellular calcium levels through hydrolysis of phosphatidylinositol phosphates and formation of diacylglycerol and inositol phosphates; (c) receptors possessing tyrosine kinase activity and assumed to act on cellular metabolism through this activity; and (d) receptors serving as ion channels, which upon interaction with their ligands, allow specific flux of ions through the plasma membrane and thereby trigger electrophysiological responses (562). Thus, on the basis of the studies reviewed, membranal receptors of ovarian cells may utilize all four known modes of signal transduction. This wide spectrum of ovarian reception mechanisms, the integrated and well-concerted function of several cell types, and the multitude of endocrine, paracrine, and autocrine mechanisms involved in ovarian physiology warrant continued interest. This may lead to new insights into ovarian biology and also form the basis for novel approaches to fertility regulation in the human and in animal husbandry.

ACKNOWLEDGMENTS

The meticulous secretarial help of Mrs. M. Kopelowitz is gratefully acknowledged. I am indebted to numerous colleagues working in this field who have generously provided published and unpublished papers; their help is most appreciated. I thank Dr. K. Ahrën, Dr. H. Billig, Dr. N. Dekel, Dr. G. S. DiZerega, Dr. E. Hazum, Dr. A. M. Kaye, Dr. Y. Koch, Dr. F. Ledwitz-Rigby, Dr. Z. Naor, Dr. L. E. Reichert, Dr. D. N. Ward, and Dr. U. Zor for their helpful comments on the manuscript. Special thanks are due to my students, past and present, S. Bar-Ami, R.H. Braw, R. Reich, and A. O. Abisogun, whose unquenched thirst for knowledge was a prime motivator and the Mrs. R. Slager and Mrs. A. Tsafriri for their expert and devoted technical help. The studies in the author's laboratory were supported by grants from the United States–Israel Binational Science Foundation (BSF), Jerusalem, and United States–Israel Binational Agricultural Research and Development Fund (BARD) and was written in part during residency at the Rockefeller Foundation Bellagio Study and Conference Center.

REFERENCES

1. Channing, C. P., Anderson, L. D., Hoover, D. J., Kolena, J., Osteen, K. G., Pomerantz, S. H., and Tanabe, K. (1982): The role of non-steroidal regulators in control of oocyte and follicular maturation. *Recent Progr. Horm. Res.*, 38:331–408.
2. Sharpe, R. M. (1984): Bibliography on intragonadal hormones. *Bibliogr. Reprod.*, 44:C1–C16.
3. Franchimont, P., and Channing, C. P., eds. (1981): *Intragonadal Regulation of Reproduction*, Academic Press, London.
4. Channing, C. P., and Segal, S. J., eds. (1982): *Intraovarian Control Mechanisms*, Plenum Press, New York.
5. Fujii, T. and Channing, C. P., eds. (1981): *Non-Steroidal Regulators in Reproductive Biology and Medicine*, Pergamon Press, Ltd., Oxford.
6. Sairam, M. R., and Atkinson, L. E., eds. (1984): *Gonadal Proteins and Peptides and Their Biological Significance*, World Scientific Publishing Co., Pte Ltd., Singapore.
7. Franchimont, P., ed. (1986): *Clinics in Endocrinology and Metabolism*, Vol. 15, No. 1, W. B. Saunders Co. Ltd., London.
8. Witschi, E. (1921): Der Hermaphroditismus der Frösche und seine Bedentung für das Geschlechts problem und Lehre von der inneren Sekretion der Keindrüsen. *Arch. Entwicklungmech. Org.*, 49:316–358.
9. Witschi, E. (1968): Biochemistry of sex differentiation in vertebrate embryos. In: *Biochemistry of Sex Differentiation in Vertebrate Embryos*, Vol. 2, edited by R. Weber, pp. 193–225. New York, Academic Press.
10. Parkes, A. S. (1966): The rise of reproductive endocrinology, 1926–1940. *J. Endocrin.*, 34:xx–xxxii.
11. Marrian, G. F. (1966): Early work on the chemistry of pregnanediol and the oestrogenic hormones. *J. Endocrin.*, 35:vi–xvi.
12. Greep, R. O. (1967): The saga and the science of the gonadotrophins. *J. Endocrin.*, 39:ii–ix.
13. Hsueh, A. J. W., Adashi, E. Y., Jones, P. B. C., and Welsh, T. H. (1984): Hormonal regulation of the differentiation of cultured granulosa cells. *Endocrine Rev.*, 5:76–127.
14. Starling, E. H. (1905): The Croonian Lectures. *Lancet*, 26:579–583.
15. Roth, J., LeRoith, D., Schiloach, J., and Rabinowitz, C. (1984): Hormones and other messenger molecules. In: *Hormonal Control of the Hypothalamo-Pituitary-Gonadal Axis*, edited by K. W. McKerns, and Z. Naor, pp. 71–87. Plenum Press, New York.
16. Roth, J., LeRoith, D., Schiloach, J., and Rubinovitz, C. (1983): Intercellular communication: an attempt at a unifying hypothesis. *Clin. Res.*,31:354–363.
17. Medawar, P. (1953): Some immunological and endocrinological problems raised by the evolution of viviparity in vertebrates. *Symp. Soc. Exp. Biol. Med.*, 7:320–338.
18. Niall, H. D. (1982): The evolution of peptide hormones. *Ann. Rev. Physiol.*, 44:615–624.
19. Feyrter, F. (1938): Über die peripheren endokrinen (parakrinen). *Drüsen des Menschen*. Ambrosius Barth, Leipzig.
20. Dockray, G. J. (1979): Evolutionary relationships of the gut hormones. *Fed. Proc.*, 38:2295–2301.
21. Sporn, M. B., and Todaro, G. J. (1980): Autocrine secretion of malignant transformation of cells. *N. Engl. J. Med.*, 303: 878–880.
22. Grossman, M. I. (1979): Chemical messengers: a view from the gut. *Federation Proc.*, 38:2341–2343.
23. Guillemin, R. (1978): Peptides of the brain: The new endocrinology of the neuron. *Science*, 202:390–402.
24. O'Malley, B. W. (1984): President's letter: endocrinology in the 1990's. *Endoc. Soc. Newsl.*, 9:1–2.
25. Ayalon, D., Tsafriri, A., Lindner, H. R., Cordova, T., and Harell, A. (1972): Serum gonadotrophin levels in pro-oestrous rats in relation to the resumption of meiosis by the oocytes. *J. Reprod. Fertil.*, 31:51–58.
26. Tsafriri, A., and Braw, R. (1984): Experimental approaches to atresia in mammals. *Oxford Rev. Reprod. Biol.*, 6:226–265.
27. Byskov, A. G. (1979): Regulation of meiosis in mammals. *Ann. Biol. Anim. Biochim. Biophys.*, 19:1251–1261.
28. Ohno, S., and Smith, J. B. (1964): Role of fetal follicular cells in meiosis of mammalian oocytes. *Cytogenetics*, 3:324–333.

29. Moor, R. M., and Trounson, A. O. (1977): Hormonal and follicular factors affecting maturation of sheep oocytes *in vitro* and their subsequent developmental capacity. *J. Reprod. Fertil.*, 49:101–109.
30. Moor, R. M., Polge, C., and Willadsen, S. M. (1980): Effect of follicular steroids on the maturation and fertilization of mammalian oocytes. *J. Embryol. Exp. Morph.*, 56:319–335.
31. Crosby, I. M., Osborn, J. C., and Moor, R. M. (1981): Follicle cell regulation of protein synthesis and developmental competence in sheep oocytes. *J. Reprod. Fertil.*, 62:572–582.
32. Vermeiden, J. P. W., and Zeilmaker, G. H. (1974): Relationship between maturation, division, ovulation and luteinization in the female rat. *Endocrinology*, 95:341–351.
33. Magnusson, C., Hillensjö, T., Tsafriri, A., Hultborn, R., and Ahrén, K. (1977): Oxygen consumption of maturing rat oocytes. *Biol. Reprod.*, 17:9–15.
34. Pincus, G., and Enzmann, E. V. (1935): The comparative behaviour of mammalian eggs *in vivo* and *in vitro*. *J. Exp. Med.*, 62:655–675.
35. Biggers, J. D. (1972): Metabolism of the oocyte. In: *Oogenesis*, edited by J. D. Biggers and A. W. Schuetz, pp. 241–251. University Park Press, Baltimore.
36. Tsafriri, A. (1978): Oocyte maturation in mammals. In: *The Vertebrate Ovary*, edited by R. E. Jones, pp. 409–433, Plenum, New York.
37. Szybek, K. (1972): *In vitro* maturation of oocytes from sexually immature mice. *J. Endocrinol.*, 54:527–528.
38. Sorensen, R. A., and Wassarman, P. M. (1976): Relationship between growth and meiotic maturation of mouse oocyte. *Dev. Biol.*, 50:532–536.
39. Bar-Ami, S., and Tsafriri, A. (1981): Acquisition of meiotic competence in the rat: role of gonadotropin and estrogen. *Gamete Res.*, 4:463–472.
40. Bar-Ami, S., Nimrod, A., Brodie, A. M. H., and Tsafriri, A. (1983): Role of FSH and oestradiol-17β in the development of meiotic competence in rat oocytes. *J. Steroid Biochem.*, 19:965–971.
41. Tsafriri, A., Lindner, H. R., Zor, U., and Lamprecht, S. A. (1972): *In vitro* induction of meiotic division in follicle-enclosed rat oocytes by LH, cyclic AMP and prostaglandin E_2. *J. Reprod. Fertil.*, 31:39–50.
42. Neal, P., and Baker, T. G. (1973): Response of mouse ovaries *in vivo* and in organ culture to pregnant mare's serum gonadotrophin and human chorionic gonadotrophin. I. Examination of critical time intervals. *J. Reprod. Fertil.*, 33:399–410.
43. Hillensjö, T. (1976): Oocyte maturation and glycolysis in isolated pre-ovulatory follicles of PMS-injected immature rats. *Acta Endocr. Copenh.*, 82:809–830.
44. Thibault, C., and Gerard, M. (1973): Cytoplasmic and nuclear maturation of rabbit oocytes *in vitro*. *Ann. Biol. Anim. Biochim. Biophys.* 13:145–155.
45. Thibault, C. (1977): Are follicular maturation and oocyte maturation independent processes? *J. Reprod. Fertil.*, 51:1–15.
46. Meinecke, B., and Meinecke-Tillman, S. (1981): Induction and inhibition of meiotic maturation of follicle-enclosed porcine oocytes *in vivo*. *Theriogenology*, 216:205–209.
47. Chang, M. C. (1955): The maturation of rabbit oocytes in culture and their maturation, activation, fertilization and subsequent development in Fallopian tube. *J. Exp. Zool.*, 128:378–399.
48. Foote, W. E., and Thibault, C. (1969): Recherches experimentales sur la maturation *in vitro* des ovocytes de truie et de veau. *Ann. Biol. Anim. Biochim. Biophys.*, 9:329–349.
49. Tsafriri, A., and Channing, C. P. (1975): Inhibitory influence of granulosa cells and follicular fluid upon porcine oocyte meiosis *in vitro*. *Endocrinology*, 96:922–927.
50. Leibfried, L., and First, N. L. (1980): Follicular control of meiosis in the porcine oocyte. *Biol. Reprod.*, 23:705–709.
51. Leibfried, L., and First, N. L. (1980): Effect of bovine and porcine follicular fluid and granulosa cells on maturation of oocytes *in vitro*. *Biol. Reprod.*, 23:699–704.
52. Downs, S. M., and Eppig, J. J. (1984): Cyclic adenosine monophosphate and ovarian follicular fluid act synergistically to inhibit mouse oocyte maturation. *Endocrinology*, 114:418–427.
53. Tsafriri, A. (1985): The control of meiotic maturation in mammals. In: *Biology of Fertilization*, Vol. 1, edited by C. B. Metz, and A. Monroy, pp. 221–252. Academic Press, New York.
54. Tsafriri, A., and Pomerantz, S. H. (1984): The control of ovum maturation in mammals: comparative aspects. In: *Gonadal Peptides and Their Biological Significance*, edited by M. R. Sairam, and L. E. Atkinson, pp. 191–206. World Scientific Publishing Co., Singapore.
55. Tsafriri, A., and Pomerantz, S. M. (1986): Oocyte maturation inhibitor. *Clin. Endocrinol. Metab.*, 15:157–170.
56. Fleming, A. D., Kuehl, T. J., and Armstrong, D. T. (1985): Maturation of pig and rat oocytes transplanted into surrogate pig follicles *in vitro*. *Gamete Res.*, 11:107–119.
57. Sato, E., and Ishibashi, T. (1977): Meiotic arresting action of the substance obtained from cell surface of porcine ovarian granulosa cells. *Jpn. J. Zootech. Sci.*, 48:22–26.
58. Centola, G. M., Anderson, L. D., and Channing, C. P. (1981): Oocyte maturation inhibitor (OMI) activity in porcine granulosa cells. *Gamete Res.*, 4:451–461.
59. Tsafriri, A., Channing, C. P., Pomerantz, S. H., and Lindner, H. R. (1977): Inhibition of maturation of isolated rat oocytes by porcine follicular fluid. *J. Endocrinol.*, 75:285–291.
60. Tsafriri, A. (1979): Mammalian oocyte maturation: model systems and their physiological relevance. In: *Ovarian Follicular and Corpus Luteum Function*, edited by C. P. Channing, J. M. Marsh, and W. A. Sadler, pp. 269–281. Plenum, New York.
61. Tsafriri, A., Pomerantz, S. H., and Channing, C. P. (1976): Follicular control of oocyte maturation. In: *Ovulation in the Human*, edited by P. G. Crosignani, and D. R. Mishell, pp. 31–39. Academic Press, New York.
62. Sato, E., Ishibashi, T., and Iritani, A. (1982): Meiotic arresting substance separated from porcine ovarian granulosa cells and hypothetical arresting mechanism of meiosis. In: *Intraovarian Control Mechanisms*, edited by C. P. Channing and S. Segal, pp. 161–173. Plenum Press, New York.
63. Sato, E., and Koide, S. S. (1984): A factor from bovine granulosa cells preventing oocyte maturation. *Differentiation*, 26:59–62.
64. Anderson, L. D., Stone, S. L., and Channing, C. P. (1985): Influence of hormones on the inhibitory activity of oocyte maturation present in conditioned media of porcine granulosa cells. *Gamete Res.*, 12:119–130.
65. Gwatkin, R. B. L., and Andersen, O. F. (1976): Hamster oocyte maturation *in vitro* inhibition by follicular components. *Life Sci.*, 19:527–536.
66. Hillensjö, T., Batta, S. K., Schwartz-Kripner, A., Wentz, A. C., Sulewski, J., and Channing, C. P. (1978): Inhibitory effect of human follicular fluid upon the maturation of porcine oocytes in culture. *J. Clin. Endocrin. Metab.*, 47:1332–1335.
67. Jagiello, G., Graffeo, J., Ducayen, M., and Prosser, R. (1977): Further studies of inhibitors of *in vitro* mammalian oocyte maturation. *Fertil. Steril.*, 28:476–481.
68. van de Wiel, D. F. M., Bar-Ami, S., Tsafriri, A., and de Jong, F. H. (1983): Oocyte maturation inhibitor, inhibin, and steroid concentrations in porcine follicular fluid at various stages of the oestrous cycle. *J. Reprod. Fertil.*, 68:247–252.
69. Channing, C. P., Liu, C. O., Jones, G. S., and Jones, H. (1983): Decline in follicular oocyte maturation inhibitor coincident with maturation and achievement of fertilizability of oocytes recovered at midcycle of gonadotropin-treated women. *Proc. Natl. Acad. Sci. U.S.A.*, 80:4184–4188.
70. Hillensjö, T., Brännström, M., Chari, S., Daume, E., Magnusson, C., Nilsson, L., Sjögren, A., and Törnel, J. (1985): Oocyte maturation as regulated by follicular factors. *Ann. N.Y. Acad. Sci.*, 442:73–79.
71. Stone, S. L., Pomerantz, S. H., Schwartz-Kripner, A., and Channing, C. P. (1978): Inhibitor of oocyte maturation from porcine follicular fluid: further purification and evidence for reversible action. *Biol. Reprod.*, 19:585–592.
72. Pomerantz, S. H., Channing, C. P., and Tsafriri, A. (1979): Studies on the purification and action of an oocyte maturation inhibitor isolated from porcine follicular fluid. In: *Peptides, Structure and Biological Function*, edited by E. Gross, and J. Meinhofer, pp. 765–774. Pierce Chemical Company, Rockford, Illinois.
73. Chari, S., Hillensjö, T., Magnusson, C., Sturm, G., and Daume, E. (1983): *In vitro* inhibition of rat oocyte meiosis by human follicular fluid fractions. *Arch. Gynecol.*, 233:155–164.

74. Downs, S. M., and Eppig, J. J. (1985): A follicular fluid component prevents gonadotropin reversal of cyclic adenosine monophosphate-dependent meiotic arrest in murine oocytes. *Gamete Res.*, 11:83–97.
75. Schuetz. A. W., and Rock, J. (1982): Stimulatory and inhibitory effects of human follicular fluid on amphibian oocyte maturation and ovulation *in vitro*. *Differentiation*, 21:41–44.
76. Cameron, I. L., Lum, J. B., Nations, C., Asch, R. H., and Silverman, A. Y. (1983): Assay for characterization of human follicular oocyte maturation inhibitor using Xenopus oocytes. *Biol. Reprod.*, 28:817–822.
77. Tsafriri, A., Pomerantz, S. H., and Channing, C. P. (1976): Inhibition of oocyte maturation by porcine follicular fluid: Partial characterization of the inhibitor. *Biol. Reprod.*, 14:511–516.
78. Downs, S. M., Schroeder, A. C., and Eppig, J. J. (1985): Developmental capacity of mouse oocytes after reversal of meiotic arrest maintained *in vitro*. *Biol. Reprod.*,32(Suppl. 1) [Abstr. 72].
79. Downs, S. M., Coleman, D. L., Ward-Bailey, P. F., and Eppig, J. J. (1985): Hypoxanthine is the principal inhibitor of murine oocyte maturation in a low molecular weight fraction of porcine follicular fluid. *Proc. Natl. Acad. Sci. U.S.A.*, 82:454–458.
80. Eppig, J. J., Ward-Bailey, P. F., and Coleman, D. L. (1985): Hypoxanthine and adenosine in murine ovarian follicular fluid: concentrations and activity in maintaining oocyte meiotic arrest. *Biol. Reprod.*, 33:1041–1049.
81. Billig, M., Bränström, M., Törnell, J., and Magnusson, C. (1985): Guanosine and hypoxanthine inhibit rat oocyte maturation. *Acta Physiol. Scand.*, 123(Suppl. 2) [Abstr. C12].
82. Miller, J. G. O., and Behrman, H. R. (1985): Adenosine—the oocyte maturation inhibitor of the follicle? *Biol. Reprod.*, 32(Suppl. 1) [Abstr. 21].
83. Hillensjö, T., Channing, C. P., Pomerantz, S. H., and Schwartz-Kripner, A. (1979): Intrafollicular control of oocyte maturation in the pig. *In Vitro*, 15:32–40.
84. Hillensjö, T., Kripner, A. S., Pomerantz, S. H., and Channing, C. P. (1979): Action of porcine follicular fluid oocyte maturation *in vitro:* possible role of the cumulus cells. In: *Ovarian Follicular and Corpus Luteum Function*, edited by C. P. Channing, J. M. Marsh, and W. A. Sadler, pp. 283–291. Plenum Press, New York.
85. Lindner, H. R., Tsafriri, A., Lieberman, M. E., Zor, U., Koch, Y., Bauminger, S., and Barnea, A. (1974): Gonadotropin action on cultured Graafian follicles: induction of maturation division of the mammalian oocyte and differentiation of the luteal cell. *Recent Prog. Horm. Res.*, 30:79–138.
86. Hillensjö, T., Ekholm, C., and Ahrén, K. (1978): Role of cyclic AMP in oocyte maturation and glycolysis in the pre-ovulatory rat follicle. *Acta Endocrinol. Copenhagen*, 87:377–388.
87. Dekel, N., and Beers, W. H. (1980): Development of rat oocyte *in vitro:* inhibition and induction of maturation in the presence or absence of the cumulus oophorus. *Dev. Biol.*, 75:247–252.
88. Dekel, N., Lawrence, T. S., Gilula, N. B., and Beers, W. H. (1981): Modulation of cell-to-cell communication in the cumulus-oocyte complex and the regulation of oocyte maturation by LH. *Dev. Biol.*, 86:356–362.
89. Cho, W. K., Stern, S., and Biggers, J. D. (1974): Inhibitory effect of dibutytyl c-AMP on mouse oocyte maturation *in vitro*. *J. Exp. Zool.*, 187:383–386
90. Nekola, M. V., and Moore-Smith, D. M. (1975): Failure of gonadotropins to induce *in vitro* maturation of mouse oocytes treated with dibutyryl cyclic AMP. *J. Exp. Zool.*, 194:529–534.
91. Dekel, N., and Beers, W. H. (1978): Rat oocyte maturation *in vitro:* relief of cyclic AMP inhibition by gonadotropins. *Proc. Natl. Acad. Sci. U.S.A.*, 75:3469–3473.
92. Moor, R. M., Smith, M. W., and Dawson, R. M. C. (1980): Measurement of intercellular coupling between oocytes and cumulus cells using intracellular markers. *Expl. Cell. Res.*, 126:15–30.
93. Schultz, R. M., Montgomery, R. R., and Belanoff, J. R. (1983): Regulation of mouse oocyte meiotic maturation: implication of a decrease in oocyte cAMP and protein dephosphorylation in commitment to resume meiosis. *Dev. Biol.*, 97:264–273.
94. Schultz, R. M., Montgomery, R. R., Ward-Bailey, P. F., and Eppig, J. J. (1983): Regulation of oocyte maturation in the mouse: possible roles of intercellular communication, cAMP, and testosterone. *Dev. Biol.*, 95:294–304.
95. Vivarelli, E., Conti, M., DeFelici, M., and Siracusa, G. (1983): Meiotic resumption and intracellular cAMP levels in mouse oocytes treated with compounds which act on cAMP metabolism. *Cell Differ.*, 12:271–276.
96. Dekel, N., Aberdam, E., and Hanski, E. (1985): Invasive bacterial adenylate cyclase maintains the meiotic arrest in isolated rat oocytes. In: *Proceeding of the Fifth Ovarian Workshop*, edited by D. O. Toft and R. J. Ryan, pp. 65–69. Ovarian Workshops, Champaign, Illinois.
97. Dekel, N., and Sherizly, I. (1983): Induction of maturation in rat follicle-enclosed oocyte by forskolin. *FEBS Lett.*, 151:153–155.
98. Dekel, N., Aberdam, E., and Sherizly, I. (1984): Spontaneous maturation *in vitro* of cumulus-enclosed rat oocytes is inhibited by forskolin. *Biol. Reprod.*, 31:244–250.
99. Racowsky, C. (1984): Effect of forskolin on the spontaneous maturation and cyclic AMP content of rat oocyte cumulus complexes. *J. Reprod. Fertil.*, 72:107–116.
100. Racowsky, C. (1985): Effect of forskolin on the spontaneous maturation and cyclic AMP content of hamster oocyte–cumulus complexes. *J. Exp. Zool.*, 234:87–96.
101. Racowsky, C. (1985): Effect of forskolin on maintenance of meiotic arrest and stimulation of cumulus expansion, progesterone and cyclic AMP production by pig oocyte-cumulus complexes. *J. Reprod. Fert.*, 74:9–21.
102. Bornslaeger, E. A., and Schultz, R. M. (1985): Regulation of mouse oocyte maturation: effect of elevating cumulus cell cAMP on oocyte cAMP levels. *Biol. Reprod.*, 33:698–704.
103. Urner, F., Herrman, W. L., Baullieu, E-E., and Schorderet-Saltkine, S. (1983): Inhibition of denuded mouse oocyte meiotic maturation by forskolin, an activator of adenylate cyclase. *Endocrinology*, 113:1170–1172.
104. Eppig, J. J., Freter, R. R., Ward-Bailey, R. F., and Schultz, R. M. (1983): Inhibition of oocyte maturation in the mouse: participation of cAMP, steroid hormones, and a putative maturation-inhibitory factor. *Dev. Biol.*, 100:39–49.
105. Olsiewski, P. J., and Beers, W. H. (1983): cAMP synthesis in the rat oocyte. *Dev. Biol.*, 100:287–293.
106. Eppig, J. J., and Downs, S. M. (1984): Chemical signals that regulate mammalian oocyte maturation. *Biol. Reprod.*, 30:1–12.
107. Törnell, J., Brännström, M., Chari, S., and Hillensjö, T. (1984): Synergistic inhibitory effects by human follicular fluid and cAMP on spontaneous rat oocyte maturation. *Biol. Reprod.*, 30(Suppl. 1) [Abstr. 228].
108. Tsafriri, A., and Bar-Ami, S. (1982): Oocyte maturation inhibitor: a 1981 perspective. In: *Intraovarian Control Mechanisms*, edited by C. P. Channing and S. J. Segal, pp. 145–149. Plenum, New York.
109. Lawrence, T. S., Dekel, N., and Beers, W. H. (1980): Binding of human chorionic gonadotropin by rat cumuli oophori and granulosa cells: a comparative study. *Endocrinology*, 106:1114–1118.
110. Channing, C. P., Bae, I-H., Stone, S. L., Anderson, L. D., Edelson, S., and Fowler, S. C. (1981): Porcine granulosa and cumulus cell properties: LH/hCG-receptors, ability to secrete progesterone and ability to respond to LH. *Mol. Cell. Endocrinol.*, 22:359–370.
111. Hillensjö, T., Pomerantz, S., Schwartz-Kripner, A., Anderson, L. D., and Channing, C. P. (1980): Inhibition of cumulus cell progesterone secretion by low molecular weight fractions of porcine follicular fluid which also inhibit oocyte maturation. *Endocrinology*, 106:584–591.
112. Nicosia, S. V., and Mikhail, G. (1975): Cumuli oophori in tissue culture: hormone production, ultrastructure and morphometry of early luteinization. *Fertil. Steril.*, 26:427–448.
113. Billig, H., Hedin, L., and Magnusson, C. (1983): Gonadotrophins stimulate lactate production by rat cumulus and granulosa cells. *Acta Endocrinologica*, 103:562–566.
114. Hillensjö, T., and Channing, C. P. (1980): Gonadotropin stimulation of steroidogenesis and cellular dispersion in cultured porcine cumuli oophori. *Gamete Res.*, 3:233–240.
115. Freter, R. R., and Schultz, R. M. (1984): Regulation of murine oocyte meiosis: evidence for a gonadotropin-induced, cAMP-dependent reduction in maturation inhibitor. *J. Cell. Biol.*, 98:1119–1128.
116. Thibault, C., Gerard, M., and Menezo, Y. (1976): Nuclear and cytoplasmic aspects of mammalian oocyte maturation *in vitro* in relation to follicle size and fertilization. *Sperm Action Prog. Reprod. Biol.*, 1:233–240.

117. Schuetz, A. W. (1985): Local control mechanisms during oogenesis and folliculogenesis. In: *Developmental Biology: Comprehensive Synthesis,* Vol. 1, *Oogenesis,* edited by L. Browder, pp. 1–83. Plenum Press, New York.
118. Rojas, F. J., Moretti-Rojas, I., De Bellabarba, G., and Bishop, W. (1981): Inhibition of ^{125}I-labeled hCG binding to gonadal receptors by a factor obtained from rat testicular tissue. *Biol. Reprod.,*25:519–529.
119. Kalla, N. R., and Zarabi, S. (1982): Presence of luteinizing hormone receptor binding inhibitor (LH-RBI) in ovine testis. *Andrologia,* 14: 265–269.
120. Dias, J. A., and Reichert, L. E. (1984): Evidence for a high molecular weight follicle-stimulating hormone binding inhibitor in bovine testis. *Biol. Reprod.,* 31:975–983.
121. Reichert, L. E., Andersen, T. T., Branca, A. A., Fletcher, P. W., and Sluss, P. M. (1984): FSH binding inhibitors of follicular fluid. In: *Gonadal Proteins and Peptides and their Biological Significance,* edited by M. R. Sairam and L. E. Atkinson, pp. 153–160. World Scientific Publishing Co., Singapore.
122. Ward, D. N. (1981): In pursuit of physiological inhibitors of and from the ovary. In: *Bioregulators of Reproduction,* edited by G. Jagiello and H. J. Vogel, pp. 371–387. Academic Press, New York.
123. Ward, D. N., Liu, W.-K., Glenn, S. D., and Channing, C. P. (1982): LH-binding inhibitors from the corpus luteum. In: *Intraovarian Control Mechanisms,* edited by C. P. Channing and S. J. Segal. Plenum Press, New York. *Adv. Exp. Med. Biol.,* 147:263–281.
124. Ward, D. N., Glenn, S. D., Liu, W.-K., and Gordon, W. L. (1983): Chemistry and physiology of gonadal peptides. In: *Factors Regulating Ovarian Function,* edited by G. S. Greenwald and P. F. Terranova, pp. 141–156. Raven Press, New York.
125. Yang, K. P., Neira, E. S., Yen, H. N., Samaan, N. A., Wong, T. S., Ward, D. N., and Channing, C. P. (1981): Corpus luteum LH-receptor binding inhibitor (LH-RBI). In: *Intragonadal Regulation of Reproduction,* edited by P. Franchimont and C. P. Channing, pp. 133–155. Academic Press, London.
126. Reichert, L. E., Jr., and Abou-Issa, H. (1977): Studies on a low molecular weight testicular factor which inhibits binding of FSH to receptor. *Biol. Reprod.,* 19:235–241.
127. Darga, N. C., and Reichert, L. E., Jr. (1978): Some properties of binding of follicle stimulating hormone to bovine granulosa cells and its inhibition by follicular fluid. *Biol. Reprod.,* 19:235–241.
128. Reichert, L. E., Jr., Sanzo, M. A., and Darga, N. S. (1979): Studies on a low molecular weight follicle-stimulating hormone binding inhibitor from human serum. *J. Clin. Endocrinol. Metabol.,* 49:866–872.
129. Dias, J. A., Treble, D. H., Bennett, A. H., and Reichert, L. E., Jr. (1981): Follicle stimulating hormone receptor binding inhibitors in human seminal fluid. *J. Androl.,* 2:239–248.
130. Sato, E., Ishibashi, T., and Iritani, A. (1982): Purification and action sites of a follicle stimulating hormone inhibitor from bovine follicle fluid. *J. Anim. Sci.,* 55:873–877.
131. Fletcher, P. W., Dias, J. A., Sanzo, M. S., and Reichert, L. E., Jr. (1982): Inhibition of FSH action on granulosa cells by low molecular weight components of follicular fluid. *Mol. Cell. Endocrinol.,* 25:303–315.
132. Sluss, P. M., Fletcher, P. W., and Reichert, L. E., Jr. (1983): Inhibition of ^{125}I-human follicle-stimulating hormone binding to receptor by a low molecular weight fraction of bovine follicular fluid: inhibitor concentration is related to biochemical parameters of follicular development. *Biol. Reprod.,* 29:1105–1113.
133. Sluss, P. M., and Reichert, L. E. (1984): Porcine follicular fluid contains several low molecular weight inhibitors of follicle-stimulating hormone binding to receptor. *Biol. Reprod.,* 30:1091–1104.
134. Andersen, T. T., and Reichert, L. E. (1982): Follitropin binding to receptors in testis: modulation by monovalent salts and divalent cations. *J. Biol. Chem.,* 257:11551–11557.
135. Andersen, T. T., and Reichert, L. E. (1984): Correlation of B coefficient of viscosity for monovalent salts with effects on binding of human follitropin to receptor. *Mol. Cell. Endocrinol.,* 35:41–46.
136. Sluss, P. M., and Reichert, L. E., Jr. (1983): Presence of bacteria in porcine follicular fluid and their ability to generate an inhibitor of follicle-stimulating hormone binding to receptor. *Biol. Reprod.,* 29:335–341.
137. Sluss, P. M., and Reichert, L. E. (1984): Secretion of an inhibitor of follicle-stimulating hormone binding to receptor by the bacteria Serretia, including a strain isolated from porcine follicular fluid. *Biol. Reprod.,* 31:520–530.
138. Sluss, P. M., Branca, A. A., and Reichert, L. E. (1985): Purification of an amine-containing substance from gonadal tissue: a putative low MW FSH binding inhibitor. *Endocrinology,* 116(Suppl. 33A) [Abst. 130].
139. Yang, K. P., Samaan, N. A., and Ward, D. N. (1976): Characterization of an inhibitor of luteinizing hormone receptor site binding. *Endocrinology,* 98:233–241.
140. Yang, K. P., Samaan, N. A., and Ward, D. N. (1976): Lutropin receptors from male and female tissues: different responses to a lutropin receptor inhibitor. *Proc. Soc. Exp. Biol. Med.,* 152:606–609.
141. Sakai, C. N., Engel, B., and Channing, C. P. (1977): Ability of an extract of pig corpus luteum to inhibit binding of ^{125}I-labelled human chorionic gonadotropin to porcine granulosa cells. *Proc. Soc. Exp. Biol. Med.,*155:373–376.
142. Kumari, G. L., and Channing, C. P. (1979): Intraovarian control of progesterone biosynthesis by granulosa cells and corpus luteum. *J. Ster. Biochem.,* 11:781–790.
143. Yang, K. P., Gray, K. N., Jardine, J. H., Yan, H. L., Samaan, N. A., and Ward, D. N. (1978): LHRBI—an inhibitor of *in vitro* luteinizing hormone binding to ovarian receptors and LH-stimulated progesterone synthesis by ovary. In: *Novel Aspects of Reproductive Physiology,* edited by C. H. Spilman and J. W. Wilks, pp. 61–80. S.P. Medical and Scientific Books, New York.
144. Iwasaki, M., Yamoto, M., Ikoma, H., and Nakano, R. (1983): LH receptor binding inhibitor in human corpora lutea and its activity. *Acta Obstet. Gynaec. Jpn.,* 35:2141 [Abst.].
145. Kumari, G. L., Kumar, N., Duraiswami, S., Datta, J. K., Vidyasagar, I. C., Vohra, S., and Roy, S. (1982): Characterization of LH/hCG receptor binding inhibitor in corpora lutea of human and sheep ovaries. In: *Intraovarian Control Mechanisms,* edited by C. P. Channing and S. J. Segal, Plenum Press, New York. *Adv. Exp. Med. Biol.,* 147:283–301.
146. Yang, K. P., Samaan, V. A., and Ward, D. N. (1979): Effects of luteinizing hormone receptor-binding inhibitor on the *in vitro* steroidogenesis by rat ovary and testis. *Endocrinology,* 104:552–558.
147. Kumari, G. L., Tucker, S., and Channing, C. P. (1979): Changes in levels of a LH binding inhibitor in aqueous extracts of porcine corpora lutea as a function of aging of the corpus luteum. *Biol. Reprod.,* 21:1043–1050.
148. Channing, C. P., Batta, S. K., and Bae, I. H. (1981): Inhibitory effect of charcoal treated aqueous porcine corpus luteum extract upon ovulation in the rabbit. *Proc. Soc. Exp. Biol. Med.,* 166: 479–483.
149. Kumari, G. L., Kumar, N., Duraiswami, S., and Roy, S. (1984): Ovarian lutropin receptor binding inhibitor. In: *Gonadal Proteins and Peptides and Their Biological Significance,* edited by M. R. Sairam and L. E. Atkinson, pp. 161–176. World Scientific Publishing Co., Singapore.
150. Behrman, H. R., and Hitchens, M. (1976): Rapid block of gonadotropin uptake by corpora lutea *in vivo* induced by prostaglandin $F_{2\alpha}$. *Prostaglandins,* 12:83–95.
151. Lintern-Moore, S., Peters, H., Moore, G. P. M., and Faber, M. (1974): Follicular development in the infant human ovary. *J. Reprod. Fertil.,* 39:53–64.
152. McNatty, K. P., Moore-Smith, D., Makris, A., Osathanondh, R., and Ryan, K. J. (1979): The microenvironment of the human antral follicle: interrelationships among the steroid levels in antral fluid, the population of granulosa cells, and the status of the oocyte *in vivo* and *in vitro. J. Clin. Endocrinol. Metab.,* 49:851–860.
153. Richards, J. S. (1980): Maturation of ovarian follicles: actions and interactions of pituitary and ovarian hormones on follicular cell differentiation. *Physiol. Rev.,* 60:51–89.
154. Peters, H., and McNatty, K. P. (1980): *The Ovary.* Granada Publishing, London.
155. May, J. V., and Schomberg, D. W. (1984): The effect of plating density on granulosa cell growth and differentiation *in vitro. Mol. Cell. Endocrinol.,* 34:201–213.
156. Rao, M. C., Midgley, A. R., and Richards, J. S. (1978): Hormonal regulation of ovarian proliferation. *Cell,* 14:71–78.

157. McNatty, K. P., and Sawers, R. S. (1975): Relationship between the endocrine environment within the Graafian follicle and the subsequent rate of progesterone secretion by human granulosa cells *in vitro*. *J. Endocrinol.*, 66:391–400.
158. Thanki, K. H., and Channing, C. P. (1976): Influence of serum, estrogen, and gonadotropin upon growth and progesterone secretion by cultures of granulosa cells from small porcine follicles. *Endocrine Res. Commun.*, 3:319–333.
159. Thanki, K. H., and Channing, C. P. (1978): Effects of follicle-stimulating hormone and estradiol upon progesterone secretion by porcine granulosa cells in tissue culture. *Endocrinology*, 103:74–80.
160. Hammond, J. M. (1981): Peptide regulators in the ovarian follicle. *Aust. J. Biol. Sci.*, 34:491–504.
161. Hammond, J. M., Yoshida, K., Veldhuis, J. D., Rechler, M. M., and Knight, A. B. (1983): Intrafollicular role of somatomedins: comparison with effect of insulin. In: *Factors Regulating Ovarian Function*, edited by G. S. Greenwald and P. F. Terranova, pp. 197–201. Raven Press, New York.
162. Adashi, E. Y., Resnick, C. E., D'Ercole, A. J., Svoboda, M. E., and Van Wyk, J. J. (1985): Insulin-like growth factors as intraovarian regulators of granulosa cell growth and function. *Endocr. Rev.*, 6:400–420.
163. Schomberg, D. W., and Gunn, E. B. (1984): Growth factors and ovarian function. In: *Gonadal Proteins and Peptides and Their Biological Significance*, edited by M. R. Sairam and L. E. Atkinson, pp. 209–214. World Scientific Publishing Co., Singapore.
164. Koos, R. D., and LeMaire, W. J. (1983): Factors that may regulate the growth and regression of blood vessels in the ovary. *Sem. Reprod. Endocrinol.*, 1:295–307.
165. Hill, D. J. (1979): Stimulation of cartilage zones of the calf costochondral growth plate *in vitro* by growth hormone-dependent rat plasma somatomedin activity. *J. Endocrinol.*, 83:219–229.
166. Chait, A., Ross, R., Albers, J. J., and Bierman, E. I. (1980): Platelet-derived growth factor stimulates activity of low density lipoprotein receptors. *Proc. Natl. Acad. Sci. U.S.A.*, 77:4084–4088.
167. Coughlin, S. R., Moskowitz, M. A., Zetter, B. R., Andoniades, H. N., and Levine, L. (1980): Platelet-dependent stimulation of prostacyclin synthesis by platelet-derived growth factor. *Nature*, 288:600–602.
168. Johnson, L. K., Baxter, J. D., Vlodavsky, I., and Gospodarowicz, D. (1980): Epidermal growth factor and expression of specific genes: effects on cultured rat pituitary cells are dissociable from the mitogenic response. *Proc. Natl. Acad. Sci. U.S.A.*, 77:394–398.
169. Tashjian, A. H., Hohmann, E. L., Antoniades, H. N., and Levine, L. (1982): Platelet-derived growth factor stimulates bone resorption via a prostaglandin-mediated mechanism. *Endocrinology*, 111:118–124.
170. Turo, K., and Florini, J. (1982): Hormonal stimulation of myoblast differentiation in the absence of DNA synthesis. *Am. J. Physiol.*, 243:C278–C284.
171. Schmid, C., Steiner, T., and Froesch, E. R. (1984): Insulin-like growth factor I supports differentiation of cultured osteoblast-like cells. *FEBS Lett.*, 173:48–52.
172. Baird, A., Morméde, P., Ying, S.-Y., Wehrenberg, W. B., Ueno, N., Ling, N., and Guillemin, R. (1985): A nonmitogenic pituitary function of fibroblast growth factor: regulation of thyrotrophin and prolactin secretion. *Proc. Natl. Acad. Sci. U.S.A.*, 82:5545–5549.
173. Cohen, S. (1962): Isolation of a mouse submaxillary gland protein accelerating incisor eruption and eyelid opening in the newborn animal. *J. Biol. Chem.*, 237:1555–1562.
174. Gospodarowicz, D., and Moran, J. S. (1976): Growth factors in mammalian cell culture. *Ann. Rev. Biochem.* 45:531–558.
175. Gospodarowicz, D., Greenburg, G., Bialecki, H., and Zetter, B. R. (1978): Factors involved in the modulation of cell proliferation *in vivo* and *in vitro:* the role of fibroblast and epidermal growth factors in the proliferative response of mammalian cells. *In Vitro*, 14:85–118.
176. Capenter, G., and Cohen, S. (1979): Epidermal growth factor. *Ann. Rev. Biochem.*, 48:193–216.
177. Gospodarowicz, D. (1975): Purification of a fibroblast growth factor from bovine pituitary. *J. Biol. Chem.*, 250:2515–2520.
178. Böhlen, P., Esch, F., Baird, A., and Gospodarowicz, D. (1985): Acidic fibroblast growth factor (FGF) from bovine brain: amino-terminal sequence and comparison with basic FGF. *EMBO J.*, 4:1951–1956.
179. Esch, F., Baird, A., Ling, N., Ueno, N., Hill, F., Denoroy, L., Klepper, R., Gospodarowicz, D., Böhlen, P., and Guillemin, R. (1985): Primary structure of bovine pituitary basic fibroblast growth factor (FGF) and comparison with the amino-terminal sequence of bovine brain acidic FGF. *Proc. Natl. Acad. Sci. U.S.A.*, 82:6507–6511.
180. Ross, R., and Vogel, A. (1978): The platelet-derived growth factor. *Cell*, 14:203–210.
181. Antonaides, H. N., Scher, C. D., and Stiles, C. D. (1979): Purification of the human platelet-derived growth factor. *Proc. Natl. Acad. Sci.*, 76:1809–1813.
182. Heldin, C.-H, Wasteson, A., and Westermark, B. (1985): Platelet-derived growth factor. *Mol. Cell Endocrinol.*, 39:169–187.
183. Froesch, E. R., Schmid, C., Schwander, J., and Zapf, J. (1985): Actions of insulin-like growth factors. *Ann. Rev. Physiol.*, 47:443–467.
184. Daughaday, W. H., Hall, K., Raben, M. S., Salmon, W. D., Van Den Brande, J. L., and Van Wyk, J. J. (1972): Somatomedin: proposed designation for sulphation factor. *Nature*, 235:107.
185. Van Wyk, J. J., Underwood, L. E., Hintz, R. L., Clemmons, D. R., Voina, S. J., and Weaver, R. P. (1974): The somatomedins: a family of insulin-like hormones under growth hormone control. *Recent Prog. Horm. Res.*, 30:259–318.
186. Van Wyk, J. J., Svoboda, M. E., and Underwood, L. E. (1980): Evidence from radioligand assays that somatomedin-C and insulin-like growth factor-I are similar to each other and different from other somatomedins. *J. Clin. Endocrinol. Metab.*, 50:206–208.
187. Svoboda, M. E., Van Wyk, J. J., Klapper, D. G., Fellows, R. E., Grissom, F. E., and Schleuter, R. J. (1980): Purification of somatomedin-C from human plasma: chemical and biological properties, partial sequence analysis and relationship to other somatomedins. *Biochemistry*, 19:790–797.
188. Klapper, D. G., Svoboda, M. E., and Van Wyk, J. J. (1983): Sequence analysis of somatomedin-C: Confirmation of identity with insulin-like growth factor I. *Endocrinology*, 112:2215–2217.
189. Rubin, J. S., Mariz, I., Jacobs, J. W., Daughaday, W. H., and Bradshaw, R. A. (1982): Isolation and partial sequence analysis of rat basic somatomedin. *Endocrinology*, 110:734–740.
190. Fett, J. W., Strydom, D. J., Lobb, R. R., Alderman, E. M., Bethune, J. L., Riordan, J. F., and Vallee, B. L. (1985): Isolation and characterization of angiogenin, an angiogenic protein from human carcinoma cells. *Biochemistry*, 24:5480–5486.
191. Strydom, D. J., Fett, J. W., Lobb, R. R., Alderman, E. M., Bethune, J. L., Riordan, J. F., and Vallee, B. L. (1985): Amino acid sequence of human tumor derived angiogenin. *Biochemistry*, 24:5486–5494.
192. Kurachi, K., Davie, E. W., Strydom, D. J., Riordan, J. F., and Vallee, B. L. (1985): Sequence of the cDNA and gene for angiogenin, a human angiogenesis factor. *Biochemistry*, 24:5494–5499.
193. Thomas, K. A., Rios-Candelore, M., Gimenez-Gallege, G., Disalvo, J., Bennett, C., Rodkey, J., and Fitzpatrick, S. (1985): Pure brain-derived acidic fibroblast growth factor is a potent angiogenic vascular endothelial cell mitogen with sequence homology to interleukin 1. *Proc. Natl. Acad. Sci. U.S.A.*, 82:6409–6413.
194. Baird, A., Esch, F., Mormede, P., Ueno, N., Ling, N., Böhlen, P., Ying, S.-Y., Wehrenberg, W. B., and Guillemin, R. (1986): Molecular characterization of fibroblast growth factor: Distribution and biological activities in various tissues. *Recent Prog. Horm. Res.*, 42:143–205.
195. McNatty, K. P., Makris, A., DeGrazia, C., Osathanondh, R., and Ryan, K. J. (1980): Steroidogenesis by recombined follicular cells from the human ovary *in vitro*. *J. Clin. Endocrinol. Metab.*, 51:1286–1292.
196. Makris, A., Yasumizu, T., and Ryan, K. J. (1982): A thecal protein growth factor which stimulates granulosa and BALBc 3T3 cell DNA synthesis. *Endocrinology*, 108 (Suppl.):110.
197. Makris, A., Klagsbrun, M. A., Yasumizu, T., and Ryan, K. J. (1983): An endogenous ovarian growth factor which stimulates BALB/3T3 and granulosa cells. *Biol. Reprod.*, 29:1135–1141.
198. Stastny, M., and Cohen, S. (1970): Epidermal growth factor. IV. The induction of ornithine decarboxylase. *Biochem. Biophys. Acta*, 204:578–589.

199. Russel, D. H. (1973): Polyamines in growth—normal and neoplastic. In: *Polyamines in Normal and Neoplastic Growth,* edited by D. H. Russel, pp. 1–13. Raven Press, New York.
200. Maudsley, D. V. (1979): Regulation of polyamine biosynthesis. *Biochem. Pharmacol.,* 28:153–161.
201. Veldhuis, J. B., Demers, L. M., and Hammond, J. M. (1979): Regulation of ornithine decarboxylase in isolated granulosa cells *in vitro* by constituents of follicular fluid. *Endocrinology,* 105:1143–1151.
202. Hammond, J. M., Veldhuis, J. D., Seale, T. W., and Rechler, M. M. (1982): Intraovarian regulation of granulosa cell replication. In: *Intraovarian Control Mechanisms,* edited by C. P. Channing and S. J. Segal, Plenum Press, New York. *Adv. Exp. Biol. Med.,* 147:341–356.
203. Gospodarowicz, D., Ill, C. R., and Birdwell, C. R. (1977): Effect of fibroblast and epidermal growth factors on ovarian cell proliferation *in vitro.* I. Characterization of the response of granulosa cells for FGF and EGF. *Endocrinology,* 100:1108–1120.
204. Gospodarowicz, D., Ill, C. R., and Birdwell, C. R. (1977): Effect of fibroblast and epidermal growth factors on ovarian cell proliferation *in vitro.* II. Proliferative response of luteal cells to FGF but not EGF. *Endocrinology,* 100:1121–1128.
205. Gospodarowicz, D., and Bialecki, H. (1979): Fibroblast and epidermal growth factors are mitogenic agents for cultured granulosa cells of rodent, porcine and human origin. *Endocrinology,* 104:757–764.
206. Vlodavsky, I., Brown, K. D., and Gospodarowicz, D. (1978): A comparison of the binding of epidermal growth factor to cultured granulosa and luteal cells. *J. Biol. Chem.,* 253:3744–3750.
207. Hsueh, A. J. W., Welsh, T. H., and Jones, P. B. C. (1981): Inhibition of ovarian and testicular steroidogenesis by epidermal growth factor. *Endocrinology,* 108:2002–2004.
208. Jones, P. B. C., Welsh, T. H., Jr., and Hsueh, A. J. W. (1982): Regulation of ovarian progestin production by EGF in cultured rat granulosa cells. *J. Biol. Chem.,* 257:11268–11273.
209. St. Arnaud, R., Walter, P., Kelly, P. A., and Labrie, F. (1983): Rat ovarian epidermal growth factor receptors: characterization and hormonal regulation. *Mol. Cell. Endocrinol.,* 31:43–52.
210. Mondschein, J. S., and Schomberg, D. W. (1981): Growth factors modulate gonadotropin receptor induction in granulosa cell cultures. *Science,* 211:1179–1180.
211. Schomberg, D. W., May, J. V., and Mondschein, J. S. (1983): Epidermal growth factor attenuates FSH-, cAMP-, or cholera toxin-mediated LH receptor induction in granulosa cell cultures. In: *Factors Regulating Ovarian Function,* edited by G. S. Greenwald and P. F. Terranova, pp. 221–224. Raven Press, New York.
212. Schomberg, D. W., May, J. V., and Mondschein, J. S. (1983): Interactions between hormones and growth factors in the regulation of granulosa cell differentiation *in vitro. J. Steroid Biochem.,* 19:291–295.
213. Knecht, M., and Catt, K. J. (1983): Modulation of cAMP-mediated differentiation in ovarian granulosa cells by epidermal growth factor and platelet-derived growth factor. *J. Biol. Chem.,* 258:2789–2794.
214. Mondschein, J. S., and Schomberg, D. W. (1984): Regulation of granulosa cell responsiveness to gonadotropins: Actions of epidermal and platelet-derived growth factors. In: *Regulation of Target Cell Responsiveness,* Vol. 1, edited by K. W. McKerns, A. Aakvag, and V. Hansson, pp. 463–485. Plenum Press, New York.
215. Channing, C. P., Garrett, R., Kroman, N., Conn, T., and Gospodarowicz, P. (1983): Ability of EGF and FGF to enhance growth of porcine granulosa cells in culture while they lead to a decrease in progesterone secretion: changes in responsiveness throughout follicular maturation. In: *Factors Regulating Ovarian Function,* edited by P. Terranova and G. S. Greenwald, pp. 215–220. Raven Press, New York.
216. Erickson, G. F., and Case, E. (1983): Epidermal growth factor antagonizes ovarian theca-interstitial cytodifferentiation. *Mol. Cell. Endocrinol.,* 31:71–76.
217. Lintern-Moore, S., Moore, G. P. M., Panaretto, B. A., and Robertson, D. (1981): Follicular development in the neonatal mouse ovary: effect of epidermal growth factor. *Acta Endocrinol.,* 96:123–126.
218. Dekel, N., and Sherizly, I. (1985): Epidermal growth factor induces maturation of rat follicle-enclosed oocytes. *Endocrinology,* 116:406–409.
219. Savion, N., Vlodavsky, I., and Gospodarowicz, D. (1981): Nuclear accumulation of epidermal growth factor in cultured bovine corneal endothelial and granulosa cells. *J. Biol. Chem.,* 1149–1154.
220. Savion, N., Lui, G. M., Laherty, R., and Gospodarowicz, D. (1981): Factors controlling proliferation and progesterone production by bovine granulosa cells in serum-free medium. *Endocrinology,* 109:409–420.
221. Mock, E. J., and Niswender, G. D. (1983): Differences in the rates of internalization of ^{125}I-labeled human chorionic gonadotropin, luteinizing hormone, and epidermal growth factor by ovine luteal cells. *Endocrinology,* 113:259–264.
222. Mondschein, J. S., and Schomberg, D. W. (1981): Platelet-derived growth factor enhances granulosa cell luteinizing hormone receptor induction by follicle-stimulating hormone and serum. *Endocrinology,* 109:325–327.
223. Veldhuis, J., Kolp, L. A., Toaff, M. E., Strauss, III, J. F., and Demmers, L. M. (1983): Mechanism subserving the trophic actions of insulin on ovarian cells. *In vitro* studies using swine granulosa cells. *J. Clin. Invest.,* 72:1046–1057.
224. May, J. V., and Schomberg, D. W. (1981): Granulosa cell differentiation *in vitro:* effect of insulin on growth and functional integrity. *Biol. Reprod.,* 25:421–431.
225. Baranao, J. L. S., and Hammond, J. M. (1984): Comparative effects of insulin and insulin-like growth factors on DNA synthesis and differentiation of porcine granulosa cell. *Biochem. Biophys. Res. Commun.,* 124:484–490.
226. Adashi, E. Y., Resnick, C. E., Svoboda, M. E., and Van Wyk, J. J. (1984): A novel role for somatomedin-C in the cytodifferentiation of the ovarian granulosa cell. *Endocrinology,* 115:1227–1229.
227. Adashi, E. Y., Resnick, C. E., Svoboda, M. E., and Van Wyk, J. J. (1985): Somatomedin-C synergizes with follicle-stimulating hormone in the acquisition of progestin biosynthetic capacity by cultured rat granulosa cells. *Endocrinology,* 116:2135–2142.
228. Veldhuis, J. D., and Furlanetto, R. W. (1985): Trophic actions of human somatomedin C/insulin-like growth factor I on ovarian cells: *in vitro* studies with swine granulosa cells. *Endocrinology,* 116:1235–1242.
229. Veldhuis, J. D. (1985): Role of estradiol as a biological amplifier of hormone action in the ovary: synergistic interaction of estradiol with insulin-like growth factor type I (IGF-I/somatomedin C). *Endocrinology,* 116(Suppl) [Abstr. 817].
230. Adashi, E. Y., Resnick, C. E., Brodie, A. M. H., Svoboda, M. E., and Van Wyk, J. J. (1985): Somatomedin-C-mediated potentiation of follicle-stimulating hormone-induced aromatase activity of cultured rat granulosa cells. *Endocrinology,* 117:2313–2320.
231. Adashi, E. Y., Resnick, C. E., Svoboda, M. E., Van Wyk, J. J., Hascall, V. C., and Yanagishita, M. (1985): Independent and synergistic actions of Somatomedin-C in the stimulation of proteoglycan biosynthesis by cultured rat granulosa cells. *Biol. Reprod.,* 32(Suppl. 1) [Abstr. 20].
232. Adashi, E. Y., Resnick, C. E., Svoboda, M. E., and Van Wyk, J. J. (1985): Somatomedin-C enhances induction of luteinizing hormone receptor by follicle-stimulating hormone in cultured rat granulosa cells. *Endocrinology,* 116:2369–2375.
233. Davoren, J. B. (1985): Binding of ^{125}I-insulin-like growth factor-I to rat granulosa cells: relation to IGF action. *Biol. Reprod.,* 32(Suppl. 1) [Abstr. 19].
234. Hammond, J. M., Baranao, J. L. S., Skaleris, D. A., Rechler, M. M., and Knight, A. P. (1984): Somatomedin (Sm) production by cultured porcine granulosa cells (GC). *J. Steroid Biochem.,* 20:1597 [Abstr. 128].
235. Hammond, J. M., Knight, A. P., and Rechler, M. M. (1984): Somatomedin secretion by porcine granulosa cells: a potential mechanism for regulating ovarian follicular growth. *Clin. Res.,* 32:485A.
236. Hammond, J. M., Lino, J., Baranao, L. S., Skaleris, D., Knight, A. B., Romanus, J. A., and Rechler, M. M. (1986): Production of insulin-like growth factors by ovarian granulosa cells. *Endocrinology,* 117:2553–2555.
237. Andersson, I., Billig, H., Fryklund, L., Hansson, H-A., Isaksson, O., Isgaard, J., Nilsson, A., Rozell, B., Skottner, A., and Stemme,

S. (1986): Localization of IGF-I in adult rats: immunohistochemical studies. *Acta Physiol. Scand.*, 126:311–312.
238. Jakob, W., Jentzsch, K. D., Mauersberger, B., and Oehme, P. (1977): Demonstration of angiogenesis-activity in the corpus luteum of cattle. *Exp. Pathol.*, 13:231–236.
239. Gospodarowicz, D., and Thakral, K. K. (1978): Production of a corpus luteum angiogenic factor responsible for proliferation of capillaries and neovascularization of the corpus luteum. *Proc. Natl. Acad. Sci. U.S.A.*, 75:847–851.
240. Heder, G., Jakob, W., Halle, W., Mauersberger, B., Kambach, G., Jentzsch, K. D., and Oehme, P. (1979): Influence of porcine corpus luteum extract on DNA synthesis and proliferation of cultured fibroblasts and endothelial cells. *Exp. Pathol.*, 17:493–497.
241. Koos, R. D., and LeMaire, W. J. (1983): Evidence for an angiogenic factor from rat follicles. In: *Factors Regulating Ovarian Function*, edited by G. S. Greenwald and P. F. Terranova, pp. 191–195. Raven Press, New York.
242. Gaede, S. D., Sholley, M. M., and Quattropani, S. L. (1985): Endothelial mitosis during initial stages of corpus luteum neovascularization in the cyclic adult rat. *Am. J. Anat.*, 172:173–180.
243. Sato, E., Ishibashi, T., and Koide, S. S. (1982): Inducement of blood vessel formation by ovarian extracts from mice injected with gonadotropins. *Experientia*, 38:1248–1249.
244. Makris, A., Ryan, K. J., Yasumizu, T., Hill, C. L., and Zetter, B. R. (1984): The nonluteal porcine ovary as a source of angiogenic activity. *Endocrinology*, 115:1672–1677.
245. Rone, J. D., and Goodman, A. L. (1985): Detection of angiotropic activity from intact rabbit follicles cultured in serum-free media. *Biol. Reprod.*, 32(Suppl. 1) [Abstr. 294].
246. Redmer, D. A., Rone, J. D., and Goodman, A. L. (1985): Detection of angiotropic activity from primate dominant follicles. *Endocrinology*, 116(Suppl. 151A) [Abstr. 604].
247. Frederick, J. L., Hoa, N., Preston, D. S., Frederick, J. J., Campeau, J. D., Ono, T., and diZerega, G. S. (1985): Initiation of angiogenesis by a porcine follicular fluid. *Am. J. Obstet. Gynecol.*, 152:1073–1078.
248. Frederick, J. L., Shimanuki, T., and diZerega, G. S. (1984): Initiation of angiogenesis by human follicular fluid. *Science*, 224:389–390.
249. Koos, R. D. (1985): Stimulation of endothelial cell proliferation by granulosa cell-conditioned medium. *Biol. Reprod.*, 32 (Suppl. 1) [Abstr. 293].
250. Goodman, A. L., and Rone, J. D. (1985): Detection of angiotropic (chemoattractant) activity released by rabbit luteal cells cultured in serum-free or serum-enriched media. *Biol. Reprod.*, 32 (Suppl. 1) [Abstr. 296].
251. Bruce, N. W., and Moor, R. M. (1976): Bibliography (with review) on ovarian blood flow and function. *J. Reprod. Fertil.*, 46:299–304.
252. Ellinwood, W. E., Nett, T. M., and Niswender, G. D. (1978): Ovarian vasculature: structure and function. In: *The Vertebrate Ovary*, edited by R. E. Jones, pp. 583–614. Plenum Press, New York.
253. Zeleznik, A., Schuller, H., and Reichert, Jr., L. E. (1981): Gonadotropin binding sites in the rhesus monkey ovary: role of the vasculature in the selective distribution of human chorionic gonadotropin to the preovulatory follicle. *Endocrinology*, 109:356–362.
254. Hay, M. F., Cran, D. G., and Moor, R. M. (1976): Structural changes occurring during atresia in sheep ovarian follicles. *Cell Tissue Res.*, 169:515–529.
255. O'Shea, J. D., Hay, M. F., and Cran, D. G. (1978): Ultrastructural changes in the theca interna during follicular atresia in sheep. *J. Reprod. Fertil.*, 54:183–187.
256. Kenney, R. M., Condon, W., Ganjam, V. K., and Channing, C. P. (1979): Morphological and biochemical correlates of equine ovarian follicles as a function of their state of viability or atresia. *J. Reprod. Fertil. Suppl.*, 27:163–171.
257. Gospodarowicz, D., Chang, J., Lui, G. M., Baird, A., Esch, F., and Böhlen, P. (1985): Corpus luteum angiogenic factor is related to fibroblast growth factor. *Endocrinology*, 117:2382–2391.
258. diZerega, G. S., Campeau, J. D., Ujita, E. L., Kling, O. R., Marrs, R. P., Lobo, R., and Nakamura, R. M. (1983): The possible role for a follicular protein in the intraovarian regulation of folliculogenesis. *Sem. Reprod. Endocrinol.*, 1:309–322.
259. diZerega, G. S., Campeau, J. D., Ujita, E. L., Schreiber, J. R., Battin, D. A., Montz, F. J., and Nakamura, R. M. (1984): Follicular regulatory proteins: paracrine regulators of follicular steroidogenesis. In: *Gonadal Proteins and Peptides and Their Biological Significance*, edited by M. R. Sairam and L. E. Atkinson, pp. 215–228. World Scientific Publishing Co., Singapore.
260. Tonetta, S. A., and diZerega, G. S. (1986): Paracrine regulation of follicular maturation in primates. *Clin. Endocrinol. Metab.*, 15:135–136.
261. Kling, O. R., Roche, P. C., Campeau, J. D., Nishimura, K., Nakamura, R. M., and diZerega, G. S. (1984): Identification of a porcine follicular fluid fraction which suppresses follicular response to gonadotropins. *Biol. Reprod.*, 30:564–572.
262. Cahill, L. P., Clarke, I. J., Cummins, J. T., Draincourt, M. A., Carson, R. S., and Findlay, J. K. (1985): An inhibitory action at the ovarian level of ovine follicular fluid on PMSG-induced folliculogenesis in hypophysectomized ewes. In: *Proceedings of the Fifth Ovarian Workshop*, edited by D. O. Toft and R. J. Ryan, pp. 35–38. Ovarian Workshops, Champaign, Illinois.
263. Hillier, S. G., van Hall, E. V., van den Boogaard, D. E., Zwart, F. A., and Key, Z. (1982): Activation and modulation of the granulosa cell aromatase system: experimental studies with rat and human ovaries. In: *Follicular Maturation and Ovulation*, edited by R. Rolland, E. V. van Hall, S. G. Hillier, K. P. McNatty, and J. Shoemaker, pp. 51–70. Elsevier, Amsterdam.
264. diZerega, G. S., Marrs, R. P., Campeau, J. D., Nakamura, R. M., and Kling, O. R. (1983): Human granulosa cell secretion of protein(s) which suppress follicular response to gonadotropins. *J. Clin. Endocr. Metab.*, 56:147–155.
265. diZerega, G. S., Goebelsmann, U., and Nakamura, R. (1982): Identification of protein(s) secreted by the preovulatory ovary which suppress follicular response to gonadotropins. *J. Clin. Endocr. Metab.*, 54:1091–1096.
266. diZerega, G. S., Marrs, R. P., Roche, P. C., Campeau, J. D., and Kling, O. R. (1983): Identification of proteins in pooled human follicular fluid which suppress follicular response to gonadotropins. *J. Clin. Endocr. Metab.*, 56:35–41.
267. diZerega, G. S., and Wilks, J. F. (1984): Inhibition of the primate ovarian cycle by a porcine follicular fluid protein. *Fertil. Steril.*, 41:635–638.
268. Cahill, L. P., Driancourt, M. A., Chamley, W. A., and Findlay, J. K. (1985): Role of intrafollicular regulators and FSH in growth and development of large antral follicles in sheep. *J. Reprod. Fertil.*, 75:599–607.
269. Ujita, E., Campeau, J. D., and diZerega, G. S. (1985): Inhibition of porcine granulosa cell adenylate activity by an ovarian protein. *Mol. Cell. Endocrinol. (in press)*.
270. diZerega, G. S., Marrs, R. P., Campeau, J. D., Nakamura, R. M., and Kling, O. R. (1983): Human granulosa cell secretion of protein(s) which suppress follicular response to gonadotropins. *J. Clin. Endocr. Metab.*, 56:147–155.
271. Schreiber, J. R., and diZerega, G. S. (1985): Porcine follicular fluid protein(s) inhibitors rat ovary granulosa cell steroidogenesis. *Biol. Reprod. (in press)*.
272. Ledwitz-Rigby, F., Rigby, B. W., Murphy, T. N., and diZerega, G. S. (1985): Enhancement of progesterone secretion by a partially purified protein fraction of follicular fluid. *Mol. Cell Endocr. (in press)*.
273. diZerega, G. S., Campeau, J. D., Lobo, R. A., Nakamura, R. M., Ujita, E. L., and Marrs, R. P. (1983): Activity of a human follicular fluid protein(s) during normal and stimulated ovarian cycles. *J. Clin. Endocrinol. Metab.*, 57:838–846.
274. diZerega, G. S., Marrs, R. P., Lobo, R., Ujita, E. L., Brown, J., and Campeau, J. D. (1984): Correlation of inhibin and follicle regulatory protein activities with follicular fluid steroid levels in anovulatory patients. *Fertil. Steril.*, 41:849–855.
275. McNatty, K. P., Hunter, W. M., McNeilly, A. S., and Sawers, R. S. (1975): Changes in the concentration of pituitary and steroid hormones in the follicular fluid of human Graafian follicles throughout the menstrual cycle. *J. Endocrinol.*, 64:555–571.
276. Hillier, S. G., Zeleznik, A. J., Knazek, R. A., and Ross, G. T. (1980): Hormonal regulation of preovulatory follicle maturation in the rat. *J. Reprod. Fertil.*, 60:219–229.
277. Hirshfield, A. N. (1985): A low dose of PMSG recruits excess follicles only during a narrowly delimited portion of the estrous cycle. *Biol. Reprod.*, 32 (Suppl. 1) [Abstr. 66].

278. Ledwitz-Rigby, F., and Rigby, B. W. (1981): Ovarian inhibitors and stimulators of granulosa cell maturation and luteinization. In: *Intragonadal Regulation of Reproduction*, edited by P. Franchimont and C. P. Channing, pp. 97–131. Academic Press, London.
279. Ledwitz-Rigby, F., and Rigby, B. W. (1983): The actions of follicular fluid factors on steroidogenesis by cultured ovarian granulosa cells. *J. Steroid Biochem.*, 19:127–131.
280. Vasilenko, P., and Mahajan, D. K. (1984): Stimulation and inhibition of granulosa cell progesterone secretion by porcine follicular fluids. In: *Gonadal Proteins and Peptides and their Biological Significance*, edited by M. R. Sairam and L. E. Atkinson, pp. 229–237. World Scientific Publishing Co., Singapore.
281. Kraiem, Z., Druker, B., and Lunenfeld, B. (1978): Inhibitory action of human follicular fluid on the ovarian accumulation of cyclic AMP. *J. Endocrinol.* 78:161–162.
282. Hillensjö, T., Chari, S., Nilsson, L., Hamberger, L., Daume, E., and Sturm, G. (1983): Inhibition of progesterone secretion in cultured human granulosa cells by a low molecular weight fraction of human follicular fluid. *J. Clin. Endocrinol. Metab.* 56:835–838.
283. Shemesh, M. (1979): Inhibitory action of follicular fluid on progesterone and PG synthesis by bovine follicles. *J. Endocrinol.* 82:27–31.
284. Bernard, J. (1973): Effect du liquide folliculaire sur la luteinisation *in vitro* des cellules granulosaires du rat. *C. R. Seances Soc. Biol. Paris*, 6:882–885.
285. Bernard, J., and Psychoyos, A. (1977): Inhibitory effect of follicular fluid on RNA synthesis of rat granulosa cells *in vitro*. *J. Reprod. Fertil.* 49:355–357.
286. Younglai, E. V. (1972): The influence of follicular fluid and plasma on the steroidogenic activity of equine granulosa cells. *J. Reprod. Fertil.* 28:95–97.
287. Channing, C. P., Batta, S. K., Condon, W., Ganjam, V. K., and Kenney, R. M. (1981): Levels of inhibin activity and of atretogenic factor(s) in follicular fluid harvested from viable and atretic mare follicles. In: *Dynamics of Ovarian Function*, edited by N. B. Schwartz and M. Hunzicker-Dunn, pp. 73–78. Raven Press, New York.
288. McLean, M. P., Rigby, B. W., and Ledwitz-Rigby, F. (1982): A morphometric analysis of the effects of follicular fluid on granulosa cells from immature antral porcine follicles. *Biol. Reprod.*, 26:89A.
289. Alexander, J. S., Rigby, B. W., and Ledwitz-Rigby, F. (1978): Ultrastructural correlates of *in vitro* inhibition of luteinization of mature porcine ovarian granulosa cells by fluid from immature porcine follicles. *Biol. Reprod.*, 19:693–700.
290. Stewart, L. E., Rigby, B. W., and Ledwitz-Rigby, F. (1982): Follicular fluid stimulation of progesterone secretion: time course, dose response and effect of inhibiting *de novo* cholesterol synthesis. *Biol. Reprod.*, 27:54–61.
291. Ledwitz-Rigby, F., and Rigby, B. W. (1979): Follicular fluid stimulation of steroidogenesis in immature granulosa cells *in vitro*. *Mol. Cell. Endocrinol.* 14:73–80.
292. Rigby, B. W., Ling, S. Y., and Ledwitz-Rigby, F. (1983): In search of the elusive follicular fluid factors. In: *Factors Regulating Ovarian Function*, edited by G. S. Greenwald and P. Terranova, pp. 179–183. Raven Press, New York.
293. Ledwitz-Rigby, F., Petito, S. H., Tyner, J. K., and Rigby, B. W. (1985): Follicular fluid effects on progesterone secretion are not due to follicle-stimulating hormone or steroids. *Biol. Reprod.*, 33:277–285.
294. Osteen, K. G., Loeken, M. R., and Channing, C. P. (1982): Intraovarian control of granulosa cell luteinization. *Endocrinol. Exp.*, 16:301–309.
295. Osteen, K., Anderson, L. D., Reichert, L. E., and Channing, C. P. (1985): Follicular fluid modulation of functional LH receptor induction in porcine granulosa cells. *J. Reprod. Fertil.* 74:407–418.
296. Bar-Ami, S., and Channing, C. P. (1984): Enhancement of granulosa cell luteinization *in vitro* by a luteinizing stimulator obtained from porcine large antral follicles. VI Workshop on Development and Function of the Reproductive Organs, The Weizmann Institute of Science, Rehovot, Israel, p. 47.
297. Ledwitz-Rigby, F., McConoughey, P. J., and Maloney, B. (1981): Follicular fluid stimulation of estrogen secretion by porcine granulosa cells *in vitro*. *Biol. Reprod.*, 24(1):83A.
298. Bar-Ami, S., Coon, T. L., and Channing, C. P. (1984): Characterization and partial purification of a luteinizing stimulator (LS) present in porcine follicular fluid. *Biol. Reprod.*, 30 (Suppl. 1) [Abstr. 13].
299. Channing, C. P., and Tsafriri, A. (1977): Mechanism of action of luteinizing hormone and follicle stimulating hormone in the ovary *in vitro*. *Metabolism*, 26:413–468.
300. Ledwitz-Rigby, F., Rigby, B. W., Gay, V.L., Stetson, M., Young, J., and Channing, C. P. (1977): Inhibitory action of porcine follicular fluid upon granulosa cell luteinization *in vitro*: assay and influence of follicular maturation. *J. Endocrinol.*, 74:175–184.
301. Bernard, J., and Chretien, F. C. (1978): Effect of follicular fluid on the surface ultrastructure of rat granulosa cells *in vitro*. *Biol. Reprod.*, 19:133–143.
302. Ledwitz-Rigby, F. (1980): Reversal of follicular inhibition of granulosa cell progesterone secretion by manipulation of intracellular cyclic AMP. *Biol. Reprod.*, 23:324–333.
303. Rigby, B. W., Ledwitz-Rigby, F., and Hunzicker-Dunn, M. (1980): Follicular fluid depression of ovarian granulosa cell adenylyl cyclase activity. *Mol. Cell. Endocrinol.*, 17:17–24.
304. Amsterdam, A., Reisel, R., Mintz, Y., Shemesh, M., and Salomon, Y. (1979): Inhibition of gonadotropin-sensitive adenylate cyclase by ovarian follicular fluid. *Biochem. Biophys. Res. Commun.*, 87:505–512.
305. Amsterdam, A., Shemesh, M., and Salomon, Y. (1979): Inhibition by follicular fluid of luteinizing hormone-sensitive adenylate cyclase in ovarian plasma membranes. In: *Ovarian Follicular and Corpus Luteum Function*, edited by C. P. Channing, J. Marsh, and W. A. Sadler, pp. 383–388. Plenum Press, New York.
306. Channing, C. P., Conn, T., Gagliano, P., and Osteen, K. (1985): Some properties of a luteinization inhibitor (LI) present in porcine follicular fluid. In: *Proceedings of the Fifth Ovarian Workshop*, edited by D. O. Toft and R. J. Ryan, pp. 39–44. Ovarian Workshops, Champaign, Illinois.
307. Channing, C. P., Gagliano, P., Conn, T., and Osteen, K. G. (1985): Luteinization inhibitor from porcine follicular fluid: partial purification and separation from inhibin activity. *Biol. Reprod.* (*in press*).
308. Channing, C. P. (1985): New developments in ovarian physiology. In: *Gamete Quality and Fertility Regulation*, edited by R. Rolland, M. J. Heineman, S. G. Hillier, and H. Vemer, pp. 3–30. Excerpta Medica, ICS658, Elsevier Science Publishers, B. V., Amsterdam.
309. Hsueh, A. J. W., and Jones, P. B. C. (1981): Extrapituitary actions of gonadotropin-releasing hormone. *Endocr. Rev.*, 2:437–461.
310. Clayton, R. N. and Catt, K. J. (1981): Gonadotropin-releasing hormone receptors: characterization, physiological regulation and relationship to reproductive function. *Endocr. Rev.*, 2:186–209.
311. Sharpe, R. M. (1982): Cellular aspects of the inhibitory actions of LHRH on the ovary and testis. *J. Reprod. Fertil.*, 64:517–527.
312. Knecht, M., Ranta, T., Naor, Z., and Catt, K. J. (1983): Direct effects of GnRH on the ovary. In: *Factors Regulating Ovarian Function*, edited by G. S. Greenwald and P. F. Terranova, pp. 225–243. Raven Press, New York.
313. Naor, Z., Molcho, J., Hermon, J., Zilberstein, M., Zakut, M., and Dekel, N. (1984): Phospholipid turnover and GnRH action in the pituitary and gonads. In: *LHRH and its Analogues: Basic and Clinical Aspects*, edited by F. Labrie, A. Belanger, and A. Dupont, pp. 245–260. International Congress Series 656, Excerpta Medica, Amsterdam.
314. Naor, Z., Molcho, J., Zilberstein, M., and Zakut, H. (1984): Phospholipid turnover in gonadotropin-releasing hormone target cells: comparative studies. In: *Hormonal Control of the Hypothalamo-Pituitary-Gonadal Axis*, edited by K. W. McKerns and Z. Naor, pp. 493–508. Plenum Press, New York and London.
315. Hazum, E. (1984): Nature of the GnRH receptors in the ovary. In: *Regulation of Target Cell Responsiveness*, edited by K. W. McKerns, A. Aakvag, and V. Hansson, pp. 23–46. Plenum Publishing Corp., New York.
316. Cooke, B. A., and Sullivan, M. H. F. (1985): The mechanisms of LHRH agonist action in gonadal tissues. *Mol. Cell. Endocrinol.* 41:115–122.
317. Birnbaumer, L., Shahabi, N., Rivier, J., and Vale, W. (1985): Evidence for a physiological role of gonadotropin-releasing hormone (GnRH) or GnRH-like material in the ovary. *Endocrinology*, 116:1367–1370.

318. Fink, G. (1976): Control of the ovarian cycle in the rat. In: *Ovulation in the Human*, edited by P. G. Crosignani and D. R. Mishell, pp. 95–114. Academic Press, New York.
319. Bauer, K., and Horsthemke, B. (1984): Degradation of LH-RH. In: *Hormonal Control of the Hypothalamo-Pituitary-Gonadal Axis*, edited by K. W. McKerns and Z. Naor, pp. 101–114. Plenum Press, New York.
320. Koch, Y., Elkabes, S., and Fridkin, M. (1984): Degradation of luteinizing hormone-releasing hormone by rat pituitary plasma membrane associated enzymes. In: *Hormonal Control of the Hypothalamo-Pituitary-Gonadal Axis*, edited by K. W. McKerns and Z. Naor, pp. 115–126. Plenum Press, New York.
321. Koch, Y., Baram, T., Hazum, E., and Fridkin, M. (1977): Resistance to enzymic degradation of LHRH analogues possessing increased biological activity. *Biochem. Biophys. Res. Commun.*, 74:488–491.
322. Rippel, R. H., and Johnson, E. S. (1976): Inhibition of hCG-induced ovarian and uterine weight augmentation in the immature rat by analogs of GnRH. *Proc. Soc. Exp. Biol. Med.*, 152:432–436.
323. Ying, S.-Y., and Guillemin, R. (1979): (D-Trp^6-Pro^9-NEt)-luteinizing hormone-releasing factor inhibits follicular development in hypophysectomized rats. *Nature (Lond.)*, 280:593–595.
324. Hsueh, A. J. W., and Erickson, G. F. (1979): Extrapituitary action of gonadotropin-releasing hormone: direct inhibition of ovarian steroidogenesis. *Science N.Y.*, 204:854–855.
325. Massicotte, J., Veilleux, R., Lavoie, M., and Labrie, F. (1980): An LHRH agonist inhibits FSH-induced cyclic AMP accumulation and steroidogenesis in porcine granulosa cells in culture. *Biochem. Biophys. Res. Commun.*, 94:1362–1366.
326. Knecht, M., Katz, M., and Catt, K. J. (1981): GnRH inhibits cyclic nucleotide accumulation in cultured rat granulosa cells. *J. Biol. Chem.*, 256:34–36.
327. Darbon, J. M., Knecht, M., Ranta, R., Dufau, M., and Catt, K. J. C. (1984): Hormonal regulation of cyclic AMP-dependent protein kinase in cultured ovarian granulosa cells. *J. Biol. Chem.*, 259:14778–14782.
328. Massicote, J., Borgus, J. P., Lachance, R., and Labrie, F. (1981): Inhibition of hCG-induced cyclic AMP accumulation and steroidogenesis in rat luteal cells by an LHRH agonist. *J. Steroid Biochem.*, 14:239–242.
329. Hsueh, A. J. W., Wang, C., and Erickson, G. F. (1980): Direct inhibitory effect of gonadotropin-releasing hormone upon follicle-stimulating hormone induction of luteinizing hormone receptor and aromatase activity in rat granulosa cells. *Endocrinology*, 106:1697–1705.
330. Dorrington, J., McKeracher, H., Munshi, S., and Gore-Langton, R. (1982): LHRH independently stimulates steroidogenic enzymes in granulosa cell cultures. *Endocrinology*, 110 (Suppl.):178.
331. Gore-Langton, R. E., Lacroix, M., and Dorrington, J. H. (1981): Differential effects of luteinizing hormone-releasing hormone on follicle-stimulating hormone-dependent responses in rat granulosa cells and Sertoli cells *in vitro*. *Endocrinology*, 108:812–818.
332. Jones, P. B. C., and Hsueh, A. J. W. (1982): Pregnenolone biosynthesis by cultured rat granulosa cells: modulation by follicle-stimulating hormone and gonadotropin-releasing hormone. *Endocrinology*, 111:713–721.
333. Jones, P. B. C., and Hsueh, A. J. W. (1981): Direct stimulation of ovarian progesterone-metabolizing enzyme by gonadotropin-releasing hormone in cultured granulosa cells. *J. Biol. Chem.*, 256:1248–1254.
334. Hsueh, A. J. W., and Ling, N. C. (1979): Effect of an antagonistic analog of gonadotropin releasing hormone upon ovarian granulosa cell function. *Life Sci.*, 25:1223–1230.
335. Navickis, R. J., Jones, P. B. C., and Hsueh, A. J. W. (1982): Modulation of prolactin receptors in cultured rat granulosa cells by FSH, LH and GnRH. *Mol. Cell. Endocrinol.*, 27:77–88.
336. Reddy, P. V., Azhar, S., and Menon, K. M. J. (1980): Multiple inhibitory actions of luteinizing hormone-releasing hormone agonist on luteinizing hormone/human chorionic gonadotropin receptor-mediated ovarian responses. *Endocrinology*, 107:930–936.
337. Hillier, S. G., Reichert, Jr., L. E., and van Hall, E. V. (1981): Modulation of FSH-controlled steroidogenesis in rat granulosa cells: direct *in vitro* effects of LHRH and ICI-118630. *Mol. Cell. Endocrinol.*, 23:193–205.
338. Magoffin, D. A., Reynolds, D. S., and Erickson, G. F. (1981): Direct inhibitory effect of GnRH on androgen secretion by ovarian interstitial cells. *Endocrinology*, 109:661–663.
339. Magoffin, D. A., and Erickson, G. F. (1982): Mechanism by which GnRH inhibits androgen synthesis directly in ovarian interstitial cells. *Mol. Cell. Endocrinol.*, 27:191–198.
340. Behrman, H. R., Preston, S. L., and Hall, A. K. (1980): Cellular mechanism of the antigonadotropic action of LHRH in the corpus luteum. *Endocrinology*, 107:656–664.
341. Clayton, R. N., Harwood, J. P., and Catt, K. J. (1979): Gonadotropin-releasing hormone analogue binds to luteal cells and inhibits progesterone production. *Nature Lond.*, 282:90–92.
342. Jones, P. B. C., and Hsueh, A. J. W. (1980): Direct inhibitory effect of gonadotropin-releasing hormone upon luteal luteinizing hormone receptor and steroidogenesis in hypophysectomized rats. *Endocrinology*, 107:1930–1936.
343. Hall, A. K., and Behrman, H. R. (1981): Culture sensitization and inhibition of luteinizing hormone responsive production of cyclic AMP in luteal cells by luteinizing hormone, prostaglandin $F_{2\alpha}$ and [D-Trp^6]-luteinizing hormone-releasing hormone. *J. Endocrinol.*, 88:27–38.
344. Harwood, J. P., Clayton, R. N., and Catt, K. J. (1980): Ovarian gonadotropin-releasing hormone receptors. I. Properties and inhibition of luteal cell function. *Endocrinology*, 107:407–413.
345. Clark, M. R., Thibier, C., Marsh, J. M., and LeMaire, W. (1980): Stimulation of prostaglandin accumulation by luteinizing hormone-releasing hormone (LHRH) and LHRH analogs in rat granulosa cells *in vitro*. *Endocrinology*, 107:17–23.
346. Clark, M. R. (1982): Stimulation of progesterone and prostaglandin E_2 accumulation by luteinizing hormone-releasing hormone (LHRH) and LHRH analogs in rat granulosa cells. *Endocrinology*, 110:146–152.
347. Sheela Rani, C. S., Ekholm, C., Billig, Magnusson, C. and Hillensjö, T. (1983): Biphasic effect of gonadotropin releasing hormone on progestin secretion by rat granulosa cells. *Biol. Reprod.*, 28:591–597.
348. Billig, H., Sheela Rani, C. S., Ekholm, C., Magnusson, C. and Hillensjö, T. (1984): Effect of a GnRH analogue on rat granulosa cell lactate production *in vitro*. *Acta Endocrinologica*, 105: 112–118.
349. Corbin, A., and Bex, F. J. (1981): Luteinizing hormone-releasing hormone agonists induce ovulation by hypophysectomized rats: direct ovarian effect. *Life Sci.*, 29:185–192.
350. Ekholm, C., Hillensjö, T., and Isaksson, O. (1981): Gonadotropin-releasing hormone agonists stimulate oocyte meiosis and ovulation in hypophysectomized rats. *Endocrinology*, 108:2022–2024.
351. Ekholm, C., Clark, M. R., Magnusson, C., Isaksson, O., and LeMaire, W. J. (1982): Ovulation induction by a GnRH analog in hypophysectomized rats involves prostaglandins. *Endocrinology*, 110:288–290.
352. Dekel, N., Sherizly, I., Tsafriri, A., and Naor, Z. (1983): A comparative study of the mechanism of action of LH and a GnRH analog on the ovary. *Biol. Reprod.*, 28:161–166.
353. Hillensjö, T., LeMaire, W. J., Clark, M. R., and Ahrén, K. (1982): Effect of GnRH and GnRH agonists upon accumulation of progesterone, cAMP and prostaglandin in isolated preovulatory rat follicles. *Acta Endocrinol. Copenh.*, 101:603–610.
354. Wang, C. (1983): Luteinizing hormone releasing hormone stimulates plasminogen activator production by rat granulosa cells. *Endocrinology*, 112:1130–1132.
355. Reich, R., Abisogun, A. O., Miskin, R., and Tsafriri, A. (1985): The mechanism(s) of LH and GnRH induced steroidogenesis and plasminogen activator in preovulatory rat follicles. *J. Steroid. Biochem.*, 23 (Suppl. 17S) [Abstr. 5].
356. Bex, F. J., and Corbin, A. (1984): Cyclic response of hypophysectomized rats to ovulation induced by LHRH agonists. Mediation by prostaglandins. *Life Sci.*, 35:969–979.
357. Koos, R. D., and LeMaire, W. J. (1985): The effects of gonadotropin-releasing hormone agonist on ovulation and steroidogenesis during perfusion of rabbit and rat ovaries *in vitro*. *Endocrinology*, 116:628–632.
358. Hillensjö, T., and LeMaire, W. J. (1980): Gonadotropin-releasing hormone agonists stimulate meiotic maturation of follicle-enclosed rat oocytes *in vitro*. *Nature Lond.*, 287:145–146.

359. Magnusson, C., and LeMaire, W. J. (1981): A gonadotrophin-releasing hormone agonist stimulates oxygen consumption and maturation of follicle-enclosed rat oocytes *in vitro*. *Acta Physiol. Scand.* 111:377–379.
360. Aberdam, E., and Dekel, N. (1985): Activators of protein kinase C stimulate meiotic maturation of rat oocytes. *Biochem. Biophys. Res. Commun.*, 132:570–574.
361. Tsafriri, A., Reich, R., and Abisogun, A. O. (1986): Ovarian regulation of oocyte maturation. In: *Gynecological Endocrinology*, edited by Genazzani, A. R., Volpe, A., and Facchinetti, F. Parthenon, 109–115.
362. Popkin, R. M., Fraser, H. M., and Jonassen, J. (1983): Stimulation of androstenedione and progesterone release by LHRH agonist from isolated rat preovulatory follicles. *Mol. Cell. Endocrinol.*, 29:169–180.
363. Hillensjö, T., Ekholm, C., and Hedin, L. (1984): Effect of gonadotrophin releasing hormone upon the pattern of steroidogenesis in isolated preovulatory rat follicles. *Acta Endocrinol.*, 105:105–111.
364. Mayar, M. Q., Tarvansky, G. K., and Reeves, J. J. (1979): Ovarian growth and uptake of iodinated D-Leu^6,desGlyNH$_2$^{10}-LHRH ethylamide in hCG-treated rats. *Proc. Soc. Exp. Biol. Med.*, 161:216–219.
365. Reeves, J. J., Seguin, C., Lefebvre, F. A., Kelly, P. A., and Labrie, F. (1980): Similar luteinizing hormone-releasing hormone binding sites in rat anterior pituitary and ovary. *Proc. Natl. Acad. Sci. U.S.A.*, 77:5567–5571.
366. Jones, P. B. C., Conn, P. M., Marian, J., and Hsueh, A. J. W. (1980): Binding of gonadotropin-releasing hormone agonist to rat ovarian granulosa cells. *Life Sci.*, 27:2125–2132.
367. Harwood, J. P., Clayton, R. N., Chen, T. T., Knox, G., and Catt, K. J. (1980): Ovarian gonadotropin-releasing hormone receptors. II. Regulation and effects on ovarian development. *Endocrinology*, 107:414–421.
368. Pieper, D. R., Richards, J. S., and Marshall, J. C. (1981): Ovarian gonadotropin-releasing hormone (GnRH) receptors: characterization, distribution and induction by GnRH. *Endocrinology*, 108: 1148–1155.
369. Smith-White, S., and Ojeda, S. R. (1983): Peripubertal decline in ovarian LHRH receptor content: characterization and distribution. *Neuroendocrinology*, 36:449–456.
370. Dalkin, A. C., Bourne, G. A., Pieper, D. R., Regiani, S., and Marshall, J. C. (1981): Pituitary and gonadal gonadotropin-releasing hormone receptors during sexual maturation in the rat. *Endocrinology*, 108:1658–1664.
371. White, S. S., and Ojeda, S. R. (1981): Changes in ovarian LHRH receptor content during the onset of puberty in the female rat. *Endocrinology*, 108:347–349.
372. Hazum, E., and Nimrod, A. (1982): Photoaffinity-labelling and fluorescence distribution studies on GnRH receptors in ovarian granulosa cells. *Proc. Natl. Acad. Sci. U.S.A.*, 79:1747–1750.
373. Hazum, E. (1981): Photoaffinity labeling of luteinizing hormone releasing hormone receptor of rat pituitary membrane preparations. *Endocrinology*, 109:1281–1283.
374. Ranta, T., Knecht, M., Kody, M., and Catt, K. J. (1982): GnRH receptors in cultured rat granulosa cells: mediation of the inhibitory and stimulatory actions of GnRH. *Mol. Cell. Endocrinol.*, 27:233–240.
375. Popkin, R. M., Fraser, H. M., and Gosden, R. G. (1983): Effect of LH-RH agonist or LH-RH immunoneutraization on pituitary and ovarian LH-RH receptors in female rats. *J. Reprod. Fertil.*, 69:245–252.
376. Naor, Z., and Yavin, E. (1982): Gonadotropin releasing hormone stimulates phospholipid labeling in cultured granulosa cells. *Endocrinology*, 111:1615–1619.
377. Davis, J. S., Farese, R. V., and Clark, M. R. (1983): Gonadotropin-releasing hormone (GnRH) stimulates phosphatidylinositol metabolism in rat granulosa cells: mechanism of action of GnRH. *Proc. Natl. Acad. Sci. U.S.A.*, 80:2049–2053.
378. Leung, P. C. K., Raymond, V., and Labrie, F. (1983): Stimulation of phosphatidic acid and phosphatidylinositol labelling in luteal cells by LHRH. *Endocrinology*, 112:1138–1140.
379. Raymond, V., Leung, P. C. K., and Labrie, F. (1983): Stimulation by prostaglandin $F_{2\alpha}$ of phosphatidic acid–phosphatidylinositol turnover in rat luteal cells. *Biochem. Biophys. Res. Commun.*, 116:39–46.
380. Leung, P. C. K. (1985): Mechanisms of gonadotropin-releasing hormone and prostaglandin action on luteal cells. *Can. J. Physiol. Pharmacol.*, 63:249–256.
381. Ranta, T., Knecht, M., Darbon, J-M., Baukal, A. J., and Catt, K. J. (1983): Calcium dependence of the inhibitory effect of GnRH on LH-induced cyclic AMP production in rat granulosa cells. *Endocrinology*, 113:427–429.
382. Eckstein, N., Eshel, A., Eli, Y., Ayalon, D., and Naor, Z. (1986): Calcium-dependent actions of gonadotropin-releasing hormone agonist and luteinizing hormone upon cyclic AMP and progesterone production in ovarian granulosa cells. *Mol. Cell. Endocrinol.*, 47:91–98.
383. Minagishi, T., and Leung, P. C. K. (1985): Luteinizing hormone stimulates arachidonic acid release in rat granulosa cells. *Endocrinology*, 117:2001–2007.
384. Michell, R. H. (1975): Inositol phospholipids and cell surface receptor function. *Biochim. Biophys. Acta*, 415:81–147.
385. Berridge, M. J., and Irvine, R. F. (1984): Inositol triphosphate, a novel second messenger in cellular signal transduction. *Nature*, 312:315–321.
386. Nishizuka, Y. (1984): Turnover of inositol phospholipids and signal transduction. *Science*, 225:1365–1370.
387. Fain, J. N. (1982): Involvement of phosphatidylinositol breakdown in elevation of cytosol Ca^{2+} by hormones and relationship to prostaglandin formation. In: *Hormone Receptors*, edited by L. D. Kohn, pp. 237–276, John Wiley & Sons Ltd.
388. Zor, U., Lamprecht, S. A., Kaneko, T., Schneider, H. P. G., McCann, S. M., Field, J. B., Tsafriri, A., and Lindner, H. R. (1972): Functional relations between cyclic AMP, prostaglandins and luteinizing hormone in rat pituitary and ovary. *Adv. Cycl. Nucl. Res.*, 1:503–520.
389. Marsh, J. M. (1976): The role of cAMP in gonadal steroidogenesis. *Biol. Reprod.*, 14:30–53.
390. Zilberstein, M., Zakut, H., Eli, Y., and Naor, Z. (1984): Regulation of prostaglandin E, progesterone and cyclic AMP production in ovarian granulosa cells by LH and GnRH: comparative studies. *Endocrinology*, 114:2374–2381.
391. Ying, S.-Y., Ling, N., Böhlen, P., and Guillemin, R. (1981): Gonadocrinins: peptides in ovarian follicular fluid stimulating the secretion of pituitary gonadotropins. *Endocrinology*, 108:1206–1215.
392. Esch, F., Ling, N., Ying, S.-Y., and Guillemin, R. (1983): Peptides of gonadal origin involved in reproductive biology. In: *Role of Peptides and Proteins in Control of Reproduction*, edited by S. M. McCann and D. S. Dhindsa, pp. 275–290. Elsevier, Amsterdam.
393. Williams, A. T., and Ulmanis, M. A. (1983): Macromolecular-bound antigonadotropin in porcine follicular fluid with LHRH immunoreactivity. *Biol. Reprod.*, 28:(Suppl. 1) [Abstr. 258].
394. Minaguchi, H., Mori, J., and Vemura, T. (1984): Partial isolation of gonadotropin releasing hormone (GnRH) like substance from the porcine ovary. In: *7th Int. Congr. Endocrinol.* Abstract No. 1560, Excerpta Medica, Amsterdam, Netherlands.
395. Aten, R. F., Wolin, D. L., and Behrman, H. R. (1985): Isolation of a GnRH-like substance from the rat ovary. *Endocrinology*, 116 (Suppl. 1) [Abstr. 31].
396. Brown, J. L., and Reeves, J. J. (1983): Absence of specific LHRH receptors in ovine, bovine, and porcine ovaries. *Biol. Reprod.*, 29:1179–1182.
397. Asch, R. H., Sickle, M. V., Rettori, V., Balmaceda, J. P., Eddy, C. P., Coy., D. H., and Schally, A. V. (1981): Absence of LHRH binding sites in corpora lutea from rhesus monkeys (*Macaca mulatta*). *J. Clin. Endocrinol. Metab.*, 53:215–217.
398. Clayton, R. N., and Huhtaniemi, I. T. (1982): Absence of gonadotropin-releasing hormone receptors in human gonadal tissue. *Nature Lond.*, 299:56–59.
399. Popkin, R. M., Bramley, T. A., Currie, A. J., Shaw, R. W., Baird, D. T., and Fraser, H. M. (1983): Specific binding of luteinizing hormone-releasing hormone to human luteal tissue. *Biochem. Biophys. Res. Commun.*, 114:750–756.
400. Milvae, R. A., Murphy, B. D., and Hansel, W. (1984): Prolongation of the bovine estrous cycle with a gonadotropin-releasing hormone analog. *Biol. Reprod.*, 31:664–670.
401. Tureck, R. W., Mastroianni, L, Jr., Blasco, L., and Strauss, J. F. (1982): Inhibition of human granulosa cell progesterone secretion by a GnRH agonist. *J. Clin. Endocrinol. Metab.*, 54:1078–1083.

402. Asch, R. H., Eddy, C. A., and Schally, A. V. (1981): Lack of luteolytic effect of D-Trp-6-LH-RH in hypophysectomized rhesus monkeys (*Macaca mulatta*). *Biol. Reprod.*, 25:963–968.
403. Casper, R. J., Erickson, G. F., Rebar, R. W., and Yen, S. S. C. (1982): The effect of LHRH and its agonist on cultured human granulosa cells. *Fertil. Steril.*, 37:406–409.
404. Tan, G. J. S., and Biggs, J. S. G. (1983): Absence of effect of LHRH on progesterone production by human luteal cells *in vitro*. *J. Reprod. Fertil.*, 67:411–413.
405. Williams, A. T., and Behrman, H. R. (1983): Paracrine regulation of the ovary by GnRH and other peptides. *Semin. Reprod. Biol.*, 1:269–277.
406. Tsafriri, A., and Eckstein, B. (1986): Changes in follicular steroidogenic enzymes following the preovulatory surge of gonadotropins and experimentally-induced atresia. *Biol. Reprod.*, 34:783–787.
407. Erickson, G. E., Hofeditz, C., and Hsueh, A. J. W. (1983): GnRH stimulates meiotic maturation in pre-antral follicles of hypophysectomized rats. In: *Factors Regulating Ovarian Function*, edited by G. S. Greenwald and P. F. Terranova, pp. 257–261. Raven Press, New York.
408. Banka, C. L., and Erickson, G. F. (1985): Gonadotropin-releasing hormone induces classical meiotic maturation in subpopulations of atretic preantral follicles. *Endocrinology*, 117:1500–1507.
409. Reich, R., Miskin, R., and Tsafriri, A. (1984): Follicular plasminogen activator: involvement in ovulation. *Endocrinology*, 116:516–521.
410. Ax, R. L., Bellin, M. E., and Grimek, H. J. (1985): Properties and regulation of synthesis of glycosaminoglycans by the ovary. In: *Proceedings of the Fifth Ovarian Workshop*, edited by D. O. Toft and R. J. Ryan, pp. 451–480. Ovarian Workshops, Champaign, Illinois.
411. Eppig, J. J., Ward-Bailey, P. F., and Schultz, R. M. (1985): The physiological functions of ovarian glycosaminoglycans. In: *Proceedings of the Fifth Ovarian Workshop*, edited by D. O. Toft and R. J. Ryan, pp. 481–491. Ovarian Workshops, Champaign, Illinois.
412. Bahr, J. M., and Ben-Jonathan, N. (1985): Ovarian catecholamines during the pre-pubertal period and reproductive cycle of several species. In: *Catecholamines as Hormone Regulators*, edited by N. Ben-Jonathan, J. M. Bahr, and R. I. Weiner, pp. 279–292. Raven Press, New York.
413. Arbogast, L., Rhoades, T., Peleg, D., and Ben-Jonathan, N. (1984): Norepinephrine synthesis by the neonatal ovary and by isolated follicles during the estrous cycle. *7th Int. Congr. Endocrinol.*, Abstr. 180, Quebec City, Canada.
414. Coleman, A. J., Paterson, D. S., and Somerville, A. R. (1979): The β-adrenergic receptor of rat corpus luteum membranes. *Biochem. Pharmacol.*, 28:1003–1010.
415. Harwood, J. P., Richert, N. D., Dufau, M. L., and Catt, K. J. (1980): Gonadotropin-induced desensitization of epinephrine action in the luteinized rat ovary. *Endocrinology*, 107:280–288.
416. Kliachko, S., and Zor, U. (1981): Increases in catecholamine-stimulated cyclic AMP and progesterone synthesis in rat granulosa cells during culture. *Mol. Cell. Endocrinol.*, 23:23–32.
417. Jordan, A. W. (1981): Changes in ovarian β-adrenergic receptors during the oestrous cycle of the rat. *Biol. Reprod.*, 24:245–248.
418. Aguado, L. I., Petrovic, S. L., and Ojeda, S. R. (1982): Ovarian β-adrenergic receptors during the onset of puberty: characterization, distribution and coupling to steroidogenic responses. *Endocrinology*, 110:1124–1132.
419. Abramowitz, J., Iyengar, R., and Birnbaumer, L. (1982): Guanine nucleotides and magnesium ion regulation of the interaction of gonadotropic and β-adrenergic receptors with their hormones: a comparative study using a single membrane system. *Endocrinology*, 110:336–346.
420. Kirchick, H. J., Iyengar, R., and Birnbaumer, L. (1983): Human chorionic gonadotropin-induced heterologous desensitization of adenylyl cyclases from highly luteinized rat ovaries: attenuation of regulatory *N* component activity. *Endocrinology*, 13:1638–1646.
421. Norjavaara, E., Rosberg, S. Gafvels, M. and Selstam, G. (1984): β-adrenergic receptor concentration in corpora lutea of different ages obtained from PMSG-treated rat. *Endocrinology*, 114:2154–2159.
422. Marsh, J. M. (1970): The stimulatory effect of luteinizing hormone on adenyl cyclase in the bovine corpus luteum. *J. Biol. Chem.*, 245:1596–1603.
423. Birnbaumer, L., Yang, P. C., Hunzicker-Dunn, M., Bockaert, J., and Duran, J. M. (1976): Adenylyl cyclase activities in ovarian tissues. I. Homogenization and conditions of assay in Graafian follicles and corpora lutea of rabbits, rats and pigs: regulation by ATP, and some comparative properties. *Endocrinology*, 99:163–184.
424. Condon, W. A., and Black, D. L. (1976): Catecholamine induced stimulation of progesterone by the bovine corpus luteum *in vitro*. *Biol. Reprod.*, 15:573–578.
425. Godkin, J. D., Black, D. L., and Duby, R. T. (1977): Stimulation of cyclic AMP and progesterone synthesis by LH, PGE_2 and isoproterenol in bovine corpus luteum *in vitro*. *Biol. Reprod.*, 17:514–518.
426. Jordan III, A. W., Caffrey, J. L., and Niswender, G. D. (1978): Catecholamine-induced stimulation of progesterone and adenosine 3′,5′-monophosphate production by dispersed ovine luteal cells. *Endocrinology*, 103:385–392.
427. Day, S. L., and Birnbaumer, L. (1980): The effect of estradiol on hormonally stimulable adenylyl cyclase activity and on progesterone production in normal and regressing corpora lutea from control and human gonadotropin-treated pseudopregnant rabbits. *Endocrinology*, 106:375–381.
428. Ratner, A., Sanborn, C. R., and Weiss, G. K. (1980): β-Adrenergic stimulation of cAMP and progesterone in rat ovarian tissue. *Am. J. Physiol.*, 239:E139–143.
429. Ratner, A., Weiss, G. K., and Sanborn, C. R. (1980): Stimulation by β_2-adrenergic receptors of the production of cyclic AMP and progesterone in rat ovarian tissue. *J. Endocrinol.*, 87:123–129.
430. Adashi, E. Y., and Hsueh, A. J. W. (1981): Stimulation of β_2-adrenergic responsiveness by follicle-stimulating hormone in granulosa cells *in vitro* and *in vivo*. *Endocrinology*, 108:2170–2178.
431. Jones, P. B. C., and Hsueh, A. J. W. (1981): Regulation of progesterone metabolizing enzyme by adrenergic agents, prolactin and prostaglandins in cultured rat ovarian granulosa cells. *Endocrinology*, 109:1347–1354.
432. Hunzicker-Dunn, M. (1982): Epinephrine-sensitive adenylyl cyclase activity in rabbit ovarian tissues. *Endocrinology*, 110:233–240.
433. Zsolnai, B., Varga, B., and Horvath, E. (1982): Increase of ovarian progesterone secretion by β2-adrenergic stimulation in oestrous rats. *Acta Endocrinol (Copenh)*, 101:268–272.
434. Rani, C. S., Nordenström, K., Norjavaara, E., and Ahrén, K. (1983): Development of catecholamine responsiveness in granulosa cells from preovulatory rat follicles—dependence on preovulatory luteinizing hormone surge. *Biol. Reprod.*, 28:1021–1031.
435. Dyer, C. A., and Erickson, G. F. (1985): Norepinephrine amplifies human chorionic gonadotropin-stimulated androgen biosynthesis by ovarian thecainterstitial cells. *Endocrinology*, 116:1645–1652.
436. Burden, H. W. (1985): The adrenergic innervation of mammalian ovaries. In: *Catecholamines as Hormone Regulators*, edited by N. Ben-Jonathan, J. M. Bahr, and R. I. Weiner, pp. 261–278. Raven Press, New York.
437. Burden, H. W., and Lawrence, I. E. (1977): The effects of denervation on the localization of Δ^5-3β-hydroxysteroid dehydrogenase activity in the rat ovary during pregnancy. *Acta Anat.*, 97:286–290.
438. Burden, H. W. (1978): Ovarian innervation. In: *The Vertebrate Ovary*, edited by R. E. Jones, pp. 616–638. Plenum Press, New York.
439. Owman, C. H., Sjöberg, N.-O., Wallach, E. E., Walles, B., and Wright, K. H. (1979): Neuromuscular mechanisms of ovulation. In: *Human Ovulation*, edited by E. S. E. Hafez, pp. 57–100. Biomedical Press, Elsevier/North-Holland.
440. Selstam, G., Norjavaara, E., Tegenfelt, T., Lundberg, S., Sandström, C., and Persson, S.-A. (1985): Partial denervation of the ovaries by transection of the suspensory ligament does not inhibit ovulation in rats treated with pregnant mare serum gonadotropin. *Anat. Rec.*, 213:392–395.
441. Deanesly, R. (1956): Cyclic function in ovarian grafts. *J. Endocrinol.*, 13:211–220.
442. Jacobowitz, D., and Laties, A. M. (1970): Adrenergic reinnervation of the cat ovary transplanted to the anterior chamber of the eye. *Endocrinology*, 86:921–924.
443. Dominguez, R., and Riboni, L. (1971): Failure of ovulation in autografted ovary of the hemispayed rat. *Neuroendocrinology*, 7:164–170.
444. Ojeda, S. R., and Aguado, L. I. (1985): Adrenergic control of the prepubertal ovary: involvement of local innervation and circulating

catecholamines. In: *Catecholamines as Hormone Regulators*, edited by N. Ben-Jonathan, J. M. Bahr, and R. I. Weiner, pp. 293–310. Raven Press, New York.

445. Gerendai, I., Marchetti, B., Maugeri, S., Amico-Roxas, M., and Scapagnini, U. (1978): Prevention of compensatory ovarian hypertrophy by local treatment of the ovary with 6-OHDA. *Neuroendocrinology*, 27:272–278.
446. Gerendai, I., and Halasz, B. (1978): Neural participation in ovarian control. *TINS*, 1:87–88.
447. Gerendai, I., and Halasz, B. (1976): Hemigonadectomy-induced unilateral changes in the protein-synthesizing activity of the rat hypothalamic arcuate nucleus. *Neuroendocrinology*, 21:331–337.
448. Curry, T. E., Lawrence, I. E., and Burden, H. W. (1984): Effect of ovarian sympathectomy on follicular development during compensatory ovarian hypertrophy in the guinea pig. *J. Reprod. Fertil.*, 71:39–44.
449. Brink, C. E., and Grob, H. (1973): Response of the denervated mouse ovary to exogenous gonadotropins. *Biol. Reprod.*, 9:108 [Abstr. 120].
450. Curry, T. E., Lawrence, I. E., and Burden, H. W. (1984): Ovarian sympathectomy in the guinea pig. I. Effects on follicular development during the estrous cycle. *Cell Tissue Res.*, 236:257–263.
451. Bahr, J. M., and Ben-Jonathan, N. (1981): Preovulatory depletion of ovarian catecholamines in the rat. *Endocrinology*, 108:1815–1821.
452. Ben-Jonathan, N., Braw, R. H., Laufer, N., Reich, R., Bahr, J. M., and Tsafriri, A. (1982): Norepinephrine in Graafian follicles is depleted by follicle-stimulating hormone. *Endocrinology*, 110:457–461.
453. Morimoto, K., Okamura, H., and Tanaka, C. (1982): Developmental and preovulatory changes of ovarian norepinephrine in the rat. *Am. J. Obstet. Gynecol.*, 143:389–392.
454. Veldhuis, J. D., Harrison, T. S., and Hammond, J. M. (1980): β_2-Adrenergic stimulation of ornithine decarboxylase activity in porcine granulosa cells *in vitro*. *Biochim. Biophys. Acta*, 627:123–130.
455. Sosa, A., Ortege-Corona, B., Chargoy, J., and Rosado, A. (1980): Presence and importance of biogenic amines in reproductive tract secretions. *Fertil. Steril.*, 33 [Abstr. suppl. 235].
456. Bahr, J. M., and Ben-Jonathan, N. (1985): Elevated catecholamines in porcine follicular fluid before ovulation. *Endocrinology*, 117:620–623.
457. Hunzicker-Dunn, M., Day, S. L., Abramowitz, J., and Birnbaumer, L. (1979): Ovarian responses of pregnant mare serum gonadotropin and human chorionic gonadotropin-primed rats: Desensitizing, luteolytic, and ovulatory effects of a single dose of human chorionic gonadotropin. *Endocrinology*, 105:442–451.
458. Norjavaara, E., Selstam, G., and Ahrén, K. (1982): Catecholamine stimulation of cyclic AMP and progesterone production in rat corpora lutea of different ages. *Acta Endocrinol.*, 100:613–622.
459. Norjavaara, E., Selstam, G., Dambar, J.-E., and Johansson, B.-M. (1983): *In vivo* effect of noradrenaline on the cyclic AMP level in rat corpora lutea. *Acta Physiol. Scand.*, 119:113–116.
460. Zor, U., and Kliachko, S. (1985): The β-adrenergic system in rat ovarian granulosa cells: hormonal and prostaglandin dependence *in vivo* and spontaneous development *in vitro*. In: *Catecholamines as Hormone Regulators*, edited by N. Ben-Jonathan, J. M. Bahr, and R. I. Weiner, pp. 311–328. Raven Press, New York.
461. Selstam, G., Norjavaara, E., Rosberg, S., Khan, I., Hamberger, B., and Hamberger, L. (1985): Norepinephrine content and stimulation of adenylate cyclase in corpora lutea of the rat. *Acta Physiol. Scand.* (*in press*).
462. Orly, J., Farkash, Y., Hershkovitz, N., Mizrahi, L., and Weinberger, P. (1982): Ovarian substance induces steroid production in cultured granulosa cells. *In Vitro*, 18:980–989.
463. Day, S. L., and Birnbaumer, L. (1980): Corpus luteum function and adenylyl cyclase stimulability in the rat after an estradiol benzoate-induced ovulatory surge of luteinizing hormone-induced ovulatory surge of luteinizing hormone: role of prolactin. *Endocrinology*, 106:382–389.
464. Abramowitz, J., and Birnbaumer, L. (1982): Temporal characteristics of gonadotropin interaction with rabbit luteal receptors and activation of adenylyl cyclase: comparison to the mode of action of catecholamine receptors. *Endocrinology*, 111:970–976.
465. Jones, P. B. C., Valk, C. A., and Hsueh, A. J. W. (1983): Regulation of progestin biosynthetic enzymes in cultured rat granulosa cells: effects of prolactin, β_2-adrenergic agonist, human chorionic gonadotropin and gonadotropin-releasing hormone. *Biol. Reprod.*, 29:572–585.
466. Lahav, M., Freud, A., and Lindner, H. R. (1976): Abrogation by prostaglandin $F_{2\alpha}$ of LH-stimulated cyclic AMP accumulation in isolated rat corpora lutea of pregnancy. *Biochem. Biophys. Res. Commun.*, 68:1294–1300.
467. Khan, I., and Rosberg, S. (1979): Acute suppression by PGF_2 on LH, epinephrine and fluoride stimulation of adenylate cyclase in rat luteal tissue. *J. Cycl. Nucl. Res.*, 5:55–63.
468. Khan, M. I., Rosberg, S., Lahav, M., Lamprecht, S. A., Selstam, G., Herlitz, H., and Ahren, K. (1979): Studies on the mechanism of action of the inhibitory effect of prostaglandin $F_{2\alpha}$ on cyclic AMP accumulation in rat corpora lutea of various ages. *Biol. Reprod.*, 21:1175–1183.
469. Thomas, J.-P., Dorflinger, L. J., and Behrman, H. R. (1978): Mechanism of the rapid antigonadotropic action of prostaglandins in cultured luteal cells. *Proc. Natl. Acad. Sci. U.S.A.*, 75:1344–1348.
470. Ahrén, K., Norjavaara, E., Rosberg, S., and Selstam, G. (1983): Prostaglandin $F_{2\alpha}$ inhibition of epinephrine stimulated cyclic AMP and progesterone production by rat corpora lutea of various ages. *Prostaglandins*, 25:839–850.
471. Capps, M. L., Lawrence, I. E., and Burden, H. W. (1978): Ultrastructure of the cells of the interstitial gland in hypophysectomized rats. *Cell Tissue Res.*, 193:433–442.
472. Krnjevitz, K. (1974): Chemical nature of synaptic transmission in vertebrates. *Physiol. Rev.*, 54:418–540.
473. Martindelrio, R., and Caballero, A. L. (1980): Presence of gamma-aminobutyric acid in rat ovary. *J. Neurochemistry*, 34:1584–1586.
474. Erdö, S. L., Rosdy, B., and Szporny, L. (1982): Higher GABA concentrations in Fallopian tube than in brain of the rat. *J. Neurochem.*, 38:1174–1176.
475. Schaeffer, J. M., and Hsueh, A. J. W. (1982): Identification of gamma-aminobutyric acid and its binding sites in the ovary. *Life Sci.*, 30:1599–1604.
476. Erdö, S. L. (1984): Alteration of GABA levels in ovary and fallopian tube of the pregnant rat. *Life Sci.*, 34:1879–1884.
477. Erdo, S. L., and Lapis, E. (1982): Bicuculline-sensitive GABA receptors in rat ovary. *Eur. J. Pharmacol.*, 85:243–246.
478. Erdö, S. L., and Lapis, E. (1982): Presence of GABA receptors in rat oviduct. *Neurosci. Lett.*, 33:275–279.
479. Apud, J. A., Tappaz, M. L., Celotti, F., Negri-Cesi, P., Masotto, C., and Racagni, G. (1984): Biochemical and immunochemical studies on the GABAergic system in the rat fallopian tube and ovary. *J. Neurochem.*, 43:120–125.
480. Apud, J., Racagni, G., Celotti, F., Negri-Cesi, P., and Martini, L. (1982): GABAergic innervation of the rat ovary: modulation and biochemical characterization. *Endocrinology*, 110 (Suppl.) [Abstr. 771].
481. Apud, J. A., Masotto, C., Cellotti, F., Negri-Cesi, P., Tappaz, M., and Racagni, G. (1983): Biochemical characterization of GABAnergic system in the fallopian tubes and in the ovary. *Endocrinology*, 112 (Suppl.) [Abstr. 381].
482. Erdo, S. L. (1983): High affinity, sodium-dependent gamma-aminobutyric acid uptake by slices of rat ovary. *J. Neurochem.*, 40:582–584.
483. Erdö, S. L., Varga, B., and Horvath, E. (1985): Effect of local GABA administration on rat ovarian blood flow, and on progesterone and estradiol secretion. *Eur. J. Pharm.*, 111:397–400.
484. Larsson, L. I., Fahrenkrug, J., and Schaffalitzky de Muckadell, O. B. (1977): Vasoactive intestinal peptide occurs in nerves of the female genitourinary tract. *Science*, 197:1374–1375.
485. Alm, P., Alumets, J., Hakanson, R., Helm, G., Owman, C., Sjoberg, N.-O., and Sundler, F. (1980): Vasoactive intestinal polypeptide nerves in the human female genital tract. *Am. J. Obstet. Gynecol.*, 136:349–351.
486. Alm, P., Alumets, J., Hakanson, R., Owman, C., Sjoberg, N.-O., Sundler, F., and Walles, B. (1980): Origin and distribution of VIP (vasoactive intestinal peptide) nerves in the genito-urinary tract. *Cell. Tissue Res.*, 205:337–347.
487. Ahmed, C. E., Dees, W. L., and Ojeda, S. R. (1985): The immature rat ovary is innervated by vasoactive intestinal peptide (VIP)- and substance P(SP)-containing fibers, but responds with steroid release only to VIP. *Endocrinology*, 116 (Suppl.) [Abstr. 821].

488. Bodner, M., Fridkin, M., and Gozes, I. (1985): Coding sequences for vasoactive intestinal peptide and PHM-27 peptide are located on two adjacent exons in the human genome. *Proc. Natl. Acad. Sci. U.S.A.*, 82:3548–3551.
489. Gozes, I., Bodner, M., Shani, Y., and Fridkin, M. (1984): Detection of mRNAs containing regulatory peptide coding sequences using synthetic oligodeoxynucleotides. *J. Cell Biochem.*, 26:147–156.
490. Davoren, J. B., and Hsueh, A. J. W. (1985): Vasoactive intestinal peptide—a novel stimulator of steroidogenesis by cultured rat granulosa cells. *Biol. Reprod.*, 33:37–52.
491. Kasson, B. G., Meidan, R., Davoren, J. B., and Hsueh, A. J. W. (1985): Identification of subpopulations of rat granulosa cells: sedimentation properties and hormonal responsiveness. *Endocrinology*, 117:1027–1034.
492. Burden, H. W., Leonard, M., Smith, C. P., and Lawrence, I. E. (1983): The sensory innervation of the ovary: a horseradish peroxidase study in the rat. *Anat. Rec.*, 207:623–627.
493. Lawrence, I. E., Burden, H. W., and Lous, T. M. (1978): Effect of abdominal vagotomy of the pregnant rat on LH and progesterone concentrations and fetal resorption. *J. Reprod. Fertil.*, 53:131–136.
494. Ojeda, S. R., White, S. S., Aguado, L. I., Advis, J. P., and Andersen, J. M. (1983): Abdominal vagotomy delays the onset of puberty and inhibits ovarian function in the female rat. *Neuroendocrinology*, 36:261–267.
495. Dees, W. L., Kozlowski, G. P., Dey, R., and Ojeda, S. R. (1985): Evidence for the existence of substance P in the prepubertal rat ovary. II. Immunocytochemical localization. *Biol. Reprod.*, 33:471–476.
496. Makris, A., Yasumizu, T., Elkind-Hirsh, K., Carraway, R., Leeman, S. E., and Ryan, K. J. (1982): Substance P and neurotensin in the ovary and pituitary of the cycling golden hamster. *Biol. Reprod.*, 26 (Suppl. 1):98A.
497. Ojeda, S. R., Costa, M. E., Katz, K. H., and Hersh, L. B. (1985): Evidence for the existence of substance P in the prepubertal rat ovary. I. Biochemical and physiologic studies. *Biol. Reprod.*, 33:286–295.
498. Sheldrick, E. L., and Flint, A. P. F. (1984): Ovarian oxytocin. In: *Gonadal Proteins and Peptides and Their Biological Significance*, edited by M. R. Sairam and L. E. Atkinson, pp. 257–272. World Scientific Publishing Co., Singapore.
499. Schaeffer, J. M., Liu, J., Hsueh, A. J. W., and Yen, S. S. C. (1984): Presence of oxytocin and arginine vasopressin in human ovary, oviduct and follicular fluid. *J. Clin. Endocrinol. Metab.*, 59:970–973.
500. Kruip, Th. A. M. Vullings, H. G. B., Schams, D., Jonis, J., and Klarenbeek, A. (1985): Immunocytochemical demonstration of oxytocin in bovine ovarian tissues. *Acta Endocrinol.*, 109: 537–542.
501. Schams, D., Kruip, Th. A. M., and Koll, R. (1985): Oxytocin determination in steroid producing tissues and *in vitro* production in ovarian follicles. *Acta Endocrinol.*, 109:530–536.
502. Khan-Dawood, F. S., and Dawood, M. Y. (1983): Human ovaries contain immunoreactive oxytocin. *J. Clin. Endocrinol. Metab.*, 57:1129–1132.
503. Khan-Dawood, F. S., Marut, E. L., and Dawood, M. Y. (1984): Presence and concentration of oxytocin in monkey corpus luteum throughout the luteal phase of the menstrual cycle. In: *Proceedings of the 7th International Congress of Endocrinology*, Abstr. 1018, Excerpta Medica, Amsterdam.
504. Robinson, G., Evans, J. J., and Forster, M. E. (1985): Oxytocin can affect follicular development in the adult mouse. *Acta Endocrinol.*, 108:273–276.
505. Rodgers, R. J., O'Shea, J. D., Findlay, J. K., Flint, A. P. F., and Sheldrick, E. L. (1983): Large luteal cells the source of luteal oxytocin in the sheep. *Endocrinology*, 113:2302–2304.
506. Niswender, G. D., Schwall, R. H., Fitz, T. A., Farin, C. E., and Sawyer, H. R. (1985): Regulation of luteal function in domestic ruminants: new concepts. *Rec. Prog. Horm. Res.*, 41:101–151.
507. Tan, G. J. S., Tweedale, R., and Biggs, J. S. G. (1982): Oxytocin may play a role in the control of the human corpus luteum. *J. Endocrinol.*, 95:65–70.
508. Tan, G. J. S., Tweedale, R. T., and Biggs, J. S. G. (1982): Effects of oxytocin on the bovine corpus luteum of early pregnancy. *J. Reprod. Fertil.*, 66:75–78.
509. Mukhopadhyay, A. K., Kumar, A., Tams, R., Bohnet, H. G., and Leidenberger, F. A. (1984): Oxytocin and vasopressin have no effect on progesterone production and cyclic AMP accumulation by rat luteal cells *in vitro*. *J. Reprod. Fertil.*, 72:137–141.
510. Wathes, D. C., Pickering, B. T., Swann, R. W., Horter, D. G., Hull, M. G. R., and Drif, G. O. (1982): Neurohyperphasial hormones in the human ovary. *Lancet*, 2:410–412.
511. Wathes, D. C., and Swann, R. W. (1982): Is oxytocin an ovarian hormone? *Nature Lond.*, 297:225–227.
512. Wathes, D. C., Swann, R. W., Hull, M. G. R., Drife, J. O., Porter, D. G., and Pickering, B. T. (1983): Gonadal sources of the posterior pituitary hormones. *Prog. Brain Res.*, 60:513–520.
513. Wathes, D. C., Swann, R. W., Birkett, S. D., Porter, D. G., and Pickering, B. T. (1983): Characterization of oxytocin, vasopressin and neurophysin from the bovine corpus luteum. *Endocrinology*, 113:693–698.
514. Lim, A. T. W., Lolait, S. J., Barlow, J. W., Autelitano, D. J., Toh, B. H., Boublik, J., Abraham, J., Johnston, C. I., and Funder, J. W. (1984): Immunoreactive arginine-vasopressin in Brattleboro rat ovary. *Nature Lond.*, 310:61–64.
515. Lolait, S. J., Lim, A. T. W., Abraham, J., Johnston, C. I., Barlow, J. W., Toh, B. H., and Funder, J. W. (1984): Arginine vasopressin in the rat and sheep ovary. In: *Proceedings of the 7th International Congress of Endocrinology*, Abst. 1292, Excerpta Medica, Amsterdam.
516. Fuller, P. J., Clements, J. A., Tregear, G. W., Nikolaidis, I., Whitfeld, P. L., and Funder, J. W. (1985): Vasopressin-neurophysin II gene expression in the ovary: studies in Sprague-Dawley, Long-Evans and Brattleboro rats. *J. Endocrinol.*, 105:317–321.
517. Tsong, S. D., Phillips, D., Halmi, N., Krieger, D., and Bardin, C. W. (1982): β-endorphin is present in the male reproductive tract of five species. *Biol. Reprod.*, 27:755–764.
518. Zimniski, S., Osteen, K., and Puett, D. (1985): Detection of β-endorphin-like components in porcine follicular fluid. *Endocrinology*, 116 (Suppl.) [Abstr. 516].
519. Krieger, D. T., Margioris, A. N., Liotta, A. S., Shaha, C., Gerendai, I., Pinter, J., and Bardin, C. W. (1984): Pro-opiomelanocortin-derived peptides in the rodent male reproductive tract. In: *Opioid Modulation of Endocrine Function*, edited by G. Delitala, M. Motta, and M. Serio, pp. 223–235. Raven Press, New York.
520. Lim, A. T., Lolait, S., Barlow, J. W., O, W-S., Zois, I., Toh, B. H., and Funder, J. W. (1983): Immunoreactive β-endorphin in sheep ovary. *Nature Lond.*, 303:709–711.
521. Shaha, C., Margioris, A., Liotta, A. S., Krieger, D. T., and Bardin, C. W. (1984): Demonstration of immunoreactive β-endorphin and γ-3-melanocyte-stimulating hormone-related peptides in the ovaries of neonatal, cyclic and pregnant mice. *Endocrinology*, 115:378–384.
522. Rothrock, M., Sarkar, D., and Erickson, G. F. (1984): Identification of β-endorphin in ovarian interstitial cells: its stimulation by LH. In: *Proceedings of the 7th International Congress of Endocrinology*, Abstr. 2111, Excerpta Medica, Amsterdam.
523. Lolait, S. J., Autelitano, D. J., Lim, A. T. W., Smith, A. I., Toh, B. H., and Funder, J. W. (1985): Ovarian immunoreactive β-endorphin and estrous cycle in the rat. *Endocrinology*, 117:161–168.
524. Chen, C.-L. C., and Chang, C.-C. (1985): Expression and regulation of pro-opiomelanocortin gene in the ovary and placenta. *Endocrinology*, 116 (Suppl.) [Abstr. 515].
525. Hamberger, L., Nordenström, K., Rosberg, S., and Sjögren, A. (1978): Acute influence of LH and FSH on cyclic AMP formation in isolated granulosa cells of the rat. *Acta Endocrinol.*, 88:567–579.
526. Hall, A. K., Preston, S. L., and Behrman, H. R. (1981): Purine amplification of luteinizing hormone action in ovarian luteal cells. *J. Biol. Chem.*, 256:10390–10398.
527. Polan, M. L., DeCherney, A. H., Haseltine, F. P., Mezer, H. C., and Behrman, H. R. (1983): Adenosine amplifies follicle stimulating hormone action in granulosa cells and luteinizing hormone action in luteal cells of rat and human ovaries. *J. Clin. Endocrinol. Metab.*, 56:288–294.
528. Billig, H., and Rosberg, S. (1986): Gonadotropin depression of ATP and interaction with adenosine in rat granulosa cells. *Endocrinology*, 118:645–652.
529. Knecht, M., Darbon, J.-M., Ranta, T., Baukal, A., and Catt, K. J. (1984): Inhibitory actions of adenosine on follicle-stimulating hormone-induced differentiation of cultured rat granulosa cells. *Biol. Reprod.*, 30:1082–1090.

530. Behrman, H. R., Hall, A. K., Preston, S. L., and Gore, S. D. (1982): Antagonistic interactions of adenosine and prostaglandin $F_{2\alpha}$ modulate acute responses of luteal cells to luteinizing hormone. *Endocrinology*, 110:38–46.
531. Behrman, H. R., Polan, M. L., Ohkawa, R., Laufer, N., Luborsky, J. L., Williams, A. T., and Gore, S. D. (1983): Purine modulation of LH action in gonadal cells. *J. Steroid Biochem.*, 19:789–793.
532. Behrman, H. R., Ohkawa, R., Preston, S. L., and MacDonald, G. J. (1983): Transport and selective utilization of adenosine as a prosubstrate for luteinizing hormone-sensitive adenylate cyclase in the luteal cell. *Endocrinology*, 113:1132–1140.
533. Brennan, T. J., Ohkawa, R., Gore, S. D., and Behrman, H. R. (1983): Adenine-derived purines increase adenosine triphosphate (ATP) levels in the luteal cell: evidence that cell levels of ATP may limit the stimulation of adenosine 3′,5′-monophosphate accumulation by luteinizing hormone. *Endocrinology*, 112:499–508.
534. Ohkawa, R., Polan, M. L., and Behrman, H. R. (1985): Adenosine differentially amplifies luteinizing hormone-over follicle-stimulating hormone-mediated effects in acute cultures of rat granulosa cells. *Endocrinology*, 117:248–254.
535. Fain, J. N., and Malbon, C. C. (1979): Regulation of adenylate cyclase by adenosine. *Mol. Cell. Biochem.*, 25:143–169.
536. Arch, J. R. S., and Newsholme, E. A. (1978): The control of the metabolism and the hormonal role of adenosine. In: *Essays in Biochemistry*, Vol. 14, edited by P. N. Campbell and W. N. Aldridge, pp. 82–123, The Biochemical Society, Academic Press, London.
537. Wolff, J., and Cook, G. H. (1977): Activation of steroidogenesis and adenylate cyclase by adenosine in adrenal and Leydig tumor cells. *J. Biol. Chem.*, 252:687–693.
538. Murphy, K. M. M., Goodman, R. R., and Snyder, S. H. (1983): Adenosine receptor localization in rat testes: Biochemical and autoradiographic evidence for association with spermatocytes. *Endocrinology*, 113:1299–1305.
539. Rommerts, F. F. G., Molenaar, R., Hoogerbrugge, J. W., and van der Molen, H. J. (1984): Development of adenosine responsiveness after isolation of Leydig cells. *Biol. Reprod.*, 30:842–847.
540. Billig, H., Rosberg, S., and Ahrén, K. (1986): Evidence for adenosine receptors in rat granulosa cells potentiating the FSH-effect on cAMP formation. Abstract submitted for presentation at the 1986 meeting of the Endocrine Society. (*Personal communication*).
541. Corey, E. J., Niwa, H., Falck, J. R., Mioskowski, C., Arai, Y., and Marfat, A. (1980): Recent studies on the chemical synthesis of eicosanoids. *Adv. Prostaglandin Thromboxane Res.*, 6:19–26.
542. Zor, U., and Lamprecht, S. A. (1977): Mechanism of prostaglandin action in endocrine glands. In: *Biochemical Actions of Hormones*, edited by G. Litwack, pp. 85–133. Academic Press, New York.
543. Behrman, H. R. (1979): Prostaglandins in hypothalamo-pituitary and ovarian function. *Ann. Rev. Physiol.*, 41:685–700.
544. Lindner, H. R., Zor, U., Kohen, F., Bauminger, S., Amsterdam, A., Lahav, M., and Salomon, Y. (1980): Significance of prostaglandins in the regulation of cyclic events in the ovary and uterus. *Adv. Prostaglandin Thromboxane Res.*, 8:1371–1390.
545. Patrono, C. (1983): Arachidonic acid metabolism in the ovary: biochemistry, methodology, and physiology. In: *The Ovary*, edited by G. B. Serra, pp. 45–56. Raven Press, New York.
546. Reich, R., Kohen, F., Naor, Z., and Tsafriri, A. (1983): Possible involvement of lipoxygenase products of arachidonic acid pathway in ovulation. *Prostaglandins*, 26:1011–1020.
547. Reich, R., Kohen, F., Slager, R., and Tsafriri, A. (1985): Ovarian lipoxygenase activity and its regulation by gonadotropin in the rat. *Prostaglandins*, 30:581–590.
548. Reich, R., Tsafriri, A., and Mechanic, G. L. (1984): The involvement of collagenolysis in ovulation in the rat. *Endocrinology*, 116:521–527.
549. Downs, S. M., and Longo, F. J. (1982): Effects of indomethacin on preovulatory follicles in immature, superovulated mice. *Am. J. Anat.*, 164:265–274.
550. Downs, S. M., and Longo, F. J. (1983): Prostaglandins and preovulatory follicular maturation in mice. *J. Exp. Zool.*, 228:99–108.
551. Salustri, A., Petrungaro, S., and Siracusa, G. (1985): Granulosa cells stimulate *in vitro* expansion of isolated mouse cumuli oophori: Involvement of prostaglandin E_2. *Biol. Reprod.*, 33:229–234.
552. Weinberger-Ohana, P., Shoshani, R., Farkash, Y., Hershkovitz, N., Goldring, N. B., Epstein-Almog, R., and Orly, Y. (1984): Low molecular weight substance from rat ovary induces steroidogenesis in cultured granulosa cells. *Mol. Cell. Endocrinol.*, 36:141–155.
553. Webley, G. E., and Luck, M. R. (1985): Melatonin directly stimulates the secretion of progesterone by human granulosa cells. *Acta Endocrinol. (Copenh.)*, 108 (Suppl. 267) [Abstr. 105].
554. Mori, T., Saito, H., Ohno, Y., Irahara, M., Hosoi, E., and Sato, S. (1984): Evidence for existence of somatostatin-like immunoreactivity with molecular heterogeneity in porcine ovaries. *Acta Endocrinol. (Copenh.)*, 106:254–259.
555. Mori, T., Irahara, M., Saito, H., Ohno, Y., and Hosoi, E. (1985): Inhibitory action of somatostatin on meiotic maturation of cultured porcine follicular ova. *Acta Endocrinol. (Copenh.)*, 110:408–412.
556. Szego, C. M., and Gitin, E. S. (1964): Ovarian histamine depletion during acute hyperaemic response to luteinizing hormone. *Nature*, 201:682–684.
557. Lipner, H. (1971): Ovulation from histamine depleted ovaries. *Proc. Soc. Exp. Biol. Med.*, 136:111–114.
558. Krishna, A., and Terranova, P. F. (1985): Alterations in mast cell degranulation and ovarian histamine in the proestrous hamster. *Biol. Reprod.*, 32:1211–1217.
559. Kirsch, T. M., Friedman, A. C., Vogel, R. L., and Flickinger, G. L. (1981): Macrophages in the corpora lutea of mice: characterization and effects on steroid secretion. *Biol. Reprod.*, 25:629–638.
560. Kirsch, T. M., Fogel, R. L., and Flickinger, G. L. (1983): Macrophages: a source of luteotropic cybernines. *Endocrinology*, 113:1910–1912.
561. Hammond, M. G., Halme, J., and Talbert, L. M. (1985): Pelvic macrophages as modulators of human granulosa cell progesterone production. In: *Gamete Quality and Fertility Regulation*, edited by R. Rolland, M. J. Heineman, S. G. Hillier, and H. Vemer, pp. 73–81. Excerpta Medica, ICS658, Amsterdam.
562. Birnbaumer, L., Codina, J., Mattera, R., Cerione, R. A., Hilderbrandt, J. D., Sunyer, T., Rojas, F. J., Caron, M. G., Lefkowitz, R. J., and Iyengar, R. (1985): Regulation of hormonal receptors and adenylyl cyclases by guanine nucleotide binding *N* proteins. *Rec. Prog. Horm. Res.*, 41:41–99.
562a. Pomerantz, S. H., and Billelo, P. A. (1987): Inhibition of progesterone-mediated maturation of oocytes of xenopus laevis by oocyte maturation inhibitor from fig follicular fluid: development of a routine assay for the inhibitor with xenopus oocytes. *Gamete Res.*, 17:267–268.

The Physiology of Reproduction,
edited by E. Knobil and J. Neill *et al.*
Raven Press, Ltd., New York © 1988.

CHAPTER 15

Inhibin

Anna Steinberger and Darrell N. Ward

The existence of a water-soluble substance of testicular origin that would regulate follicle-stimulating hormone (FSH) secretion through negative feedback was postulated more than 50 years ago. The saga of "inhibin," a term coined for this hypothetical substance by McCullagh (1), has persisted up to present-day science with considerable progress but many difficulties as well. In particular, the purification and characterization of inhibin continue to challenge the skills of many competent investigators. The major problem in the study of inhibin can be attributed to several factors: lack of specific quantitative assay methods, use of various sources of inhibin, and limited success in isolating inhibin by means of classical purification procedures. Beginning in 1985, however, substantial progress was made in resolving these problems (see section on the chemistry of inhibin).

The hypothesis for pituitary regulation by a nonsteroidal testicular substance was based on observations that injection of a water-soluble extract from bovine testis prevented the appearance of hypertrophied "castration" cells in the hypophysis (1). Clinical observations and experiments in animals indicated that damage of the seminiferous tubules following irradiation or chemotherapy and many cases of unexplained oligo- or azoospermia were often associated with selective elevation of FSH levels (2–16), which, in contrast to luteinizing hormone (LH), could not be easily suppressed by the administration of gonadal steroids (4,5). Thus, inhibin was assumed to be produced in the seminiferous tubules and to exert an inhibitory action on pituitary FSH secretion. These observations were later substantiated by more direct experiments showing that injection of steroid-free testicular extracts (12,17), rete testis fluid (18,19), or seminal plasma (20,21) into suitable animal models or their addition to pituitary cell cultures *in vitro* selectively or preferentially suppressed FSH secretion (Table 1).

Similar FSH-suppressing activity was also found to be present in steroid-free ovarian tissue and follicular fluid of several mammalian species (Table 1), suggesting that inhibin may also play a physiological role in the regulation of FSH secretion in the female. In ovariectomized rats and mice with elevated gonadotropins, administration of gonadal steroids (i.e., estrogen, progesterone, testosterone) suppresses LH but fails in most instances to suppress serum FSH to baseline, intact animal levels (22,23). In contrast, administration of steroid-free inhibin preparations (i.e., charcoal-treated ovarian extracts or follicular fluid) suppresses serum FSH, but not LH, to baseline levels (24–26). If administered at the time of castration, it can also selectively inhibit the postcastrational rise of serum FSH in rodents (24,25) as well as in the monkey (26); horse (27); and hamster (28). These observations have been elegantly reviewed by several authors (29–32) and will only briefly be summarized here.

During the normal rat estrous cycle there is a postovulatory selective rise in serum FSH (22,31,32). This postovulatory surge in FSH is not suppressible with exogenous progesterone (33), estradiol (34), or testosterone (24) but can be suppressed by administration of ovarian inhibin preparations (24,25,35–37). Furthermore, Sherman et al. (38) and Reyes et al. (39) observed that as women approach menopause, they can still have normal menstrual cycles as

TABLE 1. *Demonstration of inhibin activity from male and female sources*

Tissue or fluid	Species	Ref.
Seminal fluid	Human	8
	Bovine	20, 21, 110
Rete testes fluid	Ovine, porcine	9, 10, 18, 19, 99
Sperm extracts	Bovine	11, 16
Testicular extracts	Bovine, ovine, rat	9, 12, 17, 108, 120
Medium from Sertoli cell cultures	Rat	13, 14, 45, 48
Medium from testis organ culture	Mouse	98
Ovarian extracts	Rat, bovine	121–123
Follicular fluid	Bovine	24, 107
	Porcine	24, 25, 35, 124
	Human	125
Medium from granulosa cell cultures	Rat	51

well as normal estrogen, progesterone, and LH levels, but they have elevated serum FSH, supporting the concept of separate negative feedback regulation of FSH and LH.

It has not been known whether inhibins from different species or tissue sources are identical or dissimilar, but this question has recently been resolved for porcine and bovine inhibin (see section on the chemistry of inhibin). Moreover, although inhibin preparations of ovarian origin are effective in suppressing FSH selectively in male animals of different species and vice versa, it remains unclear whether the FSH-suppressing activities of ovarian and testicular origin differ in their structure and properties or represent the same active principle. Thus, for the sake of clarity, the studies on "testicular" and "ovarian" inhibin are considered under separate headings.

The intent of this chapter is to highlight the major findings that have contributed to our current understanding of the chemical nature and the physiology of inhibin rather than to provide a bibliographical account of all published work. Therefore, some important contributions may not have been cited herein owing to the subjective selection of references by the authors.

SOURCES OF INHIBIN

In the Male

Although inhibin in the male was believed to be produced by the testis, most probably in the seminiferous tubule, its precise cellular origin has been highly controversial. The germ cells (8,15,16,40,41) and the Sertoli cells (42–44) have separately and together (41–44) been implied as being the most likely sites of production. The germ cell origin of inhibin seemed particularly plausible, since a monotropic rise of FSH *in vivo* is often associated with germ cell depletion. Evidence from experiments *in vitro,* however, indicates that the main, and probably the only, source of inhibin in the male is the Sertoli cell (45–49).

The testis is a heterogenous organ composed of many different cell types. To delineate the cellular source of inhibin in the testis, highly enriched populations of specific cell types (Sertoli cells, germ cells, peritubular myoid cells, and interstitial cells) were isolated from rat testes and cultured *in vitro* in chemically defined media (50). The spent culture media were bioassayed for inhibin activity using monolayer cultures of rat anterior pituitary cells (see section on inhibin bioassay). The results revealed that only media from the Sertoli cell cultures selectively suppress FSH release from the pituitary cells. Similar results were reported by Labrie et al. (48); Franchimont et al. (14) and De Jong and Sharpe (49). In contrast, media from cultures of other testicular cell types of nontesticular tissues (i.e., spleen and kidney) had no effect on either FSH or LH release (45–47). Also, cocultures of Sertoli cells with pituitary cells selectively suppress FSH release compared to control cultures of pituitary cells alone (45,46). These findings clearly demonstrated that only the Sertoli cells secrete in culture an inhibin-like substance named Sertoli cell factor (SCF) (45–47) and are probably the physiologic source of inhibin in the male. SCF has been found to reduce selectively circulating FSH level *in vivo* when administered to castrated male rats.

In the Female

Ovarian inhibin appears to be produced by the granulosa cells (51), since only granulosa cells from ovarian follicles of many species [i.e., human (52,53), monkey (52,54), cow (55), rat (51,56), and pig (57)] but not cells isolated from thecal or stromal tissues secrete inhibin activity *in vitro.* The parallelism with Sertoli cells is not surprising since the Sertoli cells and granulosa cells have a similar embryologic origin.

Thus, cultures of isolated Sertoli and granulosa cells provide useful models for the study of testicular and ovarian inhibin secretion and its regulation by hormones and various other factors. Although the results from *in vitro* experiments cannot be directly extrapolated to physiological conditions, they often provide useful information that cannot be obtained using whole animals.

SITES AND MECHANISM OF ACTION OF INHIBIN

Inhibin may have several sites of action. Besides its well-documented direct effects on the anterior pituitary (6,9, 45,46,58,59), there are reports that indicate possible systemic effects of inhibin also on the hypothalamus (60–63) and the pineal gland (64), as well as local effects in the testis (65,66). These are considered under separate headings.

Pituitary

Inhibin preparations from various sources have been shown to suppress, selectively or preferentially, FSH secretion *in vivo* and *in vitro*. In some cases LH secretion is also suppressed while other pituitary hormones [i.e., growth hormone, prolactin, and thyroid-stimulating hormone (TSH)] are not affected (14). Experiments *in vitro* clearly demonstrated that inhibin can exert its effect on both FSH synthesis (13,14,67,68) and release by acting directly on the pituitary gonadotrophs (for reviews, see refs. 13,14,58,69,70).

Inhibin Effect on FSH Release

Injection of inhibin *in vivo* lowers the circulating levels of FSH. In some instances, the circulating levels of LH are also suppressed. Incubation of pituitary halves or cultures of pituitary cells with inhibin *in vitro,* in the presence or absence of gonadotropin-releasing hormone (GnRH), selectively or preferentially reduces the amount of FSH in the culture medium, providing direct evidence that inhibin suppresses both the basal and the GnRH-stimulating FSH release. A suppressing effect of inhibin on LH release has been usually observed only in the presence of GnRH and when high doses of the test material were used. In most cases the dose-response curves for LH and FSH are not parallel (for reviews, see refs. 13,14,58,69,70). It should be kept in mind that the LH suppression may be nonspecific because of unknown factors present in the impure inhibin preparations. Selective degradation of FSH during the incubation period was ruled out by demonstrating quantitative recovery of FSH following incubation with SCF (45,46) or other inhibin preparations (13,58). Moreover, it would be unlikely that a proteolytic activity would only affect FSH and not other proteinaceous hormones released by the pituitary cells.

The effect of inhibin on FSH release is relatively slow. It takes about 24 hr of contact with the pituitary cells *in vitro* to observe a significant suppression of basal or GnRH-stimulated FSH release. The degree of FSH suppression increases with additional time of exposure to inhibin, but even after 5 days of incubation, it does not reach 100% (71). The degree of FSH suppression also depends on the dose and the biological activity of the test material, providing a mean for relative measure of inhibin activity (see section on inhibin bioassay). The FSH-suppressing activity is no longer observed 24 hr after the inhibin-containing medium is replaced by fresh medium (71).

The inhibin effect is not limited to a particular species, sex, or age. Male and female pituitaries from different species and ages respond to inhibin with reduced FSH secretion; however, pituitary sensitivity to inhibin appears to increase with age during sexual maturation (72). Cultures of pituitary cells from adult animals show a greater suppression of FSH release than pituitary cells from younger animals when challenged with similar inhibin preparations.

Inhibin Effect on FSH Synthesis

Decreased medium levels of FSH following incubation of inhibin preparations with pituitary cells could be the result of suppressed FSH synthesis and/or release. The direct effect on FSH synthesis was examined *in vitro*. By measuring incorporation of ^{3}H-leucine into immunoprecipitable FSH and LH in pituitary organ cultures, Chowdhury et al. (67) demonstrated that SCF specifically suppresses FSH synthesis. The synthesis of LH was neither affected nor even stimulated. The stimulatory effect on LH synthesis could be due to the presence of a GnRH-like substance known to be secreted by cultured rat Sertoli cells. That inhibin may affect FSH synthesis was also indicated by reduced pituitary cell content of FSH following incubation with different inhibin preparations (13,14,68). The dose-dependent effect of inhibin on the cell content of FSH has been utilized by Scott et al. (68) for inhibin bioassay (see section on inhibin bioassay). Whether inhibin exerts separate actions on the synthesis and release of FSH or primarily affects only synthesis, thus reducing the amount of hormone available for release, remains to be determined.

Molecular Mechanism of Inhibin Action

The molecular mechanism by which inhibin affects FSH secretion remains to be elucidated. Binding of radiolabeled inhibin to rat anterior pituitaries has been observed *in vitro* (64,73–75) and *in vivo* (64). In analogy to other peptide hormones, the binding of inhibin to specific plasma membrane receptors in the target cell may represent the first step in its biologic action. This assumption was strengthened by demonstrating good correlation between the binding and the biologic activity of inhibin *in vitro* (75). Pituitary binding is dose related, time and temperature dependent, as well as saturable and tissue specific. Moreover, only inhibin preparations compete for the pituitary binding sites in a dose-dependent manner, and treatments that destroy the biologic activity of inhibin (i.e., trypsin and heat) also abolish, or significantly reduce, its binding (74,75). Reduced binding due to ligand degradation by tissue proteases possibly present in the inhibin preparations was ruled out. Although radiolabeled inhibin binds preferentially to the pituitary *in vivo,* some binding to the pineal gland was also observed (64), suggesting that the pineal may represent an additional site of action for inhibin.

The mechanism by which inhibin suppresses the GnRH-stimulated release of gonadotropins is not clear. Since inhibin and GnRH do not compete for pituitary binding *in vitro* (75), it appears that they may interact at some post-binding site(s). These substances have opposite effects on cyclic AMP levels. GnRH has been reported to increase endogenous cyclic AMP, whereas incubation of pituitary cell cultures with inhibin decreases the level of cyclic AMP (76). Franchimont et al. (77) observed a rapid (24 hr) dose-related increase of endogenous cyclic GMP in response to inhibin from ram rete testis fluid, which they suggested may have caused the suppression of cyclic AMP observed after 48 and 72 hr.

If, as immunocytochemical evidence indicates, both LH and FSH may be secreted by the same pituitary cells (78), it is not clear how inhibin can cause a selective suppression of FSH synthesis and release, or how these effects can be mediated by cyclic AMP or cyclic GMP. More experimental data using pure inhibin preparations are needed before the precise mechanism of inhibin action in the target cells can be fully understood.

Hypothalamus

A possible hypothalamic site of action for inhibin has been suggested by several reports. Lugaro et al. (61) and Lumpkin et al. (62) observed a selective reduction in circulating FSH levels following injection of partially purified inhibin preparation into the third ventricle; however, since in these studies the GnRH levels in the portal vessels were not measured, the decrease in peripheral FSH concentration cannot be directly ascribed to changes in GnRH secretion. Moreover, the existence of a separate hypothalamic FSH-releasing hormone has not been demonstrated. More direct evidence for a hypothalamic site of inhibin action was provided by demonstrating a decrease in GnRH content following incubation of isolated hypothalami with inhibin *in vitro* (60). The mechanism by which a reduction in GnRH content could lead to selective suppression of FSH secretion is not clear in view of the well-established stimulatory action of GnRH on the secretion of both FSH and LH. Additional studies on the effects of inhibin on the production and mode of release of GnRH (pulse frequency) may provide valuable information in this regard.

Testis

There is some evidence that inhibin may have local effects in the testis (65,66). When testicular fragments from 42-day-old rats were incubated *in vitro* for 3 hr with inhibin preparations in the presence of ^{3}H-thymidine, incorporation of the label into testicular DNA was significantly inhibited (65). Also, administration of inhibin to normal or hypophysectomized 42-day-old rats showed suppression of ^{3}H-thymidine incorporation into testicular, but not into liver, DNA. Autoradiography indicated that this effect was restricted to the germ cells, particularly the type B spermatogonia; however, since the inhibin preparations used in this study were of testicular origin (ram rete testis fluid), it remains to be determined whether this effect was caused by inhibin per se or by possible contamination of the inhibin preparations with testicular chalone, which can reduce spermatogonial DNA synthesis (79).

It has been reported that inhibin may also directly affect Leydig cell function by increasing their steroidogenic response to LH stimulation (66). The experimental evidence for this remains to be verified. It is noteworthy, however, that a GnRH-like substance, another secretory product of rat Sertoli cells, can modify Leydig cell steroid production and response to LH (80,81).

REGULATION OF INHIBIN SECRETION

Testicular Production of Inhibin

Role of Hormones

The Sertoli cells are a primary target for the action of FSH and testosterone in the testis (82,83). Cytoplasmic membrane receptors for FSH (84,85) and cytoplasmic and nuclear receptors for androgens (86,87), as well as specific chromatin acceptor sites for the androgen-receptor complex (88), have been demonstrated in the Sertoli cells. Also, many functions of the Sertoli cells, including the production of cyclic AMP (82,83,89), the secretion of androgen-binding protein (82,83), and nuclear transcriptional activity (90), are stimulated by testosterone and/or FSH. It was therefore logical to assume that inhibin secretion would also be regulated by these hormones. This assumption was investigated utilizing cultures of isolated rat Sertoli cells (47,71,74,77,91–94).

Effect of hypophysectomy. The effect of hypophysectomy on the secretion of inhibin was investigated by Steinberger (47,71,74,91) using immature (21-day-old) and mature (60-day-old) rats. At various time intervals after pituitary removal, groups of animals were sacrificed and used to initiate Sertoli cell cultures. Cultures of Sertoli cells obtained from intact animals of corresponding ages served as controls. Media collected after 3 days of incubation were bioassayed for inhibin activity. This approach was selected, since the available assay methods for inhibin are not sufficiently sensitive for direct measurements of inhibin activity in circulating blood.

The ability of Sertoli cells to secrete inhibin *in vitro* dramatically decreased following hypophysectomy in both age groups. Ten days after pituitary removal, culture media from Sertoli cells of the hypophysectomized immature animals caused only 10% suppression of FSH release, whereas those from intact controls showed 60% suppression, although both sets of cultures were comparative with respect to cell number, protein, and DNA content. In mature animals, a similar decline of inhibin secretion occurred at approximately 3 weeks after hypophysectomy.

By directly measuring inhibin activity in testicular extracts and seminiferous tubule fluid from adult rats (90-day-old) at different times following hypophysectomy, Au et al.

(93,94) reported a decline in inhibin content after 7 days and in inhibin production by 42 days. The impaired inhibin secretion following hypophysectomy is most likely due to a direct effect of hormone deprivation on Sertoli cell function rather than to germ cell depletion, since germ cells do not seem to produce inhibin or affect its secretion by Sertoli cells *in vitro* (47). The secretion of androgen-binding protein (ABP), another Sertoli cell product, also decreases after hypophysectomy (82,87).

Effect of hormonal treatments in vivo. Since inhibin secretion was dramatically reduced by pituitary removal, the effects of hormonal treatment *in vivo* were also examined in immature (47,71,74,91) and adult (93) rats. Hypophysectomized 21-day-old rats were treated for 10 days from the time of surgery with daily subcutaneous injections of either FSH (50 μg NIH-FSH-S1), LH (50 μg NIH-LH-S19), testosterone propionate [(TP) 0.5 mg], a combination of FSH plus TP, or FSH plus LH. Intact and hypophysectomized animals of similar age receiving the vehicles alone served as controls. Cultures of isolated Sertoli cells were initiated 15 to 16 hr after the last injection. Culture media collected after 3 days of incubation were bioassayed for inhibin activity using dispersed rat anterior pituitary cells. The results showed that administration of FSH, LH, or TP at the doses employed prevented the decline of inhibin secretion observed in hypophysectomized animals given the vehicles alone. Combined treatment with FSH plus LH or TP appeared more effective than either hormone administered alone. Since the effects of LH and TP were similar, the LH effect on inhibin secretion was most likely due to its stimulation of endogenous testosterone production. This assumption is reasonable in view of the fact that Sertoli cells are a primary target for the actions of FSH and testosterone and do not respond directly to LH (82–86).

In chronically (30 days) hypophysectomized adult rats, twice daily administration for 3 days of FSH (human FSH, 22 I.U. per rat per day), but not of human chorionic gonadotropin (12 I.U. per rat per day) or testosterone (5 mg per rat per day), increased testicular inhibin content (93). The lack of inhibin stimulation by human chorionic gonadotropin or testosterone in these experiments may have been due to the delay in initiating the hormone therapy.

Direct effect of hormones in Sertoli cell cultures. The effects of hormone addition to Sertoli cell cultures *in vitro* on inhibin secretion have been examined by several investigators (47,71,91–94). In some experiments, FSH (NIH-FSH-S11, 5 μg/ml), LH (NIH-LH-S19, 5 μg/ml), testosterone (10^{-7} M), cyclic AMP (0.1–1.0 mM), or 1-methyl-3-isobutyl methyl-xanthine [(MIX) 0.1 mM] were added directly to Sertoli cell cultures (47,71,91). After 2 days of incubation, the cells were rinsed and incubated for an additional 3 days in media without the above additives. Media collected after the second incubation period were bioassayed for inhibin activity. This protocol eliminated the problem of interference by the added test substances in the inhibin bioassay.

Sertoli cells preincubated with either FSH, testosterone, cyclic AMP, or MIX secreted significantly greater amounts of inhibin compared to untreated cells. Testosterone plus FSH, cyclic AMP, or MIX seemed more effective than any of these compounds tested individually. These findings are in agreement with the results obtained following the treatment with hormones *in vivo*. In contrast, LH had no effect on inhibin secretion in culture, supporting the assumption that its stimulatory effect *in vivo* was most likely mediated via enhanced endogenous production of testosterone. Increased secretion of inhibin in the presence of cyclic AMP or MIX is not surprising, since FSH is believed to exert its biological action through cyclic AMP, and many effects of FSH can be mimicked *in vitro* by cyclic AMP or MIX.

Franchimont et al. (77) and Verhoeven and Franchimont (92) also reported stimulation of inhibin production in cultures of rat Sertoli cells when either testosterone or dihydrotestosterone was added to the media, whereas FSH, human chorionic gonadotropin (HCG), or estrogen had no effect, and progesterone decreased inhibin production. These investigators concluded that only androgens acutely stimulate inhibin production by the Sertoli cells. The discrepancy with regard to FSH stimulatory effect on inhibin secretion could have been due to differences in the design of the experiments.

Although hormones can clearly influence inhibin secretion, it should be pointed out that inhibin is secreted in Sertoli cell cultures at a steady rate for at least 21 days in the absence of added hormones or serum (47,71,91). The precise role of gonadotropins and gonadal steroids in the regulation of inhibin secretion remains to be elucidated.

Effect of Elevated Temperature

Increased pituitary and circulating levels of FSH (and LH) following cryptorchidy are believed to result from impaired feedback regulation (2–5). Cryptorchidism was also shown to lower ABP production (95), suggesting that elevated temperature may impair Sertoli cell functions. The effects of elevated temperature *in vivo* (47,71,91,96,97) and *in vitro* (47,71,91,98) on inhibin secretion were investigated using cultures of rat Sertoli cells and mouse testis organ cultures.

Effects of cryptorchidy and orchidopexy. Seethalakshmi and Steinberger (97) initiated cultures of Sertoli cells from adult rats at various time intervals following surgical cryptorchidy and after 14 and 42 days of scrotal recovery (orchidopexy). The cultures were maintained at 32 to 34°C, and media collected after 3 days of incubation were assayed for inhibin activity. The data were normalized on the basis of Sertoli cell number and/or DNA content per culture dish. In these experiments, changes in circulating levels of FSH and LH and in testicular histology were also assessed to verify the effectiveness of the surgical procedures.

The results showed that cryptorchidy for 35 days severely reduces SCF secretion by Sertoli cells in culture compared to Sertoli cells from normal scrotal testes. These results support the earlier observations with Sertoli cell cultures from 25-day (47) and 14-day (96) cryptorchid animals. The decline in SCF secretion was accompanied by a rise in circulating FSH and LH levels and a progressive loss of spermatids and spermatocytes expected to occur after cryptorchidy. Impaired inhibin secretion may be one mechanism that leads to elevated pituitary and circulating levels of FSH in the cryptorchid conditions. The damaging effect of cryptorchidy on SCF secretion, however, appears to be reversible after the testes are returned to the scrotum and allowed to recover for an appropriate period of time.

When the testes of 35-day cryptorchid animals were returned to the scrotum, SCF secretion increased after 14 days and approached normal levels after 42 days (97). At the same time, the circulating levels of FSH and LH declined to near-normal values, and many seminiferous tubules contained mature spermatids. These results demonstrate that the damaging effects of cryptochidy are at least partly reversed by orchidopexy.

Effect of elevated temperature in vitro. The suppressing effect of elevated temperature on inhibin secretion was also observed *in vitro* when rat Sertoli cell cultures were incubated at 32°C and 38°C (47). While at 32°C (scrotal temperature) SCF secretion was maintained at a relatively steady rate for at least 21 days; incubation at 38°C (abdominal temperature) resulted in a progressive decline of inhibin activity to near-nondetectable level by 21 days. The damaging effect of elevated temperature *in vitro* (39°C) on inhibin secretion was also observed by Demoulin et al. (98) using mouse testis organ cultures and a different inhibin preparation. It appears from all these studies that above-scrotal temperatures *in vivo* or *in vitro* reduce the capacity of Sertoli cells to secrete inhibin.

Other Factors that Could Affect Inhibin Secretion

Developmental changes. To determine whether inhibin secretion is altered during sexual maturation, Sertoli cells isolated from rats of various ages were compared for their ability to secrete SCF in culture (47,72). The results of bioassay showed no significant differences in the amount of inhibin activity elaborated by Sertoli cells from animals between 18 and 90 days of age. Conversely, experiments in which pituitary cells from 18- to 90-day-old animals were challenged with the same inhibin preparation revealed that pituitary sensitivity to inhibin in the male rat significantly increases between 33 and 45 days (47,72). This may explain why circulating levels of FSH in the male rats decline dramatically after approximately 33 days of age (5).

Role of germ cells and peritubular cells in the secretion of inhibin. Although only the Sertoli cells appear to secrete an inhibin-like substance in culture, a possibility existed that other cell types in the testis might modulate its secretion. Both the germ cells and peritubular myoid cells were reported to influence various Sertoli cell functions (i.e., aromatization, protein, and ABP secretion). It has been suggested that inhibin secretion may depend on the interaction of Sertoli cells with germ cells, particularly the spermatids (99). To examine this possibility, enriched populations of rat germ cells (mainly spermatids or spermatocytes) were cocultured for 2 days with Sertoli cells, and their inhibin activity was compared with that of 2-day cultures of Sertoli cells alone (47,71,91). Spent media from both groups showed similar suppression of FSH release, suggesting that germ cells have no effect on the Sertoli cell secretion of SCF. Similar results were obtained when the Sertoli cells were cocultured with peritubular myoid cells. Whether a comparable situation exists *in vivo* remains to be determined; however, the equal capacity for inhibin secretion demonstrated by Sertoli cells from animals between 18 and 90 days of age (47,72), when germ cell composition changes dramatically, would argue against a significant effect of germ cells on inhibin secretion.

Although a monotropic rise of circulating FSH levels is often associated with germ cell depletion, both of these events could be interpreted as a consequence of Sertoli cell damage. Since inhibin secretion and germ cell differentiation depend on normally functioning Sertoli cells, impairment of Sertoli cell functions may result in diminished inhibin secretion, and thus in elevated FSH levels, and also in spermatogenic arrest. For example, the elevated temperature in cryptorchid conditions causes a reduction in the secretion of inhibin and ABP as well as in the number of germ cells.

Ovarian Production of Inhibin

Hormonal Control of Inhibin Secretion by Ovarian Cell Types

The granulosa cells of the ovarian follicles were shown to secrete an inhibin-like factor in culture (51) and are considered to be the source of inhibin activity in the female.

Franchimont et al. (14,77) investigated the secretion of inhibin in monolayer cultures of bovine granulosa cells. The granulosa cells were obtained from large antral follicles (78–15 mm), and inhibin activity in the culture media was assayed on the basis of inhibition of luteinizing hormone-releasing hormone (LHRH)-induced FSH secretion by dispersed pituitary cells.

The granulosa cells produced both inhibin and progesterone on the first day of culture and although progesterone secretion increased on subsequent days, presumably as a result of luteinization, inhibin production fell. These results indicate that there is an inverse relationship between progesterone and inhibin production by granulosa cells in monolayer culture. Furthermore, addition of progesterone to the granulosa cell cultures led to a decrease of inhibin secretion. Neither purified porcine FSH, LH, estrogens (estrone or estradiol-17β), or prolactin modified the inhibin secretion. Conversely, the addition of androgens, either aromatizable (androstenedione and testosterone), nonaromatizable (dihydrotestosterone), or synthetic (methyl-estrenolone and mesterolone), to the granulosa cell cultures markedly increased inhibin production without any changes in progesterone secretion. Cyproterone acetate, an antiandrogen, (35 and 350 μM) inhibited the basal and testosterone-stimulated inhibin production by granulosa cells during 24 hr of culture. Cyproterone acetate also inhibited progesterone but not estradiol-17β production by the granulosa cells.

It may be concluded from these experiments that inhibin production is decreased when the granulosa cells undergo luteinization and their progesterone secretion is increased. Also, the addition of exogenous progesterone significantly decreases inhibin secretion by cultured granulosa cells. Aromatizable, nonaromatizable, and synthetic androgens stimulate the inhibin secretion and appear to act directly without having to be aromatized. In fact, estrogens do not seem to affect inhibin production, while dihydrotestosterone, which cannot undergo aromatization, is the most potent stimulus of inhibin secretion. Furthermore, the blocking effect of cyproterone acetate provides additional evidence that androgens directly regulate inhibin production by granulosa cells and that this action may be a receptor-mediated process. Finally, the gonadotropins and prolactin do not appear to have any direct effect on inhibin secretion by granulosa cells *in vitro;* however, there are two reports that indicate that FSH stimulates inhibin production of bovine (55) and porcine (57) granulosa cells *in vitro*. The androgen enhancement of granulosa cell inhibin secretion may be responsible in part for the elevated follicular fluid levels of inhibin activity observed in women with polycystic ovarian disease (100)

Porcine, rat, and bovine granulosa cells appear to secrete more inhibin activity compared to human and monkey granulosa cells, as reflected in the inhibin content of the respective follicular fluids. It is interesting that granulosa cells isolated from porcine follicles during maturation showed an increased potential to secrete inhibin activity in culture (57). This could be due to gonadotropin exposure *in vivo,* which was adequate to mature them but not sufficient to luteinize them fully and thus decrease inhibin secretion. By contrast, inhibin activity was lower in follicular fluid from large porcine follicles compared to small follicles. This seemingly contradictory observation could be due to increased blood flow to the large follicles, which may serve to clear the inhibin more rapidly from the follicles.

Changes in Inhibin Secretion During Various Physiological States

For inhibin to qualify as a physiologically relevant hormone it should be secreted at physiologically appropriate times (i.e., when FSH is elevated, there should be generally less inhibin secreted and vice versa). It appears that ovarian inhibin fulfills this requirement. When ovarian venous blood in cycling rats was tested for inhibin activity at various times during the 4-day estrous cycle, a negative correlation was observed between the inhibin activity and circulating FSH concentrations (36,101,102). The inhibin levels are low late on the afternoon of proestrus and on the morning of estrus for the secondary rise in serum FSH. The follicular fluid inhibin activity decreases about 2 hr later than the ovarian vein levels on the afternoon of proestrus.

The levels of inhibin in follicular fluid are about 1,500 times greater than those in ovarian vein (36,54,101–104). The presence of larger amounts of inhibin activity in follicular fluid compared to ovarian vein blood could reflect the fact that the interior of the follicles is avascular and inhibin made by the granulosa cell accumulates and is only slowly cleared from the follicular atrum. Alternatively, since inhibin behaves as a high-molecular-weight complex (see below), its diffusion out of the follicle would be expected to be restricted.

Cummins et al. (105), by comparing ovarian inhibin content in two strains of ewes, observed that the strain having a higher ovulation rate also has a lower ovarian content of inhibin and a higher level of serum FSH. This observation suggests that differences in ovulation rates could be related to inhibin content of the ovarian follicles.

Inhibin activity is present in ovarian follicles of infant monkeys and humans (54). During puberty there is an increase in inhibin activity, perhaps reflecting a stimulatory action of FSH on inhibin secretion. Follicles doomed for atresia, as judged by their androgen/estrogen ratio (106), have a decreased ability to secrete inhibin (104). The physiologic significance of the decreased inhibin biosynthesis by atretic follicles may be to increase the serum FSH level at the end of the luteal phase, which may help to rescue follicular growth. The selective rise of serum FSH prior to changes in serum levels of LH, estrogen, and progesterone during the years immediately prior to menopause can best be explained by a decline in inhibin secretion, as originally proposed by Sherman et al. (38) and by Reyes et al. (39).

Changes in Follicular Inhibin Activity Associated with Various Clinical Disorders

Clinical medicine has provided unique situations that can be explained by alterations in ovarian inhibin secretion. One example is polycystic ovarian disease (PCO) in which amenorrheic women secrete elevated amounts of androgens and have numerous small follicular cysts. These women have normal or low levels of serum FSH with normal or elevated levels of LH. When challenged with GnRH, the PCO patients secrete elevated levels of LH but either normal or subnormal amounts of FSH. Tanabe et al. (100) observed that follicular fluid of these patients had a higher concentration of inhibin activity compared to similar-size follicles obtained from normal women during the follicular phase of the menstrual cycle. It is interesting that the number of granulosa cells per follicle in the polycystic follicles was considerably (tenfold) smaller compared to normal follicles of similar size. Inhibin activity was detected in the ovarian vein of three of five PCO patients, whereas in normal women, only two of 15 patients had measurable inhibin activity in the ovarian vein blood. It is tempting to conclude that the increased inhibin secretion in the PCO patients could be responsible for the altered FSH/LH ratio in the blood; however, steroid secretion in the appropriate ratio could also alter the FSH/LH secretion rate in PCO patients.

ASSAY METHODS FOR INHIBIN

A major difficulty in the studies of inhibin that has hindered progress and comparison of results from different laboratories has been the lack of uniform standard preparations and standardized methods for the detection and measurement of inhibin. Various *in vivo* (17,18,24,25,61,107–110) and *in vitro* (9,45,58,59,69,71) assay methods have been utilized to detect inhibin activity. Although many laboratories developed their own reference standards for relative potency estimates of inhibin activity, none of the standards have been sufficiently purified to provide quantitative measurements. Moreover, the available methods for inhibin assay lack the sensitivity and precision needed to measure inhibin activity in peripheral blood, thus precluding direct correlations between the circulating levels of inhibin and FSH secretion.

A general problem with the inhibin bioassays is that they are based on direct or indirect estimation of the suppression of pituitary FSH secretion. As with other bioassay methods using an inhibitory end point, the specificity of response is a major concern. Baker et al. (69) summarized this problem by stating that poorly characterized methods, where any suppression of FSH is assumed to be due to inhibin, has been the basis for most of the controversy and lack of consensus in the studies of inhibin. Specific problems encountered with the assay of inhibin have been eloquently reviewed by several investigators (13,14,58,69,70).

In Vivo Assays

Injection of biologically active inhibin preparations to intact or gonadectomized male or female animals of different species results in suppression of circulating FSH levels (10,24,25,107,108). The largest degree of suppression has been observed in acutely castrated animals. In most cases the peripheral concentrations of LH were not affected, except when large amounts of material were injected. Immature or adult rats were most commonly used as test models, but larger animals such as monkeys (26), mares (27), and castrated or cryptorchid rams (17,109) have also been used, particularly when frequent blood sampling was needed to determine the time course of FSH suppression.

In general, although various *in vivo* animal models can be used for detecting inhibin activity, none are considered optimal due to the relatively large amounts of material needed for testing. In addition there is considerable animal-to-animal variation. In some *in vivo* methods, the consequence of FSH suppression [e.g., decrease of ovarian (110) or uterine weight (111)] has been used as an end point; however, this type of assay has the additional disadvantage that any substance interfering with the interaction between FSH and its ovarian receptor will also be regarded as having inhibin-like activity. FSH-binding inhibitors have been found in follicular fluid, testicular homogenates, and seminal plasma. This binding-inhibiting activity cannot be attributed to inhibin itself, and the use of this type of assay may lead to erroneous conclusions. Other problems of nonspecificity might be encountered in the *in vivo* bioassay in which radioimmunoassay of FSH is used as an end point: Changes in the clearance of FSH, which may occur, for instance, after alteration of kidney function, or by a change in the type of FSH, which is secreted by the pituitary gland, may cause confusion.

In Vitro Assays

Bioassay

More sensitive and reproducible bioassays for inhibin activity have been developed using pituitary cell cultures *in vitro* (9,45,58,59,71,99). Most bioassays performed *in vitro* are based on the suppression of basal FSH release by pituitary cell cultures that have been incubated with the inhibin preparations. Generally, enzymatically dispersed pituitary cells are first incubated for several days at 37°C in serum-containing medium to allow formation of a cell monolayer in the culture dish. The cultures are then given fresh medium (with or without serum) containing varying concentrations of the test material or reference preparation, and the incubation is continued for an additional 1 to 3 days. After the second incubation period, the concentrations of FSH and LH in the culture medium (basal release) are measured by the respective radioimmunoassays. Addition of inhibin preparations causes a dose-related suppression of FSH release without significantly affecting the concentration of LH, except when very high doses of the test material are used.

Suppression of FSH release by inhibin is also observed in the presence of GnRH (59), provided that the GnRH is added to pituitary cell cultures that had been preincubated with the inhibin preparation for 1 to 3 days (Table 1); however, under these conditions, the release of LH is often also suppressed in a dose-related manner, although higher concentrations of inhibin are required and the regression line for LH suppression is generally not parallel to that of FSH. For example, in the assay of crude ovine testicular lymph, the LHRH-stimulated LH release is suppressed while no suppression of LH is observed in the assays utilizing basal release as an end point. Whether this effect is due to the presence of contaminating LH-inhibiting factors, as suggested by De Jong et al. (58) or to action of inhibin on the LHRH-stimulated LH release, LH synthesis or spontaneous LH release remains to be resolved. Other pituitary hormones (i.e., TSH, GH, and prolactin) are not affected by inhibin (77).

Selective suppression of FSH was also observed when pituitary cell content of FSH and LH was measured (14,58,68). The reduced cell content of FSH following a 3-day incubation with inhibin has been used as an end point for inhibin bioassay by Scott et al. (68). Whole pituitaries (110) or pituitary halves (40,70,99) have also been utilized by some investigators for detecting inhibin activity *in vitro*. Although the latter assay system is simpler and requires less time, it has not been widely accepted because it is less sensitive, less reproducible, and less precise compared with pituitary monolayer cell cultures.

The *in vitro* bioassay using dispersed pituitary cells has many advantages. It is about 1,000-fold more sensitive than the *in vivo* assays, requiring considerably lower amounts of inhibin for detection. It is also more reproducible because replicate cultures can be initiated from a single pool of pituitary cells, allowing many samples to be tested at several doses within a single assay. The assays are more economical and show a greater degree of specificity with respect to FSH response, particularly when performed in the absence of GnRH.

The main drawback of most *in vitro* assays is that they require several days for completion. In addition, various factors, such as high concentration of NaCl (112) or fetal calf serum (58), can nonspecifically suppress FSH secretion. It appears that nonspecific effects are most evident in assays based on GnRH-stimulated gonadotropin release. Therefore, it is mandatory to check the influence of test substances on the release of other pituitary hormones (i.e., LH, TSH, GH, or prolactin), as well as on the viability of the pituitary cells in culture. A generalized toxic effect on the cells can be assessed by measured changes in ^{51}Cr release from labeled pituitary cells (113).

Radioligand Assays

Attempts have been made to develop a specific and rapid radioligand assay for inhibin. Although both radioimmunoassay and radioreceptor assays have been described, they have not gained wide acceptance because of doubtful specificity.

Methods for radioimmunoassay of inhibin have been described by several investigators (14,114,115). In these assays, partly purified inhibin preparations were utilized as ligand and as antigen for generating the antibodies. The specificity of these assays has not been fully validated owing to lack of pure inhibin preparations, and no comparisons have been made between the radioimmunoassay and bioassay measurements.

There are also at least two reports on developing a receptor-binding assay for inhibin. Sairam (73) described binding of ^{125}I-inhibin from bull seminal plasma to ovine pituitary membrane that was competitively displaced in a dose-dependent manner by inhibin from bull or human seminal plasma and from bovine follicular fluid. Various non-inhibin proteins had no effect on the binding. Steinberger et al. (74) and Seethalakshmi et al. (75), using as ligand partly purified ^{3}H-SCF, secreted *in vitro* by rat Sertoli cells cultured in the presence of ^{3}H-leucine, and rat pituitary membranes or whole pituitary cells as receptor, demonstrated that the binding of ^{3}H-SCF was saturable, time and temperature dependent, and tissue specific. Unlabeled SCF and several other inhibin preparations, such as rat testis extract and ram rete testis fluid, inhibited the binding in a dose-dependent and parallel fashion, whereas other proteins, including bovine serum albumin, LH, and GnRH, did not compete with the ^{3}H-SCF binding. Moreover, good correlation was found between the pituitary binding and the biologic activity of inhibin *in vitro*, suggesting that the binding could be used as a radioreceptor assay for inhibin. The main advantage of this assay is that it can be completed within several hours; however, as with other radioligand assay methods, the use of pure inhibin as ligand would be essential to make this assay more specific and quantitative.

ISOLATION AND CHARACTERIZATION OF INHIBIN

The chemistry of inhibin was slow to develop for several reasons relating to difficulties in purification and uncertainty about the size of inhibin. These difficulties were further complicated by unreliable assay procedures, which appear to have misled several investigators in their attempts to isolate inhibin. We now know that inhibin tends to adsorb to higher molecular weight proteins, but it also appears in follicular fluid as discrete molecular forms of the molecule. The higher molecular weight forms have specific protein-processing points in them (e.g., double basic amino acid residues), which may relate to storage and secretion (this point is simply a speculation, however). (The problem of male-derived inhibin is not yet resolved.)

The variety of molecular weight forms of inhibin has been reviewed by several authors (13,14,126–128) of which we have cited only a few. Indeed, our own laboratory attempted to use the high-molecular-weight association complexes of inhibin as a means of purification (129); however, we eventually concluded that these association complexes of inhibin were not sufficiently stable to be an efficient means for isolating inhibin. The major problem was that the complexes would dissociate when submitted to various fractionation procedures, thus stringing the inhibin activity throughout the columns, etc., during the fractionation attempts. Eventually, we devised an efficient purification procedure that used quite the opposite approach. In this instance, we forced dissociation of all of the associated forms of inhibin by treating it with 95% glacial acetic acid. In summary, this procedure used an initial acetone precipitation to obtain most of the proteins and peptides in follicular fluids, according to the method of Huang and Miller (130). The acetone precipitate was then treated with 95% acetic acid at room temperature and stirred overnight. This extraction quantitatively solubilizes the inhibin and removes most of the protein. The inhibin activity was then precipitated with 90% ethanol. this precipitate was further fractionated by Sephacryl S-200 chromatography and reverse-phase high-performance liquid chromatography (HPLC) to obtain purified inhibin. The highly purified inhibin preparation thus obtained had a molecular weight of approximately 32,000 (131). The N-terminal amino acid analyses of this preparation indicate two peptide chains with an amino acid sequence that compares to that reported by Miyamoto et al. (132), Ling et al. (133), and Rivier et al. (134). In all the recent purification procedures, some form of initial dissociation was required. For the material described by Ling et al. (133), they subsequently obtained sufficient amino acid sequence data to develop a cDNA probe and from a series of studies in collaboration with the group at Genentech, Mason et al. (135) were able to propose the complete amino acid sequence for inhibin based on the cDNA sequence obtained. Their proposed sequence is shown in Fig. 1.

Alpha Subunit:

```
                        10                             20                             30         35
pS - T - A - P - L - P - W — P - W - S - P - A - A - L - R - L - L - Q - R - P - P - E - E - P - A - V - H - A - D - C - H - R - A - S - L -
h       (-)              S                                                                 A         N              V - A
                        45                             55                             65         70
pN - I - S - F - Q - E - L - G - W - D - R - W - I - V - H - P - P - S - F - I - F - H - Y - C - H - G - G - C - G - L - P - T - L - P - N
h                            E               Y                                                          H - I - P
                        80                             90                             100        105
pL - P - L - S - V - P - G - A - P - P - T - P - V - Q - P - L - L - L - V - P - G - A - Q - P - C - C - A - A - L - P - G - T - M - R - S -
h   S       P                             A           Y - S     L                                                              P
                        115                            125                     134
pL - R - V - R - T - T - S - D - G - G - Y - S - F - K - Y - E - T - V - P - N - L - L - T - Q - H - C - A - C - I.
h   H
```

Beta Subunit-A:

```
                        10                             20                             30         35
*G - L - E - C - D - G - K - V - N - I - C - C - K - K - Q - F - F - V - S - F - K - D - I - G - W - N - D - W - I - I - A - P - S - G - Y -

                        45                             55                             65         70
*H - A - N - Y - C - E - G - E - C - P - S - H - I - A - G - T - S - G - S - S - L - S - F - H - S - T - V - I - N - H - Y - R - M - R - G -
                        80                             90                             100        105
*H - S - P - F - A - N - L - K - S - C - C - V - P - T - K - L - R - P - M - S - M - L - Y - Y - D - D - G - Q - N - I - I - K - K - D - I -
                        115
*Q - N - M - I - V - E - E - C - G - C - S.
```

Beta Subunit-B:

```
                        10                             20                             30         35
pG - L - E - C - D - G - R - T - N - L - C - C - R - Q - Q - F - F - I - D - F - R - L - I - G - W - S - D - W - I - I - A - P - T - G - Y -
h                                                                                      N

                        45                             55                             65         70
*Y - G - N - Y - C - E - G - S - C - P - A - Y - L - A - G - V - P - G - S - A - S - S - F - H - T - A - V - V - N - Q - Y - R - M - R - G -
                        80                             90                             100        105
*L - N - P - G - T - V - N - S - C - C - I - P - T - K - L - S - T - M - S - M - L - Y - F - D - D - E - Y - N - I - V - K - R - D - V - P -
                        115
*N - M - I - V - E - E - C - G - C - A.
```

* These lines of sequence are identical in both species.
p=porcine sequence, h=positions that differ in the human sequence.

FIG. 1. Sequences of inhibin subunits, 32K form. (From ref. 135.)

In all of the references cited for purification of inhibin (*vide supra*) higher molecular weight forms of inhibin have been observed. In our own case (131), these were separated during the Sephacryl S-200 step. Inhibin activity in the general range of 100,000 and 60,000 molecular weight was observed. Although these higher molecular weight forms are yet to be chemically characterized, they undoubtedly relate to the higher molecular weight forms indicated from the cDNA studies of Mason et al. (135).

The historic report by Mason et al. (135) was followed shortly by a similar report for bovine inhibin. Forage et al. (136) have sequenced the cDNA for bovine inhibin and demonstrated that the two chains, which they designate A and B, are identical in the case of B to the inhibin beta-A of Mason et al. The A chain is highly homologous to the alpha subunit of Mason et al. Figure 2 compares the two predicted sequences from the cDNA studies of Forage et al. (136) and Mason et al. (135). The Australian group [Forage et al. (136)] had previously reported [Robertson et al. (137)] a purification procedure for bovine inhibin from bovine follicular fluid. The major product obtained in that study had a 56,000 molecular weight. Under reducing conditions, that material separated into two subunits of 44,000 and 14,000 molecular weight. It was subsequently shown [Robertson et al. (138)] that a 31,000-molecular-weight inhibin could also be obtained from bovine follicular fluid. This material appeared to be derived from the higher molecular weight 56,000-molecular-weight fraction.

Thus, after a long series of relatively futile attempts to fractionate and isolate inhibin, several groups appear to have converged on the true inhibin material. Moreover, studies are beginning to appear that utilize these preparations to obtain detailed information about the mechanism of action of inhibin. For example, Miller and colleagues (W. L. Miller, *personal communication*) have shown that inhibin does not decrease the expression of the FSH alpha subunit mRNA, but must act explicitly by reduction of the beta subunit expression or translation. Conversely, estradiol treatment will decrease the level of mRNA for the alpha subunit. Miller's studies were done in the sheep.

Although the definition of inhibin and inhibin action is progressing very well with the production of high-potency inhibin preparations and delineation of the proposed amino acid sequences, the story in the male is certainly less well resolved. We have reviewed the progress in the inhibin field (126) and at that time were very much encouraged by the appearance of several reports proposing sequences for inhibin-like molecules with inhibin-like activity derived from

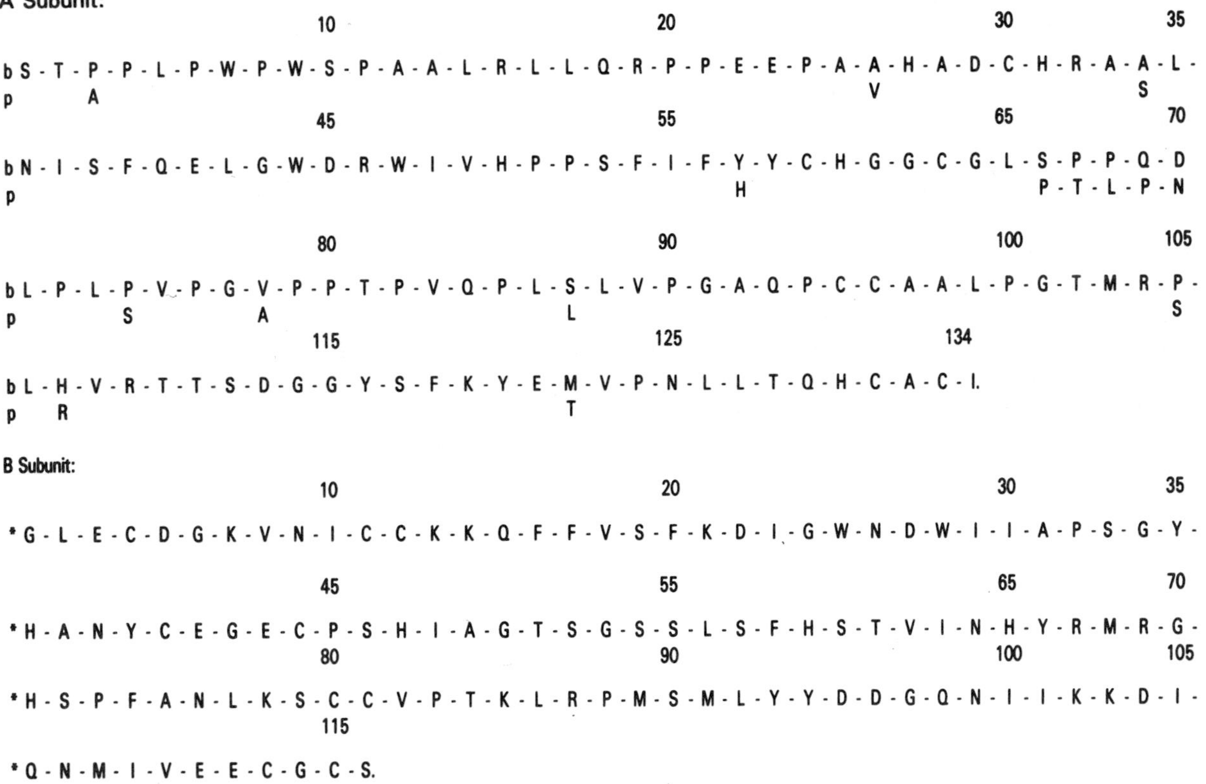

FIG. 2. Sequences of inhibin subunits, 32K form, bovine. *Note:* Letters below the sequence of the A subunit represent single-letter codes for the amino acid differences of the alpha subunit of porcine inhibin (Fig. 1). The B subunit is identical to the porcine beta subunit-A (Fig. 1). (From ref. 136.)

male sources. Two principal consortiums were involved in these proposals. The first was that of Sheth and colleagues from Bombay who collaborated with both Jornvall and colleagues in Sweden and Chretien and colleagues in Montreal to determine the amino acid sequence of a material they designated β-inhibin. The total sequence for β-inhibin was reported by Seidah et al. (139) (Montreal) and by Johansson et al. (140) (Sweden). Arbatti et al. (141) reported that the activity of this inhibin preparation resided in the C-terminal portion, which they designated β_2-inhibin. Inhibin had a molecular weight of 14,000; the β_2-inhibin had a molecular weight of 2,800. The report by Johansson et al. (140) noted that β-inhibin apparently was identical to the sperm-coating antigen designated β-microseminoprotein (MSP). β-MSP is a prostatic protein of interest in forensic medicine. The total sequence of β-MSP was subsequently reported by Akiyama et al. (142). Their sequence differed from that reported for β-inhibin by three amino acid residues. It is noted that A. R. Sheth's group was affiliated with both the Montreal group and the Sweden group for these studies. Although the sequences appear to be confirmed by the two groups, the question still remains as to whether the biological activity of these materials will be confirmed. Indeed, we have examined an authentic preparation of β-MSP in our pituitary cell culture assays and found no inhibin activity (143). Thus, we can definitely state that β-MSP has no inhibin activity. Whether the highly homologous protein, β-inhibin, has activity is yet to be confirmed. Indeed, we suspect that when two proteins are isolated from the same source and differ by only the slight differences suggested by the presently available sequence information, there is the possibility that sequencing errors could as likely be involved as protein differences. We are therefore collaborating with Dr. Akiyama and colleagues to reexamine the sequence of β-MSP, in particular, the three residues involved in the sequence differences.

Ramasharma et al. (144) also reported the amino acid sequence for a 31 amino acid peptide derived from human seminal plasma. Although they attributed inhibin-like activity to this peptide, they pointed out that their material did not have inhibin activity in the more conventional long-term pituitary cell culture assays for inhibin; rather, it required a rather shorter pituitary fragment incubation to get FSH suppression, which was only of the order of 20% suppression maximally.

In our earlier review of these sequence reports of male inhibin preparations (126), we stated "the landmark value of these studies lies in the fact that after many years investigators of inhibin are beginning to talk of exact biochemical structures that can be checked and compounds that can be used to compare results from laboratory to laboratory." Thus, 1 year later we believe that in spite of the promise concerning male inhibin, the demonstration that these structures are related to male inhibin remains to be confirmed. The structures are well established, the activity is not. Conversely, there is no reason to believe that the male does not synthesize an inhibin molecule, and in fact many of the earlier physiological studies that led to the concept of inhibin were carried out in the male. Thus, the most likely prospect at present is that male inhibin is structurally related to that reported for the female.

In summary, inhibin of proven activity is a two-polypeptide chain molecule with disulfide bonds coordinately bound between the two chains. One of these chains, the alpha or the A, as designated by the two groups reporting total structure, is glycosylated. The nature of the carbohydrate portion of this molecule must still be characterized, and the placement of the disulfide bonds in the inhibin molecule is a study that remains for the future. However, with the definition of the chemistry of inhibin well underway, the future physiological and pharmacological studies on inhibin should be more precise and informative.

PHYSIOLOGIC ROLE OF INHIBIN

Possible Role of Inhibin in the Male

The physiologic role of inhibin in the regulation of FSH secretion needs to be elucidated. Although FSH has been unequivocally shown to be essential for the maturation of spermatids during sexual maturation (2,3), its significance in the adult male has not been well defined. Thus, the consequences of over- or undersecretion of FSH in the mature male remain to be determined. In at least one study, however, suppression of circulating FSH by antibodies in the adult bonnet monkey led to impaired spermatogenesis and infertility (116). It could be inferred from these observations that production of large amounts of inhibin by the Sertoli cells could cause a delay in sexual maturation and interfere with normal spermatogenic process in the adult. Furthermore, there is considerable evidence that treatment of oligospermic patients with HCG is only effective in cases with adequate endogenous FSH production (42). Thus, suppression of inhibin secretion may be useful for increasing the circulating levels of FSH, leading to improved spermatogenesis.

The local effects of inhibin may also be of importance in regulating testicular functions. As was mentioned above, administration of inhibin preparations to male rats was reported to suppress spermatogonial DNA synthesis (65) and to increase the Leydig cell steroid production in response to LH (66).

The existence of a blood-testis barrier, which precludes entry of large molecules from the circulation into the tubule fluid, invites speculation that certain substances secreted by the Sertoli cells (possibly inhibin) may be essential for germ cell differentiation. More recent studies (117,118) indicate that Sertoli cell secretory products, such as transferrin and ABP, are specifically bound by the germ cells at certain stages of differentiation, apparently through a receptor mediated mechanism. Such transfer of Sertoli cell products could represent a possible mechanism for Sertoli cell-germ cell interaction and for providing essential substrates for germ cell metabolism. This interaction may also explain how hormones such as FSH and androgens, which are known to act in the testis primarily on the Sertoli cells, can regulate spermatogenesis.

An intriguing observation has been reported by Parvinen et al. (119) that secretion of certain Sertoli cell products (inhibin?) and their regulation by hormones vary with stages of the spermatogenic cycle. Also, a stage-related interaction between the Leydig cells and adjacent seminiferous tubules was suggested by morphometric analysis. In the rat testis, the volume of Leydig cells adjacent to tubules in stages I to VIII was smaller compared to other stages. This could potentially provide an additional fine-tuning mechanism for the local regulation of spermatogenesis. Inhibin, besides its systemic effect on FSH secretion, may play an important role in male reproductive physiology through its paracrine effects in the testis.

Possible Role of Inhibin in the Female

The observed inverse relationship between the levels of inhibin activity in the ovarian vein blood and circulating FSH implies a physiologic function for inhibin in the negative feedback regulation of FSH secretion. Since FSH plays a crucial role in follicular development and secretory functions in the ovary, inhibin can be viewed as a potential contraceptive agent. Conversely, effective methods for blocking inhibin production could provide useful means by which FSH secretion, and thus ovarian function and fertility, could be improved in the female.

Although there is no experimental evidence for the local effects of inhibin in the ovary, the possibility that inhibin may be of importance in paracrine regulation of ovarian function remains open.

ACKNOWLEDGMENTS

This work was supported in part by National Institutes of Health grants HD-15200 [A.S.], AM-9801 [D.N.W.], HD-18210 [D.N.W.], and grants from the Ford Foundation 830-0215 [D.N.W.] and the Robert A. Welch Foundation G-147 [D.N.W.].

The authors want to thank Ms. Mary Gilliland and Mrs. Harriette Young for the initial typing of the chapter.

ADDENDUM

After this chapter was submitted to the publisher, there were several significant reports concerning the chemistry of inhibin, as well as the demonstration that the dimers of the β-β subunits of inhibin possess an FSH stimulating action which can be overridden by inhibin (i.e., the α-β dimer). These reports are summarized below.

The Genentech group followed the report on the sequence of porcine inhibin with a similar report (145) on the sequence of human inhibin. These sequences are highly homologous (the differences are summarized in Fig. 1). The open reading frames for both the porcine and human inhibin genes (135,145) as well as the bovine inhibin genes (136) indicate extensive "precursor" structures on the N-terminal portion of the molecule. These protein portions are probably processed off before secretion from the follicle to produce the circulating 32K form (32,000 dalton) of inhibin shown in Figs. 1 and 2. The Australian group (146) has shown that the 54K inhibin is a putative precursor of a 31–32K form, which their studies also indicate may be derived by means of enzymes in serum.

Two groups at Salk Institute simultaneously reported that the homo- or heterodimer of the two types of beta subunit (Fig. 1) as an FSH-releasing hormone (147,148), and that the action of inhibin, on an approximately equimolar level, will override the effect of the FSH-releasing action. Thus, there is a series of hetero- or homodimers involved in the control of FSH-levels; the α-β_A (Inhibin A), the α-β_B (Inhibin B) (135), and now the β_A-β_A homodimer [designated FSH releasing protein (FRP) by Vale and colleagues (147)] or the heterodimer, β_A-β_B [designated "activin" by Ling and associates (148)].

Finally, Miyamoto and colleagues (149) have provided an excellent tool to study the high molecular weight forms of inhibin. By the combination of monoclonal antibodies for specific inhibin subunits coupled with two-dimensional electrophoresis they have been able to show that the higher molecular weight forms can be comprised of N-terminal extended (less processed) subunits as well as disulfide cross-linked trimeric and possibly higher forms.

The physiological role of these several complex forms of inhibin-related proteins is only beginning to be understood, but it promises to open an exciting new chapter in physiology.

REFERENCES

1. McCullagh, D. R. (1932): Dual endocrine activity of the testis. *Science*, 76:19–20.
2. Steinberger, E., and Duckett, G. E. (1967): Hormonal regulation of spermatogenesis. *J. Reprod. Fertil.* [*Suppl.*]2:75–87.
3. Steinberger, E., and Duckett, G. E. (1968): Studies on the mechanisms controlling the release of FSH from the pituitary gland. In: *Gonadotropins*, edited by E. Rosemberg, pp. 167–173. Geron-X, Los Altos, California.
4. Swerdloff, R. S., and Walsh, P. C. (1973): Testosterone and oestradiol suppression of LH and FSH in adult male rats: Duration of castration, duration of treatment and combined treatment. *Acta Endocrinol.* (*Copenh.*), 73:11–18.
5. Swerdloff, R. S., Walsh, P. C., Jacobs, H. S., and Odell, W. (1971): Serum LH and FSH during sexual maturation in the male rat: Effect of castration and cryptorchidism. *Endocrinology*, 88:120–128.
6. Chowdhury, M., and Steinberger, E. (1976): Differences of the effects of testosterone propionate on the production of LH and FSH. *Acta Endocrinol.* (*Copenh.*) 82:683.

7. Debeljuk, L., Arimura, A., and Schally, A. V. (1973): Pituitary and serum FSH and LH levels after massive and selective depletion of the germinal epithelium in the rat testis. *Endocrinology,* 92:48–54.
8. Franchimont, P., Millet, D., Vendrely, E., Letawe, J., Legros, J. J., and Netter, A. (1972): Relationship between spermatogenesis and serum gonadotropin levels in azoospermia and oligospermia. *J. Clin. Endocrinol. Metab.,* 34:1003–1008.
9. Baker, H. W. G., Bremner, W. J., Burger, H. G., de Kretser, D. M., Dulamanis, A., Eddie, L. W., Hudson, B., Keough, E. J., Lee, V. W. K., and Rennie, G. C. (1976): Testicular control of follicle stimulating hormone secretion. *Recent Prog. Horm. Res.,* 32:429–476.
10. Franchimont, P., Chari, S., Hazee-Hagelstein, M. T., Debruche, M. L., and Duraiswami, S. (1977): Evidence for the existence of inhibin. In: *The Testis in Normal and Infertile Men,* edited by P. Troen and H. R. Nakin, pp. 253–270. Raven Press, New York.
11. Setchell, B. P., and Main, S. J. (1974): Bibliography (with review) on inhibin. *Bibliogr. Reprod.,* 24:245–252, 361–367.
12. Lee, V. W. K., Keogh, E. J., de Kretser, D. M., and Hudson, B. (1974): Selective suppression of FSH by testis extracts. *IRCS Med. Sci.* 2:1406.
13. De Jong, F. H. (1979): Inhibin—Fact or artifact. *Mol. Cell Endocrinol.,* 13:1–10.
14. Franchimont, P., Verstraelen-Proyard, J., Hazee-Hagelstein, M. T., Renard, C. H., Demoulin, A., Bourguignon, J. P., and Hustin, J. (1979): Inhibin: From concept to reality. *Vit. Horm.,* 37:243–302.
15. Hopkinson, C. R. N., Dulisch, B., Gauss, G., Hilscher, W., and Hirschhauser, C. (1978): The effect of local testicular irradiation on testicular histology and plasma hormone levels in the male rat. *Acta Endocrinol. (Copenh.),* 87:413–423.
16. Burger, H. G., Franchimont, P., deKretser, D. M., and Hudson, B. (1974): Gonadotropins in spermatogenesis control. In: *Recent Progress in Reproductive Endocrinology,* edited by P. G. Grosignani and V. H. James, pp. 605–631. Academic Press, New York.
17. Keogh, E. J., Lee, V. W. K., Rennie, G. C., Burger, H. G., Hudson, B., and de Kretser, D. M. (1976): Selective suppression of FSH by testicular extracts. *Endocrinology,* 98:997–1004.
18. Setchell, B. P., and Jacks, F. (1974): Inhibin-like activity in rete testis fluid. *J. Endocrinol.,* 62:675.
19. Cahoreau, C., Blanc, M. R., Dacheux, J. L., Pisselet, C. L., and Courot, M. (1980): Inhibin activity in ram rete testis fluid; depression of plasma follitropin (FSH) and lutropin LH in the castrate and cryptorchid ram. *J. Reprod. Fertil. [Suppl.],* 26:97–116.
20. Franchimont, P., Chari, S., Hagelstein, M. T., and Duraiswami, S. (1975): Existence of a follicle stimulating hormone inhibiting factor "inhibin" in bull seminal plasma. *Nature,* 257:402–404.
21. Sairam, M. R., Ranganatham, M. R., and Lamothe, P. (1978): Purification and characterization of a follitropin suppressing principle from bull ejaculate. *Biol. Reprod.,* 18:53 [Abstr. 36A].
22. Campbell, C. S., Schwartz, N. B., and Firlit, M. G. (1977): The role of adrenal and ovarian steroids in the control of serum LH and FSH. *Endocrinology,* 101:162–173.
23. Bronson, F. H. (1967): Serum FSH, LH and prolactin in adult ovariectomized mice bearing silastic implants of estradiol: response to social cues. *Biol. Reprod.,* 15:147–158.
24. Welschen, R., Hermans, W. P., Dullaart, J., and DeJong, F. H. (1977): Effects of an inhibin-like factor present in bovine and porcine follicular fluid on gonadotropin levels in ovariectomized rats. *J. Reprod. Fertil.,* 50:129–131.
25. Marder, M. L., Channing, C. P., and Schwartz, N. B. (1977): Suppression of serum follicle stimulating hormone in intact and acutely ovariectomized rats by porcine follicular fluid. *Endocrinology,* 101:1639–1642.
26. Channing, C. P., Anderson, L. D., Hoover, D. J., Gagliano, P., and Hodgen, G. D. (1981): Inhibitory effects of porcine follicular fluid on monkey serum FSH levels and follicular maturation. *Biol. Reprod.,* 25:885–903.
27. Miller, K. F., Wesson, J. A., and Ginther, O. J. (1979): Changes in concentrations of circulating gonadotropins following administration of equine follicular fluid to ovariectomized mares. *Biol. Reprod.,* 21:867–872.
28. Chappel, S. C. (1979): Cyclic fluctuations in ovarian FSH-inhibiting material in golden hamsters. *Biol. Reprod.,* 21:447–458.
29. Grady, R. R., Charlesorth, M. C., and Schwartz, N. B. (1982): Characterization of the FSH-suppressing activity in follicular fluid. *Recent Prog. Horm. Res.,* 38:409–456.
30. Schwartz, N. B. (1982): Role of ovarian inhibin (folliculostatin) in regulating FSH secretion in the female rat. In: *Intra-ovarian Control Mechanisms (Adv. Exptl. Med., Vol. 147),* edited by C. P. Channing and S. Segal, pp. 193–214. Plenum Press, New York.
31. Schwartz, N. B. (1983): Selective control of FSH secretion. In: *Role of Peptides and Proteins in Control of Reproduction,* edited by S. M. McCann and D. S. Dhindsa, pp. 193–213. Elsevier Biomedical, New York.
32. Barraclough, C. (1982): New concepts on the regulation of pituitary luteinizing hormone and follicle stimulating hormone. In: *Non-steroidal Regulators in Reproductive Biology and Medicine (Adv. Biosci., Vol. 34),* pp. 1–26. Pergamon Press, Oxford.
33. Schwartz, N. B., and Talley, W. L. (1978): Effects of exogenous LH or FSH on endogenous FSH, progesterone and estradiol secretion. *Biol. Reprod.,* 18:820–828.
34. Butcher, R. L. (1977): Changes in gonadotropins and steroids associated with unilateral ovariectomy of the rat. *Endocrinology,* 101:830–838.
35. Schwartz, N. B., and Channing, C. P. (1977): Evidence for ovarian "inhibin": suppression of the secondary rise in serum follicle stimulating hormone levels in proestrous rats by injection of porcine follicular fluid. *Proc. Natl. Acad. Sci. U.S.A.,* 74:5721–5725.
36. DePaolo, L. V., Hirschfield, A. N., Anderson, L. D., Barraclough, C. A., and Channing, C. P. (1979): Suppression of pituitary secretion of FSH by porcine follicular fluid during pro-oestrus and oestrus in the rat: Effects on gonadotrophin and steroid secretion, follicular development and ovulation during the following cycle. *J. Endocrinol.,* 83:355–368.
37. Welschen, R., Hermans, W. P., and De Jong, F. H. (1980): Possible involvement of inhibin in the interrelationship between numbers of antral follicles and peripheral FSH concentrations in female rats. *J. Reprod. Fertil.,* 60:485–493.
38. Sherman, B. M., West, J. H., and Korenman, S. C. (1976): The menopausal transition: Analysis of LH, FSH, estradiol, and progesterone concentrations during menstrual cycles of older women. *J. Clin. Endocrinol. Metab.,* 42:629–636.
39. Reyes, F. I., Winter, J. S. D., and Faiman, C. (1977): Pituitary-ovarian relationships preceding the menopause. I. A cross-sectional study of serum follicle-stimulating hormone, luteinizing hormone, prolactin, estradiol, and progesterone levels. *Am. J. Obstet. Gynecol.,* 129:557–564.
40. Setchell, B. P., Davis, R. V., and Main, S. J. (1977): Inhibin. In: *The Testis, Vol. IV,* edited by A. D. Johnson and W. R. Gomez, pp. 190–238. Academic Press, New York.
41. Main, S. J., Davis, R. V., and Setchell (1978): Feedback control by the testis of gonadotrophin secretion: An examination of the inhibin hypothesis. *J. Endocrinol.,* 79:255–270.
42. Paulsen, C. A., Leonard, J. M., de Kretser, D. M., and Leach, R. D. (1972): Interrelationship between spermatogenesis and follicle stimulating hormone levels. In: *Gonadotrophins,* edited by B. B. Saxena, C. G. Beling, and H. M. Gandy, pp. 628–639. Wiley (Interscience), New York.
43. Krueger, P. M., Hodgen, G. D., and Sherins, R. J. (1974): New evidence for the role of the Sertoli cell and spermatogonia in feedback control of FSH secretion in male rats. *Endocrinology,* 95:955–962.
44. Mecklenburg, R. S., Hetzel, W. D., Gulyas, R. J., and Lipsett, M. B. (1975): Regulation of FSH secretion; use of hydroxyurea to deplete germinal epithelium. *Endocrinology,* 96:564–570.
45. Steinberger, A., and Steinberger, E. (1976): Secretion of an FSH-inhibiting factor by cultured Sertoli cells. *Endocrinology,* 99:918–921.
46. Steinberger, A., and Steinberger, E. (1977): Inhibition of FSH by a Sertoli cell factor "in vitro." In: *The Testis in Normal and Infertile Men,* edited by P. Troen and H. R. Nankin, pp. 271–279. Raven Press, New York.
47. Steinberger, A. (1980): Factors affecting *in vitro* secretion of inhibin by isolated Sertoli cells. In: *Endocrinology 1980,* edited by I. A. Cumming, J. W. Funder, and F. A. O. Mendelsohn, pp. 259–262. The Australian Academy of Science, Canberra, Australia.

48. Labrie, F., Legace, L., Ferland, L., Kelley, P. A., Drouin, J., Masicotte, J., Bonne, C., Raynaud, I. P., and Dorrington, J. (1978): Interactions between LHRH, sex steroids and inhibin in the control of LH and FSH secretion. *Int. J. Androl.* (Suppl. 2):81–101.
49. De Jong, F. H., and Sharpe, R. M. (1977): Gonadotrophins, testosterone and spermatogenesis in neonatally irradiated male rats. Evidence for role of the Sertoli cells in follicle stimulating hormone feedback. *J. Endocrinol.*, 75:209–219.
50. Steinberger, A. (1975): *In vitro* techniques for the study of spermatogenesis. In: *Hormones and Cyclic Nucleotides* (*Methods in Enzymology, Vol. 39, Part D*), edited by B. W. O'Malley and J. G. Hardman, pp. 238–296. Academic Press, New York.
51. Erickson, G. F., and Hsueh, A. J. W. (1978): Secretion of "inhibin" by rat granulosa cells "in vitro." *Endocrinology,* 193:1960–1963.
52. Channing, C. P., Anderson, L. D., Hoover, D. J., Kolena, J., Osteen, K. G., Pomerantz, S. H., and Tanabe, K. (1982): The role of nonsteroidal regulators in control of oocyte and follicular maturation. *Recent Prog. Hormone Res.*, 38:331–408.
53. Channing, C. P., Tanabe, K., Jones, H., Jones, G., and Lebeck, P. (1984): Inhibin activity of preovulatory follicles of gonadotropin-treated and untreated women. *Fertil. Steril.*, 42(2):243–248.
54. Hoover, D. J., Tanabe, K., and Channing, C. P. (1983): Inhibin secretion by the primate ovary. *Semin. Reprod. Endocrinol.*, 1:279–294.
55. Henderson, K. M., and Franchimont, P. (1983): Inhibin production by bovine ovarian tissues *in vitro* and its regulation by androgens. *J. Reprod. Fertil.*, 67:291–298.
56. Hermans, W. P., Van Leeuwen, E. C. M., Debets, H. T. H., Sander, H. J., and de Jong, F. H. (1982): Estimation of inhibin-like activity in spent medium from rat ovarian granulosa cells during long-term culture. *Mol. Cell Endocrinol.*, 27:277–290.
57. Anderson, L. D., and Hoover, D. J. (1982): Hormonal control of inhibin secretion. In: *Intraovarian Control Mechanisms,* edited by C. P. Channing and S. J. Segal, pp. 53–78. Plenum Press, New York.
58. De Jong, F. H., Smith, S. D., and Van Der Molen, H. J. (1979): Bioassay of inhibin-like activity using pituitary cells in vitro. *J. Endocrinol.*, 80:91–102.
59. Eddie, L. W., Baker, H. W., Higginson, R. E., and Hudson, B. (1979): A bioassay for inhibin using pituitary cell cultures. *J. Endocrinol.*, 81:49–60.
60. Demoulin, A., Bourguignon, J. P., and Franchimont, P. (1979): *In vitro* inhibition of hypothalamic LH-RH by human inhibin. *Acta Endocrinol.* (*Copenh.*), [Abstr.], (Suppl. 225):227.
61. Lugaro, G., Cassellato, M. M., Mazzola, G., and Fachini, G. (1973): Evidence for a peptidic factor in spermatozoa inhibiting the ovarian maturation. *Biochem. Biophys. Acta,* 304:719–724.
62. Lumpkin, M., Negro-Vilar, A., Franchimont, P., and McCann, S. (1981): Evidence for a hypothalamic site of action of inhibin to suppress FSH release. *Endocrinology,* 108:1101–1104.
63. Moodbidri, S. B., Vijayalakshmi, S., Bandivdekar, A. H., and Sheth, A. R. (1981): Inhibition of hypothalamic GnRH synthesis by inhibin. *Experientia,* 37:525.
64. Vanage, G. R., Thakur, A. N., Kadam, M. S., and Sheth, A. R. (1980): Metabolic clearance rate of inhibin in mature and immature male rats. *Biol. Reprod.*, 23:606–610.
65. Demoulin, A., Hustin, J., Lambotte, R., and Franchimont, P. (1981): Effect of inhibin on testicular function. In: *Intragonadal Regulation of Reproduction,* edited by P. Franchimont and C. P. Channing, pp. 327–342. Academic Press, London.
66. Rich, K. A., Kerr, J. B., and deKretser, D. M. (1979): Evidence for Leydig cell dysfunction in rats with seminiferous tubule damage. *Mol. Cell. Endocrinol.*, 13:123–135.
67. Chowdhury, M. A., Steinberger, A., and Steinberger, E. (1978): Inhibition of de novo synthesis of FSH by the Sertoli cell factor (SCF). *Endocrinology,* 103:644–647.
68. Scott, R. S., Burger, H., and Quigg, H. (1980): A simple and rapid *in vitro* assay for inhibin. *Endocrinology,* 107:1536–1542.
69. Baker, H. W. G., Eddie, L. W., Higginson, R. E., Hudson, B., Keogh, E. J., and Niall, H. D. (1981): Assays of inhibin. In: *Intragonadal Regulation of Reproduction,* edited by P. Franchimont and C. P. Channing, pp. 193–228. Academic Press, London.
70. Hudson, B., Baker, H. W. G., Eddie, L. W., Higginson, R. E., Burger, H. G., deKretser, D. M., Dobos, M., and Lee, V. W. K. (1979): Bioassay for inhibin: A critical review. *J. Reprod. Fertil.* [*Suppl.*], 26:17–29.
71. Steinberger, A., Seethalakshmi, L., Kessler, M., and Steinberger, E. (1983): Sertoli cell factor. In: *Role of Peptides and Proteins in Control of Reproduction,* edited by S. M. McCann and D. S. Dhindsa, pp. 215–236. Elsevier Science Publishing Co., New York.
72. Steinberger, A. (1979): Inhibin production by Sertoli cells in culture. *J. Reprod. Fertil.* [*Suppl.*] 26:31–45.
73. Sairam, M. R. (1981): Characterization of inhibin from bull seminal plasma. In: *Intragonadal Regulation of Reproduction,* edited by P. Franchimont and C. P. Channing, pp. 251–281. Academic Press, London.
74. Steinberger, A., Seethalakshmi, L., Kessler, M., and Steinberger, E. (1982): Binding of ^{3}H-Sertoli cell factor to rat anterior pituitary *in vitro*. *Endocrinology,* 111:696–698.
75. Seethalakshmi, L., Steinberger, A., and Steinberger, E. (1984): Pituitary binding of ^{3}H-Sertoli cell factor I. A possible radioreceptor assay for inhibin. *Endocrinology,* 115:1289–1294.
76. Dighe, R. R., Seethalakshmi, L., Heindel, J. J., and Steinberger, A. (1984): SCF binding and effect on FSH secretion and cAMP levels in rat anterior pituitary cells. In: *Gonadal Proteins and Peptides and Their Biological Significance,* edited by M. R. Sairam and L. E. Atkinson, pp. 9–19. World Scientific Publishing Co., Singapore.
77. Franchimont, P., Lecomte-Yerna, M. J., Henderson, K., Verhoven, G., Hazee-Hagelstein, M. T., Jaspar, J. M., Charlet-Renard, C., and Demoulin, A. (1983): Inhibin: Mechanisms of pituitary action and regulation of secretion. In: *Role of Peptides and Proteins in Control of Reproduction,* edited by S. M. McCann and D. S. Dhindsa, pp. 237–255. Elsevier Biomedical, New York.
78. Childs, G. V., and Ellison, D. G. (1980): A critique of the contributions of immunoperoxidase cytochemistry to our understanding of pituitary cell function, as illustrated by our current studies of gonadotropes, corticotropes and endogenous pituitary GnRH and TRH. *Histochem. J.*, 12:405–418.
79. Thumann, A., and Bustos-Obregon, E. (1978): An "in vitro" system for the study of rat spermatogonial proliferative control. *Andrologia,* 10:22–25.
80. Sharpe, R. M., Fraser, H. M., Cooper, I., and Rommerts, F. F. G. (1981): Sertoli-Leydig cell communication via an LHRH-like factor. *Nature,* 290:785–787.
81. Browning, J. Y., D'Agata, R., Steinberger, A., Grotjan, H. E., Jr., and Steinberger, E. (1983): Biphasic effect of gonadotropin releasing hormone and its agonist analog (HOE 766) on *in vitro* testosterone production by purified rat Leydig cells. *Endocrinology,* 113:985–991.
82. Steinberger, A., Sanborn, B. M., and Steinberger, E. (1978): FSH and the Sertoli cell. In: *Structure and Function of the Gonadotropins,* edited by K. W. McKerns, pp. 517–551. Plenum Press, New York.
83. Fritz, I. B. (1978): Sites of action of androgen and follicle stimulating hormone on the cells of the seminiferous tubules. In: *Biochemical Actions of Hormones, Vol. 5,* edited by G. Litwack, pp. 249–281. Academic Press, New York.
84. Steinberger, A., Thanki, K. H., and Siegal, B. G. (1974): FSH binding in rat testes during maturation and following hypophysectomy. Cellular localization of FSH receptors. In: *Hormone Binding and Target Cell Activation in the Testis* (*Current Topics in Molecular Endocrinology, Vol. 1*), edited by M. L. Dufau and A. R. Means, pp. 177–192. Plenum Press, New York.
85. Means, A. R., Fakunding, J. L., Huckins, C., Tindall, D. J., and Vitale, R. (1976): Follicle-stimulating hormone, the Sertoli cell and spermatogenesis. *Recent Prog. Horm. Res.*, 32:477–527.
86. Sanborn, B. M., Steinberger, A., Tcholakian, R. K., and Steinberger, E. (1977): Direct measurements of androgen receptors in cultured Sertoli cells. *Steroids,* 29:493–502.
87. Steinberger, E., Steinberger, A., and Sanborn, B. M. (1978): Molecular mechanisms concerned with hormonal control of the seminiferous epithelium. In: *Recent Progress in Andrology,* edited by A. Fabrini and E. Steinberger, pp. 143–178. Academic Press, New York.
88. Tsai, Y.-H., Sanborn, B. M., Steinberger, A., and Steinberger, E. (1977): The interaction of testicular androgen-receptor complex with rat germ cell and Sertoli cell chromatin. *Biochem. Biophys. Res. Commun.*, 75:366–372.

89. Heindel, J. J., Rothenberg, R., Robison, G. A., and Steinberger, A. (1975): LH and FSH stimulation of cyclic AMP in specific cell types isolated from the testes. *J. Cyclic Nucleotide Res.*, 1: 69–79.
90. Lamb, D. J., Tsai, Y.-H., Steinberger, A., and Sanborn, B. M. (1981): Sertoli cell nuclear transcriptional activity: Stimulation by follicle stimulating hormone and testosterone *in vitro*. *Endocrinology*, 108:1020–1026.
91. Steinberger, A. (1981): Regulation of inhibin secretion in the testis. In: *Intragonadal Regulation of Reproduction*, edited by P. Franchimont and C. P. Channing, pp. 283–298. Academic Press, New York.
92. Verhoeven, G., and Franchimont, P. (1983): Regulation of inhibin secretion by Sertoli cell-enriched cultures. *Acta Endocrinol.*, 102:136–143.
93. Au, C. L., Robertson, D. M., and de Kretser, D. M. (1984): Effects of hypophysectomy and subsequent FSH and testosterone treatment on inhibin production by adult rat testes. *J. Endocrinol.*, 105:1–6.
94. Au, C. L., Robertson, D. M., and de Kretser, D. M. (1984): An *in vivo* method for estimating inhibin production by adult rat testes. *J. Reprod. Fertil.*, 71:259–265.
95. Hagenas, L., and Ritzen, E. M. (1976): Impaired Sertoli cell function in experimental cryptorchidism in the rat. *Mol. Cell. Endocrinol.*, 4:25–34.
96. LeGac-Jegou, F., and deKretser, D. M. (1980): Studies on isolated Sertoli cells from normal and cryptorchid testes [Abstr. #684]. *Program of 6th International Congress of Endocrinology*, p. 551. Melbourne, Australia.
97. Seethalakshmi, L., and Steinberger, A. (1983): Effect of cryptorchidism and orchidopexy on inhibin secretion by rat Sertoli cells. *J. Androl.*, 4:131–135.
98. Demoulin, A., Koulischer, L., Hustin, J., Hazee-Hagelstein, M. T., Lambotte, R., and Franchimont, P. (1979): Organ culture of mammalian testis. III. Inhibin secretion. *Horm. Res.*, 10:177–190.
99. Davies, R. V., Main, S. J., and Setchell, B. (1978): Inhibin: evidence for its existence, methods of bioassay and nature of the active material. *Int. J. Androl.* [*Suppl.*] 2:102–114.
100. Tanabe, K., Gagliano, P., Channing, C. P., Nakamura, Y., Yoshimura, Y., Iizuka, R., Fortuny, A., Sulewski, J., and Rezai, N. (1983): Levels of inhibin-F activity and steroids in human follicular fluid from normal women and women with polycystic ovarian disease. *J. Clin. Endocrinol. Metab.*, 57:24–31.
101. DePaolo, L. V., Shander, D., Wise, P. M., Barraclough, C. A., and Channing, C. P. (1979): Identification of inhibin-like activity in ovarian venous plasma of rats during the estrous cycle. *Endocrinology*, 105:647–654.
102. Fujii, T., Hoover, D. J., and Channing, C. P. (1983): Changes in inhibin activity and progesterone, oestrogen and androstenedione concentrations in rat follicular fluid throughout the oestrous cycle. *J. Reprod. Fertil.*, 69:307–314.
103. Channing, C. P., Tanabe, K., Guthrie, H. D., Batta, S. K., and Hoover, D. J. (1981): Changes in inhibin-F activity (folliculostatin) in human, porcine, rat and monkey ovarian follicular fluid and ovarian vein blood during various reproductive states. In: *Intragonadal Regulation of Reproduction*, edited by P. Franchimont and C. P. Channing, pp. 365–376. Academic Press, New York.
104. Channing, C. P., Gagliano, P., Hoover, D. J., Tanabe, K., Batta, S. K., Sulewski, J., and Lebech, P. (1981): Relationship between human follicular fluid inhibin-F activity and steroid content. *J. Clin. Endocrinol. Metab.*, 52:1193–1198.
105. Cummins, L. T., O'Shea, T., Bindon, B. M., Lee, V. W., and Findlay, J. K. (1983): Ovarian inhibin content and sensitivity to inhibin in Booroola and control strain Merino ewes. *J. Reprod. Fertil.*, 67:1–7.
106. McNatty, K. P., Moore-Smith, D., Makris, A., Osathanondh, R., and Ryan, K. J. (1979): The microenvironment of the human antral follicle: Interrelationships among the steroid levels in antral fluid, the population of granulosa cells, and the status of the oocyte *in vivo* and *in vitro*. *J. Clin. Endocrinol. Metab.*, 49:851–860.
107. De Jong, F. H., and Sharpe, R. M. (1976): Evidence for inhibin-like activity in bovine follicular fluid. *Nature*, 263:71–72.
108. Nandini, S. G., Lipner, H., and Moudgal, N. R. (1976): A model system for studying inhibin. *Endocrinology*, 98:1460–1465.
109. Blanc, M. R., Cahoreau, C., Courot, M., Dacheux, J. L., Hochereau-de Reviers, M. T., and Pisselet, C. (1978): Plasma follicle-stimulating hormone (FSH) and luteinizing hormone (LH) suppression in the cryptorchid ram by a non-steroid factor (inhibin) from ram rete testis fluid. *Int. J. Androl.* (*Suppl*), 2:139–146.
110. Chari, S., Duraiswami, S., and Franchimont, P. (1978): Isolation and characterization of inhibin from bull seminal plasma. *Acta Endocrinol.*, 87:437–438.
111. Ramasharma, K., Murthy, H. M., and Moudgal, N. R. (1979): A rapid bioassay for measuring inhibin activity. *Biol. Reprod.*, 20:831–835.
112. Kao, L. W. L., Gunsalus, G. L., Williams, G. H., and Weisz, J. (1977): Response of perifused anterior pituitaries of rats to synthetic gonadotrophin releasing hormone: A comparison with hypothalamic extract and demonstration of a role for potassium in the release of luteinizing hormone and follicle-stimulating hormone. *Endocrinology*, 101:1444–1454.
113. Robertson, D. M., Au, C. L., and de Kretser, D. M. (1982): The use of ^{51}Cr for assessing cytotoxicity in an *in vitro* bioassay for inhibin. *Mol. Cell Endocrinol.*, 26:119–127.
114. Vaze, A. Y., Thakur, A. N., and Sheth, A. R. (1979): Development of a radioimmunoassay for human seminal plasma inhibin. *J. Reprod. Fertil.*, 26:135–146.
115. Sheth, A. R., Vaze, A. Y., and Thakur, A. N. (1978): Development of a radioimmunoassay for inhibin. *Indian J. Exp. Biol.*, 16:1025–1026.
116. Moudgal, N. R. (1981): A need for FSH in maintaining fertility of adult male subhuman primates. *Arch. Androlog.*, 7:117–122.
117. Holmes, S. D., Bucci, L. R., Lipshultz, L. I., and Smith, R. G. (1983): Transferrin binds specifically to pachytene spermatocytes. *Endocrinology*, 113:1916–1918.
118. Dighe, R. R., Meistrich, M., and Steinberger, A. (1986): Sertoli-germ cell interaction: Uptake of Sertoli cell secretory proteins by the germ cells during spermatogenesis. In: *Sezono Symposia Review No. 11: Development and Function of the Reproductive Organs*, edited by A. Eshkol, N. Dekel, H. Peters, and A. Tsafriri, pp. 161–170, Serone Symposia: Rome.
119. Parvinen, M. (1982): Regulation of the seminiferous epithelium. *Endocrine Rev*. 3:404–417.
120. Moodbidri, S. B., Joshi, L. R., and Sheth, A. R. (1976): Isolation of an inhibin-like substance from ram testis. *IRCS Med. Sci.*, 4:217.
121. Hopkinson, C. R. N., Daume, E., Sturm, G., Fritze, E., Kaiser, S., Hirschhauser, C. (1977): Inhibin-like activity of bovine ovarian extracts in male and female rats. *J. Reprod. Fertil.*, 50: 93–96.
122. Chappel, S. C., Acott, T., and Spies, H. G. (1979): Inhibition of "in vivo" and "in vitro" follicle-stimulating hormone secretion by steroid-free ovarian extracts. In: *Proceedings of the Workshop on Ovarian Follicular and Corpus Luteum Function*, edited by C. P. Channing, J. Marsh, and W. Sadler, pp. 361–371. Plenum Press, New York.
123. Hopkinson, C. R. N., Sturm, G., Daume, E., Fritze, E., and Hirschhauser, C. (1975): Nonsteroidal inhibition of FSH secretion by bovine ovarian fluid in male and female rats. *IRCS Med. Sci.*, 3:588.
124. Lorenzen, J. R., Channing, C. P., and Schwartz, H. B. (1978): Partial characterization of FSH suppressing activity (folliculostatin) in porcine follicular fluid using the metestrous rat as an "in vivo" bioassay model. *Biol. Reprod.*, 19:635–640.
125. Chari, S., Hopkinson, C. R., Daume, E., and Sturm, G. (1979): Purification of "inhibin" from human ovarian follicular fluid. *Acta Endocrinol* (*Copenh.*), 90:157–166.
126. Channing, C. P., Gordon, W. L., Liu, W. L., and Ward, D. N. (1985): Physiology and biochemistry of ovarian inhibin. *Proc. Soc. Exptl. Biol. Med.*, 178:339–361.
127. DeJong, F. H., and Robertson, D. M. (1985): Inhibin: 1985 update on action and purification. *Mol. Cell. Endocrinol.*, 42:95–103.
128. Ward, D. N., Glenn, S. D., Liu, W. K., and Gordon, W. L. (1983): Chemistry and physiology of gonadal peptides. In: *Factors Regulating Ovarian Function*, edited by G. S. Greenwald and P. F. Terranova, pp. 141–156. Raven Press, New York.
129. Channing, C. P., Liu, W. K., Gordon, W. L., Xue, Y. G., and Ward, D. N. (1984): Porcine inhibin: Initial fractionation as a high molecular weight complex. *Arch. Androl.*, 13:219–231.
130. Huang, E. S. R., and Miller, W. L. (1984): Porcine ovarian inhibin preparations sensitized cultured ovine gonadotroaphs to luteinizing hormone releasing hormones. *Endocrinology*, 115:513–519.
131. Gordon, W. L., Liu, W. K., and Ward, D. N. (1986): Inhibin fractionation: A comparison of human and porcine follicular fluid,

with particular reference to protease activation. *Biol. Reprod.*, 35:209–218.

132. Miyamoto, K., Hasegawa, Y., Fukuda, M., Nomura, M., Igarashi, M., Kangawa, K., and Matsuo, H. (1985): Isolation of porcine follicular fluid inhibin of 32K daltons. *Biochim. Biophys. Res. Commun.*, 129:396–403.
133. Ling, N., Ying, S. Y., Ueno, N., Esch, F., Denoroy, L., and Guillemin, R. (1985): Isolation and partial characterization of a M_r 32,000 protein with inhibin activity from porcine follicular fluid. *Proc. Natl. Acad. Sci. U.S.A.*, 82:7217–7221.
134. Rivier, J., Spiess, J., McClintock, R., Vaughan, J., and Vale, W. (1985): Purification and partial characterization of inhibin from porcine follicular fluid. *Biochem. Biophys. Res. Commun.*, 133:120–127.
135. Mason, A. J., Hayflick, J. S., Esch, F., Ueno, N., Ying, S. Y., Guillemin, R., Niall, H., and Seeburg, P. H. (1985): Complementary DNA sequences of ovarian follicular fluid inhibin show precursor structure and homology with transforming growth factor-beta. *Nature*, 318:659–663.
136. Forage, R. G., Ring, J. M., Brown, R. W., McInerney, B. V., Cobon, G. S., Gregson, R. P., Robertson, D. M., Morgan, F. J., Hearn, M. T. W., Findlay, J. K., Wettenhall, R. E. H., Burger, H. G., and deKretser, D. M. (1986): Cloning and sequence analysis of cDNA species coding for the two subunits of inhibin from bovine follicular fluid. *Proc. Natl. Acad. Sci. U.S.A.*, 83:3091–3095.
137. Robertson, D. M., Foulds, L. M., Leversha, L., Morgan, F. J., Hearn, M. T. W., Burger, H. G., Wettenhall, R. E., deKretser, D. M. (1985): Isolation of inhibin from bovine follicular fluid. *Biochem. Biophys. Res. Commun.*, 126:220–226.
138. Robertson, D. M., deVos, F. L., Foulds, L. M., McLachlan, R. I., Burger, H. G., Morgan, F. J., Hearn, M. T. W., and deKretser, D. M. (1986): Isolation of a 31 kD form of inhibin from bovine follicular fluid. *Mol. Cell. Endocrinol.*, 44:271–277.
139. Seidah, N. G., Arbatti, N. J., Rochemont, J., Sheth, A. R., and Chretien, M. (1984): Complete amino acid sequence of human seminal plasma β-inhibin: Prediction of post-Gln-Arg cleavage as a maturation site. *FEBS Lett.*, 175:349–355.
140. Johansson, J., Sheth, A., Cederlund, E., and Jornvall, H. (1984): Analysis of an inhibin preparation reveals apparent identity between a peptide with inhibin-like activity and a sperm-coating antigen. *FEBS Lett.*, 176:21–26.
141. Arbatti, N. J., Seidah, N. G., Rochemont, J., Escher, E., Sheth, A. R., and Chretien, M. (1985): β_2-Inhibin contains the active core of human seminal plasma β-inhibin: Synthesis and bioactivity. *FEBS Lett.*, 181:57–63.
142. Akiyama, K., Yoishioka, Y., Schmid, K., Offner, G. D., Troxler, R. F., Tsuda, R., and Hara, M. (1985): The amino acid sequence of human beta seminal protein. *Biochim. Biophys. Acta*, 829:288–294.
143. Gordon, W. L., Liu, W. K., Akiyama, K., Tsuda, R., Hara, M., Schmid, K., and Ward, D. N. (1987): Beta microseminoprotein (β-MSP) is not an inhibin. *Biol. Reprod.* 36:829–835.
144. Ramasharma, K., Sairam, M. R., Seidah, N. G., Chretien, M., Yamashiro, O., Li, C. H., Manjunath, P., and Schiller, P. W. (1984): Isolation, structure, and synthesis of a human seminal plasma peptide with inhibin-like activity. *Science*, 223:1199–1202.
145. Mason, A. J., Niall, H. D., and Seeburg, P. H. (1986): The structure of two human ovarian inhibins. *Biochem. Biophys. Res. Commun.*, 135:957–964.
146. Robertson, D. M., deVos, F. L., Foulds, L. M., McLachlan, R. I., Burger, H. G., Morgan, F. J., Hearn, M. T. W., and deKretser, D. M. (1986): Isolation of a 31 kDa form of inhibin from bovine follicular fluid. *Molec. Cell. Endocrinol.*, 44:271–277.
147. Vale, W., Rivier, J., Vaughan, J., McClintock, R., Corrigan, A., Woo, W., Karr, D., and Spiers, J. (1986): Purification and characterization of an FSH releasing protein from porcine ovarian follicular fluid. *Nature*, 321:776–779.
148. Ling, N., Ying, S., Veno, N., Shimasaki, S., Esch, F., Hotta, M. and Guillemin, R. (1986): Pituitary FSH is released by a heterodimer of the β-subunits from the two forms of inhibin. *Nature*, 321:779–782.
149. Miyamoto, K., Hasegawa, Y., Fukuda, M. and Igarashi, M. (1986): Demonstration of high molecular weight forms of inhibin in bovine follicular fluid (bFF) by using monoclonal antibodies to bFF 32K inhibin. *Biochem. Biophys. Res. Commun.*, 136:1103–1109.

The Physiology of Reproduction,
edited by E. Knobil and J. Neill *et al.*
Raven Press, Ltd., New York © 1988.

CHAPTER 16

Relaxin

O. David Sherwood

F. L. Hisaw's interest in modifications of the pelvic girdle that many mammalian species undergo to facilitate giving birth to their young led to the discovery of relaxin. In 1926 Hisaw reported that the injection of serum from pregnant guinea pigs or rabbits into virgin guinea pigs shortly after estrus promoted a noticeable relaxation of the pubic ligament (289). The following year the relaxative substance was found in sow corpora lutea and rabbit placentas (290). In 1930 a crude aqueous extract of the relaxative hormone was obtained from sow corpora lutea, and the hormone was named relaxin (193).

During the 1930s and most of the 1940s, there was little interest in relaxin. Not much progress was made toward the isolation of relaxin during this period; the few efforts to purify the hormone were hindered by limitations associated with the techniques available for its isolation and bioassay. Then, from the late 1940s through the 1950s, research on relaxin surged. Although impure porcine relaxin was used, pioneering discoveries concerning the biological effects of relaxin on the female reproductive tract of nonpregnant animals were made. Relaxin was found to promote elongation of the interpubic ligament in estrogen-primed mice (260,269), inhibit spontaneous contractions of the uterine myometrium in estrogen-primed guinea pigs (354), and promote cervical softening in estrogen-primed cattle (253). These biological effects, which have since been confirmed with highly purified relaxin preparations, provided valuable insight concerning probable physiological roles of relaxin during pregnancy and at parturition in several species.

Interest in relaxin lagged again during the 1960s and until the mid-1970s when straightforward techniques for isolating relaxin preparations of well-documented high purity began to be described. Since 1974, highly purified relaxin has been obtained from the pig, rat, shark, horse, and rabbit, and the availability of highly purified hormone preparations has triggered a sustained resurgence of research on relaxin. Highly purified relaxin has been used to (a) determine the primary structure of porcine, rat, and shark relaxin; (b) develop specific and sensitive homologous radioimmunoassays for porcine, rat, and equine relaxin and then determine the levels of relaxin in the blood of these species; (c) identify the source(s) and target tissues for relaxin in several species; (d) investigate the mechanism of relaxin's action on myometrial cells; (e) demonstrate that relaxin is essential for normal delivery in pigs and rats; (f) explore the possibility that relaxin may have clinical utility at birth in women; and (g) demonstrate that relaxin may have a physiological role or roles in the male. Additionally, information obtained with highly purified relaxin preparations has been used with recombinant DNA techniques to determine the putative primary structures of two forms of human relaxin as well as precursor forms of porcine, rat, and human relaxin.

No other mammalian polypeptide hormone has been demonstrated to be as rich as relaxin in the diversity of both its chemistry and physiology among species. This diversity, which includes relaxin's structure, source, regulation of synthesis and secretion, secretory profiles during pregnancy, and physiological effects during pregnancy, has influenced the organization and emphasis of this review. The review begins with a rather detailed description of both the isolation and chemistry of relaxin for the following reasons. First, only the use of highly purified relaxin preparations provides a sound basis for the study of the physiology of relaxin; therefore, the reader should know the species for which relaxin isolation procedures have been reported. Second, a good understanding of the chemistry of relaxin is needed to understand the importance of employing relaxin from homologous species wherever possible. Third, advances with the determination of the structure of relaxin and its precursors are among the most elegant studies conducted on relaxin during recent years. Finally, although superficial features of relaxin are similar to those of insulin, it is important to appreciate that detailed analysis demonstrates that marked differences exist between these two hormones.

The diversity of relaxin also influenced the organization of the biological aspects of this review. In view of the marked differences that exist among species, the descriptions of relaxin's sources, secretion, and physiological effects on the pubic symphysis and cervix are described for individual species. Relaxin has long been considered a hormone produced only in the female, but this may not be the case. This review will conclude with recent findings indicating that relaxin may also be produced in the male and have functions that enhance fertilization. Throughout the review, initial discoveries and early studies that made major contributions to an understanding of the chemistry and biology of relaxin are described; furthermore, other early studies that contributed to this understanding are cited to provide a more comprehensive reference to the relaxin literature. However, emphasis is on advances made after 1974 with highly purified preparations of relaxin. For additional descriptions of the isolation, chemistry, measurement, and physiology of relaxin, the reader is referred to other reviews (86,335,461,531,546) and conference proceedings (24, 48,89,588).

ISOLATION OF RELAXIN

Efforts to Isolate Relaxin Prior to 1974

In 1930, Fevold et al. (193) reported the first effort to isolate and characterize porcine relaxin. Corpora lutea from unselected sows were ground and extracted with hydrochloric acid (HCl) in alcohol, and the relaxin was enriched by pH adjustment and fractionations with alcohol, acetone, and ether. Although the hormone preparation was impure, these workers discovered that relaxin was probably a peptide; it was soluble in aqueous media, amphoteric, and inactivated by digestion with trypsin (192,193).

For nearly 50 years, essentially all efforts to isolate relaxin employed ovaries from pregnant pigs, since this source has a high content of relaxin bioactivity (9) and is relatively easy to acquire in large quantities. Until the late 1950s, efforts to isolate relaxin were hindered by the limited techniques available for isolating proteins: Relaxin was generally separated from other proteins on the basis of differential solubility following changes in pH, concentrations of salt, or concentrations of organic solvents (1,9,213,216). These techniques were laborious, and only modest enrichment of relaxin was generally obtained with each purification step. A second major obstacle was the lack of physicochemical techniques for determining the degree of purity of protein preparations. Instead, investigators relied heavily on the specific biological activity of relaxin preparations to assess their degree of purity. The first quantitative bioassay for relaxin employed ovariectomized, estrogen-primed guinea pigs and defined a "guinea pig unit" (GPU) as the dose of relaxin required to induce unmistakable mobility of the pubic symphysis of two-thirds of a group of 12 animals (1). This bioassay had limited utility for determining potency estimates; it was cumbersome, based on the subjective assessment of the degree of relaxin-induced mobility of the pubic symphysis, and imprecise.

During the late 1950s, improved quantitative bioassays for relaxin were developed. In 1959 Kroc et al. (356) described a bioassay based on the ability of relaxin to inhibit spontaneous contractions of the mouse uterus *in vitro,* and in 1960 Steinetz et al. (574) developed an objective bioassay in which the interpubic ligament formed in estrogen-primed female mice in response to relaxin is transilluminated and precisely measured with a dissecting microscope fitted with an ocular micrometer. Most efforts to isolate porcine relaxin after 1960 employed these two mouse bioassays to locate relaxin-containing fractions and to determine the specific bioactivity of relaxin preparations.

Bioassay reference standards that made possible determination of the relative potency (specific bioactivity) of relaxin preparations also became available during the 1950s. These standards included porcine relaxin preparations Warner-Lambert W1164-A lot 8 (150 GPU/mg), Warner-Lambert W1164, 48E-2103a (1,000 GPU/mg), and NIH-R-P1 (440 GPU/mg). These porcine relaxin reference standards enabled not only more reliable assessment of progress toward the isolation of porcine relaxin but also more reliable comparisons of the biological effects of impure relaxin preparations among laboratories.

During the 1960s, the laboratories of Frieden (210,220), Cohen (122), and Griss (256) used new protein isolation techniques such as countercurrent distribution, gel filtration, and ion-exchange chromatography to obtain preparations of porcine relaxin that contained high specific biological activity. Although the physicochemical properties of their preparations were not precisely described, these workers determined correctly that porcine relaxin is a protein with a molecular weight between 4,000 and 10,000 (122,220,256), has a basic isoelectric point (122,256), and contains disulfide bonds essential for biological activity (122,215).

Isolation of Relaxin Since 1974

Between 1974 and 1981, highly purified relaxin was isolated from the ovaries of pregnant pigs, rats, and sharks. More recently, highly purified relaxin was isolated from the placentas of horses and rabbits. Additionally, partially purified relaxin was obtained from cow corpora lutea and human corpora lutea, placentas, and decidua.

Similarities exist in the procedures developed to isolate relaxin from these species. For extraction nearly all of the isolation procedures take advantage of relaxin's stability in acidic solvents, and many also use its solubility in 60% to 70% acetone. Following extraction, relaxin is generally purified by a combination of gel filtration and either ion-exchange chromatography or isoelectric focusing. Both the mouse interpubic ligament bioassay (574) and *in vitro* mouse uterus bioassay (356) were used to locate relaxin bioactivity during the development of isolation procedures, but in some cases problems were encountered with the latter bioassay. The *in vitro* mouse uterus bioassay could not be used in the early stages of the isolation of relaxin from cow corpora lutea (194,195,200), rabbit placentas (205), or human placentas (200,201), since a small uterine "contractin factor" (thought to be oxytocin), which overrode relaxin's quiescent effect on uterine contractility, was present in the tissue extracts (200,201,205).

Yields of relaxin per kilogram of equivalent of tissue source differ greatly among species. The concentrations of relaxin in pig and rat corpora lutea are much higher than they are in tissue sources in the shark, horse, rabbit, cow, and human. Therefore, with the latter species, isolation procedures applicable to kilogram quantities of the tissue source were developed to obtain sufficient relaxin for chemical and physiological studies. Physicochemical and biological characterization studies of highly purified relaxin preparations not only revealed that superficial features of relaxin, such as its size and two-chain composition, are similar among species, but also provided early indications that the primary structure of relaxin differed markedly among species. Distinct variation was found in the isoelectric points, amino acid contents, and specific bioactivities of relaxin preparations from different species.

This section describes in the order of their publication the isolation and characterization of highly purified relaxin from the pig, rat, sand tiger shark, rabbit, and horse. Nearly all recent research on the physiology of relaxin was conducted with highly purified pig and rat relaxin. Accordingly, the isolation and characterization of relaxin from these two species are described in sufficient detail to provide a good understanding of the nomenclatures and characteristics of these hormone preparations. A summary of yields, physicochemical characteristics, and biological characteristics of highly purified porcine, rat, shark, rabbit, and equine relaxin preparations is given in Table 1. This section also contains a description of the partial purification of relaxin from the cow and human.

Isolation of Porcine Relaxin

In 1974 Sherwood and O'Byrne (555) described a procedure for isolating porcine relaxin in high yields. One kilogram of frozen ovaries from sows containing fetuses with a crown-rump length of 10 cm or greater was extracted with an acid-acetone method (0.15 N HCl, 70% acetone) patented in 1963 by Doczi (161). After gel filtration of the extract on Sephadex G-50 (Pharmacia; Piscataway, NJ), relaxin bioactivity was adsorbed to carboxymethyl cellulose

TABLE 1. *Summary of characteristics of highly purified relaxin preparations*

Species (source)	Preparation	Yield (mg/kg fresh tissue)	Molecular weight	Isoelectric point	Bioactivity (GPU/mg)	Reference
Pig (ovaries)	CMB	38	6,300	10.6	2,500–3,000[a]	555
	CMa	34	6,300	10.7	2,500–3,000	
	CMa′	36	6,300	10.8	2,500–3,000	
Rat (ovaries)	CM1	140	6,000	7.6	CM1 equivalent to CM2[a] and less than pig relaxin	538
	CM2	140	6,000	9.4		
Shark (ovaries)		2–5	6,000	—	Not detected[a,b] and less than pig relaxin[c]	484
Rabbit (placenta)		10	7,200	6.8	23[b]	177
Horse (placenta)	R1	1.5	5,600	—	28[a]	591
	R2	0.2				
	R3	0.4				

[a]Mouse interpubic ligament bioassay (574).
[b]*In vitro* mouse uterus bioassay (356,362).
[c]Guinea pig pubic symphysis palpation bioassay and *in vitro* guinea pig uterus bioassay (573).

(CMC) and then eluted as three contiguous peaks designated CMB, CMa, and CMa′ by the addition of a linear salt gradient (see Fig. 1A). The yields of each of the three relaxin preparations were about 35 mg/kg equivalent of ovarian tissue (555), and limited evidence indicated they may be increased by adding protease inhibitors to the extraction solvent (357). Characterization studies demonstrated that the three porcine relaxin preparations were essentially homogeneous and that their structures were nearly identical—that is, they were microheterogeneous (555). The specific bioactivities of CMB, CMa, and CMa′ were high and equipotent: they ranged from 2,500 to 3,000 GPU/mg when compared to Warner-Lambert Porcine Relaxin Reference Standard W1164,48E-2103a (1,000 GPU/mg) in the mouse interpubic ligament bioassay. The amino acid compositions of CMB, CMa, and CMa′ were also in close agreement, and they contained no histidine, proline, or tyrosine. Sedimentation equilibrium analysis indicated that the molecular weights of the three relaxin preparations were about 6,000 and gel filtration of reduced and carboxymethylated CMB, CMa, and CMa′ showed they consisted of two chains of similar size (designated A and B) linked by disulfide bonds. The three porcine relaxin preparations had high isoelectric points, ranging from pH 10.6 to pH 10.8.

Additional procedures for isolating multiple forms of highly purified porcine relaxin have been described since 1974. Schwabe et al. (531) described a procedure for large-scale preparation of porcine relaxin which involved acid-acetone extraction of pig ovaries according to Doczi (161) followed by ion-exchange chromatography on CMC and gel filtration on Sephadex G-50. Frieden et al. (218,219) further purified a crude preparation of porcine relaxin (NIH-R-P1; 440 GPU/mg) by means of gel filtration on Bio-Gel P-10 (Bio-Rad Laboratories; Richmond, CA) followed by column electrophoresis on Sephadex G-25 (Pharmacia; Piscataway, NJ) to obtain three microheterogeneous preparations of porcine relaxin designated A, B, and C.

A multiplicity of porcine relaxin components was observed by several workers when ovarian extracts were subjected to countercurrent distribution (220), electrophoresis (122,210,219,361,439), or ion-exchange chromatography (92,93,531,555). This multiplicity was once thought attributable to the expression of more than one relaxin gene, but this is not the case. Complete amino acid sequence analysis of porcine relaxin preparations CMB, CMa, and CMa′ obtained by the isolation procedure of Sherwood and O'Byrne (555) demonstrated that the microheterogeneity among these preparations was attributable to slight differences in the lengths of their B-chain C termini (415) (see Fig. 2). Moreover, Walsh and Niall (648) showed that the differences in lengths of the B-chain C termini were attributable to limited proteolysis of a major stored form of porcine relaxin during its isolation. By modifying an extraction procedure applicable to small, acid-resistant peptides (43), the multiplicity of forms of porcine relaxin was nearly eliminated (648). Frozen ovaries were homogenized in a strongly acidic solvent (15% trifluoroacetic acid, 5% formic acid, 1% NaCl, 1 N HCl), and after adsorption to and elution from small octadecylsilica columns, the relaxin-containing fraction was further purified by gel filtration on Sephadex G-50 and ion-exchange chromatography on CMC. Nearly all of the porcine relaxin eluted from the ion-exchange column as a single peak (see Fig. 1B). It was postulated that the strongly acidic medium minimizes proteolysis both by the low pH per se and by precipitating high-molecular-weight proteases (43). Although the procedure of Walsh and Niall (648) has the advantage of reducing the multiplicity of forms of porcine relaxin, it is not readily applied to the isolation of relaxin from kilogram batches of pig ovaries. Most of the studies conducted with highly purified porcine relaxin employed

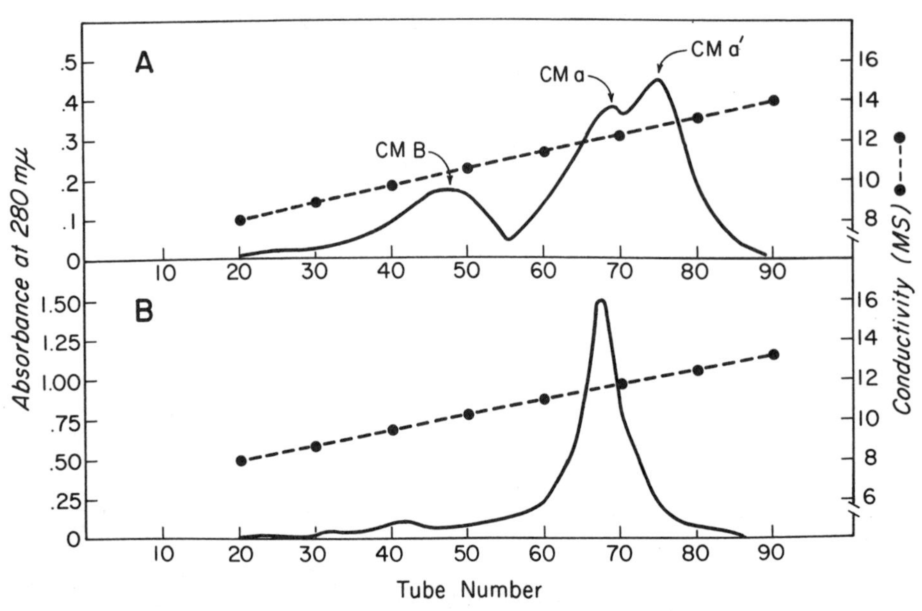

FIG. 1. Ion exchange chromatography of porcine relaxin on carboxymethyl cellulose. **A:** With the isolation procedure of Sherwood and O'Byrne (555), relaxin activity elutes in three contiguous preparations designated CMB, CMa, and CMa′ when a linear gradient of sodium chloride in equilibrating buffer is applied to the column. **B:** With the isolation procedure of Walsh and Niall (648), nearly all relaxin activity elutes in one major component, which corresponds to CMa when a linear gradient of ammonium acetate in equilibrating buffer is applied to the column. Reproduced with permission from Walsh and Niall (648).

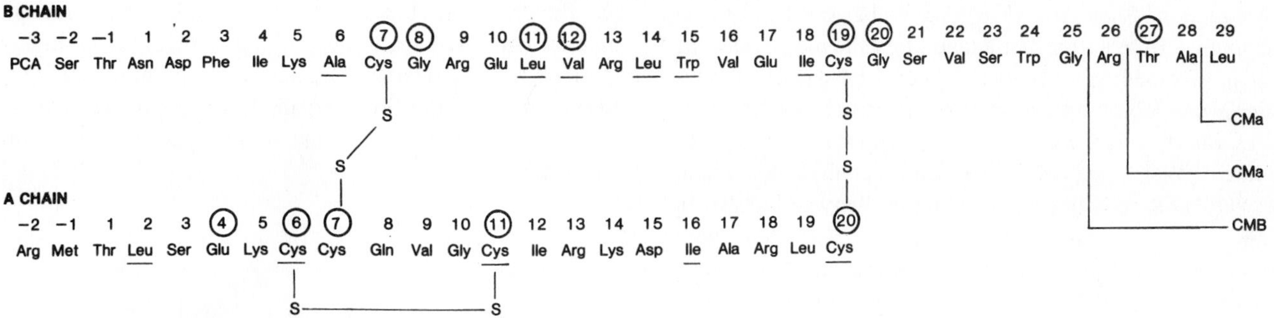

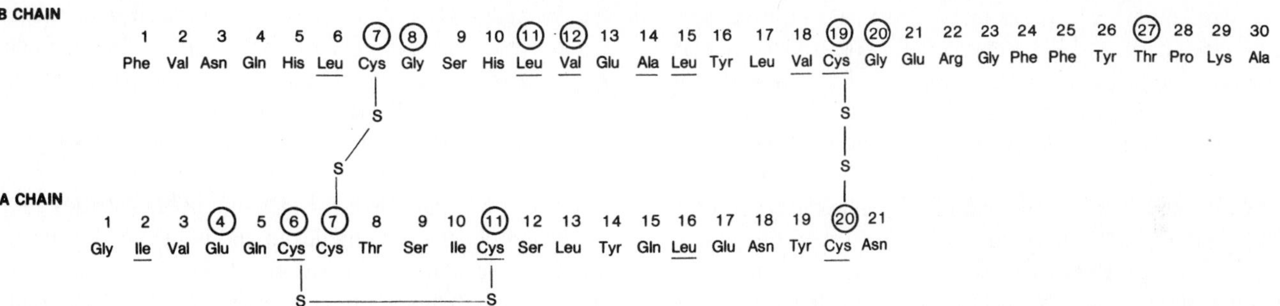

FIG. 2. Covalent structure of porcine relaxin (322,528–530) and porcine insulin (78). In this figure, residues are numbered with respect to the insulin sequence to facilitate comparison of the two hormones. The CMB, CMa, and CMa′ forms of porcine relaxin shown in Fig. 1A (555) are attributable to small differences in the lengths of their B chains as shown with the vertical lines (415). CMB, CMa, and CMa′ forms of porcine relaxin are sometimes designated B28, B31, and B29 porcine relaxin, respectively, to denote the lengths of their B chains. Numbers of the residues that are identical in relaxin and insulin are circled. Residues that contribute to the hydrophobic core of insulin and those in comparable positions in relaxin are underlined (38,39).

relaxin obtained by the procedure of Sherwood and O'Byrne (555).

Isolation of Rat Relaxin

In 1979 Sherwood described a method for the isolation of rat relaxin (538). Approximately 3 g of frozen ovaries, collected from 25 rats on day 20 of gestation, when ovarian relaxin levels are maximal (539), were extracted with phosphate-buffered saline. Following gel filtration of the extract on Sephadex G-50, the relaxin bioactivity was adsorbed to CMC and then eluted as two preparations, designated CM1 and CM2, by the addition of a linear NaCl gradient. The yields of both CM1 and CM2 were about 0.14 mg/g equivalent of ovarian tissue; therefore, the combined yield of rat relaxin was about 0.28 mg/g equivalent of ovarian tissue. Characterization studies indicated that the two rat relaxin preparations were nearly homogeneous and microheterogeneous. No difference in biological activity between CM1 and CM2 was found with the mouse interpubic ligament bioassay, and the amino acid compositions of the two preparations were similar. Superficial structural features of rat relaxin were similar to those of porcine relaxin. Sedimentation equilibrium analysis indicated the molecular weights of CM1 and CM2 to be about 6,000, and slab gel electrophoresis of reduced rat relaxin showed that it consisted of two chains of similar size linked by disulfide bonds. Other analyses, however, demonstrated differences between rat relaxin and porcine relaxin. Rat relaxin was much less bioactive, and its dose-response curve differed from that obtained with porcine relaxin in the mouse interpubic ligament bioassay (69,538). The amino acid composition of rat relaxin differed distinctly from that of porcine relaxin, and the isoelectric points of CM1 and CM2, pH 7.6 and 9.4, respectively, were lower than those of porcine relaxin preparations CMB, CMa, and CMa′.

As with porcine relaxin, the multiplicity of forms of rat relaxin appears to be attributable to limited proteolysis of a major stored form during the isolation procedure. Walsh and Niall (648) found that when ovaries obtained from pregnant rats were quickly frozen, extracted in strongly acidic solvent, enriched by adsorption to octadecylsilica, and then further purified as described above for porcine relaxin, nearly all of the rat relaxin eluted from the CMC as a single component. The yields of rat relaxin obtained with the isolation procedures of Sherwood (538) and Walsh and Niall (648) are similar. In this reviewer's laboratory the mean yields of relaxin obtained from ovaries collected on day 20 of gestation were 0.24 mg/g equivalent of ovarian tissue ($N = 6$; O. D. Sherwood, *unpublished data*) with the isolation procedure of Walsh and Niall (648), and 0.28 mg/g equivalent of ovarian tissue with the procedure of Sherwood (538). In view of the minimal microheterogeneity associated with relaxin obtained by the procedure of Walsh and Niall (648), it is the method of choice for the isolation of rat relaxin.

Isolation of Sand Tiger Shark Relaxin

Interest in the evolutionary origin of relaxin provided the motivation for its isolation from a primitive species—the shark. In 1981 Reinig et al. (484) isolated relaxin from the sand tiger shark (*Odontaspis taurus*). Ovaries obtained from pregnant sand tiger sharks were extracted with acid–70% acetone. The extract was further purified by gel filtration on Sephadex G-75, ion-exchange chromatography on CMC, and high-pressure liquid chromatography (HPLC). The yield of highly purified shark relaxin was low, 2 to 5 mg/kg equivalent of ovaries, but sufficient for chemical and biological characterization. Gel filtration indicated the molecular weight of shark relaxin to be about 6,000, and HPLC of reduced shark relaxin showed that it consisted of two chains linked by disulfide bonds. The bioactivity of the shark relaxin differed strikingly from that of porcine relaxin in both the guinea pig and the mouse. In guinea pigs, the shark relaxin was only about 4% as bioactive as porcine relaxin in the pubic symphysis palpation bioassay, and it was also less effective than porcine relaxin in inhibiting the frequency of contractions of uterine segments. Sand tiger shark relaxin appears to be inactive in the mouse, since high doses failed to either induce growth of the interpubic ligament or inhibit myometrial contractility. The amino acid composition of sand tiger shark relaxin differed distinctly from that of porcine and rat relaxin (484).

Isolation of Rabbit Relaxin

In 1985 Eldridge and Fields (177) isolated relaxin from the rabbit. Placentas obtained from rabbits of unknown stages of pregnancy were extracted with a modified acid-acetone extraction medium (256) consisting of 5.0 acetone : 2.83 H_2O : 0.17 HCl (vol/vol/vol) plus protease inhibitors. The extract was further purified by gel filtration on Sephadex G-50, ion-exchange chromatography on CMC, and gel filtration on Sepharose CL-4B (Pharmacia; Piscataway, NJ). The yield of highly purified rabbit relaxin was about 12 mg/kg equivalent of placentas. Slab gel electrophoresis of unreduced and reduced relaxin indicated that the molecular weight of rabbit relaxin was about 7,000 and that it consisted of two chains of similar size linked by disulfide bonds. Rabbit relaxin was much less active than porcine relaxin in the *in vitro* mouse uterus bioassay—23 GPU/mg for rabbit relaxin compared to 2,500 to 3,000 GPU/mg for highly purified porcine relaxin. The isoelectric point of rabbit relaxin, pH 6.8, was lower than those of porcine and rat relaxin. The amino acid composition of rabbit relaxin was not reported.

Isolation of Equine Relaxin

In 1986 Stewart (591) isolated relaxin from the horse. Relaxin was extracted from placentas obtained at term with 0.5 N HCl–85% acetone and then further purified by stepwise elution from a CMC column followed by gel filtration on Sephadex G-50. Relaxin in the fraction obtained from the Sephadex G-50 column was precipitated with 5% trichloroacetic acid, adsorbed to CMC, and then eluted in one major peak (designated R1) and two minor peaks (designated R1.5 and R2) with the addition of a linear NaCl gradient. The yield of the predominant equine relaxin preparation R1 was only about 1.5 mg/kg equivalent of placentas, but it was sufficient for characterization studies. Slab gel electrophoresis of unreduced and reduced R1 indicated that its molecular weight was about 6,000 and that it consisted of two chains of similar size linked by disulfide bonds. The specific bioactivity of R1 as determined in the mouse interpubic ligament bioassay was far lower than that of porcine relaxin—only 28 GPU/mg. The amino acid composition of equine relaxin differed from that of porcine, rat, and shark relaxin; it lacked phenylalanine and methionine.

Purification of Bovine Relaxin

Fields et al. (194–197) extracted relaxin from cow ovaries obtained during late pregnancy with a modified acid-acetone extraction medium (256) consisting of a 3 : 5 volume ratio of 0.7 N HCl: acetone. When the extract was further purified by gel filtration on Sephadex G-50, three fractions that inhibited spontaneous contractions of the mouse uterus were eluted from the column. These fractions had molecular weights of 8,000, 6,000, and 1,400. The specific bioactivity of the 6,000-dalton fraction, determined with the mouse interpubic ligament bioassay, was 71 GPU/mg, which is far lower than that of porcine relaxin. Electrofocusing of the 6,000-dalton fraction demonstrated that it contained three basic fractions which inhibited contractions of the mouse uterus and were immunologically cross-reactive with an antiserum to highly purified porcine relaxin (361). As with porcine and rat relaxin, the multiple forms of 6,000-dalton bovine relaxin appear to be attributable to limited proteolysis of a single stored form of the 6,000-dalton molecule (198). The chemical natures of the 8,000- and 1,400-dalton fractions remain largely unexplained. The curiously small, 1,400-dalton fraction showed immunological cross-reactivity with an antiserum to highly purified porcine relaxin and promoted growth of the mouse interpubic ligament (196). It was suggested that the 8,000- and 1,400-dalton molecules may be partially degraded forms of prorelaxin or 6,000-dalton relaxin, respectively; alternatively, they may be different gene products and members of a family of relaxin-like peptides (197,198). The yield of relaxin from cow ovaries was low, and the degree of purity of the bovine relaxin preparations was not described.

Purification of Human Relaxin

Efforts have been made to purify relaxin from human corpora lutea (433), placentas (176,183,184,204,673), and decidua (47,50,51). Although none of the human relaxin preparations were demonstrated to be highly purified, they displayed characteristics similar to those of porcine relaxin. Preparations from the three tissues had molecular weights of about 6,000 (50,176,204,433,673), demonstrated activity in the guinea pig pubic symphysis palpation bioassay (430) and/or mouse interpubic ligament bioassay (47,50, 183,204), and displayed immunological cross-reactivity with antisera to highly purified porcine relaxin (51,204, 430,433,673). It seems unlikely that human relaxin will be isolated in yields sufficient to enable detailed chemical and biological characterization studies in the near future. The apparent quantities of relaxin in the corpus luteum of pregnancy in women are low compared to those in the corpora lutea of pregnant pigs or rats during late pregnancy (430,433); moreover, human corpora lutea of pregnancy are not readily available. Although the placentas and decidua contain extremely small quantities of relaxin, it appears likely that it will be necessary to isolate relaxin repeatedly from one or both of these tissues to accumulate the human hormone needed for characterization studies.

CHEMISTRY OF RELAXIN

Covalent Structure of Relaxin

The amino acid sequences of the A and B chains of porcine, rat, and shark relaxin were initially determined by peptide sequence analysis of native hormone preparations (251,322,327,328,521,528–530). Later nucleotide sequence analysis not only confirmed the amino acid sequences of porcine and rat relaxin but also predicted the amino acid sequences of two forms of human relaxin (259,309–311). Locations of disulfide bonds (see Fig. 2) were determined only for porcine relaxin (528). Nevertheless, it seems certain that they are similar in rat, sand tiger shark, and human relaxin, since, in all three cases, half-cystine residues are found in positions comparable to those in porcine relaxin (see Fig. 3).

The structure of relaxin has apparently diverged considerably among species during evolution. Only 40% to 48% amino acid sequence homology exists among porcine, rat, shark, and human relaxins (see Table 2); moreover, the invariant positions are largely confined to the half-cystine residues and adjacent glycine residues (see Fig. 3). The extensive differences in amino acid residues on the surfaces

RELAXIN B CHAINS

	-7	-6	-5	-4	-3	-2	-1	1	2	3	4	(5)	6	7	8	(9)	10	11	12	(13)	14	15	16	17	18	19	20	21	22	23	24	25	26	27	28	29
Pig					PCA	Ser	Thr	Asn	Asp	Phe	Ile	Lys	Ala	Cys	Gly	Arg	Glu	Leu	Val	Arg	Leu	Trp	Val	Glu	Ile	Cys	Gly	Ser	Val	Ser	Trp	Gly	Arg	Thr	Ala	Leu
Rat	Arg	Val	Ser	Glu	Glu	Trp	Met	Asp	Gln	Val	Ile	Gln	Val	Cys	Gly	Arg	Gly	Tyr	Ala	Arg	Ala	Trp	Ile	Glu	Val	Cys	Gly	Ala	Ser	Val	Gly	Arg	Leu	Ala	Leu	
Shark$_{ST}$		PCA	Ser	Leu	Ser	Asn	Ala	Gly	Ser	Gly	Ile	Lys	Leu	Cys	Gly	Arg	Gly	Phe	Ile	Arg	Ala	Ile	Ile	Phe	Ala	Cys	Gly	Gly	Ser	Arg						
Human 1					Lys	Trp	Lys	Asp	Asp	Val	Ile	Lys	Leu	Cys	Gly	Arg	Glu	Leu	Val	Arg	Ala	Gln	Ile	Ala	Ile	Cys	Gly	Met	Ser	Thr	Trp	Ser	Lys	Arg	Ser	Leu
Human 2				Asp	Ser	Trp	Met	Glu	Glu	Val	Ile	Lys	Leu	Cys	Gly	Arg	Glu	Leu	Val	Arg	Ala	Gln	Ile	Ala	Ile	Cys	Gly	Met	Ser	Thr	Trp	Ser	Lys	Arg	Ser	Leu

RELAXIN A CHAINS

	-4	-3	-2	-1	1	2	3	4	(5)	6	7	8	9	10	11	12	(13)	(14)	15	16	17	18	19	20
Pig			Arg	Met	Thr	Leu	Ser	Glu	Lys	Cys	Cys	Gln	Val	Gly	Cys	Ile	Arg	Lys	Asp	Ile	Ala	Arg	Leu	Cys
Rat	PCA	Ser	Gly	Ala	Leu	Leu	Ser	Glu	Gln	Cys	Cys	His	Ile	Gly	Cys	Thr	Arg	Arg	Ser	Ile	Ala	Lys	Leu	Cys
Shark$_{ST}$	Ala	Thr	Ser	Pro	Ala	Met	Ser	Ile	Lys	Cys	Cys	Ile	Tyr	Gly	Cys	Thr	Lys	Lys	Asp	Ile	Ser	Val	Leu	Cys
Human 1	Arg	Pro	Tyr	Val	Ala	Leu	Phe	Glu	Lys	Cys	Cys	Leu	Ile	Gly	Cys	Thr	Lys	Arg	Ser	Leu	Ala	Lys	Tyr	Cys
Human 2	Gln	Leu	Tyr	Ser	Ala	Leu	Ala	Asn	Lys	Cys	Cys	His	Val	Gly	Cys	Thr	Lys	Arg	Ser	Leu	Ala	Arg	Phe	Cys

FIG. 3. Amino acid sequences of relaxin B and A chains for those relaxin molecules whose complete sequences have been reported. The porcine (322,529,530), rat (327), and sand tiger shark (251,521) sequences were determined by amino acid sequence analysis. The human sequences were predicted from nucleotide sequence analysis (310,311). Residues are numbered with respect to insulin as in Fig. 2. Residues common to the five sequences are boxed, and those in positions comparable to those that contribute to the hydrophobic core of insulin (38,39) are underlined. Numbers of residues postulated to be involved with the binding of relaxin to its receptor are circled (38,56,162). Nearly all of the amino acid sequence of dogfish shark relaxin has also been reported (521).

TABLE 2. *Comparison of relaxin among species*

Species	Pig	Rat	$Shark_{ST}$	Human 1	Human 2
Pig	—	40%	40%	46%	44%
Rat	21/53	—	40%	48%	44%
$Shark_{ST}$	19/48	21/53	—	42%	44%
Human 1	24/54	26/54	21/50	—	77%
Human 2	24/54	24/54	22/50	43/56	—

Ratios are the number of identical amino acids to the total number of amino acid positions shared by each pair of hormones (lower left). These values are also given as percentages (upper right).

of porcine, rat, sand tiger shark, and human relaxin form a structural basis for the observations that these relaxin preparations display different biological activities in relaxin bioassays and limited immunological cross-reactivity in radioimmunoassays.

Relaxin as a Member of the Insulin Family

Structures of Relaxin, Insulin, and Insulin-like Growth Factors

Porcine relaxin and insulin have strikingly similar superficial structural features (see Fig. 2)—namely, their A and B chains are of similar length and their disulfide bridges have the same disposition. Discovery of the comparable cystine pairings in these two hormones stimulated the view that relaxin might have a tertiary structure similar to that of insulin. The tertiary structure of insulin monomers in solution is not known with certainty; however, X-ray crystallographic analysis of porcine 2-zinc (55) and 4-zinc insulin crystals (44) showed that insulin exists as two independent molecules, designated protomers I and II, in each crystalline form. All four protomers are compact globular structures with a hydrophobic core. With the exception of protomer I of 4-zinc insulin, each protomer involves right-handed α-helical segments A2-A8, A13-A19, and B9-B19; extended regions B1-B7 and B24-B30; and turns hinging on glycines at B8, B20, and B23 as shown schematically for 2-zinc insulin I in Fig. 4 (58). Protomer I of 4-zinc insulin is much like the other protomers except that the B-chain α-helix starts at residue 2 rather than at residue 9, as shown schematically for 4-zinc insulin (see Fig. 4), and it has a more open framework.

Although the extent of homology between porcine relaxin and porcine insulin is only 12 of 49 aligned residues, the common structural features shown in Fig. 2 permit porcine relaxin a theoretical three-dimensional conformation similar to either the 2-zinc or 4-zinc structure of insulin shown in Fig. 4. Porcine relaxin has retained not only the six half-cystines but also the B8 and B20 glycines, which provide unique torsion angles for chain folding. Additionally, the residues corresponding to those packed into the hydrophobic core of insulin (indicated by underlining in Fig. 2) are nonpolar in porcine relaxin, with the exception of B15 tryptophan. Moreover, two pairs of these nonpolar residues, which would point toward the hydrophobic core from opposite sides in both insulin and relaxin (B6-B14 and A2-A16), have complimentary changes in amino acid residues which enable maintenance of core volume (38,39,58,314). Models of porcine relaxin obtained by model building (38,39,314) and interactive computer graphics (56,314,425) showed that all residues in the A chain and residues B6 to B20 in the B chain, including the burial of B15 tryptophan in the hydrophobic core, could be accommodated in a tertiary structure similar to that of 2-zinc insulin. Although the conformations of the N and C termini of porcine relaxin are presented schematically as being similar to those of 2-zinc insulin in Fig. 4 (53,54,57), they are not known.

The sequences of rat, sand tiger shark, and human relaxin (see Fig. 3) provide supporting evidence for the similar folding of relaxin and insulin. The half-cystines involved in disulfide bridge formation and glycines at B8 and B20 needed for insulin-like chain folding are common to all the relaxin molecules. Moreover, in most cases, nonpolar res-

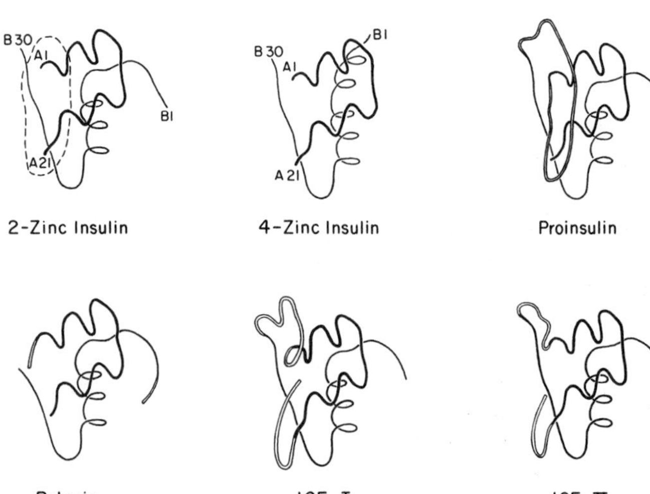

FIG. 4. Schematic representations of three-dimensional structures of protomer I forms of porcine insulin based on X-ray analysis of rhombohedral porcine 2-zinc insulin crystals (55) and 4-zinc insulin crystals (44). Proposed conformations of porcine proinsulin (565), porcine relaxin (39,313,314), and human insulin-like growth factors I and II (54,57) were determined by model building. The putative receptor binding region of insulin (472) is indicated (– – –) on the schematic 2-zinc insulin molecule. Modified and reproduced with permission from Blundell and Humbel (57).

idues are retained in positions comparable to those that contribute to the hydrophobic core of insulin.

There are indications that the hydrophobic core of relaxin may be more open than that of 2-zinc insulin. First, predictions of protein structure on the basis of amino acid sequence indicate that the region of high probability of α-helix includes residues B9 to B16 in porcine, rat, and shark relaxin (56), and this region is shorter than the α-helical region in insulin, which extends from B9 to B19. Second, chymotrypsin produces cleavages in porcine relaxin at B15 tryptophan and B11 leucine, and this indicates that at least one of these core residues is sufficiently exposed to solvent to initiate a reaction with the proteolytic enzyme (61). Finally, the ring of B15 tryptophan in porcine relaxin, although in the hydrophobic core, is sufficiently exposed to form a charge transfer complex with the chemical probe N-methyl nicotinamide chloride (321). Dodson et al. (162) suggested that the relatively open hydrophobic core of porcine relaxin may indicate that it has a tertiary structure like the relatively open 4-zinc insulin protomer I, whereas Blundell et al. (56) suggested that the loosening of the core may derive from a degree of unwinding of the B-chain helix between B16 and B19 and between A17 and A20. Whereas computer-assisted model building indicated that shark relaxin residues can be accommodated in a tertiary structure similar to 2-zinc insulin (56,251), rat relaxin cannot because of close contacts produced by B6 valine, B11 tyrosine, and B15 tryptophan. Rat relaxin residues can be better accommodated in the more open framework of the 4-zinc insulin protomer I model (162) or the 2-zinc insulin model with limited unwinding of the B-chain helix between B16 and B19 and between A17 and A20 (56).

Experimental support of the proposed insulin-like structure of relaxin is limited, since crystals suitable for determining the tertiary structure of relaxin by means of X-ray crystallography have not been obtained (335). Circular dichroic spectra of porcine insulin and porcine relaxin molecules in solution indicated that the relaxin models based on insulin coordinates are realistic: Both hormones contained about 30% α-helix (171,483,526).

Insulin-like growth factor I (IGF-I) and IGF-II are single-chain polypeptides, comprised of 70 and 67 amino acid residues, respectively, which also have structural features similar to those of insulin. The regions of structural similarity of IGF-I and IGF-II to insulin are confined to the B- and A-chain portions of the molecules where they are more homologous to insulin than is relaxin (see Fig. 5). Models for IGF-I (54) and IGF-II (57) indicate that these two growth factors may have conformations similar to that of insulin (see Fig. 4).

Evolutionary Origins of Relaxin

The similarity of their structures led to the postulation that relaxin, insulin, IGF-I, and IGF-II belong to a family of peptides (57,70); that is, that these hormones are attributable to gene duplications of a primitive, insulin-like molecule followed by gene mutations encoding molecules with different functions (39,57,322,528). Schwabe and co-workers (521,525) challenged the monophyletic hypothesis that relaxin and insulin are gene duplication products on the basis of the observation that the differences in the amino acid sequences of these two hormones remain relatively constant,

B CHAIN

	-4	-3	-2	-1	1	2	3	4	5	6	7	8	9	10	11	12	13
Relaxin 1		Lys	Trp	Lys	Asp	Asp	Val	Ile	Lys	Leu	Cys	Gly	Arg	Glu	Leu	Val	Arg
Relaxin 2	Asp	Ser	Trp	Met	Glu	Glu	Val	Ile	Lys	Leu	Cys	Gly	Arg	Glu	Leu	Val	Arg
Insulin					Phe	Val	Asn	Gln	His	Leu	Cys	Gly	Ser	His	Leu	Val	Glu
IGF-I						Gly	Pro	Glu	Thr	Leu	Cys	Gly	Ala	Glu	Leu	Val	Asp
IGF-II			Ala	Tyr	Arg	Pro	Ser	Glu	Thr	Leu	Cys	Gly	Gly	Glu	Leu	Val	Asp

	14	15	16	17	18	19	20	21	22	23	24	25	26	27	28	29	30	31
Relaxin 1	Ala	Gln	Ile	Ala	Ile	Cys	Gly	Met	Ser	Thr	Trp	Ser	Lys	Arg	Ser	Leu		
Relaxin 2	Ala	Gln	Ile	Ala	Ile	Cys	Gly	Met	Ser	Thr	Trp	Ser	Lys	Arg	Ser	Leu		
Insulin	Ala	Leu	Tyr	Leu	Val	Cys	Gly	Glu	Arg	Gly	Phe	Phe	Tyr	Thr	Pro	Lys	Thr	
IGF-I	Ala	Leu	Gln	Phe	Val	Cys	Gly	Asp	Arg	Gly	Phe	Tyr	Phe	Asn	Lys	Pro	Thr •	• •
IGF-II	Thr	Leu	Gln	Phe	Val	Cys	Gly	Asp	Arg	Gly	Phe	Tyr	Phe	Ser	Arg	Pro	Ala •	• •

A CHAIN

	-4	-3	-2	-1	1	2	3	4	5	6	7	8	9	10	11	12
Relaxin 1	Arg	Pro	Tyr	Val	Ala	Leu	Phe	Glu	Lys	Cys	Cys	Leu	Ile	Gly	Cys	Thr
Relaxin 2	Gln	Leu	Tyr	Ser	Ala	Leu	Ala	Asn	Lys	Cys	Cys	His	Val	Gly	Cys	Thr
Insulin					Gly	Ile	Val	Glu	Gln	Cys	Cys	Thr	Ser	Ile	Cys	Ser
IGF-I				• • • • • • • • •	Gly	Ile	Val	Asp	Glu	Cys	Cys	Phe	Arg	Ser	Cys	Asp
IGF-II				• • • • •	Gly	Ile	Val	Gln	Glu	Cys	Cys	Phe	Arg	Ser	Cys	Asp

	13	14	15	16	17	18	19	20	21	22	23	24	25	26	27	28	29
Relaxin 1	Lys	Arg	Ser	Leu	Ala	Lys	Tyr	Cys									
Relaxin 2	Lys	Arg	Ser	Leu	Ala	Arg	Phe	Cys									
Insulin	Leu	Tyr	Gln	Leu	Glu	Asn	Tyr	Cys	Asn								
IGF-I	Leu	Arg	Arg	Leu	Glu	Met	Tyr	Cys	Ala	Pro	Leu	Lys	Pro	Ala	Lys	Ser	Ala
IGF-II	Leu	Ala	Leu	Leu	Glu	Thr	Tyr	Cys	Ala	Thr			Pro	Ala	Lys	Ser	Glu

FIG. 5. Amino acid sequences of the human hormones relaxin H1 (310), relaxin H2 (311), insulin (416), insulin-like growth factor I (491), and insulin-like growth factor II (490). The insulin-like growth factors are single-chained peptides, and the positions of the 12 (IGF-I) and 8 (IGF-II) amino acid residues that connect the B chain–like and A chain–like regions of these molecules are indicated with dots. A gap has been placed at positions 23 and 24 of the A chain–like region of IGF-II in order to illustrate better the homology of the C termini of IGF-I and IGF-II. Residues common to the five hormones are boxed.

about 75%, with no trend toward greater relatedness in the shark, which is thought to be an ancient species. Instead, they proposed a polyphyletic "genetic potential" hypothesis which places emphasis on deterministic chemical principles to account for the origin of the insulin-like family of proteins (521,532). According to the genetic potential hypothesis, prebiotic environmental conditions brought about abiotic synthesis of large but finite numbers of nucleotide polymers which, through self-replicating capabilities, mixed and spread throughout the primeval mud flats. When cells formed, they incorporated large numbers of informational polymers (genetic potential), and some of them coded for families of proteins such as insulin. If the genetic potential hypothesis is correct, genes present in higher forms of life should be present in some, but not all, single cellular organisms. This may be the case. Schwabe et al. (527) reported the extraction of a molecule with the size and immunological properties of porcine relaxin from the protozoan *Tetrahymena pyriformis*.

Biological and Immunological Comparisons of Relaxin and Insulin

If relaxin and insulin originated from a common ancestral gene, considerable evolutionary divergence occurred between the two hormones. The limited amino acid sequence homology (about 25%) between relaxin and insulin is largely confined to the identical disposition of half-cystine residues involved in disulfide bridge formation and the glycine residues important for chain folding (see Fig. 2).

Although stringent requirements to maintain similar tertiary structures appear to exist, three lines of evidence indicate that relaxin and insulin do not share common biologically active sites. First, the amino acid residues needed for insulin bioactivity differ or are not present in relaxin. Insulin binding to its receptor involves the largely hydrophobic surface formed by the N and C termini of the A chain and the C terminus of the B chain as shown with the schematic representation of 2-zinc insulin in Fig. 4. High insulin biological activity requires conservation of residues B24, B25, A19, and A21 on the surface of the molecule (472,692). Residues in these positions differ or, in the case of A21, do not exist in relaxin (see Fig. 2). Second, competitive binding studies indicated that relaxin and insulin do not share receptor-binding domains. Porcine relaxin did not displace porcine insulin from insulin receptors on rat brain cortex (227), human or rat adipocytes (323,438), or human mononuclear leukocytes (483); furthermore, porcine insulin did not displace porcine relaxin from relaxin receptors on human skin fibroblasts or rat uterine myometrium (394,406). Third, relaxin and insulin do not demonstrate common biological activity in mammals. Unlike insulin, porcine relaxin failed to reduce blood glucose levels or increase diaphragm glucose levels in rats (632), promote collagen synthesis in fetal rat bone (355), or promote gonadotropin-stimulated progesterone secretion in pig granulosa cells (392,638). Porcine relaxin increased uterine weight and uterine glycogen content in rats, but insulin did not (632). Relaxin and insulin were reported to demonstrate a common biological activity in a lower vertebrate. Koob et al. (353) reported that both porcine relaxin and bovine insulin promoted an increase in the cross-sectional area of the cervix-like constriction separating the uterus from the urogenital sinus of the spiny dogfish; however, binding studies were not done to determine whether the two hormones have the capacity to act through a common receptor in this species.

The surfaces of porcine relaxin and porcine insulin also appear to share no immunological determinants. Studies that employed porcine relaxin (255,556) or porcine insulin radioimmunoassays (483) showed no evidence of common antigenic domains.

Structure-Activity Relationships

Structural features contributing to the activity of porcine relaxin were identified by determining the biological activity of modified native hormone and synthetic analogs. Both chains as well as the integrity of the putative hydrophobic core appear to be essential for relaxin bioactivity. Reduction and alkylation of the A and B chains (555) and oxidation of the tryptophan residue located at position B15 in Fig. 2 (524) abolished relaxin bioactivity. The basic amino acids that are invariant or that vary conservatively among species have been postulated to be involved (38,56,162,313), and these possibilities (encircled in Fig. 3) include B5 Lys (Gln), B9 Arg, B13 Arg, A5 Lys (Gln), A13 Arg (Lys), and A14 Lys (Arg). Bullesbach and Schwabe (94) found that biological activity was reduced only about 70% in a derivative of porcine relaxin ($N^{\varepsilon A5}$,$N^{\varepsilon A14}$,$N^{\varepsilon B5}$-tris[[[(methylsulfonyl)ethyl]oxy]carbonyl]-B29 relaxin) where the ε amino groups of all three lysine residues were protected.

Three lines of evidence indicate that the C terminus of the B chain is not required for biological activity. First, porcine relaxin preparations CMB, CMa, and CMa′, which lack four, one, and three amino acids, respectively, at the C terminus of their B chains (see Fig. 2) have full and equal activity in the mouse interpubic ligament bioassay (555), *in vitro* mouse uterine contractility bioassay (586), and *in vitro* rat uterine contractility bioassay (19). Second, oxidation of the tryptophan located six residues from the C terminus of the B chain (B24 in Fig. 2) did not reduce the activity of porcine relaxin in the mouse interpubic ligament bioassay (524). Third, Tregear and associates found that a form of synthetic porcine relaxin that lacked seven amino acid residues on the C terminus of the B chain retained full biological activity in the *in vitro* rat uterine contractility bioassay (625,626). Further reduction of the C terminus of the B chain by one or two amino acids, however, decreased bioactivity (625,626).

The N termini of the A and B chains of porcine relaxin

may be modified without complete loss of bioactivity. Full biological activity was retained following the addition of polytyrosine residues to the N terminus of the A chain (531,556) or alkylation of the methionine residue adjacent to the N terminus of the A chain (524). Some biological activity was retained in synthetic porcine relaxin which lacked the three N-terminal amino acids of both the A and B chains (625,626).

Biosynthesis of Relaxin

Preprorelaxin Structure

Gel filtration of sow ovarian extracts provided the first indication that relaxin is synthesized originally in precursor forms and that the putative relaxin precursors are larger than preproinsulin and proinsulin, which are 11,000 and 9,000 daltons, respectively (223,358). Frieden and Yeh (223) reported that about 5% to 10% of the relaxin bioactivity in an acid-acetone extract of porcine ovaries was associated with a biologically active fraction that had an apparent molecular weight of 42,000 as judged by its elution volume following gel filtration on Bio-Gel P-10. Similarly, Kwok et al. (358) reported that a small portion of the relaxin in an acid-acetone extract of porcine ovaries was associated with a biologically active fraction that had an apparent molecular weight of 19,000 as judged by its elution volume following gel filtration on Sephadex G-50. In both studies, treatment of the large, relaxin-like fraction with the proteolytic enzyme trypsin appeared to convert the putative precursor to 6,000-dalton relaxin: The chromatographic (223,358) and electrophoretic characteristics (223) of the proteolytic digest were indicative of 6,000-dalton relaxin formation, and relaxin bioactivity increased (223). More precise estimates of the size of the precursor(s) were obtained by synthesizing radiolabeled porcine relaxin precursors *in vitro* and then determining their size by sodium dodecylsulfate-polyacrylamide disk gel electrophoresis. Employing a cell-free system, Gast and co-workers demonstrated that pig luteal mRNA directed the synthesis of a 23,000-dalton protein immunologically related to relaxin, whereas a 20,000-dalton relaxin-related protein was obtained in the presence of ascites fluid (233–235). Gast postulated that 23,000-dalton preprorelaxin is the primary translation product and that the first step in relaxin biosynthesis is the membrane-dependent cleavage of a 3,000-dalton signal peptide to form prorelaxin (233,234) (see Fig. 6).

Niall and co-workers (259,309) conducted detailed structural studies of putative relaxin precursors, and their findings are consistent with Gast's findings. These workers determined the complete amino acid sequences of porcine (259) and rat (309) preprorelaxin by cloning of relaxin cDNA. In general, this work involved (a) amino acid sequence analysis of porcine and rat relaxin, (b) synthesis of oligoribonucleotide primers complementary to the putative mRNA sequences predicted from the amino acid sequences of porcine and rat relaxin, (c) use of these synthetic DNA primers with mRNA isolated from pig and rat corpora lutea of pregnancy for the production of radiolabeled relaxin-specific cDNA probes, and (d) the identification of relaxin-specific clones in cDNA clone banks constructed from total pregnancy-derived corpus luteum mRNA (335). Relaxin, like insulin, is initially synthesized as a single-chained preprohormone with the overall structure: signal peptide/B chain/connecting peptide/A chain as shown diagrammatically in Fig. 6. The signal peptides for porcine and rat preprorelaxin contain 24 and 26 amino acid residues, respectively (see Fig. 7).

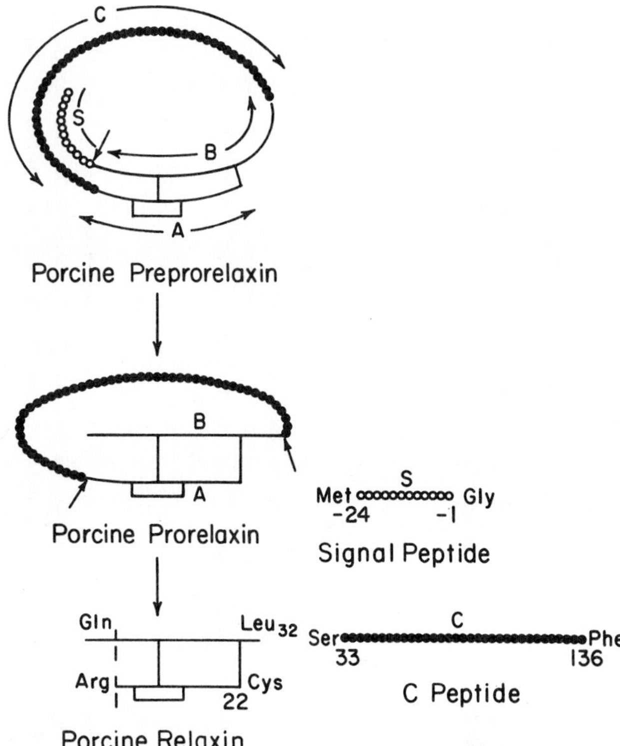

FIG. 6. Schematic summary of the processing of porcine preprorelaxin to relaxin by the successive removal of the signal peptide (S) and the connecting peptide (C) by proteolytic digestion. Modified and reproduced with permission from Kemp and Niall (335).

The size difference between relaxin and insulin precursors is largely attributable to marked differences in the lengths of the connecting (C) peptides. The C peptides in porcine (259) and rat prorelaxin (309) contain 104 and 105 residues, respectively, whereas in porcine and rat proinsulin they contain only about 30 residues (610). The function of the C peptide in relaxin is not known. One function presumably is to direct the folding of the precursors so the correct disulfide bonds are formed between the B and A chains. Additionally, its large size, variety of amino acids, and reasonable level of conservation of primary structure among species led to the postulation that the C peptide may contain peptide sequences with hormonal activities (309,335).

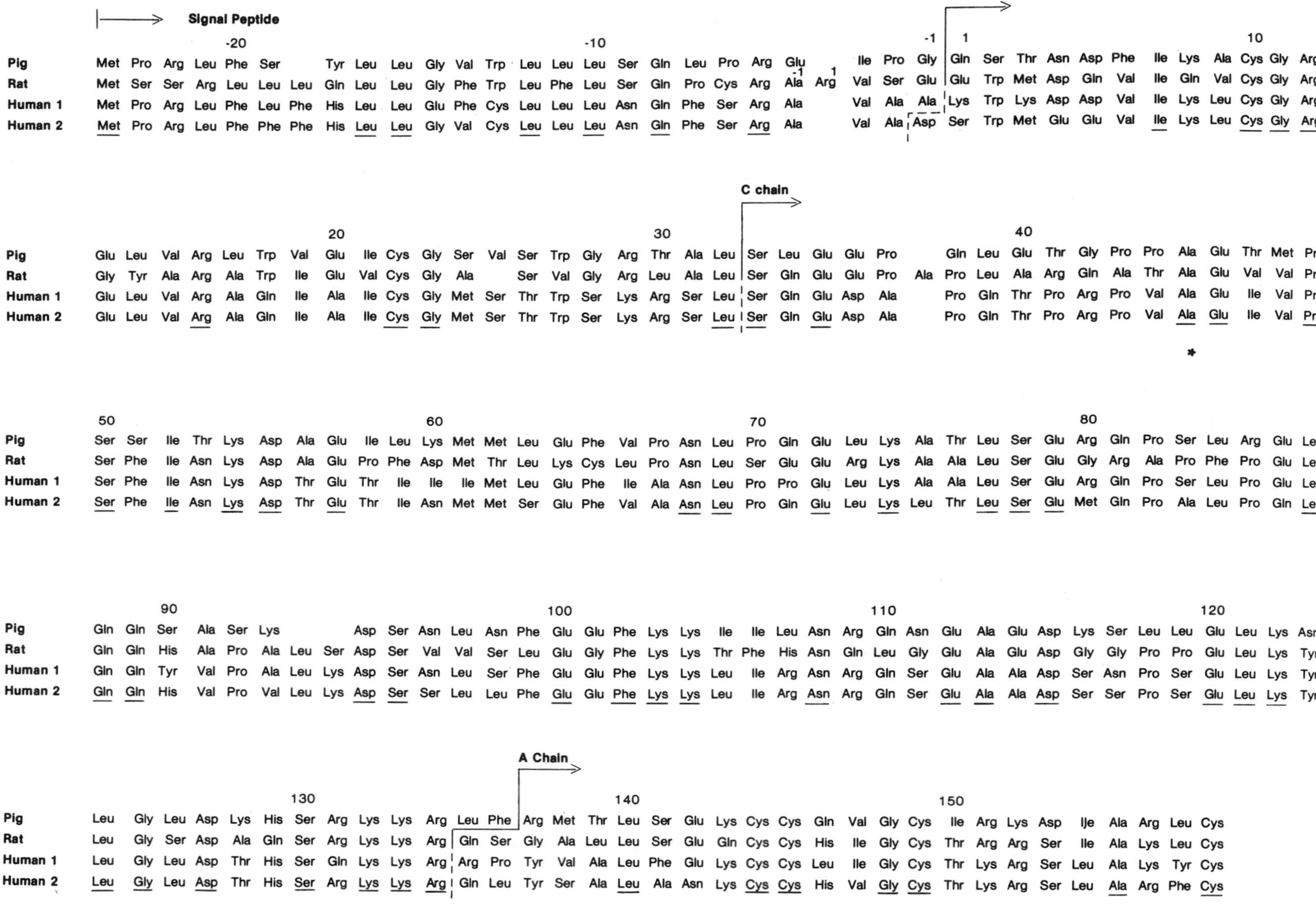

FIG. 7. Amino acid sequences of porcine (259), rat (309), human 1 (310), and human 2 (311) preprorelaxins. Sequences have been aligned to maximize homology, and amino acid identities are underscored. Amino acids are numbered from the N terminus of the porcine relaxin B chain. The cleavage sites of porcine and rat relaxin are indicated with solid vertical lines, and the putative cleavage sites for human relaxin are indicated with broken vertical lines. The asterisk beneath Ala 45 in the C peptides denotes the site of the intron in the human relaxin gene.

Knowledge of the structures of the C peptides of porcine and rat relaxin formed the basis of the strategy used by Hudson et al. (310) to determine the structure of one form of human relaxin. Human relaxin had not been isolated, and its primary structure was not known; consequently, a radiolabeled cDNA probe complementary to its putative mRNA sequence could not be synthesized. Instead, Hudson et al. (310) constructed a specific probe consisting of a short fragment of porcine relaxin cDNA corresponding to amino acids 45 to 94 of the C peptide. This region had maximal homology (71% at the nucleotide level) between porcine and rat prorelaxin sequences and was postulated to be relatively homologous among species. By utilizing this radiolabeled C peptide–specific probe to screen a human genomic library, a clone for one form of human relaxin (human 1, or H1) was obtained, and the complete coding sequence of human relaxin gene 1 was determined (310). More recently a clone for a second form of human relaxin (human 2, or H2) was identified by screening a cDNA clone bank prepared from a human corpus luteum of pregnancy with radiolabeled relaxin-specific cDNA probes corresponding to exon I and exon II of the human preprorelaxin 1 gene (311). The amino acid sequences of human preprorelaxin 1 and preprorelaxin 2 are shown in Fig. 7. Although the four to six amino acid residues on the N termini of the B and A chains of putative human relaxin 1 and human relaxin 2 differ rather markedly, both chemically synthesized forms of the hormone had relaxin-like biological activity as judged by their ability to inhibit contractions of rat uterine strips *in vitro* (310,311).

Processing of Relaxin

A schematic summary of the processing of porcine preprorelaxin to porcine relaxin is shown in Fig. 6, and the amino acids located at cleavage sites for the processing of porcine and rat preprorelaxin are shown in Fig. 7. Cleavage of the signal peptides of preprorelaxin, like that of other peptide precursors (567), occurs at an amino acid with a small side chain. Subsequent cleavage of the C peptide in prorelaxin is less well defined and appears to be less stringently controlled than with proinsulin. Proinsulin is converted to insulin by trypsin-like enzymes that cleave at pairs of basic residues at both ends of the C peptide. This is not the case with relaxin. Cleavage at the C terminus of the B chain is thought to require an enzyme with chymotrypsin-like specificity which recognizes the neutral aliphatic side chains of leucine at B32 in both porcine and rat prorelaxin (259). If this is the case with porcine relaxin, subsequent cleavage of B32 leucine must occur, since B31 (CMa) porcine relaxin (see Fig. 2), which has Ala at the C terminus, is the major form isolated from the ovaries (648). At the C peptide/A chain junction, the most likely cleavage point is carboxyl-terminal to the three basic residues in positions 132 to 134, and in rat relaxin a trypsin-like cleavage occurs in this position. If cleavage also occurs at this site in porcine relaxin, subsequent cleavage must occur, since cleavage at the Arg-Leu bond would leave an additional dipeptide (Leu-Phe) on the N terminus of the A chain. Recent evidence indicates that cleavage does occur, at least in part, at the Arg-Leu bond in position 134–135 of the C peptide of porcine relaxin. Bullesbach and Schwabe (92,93) isolated small amounts of porcine relaxin with Leu-Phe or Phe extensions on the N terminus of their A chains, and they postulated that these two forms of porcine relaxin were products of incomplete conversion of prorelaxin to relaxin.

Efforts to study the mechanisms involved with the conversion of porcine prorelaxin to relaxin are severely restricted by the limited amounts of prorelaxin present in ovarian tissue as well as the difficulty of isolating the prohormone without modification. To overcome these problems, Stewart et al. (589) prepared a gene coding for porcine prorelaxin that was cloned in the bacteria *E. coli* so that its expression was under the control of tryptophan promoter. Following individual expression of the prohormone gene, over 20% of the newly synthesized protein was associated with a molecule that appeared to be prorelaxin: Its size was about 19,000 daltons, and its antigenic determinants were similar to those of relaxin. Stewart et al. (589) reported that sufficient amounts of the apparent porcine relaxin prohormone can be isolated from *E. coli* to study the process of cleavage of the C peptide and to isolate the enzymes involved.

The cleavage sites for processing human relaxin will not be known with certainty until human relaxin is isolated. The putative cleavage sites shown with intermittent vertical lines in Fig. 7 were deduced by analogy to the processing of porcine and rat preprorelaxin (310,311).

Relaxin Genes

Partial or complete analysis of the genomic DNA from human, porcine, rat, and mouse relaxin genomic clones indicated that their general structures are consistent with that of human relaxin gene 1 shown in Fig. 8 (335). An intron interrupts the coding region at, or close to, position 45 of the C peptide as indicated in Fig. 7. The position of this intron corresponds closely to that of one of the two introns found in insulin genes (40). It is not known whether relaxin genes have a second intron corresponding to the position of the second insulin intron, which is located in the 5′ untranslated flanking region preceding the signal peptide. It was suggested that conservation of at least one intron site between relaxin and insulin genes further supports the concept that these two hormones are related through a common ancestral gene (310,335).

In view of the apparent common ancestral origin of insulin and relaxin, the genes for these two hormones were presumed to be closely linked on the same chromosome following gene duplication. In humans, and perhaps other spe-

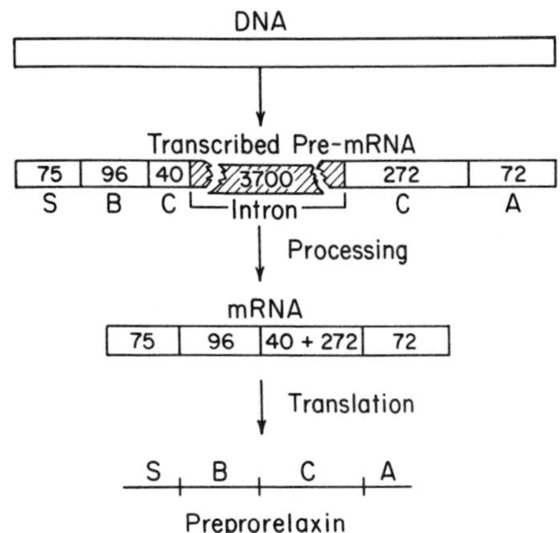

FIG. 8. Schematic illustration of the flow of information from human relaxin gene 1 to preprorelaxin. The relaxin gene is translated to give relaxin premessenger RNA which contains a 3,700-base intron. After processing, the mRNA serves as a template for the translation of preprorelaxin. Reproduced with permission from Kemp and Niall (335).

cies, this is not the case. The human insulin gene is located on the short arm of chromosome 11 (442), whereas both relaxin genes are located on the short arm of chromosome 9 (126). It was suggested that following an original gene duplication, separation of the insulin-like and relaxin-related genes may have occurred by a chromosomal translocation involving a breakpoint between the two genes and that the two nonallelic human relaxin genes evolved by a second gene duplication event (126). Presumably the second duplication occurred after the evolutionary divergence of pig, rat, and mouse genomes from the human genome, since only a single relaxin gene was found in these mammals (126).

The significance of two relaxin-related genes in the human is unknown. Human relaxin gene 2 appears to be a functional gene. Hudson et al. (311) found that human relaxin 2 is synthesized in the ovary during pregnancy. Ovarian expression of human relaxin gene 1 has not been detected. It is possible that human relaxin gene 1 is expressed in other putative sources of relaxin such as the placenta, decidua, or prostate. Preliminary experiments, however, which failed to detect any biosynthesis of relaxin in either placental or decidual tissue, do not encourage this view (311). Until human relaxin 1–specific mRNA is identified in human tissue, it remains possible that human relaxin gene 1 is a pseudogene.

MEASUREMENT OF RELAXIN

Bioassays

The three types of relaxin bioassays used throughout the past 25 years are based on the original observations that relaxin induces separation of the pubic bones in guinea pigs at estrus (289), promotes growth of the interpubic ligament in estrogen-primed mice (269), and inhibits myometrial contractility in estrogen-dominated guinea pigs, rats, and mice (354,514). Relaxin bioassays have indispensable applications. They identify and characterize relaxin preparations during the development of isolation procedures (177,194, 205,484,538,555,591), validate results obtained with radioimmunoassays (430,545,557), determine structural requirements for biological activity (94,524,555,625,626), and determine whether putative forms of relaxin whose amino acid sequences have been deduced from gene nucleotide sequences are biologically active following chemical synthesis (310,311,625).

Improved methods for the bioassay of relaxin are needed. Existing methods lack precision. Additionally, they lack the sensitivity needed to readily measure relaxin bioactivity in peripheral blood or tissue extracts where the concentrations of relaxin are low. The limit of sensitivity with both the guinea pig and mouse interpubic ligament bioassays is about 100 ng with highly purified porcine relaxin (94,555,586), and *in vitro* rat and mouse uterine contractility bioassays appear to be only moderately more sensitive (586). Responsiveness of target cells to relaxin in culture might provide precise and sensitive bioassays. It was suggested, for example, that the ability of small amounts of relaxin to enhance insulin binding and glucose uptake in adipocytes (323,438) might be utilized for such a bioassay (587).

The extensive variation in the amino acid sequences of relaxin among species has important implications for the bioassay of relaxin. First, it may be necessary to explore the bioactivity of relaxin from a given species in more than one bioassay to find a suitable response, since great differences in the bioactivity of highly purified relaxin preparations have been demonstrated in the commonly employed bioassays (see Table 1). Rat and equine relaxin have less bioactivity than porcine relaxin in the mouse interpubic ligament bioassay (538,591); furthermore, rat relaxin has a lower dose-response curve than porcine relaxin in this bioassay (69,360,538). Rabbit relaxin has less activity than porcine relaxin in the *in vitro* mouse uterine contractility bioassay (177). Shark relaxin promotes growth of the interpubic ligament and inhibits uterine contractions in guinea pigs, but neither of these activities was demonstrated in mice (484,586). Second, when *levels of relaxin bioactivity* are determined, standard and unknowns from the same species should be used, since it is unlikely that relaxin from different species will provide the parallel dose-response curves needed for valid potency estimates. Third, the extreme differences in the abilities of highly purified relaxin preparations from different species to elicit biological responses in the mouse and guinea pig bioassays preclude meaningful comparisons of their specific bioactivities in these bioassays. Reviews by Steinetz et al. (573,584,586,587) provide additional information concerning the bioassay of relaxin.

Interpubic Ligament Bioassays

Guinea pig pubic symphysis palpation bioassay. The guinea pig pubic symphysis palpation bioassay, which was first described by Fevold et al. in 1930 (193), is based on the subjective assessment by palpation of the degree to which the pubic symphysis becomes movable following relaxin-induced separation of the pubic bones. In 1944 Abramowitz et al. (1) developed the first quantitative bioassay and defined a guinea pig unit as "that amount of hormone which induces, 6 hr following injection, an unmistakable relaxation of the symphysis pubis in about two-thirds of a group of 12 castrated female guinea pigs weighing between 350 and 800 g and pretreated with 0.85 μg of estradiol daily for 4 days." This bioassay (1) has limitations. Guinea pig units based on response criteria are not valid, because of variations in the judgment of investigators (586) and marked changes in the responsiveness of the pubic symphysis that occur when guinea pigs are used repeatedly for bioassay (209,211,213,421,615,616).

Modifications of the bioassay that enabled more objective assessment of the influence of relaxin on the pubic symphysis were described in the early 1950s. Talmage and Hurst (616), using X-ray photography of the pubic symphysis, found that the interpubic distance increased linearly as the dose of relaxin increased. Catchpole et al. (108), interpreting pubic symphysis relaxation as depolymerization or solubilization of the negatively charged matrix proteoglycans, employed an electrometric method to determine the apparent density of immobile colloidal charge. Those workers (108) found that as the dose of relaxin increased there was a linear decrease in the density of negatively charged colloid in the pubic symphysis. Neither of these objective guinea pig pubic symphysis bioassays, however, has been employed. Instead, a fast and relatively simple method described by Kroc et al. in 1959 (356) has been used. These workers described a revision of the guinea pig pubic symphysis palpation bioassay which largely overcomes limitations of the original quantitative bioassay (1). In this bioassay (356) two or more doses of unknowns and graded doses of reference standard are randomized, coded, and administered to estrogen-primed intact guinea pigs. Palpation is also done under blind conditions by two or more independent operators who score the flexibility from 0 (no detectable flexibility) to 6 (extreme flexibility). Under these conditions, potency estimates with limits of error of less than 50% are obtained when 20 guinea pigs are used at each of two or more doses of standard and unknown (573). Although the guinea pig pubic symphysis palpation bioassay is cumbersome, imprecise, and expensive, it continues to be useful, since it is specific for relaxin and responsive to relaxin from a wide variety of species, including the pig, rat, shark, horse, rabbit, and human (296,430,484,531,586).

Mouse interpubic ligament bioassay. The mouse interpubic ligament bioassay is based on the original observations of Hall and Newton in the mid-1940s that the pubic symphysis of estrogen-primed mice responded to relaxin-containing extracts with a dose-dependent formation of a long interpubic ligament (260,269,271). The earliest bioassay procedures employed X-ray examination of the pelvis to obtain an assessment of the extent of growth of the interpubic ligament following relaxin treatment (163,261,347). In the late 1950s Steinetz, Kroc, and their co-workers devised a simpler direct measurement bioassay which enables objective and rapid determination of the length of the interpubic ligament (356,573,574). Rapidly growing immature female mice, weighing 18–21 g, are first primed with a single injection of long-acting estrogen. Seven days later, three or more doses of the relaxin standard or unknown(s) are injected in the repository vehicle 1% benzopurpurine-4B. Between 18 and 24 hr after the relaxin injection, the mice are killed, the pubic symphyses are cleaned of extraneous tissue, and the interpubic ligaments are measured using transillumination of the birth canal on a binocular dissecting microscope outfitted with an ocular micrometer (see Fig. 9A). There is considerable variation among animals, but when 20 mice are used per dose, potency estimates with limits of error of less than 50% can be obtained (555,573,574,586) (Fig. 9B). The repository vehicles, 5% beeswax in peanut oil (346) and 1% benzopurpurine (an azo dye) in physiological saline, potentiate the activity of porcine relaxin 100- to 300-fold and bring the mouse interpubic ligament bioassay for porcine relaxin to within the same range of sensitivity as the guinea pig pubic symphysis palpation bioassay (574). The mechanism(s) whereby the repository vehicles potentiate the activity of relaxin have not been established. Both repository vehicles may potentiate relaxin activity by mechanical retardation of absorption from the injection site (346). It was also suggested that benzopurpurine-4B may bind strongly to relaxin and protect the relaxin from degradative metabolism (39).

The mouse interpubic ligament bioassay was used extensively for the isolation and/or characterization of relaxin from the pig (112,555), rat (69,538), rabbit (205), cow (194,196), human (50,204), and horse (591). The markedly disparate abilities of relaxin from different species to promote growth of the interpubic ligament in mice may preclude the use of this bioassay with some species. Nevertheless, in view of its objectivity, specificity, and simplicity, the mouse interpubic ligament bioassay is the bioassay of choice when it can be employed.

Uterine Contractility Bioassays

Uterine contractility bioassays are based on the original discovery by Krantz et al. (354) in 1950 that relaxin-containing extracts of swine corpora lutea diminished spontaneous uterine contractility in guinea pigs. Since then, both *in vivo* and *in vitro* methods for the bioassay of relaxin based on inhibition of uterine contractility in estrogen-dom-

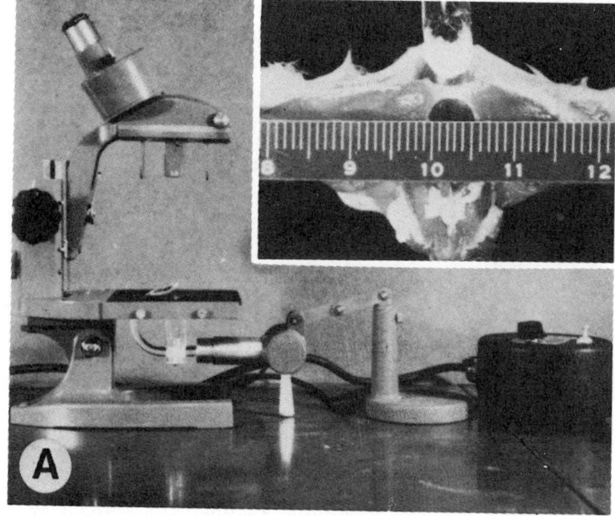

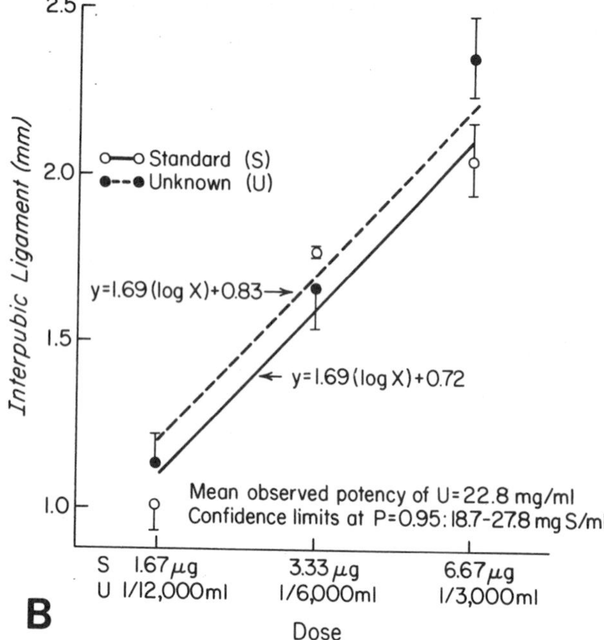

FIG. 9. A: Dissecting scope equipped with fixed transilluminating device and ocular micrometer for measurement of interpubic ligament length in mice. Inset shows the ventral view of a dissection of a mouse pelvis, showing the interpubic ligament positioned on the transilluminator. Reproduced with permission from Kroc et al. (356). **B:** Mouse interpubic ligament bioassay of an unknown porcine relaxin sample and a porcine relaxin reference standard designated Warner-Chilcott Relaxin Reference Standard W1164-A, lot 8. The unknown was made up to an estimated concentration of 20 mg reference standard per ml. Reproduced with permission from Steinetz et al. (573).

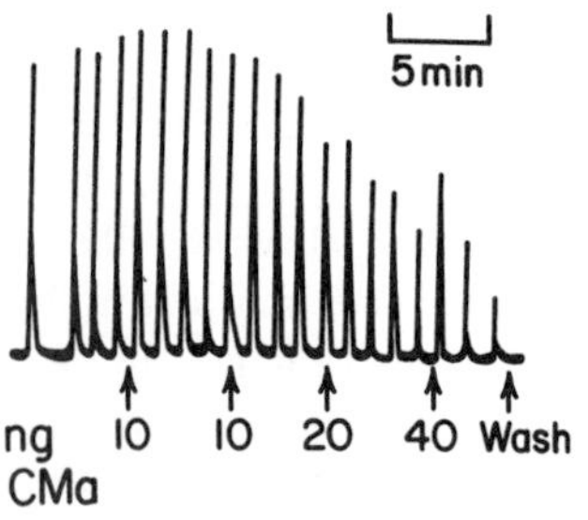

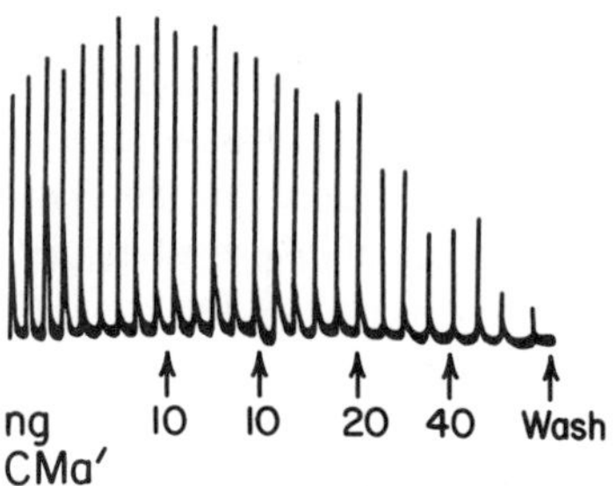

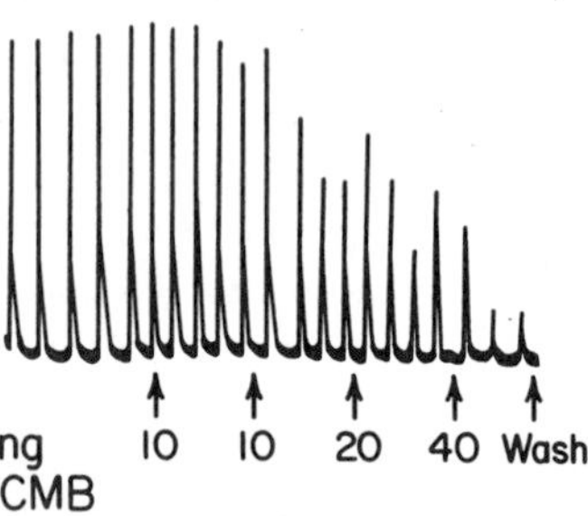

FIG. 10. Effects of increasing concentrations of highly purified porcine relaxin preparations CMa, CMa′, and CMB (555) on spontaneous contractility of estrous mouse uterine segment *in vitro.* Relaxin was added at 5-min intervals to the baths containing uterine segments in Krebs-Ringer bicarbonate-buffered medium (pH 7.4) and aerated with 95% O_2/5% CO_2. Isotonic contractions; load 1 g. Reproduced with permission from Steinetz et al. (586).

inated guinea pigs (191), rats (19,69,75,596,670), and mice (356,362) have been described. The uterine contractility bioassays have desirable features. First, relaxin-induced inhibition of uterine contractility occurs rapidly—within minutes (see Fig. 10). Second, relaxin from many species can be detected with the uterine contractility bioassays. For example, they were used for the isolation or characterization of relaxin from the pig (19,112,256,586), rat (69), shark (484), rabbit (177,205), cow (194), and human (50,176, 204,430,673). Finally, the uterine contractility bioassays may be somewhat more sensitive than the guinea pig and mouse pubic symphysis bioassays, since sensitivities lower than 100 ng/ml were reported for porcine relaxin (19,75,112, 511,512,586).

Uterine contractility bioassays also have limitations. They are not specific for relaxin. Oxytocin, which promotes uterine contractility, was present in extracts of cow corpora lutea (194,200,201), rabbit placentas (205), and human placentas (200,201) in levels sufficient to interfere with the quiescent effect of relaxin on uterine contractility. Additionally, several limitations restrict the use of these bioassays for quantitative determinations of relaxin bioactivity. First, there is considerable variation in sensitivity to relaxin among uteri; moreover, this sensitivity was reported to diminish following treatment with multiple doses of relaxin (514,668). Second, relaxin influences both the frequency and amplitude of uterine contractions, and this makes quantitation of the response difficult (670). Finally, spontaneous uterine contractions tend to be irregular, so they do not provide satisfactory baseline activity. Because of this irregularity, many of the early *in vitro* uterine contractility bioassays utilized a preliminary selection of tissue according to the frequency, regularity, and amplitude of spontaneous uterine contractions. Some investigators largely overcame the variability associated with spontaneous uterine contractions by employing only total inhibition of uterine contractility as an end point (19,256).

Recent *in vitro* uterine contractility bioassays have induced baseline uterine contractions rather than rely on irregular spontaneous uterine contractions. Nishikori et al. (418,419) induced contractions in isometrically suspended uteri from estrogen-primed rats by exposing them to a low dose of $PGF_{2\alpha}$ (0.28 μM) 10 min before the addition of relaxin. The influence of relaxin on the amplitude of the $PGF_{2\alpha}$-induced uterine contractions was determined. Bradshaw et al. (69) were the first to induce rat uterine segments to contract regularly by electrical stimulation. With this method, segments of uterine horn obtained from estrogen-dominated rats are suspended in an organ bath with one end attached to an isometric strain gauge. The uterine segments are then stimulated electrically (4–5 V, 50–60 Hz) for 4 or 5 sec at 45-sec (69) or 60-sec (73,75,371,511,512) intervals, and the influence of relaxin on the amplitude of the electrically driven base-line uterine contractions is determined (see Fig. 11A). St-Louis (596–598) described a procedure whereby a base-line tonic uterine contraction is obtained with a depolarizing solution of KCl. With this procedure segments of uterine horn obtained from estrogen-primed rats are suspended in an organ bath with one end attached to an isotonic smooth muscle transducer. A tonic contraction is then induced by partial (15% or 20%) replacement of the NaCl in physiological saline with KCl. After the first tonic contraction, and once a stable plateau is reached, relaxin is added to the organ bath. With this method the degree to which relaxin induces a relaxation of the tonic contraction is determined by planimetry (596,598) (see Fig. 11B). It is too early to know whether the recently modified uterine contractility bioassay methods which induce uterine contractility before relaxin treatment will be employed extensively.

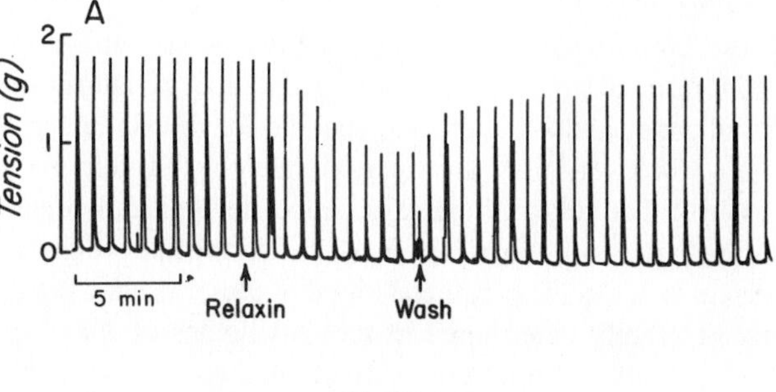

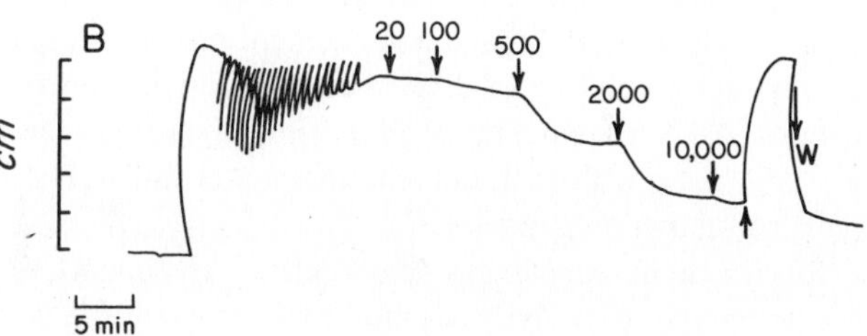

FIG. 11. A: Tension developed in a uterine strip from a proestrous rat *in vitro.* The strip was immersed in Krebs-Henseleit buffer at 37°C and stimulated electrically every 45 sec at 4 V amplitude and 50 Hz. The effect of adding 5 μg of partially purified rat relaxin and the recovery after washing out the relaxin are shown. Reproduced with permission from Bradshaw et al. (69). **B:** Experimental tracings of concentration-response curves to different concentrations of porcine relaxin (1,000 GPU/mg) ranging from 0.02 to 10 μg/ml. Arrow (↑) indicates replacement of the bathing solutions by fresh KCl-substituted saline; W indicates replacement by normal saline. Reproduced with permission from St-Louis (596).

Cervical Extensibility Bioassay

It has been known since the 1950s that porcine relaxin increases cervical extensibility (253,254,686). In 1980, Fields and Larkin (203) demonstrated that porcine relaxin promotes linear increases in cervical extensibility as well as growth of the interpubic ligament in estrogen-primed mice. Cervical extensibility, however, may not provide the basis for a useful relaxin bioassay, since slopes of dose-response curves were shallow and the correlation between cervical extensibility and interpubic ligament length ($p < 0.08$) was not highly significant.

Radioimmunoassays

The limits of sensitivity of available bioassays severely restrict their applicability for the measurement of relaxin in the blood. Determination of relaxin bioactivity levels in ovarian venous blood during late pregnancy in the pig, when relaxin levels in the blood are highest, requires the concentration of plasma to attain the limits of assay sensitivity (41). Radioimmunoassays for relaxin have been developed to measure relaxin levels in small samplings of blood. The first relaxin radioimmunoassay was developed in 1972 with the impure porcine relaxin preparation NIH-R-P1 (440 GPU/mg), which contains approximately 20% biologically active relaxin and 80% uncharacterized proteins (80,85). Employing that radioimmunoassay, relaxin was reported to be present in sera of sheep and humans under many physiological conditions (81–84,114).

When essentially pure preparations of relaxin became available, they were used for the development of homologous radioimmunoassays for porcine (8,339,377,432,485,

556,592,593,617), rat (464,544), and equine (590) relaxin. These homologous radioimmunoassays, which utilize relaxin from a single species for generation of antiserum, radioligand, and standard, are specific for relaxin and precise. Moreover, they are approximately 1,000-fold more sensitive than relaxin bioassays, since they generally detect 100 pg or less of relaxin (see Fig. 12). During late pregnancy relaxin levels in the peripheral blood of pigs, rats, and horses can be readily determined in serum volumes of 2 to 5 μl (543,545,590). Radioimmunoassays that utilize highly purified relaxin for radioligand and standard optimize the accuracy and specificity of relaxin immunoactivity determinations. All determinations of relaxin immunoactivity levels are now done with radioimmunoassays that utilize highly purified relaxin preparations.

Since radioimmunoassays detect relaxin immunoactivity but not relaxin bioactivity, caution must be exercised with physiological interpretations of relaxin immunoactivity levels. Where they were both measured, good correlations were demonstrated between levels of relaxin immunoactivity and relaxin bioactivity in the blood of pigs (41,543) and extracts of corpora lutea or ovaries from pigs (557), rats (545), and women (430).

The marked variation in the amino acid sequences of relaxin among species (Fig. 3) accounts for the limited immunological cross-reactivity of purified relaxin preparations in homologous radioimmunoassays for relaxin of other species (173,258,484,540,544,590) (see Fig. 12). It is advantageous to measure relaxin immunoactivity levels in a given species with a homologous radioimmunoassay for relaxin of that species, since there is an increased probability of a high affinity between relaxin and the relaxin antiserum. At present, however, homologous radioimmunoassays have been reported for only porcine, rat, equine, and human relaxin.

In spite of its limitations, the porcine relaxin radioimmunoassay has been used to provide useful information concerning relaxin levels in species other than pig. Antiporcine relaxin sera were shown to neutralize the biological activity of relaxin from a wide variety of species (364,575). Several investigators took advantage of the species aspecificity of antiporcine relaxin sera and used homologous porcine relaxin radioimmunoassays to detect relaxin immunoactivity in tissues from species other than the pig. Although these radioimmunoassays did not enable accurate measurement of relaxin levels, they provided an approximation of the profile of relaxin immunoactivity levels during pregnancy in the peripheral blood of the human, baboon, monkey, hamster, mouse, cat, and horse (420,429,432, 441,592,593,656).

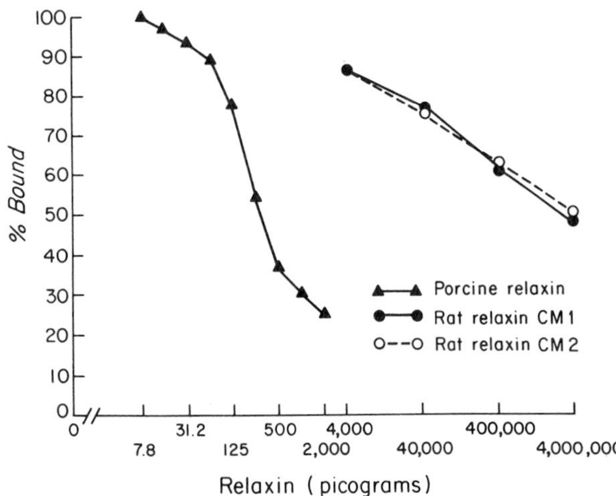

FIG. 12. Dose-response curves for highly purified porcine relaxin (555) and highly purified rat relaxin preparations CM1 and CM2 (538) in a homologous porcine relaxin radioimmunoassay (556). Reproduced with permission from Sherwood and Crnekovic (544).

Porcine Relaxin Radioimmunoassay

Table 3 summarizes the hormone preparations used, methods of radioiodination, and species applications for porcine relaxin radioimmunoassays developed with highly purified porcine relaxin. Since porcine relaxin lacks tyrosine and histidine, the commonly employed chloramine T radioiodination procedure (312) cannot be used to radiolabel unmodified hormone. Instead, three methods have been described that involve the conjugation of readily radioiodinated groups to porcine relaxin by amide bonds followed by radioiodination of the modified relaxin by the chloramine T procedure. First the reagent *N*-carboxy-L-tyrosine anhydride was used to incorporate one or more tyrosine residues primarily into the N terminus of the A chain (432,531,556). Second, the unlabeled Bolton and Hunter reagent (60) 3-(4-hydroxyphenyl) propionic acid *N*-hydroxysuccinimide ester was used to conjugate 3-(4-hydroxyphenol) propionic acid to porcine relaxin (8,407,592,617). Third, the reagent *N*-formyltyrosine-*N*-hydroxysuccinimide ester was used to incorporate *N*-formyltyrosine largely into the N terminus of the A chain (522). An additional method, in which unmodified porcine relaxin is radiolabeled directly with radioiodinated Bolton and Hunter reagent, has also been described (339,377). All four procedures provide radioligand that is suitable for porcine relaxin radioimmunoassays. The sensitivity of the porcine relaxin radioimmunoassays summarized in Table 3 are comparable—100 pg of porcine relaxin or less.

Rat Relaxin Radioimmunoassay

Two homologous radioimmunoassays for rat relaxin have been described (464,544). Sherwood and Crnekovic (544) employed equal amounts of the highly purified microheterogeneous preparations of CM1 and CM2 obtained by the isolation procedure of Sherwood (538) for radioligand, standard, and generation of the antiserum. Porter (464) employed highly purified rat relaxin obtained according to the

TABLE 3. *Porcine relaxin radioimmunoassays developed with highly purified relaxin preparations*

Development reference	Relaxin used for generation of antiserum, radioligand, and standard	Method used for preparation of the radioligand	Species applied to
556	CMB + CMa + CMa′[a] (2,500–3,000 GPU/mg)	Polytyrosyl relaxin:chloramine T	Pig
432,568	CMB + CMa + CMa′[b]	Polytyrosyl relaxin:chloramine T	Hamster, guinea pig, mouse, rat, cow, baboon, rhesus monkey, human
377	CMa′	Radioiodinated Bolton and Hunter	Human
8	CMa′	Unlabeled Bolton and Hunter:chloramine T	Pig, guinea pig
592	CMB + CMa + CMa′	Unlabeled Bolton and Hunter:chloramine T	Horse, cat
617	CMB + CMa + CMa′[c]	Unlabeled Bolton and Hunter:chloramine T	Pig
339	CMB + CMa + CMa′	Radioiodinated Bolton and Hunter	Pig
522	CMB + CMa + CMa′	Monotyrosyl relaxin:chloramine T	Pig

[a]The nomenclature of porcine relaxin preparations CMB, CMa, and CMa′ (555) is illustrated in Figs. 1 and 2.
[b]Subsequent to the original study (432) that employed an antiserum to partially purified porcine relaxin (about 1,000 GPU/mg), antiserum R6 generated with CMB, CMa, and CMa′ has been employed (568).
[c]Partially purified porcine relaxin (about 1,000 GPU/mg) was used to generate the antiserum.

isolation procedure of Walsh and Niall (648) for the radioligand and standard, and partially purified rat relaxin for generation of the antiserum. Although rat relaxin contains tyrosine, direct radioiodination of the native molecule by the chloramine T procedure (312) yields a radioligand that is not readily precipitated with antiserum (464). Accordingly, rat relaxin is either radiolabeled directly by the Bolton and Hunter procedure (544) or first conjugated with unlabeled Bolton and Hunter reagent and then radioiodinated by the chloramine T procedure (464). Both radioimmunoassays are sufficiently sensitive to measure approximately 100 pg of rat relaxin.

Equine Relaxin Radioimmunoassay

Stewart developed a homologous equine relaxin radioimmunoassay (590). Highly purified hormone (591) was used for radioligand, standard, and generation of the antiserum. Equine relaxin is radiolabeled directly by the chloramine T procedure (312). The equine relaxin radioimmunoassay is sufficiently sensitive to detect approximately 25 pg of equine relaxin.

Human Relaxin Radioimmunoassay

Eddie et al. (173) described a homologous human relaxin radioimmunoassay in 1986. An analog of human relaxin 2 was prepared by chemical synthesis and used for radioligand, standard, and generation of antiserum. The human relaxin 2 analog contained two substitutions in the B-chain to eliminate methionine residues: lysine at position −1 and alanine at position 21 in Fig. 3. The homologous human relaxin radioimmunoassay is sufficiently sensitive to detect approximately 50 pg of human relaxin per milliliter.

Enzyme Immunoassay

In 1980 Bodsch and Struck (59), in a brief report, described the development of two types of enzyme immunoassays for porcine relaxin. A rabbit antirelaxin antibody–horseradish peroxidase conjugate was used for a sandwich assay, and a mouse antirabbit Fab antibody–horseradish peroxidase conjugate was employed for a combining-site blocking assay. The sensitivity of both enzyme immunoassays was reported to be comparable to porcine relaxin radioimmunoassays, and preliminary results indicated that relaxin was detectable with both assays in the blood of pregnant women (59). There is need, however, for more rigorous characterization of enzyme immunoassays for relaxin. It is not clear that these assays are as precise or accurate as relaxin radioimmunoassays. Enzyme immunoassays for relaxin have potential advantages, since the enzyme-labeled antibody is more stable than radioiodinated hormone, and problems associated with handling and discarding radioactive waste are avoided.

SOURCES AND SECRETION OF RELAXIN IN THE FEMALE

Relaxin is produced in highest levels by female reproductive tract tissue(s) during pregnancy. The tissue that produces relaxin varies among species. It may be the corpus luteum, placenta, or uterus. In most species that have been examined, one of these tissues is the primary (and probably the sole) source of the relaxin in the peripheral blood. No clear pattern of pregnancy-related physiological factors that might predict the source of relaxin within species has emerged. With some species, such as the pig, rat, and mouse, where luteal progesterone production is required throughout pregnancy, the corpus luteum is the source of relaxin. However, in the rabbit, where luteal progesterone is required throughout pregnancy, the placenta is the source of relaxin. The human, horse, and guinea pig, species in which the corpora lutea are not the sole source of progesterone throughout pregnancy, produce relaxin in the corpora lutea, placenta, and uterus, respectively. Table 4 contains a summary of known sources of relaxin in several species. Regulation of relaxin synthesis varies extensively among species. For example, rat ovarian relaxin levels remain low unless the animal is pregnant, whereas pig ovarian relaxin can increase to high levels in the absence of pregnancy. Regulation of relaxin secretion also varies among species; consequently, the profiles of relaxin levels in the peripheral blood throughout pregnancy differ strikingly among species. In this section the sources and secretion of relaxin will be described for individual domestic species, laboratory species, and primates. Major emphasis will be on the three species studied most extensively in recent years—the pig, rat, and human.

Domestic Species

Pig

Estrous cycle. There are low levels of relaxin bioactivity in extracts of ovaries obtained during the estrous cycle, and they are maximal during the luteal phase (9,295,557). The corpora lutea are the principal source of this relaxin. Extracts of corpora lutea of the cycle contained both relaxin mRNA (233) and relaxin bioactivity (17,572). When the avidin-biotin immunoperoxidase method was used with an antiserum to purified porcine relaxin, relaxin immunostaining of the corpora lutea was most intense between days 11 and 15 of the estrous cycle (12). Additionally, when an electron microscopy immunocytochemical technique was used, relaxin immunoactivity was found associated with membrane-bound cytoplasmic granules in a small percentage of luteal cells obtained from pigs on day 14 of the estrous cycle (202).

TABLE 4. *Sources of relaxin in mammals*

Species	Ovary needed throughout pregnancy	Source of relaxin
Pig	Yes	Corpus luteum
Horse	No	Placenta
Cow	Yes	Corpus luteum
Cat	No	Placenta
Rat	Yes	Corpus luteum
Mouse	Yes	Corpus luteum
Guinea pig	No	Uterus
Rabbit	Yes	Placenta, uterus[a]
Human	No	Corpus luteum, placenta[a]

[a]Putative sources of relaxin that are not well established.

Preovulatory follicles may also produce relaxin. Although relaxin mRNA was not detected in extracts from small or large follicles (233), relaxin immunoactivity was found in follicular fluid (88,391). It is not clear whether follicular granulosa cells, theca cells, or both cell types synthesize relaxin. It was reported that granulosa cells isolated from large follicles secreted small amounts of relaxin *in vitro* when incubated for several days in the presence of luteinizing hormone (373). In contrast to these findings, it was reported that theca tissue isolated from gonadotropin-primed prepubertal pigs secreted relaxin *in vitro,* whereas granulosa cells from these animals secreted little or no detectable hormone (187).

Pregnancy. Source: The corpora lutea are the principal and, perhaps, the sole source of relaxin during the approximately 115-day gestation period. Employing immunohistochemical techniques, relaxin immunoactivity was found associated with the cytoplasm of cells from the corpora lutea but not other ovarian components (25,202,361) (see Fig. 13A). Relaxin bioactivity levels within the corpora lutea were reported to increase steadily from about day 20 of pregnancy until about day 110 and then to decline rapidly within 16 hr of birth (17,41) (see Fig. 14).

The origin(s) of the lutein cells that produce, store, and secrete relaxin in the pig are not known with certainty. It was first postulated that the granulosa and theca layers give rise to the large and small lutein cells, respectively, which are found in the corpus luteum of the pregnant pig (109,123). Relaxin has been found in the large, so-called granulosa lutein cells (41,337,361) but has yet to be reported in the small, so-called theca lutein cells. The recent observation that the theca layer from gonadotropin-primed prepubertal pigs produced more relaxin than the granulosa cells was interpreted to imply that small, theca-derived cells may ultimately become large lutein cells (187). The large lutein cells have the organelles associated with both steroid and protein synthesis (13,41,42), and it seems likely that progesterone as well as relaxin is produced by these cells.

Dense membrane-limited cytoplasmic granules (200–600 nm diameter) are observed within the lutein cells of pregnant pigs (see Fig. 13B). Two lines of evidence indicate that relaxin is stored in these granules: First, the accumulation and disappearance of the cytoplasmic granules throughout pregnancy parallels that of relaxin bioactivity (17,41). Second, relaxin immunoactivity is associated with the cytoplasmic granules (124,202,337,363) (see Fig. 13C). The amount of relaxin stored within each granule may increase during pregnancy. Fields and Fields (202) reported that the apparent quantity of relaxin immunoactivity associated with each granule increased progressively from day 17 to day 106.

Small amounts of relaxin may be produced in ovarian sites other than the corpora lutea during pregnancy. Extremely low levels of relaxin bioactivity were found in follicular and interstitial tissue (17), and relaxin immunoactivity was found in follicular fluid in ovaries of pregnant

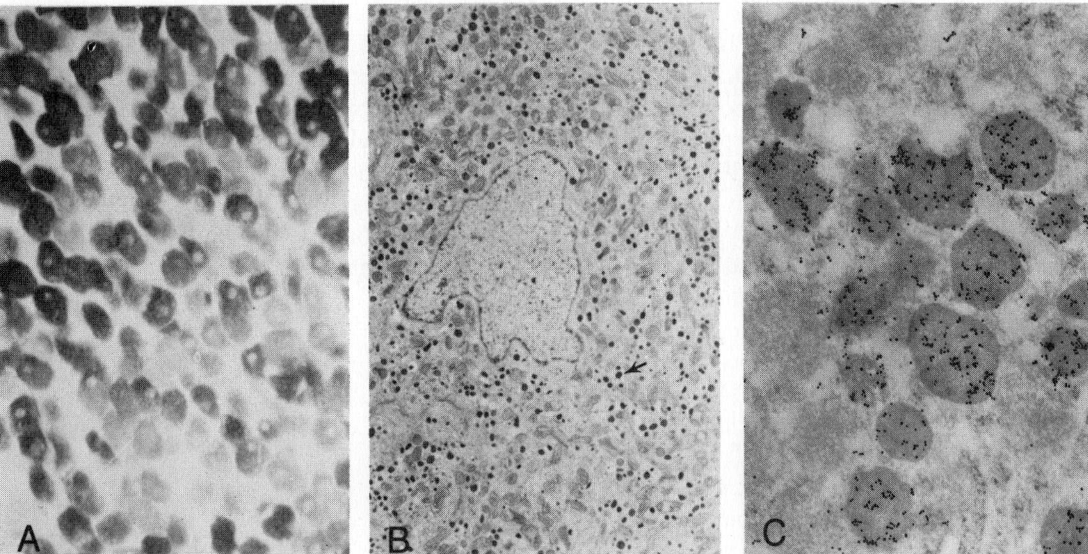

FIG. 13. A: Light microscopy immunohistochemical localization of relaxin in the cytoplasm of pig lutein cells on day 106 of pregnancy using rabbit antiporcine relaxin serum and peroxidase-antiperoxidase as marker. Note the nuclei do not stain. Reproduced with permission from Fields and Fields (202). **B:** Electron microscopy of a portion of a pig lutein cell on day 110 of pregnancy when the granule content (*arrow*) is maximal. (×2,800.) Reproduced with permission from Belt et al. (41). **C:** Electron microscopy immunocytochemical localization of relaxin in pig lutein granules (200–600 nm diameter) on day 106 of pregnancy using rabbit antiporcine relaxin serum and goat antirabbit IgG-colloidal gold (10 nm) as marker. (×37,400.) Reproduced with permission from Fields and Fields (202).

animals (88,391). It was suggested that the relaxin in the follicles may result from transport of the hormone from adjacent corpora lutea or from *de novo* synthesis within the follicle (17,88). Consistent with the latter interpretation, intact follicles obtained from pregnant pigs secreted a relaxin-immunoactive substance(s) *in vitro* (88).

Regulation of Synthesis: The corpora lutea of the pregnant pig reach maximal size (≥ 450 mg) by day 8 (17) and produce not only relaxin but also the progesterone needed to maintain pregnancy throughout the 115-day gestation period. Anderson and co-workers demonstrated that maintenance of luteal function in the pig requires the secretion of pituitary hormones (16) but not the presence of the conceptuses (14,17). In pigs in which the corpora lutea were maintained beyond 100 days following either hysterectomy or the administration of estrogen during the luteal phase of the estrous cycle, relaxin bioactivity (17) and immunoactivity (14,202) levels in the corpora lutea approached those of pregnant pigs. The observation that luteal relaxin levels are low during the estrous cycle (17,202,572) and increase as the age of the corpora lutea increases in hysterectomized pigs as well as in pregnant pigs (17,202) led to the postulation that the corpus luteum formed after ovulation is programmed for pregnancy and that luteal relaxin levels may be an indication of the luteal aging process (14,17,202). Consistent with this view, corpora lutea induced experimentally during late pregnancy had to be at least 15 days of age to release significant quantities of relaxin during the 2 days preceding birth (551).

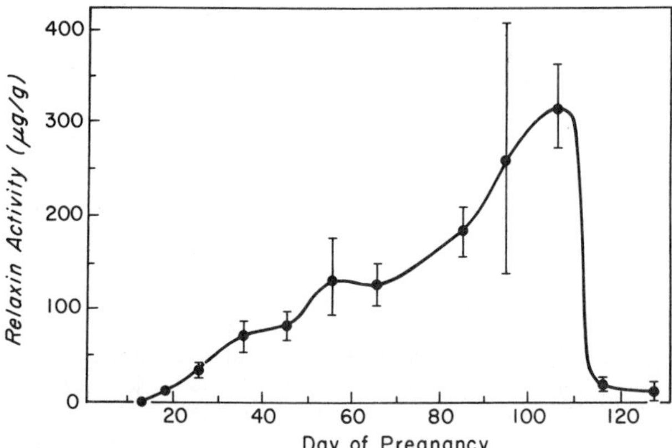

FIG. 14. Mean relaxin bioactivity levels (± SE) in pig corpora lutea throughout pregnancy. Reproduced with permission from Anderson et al. (17).

Blood Levels: The profile of relaxin levels in the peripheral blood throughout pregnancy is consistent with the view that relaxin accumulates within corpora lutea during most of pregnancy and is released during the rapid degranulation that occurs during the 2 days before birth (41). In 1971, Belt et al. (41) reported a sharp increase in relaxin bioactivity in plasma obtained from the ovarian vein between 44 and 26 hr before birth. More recently, porcine relaxin radioimmunoassays were used to determine relaxin immunoactivity levels in peripheral blood during pregnancy (14,190,248,339,543,554,617). Plasma relaxin levels remain below 2 ng/ml until about day 100 and then increase gradually to approximately 10 ng/ml 3 days before delivery

(14,543). During the 2 days before birth, relaxin levels increase markedly and attain maximal levels, which generally range from 50 to 250 ng/ml (190,248,339,541–543,553,554,558,617) (see Fig. 15). In most cases, this antepartum surge in relaxin consists of two or three sustained peaks which last 10 to 20 hr (543,554,558). The final peak, which has maximal relaxin levels, generally occurs 24 to 14 hr before delivery (543,553,554,558,617). Relaxin levels then decline rapidly to about 10 ng/ml at birth (8,554). It is not entirely clear whether delivery influences the secretion of relaxin in the pig: Whereas one study found that relaxin immunoactivity levels fluctuated considerably during delivery (8), another study did not (554). Relaxin levels decline to less than 1 ng/ml by 24 hr after delivery (543, 553,554).

Regulation of Secretion: Progress has been made toward an understanding of the regulation of the antepartum surge in blood relaxin levels in the pig. The corpora lutea undergo functional regression, as judged by a rapid fall in progesterone levels, during the 2 days that precede parturition (26,399) (see Fig. 15). Sherwood and co-workers (541, 553,554) proposed that the simultaneous surge in blood relaxin levels might be associated with luteal regression.

The factors that initiate functional luteolysis and the antepartum surge in relaxin levels are not known with certainty. There is evidence that the fetal pituitary-adrenal-placental system, which is involved with the initiation of birth in the pig, may be involved. Destruction of the fetal pituitary (62) or fecal decapitation *in utero* (121,604) prolonged pregnancy and apparently did so by preventing the rapid and sustained luteolysis that normally occurs on approximately day 113 to day 115 (121). Fetal decapitation (541) and fetal hypophysectomy (336) also disrupted the normal antepartum surge of relaxin levels—it occurred at various intervals ranging up to 10 to 12 days before birth.

Anderson and co-workers (14,190,401) provided evidence that functional luteolysis and release of relaxin may occur, at least in part, independent of fetal control. When the life-span of the corpora lutea was prolonged by hysterectomizing pigs on day 6 of the estrous cycle, the timing of a decline in progesterone levels and surge in relaxin levels in the peripheral blood resembled the timing of these events in pregnant animals. There was a decline in progesterone levels from day 108 to day 114 (401) and an increase in relaxin to maximal levels on days 112 to 114 in the hysterectomized gilts (14,190) (see Fig. 16). Anderson and co-

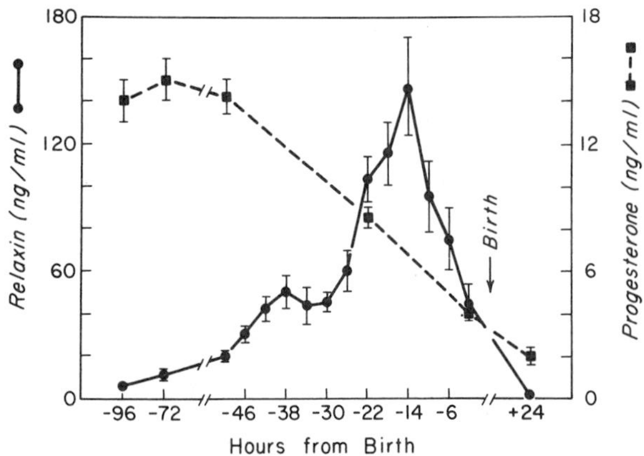

FIG. 15. Mean relaxin and progesterone immunoactivity levels (± SE) in peripheral blood plasma of pigs from 96 hr before to 24 hr after birth. Reproduced with permission from Sherwood et al. (543,553).

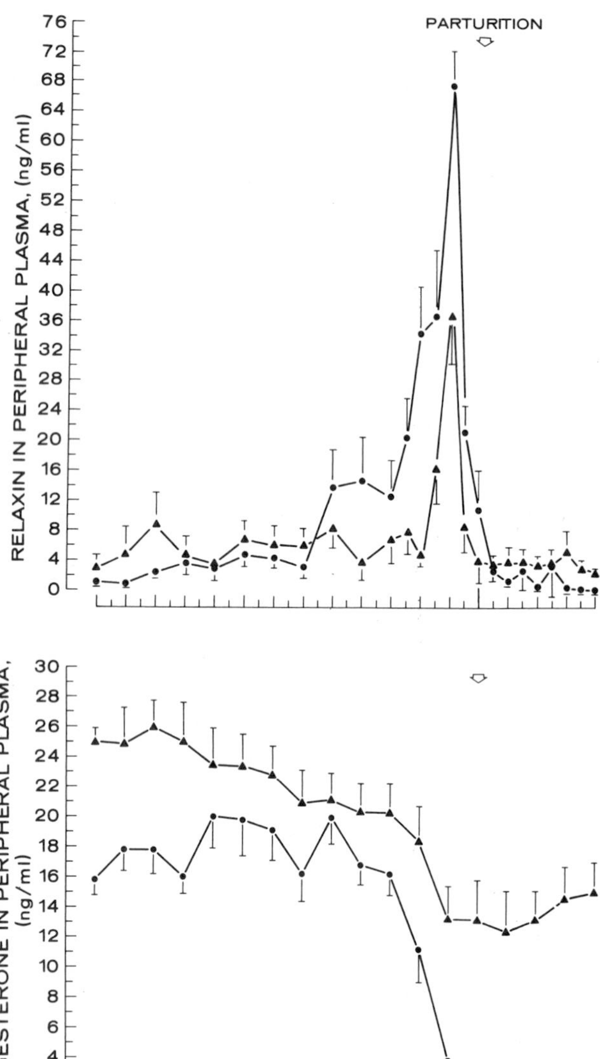

FIG. 16. Mean relaxin and progesterone concentrations (± SE) in peripheral blood plasma during pregnancy and early lactation compared with those in unmated gilts hysterectomized on day 6 of the estrous cycle. Relaxin peaked at 113.0 (± 0.7 SE) days in pregnant animals and at 113.0 (± 0.7 SE) days in hysterectomized gilts; gestation length averaged 114.0 (± 0.8 SE) days. Reproduced with permission from Felder et al. (190). ●, during pregnancy and lactation of Yorkshire gilts (n = 7). ▲, after hysterectomy of gilts (n = 9).

workers (14,190) concluded that the initiation of the disappearance of cytoplasmic granules coincident with relaxin release in aging corpora lutea may be a precisely timed, genetically controlled event related to the aging of the corpora lutea and independent of endocrine control by the conceptuses or uterus. Although genetic control may contribute to the timing of antepartum functional luteolysis and the antepartum release of relaxin, there are several indications that other factors are involved. First, the apparent amounts of relaxin released into the plasma of pregnant pigs during the 4 days before birth were greater than those released into the plasma of hysterectomized gilts during the same period (see Fig. 16). Additionally, unlike pregnant pigs, in which peripheral blood progesterone and relaxin declined abruptly to basal levels by one day postpartum on about day 116, in hysterectomized gilts, progesterone and relaxin levels declined less abruptly, to reach basal levels after day 140 (14,190,401) (see Fig. 16). Serum relaxin levels in hysterectomized gilts were higher than those in postpartum pigs until day 150 (14). Finally, the observation that there was an antepartum surge in plasma relaxin levels in pregnant pigs that contained only induced corpora lutea that were about 30 days of age supports the view that factors other than aging influence the release of relaxin from the corpora lutea during late pregnancy (551).

The putative factor(s) that promote luteolysis, the antepartum surge in relaxin levels, and birth can be carried in the systemic circulation, since these events occurred at the appropriate time in pigs whose ovaries were transplanted to the external surface of the abdominal wall (389,552). The nature of the blood-borne factor(s) that promotes the antepartum release of relaxin is not known with certainty. The antepartum surge in prolactin levels, which coincides with the antepartum surge in relaxin levels (339,617), is not required for the release of relaxin, since the administration of bromocriptine prevented the prolactin surge but not the relaxin surge (617). Likewise, the antepartum decline in serum progesterone levels does not promote the release of relaxin. Whereas administration of progesterone from day 110 to day 115 (558) or from day 111 to day 116 (617) delayed delivery, it did not delay the antepartum surge in relaxin levels. Intravenous infusion of oxytocin for 6 hr on day 110 elicited a rapid, sevenfold increase in relaxin levels in ovarian venous plasma (17). There is no evidence, however, that endogenous oxytocin promotes the release of relaxin during late pregnancy in the pig.

Two lines of evidence indicate that prostaglandins promote luteolysis and the antepartum surge in relaxin levels. First, prolonged infusion (10 hr) of sufficient $PGF_{2\alpha}$ on day 110 to induce birth on day 111 brought about a rapid drop in progesterone concentrations and a surge in relaxin levels in the peripheral plasma (553). Second, inhibition of prostaglandin synthesis by administration of the cyclooxygenase inhibitor indomethacin for 6 or 7 days during late pregnancy delayed luteolysis, the antepartum relaxin surge, and birth until 2 to 5 days after the termination of indomethacin administration (411,553,617) (see Fig. 17). Although daily administration of the prostaglandin synthesis inhibitor me-

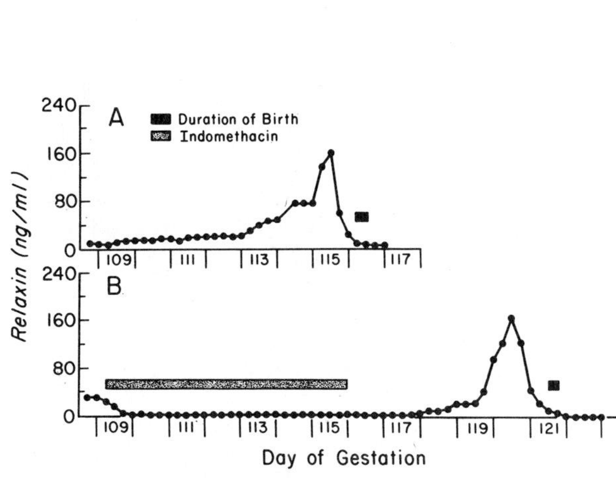

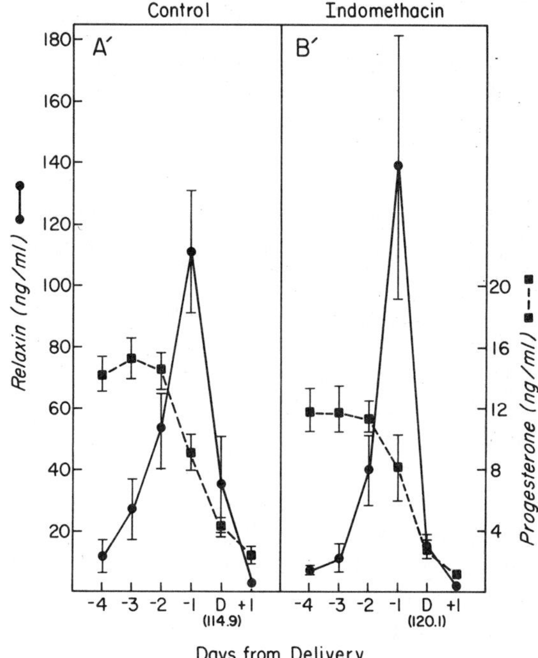

FIG. 17. Relaxin levels in peripheral blood plasma of **(A)** an untreated pig and **(B)** a pregnant pig injected intramuscularly twice each day from day 109 to day 116 with indomethacin at a dose of 4 mg/kg. Mean relaxin and progesterone concentrations (± SE; $N = 5$) in (A′) control pigs which delivered on day 114.9 ± 0.5 SE and (B′) indomethacin-treated pigs which delivered on day 120.1 ± 0.4 SE. Reproduced with permission from Sherwood et al. (553).

clofenamic acid from day 109 to day 113 failed to influence luteolysis and birth in pregnant pigs in one study, the authors concluded that a larger dose of the meclofenamic acid may have been required under the experimental conditions employed (248).

It is possible that the prostaglandin(s) associated with luteolysis is not produced in an extraovarian site and then transported to the corpora lutea via the systemic circulation. Porcine corpora lutea can synthesize $PGF_{2\alpha}$ (257,447), and perhaps they do so in response to stimulation by other blood-borne factor(s). That plasma levels of $PGF_{2\alpha}$ and its metabolite 13,14-dihydro-15-keto $PGF_{2\alpha}$ remain low until the day of birth, 1 or 2 days after functional luteolysis (248,411), supports the possibility that the natural prostaglandin that promotes luteolysis is not produced in an extraovarian site (248).

It is not known whether luteolysis and the antepartum release of relaxin are initiated by common or separate prostaglandin-mediated mechanisms. Brief (5-min) infusion of a low dose of $PGF_{2\alpha}$ on day 105 and day 108 caused an immediate surge in relaxin levels that lasted for about 1 hr but that did not influence progesterone levels (410). This may indicate that luteolysis and the release of relaxin are mediated by separate mechanisms. Alternatively, both luteolysis and the release of relaxin may be mediated by common initial steps, perhaps at the level of the plasma membrane, with divergence at subsequent steps which influence cholesterol transport or pregnenolone synthesis (410). According to this hypothesis, brief infusion of a low dose of $PGF_{2\alpha}$ would trigger the release of relaxin from a portion of the cytoplasmic storage granules but would not be adequate to influence steps associated with steroid biosynthesis.

Relaxin immunoactivity in the peripheral plasma of pregnant pigs (88,339), as well as in follicular fluid (88,391), is associated with multiple components. Neither the biological nor the structural characteristics of the relaxin-immunoactive molecules have been clearly determined. There are indications that a portion of these molecules are comparable to the bioactive molecule isolated from pig ovaries. The antepartum surge of relaxin immunoactivity coincides with the occurrence of relaxin bioactivity in the blood (41). Additionally, much of the relaxin immunoactivity is associated with a small component(s) with an apparent molecular weight of approximately 6,000 (88,90,338,556).

Lactation. Whether pigs secrete relaxin during lactation is unsettled. Two laboratories reported that relaxin levels were extremely low to nondetectable in blood samples collected from maternal pigs as frequently as 1- or 2-min intervals during lactation and that relaxin levels were not influenced by suckling (338,554). A third laboratory, however, reported that acute and transient spikes in plasma relaxin levels occur in lactating pigs (8,660). Two aspects of the studies that reported relaxin secretion in lactating pigs are difficult to reconcile with previous findings concerning porcine relaxin. First, the source of relaxin in lactating pigs is uncertain. The corpora lutea, the only known source of relaxin in the pig, contain very little relaxin following birth (17). Additionally, the apparent clearance half-time ($t_{1/2}$) for relaxin immunoactivity in lactating pigs in less than 20 sec (660), and this is exceedingly faster than the clearance $t_{1/2}$ of about 60 min reported for porcine relaxin (540,545).

Horse

The placenta is the major and, perhaps, the sole source of relaxin in the horse (591,595). Unlike corpora lutea of the pregnant pig, the placenta of the pregnant horse does not store much relaxin during pregnancy (see Table 1). Stewart and co-workers initially measured relaxin immunoactivity in the peripheral serum of horses throughout pregnancy and at parturition with a homologous porcine relaxin radioimmunoassay (592,594,595). More recently, Stewart (590) determined serum relaxin levels in pregnant horses with a homologous equine relaxin radioimmunoassay. Relaxin immunoactivity levels (see Fig. 18) are detectable by about day 80, increase to an initial peak of about 50 to 80 ng/ml between days 150 and 180, decline somewhat over the next 60 days, and then increase steadily to levels of about 60 to 100 ng/ml by the time of foaling, which normally occurs between day 300 and day 350 (590,592). A surge in relaxin levels begins a few hours before birth, reaches a maximum shortly after birth, and lasts until the placenta is expelled (590,594).

Cow

Corpora lutea produce relaxin in the pregnant cow. Luteal cells from pregnant cows stained positively for relaxin with an immunohistochemical method that employed an anti-porcine relaxin serum (194). The amount of relaxin stored by the corpora lutea in the cow, however, appears to be

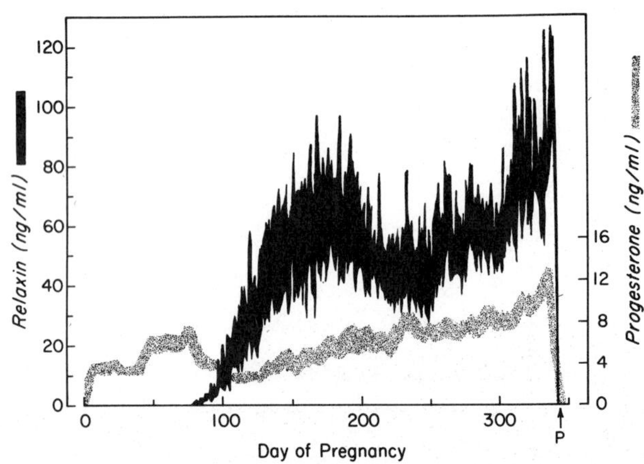

FIG. 18. Mean relaxin and progesterone immunoactivity levels (± SE; N = 4) in the peripheral blood plasma during pregnancy in the horse. Relaxin levels were determined with a homologous equine relaxin radioimmunoassay. Reproduced with permission from Stewart (590).

extremely low. There is no evidence that luteal cells in the cow contain relaxin storage granules, and the levels of relaxin bioactivity in extracts of corpora lutea obtained from pregnant cows were reported to be extremely low or nondetectable (13,194,195,198). The placenta in cows produces little if any relaxin (13,194,195).

Limitations associated with the methods available for determining relaxin levels in the peripheral blood preclude a good understanding of the secretion of relaxin during pregnancy in the cow. In 1955, Wada and Yuhara (642,643) reported that relaxin bioactivity was present in the blood of pregnant cows. Using the guinea pig pubic symphysis palpation bioassay, relaxin levels were reported to increase steadily from the first month, plateau during the last trimester, and fall rapidly to nondetectable levels within a few days after parturition, on about day 280 (642,643,646). When porcine relaxin radioimmunoassays were used, however, relaxin immunoactivity levels were reported to be low (18) or nondetectable (556) during late pregnancy. These findings may be a reflection of the limitations of the porcine relaxin radioimmunoassay for the measurement of bovine relaxin.

Sheep

It seems likely that sheep produce relaxin, since the sheep uterus is responsive to relaxin. Porter et al. (470) reported that the administration of porcine relaxin directly into the uterine artery of ovariectomized estrogen-primed ewes inhibited spontaneous uterine contractions. Nevertheless, the source of relaxin during the approximately 150-day gestation period in sheep remains uncertain. The ovary, placenta, and endometrium have been examined as possible sources of relaxin. Relaxin immunoactivity has been described in the ovary (172,470,485). It was reported that relaxin-specific immunofluorescence was observed in luteal cells of pregnant ewes (172) and that both ovarian extracts (470) and partially purified ovarian extracts (485) from pregnant ewes contained apparent low levels of a substance that cross-reacted in porcine relaxin radioimmunoassays. Investigations have not consistently found relaxin activity in the ovary. Relaxin immunoactivity was not demonstrated in sections of ovarian tissue with an immunocytochemical technique that employed an antiserum to highly purified porcine relaxin and avidin-biotin-peroxidase complex as marker; moreover, relaxin immunoactivity was not found in the ovarian vein draining the ovary containing the corpus luteum of pregnancy (485). Additionally, extracts of ovarian tissue obtained from ewes during late pregnancy demonstrated no relaxin bioactivity in mouse or rat uterine contractility bioassays (470,485). There is limited evidence that the placenta and endometrium may be sources of relaxin in sheep. Although extracts of placental and endometrial tissue obtained during pregnancy demonstrated no relaxin bioactivity in mouse or rat uterine contractility bioassays (470,485), fractions obtained following gel filtration of these extracts demonstrated apparent low levels of relaxin immunoactivity in a porcine relaxin radioimmunoassay (485).

Reports concerning the secretion of relaxin in sheep are inconsistent. Using the guinea pig pubic symphysis palpation bioassay, blood relaxin levels were reported to increase steadily from the first month, plateau during the last month, and fall rapidly to nondetectable levels within a few days after parturition, on about day 150 (644). Inconsistent with this finding, relaxin bioactivity was not found in the blood of sheep during the last 2 months of pregnancy with the mouse interpubic ligament bioassay (268). Whereas one study, which utilized a homologous porcine relaxin radioimmunoassay, found little or no relaxin immunoactivity in the serum during middle or late gestation (485), a second study, which also utilized a homologous porcine relaxin radioimmunoassay, reported surges in relaxin immunoactivity during birth and suckling (87).

Other Domestic Species

Goat. In 1956, Wada and Yuhara (644) reported that relaxin bioactivity was present in the blood of pregnant goats. Using the guinea pig pubic symphysis palpation bioassay, relaxin levels were reported to increase steadily from the first month, plateau during the last month, and fall rapidly to nondetectable levels within a few days after parturition, on about day 150 (644). A source of relaxin in the goat has not been reported.

Chicken. An early report by Hisaw and Zarrow in 1950 (296) that extracts of chicken ovaries contain relaxin-like bioactivity in the guinea pig pubic symphysis palpation bioassay has received support. In 1985, Brackett et al. (65) reported that a peptide purified from active, deyolked hen ovaries had a molecular weight similar to that of porcine relaxin, exhibited relaxin immunoactivity in a homologous porcine relaxin radioimmunoassay, and had relaxin bioactivity in the mouse uterine contractility bioassay. Moreover, an immunocytochemical localization technique that employed an antiserum to highly purified porcine relaxin demonstrated that relaxin immunoactivity was associated with granulosa cells (65).

Cat. In 1929 Hisaw (291) reported that the blood of pregnant cats contained a substance that demonstrated relaxin-like bioactivity in the guinea pig pubic symphysis palpation bioassay. In 1985 Stewart and Stabenfeldt (593) determined the general profile of relaxin immunoactivity in the peripheral blood plasma of cats throughout the approximately 65-day gestation period with a homologous porcine relaxin radioimmunoassay (see Fig. 19). Relaxin immunoactivity levels rise from about day 25 to maximal levels by about day 35, remain stable until just before parturition, and then decline sharply to undetectable levels by 24 hr following delivery. The primary source of relaxin in the cat appears to be the placenta. Relaxin immunoactivity levels were higher in extracts of placentas obtained at days 16,

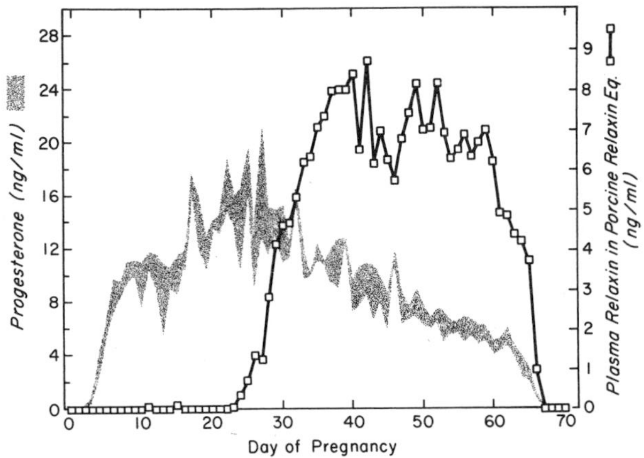

FIG. 19. Mean relaxin and progesterone immunoactivity levels (± SE; $N = 3$) in peripheral blood plasma during pregnancy in the cat. Relaxin immunoactivity was measured with a homologous porcine relaxin radioimmunoassay. Reproduced with permission from Stewart and Stabenfeldt (593).

21, 28, or 35 or near term than they were in uterine or luteal extracts (6). Moreover, ovariectomy on days 23 to 26 or days 42 to 44 did not influence relaxin levels in the peripheral blood (6).

Dog. Relaxin bioactivity (291) and immunoactivity (432) have been reported in the peripheral blood serum of pregnant dogs. Neither the source of relaxin nor the profile of relaxin levels in the blood during pregnancy has been reported.

Laboratory Species

Rat

Estrous cycle. Relaxin immunoactivity levels are extremely low, but detectable, in ovarian extracts obtained during the estrous cycle. They are maximal at estrus (557).

Pseudopregnancy. In deciduoma-bearing pseudopregnant rats, in which luteal function and elevated progesterone levels are maintained approximately 18 days, ovarian relaxin levels exceed those in cycling rats (557), but they are extremely low compared to those in the ovaries of pregnant rats after day 10 (15,545,557).

Pregnancy. Source: As with the pig, the corpora lutea are the source of both relaxin (20–22,199,247,309) and progesterone (286,628) during the approximately 23-day gestation period of the rat. Although early immunohistochemical localization studies employing antisera to impure porcine relaxin indicated that relaxin may also be found in uterine metrial glands (148) and placenta (685), studies that employed relaxin bioassays consistently demonstrated that relaxin is found only in the ovary (15,52,360,545,572). Ovarian levels of relaxin bioactivity, relaxin immunoactivity, and preprorelaxin mRNA increase from about day 10 to maximal levels 2 or 3 days before birth and then decline rapidly to low levels by 2 days postpartum (15,139,309,545) (see Fig. 20A). Immunohistochemical localization of relaxin with an antiserum to rat relaxin (247) and hybridization-histochemical localization of rat relaxin mRNA with a rat relaxin-specific cDNA probe (309) identified the corpora lutea, but not other ovarian elements, as the ovarian source of relaxin during the second half of pregnancy. It is not clear whether rat luteal cells are derived from both granulosa and theca cells (449) or only from granulosa cells (400). As in the pig, both relaxin and progesterone are probably produced by the same cell, since the luteal cells have organelles associated with both protein and steroid synthesis (374).

Rat relaxin is stored in a manner similar to that of porcine relaxin. There is conclusive evidence that rat relaxin is stored in the cytoplasm of lutein cells in small, membrane-bound granules (100–270 nm diameter). These cytoplasmic granules, which are smaller than lysosomal granules, are first observed on day 14, become more abundant during the last third of gestation, and disappear within 3 days of parturition (374). This pattern of accumulation and disappearance of the small cytoplasmic granules during pregnancy parallels that of ovarian relaxin bioactivity (15,374,545) and immunoactivity (545,557) as well as that of serum relaxin immunoactivity (241,432,545) (see Fig. 20A). Additionally, luteal cell fractionation studies demonstrated that the greatest relaxin bioactivity was in the granule-rich fraction (20). Finally, immunocytochemical studies that employed antisera to highly purified porcine relaxin (199) and rat relaxin (22) localized relaxin in the small cytoplasmic granules.

Regulation of Synthesis: Unlike in the pig, maintenance of corpora lutea throughout rat gestation requires the products of conception. After day 12, maintenance of the corpora lutea is no longer dependent on the pituitary; instead, it is dependent on the placentas (27,496). Likewise, the synthesis of high levels of relaxin in the corpora lutea of the rat is pregnancy-dependent. Each conceptus appears to contribute to the promotion of relaxin synthesis, since a direct relationship was observed between the number of conceptuses and ovarian levels of relaxin immunoactivity and preprorelaxin mRNA from day 12 to day 20 (140,244,464) (see Fig. 21).

There is evidence that it is the placentas that stimulate relaxin synthesis (241,244), as is the case with progesterone synthesis and growth of the corpora lutea (27,332). Following complete fetectomy on day 16 (241) or partial fetectomy on day 15 (244), with the placentas left undisturbed, ovarian relaxin levels and luteal weights did not differ from those in sham-operated controls. Additionally, the close temporal association of increasing ovarian relaxin levels, increasing luteal weights, and increasing serum progesterone levels between day 12 and day 15 is consistent with the view that relaxin synthesis, like the other two parameters of luteal function, is dependent on placental luteotropic support (see Fig. 20). As is the case with progesterone synthesis (237,359,436,611) and luteal weights (436,611), placental

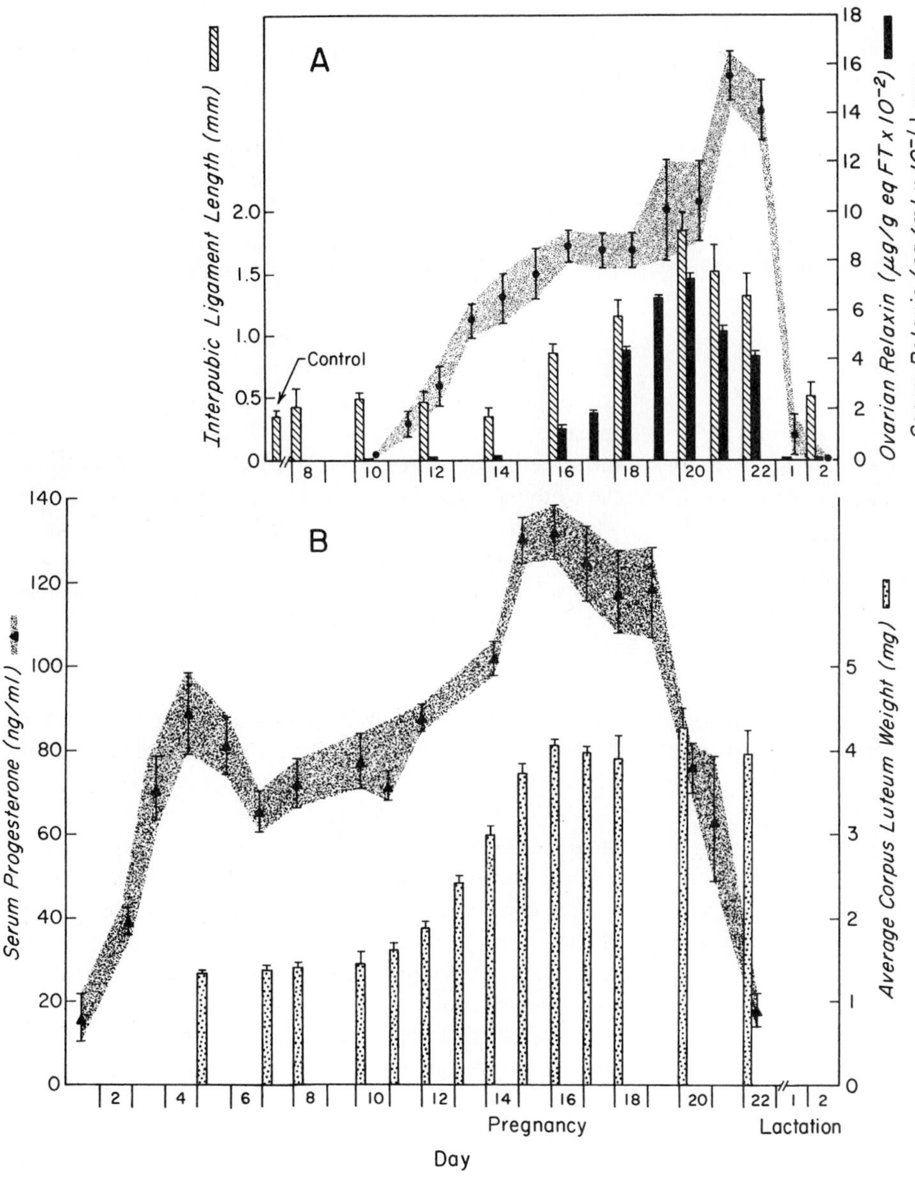

FIG. 20. A: Mean relaxin bioactivity and immunoactivity levels (+ SE) in extracts of ovaries and mean relaxin immunoactivity levels (± SE) in peripheral blood sera obtained from rats on each of the days of pregnancy and lactation shown. Reproduced with permission from Sherwood et al. (545). **B:** Mean progesterone levels in peripheral blood serum (± SE) and corpus luteum weights (+ SE) during pregnancy in rats. Modified and reproduced with permission from Pepe and Rothchild (450) and Uchida et al. (628).

support of relaxin synthesis appears to be mediated through estrogen (359).

Blood Levels from Day 10 to Day 20: Evaluation of the profile of both relaxin and progesterone immunoactivity levels in the peripheral serum throughout pregnancy led Sherwood and co-workers to postulate that the regulation of the release of relaxin from day 10 to day 20 differs from its regulation during the 3 days immediately before birth, which are designated the antepartum period (244,249,546). During the first period, relaxin immunoactivity becomes detectable in the serum by day 10, increases rapidly to 40 to 80 ng/ml by day 14, and remains relatively constant until day 20 (see Fig. 20). Serum progesterone levels also remain high, >60 ng/ml, throughout this period (244,450).

Regulation of Secretion from Day 10 to Day 20: The placenta promotes the secretion as well as the synthesis of relaxin from day 10 to day 20 (241,244). Moreover, as with relaxin synthesis, progesterone synthesis, and luteal weights, there is evidence that placental support of relaxin secretion is mediated through estrogens. The decline in serum relaxin levels that followed hysterectomy on day 12 or day 15 was attenuated by administration of estradiol-17β or the estradiol-17β precursor testosterone (239,359). Additionally, administration of the steroid biosynthesis inhibitor aminoglutethimide from day 10 to day 20 markedly reduced serum relaxin levels (583).

The placental factors that promote corpora lutea growth and activity during the second half of pregnancy in the rat

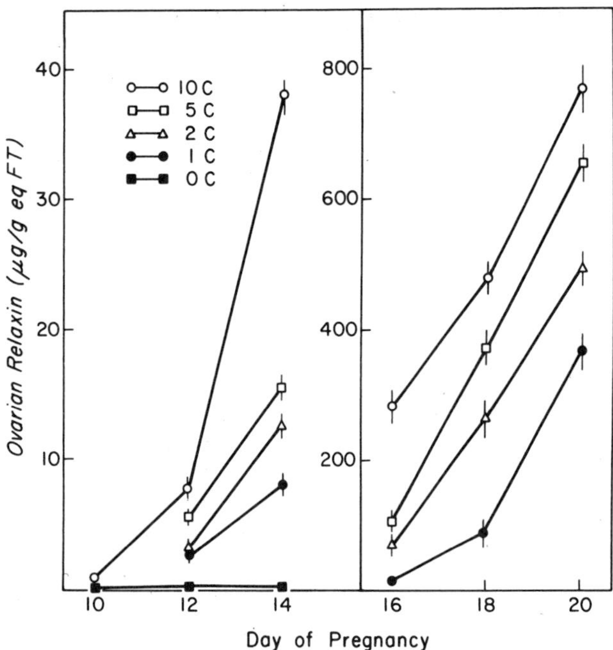

FIG. 21. Mean ovarian relaxin immunoactivity levels (± SE) in pregnant rats with 0, 1, 2, 5, or 10 or more conceptuses (C) from day 10 through day 20. Reproduced with permission from Golos and Sherwood (244).

have not been identified. Placental protein hormones may be involved. Two forms of rat placental lactogen (rPL) are secreted during the second half of pregnancy. The largest, 40,000-dalton form, designated rPL-I, is secreted from day 10 to day 15, whereas the smaller, 20,000-dalton form, designated rPL-II, is secreted maximally from day 17 to about day 22 (493,494,559). There is limited evidence that rPL-I may be luteotropic in the rat. First, its secretion from day 10 to day 15 is coincidental with the period when relaxin secretion, progesterone secretion, and corpora lutea weights increase markedly (see Fig. 20). Additionally, administration of a partially purified fraction of day 12 serum that contained rPLI, but not rPLII, sustained progesterone synthesis and maintained pregnancy in rats following suppression of the pituitary luteotropic hormone prolactin on day 6 (238). Placental steroids may also promote luteal function. The placenta is a major source of androstenedione and testosterone in the peripheral blood during the second half of pregnancy (318,566), and the capacity of the ovary to convert these androgens to estrogen increases markedly between day 12 and day 16 (318).

The mechanism whereby rat placental luteotropic factors promote relaxin synthesis, progesterone synthesis, luteal growth, and relaxin secretion are not well understood. The *in vivo* studies that demonstrated that the number of conceptuses is directly related to the rate or degree of increase of all four of these parameters of luteal function led to the postulation that placental support of these activities may be mediated, at least in part, through a common mechanism (244). Evidence obtained with *in vitro* studies, however, indicates that the secretion of relaxin and progesterone may not be mediated through a common mechanism. Although progesterone was secreted by rat luteal cell cultures treated with human chorionic gonadotropin (hCG), human placental lactogen, estradiol-17β, epinephrine, or dibutyryl cAMP individually, relaxin was secreted only when hCG and progesterone (plus various combinations of human placental lactogen, prolactin, estradiol-17β, and epinephrine) were employed in the presence of fetal calf serum (242).

The maternal pituitary first promotes and then suppresses luteal function during pregnancy in the rat. During the first half of pregnancy the pituitary is luteotropic: it provides the prolactin and luteinizing hormone (LH) required to promote the secretion of progesterone (496). After day 12, however, the maternal pituitary suppresses luteal function. From day 14 through day 20, serum relaxin levels, serum progesterone levels, and luteal weights in rats bearing one conceptus were markedly lower than those in rats with a full complement of eight or more conceptuses (244,245) (see Fig. 22). In contrast, when rats bearing one conceptus were hypophysectomized on day 13, all three parameters of luteal activity increased to values that were not significantly different from those of intact rats bearing a full complement of conceptuses (245,435) (see Fig. 22). Neither the factor(s) nor the mechanism(s) whereby the pituitary suppresses relaxin secretion, progesterone secretion, and luteal weights are known. It appears that this effect is not mediated through nonluteal ovarian components. The suppressive effect of the maternal pituitary was demonstrable in ovariectomized pregnant rats that contained ectopic corpora lutea but no other ovarian components (246).

Blood Levels During the Antepartum Period: During the antepartum period, from day 20 until birth, there is an elevation of serum relaxin immunoactivity to maximal levels, which generally range from 120 to 220 ng/ml, and this surge in relaxin levels is followed by a rapid decline throughout the approximately 24 hr before birth (249,545,547,548) (see Fig. 23A).

Regulation of Secretion During the Antepartum Period: As in the pig, the antepartum surge in relaxin levels in the rat coincides temporally with functional luteolysis. Moreover, in the rat this surge is linked to photoperiod (547). The elevation in serum relaxin to maximal mean relaxin levels (M-MRL) occurs between 36 and 24 hr before delivery, as does the marked antepartum decline in serum progesterone to basal mean progesterone levels (B-MPL) of less than 15 ng/ml (see Fig. 23A). When the times of the light:dark phases of the conventional photoperiod were advanced 18 hr on day 8, the times of occurrence of birth, M-MRL, and B-MPL were advanced; furthermore, they retained their close temporal association (cf. Fig. 23B to Fig. 23A).

The antepartum surge of relaxin levels consists of two phases, which occur at 24-hr intervals (see the vertical intermittent arrows in Fig. 23A). The first elevation (E1)

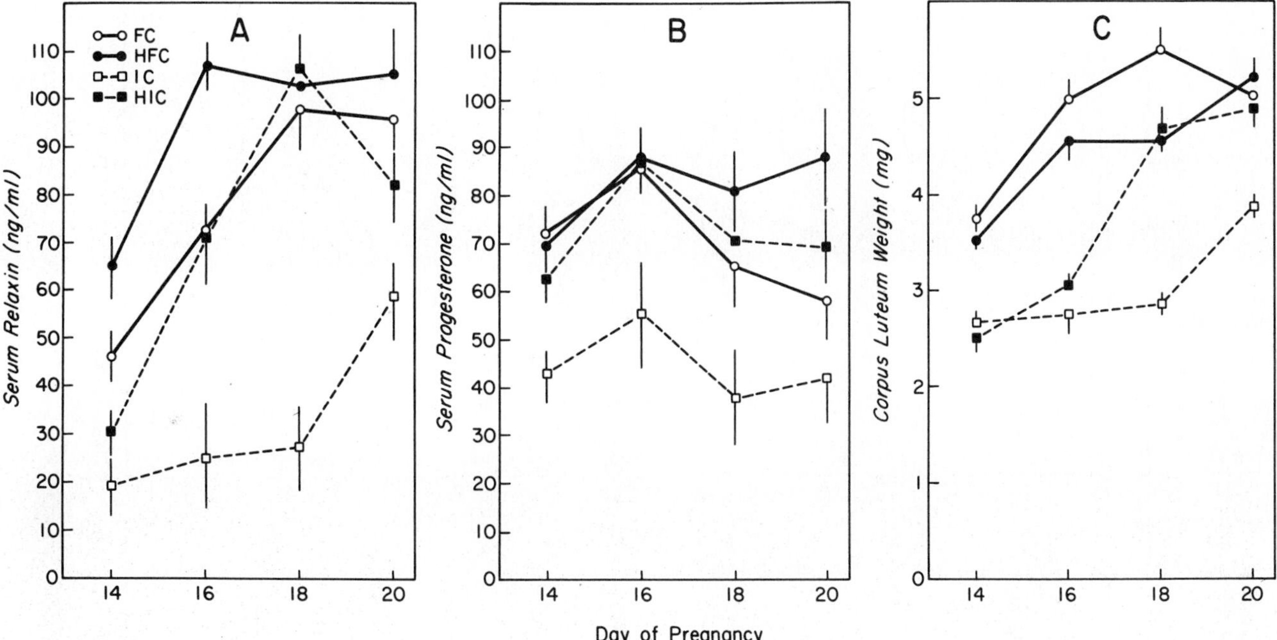

FIG. 22. Mean (± SE) levels of peripheral blood serum relaxin **(A)**, progesterone **(B)**, and corpus luteum weights **(C)** in full complement (FC), hypophysectomized full complement (HFC), one conceptus (1C) and hypophypsectomized one conceptus (H1C) bearing rats. Reproduced with permission from Golos and Sherwood (245).

begins approximately 60 hr before birth, whereas the second elevation (E2), which has maximal relaxin levels and coincides with functional luteolysis, begins 36 hr before birth. When the light:dark phases of the photoperiod were advanced, E1 and E2 were advanced; moreover, their advancement was comparable to that of birth, M-MRL, and B-MPL (see Fig. 23). Sherwood et al. (547) hypothesized that these two phases in the antepartum surge of serum relaxin levels may be indicative of an increasingly effective circadian luteolytic process whose time of occurrence is influenced by the photoperiod. That rats with small litters (3 or fewer fetuses) show a strong tendency for a 24-hr delay in the antepartum decline in serum relaxin levels, the antepartum decline in serum progesterone levels, and birth is consistent with this hypothesis (548).

The nature of the putative circadian luteolytic process is not well understood. The strong tendency for this process to be delayed 24 hr in rats with small litters indicates that the conceptuses may be involved. Four lines of evidence indicate that maternal pituitary LH may also be associated with the luteolytic process in the rat (249). First, rats experience an antepartum surge in LH levels, and an experiment conducted with intact pregnant rats indicated that this surge in LH levels may promote the antepartum surge in serum relaxin levels. Highly purified ovine LH, when administered to intact rats early on day 20, caused an immediate and marked surge in serum relaxin levels, but ovine follicle-stimulating hormone (FSH) and rat prolactin did not (see Fig. 24A). Second, when rats were hypophysectomized on day 14, the antepartum elevation in relaxin levels was disrupted and delayed, the decline in progesterone to basal levels was protracted, and birth failed to occur. When LH was administered to similarly hypophysectomized rats on day 20, however, the antepartum elevation in relaxin levels, antepartum decline in progesterone levels, and birth occurred at the normal time. Third, administration of gonadotropin-releasing hormone to intact rats on day 20 resulted in prompt and marked elevations in serum relaxin levels. Finally, reduction of endogenous serum LH levels in intact rats by injection of an LH antiserum from day 19 through day 22 delayed both luteolysis and birth.

Prostaglandins may be associated with both functional luteolysis and the antepartum surge in relaxin in rats, as they appear to be in pigs. Administration of $PGF_{2\alpha}$ during late pregnancy caused an early decline in serum progesterone levels (91,603) and an early surge in relaxin levels (250) (see Fig. 24B). Moreover, administration of indomethacin from day 19 to day 23 not only protracted luteolysis and delayed or prevented birth but also prevented the expected antepartum elevation of relaxin levels on days 21 and 22 (250).

The events within lutein cells that account for functional luteolysis and the surge in serum relaxin levels are not well understood. Levels of the enzyme 20α-hydroxysteroid dehydrogenase, which converts progesterone to a less active metabolite 20α-hydroxyprogesterone, increase during late pregnancy and appear to contribute to the reduction in progesterone levels (603). Although it seems likely that the

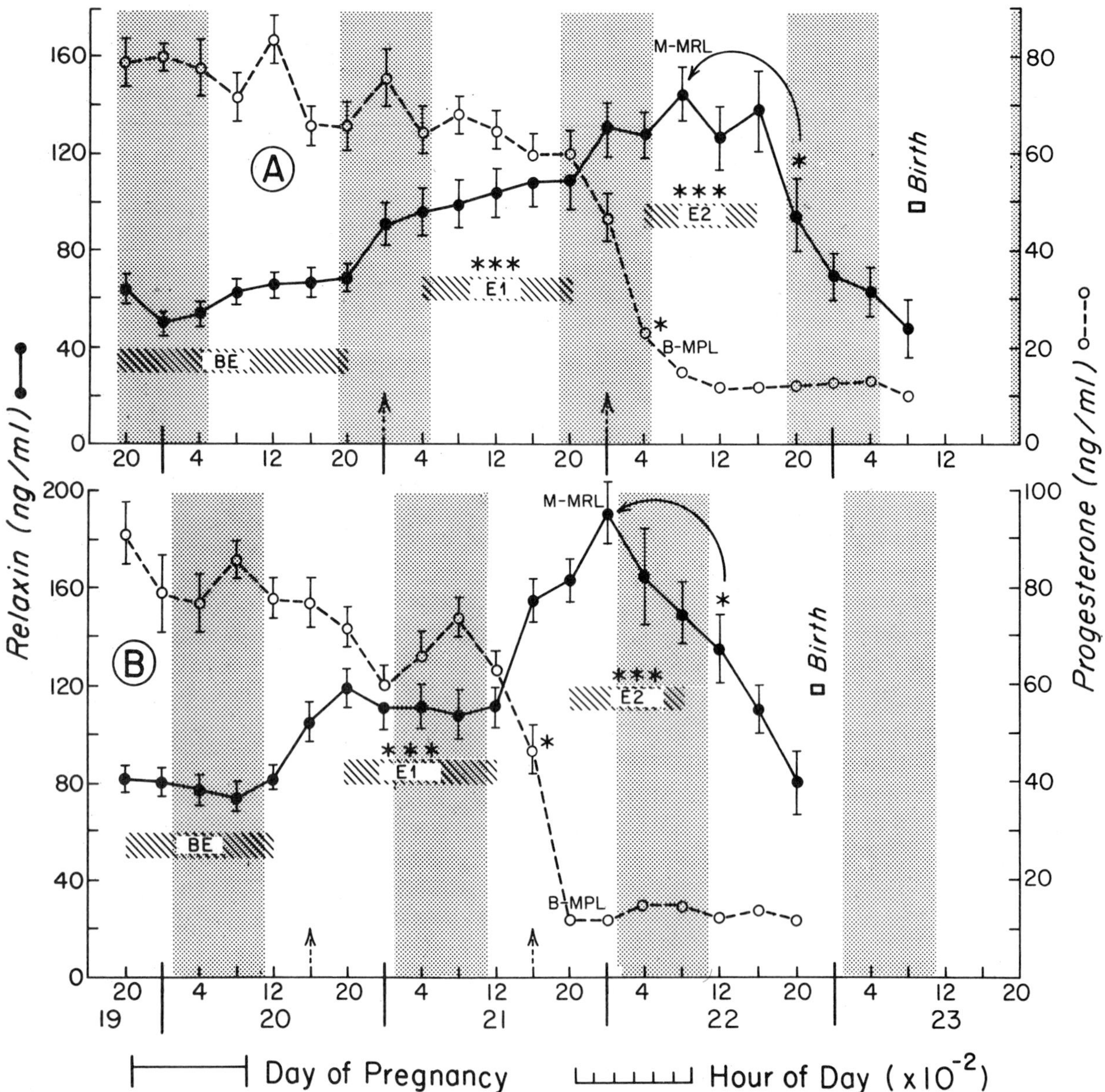

FIG. 23. Mean (± SE) relaxin and progesterone immunoactivity levels in peripheral blood serum of group A (N = 10) and group B (N = 13) pregnant rats throughout the antepartum period. The times of the light : dark phases of the photoperiod were advanced by 18 hr on day 8 in group B. The mean time of birth ± SE for both groups is given (box). Asterisks denote levels that differ significantly (*$p < 0.05$; ***$p < 0.001$) from those that immediately precede them or are indicated with an arrow. The times of occurrence of maximal mean relaxin levels (M-MRL) and basal mean progesterone levels (B-MPL) are beneath the appropriate abbreviation. The left and right vertical dashed arrows along the abscissas designate the sampling times when the first and second antepartum elevations of mean relaxin levels began, respectively. The bars containing diagonal lines indicate the before elevation (BE), elevation 1 (E1), and elevation 2 (E2) periods. Reproduced with permission from Sherwood et al. (547).

surge in serum relaxin levels is attributable to accelerated release of relaxin from cytoplasmic storage granules, the mechanism that brings this phenomenon about is not understood.

Blood Levels During Delivery: Delivery in the rat normally lasts for about 90 min. During delivery, relaxin immunoactivity levels in the peripheral serum surge markedly, and this surge lasts for an hour or more (545). Neither the factor(s) that promotes this surge in relaxin levels nor the physiological significance of the surge, if any, is known.

Multiple Forms of Relaxin in the Blood: Relaxin immunoactivity in the peripheral serum of pregnant rats is associated with three major components of different size, and the distribution of relaxin immunoactivity among these components changes in a progressive manner with the day of pregnancy (550). The three components, designated C1,

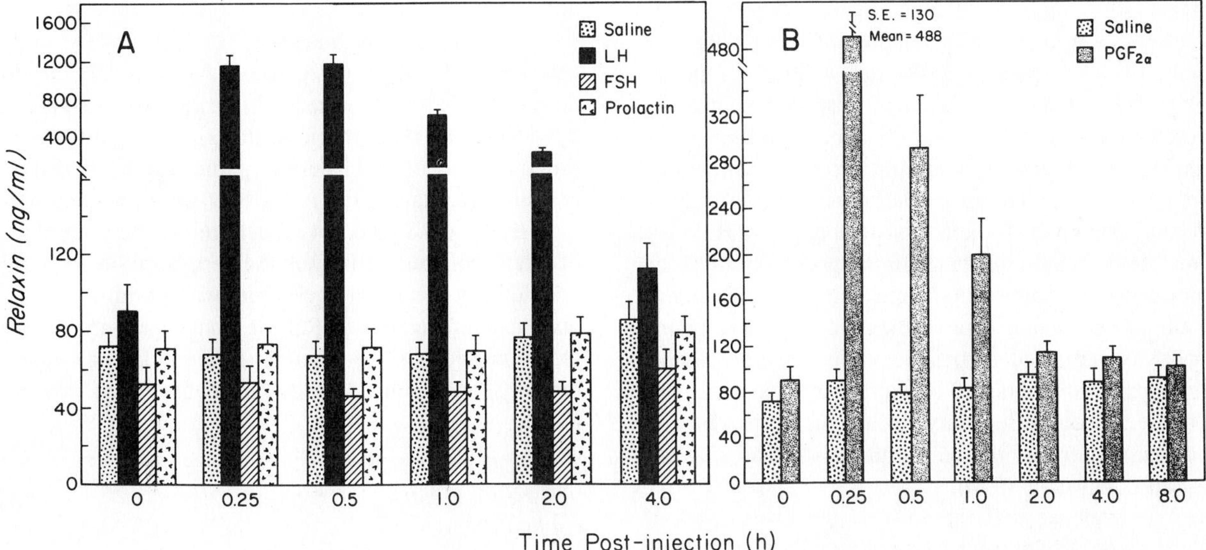

FIG. 24. Mean relaxin immunoactivity levels (+ SE) in peripheral blood serum of pregnant rats given an intravenous injection of one of the following on day 20. **A:** Saline vehicle ($N = 11$), 10 μg LH ($N = 5$), 25 μg FSH ($N = 4$), or 25 μg prolactin ($N = 5$). Reproduced with permission from Gordon and Sherwood (249). **B:** Saline vehicle ($N = 8$), or 50 μg $PGF_{2\alpha}$ ($N = 10$). Reproduced with permission from Gordon and Sherwood (250).

C2, and C3, have molecular weights of about 60,000, 13,000, and 6,500, respectively. On day 15, essentially all relaxin immunoactivity is associated with C1 (see Fig. 25). By day 17, approximately 20% of the total relaxin immunoactivity is in C2 plus C3, and by day 19 the proportion in each of these two components increases to about 25%. The nature of the three components is poorly understood. It was postulated (550) that C3 may be the 6,500-dalton, bioactive form of relaxin that has been isolated from the ovaries of rats (538,648). Insights concerning the natures of C2 and C1 are more speculative. Since the molecular weight of C2, about 13,000, is less than the 20,000 daltons reported for

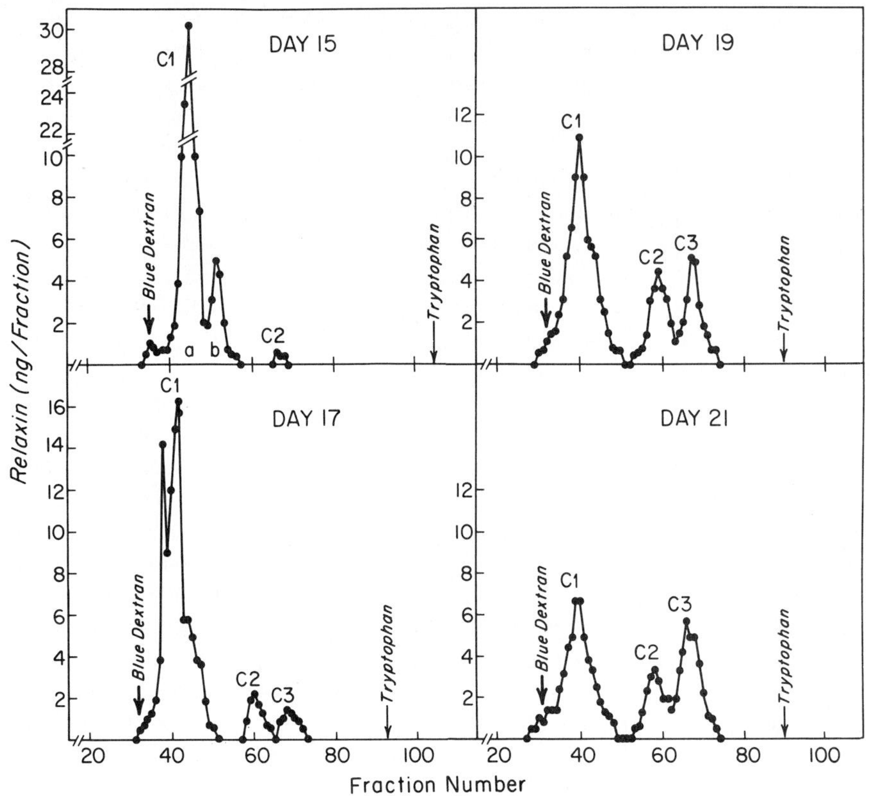

FIG. 25. Relaxin immunoactivity profiles obtained after gel filtration of peripheral blood serum from day 15, day 17, day 19, and day 21 pregnant rats on Sephacryl S-200 (Pharmacia; Piscataway, NJ). Reproduced with permission from Sherwood et al. (550).

prorelaxin (309), it may be an intermediate in the conversion of the precursor to relaxin. The nature of C1 is particularly puzzling, since its apparent molecular weight of approximately 60,000 is considerably greater than that reported for rat prorelaxin (309). Component C1 appears to possess the relaxin-like bioactivity of inhibiting uterine contractility: The frequency of intrauterine pressure cycles in nonpregnant rats declined during cross-circulation with day 15 rats, which have only the C1 component in their peripheral serum. Component C1 does not appear to be attributable to the binding of 6,000-dalton relaxin to a binding protein: Relaxin immunoactivity remained associated with the large component(s) when serum obtained on day 15 was incubated and then filtered through Sephacryl S-200 in the presence of high concentrations of the conformation-destabilizing salt potassium thiocyanate (550).

There is evidence that the shift in the distribution of relaxin immunoactivity from C1 to the smaller components C2 and C3 during late pregnancy is promoted by the conceptuses but is not influenced by the maternal pituitary (549). In rats bearing a full complement of conceptuses, only about 50% of the total relaxin immunoactivity is associated with C1 on day 19, whereas in rats bearing a single conceptus about 85% of the total, relaxin immunoactivity is associated with C1 on day 19. The physiological significance, if any, of this multiplicity of relaxin-immunoactive components is not known.

Clearance of Relaxin from the Blood: The clearance $t_{1/2}$ for rat relaxin immunoactivity appears to be similar to that of porcine relaxin (545). Following bilateral ovariectomy on day 21, the clearance $t_{1/2}$ was approximately 20 min during the first half-hour and approximately 60 min thereafter (545). Interpretation of the apparent clearance for relaxin immunoactivity during late pregnancy is complicated, since it is influenced by the relative quantities and rates of clearance of the three relaxin immunoactive components C1, C2, and C3. There is limited evidence that the rate of clearance of C1 may be slower than that of C2 and C3 (550).

Mouse

In 1959 Steinetz et al. (572) detected relaxin bioactivity in the ovaries of pregnant mice. More recent studies by Anderson and co-workers (23,636) indicate that relaxin synthesis in the mouse is similar to that in the rat. Studies that used an antiserum to highly purified rat relaxin with either the unlabeled antibody peroxidase-antiperoxidase or avidin-biotin immunoperoxidase cytochemical localization method demonstrated that immunostaining was confined to the corpora lutea of ovaries obtained during late pregnancy, and no immunostaining was demonstrated in ovaries obtained throughout the estrous cycle (23,636). An appearance and disappearance of membrane-bound cytoplasmic granules (200 nm in diameter) closely paralleled that of relaxin immunostaining of luteal cells (23). Granules appeared by day 12, were maximal between day 16 and day 18, and disappeared by 2 days postpartum. As with the rat, luteal relaxin production and secretion in the mouse may be prompted by a placental luteotropic factor(s). Hypophysectomized pregnant mice showed normal pubic relaxation if the placentas were retained but not if they were removed (414).

O'Byrne and Steinetz (432) determined the general profile of relaxin immunoactivity in the peripheral blood serum of mice during the 20-day gestation period with a porcine relaxin radioimmunoassay. Relaxin immunoactivity levels rose from about day 12 to maximal levels a day or two before delivery, and declined to low levels by 2 days postpartum (432).

Guinea Pig

Unlike the pig and rat, relaxin is produced in the uterus in the guinea pig. In 1928 Herrick (285) provided evidence that relaxin was produced in nonovarian tissue in the guinea pig when he reported that bilateral ovariectomy at midpregnancy did not prevent relaxation of the pubic symphysis during late pregnancy. Proof that the uterus was a major source of relaxin was first obtained in the 1940s, when Hisaw et al. (294,297) and Zarrow (680) demonstrated that the pelvic relaxation that occurred within 3 or 4 days following progesterone administration to castrated, estrogen-primed nonpregnant guinea pigs failed to occur if hysterectomy was performed at the same time as ovariectomy. It was not until the 1980s that the cellular source of relaxin in the guinea pig uterus was demonstrated. Employing an antiserum to highly purified porcine relaxin and the peroxidase-antiperoxidase immunocytochemical localization method, Pardo et al. (443,444) demonstrated relaxin immunostaining over only the endometrial gland cells during late pregnancy (see Fig. 26A,B). Moreover, a subsequent electron microscopy immunocytochemical localization study, which used the same relaxin antiserum and colloidal gold–goat antirabbit IgG, showed that the relaxin immunostaining was located over large (500 to 1,000 nm diameter) granules in the luminal portions of the endometrial gland cells (445) (Fig. 26C,D).

Pardo and co-workers (443,444) obtained two lines of evidence which make it seem likely that the uterine relaxin immunostaining substance is relaxin. First, a close temporal association was found between the occurrence of relaxin immunostaining in uterine sections and the ability of uterine extracts to inhibit spontaneous contractions of the mouse uterus (443). Relaxin levels were detectable by day 30, but staining was heaviest on day 45 and during the last week of pregnancy, when bioactivity levels were maximal (443). Following parturition on about day 65, uterine relaxin levels fell rapidly, and they were low by day 3 of lactation (443). Second, the biologically active substance had a molecular

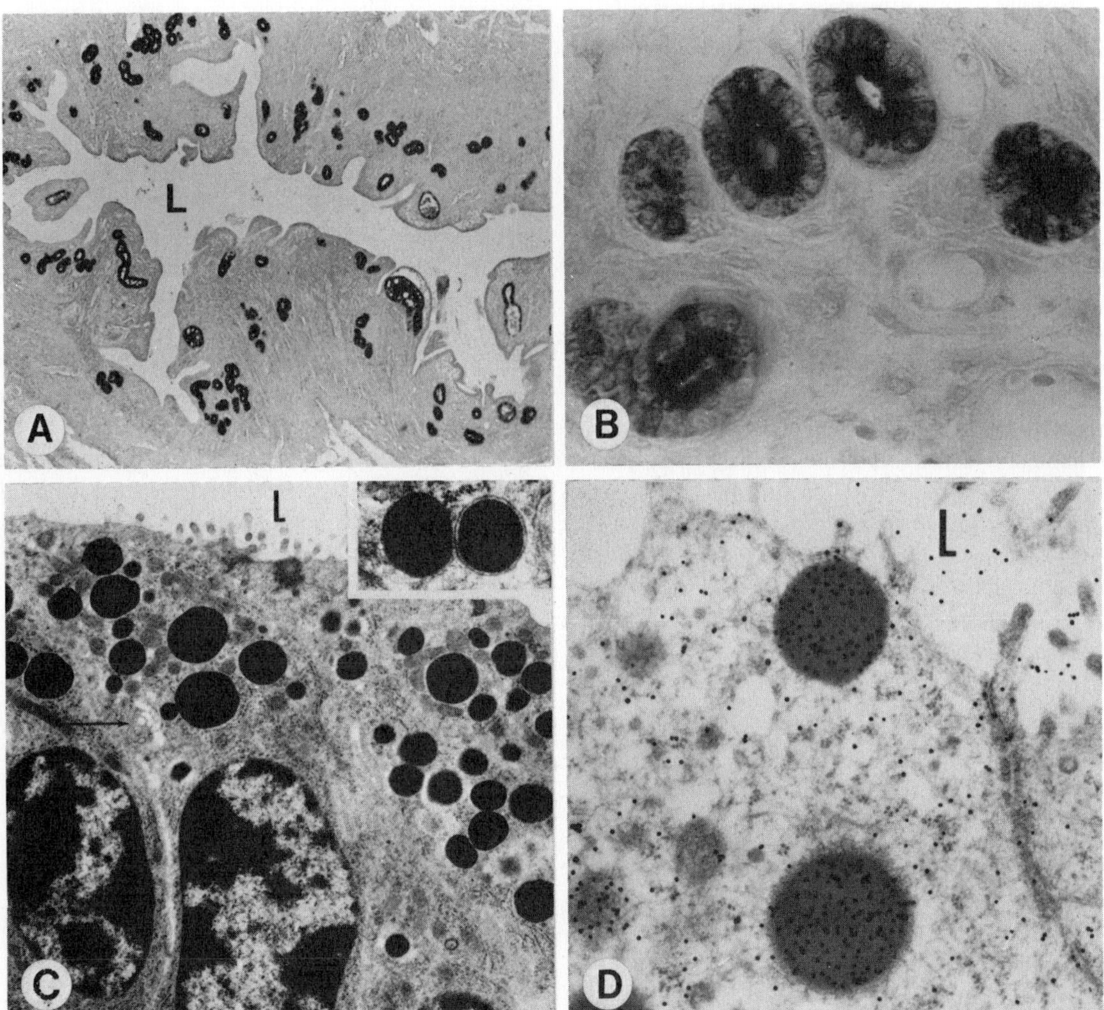

FIG. 26. A: Localization of relaxin immunoactivity in guinea pig uterus removed on day 60 of pregnancy. Light microscopy immunohistochemical localization of relaxin in a transverse section of a guinea pig uterus using rabbit antiporcine relaxin serum and peroxidase-antiperoxidase as marker. L = lumen. (×35.) **B:** A higher magnification of a section of uterus (stained as in A) showing dense relaxin immunoactivity near the luminal surfaces of the endometrial gland cells. (×455.) A and B reproduced with permission from Pardo and Larkin (443). **C:** Electron micrograph showing numerous dense granules (500–1,000 nm diameter) in the luminal portions of the endometrial gland cells. Stacks of Golgi cisterne (*arrow*) are evident. (×900.) Inset: Higher magnification of the dense granules (×17,900). **D:** Electron microscopy immunocytochemical localization of relaxin in endometrial gland cell granules using rabbit antiporcine relaxin serum and goat antirabbit immunoglobulin G–colloidal gold as marker. The granules are labeled with numerous gold particles indicating the presence of relaxin. (×30,000.) C and D reproduced with permission from Pardo et al. (445).

weight of about 6,000—similar to that of porcine relaxin (444). Consistent with these studies, Nagao and Bryant-Greenwood (409) reported that relaxin immunoactivity levels were maximal in extracts of guinea pig uteri obtained during late pregnancy and that the relaxin-immunoactive substance had a molecular weight similar to that of porcine relaxin.

The few reports describing blood levels of relaxin during pregnancy are not in close agreement. In 1947 Zarrow (679) determined relaxin bioactivity levels in the peripheral serum with the guinea pig pubic symphysis palpation assay. Relaxin bioactivity was reported to be detectable by day 21, maximal by day 28, and maintained at maximal levels until about day 63, when it began to drop gradually. Shortly after parturition, on about day 68, a precipitous decline occurred, so that by 48 hr after birth relaxin bioactivity was undetectable (679). Two studies measured relaxin immunoactivity levels in peripheral blood with porcine relaxin radioimmunoassays. In one study, which determined relaxin levels in serum samples collected at 10-day intervals throughout pregnancy, relaxin immunoactivity was detectable on about day 20, rose steadily to maximal levels on about day 50 to day 60, and did not decline by the day following parturition (432). In the second study, which determined relaxin levels in plasma samples obtained at 24-hr or 8-hr intervals from day 40 until birth, episodic surges in relaxin immunoactivity were detected, and there was no clear pattern among animals (64). Thus, a profile of relaxin levels in the peripheral blood throughout pregnancy in the guinea pig is not established.

Although the factors that normally promote the synthesis and release of relaxin from the guinea pig uterine endometrial glands during pregnancy are not well understood, it seems likely that estrogen and progesterone are involved. Following the administration of both steroids to castrated nonpregnant guinea pigs, heavy relaxin immunostaining was observed over uterine endometrial gland cells (443), levels of relaxin immunoactivity in uterine extracts increased (409), and relaxation of the pelvic ligaments occurred (297,680).

There is limited evidence that guinea pigs may also produce and secrete small amounts of relaxin from the uterus during the estrous cycle. When Bryant-Greenwood and coworkers (64,409) assayed relaxin levels in uterine extracts and peripheral blood plasma with a porcine relaxin radioimmunoassay, low levels of relaxin immunoactivity were found in both tissues throughout the estrous cycle; moreover, there was a tendency for levels to be elevated at diestrus.

Rabbit

Three lines of evidence indicate that the placenta is a major source of relaxin during pregnancy in the rabbit. First, extracts of rabbit placental tissue demonstrated relaxin-like bioactivity in the guinea pig pubic symphysis palpation bioassay (289–291,296,364,572,688), mouse uterine contractility bioassay (177,205,364), and mouse interpubic ligament bioassay (205). Second, a fivefold increase in blood levels of relaxin was measured with the guinea pig pubic symphysis palpation bioassay between day 15 and day 21, and this coincides with the time when the placenta undergoes its most rapid development (388,688). Moreover, after parturition, on about day 32, there was a rapid drop in blood relaxin levels coincident with the expulsion of the fetuses and placentas (388). Finally, Eldridge and Fields (177,178) localized relaxin in the multinucleated syncytiotrophoblast cells of placentas obtained on days 16, 23, and 30 with an immunohistochemical method which employed an antiserum to highly purified rabbit relaxin and the avidin-biotin immunoperoxidase technique as marker (see Fig. 27A). Additionally, Eldridge and Fields (179) obtained evidence at

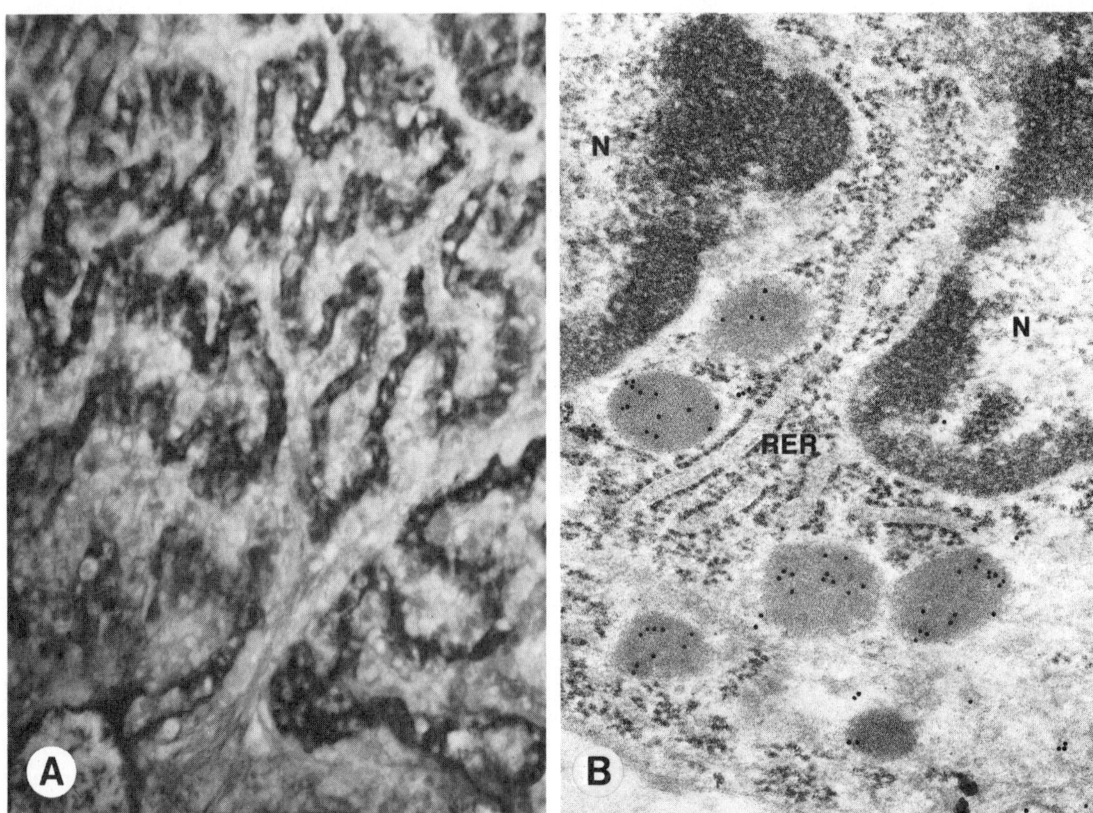

FIG. 27. A: Light microscopy immunohistochemical localization of relaxin in the syncytiotrophoblast cells of a rabbit placenta on day 23 of pregnancy using guinea pig antirabbit relaxin serum and avidin-biotin peroxidase as marker. (×218.) **B:** Electron microscopy immunocytochemical localization of relaxin in rabbit placenta granules (150–400 nm diameter) on day 23 of pregnancy using guinea pig antirabbit relaxin and goat anti–guinea pig immunoglobulin G–colloidal gold as marker. N, nucleus; RER, rough endoplasmic reticulum. (×56,600.) Reproduced with permission from Eldridge and Fields (179).

the ultrastructural level that rabbit relaxin is stored in cytoplasmic membrane-bound granules (150–400 nm diameter) which migrate to the cell membrane where they are exocytosed from the syncytiotrophoblast cells (Fig. 27B). Essentially nothing is known concerning the regulation of the synthesis or secretion of relaxin from the rabbit placenta.

The uterus may be a minor source of relaxin in the rabbit. Extracts of uterine tissue obtained from pregnant (572), pseudopregnant (688), or castrated and steroid-treated rabbits (297) were reported to demonstrate relaxin bioactivity in the guinea pig pubic symphysis palpation bioassay. Eldridge and Fields (178) found immunoreactive relaxin associated with the epithelial cells at the adluminal end of the endometrial glands between implantation sites on day 30 when the avidin-biotin immunoperoxidase method was used with an antiserum to highly purified rabbit relaxin. Eldridge and Fields (178) postulated that these endometrial epithelial cells either begin to synthesize relaxin in late pregnancy or sequester relaxin released into the venous sinusoids from the syncytiotrophoblast cells. Estrogen and progesterone may promote relaxin synthesis in the rabbit uterus. Sera obtained from castrated adult female rabbits given pharmacological doses of estradiol-17β and progesterone daily for several days promoted pelvic relaxation in guinea pigs, whereas sera obtained from castrated plus hysterectomized rabbits given the same steroid treatment did not (297).

Reports are inconsistent, but it seems unlikely that the ovaries produce relaxin during pregnancy in the rabbit. Extracts of rabbit ovaries were reported to contain little relaxin bioactivity in the guinea pig pubic symphysis palpation bioassay (296,572,688). When pregnant rabbits were ovariectomized on day 14 or day 15 and pregnancy was maintained by injecting progesterone daily, serum relaxin bioactivity levels remained similar to those in intact controls (688). Employing an immunohistochemical localization study which used an antiserum to impure porcine relaxin, Zarrow and O'Connor (687) found immunofluorescence associated with the rabbit corpora lutea on days 23 to 28. The more recent immunohistochemical localization study by Eldridge and Fields (177), however, which employed an antiserum generated with highly purified rabbit relaxin at both the light and electron microscopy levels, failed to find relaxin immunoactivity associated with the corpora lutea of pregnant rabbits.

Relaxin bioactivity levels in the peripheral blood serum of rabbits throughout pregnancy were first determined in 1944 by Marder and Money (388) employing a guinea pig pubic symphysis palpation bioassay. Relaxin levels were reported to remain low until day 12, increase about 50-fold by day 24, remain elevated and steady until delivery on day 32, and then decline precipitously. Similar results were reported in 1953 by Zarrow and Rosenberg (688). Relaxin immunoactivity levels in the peripheral blood of rabbits have not been reported.

Hamster

O'Byrne et al. (431) determined the general profile of relaxin immunoactivity in the blood of hamsters with a porcine relaxin radioimmunoassay. Relaxin immunoactivity appeared on day 8, rose to maximal levels by day 15, and dropped precipitously on day 16, which is the day before parturition. The source of relaxin in the hamster has not been established.

Primates

Human

With the isolation of porcine relaxin in 1974 (555), there came a renewal of interest in human relaxin. Between 1976 and 1986 there were many studies concerning the source(s) of relaxin, blood levels of relaxin, and regulation of relaxin secretion in women. Because human relaxin was not available during that 10-year period, antiporcine relaxin sera were used for the radioimmunoassay and immunohistochemical localization of human relaxin. A large majority of the studies employed a rabbit antiporcine relaxin serum, designated R6, which was generated by Steinetz and coworkers (585) with the three contiguous porcine relaxin peaks CMB, CMa, and CMa′ shown in Fig. 1 (555).

Three lines of evidence indicate that antiserum R6 binds human relaxin. First, R6 bound to a molecule in human luteal extracts with a molecular weight that did not differ from that of porcine relaxin—about 6,300 (375). Second, R6 inhibited the ability of crude extracts of human corpora lutea of pregnancy to promote growth of the interpubic ligament in guinea pigs (585,586). Finally, when R6 was employed with porcine relaxin radioimmunoassays, the concentration-dependent curves obtained with multiple volumes of both human corpora lutea extract and human pregnancy serum were reportedly parallel to those obtained with highly purified porcine relaxin (377,429). Unless indicated otherwise, rabbit antiporcine relaxin serum R6 was employed for the radioimmunoassays and immunohistochemical studies of human relaxin described in this section.

Menstrual cycle. Although the corpus luteum of the menstrual cycle contains insufficient relaxin to be detected with existing relaxin bioassays (429,608), there is evidence that it produces relaxin. Relaxin immunoactivity was found in luteal extracts (430), luteal cyst fluid (377), and culture medium bathing freshly dispersed luteal cells obtained during the menstrual cycle (516). Whereas a study that employed the peroxidase-antiperoxidase immunohistochemical method failed to locate relaxin immunoactivity in the corpora lutea during the early luteal phase (390), a second study, which employed the avidin-biotin immunoperoxidase method, found specific staining associated with luteinizing granulosa cells, luteal cells, and paraluteal cells (675,676,678). The amount of relaxin released from the corpora lutea during the menstrual cycle is not sufficient to be readily detected in the peripheral blood with porcine relaxin radioimmunoassays (429,477,479,620). In contrast, the peritoneal fluid, which has been reported to be mainly an exudate of the active ovary in women (352), contains detectable levels of relaxin immunoactivity during the luteal phase of the cycle (376,619) (see Fig. 28).

Evidence that relaxin may also be produced in human granulosa cells during the follicular phase of the menstrual cycle is limited and not entirely consistent. Sufficient relaxin was reported to be present in follicular fluid during the late follicular phase of the cycle to inhibit spontaneous contractions of the mouse uterus (422). Granulosa cells from medium-size cavitary follicles reportedly exhibited relaxin-specific immunofluorescence (31). Finally, detectable levels of relaxin immunoactivity were found in peripheral plasma before follicular rupture in women whose ovaries were hyperstimulated with exogenous gonadotropin treatment (620). On the other hand, the observation that long-term cultures of granulosa cells failed to release measurable relaxin in response to hCG stimulation is not consistent with the view that granulosa cells secrete relaxin (517).

There is limited and unconfirmed evidence that human relaxin may also be synthesized by the endometrium during the luteal phase of the cycle. Relaxin immunoactivity was reportedly found associated with the endometrial glands during the secretory phase, but not the proliferative phase, of the menstrual cycle using the avidin-biotin immunoperoxidase localization method (676).

Pregnancy. Source: Available evidence indicates that the corpus luteum of pregnancy is a major source of relaxin in the human. Extracts of corpora lutea obtained near parturition were reported to contain relaxin immunoactivity (375,430,654), to reduce the amplitude of spontaneous contractions of human myometrial strips (608), and to be active in the guinea pig pubic symphysis palpation bioassay (430). Relaxin immunoactivity was present in the medium bathing collagenase-dispersed cells of human corpora lutea obtained at term (240). Luteal cells displayed specific staining with immunohistochemical localization studies that employed the peroxidase-antiperoxidase and avidin-biotin immunoperoxidase localization methods (390,676).

Weiss et al. (653,655) provided evidence that the corpus luteum of pregnancy is the source of circulating relaxin in pregnant women (see Fig. 29). At term pregnancy, relaxin immunoactivity was present in the ovarian vein draining the corpus luteum in far higher concentrations than in either the ovarian vein draining the contralateral ovary or the peripheral blood (655); moreover, luteectomy produced a prompt disappearance of relaxin from the peripheral blood (653). Available evidence indicates that the levels of relaxin within the corpus luteum of pregnancy in women (430) are much lower than those in the corpora lutea of pigs (555) and rats (538). Unlike pigs (41,124,202,337), rats (22,199,374), and mice (23), there is currently no evidence of an accumulation of membrane-bound granules that store relaxin in the cytoplasm of human luteal cells during pregnancy. Cytoplasmic granules (150–200 nm diameter) were reported to be associated with the granular endoplasmic reticulum in human luteal cells obtained at term (141), but it remains to be determined whether they contain relaxin.

The corpus luteum may not be the sole source of relaxin in pregnant women. Low levels of relaxin may also be produced in decidual tissue, placental tissue, or both tissues. Four laboratories reported that extracts of term decidual tissue (47,50,51) or placental tissue (204,673) contained

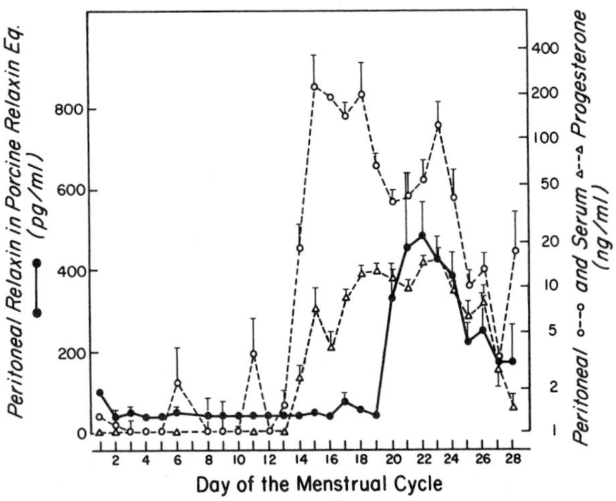

FIG. 28. Mean peritoneal progesterone concentrations, peripheral blood serum progesterone concentrations, and peritoneal relaxin concentrations (+ SE) for each day of the menstrual cycle in women. Reproduced with permission from Loumaye et al. (376).

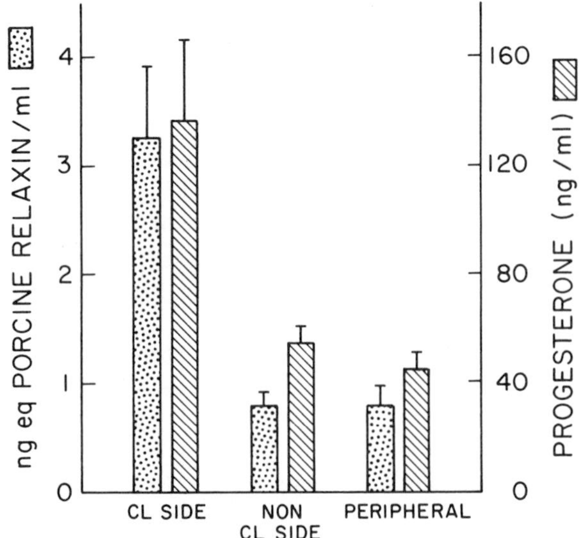

FIG. 29. Mean relaxin and progesterone immunoactivity levels (+ SE; $N = 7$) in ovarian vein and peripheral blood plasma in women after term delivery by cesarian section. Reproduced with permission from Weiss et al. (655).

sufficient quantities of a relaxin-like substance to demonstrate relaxin bioactivity. These extracts were reported to inhibit spontaneous uterine contractions in guinea pigs (50), rats (50), and mice (204,673) and also to promote growth of the interpubic ligament in mice (50,204) and guinea pigs (684). Although Schmidt et al. (518) failed to confirm the presence of sufficient relaxin in extracts of human placental or decidual tissue to promote growth of the interpubic ligament in mice or to inhibit contractions of rat uterine segments, they did report low levels of relaxin immunoactivity in extracts of these tissues. Moreover, these workers (518) found that two partially purified fractions obtained from placental extract had limited bioactivity in the guinea pig pubic symphysis palpation bioassay. Although Schmidt et al. (518) estimated the levels of relaxin immunoactivity in extracts of human decidual and placental tissue to be about 0.2 ng/g equivalent of fresh tissue, the limitations associated with the use of porcine relaxin radioimmunoassays for the measurement of relaxin from other species preclude accurate estimates of human relaxin levels. In contrast to the reports described above, two studies found very little (654) or no (377) relaxin immunoactivity in human placental extracts obtained at term.

Inconsistencies also exist with immunohistochemical efforts to locate relaxin in human placental and decidual tissue. The significance of an early immunofluorescence localization study (147,148) which indicated that granulated cells in human decidua and basal trophoblast cells of the placenta contained relaxin immunoactivity was weakened by the impurity of the porcine relaxin used to generate the antiserum. Nevertheless, several more recent immunohistochemical studies which employed a variety of antisera generated with highly purified porcine relaxin also reported the presence of relaxin immunoactivity in decidual (47,349,676) and placental tissue (204,349,674–676) (see Fig. 30). It was postulated that the low levels of relaxin found in the placenta may be produced locally, since relaxin-specific staining was observed in a term placenta obtained from a woman in whom the corpus luteum of pregnancy was removed at 16 weeks of pregnancy (674). The report that the expression of human genes was not detected in human placental or decidual tissue, however, does not support this postulate (311).

The literature is not in agreement concerning the cell type(s) in the human placenta that contains relaxin immunoactivity. One laboratory reported that relaxin was localized in the syncytiotrophoblast (674–676), whereas a second laboratory reported relaxin in the cytotrophoblast but not the syncytiotrophoblast (349). Relaxin may also be produced in trophoblastic tumors. Employing an antiserum to highly purified porcine relaxin (NIH-RXN-P1, 3,000 GPU/mg) and the avidin-biotin immunohistochemical localization method, specific staining was reportedly found in hydatidiform mole, chorioadenoma, and choriocarcinoma (675). In view of the numerous inconsistencies in the reports described above, it cannot be considered established that either the placenta or decidua is a source of relaxin in the human.

Blood Levels: Relaxin levels are elevated in the peripheral blood throughout nearly all of gestation in the human (2,173,429,457,481,515,609,684). The earliest indications

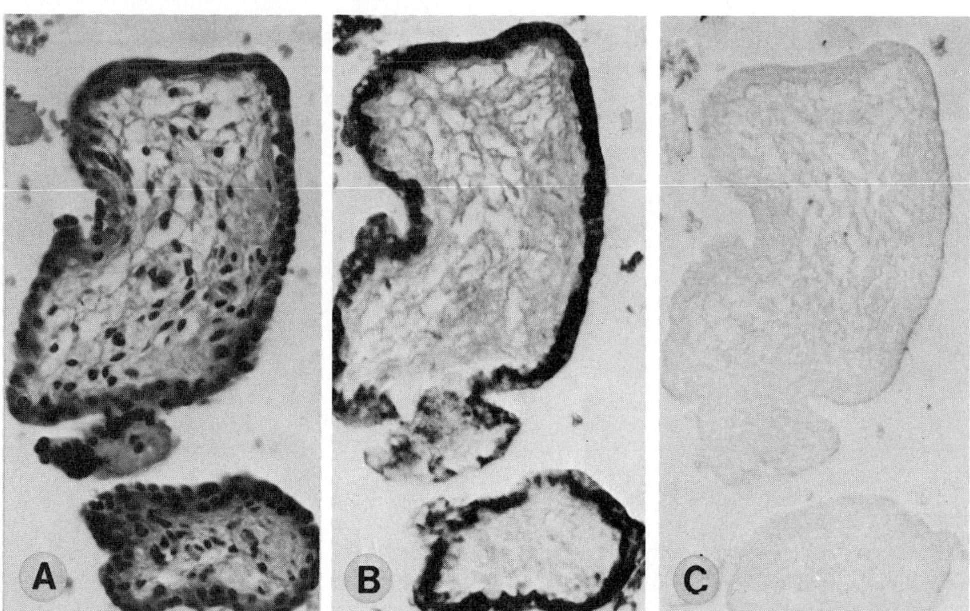

FIG. 30. Localization of relaxin in a normal human placenta removed at 6 weeks of gestation. **A:** Light microscopy of a section stained with hematoxylin and eosin. **B:** Light microscopy immunohistochemical localization of relaxin using rabbit antiporcine relaxin serum and peroxidase-antiperoxidase as a marker. The antiserum was generated with highly purified porcine relaxin (NIH-RXN-P1, 3,000 GPU/mg). **C:** Control staining of a placental section following absorption of the antiserum with porcine relaxin. (×320.) Reproduced with permission from Yki-Järvinen et al. (675).

that relaxin levels might be higher during early pregnancy than late pregnancy were obtained in the 1930s, when Pommerenke (457) and Abramson et al. (2) reported that, with advancing pregnancy, fewer and fewer human serum samples were capable of inducing pelvic relaxation in estrogen-primed guinea pigs. Consistent with these reports, subsequent radioimmunoassays, which employed antisera to either porcine relaxin (377,429,481,609) or a synthetic analog of human relaxin 2 (173), demonstrated that relaxin immunoactivity levels are higher during the first trimester than during the second or third trimester (see Fig. 31). Unlike the pig and rat, there is no antepartum surge in relaxin levels in women (429,478,481,609). Perhaps this is a reflection of the apparent low level or absence of storage of relaxin in secretory granules in the corpus luteum of women during pregnancy.

Regulation of Secretion: Four lines of evidence are consistent with the hypothesis that hCG, which is secreted by the trophoblast and which rescues the corpus luteum of the menstrual cycle, is a major stimulus for relaxin secretion during pregnancy. First, the appearance of relaxin immunoactivity in the peripheral serum about 14 days after conception (479) follows closely the appearance of hCG immunoactivity (398); moreover, the subsequent blood level profiles of the two hormones are similar throughout pregnancy (173,429,481). Second, injection of hCG during the late luteal phase of the menstrual cycle extended luteal function and induced relaxin secretion within a few days of the beginning of hCG treatment (477,620) (see Fig. 32). Third, it was reported that spontaneously aborting women with low hCG levels had low relaxin levels whereas those with normal hCG levels had normal relaxin levels (480). Finally, addition of hCG to monolayers of luteal cells collected at cesarian section increased relaxin immunoactivity levels in the media on day 2 of culture (240).

Serum relaxin levels appear to be directly related to the number of corpora lutea in pregnant women. Relaxin immunoactivity levels were reported to be greater in two trizygotic triplet pregnancies than in either a monozygotic triplet pregnancy or singleton pregnancies during the second and third trimesters (609). Consistent with these findings, relaxin immunoactivity levels were greater during the first trimester in five women bearing two to five fetuses following treatment with menotropins than in women with singleton pregnancies during the first trimester (273).

Little is known about the regulation of relaxin secretion during late pregnancy in women. As previously mentioned, there is no antepartum surge in relaxin levels (478). Moreover, efforts to induce the secretion of relaxin during late pregnancy were not successful. The administration of sufficient $PGF_{2\alpha}$ or oxytocin (298) to induce delivery did not influence serum relaxin levels. Similarly, administration of sufficient prostaglandin E2 to induce second trimester abortions did not alter serum relaxin levels (476).

Relaxin in Other Compartments During Pregnancy and Lactation: Brief reports, which require confirmation, indicate that fetal blood and milk from lactating women may contain relaxin. There is disagreement concerning the pres-

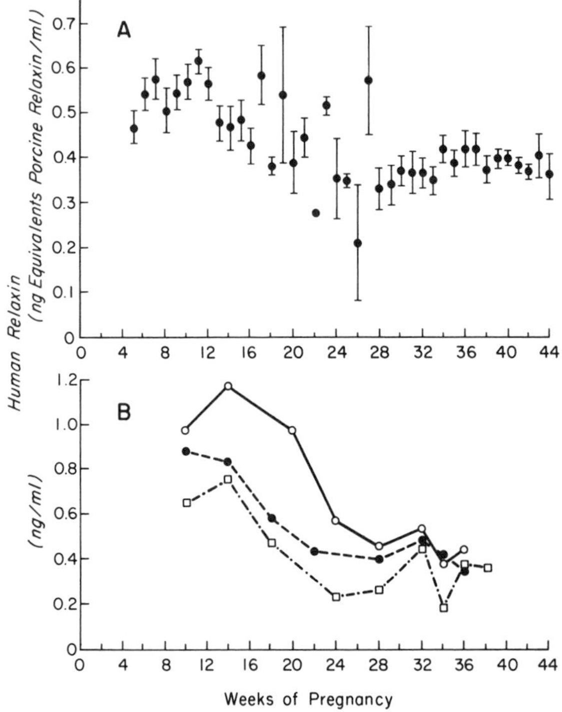

FIG. 31. Relaxin immunoactivity levels in peripheral blood of women throughout pregnancy. **A:** Relaxin levels (± SE) were determined with a homologous porcine relaxin radioimmunoassay which employed rabbit antiporcine relaxin serum R6. Reproduced with permission from O'Byrne et al. (429). **B:** Relaxin levels were determined with a homologous human relaxin radioimmunoassay which employed rabbit antihuman relaxin 2 analogue serum. Reproduced with permission from Eddie et al. (173).

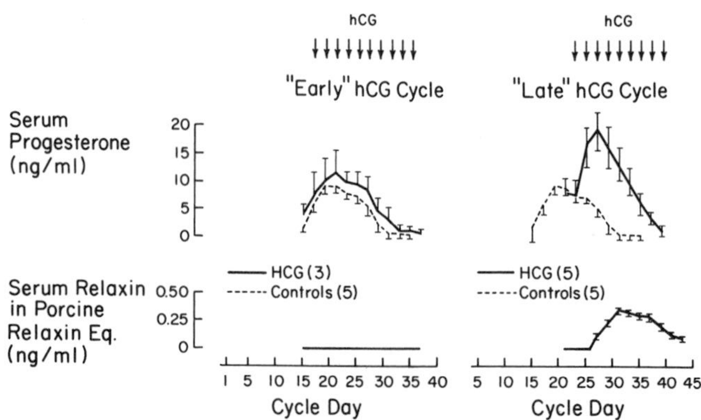

FIG. 32. Mean (± SE) peripheral blood serum progesterone and relaxin levels (± SE) in women injected intramuscularly with 2,500 IU hCG at 2-day intervals commencing 2 to 3 days after presumed ovulation (early hCG cycle) or 8 to 10 days after presumed ovulation (late hCG cycle). Numbers of women per group are in parentheses. Reproduced with permission from Quagliarello et al. (477).

ence of relaxin immunoactivity in fetal blood (182,654). Little if any relaxin immunoactivity was found in umbilical cord serum when the well-characterized rabbit antiporcine relaxin serum R6 was employed (654). The study that reported low levels of relaxin immunoactivity in the milk of lactating women from 3 days until 34 weeks after birth (372) employed antiporcine relaxin serum R6 with a porcine relaxin radioimmunoassay (377). The amnion contains little if any relaxin immunoactivity (654).

Monkeys and Baboons

The major source of relaxin, the profile of relaxin levels in the blood during pregnancy, and the control of relaxin secretion in monkeys (420,441,656) and baboons (104,106) appear similar to those in the human. The corpus luteum of pregnancy is the major source of relaxin. Following bilateral ovariectomy of the monkey *Macaca mulatta* (rhesus monkey) during the first trimester (656), luteectomy of the monkey *Macaca fascicularis* on day 150 (420), and luteectomy of baboons on day 30 (104,106), serum relaxin immunoactivity levels fell abruptly. Serum relaxin immunoactivity levels remain relatively constant in these three primates throughout most of pregnancy, with no evidence of a prelabor surge (104,420,656). As with humans, it appears that chorionic gonadotropin is a major stimulus for the initiation of relaxin secretion during early pregnancy in monkeys and baboons. When monkeys (441) and baboons (104) were administered hCG during the luteal phase of the nonfertile menstrual cycle, there was an increase in serum relaxin levels within a few days of the initiation of hCG treatment. The pattern and concentration of circulating relaxin in rhesus monkeys depend on the age of the corpus luteum at the onset of treatment (441), as in women (477,620). Relaxin levels were detectable within 5 days when hCG treatment was initiated during the late luteal phase, whereas relaxin was not detected for 9 days when hCG treatment was initiated during the early luteal phase (441). Chorionic gonadotropin is not thought to sustain relaxin production throughout pregnancy in monkeys and baboons, since serum chorionic gonadotropin levels are undetectable during late pregnancy in these species (28,104).

There is limited evidence that low levels of relaxin may be produced in nonluteal tissues in monkeys and baboons. Castration of monkeys during pregnancy did not interfere with the loosening of the pelvic ligaments near term (283). On about day 140 of the approximately 175-day gestation period, low levels of relaxin immunoactivity were found in the decidual, placental, and myometrial tissue of baboons in which the corpus luteum had been removed on day 30 (106). Since pregnancy proceeds normally after the first trimester in the absence of the corpus luteum in humans and baboons, Castracane and co-workers (106) suggested that relaxin produced in nonluteal tissue may have a physiological role during late pregnancy and at parturition.

BIOLOGICAL EFFECTS OF RELAXIN IN THE FEMALE VERTEBRATE

It was not possible to establish without doubt the biological effects of relaxin until the late 1970s, when the hormone became available in highly purified form. Nevertheless, the multitude of earlier reports demonstrating that relaxin levels are elevated in the blood and ovaries (or other portions of the reproductive tract) in a variety of mammalian species during pregnancy, coupled with the observations that impure preparations of relaxin affect connective tissue in the pubic symphysis and cervix as well as inhibit contractility of the uterus in estrogen-primed females, led to the view that relaxin was probably of considerable importance during pregnancy and at parturition (86,461,463,531,541,546,582). Recent studies with highly purified relaxin not only confirmed early findings concerning relaxin's effects on the pubic symphysis, cervix, and uterus, but demonstrated that relaxin may influence other reproductive tissues. This section places major emphasis on the effects of relaxin on the well-established target tissues, but it also describes the putative biological effects of relaxin on other reproductive tissues which have received less attention and are not well-established target tissues—the vagina, mammary gland, ovary, amnion, and chorion. It should be recognized that some biological effects of relaxin occur in certain species but not in others; for example, relaxin promotes growth of the interpubic ligament in guinea pigs (1), mice (260), Skomer bank voles (690), and bats (437) but not in rats (133). Other biological effects of relaxin such as its influence on cervical extensibility and uterine contractility appear to be generally distributed among mammals.

Nearly all recent studies of the physiology of relaxin used highly purified porcine relaxin. Since these studies confirmed earlier results obtained with impure porcine relaxin, the degree of purity of the relaxin preparations will be described only where emphasis seems important. Additionally, whenever the effects of relaxin treatment are described, it may be assumed that porcine relaxin was employed unless stated otherwise. Although the structure of porcine relaxin differs substantially from that of rat relaxin and human relaxin, it is bioactive in both of these species. Moreover, porcine relaxin is bioactive in species such as the mouse, guinea pig, sheep, and cow, where the structure of relaxin has not been determined (but probably differs from that of porcine relaxin). It seems likely that biological effects induced by highly purified porcine relaxin in species other than the pig would normally be induced by endogenous relaxin in these species.

Optimally, at least three criteria should be met to establish that relaxin has a biological effect on a putative target tissue during pregnancy. First, the putative target tissue should demonstrate the appropriate biological response following treatment with highly purified relaxin. Second, it should be demonstrated that the putative target tissue possesses finite numbers of high-affinity binding sites that are specific for relaxin. Third, a close temporal association should be demonstrated between the occurrence of the biological effect during pregnancy and elevated levels of relaxin in the blood. All three criteria are seldom met for a putative target tissue in a given species. Attainment of the second criterion has proved to be particularly difficult. Binding of porcine relaxin to putative target tissues such as the pubic symphysis and uterus has not been demonstrated consistently either *in vitro* (117,236,428) or *in vivo* (428); moreover, where binding was reported, the percentage of radioiodinated relaxin bound specifically to putative target tissues was low (117,394, 396,407). The inconsistencies among studies and the low percentage of specific binding may be attributable to (a) the employment of radioiodinated porcine relaxin with tissues from species other than the pig, (b) varying structural modifications of the porcine relaxin which are due to the different procedures used for radioiodination, (c) low numbers of relaxin receptors in target tissues, or (d) binding limitations associated with the method of preparation of the target tissue for *in vitro* studies. It has been difficult to fulfill the third criterion in some cases. The available relaxin bioassays and radioimmunoassays may lack the specificity and/or sensitivity needed to determine relaxin levels in the peripheral blood of some species during pregnancy. In spite of the present limitations associated with characterizing relaxin receptors and measuring blood levels of relaxin in most species, considerable progress has been made in recent years toward a better understanding of the biological effects of relaxin.

Pubic Symphysis

In many species, modifications of the pelvic girdle occur to enable safe delivery of their young. Examples include mammals that employ burrowing or flying for movement and that have streamlined bodies with narrow pelvic girdles or mammals whose fetal/maternal weight ratio is relatively large (461). Passage of young through the birth canal at delivery has been facilitated in many of these species by means of hormonally regulated adaptations of the pelvis. In nearly all mammals, these adaptations involve sexual dimorphism of the bony pelvis as well as increased flexibility of the sacroiliac and/or pelvic symphysis during late pregnancy. An additional adaptation that occurs in some species is transformation of pelvic joint cartilage to an elastic interpubic ligament, which enables considerable separation of the innominate bones.

A sexual dimorphism of the bony pelvis that causes the female to have a larger birth canal than the male has been described in many mammals including mice (131,228), rats (133), rabbits (378), free-tailed bats (138), and humans (132). It was demonstrated that pelvic dimorphism, which generally occurs between birth and puberty, is caused by exposure of the male pelvis to androgens during an early postnatal period. Both male and female mice and rats had female-type pelvises if they were castrated at birth, whereas treatment of both the male and female castrates with androgens led to development of male-type pelvises (45,131). Additionally, humans with testicular feminization syndrome, whose target tissues are insensitive to circulating androgens, have female-type bony pelvises (132). Although the ovary does not appear to influence prepubertal sexual dimorphism of the bony pelvis, it may have postpubertal influences on its structure. In mice, estrogens caused a partial resorption of the medial edges of the pubic bones (228).

Transformation of the pubic joint cartilage to a flexible and elastic interpubic ligament occurs during pregnancy in several species including guinea pigs, mice, bats, and humans (437,581) but not in others, such as rats (133) and sheep (36). In the rat there appears to be little adaptation of the birth canal at delivery. It was reported that the rat pelvis failed to relax during pregnancy (133,613); moreover, injections of estrogen and relaxin promoted little if any increase in flexibility of the pubic symphysis (133).

Growth of the interpubic ligament can enable marked increases in the size of the birth canal. For example, in guinea pigs the length of the interpubic ligament increases so markedly during late pregnancy that a fetus with an average head diameter twice the average diameter of the pelvic canal is delivered (461). Extensive studies of the hormonal regulation of the transformation of the interpubic ligament have been conducted with only guinea pigs and mice, and these studies demonstrated that growth of the interpubic ligament is stimulated primarily by estrogen and relaxin. Although the emphasis of this section will be on the roles estrogen and relaxin play in regulating the formation of the interpubic ligament during pregnancy, effects of other hormones will be described briefly. For additional information concerning development of the bony pelvis and hormonal regulation of the connective tissue of the pubic symphysis, see other reviews (132,215,296,581).

Guinea Pig

Structure of the pubic symphysis during pregnancy. The pubic symphysis of prepubertal male guinea pigs consists almost entirely of an uninterrupted plate of hyaline cartilage which is largely replaced by bone as adulthood is attained. Unlike in the male, the cartilaginous pubic symphysis of the maturing female is gradually replaced by fibrous connective tissue which forms a ligament between the innominate bones (501). Development of the female-type pubic symphysis requires the presence of the ovary. Castration of females soon after birth results in retention of a male-type pubic symphysis which cannot be "relaxed" by estrogen plus relaxin treatment (291). Castration of adult females not only stops the removal of cartilage but also reverses the process and starts a gradual chondrification of the symphyseal tissue (612).

The pubic symphysis of the estrogen-dominated adult female guinea pig consists largely of compact collagen fibers which are imbedded in an amorphous matrix which contains proteoglycans (120,581) (see Fig. 33A). During the last approximately 4 weeks of the 9-week gestation period, transformation of the connective tissue of the pubic symphysis occurs, and this transformation becomes most dramatic during the week before birth. Grossly, there are marked increases in the vascularity (502,613,647), weight (647), and length (647) of the interpubic ligament during the last week of pregnancy (see Fig. 34). Histologically, a rapid proliferation of connective tissue cells and resorption of the symphyseal faces of the pubic bones occur during the last 2 weeks of pregnancy (502).

Influence of hormones on the pubic symphysis. Although the roles hormones play in promoting transformation of the pubic symphysis during pregnancy have not been established, available evidence indicates that estrogen and relaxin are the key hormones. Estrogen alone promotes growth of the interpubic ligament. Prolonged treatment of intact or ovariectomized guinea pigs with estradiol caused about a two- to threefold increase in interpubic distance after 10 to 24 days of treatment (158,614,615,680). This estrogen-induced increase in interpubic ligament length was primarily attributable to proliferation of fibrous connective tissue, resorption of bone, and increased water content (296). Also important is the essential role estrogens play in conditioning the pubic symphysis for a response to relaxin. Whereas relaxin has little (217) or no (291,297) effect on symphyseal connective tissue in guinea pigs that have not been primed with estrogen, it has a marked and rapid effect in estrogen-pretreated animals. When relaxin was administered to castrated adult guinea pigs treated with estrogen for 4 or more days, the transformation of the symphyseal connective tissue was readily detected within 6 to 8 hr (214,297,613,680). The effects of relaxin on the connective tissue of the guinea pig pubic symphysis differ from those of estrogen. Following relaxin treatment, extensive dissolution and disorientation of the collagen fibers occurred (120,612,613), and the pubic symphysis became a bloody, spongy, and highly flexible structure (214) (see Fig. 33B).

There is limited evidence that relaxin brings about its effects by acting directly on the guinea pig pubic symphysis. A time-dependent concentration of radioiodinated porcine relaxin occurred in the pubic symphyses of adult guinea pigs within 90 min of the administration of the hormone (236). Although ambiguity remains concerning the profile of relaxin levels in the peripheral blood of guinea pigs throughout pregnancy (64,432,679), investigators agree that relaxin levels are elevated during late pregnancy, when growth of the interpubic ligament is most marked.

The mechanism(s) whereby relaxin promotes dissolution

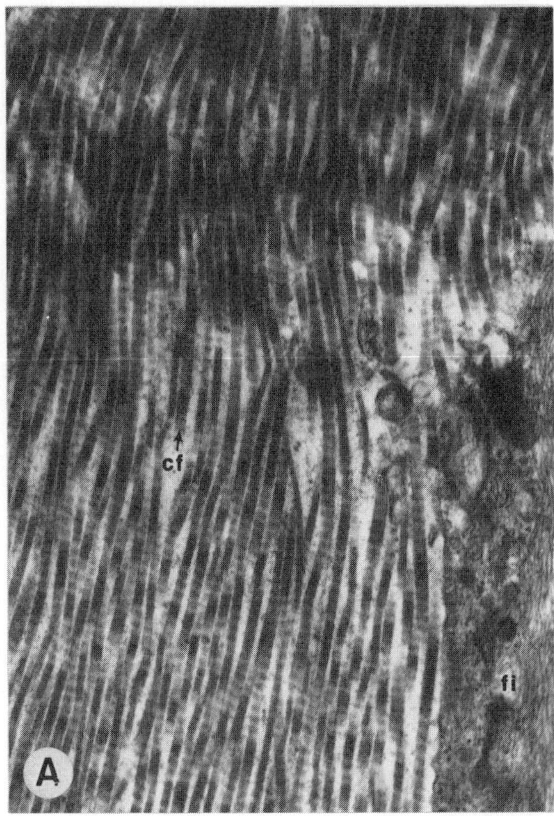

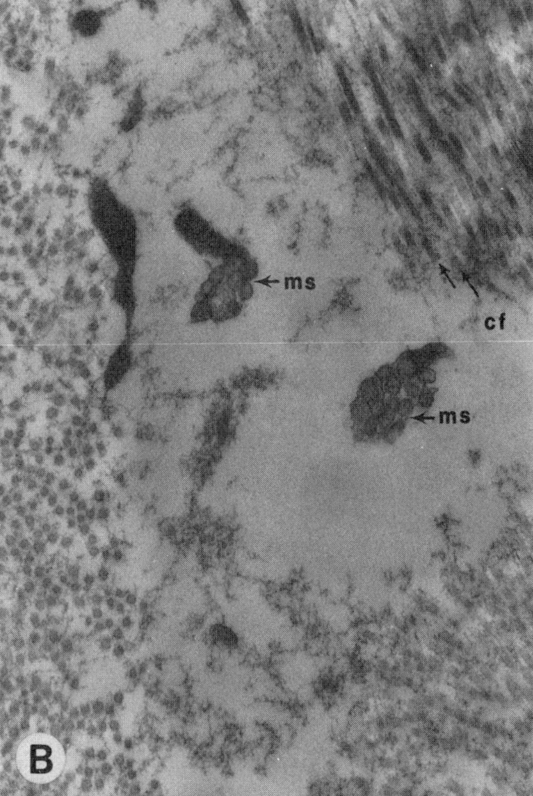

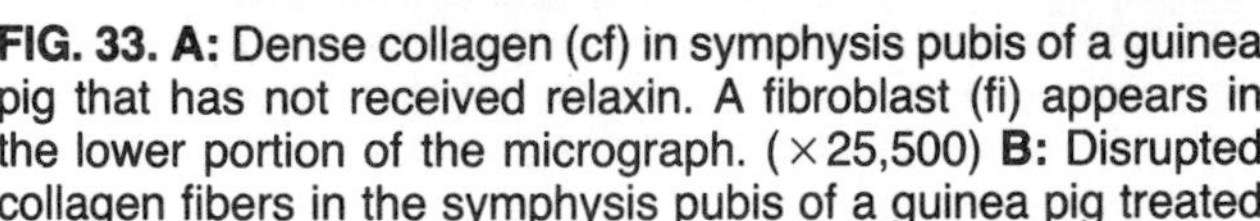
FIG. 33. A: Dense collagen (cf) in symphysis pubis of a guinea pig that has not received relaxin. A fibroblast (fi) appears in the lower portion of the micrograph. (×25,500) **B:** Disrupted collagen fibers in the symphysis pubis of a guinea pig treated with porcine relaxin. Multivesicular structures (ms) are located near sites of collagen digestion. (×23,000.) Reproduced with permission from Chihal and Espey (120).

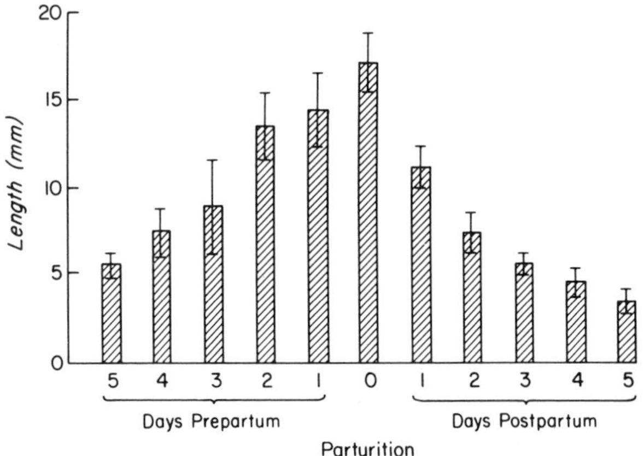

FIG. 34. Mean (± SD; $N = 8$) length of the guinea pig pubic symphysis ligament before and after parturition. Reproduced with permission from Wahl et al. (647).

and disorientation of collagen in the guinea pig pubic symphysis are poorly understood. The cell type(s) that binds relaxin in the guinea pig pubic symphysis have not been determined but it may be the fibroblasts. Chihal and Espey (120) suggested that the collagen breakdown may be caused by a substance released from multivesicular structures which protrude from fibroblasts located near sites of collagen digestion (see Fig. 33B). If this is the case, the substance does not appear to be collagenase. Wahl et al. (647) reported that collagenase levels remained low and that collagen synthesis increased about threefold during the last 5 days of pregnancy in the guinea pig. Another possibility is that relaxin exerts its effects, at least in part, by disaggregating complex proteoglycans within the matrix-ground substance. Perl and Catchpole (452) reported that highly polymerized proteoglycans in unrelaxed estrogen-dominated interpubic ligaments were insoluble in water and had little Evans blue dye associated with them. Following relaxin treatment, however, the proteoglycans became more water-soluble, and Evans blue was found in greatest concentrations in those areas of the symphyses that had been highly polymerized (452). The localization of Evans blue was attributed to both increased availability of active groups on the depolymerized molecules and increased vascular permeability. Electrometric measurements that demonstrated that the charge density of matrix colloid was reduced in relaxin-treated guinea pigs (330) are also consistent with the view that relaxin exerts its effects through disaggregation of negatively charged proteoglycan aggregates. According to this hypothesis the disaggregation of proteoglycans would somehow preclude the ordered arrangement of newly formed collagen into fibrils.

Progesterone also promotes relaxation of the interpubic ligament in guinea pigs. Unlike estrogen and relaxin, however, progesterone acts directly through the stimulation of relaxin secretion by the guinea pig uterus (296).

Mouse

Structure of the pubic symphysis during pregnancy. In adult virgin female mice the articular surfaces of the pubic bones are capped with hyaline cartilage and united by an interpubic disk of fibrocartilage (578) (see Fig. 35A). During the last week of pregnancy, the pubic bones separate (see Fig. 36). This separation of the pubic bones is attributable to resorption of the symphyseal surfaces of the pubic bones, swelling of the cartilaginous matrix, and transformation of the cartilage caps into a fibrous interpubic ligament which attains a maximum length of 3 to 6 mm at parturition (260,270,571,601). Following parturition, the length of the interpubic ligament decreases rapidly and approaches nonpregnant dimensions by day 5 postpartum (132,270,571,601).

Influence of hormones on the pubic symphysis. Although nearly all studies that have been conducted with mice used the species *Mus musculus,* the hormonal regulation of pelvic adaptations appears to be qualitatively similar among dif-

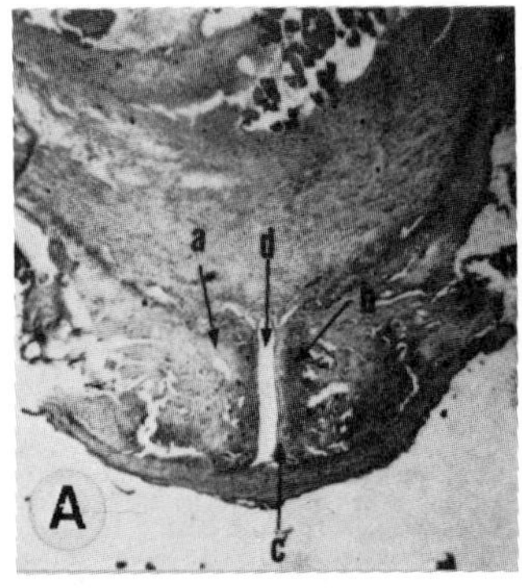

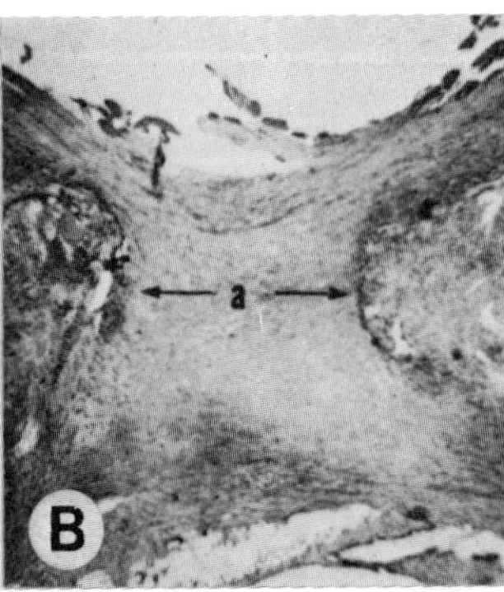

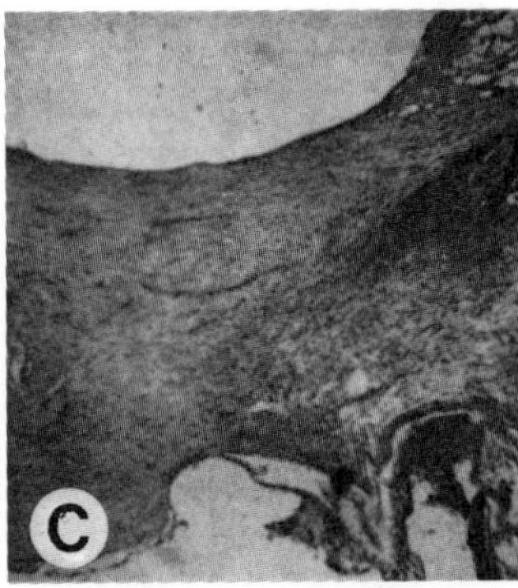

FIG. 35. A: Pubic symphysis of intact untreated control female mouse, demonstrating the articular surfaces of the pubic bones (*a*), capped with hyaline cartilage (*b*), and united by an interpubic disc of fibrocartilage (*c*). Note cleft (*d*). (×40.) **B:** Pubic symphysis of an intact mouse treated with estradiol cyclopentylpropionate. Bone and cartilage resorption occurred in area *a*, with replacement by connective tissue. (×40.) **C:** Pubic symphysis of a hypophysectomized mouse treated with estrogen, relaxin, and growth hormone. The extensive ligament formation is comparable to that found in intact mice treated only with estrogen and relaxin. (×40.) Reproduced with permission from Steinetz et al. (578).

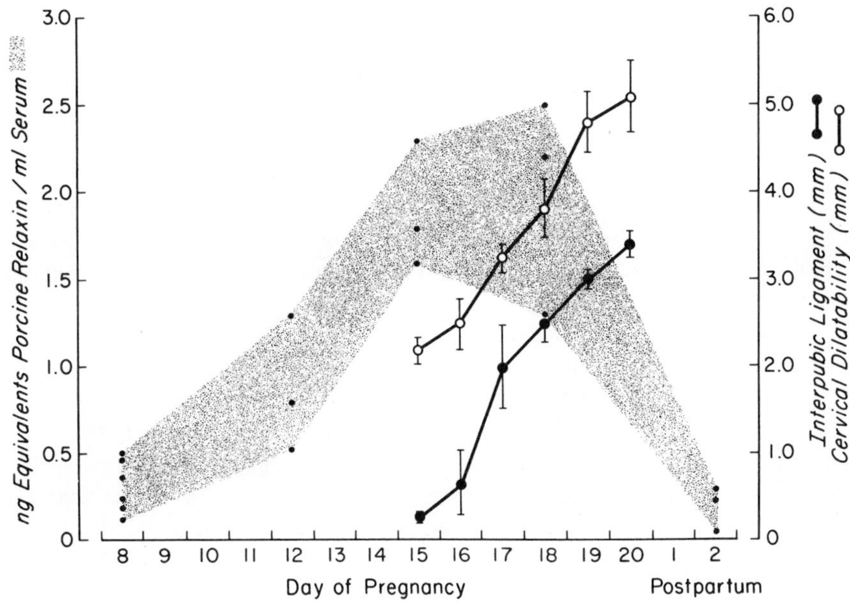

FIG. 36. Range of relaxin immunoactivity levels in sera of pregnant mice as determined with a homologous porcine relaxin radioimmunoassay and normal changes in the interpubic ligament length and cervical dilatability in pregnant mice. Modified and reproduced with permission from O'Byrne and Steinetz (432) and Steinetz et al. (571).

ferent strains and subspecies (650,683). As with guinea pigs, the combination of estrogen and relaxin promotes maximal relaxation of the pubic symphysis. Following the administration of estrogen or relaxin alone to either intact or ovariectomized, nonpregnant mice, the increase in interpubic gap was smaller than that observed during pregnancy or following the administration of estrogen plus relaxin (129,135,228,263,271,578).

Numerous studies have examined the individual and combined effects of estrogen and relaxin on the pubic symphysis in nonpregnant mice. No study, however, has demonstrated directly that relaxin promotes the marked separation of the pubic bones that occurs during late pregnancy in mice. Nevertheless, the three criteria for establishing that relaxin promotes growth of the pubic symphysis in pregnant mice are largely met. First, it was demonstrated that relaxin administration to estrogen-primed mice promotes growth of the interpubic ligament similar to that which occurs during pregnancy (264,271,574,578). Second, it was reported that the mouse pubic symphysis contains binding sites for radioiodinated porcine relaxin (407). Third, a close temporal association was demonstrated between increased pubic ligament length (260,571) and elevated levels of relaxin immunoactivity in the blood during pregnancy (432) (see Fig. 36).

In addition to conditioning the pubic symphysis to become responsive to relaxin (129), estrogen alone brings about initial stages of the transformation of the pubic symphysis (Fig. 35B). Specific actions that have been attributed to estrogen include (a) increased numbers of osteoclasts within the pubic bones (578), (b) resorption of the medial portions of the pubic bones (127,135,228,229,263,264,578,601), (c) breakdown or "depolymerization" of the matrix proteoglycans polymers with a subsequent shift to a colloid-poor, water-rich phase (132,264,578,581,601), (d) increased numbers of chondrocytes within the lacunae of both hyaline cartilage and fibrocartilage (130,578,579), and (e) swelling and transformation of hyaline cartilage caps to fibrocartilage (264,578,601). Steinetz et al. (578,581) postulated that estrogen may bring about its effects on the pubic symphysis, at least in part, by inducing cartilage and bone cells to produce catabolic enzymes that break down bone and matrix components. Following estrogen treatment, the lysosomal enzyme acid phosphatase increased markedly in the pubic joints of ovariectomized mice (577), and histochemical studies demonstrated that acid phosphatase increased in osteoclasts, osteocytes, chondroclasts, and chondrocytes (387). Likewise, the lysosomal proteases cathepsin B and dipeptidyl peptidase I, which have the potential for degrading collagen and proteoglycans, were elevated in mouse pubic symphysis following estrogen treatment (405) (see Fig. 37). Fluorescent histochemical staining indicated that both enzymes were primarily associated with chondrocytes and osteoclasts located along the periphery of the pelvic bones. Dipeptidylpeptidase I appeared to be associated with chondrocytes in the depolymerized cartilage caps and cathepsin B with osteoclastic cells inside the bone (405).

When relaxin is administered to estrogen-primed nonpregnant mice, maximal swelling of the cartilage matrix occurs, there is increased release of fibroblasts and chondrocytes from their lacunae, and extensive growth of the interpubic ligament occurs within 6 to 12 hr (264,578) (see Fig. 35C). Relaxin may bring about its effects, in part, by augmenting estrogen-stimulated processes. Levels of the lysosomal enzymes acid phosphatase, cathepsin B, and dipeptidyl peptidase I, which increase in the pubic symphysis of nonpregnant mice following estrogen treatment, were further elevated when porcine relaxin was administered to estrogen-treated mice (405,577) (see Fig. 37).

There is evidence that relaxin also affects processes that

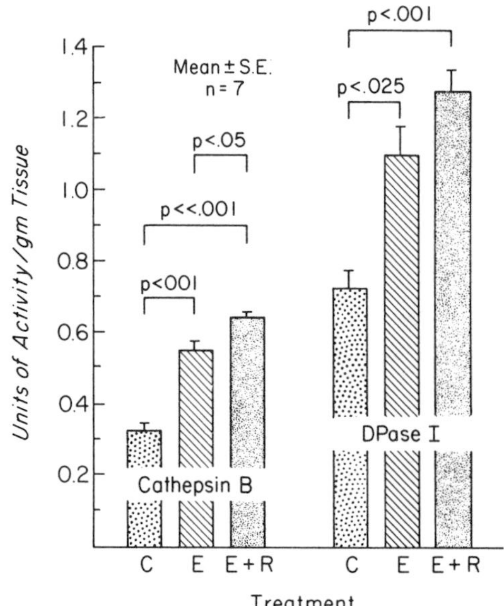

FIG. 37. Levels of the lysosomal proteases cathepsin B and dipeptidyl peptidase I in extracts of pubic symphysis taken from control (C), estrogen (E), and estrogen plus relaxin (E + R)-treated mice. Reproduced with permission from McDonald and Schwabe (405).

are not obviously influenced by estrogen alone. Estrogen plus porcine relaxin, but not estrogen alone, increased wet weight, dry weight, total collagen, and soluble collagen in pubic symphyseal tissue in immature mice (657). In addition, pubic symphyseal collagenase, serum collagen peptidase, and serum peptidase inhibitor levels were elevated following relaxin treatment in these estrogen-primed mice (657). In view of these manifestations of relaxin-induced increases in enzyme activity, Steinetz et al. (581) postulated that relaxin may cause a rapid release of lysosomal enzymes which promote the breakdown of cartilage matrix proteoglycans and also attack collagen bonds in the pubic symphyses of estrogen-primed mice; thus, the lateral forces on the pelvic girdle could pull the pelvic bones apart and give the fibrogelatinous connective tissue joining them the aspects of a ligament.

There are many isolated findings concerning the mechanisms whereby relaxin may act on the mouse pubic symphysis, but the interrelationships and significance of most of these findings as they pertain to growth of the interpubic ligament remain unclear. It is not clear whether the effects of relaxin on the pubic symphysis are mediated by chondrocytes, fibroblasts, or both cell types (379,578). McMurty et al. (406) reported that radioiodinated porcine relaxin bound to fibroblasts cultured from mouse pubic symphysis and that porcine relaxin stimulated growth of the fibroblasts *in vitro*. Braddon (66,67) demonstrated that relaxin promotes an increase in the levels of cAMP and ornithine decarboxylase in mouse pubic symphysis.

The significance of these findings is not clear, but it may be that stimulation of adenylyl cyclase and ornithine decarboxylase are early steps in the mechanism of relaxin's action on the mouse pubic symphysis. Ornithine decarboxylase promotes polyamine synthesis, and it is thought to function in the process of DNA, RNA, and protein synthesis in many hormonally stimulated tissues (66). Accordingly, ornithine decarboxylase may play a role in mediating the effects of relaxin on the mouse pubic symphysis. The mechanism whereby relaxin induces ornithine decarboxylase activity is unknown. Since ornithine decarboxylase activity is promoted by increasing cAMP levels, ornithine decarboxylase elevation in the mouse pubic symphysis following relaxin treatment may be a reflection of relaxin-induced increases in intracellular cAMP. Although estrogen priming is required for relaxin to induce a marked increase in the length of the interpubic ligament in nonpregnant mice (129), it may not be needed for initial steps in relaxin's action. Estrogen is not required for relaxin to bind to mouse pubic symphysis (407) or to increase levels of cAMP (67) and ornithine decarboxylase (66) in the tissue.

Hormones other than estrogen and relaxin influence transformation of the pubic symphysis. Whereas progesterone indirectly promotes growth of the interpubic ligament in guinea pigs by inducing secretion of relaxin from the uterus, it has an inhibitory effect on the growth of the interpubic ligament in estrogen-treated (262,264,271,627) or estrogen plus relaxin–treated nonpregnant mice (577,578,627) as well as in pregnant mice (136,571). Androgens also inhibit the symphyseal response to estrogen and relaxin in mice. Although significant pubic separation was obtained in castrate male mice given estrogen plus relaxin, the response was lower than in castrate females (128); moreover, the longer male mice retained their testes before puberty, the lower the response to hormonal treatment (134,137,274). When large doses of testosterone propionate were administered to mice during the second half of pregnancy, growth of the interpubic ligament was inhibited (230). Thyroid hormone (304,305) and growth hormone (569,578) are required for pubic symphyseal relaxation, and there is evidence that the growth hormone is needed for estrogen to bring about its "priming" effects (569,578).

Essentially nothing is known concerning hormonal control of regression of the interpubic ligament which occurs within 1 week following birth.

Other Species

Primates. Relaxation of pelvic ligaments occurs during the last of the 5½ months of pregnancy in rhesus (*Macaca mulatta*) and bonnet (*Macaca radiata*) monkeys. There is spreading of the sacroiliac joints as well as the pubic symphysis, which increases from less than 2 mm to greater than 10 mm at parturition (283,602). Unlike guinea pigs and mice, in rhesus monkeys prepartum separation of the sacroiliac joints is more pronounced than that of the pubic symphysis. It remains to be established that relaxin plays an important role in the pelvic relaxation that occurs during pregnancy in rhesus monkeys (296,461,581). Little relaxation of the pelvic ligaments occurs until the last month of pregnancy (283), even though serum relaxin levels are elevated throughout nearly all of pregnancy (656). Additionally, removal of the source of relaxin in the rhesus monkey by means of bilateral ovariectomy was reported to have no influence on relaxation of the pelvis (283). Nevertheless, that prolonged treatment with estrogen, progesterone, and porcine relaxin (but not treatment with estrogen plus progesterone) increased flexibility of the pubic joint (292) supports the possibility that relaxin induces pelvic relaxation during late pregnancy in the rhesus monkey.

Relaxation of the pelvic ligaments also occurs during pregnancy in women: The pubic symphysis separates approximately 10 mm before parturition (4,326,621). Reports concerning the possible association of relaxin with this phenomenon are limited and inconclusive. Pubic separation was reported to be detectable by the end of the first month, near maximal by the fifth to the seventh month, and relatively constant during the last 3 months of pregnancy (4,296,621). Thus, pubic separation coincides temporally with the period when relaxin immunoactivity is elevated in the peripheral serum (429,481) (see Fig. 31). Reports concerning the effects of partially purified porcine relaxin on the pubic symphysis in women are not in total agreement. It was reported that partially purified porcine relaxin relieved the pain associated with symphyseolysis during pregnancy in five women (324). When separation of the pubic symphysis was determined with the aid of X-rays, one laboratory reported that impure porcine relaxin promoted separation of the pubic symphysis in 80% of the women (151), whereas two other laboratories reported that porcine relaxin had no effect on the separation of the pubic symphysis (561,651).

Cow. In cattle, the ratio of fetal birth weight to maternal weight is high (about 11%), and the pelvic canal expands rapidly during the last 4 days of pregnancy to facilitate birth of the relatively large calf (487). Although little is known concerning secretion of relaxin in the cow, there is reason to suspect that it may influence the pelvic canal during late pregnancy. Elevation of the tail head (or "springing") is a recognized prepartum sign in cattle, and Anderson and coworkers (402,403,451) have obtained evidence that relaxin is probably implicated in that process. When 1 mg of highly purified porcine relaxin was placed in the cervical os of cattle 6 to 8 days before anticipated parturition, there was a rapid increase in pelvic height and width. Anderson and co-workers (402,403,451) interpreted these observations to mean that relaxin may loosen the pelvic joints, and particularly the sacroiliac articulations, during late pregnancy in cattle.

Cervix

Throughout most of pregnancy in mammals, the cervix increases in size but remains a relatively firm and inextensible structure, which not only protects the conceptuses from the external environment but also impedes premature delivery of the fetus. During late pregnancy, however, the consistency of the cervix changes strikingly, and it dilates rapidly in response to the uterine contractions that bring about delivery of the fetus. The term "softens" is commonly employed to refer to the changes in the tensile properties of the wall of the cervix that occur during late pregnancy. There is increased strain (increase in length divided by the original length) per unit of force, which is generally referred to as *distensibility*. During late pregnancy the cervical distensibility becomes a time-dependent process; that is to say, deformation of the tissue (strain) increases with time when a constant force (stress) is placed on the cervix (278,299). This slow deformation of the tissue under constant stress is referred to as cervical *creep* or *extensibility* (276,279). Histological studies demonstrated that the cervix contains some smooth muscle cells, but its tensile properties are largely attributable to the connective tissue, which predominates. In the firm cervix, collagen fibrils are arranged in dense parallel bands with little of the matrix, which is rich in proteoglycans, separating the collage fibrils. In the soft cervix, however, the collagen fibrils are dispersed and randomly oriented within a considerably increased matrix.

A variety of methods have been used to measure cervical tensile properties (144,299). Cervical *dilatability* has generally been measured *in vivo* by inserting conical rods (probes or sounds) of different diameters into the cervix with a constant force until a diameter is recorded where a consistent resistance is encountered. An important limitation to this method is that it does not differentiate changes that occur in the internal diameter of the cervix from changes in the compliance of the cervical wall. Cervical *distensibility* has been determined *in vitro* by a variety of stress-strain measurements. Generally, the entire cervix (or a transverse section thereof) is suspended in a buffer bath and subjected to a progressively increasing load, and the increase in the inner circumference of the cervix (strain) against load (stress or tension) is plotted. Alternatively, the circumference of the cervix is increased (strain), and the tension (stress) produced within the tissue is measured with a strain gauge transducer. Cervical *creep* or *extensibility* is generally measured by subjecting the cervix to a constant load over time and measuring the rate of increase of the internal circumference of the cervix.

This section describes studies that provide convincing evidence that relaxin plays a major role in promoting the cervical modifications that occur during late pregnancy in many mammalian species. Although there is considerable evidence that estrogen and prostaglandins also influence the tensile properties, morphology, and biochemical composition of the cervix (180,408,541), little is known concerning the mechanism(s) whereby relaxin interacts with these hormones to promote cervical softening. Accordingly, in the following account of the influence of relaxin on the cervix of individual species, little mention will be made of the effects of these hormones. It should be appreciated, however, that relaxin's effects on the cervix (like the pubic symphysis) are heavily dependent on estrogen-priming. This section presents most information according to individual species. The changes that occur in both the tensile properties and biochemical composition of the cervix during pregnancy as well as the influence of relaxin on these changes are described. The influence of relaxin on cervical softening appears to be a general phenomenon among mammalian species. Accordingly, the review of the literature concerning the mechanism of action of relaxin on the cervix combines information obtained from a variety of species to avoid redundancy and also to enable a comprehensive description of this topic in one section. The reader is referred to reviews concerning the influence of relaxin on the cervix for additional coverage of this topic (299,463,541,580,582).

Domestic Species

Pig. The three lines of evidence needed to support the view that relaxin acts directly on the pig cervix to promote the changes in its tensile properties that occur during late pregnancy appear to be met. First, partially purified porcine relaxin was demonstrated to increase cervical dilatation in both nonpregnant and pregnant pigs when examined *in vivo* with cervical rods. In the mid-1950s, Zarrow et al. (686,689) reported that three daily intramuscular injections of porcine relaxin (approximately 5 mg per day) for 4 days to ovariectomized, estrogen-primed sows caused a dilatation of the cervix which was accompanied by an increase in water content and depolymerization of cervical glycoproteins. More recently, Kertiles and Anderson (343) reported that daily intramuscular injections of partially purified porcine relaxin (approximately 250 μg relaxin) beginning on day 105 or day 107 increased cervical dilatation in pigs that were luteectomized on day 110. Second, there is evidence that pig cervical tissue contains relaxin receptors. Cervical particulate membrane preparations obtained from gonadotropin-primed prepubertal or cycling pigs were reported to bind ^{125}I-labeled highly purified porcine relaxin with the characteristics of a hormone-receptor interaction (396). Third, there is a good temporal association between the time of occurrence of the antepartum elevation of serum relaxin levels and increased cervical dilatation (see Fig. 38). This figure also illustrates that plasma levels of estrogen and $PGF_{2\alpha}$, two hormones that may interact with relaxin to influence cervical function, are also elevated near parturition.

Cow. There are reasons to suspect that relaxin influences cervical softening in the cow. In cattle, dilatation of the cervix increases strikingly during late pregnancy—about 100-fold during the 3 days before birth (451). In the early 1950s Graham and Dracy (253,254) discovered the influence of relaxin on cervical consistency in studies with nonpregnant cycling cattle. Aware of relaxin's effects on the pubic symphysis, these workers explored its use as a means of dilating the cervix for ova recovery. Employing a mechanical instrument for *in vivo* determination of cervical dilatability, they found that cervical dilatation increased within 12 hr of the injection of porcine relaxin into diethylstilbestrol-primed cattle on day 5 postestrus, whereas the cervix remained undilated in estrogen-primed controls (254). Within a year the ability of porcine relaxin to promote cervical dilatation in cattle was confirmed by Zarrow and co-workers (689), who employed ovariectomized, estrogen-primed heifers. Progesterone does not appear to inhibit relaxin-promoted cervical distensibility in cattle. When porcine relaxin was administered to nonpregnant cattle pretreated with both estrogen and progesterone, cervical dilatation occurred, and, histologically, the tissue resembled the natural condition at parturition (175). More recently, the effects of highly purified porcine relaxin on cervical dilatation in pregnant cattle were examined *in vivo* with a cervical probe (402,403,451). Anderson and co-workers (402,403,451) reported that when porcine relaxin was placed in the cervical os on day 276 or day 278, about 5 to 7 days before anticipated birth, a premature increase in dilatation of the cervix occurred within 8 to 12 hr of relaxin administration. Although the above data support the possibility that relaxin plays a key role in promoting cervical dilatation during pregnancy in the cow, the lack of knowledge concerning the physiology of relaxin in the cow precludes this conclusion.

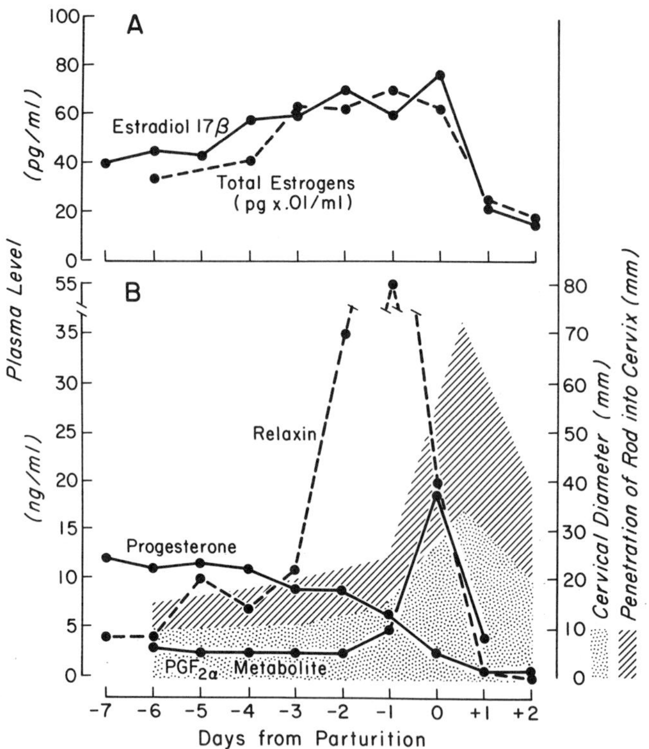

FIG. 38. Cervical diameter (343), cervical dilatation (343), and peripheral blood plasma levels of relaxin (543), progesterone (399), $PGF_{2\alpha}$ metabolite (411), estradiol 17-β (399), and total estrogens (32) near parturition in the pig. Reproduced with permission from Sherwood (541).

Sheep. In the sheep there is normally a striking increase in the compliance of the cervix at parturition (605). Failure of this process to occur in parturient ewes is called ringwomb or cervical dystocia, and the condition is of clinical interest. There is evidence that increased cervical compliance at parturition is hormone-dependent but independent of uterine contractility (605). Several studies demonstrated that prostaglandins (206,365) and estrogens (206,605,606) promote cervical softening, but the effects of relaxin on the cervix of sheep remain essentially unknown. It was reported that relaxin did not influence the depth to which an inseminating pipette could be inserted into the cervical canal 12 or 24 hr following intramuscular injection of partially purified porcine relaxin into nonpregnant ewes at estrus (504). This brief study provided little if any insight concerning the possibility that relaxin influences cervical consistency in sheep. Additionally, correlations between cervical softening and serum relaxin levels cannot be examined, since the levels of relaxin in the serum of pregnant sheep remain to be established (87,268,485).

Laboratory Species

Rat. Structural Changes in the Cervix that Occur During Pregnancy: Cervical tensile properties during pregnancy as well as the influence of relaxin on these properties have been studied most extensively in the rat. Moreover, the elegant studies of the Harknesses and their co-workers (144,275,276,278,279) in the 1950s and early 1960s not only contributed greatly to an understanding of cervical modifications in the pregnant rat but also provided reliable *in vitro* methods whereby cervical tensile properties could be measured in any species. In the rat both the size and tensile properties of the cervix change markedly during pregnancy (276,279,302,572). The inner circumference of the cervix increases approximately fivefold to be equivalent to the circumference of the fetal head at birth (302). This increase in inner circumference is attributable to both rapid cervical growth and a marked increase in cervical creep rate (279). The changes in size and tensile properties of the cervix occur during the second half of pregnancy (276,279,299,572) (see Fig. 39A). Cervical wet weight (276,302,499,691) and the inner circumference of the cervix (279) increase from about day 13 until parturition. Likewise, cervical softening increases progressively during this period, as determined by increased cervical dilatability (356,572,630,691), distensibility (499) and extensibility (279,302), and decreased cervical tensile strength (170,691). Cervical softening is a two-stage process in the rat. The first stage begins on about day 14 and increases progressively until the last day of pregnancy, when a second and more rapid stage occurs during the 3 hr before birth (279,299,300) (see Fig. 39A). During the 24 hr following parturition, a rapid reduction in cervical creep rate (276,302) and an increase in cervical tensile strength (691) occur (Fig. 39A). Hollingsworth and Gallimore (300) provided evidence that

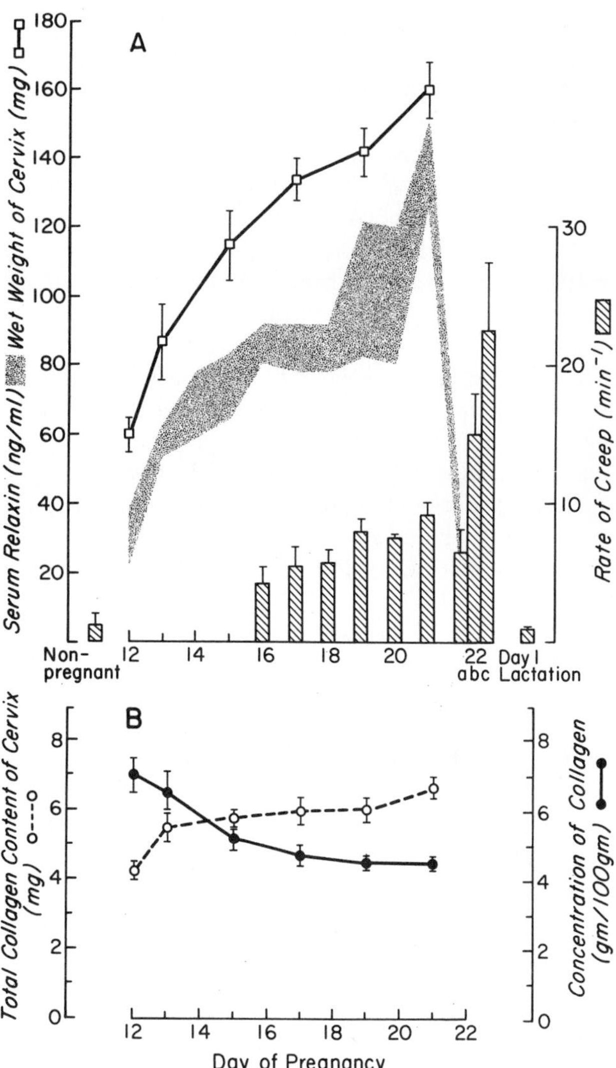

FIG. 39. Cervical changes and peripheral blood serum relaxin levels during the second half of pregnancy in the rat. **A:** Weight of the cervix in pregnant rats. Rate of creep of the cervix of nonpregnant, pregnant, and postpartum lactating rats. Day 22 rats were killed (*a*) at the onset of nesting behavior, (*b*) 10 min after the onset of continuous uterine contractility, and (*c*) 60 min after the onset of continuous uterine contractility. Serum relaxin levels in rats that gave birth on day 22. Modified and reproduced with permission from Harkness and Harkness (276), Hollingsworth (299), and Sherwood et al. (545). **B:** Total collagen content and collagen concentration of the cervix during pregnancy in rats. Reproduced with permission from Harkness and Harkness (276).

the first stage and, perhaps, the second stage of cervical softening are hormone-dependent and not dependent upon uterine contractility. Cervical softening occurred normally during the second half of pregnancy in rats in which the cervix was separated surgically from the uterine horns on day 11 (300).

Influence of Hormones on Growth of the Cervix: Maximal growth of the cervix in rats requires the combined effects of estrogen and relaxin. Administration of estrogen alone increased cervical wet weight in ovariectomized nonpregnant rats (144,356,503,691), but cervical weight was greater following combined treatment with estrogen plus porcine relaxin (144,356,691). The influence of relaxin on cervical growth is estrogen-dependent. There was little if any increase in cervical weight following treatment of ovariectomized nonpregnant rats with relaxin only (144,356,503). Progesterone has little influence on cervical weight in rats (144,356). There is also evidence that relaxin promotes cervical growth in pregnant rats (170,572). When pregnant rats were ovariectomized on day 9 and given replacement therapy throughout the remainder of pregnancy with progesterone plus estrogen in doses selected to mimic physiological levels, cervical wet weight was much lower than that of intact controls on days 18 and 22, whereas when similarly ovariectomized pregnant rats were given replacement therapy with progesterone, estrogen, and highly purified porcine relaxin, cervical wet weight did not differ from intact controls (170).

Influence of Hormones on Softening of the Cervix: Cervical softening also appears to be dependent on the combined effects of estrogen and relaxin. Whereas estrogen alone promoted *growth* of the cervix, administration of either estrogen or porcine relaxin alone to ovariectomized nonpregnant rats had little effect on cervical *softening* (144,356,691). When porcine or rat relaxin was administered to ovariectomized nonpregnant rats pretreated with estrogen (or estrogen plus progesterone), there was marked cervical softening, as judged by increased cervical dilatability (356,691), increased cervical extensibility (144), and decreased tensile strength (69,144,691). Similarly, replacement therapy with progesterone, estrogen, and relaxin was much more effective than replacement therapy with progesterone and estrogen in promoting cervical softening in rats ovariectomized during the second half of pregnancy (169,302,356,572,691). Downing and Sherwood (169) reported that when pregnant rats were ovariectomized on day 9 and given replacement therapy with progesterone and estrogen, cervical tension following extension was much greater than that of intact controls on days 18 and 22 (see Fig. 40). When the ovariectomized rats were given replacement therapy with progesterone, estrogen, and highly purified porcine relaxin, however, cervical tension following extension was similar to that of intact control pregnant rats (169).

As with cervical growth, progesterone does not appear to play a major role in promoting cervical softening in rats. The cervices of ovariectomized nonpregnant rats remained inextensible following the administration of progesterone or progesterone plus porcine relaxin (144,356). In contrast, Downing and Sherwood (169) found that cervices in ovariectomized pregnant rats that received replacement therapy with progesterone plus relaxin from day 9 were nearly as extensible on days 18 and 22 as those from ovariectomized pregnant rats that received replacement therapy with progesterone, estrogen, and relaxin (Fig. 40). This observation may not indicate that progesterone influences cervical softening in the pregnant rat. It may be that peripheral aromatization of the high levels of androgens secreted by the placentas during the second half of pregnancy (318,566) provide systemic estrogen levels sufficient to act in combination with relaxin to promote cervical softening.

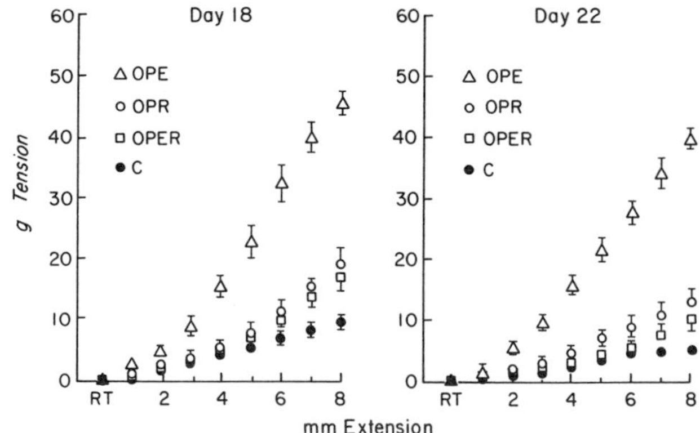

FIG. 40. Mean tension (± SE; *N* = 10 or 11) at extension in cervices from day 18 and day 22 pregnant rats. Rats were sham-ovariectomized on day 9 (C) or ovariectomized and treated with progesterone and estrogen (OPE), progesterone and highly purified porcine relaxin (OPR), or progesterone, estrogen, and relaxin (OPER). Reproduced with permission from Downing and Sherwood (169).

Prostaglandins may be associated with cervical softening in the pregnant rat. Cervical softening increased dramatically within 24 hr following the administration of PGE_2, $PGF_{2\alpha}$, or the $PGF_{2\alpha}$ analog fluprostenol to intact rats on day 18 (301,666). When pregnant rats were ovariectomized on day 16 (pregnancy was maintained by replacement therapy with progesterone and estrogen), administration of PGE_2 on day 18 promoted increased cervical extensibility by day 19, but administration of $PGF_{2\alpha}$ or fluprostenol on day 18 did not (301,666). These workers (301,666) concluded that PGE_2 may act directly on the cervix, whereas $PGF_{2\alpha}$ and fluprostenol may promote cervical softening indirectly through the ovaries by promoting luteolysis. In addition to a rapid and sustained drop in progesterone levels (91), a rapid, but transient (less than 2 hr), surge in serum relaxin immunoactivity levels occurs following the administration of $PGF_{2\alpha}$ during late pregnancy (250). Hollingsworth et al. (301) hypothesized that $PGF_{2\alpha}$-induced cervical softening might be attributable to both the decline in progesterone levels and the release of relaxin. The failure of Williams et al. (666) to observe elevated serum relaxin immunoactivity levels following fluprostenol administration on day 18 may be attributable to the long interval (≥14 hr) between administration of the $PGF_{2\alpha}$ analog and collection of the serum. The observation that indomethacin, a prostaglandin synthesis inhibitor, blocked the ability of relaxin to dilate the cervix of estrogen-primed nonpregnant rats (341,342) is consistent with the view that prostaglandins may be associated with relaxin-induced cervical softening in the rat.

Biochemical Changes that Occur in the Cervix During

Pregnancy: Studies have been conducted to gain a better understanding of the changes in the biochemical composition of the rat cervix that might be associated with the increased growth and extensibility that occur during pregnancy. Cervical water content (356,572,665,691), collagen content (97,170,243,276,665,691), and collagen solubility (170,288) increase during the second half of pregnancy, whereas cervical collagen concentration decreases (97,170, 243,276,288,499,665,691) (see Fig. 39B). Increased synthesis of matrix proteoglycans also occurs in the rat cervix during the second half of pregnancy (see Fig. 41). The combined concentration of the three primary glycosaminoglycans dermatan sulfate, hyaluronic acid, and heparan sulfate is unchanged, but there are changes in the concentrations of individual glycosaminoglycans. During late pregnancy the cervical concentration of hyaluronic acid increases markedly (97,170,243), and that of dermatan sulfate may decrease somewhat (97,243).

Influence of Hormones on the Biochemical Changes that Occur in the Cervix: Although estrogen alone has been shown to increase the water and collagen content of the cervix (144,691), studies with both ovariectomized nonpregnant rats and ovariectomized pregnant rats make it seem likely that relaxin normally plays a major role in promoting several of the changes in the biochemical composition of the cervix that occur during the second half of pregnancy. Early studies with ovariectomized estrogen-treated nonpregnant rats showed that cervical water (356,691) and collagen (144) content increased whereas cervical collagen concentration decreased (144,691) following administration of partially purified porcine relaxin. Similar results were obtained with pregnant rats. When pregnant rats were ovariectomized on day 9 and given replacement therapy throughout the remainder of pregnancy with progesterone and estrogen, cervical collagen and glycosaminoglycans parameters had not changed by day 22; that is, they resembled those of day 9 intact control rats (see Fig. 41). When similarly ovariectomized pregnant rats were administered progesterone, estrogen, and highly purified porcine relaxin, however, cervical collagen concentrations were reduced, and cervical collagen solubility was increased by day 22 to levels comparable to those of day 22 intact controls. Similarly, relaxin treatment increased glycosaminoglycans contents to levels as high as those of day 22 controls (170) (Fig. 41).

The three lines of evidence required to support the view that relaxin promotes cervical softening in the pregnant rat are largely met. First, the administration of porcine relaxin to ovariectomized pregnant rats promotes changes in the tensile properties and biochemical components of the cervix that are similar to those that occur in intact rats during late pregnancy (see Figs. 40 and 41). Second, apparent receptors for relaxin have been reported in the rat cervix (658). Finally, cervical softening occurs between day 14 and parturition in pregnant rats (279,299,572,630), when relaxin levels are elevated (545) (see Fig. 39).

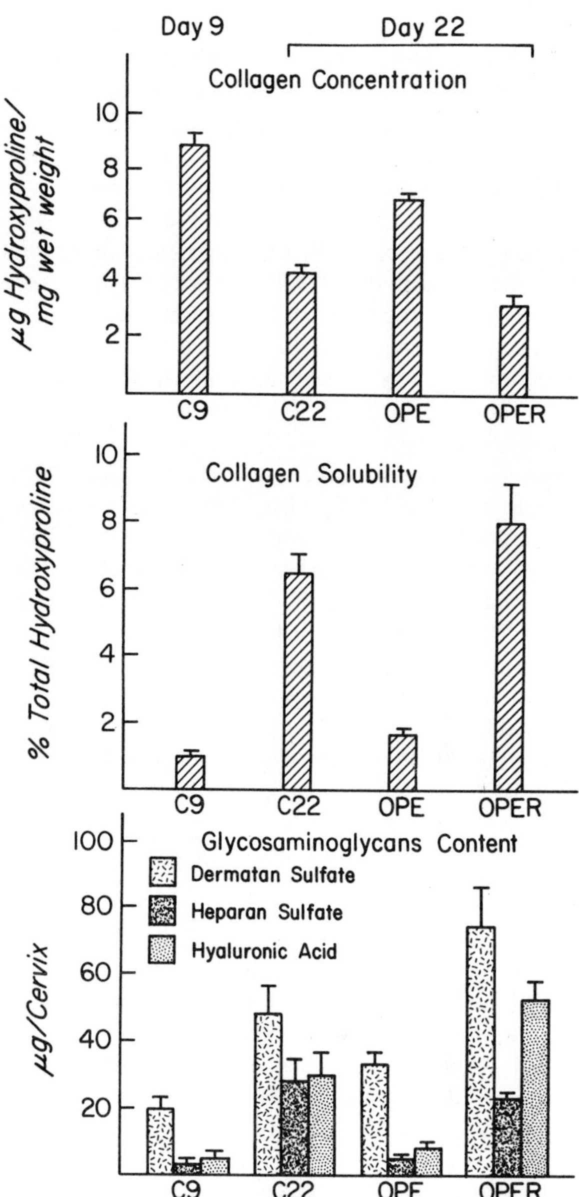

FIG. 41. Mean (+ SE) collagen concentration, collagen solubility, and glycosaminoglycans content in day 9 intact control rats (C9), day 22 intact control rats (C22), day 22 ovariectomized rats treated with progesterone and estrogen (OPE), and day 22 ovariectomized rats treated with progesterone, estrogen, and highly purified porcine relaxin (OPER). Reproduced with permission from Downing and Sherwood (170).

Mouse. Available data indicate that cervical softening and its hormonal control in the mouse are similar to those in the rat. The wet weight and dilatation of the mouse cervix increase throughout most of the second half of pregnancy, with the most pronounced increases occurring during the last 4 or 5 days before birth (366,488,571), when serum relaxin levels are maximal (432) (see Fig. 36). When porcine relaxin was administered to ovariectomized estrogen-primed mice, it synergized with the estrogen to promote maximal cervical growth and cervical dilatation (356,366). Consistent with these findings, a single injection of highly purified porcine relaxin increased cervical extensibility in intact estrogen-primed mice (203). Moreover, the response was rapid—it occurred within 24 hr (203). Biochemical studies of the mouse cervix demonstrated that the total collagen content increases, but the collagen concentration decreases, during the second half of pregnancy (488). The influence of relaxin on the biochemical composition of the mouse cervix has not been described.

Hamster. A close temporal association was reported between elevated serum relaxin levels and increased cervical dilatability during the second half of pregnancy in hamsters (432). The effects of relaxin on the hamster cervix have not been described.

Rabbit. MacLennan et al. (384) recently compared the effects of relaxin and $PGF_{2\alpha}$ on the cervix in pregnant rabbits in an effort to gain insight concerning their mechanism(s) of action. Either highly purified porcine relaxin or $PGF_{2\alpha}$ was mixed in a cellulose gel and administered intravaginally on day 27. Within 15 hr each hormone induced cervical growth and cervical softening; moreover, the histological changes in the cervix produced by the two hormones were comparable to those seen in the cervix of control rabbits in labor on day 30 (384). These workers concluded that relaxin and $PGF_{2\alpha}$ may bring about identical effects in cervical connective tissue rather than act in parallel to produce separate or complementary structural changes (384).

Human

Changes that occur in the cervix during pregnancy. Knowledge concerning the role of relaxin on cervical softening in primates is limited. The only primate in which cervical softening has been studied is the human. Data concerning cervical softening in the human are necessarily fragmentary, since cervical tensile properties must be determined *in vivo,* and analysis of cervical biochemistry is restricted to the use of small tissue samplings. Nevertheless, it appears that changes occurring in the tensile properties and biochemical composition of the human cervix during pregnancy are similar to those that occur in rats and mice. It was reported that cervical consistency decreases progressively from early pregnancy until delivery (30), whereas cervical dilatation progresses slowly from about 1 month before birth until the last few hours of pregnancy when, along with cervical effacement, it occurs rapidly (224). Cervical water content is higher (150,629), collagen concentration is lower (150,629), and collagen solubility in acetic acid is higher (316,629) in cervical tissue obtained at delivery than in tissue obtained during early pregnancy or prepregnancy. Data concerning the glycosaminoglycans composition of the human cervix during pregnancy is limited. It was reported that the total glycosaminoglycans content increases during late pregnancy (150,385) and that there is a decline in the concentrations of sulfated glycosaminoglycans including dermatan sulfate, chondroitin-4-sulfate, and chondroitin-6-sulfate (385,629).

Influence of hormones on the changes that occur in the cervix. Regulation of cervical softening in the human is complex, since several factors, including estrogens, prostaglandins, relaxin, oxytocin, catecholamines, progesterone, and uterine contractions, may be involved (98,207,287,345,368,381,383) (see Fig. 42). At the present time it is not established that relaxin plays a major role in this process in the human. It is known that relaxin levels are elevated when cervical softening occurs, since serum relaxin levels are elevated throughout pregnancy (173,429). The results of early efforts to determine the effects of impure porcine relaxin on cervical softening in the human were inconsistent. In one study, where a large dose of porcine relaxin (18,000 GPU) was administered intravenously to 16 nonpregnant women during a stage in the menstrual cycle when estrogen levels were elevated, no increase in the diameter of the internal cervical os was observed with cervical rods within 24 hr (562). Two other studies of the influence of exogenously administered impure porcine relaxin on the human cervix were clinical efforts to prepare the cervix for labor in patients who required delivery but had an inextensible (unripe) cervix (174,600), and in both cases cervical softening was reported to occur within 24 hr of parenteral administration of relaxin. However, like the study in nonpregnant women (562), these studies (174,600) were compromised not only by the impurity of the porcine relaxin preparations but also by the subjective methods used for determining cervical softening.

More recent studies, which administered highly purified porcine relaxin locally to prepare the cervix for labor induction, strengthened the view that relaxin may induce cervical softening in women. MacLennan et al. (382) conducted one double-blind study in which 2 mg of highly purified porcine relaxin was mixed in a cellulose gel and placed in the posterior vaginal fornix the evening before the surgical induction of labor. Compared to controls, the relaxin-treated group had a greater number of patients with improved cervical score; furthermore, fewer relaxin-treated women required augmentation in labor with oxytocin. In

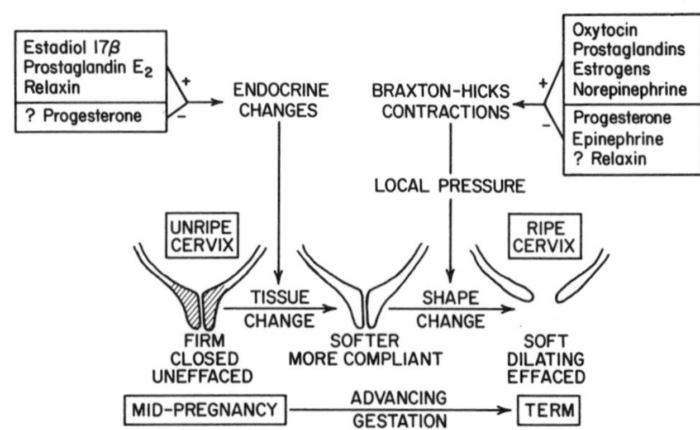

FIG. 42. Schematic representation of factors that may control cervical ripening in the human. Plus signs indicate stimulation; minus signs, inhibition. Modified and reproduced with permission from Calder (98).

that study, 10 of the 30 relaxin-treated patients, but none of the 30 control patients, spontaneously entered labor between treatment and the proposed time of induction of labor (382). In a second double-blind study, Evans et al. (189) incorporated 2 or 4 mg of highly purified porcine relaxin into polyethylene glycol pellets which were inserted as a suppository into the cervical canal at the time of the initiation of oxytocin-induced labor. Compared to controls, the relaxin-treated groups had a faster rate of both cervical effacement and dilatation as well as a shorter interval from the initiation of labor induction to delivery. In an outpatient study in which 2 or 4 mg of highly purified porcine relaxin was similarly placed in the cervical canal, 2 mg of relaxin induced greater cervical changes than the placebo control, but, for unknown reasons, 4 mg of relaxin did not (189). Although these studies provide some encouragement for the prospect that relaxin may have clinical utility, the known differences in the structure of human and porcine relaxin make it advisable to await the availability of human relaxin before conducting extensive experiments in women. The use of human relaxin in women may not only increase the efficacy of treatment but also reduce the risk of inducing the formation of relaxin antibodies.

Mechanism of Action of Relaxin on the Cervix

The early events whereby relaxin promotes cervical softening remain poorly understood. Three lines of evidence indicate that relaxin acts directly on cervical tissue. First, finite numbers of high-affinity binding sites for radioiodinated porcine relaxin were reported in cervical tissue of the pig (396), guinea pig (236,407), and rat (658). Second, levels of cyclic AMP increased in rat, pig, and human cervical tissue following *in vitro* incubation with porcine relaxin (117,331,424,506). Third, highly purified porcine relaxin inhibited ^{3}H-proline incorporation into human cervical tissue under *in vitro* incubation conditions (667). The first two lines of evidence must be interpreted with caution, since they may reflect the interaction of relaxin with smooth muscle cells, which generally comprise about 10% to 15% of cervical tissue, rather than with a cervical cell, which influences connective tissue composition. It is known that relaxin promotes increased cAMP levels in rat and pig uterine strips (117,331,506) or rat myometrial cells (306). Moreover, highly purified porcine relaxin was reported to inhibit smooth muscle cell activity in human cervical tissue *in vitro* (423). The target cells for relaxin that influence cervical connective tissue metabolism have not been identified with certainty, but they may be fibroblasts. There is limited evidence that the estrogen dependence of relaxin's effects on cervical softening may be mediated through fibroblasts. Leppi and Kinnison (367) demonstrated at the ultrastructural level that estrogen activates mouse cervical fibroblasts. Estrogen may prepare the fibroblasts for relaxin by inducing the synthesis of relaxin receptors or other molecules required for relaxin's effects.

Dramatic remodeling of the connective tissue framework of the cervix occurs during pregnancy, and the general features of the ultrastructural changes appear to be similar among those species in which they have been examined (150,367,384,446). Leppi and Kinnison (367) reported that the ultrastructural changes that occurred in the connective tissue of the mouse cervix following treatment with estrogen and relaxin were similar to those that occur during pregnancy. The cervix in control mice consisted of a compact array of interlacing collagenous fiber bundles interspersed with fibroblasts that contained little cytoplasm and appeared inactive (see Fig. 43A). Following treatment with estrogen or estrogen plus porcine relaxin, the collagen bundles were smaller and more widely scattered in the extracellular matrix, which contained the polyanionic sulfated glycosaminoglycans (Fig. 43B). The fibroblasts, which are thought to secrete the extracellular proteoglycans and collagen molecules, became more active in appearance and had an abundance of rough endoplasmic reticulum (Fig. 43C). MacLennan et al. (384) reported a similar dissolution of collagen fiber bundles and increase in extracellular matrix following the administration of highly purified porcine relaxin to rabbits during late pregnancy.

The molecular events that account for the changes in the tensile properties of the cervix are thought to involve changes that occur in both the collagen and proteoglycans components of the cervical connective tissue. The increased solubility of collagen, which occurs during pregnancy (170,288,316,629) or following relaxin treatment (170), may reflect increased collagen metabolism and/or that the collagen is present in smaller fibril bundles (170). The greater separation, reduction in size, and more random orientation of the collagen fibril bundles in the cervix may allow the fibrils to be pulled past one another so that the tissue becomes sufficiently pliable to permit the dilatation required at birth. Ideas concerning the mechanism(s) whereby increased cervical glycosaminoglycans influence the remodeling and tensile properties of the cervix are more speculative. It was postulated that the highly hydrated hyaluronic acid may accumulate in the interstices between collagen fibrils and disperse or prevent the aggregation of the fibrils (243). The sulfated glycosaminoglycans, dermatan sulfate and heparan sulfate, may also separate the collagen fibrils. These highly charged polyanions have been shown to bind to collagen (427,533) and to cause a mutual repulsion of the molecules (284).

Uterus

General Metabolic Effects of Relaxin on the Uterus

Relaxin causes several rapid changes in the biochemical composition of rat and mouse uteri. In 1957 Steinetz et al. (570) reported that uterine water content, wet weight, dry weight, glycogen content, and nitrogen content increased to maximal levels within 6 to 12 hr following the admin-

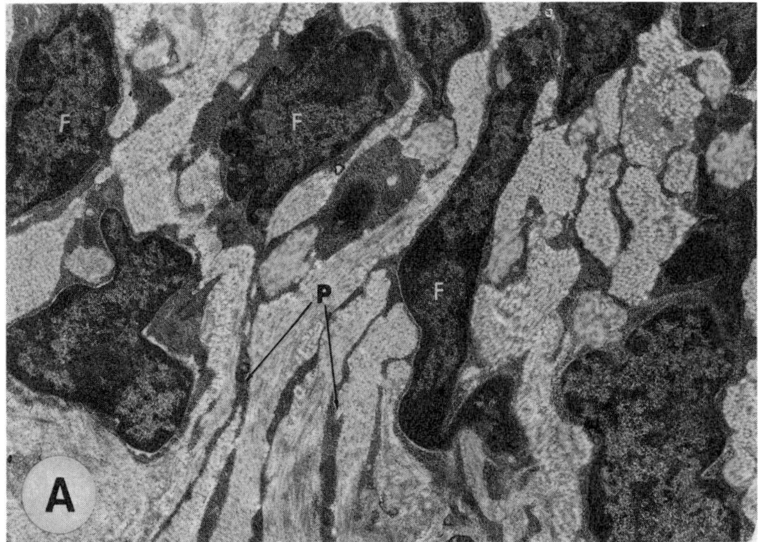

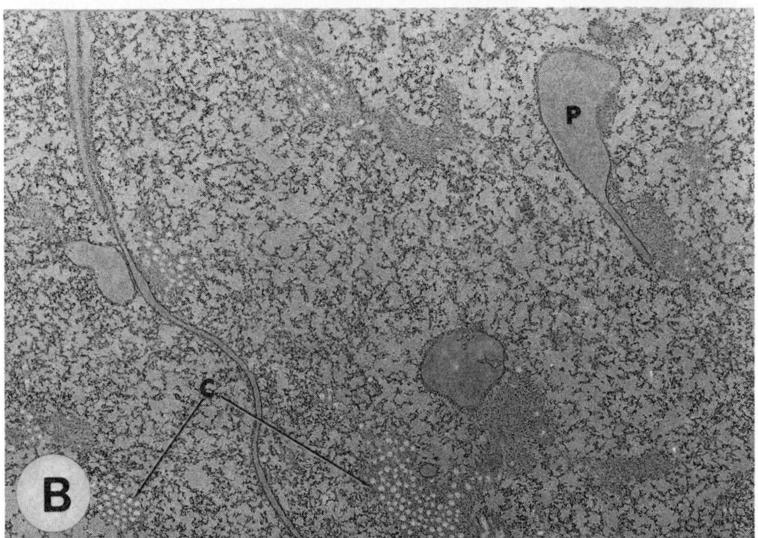

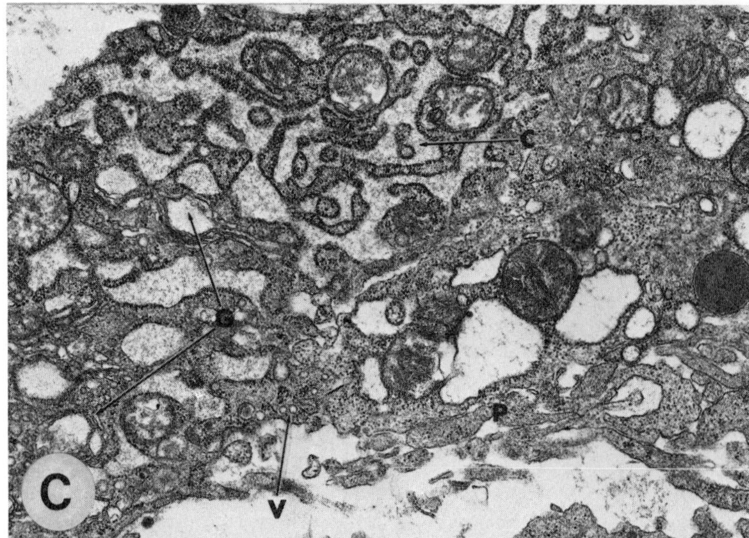

FIG. 43. A: Cervical wall of an ovariectomized control mouse showing a group of fibroblasts (F) packed tightly against bundles of collagenous fibrils (negative contrast). The "idle-looking" fibroblasts have scanty cytoplasm and few organelles. Attenuated cytoplasmic processes (P) appear throughout the extracellular space. (×7,640.) **B:** Typical stroma of the cervix of an ovariectomized mouse treated with estrogen or estrogen and relaxin. The collagenous fibrils (C) are arranged in isolated bundles throughout the expanded extracellular space which is largely filled by small aggregates of iron particles. The iron is presumed to be bound to the sulfated proteoglycans within the matrix and is not bound to the cytoplasmic processes (P). (×15,200.) **C:** Typical fibroblast from the uterine cervix of an ovariectomized mouse treated with estrogen or estrogen plus relaxin. The abundant cytoplasm is characterized by dilated cisternae (C) of rough endoplasmic reticulum. Golgi zones (G); cytoplasmic processes (P); small vesicles (V). (×15,200.) Reproduced with permission from Leppi and Kinnison (367).

istration of crude porcine relaxin to ovariectomized estrogen-primed immature rats (see Fig. 44). The general metabolic effects of relaxin have been confirmed in rats and mice with studies that employed not only partially purified porcine relaxin (72,77,266,267,317,356,519,641,681,682) and crude human relaxin extract (453) but also highly purified porcine relaxin (212,631–635). The physiological effects of relaxin on uterine metabolism appear to be less dependent on prior sensitization with estrogen than are its effects on the pubic symphysis and cervix. Relaxin treatment induced increased uterine growth, glycogen content, and protein synthesis in ovariectomized rats that were not pretreated with estrogen (5,212,633). Although estrogen pretreatment is not essential for relaxin to exert these effects on the rat uterus, a synergistic effect was obtained between the two hormones (5,212,633).

Little is known concerning either the physiological significance of the relaxin-induced changes in uterine composition or the mechanism(s) whereby these changes are brought about. Relaxin may act, at least in part, by increasing the blood flow to the uterus. Vasilenko et al. (635) reported that within 6 hr of the injection of relaxin to ovariectomized estrogen-primed rats there was a significant increase in vascularization of the vascular connective tissue layer located between the circular and longitudinal smooth muscle layers of the uterus.

Limited studies indicate that relaxin may be associated with regulation of glycogen metabolism during late pregnancy in rats and mice. Glycogen is stored primarily in the myometrium of rats during pregnancy (631) and following relaxin administration (266,267). Moreover, glycogen accumulates during late pregnancy in rats with a profile resembling that of relaxin levels in the peripheral serum (119,545,631) (see Fig. 45). Since the glycogen levels, which increase in the myometrium of rats during the second half of pregnancy, fall following birth, it was postulated that this glycogen may provide a source of energy for the strong, highly coordinated uterine contractions that occur at delivery (119,631). The mechanism(s) whereby relaxin promotes glycogen accumulation is not known. It may involve induction of enzymes associated with glycogen metabolism. Early reports indicated that crude porcine relaxin increased uterine concentrations of glycogen phosphorylase activity in estrogen-primed mice (267) and rats (489,519). A more recent report indicated that highly purified porcine relaxin, as well as partially purified relaxin obtained from human decidua, increased uterine concentrations of hexokinase, phosphoglucomutase, and glycogen phosphorylase activities in estrogen-primed mice (79). Moreover, the stimulatory effect of partially purified human relaxin on hexokinase and phosphoglucomutase activities in estrogen-primed mice was confirmed (453). It has also been postulated that relaxin may promote glycogen accumulation indirectly through a glycogen-sparing effect related to uterine quiescence (505,631).

Relaxin may also influence connective tissue remodeling of the uterine horns during pregnancy through actions that are analogous to those on the cervix. In the rat, the profile of uterine growth and involution coincides closely with the rise and fall in serum relaxin levels (545); that is, both the weight and collagen content of the uterine horns increase markedly during the second half of pregnancy and then decline rapidly following parturition (275,631) (see Fig. 45). In 1964 Cullen and Harkness (145) reported that the collagenous framework of the uterine horns of ovariectomized rats increased maximally when partially purified porcine relaxin was administered in combination with estrogen and progesterone. More recent morphometric and histological analysis of uteri obtained from immature and mature ovariectomized estrogen-primed rats are consistent with these findings. Vasilenko et al. (635) reported that, within 6 hr following relaxin treatment, the connective tissue framework of the endometrium and circular layer of the myometrium changed from dense, wavy bundles of collagen

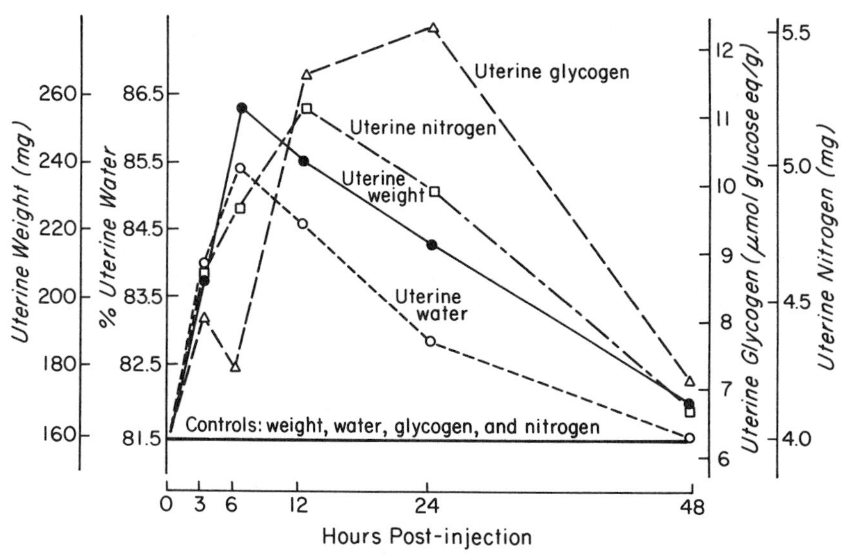

FIG. 44. Changes in uterine composition following a single injection of 100 μg of impure porcine relaxin (equivalent to approximately 5–10 μg highly purified porcine relaxin) to ovariectomized rats primed 8 days previously with 5 μg estradiol cyclopentylpropionate. Control rats received vehicle only (0.1 ml 1% benzopurpurine-4B in physiological saline). Reproduced with permission from Steinetz et al. (570).

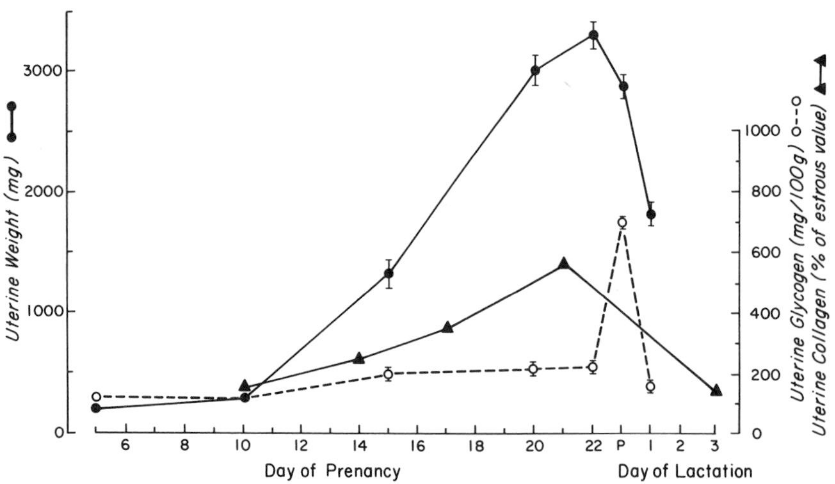

FIG. 45. Mean (± SE; N = 6) total uterine weight and uterine glycogen composition (myometrium plus endometrium) of the gravid horns of unilaterally pregnant rats. Mean (± SE; N = 6 or 7) total collagen content as a percentage of the estrous value. P = parturition. Modified and reproduced with permission from Harkness and Harkness (275) and Vasilenko et al. (631).

fibers to a more loosely arranged and widely separated collagen network which contained thinner collagen fibers and more intrafibrillar space. Cullen and Harkness (145) postulated that, independent of the distending forces exerted by the fetuses, hormone-induced cellular activity within the uterine wall may promote an increase in the collagenous framework of the uterus in the pregnant rat. Thus, relaxin might form a part of the mechanism(s) whereby pregnancy is maintained by facilitating the accommodation of the growing conceptuses. Although relaxin may influence the connective tissue framework of the uterus, it is not clear that relaxin promotes an increase in the distensibility of the uterine horns as it does the cervix. Supportive of the possibility, Wiqvist (669) reported that uterine resistance to distension with fluid was lower in ovariectomized rats treated with estrogen, progesterone, and relaxin than in animals treated with only the steroids. On the other hand, Harkness and Harkness (277) found that, in contrast to the cervix, the extensibility of the uterine horns was consistently low throughout pregnancy in rats. These workers (277) concluded that the differences in extensibility of the two portions of the reproductive tract fit their functions, since the strong contractions of the uterine horn at delivery must extend the cervix rather than its own tissue.

The mechanism whereby relaxin influences connective tissue remodeling of the rat uterine horns during pregnancy is not known. There are only a few isolated reports concerning the influence of relaxin on uterine collagen metabolism. Frieden and Adams reported that highly purified porcine relaxin not only stimulated the synthesis of uterine collagen to a greater extent than uterine noncollagen protein in ovariectomized estrogen-primed rats (212) but also inhibited uterine involution and collagenolysis in the postpartum rat (5). These workers concluded that relaxin may act as an anabolic and anticatabolic modulator of uterine collagen metabolism (212). Relaxin may promote collagen synthesis in the uterus through direct effects on fibroblasts. Porcine relaxin, as well as estrogen, increased tritiated thymidine incorporation into fibroblasts from the uteri of guinea pigs during *in vitro* culture (535). Two isolated and brief reports appear inconsistent with the hypothesis that relaxin promotes uterine collagen synthesis. Highly purified porcine relaxin was reported to decrease incorporation of tritiated proline into uterine tissue cultures obtained from women at cesarean section (667) and to increase collagenase activity in medium bathing cultures of whole uteri obtained from estrogen-primed rats (622).

Braddon (66) found that uterine levels of ornithine decarboxylase activity increased within 2 hr of the administration of highly purified porcine relaxin to mice. The physiological significance of this observation is not known. Ornithine decarboxylase may play a role in mediating the effects of relaxin on uterine growth, glycogen synthesis, and connective tissue metabolism. The mechanism whereby relaxin induces uterine ornithine decarboxylase activity is unknown. It may be a reflection of relaxin-induced increases in intracellular cAMP, since relaxin treatment was shown to increase cAMP levels in rat and pig uterine tissue (117,331,506). The influence of relaxin on uterine ornithine decarboxylase activity does not require estrogen priming, and this may mean that estrogen plays a role at a stage in the mechanism of action beyond the induction of relaxin receptors (66).

Effects of Relaxin on Myometrial Contractile Activity

The myometrium is relatively inactive throughout most of pregnancy; thus the developing fetus is maintained within a tranquil uterine cavity. Normally at term the uterine myometrium contracts rhythmically and forcefully, and this highly coordinated pattern of contractions aids in dilating the cervix and expelling the fetus and placenta. The changes in the contractile properties of the uterus during pregnancy are regulated, at least in part, by changing levels of (a) hormones which stimulate or inhibit uterine contractility, (b) hormone receptors on myometrial cells, and (c) gap junctions between adjacent myometrial cells. This section largely consists of a description of the influence of relaxin on uterine contractility in the rat, since this is the species with which most of the research has been conducted. Emphasis is placed on recent studies conducted with highly purified relaxin, studies that not only encourage the view that relaxin plays an important role in the regulation of uterine contractility during pregnancy but also provide considerable insight concerning the mechanism(s) of action of relaxin on the myometrial cells in the rat.

The effect of relaxin on uterine contractility was discovered in 1950, when Krantz et al. (354) found that intravenous administration of a crude extract of porcine relaxin to estrogen-primed guinea pigs diminished spontaneous uterine activity *in situ*. Shortly thereafter, Sawyer et al. (514) reported that crude porcine relaxin inhibited spontaneous and electrically stimulated uterine contractions in excised uteri obtained from estrogen-primed rats. Although most subsequent studies of the influence of relaxin on uterine contractility examined the effects of porcine relaxin on uterine contractility in the rat, the limited studies that examined its influence on uterine tissue obtained from other species encourage the view that relaxin's quiescent effect on uterine contractility is a generally distributed phenomenon.

Pharmacological effects of relaxin on uterine contractility. Studies of the influence of impure relaxin preparations on uterine contractility in nonpregnant mammals have contributed a great deal toward our present understanding of relaxin's role in this process. Partially purified porcine relaxin was reported to reduce the frequency and/or amplitude of uterine contractions in the rat (75,111,164,256, 371,397,462,468,469,511,512,514,596–598,645,668–670), mouse (356,514,668,669), guinea pig (191,354,458,459), hamster (344), sheep (470), and human (333,471). Partially purified rat relaxin reduced the amplitude of electrically driven contractions of rat uterine strips *in vitro* (69). Crude extracts obtained from the human corpus luteum of pregnancy reduced the amplitude of spontaneous contractions of human uterine strips *in vitro* (37,608), and a relaxin preparation obtained from human term placenta inhibited spontaneous contractions of mouse myometrial strips *in vitro* (204).

Numerous studies with highly purified porcine relaxin provided confirmation that relaxin renders the uterus quiescent in nonpregnant rats (49,112,113,118,418,419,506–508). Additionally, highly purified porcine (362) and rabbit (177) relaxin inhibited contractions of the mouse uterus *in vitro*, and highly purified shark relaxin inhibited contractions of the guinea pig uterus *in vitro* (484).

Studies with nonpregnant animals also demonstrated that relaxin can inhibit spontaneous uterine contractility over a sustained period of time. Impure porcine relaxin reduced the frequency of spontaneous uterine contractions in nonpregnant guinea pigs throughout a 20-hr infusion (459); furthermore, highly purified porcine relaxin inhibited both the frequency and amplitude of spontaneous uterine contractions in conscious and unrestrained ovariectomized rats (both estrogen-treated and steroid-untreated) throughout a 2-day infusion of the hormone (118) (see Fig. 46A).

Studies of an unphysiological nature involving the administration of porcine relaxin during early pregnancy in rats, before endogenous relaxin levels are elevated, provided indirect evidence that the uterus of the pregnant rat is responsive to relaxin. Porcine relaxin was infused intravenously for 16 hr (475) or 41 hr (495) during the periimplantation period (beginning at 1700 hr on day 4) to determine if the even distribution of implanted blastocysts

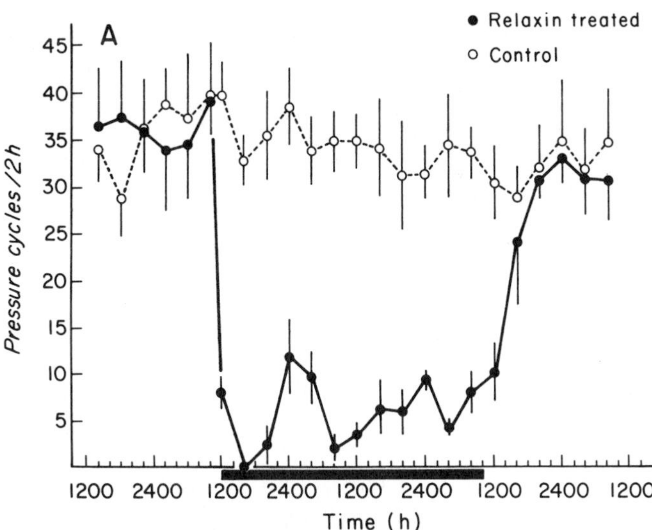

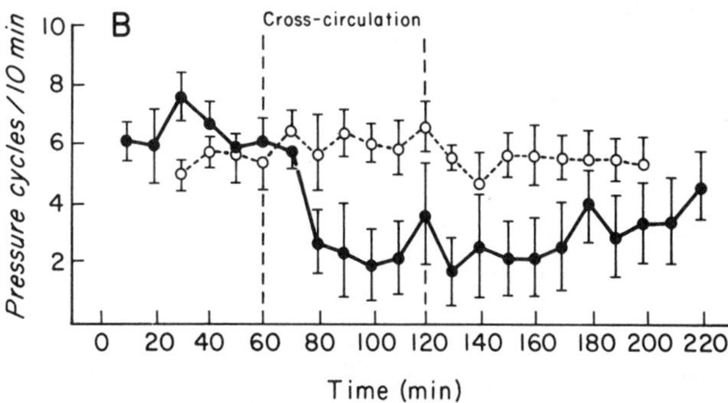

FIG. 46. A: Frequency of intrauterine pressure cycles of estrogen-dominated ovariectomized rats infused with saline ($N = 3$) or porcine relaxin (20 μg/hr; $N = 4$) for 48 hr. Reproduced with permission from Cheah and Sherwood (118). **B:** Frequency of intrauterine pressure cycles of postpartum untreated rats linked by cross-circulation to day 21 pregnant rats (——●——) ($N = 8$) or postpartum rats (- - - ○ - - -) ($N = 6$). Reproduced with permission from Porter and Downing (467).

is dependent upon spontaneous myometrial activity. Apparently it is. A preponderance of preimplantation blastocyts (475) and implantation sites (495) were found in the cranial half of the uterine horns in relaxin-treated rats. Additionally, it was observed that the implanted blastocyts were no longer invariably positioned antimesometrially within the uterine lumen and that embryonic disk orientation was frequently abnormal following prolonged infusion of relaxin from day 4 to day 6 (495). Abnormal positioning of the implantation sites may account for the high rate of fetal resorption that occurred during the second half of pregnancy, when highly purified porcine relaxin was administered to rats during the periimplantation period (576).

Reports of relaxin's quiescent effect on uterine contractility in nonpregnant mammals provided the stimulus for several clinical efforts during the late 1950s to use relaxin to prevent threatened premature labor or to inhibit the early stages of labor at term. These experiments, which generally employed (a) crude and poorly characterized porcine relaxin preparations, (b) variations in doses, routes of administration, and duration of relaxin treatment, (c) inadequate controls, and (d) inadequately described and subjective means of determining the status of labor, were confusing and in some cases conflicting. Although several investigators reported that porcine relaxin inhibited uterine contractions and/or delayed birth when given to women in premature labor (3,76,174,208,303,386,404), the most rigorous, double-blind study, which employed large numbers of women and appropriate controls, reported relaxin had little if any effect on premature labor (152). There was general agreement that relaxin had little effect on the course of term labor (152,160,181,333), and two of these studies employed internal tocometric devices for objective determination of uterine contractility (181,333).

Relaxin's effects on uterine contractility during pregnancy. Three lines of evidence support the view that relaxin restrains uterine contractile activity during pregnancy. First, studies in which the blood of a pregnant donor was cross-circulated with that of a nonpregnant recipient demonstrated the presence of a myometrial inhibitor(s) with a more rapid onset of activity than estrogen or progesterone (which require about 12 hr) in the blood of the pregnant rat, guinea pig, and rabbit (459,460,467,550) (see Fig. 46B). Second, there is evidence in rats and pigs that the uterine myometrium is relatively quiescent during the stage of pregnancy when relaxin levels are elevated. In pregnant rats the frequency of uterine contractions diminishes throughout the second half of pregnancy (168), when relaxin immunoactivity levels in the blood are elevated (432,545) (see Fig. 47A). In pregnant pigs the electrical activity of the myometrium remains low as late as the period between 24 and 10 hr before expulsion of the first piglet in spite of a decline in serum progesterone levels (618,649), and this is the time when pigs experience the antepartum surge in serum relaxin levels (543,554,617). Finally, in ovariectomized pregnant rats, replacement of endogenous relaxin with exogenous relaxin reduces the frequency of uterine contractility to levels similar to those of intact controls. When rats were ovariectomized on day 9 and given replacement therapy with progesterone and estrogen throughout the remainder of pregnancy, the frequency of intrauterine pressure cycles was considerably greater than that of intact controls, whereas when replacement therapy consisted of progesterone, estrogen, and highly purified porcine relaxin, the frequency of intrauterine pressure cycles declined to levels that did not differ from those of intact controls (168) (Fig. 47B).

Characterization of relaxin's effects on uterine contractility.

Desensitization: Desensitization of the rat uterus may occur with prolonged exposure to relaxin. Several investigators reported that the effectiveness with which porcine relaxin inhibited uterine contractility in uteri of estrogen-primed nonpregnant rats diminished following prolonged exposure to elevated relaxin levels *in vivo* (118,668) or *in vitro* (113,397,668) (see Fig. 48A). One study, however, failed to observe this tachyphylaxis. Following KCl-induced *in vitro* contraction of uterine segments obtained from estrogen-primed nonpregnant rats, the tonus of the uterine contractures declined continuously with prolonged exposure to porcine relaxin (597). It is not clear whether the uteri of pregnant rats become refractory to endogenous relaxin. It has been reported that uteri obtained from rats during late pregnancy display tachyphylaxis when treated with porcine relaxin (113,668). Nevertheless, the demonstration that hormone replacement therapy in ovariectomized pregnant rats with physiological levels of porcine relaxin from day 10 to day 23 reduced the frequency of intrauterine pressure cycles to levels found in intact controls for 13 days (see Fig. 47B) does not encourage the view that desensitization, if it exists, is a physiologically important phenomenon.

Physical Characteristics of Contractions: *In vivo* studies of the influence of relaxin on uterine contractility—which may have more physiological relevance than *in vitro* studies—demonstrated that the primary influence of relaxin is to reduce the frequency rather than the amplitude of uterine contractility. Whereas the frequency of spontaneous uterine contractions in nonpregnant guinea pigs (458,459), rabbits (460), sheep (470), and rats (118,397,467,468) was reduced dramatically during cross-circulation with pregnant animals or following administration of porcine relaxin, the reduction in the amplitude of uterine contractions in these species was less marked. Additionally, there is evidence that the coordination of rat uterine contractile activity may be improved during recovery from relaxin-induced quiescence. The rate of rise of intrauterine pressure cycles recorded from conscious (164) or anesthetized (69,164) ovariectomized rats was significantly elevated during recovery from the total myometrial quiescence imposed by treatment with porcine (164) or rat (69) relaxin.

A variety of *in vitro* methods have been used to examine the characteristics of relaxin's action on uterine contractility. In spite of the important limitation that they are relatively

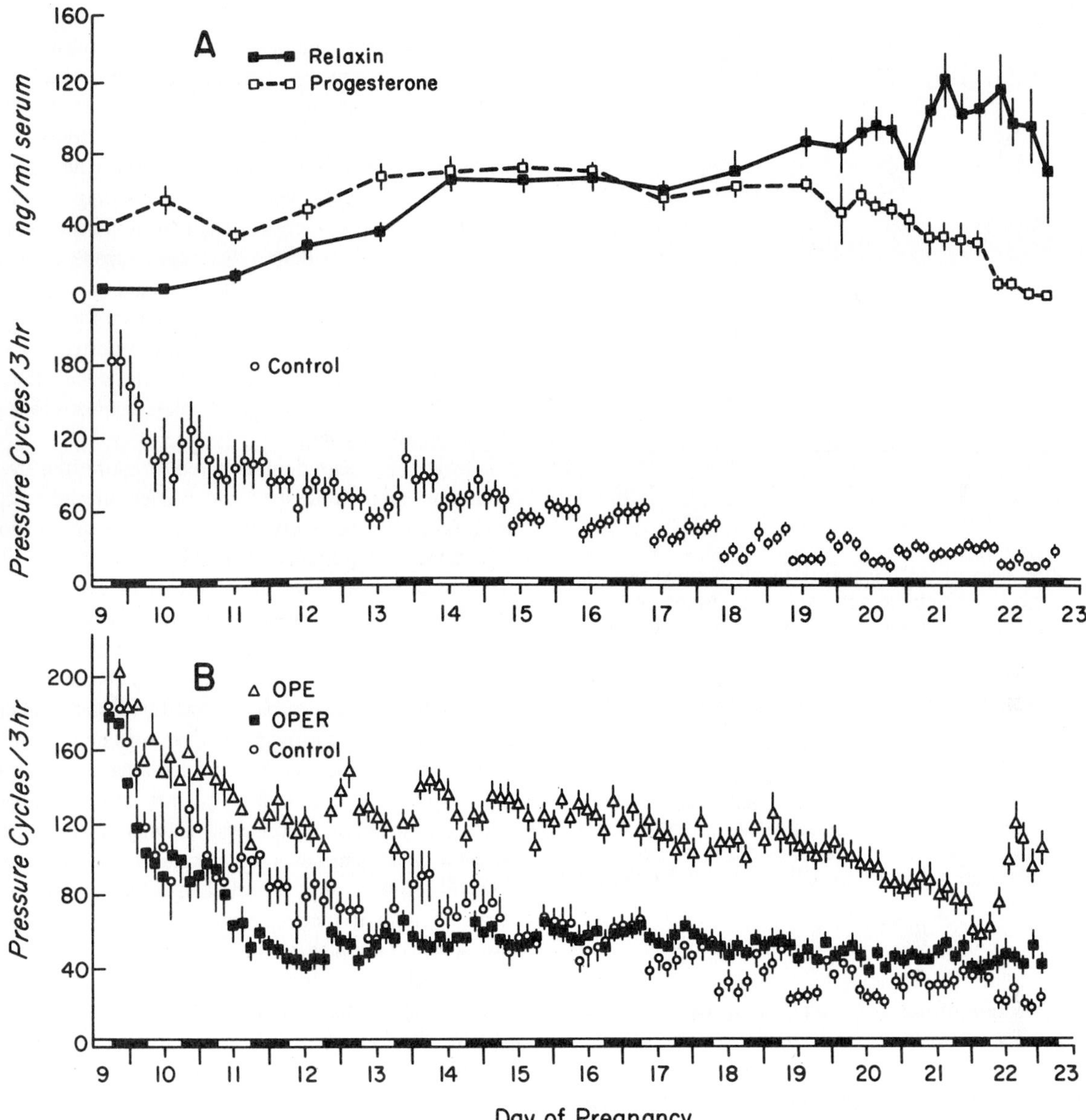

FIG. 47. A: Mean frequency of intrauterine pressure cycles ± SE from day 9 until day 23 in intact pregnant rats. Mean peripheral blood serum relaxin and progesterone levels are from the same animals. **B:** Mean frequency of intrauterine pressure cycles ± SE from day 9 until day 23 in intact pregnant rats (control), ovariectomized pregnant rats treated with progesterone and estrogen (OPE), and ovariectomized pregnant rats treated with progesterone, estrogen, and highly purified porcine relaxin (OPER). Means are from 25 or more rats. Reproduced with permission from Downing and Sherwood (168).

unphysiological, these methods have advantages over *in vivo* methods for some research objectives. For example, they require less relaxin, enable more than one treatment with uterine tissue from a single animal, permit more accurate measurement of parameters of uterine contractility, and enable direct correlations between the contractile state and biochemical composition of the uterus.

In vitro methods were used to examine the site(s) and physical characteristics of relaxin's action on the rat myometrium. A radioautographic localization study with ^{125}I-labeled porcine relaxin led Weiss and Bryant-Greenwood (658) to conclude that relaxin binding sites are present on both the longitudinal and circular smooth muscle layers of the myometrium, with the preponderance of binding sites on the circular layer. In subsequent *in vitro* studies, porcine relaxin was reported to inhibit the contractility of segments of both longitudinal and circular smooth muscle (113,465). There is evidence that relaxin may act, at least in part, through inhibition of action potentials in both smooth muscle layers. Chamley and Parkington (113) reported that when strips of uterine longitudinal smooth muscle were mounted in organ baths and stimulated electrically to induce electro-

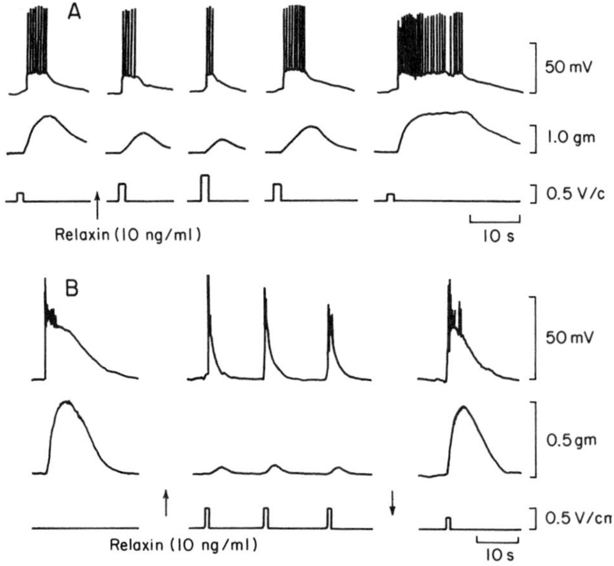

FIG. 48. The effect of the addition of highly purified porcine relaxin (↑) on the electrical activity (upper trace) and mechanical activity (middle trace) evoked by depolarizing current pulses (lower trace) in the longitudinal myometrium **(A)** and circular myometrium **(B)** of the estrogen-treated rat. In the longitudinal muscle **(A)**, the duration of electrical burst and hence the amplitude and duration of contraction were initially decreased in the presence of relaxin; however, activity recovered within 8 to 15 min despite the continual presence of relaxin. In the circular muscle **(B)**, relaxin selectively blocked the plateau component of the electrical activity, and the effect was reversed 20 to 30 min after removal of the peptide (↓). Reproduced with permission from Chamley and Parkington (113).

tonic depolarization of the membrane, bursts of spike-type action potentials occurred that outlasted the stimulus (see Fig. 48A). Addition of highly purified porcine relaxin to the electrically stimulated longitudinal muscle tissue decreased the number of action potentials per burst with a consequent decrease in the amplitude and duration of the accompanying contractions. When strips of uterine circular smooth muscle were stimulated electrically, there was an initial spike-type or short burst of spike-type action potentials followed by a long plateau of depolarization (Fig. 48B). Application of porcine relaxin to the circular muscle tissue bath eliminated the plateau component of the action potential. Consistent with these findings, the burst frequency of uterine action potentials in sheep was reduced *in vivo* following intravenous administration of highly purified porcine relaxin (473).

Interaction with Hormones Other Than Relaxin: The response of the uterus to relaxin is influenced by other hormones that act upon the uterine myometrium during pregnancy such as progesterone, estrogen, oxytocin, and prostaglandins. The way in which relaxin interacts with these hormones to influence uterine contractility is not well understood for any species, but it has been examined to some extent in the rat. Whereas progesterone alone markedly reduces the frequency or amplitude of intrauterine pressure cycles in species such as the sheep, rabbit, and pig (465), it does not in the rat (165,166,466). Instead, progesterone desynchronizes the electrical activity of the rat uterus, thus rendering the uterus unresponsive to oxytocin-induced contractions and preventing strong, highly coordinated uterine contractions like those that occur at delivery. There is limited evidence that progesterone may increase the sensitivity of the rat uterus to relaxin. Exposure of the uteri of estrogen-primed nonpregnant rats to progesterone *in vivo* (75) or *in vitro* (511,512) was reported to reduce by about half the dose of porcine relaxin needed to decrease the amplitude of electrically stimulated contractions of uterine segments *in vitro*.

Estrogen has been demonstrated to inhibit the frequency of intrauterine pressure cycles in ovariectomized postpartum rats (165). It seems likely, however, that estrogen alone has little effect on uterine contractility during most of pregnancy, since peripheral blood levels of estrogen are low until late pregnancy. Moreover, the blood levels of progesterone are elevated throughout nearly all of pregnancy, and they probably override whatever effects the low estrogen levels might have on uterine contractility. On the other hand, the low levels of estrogen may be sufficient to influence relaxin's effects on uterine contractility during the second half of pregnancy. Although relaxin has the capacity to inhibit spontaneous myometrial activity in the absence of estrogen treatment in ovariectomized nonpregnant rats (118,468,469), it was reported that the sensitivity of the uterus to relaxin increases markedly with prior estrogen treatment (397,498,668).

The mechanism whereby estrogen enhances the sensitivity of the uterus to relaxin is not known. It may do so by inducing the formation of relaxin receptors, since estrogen administration was reported to induce uterine relaxin receptors in ovariectomized rats (395) and pigs (396). It seems likely that estrogen has its most profound effects on uterine contractility during the antepartum period, when estrogen levels increase. As the uterus comes under progressively greater estrogen domination during late pregnancy, its capacity for highly coordinated contractions increases (225). In the presence of elevated estrogen levels there is an increase in gap junctions (560), uterine electrical conductivity (393), prostaglandin production (101), oxytocin receptors (10,11), and relaxin receptors (395,396).

Relaxin may influence oxytocin- and prostaglandin-stimulated uterine contractions. Both oxytocin (69,111, 118,397,458,459,467,468,470,598,669) and $PGF_{2\alpha}$ (69, 111,470,598) stimulated contractions in rat, guinea pig, and sheep uteri under the quiescent influence of relaxin. Nevertheless, evidence obtained both *in vivo* and *in vitro* indicates that relaxin inhibits oxytocin- and prostaglandin-driven uterine contractions in the rat (113,118,307,418,419, 468,469,598). The response of the uterus to relaxin or the contractile stimulants oxytocin and $PGF_{2\alpha}$ appears to depend, at least in part, on their relative concentrations in the extracellular fluid. There is limited evidence that the ability of relaxin to inhibit oxytocin- and prostaglandin-driven contractions may require prior estrogen treatment (469).

Postulated role of relaxin on uterine contractility during the antepartum period. The role of relaxin on the normal progression of antepartum and parturient uterine contractile activity has not been determined with certainty for any species. Porter (462) postulated that relaxin may provide a mechanism that protects the fetuses and placentas during the antepartum period of progesterone withdrawal in species such as rats and pigs in which high blood levels of progesterone prevent highly coordinated uterine contractility until just before birth. In these species relaxin may restrain uterine contractile activity during the antepartum period of progesterone withdrawal until overridden by stimulating agents, such as oxytocin and prostaglandins, or other mechanisms that bring about the onset of strong, highly coordinated uterine contractions and the delivery of the fetuses. Downing and Sherwood (168) obtained evidence that is consistent with this hypothesis. In the pregnant rat the myometrium is almost completely quiescent from day 20 until about 3 hr before the onset of labor, when there is an abrupt increase in uterine contractility which lasts until labor is completed (168) (see Fig. 49A). When pregnant rats were ovariectomized on day 9 and administered hormone replacement therapy with progesterone and estrogen, the frequency of intrauterine pressure cycles was greater than controls throughout

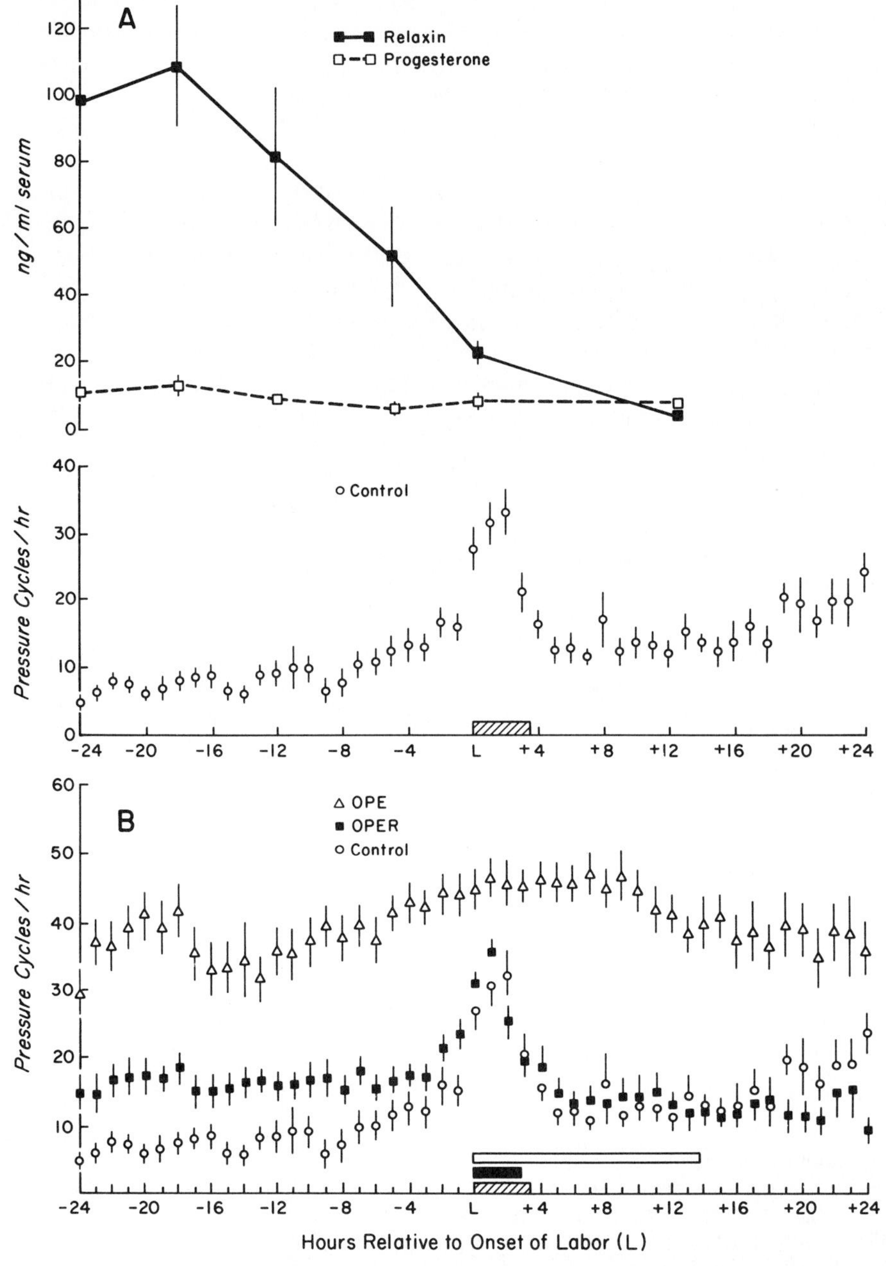

FIG. 49. A: Mean frequency of intrauterine pressure cycles (± SE; N = 18) from 24 hr before the onset of labor until 24 hr after the onset of labor in rats. Mean serum relaxin and progesterone levels ± SE are from the same animals. **B:** Mean frequency of intrauterine pressure cycles (± SE; N = 18 to 25) from 24 hr before the onset of labor until 24 hr after the onset of labor in intact pregnant rats (control), ovariectomized pregnant rats treated with progesterone and estrogen (OPE), and ovariectomized pregnant rats treated with progesterone, estrogen, and highly purified porcine relaxin (OPER). Mean durations of labor are indicated: [hatched bar], intact controls; [open bar], group OPE; [solid bar], group OPER. Reproduced with permission from Downing and Sherwood (168).

the 24-hr prelabor and postlabor periods. However, when similarly ovariectomized pregnant rats were given replacement therapy with progesterone, estrogen, and highly purified porcine relaxin, the frequency of intrauterine pressure cycles did not differ from intact controls throughout this period (168) (Fig. 49B). Although much has been learned concerning relaxin's direct effects on myometrial cells, little is known concerning the process whereby relaxin interacts with other hormones to influence the coordinated contractile activity of the entire uterus. There is limited evidence that relaxin may reduce antepartum myometrial activity in pregnant rats not only through direct effects on the uterine myometrium, but also through a central action to prevent oxytocin release (607). For additional descriptions of the possible role of relaxin on uterine contractility, the reader is referred to reviews by Porter (461,462,465).

Mechanism of action of relaxin on myometrial cells. Since 1980 considerable progress has been made at the molecular level toward an understanding of the mechanism(s) whereby relaxin inhibits contractility of the uterine myometrium, and this progress, made primarily with studies in the rat, has been reviewed in detail (335,505). It is clear that relaxin acts directly on the uterine myometrium. Studies at the whole-animal and tissue level demonstrated that relaxin receptors are present in the uterus. Finite numbers of high-affinity binding sites for radioiodinated porcine relaxin were reported in rat (394,395,407,658), guinea pig (236), and pig (396) uterine horns. Furthermore, examination of binding by radioautography demonstrated that the uterine binding sites in the rat are located in both the longitudinal and circular muscle layers (658). As with other protein hormone receptors, relaxin receptors appear to be associated with the plasma membrane. Mercado-Simmen et al. (394–396) reported that high-affinity binding sites with $K_a = 10^9$ to 10^{10} M^{-1} were located in plasma membrane–enriched particulate fractions of rat and pig uterine tissue.

These relaxin binding sites were reported to be elevated during the estrogen-dominated stages of the estrous cycle in rats (395) and following estrogen administration to ovariectomized rats and pigs (394–396). Mercado-Simmen et al. (395) postulated that modulation of relaxin receptors in the uterus may be part of the mechanism whereby estrogen increases the sensitivity of the uterus to relaxin. These workers (394,395) also reported that relaxin binding sites are elevated during the second half of pregnancy in the rat uterus and that endogenous relaxin and exogenously administered porcine relaxin may reduce their number. Relaxin receptors have not been isolated or characterized. Recent efforts to examine the mechanism of action of relaxin on the rat uterus at the cellular level are consistent with the view that relaxin acts directly on the myometrium. In 1986 Hsu and Sanborn (307) reported that relaxin promoted an increase in the length and area of oxytocin-pretreated myometrial cells in culture.

Molecular Basis for Smooth-Muscle Contraction: A brief summary of the molecular basis for the regulation of smooth-muscle contraction (7,335,505) seems appropriate to facilitate understanding the intracellular mechanism(s) whereby relaxin may inhibit uterine contractility (see Fig. 50). Contraction of smooth muscle occurs as a result of actomyosin interaction in a process that involves the hydrolysis of ATP.

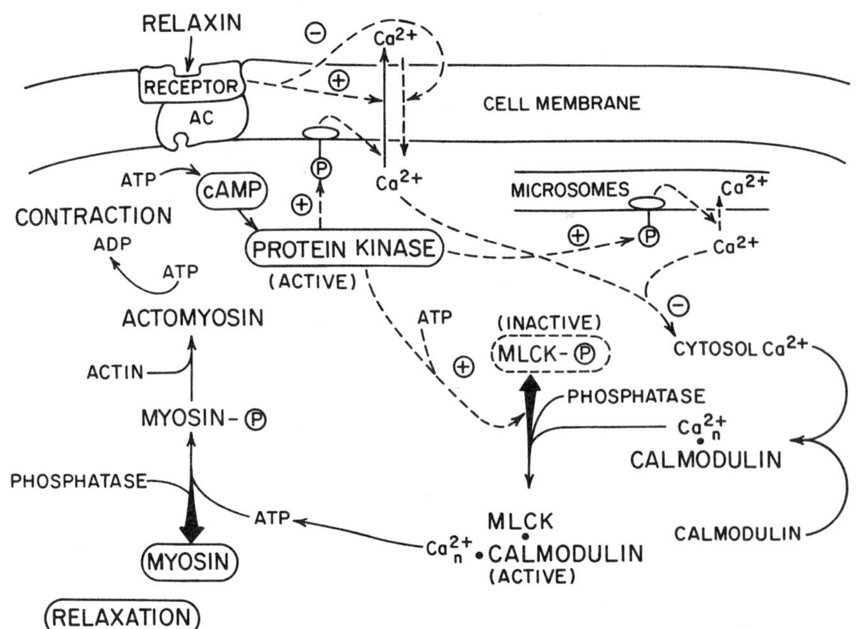

FIG. 50. Intracellular mechanisms whereby relaxin may inhibit contractions of uterine myometrial cells. The putative effects of relaxin that are supported by experimental data in rat myometrial tissue are enclosed by solid lines and preceded by solid arrows. Possible effects of relaxin that have not been demonstrated are shown with dashed lines. Abbreviations: AC, adenylyl cyclase; protein kinase, cAMP-dependent protein kinase; MLCK, myosin light chain kinase. The cAMP-dependent protein kinase dissociates in the presence of cAMP into a regulatory subunit-cAMP complex and an active protein kinase subunit that promotes the phosphorylation of intracellular proteins. Following relaxin treatment cAMP increases, protein kinase activity increases, the affinity of MLCK for the Ca^{2+} · calmodulin complex decreases, MLCK activity decreases, myosin light chain phosphorylation decreases, actomyosin ATPase activity decreases, and there is a relaxation of uterine contractility. It is not clear whether relaxin brings about its effects through the phosphorylation of MLCK. It may act, at least in part, by reducing intracellular Ca^{2+} levels, thus decreasing MLCK activity and myosin light chain phosphorylation. There is evidence that relaxin promotes increased Ca^{2+} efflux from myometrial cells in culture. References that describe these effects of relaxin are cited in the text. Modified and reproduced with permission from Sanborn (505).

This actin-activated myosin ATPase activity requires phosphorylation of the 20,000-dalton light chains that are associated with the globular head of myosin. Activation of the enzyme myosin light chain kinase (MLCK), which catalyzes myosin light chain phosphorylation, is a sequential process requiring an elevation of the intracellular calcium levels. Calcium first binds to the calcium-regulatory protein calmodulin, which is found in high concentrations and is not limiting in the uterus, to form a Ca^{2+} · calmodulin complex. The Ca^{2+} · calmodulin complex then binds to the inactive catalytic subunit of MLCK to form the active holoenzyme complex Ca^{2+} · calmodulin · MLCK. Phosphorylation of the MLCK catalytic subunit, which is catalyzed by cAMP–dependent protein kinase, reduces the capacity of the MLCK catalytic subunit to combine with Ca^{2+} · calmodulin. Thus phosphorylation of MLCK inhibits formation of the active Ca^{2+} · calmodulin · MLCK complex.

Possible Mediation through cAMP–dependent Protein Kinase: The mechanism(s) whereby relaxin brings about the inhibition of uterine contractions is not known. There is evidence, however, that it may do so through cAMP-dependent protein kinase–mediated phosphorylation of proteins within myometrial cells. Following treatment with highly purified porcine relaxin in the presence of phosphodiesterase inhibitors, there was an increase in cAMP levels in rat and pig uterine tissue (117,331,506) and rat myometrial cells (306). Moreover, in one study the effectiveness with which porcine relaxin inhibited rat uterine contractions *in vitro* was found to increase when the phosphodiesterase inhibitor theophylline was present in the organ bath (598). A preliminary experiment showed that relaxin may elevate cAMP levels by increasing adenylyl cyclase activity (507). There is limited evidence that the elevation in cAMP may activate cAMP-dependent protein kinase. Binding of cAMP to a protein presumed to be the regulatory subunit of cAMP-dependent protein kinase occurred following treatment of rat uterine tissue in the presence of a phosphodiesterase inhibitor (508). Additionally, it was reported that relaxin activated rat uterine cAMP-dependent protein kinase within 30 sec in the absence of phosphodiesterase inhibitors, and the effects of relaxin on the protein kinase paralleled those on muscle contraction in terms of time course and dose response (334). Nishikori et al. (418,419) reported that relaxin inhibited MLCK activity and myosin light chain phosphorylation in isometrically suspended strips of uteri obtained from estrogen-primed rats; furthermore, the time course and concentration response of these biochemical effects of relaxin paralleled hormone-induced inhibition of uterine contractility.

The reduction in MLCK activity was attributed to a decrease in the affinity of MLCK for its modulator Ca^{2+} · calmodulin as well as a reduction in the affinity of the active Ca^{2+} · calmodulin · MLCK complex for its substrate myosin (419). Hsu and Sanborn (308) obtained results with myometrial cells in culture that partially confirmed these effects of relaxin on MLCK. Reduction in myometrial cell MLCK activity was attributed to a decrease in the affinity of MLCK for its modulator Ca^{2+} · calmodulin (308). A decrease in the affinity of the active Ca^{2+} · calmodulin · MLCK complex for its substrate myosin was not observed with the myometrial cells in culture (308). The mechanism that accounts for the reduction in affinity of MLCK for Ca^{2+} · calmodulin is not known with certainty. There is reason to postulate that it may be attributable to phosphorylation of MLCK by cAMP-dependent protein kinase. In the absence of calmodulin, two sites on MLCK can be phosphorylated, and phosphorylation of one of these sites reduces the affinity of MLCK for calmodulin (417). Additionally, it was demonstrated that Forskolin-induced elevation of cAMP levels in tracheal smooth-muscle cells resulted in increased MLCK phosphorylation and a relaxation of the contracted muscle (156). Nevertheless, there are criteria that must be met before it can be concluded that relaxin inhibits uterine contractility through the phosphorylation of MLCK. These include demonstrating that relaxin promotes phosphorylation of MLCK and that there is a stoichiometric relationship between the degree of MLCK phosphorylation and changes in the affinity of MLCK for Ca^{2+} · calmodulin (335).

Possible Mediation through Regulation of Intracellular Ca^{2+} Levels: Another mechanism whereby relaxin may reduce MLCK activity is through regulation of intracellular Ca^{2+} levels. Formation of the Ca^{2+} · calmodulin complex needed for MLCK activation could be inhibited through the reduction of intracellular Ca^{2+} levels. Relaxin could increase sequestration of Ca^{2+} in microsomes, increase efflux of Ca^{2+} through the cell membrane, decrease influx of Ca^{2+} through the cell membrane, or promote combinations of these processes. It is possible these Ca^{2+} transport processes are mediated by cAMP-dependent protein kinase–catalyzed phosphorylation of membrane proteins, as shown schematically in Fig. 50. Consistent with these possibilities, there is evidence that intracellular Ca^{2+} can be sequestered in rat uterine microsomes; furthermore, this process, as well as phosphorylation of rat uterine microsomal proteins, is stimulated by cAMP (505). Limited evidence indicates that relaxin may influence intracellular Ca^{2+} levels. Rao and Sanborn (482) reported that relaxin increases Ca^{2+} efflux from rat myometrial cells in culture. If phosphorylation of intracellular protein(s) is a component in the molecular mechanism(s) whereby relaxin reduces MLCK activity, either by direct phosphorylation of MLCK or indirectly through the phosphorylation of proteins that influence intracellular Ca^{2+} levels, it is possible that protein kinases other than cAMP-dependent protein kinase are involved. Finally, relaxin may alter intracellular Ca^{2+} levels, at least in part, through mechanisms that do not involve the phosphorylation of cellular proteins, such as alterations of the permeability of receptor-mediated Ca^{2+} channels.

Possible Indirect Mediation through the Release of Catecholamines: Relaxin may influence uterine contractions, at least in part, through a completely different and indirect mechanism. In the early 1960s Rudzik and Miller (497,498) examined the mechanism whereby crude porcine relaxin inhibits uterine contractility in estrogen-primed rats. They concluded that relaxin may act indirectly through the release of the endogenous catecholamine epinephrine, since (a) the sensitivity of the myometrium to relaxin was parallel to the epinephrine content, (b) relaxin treatment reduced the epinephrine content, and (c) the influence of relaxin on uterine contractility was inhibited by adrenergic neuron blocking agents (497,498). Subsequent studies have in some cases been consistent with those of Rudzik and Miller (497,498). For example, the observations that β-adrenergic receptor agonists stimulate cAMP levels (306,331,506) and inhibit uterine contractility (498,506,510,597,598) are consistent with the possibility that the effects of relaxin on uterine contractility are mediated indirectly through β-adrenergic agonist activation of adenylyl cyclase. For the most part, however, studies indicate that relaxin acts independent of (or only partially through) stimulation of β-adrenergic receptors. Several studies demonstrated that levels of β-adrenergic receptor antagonists that block the effects of β-agonists do not block relaxin's inhibitory effect on uterine contractility (448,468,597,598,668) or relaxin's stimulatory effect on cAMP levels (331,506) in estrogen-dominated rats. Additionally, in contrast to the early work of Rudzik and Miller (497), Sanborn et al. (509,510) reported that highly purified porcine relaxin did not reduce uterine catecholamine levels in estrogen-primed rats; moreover, depletion of nearly all of the epinephrine from the uteri of reserpine-treated rats did not prevent relaxin from relaxing potassium-depolarized uterine strips in the absence or presence of the β-adrenergic receptor antagonist propranolol (509,510). Finally, St-Louis (597) reported that the β-adrenergic receptor antagonist propranolol abolished the relaxing effects of the β-adrenergic receptor agonist isoproterenol but that it only inhibited about 45% of the action of relaxin on potassium-contracted rat uterine strips.

Possible Medication through Prostaglandins: The prostaglandins $PGF_{2\alpha}$ and PGE_2 are potent stimulants of uterine contractility in many mammalian species. The effects of the prostaglandin prostacyclin (PGI2) on uterine contractility appear to vary among species. PGI2 was reported to stimulate uterine contractility and to potentiate the effects of oxytocin on strips of rat pregnant uterus *in vitro* (664). In contrast, PGI2 was reported to inhibit spontaneous and $PGF_{2\alpha}$-induced contractile activity in strips of human myometrium *in vitro* (440) and to reduce uterine electromyographical and contractile activity *in vivo* in nonpregnant ovariectomized sheep (380).

Circumstantial evidence indicates that increased PGI2 synthesis may be associated with the mechanisms that control uterine contractility at parturition in the rat. In pregnant rats myometrial levels of the predominant prostaglandin PGI2 increase sharply at birth, and synthesis of PGI2 is promoted by oxytocin (661,662). Williams and Tahir (663) reported that relaxin inhibited both spontaneous and oxytocin-induced synthesis of PGI2 and appeared to do so by inhibiting the enzyme phospholipase A_2, which is obligatory for the synthesis of PGI2 as well as other prostaglandins. These workers (663) concluded that relaxin might act through inhibitory effects on prostaglandin synthesis. In contrast, there are studies that indicate that relaxin's effects are not dependent on its capacity to reduce prostaglandin synthesis. Indomethacin in concentrations sufficient to block prostaglandin synthesis did not inhibit the stimulatory effects of relaxin on uterine cAMP levels (509). Moreover, the ability of relaxin to relax KCl-contracted uterine segments was reported to be potentiated by the presence of indomethacin in the organ bath (598).

Effects of Relaxin on the Endometrium

Isolated reports indicate that relaxin may have effects on the uterine endometrium in rats, but those effects remain poorly understood. In 1952 and 1960, Frieden and Velardo (221,222) reported that partially purified porcine relaxin inhibited deciduoma formation in ovariectomized pseudopregnant rats treated with progesterone; however, an effect on deciduoma formation was not confirmed when more highly purified porcine relaxin was employed (634,637,682). Nevertheless, the most recent studies indicate that relaxin may act directly on the rat endometrium and have profound effects on its growth and metabolism. There is limited evidence that the endometrium in rats may contain relaxin receptors. Weiss and Bryant-Greenwood (658) reported finite numbers of binding sites for radioiodinated porcine relaxin in the endometrium as well as the myometrium of gonadotropin-primed rats. Morphometric and histological analyses of uterine tissue obtained from ovariectomized estrogen-primed rats demonstrated that highly purified porcine relaxin had a rapid effect on the endometrium. Vasilenko et al. (635) reported that within 6 hr of the administration of 100 μg of porcine relaxin there was a dramatic increase in the volume of both the endometrium and the myometrium; moreover, the collagen network became more loosely arranged and widely scattered, resulting in more intrafibrillar space in both uterine compartments. The physiological significance of relaxin's putative effects on the growth and metabolism of the endometrium in pregnant rats during the second half of pregnancy is unknown. They may be important for uterine accommodation of the rapidly growing fetuses. Steinetz et al. (576) hypothesized that the fetal resorption that accompanies the administration of large doses of purified porcine relaxin during the periimplantation period may be attributable, at least in part, to relaxin-induced disruption of some endometrial function.

Early studies with impure porcine relaxin indicated that relaxin may influence growth of the endometrium and differentiation of its vasculature in the rhesus monkey. In the 1960s, Hisaw and co-workers (149,292,293) conducted histological studies of the influence of prolonged administration of estrogen, progesterone, and partially purified porcine relaxin on the endometrium of juvenile or ovariectomized rhesus monkeys. Growth of the endometrial stroma was reported to be maximal when the monkeys were treated with a combination of estrogen, progesterone, and relaxin (149,292). Relaxin appeared to intensify the differentiation of stromal cells into granulocytes which accumulated around the spiral arteries in the basal endometrium (149,293). Relaxin was also reported to stimulate proliferation of the endothelial cells located in the distal portions of the spiral arteries in a manner similar to the formation of sinus-like channels below an implanted embryo during early pregnancy in the rhesus monkey (149,293). This latter biological effect of relaxin, called endothelioid cytomorphosis (293), led Dallenbach-Hellweg et al. (149) to hypothesize that one of the functions of relaxin during early pregnancy in primates is to assist in the preparation of the endometrial blood vessels for implantation and fetal nourishment. An effect of highly purified relaxin on the endometrium of primates has yet to be reported.

Vagina

There are isolated reports that relatively crude preparations of relaxin have effects on the vagina. Relaxin-containing extracts obtained from the serum of pregnant rabbits or ovaries of pregnant sows were reported to potentiate the action of estrogen in inducing vaginal cornification in mice and rats (159,266,682). In addition, crude preparations of porcine relaxin were reported to induce opening of the vaginal membrane in ovariectomized or hysterectomized guinea pigs (319,320). Effects of relaxin on the vagina require confirmation with highly purified hormone preparations.

Mammary Glands

Effects of Relaxin on the Growth and Development of the Mammary Glands

The second biological effect of relaxin to be reported, its growth-promoting effect on mammary tissue, has received sporadic attention and remains poorly understood. In 1945 Hamolsky and Sparrow (272) reported that, when administered together with estrogen and progesterone, a crude preparation of porcine relaxin promoted growth and lobulation of the mammary glands of ovariectomized immature rats beyond that obtained with steroids alone. Other studies, which employed either examination of whole mounts of mammary glands or total DNA content as an index of mammary gland development in rats (280,563,671), guinea pigs (232), rabbits (232), and mice (639,640), supported the original findings of Hamolsky and Sparrow (272). Relaxin was reported to be relatively ineffective by itself (280,639,640); in fact, its effects on growth of the mammary tissue were reported to be dependent on not only ovarian mammotropic steroids but also pituitary mammotropic hormones (272,563,639) such as prolactin and growth hormone (281,282). Not all investigators, however, found that relaxin promoted growth of the mammary glands. In one study, multiple injections of crude porcine relaxin over a period of several days failed to promote alveolar growth in ovariectomized steroid-treated mice (627), and in a second study, similar treatment reportedly inhibited mammary gland growth in ovariectomized goats (125).

The most recent studies, which employed highly purified porcine relaxin, support the view that relaxin promotes growth of mammary tissue in rats and mice. Wright and Anderson (671) reported that when porcine relaxin was administered to hypophysectomized immature rats in combination with ovarian and/or pituitary mammotropins, it promoted growth of the mammary ducts, end buds, and lobule-alveoli. Similarly, Bani and co-workers (33–35,46) reported that highly purified porcine relaxin enhanced the effects of estrogen on the growth and development of both the mammary ducts and mammary stromal tissue in intact or ovariectomized estrogen-primed mice. Light and electron microscopic examination of the parenchymal cells that comprise the mammary ducts in mice indicated that relaxin stimulated the proliferation of both the epithelial cells that line the lumen of the ducts and the myoepithelial cells that lie between the inner epithelial cells and basement membrane (33–35). The primary changes observed in the mammary stroma following relaxin treatment were reported to be extensive development in the blood capillary bed and an increase in adipose tissue (34,46).

Studies of the influence of partially purified porcine relaxin on mammary tumor induction in rats have produced seemingly contradictory results which, although difficult to interpret, appear to support the view that relaxin influences mammary tissue. Cutts (146) reported that when rats bearing estrone-induced mammary tumors were administered crude porcine relaxin for a sustained period, both the growth and numbers of tumors increased markedly. Similarly, Plunkett and Gammal (454) found that crude porcine relaxin increased the induction of mammary tumors in rats when administered 6 weeks after carcinogen treatment. Paradoxically, these workers (454) reported that relaxin inhibited tumor induction when administration of the hormone was begun 1 week before carcinogen treatment. More recently Segaloff (534) reported that prolonged administration of partially purified porcine relaxin initially accelerated and then diminished the rate of mammary tumor growth in intact or ovariectomized estrogen-primed rats. The influence of highly purified relaxin on mammary tumor growth has not been reported. Another finding from a pathological study is consistent with the possibility that relaxin influences mammary gland growth and differentiation. A relaxin-like immunoactive substance was reportedly found in the mammary gland cyst fluid of women with fibrocystic disease employing a homologous porcine relaxin radioimmunoassay (413).

The mechanism(s) whereby relaxin promotes growth and differentiation of the mammary glands is not known. It may do so through effects on connective tissue remodeling. Fibroblasts obtained from rat mammary glands during late pregnancy were reported to contain sites that bound radioiodinated porcine relaxin (407). Additionally, it was reported that when fibroblasts obtained from postpuberal guinea pig mammary glands were grown in culture for 2 days with estrogen and/or highly purified porcine relaxin, both hormones (individually and in combination) promoted synthesis of DNA and RNA beyond that achieved in controls (536). The nature of the proteins synthesized by the guinea pig mammary gland fibroblasts in response to relaxin treatment is unknown. It was reported that estrogen promoted the synthesis of both collagen and noncollagen protein, whereas relaxin had no apparent effect on collagen synthesis and decreased noncollagenous protein synthesis (537).

Effects of Relaxin on the Function of the Mammary Glands

The influence, if any, of relaxin on the function of the mammary glands is not known. Several reports indicated that extended treatment over several days with partially purified porcine relaxin diminished lactational capacity. Prolonged treatment with porcine relaxin, administered in combination with ovarian steroids, reduced milk yield in ovariectomized goats (125) and depressed both milk yield and litter weights in ovariectomized rats (348). Additionally, porcine relaxin reduced nursing capabilities and litter survival to weaning when administered for an extended period during late pregnancy in both intact and luteectomized pigs (343). Cowie et al. (125) attributed the reduced milk secretion to a deficiency in growth of alveolar tissue in relaxin-treated goats. Knox and Griffith (348) suggested that the reduced milk secretion in rats may be attributable to interference with milk letdown, since the mammary glands contained copious amount of milk after the nursing period, and exogenous oxytocin had no influence on milk removal. Consistent with the latter mechanism, Summerlee et al. (607) reported that highly purified porcine relaxin inhibited reflex milk ejection in lactating rats. Moreover, these workers (607) reported that relaxin appeared to inhibit reflex milk ejection through a dual mechanism—that is, by acting centrally to reduce the release of oxytocin through a direct effect on the brain and by acting peripherally to inhibit the influence of oxytocin on the myoepithelial cells of the mammary gland. The central site of relaxin's suppression of the release of oxytocin has not been established, but there is limited evidence that it may be the neurohypophysis (434).

Local Effects of Relaxin on the Female Reproductive System

Intraovarian Effects of Relaxin in Cycling Rats

It will be recalled there is evidence that the ovaries of nonpregnant pigs and rats contain relaxin. Moreover, it appears that the relaxin is synthesized by the developing follicle, since both granulosa cells (373) and thecal cells (187) obtained from pig preovulatory follicles secrete relaxin *in vitro* in response to LH stimulation. A physiological role for the relatively low levels of relaxin in the ovaries of cycling pigs during the follicular and periovulatory period (88,391) and cycling rats during estrus (557) has not been established. Bryant-Greenwood, Too, and co-workers (86,623,624) obtained evidence that the intraovarian relaxin may act locally in the rat. These workers explored the influence of relaxin on three enzymes that may influence ovarian connective tissue remodeling during follicular development and/or ovulation—plasminogen activator (PA), collagenase, and proteoglycanase (623,624). PA is a protease that catalyzes conversion of plasminogen to plasmin, and the plasmin in turn activates latent collagenase and thereby promotes collagen breakdown. Both plasmin and proteoglycanase degrade proteoglycans. It is known that ovarian PA activity is, at least in part, regulated by the gonadotropins that are required for follicular development and ovulation. In the rat ovary, as in other mammalian tissues, there are two types of PA, designated μPA and tPA, and it was reported that ovarian μPA and tPA activities are stimulated *in vitro* by LH and FSH, respectively (100,426). Relaxin may also promote one or both of these forms of PA in cycling rats. Highly purified porcine relaxin promoted PA, as well as collagenase, and proteoglycanase activities *in vitro* when added to granulosa cells obtained from gonadotropin-primed rats (see Fig. 51). Relaxin-stimulated PA activity was maximal when granulosa cells obtained from preantral and antral follicles rather than preovulatory follicles were employed (29,623,624); therefore, it was postulated that relaxin's major paracrine function may be associated with connective tissue remodeling of the follicular wall and surrounding stroma as the antrum forms and the follicle enlarges rather than with follicular rupture (29,86,623). There is need for further work in this research area. For example, the influence of relaxin on ovarian components other than the granulosa cells has not been reported.

Intrauterine Effects of Relaxin at Parturition in the Human

Several investigators have reported low levels of intrauterine relaxin in the human near term (50,204,673). Although the source(s) of the putative intrauterine relaxin is not known with certainty, there is evidence that at least a portion of it may be produced locally. Employing immunohistochemical techniques, relaxin immunoactivity was reported to be localized in the maternal decidua (349,676), placental cytotrophoblast (349), and placental syncytiotrophoblast (674,676). The apparent localization of relaxin within the human uterus has stimulated interest in its possible function. There is evidence that it may act directly on fetal membranes. Koay and co-workers (350,351) obtained evidence that relaxin may influence connective tissue re-

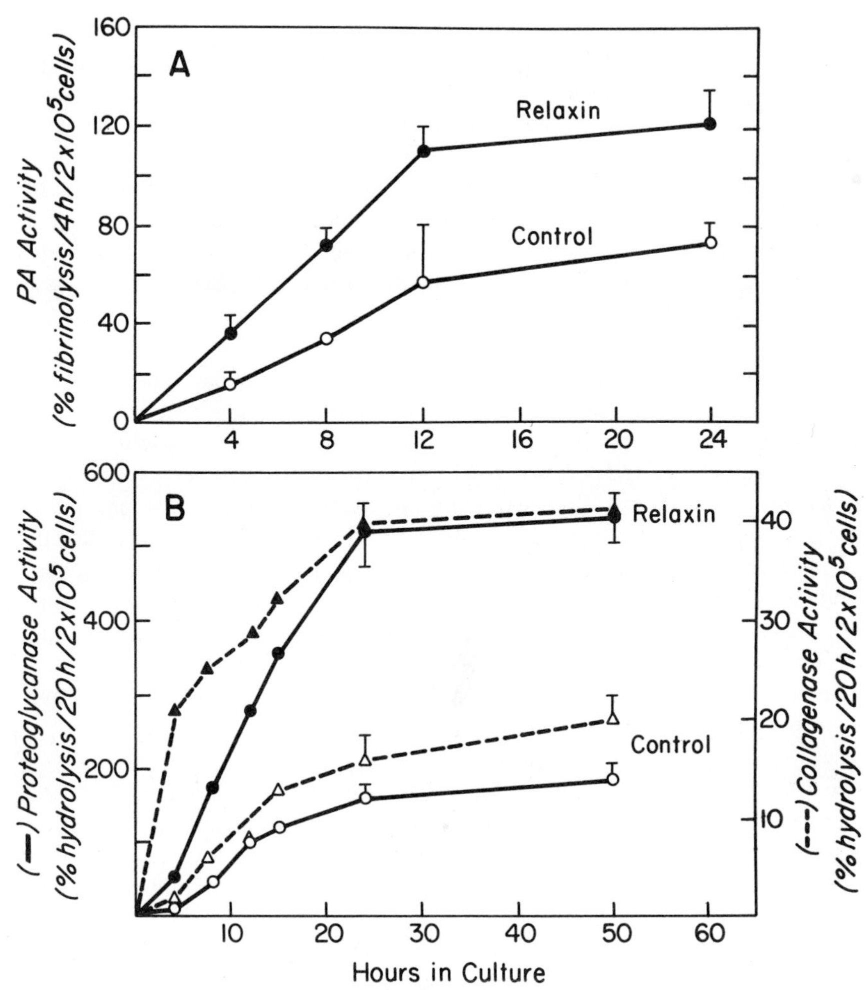

FIG. 51. Influence of relaxin on the secretion of plasminogen activator (PA) activity, proteoglycanase activity, and collagenase activity from rat granulosa cells *in vitro*. Immature rats were primed with 5 IU of pregnant mare serum gonadotropin, and the granulosa cells were harvested 48 hr later and treated with highly purified porcine relaxin (5 μg/ml) or left untreated. **A:** PA activity in the medium is shown as the mean of cumulative activities + SD ($N = 3$). **B:** Proteoglycanase and collagenase activities in the medium are shown as the mean of cumulative activities ± SD ($N = 4$). Reproduced with permission from Too et al. (623).

modeling in human fetal membranes. They reported that the secretion of PA and collagenase into the medium increased when highly purified porcine relaxin was added to cultures of human amnion and chorion cells that were dispersed from placentas obtained at elective cesarean section (350,351) (see Fig. 52). In addition, particulate fractions from the amnion and chorion contained high-affinity sites which bound radiolabeled porcine relaxin with considerable specificity (351). Koay et al. (350,351) postulated that the intrauterine relaxin may have a paracrine function on the apposed fetal membranes in weakening their connective tissue and facilitating membrane rupture at birth.

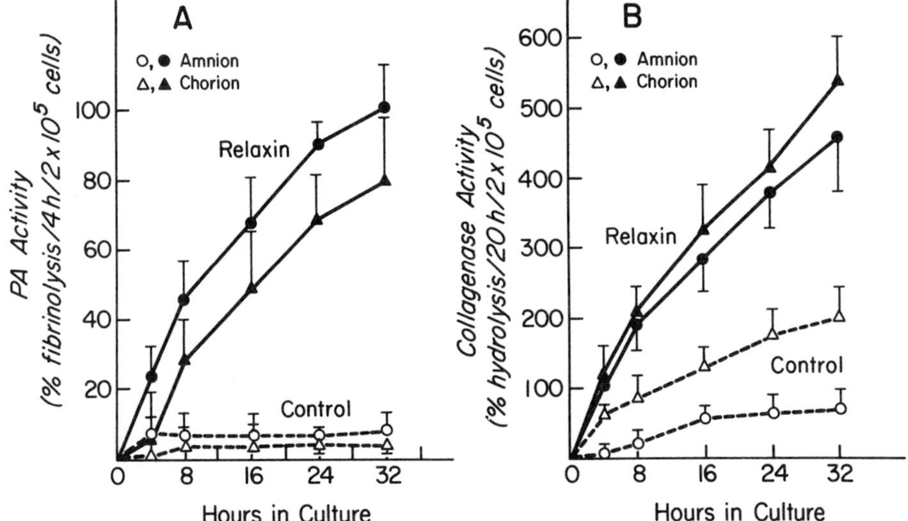

FIG. 52. A: The pattern of accumulation of plasminogen activator activity (PA) in serum-free culture medium bathing amnion cells or chorion cells treated with highly purified porcine relaxin (10 μg/ml) or untreated over a 32-hr period. Values are the mean of cumulative activities ± SD ($N = 3$). **B:** The pattern of accumulation of total collagenase (latent plus active) in serum-free culture medium bathing amnion cells or chorion cells treated with highly purified porcine relaxin (10 μg/ml) or untreated over a 32-hr period. Values are the mean of cumulative activities ± SD ($N = 3$). Reproduced with permission from Koay et al. (351).

Miscellaneous Effects of Relaxin

Diverse effects of relaxin on nonreproductive tissues including adipose, thyroid, gastric mucosa, integument, and the vasculature have been described. Olefsky et al. (438) reported that highly purified porcine relaxin enhanced the ability of porcine insulin to bind to *adipocytes* obtained from adult female rats (but not those obtained from adult male or immature female rats), and that the enhanced binding of insulin was attributable to an increase in the affinity of its receptor. It was postulated that the relaxin-induced increase in insulin-binding may have biological significance, since physiological levels of relaxin potentiated the ability of submaximal concentrations of insulin to promote glucose transport and glucose oxidation in the adipocytes (438). An enhancing effect of relaxin on both the binding and biological activity of insulin was also observed in a similar study which employed human adipocytes obtained at cesarean section (323). The mechanism(s) whereby relaxin modifies the interaction of insulin with its receptor is not known. Jarrett et al. (323) postulated that this heterologous hormone-receptor interaction may make insulin-responsive cells more sensitive to insulin during pregnancy, when women develop relative insulin resistance.

Effects of relaxin on the *thyroid* and *gastric mucosa* are not established. Claims that crude porcine relaxin increased thyroid weights, radioactive iodine uptake, and protein-bound iodine in rats (455,456) were not confirmed (71). The influence of highly purified relaxin on thyroid growth or function has not been reported. A brief report indicated that low doses of porcine relaxin activated human and rat gastric mucosal adenylyl cyclase (500); however, more extensive studies of this putative effect with highly purified relaxin are needed before the gastric mucosa can be considered a target tissue for relaxin.

Extensive clinical studies were conducted in the late 1950s and early 1960s to examine relaxin's putative effects on the *integumentary system* in humans (523). In 1956 it was reported that rats receiving prolonged administration of impure porcine relaxin showed a marked increase in the elasticity of the skin *in vivo* (63). This observation led Casten and co-workers (102,103) to explore the use of porcine relaxin in patients with two chronic debilitating connective tissue diseases characterized by severe reductions in cutaneous elasticity and blood flow to the peripheral vascular beds—namely, scleroderma and obliterative peripheral arterial disease. These workers (102,103) reported that when impure porcine relaxin was injected intramuscularly at daily or 3-day intervals for periods ranging from 6 to 30 months in combination with estrogen, dramatic curative effects were observed. Ulcers on the fingers and toes healed, the blood flow and temperature of the toes increased, and in patients with Raynaud's phenomenon the tolerance to cold increased.

Although similar curative effects were reported by several others following the administration of partially purified porcine relaxin to patients with scleroderma (68,110,188,252, 315,486,492), some investigators reported that porcine relaxin had little or no curative value (325,659). Relaxin's putative therapeutic effects on the peripheral vascular beds appeared to require continual treatment. Several workers reported that following relaxin withdrawal there was a return of the Raynaud's phenomenon and skin tightness (102,103,252,492). Treatment of patients with integumentary connective tissue disease or restrictive peripheral vascular disease has not been reported since the 1960s. Efforts to examine further the influence relaxin might have on the human integumentary connective tissue have been hindered by (a) uncertainties concerning the curative effects of relaxin, (b) uncertainties that accompany the use of impure and poorly characterized hormone preparations, (c) expense and physical discomfort associated with prolonged intramuscular administration of porcine relaxin, and (d) fear of adverse reactions to prolonged administration of the hormone. An anaphylactic shock was fatal to a patient following the intravenous administration of impure porcine relaxin (188). At the present time there are no reports of the influence of highly purified relaxin in integumentary connective tissue in any species; therefore, such an effect remains to be established.

In rats, systolic blood pressure falls during the last 3 or 4 days of gestation (599), and this coincides with the period when relaxin levels in the peripheral blood serum are elevated maximally (545). Recent reports indicate that relaxin may have effects on the *vasculature of nonreproductive tissues*. In a brief report Del Mese et al. (157) indicated that porcine relaxin and a human decidual extract exerted a prompt vasodilatory effect on the perfused microcirculation of the mesocecum. St-Louis and Massicotte (599) examined the influence of chronic intravenous infusion of low doses (approximately 100 ng/hr) of highly purified rat and porcine relaxin into spontaneously hypertensive and normotensive nonpregnant rats. These workers found that both relaxin preparations reduced systolic blood pressure in the spontaneously hypertensive rats. The infusion of relaxin did not reduce blood pressure in the normotensive rats. St-Louis and Massicotte (599) postulated that relaxin may be one of the factors responsible for decreased blood pressure during late pregnancy in the rat.

INFLUENCE OF RELAXIN ON PARTURITION

The early reports that relaxin levels are elevated in the blood of several mammals during pregnancy and that impure preparations of relaxin affect collagenous and muscular tissues in the estrogen-dominated reproductive tract of the nonpregnant female led to the view that relaxin may have an important physiological role(s) during pregnancy and/or at parturition. The most rigorous efforts to demonstrate such a role have employed ablation of the source of relaxin and subsequent hormonal replacement therapy in pregnant mice, rats, and pigs. These three species have been used because the source of relaxin, the ovaries, is readily removed. Moreover, in all three cases porcine relaxin, which is available in relatively large quantities, is bioactive. Data obtained with these three species indicate that progesterone, but not relaxin, is essential for maintenance of pregnancy, whereas relaxin in combination with estrogen is essential for normal parturition.

When pregnant mice, rats, and pigs were ovariectomized and treated with progesterone only, pregnancy was maintained, but parturition was delayed, prolonged, and difficult; furthermore, there was a low incidence of live births (167,265,356,412,564,572). When similarly ovariectomized mice and rats were treated with progesterone plus partially purified relaxin, delivery generally occurred at or near the appropriate time, but the incidence of live births remained low (356,564,572). Finally, when ovariectomized mice and rats were treated with partially purified relaxin in combination with both progesterone and estrogen, delivery was punctual, and, unlike ovariectomized animals treated with steroids only, the uterine evacuation was generally complete (265,356). In more recent studies, which employed highly purified porcine relaxin, Downing and Sherwood (167) demonstrated that relaxin is essential for normal delivery in rats. Rats were ovariectomized on day 9, before relaxin levels are detectable in the blood, and throughout the remainder of pregnancy they were given hormone replacement therapy which consisted of progesterone implants plus estrogen, relaxin, or estrogen and relaxin in doses that mimicked the normal pregnancy serum levels of these hormones (see Fig. 53A). Relaxin was found to be essential at delivery in rats, since in combination with estrogen it enabled not only a short duration of delivery but also a high incidence of live births.

Nara et al. (412) obtained similar results with pregnant pigs. The elevated levels of relaxin and progesterone normally experienced during late pregnancy were abolished by bilaterally ovariectomizing pigs on day 105. The pregnancy was maintained by progesterone administration. When parturition was induced by progesterone withdrawal on day 112, the duration of delivery was prolonged, and the incidence of live births was only 50% that of intact controls (see Fig. 53B). Replacement therapy with progesterone plus highly purified porcine relaxin restored the duration of delivery and the incidence of live births to values similar to those of controls. In comparing the results obtained with ovariectomized pregnant rats (Fig. 53A) to those obtained with ovariectomized pregnant pigs (Fig. 53B), it is important to recognize that the primary source of estrogen in the peripheral blood serum of pigs during late pregnancy is the placenta. The hormonal milieu bathing target tissues in (group OPR) pigs was most nearly like that of (group OPER) rats—thus the identical stippling of the histograms for these two groups in Fig. 53.

The importance of estrogen at parturition in rats has been clearly demonstrated (107,143,167). Since estrogen was not withdrawn following ovariectomy of pregnant pigs (412), as it was in rats (167), its importance at delivery was not clearly demonstrated. Nevertheless, it seems likely that relaxin brings about its beneficial effects on delivery in pigs, as it does in rats, by acting in concert with estrogen. A more comprehensive understanding of the processes whereby relaxin promotes normal delivery requires an appreciation of the many putative functions of estrogen at term.

In rats, several mechanisms have been postulated whereby estrogen may promote normal parturition, and many of them involve contractility of the myometrium. Estrogen induces oxytocin receptors on the rat myometrium (10,11,226) and thereby increases the responsiveness of the myometrium to the oxytocin secreted by the fetal and maternal pituitaries at parturition (226,520). It was also reported that estrogen induces relaxin receptors on both the rat and pig myometrium (395,396). Estrogen also increases the capacity of the rat myometrium and endometrium to synthesize prostaglandins (105), and there is evidence that prostaglandins may be required for luteolysis (250) and mediating oxytocin-stimulated myometrial contractility at delivery in rats (116). Additionally, estrogen treatment induces the formation of gap junctions, and these specialized contacts between adjacent myometrial cells are thought to permit coordinated and synchronized contractions during labor (231,474). Finally, estrogen promotes the formation of the contractile proteins actin and myosin which are associated with uterine myometrial activity (142). In addition to its effects on the myometrium, estrogen promotes increased cervical extensibility.

The mechanism(s) whereby estrogen promotes cervical softening is not known: It may promote relaxin receptors (396) or promote the synthesis of prostaglandins, which have been reported to reduce collagen concentrations near term in the rat cervix (288). The mechanism whereby relaxin acts in combination with estrogen to promote normal parturition (see Fig. 53) in rats is not known with certainty. Relaxin may promote normal parturition by increasing the extensibility of the cervix, preventing excessive myometrial activity until time for delivery, and enhancing the responsiveness of the uterus to oxytocics (167).

Porcine relaxin has also been reported to influence parturition following its administration to *intact* pigs, beef cattle, women, and the spiny dogfish during late pregnancy (96,189,343,353,381,382,403,451). These studies not only provide support for the view that relaxin normally promotes cervical softening and facilitates birth but also demonstrate that relaxin may influence delivery in several species. In pigs, daily intramuscular injections of partially purified porcine relaxin from day 105 or day 107 until luteectomy on day 110 reduced both the interval from surgery to the delivery of the first neonate and the duration of delivery compared to those parameters in luteectomized controls (343). The effects of the exogenous porcine relaxin may have been mediated, at least in part, through premature cervical dilatation (343). Additionally, intramuscular administration

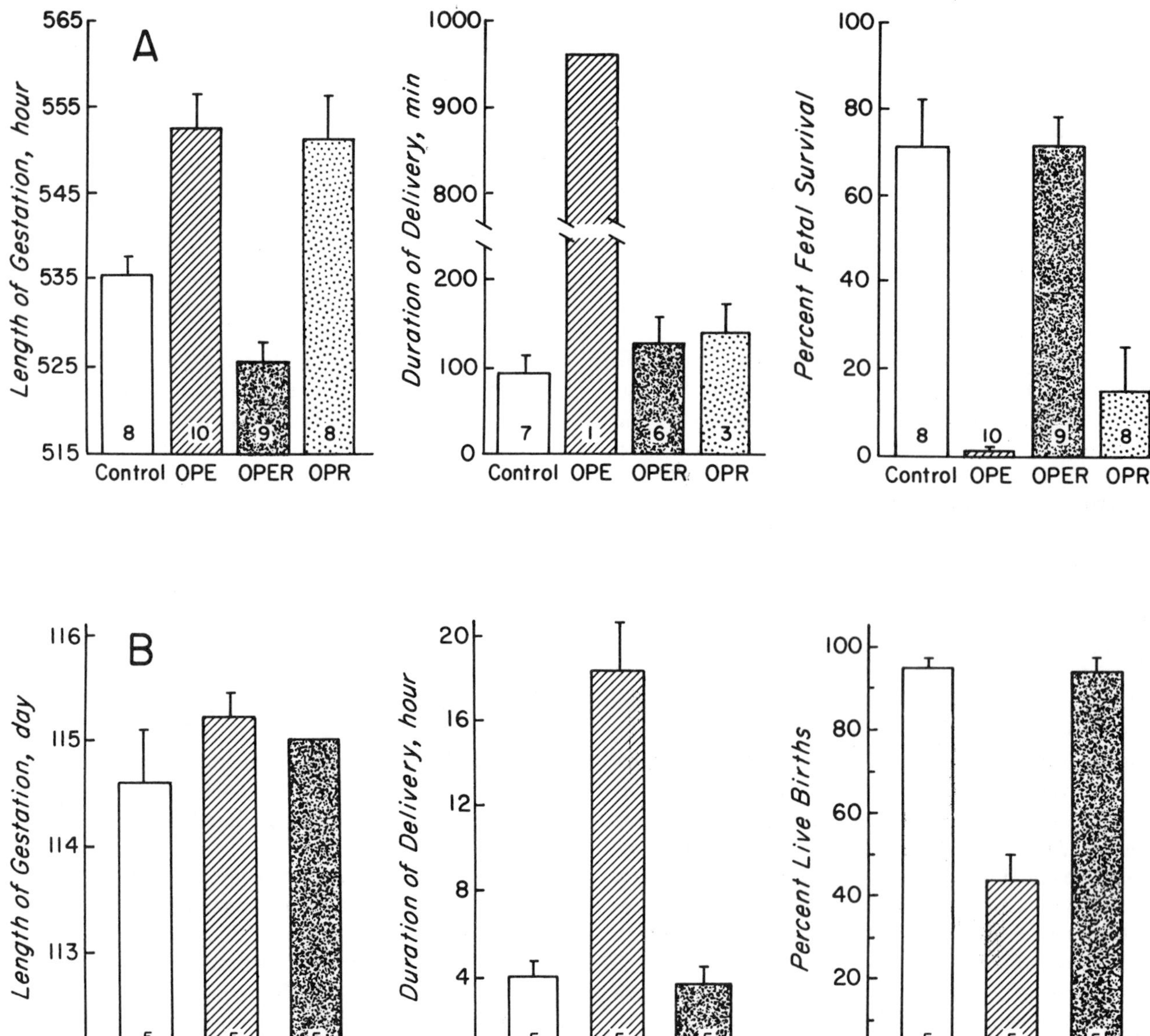

FIG. 53. A: The influence of estrogen and relaxin on birth in rats. Pregnant rats were bilaterally ovariectomized on day 9 and given progesterone (P) implants (2 silastic implants each containing 60 mg P) and, in addition, one of the following injection regimens: estrogen (E; group OPE); E and highly purified porcine relaxin (R; group OPER); or porcine relaxin (group OPR). Estrogen was administered once daily from day 9 until birth in 0.1 ml sesame oil subcutaneously, and R was administered twice daily from day 9 until birth in 0.2 ml 5% beeswax in corn oil subcutaneously. E and R were administered in various doses designed to mimic pregnancy peripheral blood serum levels of the hormones. The P implants were removed on the evening of day 21 to mimic the decline in serum levels that normally occurs at luteolysis. The control group was sham-ovariectomized on day 9 and treated with vehicle controls from day 9 until birth. Means (+ SE) are for the numbers of animals shown at the base of each histogram. Reproduced with permission from Downing and Sherwood (167). **B:** The influence of relaxin on birth in pigs. Pregnant pigs were bilaterally ovariectomized on day 105 and given 100 mg progesterone (P) intramuscularly in 4 ml of corn oil at 12-hr intervals from day 105 through day 112 and, in addition, one of the following injection regimens: highly purified porcine relaxin (R; group OPR) or R vehicle (group OP). Group OPR received 1 mg of highly purified porcine R intramuscularly in 1 ml of 0.9% saline at 6-hr intervals from day 105 until birth. The control group was sham-ovariectomized on day 105 and received the appropriate P and R vehicles thereafter. Means (+ SE) are for the five animals used for each group. Reproduced with permission from Nara et al. (412).

of highly purified porcine relaxin for 1 or 2 days before the induction of parturition with $PGF_{2\alpha}$ on day 112 reportedly improved the synchrony of onset of farrowing in pigs (96).

Anderson and co-workers (403,451) reported that intracervical administration of highly purified porcine relaxin to primiparous beef heifers 4 or 5 days before anticipated parturition induced early calving, which was accompanied by premature dilatation of the cervix and increased pelvic area. Studies demonstrating that intracervical administration of highly purified porcine relaxin to women at term increased the rate of cervical dilatation and facilitated birth were described earlier (189,381–383). Finally, when partially purified porcine relaxin was administered to estrogen-treated spiny dogfish when their pregnancy was over 75% completed, there was a premature loss of developing fetuses which was accompanied by an expansion of the cross-sectional area of the cervix-like constriction between the uterus and urogenital sinus (353). It was concluded that a relaxin-like molecule may be involved during normal parturition in the spiny dogfish (353). The spiny dogfish is the most primitive vertebrate in which relaxin has been demonstrated to influence the female reproductive tract.

The work described above indicates that elevated levels of relaxin in the peripheral blood during the antepartum period just before delivery are important, since, in combination with estrogen, relaxin promotes normal parturition. Maintenance of elevated blood levels of relaxin throughout the anticipated time of delivery, however, may interfere with normal delivery in some species. There is evidence that this is the case in rats. When highly purified porcine relaxin was infused intravenously from day 10 to day 23, gestation was prolonged; furthermore, with rats that gave birth during relaxin infusion, there was an increase in the interval between successive deliveries (329). Jones and Summerlee (329) suggested that this experiment is consistent with the hypothesis that relaxin has not only a peripheral action on the myometrium but also a central action to suppress the release of oxytocin thought to be involved with delivery of the fetuses.

RELAXIN IN THE MALE VERTEBRATE

Sources of Relaxin in the Male

Relaxin may be present in the male reproductive tract of the rooster, pig, armadillo, and human. A bioactive equivalent in rooster testicular extract was reported (572), and its growth-promoting effect on the mouse pubic symphysis was neutralized with an antiserum to impure porcine relaxin (575). In the boar, relaxin immunoactivity was first reported to be associated with both the interstitial and Sertoli cells of the testis (25,172), but when antiserum against highly purified relaxin was used, specific fluorescence was not observed in the testis (25). Additionally, the extremely low levels of relaxin immunoactivity found in tissue extracts indicates that the boar testis is probably not a source of relaxin (672). Localization of relaxin-like activity in the armadillo and human male have relied almost exclusively on techniques that used antisera to highly purified porcine relaxin. In the armadillo, relaxin may be produced only in postpuberal animals. When male reproductive tract tissues from prepuberal and adult armadillos were stained for relaxin by an immunoperoxidase technique, relaxin immunoactivity was localized only within the cells of the prostatic secretory epithelium from the adult animals (99).

Human seminal plasma was reported to contain relaxin immunoactivity levels about 10-fold higher than those in the peripheral blood of pregnant women—about 20 ng/ml (153,154,186,375,652). Limited data support the view that this substance is relaxin. At least a portion of the relaxin-like immunoactivity in human seminal extracts or human prostate extract was associated with a 6,000-dalton fraction (95,340,375). Moreover, seminal plasma extracts or partially purified fractions of these extracts reportedly displayed relaxin bioactivity in the guinea pig pubic symphysis palpation bioassay (155,186), the rat uterine *in vitro* bioassay (155,652), and on the mouse cervix (95). In only one case, however, was the claim that human seminal plasma contained relaxin bioactivity supported with data (652).

The preponderance of available evidence indicates that the prostate is the source of the relaxin-like activity in human seminal plasma; however, there is limited evidence that the seminal vesicles and ampullary part of the vas deferens may be additional sources. Elevated levels of relaxin immunoactivity were found in the seminal fluid when the ejaculated fluid was practically of pure prostatic origin—that is, following vasectomy and in cases of bilateral congenital vas deferens agenesis (153,154). In addition, low but detectable levels of relaxin immunoactivity and bioactivity were reported in adult human prostate extracts (340). Finally, when reproductive tract tissues from adult human males were stained for relaxin with an avidin-biotin immunoperoxidase method, relaxin immunoactivity was localized in the glandular epithelium of the prostate, seminal vesicles, and ampullary part of the vas deferens (677).

Biological Effects of Relaxin in the Male

The apparent presence of relaxin in human seminal plasma led workers to investigate whether this hormone influences spermatozoal physiology and the female reproductive tract after insemination. The limited studies concerning relaxin's influence on human spermatozoa motility are not entirely consistent. Weiss and co-workers reported that low levels of highly purified porcine relaxin (185) or impure porcine relaxin (369) delayed the loss of both motility and grade of forward progression of ejaculated human spermatozoa in suspension for up to 4 hr. Furthermore, an antirelaxin serum (513), but not antiinsulin serum (370), caused a rapid and marked decline of motility when added to washed human spermatozoa. In contrast to these findings, Chan and Tang (115) reported that both physiological and pharmacological concentrations of highly purified porcine relaxin failed to influence the motility of human spermatozoa at the end of a 5-hr incubation period. Relaxin does not appear to influence capacitation of the spermatozoa, since highly purified porcine relaxin did not affect human spermatozoan penetration into zona-free hamster ova (115). Finally, it was reported that the addition of physiological levels of highly purified porcine relaxin increased the ability of washed human spermatozoa to penetrate cervical mucus *in vitro* (74). It was postulated that relaxin may be an exocrine secretion in the male and that the relaxin secreted into the seminal plasma may facilitate penetration of spermatozoa through the female reproductive tract (74). Clearly, much work is needed to determine the chemical nature, source(s), and possible physiological role(s) of the putative relaxin-like substance(s) found in human seminal plasma, rooster testis, and armadillo prostate.

SUMMARY AND CONCLUSIONS

The isolation of porcine relaxin in high yields in the 1970s triggered a sustained resurgence of research on relaxin. Many advances have been made toward a better understanding of the chemistry and physiology of relaxin since then, but research on this hormone remains in its infancy. Accordingly, this section not only will summarize principal recent advances but will also include this reviewer's perception of important unsolved problems that will likely constitute a major portion of the research effort on relaxin throughout the remainder of the 20th century.

Structural studies of porcine, rat, shark, and human relaxin demonstrated that relaxin has superficial structural features similar to those of insulin. The two hormones have molecular weights of about 6,000, contain A and B chains of similar length, and contain disulfide bridges that have the same disposition. The three-dimensional structure of relaxin remains to be established, but studies that used model building and computer-assisted graphics indicated that relaxin can be accommodated into a structure similar to that of insulin. The similarities in their superficial structural features led to the postulation that relaxin and insulin (as well as IGF-I and IGF-II) evolved from a common ancestral gene. The process whereby relaxin is biosynthesized is consistent with this hypothesis. Relaxin, like insulin, is originally synthesized as a preprohormone containing the following sequence: signal peptide/B chain/connecting peptide/A chain. Following cleavage of the signal peptide, the connecting peptide is cleaved to form the active 6,000-dalton hormone. Also supportive of the view that relaxin and insulin evolved from a common gene is the observation that an intron interrupts the coding region of the connecting peptide in the human relaxin gene at a position that corresponds closely to one of two introns in the human insulin gene.

If relaxin and insulin evolved from a common ancestral gene, considerable evolutionary divergence occurred. The molecular weight of prorelaxin is 20,000, whereas that of proinsulin is only 9,000; the connecting peptides of prorelaxin contains about 100 amino acids, whereas the connecting peptide of proinsulin contains about 30 amino acids. Moreover, the primary structures of relaxin and insulin differ extensively. There is only about 25% homology in their amino acid sequences, and this homology is largely attributable to those amino acids involved in cross-linking or chain folding. The surfaces of relaxin and insulin differ markedly, and these hormones share neither immunological determinants nor biological effects. If the receptors for relaxin and insulin evolved from a common ancestral gene, they too diverged extensively during evolution (as did their function): Neither relaxin nor insulin has biologically active sites that are capable of interacting with receptors for both hormones.

The variation in the primary structure of relaxin among species is striking. Less than 50% amino acid sequence homology exists among porcine, rat, shark, and human relaxins. The apparent low degree of evolutionary constraint that permitted this divergence of relaxin's structure among species is extraordinary, and its evolutionary and physiological implications are not understood. The extreme variation of the primary structure of relaxin among species has important implications. First, in order to have anything beyond a superficial understanding of the structure of relaxin for a given species, its amino acid sequence must be determined. The recent isolation of rabbit and equine relaxin makes it seem likely that the primary structures of these two forms of relaxin will be determined in the near future. Determination of the structures of relaxin from a variety of species may provide valuable insight concerning the structural features required for biological activity.

At present little is known except that both chains and the integrity of the putative hydrophobic core of porcine relaxin are essential for full biological activity, whereas the seven amino acids at the C terminus of its B chain are not. Presumably the amino acids that contribute to relaxin's activity in a given bioassay are conserved or vary conservatively among species. Accordingly, comparisons of both the primary structures and biological activities of several forms of relaxin within a given bioassay should provide insight concerning the structural feature required for biological activity. The demonstrated or implicit variation in the structure of relaxin among species as well as the possibility that relaxin receptors have undergone evolutionary divergence may make it necessary to explore the bioactivity of relaxin from a given species in more than one bioassay to find a suitable response. Regardless of the bioassay used, when specific bioactivities are determined, standard and unknown relaxin preparations from the same species should be used to optimize the chances that parallel dose-response curves are obtained.

The marked structural variation of relaxin among species makes it advisable to determine relaxin immunoactivity levels in a given species with a homologous radioimmunoassay for relaxin in that species wherever feasible. With a totally homologous radioimmunoassay the antiserum will bind relaxin with high affinity, so the sensitivity of the radioimmunoassay will be high. Moreover, accurate measurements of relaxin immunoactivity are dependent upon the standard and unknown dose-response curves being parallel. One obvious implication is that, when rigorous studies of the secretion of relaxin in a given species are to be conducted, it may be necessary to isolate relaxin from that species so that a homologous radioimmunoassay for relaxin can be developed.

Although rapid progress has been made in recent years on many facets of relaxin research, little has been accomplished toward the development of improved methods for the bioassay of relaxin. The commonly employed guinea pig pubic symphysis palpation bioassay, mouse interpubic ligament bioassay, and mouse and rat uterine contractility bioassays continue to provide indispensable information concerning the biological activity of relaxin preparations or tissue samplings, but these bioassays have important limitations. They are neither precise nor sensitive, and they are expensive. The development of a specific, precise, and sensitive *in vitro* method(s) for the bioassay of relaxin that would have broad species applicability would be an important contribution to the relaxin field.

When considering the source of relaxin in mammalian species, it can be stated that most if not all of the hormone is produced in a single tissue in the female reproductive tract and that the highest levels are produced during pregnancy. The specific tissue that is the source of relaxin, however, varies among species. It may be the corpus luteum, placenta, or uterus. No clear pattern of pregnancy-related physiological factors that might predict the source of relaxin within a given species has emerged.

Although little is known concerning the factors that influence the synthesis of relaxin in any species, limited evidence indicates that striking differences may exist among species. The synthesis of high levels of relaxin in the corpora lutea is dependent upon placental luteotropic support in rats and women, whereas the corpora lutea appear to have an inherent capacity to produce high levels of relaxin for a period at least as long as pregnancy in pigs. Steroids have been demonstrated to promote relaxin synthesis in two species. Estrogen promotes luteal relaxin synthesis when rats are hysterectomized during the second half of pregnancy, and estrogen in combination with progesterone promotes uterine relaxin synthesis in ovariectomized nonpregnant guinea pigs. Following its synthesis, at least a portion of the relaxin is stored in dense, membrane-limited cytoplasmic granules within the source tissue in several species. These relaxin-containing granules have been identified in pig, rat, and mouse luteal cells, rabbit placental syncytiotrophoblast cells, and guinea pig uterine endometrial gland cells. It remains to be established that relaxin is stored within cytoplasmic granules in all species. The levels of relaxin that are stored in tissue sources vary tremendously among species. For example, the yields of relaxin per gram equivalent of fresh tissue from pig and rat ovaries are approximately 100-fold greater than those from shark ovaries and horse placentas. Neither the mechanisms responsible for the great differences in tissue levels of relaxin among species nor the physiological significance of these differences is understood.

Studies with the pig, rat, horse, human, and monkey have provided limited insight concerning the factors that influence relaxin secretion in these species. As with relaxin synthesis, the regulation of relaxin secretion varies greatly among species. Pigs secrete little relaxin throughout the first 100 days of the 114-day gestation period, but there is a massive release of relaxin from the corpora lutea during the 2 to 3 days before birth. There is evidence that this surge in relaxin levels, which appears to reflect both the age of the corpora lutea and the luteolytic process which precedes parturition, depends on endogenous prostaglandin biosynthesis. There is no evidence of placental involvement in the regulation of relaxin secretion in pigs.

Rats secrete little relaxin until midpregnancy. Relaxin levels in the peripheral blood rise rapidly from about day 12 until day 15 and remain elevated until day 20, when, as in the pig, there is a surge in relaxin levels during the antepartum period. Available evidence indicates that relaxin secretion during the period from day 15 to day 20 is promoted by a placental luteotropic factor (which acts in combination with estrogen) and inhibited by a pituitary suppressive factor(s). The chemical natures and mechanisms of action of the placental and pituitary factors remain completely unknown. The antepartum surge in relaxin levels in the rat is associated with an apparent luteolytic process which occurs at 24-hr intervals and is linked to the photoperiod. The factors that promote the antepartum surge in relaxin levels in the rat are not known; however, there is limited evidence that prostaglandin and LH may be involved.

In horses, relaxin levels rise from about day 80 to an initial peak near midpregnancy on about day 175, decline somewhat over the next 60 days, and then increase gradually until foaling, which occurs between day 300 and day 350. A surge in relaxin levels occurs from a few hours before birth until the placenta is expelled. The factors that influence the secretion of relaxin from the horse placenta have not been determined.

Relaxin is secreted from the corpora lutea of humans and monkeys throughout nearly all of pregnancy. Relaxin levels are higher during the first trimester than during the second or third, and, unlike the pig and rat, there is no evidence of an antepartum surge in relaxin levels in the human and monkey. It appears that chorionic gonadotropic hormones play a major role in promoting relaxin secretion in the human and monkey.

Nearly all efforts to identify the factors that influence relaxin synthesis and secretion have involved surgical or pharmacological manipulations of pregnant animals. The use of *in vivo* methods has several important advantages: *In vivo* methods can identify various organs (the placenta and pituitary, for example, in the rat) that are involved with the regulation of relaxin synthesis and secretion. Additionally, with *in vivo* methods, studies can be conducted with confidence that tissue sources for relaxin are being maintained in a viable and potentially responsive state. Finally, by employing *in vivo* methods, the chance that clear findings have physiological significance is optimized.

Nevertheless, *in vitro* methods have potential advantages: *In vitro* methods permit the examination of factors thought to act directly on source tissues to influence relaxin synthesis and secretion under much more rigidly controlled conditions than *in vivo* methods. Additionally, *in vitro* methods offer advantages for studies aimed at determining the mechanism(s) whereby factors influence relaxin synthesis and secretion. Unfortunately, there are no well-established *in vitro* methods for studying the regulation of relaxin synthesis and secretion. The development and rigorous characterization of *in vitro* methods whereby tissues that synthesize and secrete relaxin (luteal, placental, or uterine tissue) can be maintained in a clearly viable state long enough to examine the effects of various factors on relaxin synthesis or secretion would be a major contribution to the relaxin field.

Relaxin immunoactivity in the peripheral blood of rats and pigs has been demonstrated to be associated with multiple components. In rats, the relaxin immunoactivity is associated with three major components of different size during late pregnancy, and the distribution of relaxin immunoactivity among these components changes progressively with the day of pregnancy. The chemical nature and physiological significance of these multiple relaxin-immunoactive components in the rat remain to be determined.

Studies with highly purified relaxin have confirmed earlier findings that relaxin induces growth of the interpubic ligament, promotes softening of the cervix, and inhibits contractility of the uterus. Whereas relaxin's effects on the cervix and uterine contractility appear to be generally distributed among mammalian species, its effects on the interpubic ligament are not. Relaxin promotes growth of the interpubic ligament in guinea pigs and mice but not in rats, rabbits, or sheep. It cannot be concluded, however, that relaxin does not have generally distributed effects on pelvic ligament softening, of which growth of the interpubic ligament may be only one manifestation. Important fundamental questions remain unanswered concerning relaxin's biological effects on the three well-established target tissues. It is known that the biological effects of relaxin on the interpubic ligament and cervix are absolutely dependent upon estrogen priming and that relaxin's effects on contractility are maximal with the estrogen-dominated uterus. Although there is limited evidence that estrogen may act, at least in part, by inducing relaxin receptors, the mechanism(s) whereby estrogen enables relaxin to bring about its biological effects remains nearly unexplored.

Most of the studies of the effects of relaxin on the interpubic ligament and cervix have involved physical measurements of their growth and/or tensile properties as well as histological studies of the gross morphological changes that occur in their connective tissue components. Biochemical studies that examine the changes relaxin induces in the connective tissue components (collagen and proteoglycans) are in their infancy. Rigorous studies with both the pubic symphysis and the cervix that provide definitive answers to the following questions are needed. Do relaxin's effects involve the interaction with hormones other than estrogen, and, if so, what is the nature of these interactions? What is the biochemical nature of the changes relaxin induces in the connective tissue components of the pubic symphysis and cervix, and what are the mechanisms whereby relaxin induces these changes? How do relaxin-induced changes in connective tissue components contribute to growth of the interpubic ligament and cervical softening? What are the target cells for relaxin in the pubic symphysis and cervix? Can these target cells be isolated and studied in culture in an appropriately differentiated state?

Considerable progress has been made in recent years with intact uteri or uterine segments toward an understanding of relaxin's effects on uterine contractility in the rat. Available data indicate that relaxin not only inhibits the frequency and, to a lesser degree, the amplitude of spontaneous uterine contractions but also attenuates oxytocin- and prostaglandin-induced contractions when the concentrations of these contractile agents are low. The sensitivity of the uterus to the quiescent effects of relaxin is enhanced by prior estrogen treatment, but the mechanism whereby estrogen brings about this effect is largely unexplored. Advances have been made at the molecular level toward an understanding of the mechanism(s) whereby relaxin inhibits contractility of the rat uterine myometrium. There is good evidence that relaxin decreases the activity of the enzyme myosin light chain kinase (MLCK), which promotes smooth-muscle contraction by catalyzing the phosphorylation of myosin light chains. The mechanism(s) whereby relaxin decreases MLCK activity are not known with certainty. There is evidence that can be interpreted to infer that relaxin's effects are mediated through cAMP-dependent phosphorylation of MLCK (which reduces MLCK activity) or other proteins that reduce intracellular Ca^{2+} to levels inadequate to form the active Ca^{2+} • calmodulin • MLCK complex. Further studies are needed to provide a more detailed understanding of the mechanism whereby relaxin reduces MLCK activity. The recent demonstration that cultured rat myometrial cells respond to relaxin and that MLCK activity is reduced in these cells following relaxin treatment indicates that studies of the mechanism whereby relaxin acts on myometrial cells can be conducted with these cells in culture rather than in uterine tissue segments. This method has the important advantage of being able to deliver compounds of interest—such as hormones, enzyme inhibitors, radioactive metabolites, and Ca^{2+} channel blockers—to myometrial cells with efficiency.

Although it appears clear that relaxin inhibits the contractility of myometrial cells through a direct relaxin-induced reduction in MLCK activity, there continue to be isolated and conflicting reports concerning the possibility that relaxin may bring about its effects, at least in part, indirectly by activating β-adrenergic receptors (presumably through relaxin-induced release of endogenous catecholamines from myometrial cells). Studies that would establish the involvement of catecholamines—or lack thereof—with the mechanism of action of relaxin on myometrial cells would contribute substantially to this area.

Studies aimed at gaining insight into the mechanism(s) whereby relaxin influences contractility of the entire uterus are beginning to appear. Limited data indicate that relaxin acts on both the circular smooth-muscle layer and the longitudinal smooth-muscle layer in the rat myometrium and that it alters the action potentials in both smooth-muscle layers. Studies that provide insight concerning the mechanism whereby relaxin interacts with other hormones to influence the coordination of contractility of the entire uterus are needed, since they might provide valuable insight concerning the possible physiological significance of relaxin in rats and other species. It seems important to remember that nearly all studies that have been conducted concerning characterization of the effects of relaxin on uterine contractility were conducted with rats. Caution should be exercised in extrapolating the results of these studies to other species.

In addition to inhibiting myometrial contractility, relaxin has general metabolic effects on rat and mouse uteri (increased uterine water content, wet weight, glycogen content, and protein content) which are similar to changes that occur in the uterine composition during the second half of pregnancy, when relaxin levels are elevated in the peripheral blood. It was postulated that myometrial glycogen stores may provide a source of energy for the strong, highly coordinated uterine contractions that occur at birth, and that the increases in the size and collagenous framework of the uterus during the second half of pregnancy may accommodate the rapidly growing fetuses. Neither the role endogenous relaxin plays in promoting these effects in rat or mice uteri nor their physiological significance during pregnancy has been established, and further research in this area is needed. The possibility that relaxin has general metabolic effects on the uterus in species other than rats and mice remains to be determined.

There is some evidence that relaxin's effects on the uterus are not confined to the myometrium. The isolated reports that relaxin stimulates the proliferation of endothelial cells in the monkey endometrium and increases the volume of the rat endometrium require confirmation. The physiological significance of relaxin's putative effects on the endometrium, if any, are unknown.

Since the mid 1940s, sporadic, but not entirely consistent, reports indicated that the administration of relaxin, in combination with ovarian mammotropic steroids and pituitary mammotropic proteins, promoted growth and differentiation of the mammary glands in several species. Moreover, the most recent studies, which employed highly purified porcine relaxin, support the earlier claims that relaxin is mammotropic. Nevertheless, in this reviewer's judgment it has not been demonstrated beyond doubt that relaxin acts directly on mammary tissue in any species. Additionally, it remains to be demonstrated that endogenous relaxin has an important influence on either mammary gland growth and development or mammary gland function.

The putative effects of relaxin on diverse nonreproductive tissues are not established. Studies that led to claims that relaxin has effects on integumentary connective tissue in humans, integumentary vascular tissue in humans, gastric vascular tissue in rats, and thyroid tissue in rats generally arose from studies that employed crude porcine relaxin; moreover, results of studies with human integumentary connective tissue were not entirely consistent. Studies that led to claims that relaxin has effects on adipose cells in humans and rats were conducted with highly purified relaxin, but the putative effects of relaxin on adipose cells should be confirmed. Should it be established that relaxin acts upon any of these tissues, it remains to be proved that endogenous relaxin has an important influence on their function. The possibility that relaxin has effects on human integumentary connective tissue and vasculature was of considerable interest to clinicians in the late 1950s and early 1960s. Presumably there would be a resurgence of clinical interest in relaxin if its therapeutic utility could be clearly established and if human relaxin were available in large quantities at reasonable cost. Further exploration of the possible effects of relaxin on the integumentary connective tissue and peripheral vasculature seem of considerable interest. Before such studies are undertaken, however, it would be desirable to develop a method for examining the influence of relaxin on the integumentary system in a species such as the pig, where large amounts of relaxin are available and studies can be conducted with a minimum of restrictions.

In recent years the concept has emerged that relaxin may act locally to influence connective tissue remodeling in female reproductive tissues where small quantities of relaxin have been detected. Putative paracrine effects of relaxin originated with studies demonstrating that relaxin stimulates the activity of enzymes associated with collagen and proteoglycan metabolism in follicular granulosa cells obtained from nonpregnant rats and amnion and chorion cells obtained from women at cesarean section. It was postulated that relaxin may influence connective tissue remodeling associated with follicular development in rats and fetal membrane rupture at birth in humans. These putative paracrine effects of relaxin must be confirmed and demonstrated under physiological conditions before they can be considered established and physiologically important.

Although it has been widely believed for many years that relaxin has important physiological roles during pregnancy and at parturition, studies that substantiated this belief were few in number and employed crude porcine relaxin preparations. More recent studies with pregnant pigs and rats, which involved removal of the ovaries and subsequent hormonal replacement therapy with progesterone, estrogen (in rats), and highly purified porcine relaxin in doses selected to mimic physiological levels, provided strong support for the view that relaxin is essential for normal delivery in these two species. Only when relaxin was given in combination with estrogen and progesterone was there a short duration of delivery and a high incidence of live births. The principal limitation of these studies, however, was that they were not entirely physiological. The ovaries were removed for several days, and hormonal replacement therapy with combinations of hormones known to be produced and secreted by the ovary can at best approximate physiological conditions. Stronger evidence that relaxin normally plays an important role in facilitating birth in rats, pigs, and other species would be provided by experiments where the source of relaxin and other hormones is left *in situ* and the level of endogenous relaxin is selectively reduced. The mechanism whereby relaxin facilitates delivery in pigs and rats is not known with certainty. At present the most likely possibilities appear to be through its effects on uterine contractility, cervical softening, or both. It is this reviewer's opinion that relaxin's effects on the tensile properties of the cervix play an important role in facilitating birth in rats and pigs. Moreover, the recent clinical studies demonstrating that intravaginal or intracervical administration of highly purified porcine relaxin before induced delivery of women at term increased the rate of cervical effacement and dilatation encourage the view that human relaxin may have clinical utility in the future if it can be made available in sufficient quantities at reasonable cost.

Since the late 1970s several reports have challenged the long-held view that relaxin in mammals is produced only by the female. Relaxin-like immunoactivity was localized in human and armadillo prostate, and both relaxin-like immunoactivity and relaxin-like bioactivity were reported in human seminal plasma. Highly purified relaxin was reported to retard the rate of loss of human sperm motility and increase the ability of spermatozoa to penetrate the cervical mucus. It was postulated that relaxin may be an exocrine secretion in the male and that relaxin secreted into the seminal plasma may facilitate penetration of spermatozoa through the female reproductive tract. Much work is needed before it can be considered established that relaxin is of physiological importance in the male. The relaxin-like molecule must be isolated and characterized to provide more definitive evidence that relaxin is present in the male. If relaxin is present in the male, it must be demonstrated that the hormone has a physiological role. As with studies of relaxin in female mammals, caution must be exercised in extrapolating results obtained with studies in the male of one species to other species.

In conclusion, many advances have been made toward a better understanding of the chemistry and physiology of relaxin since the mid-1970s. These studies have demonstrated that relaxin has diverse and apparently essential physiological roles during pregnancy and at parturition in species such as the pig and rat. Consequently, the status of relaxin has been rapidly elevated from a poorly understood and frequently ignored hormone to one that requires substantive attention when the hormonal regulation of pregnancy and parturition in mammalian species is being considered.

The chemistry and physiology of relaxin are richly diverse among species. The primary structure, source, regulation of synthesis and secretion, quantities stored in source tissue(s), and target tissue vary extensively among species. This diversity has important implications. Sweeping statements concerning the chemistry and physiology of relaxin among species cannot be made. Understanding the chemistry and physiology of relaxin for a given species is dependent upon the detailed study of relaxin in that species. Although considerable progress has been made toward an understanding of the physiology of relaxin in a few species, accumulation of knowledge concerning this hormone is in its infancy. It is this reviewer's expectation that the numerous unexplored opportunities for further discoveries with relaxin will sustain the present high level of interest in this fascinating hormone for many years to come.

ACKNOWLEDGMENTS

I am grateful to the following persons for reviewing this manuscript and providing helpful advice for its improvement: Dr. M. B. Anderson, Dr. S. H. Cheah, Dr. S. J. Downing, Dr. R. K. Eldridge, Dr. T. G. Golos, Ms. J. J. Hwang, Dr. J. A. Jackson, Mrs. R. H. Key, Ms. M. L. Lao Guico, Ms. M. B. O'Day, and Dr. D. G. Porter. I also wish to thank Mrs. L. J. Battle for the patience and high standards she maintained in typing this manuscript. I am indebted to Mrs. A. A. Prickett for her expert help in preparing illustrations.

REFERENCES

1. Abramowitz, A. A., Money, W. L., Zarrow, M. X., Talmage, R. V. N., Kleinholz, L. H., and Hisaw, F. L. (1944): Preparation, biological assay and properties of relaxin. *Endocrinology,* 34:103–114.
2. Abramson, D., Hurwitt, E., and Lesnick, G. (1937): Relaxin in human serum as a test of pregnancy. *Surg. Gynecol. Obstet.,* 65:335–339.
3. Abramson, D., and Reid, D. E. (1955): Use of relaxin in treatment of threatened premature labor. *J. Clin. Endocrinol. Metab.,* 15:206–209.
4. Abramson, D., Roberts, S. M., and Wilson, P. D. (1934): Relaxation of the pelvic joints in pregnancy. *Surg. Gynecol. Obstet.,* 63:595–613.
5. Adams, W. C., and Frieden, E. H. (1985): Inhibition of post-partum uterine involution in the rat by relaxin. *Biol. Reprod.,* 33:1168–1175.
6. Addiego, L. A., Tsutsui, D. R., Stewart, D. R., and Stabenfeldt, G. H. (1985): Determination of the source of feline relaxin. *Program and Abstracts of the 18th Annual Meeting of the Society for the Study of Reproduction,* Montreal, Canada, abstract 231.

7. Adelstein, R. S., Pato, M. D., and Conti, M. A. (1981): The role of phosphorylation in regulating contractile proteins. *Adv. Cyclic Nucleotide Res.*, 14:361–373.
8. Afele, S., Bryant-Greenwood, G. D., Chamley, W. A., and Dax, E. M. (1979): Plasma relaxin immunoactivity in the pig at parturition and during nuzzling and suckling. *J. Reprod. Fertil.*, 56: 451–457.
9. Albert, A., Money, W. L., and Zarrow, M. X. (1947): An improved method of extraction and purification of relaxin from fresh whole ovaries of the sow. *Endocrinology*, 40:370–374.
10. Alexandrova, M., and Soloff, M. S. (1980): Oxytocin receptors and parturition. I. Control of oxytocin receptor concentration in the rat myometrium at term. *Endocrinology*, 106:730–735.
11. Alexandrova, M., and Soloff, M. S. (1980): Oxytocin receptors and parturition. II. Concentrations of receptors for oxytocin and estrogen in the gravid and nongravid uterus at term. *Endocrinology*, 106:736–738.
12. Ali, S. M., McMurtry, J. P., Bagnell, C. A., and Bryant-Greenwood, G. D. (1986): Immunocytochemical localization of relaxin in corpora lutea of sows throughout the estrous cycle. *Biol. Reprod.*, 34:139–143.
13. Anderson, L. L. (1982): Relaxin localization in porcine and bovine ovaries by assay and morphological techniques. *Adv. Exp. Med. Biol.*, 143:1–67.
14. Anderson, L. L., Adair, V., Stromer, M. H., and McDonald, W. G. (1983): Relaxin production and release after hysterectomy in the pig. *Endocrinology*, 113:677–686.
15. Anderson, L. L., Bast, J. D., and Melampy, R. M. (1973): Relaxin in ovarian tissue during different reproductive stages in the rat. *J. Endocrinol.*, 59:371–372.
16. Anderson, L. L., Dyck, G. W., Mori, H., Henricks, D. M., Melampy, R. M., (1967): Ovarian function in pigs following hypophyseal stalk transection or hypophysectomy. *Am. J. Physiol.*, 212:1188–1194.
17. Anderson, L. L., Ford, J. J., Melampy, R. M., and Cox, D. F. (1973): Relaxin in porcine corpora lutea during pregnancy and after hysterectomy. *Am. J. Physiol.*, 225:1215–1219.
18. Anderson, L. L., Perezgrovas, R., O'Byrne, E. M., and Steinetz, B. G. (1982): Biological actions of relaxin in pigs and beef cattle. *Ann. N.Y. Acad. Sci.*, 380:131–150.
19. Anderson, M. B. (1984): Bioassay of porcine relaxin components by *in vitro* inhibition of rat uterine contractions. *Endocrinology*, 114:364–368.
20. Anderson, M. B., and Long, J. A. (1978): Localization of relaxin in the pregnant rat. Bioassay of tissue extracts and cell fractionation studies. *Biol. Reprod.*, 18:110–117.
21. Anderson, M. B., Long, J. A., and Hayashida, T. (1975): Immunofluorescence studies on the localization of relaxin in the corpus luteum of the pregnant rat. *Biol. Reprod.*, 13:499–504.
22. Anderson, M. B., and Sherwood, O. D. (1984): Ultrastructural localization of relaxin immunoreactivity in corpora lutea of pregnant rats. *Endocrinology*, 114:1124–1127.
23. Anderson, M. B., Vaupel, M. R., and Sherwood, O. D. (1984): Pregnant mouse corpora lutea: Immunocytochemical localization of relaxin and ultrastructure. *Biol. Reprod.*, 31:391–397.
24. Anderson, R. R., editor (1982): *Relaxin. Adv. Exp. Med. Biol.*, Vol. 143.
25. Arakaki, R. F., Kleinfeld, R. G., and Bryant-Greenwood, F. C. (1980): Immunofluorescence studies using antisera to crude and to purified porcine relaxin. *Biol. Reprod.*, 23:153–159.
26. Ash, R. W., and Heap, R. B. (1975): Oestrogen, progesterone and corticosteroid concentrations in peripheral plasma of sows during pregnancy, parturition, lactation, and after weaning. *J. Endocrinol.*, 64:141–154.
27. Astwood, E. B., and Greep. R. O. (1938): A corpus luteum-stimulating substance in the rat placenta. *Proc. Soc. Exp. Biol. Med.*, 38:713–716.
28. Atkinson, L. E., Hotchkiss, J., Fritz, G. R., Surve, A. H., Neill, J. D., and Knobil, E. (1975): Circulating levels of steroids and chorionic gonadotropin during pregnancy in the rhesus monkey, with special attention to the rescue of the corpus luteum in early pregnancy. *Biol. Reprod.*, 12:335–345.
29. Bagnell, C. A., Domondon, M. C., and Bryant-Greenwood, G. D. (1984): Plasminogen activator (PA) activity in rat and pig follicles during follicular development. In: *Proceedings of the 5th Ovarian Workshops*, edited by R. J. Ryan and D. O. Tofts, pp. 233–238. Ovarian Workshops, Champaign, IL.
30. Bakke, T., and Gytre, T. (1980): Ultrasonic and mechanical measurement of human cervical consistency. In: *Dilatation of the Uterine Cervix*, edited by F. Naftolin and P. G. Stubblefield, pp. 219–232. Raven Press, New York.
31. Balboni, G. C., Denkova, R., Vannelli, G. B., and Zecchi, S. (1983): Immunofluorescent localization of relaxin-like molecules in the granulosa cells of cavitary follicles of human and porcine ovary. In: *Biology of Relaxin and Its Role In the Human*, edited by M. Bigazzi, F. C. Greenwood, and F. Gasparri, pp. 216–218. Excerpta Medica, Amsterdam.
32. Baldwin, D. M., and Stabenfeldt, G. H. (1975): Endocrine changes in the pig during late pregnancy, parturition and lactation. *Biol. Reprod.*, 12:508–515.
33. Bani, G., and Bigazzi, M. (1984): Morphological changes induced in mouse mammary gland by porcine and human relaxin. *Acta Anat.*, 119:149–154.
34. Bani, G., Bigazzi, M., and Bani, D. (1985): Effects of relaxin on the mouse mammary gland. I. The myoepithelial cells. *J. Endocrinol. Invest.*, 8:207–215.
35. Bani, G., Bigazzi, M., and Bani, D. (1986): The effects of relaxin on the mammary gland. II. The epithelium. *J. Endocrinol. Invest.*, 9:145–152.
36. Bassett, E. G., and Phillipps, D. S. M. (1955): Changes in the pelvic region of the ewe during pregnancy and parturition. *N. Z. Vet. J.*, 3:20–25.
37. Beck, P., Adler, P., Szlachter, N., Goldsmith, L. T., Steinetz, B. G., and Weiss, G. (1982): Synergistic effect of human relaxin and progesterone on human myometrial contractions. *Int. J. Gynaecol. Obstet.*, 20:141–144.
38. Bedarker, S., Blundell, T., Gowan, L. K., McDonald, J. K., and Schwabe, C. (1982): On the three-dimensional structure of relaxin. *Ann. N.Y. Acad. Sci.*, 380:22–33.
39. Bedarker, S., Turnell, W. G., Blundell, T. L., and Schwabe, C. (1977): Relaxin has conformational homology with insulin. *Nature*, 270:449–451.
40. Bell, G. I., Pictet, R. L., Rutter, W. J., Cordell, B., Tischer, E., and Goodman, H. M. (1980): Sequence of human insulin gene. *Nature*, 284:26–32.
41. Belt, W. D., Anderson, L. L., Cavazos, L. F., and Melampy, R. M. (1971): Cytoplasmic granules and relaxin levels in porcine corpora lutea. *Endocrinology*, 89:1–10.
42. Belt, W. D., Cavazos, L. F., Anderson, L. L., and Kraeling, R. R. (1970): Fine structure and progesterone levels in the corpus luteum of the pig during pregnancy and after hysterectomy. *Biol. Reprod.*, 2:98–113.
43. Bennett, H. P. J., Hudson, A. M., Kelly, L., McMartin, C., and Purdon, G. E. (1978): A rapid method, using octadecasilyl-silica for the extraction of certain peptides from tissues. *Biochem. J.*, 175:1139–1141.
44. Bentley, G., Dodson, E., Dodson, G., Hodgkin, D., and Mercola, D. (1976): Structure of insulin in 4-zinc insulin. *Nature*, 261:166–168.
45. Bernstein, P., and Crelin, E. S. (1967): Bony pelvic sexual dimorphism in the rat. *Anat. Rec.*, 157:517–526.
46. Bianchi, S., Bani, G., and Bigazzi, M. (1986): Effects of relaxin on the mouse mammary gland. III. The fat pad. *J. Endocrinol. Invest.*, 9:153–160.
47. Bigazzi, M., Bruni, P., Nardi, E., Petrucci, F., Pollicino, G., Franchini, M., Scarselli, G., and Farnararo, M. (1982): Human decidual relaxin. *Ann. N.Y. Acad. Sci.*, 380:87–99.
48. Bigazzi, M., Greenwood, F. C., and Gasparri, F., editors (1983): *Biology of Relaxin and Its Role in the Human*. Excerpta Medica, Amsterdam.
49. Bigazzi, M., and Nardi, E. (1981): Prolactin and relaxin: Antagonism on the spontaneous motility of the uterus. *J. Clin. Endocrinol. Metab.*, 53:665–667.
50. Bigazzi, M., Nardi, E., Bruni, P., and Petrucci, F. (1980): Relaxin in human decidua. *J. Clin. Endocrinol. Metab.*, 51:939–941.
51. Bigazzi, M., Petrucci, F., Nardi, E., and Scarselli, G. (1983): Decidua and other extraluteal sources of human relaxin. In: *Biology of Relaxin and Its Role in the Human*, edited by M. Bigazzi, F. C.

Greenwood, and F. Gasparri, pp. 377–388. Excerpta Medica, Amsterdam.
52. Bloom, G., Paul, K.-G., and Wiqvist, N. (1958): A uterine-relaxing factor in the pregnant rat. *Acta Endocrinol. (Copenh.)*, 28:112–118.
53. Blundell, T. (1979): Conformation and molecular biology of polypeptide hormones. I. Insulin, insulin-like growth factor, and relaxin. *Trends Biochem. Sci. Rev.*, 4:51–54.
54. Blundell, T. L., Bedarker, S., Rinderknecht, E., and Humbel, R. E. (1978): Insulin-like growth factor: A model for tertiary structure accounting for immunoreactivity and receptor binding. *Proc. Natl. Acad. Sci. USA*, 75:180–184.
55. Blundell, T. L., Dodson, G. G., Hodgkin, D. C., and Mercola, D. A. (1972): Insulin: The structure in the crystal and its reflection in chemistry and biology. *Adv. Protein Chem.*, 26:279–402.
56. Blundell, T., Gowan, L. K., and Schwabe, C. (1983): Relaxin—a member of the insulin family? In: *Biology of Relaxin and Its Role in the Human*, edited by M. Bigazzi, F. C. Greenwood, and F. Gasparri, pp. 14–21. Excerpta Medica, Amsterdam.
57. Blundell, T. L., and Humbel, R. E. (1980): Hormone families: Pancreatic hormones and homologous growth factors. *Nature*, 287:781–787.
58. Blundell, T., and Wood, S. (1982): The conformation, flexibility, and dynamics of polypeptide hormones. *Annu. Rev. Biochem.*, 51:123–154.
59. Bodsch, W., and Struck, H. (1980): Enzyme-immunoassay for the peptide hormone relaxin. *Fresenius Z. Anal. Chem.*, 301:133–134.
60. Bolton, A. E., and Hunter, W. M. (1973): The labelling of proteins to high specific radioactivities by conjugation to a ^{125}I-containing acylating agent. *Biochem. J.*, 133:529–539.
61. Borjesson, B. W., John, M. J., and Niall, H. D. (1981): The topographical mapping of porcine relaxin: Accessibility of hydrophobic residues and amino groups. In: *Relaxin*, edited by G. D. Bryant-Greenwood, H. D. Niall, and F. C. Greenwood, pp. 93–95. Elsevier/North-Holland, New York.
62. Bosc, M. J., du Mesnil du Buisson, F., and Locatelli, A. (1974): Mise en évidence d'un controle foetal de la parturition chez la truie. Interactions avec la fonction lutéale. *C. R. Acad. Sci. Paris*, 278:1507–1510.
63. Boucek, R. J. (1956): Biochemical and histological aspects of *in vivo* cultivated connective tissue. In: *Lectures on Orthopedics and Rheumatic Diseases*. Dedication volume, Hospital for Special Surgery, pp. 155–158. Quinnipiak Press, New Haven, CT.
64. Boyd, S., Kendall, J. Z., Mento, N., and Bryant-Greenwood, G. D. (1981): Relaxin immunoactivity in plasma during the reproductive cycle of the female guinea pig. *Biol. Reprod.*, 24:405–414.
65. Brackett, K. H., Dubois, W., Mather, F. B., Roberts, R. F., Fields, P. A., and Fields, M. J. (1985): Relaxin: An ovarian peptidyl hormone in an avian species (*Gallus domesticus*). *Program and Abstracts of the 18th Annual Meeting of the Society for the Study of Reproduction*, Montreal, Canada, abstract 11.
66. Braddon, S. A. (1978): Stimulation of ornithine decarboxylase by relaxin. *Biochem. Biophys. Res. Commun.*, 80:75–80.
67. Braddon, S. A. (1978): Relaxin-dependent adenosine 3′,5′-monophosphate concentration changes in the mouse pubic symphysis. *Endocrinology*, 102:1292–1299.
68. Bradham, G. B., Stallworth, J. M., Brailsford, L. E., and Threatt, B. A. (1962): Clinical evaluation of relaxin in ulcerative ischemic vascular or collagen diseases. *Angiology*, 13:418–420.
69. Bradshaw, J. M. C., Downing, S. J., Moffatt, A., Hinton, J. C., and Porter, D. G. (1981): Demonstration of some of the physiological properties of rat relaxin. *J. Reprod. Fertil.*, 63:145–153.
70. Bradshaw, R. A., and Niall, H. D. (1978): Insulin-related growth factors. *Trends Biochem. Sci. Rev.*, 3:274–278.
71. Braverman, L. E., and Ingbar, S. H. (1963): Effects of preparations containing relaxin on thyroid function in the female rat. *Endocrinology*, 72:337–341.
72. Brennan, D. M., and Zarrow, M. X. (1959): Water and electrolyte content of the uterus of the intact and adrenalectomized rat treated with relaxin and various steroid hormones. *Endocrinology*, 64:907–913.
73. Brenner, S. H., Lessing, J. B., D'Eletto, R. D., and Weiss, G. (1985): Relaxin-like bioactivity in pooled human pregnancy serum. *Obstet. Gynecol.*, 66:46–49.
74. Brenner, S. H., Lessing, J. B., Schoenfeld, C., Amelar, R. D., Dubin, L., and Weiss, G. (1984): Stimulation of human sperm cervical mucus penetration *in vitro* by relaxin. *Fertil. Steril.*, 42:92–96.
75. Brenner, S. H., Lessing, J. B., and Weiss, G. (1984): The effect of *in vivo* progesterone administration on relaxin-inhibited rat uterine contractions. *Am. J. Obstet. Gynecol.*, 148:946–950.
76. Bret, A. J., Coiffard, P., and Motamedi (1963): Releasine: Son emploi et ses résultats au cours de la gravidité dans les manaces d'avortement et d'accouchement prémature. *Rev. Fr. Gynecol. Obstet.*, 58:649–668.
77. Brody, S., and Wiqvist, N. (1961): Ovarian hormones and uterine growth: Effects of estradiol, progesterone, and relaxin on cell growth and cell division in the rat uterus. *Endocrinology*, 68:971–977.
78. Brown, H., Sanger, F., and Kitai, R. (1955): The structure of pig and sheep insulins. *Biochem. J.*, 60:556–565.
79. Bruni, P., Bigazzi, M., and Farnararo, M. (1982): The interaction of porcine and human relaxin with the mouse uterus: Effect on some carbohydrate-metabolizing enzymes. *Mol. Physiol.*, 2:357–362.
80. Bryant, G. D. (1972): The detection of relaxin in porcine, ovine, and human plasma by radioimmunoassay. *Endocrinology*, 91:1113–1117.
81. Bryant, G. D., and Chamley, W. A. (1976): Changes in relaxin and prolactin immunoactivities in ovine plasma following suckling. *J. Reprod. Fertil.*, 46:457–459.
82. Bryant, G. D., and Chamley, W. A. (1976): Plasma relaxin and prolactin immunoactivities in pregnancy and at parturition in the ewe. *J. Reprod. Fertil.*, 48:201–204.
83. Bryant, G. D., Panter, M. E. A., and Stelmasiak, T. (1975): Immunoreactive relaxin in human serum during the menstrual cycle. *J. Clin. Endocrinol. Metab.*, 41:1065–1069.
84. Bryant, G. D., Sassin, J. F., Weitzman, E. D., Kapen, S., and Frantz, A. (1976): Relaxin immunoactivity in human plasma during a 24-hr period. *J. Reprod. Fertil.*, 48:389–392.
85. Bryant-Greenwood, G. D. (1977): Radioimmunoassay of relaxin. In: *Handbook of Radioimmunoassay*, edited by G. E. Abraham, pp. 243–273. Marcel Dekker, New York.
86. Bryant-Greenwood, G. D. (1982): Relaxin as a new hormone. *Endocr. Rev.*, 3:62–90.
87. Bryant-Greenwood, G. D., and Greenwood, F. C. (1979): Specificity of radioimmunoassays for relaxin. *J. Endocrinol.*, 81:239–247.
88. Bryant-Greenwood, G. D., Jeffrey, R., Ralph, M. M., and Seamark, R. F. (1980): Relaxin production by the porcine ovarian Graafian follicle *in vitro*. *Biol. Reprod.*, 23:792–800.
89. Bryant-Greenwood, G. D., Niall, H. D., and Greenwood, F. C., editors (1981): *Relaxin*. Elsevier/North-Holland, New York.
90. Bryant-Greenwood, G. D., and Yamamoto, S. Y. (1983): The radioimmunoassay of relaxin, current status and future prospects. In: *Biology of Relaxin and Its Role in the Human*, edited by M. Bigazzi, F. C. Greenwood, and F. Gasparri, pp. 148–158. Excerpta Medica, Amsterdam.
91. Buckle, J. W., and Nathanielsz, P. W. (1973): The effect of low doses of prostaglandin $F_{2\alpha}$ infused into the aorta of unrestrained pregnant rats: Observations on induction of parturition and effect on plasma progesterone concentration. *Prostaglandins*, 4:443–457.
92. Bullesbach, E. E., and Schwabe, C. (1985): [Å-phenylalanyl] relaxin (porcine): An active intermediate. *Biochem. Biophys. Res. Commun.*, 126:130–135.
93. Bullesbach, E. E., and Schwabe, C. (1985): Naturally occurring porcine relaxins and large-scale preparation of B29 hormone. *Biochemistry*, 24:7717–7722.
94. Bullesbach, E. E., and Schwabe, C. (1985): Preparation and properties of α- and ε-amino-protected porcine relaxin derivitives. *Biochemistry*, 24:7722–7728.
95. Burgardt, A., Bauer, H., Lippert, T. H., and Voelter, W. (1983): Purification and biological activity of relaxin from human seminal fluid. In: *Biology of Relaxin and Its Role in the Human*, edited by M. Bigazzi, F. C. Greenwood, and F. Gasparri, pp. 399–401. Excerpta Medica, Amsterdam.
96. Butler, W. R., and Boyd, R. D. (1983): Relaxin enhances synchronization of parturition induced with prostaglandin $F_{2\alpha}$ in swine. *Biol. Reprod.*, 28:1061–1065.
97. Cabrol, D., Huszar, G., Romero, R., and Naftolin, F. (1981): Gestational changes in the rat uterine cervix: Protein, collagen, and glycosaminoglycan content. In: *The Cervix in Pregnancy and Labour*, edited by D. A. Ellwood and A. B. M. Anderson, pp. 34–39. Churchill Livingstone, New York.

98. Calder, A. A. (1981): The human cervix in pregnancy: A clinical perspective. In: *The Cervix in Pregnancy and Labour,* edited by D. A. Ellwood and A. B. M. Anderson, pp. 103–122. Churchill Livingstone, New York.
99. Cameron, D. F., Corton, G. L., and Larkin, L. H. (1982): Relaxin-like antigenicity in the armadillo prostate gland. *Ann. N.Y. Acad. Sci.,* 380:231–240.
100. Canipari, R., and Strickland, S. (1985): Plasminogen activator in the rat ovary. *J. Biol. Chem.,* 260:5121–5125.
101. Carminati, P., Luzzani, F., Soffientini, A., and Lerner, L. J. (1975): Influence of day of pregnancy on rat placental, uterine, and ovarian prostaglandin synthesis and metabolism. *Endocrinology,* 97:1071–1079.
102. Casten, G. G., and Boucek, R. J. (1958): Use of relaxin in the treatment of scleroderma. *J.A.M.A.,* 166:319–324.
103. Casten, G. G., Gilmore, H. R., Houghton, F. E., and Samuels, S. S. (1960): A new approach to the management of obliterative peripheral arterial disease. *Angiology,* 11:408–414.
104. Castracane, V. D., D'Eletto, R., and Weiss, G. (1983): Relaxin secretion in the baboon (*Papio cynocephalus*). In: *Factors Regulating Ovarian Function,* edited by G. S. Greenwald and P. F. Terranova, pp. 415–419. Raven Press, New York.
105. Castracane, V. D., and Jordon, V. C. (1975): The effect of estrogen and progesterone on uterine prostaglandin biosynthesis in the ovariectomized rat. *Biol. Reprod.,* 13:587–596.
106. Castracane, V. D., Lessing, J., Brenner, S., and Weiss, G. (1985): Relaxin in the pregnant baboon: Evidence for local production in reproductive tissues. *J. Clin. Endocrinol. Metab.,* 60:133–136.
107. Catala, S., and Deis, R. P. (1973): Effect of estrogen upon parturition, maternal behavior and lactation in ovariectomized pregnant rats. *J. Endocrinol.,* 56:219–225.
108. Catchpole, H. R., Joseph, N. R., and Engel, M. B. (1952): The action of relaxin on the pubic symphysis of the guinea-pig, studied electrometrically. *J. Endocrinol.,* 8:377–385.
109. Cavazos, L. F., Anderson, L. L., Belt, W. D., Henricks, D. M., Kraeling, R. R., and Melampy, R. M. (1969): Fine structure and progesterone levels in the corpus luteum of the pig during the estrous cycle. *Biol. Reprod.,* 1:83–106.
110. Chalmers, T. M., and Hearnshaw, J. R. (1961): A case of scleroderma treated with relaxin. *Ann. Rheum. Dis.,* 20:202.
111. Chamley, W. A., Bagoyo, M. M., and Bryant-Greenwood, G. D. (1977): *In vitro* response of relaxin-treated rat uterus to prostaglandins and oxytocin. *Prostaglandins,* 14:763–769.
112. Chamley, W. A., Bagoyo, M. M., and Bryant-Greenwood, G. D. (1981): Potencies of porcine relaxins using two bioassays. *J. Endocrinol.,* 88:89–96.
113. Chamley, W. A., and Parkington, H. C. (1984): Relaxin inhibits the plateau component of the action potential in the circular myometrium of the rat. *J. Physiol.,* 353:51–65.
114. Chamley, W. A., Stelmasiack, T., and Bryant, G. D. (1975): Plasma relaxin immunoactivity during the oestrus cycle of the ewe. *J. Reprod. Fertil.,* 45:455–461.
115. Chan, S. Y. W., and Tang, L. C. H. (1984): Lack of effect of exogenous relaxin on the fertilizing capacity of human spermatozoa. *IRCS Med. Sci.,* 12:879–880.
116. Chan, W. Y. (1983): Uterine and placental prostaglandins and their modulation of oxytocin sensitivity and contractility in the parturient uterus. *Biol. Reprod.,* 29:680–688.
117. Cheah, S. H., and Sherwood, O. D. (1980): Target tissues for relaxin in the rat: Tissue distribution of injected ^{125}I-labeled relaxin and tissue changes in adenosine 3′,5′-monophosphate levels after *in vitro* relaxin incubation. *Endocrinology,* 106:1203–1209.
118. Cheah, S. H., and Sherwood, O. D. (1981): Effects of relaxin on *in vivo* uterine contractions in conscious and unrestrained estrogen-treated and steroid-untreated ovariectomized rats. *Endocrinology,* 109:2076–2083.
119. Chew, C. S., and Rinard, G. A. (1979): Glycogen levels in the rat myometrium at the end of pregnancy and immediately postpartum. *Biol. Reprod.,* 20:1111–1114.
120. Chihal, H. J., and Espey, L. L. (1973): Utilization of the relaxed symphysis pubis of guinea pigs for clues to the mechanism of ovulation. *Endocrinology,* 93:1441–1445.
121. Coggins, E. G., and First, N. L. (1977): Effect of dexamethasone, methallibure, and fetal decapitation on porcine gestation. *J. Anim. Sci.,* 44:1041–1049.
122. Cohen, H. (1963): Relaxin: Studies dealing with isolation, purification, and characterization. *Trans. N.Y. Acad. Sci.,* 25:313–330.
123. Corner, G. W. (1919): On the origin of the corpus luteum of the sow from both granulosa and theca interna. *Am. J. Anat.,* 26:117–183.
124. Corteel, M., Lemon, M., and Dubois, M. (1977): Évolution de la réaction immunocytologique du corps jaune de Truie au cours de la gestation. *J. Physiol. (Paris),* 73:63A–64A.
125. Cowie, A. T., Cox, C. P., Folley, S. J., Hosking, Z. D., and Tindal, J. S. (1965): Relative efficiency of crystalline suspensions of hexoestrol and of oestradiol monobenzoate in inducing mammary development and lactation in the goat; and effects of relaxin on mammogenesis and lactation. *J. Endocrinol.,* 31:165–172.
126. Crawford, R. J., Hudson, P., Shine, J., Niall, H. D., Eddy, R. L., and Shows, T. B. (1984): Two human relaxin genes are on chromosome 9. *EMBO J.,* 3:2341–2345.
127. Crelin, E. S. (1954): The effect of estrogen and relaxin on intact and transplanted pubic symphyses in mice. *Anat. Rec.,* 118:380–381.
128. Crelin, E. S. (1954): The effects of androgen, estrogen, and relaxin on intact and transplanted pelves in mice. *Am. J. Anat.,* 95:47–73.
129. Crelin, E. S. (1956): Response of the pubic symphysis in castrated mice to relaxin alone. *Anat. Rec.,* 124:397.
130. Crelin, E. S. (1957): Mitosis in adult cartilage. *Science,* 125:650.
131. Crelin, E. S. (1960): The development of bony pelvic sexual dimorphism in mice. *Ann. N.Y. Acad. Sci.,* 84:481–511.
132. Crelin, E. S. (1969): The development of the bony pelvis and its changes during pregnancy and parturition. *Trans. N.Y. Acad. Sci.,* 31:1049–1058.
133. Crelin, E. S., and Brightman, M. W. (1957): The pelvis of the rat: Its response to estrogen and relaxin. *Anat. Rec.,* 128:467–484.
134. Crelin, E. S., and Grillo, M. A. (1957): The conditioning effect of puberty on the response of the pubic symphysis in mice to estrogen and relaxin. *Anat. Rec.,* 127:407.
135. Crelin, E. S., and Haines, A. L. (1955): The effects of locally applied estrogen on the pubic symphysis and knee joint in castrated mice. *Endocrinology,* 56:461–470.
136. Crelin, E. S., and Honeyman, M. S. (1957): The inhibition of interpubic ligament formation by progesterone in pregnant mice. *Anat. Rec.,* 127:407.
137. Crelin, E. S., and Levin, J. (1955): The prepuberal pubic symphysis and uterus in the mouse: Their response to estrogen and relaxin. *Endocrinology,* 57:730–747.
138. Crelin, E. S., and Newton, E. V. (1969): The pelvis of the free-tailed bat: Sexual dimorphism and pregnancy changes. *Anat. Rec.,* 164:349–358.
139. Crish, J. F., Soloff, M. S., and Shaw, A. R. (1986): Changes in relaxin precursor mRNA levels in the rat ovary during pregnancy. *J. Biol. Chem.,* 261:1909–1913.
140. Crish, J. F., Soloff, M. S., and Shaw, A. R. (1986): Changes in relaxin precursor messenger ribonucleic acid levels in ovaries of rats after hysterectomy, removal of conceptuses, and during the estrous cycle. *Endocrinology,* 119:1222–1228.
141. Crisp, T. M., Dessouky, D. A., Denys, F. R. (1973): The fine structure of the human corpus luteum of term pregnancy. *Am. J. Obstet. Gynecol.,* 115:901–911.
142. Csapo, A. I. (1950): Actomyosin formation by estrogen action. *Am. J. Physiol.,* 162:406–410.
143. Csapo, A. I., Currie, W. B., Erdos, T., and Resch, B. A. (1978): Effect of passive immunization against estradiol on the regulatory profile and character of labor in the rat. *Am. J. Obstet. Gynecol.,* 132:464–470.
144. Cullen, B. M., and Harkness, R. D. (1960): The effect of hormones on the physical properties and collagen content of the rat's uterine cervix. *J. Physiol.,* 152:419–436.
145. Cullen, B. M., and Harkness, R. D. (1964): Effects of ovariectomy and of hormones on collageneous framework of the uterus. *Am. J. Physiol.,* 206:621–627.
146. Cutts, J. H. (1966): Estrogen-induced breast cancer in the rat. *Can. Cancer Conf.,* 65:50–68.
147. Dallenbach, F. D., and Dallenbach-Hellweg, G. (1964): Immunohistologische untersuchungen zur lokalisation des relaxins in menschlicher placenta und decidua. *Virchows Arch. Pathol. Anat.,* 337:301–316.

148. Dallenbach-Hellweg, G., Battista, J. V., and Dallenbach, F. D. (1965): Immunohistological and histochemical localization of relaxin in the metrial gland of the pregnant rat. *Am. J. Anat.*, 117:433–444.
149. Dallenbach-Hellweg, G., Dawson, A. B., and Hisaw, F. L. (1966): The effect of relaxin on the endometrium of monkeys. Histological and histochemical studies. *Am. J. Anat.*, 119:61–71.
150. Danforth, D. N. (1980): Early studies of the anatomy and physiology of the human cervix—and implications for the future. In: *Dilatation of the Uterine Cervix,* edited by F. Naftolin and P. G. Stubblefield, pp. 3–15. Raven Press, New York.
151. De Camillis, L., and Pozzi, V. (1961): Radiological study of the pubic symphysis after administration of relaxin. *Minerva Ginecol.*, 13:19–21.
152. Decker, W. H., Thwaite, W., Bordat, S., Kayser, R., Harami, T., and Campbell, J. (1958): Some effects of relaxin in obstetrics. *Obstet. Gynecol.*, 12:37–46.
153. De Cooman, S., Gilliaux, P., and Thomas, K. (1983): Immunoreactive relaxin-like substance in human split ejaculates. *Fertil. Steril.*, 39:111–113.
154. De Cooman, S., Loumaye, E., and Thomas, K. (1983): IR-relaxin in human seminal plasma. In: *Biology of Relaxin and Its Role in the Human,* edited by M. Bigazzi, F. C. Greenwood, and F. Gasparri, pp. 350–360. Excerpta Medica, Amsterdam.
155. D'Eletto, R. D., Schoenfeld, C., and Weiss, G. (1983): Partial purification of relaxin from human semen plasma using only reversed-phase liquid chromatography. In: *Biology of Relaxin and Its Role in the Human,* edited by M. Bigazzi, F. C. Greenwood, and F. Gasparri, pp. 397–398. Excerpta Medica, Amsterdam.
156. De Lanerolle, P., Nishikawa, M., Yost, D. A., and Adelstein, R. S. (1984): Increased phosphorylation of myosin light chain kinase after an increase in cyclic AMP in intact smooth muscle. *Science,* 223:1415–1417.
157. Del Mese, A., Casali, R., and Novelli, G. P. (1983): Relaxin induced dilatation of the venous wall and reduction of the venous blood flow. In: *Biology of Relaxin and Its Role in the Human,* edited by M. Bigazzi, F. C. Greenwood, and F. Gasparri, pp. 291–293. Excerpta Medica, Amsterdam.
158. Dessau, F. (1935): Effect of crystalline female sex hormones on the pelvic ligaments of the guinea pig. *Act. Brev. Neerl.*, 5:138–139.
159. Dewar, A. D., Hall, K., and Newton, W. H. (1946): Potentiation of the vaginal response to oestrone by the "relaxin" fraction of pregnant rabbit serum. *J. Physiol.*, 105:37P.
160. Dill, L. V., and Chanatry, J. C. (1958): Effect of relaxin on normal labor. *J.A.M.A.*, 167:1910–1912.
161. Doczi, J. (1963): Process for the extraction and purification of relaxin. *U.S. Patent* 3,096,246.
162. Dodson, G. G., Eliopoulos, E. E., Isaacs, N. W., McCall, M. J., Niall, H. D., and North, A. C. T. (1982): Rat relaxin: Insulin-like fold predicts a likely receptor binding region. *Int. J. Biol. Macromol.*, 4:399–405.
163. Dorfman, R. I., Marsters, R. W., and Dinerstein, J. (1953): Bioassay of relaxin. *Endocrinology,* 52:204–214.
164. Downing, S. J., Bradshaw, J. M. C., and Porter, D. G. (1980): Relaxin improves the coordination of rat myometrial activity *in vivo. Biol. Reprod.*, 23:899–903.
165. Downing, S. J., Lye, S. J., Bradshaw, J. M. C., and Porter, D. G. (1978): Rat myometrial activity *in vivo:* Effects of oestradiol-17β and progesterone in relation to the concentration of cytoplasmic progesterone receptors. *J. Endocrinol.*, 75:103–117.
166. Downing, S. J., Porter, D. G., and Redstone, C. D. (1981): Myometrial activity in rats during the oestrus cycle and pseudopregnancy: Interaction of oestradiol and progesterone. *J. Physiol.*, 317:425–433.
167. Downing, S. J., and Sherwood, O. D. (1985): The physiological role of relaxin in the pregnant rat. I. The influence of relaxin on parturition. *Endocrinology,* 116:1200–1205.
168. Downing, S. J., and Sherwood, O. D. (1985): The physiological role of relaxin in the pregnant rat. II. The influence of relaxin on uterine contractile activity. *Endocrinology,* 116:1206–1214.
169. Downing, S. J., and Sherwood, O. D. (1985): The physiological role of relaxin in the pregnant rat. III. The influence of relaxin on cervical extensibility. *Endocrinology,* 116:1215–1220.
170. Downing, S. J., and Sherwood, O. D. (1986): The physiological role of relaxin in the pregnant rat. IV. The influence of relaxin on cervical collagen and glycosaminoglycans. *Endocrinology,* 118:471–479.
171. Du, Y.-C., Minasian, E., Tregear, G. W., and Leach, S. J. (1982): Circular dichroism studies of relaxin and insulin peptide chains. *Int. J. Pept. Protein Res.*, 20:47–55.
172. Dubois, M. P., and Dacheux, J. L. (1978): Relaxin, a male hormone? *Cell Tissue Res.*, 187:201–214.
173. Eddie, L. W., Bell, R. J., Lester, A., Geier, M., Bennett, G., Johnston, P. D., and Niall, H. D. (1986): Radioimmunoassay of relaxin in pregnancy with an analogue of human relaxin. *Lancet,* 1(No.8494):1344–1346.
174. Eichner, E., Waltner, C., Goodman, M., and Post, S. (1956): Relaxin, the third ovarian hormone: Its experimental use in women. *Am. J. Obstet. Gynecol.*, 71:1035–1047.
175. Eggee, C. J., and Dracy, A. E. (1966): Histological study of effects of relaxin on the bovine cervix. *J. Dairy Sci.*, 49:1053–1057.
176. Eldridge, R. K., and Fields, P. A. (1983): Isolation of human placental relaxin with octadecylsilica. In: *Biology of Relaxin and Its Role in the Human,* edited by M. Bigazzi, F. C. Greenwood, and F. Gasparri, pp. 389–391. Excerpta Medica, Amsterdam.
177. Eldridge, R. K., and Fields, P. A. (1985): Rabbit placental relaxin: Purification and immunohistochemical localization. *Endocrinology,* 117:2512–2519.
178. Eldridge, R. K., and Fields, P. A. (1985): Immunohistochemical localization of relaxin in the placenta and endometrial glands of pregnant rabbits. *Program and Abstracts of the 18th Annual Meeting of the Society for the Study of Reproduction,* Montreal, Canada, abstract 230.
179. Eldridge, R. K., and Fields, P. A. (1986): Rabbit placental relaxin: Ultrastructural localization in secretory granules of the syncytiotrophoblast using rabbit placental relaxin antiserum. *Endocrinology,* 119:606–615.
180. Ellwood, D. A., and Anderson, A. B. M., editors (1981): *The Cervix in Pregnancy and Labour.* Churchill Livingstone, London.
181. Embrey, M. P., and Garrett, W. J. (1959): The effect of relaxin on the contractility of the human pregnant uterus. *J. Obstet. Gynaecol. Br. Emp.*, 66:594–597.
182. Entenmann, A. H., Lippert, T. H., Seeger, H. M., Kieback, D. G., and Voelter, W. (1984): Identification of immunologically active relaxin in fetal blood. *IRCS Med. Sci.*, 12:881.
183. Entenmann, A. H., Lippert, T. H., and Voelter, W. (1983): Isolation of relaxin from human placenta and its biological activity. In: *Biology of Relaxin and Its Role in the Human,* edited by M. Bigazzi, F. C. Greenwood, and F. Gasparri, pp. 392–394. Excerpta Medica, Amsterdam.
184. Entenmann, A. E., Voelter, W., Lippert, T. H. (1984): Isolation and biological standardization of relaxin from human placenta. *Acta Endocrinol.* [*Suppl.*] (*Copenh.*), 105:70–71.
185. Essig, M., Schoenfeld, C., Amelar, R. D., Dubin, L., and Weiss, G. (1982): Stimulation of human sperm motility by relaxin. *Fertil. Steril.*, 38:339–343.
186. Essig, M., Schoenfeld, C., D'Eletto, R., Amelar, R., Dubin, L., Steinetz, B. G., O'Byrne, E. M., and Weiss, G. (1982): Relaxin in human seminal plasma. *Ann. N.Y. Acad. Sci.*, 380:224–230.
187. Evans, G., Wathes, D. C., King, G. J., Armstrong, D. T., and Porter, D. G. (1983): Changes in relaxin production by the theca during the preovulatory period of the pig. *J. Reprod. Fertil.*, 69:677–683.
188. Evans, J. A. (1959): Relaxin (releasin) therapy in diffuse progressive scleroderma: A preliminary report. *A.M.A. Arch. Dermatol.*, 79:150–158.
189. Evans, M. D., Dougan, M.-B., Moawad, A. H., Evans, W. J., Bryant-Greenwood, G. D., and Greenwood, F. C. (1983): Ripening of the human cervix with porcine ovarian relaxin. *Am. J. Obstet. Gynecol.*, 147:410–414.
190. Felder, K. J., Molina, J. R., Benoit, A. M., and Anderson, L. L. (1985): Relaxin's timed release from aging porcine corpora lutea during different reproductive states. *Program and Abstracts of the 67th Annual Meeting of the Endocrine Society,* Baltimore, MD, abstract 610.
191. Felton, L. C., Frieden, E. H., and Bryant, H. H. (1953): The effects of ovarian extracts upon activity of the guinea pig uterus *in situ. J. Pharmacol. Exp. Ther.*, 107:160–164.

192. Fevold, H. L., Hisaw, F. L., and Leonard, S. L. (1932): The hormones of the corpus luteum. The separation and purification of three active substances. *J. Am. Chem. Soc.*, 54:254–263.
193. Fevold, H. L., Hisaw, F. L., and Meyer, R. K. (1930): The relaxative hormone of the corpus luteum. Its purification and concentration. *J. Am. Chem. Soc.*, 52:3340–3348.
194. Fields, M. J., Fields, P. A., Castro-Hernandez, A., and Larkin, L. H. (1980): Evidence for relaxin in corpora lutea of late pregnant cows. *Endocrinology*, 107:869–876.
195. Fields, M. J., Fields, P. A., and Larkin, L. H. (1982): Chemistry of bovine relaxin. *Adv. Exp. Med. Biol.*, 143:191–207.
196. Fields, M. J., Roberts, R., and Castro-Hernandez, A. (1981): Two cow relaxins: A comparison. In: *Relaxin*, edited by G. D. Bryant-Greenwood, H. D. Niall, and F. C. Greenwood, pp. 119–125. Elsevier/North-Holland, New York.
197. Fields, M. J., Roberts, R. F., Dubois, W., Ganz, N. I., and Weber, D. M. (1983): Bovine relaxin: Isolation of luteal peptides with biological and immunological activity. In: *Biology of Relaxin and Its Role in the Human*, edited by M. Bigazzi, F. C. Greenwood, and F. Gasparri, pp. 56–58. Excerpta Medica, Amsterdam.
198. Fields, M. J., Roberts, R., and Fields, P. A. (1982): Octadecylsilica and carboxymethyl cellulose isolation of bovine and porcine relaxin. *Ann. N.Y. Acad. Sci.*, 380:36–46.
199. Fields, P. A. (1984): Intracellular localization of relaxin in membrane-bound granules in the pregnant rat luteal cell. *Biol. Reprod.*, 30:753–762.
200. Fields, P. A., Eldridge, R. K., Fuchs, A.-R., and Fields, M. J. (1983): Oxytocin contamination of bovine corpora lutea and human placental relaxin extracts: Problems encountered with the *in vitro* mouse uterus relaxin bioassay. In: *Biology of Relaxin and Its Role in the Human*, edited by M. Bigazzi, F. C. Greenwood, and F. Gasparri, pp. 185–187. Excerpta Medica, Amsterdam.
201. Fields, P. A., Eldridge, R. K., Fuchs, A.-R., Roberts, R. F., and Fields, M. J. (1983): Human placental and bovine corpora lutea oxytocin. *Endocrinology*, 112:1544–1546.
202. Fields, P. A., and Fields, M. J. (1985): Ultrastructural localization of relaxin in the corpus luteum of the nonpregnant, pseudopregnant, and pregnant pig. *Biol. Reprod.*, 32:1169–1179.
203. Fields, P. A., and Larkin, L. H. (1980): Enhancement of uterine cervix extensibility in oestrogen-primed mice following administration of relaxin. *J. Endocrinol.*, 87:147–152.
204. Fields, P. A., and Larkin, L. H. (1981): Purification and immunohistochemical localization of relaxin in the human term placenta. *J. Clin. Endocrinol. Metab.*, 52:79–85.
205. Fields, P. A., Larkin, L. H., and Pardo, R. J. (1982): Purification of relaxin from the placenta of the rabbit. *Ann. N.Y. Acad. Sci.*, 380:75–86.
206. Fitzpatrick, R. J., and Dobson, H. (1981): Softening of the ovine cervix at parturition. In: *The Cervix in Pregnancy and Labour*, edited by D. A. Ellwood and A. B. M. Anderson, pp. 40–56. Churchill Livingstone, New York.
207. Fitzpatrick, R. J., and Liggins, G. C. (1980): Effects of prostaglandins on the cervix of pregnant women and sheep. In: *Dilatation of the Uterine Cervix*, edited by F. Naftolin and P. G. Stubblefield, pp. 287–300. Raven Press, New York.
208. Folsome, C. E., Harami, T., Lavietes, S. R., and Massell, G. M. (1956): Clinical evaluation of relaxin. *Obstet. Gynecol.*, 8:536–544.
209. Frieden, E. H. (1958): Non-steroid ovarian hormones: Observations on the mechanism of the acquisition of relaxin resistance in guinea pigs. *Endocrinology*, 62:41–46.
210. Frieden, E. H. (1963): Purification and electrophoretic properties of relaxin preparations. *Trans. N.Y. Acad. Sci.*, 25:331–336.
211. Frieden, E. H., and Adams, W. C. (1977): The response to endogenous relaxin of guinea pigs refractory to porcine relaxin. *Proc. Soc. Exp. Biol. Med.*, 155:558–561.
212. Frieden, E. H., and Adams, W. C. (1985): Stimulation of rat uterine collagen synthesis by relaxin. *Proc. Soc. Exp. Biol. Med.*, 180:39–43.
213. Frieden, E. H., and Hisaw, F. L. (1950): The purification of relaxin. *Arch. Biochem. Biophys.*, 29:166–178.
214. Frieden, E. H., and Hisaw, F. L. (1951): The mechanism of symphyseal relaxation. The distribution of reducing groups, hexoseamine, and proteins in symphyses of normal and relaxed guinea pigs. *Endocrinology*, 48:88–97.
215. Frieden, E. H., and Hisaw, F. L. (1953): The biochemistry of relaxin. *Rec. Prog. Horm. Res.*, 8:333–378.
216. Frieden, E. H., and Layman, N. W. (1957): Non-steroid ovarian hormones: An improved method for the preparation of relaxin. *J. Biol. Chem.*, 229:569–573.
217. Frieden, E. H., and Martin, A. S. (1954): Uptake of glycine-1-C^{14} by connective tissue. I. Effects of estrogen and relaxin. *J. Biol. Chem.*, 207:133–142.
218. Frieden, E. H., and Rawitch, A.B. (1981): Isolation and chemical properties of relaxin subspecies. In: *Relaxin*, edited by G. D. Bryant-Greenwood, H. D. Niall, and F. C. Greenwood, pp. 21–26. Elsevier/North-Holland, New York.
219. Frieden, E. H., Rawitch, A. B., Wu, L.-H. C., and Chen, S.-W. C. (1980): The isolation of two proline-containing relaxin species from a porcine relaxin concentrate. *Proc. Soc. Exp. Biol. Med.*, 163:521–527.
220. Frieden, E. H., Stone, N. R., and Layman, N. W. (1960): Nonsteroid ovarian hormones. III. The properties of relaxin preparations purified by counter-current distribution. *J. Biol. Chem.*, 235:2267–2271.
221. Frieden, E. H., and Velardo, J. T. (1952): Effect of relaxin upon decidual reactions in the rat. *Proc. Soc. Exp. Biol. Med.*, 81:98–103.
222. Frieden, E. H., and Velardo, J. T. (1960): Reversal of the decidual-inhibiting effect of relaxin by an inactive derivitive. *Acta Endocrinol. (Copenh.)*, 34:312–316.
223. Frieden, E. H., and Yeh, L.-A. (1977): Evidence for a "pro-relaxin" in porcine relaxin concentrates. *Proc. Soc. Exp. Biol. Med.*, 154:407–411.
224. Friedman, E. A. (1980): Cervical function in human pregnancy and labor. In: *Dilatation of the Uterine Cervix*, edited by F. Naftolin and P. G. Stubblefield, pp. 17–26. Raven Press, New York.
225. Fuchs, A.-R. (1978): Hormonal control of myometrial function during pregnancy and parturition. *Acta Endocrinol. [Suppl.] (Copenh.)*, 221:1–70.
226. Fuchs, A.-R., Periyasamy, S., Alexandrova, M., and Soloff, M. S. (1983): Correlation between oxytocin receptor concentration and responsiveness to oxytocin in pregnant rat myometrium: Effect of ovarian steroids. *Endocrinology*, 113:742–749.
227. Gammeltoft, S., Staun-Olsen, P., Ottesen, B., and Fahrenkrug, F. (1984): Insulin receptors in rat brain cortex. Kinetic evidence for a receptor subtype in the central nervous system. *Peptides*, 5: 937–944.
228. Gardner, W. U. (1936): Sexual dimorphism of the pelvis of the mouse, the effect of estrogenic hormones upon the pelvis and upon the development of scrotal hernias. *Am. J. Anat.*, 59:459–483.
229. Gardner, W. U., and Pfeiffer, C. A. (1938): Skeletal changes in mice receiving estrogens. *Proc. Soc. Exp. Biol. Med.*, 37:678–679.
230. Gardner, W. U., and Van Heuverswyn, J. (1940): Inhibition of pelvic changes occurring during pregnancy in mice by testosterone propionate. *Endocrinology*, 26:833–836.
231. Garfield, R. E., Kannan, M. S., and Daniel, E. E. (1980): Gap junction formation in myometrium: Control by estrogens, progesterone and prostaglandins. *Am. J. Physiol.*, 238:C81–C89.
232. Garrett, F. A., and Talmage, R. V. (1952): The influence of relaxin on mammary gland development in guinea-pigs and rabbits. *J. Endocrinol.*, 8:336–341.
233. Gast, M. J. (1982): Studies of luteal generation and processing of the high molecular weight relaxin precursor. *Ann. N.Y. Acad. Sci.*, 380:111–125.
234. Gast, M. J. (1983): Characterization of preprorelaxin by tryptic digestion and inhibition of its conversion to prorelaxin by amino acid analogs. *J. Biol. Chem.*, 258:9001–9004.
235. Gast, M. J., Mercado-Simmen, R., Niall, H., and Boime, I. (1980): Cell-free synthesis of a high molecular weight relaxin-related protein. *Ann. N.Y. Acad. Sci.*, 343:148–154.
236. Gates, G. S., Flynn, J. J., Ryan, R. J, and Sherwood, O. D. (1981): *In vivo* uptake of ^{125}I-relaxin in the guinea pig. *Biol. Reprod.*, 25:549–554.
237. Gibori, G., Antczak, E., and Rothchild, I. (1977): The role of estrogen in the regulation of luteal progesterone secretion in the rat after day 12 of pregnancy. *Endocrinology*, 100:1483–1495.
238. Glaser, L. A., Kelly, P. A., and Gibori, G. (1984): Differential action and secretion of rat placental lactogens. *Endocrinology*, 115:969–976.

239. Goldsmith, L. T., De la Cruz, J. L., Weiss, G., and Castracane, V. D. (1982): Steroid effects on relaxin secretion in the rat. *Biol. Reprod.*, 27:886–890.
240. Goldsmith, L. T., Essig, M., Sarosi, P., Beck, P., and Weiss, G. (1981): Hormone secretion by monolayer cultures of human luteal cells. *J. Clin. Endocrinol. Metab.*, 53:890–892.
241. Goldsmith, L. T., Grob, H. S., Scherer, K. J., Surve, A., Steinetz, B. G., and Weiss, G. (1981): Placental control of ovarian immunoreactive relaxin secretion in the pregnant rat. *Endocrinology*, 109:548–552.
242. Goldsmith, L. T., Grob, H. S., and Weiss, G. (1982): *In vitro* induction of relaxin secretion in corpora lutea from nonpregnant rats. *Ann. N.Y. Acad. Sci.*, 380:60–71.
243. Golichowski, A. M., King, S. R., and Mascaro, K. (1980): Pregnancy-related changes in rat cervical glycosaminoglycans. *Biochem. J.*, 192:1–8.
244. Golos, T. G., and Sherwood, O. D. (1982): Control of corpus luteum function during the second half of pregnancy in the rat: A direct relationship between conceptus number and both serum and ovarian relaxin levels. *Endocrinology*, 111:872–878.
245. Golos, T. G., and Sherwood, O. D. (1984): Evidence that the maternal pituitary suppresses the secretion of relaxin in the pregnant rat. *Endocrinology*, 115:1004–1010.
246. Golos, T. G., and Sherwood, O. D. (1986): The suppressive effect of the maternal pituitary on relaxin secretion during the second half of pregnancy in rats does not require the presence of the nonluteal ovarian tissue. *Biol. Reprod.*, 34:595–601.
247. Golos, T. G., Weyhenmyer, J. A., and Sherwood, O. D. (1984): Immunocytochemical localization of relaxin in the ovaries of pregnant rats. *Biol. Reprod.*, 30:257–261.
248. Gooneratne, A. D., Bryant-Greenwood, G. D., Walker, F. M., Nottage, H. M., and Hartmann, P. E.(1983): Pre-partum changes in the plasma concentrations of progesterone, relaxin, prostaglandin $F_{2\alpha}$ and 13,14-dihydro-15-keto prostaglandin $F_{2\alpha}$ in meclofenamic acid–treated sows. *J. Reprod. Fertil.*, 68:33–40.
249. Gordon, W. L., and Sherwood, O. D. (1982): Evidence that luteinizing hormone from the maternal pituitary gland may promote antepartum release of relaxin, luteolysis, and birth in rats. *Endocrinology*, 111:1299–1310.
250. Gordon, W. L., and Sherwood, O. D. (1983): Evidence for a role of prostaglandins in the antepartum release of relaxin in the pregnant rat. *Biol. Reprod.*, 28:154–160.
251. Gowan, L. K., Reinig, J. W., Schwabe, C., Bedarkar, S., and Blundell, T.L. (1981): On the primary and tertiary structure of relaxin from the sand tiger shark. *FEBS Lett.*, 129:80–82.
252. Graciansky, P. de, and Boulle, S. (1961): Essais de traitement de la sclérodermie par la relaxine. *Bull. Soc. Fr. Derm. Syph.*, 68:83–86.
253. Graham, E. F., and Dracy, A. E. (1952): The effects of relaxin on the cow's cervix. *J. Dairy Sci.*, 35:499.
254. Graham, E. F., and Dracy, A. E. (1953): The effect of relaxin and mechanical dilatation of the bovine cervix. *J. Dairy Sci.*, 36:772–777.
255. Greenwood, F. C., Mercado-Simmen, R. C., and Greenwood, G. D. (1981): Insulin-related peptides examined by radioimmunoassay and radioreceptor assay: A note. In: *Relaxin*, edited by G. D. Bryant-Greenwood, H. D. Niall, and F. C. Greenwood, pp. 97–98. Elsevier/North-Holland, New York.
256. Griss, G., Keck, J., Engelhorn, R., and Tuppy, H. (1967): The isolation and purification of an ovarian polypeptide with uterine-relaxing activity. *Biochim. Biophys. Acta*, 140:45–54.
257. Guthrie, H. D., Rexroad, C. R., and Bolt, D. J. (1978): *In vitro* synthesis of progesterone and prostaglandin F by luteal tissue and prostaglandin by endometrial tissue from the pig. *Prostaglandins*, 16:433–440.
258. Gutkowska, J., St-Louis, J., and Genest, J. (1985): Solid-phase radioimmunoassay for relaxin. *Clin. Invest. Med.*, 8:133–138.
259. Haley, J., Hudson, P., Scanlon, D., John, M., Cronk, M., Shine, J., Tregear, G., and Niall, H. (1982): Porcine relaxin: Molecular cloning and cDNA structure. *DNA*, 1:155–162.
260. Hall, K. (1947): The effects of pregnancy and relaxin on the histology of the pubic symphysis of the mouse. *J. Endocrinol.*, 5:174–185.
261. Hall, K. (1948): Further notes on the action of oestrone and relaxin on the pelvis of the spayed mouse, including a single-dose test of potency of relaxin. *J. Endocrinol.*, 5:314–321.
262. Hall, K. (1949): The role of progesterone in the mechanism of pelvic relaxation in the mouse. *Q. J. Exp. Physiol.*, 35:65–75.
263. Hall, K. (1955): The effect of various combinations of progesterone and oestrogen on the symphysis pubis of ovariectomized mice. *J. Endocrinol.*, 12:247–251.
264. Hall, K. (1956): An evaluation of the roles of oestrogen, progesterone and relaxin in producing relaxation of the symphysis pubis of the ovariectomized mouse, using the technique of metachromatic staining with toluidine blue. *J. Endocrinol.*, 13:384–393.
265. Hall, K. (1957): The effect of relaxin extracts, progesterone and oestradiol on maintenance of pregnancy, parturition, and rearing of young after ovariectomy in mice. *J. Endocrinol.*, 15:108–117.
266. Hall, K. (1960): Modification by relaxin of the response of the reproductive tract of mice to oestradiol and progesterone. *J. Endocrinol.*, 20:355–364.
267. Hall, K. (1965): Histochemical investigation of the effects of oestrogen, progesterone and relaxin on glycogen, amylophosphorylase, transglycosylase, and uridine diphosphate glucose-glycogen transferase in uteri of mice. *J. Endocrinol.*, 32:245–257.
268. Hall, K., Hoare, M., and Turner, C. B. (1962): Relaxin in the blood of preparturient ewes. *J. Endocrinol.*, 28:271–278.
269. Hall, K., and Newton, W. H. (1946): The action of relaxin in the mouse. *Lancet*, 1:54–55.
270. Hall, K., and Newton, W. H. (1946): The normal course of separation of the pubes in pregnant mice. *J. Physiol.*, 104:346–352.
271. Hall, K., and Newton, W. H. (1947): The effect of oestrone and relaxin on the X-ray appearance of the pelvis of the mouse. *J. Physiol.*, 106:18–27.
272. Hamolsky, M., and Sparrow, R. C. (1945): Influence of relaxin on mammary development in sexually immature female rats. *Proc. Soc. Exp. Biol. Med.*, 60:8–9.
273. Haning, R. V., Steinetz, B. G., and Weiss, G. (1985): Elevated serum relaxin levels in multiple pregnancy after menotropin treatment. *Obstet. Gynecol.*, 66:42–45.
274. Harkey, M. E., and Crelin, E. S. (1963): Hormonal response of the pubic symphysis in adult mice gonadectomized at different times before puberty. *Anat. Rec.*, 145:323.
275. Harkness, M. L. R., and Harkness, R. D. (1954): The collagen content of the reproductive tract of the rat during pregnancy and lactation. *J. Physiol.*, 123:492–500.
276. Harkness, M. L. R., and Harkness, R. D. (1959): Changes in the physical properties of the uterine cervix of the rat during pregnancy. *J. Physiol.*, 148:524–547.
277. Harkness, M. L. R., and Harkness, R. D. (1965): The mechanical properties of the uterus compared to those of the birth canal of the rat in pregnancy. *Acta Physiol. Acad. Sci. Hung.*, 27:101–109.
278. Harkness, R. D. (1964): The physiology of the connective tissues of the reproductive tract. *Int. Rev. Connect. Tissue Res.*, 2:155–211.
279. Harkness, R. D., and Nightingale, M. A. (1962): The extensibility of the cervix uteri of the rat at different times of pregnancy. *J. Physiol.*, 160:214–220.
280. Harness, J. R., and Anderson, R. R. (1975): Effect of relaxin on mammary gland growth and lactation in the rat. *Proc. Soc. Exp. Biol. Med.*, 148:933–936.
281. Harness, J. R., and Anderson, R. R. (1977): Effects of relaxin in combination with prolactin and ovarian steroids on mammary growth in hypophysectomized rats. *Proc. Soc. Exp. Biol. Med.*, 156:354–358.
282. Harness, J. R., and Anderson, R. R. (1977): Effect of relaxin and somatotropin in combination with ovarian steroids on mammary glands in rats. *Biol. Reprod.*, 17:599–603.
283. Hartman, C. G., and Straus, W. L. (1939): Relaxation of the pelvic ligaments in pregnant monkeys. *Am. J. Obstet. Gynecol.*, 37:498–500.
284. Hascall, V. C., and Hascall, G. K. (1981): Proteoglycans. In: *Cell Biology of the Extracellular Matrix*, edited by E. D. Hay, pp. 39–63. Plenum, New York.
285. Herrick, E. H. (1928): The duration of pregnancy in guinea-pigs after removal and also after transplantation of the ovaries. *Anat. Rec.*, 39:193–200.
286. Hilliard, J. (1973): Corpus luteum function in guinea pigs, hamsters, rats, mice and rabbits. *Biol. Reprod.*, 8:203–221.
287. Hillier, K., and Wallis, R. M. (1981): Prostaglandins, steroids and the human cervix. In: *The Cervix in Pregnancy and Labour*, edited

by D. A. Ellwood and A. B. M. Anderson, pp. 144–162. Churchill Livingstone, New York.

288. Hillier, K., and Wallis, R. M. (1982): Collagen solubility and tensile properties of the rat uterine cervix in late pregnancy: Effects of arachidonic acid and prostaglandin $F_{2\alpha}$. *J. Endocrinol.*, 95:341–347.
289. Hisaw, F. L. (1926): Experimental relaxation of the pubic ligament of the guinea pig. *Proc. Soc. Exp. Biol. Med.*, 23:661–663.
290. Hisaw, F. L. (1927): Experimental relaxation of the symphysis pubis of the guinea-pig. *Anat. Rec.*, 37:126.
291. Hisaw, F. L. (1929): The corpus luteum hormone. I. Experimental relaxation of the pelvic ligaments of the guinea pig. *Physiol. Zool.*, 2:59–79.
292. Hisaw, F. L., and Hisaw, F. L. (1964): Effect of relaxin on the uterus of monkeys (*Macaca mulatta*) with observations on the cervix and symphysis pubis. *Am. J. Obstet. Gynecol.*, 89:141–155.
293. Hisaw, F. L., Hisaw, F. L., and Dawson, A. B. (1967): Effects of relaxin on the endothelium of endometrial blood vessels in monkeys (*Macaca mulatta*). *Endocrinology*, 81:375–385.
294. Hisaw, F. L., Talmage, R. V. N., Money, W. L., and Abramowitz, A. A. (1942): Relation of progesterone to the formation of relaxin. *Anat. Rec.*, 84:457.
295. Hisaw, F. L., and Zarrow, M. X. (1948): Relaxin in the ovary of the domestic sow. *Proc. Soc. Exp. Biol. Med.*, 69:395–398.
296. Hisaw, F. L., and Zarrow, M. X. (1950): The physiology of relaxin. *Vitam. Horm.*, 8:151–178.
297. Hisaw, F. L., Zarrow, M. X., Money, W. L., Talmage, R. V. N., and Abramowitz, A. A. (1944): Importance of the female reproductive tract in the formation of relaxin. *Endocrinology*, 34:122–134.
298. Hochman, J., Weiss, G., Steinetz, B. G., and O'Byrne, E. M. (1978): Serum relaxin concentrations in prostaglandin- and oxytocin-induced labor in women. *Am. J. Obstet. Gynecol.*, 130:473–474.
299. Hollingsworth, M. (1981): Softening of the rat cervix during pregnancy. In: *The Cervix in Pregnancy and Labour*, edited by D. A. Ellwood and A. B. M. Anderson, pp. 13–33. Churchill Livingstone, New York.
300. Hollingsworth, M., and Gallimore, S. (1981): Evidence that cervical softening in the pregnant rat is independent of increasing uterine contractility. *J. Reprod. Fertil.*, 63:449–454.
301. Hollingsworth, M., Gallimore, S., and Isherwood, C. N. M. (1980): Effects of prostaglandins $F_{2\alpha}$ and E-2 on cervical extensibility in the late pregnant rat. *J. Reprod. Fertil.*, 58:95–99.
302. Hollingsworth, M., Isherwood, C. N. M., and Foster, R. W. (1979): The effects of oestradiol benzoate, progesterone, relaxin, and ovariectomy on cervical extensibility in the late pregnant rat. *J. Reprod. Fertil.*, 56:471–477.
303. Holmstrom, E. G. (1958): The prevention of prematurity. *W. Va. Med. J.*, 54:343–344.
304. Horn, E. H. (1958): Effects of feeding thiouracil and/or thyroid powder upon pubic symphyseal separation in female mice. *Endocrinology*, 63:481–486.
305. Horn, E. H. (1960): Interpubic ligament regression in relaxin-treated virgin and primiparous, post-partum mice. *Endocrinology*, 67:668–673.
306. Hsu, C. J., McCormack, S. M., and Sanborn, B. M. (1985): The effect of relaxin on cyclic adenosine 3′5′-monophosphate concentrations in rat myometrial cells in culture. *Endocrinology*, 116:2029–2035.
307. Hsu, C. J., and Sanborn, B. M. (1986): Relaxin affects the shape of rat myometrial cells in culture. *Endocrinology*, 118:495–498.
308. Hsu, C. J., and Sanborn, B. M. (1986): Relaxin treatment alters the kinetic properties of myosin light chain kinase activity in rat myometrial cells in culture. *Endocrinology*, 118:499–505.
309. Hudson, P., Haley, J., Cronk, M., Shine, J., and Niall, H. (1981): Molecular cloning and characterization of cDNA sequences coding for rat relaxin. *Nature*, 291:127–131.
310. Hudson, P., Haley, J., John, M., Cronk, M., Crawford, R., Haralambidis, J., Tregear, G., Shine, J., and Niall, H. (1983): Structure of a genomic clone encoding biologically active human relaxin. *Nature*, 301:628–631.
311. Hudson, P., John, M., Crawford, R., Haralambidis, J., Scanlon, D., Gorman, J., Tregear, G., Shine, J., and Niall, H. (1984): Relaxin gene expression in human ovaries and the predicted structure of a human preprorelaxin by analysis of cDNA clones. *EMBO J.*, 3:2333–2339.
312. Hunter, W. M., and Greenwood, F. C. (1962): Preparation of iodine-131 labelled human growth hormone of high specific activity. *Nature*, 194:495–496.
313. Isaacs, N., and Dodson, G. (1981): Models of relaxin. In: *Relaxin*, edited by G. D. Bryant-Greenwood, H. D. Niall, and F. C. Greenwood, pp. 101–106. Elsevier/North-Holland, New York.
314. Isaacs, N., James, R., Niall, H., Bryant-Greenwood, G., Dodson, G., Evans, A., and North, A. C. T. (1978): Relaxin and its structural relationship to insulin. *Nature*, 271:278–281.
315. Ismay, G. (1958): Relaxin: Its effects in a case of acrosclerosis. *Br. J. Dermatol.*, 70:171–175.
316. Ito, A., Kitamura, K., Mori, Y., and Hirakawa, S. (1979): The change in solubility of type I collagen in human uterine cervix in pregnancy at term. *Biochem. Med.*, 21:267–270.
317. Jablonski, W. J. A., and Velardo, J. T. (1957): Effects of relaxin on uterine weight of immature rats. *Endocrinology*, 61:474–475.
318. Jackson, J. A., and Albrecht, E. D. (1985): The development of placental androstenedione and testosterone production and their utilization by the ovary for aromatization to estrogen during rat pregnancy. *Biol. Reprod.*, 33:451–457.
319. Jagiello, G. (1965): Effects of selected hormones on the closed vaginal membrane of the ovariectomized guinea pig. *Proc. Soc. Exp. Biol. Med.*, 118:412–414.
320. Jagiello, G. (1967): The effect of several relaxin preparations on the hysterectomized guinea-pig. *J. Reprod. Fertil.*, 13:175–177.
321. James, R., Niall, H. D., and Bradshaw, R. A. (1981): The topographical mapping of porcine relaxin: Location of the tryptophan residues. In: *Relaxin*, edited by G. D. Bryant-Greenwood, H. D. Niall, and F. C. Greenwood, pp. 85–90. Elsevier/North-Holland, New York.
322. James, R., Niall, H., Kwok, S., and Bryant-Greenwood, G. (1977): Primary structure of porcine relaxin: Homology with insulin and related growth factors. *Nature*, 267:544–546.
323. Jarrett, J. C., Ballejo, G., Saleem, T. H., Tsibris, J. C. M., and Spellacy, W. N. (1984): The effect of prolactin and relaxin on insulin binding by adipocytes from pregnant women. *Am. J. Obstet. Gynecol.*, 149:250–255.
324. Järvinen, P. A., and Luukkainen, T. (1963): Treatment of symphyseolysis with relaxin. *Ann. Chir. Gynaecol.*, 52:251–254.
325. Jefferis, J. E., and Dixon, A. St. J. (1962): Failure of relaxin in the treatment of scleroderma. *Ann. Rheum. Dis.*, 21:295–297.
326. Johanson, C.-E., and Järvinen, P. A. (1957): Factors affecting relaxation of the pelvis during normal pregnancy, delivery, and the puerperium. *Acta Obstet. Gynecol. Scand.*, 36:179–193.
327. John, M. J., Borjesson, B. W., Walsh, J. R., and Niall, H. D. (1981): Limited sequence homology between porcine and rat relaxins: Implications for physiological studies. *Endocrinology*, 108:726–729.
328. John, M. J., Borjesson, B. W., Walsh, J. R., and Niall, H. D. (1981): The amino acid sequence of rat relaxin. In: *Relaxin*, edited by G. D. Bryant-Greenwood, H. D. Niall, and F. C. Greenwood, pp. 37–43. Elsevier/North-Holland, New York.
329. Jones, S. A., and Summerlee, A. J. S. (1986): Effects of relaxin on the length of gestation and duration of parturition in the rat. *J. Endocrinol.*, 109:85–88.
330. Joseph, N. R., Engel, M. B., and Catchpole, H. R. (1952): Interaction of ions and connective tissue. *Biochim. Biophys. Acta*, 8:575–587.
331. Judson, D. G., Pay, S., and Bhoola, K. D. (1980): Modulation of cyclic AMP in isolated rat uterine slices by porcine relaxin. *J. Endocrinol.*, 87:153–159.
332. Kato, H., Morishige, W. K., and Rothchild, I. (1979): A quantitative relation between the experimentally determined number of conceptuses and corpus luteum activity in the pregnant rat. *Endocrinology*, 105:846–850.
333. Kelly, J. V., and Posse, N. (1956): The hormone relaxin in labor. *Obstet. Gynecol.*, 8:531–535.
334. Kemp, B. E. (1981): Activation of rat uterine cAMP-dependent protein kinase by relaxin. *Program and Abstracts of the 63rd Annual Meeting of the Endocrine Society*, Cincinnati, OH, abstract 471.
335. Kemp, B. E., and Niall, H. D. (1984): Relaxin. *Vitam. Horm.*, 41:79–115.
336. Kendall, J. Z., Dziuk, P. J., Nelson, D., Sherwood, O. D., Streat, C. N., and Thurmon, J. T. (1980): Aberrant parturition in pigs with hypophysectomized fetuses. *Program and Abstracts of the 13th An-*

nual Meeting of the Society for the Study of Reproduction, Ann Arbor, MI, abstract 80.

337. Kendall, J. Z., Plopper, C. G., and Bryant-Greenwood, G. D. (1978): Ultrastructural immunoperoxidase demonstration of relaxin in corpora lutea from a pregnant sow. *Biol. Reprod.,* 18:94–98.
338. Kendall, J. Z., Richards, G. E., and Shih, L.-C. N. (1983): Effect of haloperidol, suckling, oxytocin, and hand milking on plasma relaxin and prolactin concentrations in cyclic and lactating pigs. *J. Reprod. Fertil.,* 69:271–277.
339. Kendall, J. Z., Richards, G. E., Shih, L.-C. N., and Farris, T. S. (1982): Plasma relaxin concentrations in the pig during the periparturient period: Association with prolactin, estrogen, and progesterone concentrations. *Theriogenology,* 17:677–687.
340. Kendall, J. Z., Smith, R. G., Shih, L.-N., Webb, P. D., and Tate, W. H. (1983): Characterization of prostatic relaxin. In: *Biology of Relaxin and Its Role in the Human,* edited by M. Bigazzi, F. C. Greenwood, and F. Gasparri, pp. 363–366. Excerpta Medica, Amsterdam.
341. Kennedy, T. G. (1974): Effect of relaxin on oestrogen-induced uterine luminal fluid accumulation in the ovariectomized rat. *J. Endocrinol.,* 61:347–353.
342. Kennedy, T. G. (1976): Does prostaglandin $F_2\alpha$ ($PGF_2\alpha$) mediate the effect of relaxin on cervical tone in the rat? *Proc. Can. Fed. Biol. Soc.,* vol. 19, abstract 273.
343. Kertiles, L. P., and Anderson, L. L. (1979): Effect of relaxin on cervical dilatation, parturition and lactation in the pig. *Biol. Reprod.,* 21:57–68.
344. Khaligh, H. S. (1968): Inhibition by relaxin of spontaneous contractions of the uterus of the hamster *in vitro. J. Endocrinol.,* 40:125–126.
345. Kirton, K. T. (1980): Use of prostaglandins for dilatation of the cervix. In: *Dilatation of the Uterine Cervix,* edited by F. Naftolin and P. G. Stubblefield, pp. 355–361. Raven Press, New York.
346. Kliman, B., and Greep, R. O. (1958): The enhancement of relaxin-induced growth of the pubic ligament in mice. *Endocrinology,* 63:586–595.
347. Kliman, B., Salhanick, H. A., and Zarrow, M. X. (1953): The response of the pubic symphysis of the mouse to extracts of pregnant rabbit serum and pregnant sow ovaries and its application as an assay method. *Endocrinology,* 53:391–409.
348. Knox, F. S., and Griffith, D. R. (1970): Effect of ovarian hormones upon milk yield in the rat. *Proc. Soc. Exp. Biol. Med.,* 133:135–137.
349. Koay, E. S. C., Bagnell, C. A., Bryant-Greenwood, G. D., Lord, S. B., Cruz, A. C., and Larkin, L. H. (1985): Immunocytochemical localization of relaxin in human decidua and placenta. *J. Clin. Endocrinol. Metab.,* 60:859–863.
350. Koay, E. S. C., Bryant-Greenwood, G. D., Yamamoto, S. Y., and Greenwood, F. C. (1986): The human fetal membranes: A target tissue for relaxin. *J. Clin. Endocrinol. Metab.,* 62:513–521.
351. Koay, E. S. C., Too, C. K. L., Greenwood, F. C., and Bryant-Greenwood, G. D. (1983): Relaxin stimulates collagenase and plasminogen activator secretion by dispersed human amnion and chorion cells *in vitro. J. Clin. Endocrinol. Metab.,* 56:1332–1334.
352. Koninckx, P. R., Renaer, M., and Brosens, I. A. (1980): Origin of peritoneal fluid in women: An ovarian exudation product. *Br. J. Obstet. Gynaecol.,* 87:177–183.
353. Koob, T. J., Laffan, J. J., and Callard, I. P. (1984): Effects of relaxin and insulin on reproductive tract size and early fetal loss in squalus acanthias. *Biol. Reprod.,* 31:231–238.
354. Krantz, J. C., Bryant, H. H., and Carr, C. J. (1950): The action of aqueous corpus luteum extract upon uterine activity. *Surg. Gynecol. Obstet.,* 90:372–375.
355. Kream, B. E., Smith, M. D., Canalis, E., and Raisz, L. G. (1985): Characterization of the effect of insulin on collagen synthesis in fetal rat bone. *Endocrinology,* 116:296–302.
356. Kroc, R. L., Steinetz, B. G., and Beach, V. L. (1959): The effects of estrogens, progestagens, and relaxin in pregnant and nonpregnant laboratory rodents. *Ann. N.Y. Acad. Sci.,* 75:942–980.
357. Kwok, S. C. M., Bryant-Greenwood, G. D., and Niall, H. D. (1980): Evidence for proteolysis during purification of relaxin from pregnant sow ovaries. *Endocr. Res. Commun.,* 7:1–12.
358. Kwok, S. C. M., Chamley, W. A., and Bryant-Greenwood, G. D. (1978): High molecular weight forms of relaxin in pregnant sow ovaries. *Biochem. Biophys. Res. Commun.,* 82:997–1005.
359. Lao Guico, M. S., and Sherwood, O. D. (1985): Effect of oestradiol-17β on ovarian and serum concentrations of relaxin during the second half of pregnancy in the rat. *J. Reprod. Fertil.,* 74:65–70.
360. Larkin, L. H. (1974): Bioassay of rat metrial gland extracts for relaxin using the mouse interpubic ligament technique. *Endocrinology,* 94:567–570.
361. Larkin, L. H., Fields, P. A., and Oliver, R. M. (1977): Production of antisera against electrophoretically separated relaxin and immunofluorescent localization of relaxin in the porcine corpus luteum. *Endocrinology,* 101:679–685.
362. Larkin, L. H., Fields, P. A., and Pardo, R. (1981): Mouse uterus bioassay for relaxin. In: *Relaxin,* edited by G. D. Bryant-Greenwood, H. D. Niall, and F. C. Greenwood, pp. 321–328. Elsevier/North-Holland, New York.
363. Larkin, L. H., Pardo, R. J., and Renegar, R. H. (1983): Sources of relaxin and morphology of relaxin-containing cells. In: *Biology of Relaxin and Its Role in the Human,* edited by M. Bigazzi, F. C. Greenwood, and F. Gasparri, pp. 191–205. Excerpta Medica, Amsterdam.
364. Larkin, L. H., Suarez-Quian, C. A., and Fields, P. A. (1979): *In vitro* analysis of antisera to relaxin. *Acta Endocrinol. (Copenh.),* 92:568–576.
365. Ledger, W. L., Webster, M. A., Anderson, A. B. M., and Turnbull, A. C. (1985): Effect of inhibition of prostaglandin synthesis on cervical softening and uterine activity during ovine parturition resulting from progesterone withdrawal induced by epostane. *J. Endocrinol.,* 105:227–233.
366. Leppi, T. J. (1964): A study of the uterine cervix of the mouse. *Anat. Rec.,* 150:51–66.
367. Leppi, T. J., and Kinnison, P. A. (1971): The connective tissue ground substance in the mouse uterine cervix: An electron microscopic histochemical study. *Anat. Rec.,* 170:97–118.
368. Lerner, U. (1980): The uterine cervix and the initiation of labour: Action of estradiol 17-β. In: *Dilatation of the Uterine Cervix,* edited by F. Naftolin and P. G. Stubblefield, pp. 301–316. Raven Press, New York.
369. Lessing, J. B., Brenner, S. H., Schoenfeld, C., Goldsmith, L. T., Amelar, R. D., Dubin, L., and Weiss, G. (1985): The effect of relaxin on the motility of sperm in freshly thawed human semen. *Fertil. Steril.,* 44:406–409.
370. Lessing, J. B., Brenner, S. H., Schoenfeld, C., Sarosi, P., Amelar, R., Dubin, L., and Weiss, G. (1984): The effect of an anti-insulin antiserum on human sperm motility. *Fertil. Steril.,* 42:309–311.
371. Lessing, J. B., Brenner, S. H., and Weiss, G. (1984): Effect of prolactin and relaxin on *in vitro* rat uterine contractions and prolactin interaction with relaxin. *Obstet. Gynecol.,* 64:97–100.
372. Lippert, T. H., God, B., and Voelter, W. (1981): Immunoreactive relaxin-like substance in milk. *IRCS Med. Sci.,* 9:295.
373. Loeken, M. R., Channing, C. P., D'Eletto, R., and Weiss, G. (1983): Stimulatory effect of luteinizing hormone upon relaxin secretion by cultured porcine preovulatory granulosa cells. *Endocrinology,* 112:769–771.
374. Long, J. A. (1973): Corpus luteum of pregnancy in the rat—ultrastructural and cytochemical observations. *Biol. Reprod.,* 8:87–99.
375. Loumaye, E., De Cooman, S., and Thomas, K. (1980): Immunoreactive relaxin-like substance in human seminal plasma. *J. Clin. Endocrinol. Metab.,* 50:1142–1143.
376. Loumaye, E., Depreester, S., Donnez, J., and Thomas, K. (1984): Immunoreactive relaxin surge in the peritoneal fluid of women during the midluteal phase. *Fertil. Steril.,* 42:856–860.
377. Loumaye, E., Teuwissen, B., and Thomas, K. (1978): Characterization of relaxin radioimmunoassay using Bolton-Hunter reagent. *Gynecol. Obstet. Invest.,* 9:262–267.
378. Lovell, A. P. (1965): Bony pelvic dimorphism in rabbits. *Anat. Rec.,* 151:462.
379. Lowther, D. A. (1981): Molecular aspects of connective tissue remodelling. In: *Relaxin,* edited by G. D. Bryant-Greenwood, H. D. Niall, and F. C. Greenwood, pp. 277–292. Elsevier/North-Holland, New York.
380. Lye, S. J., and Challis, J. R. G. (1982): Inhibition by PGI-2 of myometrial activity *in vivo* in non-pregnant ovariectomized sheep. *J. Reprod. Fertil.,* 66:311–315.
381. MacLennan, A. H. (1981): Cervical ripening and the induction of labour by vaginal prostaglandin $F_{2\alpha}$ and relaxin. In: *The Cervix in*

Pregnancy and Labour, edited by D. A. Ellwood and A. B. M. Anderson, pp. 187–195. Churchill Livingstone, London.

382. MacLennan, A. H., Green, R. C., Bryant-Greenwood, G. D., Greenwood, F. C., and Seamark, R. F. (1980): Ripening of the human cervix and induction of labour with purified porcine relaxin. *Lancet,* 1:220–223.
383. MacLennan, A. H., Green, R. C., Bryant-Greenwood, F. C., and Seamark, R. F. (1981): Cervical Ripening with combinations of vaginal prostaglandin $F_{2\alpha}$, estradiol, and relaxin. *Obstet. Gynecol.,* 58:601–604.
384. MacLennan, A. H., Katz, M., and Creasy, R. (1985): The morphological characteristics of cervical ripening induced by the hormones relaxin and prostaglandin $F_{2\alpha}$ in a rabbit model. *Am. J. Obstet. Gynecol.,* 152:691–696.
385. Maillot, K. von (1979): Changes in the glycosaminoglycans distribution pattern in the human uterine cervix during pregnancy and labor. *Am. J. Obstet. Gynecol.,* 135:503–506.
386. Majewski, J. T., and Jennings, T. (1955): A uterine relaxing factor for premature labor. *Obstet. Gynecol.,* 5:649–652.
387. Manning, J. P., Steinetz, B. G., Butler, M. C., and Priester, S. (1965): The effect of steroids and relaxin on acid phosphatase in the pubic symphysis of the ovariectomized mouse. *J. Endocrinol.,* 33:501–506.
388. Marder, S. N., and Money, W.L. (1944): Concentration of relaxin in the blood serum of pregnant and postpartum rabbits. *Endocrinology,* 34:115–121.
389. Martin, P. A., BeVier, G. W., and Dziuk, P. J. (1978): The effect of disconnecting the uterus and ovary on the length of gestation in the pig. *Biol. Reprod.,* 18:428–433.
390. Mathieu, P., Rahier, J., and Thomas, K. (1981): Localization of relaxin in human gestational corpus luteum. *Cell Tissue Res.,* 219:213–216.
391. Matsumoto, D., and Chamley, W. A. (1980): Identification of relaxins in porcine follicular fluid and in the ovary of the immature sow. *J. Reprod. Fertil.,* 58:369–375.
392. May, J. V., and Schomberg, D. W. (1981): Granulosa cell differentiation *in vitro:* Effect of insulin on growth and functional integrity. *Biol. Reprod.,* 25:421–431.
393. Melton, C. E., and Saldivar, J. T. (1964): Impulse velocity and conduction pathways in rat myometrium. *Am. J. Physiol.,* 207:279–285.
394. Mercado-Simmen, R. C., Bryant-Greenwood, G. D., and Greenwood, F. C. (1980): Characterization of the binding of ^{125}I-relaxin to rat uterus. *J. Biol. Chem.,* 255:3617–3623.
395. Mercado-Simmen, R. C., Bryant-Greenwood, G. D., and Greenwood, F. C. (1982): Relaxin receptor in the rat myometrium: Regulation by estrogen and relaxin. *Endocrinology,* 110:220–226.
396. Mercado-Simmen, R. C., Goodwin, B., Ueno, M. S., Yamamoto, S. Y., and Bryant-Greenwood, G. D. (1982): Relaxin receptors in the myometrium and cervix of the pig. *Biol. Reprod.,* 26:120–128.
397. Miller, J. W., Kisley, A., and Murray, W. J. (1957): The effects of relaxin-containing ovarian extracts on various types of smooth muscle. *J. Pharmacol. Exp. Ther.,* 120:426–437.
398. Mishell, D. R., Nakamura, R. M., Barberia, J. M., and Thorneycroft, I. H. (1974): Initial detection of human chorionic gonadotropin in serum in normal human gestation. *Am. J. Obstet. Gynecol.,* 118:990–991.
399. Molokwu, E. C. I., and Wagner, W. C. (1973): Endocrine physiology of the puerperal sow. *J. Anim. Sci.,* 36:1158–1163.
400. Mossman, H. W., and Duke, K. L. (1973): *Comparative Morphology of the Mammalian Ovary,* pp. 209–220. University of Wisconsin Press, Madison.
401. Musah, A. I., Ford, J. J., and Anderson, L. L. (1984): Progesterone secretion as affected by 17β-estradiol after hysterectomy in the pig. *Endocrinology,* 115:1876–1882.
402. Musah, A. I., Schwabe, C., Willham, R. L., and Anderson, L. L. (1986): Pelvic development as affected by relaxin in three genetically selected frame sizes of beef heifers. *Biol. Reprod.,* 34:363–369.
403. Musah, A.I., Schwabe, C., Willham, R. L., and Anderson, L. L. (1986): Relaxin on induction of parturition in beef heifers. *Endocrinology,* 118:1476–1482.
404. McCarthy, J. J., Erving, H. W., and Laufe, L. E. (1957): Preliminary report on the use of relaxin in the management of threatened premature labor. *Am. J. Obstet. Gynecol.,* 74:134–138.
405. McDonald, J. K., and Schwabe, C. (1982): Relaxin-induced elevations of cathepsin B and dipeptidyl peptidase I in the mouse pubic symphysis, with localization by fluorescence enzyme histochemistry. *Ann. N.Y. Acad. Sci.,* 380:178–186.
406. McMurtry, J. P., Floersheim, G. L., and Bryant-Greenwood, G. D. (1980): Characterization of the binding of ^{125}I-labelled succinylated porcine relaxin to human and mouse fibroblasts. *J. Reprod. Fertil.,* 58:43–49.
407. McMurtry, J. P., Kwok, S. C. M., and Bryant-Greenwood, G. D. (1978): Target tissues for relaxin identified *in vitro* with ^{125}I-labelled porcine relaxin. *J. Reprod. Fertil.,* 53:209–216.
408. Naftolin, F., and Stubblefield, P. G., editors (1980): *Dilatation of the Uterine Cervix.* Raven Press, New York.
409. Nagao, R., and Bryant-Greenwood, G. D. (1981): Evidence for a uterine relaxin in the guinea pig. In: *Relaxin,* edited by G. D. Bryant-Greenwood, H. D. Niall, and F. C. Greenwood, pp. 61–69. Elsevier/North-Holland, New York.
410. Nara, B. S., Ball, G. D., Rutherford, J. E., Sherwood, O. D., and First, N. L. (1982): Release of relaxin by a nonluteolytic dose of prostaglandin $F_{2\alpha}$ in pregnant swine. *Biol. Reprod.,* 27:1190–1195.
411. Nara, B. S., and First, N. L. (1981): Effect of indomethacin and prostaglandin $F_{2}\alpha$ on parturition in swine. *J. Anim. Sci.,* 52:1360–1370.
412. Nara, B. S., Welk, F. A., Rutherford, J. E., Sherwood, O. D., and First, N. L. (1982): Effect of relaxin on parturition and frequency of live births in pigs. *J. Reprod. Fertil.,* 66:359–365.
413. Nardi, E., Bigazzi, M., Agrimonti, F., Dogliotti, L., Massi, G. B., Ferrari, A. M., Ciardetti, P., De Luca, V., and Angeli, A. (1983): Relaxin and fibrocystic disease of the mammary gland. In: *Biology of Relaxin and Its Role in the Human,* edited by M. Bigazzi, F. C. Greenwood, and F. G. Gasparri, pp. 417–419. Excerpta Medica, Amsterdam.
414. Newton, W. H., and Beck, N. (1939): Placental activity in the mouse in the absence of the pituitary gland. *J. Endocrinol.,* 1:65–75.
415. Niall, H. D., James, R., John, M., Walsh, J., Kwok, S., Bryant-Greenwood, G. D., Tregear, G. W., and Bradshaw, R. A. (1982): Chemical studies on relaxin. *Adv. Exp. Med. Biol.,* 143:163–169.
416. Nicol, D. S. H. W., and Smith, L. F. (1960): The amino acid sequence of human insulin. *Nature,* 187:483–485.
417. Nishikori, K., Burroughs, M., and Sanborn, B. M. (1983): cAMP-dependent phosphorylation on rat uterine myosin light chain kinase activity partially mimics the effects of relaxin treatment. *Program and Abstracts of the 65th Annual Meeting of the Endocrine Society,* San Antonio, TX, abstract 841.
418. Nishikori, K., Weisbrodt, N. W., Sherwood, O. D., and Sanborn, B. M. (1982): Relaxin alters rat uterine myosin light chain phosphorylation and related enzymatic activities. *Endocrinology,* 111:1743–1745.
419. Nishikori, K., Weisbrodt, N. W., Sherwood, O. D., and Sanborn, B. M. (1983): Effects of relaxin on rat uterine myosin light chain kinase activity and myosin light chain phosphorylation. *J. Biol. Chem.,* 258:2468–2474.
420. Nixon, W. E., Reid, R., Abou-Hozaifa, B. M., Williams, R. F., Steinetz, B. G., and Hodgen, G. D. (1983): Origin and regulation of relaxin secretion in monkeys: Effects of chorionic gonadotropin, luteectomy, fetectomy, and placentectomy. In: *Factors Regulating Ovarian Function,* edited by G. S. Greenwald and P. F. Terranova. Raven Press, New York.
421. Noall, M. W., and Frieden, E. H. (1956): Variations in sensitivity of ovariectomized guinea pigs to relaxin. *Endocrinology,* 58:659–664.
422. Noci, I., Nardi, E., Scarselli, G., Petrucci, F., Chelo, E., La Malfa, A., Tantini, C., Bruni, V., and Bigazzi, M. (1983): Immuno- and bio-active relaxin in human ovarian follicles. In: *Biology of Relaxin and Its Role in the Human,* edited by M. Bigazzi, F. C. Greenwood, and F. Gasparri, pp. 270–272. Excerpta Medica, Amsterdam.
423. Norström, A., Bryman, I., Wiqvist, N., Sahni, S., and Lindblom, B. (1984): Inhibitory action of relaxin on human cervical smooth muscle. *J. Clin. Endocrinol. Metab.,* 59:379–382.
424. Norström, A., and Wiqvist, I. (1985): Relaxin-induced changes in adenosine 3′5′-monophosphate levels in the human cervix. *Acta Endocrinol.,* 109:122–125.
425. North, A. C. T., Denson, A. K., Evans, A. C., Ford, L. O., and Willoughby, T. V. (1981): The use of an interactive computer graph-

ics system in the study of protein conformations. *Biomol. Struct. Conform. Funct. Evol. Proc. Int. Symp.*, 1:59–72.

426. Ny, T., Bjersing, L., Hseuh, A. J. W., and Loskutoff, D. J. (1985): Cultured granulosa cells produce two plasminogen activators and an antiactivator, each regulated differently by gonadotropins. *Endocrinology*, 116:1666–1668.
427. Obrink, B. (1973): A study of the interactions between monomeric tropocollagen and glycosaminoglycans. *Eur. J. Biochem.*, 33:387–400.
428. O'Byrne, E. M., Brindle, S., Quintavalla, J., Strawinski, C., Tabachnick, M., and Steinetz, B. G. (1982): Tissue distribution of injected ^{125}I-labeled porcine relaxin: Organ uptake, whole-body autoradiography, and renal concentration of radiometabolites. *Ann. N.Y. Acad. Sci.*, 380:187–197.
429. O'Byrne, E. M., Carriere, B. T., Sorensen, L., Segaloff, A., Schwabe, C., and Steinetz, B. G. (1978): Plasma immunoreactive relaxin levels in pregnant and nonpregnant women. *J. Clin. Endocrinol. Metab.*, 47:1106–1110.
430. O'Byrne, E. M., Flitcraft, J. F., Sawyer, W. K., Hochman, J., Weiss, G., and Steinetz, B. G. (1978): Relaxin bioactivity and immunoactivity in human corpora lutea. *Endocrinology*, 102:1641–1644.
431. O'Byrne, E. M., Sawyer, W. K., Butler, M. C., and Steinetz, B. G. (1976): Serum immunoreactive relaxin and softening of the uterine cervix in pregnant hamsters. *Endocrinology*, 99:1333–1335.
432. O'Byrne, E. M., and Steinetz, B. G. (1976): Radioimmunoassay of relaxin in sera of various species using an antiserum to porcine relaxin. *Proc. Soc. Exp. Biol. Med.*, 152:272–276.
433. O'Byrne, E. M., Weiss, G., and Steinetz, B. G. (1983): The isolation of human relaxin from the corpus luteum. In: *Biology of Relaxin and Its Role in the Human*, edited by M. Bigazzi, F. C. Greenwood, and F. Gasparri, pp. 370–376. Excerpta Medica, Amsterdam.
434. O'Byrne, K. T., and Summerlee, A. J. S. (1985): Relaxin suppression of oxytocin release occurs at the neurohypophysis in the rat. *J. Physiol. (Lond.)*, 365:49P.
435. Ochiai, K., Kato, H., Kelly, P. A., and Rothchild, I. (1983): The importance of a luteolytic effect of the pituitary in understanding the placental control of the rats corpus luteum. *Endocrinology*, 112:1687–1695.
436. Ochiai, K., and Rothchild, I. (1981): The relation between conceptus number and the luteotropic effect of estrogen in rats after hypophysectomy and hysterectomy on day 12 of pregnancy. *Endocrinology*, 109:1111–1116.
437. O'Conner, W. B., Cain, G. D., and Zarrow, M. X. (1966): Elongation of the interpubic ligament in the little brown bat (*Myotis lucifugus*). *Proc. Soc. Exp. Biol. Med.*, 123:935–937.
438. Olefsky, J. M., Saekow, M., and Kroc, R. L. (1982): Potentiation of insulin binding and insulin action by purified porcine relaxin. *Ann. N.Y. Acad. Sci.*, 380:200–215.
439. Oliver, R. M., Fields, P. A., and Larkin, L. H. (1978): Separation of relaxin activities in extracts of ovaries of pregnant sows by polyacrylamide gel electrophoresis. *J. Endocrinol.*, 76:517–525.
440. Omini, G., Pasargiklian, R., Folco, G. C., Fano, M., and Berti, F. (1978): Pharmacological activity of PGI2 and its metabolite 6-oxo-$PGF_{1\alpha}$ on human uterus and fallopian tubes. *Prostaglandins*, 15:1045–1054.
441. Ottobre, J. S., Nixon, W. E., and Stouffer, R. L. (1984): Induction of relaxin secretion in rhesus monkeys by human chorionic gonadotropin: Dependence on the age of the corpus luteum of the menstrual cycle. *Biol. Reprod.*, 31:1000–1006.
442. Owerbach, D., Bell, G. I., Rutter, W. J., and Shows, T. B. (1980): The insulin gene is located on chromosome 11 in humans. *Nature*, 286:82–84.
443. Pardo, R. J., and Larkin, L. H. (1982): Localization of relaxin in endometrial gland cells of pregnant, lactating, and ovariectomized hormone-treated guinea pigs. *Am. J. Anat.*, 164:79–90.
444. Pardo, R., Larkin, L. H., and Fields, P. A. (1980): Immunocytochemical localization of relaxin in endometrial glands of the pregnant guinea pig. *Endocrinology*, 107:2110–2112.
445. Pardo, R. J., Larkin, L. H., and Renegar, R. H. (1984): Immunoelectron microscopic localization of relaxin in endometrial gland cells of the pregnant guinea pig. *Anat. Rec.*, 209:373–379.
446. Parry, D. M., and Ellwood, D. A. (1981): Ultrastructural aspects of cervical softening in the sheep. In: *The Cervix in Pregnancy and Labour*, edited by D. A. Ellwood and A. B. M. Anderson, pp. 74–84. Churchill Livingstone, New York.
447. Patek, C. E., and Watson, J. (1976): Prostaglandin F and progesterone secretion by porcine endometrium and corpora lutea *in vitro*. *Prostaglandins*, 12:97–111.
448. Paterson, G. (1965): The nature of the inhibition of the rat uterus by relaxin. *J. Pharm. Pharmacol.*, 17:262–264.
449. Pederson, E. S. (1951): Histogenesis of lutein tissue of the albino rat. *Am. J. Anat.*, 88:397–427.
450. Pepe, G. J., and Rothchild, I. (1974): A comparative study of serum progesterone levels in pregnancy and in various types of pseudopregnancy in the rat. *Endocrinology*, 95:275–279.
451. Perezgrovas, R., and Anderson, L. L. (1982): Effect of porcine relaxin on cervical dilatation, pelvic area and parturition in cattle. *Biol. Reprod.*, 26:765–776.
452. Perl, E., and Catchpole, H. R. (1950): Changes induced in the connective tissue of the pubic symphysis of the guinea pig with estrogen and relaxin. *Arch. Pathol. Lab. Med.*, 50:233–239.
453. Petrucci, F., Goed, B., La Malfa, A., Nardi, E., Ciuffi, M., Scarselli, G., and Bigazzi, M. (1983): Metabolism of the uterus after administration of relaxin from human decidua. In: *Biology of Relaxin and Its Role in the Human*, edited by M. Bigazzi, F. C. Greenwood, and F. Gasparri, pp. 137–139. Excerpta Medica, Amsterdam.
454. Plunkett, E. R., and Gammal, E. B. (1967): The effect of relaxin upon DMBA-induced mammary cancer in female rats. *Br. J. Cancer*, 21:592–600.
455. Plunkett, E. R., Squires, B. P., and Heagy, F. C. (1963): Effect of relaxin on thyroid function in the rat. *J. Endocrinol.*, 26:331–338.
456. Plunkett, E. R., Squires, B. P., and Richardson, S. J. (1960): The effect of relaxin on thyroid weights in laboratory animals. *J. Endocrinol.*, 21:241–246.
457. Pommerenke, W. T. (1934): Experimental ligamentous relaxation in the guinea pig pelvis. *Am. J. Obstet. Gynecol.*, 27:708–713.
458. Porter, D. G. (1971): The action of relaxin on myometrial activity in the guinea-pig *in vivo*. *J. Reprod. Fertil.*, 26:251–253.
459. Porter, D. G. (1972): Myometrium of the pregnant guinea pig: The probable importance of relaxin. *Biol. Reprod.*, 7:458–464.
460. Porter, D. G. (1974): Inhibition of myometrial activity in the pregnant rabbit: Evidence for a "new" factor. *Biol. Reprod.*, 10:54–61.
461. Porter, D. G. (1979): Relaxin: Old hormone, new prospect. In: *Oxford Reviews of Reproductive Biology*, edited by C. A. Finn, pp. 1–57. Clarendon Press, Oxford.
462. Porter, D. C. (1979): The myometrium and the relaxin enigma. *Anim. Reprod. Sci.*, 2:77–96.
463. Porter, D. G. (1981): Relaxin and cervical softening: A review. In: *The Cervix in Pregnancy and Labour*, edited by D. A. Ellwood and A. B. M. Anderson, pp. 85–99. Churchill Livingstone, New York.
464. Porter, D. G. (1982): Unsolved problems of relaxin's physiological role. *Ann. N.Y. Acad. Sci.*, 380:151–162.
465. Porter, D. G. (1983): The possible involvement of relaxin in the regulation of uterine contraction. In: *Biology of Relaxin and Its Role in the Human*, edited by M. Bigazzi, F. C. Greenwood, and F. Gasparri, pp. 114–124. Excerpta Medica, Amsterdam.
466. Porter, D. G., and Challis, J. R. G. (1974): Failure of high uterine concentrations of progesterone to inhibit myometrial activity *in vivo* in the postpartum rat. *J. Reprod. Fertil.*, 39:157–162.
467. Porter, D. G., and Downing, S. J. (1978): Evidence that a humoral factor possessing relaxin-like activity is responsible for uterine quiescence in the late pregnant rat. *J. Reprod. Fertil.*, 52:95–102.
468. Porter, D. G., Downing, S. J., and Bradshaw, J. M. C. (1979): Relaxin inhibits spontaneous and prostaglandin-driven myometrial activity in anaesthetized rats. *J. Endocrinol.*, 83:183–192.
469. Porter, D. G., Downing, S. J., and Bradshaw, J. M. C. (1981): Inhibition of oxytocin- or prostaglandin $F_2\alpha$-driven myometrial activity by relaxin in the rat is oestrogen-dependent. *J. Endocrinol.*, 89:399–404.
470. Porter, D. G., Lye, S. J., Bradshaw, J. M. C., and Kendall, J. Z. (1981): Relaxin inhibits myometrial activity in the ovariectomized non-pregnant ewe. *J. Reprod. Fertil.*, 61:409–414.
471. Posse, N., and Kelly, J. V. (1956): A study of the effect of relaxin on contractility of the non-pregnant uterus by internal tocometry. *Surg. Gynecol. Obstet.*, 103:687–694.
472. Pullen, R. A., Lindsay, D. G., Wood, S. P., Tickle, I. J., Blundell, T. L., Wollmer, A., Krail, G., Brandenburg, D., Zahn, H., Glei-

mann, J., and Gammeltoft, S. (1976): Receptor-binding region of insulin. *Nature,* 259:369–373.

473. Prud'Homme, M.-J., Martinat, N., and Picaper, G. (1983): The effect of relaxin on *in vivo* uterine electromyographic activity in the conscious ovariectomized ewe is oestrogen-dependent. *Reprod. Nutr. Dev.,* 23:493–499.
474. Puri, C. P., and Garfield, R. E. (1982): Changes in hormone levels and gap junctions in the rat uterus during pregnancy and parturition. *Biol. Reprod.,* 27:967–975.
475. Pusey, J., Kelly, W. A., Bradshaw, J. M. C., and Porter, D. G. (1980): Myometrial activity and the distribution of blastocysts in the uterus of the rat: Interference by relaxin. *Biol. Reprod.,* 23:394–397.
476. Quagliarello, J., Cederqvist, L., Steinetz, B., and Weiss, G. (1978): Serum relaxin levels in prostaglandin E_2 induced abortions. *Prostaglandins,* 16:1003–1006.
477. Quagliarello, J., Goldsmith, L., Steinetz, B. G., Lustig, D. S., and Weiss, G. (1980): Induction of relaxin secretion in nonpregnant women by human chorionic gonadotropin. *J. Clin. Endocrinol. Metab.,* 51:74–77.
478. Quagliarello, J., Lustig, D. S., Steinetz, B. G., and Weiss, G. (1980): Absence of a prelabor relaxin surge in women. *Biol. Reprod.,* 22:202–204.
479. Quagliarello, J., Steinetz, B. G., and Weiss, G. (1979): Relaxin secretion in early pregnancy. *Obstet. Gynecol.,* 53:62–63.
480. Quagliarello, J., Szlachter, N., Nisselbaum, J. S., Schwartz, M. K., Steinetz, B. G., and Weiss, G. (1981): Serum relaxin and human chorionic gonadotropin concentrations in spontaneous abortions. *Fertil. Steril.,* 36:399–401.
481. Quagliarello, J., Szlachter, N., Steinetz, B. G., Goldsmith, L. T., and Weiss, G. (1979): Serial relaxin concentrations in human pregnancy. *Am. J. Obstet. Gynecol.,* 135:43–44.
482. Rao, M. R., and Sanborn, B. M. (1985): Relaxin increases Ca^{2+} efflux from rat myometrial cells in culture. *Program and Abstracts of the 67th Annual Meeting of the Endocrine Society,* Baltimore, MD, abstract 736.
483. Rawitch, A. B., Moore, W. V., and Frieden, E. H. (1980): Relaxin-insulin homology: Predictions of secondary structure and lack of competitive binding. *Int. J. Biochem.,* 11:357–362.
484. Reinig, J. W., Daniel, L. N., Schwabe, C., Gowan, L. K., Steinetz, B. G., and O'Byrne, E. M. (1981): Isolation and characterization of relaxin from the sand tiger shark (*Odontaspis taurus*). *Endocrinology,* 109:537–543.
485. Renegar, R. H., and Larkin, L. H. (1985): Relaxin concentrations in endometrial, placental, and ovarian tissues, and in sera from ewes during middle and late pregnancy. *Biol. Reprod.,* 32:840–847.
486. Reynolds, H., and Livingood, C. S. (1959): Use of relaxin in management of ulceration and gangrene due to collagen disease. *A.M.A. Arch. Dermatol.,* 80:407–409.
487. Rice, L. E., and Wiltbank, J. N. (1972): Factors affecting dystocia in beef heifers. *J.A.M.A.,* 161:1348–1358.
488. Rimmer, D. M. (1973): The effect of pregnancy on the collagen of the uterine cervix of the mouse. *J. Endocrinol.,* 57:413–418.
489. Rinard, G. A. (1970): Phosphorylase a activity in rat uterine homogenates: Loss of activity related to *in vivo* treatment with estrogen, progesterone, relaxin, and CaEDTA. *Biochim. Biophys. Acta,* 222:455–464.
490. Rinderknecht, E., and Humbel, R. E. (1978): Primary structure of human insulin-like growth factor II. *FEBS Lett.,* 89:283–286.
491. Rinderknecht, E., and Humbel, R. E. (1978): The amino acid sequence of human insulin-like growth factor I and its structural homology with proinsulin. *J. Biol. Chem.,* 253:2769–2776.
492. Rivelis, A. L., Traeger, C., and Rogoff, B. (1965): The use of relaxin in progressive systemic sclerosis and other connective tissue diseases. A clinical study. *Arch. Interam. Rheumatol.,* 8:19–31.
493. Robertson, M. C., and Friesen, H. G. (1981): Two forms of rat placental lactogen revealed by radioimmunoassay. *Endocrinology,* 108:2388–2390.
494. Robertson, M. C., Gillespie, B., and Friesen, H. G. (1982): Characterization of the two forms of rat placental lactogen (rPL): rPL-I and rPL-II. *Endocrinology,* 111:1862–1866.
495. Rogers, P. A. W., Murphy, C. R., Squires, K. R., and MacLennan, A. H. (1983): Effects of relaxin on the intrauterine distribution and antimesometrial positioning and orientation of rat blastocysts before implantation. *J. Reprod. Fertil.,* 68:431–435.
496. Rothchild, I. (1981): The regulation of the mammalian corpus luteum. *Rec. Prog. Horm. Res.,* 37:183–283.
497. Rudzik, A. D., and Miller, J. W. (1962): The mechanism of uterine inhibitory action of relaxin-containing ovarian extracts. *J. Pharmacol. Exp. Ther.,* 138:82–87.
498. Rudzik, A. D., and Miller, J. W. (1962): The effect of altering the catecholamine content of the uterus on the rate of contractions and the sensitivity of the myometrium to relaxin. *J. Pharmacol. Exp. Ther.,* 138:88–95.
499. Rundgren, A. (1974): Physical properties of connective tissue as influenced by single and repeated pregnancies in the rat. *Acta Physiol. Scand. [Suppl. 417],* 92:1–138.
500. Ruoff, H. J., Lippert, T. H., Seeger, H., and Voelter, W. (1984): Immunoreactive relaxin-like substance and relaxin sensitive adenylate cyclase in the gastric mucosa. *IRCS Med. Sci.,* 12:224–225.
501. Ruth, E. B. (1936): Metamorphosis of the pubic symphysis. II. The guinea pig. *Anat. Rec.,* 67:69–79.
502. Ruth, E. B. (1937): Metamorphosis of the pubic symphysis. III. Histological changes in the symphysis of the pregnant guinea pig. *Anat. Rec.,* 67:409–421.
503. Saito, Y., Takahashi, S., and Maki, M. (1981): Effects of some drugs on ripening of uterine cervix in nonpregnant castrated and pregnant rats. *Tohoku J. Exp. Med.,* 133:205–220.
504. Salamon, S., and Lightfoot, R. J. (1970): Fertility of ram spermatozoa frozen by the pellet method. III. The effects of insemination technique, oxytocin and relaxin on lambing. *J. Reprod. Fertil.,* 22:409–423.
505. Sanborn, B. M. (1986): The role of relaxin in uterine function. In: *Physiology and Biochemistry of the Uterus in Pregnancy and Labor,* edited by G. Huszar, pp. 225–238. CRC Press, Boca Raton, FL.
506. Sanborn, B. M., Kuo, H. S., Weisbrodt, N. W., and Sherwood, O. D. (1980): The interaction of relaxin with the rat uterus. I. Effect on cyclic nucleotide levels and spontaneous contractile activity. *Endocrinology,* 106:1210–1215.
507. Sanborn, B. M., Kuo, H. S., Weisbrodt, N. W., and Sherwood, O. D. (1982): Effect of relaxin on cyclic nucleotide levels and spontaneous contractions of the rat uterus. *Adv. Exp. Med. Biol.,* 143:273–282.
508. Sanborn, B. M., and Sherwood, O. D. (1981): Effect of relaxin on bound cAMP in rat uterus. *Endocr. Res. Commun.,* 8:179–192.
509. Sanborn, B. M., Sherwood, O. D., and Kuo, H. S. (1980): Evidence against the primary role for catecholamine release or prostaglandin synthesis in the effect of relaxin on uterine cyclic AMP levels. *Program and Abstracts of the 62nd Annual Meeting of the Endocrine Society,* Anaheim, CA, abstract 42.
510. Sanborn, B. M., Weisbrodt, N. W., and Sherwood, O. D. (1981): Evidence against an obligatory role for catecholamine release in the effects of relaxin on the rat uterus. *Biol. Reprod.,* 24:987–992.
511. Sarosi, P., Schmidt, C. L., Essig, M., Steinetz, B. G., and Weiss, G. (1983): The effect of relaxin and progesterone on rat uterine contractions. *Am. J. Obstet. Gynecol.,* 145:402–405.
512. Sarosi, P., Schmidt, C. L., Steinetz, B. G., and Weiss, G. (1983): Progesterone relaxin synergism and $PGF_{2\alpha}$-relaxin antagonism in electrostimulated isolated rat uterine horn segments. In: *Biology of Relaxin and Its Role in the Human,* edited by M. Bigazzi, F. C. Greenwood, and F. Gasparri, p. 180. Excerpta Medica, Amsterdam.
513. Sarosi, P., Schoenfeld, C., Berman, J., Basch, R., Randolph, G., Amelar, R., Dubin, L., Steinetz, B. G., and Weiss, G. (1983): Effect of anti-relaxin antiserum on sperm motility *in vitro*. *Endocrinology,* 112:1860–1861.
514. Sawyer, W. H., Frieden, E. H., and Martin, A. C. (1953): *In vitro* inhibition of spontaneous contractions of the rat uterus by relaxin-containing extracts of sow ovaries. *Am. J. Physiol.,* 172:547–552.
515. Scarselli, G., Bigazzi, M., Acanfora, L., Cozzi, C., Branconi, F., and Nardi, M. (1983): RIA assay of relaxin in human pregnancy. In: *Biology of Relaxin and Its Role in the Human,* edited by M. Bigazzi, F. C. Greenwood, and F. Gasparri, pp. 318–320. Excerpta Medica, Amsterdam.
516. Schmidt, C. L., Black, V. H., and Weiss, G. (1982): Hormonal and ultrastructural studies of longterm monolayer cultures of human luteal cells. *Program and Abstracts of the 64th Annual Meeting of the Endocrine Society,* San Francisco, abstract 758.
517. Schmidt, C. L., Kendall, J. Z., Dandekar, P. V., Quigley, M. M., and Schmidt, K. L. (1984): Characterization of long-term monolayer

cultures of human granulosa cells from follicles of different size and exposed *in vivo* to clomiphene citrate and hCG. *J. Reprod. Fertil.*, 71:279–287.
518. Schmidt, C. L., Sarosi, P., Steinetz, B. G., O'Byrne, E. M., Tyson, J. E., Horvath, K., Sas, M., and Weiss, G. (1984): Relaxin in human decidua and term placenta. *Eur. J. Obstet. Gynaecol. Reprod. Biol.*, 17:171–182.
519. Schmidt, J. E., and Leonard, S. L. (1960): The effect of relaxin on uterine phosphorylase in the rat. *Endocrinology*, 67:663–667.
520. Schreifer, J. A., Lewis, P. R., and Miller, J. W. (1982): Role of fetal oxytocin in parturition in the rat. *Biol. Reprod.*, 27:362–368.
521. Schwabe, C. (1983): Relaxin sequences. In: *Biology of Relaxin and Its Role in the Human*, edited by M. Bigazzi, F. C. Greenwood, and F. Gasparri, pp. 22–31. Excerpta Medica, Amsterdam.
522. Schwabe, C. (1983): N-α-formyl-tyrosyl-relaxin. A reliable tracer for relaxin radioimmunoassays. *Endocrinology*, 113:814–815.
523. Schwabe, C. (1983): Relaxin in connective tissue diseases. In: *Biology of Relaxin and Its Role in the Human*, edited by M. Bigazzi, F. C. Greenwood, and F. Gasparri, pp. 402–409. Excerpta Medica, Amsterdam.
524. Schwabe, C., and Braddon, S. A. (1976): Evidence for one essential tryptophan residue at the active site of relaxin. *Biochem. Biophys. Res. Commun.*, 68:1126–1132.
525. Schwabe, C., Gowan, L. K. and Reinig, J. W. (1982): Evolution, relaxin, and insulin: A new perspective. *Ann. N.Y. Acad. Sci.*, 380:6–12.
526. Schwabe, C., and Harmon, S. J. (1978): A comparative circular dichroism study of relaxin and insulin. *Biochem. Biophys. Res. Commun.*, 84:374–380.
527. Schwabe, C., LeRoith, D., Thompson, R. P., Shiloach, J., and Roth, J. (1983): Relaxin extracted from protozoa (*Tetrahymena pyriformis*). *J. Biol. Chem.*, 258:2778–2781.
528. Schwabe, C., and McDonald, J. K. (1977): Relaxin: A disulfide homolog of insulin. *Science*, 197:914–915.
529. Schwabe, C., McDonald, J. K., and Steinetz, B. G. (1976): Primary structure of the A chain of porcine relaxin. *Biochem. Biophys. Res. Commun.*, 70:397–405.
530. Schwabe, C., McDonald, J. K., and Steinetz, B. G. (1977): Primary structure of the B chain of porcine relaxin. *Biochem. Biophys. Res. Commun.*, 75:503–510.
531. Schwabe, C., Steinetz, B. G., Weiss, G., Segaloff, A., McDonald, J. K., O'Byrne, E. M., Hochman, J., Carriere, B., and Goldsmith, L. (1978): Relaxin. *Recent Prog. Horm. Res.*, 34:123–199.
532. Schwabe, C., and Warr, G. W. (1984): A polyphyletic view of evolution: The genetic potential hypothesis. *Perspect. Biol. Med.*, 27:465–485.
533. Scott, J. E., and Orford, C. R. (1981): Dermatan sulphate-rich proteoglycan associates with rat tail-tendon collagen at the d band in the gap region. *Biochem. J.*, 197:213–216.
534. Segaloff, A. (1983): The role of the ovary in the synergism between radiation and estrogen in the production of mammary cancer in the rat. In: *Biology of Relaxin and Its Role in the Human*, edited by M. Bigazzi, F. C. Greenwood, and F. Gasparri, pp. 410–416. Excerpta Medica, Amsterdam.
535. Sheffield, L. G., and Anderson, R. R. (1983): Effect of porcine relaxin and estradiol-17β on the incorporation of tritiated thymidine by fibroblasts isolated from guinea pig uteri. *Life Sci.*, 33:543–546.
536. Sheffield, L. G., and Anderson, R. R. (1984): Effect of estradiol and relaxin on growth of fibroblastic cells isolated from guinea pig mammary glands. *Biol. Reprod.*, 30:338–343.
537. Sheffield, L. G., and Anderson, R. R. (1984): Effect of estradiol and relaxin on collagen and non-collagen protein synthesis by mammary fibroblasts. *Life Sci.*, 35:2199–2203.
538. Sherwood, O. D. (1979): Purification and characterization of rat relaxin. *Endocrinology*, 104:886–892.
539. Sherwood, O. D. (1982): Isolation and characterization of porcine and rat relaxin. *Adv. Exp. Med. Biol.*, 143:115–147.
540. Sherwood, O. D. (1982): Radioimmunoassay of relaxin. *Adv. Exp. Med. Biol.*, 143:221–248.
541. Sherwood, O. D. (1982): Relaxin at parturition in the pig. In: *Control of Pig Reproduction*, edited by D. J. A. Cole and G. R. Foxcraft, pp. 343–375. Butterworth Scientific, London.
542. Sherwood, O. D., Chang, C. C., BeVier, G. W., Diehl, J. R., and Dziuk, P. J. (1976): Relaxin concentrations in pig plasma following the administration of prostaglandin $F_2\alpha$ during late pregnancy. *Endocrinology*, 98:875–879.
543. Sherwood, O. D., Chang, C. C., BeVier, G. W., and Dziuk, P. J. (1975): Radioimmunoassay of plasma relaxin levels throughout pregnancy and at parturition in the pig. *Endocrinology*, 97: 834–837.
544. Sherwood, O. D., and Crnekovic, V. E. (1979): Development of a homologous radioimmunoassay for rat relaxin. *Endocrinology*, 104:893–897.
545. Sherwood, O. D., Crnekovic, V. E., Gordon, W. L., and Rutherford, J. E. (1980): Radioimmunoassay of relaxin throughout pregnancy and during parturition in the rat. *Endocrinology*, 107:691–698.
546. Sherwood, O. D., and Downing, S. J. (1983): The chemistry and physiology of relaxin. In: *Factors Regulating Ovarian Function*, edited by G. S. Greenwald and P. F. Terranova, pp. 381–410. Raven Press, New York.
547. Sherwood, O. D., Downing, S. J., Golos, T. G., Gordon, W. L., and Tarbell, M. K. (1983): Influence of light-dark cycle on antepartum serum relaxin and progesterone immunoactivity levels and on birth in the rat. *Endocrinology*, 113:997–1003.
548. Sherwood, O. D., Downing, S. J., Rieber, A. J., Fraley, S. W., Bohrer, R. E., Richardson, B. C., and Shanks, R. D. (1985): Influence of litter size on antepartum serum relaxin and progesterone immunoactivity levels and on birth in the rat. *Endocrinology*, 116:2554–2562.
549. Sherwood, O. D., Golos, T. G., and Key, R. H. (1986): Influence of the conceptuses and the maternal pituitary on the distribution of multiple components of serum relaxin immunoactivity during pregnancy in the rat. *Endocrinology*, 119:2143–2147.
550. Sherwood, O. D., Key, R. H., Tarbell, M. K., and Downing, S. J. (1984): Dynamic changes of multiple forms of serum immunoactive relaxin during pregnancy in the rat. *Endocrinology*, 114:806–813.
551. Sherwood, O. D., Martin, P. A., Chang, C. C., and Dziuk, P. J. (1977): Plasma relaxin levels in pigs with corpora lutea induced during late pregnancy. *Biol. Reprod.*, 17:97–100.
552. Sherwood, O. D., Martin, P. A., Chang, C. C., and Dziuk, P. J. (1977): Plasma relaxin levels during late pregnancy and at parturition in pigs with altered utero-ovarian connections. *Biol. Reprod.*, 17:101–103.
553. Sherwood, O. D., Nara, B. S., Crnekovic, V. E., and First, N. L. (1979): Relaxin concentrations in pig plasma after the administration of indomethacin and prostaglandin $F_2\alpha$ during late pregnancy. *Endocrinology*, 104:1716–1721.
554. Sherwood, O. D., Nara, B. S., Welk, F. A., First, N. L., and Rutherford, J. E. (1981): Relaxin levels in the maternal plasma of pigs before, during, and after parturition and before, during, and after suckling. *Biol. Reprod.*, 25:65–71.
555. Sherwood, O. D., and O'Byrne, E. M. (1974): Purification and characterization of porcine relaxin. *Arch. Biochem. Biophys.*, 160:185–196.
556. Sherwood, O. D., Rosentreter, K. R., and Birkhimer, M. L. (1975): Development of a radioimmunoassay for porcine relaxin using ^{125}I-labeled polytyrosyl-relaxin. *Endocrinology*, 96:1106–1113.
557. Sherwood, O. D., and Rutherford, J. E. (1981): Relaxin immunoactivity levels in ovarian extracts obtained from rats during various reproductive states and from adult cycling pigs. *Endocrinology*, 108:1171–1177.
558. Sherwood, O. D., Wilson, M. E., Edgerton, L. A., and Chang, C. C. (1978): Serum relaxin concentrations in pigs with parturition delayed by progesterone administration. *Endocrinology*, 102:471–475.
559. Shiu, R. P. C., Kelly, P. A., and Friesen, H. G. (1973): Radioreceptor assay for prolactin and other lactogenic hormones. *Science*, 180:968–971.
560. Sims, S. M., Daniel, E. E., and Garfield, R. E. (1982): Improved electrical coupling in uterine smooth muscle is associated with increased numbers of gap junctions at parturition. *J. Gen. Physiol.*, 80:353–375.
561. Slate, W. G. (1960): Pelvic girdle relaxation. *Obstet. Gynecol.*, 16:625–627.
562. Slate, W. G. (1961): Effect of relaxin on the cervix of nonpregnant women. *Obstet. Gynecol.*, 17:294–296.
563. Smith, T. C. (1954): The action of relaxin on mammary gland growth in the rat. *Endocrinology*, 54:59–70.

564. Smithberg, M., and Runner, M. (1956): The induction and maintenance of pregnancy in prepuberal mice. *J. Exp. Zool.*, 133:441–457.

565. Snell, C. R., and Smyth, D. G. (1975): Proinsulin: A proposed three-dimensional structure. *J. Biol. Chem.*, 250:6291–6295.

566. Sridaran, R., Basuray, R., and Gibori, G. (1981): Source and regulation of testosterone secretion in pregnant and pseudopregnant rats. *Endocrinology,* 108:855–861.

567. Steiner, D. F., Quinn, P. S., Chan, S. J., Marsh, J., and Tager, H. S. (1980): Processing mechanisms in the biosynthesis of proteins. *Ann. N.Y. Acad. Sci.*, 343:1–16.

568. Steinetz, B. G. (1982): Specificity and reliability of radioimmunoassays, radioreceptor assays, and bioassays: Round table discussion summary. *Ann. N.Y. Acad. Sci.*, 380:51–59.

569. Steinetz, B. G., and Beach, V. L. (1963): Hormonal requirements for interpubic ligament formation in hypophysectomized mice. *Endocrinology,* 72:771–776.

570. Steinetz, B. G., Beach, V. L., Blye, R. P., and Kroc, R. L. (1957): Changes in the composition of the rat uterus following a single injection of relaxin. *Endocrinology,* 61:287–292.

571. Steinetz, B. G., Beach, V. L., and Kroc, R. L. (1957): The influence of progesterone, relaxin and estrogen on some structural and functional changes in the pre-parturient mouse. *Endocrinology,* 61:271–280.

572. Steinetz, B. G., Beach, V. L., and Kroc, R. L. (1959): The physiology of relaxin in laboratory animals. In: *Recent Progress in the Endocrinology of Reproduction,* edited by C. W. Lloyd, pp. 389–423. Academic Press, New York.

573. Steinetz, B. G., Beach, V. L., and Kroc, R. L. (1969): Bioassay of relaxin. In: *Methods in Hormone Research,* edited by R. I. Dorfman, pp. 481–513. Academic Press, New York.

574. Steinetz, B. G., Beach, V. L., Kroc, R. L., Stasilli, N. R., Nussbaum, R. E., Nemith, P. J., and Dun, R. K. (1960): Bioassay of relaxin using a reference standard: A simple and reliable method utilizing direct measurement of interpubic ligament formation in mice. *Endocrinology,* 67:102–115.

575. Steinetz, B. G., Beach, V. L., Tripp, L. V., and DeFalco, R. J. (1964): Reactions of antisera to porcine relaxin with relaxin-containing tissues of other species *in vivo* and *in vitro. Acta Endocrinol.*, 47:371–384.

576. Steinetz, B. G., Butler, M. C., Sawyer, W. K., and O'Byrne, E. M. (1976): Effects of relaxin on early pregnancy in rats. *Proc. Soc. Exp. Biol. Med.*, 152:419–422.

577. Steinetz, B. G., and Manning, J. P. (1967): Influence of growth hormone, steroids and relaxin on acid phosphatase activity of connective tissue. *Proc. Soc. Exp. Biol. Med.*, 124:180–184.

578. Steinetz, B. G., Manning, J. P., Butler, M., and Beach, V. (1965): Relationships of growth hormone, steroids and relaxin in the transformation of pubic joint cartilage to ligament in hypophysectomized mice. *Endocrinology,* 76:876–882.

579. Steinetz, B. G., Matthews, J. R., Butler, M. T., and Thompson, S. W. (1973): Inhibition by thyrocalcitonin of estrogen-induced bone resorption in the mouse pubic symphysis. *Am. J. Pathol.*, 73:735–741.

580. Steinetz, B. G., and O'Byrne, E. M. (1983): Speculations on the probable role of relaxin in cervical dilation and parturition in rats. *Semin. Reprod. Endocrinol.*, 1:335–342.

581. Steinetz, B. G., O'Byrne, E. M., Butler, M. C., and Hickman, L. B. (1983): Hormonal regulation of the connective tissue of the symphysis pubis. In: *Biology of Relaxin and Its Role in the Human,* edited by M. Bigazzi, F. C. Greenwood, and F. Gasparri, pp. 71–92. Excerpta Medica, Amsterdam.

582. Steinetz, B. G., O'Byrne, E. M., and Kroc, R. L. (1980): The role of relaxin in cervical softening during pregnancy in mammals. In: *Dilation of the Uterine Cervix,* edited by F. Naftolin and P. G. Stubblefield, pp. 157–177. Raven Press, New York.

583. Steinetz, B. G., O'Byrne, E. M., Sawyer, W. K., Butler, M. C., Munigle, J., and Steele, R. E. (1985): Effects of aminoglutethimide on cervical dilatability and serum immunoreactive relaxin in pregnant rats. *Proc. Soc. Exp. Biol. Med.*, 178:101–104.

584. Steinetz, B. G., O'Byrne, E. M., and Schwabe, C. (1981): Specificity and applications of biological assays for porcine relaxin. In: *Relaxin,* edited by G. D. Bryant-Greenwood, H. D. Niall, and F. C. Greenwood, pp. 331–335. Elsevier/North-Holland, New York.

585. Steinetz, B. G., O'Byrne, E. M., and Weiss, G. (1981): Measurement of "relaxin" in human plasma and serum samples using a homologous porcine radioimmunoassay. In: *Relaxin,* edited by G. D. Bryant-Greenwood, H. D. Niall, and F. C. Greenwood, pp. 373–375. Elsevier/North-Holland, New York.

586. Steinetz, B. G., O'Byrne, E. M., Weiss, G., and Schwabe, C. (1982): Bioassay methods for relaxin: Uses and pitfalls. *Adv. Exp. Med. Biol.*, 143:79–104.

587. Steinetz, B. G., O'Byrne, E. M., Sarosi, P., and Weiss, G. (1983): Bioassay of relaxin: Present status and future prospects. In: *Biology of Relaxin and Its Role in the Human,* edited by M. Bigazzi, F. C. Greenwood, and F. Gasparri, pp. 140–147. Excerpta Medica, Amsterdam.

588. Steinetz, B. G., Schwabe, C., and Weiss, G., editors (1982): *Relaxin: Structure, Function, and Evolution. Ann. N.Y. Acad. Sci.*, vol. 380.

589. Stewart, A. G., Richards, H., Roberts, S., Warwick, J., Edwards, K., Bell, L. Smith, J., and Derbyshire, R. (1983): Cloning and expression of porcine prorelaxin gene in *E. coli. Nucleic Acids Res.*, 11:6597–6609.

590. Stewart, D. R. (1986): Development of a homologous equine relaxin radioimmunoassay. *Endocrinology,* 119:1100–1104.

591. Stewart, D. R., and H. Papkoff (1986): Purification and characterization of equine relaxin. *Endocrinology,* 119:1093–1099.

592. Stewart, D. R., and Stabenfeldt, G. (1981): Relaxin activity in the pregnant mare. *Biol. Reprod.*, 25:281–289.

593. Stewart, D. R., and Stabenfeldt, G. (1985): Relaxin activity in the pregnant cat. *Biol. Reprod.*, 32:848–854.

594. Stewart, D. R., Stabenfeldt, G. H., and Hughes, J. P. (1982): Relaxin activity in foaling mares. *J. Reprod. Fertil.* [*Suppl.*], 32:603–609.

595. Stewart, D. R., Stabenfeldt, G. H., Hughes, J. P., and Meagher, D. M. (1982): Determination of the source of equine relaxin. *Biol. Reprod.*, 27:17–24.

596. St-Louis, J. (1981): Relaxin inhibition of KCl-induced uterine contractions *in vitro:* An alternative bioassay. *Can. J. Physiol. Pharmacol.*, 59:507–512.

597. St-Louis, J. (1982): Pharmacological studies on the action of relaxin upon KCl-contracted rat uterus. *Pharmacology,* 25:327–337.

598. St-Louis, J. (1983): Pharmacological studies of the effect of porcine relaxin on rat uterus *in vitro.* In: *Biology of Relaxin and Its Role in the Human,* edited by M. Bigazzi, F. C. Greenwood, and F. Gasparri, pp. 128–133. Excerpta Medica, Amsterdam.

599. St-Louis, J., and Massicotte, G. (1985): Chronic decrease of blood pressure by rat relaxin in spontaneously hypertensive rats. *Life Sci.*, 37:1351–1357.

600. Stone, M. L. (1959): Effects of relaxin in the human. In: *Recent Progress in the Endocrinology of Reproduction,* edited by C. W. Lloyd, pp. 429–439. Academic Press, New York.

601. Storey, E. (1957): Relaxation in the pubic symphysis of the mouse during pregnancy and after relaxin administration, with special reference to the behavior of collagen. *J. Pathol. Bacteriol.*, 74:147–162.

602. Straus, W. T. (1932): Pelvic relaxation in the pregnant rhesus macaque. *Anat. Rec.*, 52:38.

603. Strauss, J. F., and Stambaugh, R. L. (1974): Induction of 20α-hydroxysteroid dehydrogenase in rat corpora lutea of pregnancy by prostaglandin $F_{2}\alpha$. *Prostaglandins,* 5:73–85.

604. Stryker, J. L., and Dziuk, P. J. (1975): Effects of fetal decapitation on fetal development, parturition, and lactation in pigs. *J. Anim. Sci.*, 40:282–287.

605. Stys, S. J., Clark, K. E., Clewell, W. H., and Meschia, G. (1980): Hormonal effects on cervical compliance in sheep. In: *Dilatation of the Uterine Cervix,* edited by F. Naftolin and P. G. Stubblefield, pp. 147–156. Raven Press, New York.

606. Stys, S. J., Dresser, B. L., Otte, T. E., and Clark, V. E. (1981): Effect of prostaglandin E_2 on cervical compliance in pregnant ewes. *Am. J. Obstet. Gynecol.*, 140:415–419.

607. Summerlee, A. J. S., O'Byrne, K. T., Paisley, A. C., Breeze, M. F., and Porter, D. G. (1984): Relaxin affects the central control of oxytocin release. *Nature,* 309:372–374.

608. Szlachter, N., O'Byrne, E., Goldsmith, L., Steinetz, B. G., and Weiss, G. (1980): Myometrial inhibiting activity of relaxin-containing extracts of human corpora lutea of pregnancy. *Am. J. Obstet. Gynecol.*, 136:584–586.

609. Szlachter, B. N., Quagliarello, J., Jewelewicz, R., Osathanondh, R., Spellacy, W. N., and Weiss, G. (1982): Relaxin in normal and pathogenic pregnancies. *Obstet. Gynecol.*, 59:167–170.
610. Tager, H. S., and Steiner, D. F. (1972): Primary structures of the proinsulin connecting peptides of the rat and the horse. *J. Biol. Chem.*, 247:7936–7940.
611. Takayama, M., and Greenwald, G. S. (1973): Direct luteotropic action of estrogen in the hypophysectomized-hysterectomized rat. *Endocrinology*, 92:1405–1413.
612. Talmage, R. V. (1947): Changes produced in the symphysis pubis of the guinea pig by the sex steroids and relaxin. *Anat. Rec.*, 99:91–113.
613. Talmage, R. V. (1947): A histological study of the effects of relaxin on the symphysis pubis of the guinea pig. *J. Exp. Zool.*, 106:281–297.
614. Talmage, R. V. (1950): The role of estrogen in the estrogen-relaxin relationship in symphyseal relaxation. *Endocrinology*, 47:75–82.
615. Talmage, R. V., and Garrett, F. A. (1951): Effects of repeated injections of the steroids and relaxin on the symphisis pubis of the guinea pig as studied by X-ray. *Endocrinology*, 48:162–168.
616. Talmage, R. V., and Hurst, W. R. (1950): Variability in the response of the symphysis pubis of the guinea-pig to relaxin. *J. Endocrinol.*, 7:24–30.
617. Taverne, M., Bevers, M., Bradshaw, J. M. C., Dieleman, S. J., Willemse, A. H., and Porter, D. G. (1982): Plasma concentrations of prolactin, progesterone, relaxin, and oestradiol-17β in sows treated with progesterone, bromocriptine or indomethacin during late pregnancy. *J. Reprod. Fertil.*, 65:85–96.
618. Taverne, M. A. M., Naaktgeboren, C., Elsaesser, F., Forsling, M. L., Van der Weyden, G. C., Ellendorff, F., and Smidt, D. (1979): Myometrial electrical activity and plasma concentrations of progesterone, estrogens and oxytocin during late pregnancy and parturition in the miniature pig. *Biol. Reprod.*, 21:1125–1134.
619. Thomas, K., Loumaye, E., and Donnez, J. (1982): Immunoreactive relaxin in the peritoneal fluid during spontaneous menstrual cycle in women. *Ann. N.Y. Acad. Sci.*, 380:126–130.
620. Thomas, K., Loumaye, E., and Ferin, J. (1980): Relaxin in non-pregnant women during ovarian stimulation. *Gynecol. Obstet. Invest.*, 11:75–80.
621. Thoms, H. (1936): Relaxation of the symphysis pubis in pregnancy. *J.A.M.A.*, 106:1364–1366.
622. Too, C. K. L., Bryant-Greenwood, G. D., and Greenwood, F. C. (1982): The effect of relaxin on the release of collagenase from rat uterine and granulosa cells *in vitro*. *Program and Abstracts of the 64th Annual Meeting of the Endocrine Society*, San Francisco, abstract 329.
623. Too, C. K. L., Bryant-Greenwood, G. D., and Greenwood, F. C. (1984): Relaxin increases the release of plasminogen activator, collagenase, and proteoglycanase from rat granulosa cells *in vitro*. *Endocrinology*, 115:1043–1050.
624. Too, C. K. L., Weiss, T. J., and Bryant-Greenwood, G. D. (1982): Relaxin stimulates plasminogen activator secretion by rat granulosa cells *in vitro*. *Endocrinology*, 111:1424–1426.
625. Tregear, G. W., Du, Y.-C., Wang, K.-Z., Southwell, C., Jones, P., John, M., Gorman, J., Kemp, B., and Niall, H. D. (1983): The chemical synthesis of relaxin. In: *Biology of Relaxin and Its Role in the Human*, edited by M. Bigazzi, F. C. Greenwood, and F. Gasparri, pp. 42–55, Excerpta Medica, Amsterdam.
626. Tregear, G. W., Fagan, C., Reynolds, H., Scanlon, D., Jones, P., Kemp, B., and Niall, H. D. (1982): Porcine relaxin: Synthesis and structure activity relationships. In: *Peptides, Synthesis, Structure, Function: Proceedings of the Seventh American Peptide Symposium*, pp. 249–252. Pierce Chemical Co., Rockford, IL.
627. Trentin, J. J. (1951): Relaxin and mammary growth in the mouse. *Proc. Soc. Exp. Biol. Med.*, 78:9–11.
628. Uchida, K., Kadowaki, M., Nomura, Y., Miyata, K., and Miyake, T. (1970): Relationship between ovarian progestin secretion and corpora lutea function in pregnant rats. *Endocrinol. Jpn.*, 17: 499–507.
629. Uldbjerg, N., Ulmsten, U., and Ekman, G. (1983): The ripening of the human uterine cervix in terms of connective tissue biochemistry. *Clin. Obstet. Gynecol.*, 26:14–26.
630. Uyldert, I. E., and De Vaal, O. M. (1947): Relaxation of the rat's uterine ostium during pregnancy. *Acta Brev. Neerl. Physiol.*, 15:49–53.
631. Vasilenko, P., Adams, W. C., and Frieden, E. H. (1981): Urterine size and glycogen content in cycling and pregnant rats: Influence of relaxin. *Biol. Reprod.*, 25:162–169.
632. Vasilenko, P., Adams, W. C., and Frieden, E. H. (1982): Comparison of systemic and uterine effects of relaxin and insulin in alloxan-treated, hyperglycemic rats. *Proc. Soc. Exp. Biol. Med.*, 169:376–379.
633. Vasilenko, P., Frieden, E. H., and Adams, W. C. (1980): Effect of purified relaxin on uterine glycogen and protein in the rat. *Proc. Soc. Exp. Biol. Med.*, 163:245–248.
634. Vasilenko, P., and Mahajan, D. K. (1983): Anabolic effects of relaxin in the uterus and cervix of the rat: Comparison with insulin, estrogen, and progesterone. In: *Biology of Relaxin and Its Role in the Human*, edited by M. Bigazzi, F. C. Greenwood, and F. Gasparri, pp. 134–136. Excerpta Medica, Amsterdam.
635. Vasilenko, P., Mead, J. P., and Weidmann, J. E. (1986): Uterine growth promoting effects of relaxin: A morphometric and histological analysis. *Biol. Reprod.*, 35:987–995.
636. Vaupel, M. R., Sherwood, O. D., and Anderson, M. B. (1985): Immunocytochemical Studies of relaxin in ovaries of pregnant and cycling mice. *J. Histochem. Cytochem.*, 33:303–308.
637. Velardo, J. T. (1958): Inability of purified relaxin to inhibit progesterone in decidual tissue formation. *Anat. Rec.*, 130:445–446.
638. Veldhuis, J. D., Kolp, L. A., Toaff, M. E., Strauss, J. F., and Demers, L. M. (1983): Mechanisms subserving the trophic actions of insulin on ovarian cells. *J. Clin. Invest.*, 72:1046–1057.
639. Wada, H., and Turner, C. W. (1958): Role of relaxin in stimulating mammary gland growth in mice. *Proc. Soc. Exp. Biol. Med.*, 99:194–197.
640. Wada, H., and Turner, C. W. (1959): Effect of relaxin on mammary gland growth in female mice. *Proc. Soc. Exp. Biol. Med.*, 101:707–709.
641. Wada, H., and Turner, C. W. (1961): Interaction of relaxin and ovarian steroid hormones on uterus of rat. *Endocrinology*, 68:1059–1063.
642. Wada, H., and Yuhara, M. (1955): Studies on relaxin in ruminants. (1) Relaxin content of the blood serum of pregnant and postpartum dairy cows. *Jpn. J. Zootech. Sci.*, 26:215–220.
643. Wada, H., and Yuhara, M. (1955): Studies on relaxin in ruminants. (2) Relaxin content of the blood serum of pregnant and postpartum cows of the Japanese black breed of cattle. *Sci. Rep. Fac. Agric. Okayama Univ.*, 7:13–21.
644. Wada, H., and Yuhara, M. (1956): Studies on relaxin in ruminants. (4) Concentration of relaxin in the blood serum of pregnant and postpartum goats and ewes. *Sci. Rep. Fac. Agric. Okayama Univ.*, 8:31–37.
645. Wada, H., and Yuhara, M. (1956): Inhibitory effect of relaxin preparation upon spontaneous uterine contractions of the rat and guinea pig *in vitro*. *Sci. Rep. Fac. Agric. Okayama Univ.*, 9:11–20.
646. Wada, H., and Yuhara, M. (1961): Concentration of relaxin in the blood serum of pregnant cow and cow with ovarian cyst. *Proc. Silver Jubilee Lab. Anim. Husbandry*, Kyoto University, pp. 61–66.
647. Wahl, L. M., Blandau, R. J., and Page, R. C. (1977): Effect of hormones on collagen metabolism and collagenase activity in the pubic symphysis ligament of the guinea pig. *Endocrinology*, 100:571–579.
648. Walsh, J. R., and Niall, H. D. (1980): Use of an octadecylsilica purification method minimizes proteolysis during isolation of porcine and rat relaxins. *Endocrinology*, 107:1258–1260.
649. Watts, A., Jones, R. G., Flint, A. P. F., Foxcroft, G. R., and Porter, D. G. (1984): The relationship between electrical and mechanical uterine activity and changes in plasma hormone titres in the prepartum mini pig. *Programme and Abstracts of the Annual Conference for the Society for the Study of Fertility*, abstract 90.
650. Wedemeyer, P. P. (1964): Response of four inbred types of mice to relaxin. *Yale J. Biol. Med.*, 37:153–157.
651. Weinberg, A. (1956): An X-ray pelvimetric study of relaxin extract in pelvic expansion. *Surg. Gynecol. Obstet.*, 103:303–306.
652. Weiss, G., Goldsmith, L. T., Schoenfeld, C., and D'Eletto, R. (1986): Partial purification of relaxin from human seminal plasma. *Am. J. Obstet. Gynecol.*, 154:749–754.
653. Weiss, G., O'Bryne, E. M., Hochman, J. A., Goldmith, L. T., Rifkin, I., and Steinetz, B. G. (1977): Secretion of progesterone and relaxin by the human corpus luteum at midpregnancy and at term. *Obstet. Gynecol.*, 50:679–681.

654. Weiss, G., O'Byrne, E. M., Hochman, J., Steinetz, B. G., Goldsmith, L., and Flitcraft, J. G. (1978): Distribution of relaxin in women during pregnancy. *Obstet. Gynecol.*, 52:569–570.
655. Weiss, G., O'Byrne, E. M., and Steinetz, B. G. (1976): Relaxin: A product of the human corpus luteum of pregnancy. *Science*, 194:948–949.
656. Weiss, G., Steinetz, B. G., Dierschke, D. J., and Fritz, G. (1981): Relaxin secretion in the rhesus monkey. *Biol. Reprod.*, 24:565–567.
657. Weiss, M., Nagelschmidt, M., and Struck, H. (1979): Relaxin and collagen metabolism. *Horm. Metab. Res.*, 11:408–410.
658. Weiss, T. J., and Bryant-Greenwood, G. D. (1982): Localization of relaxin binding sites in the rat uterus and cervix by autoradiography. *Biol. Reprod.*, 27:673–679.
659. Wells, R. S. (1963): Relaxin in the treatment of localized scleroderma. *Trans. St. John Hosp. Derm. Soc.*, 49:149–151.
660. Whitely, J., Willcox, D. L., Hartmann, P. E., Yamamoto, S. Y., and Bryant-Greenwood, G. D. (1985): Plasma relaxin levels during suckling and oxytocin stimulation in the lactating sow. *Biol. Reprod.*, 33:705–714.
661. Williams, K. I., and El Tahir, K. E. H. (1980): Spatial and temporal variations in prostacyclin production by the pregnant rat uterus. *Adv. Prostaglandin Thromboxane Res.*, 8:1413–1417.
662. Williams, K. I., and El Tahir, K. E. H. (1980): Effect of uterine stimulant drugs on prostacyclin production by the pregnant rat myometrium. I. Oxytocin, bradykinin and $PGF_{2\alpha}$. *Prostaglandins*, 19:31–38.
663. Williams, K. I., and El Tahir, K. E. H. (1982): Relaxin inhibits prostacyclin release by the rat pregnant myometrium. *Prostaglandins*, 24:129–136.
664. Williams, K. I., El Tahir, K. E. H., and Marcinkiewicz, E. (1979): Dual actions of prostacylin (PGI2) on the rat pregnant uterus. *Prostaglandins*, 17:667–672.
665. Williams, L. M., Hollingsworth, M., and Dixon, J. S. (1982): Changes in the tensile properties and fine structure of the rat cervix in late pregnancy and during parturition. *J. Reprod. Fertil.*, 66:203–211.
666. Williams, L. M., Hollingsworth, M., Dukes, M., and Morris, I. D. (1983): Fluprostenol-induced softening of the cervix of the pregnant rat. *J. Endocrinol.*, 97:283–290.
667. Wiqvist, I., Norström, A., O'Byrne, E., and Wiqvist, N. (1984): Regulatory influence of relaxin on human cervical and uterine connective tissue. *Acta Endocrinol. (Copenh.)*, 106:127–132.
668. Wiqvist, N. (1959): Desensitizing effect of exo- and endogenous relaxin on the immediate uterine response to relaxin. *Acta Endocrinol. [Suppl.] (Copenh.)*, 46:3–14.
669. Wiqvist, N. (1959): The effect of prolonged administration of relaxin on some functional properties of the non-pregnant mouse and rat uterus. *Acta Endocrinol. [Suppl.] (Copenh.)*, 46:15–32.
670. Wiqvist, N., and Paul, K.-G. (1985): Inhibition of the spontaneous uterine motility *in vitro* as a bioassay of relaxin. *Acta Endocrinol. (Copenh.)*, 29:135–146.
671. Wright, L. C., and Anderson, R. R. (1982): Effect of relaxin on mammary growth in the hypophysectomized rat. *Adv. Exp. Med. Biol.*, 143:341–353.
672. Yamamoto, S., and Bryant-Greenwood, G. D. (1981): The isolation of relaxin from boar testis. In: *Relaxin*, edited by G. D. Bryant-Greenwood, H. D. Niall, and F. C. Greenwood, pp. 71–74. Elsevier/North-Holland, New York.
673. Yamamoto, S., Kwok, S. C. M., Greenwood, F. C., and Bryant-Greenwood, G. D. (1981): Relaxin purification from human placental basal plates. *J. Clin. Endocrinol. Metab.*, 52:601–604.
674. Yki-Järvinen, H., and Wahlström, T. (1984): Immunohistochemical demonstration of relaxin in the placenta after removal of the corpus luteum. *Acta Endocrinol. (Copenh.)*, 106:544–547.
675. Yki-Järvinen, H., Wahlström, T., and Seppälä, M. (1983): Immunohistochemical demonstration of relaxin in gynecological tumors. *Cancer*, 52:2077–2080.
676. Yki-Järvinen, H., Wahlström, T., and Seppälä, M. (1983): Immunohistochemical demonstration of relaxin in the genital tract of pregnant and nonpregnant women. *J. Clin. Endocrinol. Metab.*, 57:451–454.
677. Yki-Järvinen, H., Wahlström, T., and Seppälä, M. (1983): Immunohistochemical demonstration of relaxin in the genital tract of men. *J. Reprod. Fertil.*, 69:693–695.
678. Yki-Järvinen, H., Wahlström, T., Tenhunen, A., Koskimies, A. I., and Seppälä, M. (1984): The occurrence of relaxin in hyperstimulated human preovulatory follicles collected in an *in vitro* fertilization program. *J. In Vitro Fertil. Embryo Transf.*, 1:180–182.
679. Zarrow, M. X. (1947): Relaxin content of blood, urine and other tissues of pregnant and postpartum guinea pigs. *Proc. Soc. Exp. Biol. Med.*, 66:488–491.
680. Zarrow, M. X. (1948): The role of steroid hormones in the relaxation of the symphysis pubis of the guinea pig. *Endocrinology*, 42:129–140.
681. Zarrow, M. X., and Brennan, D. M. (1957): Increased concentration of water in uterus of the rat following treatment with relaxin. *Proc. Soc. Exp. Biol. Med.*, 95:745–747.
690. Zarrow, M. X., and Wilson, E. D. (1963): Hormonal control of the pubic symphysis of the Skomer bank vole (*Clethrionomys skomerensis*). *J. Endocrinol.*, 28:103–106.
683. Zarrow, M. X., Eleftheriou, B. E., Whitecotten, G. L., and King, J. A. (1961): Separation of the pubic symphysis during pregnancy and after treatment with relaxin in two subspecies of *Peromyscus maniculatus*. *Gen. Comp. Endocrinol.*, 1:386–391.
684. Zarrow, M. X., Holmstrom, E. G., and Salhanick, H. A. (1955): The concentration of relaxin in the blood serum and other tissues of women during pregnancy. *J. Clin. Endocrinol. Metab.*, 15: 22–27.
685. Zarrow, M. X., and McClintock, J. A. (1966): Localization of ^{131}I-labelled antibody to relaxin. *J. Endocrinol.*, 36:377–387.
686. Zarrow, M. X., Neher, G. M., Sikes, D., Brennan, D. M., and Bullard, J. F. (1956): Dilatation of the uterine cervix of the sow following treatment with relaxin. *Am. J. Obstet. Gynecol.*, 72:260–264.
687. Zarrow, M. X., and O'Connor, W. B. (1966): Localization of relaxin in the corpus luteum of the rabbit. *Proc. Soc. Exp. Biol. Med.*, 121:612–614.
688. Zarrow, M. X., and Rosenberg, B. (1953): Sources of relaxin in the rabbit. *Endocrinology*, 53:593–598.
689. Zarrow, M. X., Sikes, D., and Neher, G. M. (1954): Effect of relaxin on the uterine cervix and vulva of young, castrated sows, and heifers. *Am. J. Physiol.*, 179:687.
690. Zarrow, M. X., and Wilson, E. D. (1963): Hormonal control of the pubic symphysis of the Skomer bank vole (*Clethrionomys skomerensis*). *J. Endocrinol.*, 28:103–106.
691. Zarrow, M. X., and Yochim, J. (1961): Dilation of the uterine cervix of the rat and accompanying changes during the estrous cycle, pregnancy and following treatment with estradiol, progesterone, and relaxin. *Endocrinology*, 69:292–304.
692. Zimmerman, A. E., Moule, M. L., and Yip, C. C. (1974): Guinea pig insulin. II. Biological activity. *J. Biol. Chem.*, 249:4026–4029.

The Physiology of Reproduction,
edited by E. Knobil and J. Neill *et al.*
Raven Press, Ltd., New York © 1988.

CHAPTER 17

Actions of Ovarian Steroid Hormones

James H. Clark and Barry M. Markaverich

Ovarian steroid hormones, estrogen and progesterone, control or influence every aspect of reproductive function. The purpose of this chapter is to discuss the mechanisms by which these two hormones accomplish these tasks. In order to provide some perspective and to set the stage for a contemporary discussion of this problem, it is important to examine the steps that form the historical background for our current understanding of ovarian hormone action.

DISCOVERY AND IDENTIFICATION

It has been known from ancient times that removal of the ovaries from animals results in the loss of sexual activity and infertility. However, many hundreds of years passed before the concept evolved that the ovary was producing hormones that controlled these processes. Knauer (249) demonstrated this convincingly by removing the ovaries from guinea pigs and grafting ovarian pieces back to the same animals at new sites. He noted that this prevented the occurrence of castrate atrophy and concluded that the ovary was secreting substances responsible for uterine growth. Marshall and Jolly (313) demonstrated that estrus could be induced in ovariectomized dogs by injecting extracts of the ovary removed from another dog during estrus. These investigators recognized that the ovary produced two different hormones and that the secretion that caused estrus was different from that of the corpora lutea. The work of Allen and Doisy (5,6), who discovered that follicular fluid from the pig ovary caused vaginal cornification in the rat, led the way to the isolation and identification of estrone (54,101). This was followed by the demonstration by Corner and Allen (91) that extracts from the corpora lutea of pigs would cause progestational proliferation of the rabbit uterus. This observation opened the way for the isolation and identification of progesterone (9,55,176,177,481)

EARLY STUDIES

Permeability and Enzymatic Activity

During the years that followed these extremely important findings many investigators engaged in descriptive studies that defined the multiple functions of the ovarian hormones. Much of the work on the actions of estrogen and progesterone centered on the uterus, and it became clear that these two hormones regulated the growth of this organ by stimulating hypertrophy and hyperplasia of uterine cells (7,53,93,427). It was also established that progesterone was effective only when the uterus had been activated by previous exposure to estrogen (53,185,426). The ability of ovarian steroids to regulate the growth and development of all female sex accessory organs and tissues was carefully documented by many investigators during the two decades following their discovery (for reviews see refs. 53,426,427). Early work on the mechanism of action of ovarian steroids suggested that the hyperemia and vasodilation that occurred after estrogen treatment might be involved with the stimulation of uterine growth (311,312). Although many investigators considered such mechanisms, Szego and Roberts (516) were the first to suggest that alterations in uterine vascularity and permeability might play a role in the primary events that result in uterotropic responses. Such changes in permeability were thought to be caused by the local mobilization and release of histamine (491–493). There is no question that such changes in uterine permeability occur and undoubtedly are important for the full expression of estrogen-induced uterine growth. However, these changes do not appear to be the primary cause of uterine growth, but instead provide the optimal environment for growth by maximizing substrate availability and ionic constituents. The relationships between these early supportive events and the biosynthetic evens that result in true uterine growth will be discussed in detail in Control of Gene Expression and Growth, below.

The increased metabolic activity stimulated by estrogen was considered by some investigators to result from direct effects of estrogen on enzymes. Villee (550) proposed that estrogen interacted with transhydrogenase in the placenta to stimulate the formation of high-energy phosphates and thioesters that were used in the biosynthesis of proteins, lipids, and nucleic acids. Talalay (519,520) proposed that the oxidation-reduction of estradiol and estrone by estradiol dehydrogenase was involved in the production of triphosphopyridine nucleotides, which were responsible for the physiological effects of estrogen. Although the concepts of Villee and Talalay created considerable interest and investigation, their hypothesis that such enzymatic interactions were the primary cause of estrogenic stimulation has not received support. The studies on transhydrogenase were done in the placenta and it was subsequently demonstrated that this enzyme was not found in other estrogen target organs (351). Also, low levels of diethylstilbestrol (DES), a very potent estrogen, had no effect on this enzyme (143); therefore, direct interaction of estrogen with transhydrogenase seemed not to be a primary event in estrogen action.

It is clear that estrogens do undergo oxidation-reduction reactions during their metabolism; however, these reactions do not appear to be directly involved in the mechanism of action of estrogens. One of the first experiments with [^{3}H]estradiol demonstrated that no conversion to estrone took place in the rat uterus, and that [^{3}H]estradiol could be recovered from uterine tissue (215). Since uterotropic stimulation was observed under these conditions, it was concluded that metabolism is not involved in any primary or direct way.

Stimulation of Biosynthetic Activity

Although the concept of estrogen action via direct enzyme interaction appeared to be an unlikely primary event in the mechanism of action of estrogen, it was clear that estrogen administration elevated enzyme activity in target tissues. Mueller and his colleagues (2,322,349,353,573) demonstrated that estrogen enhanced the synthesis of phospholipids, nucleic acids, and proteins in the rat uterus. They proposed that estrogen controlled the production of templates composed of nucleic acids and that estrogen may act as an inducer or antiinducer of this biosynthetic activity (350,353). These important studies were followed by experiments that demonstrated that puromycin, an inhibitor of protein synthesis, blocked the stimulatory effects of estrogen (169,170,352). Thus, the concept evolved that estrogen increased enzymatic activity in the uterus by stimulating the synthesis of enzymes. Further experiments demonstrated that the incorporation of [^{3}H]RNA precursors into all classes of RNA was elevated during the first few hours after estrogen treatment and that actinomycin-D, an RNA synthesis inhibitor, would block this effect (150,169–171,376,578). Estrogen and progesterone were also shown to regulate RNA and protein synthesis in the chick oviduct (385). These experiments, plus others that will be discussed later in this chapter, led to the conclusion that estrogens had a direct effect at the level of RNA transcription that resulted in increased synthesis of specific proteins (172,385).

THE RECEPTOR HYPOTHESIS

The actions of ovarian hormones on specific target organs imply that these organs contain receptors for the hormones. The concept of receptors for drugs and hormones is an old one and was first proposed by Langley (272) and extended by Ehrlich (108), who stated "drugs do not act unless they bind." However, no experimental evidence existed for this concept until the demonstration by Glasscock and Hoekstra (144) and Jensen and Jacobson (215) that [^{3}H]estrogens were preferentially accumulated and retained by target organs. Jensen's laboratory succeeded in synthesizing [^{3}H]estradiol labeled to a high specific activity and showed that the uterus, vagina, and pituitary retained significant quantities of the hormone against a marked concentration gradient. Since nontarget tissues such as diaphragm, muscle, and kidney did not retain [^{3}H]estradiol, the assumption was made that specific molecules that bind estradiol must be present in target tissues. The concept of steroid receptors was extended by King et al. (243), who proposed that [^{3}H]estradiol was localized in nuclei of target cells and was in association with chromatin (239,240,241,242,244,377). That specific steroid receptors existed was verified by Talwar et al. (521) and Toft and Gorski (541) when they showed that cytosol fractions of the rat uterus contained a macromolecule that had the characteristics expected of an estradiol receptor. Experiments with [^{3}H]progesterone established that receptors with similar characteristics also exist for this hormone (92,274,391,458,470,574).

The important demonstration of specific receptors present in target organs for ovarian hormones and the growing knowledge concerning the ability of estrogen to stimulate RNA and protein synthesis led to the concept that these hormones were acting at the gene level through a receptor-mediated mechanism. During the intervening years many laboratories have been devoted to the further refinement and elaboration of this basic model and their work forms the basis for the remainder of this chapter.

RECEPTORS AND HORMONE ACTION

The steroid receptor concept that emerged from the studies discussed above was an important step in our understanding of the mechanism of action of ovarian hormones. The binding of a steroid hormone to a receptor and the subsequent interactions of this receptor-hormone complex with cellular components is considered to be a primary event in the mechanism of action of ovarian steroids. Thus a knowledge of ovarian steroid hormone receptors forms the foundation for understanding the action of these hormones.

Definition and Characteristics of Steroid Receptors

Steroid hormone receptors are expected to display certain characteristics on the basis of theoretical considerations. These were first formalized by Clark (68), who outlined the basic mathematical formulation that describes receptor binding characteristics. These considerations, along with others which will be discussed later, constitute the basic criteria for ovarian hormone receptors.

Finite Binding Capacity

The biological response to steroid hormones is a saturable phenomenon. Assuming that the formation of receptor-hormone complexes is obligatory for the production of biological responses, then the number of receptors per unit mass of tissue should be limited; hence there should exist a finite number of receptor sites. This criterion is met by the demonstration that the steroid-binding system under study can be saturated. This is usually accomplished by exposing the receptor to various concentrations of radioactive steroid and subsequently measuring the amount of bound and/or free steroid after equilibrium is achieved. In such a system, the total amount of receptor (R_t) is determined under equilibrium conditions by adding steroid (S) until saturation or near saturation is obtained (Fig. 1). The amount of bound ligand (RS) which is observed in this system can be related mathematically to free ligands(s), total receptor (R_t) and the dissociation constant (K_d) of the receptor-ligand complex in the following way:

$$[RS] = \frac{[R_t]\,[S]}{K_d + [S]}$$

This is the classic formulation of rapid equilibrium kinetics employed in the derivation of the Michaelis-Menton equation and applies equally well to studies of ligand binding as long as conditions of equilibrium exist. In Fig. 1 it can be seen that as steroid is added to the system the receptor sites become saturated. The actual point of saturation is equal to the number of receptor sites (n) or R_t. The dissociation constant (K_d) is the concentration of steroid at which 50% of the receptor sites are bound. This value in Fig. 1 is 1 nM. Although one can make reasonable estimates of R_t and K_d from saturation plots, these parameters should be obtained by Scatchard (449a) analysis as shown in Fig. 1B and discussed in the following section.

High Affinity

Steroid receptors should possess a high affinity for their respective hormones. This is expected because the circulating levels of steroid are usually 10^{-10} to 10^{-8} M. Thus the existence of receptor-mediated responses of physiologic importance demands that the receptor have an affinity for the hormone that is in the range of the blood hormone levels; otherwise the response would not occur. These considerations have proven true for a variety of target tissue receptors;

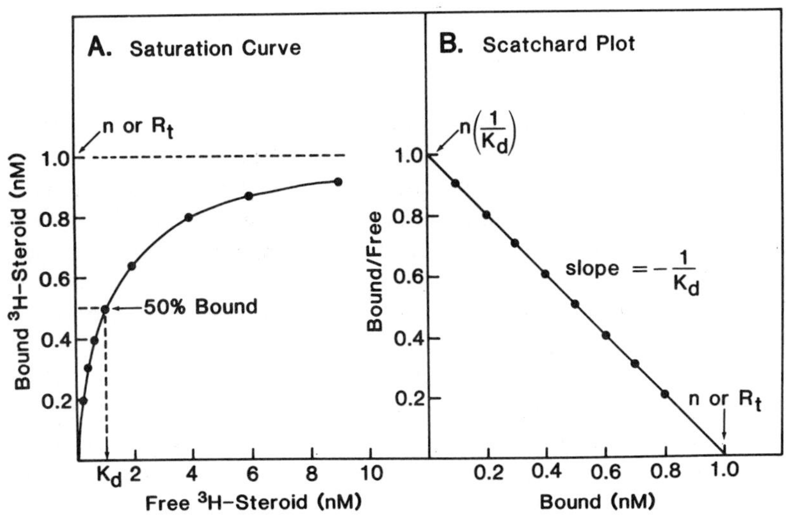

FIG. 1. Saturation and Scatchard analyses of receptor steroid binding. Abbreviations: n or R_t, number of receptor sites; K_d, dissociation constant.

however, they do not preclude receptor interactions of weaker affinity if blood or tissue levels of steroids or receptors are elevated.

Affinity or association constants (K_a) or their reciprocal, dissociation constants (K_d), can be obtained from the Scatchard plot shown in Fig. 1B. The Y intercept equals $n(K_a)$ or $(1/K_d)$ and the X intercept equals number of receptor sites (n or R_t). The slope of the Scatchard plot is equal to $-K_a$ or $-1/K_d$.

The affinity of a receptor for a hormone is in general an indication of the relative potency of the hormone; however, a number of factors determine the ultimate expression of hormonal activity and these considerations will be discussed later in this chapter.

Hormone Specificity

Generally speaking, receptors are expected to display high affinities for a specific hormone or class of hormones. This "specificity" enables a given target cell to respond to a hormonal signal without interference from other signals. Thus, hormones of the same class as well as their agonists and antagonists should compete effectively for a given class of receptor while not affecting other receptor systems.

It should be noted that steroid receptor sites do not display absolute stereospecificity; that is, the binding or recognition site on the receptor has a limited capacity for the recognition and differentiation of various steroid structures. Estrogen receptors have some affinity for all steroids, as has been shown for androgens (137,138,432,441,591). These *in vitro* and *in vivo* studies have demonstrated that extremely high concentrations of androgen (3–10 mg *in vivo;* 1–10 μM *in vitro*) will promote nuclear accumulation of the estrogen receptor as well as stimulate both general protein synthesis and the synthesis of the so-called IP, or induced proteins. Under these conditions testosterone also binds to androgen receptors which are present in the uterus. These receptors are distinct from the estrogen receptor and do not appear to be involved in the observed estrogenic stimulation (433).

The binding of progesterone to its receptor appears to be less specific than that of estrogen. Progesterone binds to both androgen and glucocorticoid receptors (292,436); in addition, glucocorticoids are known to bind to progesterone receptors (553). Therefore, the progesterone receptor must be measured with particular attention to competitive binding analysis.

Tissue Specificity

Only certain tissues and organs appear to be stimulated by the sex steroids. Classically these have been termed target organs, e.g., uterus, vagina, mammary gland, etc. It is generally accepted that if responses of these target organs result from receptor-steroid interactions, then the number of receptors in these tissues should be higher than that of nontarget tissues. Although there is no established minimum for the number of receptors required to define a target cell, tissue specificity should be part of any receptor validation scheme. For example, the number of cytoplasmic estrogen receptors is very high in uterus, vagina, and pituitary, and low, but not totally absent, in other tissues (82). Some target tissues, such as hypothalamus, possess low densities of receptor because of the heterogeneity of cell types within their anatomic boundary. Thus not all cells in the hypothalamus are estrogen targets but those which are estrogen responsive probably possess receptors in numbers equivalent to other target cells. In those cases where receptors are fewer than one per cell, one must presume either that the tissue is not a target or that the target is more circumscribed than the tissue.

Correlation with Biological Response

Implicit in all studies of macromolecules that bind steroids and meet the above criteria is the assumption that this binding results in a biological response. Thus binding of hormone to putative receptors must precede or accompany tissue responses and the extent of response should relate to some function of receptor occupancy. The relationship between receptor occupancy and response will be discussed further in subsequent portions of this chapter.

The preceding discussion of receptor characteristics and criteria provides only the basic principles for defining receptors. A complete consideration of these concepts and the complex interactions of hormones with other binding sites and the methods that can be used to resolve these interactions is presented elsewhere (82).

Hormone Uptake and Cellular Localization of Receptors

The uptake of ovarian steroids is a necessary step before hormone-receptor binding can occur. Consideration of how this occurs in relation to cellular localization of receptors has been and still is a much discussed area of research.

Cellular Uptake

The experiments of Jensen and Jacobson (215) demonstrated that [^{3}H]estradiol was taken up very rapidly after hormone injection by both target and nontarget organs in the rat. Retention of the [^{3}H]hormone for several hours was noted only in the target organs while the hormone was lost rather rapidly from nontarget organs. This initial and very important observation not only provided evidence for the presence of receptors in target organs but also demonstrated that all tissues could take up the hormone readily. Thus, there appears to be no impediment to cellular uptake by any cell and the retention of the hormone in target cells is due to the presence of receptors. Also, since the uptake is rapid (within minutes) by all organs, it seems unlikely that any active uptake process is involved. However, the mechanism of cellular uptake and its possible involvement with receptors has concerned several investigators.

Some of the confusion in early studies concerning cellular uptake arose from a failure to differentiate between uptake and retention. Uptake is defined as the initial rate of movement of steroid into cells, whereas retention is defined by the amount of steroid found in the cells under equilibrium conditions. Two experimental approaches have been employed to counter the difficulty of entry versus retention. In an elegant series of experiments employing steady-state perfusion of two isotopes, Gurpide and co-workers (165,166) showed that various steroids can enter target and nontarget cells with equal facility at rates linearly related to their steady-state concentration over a rather wide range of concentrations (0.2–5,000 ng/ml). Although it is not possible to completely rule out a carrier-mediated process, these results are most easily interpreted in terms of the diffusion of steroid across cell membranes.

The more direct approach to this problem is to examine the initial rate of uptake of the steroid. Peck et al. (404) demonstrated that the uptake of [^{3}H]estradiol under initial velocity conditions was linear over a wide range of steroid concentrations at physiological temperatures. In addition, this rate was the same for both target and nontarget tissues in the presence or absence of *N*-ethylmaleimide or excess DES. Either of these compounds would interfere with carrier-mediated transport and/or processes employing cytoplasmic receptor as a carrier. The entry of steroid is not dependent on metabolic energy as demonstrated by preincubation with 2,4-dinitrophenol for 30 min at 37°C prior to the study of uptake. Thus, estradiol enters uterine cells by passive diffusion. The same conclusion was reached by Müller and Wotiz (360), who performed similar experiments with rat uterine cell suspensions. Also, these investigators found no evidence for estrogen receptors in purified uterine plasma membranes (358), as had been proposed by Pietras and Szego (411). Recent work by King and Greene (245) using monoclonal antibodies to the estrogen receptor demonstrates that estrogen receptors are absent from plasma membranes. Therefore it appears that estradiol is not taken up by a plasma-membrane-mediated process in uterine cells. However, membrane-mediated effects of estrogens cannot be excluded in the central nervous system. Electrophysiological responses induced by direct application of steroid hormones have latencies that are too short to be the result of nuclear-mediated events (238), and steroids are known to have anesthetic properties that probably result from steroid-membrane interactions (190). Whether these effects on the nervous system are membrane-receptor-mediated or the consequence of non-receptor-membrane interactions remains to be resolved.

The studies of initial rate of uptake discussed above were done at 37°C and appear to reflect the rapid uptake *in vivo* by target and nontarget tissues as first shown by Jensen and Jacobson (215). Several investigators have suggested a pump or carrier-mediated uptake because steroid uptake is a temperature-dependent process (341,536,575). That is, at low temperatures estradiol enters cells very slowly; however, when the temperature is increased rapid uptake takes place. This finding is consistent with a carrier-mediated transport process; however, it is not sufficient to establish the same. In fact, activated diffusion (as opposed to facilitated diffusion) may result from the chemical properties of solutes and their affinities for the lipid matrix of the cellular membrane (142). In activated diffusion, transport rate is linearly related to solute concentration and shows a temperature dependence indicative of activated states (kinetic properties similar to carrier-mediated diffusion or transport). The diffusion of steroids is expected to be "activated" since they are lipophilic and likely to encounter a diffusional barrier before entering the aqueous environment of the cytoplasm from the hydrophobic environ of the membrane matrix. In addition, the state of lipid bilayers is temperature dependent, undergoing transition from a liquid to a more solid state with decreasing temperature (393,479). Finally, the mobility within bilayers of optical probes is restricted by these phase transitions (546,547). Thus transitions of membrane state may impose a temperature dependence on estrogen entry. However, such observations appear to have little application to the *in vivo* situation, since, as discussed above, uptake is by passive diffusion at 37°C. Therefore, it is generally believed that ovarian steroid hormones enter cells by passive diffusion and bind to receptors present inside the cell.

Cellular Localization of Receptors and the Nuclear Translocation Model

The exact subcellular localization of receptors for steroid hormones may never be known with certainty because the exposure of tissues to experimental manipulations is likely to alter the distribution of the receptor. However, early experiments indicated that the estrogen receptor existed as a macromolecule with a sedimentation coefficient of 8S in the high-speed cytosol prepared from non-estrogen-treated rat uteri (541). Following exposure to estrogen, the receptor was found predominantly in the uterine nuclear fraction which could be partially extracted with 0.4 M KCl to yield a macromolecule with a sedimentation coefficient of 5S (217,475,543). Jensen et al. (217) proposed that the 8S form of the receptor was made up of 4S subunits and that the binding of estradiol to the 4S form of the receptor resulted in a transformed 5S receptor hormone complex that migrated (translocated) to the nucleus. Similar, but not identical, generalizations concerning the progesterone receptor were also made by O'Malley et al. (391) and Schrader and O'Malley (458). In contrast to these findings, Siiteri et al. (476) and Linkie and Siiteri (289) suggested that the 4 to 5S transformation was an intranuclear event and that estrogen first binds to a 4S form of the receptor, which undergoes translocation to the nucleus before the transformation step takes place.

The nuclear translocation or two-step model of Jensen et al. (217) and Gorski et al. (151) was widely accepted and appeared to be applicable to all steroid hormone receptors (286,390,545,579). The two-step model is shown in Fig. 2A. Notable and important studies that support this hypothesis were done in the laboratories of Munck and Katzenellenbogen. In these experiments the kinetics of the formation of the cytosol receptor-steroid complex were compared with the kinetics of nuclear accumulation of the complex (363,402,582). These authors concluded that the cytosol receptor-hormone complex forms before nuclear accumulation takes place. Even though these experiments were done under conditions that seemed to preclude an artifactual relocation of the receptor, such an artifact cannot be excluded and will be discussed in the following section.

Williams and Gorski (575) made the important observation that the amount of occupied nuclear bound receptor relative to the amount of occupied cytosol receptor maintained a constant ratio of approximately 95% to 5% respectively over a wide range of [^{3}H]estradiol concentrations. These authors suggested that these results probably reflected an equilibrium state of the receptor in which most of the unoccupied receptor was nuclear and very little was cytoplasmic. Such a proposal was a prelude to the work discussed below, which suggested that unoccupied receptors are found exclusively in the nuclear compartment.

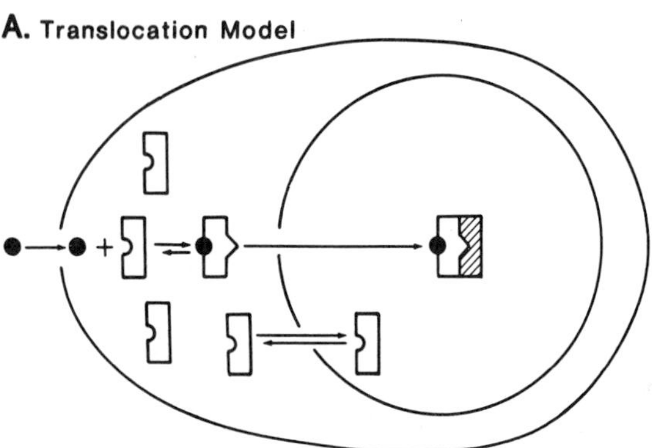

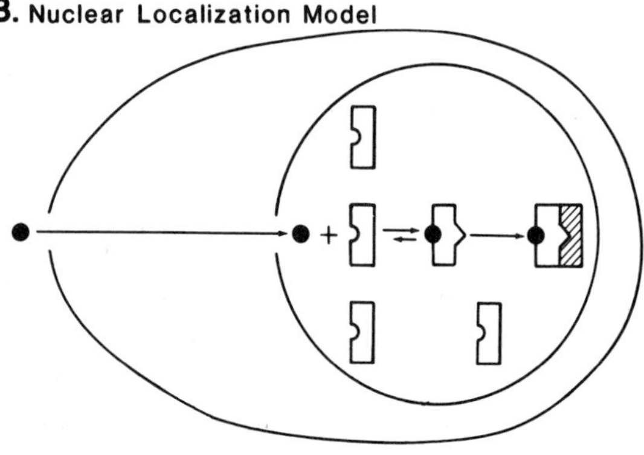

FIG. 2. Cellular localization of steroid receptors.

The Nuclear Localization Model

The experiments cited above suggest that receptor-steroid complexes undergo translocation to the nucleus of target cells; however, they do not prove that such translocation occurs. Indeed, it has been suggested that steroid receptors reside predominantly in the nucleus *in vivo* and that cytoplasmic receptor may represent an artifact found only after cellular disruption during homogenization of tissues (468). According to this hypothesis, which is illustrated in Fig. 3, cytoplasmic receptor (R_c) is observed in cytosol fraction after homogenization because it is readily solubilized from the nucleus where it resides as unoccupied nuclear receptor (R_n) *in vivo*. Steroid treatment would result in an apparent translocation because nuclear receptor estrogen complexes (R_nE) are tightly bound or stabilized in the nucleus and are not readily dislodged on homogenization. In this manner exposure to steroid would appear to decrease the quantity of R_c while increasing the quantity of R_nE.

The presence of unoccupied nuclear estrogen receptors has been reported by several investigators (3,209,321,335, 337,396,412,449,468,487,590). Nuclear localization of estrogen receptors has been reported by Martin and Sheridan (317), who used autoradiography to detect receptors in uteri incubated *in vitro* at 4°C. Under these conditions the temperature-dependent transformation step (4 to 5S transition) would not take place. Also, unoccupied nuclear receptors have been reported for thyroxine, ecdysteroids, and vitamin D (392,558,559,586).

Two important experimental approaches have been taken recently to attempt to resolve the cellular localization problem. Welshons et al. (568) have shown that cytochalasin enucleation of GH_3 cells results in the formation of cytoplasts (cytoplasm plus intact plasma membrane) which contain few unoccupied estrogen receptors, whereas the majority of the receptors were found in the nucleoplasts (nuclei plus small amounts of cytoplasm surrounded by intact membrane). In contrast, unoccupied receptors were found predominantly in the cytosol fraction following homogenization and fractionation of GH_3 cells. These authors conclude that unoccupied estrogen receptors are found *in situ* predominantly in the nucleus and that the homogenization artifact (discussed above and shown in Fig. 3) accounts for the previous observations of unoccupied receptors in the cytosol. A comparison of the translocation and nuclear localization models is shown in Fig. 2.

In another approach to this problem King and Greene (245) used immunocytochemistry with monoclonal antibodies to the estrogen receptor and reached the same conclusion. They showed that unoccupied receptor could be found only in the nuclei and not in the cytoplasm of human and rabbit endometrium, human breast tumor, and MCF-7

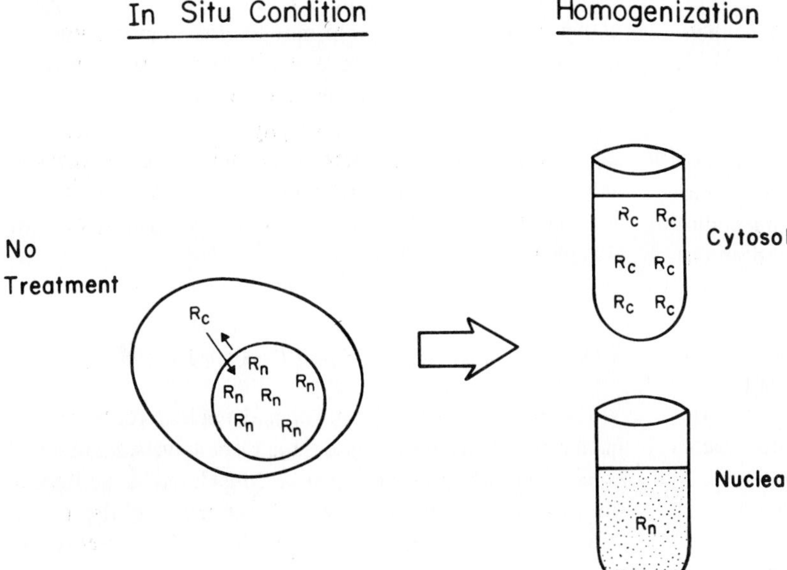

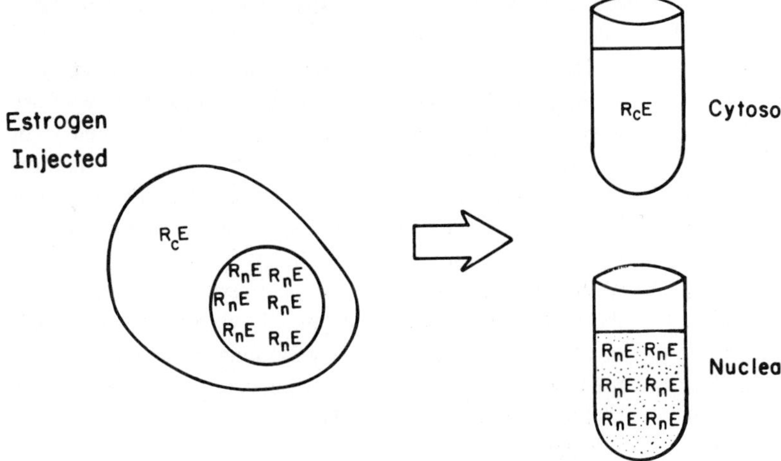

FIG. 3. Receptor distribution *in situ* and after homogenization.

cells. Also their studies indicate that the estrogen receptor is distributed throughout the nucleus and is not localized on the nuclear membrane or any specific nuclear compartment. Similar observations have been made in the reproductive tract of the macaque (320).

The progesterone receptor also appears to be localized in the nucleus of target cells. Perrot-Applanat et al. (407) demonstrated nuclear localization in several target tissues of the rabbit and guinea pig by immunocytochemical methods using monoclonal antibodies to the progesterone receptor.

These recent experiments lead one to the tentative conclusion that unoccupied estrogen receptors are loosely bound to nuclear sites *in situ* prior to hormone exposure and become tightly bound following the hormone binding and transformation interaction. Such a new model of receptor localization has perplexed many investigators because of the widely held belief that cytoplasmic receptors were necessary for the transport of hormones to the nucleus. However, as pointed out earlier, there appears to be no barrier to estradiol uptake by target or nontarget cells or tissues. Likewise, no impediment exists to nuclear accumulation in nontarget organs. Peck et al. (404) showed that nonspecific accumulation of [^{3}H]-estradiol by diaphragm and uterine nuclei is identical. Also, nonspecific nuclear localization of [^{3}H]-estradiol has been demonstrated by autoradiography (469). Therefore, estradiol appears to be able to diffuse readily into the nuclear compartment of all cells, but is accumulated and retained in this compartment only when receptors are present.

Although the evidence for nuclear localization of the estrogen receptor is persuasive, the question is still open for debate and it is difficult to reconcile this concept with existing conflicting data. The finding that most of the receptor is found in nucleoplast after cytochalasin exposure could reflect some unknown effect of this drug on redistribution of the receptor. Unpublished data from the laboratory of Gorski indicate that nuclear localization of steroid hormone receptor can be obtained by centrifugation of intact cells without exposure to cytochalasin (*personal communication*). Such results would argue against a drug-induced artifact; however, one can still argue about the possible effects of centrifugation on receptor redistribution.

The nuclear localization of receptor with antibodies would appear to be free of the above-mentioned experimentally induced artifacts. However, the results of King and Greene (245) are in conflict with several reports including one from their own laboratory which showed cytoplasmic or perinuclear localization (214). Cytoplasmic localization of receptor has been reported by Lee (280), Perschuk et al. (408), and Rao et al. (416), who used histochemical methods, and by Perschuk et al. (409) and Nenci et al. (374), who used immunohistochemical methods. These studies have all been criticized on the basis that the estrogen derivatives used in these studies were binding to lower affinity or type II estrogen binding sites and thus do not reflect an accurate measurement of estrogen receptors (334).

It is difficult to imagine the thermodynamic properties that would permit exclusive nuclear localization of loosely associated receptor molecules. Therefore, it is likely that an equilibrium exists between unoccupied receptor that maintains most but not all receptors in the nucleus. Such an equilibrium state was first suggested by Williams and Gorski (575,576) and extended by Sheridan et al. (469). Such a circumstance may explain why a small number of receptors (5–10%) was observed in cytoplast in the enucleation studies of Welshons et al. (568). Therefore, it seems likely that unoccupied receptors are present predominantly in the nucleus loosely bound to nuclear sites (a more detailed discussion of this topic can be found in Nuclear Binding of Receptor-Hormone Complexes, *below*). The nuclear sites are in a state of equilibrium with the cytoplasmic compartment, which results in a small percentage of receptors being located in the cytoplasm. The controversy concerning cellular localization of estrogen receptors remains a hot topic for debate and the reader is referred to the following articles for interesting discussions of this problem (149, 155, 213, 454,515,560).

It has been suggested that unoccupied nuclear receptors are active and that binding of hormone simply increases their activity. It is well known that antiestrogens suppress the activity of MCF-7 cells in the absence of estrogen, and thus the unoccupied estrogen receptor may be active in maintaining basal cell regulation (235,291). The concept of active unoccupied receptors may at first glance seem surprising; however, it is generally held that hormones are substances that do not initiate new events, but instead, act as modulators or regulators of physiological processes already in operation. Therefore, unoccupied nuclear receptors may be involved in the control of basal cellular activity and are able to stimulate enhanced activity when they become occupied by hormone.

Receptor States: Occupied and Unoccupied Binding Sites

The measurement of cytosol and nuclear receptors has been used extensively to assess the responsive state of target cells. These observations must be considered in the light of the discussions above concerning the true cellular localization of receptor; however, regardless of the precise localization, it is clear that receptors exist in at least two binding states in the cell: occupied and unoccupied sites. Unoccupied sites are measured by exposing the receptor to [^{3}H]steroid and assessing the amount of bound and free [^{3}H]steroid (115,257). Occupied receptors are measured by [^{3}H]steroid exchange assays which employ methods that result in the dissociation of the bound ligand from occupied receptor sites and the reassociation of [^{3}H]steroid (11,237,341,553–555). For a review of these various methods see Clark and Peck (82).

The actual binding state *in situ* and relationship between occupied and unoccupied estrogen receptor sites was first demonstrated by Williams and Gorski (575) in their study of the cytoplasmic estrogen receptor. This investigation, since confirmed by our own laboratory (82), demonstrated that a constant and very low percentage of total occupied estrogen receptors remains in the cytoplasmic compartment of uterine cells despite the level of estrogen present. Furthermore, the number of occupied cytoplasmic sites could be artifactually high unless precautions are taken to prevent the association of estrogen with unoccupied cytosol receptors following tissue disruption.

Target tissue contains several pools of estrogen: free hormone in the intercellular and intracellular spaces, loosely associated hormone bound to nonspecific sites (lipids, hydrophobic proteins), hormone bound to higher affinity type II sites, and hormone bound to receptor. Occupied receptors are present primarily in the nuclear compartment and unoccupied sites are found primarily in the cytosol fraction (82,575). If tissues are homogenized, estrogen previously in the intercellular space and unavailable for interaction with the cytosol receptor is free to occupy previously unoccupied sites. In addition, estrogen previously bound to nonspecific, low-affinity sites is likely to dissociate and be available for interaction with unoccupied receptor sites. Thus, the act of homogenization with its attendant disruption of cellular compartments and dilution of pools results in an artifactually high estimate of occupied cytosol sites. The correction introduced by Williams and Gorski (575) to avoid this artifact consisted of tissue homogenization in the presence of excess unlabeled estrogen. This manipulation allows the estimation of receptor sites occupied with [^{3}H]estradiol under various *in vitro* conditions. The procedure has been modified for *in vivo* studies (82).

These experimental manipulations are absolutely required for valid assessment of the binding state of steroid receptors, and since they are rarely performed, most studies concerning this point must be viewed with caution. This stipulation, plus the problems involved with the determination of the *in situ* localization of receptor, make it difficult to draw concrete conclusions about receptor localization and receptor binding state in most studies.

Structural and Biochemical Characteristics of Receptors

The structural and biochemical characteristics of estrogen and progesterone receptors are complex and not fully understood. The purpose of this section is to discuss the current state of the art and to put these observations in perspective with relation to the topics discussed in the previous section.

Receptor Structure

Although there are structural and biochemical similarities between estrogen and progesterone receptors, sufficient differences exist to warrant separate discussion of these receptors.

Estrogen receptor. The estrogen receptor is found in the cytosol of estrogen target tissues as a proteinacous macromolecule with a sedimentation coefficient of 8S as determined by sucrose density gradient centrifugation in low ionic strength buffer (217,541). This 8S form of the receptor is generally considered to be an aggregate consisting of 4S subunits, which can be observed when high-salt (0.4 M KCl) buffers are used (258). However, the sedimentation coefficient of the estrogen receptor is known to vary with the experimental conditions. Various sedimentation values, ranging from 4 to 8S, for the cytosol estrogen receptor can be obtained by changing the salt concentration in the gradients (64,500). Physiological salt concentrations of 0.15 to 0.2 M KCl yield a 6S form (64,425). In addition, Chamness et al. (64) and Stancel et al. (500) have shown that various S values can be obtained by varying the quantity of protein and by including heparin in the gradient. Conformational changes in the receptor that have no effect on the molecular weight of the molecule could result in changes in the sedimentation coefficient (380). Undoubtedly the addition of ethylenediaminetetraacetate (EDTA), proteolysis inhibitors, sulfhydryl reagents, etc. by some investigators and not by others has resulted in many of the differences reported in the literature. Endogenous proteases exist in cytosol preparations and can give rise to several proteolytic fragments of receptors (470). In addition, as discussed below, binding sites that are not receptors have undoubtedly contributed to this confusion.

The problem of variable sedimentation coefficients has been overcome by the addition of sodium molybdate (20 mM) to hypotonic buffers. Sherman et al. (474) and Sherman and Stevens (471,472) have shown that cytosol estrogen receptors sediment as 9 to 10S asymmetric structures which have a Stokes radius of 7.8 nm and molecular weight of 316,000. The possible forms of the receptor and the way in which they combine to form these large multimers have been described by Sherman and Stevens (472), and these relationships will be discussed further in the next section.

Puca et al. (414) purified the estrogen receptor from calf uterine cytosol by affinity chromatography and detected a single protein band by gel electrophoresis of 70,000 molecular weight. This purified receptor sedimented as an 8S form in low ionic strength sucrose gradients and 4S in high-salt gradients. Estrogen receptors purified by affinity chromatography from MCF-7 cells have a 4.5 sedimentation coefficient and molecular weight of 65,000 (154). Similar values have also been obtained by studies utilizing covalent attachment of tamoxifen aziridine to the estrogen receptor in MCF-7 cells (347) and rat and lamb uterine cytosol (236). These authors were not able to observe any higher molecular weight forms of the receptor even when cells were directly homogenized in sodium dodecyl sulfate (SDS) (347). These results do not completely rule out the possibility that the receptor exists *in situ* as a large multimeric structure, but they clearly define a basic form of the receptor.

Until recently it has been assumed that the 8S form of the receptor was made up of 4S subunits, each of which binds estrogen; however, Joab et al. (219) have suggested that a non-hormone-binding subunit with a molecular weight of 90,000 may combine with a hormone-binding 4S subunit to form the 8S complex of estrogen and progesterone receptors. The rabbit uterine progesterone receptor also has a non-steroid-binding component (59,000 daltons) associated with larger steroid-binding subunits (518). Murayama (366) has suggested that there are two different macromolecular components that combine with the 4S to receptor to form 5, 6, and 8S receptor forms.

The native state (*in situ* structure) of the cytosol form of the receptor may never be known because of the nonphysiological and potentially artifactual conditions under which the analyses must be done. In addition, as discussed in the previous section, it is possible that cytoplasmic receptors do not exist *in situ*, but are a result of the homogenization procedure that dislodges them from the nucleus.

In the chick oviduct and human uterus two forms of the estrogen receptor have been described (484). These components are specific for estrogens and have equilibrium dissociation constants of 0.1 and 1.0 nM. Both forms of the receptor can be found in nuclei; therefore, the lower-affinity form (K_d 1.0 nM) does not appear to be analogous to type II binding sites described for rat uterine preparations (see below for discussion of type II sites). These two forms have been called X and Y and at the present time their relationship to the estrogen receptor from the rat uterus is unknown.

Progesterone receptor. The original work on the progesterone receptor was done by sucrose density gradient centrifugation and these results are subject to the various problems discussed above for the estrogen receptor. Sedimentation values ranging from 3.5 to 8S have been reported depending on conditions and species (119,120,126, 340,387,422,443,459,470) Schrader et al. (457) have shown that the progesterone receptor in the chick oviduct exists as a 6S dimer which is composed of two nonidentical 4S subunits (A and B). Other investigators have proposed a similar subunit relationship in the guinea pig uterus (119,340) and in the rabbit uterus (120). Sherman et al. (471,473) showed that at least five forms of the receptor can be obtained from chick oviduct cytosol and that two of these are similar to the A and B nonidentical subunits that make up a 6S form of the receptor. A heavier multimeric form (~ 300,000 molecular weight), which is stabilized by the addition of molybdate to buffers, is probably made up of 4S subunits (472). An endogeneous protease exists in oviduct cytosol that cleaves both A and B subunits into two fragments that contain the hormone-binding site: form IV (43,000 molecular weight) containing a DNA-binding site and the mero receptor (23,000 molecular weight) (40,473).

Much of the work on the progesterone receptor has centered on the 6S form and its two 4S subunits. These subunits have been shown by photoaffinity labeling to consist of two proteins; form A, molecular weight 80,000, and form B, molecular weight 108,000 (103). Similar findings have been reported for progesterone receptors from MCF-7 cells and rabbit uterus (192,269,285). Although the evidence is substantial that the A and B forms of receptor are different, some evidence exists to suggest that they are similar. Peptide maps of photoaffinity-labeled progesterone receptor form A and B show considerable similarity, and the suggestion has been made that form A may be derived from form B by proteolysis (157). These investigators also demonstrated that polyclonal antibodies to forms A and B interact with each of the forms of the receptor (157). Although Schrader et al. (455) believe that the 6S form is made up of A and B subunits, Dougherty and Toft (102) have reported that the 8S receptor can be resolved into two populations, one consisting only of the A subunit and the other containing the B subunit. A non-hormone-binding form of the progesterone receptor (form B) has also been described (107,405); however, the functional relationships between the two proteins have not been established.

Analysis of the mammalian receptor has yielded variable results. Several forms of the receptor from rabbit uterus have been described, which have molecular weights ranging from 65,000 to 100,000 (211,572). This heterogeneity may be due to proteolysis, since Lamb and Bullock (269) were able to show similar multiple forms of the receptor before proteolytic activity was removed from rabbit uterine cytosol. After removal of proteolytic activity the receptor appeared as 78,000 and 102,000 molecular weight forms. In contrast to these findings, a single form of the receptor has been described by Milgrom et al. (341) from the rabbit uterus and by Smith et al. (485) from the human. Recently Loosfelt et al. (295) demonstrated that a single 110,000-dalton protein was detected by monoclonal antibodies in cytosol from the rabbit uterus. Smaller forms were observed if precautions were not taken to block proteolysis. When poly(A)+ RNA from the rabbit uterus was translated in a reticulate lysate, a 110,000-dalton protein was present and could be precipitated by antibodies to the progesterone receptor.

At the present time it is not possible to resolve these ambiguities concerning the precise nature of the progesterone receptor; however, some of the confusion may originate from the observation that a non-hormone-binding subunit with a molecular weight of 90,000 is a component of 8S complexes (423). Since this protein is present in excess, it is not certain whether 8S complexes are a true *in vivo* form or the result of an artifactual association of proteins (40,415).

Another possible cause for these uncertainties concerning the molecular weight form of the progesterone receptor resides in the definition of the receptor. That is, the identification of a protein that binds progesterone does not define it as a receptor. It is necessary to establish that the protein in question conforms to the criteria listed in Definition and Characteristics of Steroid Receptors. Such validations require extensive experimentation and in most cases have not been done. Some of the hormone-binding forms may be other steroid-binding proteins that are not receptors but function in different capacities. These are discussed in DNA Binding and Acceptor Sites, below.

Receptor Transformation and Nuclear Binding

The binding of the receptor-hormone complex to nuclear components is assumed to be an important step in the sequence of reactions that leads to the stimulation of biosynthetic events. As discussed in previous sections, unoccupied receptors have a low affinity for nuclear sites and are easily solubilized, whereas occupied receptors have a high affinity for nuclear sites. This change from low affinity to high affinity has been called activation or transformation. These reactions occur for all steroid receptors; however, because several important differences exist between estrogen and progesterone receptors, these will be discussed separately.

Estrogen receptor. Jensen et al. (217) suggested that the 4S form of the estrogen receptor was converted to a 5S form that had a high affinity for nuclear binding sites. This reaction was thought to occur in the cytosol, but as pointed out earlier, it probably occurs in the nucleus (476). Regardless of the cellular localization of this reaction, it is clear that receptor-estrogen complexes undergo a change in affinity for nuclear sites. This receptor activation or transformation reaction has been examined in detail by several investigators. Notides and Nielson (379) have suggested that the formation of the 5S complex (molecular weight 130,000–140,000) involves the dimerization of two 4S subunits (~ 75,000 molecular weight). When transformation occurs, the dissociation of estradiol from the receptor changes from a rapid to a slow rate (564). Thus, the transformed receptor is a dimer of 4S subunits that binds estradiol with high affinity (slow dissociation rate) and has a high affinity for nuclear binding sites (Fig. 4A). Bailly et al. (22) suggested that the 4 to 5S conversion step was not synonymous with transformation but instead represented a second-order dimerization that takes place after the transformation step. The exact molecular interactions involved in these conversions are a matter of debate, and the model proposed by Müller et al. (357,359) is presented in Fig. 4B for comparison. In this model the 4S monomers undergo a pretransformation step that results in a shift from a low-affinity 4S form to a high-affinity 4S form. The high-affinity 4S monomers then combine to form a 5S dimer. Evidence for this model is based on the observation that 4S monomers immobilized on hydroxylapatite undergo a temperature-induced transition from a rapidly dissociating to a slowly dissociating state which remains as a 4S form when it is eluted from the hydroxylapatite and analyzed by sucrose density centrifugation (359). Similar findings have been reported by Sakai and Gorski (444).

Notides et al. (378) have shown that estradiol-modulated equilibrium between low- (4S) and high- (5S) affinity states of the cytosol receptor results in a positively cooperative equilibrium binding of estradiol. This finding is in contrast to the findings of others who showed that estradiol binding is noncooperative in intact tissues and cells (230,404,575,576). In addition, 4S receptor immobilized on hydroxylapatite does not display this cooperative binding behavior. The immobilized 4S forms of the receptor are not free to form dimers; therefore, dimerization is not required for transformation of receptor from a low-affinity to a high-affinity form. Gorski et al. (152) suggest that these divergent results can be explained if the unoccupied receptor is immobilized in the nuclear compartment and as such would not display cooperative behavior. However, when receptors are solubilized, as they were in the case of Notides's studies, they are free to form dimers and to undergo a shift from a lower to higher affinity state, and this is observed as cooperative binding.

Although these suggestions by Gorski et al. (152) may account for the differences observed between soluble and immobilized receptor, the question of whether cooperative binding exists in solution is open. Notides et al. (378) observed apparent cooperativity only when the concentration of receptor was relatively high. Under such conditions the concentration of receptor is equal to or greater than the K_d

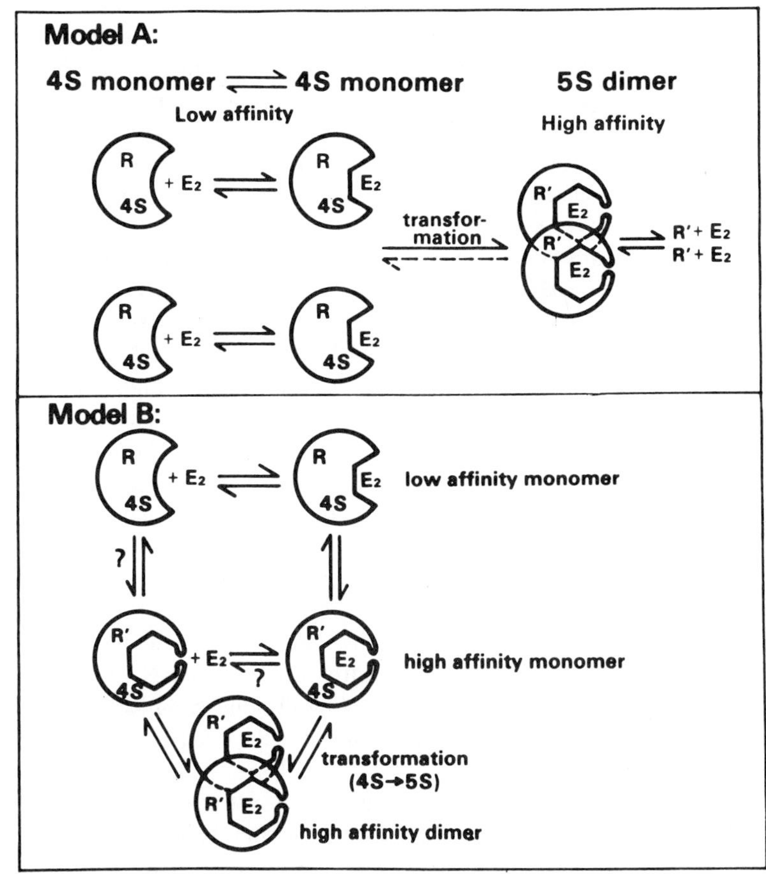

FIG. 4. Models for the molecular mechanism of the transition of the estrogen receptor from a state with fast dissociation rates (R, RE_2; low-affinity 4S monomers) to a state with slow dissociation rates ($R'E_2$; high-affinity 4S monomers). See text for details. (From ref. 357.)

of the binding reaction, and will result in a linear saturation curve at the lowest concentrations of ligand, which becomes curvilinear at higher concentrations. Such saturation data when transformed by Scatchard analysis will give a straight line that is parallel to the X axis at low concentrations of bound ligand and that gradually curves downward at higher concentration of bound ligand. Such a curve can be mistakenly considered to represent a cooperative binding interaction. For further consideration of artifacts and problems concerning ligand binding interactions see Clark and Peck (82).

Progesterone receptor. Transformation of the progesterone receptor from chick oviduct involves a dissociation of subunits rather than an association, as with the estrogen receptor. The native progesterone receptor is thought to exist as a 6 to 8S dimer which is made up of two nonidentical subunits (see previous section on Receptor Structure for details). The complex can be dissociated to 4S A and B monomers by any of the treatments known to cause transformation of other receptors, i.e., heat, salt, dialysis, etc. (456,457). The A monomer exhibits high-affinity binding to DNA, and its binding site is apparently occluded when it is complexed with the B monomer (387,389). Thus, transformation appears to involve the dissociation of the A-B dimer as an obligatory step before the binding of the A monomer to DNA can take place. Under some conditions the B form of the receptor from oviduct can bind to DNA (157), and both A and B forms of the receptor from rabbit uterus and MCF-7 cells bind to DNA (192,269).

These considerations of transformation of the progesterone receptor are based on DNA binding as an endpoint, and it should be pointed out that, unlike the estrogen receptor, the 6S dimer of the progesterone receptor will bind to nuclei without transformation (459). That is, the 6S dimer binds to nuclei at 4°C under low salt conditions. Therefore it appears that the 6S dimer is already in a transformed state with respect to its ability to bind to nuclei. It is possible that the 6S dimer does not represent the native nontransformed receptor but instead a dissociated product of larger aggregates which are not transformed (156). The topic of nuclear binding is discussed in detail in Specificity of Nuclear Binding *In Vitro,* below.

Additional factors may be involved in receptor transformation. These include translocation inhibitor macromolecules, translocation promoters or modulator factors, and a host of other poorly characterized substances that interfere with or facilitate transformation. These have recently been reviewed by Isohashi and Sakamoto (206) and Sato et al. (448) and are beyond the scope of this chapter.

Nuclear Binding of Receptor-Hormone Complexes

The binding of occupied receptor-hormone complexes to nuclear sites is generally assumed to be an important step in the mechanism of action of steroid hormones. This concept has been derived from studies of nuclear binding done *in vivo* and *in vitro*. The purpose of this section is to describe these studies and to examine the problems attendant to their interpretation.

Nuclear Binding In Vivo

Studies of nuclear binding of steroid receptor complexes *in vivo* have revealed complexities that require consideration and that will eventually have to be integrated into our understanding of *in vitro* analyses of nuclear-receptor interactions.

Estrogen receptor. An injection of estradiol results in the rapid accumulation of the estrogen-receptor complex in rat uterine nuclei (Fig. 5; 11,12,16,215,217,242,243,270). This is accompanied by a stoichiometric depletion of cytosol receptors and probably reflects increased nuclear affinity of occupied receptor for nuclear binding sites. Following nuclear accumulation 10 to 20% of the estrogen receptor is occupied for several hours in the nuclear compartment. Thus *in vivo* nuclear binding has a temporal as well as a quantitative aspect that requires consideration.

The most straightforward relationship that could exist between nuclear binding of receptor-steroid complexes and biological response would be that these parameters were proportional and that occupancy of all receptors would be correlated with maximal response. Such relationships have been shown for several responses but not for others. For example, early uterotropic responses, such as water inhibition, stimulation of uterine induced protein (IP), and early activation of RNA polymerase are proportional to receptor occupancy (12,13,16,173,233). In contrast, glucose oxidation is maximal in the rat uterus when only 5 to 10% of the receptors are occupied (13). Late uterotropic responses, such as sustained RNA polymerase activity, cellular hypertrophy, and hyperplasia, are correlated with the nuclear occupancy of 10 to 20% of the total number of receptors present (for review see 82). These receptor-hormone complexes, which are occupied for long periods of time (6 hr and longer), are resistant to extraction by high salt and probably represent a population of complexes that are tightly bound to nuclear acceptor sites (Fig. 5; 82,437). The complexes that are extractable with salt may represent more loosely attached complexes that are either bound to nonspecific nuclear sites or are only associated with the stimulation of early uterotropic responses.

Barrack et al. (33) have suggested that salt-insoluble receptor sites are bound to the nuclear matrix and that they may be involved in the control of DNA and RNA synthesis (32). The binding of receptor-hormone complexes to the nuclear matrix is discussed in more detail in Nuclear Matrix, below.

Long-term nuclear occupancy of estrogen receptors has also been described for the mouse uterus; however, an additional second nuclear elevation occurs between 7 and 8

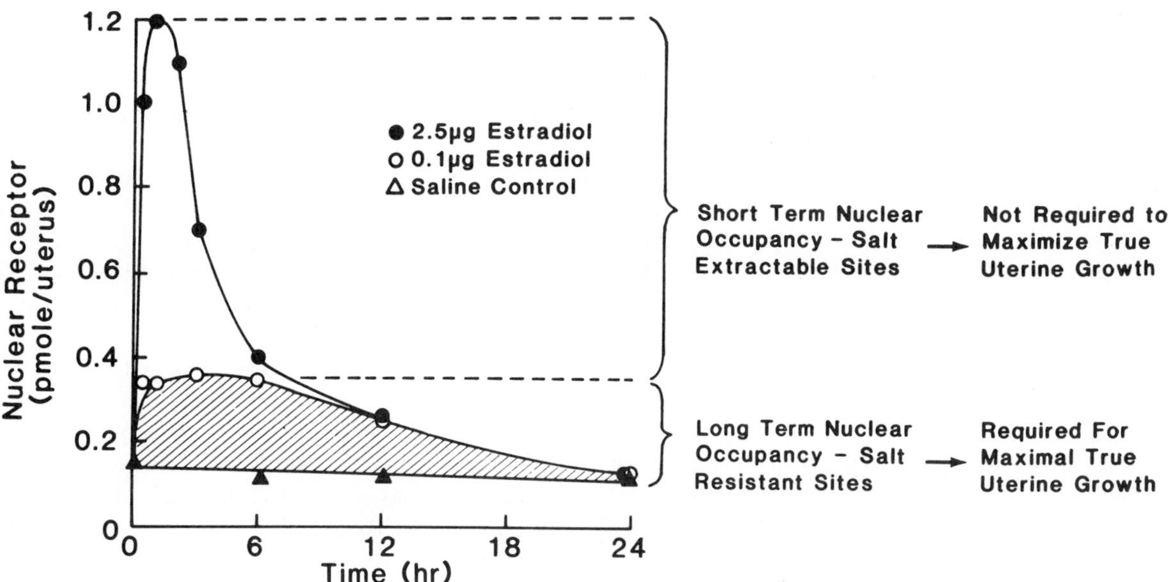

FIG. 5. Relationship between nuclear occupancy of the estrogen receptor and uterine growth.

hr after an injection of estradiol (255). Although the reason for this second nuclear peak of receptor occupancy is not clear, it is also correlated with true uterine growth in the mouse (256). The relationship between long-term nuclear occupancy and secondary elevations of nuclear binding is discussed in more detail in Hormone Effects on Protein and RNA Synthesis.

Subsequent to the initial accumulation of receptor-hormone complexes in nuclei there is a gradual loss of receptor from the nucleus, which may involve an active processing step rather than a simple dissociation of the complex and the hormone from nuclear sites (194). This processing step may involve the inactivation of the receptor by a specific nuclear phosphatase (20). Whether receptor loss occurs under all experimental circumstances is debatable. Jakesz et al. (210) have suggested that no receptor loss occurs following continuous estrogen exposure in the rat uterus and that a portion of cytosol receptors and salt-resistant receptor estrogen complexes do not dissociate over time. Although we have never observed nondissociable receptor forms, we have shown that continuous estrogen exposure leads to receptor loss after 24 hr of exposure, but not before (306). During the period of receptor loss uterine growth becomes maximal and this response is maintained for up to 16 days. Whether this receptor loss is due to the formation of nonexchangeable receptor forms is unknown. As explained in the following two sections, all studies of receptor processing or loss are compounded by the failure of most investigators to assess the loss of nuclear-bound receptors during the preparation of nuclei. In addition, artifactual loss of receptors can be observed in crude nuclear fractions due to endogenous nuclease activity, which results in the release of receptors from nuclear sites (452).

In the chick oviduct system an injection of estradiol is followed by nuclear accumulation of the estrogen receptor (225). If occupancy is maintained by long-acting estrogens, such as estradiol benzoate, the rate of conalbumin mRNA production is directly proportional to the concentration of nuclear receptors, with a half-maximal induction occurring at 50% occupancy. In contrast, half-maximal induction of ovalbumin mRNA occurs when nuclear receptor levels are 80% of maximum (361). These authors suggest that these differential responses may be related either to different numbers of specific binding sites regulating the production of each mRNA, or to different affinities of regulatory sites for estrogen receptors.

Nuclear binding and response in the chick oviduct system requires the interaction of two forms of the estrogen receptor. The higher-affinity receptor (X, K_d 0.1 nM) increases RNA polymerase II activity directly (528,529), and the lower-affinity form (Y, K_d 1.0 nM) seems to be necessary to confer specificity to transcription of estrogen-dependent genes (486).

Progesterone receptor. An injection of [^{3}H]progesterone in estrogen-primed chicks will result in the nuclear binding of receptor progesterone complexes in the oviduct (336,391). In contrast to the long-term nuclear occupancy of the receptor estrogen, progesterone receptor complexes accumulate rapidly (peak at 8 min) and decline significantly by 45 min after the injection. In addition, a large proportion of the total receptor remains in the cytosol during the entire time following injection. Apparently receptor-progesterone complexes are readily solubilized from their nuclear sites during the preparation of nuclei. Although this possibility has not been examined in the chick oviduct, it is likely in view of the results that have been obtained from studies in the rat uterus. In contrast to these observations, progesterone-receptor occupancy in oviduct nuclei can be observed for several hours after large doses of progesterone in oil

(362). However, even under these circumstances only 15 to 20% of the cytosol receptors are recovered in the nuclear fraction. Within 30 min after the injection the number of nuclear receptors increases fivefold (1,500 molecules/cell); however, the induction of ovalbumin and conalbumin mRNA is delayed for 2 hr. Half-maximal induction of conalbumin mRNA occurs when nuclear occupancy is 50% of maximum, whereas half-maximal induction of ovalbumin mRNA occurs at 80% occupancy. Mulvihill and Palmiter (362) suggest that the lag period in mRNA induction is due to intermediate events between receptor localization in the nucleus and activation of transcription and that different numbers of regulatory sites account for the differences in receptor numbers required to give half-maximal responses.

Rat uterine nuclei also show a rapid accumulation of the progesterone receptor; however, the number of nuclear receptors accumulated is considerably lower than the number of depleted cytosol receptors (342,554). This lack of stoichiometry is due to the loss of loosely bound receptor complexes during nuclear preparation and washing (555,557). These results indicate that progesterone-receptor complexes are less tightly associated with nuclear binding sites and do not undergo long-term nuclear occupancy as do estrogen-receptor complexes. Therefore, it is likely that nuclear binding of progesterone- and estrogen-receptor complexes may differ in significant ways.

In T47D human breast cancer cells, exposure to micromolar levels of progesterone does cause a stoichiometric nuclear accumulation and cytosol depletion of the progesterone receptor (345). This is also a very rapid process (5 min) and is followed by a loss of receptors in both cellular compartments. This loss has been attributed to nuclear processing of the receptor; however, it is also possible that loosely bound nuclear receptor is being lost during the nuclear washing procedures.

Specificity of Nuclear Binding In Vitro

A great deal of effort has gone into the analysis of receptor binding to cellular components *in vitro*. These experiments have been done in order to define the specific acceptors for receptor-hormone complexes. Most investigators have concentrated on the examination of acceptor sites in nuclei, chromatin, DNA, and the nuclear matrix. Each of these will be discussed below; however, before detailing these findings a general discussion of the specificity of acceptor site binding will be presented.

The demonstration of acceptor sites in the nucleus has been the subject of considerable controversy (52,62,63). Several investigators have shown that nuclear binding of receptor-steroid complexes is a saturable phenomenon, thus suggesting that specific acceptor sites exist (3,52,122,183, 225,240,279,301,388,494), whereas others claim that limited numbers of specific nuclear sites do not exist and that nuclear saturation is an artifact (62,63,576). Much of this conflict probably stems from the difficulties inherent in the detection of a low number of specific binding sites in the presence of a large number of nonspecific sites (585). This is especially true in view of the very "sticky" nature of the receptor-estrogen complex after it has been exposed to elevated temperatures (20–30°C) at physiological salt concentrations (72). This process has been observed by many investigators and is generally called transformation, a topic discussed previously in Receptor Transformation and Nuclear Binding. Thus, studies of the binding of the receptor-estrogen complex to nuclei, chromatin, and/or DNA in cell-free systems are susceptible to the error introduced by the masking effect on nonspecific binding to many surfaces. The problem of nonspecific binding is not easily overcome; however, certain basic criteria and principles outlined in the following discussion should be followed.

The principles involved in the study of specific binding of receptor-steroid complexes (*RS*) to acceptor sites are identical to those encountered in the examination of the binding of a steroid to its receptor. These principles have been carefully worked out and criteria for specific binding have been established. Although these principles and concepts have been discussed for receptor-hormone interactions in Definition and Characteristics of Steroid Receptors, they will be reiterated here as they apply to receptor-steroid complex binding to acceptor sites.

The binding of *RS* to acceptor sites should be a saturable function from which a dissociation constant (K_d) can be determined. Such analysis must be done under conditions that maintain the concentration of DNA sequences at approximately the K_d of the binding interaction. If the DNA concentration greatly exceeds the K_d of the interaction, which is likely to be the case, then DNA binding sites will act as a "sink" for *RS* binding and a normal saturation curve will not be obtained. Therefore, no determination of K_d can be made.

The binding of *RS* to acceptor sites should be a specific interaction. That is, labeled complexes (*RS**) should be competitively inhibited by nonlabeled complexes (*RS*). This can be accomplished by adding increasing concentrations of nonlabeled *RS* complexes to a fixed quantity of *RS** plus acceptor sites or by saturation analysis with different concentrations of nonlabeled *RS* complexes. These two methods provide data that can be analyzed via competitive inhibition curves or by double reciprocal analysis, respectively. Usually the only assessment of specificity that is performed consists of adding nonlabeled steroid to the *RS** plus acceptor sites mixture with subsequent analysis of the amount of *RS** bound to acceptor sites. This procedure only tests the specificity of *RS** interaction, *not* the specificity of the *RS** binding to acceptor sites.

Chromatin Binding and Chromatin Proteins

The specific binding of receptor-steroid complexes to acceptor sites probably involves binding interactions between chromosomal proteins, DNA, and the receptor-steroid complex. Such interactions were first suggested by Schrader et al. (459), who showed that the A subunit of the progesterone receptor binds to DNA and the B subunit binds to chromatin. These authors have suggested that the A-B dimeric form of the receptor first binds to chromatin protein acceptors, probably specified by the B component, and results in the dissociation of the A subunit, which subsequently binds to DNA (156).

Putative chromatin acceptor proteins have been studied extensively by Spelsberg and his collaborators (46,494,496–498). These acceptor proteins, which are acidic and bound to DNA, are referred to as nucleoacidic proteins (NAP). NAP bind the progesterone receptor in a saturable fashion with a dissociation constant of one nanomole (495). Similar acceptor sites have been described for the estrogen-receptor complex from the avian oviduct (254,439).

Whether these NAP are true nuclear acceptors for the progesterone receptor is open to question, and indeed, Littlefield and Spelsberg (293) have recently discussed several of the problems and artifacts that can arise from such binding analyses. For example, highly purified receptor loses its capacity to bind to NAP under some conditions, assay conditions employing pH of 6.0 to 6.5 greatly increase the binding to NAP, and unmasking of chromatin by high salt exposure increases the number of apparent NAP. Thus, one can obtain false estimates of acceptor site binding depending on assay conditions and receptor preparation. A major consideration in all acceptor site studies, which is usually not addressed, is the evaluation of the specificity of acceptor site interactions, as explained in Specificity of Nuclear Binding *In Vitro*. In any evaluation of putative acceptor sites, the specificity of binding must be examined by competitive inhibition analysis with nonlabeled receptor-steroid complexes. If this were done many of the artifacts might disappear.

DNA Binding and Acceptor Sites

As explained in the previous section, the binding of receptor-steroid complexes to chromatin probably results in binding interactions of the receptor with DNA. It has been recognized for several years that transformed receptor-steroid complexes have a high affinity for DNA from target and nontarget tissues (540), and therefore, the determination of specific DNA sequences that might recognize receptor-steroid complexes in a specific way would be a difficult task (585). Steroid receptors do recognize different nucleotide base structures and have the highest affinity for guanine, with intermediate to lower affinities for the pyrimidines and adenine (263). Such preferential binding may reflect structural components of target DNA that enables the receptor to recognize regulatory elements. With the advent of new methods provided by molecular biology, such studies of receptor binding to regulatory elements of genes have become possible.

The A protein of the chick oviduct progesterone receptor has been tested for its interaction with the 5′-flanking sequence of the chicken ovalbumin gene, cloned in bacterial plasmids (87). In the experiments, receptors were incubated with specific fragments of DNA excised from the plasmids with restriction endonucleases. The DNA fragments were labeled with ^{32}P, and the receptor-[^{32}P]DNA complexes formed were isolated by adsorption to nitrocellulose. Receptor-bound [^{32}P]DNA was eluted from the nitrocellulose with NaCl, and the absorbed fragment was identified by its unique size during gel electrophoresis. In this manner, a strong receptor-binding site has been identified upstream of the gene approximately 150 to 200 base pairs from the start of ovalbumin gene transcription. This region of DNA is depicted in Fig. 6, which also shows other features of receptor interaction that suggest that this location is of importance in gene induction *in vivo* (97).

When a test ovalbuminglobin fusion gene was transfected into chicken oviduct cells in culture, the region between 95 and 222 base pairs upstream of the ovalbumin gene was required for progesterone induction. Thus, this region has the biologic activity in cells predicted from the DNA sequence preference tests. The degree of sequence preference observed *in vitro* by receptor A is only about 10- to 20-fold i.e., receptor binds DNA containing the strong site about 10–20 times better than other DNAs of similar size lacking the sequence.

Although these studies concerning preferential binding of the receptor A protein to DNA are interesting, other investigators have noted that both A and B proteins will bind to DNA (157,158,160,192,269). Obviously the experimental conditions, such as those mentioned in the previous section, are involved in these determinations. Likewise, the true specificity of these binding interactions has not been determined by competitive inhibition with nonlabeled steroid-receptor complexes.

Several hormone-inducible genes appear to contain similar 5′ flanking sequences that bind several different steroid hormone receptors. Glucocorticoid- and progesterone-receptor complexes bind to similar nucleotide sequences in the regulatory region of the mouse mammary tumor virus (MMTV) and the chicken lysozyme gene (403,552). Since glucocorticoids, and not progesterone, induce MMTV transcription and both hormones induce the lysozyme gene, the significance of this preferential binding must await further analysis. Similar preferential binding sequences have also been described in the genes for ovalbumin, vitellogenin, and androgen-dependent prostatic protein (97,224,399). Therefore, it is possible that steroid hormone-inducible genes may contain a common nucleotide sequence that recognizes all steroid hormone receptors.

Nuclear Matrix

The nuclear matrix is a fibrillar network of proteins that contains the residual nucleolus and lies within the nuclear membrane (32). Several actively transcribed genes and re-

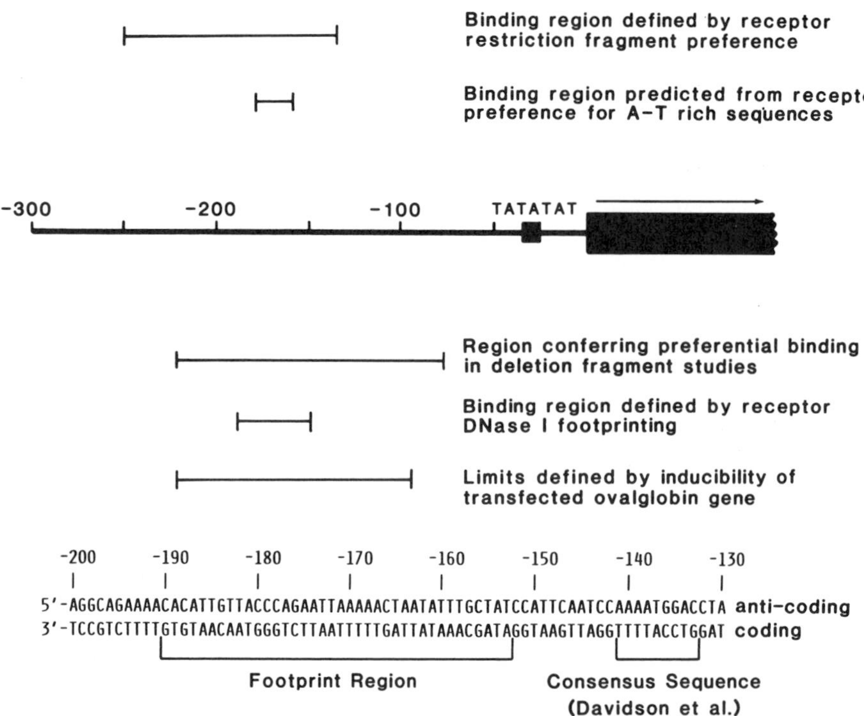

FIG. 6. Location of DNA sequences implicated in progesterone receptor interaction with the chicken oviduct ovalbumin gene. The gene map shows the 300 bp of DNA flanking the ovalbumin gene on its 5′ (upstream) side. The *wide block* shows the start of the gene itself, with the *arrow* indicating the direction of transcription *in vivo.* The control sequence T A T A T A T is located in the *small box.* Key receptor interaction regions have been delimited by several methods and their limits of resolution are shown. The most important region is the "footprint region," where receptor *in vitro* alters the DNA susceptibility of deoxyribonuclease I. The nucleotide sequence of this region is shown at the bottom. A highly AT-rich region is present at this location, from bases 155 to 175. The consensus sequence on the right is present with few changes in a number of hormone-regulated chicken genes.

peated DNA sequences are anchored to the nuclear matrix and it is the site of synthesis and processing of heterogeneous nuclear RNA and DNA replication (67,208,398,429,482, 551). Barrack et al. (33) demonstrated that the estrogen receptor is tightly bound to the nuclear matrix of rat uterine nuclei after an injection of estradiol. These matrix-bound receptor-estrogen complexes are probably identical to the fraction of receptor complexes that are not extractable with high salt and have correlated with true growth of the uterus (82).

The binding of estrogen- and androgen-receptor complexes to the nuclear matrix from several hormone-responsive tissues has been demonstrated *in vivo* (30,31,478) and *in vitro* (29,56). Nuclear type II estrogen-binding sites are also tightly associated with the nuclear matrix of uterine, prostatic, and liver nuclei (78,109,507). Since both the nuclear binding of the estrogen receptor and the elevation of type II binding site are thought to be involved in the regulatory mechanisms that control biosynthetic activity of target tissues, it is tempting to conclude that nuclear matrix-receptor binding is involved in this mechanism. This point is discussed further in Organization of Chromosomes and Genes.

Synthesis and Replenishment of Receptors

The intracellular concentration of steroid receptors is an important factor in determining the responsive state of the target cells. The control of the cellular concentration of steroid receptors is influenced by several interacting factors, which are discussed in this section. As in previous sections of this chapter, the term cytosol receptor is used to define the soluble unoccupied form of the receptor regardless of its actual site of cellular localization.

Although many aspects of receptor replenishment and control are not known, a general picture of the possible pathways will be discussed and in subsequent sections specific receptor control mechanism will be examined. Following transformation and nuclear binding, there are at least three ways that receptor regulation may occur (Fig. 7). The receptor-steroid complex may stimulate the transcription of its own mRNA, which will result in the synthesis of new receptor molecules. These may be either hormone-binding forms (R_b) or non-hormone-binding forms (R_{nb}) which have to be converted to R_b. The *RS* complex may be reutilized either by being converted to a non-binding form that is subsequently activated to a binding form, or by being re-

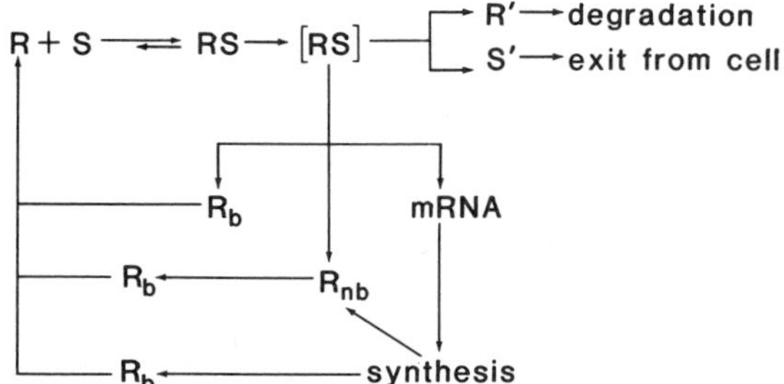

FIG. 7. Possible pathways for the regulation of synthesis, replenishment, and degradation of steroid receptors.

cycled directly as an activated binding form. In addition to these replenishment mechanisms the receptor may undergo degradation to an inactive form (R'). Associated with each of these receptor pathways is the loss or elimination of the steroid from the cell (S').

Control of Estrogen Receptor Concentration

Estrogen-responsive cells in the uterus of a castrated rat maintain levels of receptor that enable it to respond to administered estrogen. This basal level of receptor is probably controlled by genetic mechanisms that are programmed for the constitutive synthesis of the cytosol receptor. Thus estrogen target tissues can usually detect and respond to estrogens. This is also true of estrogen target tissues in the male animal, which will respond readily to exogenous estrogen and which have estrogen receptor levels equal to those of the female (14,65,66,71,355,356).

Although estrogen target cells appear capable of maintaining a constitutive level of cytosol receptor, this does not imply that sex hormones have no influence on the level of cytosol receptor. To the contrary, it is well known that steroid receptor levels are influenced by endogenous and exogenous steroids. As pointed out earlier, an injection of estradiol causes a rapid depletion of cytosol receptors, which bind tightly in the nucleus as receptor-estrogen complexes. This is followed by a period during which the cytosol receptor is replenished. This replenishment involves at least two processes, the reactivation or reutilization of nuclear bound receptor and the *de novo* synthesis of receptor molecules. In tissues that do not grow in response to hormone, replenishment may involve only reactivation or recycling. This was first suggested by Munck et al. (364) for glucocorticoid receptors in thymus cells. In fact, replenishment of cytosol receptors for glucocorticoids does not depend on protein and RNA synthesis (205,339,436).

Reactivation of a nonbinding form of the estrogen receptor in the chick oviduct has been observed (419). The Y form (R_d 1.0 nM) exists in a binding and nonbinding form in oviduct cytosol. Addition of ATP or ADP to the nonbinding form converts it to the binding form, and this process can be reversed by dialysis. How these interconversions relate to replenishment of the estrogen receptor is not known; however, they provide evidence that nonbinding (nonactivated) receptor forms exist and suggests the possibility that such interactions may occur *in vivo*.

In tissues that grow in response to hormone stimulation, such as uterus, vagina, and mammary gland, it is easy to envision the involvement of both reactivation and synthesis in the replenishment process. It follows that synthesis of more cytosol receptor molecules is required in cells that will undergo cell division after hormone stimulation. In this manner a constant amount of receptor per cell is maintained. Cells that grow in size and do not divide may also require receptor synthesis to counteract the dilution effect brought about by cellular hypertrophy. The involvement of protein synthesis in the replenishment process has been suggested by several investigators (65,66,218,336,338,447). In these experiments protein synthesis inhibitors, such as cycloheximide, were shown to partially block replenishment of the estrogen receptor. All of these results are subject to question, since long periods of cycloheximide exposure are required to produce observed inhibitory effects, and nonspecific toxic side effects of this drug cannot be ruled out. Kassis and Gorski (229) demonstrated that the short-acting estrogen, 16α-estradiol, will cause complete replenishment of cytosol receptor within 4 hr after an injection, which is not blocked by cycloheximide. Thus, reutilization or recycling of the estrogen receptor can occur when short-acting estrogens are used to cause nuclear accumulation. Such short-acting estrogens do not cause true uterine growth and therefore may not stimulate the necessary biosynthetic events associated with cell hypertrophy and hyperplasia. This point will be discussed in more detail in Antagonism of Hormone Action.

The replenishment of cytosol receptors following hormone-induced depletion is an important factor in determining the ability of the uterus to respond to subsequent hormone stimulation. Within the first 6 hr after an injection of estradiol, a time during which very little replenishment has taken place, a second injection of estradiol does not stimulate uterotropic responses above those obtained with the first injection (15). A second injection at 12 hr, however, when cytosol receptors have been replenished, will cause nuclear accumulation of the newly replenished receptor and elevated uterotropic responses.

Control of the Progesterone Receptor by Estrogen

The uterus is relatively insensitive to progesterone unless first exposed to estrogen. Thus progesterone treatment in the nonestrogenized uterus will not produce a secretory uterine epithelium (427); however, with estrogen priming, progesterone treatment has dramatic effects on the production of secretory responses. These observations may be explained *a priori* by assuming that estrogen priming stimulates the synthesis of the progesterone receptor, thereby enhancing the ability of the uterus to respond to progesterone. Several investigators have shown that estrogen treatment does increase the quantity of progesterone receptors (119,127,133,197,198,278,296,341,416,417,422,542, 549). These effects of estrogen occur in both the endometrium and myometrium of the guinea pig uterus and hence there does not appear to be any differential cell effect of estrogen (296,561). The ability of estradiol to increase the level of the cytosol progesterone receptor also occurs in the neurons of hypothalamus (232,323,446).

Other investigators have observed that not only does estrogen treatment increase the quantity of cytosol progesterone receptor, but it also causes a shift in the sedimentation coefficient. Castrated animals contain primarily the 4S form of the receptor and estrogen treatment causes a shift to the 7 to 8S form. This observation has been made in endometrium and myometrium of the monkey (110,204), in the human uterus (212), in the guinea pig uterus (133), and the chick oviduct (542). From these observations it can be concluded that estrogen stimulates the uterus to produce qualitative, as well as quantitative, changes in the cytosol progesterone receptor, probably by *de novo* synthesis. Thus, estrogen sets the stage for the binding of progesterone, which is prerequisite for progesterone action.

Leavitt et al. (277) have also shown this effect *in vitro*. Uterine strips from the hamster were incubated *in vitro* with estradiol, and the quantity of cytoplasmic progesterone receptor increased dramatically over a 24-hr period of incubation. The increased quantity of uterine cytosol receptor is blocked by the addition of cycloheximide and actinomycin D, both *in vitro*, to hamster uteri (277) and *in vitro* in the guinea pig (341). Thus, estrogenic stimulation of cytosol progesterone receptor probably involves RNA and protein synthesis.

Effects of Progesterone on Progesterone Receptors

Milgrom et al. (341) and Freifeld et al. (133) demonstrated that progesterone has the paradoxical effect of causing a rapid decline in the quantity of cytosol progesterone receptor in the guinea pig uterus. These authors suggested that this decline was not simply the result of receptor accumulation in the nucleus, although this mechanism is clearly functioning immediately after an injection of progesterone (533), but that instead the decline in receptors was due to receptor loss in both cytosol and nuclear fractions. The interpretation of this decline in progesterone receptors is complicated by the fact that nuclear bound receptor-progesterone complexes are loosely bound and are lost during cell fractionation and washing procedures (555,558). Since most of the studies on progesterone-induced receptor decline have not assessed this loss during cell fractionation, it is difficult to make definitive statements concerning these results.

Regardless of the precise interpretation of progesterone-induced receptor decline, it is clear that the presence of estrogen is required to maintain progesterone receptor levels (558). If rats are maintained on estrogen, no decline of progesterone receptors occurs after progesterone administration, whereas in estrogen-withdrawn animals a rapid decline appears to take place.

Estrogen withdrawal implies a lack of estrogen action, which could result from either declining serum levels of estrogen or declining levels of estrogen receptor. Since progesterone suppresses the synthesis of the estrogen receptor (see below) and since the synthesis of the progesterone receptor is dependent on the action of estrogens via the estrogen receptor, it is possible for progesterone to suppress the synthesis of its own receptor by desensitizing the uterus to estrogen.

The level of cytosol progesterone receptor is correlated with the ability of the uterus to respond to progesterone. When cytosol progesterone receptors are low an injection of progesterone has no antagonistic effect on estrogen-induced early uterotropic events (556). Thus, the ability of the uterus to respond to progesterone depends on the presence of its receptor.

Control of the Estrogen Receptor by Progesterone

Progesterone acts on the estrogen-primed uterus to alter cell function and reproductive competence. Often this ability of progesterone is considered to be antagonistic to estrogen; however, it probably should be referred to as a modifier of estrogen action. Nevertheless, progesterone will reduce the ability of estrogens to cause uterine growth and vaginal cornification (for reviews see 199,283). This ability of progesterone to modify or antagonize estrogen action is generally considered to involve receptor mechanisms.

Progesterone does not interfere with the initial binding of estradiol to the cytosol estrogen receptor or to the subsequent nuclear binding of the complex (11,80,541). Thus, the source of its antagonism does not lie at these levels. Instead, progesterone has the ability to decrease the level of cytosol estrogen receptor concentration (49,76, 197,336,401). This decline in receptor level is correlated with a decreased ability of estradiol to stimulate uterine growth (197). In addition to this decrease in cytosol estrogen receptors, progesterone also reduces the level of nuclear bound receptor-estrogen complexes in the hamster uterus (382,383,569). This reduction in nuclear bound receptor-estrogen complexes may be due to the induction of an estrogen receptor regulatory factor by progesterone (297,298,382,383). Such a factor may be involved in the dephosphorylation-inactivation mechanisms reported by Aurrichio et al. (20). Under conditions of continuous exposure of the animal to estrogen, progesterone causes a temporary reduction of nuclear estrogen-receptor complexes, which is followed by a return to elevated levels (381). The involvement of the control of estrogen receptor levels by progesterone, as well as other proposed antagonistic functions of progesterone, is discussed in more detail in Antagonism of Hormone Action.

In the chick oviduct acute administration of progesterone to estrogen-stimulated chicks causes a preferential destruction of the Y form (K_d 1.0 nM) of the estrogen receptor and has no effect on the X form (K_d 0.1 nM) (331). This is accompanied by an interruption of ovalbumin gene expression. Since both X and Y forms of the receptor are thought to be necessary for estrogen action, it is possible that progesterone antagonizes estrogenic effects by this mechanism.

Non-Receptor-Binding Proteins

In addition to steroid hormone receptors, there are several nonreceptor proteins that bind estrogen and progesterone. These are found in both cytosol and nuclear fractions.

Cytosol Non-Receptor-Binding Sites

The cytosol from immature rat uteri contains a proteinaceous macromolecule, which is observed when saturation analysis by [^{3}H]estradiol exchange is performed on uterine cytosol obtained from immature rats. These type II estrogen binding sites have a 4S sedimentation coefficient on post-labeled sucrose density gradients, and unlike the estrogen receptor, they do not appear to undergo translocation to the nucleus (75,117). That is, an injection of estradiol that causes cytoplasmic depletion and concomitant nuclear accumulation of the estrogen receptor does not deplete type II sites from the cytosol. Type II sites have a somewhat lower affinity ($K_d \sim$ 20 nM) than the receptor ($K_d \sim$ 1 nM) but the number of sites may greatly exceed type I sites. Type II sites display stereospecificity for estrogenic compounds and are present in other estrogen targets such as the vagina (75), mouse (562), and human mammary tumors (397), in MCF-7 cells (334), rabbit endometrial cells (365), and Mullerian ducts of the chick embryo (299). Similar secondary binding sites have been observed in the prostate (109,507), seminal vesicle (565), and rabbit corpus luteum (589). Thus, the presence of secondary binding sites for estrogenic hormones appears to be a general phenomenon.

Although the function of cytosol type II sites is not known, their presence complicates the interpretation of receptor assays. The quantity of these sites varies with many factors and may range from two to 10 times the quantity of estrogen receptor. The influence of these kinds of variation on the determination of the type I receptor can be significant. As the quantity of type II sites increases, the error introduced in the estimation of the K_d and the number of type I sites progressively increases. This only becomes apparent when saturation analysis is run over a wide range of hormone concentrations. Consequently, assays that are limited to a single concentration of hormone (1–10 nM) will measure both sites and may lead to overestimates of the affinity and numbers of type I sites. These points have been discussed in detail by Clark and Peck (82).

A steroid-binding protein that is somewhat similar to cytosol type II sites has been reported from the chick oviduct (529). This protein, which is called the Z protein, does not display stereospecificity for estrogen, but instead, binds estrogens, progestins, and androgens with similar affinities. Therefore, the Z protein is different from cytosol type II sites; however, it is similar in that it does not undergo translocation to the nucleus and has approximately the same affinity for estradiol (K_d 20 nM). Also the Z protein is in excess ($\sim$ 15-fold) of the estrogen receptor in the oviduct cytosol (440).

The relationship of the Z protein to steroid receptor is unknown; however, they do have certain characteristics in common. These include a sedimentation coefficient of ~8S, tissue specificity, stabilization by molybdate, and similar chromatographic behavior on diethylaminoethyl (DEAE) cellulose (440,529). Thus, it is possible that this protein may be a precursor of other sex steroid receptors in the oviduct (529). It is also possible that the Z protein could act as a general mechanism for concentrating steroids in oviduct tissue. This function has also been suggested for type II sites (82). However, currently it is thought that type II sites are more likely involved in binding an endogenous ligand that is involved in the control of cell proliferation (see Physiological Estrogen Antagonists for discussion of this point).

Nuclear Type II Estradiol-Binding Sites

In addition to nuclear bound estrogen receptor (type I sites), a second estrogen-binding site is found in nuclei of various tissues. These are called nuclear type II estradiol-binding sites and are located on the nuclear matrix (78,116,304). The relationship between cytosol and nuclear type II sites is not known; however, as explained above, cytosol type II sites do not appear to undergo nuclear translocation and therefore the cytosol and nuclear forms may be separate forms of related macromolecules. Nuclear type II sites are specific for estrogenic molecules and are elevated by estrogen treatment (309,310).

Nuclear type II sites appear to bind estrogen in a cooperative manner and display a sigmoid saturation curve. Figure 8 shows an example of this type of curve and its relationship to the type of curve obtained with the estrogen receptor (type I). Type I sites display the usual saturation curve, which has the shape of a rectangular hyperbola and can be analyzed by a Scatchard plot to yield a linear component. Nuclear type II sites, however, have a more complex binding function, which is sigmoidal and curvilinear by saturation and Scatchard analysis, respectively (Fig. 8A and B). Complex curves such as these are difficult to resolve into their individual components: however, we have observed that dithiothreitol (DTT) exposure causes the disap-

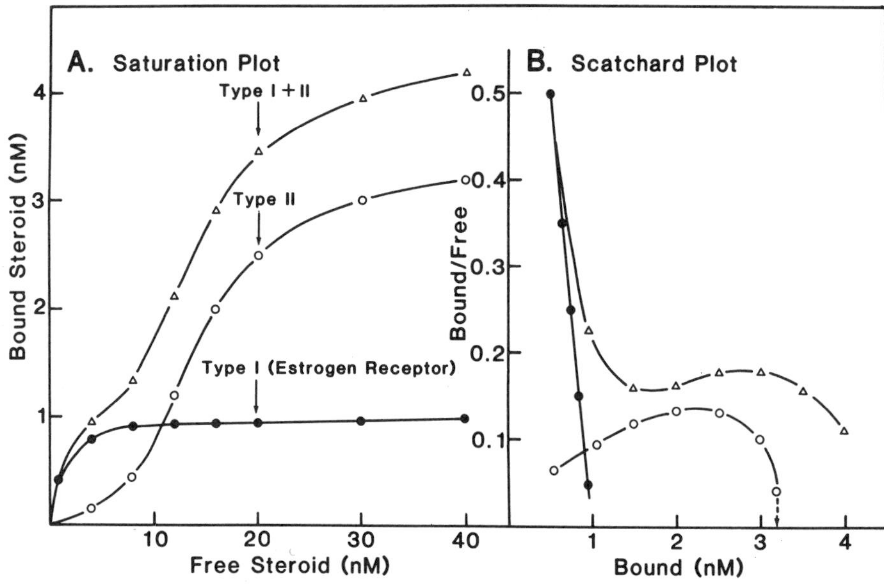

FIG. 8. Saturation and Scatchard analyses of type I and II binding sites. △, Total specific binding; ●, binding due to type I site (estrogen receptor); ○, specific binding due to type II sites; *arrow* in B indicates number of type II sites.

pearance of type II sites and permits the independent measurement of the estrogen receptor (308).

The physiological role of nuclear type II sites and their relationship to cytosol type II sites is discussed in Physiological Estrogen Antagonists.

CONTROL OF GENE EXPRESSION AND GROWTH

Estrogen and progesterone stimulate many biosynthetic events in their respective target organs. As discussed at the beginning of this chapter, early work by several investigators suggested that ovarian steroids stimulated RNA and protein synthesis in the uterus and chick oviduct. This stimulation of biosynthetic events that leads to changes in cell function and proliferation is thought to involve the interactions of receptor hormone complexes with the genome. The purpose of this section is to discuss these interactions and to present the more recent work on the control of gene expression and growth by ovarian steroids.

Hormone Effects on Protein and mRNA Synthesis

Studies in the 1960s revealed that all major RNA fractions were stimulated by steroid hormones (for reviews see 172,385). These observations cast some doubt on the specificity of the role of new RNA molecules. The early evidence favoring mRNA accumulation as the mechanism for regulating protein synthesis was based on general observations such as hormonal stimulation of nuclear RNA polymerase activity and inhibition of steroid effects on protein synthesis by the RNA synthesis inhibitor actinomycin D. The concept was stimulated further by "nearest-neighbor analysis" (dinucleotide composition analysis) of RNA synthesized from the chromatin template isolated from tissues prior to and following sex steroid hormone administration, which showed a qualitative hormone-mediated change in nuclear gene transcription (385). The advent of DNA-RNA hybridization technology permitted the demonstration that estrogen or progesterone stimulated the production of new species of nuclear hybridizable RNA and strongly suggested that steroid hormones could exert a qualitative influence on the transcription of eukaryotic DNA.

Regulation of mRNA Levels

The initial indication that steroid hormones lead to elevated cellular mRNA levels was the result of several studies in the chicken oviduct where cellular RNA was isolated and mRNA was translated on heterologous reticulocyte ribosomes *in vitro*. In these studies the synthesis of radiolabeled ovalbumin was shown to be dependent on prior administration of estrogen (281,330,332,428). Following purification of the ovalbumin mRNA to near homogeneity, a radioactive complementary DNA (cDNA) probe was synthesized using reversed transcriptase and employed in hybridization studies to accurately quantify the number of ovalbumin mRNA molecules per cell (175). These results showed that in the absence of hormone oviduct cells contained less than five copies of ovalbumin mRNA, whereas within 4 hr following stimulation with sex steroid hormone (DES) the mRNA reached levels greater than 2,000 molecules/cell. By 24 hr the level approached 20,000 molecules/cell. The accumulation curves were consistent with an effect of steroid hormones on ovalbumin gene transcription.

Effects on the Rate of mRNA Synthesis

Although these and other results were consistent with the primary effect of steroid hormones being at the level of gene transcription, it could be argued that the rate of transcription remains relatively constant during induction and that the accumulation of mRNA is due simply to the prevention of RNA degradation by steroid hormone. In fact, evidence exists that in certain cases sex steroid hormones can indeed decrease the turnover rate of mRNA. Definitive answers to these questions required synthetic analyses of pulse-labeled RNA obtained in "nuclear run-off assays."

In studies using the chick oviduct, nuclei were obtained prior to and following hormonal stimulation of target cells. The nuclei were incubated with radioactive precursors to RNA, and the labeled RNA was hybridized to cloned ovalbumin cDNA or natural gene fragments. In the absence of hormone, no detectable synthesis of radiolabeled mRNA was detected, but within 1 hr following the exposure of cells to steroid hormones, an induction of synthesis was observed. Under these conditions, an accurate assessment of the rate of mRNA synthesis could be obtained (281,508). In the rat uterus, estradiol also increases the amount of mRNA for glucose-α-phosphate dehydrogenase and also increases the rate of translation of the mRNA (25).

The accumulation of mRNA is due to increased rates of synthesis as well as decreased rates of turnover. For example, the induction of ovalbumin and vitellogenin by estrogens is due to synthesis and stabilization of mRNA coding for these proteins (23,123,394,395,461,463). Hormonal stabilization of milk protein mRNA also occurs in the mammary gland (167,186).

It should be noted, however, that all steroid hormone responses at the level of DNA may not be inductive. For example, evidence exists that the action of estrogen in pituitary cells on mRNA for gonadotropins may be depressive, that is to say, transcription of specific mRNAs may be decreased in the presence of hormone (4).

Regulatory Elements and Transcriptional Control

During the course of transcription of eukaryotic genes, RNA polymerase must initiate and terminate at specific sites on DNA. The initiation reaction requires the formation of a tightly bound complex between RNA polymerase and DNA at a site that surrounds the first base to be transcribed into RNA. The complete sequence of DNA that is necessary for the formation of this initiation complex is called the promoter. The promoter appears to act as a thermostat to regulate the rate and accuracy of transcription. Additional regulatory elements may be located adjacent to the promoter region and may act as activators to turn on (or turn off) functional promoters. Hormone control elements are one example of this latter class of regulators (50,90,329,330).

Promoters

The basic promoter for eukaryotic genes transcribed by RNA polymerase II appears to consist of at least two main parts (Fig. 9). Beginning at −32 nucleotides (32 bases upstream) prior to the start site of transcription is a 7-base-pair (bp) AT-rich sequence called the "TATA" or "Hogness box." A consensus sequence for all TATA boxes can be described as T A T A T/A A. The TATA box may contain either an A or a T in positions 5 and 7 but in only a minority of cases is a GC pair present within the box. This sequence seems to be primarily concerned with directing accurate initiation at nucleotide +1 of the structural gene. Changing only one interior nucleotide pair within the sequence to a GC residue is sufficient to eliminate 80% of the appropriate transcription from that gene (90).

Further upstream (to the left) of the structural gene there is an additional sequence within the promoter that has been conserved in many instances. The sequence lies at approximately −75 nucleotides from the gene itself and has a consensus sequence of G G C/T C A A T C T. This sequence is commonly referred to as a CAAT box and is thought to be important in modifying the basal *rate* of transcription as determined for a given promoter (21,329).

Hormone Control

Control of the rate of gene transcription is of ultimate importance to the eukaryotic cell. Following differentiation, it is not only important to have cell specific expression of genetic information, but also to have the appropriate intracellular concentration of a protein required for maintenance of the physiological state of an organism. Since the levels of intracellular proteins are dependent usually on the intracellular concentration of their messenger RNAs, and since messenger RNA concentration appears to be controlled primarily at the level of gene transcription, it is likely that regulatable genes have an additional DNA sequence that is required for inductive (or perhaps suppressive) regulation of gene expression. The existence of such regulatory elements has been demonstrated in three steroid hormone regulatable systems.

The first of these systems involves the regulation of the rate of transcription of MMTV DNA by glucocorticoids such as dexamethasone (159,403). The initiation and regulatory regions for this gene exist in a long terminal repeat (LTR) sequence that exists at the 5′ side of the gene. Hormonal regulation of this gene by glucocorticoids is maintained when cloned DNA fragments containing the MMTV LTR are introduced into cultured cells by transfection methods. The transfection technique involves (a) the incubation of cloned genes with cultured cells, (b) the short-term uptake of such DNA into cells, and (c) the transient transcription of these test genes without their being integrated into the cellular genome. The simplicity of this technique allows the rapid analysis of a series of "modified" genes in which portions of the regulatory element have been deleted or perhaps moved to other locations relative to the gene. In such studies, glucocorticoids have been shown to stimulate transcriptional initiation within mammary tumor virus DNA sequences present in the infected cells. It was concluded that the MMTV promoter region (LTR) contains a "glucocorticoid response element" that can be separated from a second element (the promoter) essential for MMTV transcription initiation. The hormone response element was mapped to within a 340-bp MMTV DNA fragment that also contained specific binding sites for purified glucocorticoid receptor protein *in vitro*. Comparison of several different recombinant constructions indicated that the location and orientation of the glucocorticoid response element relative to the transcription start site was not rigidly constrained. Importantly, the capacity of the glucocorticoid response element to function independently of stringent spacing and orientation requirements implied that the mechanism by which this element acts, presumably in conjunction with a bound hormone receptor complex, might not involve direct interaction with RNA polymerase II or other components in the basal promoter region.

Similar studies have been done with the regulation of the chicken ovalbumin gene or lysozyme gene by steroid hormones (97,424). In contrast to the MMTV system described above, the regulatable expression of these genes is markedly cell specific. These experiments have involved construction of a "fusion gene" which is composed of a structural gene such as that for globin or a viral gene fused to the 5′ regulatory elements and first few nucleotides of the ovalbumin gene. This gene can respond to steroid hormones after transfection into homologous oviduct cells in culture. Studies of a series of recombinant genes that have successively greater portions of the 5′ flanking region deleted indicate that sequences located between −220 and −100 upstream from the gene are required for hormonal induction of gene expression. The results demonstrate that the hormone regulatory region and the basal promoter for the ovalbumin gene are distinct sequences with no obvious overlap. Similar results were obtained when the 5′ flanking region of a lysozyme fusion gene was subjected to deletion analysis, and again indicated the presence of an estrogen control element upstream (between −220 and −100) from the lysozyme gene. Results of these studies are in good agreement with the results for glucocorticoid induction of the MMTV gene.

The relative locations of the hormone control site and the promoter site for the chicken ovalbumin gene are displayed in Fig. 9. The promoter is composed of two major parts and is located within the 100-bp region immediately adjacent to the gene itself. The so-called CAAT box is located at about −75 and the TATA box at about −32 bp upstream from the gene. The hormone control site is located within the region −220 and −100 bp nucleotides upstream from the gene. Although less well defined, this control region also appears to be composed of two parts. The receptor-binding site is located at about −195 to −150 bp from the gene. Also at about −140 bp from the gene, a conserved 9-nucleotide sequence has been observed to exist at a similar location for all six steroid hormone regulatable genes of the chicken but has not been found to be present in the case of four nonregulatable genes (Fig. 9). This association is statistically significant but its precise role remains to be elucidated.

An additional question can be raised as to the mechanism by which more than one steroid hormone can activate the same structural gene. Again, the ovalbumin gene provides a suitable model to define such a phenomenon since the ovalbumin gene can be regulated by three steroid hormones, namely, progesterone, estrogen, and glucocorticoid (86, 327,445,544). Using the identical set of gene deletions described above, it was found that removal of sequences in the region of −220 to −100 bp leads to a simultaneous diminished response to all three hormones.

Nucleotide sequences that bind glucocorticoid and progesterone receptors have been described in the mouse mammary tumor virus and chicken lysozyme genes (403,552). These sequences occur in the same location of the 5′ flanking region of the ovalbumin gene, and it has been suggested that these three genes, as well as other steroid hormone-inducible genes, contain a common nucleotide sequence that recognizes progesterone, glucocorticoid, androgen, and estrogen receptors (552). Since egg white protein genes are induced *in vivo* by these four hormones and this induction appears to be mediated by four separate receptors, it is possible that each of the four steroid-receptor complexes is recognized by the same nucleotide sequence (346,552). Even though such commonality of binding may be associated with receptor-mediated transcriptional activity, it should be noted that progesterone does not induce MMTV genes, yet the

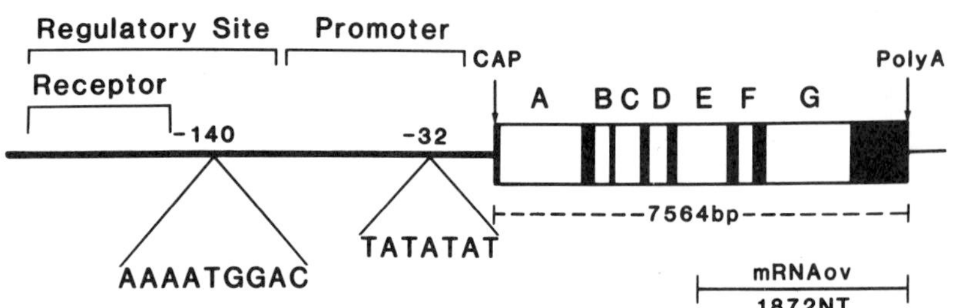

FIG. 9. Transcriptional control regions of the ovalbumin gene of chicken.

progesterone receptor binds to the same nucleotide sequence as does the glucocorticoid receptor (552).

Organization of Chromosomes and Genes

The human cell contains ~ 3×10^9 bp of DNA and contains information for approximately 1 to 2×10^5 functional genes. This extraordinary length of DNA must fit into the nucleus of a cell whose diameter may be only 6 μm. In addition, the majority (90%) of the DNA in most cells is not called into action for cellular functions. For these reasons, it seems logical to package the majority of the DNA into inaccessible higher-order chromosomal structures such that the length of the DNA is greatly reduced. Genes and segments of DNA that will be expressed in the lifetime of a given cell must obviously be in a different and more accessible structure (261,567).

Higher-Order Structure

The primary structural interaction for the formation of eukaryotic chromosomes is that between histone and DNA (248,273). There are five basic histones (H1, H2A, H2B, H3, and H4). All the histones except H1 interact directly with DNA to form a first-level organization of particles in chromatin. This basic level of organization of chromatin is the histone octamer, which in combination with about 200 bp of DNA forms a beadlike structure (nucleosomes) along the DNA, which increases the fiber width to 10 nm and now creates a length compaction ratio of 6. The DNA is wound around the outside of the core histone particles and may be available to interact with regulatory proteins or RNA polymerase. This nucleosomal level of organization is now supercoiled upon itself like a giant "slinky" into a structure referred to as a "solenoid" (324). H1 histone plays a role in linking the nucleosomal strands to produce the solenoid. The fiber now becomes thicker (30 nm) and the compaction ratio reaches approximately 40. The final structural organization of chromatin is not well understood but probably it involves a further supercoiling of the solenoid so that one achieves a final compaction ratio of approximately 1,000 in interphase chromosomes. The mitotic chromosomes are packaged even more tightly to a compaction ratio of approximately 10,000.

The second group of important proteins that are involved in chromosomal organization are the nonhistone proteins (324,566). There are many different species of nonhistone proteins, perhaps more than 500. They contain all of the proteins necessary for replicating and transcribing DNA and enzymes that are involved in structural and covalent modifications or degradations. Most important, however, are the regulatory proteins that play a role in determining the appropriate structures for gene expression, or in aiding or retarding the initiation of transcription. As discussed in Nuclear Binding of Receptor-Hormone Complexes, nonhistone proteins have been suggested to be acceptor sites for receptor-hormone complexes (495).

Active Domains in Chromosomes

Steroid hormones increase the chromatin template activity of target cell nuclei, and the suggestion was made by many investigators that steroid hormones modified chromatin structure to allow a preferential activation of genes that code for ovalbumin and other egg white proteins (reviewed in 386). More recent studies have firmly established that expressible genes are packaged into chromatin differently when compared to regions of the DNA that are genetically repressed (275,566). In particular, genes that are transcriptionally active, or that have the potential for rapid expression in response to appropriate inducers, have been shown to exhibit a preferential susceptibility to cleavage by nucleases.

The ovalbumin gene, as well as genes coding for other egg white proteins, becomes highly susceptible to digestion by DNase I in oviduct nuclei, but not in nuclei from other tissues (35,140,395,464,566). After estrogen and progesterone treatment the ovalbumin gene becomes nuclease sensitive, whereas prior to hormone exposure this gene exists in a nuclease insensitive conformation (41,42,549). This observation by Anderson et al. (17) that the rapidly transcribed ovalbumin gene in hen oviduct nuclei is cleaved selectively by micrococcal nuclease, whereas the transcriptionally inactive sequences adjacent to this gene are not, suggests that the chromosomal state attacked by this enzyme is related to the transcriptional rate in the oviduct system. Such studies further suggest that the transcribed ovalbumin gene is packaged into a hormone-dependent subdomain of chromatin structure (for a review see 10).

The exact relationship between the nuclease-sensitive regions of chromatin described above and the mechanisms of ovarian steroid action is not understood. However, nuclease treatment does result in the release of nucleosomes that are associated with receptor-estrogen complexes (319,462,465). Receptor-associated nucleosomes containing transcribed genes are preferentially excised from chromatin during mild digestion of nuclei with micrococcal nuclease, and the kinetics of this release are similar to the release of mononucleosomes containing transcribed gene (41,42).

The quantitative relationships between nuclear estrogen-receptor binding and nuclease-sensitive sites have been examined in the rat uterus (453). Following an injection of estradiol, which is sufficient to cause nuclear accumulation of all receptors, only 30% of the receptors are solubilized by nuclease digestion. This finding suggests that only a fraction of the receptors that accumulate in the nucleus are associated with active chromatin sites; the remainder may associate with other non-chromatin-binding sites. The quantity of nuclease-sensitive receptor sites shows a relatively small decrease during the first 12 hr after injection of estradiol. This pattern of nuclear binding corresponds to the quantitative and temporal relationships between salt-resistant nuclear bound receptors that have been correlated with true uterine growth (81,82).

DNase I sensitivity appears to reflect a region of more accessible chromatin structure that in turn relates to the developmental capacity of a cell to express the gene in question. It can be viewed as a necessary but not wholly sufficient step in the prior commitment of the cell to allow a certain gene to be transcribed. Such a mechanism would make it possible for distinct cell types to respond to a single inducer each in its own individual and distinctive manner. In other words, all genes that are ever to be transcribed in a given cell must be contained within these accessible regions of chromatin at the time of terminal differentiation. The chromosomal domains appear to be related to molecular differentiation since they are not only tissue-specific but irreversible. Once included in this "expressible" domain, genes would be accessible then to regulatory factors such as hormone-receptor complexes. The DNA that is not contained in these domains appears to be passively packaged into a more complex chromatin structure by histones. The DNA in such higher-order structures, the majority of DNA in each cell type, would be unavailable for interactions with regulatory molecules.

Nuclear Matrix

Finally, it is appropriate to conclude a discussion of higher-order structure by consideration of an even more complex structural interaction of cellular genes and genomic domains with the nuclear matrix (32). The nuclear matrix is a dense fibrillar network of proteins that contains a residual nucleolus and lies within the nuclear membrane. This structure acts as a nuclear skeleton and may form a continuous communication network with the cytoskeleton proteins. The structure of the matrix fibrils is not yet understood, although we do know that it is rather complex since it is composed of a large number of different proteins. The chromatin itself is intermittently attached to the nuclear matrix, and it is likely that the primary RNA transcripts of genes become attached soon after or even during their transcription. Evidence exists that RNA processing and DNA replication also may take place on the matrix (67,208,303,398,429,482,551).

The nuclear matrix is prepared by repeated high-salt (2 N NaCl) extraction of nuclei. Approximately 10 to 15% of the nuclear protein remains. This virtually strips the nucleus of all histone and a great deal of the loosely bound non-histone protein. This preparation has been analyzed by investigators using electron microscopy and sedimentation analysis. The dehistonized and uncoiled DNA is attached to the residual protein matrix in short regions interspersed with unattached "loops" of DNA that are an average size of 30 to 100 kilobases (kb) in length. If the dehistonized unattached DNA present in the loops is digested with a site-specific restriction endonuclease, 85% of the DNA can be released from the preparation. The residual matrix-bound DNA, representing 15% of the total, can be purified and analyzed for the presence of specific sequences.

In the chicken, it has been shown that actively transcribed genes are firmly bound to the proteinaceous nuclear matrix (67,429). All genes not expressed are found in the released DNA fraction after restriction enzyme treatment, since they are not attached to the matrix. During hormone stimulation the ovalbumin gene is attached to the nuclear matrix, and when the hormone is withdrawn from the tissue and ovalbumin gene transcription ceases, the gene is no longer found attached to the matrix. Constitutively expressed genes are always attached to the matrix, and the attachment is independent of the absolute rate of transcription. This close relationship between the transcription of genes and their association with the nuclear matrix indicate that the nuclear matrix is a likely site for cellular DNA transcription. This conclusion is consistent with the idea that the nucleus is a highly organized organelle and that transcription does not occur free in solution to the eukaryotic nucleus but rather on a fixed protein skeleton. Such attachment to the matrix could either facilitate transcription of DNA by RNA polymerase or could constitute an obligatory interaction that is necessary for transcription. Cessation of transcription in the presence of actinomycin D does not itself lead to release of genes from the matrix.

As explained in Nuclear Binding of Receptor-Hormone Complexes, steroid hormone receptors have been found associated with the nuclear matrix (31,32,477,478). Upon hormonal withdrawal, the cellular receptors are no longer associated with the nuclear matrix. When the nuclear matrix is prepared by first exposing nuclei to DNase I and then to high salt extraction, no preferential binding of receptors to the matrix is observed (56). These results suggest that DNase I treatment has destroyed the active DNA associated with the matrix and as a consequence also eliminated the acceptor-like properties of the matrix. In addition Buttyan et al. (56) showed that DNA extracted from the matrix was an effective competitor for receptor binding to DNA cellulose, suggesting that matrix-bound DNA is a component of the matrix-acceptor complex. Type II estrogen binding sites are also localized on the nuclear matrix (78,109,477,478,507). Since the elevation of nuclear type II sites is observed in tissues undergoing hypertrophy and hyperplasia, it is possible that these sites are also involved in matrix-bound biosynthetic machinery involved in DNA and RNA synthesis (see section on physiological estrogen antagonists for more discussion of this point). Estrogen also stimulates the association of calmodulin and myosin light chain kinase with the nuclear matrix of chicken liver (478). These associations with the nuclear matrix suggest that such interactions may be important in the control of hormone-induced gene transcription.

Structural Requirements for Gene Expression

In conclusion, it is fair to speculate that the cellular forces involved in steroid hormone induction of transcription are complex indeed, but appear to involve the following interactions:

1. The steroid receptor binds to chromatin proteins and DNA and is the obligatory and active intermediate required for steroid hormone action. It acts as a transducer to transfer the informational signal inherent in a steroid hormone molecule to the regulatable gene. It is likely that hormone receptors are only members of a larger, and as yet undefined, class of nuclear regulatory proteins.
2. The primary sequence of the gene itself is of obvious importance since it not only contains the inherited structural code for the protein, but it appears to contain distinct "promoter" and "regulatory" elements, the latter of which both binds receptor and determines the maximal rate of hormone-induced gene expression.
3. Inducible genes are contained within large, structurally distinct (DNAse-I-sensitive) domains that are an index of molecular differentiation and that are likely to maintain the capacity of genes to respond to inductive influences.
4. The chromatin itself undergoes a specific attachment to the nuclear matrix so that the actively expressed regions of these domains appear to be more firmly bound, and perhaps more easily transcribed by the nuclear transcriptive apparatus. Matrix-bound estrogen-binding sites may be involved in the specific attachment of expressed genes or in interactions that stimulate their transcription.

Hormone-Induced Response Patterns and Cellular Growth

In the preceding section of this chapter the mechanism of action of ovarian steroids has been discussed from the molecular biological or reductionist approach. It is clear from the work of many investigators that these hormones have a multiplicity of effects, not all of which may be mediated by genomic interactions. In addition, the biological responses of a target organ to an ovarian hormone involve interactions at many levels of biological organization. The purpose of this section is to present a more integrated synthesis of the existing data on these complex interactions.

Early and Late Responses

Many hormones induce responses that occur within minutes after hormone exposure (82). The relationship between these early responses and later events that culminate in cellular hypertrophy and hyperplasia (true growth) has received considerable study. Uterotropic responses to estrogen will be used as an example of such relationships. Other growth-promoting hormones also stimulate similar pleiotropic response patterns and these have been reviewed by Tata (522).

Uterotropic responses to estrogen can be classified according to their time of appearance and functional relationship (Tables 1 and 2). Early responses include both biosynthetic and metabolic activities. The relationship between these events can be visualized in the following way. Hyperemia, calcium influx, histamine release, eosinophil infiltration, increased RNA and protein precursor uptake, and enhanced glucose oxidation are due to the ability of estrogen to mobilize many physiological functions in order to optimize biosynthetic activity. Early responses also include increased RNA and protein synthesis, which are components of the biosynthetic machinery that eventually causes the uterus to grow. However, as discussed below, the stimulation of these biosynthetic events is not necessarily obligatory in the stimulation of uterine growth. Late responses, some of which are simply extensions of those which were begun during the early period, include increased and sustained RNA and protein synthesis. This biosynthetic activity results in cellular hypertrophy and eventual DNA synthesis and hyperplasia. These late responses are considered to be true growth responses of the uterus. Obviously true growth would occur most readily in an environment in which substrate availability has been optimized. This environment is provided by the increased blood flow and other supportive events that are listed in Tables 1 and 2.

Very rapid elevations in cyclic AMP levels have been reported following estrogen treament in the uterus, and it has been suggested that cyclic AMP is a mediator of estradiol effects (512,513). Other investigators have not confirmed this effect, and it remains to be shown that activation of adenylate cyclase is involved in estrogen action (259,592). Several investigators have demonstrated that estrogen treatment *in vivo* and *in vitro* stimulates cyclic GMP accumulation in the rat uterus (128,129,262). This response appears to depend on RNA and protein synthesis, since it can be blocked by cycloheximide and actinomycin D administration (130,131,375). Szego (511) has suggested that estrogen causes nuclear accumulation of lysosomes and that enzymes that are released into the nucleus control gene activity. Because of the uncertain role of lysosomes in the mechanism of hormone action, they have been included in both categories of early responses. Tchernitchin and Tchernitchin (533) have suggested that estrogen causes eosinophils to be attracted to uterine capillaries where they migrate into the extracellular spaces of the uterus. The eosinophils then release hydrolytic enzymes that depolymerize the uterine ground substance (534). Eosinophils may also cause mast cells to release histamine, and this, coupled with the hydrolysis of mucopolysaccharides, increases vascular permeability and creates an osmotic environment that favors water inhibition and precursor uptake.

It has been suggested that some of these early events are involved in the primary mechanism of action of estrogen.

TABLE 1. *Early uterotropic responses*

Supportive or metabolic	Refs.
Hyperemia	132,294,300,311,312
Histamine mobilization	467,510
Eosinophil infiltration	530,531
Water imbibition	19,516
Albumin accumulation	226,491
Increased electrolytes	226,493
Lysosome labilization	511
Increased cyclic nucleotides, prostaglandins, and associated enzyme activation	130,131,168,262,512
Increased glucose metabolism and associated enzyme activity	348,516
Increased uptake of RNA	181,333
Calcium influx	410
Ornithine decarboxylase	51,434,442
Biosynthetic	
Increased lipid synthesis	2
Increased activity of RNA	145,148,173
Synthesis of the induced protein (IP) and its mRNA	27,98,233
Increased synthesis of glucose-6-phosphate dehydrogenase	483
Increased chromatin template activity and RNA polymerase initiation sites	26,145,305
Increased synthesis of histone and nonhistone proteins	24,145

Spaziani and Szego (492,493) and Szego and Lawson (514) have suggested that uterine growth is mediated by estrogen-induced histamine release that causes increased capillary permeability and hyperemia. Although these events undoubtedly maximize the ability of the uterus to grow, most investigators do not consider them as primary events. Eosinophil infiltration and its attendant responses can be blocked with glucocorticoids without having any significant effect on DNA, RNA, and protein synthesis in the uterus (532,534). Early uterotropic responses can be included by estradiol in rats pretreated with nafoxidine, an antiestrogen that blocks late responses; however, no stimulation of late responses is observed (135,139). Zor et al. (592) showed the estrogen-induced uterine growth was independent of cyclic AMP, prostaglandins and β-adrenergic mediation. Even the estrogen-induced elevation in the activity of ornithine decarboxylase, an enzyme assumed to be involved in cell proliferation, can be blocked and estrogen-induced uterine growth still takes place (434).

TABLE 2. *Late uterotropic responses*

Supportive or metabolic	
Many of the functions that are listed in Table 1 continue for many hours after estrogen administration.	
Biosynthetic	Refs.
Increased general and specific protein and RNA synthesis	2,25,250,483
Continued stimulation of RNA polymerase activity	145,173
DNA synthesis and mitosis	2,114,174
Cellular hypertrophy and hyperplasia	7,8,184
Increased synthesis or changes in histone and nonhistone proteins	24,145

Additional evidence that these early events are not the primary ones involved in stimulating true uterine growth comes from the observation that estriol and other short-acting estrogens do not cause true uterine growth after a single injection (16,82,174,270). Estriol causes transient nuclear binding of the estrogen receptor and stimulates all the early uterotropic responses; however, it fails to stimulate uterine hyperplasia and growth. Estriol apparently fails in this regard because it does not maintain the estrogen receptor in an occupied state for a sufficient length of time, and as a consequence, it does not maintain the necessary biosynthetic events (late responses) that culminate in cell proliferation and growth.

From the above results it is concluded that early uterotropic responses are supportive, but are not obligatory for the stimulation of uterine hypertrophy and hyperplasia. Also, it is likely that separate regulatory mechanisms are involved in the control of some early and late events in the rat uterus (136,139,534,535).

The sustained stimulation of RNA and protein synthesis that ultimately culminates in cell proliferation appears to depend on the nuclear occupancy by 10 to 20% of estrogen receptors for longer than 4 to 6 hr (12,16,82,270). This long-term nuclear occupancy of receptor is correlated with elevations in total cellular RNA, sustained RNA polymerase I and II activity, sustained chromatin template activity, DNA synthesis, and cellular growth (see Table 2 for references).

Sustained levels of estrogen are required for mRNA stability and continued synthesis of several proteins (23,123,167, 186,394,395,461,463,509). Long-term nuclear occupancy of estrogen receptors is also associated with an elevation of nuclear type II estrogen binding sites, which is correlated with the late uterotropic growth responses (304,308–310).

These results suggest that a sustained occupancy of estrogen receptors is required for the complete sequence of events that ultimately produce uterine hypertrophy and hyperplasia. Therefore the examination of initial binding interactions of hormone-receptor complexes with acceptor sites may give only a limited amount of information concerning the full sequence of events necessary to elicit growth responses. Also the number of receptor-acceptor sites appears to be small and involves only 10 to 20% of the total number of receptors available. This observation will also eventually have to be integrated into the overall scheme of binding and response studies done at the molecular level.

Direct and Indirect Actions of Ovarian Steroids

In addition to the direct hormone-receptor pathway that leads to changes in cellular function and proliferation, indirect pathways have been suggested to account for some of the actions of ovarian steroids.

In vivo *studies.* Kirkland et al. (246) and Sonnenschein and Soto (488) proposed that a factor from the pituitary was necessary to obtain a full growth response of the oviduct and uterus. In their experiments a single injection of estradiol failed to stimulate the complete growth response in the absence of the pituitary. However, Huggins and Jensen (199) showed that a full uterotropic response could be obtained in hypophysectomized rats if estradiol was given for several days. Therefore, it seems that the pituitary plays a permissive role, probably because growth hormone and perhaps other pituitary hormones are required to maintain the integrity of the metabolic machinery necessary to maximize response to a single estrogen injection. Other experiments that make it unlikely that pituitary factors or other extrauterine factors are involved include the stimulation of epithelial proliferation following direct local application of estrogen to the vagina (430). These and other experiments involving direct applications to target organs will be discussed below.

It has also been proposed that the liver responds to estrogen and acts as an intermediary in the stimulation of the quail oviduct (271). In these experiments estradiol was infused into the hepatoportal circulation and was completely metabolized by the liver. Under these circumstances no estrogen receptor accumulation by oviduct nuclei was observed, yet the DNA content of the oviduct was elevated to the same extent as in animals receiving systemic treatment with estradiol. Although these are interesting findings, the same investigators did not observe a similar liver-mediated effect on the rat uterus (451). Therefore, the general applicability of this liver-mediated effect is questionable.

Sirbasku and Benson (480) have proposed that estrogens stimulate the synthesis of specific polypeptide growth factors that act as mitogens on estrogen-responsive cells. These growth factors are produced by the rat uterus and kidney and have been proposed to act in one of three ways: (a) as endocrine factors that are secreted into the circulation; (b) as paracrine factors that are produced by cells in close proximity to the target cell; and (c) as autocrine factors produced by the same cell in which they act (Fig. 10). Certainly there is evidence for a paracrine function of uterine stromal tissue on the epithelium of this organ (94). Whether these stromal-epithelial interactions involve specific factors remains to be determined. Also there is evidence that epidermal growth factor (EGF) and its receptor are present in the uterus of several species and in the mammary gland of the mouse (104,147,187,354). Although the physiological role of EGF in the uterus is not known, EGF is known to be mitogenic in many cell types (60,188). Perhaps EGF is similar to the growth factor purified from the uterus by Ikeda and Sirbasku (203) and may be involved in the autocrine or paracrine stimulation of cell proliferation in the uterus.

The stimulation of autocrine or paracrine factors by estradiol in the uterus seems much more likely to be of physiological significance than the stimulation of endocrine factors. As mentioned earlier, local application of estrogen to the vagina causes cellular proliferation and cornification. These experiments were first done by Robson and Adler (430), who surgically formed two separate vaginal sacs in mice. They placed small amounts of estradiol in one vaginal sac and observed typical epithelial proliferation and cornification. No estrogenic effect was observed in the nontreated vaginal sac. Thus, they concluded that estradiol was having a direct effect on the vaginal cells and not acting systemically in some indirect way. Several investigators have applied estradiol locally to the vagina and uterus and have drawn similar conclusions (36,37,111,121,247,316,499). Although these experiments rule out an endocrine or systemic effect of estradiol, they do not rule out cell-cell interactions (paracrine) or autocellular stimulation (autocrine). It seems likely that ovarian steroids act via cellular receptors to stimulate cellular growth directly as well as by elevating

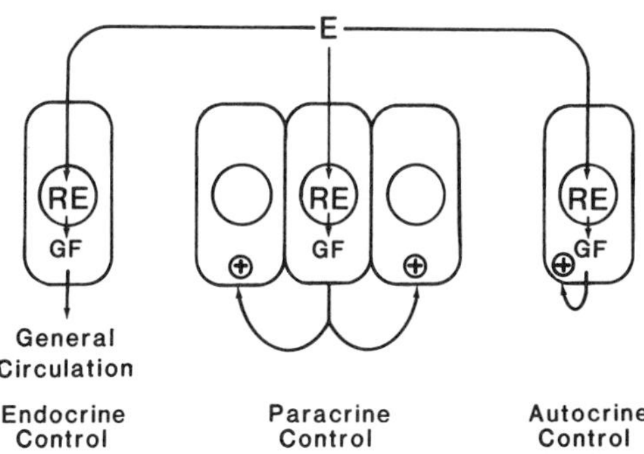

FIG. 10. Various indirect mechanisms by which estrogen can stimulate cell proliferation. Abbreviations: E, estrogen; RE, estrogen receptor complex; GF, growth factor.

the local production of growth factors which may act on surrounding cells or on the cell producing them.

In vitro *studies*. The question of direct effect of estrogen has been addressed by many investigators in cell culture systems. As an example, MCF-7 cells are dependent on estrogen for growth in athymic nude mice, but the estrogenic effects on cell proliferation in cell culture have not been consistently demonstrated (290,466,489,490,587). MCF-7 and normal epithelial cells will grow exponentially in defined serumless media and the addition of estradiol does not significantly alter this growth response (28,201,372,489). Sato and Sonnenschein (489) observed that the presence of serum in the culture medium inhibits cell proliferation and that estradiol overcomes this inhibition and stimulates cell proliferation. These authors believe that estradiol is acting indirectly by binding to a serum macromolecule that in its unoccupied state is an inhibitor of cell proliferation. From these observations Sato and Sonnenschein (489) concluded that estrogens are not directly mitogenic. However, it should be noted that placing isolated epithelial cells in a culture medium that maximizes their ability to proliferate may eliminate the need for estrogen as a mitogen. The inhibition of cell proliferation by serum may result from the presence of other types of inhibitors, such as the endogenous ligand for type II sites (306,307). This point is discussed further in Antagonism of Hormone Action. Also such cultures do not permit the normal cell-cell interactions that may take place *in vivo*. McGrath (325) demonstrated that estradiol did have a direct mitogenic effect on normal mammary epithelium when both epithelial and stromal cells were present in the culture system.

ANTAGONISM OF HORMONE ACTION

The subject of ovarian steroid hormone antagonism is very broad and complex; therefore, no attempt will be made in this section to present a comprehensive treatment of this subject (for reviews see 77,79,134,220). Instead, the salient features of hormone antagonism and their relationship to reproductive function will be presented.

Short-Acting Estrogen Antagonists

Short-acting estrogens are estrogenic compounds that display mixed agonist-antagonistic properties when they are injected in saline. Such a mixed estrogenic function results from the rapid clearance of these compounds from target tissues. In contrast, when short-acting estrogens are administered by pellet implant, which results in sustained blood and tissue levels, they act as full agonists.

Uterotropic Responses

Short-acting estrogens have the ability to stimulate early uterotropic responses while having little effect on true uterine growth when they are administered in saline by injection (Fig. 11, Table 1, and Hormone-Induced Response Patterns and Cellular Growth). This pattern of activity was first observed by Hisaw (184) for estriol and has been shown to occur for other estrogens such as dimethystilbestrol (DMS) and estradiol-17α (12,57,80,270). Early uterotropic responses are usually made by simply measuring the 4- to 6-hr gain in wet weight of the uteri, following an injection. This parameter is easy to measure and seems to reflect a multitude of complex events.

The activities of RNA polymerase I and II increase during early periods following an injection of either estradiol or estriol (Fig. 12) (173). However, estriol fails to sustain the stimulation of RNA polymerase I and to cause a secondary stimulation in RNA polymerase II, whereas estradiol maintains both of these parameters over long periods of time. A similar pattern of differences was also observed for RNA polymerase initiation sites (305). We concluded from these experiments that estriol is able to initiate the early biosynthetic events but is not able to maintain them; consequently, early uterotropic events are stimulated but late events are not.

Such a pattern of early stimulation followed by minimal

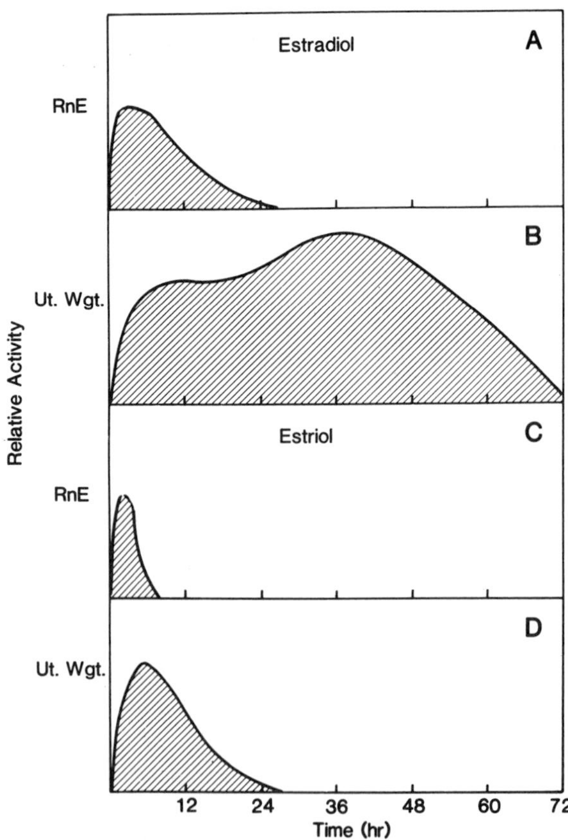

FIG. 11. Comparison of the effects of estradiol and estriol on the activities of RNA polymerase and template activity in the rat uterus. Animals were injected at time zero with 1 μg of estradiol or estriol.

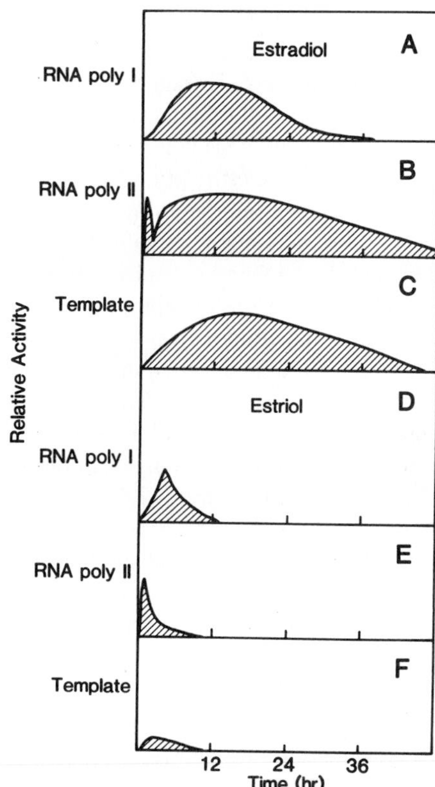

FIG. 12. Comparison of the effects of estradiol and estriol on the nuclear binding of the estrogen receptor and uterine weight. Animals were treated as in Fig. 11.

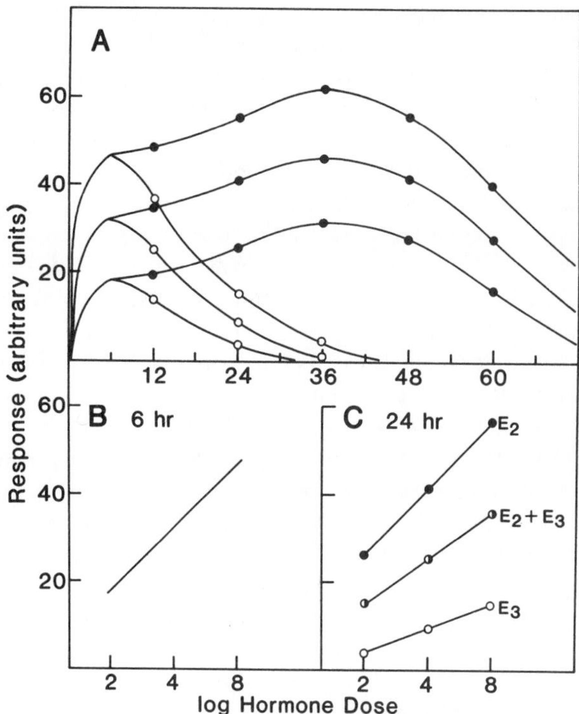

FIG. 13. The relationship between the uterotropic response and dose response curves obtained with estradiol (E_2, ● and estriol E_3, ○). See text for discussion.

to no long-term stimulation produces dose-response curves in the classical uterine growth assay that are attenuated and not similar to those obtained with estradiol (537). Uterine growth assays are usually done after 3 to 4 days of daily injections of the hormone and thus involve primarily the late uterotropic events. Under such conditions short-acting estrogens will not produce similar dose-response curves. However, during the first few hours after injection the dose-response curves for long- and short-acting estrogens will be identical. The point is examined further in Antagonistic Action of Short-Acting Estrogens and is shown in Fig. 13. Such differences in response pattern and intensity have often been ignored and have led to considerable confusion concerning relative potencies and biological activity. It should be noted that the differentiation of early and late responses depends on the administration of the hormone in saline or some vehicle that permits rapid absorption and dissemination. If oil is used as an injection vehicle, the hormone will be absorbed and cleared more slowly and hence will act as an intermediate to long-acting hormone. This probably explains the observation of Fagg and Martin (121) that estriol injected in oil will cause late uterotropic events such as DNA synthesis and cell division with half the effectiveness of estradiol (see Antagonistic Action of Short-Acting Estrogens for further discussion).

Receptor Interactions and Uterotropic Responses

Short-acting estrogens, such as estriol and DMS, bind to the cytosol form of the estrogen receptor with an affinity that is similar to or slightly less than estradiol (K_d 1–10 nM) (15,257). Therefore, it is possible that if they formed a receptor complex that did not undergo nuclear binding they would act as estradiol antagonists. This does not appear to be the case, since it has been shown by many investigators that short-acting estrogens are very effective in this regard (12,57,270). The mechanism of action of short-acting estrogens as agonist and antagonist appears to involve steps subsequent to nuclear binding and these interactions are the subject of the following discussion.

Pollard and Martin (413), Martin (314), Miller and Emmens (343) and Terenius and Ljungkvist (538) were the first to suggest that the pattern of estrogenic response observed with short-acting estrogens was due to a failure of these compounds to occupy receptors for sufficient periods of time to elicit full responses. This concept has been confirmed and extended by several investigators. The uterotropic response patterns observed with estriol are correlated with short-term occupancy of estrogen receptors in uterine nuclei (12,16). Estriol and estradiol are equally capable of causing early nuclear accumulation of receptor-hormone complexes; however, the quantity of receptor-estriol complexes declined rapidly following the initial accumulation (Fig. 11). In contrast, the quantity of receptor-estradiol complexes was maintained for considerably longer periods of time. Similar findings have been observed in the mouse uterus by Korach et al. (256); however, in these studies a second small elevation in nuclear bound receptor estradiol sites was noted between 7 and 9 hr after hormone treatment. These observations lead to the conclusion that long-term retention of the receptor in the nucleus is required for the late uterotropic response that involve true uterine growth (82). These observations have been confirmed by several investigators in the rat (174,270,318) and in the guinea pig (164,400). This concept predicts that short-acting estrogens would be full agonists if they were administered in a continuous fashion (see Agonistic Effects of Short-Acting Estrogens for further discussion of this point).

The reasons why short-acting estrogens occupy nuclear bound receptors for short periods of time following an injection are manifold and not completely clear. It is known that the dissociation rate of estriol from the receptor is more rapid than estradiol (48), and Bouton and Raynard (44) have suggested that this differential in dissociation rate accounts for short-term nuclear retention. Estriol is also cleared from the body more rapidly than estradiol (216). Therefore, the equilibrium between tissue and blood levels would result in more rapid dissociation of nuclear bound receptor-estriol complexes. It is also possible that receptor-estriol complexes dissociate from their nuclear binding sites more rapidly than receptor-estradiol complexes. This could result in a more rapid turnover or processing of receptor and loss of hormone from the tissues.

Antagonistic Action of Short-Acting Estrogens

As explained in the previous sections, short-acting estrogens have the ability to stimulate early uterotropic responses while having little effect on true uterine growth when they are administered by injection in saline. This explains why they have no antagonistic action when examined by short-term uterotropic assays but display partial antagonism when long-term uterine growth assays are used. This dichotomy is easily explained by examining the idealized data shown in Fig. 13. The response patterns for estradiol and estriol at three dose levels are plotted as a function of time after a single injection. If uterotropic responses are measured at 6 hr after an injection of either estradiol or estriol, they are identical (Fig. 13B), and therefore no antagonism will be noted. However, measurements at 24 hr do show antagonism (Fig. 13C). This inhibition is shown in the form of dose-response curves and results from the reduced capacity of estriol to stimulate true uterine growth. When the effects of estradiol and estriol are summed at 24 hr the overall uterotropic effect is reduced.

The antagonistic effects of short-acting estrogens do not appear to be due to a failure of these hormones to induce the replenishment of cytosol receptors (57,80,83,229,234). Instead, the antagonistic effects are due to competitive interaction of the estriol- and estradiol-receptor complexes at the nuclear level. Both estrogens cause a rapid accumulation of receptor by the nucleus. Estradiol treatment results in long-term nuclear reaction of the receptor, whereas a rapid decline in nuclear bound receptor is observed following estriol. When estradiol and estriol are given simultaneously, the quantity of receptor exhibiting long-term nuclear retention is reduced (80). These results indicate that the partial antagonist effects of estriol probably result from competition between estradiol- and estriol-receptor complexes for nuclear acceptor sites and from the rapid clearance of estriol from uterine tissue (216). Thus estradiol and estriol promote the nuclear binding of receptors and receptor-estriol complexes compete with receptor-estradiol complexes for those nuclear sites that are involved in long-term occupancy and promotion of uterotropic response (12,13,16). Since estriol is cleared rapidly and estriol-receptor complexes are in equilibrium with receptor and estriol, the competition between estradiol- and estriol-receptor complexes reduces the number of receptor-estrogen complexes retained in the nuclear compartment. Because long-term retention of estrogen-receptor complexes is related to the stimulation of true uterine growth, this reduction in the number of effective receptor-estrogen complexes could account for the observed antagonism. These pharmacokinetic properties of estriol explain why some investigators have considered this hormone to be impeded or inadequate (85,199,282,584). The rapid loss of estriol-receptor complexes from the nuclear compartment may be due in part to the rapid rate of dissociation of estriol-receptor complexes when compared to estradiol-receptor complexes. Bouton and Raynand (44) have suggested that the degree of antagonism observed with any estrogen antagonist is related to the dissociation rate of the hormone from the receptor. This is probably true for short-acting estrogens of the estriol type; however, it does not seem to be the case with triphenylethylenes such as tamoxifen and clomiphene (77,433).

Agonistic Effects of Short-Acting Estrogens

The results discussed above suggest that short-acting estrogens would not be antagonists if they were present in a continuous fashion that would result in constant or long-term occupancy of the estrogen receptor. Pollard and Martin (413) showed that frequent administration of DMS stimulated full estrogenic responses in the mouse vagina. They suggested that this effect was the result of continuous occupancy of receptors. This suggestion was confirmed in the rat by injecting estriol every 3 hr for 15 hr or implanting estriol (16,80). These treatments stimulated full uterine growth and continuous occupancy of nuclear estrogen receptors. No antagonism was observed in animals that were implanted with estriol plus estradiol. Martucci and Fishmann (318) have confirmed these observations with estriol and demonstrated that estrone is also capable of causing true uterine growth under these conditions. Gulino et al. (164) have made similar observations with repeated estriol administration in the fetal guinea pig uterus. A similar effect has been observed by Lan and Katzenellenbogen (270) with 17α ethinyl estriol and estriol cyclopentylether. These steroid derivatives extend the biological half-life of the estrogen and result in long-term nuclear occupancy and true uterine growth. Thus they are analogous to the hormone implant system. Likewise, DMS acts as a full uterotropic agent when its biological half-life is extended by derivitizing it with the dimethyl ether (234). DMS is also an agonist when injected in oil, which acts to extend its half-life (177). Continuous administration of estriol has also been shown to cause implantation in the rat (228), whereas a single injection will block this process (583). Implantation in the rat is dependent on elevated levels of estradiol on days 3 to 4 of pregnancy, and a bolus administration of estriol apparently interferes with estradiol action by reducing the effective level of receptor-estradiol complexes. However, if estriol is given continuously it acts as an estrogen and causes implantation.

In addition to these animal studies, Lippman et al. (292) have shown that estriol is fully capable of stimulating metabolic activity of human breast cancer cells (MCF-7) in culture. Likewise, estradiol-17α has been shown to elicit full estrogenic responses in MCF-7 cells (105). In these experiments the hormone was maintained at a constant level in the culture medium which results in continuous occupancy of the estrogen receptor, thereby stimulating pellet implant conditions in the animal.

These results demonstrate that short-acting estrogens are neither ineffectual nor antagonistic when present in a continuous or chronic fashion. However, estriol does manifest these properties when injected. This paradox relates to the concept, previously suggested by Emmens and Miller (113), Martin (314), and Miller and Emmens (343), that "weak" estrogenicity correlates with short-term nuclear receptor occupancy. What is clear from the present results is that "weak" estrogenicity in the case of estriol arises from competition between estradiol- and estriol-receptor complexes for nuclear retention sites and from the rapid clearance of estriol from uterine tissue (216). Thus, estradiol and estriol promote the accumulation of receptors in the nuclear compartment where estriol-receptor complexes compete with estradiol-receptor complexes for those nuclear sites involved in long-term occupancy and promotion of uterotropic responses (12,13,16). The competition between estradiol- and estriol-receptor complexes reduces the number of receptor-estrogen complexes retained in the nuclear compartment. Because long-term retention appears to be necessary for the simulation of true uterine growth, this reduction in the number of effective receptor-estradiol complexes could account for the observed antagonism. However, when estriol is present in a continuous fashion, as in the pellet implant experiments presented here, estriol by continually binding to receptor sites promotes long-term nuclear retention and true uterine growth equivalent to that of estradiol. Since long-term retention of the receptor-estrogen complex by the nucleus appears to cause true growth regardless of the estrogen occupying the receptor, estriol acts as an estrogen agonist under these conditions.

Nonsteroidal Antiestrogens

Nonsteroidal antiestrogens are triphenylethylene derivatives, such as tamoxifen and clomiphene (Fig. 14). These drugs have been used extensively in women for the induction of ovulation (clomiphene) or in the treatment of breast cancer (tamoxifen) (77,134,220). They are generally considered to be antiestrogens; however, their agonistic or antagonistic properties depend on the species, organ, tissue, and experimental condition used to test those activities.

Agonistic and Antagonistic Properties

Mixed agonism-antagonism is very common among the antisteroid hormones; therefore, an explanation of this term will be offered here as a general example. An agonist is a compound that stimulates a response (Fig. 15A), whereas an antagonist will completely inhibit the action of an agonist. A mixed agonist-antagonist will partially inhibit the action of an agonist, but because it has inherent agonistic properties it will partially mimic the response of the agonist. The degree of agonist or antagonist activity observed depends on the species, organ, tissue, or cell type that is being examined and on the endpoint assay chosen (77). For example, clomiphene and tamoxifen stimulate the rat uterus to grow when administered alone, but they inhibit the growth-promoting effects of estradiol when both substances are given simultaneously (Fig. 15) (82,221,227). These stimulatory and inhibitory functions are the result of the ability of these drugs to stimulate cellular hypertrophy of the ep-

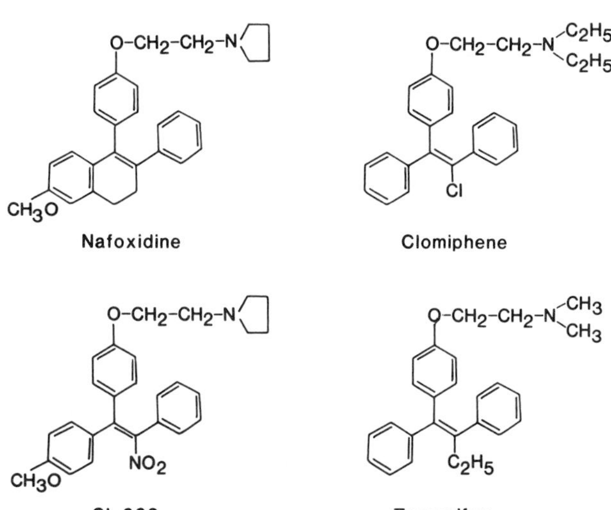

FIG. 14. Chemical structures of antiestrogens of the triphenylethylene type.

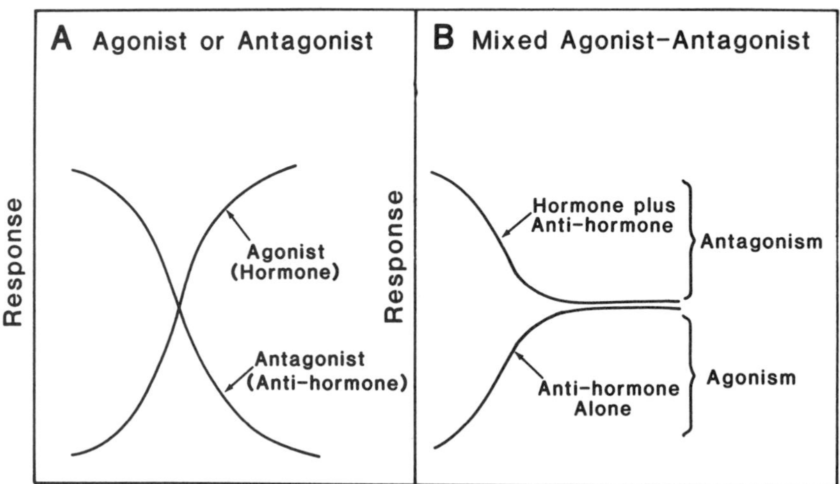

FIG. 15. Comparison of dose-response curves for agonists, antagonists and mixed agonist-antagonists.

ithelial cells of the endometrium while having little effect on hypertrophy of the stromal or myometrial cells. Estradiol, on the other hand, stimulates cellular hypertrophy and hyperplasia in all three tissue layers and hence produces a uterus that is considerably larger than that seen with clomiphene alone. The elevation in uterine weight caused by clomiphene or tamoxifen alone is due primarily to the hypertrophy of epithelial cells and some slight, but significant, stimulation of the stroma and myometrium. The inhibition of estradiol action on uterine growth results from the antagonism of cellular hypertrophy in the stromal and myometrial compartments. Therefore, triphenylethylene drugs act like partial estrogen agonists in the epithelial cells and primarily as estrogen antagonists in other uterine cells *in vivo*.

The estrogenic properties of clomiphene have also been observed in vaginal epithelium. Both the cis and trans isomers of clomiphene stimulate vaginal epithelial cell proliferation and keratin synthesis comparable to that seen with estradiol during the first 24 hr after treatment (261). No further stimulation is observed with longer exposure to clomiphene, whereas longer estradiol exposure stimulates full vaginal cornification and keratin synthesis.

The ability of triphenylethylene drugs to manifest any estrogen antagonism is difficult to understand in light of their estrogen-like actions during the first 12 to 24 hr after administration in the rat. During this time, these drugs cause nuclear binding of the estrogen receptor and stimulate RNA and protein synthesis, specific uterine induced protein (IP), RNA polymerase I and II activity, and DNA synthesis (34,70,141,173,260,264,302,305,309,315). Thus the uterus and vagina of the rat display a response profile as though they had been exposed to an estrogen. It is only after 24 hr that antiestrogens begin to exert their antagonistic effects, even though they maintain a significant level of estrogenic stimulation (approximately 2 × control, Fig. 16). Thus by 3 to 4 days after the beginning of such treatment, both antagonistic and agonistic effects can be observed. Obviously triphenylethylene drugs must have some indirect action that accounts for their antagonistic effects and these

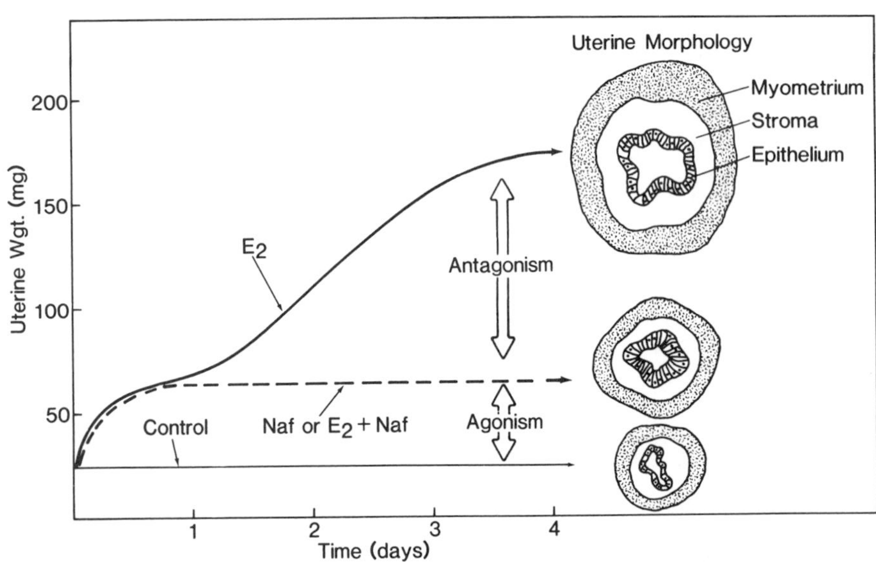

FIG. 16. The differential response pattern of the uterus to estradiol (E_2) and nafoxidine (NAF).

are associated with events that require at least 24 hr. At the present time the mechanisms involved are not known but some suggestions are presented in Antiestrogen Binding Sites, below.

In contrast to the mixed agonistic-antagonistic function of nonsteroidal antiestrogens in the rat, in the adult mouse these compounds are estrogenic with little if any antiestrogenic activity (112,413,537). In the chick oviduct and liver, however, these compounds are estrogen antagonists with virtually no detectable agonist activity under most circumstances (38,59,276,502,504). However, it has been shown by Binart et al. (39) that tamoxifen when administered with progesterone will induce cytodifferentiation of oviduct tubular gland cells and stimulate the synthesis of conalbumin and ovalbumin, whereas tamoxifen alone has no effect. The interactions of these two compounds that bring about these effects are not known. In primates, clomiphene and tamoxifen are primarily antiestrogenic; however, estrogenicity has been noted depending on the species and endpoint used (77,373). The effects of clomiphene at the hypothalamic-hypophyseal level in primates are discussed in the next section. Other species manifest a broad spectrum of agonistic-antagonistic responses to nonsteroidal antiestrogens, discussion of which goes beyond the scope of this chapter (for review see 77,134).

These species differences in response to nonsteroidal antiestrogens essentially disappear when these compounds are tested in cell culture. Tamoxifen and 4-hydroxytamoxifen block the estrogen-stimulated increases in several specific proteins in MCF-7 cells and have no agonistic activity (570,571). Tamoxifen and nafoxidine inhibit [^{3}H]thymidine incorporation and DNA polymerase activity, and reduce cell number in MCF-7 cell cultures (84,106,291). Estrogen-stimulated prolactin synthesis is inhibited by tamoxifen and no agonistic effect is seen with the drug alone (287,288).

Ovulation and Hypothalamic-Hypophyseal Interactions

Clomiphene and its closely related analog ethamoxytriphetol (MER-25) were initially described as inhibitors of gonadotropin secretion in the rat (189) and were considered to be likely candidates for agents that would block fertility. However, when they were tried in women the opposite situation was observed (153). This difference between the effects of clomiphene in the rodent and human may be due to species differences; however, it is more likely to be due to differences in treatment protocols (reviewed in 77).

As originally observed by Holtkamp et al. (189), clomiphene inhibits reproduction in the cycling rat. This inhibition was attributed to decreased secretion of gonadotropins; however, these studies were done with high doses of clomiphene and over long periods of time relative to the short cycle length of the rat. Schally et al. (450) suggested that high doses of clomiphene inhibit FSH and LH release and lower doses stimulate either release or facilitate LH-RH action. Recently Hseuh et al. (196) have shown that enclomiphene sensitizes the pituitary to LH-RH. Several studies have shown that low doses of clomiphene increase gonadotropin secretion and cause ovulation in the intact rat (89,252,371). As pointed out by Docke (99), the cycling rat is not comparable to an ovulatory woman, and he demonstrated that clomiphene did induce ovulation in either androgen-sterilized rats or in rats in persistent estrus due to constant light.

In humans, clomiphene induces ovulation in anovulatory women (153). The drug is usually administered for 5 days beginning on the fifth day of cycle following either spontaneous or progesterone-induced menstrual bleeding. The blood levels of gonadotropins increase during the time of clomiphene treatment, and this is correlated with follicular growth and a gradual elevation in estrogen secretion (421,435,588). Ovulation occurs approximately 7 days after the end of treatment.

The mechanisms and sites of action of clomiphene are not completely understood. Igarashi et al. (200) showed that implantation of clomiphene directly into the anterior hypothalamus or median eminence caused increased gonadotropin levels in the blood of rats, which suggested that the hypothalamus was the site of action. Indirect evidence for a central nervous system effect was shown by Coppola et al. (88), who demonstrated that phenobarbital would block gonadotropin secretion in clomiphene-treated pregnant mare serum (PMS)-primed immature rats. Likewise, clomiphene was shown to cause ovulation when implanted in the hypothalamus, implying a direct stimulatory effect in the brain (100).

In addition to the effects of clomiphene at the hypothalamic level, the pituitary also appears to be a primary target of this compound. The work of Docke (100) with bilateral implants of clomiphene in the brain indicates that the drug blocks ovulation induction by estrogen at the pituitary level. The pituitary is much more sensitive to clomiphene than the hypothalamus (1,231,265). In addition, Hseuh et al. (196) have shown that enclomiphene sensitizes the pituitary to LH-RH in a fashion similar to estradiol (266). Enclomiphene also stimulates the secretion of prolactin and suppresses growth hormone secretion in pituitary cell cultures (GH-cells), whereas zuclomiphene is without effect (96). Suppression of blood levels of growth hormone has also been reported in normal men (406).

From the above discussion it can be concluded that both the hypothalamus and pituitary are involved in the action of clomiphene. The mechanisms by which clomiphene exerts its effects are not fully understood and are undoubtedly more complex than the normal mechanisms by which endogenous hormones function. The usual explanation given, however, is based on the antiestrogenic properties of the drug and is focused on the ability of clomiphene to bind to estrogen receptors, thus blocking the negative feedback effects of estrogen. This inhibition of negative feedback presumably results in gonadotropin secretion and ovulation.

This explanation seems to hold for some circumstances; however, it is incomplete and ignores some of the basic pharmacology of clomiphene.

It should be remembered that clomiphene is both estrogenic and antiestrogenic to varying degrees in all mammals including humans; therefore, this mixed function must be considered in any model. As mentioned above, some investigators have attempted to explain these mixed agonistic/antagonistic properties by proposing that clomiphene is antagonistic at low concentrations and agonistic at high concentrations (45,252,371,450,460). In this scheme, clomiphene binds to estrogen receptors at low doses and blocks the negative feedback of endogenous estrogens. This results in the release of gonadotropins and subsequent ovulation. At high doses the drug also binds estrogen receptors but acts as an estrogen and blocks gonadotropin secretion because of its inherent estrogenicity at these high levels. However, clomiphene is estrogenic and antiestrogenic over the same dose range in uterotropic assays (73). Therefore, unless one is willing to invoke a special case for the brain, the above explanation of positive and negative effects on gonadotropic secretion does not hold. It is possible, however, to propose a scheme whereby stimulatory and inhibitory effects could be observed. Perhaps clomiphene at low doses interacts only with estrogen receptors in the pituitary and this effect is positive, i.e., gonadotropin secretion is stimulated. At higher doses the drug binds to hypothalamic estrogen receptor sites, which has a negative effect on gonadotropin-releasing hormone secretion. These differential effects seem quite likely in view of the previously noted steroid-binding affinity of pituitary and hypothalamic estrogen receptors for clomiphene (1,231,265).

A positive feedback effect of clomiphene on gonadotropin release in humans is not usually considered; however, it seems as likely an explanation as the inhibition of the negative feedback effects of estrogens. Indeed, it has been demonstrated that estradiol administration for 3 days of the menstrual cycle results in an increase in blood levels of LH and FSH (539,588). These changes in gonadotropin secretion are very similar, although not identical, to those seen following clomiphene administration. These changes in gonadotropin levels have been attributed to the positive feedback effects of estrogens and are similar to those described for the rat (for review see 251).

Therefore, it is possible to envision clomiphene acting, at least in some anovulatory syndromes, as an extraestrogenic positive stimulus to gonadotropin secretion. This action may explain the ability of zuclomiphene to cause ovulation in patients with Chiari-Frommel syndrome who have very low to nondetectable levels of estrogen (373). It is difficult to fit this finding with the concept of a blockade of the negative feedback of endogenous estrogen, since zuclomiphene is considered to be primarily estrogenic. A positive action of clomiphene is also possible in women with polycystic ovarian disease. The ovarian follicles of these women synthesize large quantities of androstenedione but fail to convert this precursor to estradiol. Since clomiphene can be estrogenic under some circumstances, perhaps the drug is acting directly at the ovarian level as an estrogen. This estrogenicity of clomiphene may be a necessary requirement for ovulation in these patients.

Ethynyl estradiol is known to have negative feedback effects on gonadotropin secretion in humans, and clomiphene will block this effect under some circumstances (548). These results are usually cited as evidence that clomiphene acts by blocking the negative feedback effects of estrogen. However, it is also known that clomiphene will suppress gonadotropin secretion in ovariectomized or postmenopausal women (95,178,418). Therefore, under some circumstances, clomiphene can mimic the negative feedback effects of estrogens. In addition to these estrogenic effects of clomiphene, it has been shown that high doses of ethynyl estradiol do not interfere with the ovulation-inducing effects of clomiphene (527). If clomiphene were acting only to block the negative feedback effects of estrogens, then high doses of ethynyl estradiol should overcome this effect and block gonadotropin secretion.

These observations appear contradictory and difficult to reconcile; however, it must be remembered that the various effects of estrogen or clomiphene on ovulation are being observed under two different physiological circumstances. Negative feedback effects are seen after castration or menopause when gonadotropin blood levels are very high. Conversely, the positive effects are observed when gonadotropin secretion is operating at a much reduced level and is under the control of endogenous steroids. These two hypothalamic-hypophyseal states are probably not comparable with respect to control mechanisms. For example, in the ovariectomized animal the gonadotropin control centers in the brain have been operating in the absence of estrogen for several days to weeks before experiments are performed. Thus, it is possible that a positive feedback center might not operate optimally under these conditions and only the negative functions would be intact. A decline in the function of a positive center could reflect a dependency on continuous exposure to some level of estrogen. Therefore, when either estradiol or clomiphene is given to a castrated animal or postmenopausal woman a suppression of gonadotropin secretion is observed. However, under normal physiological circumstances, the presence of estrogen maintains the positive feedback control centers at an operative level, and when a sufficient estrogenic stimulus is detected, ovulatory levels of gonadotropins are secreted. Czygan and Schulz (95) demonstrated that clomiphene had a positive effect on gonadotropin secretion in the presence of estrogen, whereas as mentioned earlier, it suppressed gonadotropin in the absence of estrogen. These results support the concept that estrogen is required for maintenance of the positive control centers.

Receptor Binding

Nonsteroidal antiestrogens bind to the cytosol form of the estrogen receptor and will cause nuclear accumulation of the receptor-antiestrogen complex (58,69,222,223,234,433). This is expected because, as discussed previously, these compounds stimulate biosynthetic activity in target tissues during the first 24 hr in a fashion similar to estradiol. Obviously there is paradox, since one would expect that antiestrogens would block the action of estrogens, yet during these initial hours of interaction they appear to be estrogenic. Therefore, differences must exist at some level or at some time that account for the mixed agonistic and antagonistic properties of these drugs.

One difference is that triphenylethylene antiestrogens, such as nafoxidine, clomiphene, and tamoxifen cause long-term occupancy of the nuclear bound receptor and a sustained depletion of cytosol receptors (69). Such an effect could be caused by the long half-life of these compounds with the resultant continuous nuclear occupancy of receptors or a defect in nuclear receptor processing (82). Defective nuclear processing of the receptor-nafoxidine complex has been observed in MCF-7 cells (193–195). In these experiments the long-term occupancy of the nuclear receptor induced by nafoxidine continued in the absence of nafoxidine in the culture media, thus eliminating the possibility that sustained occupancy results from the continuous presence of nafoxidine as might be the case *in vivo*. Continuous occupancy of nuclear estrogen receptor by estradiol does not produce inhibitory effects on uterine growth responses (80,83). Therefore, it is likely that defective nuclear processing is somehow involved in the failure of these nonsteroidal antiestrogens to elicit the entire spectrum of true uterine growth.

Some investigators have reported specific but subtle differences in the physicochemical characteristics of receptor antiestrogen and receptor estradiol complexes (118,431, 524,525). However, it is not clear how such differences relate to hormone antagonism. No difference between receptor-antiestrogen and receptor-estradiol complexes has been found with respect to their recognition by monoclonal antibodies to the receptor, or binding to their DNA or polynucleotides (43,368,523). Evans et al. (118) did show that estradiol-receptor complexes bind more tightly to calf thymus DNA than antiestrogen-receptor complexes. Perhaps this observation relates to the finding that nuclear bound receptor-antiestrogen complexes can be readily extracted by high salt, whereas a portion of estrogen-receptor complexes cannot (437). These salt-extracted forms of the receptor do not differ significantly from those of the estradiol-receptor complex (438,524,526). Differential extraction of estrogen and tamoxifen receptors has also been observed with the nonionic detergent Nonidet P-40 (202). All of the nuclear tamoxifen-receptor complex from MCF-7 cells is extracted with this detergent and sediments as 7 and 5S peaks on sucrose density gradients. In contrast, nuclear estradiol complexes resist extraction. These results suggest that the interactions of these two receptor complex forms with chromatin differ in some way.

Although there are some differences between the receptor-binding interactions of estrogens and antiestrogens, it is difficult to fit these into a unifying scheme to explain the antagonistic activity of these compounds. Considering the ability of these compounds to cause nuclear accumulation of the estrogen receptor and to stimulate uterine DNA, RNA, and protein synthesis during the first 24 hr after exposure, it seems likely that mechanisms other than those mediated by the estrogen receptor may be involved. Some of these mechanisms will be discussed in the following sections.

Antiestrogen Binding Sites

In addition to the estrogen receptor, many tissues contain triphenylethylene antiestrogen binding sites (TABS) that bind antiestrogens, such as tamoxifen and clomiphene, with high affinity ($K_d \sim 1$ nM) and are present in estrogen target and nontarget tissues (503,506). In addition, somewhat similar sites with lower affinity ($K_d \sim 10$ nM) are associated with low-density lipoprotein in rat serum (581). The binding specificity of TABS spans a rather broad range; however, it is generally agreed that triphenylethylene derivatives that contain the alkylaminoethoxy side chain are bound with the highest affinity and steroids are not bound by these sites (162,501,506,580). Other compounds, such as chlorpromazine, ketocholesterol, and cholesterol, have a reduced affinity; however, as discussed below these may be significant (369).

The subcellular localization of TABS appears to vary with species and/or cell type. Several laboratories have reported the presence of TABS in high-speed cytosols of the chick oviduct, guinea pig and rat uterus, human mammary carcinoma, and in nontarget human tissues (125, 161,253,367,503,505,506), and Sudo et al. (501) found TABS predominantly in the microsomal fraction of tissues from the rat. Cytosol and nuclear localization in the guinea pig uterus has been reported by Gulino and Pasquilini (162), and it has been suggested that the level of these sites is modulated by estradiol and progesterone (163,581). Nuclear localization has also been reported in human breast cancer tissue and chicken and rat liver (74,253,369).

The physiological function of TABS has not been defined, and although it is tempting to suggest that these sites are antiestrogen receptors, in general the data do not support this hypothesis. The estrogenic and antiestrogenic properties of nonsteroidal antiestrogens correlate with their relative binding affinities for the estrogen receptor and not for TABS (69,368). The cis and trans isomers of clomiphene bind to TABS with similar affinities, yet they have dissimilar agonist-antagonist profiles (501,581). Tamoxifen resistance has been described in a cell line of MCF-7 breast cancer cells that contained very low levels of TABS and normal levels of estrogen receptor (124). However, Miller and Katzenellenbogen (344) were unable to relate the levels of TABS to tamoxifen sensitivity but instead showed that sensitivity was correlated with estrogen receptor levels. Some indication that TABS are involved in antiestrogen action comes from the work of Brandes (47), who showed that a diphenylmethane derivative that binds to TABS, but not to the estrogen receptor, inhibits the growth of MCF-7 cells.

The possible involvement of TABS in the mechanism of action of antiestrogen is suggested by the observation that estrogen administration and the physiological state of the ovary have effects on the level of TABS in both liver and uterus (580). At the time of puberty, the liver TABS concentration increased significantly in the female when compared to both mature males or immature females. TABS levels in rat uterine cytosol increase significantly in mature females when compared to either castrated or younger animals. In addition, both uterine and liver TABS levels fluctuated throughout the estrous cycle and reached a peak approximately on the day of estrus. Treatment of ovariectomized rats with physiological amounts of estradiol caused a twofold increase in TABS levels in the uterus, thus mimicking the midcycle peak of TABS. Gulino and Pasqualini (163) have shown that the level of TABS is modulated in the guinea pig uterus by estradiol and progesterone.

The presence of TABS associated with the serum low-density lipoprotein (LDL) fraction from the rat is of interest since LDL-cholesterol is involved in the control of cellular cholesterol synthesis (146,581). Triphenylethylene antiestrogens are inhibitors of cholesterol synthesis, and Tabacik et al. (517) showed that tamoxifen inhibited cholesterol synthesis in MCF-7 cells. Murphy et al. (369,370) demonstrated that 7-ketocholesterol acts as an endogenous ligand that binds to tissue TABS. 7-Ketocholesterol is a potent inhibitor of cholesterol synthesis and cell growth in human fibroblasts (146), and its half-maximal concentration (1 μM) for inhibition is in the range of its binding affinity for TABS (369). These results suggest that TABS may be involved in some aspect of cholesterol synthesis or metabolism. Since cellular growth is dependent on cholesterol synthesis, it is possible that these sites are somehow involved. However, triparanol (MER-25) is a potent inhibitor of cholesterol synthesis, yet it has little to no antiestrogenic properties (*unpublished observations*).

The binding of 7-ketocholesterol to TABS may be fortuitous, since many other compounds inhibit the binding of [^{3}H]tamoxifen with the same relative affinities. Cholesterol, chlorpromazine, various ligands, and W-13, a calmodulin inhibitor, act as competitive inhibitors of the binding of [^{3}H]tamoxifen to TABS (*unpublished observations*). The inhibition by W-13 is of special interest, since it has been demonstrated that tamoxifen is an inhibitor of calmodulin-mediated phosphodiesterase activity (268). Calmodulin is thought to be involved in the control of cell proliferation, and inhibitors of calmodulin will block the cell cycle at the G1 phase (61,207,563,577). Since nonsteroidal antiestrogens block cellular proliferation, it is possible that calmodulin inhibition is involved in this effect. However, such an inhibition of cell proliferation appears to occur primarily in estrogen-responsive cells, and therefore must somehow be linked to estrogen sensitivity.

Physiological Estrogen Antagonists

The blood levels of estrogen fluctuate according to the stage of the reproductive cycle, and this is accompanied by changing levels of estrogen-receptor binding (71,569). Thus the effects of estrogen wax and wane as a result of these changes in ovarian secretion of estrogens. In addition to these influences of estrogen alone, other hormones act to alter the actions of estrogen at the cellular level and modify estrogen-directed functions.

Progesterone

Progesterone acts on the estrogen-primed uterus to alter cell function and reproductive competence. Often this ability of progesterone is considered to be antagonistic to estrogen; however, it probably should be referred to as a modifier of estrogen action rather than an antagonist. Nevertheless, progesterone will reduce the ability of estrogens to cause uterine growth and vaginal cornification (199,283). This ability of progesterone to modify or antagonize estrogen action is generally considered to involve receptor mechanisms that have been discussed previously in Synthesis and Replenishment of Receptors. These effects of progesterone involve decreasing the number of cytosol and nuclear bound estrogen-receptor complexes. Such reductions in receptor number have been correlated with a reduced sensitivity of the uterus to estradiol (80,198).

Most of the studies concerned with progesterone effects on estrogen receptor levels have been done under nonphysiological circumstances. However, in the elegant studies of Brenner et al. (49), physiological conditions were maintained by creating artificial menstrual cycles in ovariectomized rhesus monkeys. Under these conditions estradiol blood levels were maintained at a constant level throughout the cycle and progesterone was elevated during the second half of the cycle. Cytosol estrogen receptor levels were elevated during the first half of the cycle and dramatically decreased during the second half. These data suggest that progesterone does lower cytosol estrogen receptor even when estradiol is present. Although nuclear estrogen receptors were not examined in this study, progesterone does decrease their level in the hamster uterus under physiological circumstances (569).

Modulated estrogen receptor levels are correlated with striking changes in the morphology of the uterine luminal epithelium (569). When nuclear receptor levels are elevated, the epithelium is hypertrophied and mitotic, whereas when receptor levels are suppressed, the epithelium is atrophied and shows degenerative changes. Such changes in morphology and functional state of uterine cells probably reflect the normal cyclic interaction of estrogen and progesterone on the reproductive tract.

In addition to these effects on the estrogen receptor, progesterone also inhibits the stimulation of nuclear type II estrogen-binding sites (309). This inhibition of nuclear type

II sites is correlated with reduced uterotropic response to estrogen, and does not appear to be related to any effects of progesterone on estrogen receptor levels. The inhibitory effects of progesterone do appear to be mediated by the progesterone receptor, since estrogen priming is necessary in order to observe the inhibitory effects of progesterone.

Androgens

Androgenic steroids are known to inhibit the actions of estrogen on the growth of estrogen target tissues (432). Indeed, androgen therapy is used in the treatment of estrogen-dependent breast cancer (326). This treatment is based on the rationale that androgens should block or antagonize the estrogen-stimulated growth of breast cancer cells. The mechanisms by which androgens antagonize estrogenic functions are not known; however, it is known that androgen receptors are present in estrogen target tissues (138). Physiological concentrations of androgens do not cause growth or stimulate other known functions of MCF-7 breast cancer cells, even though nuclear binding of the receptor-androgen complex is readily observed (432). Likewise in the rat uterus there appears to be no biological response to nuclear binding of the receptor-androgen complex. However, chronic exposure to physiological levels of androgens in the rat does depress uterine weight, an indication that androgens are antiestrogenic by some mechanism (432).

In contrast, high doses of androgens stimulate growth of the rat uterus, mammary tumors, and MCF-7 cells (137, 180,284,291,591). Thus, androgens appear to have the capacity to both inhibit and stimulate estrogen target tissues depending on the dose used. The low-dose inhibition may be mediated directly by the androgen receptor or it may operate indirectly via interactions at the hypothalamic-pituitary level or some other pathway. The high-dose stimulation effect is mediated by the estrogen receptor, since it is known that high concentrations of androgens will bind to the estrogen receptor, cause nuclear accumulation, and produce an estrogen-like response (433,441).

Type II Estrogen-Binding Sites and Estrogen Antagonism

One of the pleiotropic events stimulated by exposure to estrogen is an elevation of type II estrogen-binding sites (304). These sites are present in the cytosol and nuclei and are different from the estrogen receptor (type I; see 75 for reviews). Nuclear type II sites are occupied by an endogenous ligand that appears to be an inhibitor of cell proliferation, and as such, may constitute a new class of antiestrogen (307). Since estrogen-induced uterine cell proliferation is observed only when nuclear type II sites are elevated, this may mean that the inhibitory ligand has dissociated from these sites. Such dissociation would open up sites that are measured by the binding of labeled estradiol. Nuclear type II sites are tightly associated with the nuclear matrix and may be coupled to the regulatory components involved with DNA synthesis. Therefore, the dissociation of an inhibitory ligand from these sites may act as a positive regulation signal that initiates DNA synthesis and cell proliferation.

Inhibitors of Progesterone Action

Although there are several exogenous and endogenous antiestrogens, antiprogestational compounds are rare. Many progesterone derivatives have been synthesized; however, only one compound appears to have antagonistic properties (18,182,420). 17β-Hydroxy-11β-[-4-dimethylamino-phenyl]-17α-[1-propynyl] estra-4, 9-dien-3-one (RU 38486), which was synthesized by Roussel Uclaf, has been shown to interrupt the luteal phase of the menstrual cycle and terminate pregnancy in women (182). RU 38486 induces early onset of vaginal bleeding when administered during the luteal phase of cycling monkeys (18,179). Such actions are considered to be due to a direct antagonistic effect of RU 38486 at the receptor level in the uterine endometrium. This compound binds to progesterone receptors in the rabbit uterus and glucocorticoid receptors in the thymus where it acts as an antiglucocorticoid (182). In T47D cells RU 38486 binds to the progesterone receptor and inhibits cellular proliferation, as does R5020, a synthetic progesterone (191). Thus, RU 38486 is an agonist by this criterion; however, it does antagonize the stimulation of insulin receptors by R5020. Therefore, in T47D cells RU 38486 manifests mixed agonist-antagonist properties.

As pointed out earlier for antiestrogens, the actions of antisteroid hormone drugs *in vitro* are not necessarily identical to their actions *in vivo*. Obviously more work *in vivo* is needed on this important class of antiprogestins before definitive statements can be made regarding their mechanism of action and their true pharmacologic and physiologic actions.

An inhibitor of progesterone-receptor binding has been described in the cytosol from rat placenta (384). This inhibitor is a macromolecule that decreases the affinity of the receptor for progesterone but has no effect on the number of receptor sites. The function of this inhibitor is not known; however, inhibitory activity in trophoblast cytosol is greatest on days 9 and 12 of pregnancy and declines thereafter (384). By day 18 inhibitory activity is no longer detectable and this coincides with a sharp decrease in the progesterone receptor. The presence of such inhibitors in other systems has not been described; however, their potential physiological significance in the regulation of progesterone action is considerable.

ACKNOWLEDGMENTS

This work was supported by NIH grants HD 08436, CA 26112, and CA 35480. We thank Georgietta Brown, David

Scarf, Sylvia Guthrie, and Bill Mitchell for their help in the preparation of this manuscript.

REFERENCES

1. Adashi, E. V., Hsueh, A. J. W., and Yen, S. S. C. (1980): Alterations induced by clomiphene in the concentrations of oestrogen receptors in the uterus, pituitary gland and hypothalamus of female rats. *J. Endocrinol.*, 87:383–392.
2. Aizawa, Y., and Mueller, G. C. (1961): The effect *in vivo* of estrogens on lipid synthesis in the rat uterus. *J. Biol. Chem.*, 236:281–286.
3. Alberga, A., Massol, N., Raynaud, J.-P., and Baulieu, E.-E. (1971): Estradiol binding of exceptionally high affinity by a nonhistone chromatin fraction. *Biochemistry*, 10:3835–3843.
4. Alexander, D. C., and Miller, W. L. (1982): Regulation of ovine follicle stimulating hormone β-chain mRNA by 17β-estradiol *in vivo* and *in vitro*. *J. Biol. Chem.*, 267:2282–2286.
5. Allen, E., and Doisy, E. A. (1923): An ovarian hormone. *JAMA*, 81:819–821.
6. Allen, E., and Doisy, E. A. (1924): The induction of a sexually mature condition in immature females by injection of the ovarian follicular hormone. *Am. J. Physiol.*, 69:577–588.
7. Allen, E., Smith, G. M., and Gardner, W. V. (1937): Accentuation of the growth effect of theelin on genital tissues of the ovariectomized mouse by arrest of mitosis with colchicine. *Am. J. Anat.*, 61:321–341.
8. Allen, E., Smith, G. M., and Reynolds, S. R. M. (1973): Hyperplasia in uterine muscle. *Proc. Soc. Exp. Biol. Med.*, 37:257–259.
9. Allen, W. M., and Wintersteiner, O. S. (1934): Crystalline progestin. *Science*, 80:190–191.
10. Anderson, J. N. (1984): The effect of steroid hormones on gene expression. In: *Biological Regulation and Development*, edited by R. F. Goldberger and K. R. Yamamoto, pp. 169–212. Plenum Press, New York.
11. Anderson, J. N., Clark, J. H., and Peck, E. J., Jr. (1972): Oestrogen and nuclear binding sites: Determination of specific sites by ^{3}H-oestradiol exchange. *Biochem. J.*, 126:561–567.
12. Anderson, J. N., Clark, J. H., and Peck, E. J., Jr. (1972): The relationship between nuclear receptor estrogen binding and uterotrophic responses. *Biochem. Biophys. Res. Commun.*, 48:1460–1468.
13. Anderson, J. N., Peck, E. J., Jr., and Clark, J. H. (1973): Nuclear receptor estrogen complex: Relationship between concentration and early uterotrophic responses. *Endocrinology*, 92:1488–1495.
14. Anderson, J. N., Peck, E. J., and Clark, J. H. (1973): Nuclear receptor estrogen complex: Accumulation, retention and localization in the hypothalamus and pituitary. *Endocrinology*, 93:711–717.
15. Anderson, J. N., Peck, E. J., Jr., and Clark, J. H. (1974): Nuclear receptor estradiol complex: A requirement for uterotropic responses. *Endocrinology*, 95:174–178.
16. Anderson, J. N., Peck, E. J., Jr., and Clark, J. H. (1975): Estrogen-induced uterine responses and growth: Relationship to receptor estrogen binding by uterine nuclei. *Endocrinology*, 96:160–167.
17. Anderson, J. N., Vanderbilt, J. N., Lawson, G. M., Tasai, M.-J., and O'Malley, B. W. (1983): Chromatin structure of the ovalbumin gene family in the chicken oviduct. *Biochemistry*, 22:21–30.
18. Asch, R. H., and Rojas, F. J. (1985): The effects of RW 486 on the luteal phase of the rhesus monkey. *J. Steroid Biochem.*, 22:227–230.
19. Astwood, E. B. (1938): A six-hour assay for the quantitative determination of estrogen. *Endocrinology*, 23:25–31.
20. Aurricchio, F., Migliaccio, A., Castoria, G., Rotondi, A., and Lastoria, S. (1984): Direct evidence of *in vitro* phosphorylation-dephosphorylation of the estradiol-17β receptor, role of Ca^{2+}-calmodulin in the activation of hormone binding sites. *J. Steroid Biochem.*, 20:31–35.
21. Axel, R., Maniatis, T., and Fox, C. F. (1979): Eucaryotic gene regulation. In: *Proceedings of ICN-UCLA Symposia on Molecular and Cellular Biology, Vol. XIV*. Academic Press, New York.
22. Bailly, A., Le Fevre, B., Savouret, J. F., and Milgrom, E. (1980): Activation and changes in sedimentation properties of steroid receptors. *J. Biol. Chem.*, 10:2729–2734.
23. Baker, H. J., and Shapiro, D. J. (1977): Kinetics of estrogen induction of *Xenopus laevis* vitellogenin messenger RNA as measured by hybridization to complementary DNA. *J. Biol. Chem.*, 252:8428–8434.
24. Barker, K. L. (1971): Estrogen-induced synthesis of histones and a specific non-histone protein in the uterus. *Biochemistry*, 10:284–291.
25. Barker, K. L., Adams, D. J., and Donohue, T. M., Jr. (1981): Regulation of the levels of mRNA for glucose-6-phosphate dehydrogenase and its rate of translation in the uterus by estradiol. In: *Cellular and Molecular Aspects of Implantation*, edited by S. R. Glasser and D. W. Bullock, pp. 269. Plenum Press, New York.
26. Barker, K. L., and Warren, J. C. (1966): Template capacity of uterine chromatin: Control by estradiol. *Proc. Natl. Acad. Sci. USA*, 56:1298–1302.
27. Barnea, A., and Gorski, J. (1970): Estrogen-induced protein: Time course of synthesis. *Biochemistry*, 9:1899–1904.
28. Barnes, D., and Sato, G. (1979): Growth of a human mammary tumour cell line in a serum-free medium. *Nature*, 281:388–389.
29. Barrack, E. R. (1983): The nuclear matrix of the prostate contains acceptor sites for androgen receptors. *Endocrinology*, 113:430–432.
30. Barrack, E. R., Bujnovszky, P., and Walsh, P. C. (1983): Subcellular distribution of androgen receptors in human normal, benign hyperplastic, and malignant prostatic tissues: Characterization of nuclear salt-resistant receptors. *Cancer Res.*, 43:1107–1116.
31. Barrack, E. R., and Coffey, D. S. (1980): The specific binding of estrogens and androgens to the nuclear matrix of sex hormone responsive tissues. *J. Biol. Chem.*, 255:7265–7275.
32. Barrack, E. R., and Coffey, D. S. (1982): Biological properties of the nuclear matrix: Steroid hormone binding. *Recent Prog. Horm. Res.*, 38:133–195.
33. Barrack, E. R., Hawkins, E. F., Allen, S. L., Hicks, L. L., and Coffey, D. S. (1977): Concepts related to salt resistant estradiol receptors in rat uterine nuclei: Nuclear matrix. *Biochem. Biophys. Res. Commun.*, 79:829–836.
34. Baudendistel, L. J., Ruh, M. F., Nadel, E. M., and Ruh, T. S. (1978): Cytoplasmic oestrogen receptor replenishment: Oestrogens versus antioestrogens. *Acta Endocrinol.*, 89:599–611.
35. Bellard, M., Gannon, F., and Chambon, P. (1978): Nucleosome structure III: The structure and transcriptional activity of the chromatin containing the ovalbumin and globin genes in chick oviduct nuclei. *Cold Spring Harbor Symp. Quant. Biol.*, 42:779–791.
36. Biggers, J. D. (1951): Observations on the intravaginal assay of natural oestrogens using aqueous egg albumin as the vehicle of administration. *J. Endocrinol.*, 7:163–171.
37. Biggers, J. D., and Claringbold, P. J. (1955): Mitotic activity in the vaginal epithelium of the mouse following local oestrogenic stimulation. *J. Anat.*, 89:124–131.
38. Binart, N., Catelli, M. H., Geynet, C., Puri, V., Hahnel, R., Mester, J., and Baulieu, E. E. (1979): Monohydroxytamoxifen: An antiestrogen with high affinity for the chick oviduct oestrogen receptor. *Biochem. Biophys. Res. Commun.*, 91:812–818.
39. Binart, N., Mester, J., Baulieu, E. E., and Catelli, C. G. (1982): Combined effects of progesterone and tamoxifen in the chick oviduct. *Endocrinology*, 111:7–16.
40. Birnbaumer, M., Bell, R. C., Schrader, W. T., and O'Malley, B. W. (1984): The putative molybdate-stabilized progesterone receptor subunit is not a steroid binding protein. *J. Biol. Chem.*, 259:1091–1098.
41. Bloom, K. S., and Anderson, J. N. (1978): Fractionation of hen oviduct chromatin into transcriptionally active and inactive regions after selective micrococcal nuclease digestion. *Cell*, 15:141–150.
42. Bloom, K. S., and Anderson, J. N. (1979): Conformation of ovalbumin and globin genes in chromatin during differential gene expression. *J. Biol. Chem.*, 254:10532–10539.
43. Borgna, J. L. and Rochefort, H. (1980): High affinity binding to the estrogen receptor of [^{3}H]4-hydroxytamoxifen, an active antiestrogen metabolite. *Mol. Cell Endocrinol.*, 20:71–85.
44. Bouton, M., and Raynaud, J. P. (1979): The relevance of interaction kinetics in determining biological responses to estrogens. *Endocrinology*, 105:509–515.
45. Boyar, R. M. (1970): Effects of clomiphene citrate on pituitary FSH, FSH-RF, and release of LH in immature and mature rats. *Endocrinology*, 86:629–633.

46. Boyd-Leinen, P., Gosse, B., Rasmussen, K., Martin-Dani, G., and Spelsberg, T. C. (1984): Regulation of nuclear binding of the avian oviduct progesterone receptor. Changes during estrogen-induced oviduct development, withdrawal, and secondary stimulation. *J. Biol. Chem.*, 259:2411–2421.
47. Brandes, L. J. (1984): A diphenylmethane derivative selective for the antiestrogen binding site may help define its biological role. *Biochem. Biophys. Res. Commun.*, 124:244–249.
48. Brecher, P. I., and Wotiz, H. H. (1968): *Proc. Soc. Exp. Biol. Med.*, 128:470–472.
49. Brenner, R. M., Resko, J. A., and West, N. B. (1974): Cyclic changes in oviductal morphology and residual cytoplasmic estradiol binding capacity induced by sequential estradiol-progesterone treatment of spayed rhesus monkeys. *Endocrinology*, 95: 1094–1104.
50. Brown, D. D. (1981): Gene expression in eucaryotes. *Science*, 211:667–674.
51. Bulger, W. H., and Kupfer, D. (1977): Induction of uterine ornithine decarboxylase [ODC] by antiestrogens: Inhibition of estradiol-mediated induction of ODC: A possible mechanism of action of antiestrogens. *Endocr. Res. Commun.*, 3:209–218.
52. Buller, R. E., Schrader, W. T., and O'Malley, B. W. (1975): Progesterone-binding components of chick oviduct. IX. The kinetics of nuclear binding. *J. Biol. Chem.*, 250:809–818.
53. Burrows, H. (1949): *Biological Actions of Sex Hormones*, 2d ed. Cambridge University Press, London.
54. Butenandt, A. (1929): Untersuchungen über das weibliche Sexualhormon. *Dtsch. Med. Wochenschr.*, 55:2171–2173.
55. Butenandt, A., and Dannenbaum, H. (1934): Uber Androsteron: Isolierung eines neuen, physiologisch unwirksamen Sterioderivatives ans Mannernarn, seine verknutsung mit Dehydroandrosterone und Androsterone bin Beitrag vurk Constitution des Androsterone. *Z. Physiol. Chem.*, 229:192–208.
56. Buttyan, R., Olsson, C. A., Sheard, B., and Kallos, J. (1983): Steroid receptor-nuclear matrix interactions: The role of DNA. *J. Biol. Chem.*, 258:14366–14370.
57. Capony, F., and Rochefort, H. (1977): *In vitro* and *in vivo* interaction of ^{3}H-dimethylstilbestrol with the estrogen receptor. *Mol. Cell Endocrinol.*, 8:47–64.
58. Capony, F., and Rochefort, H. (1978): High affinity binding of the antiestrogen [^{3}H]tamoxifen to the 8S estradiol receptor. *Mol. Cell Endocrinol.*, 11:181–198.
59. Capony, F., and Williams, D. L. (1981): Antiestrogen action in avian liver: The interaction of estrogens and antiestrogens in the regulation of apolipoproteins β synthesis. *Endocrinology*, 108:1862–1868.
60. Carpenter, G., and Cohen, S. (1979): Epidermal growth factor. *Annu. Rev. Biochem.*, 48:193–216.
61. Chafouleas, J. G., Lagace, L., Boulton, W. E., Boyd, A. E., and Means, A. R. (1984): Changes in calmodulin and its mRNA accompany re-entry of quiescent (G_0) cells in the cell cycle. *Cell*, 36:73–81.
62. Chamness, G. C., Jennings, A. W., and McGuire, W. L. (1973): Oestrogen receptor binding is not restricted to target nuclei. *Nature*, 241:458–460.
63. Chamness, G. C., Jennings, A. W., and McGuire, W. (1974): Estrogen receptor binding to isolated nuclei. A nonsaturable process. *Biochemistry*, 13:327–331.
64. Chamness, G. C., and McGuire, W. L. (1972): Estrogen receptor in the rat uterus, physiological forms and artifacts. *Biochemistry*, 11:2466–2472.
65. Cidlowski, J. A., and Muldoon, T. G. (1974): Estrogenic regulation of cytoplasmic receptor populations in estrogen-responsive tissues of the rat. *Endocrinology*, 95:1621–1629.
66. Cidlowski, J. A., and Muldoon, T. G. (1976): Sex-related differences in the regulation of cytoplasmic estrogen receptor levels in responsive tissues of the rat. *Endocrinology*, 94:833–841.
67. Ciejek, E. M., Nordstrom, J. L., Tsai, M.-J., and O'Malley, B. W. (1982): Ribonucleic acid precursors are associated with the chick oviduct nuclear matrix. *Biochemistry*, 21:4945–4953.
68. Clark, A. J. (1937): *The Mode of Action of Drugs on Cells*. Williams and Wilkins, Baltimore.
69. Clark, J. H., Anderson, J. N., and Peck, E. J., Jr. (1973): Estrogen receptor-antiestrogen complex: Atypical binding by uterine nuclei and effects on uterine growth. *Steroids*, 22:707–718.
70. Clark, J. H., Anderson, J. N., and Peck, E. J., Jr. (1974): Oestrogen receptors and antagonism of steroid hormone action. *Nature*, 251:446–448.
71. Clark, J. H., Campbell, P. S., and Peck, E. J., Jr. (1972): Receptor estrogen complex in the nuclear fraction of the pituitary and hypothalamus of male and female immature rats. *Neuroendocrinology*, 77:218–228.
72. Clark, J. H., and Gorski, J. (1969): Estrogen receptors: An evaluation of cytoplasmic-nuclear interactions in a cell-free system and a method
73. Clark, J. H., and Guthrie, S. C. (1981): The agonistic and antagonistic effects of clomiphene citrate and its isomers. *Biol. Reprod.*, 25:667–672.
74. Clark, J. H., and Guthrie, S. C. (1986): Subcellular localization of triphenylethylene and antiestrogen binding sites (TABS) in rat liver. *J. Steroid Biochem.*, 26:433–437.
75. Clark, J. H., Hardin, J. W., Upchurch, S., and Eriksson, H. (1978): Heterogeneity of estrogen binding sites in the cytosol of the rat uterus. *J. Biol. Chem.*, 253:7630–7634.
76. Clark, J. H., Hseuh, A., and Peck, E. J., Jr. (1977): Regulation of estrogen receptor relenishment by progesterone. *Biochemical Actions of Progesterone and Progestins, Ann. NY Acad. Sci.*, 286:161–179.
77. Clark, J. H., and Markaverich, B. M. (1982): Agonist and antagonist properties of clomiphene: A review. *Pharmacol. Ther.*, 15:467–519.
78. Clark, J. H., and Markaverich, B. M. (1982): Heterogeneity of estrogen binding sites and the nuclear matrix. In: *The Nuclear Envelope and the Nuclear Matrix*, edited by B. Manul, pp. 259–269. Liss, New York.
79. Clark, J. H., and Markaverich, B. M. (1983): The agonistic and antagonistic effects of short acting estrogens: A review. *Pharmacol. Ther.*, 21:429–453.
80. Clark, J. H., Paszko, Z., and Peck, E. J., Jr. (1977): Nuclear binding and retention of the receptor estrogen complex: Relation to the agonistic and antagonistic properties of estriol. *Endocrinology*, 100:91–96.
81. Clark, J. H., and Peck, E. J., Jr. (1976): Nuclear retention of receptor-oestrogen complex and nuclear acceptor sites. *Nature*, 260:635–647.
82. Clark, J. H., and Peck, E. J., Jr. (1979): *Female Sex Steroids: Receptors and Function*. Springer-Verlag, Berlin.
83. Clark, J. H., Williams, M., Upchurch, S., Eriksson, H., Helton, E., and Markaverich, B. M. (1982): Effects of estradiol 17α on nuclear occupancy of the estrogen receptor stimulation of nuclear type II sites and uterine growth. *J. Steroid Biochem.*, 16:323–328.
84. Coezy, E., Borgna, J. L., and Rochefort, H. (1982): Tamoxifen and metabolites in MCF-7 cells: Correlations between binding to estrogen and cell growth inhibition. *Cancer Res.*, 42:317–323.
85. Cole, P., and MacMahon, B. (1969): Oestrogen fractions during early reproductive life in the etiology of breast cancer. *Lancet*, 1:604–606.
86. Compere, S. J., McKnight, G. S., and Palmiter, R. D. (1981): Androgens regulate ovomucoid and ovalbumin gene expression independently of estrogen. *J. Biol. Chem.*, 256:6341–6347.
87. Compton, J. G., Schrader, W. T., and O'Malley, B. W. (1983): DNA sequence preference of the progesterone receptor. *Proc. Natl. Acad. Sci. USA*, 80:16–20.
88. Coppola, J. A., Leonardi, R. G., and Ringler, I. (1966): Reversal of the effects of anti-oestrogens and norethynodrel on gonadotropin-induced ovulation in rats. *J. Reprod. Fertil.*, 11:65–71.
89. Coppola, J. A., and Perrine, J. W. (1965): Influence of two nonsteroidal antiestrogens on vaginal opening and PMS-induced ovulation in rats. *J. Reprod. Fertil.*, 13:373–374.
90. Corden, J., Wasylyk, B., Buchwalder, A., Sassone-Corsi, P., Kedinger, C., and Chambon, P. (1980): Promoter sequences of eukaryotic protein-coding genes. *Science*, 209:1406–1414.
91. Corner, G. W., and Allen, W. M. (1929): Physiology of the corpus luteum. *Am. J. Physiol.*, 88:326–339.
92. Corvol, P., Falk, R., Friefeld, M., and Bardin, C. W. (1972): *In vitro* studies of progesterone binding proteins in guinea pig uterus. *Endocrinology*, 90:1464–1469.
93. Crandall, W. R. (1938): Effect of progesterone on cell division in circular muscle of rabbit's uterus. *Anat. Rec.*, 72:195–210.
94. Cunha, G. R., Chung, L. W. K., Shannon, J. M., Taguchi, O., and Fujii, H. (1983): Hormone induced morphogenesis and growth: Role

of mesenchymal-epithelial interactions. *Recent Prog. Horm. Res.*, 39:559–598.

95. Czygan, P.-J., and Schulz, K. D. (1972): Studies on the anti-oestrogenic and oestrogen-like action of clomiphene citrate in women. *Gynecol. Invest.*, 3:126–134.
96. Dannies, P. S., Yen, P. N., and Tashjian, A. H., Jr. (1977): Antiestrogenic compounds increase prolactin and growth hormone synthesis in clonal strains of rat pituitary cells. *Endocrinology,* 101:1151–1156.
97. Dean, D. C., Knoll, B. J., Riser, M. E., and O'Malley, B. W. (1983): A 5′-flanking sequence essential for progesterone regulation of an ovalbumin fusion gene. *Nature,* 305:551–554.
98. DeAngelo, A. B., and Gorski, J. (1970): The role of RNA synthesis in the estrogen induction of a specific uterine protein. *Proc. Natl. Acad. Sci. USA,* 66:693–700.
99. Docke, F. (1969): Ovulation-inducing action of clomiphene citrate in the rat. *J. Reprod. Fertil.*, 18:135–139.
100. Docke, F. (1971): Studies on the anti-ovulatory action of clomiphene citrate in the rat. *J. Reprod. Fertil.*, 24:45–54.
101. Doisy, E. A., Veler, C. D., and Thayer, S. (1929): Folliculin from urine of pregnant women. *Am. J. Physiol.*, 90:329–330.
102. Dougherty, J. J., and Toft, D. O. (1982): Characterization of two 8-S forms of chick oviduct progesterone receptor. *J. Biol. Chem.*, 257:3113–3119.
103. Dure, L. S., Schrader, W. T., and O'Malley, B. W. (1980): Covalent attachment of a progestational steroid to chick oviduct progesterone receptor by photoaffinity labelling. *Nature,* 283:784–786.
104. Edery, M., Pang, K., Larson, L., Colosi, T., and Naudi, S. (1985): Epidermal growth factor receptor levels in mouse mammary glands in various physiological states. *Endocrinology,* 117:405–411.
105. Edwards, D. P., and McGuire, W. L. (1980): 17α-Estradiol is a biologically active estrogen in human breast cancer cells in tissue culture. *Endocrinology,* 107:884–891.
106. Edwards, D. P., Murphy, S. R., and McGuire, W. L. (1980): Effects of estrogen and antiestrogen on DNA polymerase in human breast cancer. *Cancer Res.*, 40:1722–1726.
107. Edwards, D. P., Weigel, N. L., Schrader, W. L., O'Malley, B. W., and McGuire, W. L. (1984): Structural analysis of chicken oviduct progesterone receptor using monoclonal antibodies to the subunit B protein. *Biochemistry,* 23:4427–4435.
108. Ehrlich, P. (1913): Chemotherapeutics: Scientific principles, methods, and results. *Lancet,* 2:445–451.
109. Ekman, P., Barrack, E. R., Greene, G. L., Jensen, E. V., and Walsh, P. C. (1983): Estrogen receptors in human prostate: Evidence for multiple binding sites. *J. Clin. Endocrinol. Metab.*, 57:166–176.
110. Elsner, C. W., Illingworth, D. V., De Groot, K., Flickinger, G. L., and Mikhail, G. (1977): Cytosol and nuclear estrogen receptor in the genital tract of the rhesus monkey. *J. Steroid Biochem.*, 8:151–155.
111. Emmens, C. W. (1942): The differentiation of oestrogens from prooestrogens by the use of spayed mice possessing two separate vaginal sacs. *J. Endocrinol.*, 3:174–177.
112. Emmens, C. W. (1965): Oestrogenic, anti-oestrogenic and anti-fertility activity. *Acta Med. Philip.*, 1:220–224.
113. Emmens, C. W., and Miller, B. G. (1969): Estrogens, progestogens and antiestrogens. *Steroids,* 13:723–750.
114. Epifanova, O. I. (1966): Mitotic cycles in estrogen-treated mice: A radiographic study. *Exp. Cell Res.*, 42:562–577.
115. Erdos, T., Best-Belpomme, M., and Bessada, R. (1970): A rapid assay for binding estradiol to uterine receptor(s). *Anal. Biochem.*, 37:244–252.
116. Eriksson, H., Upchurch, S., Hardin, J. W., Peck, E. J., Jr., and Clark, J. H. (1978): Heterogeneity of estrogen receptors in the cytosol and nuclear fractions of the rat uterus. *Biochem. Biophys. Res. Commun.*, 81:1–7.
117. Etgen, A. M., and Whalen, R. E. (1978): Dimethystilbestrol is not antiestrogenic for rat sexual behavior or gonadotropin secretion. *Biol. Reprod.*, 19:454–458.
118. Evans, E., Baskevitch, P. P., and Rochefort, H. (1982): Estrogen receptor DNA interactions: Difference between activation by estrogen and antiestrogen. *Eur. J. Biochem.*, 128:185–191.
119. Faber, L. E., Sandmann, M. L., and Stavely, H. E. (1972): Progesterone-binding proteins of the rat and rabbit uterus. *J. Biol. Chem.*, 247:5648–5649.
120. Faber, L. E., Sandmann, M. L., and Stavely, H. E. (1973): Progesterone and corticosterone binding in rabbit uterine cytosols. *Endocrinology,* 93:74–80.
121. Fagg, B., and Martin, L. (1979): Oestrogen content of the uterine tissues of mice and their relationship to epithelial cell proliferation after subcutaneous and intraluminal administration of hormones. *J. Endocrinol.*, 83:295–304.
122. Fang, S., and Liao, S. (1979): Steroid and tissue specific retention of a 17β-hydroxy-5α-androstan-3-one-protein complex by the cell nuclei of ventral prostate. *J. Biol. Chem.*, 246:16–24.
123. Farmer, S. R., Henshaw, E. C., Berridge, M. V., and Tata, J. R. (1978): Translation of *Xenopus* vitellogenin mRNA during primary and secondary induction. *Nature,* 273:401–403.
124. Faye, J. C., Jozan, S., Redewith, G., Baulieu, E. E., and Bayard, F. (1983): Physicochemical and genetic evidence for specific antiestrogen binding sites. *Proc. Natl. Acad. Sci. USA,* 80:3158–3162.
125. Faye, J. C., Lasserre, B., and Bayard, F. (1980): Antiestrogen specific, high affinity saturable binding sites in rat uterine cytosol. *Biochem. Biophys. Res. Commun.*, 93:1225–1231.
126. Feil, P. D., and Bardin, C. W. (1975): Cytoplasmic and nuclear progesterone receptors in the guinea pig uterus. *Endocrinology,* 97:1398–1407.
127. Feil, P. D., Glasser, S. R., Toft, D. O., and O'Malley, B. W. (1972): Progesterone binding in the mouse and rat uterus. *Endocrinology,* 9:738–746.
128. Flandroy, L., Fastrez-Boute, A., and Galand, P. (1976): Oestrogen induced changes in uterine cGMP: Relationship with other parameters of hormonal stimulation. *Arch. Int. Physiol. Biochim.*, 84:1072–1078.
129. Flandroy, L., and Galand, P. (1975): Oestrogen related changes in uterine and vaginal cAMP and cGMP. *Arch. Int. Physiol. Biochim.*, 83:965–971.
130. Flandroy, L., and Galand, P. (1978): Changes in cGMP and cAMP content in the estrogen stimulated rat uterus: Temporal relationship with other parameters of hormonal stimulation. *J. Cyclic Nucleotide Res.*, 4:145–151.
131. Flandroy, L., and Galand, P. (1980): *In vitro* stimulation by estrogen of guanosine 3′,5′-monophosphate accumulation in incubated rat uterus. *Endocrinology,* 106:1187–1192.
132. Freiderici, H. H. R. (1967): The early response to uterine capillaries to estrogen stimulation. An electron microscopic study. *Lab. Invest.*, 17:322–333.
133. Freifeld, M. L., Feil, P. D., and Bardin, C. W. (1974): The *in vivo* regulation of the progesterone "receptor" in guinea pig uterus: Dependence on estrogen and progesterone. *Steroid,* 23:93–103.
134. Furr, B. J. A., and Jordon, V. C. (1984): The pharmacology and clinical uses of tamoxifen. *Pharmacol. Ther.*, 25:127–205.
135. Galand, P., Mairesse, N., Roorijck, J., and Fandroy, L. (1983): Differential blockade of estrogen induced uterine responses by the antiestrogen nafoxidine. *J. Steroid Biochem.*, 19:1259–1263.
136. Galand, P. N., Tchernitchin, X., and Tchernitchin, A. N. (1984): Time course of the effects of nafoxidine and oestradiol on separate groups of responses in the uterus of the immature rat. *J. Steroid Biochem.*, 21:43–47.
137. Garcia, M., and Rochefort, H. (1978): Androgen effects mediated by estrogen receptor in 7,12-dimethylbenz(a)anthracene-induced rat mammary tumors. *Cancer Res.*, 38:3922–3929.
138. Garcia, M., and Rochefort, H. (1979): Evidence and characterization of the binding of two ^3H androgens to the estrogen receptor. *Endocrinology,* 104:1797–1804.
139. Gardner, R. M., Kirkland, J. L., and Stancel, G. M. (1978): Selective blockade of estrogen induced uterine responses by the antiestrogen nafoxidine. *Endocrinology,* 103:1583–1589.
140. Garel, A., and Axel, R. (1978): The structure of the transcriptionally active ovalbumin genes in chromatin. *Cold Spring Harbor Symp. Quant. Biol.*, 42:701–708.
141. Gasde, K., Kramer, G., and Schulz, K. O. (1971): Effects of oestradiol-17β on uterine ribosomes: Altered sedimentation profile and enhanced protein-synthesizing activity. *Hoppe Seylers Z. Physiol. Chem.*, 352:318–320.
142. Giese, A. C. (1973): *Cell Physiology,* 4th ed., pp. 289–292. W. B. Saunders Co., Philadelphia.
143. Glass, R., Loring, J., Spencer, J., and Villee, C. A. (1961): The estrogenic properties *in vitro* of diethylstilbestrol and substances related to estradiol. *Endocrinology,* 68:327–333.

144. Glasscock, R. F., and Hoekstra, W. G. (1959): Selective accumulation of tritium-labeled hexosterol by the reproductive organs of immature female goats and sheep. *Biochem. J.*, 72:673–682.
145. Glasser, S. R., Chytil, F., and Spelsberg, T. C. (1972): Early effects of oestradiol-17 on the chromatin and activity of the deoxyribonucleic acid-dependent ribonucleic acid polymerases I and II of the rat uterus. *Biochem. J.*, 130:947–957.
146. Goldstein, J. L., and Brown, M. S. (1979): The LDL receptor locus and the genetics of familial hypercholesterolemia. *Annu. Rev. Genetics*, 13:259–291.
147. Gonzalez, F., Lakshmanan, J., Hoath, S., and Fisher, D. A. (1984): Effect of oestradiol-17β on uterine epidermal growth factor concentration in immature mice. *Acta Endocrinol.*, 105:425–428.
148. Gorski, J. (1964): Early estrogen effects on the activity of uterine ribonucleic acid polymerase. *J. Biol. Chem.*, 239:889–892.
149. Gorski, J. (1985): Gorski replies. *Nature*, 318:89.
150. Gorski, J., and Mueller, G. C. (1963): Early effects of estrogen and acid soluble nucleotides on the rat uterus. *Arch. Biochem. Biophys.*, 102:21–25.
151. Gorski, J., Toft, D., Shyamala, G., Smith, D., and Notides, A. (1968): Hormone receptors: Studies on the interaction of estrogen with the uterus. *Recent Prog. Horm. Res.*, 24:45–80.
152. Gorski, J., Welshons, W., and Sakai, D. (1984): Remodeling the estrogen receptor model. *Mol. Cell. Endocrinol.*, 36:11–15.
153. Greenblatt, R. B., Barfield, W. E., Jungck, E. C., and Ray, A. W. (1961): Induction of ovulation with MRL/41. Preliminary report. *JAMA*, 178:101–104.
154. Greene, G. L. (1984): Immunochemical studies of estrogen receptor. In: *Gene Regulation by Steroid Hormones II*, edited by A. K. Roy and J. H. Clark, pp. 191–200. Springer-Verlag, New York.
155. Greene, G. L., and King, W. J. (1985): Greene and King reply. *Nature*, 317:88–89.
156. Grody, W. W., Schrader, W. T., and O'Malley, B. W. (1982): Activation, transformation and subunit structure of steroid hormone receptors. *Endocr. Rev.*, 3:141–163.
157. Gronemeyer, H., Govindan, M. V., and Chambon, P. (1985): Immunological similarity between the chick oviduct progesterone receptor forms A and B. *J. Biol. Chem.*, 260:6916–6925.
158. Gronemeyer, H., Harry, P., and Chambon, P. (1983): Evidence for two structurally related progesterone receptors in chick oviduct cytosol. *FEBS Lett.*, 156:287–292.
159. Groner, B., Kennedy, N., and Rahmsdorf, R. (1982): Introduction of a proviral mouse mammary tumor virus gene and a chimeric MMTV-thymidine kinase gene into L cells results in their glucocorticoid responsive expression. In: *Hormones and Cell Regulation, Vol. 6*, edited by J. E. Dumont, J. Nunez, and G. Shutz, pp. 217–228. Elsevier-North Holland, New York.
160. Gschwendt, M. (1980): The general validity of the subunit model of the progesterone receptor from chick oviduct appears questionable. *Mol. Cell. Endocrinol.*, 19:57–67.
161. Gulino, A., and Pasqualini, J. R. (1980): Specific binding and biological response of antiestrogens in the fetal uterus of the guinea pig. *Cancer Res.*, 40:3821–3826.
162. Gulino, A., and Pasqualini, J. R. (1982): Heterogeneity of binding sites for tamoxifen and tamoxifen derivatives in estrogen target and nontarget fetal organs of guinea pig. *Cancer Res.*, 42:1913–1921.
163. Gulino, A., and Pasqualini, J. R. (1983): Modulation of tamoxifen specific binding sites and estrogen receptors by estradiol and progesterone in the neonatal uterus of guinea pig. *Endocrinology*, 112:1871–1873.
164. Gulino, A., Sumida, C., Gelley, C., Giambiagi, N., and Pasqualini, J. R. (1981): Comparative dynamic studies of the biological responses to estriol and estradiol in the fetal uterus of guinea pig: Relationship to circulating estrogen concentration. *Endocrinology*, 109:748–756.
165. Gurpide, E., Stolee, A., and Tseng, L. (1971): Quantitative studies of tissue uptake and disposition of hormones. In: *Karolinksa Symposia on Research Methods in Reproductive Endocrinology: 3rd Symposium:* In vitro *Methods in Reproductive Cell Biology*, pp. 247–278.
166. Gurpide, E., and Welch, M. (1969): Dynamics of uptake of estrogens and androgens by human endometrium. *J. Biol. Chem.*, 224: 5159–5167.
167. Guyette, W. A., Matusik, R. J., and Rosen, J. M. (1979): Prolactin-mediated transcriptional and post-transcriptional control of casein gene expression. *Cell*, 17:1013–1023.
168. Ham, E. A., Cirillo, V. J., Zanetti, M. E., and Kuehl, F. A. (1975): Estrogen directed synthesis of specific prostaglandins in uterus. *Proc. Natl. Acad. Sci. USA*, 72:1420–1424.
169. Hamilton, T. H. (1962): Inhibition of protein synthesis and some quantifications of early estrogen action and response. *Science*, 138:989.
170. Hamilton, T. H. (1963): Isotopic studies on estrogen-induced accelerations of ribonucleic acid and protein synthesis. *Proc. Natl. Acad. Sci. USA*, 49:373–379.
171. Hamilton, T. H. (1964): Sequences of RNA and protein synthesis during early estrogen action. *Proc. Natl. Acad. Sci. USA*, 51:83–89.
172. Hamilton, T. H. (1968): Control by estrogen of genetic transcription and translation. *Science*, 161:649–660.
173. Hardin, J. W., Clark, J. H., Glasser, S. R., and Peck, E. J., Jr. (1976): Estrogen receptor binding by uterine nuclei: Relationship to endogenous nuclear RNA polymerase activity. *Biochemistry*, 15:1370–1374.
174. Harris, J., and Gorski, J. (1978): Evidence for a discontinuous requirement for estrogen in stimulation of deoxyribonucleic acid synthesis in the immature rat uterus. *Endocrinology*, 103:240–245.
175. Harris, S. E., Rosen, J. M., and Means, A. R. (1975): Use of a specific probe for ovalbumin mRNA to quantitate estrogen-induced gene transcripts. *Biochemistry*, 14:2072.
176. Hartmann, M., and Wettstein, A. (1934): Zur Kenntnis der Corpus-luteum Hormone. *Helv. Chim. Acta*, 17:1365–1372.
177. Hartmann, M., and Wettstein, A. (1934): Ein krystallisiertes Hormon aus Corpus luteum. *Helv. Chim. Acta*, 17:878–882.
178. Hashimoto, T., Miyai, K., Izumi, K., and Kumahara, Y. (1976): Effect of clomiphene citrate on basal and LRH-induced gonadotropin secretion in postmenopausal women. *J. Clin. Endocrinol. Metab.*, 42:593–594.
179. Healy, D. L., Baulieu, E. E., and Hodgen, G. D. (1983): Induction menstruation by an antiprogesterone steroid (RU 486) in primates: Site of action, dose-response relationships, and hormonal effects. *Fertil. Steril.*, 40:253–257.
180. Heise, E., and Gorlich, M. (1966): Growth and therapy of mammary tumors induced by 7,12-dimethylbenzanthracene in rats. *Br. J. Cancer*, 20:539–545.
181. Herranen, A., and Mueller, G. C. (1956): Effect of estradiol on the metabolism of serine-3-C^{14} in surviving uterine segments. *J. Biol. Chem.*, 223:369–375.
182. Herrmann, W., Wyss, R., Riondel, A., Philibert, D., Teutsch, G., Sakiz, E., and Baulieu, E. E. (1982): The effects of an antiprogesterone steroid in women: Interruption of the menstrual cycle and of early pregnancy. *C. R. Sciences Acad. Sci. (III)*, 294:933–938.
183. Higgins, S. J., Rousseau, G. G., Bacter, J. D., and Tomkins, G. M. (1973): Nature of nuclear acceptor sites for glucocorticoid- and estrogen-receptor complexes. *J. Biol. Chem.*, 248:5873–5879.
184. Hisaw, F. L., Jr. (1959): Comparative effectiveness of estrogens on fluid inhibition and growth of the rat's uterus. *Endocrinology*, 64:276–289.
185. Hisaw, F. L., Greep, R. O., and Ferold, H. L. (1937): Effects of progesterone on female genital tract after castration atrophy. *Proc. Soc. Exp. Biol. Med.*, 36:840–842.
186. Hobbs, A. A., Richards, D. A., Kessler, D. J., and Rosen, J. M. (1982): Complex hormonal regulation of rat casein gene expression. *J. Biol. Chem.*, 257:3598–3605.
187. Hofmann, G. E., Rao, C. H. V., Barrows, G. H., Schultz, G. S., and Sanfilippo, J. S. (1984): Binding sites for epidermal growth factor in human uterine tissues and leiomyomas. *J. Clin. Endocrinol. Metab.*, 58:880–884.
188. Hollenberg, M. D. (1979): Epidermal growth factor—Urogastrone, a polypeptide acquiring hormone status. *Vitam. Horm.*, 37:69–110.
189. Holtkamp, D. E., Greslin, J. G., Root, C. A., and Lerner, L. J. (1960): Gonadotrophin inhibiting and anti-fecundity effect of chloramiphene. *Proc. Soc. Exp. Biol. Med.*, 105:197–201.
190. Holzbauer, M. (1976): Physiological aspects of steroids with anesthetic properties. *Med. Biol.*, 54:227–242.
191. Horwitz, K. B. (1985): The antiprogestin RW 38486: Receptor-mediated progestin versus antiprogestin actions screened in estrogen-insensitive T47D human breast cancer cells. *Endocrinology*, 116:2236–2245.
192. Horwitz, K. B., and Alexander, P. S. (1983): *In situ* photolinked nuclear progesterone receptors of human breast cancer cells: Subunit

molecular weights after transformation and translocation. *Endocrinology*, 113:2195–2201.
193. Horwitz, K. B., Koseki, Y., and McGuire, W. L. (1978): Estrogen control of progesterone receptor in human breast cancer: Role of estradiol and antiestrogen. *Endocrinology*, 103:1742–1751.
194. Horwitz, K. B., and McGuire, W. L. (1978): Actinomycin D prevents nuclear processing of estrogen receptor. *J. Biol. Chem.*, 253:6319–6322.
195. Horwitz, K. B., and McGuire, W. L. (1978): Nuclear mechanisms of estrogen action. Effects of estradiol and anti-estrogens on estrogen receptors and nuclear receptor processing. *J. Biol. Chem.*, 253:8185–8191.
196. Hsueh, A. J. W., Erickson, G. F., and Yen, S. S. C. (1978): Sensitization of pituitary cells to luteinizing hormone releasing hormone by clomiphene citrate *in vitro*. *Nature*, 273:57–59.
197. Hsueh, A. J., Peck, E. J., Jr., and Clark, J. H. (1975): Progesterone antagonism of the oestrogen receptor and oestrogen-induced uterine growth. *Nature*, 254:337–339.
198. Hsueh, A. J., Peck, E. J., Jr., and Clark, J. H. (1976): Control of uterine estrogen receptor levels by progesterone. *Endocrinology*, 98:438–444.
199. Huggins, C., and Jensen, E. V. (1955): The depression of estrone-induced uterine growth by phenolic estrogens with oxygenated functions at positions 6 or 16: The impeded estrogens. *J. Exp. Med.*, 102:335–346.
200. Igarashi, M., Ibuki, Y., Kubo, H., Kamioka, J., Yokota, N., Ebara, Y., and Matsumoto, S. (1967): Mode and site of action of clomiphene. *Am. J. Obstet. Gynecol.*, 97:120–123 (Abstr. in *Obstet. Gynecol.*, 9:47).
201. Iguchi, T., Uchima, F.-D., Ostrander, P. L., and Beru, H. A. (1983): Growth of normal mouse vaginal epithelial cells in and on collagen gels. *Proc. Natl. Acad. Sci. USA*, 80:3743–3747.
202. Ikeda, M., Omukai, Y., Hosokawa, K., and Senoo, T. (1984): Differences in extractability of estradiol and tamoxifen receptor complex in the nuclei from MCF-7 cells with Nonidet P-40. *Steroids*, 43:481–489.
203. Ikeda, T., and Sirbasku, D. A. (1984): Purification and properties of a mammary-uterine-pituitary tumor cell growth factor from pregnant sheep uterus. *J. Biol. Chem.*, 259:4049–4064.
204. Illingworth, D. V., Elsner, C., De Groot, K., Flickinger, G. L., and Mikhail, G. (1977): A specific progesterone receptor of myometrial cytosol from the rhesus monkey. *J. Steroid Biochem.*, 8:157–160.
205. Ishii, D. N., and Aronow, L. (1973): *In vitro* degradation and stabilization of the glucocorticoid binding component from mouse fibroblasts. *J. Steroid Biochem.*, 4:593–603.
206. Isohashi, F., and Sakamoto, Y. (1985): Low molecular weight and macromolecular translocation modulators affecting the binding of activated receptor glucocorticoid complex to nuclei, chromatin and DNA. In: *Molecular Mechanism of Steroid Hormone Action* edited by V. K. Moudgil, pp. 225–247. Walter deGrunter, Berlin.
207. Ito, H., and Hidaka, H. (1983): Antitumor effect of a calmodulin antagonist on the growth of solid sarcoma-180. *Cancer Lett.*, 19:215–220.
208. Jackson, D. A., McCready, S. J., and Cook, P. R. (1981): RNA is synthesized at the nuclear cage. *Nature*, 292:552–555.
209. Jackson, V., and Chalkley, R. (1974): The binding of estradiol-17β to the bovine endometrial nuclear membrane. *J. Biol. Chem.*, 249:1615–1626.
210. Jakesz, R., Kasid, A., and Lippman, M. E. (1983): Continuous estrogen exposure in the rat does not induce loss of uterine estrogen receptor. *J. Biol. Chem.*, 258:11798–11806.
211. Jänne, O. A. (1982): Purification and photoaffinity labeling of rabbit uterine progesterone receptor. *Endocrinology*, 110:A141.
212. Jänne, O., Kontula, K., and Vihko, R. (1976): Progestin receptors in human tissues: Concentrations and binding kinetics. *J. Steroid Biochem.*, 7:1061–1068.
213. Jensen, E. V. (1984): Editorial: Intracellular localization of estrogen receptors, implications for interaction mechanism. *Lab. Invest.*, 51:11.
214. Jensen, E. V., Greene, G. L., Closs, L. E., DeSombre, E. R., and Nadji, M. (1982): Receptors reconsidered: A 20-year perspective. *Recent Prog. Horm. Res.*, 38:1–40.
215. Jensen, E. V., and Jacobson, H. I. (1962): Basic guides to the mechanism of estrogen action. *Recent Prog. Hormone Res.*, 18:387–414.
216. Jensen, E. V., Jacobson, H. I., Flesher, J. W., Saha, N. N., Gupta, G., Smith, S., Colucci, V., Shiplacoff, D., Neumann, H. G., DeSombre, D. R., and Jungblut, P. W. (1966): Estrogen receptors in target issues. In: *Steroid Dynamics*, edited by G. Pincus, T. Nakao, and J. F. Tait, pp. 133–157. Academic Press, New York.
217. Jensen, E. V., Suzuki, T., Kawashima, T., Stumpf, W. E., Jungblut, P., and DeSombre, E. R. (1968): A two-step mechanism for the interaction of estradiol with rat uterus. *Proc. Natl. Acad. Sci. USA*, 59:623–638.
218. Jensen, E. V., Suzuki, T., Numata, M., Smith, S., and DeSombre, E. R. (1969): Estrogen binding substances of target tissues. *Steroids*, 13:417–427.
219. Joab, I., Radanyi, C., Renoir, M., Buchou, T., Catelli, M. G., Binart, N., Mester, J., and Baulieu, E. E. (1984): Common non-hormone binding component in non-transformed chick oviduct receptors of four steroid hormones. *Nature*, 308:850–853.
220. Jordan, V. C. (1984): Biochemical pharmacology of antiestrogen action. *Pharmacol. Rev.*, 36:245–276.
221. Jordan, V. C., Dix, C. J., and Prestwich, G. (1979): Inhibition of cell division and stimulation of progesterone receptor synthesis in rat oestrogen target tissues by non-steroid anti-oestrogens. In: *Steroid Hormone Receptor Systems*, edited by W. W. Leavitt and J. H. Clark, pp. 133–156. Plenum Press, New York.
222. Jordan, V. C., and Naylor, K. E. (1979): The binding of ^{3}H-oestradiol in the immature rat uterus during the sequential administration of antioestrogens. *Br. J. Pharmacol.*, 65:167–173.
223. Jordan, V. C., and Prestwich, G. (1977): Binding of [^{3}H]tamoxifen in rat uterine cytosols: A comparison of swinging bucket and vertical tube rotor sucrose density gradient analysis. *Mol. Cell Endocrinol.*, 8:179–188.
224. Jost, J. P., Seldran, M., and Geiser, M. (1984): Preferential binding of estrogen-receptor complex to a region containing the estrogen-dependent hypothylation site preceding the chicken vitellogenin II gene. *Proc. Natl. Acad. Sci. USA*, 81:429–433.
225. Kalimi, M., Beato, M., and Feigelson, P. (1973): Interaction of glucocorticoids with rat liver nuclei I. role of the cytosol proteins. *Biochemistry*, 2:3365–3371.
226. Kalman, S. M., and Lowenstein, J. M. (1958): The effect of estrogens on the uptake of albumin and electrolytes by the rat uterus. *J. Pharmacol. Exp. Ther.*, 122:163–167.
227. Kang, Y.-H., Anderson, W. A., and DeSombre, E. R. (1975): Modulation of uterine morphology and growth by estradiol-17β and an estrogen antagonist. *J. Cell Biol.*, 64:682–691.
228. Kapetanakis, M., Dnowski, W. P., and Scommegna, A. (1980): Induction of delayed implantation in rats with continuous but not with bolus administration of estriol. *Biol. Reprod.*, 23:88–91.
229. Kassis, J. A., and Gorski, J. (1984): Estrogen receptor replenishment: Evidence for receptor recycling. *J. Biol. Chem.*, 256:7378–7382.
230. Kassis, J. A., Walent, J. H., and Gorski, J. (1984): Estrogen receptors in rat uterine cell cultures: Effects of medium on receptor concentration. *Endocrinology*, 115:762–769.
231. Kato, J., Kobayashi, T., and Villee, C. A. (1968): Effect of clomiphene on the uptake of estradiol by the anterior hypothalamus and hypophysis. *Endocrinology*, 82:1049–1052.
232. Kato, J., and Onouchi, T. (1977): Specific progesterone receptors in the hypothalamus and anterior hypophysis of the rat. *Endocrinology*, 101:920–928.
233. Katzenellenbogen, B. S., and Gorski, J. (1972): Estrogen action *in vitro:* Induction of the synthesis of specific uterine protein. *J. Biol. Chem.*, 247:1299–1305.
234. Katzenellenbogen, B. S., Katzenellenbogen, J. A., Ferguson, E. R., and Krauthammer, N. (1978): Antiestrogen interaction with uterine estrogen receptors: Studies with a radiolabeled anti-estrogen (CI 628). *J. Biol. Chem.*, 253:697–707.
235. Katzenellenbogen, B. S., Norman, M. J., Eckert, R. L., Peltz, S. W., and Mangel, W. F. (1984): Bioactivities, estrogen receptor interactions, and plasminogen activator-inducing activities of tamoxifen and hydroxy-tamoxifen isomers in MCF-7 human breast cancer cells. *Cancer Res.*, 44:112–119.
236. Katzenellenbogen, J. A., Carlson, K. E., Heiman, D. F., Robertson, D. W., Wai, L. L., and Katzenellenbogen, B. S. (1983): Efficient and highly selective covalent labeling of the estrogen receptor with [^{3}H]tamoxifen aziridine. *J. Biol. Chem.*, 258:3487–3495.
237. Katzenellenbogen, J. A., Johnson, H. J., and Carlson, K. E. (1973): Studies on the uterine, cytoplasmic estrogen binding protein. Thermal

stability and ligand dissociation rate. An assay of empty and filled sites by exchange. *Biochemistry,* 12:4092–4099.
238. Kelly, M. J., Moss, R. L., Dudley, C. A., and Fawcett, C. P. (1977): The specificity of the response of preoptic-septal area neurons to estrogen: 17β-Estradiol versus 17α-estradiol and the response of extra hypothalamic neurons. *Exp. Brain Res.,* 30:43–52.
239. King, R. J. B., Cowan, D. M., and Inman, D. R. (1965): The uptake of ^{3}H-oestradiol by dimethyl-benzanthracene in induced rat mammary tumors. *J. Endocrinol.,* 32:83–90.
240. King, R. J. B., and Gordon, J. (1966): The localization of ^{3}H-oestradiol-17β in rat uterus. *J. Endocrinol.,* 34:431–437.
241. King, R. J. B., and Gordon, J. (1972): Involvement of DNA in the acceptor mechanism for uterine oestradiol receptor. *Nature New Biol.,* 240:185–187.
242. King, R. J. B., Gordon, J., Cowan, D. M., and Inman, D. R. (1966): The intranuclear localization of ^{3}H-oestradiol in dimethylbenzanthracene induced rat mammary adenocarcinoma and other tissues. *J. Endocrinol.,* 36:139–150.
243. King, R. J. B., Gordon, J., and Inman, D. R. (1965): The intracellular localization of oestrogen in rat tissues. *J. Endocrinol.,* 32:9–15.
244. King, R. J. B., Gordon, J., and Martin, L. (1965): The association of (6,7-$^3H_2$) oestradiol with nuclear chromatin. *Biochem. J.,* 97:28P.
245. King, W. J., and Greene, G. L. (1984): Monoclonal antibodies localize oestrogen receptor in the nuclei of target cells. *Nature,* 307:745–747.
246. Kirkland, J. L., Gardner, R. M., Ireland, J. S., and Stancel, G. M. (1977): The effect of hypophysectomy on the uterine response to estradiol. *Endocrinology,* 101:403–410.
247. Kirkland, J. L., Mukku, V. R., Hardy, M., and Stancel, G. M. (1984): Hormonal control of uterine growth: Alterations in luminal epithelial deoxyribonucleic acid synthesis after intraluminal application of estrogen. *Endocrinology,* 114:969–973.
248. Klug, A., Rhodes, D., and Smith, J. (1980): A low resolution structure for the histone core of the nucleosome. *Nature,* 287: 509–516.
249. Knauer, E. (1900): Die Ovarientransplantation. *Arch. Gynakol.,* 60:322–376.
250. Kneifel, M. A., Leytus, S. P., Fletcher, E., Weber, T., Mangel, W. F., and Katzenellenbogen, B. S. (1982): Uterine plasminogen activator activity: Modulation by steroid hormones. *Endocrinology,* 111:493–399.
251. Knobil, E. (1980): The neuroendocrine control of the menstrual cycle. *Rec. Prog. Horm. Res.,* 36:53–88.
252. Koch, Y., Dikstein, S., Superstine, E., and Sulman, F. G. (1971): The effect of promethazine and clomiphene on gonadotrophin secretion in the rat. *J. Endocrinol.,* 49:13–17.
253. Kon, O. L. (1983): An antiestrogen-binding protein in human tissues. *J. Biol. Chem.,* 258:3173–3177.
254. Kon, O. L., and Spelsberg, T. C. (1982): Nuclear binding of estrogen-receptor complex: Receptor-specific nuclear acceptor sites. *Endocrinology,* 111:1925–1935.
255. Korach, K. S., and Ford, E. B. (1978): Estrogen action in the mouse uterus: An additional nuclear event. *Biochem. Biophys. Res. Commun.,* 83:327–333.
256. Korach, K. S., Fox-Davies, C., and Baker, V. (1980): Differential response to estriol and estradiol in the mouse uterus: Correlation to an additional nuclear event. *Endocrinology,* 106:1900–1906.
257. Korenman, S. G., Perrin, L. E., and McCallum, T. P. (1969): A radio-ligand binding assay system for estradiol measurement in human plasma. *J. Clin. Endocrinol.,* 29:879–883.
258. Korenman, S. G., and Rao, B. R. (1968): Reversible disaggregation of the cytosol-estrogen binding protein of uterine cytosol. *Proc. Natl. Acad. Sci. USA,* 61:1028–1033.
259. Korenman, S. G., Sanborn, B. M., and Bhalla, R. C. (1973): Adenyl cyclase and the cyclic AMP responsive systems in the uterus. In: *Receptors for Reproductive Hormones,* edited by B. W. O'Malley and A. R. Means, pp. 241–262. Plenum Press, New York.
260. Korenberg, M. S., and Clark, J. H. (1985): Changes in keratin expression during the estrogen mediated differentiation of rat vaginal epithelium. *Endocrinology,* 117:1480–1489.
261. Kornberg, R. D. (1977): Structure of chromatin. *Annu. Rev. Biochem.,* 46:931.
262. Kuehl, F. A., Ham, E. A., Zanetti, M. E., Sanford, C., Nicol, S. E., and Goldberg, N. D. (1974): Estrogen-related increases in uterine guanosine 3′:5′-cyclic monophosphate levels. *Proc. Natl. Acad. Sci. USA,* 71:1866–1870.
263. Kumar, S. A., and Dickerman, H. W. (1985): Steroid receptor-DNA interactions. In: *Molecular Mechanism of Steroid Hormone Action: Recent Advances,* edited by V. K. Moudgil, pp. 505–538. De Gruyter, Berlin.
264. Kurl, R. N., and Borthwick, N. M. (1980): Clomiphene and tamoxifen action in the rat uterus. *J. Endocrinol.,* 85:519–524.
265. Kurl, R. N., and Morris, I. D. (1978): Differential depletion of cytoplasmic high affinity oestrogen receptors after the *in vitro* administration of the antioestrogen clomiphene, MER-25 and tamoxifen. *Br. J. Pharmacol.,* 62:487–493.
266. Labrie, F., Drouin, J., Ferland, L., Lagace, L., Beaulieu, M., DeLean, A., Kelly, P. A., Caron, M. G., and Raymond, V. (1978): Mechanism of action of hypothalamic hormones in the anterior pituitary gland and specific modulation of their activity by sex steroids and thyroid hormones. *Recent Prog. Horm. Res.,* 34: 25–93.
267. Labrie, F., Simard, J., and Luthy, I. (1986): Unoccupied androgen receptors are biologically active in pituitary gonadotrophs. *Science* 23X:525–526.
268. Lam, P.H.-Y. (1984): Tamoxifen is a calmodulin antagonist in the activation of cAMP phosphodiesterase. *Biochem. Biophys. Res. Commun.,* 118:27–32.
269. Lamb, D. L., and Bullock, S. W. (1984): Heterogeneous deoxyribonucleic acid-binding forms of rabbit uterine progesterone receptor. *Endocrinology,* 114:1833–1840.
270. Lan, N. C., and Katzenellenbogen, B. S. (1976): Temporal relationships between hormone receptor binding and biological responses in the uterus: Studies with short- and long-acting derivatives of estriol. *Endocrinology,* 98:220–227.
271. Langier, C., Pageaux, J. F., Soto, A. M., and Sonnenschein, C. (1983): Mechanisms of estrogen action: Indirect effect of estradiol on proliferation of quail oviduct cells. *Proc. Natl. Acad. Sci. USA,* 80:1621–1625.
272. Langley, J. N. (1905): On the reaction of cells and of nerve-endings to certain poisons chiefly as regards the reaction of striated muscle to nicotine and to curari. *J. Physiol. (Lond.),* 33:374–413.
273. Laskey, R. A., and Earnshaw, W. C. (1980): Nucleosome assembly. *Nature,* 286:763–767.
274. Laumas, K. R., and Farooq, A. (1966): The uptake *in vivo* of [1,2,-^{3}H]progesterone by the brain and genital tract of the rat. *J. Endocrinol.,* 36:95–96.
275. Lawson, G. M., Knoll, B. J., March, C. J., Woo, S. L. C., Tsai, M.-J., and O'Malley, B. W., (1982): Definition of 5′ and 3′ structural boundaries of the chromatin domain containing the ovalbumin multigene family. *J. Biol. Chem.,* 257:1501.
276. Lazier, C. B., Capony, F., and Williams, D. L. (1981): Antioestrogen action in chick liver: Effects on oestrogen receptors and oestrogen-induced proteins. In: *Non-Steroidal Antioestrogens,* edited by R. L. Sutherland and V. C. Jordan, pp. 215–230. Academic Press, Sydney.
277. Leavitt, W. W., Chen, T. J., Do, Y. S., Carlton, B. D., and Allen, T. C. (1978): Biology of progesterone receptors. In: *Receptors and Hormone Action,* edited by B. W. O'Malley and L. Birnbaumer, pp. 157–188. Academic Press, New York.
278. Leavitt, W.W., Toft, D. O., Strott, C. A., and O'Malley, B. W (1974): A specific progesterone receptor in the hamster uterus: Physiologic properties and regulation during the estrous cycle. *Endocrinology,* 94:1041–1053.
279. Leclercq, G., Hulin, N., and Heuson, J. C. (1973): Interaction of activated estradiol-receptor complex and chromatin in isolated uterine nuclei. *Eur. J. Cancer,* 9:681–685.
280. Lee, S. H. (1978): Cytochemical study of estrogen receptor in human mammary cancer. *Am. J. Clin. Pathol.,* 70:197–203.
281. LeMeur, M., Glanville, N., and Mandel. J. L. (1981): The ovalbumin gene family: Hormonal control of X and Y gene transcription and mRNA accumulation. *Cell,* 23:561–571.
282. Lemon, H. (1980): Pathophysiologic considerations in the treatment of menopausal patients with oestrogens; the role of oestriol in the prevention of mammary carcinoma. *Acta Endocrinol. (Suppl.),* 23:17–27.
283. Lerner, L. J. (1964): Hormone antagonists: Inhibitors of specific activities of estrogen and androgen. *Recent Prog. Horm. Res.,* 20:435–490.

284. Lerner, L. J., Hilf, R., Turkheimer, A. R., Michel, I., and Engle, S. L. (1966): Effects of hormone antagonists on morphological and biochemical changes induced by hormonal steroids in the immature rat uterus. *Endocrinology*, 78:111–124.

285. Lessey, B. A., Alexander, P. S., and Horwitz, K. B. (1983): The subunit structure of human breast cancer progesterone receptors: Characterization by chromatography and photoaffinity labeling. *Endocrinology*, 112:1267–1274.

286. Liao, S., and Fang, S. (1970): Receptor-proteins for androgens and the mode of action of androgens on gene transcription in ventral prostate. *Vitam. Horm.*, 27:17–90.

287. Lieberman, M. E., Gorski, J., and Jordan, V. C. (1983): An estrogen receptor model to describe the regulation of prolactin synthesis by antiestrogens *in vitro*. *J. Biol. Chem.*, 258:4741–4745.

288. Lieberman, M. E., Jordan, V. C., Fritsch, M., Santos, M. A., and Gorski, J. (1983): Direct and reversible inhibition of estradiol-stimulated prolactin synthesis by antiestrogen *in vitro*. *J. Biol. Chem.*, 258:4734–4740.

289. Linkie, D. M., and Siiteri, P. K. (1978): A re-examination of the interaction of estradiol with target cell receptors. *J. Steroid Biochem.*, 9:1071–1078.

290. Lippman, M. (1981): Hormonal regulation of human breast cancer cells *in vitro*. *Banbury Rep.*, 8:171–184.

291. Lippman, M., Bolan, G., and Huff, K. (1976): The effects of androgens and anti-androgens on hormone-responsive human breast cancer in long term tissue culture. *Cancer Res.*, 36:4595–4601.

292. Lippman, M., Monaco, M. E., and Bolan, G. (1977): Effects of estrone, estradiol and estriol on hormone-responsive human breast cancer in long-term tissue culture. *Cancer Res.*, 37:1901–1907.

293. Littlefield, B. A., and Spelsburg, T. C. (1985): Problems and artifacts in the identification of nuclear acceptor sites for avian oviduct progesterone receptor. *Endocrinology*, 17:412–414.

294. Loeb, L., and Kountz, W. B. (1928): The effect of injection of follicular extract on the sex organs in the guinea pig and the interaction between the follicular substances and substances given off by the corpus luteum. *Am. J. Physiol.*, 84:283–306.

295. Loosfelt, H., Logeat, F., Vu Hai, M. T., and Milgrom, E. (1984): The rabbit progesterone receptor: Evidence for a single steroid binding subunit and characterization of receptor mRNA. *J. Biol. Chem.*, 259:14196–14202.

296. Luu Thi, M. T., Baulieu, E. E., and Milgrom, E. (1975): Comparison of the characteristics and of the hormonal control of endometrial and myometrial progesterone receptors. *J. Endocrinol.*, 66:349–356.

297. MacDonald, R. G., Okulicz, W. C., and Leavitt, W. W. (1982): Progesterone-induced inactivation of nuclear estrogen receptor in the hamster uterus is mediated by acid phosphatase. *Biochem. Biophys. Res. Commun.*, 104:570–576.

298. MacDonald, R. G., Rosenberg, S. P., and Leavitt, W. W. (1983): Localization of estrogen receptor regulatory factor in the uterine nucleus. *Mol. Cell. Endocrinol.*, 32:301–313.

299. MacLaughlin, D. T., Hudson, J. M., and Donoahue, P. M. (1983): Specific estradiol binding in embryonic mullerian ducts: A potential modulator of regression in the male and female chick. *Endocrinology*, 113:144–145.

300. MacLeod, J., and Reynolds, S. R. M. (1938): Vascular, metabolic, and motility responses of uterine tissue following administration of oestrin. *Proc. Soc. Exp. Biol. Med.*, 37:666–668.

301. Mainwaring, W.I. P., and Peterken, B. M. (1971): A reconstituted cell-free system for the specific transfer of steroid-receptor complexes into nuclear chromatin isolated from rat ventral prostate gland. *Biochem. J.*, 125:285–295.

302. Mairesse, N., and Galand, P. (1979): Comparison between the action of estradiol and that of the antiestrogen U11-100A on the induction in the rat uterus of a specific protein (the induced protein). *Endocrinology*, 105:1248–1253.

303. Mariman, E. C. M., van Eekelen, C. A. G., Reinders, R. J., Berns, A. J. M., and van Venrooiji, W. J. (1982): Adenoviral heterogeneous nuclear RNA is associated with the host nuclear matrix during splicing. *J. Mol. Biol.*, 154:103–119.

304. Markaverich, B. M., and Clark, J. H. (1979): Two binding sites for estradiol in rat uterine nuclei: Relationship to uterotropic response. *Endocrinology*, 105:1458–1462.

305. Markaverich, B. M., Clark, J. H., and Hardin, J. W. (1978): RNA transcription and uterine growth: Differential effects of estradiol, estriol and nafoxidine on chromatin RNA initiation sites. *Biochemistry*, 17:3146–3152.

306. Markaverich, B. M., Roberts, R. R., Alejandro, M., and Clark, J. H. (1984): The effect of low dose continuous exposure to estradiol on the estrogen receptor (type I) and nuclear type II sites. *Endocrinology*, 114:814–820.

307. Markaverich, B. M., Roberts, R. R., Finney, R. W., and Clark, J. H. (1983): Preliminary characterization of an endogenous inhibitor of [^{3}H]estradiol binding in rat uterine nuclei. *J. Biol. Chem.*, 258:11663–11671.

308. Markaverich, B. M., Upchurch, S., and Clark, J. H. (1981): Progesterone and dexamethasone antagonism of nucleus growth: A role for a second nuclear binding site for estradiol in estrogen action. *J. Steroid Biochem.*, 14:125–132.

309. Markaverich, B. M., Upchurch, S., McCormack, S. A., Glasser, S. R., and Clark, J. H. (1981): Differential stimulation of uterine cells by nafoxidine and clomiphene: Relationship between nuclear estrogen receptors and type II estrogen binding sites and cellular growth. *Biol. Reprod.*, 24:171–181.

310. Markaverich, B. M., Williams, M., Upchurch, S., and Clark, J. H. (1981): Heterogeneity of nuclear estrogen-binding sites in the rat uterus: A simple method for the quantitation of the Type I and Type II sites by [^{3}H]estradiol exchange. *Endocrinology*, 109:62–69.

311. Markee, J. E. (1932): Rhythmic vascular uterine changes. *Am. J. Physiol.*, 100:32–39.

312. Markee, J. E. (1932): Analysis of rhythmic vascular changes in uterus of rabbit. *Am. J. Physiol.*, 100:374–382.

313. Marshall, F. H. A., and Jolly, W. A. (1905): Contributions to the physiology of mammalian reproduction. *Phil. Trans. Roy. Soc. B*, 198:99–142.

314. Martin, L. (1969): Dimethylstilbestrol and 16-oxo-estradiol: Antiestrogens or estrogens. *Steroids*, 13:1–10.

315. Martin, L. (1980): Estrogens, anti-estrogens and the regulation of cell proliferation in the female reproductive tract *in vivo*. In: *Estrogens in the Environment*, edited by J. McLachlan, pp. 103–130. Elsevier/North Holland, Amsterdam.

316. Martin, L., and Claringbold, P. J. (1960): The mitogenic action of oestrogens in the vaginal epithelium of the ovariectomized mouse. *J. Endocrinol.*, 20:173–186.

317. Martin, P. M., and Sheridan, P. J. (1982): Towards a new model for the mechanism of action of steroids. *J. Steroid Biochem.*, 16:215–229.

318. Martucci, C., and Fishman, J. (1977): Direction of estradiol metabolism as a control of its hormonal action—Uterotrophic activity of estradiol metabolites. *Endocrinology*, 101:1709–1715.

319. Massol, N., Lebeau, M.-C., and Baulieu, E.-E. (1978): Estrogen receptor in hen oviduct chromatin, digested by micrococcal nuclease. *Nucleic Acids Res.*, 5:723–738.

320. McClellan, M. C., West, N. B., Tacha, D. E., Greene, G. L., and Brenner, R. M. (1984): Immunochemical localization of estrogen receptors in the macaque reproductive tract with monoclonal antiestrophilins. *Endocrinology*, 114:2002–2014.

321. McCormack, S. A., and Glasser, S. R. (1980): Differential response of individual uterine cell types from immature rats treated with estradiol. *Endocrinology*, 106:1634–1649.

322. McCorquodale, D. J., and Mueller, G. C. (1958): Effect of estradiol on the level of amino acid-activating enzymes in the rat uterus. *J. Biol. Chem.*, 232:31–42.

323. McEwen, B. S. (1978): Gonadal steroid receptors in neuroendocrine tissues. In: *Receptors for Hormones, Vol. II*, edited by B. W. O'Malley and L. Birnbaumber, pp. 353–400. Academic Press, New York.

324. McGhee, J. D., and Felsenfeld, G. (1980): Nucleosome structure. *Annu. Rev. Biochem.*, 49:1115–1156.

325. McGrath, C. M. (1983): Augmentation of the response of normal mammary epithelial cells to estradiol by mammary stroma. *Cancer Res.*, 43:1355–1360.

326. McGuire, W. L., Carbone, P. P., Sears, M. E., and Escher, G. C. (1975): Estrogen receptors in human breast cancer: An overview. In: *Estrogen Receptors in Human Breast Cancer*, edited by W. L. McGuire, P. P. Carbone, and E. P. Vollmer, pp. 1–7. Raven Press, New York.

327. McKnight, G. S. (1978): The induction of ovalbumin and conalbumin mRNA by estrogen and progesterone in chick oviduct explant cultures. *Cells*, 14:403–413.

328. McKnight, G. S., Gavis, E. R., and Kingsbury, R. (1981): Analysis of transcriptional regulatory signals of the HSV-thymidine kinase gene: Identification of an upstream control region. *Cell,* 25: 385–398.
329. McKnight, G. S., and Kingsbury, R. (1982): Transcriptional control signals of a eucaryotic protein-coding gene. *Science,* 217:316–324.
330. McKnight, G. S., and Palmiter, R. D. (1979): Transcriptional regulation of the ovalbumin and conalbumin genes by steroid hormones in chick oviduct. *J. Biol. Chem.,* 254:9050.
331. McNaught, R. W., Raymoure, W. J., and Smith, R. G. (1983): Separation and progesterone regulation of two chick estrogen receptors. *Endocrinology,* 112(*suppl*):342.
332. Means, A. R., Comstock, J. P., and Rosenfeld, G. C. (1972): Ovalbumin messenger RNA of chick oviduct: Partial characterization, estrogen dependence and translation *in vitro. Proc. Natl. Acad. Sci. USA,* 69:1146.
333. Means, A. R., and Hamilton, T. H. (1966): Evidence for depression of nuclear protein synthesis and concomitant stimulation of nuclear RNA synthesis during early estrogen action. *Proc. Natl. Acad. Sci. USA,* 56:686–693.
334. Mercer, W. D., Edwards, D. P., Chamness, G. C., and McGuire, W. L. (1981): Failure of estradiol immunofluorescence in MCF-7 breast cancer cells to detect estrogen receptors. *Cancer Res.,* 41:4644–4652.
335. Mester, J., and Baulieu, E. E. (1972): Nuclear estrogen receptor of chick liver. *Biochim. Biophys. Acta,* 261:236–244.
336. Mester, J., and Baulieu, E. E. (1975): Dynamics of oestrogen-receptor distribution between the cytosol and nuclear fractions of immature rat uterus after oestradiol administration. *Biochem. J.,* 146:617–623.
337. Mester, J., Brunelle, R., Tung, I., and Sonnenschein, C. (1973): Estrogen-sensitive cells. *Exp. Cell Res.,* 81:447–452.
338. Mester, J., Martel, D., Psychoyos, A., and Baulieu, E. E. (1974): Hormonal control of oestrogen receptor in uterus and receptivity for ovoimplantation in the rat. *Nature,* 250:776–778.
339. Middlebrook, J. L., Wong, M. D., Ishii, D. N., and Aronow, L. (1975): Subcellular distribution of glucocorticoid receptors in mouse fibroblasts. *Biochemistry,* 14:180–186.
340. Milgrom, E., Atger, M., and Baulieu, E. E. (1970): Progesterone in uterus and plasma. IV. Progesterone receptors in guinea pig uterus cytosol. *Steroids,* 16:741–764.
341. Milgrom, E., Thi, L., Atger, M., and Baulieu, E. E. (1973): Mechanisms regulating the concentration and the conformation of progesterone receptor(s) in the uterus. *J. Biol. Chem.,* 248:6366–6374.
342. Milgrom, E., Vu Hai, M. T., and Logeat, F. (1977): Use of ^{3}H-R5020 for the assay of cytosol and nuclear progesterone receptor in the rat uterus. In: *Progesterone Receptors in Normal and Neoplastic Tissues,* edited by W. L. McGuire, M.-P. Raynaud, and E.-E. Baulieu, pp. 261–270. Raven Press, New York.
343. Miller, B. G., and Emmens, C. W. (1969): The oestrogenic potency in the mouse of several substances closely related to diethylstilboestrol and mesohexoestrol. *J. Endocrinol.,* 45:9–15.
344. Miller, M. A., and Katzenellenbogen, B. S. (1983): Characterization and quantitation of antiestrogen binding sites in estrogen receptor-positive and -negative human breast cancer cell lines. *Cancer Res.,* 43:3094–3100.
345. Mockus, M. B., and Howitz, K. B. (1983): Progesterone receptors in human breast cancer. Stoichiometric translocation and nuclear receptor processing. *J. Biol. Chem.,* 258:4778–4783.
346. Moen, R. C., and Palmiter, R. D. (1980): Changes in hormone responsiveness of chick oviduct during primary stimulation with estrogen. *Dev. Biol.,* 78:450–463.
347. Monsma, F. J., Jr, Katzenellenbogen, B. S., Miller, M. A., Ziegler, Y. S., and Katzenellenbogen, J. A. (1984): Characterization of the estrogen receptor and its dynamics in MCF-7 human breast cancer cells using a covalently attaching antiestrogen. *Endocrinology,* 115:143–153.
348. Moulton, B. C., and Barker, K. L. (1971): Synthesis and degradation of glucose-6-phosphate dehydrogenase in the rat uterus. *Endocrinology,* 89:1131–1136.
349. Mueller, G. C. (1957): A discussion of the mechanism of action of steroid hormones. *Cancer Res.,* 17:490–506.
350. Mueller, G. C. (1960): Biochemical parameters of estrogen action. In: *Biological Activities of Steroids in Relation to Cancer,* edited by G. Pincus and E. P. Vollmer, pp. 129–145. Academic Press, New York.
351. Mueller, G. C. (1961): Discussion of a paper: Hagerman, D. D., and Villee, C. A., A mechanism of action for estrogenic steroid hormones, pp. 169–181. In: *Mechanism of Action of Steroid Hormones,* edited by C. A. Villee and L. L. Engel, pp. 181–187. Pergamon Press, New York.
352. Mueller, G. C., Gorski, J., and Aizawa, Y. (1961): The role of protein synthesis in early estrogen action. *Proc. Natl. Acad. Sci. USA,* 47:164–169.
353. Mueller, G. C., Herranen, A. M., and Jervell, K. (1958): Studies on the mechanisms of action of estrogens. *Recent Prog. Horm. Res.,* 14:95–139.
354. Mukku, V. R., and Stancel, G. M. (1985): Receptors for epidermal growth factor in the rat uterus. *Endocrinology,* 117:149–154.
355. Muldoon, T. G. (1981): Regulation of steroid hormone receptor activity. *Endocr. Rev.,* 1:339–364.
356. Muldoon, T. G. (1981): Role of receptors in the mechanism of steroid hormone action in the brain. In: *The Endocrine Functions of the Brain,* edited by M. Motta, pp. 51–93. Raven Press, New York.
357. Müller, R. E., Beebe, D. M., Bercel, E., Traish, A. M., and Wotiz, H. H. (1984): Estriol and estradiol interactions with the estrogen receptor *in vivo* and *in vitro. J. Steroid Biochem.,* 20:1039–1046.
358. Müller, R. E., Johnston, T. C., and Wotiz, H. H. (1979): Binding of estradiol to purified uterine plasma membranes. *J. Biol. Chem.,* 254:7895–7900.
359. Müller, R. E., Traish, A. M., Hirota, T., Bercel, E., and Wotiz, H. H. (1985): Conversion of estrogen receptor from a state with low affinity for estradiol into a state of higher affinity does not require 4S to 5S dimerization. *Endocrinology,* 116:337–345.
360. Müller, R. E., and Wotiz, H. H. (1979): Kinetics of estradiol entry into uterine cells. *Endocrinology,* 105:1107–1114.
361. Mulvihill, E. R., and Palmiter, R. D. (1977): Relationship of nuclear estrogen receptor levels to induction of ovalbumin and conalbumin mRNA and chick oviduct. *J. Biol. Chem.,* 252:2060–2068.
362. Mulvihill, E. R., and Palmiter, R. D. (1980): Relationship of nuclear progesterone receptors to induction of ovalbumin and conalbumin mRNA in chick oviduct. *J. Biol. Chem.,* 255:2085–2091.
363. Munck, A., and Foley, R. (1976): Kinetics of glucocorticoid-receptor complexes in rat thymus cells. *J. Steroid Biochem.,* 7:1117–1122.
364. Munck, A., Wira, C., Young, D. A., Mosher, K. M., Hallahan, C., and Bell, P. A. (1972): Glucocorticoid-receptor complexes and the earliest steps in the action of glucocorticoids on thymus cells. *J. Steroid Biochem.,* 3:567–578.
365. Murai, J. T., Lieberman, R. C., Yang, J. J., and Gerschenson, L. E. (1979): Decrease of estrogen receptors induced by 17β-estradiol and progesterone in cultured rabbit endometrial cells. *Endocrinol. Res. Commun.,* 6:235–247.
366. Murayama, A. (1985): Molecular organization of the estrogen receptor system. In: *Molecular Mechanism of Steroid Hormone Action,* edited by V. K. Moudgil, pp. 1–30. W. deGrunter, Berlin.
367. Murphy, L. C., and Sutherland, R. L. (1981): A high-affinity binding site for the antioestrogen, tamoxifen and CI628, in immature rat uterine cytosol which is distinct from the oestrogen receptor. *J. Endocrinol.,* 91:155–161.
368. Murphy, L. C., and Sutherland, R. L. (1983): Antitumor activity of clomiphene analogs *in vitro:* Relationship to affinity for the estrogen receptor and another high affinity antiestrogen-binding site. *J. Clin. Endocrinol. Metab.,* 57:373–379.
369. Murphy, P. R., Breckenridge, W. C., and Lazier, C. B. (1985): Binding of oxygenated cholesterol metabolites to antiestrogen binding sites from chicken liver. *Biochem. Biophys. Res. Commun.,* 127:786–792.
370. Murphy, P. R., Butts, C., and Lazier, C. B. (1984): Triphenyethylene antiestrogens binding sites in cockerel liver nuclei: Evidence for an endogenous ligand. *Endocrinology,* 115:420–426.
371. Nagel, S., Baier, H., and Taubert, H.-D. (1970): Contrasting actions of cis and trans-clomiphene on the release of FSH and FSH-RF in the female rat. *Horm. Metab. Res.,* 2:344–348.
372. Nandi, S., Imagawa, W., Tomooka, Y., McGrath, M. F., and Edery, M. (1984): Collagen gel culture system and analysis of estrogen effects on mammary carcinogenesis. *Arch. Toxicol.,* 55:91–96.
373. Natrajan, P. K., and Greenblatt, R. B. (1979): *Clomiphene Citrate: Induction of Ovulation,* pp. 35–76. Lea and Febiger, Philadelphia.

374. Nenci, I., Beccatti, M. D., Piffanelli, A., and Lanza, G. (1976): Detection and dynamic localization of estradiol-receptor complexes in intact target cells by immunofluorescent technique. *J. Steroid Biochem.*, 7:505–510.
375. Nicol, S. E., and Goldberg, N. D. (1976): Inhibition of estrogen induced changes in uterine cGMP: Relationship with other parameters of hormonal stimulation. *Arch. Int. Physiol. Biochim.*, 84:1072–1078.
376. Noteboom, W. D., and Gorski, J. (1963): An early effect of estrogen on protein synthesis. *Proc. Natl. Acad. Sci. USA*, 50:250–255.
377. Noteboom, W. D., and Gorski, J. (1965): Stereospecific binding of estrogens in the rat uterus. *Arch. Biochem. Biophys.*, 11:559–568.
378. Notides, A. C., Lerner, N., and Hamilton, D. E. (1981): Positive cooperativity of the estrogen receptor. *Proc. Natl. Acad. Sci. USA*, 78:4926–4930.
379. Notides, A. C., and Nielsen, S. (1974): The molecular mechanism of the *in vitro* 4S to 5S transformation of the uterine estrogen receptor. *J. Biol. Chem.*, 249:1866–1873.
380. Notides, A. C., and Nielsen, S. (1975): A molecular and kinetic analysis of estrogen receptor transformation. *J. Steroid Biochem.*, 6:483–486.
381. Okulicz, W. C. (1985): Temporal limitation of progesterone inhibition of occupied nuclear estrogen receptor retention in the rat uterus. *Program Endocr. Soc.*, p. 81, Astr. 322.
382. Okulicz, W. C., Evans, R. W., and Leavitt, W.W. (1981): Progesterone regulation of estrogen receptor in the rat uterus: A primary inhibitory influence on the nuclear fraction. *Steroids*, 37: 463–470.
383. Okulicz, W. C., Evans, R. W., and Leavitt, W. W. (1981): Progesterone regulation of the occupied form of nuclear estrogen receptor. *Science*, 213:1503–1505.
384. Olge, F. F. (1981): Kinetic and physiochemical characteristics of an endogenous inhibitor to progesterone-receptor binding in rat placental cytosol. *Biochem. J.*, 199:371–381.
385. O'Malley, B. W., McGuire, W. L., Kohler, P. O., and Korenman, S. G. (1969): Studies on the mechanism of steroid hormone regulation of synthesis of specific proteins. *Recent Prog. Horm. Res.*, 25:105–160.
386. O'Malley, B. W., Roop, D. R., Lai, E. C., Nordstrom, J. L., Catterall, J. F., Swaneck, G. E., Colbert, D. A., Tsai, M. J., Dugaiczyk, A., and Woo, S. (1979): The ovalbumin gene: Organization, structure, transcription and regulation. *Recent Prog. Horm. Res.*, 35:1–46.
387. O'Malley, B. W., and Schrader, W. T. (1972): Progesterone receptor components: Identification of subunits binding to the target-cell genome. *J. Steroid Biochem.*, 3:617–629.
388. O'Malley, B. W., Schrader, W. T., and Spelsberg, T. C. (1973): Hormone receptor interactions with the genome of eukaryotic target cells. *Adv. Exp. Med. Biol.*, 36:174–196.
389. O'Malley, B. W., Sherman, M. R., and Toft, D. O. (1970): Progesterone "receptors" in the cytoplasm and nucleus of chick oviduct target tissue. *Proc. Natl. Acad. Sci. USA*, 67:501–511.
390. O'Malley, B. W., Spelsberg, T. C., Schrader, W. T., Chytil, F., and Steggles, A. W. (1972): Mechanisms of interaction of a hormone-receptor complex with the genome of a eukaryotic target cell. *Nature*, 235:141–144.
391. O'Malley, B. W., Toft, D. O., and Sherman, M. R. (1971): Progesterone binding components of chick oviduct. II. Nuclear components. *J. Biol. Chem.*, 246:1117–1122.
392. Oppenheimer, J. H., Schwartz, H. L., Surks, M. I., Koeruer, D., and Dillman, W. H. (1976): Nuclear receptors and the initiation of thyroid hormone action. *Recent Prog. Horm. Res.*, 32:529–565.
393. Overath, P., and Trauble, H. (1973): Phase transitions in cells, membranes, and lipids of *Escherichia coli*. Detection by fluorescent probes, light scattering, and dilatometry. *Biochemistry*, 12: 2625–2634.
394. Palmiter, R. D. (1975): Quantitation of parameters that determine the rate of ovalbumin synthesis. *Cell*, 4:189–197.
395. Palmiter, R. D., Mulvihill, E. R., McKnight, G. S., and Senear, A. W. (1978): Regulation of gene expression in the chick oviduct by steroid hormones. *Cold Spring Harbor Symp. Quant. Biol.*,42:639–647.
396. Panko, W. B., and Macleod, R. M. (1978): Uncharged nuclear receptors for estrogen in breast cancers. *Cancer Res.*, 38:1948–1951.
397. Panko, W. B., Watson, C. S., and Clark, J. H. (1981): The presence of a second, specific estrogen binding site in human breast cancer. *J. Steroid Biochem.*, 14:1311–1316.
398. Pardoll, D. M., Vogelstein, B., and Coffey, D. S. (1980): A fixed site of DNA replication in eukaryotic cells. *Cell*, 19:527–536.
399. Parker, M., Hurst, H., and Page, M. (1984): Organization and expression of prostatic steroid binding protein genes. *J. Steroid Biochem.*, 20:67–71.
400. Pasqualini, J. R., Gulino, A., Nguyen, B. L., and Partois, M. C. (1980): Receptor and biological response to estriol in the fetal uterus of guinea pig. *J. Receptor Res.*, 1–261.
401. Pavlik, E. J., and Coulson, P. B. (1976): Modulation of estrogen receptors in four different target tissues: Differential effects of estrogen vs. progesterone. *J. Steroid Biochem.*, 7:369–376.
402. Pavlik, E. J., Rutledge, S., Eckert, R. L., and Katzenellenbogen, B. S. (1979): Localization of estrogen receptors in uterine cells: An appraisal of translocation. *Exp. Cell Res.*, 123:177–189.
403. Payvar, R., DeFranco, D., and Firestone, G. L. (1983): Sequence-specific binding of glucocorticoid receptor to MTV DNA at sites within and upstream of the transcribed region. *Cell*, 35:381–392.
404. Peck, E. J., Jr., Burgner, J., and Clark, J. H. (1973): Estrophilic binding sites of the uterus. Relation to uptake and retention of estradiol *in vitro*. *Biochemistry*, 12:4596–4603.
405. Peleg, S., Schrader, W. T., Edwards, D. P., McGuire, W. L., and O'Malley, B. W. (1985): Immunologic detection of a protein homologous to chicken progesterone receptor B subunit. *J. Biol. Chem.*, 260:8492–8501.
406. Perlow, M., Sassin, J., Boyar, R., Hellman, L., and Weitzman, E. D. (1973): Reduction of growth hormone secretion following clomiphene administration. *Metabolism*, 22:1269–1275.
407. Perrot-Applanat, M., Logeat, F., Groyer-Picard, M. T., and Milgrom, E. (1985): Immunocytochemical study of mammalian progesterone receptor using monoclonal antibodies. *Endocrinology*, 116:1473–1484.
408. Pertschuk, L. P., Gatejens, E. G., Carter, A. C., Brigati, D. J., Kim, D. S., and Fealey, T. E. (1979): An improved histochemical method for detection of estrogen receptors in mammary cancer. *Am. J. Clin. Pathol.*, 71:504–508.
409. Pertschuk, L. P., Tobin, E. H., Brigati, D. J., Kim, D. S., Bloom, N. D., Guetjens, E., Beman, P. J., Carter, A. C., and Deyenshein, G. A. (1978): Immunofluorescent detection of estrogen receptors in breast cancer. *Cancer*, 41:907–911.
410. Pietras, R. J., and Szego, C. M. (1976): Endometrial cell calcium and oestrogen action. *Nature*, 253:357–359.
411. Pietras, R. J., and Szego, C. M. (1977): Specific binding sites for oestrogen at the outer surfaces of isolated endometrial cells. *Nature*, 265:68–71.
412. Pietras, R. J., and Szego, C. M. (1980): Partial purification and characterization of oestrogen receptors in subfractions of hepatocyte plasma membranes. *Biochem. J.*, 191:743–760.
413. Pollard, I., and Martin, L. (1968): The oestrogenic and anti-oestrogenic activity of some synthetic steroids and non-steroids. *Steroids*, 11:897–907.
414. Puca, G. A., Sica, V., Nola, E., and Bresciani, F. (1979): Purification and properties of native oestradiol estrogen. *J. Steroid Biochem.*,11:301–306.
415. Puri, R. K., Grandics, P., Dougherty, J. J., and Toft, D. D. (1982): Purification of nontransformed avian progesterone receptor and preliminary characterization. *J. Biol. Chem.*, 257:10831–10837.
416. Rao, B. R., Fry, G. C., Hunt, S., Kuhnel, R., and Dandliker, W. B. (1980): A fluorescent probe for rapid detection of estrogen receptors. *Cancer*, 46:2902–2906.
417. Rae, B. R., Wiest, W. G., and Allen, W. M. (1973): Progesterone "receptor" in rabbit uterus. I. Characterization and estradiol-17beta augmentation. *Endocrinology*, 92:1229–1240.
418. Ravid, R., Jedwab, G., Persitz, E., David, M. P., Karni, N., Gil, S., Cordova, T., Harell, A., and Ayalon, D. (1977): Gonadotrophin release in ovariectomized patients. I. Suppression by clomiphene or low doses of ethinyl oestradiol. *Clin. Endocrinol.*, 6:333–338.
419. Raymoure, W. J., McNaught, R. W., and Smith, R. G. (1985): Reversible activation of non-steroid binding oestrogen receptor. *Nature*, 314:745–747.
420. Raynaud, J.-P., and Ojasco, T. (1983): The relevance of structure affinity relationships in the study of steroid hormone action. In:

Steroid Hormone Receptors: Structure and Function, edited by H. Eriksson and J. A. Gustafsson, pp. 141–170. Elsevier, Amsterdam.

421. Rebar, R., Judd, H. L., Yen, S. S. C., Rakoff, J., Vandenberg, G., and Naftolin, F. (1976): Characterization of the inappropriate gonadotropin secretion in polycystic ovary syndrome. *J. Clin. Invest.,* 57:1320–1329.
422. Reel, J. R., and Shih, Y. (1975): Oestrogen-inducible uterine progesterone receptors. Characteristics in the ovariectomized immature and adult hamster. *Acta Endocrinol.,* 80:344–354.
423. Renior, M., Yang, C.-R., Formstecher, P., Lustenberger, P., Wolfsou, A., Redeuilh, B., Mester, J., Richard-Foy, H., and Baulieu, E. E. (1982): Progesterone receptor from chick oviduct: Purification of molybdate stabilized form and preliminary characterization. *Eur. J. Biochem.,* 127:71–79.
424. Renkawitz, R., Bueg, H., Graf, T., Matthias, P., Grez, M., and Schütz, G. (1982): Expression of a chicken lysozyme recombinant gene is regulated by progesterone and dexamethasone after microinjection into oviduct cells. *Cell,* 31:167–176.
425. Reti, I., and Erdos, T. (1971): On the "native state" of the uterine estradiol "receptor." *Biochimie,* 53:435–437.
426. Reynolds, S. R. M. (1949): *Physiology of the Uterus,* 2d ed. Hoeber, New York.
427. Reynolds, S. R. M. (1951): Determinants of uterine growth and activity. *Physiol. Rev.,* 31:244–273.
428. Rhoads, R. E., McKnight, G. S., and Schimke, R. T. (1971): Synthesis of ovalbumin in a rabbit reticulocyte cell-free system programmed with hen oviduct ribonucleic acid. *J. Biol. Chem.,* 246:7407–7410.
429. Robinson, S. I., Nelkin, B. D., and Vogelstein, B. (1982): The ovalbumin gene is associated with the nuclear matrix of chicken oviduct cells. *Cell,* 28:99–106.
430. Robson, J. M., and Adler, J. (1940): Site of action of oestrogens. *Nature,* 146–160.
431. Rochefort, H., and Borgna, J. L. (1981): Differences between oestrogen receptor activation by oestrogen and antioestrogen. *Nature,* 292:257–259.
432. Rochefort, H., and Garcia, G. (1984): The estrogenic and antiestrogenic activities of androgens in female target tissues. *Pharmacol. Ther.,* 23:193–216.
433. Rochefort, H., Lignon, F., and Capony, F. (1972): Formation of estrogen nuclear receptor in uterus: Effects of androgen, estrone and nafoxidine. *Biochem. Biophys. Res. Commun.,* 47:662–670.
434. Rorke, E. A., and Katzenellenbogen, B. S. (1984): Dissociated regulation of growth and ornithine decarboxylase activity by estrogen in the rat uterus. *Biochem. Biophys. Res. Commun.,* 122:1186–1193.
435. Ross, G. T., Cargille, C. M., Lipsett, M. B., Rayford, P. L., Marshall, J. R., Strott, C. A., and Rodbard, D. (1970): Pituitary and gonadal hormones in women during spontaneous and induced ovulatory cycles. *Recent Prog. Horm. Res.,* 26:1–62.
436. Rousseau, G. G., Baxter, J. D., Higgins, S. J., and Tomkins, G. M. (1973): Steroid-induced nuclear binding of glucocorticoid receptors in intact hepatoma cells. *J. Mol. Biol.,* 79:539–544.
437. Ruh, T. S., and Baudendistel, L. J. (1977): Different nuclear binding sites for antiestrogen and estrogen receptor complexes. *Endocrinology,* 100:420–426.
438. Ruh, T. S., and Ruh, M. F. (1983): The agonistic and antagonistic properties of the high affinity antiestrogen H1285. *Pharmacol. Ther.,* 21:247–264.
439. Ruh, T. S., and Spelsberg, T. C. (1983): Acceptor sites for the oestrogen receptor in hen oviduct chromatin. *Biochem. J.,* 210:905–912.
440. Ruh, M. F., and Toft, D. O. (1984): Characterization of an unusual sex steroid binding component from the chicken oviduct. *J. Steroid Biochem.,* 21:1–8.
441. Ruh, T. S., Wassilak, S. G., and Ruh, M. F. (1975): Androgen-induced nuclear accumulation of the estrogen receptor. *Steroids,* 25:257–273.
442. Russell, D. H., and Taylor, R. L. (1971): Polyamine synthesis and accumulation in the castrated rat uterus after estradiol-17β stimulation. *Endocrinology,* 88:1397–1403.
443. Saffranj, J., Loesser, B. K., Bohnett, S. A., and Faber, L. E. (1976): Binding of progesterone receptor by nuclear preparations of rabbit and guinea pig uterus. *J. Biol. Chem.,* 251:5607–5613.
444. Sakai, D., and Gorski, J. (1984): Estrogen receptor transformation to a high-affinity state without subunit-subunit interactions. *Biochemistry,* 23:3541–3547.
445. Sanders, M. M., and McKnight, G. S. (1985): Chicken egg white genes: Multihormonal regulation in a primary cell culture system. *Endocrinology,* 116:398–405.
446. Sar, M., and Stumpf, W. E. (1973): Neurons of the hypothalamus concentrate (^{3}H)progesterone on its metabolites. *Science,* 182:1266–1268.
447. Sarff, M., and Gorski, J. (1971): Control of estrogen-binding protein concentration under basal conditions and after estrogen administration. *Biochemistry,* 10:2557–2563.
448. Sato, B., Nishizawa, Y., Noma, K., Nakao, M., and Kishimoto, S. (1985): The important role of cytoplasmic modulators in the pathway for steroid receptor to be converted to the biologically active form. In: *Molecular Mechanism of Steroid Hormone Action,* edited by J. K. Mondgil pp. 249–278. Walter de Grunter, Berlin.
449. Satysaswaroop, P. G., Fleming, H., Bressler, R. S., and Gurpide, E. (1978): Human endometrial cancer cell cultures for hormonal studies. *Cancer Res.,* 38:4367–4375.

449a. Scatchard, G. (1949): The attractions of proteins for small molecules and ions. *Ann. N.Y. Acad. Sci.,* 51:660–672.

450. Schally, A. V., Carter, W. H., Parlow, A. F., Saito, M., Arimura, A., Bowers, C. Y., and Holtcamp, O. E. (1970): Alteration of LH and FSH release in rat treated with clomiphene and its isomers. *Am. J. Obstet. Gynecol.,* 107:1156–1167.
451. Schatz, R., Soto, A. M., and Sonnenschein, C. (1984): Estrogen induced cell multiplication: Direct or indirect effect on rat uterine cells. *Endocrinology,* 115:501–506.
452. Schoenberg, D. R., and Clark, J. H. (1979): Effect of intercalating drugs on the release of uterine nuclear estrogen receptors. *J. Biol. Chem.,* 254:8270–8275.
453. Schoenberg, D. R., and Clark, J. H. (1981): Nuclear association sites of rat uterine oestrogen receptors as probed by nuclease digestion. *Biochem. J.,* 196:423–432.
454. Schrader, W. T. (1984): New model for steroid hormone receptors? *Nature,* 308:17.
455. Schrader, W. T., Birnbaumer, M. E., Hughes, M. R., Weigel, N. C., Grody, W. W., and O'Malley, B. W. (1981): Studies on the structure and function of the chick progesterone receptor. *Recent Prog. Horm. Res.,* 37:583–633.
456. Schrader, W. T., Coty, W. A., Smith, R. G., and O'Malley, B. W. (1977): Purification and properties of progesterone receptors from chick oviduct. *Ann. NY Acad. Sci.,* 286:64–80.
457. Schrader, W. T., Heuer, S. S., and O'Malley, B. W. (1975): Progesterone receptors of chick oviduct: Identification of 6S receptor dimers. *Biol. Reprod.,* 12:134–142.
458. Schrader, W. T., and O'Malley, B. W. (1972): Progesterone-binding components of chick oviduct. IV. Characterization of purified subunits. *J. Biol. Chem.,* 247:51–59.
459. Schrader, W. T., Toft, D. O., and O'Malley, B. W. (1972): Progesterone-binding protein of chick oviduct: VI. Interaction of purified progesterone-receptor components with nuclear constituents. *J. Biol. Chem.,* 247:2401–2407.
460. Schulz, K. D., August, S., Gasde, K., and Kramer, G. (1972): Studies on the anti-oestrogenic and oestrogen-like action of clomiphene citrate. Animal experiments. *Gynecol. Invest.,* 3:135–141.
461. Schutz, G., Nguyen-Huu, M. C., Giesecke, K., Hynes, N. E., Groner, B., Wurtz, T., and Sippel, A. E. (1977): Hormonal control of egg white protein messenger RNA synthesis in the chicken oviduct. *Cold Spring Harbor Symp. Quant. Biol.,* 42:617–624.
462. Scott, R. W., and Frankel, F. R. (1980): Enrichment of estradiol-receptor complexes in a transcriptionally active fraction of chromatin from MCF-7 cells. *Proc. Natl. Acad. Sci. USA,* 77:1291–1295.
463. Searle, P. F., and Tata, J. R. (1981): Vitelloginin gene expression in male *Xenopus* hepatocytes during primary and secondary stimulation with estrogen in cell cultures. *Cell,* 23:741–746.
464. Searn, A. W., and Paliter, R. D. (1981): Multiple structural features are responsible for the nuclease sensitivity of the active ovalbumin gene. *J. Biol. Chem.,* 256:1191–1198.
465. Senior, M. B., and Frankel, F. R. (1978): Evidence for two kinds of chromatin binding sites for the estradiol-receptor complex. *Cell,* 14:857–863.

466. Shafie, S. M. (1980): Estrogen and the growth of breast cancer: New evidence suggests indirect action. *Science,* 209:701–702.
467. Shelesnyak, M. C. (1959): Effect of estrogens on histamine release in the rat uterus. *Proc. Soc. Exp. Biol. Med.,* 100:739–742.
468. Sheridan, P. J. (1975): Is there an alternative to the cytoplasmic receptor model for the mechanism of action of steroids? *Life Sci.,* 17:497–502.
469. Sheridan, P. J., Buchanan, J. M., Anselmo, V. C., and Martin, P. M. (1979): Equilibrium: The intracellular distribution of steroid receptors. *Nature,* 282:579–582.
470. Sherman, M. R., Corval, P. L., and O'Malley, B. W. (1970): Progesterone-binding components of chick oviduct. I. Preliminary characterization of cytoplasmic components. *J. Biol. Chem.,* 245:6085–6096.
471. Sherman, M. R., Pickering, L. A., Rollwagen, F. M., and Miller, L. K. (1978): Mero-receptors: Proteolytic fragments of receptors containing the steroid-binding site. *Fed. Proc.,* 37:167–173.
472. Sherman, M. R., and Stevens, J. (1984): Structure of mammalian steroid receptors: Evolving concepts and methodological developments. *Annu. Rev. Physiol.,* 46:83–105.
473. Sherman, M. R., Tuazon, F. B., Diaz, S. C., and Miller, L. K. (1976): Multiple forms of oviduct progesterone receptors analyzed by ion exchange filtration and gel electrophoresis. *Biochemistry,* 15:980–989.
474. Sherman, M. R., Tuazon, F. B., Stevens, Y.-W., and Niu, E. M. (1983): Oligomeric steroid receptor forms and the products of their dissociation and proteolysis. In: *Steroid Hormone Receptors: Structure and Function,* edited by H. Eriksson and J. A. Gustafsson, pp. 3–24. Elsevier, Amsterdam.
475. Shyamala, G., and Gorski, J. (1967): Estrogen receptors in the rat uterus. Studies on the interaction of cytosol and nuclear binding sites. *J. Biol. Chem.,* 244:1097–1103.
476. Siiteri, P. K., Schwartz, B. E., Moriyama, I., Ashby, R., Linkie, D., and MacDonald, P. C. (1973): Estrogen binding in the rat and human. In: *Receptors for Reproductive Hormones,* edited by B. W. O'Malley and A. R. Means, pp. 97–112. Plenum Press, New York.
477. Simmen, R. C. M., Dunbar, B. S., Guerriero, V., Chafouleaus, J. G., Clark, J. H., and Means, A. R. (1984): Estrogen stimulates the transient association of calmodulin and myosin light chain kinase with the chicken liver nuclear matrix. *J. Cell Biol.,* 99:5588–5593.
478. Simmen, R. C. M., Means, A. R., and Clark, J. H. (1984): Estrogen modulation of nuclear matrix associated steroid hormone binding. *Endocrinology,* 115:1197–1202.
479. Singer, S. J. (1974): The molecular organization of membranes. *Annu. Rev. Biochem.,* 43:805–833.
480. Sirbasku, D. A., and Benson, R. H. (1979): Estrogen-inducible growth factors that may act as mediators (estromedins) of estrogen promoted tumor cell growth. *Cold Spring Harbor Conf. Cell Prolif.,* 6:477–497.
481. Slotta, K. H., Ruschig, H., and Fels, E. (1934): Die reindarstellung der hormone aus dem corpus luteum. *Bev. Deutsch. Chem. Ges.,* 67:1207–1208.
482. Small, D., Nelkin, B., and Vogelstein, B. (1982): Nonrandom distribution of repeated DNA sequences with respect to supercoiled loops and the nuclear matrix. *Proc. Natl. Acad. Sci. USA,* 79:5911–5915.
483. Smith, E. R., and Barker, K. L. (1974): Effects of estradiol and nicotinamide adenine dinucleotide phosphate on the rate of synthesis of uterine glucose 6-phosphate dehydrogenase. *J. Biol. Chem.,* 249:6541–6547.
484. Smith, R. G., Clarke, S. G., Zalta, E., and Taylor, R. N. (1979): Two estrogen receptors in reproductive tissue. *J. Steroid Biochem.,* 10:31–35.
485. Smith, R. G., d'Istria, M., and Van, N. T. (1981): Purification of a human progesterone receptor. *Biochemistry,* 20:5557–5565.
486. Smith, R. G., and Taylor, R. N. (1981): Estrogen receptors as mediators of gene transcription. *J. Steroid Biochem.,* 15:321–328.
487. Snow, L. D., Eriksson, H., Hardin, J. W., Chan, L., Jackson, R. L., Clark, J. H., and Means, A. R. (1978): Nuclear estrogen receptor in the avian liver: Correlation with biologic response. *J. Steroid Biochem.,* 9:1017–1026.
488. Sonnenschein, C., and Soto, A. M. (1978): Pituitary uterotrophic effect in the estrogen-dependent growth of the rat uterus. *J. Steroid Biochem.,* 9:533–537.
489. Soto, A. M., and Sonnenschein, C. (1985): The role of estrogens on the proliferation of human breast tumor cells (MCF-7). *J. Steroid Biochem.,* 23:87–94.
490. Soule, H. D., and McGrath, C. M. (1980): Estrogen responsive proliferation of clonal human breast carcinoma cells in athymic mice. *Cancer Lett.,* 10:177–189.
491. Spaziani, E. (1963): Relationship between early vascular responses and growth in the rat uterus: Stimulation of cell division by estradiol and vasodilating amines. *Endocrinology,* 72:180–191.
492. Spaziani, E., and Szego, C. M. (1958): The influence of estradiol and cortisol on uterine histamine of the ovariectomized rat. *Endocrinology,* 63:669–678.
493. Spaziani, E., and Szego, C. M. (1958): Early effects of estradiol and cortisol on water and electrolyte shifts in the uterus of the immature rat. *Am. J. Physiol.,* 197:355–359.
494. Spelsberg, T. C. (1976): Nuclear binding of progesterone in chick oviduct: Multiple binding sites *in vivo* and transcriptional response. *Biochem. J.,* 156:391–398.
495. Spelsberg, T. C., Littlefield, B. A., Seelke, R., Dani, G. M., Toyoda, H., Boyd-Leinen, P., Thrall, C., and Kon, O. L. (1983): Role of specific chromosomal proteins and DNA sequences in the nuclear binding sites for steroid receptors. *Recent Prog. Horm. Res.,* 39:463–517.
496. Spelsberg, T. C., Steggles, A. W., Chytil, F., and O'Malley, B. W. (1972): Progesterone binding components of chick oviduct. V. Exchange of progesterone binding capacity from target to nontarget tissue chromatin. *J. Biol. Chem.,* 247: 1368–1374.
497. Spelsberg, T. C., Steggles, A. W., and O'Malley, B. W. (1971): Progesterone-binding components of chick oviduct. *J. Biol. Chem.,* 246:4188–4197.
498. Spelsberg, T. C., Webster, R., Pickler, G., Thrall, C., and Wells, D. (1976): Role of nuclear proteins as high affinity sites ("acceptors") for progesterone in the avian oviduct. *J. Steroid Biochem.,* 7:1091–1101.
499. Stack, G., and Gorski, J. (1984): Direct mitogenic effect of estrogen on the prepuberal rat uterus: Studies on isolated nuclei. *Endocrinology,* 115:1141–1150.
500. Stancel, G. M., Leung, K. M. T., and Gorski, J. (1973): Estrogen receptors in the rat uterus. Multiple forms produced by aggregation. *Biochemistry,* 12:2130–2136.
501. Sudo, K., Monsma, F. J., Jr., and Katzenellenbogen, B. S. (1983): Anti-estrogen-binding sites distinct from the estrogen receptor: Subcellular localization, ligand specificity, and distribution in tissues of the rat. *Endocrinology,* 112:425–434.
502. Sutherland, R. L. (1981): Estrogen antagonists in chick oviduct: Antagonist activity of eight synthetic triphenylethylene derivatives and their interactions with cytoplasmic and nuclear estrogen receptors. *Endocrinology,* 109:2061–2068.
503. Sutherland, R. L., and Foo, M. S. (1979): Differential binding of anti-estrogens by rat uterine and chick oviduct cytosol. *Biochem. Biophys. Res. Commun.,* 91:183–191.
504. Sutherland, R. L., Mester, J., and Baulieu, E. E. (1977): Tamoxifen is a potent "pure" antioestrogen in the chick oviduct. *Nature,* 267:434–435.
505. Sutherland, R. L., and Murphy, L. C. (1980): The binding of tamoxifen to human mammary carcinoma cytosol. *Eur. J. Cancer,* 16:1141–1148.
506. Sutherland, R. L., Murphy, L. C., Foo, M. S., Green, M. D., Whybourne, A.M., and Krozowski, A. S. (1980): High affinity antioestrogen binding site distinct from the oestrogen receptor. *Nature,* 288:273–275.
507. Swaneck, G. E., Alvarez, J. M., and Sufrin, G. (1982): Multiple species of estrogen binding sites in the nuclear fraction of the rat prostate. *Biochem. Biophys. Res. Commun.,* 106:1441–1447.
508. Swaneck, G. E., Nordstrom, J. L., Kreuzaler, F., Tsai, M.-J., and O'Malley, B. W. (1979): Effect of estrogen on gene expression in chicken oviduct: Evidence for transcriptional control of ovalbumin gene. *Proc. Natl. Acad. Sci. USA.,* 76:1049.
509. Swanson, L. V., and Barker, K. L. (1983): Antagonistic effects of progesterone on estradiol-induced synthesis and degradation of uterine glucose-6-phosphate dehydrogenase. *Endocrinology,* 112:459–465.
510. Szego, C. M. (1965): Role of histamine in mediation of hormone action. *Fed. Proc.,* 24:1343–1352.

511. Szego, C. M. (1971): The lysosomal membrane complex as a proximate target for steroid hormone action. In: *The Sex Steroids*, edited by K. W. McKerns, pp. 1–51. Appleton-Century-Crofts, New York.
512. Szego, C. M., and Davis, J. S. (1967): Adenosine 3′5′-monophosphate in rat uterus: Acute elevation by estrogen. *Proc. Natl. Acad. Sci. USA*, 58:1711–1718.
513. Szego, C. M., and Davis, J. S. (1969): Inhibition of estrogen-induced elevation of cyclic 3′,5′-adenosine monophosphate in rat uterus. I. By β-adrenergic receptor blocking drugs. *Mol. Pharmacol.*, 5:470–480.
514. Szego, C. M., and Lawson, D. A. (1964): Influence of histamine on uterine metabolism: Stimulation of incorporation of radioactivity from amino acids into protein, lipid and purines. *Endocrinology*, 74:372–381.
515. Szego, C. M., and Pietras, R. J. (1985): Subcellular distribution of oestrogen receptors. *Nature*, 317:88.
516. Szego, C. M., and Roberts, S. (1953): Steroid action and interaction in uterine metabolism. *Recent Prog. Horm. Res.*, 8:419–469.
517. Tabacik, C., Cypriani, B., Alian, S., and Crastes de Paulet, A. (1984): Cholesterol biosynthesis in MCF-7 cell line in relation to cell division: Stimulation by estradiol and inhibition by tamoxifen. In: *Progress in Cancer Research and Therapy, Vol. 31*, edited by F. Bresciani, R. J. B. King, M. E. Lippman, M. Namer, and J.-P. Raynaud, pp. 213–222. Raven Press, New York.
518. Tai, P.-K. K., and Faber, L. L. (1985): Isolation of dissimilar components of the 8.5S nonactivated uterine progestin receptor. *Can. J. Biochem. Cell Biol.*, 63:41–49.
519. Talalay, P. (1961): Enzymatic interactions between steroid hormones and pyridine nucleotides. In: *Biological Approaches to Cancer Chemotherapy*, edited by R. J. C. Harris, pp. 59–75. Academic Press, New York.
520. Talalay, P. (1962): Studies on the placental 17β-hydroxysteroid dehydrogenase. In: *On Cancer and Hormones: Essays in Experimental Biology*, pp. 271–289. University of Chicago Press, Chicago.
521. Talwar, G. P., Segal, S. J., Evans, A., and Davidson, O. W. (1964): The binding of estradiol in the uterus: A mechanism for derepression of RNA synthesis. *Proc. Natl. Acad. Sci. USA*, 52:1059–1066.
522. Tata, J. R. (1984): The action of growth and developmental hormones: Evolutionary aspects. In: *Biological Regulation and Development*, edited by R. F. Goldberger and K. R. Yamamoto, pp. 1–58. Plenum Press, New York.
523. Tate, A. C., DeSombre, E. R., Greene, G. L., Jensen, E. V., and Jordan, V. C. (1983): Interaction of [^{3}H]monohydroxytamoxifen-estrogen receptor complexes with a monoclonal antibody. *Breast Cancer Res. Treat.*, 3:267–277.
524. Tate, A. C., Greene, G. L., DeSombre, E. R., Jensen, E. V., and Jordan, V. C. (1984): Differences between estrogen- and antiestrogen-estrogen receptor complexes from human breast tumors identified with an antibody raised against the estrogen receptor. *Cancer Res.*, 44:1012–1018.
525. Tate, A. C., and Jordan, V. C. (1984): Nuclear [^{3}H]4-hydroxytamoxifen (4-OHTAM)- and [^{3}H]estradiol (E_2)-estrogen receptor complexes in the MCF-7 breast cancer and GH_3 pituitary tumor cell lines. *Mol. Cell. Endocrinol.*, 36:211–219.
526. Tate, A. C., Lieberman, M. E., and Jordan, V. C. (1984): The inhibition of prolactin synthesis in GH_3 rat pituitary tumor cells by monohydroxytamoxifen is associated with changes in the properties of the estrogen receptor. *J. Steroid Biochem.*, 20:391–395.
527. Taubert, H.-D., and Dericks-Tan, J. S. E. (1976): High doses of estrogens do not interfere with the ovulation-inducing effect of clomiphene citrate. *Fertil. Steril.*, 27:375–382.
528. Taylor, R. N., and Smith, R. G. (1982): Effects of highly purified estrogen receptors on gene transcription in isolated nuclei. *Biochemistry*, 21:1781–1787.
529. Taylor, R. N., and Smith, R. G. (1982): Identification of a novel sex steroid binding protein. *Proc. Natl. Acad. Sci. USA*, 79:1742–1746.
530. Tchernitchin, A. (1972): Radioautographic study of the effect of estradiol-17β, estrone, estriol, progesterone, testosterone and corticosterone on the *in vitro* uptake of 2,4,6,7,-^{3}H estradiol-17β by uterine eosinophils of the rat. *Steroids*, 19:575–586.
531. Tchernitchin, A. (1976): Effect of progesterone on the *in vivo* binding of estrogens by uterine cells. *Experientia*, 32:1069–1071.
532. Tchernitchin, A., Roorijck, J., Tchernitchin, X., Vanden hende, J., and Galand, P. (1976): Effects of cortisol on uterine eosinophilia and other oestrogenic responses. *Mol. Cell Endocrinol.*, 2:331–337.
533. Tchernitchin, A., and Tchernitchin, X. (1977): Characterization of the estrogen receptors in the uterine and blood eosinophil leukocytes. *Experientia*, 32:1240–1242.
534. Tchernitchin, A., Tchernitchin, X., and Galand, P. (1976): New concepts on the actions of oestrogens in the uterus and the role of the eosinophil receptor system. *Differentiation*, 5:145–150.
535. Tchernitchin, A., Tchernitchin, X., and Galand, P. (1983): Dissociation of separate mechanisms of estrogen action by actinomycin D. *Experientia*, 38:511–512.
536. Terenius, L. (1968): Oestrogen binding in the mouse uterus. *Acta Endocrinol.*, 57:669–682.
537. Terenius, L. (1971): Structure-activity relationships of anti-oestrogens with regard to interaction with 17beta-oestradiol in the mouse uterus and vagina. *Acta Endocrinol.*, 66:431–447.
538. Terenius, L., and Ljungkvist, I. (1972): Aspects on the mode of action of anti-estrogens and anti-progestogens. *Gynecol. Invest.*, 3:96–107.
539. Thompson, I. E., Karam, K. S., and Taymor, M. L. (1974): Positive feedback effects of estrogen in amenorrheic women. *Am. J. Obstet. Gynecol.*, 118:788–792.
540. Toft, D. O. (1972): The interaction of uterine estrogen receptors with DNA. *J. Steroid Biochem.*, 3:515–522.
541. Toft, D., and Gorski, J. (1966): A receptor molecule for estrogens: Isolation from the rat uterus and preliminary characterization. *Proc. Natl. Acad. Sci. USA*, 55:1574–1581.
542. Toft, D., and O'Malley, B. W. (1972): Target tissue receptors for progesterone: The influence of estrogen treatment. *Endocrinology*, 9:1041–1045.
543. Toft, D., Shyamala, G., and Gorski, J. (1967): A receptor molecule for estrogens: Studies using a cell-free system. *Proc. Natl. Acad. Sci. USA*, 57:1740–1743.
544. Tokarz, R. R., Harrison, R. W., and Seaver, S. S. (1979): The mechanism of androgen and estrogen synergism in the chick oviduct. *J. Biol. Chem.*, 254:9178.
545. Tomkins, G. M., Martin, D. W., Stillwagen, R. H., Baxter, J. D., Mamont, P., and Levinson, B. B. (1970): Regulation of specific protein synthesis in eucaryotic cells. *Cold Spring Harbor Symp. Quant. Biol.*, 35:635–640.
546. Tsong, T. W. (1975): Effect of phase transition on the kinetics of dye transport in phospholipid bilayer structures. *Biochemistry*, 14:5409–5414.
547. Tsong, T. W. (1975): Transport of 8-Anilino-1-papthalenesulfunate as a probe of the effect of cholesterol on the phospholipid bilayer structure. *Biochemistry*, 14:5415–5417.
548. Vaitukaitis, J. L., Bermudez, J. A., Cargille, C. M., Lipdryy, M. B., and Ross, G. T. (1971): New evidence for an anti-estrogenic action of clomiphene citrate in women. *J. Clin. Endocrinol.*, 32:503–508.
549. Vanderbilt, J. N., Bloom, K. S., and Anderson, J. N. (1982): Endogenous nuclease: Properties and effects on transcribed genes in chromatin. *J. Biol. Chem.*, 257:13009–13017.
550. Villee, C. A. (1962): The role of steroid hormones in the control of metabolic activity. In: *The Molecular Control of Cellular Activity*, edited by J. M. Allen, pp. 297–318. McGraw-Hill, New York.
551. Vogelstein, B., Pardoll, D. M., and Coffey, D. S. (1980): Supercoiled loops and eukaryotic DNA replication. *Cell*, 22:79–85.
552. vonder Ahe, D., Janich, S., Scheidereit, C., Renkawitz, R., Schutz, G., and M. Beato (1985): Glucocorticoid and progesterone receptors bind to the same sites in two hormonally regulated promoters. *Nature*, 313:706–709.
553. Walters, M. R., and Clark, J. H. (1977): Cytosol progesterone receptors of the rat uterus: Assay and receptor characterizatics. *J. Steroid Biochem.*, 8:1137–1144.
554. Walters, M. R., and Clark, J. H. (1978): Cytosol and nuclear compartmentalization of progesterone receptors of the rat uterus. *Endocrinology*, 103:601–609.
555. Walters, M. R., and Clark, J. H. (1978): Stoichiometric translocation of the rat uterine progesterone receptor. *Endocrinology*, 103:1952–1955.
556. Walters, M. R., and Clark, J. H. (1979): Relationship between the quantity of progesterone receptor and the antagonism of estrogen induced uterotropic response. *Endocrinology*, 105:382–386.

557. Walters, M. R., and Clark, J. H. (1980): Estrogen and progesterone modulation of progesterone receptor content in the rat uterus. In: *Steroid Induced Proteins*, edited by M. Beato, pp. 1873–1896. Elsevier/North-Holland.
558. Walters, M. R., Hunziker, W., and Clark, J. H. (1980): Hydroxylapatite prevents nuclear receptor loss during the exchange assay of progesterone receptors. *J. Steroid Biochem.*, 13:1129–1132.
559. Walters, M. R., Hunziker, W., and Norman, A. W. (1980): Unoccupied 1,25-dihydroxy vitamin D_3 receptors. *J. Biol. Chem.*, 255:6799–6805.
560. Walters, M. R., Hunziker, W., and Norman, A. W. (1981): A mathematical model describing the subcellular localization of nonmembrane bound steroid, seco-steroid and thyronine receptors. *J. Steroid Biochem.*, 15:491–495.
561. Warembourg, M., and Milgrom, E. (1977): Radioautography of the uterus before and after [^{3}H] progesterone injection into guinea pigs at various periods of the estrous cycle. *Endocrinology*, 100:175–181.
562. Watson, C. S., and Clark, J. H. (1980): Heterogeneity of estrogen binding sites in mouse mammary cancer. *J. Receptor Res.*, 1:91–111.
563. Wei, J. W., Hickie, R. A., and Klaessen, D. J. (1983): Inhibition of human breast cancer colony formation by anticalmodulin agents: Trifluoperazine, W-7 and W-13. *Cancer Chemother. Pharmacol.*, 11:86–90.
564. Weichman, B. M., and Notides, A. C. (1977): Estradiol-binding kinetics of the activated and nonactivated estrogen receptor. *J. Biol. Chem.*, 252:8856–8862.
565. Weinberger, M. J. (1984): Heterogeneity and distribution of estrogen binding sites in guinea pig seminal vesicle. *J. Steroid Biochem.*, 20:1327–1332.
566. Weintraub, H., and Groudine, M. (1976): Chromosomal subunits in active genes have an altered conformation. *Science*, 193:848.
567. Weisbrod, S. (1982): Active chromatin. *Nature*, 297:289.
568. Welshons, W. V., Lieberman, M. E., and Gorski, J. (1984): Nuclear localization of unoccupied estrogen receptors: Cytochalasin enucleation of GH_3 cells. *Nature*, 307:747–749.
569. West, N. B., Norman, R. L., Sandow, B. A., and Brenner, R. M. (1978): Hormonal control of nuclear estradiol receptor content and the luminal epithelium in the uterus of the golden hamster. *Endocrinology*, 103:1732–1741.
570. Westley, B. R., and Rochefort, H. (1979): Estradiol-induced proteins in the MCF-7 human breast cancer cell line. *Biochem. Biophys. Res. Commun.*, 90:410–416.
571. Westley, B., and Rochefort, H. (1980): A secreted glycoprotein—Induced by estrogen in human breast cancer cell lines. *Cell*, 20:353–362.
572. Westphal, H. M., Fleischmann, G., and Beato, M. (1981): Photoaffinity labeling of steroid binding proteins with unmodified ligands. *Eur. J. Biochem.*, 119:101–106.
573. Wi, H., and Mueller, G.C. (1963): The role of RNA synthesis in early estrogen action. *Proc. Natl. Acad. Sci. USA*, 50:256–260.
574. Wiest, W. G., and Rao, B. R. (1971): Progesterone binding proteins in rabbit uterus and human endometrium. In: *Advances in the Biosciences, 7*. edited by G. Raspe, pp. 251–266. Pergamon Press, Vieweg.
575. Williams, D., and Gorski, J. (1971): A new assessment of subcellular distribution of bound estrogen in the uterus. *Biochem. Biophys. Res. Commun.*, 45:258–264.
576. Williams, D., and Gorski, J. (1974): Equilibrium binding of estradiol by uterine cell suspensions and whole uteri *in vitro*. *Biochemistry*, 13:5537–5542.
577. Willingham, M. C., Wehland, J., Klee, C. B., Richert, N. O., Rutherford, A. V., and Pastan, I. H. (1984): Ultrastructural immunocytochemical localization of calmodulin in cultured cells. *J. Histochem. Cytochem.*, 31:445–461.
578. Wilson, J. D. (1963): The nature of the RNA response to estradiol administration by the uterus of the rat. *Proc. Natl. Acad. Sci. USA*, 50:93–100.
579. Wilson, J. D., and Glozna, R. E. (1970): The intra nuclear metabolism of testosterone in the accessory organs of reproduction. *Recent Prog. Horm. Res.*, 26:309–336.
580. Winneker, R. C., and Clark, J. H. (1983): Estrogen stimulation of the antiestrogen specific binding site in rat uterus and liver. *Endocrinology*, 112:1910–1915.
581. Winneker, R. C., Guthrie, S. C., and Clark, J. H. (1983): Characterization of a triphenyethylene-antiestrogen-binding site on rat serum low density lipoprotein. *Endocrinology*, 112:1823–1827.
582. Wira, C. R., and Munck, A. (1974): Glucocorticoid receptor complexes in rat thymus cells. *J. Biol. Chem.*, 249:5328–5336.
583. Wotiz, H. H., and Scublinksy, A. (1971): The contraceptive action of impeding oestrogens. *J. Reprod. Fertil.*, 26:143–148.
584. Wotiz, H. H., Sjhane, J. A., Vigersky, R., and Brecher, P. I. (1968): The regulatory role of estradiol in the proliferative action of estradiol. In: *Prognostic Factors in Breast Cancer*, edited by A. P. M. Forrest and P. B. Kunkler, pp. 368–376. Livingston Press, Edinburgh.
585. Yamamoto, K., and Alberts, B. (1975): The interaction of estradiol-receptor protein with the genome: An argument for the existence of undetected specific sites. *Cell*, 4:301–310.
586. Yand, M. A., King, D. S., and Fristrom, P. (1978): Ecdysteroid receptors in imaginal discs of *Drosophila melanogaster*. *Proc. Natl. Acad. Sci. USA*, 75:6039–6043.
587. Yang, J., Guzman, R., Richards, J., Imagawa, W., McCormick, K., and Nandi, S. (1980): Growth factor- and cyclic nucleotide-induced proliferation of normal and malignant mammary epithelial cells in primary culture. *Endocrinology*, 107:35–41.
588. Yen, S. S. C., Vela, P., and Ryan, K. J. (1970): Effect of clomiphene citrate in polycystic ovary syndrome: Relationship between serum gonadotropin and corpus luteum function. *J. Clin. Endocrinol.*, 31:7–13.
589. Yuh, K.-C., and Keyes, P. L. (1979): Properties of nuclear and cytoplasmic estrogen receptor in the rabbit corpus luteum: Evidence for translocation. *Endocrinology*, 105:690–696.
590. Zava, D. T., Chamness, G. C., Horwitz, K. B., and McGuire, W. L. (1977): Human breast cancer: Biologically active estrogen receptor in absence of estrogen. *Science*, 196:663–664.
591. Zava, D. T., and McGuire, W. L. (1978): Androgen action through estrogen receptor in a human breast cancer cell line. *Endocrinology*, 103:624–631.
592. Zor, U., Koch, Y., Lamprecht, S. A., Ausher, J., and Lindner, H. R. (1973): Mechanism of oestradiol action on the rat uterus: Independence of cyclic AMP, prostoglandin E_2 and β-adrenergic mediation. *J. Endocrinology*, 58:525–533.

THE REPRODUCTIVE SYSTEMS

The Male

The Physiology of Reproduction,
edited by E. Knobil and J. Neill *et al.*
Raven Press, Ltd., New York © 1988.

CHAPTER 18

Perspectives in the Male Sexual Physiology of Eutherian Mammals

H. G. Williams-Ashman

The aim of this introductory essay is to place in perspective certain fundamental concepts of sexual development and adult reproductive functions in eutherian males. Considerable emphasis is placed on gene expression and hormone action mechanisms germane to these processes, and on the possible evolutionary adaptive value of some of the huge species variations in the structure and physiology of male reproductive tracts, gametes, and secondary sexual tissues. The choice of topics presented is highly selective with omission of many important subjects, notably male sex behavior. Following a brief consideration of the evolution of mammalian reproductive mechanisms, the rest of this chapter is confined to generalizations about masculinity in eutherian mammals, so as to preclude quoting exceptions related to unique sexual attributes of the evolutionarily more primitive monotremes and marsupials. More detailed accounts of observations and experiments in support of many salient conclusions presented below are provided in other appropriate chapters in this volume.

Sexually mature males and females differ profoundly in countless features of their anatomy, physiology, and behavior in all species of eutherian mammals. Yet zygotes and very early embryos cannot be distinguished as masculine or feminine except on the basis of their sex chromosomes. Our comprehension of how these differences between the two sexes are gradually brought about during ontogeny has undergone radical changes over the last 40 years. The four most fundamental sequential stages in eutherian sexual development are as follows.

1. *Establishment of the genetic sex*. This normally occurs at fertilization. The sex karyotype of somatic cells is nearly always XY in males and XX in females. The male is invariably the heterogametic sex, and there are only extremely few exceptions to the rule that the female is homogametic. In comparison with nearly all the autosomes, the eutherian Y chromosome is usually strikingly small and apparently harbors only a tiny complement of expressible genes. By contrast, the X chromosome is of intermediate size, frequently comprises roughly 5% of the total haploid female genome, and contains well over 100 genes, the majority of which are not proximally implicated in sex determination or differentiation. The huge preponderance of genes on the X versus the Y chromosome underscores that remarkably little extra genetic information is required for the genesis of a masculine phenotype, especially considering that most

of the genes on one of the X chromosomes in normal female somatic cells become permanently inactivated (i.e., non-transcribable) very early in embryonic development on a random basis among adjacent cells with respect to the maternal or paternal origin of the X chromosome.

2. *Differentiation of the gonads.* When first evident in embryos of both sexes, the gonadal anlagen (genital ridges) that differentiate into testes in males or ovaries in females are morphologically identical. The genetic sex primarily determines the gonadal sex. The presence of a Y chromosome generally seems to be necessary for the initially indifferent gonadal primordium to develop into a testis and its absence to be required for ovarian differentiation, regardless of the complement of X chromosomes. (Rare exceptions to this XX/XY mode of eutherian chromosomal sex determination are considered later.) The production of the minor histocompatibility H-Y antigen under the influence of the Y chromosome has been implicated in the mechanisms of eutherian testicular differentiation, although recently this notion has been increasingly challenged.

3. The subsequent *differentiation of extragonadal reproductive organs* from precursor tissues that initially appear the same in fetuses of both sexes is normally controlled by hormones from the fetal testis in males but is not dependent on hormones produced by the fetal ovary. The pioneering experiments of Jost (1,2) demonstrated that development of a primitive female urogenital tract proceeds on schedule whether or not the fetal ovaries are extirpated. By contrast, if the fetal testes are excised before the beginning of male reproductive tract differentiation, then a female, rather than a sexually indifferent, tract results. Formation of a normal male reproductive tract has been shown to require two types of fetal testicular hormones: the steroidal androgen testosterone and a glycoprotein müllerian duct involuting hormone. The virilizing effects of testosterone on the fetal urogenital sinus and external genital primordia, but not on the wolffian duct, are amplified by conversion of testosterone to 5α-dihydrotestosterone in the anlagen (3). Several lines of evidence indicate that differentiation of reproductive tracts in eutherian fetuses is genetically programmed to proceed in a feminine direction regardless of the genetic sex, unless testicular hormones, produced and acting on their target cells at critical and restricted period of development, effectively prevent expression of this female program and irreversibly impress masculinity. In some species, it appears that testicular androgens acting in the fetus or neonatally also instigate long-lasting changes in certain neurons in the central nervous system, and cells in certain other regions of the body, that influence the responsivity of such tissues to steroid sex hormones in adulthood.

4. *Onset of the full gametogenic and endocrine functions of the gonads* that are essential for breeding are not attained until puberty, with the establishment of adult modes of gonadotrophin output. The patterns of FSH and LH secretion required for reproduction are quite different in the two sexes and depend critically on complex feedback influences of circulating gonadal hormones on appropriate cells in the hypothalamus and anterior pituitary.

EVOLUTION OF REPRODUCTIVE MECHANISMS IN MAMMALS

It is widely accepted that the first mammals evolved from therapsid reptiles well over 200 million years ago, in the late Triassic and Jurassic periods of the Mesozoic era (4,5). Mammals are conventionally classified into two subclasses: the Protheria and the Theria. Extant protherians represented by the order Monotremata—the duck-billed platypus and the spiny anteaters—are true mammals, since the mothers have functional, though nippleless, mammary glands for feeding infants, but they retain certain reptilian characteristics not found in other mammals, such as the laying of shelled eggs and the presence in both sexes of a cloaca without separate anal and urogenital openings. The recent Theria are subdivided into two infraclasses. The first of these is the Metatheria, all of which belong to the order Marsupalia, whose offspring are born in an extremely immature state and then develop extensively in the marsupium (pouch) on the mother's abdomen. In marsupials, placenta is relatively primitive in design and pregnancy is quite short. The marsupial female genital tract usually is equippped with two lateral vaginas utilized for sperm ascent (which are negotiated in some species by a bifurcated penis) plus a central pseudovaginal canal involved in parturition. The second therian infraclass is the Eutheria, comprised of 16 orders that collectively subsume the great majority of the more than 4,000 species of modern mammals. Eutherians, which are sometimes infelicitously called placental mammals, generally have quite long pregnancies, during which extensive fetal development takes place, and advanced chorioallantoic placentas. Archaic marsupials and eutherians originated during the Cretaceous period more than 100 million years ago. But large-scale divergent evolution of therian creatures, and especially of larger species, did not begin until the Paleocene epoch of the Tertiary period less than 65 million years before now, following massive extinction of the giant reptiles. Most contemporary species of mammals or their immediate evolutionary ancestors probably evolved only within the last several million years (4,5).

Extensive coevolution of many male and female characteristics has obviously played a vital role in all successful eutherian speciations. Species differences in the morphology and functions of cells and organs involved in reproduction have inevitably been looked upon in the light of their possible adaptive value to evolution by natural or sexual selection. Nevertheless, as Austin (6) has pointed out in the context of mammalian gametes, whereas many of their morphological and biochemical attributes are obviously meaningful in relation to function in a given species, some of the interspecific variations in the structure and physiology of eggs and sperms seem to have no advantageous adaptive value. As Austin (6) puts it, "The drive towards adaptive fitness must involve a response of the animal or gamete as a whole to selective pressure. Under the circumstances, it is really no less than logical that gametic (and somatic) characters of different species should differ to some degree in every little particular without serious positive or negative influence on total fitness or adaptive value." Indeed, recent studies on DNA sequencing in relation to evolution increasingly hint that point mutations due to nucleotide substitutions can sometimes become fixed by random genetic drift, rather than always becoming fixed as a result of Darwinian selection acting on advantageous mutations (7,8). Or as Ohno (9) has stated, "The notion that all still functioning genes in the genome must be indispensable for the well being of the host should be abandoned once and for all." However, biologists have tended to eschew invoking selective neutrality for characteristics at a higher level of organization, such as organ size and function (more on this in later discussions of species differences in eutherian male external genitalia and male accessory sex glands). It may be fitting to conclude these general evolutionary considerations by briefly comparing and contrasting the development of the genitourinary tracts of eutherian females and males (10).

In female fetuses, the müllerian ducts differentiate cranially into bilateral oviducts, fuse caudally to form the upper region of the vagina, and from their middle segments there develops a uterus that, depending on the species, exhibits varying degrees of fusion of the original bilateral structures. The wolffian ducts almost completely involute, the urogenital sinus develops into a female type of urethra and the lower vagina (vestibule), and morphogenesis of the vulva involves formation of a clitoris from the genital tubercle plus sets of labia from the genital swellings and folds, which do not fuse. In nearly all species the eutherian clitoris is normally minuscule in comparison with the male phallus, and the feminine urethra terminates below the clitoris. In female eutherians, a rudimentary mammary duct system leading into a primitive nipple is formed before birth. Meiosis of female germ cells begins in the fetal ovary, but the oocyte becomes arrested in the dictyotene of the first meiotic prophase; the first meiotic division is usually completed at ovulation, and the second meiotic division takes place at fertilization. At puberty, the eutherian female tract under the influence of cyclically secreted ovarian steroid hormones undergoes full functional differentiation that is well adapted for periodic ovulation, zygote cleavage and transport, implantation of blastocysts into the uterine endometrium, the formation of intricate placentas and extensive growth of the conceptus during pregnancy, expulsion of newborns from the uterus at parturition, and sperm transport from the vagina through the uterus and up to the ampullary region of the oviduct.

By contrast, in the male, as illustrated in Fig. 1, the genital ducts and accessory sex glands differentiate from the Wolffian duct and urogenital sinus under the influence of fetal testicular androgen, which also triggers the morphogenesis of the male external genitalia, while the mullerian ducts essentially disappear as a result of the action of a glycoprotein hormone from the fetal testis. Normally the relatively long male urethra terminates close to the tip of the phallus. Two other types of masculine reproductive structures are unique to mammals. These are, first, the prostate and bulbourethral glands, and also the seminal vesicles, which are found only in certain species. These androgen-dependent male accessory sex glands function to secrete the bulk of the seminal plasma, which in mammals is generally quite voluminous. Also, most, though by no means all, male mammals have scrotums formed by fusion of the fetal genital swellings and into which the testes come to lie at times that males are capable of breeding. Scrotums are absent from nonmammalian vertebrates. Spermatogenesis in eutherians that possess scrotums can proceed only if the temperature of the testis is kept significantly lower than that of all other internal organs.

THE Y CHROMOSOME, THE H-Y ANTIGEN, AND TESTIS DIFFERENTIATION IN EUTHERIANS

Various hypotheses have been put forward to explain how the presence of a Y chromosome nearly always vouchsafes the differentiation of only testicular tissue from gonadal primordia in eutherian fetuses. Evaluation of these proposed mechanisms of genetic control of eutherian testis differentiation is currently in the melting pot, so this topic will now be considered in some detail. It is a general rule that in all eutherian species that have been examined, a structure clearly recognizable as a testis is formed in normal male embryos well before a definitive ovary is first detectable during normal female development. After male gonadal differentiation is established in eutherian fetuses, it cannot be reversed before or after parturition by treatment with any types of sex steroid or other hormones (10,11).

Consideration of putative genes on the Y chromosome that are believed to be involved in testis differentiation is prefaced by discussion of certain aberrancies of chromosomal determination of gonadal sex in eutherian mammals.

Aberrations of Chromsomal Sex Determination in Eutherians

In a penetrating review, Fredga (12) has discussed some rare exceptions to the rule of the XX/XY modality of sex determination in eutherian animals. The creeping vole *Microtus oregoni*, as Ohno et al. (13) first showed, is a gonosomic mosaic: The female is normally XO in her somatic cells but exhibits a XX karyotype in her germ cells, which produce X-bearing gametes. The male of this species develops from a XY zygote and remains XY in the soma, but the testes have XXY plus OY spermatozoa. Since the female creeping vole produces only one type of ovum, heterogamety of both sexes is avoided. Fredga (12) has suggested that

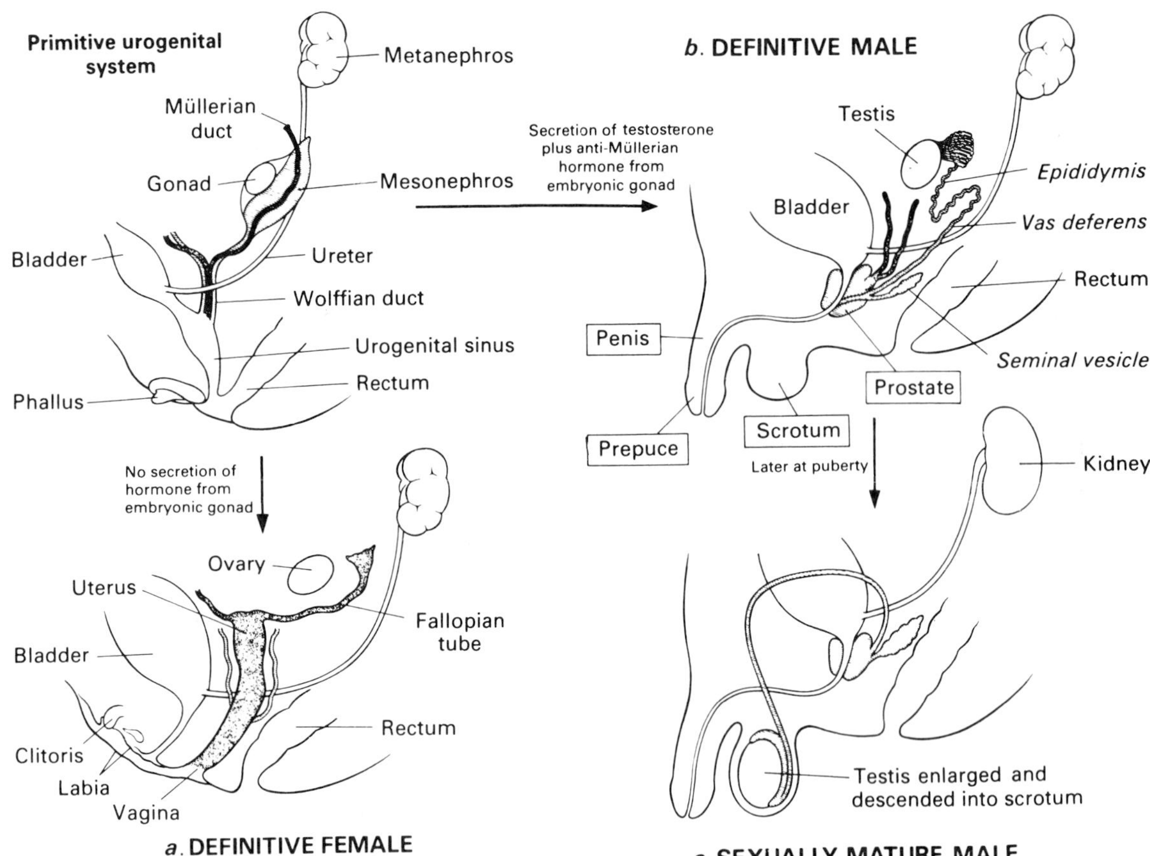

FIG. 1. Differentiation of male and female genitourinary tracts in eutherian mammals, as illustrated for the human species. In the process of differentiation in the fetal male (**b**), structures requiring testosterone are indicated in italics, those requiring 5α-dihydrotestosterone are boxed. (From ref. 66.)

this odd sort of chromosomal sex determination may be related to two factors. The first involves the loss of a gene regulating X-inactivation; since mammals with two active X chromosomes in the soma have not been found, the latter situation is presumed to be lethal, so that one of the two X chromosomes may have been eliminated from female somatic cells. Second, a gene (or genes) controlling separation of X chromosomes during mitosis in primordial germ cells may have been lost; thus in the ovary XX and OO cells are formed, but the OO cells die off and only the XX cells undergo meiosis, whereas in the testis, XXY and YO germ cells are produced, but only the YO cells undergo meiosis and differentiate into spermatozoa.

In the mole vole *Ellobius rutescens,* somatic cells of both sexes, and also male germ cells, are XO, and there are indications that this is also the case for female germ cells. A likely explanation for this is that there occurred a translocation of testis-determining loci from an original Y chromosome to the male X, which might thus be designated as X^Y (12). It is believed that male germ cells are X^YO and serve as progenitors for both X^Y and O spermatozoa, and also that female XO germ cells produce both X and O oocytes, so that both sexes are heterogametic. It is noteworthy that an XYY sex genotype in the human, which is evident in roughly 0.1% of newborn boys and can occur in mice, is associated with abnormalities of testicular histology, even though many XYY individuals are fertile, presumably because the surplus Y chromosome gets lost, so that meiosis in the testis is not compromised.

Fertile XY females have been encountered in some eutherian species. The pioneering studies of Fredga (12) indicated that in the wood lemming *Myopus schisticolor,* three types of sex genotypes can be present in females: XX, X*X, and X*Y, where the asterisk indicates a mutated X chromosome that causes X*Y animals to develop as females. The mutated X* chromosome is morphologically distinct from the wild-type X in exhibiting a smaller short arm with a different Giemsa-banding pattern. All normal male wood lemmings are XY, whereas females can be homozygous XX, heterozygous X*X, or X*Y, which are in all instances fertile and phenotypically of the same feminine appearance. The offspring of mating between XY males and XX females are produced in a 1:1 sex ratio; breeding males with X*X females gives a ratio of 3 females:1 male; and X*Y mothers produce a vast preponderance of daughters (perhaps because only X*-carrying ova are formed in X*Y females owing to double nondisjunction in primordial germ cells). Interestingly, abnormal numbers of sex chromosomes are quite frequently evident in the wood lemming, including XXY sterile males; X*XY sterile males, fertile females, and true hermaphrodites; X*YY fertile females; and XO as well as X*O fertile females. In X*XY wood lemmings the wild-type X chromosome is late replicating (i.e., inactivated) in all cells of X phenotypic females, whereas the mutated X* was late replicating in all somatic cells in animals with a male phenotype (14). It was concluded (12) that the mutated X* chromosome in wood lemmings has lost genes required for testis differentiation, for which both an active wild-type X and a Y chromosome are mandatory; this fits in with observations that X*YY individuals of this species develop into fertile females.

These unusual modes of sex determination in wood lemmings may be compared instructively with sex reversal in mice that contain the *Sxr* gene discovered by Cattanach et al. (15). The sex reversing *Sxr* gene originally was thought to be transmitted as an autosomal dominant, its presence giving rise to equal proportions of normal XY males, XY *Sxr*-carrying males, normal XX females, and sterile XX *Sxr* males (16). However, later studies did not point to an autosomal linkage or to any transfer of material from the Y chromosome to an autosome. It appears more likely that in XY *Sxr* mice, sequences on the Y chromosome concerned with testis determination are duplicated to yield an extra fragment on the end of the short arm of the Y, which can be transferred by nonreciprocal genetic recombination that occurs between limited regions of the sex chromosomes during meiosis in male mice (16–18). Hence the *Sxr* gene may be inherited pseudoautosomally. In eutherians, some smaller creatures such as mice with an XO sex genotype develop as fertile females, whereas larger animals (horse, pig, rhesus monkey, and human) that are XO are phenotypically female but immature and sterile in adulthood because of gonadal dysgenesis. If the *Sxr* gene is incorporated into XO mice, some of the germ cells are sex-reversed, and a minority of the males are capable of spermatogenesis and producing motile spermatozoa (many of which are abnormal). If female mice heterozygous for Searle's (19) X-autosome translocation known as T(X;16)H (or T16H) are crossed with male carriers of the *Sxr* gene duplicated on the Y chromosome (X/Y*Sxr*), all of the XX*Sxr* progeny that inherited the normal X chromosome were sterile males. But among the T16H/X*Sxr* offspring, only 50% were sterile males, 30% were male intersexes, and 20% were fertile females (16). The translocated T16H X chromosome is preferentially active, so in its presence, genes on the normal X are not expressed, and this may account for the finding of female *Sxr* carriers among the progeny when the T16H translocation is present (16).

XX and XY gonadal dysgenesis is encountered clinically: The patients have streak gonads and, as only to be expected, an immature female phenotype. Human 46,XX males have been described, with a frequency of about 1 in 20,000. Among the explanations that have been proposed for human XX males are hidden sex chromosome mosaicism, Y-X or Y-autosome interchanges or translocations, and mutated X chromosomes. Human XX males often have poor masculine development, resembling that seen in Klinefelter's syndrome [XXY, XXXY, or other variants of the presence of Y chromosome(s) alongside supernumerary X chromosomes], usually with defective spermatogenesis. The condition of true hermaphroditism, in which elements of testicular and ovarian tissue are present in the same individual and often accompanied by markedly intersexual development of the genitourinary tracts, can occur in a number of mammalian species; the incidence is very low in the human but not inconsiderable in some strains of pigs. The commonest somatic karyotype in human true hermaphroditism is 46,XX, although a 46,XY karyotype, or sex chromosome mosaicism (45,XO/46,XY; 46,XX/46,XY), as well as chimerism, is encountered less frequently (20).

Genes and Nucleotide Sequences Associated with the Y Chromosome

In most eutherian species, the Y chromosome is relatively minute, and in man is smaller than all the autosomes except chromosomes 22 and 23. Yet the DNA of the human Y chromosome contains more than 3×10^7 base pairs, which in theory could hold information for more than 10,000 structural genes. However, as indicated by cytogenetic studies on partial deletions, most of the long arm of the human Y chromosome is heterochromatic and is not required for testis differentiation. Two repeated sequences account for roughly 70% of the DNA of the long arm of the human Y; these sequences are located in the heterochromatin and presumably have no genetic function because patients lacking them are phenotypically normal males (21). At various times it has been proposed, on the basis of indirect evidence, that the human Y contains loci that specify (a) testis differentiation (*Tdy*), (b) production of the H-Y antigen (*Hy*), (c) regulation of spermatogenesis, (d) male body stature, (e) male tooth size, and (f) very hairy ears in males (22). However, as reviewed by Goodfellow et al. (23), extremely few expressible structural genes had been convincingly shown to reside on the human Y chromosome by the end of 1985, although by this time an increasing wealth of information had accumulated about defined base sequences on the Y, including Y-specific repeats, low copy number Y-specific base sequences, and sequences present outside or within the restricted pairing regions that apparently are shared by the X and Y chromosomes.

The Y chromosome contains an expressed structural gene that codes for a cell-surface antigen that is detected by its reactivity with the monoclonal antibody 12E7; the Y-linked locus (*MIC2Y*) for this gene is homologous with a locus on the X chromosome (*MIC2X*) that escapes X-inactivation (24). A complementary DNA sequence that hybridized with the *MIC2* gene was used as a probe to demonstrate that the *MIC2X* and *MIC2Y* loci are very similar, if not identical, and are localized close to the tips of the short arms of the human X and Y chromosomes (25). These pairing regions of the human sex chromosomes also contain noncoding repetitive nucleotide seqquences that are highly polymorphic, exhibit a "pseudoautosomal" pattern of inheritance (26,27), and are telomeric, i.e., are present at the molecular ends of linear chromosomes and are required for chromosomal replication and stability (28). Of related interest are studies on hybridization of mammalian sex chromosomes with so-called *Bkm* DNA (or cloned fragments thereof), a *m*inor satellite DNA obtained from the W chromosome of the Indian *b*anded *k*rait *Bungarus fasciatus*. (The latter snake species has heterologous Z and W sex chromosomes: The males are ZZ homogametic and the females are ZW heterogametic.) *Bkm* sequences, which have been strongly conserved during vertebrate evolution and are also detectable in the genome of many invertebrates and primitive eukaryotes, contain a large preponderance of tetranucleotide GATA repeats, which can be transcribed in male but not female mice, as indicated by hybridization of cloned *Bkm* fragments with total poly(A) RNA preparations from various murine tissues (29). (Whether transcriptions of *Bkm* sequence repeats result in the synthesis of functional proteins has not been proven.) *Bkm* sequences are quantitative (but not qualitative) indicators not of the sex of species that exhibit genetic control of primary sex determination, but rather of the heterogametic sex, even when gonadal organizing mechanisms have become aberrant for mutational reasons (30). Comparable investigations on evolutionarily conserved heterogametic sex-specific satellite DNA repeated sequences have been carried out with appropriate DNA preparations isolated from another snake species, *Elaphe radiata* (31); in this instance, the simple repeated sequence is GATAGACA, which again can be transcribed into RNA in animal systems and translated in cell-free bacterial protein-synthesizing systems. Although such highly conserved snake DNA repetitive sequences are preferentially associated with the heterogametic sex in various vertebrates and have been useful in identifying male-determining chromosomal *Sxr* fragments in mice, their genetic functions (if any) are unknown (29–31). Moreover, according to Kiel-Metzger et al. (32), few *Bkm* sequences are present on the Y chromosome of man, although these sequences are concentrated on the human X and two autosomes. It may be added that both the X and Y chromosomes of man contain pseudogenes for arginosuccinate synthetase (22,23), though these sequences are not, of course, transcribed.

The H-Y Antigen and Eutherian Testis Organization

In 1955, Eichwald and Silmser (33) discovered that in syngeneic mice, male skin grafts were rejected by females, whereas grafting male skin to other males or female skin to either females or males did not result in transplant rejection. These findings were attributed to a cell surface minor histocompatibility antigen (H-Y) whose production was postulated to depend on a locus on the Y chromosome. Determination of the H-Y antigen status of tissues by classical transplantation procedures is often tedious and imprecise, and in some instances impossible. The demonstration in 1971 by Goldberg et al. (34) that the H-Y antigen can be determined with serological methods was therefore an important advance that stimulated much research on correlations between serologically estimated H-Y antigen and the sex chromosomal status of cells. In 1975, Wachtel et al. (35) provided evidence that the H-Y antigen has been strongly conserved during mammalian evolution; shortly thereafter, in another contribution together with Ohno (36), they proposed that in eutherians, the H-Y antigen acts in a hormonelike fashion to direct the embryonic genital ridges to develop into testes and to suppress formation of ovarian tissue. Later comparative studies (37) indicated that high titers of H-Y antigen are indicative not of maleness as such, but rather of the heterogametic sex. Thus, in birds, for example, it was found that homogametic ZZ males rejected isologous female grafts and that normal ZW females are H-Y antigen positive. In mammals with normal sex chromosomal sex-determining mechanisms, H-Y antigen is produced by many types of male, but not female, cells, as is evident very early in embryonic development (38). It was proposed that H-Y antigen can bind to cell surface via two modes of attachment: (a) to anchorage sites related to dimers of the major histocompatibility complex (MHC) and β_2-microglobulin (gene loci for MHC are known as HLA-A, -B, and -C in man, and H-2D and H-2K in mice); or (b) to gonad-specific receptors for the H-Y antigen (37).

The idea that the eutherian male-determining locus on the Y chromosome (*Tdy*) is related to the structural gene for the H-Y antigen (*Hy*) that directs testis differentiation has been quite widely championed and has prompted many productive investigations, which have been amply reviewed (37,39–41). However, over the last few years the role of H-Y antigen in eutherian testicular morphogenesis has been increasingly questioned, and doubt has been cast on whether the transplantation and the serologically determined methods used for H-Y antigen assay actually measure the same substance. Furthermore, although preparations that apparently are enriched in H-Y antigen have been obtained from certain cells, the molecular structure of this antigen has not been fully elucidated. And it is debatable whether the chromosomal locus for the structural gene for the H-Y antigen is normally present on the eutherian Y chromosome or that the *Hy* locus is the same as the *Tdy* locus. It is often presumed quite reasonably that the H-Y antigen influences the differentiation of eutherian gonadal anlagen in a testicular direction by the antigen first combining with a gonad-specific receptor for this entity (37,40,41). Virtually nothing is known about this putative gonadal H-Y antigen receptor, or the proximal biochemical processes that amplify the signals generated when the H-Y antigen combines with this receptor molecule.

Silvers et al. (42) concluded that H-Y antigen titers measured serologically define a different entity from the H-Y antigen assayed by transplantation techniques. However, Ohno (39) has pointed out that immune responses to minor histocompatibility antigens such as the H-Y are likely to occur only if the donor and recipient animals possess identical major histocompatibility antigens. On these and other technical grounds, Ohno (39) has questioned the views of Silvers et al. (42). Monoclonal antibodies directed against determinants on the H-Y antigen have been prepared in several laboratories (39–41), and Brunner et al. (43) used one such monoclonal antibody to develop an enzyme-linked immunoabsorption assay for H-Y antigen. However, H-Y antigen assays based on reactivity with monoclonal antibodies are still in their infancy, and as Ohno (39) emphasizes, whether these tests can be applied unambiguously to human materials may depend critically on how far Class I MHC antigens influence recognition of H-Y antigen determinants, since many HLA haplotypes may not respond to the H-Y antigen. Likewise, the validity of H-Y antigen assays based on T-cell responses may vary with the frequency of H-Y responders in a given population. Moreover, if the putative gonadal anlagen-specific H-Y antigen receptor was nonfunctional for genetic or epigenetic reasons, then correlations between a positive H-Y antigen status and testis formation might not be expected. More incisive investigations on the reliability of various quantitative assay procedures for H-Y antigen, and for estimating the status of gonad-specific H-Y receptors, will have to be accomplished before many contradictory results in this field can be resolved.

Simpson et al. (44) reported that some X/X*Sxr* animals obtained by coupling of the *Sxr* mutation with the T16H translocation (see above) were fertile females with normal male levels of H-Y antigen. However, Ohno (39) has argued that the occasional finding of fertile female T16H-X/X*Sxr* mice whose positive H-Y antigen status was assigned on the basis of measurements on spleen cells cannot be regarded as evidence that the *Tdy* and *Hy* loci are different from one another. A more serious discrepancy arises from the report by McLaren et al. (45) that a few X/X*Sxr* males were among the progeny of apparently H-Y antigen negative T16H-X/X*Sxr* females mated with non-*Sxr*-carrying male mice. If truly authentic, the existence of H-Y antigen-negative males would seriously question the idea that H-Y antigen induces fetal testicular organization. In a critique of the latter notion, Ohno (39) admits that the apparent lack of H-Y antigen production in the male mice described by McLaren et al. (45) probably cannot be accounted for in terms of artifacts that might have interfered with the method of H-Y antigen assay employed. However, Ohno (39) suggested that considerable shortening of the pairing segment of the X*Sxr* chromosome of the foundation mother might have occurred during meiosis in her ovaries, and, if so, this could permit inactivation of the X chromosome to extend more frequently, so as to suppress expression of the X*Sxr* locus. Thus, under such circumstances, some of the T16h–X/X*Sxr* progeny might be anticipated to develop as males, especially considering McLaren's (46) earlier demonstration that XX/XY mouse blastocyst fusion chimeras with a 4:1 proportion of XX and XY cells in their gonads can still develop as males.

In addition to the aforementioned anomalous T16H–X/X*Sxr* fertile female mice with high H-Y antigen titers, there are other examples of equivalent XY fertile females of positive H-Y antigen status. This condition is found occasionally among wild populations of the wood lemming *Myopus schisticolor,* in this instance being associated with rearrangements of the short arm of the X chromosome (47); an earlier report that these creatures were H-Y antigen negative (48) was later shown to be in error (49). Ohno (39) has proposed that the X chromosome short-arm rearrangement prevents expression of the gonad-specific H-Y antigen receptor gene. XY females with high H-Y antigen levels have also been reported among progeny resulting from continuous back-crossing of feral *Mus poschiavanus* with laboratory mice with a C57BL/6J genome (50), which again might be accounted for in terms of interspecific incompatibility of recognition of H-Y antigen receptors (39).

In human patients, high levels of H-Y antigen have accorded with the presence of testicular tissue in normal XY men; XY male pseudohermaphrodites with varying manifestations of a feminine external phenotype; true hermaphrodites (including those with 46,XX or 46,XY karyotypes or with XX/XY mosaicism); sex chromosome mosaics exhibiting mixed gonadal dysgenesis; and 45,X males. Comparably, sex-reversed mouse XX males, XY individuals with testes showing a female phenotype due to androgen-insensitivity, XX/XY chimeras, and XO males (51) are antigen positive. The demonstration of H-Y antigen positive XO males in mice and humans (51) without evidence of sex chromosomal mosaicisms or the presence of Y-chromosomal material suggests that the structural gene for the H-Y antigen cannot be located on the Y chromosome. Moreover, human XO females with gonadal dysgenesis (Turner syndrome) apparently have intermediate levels of H-Y antigen as determined serologically (52) or by transplantation techniques (53). Human XYY males were reported to have roughly twice as much H-Y antigen as normal XY men (54). Normal XX females of the human and a variety of other eutherian species are H-Y antigen negative.

Meck (40), Muller and Schindler (51), and Ohno (37,39) have reviewed experimental disaggregation–reaggregation studies on newborn gonadal cells that indicate the following: (a) Addition of H-Y antigen-rich extracts of certain tissues evokes reorganization of testicular tubules from dispersed ovarian cells; and (b) free cells from the testes of neonates that were lysostripped of H-Y antigen can apparently reaggregate into structures resembling ovarian follicles. Nevertheless, until H-Y antigen(s) preparations that have been purified to homogeneity are available, interpretation of the latter findings will remain equivocal.

Hypothetical Mechanisms of Genetic Control of Eutherian Gonadal Differentiation

Genes located on the X chromosome and autosomes are clearly required for differentiation of both testes and ovaries in eutherians, and in normal XY males, nucleotide sequences on the DNA of the Y chromosome seem to be required for testis organization in the embryo. It must be emphasized that there is abundant evidence for Ohno's (55) generalization that the genetic complement of the X chromosome has been strongly conserved during eutherian evolution. The gene for the androgen receptor, which plays a paramount role in male sex differentiation processes that take place after the eutherian testis is formed, is clearly present on the X chromosome, as considered below.

The evidence summarized in the preceding section indicates that there is no compelling evidence that the structural gene(s) for the H-Y antigen (*Hy*) are Y-linked and that the role of H-Y antigen in testis differentiation is problematic. Ohno et al. (56) proposed that *Hy* loci are on the X chromosome and that such loci are not normally expressed in the absence of functional Y-linked inducer gene(s). Contrariwise, Wolf et al. (52,57) suggested that *Hy* gene(s) are autosomally located and that their expression is attenuated by an X-linked repressor whose actions are overcome by Y-linked deprepressor factor. [Wolf (57) considers that the gene for the H-Y antigen receptor is X-linked.] All ideas concerning the mechanisms of genetic control of eutherian gonadal differentiation proposed heretofore must be regarded as tentative. Very recently, Chandra (58) has advanced an hypothesis that assumes that there is no Y-linked *structural* gene with male-determining properties, and he does not invoke a role of H-Y antigen in testis organization. An essential feature of Chandra's (58) model is the supposition of a multicopy *noncoding* nucleotide sequence on the Y chromosome, the function of which is to bind a repressor substance coded for by autosome(s) that is formed in limiting concentrations. It is assumed that this repressor has a high affinity for the putative noncoding sequence on Y-DNA and a lower affinity for a testis-determining gene on the X chromosome, which is designated for obvious reasons as *Tdx* rather than *Tdy*. A consequence of this hypothesis would be that the *Tdx* gene would normally be transcribed in XY cells but not in XX cells because the presumptive Y-linked noncoding sequence would act as a sink for the autosomally coded repressor; thus, in the absence of a Y chromosome, the *Tdx* gene would not be expressed. Chandra (58) emphasizes that this model is not dependent on any protein synthesized under the direction of *Bkm* sequences that might be related to any *Sxr* gene (see above). In another very recent contribution, Chandra (59) suggests that X chromosome-inactivation in eutherians is more concerned with sex determination (by bringing about a reduction in the copy number of putative X-linked *Tdx* gene) than with dosage compensation of X-linked genes in cells that contain more than one X chromosome.

MECHANISTIC ASPECTS OF STEROID SEX HORMONE ACTION

Androgens play a paramount role in the development and maintenance of masculine characteristics in eutherians. These hormones are essential for the fetal differentiation of the extragonadal organs of the male genitourinary tract, the complete development of the male tract and secondary sexual tissues that begins at puberty, the establishment of male courtship and coital behavior patterns, and no less importantly, spermatogenesis. From the standpoint of vertebrate phylogeny, the stimulation of spermatogenesis by androgens via their actions on Sertoli cells is probably the most fundamental function of these hormones. The output of testosterone by Leydig cells is controlled postnatally by luteinizing hormone (LH), and the secretion of LH is, in turn, enhanced by the hypothalamic gonadotrophins releasing hormone (GnRH). The actions of LH on Leydig cells, of follicle-stimulating hormone (FSH) on Sertoli cells, and of GnRH on pituitary gonadotroph cells are in each instance mediated by specific receptors present predominantly on the plasmalemma with their hormone-binding sites exposed on the outer surfaces of the responsive cells, via mechanisms discussed in chapters 21, 22 and 30.

Testosterone is the principal circulating androgen of testicular origin in sexually mature eutherian males (3,60,61). A variety of tissues (including many but not all structures that are highly androgen responsive) can convert testosterone to 5α-dihydrotestosterone (DHT), which as considered later is the intracellular mediator of certain actions of testosterone. The concentrations of DHT in blood plasma are usually less than a tenth of those of testosterone, most of the circulating DHT being derived by peripheral conversion from plasma testosterone since the testes secrete relatively little DHT. Testosterone and the weaker androgens androstenedione and dehydroepiandrosterone (which are secreted in small amounts by the testes and in larger amounts by the adrenal cortex) also serve a precursors in males for the phenolic estrogens 17β-estradiol and estrone. In men, the majority of these estrogens in the circulation normally arise by aromatization of androgens in peripheral tissues, but if LH output is abnormally high, then the testes may secrete more than the low amounts of estrogens they normally supply to blood plasma (3). Whether estrogens have important functions in normal eutherian male sexual physiology is a rather open question, although estrogen formation from testosterone in the hypothalamus is thought to be involved, together with conversion of testosterone to DHT, in some of the behavioral and other effects of testosterone operating at a hypothalamic level (62,63). It is noteworthy that the steroid 5α-reductase reaction in which testosterone is reduced to DHT is essentially irreversible and that DHT is not a substrate for the aromatase system that converts testosterone or androstenedione to estrogens. Thus, DHT once formed from testosterone cannot be transformed into estrogens. However, DHT produced in androgen target cells can be converted by the action of reversible reactions catalyzed by appropriate hydroxysteroid dehydrogenases into the two isomeric 3α- and 3β-5α-androstanediols. The latter androstanediols exhibit significant androgenic activity in certain bioassays, which in most instances is probably attributable to their enzymatic conversion back to DHT (61). Testosterone and DHT can be enzymatically converted into several other derivatives with diminished or altered types of biological activities in many tissues, including those that are androgen responsive (64–66); the possible roles of some of the latter metabolites in the inactivation and turnover of androgens in living cells are discussed by Coffey in Chapter 24.

Role of Receptors in Androgen and Estrogen Action in Males

There is abundant evidence that the major physiological effects of all six classes of vertebrate steroid hormones (androgens, estrogens, progestins, glucocorticoids, mineralocorticoids, and 1α,25-dihydroxyvitamin D) are mediated by corresponding specific receptor proteins. The properties and biological significance of steroid sex hormone receptors have been reviewed extensively (e.g., refs. 64–69), and only a few very fundamental aspects of the nature and functions of androgen and estrogen receptors are outlined in the following paragraphs.

The separate receptors for androgens and estrogens are proteins that are present mainly in the interior of responsive cells, in marked contrast to the multitude of receptors for polypeptide and catecholamine hormones, which are found predominantly in plasma membranes with their hormone-binding sites exposed to the exterior of their target cells. It is widely believed that free steroid sex hormones in extracellular fluids penetrate their target cells by passive diffusion through the lipid bilayer of the plasmalemma, although more complex mechanisms for the entry of these hormones into cells have occasionally been postulated. [The androgen-binding protein of Sertoli cells, which is entirely distinct from the androgen receptor, is a special case in that this protein does seem to play an important role in the sequestration of testosterone of Leydig cell origin in the cytoplasm of Sertoli cells (70).] Once they have entered cells, androgens and estrogens are bound to their corresponding receptors. The resulting hormone–receptor complexes eventually become associated primarily with the chromatin in nuclei. An overall scheme of estrogen action originally proposed by Jensen (69) on the basis of studies on immature uterus has been widely considered as a paradigm for the intracellular dynamics of receptors for all classes of steroid hormones. According to this hypothesis, the steroid hormone first combines with a cytoplasmic form of its specific receptor and the steroid–receptor complex then undergoes a temperature-dependent "transformation" that increases its capacity to be sequestered by cell nuclei and associated with the chromatin therein. There is indeed ample evidence that the major fraction of occupied steroid receptors is present in the nuclei of living cells. However, whether an initial formation of steroid–receptor complexes and their transformation occur mainly in the cytoplasm and represent a mandatory step in promoting extensive nuclear localization of steroid receptors *in vivo* has been increasingly questioned recently, with the demonstration of a predominance of both unoccupied as well as occupied forms of the receptors in target cell nuclei (71,72).

Receptors for androgens and estrogens are often present together in responsive cells, and in very low abundance (less than 30,000 receptor molecules per cell). These receptors contain hormone-binding sites that exhibit extremely high affinities for their steroid ligands; once the active hormones are bound, they probably become enveloped in a hydrophobic pocket in the receptor proteins. However, the complete amino acid sequence of the human estrogen receptor was recently deduced from the nucleotide sequences of cDNA clones complementary to the messenger RNA for this receptor (73–75). Using comparable experimental strategies, the complete primary structure of the human glucocorticoid receptor has also been elucidated (76). There are some tantalizing homologies between the human estrogen and glucocorticoid receptors, both of which are single-chain proteins. In each case, there are strong indications that the specific steroid-binding domain is in the carboxyl-terminal region. Also, both receptors contain domains closer to the N-terminus that are rich in cysteine, arginine, and lysine, and which are implicated in the interactions of the steroid-occupied receptors with DNA. Interestingly, the latter regions in both the estrogen and the glucocorticoid receptor have striking homologies with the sequences of the putative product of the v-*erb*A oncogene of avian erythroblastosis virus (74,75).

Androgen receptors have not yet been purified to a high degree, nor have cDNA or genomic clones cognate to the androgen receptors been obtained, so that nothing is known about their primary structures. The gene for mammalian androgen receptor clearly resides on the X chromosome (77), whereas the genes for all other types of steroid hormone receptors apparently are autosomally linked [the genes for the glucocorticoid (78) and estrogen (73) receptors appear to be present on human chromosomes 5 and 6, respectively]. Both androgen and estrogen receptors are detectable in a wide variety of cell types found in the reproductive tracts of both sexes and in many other locations in eutherian organisms. The expression of the androgen and estrogen receptor genes, and hence the tissue contents of these receptors, are regulated differentially in various tissues by a large number of factors, including developmental status, age, and many sorts of homologous and heterologous hormones (65,66,68,79). Steroid sex hormone receptors are both synthesized and degraded in the cells that contain them. In many cells responsive to these hormones, occupied receptors for androgens and estrogens disappear from nuclei after the cells are deprived of the steroids. Some of this receptor loss may not be due solely to irreversible receptor degradation, but may also entail a recycling process in which the receptor is inactivated to a form that is unable to bind the hormone or associate firmly with chromatin and then can be reactivated by energy-dependent reactions (65).

Sites on androgen and estrogen receptors that firmly bind natural and synthetic strong hormonal agonists represent the locus of action of a variety of drugs that act as specific antiandrogens or antiestrogens *in vivo* to attenuate the effects of the natural hormones at an end-organ level. Synthetic substances are available that apparently serve as pure antagonists for only one type of steroid hormone receptor, presumably as a result of interacting with the receptor's hormone binding site nonproductively (i.e., the bound antagonist may not evoke a conformational change in the receptor that permits the receptor complex to instigate biochemical changes in a responsive cell, but antagonist binding will prevent or displace hormone agonists from interacting with the receptor). Other substances that can antagonize the action of strong hormone agonists on living cells may actually exhibit weak or partial agonist activities when given *in vivo* or may cross-react with other types of receptor either productively or nonproductively. For example, the synthetic steroid Cyproterone is a fairly powerful androgen antagonist that has insignificant progestational activity, whereas the related compound Cyproterone acetate is a very potent antiandrogen that binds nonproductively with the androgen receptor but is also a powerful progestin agonist because it is bound productively to the progestin receptor (65,66,79). Jänne and Bardin (80) have reviewed the mechanisms of actions of various synthetic antiandrogens, some of which have been fruitfully applied to experimental analysis of the role of testosterone in eutherian male sex differentiation. Mechanistic studies on antiestrogenic drugs, some of which exhibit weak partial agonist activities, are discussed by Liao and Hiipakka (65) and Jensen (69). It must be stressed that natural and synthetic strong estrogen agonists bind only poorly to androgen receptors and are at best only feeble antagonists of the formation and functions of androgen-receptor complexes (65,66,79). Relatively high circulating levels of estrogens are well known to exert marked demasculinizing and feminizing effects in eutherian males, which are largely brought about by estrogens: (a) inhibiting LH output via negative-feedback influences on the hypothalamus and anterior pituitary, (b) directly depressing steroidogenesis at a Leydig cell level, and (c) stimulating various female heterosexual remnant tissues in the male organism (e.g., rudimentary mammary glands) and also other tissues such as the fibromuscular stroma of male accessory sex glands. By mechanisms which remain foggy, testosterone in the concentrations present in the circulation in sexually mature males exert depressive influences on the feminizing actions of low concentrations of plasma estrogens on masculine structures (66,79).

When extracted into solution from homogenates or subcellular fractions from many tissues, androgen and estrogen receptors are often present in several forms, as evident from measurements of their molecular size (sedimentation coefficients, etc.) and other properties. A large number of factors influence this heterogeneity of receptors for a given class of steroid sex hormones in a particular tissue, including endocrine status, state of cell differentiation of the cells, and ionic strength, divalent metal ion content, pH, and temperature of the extraction media, as well as the action of various proteolytic enzymes present in relatively crude tissue extracts (68,80,81). Steroid sex hormone receptors appear to be single polypeptide chains. Functional receptor monomers, dimers, and tetramers sediment at roughly 4, 6, and 8–9 S, respectively. Forms of these receptors that apparently sediment at 3 S have been designated as "meroreceptors," which are polypeptide chains containing the hormone-binding sites that have been sundered proteolytically from other domains of the receptor molecules that are concerned with the cell regulatory functions of the hormone-occupied receptor protein (81). Various procedures such as mild warming and exposure to monovalent salt concentrations of 0.4 M or higher can effect "transformation" of occupied androgen and estrogen receptors to forms that have increased affinity for naked DNA, chromatin, and various polyanions like ADP- or ATP–Sepharose and phosphocellulose. These reactions, which presumably involve changes in hormone–receptor conformations but are not understood in depth, are impeded by fairly high concentrations (10–20 mM) of sodium molybdate and related oxyanions (81). Steroid sex hormone receptors also bind firmly to various RNA molecules and ribonucleoprotein particles to produce large aggregates (65,66,69). There are hints that RNAs and ribonucleoprotein particle can effectively release transformed steroid receptors from DNA or chromatins, which may perhaps play a role in the previously mentioned recycling of nuclear receptors in intact cells. A significant proportion of nuclear androgen and estrogen receptors in various reproductive tissues cannot be extracted into solution by high-molarity salt concentrations with nucleolytic cleavage; this seems to reflect firm associations of the insoluble receptor complexes with the proteinaceous nuclear matrix (82), which is known to act as a framework for anchorage sites for supercoiled DNA, and major loci for initiation of DNA replication and RNA transcription (83,84).

According to current dogma, most of the receptor-mediated physiological actions of androgens and estrogens primarily depend on differential changes in the transcription of subsets of genes (65,69). Steroid sex hormone–receptor complexes certainly can influence the formation and abundance of mRNA copies of certain structural genes (usually positively but in some instances negatively). Many lines of evidence indicate that the majority of the cellular effects of these hormones can ultimately be accounted for by alterations in the production and accumulation of intracellular or secretory enzymes and structural proteins. However, androgens and estrogens can also profoundly affect the abundance and turnover of ribosomal and transfer RNAs in certain tissues, probably because the sex steroids instigate changes in transcription of the genes that specify these polynucleotides (65,66). There are many examples of gonadal hormones regulating the expression of certain structural genes in some but not in other receptor-replete tissues of the same organism at a given state of development. These selective effects of sex steroids are not fundamentally related to direct hormonal perturbations of nuclear RNA polymerases but perhaps relate to the abundance of tissue-specific factors needed for the operation of stable transcription complexes that produce RNA copies of selected genes (85) or post-translational modifications of certain of the large number of proteins involved in transcription processes. Only very recently have substantial inroads been made into precise definition of the many factors required for steroid–receptor complexes to influence directly the transcription of specific genes in cell-free nuclear systems (e.g., refs. 85, 86). Furthermore, it has not been ruled out that steroid receptors can also proximally influence the complex intranuclear processing of initial nuclear RNA transcripts of most genes, involving postsynthetic modifications to remove introns and add 5′-caps and 3′poly(A) tails for the production of mature, functional mRNA molecules (87). Although it has occasionally been suggested on the basis of indirect evidence that certain sex steroid receptors may somehow directly influence the translation of mRNAs by cytoplasmic polyribosomal systems, the available evidence in support of this is not compelling despite the fact that transcriptional activity in the nucleus is often tightly coordinated with translational events in the cytoplasm (65,66,88,89).

Increasingly, two experimental approaches have been employed to probe into the mechanisms of sex hormone control of specific gene transcription: studies on (a) changes evoked by steroids *in vivo* of higher organizational levels of the nuclear chromatin that may render certain sets of genes expressible, and (b) direct selective interactions of hormone–receptor complexes with discrete nucleotide sequences of refined structural gene fragments that are implicated in the control of initiation of transcription. The chromatin of higher animals is largely comprised of DNA, histones, and nonhistone proteins. Most of the DNA is wrapped up into nucleosomes with a core structure comprised of two copies each of the histones H2a, H2b, H3, and H4. The chromatin also contains H1 (lysine-rich) histones, which are not in the nucleosome core structure, plus a large number of nonhistone proteins. The nucleosomes are arranged like beads on a long string of DNA. Application to isolated nuclei or chromatin of deoxyribonucleases from various sources has shown that expressible genes are generally more susceptible to digestion with these enzymes and that treatment with sex steroid hormones *in vivo* can alter chromatin structure in ways that render certain genes more readily digestible by pancreatic DNase I (86). Experiments involving selective removal of chromatin proteins, followed by reconstitution of chromatins with various nonhistone protein fractions, have hinted that certain of the latter proteins might serve as "acceptor" sites for sex steroid receptors (65,66,69,88,89). Whether such putative acceptor sites directly mask adjacent DNA nucleotide sequences of genes whose transcription is regulated by the appropriate hormones or, alternatively, may be involved in directing chromatin-associated receptors to more distal genomic regions is far from established.

Recent studies have indicated that glucocorticoid receptors can selectively interact directly with certain regions of a variety of viral, as well as eutherian cellular, genes whose transcriptions are stimulated by this class of hormones (for literature, see refs. 76 and 90). These receptor binding genomic nucleotide sequences, which usually are in flanking regions 5′-upstream from the transcription-initiation sites, have been postulated to be enhancer regions that regulate the function of promotor sequences involved in transcription initiation. [In the case of the human growth hormone gene, glucocorticoid receptors bind selectively to a downstream sequence in the first intron (90).] A similar 5′-flanking region in the ovalbumin gene is apparently required for both the estrogen and progesterone receptor-mediated induction of this protein in chick oviduct cells (91). Selective binding of 4.5-S androgen–receptor complexes to nucleotide sequences 5′-upstream from the transcription-initiation site of the gene for the C3(1) subunit of a prostate protein known as prostatein (90) or α-protein (65), which is strongly induced by androgens *in vivo,* has been reported by Perry et al. (92). The failure of Mulder et al. (93) to demonstrate selective binding of a 3-S androgen–receptor preparation to a cloned gene fragment containing the aforementioned receptor-binding nucleotide sequence was ascribed by others (92) to the absence of a necessary functional domain in the androgen receptor of smaller size. Further studies on the binding of androgen and estrogen receptors to specific regions of individual genes that may control transcription initiation are undoubtedly warranted. However, the selective strength of all reported associations of various steroid receptors with discrete genomic sequences is not exceptionally striking in comparison with the very tight binding of repressors to bacterial gene promotor regions (*cf.* ref. 87), and it is difficult to see how such direct interactions of receptors with certain gene regions could account solely for the sex hormone regulation of specific gene transcription, which can vary greatly among different tissues of the same organism.

From the foregoing it is evident that our understanding of the mechanisms by which steroid sex hormone receptors influence the expression of genes remains woefully inadequate. Future progress in this area will most likely depend heavily on development of greater insight into the complex basic biochemistry of RNA transcription and processing in eutherian cell nuclei.

Role of 5α-Dihydrotestosterone in the Action of Testosterone on Various Cells

Steroid 5α-reductases catalyzing the irreversible reduction by NADPH of testosterone to DHT are present in many but not all eutherian tissues. The 5α-reductase in the prostate gland has been studied in depth (94). Progesterone is a somewhat more effective substrate than testosterone. Most of the enzyme in homogenates is associated with the nuclear fraction and endoplasmic reticulum membranes; less than 15% of the total activity is in the cytosol. The 5α-reductase activity is greater in stromal than in epithelial cells; the stromal cell enzyme has a relatively higher K_m for testosterone or progesterone and may represent an isoenzymic form. A number of powerful and apparently specific inhibitors of 5α-reductase have been synthesized (e.g., *N,N*-diethylcarbamoyl-4-methyl-4-aza-5α-androstane-3-one and 6-methylene testosterone are potent competitive and noncompetitive inhibitors, respectively). Testosterone is reduced to DHT in prostate cells, and the DHT then binds more firmly than testosterone to the androgen receptor. There is no convincing evidence for the existence of separate receptors for testosterone and DHT. DHT is a considerably more potent androgen than testosterone in several bioassay systems. There is evidence that when the androgen receptor is saturated with DHT and undergoes transformation, it binds more firmly to naked DNA or other polyanionic substances than does the corresponding testosterone–receptor complex (95,96). Thus, it is considered that in those tissues with a capacity to reduce testosterone to DHT, the latter derivative serves to amplify the androgenic potency of the circulating hormone. A minority of androgen-sensitive tissues (e.g., the wolffian duct at the time of embryonic male sex differentiation and the kidney and certain muscles in adult eutherians) are essentially devoid of steroid 5α-reductase, and in these tissues, testosterone forms complexes with the androgen receptor as such and acts in the nucleus (3,61,97). The 5α-reductase activity of the prostate of sexually mature animals declines swiftly and extensively after orchiectomy, and the low activity in castrated animals is increased many fold by administration of testosterone (61). Unlike the X-linked androgen receptor, the gene for steroid 5α-reductase clearly is autosomally located.

HEREDITARY DEFECTS OF TESTOSTERONE ACTION

One cannot overestimate the importance for all hormonal regulations not only of the arrival at target cells of adequate amounts of a given hormone (and in some cases its conversion in the responding cell to more biologically active derivatives), but also of (a) the presence of sufficient numbers of the corresponding functional receptors in appropriate intracellular locations, and (b) an intact postreceptor biochemical machinery that amplifies the hormone–receptor signal. If either the receptor or postreceptor mechanisms are rendered ineffective for genetic or other reasons, then cellular responses to the hormone will be compromised. A number of genetically determined syndromes in which the virilizing actions of testosterone are attenuated to varying degrees have been described in several mammalian species, including man. These disorders, most of which appear to result from single gene defects, are primarily due to dysfunctions of either androgen receptors or steroid 5α-reductase. Such congenital androgen insensitivities can give rise to a wide spectrum of mishaps in the development of a normal masculine phenotype in XY males with endocrinologically functional testes but devoid of ovarian tissue (3). Studies on these types of hereditary male pseudohermaphroditisms have been most instructive from the standpoint of understanding the critical roles of testosterone and DHT in normal male sex differentiation. Phenocopies of some of these can be induced by application of specific antagonists of androgen receptors or inhibitors of steroid 5α-reductase at suitable stages of fetal sexual development in normal males.

Before considering the developmental abnormalities associated with genetic brakes on androgen action, it should be pointed out that other types of gene defects can result in symptoms of male pseudohermaphroditism. Disturbances in the production and/or functions of five of the enzymes involved in the biosynthesis of testosterone are well known to be associated with impaired virilization and the appearance of certain female phenotypic characteristics (98). And as already mentioned, the müllerian duct involuting hormone (MDIH) secreted by fetal testicular Sertoli cells is essential for prevention during normal male sexual development of morphogenesis of oviductal, uterine, or upper vaginal structures. In the extremely rare persistent müllerian duct syndrome, miniature müllerian structures are formed alongside a normal male reproductive tract in XY men with testes that secrete ample testosterone but who have no ovaries (99). This situation could obviously arise from genetic defects in either the production of MDIH or the function of the putative MDIH receptor during embryonic male sex differentiation.

Syndromes of Androgen Resistance

Androgen Receptor Disorders

A variety of syndromes attributable to mutations of the androgen receptor and that present varying degrees of disordered masculine phenotypic development and function have been described, as admirably reviewed by Wilson et al. (3). All of the afflicted patients or animals are XY males with testes but also a spectrum of feminine characteristics. In adulthood, these male pseudohermaphrodites have normal or higher plasma concentrations and production rates of testosterone, greater than normal levels of circulating estrogens, and elevated LH in blood plasma. The inheritance of these conditions is X-linked recessive.

In the so-called complete form of human testicular feminization (or androgen-insensitivity) syndrome, the testes are abdominal or inguinal in location. Externally there is a vulva, with unfused labia that may be underdeveloped and usually a minuscule clitoris, and the introitus leads into a short, blind-ending vagina. Internally there are no organs derived from the wolffian and müllerian ducts, and a typically female urethra terminates below the clitoris as in normal women. At puberty, facial, pubic, and axillary hair hardly develops, yet breast development is florid. The testes are incapable of spermatogenesis, and the seminiferous tubules resemble those found in cryptorchid male gonads; for obvious reasons the patients never menstruate. In the much less frequent incomplete form of testicular feminization, the clinical picture resembles that of the complete form of the syndrome except that the external genitalia are often ambiguous, with cliteromegaly and fusion of the labioscrotal folds; a slight development of wolffian duct-derived structures may also occur. At puberty there ensues some degree of virilization (facial and pubic hair) and feminization (enlarged mammary glands). In the less severe Reifenstein syndrome, intersexuality of external or internal reproductive organs is apparent, though organs derived from the müllerian ducts are lacking. Patients with complete testicular feminization are entirely refractory to masculinizing influence of their high endogenous circulating androgens or to either testosterone or DHT given exogenously, even in very high doses. In incomplete testicular feminization and the Reifenstein syndrome, there is partial resistance to testosterone and DHT. Recent investigations (3) suggest that what has been designated as the infertile male syndrome (100) is the mildest form of genetically determined androgen insensitivity in man. These patients are essentially phenotypic males, though they tend to have minimum male facial and bodily hair and sometimes exhibit gynecomastia. The resistance to androgens is manifest mainly in the testicular seminiferous tubules, with infertility due to extensive deficiency in spermatogenesis. It is thought that this condition accounts for as much as a quarter of all cases of male infertility associated with idiopathic azoospermia or oligospermia (3).

Comparable male pseudohermaphroditisms with androgen insensitivity and X-linked inheritance have been described in the cow, rat, mouse, horse, chimpanzee, and dog (3). First described by Lyon and Hawkes (101), testicular feminization in the mouse, which is redolent of complete testicular feminization in man, has been the most thoroughly studied of these animal conditions.

Investigations on biochemical defects of animals and patients with androgen insensitivities have been aided greatly by studies on cultured fibroblasts, which provide sufficient amounts of cells for in-depth analyses of androgen receptor and steroid 5α-reductase functions, the deranged biochemical phenotypes usually being retained under the conditions of cell culture (3). Fibroblasts from genital skin of normal men (penile foreskin and scrotum) and women (labia) are compared with fibroblasts from labial skin or clitoral foreskin of the androgen-insensitive mutants. (In normal men and women, the androgen receptor content of genital skin fibroblasts is generally greater than that of fibroblasts from nongenital sites.) As estimated by binding of various radioactively labeled androgen agonists, a majority of patients with complete testicular feminization have very little or no androgen receptor, as estimated at 37 or 42°C, while a significant fraction of patients exhibit receptors with intermediate binding at 37°C and very low binding of DHT at 42°C. Individuals with incomplete testicular feminization, or the Reifenstein or infertile male syndromes, usually have receptors that bind DHT but with a diminished capacity and/or various qualitative defects, as evidenced by thermolability or decreased stabilization of the cytosol receptor by molybdate (3). Another abnormality of androgen receptors in some patients afflicted with one of the hereditary androgen insensitivities is a decrease in temperature-dependent transformation of the DHT– or testosterone–receptor complexes to a DNA-binding state (96), which with normal androgen receptors (95) and the abnormal mutant receptors (96) occurs more readily when DHT rather than testosterone is the hormonal ligand. It seems probable that if more is found out about the functional architecture of androgen receptor proteins, then more subtle tests for deranged mutant androgen receptor proteins will be devised. Although androgen insensitivities due to androgen receptor defects all appear to be caused by mutations of the X-linked gene for this receptor, this does not necessarily mean that a single mutation is responsible for all of the aforementioned syndromes. A minority of patients with complete testicular feminization apparently have androgen receptors that are often normal both quantitatively and qualitatively, as evidenced by affinities for testosterone and DHT, turnover rates, nuclear localization, and thermal stability. Although it is conceivable that the defect in these instances is related to some postreceptor dysfunction in androgen action (102), it could well be that there are some more subtle mutations of the androgen receptor gene that cannot be detected with available methods.

In contrast to the various androgen receptor malfunctions characteristic of testicular feminization and the Reifenstein or infertile male syndromes, conversion of testosterone to DHT is normal or only somewhat diminished in these patients, as evidenced by measurements of 5α-reductase activities in skin biopsies and DHT excretion; normal DHT formation is observed in cultured fibroblasts, however (3). These disorders are therefore clearly different from androgen insensitivities resulting from mutations of steroid 5α-reductase now to be considered.

Steroid 5α-Reductase Deficiencies

A condition known as pseudovaginal perineoscrotal hypospadias, and now usually designated as steroid 5α-reductase deficiency, is a form of male pseudohermaphroditism that results from defects in testosterone action but is not primarily related to mutations of the androgen receptor (3). The syndrome is found in XY males with testes and no ovaries and is inherited as an autosomal recessive. Among the clinical features are a pronounced perineoscrotal hypospadias with a large clitoral-like phallus, frequently a small vulval structure opening into a blind vaginal pouch, and internally well-developed wolffian duct-derived structures (epididymis, vas deferens, and seminal vesicles) but only tiny, if any, prostate and bulbourethral glands (which originate embryologically from the urogenital sinus). There is no upper vagina, uterus, or oviducts. At puberty, these individuals may undergo extensive masculinization (phallic growth, appearance of some facial and pubic hair, manifestation of male sex behavior patterns, etc.) but do not develop gynecomastia. The production and plasma levels of testosterone and estrogens are usually close to those in normal men, as are plasma LH levels (3).

Investigations on biopsies of genital skin and fibroblasts cultured therefrom have revealed a variety of defects in steroid 5α-reductase in patients with pseudovaginal perineoscrotal hypospadias: (a) very low enzyme activity, with the residual 5α-reductase having a high apparent K_m for testosterone and an apparently normal K_m for NADPH; (b) diminished but measurable activities with abnormally large K_m values for NADPH but not for testosterone, the enzyme in cultured fibroblasts from some of these patients exhibiting a greatly decreased half-life, as evidenced by a much faster than normal rate of decline in activity after exposure of the cells to the protein biosynthesis inhibitor cycloheximide; and (c) an enzyme variant with apparently normal K_m values for both substrates whose activity in cultured cells is within the normal range but is very unstable when the cells are treated with cycloheximide (3). A simple explanation for these diverse findings is that a variety of mutations of the steroid 5α-reductase gene can occur. It should be emphasized that all reported human steroid 5α-reductase deficiencies are partial—there is always some detectable residual enzyme activity—and androgen receptor levels in tissues of these patients are nearly always within the normal range (3).

The clinical pictures in human steroid 5α-reductase deficiencies accord with experimental evidence that, in a number of eutherian species, DHT produced in the anlagen is the active form of circulating testosterone that in combination with androgen receptor directs a masculine mode of differentiation of the fetal urogenital sinus (UGS) and external genital primordia, whereas differentiation of the wolffian duct into male structures is evoked by testosterone–receptor complexes. Defects of either androgen receptor or steroid 5α-reductase presumably do not influence the production or actions of fetal testicular MDIH, which would account for absence of müllerian duct-derived structures in the syndromes of testicular feminization and 5α-reductase deficiency.

Phenocopies of Congenital Androgen Insensitivities

Studies by Neumann et al. (103) using the androgen-receptor antagonists Cyproterone and Cyproterone acetate showed that phenocopies of testicular feminization—in which XY males with testes and no ovaries have female external genitalia but no internal reproductive organs of either sex—can be induced by application to dog and rabbit male fetuses of these antiandrogens, which cross the placenta when administered to the mothers. However, Cyproterone acetate, which blocks wolffian duct differentiation evoked by exogenous testosterone in female fetal rats, did not depress morphogenesis of epididymis, vas deferens, and seminal vesicles in the fetal male rat, whereas the antiandrogen was active in the latter respect in dog and rabbit fetuses. The latter conflicting findings may possibly reflect species differences in the pharmacokinetics of Cyproterone acetate in the fetus and/or the mother. The aforementioned observations are of interest in the light of recent studies by Imperato-McGinley and Guerro—who independently discovered steroid 5α-reductase deficiency in man (104)—concerning the induction of male pseudohermaphroditism in rats by treating the mothers during pregnancy with 4-methyl-4-aza-5-pregnane-3-one-20[s]carboxylate, a very powerful inhibitor of steroid 5α-reductase with only negligible affinity for the androgen receptor (105). This drug elicited complete and irreversible feminization of the external genitalia of male fetal rats with formation of a pseudovagina; epididymides, vasa deferentia, and seminal vesicles were well developed, which would accord with testosterone, rather than DHT, being the stimulus to wolffian duct differentiation. However, male rat fetuses exposed to the 4-methyl-4-aza steroid inhibitor did develop prostatic buds, which might be accounted for by failure of the drug to inhibit DHT formation completely during fetal male sex differentiation, if it is assumed that prostate differentiation has a lower threshold for DHT than male development of the external genital anlagen. In any event, these studies of Imperato-McGinley et al. (105) emphasize the key role of DHT formation in the fetal differentiation of eutherian male external genitalia and represent the chemical induction of a partial phenocopy of the syndrome of steroid 5α-reductase deficiency. To my knowledge, mutations of the 5α-reductase gene have not been described in any eutherian species except man.

Cellular Sites of Androgen Action in Epithelial–Mesenchyme Interactions During Prostate Morphogenesis

The development of prostate glands from the embryonic UGS is utterly dependent on androgens produced by the fetal testis (1,10,87,106). Cunha et al. (107) have investigated the role of androgenic influences on the mesenchyme of the UGS in the fetal differentiation of the prostate, which appears to involve the following phases. The mesenchymal elements of the UGS promote the endodermal epithelium of this primordium to differentiate into prostate secretory cells, the initial morphogenesis of which entails formation of a branched ductal-acinar architecture. The dimensions of the emerging prostate increase in the fetus, and secretory cytodifferentiation of the epithelial cells begins postnatally, culminating in full prostatic growth and secretory activity at puberty in response to high levels of circulating testosterone. Cunha et al. (107,108) demonstrated that in the presence of androgens, the epithelium of the fetal or adult bladder (or BLE, which also derives from the UGS) can develop into prostate buds when grown in the presence of UGS mesenchyme, with extensive growth of typically prostatic epithelial cells. Androgens appear to stimulate the latter processes by acting on mesenchyme, eventually resulting in extensive growth of typically prostatic epithelial cells. One line of evidence supporting this notion stems from recombinant tissue experiments in male athymic nude mice, in which wild-type UGS mesenchyme from androgen-sensitive mouse embryos was shown to induce differentiation of prostate epithelial cells from androgen-insensitive and receptor-negative explants of BLE originating from mice with testicular feminization (Tfm). Growing wild UGM plus Tfm BLE recombinant explants grown for one week in intact mice of normal androgenic status resulted in formation of a branched network of prostatic ducts that underwent secretory cytodifferentiation (107). These and other results (108) hint that epithelial cell responses to androgens during prostate morphogenesis are largely, if not exclusively, mediated by trophic factors emanating from the androgen-sensitive mesenchyme. [There is no doubt that adult prostate epithelia are replete with androgen receptors and are directly influenced by androgenic hormones (66).] Shannon and Cunha (108) are of the opinion that the aforementioned findings lend credence to the hypothesis of McNeal (109) that human benign prostatic hyperplasia is caused by a reawakening of embryoniclike induction of adult epithelial cell growth by stimuli from the mesenchyme of this gland.

PRODUCTION, MATURATION, TRANSPORT, AND FUNCTIONS OF SPERMATOZOA

At times when eutherians are capable of breeding, the continual daily production of prodigious quantities of spermatozoa by males stands in marked contrast to the only periodic ovulation of relatively very small numbers of eggs by females. Spermatogenesis and the physiology of spermatozoa are considered at length elsewhere in this text (chapters 2 and 20), so that only a few basic aspects of these topics are highlighted in this section.

Eutherian Spermatogenesis

Spermatogenesis with the production of free testicular spermatozoa does not commence until puberty in mammals, when sufficiently high circulating levels of LH and FSH are attained. The targets for FSH and LH are Sertoli and Leydig cells, respectively. The effect of LH on spermatogenesis is indirect because the function of this gonadotrophin in the male is to stimulate *de novo* synthesis by Leydig cells of testosterone, high concentrations of which must be present in Sertoli cells (which lack LH receptors) for sperm production to occur. The two hormones that are proximally required by Sertoli cells to support spermatogenesis in all of its phases are FSH and testosterone. Androgen and FSH receptors are present in Sertoli cells but are apparently lacking in all differentiating male germ cells, which are thus not directly affected by these hormones (110). Circulating testosterone exerts negative-feedback influences on the output of LH via the hypothalamicopituitary axis. The mature eutherian testis exerts negative influences over FSH secretion; these actions are probably mediated by polypeptide "inhibin(s)," which have been purified from seminal plasma and partially characterized (111). However whether inhibin-like substances in the male originate from the testis or perhaps from androgen-dependent male accessory sex glands has not yet been completely settled. (Female inhibins, that differ structurally from those obtained from seminal fluid, are found in ovarian follicular fluid (112).]

Meiosis leading to the formation of haploid spermatids in the eutherian testis does not proceed completely before puberty, although in some species male germ cells have a very limited ability to embark on the early stages of meiosis in late fetal or neonatal life. There are suggestions that a specific meiosis-preventing substance is present in testicular cords in juvenile animals, but the nature and physiological importance of this material is uncertain (113). In almost all eutherians, meiosis normally seems to yield equal proportions of X- and Y-chromosome-bearing spermatozoa and presumably spermatids, and deviations of the sex ratio at birth from exact unity are commonly ascribed to differential mortality of embryos of the two sexes.

Spermiogenesis—the differentiation of spermatozoa from haploid spermatids—differs greatly in detail among eutherian species, as does the morphology of testicular, epididymal, and ejaculated spermatozoa. No *de novo* synthesis of nuclear DNA occurs in spermatids or spermatozoa (very low rates of thymidine incorporation into DNA reported to occur in sperm cells are almost certainly due to mitochondrial DNA replication (114)]. If any haploid nuclear gene expression occurs during spermiogenesis, it seems to relate to very few genes, despite evidence that round (early) spermatids seem to synthesize ribosomal and polyadenylated RNA, which ceases as the spermatids later move into luminal crypts (110). Differentiation of spermatozoa from early spermatids involves, of course, selective breakdown of many macromolecules held over from secondary spermatocytes, as well as the new formation of a large number of sperm-specific proteins.

An apparently unique attribute of spermiogenesis in therian mammals is that the species-specific sperm nuclear basic proteins are rich in arginine, serine, and cysteine, and gradually become cross-linked via disulfide bridges during sperm maturation. As nuclear histones are destroyed during spermiogenesis they are not replaced immediately by the cysteine-rich sperm head proteins but are first replaced transiently by intermediary basic proteins devoid of cysteine and containing considerable amounts of both lysine and arginine (115). The species-specific, cysteine-rich mammalian sperm head proteins almost certainly play an important role in determining the morphogenesis of the sperm head, and the gradual formation of disulfide cross-bridges helps to impart a greater rigidity to the sperm head in comparison with nontherian vertebrates. A comparable cross-linking of protein-bound sulfhydryl groups of spermatozoal dense fibers, mitochondrial membranes, and sheaths during therian sperm maturation may also stabilize the head and tail components. Bedford (116) has proposed that the aforementioned rigidification of therian spermatozoa may represent an evolutionary adaptation of the sperm head of therians to increasing difficulty of penetration of their peculiarly extensive egg vestments (especially the zona pellucida), which are less frail than in other vertebrates.

The timing of each stage of spermatogenesis does not seem to depend on hormones but rather to be genetically determined, even though FSH and androgens obviously control the numbers of spermatogonial stem cells that eventually enter spermatogenic cycles. In the majority of eutherians, spermatogenesis will not proceed to completion unless the temperature of the testis is a few degrees lower than that of all other internal organs of the body. Two structures are responsible for keeping eutherian testicular temperatures below normal body temperature at periods when spermatogenesis occurs: the scrotum and the pampiniform plexus of testicular veins (110). Scrotums are not found in nontherian vertebrates. The potential evolutionary value of the scrotum is considered in the last section of this chapter. Scholarly accounts of species variations in the functional anatomy of eutherian spermatozoa are provided by Austin (6) and in two cyclopedic treatises (114,117). Some salient features of this topic may be summarized as follows, remembering that certain characteristics of testicular spermatozoa become modified during maturation in the epididymis and also as a result of contact of sperms with seminal plasma at ejaculation. There exists remarkable diversity in the size, shape, and biochemical properties of sperm head-pieces, acrosomes (especially their enzymes), nuclear envelopes, mitochondria, and flagella among various eutherians; striking similarities in these components are often evident between closely related species but sometimes also between evolutionarily quite distant creatures. All eutherian spermatozoa have a 9 + 2 microtubular axonemal complex, and morphologically more species-variable coarse fibers, in their flagella. There are large species differences in the energy metabolism of ejaculated spermatozoa. In general, all eutherian sperms exhibit high rates of anaerobic lactate production from hexoses and lesser, but still considerable, glycolysis in the presence of oxygen. Eutherian spermatozoa do not store carbohydrates in the form of glycogen or other polymers. Fructose is the principal sugar in the seminal plasma of most eutherians and serves as the major exogenous source of substrate for lactate production by sperm glycolytic enzymes. Seminal fructose is formed in male accessory glands (most frequently the seminal vesicles) by a nonphosphorylative pathway in which glucose is enzymatically reduced by NADPH to sorbitol and then oxidized to fructose by NAD (114,118). The very slow rates of incorporation of labeled amino acids into proteins and nucleoside precursors into nucleic acids demonstrable in spermatozoa almost certainly occur only in the mitochondria, and eutherian ejaculated sperms are normally devoid of extramitochondrial polyribosomes (114). In some species, sperm have a considerable capacity to oxidize their endogenous phospholipid fatty acids by oxygen, although in certain eutherians (e.g., man) sperm respiration is feeble. The relatively large contribution of glycolysis to ATP production by spermatozoa is probably of adaptive value in sperm transport to the sites of fertilization through uterine and oviductal fluids, the oxygen content of which may be quite low in the female genital tract.

Whereas many spermatozoal characteristics are obviously of functional value, there are, as Austin (6) points out, a variety of conspicuous peculiarities of spermatozoal architecture in certain eutherians that seem to be devoid of biological advantage, e.g., the relatively enormous length of the Chinese hamster's sperm flagellum; there is also a wide spectrum of species differences in the size and shape of spermatozoal head-pieces, which seem to be of no value for sperm transport or survival in the male or female genital tracts or for egg negotiation at fertilization. These seemingly valueless properties of spermatozoa occasionally perhaps represent evolutionary vestiges, but in most instances probably reflect mutations of genes whose expression during spermiogenesis are of neutral selective value.

Sperm Transport and Maturation in the Epididymis

When therian spermatozoa are released from the rete testis, they are devoid of the capacity for motility or fertilization but acquire these attributes during their transit through the lumen of the epididymis, which takes place in the course of a few weeks. Bedford (116) avers that, although testicular spermatozoa of many subtherian vertebrates in which internal fertilization occurs may develop a capability for motility during their passage through the wolffian duct, "there seems to be an almost quantum leap in complexity of epididymal function with the evolutionary emergence of marsupials and eutherian mammals, in which maturation of fertilizing ability involves several additional changes in the sperm cell." Eutherian epididymal epithelia secrete fluids whose composition varies with the species. Some of the components of epididymal plasma may contribute to sperm maturation by affecting the cell surface and in other ways, and also can enter the seminal plasma. When ejaculation is not exceptionally frequent, virtually all of the sperms in eutherian semen originate from the cauda of the epididymis and the vas deferens. For an authoritative and comprehensive review of the chemical physiology of the epididymis and its secretions, the reader should consult the book by Mann and Lutwak-Mann (114). Epididymal development and function are strictly regulated by androgens. Although the eutherian epididymis lies in close proximity to the testis, there is experimental evidence that in those species in which the testes reside in a scrotum during male breeding seasons, the maturation of spermatozoa in the epididymis can proceed just as well at the temperature of all internal organs in other bodily locations as it normally does at the lower intrascrotal temperature. For more information on the transport and maturation of sperms in the epididymis, see chapter 23.

MALE ACCESSORY SEX GLANDS AND THE FORMATION AND FUNCTIONS OF SEMINAL PLASMA

All male mammals develop a series of specialized secretory organs from the fetal UGS (the prostate and bulbourethral glands), and in some species the wolffian duct develops into seminal vesicles and a secretory ampulla of the vas deferens (106,114,118). Each of these glands contains a secretory epithelium that is greatly increased by villous infoldings or a compound tubuloalveolar structure, a lamina propria, and a fibromuscular stroma. The differentiation of these structures in the fetus, as well as their extensive growth and secretory activity initiated at puberty, is utterly dependent on androgens. The male accessory gland secretions are stored in the glandular alveoli and are delivered out of the ducts into the urethra at seminal emission. The secretions of the prostate and bulbourethral glands, together with those of the seminal vesicles in those species that possess the latter organs, make up the bulk of the seminal plasma, which also contains components of rete testis and epididymal fluids. Secretion by some male accessory sex glands is enhanced during sexual excitement in the male. The only important function of these glands is to produce the bulk of the seminal plasma (106,114,118,119).

Male accessory sex glands are not found in nonmammalian vertebrates. These glands probably developed very early in mammalian evolution (106). In comparison with nontherian vertebrates, the semens of the great majority of eutherian species are relatively dilute because of the large proportion of seminal plasma. The volume of a normal ejaculate varies considerably among different species, as do seminal plasma volumes in different ejaculates of the same individual, even when seminal emission is not too frequent; this is because of short-term vagaries in the degree of emptying of preformed secretions from the various accessory glands during the ejaculatory process, the extent and duration of precoital male sexual excitement, and fluctuations in the levels of circulating testosterone (114,119). A minority of male eutherians produce copious amounts of pre-ejaculatory secretions prior to true seminal emission. These are largely derived from the bulbourethral glands, e.g., the boar (114), and effectively lubricate the penis and even the vagina; additionally, they may serve a pheromonal function by virtue of their containing volatile odoriferous substances that could attract females. However, in most species, male pre-ejaculatory secretions are sparse, and their function, if any, may be to lubricate the penile urethra to protect it against any deleterious constituents of prostate or seminal vesicle secretions present in semen.

Modern reptiles have no prostates or seminal vesicles, and the low volumes of seminal plasma they produce originate mainly from the epididymis and the sexual segment of the long, lobulated kidney. Comparably, in birds the small amounts of seminal plasma are apparently secreted almost entirely by the seminiferous tubules and vasa efferentia (106,114). Price and Williams-Ashman (106) proposed that the evolution of large and complex male accessory glands in eutherian mammals may have compensated for the loss of a functional sexual segment of the kidney found in male reptiles. Noteworthy in this regard is the retention by the metanephric kidney of both sexes of certain eutherian species (notably mice and certain other rodents) of marked responsivity to the growth-promoting actions of testosterone (97), even though fluids from the kidneys do not contribute to mammalian seminal plasma.

In some eutherian animals, the prostate glands are subdivided into several distinct lobes, each of which differs markedly in morphology, quantitative response to testosterone, and composition of the secretions produced (106,114,119). The anterior lobe of the prostate in certain species (particularly in many rodents) lies alongside the seminal vesicles and is known as the coagulating gland. The coagulating gland contains powerful transglutaminases in its secretion that catalyze cross-linking of certain bulk proteins in seminal vesicle secretion via formation of γ-glutamyl-ε-lysine cross-bridges; this process is responsible for the postejaculatory formation of very insoluble semen clots, vaginal plugs, in various eutherian females after coitus (119,120).

The principal substance in seminal plasma is water. There can be no doubt that the overriding function of eutherian seminal plasma is a hydrodynamic one, to ensure that the semen is effectively ejaculated into the female genital canal. There are two main mechanisms of delivery of semen into females in mammals: Either most of the semen is deposited as a pool in the upper vagina of species with a large cervix that may be filled with a secretory mucus (e.g., in cows and women), or alternatively, much of the ejaculated semen is swiftly forced through a relatively short cervix directly into the uterine lumen (as in rats and mice). Nevertheless, it must be remembered that in most eutherians, of the many hundreds of millions or more of spermatozoa that males deposit in females in a single ejaculate, a substantial proportion never pass beyond the cervix, and only a very tiny number (usually several hundred) arrive near the surface of a newly ovulated ovum in the ampulla of the oviduct where fertilization takes place (114). Moreover, almost none of the constituents of seminal plasma reaches the upper oviduct since the concentrations of the substances that ever enter into the uterus are enormously diluted by uterine and oviductal secretions. It is thus extremely unlikely that any of the biomolecules in seminal plasma directly participate in the fertilization process.

As considered in detail by Mann and Lutwak-Mann (114), and by me (106,118,119), there are huge species variations in the chemical composition of the secretions of the individual male accessory sex glands, and hence of seminal plasma. Some of these accessory gland secretion constituents undoubtedly serve significant reproductive functions. The high concentrations of fructose in the seminal plasma of many eutherians almost certainly supports the energy metabolism of spermatozoa during their residence in the vaginal barrel, perhaps to a lesser extent in the distal end of the uterus. Certain of the bulk proteins in seminal plasma (the vast majority of which are synthesized *de novo* by secretory epithelial cells of the male genital ducts and glands rather than being abstracted from blood plasma prior to secretion) may significantly affect sperm survival or transport in the female. For example, in the human, the buffering power of some of the major seminal proteins derived from vesicular secretion may contribute to alkalinization of the quite acid (pH 5 or less) vaginal secretions, that, as such, are deleterious to the motility of unbuffered suspensions of washed sperms (114). The possible functions of vaginal plugs of semen in certain species have been discussed elsewhere (119,120). Again, some of the many types of prostaglandins in human seminal plasma may conceivably assist transport of spermatazoa in the female reproductive tract. However, many major components of seminal plasma seem to play no role in sperm transport or fertilization, e.g., the very high levels of divalent zinc ions, citric acid, inositol, and many of the proteinases and other hydrolytic enzymes secreted by various male accessory glands (114). Although precluding the possibility that any particular seminal plasma constituent, other than water and the inorganic ions that render the plasma roughly iso-osmotic with blood serum, may have some physiological value is patently absurd, it is no less unreasonable to assume that every substance found in appreciable amounts in the seminal plasma must somehow be of reproductive importance, any more than imagining that every chemical substance in blood plasma should be of significance to the physiology of red or white blood cells (114,121).

EVOLUTION OF THE FUNCTIONAL MORPHOLOGY OF EUTHERIAN MALE EXTERNAL GENITALIA

Among extant species of eutherian mammals, there is a striking diversity in the architecture and size of the normal external genitalia of sexually mature males. Considerably less interspecific variations are evident in the female with respect to the fundamental design (though not, of course, the overall dimensions) of the homologous vulva, but not with regard to the nonhomologous müllerian duct-derived structures (vagina, uterine cervix) that accommodate the penis during copulation. Furthermore, the topography of the external genital primordia before the onset of fetal sex differentiation in a given species is essentially the same in both sexes, being remarkably similar among different eutherian species. As considered above, morphogenesis of the male external genital apparatus from fetal primordia is utterly androgen dependent, and if the actions of testicular androgens in the fetus are attenuated because of mutations of the androgen receptor, steroid 5α-reductase, or other reasons, then virilization of the fetal external genital anlagen will be compromised or abrogated. In normal individuals of nearly all eutherian species, there is obvious sexual dimorphism of the external genitalia. However, a striking exception to this rule is provided in the odd case of the spotted hyena, *Crocuta crocuta*. As illustrated in Fig. 2, the sexually mature female of this species has large, empty pseudoscrotum and a gigantic highly erectile clitoris that appears similar to the penis of the male. The female lower vagina opens at the distal end of the clitoris, with a female type of urethra opening near the glans clitoridis; at copulation, the male intromits his penis into the female phallus (122). Considering that the ovary of the sexually mature female spotted hyena atypically secretes very high amounts of testosterone into the blood plasma, and also that blood from fetal females of this species is remarkably rich in testosterone (123), it is not surprising in the light of androgenic influences on external genitalic morphogenesis and growth (see above) that this condition pertains.

Functions of the Eutherian Penis

The eutherian penis has two obvious functions: (a) by virtue of the penile shaft surrounding the distal part of the male urethra that terminates close to the tip of the glans, the organ serves as a conduit for urine; and (b) since all components of semen are eventually emitted from the male urethra, the penis serves to inseminate females. Some degree of penile erection is a necessary prelude to the normal ejaculatory process. Micturition and semen ejaculation are usually mutually exclusive phenomena, since full penile tumescence prohibits urination, and the internal sphincter of the bladder contracts during seminal emission. The central and peripheral neuronal events that provoke penile erection and seminal emission (see Chapter 24) remain poorly understood, especially from the standpoints of the complexities of the pertinent sensory and motor neuronal circuitries, as well as the participation of various neurotransmitters in, and influences of sex steroid and other hormones on, these processes (124–126). Only very recently, for example, has evidence accrued to suggest that vasoactive intestinal polypeptide serves a peripheral neurotransmitter function in re-

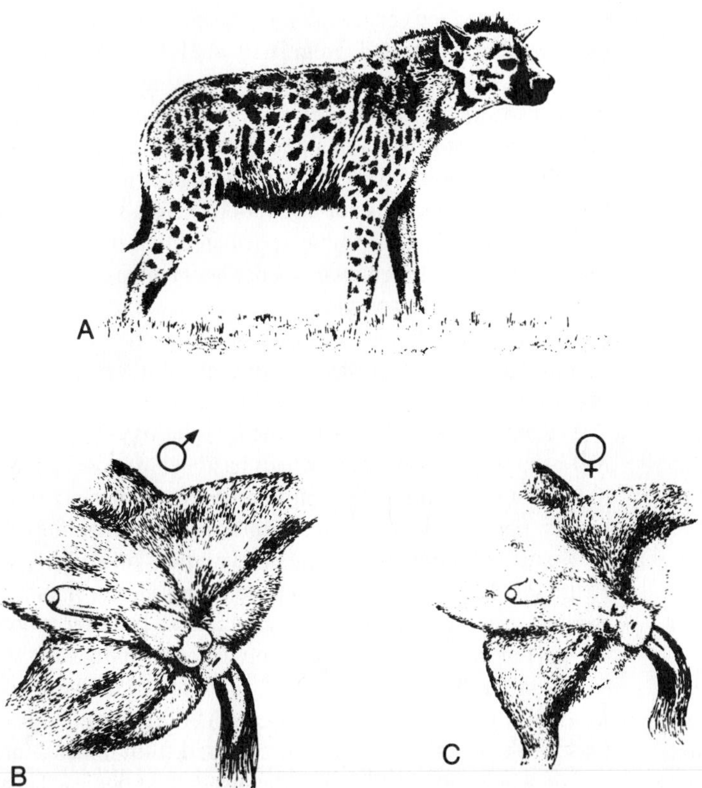

FIG. 2. A: Sexual mimicry in the external genitalia of the spotted hyena *Crocuta crocuta.* **B:** Ventral view of the external genitalia of an adult male spotted hyena, showing the penis within its prepuce, and the scrotum and anus. **C:** Ventral view of the external genitalia of a pubertal female spotted hyena, showing the clitoris within its prepuce (very similar in size, shape, and location to the male penis) and the "false" scrotum, which is smaller than that of the male because it does not contain any gonadal tissue. (From ref. 10.)

lation to the vascular changes in the penis associated with erection in some species (127,128), or has much insight been obtained into the roles of serotonin, dopamine, and norepinephrine (129–131) as neurotransmitters in neuronal pathways in the brain related to penile erection, ejaculation, and the postejaculatory period of sexual inadequacy observed in most, if not all, eutherian males.

Among different eutherian species, average normal penile dimensions, whether measured in the stretched flaccid or erect states, do not bear any simple linear relationship to body weight or size. This is well illustrated by Short's (132) in-depth analysis of the dimensions and functions of the penis in various species of the primate subfamily Ponginae (the great apes) and man. The male gorilla (the largest and heaviest species) has a tiny penis, which is quite difficult to discern amidst the extensive abdominal hair when it is fully retracted into its prepuce in the flaccid state and is only about 3 cm long when erect. Comparably, the penis of the orangutan is almost inconspicuous when not erect and short when it is. By contrast, the penis of the adult African pygmy chimpanzee, a much smaller creature, is remarkably long and thin, often attaining a length of 8 cm or more on erection. In the latter species, prolonged display of the erect penis to females in estrus is a standard maneuver of male courtship, in contrast to the great majority of eutherians. The human male has the largest penis of all of the primates, whose length when flaccid but stretched is 13 cm on the average. Clinical observations of patients with micropenis and animal experimental studies (133) indicate that, in addition to the paramount requirement for androgens, there is a significant contribution of pituitary growth hormone (probably mediated via production of somatomedin C) to penile growth. Full growth of the human penis is usually completed by the end of puberty, and adult penile size is normally not correlated with body build or the frequency of erection or copulation.

Some examples of the extraordinary species variations in eutherian penile anatomy follow. In all dogs and various other carnivores, sea lions, Mustelidae (minks, weasels, etc.), and many rodents, bats, and nonhuman primates, part of the penile corpus cavernosum ossifies to produce an os penis, or baculum, comprised of true bone (134–137). In some species, the os penis does seem to facilitate negotiation of the vagina by the erect penis and its retention therein. A spectacular example of this concerns the complementary relationships between the architecture of the penis and the vagina in two related species of macaque monkeys (136). In the rhesus monkey, *Macaca mulatta mulatta,* and most other macaques, the glans penis is less than 2.5 cm long and is shaped rather like a helmet or mushroom, approximating that of man. The rhesus monkey penis fits nicely into the introitus and vagina of the female of this species so as to allow facile deposition of a pool of semen close to the uterine cervix. In the red-faced, stump-tailed bear macaque, *M. arctoides,* however, the glans of the penis is relatively long (5–7 cm), slender, lance-shaped, rather than being short, blunt, and rounded as in other macaques. This evolutionary quirk of penile morphology complements the relatively longer vagina of the female partner, the introitus of which is obstructed by a large middorsal ellipsoid mass comprising a dorsal vestibular colliculus; thus, the penis of the male of this species, but not that of other macaques, can be readily inserted deep into the long vaginal barrel. The os penis of *M. arctoides* is about 6 cm long, about twice the length observed in other macaques. Parenthetically, an os clitoridis, a minuscule bone inside the clitoris that is the female homolog of the penis, is found in a variety of eutherian animals, though there are some species in which the male has an os penis but the female does not possess an os clitoridis (134,137). The genesis of os penes and clitorides is unquestionably androgen dependent. It is a tribute to the amazing morphogenetic powers of testosterone that this androgen, when administered in large doses to neonates, can induce the appearance of an os clitoridis in certain species in which the female normally does not have this structure (138). It is commonly believed that the os clitoridis is of no functional value, although Meczynski (139) suggests that the "teeth" of the os clitoris in sousliks might contact the intromitted penis during coitus.

Among eutherian mammals there are large species variations in the architecture of the penis with respect to the relative proportions of fibroelastic and vascular cylinder (corpora cavernosa and corpus spongiosum) elements and the mechanics of penile erection. The glans penis that caps the corpora cavernosa assumes a variety of forms. In man it is somewhat mushroom-shaped; in the boar it is corkscrew-shaped, as it is in the bull, though with a less pronounced twist. In some species, such as the rat and the cat, there are cornified papillae or penile spines embedded in the epithelial folds of the glans; growth of these spines is stimulated by androgens, and they regress greatly after castration of adult animals (140,141). When stimulated on contact with the vaginal wall, these penile spines, via neural connections to touch corpuscles located at the base of each spine, enhance sensory input from the penis to the brain, and it is believed that this contributes to male sexual arousal (140). In the goat, ram, and various other hoofed animals, there are thin structures (urethral or vermiform processes) that extend several centimeters beyond the tip of the penile glans, and are thought in some species to flip forward in the vaginal canal and thus stimulate female sensory nerve endings (142). Species differences in sexually mature male phallic morphology may in some instances correlate with patterns of copulatory behavior. For example, Estep and Dewsbury (143) discuss evidence favoring the hypothesis that muroid rodent species that display a lock (i.e., a mechanical tie between penis and vagina during coitus) may differ from nonlocking species in possessing (a) a penile glans that is thicker relative to its length, (b) more prominent penile spines, and (c) a relatively reduced complement of male accessory sex glands. Again, spines or other protuberances on the penis may stimulate sensory nerve endings in the vulvovaginal area of the female partner and thereby elicit neuroendocrine changes that result in ovulation and/or maintenance of the corpus luteum required for establishment of pregnancy or pseudopregnancy (141,144–148). Noteworthy in the latter context is the phenomenon in several rodents species of males briefly inserting their penes a number of times into the vagina and then withdrawing without ejaculating prior to a final, more prolonged intromission that results in seminal emission (125,141,145–148). It may be added that Milligan (149) has speculated that penile spines may facilitate male removal of copulatory plugs, deposited in the vagina during previous ejaculations, and so promote the fertility of the latest ejaculate (see discussion by Williams-Ashman (120) of the possible roles of vaginal plugs in fertility in certain mammalian species).

The extravagant diversity of the morphology of the penis and baculum in eutherians, which has been of considerable aid in the taxonomy of certain families and genera of some orders, poses some interesting problems concerning the role of sexual selection in divergent evolution of species, as Eberhard (150) discusses in his penetrating survey of animal external genitalia in an evolutionary context. Worthy of note is that females of animals utilizing internal modes of fertilization hardly ever possess intromittent organs designed to transfer their gametes to the male. Yet there is no logical reason why eggs could not be transferred from females into males, who could then fertilize the ova in their bodies. There is only one authentic exception to the general rule that males of species having internal fertilization transfer gametes to females rather than vice versa, viz., the females of the syngathid fish (sea horses and pipefish) have intromittent structures used to introduce eggs into a cavity in the male, where they are fertilized by sperms, who then broods the zygotes (150). As Eberhard (150) discusses, the almost universal prerogative of male animals to inseminate females is a facet of the general rule that males have a smaller investment in their offspring than females, with the consequence that reproduction in the male is constrained more by sexual access to contrasexual mates than it is in the female. In other words, competition between males for giving service to females may be responsible for intromittent organs being confined almost exclusively to the male.

What explanations can be provided to explain how male external genitalia have so often been subject to unusually rapid and divergent changes during evolution? Eberhard (150) discusses several hypotheses. The "*lock and key*" hypothesis, the most time-honored notion, proposes that evolution of male intromittent organs that act as a "key" to fit the female vulvovaginal "lock" tends to prohibit females getting their eggs fertilized by males of another species. This idea, which implies that new eutherian species are likely to develop unique female vulvovaginal locks and male penile keys, is in accord with such observations as the mechanics of coitus in two species of macaques with strikingly different penile and vaginal morphologies (mentioned above) but not with other facts. For example, there are many invertebrate and vertebrate species in which the female genitalia can easily accommodate the male copulatory organ of other species, yet in which the male genitalic structures exhibit wide interspecific variations. Furthermore, there exist creatures that almost certainly evolved in complete isolation from all close relatives yet exhibit large species-specific variations in their male genital morphologies. There are comparable difficulties in completely accepting the *genitalic recognition* hypothesis, which presumes that features of male external genitalia that are stimulatory to the female can be selected by females to identify males of the same species.

The *pleiotropic* hypothesis put forward by Mayr (151) propounds that species differences in male genitalic morphology are essentially of neutral value in sexual selection and that the male organs vary divergently because their development is pleiotropically influenced by genes that are also responsible for entirely different and selectively important characteristics.

Eberhard (150) emphasizes another hypothesis: *sexual selection by female choice*. In essence, this postulates that females can discriminate among males of their own species on the basis of their genitalia, with the result that males with favorable external genitals produce more offspring than others. In this respect, male genital organs might be conceived as "internal courtship" devices. Eberhard (150) considers two criteria by which a female could discriminate among male genitalia: stimuli she may receive directly from the male genital structures and the extent of the "fit" between the male and female copulatory organs. Virtually all of the evidence culled by Eberhard (150) in favor of the sexual selection by female choice hypothesis comes from observations on intromittent organs in invertebrates or fish (e.g., claspers, pedipalps) rather than on mammalian external genitalia.

The Scrotum

The scrotum, the male homolog of the major labia of the female vulva, is found in only some eutherian species. It is absent in armadillos, sloths, elephants, dolphins, and whales, yet spermatogenesis readily proceeds in the intra-abdominal testicles at normal body temperature. The scrotum lies against the ventral abdominal wall and is somewhat inconspicuous in hedgehogs and some other insectivores. The scrotum lies at the base of the tail in moles, shrews, and certain bats. Pigs, horses, rats, rabbits, and carnivores have nonpendulous scrotums underneath the anus. Strikingly pendulous scrotums are found in sheep, cattle, and other ruminants, and also in certain primates, notably man (110). The time of descent of the testes into the scrotum is species dependent: in man this usually occurs just before birth, in some other species it takes place postnatally or at puberty. In some eutherians the testes come to reside in the scrotum only during the male breeding season, in contrast to man, for example, in which the testicles remain permanently in this pocket of skin. The differentiation and maintenance of scrotal morphology is highly dependent on androgenic hormones.

Scrotums facilitate maintenance of the testis at a temperature several degrees centigrade lower than that of the internal organs of the abdomen. Eutherians with scrotums cannot carry out spermatogenesis if the testis is exposed to normal body temperatures (110,152). The cooling effect of the scrotum on the testis is in good part due to evaporative heat loss effected by the luxuriant population of sweat glands in the scrotal skin; this occurs even in species such as sheep in which sweating from other parts of the organism is not important for maintenance of homoiothermia (110,152). For a detailed discussion of regulation of testicular temperatures in mammals, see Chapter 2 and Waites (152).

Are there evolutionary advantages to the scrotum? It is easy to imagine disadvantages for animals that can breed only if the testicles are in a scrotal location (especially if the scrotum is very pendulous) with regard to testicular injury, e.g., inter- or intraspecies fighting. Two hypotheses have featured prominently in attempts to explain the biological value of a low-temperature requirement for spermatogenesis in many eutherians: (a) the rate of spontaneous mutations in testicular germ cells may be reduced in the cooler environment of the scrotum (153,154); and (b) it may prevent spermatogenesis at times other than those restricted periods of each year when the males of certain species breed. (Note, however, that scrotums are prominent in many species in which the male can breed continually from puberty to senescence.) It should be emphasized that in many species, testosterone secretion by Leydig cells is much less deleteriously affected by exposure of the testis to body temperatures than is spermatogenesis, so that cryptorchid animals or patients may develop and maintain many androgen-dependent masculine characteristics other than a capacity of the seminiferous tubules to produce spermatozoa. Other functions of the scrotum have been postulated. Portman's (155) thesis that the scrotum is exclusively an organ of male sexual adornment that attracts females to coital negotiations is clearly absurd (156,157). It is conceivable that the sebaceous glands in the scrotums of some species discussed by Wislocki (158) could produce secretions that contain pheromonally active constituents.

CONCLUDING COMMENTS

The essence of male sexual development in eutherian mammals may be summarized as follows. The attributes of masculinity are impressed at critical periods of development upon an ontogenetic substratum that has a fundamental tendency to differentiate in a feminine direction. The presence of a Y chromosome nearly always determines that the primitive indifferent gonad of the eutherian embryo will become a testis; in the absence of a Y chromosome an ovary normally develops. The fetal testis directs the formation of a male phenotype by virtue of producing: (a) testosterone, which is essential for the differentiation of male reproductive tracts, and secondary sexual tissues, as well as of masculine characteristics of the central nervous system and many other tissues; and (b) the anti-müllerian MDIH, which prohibits the formation of oviductal, uterine, and upper vaginal tissues. Thus, the establishment of an extragonadal male phenotype is entirely dependent on testicular hormones and does not entail expression of any additional genetic information that may be harbored by a Y chromosome. The most outstanding unsolved problems in eutherian male sexual physiology concern the mechanisms by which (a) nucleotide base sequences on the Y chromosome influence the differentiation of fetal testes and suppress the formation of ovarian tissue and (b) testosterone and MDIH exert their respective actions that determine the formation of male structures and "kill off" the embryonic mullerian ducts so as to prevent the differentiation of the principal internal extragonadal organs of a female reproductive tract. The chemical nature of testosterone, its mode of biosynthesis and secretion by the testis, and the importance of the conversion of testosterone to DHT in many androgen-sensitive tissues for the virilizing effects of this hormone have long since been established. However, the structure of the gene for the androgen receptor and the mechanisms responsible for the expression of this gene at various stages of development, as well as the mode of interaction of this receptor with chromatin, remain wrapt in mystery. It seems likely that cloning and sequencing of the androgen receptor gene will be accomplished before long, and, if so, the way will be opened to much greater understanding in molecular terms of innumerable features of the phenomenology of androgen action at the cellular and organ levels. The enormous powers of recently developed recombinant DNA technologies to gain insight into the structure of specific genes is illustrated by the very recent isolation of the bovine and human genes for MDIH and the determination of the mRNA nucleotide sequence (and hence the primary structure) of bovine MDIH (159), which has just been reported at the time of writing. Yet until the nature of the corresponding receptor for MDIH is elucidated, insight into its actions, which play such an important role in normal eutherian male sex development, is bound to remain very limited.

REFERENCES

1. Jost, A. (1970): Hormonal factors in the sex differentiation of the mammalian fetus. *Phil. Trans. R. Soc. London, Ser. B,* 259:119–130.
2. Jost, A. (1973): A new look at the mechanisms controlling sex differentiation in mammals. *Johns Hopkins Med. J.,* 130:38–53.
3. Wilson, J. D., Griffin, J. E., Leshin, M., and MacDonald, P. C. (1983): The androgen resistance syndromes: 5α-reductase deficiency, testicular feminization, and related disorders. In: *The Metabolic Basis of Inherited Disease,* 5th ed., edited by J. B. Stanbury, J. B. Wyngaarden, D. S. Frederickson, J. L. Goldstein, and M. S. Brown, pp. 1001–1026. McGraw-Hill, New York.
4. Colbert, E. H. (1969): *Evolution of the Vertebrates,* 2nd. ed. Wiley, New York.
5. Vaughn, T. A. (1978): *Mammalogy.* Saunders, Philadelphia.
6. Austin, C. R. (1976): Specialization of gametes. In: *Reproduction in Mammals, Book 6: The Evolution of Reproduction,* 1st ed., edited by C. R. Austin and R. V. Short, pp. 149–182. Cambridge University Press, Cambridge, U.K.
7. Kimura, M. (1983): *The Neutral Theory of Molecular Evolution.* Cambridge University Press, Cambridge, U.K.
8. Jukes, T. H., and Kimura, M. (1984): Evolutionary constraints and the neutral theory. *J. Mol. Evol.,* 21:90–92.
9. Ohno, S. (1985): Dispensable genes. *Trends Genet.,* 1:160–164.
10. R. V. Short (1982): Sex determination and differentiation. In: *Reproduction in Mammals, Book 2: Embryonic and Fetal Development,* 2nd. ed., edited by C. R. Austin and R. V. Short, pp. 70–113. Cambridge University Press, Cambridge, U.K.
11. Burns, R. K. (1961): Role of hormones in the differentiation of sex. In: *Sex and Internal Secretions,* Vol. 1, 3rd ed., edited by W. C. Young, pp. 76–158. Williams and Wilkins, Baltimore.
12. Fredga, K. (1983): Aberrant sex chromosome mechanisms in mammals: Evolutionary aspects. *Differentiation,* 23(Suppl. 1):23–30.
13. Ohno, S., Jainchill, J., and Stenius, C. (1963): The creeping vole (*Microtus oregoni*) as a gonosomic mosaic. I. The OY/XY constitution of the male. *Cytogenetics,* 2:232–239.
14. Schempp, W., Wiberg, U., and Fredga, K. (1985): Correlation between sexual phenotype and X-chromosome inactivation pattern in the X*XY wood lemming. *Cytogenet. Cell Genet.,* 39:30–34.
15. Cattanach, B. M., Pollard, C. E., and Hawkes, S. G. (1971): Sex-reversed mice: XX and XO males. *Cytogenetics,* 10:318–327.
16. McLaren, A. (1983): Sex reversal in the mouse. *Differentiation,* 23:(Suppl. 1):93–98.
17. Burgoyne, P. S. (1982): Genetic homology and crossing over in the X and Y chromosomes. *Human Genet.,* 61:85–90.
18. Evans, E. P., Burtenshaw, M. D., and Cattanach, B. M. (1982): Meiotic crossing-over between the X and the Y chromosomes of male mice carrying the sex-reversing *(Sxr)* factor. *Nature,* 300:443–445.
19. Lyon, M. F., Searle, A. G., Ford, C. E., and Ohno, S. (1964): A mouse translocation suppressing sex-linked variegation. *Cytogenetics,* 3:306–323.
20. Conte, F. A., and Grumbach, M. M. (1979): Pathogenesis, classification, diagnosis and treatment of anomalies of sex. In: *Endocrinology,* Vol. 3, edited by L. J. DeGroot, G. F. Cahill, L. Martini, et al., pp. 1309–1351. Grune & Stratton, New York.
21. Cooke, H., Fantes, J., and Green D. (1983): Structure and evolution of human Y chromosomal DNA. *Differentiation,* 23(Suppl. 1):48–55.
22. McKusick, V. A. (1985): The human gene map. 1 December, 1985. *Clinical Genet.* 27:207–239.
23. Goodfellow, P. N., Davies, K. E., and Ropers, H.-H. (1985): Report of the committee on the genetic constitution of the X and Y chromosomes. *Cytogenet. Cell. Genet.,* 40:296–353.
24. Goodfellow, P. N., Pym, B., Mohandas, T., and Shapiro, L. T. (1984): The cell surface antigen locus, *MIC24,* escapes X-inactivation. *Am. J. Human Genet.,* 36:777–782.
25. Buckle, V., Mondello, C., Darling, S., Craig, I. W., and Goodfellow, P. N. (1985): Homologous expressed genes in the human sex chromosome pairing region. *Nature,* 317:739–741.
26. Cooke, H. J., Brown, W. R. A., and Rappold, G. A. (1985): Hypervariable telomeric sequences from the human sex chromosomes are pseudoautosomal. *Nature,* 317:687–692.
27. Simmler, M. C., Rouyer, F., Vergnaud, G., et al. (1985): Pseudoautosomal DNA sequences in the pairing region of the human sex chromosomes. *Nature,* 317:692–697.
28. Blackburn, E. H., and Szostak, J. W. (1984): The molecular structure of centromeres and telomeres. *Annu. Rev. Biochem.,* 53:163–194.
29. Singh, L., Phillips, C., and Jones, K. W. (1984): The conserved nucleotide sequences of *Bkm,* which define *Sxr* in the mouse, are transcribed. *Cell,* 36:111–120.
30. Jones, K. W. (1983): Evolutionary conservation of sex specific DNA sequences. *Differentiation* 23(Suppl. 1):60–63.
31. Epplen, J. T., Cellini, A., Shorte, M., and Ohno, S. (1983): On evolutionary conserved simple repetitive DNA sequences: Do "sex-specific" satellite components serve any sequence dependent function? *Differentiation,* 23(Suppl. 1):60–63.

32. Kiel-Metzger, K., Warren, G., Wilson, G. N., and Erickson, R. P. (1985): Evidence that the human Y chromosome does not contain clustered DNA sequences *(Bkm)* associated with heterogenetic sex determination in other vertebrates. *N. Engl. J. Med.*, 313:242–245.
33. Eichwald, E. J., and Silmser, C. R. (1955): Communication. *Transplant Bull.*, 2:148–149.
34. Goldberg, E. H., Boyse, E. A., Bennett, D., Scheid, M., and Carswell, E. A. (1971): Serological demonstration of H-Y (male) antigen on mouse sperm. *Nature*, 232:378–380.
35. Wachtel, S. S., Koo, G. C., and Boyse, E. A. (1975): Evolutionary conservation of the H-Y (male) antigen. *Nature*, 254:270–272.
36. Wachtel, S. S., Ohno, S., Koo, G. C., and Boyse, E. A. (1975): Possible role of H-Y antigen in primary sex determination. *Nature*, 257:235–236.
37. Ohno, S. (1979): *Major Sex-Determining Genes*. Springer-Verlag, New York.
38. Krco, C. J., and Goldberg, E. H. (1976): H-Y (male) antigen: detection on eight-cell mouse embryos. *Science*, 193:1134–1135.
39. Ohno, S. (1985): The Y-linked determining gene and H-Y plasma membrane antigen: Are they one and the same? *Endocrinol. Rev.*, 6:421–431.
40. Meck, J. M. (1984): The genetics of the H-Y antigen system and its role in sex determination. *Perspect. Biol. Med.*, 27:560–584.
41. Wachtel, S. S. (1982) *H-Y Antigen and the Biology of Sex Determination*. Grune & Stratton, New York.
42. Silvers, W. K., Gasser, P. L., and Eicher, E. M. (1982): H-Y antigen, serologically determined male antigen and sex determination. *Cell*, 28:439–445.
43. Brunner, M., Moreira-Filho, C. A., Wachtel, and Wachtel, S. (1984): On the secretion of H-Y antigen. *Cell*, 37:615–621.
44. Simpson, E., McLaren, A., Chandler, P., and Tomonari, K. (1984): Expression of H-Y antigen by female mice carrying *Sxr*. *Transplantation*, 37:17–21.
45. McLaren, A., Simpson, E., Tomonari, K., Chandler, P., and Hogg, H. (1984): Male sexual differentiation in mice lacking H-Y antigen. *Nature*, 312:552–555.
46. McLaren, A. (1976): *Mammalian Chimeras*. Cambridge University Press, Cambridge, U.K.
47. Gropp, A., Winking, H., Frank, F., Noack, G., and Fredga, K. (1976): Sex-chromosome aberrations in wood lemmings (*Myopus schisticolor*). *Cytogenet. Cell. Genet.*, 17:343–358.
48. Wachtel, S. S., Koo, G. C., Ohno, S., et al. (1976): H-Y antigen and the origin of XY female wood lemmings. *Nature*, 264:638–640.
49. Wiberg, V., Mayerova, A., Muller, V., Fredga, K., and Wolf, V. (1982): X-linked genes of the H-Y antigen system in the wood lemming (*Myopus Schisticolor*). *Hum. Genet.*, 60:163–173.
50. Eicher, R. M., Washinburn, L. L., Whitney III, J. B., and Morrow, K. E. (1982): *Mus poschiavanus* Y chromosome in the C57BL/6J murine genome causes sex reversal. *Science*, 217:535–538.
51. Muller, U., and Schindler, H. (1983): Testicular differentiation—A developmental cascade. Morphogenetic affects of H-Y antigen and testosterone in the male mammalian gonad. *Differentiation* (Suppl. 1), 23:99–103.
52. Wolf, V., Fraccaro, M., Mayerova, A., Hecht, T., Zuffardi, O., and Hameister, H. (1980): Turner syndrome patients are H-Y positive *Hum. Genet.*, 54:315–318.
53. Wiberg, U. H. (1985): H-Y transplantation antigen in human XO females. *Hum. Genet.*, 69:15–18.
54. Wachtel, S. S., Koo, G. C., Breg, R., Elias, S., Boyse, E. A., and Miller, O. J. (1975): Expression of H-Y antigen in human males with two Y chromosomes. *N. Engl. J. Med.*, 293:1070–1072.
55. Ohno, S. (1967): *Sex Chromosomes and Sex-linked Genes*. Springer-Verlag, New York.
56. Ohno, S., Epplen, J. T., and Sutou, S. (1981): Testis-organizing H-Y antigen as a discrete protein; its MHC restricted immune recognition and the genomic environment in which H-Y genes operate. *Hum. Genet.*, 58:37–45.
57. Wolf, U. (1983): X-linked genes and gonadal differentiation. *Differentiation*, 23(Suppl. 1):104–106.
58. Chandra, H. S. (1985): Sex-determination: A hypothesis based on noncoding DNA. *Proc. Natl. Acad. Sci. USA*, 82:1165–1169.
59. Chandra, H. S. (1985): Is human X chromosome inactivation a sex-determining device? *Proc. Natl. Acad. Sci. USA*, 82:6947–6949.
60. Ewing, L. L., and Zirkin, B. R. (1983): Leydig cell structure and function. *Recent Prog. Horm. Res.*, 39:599–635.
61. Wilson, J. D. (1975): Metabolism of testicular androgens. In: *Handbook of Physiology, Sect. 7: Endocrinology, Vol. 5, Male Reproductive System*, edited by R. O. Greep and E. B. Astwood, pp. 491–508. American Physiological Society, Washington, D. C.
62. McEwen, B. S. (1981): Neural gonadal steroid action. *Science*, 211:1303–1311.
63. Mac Luskey, N. J., and Naftolin, F. (1981): Sexual differentiation of the central nervous system. *Science*, 211:1294–1303.
64. Williams-Ashman, H. G., and Reddi, A. H. (1971): Actions of vertebrate sex hormones. *Annu. Rev. Physiol.*, 33:31–82.
65. Liao, S., and Hiipakka, R. A. (1984): Mechanism of action of steroid hormones at the subcellular level. In: *Biochemistry of Steroid Hormones*, edited by H. L. J. Mulkin, pp. 633–680. Blackwell, Oxford, U.K.
66. Mainwaring, W. I. P. (1977): *The Mechanism of Action of Androgens*. Springer-Verlag, New York.
67. Jensen, E. V., and DeSombre, E. S. (1972): Mechanism of action of female sex hormones. *Annu. Rev. Biochem.*, 41:203–230.
68. Gorski, J., and Gannon, F. (1976): Current models of steroid hormone action: A critique. *Annu. Rev. Physiol.*, 38:425–450.
69. Jensen, E. V. (1979): The oestrogens. In: *Reproduction in Mammals, Book 7: Mechanisms of Hormone Action,* 1st ed., edited by C. R. Austin and R. V. Short, pp. 157–184. Cambridge University Press, Cambridge, U.K.
70. Tindall, D. J., and Means, A. R. (1980): Properties and hormonal regulation of androgen-binding proteins. *Adv. Sex Horm. Res.*, 4:636–652.
71. King, W. J., and Greene, G. L. (1984): Monoclonal antibodies localize oestrogen receptor in the nuclei of target cells. *Nature*, 307:745–747.
72. Welshons, W. V., Krumme, B. M., and Gorski, J. (1985): Nuclear localization of unoccupied estrogens and progesterone in GH3 cells. *Endocrinology*, 117:2140–2167.
73. Walter, P., Green, S., Greene, G., et al. (1985): Cloning of the human estrogen receptor cDNA. *Proc. Natl. Acad. Sci. USA*, 82:7889–7893.
74. Greene, G. L., Gilna, P., Waterfield, M., Baker, A., Hort, Y., and Shine, J. (1986): Sequence and expression of human estrogen receptor complementary DNA. *Science*, 231:1150–1154.
75. Green, S., Walter, P., Kumar, V., et al. (1986): Human oestrogen receptor cDNA: sequence, expression and homology to v-*erb*-A. *Nature*, 320:134–139.
76. Hollenberg, S. M., Weinberger, C., Ong, E. S., et al. (1985): Primary structure and expression of a functional human glucocorticoid receptor cDNA. *Nature*, 318:635–640.
77. Meyer, W. J. III, Migeon, B. R., and Migeon, J. (1975): Locus on human X chromosome for dihydrotestosterone receptor and androgen insensitivity. *Proc. Natl. Acad. Sci. USA*, 72:1469–1472.
78. Gehring, U., Segnitz, B., Foellmer, B., and Francke, U. (1985): Assignment of the human gene for the glucocorticoid receptor to chromosome 5. *Proc. Natl. Acad. Sci. USA*, 82:3751–3755.
79. Katzenellenbogen, B. S. (1980): Dynamics of steroid hormone receptor action. *Annu. Rev. Physiol.*, 42:17–35.
80. Jänne, O. A., and Bardin, C. W. (1984): Androgen and antiandrogen receptor binding. *Annu. Rev. Physiol.*, 46:107–118.
81. Sherman, M. R., and Stevens, J. (1984): Structure of mammalian steroid receptors: Evolving concepts and methodological developments. *Annu. Rev. Physiol.*, 46:107.
82. Barrack, E. R., and Coltey, D. S. (1980): The specific binding of estrogens and androgens to the nucleas matrix of sex hormone responsive tissues. *J. Biol. Chem.*, 255:7265.
83. Pardoll, D. M., Vogelstein, B., and Coffey, D. S. (1980): A fixed site of DNA replication in eucaryotic cells. *Cell*, 19:527–536.
84. Shaper, J. H., Pardoll, D. M., Kaufmann, S. H., Barrack, E. R., Vogelstein, B., and Coffey, D. S. (1979): The relationship of the nuclear matrix to cellular structure and function. *Adv. Enzyme Regul.*, 17:213–248.
85. Brown, D. D. (1984): The role of stable complexes that repress and activate eucaryotic genes. *Cell*, 37:359–365.
86. Jost, J. P., Moncharmont, B., Jiricny, J., Saluz, H., and Hertner, S. (1986): *In vitro* secondary activation (memory effect) of avian

vitellogenin II gene in isolated liver nuclei. *Proc. Natl. Acad. Sci. USA,* 83:43–47.
87. Weisberg, R. A., and Leder, P. (1983): Fundamentals of molecular genetics. In: *The Metabolic Basis of Inherited Disease,* 5th ed., edited by J. B. Stanbury, J. B. Wyngaarden, D. S. Frederickson, J. L. Goldstein and M. S. Brown, pp. 61–76. McGraw-Hill, New York.
88. Tata, J. R. (1980): The action of growth and developmental hormones. *Biol. Rev.,* 55:285–319.
89. Williams-Ashman, H. G. (1975): Metabolic effects of testicular androgens. In: *Handbook of Physiology, Sect. 7: Endocrinology, Vol. 5: Male Reproductive System,* ed. by R. O. Greep and E.B. Astwood, pp. 473–490. American Physiological Society, Washington, D. C.
90. Moore, D. D., Marks, A. R., Buckley, D. I., Kapler, G., Payvar, F., and Goodman, H. M. (1985): The first intron of the human growth hormone contains a binding site for glucocorticoid receptor. *Proc. Natl. Acad. Sci. USA,* 82:699–702.
91. Dean, D. C., Gope, R., Knoll, B. J., Riser, M. E., and O'Malley, B. M. (1984): A similar 5'-flanking region is required for estrogen and progesterone induction of ovalbumin gene expression. *J. Biol. Chem.,* 259:9967–9970.
92. Perry, S. T., Viskochil, D. H., Ho, Fong, K., Stafford, D. W., Wilson, E. M., and French, F. S. (1985): Androgen receptor binding to the C3(1) subunit gene of rat prostatein. In: *Regulation of Androgen Action,* edited by N. Bruchovsky, A. Chapdelaine, and F. Neumann, pp. 162–173. Congressdruck R. Bruckner, Berlin.
93. Mulder, E., Vrij, A. A., Brinkman, A. O., Van der Molen, H. J., and Parker, M. G. (1984): Interaction of rat prostate androgen receptors with polynucleotides, RNA, DNA and cloned DNA fragments. *Biochem. Biophys. Acta,* 781:121–129.
94. Rennie, P. S., Bruchovsky, N., McLoughlin, M. G., Batzhold, F. H., and Dunstan-Adams, E. (1983): Kinetic analysis of 5α-reductase isoenzymes in benign prostatic hyperplasia. *J. Steroid Biochem.,* 19:169–173.
95. Kovacs, W., Griffin, J. F., and Wilson, J. D. (1983): Transformation of human androgen receptors to the deoxyribonucleic acid-binding state. *Endocrinology,* 113:1574–1581.
96. Kovacs, W. J., Griffin, J. E., Weaver, D. D., Carlson, B. R., and Wilson, J. D. (1984): A mutation that causes lability of the androgen receptor under conditions that normally promote transformation to the DNA-binding state. *J. Clin. Invest.,* 73:1095–1104.
97. Bardin, C. W., and Catterall, J. F. (1981): Testosterone: A major determinant of extragenital sexual dimorphism. *Science,* 211:1285–1294.
98. Conte, F. A., and Grumbach, M. M. (1979): Pathogenesis classification diagnosis and treatment of anomalies of sex. In: *Endocrinology,* Vol. 3, edited by L. J. DeGroot, G. F. Cahill, L. Martini, et al., pp. 1317–1351. Grune & Stratton, New York.
99. Sloan, W. R., and Walsh, P. C. (1976): Familial persistent mullerian duct syndrome. *J. Urol.,* 115:454–465.
100. Aiman, J., Griffin, J. E., Grazak, J. M., Wilson, J. D., and MacDonald, P. C. (1974): Androgen insensitivity as a cause of infertility in otherwise normal men. *N. Engl. J. Med.,* 300:223–230.
101. Lyon, M. E., and Hawkes, S. G. (1970): X-linked gene for testicular feminization in the mouse. *Nature,* 227:1217–1219.
102. Amrhein, J. A., Meyer, W. J. III, Jones, H. W., and Migeon, C. J. (1970): Androgen insensitivity in man: evidence for genetic heterogeneity. *Proc. Natl. Acad. Sci. USA,* 73:891–895.
103. Neumann, F., Von Berswardt-Wallrabe, R., Elger, W., Steinbeck, H., Hahn, J. D., and Dramer, M. (1970): Aspects of androgen-dependent events as studied by antiandrogens. *Recent Prog. Horm. Res.,* 26:337–365.
104. Imperato-McGinley, J., and Guerro, L. (1974): Steroid 5α-reductase deficiency in man: an inherited form of male pseudohermaphroditism. *Science,* 186:1213–1215.
105. Imperato-McGinley, J., Binienda, Z., Arthur, A., Mininberg, D. T., Vaughn, E. D., and Quimby, F. W. (1985): The development of a male pseudohermaphroditic rat using an inhibitor of the enzyme 5α-reductase. *Endocrinology,* 116:807–812.
106. Price, D., and Williams-Ashman, H. G. (1961): The accessory reproductive glands of mammals. In: *Sex and Internal Secretions,* Vol. 1, 3rd ed., edited by W. C. Young, pp. 366–448. Williams & Wilkins, Baltimore.
107. Cunha, G. R., Sugimura, Y., and Bigsby, R. M. (1985): Androgenic response in the prostate: Role of stromal-epithelial interactions. In: *Regulation of Androgen Action,* edited by N. Bruchovsky, A. Champelaine, and F. Neumann, pp. 191–197. Congressdruck R. Bruckner, Berlin.
108. Shannon, J. M., and Cunha, G. R. (1984): Characterization of androgen binding and deoxyribonucleic acid synthesis in prostate-like structures induced in the urothelium of testicular feminized (Tfm/Y) mice. *Biol. Reprod.,* 31:175–183.
109. McNeal, J. E. (1978): Origin and evolution of benign prostatic enlargement. *Invest. Urol.,* 15:340–345.
110. Setchell, B. P. (1982): Spermatogenesis and spermatozoa. In: *Reproduction in Mammals, Book I: Germ Cells and Fertilization,* 2nd. ed., edited by C. R. Austin and R. V. Short, pp. 63–101. Cambridge University Press, Cambridge, U.K.
111. Li, C. H., Hammonds, R. G., Ramarsharma, K., and Chung, D. (1985): Human seminal inhibins. Isolation, characterization, and structure. *Proc. Natl. Acad. Sci. USA,* 82:4041–4044.
112. Ling, N., Ying, S.-H., Veno, N., Esch, F., Denoroy, L., and Guillemin, R. (1985): Isolation and partial characterization of a M_r 32,000 protein with inhibin activity from porcine follicular fluid. *Proc. Natl. Acad. Sci. USA,* 82:7217–7221.
113. Byskov, A. G. (1982): Primordial germ cells and regulation of meiosis. In: *Reproduction in Mammals, Book I: Germ Cells and Fertilization,* 2nd ed., edited by C. R. Austin and R. V. Short, pp. 1–16. Cambridge University Press, Cambridge, U.K.
114. Mann, T., and Lutwak-Mann, C. (1981): *Male Reproductive Function and Semen.* Springer-Verlag, New York.
115. Kistler, W. S., and Williams-Ashman, H. G. (1975): On three varieties of specific basic proteins with mammalian spermatogenesis. In: *Hormonal Regulation of Spermatogenesis,* edited by F. S. French, V. Hansson, E. M. Ritzen, and S. N. Nayfeh, pp. 423–432. Plenum, New York.
116. Bedford, J. M. (1982): Fertilization. In: *Reproduction in Mammals, Book I: Germ Cells and Fertilization,* 2nd ed., edited by C. R. Austin and R. V. Short, pp. 128–162. Cambridge University Press, Cambridge, U.K.
117. Afzelius, B. A., ed. (1975): *The Functional Anatomy of the Spermatozoa.* (Wenner-Gren Center International Symposium Series No. 23). Pergamon Press, Oxford, U.K.
118. Williams-Ashman, H. G. (1983): Regulatory features of seminal vesicle development and function. *Curr. Top. Cell. Regul.,* 22:202–273.
119. Williams-Ashman, H. G. (1962): Chemical approaches to the function of the prostate gland and seminal vesicles. In: *On Cancer and Hormones,* pp. 325–346. University of Chicago Press, Chicago.
120. Williams-Ashman, H. G. (1984): Transglutaminases and the clotting of mammalian seminal fluids. *Mol. Cell. Biochem.,* 58:51–61.
121. Williams-Ashman, H. G., and Lockwood, D. H. (1970): Role of polyamines in reproductive physiology and sex hormone action. *Ann. NY Acad. Sci.,* 171:882–894.
122. Neaves, W. B., Griffin, J. E., and Wilson, J. D. (1980): Sexual dimorphism of the phallus in spotted hyena (*Crocuta crocuta*). *J. Reprod. Fertil.,* 59:509–513.
123. Racey, P. A., and Skinner, J. D. (1979): Endocrine aspects of sexual mimicry in spotted hyenas *Crocuta crocuta. J. Zool.,* 187:315–326.
124. Karacan, I., Aslan, C., and Hirshkowitz, M. (1983): Erectile mechanisms in man. *Science,* 220:1080–1082.
125. Sachs, B., and Barfield, R. (1977): Functional analysis of masculine copulatory behavior in the rat. In: *Adv. Study Behav.,* 7:91–154.
126. Kaverne, E. B. (1985): Reproductive behavior. In: *Reproduction in Mammals, Vol. 4: Reproductive Fitness,* 2nd ed., C. R. Austin and R. V. Short, eds., pp. 133–175. Cambridge University Press, Cambridge, U.K.
127. Dixon, A. F., Kendrick, K. M., Blank, M. A., and Bloom, S. R. (1984): Effects of tactile and electronic stimuli upon release of vasoactive intestinal polypeptide in the mammalian penis. *J Endocrinol.,* 100:249–252.
128. Ottesoen, B., Wagner, G., Virag, R., and Fahrenburg, J. (1984): Penile erection: possible role for vasoactive intestinal polypeptide as a neurotransmitter. *Br. Med. J.,* 288:9–11.
129. McIntosh, M., and Barfield, R. J. (984): Brain monoaminergic control of male reproductive behavior. I. Serotonin and the post-ejaculatory refractory period. *Behav. Brain Res.,* 12:255–265.

130. McIntosh, M., and Barfield, R. J. (1984): Brain monoaminergic control of male reproductive behavior. II. Dopamine and the post-ejaculatory refractory period. *Behav. Brain Res.*, 12:267–273.
131. McIntosh, M., and Barfield, R. J. (1984): Brain monoaminergic control of male reproductive behavior. III. Norepinephrine and the post-ejaculatory refractory period. *Behav. Brain Res.*, 12:275–281.
132. Short, R. V. (1979): Sexual selection and its component parts, somatic and genital selection, as illustrated by man and the great apes. *Adv. Study Behavior*, 9:131–158.
133. Danish, R. K., Lee, P. A., Mazur, T., Amrhein, J. A., and Migeon, C. J. (1980): Micropenis. II. Hypogonadotropic hypogonadism. *Johns Hopkins Med. J.*, 146:177–184.
134. Long, C. A., and Frank, T. (1968): Morphometric variation and function in the baculum, with comments on correlation of the parts. *J. Mammalogy*, 49:32–43.
135. Fooden, J. (1971): Male external genitalia and systematic relationships of the Japanese macaque (*Macaca fuscata* BLYTH, 1975). *Primates*, 12:305–311.
136. Fooden, J. (1967): Complementary specialization of male and female reproductive structures in the bear macaque, *Macaca arctoides*. *Nature*, 214:939–941.
137. Patterson, B. D., and Thaeler, C. S. (1982): The mammalian baculum: hypotheses on the nature of bacular variability. *J. Mammal.*, 63:1–15.
138. Yoshida, H., and Huggins, C. B. (1980): Induction of ossification in the clitoris of neonatal female rats by administration of androgens. *Endocrinology*, 106:1956–1959.
139. Meczynski, S. (1974): Morphohistological structure of the female genital organs in sousliks. *Acta Theriol.*, 19:91–106.
140. Aronson, L. R., and Cooper, M. L. (1969): Mating behavior in sexually inexperienced cats after densensitization of the glans penis. *Anim. Behav.*, 17:208–212.
141. Sachs, B., Glater, G. B., and O'Hanlon, T. K. (1984): Morphology of the erect glans penis in rats under various gonadal hormone conditions. *Anat. Rec.*, 210:45–52.
142. Walton, A. (1960): Copulation and natural insemination. In: *Marshall's Physiology of Reproduction*, Vol. 2, 3rd ed., edited by A. S. Parkes. Longmans, London.
143. Estep, D. Q., and Dewsbury, D. A. (1976): Copulatory behavior of *Neotoma lepida* and *Biormys taylori:* relationships between penile morphology and behavior. *J. Mammal.*, 57:570–573.
144. Baumgardner, D. J., and Dewsbury, D. A. (1980): Pseudopregnancy in female rats: effects of hormonal manipulation of the male. *Horm. Behav.*, 16:208–223.
145. Taylor, G. T., Weiss, J., and Komitowski, D. (1983): Penile morphology and penile papillae morphology of rats after sexual experience. *J. Endocrinol.*, 98:155–163.
146. Terkel, J., and Sawyer, C. H. (1978): Male copulatory behavior triggers nightly prolactin surges resulting in successful pregnancy in rats. *Horm. Behav.*, 11:304–309.
147. Beach, F. A. (1967): Cerebral and hormonal control of reflexive mechanisms involved in male copulatory behavior. *Physiol. Rev.*, 47:289–316.
148. Wilson, J. R., Adler, N., and LeBoef, B. (1965): The effects of intromission frequency on successful pregnancy in the female rat. *Proc. Natl. Acad. Sci. USA*, 53:1392–1395.
149. Milligan, S. R. (1979): The copulatory patterns of the Bank vole *Clethrionomys glareolus* and speculation on the role of penile spines. *J. Zool.*, 188:279–283.
150. Eberhard, W. G. (1985): *Sexual Selection and Animal Genitalia*. Harvard University Press, Cambridge, Mass.
151. Mayr, E. (1963): *Animal Species and Evolution*. Harvard University Press, Cambridge, Mass.
152. Waites, G. M. H. (1970): Temperature regulation and the testis. In: *The Testis*, Vol. 1, edited by A. D. Johnson, W. R. Gomes, and N. L. Vandemark, pp. 241–279. Academic, New York.
153. Ehrenberg, L., von Ehrenstein, G., and Hedgran, A. (1957): Gonadal temperatures and spontaneous mutation rates in man. *Nature*, 180:1433–1434.
154. Cowles, R. B. (1965): Hyperthermia, aspermia, mutation rates and evolution. *Q. Rev. Biol.*, 40:341–367.
155. Portman, A. (1952): *Animal Forms and Evolution*. Faber and Faber, London.
156. Ruibal, R. (1957): The evolution of the scrotum. *Evolution*, 11:376–377.
157. Cowles, R. B. (1958): The evolutionary significance of the scrotum. *Evolution*, 12:417–418.
158. Wislocki, G. B. (1936): The external genitalia of the simian primates. *Human Biol.*, 8:311–347.
159. Cate, R. L., Mattaliano, R. J., Hession, C., et al. (1986): Isolation of the bovine and human genes for Mullerian inhibiting substance and expression of the human gene in animal cells. *Cell*, 45:685–698.

The Physiology of Reproduction,
edited by E. Knobil and J. Neill *et al.*
Raven Press, Ltd., New York © 1988.

CHAPTER 19

Anatomy, Vasculature, Innervation, and Fluids of the Male Reproductive Tract

B. P. Setchell and D. E. Brooks

ANATOMY

The male reproductive tract consists of two testes, two epididymides, each with its ductus deferens, and the accessory glands (Figs. 1,2). The reproductive organs of the male rat, which is a species in which all the major accessory glands are present, are shown in Fig. 3. The testes are formed from the primordial germ cells which migrate from the yolk sac to the genital ridge of the mesonephros, where they form the primary epithelial or medullary cords in association with somatic cells from the genital ridge. This gonad then appropriates the duct system of the degenerating mesonephros or Wolffian duct to form the epididymis, ductus deferens, ampulla, and seminal vesicles (vesicular glands). The prostate and bulbourethral (Cowper's glands) are derived from the urogenital sinus or urethra. The major portion of the Wolffian duct develops into the epididymis, a single tubule of considerable length which is coiled upon itself and comes to lie around one margin of the testis. It leads sperm from the efferent ducts of the testis to the ductus deferens. The lower end of the ductus deferens may possess a glandular wall to form the ampullary gland. In primates, the seminal vesicle is associated with the ductus deferens which drains by a common duct, the ejaculatory duct, into the urethra. However, in most mammals the seminal vesicles have separate openings into the urethra, close to the openings of the deferent ducts. The prostate glands are associated with the proximal urethra and generally drain into it via multiple ducts at the level of the colliculus seminalis. The bulbourethral glands drain into the distal urethra in the region of the urethral bulb. In addition to these principal male accessory glands, there are small mucus-secreting glands (glands of Littré) which open into the urethra along its length, as well as preputial glands which are modified sebaceous glands, of ectodermal origin, emptying into the prepuce.

There is considerable variation between and within orders of mammals with respect to the range of accessory glands which are represented (Table 1). Apart from the excurrent duct system of the testis (i.e., the epididymis and ductus deferens) which is present in all species, the only other accessory gland present in virtually all mammals is the prostate gland. In some mammals, such as cetaceans and carnivores, the prostate is the only male accessory gland. Practically all other mammals have at least one pair of bulbourethral glands, which are especially well developed in certain insectivores (e.g., moles) and in squirrels.

However, it should be remembered that nomenclature of glands in early descriptive studies was based on anatomical relationships and gross morphological appearance and does

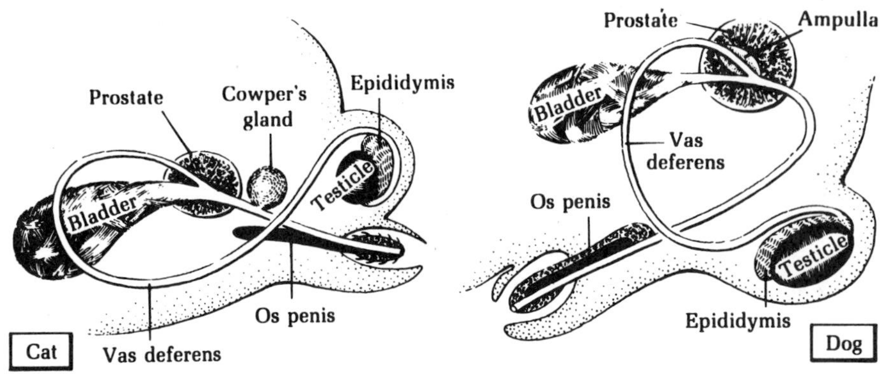

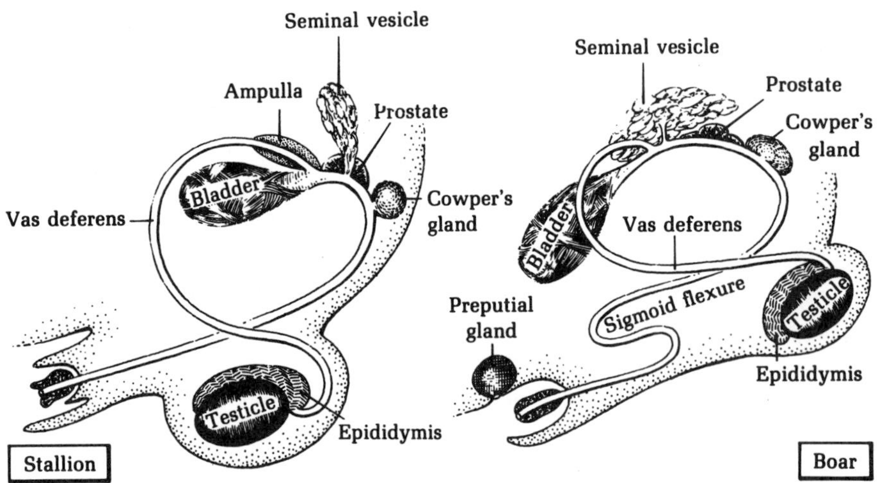

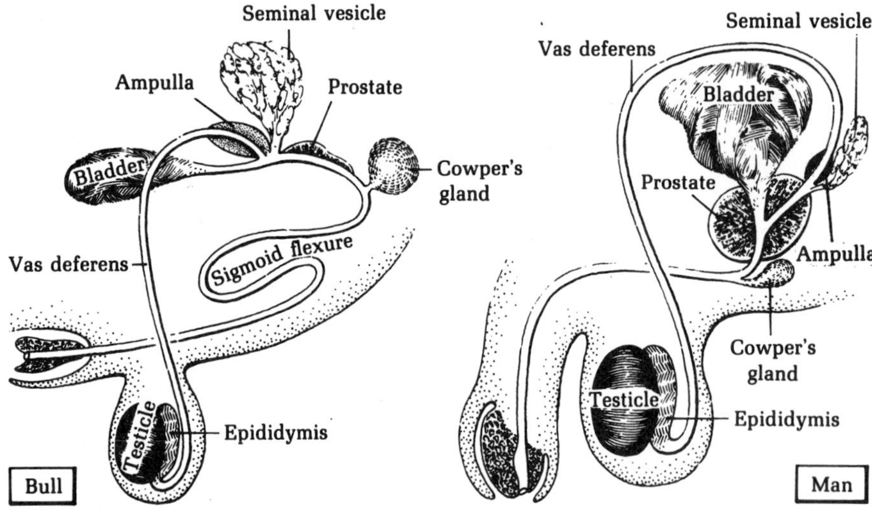

FIG. 1. Schematic representation of the genital tracts of man, dog, stallion, boar, bull, and tom cat. Where a common duct drains the contents of the ductus deferens and the seminal vesicles into the urethra, as occurs in man, it is known as the ejaculatory duct. (From ref. 840.)

not necessarily reflect the functional relationships of the glands. This is exemplified by somewhat confusing differences in chemical composition of secretions from similarly named glands in various species (1).

Testis

The testes in all mammals are paired encapsulated ovoid organs consisting of seminiferous tubules separated by interstitial tissue. Their size varies depending on the species; in rodents and ungulates they can be as much as 1% or more of body weight (see ref. 2), whereas in the human and some apes, they are considerably smaller (3). The largest testes, as a proportion of body weight, are to be found in a gerbil, *Tatera afra,* whose two testes can reach 8% of body weight (4). There are two similar, closely related genera of Australian rodents (*Pseudomys* and *Notomys*) whose testes differ in size by a factor of 20! (5).

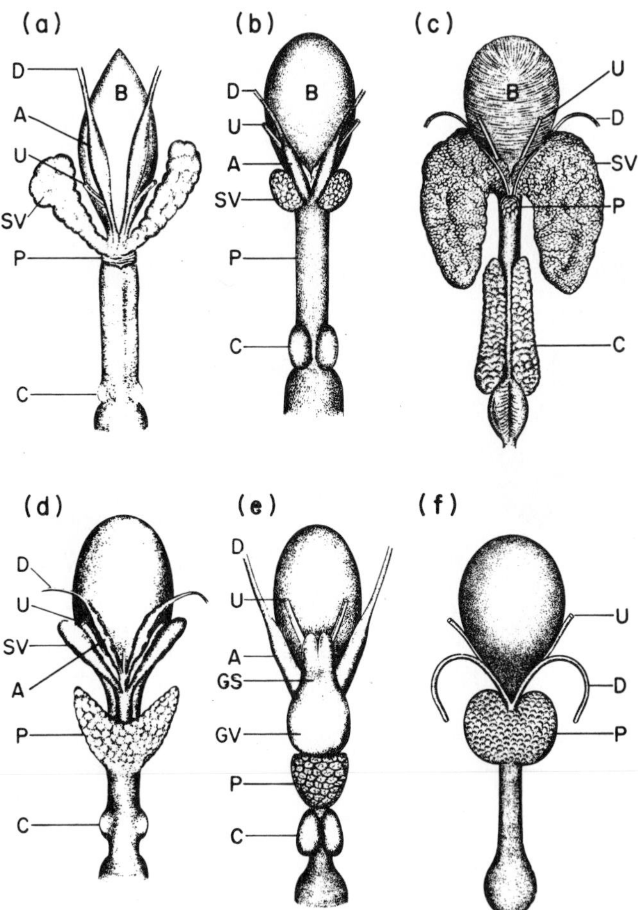

FIG. 2. Diagrammatic view of the dorsal aspect of the male accessory glands in various species. **(a):** bull; **(b):** ram; **(c):** boar; **(d):** stallion; **(e):** rabbit; **(f):** dog. SV, seminal vesicle; P, prostate (disseminate in ram); C, Cowper's glands; A, ampulla; D, ductus deferens; U, ureter; B, bladder; GS, glandula seminalis; GV, glandula vesicularis. (From ref. 813.)

Descent of the Testis

In most mammals, the testes migrate from their original site and, in many, they pass through the abdominal wall into an evagination of the peritoneum to form a scrotum. In some species, e.g., sheep and cattle, the testis has reached the scrotum by the time of birth, but in others, such as rats and dogs, the testis reaches its final position only after birth. This process of testicular descent has been divided into three stages, nephric displacement, transabdominal movement, and inguinal passage (6). The last phase involves a structure known as the gubernaculum, which develops in the caudal end of the nephrogenic cord. It was formerly believed that the gubernaculum played no active role in testicular descent, merely providing a space into which the testis descended (7,8), but later evidence suggests that outgrowth of the gubernaculum through the inguinal canal and its enlargement in what is effectively a nondistensible tube force it outwards, with the testis following; regression of the gubernaculum completes the process of testicular descent (Fig. 4) (9–12). It is probably incorrect to speak of contraction of the gubernaculum, as it contains no contractile elements and, in any case, its distal insertion into the subcutaneous tissue is hardly a secure base from which to apply traction. Some authors believe that an intact hypothalamic-pituitary-testis axis is necessary for descent (13), but in pigs decapitated *in utero* before testicular descent has begun, the gubernaculum develops normally, and initially the testis descends normally (14). Outgrowth of the gubernaculum in the dog certainly requires the presence of a testis (15), but it does not appear to involve androgens in this species (16), although it may in the rabbit (17). There is no doubt that regression of the gubernaculum, and hence the final stage of testicular descent, does involve androgens (16). If the gubernaculum is cut near its cutaneous end in newborn rats, the testis on that side never descends, whereas if the cut is made nearer the testis, the vaginal process of the peritoneum forms normally, but it often remains empty as there is nothing to hold the testis and epididymis in the scrotum (18,19).

Cryptorchism occurs spontaneously in many mammals, and is relatively common in pigs, horses, and humans. When the testis does not descend properly, spermatogenesis does not proceed, and although some androgens are produced, the secretion rate is lower than normal (see ref. 2), particularly if the condition is unilateral (20), because then there is no compensatory stimulation by the increased levels of luteinizing hormone (LH) (21). Spermatogenesis can be initiated in an abdominal testis by cooling it artificially, so it appears that temperature is the key (22).

The reason for the testis making this remarkable journey is not clear. Although the scrotal testis is sensitive to warming to body temperature, movement to a cooler environment cannot be the prime motive, since testicular migration within the abdominal cavity occurs in many mammals without any change in temperature (23). It has been suggested that the epididymis initiates the process and the testis just follows (24), but experiments in which the epididymis was returned to the abdominal cavity leaving the testis in the scrotum gave somewhat equivocal results (25), and, in any case, these results are open to alternative explanation because of the disruption of lymphatic communications between the testis and epididymis during this procedure (26).

Capsule

The capsule of the testis is often referred to as the tunica albuginea. It is a tough fibrous covering that is really composed of three layers, an outer layer of visceral peritoneum, the tunica vaginalis, then the tunica albuginea proper, and on the inside, the tunica vasculosa (Fig. 5), which is really a subtunical extension of the interstitial tissue, consisting of blood vessels and some Leydig cells in a loose connective tissue (see ref. 2). The tunica albuginea itself consists of fibroblasts and bundles of collagen, but in some species

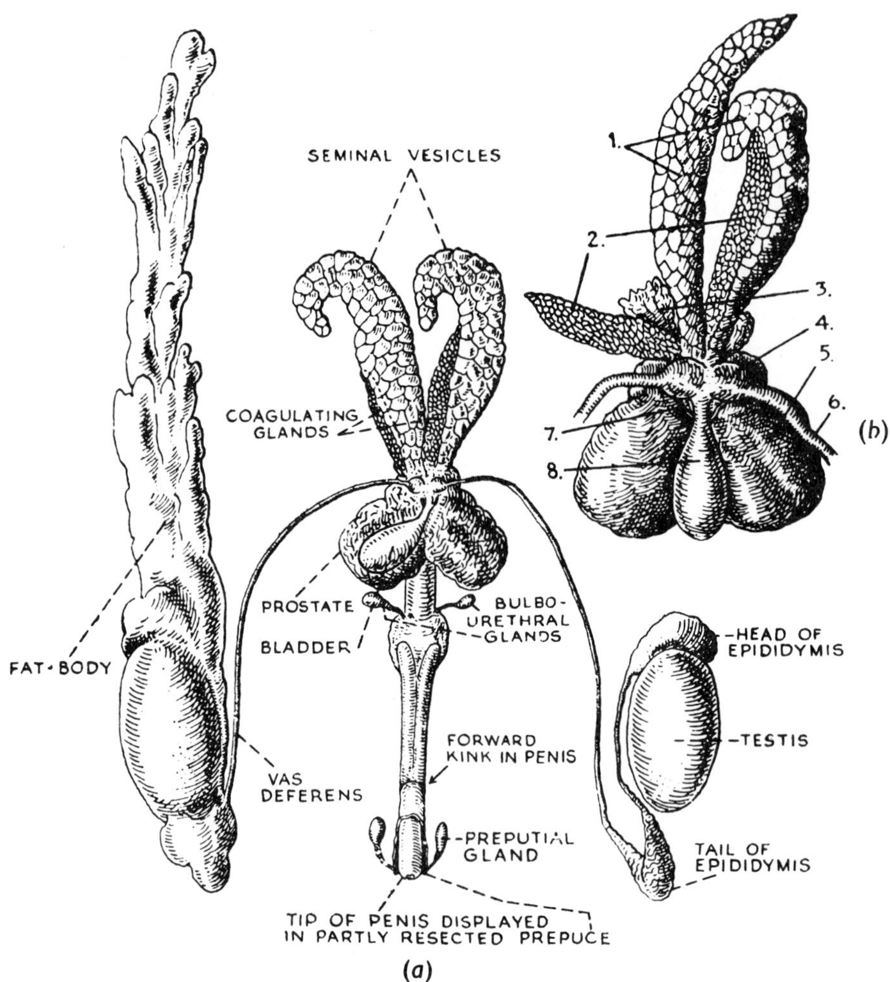

FIG. 3. Reproductive organs of the male rat. **(a):** Anterior view with the epididymal fat body removed on the left side; **(b):** magnified view of the prostatic lobes and seminal vesicles with the right lobe of the coagulating gland drawn away from the seminal vesicle to display the dorsolateral lobe of the prostate. 1, Seminal vesicles; 2, coagulating glands; 3, lobe of dorsolateral prostate; 4, ampullary gland; 5, lobe of ventral prostate; 6, ductus deferens; 7, ureter; 8, bladder (displaced downwards). (From ref. 195.)

TABLE 1. *Occurrence of male accessory reproductive glands in various mammalian orders*[a]

Mammalian order	Ampulla	Seminal vesicle	Prostate	Bulbourethral
Monotremata	–	–	–[b]	+
Marsupiala	–	–	+	+
Insectivora	±	±	+	+
Chiroptera	±	±	+	+
Primates	±	±	+	+
Carnivora	±	–	+	±
Perissodactyla	+	+	+	+
Artiodactyla	±	+	+	+
Hyraciodea	–	+	+	+
Proboscidea	+	+	+	+
Sirenia	–	+	+	–
Cetacea	–	–	+	–
Edentata	–	+	+	±
Pholidota	–	+	+	–
Rodentia	±	+	+	+
Lagomorpha	+	±	+	+

[a]+ = The presence of a well-developed functioning gland; – = either a small vestigial gland or the absence of any rudiment.

[b]More recent opinion considers that glands lining the urethra of monotremes corresponds to the disseminate prostate found in marsupials and many eutherian mammals (824).

From ref. 823.

there are appreciable numbers of smooth muscle cells. These cells are particularly well developed in the rabbit (27,28) and horse (29) (Fig. 6), but can also be found in the dog and cat (30), man (27,31), and pig (29). In the rat (32,33) and sheep (29), these cells are mainly "myofibroblasts" rather than typical smooth muscle cells. In the boar, the large and medium-sized vessels are sandwiched between two layers, the outer consisting of dense collagenous tissue and the inner layer of collagen fibers, fibroblasts, Leydig cells, and small blood and lymph vessels; in this layer near the epididymal margin of the testis, myoid cells can be found (34). The tunic is well innervated (35,36), although there appear to be few nerve terminals among the actual muscle cells (30), and the contractile activity is probably myogenic (37).

The muscle cells are capable of rhythmic contractions (38,39), which seem to be more important in the rabbit than in the rat, mouse, hamster, or squirrel. These contractions may be important for the transport of spermatozoa out of the testis into the epididymis (40), although in the rat, the flow of fluid from the rete testis is unaffected by removal of the capsule (41). Capsular contractions in the rabbit are maximal at a temperature of 32°C, and are inhibited at higher or lower temperatures (42). The capsule contracts in response to acetylcholine, norepinephrine, epinephrine, and

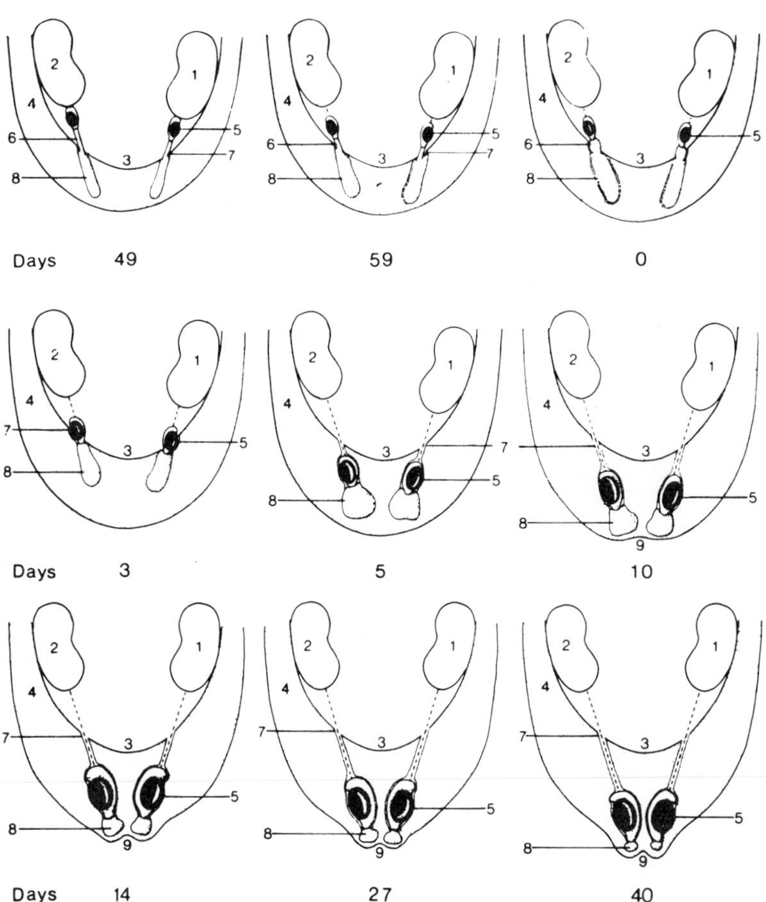

FIG. 4. Schematic diagram of testicular descent in the dog. The drawing illustrates a ventral view of the caudal part of the abdomen showing the normal sequence of testicular descent in the dog between day 53 p.c. and day 40 after birth. 1, Left kidney; 2, right kidney; 3, abdominal wall; 4, subcutaneous tissue; 5, testis; 6, gubernaculum, intra-abdominal part; 7, inguinal canal; 8, gubernaculum, extra-abdominal part; 9, scrotum. (From ref. 15.)

prostaglandin F_1, as well as to sympathetic nerve stimulation, and it relaxes when exposed to isopropylnorepinephrine and prostaglandin E_1 (39,43–49). Histamine also stimulates contraction of the capsule, probably due, at least in part, to the secondary release of prostaglandins (50). In man, the capsule contracts spontaneously at a frequency of approximately once every 14 min, and in response to acetylcholine, norepinephrine, tetramethylammonium, and barium salts (38,51). In the pig, there were regular spontaneous contractions (5–30/10 min) and norepinephrine, acetylcholine, and oxytocin all produced an increase in contractility (Fig. 7), mainly in the form of a rise in tone (34). The

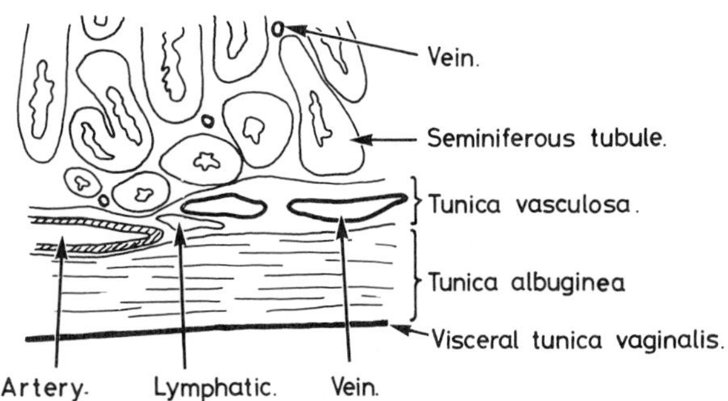

FIG. 5. Diagram (based on an actual section) of the tunics of the testis of a ram. The parenchyma of the testis is at the top of the drawing. (From ref. 2.).

myoid cells in the capsule are not apparent at birth, but appear in the rat shortly before and in the rabbit at about the time of puberty (33,52).

As well as its influence on sperm transport, the capsule probably plays an important role in maintaining the interstitial pressure inside the testis. This pressure has been measured in rats (53), and it increases after the administration of cadmium salts (54), but otherwise, little attention has been directed to this particular aspect. It was also suggested many years ago that the capsule may control the flow of blood through the testis because the testicular artery passes through the capsule at a very oblique angle (55), but this interesting suggestion does not appear to have been followed up. In the capsule of the testis, particularly in the vicinity of the testicular artery, there are appreciable numbers of mast cells (56,57), which may release vasoactive materials to influence the blood vessels of the testis.

Interstitial Tissue

The interstitial tissue (Fig. 8) fills up the spaces between the seminiferous tubules, and contains all the blood and lymph vessels and nerves of the testicular parenchyma (58–61). Also found there are the hormone-secreting Leydig cells, as well as appreciable numbers of mast cells (56,62,63) and macrophages (Fig. 9) (64–66,106,513). The macro-

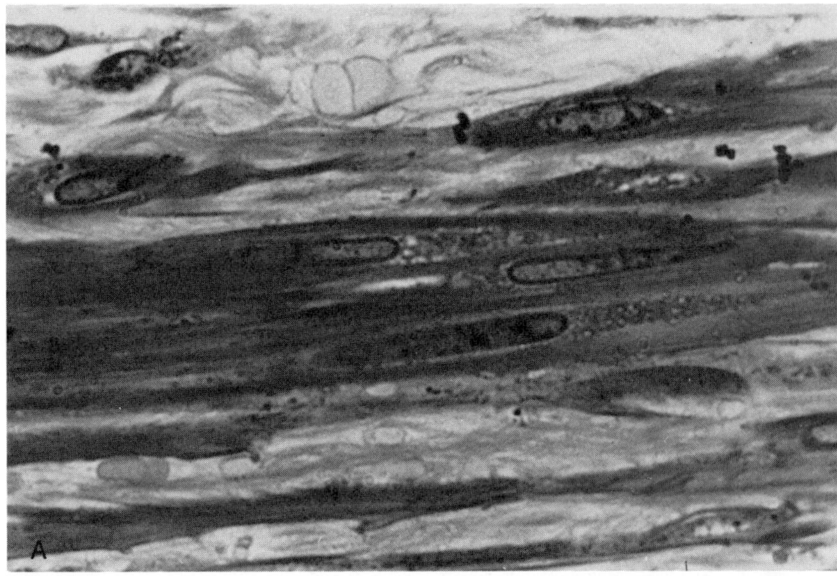

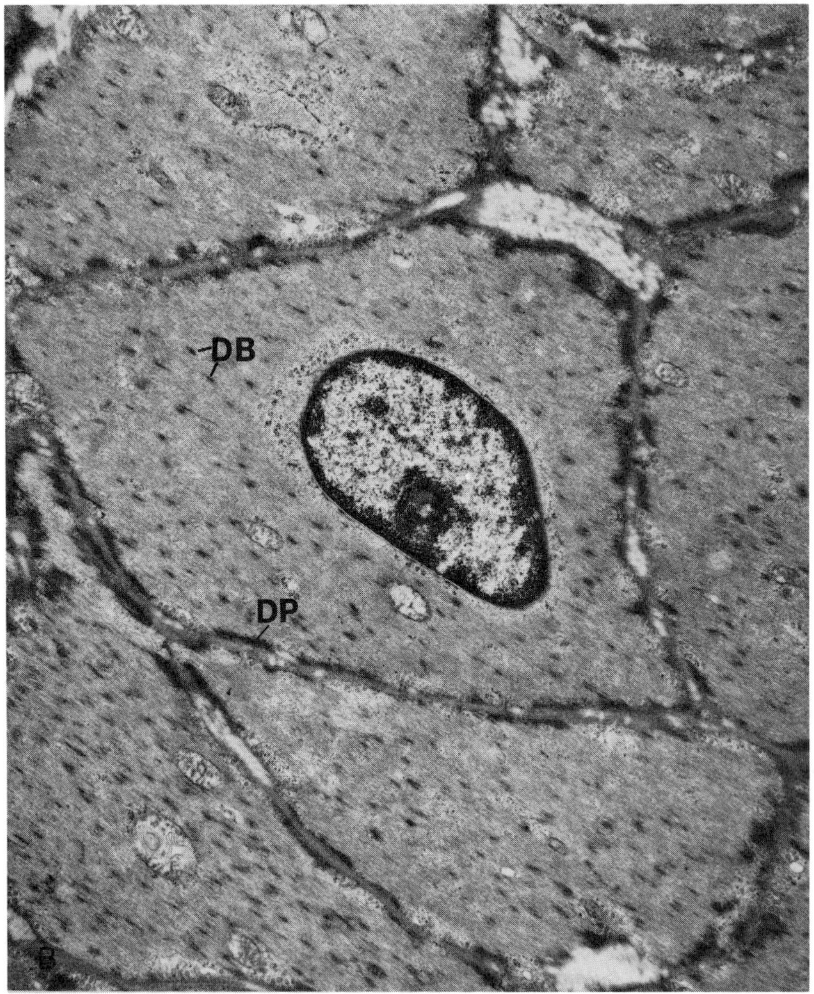

FIG. 6. The structure of the testicular capsule of the horse. **(A):** Section at right angles to the surface of the capsule showing a group of smooth muscle cells lying somewhat obliquely to the longitudinal axis. The cytoplasm beyond the poles of the nuclei is characteristically more granular. (Toluidine blue stain, × 1,120.) **(B):** Section parallel to the surface, showing the typical distribution of organelles including dense bodies (DB) and dense plaques (DP). There are numerous intercellular junctions involving opposing dense plaques with an intervening condensation of extracellular matrix; no gap junctions could be found. (× 992.) (From ref. 29.)

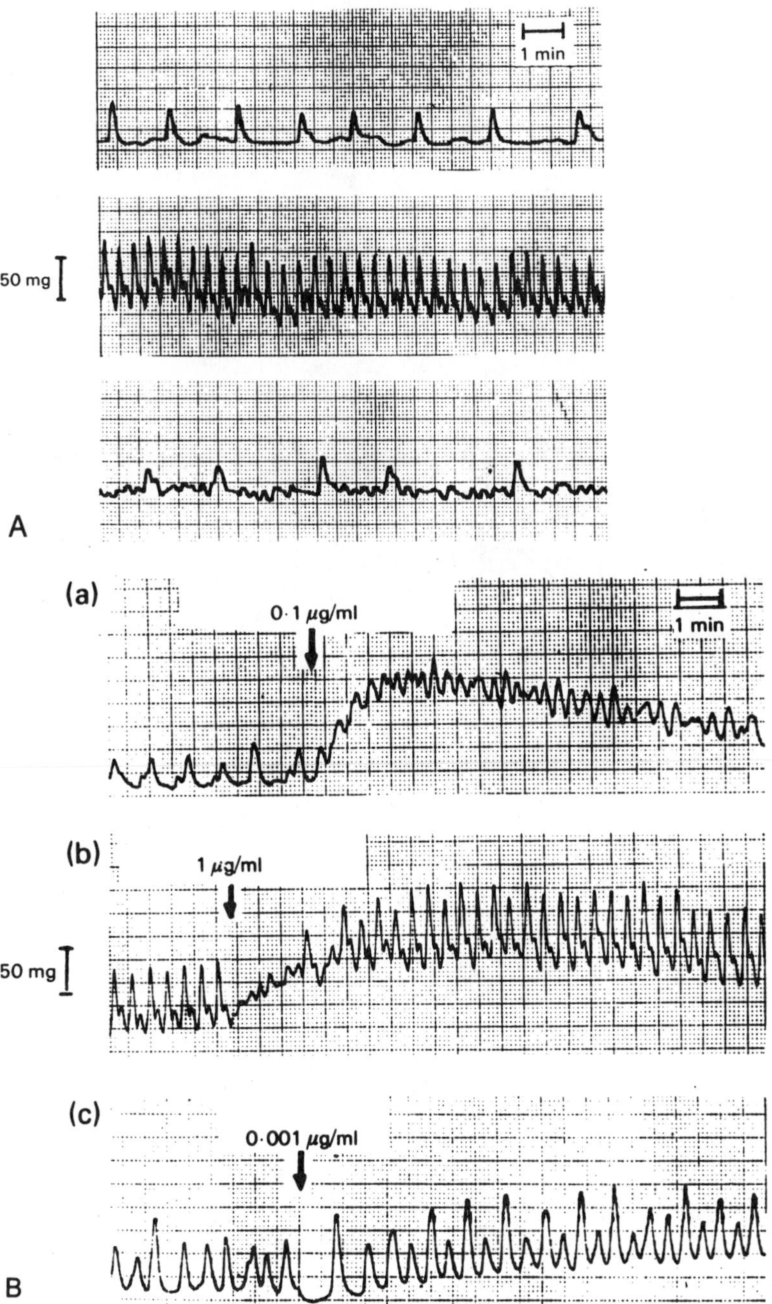

FIG. 7. Contractions of the testicular capsule of the boar. **A:** Different patterns of spontaneous contractions of part of the capsule from the midposterior border. **B:** The effect of (a) norepinephrine, (b) acetylcholine, and (c) oxytocin on the contractions. (From ref. 34.)

phages endocytose foreign material, but they are also in close association with the Leydig cells and can be seen to endocytose portions of Leydig cell cytoplasm (67); they have receptors for follicle-stimulating hormone (FSH) (68) and increase their production of lactate and other biochemical activities when stimulated with this hormone (69–71). In unilaterally cryptorchid rats, macrophage and Leydig cell size are both reduced (72). Some of the Leydig cells appear to be associated with blood vessels (58,60); others are found nearer to the walls of the seminiferous tubules, and these latter cells show variations in size and structure depending on the spermatogenic stage of the adjacent tubules (73,74). The connective tissue of the interstitial tissue, as well as the peritubular tissue is rich in fibrinonectin (75).

The amount of interstitial tissue varies between species (Fig. 8) (76), from approximately 10% of the tissue in guinea pigs and dogs, approximately 15% in rats and sheep, 25 to 30% in man, to almost 40% in pigs (77–79) and some marsupials (see ref. 80). In the pig, Leydig cells occupy almost the entire space between the tubules (58), whereas in rats they account for only 17% of the interstitial tissue (79). No explanation has been advanced for this difference

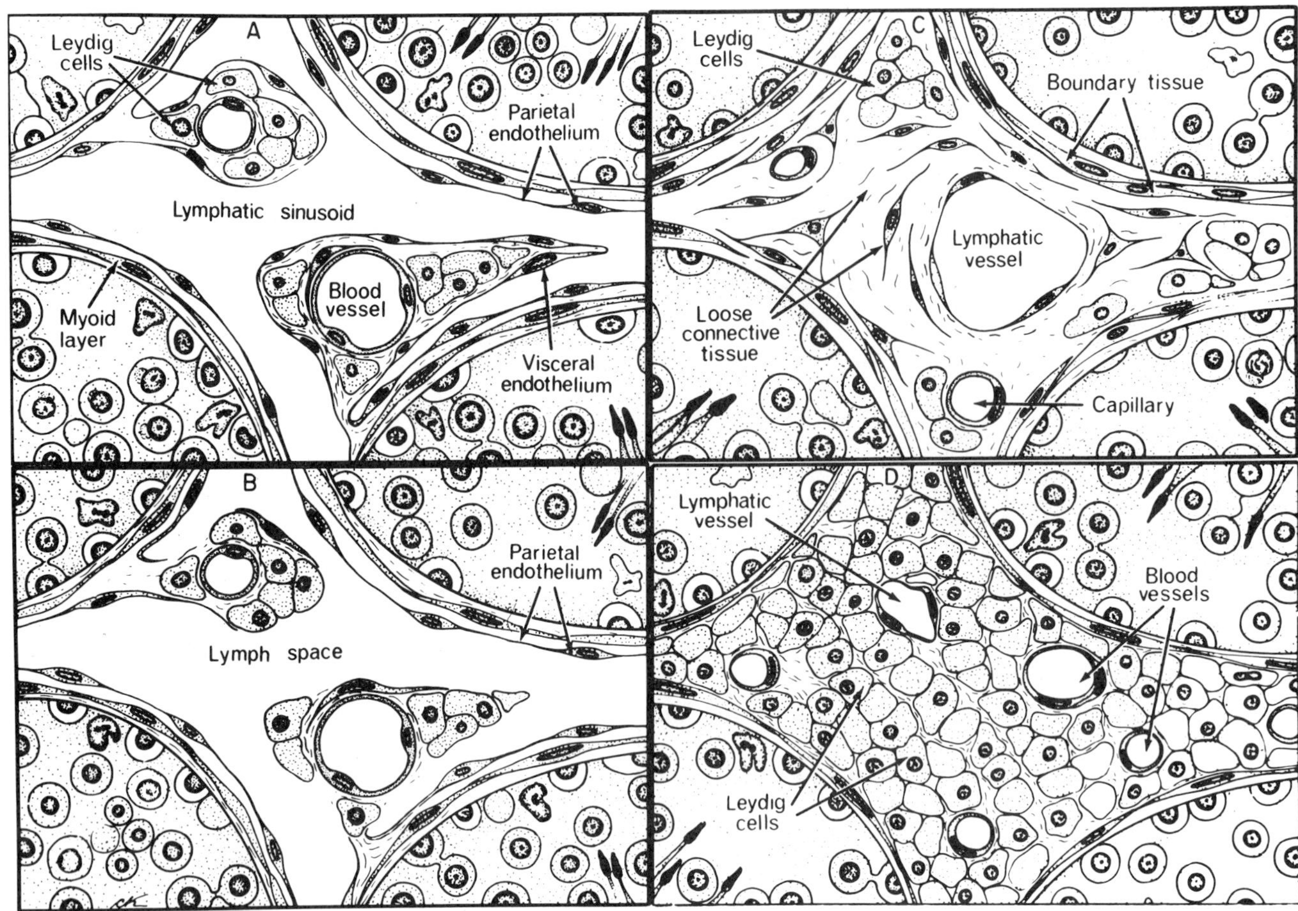

FIG. 8. Diagram of the interstitial tissue of various species. **A:** Guinea pig, showing the Leydig cells clustered around the blood vessels, with the groups of cells completely surrounded by endothelial cells and "floating" in a fluid-filled lymphatic sinusoid. **B:** Rat, similar to the guinea pig, but with an incomplete investment of endothelial cells around the groups of Leydig cells. **C:** Sheep and man, with the Leydig cells either in groups near a blood vessel or in a loose connective tissue. **D:** Pig, with the interstitial tissue packed with numerous Leydig cells, with very inconspicuous blood and lymph vessels. (From ref. 76.)

in Leydig cell numbers, but it is interesting that in two species with abundant Leydig cells, the pig and the horse, the testis secretes large amounts of estrogens (81,82).

Seminiferous Tubules

The majority of the testis is made up by the seminiferous tubules (Fig. 10), where the spermatozoa are formed. In most species, these tubules are between 200 and 250 μm in diameter. In the rat, there are approximately 12 m of tubules per gram of testis, with a surface area of approximately 120 cm/g (83). In man, the tubules are slightly smaller in diameter, and there are between 20 and 25 m/g of testis (77,78). However, in some Australian marsupials, in particular the dasyurids and peramelids, the tubules are almost twice this diameter (80,84), but the significance of this difference is obscure.

In most mammalian species, the tubules are two-ended, convoluted loops, with both ends opening into the rete testis (Fig. 11). In rats, it has been shown that there are normally approximately 30 tubules (85), but there may be as few as five tubules in some of the dasyurid marsupials (84), and many more in humans and in farm animals. In humans, the tubules are arranged in approximately 300 lobules, each containing between one and four tubules (86), but lobulation is much less obvious in some other animals. It has been suggested that in humans, hypercurvature of the seminiferous tubules may be a cause of infertility (87,88).

In mature rats, each tubule has a lumen with a diameter of approximately 50 μm along most of its length, although this value does increase to approximately double in the area where the spermatozoa are just about to be released (83). For some unexplained reason, successive stages of the spermatogenic cycle are arranged in descending order along the tubule, beginning at the rete (Fig. 12). Consequently, these two "waves" meet at a point along the length of the tubule, the "site of reversal," and there are modulations of the wave

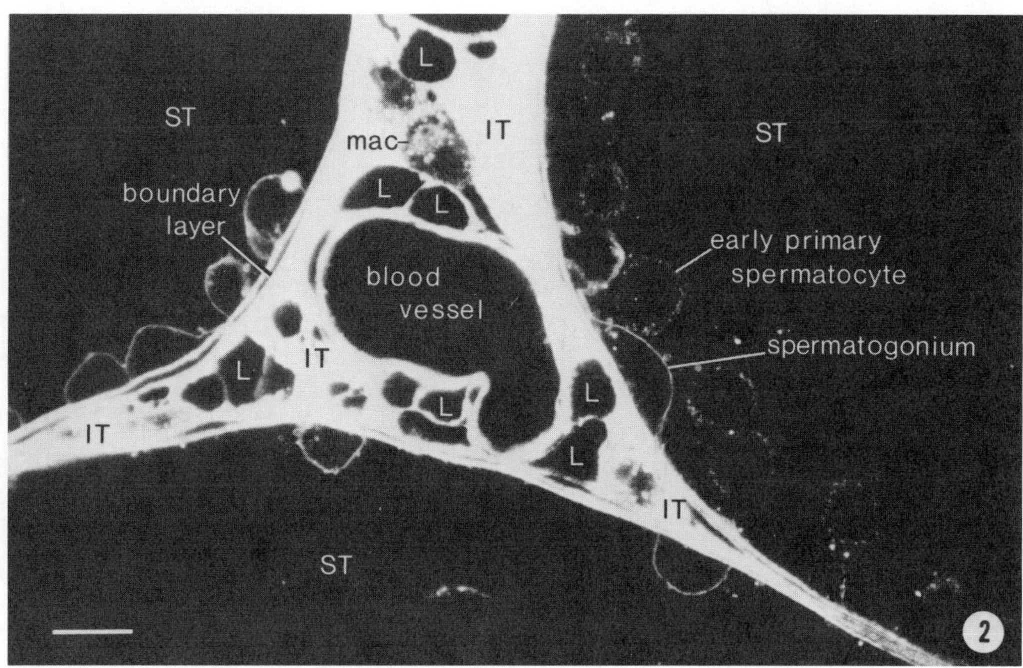

FIG. 9. A fluorescent light micrograph of the interstitial tissue of a frozen section of a rat testis which had been treated with a fluorescein-coupled antibody to rat serum albumin. Albumin fills the interstitial tissue (IT) except for the Leydig cells (L); a macrophage (mac) has taken up some of the albumin. The seminiferous tubules (ST) contain no detectable albumin, except around the spermatogonia and early primary spermatocytes. (From ref. 62.)

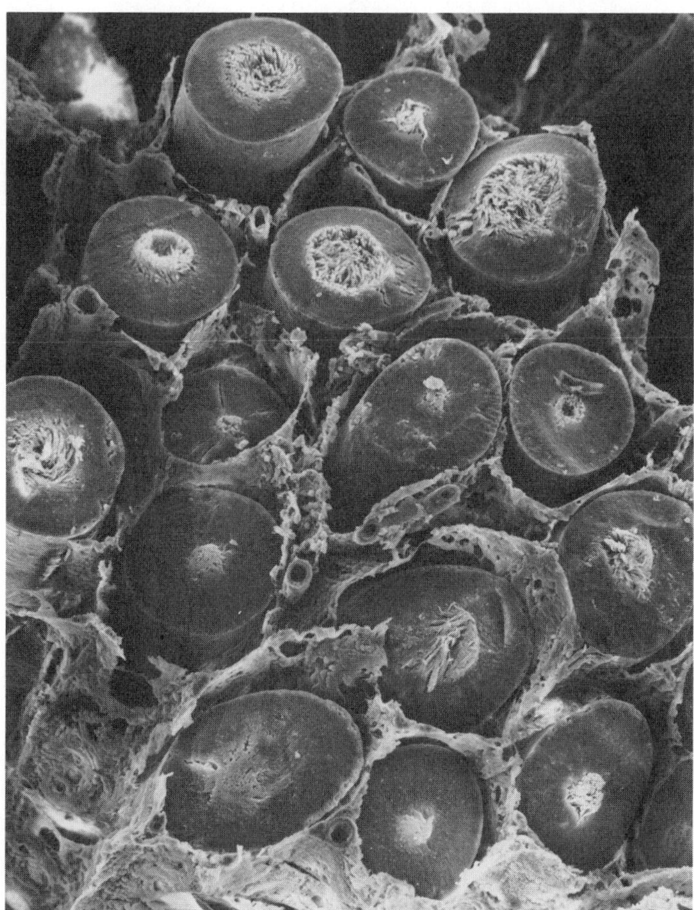

FIG. 10. A scanning electron micrograph of a cut surface of a rat testis. Note the individual seminiferous tubules embedded in the interstitial tissue. (Electron micrograph supplied by Dr. A. K. Christensen, Department of Anatomy and Cell Biology, The University of Michigan Medical School, Ann Arbor, MI.)

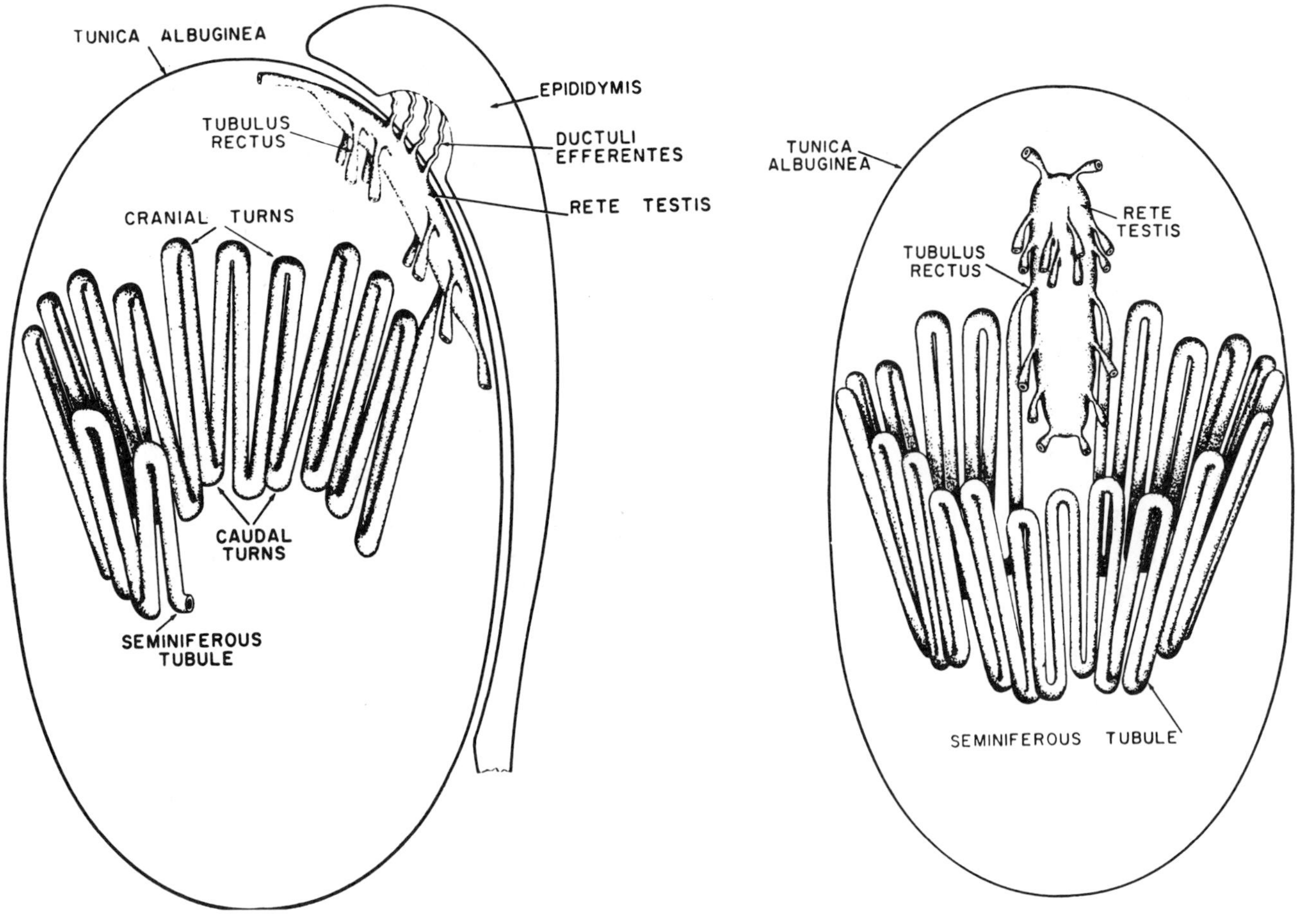

FIG. 11. A diagram of the anatomy of an individual seminiferous tubule and the rete testis of a rat. **Left:** Only part of one tubule is shown, and only some of the junctions of seminiferous tubules with the rete testis are depicted. (From ref. 85.)

where, for short stretches, the order of the stages is reversed (89,90). In man, the wave is arranged helically (91).

The walls of the tubules of rodents are composed of four layers, an innermost layer of noncellular material, surrounded by a layer of smooth muscle-like or myoid cells, which are probably responsible for the peristaltic movements of the tubules (92,93); then there is a layer of collagen fibers, and finally, on the outside, a layer of endothelial cells which line the lymphatic sinusoids in the interstitial tissue (93; see ref. 2 for earlier references). The myoid cells are extremely flat, and are arranged in a single virtually continuous layer (94). A similar arrangement is found in

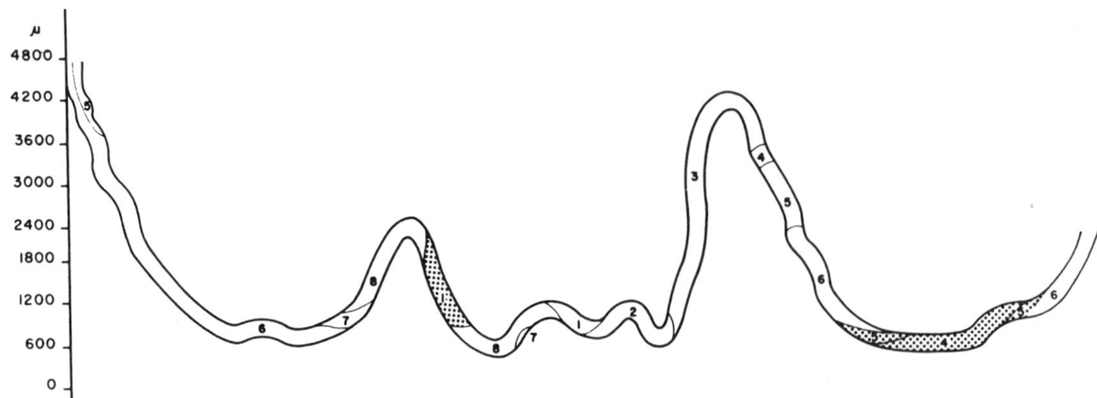

FIG. 12. A diagram of seminiferous tubule of a rat, showing a complete spermatogenic wave. The stages are arranged from left to right, and the wave includes two modulations (*dotted shading*). (From ref. 90.)

rabbits (52,95), but in humans and monkeys (Fig. 13) there are several layers of myoid cells interspersed with layers of connective tissue fibrils (97–100). There are also several layers of myoid cells in the ram (101) and cat (102), and, in the ram and boar, the inner noncellular layer consists of a number of concentric layers (101,103). In the ram lamb, the myoid cells are apparent as early as a week after birth (101), but in the mouse (104), rat (105,118), and rabbit (52) they do not appear until approximately the time of puberty. The development of the myoid cells in the mouse depends on the presence of pituitary hormones (107), but it is not clear whether these hormones act directly. Testosterone receptors seem to be present in these cells (108), and the contractility in organ culture of tubules from immature rats was enhanced by the addition of testosterone and inhibited by the antiandrogen, cyproterone acetate (109). In adult animals, testosterone, dihydrotestosterone, and estradiol added *in vitro* inhibited tubular contractions at low concentrations, whereas higher concentrations were without effect; pretreatment of the rats had a similar effect except that estradiol was inhibitory at all doses used (110). Cyproterone acetate also impaired differentiation and the appearance of alkaline phosphatase in the myoid cells, whereas treatment with human chorionic gonadotropin stimulated their division; this latter effect was not produced by testosterone (111). Myoid cells persist in hypophysectomized adult rodents (107,112), suggesting that the hormonal control of their differentiation may be different from that of their maintenance.

Actin, myosin, and fibronectin have been demonstrated in peritubular cells (75,113–116), and actin-like proteins have been demonstrated in these cells in human, mouse, and pig testis (117). Isolated tubules from rats more than 15 days old contract spontaneously *in vitro* (118) and respond to oxytocin (119); in very young rats at approximately the age when oxytocin levels in the testis are at a peak, there are no spontaneous contractions, but the response to oxytocin is increased (120). Melatonin, cyclic AMP, and theophylline decreased the frequency and depth of the contractions. Prostaglandin E_1 had a stimulatory effect at low concentrations, but was inhibitory at higher levels (121). The frequency and depth of contraction do not appear to be associated with any particular stages of the seminiferous cycle (122), but increase if the temperature of incubation is increased (123).

Contractility persists for approximately 3 weeks in cultured fragments of seminiferous tubules from adult rats, as does the enzyme alkaline phosphatase which appears at approximately the age when tubules begin to contract (118,124). However, addition of cyproterone acetate to the culture medium eliminates contractions within 1 week, without affecting the enzyme levels (109). Contractions disappear from the fifth day after the testis has been made cryptorchid (123), and the peritubular tissue becomes noticeably thickened as spermatogenesis becomes affected (123,125–127), as seen after hypophysectomy and seminiferous tubule failure, but not after irradiation (99,128,129). Myoid cells have been kept in culture, and under these conditions secrete a number of proteoglycans and extracellular matrix, especially when cocultured with Sertoli cells (115,130,131); the myoid cells also exercise important influences on Sertoli cells in cocultures (131,132).

Transitional Zone and Tubuli Recti

At each end of the seminiferous tubules, where they open into the rete testis (Fig. 14a,b), there is a short transitional

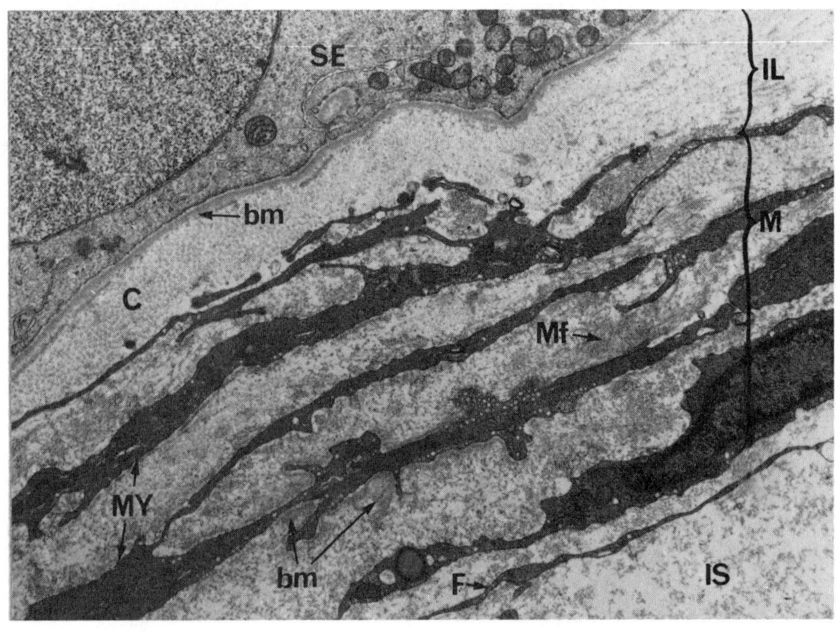

FIG. 13. A low-power electron micrograph of the peritubular tissue in a human testis. The seminiferous epithelium (SE) is towards the *top* and the interstitial tissue (IS) towards the *bottom.* The peritubular tissue shows three distinct zones; a thick inner lamella (IL) containing a large amount of collagen (C), poorly stained in this preparation; a myoid layer (M) composed of several layers of myoid cells (MY) interspersed with connective tissue lamellae, and an adventitial layer of fibrocytes (F). The myoid cells contain many more filaments than the fibrocytes, which show only a few caveolae associated with the plasma membrane. The connective tissue lamellae contain abundant microfibrils (Mf) as well as collagen. There is a continuous basement membrane (bm) underlying the seminiferous epithelium, and similar material (bm) is also seen over small areas of the surfaces of the myoid cells. (From ref. 100.)

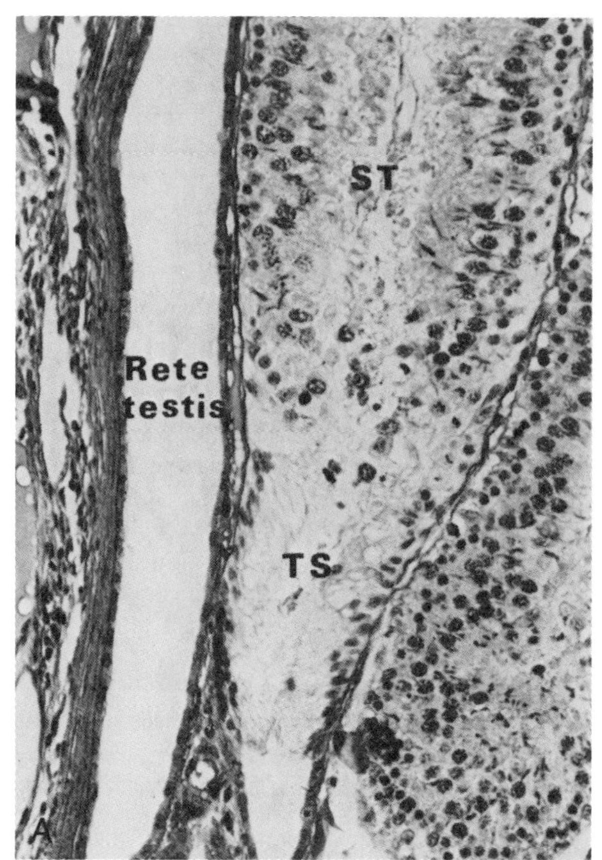

FIG. 14. The structure of the terminal segment of the seminiferous tubule. **A:** Photomicrograph (× 300) of a longitudinal section through the terminal segment (TS) of a seminiferous tubule (ST) in a rat testis. The lumen appears to be completely occluded by vacuolated cytoplasmic processes of modified Sertoli cells. (From ref. 137.)

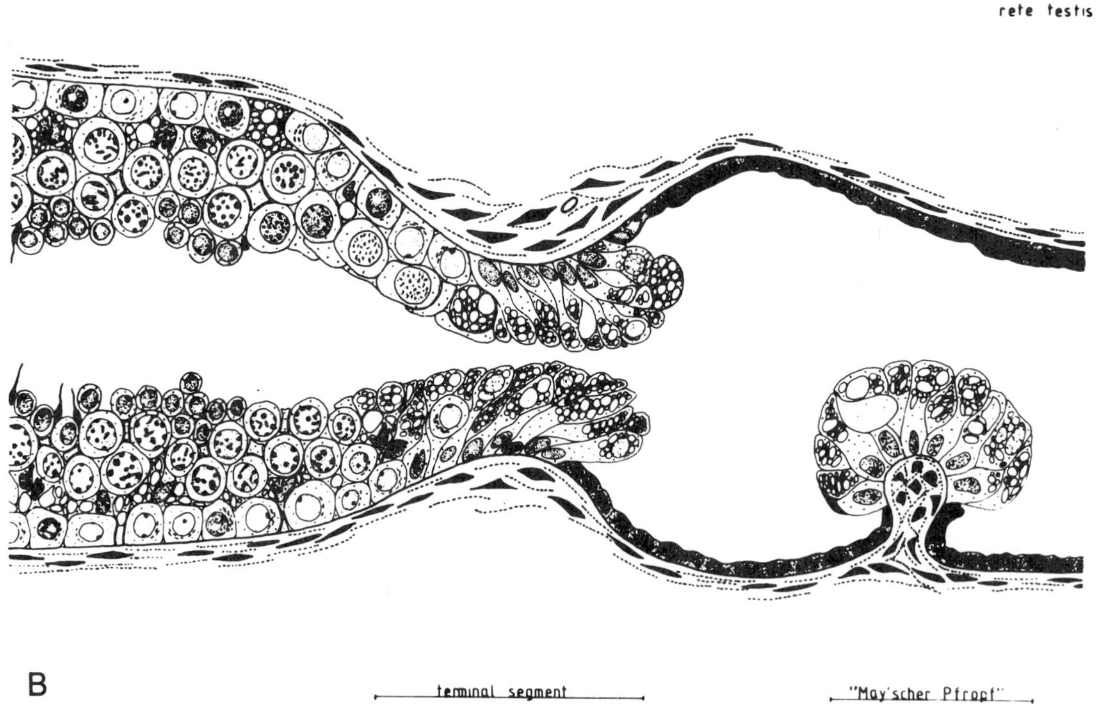

B: Semi-schematic drawing of the transitional zone of a seminiferous tubule in a human, based on numerous semi-thin sections, with a similar valve-like structure formed by modified Sertoli cells, and a May'scher Pfropf consisting of a basal lamina and myoid cells protruding into the lumen of the tubulus rectus. (From ref. 141.)

zone lined only with cells resembling Sertoli cells (133–141). These cells appear to form a valve or plug (see refs. 142 and 143 for early references) which may prevent the passage of fluid from the rete into the tubules (144), although the effectiveness of this valve would depend on the state of the cells in the living animal. In later studies, it was found that in most of the tubules, there was a narrow open channel (134,145), and the passage of injected dyes from the rete into the tubules (146) and the opening up of the channels after efferent duct ligation (147,148) would suggest that, if they do act as valves, they are reasonably ineffective. The transitional zone is joined to the rete testis by a tubulus rectus, which is really a narrow extension of the rete proper and is lined with similar cells (148). In the human, up to six seminiferous tubules can join a single tubulus rectus (149). In the horse, junctions between seminiferous epithelium and transitional tubules can be found throughout the parenchyma (150).

Some dyes and horseradish peroxidase infused into an individual seminiferous tubule appear to be taken up by the cells of the tubulus rectus (151,152). The cells of the tubuli recti and the proximal part of the rete testis in the guinea pig are rich in glycogen (153).

Rete Testis

The rete testis is a complicated network of intercommunicating channels lined with cells which range from squamous to columnar, with comparatively few organelles; the cells are joined near their luminal boundaries by specialized junctions (143,149,154–161). The rete in the buffalo has a stratified epithelium (162), and the cells lining the bull rete show an unusually high leucine aminopeptidase activity (163). The cells lining the rete in the rat are involved in both adsorptive and fluid-phase endocytosis (164).

Through this network, the spermatozoa and the fluid in which they are suspended are carried to the epididymis. In humans and monkeys, the rete lies along the epididymal edge of the testis (149,158). In the rat, it is a fairly simple sac just under the tunica albuginea near where the efferent ducts run to the epididymis (144). In some marsupials, it extends down both surfaces of the testis under the superficial arteries and veins (80), whereas in ungulates, carnivores, rabbits, and guinea pigs the rete is located near the center of the testis (Fig. 15), extending along approximately two-thirds of its long axis (see refs. 142,143,154). In the horse, there is a recognizable rete adjacent to the central vein, but other tubuli recti lead individually to the dorsocranial pole of the testis, where they join the rete (150).

In all species, the rete testis appears to be located close to the testicular artery in part of its course on the surface of the testis, or where the main branches of the testicular artery turn back into the parenchyma and begin to branch (142), and in the rat, it is covered by the veins of the intraalbugineal plexus (165). The significance of this arrangement is not yet understood.

Efferent Ducts

The rete testis is linked to the epididymis by the efferent ducts. The position and dimensions of these depend on the relationship between the testis and epididymis; in rats and marsupials, the ducts are comparatively long because the epididymis is only loosely attached to the testis, whereas in man and the domestic animals, the epididymis is much more closely applied and the efferent ducts are correspondingly shorter. In the rat there are between two and nine ducts (154,158,166–168), whereas in monkeys, there are between eight and 16 (169). In the domestic animals, there are between 13 and 20 efferent ducts (170), which show evidence of fluid resorption and acid phosphatase, esterase, β-glucuronidase, and carbonic anhydrase activity (171,172). Some of these ductules may coalesce before they join the epididymal duct proper (Fig. 16). Blind-ending ducts and other ducts which make no connection with the rete testis (aberrant ductuli) are not uncommon (170). At the testicular end, the ducts are only slightly convoluted but then become more convoluted to form the bulbous coni vasculosi, which then extend by a narrow isthmus to connect with the epididymal duct (Figs. 16,17).

The epithelium of the efferent ducts is comprised of two main cells types in most species, namely principal and ciliated cells; these cells are columnar, with prominent intercellular junctions near their luminal borders. Some cells are ciliated and there is a thick basal lamina. Their ultrastructural features suggest only a low capacity for protein synthesis and secretion, but the nonciliated cells appear to be actively involved in fluid resorption (155,161,169,172–177). The nonciliated cells are also actively involved in fluid-phase and adsorptive endocytosis (178). In the horse, there is a sharp transition between the simple cuboidal cells of the rete and the columnar epithelium of the ducts; the efferent ducts are also surrounded by many more peritubular capillaries (150).

Epididymis

The ductus epididymidis is a single highly convoluted duct, closely applied to the surface of the testis extending from the anterior to the posterior pole of that organ and held more or less firmly, depending on species, to the tunica albuginea by connective tissue. The duct is coiled into segments demarcated by connective tissue septula (Fig. 18), and the organ is contained within a fibrous tissue capsule. The segment into which the ductuli efferentes empty is usually referred to as the initial segment and the remainder of the epididymis is loosely defined into three parts termed the caput, corpus, and cauda epididymidis. An alternative

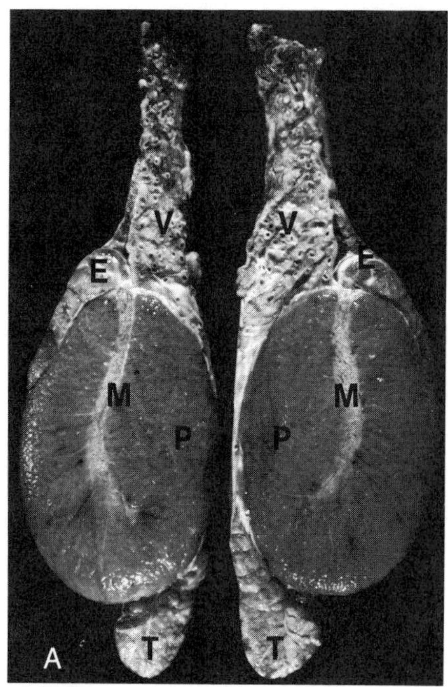

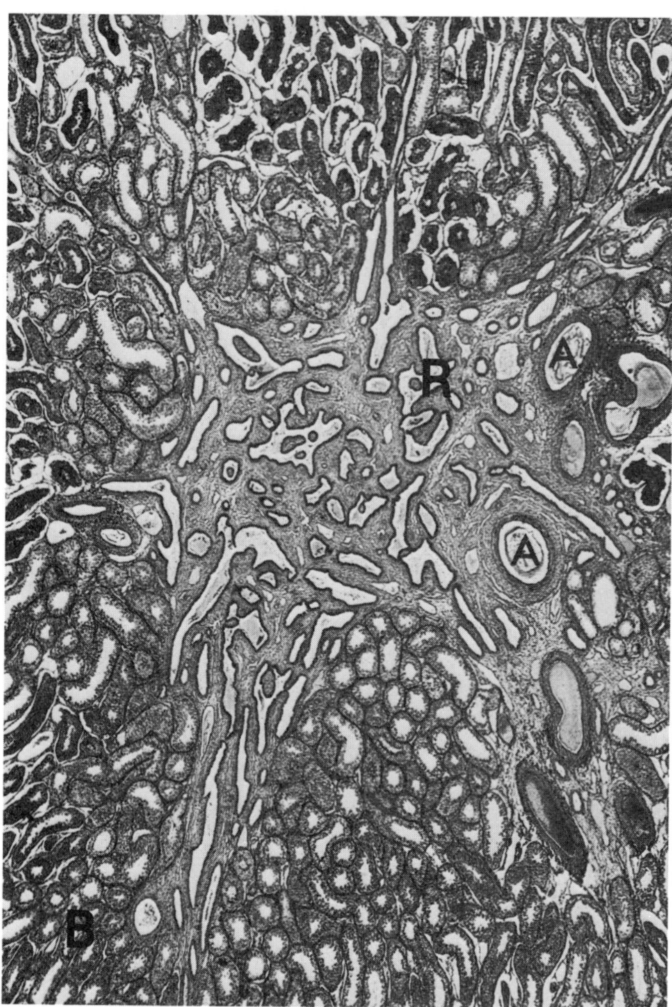

FIG. 15. The anatomy of the rete testis in the ram. **A:** A ram testis has been cut longitudinally to show the rete testis, which is situated in a fibrous mediastinum (M) along the long axis of the testis, surrounded by parenchyma (P); E: head of epididymis; T: tail of epididymis; V: vascular cone. **B:** A transverse section through a ram testis, showing the multiple channels of the rete (R) in a fibrous mediastinum, with arterial branches (A) cut in cross-section where they run near the rete. (From ref. 2.)

subdivision, based on histological and functional criteria has been proposed (179). In this system the epididymis is subdivided into three regions, the initial, middle, and terminal segments (Fig. 19). The initial and middle segments are primarily concerned with sperm maturation, whereas the terminal segment coincides with the region where mature sperm are stored prior to ejaculation or voidance into the urine.

The subdivisions of Glover and Nicander (179) do not necessarily coincide with the more traditional subdivision of caput, corpus, and cauda. This is particularly apparent in the case of the guinea pig in which the corpus region should be more correctly classified as part of the initial segment (Fig. 19). In certain rodents, such as the rat, large accumulations of fat surround the proximal regions of the epididymis and constitute the "epididymal fat pad" (Fig. 3). The location of the epididymis together with the testis in the scrotum results in the maintenance of epididymal temperature several degrees below that of core body temperature (180–183).

Perhaps the most comprehensive histological descriptions of the epididymis have been carried out in the rat (184), the rabbit (185), and the stallion, ram, and bull (186). These descriptions subdivided the epididymis into between six and eight histological zones. The epididymal epithelium is complex in that it contains a variety of cell types (177,184), each cell type varying as a proportion of the total population at different points along the duct. In contrast to the ductuli efferentes, ciliated cells are absent from the epithelium of the epididymal duct. The predominant cell type is the principal cell which bears apical stereocilia. Other cell types described include apical cells, basal cell, clear cells, and halo cells (intraepithelial lymphocytes). Many detailed descriptions of the ultrastructure of these cells have been pub-

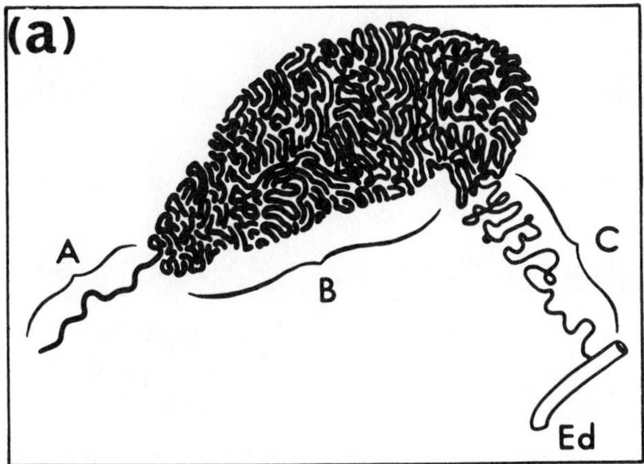

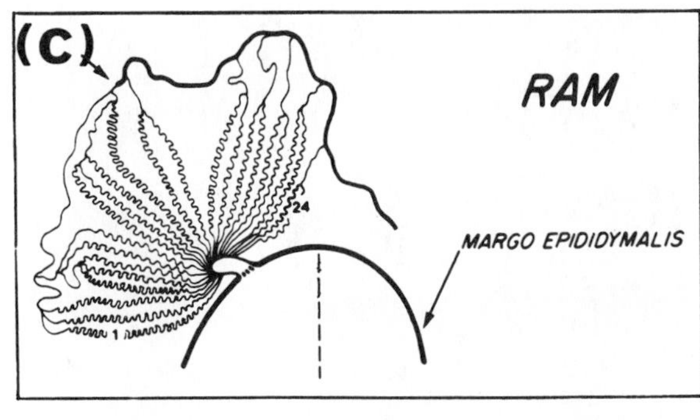

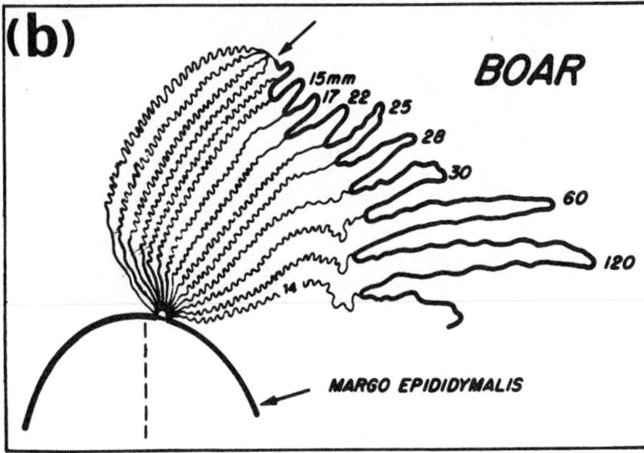

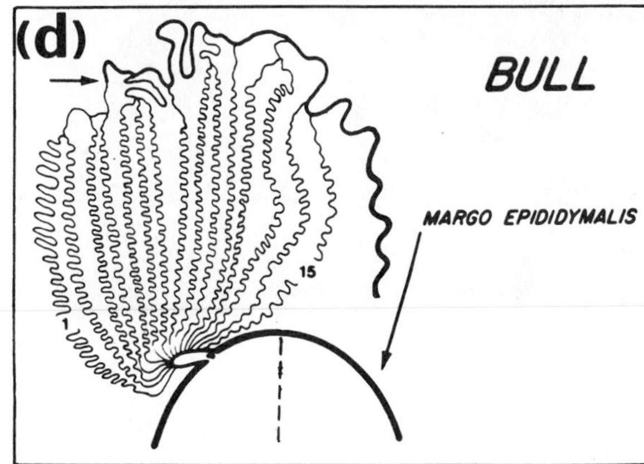

FIG. 16. Arrangement of ductuli efferentes in various species. **(a):** A single efferent ductule of a bull showing the slightly undulating testicular segment (A); the highly coiled cone segment (B); the moderately coiled epididymal segment (C); the epididymal duct (Ed). **(b), (c),** and **(d)** show the ductuli efferentes of the boar, ram, and bull, respectively. The ductuli are drawn to scale to show the relative coiled lengths of the ductuli. The first and last ductuli have numerals and the *arrow* marks the beginning of the epididymal duct. (From ref. 814.)

lished [e.g., rat (177), mouse (187), hamster (188), rabbit (161), monkey (189), bull (190)]. In general terms, the first part of the epididymis or initial segment is characterized by a high epithelium with long straight stereocilia which almost obliterate the lumen which is sparsely populated with spermatozoa. The middle segment has a wider lumen and the stereocilia are usually bent and sometimes branched, while supranuclear vacuoles are prominent in the epithelium. The terminal segment has a lower epithelium; stereocilia are shorter and less dense and the lumen of the tubule is wider and densely packed with sperm. The epididymis of testicond mammals, such as the elephant, follows the same basic structure as that of the scrotal mammals (191).

The epididymal tubule is surrounded by connective tissue which contains fibroblasts, collagen, elastic fibers, blood vessels, lymphatic vessels, nerve fibers, macrophages, wandering leucocytes, and concentric layers of smooth muscle fibers. The amount of intertubular connective tissue varies considerably between species. Within a species the thickness of the smooth muscle layer surrounding the tubules increases from the initial segment to the terminal segment.

Ductus Deferens

The ductus (vas) deferens is a continuation of the epididymal duct beginning at the point where the ductus epididymidis straightens and reverses direction towards the inguinal canal. The duct is approximately 25 cm long in the adult human male and 6 cm in the rat, and is suspended in a mesentery that is continuous with that over the epididymis. The ductus deferens should not be considered as a simple conduit leading sperm from the epididymis to the urethra, since it has a complex epithelium which has both absorptive and secretory functions.

In the rat, the ductus deferens can be subdivided into three sections (192). The proximal vas deferens, located primarily in the scrotum, is flattened due to an asymmetric

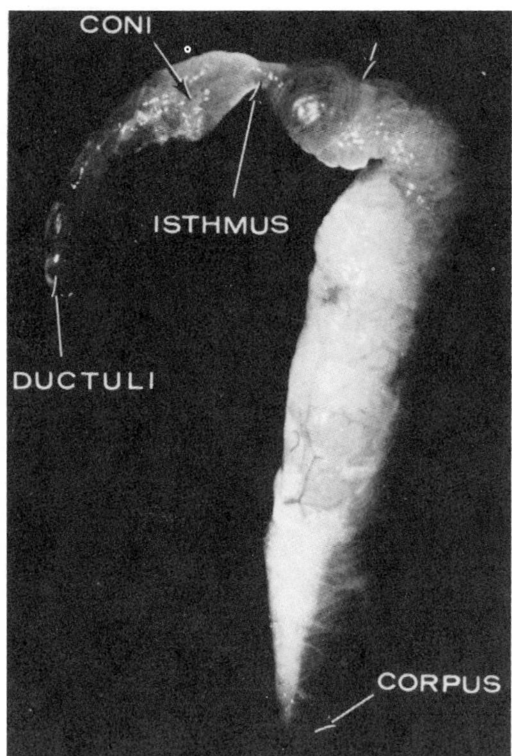

FIG. 17. Gross structure of the ductuli efferentes, initial segment of the epididymis, and caput epididymidis of the rat. The epididymal fat pad has been dissected away and the testis removed. The convoluted region of the ductuli efferentes forms the coni vasculosi. The ductuli straighten to form the isthmus where the ductuli join the initial segment of the epididymis. The initial segment begins at the isthmus and terminates at the single *arrow* and characteristically has a reddish color indicating a greater degree of vascularization than the caput epididymidis which lies distal to it. (From ref. 177.)

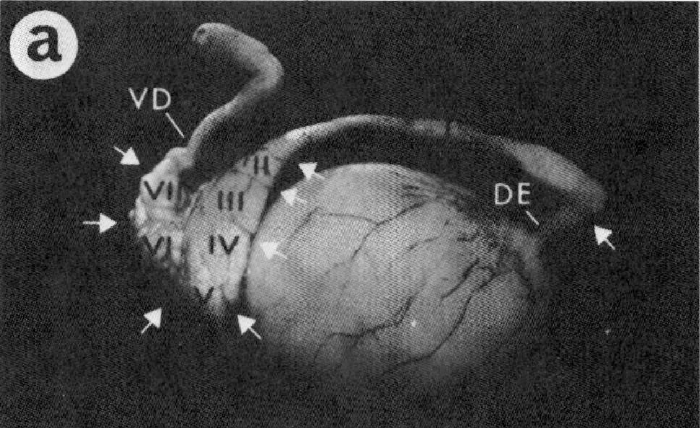

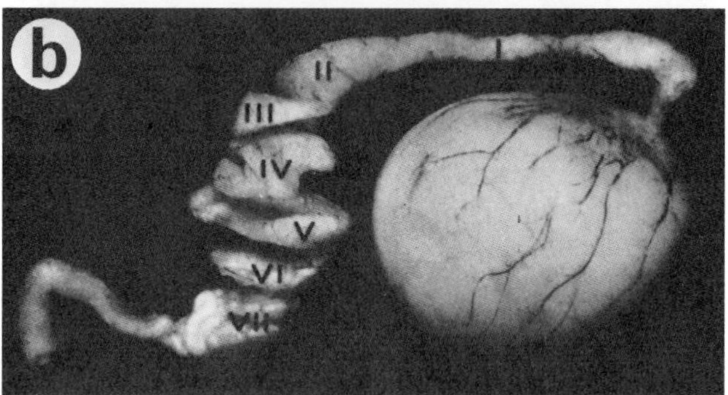

FIG. 18. Guinea pig testis and epididymis showing subdivision of the epididymis into segments dermarcated by connective tissue septula. **(a):** The epididymis, which leads from the ductuli efferentes (DE) to the vas deferens (VD), is divided into seven segments demarcated by connective tissue septula. The epididymal fat pad has been removed to expose details of the epididymis. **(b):** Partial unraveling of the epididymal tubule following removal of the organ capsule and separation of segments along natural planes of cleavage. (From ref. 815.)

distribution of longitudinal muscle layers, but contains a tubule which is circular in cross-section. The distal vas deferens, in the inguinal region, is circular in cross-section due to the presence of thick longitudinal layers, but the epithelium of the duct becomes crenelated with two to six infoldings, and the structural features of the epithelial cells differ from those in the proximal vas. The terminal region of the vas deferens lies in the abdominal pelvis and terminates at the point where it is joined by the duct of the seminal vesicles to form the short ejaculatory duct. It is characterized by replacement of columnar principal cells, in some areas, by pockets of smaller cells which can be seen actively to phagocytose spermatozoa.

The epithelium of the human vas deferens is crenelated in more distal regions as in the rat and this produces a stellate shape in cross-section (Fig. 20a). Four different cell types are recognized in the epithelium, namely principal cells, pencil cells, mitochondrion-rich cells, and basal cells (193). The muscle coat is composed of three layers, an inner longitudinal layer, a middle oblique or circular layer, and an outer longitudinal layer (Fig. 20a). In contrast to the rat, there is a progressive decrease in the development of the epithelium and muscle layers in moving from the proximal to terminal regions. Elastic fibers are prominent in the lamina propria where they form two layers and they are also present among the smooth muscle cells of the inner muscle layer (194).

Ampulla

The ampulla, when present, exists as a spindle-shaped thickening of the terminal portion of the ductus deferens. It is particularly well developed in the stallion where it may measure 25 cm long and 2 cm in diameter. Dimensions in other species have been reported as follows: bull (10 × 1.5 cm), ram (7 × 0.6 cm), red deer (6 × 0.6 cm), elephant (8 × 6 cm), and camel (13 × 0.5 cm) (195–198). Details of the structure of the ampulla are scant. In the human, the epithelium lining the ampulla is thrown into numerous, irregular branching folds (Fig. 20b). Between the folds there

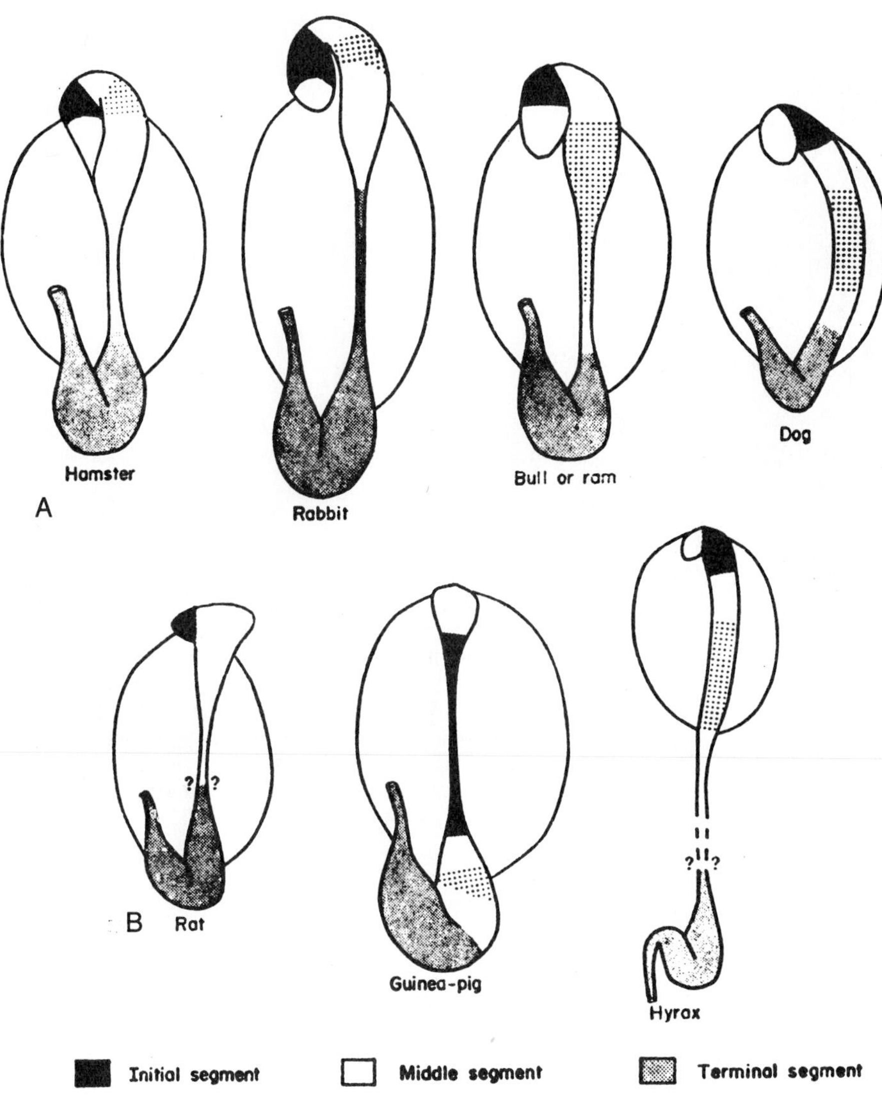

FIG. 19. Diagrammatic representation of a scheme for the subdivision of the epididymis into three segments in a variety of species. The subdivision into initial, middle, and terminal segments is based on histological and cytological features which do not necessarily occupy the same gross morphological position in different species. (From ref. 179.)

are many branched outpocketings that reach deep into the surrounding muscular layer which is less regularly arranged than in the rest of the ductus deferens. A single layer of columnar cells with secretory function line the surface of the ampullary glands. A similar arrangement appears to exist in the bull (199), red deer (197), and rabbit (200,201). In the last-mentioned species the glands consist of large fluid-filled vesicles connecting with the lumen where the mucosa is thrown into irregular folds. The ampulla in the elephant consists of numerous, simple tubular glands containing large eosinophilic bodies of homogenous but concretionary appearance, as well as spermatozoa (196). In the camel, two types of ampullary glands are present (202). Central submucosal glands are relatively small with narrow lumina lined by a low columnar epithelium; larger peripheral glands with wide lumina are lined by tall slender columnar cells with a brush border. The luminal fluid contains globular bodies, oval concretions, and spermatozoa. Ampullary glands have been described in the rat, mouse, and hamster where they are located on the dorsal wall of the urethra. They consist of acini lined with cuboidal to columnar epithelial cells with the epithelium being thrown into deep longitudinal folds (203,204). Tubules leading from the acini to the wide vestibule of the ampulla are surrounded by a thin layer of smooth muscle cells and are held together by a thin connective tissue membrane.

Seminal Vesicles

Seminal vesicles are so-named because of an early misconception that they were receptacles or reservoirs for sperm (467). The glands are absent from monotremes, marsupials, carnivores, cetaceans, and from some insectivores, chiropterans, primates, and lagomorphs (195) (Table 1). Some confusion originally surrounded the homology of the vesicular glands in the rabbit, but it is now considered that the glandula seminalis and glandula vesicularis, being both de-

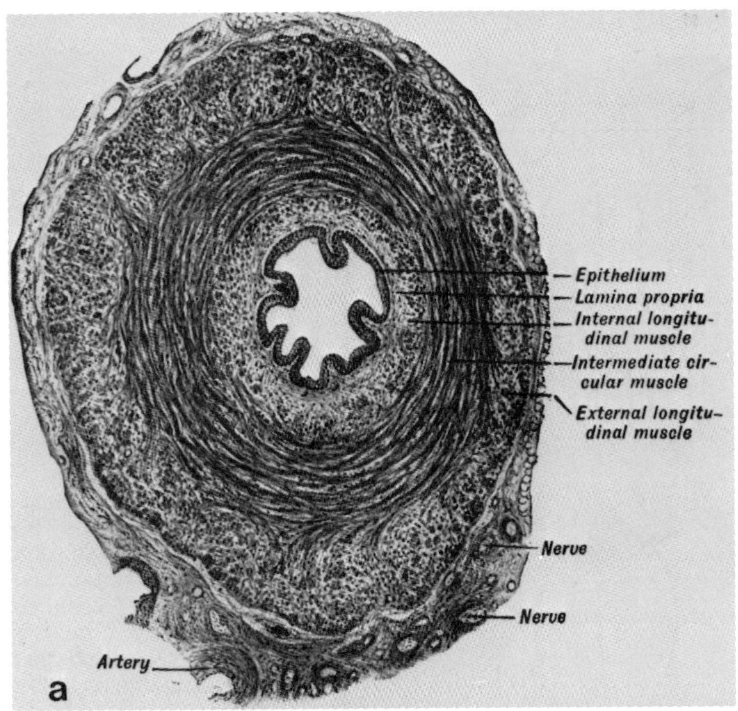

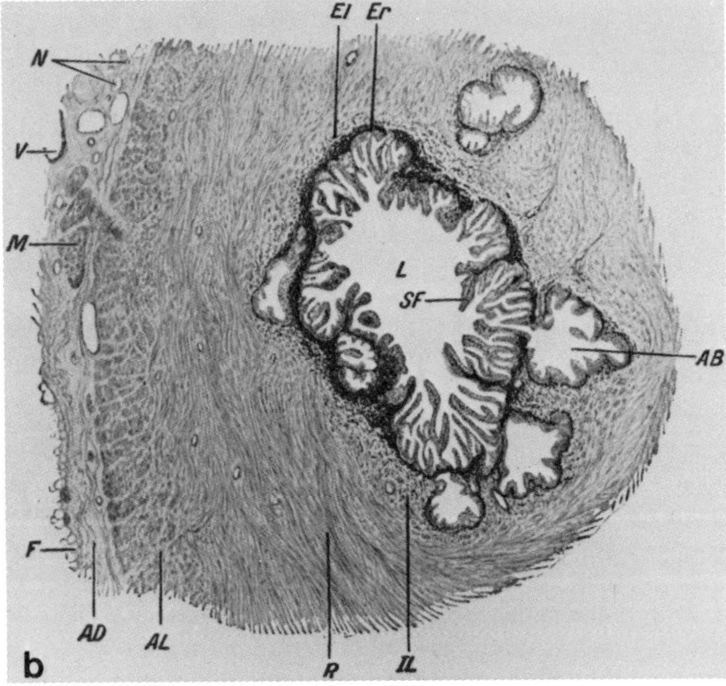

FIG. 20. Cross-section of **(a)** the ductus deferens, and **(b)** a portion of the ampulla of man. F, fat tissue; M, smooth muscle bundles in adventitia; N, nerves; V, veins; AD, adventitia; AL, external longitudinal muscle; R, intermediate circular muscle; IL, internal longitudinal muscle; El, longitudinal elastic fibers; Er, ring-shaped elastic fibers; L, main lumen; AB, gland-like outpouching of the main lumen; SF, folds of mucosa. (From ref. 816.)

rived from the Wolffian duct, correspond to the seminal vesicles (205).

The seminal vesicles are paired, bag-shaped glands in man, stallion, rat, and guinea pig, although the internal surface may be thrown into an intricate system of folds to form irregular diverticula (Fig.21). In other mammals, such as the bull, ram, and boar (206), the seminal vesicles consist of compact glandular tissue arranged in multiple lobes and containing a system of ramified secretory ducts. The epithelium is generally pseudostratified, consisting of a row of round basal cells and a row of larger low columnar cells. The remainder of the gland is completed by loose connective tissue, a layer of smooth muscle, and an external sheet of connective tissue. The guinea pig seminal vesicle has been used as a model system for studies of the differential action of hormones on the epithelium versus the stroma, due to the ease of stripping the epithelium from the underlying tissue (207,208).

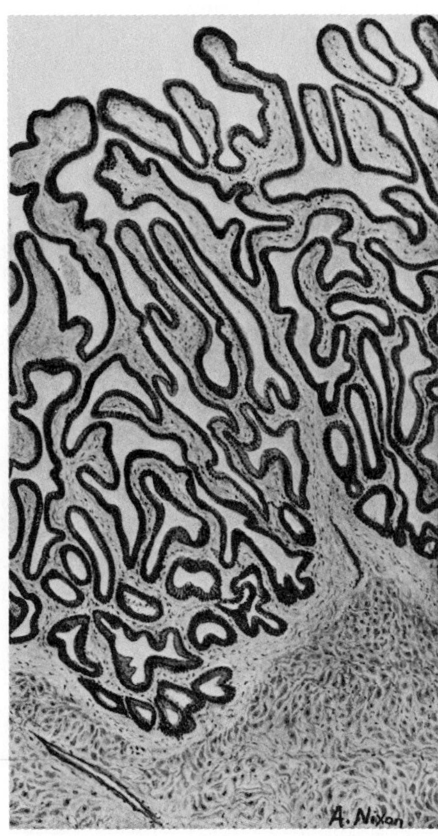

FIG. 21. Section through the wall of the human seminal vesicle. The mucosa is thrown into an intricate system of folds with the epithelium overlying the lamina propria. The smooth muscle layer occupies the lower part of the tissue section. (From ref. 816.)

Prostate

The prostate, apparently so named due to its location anterior to the bladder and seminal vesicles, is present in essentially all mammalian species (Table 1), but has a widely varying morphology. It is not our intention to make an exhaustive review of the prostate in all species and the reader is referred to the more extensive systematic coverage of Eckstein and Zuckerman (195).

The prostate is a compound tubuloalveolar gland. It is classified as disseminate or diffuse if the glandular acini remain within the lamina propria around the urethra without penetrating the surrounding voluntary muscle. On the other hand, if the gland forms a definite body outside the urethral muscle, it is classified as discrete. In some species, such as the bull and boar, both types of prostatic tissue may be present. The prostate may frequently be referred to as "lobed," although some confusion surrounds the use of this term. It may refer to separate and distinct anatomical structures, to histologically discrete areas within a given structure, to zones that respond differentially to hormones, or to zones with differential propensity to metastasis.

The human prostate is frequently described as a compact gland about the size of a chestnut, weighing approximately 20 g. It surrounds the urethra at the base of the bladder with the two ejaculatory ducts penetrating the gland through its posterior surface close to its upper border. The organ contains between 30 and 50 tubuloalveolar glands which empty into the prostatic urethra via 15 to 30 ducts. Calcified concretions which may exceed 1 mm in diameter exist in the secretion within the lumen of the acini (Fig. 22). The gland was considered by early anatomists to be reasonably homogeneous, but more recent studies have shown this not to

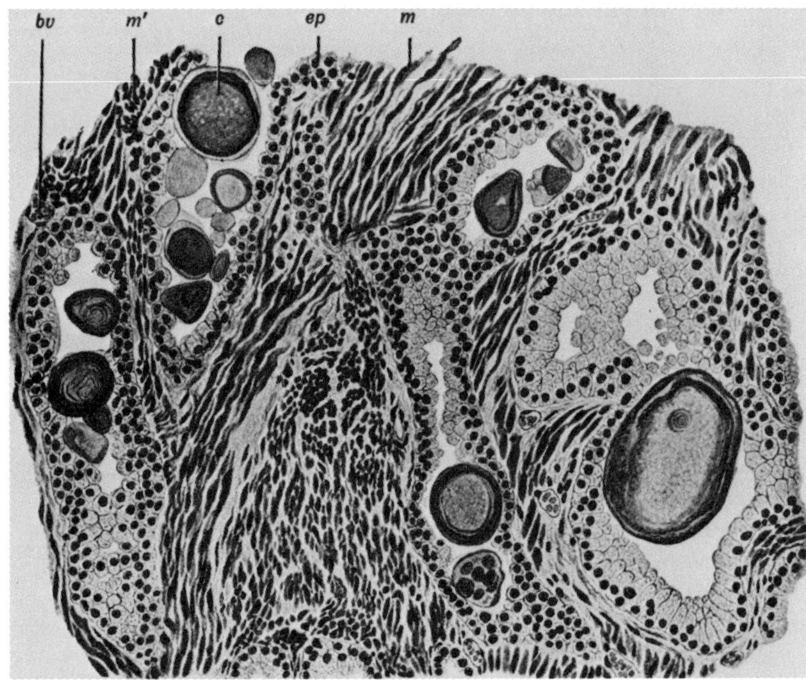

FIG. 22. Section through portion of the human prostate. bv, Blood vessels; c, concretions; ep, epithelium lining the glandular acini; m, smooth muscle in longitudinal section; m′, smooth muscle in cross-section. (From ref. 816.)

be correct. There is, nevertheless, still some dispute as to the precise subdivision of the gland (e.g., ref. 209). A detailed anatomical study (210) recognizes three glandular regions, the peripheral zone, central zone, and preprostatic region surrounded by a thick anterior fibromuscular stroma. Benign prostatic hyperplasia is specifically restricted to the preprostatic region.

The dog prostate has been a popular experimental system for studies of prostatic function for several reasons. It is the only accessory gland in this species, and when stimulated with pilocarpine hydrocholoride, large quantities of pure prostatic secretion can be obtained (211,212). Moreover, the canine prostate has a tendency to hypertrophy, and thus provides a suitable model system in which to study this aspect of human pathology.

The rat prostate is also a popular experimental system, particularly for studies of androgenic control of male accessory glands. The rat prostate is a complex structure with several distinct anatomical lobes (Fig. 3). Some confusion surrounded the classification of these lobes in early descriptions. The currently accepted classification encompasses the ventral prostate, which is a bilobed structure situated ventral to the urethra, and the dorsolateral prostate, which is comprised of a clearly separate medial portion and two lateral lobes located over the dorsolateral aspect of the urethra. The coagulating gland is an additional lobe of the prostate and was previously known as the anterior prostate. It lies adjacent to the seminal vesicles, with which it shares a common peritoneal sheath. A detailed morphological and histological study of the rat prostatic complex has been made recently (204). The ventral, lateral, and dorsal lobes of the prostate are each drained into the urethra by multiple ducts, whereas each coagulating gland is drained by a single duct.

The guinea pig contains a prostatic complex and coagulating gland complex, each consisting of six to seven lobes bound closely together by loose areolar tissue and entering by individual ducts into a common ejaculatory chamber (213). Each major lobe is subdivided peripherally into finger-like lobules. The authors consider that subdivision of the prostatic lobes into discrete dorsal, ventral, and lateral entities cannot be justified. Histologically, the prostatic lobes can be seen to be simple tubular glands, whereas the coagulating glands are tubuloalveolar in type. The epithelium is described as stratified, consisting of a superficial columnar secretory layer overlying a basal layer. In all probability, fine structural studies may reveal that the superficial columnar cells extend to the basement membrane, in which case the epithelium would be more correctly described as pseudostratified.

The disseminate prostate of marsupials is generally carrot-shaped, except in bandicoots and the koala in which it is described as heart-shaped and surrounded by a thick striated muscle coat (80,214). The prostate may attain considerable size during the breeding season when it may be the largest organ in the body cavity after the liver (215). Histologically, the prostate can be divided into two to three segments arranged along the urethra or ventral and dorsal to it (214). The segments contain numerous simple branched tubular glands lined by a single layer of columnar cells and empty via collecting ducts into the urethra.

Bulbourethral Glands

Bulbourethral glands or Cowper's glands are multilobular compound, tubular, or tubuloalveolar glands (216) present in the majority of mammals, but absent in aquatic mammals, mustelids, bears, and dogs (195) (Table 1). The glands are especially large in the boar (217). A single pair of glands is usually present, but there may be as many as three pairs in some marsupials (80,214,218). The glands are compact and smooth-surfaced being located near the bulb of the penis and connected to the urethra by a duct (219). The glands are divided by connective tissue septa containing a net of elastic fibers together with both smooth and striated muscle fibers, and the whole gland is surrounded by a fibroelastic capsule and a thick striated compressor muscle. Striated muscle fibers are apparently absent from the septa in ruminants (cattle, goats, and sheep) which also have an exceptionally thick collagenous capsule (216). The alveoli of the glands are lined with mucous-like cells (Fig. 23), and the ducts by a single layer of cuboidal or squamous cells (220,221).

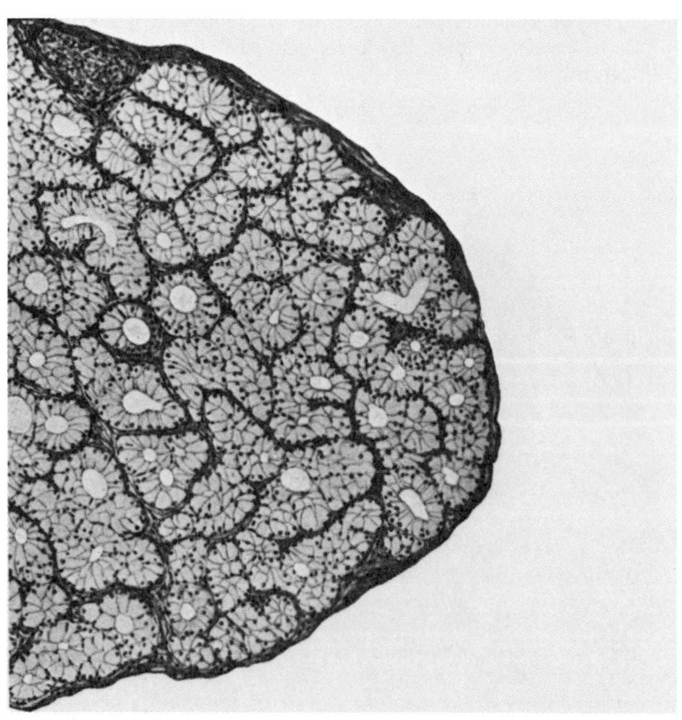

FIG. 23. Section through portion of the human bulbourethral (Cowper's) gland. The gland in man is about the size of a pea and is divided into lobules, a portion of which is shown in the figure. The section shows individual acini surrounded by a thin layer of smooth muscle. (From ref. 816.)

Urethral Glands

The urethral glands or glands of Littré are multiple mucosal glands opening into the cavernous portion of the urethra in man (Fig. 24). Some of the glands are simple outpocketings of the urethral mucosa, whereas others are more globular and connected to the urethra by a short duct. Earlier reports of the presence of urethral glands in the bull have since been refuted (199), but they are clearly present in the boar (217).

Preputial Glands

Preputial glands are found in rodents, where they lie beneath the preputial skin, and open, each by a main secretory duct, into the preputial sac near its free margin (Fig. 3). A homologous gland occurs in female rodents. The gross morphology of the gland has been described as "flask-like" in the rat and "leaf-like" in the mouse. The gland is usually regarded as a hypertrophied and modified sebaceous gland, but on a histological basis this may be an oversimplification. Histological studies (222–224) show the gland to contain dense epithelioid acini supported by thin connective tissue trabeculae, which are continuous with the capsule of the organ. The rat gland has a dense parenchyma and a ramifying system of ductules (Fig. 25a). In comparison, the parenchyma of the mouse gland is much less dense with fewer acini and large cavernous ductular spaces (Fig. 25b). There is evidence that the preputial gland of the rat, but not the mouse, produces a nonlipid secretion in addition to the normal lipid secretion characteristic of sebaceous glands. Smaller glands, but of similar structure, can be found surrounding the prepuce of the rabbit (201).

BLOOD VASCULAR SYSTEM

Spermatic Cord and Pampiniform Plexus

In those mammals whose testes descend into a scrotum, the testicular arteries retain their origin from the abdominal aorta and become elongated as the testes migrate. The elongation is greater than is necessary to allow for the movement of the testis, with the result that, in the eutherian mammals, the artery also becomes extensively coiled, particularly in the section outside the inguinal canal (Fig. 26,27a). In the large domestic ruminants and in the pig, as much as 5 m of artery can be tightly coiled up into approximately 10 cm of spermatic cord (see refs. 2,142,225,226). The thickness of the wall and the number of layers of smooth muscle cells decreases along the length of the artery (227). In marsupials, as the testicular artery passes through the inguinal canal, it divides into an arterial rete of up to 200 parallel branches, which run in the spermatic cord to the testis, where they reunite to form two or three arterial trunks which supply the testis (80,228).

The veins leaving the testis divide near the dorsal pole to form a venous plexus, called the pampiniform plexus (Fig. 27b) from its resemblance to a mass of vine tendrils. These venous branches surround the coiled artery in the eutherian mammals, and lie interspersed among the branches of the arterial rete in the marsupials, until approximately the level of the inguinal canal, where they reunite progres

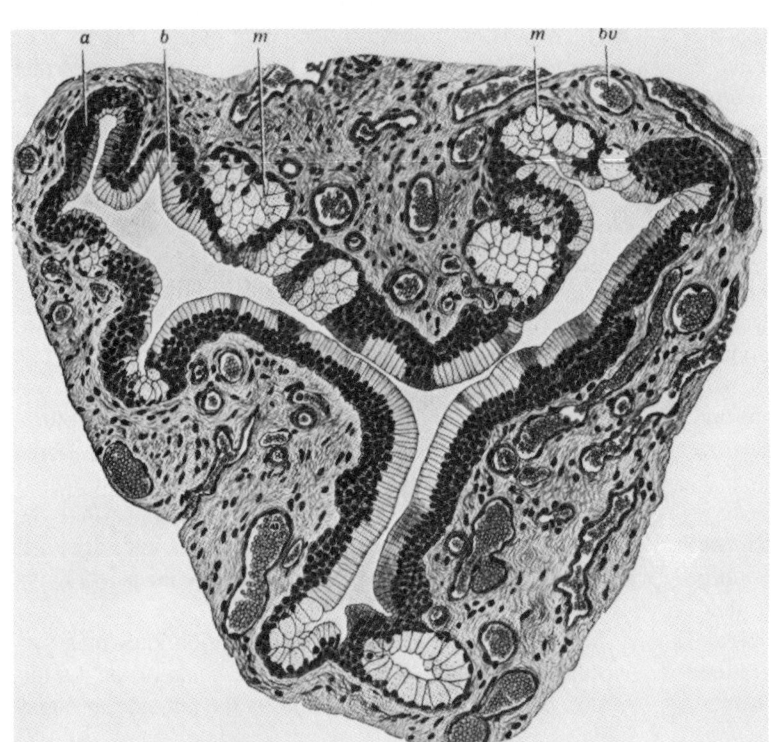

FIG. 24. Section through human urethral glands (glands of Littré) from the cavernous part of the urethra. The glands run obliquely in the lamina propria and may penetrate deep into the spongy body of the penis. The lumen is lined with the same epithelium as the mucus membrane of the urethra, but containing intraepithelial nests of clear mucous cells. a, Darkly staining stratified columnar epithelium; b, epithelium with clear cells; bv, blood vessels; m, outpocketings with clear mucous cells. (From ref. 816.)

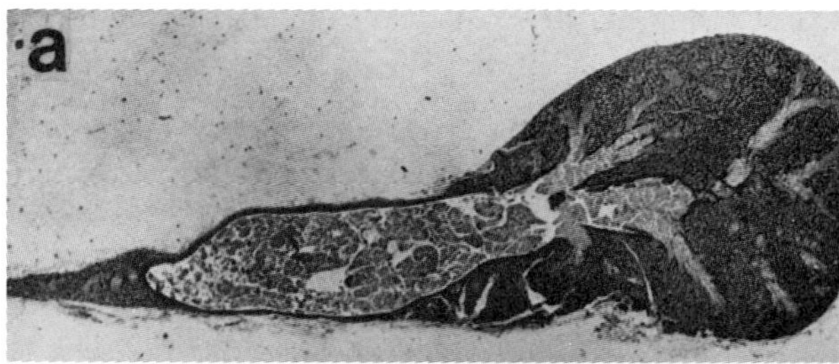

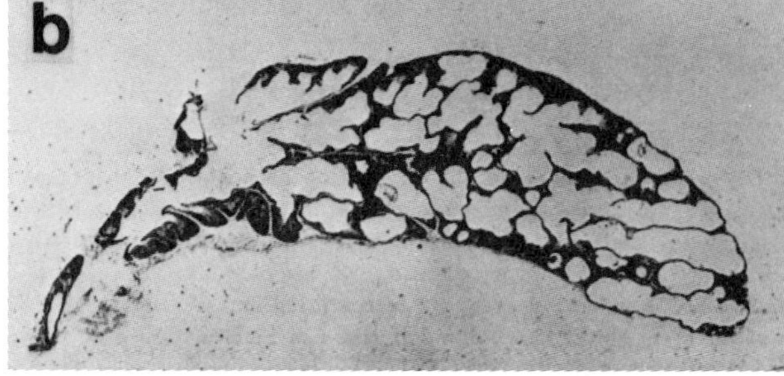

FIG. 25. Longitudinal section of the preputial gland of **(a)** rat and **(b)** mouse. (From ref. 817.)

sively to form several large venous trunks, which eventually empty either into the vena cava, the renal vein, the hypogastric, or common iliac vein (see Fig. 39; refs. 2,142, 229,230). Within the plexus in bulls, there are three classes of veins; the first type are large (approximately 200 μm diameter), with four to six layers of smooth muscle cells in their walls, and run parallel to one another, surrounding the testicular artery. The second class are smaller (40–70 μm), lack smooth muscle cells, and are arranged in a less organized pattern. The third class of veins occupy a periarterial or intramural location, often at the junction between the media and adventitia of the artery (Fig. 28a–c). Veins of the three classes communicate with one another, and none of the veins in the plexus have valves (227), in contrast to those immediately above it (433). A slightly simpler but similar arrangement is found in the rat, with the larger veins showing sac-like pouching and constriction bands in the wall; there are two types of venules, long smooth-surfaced and short saccular ones (230,231). Around the outside of this vascular complex, there are a number of sizable lymphatic vessels that originate from the testis and epididymis. The whole cord is encased in a peritoneal covering, with the cremaster muscle on one side. The ductus deferens and its associated deferential artery and veins run in a separate fold of peritoneum into the abdominal cavity.

This curious arrangement has a number of consequences (Fig. 29). First, the pulse is almost eliminated from the arterial blood as it flows through the cord, with only minor changes in mean pressure (232,233). Second, the spermatic cord acts as a very efficient counter-current heat exchanger, so that the arterial blood is cooled from body temperature to scrotal temperature by the venous blood, which leaves the testis at a temperature similar to that under the scrotal skin; at the same time the venous blood is warmed to body temperature by the arterial blood (233–235). A similar arrangement is found in the extremities of a number of animals living in cold environments, but, in these cases, the function is clearly to prevent heat loss to the surroundings (see ref. 142). In the testis, it is probably more to maintain the testis and epididymis at a temperature lower than that of the abdominal cavity, though why this should be an advantage is not clear. The system does ensure that an even temperature is maintained throughout the testis, and there is no doubt that the function of the testis is deranged if its temperature is raised to body temperature for more than a short period (see ref. 2). There is also evidence that substances can cross from the arterial blood to the venous blood by diffusion or transport through the vessel walls. Whereas this undoubtedly occurs for a number of marker substances such as inert gases (236,237) and tritiated water (238), it appears to be of trivial quantitative significance for all the physiologically important substances so far studied. Unless active transport against a concentration gradient is invoked, the system would only operate for a substance produced or utilized by the testis, producing a locally increased or decreased concentration in the tissue, respectively. An obvious candidate is testosterone, but the increase in the concentration in the arterial blood as it passes through the cord (239) is insignificant when compared with the difference between venous and arterial blood (see Testis Blood Flow and Composition, p. 797). However, the transfer of testosterone to the epididymis or the fat pad may be of much greater importance.

One of the most interesting findings of recent years has been the demonstration of arteriovenous anastomoses in the spermatic cord of sheep and pigs. Experimental evidence for these was first sought by de Graaf over 300 years ago, but he could find none. Several later authors suggested that these anastomoses did exist (see ref. 142 for early references), but it was only recently that conclusive anatomical (227,240) and functional evidence for their existence has been obtained. It now seems that as much as 40% of the blood flowing through the testicular artery into the cord may return to the venous system without passing through the testis, even when all the vessels to the epididymis are ligated (241,242). The significance and control of these anastomoses require further study and they cannot be found in rats (231).

In mammals whose testes do not descend into a scrotum, there is no spermatic cord, but the artery does show some elongation and coiling in those species in which the testis migrates within the abdominal cavity. In animals like the elephant and hyrax, in which the testis does not migrate at all, the artery is simple and runs straight into the parenchyma of the testis (see ref. 142).

In humans, there is a common condition known as varicocoele, which is a varicosity of the veins of the pampiniform plexus. It is usually found on the left side, but may

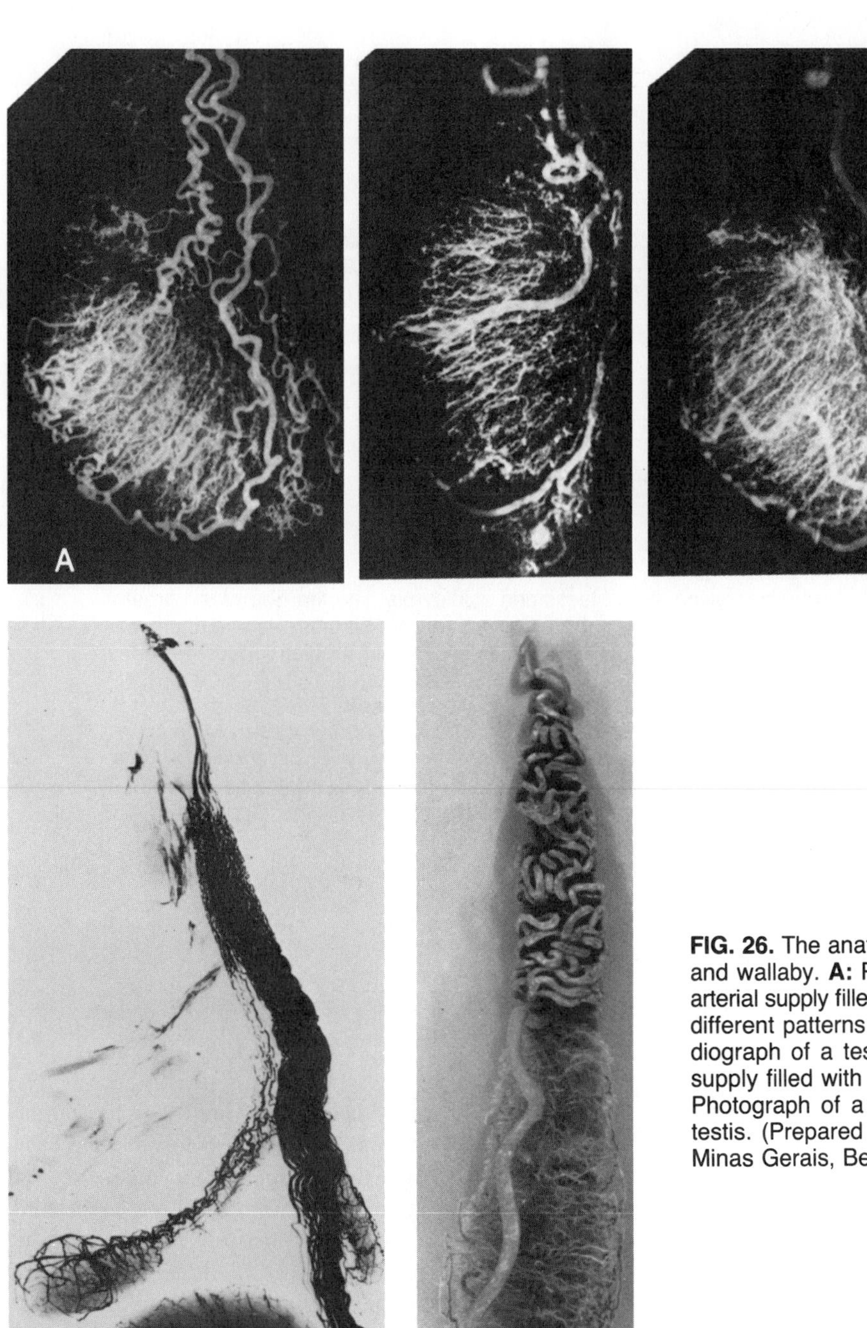

FIG. 26. The anatomy of the testicular artery of human, bull, and wallaby. **A:** Radiograph of three human testes with the arterial supply filled with radio-opaque medium, showing some different patterns of arterial supply. (From ref. 818.) **B:** Radiograph of a testis of a tammar wallaby, with the arterial supply filled with radio-opaque medium. (From ref. 819.) **C:** Photograph of a resin cast of the arterial supply to a bull testis. (Prepared by Professor H. P. Godinho, University of Minas Gerais, Belo Horizonte, Brazil.)

be bilateral and is probably due to incompetence of the valves in the main vein near where it opens into the renal vein. This can lead to retrograde flow of blood down the plexus, returning to the general circulation through anastomoses with the cremasteric or scrotal vessels. Many authors believe that this condition is associated with lowered fertility (see refs. 243–247), but a recent detailed statistical study of the fertility of normal men and men with varicocoele found no evidence that men with varicocoele were less fertile or that their fertility was improved by ligation of the varicocoele (248). Why varicocoele should cause infertility is not certain, although a number of possible

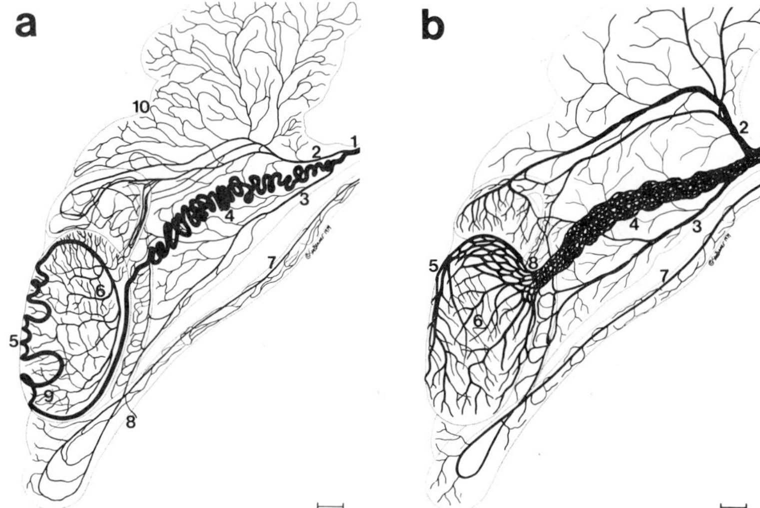

FIG. 27. Arrangement of arteries and veins supplying the rat testis and epididymis. The margins of the organs are shown in *stippled outline.* Blood vessels are drawn to accurately reflect relative dimensions and to provide a three-dimensional view. *Solid black lines* designate blood vessels closest to the medial surface whereas vessels coursing near the lateral surface appear as *discontinuous lines.* **a:** Arterial system: 1, spermatic artery; 2, superior epididymal artery; 3, inferior epididymal artery; 4, testicular artery; 5, capsular artery; 6, intratesticular artery; 7, vas deferential artery; 8, cremasteric artery; 9, intratesticular artery-artery anastomosis; 10, epididymal fat pad artery-artery anastomosis. **b:** Venous system: 1, spermatic vein; 2, superior epididymal vein; 3, inferior epididymal vein; 4, pampiniform plexus; 5, testicular surface vein; 6, intratesticular vein; 7, vas deferential vein; 8, anastomosis between testicular surface and efferent ductule veins. Scale bar = 2.7 mm. (From ref. 250.)

mechanisms have been suggested; the most recent suggestion is that dilated veins in the mediastinum cause obstruction to the excurrent ducts (249).

Testis

Testicular Artery

By the time the artery reaches the surface of the scrotal testis, it is comparatively thin-walled, so that in its course along the surface of the testis, it has a flattened profile. Instead of penetrating directly into the parenchyma, in many species the artery runs for a considerable distance in the tunic, often running along the epididymal margin to the caudal pole before branching. In the rabbit, the artery encircles the testis completely before branching, and the two initial branches then make a further half-circuit before branching again. In the rat, the artery runs straight down the epididymal margin of the testis, around the caudal pole, and then winds along the free surface (Fig. 27a) to enter the parenchyma near the rete before beginning to branch (see refs. 2,142,250). In many larger animals, the artery begins to branch near the caudal pole, and the convoluted branches run along the surface for some distance before turning sharply to run without further branching to near the rete; there they often form a tight coil before turning back on themselves to begin branching. In marsupials, several arteries are formed at the end of the arterial rete in the cord and these run down one face of the testis, on the opposite side to the veins (see refs. 2,80,142). In the rat, there are frequent arterioarterial anastomotic arcades and occasional arteriovenous anastomoses within the testis (231).

The sensitivity of the arterial wall to the vasoconstrictor activity of norepinephrine decreases along the length of the testicular artery in the ram, with the artery on the surface of the testis being almost unresponsive even to very large doses (251). The endothelial cells of the artery in the spermatic cord and on the surface of the postpubertal rat testis, as well as those lining the arterioles inside the testis, contain a high concentration of the enzyme γ-glutamyl transpeptidase (252); in other tissues, this enzyme is associated with amino acid transport, and the endothelial cells of the arterioles within the testis have been shown to transport leucine in a selective and saturable manner (253).

When the testicular artery was transected above the spermatic cord in young pigs, anastomoses between the testic-

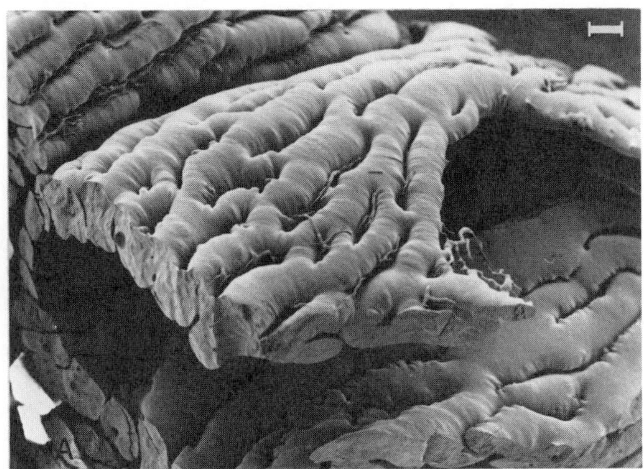

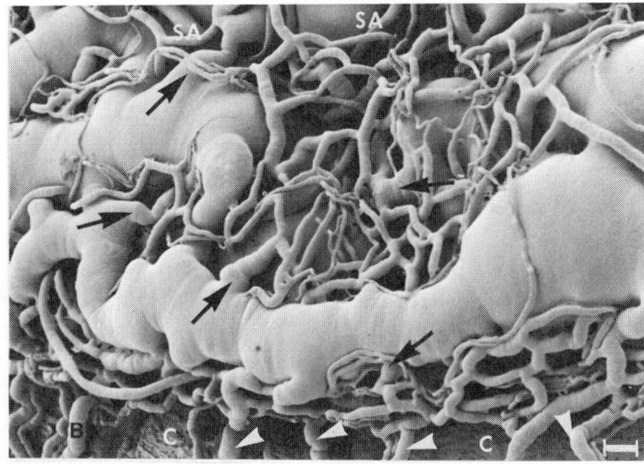

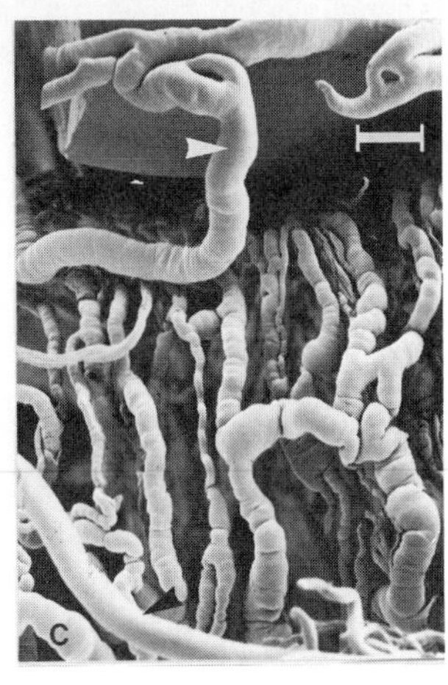

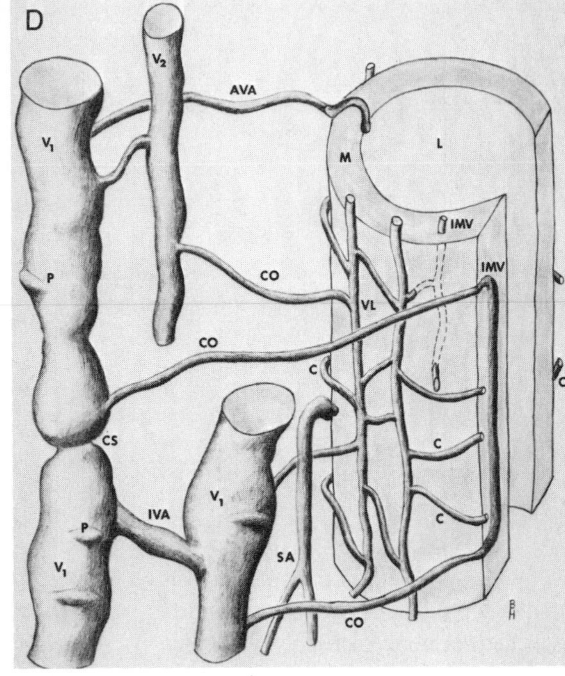

FIG. 28. The anatomy of the veins of the pampiniform plexus in the bull. **A:** Cast of the large veins of the first network, which run parallel and anastomose frequently, forming a venous covering to the testicular artery, which lies in the central empty space. Where the artery reaches the surface of the spermatic cord, the covering of veins is absent. Bar = 200 μm. **B:** Venous cast showing the first and intermediate networks of the pampiniform plexus. The large veins show varicose pouches. The *arrows* indicate connections between the two networks and the *arrowheads* point to connecting veins joining the periarterial venous network (C), seen faintly in the background. SA, small branches of the testicular artery. Bar = 100 μm. **C:** Cast of the third periarterial venous network, consisting of venules and venous capillaries. The venules show characteristic constrictions along their course. The *arrowhead* shows a connecting vein running from the periarterial network to the first venous network at the top. Bar = 100 μm. **D:** A diagram illustrating the arrangement of the three venous networks (V1, V2, and VL, respectively). A small arterial branch (SA) of the testicular artery and an arteriovenous anastomosis (AVA) are also shown. L, lumen of testicular artery; M, media of wall of testicular artery; C, venous capillaries of the third venous network; CO, connecting veins linking the periarterial and the other venous networks; IVA, anastomosis between veins of the first and second network; IMV, intramural venule of the periarterial network; P, pouches; and CS, constrictions in the veins. (From ref. 227.)

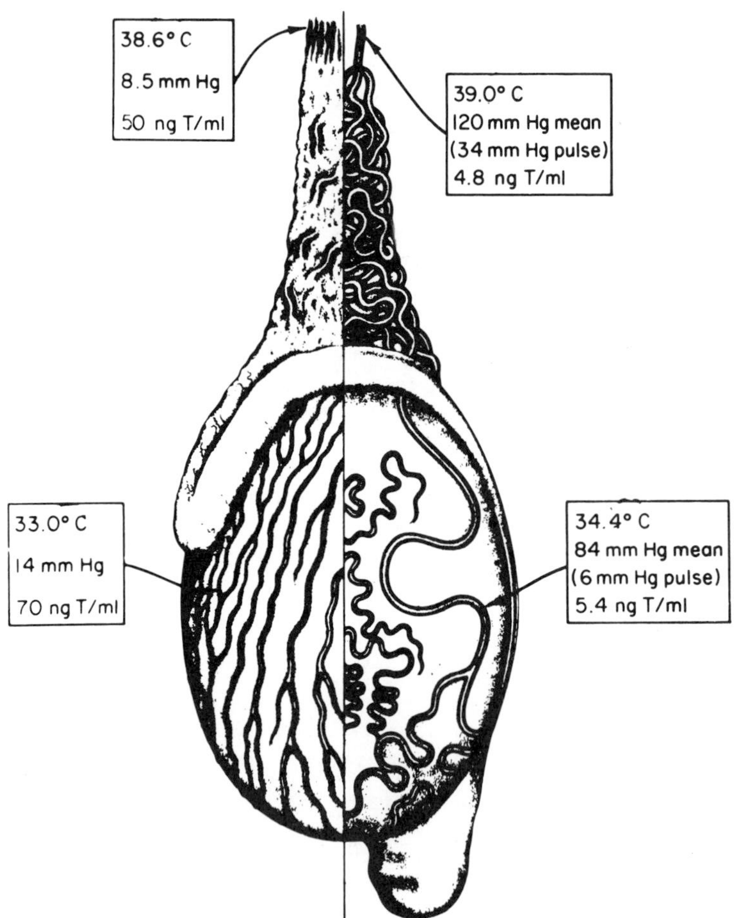

FIG. 29. The effects of the spermatic cord on blood temperature, pressure, and concentrations of testosterone. A composite diagram with the arterial system shown on the *right* and the venous drainage on the *left*. The figures in the boxes give the values for blood at the point in the vascular system indicated by the *arrow tip*. (From ref. 813.)

ular and vasal arteries opened up, both in the cord and on the surface of the testis. When the animals were examined 4 months later, the testes had developed normally, testicular blood flow was only slightly reduced, and testosterone concentrations in peripheral blood were normal (254). This suggests that during orchidopexy for treatment of cryptorchidism in boys, transection of the artery might be an acceptable alternative to imposing excessive tension on the artery.

Testicular Capillaries

The capillaries of the rat testis are of two types (Fig. 30), the Zwickelcapillaren which run parallel to the seminiferous tubules and the Quercapillaren, which run around the tubular walls at approximately right angles to their long axes (231,255–258). This arrangement appears only at puberty, as does the high level of alkaline phosphatase activity seen in this species (259). The walls of the testicular capillaries, in contrast to those of all other endocrine tissues, are unfenestrated, being of the A-1-αtype (260,261), similar to those found in muscle (58). The capillaries and postcapillary venules comprise 6.2% of the interstitial tissue, 0.6% of the whole rat testis, have a total volume of 5.8 μl/g, and an endothelial surface area of 27 cm^2/g (262). The total blood volume in the rat testis is approximately 10 μl/g (263).

The permeability of the capillaries in the perfused rat testis to sodium, mannitol, chromium-ethylenediaminetetraacetic acid (Cr-EDTA), (264), and albumin (265) does not appear to be very different from that of other capillaries, but cadmium salts in subtoxic doses cause a catastrophic increase (266–268), which in a few hours leads to a virtual stoppage of blood flow (269). Ultrastructural changes in the endothelial cells can be seen within hours of the administration of cadmium (270–272), and again it is only the capillaries of the postpubertal testis that show this peculiarity (273). The permeability to albumin of the blood vessels in the rat testis increases after an injection of human chorionic gonadotropin (Fig. 31), beginning at approximately 8 hr after injection (263) and reaching a maximum after approximately 30 hr. This effect seems to be mediated to some extent by 5-hydroxytryptamine (57), but does not appear to involve androgens, estrogens, prostaglandins, histamine, or bradykinin (57,274), although it is abolished if the Leydig cells are eliminated from the testis with ethylene dimethane sulphonate (275).

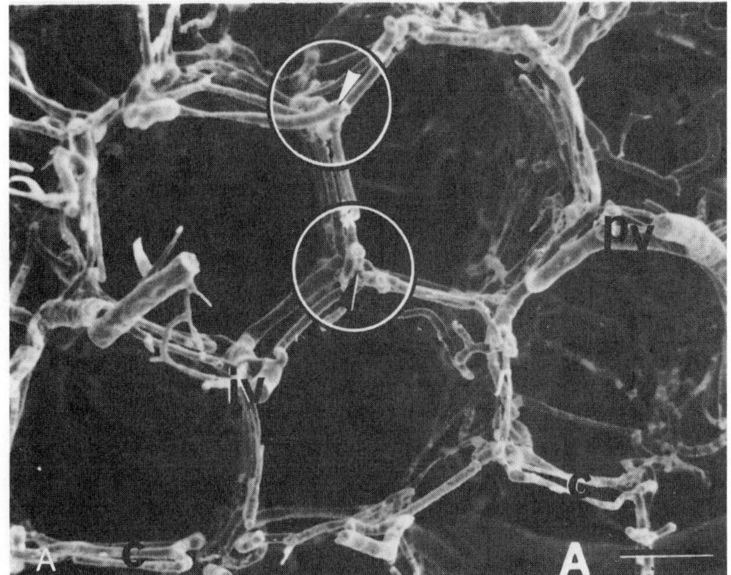

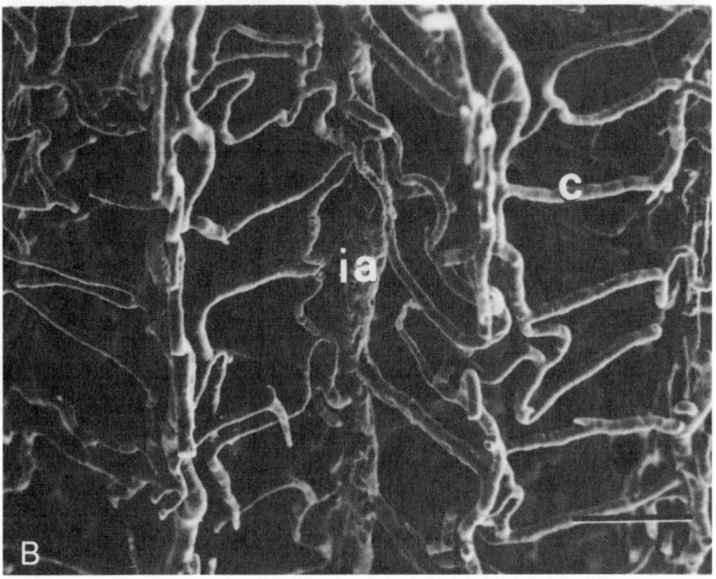

FIG. 30. The anatomy of the blood vessels in the rat testis. **A:** Cast of the blood vessels inside the testis sectioned at right angles to the seminiferous tubules, showing the three-dimensional arrangement of the intertubular and peritubular vessels. Note the clear hexagonal pattern of the vessels, with only one intertubular vessel (*arrowhead*) at each interstitial space (*circled*). iv, Intertubular venule; pv, peritubular venule; c, peritubular capillaries; A, artery. Bar = 100 μm. **B:** Cast of the blood vessels cut parallel to the seminiferous tubules. Note the wavy intertubular vessels connected by short peritubular capillaries (c) to give the appearance of a rope-ladder. ia, Intertubular arteriole. Bar = 100 μm. (From ref. 231.)

Testicular Veins

The veins of the testis are also unusual in that they do not run with a corresponding artery. The small veins in the parenchyma open either into small veins on the surface of the testis (Fig. 32) or into a group of veins near the mediastinum. The balance between these two routes depends on species, for example, the capsular veins take the majority of the blood in the ram; whereas in the stallion, the mediastinal veins are more important; in human, the two routes are of approximately equal importance. In the rat, there are two large veins on the free face of the testis that unite just where the artery enters the parenchyma; they then divide again to form over the rete a small plexus which is really an extension of the pampiniform plexus. Veins from the epididymal face join this plexus near the point where the testicular artery reaches the testis to form the pampiniform plexus proper (2,142,231,250). In marsupials, the veins drain to several main veins on the opposite side of the testis to the arteries (2,80,142).

The mean pressure in the veins on the surface of the testes of rams and boars was approximately twice that in the testicular vein above the spermatic cord (276).

Epididymis

The epididymis receives its blood from two main arterial routes (Fig. 27a). The caput, corpus, and proximal cauda epididymidis are supplied by arteries that branch from the spermatic artery just before, or soon after, it reaches the pampiniform plexus [e.g., mouse (250,257,277), rat (230,

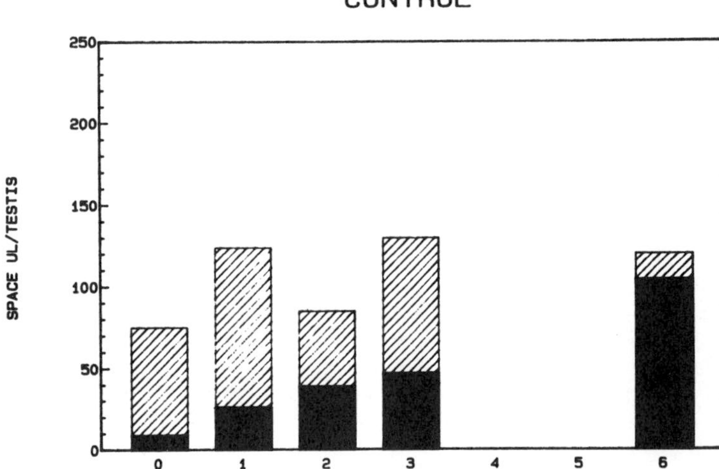

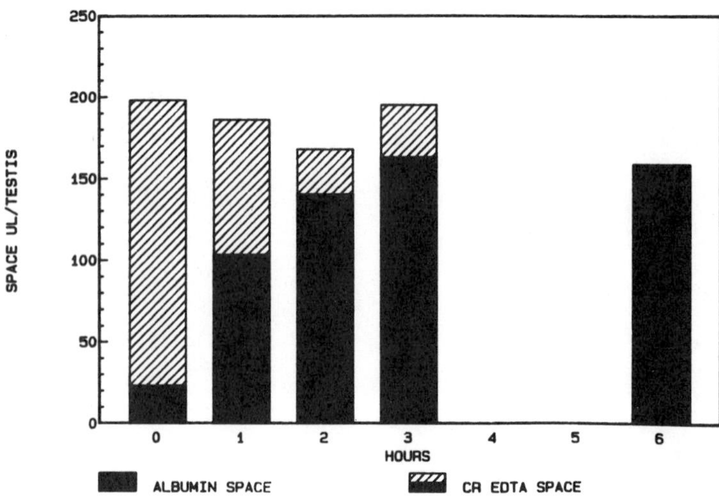

FIG. 31. The Cr-EDTA and albumin spaces in the testes of rats, and the effect of injection with hCG. The markers were injected intravenously after cutting the ureters to prevent excretion of the Cr-EDTA. At the times shown (0 hr was actually 3 min), testes and blood plasma were counted, and the spaces in μl/g calculated by dividing cpm/g testis by cpm/μl plasma. Note that the albumin space (Valb) has almost equalled the Cr-EDTA space (VCr) by 6 hr in the control rats, but that after hCG, although the Cr-EDTA space is greater, the albumin space equals it much sooner. The rate at which the alumin space approaches the Cr-EDTA space (determined from the slope of the line log) (1 − Valb/VCr) is a measure of vascular permeability to albumin. (From ref. 263.)

250,278,279), rabbit (250,280), dog (278), ram (281), camel (282), and man (278,283)], whereas the cauda epididymidis is supplied from the deferential artery, a branch from the internal iliac (hypogastric) artery. The lemur does not conform to this general pattern in that vessels supplying the caput and corpus epididymidis branch from the testicular artery after it has gained the surface of the testis rather than branching from the spermatic cord (225). There are usually two branches of the epididymal artery (Fig. 27a). The superior epididymal artery supplies the ductuli efferentes, caput and proximal corpus, whereas the inferior epididymal artery serves the corpus and proximal cauda epididymidis. Anastomoses exist between the epididymal arteries and deferential artery at the level of the surface of the epididymis (250,257,277–280,282–286). Functional anastomoses between the superior epididymal artery and the testicular artery and between the deferential artery and the testicular artery have also been reported (256,278,283,285,287,288). The epididymal arteries ramify on the surface of the epididymis and enter the organ centripetally within the connective tissue septula which divide the epididymis into zones. Each septal artery provides branches to both adjacent zones to form capillary networks around the tubule.

The epididymal veins follow the same route as their respective arteries (Fig. 27b). As with the arterial system, extensive anastomoses occur among the epididymal veins. In the rat, the inferior epididymal vein forms a plexus which completely surrounds the proximal portion of the inferior epididymal artery (230). A similar arrangement has been described in the rabbit for the superior and inferior epididymal veins and the deferential vein (250). These plexus systems may function as a countercurrent heat exchange system to cool the epididymal blood supply in an analogous fashion to the pampiniform plexus. Veins have also been shown to form vascular connections between the testis and ductuli efferentes in the mouse, rat, and rabbit (250); in the rat and rabbit there is also a venous connection between the posterior pole of the testis and the cauda epididymidis (250,256).

The microvasular structure of the epididymis has been

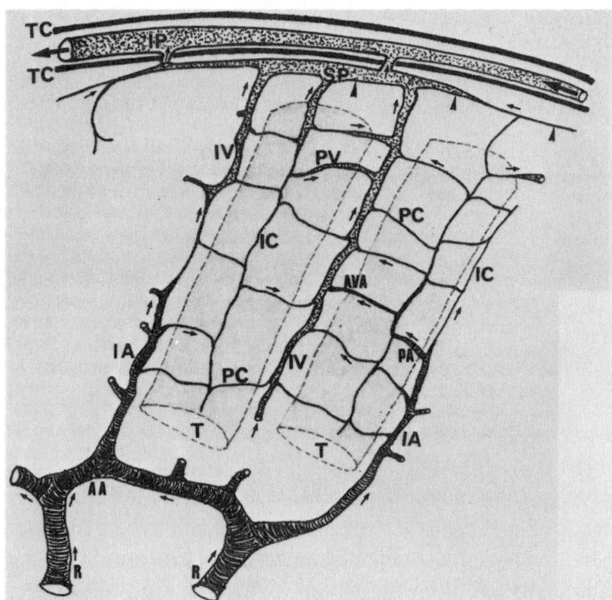

FIG. 32. A diagram of the blood vessels in the testis of a rat, in a plane parallel to the seminiferous tubules. The direction of blood flow is indicated by the *arrows.* T, seminiferous tubules; R, radiate arteries; AA, arterioarterial anastomotic arcade; IA, intertubular arteriole; IC, intertubular capillary; PA, peritubular arteriole; PC, peritubular capillary; PV, peritubular venule; AVA, arteriovenous anastomosis; IP, intra-albugineal plexus within the testicular capsule (TC); SP, subalbugineal plexus, with *arrowheads* indicating its component vein, venule, and capillary, respectively, from left to right. Venovenous anastomoses in this area are not shown. (From ref. 231.)

the subject of a number of studies using a variety of techniques. In the now classical study of Kormano (279), the microangiographic technique revealed significant differences in the capillary arrangement in different regions of the epididymis. In the initial segment of the epididymis, capillaries form a dense and tortuous network around the tubules. In the middle segment of the epididymis, the density and tortuosity of the capillaries is reduced and the capillaries follow the wall of the epididymal duct more closely. As the muscle wall thickens in the terminal segment of the epididymis, the capillaries tend to form two separate networks around the epididymal duct. One network is located in the interductular connective tissue and this sends branches to a second network surrounding the lamina propria. A similar study of the human epididymis (289) reveals some differences when compared to the rat. The principal differences concern a thick densely vascularized connective tissue sheath surrounding the human epididymis and an extensive degree of coiling of the arteries which penetrate into the organ among the connective tissue septula. Few branches are given off before the septal arteries disperse into the fine microvascular bed. The human ductuli efferentes are supplied by a relatively dense subepithelial capillary bed. The capillary bed of the epididymis is less extensive and, in contrast to the rat, the organization of the capillary network does not show much variation along the length of the epididymis.

A more recent technique of casting coupled with scanning electron microscopy has been applied to examine the microvasculature of the mouse epididymis (257), which largely confirms the features described in the rat (279). The ductuli efferentes are supplied with vessels that run longitudinally and give off peritubular capillaries analogous to the arrangement seen within the testis (Fig. 30). A similar arrangement is present in the middle segment of the epididymis (Figs. 33a,34a). By contrast, in the initial segment, peritubular capillaries penetrate the thin muscular layer and form a dense

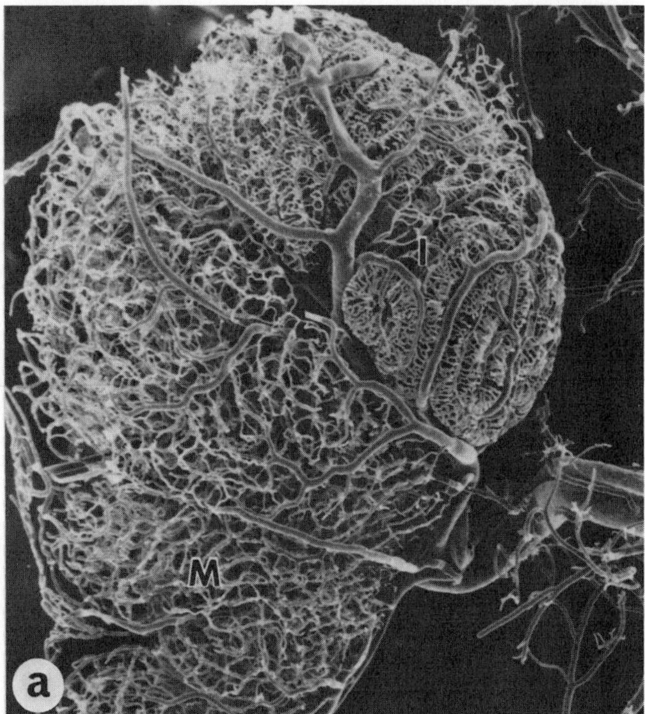

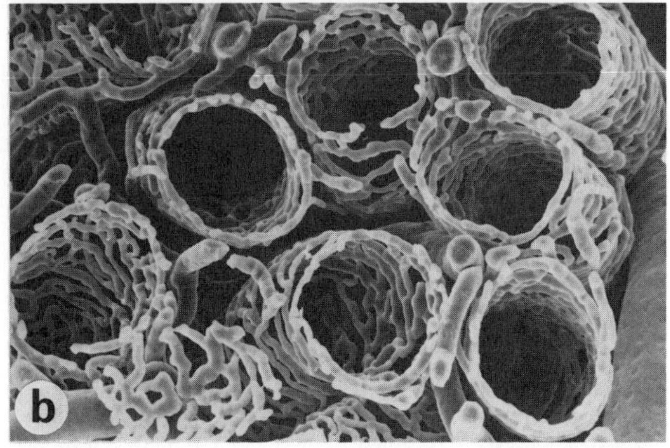

FIG. 33. Microvasculature of the initial and middle segments of the mouse epididymis. **a:** In the initial segment (I) peritubular capillaries form a dense cylindrical subepithelial network with frequent interconnections, while in the middle segment (M) peritubular capillaries branch from longitudinal vessels and do not interconnect. **b:** View of the cut surface of the initial segment to reveal the dense network of interconnected peritubular capillaries. Larger vessels can be seen running in the interstitial spaces. (From ref. 257.)

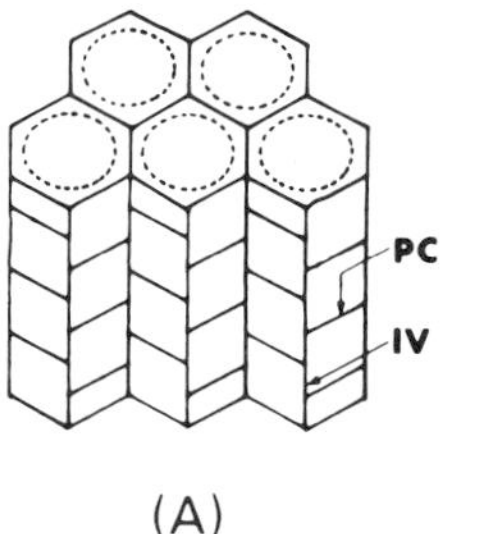

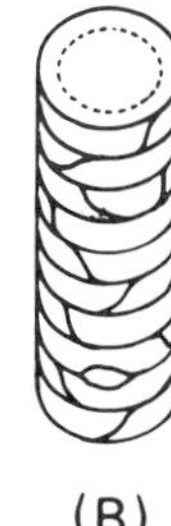

FIG. 34. Diagrammatic representation of the two fundamental types of peritubular capillaries seen in the mouse testis and excurrent duct system. The arrangement in the testis and middle segment of the epididymis is depicted in **(A),** whereas **(B)** represents the arrangement in the initial segment and ductus deferens. The tubule is depicted by the *dotted line* and the intertubular vessels (IV) are simplified as a single straight line joined by peritubular capillars (PC). (From ref. 257.)

cylindrical subepithelial network with frequent interconnections (Figs. 33a,b, and 34b).

Ultrastructural analysis reveals that the capillaries of the initial segment are fenestrated, whereas those in the remainder of the epididymis are not (257,277). The presence of fenestrated capillaries in the initial segment may be an adaptation to the specific role of this region of the epididymis in the reabsorption of the bulk of the rete testis fluid which enters the epididymis. Indeed, the development and continued presence of fenestrated capillaries is dependent on the efferent ducts being patent, since the fenestrations are markedly reduced following section of the ducts (277). This specific role of the initial segment in fluid reabsorption is also reflected by the fact that the blood flow to this region is substantially greater than in any other part of the epididymis (290,291). Moreover, the enhanced blood flow in the initial segment is abolished after efferent duct ligation or castration (291).

Ductus Deferens

Blood travels to the ductus deferens by way of the internal iliac, hypogastric, and finally the deferential artery. The returning venous blood travels in the deferential vein which returns along the ductus deferens and empties into the hypogastric vein. It is clear from microangiographic studies that the microvascular bed surrounding the ductus deferens forms two separate networks (279,289). The outer network is located within the connective tissue surrounding the muscle layers and from this small arteries penetrate through the muscle to the lamina propria, where they form a dense subepithelial capillary network. More sophisticated corrosion casting and scanning electron microscopy have confirmed this arrangement and revealed additional features (192,257,286). In the distal two-thirds of the rat ductus deferens and also in the mouse ductus deferens, a sinusoidal layer is found beneath the muscle layer (Fig. 35a). Arterial branches penetrate from the adventitial layer centripetally through the muscle layer supplying capillaries to the muscular tissue *en route*. When they reach the lamina propria these arteries break up into arterioles, some of which end in a sinusoidal layer while others penetrate through this network to form a subepithelial capillary network (Fig. 34b) reminiscent of that seen in the initial segment of the epididymis (Fig. 33). The subepithelial capillary network drains into the sinusoidal network, which is in turn drained by venules that pass through the muscle layers, collecting capillaries from the muscle layers on the way, and joining veins in the adventitia. Conspicuous constrictions are present in the venules at the point at which they leave the sinusoidal network (Fig. 35b).

The exact function of the sinusoidal layer in the ductus deferens is unknown at present. It is possible that engorgement of the sinusoidal network could be achieved by further contraction of the sphincter-like constrictions present in the venules which drain the system. Thus the sinusoidal layer may function as a device to increase pressure within the lumen of the ductus deferens during ejaculation.

Prostate and Seminal Vesicles

The blood supply to the accessory glands of the rat has been described by Jesik et al. (204). The arterial supply can be traced from the aorta to the common iliac arteries, which divide to form the internal and external iliac arteries. The internal iliac artery, otherwise known as the hypogastric artery, supplies the prostate, bladder, coagulating glands, seminal vesicles, and vasa deferentia (Fig. 36). The superior vesical artery leaves from the ventral surface of the internal iliac and supplies branches to the seminal vesicles and coagulating glands, and continues to supply branches to the dorsal, lateral, and ventral prostatic lobes, and to the vasa deferentia (deferential arteries) and ureters (ureteral arteries). The inferior vesical artery leaves the superior vesical artery at the point where it meets the urinary bladder. It supplies blood to the dorsal surface of the prostate and the bladder, anastomosing with the superior vesical artery.

The venous drainage of the rat accessory glands has been studied in detail by Lewis and Moffat (229), and the organization described by them has been largely confirmed by Ohtani and Gannon (286). The general arrangement is depicted in Fig. 37. The deferential vein draining the cauda epididymidis and ductus deferens empties into the hypogastric vein, as does the left spermatic vein from the testis and veins from the seminal vesicle and coagulating gland. The hypogastric vein drains at one end into the external iliac vein, but at its other end it joins a single large circular anastomosis formed by dorsal and ventral veins surrounding the base of the bladder. The ventral prostatic lobes drain by straight veins directly into this venous circle around the bladder and the term "prostatic veins" has been suggested for them. Lewis and Moffat (229) considered that veins

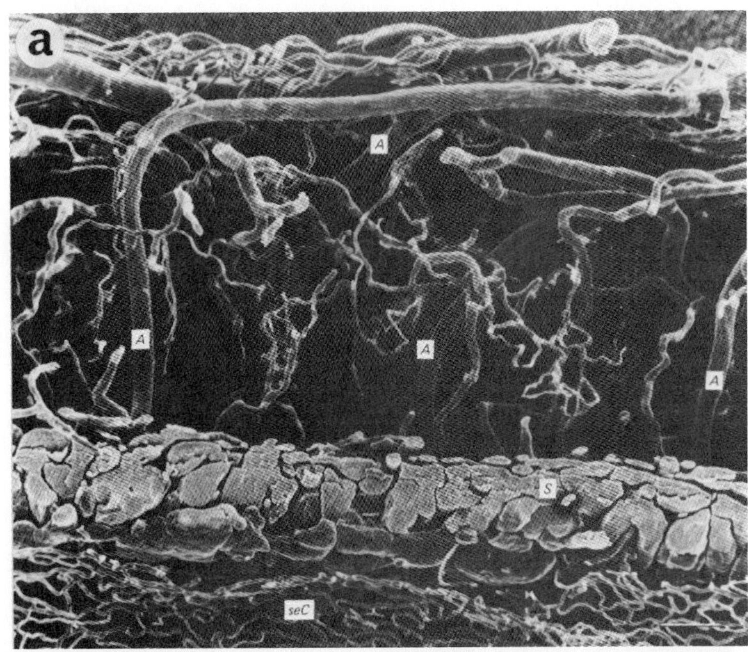

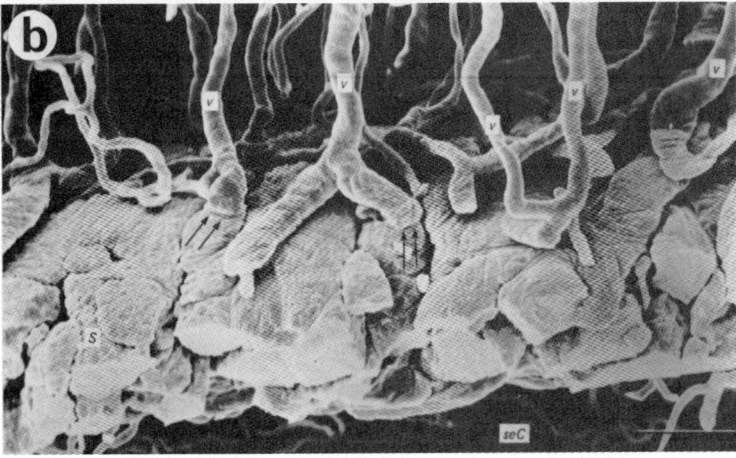

FIG. 35. Corrosion cast of the vascular supply to the rat ductus deferens. **a:** The major blood vessels run in the adventitia and send arterial branches (A) through the muscle layer where they supply a sinusoidal layer (S) and a subepithelial network (seC). **b:** Detailed view of the sinusoidal layer (S) being drained by venules (V) with prominent constrictions (*arrows*) located at the point of departure of these vessels from the sinusoidal layer. (From ref. 286.)

from the dorsolateral prostate also drain into the venous circle, but Ohtani and Gannon (286) claim that the drainage of this gland and of the distal vas deferens is into the vein leaving the seminal vesicle. The particular anatomy of the venous system may allow intermittent reversed flow from the hypogastric vein, thus carrying the drainage from the cauda epididymidis and ductus deferens into the prostatic complex. A similar vascular arrangement would allow retrograde flow from the deferential vein into the canine prostate (292). Such an event may explain the observed local control of the accessory sex glands by the epididymis and ductus deferens (293). It is assumed that the local factors responsible are androgens traveling in the deferential vein. In fact the concentration of steroid hormones measured in the deferential vein of the dog are an order of magnitude greater than in peripheral plasma (294).

The arterial supply to the seminal vesicles and prostate of man has been the subject of a number of studies (295–297). There is considerable variation between specimens in the arrangement of the blood vessels and some confusion has arisen due to differences in the nomenclature used to describe the vessels. It seems that the main arterial supply is derived from the anterior division of the internal iliac (hypogastric) artery. From this vessel arise the umbilical, vesiculodeferential and prostatovesical arteries. The superior vesical branches from the umbilical artery near its junction with the internal iliac artery, whereas the origin of the vesiculodeferential and prostatovesical arteries is variable. The seminal vesicles and ductus deferens are supplied by branches from the vesiculodeferential artery, whereas the prostatovesical artery divides to form the inferior vesical and prostatic arteries. The prostatic artery further subdivides into a urethral and capsular group of blood vessels. The urethral group supplies the periurethral regions of the prostate and the urethra, whereas the capsular group supplies the ventral and dorsal regions of the prostatic capsule and approximately two-thirds of the parenchyma. A particular feature of the prostatic arteries is a tortuosity or "corkscrew"

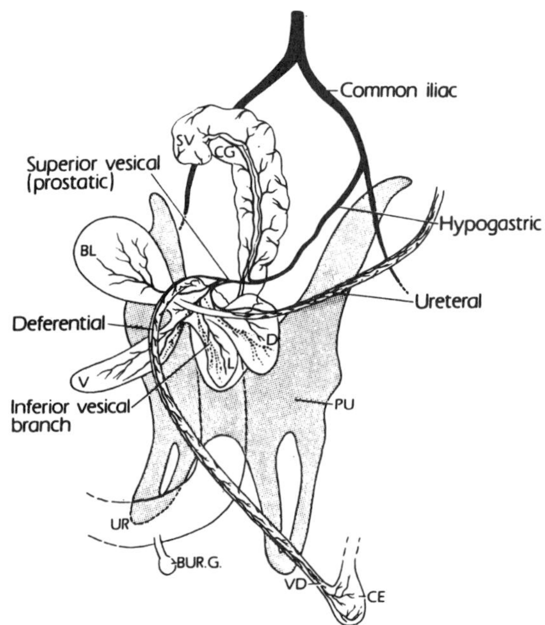

FIG. 36. Arterial supply to the male accessory glands of the rat. SV, seminal vesicle; CG, coagulating gland; V, ventral prostate; L, lateral prostate; D, dorsal prostate; BL, bladder; UR, urethra; PU, pubic bones; BUR.G., bulbourethral gland; VD, vas deferens; CE, cauda epididymidis. (From ref. 204.)

pattern on the surface of the organ and also in the stroma (296). Greater detail of the arrangement of vessels within the gland can be found in the article by Clegg (297). Venous blood leaves the prostate via a plexus (plexus of Santorini) situated at the base of the gland, particularly on the anterior and lateral surface. The seminal vesicle also drains into the prostatic plexus and the inferior vesical plexus. Blood from these plexuses then enters the internal iliac veins.

The arterial supply to the prostate of the dog differs from that in man in that the glandular tissue of the prostate is supplied solely from the capsular group of arteries (29). The capsular arteries are derived from branches of the umbilical artery, urogenital artery, and internal pudendal arteries, which are ultimately derived from the internal iliac artery. The venous drainage takes the form of a densely branching network within the radial septa of the gland which converge to form larger vessels within the septa and pass towards the periphery to form a venous plexus beneath the capsule. Prostatic veins leave this plexus accompanying prostatic arteries and unite to form the prostatica-vesical vein which may unite with the prostatica-urethral vein to become the urogenital vein which drains into the external iliac vein (292,298).

Bulbourethral Glands

The main arterial supply to the human bulbourethral glands is derived from the artery to the bulb of the penis with subsidiary supplies from the internal pudendal artery, the urethral artery, the perineal artery, or an anastomosis between the cystic inferior artery and the internal pudendal artery (299). Arteries within the capsule of the gland send arterioles into the septa between the lobules of the gland.

LYMPHATIC DRAINAGE

The general arrangement of the lymphatic drainage from the testis and accessory glands is shown in Fig. 38. Lymphatic vessels which originated from the testis and epididymis run in the spermatic cord to the lumbar or para-aortic lymph nodes (300–303). In pigs, there may sometimes be a small lymph node in the spermatic cord itself. In rats, it was claimed that testicular lymph reached the thoracic duct without passing through a lymph node (304), but later studies using the movement of carbon particles or fluorescein-labeled lymph node cells injected into the testis showed that the lymphatic vessels in the cord run to iliac and renal lymph nodes, with some drainage to para-aortic, lumbar, and posterior gastric nodes. These findings were supported by observations on regional hypertrophy of draining lymph nodes following a graft-versus-host reaction induced by the injection of foreign lymph node cells into the testis (305).

Testis

The lymphatic drainage of the testis was described and illustrated by the early anatomists (see refs. 142,306), but there was a lively controversy about the nature of the system inside the testis. One group believed that there were no true lymphatic vessels there, but only lymphatic spaces surrounding the tubules. Another series of authors believed that in the interstitial spaces they could see discrete lymphatic vessels, which joined larger vessels in the septa and a network of vessels in the capsule giving rise to the lymphatic trunks in the spermatic cord. Later studies with the electron microscope showed that in rodents, there were indeed large lymphatic sinusoids surrounding the tubules, so that these were virtually floating in a sea of lymph; on the other hand, in man and in many of the larger mammals, there were definite lymphatic vessels which lay in a fibrous interstitial tissue (Figs. 8,9) (58,60).

The lymphatic vessels of the rabbit testis run in the tunica albuginea towards the epididymal margin and over the epididymis to join the epididymal lymphatics and form large lymphatic vessels in the cord (307). The lymphatic drainage of the rat testis has recently been re-examined (308,309). There are three groups of lymphatic vessels leaving the surface of the testis, from the cranial pole, the epididymal margin, and the caudal pole (Fig. 39), but all three join the epididymal lymphatics in the spermatic cord (Figs. 40,41). Recent studies have confirmed that the lymphatic vessels leaving the rat testis pass over the surface of the epididymis, and showed that, in the ram, much of the lymphatic drainage from the caudal pole of the testis runs in a vessel which

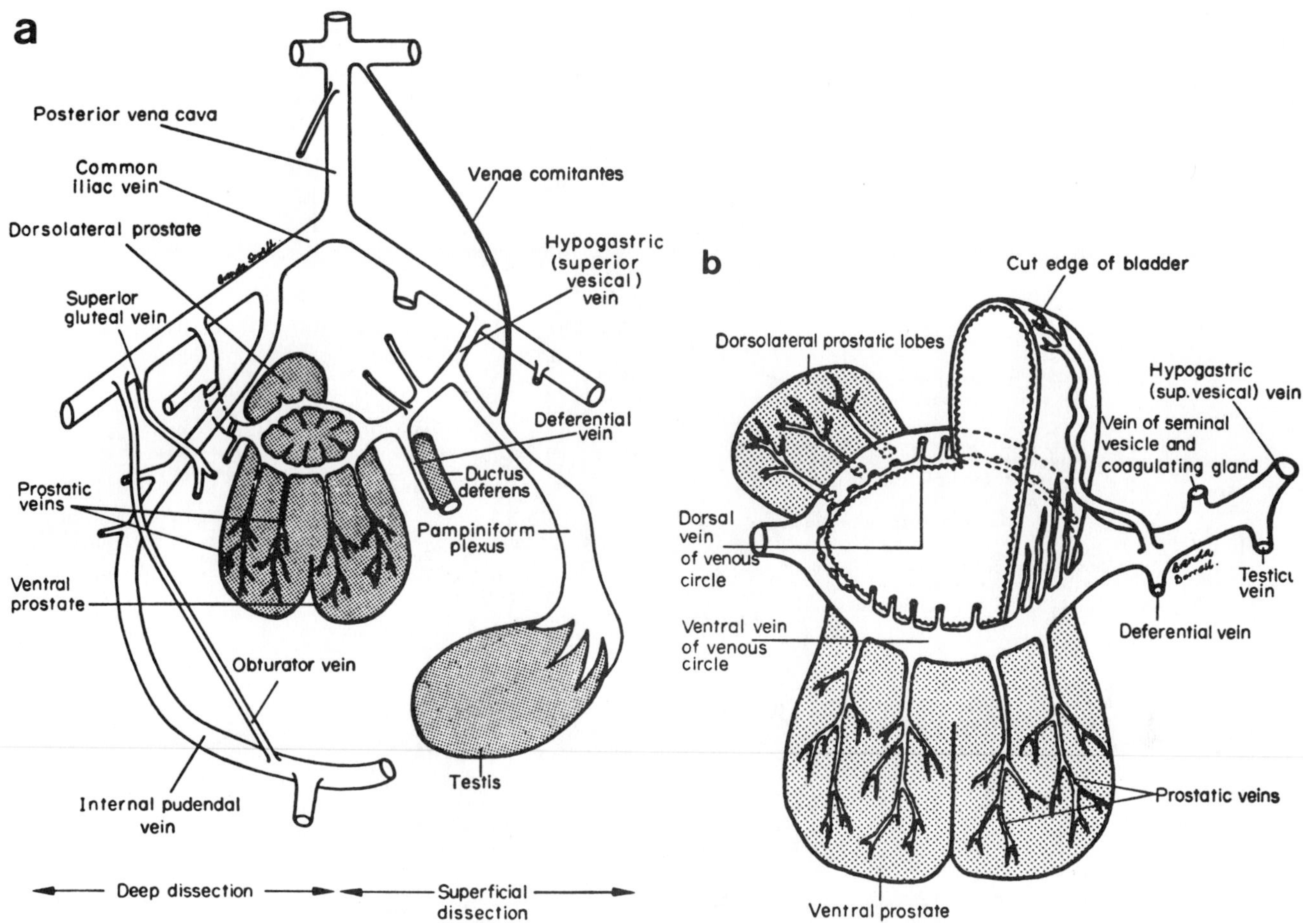

FIG. 37. Venous drainage of the male accessory glands of the rat. **(a):** General representation of the pelvic venous system showing vessels seen by superficial dissection on the right and deep dissection on the left. **(b):** Details of the venous drainage from the bladder and prostatic lobes. (From ref. 229.)

passes under the tail of the epididymis and then between the ductus deferens and the body of the epididymis (Fig. 39) to the spermatic cord (26). This arrangement has important physiological implications in the transfer of substances from the testis to the epididymis (see Significance of Testicular Lymph, p. 801).

Ligation of the testicular lymphatic vessels in the rabbit led to degenerative changes in the testis and substantial falls in the testosterone levels in blood from the internal spermatic vein (310). In the rat, less obvious, but nonetheless appreciable changes in the testis and epididymis have been reported following interruption of the lymphatic drainage (311).

Epididymis

Lymphatic sinusoids can be seen in the intertubular spaces in tissue sections prepared for electron microscopy (e.g., refs. 177,312). Details of the arrangement of lymphatic vessels within the organ as a whole have not, however, been elucidated. The only species in which there has been any detailed investigation of the lymphatic drainage system leaving the epididymis has been the rat (309). Lymphatic vessels leave the epididymis at various points along its length. The caput epididymidis has the greatest number of vessels leaving it, one or two vessels leave the corpus, and a single vessel emanates from the cauda. There is little anastomosis between the vessels with the exception of a channel running along the medial face of the caput and proximal corpus, but the vessels gradually coalesce and join the main testicular lymphatic trunk, which accompanies the spermatic artery to reach the para-aortic group of lymph nodes. The lymphatic vessels leaving the epididymis form a so-called "lymphatic triangle" (Fig. 40) occupying a plane posterolateral to the testicular vascular bundle, which intervenes between the lymphatic drainage system of the testis and the epididymis. Nevertheless, there are several connections between the lymphatic drainage of the testis and epididymis, apart from the final convergence of the main testicular and lymphatic trunks (Fig. 41).

Prostate

The only male accessory organ that has received any attention with regard to lymphatic drainage is the prostate. The lymphatic drainage system is conceived as a possible

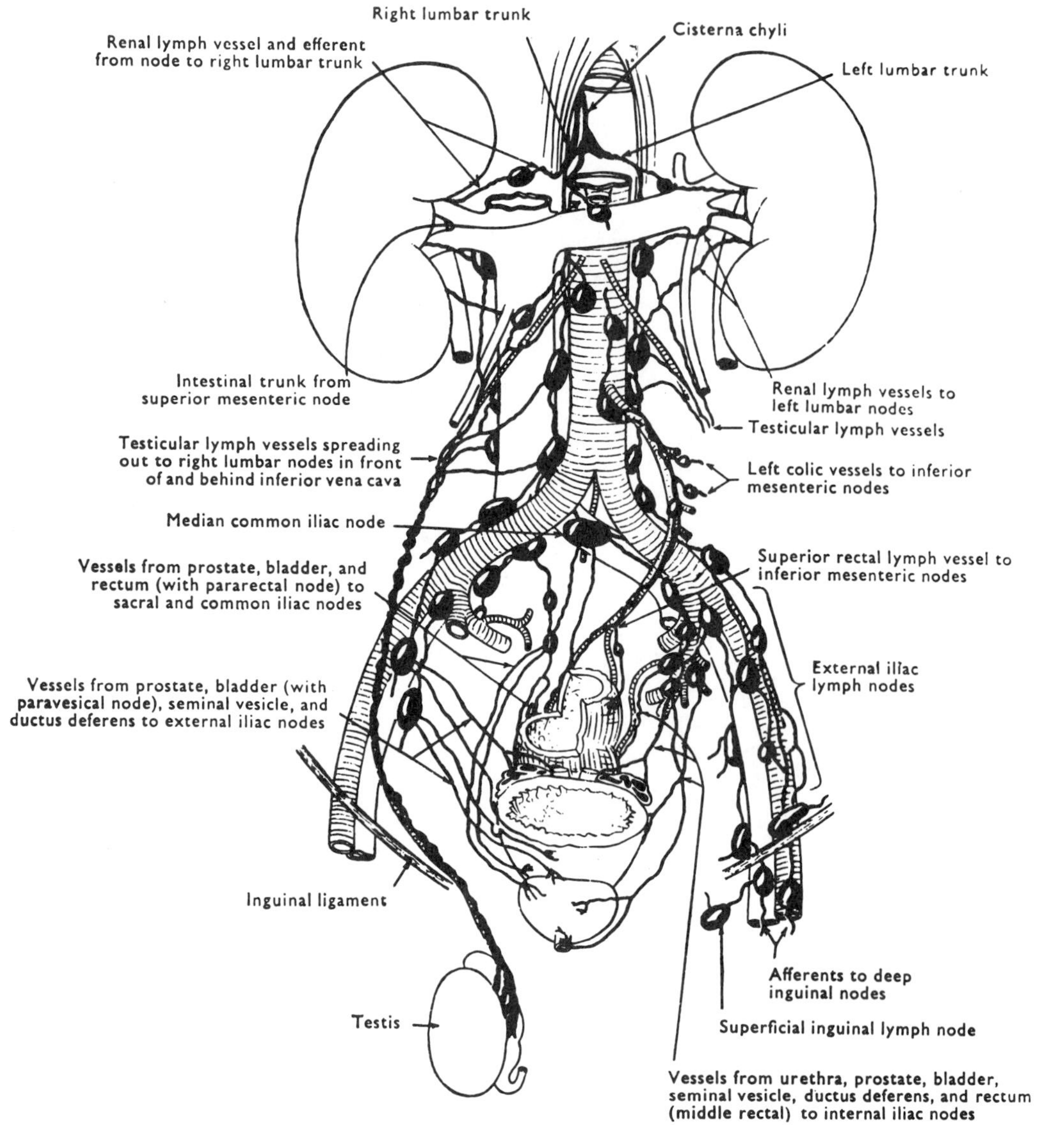

FIG. 38. Distribution of lymph vessels and lymph nodes in the human pelvis and abdomen. (From ref. 820.)

route for the spread of tumor cells derived from carcinoma of the prostate, while the possible absence of intraprostatic lymphatics could render the prostate an immunologically privileged site favoring growth of malignantly transformed cells. The existence of a pericapsular lymphatic system which drains towards the external iliac, internal iliac, and common iliac lymph nodes is well established (Fig. 38), but the existence of intraprostatic lymphatics has been open to more controversy (313). The debate has perhaps arisen because the methods chosen to demonstrate intraprostatic lymphatics have not always been appropriate, such as the use of vital stains which leach out during processing of tissue for light microscopy (314). There has also been some confusion as to whether spaces which are observed to surround some prostatic neurons in tissue sections are perineural spaces or lymphatic channels (315), but the absence of an endothelium indicates that such spaces are not lymphatic vessels. However, the weight of evidence from studies using precipitable dyes and direct ultrastructural studies (316–320) would support the existence of intraprostatic lymphatics located in the connective tissue of the gland parenchyma and radiating to the capsule of the organ through the fibrous trabeculae.

INNERVATION

For an historical account of the study of the innervation of the internal male genital organs the reader is referred to the article by Sjöstrand (321). The testis, epididymis, and male accessory glands are devoid of somatic innervation, but receive dual innervation from branches of the autonomic nervous system and possess, in addition, a sensory afferent system. The visceral efferent (motor) supply to these organs is derived from prevertebral nerve plexuses surrounding the

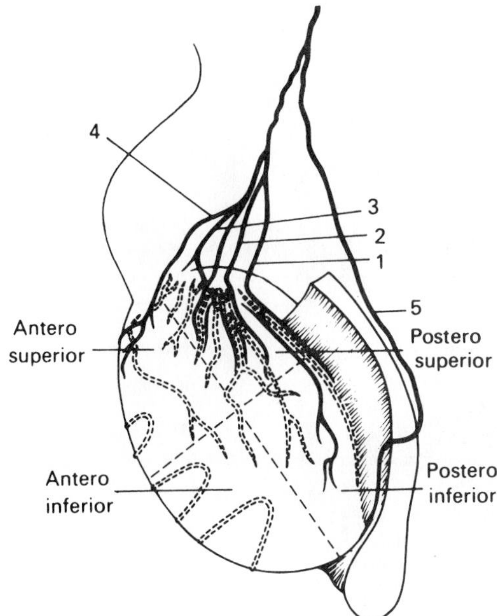

FIG. 39. The lymphatic drainage of the testis of a rat. This drawing was made from a rat that had received an intratesticular injection of India ink. The testicular artery and veins are shown by *dotted lines,* and the testis has been divided into four quadrants. The superficial lymphatic vessels are shown draining the anterosuperior, posterosuperior, and posteroinferior quadrants. The numbers on the diagram show the order in which the vessels were filled with the ink when injection was made into the lower pole of the testis. (From ref. 308.)

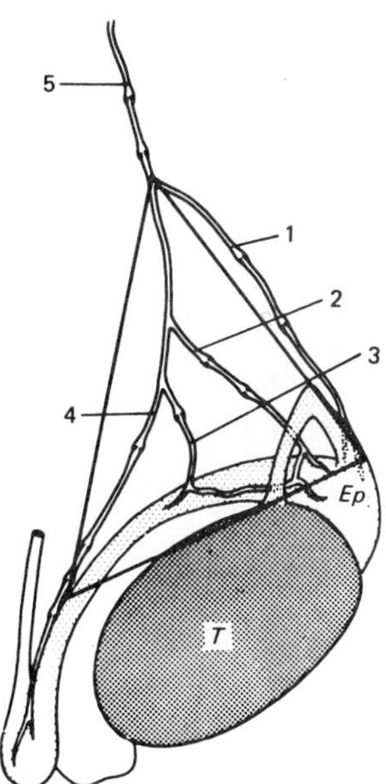

FIG. 40. Diagrammatic representation of the basic pattern of lymphatic drainage of the rat epididymis. 1, Ductular lymphatic trunk; 2, superior epididymal trunk; 3, corporeal epididymal trunk; 4, inferior epididymal trunk; 5, main testicular lymphatic trunk; T, testis; Ep, epididymis. Note the epididymal "lymphatic triangle" subtended on the epididymis and bounded by the lymphatic trunk (1) and the inferior epididymal trunk (4). (From ref. 309.)

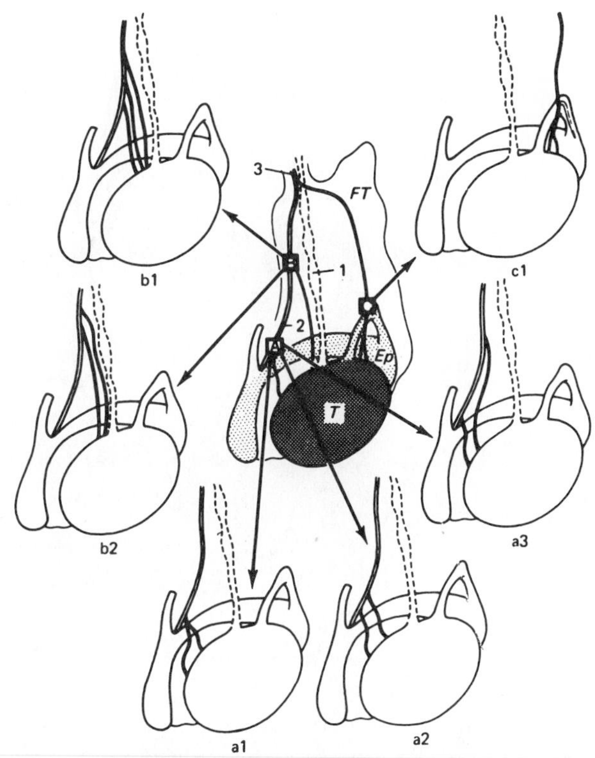

FIG. 41. Diagrammatic representation of various patterns of communication between the lymphatic drainage of the testis and the lymphatic drainage of the epididymis in the rat. T, testis; Ep, epididymis; FT, epididymal fat pad. In the central drawing, note (1) the pampiniform plexus in *dotted outline,* (2) the inferior epididymal trunk, (3) the main testicular lymphatic trunk and other testicular lymphatics in *black.* Sites at which testicular lymphatics join epididymal lymphatics are indicated by A, B, and C; variations in the communication of testicular lymphatics with epididymal lymphatics at the three sites are depicted in the peripheral drawings (a_1, a_2, a_3, b_1, b_2, c_1). (From ref. 309.)

arteries. There are five main interconnecting prevertebral plexuses. These are the celiac (solar), intermesenteric (aortic), caudal (inferior, posterior) mesenteric, hypogastric, and pelvic plexuses (Fig. 42a,b). The celiac plexus obtains its sympathetic supply from the thoracic and lumbar splanchnic nerves, whereas the other plexuses receive only lumbar splanchnics. The celiac plexus also receives a parasympathetic supply from the vagus nerve. The intermesenteric plexus, which lies on the ventral and ventrolateral aspects of the aorta, connects the celiac plexus with the more caudal plexuses (caudal mesenteric, hypogastric, and pelvic plexuses). In most species the majority of the nerves pass from the intermesenteric plexus to the caudal mesenteric plexus, but in man some of the outermost nerves pass directly to the hypogastric plexus. The caudal mesenteric plexus surrounds the caudal mesenteric artery and contains one or more ganglia. A net of nerves located distal to the bifurcation of the aorta constitutes the hypogastric plexus in man, but in other species the hypogastric nerve is a single discrete nerve arising from the posterior border of the caudal mes-

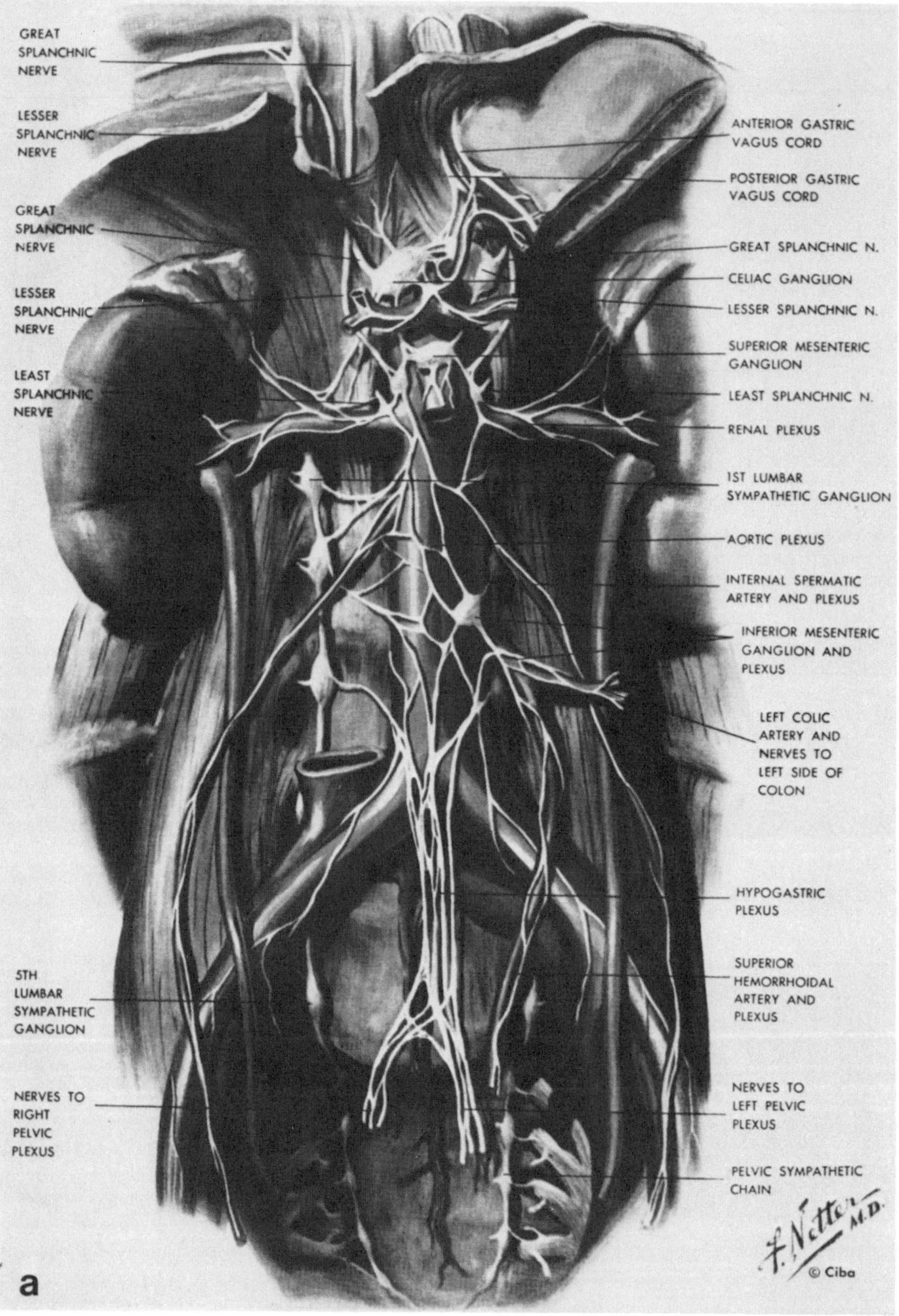

FIG. 42. Arrangement of autonomic nerves and ganglia in the abdomen **(a)** and pelvis **(b)** of man. (From ref. 821.)

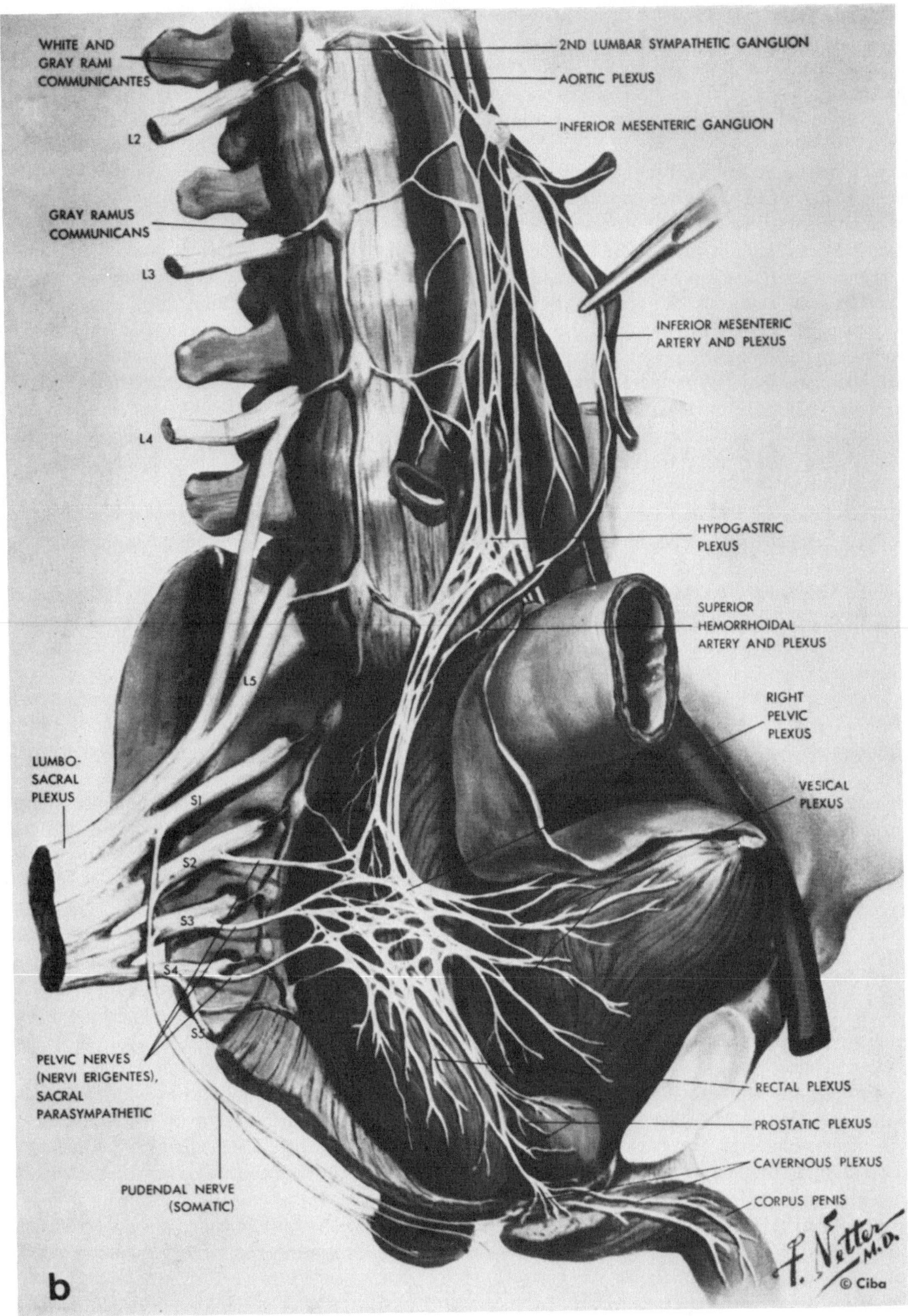
WHITE AND
GRAY RAMI
COMMUNICANTES
L2
GRAY RAMUS
COMMUNICANS
L3
L4
L5
LUMBO-
SACRAL
PLEXUS
S1
S2
S3
S4
S5
PELVIC NERVES
(NERVI ERIGENTES),
SACRAL
PARASYMPATHETIC
PUDENDAL NERVE
(SOMATIC)
2ND LUMBAR SYMPATHETIC GANGLION
AORTIC PLEXUS
INFERIOR MESENTERIC GANGLION
INFERIOR MESENTERIC
ARTERY AND PLEXUS
HYPOGASTRIC
PLEXUS
SUPERIOR
HEMORRHOIDAL
ARTERY AND PLEXUS
RIGHT
PELVIC
PLEXUS
VESICAL
PLEXUS
RECTAL PLEXUS
PROSTATIC PLEXUS
CAVERNOUS PLEXUS
CORPUS PENIS
F. Netter M.D.
© Ciba
b

enteric ganglion. The hypogastric nerves which are fused for a short distance in the rabbit supply the right and left pelvic plexuses. In addition to the sympathetic supply from the hypogastric nerve, the pelvic plexus receives parasympathetic fibers from the pelvic nerve which arises from the sacral nerves (Fig. 42b).

Various peripheral ganglia have been recognized in different species (322). There is often a small ganglion, the spermatic ganglion, near the origin of the testicular artery from the aorta; this ganglion is supplied by branches from a number of other ganglia, the intermesenteric and celiac plexuses, and in many mammals, but not man, the caudal mesenteric plexus. The spermatic ganglion also receives fibers directly from the lumbar sympathetic nerves. In some species, the spermatic ganglion is fused with the caudal mesenteric plexus (323). The "hypogastric ganglion" occurs only in man and monkey and is located at the junction of the hypogastric and pelvic nerve trunks. In the rat, the "major pelvic ganglion" lies on the posterosuperior surface of the lateral prostatic lobe. Its equivalent in the guinea pig is the "anterior pelvic ganglion" located on the posterolateral aspect of the coagulating gland and a smaller "posterior pelvic ganglion" behind the caudal portion of the gland. The "pelvic plexus ganglia" are present in all species associated with branch nerves of the pelvic plexus but can only be seen under magnification. The ganglia vary in number being most numerous in the cat and are freely interconnected.

Visceral afferent (sensory) fibers are present among all the nerve tracts described above. These fibers either travel in the pelvic nerve to enter the spinal cord via the sacral nerves, or pass by way of the hypogastric nerve and more proximal prevertebral plexuses, and thence through the splanchnic nerves and sympathetic chain ganglia to enter the spinal cord through the dorsal roots of the spinal nerves.

Testis

The nerves to the testis run from the spermatic ganglion alongside the testicular artery, in some species as a sheath of nerves (spermatic plexus) surrounding the artery, and in others as a discrete nerve, the superior spermatic nerve (323). In the testis, adrenergic nerves can be found in the interstitial tissue in association with blood vessels, particularly in and near the capsule; the cat and man have a much greater density of nerves than the other species studied (rats, rabbits, and guinea pigs) (35,324–326). There is no doubt that vascular tone in the testis is under nervous control, as stimulation of the nerves in the spermatic cord of isolated perfused ram testes led to sudden increases in pressure during isovolumetric perfusions (327).

It was originally believed that the testis had no cholinergic fibers (328), but later studies revealed that there were acetylcholinesterase-containing fibers in the testicular capsule of several species of mammal, including monkey, rat, rabbit, and ram (35,36). In the cat there are also vasoactive intestinal polypeptide (VIP)-containing terminals in the capsule and around the blood vessels of the cat and guinea pig, but not in the rat (329,330). There may be associations between the nerve fibers and the cells of the peritubular tissue (324,331), and some authors have suggested that the Leydig cells may also be in contact with nerve terminals (324,332–334). It is probably relevant that Leydig cells appear to have β-adrenergic binding sites (335), and that cultured Leydig cells increase their production of testosterone when stimulated with catecholamines (336–338). Furthermore, nicotinic cholinergic agonists inhibit androgen biosynthesis by cultured testicular cells from hypophysectomized rats (339). Catecholamines also stimulate cyclic AMP production and aromatization in Sertoli cells (340), and these cells also contain β-adrenergic receptors (341).

Sensory receptors with fibers in the spermatic nerve are probably responsible for the sensation of the pain commonly experienced following trauma to the testis. Studies with local anesthetics applied to the outside of the testis suggest that these receptors are present in the parenchyma as well as in the capsule (342), but there is a higher density of receptors near the surface (343). In the cat and dog, the receptors appear to be of three types: mechanoreceptors, chemical receptors, and thermal receptors. As judged by electrical recording from fibers in the superior spermatic nerve, the mechanical receptors respond to a degree of compression of the testis that does not invoke a pseudoaffective response in lightly anesthetized subjects, but a different response, possibly from different receptors, is obtained if the intensity of the stimulus is increased. The chemical receptors respond to hypertonic sodium chloride, potassium chloride, bradykinin, sodium citrate, substance P, acetylcholine, and histamine (Fig. 43), and their sensitivity is increased when the temperature is raised; the response to bradykinin is blocked by indomethacin, so prostaglandins are probably involved. The discharge from the thermal receptors increased roughly in parallel to the temperature rise, with an average threshold of approximately 42°C. However, more than 90% of the receptors respond to all three stimuli, and therefore probably should be classified as polymodal receptors (342,344–348).

The fibers in the spermatic nerve are largely unmyelinated, but the myelinated fibers have diameters ranging from 1.4 to 6 μm, with conduction velocities of electrically evoked potentials typical of A-fibers, ranging from 3 to 52 m/sec (Fig. 44). A large compound potential representing C-fibers could also be evoked, with conduction velocities ranging from 0.5 to 2.3 m/sec (342,344,345,347,348).

There were some suggestions in the early literature that removal of part of the lumbar sympathetic chain and/or the thoracic splanchnic nerves, or the celiac plexus, or the caudal mesenteric ganglion and spermatic plexus caused vasodilatation and degeneration in the testis. (see refs. 2,323). However, the effects were slow to appear and the degeneration may have been secondary to the vascular effects or

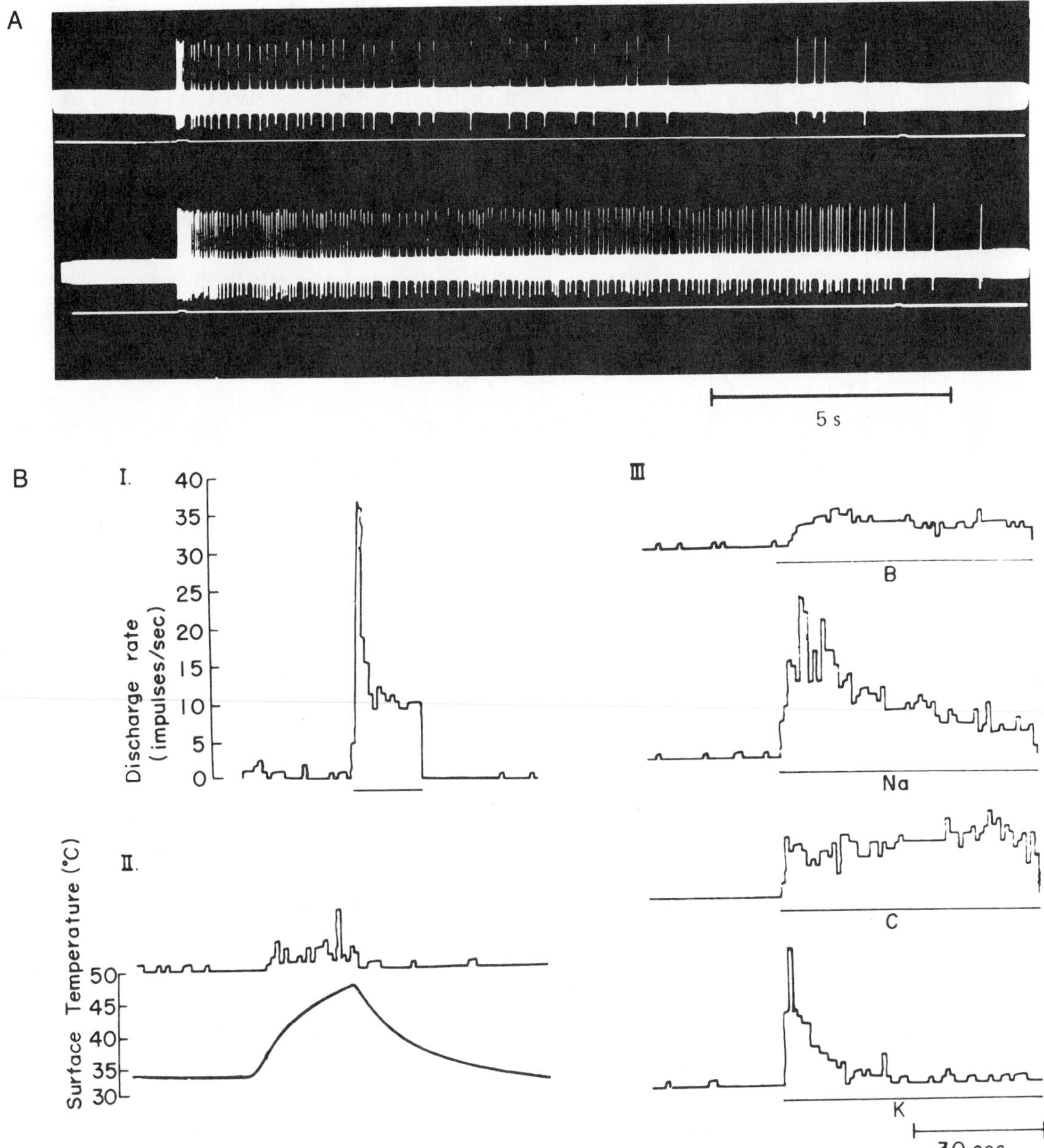

FIG. 43. Response of nerve bundles or filaments in the superior spermatic nerve in the abdominal cavity of dogs to mechanical, chemical, and thermal stimuli. **A:** Discharge pattern in response to mechanical stimulation of a polymodal unit with a conduction velocity of 10.5 m/sec. During the period between the two upward deflections of the lower line, a weight was applied to the testis using a falling type mechanostimulator, 500 g in the *upper panel* and 1,000 g in the *lower;* the upper line shows the action potential. **B:** Response of an Ad fiber unit with a conduction velocity of 5.6 m/sec to various stimuli. I: the receptive point was pressed with a von Frey hair (2 g, 420-μm diameter), for the period shown by the lower line. II: the surface of the testis around the receptive area was heated by radiant heat, while the surface temperature (*lower trace*) was recorded with a thermistor. III: Chemical stimulation was applied to the receptive area by applying a cotton ball (1.5-mm diameter) soaked in bradykinin (10 μg/ml, B), sodium chloride (4.5%, Na), sodium citrate (18%, C) or potassium chloride (60 mM, K) for the period shown by the lower line. (From refs. 346 and 344, respectively.)

to interference with transport of sperm and fluid through the epididymis. Transection of the main vascular and nervous supply to the testes of young pigs had no effect on their subsequent development (349), although re-innervation could not be excluded. Similarly, section of the testicular nerves to the testes of adult rams caused no deterioration in seminal characteristics for the next 6 weeks (350). Testicular denervation in young rats caused severe degeneration and reduced testis weight, and a similar effect was produced by local injection of 6-hydroxydopamine, which induces local destruction of sympathetic nerve terminals (351). Testicular innervation is necessary for the response of plasma testos-

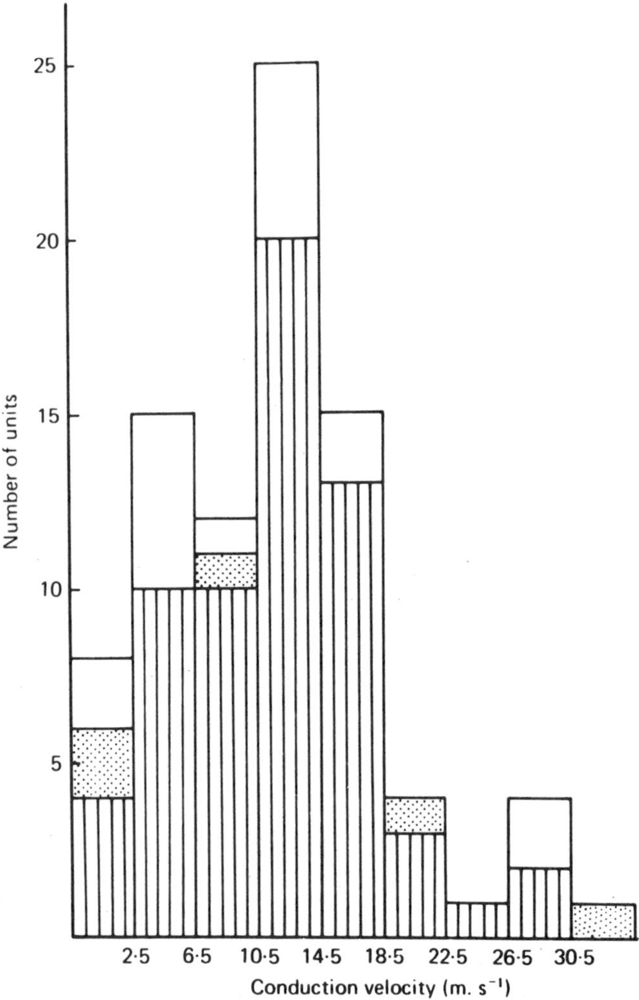

FIG. 44. The conduction velocities of all units responding to mechanical stimulation studied in the superior spermatic nerves of dogs. The histograms show the total number of units with conduction velocities in the ranges shown. The *hatched columns* represent units which were also sensitive to heat, the *stippled columns* the units which were not also sensitive to heat, and the *open columns* units whose response to heat was not tested. (From ref. 347.)

terone concentrations to acute stress in rats (352), and although denervation has no effect of the endocrine response to hemicastration (353,354), this is suppressed by vasectomy on the side of the remaining testis, suggesting that the inferior spermatic nerves may be involved (355). It has recently been suggested that the short-term effects of vasoligation or unilateral castration on plasma FSH, LH, and prolactin provide evidence for a direct neural connection between the testes and the central nervous system (356,357).

Epididymis and Ductus Deferens

The epididymis is supplied by the middle spermatic and inferior spermatic nerves (323). The route of the middle spermatic nerves depends on species. In man and cat (325), the nerves originate from the hypogastric plexus and accompany the spermatic artery to the epididymis, whereas in other species a group of nerves leaves the termination of the hypogastric nerve and pass to a group of ganglia located near the termination of the ductus deferens from where they travel to the epididymis along the ductus deferens. The inferior spermatic nerves arise from the pelvic plexus and contain both sympathetic and parasympathetic fibers. These nerves form a plexus around the ductus deferens after synapsing with a group of ganglia near the prostate (358). The nerves supply the muscle of the ductus deferens and continue to the cauda epididymidis.

Throughout the epididymis there are rich adrenergic and cholinergic perivascular plexuses (359). The distribution of interstitial and peritubular adrenergic and cholinergic nerves, however, varies considerably in different anatomical regions of the epididymis and in different species. Thus, the ductuli efferentes and the caput and corpus epididymidis are sparsely innervated in the rat, rabbit, guinea pig, and man (325,326,359,360), but a richer innervation exists in these regions in the cat and dog (359). The innervation of the cauda epididymidis becomes progressively more prominent as the layer of smooth muscle increases towards the ductus deferens. Ganglia have been seen only in the caput epididymidis of the cat, whereas cholinergic and adrenergic fibers have been reported in the lamina propria and epithelium by light microscopy in the caput and cauda, but not the corpus of all species studied except the rat (325,359). However, intraepithelial localization of neurons has never been observed in ultrastructural studies (361).

The ductus deferens has been a favorite system for neuropharmacological studies, for which a voluminous literature exists. The extensive adrenergic innervation of the smooth muscle layers which becomes prominent in the cauda epididymidis continues in the three layers of the ductus deferens (321). The particular exception appears to be the dog, and possibly the fox, in which the outer and middle muscle layers of the proximal portion of the duct lack a rich adrenergic innervation (321,362); the smooth muscle of the terminal portion of the duct has a more normal adrenergic innervation (362). The adrenergic innervation to the human vas deferens is also relatively sparse in comparison with most other species (363). The presence of cholinergic neurons in the ductus deferens has been adequately demonstrated by histochemical and ultrastructural techniques in a number of species (328,362,364–367). The cholinergic innervation of the human vas deferens is largely confined to the subepithelial mucosa. Specific purinergic terminals which may utilize ATP or other purines as a cotransmitter with norepinephrine have also been described (363,368,369).

Scrotum

The nervous supply of the scrotal skin is quite separate from that of the testis and epididymis, but in view of the importance of the scrotum in keeping the testis and epididymis cool, some consideration of its nerve supply seems appropriate. The scrotum is supplied by fibers in the pudendal, inguinal, and ilioinguinal nerves, and these contain sensory, sympathetic (vasomotor, sudomotor, and piloerector), and somatic efferent fibers (see ref. 2, p. 323). Scrotal skin also contains a large number of thermal receptors that transmit information about the temperature of the scrotal skin through the spinal cord to the thalamus, the hypothalamus, and cortex via the raphe magnus. Some neurons increase their firing rate dramatically as scrotal skin temperature rises by approximately 2°C, whereas other neurons increase their firing rate as the temperature falls by a similar amount, although different neurons have different transition temperatures; above and below those temperatures the rate of firing is reasonably constant (370–380).

These thermal receptors provide the input through the pudendal nerve which enables the brain to control the important systemic responses (381), the increase in scrotal sweating (382), and the relaxation of the tunica dartos (383) which follow an increase in scrotal skin temperature. The response of the dartos muscle was not dependent on the normal functioning of these scrotal nerves, because contraction of the dartos muscle could still be induced by exposure to low temperatures in rams with denervated scrotal skin (350). The pudendal nerve also carries the efferent fibers to the tunica dartos (383) and the sweat glands, although the latter also respond to catecholamines in the blood (382).

Accessory Glands

Nerves supplying the accessory glands arise on each side from the pelvic plexus (Fig. 42b). The nerves supply the ipsilateral organs, but there is also crossing of the midline ventrally and dorsally to provide innervation to the contralateral organ. Peripheral ganglia are located along the neural pathway to the accessory organs distal to the pelvic plexus and at a short distance from, adjacent to, or within the organs they innervate (Fig. 45). The existence of short postganglionic fibers with their cell bodies located in ganglia close to the innervated organ is a feature of the male accessory organs which differs from that associated with the sympathetic adrenergic innervation of most other organs. Collectively these nerves have been termed the "short adrenergic neuron system" (321) or the "urogenital short neuron system" (322). The existence of the short adrenergic neuron system is revealed by the persistence of unchanged neurons following total extrinsic denervation (e.g., refs. 321,384). The short adrenergic neuron system seems largely to be responsible for innervation of the smooth muscle. The vasculature would appear to be supplied by long postganglionic nerves which travel with the blood vessels and bypass the short adrenergic neuron system, since lumbosacral sympathectomy results in marked depletion of adrenergic vascular neuroplexuses within the accessory glands (321).

Numerous "intrinsic preterminal ganglia" are present in

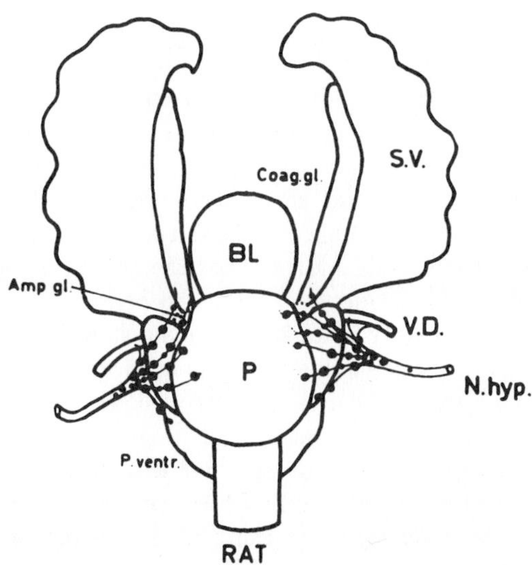

FIG. 45. Diagrammatic representation of the localization of sympathetic ganglia innervating the male accessory glands of the rat. Dorsal view with adrenergic ganglia indicated by *black dots.* BL, bladder; S.V., seminal vesicle; Coag. gl., coagulating gland; Amp. gl., ampullary gland; V.D., vas deferens; P, dorsal prostate with lateral lobes at each side; P. ventr., ventral prostate; N. hyp., hypogastric nerve. (From ref. 321.)

most species. These individual or clustered ganglion cells are associated with intrinsic nerves supplying the terminal ramifications of the nerve fibers within the accessory glands. They are particularly abundant in the organ capsule or adventitia, some are present in the muscle layer, and a few are located in the subepithelial connective tissue. These ganglia may also be classified as "epineural" or "intraneural" (beside or within major nerve bundles), "paravascular" (next to major intrinsic blood vessels), or "neuroterminal" (within neuroplexuses such as those supplying the smooth muscle of the organ).

Catecholamine-containing neurons are distinguishable by fluorescence microscopy of formaldehyde-fixed tissue, whereas cholinergic neurons are detected by histochemical staining for acetylcholinesterase. The adrenergic neurons are postganglionic sympathetic fibers characterized by many intracytoplasmic granules of moderate fluorescence. The nonadrenergic neurons are nonfluorescent, but most are acetylcholinesterase-positive, and represent postganglionic parasympathetic fibers. Persistence of the staining reactions after extrinsic denervation has frequently been used to confirm the identity of neurons as postganglionic elements of the short neuron system (e.g., ref. 321). A third type of neuronal element, termed the small intensely fluorescent cell (SIF) or chromaffin cell, is also present in the male accessory glands. These cells are characterized by an intense homogeneous cytoplasmic fluorescence due to their content of both epinephrine and norepinephrine. The SIF cells are believed to be interneurons which establish efferent synapses with juxtaposed sympathetic or parasympathetic neurons.

The different types of neurons can also be distinguished by their ultrastructure (385).

The general structure and arrangement of the intrinsic innervation of the male accessory glands is similar to that of the excurrent duct system (322,359). Nerve bundles, containing both adrenergic and cholinergic fibers, travel in the adventitia or capsule of the organ or gland in association with blood vessels and their perivascular neuroplexuses. These adventitial nerves branch and penetrate the gland, where they ramify in the fibromuscular stroma to form adrenergic and cholinergic perivascular plexuses around arteries and veins. Some stromal nerves do not associate with blood vessels but innervate smooth muscle of the glandular and ductal components of the gland. In addition, prominent neuroplexuses may also form below the epithelium lining the ducts and acini. These neuroplexuses are predominantly cholinergic while the innervation to the musculature is mainly adrenergic. The density of the adrenergic innervation is very variable in different glands and in different species, but correlates to a large degree with the extent of the development of the smooth musculature (321). The extent of the sparse cholinergic innervation of the smooth muscle is also variable, but is unrelated to the amount of smooth muscle (322).

Adrenergic innervation of the smooth muscle in the seminal vesicles has been clearly demonstrated in several species (321,325), the innervation being particularly rich in the case of the rabbit. Ultrastructural identification of fibers with the characteristics of adrenergic and cholinergic neurons has been made in the guinea pig (367,386). The smooth muscle of the proximal 1.5 cm of the gland is in two layers, an outer longitudinal and inner circular layer. Adrenergic neurons are abundant throughout both muscle layers, whereas cholinergic neurons are largely restricted to the inner circular layer. Both types of neurons arise from mixed ganglia located in the adventitia located on the lateral sides of the proximal part of the seminal vesicle. Below the muscle layers acetylcholinesterase-positive neurons form a rich submucosal complex and the presence of a few intraepithelial fibers has been reported (367). Catecholamine-containing neurons are rare in the submucosa, and those which are present are associated with blood vessels, occasionally forming perivascular plexuses.

The pattern of adrenergic innervation of the prostate is similar to that observed in the other accessory glands (321). The extent of innervation is proportional to the amount of smooth muscle present in the organ. This is evident both in cases where there are separate and distinct morphological lobes (e.g., rat) as well as histologically demonstrable lobes (e.g., dog, monkey). Dual innervation of the rat and human prostate has been confirmed by Vaalasti and Hervonen (387–389). Cholinergic neurons are more sparsely distributed than the adrenergic neurons in the rat prostate, and do not make such intimate contact with the smooth muscle cells. Cholinergic neurons are more numerous in the human compared with the rat prostate. They outnumber adrenergic neurons in the fibrous capsule and fibromuscular stroma. Some cholinergic neurons are present near the base of the epithelium. However, no evidence has been found for direct contact of neurons with epithelial cells in either the rat or human prostate.

The adrenergic innervation of the bulbourethral glands, which has been examined in the rabbit and guinea pig, is relatively sparse commensurate with the thin layer of smooth muscle (321,384). Innervation of the vasculature is unexceptional. The preputial gland of the rat has been shown to contain both adrenergic and cholinergic fibers located in the connective tissue capsule and in the trabeculae that separate the acini; some association of neurons with blood vessels has also been demonstrated (390).

Little is known about the afferent (sensory) innervation of the male accessory glands because there is currently no way to identify unequivocally afferent neurons by their morphology in autonomically innervated visceral organs. One can merely make predictions that free terminals located in a subepithelial position and separate from blood vessels could serve a sensory function. Fibers of this type have been shown to degenerate in the rabbit seminal vesicle after extrinsic denervation (391), although this was not the case for other fibers presumably belonging to the short adrenergic neuron system. The variety of sensory functions that might be represented include pressure, pain, and temperature.

Peptidergic Neurons

Peptide neurotransmitter substances have been extracted from various parts of the male reproductive tract (e.g., refs. 392–395), and immunohistochemical techniques have been used to localize putative peptidergic neurons within these structures. It is possible that the peptide transmitters are costored in adrenergic or cholinergic neurons (361). Alternatively, the peptidergic neurons may correspond to the nonadrenergic noncholinergic neurons, which are characterized by a predominance of large granular vesicles when viewed in the electron microscope (389), but such an assignation remains entirely speculative at present.

Within the human genital tract, neuropeptide Y is found in highest concentration in the seminal vesicles (396). Immunohistochemical staining showed this substance to be associated primarily with the connective tissue in the seminal vesicles and prostate, and with the smooth muscle layer and vascular smooth muscle of the ductus deferens. Enkephalin immunoreactive nerves have been demonstrated in the distal ductus deferens and in the prostate of man in close relation to smooth muscle cells, but these fibers are absent or very rare in the ampulla and seminal vesicles (397,398) and have not been detected in guinea pig ductuli efferentes or epididymis (361). Nerves positive for methionine-enkephalin are more numerous than those which stain for leucine-enkephalin in the human prostate (397). On the other hand, Gu et al. (399) have been unable to demonstrate enkephalin-positive fibers in any of the human accessory glands. A few nerves staining for somatostatin have been found in the interstitium and smooth muscle of the human prostate and in the muscle of the vas deferens (399). Scattered fibers staining for gastrin-releasing peptide have been found in the vas deferens and seminal vesicles of mice, guinea pigs, and rabbits (400).

Nerves containing substance P have been found in parts of the male reproductive tract of the mouse, guinea pig, rabbit, and cat, but are totally absent from the rat (361, 400,401). In man, the ductus deferens is devoid of fibers (363), but occasional nerves have been found in the connective tissue of the seminal vesicle (399). In the ductuli efferentes and epididymis of the guinea pig, fibers are present in the interstitial connective tissue mostly adjacent to blood vessels and also in muscle layers of more distal regions of the epididymis (361). The ductus deferens of the guinea pig and cat has fibers beneath the epithelium, in the muscle layer, and in the adventitia (330). Positive fibers have been located in the seminal vesicle of the mouse, guinea pig, and rabbit, particularly in the smooth muscle, but not in the seminal vesicle of rat or cat, nor in the prostate of any of these species (330,400).

Vasoactive intestinal polypeptide (VIP) nerves have been demonstrated in the testis, epididymis, ductus deferens, seminal vesicles, prostate, and bulbourethral glands of several species (329,330,361,397,399,402). However, the distribution of VIP-positive fibers within any particular organ or gland is somewhat variable between species, and in some instances conflicting results have been reported by different authors. In the testis, VIP fibers are associated almost exclusively with the organ capsule in the guinea pig and cat, but are totally absent in the rat (329,330). In the cat epididymis, fibers are much more numerous than in the testis and are located immediately below the basement membrane and in the connective tissue between the tubules (329). A similar localization below the basement membrane exists in the human epididymis (399); in the guinea pig, positive fibers are found only in the terminal segment where they are present in large numbers in the subepithelial and muscular layers (361). The distribution of VIP fibers in the ductus deferens of rat, guinea pig, cat, and man is predominantly in the submucosa with a few scattered fibers in the smooth muscle and around blood vessels in the adventitia (330,363,399). However, Larsson et al. (329) reported that in the cat they are mainly associated with the smooth muscle with only a few fibers in the submucosa and around adventitial blood vessels, although Alm et al. (402) found an approximately equal density of fibers in the submucosa and muscle. The seminal vesicles of man and guinea pig contain a dense plexus of VIP fibers just below the epithelium with other fibers in the muscle layer (330,397,399). In the cat prostate, fibers are present in the smooth muscle, connective tissue, and around adventitial arteries (329,402). In man, the distribution is rather variable in different regions of the prostate, but fibers with a thin-beaded appearance can be found around the acini, in the interstitial tissue, and in the perivascular plexuses of arteries (397). In the cat, VIP nerves form a dense plexus in the prostatic capsule and give off branches to the stroma (330). VIP fibers are less numerous in the guinea pig prostate, whereas they are absent from the rat prostate (330).

Functional Significance of Innervation to the Male Accessory Organs

Motor innervation to the male accessory glands can be considered as subserving the following principal functions, namely, motor control of smooth muscle contraction, vascular activity, and epithelial secretory activity (Fig. 46).

Most visceral organs are considered to be in a state of tonic activity, which can be excited or inhibited by activity of the autonomic nervous system. Thus, smooth muscle systems exhibit spontaneous activity, have extensive electrotonic coupling and abundant muscle to muscle nexus-type close contact, and demonstrate slow, graded responses to neural stimulation. By contrast, the smooth muscle of the male accessory glands, as typified by the vas deferens, does not establish nexus-like close contacts and shows limited electrotonic coupling. Direct innervation of individual muscle cells allows for limited or no spontaneous activity but a fast, powerful, and coordinated response to neural stimulation. A gradation between the two forms of smooth muscle activity can be observed along the male excurrent duct system (360,403,404). Thus, the ductuli efferentes and proximal regions of the epididymis, which are sparsely innervated, display spontaneous contraction (405–407) which can be increased by adrenergic agents acting on α-receptors (408–411), whereas the distal cauda epididymidis and vas deferens are normally quiescent until neural stimulation is received during the ejaculatory process (410,412).

Contraction of the smooth muscle of the cauda epididymidis, vas deferens, and accessory sex glands occurs in response to stimulation of the hypogastric nerve (413). The response is adrenergic since seminal emission can be induced by intravenous injection of epinephrine (413) and inhibited by selective chemical sympathectomy (414). The bulbourethral glands may be an exception to this generalization since atropine, which acts as a blocker of muscarinic receptors, selectively and substantially reduces the liberation of bulbourethral gland secretion during ejaculation in the boar (415).

There is evidence that release of norepinephrine at the neuromuscular junction in the vas deferens is subject to inhibitory or braking influences at the postganglionic synapse and the neuromuscular junction (322). The role of parasympathetic innervation to the musculature of the ex-

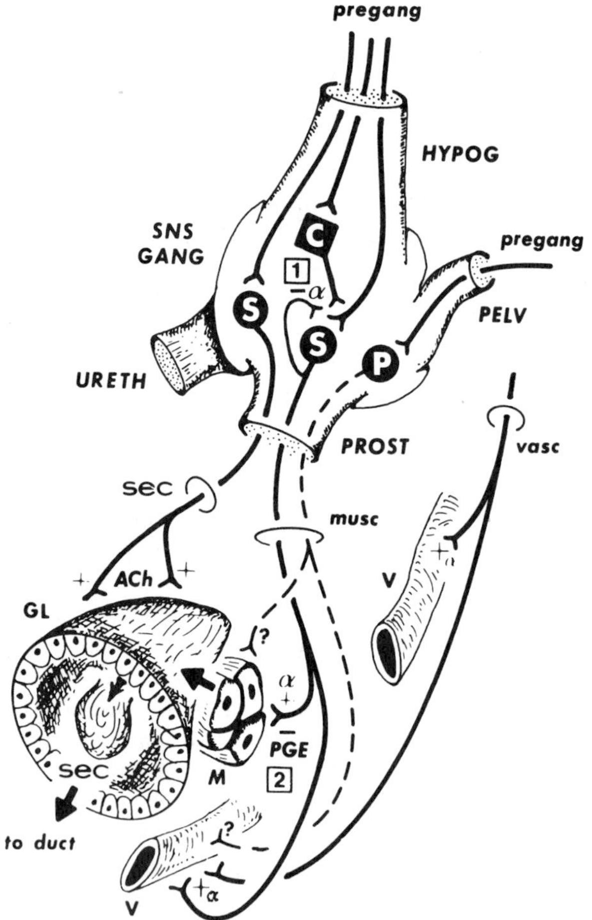

FIG. 46. Model of proposed pathways involved in the neural control of glands (GL), muscle (M), and vasculature (V) of the prostate. Prostatic nerves (PROST) originate together with urethral nerves (URETH) from ganglia of the short neuron system (SNS GANG). Sympathetic and parasympathetic preganglionic nerve fiber (*pregang*) input to the ganglion is provided by pelvic plexus branches of the hypogastric (HYPOG) and pelvic (PELV) nerves, respectively. Prostatic nerves are composed of sympathetic secretory nerves (*sec*) which supply the glands (GL), and muscular nerves (musc) which innervate both musculature (M) and vessels (V). These nerves are derived from cell bodies of postganglionic sympathetic (S) and parasympathetic (P) neurons located within the short neuron system ganglion. Sympathetic secretory nerves are cholinergic, stimulating secretion by release of acetylcholine (ACh). The secretion is expelled into the draining duct by contraction of related musculature (*arrows*) under the α-adrenergic excitatory effect of sympathetic adrenergic muscular nerves, which also have an α-adrenergic excitatory effect on blood vessels. The functional significance of parasympathetic cholinergic muscular nerves (*dashed line*) is still not fully resolved (?). Prostatic vessels are also supplied by vascular nerves (*vasc*), which are derived directly from the sympathetic chain and reach the organ along its vessels, independently of the pelvic plexus and short neuron system ganglia. Two inhibitory mechanisms probably modulate sympathetic muscular action: 1, α-adrenergic influence of SIF cell (C) terminals and/or collateral postganglionic adrenergic fibres on the sympathetic ganglion cell (S); and 2; prostaglandin E (PGE) released indigenously in the vicinity of the sympathetic neuromuscular junction. (From ref. 322.)

current ducts and accessory glands is not entirely clear. It is suggested that it is preferentially involved in basal muscular activity in the parasympathetic-dependent erection phase prior to ejaculation and during the process of urination (322).

Regulation of vascular tonus of the male accessory glands is probably mediated both by direct neural stimulation and by indirect humoral control from the adrenal gland. This dual control is indicated by the demonstration that either direct nervous stimulation or intravenous injection of epinephrine can decrease testicular and epididymal oxygen tension due presumably to reduction in capillary blood flow (416). Further evidence for neural control of the vascular system in the excurrent duct system is seen by removal of the lumbar sympathetic chain together with the posterior mesenteric ganglion and the hypogastric nerves from rabbits, which results in considerable vasodilation and vascular stagnation in certain regions of the epididymis and ductus deferens (417).

The effect of autonomic innervation on secretory activity of the male accessory glands has been studied extensively in the dog prostate (418). Copious secretion can be induced above the low basal rate, which is independent of the autonomic nervous system, by electrical stimulation of the hypogastric nerve of intact or decentralized animals. The secretory rate is in direct proportion to the frequency of stimulation (419). Pilocarpine, which is a powerful cholinomimetic drug, can also induce the formation of copious amounts of secretion when administered systemically. Other cholinomimetics also induce secretion, although sympathomimetics and cholinesterase inhibitors have only a weak effect. The use of a variety of blocking drugs and the absence of any involvement of the pelvic nerve indicate that the nerves responsible for stimulating secretion are postganglionic cholinergic sympathetic neurons and not parasympathetic neurons (322,418).

The role of nerves in regulating the secretory activity of glandular epithelia in the accessory glands of other species is far from clear. Removal of the posterior mesenteric ganglion plus hypogastric nerves, or removal of the lumbar sympathetic chain has no effect on the secretory activity of the prostate and seminal vesicles in the rabbit (420). However, when all these components are removed, secretory activity is markedly disrupted (417). Although this result may implicate direct neuronal involvement in secretion, the observation may also be explained as an indirect consequence of reduced testosterone synthesis by the concomitantly damaged testes (417).

The urethral glands, or glands of Littré, do not store secretion but produce it during coitus. Control of secretion by these glands has been studied in the boar (415) which has a protracted ejaculatory period of 15 to 30 min. Secretory activity appears to be under cholinergic control since administration of atropine, a muscarinic receptor antagonist, causes marked inhibition of secretion from these glands.

FLUIDS OF THE MALE REPRODUCTIVE TRACT

Testis

Blood Flow and Composition

In any organ, the amount of arterial blood entering must equal the sum of the amount of venous blood and lymph leaving, otherwise the size of the organ would change. Under most circumstances, the flow of lymph is small compared to blood flow, and therefore it is usual to equate arterial and venous blood flow. It is also important to make a distinction between total blood flow and nutrient blood flow: that is, the fraction of the total that exchanges with the tissue via the capillaries. Each of these components can be measured and the testis has the added complication of the spermatic cord, which can introduce errors in some of the measurements.

Arterial inflow can be measured by an electromagnetic flowmeter, either applied to the outside of the vessel or introduced into the circuit by cannulation of the vessel. It is difficult with either procedure to ensure that measurements are made under physiological conditions, but it is a useful technique for following rapid changes in flow and can be useful for calibrating other methods (241,242,422). A friction flowmeter introduced into the course of the vessel has also been used (423). The flow-velocity of arterial blood can be measured using a Doppler flowmeter (424–426), but estimation of volume flow depends on measurement of the cross-sectional area of the vessel and this can be difficult. Again, this method is probably most useful for recording rapid changes in flow. Arterial inflow can also be measured by dilution of a suitable marker infused into the arterial system, knowing the amount infused and its concentration in venous blood when equilibrium has been attained. Suitable markers used have been iodinated albumin, Cr-EDTA, sodium, and glucose. Usually, radioactively labeled material is used (241,427,428), but with Cr-EDTA, the chromium can be measured by atomic absorption spectroscopy (429). Paraaminohippuric acid (PAH), which is a suitable marker for venous infusion, does not appear to be suitable for intra-arterial infusion, presumably because it is metabolized to some extent in the tissue. Unless an arterial catheter is being introduced for some other reason, probably the most physiological way of measuring total testicular blood flow is to infuse a suitable marker into a testicular vein on the surface of the testis and to measure its concentration in blood from the testicular or internal spermatic vein above the spermatic cord. This uses the pampiniform plexus as a mixing unit and can give successive measurements of venous flow every minute, or even more frequently depending on how little blood is necessary for the estimation of the marker. In this instance, PAH is probably the best marker to use, as it does not build up in the arterial blood because it is cleared from the circulation by the kidneys (430–432). The marker must not cross from the vein to the artery in the spermatic cord, otherwise an overestimate would result. Overestimation from this source is a problem in the use of tritiated water and the Fick principle, which states that the amount of a marker taken up or produced by a tissue is a product of blood flow and the integrated arteriovenous difference over the period of study. The amount of tritiated water taken up is derived from the equilibrium concentration at the end of a 20-min infusion of the marker into the jugular or any other suitable peripheral vein, and the arteriovenous difference calculated from the concentrations in a series of testicular venous and peripheral arterial blood samples (433–435). As well as being difficult to carry out, and being possible only once, or at most twice, in any one animal due to accumulation of the marker, this method gives a slight overestimate because tritiated water does cross from artery to vein and vice-versa in the spermatic cord. A marker that did not do so would probably not come into equilibrium quickly enough with the tissue. In measurements of total blood flow, there is still a place for the simplest method of all, the collection of the total venous outflow over a given time. This is obviously unphysiological because of the surgery involved and disturbances to venous pressure, but it does have value for calibration of more physiological methods.

Total blood flow is what should be measured if production or uptake is being estimated, but if one is interested in the fluid dynamics in the tissue, then a measurement of nutrient or capillary blood flow is probably more appropriate. One technique for this depends on measurement of the rate of clearance or accumulation of a suitable marker in the tissue. The markers used have been radioactive inert gases (436–448) and radioactive sodium (428), but the former suffer from difficulty in knowing their lipid solubility and therefore their partition coefficient, and also give a slight underestimate because they cross readily from vein to artery and therefore recirculate back to the testis; with sodium, the difficulty is to determine its volume of distribution accurately. Alternatively, one can measure the amount of microspheres or an appropriate soluble marker which lodges in the tissue following introduction into the circulation. Microspheres have become very popular recently (263,422, 447,449–451), but their use does require cannulation either of the left side of the heart or the aorta above the testicular arteries for their injection; and if absolute values are to be obtained instead of a fraction of the cardiac output, then this must be measured separately or arterial blood must be sampled at a known and constant rate from an artery near the tissue under investigation. Furthermore, although several estimates can be made in an individual animal by using microspheres labeled with different isotopes, the method is expensive and does not lend itself to repeated measurements. Although the earlier technique using soluble markers (269,452–456) is easier to use, requiring only intravenous injection of marker, the animal must be killed or the tissue removed within 1 min of injection, and there is some doubt about the precision of the values obtained because of the loss of marker from the tissue back into the circulation. As with micropheres, it is necessary to measure cardiac output at the same time if the values are to be in absolute terms. Nevertheless, this technique has been useful in demonstrating differences within a tissue or between organs.

Representative values for testicular blood flow obtained by the various techniques in a variety of species are given in Table 2. Compared with other tissues, testicular blood flow is comparatively low, but this may be due at least in part to a physical limitation imposed by the dimensions of the testicular artery in the spermatic cord (142,239). Testicular blood flow (TBF) does not show any immediate increase when the testis is stimulated by tropic hormones (see refs. 2,142,424) or shows only a small rise (457), in contrast to other endocrine tissues such as ovary, adrenal cortex, and thyroid. However, when the stimulation is prolonged, as by the use of human chorionic gonadotropin (hCG) instead of LH, TBF does increase (96,263,458) and a hyperemia, presumably due to dilatation of the testicular veins, becomes apparent (459). As already discussed, this is preceded by a dramatic change in vascular permeability.

Vasodilatory drugs such as acetylcholine and isopropylnorepinephrine are without marked effects (422,436), whereas there is a marked vasodilation after adenosine (241). The response to vasoconstrictors seems to depend on the mode of administration. When epinephrine or norepinephrine were given into the testicular artery, a marked reduction in TBF followed in rams and rats (423,436); if the drug was administered peripherally, a reduction was reported in some studies but not in others (422,423,449). Prostaglandins (460) and 5-hydroxytryptamine (461) produce reductions in blood flow. The testis shows a reactive hyperemia after a short period of ischemia (241,462) but the testis does not vary its blood flow with temperature (435,436,456,463–465), unless the heating is frankly unphysiological. Cadmium salts in subtoxic doses cause a catastrophic fall in blood flow (268,269), which is probably secondary to an increase in vascular permeability (see earlier section). If spermatogenesis is disrupted by heat, irradiation, or following efferent duct ligation, testicular blood flow falls proportionately with testis weight; it therefore appears that the seminiferous tubules, because of their greater mass, are a more important determinant of testicular blood flow than are the Leydig cells (466).

Changes in composition of the blood passing through the testis are caused both by the production and uptake of substances by the testis. The only substances known to be produced by the testis are hormones, steroid and peptide. If the peptides are larger than a few amino acids, they will probably leave the testis largely in the lymph, so here we will concentrate attention on the steroid hormones secreted by the testis into the venous blood. The one usually associated with the testis is testosterone, first isolated from the testis in 1935 and shown to be secreted into the blood in the mid-50s (see ref. 467), but a number of other steroids, including some like pregnenolone which do not appear to be androgens, are secreted by the testis, the exact pattern depending on the species (Tables 3,4). Testosterone is the steroid secreted in largest amount by most mammalian testes into the testicular venous blood (468–479,514), with the exception of the pig testis, which secretes as much of the "boar-taint" steroid, 5α-androstenone as testosterone (480,481) and almost as much dehydroepiandrosterone sulphate and estrone sulphate (81,481) into the venous blood (Fig. 47). Sulphated steroids are also secreted by the human testis into venous blood (479,482), but in the pig, the lymph appears to be a more important route than the venous blood for the secretion of conjugated steroids (see Lymph Flow and Composition, p. 800) (81). The concentration of testosterone in the testicular venous blood varies by a factor of ten between species; the human with a small testis in relation to body size has the highest reported concentration

TABLE 2. *Blood flow through the testes of various mammals estimated by different techniques*[a]

Techniques	Rat	Rabbit	Dog	Monkey	Ram	Boar
Direct collection	6	15	7–20		10	
Friction flowmeter	22					
Electromagnetic flowmeter					12	12
Dilution of intra-arterial marker					11	
Dilution of intravenous marker					11–26	4–18
Fick principle with TOH or iodoantipyrine					10	
Microspheres	14–38	28				9
Indicator fractionation	23	24			9	
Inert gas clearance	18–24		22	16	8	

[a]Blood flow in ml/100 g/min.

TABLE 3. *Differences between the concentrations (ng/ml) of steroids in the spermatic venous blood and arterial blood in various species*

Steroid	Rat	Rabbit	Man	Sheep	Bull	Pig	Horse
Pregnenolone			10				
Progesterone			5–23		3–7		
17α-Hydroxyprogesterone			60–340				
Dehydroepiandrosterone			38			0.3–0.8	1.5
Androstenedione			10–40		1.8–8		
Androstenediol			47		5–23		
Testosterone	50–200	140	200–680	30–80	75–340	40–60	4-26
Dihydrotestosterone	6	40	3.5–22				
3α-Androstanediol	25	5	0.9–1.7		2–11		
3β-Androstanediol	4	25	7.5		4–16		
Estradiol-17β			0.6–3.4	}	0.003–0.015	0.25	
Estrone			49			62	
5α-Androstenone						62	
Pregnenolone sulphate			140				
Dehydroepiandrosterone sulphate			96–155			34–120	2.7
Dehydroepiandrosterone glucuronide						2	
5-Androstene-3β,17β-diol sulphate			34–102				
Testosterone sulphate			28–53				
Testosterone glucosiduronate							
Estrone sulphate						0.53	200

References are given in the text.

of testosterone in testicular venous blood. Testosterone is also the major steroid secreted by the maximally stimulated perfused testis of a number of species, although the rabbit testis secreted appreciable amounts of 5α-reduced androgens and the rat testis produces almost as much pregnenolone as testosterone under these conditions (473,483–488).

In some species, the pattern of steroid secretion changes with age. The greatest rises in secretion during puberty in boys are found in testosterone and androstenediol, but a substantial part of these rises takes place in the early stages of puberty, so that dehydroepiandrosterone and androstenedione show the greatest difference between midpuberty and adulthood (489). In young bulls, there is more androstenedione secreted than testosterone, but as the animal matures, the arteriovenous difference for androstenedione falls and that for testosterone rises, so that in mature bulls, more than 90% of the androgen secreted by the testis is testosterone (468,474,490). In the rat, the ratio between 3α-androstanediol and testosterone falls as the animal matures (478), whereas in the rabbit, whose testes also secrete appreciable amounts of 5α-reduced androgens, the proportion does not change with age (491,492). In the pig, testosterone secretion approximately doubles at puberty, compared with increases of approximately fivefold in the sulphated steroids (81).

Testicular venous blood contains approximately half as much oxygen as arterial blood (433,493), so that if metab-

TABLE 4. *Difference between the concentrations (ng/ml) of steroids in perfusion fluid leaving and entering the maximally stimulated testis in varous species*

Steroid	Rat	Rabbit	Mouse	Hamster	Guinea Pig	Dog
Pregnenolone	135	100	20			
Progesterone	20	4	10			
17α-Hydroxypregnenolone	130	60	50			
17α-Hydroxyprogesterone	40	45	6			
Dehydroepiandrosterone	10	65	53			
Androstenedione	5	20	100			
Androstenediol	undetectable	65	10			
Testosterone	165–180	370–660	600	40	450	370–400
Dihydrotestosterone	0.5	210	5			6
3α-Androstanediol	0.5	17	10			4.5
3β-Androstanediol	0.5	40	5			55

References are given in the text.

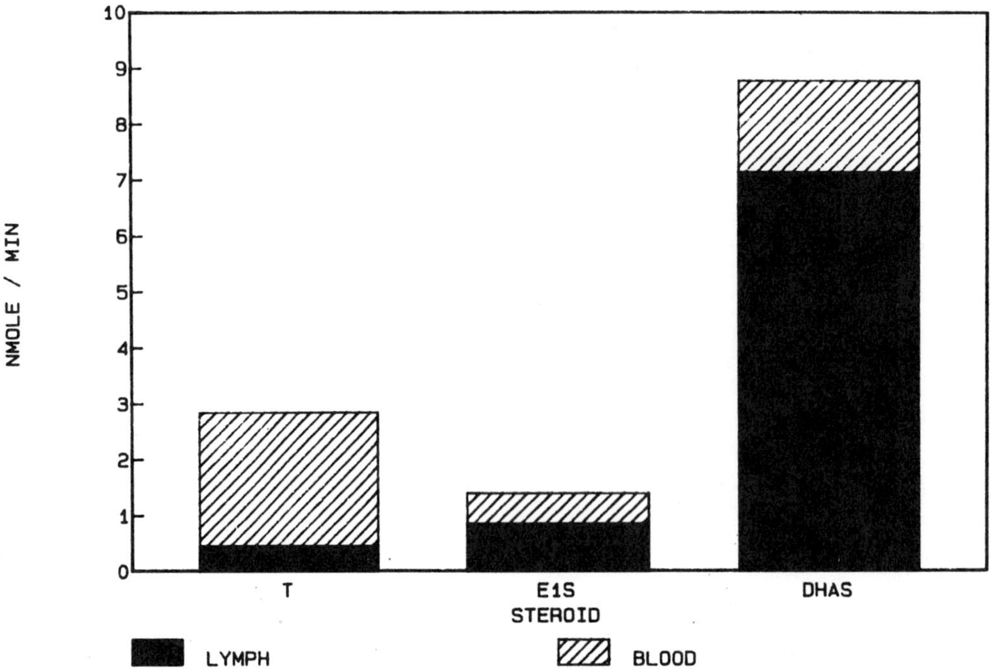

FIG. 47. The secretion of free and conjugated steroids into venous blood and lymph by the pig testis. The steroids shown are testosterone (T), estrone sulphate (E1S), and dehydroepiandrosterone sulphate (DHAS); the secretion rates were calculated from measurements of blood and lymph flow and the concentrations of these steroids in testicular lymph and venous blood and in arterial blood. (From ref. 81.)

olism increases without a corresponding increase in blood flow, the testis can become hypoxic; this may happen if the temperature of the testis is increased (435). The testis releases significant amounts of carbon dioxide and lactate into the venous blood, and removes approximately 20% of the glucose and ketone bodies and approximately one-third of the acetate from the arterial blood (142,427).

Lymph Flow and Composition

Flow of testicular lymph has been estimated in three ways, by cannulation of one or more of the lymphatic vessels in the spermatic cord and ligation of the rest, by measuring the degree of hemoconcentration as the blood passes through the testis, or by measuring the half-time of clearance of radioactive albumin injected directly into the testis, when this marker will be removed almost entirely in the lymph. There is considerable variation between species in the flow of lymph, with animals like the rat with the largest lymphatic sinusoids in the testis having the slowest flow (approximately 0.5 μl/g/hr), the ram and ferret being intermediate (approximately 1 μl/g/hr), while the boar, which has very inconspicuous lymphatic vessels in the testis, has the highest lymph flow of up to 10 μl/g/hr. (81,263,300,302,494–498). Lymph flow can be increased by increasing venous pressure (498), by warming the testis, and during exercise; flow is decreased by cooling the scrotum (494).

Testicular lymph collected from a catheter in a lymphatic vessel in the spermatic cord of rams (494,499) and boars (498) is, in general, very similar to testicular venous blood plasma; the ionic composition is virtually identical while the glucose concentration is somewhat lower, presumably because of utilization by the testis. The protein concentration is between two-thirds and three-quarters as high as blood plasma, and surprisingly does not vary with lymph flow; the difference in the protein concentration between lymph and blood plasma is much less for testicular lymph than for lymph from other sites in the body, with the exception of liver lymph. The proteins in blood plasma and testicular-lymph are similar, although the albumin/globulin ratio in lymph is higher (495,500), and there is a lower concentration of α_2-macroglobulin there (300). The amino acid composition of testicular lymph is very similar to that of blood plasma (501). There are no red cells in testicular lymph, but there are between 100 and 400 white cells/μl, of which approximately 80% are lymphocytes (499,502). Following vasectomy, significant numbers of spermatozoa can be found in lymph collected from a vessel in the spermatic cord of sheep and pigs (503).

The concentration of testosterone and androstenedione in testicular lymph from rams was approximately two-thirds of that in testicular venous blood, even when the animals were injected with hCG (300,490,504,505). In men, the fluid within the tunica vaginalis contained approximately 20 times as much testosterone as peripheral blood (506); this ratio is probably lower than the testicular vein to peripheral ratio which was not measured in these individuals, and the fluid is probably derived from a number of sources besides testicular lymph. In pigs and horses, there is appreciably more testosterone, dehydroepiandrosterone, and total unconjugated estrogens in lymph than in venous blood, and very much more estrone sulphate and dehydroepiandrosterone sulphate (81,507). Because lymph flow is also high in pigs, this means that in this species the majority of these conjugated steroids are secreted via the lymph. Lymph also contains a much higher concentration of inhibin than testicular venous blood, and has been used as a standard preparation of this substance (508).

Significance of Testicular Lymph

With its comparatively high concentration of steroids, testicular lymph probably exerts an important influence on the lymph nodes to which it drains. This may be at least a partial explanation for the persistence of grafts in the rodent testis (509). However, the testes of sheep are not immunologically privileged sites (510), so this cannot be the entire explanation. Spermatozoa in the lymph (503) and in abdominal lymph nodes (511) after vasectomy will obviously be an important source of antigen in the immunological reactions seen under these conditions (512). Evidence for another target for testicular lymph has recently come to light. Radioactive albumin injected into one testis or into a lymphatic vessel on the surface of a testis is preferentially transferred to the ipsilateral epididymis (and to the ipsilateral fat pad in rats) (Fig. 48) (26). This provides an alternative route by which hormones could reach the epididymis, and may provide another explanation for the seminal abnormalities seen in rabbits whose epididymides were separated from the testes and reflected into the inguinal canal (25), since effects were also seen in rams in which the testis and epididymis were separated but left in the scrotum (26). Transfer via the fluid in the tunica vaginalis may also be important, especially in men where this cavity becomes separate from the peritoneal cavity.

There have also been several studies on the effects on the testis of lymphatic obstruction. Ligature of the lymphatics accompanying the spermatic artery and vein at the level of the common iliac artery in rabbits was followed by a fall in the testosterone levels in testicular venous blood and serious degenerative changes in the seminiferous epithelium (310). In rats, ligature of the lymphatic vessels either near or at a distance from one testis produced degeneration of the tubules and interstitial edema, with some abnormalities on the control side; the latter were attributed to immunological damage (311). The lymphatics are an important route for the spread of metastases from testicular tumors (515,516).

Interstitial Fluid of the Testis: Volume, Turnover Rate, and Composition

The seminiferous tubules and the cells of the interstitial tissue are surrounded by interstitial fluid, which appears to be rich in albumin (64). The volume of this fluid can be estimated from the volume of distribution or "space" in the testis of a marker for interstitial fluid such as Cr-EDTA infused intravenously. As radioactive albumin introduced into the bloodstream reaches equilibrium with lymph from a lymphatic vessel in the spermatic cord within 2 to 3 hr (494), and its volume of distribution within the rat testis reaches values similar to those for the usual markers for interstitial fluid within 3 to 6 hr (263), albumin space also gives a reasonable estimate of the volume of interstitial fluid and is much simpler to use, not requiring a continuous intravenous infusion or severing of the ureters as Cr-EDTA does.

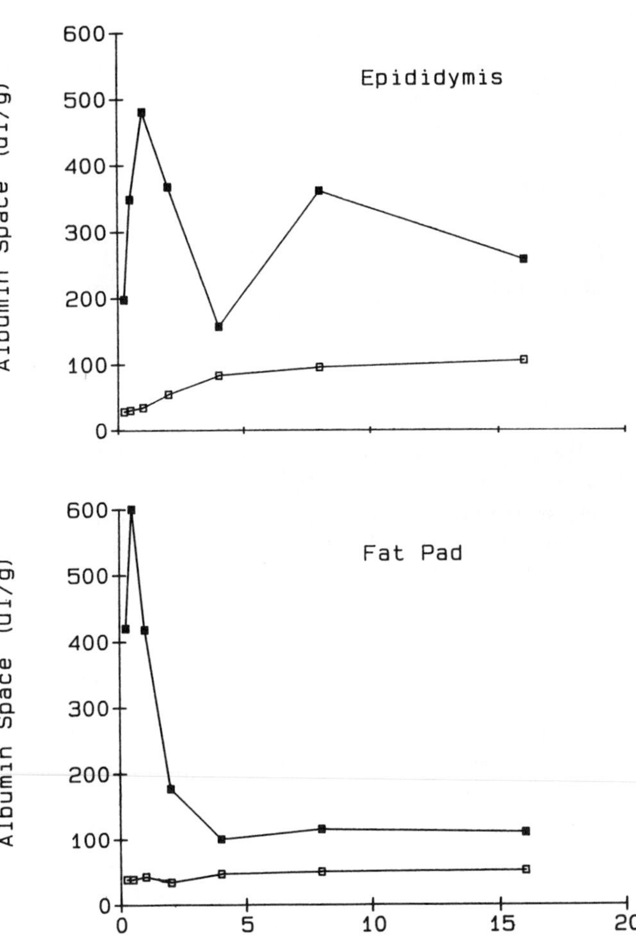

FIG. 48. The albumin "spaces" in the epididymides and epididymal fat pads of rats which had been given an injection of radioactive iodinated human serum albumin into one testis at time 0. The "spaces" in μl/g were calculated by dividing the radioactivity in the tissue in dpm/g by the radioactivity in blood plasma in dpm/μl. As the tissue on both sides would have received blood containing the same amount of radioactive albumin, the higher spaces on the injected side (*solid symbols*) indicate that albumin was reaching the tissue directly from the injected testis, presumably in the lymph. (From ref. 26.)

Knowing the volume of the interstitial fluid, its turnover rate can be estimated from the half-time of clearance of albumin injected directly into the testis, as albumin injected in this way is almost exclusively removed in the lymph (497). The results obtained with this technique have already been discussed in the section on lymph flow.

Interstitial fluid can be collected from isolated testes for analysis by making an incision in the capsule and allowing the fluid to drip out into a container in the cold room (517–520) or collecting it by gentle centrifugation (521–523), and the volume of fluid collected in this way is well related to the volume of fluid in the testis, as determined with radioactive albumin (524–526). A more physiological approach is to use a push-pull cannula in anesthetized animals, the degree of dilution of the infused fluid with interstitial fluid being determined by loading the animal previously with an appropriate marker (527). When the "drip" technique was used, interstitial fluid appeared to contain higher concentrations of potassium and certain intracellular enzymes than blood plasma, and approximately twice the level of testosterone as testicular venous blood plasma. This would imply that testosterone was not crossing the endothelial lining of the capillaries as readily as one would expect (see ref. 528), but analysis of fluid collected with the push-pull cannula indicates that the testosterone concentration is certainly no higher than that in venous blood plasma and may be somewhat lower; the protein concentration is, as expected, similar to plasma, and the potassium and sodium concentrations, determined with ion-sensitive electrodes, are also similar to plasma (421).

Interstitial fluid collected by the drip technique contains a luteinizing-hormone-releasing-hormone (LHRH)-like substance (529–531) which may influence testosterone secretion by the Leydig cells (526,532–535). There is also a report that testicular interstitial fluid contains more than ten times as much androgen-binding protein (ABP) as testicular venous blood (522), but again these values may be somewhat suspect because of the unphysiological technique used for its collection. The Leydig cells of several species have also been shown to contain β-endorphin or other pro-opiomelanocortin-derived peptides (536–541), and as judged by the localization of the mRNA, the highest concentrations are found in the Leydig cells adjacent to tubules in which a generation of spermatozoa had just been shed (542). It has been suggested that this peptide may exert a paracrine effect on the function of Sertoli cells or an autocrine effect on the Leydig cells themselves, presumably by secretion into the interstitial fluid; however, its presence in this fluid has not been reported.

The amount of interstitial fluid in the rat testis is increased if the animal is treated with hCG (263,520) or LHRH (534), and in conditions where the spermatogenic function of the tubules is decreased, such as cryptorchidism (262,543) and following irradiation (450) or local heating of the testes (544).

Seminiferous Tubule Fluid: Flow and Composition

The lumina of the seminiferous tubules are filled with a fluid which carries the spermatozoa away when they have been released. Some studies have been made of the electrophysiology of isolated tubules in relation to fluid secretion (545,546), and a technique has been described for measuring fluid secretion *in vitro;* the rates found were approximately three times higher than those for the whole testis, and could be reduced by cooling, removal of glucose or potassium from the bathing medium, or the addition of the inhibitors 2,4-dinitrophenol, ouabain, or acetazolamide; removal of calcium from the bathing fluid caused an increase in secretory rate (547).

The amount of fluid being secreted *in vivo* by all the tubules plus the rete testis can be estimated by measuring the weight gain of a testis following ligation of the efferent ducts; the weight of the testis increases linearly for approximately 36 hr in rats and hamsters and for approximately 72 hr in sheep and goats, and histological examination of the ligated testes shows that the increase is due to distention of the seminiferous tubules and rete testis (548,549). Fluid secretion begins just after puberty in the rat, before the first spermatozoa are shed, with a sharp increase at approximately 30 days of age, reaching adult rates of approximately 15 μl/g of testis at approximately 40 days (528,548,550). Hypophysectomy has no immediate effect on fluid secretion (548), although there may be a small decrease before the testis begins to shrink (551). Treatment of young rats with FSH produced a small increase in fluid production, whereas LH, prolactin, growth hormone, or testosterone were without effect (549,550). LH injected into intact adult rats had no immediate effect (549,552), but repeated treatment of intact or hypophysectomized rats with LH or testosterone propionate did produce a small increase in fluid secretion (551). Fluid secretion continued in rats and rams made aspermatogenic by locally heating the testis (553,554), but fluid secretion decreased if the testis was made cryptorchid (548,550) and actually increased after treatment of adult rats with the antimitotic agent, busulphan (555). Fluid secretion can also be demonstrated in the testes of rats treated prenatally with busulphan or irradiation to destroy the germ cells (refs. 556; B.P. Setchell and B.T. Hinton, *unpublished results*) and in the testes of rats treated with ethanedimethane sulphonate to eliminate the Leydig cells (557). Fluid secretion is reduced if the rats were treated with inhibitors of carbonic anhydrase (558).

The dynamics of fluid flow in individual tubules is more difficult to study, but from the infusion of concentrated dye solutions into individual superficial tubules, or the introduction of small droplets of colored oil, it appears that the flow is irregular both in rate and direction. Each tubule did appear to have a preferred direction of flow, but whether this was towards or away from the rete testis could not be determined. By sampling as much fluid as possible from a single tubule over approximately 1 hr and by estimating the degree of dilution of infused dye, it did appear that the flow along each tubule is probably between 0.5 and 1 μl/hr (151), and as there are approximately 30 tubules in the rat, this would correspond reasonably well with the estimates of total flow.

Small samples of fluid can be removed by micropuncture from individual tubules for analysis, although the samples are so small that the range of possible analyses is limited (Tables 5 and 6). Originally it was believed that there was a higher concentration of spermatozoa in seminiferous tubule fluid (STF) than in rete testis fluid (560), but when the numbers were obtained by counting the cells (151) rather than centrifuging the samples, it became clear that the "spermatocrit" values for STF were too high (spermatocrit is analogous to hematocrit and measures the proportion of the luminal fluid occupied by spermatozoa following centrifugation in a small capillary tube). STF is appreciably hypertonic in the hamster (561), but not in the rat (560). There is almost ten times as much potassium in STF as in blood

TABLE 5. *Concentration (mM) of ionic constitutents in secretions of the male reproductive tract*[a]

Male reproductive tract secretions	Sodium	Potassium	Calcium	Magnesium	Chloride	Phosphate	Bicarbonate
Seminiferous tubule fluid							
Rat	108 (±7)	50 (±5)	0.44 (±0.02)	1.2 (±0.18)	120 (±5)	<0.1	20
Rete testis fluid							
Wallaby	118	14			137		
Rat	143 (±4)	14 (±1)	0.81 (±0.09)	0.39 (±0.09)	140 (±2)	<0.1	21
Rabbit	147	7.8	0.8	0.5			
Ram	121	11.2	1.0	0.4	128	0.025	8
Bull	133	9.1	0.4	0.4	122	0.017	7
Boar	116	8.8	1.2		134	0.22	
Monkey	136	7.4					
Cauda epididymidis or ductus deferens							
Rat	26 (15–37)	47 (43–55)	0.18 (0.11–0.25)	1.1 (0.9–1.3)	24 (20–27)	13 (9.5–16)	6.7
Hamster	16 (6.1–25)	31 (24–38)	0.1	1.3	11	29	
Guinea pig	17	18	0.1	2.2	10	5.4	
Rabbit	17 (15–20)	22 (18–25)	0.47	7.2	14 (8–23)	3.9	
Dog	22	38	0.85	1.1	16	7.2	
Goat	56	38	1.3				
Ram	40 (22–57)	29 (24–39)	0.61 (0.48–0.95)	0.7 (0.3–1.3)	22 (9.4–34)	8.3 (7.6–9)	
Bull	34 (30–38)	26 (22–28)	1.35 (0.35–1.1)	1.2	30 (12–65)	17.5 (14–21)	0
Boar	30 (24–38)	35 (35–48)	1.8 (0.9–2.8)	0.8 (0–1.2)	13 (3.4–23)	5.3 (2.2–12)	4
Stallion	41	32	0.55	1.2	12	4.3	
Elephant	103	37					
Monkey	18	49		2	10.5	1.7	
Man	30	111			103	24	
Ampulla							
Goat	50	31	1.9				
Bull	84 (60–108)	28	8.8 (8–9.6)	3.1 (2.7–3.5)			
Stallion					36		

continued

TABLE 5. *Continued*

Male reproductive tract secretions	Sodium	Potassium	Calcium	Magnesium	Chloride	Phosphate	Bicarbonate
Seminal vesicles							
Rat						4.8	
Guinea pig						1.6	
Goat	87	61	3				
Ram	93	37	3.4	3.2			
Bull	109	64 (27–100)	15 (12.6–17.5)	5.6 (3.9–7.2)		2.3	
Boar	26 (22–30)	126 (24–300)	3	28	12 (3–20)	1 (0.7–1.3)	
Stallion					59		
Man		19 (18–20)			28	8.9 (3.2–14.5)	
Prostate							
Dog	157 (154–159)	6.3 (5.1–8.7)	0.5 (0.3–1.1)	0.6	160	1	4.2
Man	155 (153–157)	53 (45–67)	26 (15–32)	19 (17–20)	45 (38–61)	1	8
Cowper's gland							
Boar	90	28			105	2.3	

[a]Where several values were available, the mean was calculated and the SEM or the range is shown in parentheses. From refs. 651 and 142.

plasma (560,562,563). However, in rats made aspermatogenic by treatment *in utero* with busulphan or irradiation, the potassium concentration in STF was serum-like (151,564,565; but cf. ref. 566). Chloride concentration in STF is similar to plasma (560,563) and so is calcium and sulphur, whereas magnesium and total phosphorus are higher in STF (563). The protein concentration is less in STF than in blood plasma or interstitial fluid (151,152), but there are a number of proteins in tubular fluid which cannot be seen in blood plasma (567–570) and high concentrations of androgen-binding protein (522,571). There are also low concentrations of transferrin in STF, approximately 25 times less than in blood plasma or testicular interstitial fluid (572). Glucose cannot be detected in STF, but there is more than 100 times as much inositol as in blood plasma (573). The concentration of testosterone in STF (Table 7) is slightly lower than that in interstitial fluid, and both increase similarly if the animal is stimulated for 4 days with hCG (574).

Larger samples of less pure fluid can be collected by decapsulating the testis, disrupting the seminiferous tubules by forcing the parenchyma through a hypodermic needle, and centrifuging the cell dispersion. Contamination with interstitial fluid can be minimized by rinsing the tubules before disrupting them (522), or by applying a correction obtained by ligating the efferent ducts of one testis 16 hr previously to increase the proportion of tubular fluid in that testis, and assuming that both have the same amount of interstitial fluid (575–577). With the latter variant, the potassium and inositol content of the fluid are identical to those of fluid obtained by micropuncture, and with both variants, the testosterone concentrations are similar. However, with the former variant, the protein content is clearly higher, suggesting that there is appreciable contamination with cell contents or interstitial fluid; androgen-binding protein concentrations, on the other hand, are appreciably lower than in micropuncture fluid. When the testosterone concentration in the blood was raised by parenteral injection of the steroid in oil or hCG, the concentration of testosterone in tubular fluid did increase, but not to the same extent; this was taken as evidence that testosterone was entering the tubules by a process involving facilitated diffusion (577,578).

Rete Testis Fluid: Flow and Composition

Rete testis fluid (RTF) has been collected from catheters chronically implanted into the rete testis of rams (579,580), bulls (581), and boars (582,583), and acutely from rats (560,584), rhesus monkeys (585), rabbits (586–589), and wallabies (590). In some studies, the efferent ducts were ligated for some hours beforehand to allow some fluid to accumulate, but this does not appear to make much difference to the flow of the fluid once the accumulated fluid has gone (584).

Flow rate of fluid from a catheter was usually in the range of 4 to 20 μl/g/hr, with the smaller animals tending to have faster flows (see refs. 2,142,591–593). The flow of fluid in rams is steady and shows no apparent diurnal rhythm. Administration of gonadotropins does not have any obvious effect, nor did atropine or pilocarpine. Oxytocin had no

TABLE 6. *Concentration (mM) of low-molecular-weight organic compounds and of total protein (mg/ml) in secretions of the male reproductive tract*[a]

Male reproductive tract secretions	Glucose	Fructose	Inositol	Citric acid	Carnitine	Glycero-phospho-choline	Phospho-choline	Ergo-thioneine	Ascorbic acid	Protein
Seminiferous tubule fluid										
Rat	<1		1.8		<1	<0.1	<0.1			6
Hamster			3.2		<1					
Rabbit			2.1							
Rhesus monkey			9.5							
Rete testis fluid										
Rat	<0.1		2.5		<1	<0.1	<0.1			
Hamster			3.1		<1					
Ram	0.1		5.7		0.028					1
Boar			5.7		0.012					1.1
Cauda epididymidis or ductus deferens										
Rat			31		54 (16–82)	32 (21–41)	20			32 (27–41)
Hamster			90		30 (11–48)	41				37 (24–49)
Guinea pig					67	39 (27–51)				34 (25–42)
Rabbit		0	0		43 (19–69)	41 (19–59)				42 (35–62)
Dog					20	34				30
Ram			2.1 (1–3.2)		17 (15–19)	65 (21–97)				19 (13–27)
Bull			2.5	0	2	36 (17–54)				31 (29–33)
Boar		0.2								
			2.8 (1–5.3)	0.3 (0–0.6)	11 (6–16)	72 (48–111)		0.06 (0–0.13)		35 (19–100)
								0		
Jackass				0						
Stallion					11	45 (43–46)				32
Elephant										36
Monkey			17		80	87				74
Man			5.9		5.8 (5.5–6)	< 5	< 5			29

continued

TABLE 6. *Continued*

Male reproductive tract secretions	Glucose	Fructose	Inositol	Citric acid	Carnitine	Glycero-phospho-choline	Phospho-choline	Ergo-thioneine	Ascorbic acid	Protein
Ampulla										
Rat				0						
Bull				29		3.4				
Jackass				0				3.8 (2.2–5)		
Zebra			0	0						
Stallion		0.15	1.1	0.04 (0.02–0.05)				3.6 (1.9–6.1)		
Elephant		4.3		0						
Seminal vesicles										
Hedgehog		28		0				2		
Rat	0.4	0.2		6		22 (16–25)		0	0.23	250 (200–300)
Mouse	1.1	31								
Vole	0.3	0								
Hamster	trace	0								
Guinea pig	9 (6.5–11)	5.8 (3.5–6.9)	1.1 (6–18)	12		10		0	0.5	
Coypu		3		5						
Rabbit				43						
Ram		99								55
Bull		46	1.6	35		trace		0	0.8	
Buffalo		54		15						
Boar		4.3 (3.1–6.2)	117 (100–134)	30 (29–32)		6.9		2.9 (1.8–3.8)	0.23	99 (80–112)
Jackass				3.3 (2.7–3.8)				0.09		
Stallion		trace		13 (6.6–19)		trace		0.49 (0.26–0.71)		
Zebra				27						
Elephant		4		0.01						
Monkey			8.1			0				
Man		22		3.8 (1–6.5)				0	0.28	

TABLE 6. *Continued*

Male reproductive tract secretions	Glucose	Fructose	Inositol	Citric acid	Carnitine	Glycero-phospho-choline	Phospho-choline	Ergo-thioneine	Ascorbic acid	Protein
Coagulating glands										
Rat	9	28 (23–34)		0						240
Guinea pig		0		0						
Coypu		0.2		19						
Prostate										
Rat		0				0				95
Guinea pig		0								
Dog				0.14					0.04	8
Boar								0		44
Jackass				0				0		
Stallion				trace				trace		
Elephant		2.1		0.15						
Man	0.9	0	8.2	91 (45–176)					0.03	24 (22–26)
Cowper's glands										
Coypu		0.1		0.2						
Hedgehog		0		4.5				0		
Rabbit		0								
Boar		0	0	0				0		5
Elephant		0.06		0.26						

[a]Where several values were available, the mean was calculated and the range is shown in parentheses.
From refs. 651 and 142.

TABLE 7. *Concentration (ng/ml) of steroids in the testicular excurrent duct system*[a]

Steroid	Peripheral blood plasma	Seminiferous tubule fluid	Rete testis fluid	Caput epididymal fluid	Cauda epididymal fluid
Pregnenolone					
Rabbit	2.8		3.3–22.4		
Ram			0.85		9.9
Progesterone					
Rabbit			1.2		
Bull	0.3–0.6		3.7		7.4
Dehydroepiandrosterone					
Rabbit	0.4		0.5–4.2	4.2	
Ram			6.4	33.8	25.8
Bull	0.65–0.71		21	8	
5-Androstene-3,17-dione					
Rabbit	0.1		1.1–5.2		
Dog				2	
Ram			1.5		1.3
Bull	0.38–0.57		7.6–17		1.7
Testosterone					
Rat	0.8–7.7	40–115	22–46.5	5	2–4
Rabbit	0.5–10		47.8–69		
Dog	0.8–1.9				2.5
Ram	0.7–26		3–88	24.8	10.8
Bull	2–24		20.4–33		6.2–11.5
Boar	2.9–7		13.3		
Monkey	3.2–10.3		2.5–10.5		
Dihydrotestosterone					
Rat	0.24	1.0–1.5	1.9–32.7	40	5–7
Rabbit	0.5		11.2–28.5		
Dog				3	
Ram	0.14		1		4.4–17
Bull	<0.03–0.10		1.3		13.6–20.3
5α-Androstan-3α,17β-diol					
Rat			26		9.2
Dog					2.1
Bull	< 0.03		1.6		4.0
5α-Androstan-3β,17β-diol					
Rat			8		7.8
Dog					1.8
Bull	< 0.03		2.4		6.5
5-Androstene-3β,17β-diol					
Bull	0.12–0.16		4.0		4.2
Estradiol or total estrogens					
Rat			0.248		
Rabbit			<0.02–0.027		
Bull	0.009–0.010		0.012		0.026
Boar	0.050		0.10		
Monkey			0.066		

[a]From ref. 651. Values for peripheral blood plasma are from refs. 81 and 825–829.

effect in one study (594), although there was a small short-lived increase in another (595). Reducing the concentration of spermatozoa by locally heating the testis had no effect on the flow of fluid (553), and fluid flow increased first, followed by sperm concentration, at the beginning of the breeding season of rams in France (596).

RTF is a dilute suspension of immature, immotile spermatozoa, the concentration ranging from approximately 30 million/ml in rats and rabbits to between 100 and 300 million/ml in rams, boars, and monkeys (see refs. 2,142,591–593,597). In rams, there is a seasonal variation in concentration (596), and locally heating the testis causes a drop in sperm concentration approximately 20 days later, without any apparent effect on flow or composition of the fluid (553). In rats, a similar but slightly earlier fall in sperm concentration can be detected (554). As well as being immotile, the testicular spermatozoa differ from sperm from the tail of the epididymis in composition, metabolism, and surface properties (see Chapter 23, *these volumes*).

The ionic composition of RTF is different from blood plasma, lymph, and testicular interstitial fluid on the one hand, and from STF on the other; its potassium and sodium concentrations are intermediate, and it contains more chloride and less bicarbonate than any of the other fluids (Table 5). The concentrations of calcium and magnesium in ram RTF are about half of the total in blood plasma, but similar to the concentrations of the free ions (see refs. 2,142,591, 592,597), although measurements in rats using electron probe microanalysis gave serum-like values for magnesium and higher than serum for calcium, with calcium higher and magnesium less than in STF (563). Inorganic phosphate was undetectable in rat RTF (598), and much lower than blood plasma in the rat (597); total phosphorus was slightly lower in RTF than in serum, but much lower than in STF. Total sulphur concentrations were comparable in all three fluids (563). There is practically no glucose in RTF, but inositol is to be found there in concentrations up to 100 times those in blood plasma (573,599) (Table 6). The inositol appears to be formed by synthesis within the tubules from glucose, not accumulated as such from the blood (600), and if rats are given galactose in their diet, RTF contains galactitol as well as inositol (601). Ram RTF contains about as much glycerol as does testicular venous blood, and this substrate, in contrast to inositol can be used by testicular spermatozoa (602). Lactate and pyruvate are present in RTF in similar concentrations to those in blood plasma, and there are slightly lower concentrations of acetate (142). Most of the free amino acids are found in RTF in lower concentrations than in blood, but glutamate, aspartate, glycine, and alanine are present in much higher concentrations (327,501).

RTF contains very little protein (Table 6), approximately 1 mg/ml, even less than STF, although the reason for this latter difference is not clear (151,152). Many of the proteins of blood plasma appear to be present in RTF, but this fluid is proportionately richer in α_2-macroglobulin, which is less abundant in lymph (see Lymph Flow and Composition, p. 800), although immunoglobulins are proportionately even lower than total protein (603,604). Using step-gel electrophoresis, it was shown that a number of blood plasma proteins were not present in RTF, and, conversely, there were proteins in RTF that could not be found in blood plasma; however, the concentrations of these specific proteins appeared to be less in RTF than in STF (567). Using polyvalent antisera, it was found that RTF contained nine specific proteins and 12 proteins identical to those in serum; however, even the latter were probably also synthesized by the Sertoli cells and not derived from the blood (605). Rat RTF contains an ABP (606,607), which can only be detected in blood at very much lower concentrations, and is probably derived from the testis (608,609); the concentration in RTF is very similar to that found in micropuncture samples of STF (522). ABP is also present in ram RTF, but in this species a very similar protein is found in blood plasma even in castrated animals (610). Boar RTF contains no detectable ABP (B. Jegou and J.-L. Dacheux, quoted in ref. 610). Transferrin is found in rat RTF in concentrations approximately one-third of those in STF, and approximately 75 times less than those in blood plasma and lymph (572). A number of enzymes are found in higher concentrations in ram RTF than in blood plasma, and one isozyme of malate dehydrogenase and one of aspartate aminotransferase are found in RTF but not in blood plasma; the isozymes of lactate dehydrogenase found in RTF are those found in many tissues, but isozyme X, which is specific to the testis, is not present in RTF (611). Rat RTF also contains different forms of esterase, acid phosphatase (568) and uridine 5′-diphosphate (UDP)-galactose: *N*-acetylglucosamine galactosyltransferase (612) from those found in blood serum; this last enzyme is believed to transfer galactose from UDP-galactose to glycoproteins in epididymal fluid or spermatozoa and its receptor specificity is changed from *N*-acetylglucosamine to glucose or inositol by an α-lactalbumin-like material in epididymal fluid (613). RTF from rams and boars contains high concentrations of a peptide inhibitor of trypsin and acrosin, which may be important in neutralizing the effect of any of the latter enzyme released prematurely from the spermatozoa (611,614).

A nonglycosylated peptide mitogenic growth factor, which stimulates the division of mouse 3-T-3 cells in culture has been found in ram RTF; this factor appears to be different from other better-known growth factors (615), and from the growth factor derived from Sertoli cells (616). Another peptide has been described in RTF which inhibits spermatogonial mitoses (617). There is also a highly acidic glycoprotein there which has been named "clusterin" and which elicits clustering of Sertoli and other cells in culture; this substance comprises approximately 18% of the total protein in ram RTF and may be involved in influencing cell interactions in the testis or epididymis at some stage of germ cell development or maturation (618,619). Ram RTF is a potent source of inhibin-like activity (620,621), although the endocrinological significance of this hormone to the male animal is still obscure; and Mullerian duct inhibiting factor, usually considered to be a secretory product of fetal Sertoli cells, can be found in boar RTF (622).

Testosterone was shown to be present in some of the first samples of RTF collected from conscious rams (579), and since then a number of analyses of fluids from a variety of species have been reported (Table 7). In general, most of the free steroids present in interstitial fluid or testicular venous blood are present in RTF, though usually in slightly lower concentrations if the concentrations outside the tubules are normal or elevated (81,522,553,574,577, 581,585, 588,589,623–632). Conjugated steroids are present in much lower concentrations in RTF than in venous blood or lymph (81). On the other hand, in hypophysectomized rats, especially if they were treated with pregnenolone, 17-hydroxypregnenolone, progesterone, or 17-hydroxyprogesterone, the concentrations of androgens in the RTF are higher than those in testicular venous blood (523,626). The concentration of testosterone in RTF is lower than that in STF, whereas the concentration of DHT is higher in RTF (522,574). The concentration of testosterone is similar in fluid collected after ligation of the efferent ducts and in fluid collected without ligation, whereas estradiol concentrations are much higher in samples collected from unligated testes (584).

The earlier observations on ionic composition and on spermatocrit (560,633) were interpreted as evidence for two types of secretion, one in the tubules and one in the rete. However, later evidence on the similar numbers of spermatozoa and the similar concentrations of inositol in the two fluids, led to a revision of this two-fluid theory, and it was suggested that the composition of tubular fluid was altered when it reached the rete (151). This conclusion has been supported by the observation that the concentration of ABP was similar in the two fluids (522), but is difficult to reconcile with the differences in total protein and steroids, although it is possible that these compounds and others may be resorbed in the rete. There is some evidence that the rete and the tubules may have different permeabilities to sodium and potassium ions (151), and it has been suggested that substances can exchange directly between the superficial testicular veins and the fluid in the rete (634).

Whereas the STF is of interest primarily as a reflection of the complex cell interaction involved in spermatogenesis, RTF has the added interest of being a possible route of communication between the testis and epididymis, although many of the functions of the epididymis are unaffected by interrupting the flow of RTF by ligating the efferent ducts (see ref. 635). However, the cells in the first part of the epididymis do appear to alter after efferent duct ligation (277,636–640), and specific changes in intermediary metabolism (641) and in protein synthesis (642–644) are evident. Thus further investigation on the significance of RTF in the control of epididymal function would appear to be warranted.

Epididymis

The RTF which passes to the epididymis by way of the ductuli efferentes is the initial source of luminal fluid for the epididymis. A cilio-peristaltic model for the flow of the fluid and spermatozoa through the efferent ducts has been proposed (645). It is now well established that the epididymis has both a secretory and absorptive function and thus the composition of the RTF is extensively modified as it makes its progress through the epididymal duct. Originally the extent of these modifications was assessed by cannulating the rete testis and distal cauda epididymidis or vas deferens and comparing the composition of the fluids thus obtained. Greater insight into which regions of the epididymis are responsible for making specific changes to the composition of the intraluminal fluid has been gained by the use of the micropuncture technique. The most extensive studies of this type have been carried out in the laboratory rat and are presented in Fig. 49.

The absorptive capacity of the epididymal epithelium, which results in the bulk removal of fluid, is reflected by the increase in spermatocrit (Fig. 49). The proximal caput is the principal region involved in fluid resorption, but due to the technical difficulties of cannulating this region of the epididymal duct, the cauda epididymidis has been used more extensively to study the mechanism of fluid resorption. Here, it has been shown that resorption is an energy-dependent process which can be modified by hormones and sympathetic agents (646–650). It has been suggested that sodium ions are passively transported from the luminal fluid at the luminal surface of the epithelial cells, and actively transported at the serosal surface to establish a standing osmotic gradient which draws water and chloride ions from the luminal fluid. In contrast, potassium and phosphate ions are retained or secreted into the luminal fluid with the result that their concentration increases as the fluid travels down the epididymal duct (Fig. 49). However, the bulk of the replacement of sodium chloride is with various low molecular weight organic molecules which, together with the remaining ions, sustain a constant fluid osmolarity. The principal organic molecules involved in this replacement are glycerophosphocholine, phosphocholine, carnitine, and inositol (Fig. 49). The other feature brought out in Fig. 49 is the marked acidification of the epididymal fluid, which occurs in the proximal portion of the epididymis. This is achieved by the removal of bicarbonate and is possibly aided by the addition or retention of substantial quantities of glutamic acid (651). It is now recognized that the low pH of epididymal fluid, and the presence of permeant organic acids are important contributing factors to the maintenance of sperm in a quiescent condition within the epididymal environment (652,653).

There is a general lack of reducing sugar in epididymal fluid. However, a facilitated transport system for glucose does exist in epididymal cells (654) and glucose can be shown to appear in the epididymal lumen when the normal luminal contents are removed (655,656). Transport of the nonmetabolizable glucose analog 3-*O*-methylglucose from the bloodstream to the epididymal lumen *in vivo* has also been demonstrated (657). It has been suggested that metabolic disposal of glucose by sperm within the epididymal lumen normally accounts for the failure of reducing sugar to accumulate in the epididymal fluid (658).

The high concentration of inositol in cauda epididymal fluid is a specific feature of the rat, hamster, and monkey (573) (Table 6); in other species, such as bull and rabbit, inositol concentrations are greater in proximal than in distal regions of the duct (659). The testis actively synthesizes inositol from glucose (660,661) and the secreted inositol passes into the epididymis with the RTF (560,573,599,659). It has been calculated that additional inositol must be added

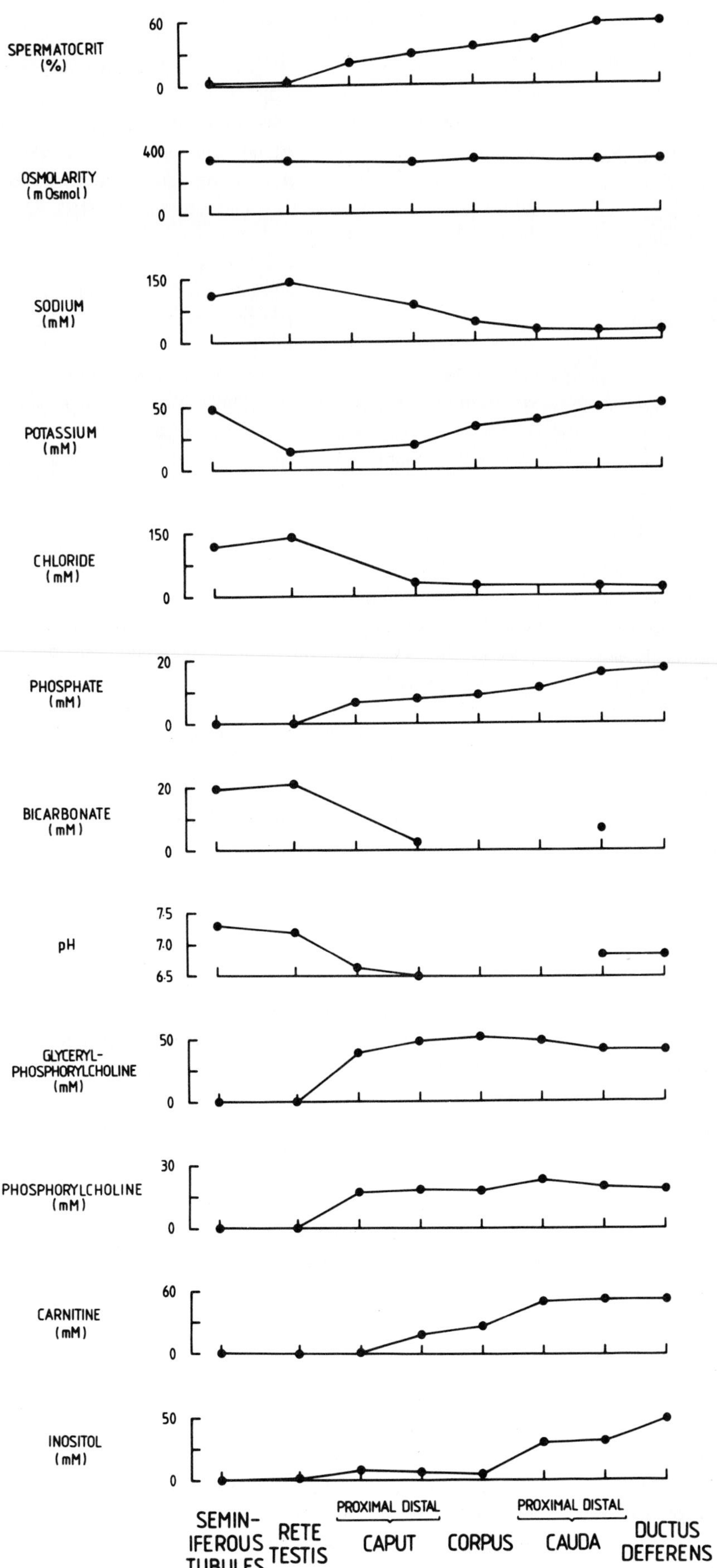

FIG. 49. Characteristics of the fluid sampled at various points within the testis and excurrent duct system of the rat. (From ref. 679.)

to the epididymal fluid (662). This could occur by synthetic activity of the epididymal tissue (663,664) and by transport from the bloodstream (656,665–668).

High concentrations of glycerophosphocholine are encountered in the epididymal plasma of all species studied except man (Table 6). Epididymal tissue itself is responsible for the synthesis of this compound (669,670). Current evidence favors epididymal lecithin as the immediate precursor (669,671,672), which may in turn be derived from lecithin associated with blood lipoproteins (673).

Another major constituent of epididymal fluid, except in the bull, is carnitine (Table 6). This compound is transported into the epididymal lumen against a concentration gradient of over 2000:1 (674–677) by a saturable uptake process (678,679). The epididymis itself appears unable to synthesize carnitine (680).

Epididymal fluid contains a broad range of amino acids (501,681–684) with particularly high levels of glutamic acid (10–30 mM) in the ram, bull, and boar; asparagine plus glutamine (21 mM) in the ram; and taurine plus hypotaurine (50 mM) in the boar and rabbit. The concentration of urea is in the range of 7 to 19 mM (682,684), which is comparable to the concentration in blood serum (1–10 mM) (685).

Epididymal fluid contains substantial quantities of steroid hormones and their metabolites (Table 7). The RTF entering the epididymis is undoubtably a major source of these steroids, at least for fluid from proximal regions of the epididymal duct (Table 7). Testosterone is the predominant androgen in RTF, but is converted to the reduced form of dihydrotestosterone on entering the epididymal duct, due presumably to the activity of 5α-reductase in the epididymal epithelium. The bloodstream is the other major route for the supply of androgens to the epididymis; uptake of systemic androgens into the epididymal lumen has been amply demonstrated (686–689).

It is not our intention to discuss in any depth the protein components of epididymal fluid; for this the reader is referred to in Chapter 23 and the review by Brooks (651). Suffice it to say that there has been a particular interest in recent years in analyzing various androgen-dependent secretory proteins (690) which are synthesized and secreted by the epididymal epithelium, and which are implicated in effecting the functional maturation of sperm during their passage through the epididymis. This functional maturation is thought to be brought about by an incorporation of the proteins into the sperm plasma membrane or through enzymatic activity of the proteins producing changes to existing membrane components. The most intensively studied species has been the rat in which several of these epididymal proteins have been purified (644,691–696), and for two of the proteins the complete amino acid sequence has been derived by cloning their cDNA (697,698). The use of antibody and cDNA probes has in general established that the secretory proteins are tissue-specific and species-specific (697–699). The precise physiological role of any particular protein, however, remains to be established.

Fluids of the Accessory Glands

The male accessory glands contain a rather bewildering array of chemical constituents and we still remain rather ignorant of the specific physiological function of many of the components. Accessory glands were originally classified on the basis of their gross morphology and anatomical relationship to other parts of the male reproductive tract. Unfortunately, this classification does not always coincide with functional relationships from the point of view of the nature of the chemical constituents present in the secretion (1).

For instance, fructose, which is the principal glycolyzable substrate for sperm in seminal plasma, may, depending on species, have its origin in either the seminal vesicles, coagulating glands, or ampullary glands. Moreover, particular chemical constituents are present almost universally in mammalian semen, but are notably absent from the semen of certain species without any obvious physiological explanation. This is the case with fructose, for example, which is completely lacking in the semen of the dog, stallion, and jackass. For these reasons a global description of the composition of the chemical constituents of the secretions of the male accessory glands is difficult. However, a comprehensive catalog of the concentration of identified constituents in the accessory gland secretions of various animals is presented in Tables 5 and 6, and a description of the more salient features is attempted. For more detailed and comprehensive historical accounts, and in particular for a review of the protein components of these fluids, the reader is referred to Mann (700), Mann and Lutwak-Mann (701), Brooks (651), and Chapter 24.

Ampulla

There have been only scattered reports on the composition of the secretion of the ampulla due perhaps to the problem of obtaining pure ampullary secretion without contamination from fluid arriving at the ampulla from the ductus deferens. In the goat there is little difference in fluid composition between the epididymis and ampulla (Table 5) but, in the bull, the concentration of sodium, calcium, and magnesium ions are two to ten times greater in fluid from the ampulla then from the epididymis (702,703). Fluid from the bovine ampulla contains a high concentration of citric acid (704), whereas the stallion and jackass are noted for the substantial quantities of ergothionine present in this secretion (705–708).

Seminal Vesicles

Sodium and potassium are the predominant cations in seminal vesicle secretion (Table 5). Unusually high concentrations of calcium and magnesium are found in the vesicular secretion of bull and boar, respectively (702, 703,709). Chloride and phosphate concentrations are relatively low (Table 5), indicating that some other moiety must be the major anion. The usual alkaline pH of vesicular secretion may indicate that bicarbonate is an important anion, and undoubtably citrate also fulfils a role as a major anion (Table 6).

The seminal vesicle is the principal accessory gland responsible for synthesis of fructose from blood glucose in the majority of species. Glucose itself is also present in the vesicular secretion of some species, attaining a concentration equivalent to that of blood plasma in the guinea pig (710,711). Fructose is lacking in stallion and jackass semen which implies that these sugars are not secreted by the seminal vesicles (or any other gland) in these species. The synthesis of fructose, like many other secretory products of the male accessory glands, is strictly regulated by androgenic hormones, and the concentration of seminal fructose can serve as a simple test of the androgenic status of an animal.

Inositol, a cyclic polyol, is present in the vesicular secretion of several species (Table 6) attaining extraordinarily high concentrations in the case of the boar (709,712). High concentrations are also found in extracts of rat seminal vesicles (661,713). Most of the inositol is present as *myo*-inositol, but approximately 6% of the total occurs as scylloinositol (714). Other compounds that are present in high concentrations in a few species include glycerophosphocholine [rat, guinea pig, and boar (671,715,716)], ergothioneine [boar, stallion, and hedgehog (705,707,712,717)], and hypotaurine and taurine [guinea pig (718)]. The prostaglandin content of seminal plasma, which is particularly high in the case of man and the ram, is probably derived principally from the seminal vesicle secretion (719,720).

Coagulating Glands

In the rat, the coagulating glands, rather than the seminal vesicles, are responsible for fructose secretion (704, 710,721,722). In the mouse, this activity is shared by the coagulating glands and the seminal vesicles, whereas the coagulating gland secretion is devoid of fructose in the guinea pig and coypu (723,724). Glucose and citric acid are found in the secretions of the rat and coypu, respectively (704,710, 722,725).

Prostate

The composition of prostatic secretion has largely been gleaned from the dog since in this species neither seminal vesicles nor bulbourethral glands are present. A surgical procedure has been developed to divert the urinary outflow which allows pure prostatic secretion to be collected directly from the urethra (212,726). Moreover, the rate of production of secretion can be enhanced from 0.1 to 2 ml/hr to 60 ml/hr by administration of pilocarpine hydrochloride (211,212). However, there are significant differences in the composition of canine prostatic secretion when "resting fluid" is compared with "active secretion" produced under the influence of pilocarpine, hypogastric nerve stimulation, or during ejaculation (418). The predominant ionic constituents of canine prostatic active secretion are sodium and chloride (Table 5). In contrast, human prostatic secretion contains considerably more calcium and potassium, and the principal anion is citrate rather than chloride. Prostatic secretion is usually slightly acid with a pH of about 6.5 (212). Citric acid also occurs in the prostate of rat, mole, and hedgehog (704,717,721), whereas inositol is an important component of the rat prostate (713) and possibly the human prostate (727).

The prostate in man and rat is also a rich source of polyamines, particularly spermine and spermidine (728–731). The concentration of spermine and spermidine in rat prostatic secretion has been measured as 6 mM and 7 mM, respectively (725), whereas in blood serum these compounds are essentially undetectable.

Bulbourethral Glands

The ionic composition of the secretion of the bulbourethral glands has been reported only for the boar (Table 5). The secretion generally lacks any of the unusual low-molecular-weight organic compounds encountered in the other accessory glands (Table 6). The principal component of the secretion is a sialomucin which is responsible for the gelation reaction in boar semen (732,733). The composition of the mucin has been analyzed (732,734) and found to contain on a dry weight basis 27% sialic acid, 13% galactose (probably as *N*-acetylgalactosamine), and 4% neutral sugars. The extraordinarily high content of sialic acid accounts for the very low isoelectric point ($pI = 1.1$) of the mucin. The approximate molecular weight of the mucin has been estimated as 6.5×10^6 daltons.

Preputial Glands

Preputial glands differ from other accessory glands in that they do not produce a copious watery secretion. Rather, these glands are modified sebaceous glands, and as such they produce a fatty secretion which seems to be primarily associated with pheromonal functions (e.g., refs. 735–737). The precise structure of these pheromones has not been determined but in the rat they are possibly volatile seven- and eight-carbon alcohols (738).

Seminal Plasma

Seminal plasma is the fluid portion of the ejaculate and results from the admixture of secretions from the various male accessory glands during seminal emission. Several points should be borne in mind when analyzing the composition of seminal plasma. For instance, there is a temporal sequence among the glands with respect to voidance of their respective secretions; complete mixing of the secretions may not take place for semen deposited normally within the female reproductive tract. In the case of semen collected artificially by electroejaculation, the contribution of any particular accessory gland is critically dependent on the positioning of the stimulating electrodes. There is also considerable variation in seminal plasma composition between individual males as well as for the same individual between successive ejaculates, which may reflect seasonal differences and the time intervening since the previous ejaculation. Apart from this form of variability, there are also changes brought about in seminal plasma composition following ejaculation through the agency of enzymes in the seminal plasma and metabolic activity of the sperm suspended in the seminal plasma. Particular examples of enzymatic activity in seminal plasma include proteolytic activity which results in liberation of peptides and amino acids, and, in human seminal plasma, the hydrolysis of phosphocholine to release free phosphate which interacts with spermine to form insoluble crystals of spermine phosphate. The most obvious change induced by spermatozoa is the metabolic conversion of fructose to lactic acid.

A detailed account of the composition of seminal plasma can be found in the monographs by Mann (700) and Mann and Lutwak-Mann (701). A summary of the most salient features is presented in Table 8. Our coverage is restricted to inorganic ions and low-molecular-weight organic molecules.

Sodium is the principal cation in seminal plasma, but its concentration is considerably below that encountered in blood plasma and interstitial fluid. The deficit is to some extent accounted for by potassium. Calcium and magnesium concentrations in seminal plasma are generally similar to those of blood plasma, although there are exceptions, such as the high concentration of calcium in the case of bull, stallion, and man, and of magnesium in rabbit and boar (Table 8). However, the proportion of these ions which are free in solution as against that proportion which is complexed with low-molecular-weight organic molecules (e.g., citrate) and proteins has not generally been ascertained. Chloride is the principal anion and bicarbonate concentrations are relatively low, although postejaculatory changes in bicarbonate concentration have generally not been taken into account.

TABLE 8. *Concentration of various substances in the seminal plasma of several species*[a]

Seminal plasma	Rabbit	Dog	Ram	Goat	Boar	Bull	Stallion	Man
Volume (ml)	0.4–6	2–15	0.7–2	0.2–2.5	150–500	2–10	30–300	2–6
Sperm concentration ($\times 10^{-6}$/ml)	50–350	60–300	2,000–5,000	1,000–5,000	25–300	300–2,000	30–800	50–150
Sodium	61–82	72–180	77		125–252	65–161	112	43–112
Potassium	20–29	8	23		17–46	13–97	26	14–28
Calcium	1.5–2	0.2–1.2	1.6–2.3		1.5–4.6	6–15	6.5	5–7
Magnesium	11	0.15–1.5	2.4		2.5–24	3.3	3.7	1.2–5
Chloride	99	152	51		85–105	42–110	23–113	28–56
Phosphate		0.3	2.5		0.4	2.8	0.6	
Bicarbonate		2.9	7			7	11	8
Fructose	2.2–18	<0.03	8–37		0.5	17–56	<0.06	2–33
Glucose	1.6				0.06–0.3		0.7	0.4
Sorbitol	4.4	<0.05	1.4–6.6		0.4	0.6–7.5	1.1–3.3	0.6
Inositol			0.6–0.8		28	1.3–2.6	1.1–2.6	3–3.5
Lactic acid		1.2–3.3	3.9		2.2	2.2–5.6	1–2.8	2.2–5.6
Pyruvic acid			1.1			0.6	0.3	3.4
Citric acid	5.2–26		16–42		2.6–10.4	18–52	0.5–2.6	5.2–73
Glutamic acid			4.5–5.2		2	1–8		6.5
Ascorbic acid			0.3			0.3	0.3	0.6
Carnitine			4.5					0.2–1.3
Acetylcarnitine			2.8					0.06–0.28
Glycerophosphocholine	7.6–14	6.6	58–73	51–58	4	4–18	1.4–4	2.0–3.3
Phosphocholine	0		0	0	0	0	0	14–21
Glycerophosphoinositol			1.5		0.26	1.4	0.25	
Spermine						0.1		3
Spermidine								0.1
Putrescine								0.2
Creatine	0.15	0	0.15–1.2			0.9	0.4	1.5
Arginine	0	0.11	0.53–1.2		0.01	0.2		5.2
Creatine					0.03	1.1	0.3	
Ergothionine			trace	absent	0.7	trace	0.2–0.7	trace
Uric acid			0.24–1.4					0.1–0.4
Protein (mg/ml)	22	24			30	55		35–50

[a]Concentration is given in mM unless stated otherwise.
From refs. 501, 676, 682, 683, 700–702, 754, and 830–839.

Fructose rather than glucose is the principal reducing sugar in seminal plasma, although small amounts of glucose are also encountered. It thus serves as the major glycolyzable substrate for spermatozoa in semen. Fructose concentrations are particularly high in bull and ram seminal plasma, but are considerably lower in other species, whereas fructose is essentially absent from dog and stallion semen (Table 8). In certain Australian marsupials, the chief seminal carbohydrate is not fructose, but *N*-acetylglucosamine (739,740). The concentration of *N*-acetylglucosamine in kangaroo seminal plasma is in the range of 15 to 23 mM; glucose is also present at a concentration of 1.6 to 6.2 mM (740). The origin of the *N*-acetylglucosamine in marsupial semen is the prostate (741). *N*-acetylglucosamine may not, however, be the characteristic sugar of the semen of all marsupials (218). Sorbitol also occurs in seminal plasma. The sperm of some species such as rams, but not boars, possess a sorbitol dehydrogenase which enables sorbitol to be converted to fructose and used as a metabolic substrate (742,743). Inositol is another polyol which is present in seminal plasma, particularly in the boar where it is derived from the seminal vesicle secretion. However, unlike sorbitol, inositol cannot be used as a metabolic substrate for spermatozoa.

Both lactic and pyruvic acids, which are the end-products of glycolysis, are found in seminal plasma. These acids presumably accumulate in accessory gland secretions due to glycolytic activity within the glandular tissue. Additional lactic acid accumulates in seminal plasma due to the fructolytic activity of the spermatozoa after ejaculation. Spermatozoa are also capable of carrying out a dismutation reaction with pyruvate under aerobic and anaerobic conditions. The products of this reaction under anaerobic conditions include lactate, acetate, succinate, acetoacetate, and CO_2 (744). The other organic acids that occur in seminal plasma cannot, in general, serve as metabolic substrates for spermatozoa. Citric acid is the principal organic acid and is usually derived from the seminal vesicle secretion, except in man where it is produced in the prostate (Table 6); its function still remains obscure. There is a broad range of amino acids in seminal plasma and their concentration increases after ejaculation due to the extensive proteolytic activity that takes place in semen. Glutamic acid is particularly notable for its relatively high concentration in RTF, epididymal plasma, and seminal plasma.

The carnitine and acetylcarnitine found in seminal plasma is derived entirely from the epididymal secretion (745), except possibly in man, where other accessory glands may contribute up to half of the carnitine in seminal plasma (746,747). The acetylcarnitine in seminal plasma, unlike that within the sperm, cannot be used as a metabolic substrate (745) owing to its inability to permeate the sperm plasma membrane (748–750). There is some suggestion that exogenous acetylcarnitine can influence sperm motility through a pharmacological effect (751–753).

Glycerophosphocholine is a common constituent of seminal plasma, attaining substantial concentrations, particularly in ram seminal plasma (Table 8). Like carnitine, glycerophosphocholine is derived principally from the epididymal fluid, but other accessory glands, especially the seminal vesicles, also make a contribution in some species (e.g., rat, man). A related compound, glycerophosphoinositol, has been found at somewhat lower concentrations in the seminal plasma of domestic livestock (754). Whereas choline exists in bound form in seminal plasma principally as glycerophosphocholine, in human seminal plasma the predominant form is phosphocholine (716). In contrast to glycerophosphocholine, which is relatively stable in seminal plasma, phosphocholine is rapidly degraded after ejaculation to free choline and inorganic phosphate, owing to its exposure to phosphatase enzymes. The liberated phosphate can complex with spermine to form insoluble crystals of spermine phosphate (Boettcher's crystals). The concentration of spermine is normally approximately 1 to 3 mM in human seminal plasma while the concentration of the other polyamines (spermidine, putrescine) are at least ten times lower (755,756). Seminal plasma polyamines in men and rats are derived from the prostatic secretion (725,729). Polyamines are involved in the clotting reaction of rat and guinea pig seminal plasma (757). A variety of other functions have been ascribed to the polyamines with regard to their influence on spermatozoa (see ref. 651). Whereas spermine can considerably enhance the glycolytic rate of epididymal rat sperm (758), oxidized spermine is extremely toxic to spermatozoa (759–761). Oxidation of the polyamines is brought about by a polyamine oxidase which is particularly active in human seminal plasma (756).

A variety of reducing substances such as ascorbic acid, ergothioneine, hypotaurine, and uric acid is found in seminal plasma. Ascorbic acid is present in ram, bull, stallion, and human seminal plasma (Table 8). Ergothioneine occurs predominantly in the seminal plasma of boar, stallion, jackass, and zebra (700). Hypotaurine has been identified in boar, bull, and dog seminal plasma (682,762), but undoubtedly occurs in the seminal plasma of other species as it has been found in epididymal plasma (e.g., ram and rabbit) (684) and in seminal vesicles and prostate (guinea pig) (718). Uric acid exists in ram, bull, boar, and human seminal plasma (700); in the bull it is derived from the seminal vesicle secretion (763).

The seminal plasma of some primates contains the highest concentration of prostaglandins of any biological fluid, principally 19-hydroxylated derivatives of the E series: 19-OH PGE_1 + 19-OH PEG_2 amounts to 53 to 1,094 μg/ml in man (764) and 474, 504, and 930 μg/ml in the semen of chimpanzee, rhesus monkey, and stump-tailed monkey, respectively (765). However, these high levels of 19-OH PGEs are not found in gorilla or orangutan semen or in the semen of various nonprimates (stallion, bull, ram, boar, rabbit) (765). Quantitatively the next most important prostaglandins in man are PGE_1 + PGE_2, 19-OH PGFs, and $PGF_{1\alpha}$ + $PGF_{2\alpha}$. The concentration of prostaglandins in ram seminal plasma is somewhat less than for the primates (766), whereas the concentration in other species is very much lower (< 1 μg/ml) (767). It seems unlikely that prostaglandins have any direct effect on spermatozoa (768), and suggestions that they aid in sperm transport within the female reproductive tract by stimulating smooth muscle activity likewise has no firm foundation (701).

BLOOD-TESTIS AND BLOOD-EPIDIDYMAL BARRIERS

The remarkable differences in composition between STF and RTF on the one hand and blood plasma, testicular lymph, and interstitial fluid on the other imply that substances do not diffuse readily into or out of the seminiferous tubules and rete, otherwise these concentration differences would be dissipated. This suggestion has been abundantly substantiated by measurements of the rates at which a range of marker substances infused into the circulation appear in the fluids. Studies of this nature have been done for RTF in rams (600,604,769–771), boars (772), and rats (151,575, 577,773–778), and for STF in rats using micropuncture (779) and the difference technique (151,575, 576, 577,778). Various markers enter the fluids at widely differing rates, ranging from almost instantaneous entry to virtual exclusion. The main factor that determines the entry rate is lipid solubility; molecular size is much less important (Fig. 50). Lipid-soluble substances probably pass through the cells, whereas water-soluble compounds would enter via the spaces between them (see refs. 142,528,578,592,780). Two substances enter STF and RTF more rapidly than one would predict from their lipid solubility, glucose (or rather its nonmetabolized analog, 3-*O*-methylglucose) and testosterone. Glucose enters many cells by facilitated diffusion, and therefore it is perhaps not surprising that it should enter the luminal fluids of the testis in a similar way (781). However, it is usually assumed that steroids enter cells readily, and it was rather surprising to find that testosterone entered the luminal fluids more rapidly than dihydrotestosterone, which is marginally more lipid-soluble (575,689,775). Furthermore, the entry rate of radioactive testosterone was depressed by injecting the animal with hCG to stimulate testosterone production, or with nonradioactive testosterone, but not dihydrotestosterone (577,782). In contrast to glucose, the entry of radioactive testosterone into tubules incubated *in vitro* cannot be depressed by the addition of the nonradioactive form, so details of the transport mechanism have not yet been elucidated. The situation with urea is rather puzzling. In rams, this substance passes reasonably freely from blood to RTF, reaching equilibrium in approximately 2 hr (770). In hamsters, the level of ^{14}C-urea in STF never exceeds 25% of blood levels even during experiments lasting up to 4 hr (779). In nephrectomized rats on the other hand, radioactivity in STF reached values comparable to those in blood by 90 min but then continued to increase, reaching 150% of blood levels after 19 hr; this apparent concentration of urea inside the tubules was inhibited by dinitrophenol and ouabain, suggesting that urea was being actively transported into the tubules (783), but the identity of the radioactivity was not established.

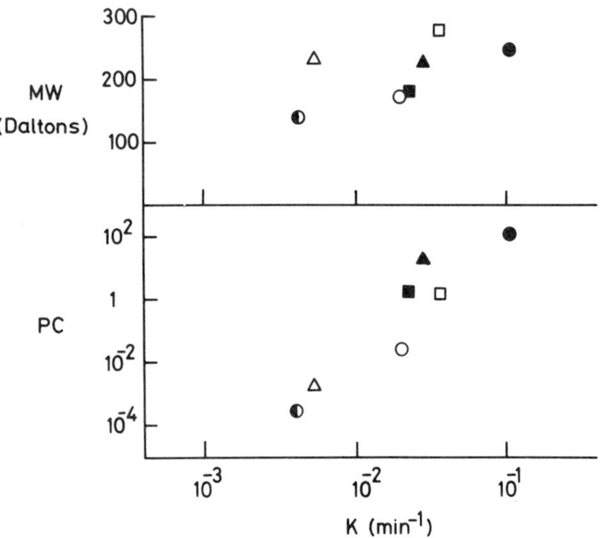

FIG. 50. The relationships between lipid solubility or molecular size and the rate of entry of some barbiturates and sulphonamides into rete testis fluid of rats. The entry rate has been calculated as a transfer constant ($K = -(l/t)$ log e[Cp − (C_{rtf}/C_p) where C_p and C_{rtf} are the concentrations in plasma and rete testis fluid, respectively, at time t. The lipid solubility is given as a partition coefficient between chloroform and phosphate buffer and the molecular weight (MW) is given in Daltons. The compounds shown are thiopental (*solid circle*), pentobarbital (*solid triangle*), barbital (*solid square*), sulphanamide (*open circle*), sulphaguanidine (*open triangle*), sulphamethoxypyridazine (*open square*), and salicylic acid (*half-filled circle*). [From ref. 774 as plotted by Setchell (578)].

Some studies have also been conducted in which the marker substances were infused into the lumen of one seminiferous tubule by micropuncture, and the appearance of radioactivity measured in the circulating blood. Using this technique, it was confirmed that albumin did not cross the tubular wall, but the rate of appearance of inositol and testosterone in the blood was much reduced if the efferent ducts were ligated, suggesting that these markers were leaving the tubules rapidly and being resorbed in the efferent ducts or the epididymis. The exit rates for testosterone, with the ducts ligated or not, were reduced by the inclusion of nonradioactive compound in the infusate, supporting the idea of a saturable transport system (784,785).

The location of the barrier was established in a series of studies, first with dyes (259,786; see ref. 780 for early references), then with labeled proteins (64,267,787–789), and finally, and most precisely, with electron-opaque markers (59,790,791). There is some slight restriction of movement at the capillary wall, and some at the peritubular myoid cells, but the most complete barrier to these molecules is at the junctions between pairs of adjacent Sertoli cells (Fig. 51). These junctions have a very elaborate structure and

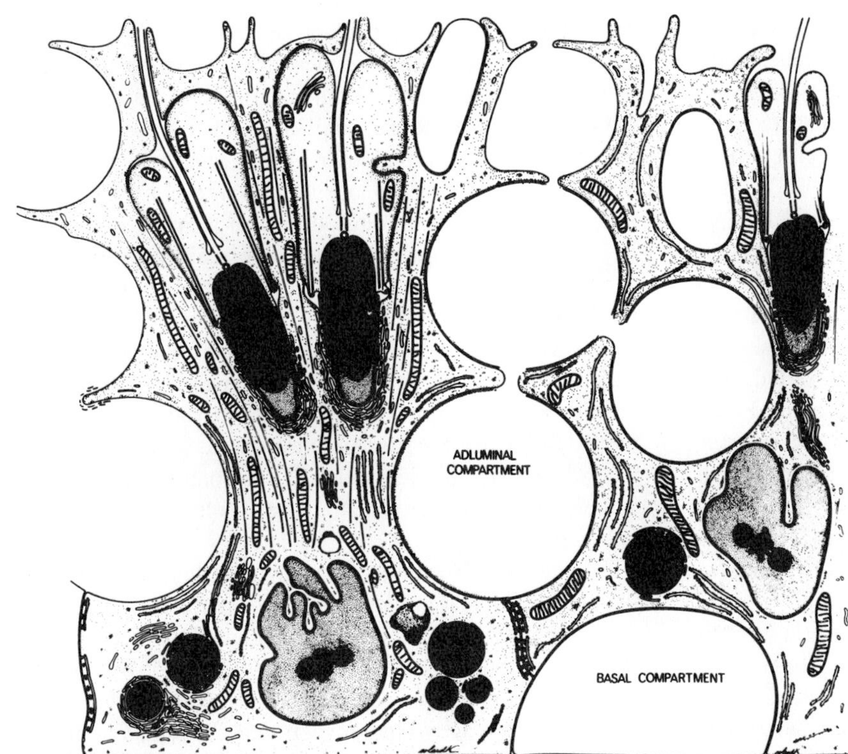

FIG. 51. A diagram of the junctional complexes between Sertoli cells and their role in forming the blood-testis barrier. A section of the wall of a seminiferous tubule is represented, with the lumen at the top and the peritubular tissue at the bottom. Late spermatids embedded in the luminal surfaces of the Sertoli cells are the only germ cells shown. The basal compartment between the Sertoli cells and the peritubular tissue is filled with spermatogonia and preleptotene primary spermatocytes, and the adluminal compartment between adjacent pairs of Sertoli cells is filled with later primary and secondary spermatocytes and round spermatids. The junctional complexes between the Sertoli cells prevent electron-opaque markers from penetrating any further into the tubule. (From ref. 822.)

form only at puberty when the barrier is established (792–795). However, it should be stressed that all the molecules that can be visualized either under the light or the electron microscope are fairly large hydrophilic molecules, which must enter the tubules by a paracellular route. Smaller, lipophilic molecules enter through the cells and their entry is regulated by the cells themselves, not by the junctions between them.

As already stated, the junctions form at about the time of puberty, in the rat at approximately 18 days of age (792,793), and it is at this age that the barrier to dyes develops (259). However, the establishment of a functional barrier to smaller molecules is less sudden, and the barrier to Cr-EDTA is still not complete even at 25 days of age in rats (796). This gradual development of a barrier is consistent with the pattern of fluid secretion, which rises suddenly at approximately 30 days, but only reaches adult levels at 40 days of age (see Seminiferous Tubule Fluid: Flow and Composition, p. 802) (528). A lumen first appears in the tubules at approximately 20 days, but continues to enlarge beyond 40 days of age (797). Androgen-binding protein concentrations in the testes of rats peaks at 20 days of age, then falls away to reach adult levels at approximately 40 days of age, whereas epididymal levels rise steadily until approximately 50 days of age (797,798). Plasma ABP concentrations also peak at 20 days of age and then fall away again, but the concentrations at 40 days of age are still considerably higher than adult levels (608,609,798), suggesting that the barrier is still not fully functional even at that age.

Once established, the blood-testis barrier apparently cannot be easily disrupted. Heat (770,777) or irradiation (450) are without effect, and the only treatments which do appear to cause a breakdown are treatment with cadmium salts (268,799) and distention of the tubules following efferent duct ligation; in the latter case, evidence includes an increase in the space of distribution of Cr-EDTA to values greater than the volume of the interstitial tissue (528), and in increased levels of ABP in blood (608). Both treatments are certainly followed by degeneration of the seminiferous epithelium, but cadmium salts also produce virtual cessation of blood flow within 8 hr. Interpretation of the effects of ligation of the efferent ducts is complicated by the very similar tubular lesions seen if the lumen of a single tubule is blocked with a plug of nontoxic latex (800); it is likely that efferent duct ligation and the consequent turgidity of the testis would also interfere with fluid movement along the tubules. The barrier is deficient in the testes of mice with testicular feminization and sex reversal, but not in a number of other genetically defective mice (801).

The significance of the barrier is difficult to define, but it seems likely that it is involved in creating the right conditions for meiosis in the tubules. The barrier develops at approximately the time the first cells are entering the meiotic prophase, and the exclusion of lanthanum is clearest in those parts of the seminiferous tubules of 15-day-old rats where the germ cells have reached pachytene (795). Meiosis fails in cultured fragments of seminiferous tubules (802), in which the barrier is not maintained (I. B. Fritz, *personal communication*). However, it is difficult to say just what the right conditions are, as complete spermatogenesis has never been achieved *in vitro* with mammalian cells. Some progress has recently been reported (803,804), but there are still several steps that apparently cannot progress outside the animal. However, a blood-testis barrier has been described in a number of vertebrate and invertebrate animals (see ref. 805), and a close association of somatic and germ cells is found in a wide range of animals (806).

Other consequences of the blood-testis barrier, although not its primary function, may nevertheless be of considerable significance (see refs. 578,780). The barrier ensures that the body does not recognize the haploid germ cells, or the spermatocytes from midpachytene onwards as self. A male animal can therefore become immune to his own spermatozoa, and this does often happen in vasectomized men (512). This could be due to the spermatozoa found in spermatic cord lymph after vasectomy (503), or to spermatozoal proteins absorbed from the ligated portion of the ductus deferens, where many of the sperm break down. The barrier also regulates the movement of peptide hormones such as inhibin and the gonadotropins, maintaining a high concentration of the former in the luminal fluids and excluding the latter (576), although the major site of action of FSH is the Sertoli cell. It was, therefore, of considerable interest that the receptors for FSH appear to be on the basal surfaces of these cells (68). Other peptides formed inside the tubules would be largely retained there, as indeed are smaller molecules such as inositol. The blood-testis barrier should also be considered in any toxicological investigations involving the testis. The entry of a substance into the tubule is an essential first step for it to have a direct effect on the later germ cells (see ref. 778). For example, it has recently been shown that although colchicine and vinblastine have similar effects in arresting mitosis in many tissues, colchicine is much more effective in the testis (807). It would be interesting to know whether both compounds enter the tubules.

From immunological studies, it has been claimed that the barrier in the rete is less complete than in the tubules (808,809), and the permeability of the rete to potassium, but not sodium, is higher than that of the tubules (151). The even greater concentration difference between epididymal luminal fluid and blood plasma suggests that a permeability barrier exists there, as well as in the seminiferous tubules, and again this suggestion has been confirmed in studies with suitable tracers. Two preparations have been used. With micropuncture techniques, it is possible to remove samples of luminal fluid during intravenous infusion of suitable markers in rats and hamsters; tritiated water enters the epididymal luminal fluid (ELF) readily, urea enters only slightly slower, whereas inulin, polyethylene glycol, and iodinated bovine serum albumin are virtually excluded (779,810). The entry of 3-*O*-methylglucose into ELF from the caput is much faster than that of L-glucose, and can be reduced by making the animal hyperglycemic either with streptozotocin or urethane; saturable carriers can also be demonstrated for the nonmetabolized amino acid α-aminobutyric acid and inositol (668), although the difference in level of inositol between RTF and ELF from the caput could be explained by concentration of the fluid by absorption (662), and the epididymis also contains the enzymes for synthesizing this compound from glucose (663). With both markers, fluid to plasma ratios greater than one are found in the caput, (inositol values greater than 10 are found after 24 hr), whereas much lower fluid to plasma ratios for inositol (0.3 after 3 hr) are found in the cauda (668), although this is an area where the rise in inositol concentration cannot be explained by fluid resorption (662). Radioactivity appears in ELF from the cauda when labeled testosterone, dihydrotestosterone, or progesterone was infused into the blood stream, but as less than half of the radioactivity in the blood was associated with 5α-dihydrotestosterone (DHT) and progesterone, respectively, when these steroids were infused, and only 4% of the radioactivity in the caudal ELF chromatographed with authentic testosterone (689), these results are difficult to interpret.

An alternative technique to study the entry of substances into the epididymal lumen involves the perfusion of sections of the epididymal duct during infusion of marker into the blood or its incorporation in the perfusate (655). Unfortunately this technique can be applied only to the cauda, which is probably less active in transport than the caput or corpus; but it has been shown that tritiated water in the perfusate reaches values almost equal to blood within 30 min, no radioactivity was detected when inulin or carboxydextran were infused into the bloodstream, and no cholesterol, protein, or sialic acid appeared in the perfusate, although appreciable amounts were present in the blood. Small amounts of radioactivity appeared in the perfusate when radioactive glucose or 3-*O*-methylglucose were infused into the blood (655). Radioactive inositol entered the perfusate, reaching 26% of blood levels after 3 hr of perfusion without reaching a plateau, and this value was not affected by the inclusion of nonradioactive inositol in the perfusate; radioactive inositol perfused through the lumen was not absorbed by the tissue. Inositol could be detected in perfusate at concentrations approximately five times those in blood, suggesting either that there is a large intracellular pool of inositol accumulated from the blood, or that local synthesis from glucose is an important source (656). Using this technique, it was also shown that the entry of testosterone into the cauda depended very much on the protein content of the perfusate; the inclusion of albumin (38 mg/ml) increased entry rate by approximately ten times, and the addition of protein from ovine RTF increased it even further (655). Radioactive DL-carnitine also appears in perfusate, reaching a plateau after 2 to 4 hr of approximately 0.5% of blood values per centimeter of duct perfused in the distal cauda, 1%/cm for proximal cauda, and 2%/cm for corpus. The addition of DL- or L-carnitine, phosphocholine, or inositol was without effect on these values, but the addition of glycerophosphocholine, choline, or betaine to the perfusion fluid increased carnitine entry, whereas the addition of albumin decreased it; glycine and γ-butyrobetaine were without effect. L-carnitine entered the perfusate 14 times faster than D-carnitine

(677). However, it should be emphasized that it is only in the caput where it is necessary to invoke carnitine transport to explain the differences in concentration in the luminal fluid (662), and therefore these studies using the cauda should be extended with experiments on the caput. Radioactive inositol enters a section of epididymal duct from the cauda or corpus in which the lumen was perfused *in vitro;* the rate of entry could be reduced by the inclusion of nonradioactive inositol in the bath fluid, but was unaffected by increasing the luminal concentration to physiological levels. The amount of radioactivity in the perfusate reached approximately 25% of bath values after 3 hr of perfusion (811).

The site of the barrier to intravascularly perfused lanthanum nitrate was located at the zonula occludens at the apicolateral surface of the epididymal epithelial cells; the movement of the marker was not impeded by the vascular endothelium, the peritubular myoid layer, or other lateral cell surface specializations (812).

REFERENCES

1. Mann, T., and Lutwak-Mann, C. (1976): Evaluation of the functional state of male accessory glands by the analysis of seminal plasma. *Andrologia,* 8:237–242.
2. Setchell, B. P. (1978): *The Mammalian Testis,* Elek Books, London, and Cornell University Press, Ithaca.
3. Harcourt, A. H., Harvey, P. H., Larson, S. G., and Short, R. V. (1981): Testis weight, body weight and breeding systems in primates. *Nature,* 293:55–57.
4. Kenagy, G. J. and Trombulak, S. C. (1986): Size and function of mammalian testes in relation to body size. *J. Mammalogy,* 67:1–22.
5. Breed, W. G. (1982): Morphological variation in the testes and accessory sex organs of Australian rodents in the genera *Pseudomys* and *Notomys. J. Reprod. Fertil.,* 66:607–613.
6. Gier, H. T., and Marion, G. B. (1970): Development of the mammalian testis. In: *The Testis,* edited by A. D. Johnson, W. R. Gomes, and N. L. Vandemark, pp. 1–45. Academic Press, New York.
7. Backhouse, K. M., and Butler, H. (1960): The gubernaculum testis of the pig (*Sus scrofa*): *J. Anat.,* 94:107–120.
8. Backhouse, K. M. (1964): The gubernaculum testis Hunteri, testicular descent and maldescent. *Ann. R. Coll. Surg. Engl.,* 35:15–32.
9. Wensing, C. J. G. (1968): Testicular descent in some domestic mammals. I. Anatomical aspects of testicular descent. *Proc. Kon. Ned. Akad. Wetensch.,* C71:423–434.
10. Wensing, C. J. G. (1973): Testicular descent in some domestic mammals. II. The nature of the gubernacular change during the process of testicular descent in the pig. *Proc. Kon. Ned. Akad. Wetensch.,* C76:190–195.
11. Wensing, C. J. G. (1973): Testicular descent in some domestic mammals. III. Search for the factors that regulate the gubernacular reaction. *Proc. Kon. Ned. Akad. Wetensch.,* C76:196–202.
12. Wensing, C. J. G., Colenbrander, B., and van Straaten, H. W. M. (1980): Normal and abnormal testicular descent in some mammals. In: *Descended and Cryptorchid Testis,* edited by E. S. E. Hafez. pp. 125–137. Nijhoff, Boston.
13. Rajfer, J., and Walsh, P. C. (1977): Hormonal regulation of testicular descent: experimental and clinical observations. *J. Urol.,* 118:985–990.
14. Colenbrander, B., van Rossum-Kok, C. M. J. E., van Straaten, H. W. M., and Wensing, C. J. G. (1979): The effect of fetal decapitation on the testis and other endocrine organs in the pig. *Biol. Reprod.,* 20:198–204.
15. Baumans, V., Dijkstra, G., and Wensing, C. J. G. (1982): The effect of orchidectomy on gubernacular outgrowth and regression in the dog. *Int. J. Androl.,* 5:387–400.
16. Baumans, V., Dijkstra, G., and Wensing, C. J. G. (1983): The role of a non-androgenic testicular factor in the process of testicular descent in the dog. *Int. J. Androl.,* 6:541–552.
17. Elder, J. S., Isaacs, J. T., and Walsh, P. C. (1982): Androgenic sensitivity of the gubernaculum testis: evidence for hormonal/mechanical interactions in testicular descent. *J. Urol.,* 127:170–176.
18. Bergh, A., Helander, H. F., and Wahlqvist, L. (1982): Studies on factors governing testicular descent in the rat—particularly the role of gubernaculum testis. *Int. J. Androl.,* 1:42–356.
19. Frey, H. L., and Rajfer, J. (1984): Role of the gubernaculum and intraabdominal pressure in the process of testicular descent. *J. Urol.,* 131:574–579.
20. Damber, J. E., Bergh, A., and Janson, P. O. (1978): Testicular blood flow and testosterone concentration in the spermatic venous blood in rats with experimental unilateral cryptorchidism. *Acta Endocrinol.,* 88:611–618.
21. Risbridger, G. P., Kerr, J. B., and de Kretser, D. M. (1981): Evaluation of Leydig cell function and gonadotropin binding in unilateral and bilateral cryptorchidism: evidence for local control of Leydig cell function by the seminiferous tubule. *Biol. Reprod.,* 24:534–540.
22. Frankenhuis, M. T., and Wensing, C. J. G. (1979): Induction of spermatogenesis in the naturally cryptorchid pig. *Fertil. Steril.,* 31:428–433.
23. Carrick, F. N., and Setchell, B. P. (1977): The evolution of the scrotum. In: *Reproduction and Evolution,* edited by J. H. Calaby and C. H. Tyndale-Biscoe, pp. 165–170. Australian Academy of Sciences, Canberra.
24. Bedford, J. M. (1978): Anatomical evidence for the epididymis as the prime mover in the evolution of the scrotum. *Am. J. Anat.,* 152:483–508.
25. Bedford, J. M. (1978): Influence of abdominal temperature on epididymal function in the rat and rabbit. *Am. J. Anat.,* 152:509–522.
26. Setchell, B. P. (1986): Physiological communications between the testis and epididymis. *Proceedings of the International Union of Physiological Sciences,* 16:494.
27. Holstein, A. F. (1967) Die glatte Muskulatur in der Tunica albuginea des Hodens und ihr Einfluss auf den Spermatozoentransport in den Nebenhoden. *Anat. Anz. Ergeb.,* 121:10–108.
28. Davis, J. R., Langford, G. A., and Kirby, P. J. (1970): The testicular capsule. In: *The Testis, Vol. I,* edited by A. D. Johnson, W. R. Gomes, and Vandemark, N. L., pp. 281–337. Academic Press, New York.
29. Chacon-Arellano, J. T., and Woolley, D. M. (1980): Smooth muscle in the testicular capsule of the horse, pig and sheep. *J. Anat.,* 131:263–273.
30. Leeson, T. S., and Cookson, F. B. (1974): The mammalian testicular capsule and its muscle elements. *J. Morphol.,* 14:237–254.
31. Langford, G. A., and Heller, C. G. (1973): Fine structure of muscle cells of the human testicular capsule: basis of testicular contractions. *Science,* 179:573–575
32. Gorgas, K., and Bock, P. (1974): Myofibroblasts in the rat testicular capsule. *Cell. Tiss. Res.,* 154:533–541.
33. Leeson, T. S. (1975): Smooth muscle cells in the rat testicular capsule: a developmental study. *J. Morphol.,* 147:171–186.
34. Ohanian, C., Rodriguez, H., Piriz, H., Martino, I., Rieppi, G., Garafalo, E. G., and Roca, R. A. (1979): Studies on the contractile activity and ultrastructure of the boar testicular capsule. *J. Reprod. Fertil.,* 57:79–85.
35. Bell, C., and McLean, J. R. (1973): The autonomic innervation of the rat testicular capsule. *J. Reprod. Fertil.,* 32:253–258.
36. Langford, G. A., and Silver, A. (1974): Histochemical localization of acetylcholinesterase-containing nerve fibres in the testis. *J. Physiol.,* 242:9P–10P.
37. Hargrove, J. L., and Ellis, L. C. (1976): Autonomic nerves versus prostaglandins in the control of rat and rabbit testicular capsular contractions *in vivo* and *in vitro. Biol. Reprod.,* 14:651–657.
38. Davis, J. R., and Langford, G. A. (1970): Pharmacological studies on the testicular capsule in relation to sperm transport. *Adv. Exp. Med. Biol.,* 10:495–514.
39. Davis, J. R., and Langford, G. A. (1971): Comparative responses of the isolated testicular capsule and parenchyma to autonomic drugs. *J. Reprod. Fertil.,* 26:241–246.
40. Ellis, L. C., Buhrley, L. E., and Hargrove, J. L. (1978): Species differences in contractility of seminiferous tubules and tunica albu-

ginea as related to sperm transport through the testis. *Arch. Androl.*, 1:139–146.

41. Free, M. J., Jaffe, R. A., and Morford, D. E. (1980): Sperm transport through the rete testis in anaesthetized rats: role of the testicular capsule and effect of gonadotropins and prostaglandins. *Biol. Reprod.*, 33:1073–1078.
42. Davis, J. R., and Horowitz, A. M. (1979): Effect of various exposure times to hyperthermia and hypothermia on spontaneous contractions of the adult rabbit isolated testicular capsule. *Biol. Reprod.*, 21:413–417.
43. Davis, J. R., and Langford, G. A. (1969): Response of the testicular capsule to acetylcholine and noradrenaline. *Nature*, 222:386–387.
44. Davis, J. R., and Langford, G. A. (1969): Response of the isolated testicular capsule of the rat to autonomic drugs. *J. Reprod. Fertil.*, 19:595–598.
45. Hargrove, J. L., Johnson, J. M., and Ellis, L. C. (1971): Prostaglandin E1 induced inhibition of rabbit testicular contractions *in vitro*. *Proc. Soc. Exp. Biol. Med.*, 136:958–961.
46. Johnson, J. M., Hargrove, J. L., and Ellis, L. C. (1971): Prostaglandin F-1α induced stimulation of rabbit testicular contractions *in vitro*. *Proc. Soc. Exp. Biol. Med.*, 138:378–381.
47. Hargrove, J. L., Seeley, R. R., Johnson, J. M., and Ellis, L. C. (1973): Prostaglandin-like substances: initiation and maintenance of rabbit testicular contraction *in vitro*. *Proc. Soc. Exp. Biol. Med.*, 142:205–209.
48. Hargrove, J. L., Seeley, R. R., and Ellis, L. C. (1975): Rabbit testicular contractions: bimodal interaction of prostaglandin E-1 with other agonists. *Am. J. Physiol.*, 228:810–814.
49. Tso, E. C. F., and Lacy, D. (1975): Effects of prostaglandin F-2 on the reproductive system of the male rat. *J. Reprod. Fertil.*, 44:545–550.
50. Nemetallah, B. R., Howell, R. E., and Ellis, L. C. (1983): Histamine H1 receptors and prostaglandin-histamine interactions modulating contractility of rabbit and rat testicular capsules *in vitro*. *Biol. Reprod.*, 28:632–635.
51. Firlit, C. F., King, L. R., and Davis, J. R. (1975): Comparative responses of the isolated human testicular capsule to autonomic drugs. *J. Urol.*, 113:500–504.
52. Leeson, C. R., and Forman, D. E. (1981): Postnatal development and differentiation of contractile cells within the rabbit testis. *J. Anat.*, 132:491–511.
53. Holstein, A. F., and Weiss, C. (1967): Uber die Wirkung der glatten Muskulatur in der Tunica Albuginea im Hoden des Kaninchens; Messungen des interstitiellen Druckes. *Z. Ges. Exp. Med.*, 142:334–337.
54. Kormano, M., and Suvanto, O. (1968): Cadmium-induced changes in the intratesticular pressure in the rat. *Acta Pathol. Microbiol. Scand.*, 72:444–445.
55. Schweitzer, R. (1929): Uber die Bedeutung der Vascularisation, der Binnendruckes und der Zwischenzellen fur die Biologie des Hodens. *Z. Anat. Entwickl.*, 89:775–796.
56. Nistal, M., Santamaria, L., and Paniagua, R. (1984): Mast cells in the human testis and epididymis from birth to adulthood. *Acta Anat.*, 119:155–160.
57. Sowerbutts, S. F., Jarvis, L. G., and Setchell, B. P. (1986): The increase in testicular vascular permeability induced by human chorionic gonadotrophin involves 5-hydroxytryptamine and possibly oestrogens, but not testosterone, prostaglandins, histamine or bradykinin. *Aust. J. Exp. Biol. Med. Sci.*, 64:137–147.
58. Fawcett, D. W., Heidger, P. J., and Leak, L. V. (1969): The lymph-vascular system of the interstitial tissue of the testis as revealed by electron microscopy. *J. Reprod. Fertil.*, 19:109–119.
59. Fawcett, D. W., Leak, L. V., and Heidger, P. M. (1970): Electron microscopic observations on the structural components of the blood-testis barrier. *J. Reprod. Fertil.*, Suppl. 10:105–119.
60. Fawcett, D. W., Neaves, W. B., and Flores, M. N. (1973): Comparative observations on intertubular lymphatics and the organization of the interstitial tissue of the mammalian testis. *Biol. Reprod.*, 9:500–512.
61. Clark, R. V. (1976): Three-dimensional organization of testicular interstitial tissue and lymphatic space in the rat. *Anat. Rec.*, 184:203–226.
62. Christensen, A. K., Komorowski, T. E., Wilson, B., Ma, S. F., and Stevens, R. W. (1985): The distribution of serum albumin in the rat testis, studied by electron microscope immunocytochemistry on ultrathin sections. *Endocrinology*, 116:1983–1996.
63. Hermo, L., and Lalli, M. (1978): Monocytes and mast cells in the limiting membrane of human seminiferous tubules. *Biol. Reprod.*, 19:92–100.
64. Christensen, A. K., and Gillim, S. W. (1969): The correlation of fine structure and function in steroid-secreting cells, with emphasis on those of the gonads. In: *The Gonads*, edited by K. W. McKerns, pp. 415–488. Appleton-Century Crofts, New York.
65. Christensen, A. K. (1975): Leydig cells. In: *Handbook of Physiology, Vol. V*, edited by D. W. Hamilton and R. O. Greep, pp. 57–94. American Physiological Society, Washington, D.C.
66. Maseki, Y., Miyake, K., Mitsuya, H., Kitamura, H., and Yamada, K. (1981): Mastocytosis occurring in the testes from patients with idiopathic male infertility. *Fertil. Steril.*, 36:814–817.
67. Miller, S. C., Bowman, B. M., and Rowland, H. G. (1983): Structure, cytochemistry, endocytotic activity and immunoglobulin (Fc): receptors of rat testicular interstitial-tissue macrophages. *Am. J. Anat.*, 168:1–13.
68. Orth, J., and Christensen, A. K. (1977): Localization of 125-I-labelled FSH in the testes of hypophysectomized rats by autoradiography at the light and electronmicroscope levels. *Endocrinology*, 101:262–278.
69. Yee, J. B., and Hutson, J. C. (1983): Testicular macrophages: isolation, characterization and hormonal responsiveness. *Biol. Reprod.*, 29:1319–1326.
70. Yee, J. B., and Hutson, J. C. (1985): Biochemical consequences of follicle-stimulating hormone binding to testicular macrophages in culture. *Biol. Reprod.*, 32:872–879.
71. Yee, J. B., and Hutson, J. C. (1985): *In vivo* effects of follicle-stimulating hormone on testicular macrophages. *Biol. Reprod.*, 32:880–883.
72. Bergh, A. (1985): Effect of cryptorchidism on the morphology of testicular macrophages: evidence for a Leydig cell-macrophage interaction in the rat testis. *Int. J. Androl.*, 8:86–96.
73. Bergh, A. (1982): Local differences in Leydig cell morphology in the adult rat testis: evidence for a local control of Leydig cells by adjacent seminiferous tubules. *Int. J. Androl.*, 5:325–330.
74. Bergh, A. (1983): Paracrine regulation of Leydig cells by the seminiferous tubules. *Int. J. Androl.*, 6:57–65.
75. Stenman, S., and Vaheri, A. (1978): Distribution of a major connective tissue protein, fibronectin, in normal human tissues. *J. Exp. Med.*, 147:1054–1064.
76. Fawcett, D. W. (1973): Observations on the organization of the interstitial tissue of the testis and on the occluding cell junctions in the seminiferous epithelium. *Adv. Biosci.*, 10:83–99.
77. Bascom, K. F., and Osterud, H. L. (1925): Quantitative studies of the testicle. II. Pattern and total tubule length in the testicles of certain common mammals. *Anat. Rec.*, 31:159–169.
78. Lennox, B., Ahmad, K. N., and Mack, W. S. (1970): A method for determining the relative total length of the tubules in the testis. *J. Pathol.*, 102:229–238.
79. Mori, H., and Christensen, A. K. (1980): Morphometric analysis of Leydig cells in the normal rat testis. *J. Cell Biol.*, 84:340–354.
80. Setchell, B. P. (1975): Reproduction in male marsupials. In: *The Biology of Marsupials*, edited by B. Stonehouse and D. Gilmore, pp. 411–457. Macmillan, London.
81. Setchell, B. P., Laurie, M. S., Flint, A. P. F., and Heap, R. B. (1983): Transport of free and conjugated steroids from the boar testis in lymph, venous blood and rete testis fluid. *J. Endocrinol.*, 96:127–136.
82. Setchell, B. P., and Cox, J. E. (1982): Secretion of free and conjugated steroids by the horse testis into lymph and venous blood. *J. Reprod. Fertil.*, Suppl. 32:123–127.
83. Wing, T. Y., and Christensen, A. K. (1982): Morphometric studies on rat seminiferous tubules. *Am. J. Anat.*, 165:13–25.
84. Woolley, P. (1975): The seminiferous tubules in Dasyurid marsupials. *J. Reprod. Fertil.*, 45:255–261.
85. Clermont, Y., and Huckins, C. (1961): Microscopic anatomy of the sex cords and seminiferous tubules in growing and adult male albino rats. *Am. J. Anat.*, 108:79–97.
86. Lauth, E. A. (1830): Memoire sur le testicule humaine. *Mem. Soc. Hist. Nat. (Strasbourg)*, 1:1–42.

87. Averback, P., and Wight, D. G. D. (1979): Seminiferous tubule hypercurvature: a newly recognized common syndrome of human male infertility. *Lancet,* I:181–183.
88. Averback, P. (1980): Histopathological diagnosis of hypercurved seminiferous tubules. *Histopathology,* 4:75–82.
89. Perey, B., Clermont, Y., and Leblond, C. P. (1961): The wave of the seminiferous epithelium in the rat. *Am. J. Anat.,* 108:47–77.
90. Hochereau, M. T. (1963): Etude comparée de la vague spermatogénetique chez le taureau et chez le rat. *Ann. Biol. Anim. Biochim. Biophys.,* 3:5–20.
91. Schulze, W. (1982): Evidence of a wave of spermatogenesis in human testis. *Andrologia,* 14:200–207.
92. Roosen-Runge, E. C. (1951): Motions of the seminiferous tubules of rat and dog. *Anat. Rec.,* 109:413.
93. Clermont, Y. (1958): Contractile elements in the limiting membrane of the seminiferous tubules of the rat. *Exp. Cell Res.,* 15: 438–440.
94. Muramaki, M., Hamasaki, M., Okitas, S., and Abe, J. (1979): SEM surface morphology of the contractile cells in the rat seminiferous tubules. *Experientia,* 35:1099–1101.
95. Crabo, B. (1963): Fine structure of the interstitial cells of the rabbit testis. *Z. Zellforsch. Mikroskop. Anat.,* 61:587–604.
96. Daehlin, L., Damber, J. E., Selstam, G., and Bergman, B. (1985): Effects of human chorionic gonadotrophin, oestradiol and estromustine on testicular blood flow in hypophyectomized rats. *Int. J. Androl.,* 8:58–68.
97. Ross, M. H., and Long, I. R. (1966): Contractile cells in human seminiferous tubules. *Science,* 153:1271–1273.
98. Bustos-Obregon, E., and Holstein, A. F. (1973): Ultrastructure and function of the lamina propria of human seminiferous tubules. *Z. Zellforsch.,* 141:413–425.
99. de Kretser, D. M., Kerr, J. B., and Paulsen, C. A. (1975): The peritubular tissue in the normal and pathological human testis. An ultrastructural study. *Biol. Reprod.,* 12:317–324.
100. Hermo, L., Lalli, M., and Clermont, Y. (1977): Arrangement of connective tissue components in the walls of seminiferous tubules of man and monkey. *Am. J. Anat.,* 148:433–446.
101. Bustos-Obregon, E., and Courot, M. (1974): Ultrastructure of the lamina propria in the ovine seminiferous tubule. *Cell Tiss. Res.,* 150:481–492.
102. Burgos, M. H., Vitale-Calpe, R., and Aoki, A. (1970): Fine structure of the testis and its functional significance. In: *The Testis, Vol. I,* edited by A. D. Johnson, W. R. Gomes, and N. L. Vandemark. pp. 551–649. Academic Press, New York.
103. Dierachs, R., and Wrobel, K. H. (1973): Licht- und elektronenenmikroskopische Untersuchungen an der peritubularen Zellen des Schweinhodens wahrend der postnatalen Entwicklung. *Z. Anat. Entwickl.,* 143:49–64.
104. Ross, M. H. (1967): The fine structure and development of the peritubular contractile cell component in the seminiferous tubules of the mouse. *Am. J. Anat.,* 121:523–558.
105. Leeson, C. R., and Leeson, T. S. (1963): The postnatal development and differentiation of the boundary tissue of the seminiferous tubule of the rat. *Anat. Rec.,* 147:243–259.
106. Niemi, M., Sharpe, R. M., and Brown, W. R. A. (1986): Macrophages in the interstitial tissue of the rat testis. *Cell Tiss. Res.,* 243:337–344.
107. Bressler, R. S., and Ross, M. H. (1972): Differentiation of peritubular myoid cells of the testis: effects of intratesticular implantation of newborn mouse testes into normal and hypophysectomised adults. *Biol. Reprod.,* 6:148–159.
108. Sar, M., Stumpf, W. E., McLean, W. S., Smith, A. A., Hansson, V., Nayfeh, S. N., and French, F. S. (1975): Localization of androgen target cells in the rat testis: autoradiographic studies. *Curr. Top. Mol. Endocrinol.,* 2:311–319.
109. Hovatta, O. (1972): Effect of androgens and antiandrogens on the development of the myoid cells of the rat seminiferous tubules (organ culture): *Z. Zellforsch.,* 131:299–308.
110. Urry, R. L., Asay, R. W., and Cockett, A. T. K. (1976): Hormonal control of seminiferous tubule contractions; a hypothesis of sperm transport from the testicle. *Invest. Urol.,* 14:194–197.
111. Santiemma, V., Francavilla, S., Santucci, R., Onori, D., Bellocci, M., and Fabbrini, M. (1978): Development and hormone dependence of peritubular smooth muscle cells of the rat testis. In: *Recent Progress in Andrology,* edited by A. Fabbrini and E. Steinberger, pp. 185–199. Academic Press, London.
112. Ross, M. H., and Grant, L. (1968): On the structural integrity of the basement membrane. *Exp. Cell Res.,* 50:277–285.
113. Archer, F. L., Beck, J. S., and Melvin, J. M. O. (1971): Localization of smooth muscle protein in myoepithelium by immunofluorescence. *Am. J. Pathol.,* 63:109–118.
114. Groschel-Stewart, U., and Unsicker, K. (1977): Direct visualization of contractile proteins in peritubular cells of the guinea-pig testis using antibodies against highly purified actin and myosin. *Histochemistry,* 51:315–319.
115. Tung, P. S., Skinner, M. K., and Fritz, I. B. (1984): Fibronectin synthesis is a marker for peritubular cell contaminants in Sertoli cell-enriched cultures. *Biol. Reprod.,* 30:199–211.
116. Vogl, A. W., Soucy, L. J., and Lew, G. J. (1985): Distribution of actin in isolated seminiferous epithelia and denuded tubule walls of the rat. *Anat. Rec.,* 213:63–71.
117. Toyama, Y. (1977): Actin-like filaments in the myoid cell of the testis. *Cell Tiss. Res.,* 177:221–226.
118. Kormano, M., and Hovatta, O. (1972): Contractility and histochemistry of the myoid cell layer of the rat seminiferous tubules during postnatal development. *Z. Anat. Entwickl.,* 137:239–248.
119. Niemi, M., and Kormano, M. (1965): Contractility of the seminiferous tubule of the postnatal rat testis and its response to oxytocin. *Ann. Med. Exp. Fenn.,* 43:40–42.
120. Worley, R. T. S., Nicholson, H. D., and Pickering, B. T. (1984): Testicular oxytocin: an initiator of seminiferous tubule movement? *Coll. INSERM,* 123:205–212.
121. Ellis, L. C., and Buhrley, L. E. (1978): Inhibitory effects of melatonin, prostaglandin E-1, cyclic AMP, dibutyryl cyclic AMP and theophyline on rat seminiferous tubular contractility in vitro. *Biol. Reprod.,* 19:217–222.
122. Suvanto, O., and Kormano, M. (1970): The relation between *in vitro* contractions of the rat seminiferous tubules and the cyclic stage of the seminiferous epithelium. *J. Reprod. Fertil.,* 21: 227–232.
123. Suvanto, O., and Kormano, M. (1970): Effect of experimental cryptorchidism and cadmium injury on the spontaneous contractions of the seminiferous tubules of the rat testis. *Virchows Arch. Abt. B. Zellpath.,* 4:217–224.
124. Hovatta, O. (1972): Contractility and structure of adult rat seminiferous tubules in organ culture. *Z. Zellforsch.,* 130:171–179.
125. Leeson, T. S., and Leeson, C. R. (1970): Experimental cryptorchidism in the rat. A light and electron microscope study. *Invest. Urol.,* 8:127–144.
126. Saba, P., Gori, Z., Carnicelli, A., Todeschini, G., and Marescotti, V. (1972): An electron microscopic study of the rat testis in experimental cryptorchidism. *Endokrinologie,* 60:103–116.
127. Kerr, J. B., Rich, K. A., and de Kretser, D. M. (1979): Effects of experimental cryptorchidism on the ultrastructure and function of the Sertoli cell and peritubular tissue of the rat testis. *Biol. Reprod.,* 21:823–838.
128. Tonutti, E. (1955): Uber die Strukturelemente des Hodens und ihr Verhalten unter experimentellen Bedingungen. In: *1. Symposion Deutsche Gesellschaft Endokrinologie,* Hamburg, 1953, pp. 146–158. Springer, Berlin.
129. Lacy, D., and Rotblat, J. (1960): Study of normal and irradiated boundary tissue of the seminiferous tubules of the rat. *Exp. Cell Res.,* 21:49–70.
130. Skinner, M. K., and Fritz, I. B. (1985): Structural characterization of proteoglycans produced by testicular peritubular cells and Sertoli cells. *J. Biol. Chem.,* 260:11874–11883.
131. Skinner, M. K., Tung, P. S., and Fritz, I. B. (1985): Cooperativity between Sertoli cells and testicular peritubular cells in the production and deposition of extracellular matrix components. *J. Cell Biol.,* 100:1941–1947.
132. Tung, P. S., and Fritz, I. B. (1980): Interactions of Sertoli cells with myoid cells *in vitro. Biol. Reprod.,* 23:207–217.
133. Vitale-Calpe, R., and Aoki, A. (1969): Fine structure of the intratesticular excretory pathway in the guinea pig. *Z. Anat. Entwicklung.,* 129:135–153.
134. Dym, M. (1974): The fine structure of monkey Sertoli cells in the transitional zone at the junction of the seminiferous tubules with the tubuli recti. *Am. J. Anat.,* 140:1–26.

135. Cavicchia, J. C., and Burgos, M. H. (1977): Tridimensional reconstruction and histology of the intratesticular seminal pathway in the hamster. *Anat. Rec.*, 187:1–10.
136. Osman, D. I. (1978): On the ultrastructure of modified Sertoli cells in the terminal segment of seminiferous tubules in the boar. *J. Anat.*, 127:603–613.
137. Osman, D. I., and Ploen, L. (1978): The terminal segment of the seminiferous tubules and the blood-testis barrier before and after efferent ductule ligation in the rat. *Int. J. Androl.*, 1:234–249.
138. Osman, D. I., and Ploen, L. (1979): Fine structure of the modified Sertoli cells in the terminal segment of the seminiferous tubules of the bull, ram and goat. *Anim. Reprod. Sci.*, 2:343–351.
139. Osman, D. I., Ploen, L., and Hagenas, L. (1979): On the postnatal development of the terminal segment of the seminiferous tubules in normal and germ cell depleted rat testes. *Int. J. Androl.*, 2: 419–431.
140. Wrobel, K. H., Sinowatz, F., and Mademann, R. (1982): The fine structure of the terminal segment of the bovine seminiferous tubule. *Cell Tiss. Res.*, 225:29–44.
141. Lindner, S. G. (1982): On the morphology of the transitional zone of the seminiferous tubule and the rete testis in man. *Andrologia*, 14:352–362.
142. Setchell, B. P. (1970): Testicular blood supply, lymphatic drainage and secretion of fluid. In: *The Testis, Vol. I*, edited by A. D. Johnson, W. R. Gomes, and N. L. Vandemark, pp. 101–239. Academic Press, New York.
143. Kormano, M. (1977): The rete testis. In: *The Testis, Vol. IV*, edited by A. D. Johnson and W. R. Gomes, pp. 461–479. Academic Press, New York.
144. Roosen-Runge, E. C. (1961): The rete testis in the albino rat: its structure, development and morphological significance. *Acta Anat.*, 45:1–30.
145. Nykanen, M. (1979): Fine structure of the transitional zone of the rat seminiferous tubule. *Cell Tiss. Res.*, 198:441–454.
146. Clegg, E. J., and MacMillan, E. W. (1965): The uptake of vital dyes and particulate matter by the Sertoli cells of the rat testis. *J. Anat.*, 99:219–229.
147. Nykanen, M., and Kormano, M. (1978): Early effects of efferent duct ligation on the rat rete testis. *Int. J. Androl.*, 1:225–234.
148. Osman, D. I., and Ploen, L. (1978): The mammalian tubuli recti: ultrastructural study. *Anat. Rec.*, 192:1–18.
149. Roosen-Runge, E. C., and Holstein, A. F. (1978): The human rete testis. *Cell Tiss. Res.*, 189:409–433.
150. Amann, R. P., Johnson, L., and Pickett, B. W. (1977): Connection between the seminiferous tubules and the efferent ducts in the stallion. *Am. J. Vet. Res.*, 38:1571–1579.
151. Setchell, B. P., Davies, R. V., Gladwell, R. T., Hinton, B. T., Main, S. J., Pilsworth, L., and Waites, G. M. H. (1978): The movement of fluid in the seminiferous tubules and rete testis. *Ann. Biol. Anim. Biochim. Biophys.*, 18:623–632.
152. Hinton, B. T., and Keefer, D. A. (1983): Evidence for protein absorption from the lumen of the seminiferous tubule and rete of the rat testis. *Cell Tiss. Res.*, 230:367–375.
153. Fawcett, D. W., and Dym, M. (1974): A glycogen-rich segment of the tubuli recti and proximal portion of the rete testis in the guinea pig. *J. Reprod. Fertil.*, 38:401–409.
154. Benoit, J. (1926): Recherches anatomiques, cytologiques et histophysiologiques sur les voies excrétrices du testicule chez les mammifères. *Arch. Anat. Histol. Embryol.*, 5:173–414.
155. Ladman, A. J., and Young, W. C. (1958): An electron microscopic study of the ductuli efferentes and rete testis of the guinea pig. *J. Biophys. Biochem. Cytol.*, 4:219–226.
156. Leeson, T. S. (1962): Electron microscopy of the rete testis of the rat. *Anat. Rec.*, 144:57–67.
157. Buston-Obregon, E., and Holstein, A. F. (1976): The rete testis in man: ultrastructural aspects. *Cell Tiss. Res.*, 175:1–15.
158. Dym, M. (1976): The mammalian rete testis—a morphological examination. *Anat. Rec.*, 186:493–524.
150. Osman, D. I. (1978): The ultrastructure of the rete testis and its permeability barrier before and after efferent duct ligation. *Int. J. Androl.*, 1:357–370.
160. Wrobel, K. H., Sinowatz, F., and Kugler, P. (1978): Zur funktionellen Morphologie des Rete testis, der Tubuli recti und der Terminalsegmente der Tubuli seminiferi des geschlechtsreifen Rindes. *Anat. Histol. Embryol.*, 7:320–335.
161. Jones, R., Hamilton, D. W., and Fawcett, D. W. (1979): Morphology of the epithelium of the extratesticular rete testis, ductuli efferentes and ductus epididymidis of the adult male rabbit. *Am. J. Anat.*, 156:373–400.
162. Dhingra, L. D. (1977): Mediastinum testis. In: *The Testis, Vol. IV*, edited by A. D. Johnson and W. R. Gomes, pp. 451–460. Academic Press, New York.
163. Wrobel, K. H., and El Etreby, M. F. (1971): Enzymhistochemie an der mannlichen Keimdruse des Rindes wahrend ihres fetalen und postnatalen Entwicklung. *Histochemie*, 26:160–179.
164. Morales, C., Hermo, L., and Clermont, Y. (1984): Endocytosis in epithelial cells lining the rete testis of the rat. *Anat. Rec.*, 209:185–195.
165. Free, M. J. (1980): "Leaky" membranes in the male reproductive tract: a discussion of unusual molecular exchanges between different fluid compartments. In: *Testicular Development, Structure and Function*, edited by A. Steinberger and E. Steinberger, pp. 281–290. Raven Press, New York.
166. Cooper, E. R. A., and Jackson, H. (1972): The vasa efferentia in the rat and mouse. *J. Reprod. Fertil.*, 28:317–319.
167. Talo, A. (1981): *In vitro* spontaneous electrical activity of rat efferent ductules. *J. Reprod. Fertil.*, 63:17–20.
168. Lewis-Jones, D. I., Harrison, R. G., and MacMillan, E. W. (1982): A reexaminiation of rat ductuli efferentes. *Anat. Rec.*, 203:461–462.
169. Ramos, A. S., and Dym, M. (1977): Ultrastructure of the ductuli efferentes in monkeys. *Biol. Reprod.*, 17:339–349.
170. Hemeida, N. A., Sack, W. O., and McEntee, K. (1978): Ductuli efferentes in the epididymis of boar, goat, ram, bull and stallion. *Am. J. Vet. Res.*, 39:1892–1900.
171. Wrobel, K. H. (1972): Zur Morphologie der Ductuli efferentes des Bullen. *Z. Zellforsch.*, 135:129–148.
172. Goyal, H. O., and Hrudka, F. (1981): Ductuli efferentes of the bull—a morphological, experimental and developmental study. *Andrologia*, 13:292–306.
173. Holstein, A. F. (1964): Elektronenemikroskopische Untersuchungen an den Ductuli-Efferentes des normalen und kastrieten Kaninchens. *Z. Zellforsch.*, 64:767–777.
174. Morita, I. (1966): Some observations on the fine structure of the human ductuli efferentes testis. *Arch. Histol. Jpn.*, 6:341–365.
175. Ladman, A. J. (1967): The fine structure of the ductuli efferentes of the opossum. *Anat. Rec.*, 157:559–576.
176. Hoffer, A. P. (1972): The fine structure of the ductuli efferentes in mouse and rat. *Anat. Rec.*, 172:331–332.
177. Hamilton, D. W. (1975): Structure and function of the epithelium lining the ductuli efferentes, ductus epididymidis and ductus deferens in the rat. In: *Handbook of Physiology, Vol. V*, edited by D. W. Hamilton and R. O. Greep, pp. 259–301. American Physiological Society, Washington, D.C.
178. Hermo, L., and Morales, C. (1984): Endocytosis in non-ciliated cells of the ductuli efferentes in the rat. *Am. J. Anat.*, 171:59–64.
179. Glover, T. D., and Nicander, L. (1971): Some aspects of structure and function in the mammalian epididymis. *J. Reprod. Fertil. (Suppl.)*, 13:39–50.
180. Leidl, W., and Schefels, W. (1970): Thermographische Registrierung der Temperaturveteilung am Skrotum. *Fortpfl. Haust.*, 6:207–212.
181. Brooks, D. E. (1973): Epididymal and testicular temperature in the unrestrained conscious rat. *J. Reprod. Fertil.*, 35:157–160.
182. Stone, B. A. (1981): Thermal characteristics of the testis and epididymis of the boar. *J. Reprod. Fertil.*, 63:551–557.
183. Foster, M. E., Jones, A. S., and Eccles, R. (1983): Epididymal and testicular temperature in the anaesthetized rat. *IRCS Med. Sci.*, 11:234–235.
184. Reid, B. L., and Cleland, K. W. (1957): The structure and function of the epididymis. I. The histology of the rat epididymis. *Aust. J. Zool.*, 5:223–246.
185. Nicander, L. (1957): On the regional histology and cytochemistry of the ductus epididymidis in rabbits. *Acta Morphol. Neerl. Scand.*, 1:99–118.
186. Nicander, L. (1957): Studies on the regional histology and cytochemistry of the ductus epididymidis in stallions, rams and bulls. *Acta Morphol. Neerl. Scand.*, 1:337–362.
187. Abe, K., Takano, H., and Ito, T. (1983): Ultrastructure of the mouse epididymal duct with special reference to the regional differences of the principal cells. *Arch. Histol. Jpn.*, 46:51–68.

188. Flickinger, C. J., Howards, S. S., and English, H. F. (1978): Ultrastructural differences in efferent ducts and several regions of the epididymis of the hamster. *Am. J. Anat.*, 152:557–586.
189. Ramos, A. S., and Dym, M. (1977): Fine structure of the monkey epididymis. *Am. J. Anat.*, 149:501–532.
190. Goyal, H. O. (1985): Morphology of the bovine epididymis. *Am. J. Anat.*, 172:155–172.
191. Jones, R. C., and Brosnan, M. F. (1981): Studies of the deferent ducts from the testis of the African elephant, *Loxodonta africana*. I. Structural differentiation. *J. Anat.*, 132:371–386.
192. Hamilton, D. W., and Cooper, T. G. (1978): Gross and histological variations along the length of the rat vas deferens. *Anat. Rec.*, 190:795–810.
193. Paniagua, R., Regadera, J., Nistal, M., and Abaurrea, M. A. (1981): Histological, histochemical and ultrastructural variations along the length of the human vas deferens before and after puberty. *Acta Anat.*, 111:190–203.
194. Paniagua, R., Regadera, J., Nistal, M., and Santamaría, L. (1983): Elastic fibres of the human ductus deferens. *J. Anat.*, 137:467–476.
195. Eckstein, P., and Zuckerman, S. (1956): Morphology of the reproductive tract. In: *Marshall's Physiology of Reproduction, 3rd ed., Vol. 1,* edited by A. S. Parkes, pp. 43–155. Longmans, London.
196. Short, R. V., Mann, T., and Hay, M. F. (1967): Male reproductive organs of the African elephant, *Loxodonta africana*. *J. Reprod. Fertil.*, 13:517–536.
197. Aughey, E. (1969): Histology and histochemistry of the male accessory glands of the red deer, *Cervus elaphus* L. *J. Reprod. Fertil.*, 18:399–407.
198. Elwishy, A. B., Mobarak, A. M., and Fouad, S. M. (1972): The accessory genital organs of the one-humped male camel (*Camelus dromedarius*). *Anat. Anz.*, 131:1–12.
199. Kainer, R. A., Faulkner, L. C., and Abdel-Raouf, M. (1969): Glands associated with the urethra of the bull. *Am. J. Vet. Res.*, 30:963–974.
200. Bern, H. A., and Krichesky, B. (1943): Anatomic and histological studies of the sex accessories of the male rabbit. *Univ. Calif. Publ. Zool.*, 47:175–196.
201. Holtz, W., and Foote, R. H. (1978): The anatomy of the reproductive system in male dutch rabbits (*Oryctolagus cuniculus*) with special emphasis on the accessory sex glands. *J. Morphol.*, 158:1–20.
202. Ali, H. A., Tingari, M. D., and Moniem, K. A. (1978): On the morphology of the accessory male glands and histochemistry of the ampulla ductus deferentis of the camel (*Camelus dromedarius*). *J. Anat.*, 125:277–292.
203. Hummel, K. P., Richardson, F. L., and Fekete, E. (1966): Anatomy. In: *Biology of the Laboratory Mouse, 2nd ed.*, edited by E. L. Green, pp. 247–307. McGraw-Hill, New York.
204. Jesik, C. J., Holland, J. M., and Lee, C. (1982): An anatomic and histologic study of the rat prostate. *Prostate,* 3:81–97.
205. Davies, D. V., and Mann, T. (1947): Functional development of accessory glands and spermatogenesis. *Nature*, 160:295.
206. Mann, T., Davies, D. V., and Humphrey, G. F. (1949): Fructose and citric acid assay in the secretions of the accessory glands of reproduction as indicator tests of male sex hormone activity. *J. Endocrinol.*, 6:75–85.
207. Levey, H. A., and Szego, C. M. (1955): Metabolic characteristics of the guinea-pig seminal vesicle. *Am. J. Physiol.*, 182:507–512.
208. Mariotti, A., and Mawhinney, M. (1982): The hormonal maintenance and restoration of guinea pig seminal vesicle fibromuscular stroma. *J. Urol.*, 128:852–857.
209. Tisell, L. E., and Salander, H. (1984): Anatomy of the human prostate and its three paired lobes. *Prog. Clin. Biol. Res.*, 145:55–65.
210. McNeal, J. E. (1981): The zonal anatomy of the prostate. *Prostate,* 2:35–49.
211. Huggins, C. (1945): The physiology of the prostate gland. *Physiol. Rev.*, 25:281–295.
212. Huggins, C. (1947). The prostatic secretion. *Harvey Lect.*, 42:148–193.
213. Davies, J., and Danzo, B. J. (1981): Hormonally responsive areas of the reproductive system of the male guinea pig. 1. Morphology. *Biol. Reprod.*, 25:1135–1147.
214. Rodger, J. C., and Hughes, R. L. (1973): Studies of the accessory glands of male marsupials. *Aust. J. Zool.*, 21:303–320.
215. Bolliger, A. (1946): Presidential address. *Proc. R. Soc. N.S.W.*, 80:1–13.
216. Bharadwaj, M. B., and Calhoun, M. L. (1962): Histology of the bulbo-urethral gland of the domestic animals. *Anat. Rec.*, 142:216.
217. McKenzie, F. F., Miller, J. C., and Bauguess, L. C. (1938): The reproductive organs and semen of the boar. *Bull. Univ. Miss. Agric. Exp. Sta.*, No. 279.
218. Brooks, D. E., Gaughwin, M., and Mann, T. (1978): Structural and biochemical characteristics of the male accessory organs of reproduction in the hairy-nosed wombat (*Lasiorhinus latifrons*). *Proc. R. Soc. London. (B.)*, 201:191–207.
219. Sikorski, A. (1978): Comparative anatomy of the bulbourethral glands. *Folia Morphol. (Warsz.)*, 37:151–156.
220. Aitken, R. N. C. (1960): A histochemical study of the accessory genital glands of the boar. *J. Anat.*, 94:130–142.
221. Nielsen, E. H. (1976): The bulbourethral gland of the rat. Fine structure and histochemistry. *Anat. Anz.*, 139:254–263.
222. Schaffer, J. (1933): Die Vorhautdrüsen von Maus und Ratte. *Z. Mikrosk. Anat. Forsch.*, 34:1–22.
223. Montagna, W., and Noback, C. R. (1946): The histology of the preputial gland of the rat. *Anat. Rec.*, 96:111–128.
224. Pannese, E. (1954): Osservazioni morfologiche e istochemiche sulle ghiandole preputiale del ratto. *Arch. Ital. Anat. Embriol.*, 59:57–82.
225. Harrison, R. G. (1949): The comparative anatomy of the blood supply of the mammalian testis. *Proc. Zool. Soc. Lond.*, 19:325–343.
226. Hofmann, R. (1960): Die Gefassarchitektur des Bullenhodens, zugleich ein Versuch ihrer funktionellen Deutung. *Zentrabl. Veterinaermed.*, 7:59.
227. Hees, H., Leiser, R., Kohler, T., and Wrobel, K. H. (1984): Vascular morphology of the bovine spermatic cord and testis I. Light- and scanning electron-microscopic studies on the testicular artery and pampiniform plexus. *Cell Tiss. Res.*, 237:31–38.
228. Harrison, R. G. (1948): Vascular patterns in the testis, with particular reference to *Macropus*. *Nature,* 161:399–400.
229. Lewis, M. H., and Moffat, D. B. (1975): The venous drainage of the accessory reproductive organs of the rat with special reference to prostatic metabolism. *J. Reprod. Fertil.*, 42:497–502.
230. Ohtsuka, A. (1984): Microvascular architecture of the pampiniform plexus-testicular artery system in the rat: a scanning microscope study of corrosion casts. *Am. J. Anat.*, 169:285–293.
231. Weerasooriya, T. R., and Yamamoto, T. (1985): Three-dimensional organization of the vasculature of the rat spermatic cord and testis. A scanning electron-microscopic study of vascular corrosion casts. *Cell Tiss. Res.*, 241:317–323.
232. Waites, G. M. H., and Moule, G. R. (1960): Blood pressure in the internal spermatic artery of the ram. *J. Reprod. Fertil.*, 1:223–229.
233. Setchell, B. P., and Waites, G. M. H. (1969): Pulse attenuation and counter-current heat exchange in the internal spermatic artery of some Australian marsupials. *J. Reprod. Fertil.*, 20:165–169.
234. Dahl, E. V., and Herrick, J. F. (1959): A vascular mechanism for maintaining testicular temperature by counter-current exchange. *Surg. Gynecol. Obstet.*, 108:697–705.
235. Waites, G. M. H., and Moule, G. R. (1961): Relation of vascular heat exchange to temperature regulation in the testis of the ram. *J. Reprod. Fertil.*, 2:213–224.
236. Einer-Jensen, N. (1974): Local recirculation of 133-xenon and 85-krypton to the testes and caput epididymidis in rats. *J. Reprod. Fertil.*, 37:55–60.
237. Einer-Jensen, N., and Waites, G. M. H. (1977): Testicular blood flow and a study of the testicular venous to arterial transfer of radioactive krypton and testosterone in the rhesus monkey. *J. Physiol.*, 267:1–15.
238. Jacks, F. and Setchell, B. P. (1973): A technique for studying the transfer of substances from venous to arterial blood in the spermatic cord of wallabies and rams. *J. Physiol.*, 233:17P–18P.
239. Free, M. J. (1977): Blood supply to the testis and its role in local exchange and transport of hormones. In: *The Testis, Vol. IV,* edited by A. D. Johnson and W. R. Gomes, pp. 39–90. Academic Press, New York.
240. Wensing, C. J. G., Dijkstra, G., and Frankenhuis, M. T. (1981): The intricate morphological relations between testicular artery and pampiniform plexus. *Int. J. Androl.*, Suppl.3:77–78.
241. Fleet, I. R., Laurie, M. S., Noordhuizen-Stassen, E. N., Setchell, B. P., and Wensing, C. J. G. (1982): The flow of blood from artery to vein in the spermatic cord of the ram, with some observations on reactive hyperaemia in the testis and the effects of adenosine and noradrenaline. *J. Physiol.*, 332:44P–45P.

242. Noordhuizen-Stassen, E. N., Charbon, G. A., de Jong, F. H., and Wensing, C. J. G. (1985): Functional arterio-venous anastomoses between the testicular artery and the pampiniform plexus in the spermatic cord of rams. *J. Reprod. Fertil.*, 75:193–201.
243. Verstoppen, G. R., and Steeno, O. P. (1977): Varicocele and the pathogenesis of the associated subfertility: a review of the various theories. I. Varicocelogenesis. *Andrologia,* 9:133–140.
244. Verstoppen, G. R., and Steeno, O. P. (1977): Varicocele and the pathogenesis of the associated subfertility: a review of the various theories. II. Results of surgery. *Andrologia,* 9:293–305.
245. Saypol, D. C. (1981): Varicocele. *J. Androl.*, 2:61–71.
246. Comhaire, F. H. (1983): Varicocele infertility: an enigma. *Int. J. Androl.*, 6:401–404.
247. Turner, T. T. (1983): Varicocele: still an enigma. *J. Urol.*, 129:695–699.
248. Baker, H. W. G., Burger, H. G., De Kretser, D. M., Hudson, B., Rennie, G. C., and Straffon, W. G. E. (1985): Testicular vein ligation and fertility in men with varicoceles. *Br. Med. J.*, 291:1678–1680.
249. Nistal, M., Paniagua, R., Regadera, J., and Santamaria, L. (1984): Obstruction of the tubuli recti and ductuli efferentes by dilated veins in the testes in men with variococele and its possible role in causing atrophy of the seminiferous tubules. *Int. J. Androl.*, 7:309–323.
250. Chubb, C., and Desjardins, C. (1982): Vasculature of the mouse, rat and rabbit testis-epididymis. *Am. J. Anat.*, 165:357–372.
251. Waites, G. M. H., Archer, V., and Langford, G. A. (1975): Regional sensitivity of the testicular artery to noradrenaline in the ram, rabbit, rat and boar. *J. Reprod. Fertil.*, 45:159–163.
252. Niemi, M., and Setchell, B. P. (1987): Gamma-glutamyl transpeptidase in the vasculature of the rat testis. *Biol. Reprod.*, 35:385–391.
253. Bustamante, J. C., Jarvis, L. G., and Setchell, B. P. (1982): Role of the endothelium in the uptake of amino acids by the isolated perfused testis. *J. Physiol.*, 330:62P–63P.
254. Noordhuizen-Stassen, E. N., Dijkstra, G., Schanhardt, H. C., and Wensing, C. J. G. (1983): Compensatory development of a patent vascular supply to the testis after intra-abdominal transection of its main blood vessels. *Int. J. Androl.*, 6:509–519.
255. Muller, I. (1957): Kanalchen- und Capillararchitektonik des Rattenhodens. *Z. Zellforsch.*, 45:522–537.
256. Kormano, M. (1967): An angiographic study of the testicular vasculature in the postnatal rat. *Z. Anat. Entwickl.*, 126:138–153.
257. Suzuki, F. (1982): Microvasculature of the mouse testis and excurrent duct system. *Am. J. Anat.*, 163:309–325.
258. Takayama, H., and Tomoyoshi, T. (1981): Microvascular architecture of rat and human testes. *Invest. Urol.*, 18:341–344.
259. Kormano, M. (1967): Dye permeability and alkaline phosphatase activity of testicular capillaries in the postnatal rat. *Histochemie,* 9:327–338.
260. Wolff, J., and Merker, H. J. (1966): Ultrastruktur und Bildung von Poren im Endothel von porosen und geschlossen Kapillaren. *Z. Zellforsch.*, 73:174–191.
261. Hundeiker, M. (1971): Die Capillaren im Hodenparenchym. *Arch. Klin. Exp. Dermatol.*, 239:426–435.
262. Damber, J. E., Bergh, A., and Daehlin, L. (1985): Testicular blood flow, vascular permeability and testosterone production after stimulation of unilaterally cryptorchid adult rats with human chorionic gonadotropin. *Endocrinology,* 117:1906–1913.
263. Setchell, B. P., and Sharpe, R. M. (1981): Effect of injected human chorionic gonadotrophin on capillary permeability, extracellular fluid volume and the flow of lymph in the testes of rats. *J. Endocrinol.*, 91:245–254.
264. Bustamante, J. C., and Setchell, B. P. (1981): Measurement of capillary permeability-surface area products in the isolated perfused rat testis. *J. Physiol.*, 319:16P–17P.
265. Setchell, B. P., Bustamante, J. C., and Niemi, M. (1984): The microcirculation of the testis. In: *Progress in Microcirculation Research, II,* edited by F. C. Courtice, D. G. Garlick, and M. A. Perry, pp. 291–296. Committee in Postgraduate Medical Education, University of New South Wales, Sydney.
266. Clegg, E. J., and Carr, I. (1966): Increased vascular permeability in the reproductive organs of cadmium chloride-treated male rats. *J. Anat.*, 100:696–697.
267. Gupta, R. K., Barnes, G. W., and Skelton, F. R., (1967): Light-microscopic and immunopathologic observations of cadmium chloride-induced injury in mature rat testis. *Am. J. Pathol.*, 51:191–205.
268. Setchell, B. P., and Waites, G. M. H. (1970): Changes in the permeability of the testicular capillaries and of the "blood-testis barrier" after injection of cadmium chloride in the rat. *J. Endocrinol.*, 47:81–86.
269. Waites, G. M. H., and Setchell, B. P. (1966): Changes in blood flow and vascular permeability of the testis, epididymis and accessory reproductive organs of the rat after the administration of cadmium chloride. *J. Endocrinol.*, 34:329–342.
270. Chiquoine, A. D. (1964): Observations on the early events of cadmium necrosis of the testis. *Anat. Rec.*, 149:23–35.
271. Clegg, E. J., and Carr, I. (1967): Changes in the blood vessels of the rat testis and epididymis produced by cadmium salts. *J. Pathol. Bacteriol.*, 94:317–322.
272. Aoki, A., and Hoffer, A. P. (1978): Reexamination of the lesions in rat testis caused by cadmium. *Biol. Reprod.*, 18:579–591.
273. Clegg, E. J., Niemi, M., and Carr, I. (1969): The age at which the blood vessels of the rat testis become sensitive to cadium salts. *J. Endocrinol.*, 43:445–449.
274. Veijola, M., and Rajaniemi, H. (1985): The hCG-induced increase in hormone uptake and interstitial fluid volume in the rat testis is not mediated by steroids, prostaglandins or protein synthesis. *Int. J. Androl.*, 8:69–79.
275. Setchell, B. P., and Rommerts, F. F. G. (1986): The importance of the Leydig cells in the vascular response to hCG in the rat testis. *Int. J. Androl.*, 8:436–440.
276. Noordhuizen-Stassen, E. N., Buwalda, G., and Wensing, C. J. G. (1984): Testicular, arterial, and venous blood pressure patterns in ram and boar. In: *Functional and Morphological Aspects of Testicular Blood Supply* [Doctoral thesis]. E. N. Noordhuizen-Stassen. Utrecht, Netherlands: Rijksuniversiteit, pp. 73–80. Offsetdrukkerij Kanters BV, Amsterdam.
277. Abe, K., Takano, H., and Ito, T. (1984): Microvasculature of the mouse epididymis, with special reference to fenestrated capillaries localized in the initial segment. *Anat. Rec.*, 209:209–218.
278. Harrison, R. G. (1949): The distribution of the vasal and cremasteric arteries to the testis and their functional importance. *J. Anat.*, 83:267–282.
279. Kormano, M. (1968): Microvascular structure of the rat epididymis. *Ann. Med. Exp. Fenn.*, 46:113–118.
280. Clavert, A., Cranz, C., and Brun, B. (1980): Etude de la vascularisation de l'épididyme. *Bull. Assoc. Anat.*, 64:539–546.
281. Jantošovičová, J. (1977): Topographisch-anatomische Angaben über die A. testicularis, A. ductus deferentis und A. cremasterica beim Widder. *Gegenbaurs Morphol. Jahrb.*, 123:914–923.
282. Osman, D. I., Tingari, M. D., and Moniem, K. A. (1979): Vascular supply of the testis of the camel (*Camelus dromedarius*). *Acta Anat.*, 104:16–22.
283. MacMillan, E. W. (1954): The blood supply of the epididymis in man. *Br. J. Urol.*, 26:60–71.
284. Harrison, R. G., and Barclay, A. E. (1948): The distribution of the testicular artery (internal spermatic artery) to the human testis. *Br. J. Urol.*, 20:5–66.
285. Fehlings, K., and Pohlmeyer, K. (1978): Die Arteria testicularis und ihre Aufzweigung im Hoden und Nebenhoden des Esels (*Equus africanus f. asinus*). Korrosionsanatomische und röntgenologische Untersuchungen. *Anat. Histol. Embryol.*, 7:74–78.
286. Ohtani, O., and Gannon, B. J. (1982): The microvasculature of the rat vas deferens: a scanning electron and light microscopic study. *J. Anat.*, 135:521–529.
287. Joranson, Y., Emmel, V. E., and Pilka, H. J. (1929): Factors controlling the arterial supply of the testis under experimental conditions. *Anat. Rec.*, 41:157–176.
288. Niemi, M., and Kormano, M. (1965): An angiographic study of cadmium-induced vascular lesions in the testis and epididymis of the rat. *Acta Pathol. Microbiol. Scand.*, 63:513–521.
289. Kormano, M., and Reijonen, K. (1976): Microvascular structure of the human epididymis. *Am. J. Anat.*, 145:23–32.
290. Setchell, B. P., Waites, G. M. H., and Till, A. R. (1964): Variations in flow of blood within the epididymis and testis of the sheep and rat. *Nature,* 203:317–318.
291. Brown, P. D. C., and Waites, G. M. H. (1972): Regional blood flow in the epididymis of the rat and rabbit: effect of efferent duct ligation and orchidectomy. *J. Reprod. Fertil.*, 28: 221–233.

292. Dhabuwala, C. B., and Pierrepoint, C. G. (1977): Venous drainage and functional control of the canine prostate gland. *J. Endocrinol.*, 75:105–108.
293. Pierrepoint, C. G., Davies, P., Lewis, M. H., and Moffat, D. B. (1975): Examination of the hypothesis that a direct control system exists for the prostate and seminal vesicles. *J. Reprod. Fertil.*, 44:395–409.
294. Boulanger, P., Desaulniers, M., Bleau, G., Roberts, K. D., and Chapdelaine, A. (1983): Sex steroid concentrations in plasma collected from the canine deferential vein. *J. Endocrinol.*, 96:223–228.
295. Flocks, R. H. (1937): The arterial distribution within the prostate gland: its role in transurethral prostatic resection. *J. Urol.*, 37:524–548.
296. Clegg, E. J. (1955): The arterial supply of the human prostate and seminal vesicles. *J. Anat.*, 89:209–216.
297. Clegg, E. J. (1956): The vascular arrangements within the human prostate gland. *Br. J. Urol.*, 28:428–435.
298. Hodson, N. (1968): On the intrinsic blood supply to the prostate and pelvic urethra in the dog. *Res. Vet. Sci.*, 9:274–280.
299. Lasinski, W., and Sikorski, A. (1975): La vascularisation arterielle des glandes bulbo-uretrales humaines. *Bull. Assoc. Anat.*, 59:911–918.
300. Lindner, H. R. (1963): Partition of androgen between the lymph and venous blood of the testis in the ram. *J. Endocrinol.*, 25: 483–494.
301. McIntosh, G. H. (1969): Lymphatics of the urogenital system of the sheep. *Ph.D. Thesis,* Australian National University, Canberra.
302. Morris, B., and McIntosh, G. H. (1971): Techniques for the collection of lymph with special reference to the testis and ovary. *Acta Endocrinol.*, Suppl. 158:145–168.
303. Moller, R. (1980): Arrangement and fine structure of lymphatic vessels in the human spermatic cord. *Andrologia,* 12:564–576.
304. Engeset, A. (1959): The route of peripheral lymph to the blood stream. An X-ray study of the barrier theory. *J. Anat.*, 93:96–100.
305. Head, J. R., Neaves, W. B., and Billingham, R. E. (1983): Reconsideration of the lymphatic drainage of the rat testis. *Transplantation,* 35:91–95.
306. Hundeiker, M., and Keller, L. (1963): Die Gefassarchitektur des menschlichen Hodens. *Morphol. Jb.*, 105:26–73.
307. Clavert, A., Cranz, C., and Brun, B. (1981): Epididymal vascularization and microvascularization. *Prog. Reprod. Biol.*, 8:48–57.
308. Perez-Clavier, R., and Harrison, R. G. (1978): The pattern of lymphatic drainage of the rat testis. *J. Anat.*, 127:93–100.
309. Perez-Clavier, R., Harrison, R. G., and MacMillan, E. W. (1982): The pattern of the lymphatic drainage of the rat epididymis. *J. Anat.*, 134:667–675.
310. Kotani, M., Seiki, K., and Hattori, M. (1974): Retardation of spermatogenesis and testosterone secretion after ligature of lymphatics draining the testes of rabbits. *Endocrinol. Jpn.*, 21:1–8.
311. Perez-Clavier, R., and Harrison, R. G. (1978): The effect of interruption of lymphatic drainage from the rat testis. *J. Pathol.*, 124:219–225.
312. Kazeem, A. A. (1983): The assessment of epididymal lymphatics within the concept of immunologically privileged sites. *Lymphology,* 16:168–171.
313. McCullough, D. L. (1975): Experimental lymphangiography. Experience with direct medium injection into the parenchyma of the rat testis and prostate. *Invest. Urol.*, 13:211–219.
314. Smith, M. J. V. (1966): The lymphatics of the prostate. *Invest. Urol.*, 3:439–444.
315. Rodin, A. E., Larson, D. L., and Roberts, D. K. (1967): Nature of the perineural space invaded by prostatic carcinoma. *Cancer,* 20:1772–1779.
316. Connolly, J. G., Thomson, A., Jewett, M. A. S., Hartman, N., and Webber, M. (1968): Intraprostatic lymphatics. *Invest. Urol.*, 5:371–378.
317. Uemura, Y. (1976): The fine distribution of the lymph vessels in the prostate of the dog. *Acta Anat. Nippon.*, 51:17–31.
318. Menon, M., Menon, S., Strauss, H. W., and Catalona, W. J. (1977): Demonstration of the existence of canine prostatic lymphatics by radioisotope techniques. *J. Urol.*, 118:274–277.
319. Neaves, W. B., and Billingham, R. E. (1979): The lymphatic drainage of the rat prostate and its status as an immunologically privileged site. *Transplantation,* 27:127–132.
320. Furusato, M., and Mostofi, F. K. (1980): Intraprostatic lymphatics in man: light and ultrastructural observations. *Prostate,* 1:15–23.
321. Sjöstrand, N. O. (1965): The adrenergic innervation of the vas deferens and the accessory male genital glands. *Acta Physiol. Scand.*, 65,Suppl. 257:1–82.
322. Elbadawi, A., and Goodman, D. C. (1980): Autonomic innervation of accessory male genital glands. In: *Male Accessory Sex Glands,* edited by E. Spring-Mills and E. S. E. Hafez, pp. 101–128. Elsevier/North-Holland, Amsterdam.
323. Hodson, N. (1970): The nerves of the testis, epididymis, and scrotum. In: *The Testis, Vol. I,* edited by A. D. Johnson, W. R. Gomes, and N. L. Vandemark, pp. 47–99. Academic Press, New York.
324. Baumgarten, H. G., and Holstein, A. F. (1967): Catecholaminhaltige Nervenfasern im Hoden des Menschen. *Z. Zellforsch.*, 79:389–395.
325. Norberg, K. A., Risley, P. L., and Ungerstedt, U. (1967): Adrenergic innervation of the male reproductive ducts in some mammals. I. The distribution of adrenergic nerves. *Z. Zellforsch.*, 76:278–286.
326. Baumgarten, H. G., Falck, B., Holstein, A.-F, Owman, C., and Owman, T. (1968): Adrenergic innervation of the human testis, epididymis, ductus deferens and prostate: A fluorescence microscopic and fluorimetric study. *Z. Zellforsch.*, 90:81–95.
327. Linzell, J. L., and Setchell, B. P. (1969): Metabolism, sperm and fluid production of the isolated perfused testis of the sheep and goat. *J. Physiol.*, 201:129–143.
328. Risley, P. L., and Skrepetos, C. N. (1964): Histochemical distribution of cholinesterases in the testis, epididymis and vas deferens of the rat. *Anat. Rec.*, 148:231–249.
329. Larsson, L. I., Fahrenkrug, J., and Schaffalitsky de Muckadell, O. B. (1977): Occurrence of nerves containing vasoactive intestinal polypeptide immunoreactivity in the male genital tract. *Life Sci.*, 21:503–508.
330. Alm, P., Alumets, J., Håkanson, R., Owman, Ch., Sjöberg, N.-O., Sundler, F., and Walles, B. (1980): Origin and distribution of VIP (vasoactive intestinal polypeptide)-nerves in the genito-urinary tract. *Cell Tiss. Res.*, 205:337–347.
331. Shioda, T., and Nishida, S. (1966): Innervation of the bull testis. *Jpn. J. Vet. Sci.*, 28:251–257.
332. Okkels, H., and Sand, K. (1940): Morphological relationship between testicular nerves and Leydig cells in man. *J. Endocrinol.*, 2:38–46.
333. van Campenhout, E. (1949): Les relations nerveuses de la glande interstitielle des glandes genitales chez les mammiferes. *Rev. Can. Biol.*, 8:374–429.
334. Holstein, A. F. (1985): Die mannlichen Geschlechtsorgane. In: *Benninghoff Anatomie. Makroskopische und mikroskopische Anatomie des Menschen, Band 2. Kreislauf ind Eingeweide,* edited by K. Fleischhauer, pp. 460–514. Urban & Schwarzenberg, Munich.
335. Anakwe, O. O., Murphy, P. R., and Moger, W. H. (1985): Characterization of β-adrenergic binding sites on rodent Leydig cells. *Biol. Reprod.*, 33:815–826.
336. Cooke, B. A., Golding, M., Dix, C. J., and Hunter, M. G. (1982): Catecholamine stimulation of testosterone production via cyclic AMP in mouse Leydig cells in monolayer culture. *Mol. Cell. Endocrinol.*, 27:221–231.
337. Moger, W. H., Murphy, P. R., and Casper, R. F. (1982): Catecholamine stimulation of androgen production by mouse interstitial cells in primary culture. *J. Androl.*, 3:227–231.
338. Moger, W. H., and Murphy, P. R. (1983): β-Adrenergic agonist induced androgen production during primary culture of mouse Leydig cells. *Arch. Androl.*, 10:135–142.
339. Kasson, B. G., and Hsueh, A. J. W. (1985): Nicotinic cholinergic agonists inhibit androgen biosynthesis by cultured rat testicular cells. *Endocrinology,* 117:1874–1880.
340. Verhoeven, G., Dierickx, P., and de Moor, P. (1979): Stimulation effect of neurotransmitters on the aromatization of testosterone by Sertoli cell-enriched cultures. *Mol. Cell. Endocrinol.*, 13:241–253.
341. Heindel, J. J., Steinberger, A., and Strada, J. J. (1981): Identification and characterization of a β_1-adrenergic receptor in the rat Sertoli cell. *Mol. Cell. Endocrinol.*, 22:349–358.
342. Peterson, D. F., and Brown, A. M. (1973): Functional afferent innervation of testis. *J. Neurophysiol.*, 36:425–433.
343. Yamashita, K. (1939): Histological studies on the innervation of human testis and epididymis (in Japanese). *J. Orient. Med.*, 30:367–394.

344. Kumazawa, T., and Mizumura, K. (1977): The polymodal receptors in the testis of dog. *Brain Res.*, 136:553–558.
345. Kumazawa, T., and Mizumura, K. (1979): Effects of synthetic substance P on unit-discharges of testicular nociceptors of dogs. *Brain Res.*, 170:553–557.
346. Kumazawa, T., and Mizumura, K. (1980): Mechanical and thermal responses of polymodal receptors recorded from the superior spermatic nerve of dogs. *J. Physiol.*, 299:233–245.
347. Kumazawa, T., and Mizumura, K. (1980): Chemical responses of polymodal receptors of the scrotal contents in dogs. *J. Physiol.*, 299:219–231.
348. Kumazawa, T., and Mizumura, K. (1983): Temperature dependency of the chemical responses of the polymodal receptor units in vitro. *Brain Res.*, 278:305–307.
349. Noordhuizen-Stassen, E. N., and Wensing, C. J. G. (1983): The effect of transection of the main vascular and nervous supply of the testis on the development of spermatogenic epithelium in the pig. *J. Pediatr. Surg.*, 18:601–606.
350. Martin, I. C. A., Lapwood, K. R., and Kitchell, R. L. (1984): The effects of specific neurectomies and cremaster muscle sectioning on semen characteristics and scrotal thermoregulatory responses of rams. In: *Reproduction in Sheep*, edited by D. R. Lindsay and D. T. Pearce, pp. 73–75. Australian Academy of Science, Canberra.
351. Nagai, K., Murano, S., Minokoshi, Y., Okuda, H., and Kinutani, M. (1982): Effects of denervation and local 6-hydroxydopamine injection on testicular growth in rats. *Experientia*, 38:592–594.
352. Frankel, A. I., and Ryan, E. L. (1981): Testicular innervation is necessary for the response of plasma testosterone levels to acute stress. *Biol. Reprod.*, 24:491–495.
353. Frankel, A. I., and Mock, E. J. (1982): A study of the first eight hours in the stabilization of plasma testosterone concentration in the hemicastrated rat. *J. Endocrinol.*, 92:225–229.
354. Mock, E. J., and Frankel, A. I. (1982): Response of testosterone to hemicastration in the testicular vein of the mature rat. *J. Endocrinol.*, 92:231–236.
355. Frankel, A. I., Mock, E. J., and Chapman, J. C. (1984): Hypophysectomy and hemivasectomy can inhibit the testicular hemicastration response of the mature rat. *Biol. Reprod.*, 30:804–808.
356. Mizunuma, H., Palatis, L., and McCann, S. M. (1983): Effect of unilateral orchidectomy on plasma FSH concentration: evidence for a direct neural connection between testes and CNS. *Neuroendocrinology*, 37:291–296.
357. Preslock, J. P., and McCann, S. M. (1985): Short-term effects of vasoligation upon plasma follicle-stimulating hormone, luteinizing hormone and prolactin in the adult rat: further evidence for a direct neural connection between the testes and the central nervous system. *Biol. Reprod.*, 33:1120–1125.
358. Kuntz, A., and Morris, R. E. (1946): Components and distribution of the spermatic nerves and the nerves of the vas deferens. *J. Comp. Neurol.*, 85:33–44.
359. El-Badawi, A., and Schenk, E. A. (1967): The distribution of cholinergic and adrenergic nerves in the mammalian epididymis. A comparative histochemical study. *Am. J. Anat.*, 121:1–14.
360. Baumgarten, H. G., Holstein, A. F., and Rosengren, E. (1971): Arrangement, ultrastructure, and adrenergic innervation of smooth musculature of the ductuli efferentes, ductus epididymidis and ductus deferens of man. *Z. Zellforsch.*, 120:37–79.
361. Greenberg, J., Schubert, W., Metz, J., Yanaihara, N., and Forssmann, W.-G. (1985): Studies of the guinea-pig epididymis. III. Innervation of epididymal segments. *Cell Tiss. Res.*, 239: 395–404.
362. Bell, C., and McLean, J. R. (1970): The distribution of cholinergic and adrenergic nerve fibres in the retractor penis and vas deferens of the dog. *Z. Zellforsch.*, 106:516–522.
363. Alm, P. (1982): On the autonomic innervation of the human vas deferens. *Brain Res. Bull.*, 9:673–677.
364. Jacobowitz, D., and Koelle, G. B. (1965): Histochemical correlations of acetylcholinesterase and catecholamines in postganglionic autonomic nerves of the cat, rabbit, and guinea pig. *J. Pharmacol. Exp. Ther.*, 148:225–237.
365. Furness, J. B., and Iwayama, T. (1972): The arrangement and identification of axons innervating the vas deferens of the guinea-pig. *J. Anat.*, 113:179–196.
366. Gosling, J. A., and Dixon, J. S. (1972): Differences in the manner of autonomic innervation of the muscle layers of the guinea-pig ductus deferens. *J. Anat.*, 112:81–91.
367. Al-Zuhair, A., Gosling, J. A., and Dixon, J. S. (1975): Observations on the structure and autonomic innervation of the guinea-pig seminal vesicle and ductus deferens. *J. Anat.*, 120:81–93.
368. Fedan, J. S., Hogaboom, G. K., O'Donnell, J. P., Colby, J., and Westfall, D. P. (1981): Contribution by purines to the neurogenic response of the vas deferens of the guinea pig. *Eur. J. Pharmacol.*, 69:41–53.
369. McConnell, J., Benson, G. S., and Wood, J. G. (1982): Autonomic innervation of the urogenital system: adrenergic and cholinergic elements. *Brain Res. Bull.*, 9:679–694.
370. Iggo, A. (1969): Cutaneous thermoreceptors in primates and subprimates. *J. Physiol.*, 200:403–430.
371. Hellon, R. F., and Misra, N. K. (1973): Neurones in the dorsal horn of the rat responding to scrotal skin temperature changes. *J. Physiol.*, 232:375–388.
372. Hellon, R. F., and Misra, N. K. (1973): Neurones in the ventrobasal complex of the rat responding to scrotal skin temperature changes. *J. Physiol.*, 232:389–399.
373. Hellon, R. F., Misra, N. K., and Provins, K. A. (1973): Neurones in the somatosensory cortex of the rat responding to scrotal skin temperature changes. *J. Physiol.*, 232:401–411.
374. Hellon, R. F., Hensel, H., and Schafer, K. (1975): Thermal receptors in the scrotum of the rat. *J. Physiol.*, 248:349–357.
375. Hellon, R. F., and Mitchell, D. (1975): Convergence in a thermal afferent pathway in the rat. *J. Physiol.*, 248:359–376.
376. Hellon, R. F., and Taylor, D. C. M. (1973): An analysis of a thermal afferent pathway in the rat. *J. Physiol.*, 326:319–328.
377. Nakayama, T., Ishikawa, Y., and Tsurutani, T. (1979): Projection of scrotal thermal afferents to the preoptic and hypothalamic neurons in rats. *Pfluegers Arch.*, 380:59–64.
378. Pierau, F. K., Torrey, P., and Carpenter, D. O. (1975): Afferent nerve fiber activity responding to temperature changes of scrotal skin of the rat. *J. Neurophysiol.*, 38:601–612.
379. Schingnitz, G., and Werner, J. (1980): Responses of thalamic neurons to thermal stimulation of the limbs, scrotum and tongue in the rat. *J. Therm. Biol.*, 5:53–61.
380. Taylor, D. C. M. (1982): The effects of nucleus raphe magnus lesions on an ascending thermal pathway in the rat. *J. Physiol.*, 326:309–318.
381. Waites, G. M. H. (1962): The effect of heating the scrotum of the ram on respiration and body temperature. *Q. J. Exp. Physiol.*, 47:314–323.
382. Waites, G. M. H., and Voglmayr, J. K. (1963): The functional activity and control of the apocrine sweat glands of the scrotum of the ram. *Aust. J. Agric. Res.*, 14:839–851.
383. Fowler, D. G. (1969): The relationship between air temperature and scrotal surface area and testis temperature in rams. *Aust. J. Exp. Agric. Anim. Husb.*, 9:258–261.
384. Owman, C., and Sjöstrand, N. O. (1965): Short adrenergic neurons and catecholamine-containing cells in vas deferens and accessory male genital glands of different mammals. *Z. Zellforsch.*, 66:300–320.
385. Richardson, K. C. (1966): Electron microscopic identification of autonomic nerve endings. *Nature*, 210:756.
386. Clementi, F., Naimzada, K. M., and Mantegazza, P. (1969): Study of the nerve endings in the vas deferens and seminal vesicle of the guinea pig. *Int. J. Neuropharmacol.*, 8:399–403.
387. Vaalasti, A., and Hervonen, A. (1979): Innervation of the ventral prostate of the rat. *Am. J. Anat.* 154: 231–244.
388. Vaalasti, A., and Hervonen, A. (1979): Autonomic innervation of the human prostate. *Invest. Urol.*, 17:293–297.
389. Vaalasti, A., and Hervonen, A. (1980): Nerve endings in the human prostate. *Am. J. Anat.*, 157:41–47.
390. Ambadkar, P. M., and Vyas, D. M. (1981): Innervation of the rat preputial gland. *Acta Anat.*, 110:98–102.
391. Dent, J., Hodson, N., and Selhi, H. (1971): Ultrastructural differentiation of fibre types in rabbit seminal vesicles. *J. Physiol.*, 217:7P–9P.
392. Larsen, J-J., Ottesen, B., Fahrenkrug, J., and Fahrenkrug, L. (1981): Vasoactive intestinal polypeptide (VIP) in the male genitourinary tract. Concentration and motor effect. *Invest. Urol.*, 19:211–213.

393. Polak, J. M., Gu, J., Mina, S., and Bloom, S. R. (1981): VIPergic nerves in the penis. *Lancet*, 2:217–219.
394. Sastry, B. V. R., Janson, V. E., Owens, L. K., and Tayeb, O. S. (1982): Enkephalin- and substance P-like immunoreactivities of mammalian sperm and accessory sex glands. *Biochem. Pharmacol.*, 31:3519–3522.
395. Pekary, A. E., Yamada, T., Sharp, B., Bhasin, S., Swerdloff, R. S., and Hershman, J. M. (1984): Somatostatin-14 and -28 in the male rat reproductive system. *Life Sci.*, 34:939–945.
396. Adrian, T. E., Gu, J., Allen, J. M., Tatemoto, K., Polak, J. M., and Bloom, S. R. (1984): Neuropeptide Y in the human male genital tract. *Life Sci.*, 35:2643–2648.
397. Vaalasti, A., Linnoila, I., and Hervonen, A. (1980): Immunohistochemical demonstration of VIP, [Met^5]- and [Leu^5]-enkephalin immunoreactive nerve fibres in the human prostate and seminal vesicles. *Histochemistry*, 66:89–98.
398. Del Fiacco, M. (1982): Enkephalin-like immunoreactivity in the human male genital tract. *J. Anat.*, 135:649–656.
399. Gu, J., Polak, J. M., Probert, L., Islam, K. N., Marangos, P. J., Mina, S., Adrian, T. E., McGregor, G. P., O'Shaughnessy, D. J., and Bloom, S. R. (1983): Peptidergic innervation of the human male genital tract. *J. Urol.*, 130:386–391.
400. Stjernquist, M., Håkanson, R., Leander, S., Owman, C., Sundler, F., and Uddman, R. (1983): Immunohistochemical localization of substance P, vasoactive intestinal polypeptide and gastrin-releasing peptide in vas deferens and seminal vesicle, and the effect of these and eight other neuropeptides on resting tension and neurally evoked contractile activity. *Reg. Pep.*, 7:67–86.
401. Alm, P., Alumets, J., Brodin, E., Håkanson, R., Nilsson, G., Sjöberg, N.-O., and Sundler, F. (1978): Peptidergic substance P nerves in the genitourinary tract. *Neuroscience*, 3:419–425.
402. Alm, P., Alumets, J., Håkanson, R., and Sundler, F. (1977): Peptidergic (vasoactive intestinal peptide) nerves in the genito-urinary tract. *Neuroscience*, 2:751–754.
403. Melin, P. (1970): *In vivo* recording of contractile activity of male accessory genital organs in rabbits. *Acta Physiol. Scand.*, 79:109–113.
404. Talo, A., Jaakkola, U.-M., and Markkula-Vittanen, M. (1979): Spontaneous electrical activity of the rat epididymis *in vitro*. *J. Reprod. Fertil.*, 57:423–429.
405. Risley, P. L. (1958): The contractile behavior *in vivo* of the ductus epididymidis and vasa efferentia of the rat. *Anat. Rec.*, 130:471.
406. van de Velde, R. L., and Risley, P. L. (1963): The origin and development of smooth muscle and contractility in the ductus epididymidis of the rat. *J. Embryol. Exp. Morphol.*, 11:369–382.
407. Talo, A. (1981): *In-vitro* spontaneous electrical activity of rat efferent ductules. *J. Reprod. Fertil.*, 63:17–20.
408. Muratori, G. (1956): Osservazioni preliminari sull'azione dell' adrenalina e dell'acetilcolina sui movimenti del canale dell'epididimo del ratto. *Boll. Soc. Ital. Biol. Sper.*, 32:248–249.
409. Muratori, G. (1961): Bewegungen des Ductus epididymidis der Ratte (film). *Acta Anat.*, 47:393.
410. Knight, T. W. (1974): A qualitative study of factors affecting the contractions of the epididymis and ductus deferens of the ram. *J. Reprod. Fertil.*, 40:19–29.
411. Pholpramool, C., and Triphrom, N. (1984): Effects of cholinergic and adrenergic drugs on intraluminal pressures and contractility of the rat testis and epididymis *in vivo*. *J. Reprod. Fertil.*, 71:181–188.
412. Hib, J., Ponzio, R., and Vilar, O. (1982): Contractility of the rat cauda epididymidis and vas deferens during seminal emission. *J. Reprod. Fertil.*, 66:47–50.
413. Cross, B. A., and Glover, T. D. (1958): The hypothalamus and seminal emission. *J. Endocrinol.*, 16:385–395.
414. Hepp, R., and Kreye, V. A. W. (1973): Effect of long-term treatment with high doses of guanethidine on sperm transport and fertility of rats. *Br. J. Pharmacol.*, 48:30–35.
415. Dziuk, P. J., and Mann, T. (1963): Effect of atropine on the composition of semen and secretory function of male accessory organs in the boar. *J. Reprod. Fertil.*, 5:101–108.
416. Cross, B. A., and Silver, I. A. (1962): Neurovascular control of oxygen tension in the testis and epididymis. *J. Reprod. Fertil.*, 3:377–395.
417. Hodson, N. (1965): Sympathetic nerves and reproductive organs in the male rabbit. *J. Reprod. Fertil.*, 10:209–220.
418. Smith, E. R. (1975): The canine prostate and it secretion. In: *Molecular Mechanisms of Gonadal Hormone Action, Vol. 1*, edited by J. A. Thomas and R. L. Singhal, pp. 167–204. University Park Press, Baltimore.
419. Smith, E. R., and Lebeaux, M. I. (1970): The mediation of the canine prostatic secretion provoked by hypogastric nerve stimulation. *Invest. Urol.*, 7:313–318.
420. Hodson, N. (1964): Role of the hypogastric nerves in seminal emission in the rabbit. *J. Reprod. Fertil.*, 7:113–122.
421. Maddochs, S. and Setchell, B. P. (1987): The composition of the extracellular interstitial fluid in the rat testis. *J. Physiol.*, (*in press*).
422. Noordhuizen-Stassen, E. N., Beijer, H. J. M., Charbon, G. A., and Wensing, C. J. G. (1983): The effect of norepinephrine, isoprenaline and acetylcholine on the testicular and epididymal circulation in the pig. *Int. J. Androl.*, 6:44–56.
423. Free, M. J., and Jaffe, R. A. (1972): Dynamics of circulation in the testis of the conscious rat. *Am. J. Physiol.*, 223:241–248.
424. Amann, R. P., Nett, T. M., and Niswender, G. D. (1978): Effects of LH, FSH, prolactin and $PGF_{2\alpha}$ on testicular blood flow and testosterone secretion in the ram. *J. Anim. Sci.*, 47:1307–1313.
425. Damber, J. E., Lindahl, O., Selstam, G., and Tenland, T. (1982): Testicular blood flow measured with a laser Doppler flowmeter: acute effects of catecholamines. *Acta Physiol. Scand.*, 115: 209–215.
426. Damber, J. E., Lindahl, O., Selstam, G., and Tenland, T. (1983): Rhythmical oscillations in rat testicular microcirculation as recorded by laser Doppler flowmetry. *Acta Physiol. Scand.*, 118: 117–123.
427. Setchell, B. P., and Hinks, N. T. (1967): The importance of glucose in the oxidative metabolism of the testis of the conscious ram and the role of the pentose cycle. *Biochem. J.*, 102:623–631.
428. Godinho, H. P., and Setchell, B. P. (1975): Total and capillary blood flow through the testes of anaesthetized rams. *J. Physiol.*, 251:19P–20P.
429. Cox, J. E., Maddocks, S., and Setchell, B. P. (1987): The effect of cortisol and adrenocorticotrophic hormone on testosterone production in the bull and ram. *J. Endocrinol.* (*in press*).
430. Laurie, M. S., and Setchell, B. P. (1979): The continuous measurement of testicular blood flow in the ram, in relation to the pulsatile secretion of testosterone. *J. Physiol.*, 287:10P.
431. Chandrasekhar, Y., Holland, M. K., D'Ochhio, M. J., and Setchell, B. P. (1985): Spermatogenesis, seminal characteristics and reproductive hormone levels in mature rams with induced hypothyroidism and hyperthyroidism. *J. Endocrinol.*, 105:39–46.
432. Chandrasekhar, Y., D'Ochhio, M. J., Holland, M. K., and Setchell, B. P. (1985): Activity of the hypothalamo-pituitary axis and testicular development in prepubertal ram lambs with induced hypothyroidism or hyperthyroidism. *Endocrinology*, 117:1645–1651.
433. Setchell, B. P., and Waites, G. M. H. (1964): Blood flow and the uptake of glucose and oxygen in the testis and epididymis of the ram. *J. Physiol.*, 171:411–425.
434. Setchell, B. P., Waites, G. M. H., and Lindner, H. R. (1965): Effect of undernutrition on testicular blood flow and metabolism and the output of testosterone in the ram. *J. Reprod. Fertil.*, 9: 149–162.
435. Waites, G. M. H., and Setchell, B. P. (1964): Effect of local heating on blood flow and metabolism of the testes of the conscious ram. *J. Reprod. Fertil.*, 8:339–344.
436. Setchell, B. P., Waites, G. M. H., and Thorburn, G. D. (1966): Blood flow in the testis of the conscious ram measured with krypton-85; effects of heat catecholamines and acetylcholine. *Circ. Res.*, 18:755–765.
437. Wax, S. H., and Peterson, N. (1967): Measurement of testicular blood flow by intratesticular injection of xenon-133. *Surg. Forum.*, 18:544–546.
438. Sand, R. S., Dutt, R. H., and Preston, D. F. (1971): Effects of local heating on ram testis blood flow. *J. Anim. Sci*, 32:391.
439. Joffre, J., and Joffre, M. (1973): Seasonal changes in the testicular blood flow of seasonally breeding mammals: dormouse (*Glis glis*), ferret (*Mustela furo*) and fox (*Vulpes vulpes*). *J. Reprod. Fertil.*, 34:227–233.
440. Joffre, M., (1977): Relationship between testicular blood flow, testosterone secretion and spermatogenic activity in young and adult wild red foxes (*Vulpes vulpes*). *J. Reprod. Fertil.*, 51:35–40.

441. Jones, T., (1971): Blood flow and volume measurements in the radiation depopulated testis of the rat. *Br. J. Radiol.*, 44:841–849.

442. Fritjofsson, A., Persson, J. E., and Pettersson, S. (1969): Testicular blood flow in man measured with xenon-133. *Scand. J. Urol. Nephrol.*, 3:276–280.

443. Einer-Jensen, N., and Soofi, G. (1974): Decreased blood flow through rat testis after intratesticular injection of PGF-2. *Prostaglandins*, 7:377–382.

444. Einer-Jensen, N., and Waites, G. M. H. (1977): Testicular blood flow and a study of the testicular venous to arterial transfer of radioactive krypton and testosterone in the rhesus monkey. *J. Physiol.*, 267:1–15.

445. Damber, J. E., Lindgren, S., and Nasman, B. (1977): Testicular blood flow and oxygen tension in unilaterally orchidectomized rats. *Experientia*, 33:635–636.

446. Damber, J. E., and Janson, P. O. (1977): Methodological aspects of testicular blood flow measurements in rats. *Acta Physiol. Scand.*, 101:278–285.

447. Pirke, K. M., Bofilas, I., Sintermann, R., Langhammer, H., Wolf, I., and Pabst, H. W. (1979): Relative capillary blood flow and Leydig cell function in old rats. *Endocrinology* 105:842–845.

448. Pirke, K. M., Bofilas, I., Spyra, B., Langhammer, H., and Pabst, H. W. (1982): Capillary blood flow in the testes and testosterone secretion in the starved rat. *Experientia*, 38:516–517.

449. Damber, J. E., and Janson, P. O. (1978): Testicular blood flow and testosterone concentrations in spermatic venous blood of anaesthetized rats. *J. Reprod. Fertil.*, 52:265–269.

450. Wang, J., Galil, K. A. A., and Setchell, B. P. (1983): Changes in testicular blood flow and testosterone production during aspermatogenesis after irradiation. *J. Endocrinol.*, 98:35–46.

451. Punjabi, U., Van Hoecke, L., Verdonck, L., and Vermeulen, A. (1984): Testicular blood flow in young and old rats and influence of hCG. *J. Androl.*, 5:223–226.

452. Setchell, B. P., Waites, G. M. H., and Till, A. R. (1964): Variations in flow of blood within the epididymis and testis of the sheep and rat. *Nature*, 203:317–318.

453. Fowler, D. G., and Setchell, B. P. (1971): Selecting Merino rams for ability to withstand infertility caused by heat. 2. Effect of heat on scrotal and testicular blood flow. *Aust. J. Exp. Agric. Anim. Husb.*, 11:143–147.

454. Brown, P. D. C., and Waites, G. M. H. (1972): Regional blood flow in the epididymis of the rat and rabbit: effect of efferent duct ligation and orchidectomy. *J. Reprod. Fertil.*, 28:221–233.

455. Bindon, B. M., and Waites, G. M. H. (1968): Discrepancy in weight and blood flow of the testis and epididymis of the mouse before and after hypophysectomy. *J. Endocrinol.*, 40:385–386.

456. Waites, G. M. H., Setchell, B. P., and Quinlan, D. (1973): The effect of local heating of the scrotum, testes and epididymides on cardiac output and regional blood flow. *J. Reprod. Fertil.*, 34:41–49.

457. Damber, J. E., and Janson, P. O. (1978): The effects of LH, adrenaline and noradrenaline on testicular blood flow and plasma testosterone concentrations in anaesthetized rats. *Acta Endocrinol.*, 88:390–396.

458. Damber, J. E., Selstam, G., and Wang, J. (1981): Inhibitory effect of estradiol-17β on human chorionic gonadotropin-induced increment of testicular blood flow and plasma testosterone concentrations in rats. *Biol. Reprod.*, 25:555–559.

459. Hartmann, C. G., Millman, N., and Stavorski, J. (1950). Vasodilatation of the rat testis in response to human chorionic gonadotropin. *Fertil. Steril.*, 1:443–453.

460. Free, M. J., and Jaffe, R. A. (1972): Effect of prostaglandins on blood flow and pressure in the testis of the conscious rat. *Prostaglandins*, 1:483–498.

461. Free, M. J., and Nguyen Duc Kien, (1973): Venous arterial interactions involving serotonin in the pampiniform plexus of the rat. *Proc. Soc. Exp. Biol. Med.*, 143:284–288.

462. Blombery, P. A., and Waites, G. M. H. (1968): Non-uniform blood flow in the testis of sheep and dog and preliminary observations on reactive hyperaemia. *Aust. J. Exp. Biol. Med. Sci.*, 46:25.

463. Glover, T. D. (1965): Changes in blood flow in the testis and epididymis of the rat following artificial cryptorchidism. *Acta Endocrinol.* (*Suppl.*), 100:38.

464. Glover, T. D. (1966): The influence of temperature on flow of blood in the testis and scrotum of rats. *Proc. R. Soc. Med.*, 59:765–766.

465. Glode, L. M., Robinson, J., and Horwitz, L. D. (1984): Scrotal hypothermia and testicular blood flow in the dog. *J. Androl.*, 5:227–229.

466. Setchell, B. P., and Galil, K. A. A. (1983): Limitations imposed by testicular blood flow on the function of Leydig cells in rats *in vivo*. *Aust. J. Biol. Sci.*, 36:285–293.

467. Setchell, B. P. (1984): Male Reproduction. In: *Benchmark Papers in Human Physiology, Vol. 17*, pp. 1–401. Van Nostrand Reinhold, New York.

468. Lindner, H. R. (1961): Androgens and related compounds in the spermatic vein blood of domestic animals I. Neutral steroids secreted by the bull testis. *J. Endocrinol.*, 23:139–159.

469. Lindner, H. R. (1961): Androgens and related compounds in the spermatic vein blood of domestic animals IV. Testicular androgens in the ram, boar and stallion. *J. Endocrinol.*, 23:171–178.

470. Tcholakian, R. K., and Eik-Nes, K. B. (1971): Δ^5-Pregnenolone and testosterone in spermatic venous blood of anaesthetized dogs. *Am. J. Physiol.*, 221:1824–1826.

471. Kelch, R. P., Jenner, M. R., Weinstein, R., Kaplan, S. L., and Grumbach, M. M. (1972): Estradiol and testosterone secretion by human, simian and canine testes, in males with hypogonadism and in male pseudohermaphrodites with the feminizing testes syndrome. *J. Clin. Invest.*, 51:824–830.

472. Scholler, R., Nahoul, K., Grenier, J., Charles, J. F., and Netter, A. (1975): Concentrations de sept stéroïdes dans la veine spermatique de l'homme. Comparaison aux taux peripheriques. *Ann. Endocrinol.*, 36:353–354.

473. Ewing, L., Brown, B., Irby, D. C., and Jardine, I. (1975): Testosterone and 5α-reduced androgen secretion by rabbit testes-epididymides perfused *in vitro*. *Endocrinology*, 96:610–617.

474. Amann, R. P., and Ganjam, V. K. (1976): Steroid production by the bovine testis and steroid transfer across the pampiniform plexus. *Biol. Reprod.*, 15:695–703.

475. Carrick, F. N., and Cox, R. I. (1977): Testicular endocrinology of marsupials and monotremes. In: *Reproduction and Evolution*, edited by J. H. Calaby and C. H. Tyndale-Biscoe, pp. 137–141. Australian Academy of Sciences, Canberra.

476. Hammond, G. L., Ruokonen, A., Kontturi, M., Koskela, E., and Vikho, R. (1977): The simultaneous radioimmunoassay of seven steroids in human spermatic and peripheral venous blood. *J. Clin. Endocrinol.*, 45:16–24.

477. Moneti, G., Pazzagli, M., Fiorelli, G., and Serio, M. (1980): Measurement of 5α-androstane-3α,17β-diol in human spermatic venous plasma by mass-fragmentography. *J. Steroid Biochem.*, 13:623–627.

478. Foldesy, R. G., and Leathem, J. H. (1980): Simultaneous measurements of testosterone and three 5α-reduced androgens in the venous effluent of immature rat testes *in situ*. *Steroids*, 35:621–631.

479. Leinonen, P., Ruokonen, A., Kontturi, M., and Vikho, R. (1981): Effects of estrogen treatment on human testicular unconjugated steroid and steroid sulfate production *in vivo*. *J. Clin. Endocrinol. Metabol.*, 53:569–573.

480. Gower, D. B., Harrison, F. A., and Heap, R. B. (1970): The identification of C19-16-unsaturated steroids and estimation of 17-oxosteroids in boar spermatic vein plasma and urine. *J. Endocrinol.*, 47:357–368.

481. Claus, R., and Hoffmann, B. (1980): Oestrogens, compared to other steroids of testicular origin, in bloodplasma of boars. *Acta Endocrinol.*, 94:404–411.

482. Ruokonen, A., Lukkarinen, O., and Vihko, R. (1981): Secretion of steroid sulphates from human testis and their response to a single intramuscular injection of 5000 IU hCG. *J. Ster. Biochem.*, 14:1357–1360.

483. Chubb, C., and Ewing, L. L. (1979): Steroid secretion by *in vitro* perfused testes: secretions of rabbit and rat testes. *Am. J. Physiol.*, 237:E231–E238.

484. Chubb, C., and Ewing, L. L. (1979): Steroid secretion by *in vitro* perfused testes: testosterone biosynthetic pathways. *Am. J. Physiol.*, 237:E247–E254.

485. Ewing, L. L., Zirkin, B. R., Cochran, R. C., Kromann, N., Peters, C., and Ruiz-Bravo, N. (1979): Testosterone secretion by rat, rabbit, guinea pig, dog, and hamster testes perfused *in vitro:* correlation with Leydig cell mass. *Endocrinology*, 15:1135–1142.

486. Zirkin, B. R., Ewing, L. L., Kromann, N., and Cochran, R. C. (1980): Testosterone secretion by rat, rabbit, guinea pig, dog, and hamster testes perfused in vitro: correlation with Leydig cell ultrastructure. *Endocrinology,* 107:1867–1874.
487. Chubb, C., and Desjardins, C. (1983): Steroid secretion by mouse testes perfused *in vitro*. *Am. J. Physiol.,* 244:E575–E580.
488. Ewing, L. L., Thompson, D. L., Cochran, R. C., Lasley, B. L., Thompson, M. A., and Zirkin, B. R. (1984): Testicular androgen and estrogen secretion and benign prostatic hyperplasia in the beagle. *Endocrinology,* 114:1308–1314.
489. Forti, G., Toscano, V., Casilli, D., Maroder, M., Balducci, R., Adamo, M. V., Santoro, S., Grisolia, G. A., Pampaloni, A., and Serio, M. (1985): Spermatic and peripheral venous plasma concentrations of testosterone, 17-hydroxyprogesterone, androstenedione, dehydroepiandrosterone, Δ5-androstene-3β,17β-diol, dihydrotestosterone, 5α-androstane-3α,17β-diol, 5α-androstane-3β,17β-diol, and estradiol in boys with idiopathic varicocele in different stages of puberty. *J. Clin. Endocrinol. Metabol.,* 61:322–327.
490. Lindner, H. R. (1969): The androgenic secretion of the testis in domestic ungulates. In: *The Gonads,* edited by K. W. McKerns, pp. 615–648. Appleton-Century-Crofts, New York.
491. Chubb, C., Ewing, L., Irby, D., and Desjardins, C. (1978): Testicular maturation in the rabbit: secretion of testosterone, dihydrotestosterone, 5α-androstan-3α,17β-diol and 5α-androstan-3β,17β-diol by perfused rabbit testes-epididymides and spermatogenesis. *Biol. Reprod.,* 18:212–218.
492. Chubb, C., and Ewing, L. L. (1981): Steroid secretion by sexually immature rat and rabbit testes perfused *in vitro*. *Endocrinology,* 109:1999–2003.
493. Himwich, H. E., and Nahum, L. H. (1929): The respiratory quotient of the testicle. *Am. J. Physiol.,* 88:680–685.
494. Cowie, A. T., Lascelles, A. K., and Wallace, J. C. (1964): Flow and protein content of testicular lymph in conscious rams. *J. Physiol.,* 171:176–187.
495. Morris, B., and McIntosh, G. H. (1970): The lymphatic drainage of the testis and scrotal serous cavity in the ram. In: *Progress in Lymphology II,* edited by M. Viamonte, P. R. Kochler, M. Witte, and C. Witte, pp. 173–176. Georg Thieme Verlag, Stuttgart.
496. Main, S. J. (1976): The blood-testis barrier and temperature. *Ph. D. Thesis,* University of Reading, Reading, England.
497. Galil, K. A. A., Laurie, M. S., Main, S. J., and Setchell, B. P. (1981): The measurement of the flow of lymph from the testis. *J. Physiol.,* 319:17P.
498. Setchell, B. P. (1982): The flow and composition of lymph from the testes of pigs with some observations on the effect of raised venous pressure. *Comp. Biochem. Physiol.,* 73A:201–205.
499. Wallace, J. C., and Lascelles, A. K. (1964): Composition of testicular and epididymal lymph in the ram. *J. Reprod. Fertil.,* 8:235–242.
500. Beh, K. J., Watson, D. L., and Lascelles, A. K. (1974): Concentrations of immunoglobulins and albumin in lymph collected from various regions of the body of the sheep. *Aust. J. Exp. Biol. Med. Sci.,* 52:81–86.
501. Setchell, B. P., Hinks, N. T., Voglmayr, J. K., and Scott, T. W. (1967): Amino acids in ram testicular fluid and semen and their metabolism by spermatozoa. *Biochem. J.,* 105:1061–1065.
502. Smith, J. B., McIntosh, G. H., and Morris, B. (1970): The traffic of cells through tissues: a study of peripheral lymph in sheep. *J. Anat.,* 107:87–100.
503. Ball, R. Y., and Setchell, B. P. (1983): The passage of spermatozoa to regional lymph nodes in testicular lymph following vasectomy in rams and boars. *J. Reprod. Fertil.,* 68:145–153.
504. Lindner, H. R. (1967): Participation of lymph in the transport of gonadal hormones. *Excerpta Med. Found. Int. Congr. Ser.,* 132:821–827.
505. Daniel, P. M., Gale, M. M., and Pratt, O. E. (1963): Hormones and related substances in the lymph leaving four endocrine glands—the testis, ovary, adrenal and thyroid. *Lancet,* I:1232–1234.
506. Karpe, B., Fredricsson, B., Svensson, J., and Ritzen, E. M. (1982): Testosterone concentration within the tunica vaginalis of boys and adult men. *Int. J. Androl.,* 5:549–556.
507. Setchell, B. P., and Cox, J. E. (1982): Secretion of free and conjugated steroids by the horse testis into lymph and venous blood. *J. Reprod. Fertil. (Suppl.),* 32:123–127.
508. Hudson, B., Baker, H. W. G., Eddie, L. W., Higginson, R. E., Burger, H. G., De Kretser, D. M., Dobos, M., and Lee, V. W. K. (1979): Bioassays for inhibin: a critical review. *J. Reprod. Fertil. (Suppl.),* 26:17–29.
509. Maddocks, S., Oliver, J. R., and Setchell, B. P. (1984): The survival and function of isolated pancreatic islets of Langerhans transplanted into the testis of adult rats and their effect on the testis. *Coll. INSERM.,* 123:497–502.
510. Maddocks, S., Cormack, J., and Setchell, B. P. (1985): The failure of thyroid allografts in the ovine testis. *Proc. Aust. Soc. Reprod. Biol.,* 17:51.
511. Ball, R. Y., Naylor, C. P. E., and Mitchinson, M. J. (1982): Spermatozoa in an abdominal lymph node after vasectomy in a man. *J. Reprod. Fert.,* 66:715–716.
512. Alexander, N. J. (1977): Immunological aspects of vasectomy. In: *Immunological Influences on Human Fertility,* edited by B. Boettcher, pp. 25–46. Academic Press, Sydney.
513. Miller, S. C., Bowman, B. M., and Roberts, L. K. (1984): Identification and characterization of mononuclear phagocytes isolated from rat testicular interstitial tissues. *J. Leucocyt. Biol.,* 36:679–687.
514. Tamm, J., Volkwein, U., Becker, H., and Klosterhalfen, H. (1982): Comparison of steroid concentrations in venous and arterial blood across the human testis. Unconjugated 5-androstane-3,17-diol: an important androgen metabolite of the human testicular-epididymal unit. *J. Steroid Biochem.,* 16:567–571.
515. Mostofi, F. K. (1973): Testicular tumors. *Cancer,* 32:1186–1201.
516. Pugh, R. C. B. (1976): *Pathology of the Testis*. Blackwells, Oxford.
517. Pande, J. K., Chowdhury, S. R., Dasgupta, P. R., Chowdhury, A. R., and Kar, A. B. (1966): Biochemical composition of the rat testis fluid. *Proc. Soc. Exp. Biol. Med.,* 121:899–902.
518. Pande, J. K., Dasgupta, P. R., and Kar, A. B. (1967): Biochemical composition of human testicular fluid collected post mortem. *J. Clin. Endocrinol. Metabol.,* 27:892–894.
519. Pande, J. K., Dasgupta, P. R., and Kar, A. B. (1967): Chemical composition of fluid collected from testis of the rhesus monkey and goat. *Ind. J. Exp. Biol.,* 5:65–67.
520. Sharpe, R. M. (1979): Gonadotrophin-induced accumulation of 'interstitial fluid' in the rat testis. *J. Reprod. Fertil.,* 55:365–371.
521. Hagenas, L., Ritzen, E. M., and Suginami, H. (1978): Hormonal milieu of the seminiferous tubules in the normal and cryptorchid rat. *Int. J. Androl.,* 1:477–484.
522. Turner, T. T., Jones, C. E., Howards, S. S., Ewing, L. L., Zegeye, B., and Gunsalus, G. L. (1984): On the androgen microenvironment of maturing spermatozoa. *Endocrinology,* 115:1925–932.
523. Turner, T. T., Ewing, L. L., Jones, C. E., Howards, S. S., and Zegeye, B. (1985): Androgens in male reproductive tract fluids: hypophysectomy and steroid replacement. *Am. J. Physiol.,* 248:E274–E280.
524. Sharpe, R. M., (1981): The importance of testicular interstitial fluid in the transport of injected hCG to the Leydig cells. *Int. J. Androl.,* 4:64–74.
525. Sharpe, R. M., and Cooper, I. (1983): Testicular interstitial fluid as a monitor for changes in the intratesticular environment in the rat. *J. Reprod. Fertil.,* 69:125–135.
526. Sharpe, R. M., and Bartlett, J. M. S. (1985): Intratesticular distribution of testosterone in rats and the relationship to the concentrations of a peptide that stimulates testosterone secretion. *J. Reprod. Fertil.,* 73:223–236.
527. Maddocks, S., and Setchell, B. P. (1986): The composition of the interstitial fluid of the rat testis. *Proceedings: 4th European Testis Workshop,* Capri, p. 154.
528. Setchell, B. P. (1987): The movement of fluids and substances in the testis. *Aust. J. Biol. Sci.,* 39:193–207.
529. Sharpe, R. M., and Fraser, H. M. (1980): HCG stimulation of testicular LHRH-like activity. *Nature,* 290:642–643.
530. Sharpe, R. M., Fraser, H. M., Cooper, I., and Rommerts, F. F. G. (1981): Sertoli-Leydig cell communications via an LHRH-like factor. *Nature,* 290:785–787.
531. Sharpe, R. M., Fraser, H. M., Cooper, I., and Rommerts, F. F. G. (1982): The secretion, measurement and function of a testicular LHRH-like factor. *Ann. NY Acad. Sci.,* 383:272–294.
532. Sharpe, R. M. (1983): Local control of testicular function. *Q. J. Exp. Physiol.,* 68:265–287.

533. Sharpe, R. M. (1984): Intratesticular factors controlling testicular function. *Biol. Reprod.*, 30:29–49.
534. Sharpe, R. M., Doogan, D. G., and Cooper, I. (1983): Direct effects of a luteinizing hormone-releasing hormone agonist on intratesticular levels of testosterone and interstitial fluid formation in intact male rats. *Endocrinology*, 113:1306–1313.
535. Sharpe, R. M., and Cooper, I. (1984): Intratesticular secretion of a factor(s) with major stimulatory effects on Leydig cell testosterone secretion *in vitro*. *Mol. Cell. Endocrinol.*, 37:159–168.
536. Sharp, B., Pekary, A. E., Meyer, N. V., and Hershman, J. M. (1980): β-Endorphin in male rat reproductive organs. *Biochem. Biophys. Res. Commun.*, 95:618–623.
537. Tsong, S. D., Phillips, D. M., Halmi, N., Krieger, D., and Bardin, C. W. (1982): β-Endorphin is present in the male reproductive tract of five species. *Biol. Reprod.*, 27:755–764.
538. Tsong, S. D., Phillips, D., Halmi, N., Liotta, A. S., Margioris, A., Bardin, C. W., and Krieger, D. (1982): ACTH and β-endorphin-related peptides are present in multiple sites in the reproductive tract of the male rat. *Endocrinology*, 110:2204–2206.
539. Margioris, A. N., Liotta, A. S., Vaudry, H., Bardin, C. W., and Krieger, D. T. (1983): Characterization of immunoreactive propiomelanocortin-related peptides in rat testes. *Endocrinology*, 113:663–671.
540. Gerendai, I., Shaha, C., Thau, R., and Bardin, C. W. (1984): Do testicular opiates regulate Leydig cell function? *Endocrinology*, 115:1645–1647.
541. Bardin, C. W., Shaha, C., Mather, J., Salomon, Y., Margioris, A. N., Liotta, A. S., Gerendai, I., Chen, C. L., and Krieger, D. T. (1984): Identification and possible function of pro-opiomelanocortin-derived peptides in the testis. *Ann. NY Acad. Sci.*, 438:346–364.
542. Gizang-Ginsberg, E., and Wolgemuth, D. J. (1985): Localization of mRNAs in mouse testes by *in situ* hybridization: distribution of α-tubulin and developmental stage specificity of pro-opiomelanocortin transcripts. *Dev. Biol.*, 111:293–305.
543. Sharpe, R. M. (1983): Impaired gonadotrophin uptake *in vivo* by the cryptorchid rat testis. *J. Reprod. Fertil.*, 67:379–387.
544. Galil, K. A. A. (1982): Effects of high environmental temperature on the testis. *Ph.D. Thesis*, University of Cambridge, Cambridge.
545. Cuthbert, A. W., and Wong, P. Y. D. (1975): Intracellular potentials in cells of seminiferous tubules of rats. *J. Physiol.*, 248:173–191.
546. Gladwell, R. T. (1977): The effect of temperature on the potential difference and input resistance of rat seminiferous tubules. *J. Physiol.*, 268:111–121.
547. Cheung, Y. M., Hwang, J. C., and Wong, P. Y. D. (1977): *In vitro* measurement of rate of fluid secretion in rat isolated seminiferous tubules: effects of metabolic inhibitors and ions. *J. Physiol.*, 269:1–15.
548. Setchell, B. P., (1970): The secretion of fluid by the testes of rats rams, and goats with some observations on the effect of age, cryptorchidism and hypophysectomy. *J. Reprod. Fertil.*, 23:79–85.
549. Setchell, B. P., Duggan, M. C., and Evans, R. W. (1973): The effects of gonadotrophins on fluid secretion and production of spermatozoa by the rat and hamster testis. *J. Endocrinol.*, 56:27–36.
550. Jegou, B., Le Gac, F., and De Kretser, D. M. (1982): Seminiferous tubule fluid and interstitial fluid production. I. Effects of age and hormonal regulation in immature rats. *Biol. Reprod.*, 27: 590–595.
551. Jegou, B., Le Gac, F., Irby, D. C., and De Kretser, D. M. (1983): Studies on seminiferous tubule fluid production in the adult rat: effect of hypophysectomy and treatment with FSH, LH and testosterone. *Int. J. Androl.*, 6:249–260.
552. Free, M. J., Jaffe, R. A., and Morford, D. E. (1980): Sperm transport through the rete testis of anesthetized rats: role of the testicular capsule and effect of gonadotropins and prostaglandins. *Biol. Reprod.*, 22:1073–1078.
553. Setchell, B. P., Voglmayr, J. K., and Hinks, N. T. (1971): The effect of local heating on the flow and composition of rete testis fluid in the conscious ram. *J. Reprod. Fertil.*, 25:81–89.
554. Setchell, B. P., and Waites, G. M. H. (1972): The effects of local heating of the testis on the flow and composition of rete testis fluid in the rat, with some observations on the effects of age and unilateral castration. *J. Reprod. Fertil.*, 30:225–233.
555. Laporte, P., and Gillet, J. (1975): Influence de la spermatogenese sur la secretion du fluide testiculaire chez le rat adulte. *C. R. Acad. Sci. (Paris)*, 281:1397–1400.
556. Setchell, B. P. (1969): Do Sertoli cells secrete fluid into the seminiferous tubules? *J. Reprod. Fertil.*, 19:391–392.
557. Morris, I. D., (1979): Effect on gonadotrophin secretion of blockage of ductuli efferentes in the normal and androgen-deprived rat. *J. Reprod. Fertil.*, 57:469–475.
558. Setchell, B. P., and Brown, B. W. (1972): The effect of metabolic alkalosis, hypotension and inhibitors of carbonic anhydrase on fluid secretion by the rat testis. *J. Reprod. Fertil.*, 28:235–240.
559. Setchell, B. P., Davies, R. V., Gladwell, R. T., Hinton, B. T., Main, S. J., Pilsworth, L., and Waites, G. M. H. (1978): The movement of fluid in the seminiferous tubules and rete testis. *Ann. Biol. Anim. Biochim. Biophys.*, 18:623–632.
560. Tuck, R. R., Setchell, B. P., Waites, G. M. H., and Young, J. A. (1970): The composition of fluid collected by micropuncture and catheterization from the seminiferous tubules and rete testis of rats. *Pfluegers Arch.*, 318:225–243.
561. Johnson, A. L., and Howards, S. S. (1977): Hyperosmolarity in intraluminal fluids from hamster testis and epididymis: a micropuncture study. *Science*, 195:492–493.
562. Levine, N., and Marsh, D. J. (1971): Micropuncture studies of the electrochemical aspects of fluid and electrolyte transport in individual seminiferous tubules, the epididymis and vas deferens in rats. *J. Physiol.*, 213:557–570.
563. Jenkins, A. D., Lechene, C. P., and Howards, S. S. (1980): Concentration of seven elements in the intraluminal fluids of the rat seminiferous tubules, rete testis and epididymis. *Biol. Reprod.*, 23:981–987.
564. Tuck, R. R. (1969): An investigation of the fluid secreted by the seminiferous tubules and the rete testis of the rat. *B. Sc. Thesis*, University of Sydney, Sydney.
565. Levine, N., and Marsh, D. J. (1975): Micropuncture study of the fluid composition of 'Sertoli cell-only' seminiferous tubules in rats. *J. Reprod. Fertil.*, 43:547–549.
566. Muffly, K. E., Turner, T. T., Brown, M., and Hall, P. F. (1985): Content of K^+ and Na^+ seminiferous tubule and rete testis fluids from Sertoli cell-enriched testes. *Biol. Reprod.*, 33:1245–1251.
567. Kormano, M., Koskimies, A. I., and Hunter, R. L. (1971): The presence of specific proteins in the absence of many serum proteins in the rat seminiferous tubule fluid. *Experentia*, 27:1461–1463.
568. Koskimies, A. I., and Kormano, M. (1973): Proteins in fluids from the seminiferous tubules and rete testis in the rat. *J. Reprod. Fertil.*, 34:433–444.
569. Koskimies, A. I., Kormano, M., and Lahti, A. (1971): A difference in the immunoglobulin content of seminiferous tubule fluid and rete testis fluid of the rat. *J. Reprod. Fertil.*, 27:463–465.
570. Koskimies, A. I., Kormano, M., and Alfthan, O. (1973): Proteins of the seminiferous tubule fluid in man—evidence for a blood-testis barrier. *J. Reprod. Fertil.*, 32:79–86.
571. Turner, T. T., Plesums, J. L., and Cabot, C. L. (1979): Luminal fluid proteins of the male reproductive tract. *Biol. Reprod.*, 21:883–890.
572. Sylvester, S. R., and Griswold, M. D. (1984): Localization of transferrin and transferrin receptors in rat testes. *Biol. Reprod.*, 31:195–203.
573. Hinton, B. T., White, R. W., and Setchell, B. P. (1980): Concentrations of *myo*-inositol in the luminal fluid of mammalian testes and epididymides. *J. Reprod. Fertil.*, 58:395–399.
574. Comhaire, F. H., and Vermeulen, A. (1976): Testosterone concentration in the fluids of seminiferous tubules, the interstitium and the rete testis of the rat. *J. Endocrinol.*, 70:229–235.
575. Setchell, B. P., and Main, S. J. (1975): The blood-testis barrier and steroids. *Curr. Top. Mol. Endocrinol.*, 2:223–233.
576. Setchell, B. P., Hinton, B. T., Jacks, F., and Davies, R. V. (1976): Restricted penetration of iodinated follicle-stimulating and luteinizing hormone into the seminiferous tubules of the rat testis. *Mol. Cell. Endocrinol.*, 6:59–69.
577. Setchell, B. P., Laurie, M. S., Main, S. J., and Goats, G. C. (1978): The mechanism of transport of testosterone through the walls of the seminiferous tubules of the rat testis. *Int. J. Androl. (Suppl.)*, 2:506–512.

578. Setchell, B. P. (1980): The functional significance of the blood-testis barrier. *J. Androl.*, 1:3–10.
579. Voglmayr, J. K., Waites, G. M. H., and Setchell, B. P. (1966): Studies on spermatozoa and fluid collected directly from the testis of the conscious ram. *Nature,* 210:861–863.
580. Voglmayr, J. K., Scott, T. W., Setchell, B. P., and Waites, G. M. H. (1967): Metabolism of testicular spermatozoa and characteristics of testicular fluid collected from conscious rams. *J. Reprod. Fertil.*, 14:87–99.
581. Voglmayr, J. K., Larsen, L. H., and White, I. G. (1970): Metabolism of spermatozoa and composition of fluid collected from the rete testis of living bulls. *J. Reprod. Fertil.*, 21:449–460.
582. Dacheux, J. L., O'Shea, T., and Paquinon, M. (1979): Effects of osmolality, bicarbonate and buffer on the metabolism and motility of testicular, epididymal and ejaculated spermatozoa of boars. *J. Reprod. Fertil.*, 55:287–296.
583. Evans, R. W., and Setchell, B. P. (1979): Lipid changes in boar spermatozoa during epididymal maturation, with some observations on the flow and composition of boar rete testis fluid. *J. Reprod. Fertil.*, 57:189–196.
584. Free, M. J., and Jaffe, R. A. (1979): Collection of rete testis fluid from rats without previous efferent duct ligation. *Biol. Reprod.*, 20:269–278.
585. Waites, G. M. H., and Einer-Jensen, N. (1974): Collection and analysis of rete testis fluid from Macaque monkeys. *J. Reprod. Fertil.*, 41:505–508.
586. Lambiase, J. T., and Amann, R. P. (1973): Infertility of rabbit testicular spermatozoa collected in their native fluid environment. *Fertil. Steril.*, 24:65–67.
587. Cooper, T. G., and Orgebin-Crist, M. C. (1975): The effect of epididymal and testicular fluids on the fertilising capacity of testicular and epididymal spermatozoa. *Andrologia,* 7:85–93.
588. Cooper, T. G., Danzo, B. J., Dipietro, D. L., McKenna, T. J., and Orgebin-Crist, M. C. (1976): Some characteristics of rete testis fluid from rabbits. *Andrologia,* 8:87–94.
589. Guerrero, R., Ritzen, E. M., Purvis, K., Hansson, V., and French, F. S. (1975): Concentration of steroid hormones and androgen binding protein (ABP) in rabbit efferent duct fluid. *Curr. Top. Mol. Endocrinol.*, 2:213–221.
590. Setchell, B. P. (1970): Fluid secretion by the testes of an Australian marsupial *Macropus eugenii. Comp. Physiol. Biochem.*, 36:411–414.
591. Waites, G. M. H. (1977): Fluid secretion. In: *The Testis, Vol. IV,* edited by A. D. Johnson and W. R. Gomes, pp. 91–123. Academic Press, New York.
592. Waites, G. M. H., and Gladwell, R. T. (1982): Physiological significance of fluid secretion in the testis and blood-testis barrier. *Physiol. Rev.*, 62:624–671.
593. Waites, G. M. H., and Setchell, B. P. (1987): Physiology of the mammalian testis. In: *Marshall's Physiology of Reproduction, Vol. B,* edited by G. E. Lamming. Churchill Livingstone, London (*in press*).
594. Setchell, B. P., and Linzell, J. L. (1968): Effects of some drugs, hormones and physiological factors on the flow of rete testis fluid in the ram. *J. Reprod. Fertil.*, 16:320–321.
595. Voglmayr, J. K. (1975): Output of spermatozoa and fluid by the testis of the ram and its response to oxytocin. *J. Reprod. Fertil.*, 43:119–122.
596. Dacheux, J. L., Pisselet, C., Blanc, M. R., Hochereau-de Reviers, M. T., and Courot, M. (1981): Seasonal variations in rete testis fluid secretion and sperm production in different breeds of ram. *J. Reprod. Fertil.*, 61:363–371.
597. Setchell, B. P., Scott, T. W., Voglmayr, J. K., and Waites, G. M. H. (1969): Characteristics of testicular spermatozoa and the fluid which transports them into the epididymis. *Biol. Reprod.* (*Suppl.*), 1:40–66.
598. Hinton, B. T., and Setchell, B. P. (1980): Concentration of glycerophosphocholine, phosphocholine and free inorganic phosphate in the luminal fluid of the rat testis and epididymis. *J. Reprod. Fertil.*, 58:401–406.
599. Setchell, B. P., Dawson, R. M. C., and White, R. W. (1968): The high concentration of free *myo*-inositol in rete testis fluid from rams. *J. Reprod. Fertil.*, 17:219–221.
600. Middleton, A., and Setchell, B. P. (1972): The origin of inositol in rete testis fluid. *J. Reprod. Fertil.*, 30:473–475.
601. Middleton, A. (1973): Glucose metabolism in rat seminiferous tubules. *Ph.D. Thesis.*, pp. 1–90. University of Cambridge, Cambridge.
602. Dacheux, J. L. (1980): Interactions de l'environment sur l'activité métabolique, la motilité et le pouvoir fécondant des spermatozoïdes en fonction de leur état de maturation. *D. Sc. Thesis,* Université Francois-Rabelais, Tours, France.
603. Johnson, M. H., and Setchell, B. P. (1968): Protein and immunoglobulin content of rete testis fluid of rams. *J. Reprod. Fertil.*, 17:403–406.
604. Setchell, B. P. (1974): Secretions of the testis and epididymis. *J. Reprod. Fertil.*, 37:165–177.
605. Wright, W. W., Musto, N. A., Mather, J. P., and Bardin, C. W. (1981): Sertoli cells secrete both testis-specific and serum proteins. *Proc. Natl. Acad. Sci. USA,* 78:7565–7569.
606. French, F. S., and Ritzen, E. M. (1973): Androgen-binding protein in efferent duct fluid of rat testis. *J. Reprod. Fertil.*, 32:479–483.
607. French, F. S., and Ritzen, E. M. (1973): A high affinity androgen-binding protein (ABP) in rat testis. Evidence for secretion into efferent duct fluid and absorption by the epididymis. *Endocrinology,* 93:88–95.
608. Gunsalus, G. L., Musto, N. A., and Bardin, C. W. (1978): Factors affecting blood levels of androgen binding protein in the rat. *Int. J. Androl.* (*Suppl.*), 2:482–493.
609. Gunsalus, G. L., Musto, N. A., and Bardin, C. W. (1980): Bidirectional release of a Sertoli cell product, androgen binding protein, into the blood and seminiferous tubule. In: *Testicular Development, Structure and Function,* edited by A. Steinberger and E. Steinberger, pp. 291–297. Raven Press, New York.
610. Jegou, B., Dacheux, J. L., Garnier, D. H., Terqui, M., Colas, G., and Courot, M. (1979): Biochemical and physiological studies of androgen-binding protein in the reproductive tract of the ram. *J. Reprod. Fertil.*, 57:311–318.
611. Suominen, J., and Setchell, B. P. (1972): Enzymes and trypsin inhibitor in the rete testis fluid of rams and boars. *J. Reprod. Fertil.*, 30:235–245.
612. Hamilton, D. W. (1980): UDP-galactose: *N*-acetylglucosamine galactosyltransferase in fluids from rat rete testis and epididymis. *Biol. Reprod.*, 23:377–385.
613. Hamilton, D. W. (1981): Evidence for α-lactalbumin-like activity in rat male reproductive fluids. *Biol. Reprod.*, 25:385–392.
614. Suominen, J. J. O., and Setchell, B. P. (1976): Proteinase inhibitors in testicular and epididymal fluid. In: *Protides of the Biological fluids.*, edited by H. Peeters, pp. 171–175. Pergamon Press, Oxford.
615. Brown, K. D., Blakely, D. M., Henville, A., and Setchell, B. P. (1982): Rete testis fluid contains a growth factor for cultured fibroblasts. *Biochem. Biophys. Res. Commun.*, 105:371–379.
616. Feig, L. A., Bellve, A. R., Erickson, N. H., and Klagsburn, M. (1980): Sertoli cells contain a mitogenic polypeptide. *Proc. Natl. Acad. Sci. USA,* 77:4774–4778.
617. Bolonge, R., Demoulin, A., Hustin, J., Verstraelen-Proyard, J., Gysen, P., and Franchimont, P. (1979): Etude de l'incorporation de la thymidine tritieé dans l'acide desoxyribonucleique testiculaire du rat. Influence de l'inhibine. *C. R. Soc. Biol.*, 173:654–659
618. Fritz, I. B., Burdzy, K., Setchell, B. P., and Blaschuk, O. (1983): Ram rete testis fluid contains a protein (clusterin) which influences cell-cell interactions *in vitro*. *Biol. Reprod.*, 28:1173–1188.
619. Blaschuk, O., Burdzy, K., and Fritz, I. B. (1983): Purification and characterization of a cell-aggregating factor (clusterin), the major glycoprotein in ram rete testis fluid. *J. Biol. Chem.*, 258:7714–7720.
620. Setchell, B. P., and Jacks, F. (1974): Inhibin-like activity in rete testis fluid. *J. Endocrinol.*, 62:675–676.
621. Davies, R. V., Main, S. J., and Setchell, B. P. (1979): Inhibin in ram rete testis fluid. *J. Reprod. Fertil.* (*Suppl.*), 26:87–95.
622. Josso, N., Picard, J. Y., Dacheux, J. L., and Courot, M. (1979): Detection of anti-Mullerian activity in boar rete testis fluid. *J. Reprod. Fertil.*, 57:397–400.
623. White, I. G., and Hudson, B. (1968): The testosterone and dehydroepiandrosterone concentration in fluids of the mammalian male reproductive tract. *J. Endocrinol.*, 41:291–292.
624. Cooper, T. G., and Waites, G. M. H. (1974): Testosterone in rete testis fluid and blood of rams and rats. *J. Endocrinol.*, 62:619–629.

625. Harris, M. E., and Bartke, A. (1974): Concentration of testosterone in testis fluid of the rat. *Endocrinology,* 95:701–706.
626. Harris, M. E., and Bartke, A. (1975): Maintenance of rete testis fluid testosterone and dihydrotestosterone level by pregnenolone and other C21 steroids in hypophysectomized rats. *Endocrinology,* 96:1396–1402.
627. Vreeburg, J. T. M. (1975): Distribution of testosterone and 5α-dihydrotestosterone in rat epididymis and their concentrations in efferent duct fluid. *J. Endocrinol.,* 67:203–210.
628. Ganjam, V. K., and Amann, R. P. (1976): Steroids in fluids and sperm entering and leaving the bovine epididymis, epididymal tissue and accessory sex gland secretions. *Endocrinology,* 99:1618–1630.
629. Ritzen, E. M., Hagenas, L., Purvis, K., Guerrero, T., Johnsonbaugh, R. E., Dym, M., French, F. S., and Hansson, V. (1976): Androgens and androgen binding protein (ABP) in testicular fluids. In: *Maldescensus Testis,* edited by J. R. Bierich, K. Raher, and M. B. Ranke, pp. 79–97. Urban and Schwarzenberg, Heidelberg.
630. Lau, I. F., and Saksena, S. K. (1979): Steroids in the rete testis fluid of fertile male rabbits. *Arch. Androl.,* 2:49–52.
631. Voglmayr, J. K., Roberson, C., and Musto, N. A. (1980): Comparison of androgen levels in ram rete testis fluid, testicular lymph and spermatic venous blood plasma: evidence for a regulatory mechanism in the seminiferous tubules. *Biol. Reprod.,* 23:29–39.
632. Foldesy, R. G., and Leathem, J. H. (1981): Pubertal changes in androgen composition of rat rete testis and cauda epididymal fluids. *J. Ster. Biochem.,* 14:109–110.
633. Henning, R. D., and Young, J. A. (1971): Electrolyte transport in the seminiferous tubules of the rat studied by the stopped-flow microperfusion technique. *Experientia,* 27:1037–1039.
634. Free, M. J. (1980): "Leaky" membranes in the male reproductive tract: a discussion of unusual molecular exchanges between different fluid compartments. In: *Testicular Development, Structure and Function,* edited by A. Steinberger and E. Steinberger, p. 281. Raven Press, New York.
635. Pholpramool, C., White, R. W., and Setchell, B. P. (1982): Influence of androgens on inositol secretion and sperm transport in the epididymis of rats. *J. Reprod. Fertil.,* 66:547–553.
636. Danzo, B. J., Cooper, T. G., and Orgebin-Crist, M. C. (1977): Androgen binding protein (ABP) in fluids collected from the rete testis and cauda epididymis of sexually mature and immature rabbits and observations on morphological changes in the epididymis following ligation of the ductuli efferentes. *Biol. Reprod.,* 17:64–77.
637. Moniem, K. A., Glover, T. D., and Lubicz-Nawrocki, C. W. (1978): Effect of duct ligation and orchidectomy on histochemical reactions in the hamster epididymis. *J. Reprod. Fertil.,* 54:173–176.
638. Fawcett, D. W., and Hoffer, A. P. (1979): Failure of exogenous androgen to prevent regression of the initial segments of the rat epididymis after efferent duct ligation or orchidectomy. *Biol. Reprod.,* 20:162–181.
639. Gray, B. W., Brown, B. G., Ganjam, V. K., and Whitesides, J. F. (1983): Effect of deprival of rete testis fluid on the morphology of efferent ductules. *Biol. Reprod.,* 29:525–534.
640. Nicander, L., Osman, D. I., Ploen, L., Bugge, H. P., and Kvisgaard, K. N. (1983): Early effects of efferent ductule ligation on the proximal segment of the rat epididymis. *Int. J. Androl.,* 6:91–102.
641. Brooks, D. E. (1979): Influence of testicular secretions on tissue weight and on metabolic and enzyme activities in the epididymis of the rat. *J. Endocrinol.,* 82:305–313.
642. Brooks, D. E., and Higgins, S. J. (1980): Characterization and androgen-dependence of proteins associated with luminal fluid and spermatozoa in the rat epididymis. *J. Reprod. Fertil.,* 59:363–375.
643. Jones, R., von Glos, K. I., and Brown, C. R. (1980): The synthesis of a sperm-coating protein in the initial segment of the rat epididymis is stimulated by factors in testicular fluid. *IRCS Med. Sci.,* 8:56.
644. Jones, R., Brown, C. R., von Glós, K. I., and Parker, M. G. (1980): Hormonal regulation of protein synthesis in the rat epididymis. Characterization of androgen-dependent and testicular fluid-dependent proteins. *Biochem. J.,* 188:667–676.
645. Winet, H. (1980): On the mechanism of flow in the efferent ducts. *J. Androl.,* 1:304–311.
646. Wong, P. Y. D., and Yeung, C. H. (1976): Inhibition by amiloride of sodium-dependent fluid reabsorption in the rat isolated caudal epididymis. *Br. J. Pharmacol.,* 58:529–531.
647. Wong, P. Y. D., and Yeung, C. H. (1977): Fluid reabsorption in the isolated duct of the rat cauda epididymis. *J. Reprod. Fertil.,* 49:77–81.
648. Wong, P. Y. D., and Yeung, C. H. (1978): Absorptive and secretory functions of the perfused rat cauda epididymidis. *J. Physiol.,* 275:13–26.
649. Wong, P. Y. D., and Yeung, C. H. (1978): Effects of catecholamines and adrenergic blockage on fluid reabsorption in isolated rat cauda epididymidis. *Jpn. J. Pharmacol.,* 28:115–123.
650. Au, C. L., Ngai, H. K., Yeung, C. H., and Wong, P. Y. D. (1978): Effect of adrenalectomy and hormone replacement on sodium and water transport in the perfused rat cauda epididymidis. *J. Endocrinol.,* 77:265–266.
651. Brooks, D. E. (1987): Biochemistry of the male accessory glands. In: *Marshall's Physiology of Reproduction, Vol. 2,* edited by G. E. Lamming. Churchill Livingstone, Edinburgh (*in press*).
652. Carr, D. W., and Acott, T. S. (1984): Inhibition of bovine spermatozoa by caudal epididymal fluid: I. Studies of a sperm motility quiescence factor. *Biol. Reprod.,* 30:913–925.
653. Acott, T. S., and Carr, D. W. (1984): Inhibition of bovine spermatozoa by caudal epididymal fluid: II. Interaction of pH and a quiescence factor. *Biol. Reprod.,* 30:926–935.
654. Brooks, D. E. (1979): Carbohydrate metabolism in the rat epididymis: evidence that glucose is taken up by tissue slices and isolated cells by a process of facilitated transport. *Biol. Reprod.,* 21:19–26.
655. Cooper, T. G., and Waites, G. M. H. (1979): Investigation by luminal perfusion of the transfer of compounds into the epididymis of the anaesthetized rat. *J. Reprod. Fertil.,* 56:159–164.
656. Cooper, T. G. (1982): Secretion of inositol and glucose by the perfused rat cauda epididymidis. *J. Reprod. Fertil.,* 64:373–379.
657. Turner, T. T., D'Addario, D. A., and Howards, S. S. (1980): [^{3}H]3-*O*-methyl-D-glucose transport from blood into the lumina of the seminiferous and epididymal tubules in intact and vasectomized hamsters. *J. Reprod. Fertil.,* 60:285–289.
658. Brooks, D. E. (1979): Biochemical environment of sperm maturation. In: *The Spermatozoon,* edited by D. W. Fawcett and J. M. Bedford, pp. 23–34. Urban & Schwarzenberg, Baltimore.
659. Voglmayr, J. K., and Amann, R. P. (1973): The distribution of free *myo*-inositol in fluids, spermatozoa, and tissues of the bull genital tract and observations on its uptake by the rabbit epididymis. *Biol. Reprod.,* 8:504–513.
660. Eisenberg, F., and Bolden, A. H. (1963): Biosynthesis of inositol in rat testis homogenate. *Biochem. Biophys. Res. Commun.,* 12:72–77.
661. Eisenberg, F., and Bolden, A. H. (1964): Reproductive tract as site of synthesis and secretion of inositol in the male rat. *Nature,* 202:559–560.
662. Setchell, B. P., and Hinton, B. T. (1981): The effects of spermatozoa of changes in the composition of luminal fluid as it passes along the epididymis. *Prog. Reprod. Biol.,* 8:58–66.
663. Robinson, R., and Fritz, I. B. (1979): Myoinositol biosynthesis by Sertoli cells, and levels of myoinositol biosynthetic enzymes in testis and epididymis. *Can. J. Biochem.,* 57:962–967.
664. Hasegawa, R., and Eisenberg, F. (1981): Selective hormonal control of *myo*-inositol biosynthesis in reproductive organs and liver of the male rat. *Proc. Natl. Acad. Sci.,* 78:4863–4866.
665. Lewin, L. M., and Sulimovici, S. (1975): The distribution of radioactive myoinositol in the reproductive tract of the male rat. *J. Reprod. Fertil.,* 43:355–358.
666. Lewin, L. M., Yannai, Y., Sulimovici, S., and Kraicer, P. F. (1976): Studies on the metabolic role of *myo*-inositol. Distribution of radioactive *myo*-inositol in the male rat. *Biochem. J.,* 156:375–380.
667. Lewin, L. M., Yannai, Y., and Kraicer, P. (1979): The effect of cyproterone acetate on *myo*-inositol uptake and secretion in the reproductive tract of the male rat. *Int. J. Androl.,* 2:171–181.
668. Hinton, B. T., and Howards, S. S. (1982): Rat testis and epididymis can transport [^{3}H]3-*O*-methyl-D-glucose, [^{3}H]inositol and [^{3}H]α-aminoisobutyric acid across its epithelia *in vivo. Biol. Reprod.,* 27:1181–1189.
669. Scott, T. W., Wales, R. G., Wallace, J. C., and White, I. G. (1963): Composition of ram epididymal and testicular fluid and the biosynthesis of glycerylphosphorylcholine by the rabbit epididymis. *J. Reprod. Fertil.,* 6:49–59.

670. Wallace, J. C., Wales, R. G., and White, I. G. (1966): The respiration of the rabbit epididymis and its synthesis of glycerylphosphorylcholine. *Aust. J. Biol. Sci.*, 19:849–856.
671. Dawson, R. M. C., and Rowlands, I. W. (1959): Glycerylphosphorylcholine in the male reproductive organs of rats and guinea-pigs. *Q. J. Exp. Physiol.*, 44:26–34.
672. Scott, T. W., Dawson, R. M. C., and Rowlands, I. W. (1963): Phospholipid interrelationships in rat epididymal tissue and spermatozoa. *Biochem. J.*, 87:507–512.
673. Hammerstedt, R. H., and Rowan, W. A. (1982): Phosphatidylcholine of blood lipoprotein is the precursor of glycerophosphorylcholine found in seminal plasma. *Biochim. Biophys. Acta*, 710:370–376.
674. Brooks, D. E., Hamilton, D. W., and Mallek, A. H. (1973): The uptake of L-[methyl-^{3}H]carnitine by the rat epididymis. *Biochem. Biophys. Res. Commun.*, 52:1354–1360.
675. Hinton, B. T., Snoswell, A. M., and Setchell, B. P. (1979): The concentration of carnitine in the luminal fluid of the testis and epididymis of the rat and some other mammals. *J. Reprod. Fertil.*, 56:105–111.
676. Brooks, D. E. (1980): Carnitine in the male reproductive tract and its relation to the metabolism of the epididymis and spermatozoa. In: *Carnitine Biosynthesis, Metabolism, and Functions,* edited by R. A. Frenkel and J. D. McGarry, pp. 219–235. Academic Press, New York.
677. Yeung, C. H., Cooper, T. G., and Waites, G. M. H. (1980): Carnitine transport into the perfused epididymis of the rat: regional differences, stereospecificity, stimulation by choline, and the effect of other luminal factors. *Biol. Reprod.*, 23:294–304.
678. James, M. J., Brooks, D. E., and Snoswell, A. M. (1981): Kinetics of carnitine uptake by rat epididymal cells. Androgen-dependence and lack of stereospecificity. *FEBS Lett.*, 126:53–56.
679. Brooks, D. E. (1983): Epididymal functions and their hormonal regulation. *Aust. J. Biol. Sci.*, 36:205–221.
680. Casillas, E. R., and Erickson, B. J. (1975): Studies on carnitine synthesis in the rat epididymis. *J. Reprod. Fertil.*, 44:287–291.
681. Sexton, T. J., Amann, R. P., and Flipse, R. J. (1971): Free amino acids and protein in rete testis fluid, vas deferens plasma, accessory sex gland fluid, and seminal plasma of the conscious bull. *J. Dairy Sci.*, 54:412–416.
682. Johnson, L. A., Pursel, V. G., Gerrits, R. J., and Thomas, C. H. (1972): Free amino acid composition of porcine seminal, epididymal and seminal vesicle fluids. *J. Anim. Sci.*, 34:430–434.
683. Brown-Woodman, P. D. C., and White, I. G. (1974): Amino acid composition of semen and the secretions of the male reproductive tract. *Aust. J. Biol. Sci.*, 27:415–422.
684. Jones, R. (1978): Comparative biochemistry of mammalian epididymal plasma. *Comp. Biochem. Physiol.*, 61B:365–370.
685. Altman, P. L., and Dittmer, D. S. (editors) (1974): *Biology Data Book, 2nd ed., Vol. III,* pp. 1433–2123. Federation of American Societies for Experimental Biology, Bethesda.
686. Back, D. J. (1975): The presence of metabolites of ^{3}H-testosterone in the lumen of the cauda epididymidis of the rat. *Steroids,* 25:413–420.
687. Cooper, T. G., and Waites, G. M. H. (1979): Factors affecting the entry of testosterone into the lumen of the cauda epididymis of the anaesthetized rat. *J. Reprod. Fertil.*, 56:165–174.
688. Cooper, T. G. (1980): The general importance of proteins and other factors in the transfer of steroids into the rat epididymis. *Int. J. Androl.*, 3:333–348.
689. Turner, T. T., Cochran, R. C., and Howards, S. S. (1981): Transfer of steroids across the hamster blood testis and blood epididymal barrier. *Biol. Reprod.*, 25:342–348.
690. Brooks, D. E. (1981): Metabolic activity in the epididymis and its regulation by androgens. *Physiol. Rev.*, 61:515–555.
691. Lea, O. A., Petrusz, P., and French, F. S. (1978): Purification and localization of acidic epididymal glycoprotein (AEG): a sperm coating protein secreted by the rat epididymis. *Int. J. Androl. (Suppl.)*, 2:592–607.
692. Garberi, J. C., Kohane, A. C., Cameo, M. S., and Blaquier, J. A. (1979): Isolation and characterization of specific rat epididymal proteins. *Mol. Cell. Endocrinol.*, 13:72–82.
693. Faye, J. C., Duguet, L., Mazzuca, M., and Bayard, F. (1980): Purification, radioimmunoassay, and immunohistochemical localization of a glycoprotein produced by the rat epididymis. *Biol. Reprod.*, 23:423–432.
694. Brooks, D. E. (1981): Secretion of proteins and glycoproteins by the rat epididymis: regional differences, androgen-dependence, and effects of protease inhibitors, procaine, and tunicamycin. *Biol. Reprod.*, 25:1099–1117.
695. Brooks, D. E. (1982): Purification of rat epididymal proteins 'D' and 'E', demonstration of shared immunological determinants, and identification of regional synthesis and secretion. *Int. J. Androl.*, 5:513–524.
696. Brooks, D. E. (1985): Characterization of a 22kDa protein with widespread tissue distribution but which is uniquely present in secretions of the testis and epididymis and on the surface of spermatozoa. *Biochim. Biophys. Acta,* 841:59–70.
697. Brooks, D. E., Means, A. R., Wright, E. J., Singh, S. P., and Tiver, K. K. (1986): Molecular cloning of the cDNA for two major androgen-dependent secretory proteins of 18.5 kilodaltons synthesized by the rat epididymis. *J. Biol. Chem.*, 261:4956–4962.
698. Brooks, D. E., Means, A. R., Wright, E. J., Singh, S. P., and Tiver, K. K. (1986): Molecular cloning of the cDNA for androgen-dependent sperm-coating glycoproteins secreted by the rat epididymis. *Eur. J. Biochem.*, 161:13–18.
699. Kohane, A. C., Garberi, J. C., Cameo, M. S., and Blaquier, J. A. (1979): Quantitative determination of specific proteins in rat epididymis. *J. Steroid Biochem.*, 11:671–674.
700. Mann, T. (1964): *The Biochemistry of Semen and of the Male Reproductive Tract,* pp. 1–493. Methuen, London.
701. Mann, T., and Lutwak-Mann, C. (1981): *Male Reproductive Function and Semen,* pp. 1–495. Springer-Verlag, Berlin.
702. Quinn, P. J., White, I. G., and Wirrick, B. R. (1965): Studies of the distribution of the major cations in semen and male accessory secretions. *J. Reprod. Fertil.*, 10:379–388.
703. Cragle, R. G., Salisbury, G. W., and Muntz, J. H. (1972): Distribution of bulk and trace minerals in bull reproductive tract fluids and semen. *J. Dairy Sci.*, 41:1273–1277.
704. Humphrey, G. F., and Mann, T. (1949): Studies on the metabolism of semen. 5. Citric acid in semen. *Biochem. J.*, 44:97–105.
705. Leone, E. (1954): Ergothioneine in the equine ampullar secretion. *Nature,* 174:404–405.
706. Mann, T., Leone, E., and Polge, C. (1956): The composition of the stallion's semen. *J. Endocrinol.*, 13:279–290.
707. Mann, T., Short, R. V., Walton, A., Archer, R. K., and Miller, W. C. (1957): The 'tail-end sample' of stallion semen. *J. Agric. Sci. (Camb.)*, 49:301–312.
708. Mann, T., Minotakis, C. S., and Polge, C. (1963): Semen composition and metabolism in the stallion and jackass. *J. Reprod. Fertil.*, 5:109–122.
709. Einarsson, S. (1971): Studies on the composition of epididymal content and semen in the boar. *Acta Vet. Scand. (Suppl.)*, 36:1–80.
710. Fouquet, J. P. (1971): Secretion of free glucose and related carbohydrates in the male accessory organs of rodents. *Comp. Biochem. Physiol.*, 40A:305–317.
711. Prendergast, F. G., and Veneziale, C. M. (1975): Control of fructose and citrate synthesis in guinea pig seminal vesicle epithelium. *J. Biol. Chem.*, 250:1282–1289.
712. Mann, T. (1954): On the presence and role of inositol and certain other substances in the seminal vesicle secretion of the boar. *Proc. R. Soc. Lond. (Biol.)*, 142:21–32.
713. Melampy, R. M., and Mason, R. B. (1957): Androgen and the *myo*-inositol content of male accessory organs of the rat. *Proc. Soc. Exp. Biol. Med.*, 96:405–408.
714. Seamark, R. F., Tate, M. E., and Smeaton, T. C. (1968): The occurrence of scylloinositol and D-glycerol 1-(L-myoinositol 1-hydrogen phosphate) in the male reproductive tract. *J. Biol. Chem.*, 243:2424–2428.
715. Williams-Ashman, H. G., and Banks, J. (1956): Participation of cytidine coenzymes in the metabolism of choline by seminal vesicle. *J. Biol. Chem.*, 223:509–521.
716. Dawson, R. M. C., Mann, T., and White, I. G. (1957): Glycerylphosphorylcholine and phosphorycholine in semen, and their relation to choline. *Biochem. J.*, 65:627–634.
717. Mann, T. (1956): Male sex hormone and its role in reproduction. *Rec. Prog. Horm. Res.*, 12:353–376.

718. Kochakian, C. D. (1973): Hypotaurine: regulation of production in seminal vesicles and prostate of guinea-pig by testosterone. *Nature,* 241:202–203.
719. Eliasson, R. (1959): Studies on prostaglandin. Occurrence, formation and biological actions. *Acta Physiol. Scand. (Suppl.),* 46, 158:1–73.
720. Gerozissis, K., Jouannet, P., Soufir, J. C., and Dray, F. (1982): Origin of prostaglandins in human semen. *J. Reprod. Fertil.,* 65:401–404.
721. Humphrey, G. F., and Mann, T. (1948): Citric acid in semen. *Nature,* 161:352–353.
722. Lutwak-Mann, C., Mann, T., and Price, D. (1949): Metabolic activity in tissue transplants. Hormone-induced formation of fructose and citric acid in transplants from accessory glands of reproduction. *Proc. Roy. Soc. Lond. (Biol.),* 136:461–471.
723. Ortiz, E., Price, D., Williams-Ashman, H. G., and Banks, J. (1956): The influence of androgen on the male accessory reproductive glands of the guinea pig: studies on growth, histological structure and fructose and citric acid secretion. *Endocrinology,* 59:479–492.
724. Mann, T., and Wilson, E. D. (1962): Biochemical observations on the male accessory organs of nutria, *Myocastor coypus* (Molina). *J. Endocrinol.,* 25:407–408.
725. Levy, B. J., and Fair, W. R. (1973): The location of antibacterial activity in the rat prostatic secretions. *Invest. Urol.,* 11:173–177.
726. Huggins, C., Masina, M. H., Eichelberger, L., and Wharton, J. D. (1939): Quantitative studies of prostatic secretion. I. Characteristics of the normal secretion; the influence of thyroid, suprarenal, and testis extirpation and androgen substitution on the prostatic output. *J. Exp. Med.,* 70:543–556.
727. Lewin, L. M., and Beer, R. (1973): Prostatic secretion as the source of *myo*-inositol in human seminal fluid. *Fertil. Steril.,* 24:666–670.
728. Harrison, G. A. (1931): Spermine in human tissues. *Biochem. J.,* 25:1885–1892.
729. Harrison, G. A. (1933): The approximate determinations of spermine in single human organs. *Biochem. J.,* 27:1152–1156.
730. Rosenthal, S. M., and Tabor, C. W. (1956): The pharmacology of spermine and spermidine. Distribution and excretion. *J. Pharmacol. Exp. Ther.,* 116:131–138.
731. Pegg, A. E., Lockwood, D. H., and Williams-Ashman, H. G. (1970): Concentrations of putrescine and polyamines and their enzymic synthesis during androgen-induced prostatic growth. *Biochem. J.,* 117:17–31.
732. Boursnell, J. C., Hartree, E. F., and Briggs, P. A. (1970): Studies of the bulbo-urethral (Cowper's)-gland mucin and seminal gel of the boar. *Biochem. J.,* 117:981–988.
733. Boursnell, J. C., and Butler, E. J. (1973): Studies on properties of the seminal gel of the boar using natural gel and gel formed *in vitro. J. Reprod. Fert.,* 34:457–465.
734. Hartree, E. F. (1962): Sialic acid in the bulbo-urethral glands of the boar. *Nature,* 196:483–484.
735. Bronson, F. H., and Caroom, D. (1971): Preputial gland of the male mouse: attractant function. *J. Reprod. Fertil.,* 25:279–282.
736. Orsulak, P. J., and Gawienowski, A. M. (1972): Olfactory preferences for the rat preputial gland. *Biol. Reprod.,* 6:219–223.
737. Chipman, R. K., and Albrecht, E. D. (1974): The relationship of the male preputial gland to the acceleration of oestrus in the laboratory mouse. *J. Reprod. Fertil.,* 38:91–96.
738. Gawienowski, A. M., Orsulak, P. J., Stacewicz-Sapuntzakis, M., and Joseph, B. M. (1975): Presence of sex pheromone in preputial glands of male rats. *J. Endocrinol.,* 67:283–288.
739. Rodger, J. C., and White, I. G. (1974): Free *N*-acetylglucosamine in marsupial semen. *J. Reprod. Fertil.,* 39:383–386.
740. Rodger, J. C., and White, I. G. (1975): Electroejaculation of Australian marsupials and analyses of the sugars in the seminal plasma from three macropod species. *J. Reprod. Fertil.,* 43:233–239.
741. Rodger, J. C., and White, I. G. (1976): Source of seminal *N*-acetylglucosamine in Australian marsupials and further studies of free sugars of the marsupial prostate gland. *J. Reprod. Fertil.,* 46:467–469.
742. King, T. E., and Mann, T. (1959): Sorbitol metabolism in spermatozoa. *Proc. R. Soc. Lond. (Biol.),* 151:226–243.
743. Brooks, D. E., and Mann, T. (1972): Relation between the oxidation state of nicotinamide-adenine dinucleotide and the metabolism of spermatozoa. *Biochem. J.,* 129:1023–1034.
744. Brooks, D. E., and Mann, T. (1973): Pyruvate metabolism in boar spermatozoa. *J. Reprod. Fertil.,* 34:105–119.
745. Brooks, D. E. (1979): Carnitine, acetylcarnitine and the activity of carnitine acyltransferases in seminal plasma and spermatozoa of men, rams and rats. *J. Reprod. Fertil.,* 56:667–673.
746. Frenkel, G., Peterson, R. N., Davis, J. E., and Freund, M. (1974): Glycerylphosphorylcholine and carnitine in normal human semen and in postvasectomy semen: differences in concentrations. *Fertil. Steril.,* 25:84–87.
747. Fahimi, F., Bieber, L., and Lewin, L. M. (1981): The sources of carnitine in human semen. *J. Androl.,* 2:339–342.
748. Calvin, J., and Tubbs, P. K. (1976): A carnitine : acetylcarnitine exchange system in spermatozoa. *J. Reprod. Fertil.,* 48:417–420.
749. Bøhmer, T., Johansen, L., and Kjekshus, E. (1978): Carnitine-acetyl-transferase transferase in human spermatozoa and seminal plasma determined by a sensitive radioisotope method. *Int. J. Androl.,* 1:262–269.
750. Bøhmer, T., and Johansen, L. (1978): Inhibition of sperm maturation through intervention of the carnitine system. *Int. J. Androl. (Suppl.),* 2:565–573.
751. Tanphaichitr, N. (1977): *In vitro* stimulation of human sperm motility by acetylcarnitine. *Int. J. Fertil.,* 22:85–91.
752. Hinton, B. T., Brooks, D. E., Dott, H. M., and Setchell, B. P. (1981): Effects of carnitine and some related compounds on the motility of rat spermatozoa from the caput epididymidis. *J. Reprod. Fertil.,* 61:59–64.
753. Jeulin, C., Soufir, J. C., and Jouannet, P. (1981): The effects of L-carnitine and D,L-acetylcarnitine on human sperm motility as measured by laser doppler velocimetry. *IRCS Med. Sci.,* 9:722–723.
754. Brooks, D. E. (1970): Acid-soluble phosphorus compounds in mammalian semen. *Biochem. J.,* 118:851–857.
755. Fair, W. R., Clark, R. B., and Wehner, N. (1972): A correlation of seminal polyamine levels and semen analysis in the human. *Fertil. Steril.,* 23:38–42.
756. Jänne, J., Hölttä, E., Haaranen, P., and Elfving, K. (1973): Polyamines and polyamine-metabolizing enzyme activities in human semen. *Clin. Chim. Acta,* 48:393–401.
757. Williams-Ashman, H. G., and Canellakis, Z. N. (1979): Polyamines in mammalian biology and medicine. *Perspect. Biol. Med.,* 22:421–453.
758. Pulkkinen, P., Sinervirta, R., and Jänne, J. (1975): Modification of the metabolism of the rat epididymal spermatozoa by spermine. *Biochem. Biophys. Res. Commun.,* 67:714–722.
759. Tabor, C. W., and Rosenthal, S. M. (1956): Pharmacology of spermine and spermidine. Some effects on animals and bacteria. *J. Pharmacol. Exp. Ther.,* 116:139–155.
760. Pulkkinen, P., Sinervirta, R., and Jänne, J. (1977): Mechanism of action of oxidized polyamines on the metabolism of human spermatozoa. *J. Reprod. Fertil.,* 51:399–404.
761. Pulkkinen, P. (1978): Specific inhibition of spermatozoal energy metabolism by oxidized spermine. *Contraception,* 17:423–433.
762. Van der Horst, C. J. G., and Grooten, H. J. G. (1966): The occurrence of hypotaurine and other sulfur-containing amino acids in seminal plasma and spermatozoa of boar, bull and dog. *Biochim. Biophys. Acta,* 117:495–497.
763. Leone, E. (1953): Acido urico e xantinossidasi in vescichette seminali. *Boll. Soc. Ital. Biol. Sper.,* 29:513–516.
764. Templeton, A. A., Cooper, I., and Kelly, R. W. (1978): Prostaglandin concentrations in the semen of fertile men. *J. Reprod. Fertil.,* 52:147–150.
765. Kelly, R. W., Taylor, P. L., Hearn, J. P., Short, R. V., Martin, D. E., and Marston, J. H. (1976): 19-Hydroxyprostaglandin E_1 as a major component of the semen of primates. *Nature,* 260:544–545.
766. Bygdeman, M., and Holmberg, O. (1966): Isolation and identification of prostaglandins from ram seminal plasma. *Acta Chem. Scand.,* 20:2308–2310.
767. Poyser, N. L. (1974): Some aspects of prostaglandins in reproduction. *Biochem. Soc. Trans.,* 2:1196–1200.
768. Cenedella, R. J. (1975): Prostaglandins and male reproductive physiology. In: *Molecular Mechanisms of Gonadal Hormone Action,* edited by J. A. Thomas and R. L. Singhal, pp. 325–328. University Park Press, Baltimore.
769. Setchell, B. P. (1967): The blood-testicular fluid barrier in sheep. *J. Physiol.,* 189:63P.

770. Setchell, B. P., Volglmayr, J. K., and Waites, G. M. H. (1969): A blood-testis barrier restricting passage from blood into rete testis fluid but not into lymph. *J. Physiol.*, 200:73–85.
771. Setchell, B. P., and Wallace, A. L. (1972): The penetration of iodine-labelled FSH and albumin into the seminiferous tubules of sheep and rats. *J. Endocrinol.*, 54:67–77.
772. Setchell, B. P. (1974): The entry of substances into the seminiferous tubules. In: *Male Fertility and Sterility,* edited by R. E. Mancini and L. Martini, pp. 37–57. Academic Press, New York.
773. Waites, G. M. H., Jones, A. R., Main, S. J., and Cooper, T. G. (1973): The entry of antifertility and other drugs into the testis. *Adv. Biosci.*, 10:101–116.
774. Okumura, K., Lee, I. P., and Dixon, R. L. (1975): Permeability of selected drugs and chemicals across the blood testis barrier of the rat. *J. Pharmacol. Exp. Ther.*, 194:89–95.
775. Cooper, T. G., and Waites, G. M. H. (1975): Steroid entry into rete testis fluid and the blood-testis barrier. *J. Endocrinol.*, 65:195–205.
776. Edwards, E. M., Jones, A. R., and Waites, G. M. H. (1975): The entry of α-chlorhydrin into body fluids of male rats and its effect upon incorporation of glycerol into lipids. *J. Reprod. Fertil.*, 43:225–232.
777. Main, S. J., and Waites, G. M. H. (1977): The blood-testis barrier and temperature damage to the testis of the rat. *J. Reprod. Fertil.*, 51:439–450.
778. Setchell, B. P., and Main, S. J. (1978): Drugs and the blood-testis barrier. *Environ. Health Perpect.*, 24:61–64.
779. Howards, S. S., Jesse, S. J., and Johnson, A. L. (1976): Micropuncture studies of the blood-seminiferous tubule barrier. *Biol. Reprod.*, 14:264–269.
780. Setchell, B. P., and Waites, G. M. H. (1975): The blood-testis barrier. In: *Handbook of Physiology, Vol. V,* edited by D. W. Hamilton and R. O. Greep, pp. 143–172. American Physiological Society, Washington, D.C.
781. Middleton, A., and Setchell, B. P. (1987): The entry of 3-*O*-methylglucose into the seminiferous tubules of rats and rams (*in press*).
782. Main, S. J., and Setchell, B. P. (1978): The facilitated diffusion of testosterone into the rete testis of the ram. *J. Physiol.*, 284: 17P–18P.
783. Turner, T. T., Hartmann, P. K., and Howards, S. S. (1979): Urea in the seminiferous tubule: evidence for active transport. *Biol. Reprod.*, 20:511–515.
784. Burrow, P., and Setchell, B. P. (1980): The fate of radioactive substances infused into a single seminiferous tubule in anaesthetised rats. *Proceedings of the Winter Meeting of the Society for the Study of Fertility,* Abstract 32, London.
785. Burrow, P. V., Pholpramool, C., and Setchell, B. P. (1981): The movement of substances out of the seminiferous tubules and epididymal duct during microinfusion. *J. Physiol.*, 319:15P–16P.
786. Kormano, M. (1968): Penetration of intravenous trypan blue into the rat testis and epididymis. *Acta Histochem.*, 30:133–136.
787. Mancini, R. E., Vilar, O., Alvarez, B., and Seiguer, A. C. (1965): Extravascular and intratubular diffusion of labelled serum proteins in the rat testis. *J. Histochem. Cytochem.*, 13:376–385.
788. Mancini, R. E., Castro, A., and Seiguer, A. C. (1967): Histological localization of follicle-stimulating and luteinizing hormones in the rat testis. *J. Histochm. Cytochem.*, 15:516–525.
789. Johnson, M. H. (1972): The distribution of immunoglobulin and spermatozoal autoantigen in the genital tract of the male guinea pig. *Fertil. Steril.*, 23:383–392.
790. Dym, M., and Fawcett, D. W. (1970): The blood-testis barrier in the rat and the physiological compartmentation of the seminiferous epithelium. *Biol. Reprod.*, 3:308–326.
791. Dym, M. (1973): The fine structure of the monkey (*Macaca*) Sertoli cell and its role in maintaining the blood-testis barrier. *Anat. Rec.*, 175:639–656.
792. Gilula, N. B., Fawcett, D. W., and Aoki, A. (1976): The Sertoli cell occluding junctions and gap junctions in mature and developing mammalian testes. *Dev. Biol.*, 50:142–168.
793. Vitale-Calpe, R., Fawcett, D. W., and Dym, M. (1973): The normal development of the blood-testis barrier and the effects of clomiphene and estrogen treatment. *Anat. Rec.*, 176:333–344.
794. Hatier, R., and Grignon, G. (1980): Ultrastructural study of Sertoli cells in rat seminiferous tubules during intrauterine life and the postnatal period. *Anat. Embryol.*, 160:11–27.
795. Bergmann, M., and Dierichs, R. (1983): Postnatal formation of the blood-testis barrier in the rat with special reference to the initiation of meiosis. *Anat. Embryol.*, 168:269–275.
769. Setchell, B. P., Laurie, M. S., and Jarvis, L. G. (1981): The blood-testis barrier at puberty. *Excerpta Med. Int. Cong. Ser.*, 559:186–190.
797. Tindall, D. J., Vitale, R., and Means, A. R. (1975): Androgen binding protein as a biochemical marker of formation of the blood-testis barrier. *Endocrinology,* 97:636–648.
798. Danzo, B. J., and Eller, B. C. (1985): The ontogeny of biologically active androgen-binding protein in rat plasma, testis and epididymis. *Endocrinology,* 117:1380–1388.
799. Johnson, M. H. (1969): The effect of cadmium chloride on the blood-testis barrier of the guinea-pig. *J. Reprod. Fertil.*, 19:551–553.
800. Pilsworth, L. M. C., Hinton, B. T., and Setchell, B. P. (1981): Effects of obstruction of the flow of seminiferous tubule fluid on the germinal epithelium of the rat. *J. Reprod. Fertil.*, 63:347–353.
801. Fritz, I. B., Lyon, M. F., and Setchell, B. P. (1983): Evidence for a defective seminiferous tubular barrier in the testes of Tfm and Sxr mice. *J. Reprod. Fertil.*, 67:359–363.
802. Steinberger, A. (1975): *In vitro* techniques for the study of spermatogenesis. *Meth. Enzymol.*, 39:283–296.
803. Parvinen, M., Wright, W. W., Phillips, D. M., Mather, J. P., Musto, N. A., and Bardin, C. W. (1983): Spermatogenesis *in vitro:* completion of meiosis and early spermiogenesis. *Endocrinology,* 112:1150–1152.
804. Toppari, J., and Parvinen, M. (1985): *In vitro* differentiation of rat seminiferous tubular segments from defined stages of the epithelial cycle: morphological and immunolocalization analysis. *J. Androl.* 6:334–343.
805. Pilsworth, L. M., and Setchell, B. P. (1980): Spermatogenic and endocrine functions of the testes of invertebrate and vertebrate animals. In: *The Testis,* edited by H. Burger and D. M. de Kretser, pp. 9–38. Raven Press, New York.
806. Roosen-Runge, E. C. (1977): *The Process of Spermatogenesis in Animals,* pp. 1–214. Cambridge University Press, Cambridge.
807. Liang, J. C., Hsu, T. C., and Gay, M. (1985): Response of murine spermatocytes to the metaphase-arresting effect of several mitotic arrestants. *Experientia,* 41:1586–1588.
808. Waksman, B. H. (1959): A histologic study of the auto-allergic testis lesion in the guinea-pig. *J. Exp. Med.*, 109:311–324.
809. Johnson, M. H. (1970): Changes in the blood-testis barrier of the guinea-pig in relation to histological damage following isoimmunization. *J. Reprod. Fertil.*, 22:119–127.
810. Hinton, B. T., and Howards, S. S. (1981): Permeability characteristics of the epithelium in the rat caput epididymidis. *J. Reprod. Fertil.*, 63:95–99.
811. Cooper, T. G., Yeung, C. H., Lui, W., and Yang, C. Z. (1985): Luminal secretion of *myo*-inositol by the rat epididymis perfused in vitro. *J. Reprod. Fertil.*, 74:135–144.
812. Hoffer, A. P., and Hinton, B. T. (1984): Morphological evidence for a blood-epididymis barrier and the effects of gossypol on its integrity. *Biol. Reprod.*, 30:991–1004.
813. Setchell, B. P. (1977): Male reproductive organs and semen. In: *Reproduction in Domestic Animals, 3rd ed.*, edited by H. H. Cole and P. T. Cupps, pp. 229–256. Academic Press, New York.
814. Hemeida, N. A., Sack, W. O., and McEntee, K. (1978): Ductuli efferentes in the epididymis of boar, goat, ram, bull, and stallion. *Am. J. Vet. Res.*, 39:1892–1900.
815. Hoffer, A. P., and Greenberg, J. (1978): The structure of the epididymis, efferent ductules and ductus deferens of the guinea pig: a light microscope study. *Anat. Rec.*, 190:659–678.
816. Bloom, W., and Fawcett, D. W. (1962): *A Textbook of Histology, 8th ed.* Saunders, Philadelphia.
817. Brown, J. C., and Williams, J. D. (1972): A histochemical study of the preputial glands of male laboratory rat and mouse. *Acta Anat.*, 81:270–285.
818. Sasano, N., and Ichijo, S. (1969): Vascular patterns of the human testis with special reference to its senile changes. *Tohoku J. Exp. Med.*, 99:269–280.
819. Harrison, R. G. (1951): Applications of microradiography: The testis. In: *Microarteriography,* edited by A. E. Barclay, pp. 89–90. Blackwell, Oxford.

820. Walls, E. W. (1981): The blood vascular and lymphatic systems. In: *Cunningham's Textbook of Anatomy, 12th ed.*, edited by G. J. Romanes, pp. 871–1037. Oxford University Press, Oxford.
821. Netter, F. H. (1953): *The CIBA Collection of Medical Illustrations. Vol. 1. The Nervous System*, pp. 1–168. Colorpress, New York.
822. Fawcett, D. W. (1975): Ultrastructure and function of the Sertoli cell. In: *Handbook of Physiology, Vol. 5.*, edited by D. W. Hamilton and R. O. Greep, pp. 21–55. American Physiological Society, Washington, D.C.
823. Price, D., and Williams-Ashman, H. G. (1961): The accessory reproductive glands of mammals. In: *Sex and Internal Secretions, 3rd ed., Vol. 1*, edited by W. C. Young, pp. 366–448. Williams & Wilkins, Baltimore.
824. Carrick, F. N., and Hughes, R. L. (1978): Reproduction in male monotremes. *Aust. Zool.*, 20:211–231.
825. Gustafson, A. W., and Shemesh, M. (1976): Changes in plasma testosterone levels during the annual reproductive cycle of the hibernating bat, *Myotis lucifugus lucifugus* with a survey of plasma testosterone levels in adult male vertebrates. *Biol. Reprod.*, 15:9–24.
826. Lau, I. F., and Saksena, S. K. (1979): Steroids in the rete testis fluid of fertile male rabbits. *Arch. Androl.*, 2:49–52.
827. Pujol, A., Bayard, F., Louvet, J.-P., and Boulard, C. (1976): Testosterone and dihydrotestosterone concentrations in plasma, epididymal tissues, and seminal fluid of adult rats. *Endocrinology*, 98:111–113.
828. Ganjam, V. K., and Amann, R. P. (1976): Steroids in fluids and sperm entering and leaving the bovine epididymis, epididymal tissue, and accessory sex gland secretions. *Endocrinology*, 99:1618–1630.
829. Schanbacher, B. D. (1976): Rapid chromatography for quantitation of radioimmunoassayable 5α-androstane-17β-ol-3-one and testosterone in ram, bull and boar serum. *Endocr. Res. Commun.*, 3:71–82.
830. Mann, T., and Parsons, U. (1950): Studies on the metabolism of semen. 6. Role of hormones, effect of castration, hypophysectomy and diabetes. Relation between blood glucose and seminal fructose. *Biochem. J.*, 46:440–450.
831. White, I. G., and Griffiths, D. E. (1958): Guanidines and phosphagens of semen. *Aust. J. Exp. Biol. Med. Sci.*, 36:97–102.
832. Bartlett, D. T. (1962): Studies on dog semen. II. Biochemical characteristics. *J. Reprod. Fertil.*, 3:190–205.
833. Mann, T. (1969): Physiology of semen and of the male reproductive tract. In: *Reproduction in Domestic Animals, 2nd ed.*, edited by H. H. Cole and P. T. Cupps, pp. 277–312. Academic Press, New York.
834. Baronos, S. (1971): Seminal carbohydrate in boar and stallion. *J. Reprod. Fertil.*, 24:303–305.
835. Eliasson, R. (1965): Accurate determination of glucose in human semen. *J. Reprod. Fertil.*, 9:325–330.
836. Einarsson, S., Crabo, B., and Ekman, L. (1970): A comparative study on the chemical composition of plasma from the cauda epididymidis, semen fractions, and whole semen in boars. *Acta Vet. Scand.*, 11:156–180.
837. Fjellström, D., and Kihlström, J. E. (1975): On the concentrations of some inorganic ions and protein nitrogen in rabbit seminal fluid. *J. Reprod. Fertil.*, 44:559–560.
838. Oltjen, R. R., Bond, J., Gerrits, R. J., and Johnson, L. A. (1971): Growth and reproductive performance of bulls and heifers fed purified and natural diets. V. Free amino acids in the semen and blood plasma of bulls (puberty to 148 weeks of age). *J. Anim. Sci.*, 33:814–818.
839. Holtz, W., and Foote, R. H. (1978): Composition of rabbit semen and the origin of several constituents. *Biol. Reprod.*, 18:286–292.
840. Nalbandov, A. V. (1976): *Reproductive Physiology of Mammals and Birds*, 3rd ed., pp. 1–334. W. H. Freeman and Company, San Francisco.

The Physiology of Reproduction,
edited by E. Knobil and J. Neill *et al.*
Raven Press, Ltd., New York © 1988.

CHAPTER 20

The Cytology of the Testis

D. M. de Kretser and J. B. Kerr

HISTORICAL ASPECTS

Although the effects of castration were recognized in antiquity, probably as far back as Neolithic times (ca. 7000 B.C.) (1), the association between the testis and fertility was not revealed until the seventeenth century. Reasonably accurate diagrammatic representations of the testicular anatomy can be attributed to Aristotle in 400 B.C. (2), but the necessity of the testes for fertility was not recognized at that time. A treatise by de Graaf (3) recorded accurately the general structure and functions of the testis, and his observations were soon followed by the observation of spermatozoa in seminal fluid by van Leeuwenhoek in 1667 (4). The link between the seminiferous tubules and the production of spermatozoa was not fully revealed until the studies of von Kölliker (5), who concluded that spermatozoa were formed by a process of cellular development within the tubules. The cellular changes resulting in the production of spermatozoa thus constituted spermatogenesis.

Accurate descriptions of the hormonal effects of castration were also available in Aristotle's time, but experimental proof emerged from the studies of Berthold (6), who showed that the decrease in comb size and absence of crowing that occurred in roosters after castration could be reversed by transplantation of testes. The site of production of the masculinizing factor was subsequently attributed to the Leydig cells by Bouin and Ancel (7), but the isolation of testosterone by David *et al.* (8) did not occur until 1935.

The improvements in microscopy in the late nineteenth century expanded our knowledge of the light-microscopic features of spermatogenesis, and identification of chromosomes and the processes of mitosis and meiosis greatly improved our understanding of gamete production in the male. The results of those studies provide the foundation of our knowledge.

GENERAL STRUCTURE OF THE TESTIS

The testis is surrounded by a dense connective-tissue capsule, the tunica albuginea, that is covered on its anterior and lateral aspects with the remnants of the processus vaginalis, forming the visceral and parietal layers of the tunica vaginalis (9). From the internal surface of the tunica albuginea, connective-tissue septa extend posteriorly toward a region of the testis termed the mediastinum. This area consists of connective tissue within which an anastomotic network of ducts can be identified: the rete testis.

The tunica albuginea is formed by dense connective tissue within which smooth-muscle fibers can be found (10), the latter being responsible for the capacity of the capsule to contract in response to pharmacological stimuli (11). The inner surface of the tunica albuginea is apposed to loose, highly vascular connective tissue sometimes termed the tunica vasculosa. The degree of lobulation of the testis varies between species, and within these lobules lie the seminiferous tubules, within which spermatogenesis occurs. The tubules extend as loops from the mediastinum testis, both ends of each loop communicating via single straight tubules, the tubuli recti (12). In the majority of mammals this simple arrangement is obscured in the adult testis (Fig. 1), because the tubule forming each loop becomes extensively folded, thereby extending its surface area (13–15). The extensive lengthening of the tubule loops that occurs during development is the result principally of the mitotic activity of immature Sertoli cells.

The organization of the intertubular tissue varies dramatically between species (16), but contains the blood vessels, lymphatics, and nerve fibres (*vide infra*). The Leydig cells are scattered in groups in the intertubular tissue in relation to the vasculature and the lamina propria of the seminiferous tubules, the outer layers of which consist of modified smooth-muscle cells termed myoid cells (Fig. 1).

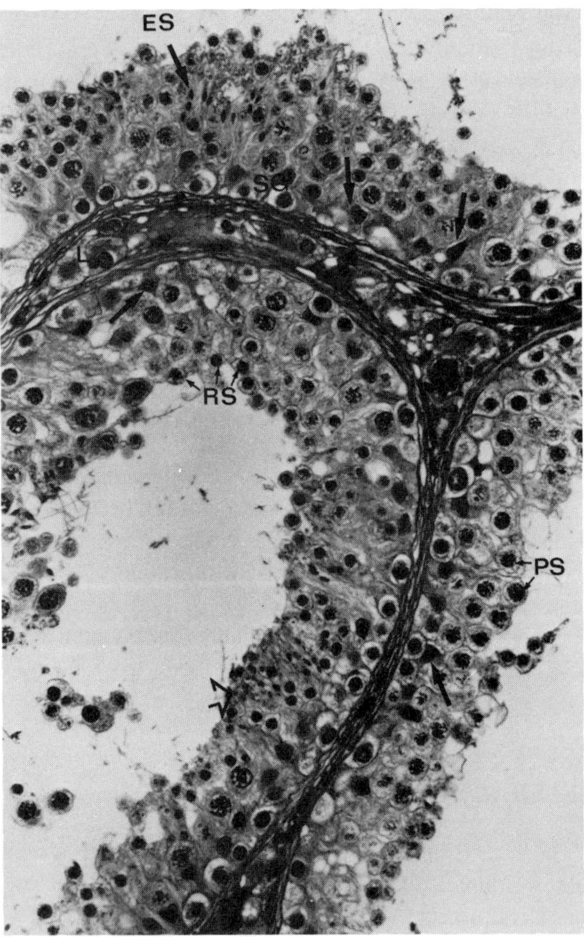

FIG. 1. This light micrograph of the normal human testis illustrates spermatogonia (SG), primary spermatocytes (PS), round spermatids (RS), and elongating spermatids (ES). Note residual bodies (*open arrow*), Sertoli cells (*arrows*), and Leydig cells (L).

INTRATESTICULAR DUCTS

Transitional Distal Segment of Seminiferous Tubule

The segment of the seminiferous tubule that establishes continuity with the rete testis is lined by an epithelium devoid of germ cells. This segment, termed the transitional distal seminiferous segment (Fig. 2), narrows, forming an "epithelial plug" that projects slightly into the tubuli recti, which has a wider lumen. The epithelium consists of Sertoli

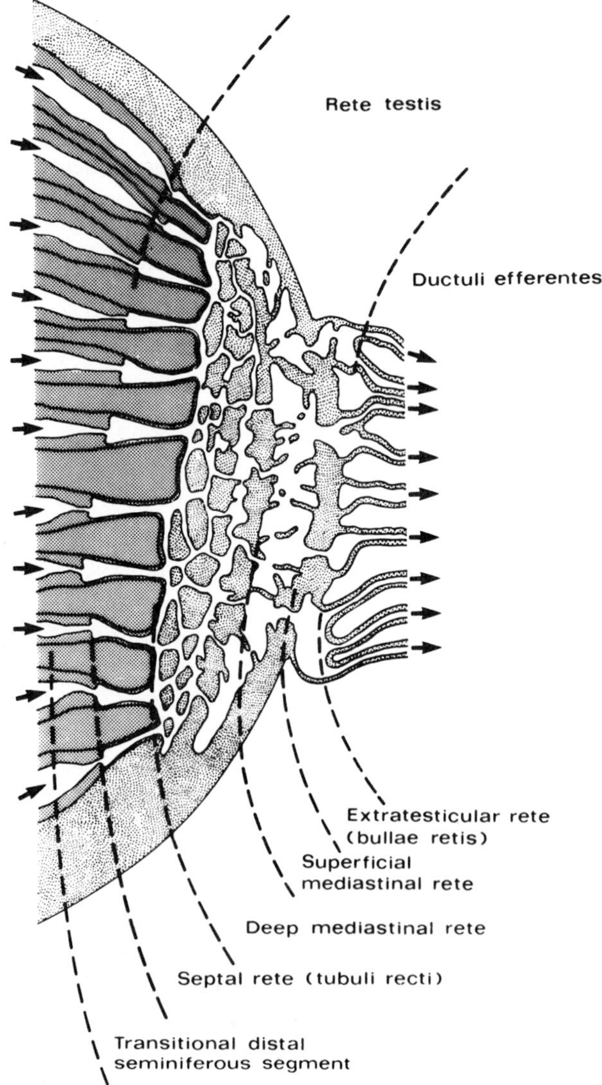

FIG. 2. Method by which seminiferous tubules terminate in the rete testis. The zones of the rete testis are denoted. (From ref. 773.)

cells that contain more extensive rough endoplasmic reticulum and lipid inclusions, but less smooth endoplasmic reticulum. Prominent bundles of filaments are present in the cells and may confer some structural rigidity to this region, which may function as a plug to regulate the movement of cells and fluid into the rete testis (14). Dym (17) suggested that the slope of the apices of the cells toward the rete testis made it unlikely that reflux could occur into the seminiferous tubules.

Rete Testis

This represents an anastomotic series of ducts into which the transitional distal segments of the seminiferous tubules open and that drain at their cranial pole via the ductuli efferentes to form the duct of the epididymis. It lies in the mediastinum of the testis parallel to the axis of the epididymis and has been divided into several zones (Fig. 2) by Roosen-Runge and Holstein (18): (a) septal rete, (b) mediastinal rete, and (c) extratesticular rete. The septal rete consists of the zone of the straight ducts, the tubuli recti that drain the seminiferous tubules. The mediastinal rete can be subdivided further into a deep zone consisting of an anastomotic maze of tubules draining the septal rete and opening into a superficial zone—a series of relatively wide longitudinal channels emptying into the extratesticular rete or bullae retis. The latter is characterized by macroscopically visible dilated spaces drained by the ductuli efferentes.

The region of the mediastinal rete is characterized by an irregular network of cylindrical strands, the chordae retis, which range in diameter from 5 to 40 μm (18). The thinner cords are avascular, but each contains a fibroelastic matrix containing myofibroblastic cellular elements, the myoid cells showing similar features as those surrounding the seminiferous tubules. It is postulated that their strut-like features may prevent overdistension of the thin-walled rete channels and together with the contractile properties of the myoid elements may provide a mechanism for raising intra-rete pressure, thereby forcing fluid into the extratesticular ducts.

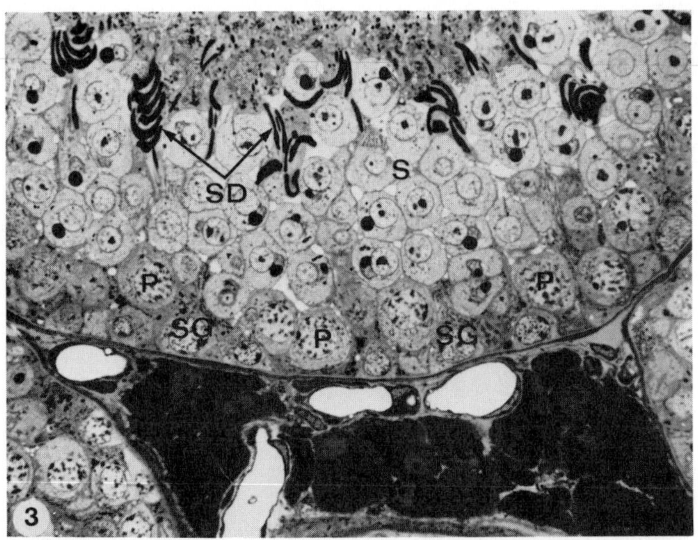

FIG. 3. Guinea pig seminiferous epithelium showing spermatogonia (SG), primary spermatocytes (P), round spermatids (S), and mature spermatids (SD).

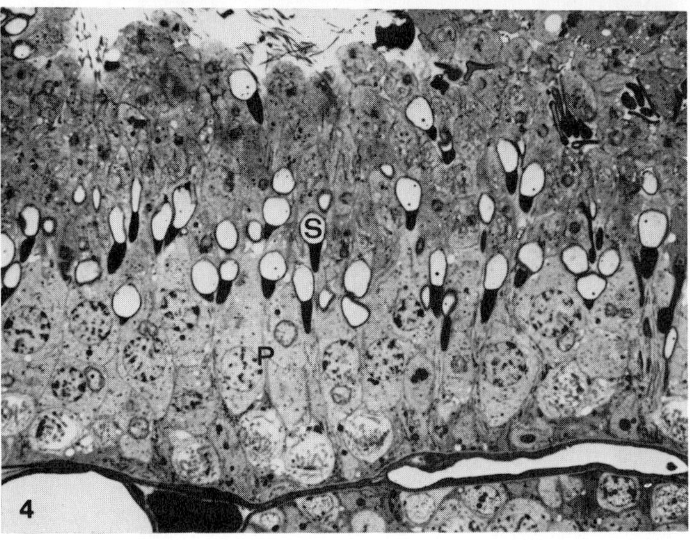

FIG. 4. Guinea pig seminiferous epithelium showing pachytene primary spermatocytes (P) and elongated spermatids (S).

Two distinct cell types are present: the squamous cells lining most of the rete, and the prismatic cells that occur in clusters at bends and corners in the channels (19). The squamous cells are studded with short microvilli, and each contains a long single cilium, their cytoplasm containing lipid inclusions, glycogen, and a few areas of smooth endoplasmic reticulum. The prismatic cells stain lightly; each contains an irregular nucleus with fine granular chromatin and also a single cilium. Their cytoplasmic organelles are polarized, with prominent basal collections of lipid and glycogen and a supranuclear Golgi complex, the surface showing a few thick microvilli that are shorter than the squamous cells. External to the epithelium is a connective-tissue layer containing fibroblasts and smooth-muscle cells and bundles of collagen and elastin fibers.

The extratesticular rete is characterized by vesicular dilatations that are visible macroscopically and act as the vestibules for the excurrent duct system that extends as the ductuli efferentes.

SPERMATOGENESIS

The sequence of cytological events that result in the formation of mature spermatozoa from precursor cells is known as spermatogenesis (Figs. 3 and 4). In many mammals this process takes place within the seminiferous tubule throughout the reproductive life-span of the male. In some species it is interrupted or subdivided into a series of distinct phases based on environmental cues that are transduced into hormonal signals stimulating or inhibiting spermatogenesis, i.e., seasonal breeders (20). In others, somewhat unusual processes occur such that a single wave of spermatogenic development is seen within the testis, subsequent to which the animal is sterile; such a process occurs in the marsupial mouse *Antechinus stuartii* and *A. swainsonii,* whose stem cells, after a burst of mitotic activity, differentiate and proceed through the spermatogenic process, resulting in a single wave of reproductive activity (21). Thus, it is possible to see within a seminiferous tubule spermatids of varying ma-

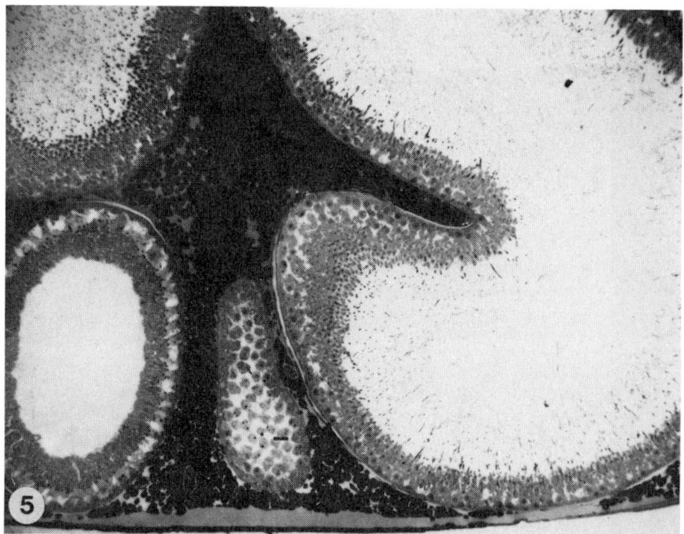

FIG. 5. *Antechinus* testis, illustrating the shallow depth of the seminiferous epithelium in relation to the dimensions of the seminiferous tubules.

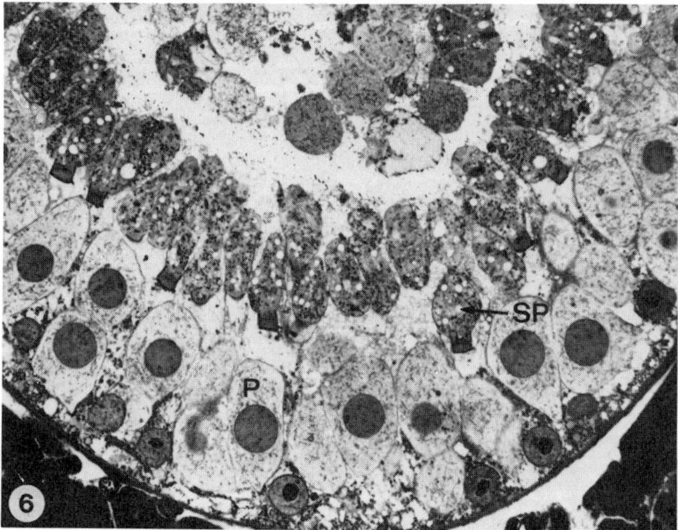

FIG. 6. *Antechinus* seminiferous epithelium in May, showing Sertoli cells, pachytene primary spermatocytes (P), and elongating spermatids (SP). Spermatogonia and early primary spermatocytes are not commonly observed.

turity without any other basally placed germ cells (Figs. 5–10).

Spermatozoa can be viewed as the "secretory product" of the spermatogenic process. To enable continuous production of cells as a product, the process of spermatogenesis must involve a continuous replication of stem cells to produce cohorts of cells that can proceed through the subsequent changes. Furthermore, because the nucleus of the sperm fuses with that of the oocyte to form the zygote, a reduction in the number of chromosomes to the haploid state must occur in gametogenesis such that the diploid state is restored on syngamy. There are three major elements that together constitute spermatogenesis: (a) stem cell renewal by the process of mitosis, (b) reduction of chromosomal number by meiosis, and (c) the transformation of a conventional cell into the complex structure of the spermatozoon by a series of changes involving no further cell division, but representing a metamorphic process termed spermiogenesis. The stem cells for the spermatogenic process are termed spermatogonia, which undergo mitotic division (Figs. 1 and 3). Groups of spermatogonia then proceed to enter meiosis, the cells being termed primary spermatocytes and secondary spermatocytes. The latter divide to form spermatids, which are transformed during spermiogenesis into spermatozoa.

The conditions under which spermatogenesis is successfully completed are relatively specialized and necessitate the creation of a unique environment within the seminiferous tubule. This is achieved by the organization of the non-germ-cell elements within the tubules, namely, the Sertoli cells (Fig. 11), which form the blood-testis barrier (22) (*vide infra*). Furthermore, the unusual cellular nature of the product of spermatogenesis, namely, spermatozoa, creates a specific requirement within the epithelium, namely, the support of a migratory population of cells that proliferate at the base of the tubule and move progressively toward the lumen of the tubule as the cells differentiate (Figs. 12 and 13). Again, this is achieved by the nature of the nondividing or stable population of Sertoli cells.

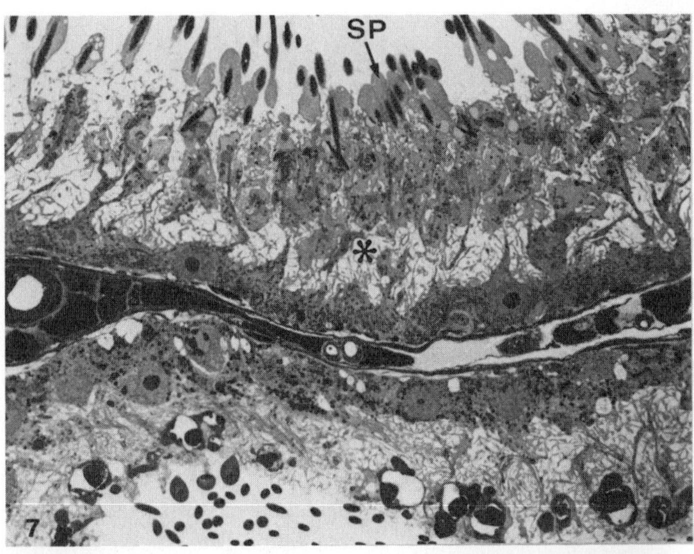

FIG. 7. *Antechinus* seminiferous epithelium in July, indicating Sertoli cell cytoplasmic processes (*asterisk*) supporting mature spermatids (SP).

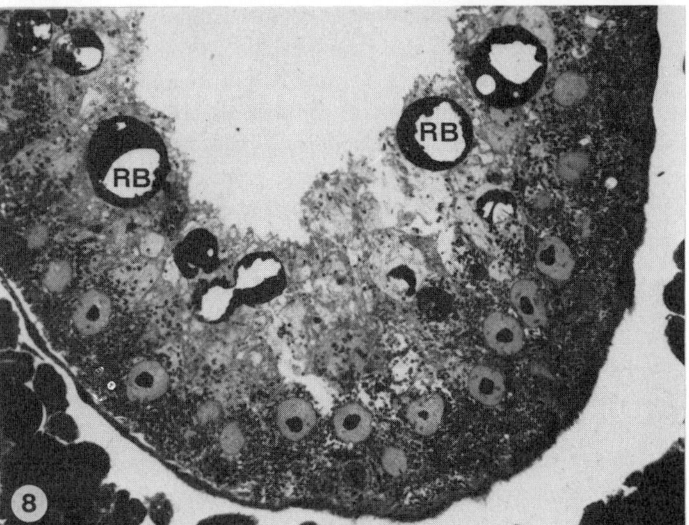

FIG. 8. *Antechinus* seminiferous epithelium late in July, showing Sertoli cell nuclei with prominent nucleoli and numerous residual bodies (RB) at the apex of the Sertoli cell cytoplasm.

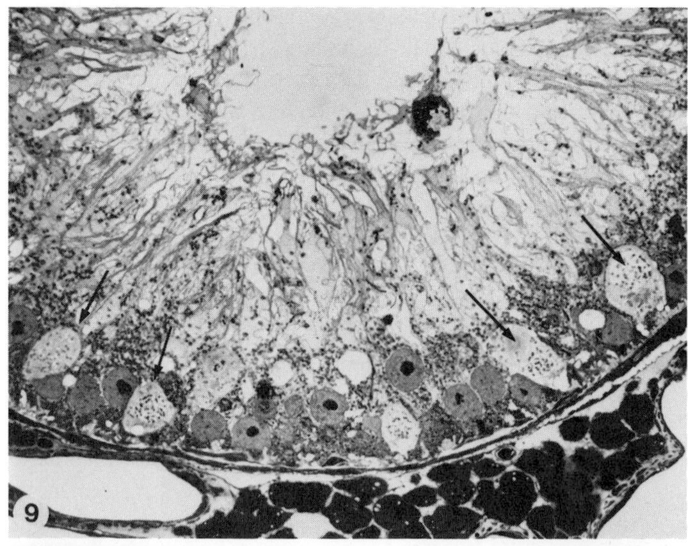

FIG. 9. *Antechinus* seminiferous epithelium in early August, illustrating disappearance of most germ cells. A few early primary spermatocytes are indicated (*arrows*).

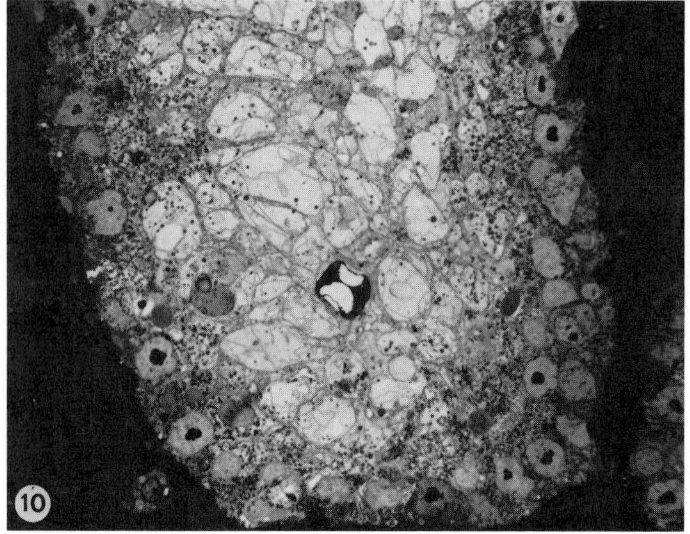

FIG. 10. *Antechinus* seminiferous epithelium in late August at the height of the mating period. The seminiferous tubule is filled with Sertoli cell cytoplasm.

DEVELOPMENTAL CONSIDERATIONS

Although the detailed development of the testis is the subject of another chapter, a brief consideration is of value in understanding the relationships of the two populations of cells: the germ cells and Sertoli cells. The development of the testis is associated with the formation of a series of sex cords, arranged as a series of C-shaped arches running at right angles to the long axis of the testis, each end of the arch connecting with developing rete testis (12,13). With further development, the orientation of the plane of the cords perpendicular to the longitudinal axis of the testis changes, and elongation is achieved by infolding of the cords to form a series of convolutions mostly in a craniocaudal orientation (12). The mechanisms by which these cords arise from their mesenchymal precursors is complex and is still a subject of debate (23). Nevertheless, there is general agreement that the cords are composed of two types of cells, the supporting cells and the primordial germ cells (Fig. 14). Though it is now accepted that these two cell types remain distinct in terms of origin and subsequent development, earlier studies suggested that the germ cells degenerated in fetal life and were reestablished by differentiation from the supporting cells (24–27). However, the detailed studies of Clermont and Perey (28) provided strong evidence to support the view that the Sertoli cells are formed by differentiation of the supporting cells and that the primordial germ cells give rise to spermatogonia. The supporting cells in the fetal testis greatly outnumber the primordial germ cells. Though this balance changes because of mitotic multiplication of the primordial germ cells, even at birth, in the majority of mammalian species, the number of supporting cells is considerably greater than the number of germ cells (28).

Before birth, the primitive Sertoli cells are predominantly arranged adjacent to the boundary tissue of the seminiferous cords, although some are displaced more centrally because of the close packing of cells within the cords (23,29–37). Primitive Sertoli cells exhibit a conical or polygonal shape, with their cytoplasm often oriented radially within the seminiferous cord (Fig. 14). Their nuclei are variable in shape

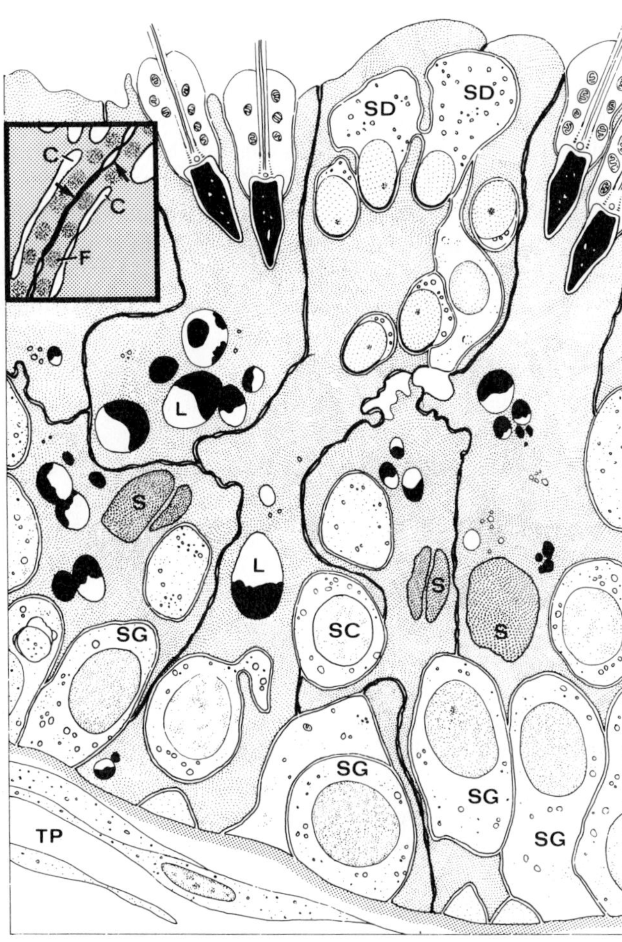

FIG. 11. Relationships between germ cells and Sertoli cells are shown for the human seminiferous epithelium. Note spermatogonia (SG), primary spermatocytes (SC), spermatids (SD), Sertoli cells (S), and their cytoplasm containing lipids (L). The specialized inter-Sertoli-cell junctions are shown by a *heavy line* and diagrammatically illustrated at higher magnification in the inset; C, cisternae; F, fibrils.

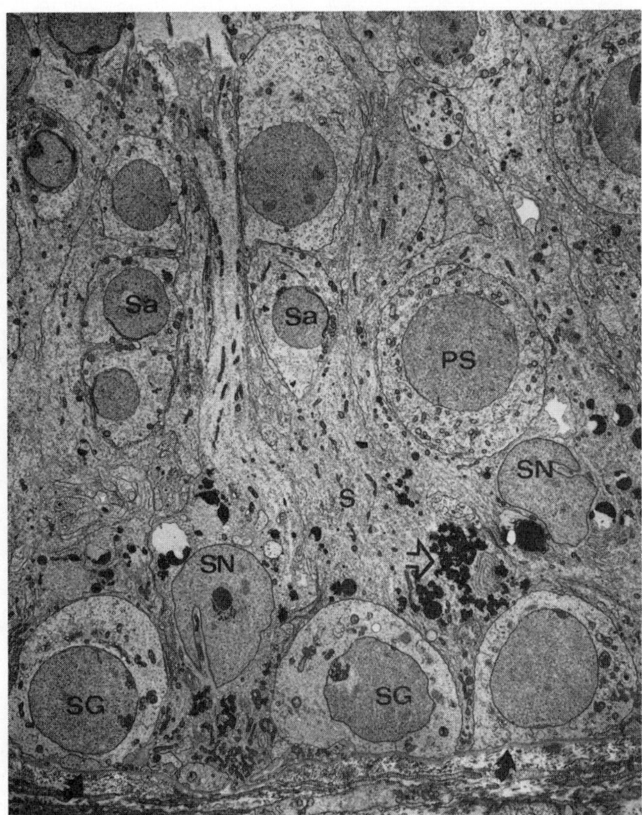

FIG. 12. Low-power electron micrograph of the human seminiferous epithelium showing the following features: spermatogonia (SG), primary spermatocytes (PS), spermatids at the Sa stage, Sertoli cell nuclei (SN), and cytoplasm (S) collections of lipid (*open arrow*) and the basement membrane (*arrows*).

and seldom show deep indentations. A nucleolus is often present, together with peripheral clumps of heterochromatin associated with the nuclear membrane. The cytoplasm of primitive Sertoli cells in the fetus is unremarkable, but tubular membranes of endoplasmic reticulum are well represented, often bearing variable amounts of ribosomes (29,38), and for this reason these organelles are referred to as a transitional form between conventional smooth and rough endoplasmic reticulum.

A gradual expansion in the diameter of seminiferous cords during fetal life is a reflection of the changing internal organization due to proliferation of primitive Sertoli cells and the gonocytes (38). As the gonocytes proliferate and differentiate into spermatogonia, they often form groups of cells that are accommodated in recesses provided by the Sertoli cells, indicating that the fetal Sertoli cells are deformable. This presumably allows the immature germ cells to gain attachment to the boundary tissues of the seminiferous cords, a location that in postnatal life becomes their exclusive domain. Information on the proliferative behavior of Sertoli cells in the fetus has been gained from morphometric assessment of their numbers in the pig and from autoradiographic studies in rats examining the incorporation of tritiated thymidine into the DNA of primitive Sertoli cell nuclei (30,31,38). It was found that the numbers of fetal Sertoli cells increased steadily until shortly before birth, and thereafter their proliferative capacity declined to produce a stable population of nondividing Sertoli cells. Cessation of Sertoli cell proliferation has been much studied in laboratory rodents and occurs on days 10 to 12 after birth in the mouse (28,39–44) and on days 14 to 16 in the immature rat.

The peak of proliferative activity of Sertoli cells just prior to parturition has implicated the production of mitogenic factors capable of controlling expansion of the fetal Sertoli cell population. Not unexpectedly, the involvement of gonadotropic hormones has been favored as the mechanism governing the mitotic activity of fetal Sertoli cells. This idea has gained support not only by inference from the known trophic actions of follicle-stimulating hormone (FSH) on the seminiferous epithelium in postnatal life (45) but also from evidence gained from studies of the male fetus suggesting

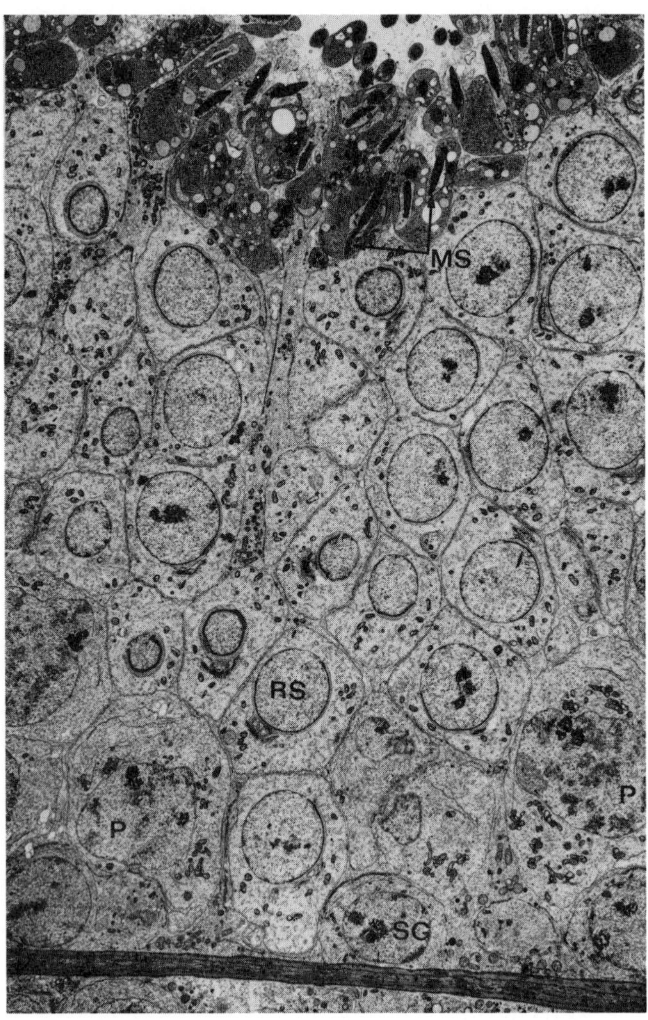

FIG. 13. Mouse seminiferous epithelium showing spermatogonia (SG), pachytene primary spermatocytes (P), and round (RS) and mature (MS) spermatids.

a functional relationship between the fetal pituitary and testis. The pituitary-testicular axis appears to be activated by day 17 of fetal life in the rat, because at or before that time the hypothalamus contains gonadotropin-releasing hormone (GnRH) (46), and FSH and luteinizing hormone (LH) are detectable in the pituitary (46–48). The role of FSH in development of fetal Sertoli cells has been highlighted further by demonstration of maximum FSH binding to fetal testes at precisely the time of maximum proliferation of Sertoli cells (49). Furthermore, addition of FSH to cultures of Sertoli cells derived from postnatal testes results in increased mitotic activity (50,51).

A significant step forward in elucidation of the factors that control proliferation of fetal Sertoli cells was provided by Orth (31), who showed that removal of the fetal pituitary or treatment with an antiserum to FSH both produced dramatic reduction in Sertoli cell mitosis. She further showed that this effect, at least *in vitro,* was mediated via cyclic AMP. Another collection of data indicates that local interactions within the fetal testis may be involved with cell proliferation prior to birth. Coincident with maximum mitoses of fetal Sertoli cells shortly before parturition, the fetal Leydig cells attain their maximum numbers at or slightly prior to this time (52,53). Levels of circulating testosterone (54), the activity of Leydig cell steroidogenic enzymes (55), and the production of testicular testosterone and total steroid content per Leydig cell are greatest during this period (53,56,57). These data raise the possibility that a paracrine relationship exists between fetal Sertoli cells and Leydig cells and emphasize that in addition to the demonstrated role of FSH, other factors may be of importance in influencing the expansion of the Sertoli cell population.

During postnatal growth of the testis, the immature Sertoli cells continue to proliferate, albeit at a steadily declining rate, until the adult population is established. The appearance of pachytene primary spermatocytes in the rat testis is

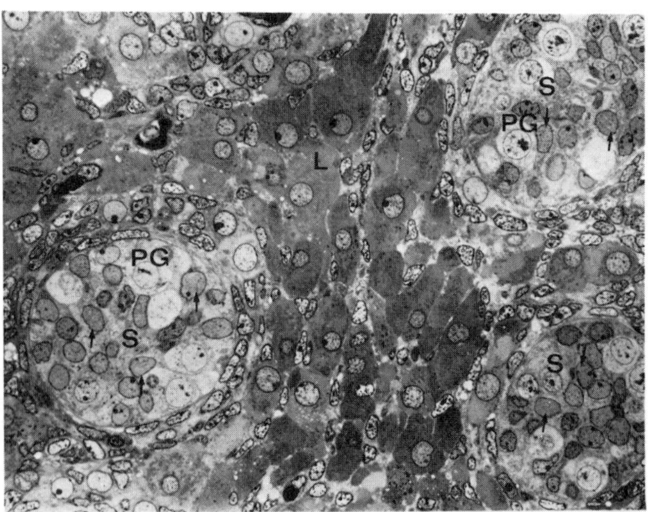

FIG. 14. Leydig cells (L) and seminiferous cords (S) from a 16-week human fetus. Note primordial germ cells (PG) and immature Sertoli cells (*arrows*).

associated with this restriction of Sertoli cell division, which, according to numerous studies, provides for a stable Sertoli cell population during adult life (58–60). With the initiation of spermatogenesis soon after birth in rodents and at various later times in domestic, ruminant, and primate species, the immature Sertoli cells undergo morphological maturation to attain the adult-type structural features seen in the mature testis (60–64). These changes include a large increase in cell size, movement of the nucleus to a basal position within the cell, development of a complex nuclear shape and a tripartite nucleolus, and proliferation of organelles, particularly the smooth endoplasmic reticulum.

A much-studied aspect of Sertoli cell maturation in the developing testis has focused on the morphological differentiation of the blood-testis barrier. Light-microscopic analysis had earlier indicated that the barrier (detected by the admittance or exclusion of acridine dyes) appears at the onset of spermatogenesis (65). Electron-microscopic studies (61,64–69) have confirmed that electron-opaque tracers freely penetrate into the seminiferous cords of newborn animals, but are subsequently restricted from entry concurrent with the appearance of inter-Sertoli-cell junctional complexes. In the immature rat the barrier forms during the 16th to 19th postnatal days, which is after cessation of Sertoli cell mitoses and commencement of the meiotic maturation of germ cells. Because pachytene primary spermatocytes are formed prior to the effective establishment of the blood-testis barrier (64), it seems that the meiotic maturation process during the initiation of spermatogenesis is not dependent on the formation of an adluminal epithelial compartment.

The factors controlling the formation of the blood-testis barrier are not known, although the possible involvement of gonadotropins remains under discussion. Certainly the appearance of inter-Sertoli-cell junctions is not dependent on spermatogenesis, because elimination of germ cells from the testis (45,70–72) did not prevent development of the junctions. However, the appearance of the blood-testis barrier in immature rats was delayed when rats were treated daily from birth with clomiphene citrate or estradiol benzoate, agents that are thought to suppress gonadotropin secretion (64). This finding has remained difficult to evaluate, because measurements of gonadotropin levels were not available, and the possible direct effects of clomiphene or estradiol on the testis were not considered. It was concluded that the formation of inter-Sertoli-cell junctions was not directly dependent on gonadotropins. Similar views were expressed when it was found that long-term hypophysectomy failed to disrupt the blood-testis barrier in rats (73–76). In the human testis, however, it has been shown (77) that the formation of inter-Sertoli-cell junctions in men with hypogonadotropic hypogonadism is related to administration of exogenous gonadotropins. The morphological changes that appear in the Sertoli cells during sexual maturation require further study, with particular emphasis on the roles of the gonadotropic and steroid hormones.

The primordial germ cells migrate from endoderm and dorsal yolk sac epithelium via the dorsal mesentery into the gonadal ridge (78,79). Whether they arise from endoderm or from the underlying mesoderm is still in question. Clark and Eddy (80) noted that their fine structural features resembled those of underlying mesodermal cells rather than the surrounding endoderm. The histochemical presence of alkaline phosphatase in these primordial germ cells permits their identification during this migratory phase (81). These germ cells become associated with the precursors of the Sertoli cells to form primitive testicular cords, an association thought to be important in establishing the different behaviors of male primordial germ cells and those in the female. Evidence exists that if the structure of the cords is disrupted, or if male germ cells lodge in aberrant sites such as the adrenal gland (82), they will commence meiosis during fetal life—a characteristic of germ cells in the developing ovary (83).

Subsequently, the primordial germ cells undergo a defined period of mitotic cell division during which daughter cells remain connected by intercellular bridges (84,85). In the rat, the period of cell division occurs for 48 hr from day 14 to day 16 of fetal life, and because the daughter cells differ slightly in structure from the primordial germ cells, they have been called M prospermatogonia (86). Hilscher and colleagues identified yet another period of fetal mitotic activity that gave rise to prospermatogonia, in turn giving rise to the adult A spermatogonial stage. In other species the sequence of changes is less well defined and the terminology confusing, but general agreement exists that there is a period of mitotic activity within the prenatal testis that increases germ cell numbers, but they still remain the minority cell population within the seminiferous cords, usually lying in a central position. The numbers of gonocytes and spermatogonia decrease in fetal life because of a degenerative process that has been estimated to reduce numbers 30% to 40% (87). The degenerating cells are phagocytosed by the immature Sertoli cells.

Gondos (88) has suggested a more simple terminology, dividing the germ cells in the fetal testis into (a) primitive germ cells that are part of the undifferentiated gonad and (b) gonocytes when the germ cells are located within the seminiferous cords in a central position and (c) spermatogonia when they move to the periphery of the tubule. The primordial germ cell is a relatively large, rounded cell with an irregular horseshoe-shaped nucleus and filamentous, centrally placed nucleolus (80). The mitochondria are large and rounded and contain few cristae. There is sparse endoplasmic reticulum, plentiful free ribosomes, and characteristic membrane-bounded granules with a central dense core separated from the membrane by a flocculent zone (80). In the human, the gonocytes have features similar to those of globular mitochondria whose cristae are dilated (89). Apart from perinuclear smooth-membraned vesicles, there is a paucity of other organelles. Gondos and colleagues (84,89) noted that processes extended from the gonocytes as they migrated toward the basement membrane of the cords to become spermatogonia. The processes contained microtubules presumably aiding the migratory process. The spermatogonia have similar cytological features during fetal life, but differ in being peripherally placed and being interconnected by cytoplasmic bridges due to incomplete cytokinesis during mitosis.

The pattern of development in the sex cords after birth varies considerably in mammals depending on the time span between birth and the acquisition of sexual maturity. In species such as the rat, spermatogenesis effectively commences at birth, because the duration of spermatogenesis in this species is 49 days (90), and spermatozoa are present in the testis at about 50 days (91). Hence, the seminiferous tubules undergo rapid development after birth, sequentially demonstrating the stages of germ cell development constituting spermatogenesis. In other species, such as humans, there is an extensive prepubertal period during which the testes show little change from their appearance at birth. Recent detailed morphometric studies of testes from children who died suddenly have shown that little change occurs until 7 to 9 years, following which mitotic activity of the gonocytes occurs, populating the bases of the seminiferous tubules with spermatogonia in numbers equal to those of the Sertoli cells (92). The spermatogonia subsequently undergo the spermatogenic process, with spermatozoa being released into the lumen between 11 and 13 years.

SPERMATOGONIA

The cells that divide by mitosis and constitute the pool of cells from which meiosis and spermiogenesis proceed are termed spermatogonia. They were first identified as entities separate from the Sertoli cells by von Ebner (93) in 1871, but the term spermatogonia was first applied to this class of cells by von La Valette St. George (94) in 1876. The first detailed study of these cells was performed by Regaud (27), who defined two types of spermatogonia in the rat, the "dusty" cells and "crusty" cells, on the basis of differences in the chromatin patterns of their nuclei. The dusty cells showed a nuclei with fine, palely stained chromatin granulation, whereas the crusty cells had nuclei with coarse granules of heavily stained chromatin close to the nuclear membrane. Regaud (27) subdivided the dusty spermatogonia into two classes based on nuclear morphology and staining with safranin and also clearly distinguished early primary spermatocytes from the crusty spermatogonia.

Allen (25) used a different terminology that persists today, calling the equivalent of dusty spermatogonia type A spermatogonia, and the crusty cells type B spermatogonia. In the rat, spermatogonia with nuclear characteristics intermediate between type A and type B could be identified principally by the presence of fine plaques of chromatin close to the nuclear membrane, and they were termed intermediate spermatogonia (40). Similar subtypes can be identified in other species, such as the mouse (95), ram (41), bull (96), and guinea pig (97). More recent studies in the rat have identified further spermatogonial types on the basis of their nuclear morphology, separating four classes of type A spermatogonia as well as the intermediate and type B (98). Similar types of observations are now available for other species, with the number of generations of spermatogonia varying significantly, as reviewed by Clermont (90).

The ability to differentiate different classes of spermatogonia is critically dependent on the fixation employed, because identification is based on the morphological characteristics of the nuclei. The type of fixation precipitates chromatin to varying degrees, with Zenker formol providing optimal chromatin patterns for identification because the chromatin remains widely dispersed (90). On the other hand, Bouin's fixative creates larger chromatin clumps close to the nuclear membrane, rendering spermatogonial classification more difficult. Additionally, the characteristic features of the nuclei that are used to identify each type are present only at certain phases of the cell cycle, usually acquiring the typical nuclear morphology at the S and G_2 phases (40,99).

In humans and in some primate species, somewhat different nuclear characteristics have been noted. Branca (100) noted great variability in the morphology of human spermatogonia, describing palely staining areas in some nuclei termed nuclear vacuoles. Subsequently, types A and B spermatogonia were identified in humans, with the type A being subdivided into the dark and pale types (101–103). The type A dark spermatogonia are characterized by a densely staining chromatin, usually containing a central pale-stained area termed the nuclear vacuole. Close to the nuclear membrane, one or more nucleoli are found. In contrast, the type A pale spermatogonium contains an ovoid nucleus, with palely staining granular chromatin and exhibiting one or two nucleoli lying close to the nuclear membrane. The type B spermatogonia exhibit the characteristics described for other species, though the human cells are somewhat smaller. Similar spermatogonial types have been identified in monkeys (*Macacus rhesus, Cercopithecus aethiops*), but do not show the nuclear vacuole (104,105).

It is self-evident that to enable spermatogenesis to proceed as a continuous process, the spermatogonia not only must provide the precursors for the meiotic process but also must renew themselves. The mechanisms by which this is achieved are discussed later in this review, together with the cycle of spermatogenesis.

The cytoplasmic features of spermatogonia on light microscopy are relatively unremarkable. They have a poorly staining cytoplasm, and studies of whole mounts of seminiferous tubules have demonstrated that they remain connected by intercellular bridges such that large numbers are effectively linked together (106–108). Using the periodic acid Schiff (PAS) reaction, glycogen is found in the A type dark spermatogonia.

Fine Structure: There have been relatively few detailed ultrastructural studies of spermatogonia, and investigators often have had difficulty in identifying the ultrastructural counterparts of the subclasses of spermatogonia identified by light microscopy. The basal position of spermatogonia within the epithelium (Figs. 12, 13, and 15) and their extensive contact with the basement membrane of the tubule are clearly evident by electron microscopy (109,110). The extent of this contact decreases in type B spermatogonia, which will eventually lose all contact with the basement membrane to become preleptotene primary spermatocytes (111). All types of spermatogonia are characterized by a relatively electron-lucent cytoplasm and a paucity of cytoplasmic organelles (110–113). Furthermore, because of incomplete cytokinesis during mitosis, spermatogonia remain connected by intercellular bridges originally identified by Watson (114). These bridges are 2 to 3 μm in width and usually do not contain organelles or microtubules; they are limited by the cell membrane, which is more electron-dense in this region and is separated from the adjacent Sertoli cell membrane by an intercellular space of approximately 200 Å (108,115). Occasionally, microtubules can be observed crossing these intercellular bridges, and Fawcett (116) has observed membranous partitions that can appear transiently across the bridge separating the cells without breaking down the connections.

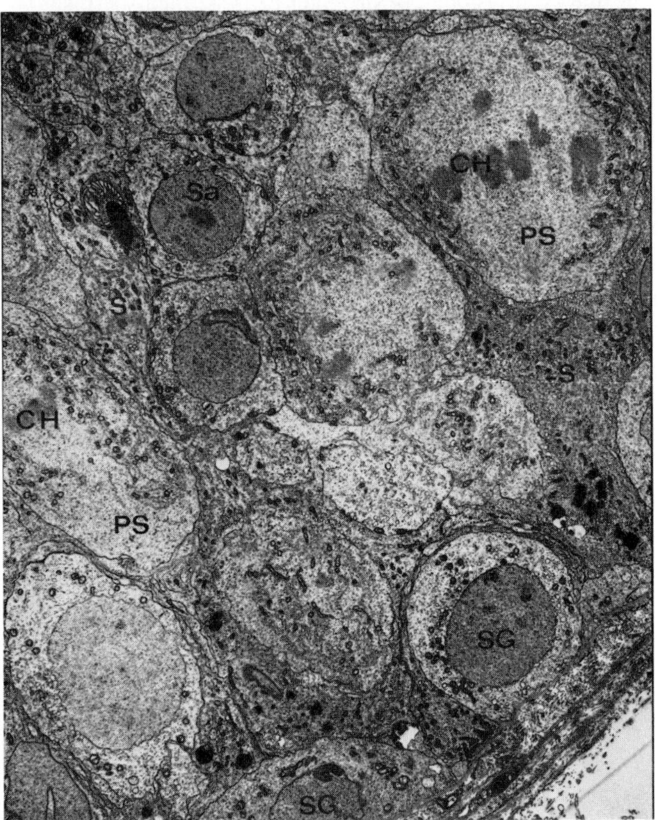

FIG. 15. Micrograph illustrating the epithelium at stage VI of the human seminiferous cycle. Note spermatogonia (SG), dividing primary spermatocytes (PS) containing chromosomes (CH), spermatids (Sa), and the Sertoli cell cytoplasm (S).

Attempts have been made to classify spermatogonia at the electron-microscopic level, particularly in the human (111,117,118). Most investigators agree that it is possible in humans to identify the type A dark, type A pale, and type B spermatogonia, though intermediate forms have been noted to occur (119). The classification (111) is based on (a) the nuclear and nucleolar features, (b) the presence of aggregations of mitochondria, (c) the presence or absence of glycogen granules, and (d) the presence of crystalloids known as the Lubarsch crystal found in human spermatogonia (120).

Type A Dark Spermatogonia: These cells have an oval-shaped nucleus and demonstrate a relatively electron-translucent region consistent with the appearance of the nuclear vacuole on light microscopy. The nucleoli are small and peripherally placed adjacent to the nuclear membrane and consist of a nucleolonema; occasionally they are surrounded by nuclear vacuole. The decreased electron density of these regions is due to the absence of chromatin fibrils in the area. The mitochondria lie close to the nucleus, and between the mitochondria there is finely granular, moderately electron-dense material. The cristae extend transversely across the matrix, though some areas of the mitochondria are devoid of cristae; in some mitochondria the intracristal space is dilated. Profiles of rough endoplasmic reticulum are largely seen, though some smooth-membraned vesicles are present. The Golgi complex is poorly developed. Glycogen granules are present, often forming aggregations (111). The crystalloids of Lubarsch are present, represented by collections of fibrils and tubules aligned along the long axis of the structure, which may be up to 3 μm in length. Linear arrays of small electron-dense granules separate the fibrillar elements, and small collections of similar granular material are sometimes present in the adjacent cytoplasm (113,121,122). Their function is unknown, though they show some similarities to the structure of the crystals of Charcot-Böttcher found in Sertoli cells.

Type A Pale Spermatogonia: These have less extensive contact with the basement membrane of the tubule, and their nuclei do not show nuclear vacuoles (Fig. 16). Their nucleoli are peripherally placed and consist of a nucleolonema and pars amorpha. The mitochondria rarely form perinuclear collections, often lying together as pairs separated by the granular intermitochondrial material found in type A dark spermatogonia. Glycogen granules are infrequently found, though Lubarsch crystals can be present.

Type B Spermatogonia: These cells have the least contact with the basement membrane and contain peripherally placed nuclear chromatin aggregations that, because of the thin sections, are not as prominent as visualized by light microscopy. The nucleolus is centrally placed and consists of nucleolonema and pars amorpha. The mitochondria are scattered singly in the cytoplasm, with an apparent disappearance of the intermitochondrial material seen in type A cells. This is of interest because it reappears in primary spermatocytes and has been linked to the perinuclear dense bodies

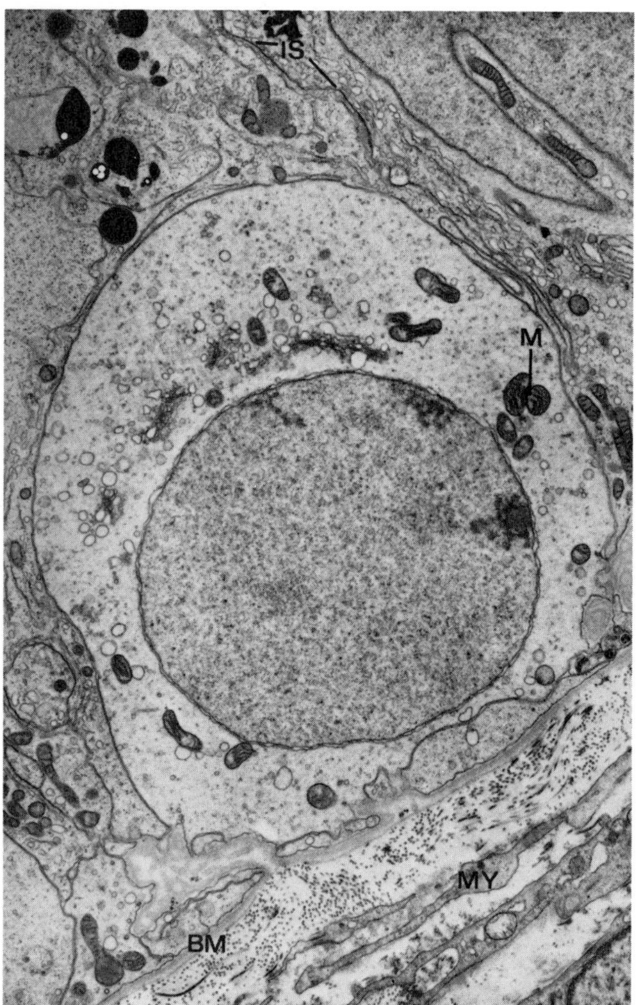

FIG. 16. Electron micrograph illustrating a type A pale spermatogonium situated on the basement membrane (BM) of a seminiferous tubule from the human testis. Note the paucity of organelles and the mitochondria (M) sometimes clustered around an intermitochondrial electron-dense matrix. The adjacent Sertoli cells show specialized inter-Sertoli-cell junctions (IS). Note myoid cell processes (MY).

or nuage of invertebrate and amphibian oogenesis, as reviewed by Fawcett (123). Scanty profiles of smooth and rough endoplasmic reticulum are present, and the Golgi complex, though not dramatic, is better developed than in type A spermatogonia.

Type A Long Spermatogonia: Rowley *et al.* (111) identified yet another type characterized by its shape: long and very flat, with contact to the basal lamina extending up to 30 μm in length. The nucleus was irregular in shape, with a peripherally placed nucleolus. The mitochondria occurred in large collections (up to 10) in the perinuclear region and were joined together by the granular intermitochondrial material. Glycogen and Lubarsch crystalloids were noted. They commented that this type may correspond to the A_0 spermatogonial type of other species (99).

SPERMATOCYTES

The cells in the spermatogenic process that are involved in meiosis are the primary and secondary spermatocytes. The term spermatocyte was first used by von La Valette St. George (94) to designate the cells previously termed "growing cells" by other investigators. Although the drawings by Brown (124) are remarkably accurate in depicting the nuclear patterns in these cells, their true significance did not become apparent until the studies of Winiwater (125) and Montgomery (126).

The process of meiosis actually involves two cell divisions (Fig. 17). In the first, which involves the primary spermatocytes, the chromosomes appear each as a pair of chromatids, subsequent to which heterologous chromosomes pair by synapsis to form bivalents. Each member of the bivalent pair subsequently moves to the daughter cells, termed secondary spermatocytes, which contain half the number of chromosomes (haploid number), but because each chromosome is composed of a pair of daughter chromatids, the actual total DNA content is equivalent to that of somatic cells.

The second division occurs after a relatively short duration, and during this the chromatids of each chromosome separate to daughter cells by mechanisms similar to those of mitotic division. The daughter cells, termed spermatids, contain the haploid number of chromosomes and half the DNA content of somatic cells.

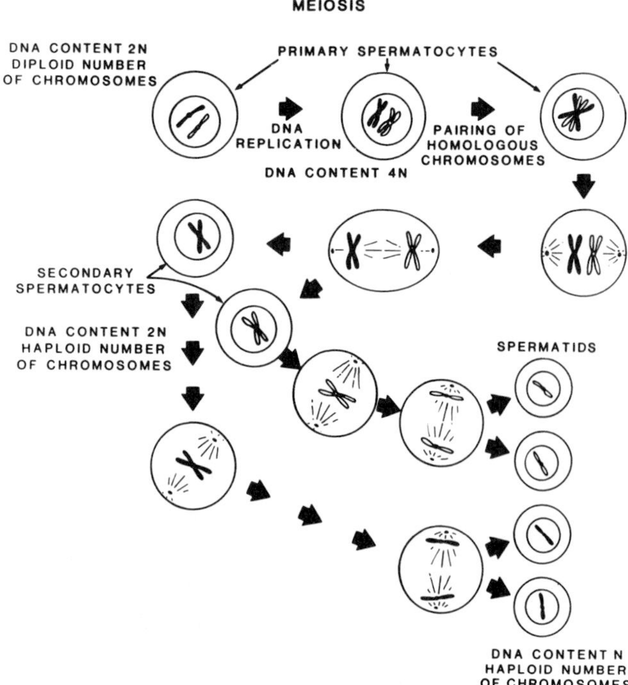

FIG. 17. Diagram illustrating the changes occurring during the meiotic divisions involving the primary and secondary spermatocytes.

Primary Spermatocytes

These cells demonstrate the features of the first meiotic division in terms of nuclear morphology. Early studies by Montgomery (126) showed that distinct pairs of chromosomes were visible in primary spermatocytes and suggested that each pair was composed of a chromosome of maternal or paternal origin. Their pairing was originally suggested to be end to end (126,127), but subsequently was shown to be side to side (125).

The primary spermatocytes arise from type B spermatogonia that lose contact with the basement membrane of the seminiferous tubule. They are characterized by a spherical nucleus with features similar to those of the type B spermatogonia, lacking any details of chromosomal structure. During this phase they are termed preleptotene spermatocytes and are actively engaged in DNA synthesis (128). This DNA synthesis is the mechanism by which each chromosome, when it condenses, is composed of a pair of chromatids, the total DNA content representing twice the diploid content (Fig. 17). The period of DNA synthesis represents the last in the process of spermatogenesis, and these cells represent the most mature cells capable of being labeled with markers such as ^{3}H-thymidine, which is incorporated into the DNA.

Because the primary spermatocytes are the cells that undergo the first meiotic division, their nuclear morphology reflects the events associated with this process. The prophase of the first division is characteristically of long duration, and cells in the phases of this process demonstrate nuclear features based on the appearance and morphology of the chromosomes. Condensation of chromosomes results in their appearance in the leptotene stage (Fig. 18) as single filamentous strands that have been shown by electron-microscopic studies to be attached at each end to the nuclear membrane by attachment plaques (129). These attachments probably represent the reasons for the "bouquet" arrangement of chromosomes seen in leptotene. Though at this stage the chromosomes are already composed of two chromatids, these do not become evident until later in prophase. The zygotene stage is characterized by thickening of the chromosomal elements that commence the process of pairing known as synapsis (Fig. 18). The mechanisms whereby homologous chromosomes recognize each other to pair as bivalents are still unknown.

The long pachytene stage commences with the completion of synapsis and is associated with further thickening and shortening of the chromosomes, which by careful study can be shown to be paired (130). During this phase, exchange of chromosomal material between maternal and paternal homologous chromosomes occurs by a "crossing-over," the chromosomes being linked at such sites by chiasmata. The pachytene phase is characterized by nuclear and cytoplasmic growth, resulting in these cells becoming the largest of the germ cell line. As desynapsis occurs during the next phase, known as diplotene, the paired chromosomes partially separate, but remain joined at their chiasmata. Subsequently, in the diakinetic phase, further shortening of chromosomes occurs, and they detach from the nuclear membrane. It is at this stage that each chromosome can be seen to be composed of two chromatids.

Diakinesis is rapidly followed by dissolution of the nuclear membrane, appearance of the spindle, and attachment of the bivalents to the equator of the spindle during metaphase. Anaphase subsequently results in the movement of each member of the bivalent to the opposite pole of the spindle, resulting in daughter cells, termed secondary spermatocytes, that contain the haploid number of chromosomes, each composed of two chromatids.

Fine Structure: Electron microscopy has added greatly to our knowledge of events in these cells. Moses (131) and Fawcett (132) independently described the existence of elements termed synaptinemal complexes in the nuclei of primary spermatocytes from a number of species. This complex consisted of two lateral elements that appeared as electron-dense fibrils equidistant from a central element consisting of a delicate linear region of increased electron density (Figs. 18 and 19). Woolam and Ford (133) suggested that the lateral elements represented cores of the paired chromosomes and that the central element was composed of microfibrillar processes that extended inward from each lateral element. These views were supported by the observation, from serial electron-microscopic reconstructions of the spermatocyte nucleus, that the number of synaptinemal complexes was equal to the number of bivalents (129).

Each lateral element first appears in the leptotene stage,

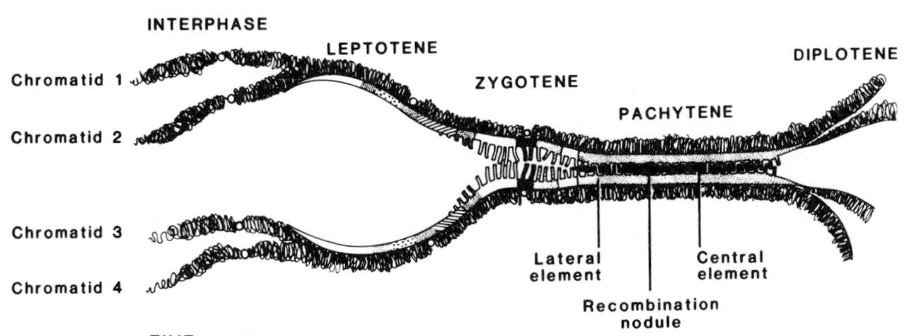

FIG. 18. The manner in which pairs of homologous chromosomes undergo synapsis during meiosis. Note how the lateral elements of the synaptinemal complex come together at pachytene, separating at the diplotene stage.

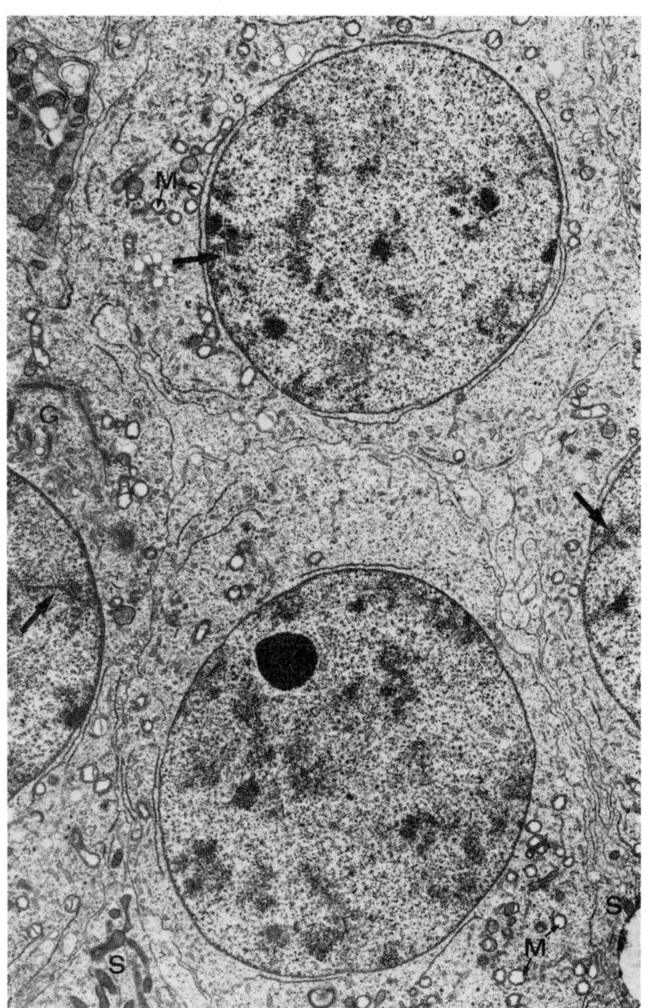

FIG. 19. Two human primary spermatocytes. Note mitochondria (M), Golgi complex (G), leptotene synaptinemal threads (*arrows*), and Sertoli cell cytoplasm (S).

representing elements of the single unpaired chromosomes that attach to the nuclear membrane at each end (134,135). Pairing of the elements commences in the zygotene stage, and fully formed synaptinemal complexes over the entire length of the chromosomes are seen in the pachytene stage. Study of these events has been greatly facilitated by the observation that the protein that forms the lateral elements of the complex stains with silver (136). The DNA of each chromosome forms a series of loops extending away from the lateral element, and the process of synapsis is associated with the assembly of the central component, probably by a recognition process involving proteins of the microfibrillar elements projecting centrally from the lateral elements (137,138). Though the synaptinemal complex provides the framework necessary for synapsis, it is thought that the recombination nodules are the vital components in the crossing-over of genetic material. These represent ellipsoidal-to-spherical protein globules approximately 90 nm in diameter that sit along the central portion of the synaptinemal complexes at a number of sites consistent with the number of chiasmata (Fig. 18). Events in the diplotene stage result in disruption of the synaptinemal complexes and separation of the bivalents, which still remain connected at chiasmata.

During meiosis, the sex chromosomes were noted by Painter (130) to be associated with a "chromatin nucleolus," a structure subsequently termed the sex vesicle, because it was shown not to represent a true nucleolus (139). It is formed at the end of leptotene and disappears after diakinesis, being ovoid in shape, with a diameter of 2 to 3 μm. It consists of an area of increased electron density composed of chromatin fibrils through which linear elements similar in appearance to the lateral elements of synaptinemal complexes are scattered (140–143). These take the form of linear arrays or circular profiles, and only occasional short full-formed synaptinemal complexes are seen. This is consistent with the behavior of the sex chromosomes, which pair only over relatively short portions of their length (144).

Nucleoli are frequently seen in primary spermatocytes and consist of peripherally placed collections of granules that are extremely electron-dense. These are sometimes associated with chromatin collections close to synaptinemal complexes.

A structure termed the "round body" has been found in spermatocyte nuclei (141,145), occurring as a spherical electron-dense structure adjacent to the nuclear membrane. It is composed of nonhistone protein; it appears in the leptotene stage and increases in size to 1.6 μm in diameter in the diplotene stage. It persists in secondary spermatocytes and spermatids, decreasing in size progressively, and disappearing at step 8 spermatids (145). Schultz and colleagues noted that nucleoli actively incorporated ^{3}H-thymidine while they were associated with a round body that was increasing in size, but not during its decline, thereby suggesting that the round body may be a controller of nucleolar activity in meiotic cells.

The cytoplasm of primary spermatocytes is more electron-dense than that of spermatogonia and contains evenly scattered polysomes and ribosomes (146). Profiles of rough or smooth endoplasmic reticulum are sparse, though as prophase progresses, the Golgi complex progressively enlarges. It is perinuclear in position and consists of concentric arrays of membranous lamellae and vesicles, some of which contain prominent electron-dense cores.

The mitochondria are ovoid (Fig. 19) and in the leptotene and zygotene stages are frequently aggregated into groups of two or three, with electron-dense mitochondrial material similar to that seen in spermatogonia (147,148). The intracristal spaces are dilated, and later in meiosis the cristae often are displaced toward the periphery as concentric membranous layers, leaving a central electron-lucid area.

Other types of collections of finely granular electron-dense material have been seen in spermatocytes and have been termed "nuage." Russell and Frank (148) have identified six types. Their exact role remains unclear, though one type is similar in appearance to the chromatid body

(149), and Russell and Frank have suggested that this structure disappears in the late diplotene stage, reforming by coalescence in secondary spermatocytes.

Unusual aggregations of parallel membranous lamellae or cisternae are seen, with the adjacent lamellae sometimes joined to each other at regular intervals by annuli. These resemble the structures termed annulate lamellae that are found in oocytes of many species (150). Similar aggregations have been observed adjacent to or often attached to the nuclear membrane, supporting the view that they originate from that site (151,152).

Primary spermatocytes are joined to each other by intercellular bridges similar to those found between spermatogonia. They are separated from adjacent Sertoli cells by distinct intercellular spaces that are modified in some regions by desmosome-like structures (153,154). As preleptotene spermatocytes lose their contact with the basement membrane, the processes of Sertoli cell cytoplasm that intervene develop specialized inter-Sertoli-cell junctions, as discussed later in this review (155).

Secondary Spermatocytes

These are the cells that undertake the second meiotic division. The first description of their characteristics is credited to von Ebner (156). The relatively infrequent appearances of these cells in sections of the testis and labeling studies with ^{3}H-thymidine (157) have shown that they have a short life-span before they complete meiosis to form spermatids. Montgomery (158) correctly noted that the secondary spermatocytes have the haploid number of chromosomes, though their DNA content is still diploid (Fig. 17), and when they complete meiosis the resultant spermatids have both the haploid DNA and haploid chromosomal content.

The cells are spherical, intermediate in size between primary spermatocytes and spermatids, with a diameter of 10 to 12 μm. They are situated close to the lumen of the seminiferous tubules, and their spherical nuclei contain a homogeneous chromatin network throughout which large globular chromatin masses are dispersed. Centrally placed nucleoli are often seen. Light- and electron-microscopic studies have shown that these cells are joined by intercellular bridges identical with those found between other germ cells (108,159,160).

Fine Structure: There have been few detailed studies of the ultrastructure of secondary spermatocytes, partly because of the difficulty of identifying sections of tubules within which they are present (147,160,161). Their cytoplasm contains scattered cisternal profiles of endoplasmic reticulum arranged concentrically around the nucleus. The Golgi complex is prominent and often contains vesicles demonstrating electron-dense granules. Collections of membranes with the features of annulate lamellae are found sometimes embedded in electron-dense granular material (151,160). The mitochondria are dispersed within the cytoplasm and show dilated intracristal spaces that result in the cristal membranes being pushed to the periphery of the organelle.

SPERMIOGENESIS

The transformation of spermatids to spermatozoa involves a fascinating but complex sequence of events that constitute the process of spermiogenesis. No cell division is involved, but the process is in essence a metamorphosis in which a conventional cell is converted into a highly organized motile structure. The major features of spermiogenesis are common to all species, but the details vary for each species because there are distinguishing morphological features between spermatozoa determined by genetic factors. Many aspects are visible by light microscopy, but the finer details require the magnification of the electron microscope. Hence, in this section of the review, the light- and electron-microscopic features are described together (Figs. 20 and 21). For convenience, it is possible to divide the cytological changes during spermiogenesis into a series of developmental steps involving different cellular organelles, but it is important to recognize that some steps occur contemporaneously. The changes can be grouped into (a) formation of the acrosome, (b) nuclear changes, (c) development of the flagellum, (d) reorganization of the cytoplasm and cell organelles, and (e) spermiation relationships of the Sertoli cells and spermatids.

Spermatids, like other germ cells, were named by von La Valette St. George (162), and some investigators use the term "spermateliosis" as an alternative to "spermiogenesis." A number of early studies described the general changes characterizing spermiogenesis (100,126,163–165), and these were expanded and utilized by Clermont (166–168) in developing a classification for the stages of spermiogenesis. This classification was aided by the demonstration that the acrosome stained clearly with the PAS reaction.

Recently formed spermatids are spherical cells that are smaller in size than secondary spermatocytes and are found at the luminal aspect of the seminiferous epithelium. The spermatid has a centrally placed spherical nucleus, a well-developed Golgi complex, and adjacent centrioles. The mitochondria are dispersed and lie peripherally close to the plasma membrane. Additionally, a chromophilic, electron-dense mass, the chromatid body, can be observed adjacent to the Golgi complex in a perinuclear location (166,169).

Formation of the Acrosome

This structure arises from the Golgi complex, a fact established in this century by Bowen (170,171) from studies in mammals and other classes. Gatenby and Beams (165) identified "proacrosomic" granules in the Golgi regions of primary spermatocytes, though it is still unclear today whether or not the granules in these cells are transmitted to daughter

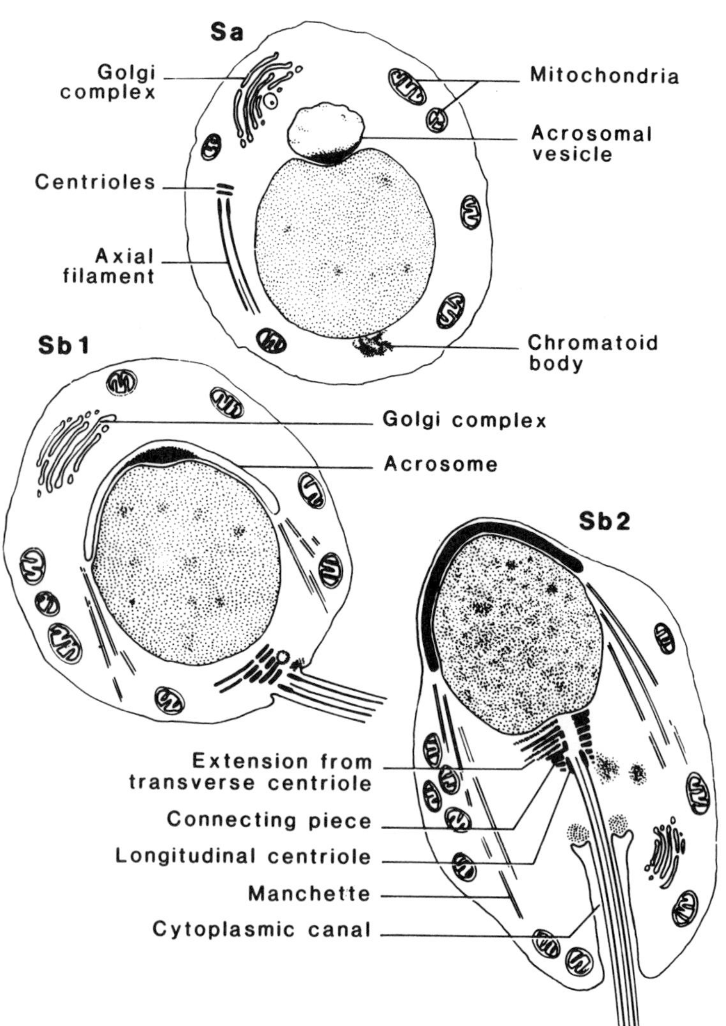

FIG. 20. Electron-microscopic features of the stages of human spermiogenesis (Sa to Sb_2). (From ref. 774.)

cells; more likely they represent some form of secretory protein that is packaged in the Golgi complex (Figs. 22 and 23). These investigators noted that similar granules were elaborated in the Golgi apparatus of newly formed spermatids, and the vacuole and granule were deposited at one pole of the nucleus, where they spread out to form the acrosome cap. Gatenby and Beams (165) noted that once the acrosomal cap had been formed, the remainder of the Golgi complex passed to the opposite pole of the spermatid.

This view concerning the formation of the acrosome was confirmed by early electron-microscopic studies (172–174). Several proacrosomic granules are often elaborated in the Golgi complex, coalescing to form a single large granule that comes into contact with the nuclear membrane (Fig. 22). It is closely applied as a cap-like structure spreading over approximately 25% to 60% of the nuclear surface. During this phase, additional material appears to be transferred from the Golgi complex to the acrosome by vesicles, a process recently analyzed in considerable detail (175–177). The Golgi complex has been divided into cortical and medullary zones, the cortex being limited externally by cisternae of rough endoplasmic reticulum. The transition from cortex to medulla is marked by a change from cisternal profiles to vesicles, and it is from this aspect that vesicles are transported to the acrosomal cap. Clermont and Tang (177) showed that glycoproteins are transferred from the Golgi complex to the acrosome, and this accumulation occurs slowly (1 hr) in comparison with other cells (2–10 min) (178,179).

For a time, the acrosome contains a centralized electron-dense granule and a less electron-dense periphery, but in the human this difference is progressively lost as the cap spreads over the nuclear surface (Fig. 24). In other species, this zonal arrangement persists for a longer period of time. In many species, such as the guinea pig, chinchilla, and ground squirrel, a conspicuous thickening of the acrosomal cap extends beyond the nucleus (Fig. 25) and is termed the apical segment (180), but the reasons for this specialization remain unknown. Similarly, the caudal region of the acrosome in many species is partly attenuated and is termed the equatorial segment, and in the human some lamination has been noted in this area (181,182). Though the reason for this specialization is unknown, this region of the acrosome persists after the remainder of the acrosomal contents

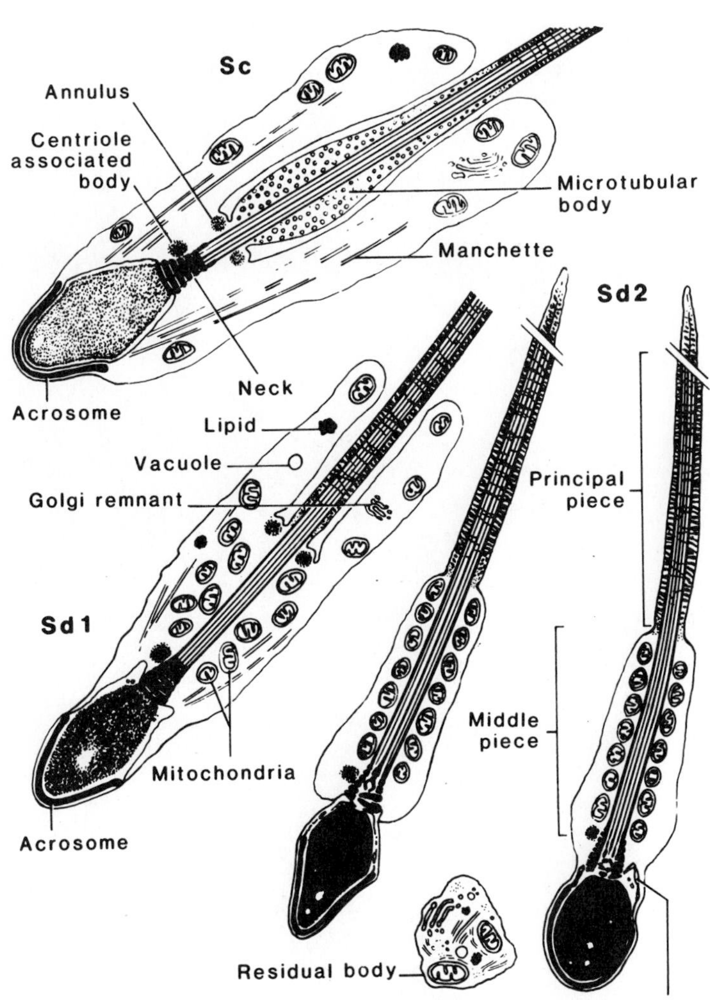

FIG. 21. Electron-microscopic features of the stages of human spermiogenesis (Sc to Sd_2). (From ref. 774.)

are lost following the acrosomal reaction (183). Furthermore, it represents the region in which binding occurs to the cell membrane of the oocyte during fertilization (184). The size of the acrosome varies significantly between species, being closely applied to the nucleus in humans, but being very large and elaborate in species such as the guinea pig (185,186). Furthermore, modifications to this structure may occur after spermatozoa leave the epithelium and pass through the epididymis (185). The glycoprotein nature of the acrosome is consistent with the observation that it contains a variety of lysosomal enzymes important for penetration of the zona pellucida of the ovum and other specific proteins such as acrosin (187,188).

With subsequent changes in nuclear position, the acrosome is closely applied to the cell membrane of the spermatid. Between the inner acrosomal membrane and nuclear membrane, the human spermatid contains a thin layer of moderately electron-dense material (Fig. 24) that Bedford (189) has suggested represents the perforatorium. The subacrosomal space contains a variable amount of electron-dense material whose organization differs markedly between species. In rodents, this space is extensive, particularly at the cranial aspect, and the material is organized to form a rod-like perforatorium that appears to be prolonged backward over the nucleus as three prongs, possibly thickenings of the nuclear membrane (190,191) (Figs. 26 and 27). In the toad, the perforatorium consists of strands of electron-dense material in the subacrosomal space (192), and a similar structure has since been found in many species (193,194). Some investigators have postulated a mechanical role for the perforatorium, and others have suggested that it carries a lysin distinct from that found in the acrosome (195). Recently, actin has been identified as a component of the subacrosomal space (196).

Nuclear Changes

In the majority of species, the nucleus changes position during spermiogenesis from a central to an eccentric position. The region of the nucleus that first comes into close apposition with the cell membrane is that segment covered with the developing acrosomal cap. Subsequently, during the rearrangement of spermatid cytoplasm, larger segments

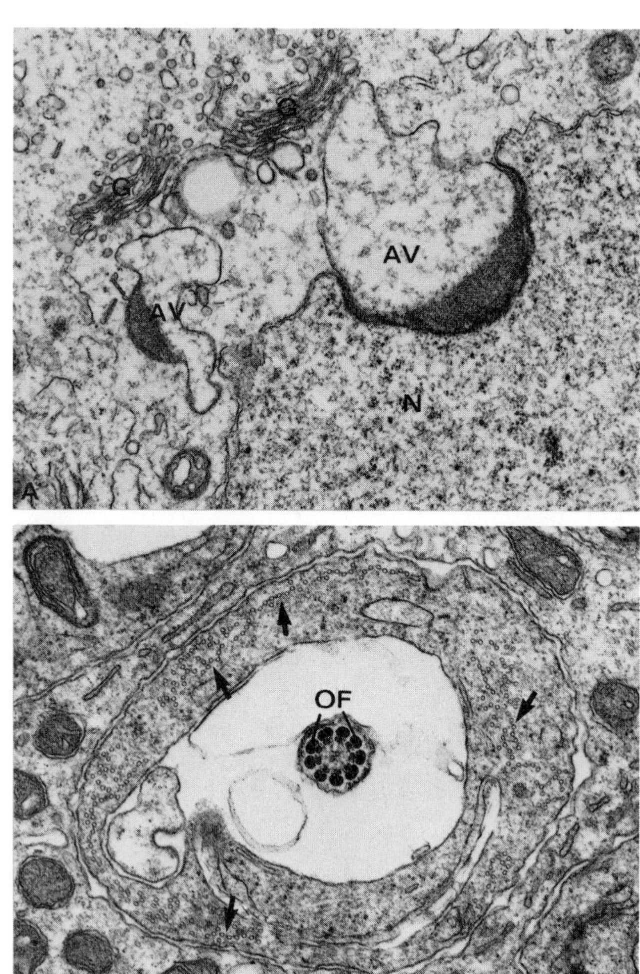

FIG. 22. A: Developing acrosomal cap of a human spermatid. Note nucleus (N), Golgi complex (G), and acrosomal vesicle (AV). B: Axial filament of a spermatid. Note outer dense fibers (OF) surrounding the 9 + 2 microtubular structure. The surrounding spermatid cytoplasm contains the microtubules of the manchette (*arrows*).

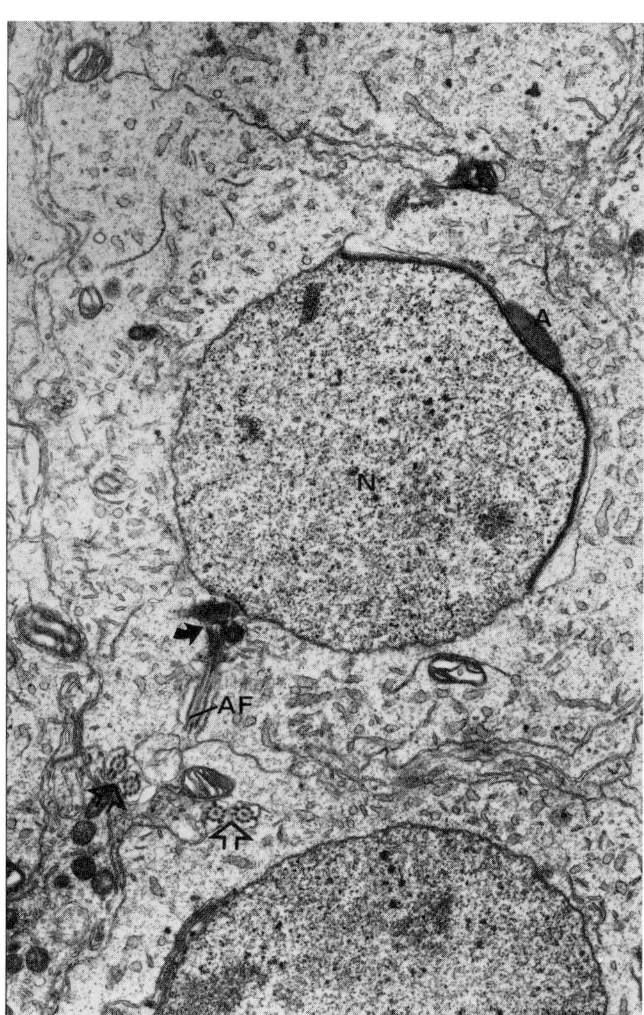

FIG. 23. A human spermatid (Stage Sb_1) shows acrosome (A), nucleus (N), developing connecting piece (*arrow*), and axial filament (AF and *open arrow*).

of the nucleus come into close association with the plasma membrane.

Associated with the change in nuclear position there is a progressive condensation of chromatin to form larger and more electron-dense granules. These increase in number and condense to eventually form an osmiophilic electron-dense homogeneous mass. The degree of condensation can vary with species and is particularly variable in human spermiogenesis (175,197,198). In the rat there is a progressive pattern of development that is not complete until late in spermiogenesis (Figs. 26 and 27). Together with the acrosomal modifications, the final structure of the head of the rat spermatid takes some time to evolve (191). Additionally, in humans, electron-lucid spaces occur within the nucleus that, though not limited by a membrane, are termed nuclear vacuoles (192).

The coalescence of chromatin granules is associated with

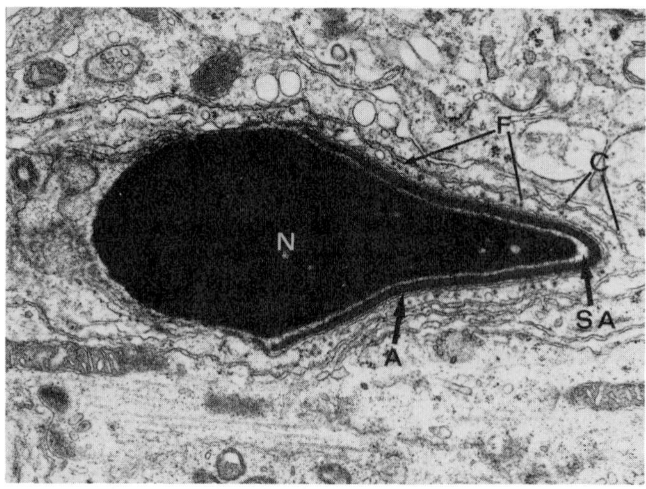

FIG. 24. The human spermatid head is composed of the nucleus (N), acrosome (A), and subacrosomal space (SA). Note the cisternae (C) delineating a zone of Sertoli cell cytoplasm containing fibrils (F).

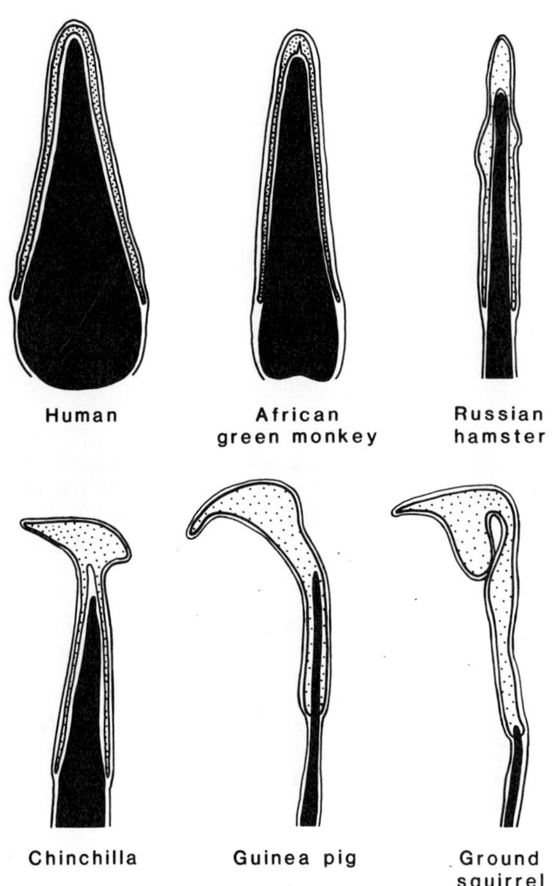

FIG. 25. Variations in shape of the components of the heads of spermatozoa from a number of species. (Some views from refs. 189 and 204.)

ill-defined chemical changes in the DNA, which is stabilized and is resistant to digestion by the enzyme DNAase (169,199). This stabilization occurs at a time when lysine-rich histones are being replaced by arginine-rich histones in the spermatid nuclei, the lysine-rich protein accumulating subsequently in the sphere chromatophile, a component of the residual body of spermatids (200). More extensive studies of nuclear proteins have shown dramatic changes: the presence of a single species of species-specific protamine, rich in arginine and cysteine, the presence of a number of nonprotamine proteins, and the transient appearance of several basic nuclear proteins, the latter of which may be associated with the initiation of chromatin condensation of spermatids (201–203). These changes and the loss of virtually all nonhistone nuclear proteins late in spermiogenesis occur at a time of complete repression of gene transcription and shaping of the sperm nucleus (204,205).

During the chromatin condensation there are progressive reductions in nuclear volume and, in some species, dramatic changes in shape to result in sperm heads with shapes characteristic for each species (204,206). These striking differences in head shape have prompted investigators to seek the mechanisms responsible. The appearance of a microtubular sheath termed the manchette (*vide infra*) close to the nucleus at a time when significant elongation and shaping occur (Fig. 28) led a number of investigators to suggest a causal relationship (207,208). However, on the basis of their detailed studies, Fawcett et al. (204) could not support this view. They noted that significant variations in the form of the manchette did not occur, a fact that would be necessary to explain the nuclear changes if they were causally related. They noted the observations of Beatty (209) that head shape could vary between strains of the same species and could be varied experimentally by selective breeding. In view of this and their own observations, they proposed that the remarkable diversity of head shape is the result of genetically determined patterns of the molecular aggregation that takes place during chromatin condensation.

The reduction in nuclear volume is associated with a probable loss of materials from the nucleus via nuclear poles (197) and also results in the formation of redundant folds of nuclear membrane (198,210). This is most evident at the abacrosomal pole of the nucleus, where these folds are separated from the condensed chromatin by an electron-lucid zone containing flocculent material. In this region the nuclear membrane is studded with nuclear pores and frequently exhibits the formation of lamellae and vesicles, the latter containing flocculent material (Fig. 24).

Formation of the Tail

The concept that the sperm tail arose from the centrioles of the spermatid was recognized by Meves (163,164), who noted that the two centrioles moved to the periphery of the cell, where the axial filament arose from the more peripherally placed centriole. These observations were substantiated by other investigators early in this century (100, 158,165). However, Gatenby and Beams (165) implicated both centrioles in the formation of the axial filament and noted that the flagellum moved inward toward the nucleus, where the complex lodged at its caudal pole opposite the developing acrosome. Some confusion, however, arose from these early studies, because the structures involved in development of the tail were difficult to observe because they are near the limit of resolution of the light microscope.

The early electron-microscopic studies confirmed that the central core of the sperm tail, the axial filament, arose from the pair of centrioles lodged at the periphery of the spermatid cytoplasm and subsequently moved centrally to be lodged at the caudal pole of the nucleus (192). Both Anberg (211) and Fawcett (212) noted the presence of a centriole within the connecting piece of the neck in human spermatozoa and termed it the proximal or transverse centriole. However, they failed to find evidence of the distal or longitudinal centriole. Fawcett (212) also showed that the structure termed the ring centriole by light microscopists is represented in ultrastructural studies as the annulus that marks the caudal limit of the middle piece of the tail.

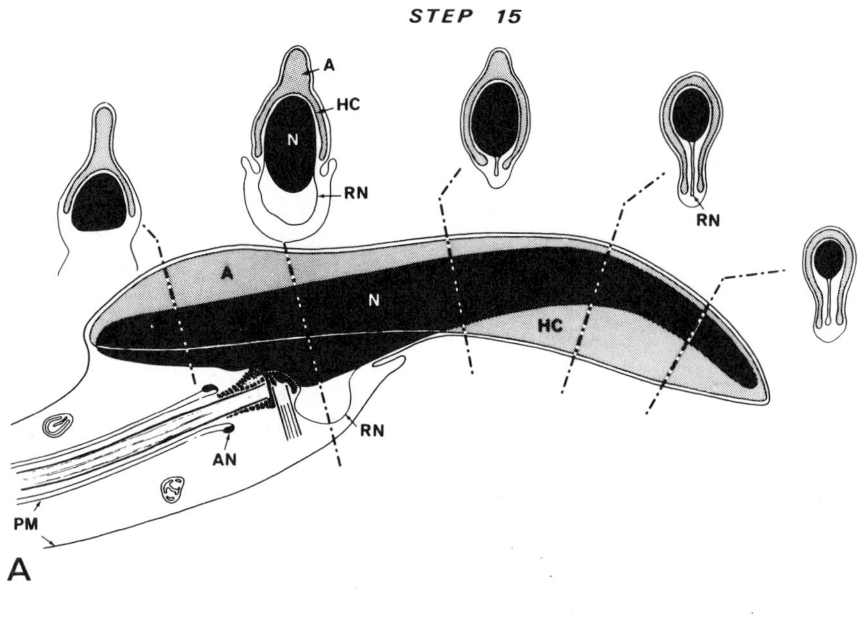

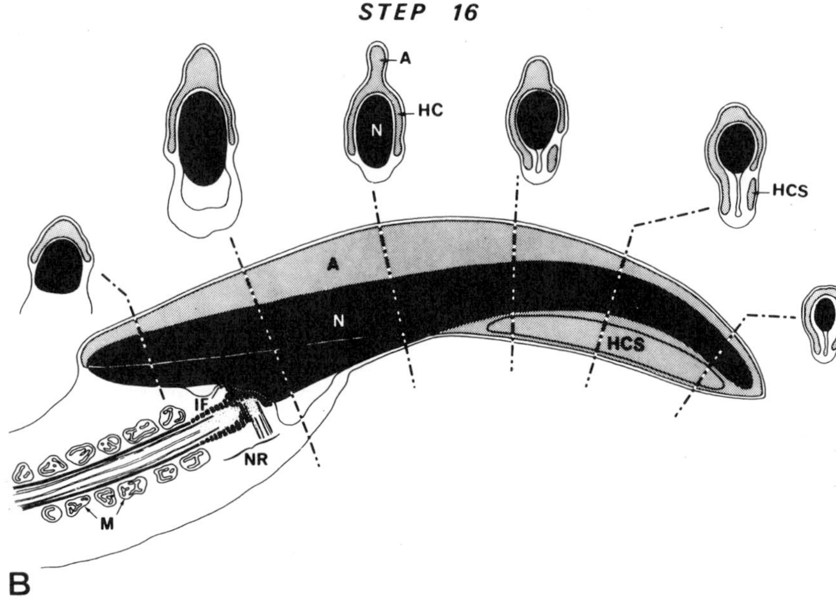

FIG. 26. Diagram demonstrating the changes occurring in the relationships and shapes of the structures composing the head of the rat spermatid during spermiogenesis at stages 15 and 16: A, acrosome; AN, annulus; AX, axoneme; HC, head cap; HCS, separated head-cap segment; IF implantation fossa; M, mitochondria; N, nucleus; NR, neck region; PM, plasma membrane; RN, redundant nuclear envelope. (From ref. 191.)

More recent studies have confirmed that the axial filament arises from the distal or longitudinal centriole and that this basic structure is modified by specialization in the different regions of the sperm tail. The subsequent description of cytological events is most easily subdivided into (a) development of the axial filament, (b) formation of the neck or connecting piece, (c) formation of the dense fiber system, (d) development of the principal piece, and (e) formation of the middle piece.

Development of the Axial Filament

Several studies have shown that axial filament develops from the centriole, which is aligned to the axis of the flagellum and is termed the longitudinal or distal centriole (198,213,214). The other centriole is oriented perpendicular to the axial filament and is termed the proximal or transverse centriole. The basic structure of the axial filament is common to flagella and cilia and consists of nine peripheral doublet microtubules arranged equidistant from each other around a circle at whose center two single microtubules are found (Figs. 22 and 29).

The doublets consist of two subfibers, one of which (subfiber A) is a complete microtubule and is circular in cross section, whereas the other (subfiber B) is C-shaped, the concavity of the C being attached to subfiber A (206). The walls of both subfibers are composed of protofilaments of tubulin (215–217). The axoneme demonstrates a highly organized substructure that is described in more detail by

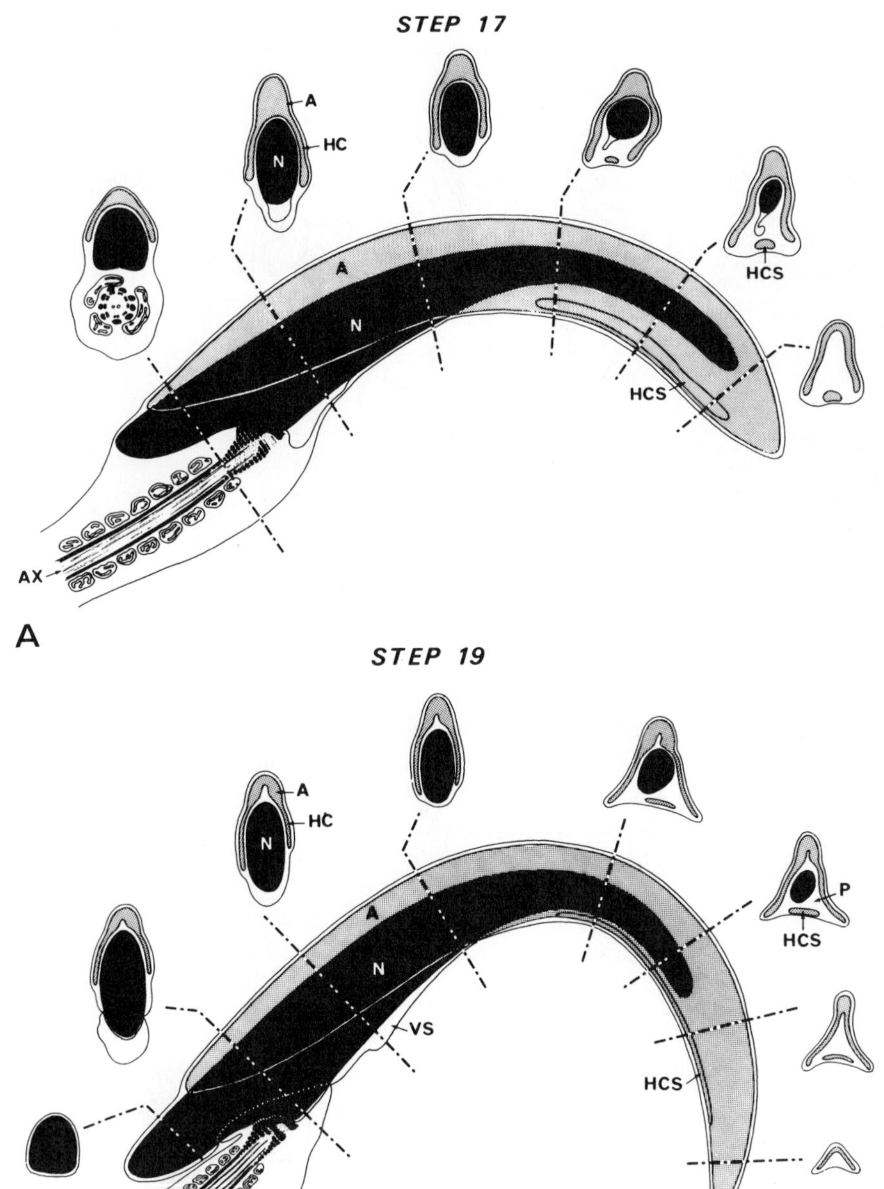

FIG. 27. Diagram demonstrating the changes occurring in the relationships and shapes of the structures composing the head of the rat spermatid during spermiogenesis at stages 17 and 19: A, acrosome; AX, axoneme; HC, head cap; HCS, separated head-cap segment; M, mitochondria; N, nucleus; P, perforatorium; PM, plasma membrane; VS, ventral spur. (From ref. 191.)

E. M. Eddy (Chapter 2, *these volumes*). Briefly, subfiber A extends a pair of hook-like arms that project toward subfiber B of the adjacent doublet; these extensions, termed dynein arms, are composed of a protein, dynein, with ATPase activity (218).

Additional links between the doublets are provided by nexin links (219), and the doublets are connected to the helical sheath surrounding the two central microtubules by radial spokes (220). The nature of the substructure of the flagellum has taken on additional significance because of genetically determined abnormalities in its structure that result in immotility of sperm and consequent infertility (221,222).

Fawcett (206) proposed a numbering system for the doublets, designating the doublet bisected by a plane passing between the central two microtubules as doublet 1 and the other sequentially in a clockwise direction.

Development of the axial filament commences early in spermiogenesis, and it projects from the surface of a round spermatid, the microtubular core being separated from a finger-like protrusion of the cell membrane by a thin layer of cytoplasm. An invagination of the cell membrane forms a cleft, the cytoplasmic canal, which surrounds the proximal portion of the axial filament and whose proximal limit is formed by the attachment of the annulus (213). Later, the centriolar complex and axial filament become lodged at the

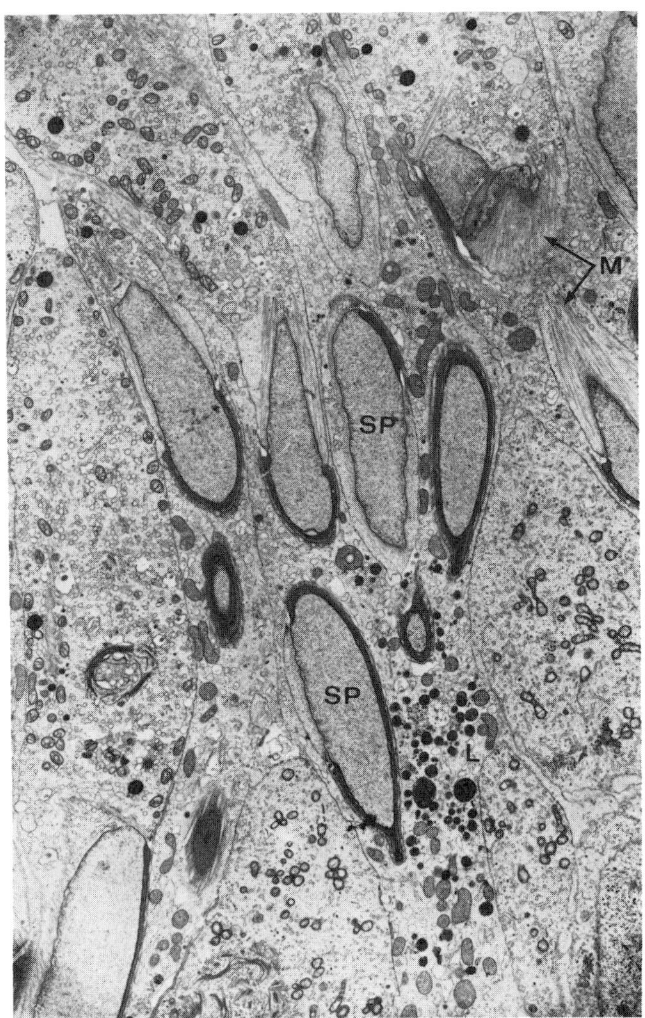

FIG. 28. Rat seminiferous epithelium, illustrating elongated spermatids (SP) and the manchette (M). The Sertoli cell cytoplasm contains numerous lysosomes (L).

abacrosomal pole of the nucleus to form the neck or connecting piece, the complex articulation of the future head and tail of the spermatozoon (Fig. 23). Recently, flagellum formation has been successfully initiated by *in vitro* culture of spermatids (223).

Formation of the Neck or Connecting Piece

The final form of the connecting piece varies significantly between species, but in all mammalian forms a basic structural organization can be discerned. The connecting piece can be regarded as a truncated cone, modified to contain the proximal and distal centrioles (Fig. 30). The truncated apex points distally, and from it emerges the tail of the sperm. The base forms an arched sheet, termed the capitulum, composed of electron-dense material, that is lodged

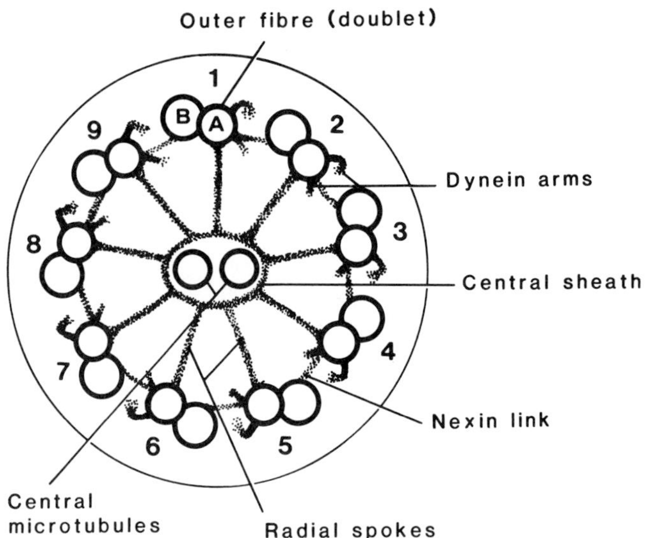

FIG. 29. Diagram illustrating the components of the axial filament when cut in perfect cross section.

in a shallow depression called the implantation fossa in the caudal pole of the nucleus. The truncated apex of the cone surrounds the distal or longitudinal centriole from which the axial filament of the tail is derived. Superior or rostral to the distal centriole, the conical structure surrounds the proximal centriole, which lies at an angle of 75° to 90° to the longitudinal axis of the sperm tail, except in one region opposite its distal end, from which an extension, termed the centriolar adjunct, emerges (Figs. 30 and 31). The actual

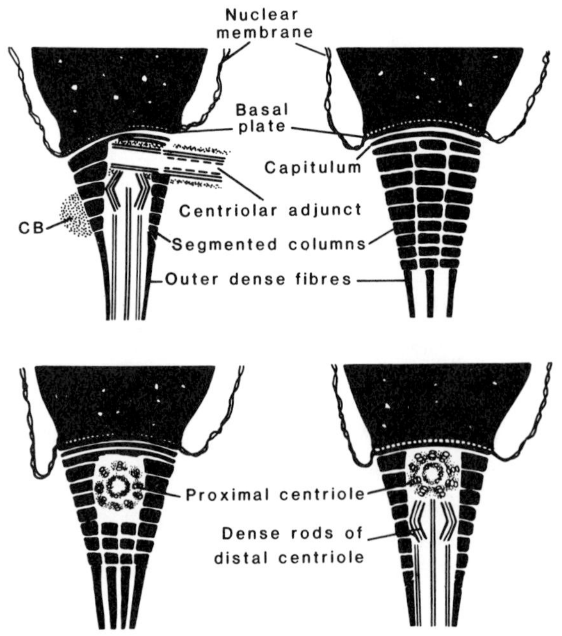

FIG. 30. Diagram illustrating the relationships of the components of the neck of the human spermatid during spermiogenesis. The different appearances indicate the views seen depending on the plane of section.

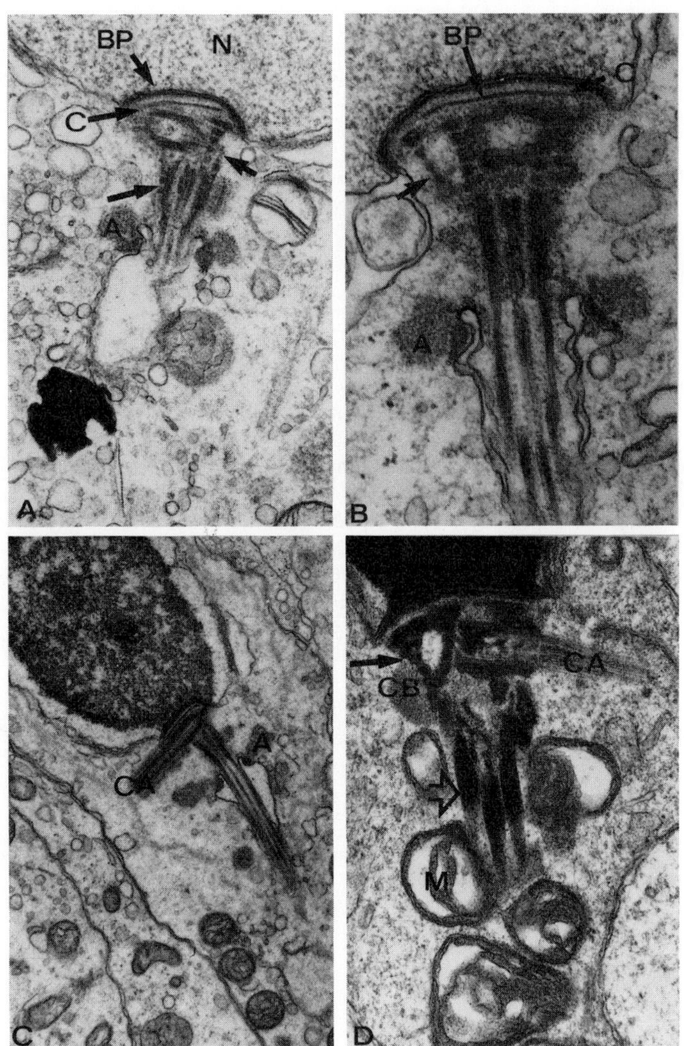

FIG. 31. Developing connecting piece of the human spermatid shown at the Sb_2 **(A, B)**, Sc **(C)**, and Sd_2 stages **(D)**. Note progressive condensation of the nucleus (N). Also shown are basal plate (BP), capitulum (C), segmented columns of connecting piece (*arrows*), annulus (A), centriolar adjunct (CA), centriole-associated body (CB), mitochondrial sheath (M), and outer dense fibers of the middle piece (*open arrow*).

structure of the wall of the truncated cone is dependent on the level at which it is examined. The truncated apex at the level of the distal centriole is composed of nine longitudinal cross-striated columns, which cranially fuse to varying degrees. Those columns opposite the centriolar extension coalesce and lose their individuality and together with the others, except those interrupted by the centriolar adjunct on extension, extend cranially to fuse with the capitulum.

The development of the connecting piece commences in round or Golgi-phase spermatids prior to the association of the developing axial filament with the nucleus. Although the ultimate structure of the connecting piece varies considerably between species, there is general agreement as to the roles played by the proximal and distal centrioles during its formation, based on detailed studies of this region during spermiogenesis in a number of different species (160, 198,214). During formation of the connecting piece, the nine cross-striated columns arise from electron-dense material that accumulates adjacent to the triplets of the distal centriole (Fig. 32). This material is augmented by material of similar appearance that develops adjacent to the triplets of the proximal centriole and also extends to contribute to the capitulum. The cross-banding of these fibers is relatively imprecise early in spermiogenesis, but becomes quite evident later in the process (214). The dimensions of the cross-striated columns usually are smaller in the region of the distal centriole, expanding to varying degrees, depending on the species, as they pass rostrally to insert into the basal plate of the implantation fossa. The latter occurs except for those columns that are interrupted by the extension from the proximal centriole, termed the centriolar adjunct, which takes the form of a "miniflagellum" extending into the cytoplasm adjacent to the neck of the spermatid (Fig. 33). The cross-striated columns adjacent to the proximal centriole opposite the centriolar adjunct tend to lose their individuality, fusing together to variable degrees.

"Centriolar adjunct" is preferred as the term to denote the structure that emerges from the distal end of the proximal centriole, because it is not a direct extension of the triplet structure of the centriole (214). The centriolar adjunct extends into the cytoplasm adjacent to the neck of the spermatid (198). This extension retains the basic organiza-

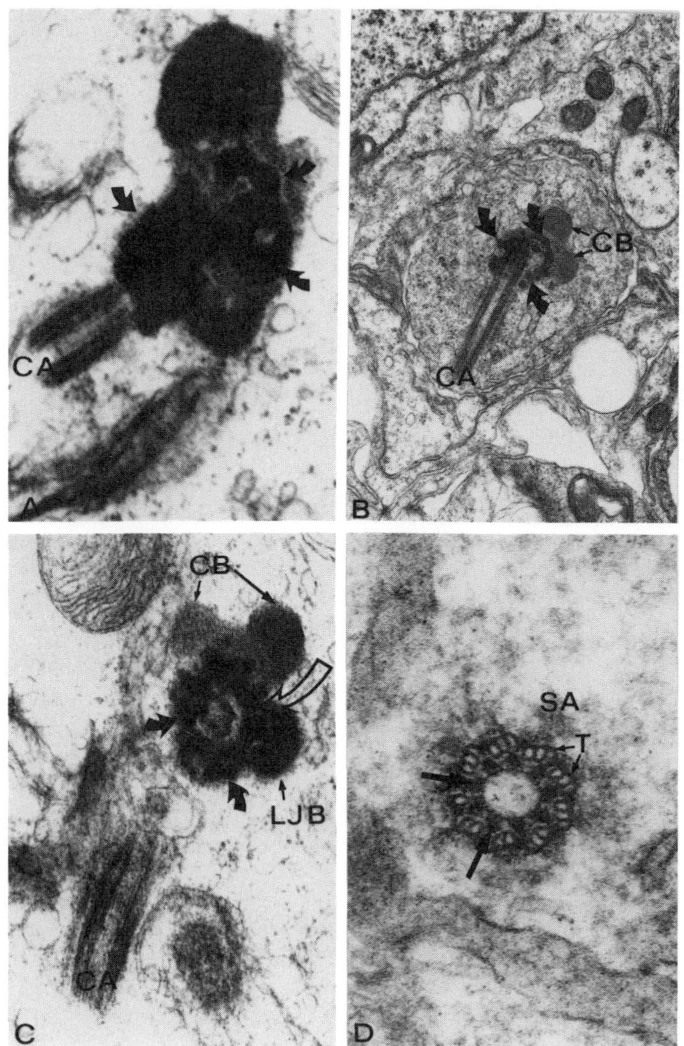

FIG. 32. Micrographs **(A–C)** illustrating sections taken at approximately right angles to the axial filament, at progressively descending levels of the connecting piece of the spermatid. Note the columns of the connecting piece (*large arrows*), centriolar adjunct (CA), triplets of longitudinal centriole (*open arrow,* **C**), centriole-associated body (CB), and lateral junctional body (LJB). **D:** Section at right angles through the centriolar adjunct showing triplets (T) of proximal centriole (T), satellite arms (SA), and the inner ring (*arrows*).

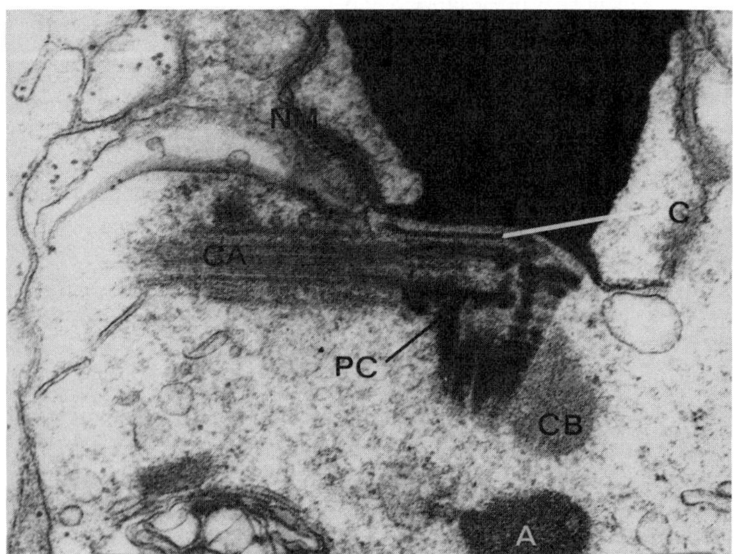

FIG. 33. The neck of the developing human spermatid at the Sd_1 stage shows the proximal centriole (PC), centriolar adjunct (CA), capitulum (C), centriole-associated body (CB), annulus (A), and nuclear membrane (NM).

tion of the centriole, with the nine triplets forming a major part of the adjunct (Figs. 32 and 33). However, the outer pair of subunits, termed B and C, of the triplets are incomplete, presenting a J-shaped profile (214). Within this ring of nine modified triplets, a second ring of nine collections of minute tubular units is found (160,198). These collections are not continuous, because longitudinal views of the centriolar adjunct demonstrate distinct breaks, suggesting a series of 10 to 14 rings in human spermatids (160). Internal to these collections, a circular rim of tubular profiles surrounds an empty cylindrical space.

External to the modified triplets, moderately electron-dense material is organized to form satellite arms (160). Despite its structural similarity to a centriole, the centriolar adjunct appears to lack the capacity to organize cross-striated material (214). The purpose of forming a centriolar adjunct remains obscure, but it may represent a response of the proximal centriole to influences that cause the distal centriole to form the axial filament. Later in spermatogenesis, the adjunct disappears, and it is only occasionally observed in ejaculated spermatozoa.

The structure of the distal centriole is significantly modified during spermiogenesis, and in some species no evidence of its structure is discernible in mature spermatozoa (224). Early in spermiogenesis, periodic densities can be observed in the walls of the distal centriole and adjacent cytoplasm that are the precursors of the distal ends of the longitudinal cross-striated columns of the connecting piece (Fig. 23). The electron-dense material accumulates around the triplets of the centriole and appears to expand the diameter of the centriole (214). The dense material extends outward between the triplets forming the longitudinal columns of the connecting piece (Fig. 32). Additionally, two paired rod-like masses develop between the centriole wall and the central pair of microtubules of the axial filament that traverse this region to make contact with the proximal centriole (214). In humans, these dense rods appear to consist of two electron-dense laminae separated by an electron-lucent region, and they bow symmetrically (160).

There is general agreement that the distal centriole does not give rise to the nine outer dense fibrils that characterize the middle piece of the spermatozoon (214,225). They arise in continuity with the doublet microtubules of the axial filament and diverge cranially to appear as separate entities (214,226). They develop out of synchrony with the longitudinal striated columns of the connecting piece, but the two systems are closely apposed at an oblique junction at the level of the distal centriole.

Although the method of formation of the connecting piece has been elucidated, the actual mechanisms remain unknown. Fawcett and Phillips (214) proposed that the centrioles act as sites of assembly of precursor molecules formed by normal mechanisms of ribosomal protein synthesis and that the nine striated columns originally present in the developing connecting piece are an expression of the nine-part symmetry of the centriole established by the nine triplets. Fawcett and Phillips (214) have suggested that the cross-striated appearance of the columns is due to the alignment of successive segments of cross-straited fibers composed of a fibrous protein, with a repeating period of 665 Å measured from the middle of one light band to the corresponding next light band. The dark segments demonstrate less obvious banding, each exhibiting 10 minor bands similar to the cross-striated elements of goshopod spermatozoa (227). The source of precursor material remains conjectural, but several electron-dense aggregations of fibrillar-granular material are seen in the vicinity of the developing connecting piece. In human spermatozoa, one of these consists of electron-dense granular material that is found associated with one side of the distal centriole and often exhibits a less dense central zone (198). It is also present in bandicoot (*Perameles nasuta*) spermatids and was termed the lateral junctional body by Sapsford et al. (213).

The lateral junctional body appears early in spermiogenesis prior to the articulation of the developing tail with the nucleus (Figs. 30–32). A second, roughly spherical body, slightly less electron-dense than the lateral junctional body, is seen at the same level, closely associated with the distal centriole, and it has been termed the centriole-associated body (198). In some views, the finely granular material demonstrates periodicity, giving the appearance of linear arrays (160). Both the centriole-associated body and lateral junctional body disappear very late in spermiogenesis.

A third structure of moderate electron density is the annulus, which also appears early in spermiogenesis at the stage in which the intracytoplasmic portion of the axial filament is largely exteriorized. This occurs by the formation of a cleft termed the cytoplasmic canal, which results in an invagination of the cell membrane around the flagellum. The annulus forms a ring-shaped structure that limits the proximal boundary of the cytoplasmic canal. Early in spermiogenesis it is relatively small, but it is augmented later by yet another structure, the chromatid body, which has migrated from the vicinity of the Golgi complex to the region of the annulus (149). Here it forms a relatively large ring-shaped electron-dense granular structure that is in contact with the annulus and in some views appears to contribute material to that structure. The combined annulus and ring-shaped chromatid body correspond to what was termed by early investigators the "ring centriole." Fawcett et al. (149) noted a progressive decrease in size of the chromatid body, with its eventual disappearance, whereas others suggested that it was lost in the residual body (228). The actual nature of the chromatid body is under debate. Early work suggested that it contained basic proteins and might be a source of RNA (169,229,230); however, Eddy (231) was not able to confirm this conclusion. More recently, Walt and Armbuster (232) again proposed that RNA is found in the chromatid body and also demonstrated that it contains actin, perhaps reflecting its remarkable motility in spermatids.

The form of the annulus varies among species (225). In some, such as humans, guinea pig, chinchilla, mouse, and ram, the ring-shaped electron density has a convex outer border in contact with the cell membrane in a fold at the proximal limit of the cytoplasmic canal (Fig. 34). Its free edge is in contact rostrally with the lower edge of the mitochondrial helix of the middle piece. In other species (dormouse, Chinese hamster, suni antelope) the annulus is wedge-shaped, located at the proximal limit of the cytoplasmic canal, and its apex extends toward the axial filament.

The articulation of the connecting piece with the nucleus occurs at the implantation fossa. In this region the nuclear membranes are closely apposed, separated by a space of 60 to 80 Å that in favorable views is crossed by uniformly spaced densities perhaps indicating structures that bind the membranes together (225). The outer nuclear membrane appears thickened by the deposition of electron-dense material to form the basal plate (Figs. 30 and 31). The anlage of the connecting piece lodges in the implantation fossa in such a manner that the capitulum is aligned parallel to the basal plate, but separated from it by an electron-lucent space approximately 400 Å wide. Fawcett and Phillips (214) observed many fine filaments traversing this zone, oriented perpendicular to the capitulum and basal plate, and they suggested that these were responsible for attaching the flagellum to the head.

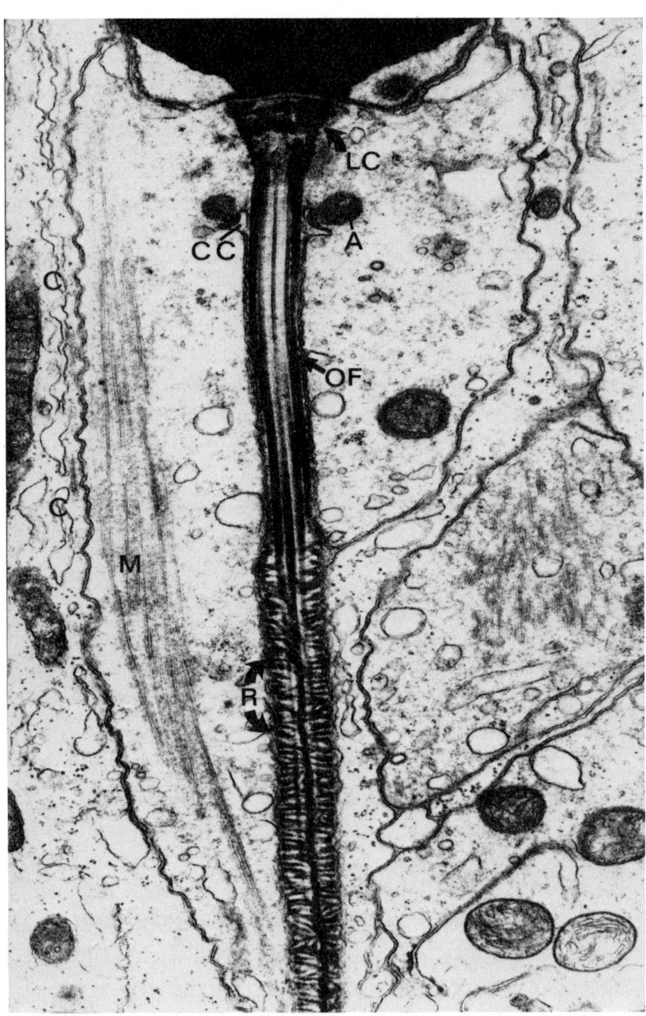

FIG. 34. The structure of the developing human spermatid at the Sd_1 stage is shown, illustrating the longitudinal segmented columns (LC), annulus (A), cytoplasmic canal (CC), outer dense fibers (OF), ribs (R) of principal piece, and manchette (M). Note the cisternae (C) delineating a mantle of Sertoli cell cytoplasm containing fibrils.

Formation of the Dense Fiber System

Over a large portion, the axial filament is modified by the development of a set of nine electron-dense fibers termed the outer dense fiber system (Figs. 22 and 34). They appear to develop as very thin fibers that are attached to the outer wall of the doublet microtubules of the axial filament (214). They appear to separate proximally to develop further as independent fibers by further accretion of material. This relationship to the doublets of the axoneme persists, with the outer dense fibers being separated by a greater distance from the doublets cranially, whereas distally they retain their close association with the doublets and taper to eventually disappear. Recently, Irons and Clermont (233) have shown that ^{3}H-proline and ^{3}H-cystine are incorporated into the outer dense fiber system over an extensive period of spermatid development from step 8 to step 19, indicating the presence of a peak of protein synthetic activity in midspermiogenesis. This view is supported by the studies of O'Brien and Bellve (234), who approached the problem in the mouse by different techniques.

There are significant differences in regard to size and length of the outer dense fiber system between species (206,211). In human sperm, the outer fibers end in the proximal part of the principal piece, fibers 3 and 8 being the first to terminate. In some, they are prominent and extend throughout the middle piece and principal piece, whereas in others they terminate more proximally. Unlike the doublets of the axial filament, which are similar in size and appearance, the outer dense fiber system, numbered according to the adjacent doublet, shows significant differences in size (206). Fibers 1, 5, and 6 are usually larger in many species.

Telkka et al. (235) showed that the outer dense fibers possess cortical and central zones that differ in electron density. The portion of the cortical zone immediately adjacent to the axial filament consists of electron-dense punctate granules in guinea pig spermatozoa, leading Fawcett (206) to call them satellite fibrils. The outer dense fiber system must be considered as a set of structures independent of the striated fibers of the connecting piece, because they develop independently and asynchronously (214). However, they do join each other at the lower level of the connecting piece at an oblique junction.

Development of the Principal Piece

The region of the tail between the annulus and the termination of the fibrous sheath or tail helix is termed the principal piece (212). The presence of a fibrous sheath is peculiar to mammalian spermatozoa, and early ultrastructural studies demonstrated that the sheath was not helical, but consisted of a series of rib-like structures joined to two longitudinal columns (212,236) (Fig. 35). The closely spaced ribs sometimes branch, attaching to adjacent ribs. Proximally the longitudinal columns consist of the outer dense fibers 3 and 8, but these terminate distally, and the ribs are attached to a thin electron-dense ridge that projects from doublets 3 and 8. The longitudinal columns vary in prominence with species, being well developed in rodents but insignificant in humans (211,212,235).

In the human, the anlage of the fibrous sheath appears to be a system of transversely oriented microtubules (198). The hollow cores of these tubules are progressively obliterated by an electron-dense material, a process that gives rise to the transversely oriented ribs (Fig. 36). Progressive addition of electron-dense material thickens the ribs. More extensive studies of the development of the principal piece in human spermatids have confirmed the microtubular origin of the ribs (237), showing that a large accumulation of microtubules occurs in the region of the developing principal piece (Fig. 37) to form a "microtubular body" at the equivalent of Sc spermatids (168). Subsequently, with elongation of the axial filament and distal migration of the annulus, this collection of microtubules is diminished and eventually disappears (160). A microtubular body similar to that in human spermatids was described by Nicander (238) in cat and rabbit spermatids; it occurred at the anterior extremity of the principal piece and eventually disappeared.

An alternative method of formation of the ribs of the principal piece was proposed by Sapsford et al. (239) from their studies of the bandicoot (*P. nasuta*). They could find no evidence of microtubules forming the anlage of the ribs; instead, they observed that a series of fine filaments joined the longitudinal columns that had appeared as electron-dense

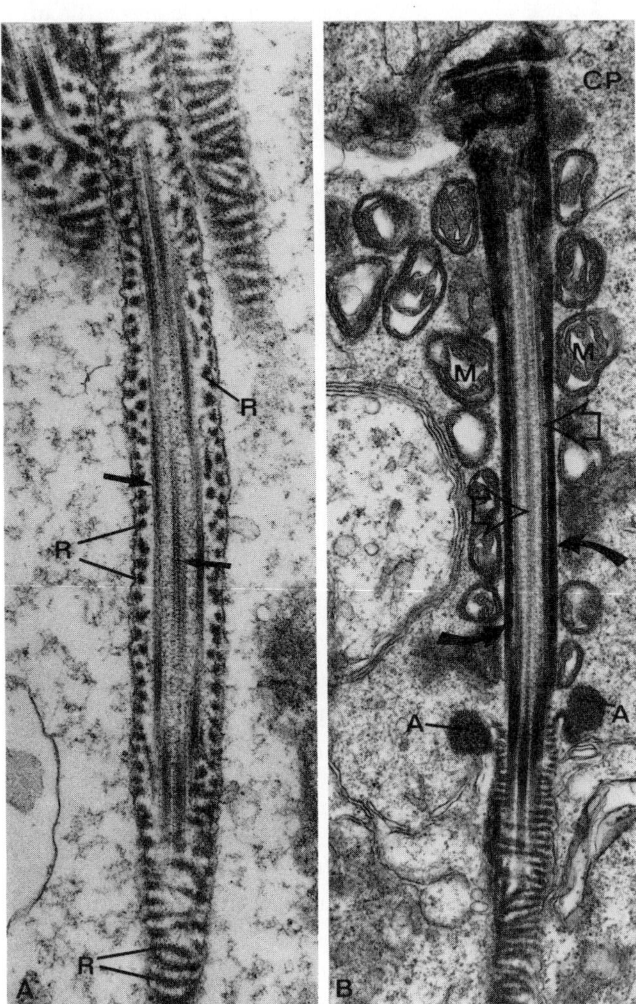

FIG. 35. Two longitudinal sections through developing spermatid tails in the region of the middle piece **(B)** and principal piece **(A).** Note the ribs (R), microtubules of axial filament (*arrows,* **A;** *open arrows,* **B**), annulus (A), connecting piece (CP), mitochondria (M), and outer dense fibers (*arrows,* **B**).

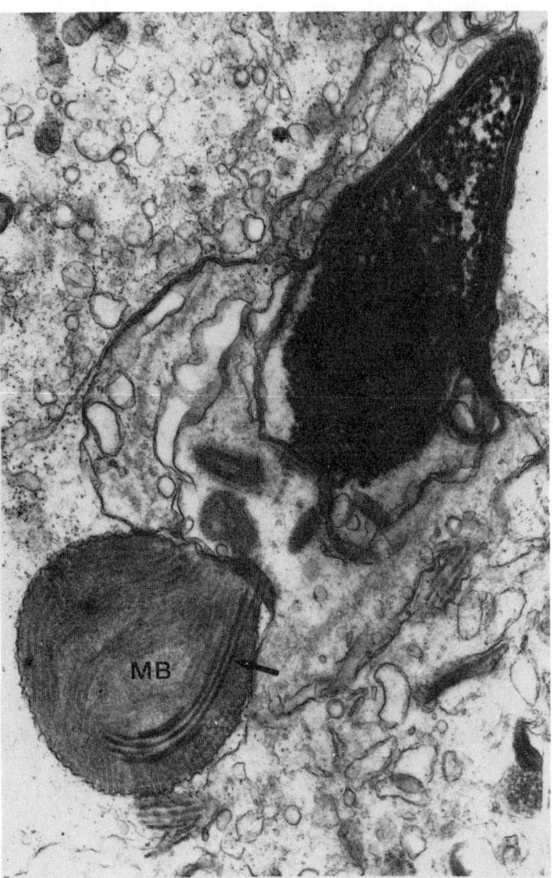

FIG. 36. Human spermatid at the Sc stage shows the axial filament (*arrow*) surrounded by the microtubular body (MB).

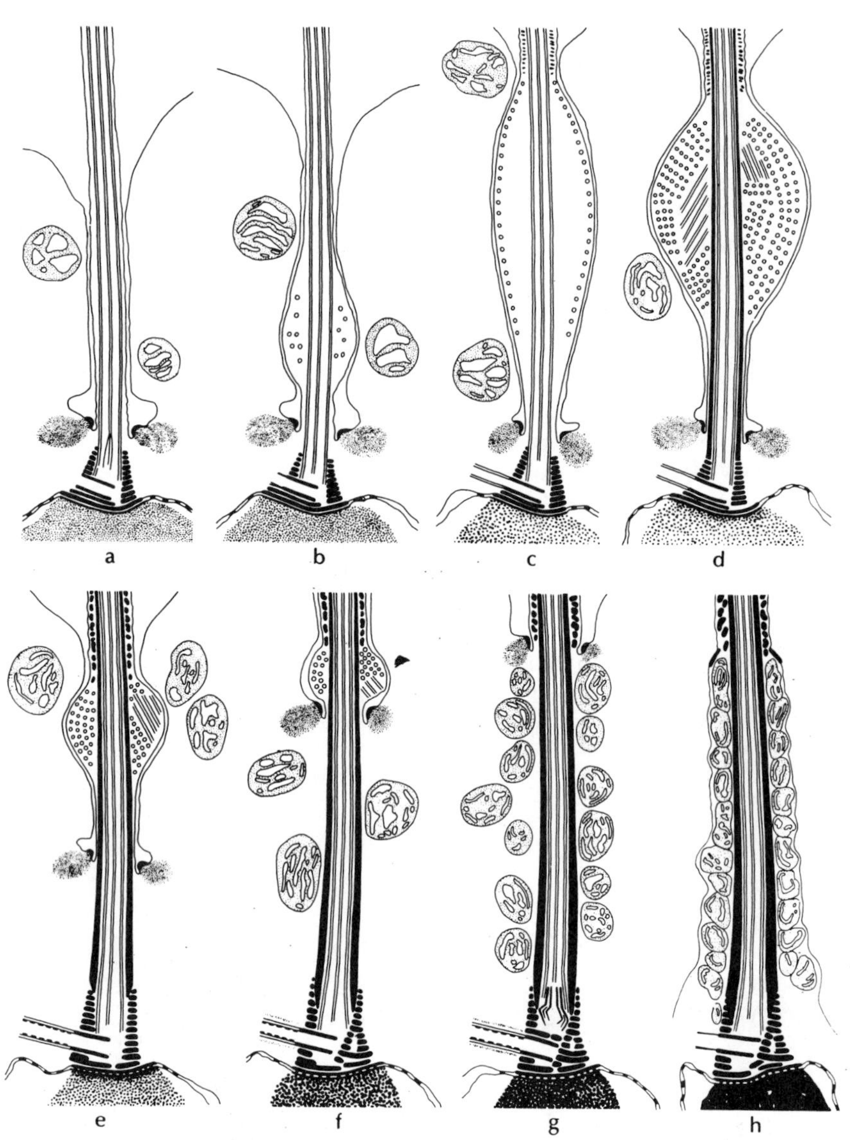

FIG. 37. Diagram illustrating the contribution of the microtubular body to the formation of the principal piece in human spermiogenesis. (From ref. 160.)

thickenings adjacent to doublets 5 and 8. These filaments aggregate and converge to form the definitive ribs. Similar fine filaments have been noted in the lizard (240) and mouse (241). The two methods of rib formation are strikingly dissimilar, and further studies will be required in other species to determine which process is more common. Recently, Irons and Clermont (242) demonstrated by the use of ^{3}H-proline incorporation into proteins that the longitudinal columns of the principal piece take 15 days to be formed. They also showed that in the rat, the ribs develop asynchronously and independent of the longitudinal columns over a period of 4 to 5 days from proteinaceous filaments.

The Mitochondrial Sheath

Jensen (243) and Benda (244) described aggregation of mitochondria in spermatids around the axial filament in the region now called the middle piece. Similar findings were noted for the human testis. Early ultrastructural studies demonstrated that the mitochondria actually form a spiral sheath that in mammalian spermatozoa is of variable length (212,245). The number of spirals forming the sheath varies from 5 to 14 for humans (246,247) and up to 40 in the guinea pig (206). The mouse, with 90, the bat, with 15, and the rat, with 350, have the largest numbers of spirals encountered (180). Andre (147) has drawn attention to the fact that the helical configuration provides the least resistance to bending.

The actual formation of the middle piece occurs late in spermiogenesis (213). Earlier, the mitochondria are distributed evenly in the cytoplasm in some species; in others, such as humans, they are peripherally placed close to the cell membrane (172,197). Formation of the mitochondrial sheath is preceded by caudal migration of the annulus, and the mitochondria associated with the axial filament between the connecting piece and the annulus (Figs. 34 and 35). The mechanisms involved in the migration and aggregation of mitochondria remain unknown. However, the organization of the manchette, a cylindrical collection of microtubules extending from the nuclear region to the caudal region of the spermatid, excludes the mitochondria from the region of the flagellum. When this collection of microtubules disperses late in spermiogenesis, the mitochondria are free to aggregate to form helical arrays (204). The end-to-end arrangement of mitochondria is unusually random, but Fawcett (180) has drawn attention to the observation that in some species there is a remarkable regularity in spacing (226,248).

In many species the organization of the cristae of mitochondria in germ cells takes on certain unique features. As described earlier, the intracristal space of mitochondria in primary and secondary spermatocytes is dilated, often giving a vacuolated appearance to these organelles (147). This process persists in spermatids and results in peripheral margination of the cristae such that in some species a central clear zone appears in the mitochondria (245). In other species, the entire mitochondrion appears to be filled by membranes that are concentrically oriented (225,248).

Reorganization of Cytoplasm and Organelles and Spermiation

The process of spermiogenesis is characterized by dramatic changes in the relationship of the nucleus and the cytoplasm and remarkable movements of organelles within spermatids. Many of these changes were described by the classic cytologists and were used by Le Blond and Clermont (166) to stage the process of spermiogenesis. The changes in nuclear shape and position were described earlier, but the movement of cytoplasm toward the caudal end of the spermatid requires some discussion.

It was noted that when the caudal movement of cytoplasm occurred, a system of cytoplasmic filaments appeared, extending from the nuclear membrane and terminating freely in the caudal cytoplasm (164). This system was given the name manchette by von Lenhossek (249). Subsequently, Zlotnik (250) described the origin of the manchette as the nuclear membrane caudal to the acrosome, a view confirmed by later electron-microscopic studies. These early studies also demonstrated that the manchette disappeared later in spermiogenesis.

McIntosh and Porter (207) demonstrated that the manchette actually was composed of a cylindrical array of microtubules that was noted to arise from a ring-like structure surrounding the postacrosomal region of spermatids in the cat (172). This nuclear ring, originally described by Gresson and Zlotnik (251), consists of electron-dense material that appears to thicken the cell membrane adjacent to the postacrosomal region of the nuclear membrane (204). The proximal ends of the microtubules of the manchette are embedded in this dense fibrillar material. However, this electron-dense deposit has not been observed in all species, being absent from humans and the bandicoot (198,213).

The microtubular nature of the manchette (Figs. 24,28) has led numerous investigators to suggest that it is responsible for shaping of the nucleus and reorganization of the cytoplasm (207,241). However, in a detailed study of spermiogenesis in a number of species, Fawcett et al. (204) produced evidence to indicate that nuclear shape was dependent on genetic factors rather than on the manchette. They also suggested that rather than being involved in the physical movement of cytoplasm, the microtubules of the manchette might act as a framework or conveyor for transport of cytoplasmic vesicles. These vesicles were closely associated with the manchette and sometimes were physically linked by slender linear densities (204). These linear densities are similar in appearance to those linking adjacent microtubules composing the manchette (Fig. 24). The fate of the manchette were unclear, but de Kretser (198) suggested that the microtubules were incorporated in the residual body, a view recently confirmed by studies of equine spermiogenesis (252).

Associated with the caudal movement of the cytoplasm, the Golgi complex and chromatid body migrate to the abacrosomal pole. The former can be identified as a component of the residual body, that portion of the spermatid cytoplasm that is shed when the spermatid leaves the seminiferous epithelium (Fig. 38), the latter process being called spermiation. Early studies demonstrated that the greater part of the spermatid cytoplasm is "shed" as the residual body, which, in the majority of instances, is phagocytosed by the adjacent Sertoli cells (253,254). The term "residual body" (corps residuel) was originally applied to these structures by Regaud (27), who noted their formation. Some cytoplasm remains to form a droplet that surrounds the middle piece and contains a few vesicular profiles. Lacy (254) noted that the residual body contained remnants of the Golgi complex and endoplasmic reticulum, and a number of studies have confirmed their phagocytosis by Sertoli cells (255–258).

The method by which the spermatid sheds the residual body and leaves the epithelium has been determined from the results of a number of ultrastructural studies (198,259,260). It was noted (198) that late in spermiogenesis the caudal spermatid cytoplasm is invaginated by processes of Sertoli cell cytoplasm, and it was postulated that these processes actually were responsible for "pulling off" the residual body (Figs. 38 and 39). Similar processes of Sertoli cell cytoplasm within spermatids have been observed in studies of rat spermiogenesis by Morales and Clermont (260). The residual cytoplasm, in addition to containing remnants of the Golgi complex, contains ribosomes, lipid inclusions, mitochondria, microtubular remnants of the manchette, and electron-dense remnants of the chromatid body. The residual bodies from human spermatids have also been noted to contain

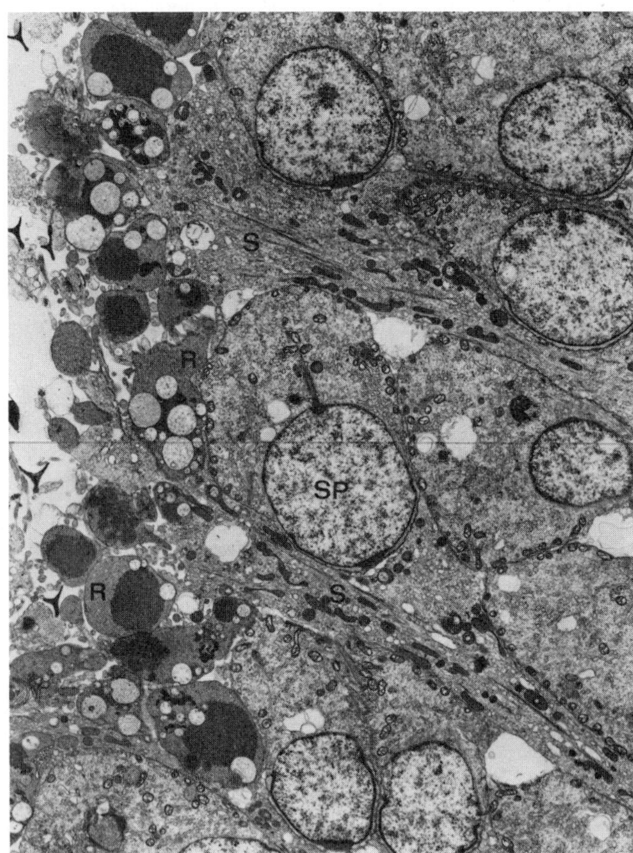

FIG. 38. Adluminal aspect of the seminiferous epithelium of the rat testis, illustrating Sertoli cell cytoplasm (S), spermatids (SP), and lobes of residual cytoplasm (R).

"flower-like" structures, noted in the cytoplasm of spermatids earlier in spermiogenesis (261). These consist of a core of densely packed osmiophilic granules surrounded by translucent vesicles and originally appear near the nucleus in association with the chromatid body. Their function within the spermatid remains unclear. Associated with the invagination of spermatid cytoplasm by Sertoli cell processes there is progressive movement of the spermatid toward the lumen; the cytoplasm, attached to the Sertoli cell, is linked to the spermatid by progressively attenuating connections (259). All connections are lost eventually, the majority of the residual bodies being retained with the Sertoli cell. Breucker et al. (262), however, suggested that in the human, many residual bodies are shed into the tubule lumen.

The mechanisms involved in spermiation remain unclear. In mammals, the late spermatids appear to progressively lose their contact with the Sertoli cell, being anchored by a special device in the region of the head described originally in the rat by Russell and Clermont (263). The structure of this device is described later, but it represents the final attachment device by which the spermatid retains contact with the Sertoli cell. Though originally described in the rat, it has also been found in humans (160). Loss of this final contact represents the completion of spermiogenesis, and

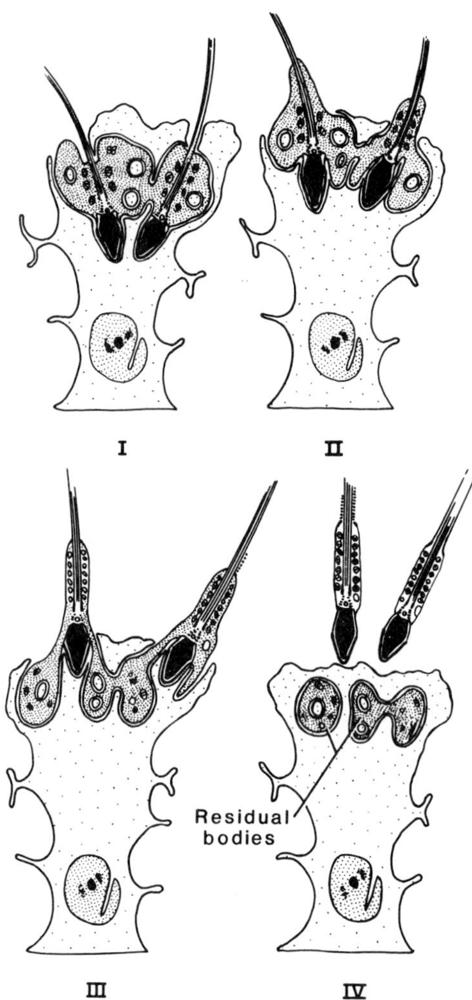

FIG. 39. The final stages of human spermiogenesis are illustrated diagrammatically and show the manner in which processes of Sertoli cell cytoplasm essentially "pull off" the residual cytoplasm (residual body) and retain it within their cytoplasm.

by definition the cell is now termed a spermatozoon (259,264). In amphibians, Burgos and Vitale-Calpe (265,266) suggested that spermiation resulted in a swelling of the terminal cytoplasmic processes of the Sertoli cells, resulting in evagination of the lacunae that housed the spermatids, thereby shedding them into the lumen of the tubule. This was suggested to be a response to human chorionic gonadotropin (hCG) or LH, but similar actions have not been confirmed in mammals.

Relationships of Sertoli Cells and Spermatids

During the early stages of spermiogenesis, the spermatids lie centrally, immediately adjacent to the lumen of the seminiferous tubules, surrounded by processes of Sertoli cell cytoplasm. At this time, small punctate desmosome-like cell junctions occur with the adjacent Sertoli cell (153). The spermatids do not demonstrate any specific orientation to the Sertoli cell, but in later stages they are deeply embedded within the epithelium, oriented such that their heads, covered by the acrosomal cap, point toward the basement membrane of the tubule. Subsequently, as described earlier, they are progressively moved toward the lumen of the tubule, eventually to lose all contact after spermiation. Studies in procarbazine-treated rats have shown that acrosome formation is disrupted, but that this process does not alter the movement of the nucleus into its eccentric position (267). However, the altered acrosome formation disrupts alignment of the heads of the spermatid within the epithelium, possibly by altering the distribution of the Sertoli-cell–spermatid junctional specializations described later.

The formation of certain specialized junctions with the adjacent Sertoli cell is probably related to the specific orientation taken by the spermatids in midspermiogenesis. Early studies noted that the cytoplasm of the Sertoli cell adjacent to the heads of spermatids late in spermiogenesis (Fig. 24) was separated into a mantle layer by the presence of an array of vesicles (197,268). Nagano (269) confirmed these findings and noted the presence of thick filaments in this mantle layer of Sertoli cell cytoplasm. A number of studies in different species have demonstrated the existence of these specialized cell attachments, in which there is no reduction in the intercellular space, but the demarcation of a thin zone of Sertoli cell cytoplasm by the presence of a series of cisternae, the cytoplasmic layer so defined demonstrating the presence of numerous fibrils (159,269,270). The cell junctions have some similarity to the inter-Sertoli-cell junctions, but there is no modification of the intercellular space. In many species, these specialized Sertoli-cell–spermatid-cell junctions are located only in the region of the head, but in the human they can be demonstrated over larger areas of the spermatid cell surface (Fig. 34). The cell junctions first appear when the spermatid nucleus takes up an eccentric position with the cell coming into close association with the cell membrane.

A further junctional specialization occurs between late spermatids and the Sertoli cells wherein the cell membrane in the region of the head of the spermatid projects into the surrounding Sertoli cell cytoplasm (263). These tubulobulbar processes provide a mechanism of anchoring spermatids immediately prior to spermiation (Fig. 40). In the rat, they appear to be limited to the cell membrane in relation to the concave portion of the nucleus (271,272), but in humans they are more irregularly distributed (160).

Reference was made earlier to the processes of Sertoli cell cytoplasm that appear to invaginate the caudal spermatid cytoplasm immediately preceding spermiation. Recently, Morales and Clermont (260) have described two types of Sertoli cell processes in the rat, one that is essentially devoid of organelles, and one that contains vesicles. From these observations they have proposed that the latter may represent a mechanism of transferring materials between these two cell types.

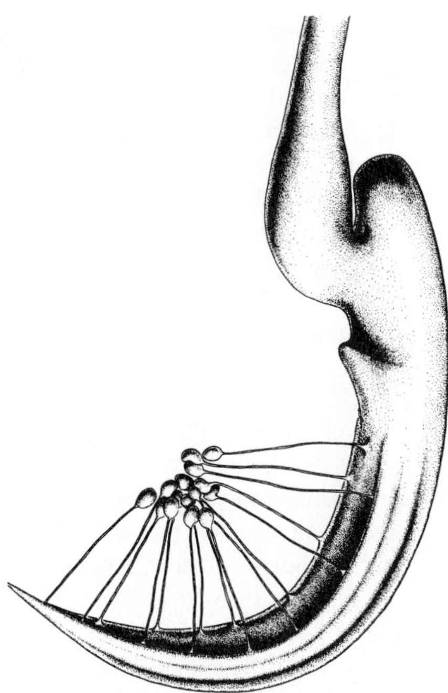

FIG. 40. Diagrammatic representation of the three-dimensional features of a step-19 spermatid of the rat. The concave aspect of the sperm head extends elaborate tubulobulbar complexes into the surrounding Sertoli cell cytoplasm, the latter not shown here. The complexes are congregated together and form bulbous terminal dilations. They are said to act as an anchoring device to temporarily retain the spermatid head within apical extensions of Sertoli cell cytoplasm. (From ref. 263.)

SERTOLI CELLS

The nongerminal component of the seminiferous epithelium was originally described in 1865 by the Italian physiologist Enrico Sertoli (273). He identified the cells that now bear his name as being individual elements extending from the basement membrane to the lumen of the seminiferous tubule and, in doing so, enveloping the many clusters of associated germ cells. Within the mammalian testis the Sertoli cell is a tall columnar cell extending perpendicularly through the seminiferous epithelium (Fig. 11), and von Ebner (93,156) first proposed that a physiological relationship existed between the Sertoli cells and the germ cells.

Without the advantage of modern optical equipment and methods of tissue preservation, Sertoli (274) and Brown (124) constructed diagrams of the shape of Sertoli cells indicating the pronounced length of the centripetal axis compared with the circumferential axis. Although further investigations of the topography of the Sertoli cell by Regaud (77) and von Ebner (275) verified Sertoli's observations that these cells presented a highly irregular nucleus and elaborate ramifying cytoplasmic processes, the limited resolution of their light microscopes raised a point of controversy regarding the existence of the Sertoli cell as a syncytium or as an individual cell. It had been Sertoli's earlier contention that the Sertoli cells were independent cellular units and did not form a syncytial relationship with each other, but von Ebner (93) put forward the notion that a symbiotic relationship existed between the Sertoli cells and the more mature generations of germ cells, thereby forming a functional unit he termed the spermatoblast. In the same study, he also considered the Sertoli cells to form a complex syncytium, a concept he later discarded (156) in favor of their independent existence.

The precise morphological organization of the Sertoli cell remained poorly understood for many years thereafter (114,276–280). With the greatly improved resolution of the electron microscope, Watson (114,281) and Challice (282) provided the first descriptions of the fine structure of the seminiferous epithelium, but it was not until 1956 that Fawcett and Burgos demonstrated that each Sertoli cell had distinct cellular boundaries. The recent ultrastructural investigations of Fawcett (283–287) have greatly increased our appreciation of the central role played by this cell in the regulation of spermatogenesis. Detailed studies of the topography of the Sertoli cell, its relationship to germ cells, and the changes in Sertoli cell morphology in health and disease (289–295) have added substantially to a deeper understanding of Sertoli cell biology.

Shape

The early histologists recognized that the unusual columnar shape of the Sertoli cell reflected a three-dimensional configuration of great complexity (124,274). In their studies defining the seminiferous cycle, Le Blond and Clermont (167) noted that the Sertoli cells alter their shape in relation to the 14 stages of the spermatogenic cycle. With a silver-staining method applied to paraffin sections, Elftman (296) concluded that in the rat testis the Sertoli cells were tall and columnar in shape, and their distribution within the seminiferous epithelium resembled the pattern of trees planted in an orchard. On the basis of earlier studies on the mouse testis (280), the basal aspect of the Sertoli cell, most readily visible by light microscopy, was likened to the trunk of a tree (Fig. 41), the many cytoplasmic ramifications between the surrounding germ layer being analogous to the branches of a tree. This simple description has largely stood the test of time, and many subsequent ultrastructural studies of thin sections have confirmed that although this appealing topographic description may not be entirely applicable to all species thus far studied, a better portrayal has not emerged.

The strategic position of the Sertoli cell within the seminiferous epithelium and its intrinsic relationships to neighboring Sertoli cells and germ cells (Figs. 41–45) have repeatedly been emphasized in fine-structural analysis of a great variety of vertebrate and invertebrate species (285,297–302). Recent ultrastructural studies in the rat have shown that Sertoli cell shape is more complex than was appreciated previously and have stressed that the cytoplasmic extensions of the Sertoli cell characterize the topography of the cell as possibly the most complex yet described in any epithelium. The Sertoli cells must continually alter their shape to accommodate the structural transformations and mobilization

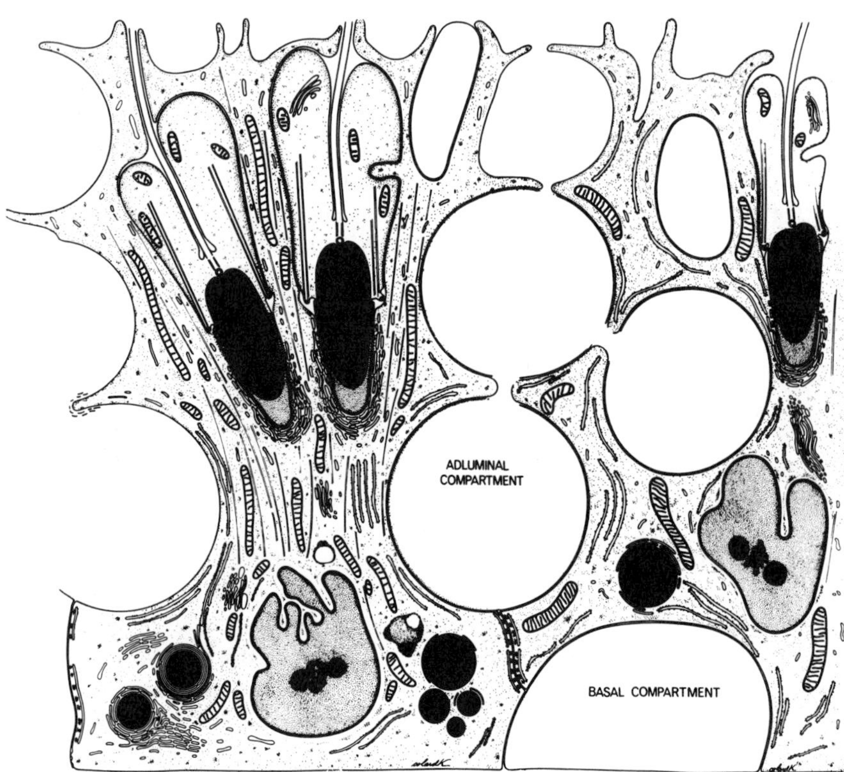

FIG. 41. Diagram illustrating how the occluding inter-Sertoli-cell junctions divide the seminiferous epithelium into a basal compartment (containing spermatogonia and early primary spermatocytes) and an adluminal compartment (containing more advanced germ cells). (From ref. 285.)

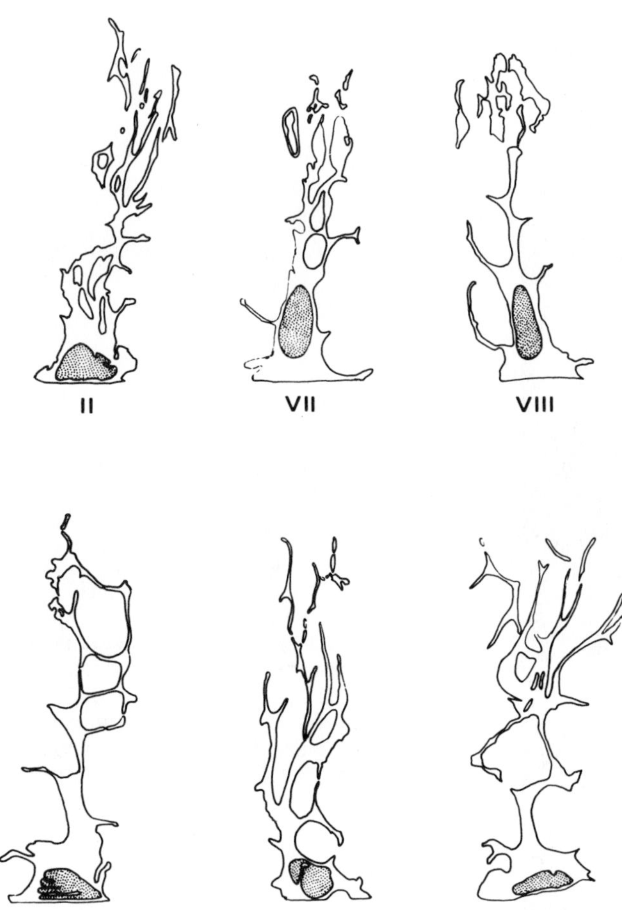

FIG. 42. India-ink tracings of plasma membranes of individual Sertoli cells at various stages of the rat spermatogenic cycle. The surface of each Sertoli cell was identified from assembled electron-micrograph montages and emphasizes the complex and varying shape of the Sertoli cell.

of germ cells from the base to the free surface of the seminiferous epithelium. Wong and Russell (291) serially sectioned a single Sertoli cell from a stage V rat seminiferous tubule and showed that the cell was best characterized as a short body resting on the basal lamina, with many upward-projecting sheet-like cytoplasmic extensions forming cone, cup, and cylindrical configurations in relation to germ cells and adjacent Sertoli cells. When the seminiferous epithelium was viewed perpendicular to the basal lamina, the Sertoli cells were reported to form a hexagonal array, i.e., they presented six membrane surfaces near their bases (274,279,303). Most recent studies suggest that the basal regions of the Sertoli cells are more likely packed in the seminiferous tubule in a pentagonal arrangement (292,304).

Ultrastructural studies of rat Sertoli cells at stages II, VII, VIII, IX–XI, and XIII–XIV of the spermatogenic cycle depicted variations in shape (Fig. 42) that seemed at first to indicate highly irregular and disordered configurations (305). However, the margins of the Sertoli cell are obliged to undergo transformations to remain in association with (a) the expanding spherical volumes exemplified by spermatogonia, spermatocytes, and spermatids, (b) mature spermatids, (c) spermatogonial mitoses and the meiotic maturation divisions, and (d) the formation and subsequent release of the excess spermatid residual cytoplasm. Reconstruction of entire profiles of Sertoli cells from many smaller micrographs of each cell reveal that for the major proportion of the rat spermatogenic cycle (Figs. 43–45), the overall shape of the cell is best described as tall, irregularly columnar, and possessing numerous very thin lateral processes and cylindrical recesses to accommodate the penetration of elongated spermatids. Similar findings were noted by Wong and Russell (291), who emphasized that for the remainder of the spermatogenic cycle, these extremely attenuated cytoplasmic processes are absent because of the elongated spermatids adopting positions at the extreme apical margins of the Sertoli cells and their subsequent release from the seminiferous epithelium (stages VII–IX).

Cyclic variations in Sertoli cell shape commensurate with the changing composition and cross-sectional area of the seminiferous epithelium (306) logically lead to a consideration of changes in Sertoli cell volume that may also reveal morphological alterations in the internal composition of the Sertoli cell, a subject dealt with in detail later in this section. Although morphometric techniques have been used to estimate the numerical density and total number of Sertoli cells in the perfused-fixed rat testis (306), efforts to obtain additional quantitative information on Sertoli cell shape and volume during the spermatogenic cycle have met with considerable difficulty because of the intricate topography of the Sertoli cells. Earlier quantitative studies on rat seminiferous tubules reported 10% to 13% occupancy of the seminiferous epithelium by the Sertoli cells (307). In the human testis and rat testis, Sertoli cells were reported to occupy 36% and 11%, respectively, of the seminiferous epithelium (308). However, these data are difficult to evaluate, because they were based on light-microscopic analysis of Sertoli cells in semithin sections of seminiferous tubules, where the limits of optical resolution possibly fail to detect the thin ramifying processes of the Sertoli cell. Ultrastructural examination of monkey Sertoli cells revealed that the relative volume of Sertoli cells within the seminiferous epithelium ranged from 24% at stage I to 32% at stage VII of the monkey spermatogenic cycle (309,310). Morphometric analysis of the rat seminiferous epithelium in our laboratory has shown that the proportion occupied by Sertoli cells during the spermatogenic cycle ranges from 19% to 28%, representing a cyclical volume change, lowest during stage VII (approximately 2,000 μm^3). When a single stage V rat Sertoli cell was photographed by electron microscopy and reconstructed as a plexiglas model, its volume was estimated at 6,000 μm^3 (291). Taken together, these advances in our appreciation of the changing shape and volume of the Sertoli cell suggest that the cell engages in continual motor activity and exhibits a high degree of plasticity synchronized with the ever mobile population of germ cells.

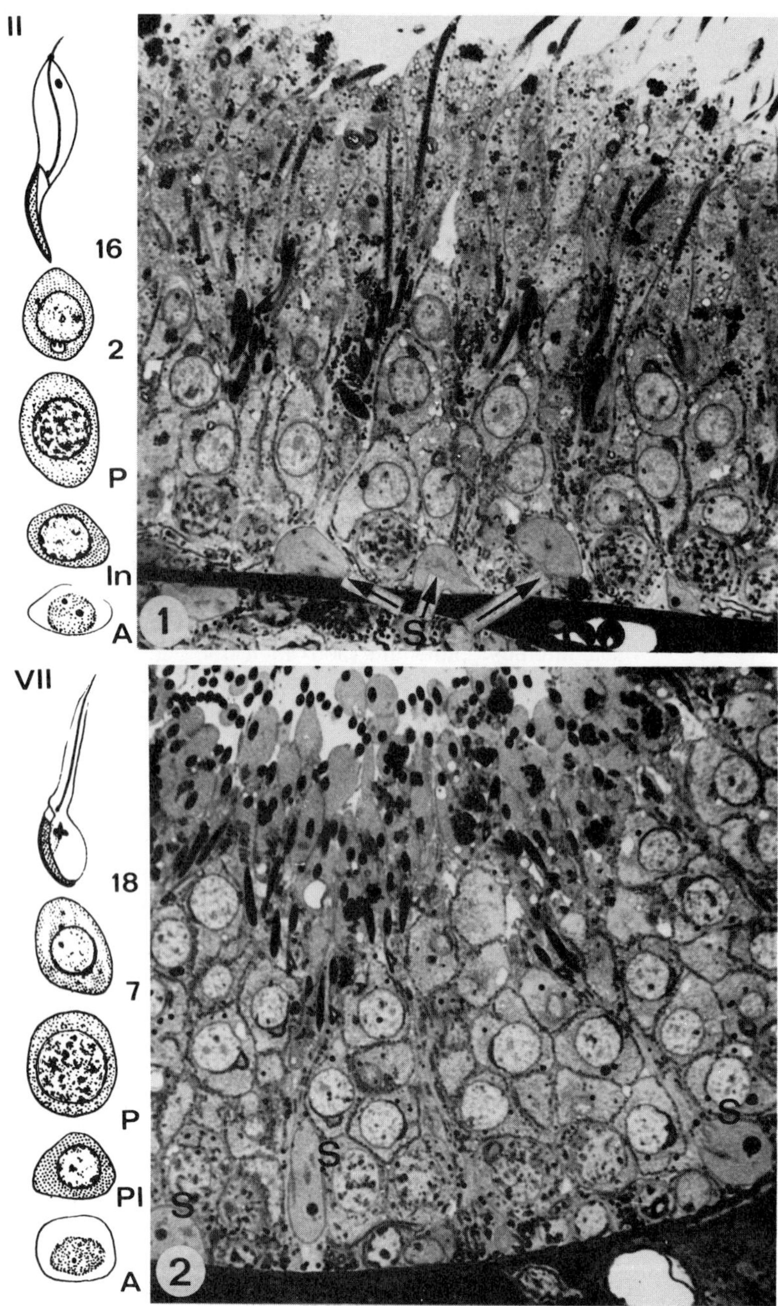

FIG. 43. Cell associations forming stages II and VII of the rat seminiferous cycle. Note Sertoli cells (S). A: type A spermatogonia; In: intermediate type spermatogonia; Pl: preleptotene primary spermatocytes; L: leptotene; Z: zygote; P: pachytene; Di: diplotene-diakinesis; L–19 represent steps in spermiogenesis. Explanation of symbols adapted from Leblond and Clermont (1952).

Ultrastructural Features

Nucleus

For a wide variety of animals, the nucleus of the Sertoli cell exhibits a characteristic morphology readily visible within the basal aspect of the seminiferous epithelium. Detailed accounts of nuclear cytology in the adult testis are available for rodents (285,286,311), monkeys (17,313), human (113,288,289,314–318), and other species (285,294). The Sertoli cell nucleus is large and irregular and usually occupies a position within the basal aspect of the cell that rests on the basement membrane of the seminiferous tubule (Figs. 12, 13, and 46). Usually they form a single row, although at times they are displaced toward the luminal regions of the seminiferous tubule (Figs. 43–45). Often the nuclear membrane is highly infolded, a feature recognized by light microscopy of plastic-embedded sections, and numerous electron-microscopic studies of many divergent species have revealed extensive nuclear membrane infoldings (285,294, 313,316,318).

Neither the position nor the many lobulations of the monkey Sertoli cell nucleus have exhibited any variations throughout the spermatogenic cycle (313). Similar results have been reported for the human Sertoli cell (288,314,315). However, in rodents, the shape and position of the Sertoli

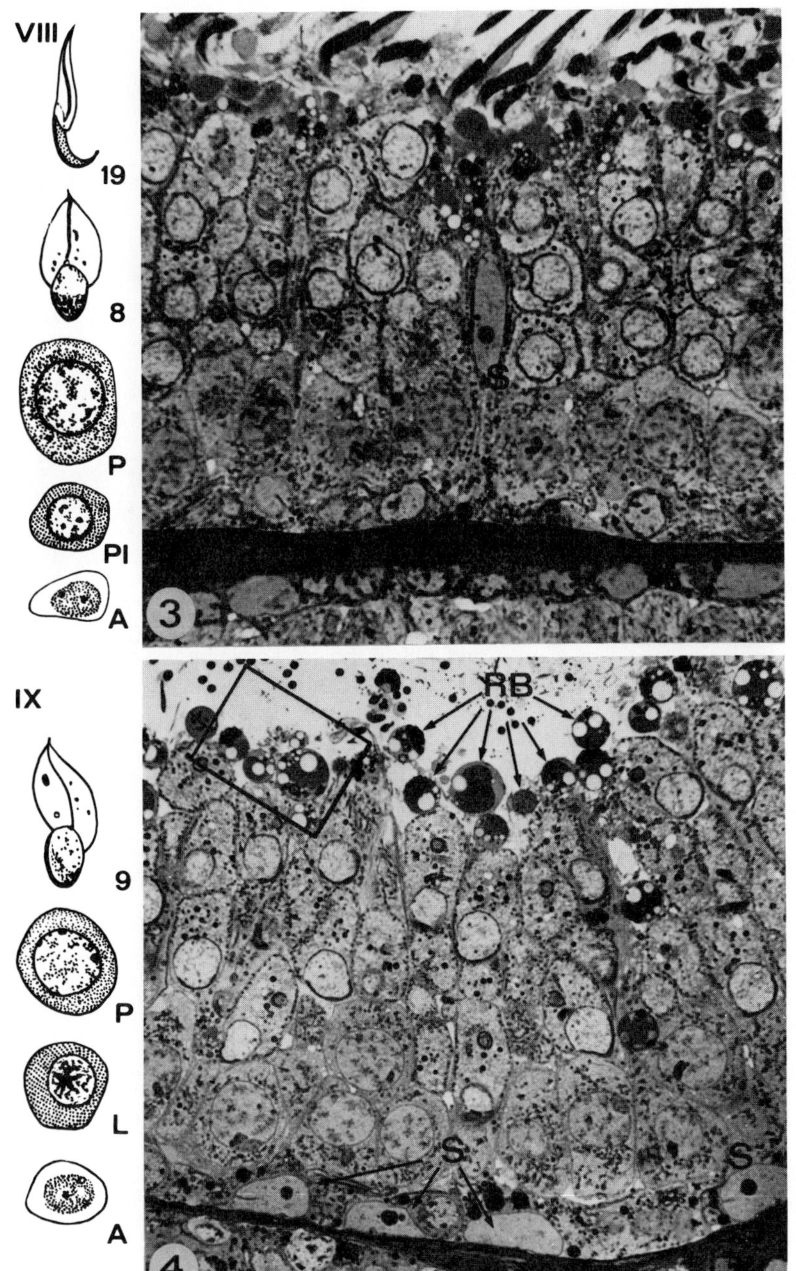

FIG. 44. Cell associations forming stages VIII and IX of the rat seminiferous cycle. Note Sertoli cells (S) and residual bodies (RB). For symbols, see Fig. 43. Area denoted by rectangle shown in Fig. 54.

cell nucleus vary according to the stages of the spermatogenic cycle. The nucleus often may be triangular or polygonal in appearance following release of mature spermatids; alternatively, they may appear elongated as the developing elongate spermatids penetrate deep into the basal aspects of the epithelium (280) (Figs. 43–45). Generally, most of the Sertoli cell nuclei remain flattened along the basal lamina of the seminiferous tubule throughout the spermatogenic cycle (167). Within the terminal portions of the seminiferous tubules, near their junctions with the tubuli recti, the Sertoli cells exclusively occupy these terminal segments, where their nuclei become closely packed, elongated, and highly irregular in profile (17,319).

The fine structure of the adult Sertoli cell nucleoplasm in all species thus far studied reveals a homogeneous distribution of euchromatin with a fine fibrillar-granular texture. Clumps of more densely stained and compact masses of the heterochromatin are principally confined to the region of the nucleolar complex, although on rare occasions small heterochromatic masses may occur elsewhere within the nucleoplasm or associated with the nuclear membrane (61,291,305,313). Sertoli cells of the human testis contain a relatively large nucleolus, and its intense staining with basophilic dyes facilitates identification of Sertoli cell nuclei within the seminiferous epithelium (Fig. 12). Its usual configuration (289,320) resembles a tripartite structure, with a

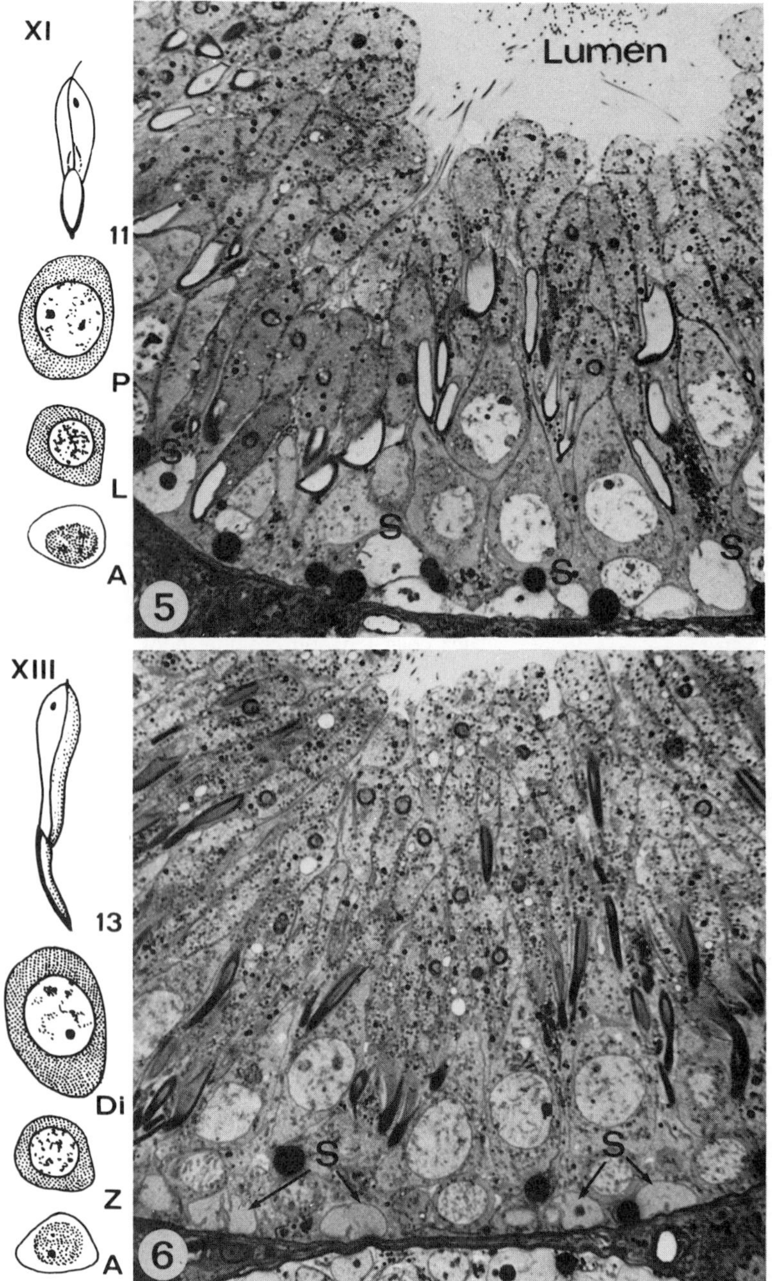

FIG. 45. Cell associations forming stages XI and XIII of the rat seminiferous cycle. Note Sertoli cells (S). For symbols, see Fig. 43.

central dense, compact nucleolar mass, the nucleolonema proper. From this body, variable projections often extend outward to gain association with two patches of heterochromatin material that flank the central nucleolonema in a symmetrical relationship. These two laterally associated bodies are at times referred to as the pars amorpha, perinucleolar spheres, satellite karyosomes, or heteropyknotic bodies; they stain positively for DNA with the Feulgen reaction, whereas the nucleolonema material remains negative (60,285).

Although the tripartite arrangement of the Sertoli cell nucleolus is maintained in rodents and other laboratory species, no close association or contact is established between the central nucleolonema and the satellite heterochromatin. Nevertheless, the nucleolus is readily identified in rat Sertoli cell nuclei and attains special prominence in size and electron density in mouse, guinea pig, and hamster Sertoli cells (285) (Fig. 41). In mouse Sertoli cell nucleoli, the nucleolonema contains serial ring-shaped fibrillar components (321) that were shown to rapidly incorporate ^{3}H-uridine, indicating sites of RNA synthesis. With the passage of time, the incorporation of labeled uridine occurred within clusters of interchromatin granules at sites distant from the nucleolus, and at later intervals evidence of labeling disappeared from the nucleus. More recent studies of mouse Sertoli cell nucleoli (322) have shown that hybridization with ^{3}H-rRNA is localized to the central nucleolar mass, within which are many fibrillar centers (26 to 41 per cell). The latter, together with an interconnecting nucleolar fibrillar network, constitute the site of nucleolus-organizing regions. Autoradiographic studies after ^{3}H-uridine incorporation indicated that rDNA transcription occurred only in the fibrillar nucleolar network, implying that the aforementioned fibrillar centers are not sites of rRNA gene transcription. Bustos-Obregon and Esponda (315) described unusual granular nuclear bodies, termed "sphaeridia," in human Sertoli cells, 0.4 to 1.9 μm in diameter and surrounded by a clear halo 0.08 to 0.1 μm in width. Their functional significance remains unknown.

A highly unusual nucleolar morphology has been described for the Sertoli cells of the bull (323–325), which display an aggregation of many membrane-limited vesicles, averaging 0.2 to 0.35 μm in diameter and bearing 150-Å granules on their outer surfaces. Similar structures have been noted in the Sertoli cells of the ram, African buffalo, and gerenuk (a rare antelope of East Africa), and it has been suggested (285) that other ruminant species may display these multivesicular nucleolar bodies. Although these membranous forms of the nucleolus in Sertoli cells resemble those observed in the human endometrium (326) and type A dark spermatogonia (111), their functional duties remain unclarified. Many nuclear pores traverse the nuclear membrane (327), which itself is invested with a thin zone of 70-Å cytoplasmic filaments forming a sheath 150 to 250 nm in thickness, thought to confer structural rigidity to the nucleus and prevent close incursion of cytoplasmic organelles.

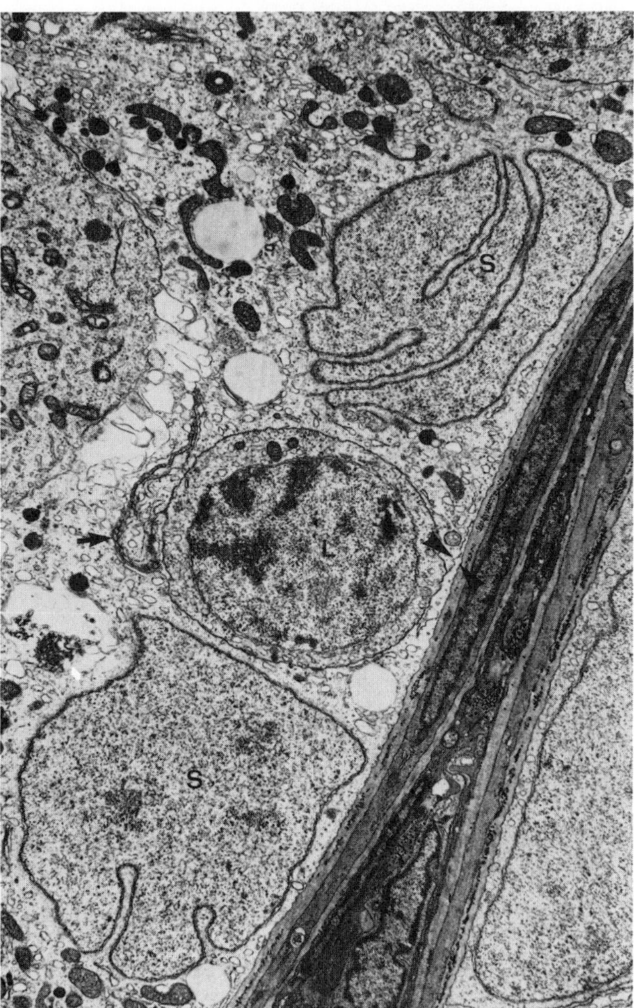

FIG. 46. Basal aspects of two Sertoli cells (S) showing an inter-Sertoli-cell tight junction (*arrow*) above a leptotene primary spermatocyte (L). Note that below the germ cell, the opposing surfaces of the Sertoli cells are not associated with specialized junctional complexes (*arrowheads*).

Cytoplasm

In general, the cytoplasmic components of the Sertoli cell show a polarized distribution; the basal and lower trunk regions of the cytoplasm contain an abundance of organelles and inclusions, whereas the apical extensions usually exhibit a paucity of such structures. Exceptions to this rule can be illustrated by preferential distributions of mitochondria, smooth endoplasmic recticulum, and glycogen to the uppermost apical extensions of the Sertoli cell cytoplasm in the mouse, squirrel, and human (288,328,329), although it must be emphasized that these arrangements are not often encountered. Sertoli cell mitochondria in the past have been considered to adopt slender or spherical shapes in ultrathin sections (285,286,288), although cup-shaped forms have been noted (288). Analysis of Sertoli cells throughout the rat spermatogenic cycle reveals a greater diversity of mitochondrial forms than was previously described (Fig. 46). The mitochondria of this species exhibit S shapes and irregular dumbbell or doughnut-type profiles in addition to the usual elongated and round forms. In all of the species thus far examined, the mitochondria have had transversely oriented foliate cristae, but the tubular form is often encountered, particularly in the spherical varieties.

Detailed ultrastructural studies of the three-dimensional morphology of the Golgi apparatus have been achieved by high-voltage electron-microscopic analysis of semithin and thick (1–7 μm) sections stained with a variety of heavy-metal salts (330,331). In rat and mouse testes, the Sertoli cell Golgi apparatus consists of a primary network, visible only by electron microscopy, of perforated membrane sheets, interconnected by narrow bridges. When considered in its entirety, the secondary network, detectable by light microscopy, forms a large, three-dimensional structure, adopting the overall shape of a cylinder, that extends in the main body of Sertoli cell cytoplasm from the juxtanuclear region toward the lumen of the seminiferous epithelium. These findings have been chiefly confined to stages V to VIII of the spermatogenic cycle, making it possible that the general architecture of the Golgi apparatus is modified in other stages.

Despite these elegant descriptions of the Golgi membranes of the Sertoli cell, they appear to be devoid of any appreciable numbers of vesicles or condensing vacuoles usually associated with cells actively engaged in the synthesis of proteins destined for transport or secretion (285,286). Similarly, the Sertoli cells contain only limited amounts of rough or granular endoplasmic reticulum, which occurs as several short lengths of parallel cisternae or, alternatively, taking the form of small individual tubules principally in the base or trunk of the Sertoli cell cytoplasm (288,289, 313,320). This is surprising in view of the increasing evidence that the Sertoli cells produce numerous proteins (179,332–334), some of which, such as androgen-binding protein, are secreted into the lumen of the tubule. Others, such as the glycoprotein hormone inhibin, must be secreted by the Sertoli cell to circulate in plasma and influence FSH secretion (335–338).

The occurrence of smooth or agranular endoplasmic reticulum has been exhaustively described in studies of the fine structure of the Sertoli cell in vertebrate and invertebrate animals (285,286,294,297,301,313,316). There is no general morphological pattern that can be used for a description of the Sertoli cell smooth endoplasmic reticulum, because it has variously been referred to as vesicular, tubular, cisternal, fenestrated, or lamellar (Figs. 46–48). Species differences may account for such variations in fine structure, but equally, the differential effects of tissue fixation probably contribute substantially to the observed changes in vesicular structure. The true morphology of smooth endoplasmic reticulum often is difficult to preserve faithfully (339–342), making it likely that the descriptions of this organelle in some studies reflect merely random ultrastructural alterations.

The most striking arrangements of Sertoli cell smooth endoplasmic reticulum occur in several artiodactyl species (even-toed quadrupeds such as the bull, boar, ram, antelope, and gazelle), in which large compacted masses of smooth membranes invest and surround the developing heads of elongating spermatids (285,286). A remarkable development of the smooth endoplasmic reticulum in relation to the maturation of spermatids is illustrated by the squirrel, in which, just prior to sperm release, the spermatid head is retained by the Sertoli cell via its association with very large bulbous projections of Sertoli cell cytoplasm filled with smooth endoplasmic reticulum. After spermiation, these membranous masses are transported toward the base of each Sertoli cell (329,343). Multiple concentric layers of smooth endoplasmic reticulum have also been described in the basal aspects of ruminant Sertoli cells, where they surround lipid inclusions (285). In rat Sertoli cells, smooth endoplasmic reticulum undergoes cyclic change in morphology, from tubular to vesicular, in association with the spermatogenic cycle (344,345). To date, however, nothing is known about the functional significance of the often rich supplies of smooth endoplasmic reticulum within the Sertoli cells. However, the ubiquitous occurrence of many or large lipid inclusions within the Sertoli cell cytoplasm has reinforced a longstanding view that in some way the metabolism or synthesis of certain steroid compounds known to occur in isolated Sertoli cells (346,347) is mediated via their distinctive cytoplasmic components, characteristically found in accredited steroidogenic cells.

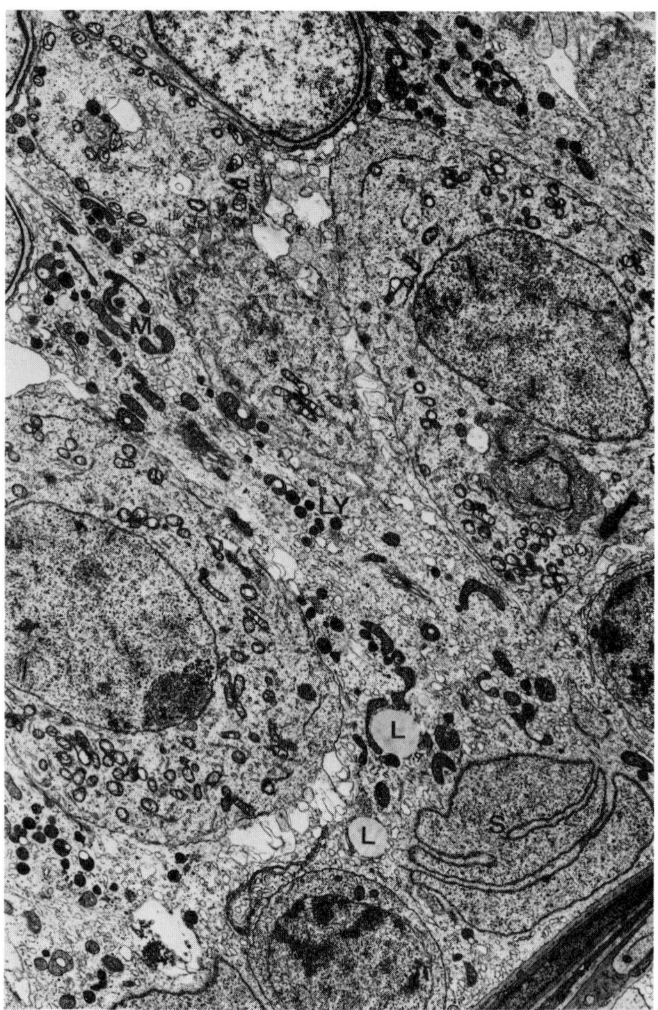

FIG. 47. Stage IX of the rat spermatogenic cycle illustrating Sertoli cell nucleus (S) and the columnar trunk of the Sertoli cell containing lysosomes (LY), mitochondria (M), and lipid inclusions (L).

In parallel to the general uncertainty regarding the role of smooth endoplasmic reticulum in the Sertoli cell, some confusion exists as to the formation, distribution, and fate of Sertoli cell lipid inclusions. Readily recognizable and striking variations in Sertoli cell morphology between different species and between Sertoli cells in different stages of the spermatogenic cycle in a given species are seen in the size and content of their cytoplasmic lipid inclusions (Figs. 43–45). Von Ebner (156) was the first to suggest that the seminiferous epithelium exhibited a cyclic variation in lipid content, and Sertoli cell lipids have received increasing attention in more recent investigations (254,258,285,288, 348–351). Recently, these observations have been confirmed by morphometric analysis of Sertoli cells during the

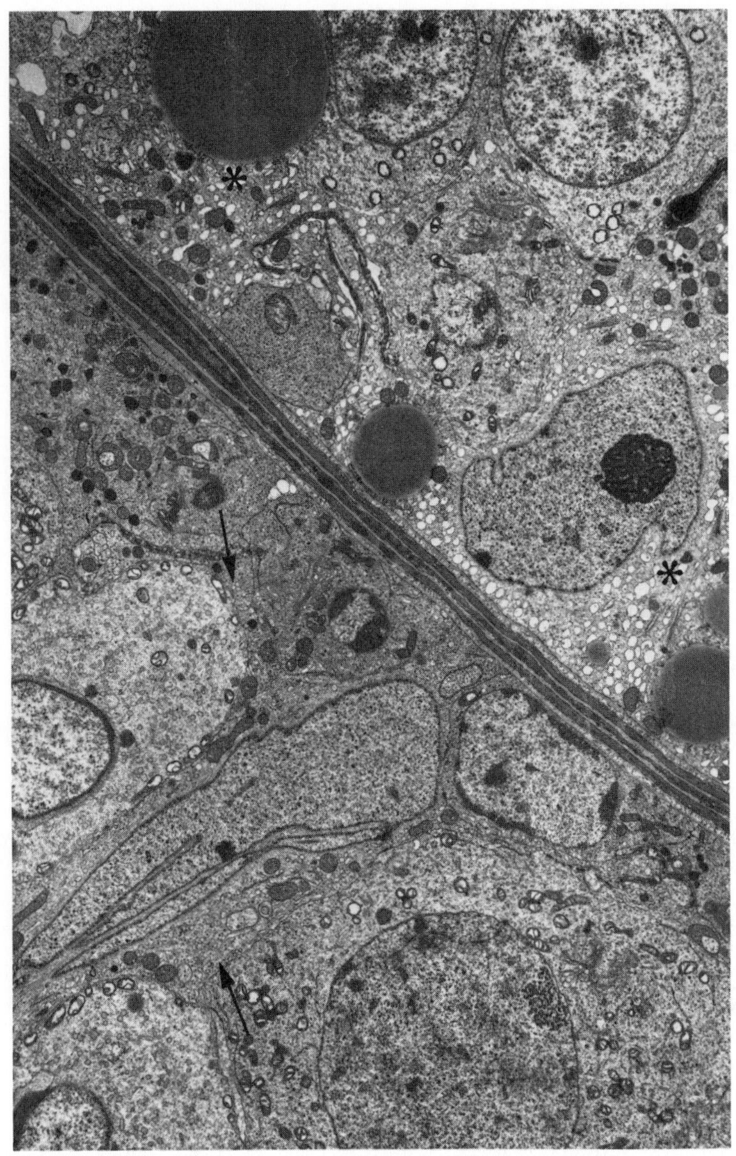

FIG. 48. Rat seminiferous epithelium showing stage 1 **(upper),** with dilated Sertoli cell smooth endoplasmic reticulum (*asterisks*), and stage VII **(lower),** exhibiting tubulovesicular profiles (*arrows*) of Sertoli cell smooth endoplasmic reticulum.

spermatogenic cycle in the rat, in which a cycle of accumulation and decline in Sertoli cell lipid inclusions has been described (305). Dramatic increases in Sertoli cell lipid content are evident in situations of spermatogenic arrest (e.g., seasonal breeders) or under conditions that cause germ cell damage (20,297,352–354), but with the reinitiation of spermatogenesis, the lipids gradually disappear, to return to their normal size and number.

Degenerating germ cells and the end products of degenerate lobes of spermatid residual cytoplasm have been considered to provide the source of lipid inclusions (Fig. 49) that accumulate within the Sertoli cell (254,352,355). However, no definite link between the phagocytosis of residual cytoplasm and the content of Sertoli cell lipid inclusions has been demonstrated. In the mouse (255), rat (356), bandicoot (256), human (288), and other species (285), the lipid components of degenerating residual bodies do not appear to be released into the Sertoli cell, but are probably degraded entirely. Following the destruction of residual bodies, Sertoli cells in the rat testis actually begin to accumulate lipid inclusions (305).

In support of the notion that cyclic variations in Sertoli cell lipid inclusions represent a balance between lipolysis and synthesis, Bergh (71) found that an increase in Sertoli cell lipid inclusions in the cryptorchid rat testis preceded the phase of germ cell degeneration. Accumulation of Sertoli cell lipid also occurred following induction of cryptorchidism in testes lacking germ cells as a result of prior fetal irradiation (71). It therefore seems that Sertoli cells are capable of synthesizing lipid in the absence of a contribution of substrates from degenerating germ cells. In this connection, the smooth endoplasmic reticulum enzymes are perhaps responsible for lipid synthesis from glycerol and fatty acids that on esterification within the Sertoli cell becomes visible as lipid inclusions. This hypothesis is supported by the finding that in mammalian and a variety of vertebrate

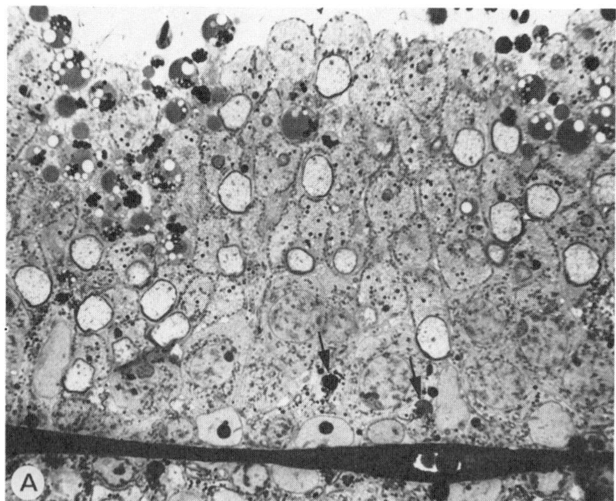

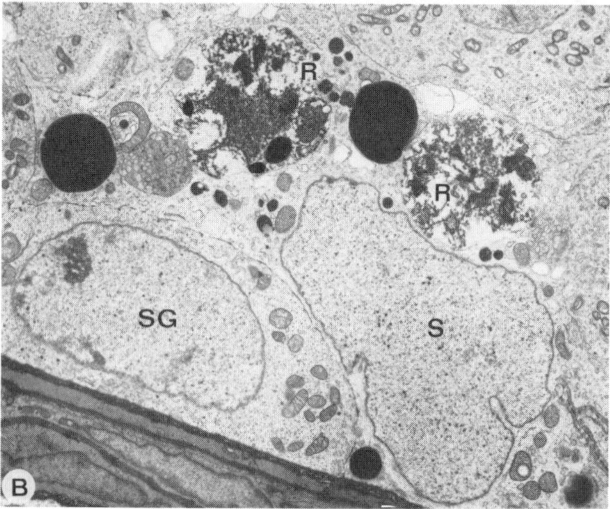

FIG. 49. A: Stage IX of the rat spermatogenic cycle showing descent of residual bodies into the basal aspect of the Sertoli cell. Final dissolution of residual bodies occurs within the Sertoli cells (*arrows*). **B:** Basal aspect of the Sertoli cell showing degenerated residual bodies (R). Sertoli cell nucleus (S) and spermatogonium (SG) are also shown.

species, Sertoli cell lipid inclusions contain a higher ratio of esterified-to-unesterified cholesterol than do germ cells (297,357,358). However, none of the foregoing studies has determined a role for lipid within the Sertoli cell, and there is a need for further work to clarify its function.

An unusual type of inclusion body found within the human Sertoli cell is the Charcot-Böttcher crystal. Such filamentous inclusions are of two main types, originally classified according to their length and thickness. Stieve (359) reported that Lubarsch (120) discovered large crystals up to 25 μm in length within the Sertoli cell cytoplasm that he termed crystals of Charcot-Böttcher. Later, Spangaro (360) observed much smaller crystals within the Sertoli cell, and all of these inclusions are now collectively referred to as Charcot-Böttcher crystals (113,121,314,320,361,362). Readily visible by light microscopy, their ultrastructural features can be summarized as follows: (a) they are perinuclear, often obliquely oriented in relation to the basal lamina; (b) they have an elongated, fusiform shape, up to 5 μm in width and 10 to 25 μm long; (c) they often form simple bifurcations, between which are found glycogen or 10-nm filaments; (d) they consist of dense parallel filaments, approximately 150 Å in diameter, that in cross section exhibit zigzag or meandering profiles; (e) their terminal spike-like ends may be continuous with 9- to 12-nm cytoplasmic filaments (285,286,289). Crystalloids are also found in Sertoli cells of the pig (363), although they are smaller than those seen in the human and consist of parallel filaments 50 Å in diameter. These filaments contain actin (364) and thus may be derivatives of the cytoskeleton of the Sertoli cell.

Rod-like crystalloid inclusions have also been described in Sertoli cells of some marsupials, notably the koala (365–367) and the American opossum (368). Recently, ultrastructural analysis of koala Sertoli cells (369) has confirmed these earlier observations and shown that koala Sertoli cells exhibit extraordinary cytoplasmic crystals, often aligned perpendicular to the basal lamina and in the vicinity of the Sertoli cell nucleus. They are easily visible by light microscopy and occur in prepubertal and adult specimens (Figs. 50 and 51). Ultrastructurally they resemble human Charcot-Böttcher crystals, although they exhibit a more highly ordered substructure in which the filaments are arranged in tubules, thereby forming a regular latticework (Fig. 52). Although crystalloids of koala Sertoli cells are at times associated with cytoplasmic filaments in various configurations suggesting assembly of or dissociation from the major crystalloid body, their functional duties in this species, the pig, and the human are not clear.

Sertoli cells contain variable amounts of dense bodies usually referred to as collections of lysosomes, multivesicular bodies, and heterophagic vacuoles (285,286,288, 289,294,313,316). Often these components of the lysosomal system are sequestered in the deepest regions of the Sertoli cell, where they flank the nucleus (Figs. 46, 47, and 49), but, alternatively, they are seen in large numbers within the upward columnar trunk of the Sertoli cell, where they lie close to developing spermatids.

Historically, Maximow (370) originally suggested that the Sertoli cell is active in the phagocytosis of germ cells, and more recent histochemical analysis has revealed the presence of strong hydrolytic enzyme activity in the Sertoli cell (356,371–376) that is principally localized within membrane-limited dense bodies (lysosomes) (356). Sertoli cells are thus equipped with a well-developed cytoplasmic digestive system capable of ingesting injected dyes and certain foreign particulate matter (377–379) and participating in the removal of degenerating germ cells (95,256).

The disposal of the excess spermatid cytoplasm left behind by the mature sperm as they are released from the luminal surface of the Sertoli cells has received much attention ever since it was recognized by Regaud (27) in 1901

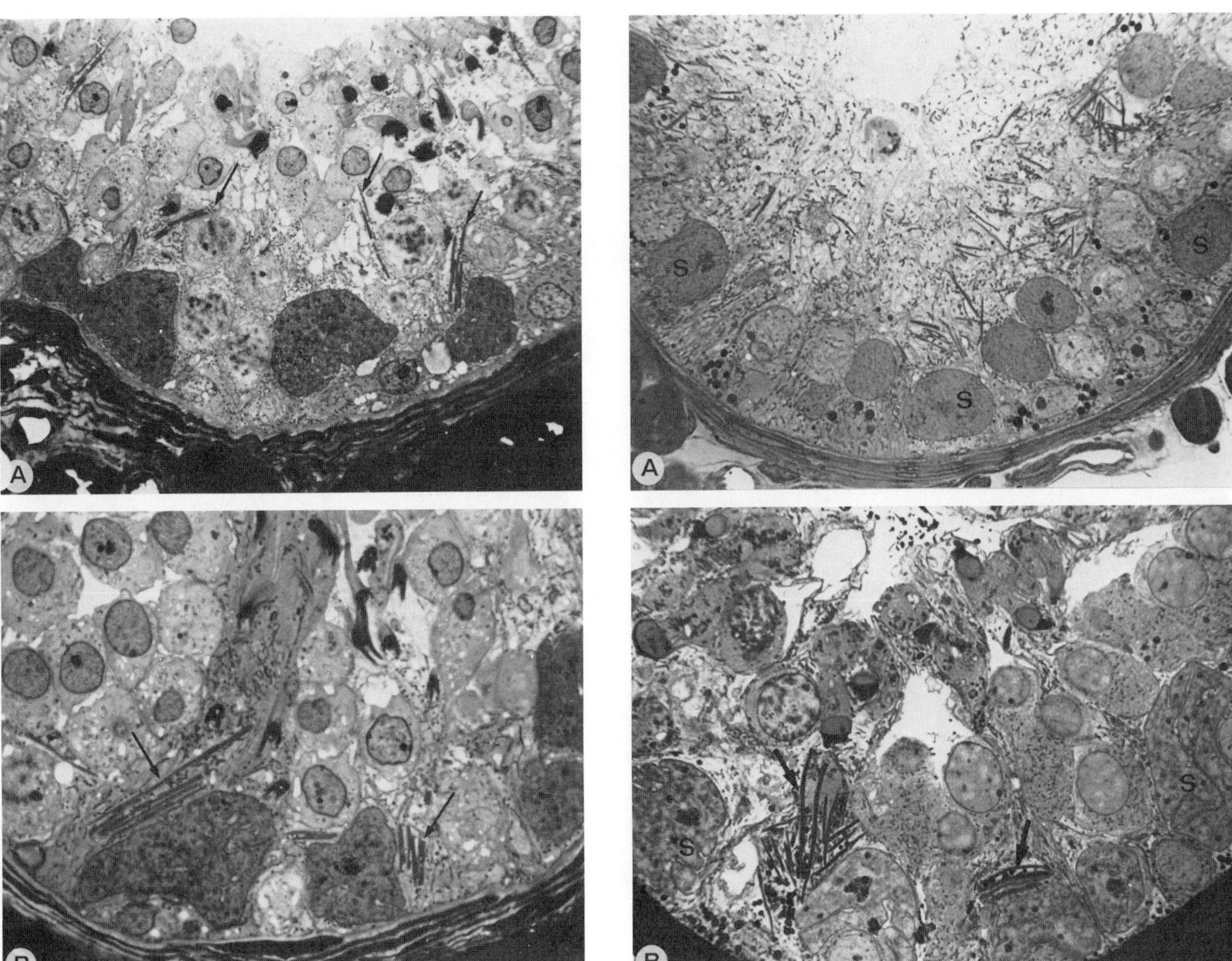

FIG. 50. A: Adult koala testis, illustrating giant Sertoli cell nuclei and needle-shaped cytoplasmic inclusions (*arrows*). **B:** Numerous crystalloid inclusions are commonly found in the basal aspects of the Sertoli cells of the adult koala (*arrows*).

FIG. 51. A: Juvenile koala testis, showing oval-shaped Sertoli cell nuclei (S) and numerous needle-type inclusions in the adluminal cytoplasm. **B:** Pubertal koala testis, indicating giant Sertoli cell nuclei with many indentations (S). Cytoplasmic crystalloid inclusions occur in association with the Sertoli cell nuclei (*arrows*).

that the Sertoli cells probably were responsible for the phagocytosis and destruction of the excess residual cytoplasm. Regaud described their disposal in four steps: (a) release into the lumen; (b) resorption within the Sertoli cells; (c) peripheral migration deep into the epithelium; (d) transformation into "Sertoli hyaline" spheres that blackened in the presence of osmic acid. Since then, the formation (Figs. 53–57) and fate of residual bodies have been studied by light and electron microscopy (253–255,257,258, 262,285,305,313,344,380), but the mechanisms by which the residual bodies are eliminated by the Sertoli cells were not resolved by these studies.

Recent examination of the lysosomal apparatus of the Sertoli cells has now shed light on this process. When electron-dense tracers were introduced into the lumen in seminiferous tubules, they were actively incorporated into the apical regions of the Sertoli cells by means of small vesicles formed at the cell surface (381,382), suggesting a process of fluid-phase endocytosis (pinocytosis). The tracers internalized by this process are eliminated by the lysosomes in the columnar and basal regions of Sertoli cell cytoplasm (383). These studies have been extended (384) to an investigation of the endocytic and phagocytic properties of the Sertoli cell using native ferritin and protein-gold complexes to demonstrate fluid-phase endocytosis, and cationic ferritin and concanavalin-A-ferritin to identify adsorptive endocytosis. The latter process occurs when molecules initially bind to the cell surface prior to internalization by small vesicles. The results indicate that fluid-phase endocytosis by rat Sertoli cells occurs in all stages of the spermatogenic cycle. At stages VIII and IX, the lysosomes formed as a consequence of this process fuse with the newly formed residual bodies and transform them into phagolysosomes,

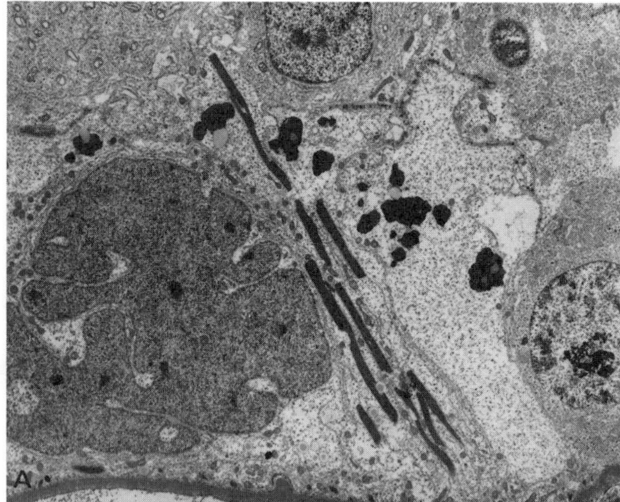

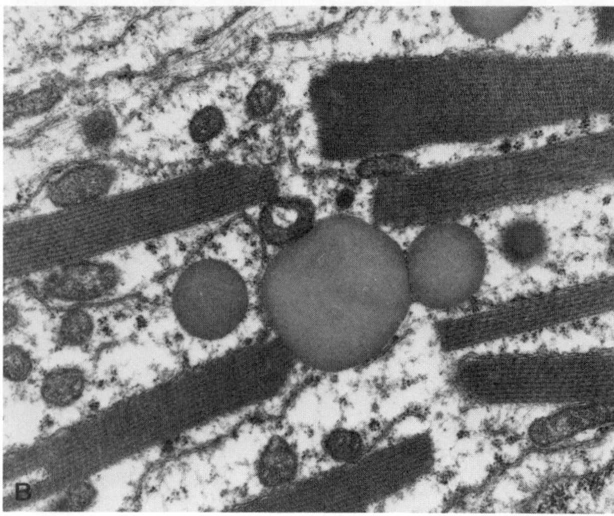

FIG. 52. A: Ultrastructure of adult koala Sertoli cell, showing a highly irregular nucleus and bundles of cytoplasmic crystalloids. **B:** Crystalloids of koala Sertoli cells exhibit a regular lattice-type substructure.

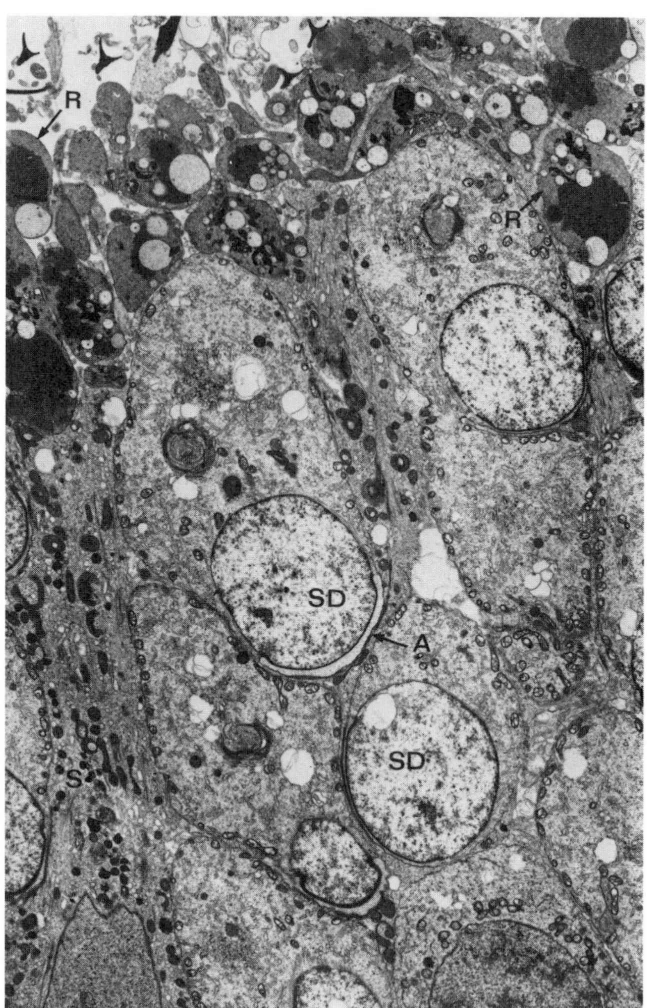

FIG. 53. Stage VIII of the rat spermatogenic cycle, illustrating a tall columnar Sertoli cell (S), spermatids (SD) with acrosomal caps (A), and many lobes of residual cytoplasm (R).

whereupon they disintegrate at the base of the Sertoli cell (Fig. 58). The formation of lysosomes and their participation in the dissolution of residual bodies thus provide a link between the endocytic and phagocytic activities of the Sertoli cell. Adsorptive endocytosis occurs principally during stage VII, when various phagocytic vacuoles form close to the heads of late spermatids, where they probably play a role in resorption of the specialized tubulobulbar complexes that anchor the spermatid head to the apical cytoplasmic processes of the Sertoli cells.

Scant attention has been accorded to the presence of concentric layers of smooth membranes usually confined to the basal aspects of the human Sertoli cell (197,288,289,316,362). Because of the presence of pore-like complexes that form a bridgework between parallel profiles of these membranes (288,289,316), they have been likened to annulate lamellae that have been described in other tissues (385–388). Although their function in the Sertoli cell remains unknown, the annulate lamellae have been implicated in RNA transport from the nucleus (389), in protein synthesis (387,388,390), and as site of tubulin synthesis or polymerization of microtubules (391).

As would be expected for a cell that is obliged to radically alter its shape in conforming to the ever changing events within the seminiferous epithelium, all Sertoli cells thus far studied have been endowed with an elaborate cytoskeleton together with contractile elements occupying most parts of the cytoplasmic matrix (285,286). The former component, responsible for maintenance of cell shape and the redistribution of the cytosolic gel matrix to the cell, is attributed to an often extensive and intricate system of microfilaments (60–70 Å) and intermediate filaments (100 Å). Together these dense filamentous networks are thought to play a major role in structural support of the Sertoli cell when rigidity is necessary, and at other times it is thought that they engineer changes in cell matrix viscosity, allowing variable degrees

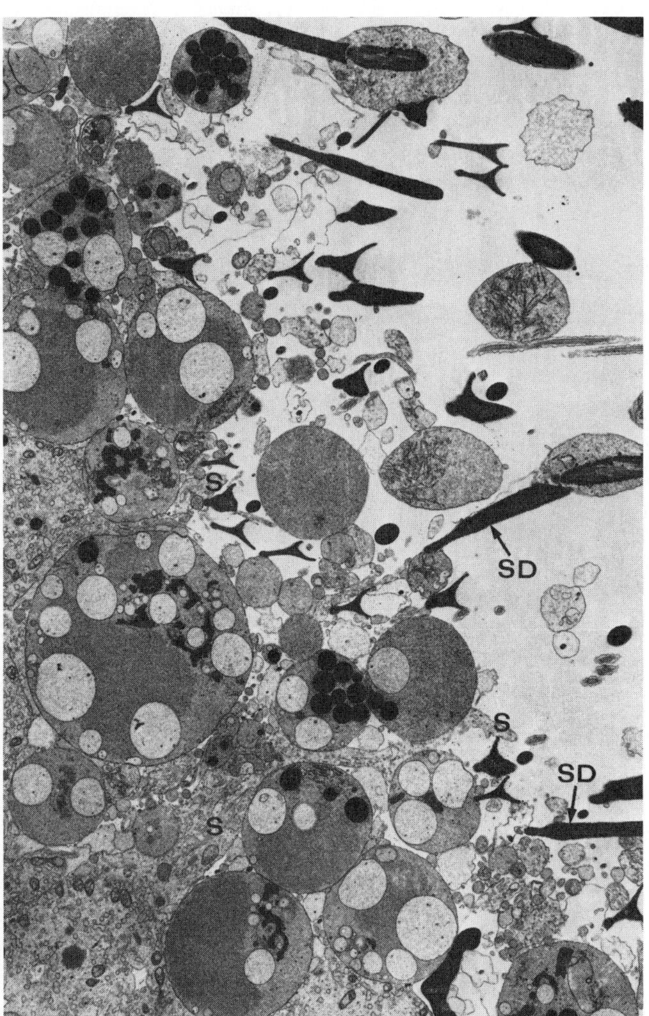

FIG. 54. Stage VIII of the rat spermatogenic cycle, illustrating large spherical residual bodies (R) and mature spermatids (SD) being released from the Sertoli cell cytoplasm (S).

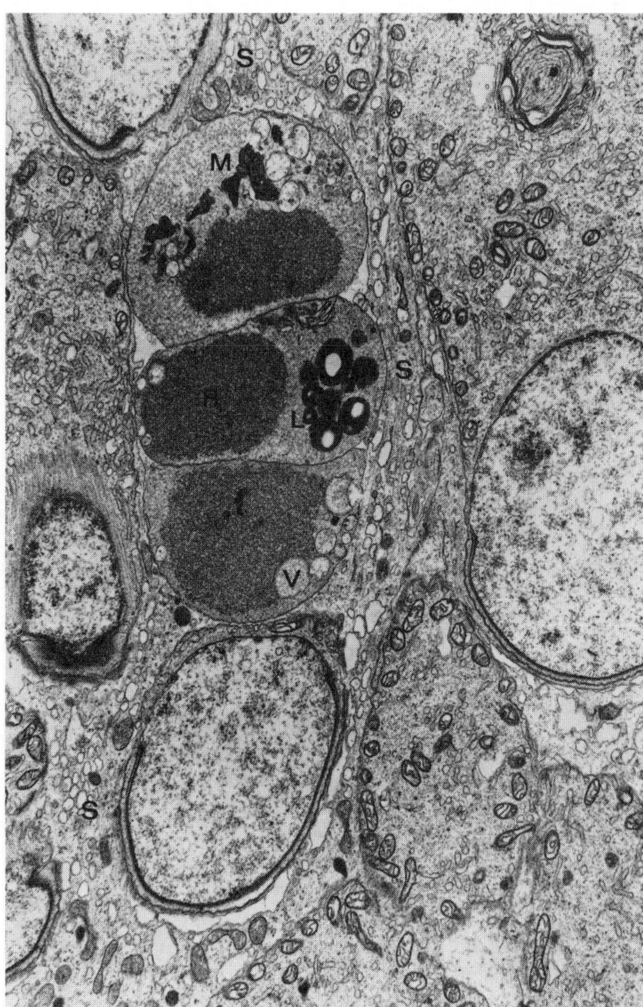

FIG. 55. A residual body composed of three lobes, containing ribosomes (R), vacuoles (V), lipid inclusions (L), and condensed mitochondria (M). Note that the residual body is surrounded by Sertoli cell cytoplasm (S).

of plasticity that are essential to accommodate the constant mobility of the germ cells. These filaments are rich in actin (392,393) and vimentin (393,394). Concentrations of filaments occur at the very base of the Sertoli cell adjacent to the basal lamina, around the Sertoli cell nucleus and in the columnar cytoplasm, where they course parallel to the cell axis, and also in association with numerous ectoplasmic specializations. The latter attain close proximity to developing spermatids and form junctional complexes between neighboring Sertoli cells in the basal aspects of the epithelium.

Especially rich supplies of filaments are seen to fill the cytoplasm of many monkey Sertoli cells in the terminal segments of the seminiferous tubules (17), although the reason for their abundance is not clear. Study of the structure-function relationships of the Sertoli cell cytoskeleton in the ground squirrel has added much to an understanding of the mechanisms underlying shape change (304). The Sertoli cells of the squirrel were chosen for investigation because the seminiferous epithelium contains relatively small numbers of germ cells, compared with other species (287), and the Sertoli cells undergo dramatic shape changes. It now seems likely, based on the results obtained from squirrel Sertoli cells (304,343), that actin-rich filaments in ectoplasmic specializations are devoid of myosin, and rather than fulfilling a contractile role, they probably stabilize the cortical cytoplasm of Sertoli cells at the sites where they occur. Perhaps the filaments maintain the shape of Sertoli cell crypts embracing the penetrating clones of spermatids (290,395) and may add reinforcement to the zone of Sertoli cell ectoplasm at the level of the basal junctional complexes between adjacent Sertoli cells.

If filaments associated with ectoplasmic specializations are not contractile, then what generates the forces necessary for alterations in Sertoli cell shape? New light has been shed on this problem following the recent demonstration that exposure of Sertoli cells to colchicine causes severe dis-

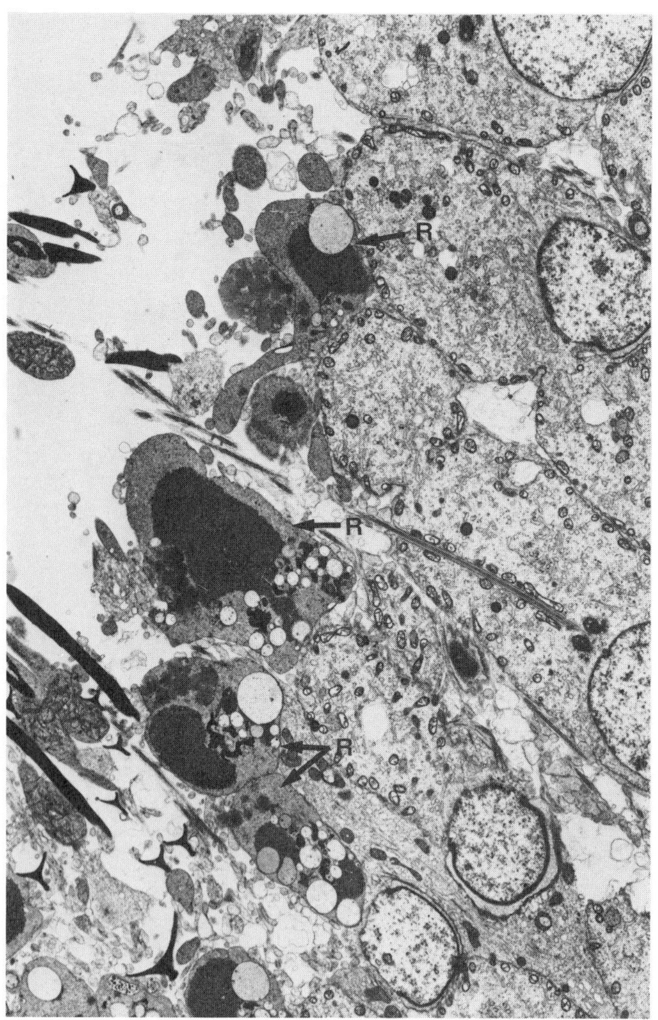

FIG. 56. Stage VIII of the rat spermatogenic cycle, showing large irregular lobes of residual cytoplasm (R).

FIG. 57. Degenerated residual bodies (R) deep within the Sertoli cell cytoplasm (S). The lipid component (L) of the residual body is resistant to the phagocytic action of the Sertoli cell.

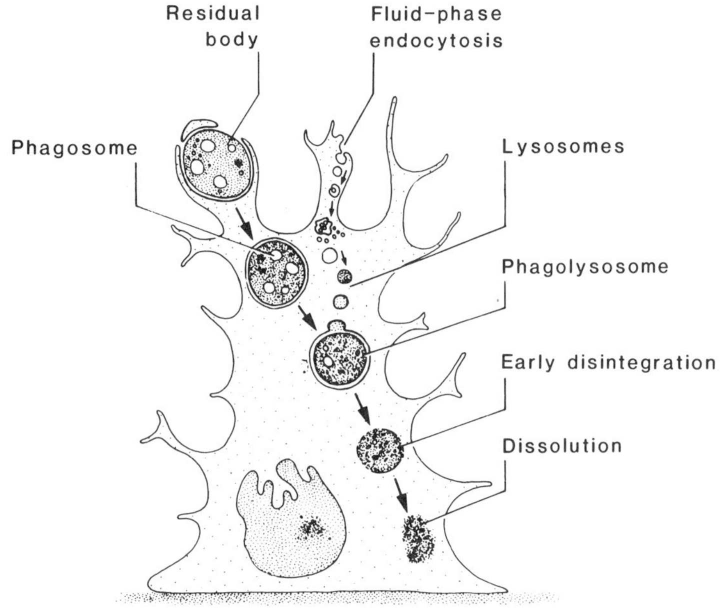

FIG. 58. Representation of phagocytosis of residual bodies and fluid-phase endocytosis by the Sertoli cell. These processes may be integrated to allow disintegration of the residual bodies as they proceed through the body of the Sertoli cell. (Adapted from ref. 384.)

ruption of germ cell movements and blocks intracellular transport of membranous organelles (329). Administration of colchicine *in vivo* destroyed virtually all Sertoli cell microtubules, indicating that they play a significant part in molding and sculpturing the Sertoli cell cytoplasm to facilitate upward and downward movements of germ cells. Additionally, these studies offered a new interpretation of the mechanism by which Sertoli cells participate in sperm release. Earlier studies (396–398) favored the view that microtubules were involved with shedding of spermatids from the apex of the Sertoli cell. Others (399) proposed that the sloughing of many spermatids into the lumen of the seminiferous tubule after colchicine treatment was due to Sertoli cell disruption rather than to a selective interference with Sertoli cell microtubules. When the effects of colchicine were reinvestigated (329), late spermatids were not shed from the Sertoli cells, and the special ectoplasmic regions adjacent to spermatid heads remained intact, as did those subjacent to basal tight junctions between Sertoli cells. As yet, no adequate explanation has been offered to account for the role of those filaments that are found in random orientations throughout the Sertoli cell cytoplasm.

Surface Specializations

A well-recognized property of the testis is the maintenance, within the seminiferous tubules, of a highly specialized microenvironment created by the Sertoli cells that partitions young and more mature germ cells into two compartments within the seminiferous epithelium. At this point it is pertinent to acknowledge the contribution of earlier studies to this topic. Together these numerous observations led to the discovery of a blood-testis barrier that exists in the testes of phylogenetically distant species and thus reinforces the fundamental importance of the Sertoli cell in the regulation of spermatogenesis.

Early in this century, physiological studies by Ribbert (400), Bouffard (401), and Pari (402) indicated that the testis was one of the few organs into which intranvenously injected dyes did not gain entry. No significance was assigned to these initial observations or to more recent work reporting similar results (403,404). The vascular network of the testicular interstitial tissue is highly permeable to large molecules, as demonstrated by Everett and Simmons (405) when they noted that intravenously injected serum albumin had a rapid rate of extravascular transfer and readily permeated into the interstitium. Many other substrates were found to readily diffuse from the testicular blood vessels into the interstitial lymphatics, but did not appear in the fluid collected from the rete testis. Thus, the blood-testis permeability barrier seemed to be anatomically located either surrounding or actually within the wall of the seminiferous tubules (65,406–410).

In common laboratory rodents, penetration of electron-dense markers from the blood vasculature into the seminiferous tubules is partly retarded by peritubular myoid cells. This incomplete barrier is not found in the ram, bull, boar, or primate (285,286), and in all species the effective component of the blood-testis barrier resides within the seminiferous epithelium. In the light of this evidence, closer examination of the ultrastructural features of the seminiferous epithelium revealed the presence of various types of tight junctions or desmosome-like structures associated with the plasma membrane of the Sertoli cell (161,197,323,362). Brökelmann (173) originally provided a clear illustration of these inter-Sertoli-cell junctions in a variety of animals. He noted that whenever the boundaries of the Sertoli cell were apposed, they formed complex cytoplasmic membranes immediately adjacent to and parallel with the limiting plasma membrane. These profiles were apparently cisternae of endoplasmic reticulum, and in a study of postnatal development of the mouse testis, Flickinger (62) again observed a similar type of junction and noted that these specializations between Sertoli cells increased in numbers with the onset of meiosis and the formation of a tubule lumen.

Junctional specializations were not seen in the testes of fetal or neonatal cattle or dogs, and Nicander (159) proposed that in adult testes the junctions might restrict intercellular passage of substances to germ cells. These morphological studies were complemented by physiological work indicating that the barrier was absent at birth, but with sexual maturation the previously unrestricted transport of acriflavine dyes was prevented concomitant with meiotic maturation of the primary spermatocytes (65). Since then, the ultrastructural features of inter-Sertoli-cell junctions have been documented in many excellent descriptions (66,270,284–286,313,411–414) and are summarized in Figs. 59 to 61 as follows: (a) Junctional specializations between Sertoli cells are particularly prominent in the basal regions of the seminiferous epithelium, and usually occur when adjacent Sertoli cell cytoplasmic processes meet. (b) Sometimes, at the very base of the Sertoli cell adjacent to the basal lamina, the meeting of two apposed Sertoli cell cytoplasmic processes may be devoid of junctional specialization. (c) The basal location of junctional specializations circumscribing the lateral margins of Sertoli cells is anatomically reversed compared with the tight junctional specializations present in many other epithelia. (d) Normally, a space of 150 to 200 Å separates the outer leaflets of adjacent Sertoli cell membranes. (e) Occasionally this space is narrowed to 20 Å, similar to the traditional gap junction or nexus of other cells. (f) In thin sections studied by transmission electron microscopy, multiple sites of fusion of the outer membrane leaflets are seen at regular intervals along the cell-to-cell interfaces. (g) Sertoli cell junctions are often flanked by parallel cisternae of endoplasmic reticulum, irregularly fenestrated and exhibiting ribosomes toward the cell body, but agranular on the ectoplasmic face. (h) Sandwiched between the cisternae and cell surface, bundles of fine filaments are oriented parallel to the cell surface and, in transverse views, are packed in hexagonal arrays.

With the advent of freeze-cleaving methods, the multiple focal sites of fusion between Sertoli cell membranes were

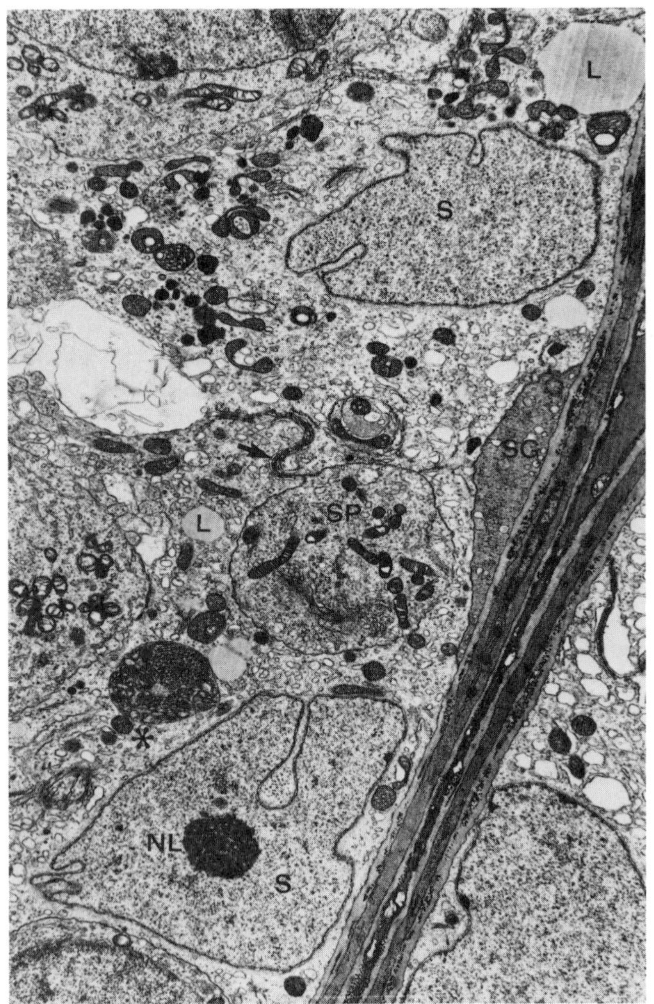

FIG. 59. Basal aspect of the rat seminiferous epithelium, illustrating two Sertoli cells (S), one containing a large nucleolus (NL). Note inter-Sertoli-cell junction (*arrow*) and cytoplasm of an early primary spermatocyte (SP) and a basally situated spermatogonium (SG). A degenerated residual body (*asterisk*) and lipid inclusions (L) are shown.

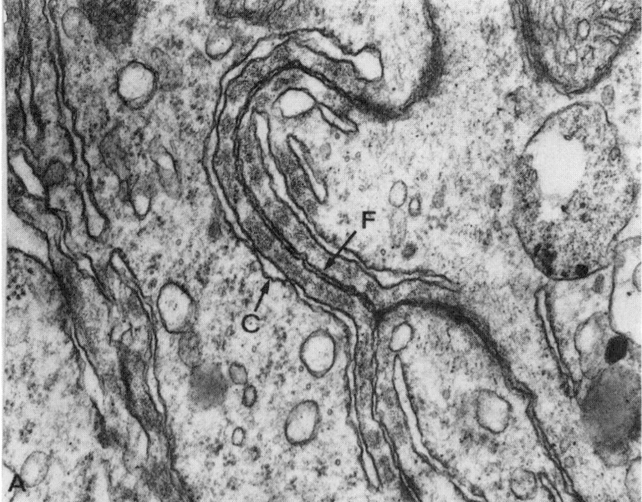

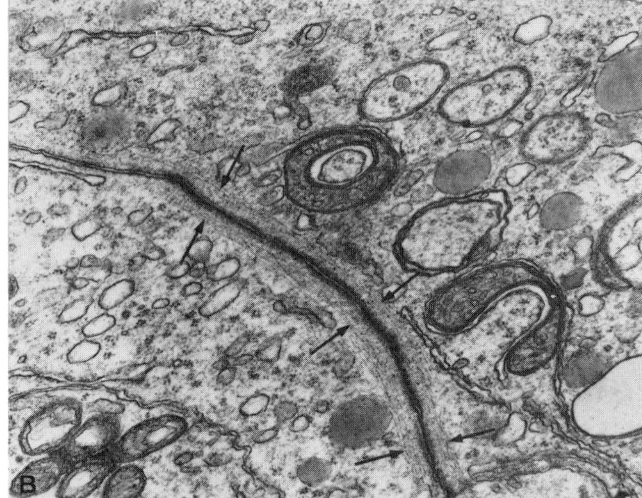

FIG. 60. A: Inter-Sertoli-cell junction, illustrating bundles of filaments (F) adjacent to the Sertoli cell plasma membrane. Smooth-surfaced cisternae (C) run parallel to the opposed surfaces of the Sertoli cells. **B:** Longitudinal profile of an inter-Sertoli-cell junction showing parallel arrays of filaments (*arrows*).

shown to extend entirely around the circumference of the cell and to consist of long parallel rows of intramembranous particles intercalated with matching grooves (66,284–286, 327,415,416). This collar of junctional specialization occupies approximately 4% of the surface area of the plasma membrane in the rat Sertoli cell (292). Up to 50 parallel lines of membrane fusion between adjacent surfaces of Sertoli cells together constitute a highly effective barrier against the intraepithelial penetration of the spaces between cells residing in the base of the seminiferous epithelium (313,411,413). The capacity of inter-Sertoli-cell junctions in maintaining cell adhesion has been convincingly demonstrated after ligation of the efferent ductules, a procedure causing marked distention of the seminiferous tubules. Junctions between Sertoli cells fail to separate regardless of the degree of tubular distention (412). Recent studies of the permeability properties of inter-Sertoli-cell tight junctions have shown a progressive loss of impermeability from the base to the lumen of the seminiferous tubule that is correlated with an increasing incidence of disintegration of the junctional complex (67).

The strategic and unusual location of Sertoli cell tight junctions in relation to the germ cells has given rise to the concept of an anatomic and functional subdivision of the seminiferous epithelium into (a) a basal compartment containing spermatogonia and preleptotene and leptotene primary spermatocytes and (b) an adluminal component beyond the level of the tight junctions that sequesters the more differentiated germ cells into a unique physiological environment (284,313,413). Some species differ in the precise manner in which germ cells ascend from the basal to the

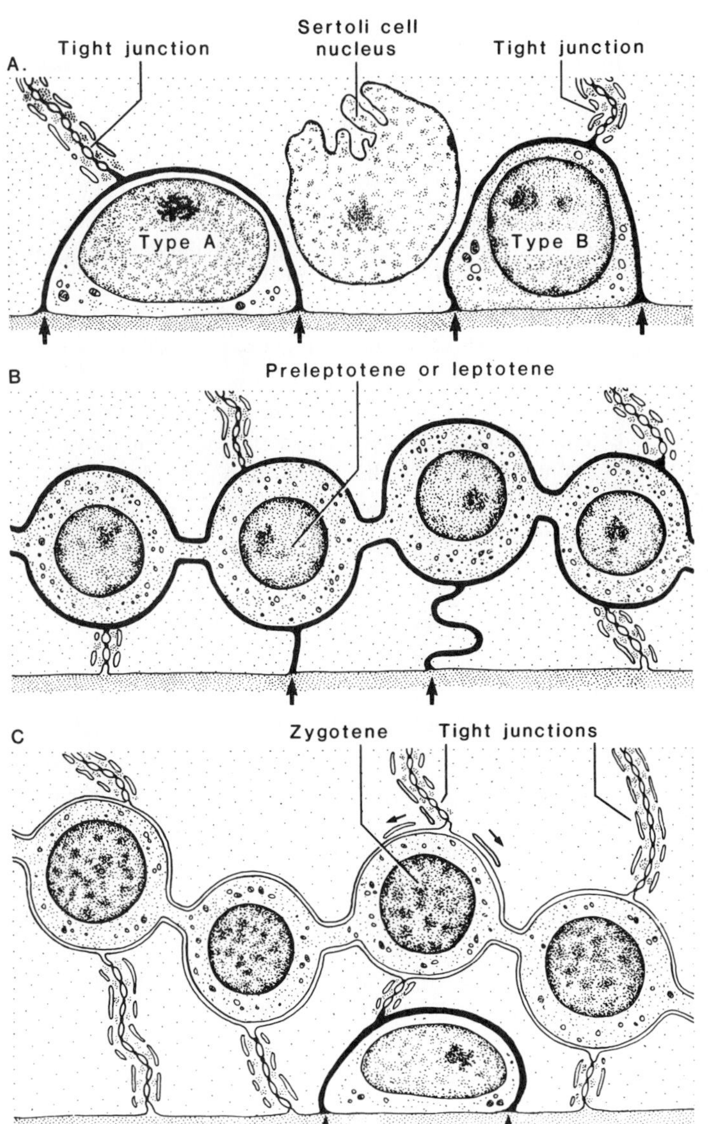

FIG. 61. Diagrams illustrating the upward migration of germ cells from the basal aspect of the seminiferous epithelium toward the lumen. In each diagram, tracer entry into the intercellular spaces is shown by *large arrows.* (Adapted from ref. 417.) **A:** Entry of tracers into the seminiferous epithelium is prevented by the occluding inter-Sertoli-cell tight junctions. **B:** Preleptotene and leptotene primary spermatocytes are displaced above the basal lamina. Tight junctions are seen below, above, or both below and above these forms of cells, and consequently tracers are able to surround the interconnected cells via cytoplasmic bridges. Tight junctions above the germ cells prevent further passage of tracers into the seminiferous epithelium. **C:** When leptotene primary spermatocytes enter the zygotene phase of meiotic prophase, tracers do not surround zygotene spermatocytes, because tight junctions are formed beneath these cells. Dissociation of inter-Sertoli-cell junctions into hemijunctions has been suggested and is indicated by *small arrows.*

adluminal compartment, thereby breaching the barrier maintained by the Sertoli cell tight junctions. In the macaque testis, leptotene primary spermatocytes reside in the basal subdivision and, following upward mobilization, mature into zygotene primary spermatocytes on reaching the adluminal compartment (417). For the rat, the transition from basal region to adluminal region has been suggested to occur through the agency of a short-lived intermediate compartment, embodying some leptotene primary spermatocytes (418). This transit chamber is flanked above and below by tight junctional complexes, i.e., neither truly basal (permeable to blood-borne substances) nor adluminal (impermeable to blood-borne substances). Further research will be necessary to determine if the so-called intermediate compartment provides a special physiological milieu different from either the basal or adluminal compartment.

Whatever the histological organization of the testis, some form of intraepithelial junctional specialization is always localized in the somatic cells surrounding the germ cells, suggesting that the blood-testis barrier is an ancient evolutionary trait of central importance for successful development of viable gametes. In broad terms, the ultrastructural organization of the inter-Sertoli-cell junctions can be classified into three main types based principally on the type of membrane specialization. The testes of mammals show a complex organization of the blood-testis barrier, and in species described to date, the arrangement described earlier is virtually unchanged. Examples can be found in studies of rodents (mouse, rat, guinea pig, squirrel), ruminants (bull, ram, goat), domesticated carnivores (dog), and primates (macaque and human). A group exhibiting somewhat simpler organization of the junctional complexes, in that they often lack the bundles of actin-rich filaments and subsurface membranous cisternae, can be illustrated by birds and reptiles (299,301,419). A simple arrangement serving the function of a blood-testis barrier is peculiar to amphibians and fishes, where only desmosome-like and short tight junctions are observed between Sertoli cells (266,298,420–425). In other groups, however, the form of barrier is less well defined, and in nematodes and insects, small septate, desmosome-like and tight junctions are regarded as the structural entities of the blood-testis barrier (422,426–429).

Despite the aforementioned studies, little is known about the actual physiological role of the blood-testis barrier (73). The formation of inter-Sertoli-cell junctions coincides with the cessation of Sertoli cell proliferation in the immature testis (43), and junctions make their appearance as germ cells proceed through the zygotene to pachytene steps of meiotic maturation (64,66,68,417). However, the junctions also appear in the absence of germ cells (45,70,71) or in response to gonadotropic stimulation of the Sertoli cells (77), but their formation is dependent on transformation of Sertoli cells from an immature to adult-type morphology. Because early primary spermatocytes (leptotene or zygotene) reside in the basal compartment of the mammalian seminiferous epithelium, and similar observations have been reported in lower orders of animals (298), then evidently the initiation of meiotic maturation does not require the specialized intratubular milieu provided within the confines of the adluminal epithelial compartment. In the rat testis, as the primary spermatocytes enter prophase, cell surface antigens specific to germ cells appear on pachytene primary spermatocytes and all subsequent stages of germ cell differentiation (430–433). Specific antigens also appear on the surfaces of Sertoli cells (434) and it has been suggested that the processes of meiotic maturation and differentiation of spermatids occur in an immunologically privileged adluminal microenvironment sustained via the inter-Sertoli-cell tight junctions (73,435). Isolation of these germ cells by the blood-testis barrier either restricts leakage of antigen or prevents entry of antibodies or immune cells from the vascular system. That the germ cells are not absolutely dependent on an intact blood-testis barrier has recently been demonstrated in the seasonally breeding mink, in which the blood-testis barrier appears to undergo cyclic formation and decay in association with respective periods of activity and inactivity of the seminiferous epithelium (436).

The upward movement of early spermatocytes into the adluminal compartment requires that some mechanism be available to allow the migrating germ cells to traverse the specialized inter-Sertoli-cell junctions. These junctions have been observed both above and below young spermatocytes (159,417), and an orderly process of breakdown and formation of tight junctions has been proposed to permit cell transfer from the basal to the adluminal compartment (159,413). Further studies have indicated that new tight junctions between Sertoli cells form below young spermatocytes, whereas those previously above these cells are thought to dissociate, thus ensuring the patency of the permeability barrier (395,417,418). Thus, the barrier is flexible and deformable and compatible with the movements of migrating germ cells. Early stages of formation of tight junctions beneath migrating germ cells are characterized by increasing numbers of intramembranous junctional strands that increase in length and begin to assume parallel orientations, thus collectively contributing to an increasing degree of continuity, culminating into a typical junctional complex (67).

The complex, yet highly ordered, arrangement of multiple clones of germ cells, each embraced by the highly branched Sertoli cell, demands that the Sertoli cell not only be capable of conforming to the remarkable shape changes of the germ cells but also play a role in conferring stability throughout the seminiferous epithelium. In reviewing this topic, a wealth of morphological information is now available from comparative studies of Sertoli-cell–germ-cell relationships that together indicates the central role played by the Sertoli cell in maintaining an attachment to germ cells, in addition to providing potential avenues of intercellular communication. The literature concerned with this aspect of the biology of Sertoli cells is voluminous, but the reader is directed to a number of excellent studies that provide the basis for our present understanding (259,263,285,290,292,304,328, 329,343,414,437–439).

Prevention of premature disengagement and sloughing of germ cells into the lumen of the seminiferous tubule is thought to rely, at least in part, on regions of ectoplasmic specializations of the Sertoli cell that face the surfaces of certain germ cells. These structures consist of a dense band of actin-rich filaments sandwiched between the Sertoli cell plasma membrane and a cistern of endoplasmic reticulum, and thus resemble one half of the paired ectoplasmic specializations that constitute the inter-Sertoli-cell tight junctions at the base of the Sertoli cells. Originally described between adjacent Sertoli cells and spermatids in the rat testis (173,268), their widespread occurrence in other species has subsequently been confirmed (154,159,270,285,302,328, 393,395,440,441).

Visualization of the sites of apposition of germ cells to ectoplasmic specializations at the lateral and apical surfaces of the Sertoli cell is dependent on the orientation and plane of section when the seminiferous epithelium is examined with the electron microscope. This limitation restricts an objective appraisal of what type and how many germ cells are associated with ectoplasmic specializations, and it also seems likely that this relationship is variable between different species. In hamster, monkey, and human testes, regions of ectoplasmic specialization have been reported facing zygotene primary spermatocytes (84,289,313,441), but other studies of a number of species have suggested that this association occurs only rarely (440). Where most reports seem to be in agreement is in the occurrence of ectoplasmic specializations facing midpachytene primary spermatocytes (Fig. 62) and round spermatids, but as the spermatids begin to elongate (Figs. 24 and 62) and undergo their final phase of maturation, a mantle of ectoplasmic specialization is always positioned around the spermatid head (290,395,440). Whenever elongated spermatids are seen to deeply penetrate the Sertoli cell, the resultant recess that contains the sper-

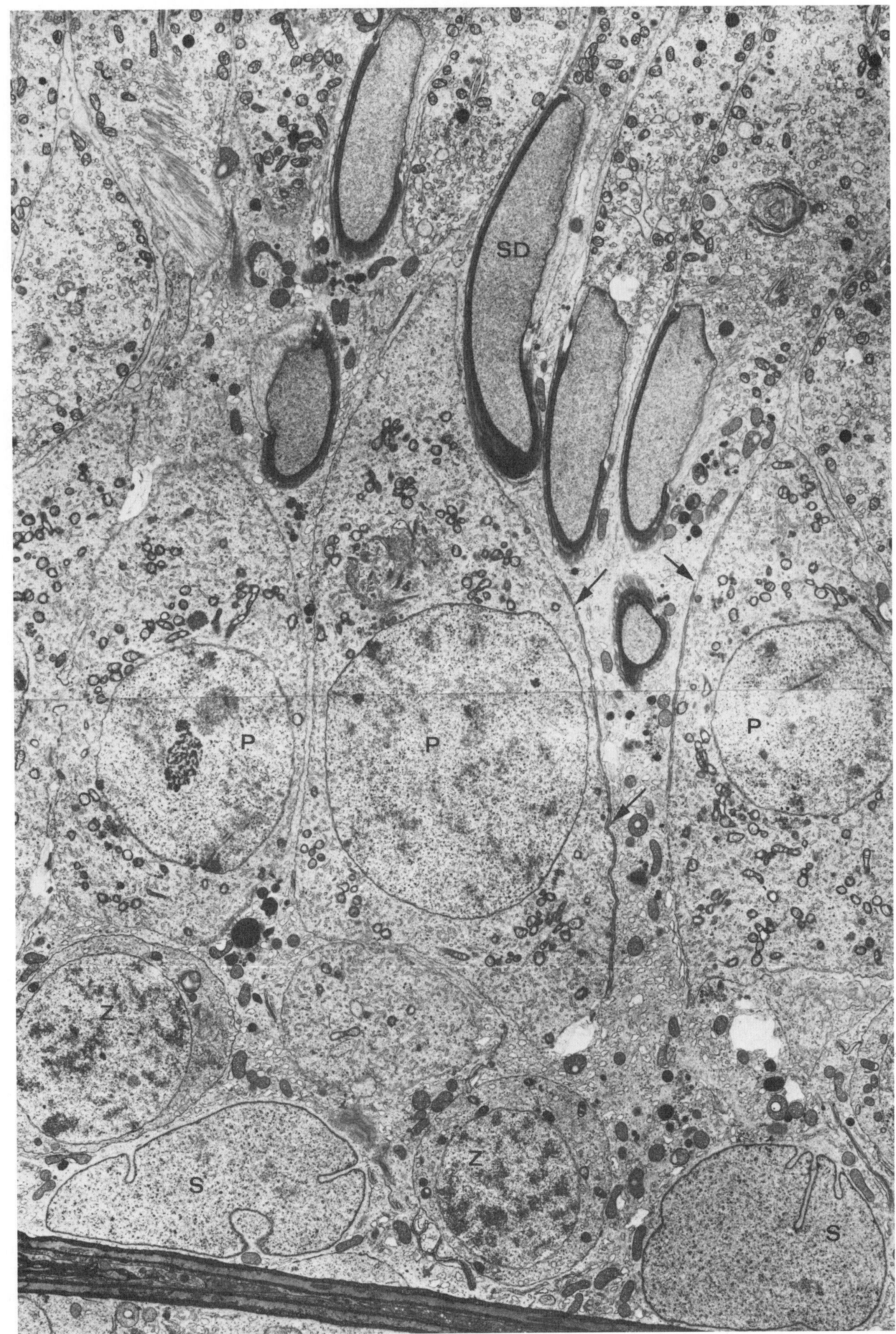

FIG. 62. Stage XI of the rat spermatogenic cycle, illustrating Sertoli cells (S), zygotene primary spermatocytes (Z), pachytene primary spermatocytes (P), and elongated spermatids (SD). Note hemijunctions (*arrows*) associated with the plasma membranes of the pachytene primary spermatocytes.

matid head is lined by ectoplasmic specialization that is preferentially associated with the acrosome.

The function of Sertoli cell ectoplasmic specializations adjacent to germ cells is, however, unknown. Differences in adhesive properties between Sertoli cells and various germ cells have provided circumstantial evidence that ectoplasmic specializations may actually bind to adjacent germ cells. Round germ cells (spermatocytes and early round spermatids) are easily separated from Sertoli cells (393, 395,442), but elongate germ cells (maturing spermatids) are more resistant to dislodgement, and enzymatic digestion with trypsin is required to separate them away from the Sertoli cell (60,442). Because desmosomes are not observed between elongate spermatids and Sertoli cells (290), the adhesive property that exists between them has implicated the ectoplasmic specialization in partly fulfilling this role. Additional suggested activities for the ectoplasmic specializations include (a) structural support for the Sertoli cell during germ cell mobilization (290,395), (b) participation in sperm release and acrosome shaping (287,328,437,442), (c) a contractile role (392,443), and (d) sites of intercellular attachment (328,393,442,444).

A general concept of the origin of ectoplasmic specializations and their role in sperm release was put forward by Ross and Dobler (302,328). Based on their observations on the mouse Sertoli cell, they suggested that as primary spermatocytes begin to ascend through the area of the blood-testis barrier, the inter-Sertoli-cell tight junctions disengage, and each intact, free ectoplasmic specialization thus formed will gain attachment to the spermatocyte on entering the adluminal compartment of the seminiferous epithelium. This hypothesis has been questioned (290) on the grounds that (a) in the rat testis, no ectoplasmic specializations are observed in association with the ascending young spermatocytes, and (b) such round germ cells are not actually attached to ectoplasmic specializations, as discussed earlier. Further studies will be necessary to clarify the origin and early location of ectoplasmic specializations.

There is no doubt that ectoplasmic specializations are seen facing midpachytene primary spermatocytes and round spermatids (289,290,328,417), where they occupy approximately 1% of the surface area of the Sertoli cell in the rat testis at stage V of the spermatogenic cycle (292). All elongate and maturing spermatids are associated with ectoplasmic specializations, comprising approximately 3% of Sertoli cell membrane surface area. The participation in sperm release and ultimate fate of ectoplasmic specializations are subjects of some discussion. Following elongation of mature spermatids and their ascent toward the lumen of the seminiferous tubule, the spermatid head disengages from the ectoplasmic specializations and allows for release of sperm from the apical surface of the Sertoli cells. Profiles of ectoplasmic specialization are retained by the Sertoli cell, and in studies of the mouse Sertoli cell (328) they were seen facing the engulfed lobes of excess spermatid residual cytoplasm and were also found free at the surface of the Sertoli cell or as isolated nonsurface elements within the cytoplasm. It was inferred from these observations that the occurrence of ectoplasmic specializations free within the cytoplasm signaled an early stage in their disintegration and subsequent disappearance. These findings have provided the basis for additional study of the ectoplasmic specializations (395, 418,437,440,445), and three theories have been advanced to account for the origin, behavior, and fate of ectoplasmic specializations, as depicted in Fig. 63: (a) They may degenerate and, following internalization by the Sertoli cell, then disappear (328,440,443,446,447). (b) They become adherent to the cytoplasmic lobe of the sperm and thus selectively retain the lobes of residual cytoplasm (441). (c) They are removed intact from the Sertoli cell surface and, when free in the cytoplasm, became available for reutilization by the next generation of germ cells. Recycling of ectoplasmic specializations could occur by their distribution from a common pool or by intercellular transfer, e.g., from round spermatids to pachytene spermatocytes (395,440,448). As yet, the factors regulating the formation and degradation of ectoplasmic specializations and their suggested role in germ cell movement, sperm release, and structural support of the Sertoli cell remain to be determined.

As the mature spermatids are released from their attachments to Sertoli cell ectoplasmic specializations, they are retained at the surface of the seminiferous epithelium via very slender upward projections of the apical Sertoli cell cytoplasm. In this position they await their release into the lumen of the seminiferous tubule (Figs. 40 and 64). In favorable semithin sections examined by light microscopy, the spermatid head lies at the very tip of the seminiferous epithelium, with the flagellum projecting into the lumen. The sperm appear to retain contact with the seminiferous epithelium via two structures. First, and well illustrated in the rat, the apical stalk of Sertoli cell cytoplasm balloons out within the concave aspect of the spermatid head; second, the cytoplasm of the elongate spermatid becomes progressively attenuated along the long axis of the sperm and thus forms a slender cytoplasmic lobe (future residual cytoplasm) extending from the neck of the spermatid and coursing toward the apical regions of the Sertoli cell.

Returning to the delicate Sertoli cell cytoplasmic stalk associated only with the head and neck of the spermatid, faint striations are observed within the concave recess of Sertoli cell cytoplasm. In a series of excellent studies of this relationship between the two cells (263,271,272, 290,437,438), these radially oriented spokes (Figs. 40 and 65) have been seen to form a so-called tubulobulbar complex. This region of specialization consists of a series of long narrow cytoplasmic stalks that protrude, in the case of rat spermatids, from the spermatid head and invaginate the recess of Sertoli cell cytoplasm that fills out the concave environs of the spermatid head (Fig. 65). As the spermatid tubular evaginations penetrate into the Sertoli cell, the Sertoli cell plasma membrane closely conforms to that of the spermatid, except at the tips of the projections, where small

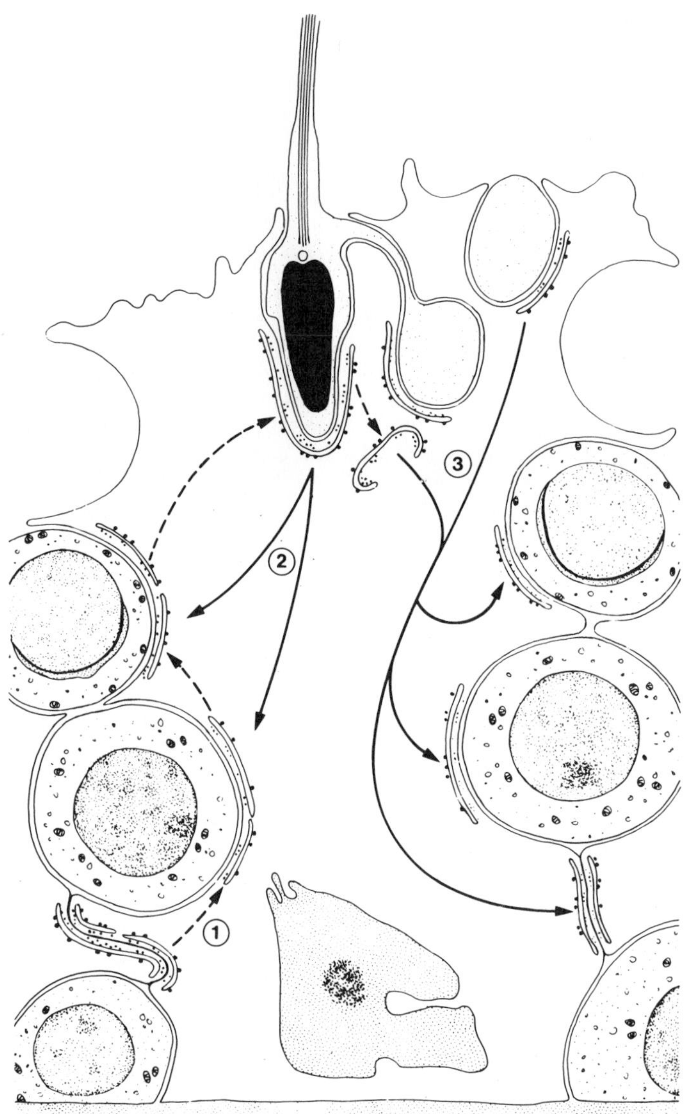

FIG. 63. Diagram demonstrating possible pathways for redistribution of inter-Sertoli-cell junctions. In route 1, basally situated junctions may separate to form hemijunctions associated with the surfaces of primary spermatocytes and early and late spermatids. Route 2 indicates proposed recycling of crypt-shaped hemijunctions from the late spermatids back to earlier generations of germ cells. Route 3 illustrates possible formation of pools of free hemijunctions that recycle to earlier germ cells and may be involved in the formation of basal inter-Sertoli-cell junctions. (Adapted from refs. 328 and 440.)

bulbous knobs are formed. Tubulobulbar complexes have been described in numerous mammals (438), their numbers ranging from 4 to 24 per spermatid head and attaining lengths of 1 to 8 μm. The complexes are not formed from round spermatids, nor are they seen emanating from elongate spermatids located deep within recesses of Sertoli cell cytoplasm. However, when spermatids rise to the very tips of the Sertoli cell, they lose their relationship to ectoplasmic specializations, whereupon tubulobulbar complexes make their initial appearance. As the Sertoli cell gradually withdraws from the spermatid head, these complexes are maintained until only the extreme tip of the late spermatid head is related to the slender processes of the Sertoli cell. This finding has led to the suggestion that the complexes anchor the spermatid head and participate in its stabilization.

Because several generations of tubulobulbar complexes are formed and then degraded in succession by the Sertoli cells (272), it seems plausible that a proportion of spermatid cytoplasm is resorbed through the degradation of numerous tubulobulbar complexes. The flow of spermatid cytoplasm into these complexes has also been suggested to trigger the sperm release mechanism (448). Although the mechanism by which the Sertoli cell is able to selectively retain, sculpture, and engulf the excess residual cytoplasm remains unclear, Russell (272) has advanced the concept that the tubulobulbar complexes indirectly engineer the formation of the residual bodies. This suggestion is based on his observation that in the period immediately preceding sperm release, the volume of the spermatid cytoplasm is reduced as much as 70%, and this disposal of cytoplasm coincides with the successive formation and degradation of tubulobulbar complexes. The cytoplasm eliminated with the resorption of the tubulobulbar complexes by the Sertoli cell is usually "watery" and lacks organelles, suggesting that the remaining spermatid cytoplasm could become progressively more condensed and filled with spermatid organelles and inclusion

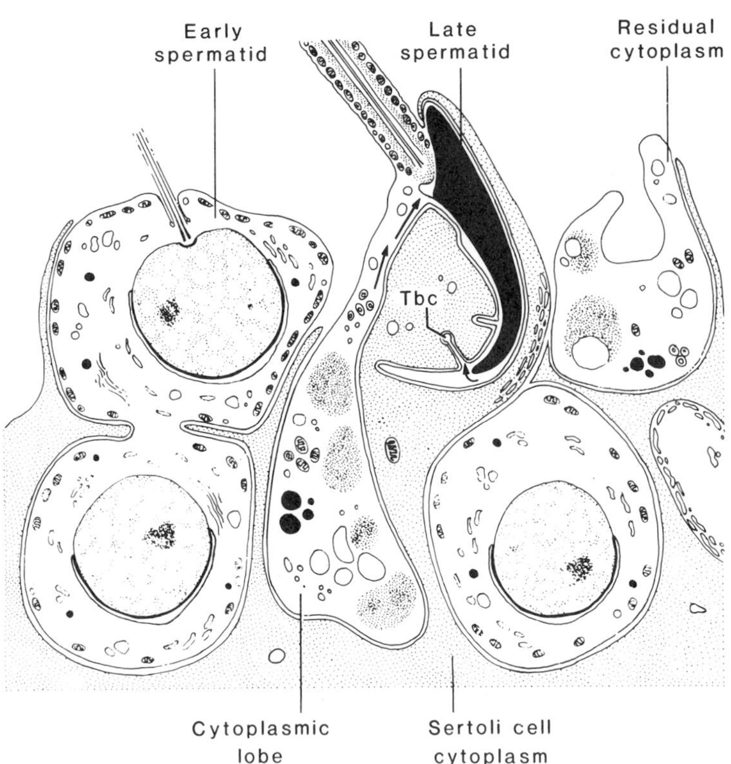

FIG. 64. Relationship between the mature generation of spermatids and the apical surface of the Sertoli cell. Tubulobulbar complexes (Tbc) extend from the concave surface of the spermatid head into the Sertoli cell cytoplasm. Cytoplasm within the cytoplasmic lobe of the spermatid is thought to flow into tubulobulbar complexes, as indicated by *arrows*. (Adapted from ref. 271.)

bodies. In all species thus far studied, the excess cytoplasmic lobes always exhibit these features, and after the sperm are shed, they form deeply staining residual bodies (Figs. 58 and 64). It is not yet known how the Sertoli cell releases the sperm but selectively retains the excess residual cytoplasm, although a recent report (329) has shown that the Sertoli cell cytoplasmic projections that surround and invaginate the residual cytoplasm are richly supplied with filaments and microtubules, which probably pull the residual cytoplasm from the lumen to the apical trunk of the Sertoli cell.

Tubulobulbar complexes also occur between adjacent Sertoli cells at the level of the blood-testis barrier and occasionally give rise to tight and gap junctions in the region of interdigitation (263,445). The tubulobulbar complex is a protrusion of cytoplasm of one Sertoli cell into a neighboring Sertoli cell and resembles a narrow tube 2 to 4 μm in length terminating in a bulbous dilation. The complexes undergo a cyclic variation in number during the spermatogenic cycle in the rat, and their degradation and disappearance at stages VI to VII may represent a mechanism for the development or turnover of junctional contacts between the Sertoli cells.

Other types of specialized junctional regions found within the seminiferous epithelium include desmosomes, hemidesmosomes, and gap junctions. Desmosomes (or macula adherens) are traditionally recognized as small apposed plaques on adjacent cells flanked by a thin dense layer just beneath the plaque and represent strong adhesion sites between cells. They have been described between Sertoli cells and all round germ cells, but are absent from the interface with elongate spermatids (67,153,154,159,173,289,449). In the rat, they are oriented toward the body of the Sertoli cell and often are seen toward the base of the seminiferous tubule, suggesting that they could resist any force tending to dislodge germ cells into the lumen (293). Their general function is believed to be to assist the surface of the Sertoli cell in the orderly upward movement of germ cells during their maturation.

Hemidesmosomes occupy the site where the base of the Sertoli cell rests on the basal lamina of the seminiferous tubule (418,450) and probably confer firm anchoring of the Sertoli cells necessary for them to maintain their pentagonal or hexagonal relationships to each other. Gap junctions (or nexus) are represented as extremely close sites of apposition (20 Å) between adjacent cell membranes and are thought to offer the capability of ionic flux and exchange of small molecules. They also confer sites of firm adhesion between cells. Gap junctions occur between Sertoli cells in laboratory species (66,285,413,451), but are not present on human Sertoli cells (289,327). Their presence has also been noted between Sertoli cells and round germ cells (205,452), although they are often seen in association with desmosomes and are occasionally referred to as desmosome–gap-junctional complexes (293). Gap junctions are not observed between Sertoli cells and elongating spermatids. At present their function is unknown, although potentially they could play a role in intercellular communication.

Changes Associated with Seasonal Breeding and Age

The great majority of mammals are subjected to wide variations in the environmental conditions in which they

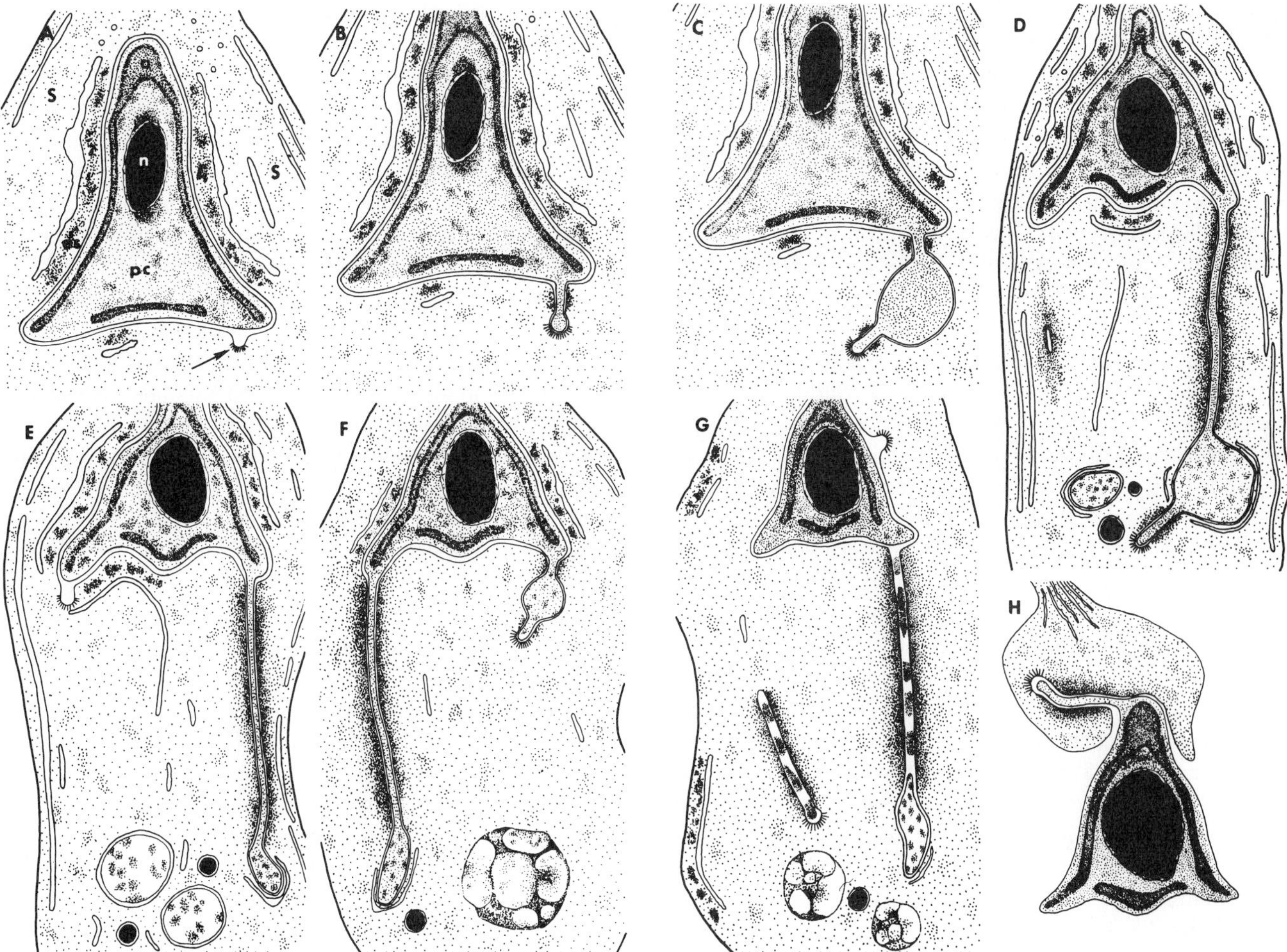

FIG. 65. Illustrations of the temporal sequence in the formation and disappearance of tubulobulbar complexes in the rat testis. Sertoli cell cytoplasm is stippled; spermatid head is drawn in transverse section. **A:** A coated pit (*arrow*) of the Sertoli cell occurs in areas devoid of junctional specialization. Perinuclear cytoplasm (pc) is indicated. **B:** A tube forms by evagination of spermatid into the Sertoli cell. **C:** Midportion of the tube develops a bulbous dilatation. **D:** Proximal elongation of the tube, with the distal portion associated with lysosomes. **E:** Separation of bulbs from the tube, with an associated increase in their watery consistency. **F:** Individual bulbs sequestered into Sertoli cell phagocytic vacuoles. New tubulobulbar complexes form. **G:** Dissolution of tubular portions. **H:** Prior to sperm release, the Sertoli cell cytoplasm withdraws from the spermatid head, and new tubulobulbar complexes develop at the convex margin of the spermatid head. These are subsequently resorbed, and the sperm is released. (From ref. 290.)

live, and thus seasonal variations in photoperiod, ambient temperatures, and availability of food and water together contribute to seasonal cycles of reproductive activity of many wild and domestic animals. Seasonally breeding animals, unlike their laboratory-bred counterparts, provide an opportunity to investigate the structure and function of the Sertoli cell during the cyclic waxing and waning of spermatogenesis. A great deal of information has accumulated over many years attesting to the annual regression and recovery of spermatogenic activity within the testes of a wide range of vertebrates (20,297,352,453–456).

Histological investigations of the changes in testicular activity among seasonally breeding fish, amphibians, reptiles, birds, and mammals have demonstrated that regression of the seminiferous epithelium is often accompanied by an accumulation of lipid inclusions within the Sertoli cells (297). With reactivation of spermatogenesis, the Sertoli cell lipid inclusions disappear, although the precise role of lipid in the presumed alterations of Sertoli cell function remains unknown. The changing structure of the Sertoli cell in a seasonally breeding wild rat has been documented at the light- and electron-microscopic levels (353,457,458). In seasonally breeding mammals, arrest of spermatogenesis is accompanied by marked reductions in Sertoli cell volume and its content of organelles, although simultaneous accumulation of lipid inclusions is also a common feature, possibly relating to deposition and storage of lipid-rich substances contributed in part from the degeneration of many germ cells (459–461). These structural changes to Sertoli cells during the nonbreeding season are thought to occur in response to declines in levels of FSH, LH, and testosterone (462–464) and to resemble the morphological changes to Sertoli cells seen after hypophysectomy (465).

Little is known concerning the integrity of the blood-testis barrier in seasonally breeding mammals, and although the inter-Sertoli-cell junctions remain during the regression of the seminiferous epithelium (443,457,466), their effectiveness as a permeability barrier requires additional study. However, in lower orders of vertebrates, such as reptiles and amphibians (298,301), tight junctions between Sertoli cells disappear during the nonbreeding season. In testes exhibiting regional differences in spermatogenic activity, germ cell maturation is accompanied by Sertoli cell junctions, whereas in regressive zones of the testis not associated with germ cell activity, tight junctions disappear. Thus, at least in some species, formation of the barrier is correlated with spermatogenic activity.

The basic tenet that Sertoli cell numbers remain stable in the adult testis (28,43) has in recent years been brought into question. Given the fact that sperm production in many animals may vary with season, together with the observation that daily sperm production is subject to an age-related decline, the effect of variation in Sertoli cell numbers offers a theoretical mechanism to allow these changes to occur. Variation in the Sertoli cell population has been documented, although this phenomenon has in the past attracted little attention, possibly because of lack of statistical significance or because of large changes in the dimensions of the seminiferous tubules. Nevertheless, when mice testes were X-irradiated to partially destroy the germ cell population, the restoration of testicular function was associated with an increased number of Sertoli cells per seminiferous tubule cross section (467).

When rat testes were made artificially cryptorchid (468,469), the Sertoli cells were reported to transiently increase in number, and with prolonged periods of cryptorchidism, Sertoli cells disappeared from the seminiferous tubules (470). Sertoli cells of the immature rat testis apparently continue their division processes for longer than is otherwise indicated by their mitotic index (471), and in the absence of germ cells, Sertoli cells in prepubertal rats continue to proliferate beyond day 20, when their numbers normally stabilize (71). Increases in the Sertoli cell population have been reported to occur during FSH treatment of rats following hypophysectomy (472). The lack of rigid quantitative assessment of Sertoli cell numbers in some of these and other studies has been advanced as a criticism of their conclusions. However, other studies of seasonally breeding red deer (473) and stallions (474,475) have presented clear evidence that the Sertoli cell population is capable of increasing in the adult by fluctuating with season. Seasonal differences in Sertoli cell numbers of 60 adult stallions were characterized by a 36% increase in the breeding versus nonbreeding season. Because horse Sertoli cells have only a limited capacity to alter the ratio of germ cells to single Sertoli cells, a seasonal variation in total numbers of Sertoli cells provides an additional mechanism for increased daily sperm production per testis known to occur in the breeding season. The source of additional Sertoli cells found in the breeding season and the factors promoting their appearance and disappearance remain unclear. Mitotic figures at the base of the seminiferous epithelium in the stallion were seen at stages II and III of the spermatogenic cycle, whereas spermatogonia are thought to divide only between stages V and VIII. Concentrations of FSH, LH, and testosterone measured in the same study (475) were altered not only by season but also with age, and no clear relationship has emerged to link hormone changes with Sertoli cell numbers. The numbers of type A spermatogonia also exhibit changes with season in adult stallions (476), and it seems possible that the Sertoli cells may influence these cells through hormonal action (477) or perhaps directly via mitogenic peptides secreted by the Sertoli cells (478). Although the adult stallion appears to be an exception to the rule that Sertoli cell numbers remain stable after puberty, additional research may well indicate that Sertoli cells are a dynamic rather than sessile population.

A very different account of the biology of Sertoli cells is revealed when their numbers are related to increasing age. Using morphometric techniques to evaluate cell numbers (479), it was shown that the number of Sertoli cells in the human testis exhibits an age-related decline. In a study of men aged 20 to 85 years who were in apparent good health prior to sudden death, young adult men (20–48 years, $N = 37$) had approximately 500 million Sertoli cells per testis, and this number declined significantly to a mean of 300 million per testis for older men (50–85 years, $N = 34$). When the relationship between age and numbers of Sertoli cells per testis was examined, there was a significant age-related decline in the Sertoli cell population (317). In addition, the same study reported a significant correlation between Sertoli cell numbers and daily sperm production, although the numbers of germ cells accommodated by the Sertoli cells at any age remain unchanged. Taken together, the analysis of changes in spermatogenesis and Sertoli cell numbers in the special examples of old age and in seasonal breeders indicates that variation in daily sperm production can be attributable to alterations in the total numbers of Sertoli cells and/or changes in the numbers of germ cells that are associated with an individual Sertoli cell.

Response to Injury

In the past, the persistence of Sertoli cells following damage or elimination of the germ cells was taken to indicate that the Sertoli cells were resistant to a wide variety of treatments that otherwise caused spermatogenic disruption. This belief was based on light-microscopic observations of Sertoli cells following testicular damage in which their morphology appeared little changed from normal. However, as pointed out by Fawcett (285,286), the availability of semithin sections of testicular tissues embedded in plastic has revealed far more morphological details of the Sertoli cell than previously appreciated from studies on paraffin sections. The sensitivity of the Sertoli cell to damage has been emphasized by the early ultrastructural and functional changes in this cell in response to a great range of unrelated treatments that exert adverse effects on the testis (354).

The literature relating to morphological alterations of Sertoli cells is voluminous and encompasses a wide range of treatments too numerous to describe in this chapter. We have chosen, therefore, to discuss and illustrate changes in Sertoli cell structure in a general manner, because it seems likely that the reaction of this cell to injury is often reflected by very similar morphological alterations. An early indication of altered Sertoli cell cytology is the appearance of many clear, watery vacuoles or vesicles within the basal aspects of the cell. These are readily visible by light microscopy (Fig. 66), and when examined by electron microscopy, they consist of membrane-limited vacuoles arising from three locations. First, the basal cytoplasm exhibits intracellular vacuoles of variable configuration (Fig. 66), but whether these form by dilation of endoplasmic reticulum or endocytosis of fluids has not been clarified. Second, vacuoles occasionally appear in the intercellular spaces between Sertoli cells and neighboring germ cells. Third, vacuoles clearly visible by light microscopy are associated with the regions of junctional specialization between adjacent Sertoli cells (Fig. 67). These vacuoles are of particular interest because they involve radical disorganization of the inter-Sertoli-cell junctions in which progressive expansion of the intercellular spaces at the sites of junctional complexes gives rise to multiple extracellular vacuoles along the pathway of each junctional complex. The formation of these vacuoles in relation to seminiferous tubule damage has been closely studied after induction of experimental cryptorchidism (480), and it was suggested that they contribute to complex membranous bodies within the Sertoli cells. The sequence of morphological changes to the inter-Sertoli-cell junctions during cryptorchidism is illustrated by light and electron micrographs (Fig. 68) and summarized diagrammatically in Fig. 69. Vacuolization is probably a nonspecific response of the Sertoli cells to injury, because it occurs in unrelated conditions of experimental damage to the seminiferous epithelium (71,74,399,481–487).

An additional sign of morphological disturbance to the Sertoli cell is the rapid accumulation of cytoplasmic lipid droplets that often accompany impairment of spermatogenesis. Although lipid inclusions are a common feature of Sertoli cells in the normal testis, they appear to increase in size and number coincident with morphological evidence of germ cell degeneration, suggesting that the degradation products of effete germ cells contribute to ever increasing numbers of Sertoli cell lipid inclusions. However, autolysis and phagocytosis of germ cells by Sertoli cells may not be the exclusive source of these lipid droplets, because they are known to accumulate within the Sertoli cell in the absence of germ cells (71). In conditions of prolonged atrophy of the seminiferous tubules, some Sertoli cells retain their content of lipid, whereas others exhibit few, if any, lipid inclusions. The latter situation of complete degeneration and disappearance of germ cells from the seminiferous epithelium results in further structural modifications to the Sertoli cells that involve retraction and convolution of their apical cytoplasm. Such seminiferous tubules exhibit a thin rim of flattened Sertoli cells. Alternatively, removal of the germ cells allows for shrinkage of the seminiferous tubule, whereupon the Sertoli cell cytoplasm becomes interdigitated as the cells are closely packed into the reduced volume of the atrophic tubule. Destruction of Sertoli cells has not often been reported, although this was clearly demonstrated some years ago (488) when it was shown that cadmium salts were acutely toxic to the seminiferous epithelium, causing destruction of germ cells and Sertoli cells. Other agents that

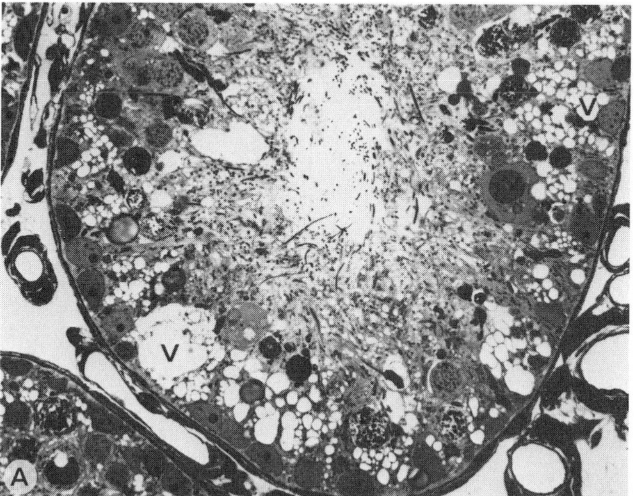

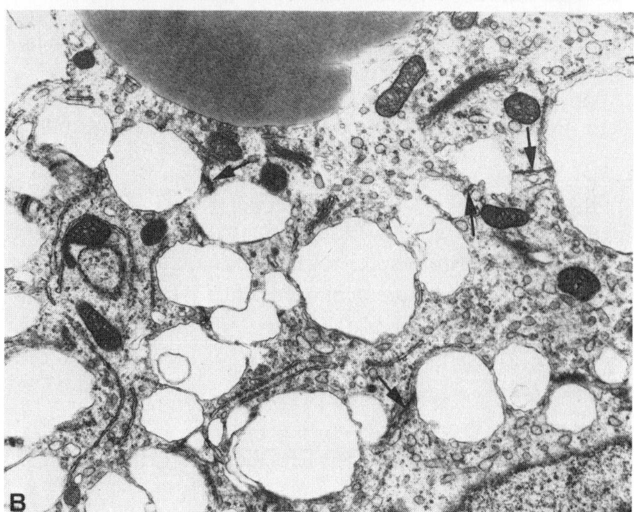

FIG. 66. A: Five-day experimentally cryptorchid rat testis showing many vacuoles (V) within the seminiferous epithelium. **B:** Many of these vacuoles in the 5-day cryptorchid testis are interconnected (*arrows*) by junctional specializations between adjacent Sertoli cells.

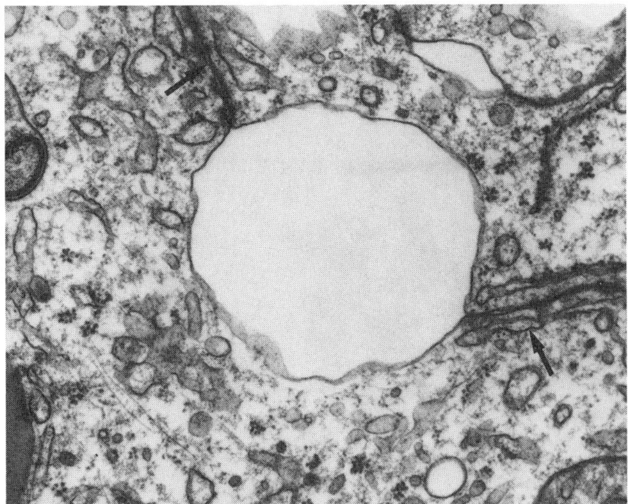

FIG. 67. Five-day experimentally cryptorchid testis showing a dilation of the intercellular space between two Sertoli cells. At opposite sides of the extracellular space, the pathway of inter-Sertoli-cell junctional complexes can be noted (*arrows*).

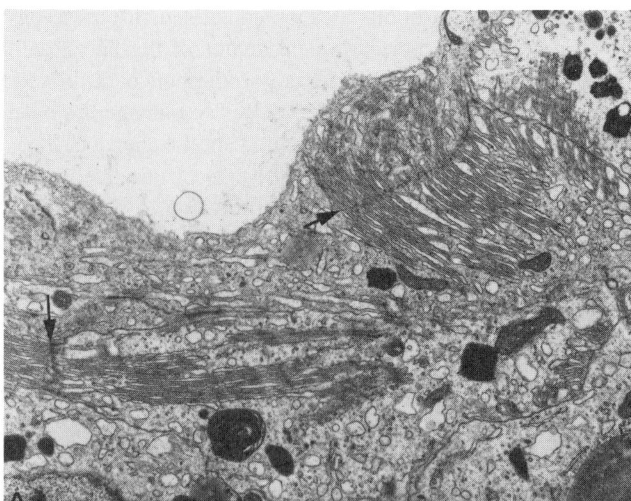

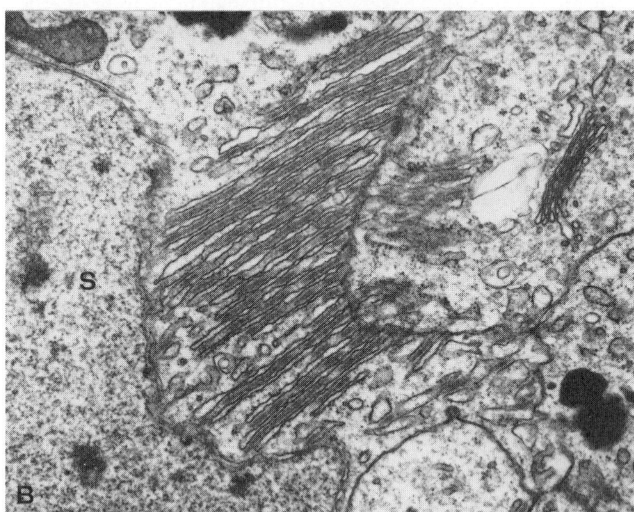

FIG. 68. A: Four-week experimentally cryptorchid testis showing complex membranous bodies within the Sertoli cell cytoplasm. The membranes are arranged perpendicular to a central axis (*arrows*). **B:** Sertoli cell membranous complex illustrating parallel cisternae of smooth membranes, occasionally bearing ribosomes, and electron-dense materials representing bundles of filaments. Sertoli cell nucleus (S).

bring about Sertoli cell necrosis include LH, LH plus LHRH agonists, and hCG (489,490), although the mechanisms by which these hormones destroy Sertoli cells have not been studied. All of the aforementioned alterations to the Sertoli cell have been described in disorders of the human testis (289,318,320,491–493) and in testes of men of advanced age (479,494).

CYCLE OF THE SEMINIFEROUS EPITHELIUM

The organization of the cell types that contribute to the process of spermatogenesis within the seminiferous epithelium is not random, but in fact highly organized. This fact was elucidated toward the end of the nineteenth century by a number of investigators (27,93,124,156,495). They noted that the germ cells at different developmental phases formed easily identifiable collections termed cell associations. Subsequent studies (496,497) were extended by the detailed studies of Le Blond and Clermont (166,167), who defined the cycle of the seminiferous epithelium as "the series of changes in a given area of the seminiferous epithelium between two appearances of the same developmental stage." These studies used the PAS reaction to stain the acrosomes of spermatids and on the basis of this structure and nuclear morphology divided spermatogenesis in the rat into 14 stages or cell associations (Fig. 70). The complete sequence of 14 stages or cell associations constitutes one cycle of the seminiferous epithelium. Should we have the ability to observe a segment of the seminiferous epithelium by time-lapse photography over a period of days, the organization of spermatogenesis in this cyclic manner would result in the epithelium passing through the 14 stages, with the eventual appearance of stage 1. They also established that the transformation of a type A spermatogonium into a mature spermatid that is released at stage 8 of the cycle occupied four such cycles. In the rat, the entire tubule cross section is in the same stage of the seminiferous cycle, which in fact extends over several millimeters of adjacent seminiferous tubule.

Investigation in other mammals subsequently established a seminiferous cycle in the mouse (95,498), the ram (498), and the monkey (104). Because spermatogenesis is a continuous sequence of changes, the subdivision into stages is artificial, and the number of stages will depend on the criteria used. The more extensive the criteria used, the more specific and detailed become the stages that can be identified. For light-microscopic studies, the conventional staging of Clermont (90) is usually applied to kinetic studies of the seminiferous epithelium. The cycle has been studied and defined in a number of mammalian species, each of which has a characteristic pattern and number of stages (Table 1).

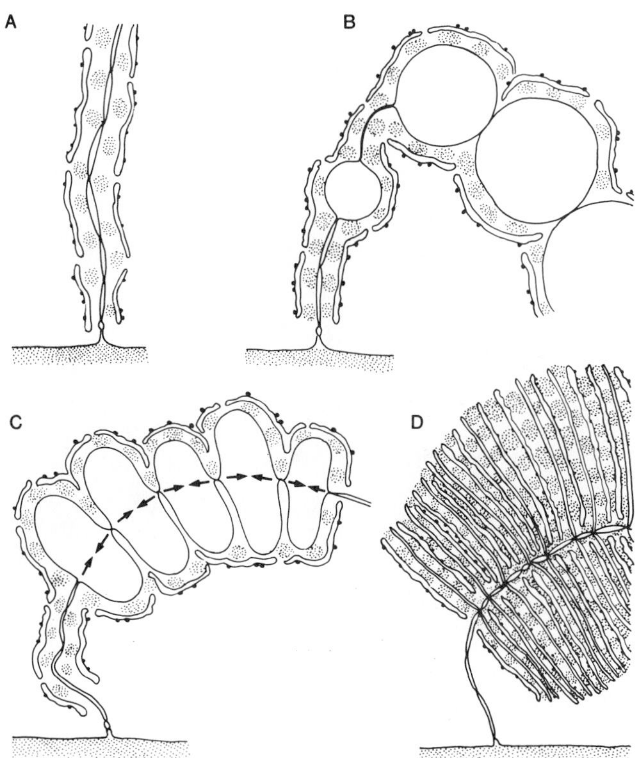

FIG. 69. Suggested sequence of formation of extracellular vacuoles and complex membranous cisternae in the seminiferous epithelium of the experimentally cryptorchid rat testis. **A:** Inter-Sertoli-cell junction in normal testis. **B:** In short-term cryptorchidism, vacuoles develop in the intercellular regions between sites of membrane occlusion. **C:** At later time intervals, degeneration of germ cells allows shrinkage of the seminiferous tubule and progressive collapse of the vacuoles, as indicated by *arrows.* **D:** With continued compression of the Sertoli cells, it is suggested that the rows of collapsing vacuoles undergo a concertina-type compression, forming elaborate parallel stacks of flattened vacuoles interposed between the cisternae associated with the tight junctions.

In the human, considerable difficulty was experienced in identifying the cell associations or stages because of the fact that multiple stages could be seen in a single cross section of a tubule and because of inadequate care in the fixation and handling of tissue. However, by detailed studies, Clermont (168) identified six cell associations as stages that formed the cycle of the human seminiferous epithelium (Fig. 71). Of the species examined to date, the only one demonstrating multiple stages in a seminiferous tubule cross section is the baboon, *Papio anubis* (500).

Recently, Schulze and Rehder (501) analyzed the human seminiferous epithelium in a different manner and proposed that germ cells at the same stage of development are distributed in a helical pattern. As they progress through spermatogenesis, the diameter of the helix decreases such that they are overlapped on the external surface by a gyration from another helical sequence (Fig. 72). They proposed that this concept of an Archimedian spiral provides the best explanation of the human data. They also suggested that the greater spermatogonal mitotic rate in species other than humans provides a larger spermatocyte population and hence the conventional appearance of stages of a seminiferous cycle. Further studies clearly will be necessary to demonstrate whether this concept extends to all species or whether it may be limited to species such as the baboon, which has a seminiferous epithelium similar to that of humans (500).

Duration of Spermatogenesis

Studies to determine the duration of spermatogenesis centered initially on attempts to destroy sensitive germ cell stages and analyze the rate of depletion of the seminiferous epithelium. Such approaches defined the duration of the cycle in the mouse as 8.6 days, with the entire process taking 34.6 days (498). Alternative approaches emerged with the availability of radioactive tracers such as ^{32}P and ^{3}H-labeled thymidine. Using ^{32}P, Ortavant (502,503) demonstrated that the cycle in the ram lasted 10.4 days, the entire process occupying 49 days. Subsequently, incorporation of tritiated thymidine into the DNA of dividing cells has been used in studies of spermatogenesis in a number of species and has demonstrated a specific duration for each species (Table 1). The duration of spermatogenesis appears to be specific for each species, and attempts to influence this biological constant by numerous factors have been unsuccessful. Ortavant (499) showed that although photoperiod could affect the yield of spermatozoa, it could not affect the rate of spermatogenesis. Removal of the pituitary to assess the influence of the hypophyseal hormones was shown to be without effect (504), and similar conclusions were reached in studies in the ram (505). It appears that the germ cells progress through the spermatogenic process at predetermined rates or subsequently degenerate. This view has recently been challenged by Russell et al. (506), who noted that spermatids in procarbazine-treated rats were found out of phase with the normal cycle of the seminiferous epithelium. The existence of a fixed rate of development of the germ cells results in an important corollary, namely, the volume occupancy (or absolute volume, if referring to the testis) of a germ cell in sections of the epithelium is a reflection of the length that that cell occupies in the spermatogenic process. Thus, secondary spermatocytes have a short life-span, and they and the stage of the cycle at which they are seen (stage 14 in the rat, stage 6 in humans) are represented infrequently in sections of the seminiferous epithelium.

Coordination Within Seminiferous Epithelium

The remarkable organization of the seminiferous cycle and the demonstration that the duration of spermatogenesis in many species is a biological constant have led to speculation as to the method by which this coordination is achieved. Two basic concepts of the method of synchronization were proposed by Roosen-Runge and Giesel (497): (a) that the

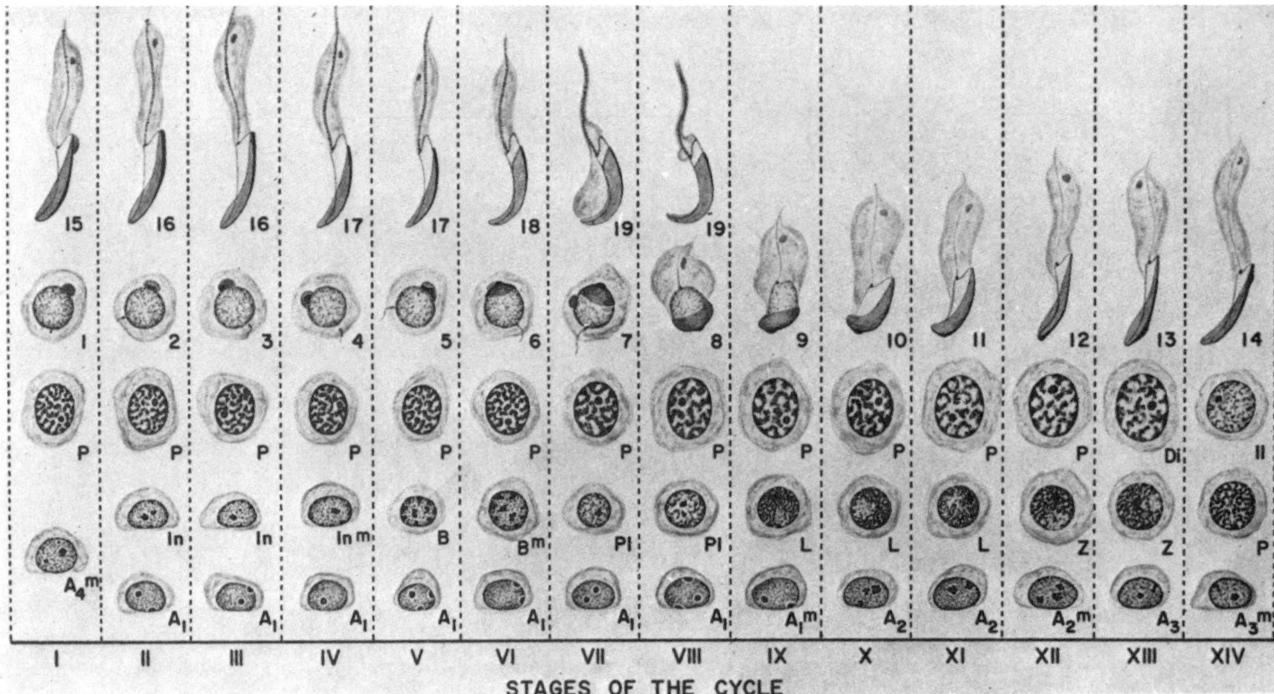

FIG. 70. Diagram illustrating the stages of the rat seminiferous cycle and the cell associations composing them. (From ref. 510.)

regulated development depends on the precise rate of each stage of cell development due to inherent timing devices or (b) that synchronization is dependent on external factors.

Of external factors, the Sertoli cell has emerged as a potential candidate for coordination, though one of the earliest suggestions (507) of such a role was based on the concept that the Sertoli cells formed a syncytium, now known to be a false assumption. The demonstration of the existence of specialized inter-Sertoli-cell junctions (270) forming the blood-testis barrier (413) emphasizes the close relationship of this cell to the germ cells, particularly those located on the luminal side of the barrier. Though favorably placed to exert a coordinating influence based in a radial direction in the epithelium, the Sertoli cell is less able to extend its coordinating influence along the length of the tubule unless the specialized inter-Sertoli-cell junctions facilitate communication between adjacent Sertoli cells. The extensive arborization of the Sertoli cell extends a potential influence over a number of germ cells in various phases of development, raising the potential of it influencing these cells by the secretion of local regulators, a hypothesis put forward many years ago, but still lacking evidence (254). The phagocytosis of the residual bodies of spermatids led numerous investigators to suggest that this action constitutes a signal to the Sertoli cell that may be important in controlling spermatogenesis (254,508).

Clermont (90), however, discounted the Sertoli cell as a factor, based on (a) the fact that cyclic activity is established within the epithelium prior to the Sertoli cells attaining their mature cytological characteristics (509) and (b) the observation that in hypophysectomized rats, the Sertoli cells are regressed, yet the germ cell stages that are present in the epithelium maintain their characteristic cell associations (504). Furthermore, he noted that coordination within the epithelium also existed in the absence of residual bodies either prior to their formation (509) or subsequent to irradiation (510). He concluded that the "cycle of the epithelium is the direct consequence of the entrance, at fixed intervals, of spermatogonial stem cells in spermatogenesis and of the fixed duration of the various steps of spermatogenesis."

The nature of such inherent timing devices has not been resolved, but more recent studies have emphasized the extensive links between synchronously developed germ cells because of the formation of cytoplasmic bridges associated with incomplete cytokinesis (108). These bridges, which

TABLE 1. *Duration of seminiferous cycle*

Species	Days	References
Mouse	34–35	498,763
Hamster (*Cricetus auratus*)	35–36	763,764
Boar	34–35	765
Rat	48–53	766,767
Ram	49	503,768
Bull	54	523
Rabbit	48–51	769,770
Monkey		
Macaca speciosa	45	771
Macaca mulatta	70	772
Human	64	157

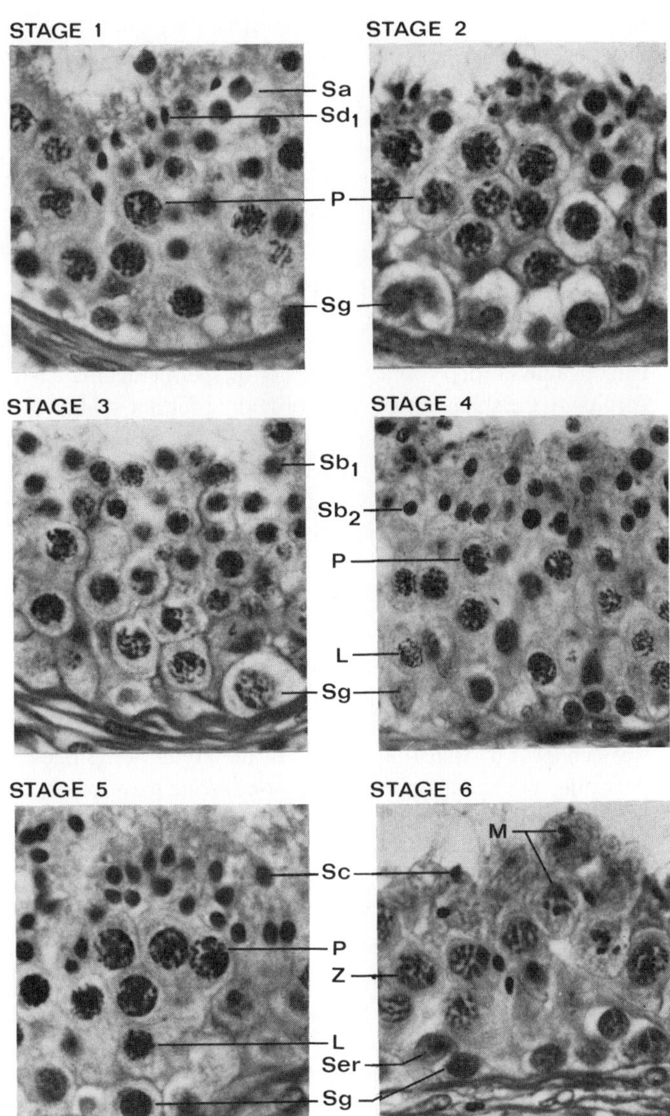

FIG. 71. Light micrographs illustrating the six stages of the human seminiferous cycle, as defined by Clermont (168). (From ref. 107.) Explanation of symbols: Ser, Sertoli cells; Sg, spermatogonia; M, meiotic division; Sa, Sb, Sc, Sd, spermatids. Other symbols as in Fig. 72.

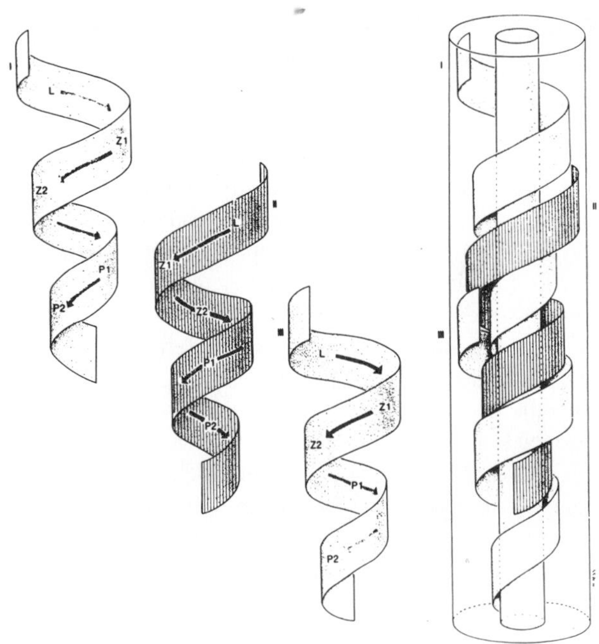

FIG. 72. Proposed three-dimensional model for arrangement of primary spermatocytes in the human seminiferous tubule. Populations of subsequent degrees of development occupy helically running strip-shaped areas of the epithelium. As development proceeds, the strip approaches the lumen. L, leptotene; Z, early zygotene; Z_2, late zygotene; P, early/middle pachytene; P_2, late pachytene. (From ref. 501.)

link adjacent cells at all stages of germ cell development, effectively create a syncytium, and, based on calculations, up to 512 spermatids may be linked in such a manner (108). The existence of large numbers of cells joined in this manner was amply demonstrated by Moens and Hugenholtz (511), who observed 80 spermatocytes joined by cytoplasmic bridges. Because of incomplete cytokinesis of spermatogonial stem cells, cohorts of cells remain linked in a syncytium, enabling coordinated subsequent cell division.

Spermatogonial or Stem Cell Renewal

Because it seems likely that one of the major factors responsible for the coordination seen in spermatogenesis is the regular division of spermatogonia, it seems pertinent to consider their pattern of division in more detail. Spermatogonial renewal is also of importance for the continuation of spermatogenesis throughout adult life, as there must be a mechanism by which they are renewed and yet provide a pool of cells to enter the later stages of the process. Early studies proposed that this was achieved by the products of spermatogonial division being different, i.e., bivalent, with one daughter cell remaining a spermatogonium and the other a primary spermatocyte (512). This concept ignored the fact that there are different types of spermatogonia, as described by Regaud (27). Further studies by Roosen-Runge and Giesel (497) recognized that multiple spermatogonial divisions occurred throughout the seminiferous cycle. Subsequently, Clermont and Le Blond (40) proposed a scheme to account for the five peaks of mitosis observed in the epithelium during the seminiferous cycle. In their view, some type A spermatogonia divided in "bivalent" fashion, to form stem cells that remained dormant throughout the cycle and type A spermatogonia, which entered the cycle.

The subsequent development of concepts in this field was a direct result of improved methods of identifying spermatogonial cell types and the study of spermatogonia in whole mounts of seminiferous tubules (98,99,107). In the rat, five different types of spermatogonia were identified, A_0, A_1, . . . , A_4, the A_0 being viewed as a reserve stem cell that did not divide unless the epithelium was damaged by agents such as irradiation (98,99). The renewing stem cells were proposed to arise by one of the A_4 spermatogonia dividing to form two A_1 spermatogonia. This proposal seemed unlikely in view of the observation that groups of dividing spermatogonia remained linked by cytoplasmic bridges, making it difficult to accept that one member of such a cohort could act independent of the rest (108).

A new theory emerged from the studies of Huckins (107,513–515), using whole mounts of rat seminiferous tubules in combination with autoradiography using ^{3}H-thymidine. She recognized three spermatogonial compartments (Fig. 73), the stem cells (A_s), the proliferating cells (A_{pr} and A_{al}), and the differentiating cells (A_{1-4}, In, B). The stem cells, A_s, divide sporadically to replicate themselves as isolated entities and to provide pairs of spermatogonia (A_{pr}). The latter engage in a series of synchronous divisions leading to the formation of chains of spermatogonia joined by intercellular bridges, the aligned spermatogonia (A_{al}). The proliferating compartment, on approaching its final size, ceases mitotic division, and the A_{al} cells differentiate synchronously into A_1 spermatogonia, which resume, again synchronously, their maturation into the more differentiated spermatogonial types (A_2, A_3, A_4, In, B). The type B subsequently differentiate to form preleptotene spermatocytes. This view has been supported by studies in the mouse (516,517), the Chinese hamster (518,519), and the ram (520). The concept proposed by Huckins (107) fits well with the observed data of increased numbers of proliferating cells joined by intercellular bridges (108).

Numerous studies were performed in the decade 1960 to 1970 in different species, quantifying the number of spermatogonial divisions and proposing schemes of spermatogonial multiplication (Table 1). These have been extensively reviewed by Clermont (90), and readers are referred to that study for details. Though they may be inaccurate in terms of the method of stem cell renewal, they do provide a data base for each species.

Spermatogonial Wave

Von Ebner (93) recognized that the stages of the seminiferous cycle were distributed along the length of the seminiferous tubule in an orderly sequence, thus introducing the concept of the "spermatogenic wave." Regaud (27) correctly interpreted the significance of this wave by the statement "the wave is in space what the cycle is in time." Detailed histological studies have analyzed the distribution of stages along the length of the seminiferous tubule (Fig. 74) and found that the subdivisions between each stage are irregular but distinct (509). Each rat seminiferous tubule contains approximately 12 complete spermatogenic waves, each approximately 2 to 6 cm in length (509). Studies using autoradiography of whole mounts of seminiferous tubules demonstrated orderly mitotic activity of spermatogonia according to the stage of the cycle, providing further evidence to support the concept that the cycle of the seminiferous epithelium is coordinated by the mitotic activity of the spermatogonia (521). The wave has been identified in a number of mammalian species, such as the mouse, bull, mink, guinea pig, rabbit, boar, dog, cat, and marsupials (495,509,522–524).

The orderly distribution of stages of the seminiferous cycles along the tubule is the basis for the innovative studies of Parvinen (525), which involved dissection of the tubule into lengths according to the stage of the cycle present. This was achieved by transillumination of the tubule, the stages providing particular appearances based principally on the light scattering achieved by the condensing spermatid nucleus. The studies of Parvinen (525) have demonstrated that the nature of the germ cells surrounding the Sertoli cell can significantly influence certain metabolic activities of the Sertoli cells. Additional evidence has been provided by the studies of Jegou et al. (526), which showed that modification of Sertoli cell function following exposure of the rat testis to a single episode of heat did not occur until a loss of spermatids occurred. During recovery, Sertoli cell function remained abnormal until the return of spermatids. Further-

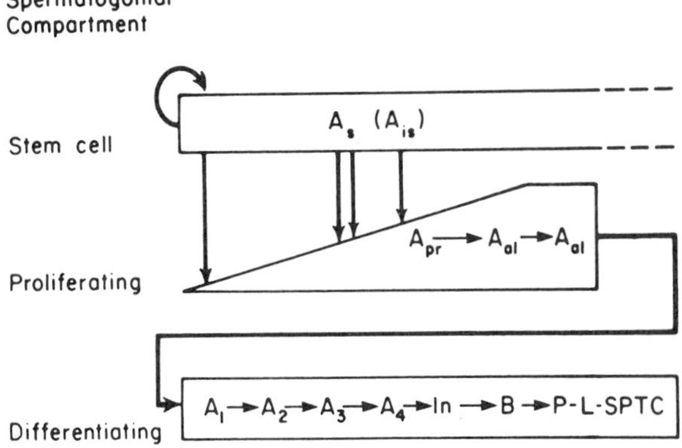

FIG. 73. Proposed model for renewal and differentiation of spermatogonia. (From ref. 107.)

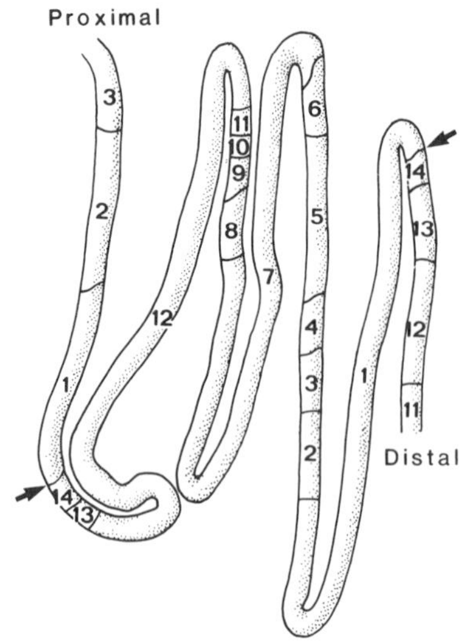

FIG. 74. Distribution of the stages of the rat seminiferous cycle that constitute the seminiferous wave along the tubule. (Adapted from ref. 509.)

more, the studies of Kerr and colleagues (258,305) have shown significant changes in the morphology of the Sertoli cell according to the stage of the cycle in the rat. These studies emphasize the fact that the seminiferous tubule compartment cannot be viewed as homogeneous tissue in terms of either structure or function.

LEYDIG CELLS

In reviewing the cytology of the Leydig cells and the intertubular tissues in which they reside, we recognized that for the purposes of this chapter it was not possible to acknowledge the work supplied by every contributor to this field of study. One can appreciate the difficulties faced when one considers that a review of the same topic in 1921 by Stieve (527) was based on approximately 1,000 earlier studies. Thus, the literature on Leydig cell morphology and its functional significance is vast. Our objectives are subsequently directed toward two major topics: First, we provide a review of Leydig cells based on authoritative accounts that together form an accurate survey of the light- and electron-microscopic features of the Leydig cells and the interstitial tissue. Particularly useful dissertations are available (16,341,359,411,527–537). Second, we discuss and provide new illustrations of the morphology of Leydig cells that we hope will add to an increased understanding of the biology of these cells.

Historical Background

The earliest description of the histology of the intertubular tissue of the testis was provided in 1850 by Leydig (538), who reported that the spaces between the seminiferous tubules were occupied by conspicuous masses of cells containing fatty vacuoles and pigment inclusions. Another student of testicular histology, Kölliker, who some years earlier had concluded that spermatozoa originate from the seminiferous tubules, also provided a similar description of the cellular composition of the intertubular tissue (5). Both investigators considered the cells to be a specialized form of connective tissue.

Although Berthold (6) demonstrated that the testis secreted substances into the bloodstream to influence the growth of anatomically distant tissues, the question of which tissue in the testis contributed to this secretion remained unanswered for many years. The prevailing view of Leydig cells as connective tissue was extended by von Ebner (93) and Hofmeister (539). But thereafter, a new concept gained favor in which Leydig cells were thought to produce fats, nutrients, or other substances for consumption by the seminiferous tubules (27,540,541). Because of the well-recognized occurrence of lipid inclusions within the Leydig cells of many species, Loisel (542) and Ganfini (543) put forward the view that Leydig cell lipid droplets provided the substrate from which testicular hormones were synthesized. This idea received support from the studies of Bouin and Ancel (7,544,545), who coined the term "la glande interstitielle" and offered convincing evidence that the Leydig cells of both normal and cryptorchid testes provided the hormonal stimulus for production of sperm and for maintenance of secondary sexual characteristics.

Leydig cell lipid inclusions later were shown to contain cholesterol esters (546–548), leading to the demonstration by McGee (549) that lipid extracts from bovine testes could stimulate masculine development when administered to other animals. Testosterone was finally identified in these extracts (8,550) and soon was synthesized using cholesterol as the starting material (551,552). Pathways for steroidogenesis and their control by various hormones are reviewed elsewhere in this volume, although it is important to emphasize that many years passed before it became clear that the Leydig cells represented the predominant site for steroidogenic enzymes (553–555) and the chief source of testicular androgens (556,557).

Organization of Intertubular Tissue

In routine histological sections of the testes of common laboratory rodents (rat, mouse, guinea pig, hamster), a clear space of variable extent is commonly observed separating individual seminiferous tubules. Within this space are found numerous blood vessels of variable caliber, often forming a central core around which are deployed numerous Leydig cells and other cellular constituents of the intertubular tissue. Thus, a cursory examination of the intertubular tissue confirms that its histological organization is consistent with an endocrine function, namely, a rich vascular supply and a close association between Leydig cells and blood vessels, the latter facilitating passage of steroids into the circulation. Empty spaces surrounding the seminiferous tubules have often been interpreted as preparation artifacts brought about by shrinkage during tissue fixation and dehydration prior to paraffin embedding. Although this is no doubt correct, we now recognize that these clear spaces, at least in the previously mentioned species, are not entirely exaggerated in their extent, but in fact represent species variation in the size and architecture of intertubular lymphatic vessels. For many years the intertubular tissue was regarded simply as loose connective tissue, harboring Leydig cells, fibroblasts, and extracellular elements. The concept of a system of lymphatic channels penetrating beyond the regions of the septula, rete, and tunica albuginea and into the interior of the testis had long been supported (558–564), but was doubted (565–568). Improvements in tissue preservation for subsequent ultrastructural examination have shown that the intertubular tissue is in fact supplied by a lymph vascular system, and its relative volume, architecture, and relationship to Leydig cells are unique for a given species (287,411,535,569,570).

The claim that in the mammalian testis Leydig cells are usually clustered around blood vessels is somewhat misleading in light of an excellent comparative study by Fawcett et al. (16) of the organization of the testicular intertubular tissue in 14 species of mammals. Four more-or-less distinct patterns of organization were distinguished (Figs. 75 and 76). In rodents, such as the guinea pig (Fig. 81) and chinchilla, only a small fraction of the testicular volume is taken up by the Leydig cells, which are commonly clustered together around blood vessels. The remaining and greater part of the intertubular area is occupied by extensive peritubular lymphatic sinusoids, whose limiting walls consist of a delicate layer of endothelium. To accommodate the intervening blood vessels and Leydig cells, the lymphatic endothelium invests the perivascular Leydig cells in what has been termed "visceral" (16) or "interstitial" (569) endothelium. Closely applied and coursing parallel to the boundary tissues of the seminiferous tubules, the lymphatic endothelial wall here is termed "parietal" (16) or "peritubular" (569) endothelium (Figs. 77 and 78). In general, the endothelial walls of the lymphatic sinusoids are continuous, although on some occasions small gaps or discontinuities have been noted in the visceral wall flanking the Leydig cells. Structural support between the seminiferous tubules and the Leydig-cell–vascular entities is provided by bundles of collagen fibers and occasional fibroblast-like cells forming a bridge linking the clusters of Leydig cells with the peritubular tissues.

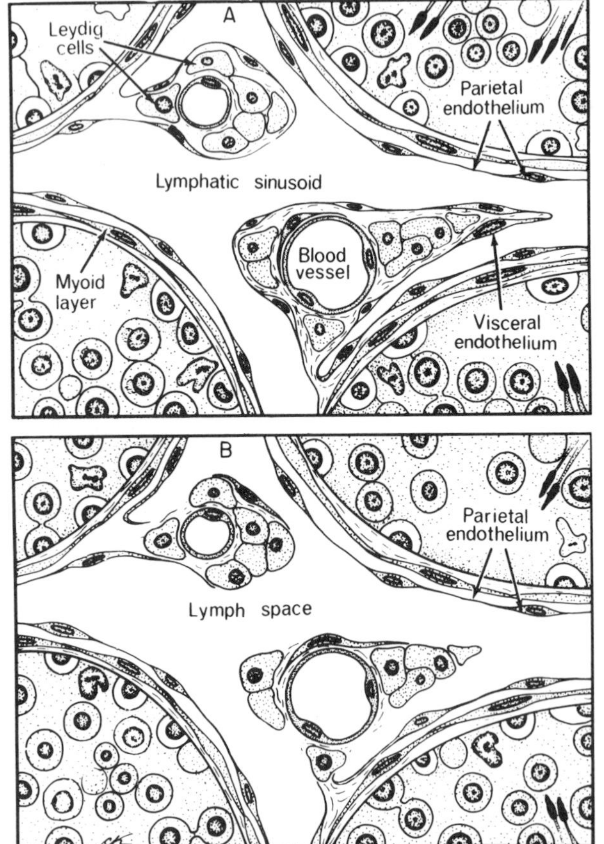

FIG. 75. Architecture of intertubular tissues from a variety of species. **A:** Chinchilla and guinea pig. Leydig cells associated with blood vessels and enclosed by lymphatic endothelium. **B:** Rat and mouse, showing discontinuities of the lymphatic endothelium, thus partly surrounding perivascular Leydig cells. (From ref. 284.)

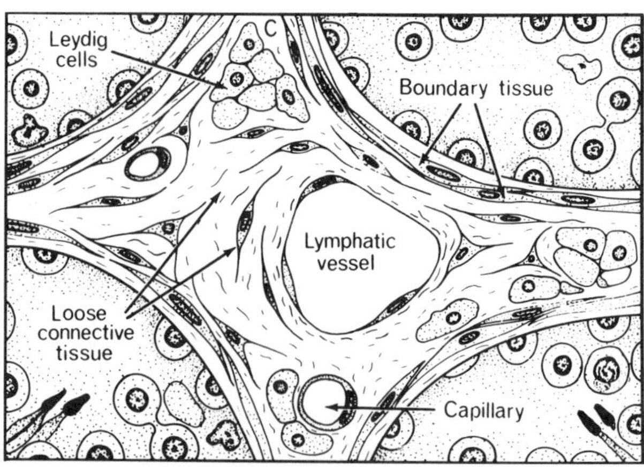

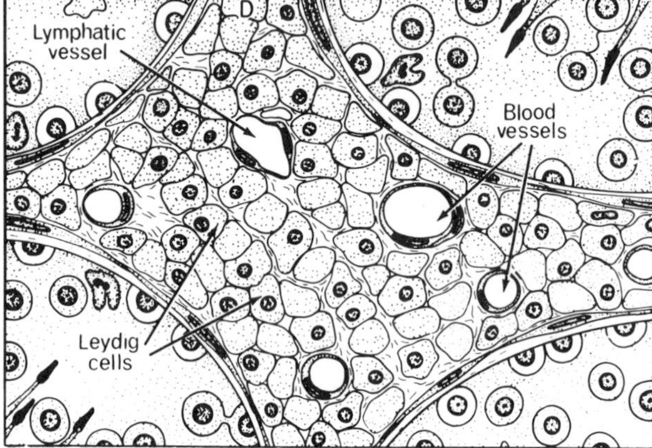

FIG. 76. Architecture of intertubular tissues from a variety of species. **Top:** Larger mammals, including ram, bull, monkey, and human. Randomly scattered clusters of Leydig cells appear within loose connective tissue rich in interstitial fluid. Lymphatic vessels are also demonstrated. **Bottom:** Boar, wart hog, zebra, naked mole rat, and numerous marsupial species. Many large Leydig cells occupy the intertubular space. Connective tissue and lymphatic vessels are not prominent. (From ref. 284.)

A similar organization of the intertubular tissue is seen in the rat and mouse, although a significant difference occurs in the extent to which Leydig cells are exposed to the fluids within the lymphatic sinusoids. Thus, the visceral layer of lymphatic endothelium is usually absent from the surfaces of Leydig cell clusters, permitting direct communication between loose connective tissues containing collagen and the lymph space (Figs. 79 and 80). In these species, the architecture of the intertubular lymphatic channels has been aptly classified as lymphatic sinusoids, implying a continuous admixture of lymph fluids and the ground substance of perivascular connective tissues. It should be mentioned here that in addition to the schema described (16), Leydig cells of the rat and mouse are not constantly confined to perivascular locations, but often are seen in peritubular positions or, alternatively, in more central regions of the in-

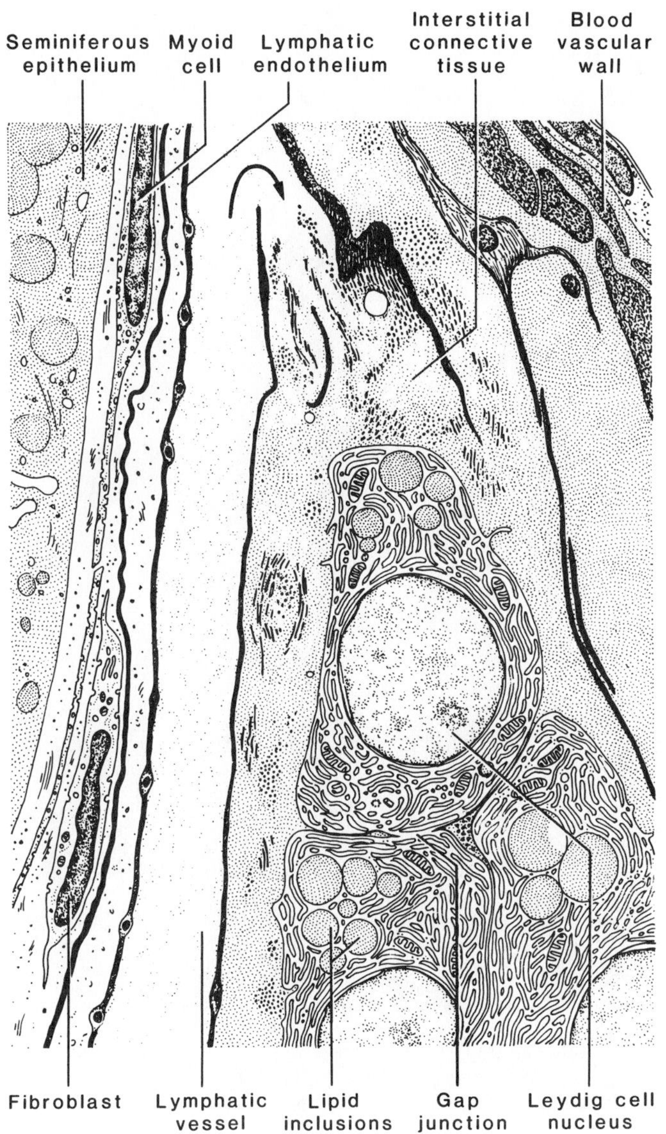

FIG. 77. Schematic representation of the intertubular tissue of the testis. Note the discontinuity in the endothelial wall of a lymphatic vessel, allowing its content of interstitial fluid to gain access to the loose connective tissues containing the Leydig cells. (Adapted from refs. 411 and 535.)

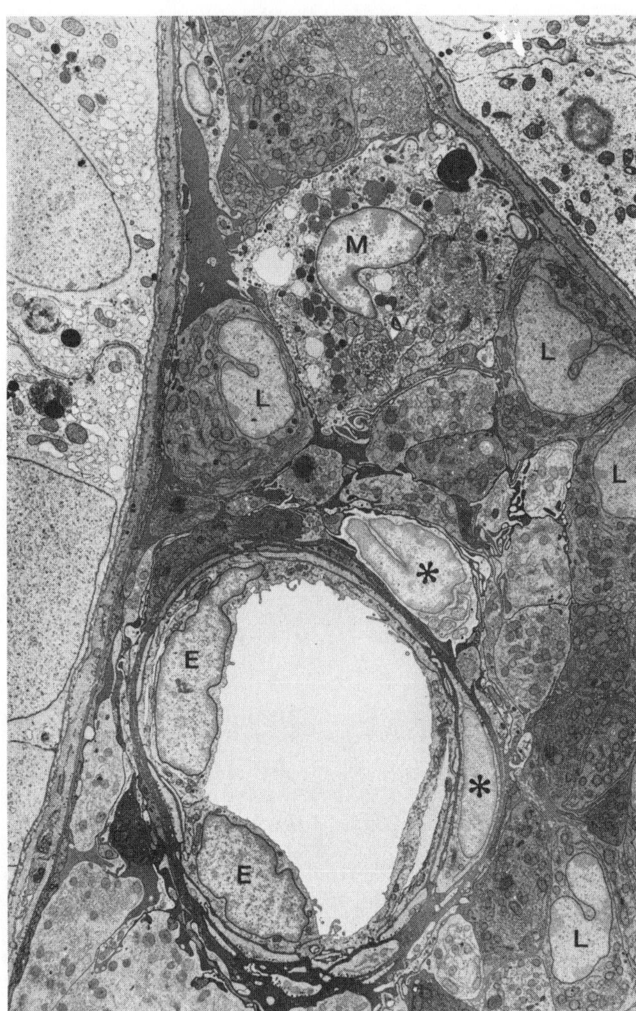

FIG. 78. Ultrastructure of the intertubular tissue of the adult rat testis, showing Leydig cell nuclei (L), a macrophage (M), vascular endothelial cell nuclei (E), and perivascular interstitial cells (*asterisks*) traditionally classified as pericytes or adventitial cells. Tissue fixed with collidine-buffered glutaraldehyde.

tertubular tissue, where they appear to lack any association with connective tissue and are in fact almost entirely bathed by lymph (Fig. 80). This observation emphasizes the role played by the lymphatic sinusoids in providing the medium by which Leydig cells receive and secrete substances carried by the bloodstream. However, these special features of the histology of intertubular tissues in the rat and mouse are quite different from those of many other mammals and raise a note of caution in regard to extrapolating their associated physiological properties to cover other species in general.

In the second category described by Fawcett et al. (16), the intertubular tissue is characterized by large areas of very loose connective tissue containing small aggregations of Leydig cells, often associated with blood vessels, or less often occupying positions rather distant from the vascular supply. Lymphatic drainage is achieved through prominent lymphatic vessels placed centrally or eccentrically within each intertubular area. These lymphatic vessels are bounded by continuous, unbroken endothelial cells and, together with the Leydig cells, are supported by variable quantities of collagen and fibroblasts. To this broad but distinct category belong species such as the ram, bull, hyrax, elephant, monkey, and human (Fig. 76). The relative paucity of Leydig cells in this group, together with their often wide separation from blood vessels, suggests that steroids secreted from the Leydig cells must gain access to the seminiferous tubules and venous system via diffusion through the edematous loose connective tissue. When the intertubular architecture in the rat and mouse (with extensive lymphatic sinusoids) is compared with that found in these larger mammals (ex-

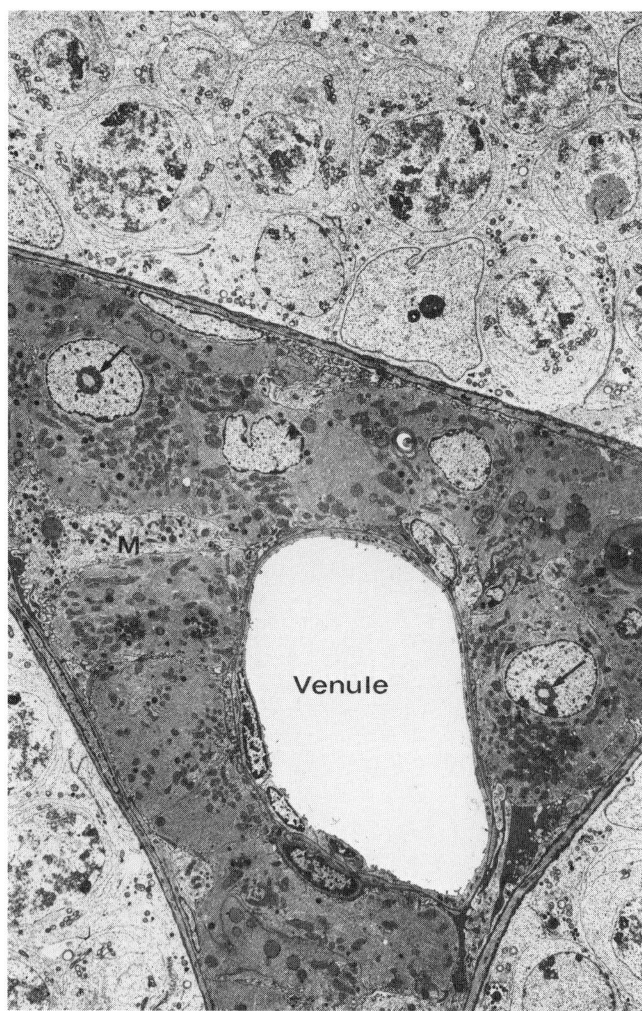

FIG. 79. Ultrastructural features of the intertubular tissue of the adult mouse testis. Leydig cells are closely packed, some showing annular nucleoli (*arrows*). Note the close association between macrophage (M) and Leydig cell. The venule appears empty because of perfusion fixation.

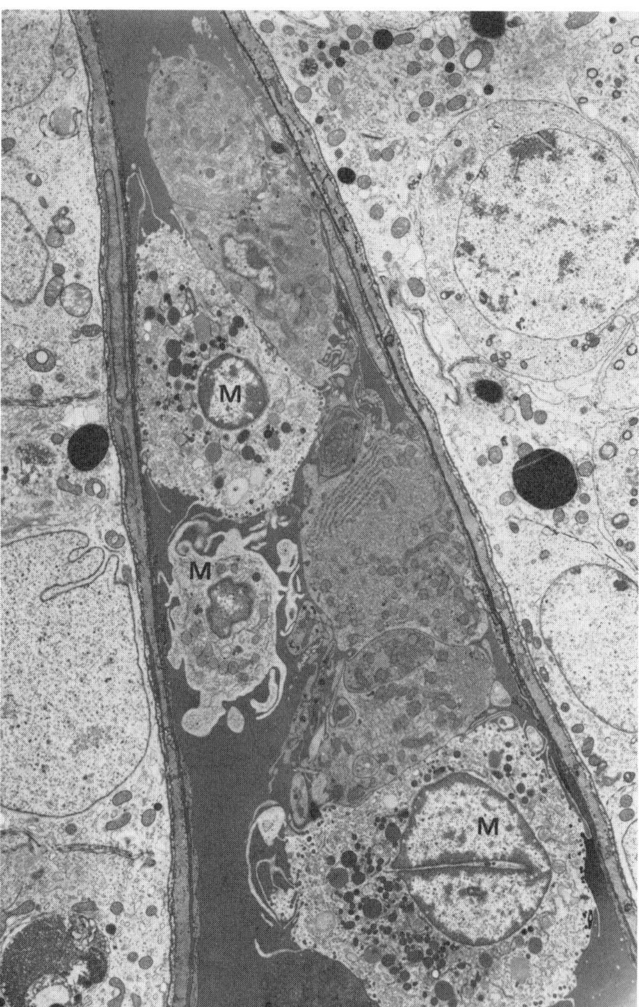

FIG. 80. Ultrastructure of macrophages in the intertubular tissue of the rat testis. The macrophages (M) show many cytoplasmic organelles and inclusions and possess numerous filopodial surface extensions. Tissue fixed with collidine-buffered glutaraldehyde.

hibiting much connective tissue), it can be appreciated why Christensen and Mason (556) found that manual separation of seminiferous tubules in rats and mice could be achieved with ease, whereas they were unsuccessful in their attempts to tease out fresh specimens obtained from the cat and the human. The lack of extensive peritubular sinusoids in the latter examples thus prevents a clean separation of the two testicular compartments.

A third variation in the composition of intertubular tissue is exemplified by those animals displaying an extraordinary abundance of Leydig cells, but very little intertubular connective tissue. Examples in this category include the zebra, domestic boar, wart hog, dog, opossum, and naked mole rat, in which Leydig cells occupy 20% to 60% of the testis volume (Fig. 81). To this group we can now add some Australian marsupials, the brush and ring-tailed opossums, two marsupial mice, *Antechinus stuartii* and *A. swainsonii*, belonging to the dasyurid group, and the koala (Fig. 82). In these species, small lymphatic vessels are encountered infrequently, and it is remarkable that many Leydig cells, by virtue of their large numbers and close packing, are often positioned at considerable distances from the nearest blood vessel. Why these animals develop large masses of Leydig cells is not understood, although some interesting speculations have been put forward by Fawcett et al. (16,284). These authors suggest that it is unlikely that such a large volume of endocrine tissue is necessary to offset a relative insensitivity of the seminiferous epithelium or to compensate for relatively inefficient mechanisms for delivery of androgens to the tubules. In their view, the appreciable amounts of Leydig cells may be related to a systemic requirement for products of the interstitial tissue other than testosterone, such as the secretion of hormone-binding globulins or pheromones. A further possibility of an androgen-

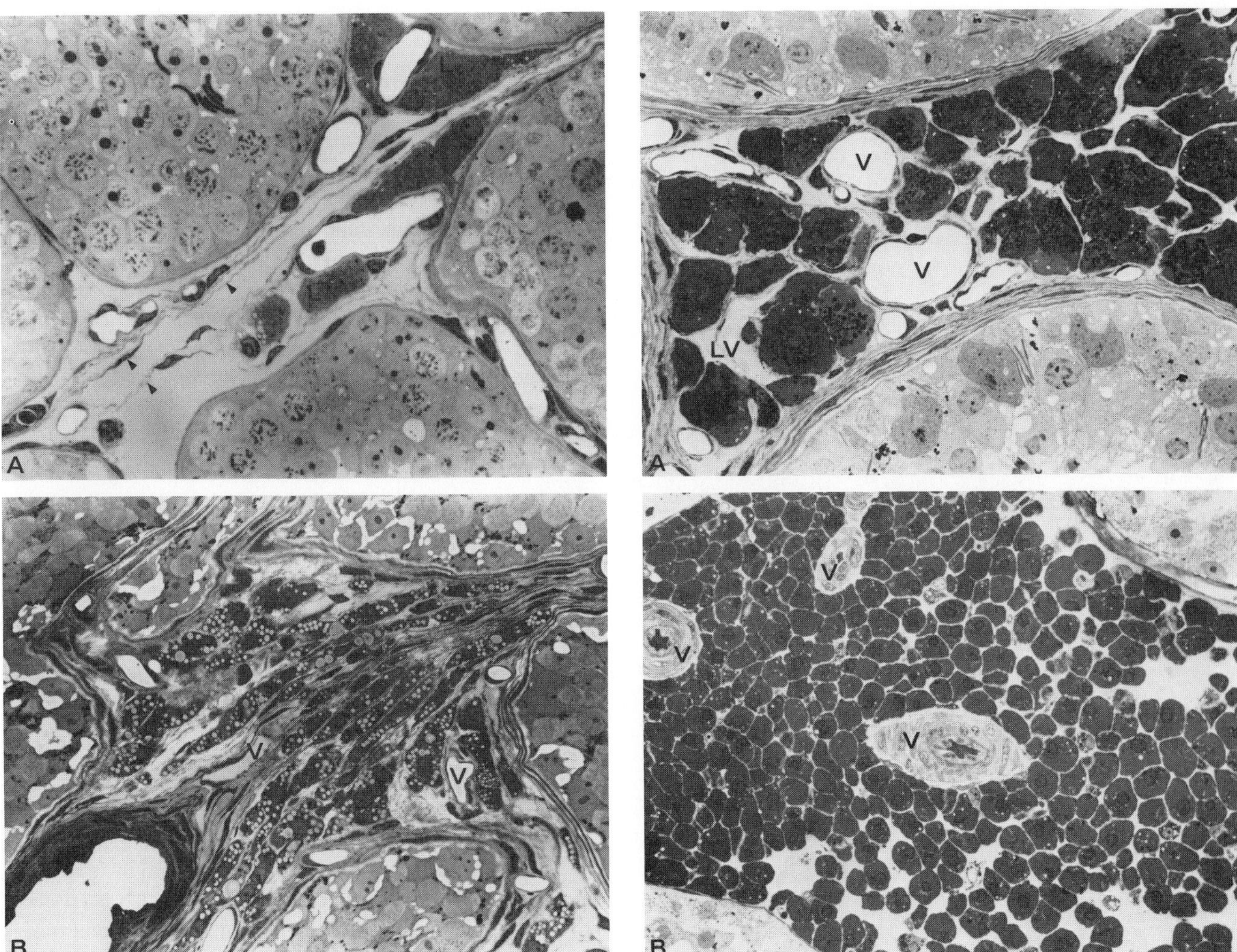

FIG. 81. A: Guinea pig testis, illustrating lymphatic endothelium (*arrowheads*) and perivascular Leydig cells (L). **B:** Dog testis, showing large clusters of lipid-rich Leydig cells embedded in loose connective tissue. Note small lymphatic vessels (V).

FIG. 82. A: Koala testis, showing large Leydig cells, intertubular blood vessels (V), and a lymphatic vessel (LV). **B:** Marsupial mouse testis, illustrating the dense-packed arrangement of the Leydig cells. Intertubular blood vessels (V).

dependent enhancement of aggression and courtship behavior exhibited by male marsupial mice has also been considered (21).

Turning now to other cytological features of the intertubular tissue, the presence of macrophages, fibroblasts, lymphocytes, plasma cells, and, more rarely, mast cells has been recognized for many years, but very little is known of their function. Because of their capacity for phagocytosis, macrophages have been readily identified in the interstitial tissue following application of various dyes such as pyrrol blue, chlorazol fast pink, and acid fuchsin and thionin (571,572). Subcutaneous injection of trypan blue had been a favored method with which to identify macrophages (537,573–576). Additional methods have recently become available to demonstrate macrophages using nonspecific esterase histochemistry (577) and the uptake of latex beads (578). Numerous ultrastructural descriptions of testicular macrophages (Figs. 78–80) (579) have stimulated renewed interest in their function, and it is known that testicular macrophages are endocytically active, avidly incorporating a variety of exogenous dyes, radiolabeled plutonium, and FSH (579–582). Recently, macrophages in rat intertubular tissue were shown to take up albumin (583). The presence of coated vesicles beneath the surface membrane in macrophages (Fig. 83) has been linked to receptor-mediated transport of specific proteins, because plutonium is known to bind to transferrin. Alternatively, fluid-phase endocytosis (pinocytosis) is thought to be the mechanism by which macrophages incorporate albumin from the interstitial lymphatics (538). Specialized contacts have been noted between Leydig cells and macrophages (579), and Bergh (584) has shown that an approximate ratio of 4:1 between these cells occurs in the normal rat testis and following destruction of the seminiferous epithelium induced by artificial cryptor-

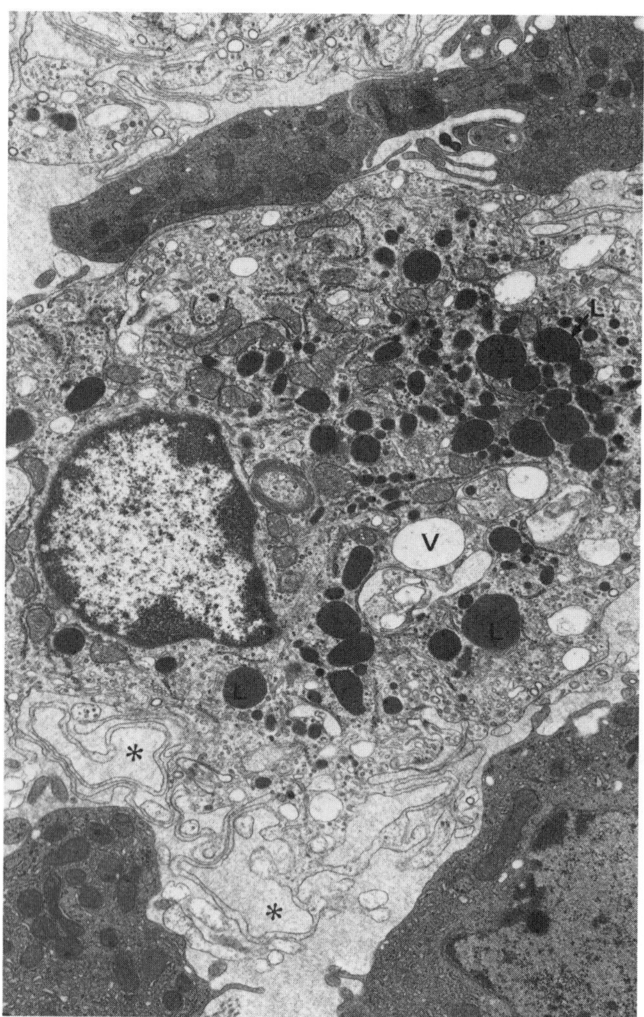

FIG. 83. Intertubular macrophage from the rat testis, showing cytoplasmic lysosomes and dense bodies (L), vacuoles (V), and long surface filopodia and lamellipodia (*asterisks*).

chidism. These findings suggest a functional coupling of these cell types.

Additional data on the function of interstitial macrophages has indicated that under special circumstances, they engulf and phagocytose Leydig cells (585,586). Participation of macrophages in destruction of Leydig cells has been verified by ultrastructural studies (587) showing that once this activity has commenced, all Leydig cells disappear from the testis, leaving the interstitium practically empty save for the presence of the macrophages and connective-tissue cells. These findings are discussed more fully in the section dealing with the response of Leydig cells to testicular damage.

The supporting connective tissues of the interstitial space have received little attention in the past, principally because of their unremarkable morphology and relative scarcity as compared with the often much larger sizes and numbers of Leydig cells (537). However, their importance is highlighted when consideration is given to the mechanisms by which Leydig cells develop within the testis and the question of dedifferentiation of Leydig cells into fibroblast-like cells (289,537). A fuller account of the morphology of fibroblastic tissues and their proposed relationships to Leydig cell differentiation is given later in the section concerned with the life history of Leydig cells.

Mononucleated wandering cells such as monocytes, together with infrequently encountered lymphocytes and plasma cells, have been accorded scant attention in studies of the morphology of the intertubular tissue. At present we can add little to this topic beyond mentioning that severe insults to the testis are unmistakably accompanied by increased numbers of these cells (585,588). Mast cells are occasionally observed in human intertubular tissues (589,590), but rarely encountered in species such as the rat, except in the peripheral margins of the intertubular tissues, where it joins within the subtunical areolar tissues. In the normal testis, their functional significance remains obscure, but their plentiful occurrence in rat interstitial tissue following recovery of testicular function after earlier impairment indicates a hitherto unsuspected role in the restoration of normal activity.

Although this review of the organizational patterns of intertubular tissues has been confined to mammalian species, a substantial body of information on this topic is available for nonmammalian vertebrates and many invertebrates (454,591–597).

Ultrastructure

Detailed descriptions of Leydig cell structure in relation to function are available in excellent reviews by Christensen and Gillim (341,537), in which information on some 46 mammalian species is presented. Since then, additional ultrastructural studies of Leydig cells in the adult mammalian testis have emerged emphasizing the diversity of their internal composition (Table 2). Accordingly, detailed reiter-

TABLE 2. *Selected examples of Leydig cell ultrastructure in adult mammalian testes since 1975*

Species	References
Mouse	608,616,622
Rat	603,604,620,638
Bush rat	458,656
Guinea pig	605,754,755
Hamster	605,716,756,757
Squirrel	460
Hare	758
Hyrax	713
Mole	717
Armadillo	610
Iranian vole	759
Bat	634
Seal	760
Boar	761
Ox	623
Dog	536,609
Monkey	683
Human	289,316,607,762

ation of the many subtle ultrastructural features of Leydig cells unique to a given species would be largely redundant and add little to advance our understanding or identify gaps in our knowledge of the biology of these cells. Therefore, emphasis is directed toward a review of the subcellular structure of Leydig cells in relation to known or suggested physiological activities.

Nucleus

Leydig cell nuclei often are eccentrically placed within the cell and usually display a round or irregularly oval shape. Alternatively, the nucleus may present as irregularly polygonal in thin sections, with numerous indentations of the nuclear envelope. When seen in proximity to the walls of blood vessels or the tunica propria of the seminiferous tubules, the nucleus usually conforms to the elongated configuration of the cell by displaying an elliptical profile. In the human testis, Leydig cells with two or more nuclei have been noted (289). An inner mantle of peripheral heterochromatin associated with the nuclear envelope is a universal feature of Leydig cells, at times forming small dense clumps of electron-dense material at irregularly spaced intervals along the inner aspect of the nuclear membrane (Fig. 84). The nucleolus is usually conspicuous and exhibits a conventional fine structure comprising the nucleolonema and dense granular and amorphous areas. Leydig cells of the human testis frequently show duplicate nucleoli, and in the nuclei of adult mice Leydig cells, an annular nucleolus is commonly noted (598). This unusual configuration in mouse Leydig cells has been correlated with Leydig cell development, because they do not appear in immature animals. Extrapolating from their occurrence in other cell types (599), it has been suggested that the central core of annular nucleoli is associated with partial cessation of RNA synthesis. Suppression of RNA synthesis in the annular nucleolus may be reflected by a maturational shift in the conversion of rough to smooth endoplasmic reticulum in the cytoplasm, because the cistrons of rRNA exist in the nucleolus.

Cytoplasm

The dominant organelle within the cytoplasm of mammalian Leydig cells is the smooth endoplasmic reticulum, which on its surface provides binding sites for numerous enzymes necessary for a variety of steroidogenic conversions. Great diversity in the architecture of the smooth endoplasmic reticulum has been indicated in reviews of its ultrastructure (341,537). The qualitative and quantitative differences in the morphology of membranes of smooth endoplasmic reticulum have been described in common laboratory species such as the guinea pig and mouse, in which it is most abundant (537,600), and the rat and human, where it is moderately abundant (341,601,602). Examples of these between-species ultrastructural differences are illustrated in Figs. 84–86.

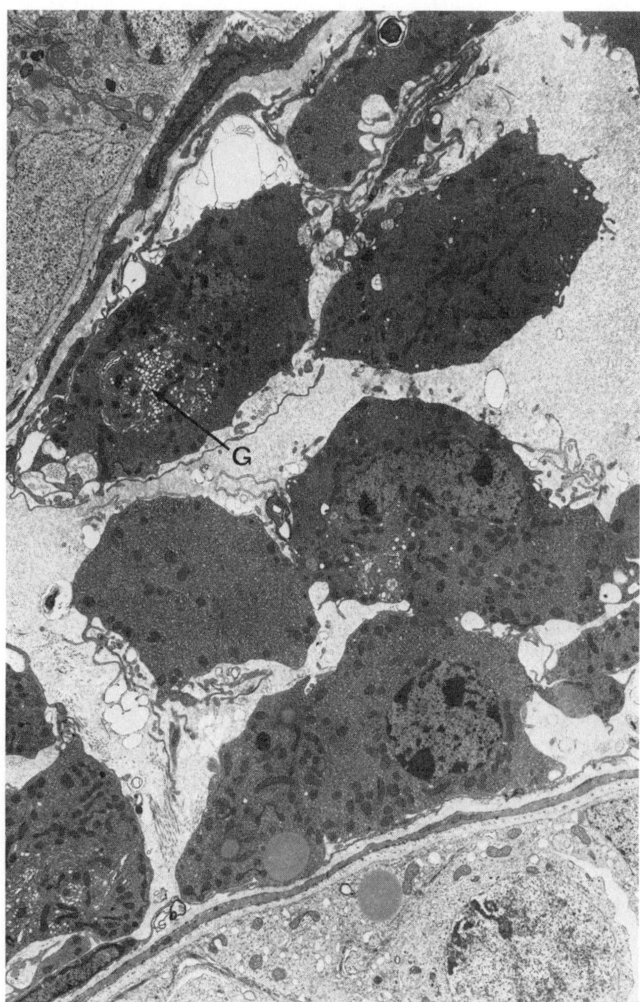

FIG. 84. Ultrastructure of Leydig cells of the normal adult rat testis. The cytoplasm is richly supplied with smooth endoplasmic reticulum. At times, the Golgi apparatus (G) is associated with numerous vesicles.

Our own studies of the internal organization of the Leydig cell were the first to quantitatively examine the proportion of cytoplasm occupied by smooth endoplasmic reticulum (603), and for the rat, approximately 39% of Leydig cell volume was taken up by the internal cavities of this organelle. Since then, the volume occupancy and surface area for this and all other cytoplasmic components in Leydig cells of the rat, mouse, hamster, dog, rabbit, guinea pig, and human have been documented (604–608). All of these studies indicate that the surface area of smooth endoplasmic reticulum is vast. For example, if a single rat Leydig cell were represented as a golf ball, then an unraveling of its membranes of smooth endoplasmic reticulum would generate a square approximately 3 feet on a side. *In situ,* therefore, the membranes of smooth endoplasmic reticulum appear as a vast concentration of tubules interconnected in various patterns to form a meshwork extending throughout the entire cytoplasm of the Leydig cell. The membranes thus enclose a cavity constituting an intracellular compart-

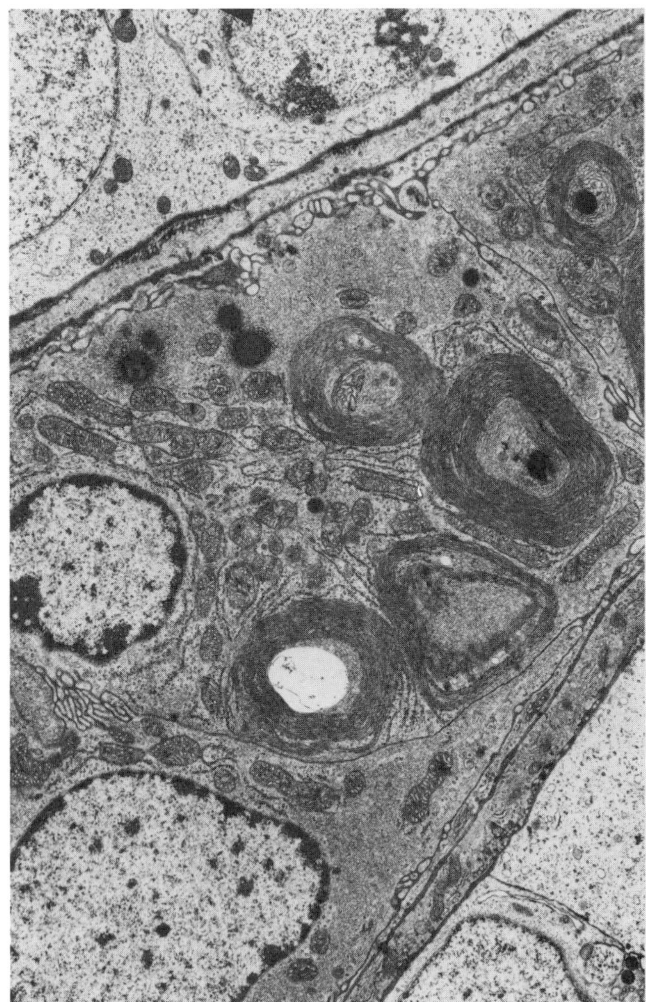

FIG. 85. Mouse Leydig cells, illustrating compact whorls of concentric membranes.

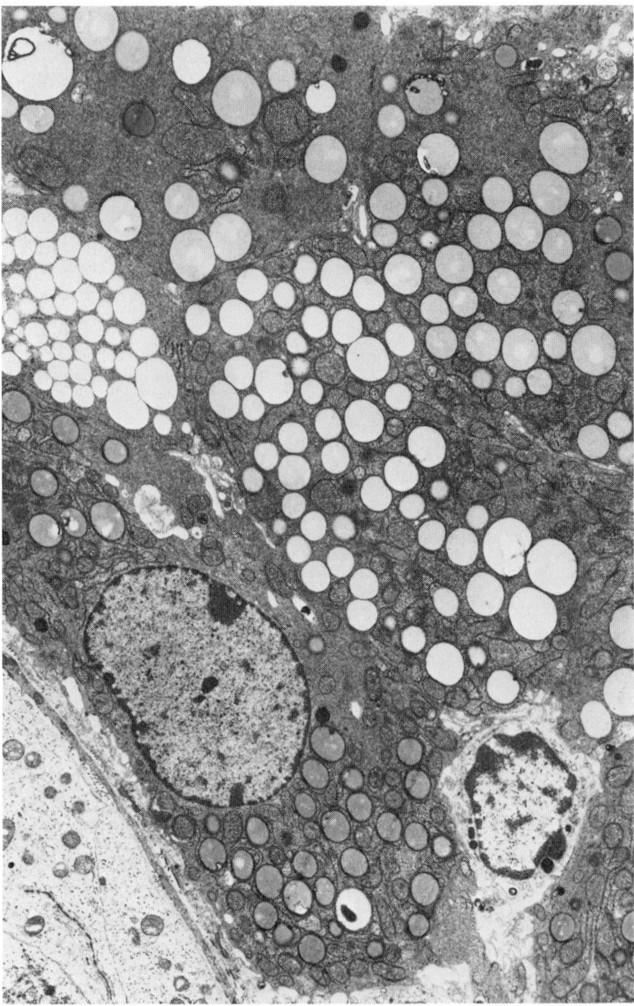

FIG. 86. Mouse Leydig cells, illustrating large numbers of cytoplasmic lipid inclusions that exhibit various densities because of extraction during their fixation and preparation for electron microscopy.

ment separated from the ground cytoplasm. A scheme suggesting possible interconversions of the different ultrastructural configurations of smooth endoplasmic reticulum was based on electron-microscopic analysis of guinea pig Leydig cells (339). The common form of smooth endoplasmic reticulum consists of a random network of interconnected tubules that may transform into loosely packed sheets of tubules or form more regular arrays of fenestrated cisternae. Leydig cells of the mouse exhibit all these various forms and in addition show a marked segregation of their cytoplasmic membranes, a spectacular example being seen in the appearance of extensive concentric whorls of smooth membranes (Fig. 85). These may surround lipid inclusions, mitochondria, or dense membrane-bound bodies, and similar whorls are observed in the guinea pig, rat, dog, armadillo, and monkey (341,480,609–611). The absence of these whorled membranes from many other species raises the possibility that they provide a specific function to meet the biochemical requirements of those particular cells.

A similar concept could be used to explain the infrequent occurrence of other unusual membranous bodies such as single- or double-walled tubules that occur in the mouse, opossum, and rat (598,600,612,613) and structures resembling annulate lamellae seen in adult mouse and rabbit Leydig cells (612–616). The functional significance of these organelles remains unknown. However, the morphological diversity of Leydig cell smooth membranes emphasizes the role of quantitative methods designed to estimate what proportion of the cytoplasm is occupied by a particular organelle. A major objective of stereological analysis of the Leydig cell has been to correlate the relative abundance of cellular components with the amounts of steroid compounds synthesized and secreted by the same cells (604). An approach adopted by Ewing and associates has attempted to link Leydig cell ultrastructure and various pathways of steroidogenesis. They have examined changes in Leydig cell morphology and the capacity to synthesize various steroids by manipulating the degree to which LH is available to act on the Leydig cell (605,617–619). A summary of their findings is presented: When different species were examined, the production of testosterone after LH stimulation varied significantly between species, but was not related to the total mass of Leydig cells within the testis. Instead, they found a strong correlation between testosterone secretion and the amounts of smooth endoplasmic reticulum and Golgi membranes within the Leydig cell cytoplasm, indicating the central role played by these organelles in determining how much testosterone is provided by a single Leydig cell. Furthermore, they have shown that there is a subdivision of enzyme function in the steroidogenic pathway that exists within the membranes of smooth endoplasmic reticulum, raising the interesting possibility that certain conversions such as pregnenolone to progesterone may be sequestered to specialized regions of the Leydig cell. These findings implicate the concentric whorls and other varieties of smooth cytoplasmic membranes in subserving this function.

Mitochondria vary in size and form both in a given Leydig cell and between different species, and their ultrastructure has been well described in earlier studies (341,537,620). Cholesterol is known to undergo side-chain cleavage within the mitochondrion, possibly on the surfaces of the cristae, which exhibit various profiles ranging from foliate to tubular or intermediate forms, and details of the reactions and enzyme systems with Leydig cell mitochondria appear elsewhere in these volumes. Electron-dense mitochondrial granules often occur within the matrix of the mitochondrion, but that function is obscure (341,537,620).

Depending on the species, Leydig cells may exhibit an abundance of lipid inclusions, or they may be only rarely observed. Some confusion may exist about the occurrence of lipid inclusions in Leydig cells, because even within a single section of a testis, Leydig cells may show differing amounts of lipid (Fig. 87) (602), suggesting variable degrees of functional activity. When an estimation of the lipid content of mouse Leydig cells was averaged over many cells (607), each Leydig cell contained about 147 lipid inclusions, with diameter approximately 1 μm and collectively occupying about 6% of cytoplasmic volume. However, when mouse Leydig cells are centrifuged in Percoll density gradients (622), they separate according to buoyant density, and cells of low and high specific gravity show, respectively, a great many or very few cytoplasmic lipid inclusions (Fig. 87). Similar observations may be made for rat Leydig cells, of which the far greater majority is devoid of lipid inclusions, although occasionally some Leydig cells contain an abundance of these inclusions.

Obvious differences in the extent of lipid inclusions occur between species. The Leydig cells of the dog, cat, mole, mouse, elephant, and rhesus monkey often contain a high proportion of lipid (Figs. 81 and 87) (16,605,609); those of the guinea pig, rabbit, and boar exhibit somewhat less Fig. 81) (16,339,605); those of the human, rat, hamster, opossum, ox, African green monkey, squirrel monkey, and several marsupial species found in Australia contain very few lipid inclusions (Fig. 82) (604,605,607,611, 623,624). Studies of the likely functional role of Leydig cell lipid inclusions (341,537) have reviewed the evidence that they represent sites of cholesterol storage and/or synthesis. The belief that lipid inclusions are intimately involved in fatty acid metabolism and, by inference, certain steroidogenic reactions has been supported by morphological data. In rat fetuses, for example, one of the principal structural features enabling identification of the fetal Leydig cells is their rich supply of lipid inclusions, but in postnatal life, adult Leydig cells rarely contain lipid. That these changes in lipid content reflect alterations in Leydig cell function is further emphasized by the finding that trophic stimulation (with LH/hCG) of Leydig cells rapidly depletes their stores of morphologically recognizable lipid droplets (625–629) and heralds an increase in testosterone secretion. Animals fed a cholesterol-rich diet showed significant depletion of lipid inclusions in the Leydig cells, indicating that, if avail-

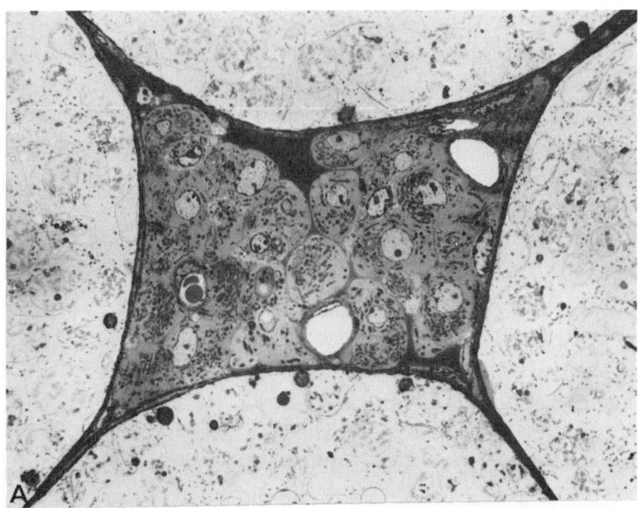

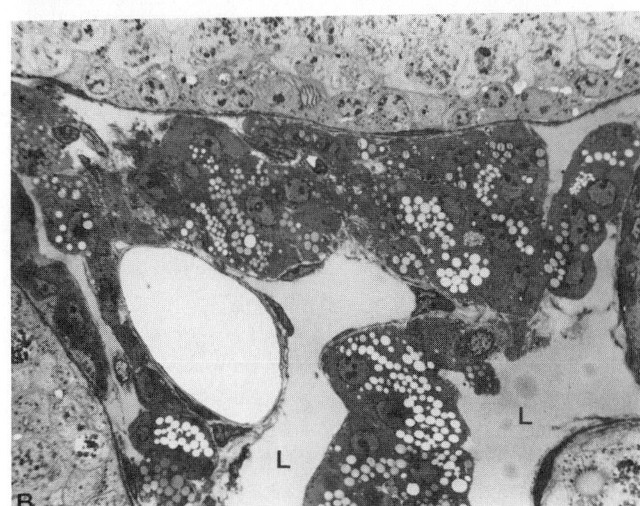

FIG. 87. A: Adult mouse testis, showing Leydig cells that contain many cytoplasmic granules representing mitochondria and lysosomes. **B:** Adult mouse testis, illustrating lipid-rich Leydig cells. Lymphatic channels (C).

able, cholesterol is taken up by the Leydig cell and thus obviates the need for lipid storage in the cytoplasm (606). Opposite changes occurred when Leydig cells were examined after withdrawal of gonadotropins, with lipid inclusions becoming plentiful (621,630), but replacement therapy with exogenous LH resulted in marked depletion of the accumulated lipid.

The Golgi apparatus of Leydig cells is moderately well developed, and although its peripheral vesicles are usually devoid of any internal material, under conditions of Leydig cell hyperactivity the saccules of the Golgi complex often appear swollen and contain distinct electron-dense flocculent material (Fig. 96). Nothing is known at present about the role played by the Golgi apparatus, except its participation in the intracellular passage of radiolabeled fucose, traced by electron-microscope autoradiography (631). It was tentatively concluded from a brief summary of this study that Leydig cells secrete glycoproteins, with the Golgi complex featuring prominently in their early synthesis.

The uncertainty that surrounds the precise functional duties of Leydig cell organelles is nowhere more apparent than in relation to the question, often posed, of the mechanism by which testosterone or any other secretory product is transposed through the cytoplasm and released into the extracellular space. This intriguing topic has been discussed many times (537), but at present remains only speculative. However, in other steroid-secreting tissues, such as the luteal cells of the ovary, evidence has been put forward to suggest that progesterone is secreted in granule form (632). Secretion of corticosteroids from the adrenal tissue is thought to occur in a similar fashion (633). For most species, Leydig cells do not exhibit typical secretory granules or vacuoles in the cytoplasm. However, in a species of seasonally breeding bat, maximum testosterone secretion in the breeding season is accompanied by a marked increase in the abundance of small, dense, membrane-bound granules, whereas in periods of Leydig cell quiescence, the granules largely disappear from the cytoplasm (634). Because the majority of these granules do not share the enzymatic or morphological properties attributable to lysosomes or peroxisomes, they were thought to be involved in the transport of testosterone through the cytoplasm prior to its secretion. More recent studies (635) on cytoplasmic granules in luteal cells of guinea pigs failed to detect granule exocytosis and could show no relationship between the abundance of small granules and maximum progesterone secretion. The functional significance of Leydig cell granules in particular species thus requires further clarification. Furthermore, there is increasing evidence that the ovary secretes relaxin and oxytocin, which, being peptides, are more likely to be stored as secretory granules (636,637).

Lysosomes are commonly observed in Leydig cells. These organelles are about 0.5 μm in diameter, bounded by a single membrane, and show circular or irregular profiles on electron microscopy. They are also referred to as dense bodies because of their notable staining properties. The lysosomes present in Leydig cells conform to their usual pleomorphic occurrence in other cells, exhibiting various states of fusion with cytoplasmic vacuoles, thus categorizing them as secondary lysosomes as distinct from the individual primary lysosome (537). Multivesicular bodies are regarded as structural variations within the lysosomal system and probably represent packaging of recently internalized vesicles destined for lysosomal disposal. The involvement of elements of the lysosomal family of organelles within the Leydig cell has been investigated by studying the responses of Leydig cells to exogenous tracers known to be incorporated into lysosomes of other cell types (638). In this study, Leydig cells were active endocytic cells using both fluid-phase and adsorptive endocytic mechanisms to take up extracellular macromolecules. The destruction of the internalized tracers followed different routes of transport within the Leydig cell cytoplasm, depending on the ionic charges of individual tracers. As seen diagrammatically in Fig. 88, fluid-phase endocytosis involved the lysosomal tracers following this same route or, alternatively, being carried to the Golgi region, whereupon they ultimately disappeared. The existence of these separate pathways for internalized macromolecules suggests that the disposal of unwanted material can be dealt with in a variety of ways.

Poorly digested substances often remain within the Leydig cell lysosomal system and are recognized as dense membrane-bound granules referred to as lipofuscin pigment granules. They are commonly seen in human Leydig cells as heterogeneous conglomerates of myelin figures and particulate matter (537,601,639–641). Stimulation of Leydig cells with hCG tends to increase their abundance (602,629). Although the biochemistry of lipofuscin granules is unclear, they contain acid phosphatases (602,629), suggesting a derivation from lysosomes. Their appearance in other species has been reviewed by Ohata (616). The studies of Reddy and Svoboda (642) and Hruban et al. (643) identified the peroxisome within the Leydig cell as a homogeneous pale-staining granule approximately 0.2 μm in diameter. These organelles contain catalase and oxidases, and although they increase in number following hCG stimulation (626), their functional role is unknown. Centrioles at times associated with the Golgi complex have been identified, and cilia may be noted developing from the paired centrioles (609,616,644). Because the fibril pattern of the cilium has a 9 + 0 pattern, it could reflect a sensory or chemoreceptor property (645).

Microtubules and filaments are present within the Leydig cell cytoplasm, the latter occurring throughout the cytoplasm, and at times forming a network subjacent to the plasma membrane (289). When microtubular systems of steroid-secreting cells are disrupted with inhibitors such as colchicine or vinblastine (646,647), an increase in steroidogenesis is observed. In isolated rat Leydig tumor cell lines, the resting cells exhibit tubulin in discrete granular units distributed throughout the cytoplasm, but when steroidogenesis is induced by treatment with cAMP, vast microtubular networks appear, forming radial patterns around the

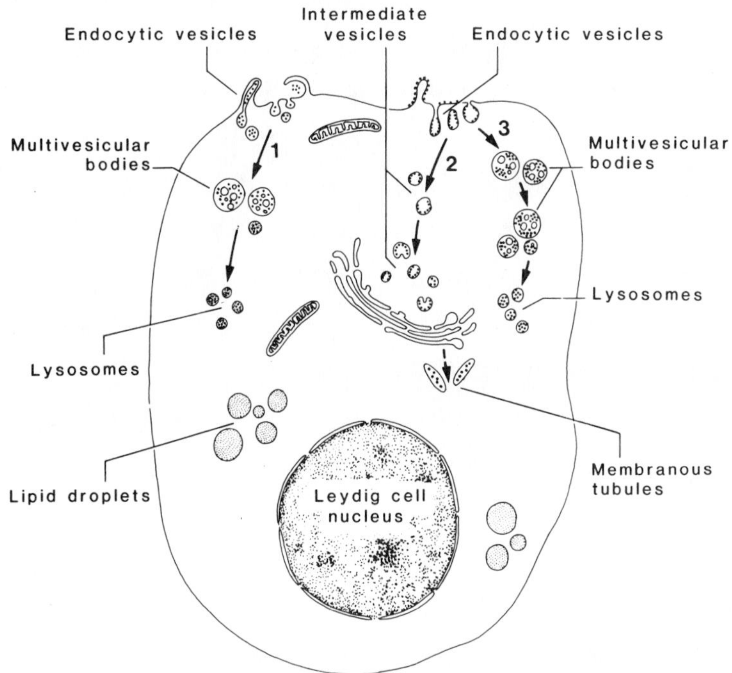

FIG. 88. Intracellular pathways of endocytosed tracers in the Leydig cell. Pathway 1 shows tracers destined for lysosomal incorporation. Pathway 2 illustrates adsorptive endocytosis of molecules initially bound to the cell surface, and ultimately transported to the Golgi region via intermediate vesicles. In pathway 3, these molecules follow an intracellular route involving only the lysosomes. Some tracer molecules also appear in membranous tubules associated with the Golgi membranes, although their subsequent fate is not known. (Data from ref. 638.)

central cell nucleus (648). The small cytoplasmic granules in unstimulated cells are rich in tubulin and cholesterol, indicating that one role of microtubular organization is to make intracellular cholesterol freely available for conversion into pregnenolone. An additional role of microtubular-microfilamentous systems in Leydig cells is in the process of LH/hCG receptor down-regulation, which does not occur following treatment with microtubule inhibitors (649). When vinblastine was administered, the Leydig cells showed remarkable increases in Golgi-associated vesicles and cytoplasmic filamentous material, suggesting alterations of the transport mechanisms within the cytoplasm. Filaments with diameters of 5 to 7 nm or 10 to 12 nm are always seen in Leydig cells, and their ultrastructure has been reviewed elsewhere (537,609).

A remarkable specialization of human Leydig cells is the crystal of Reinke (650). Readily visible by light microscopy, they frequently present as rod-shaped structures up to 20 μm in length, although they may exhibit triangular, rhombic, or polygonal shapes (Fig. 89). Not every Leydig cell contains these crystals. Their ultrastructure and crystalline nature have been repeatedly documented (601,602,639, 640,651,652), and although they are known to contain protein (653) and to increase in size and number in aging testes (654), their functional role is unclear. Various other crystalline structures, termed paracrystalline inclusions, have also been noted in human Leydig cells (289). Because the subunits of Reinke crystals are similar to the paracrystalline inclusions, the latter have been considered as precursors of the much larger Reinke crystals (601). Occasionally, either type of crystalline material may occur in the Leydig cell nucleus (601,652,655).

Reinke crystals were commonly believed to be unique to human Leydig cells until similar cytoplasmic crystalloids were described in Leydig cells of the sexually regressed wild bush rat, *Rattus fuscipes* (353). These rats are seasonal breeders, and in the nonbreeding season their serum gonadotropins and testosterone are decreased. Using modified laboratory conditions mimicking the natural environment of the nonbreeding season, Irby et al. (458) induced Leydig cell atrophy in the same species, whereupon many large crystalloid inclusions made their appearance in the Leydig cell cytoplasm (Figs. 90 and 91). Again serum hormone levels declined significantly, as compared with breeding rats, which do not display these crystalloid inclusions. When gonadotropin secretion was experimentally suppressed by hypophysectomy or testosterone implants (656), the Leydig cells atrophied, and many crystalloids appeared in the cytoplasm (Fig. 92). Formation of nuclear vesicles, their subsequent transfer to the Leydig cell cytoplasm, and concurrent development of paracrystalline material within the vesicles have been suggested as mechanisms to explain the growth of crystalloids by assembly and fusion of smaller subunits (Fig. 91). Because these crystals occur only in regressive forms of Leydig cells producing very little testosterone, they may represent a storage facility of steroid precursors and enzymes, although further work will be necessary to elucidate their precise function.

The surface area of Leydig cell plasma membrane is very large because of extensive surface projections of filopodia

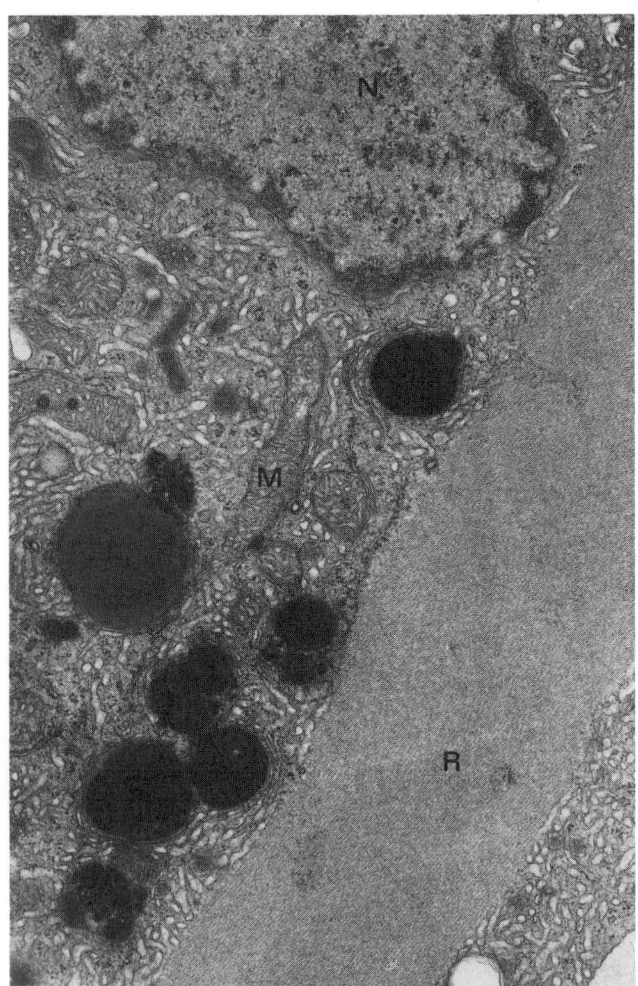

FIG. 89. A Leydig cell in the human testis, illustrating a large Reinke crystal (R). Note nucleus (N), smooth endoplasmic reticulum, mitochondria (M), and lipid (L).

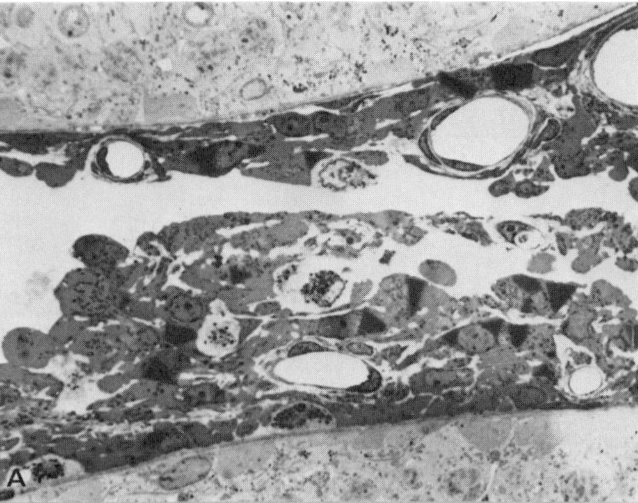

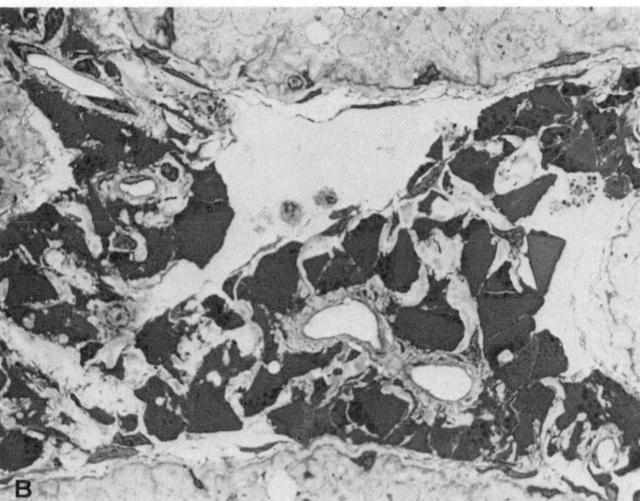

FIG. 90. A: Leydig cells in the testis of the bush rat, *R. fuscipes,* showing triangular and polygonal crystalloid inclusions that appear as the process of spermatogenesis begins to undergo regression. **B:** In the fully regressed testis of *R. fuscipes,* the Leydig cells develop large crystalloid inclusions.

and microvilli (536,537,616,621). In a morphometric analysis of rat Leydig cells (604), their volume was estimated to be about 1,200 μm^3, and if considered to be spherical, their surface area would have been approximately 500 μm^2. However, the actual figure was 1,500 μm^2, reflecting the complex topography of their surfaces. Leydig cells found in clusters form junctions with neighboring Leydig cells and occasionally form junctions with themselves (536). Gap junctions are frequently observed where the intercellular space is narrowed to 20 Å (537,609). These junctions are normally 0.2 to 2 μm in greatest diameter (327) and in thin sections appear as ring-shaped circular or double-circle structures (Fig. 93). Septate-like junctions have occasionally been described (536), and these are partially permeable to electron-dense tracers such as lanthanum. Tight junctions or desmosomes are generally not considered to form between Leydig cells, although rudimentary desmosomes have been observed in canine Leydig cells (609).

Special sites of contact between Leydig cells and macrophages occur frequently (579) and consist of short projections of Leydig cell cytoplasm that invaginate nearby macrophages. The plasma membrane of the macrophage develops an inner bristle coat, suggesting the possibility that small amounts of Leydig cell cytoplasm may be endocytosed by the macrophage. A thin, discontinuous layer of basal-lamina-type material may partly surround the surface of the Leydig cell (537,609,616,640) and may provide structural support to the cell in conjunction with scattered bundles of collagen fibers.

Life History

The origin, differentiation, proliferation, and attrition of Leydig cells have been subjects of hundreds of investigations, and yet many unsolved problems remain. A comprehensive review of the morphology and function of Leydig

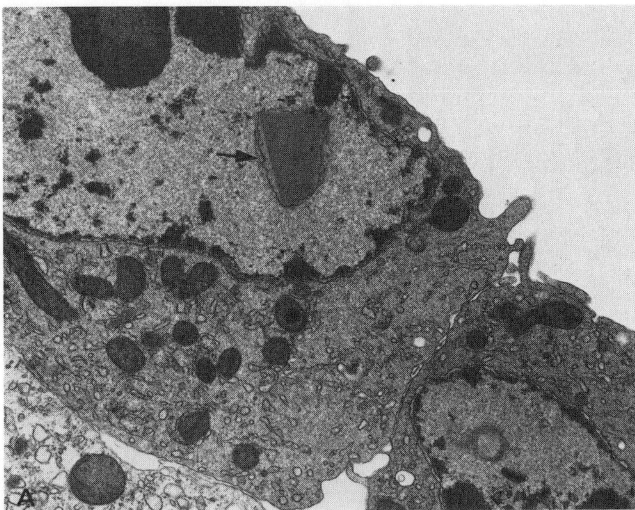

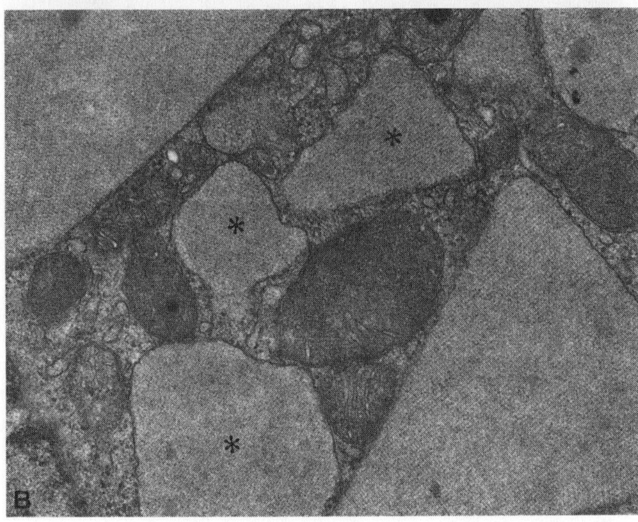

FIG. 91. A: *R. fuscipes* Leydig cells illustrating intranuclear formation of a crystalloid (*arrow*). **B:** *R. fuscipes* Leydig cell showing angular and pleomorphic (*asterisks*) cytoplasmic crystalloid inclusions.

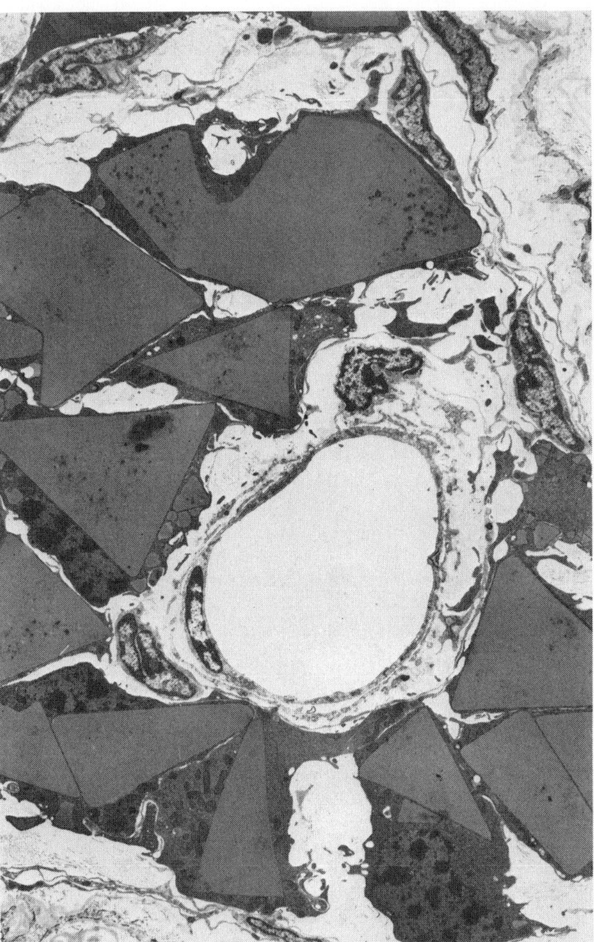

FIG. 92. Leydig cells in the testis of the hypophysectomized bush rat, *R. fuscipes,* showing the striking formation of crystalloid inclusions.

cells from initiation of testicular differentiation proceeding through puberty and adult life and terminating with the senescent testis is quite beyond the range of this review, and therefore it is intended to emphasize some of the fundamental aspects of Leydig cell biology available from selected earlier studies and some recent investigations. The history of Leydig cell life in the normal mammalian testis can be temporally subdivided into six categories: (a) the development of fetal Leydig cells, (b) changes in Leydig cells at birth, (c) pubertal development, (d) the adult population, (e) seasonal alterations in Leydig cell biology, and (f) the status of Leydig cells in old age.

In those species thus far studied, the fetal testis develops a spectacularly high proportion of active Leydig cells whose morphology and secretory function are unique to this phase of their growth. The debate concerning the precise embryological derivation of fetal Leydig cells has been amply discussed in the past (23,657–662), with two concepts being put forward to explain their origin. First, the most generally accepted theory favors a mesenchymal origin, although alternative evidence is available (663) favoring their derivation from mesonephric cells. A good deal of uncertainty surrounds the validity of each of these theories, because the process of gonadal differentiation is extremely complex, and repeated attempts to identify the origin and cell type giving rise to histologically recognizable Leydig cells have fallen short of providing clear answers. A useful review of this problem has recently been provided (23).

The notion of a mesenchymal origin of Leydig cells has gained acceptance on a number of grounds. Ultrastructural analysis of the early fetal testis reveals numerous mesenchymal-like interstitial cells between the seminiferous cords that are believed to differentiate into fetal Leydig cells (Figs. 14 and 94) (29,35,664,665). Similar observations have been presented many times for the postnatal development of Leydig cells, whereby they are thought to arise chiefly by differentiation from simple bipolar interstitial cells within the interstitial tissue and, to a lesser extent, by mitotic prolif-

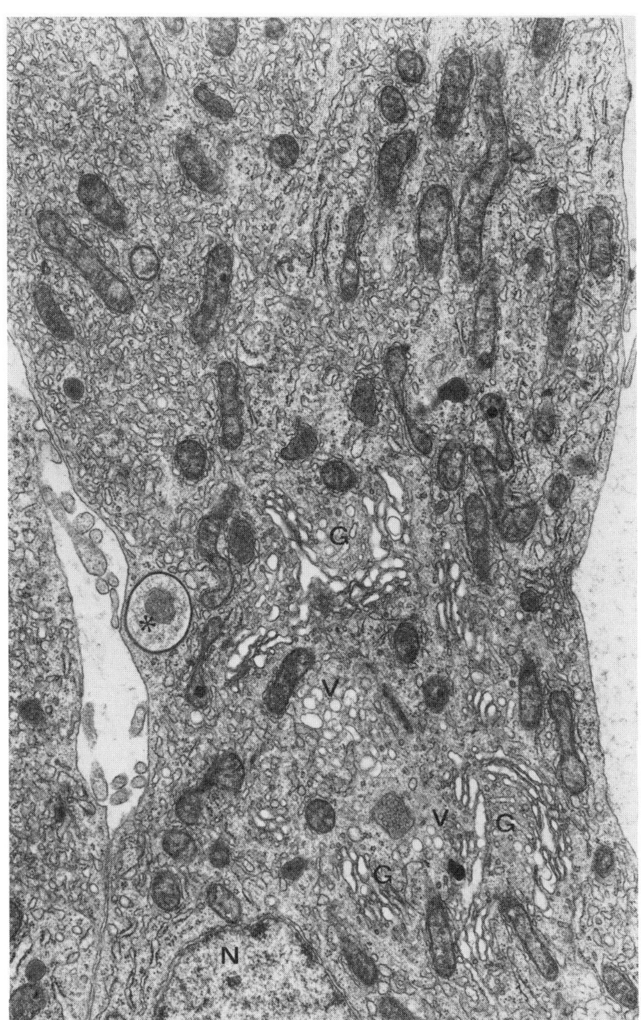

FIG. 93. Leydig cell from a 4-week experimentally cryptorchid rat testis, illustrating numerous stacks of Golgi membranes (G) and associated vesicles (V). Note circular junctional specialization (*asterisk*) formed by a penetrating piece of cytoplasm. Leydig cell nucleus (N).

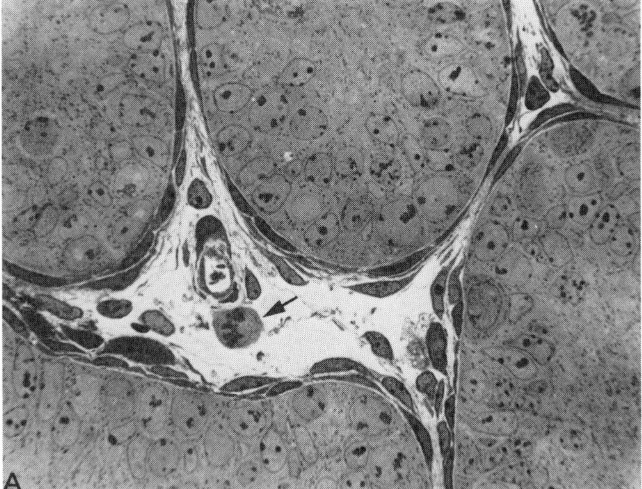

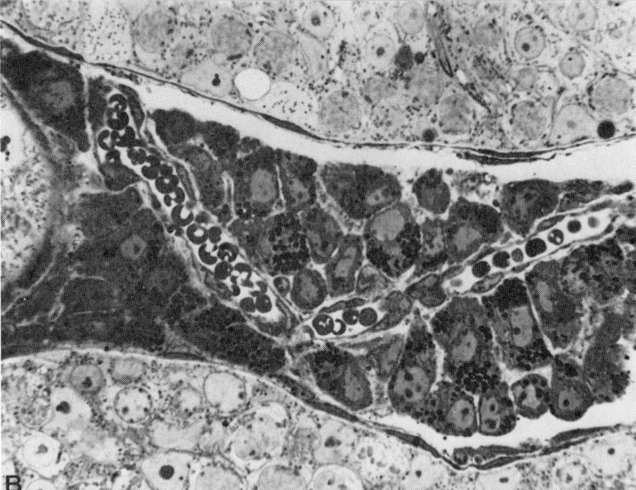

FIG. 94. A: Seven-day-old mouse testis, illustrating numerous spindle-shaped interstitial cells and a metaphase figure (*arrow*). **B:** Five-week-postnatal mouse testis, showing abundant lipid-rich Leydig cells.

eration of fully formed Leydig cells (341,531,532,537, 659,666–669). Some confusion still exists as to the precise histological classification of these Leydig stem cells (669,670). They have been variously designated as pure mesenchymal cells (especially in the fetus) or fibroblasts, myofibroblasts (having affinity with peritubular smooth-muscle contractile cells), fibroblastic mesenchymal cells, and many other classifications. A further complication pertaining to Leydig cell differentiation concerns the dual sites of their origin, some arising in peritubular positions and others developing in association with capillaries and in more central regions of the interstitial tissue, a feature well illustrated in the pig testis (671–674).

Which cell type(s) represents the Leydig cell precursor? The answer to this question is not yet available, but here we return to the alternative theory of Leydig cell differentiation, namely, their development from mesonephrogenic tissues. During early gonadal differentiation, mesenchyme-like cells of mesonephric origin invade the entire testis and occupy the presumptive interstitial tissue (23). These cells, together with others migrating in from the gonadal blastema, could thus form the stem cells for later development of Leydig cells. Because mesonephric cells exhibit the capacity to "transdifferentiate" into completely different cells during fetal life, then in theory this behavior may be retained by the intertubular tissue beyond intrauterine life. Examples of transdifferentiation of testicular interstitial cells are available. At birth, the seminiferous cords are surrounded by a homogeneous population of fibroblasts, but as the tubules expand during testicular enlargement, these cells transform into an inner peritubular myoid cell, acquiring epithelioid characteristics, and an outer fibroblastic layer with ultrastructure similar to that in the newborn situation (675). Alternatively, cells lining the seminiferous tubules are known to differentiate into Leydig cells (676), and intermediate steps in the route of differentiation have been suggested (112,609,639,677–679).

This intriguing topic of Leydig cell differentiation is intimately related to another well-known feature of the Leydig cell population in late fetal life and shortly after birth, namely, their disappearance from the testis. A biphasic pattern of Leydig cell growth has been recognized for many years. Among the first to describe peaks of Leydig cell development in the fetus and in postnatal life was Whitehead (680,681), who studied the pig testis. In fact, the pig testis is a special case, because it exhibits three consecutive stages of Leydig cell development—fetal, perinatal, and postpubertal—whereas the common laboratory rodents and other species show a spurt of Leydig cell proliferation in late fetal life and postnatally coincident with initiation of spermatogenesis (52,669,670,682,683). The stimulus for rapid proliferation of fetal Leydig cells is chorionic gonadotropin, and possibly, to a lesser extent, pituitary LH, which results in large elevations of intratesticular testosterone and other steroids, reflected a short time later by raised serum levels of testosterone (53,684,685). A sharp decline in the amount of steroids secreted by each fetal Leydig cell occurs just before birth in the rat, and thereafter a further fall is a reflection of a considerable loss of Leydig cells from the testis (53). Two suggestions have been offered to account for the dramatic perinatal decline in Leydig cell numbers: (a) a process of cell death (35,659,677,678,686) or (b) dedifferentiation back to fibroblastic-type cells (687,688). Although the morphology of fetal Leydig cells is well recognized (Fig. 14), no evidence favoring either theory has been available. At this time it is also not clear if changes in the pituitary-testicular hormonal axis and/or alterations in the cellular composition of the fetal testis may influence this pattern of Leydig cell attrition.

A great many studies have concentrated on the morphological features of the intertubular tissue during the period between birth and puberty. The point of interest here has been to characterize, in morphological terms, the process of Leydig cell differentiation and proliferation that parallels the establishment of spermatogenesis and to ascertain the identity and mechanisms of action of hormones that support renewed growth of Leydig cells at puberty, as reviewed by Sharpe (689,691). When the developing testis is studied by light and electron microscopy, there is general agreement that the resident population of interstitial fibroblasts or mesenchymal cells is stimulated by LH to differentiate into the adult-type generation of Leydig cells (537,601,666,667, 670,674). Differentiation of adult-type Leydig cells in postnatal life is thought to occur as the numbers of mes enchymal cells decline (659,666,667), with the latter signaling their transformation into Leydig cells by synthesizing increasing amounts of smooth endoplasmic reticulum (666,669,670,692). The complex hormonal control of sexual maturation has been a subject of intensive clinical and experimental investigation that has been continually updated as new information has become available (693–697). However, some data relating to the physiology of testicular maturation have been difficult to interpret. First, the mature or partly differentiated Leydig cells in humans are thought to be absent from the testis from about 1 year after birth until puberty (23,35,677,678,698–700). However, the concentration of testosterone in spermatic venous blood in boys is five times higher than in peripheral blood (701). Second, acute hCG treatment of prepubertal boys induces rapid increases in serum testosterone levels (702). Third, elevation of serum FSH levels during sexual maturation is known to increase testis weight via stimulation of spermatogenesis. However, it is not clear how spermatogenesis is supported without a supply of testosterone from the Leydig cells. Some data favoring a stimulatory effect of FSH on the interstitial tissue have demonstrated FSH-induced enhancement of LH receptors (703–705) and increased testosterone secretion in response to LH *in vivo* and *in vitro* (703,706–708). Furthermore, these findings have been difficult to evaluate because Leydig cells and the primitive mesenchymal cells lack receptors for FSH. The results of recent investigations have provided additional information on the structure-function relationships of Leydig cells in the immature testis. Ultrastructural analysis of testicular biopsies collected from 30 boys aged 3 to 8 years has revealed the presence of immature Leydig cells composing about 9% of the total interstitial cell population (669). Furthermore, acute hCG stimulation of the testes of cryptorchid boys caused a precocious secretion of testosterone within the testis and induced rapid differentiation of immature Leydig cells from primitive fibroblastic cells (670). The role of FSH in induction of Leydig cell function during testicular maturation has been studied in immature rats, in which FSH treatment induced rapid hypertrophy and hyperplasia of interstitial cells, which became transformed into mature Leydig cells (709,710). These effects could not be duplicated with LH. With FSH treatment, numerous Leydig cells appeared to arise from the peritubular tissues, again implicating a reserve stock of mesenchymal or fibroblastic cells capable of differentiation into Leydig cells. Because the target tissue for FSH is the seminiferous epithelium, the effects of FSH treatment on Leydig cells suggest that secretion of factors by the seminiferous tubules may mediate the maturation of Leydig cells.

Very recently, studies with a single dose of the substance ethane dimethane sulfonate have demonstrated that the Leydig cells in the adult rat testis can be totally destroyed, but they regenerate 3 weeks later (585,586). This regeneration appears to occur from a multifocal differentiation of connective-tissue cells consisting of pericytes, fibroblasts, and lymphatic endothelial cells. These data indicate that with appropriate stimulation, the connective tissue of the intertubular region and the testis can be induced to develop into Leydig cells (586).

Little is known about the dynamics of the total Leydig cell population during adult life, because in the common laboratory species (mouse, rat, guinea pig) the histology of the interstitial tissue appears unchanged during the reproductive lifetime of the animal. However, most mammalian species do not remain reproductively active throughout the year, showing varying degrees of seasonal regression of spermatogenesis and Leydig cell function (20,456). Studies of the morphological and functional changes in Leydig cells of pronounced seasonal breeders have not been prolific, and additional work is warranted. Examples of combined ultrastructural-functional investigations of changes in the Leydig cells of seasonal breeders include amphibians (597), rock hyrax (711,712,713), wild rats (353,458,656), bats (634,714), hamster (715), squirrel (460), mole (716), and monkey (624).

It is known that Leydig cells usually undergo some degree of atrophy during periods of diminished sperm production, but whether or not they decline in numbers at this time and later reestablish an active cell population is not known. Involution of the Leydig cells often is marked by accumulation of cytoplasmic lipid inclusions, suggestive of Leydig cell inactivity (624,712), whereas in seasonally breeding white-tailed deer and European moles, Leydig cell lipid content is maximal in the sexually active phase (717,718). Clearly, the morphological features of Leydig cells in seasonal-breeding species represent a spectrum of changes that emphasize caution in extrapolating observations from one species to another. The effects of season on numerous Leydig cell parameters were recently reported in adult stallions (474), 48 of which were selected at the onset and during the midphase of the breeding season. The latter stallions exhibited a 30% increase in testis weight and 50% increase in daily sperm production per testis, as compared with the values obtained in the nonbreeding period. When the interstitial compartment was analyzed by quantitative light microscopy and electron microscopy, the total volume of Leydig cells per testis also showed a corresponding 50% increase, yet the numbers of Leydig cells remained unchanged, indicating, at least for this species, that hypertrophy rather than hyperplasia characterizes the Leydig cell response to seasonal changes in testis function.

The fate of Leydig cells with increasing age has been discussed for many years (289,529). A considerable degree of controversy over the morphological and functional status of the Leydig cell population, particularly in the human, has been evident from the conflicting reports claiming an age-related increase (719,720) or decline in Leydig cell numbers or mass (479,721,722). Other claims have been put forward favoring no change in Leydig cell abundance with increasing age (677,723) or a progressive atrophy in elderly men (724), commonly characterized by increasing degrees of vacuolization, lipid accumulation, and pigmentation (289). In a reinvestigation of this subject in 25 men ranging from 18 to 87 years of age in which spermatogenesis was normal, it was shown that a significant negative correlation existed between age and total Leydig cell number (725). Young adult men, 20 years of age, on average, contained over 700 million Leydig cells in paired testes; by years 70 to 80, this figure had declined to about 200 million per paired testes, representing a loss of 8 million Leydig cells per annum beyond the age of 20 years. These findings were confirmed and extended (726) in a subsequent study of 30 men aged 20 to 76 years, in which the average 60-year-old man had less than half as many Leydig cells as an average 20-year-old individual. However, the question remained as to the mechanism of attrition, either through Leydig cell death or alternatively via dedifferentiation back to a primitive interstitial cell. If the latter process occurred, then the abundance of primitive (or fibroblastic-type) cells might be expected to increase as the Leydig cells declined. When this idea was tested by morphometric examination of cell types in the interstitial tissue of testes from the previously mentioned group (727), the population of interstitial cells (not being Leydig cells or macrophages) decreased significantly with increasing age. This finding thus makes it unlikely that the loss of Leydig cells from aging is due to Leydig cell regression into other interstitial cells. Still unresolved, however, is the process by which Leydig cells undergo a slow but continual loss from the testis.

Although Leydig cells in the aging human testis may develop abundant lipid inclusions, lysosomes, and lipofuscin bodies (289), there is no evidence to suggest that these morphological features reflect an exhausted functional state, nor have there been any data to show that the disappearance of Leydig cells might occur by autolysis, culminating in self-destruction. It would seem more likely that dysfunctional Leydig cells would be disposed of by cells equipped to fulfill this role, namely, the interstitial macrophages. At present, nothing is known about the functional duties of testicular macrophages, but from evidence to be reviewed in the next section, it is clear that their phagocytic capacity can be directed toward the Leydig cells. These observations may help in explaining the age-related disappearance of the Leydig cell.

No such attrition of the Leydig cell population has been recorded in aging rats (728), but in distinct contrast to this species and to humans, the testes of aging stallions show a striking increase in Leydig cell numbers (474). A twofold to threefold increase in Leydig cell number per testis occurred in stallions between 2 to 3 years and 20 years of age, yet in the examination of 48 testes in this study, no mitotic figures were observed. A similar failure to observe mitotic figures in the interstitial tissue of rats was reported in a study in which Leydig cell number per testis tripled during 5 weeks of chronic hCG stimulation (576). However, as mentioned in the study of Leydig cells in stallions (474), if mitosis were responsible for Leydig cell proliferation at the measured rate, no more than 1 Leydig cell of every 20,000 observed should exhibit a mitotic figure. Hence, failure to detect mitosis of Leydig cells was not considered as supporting the notion that cell division does not occur. An alternative mechanism of Leydig cell proliferation from other interstitial cells was reviewed earlier in this section and remains a viable possibility to account for these age- and treatment-related changes in Leydig cell populations.

Response to Testicular Damage

Impairment of testicular function can be manifested by changes in either seminiferous tubules or interstitial tissue, and for many years it was thought that treatments compromising one particular compartment of the testis were virtually without harmful effect on the adjacent compartment. This conclusion seemed valid at the time, because microscopists had to rely heavily on the relatively imprecise technique of histological evaluation of the testis in paraffin section, and, in addition, biochemists and physiologists interested in pathological changes to the testis had few methods available with which to monitor alterations in testicular function. Significant advances in the morphological sciences, together with increasing numbers of sensitive and specific assays for cell and tissue function in the testis, have together greatly improved our understanding of testicular pathology (354,729–732). In this section we present an overview of the morphological changes of Leydig cells in three broad areas in which testicular damage is sustained. First, we discuss nonspecific and unrelated treatments that precipitate impairment of spermatogenesis of varying degrees of severity; second, the deleterious effects on spermatogenesis of endogenous hormones or their synthetic analogues are contrasted with alterations of the Leydig cell population; third, the extreme sensitivity of Leydig cells to selected toxic compounds is reviewed.

A considerable body of evidence is now available clearly indicating that disruption of spermatogenesis induced by unrelated agents is accompanied by morphological and function changes of the Leydig cells indicative of a state of stimulation (Figs. 95 and 96). Those treatments that result in this peculiar response of the Leydig cells share a common feature, namely, the induction of varying degrees of seminiferous tubule damage. Some examples of these experimental models of spermatogenic damage include surgical cryptorchidism, ligation of the efferent ducts, temporary heat treatment, a vitamin-A-deficient diet, treatment with the cytostatic agent hydroxyurea, and irradiation *in utero*; the details of these experiments have been reviewed elsewhere (354,525,526,690,691,733). The stimulated condition of Leydig cells is reversible (526) and can occur independent of any involvement by their known endogenous trophic hormone, LH (734–736), and, in addition, this same response is confined to only the immediate vicinity of damaged seminiferous tubules (737). Thus, the concept has emerged of a paracrine relationship between the seminiferous tubules and the Leydig cells, a subject that is attracting increasing attention (691,738,739). Judging from the morphological response of the Leydig cells to spermatogenic damage, it seems likely that their enlargement and proliferation of organelles are reflections of the actions of some potent intratesticular factor or factors that, for reasons not yet understood, constitute a pathway for a short-loop feedback mechanism within the testis.

It is a little-known fact that the naturally occurring gonadotropic hormones LH and hCG can exert deleterious effects on the testis, in direct contrast to their usual mode of action, namely, the stimulation of intertubular tissue, with subsequent support or enhancement of spermatogenesis. The data in support of these findings are not new, and examples of the toxic effects of hCG on spermatogenesis in immature rats and guinea pigs are available (629,740). However, the impairment of spermatogenesis in these experimental situations is again accompanied by hypertrophy and/or hyperplasia of the Leydig cells, an effect similar to that described earlier for nonspecific induction of spermatogenic damage. This phenomenon is not confined to hCG treatment, because hCG and PMSG given to adult rats for 1 to 2 weeks caused degeneration of the seminiferous epithelium (740), and in investigations of the antispermatogenic effects of LH and LHRH agonists in adult hypophysectomized rats (489) it was shown that LH alone or in combination with LHRH agonist can focally inhibit spermatogenesis and, in certain

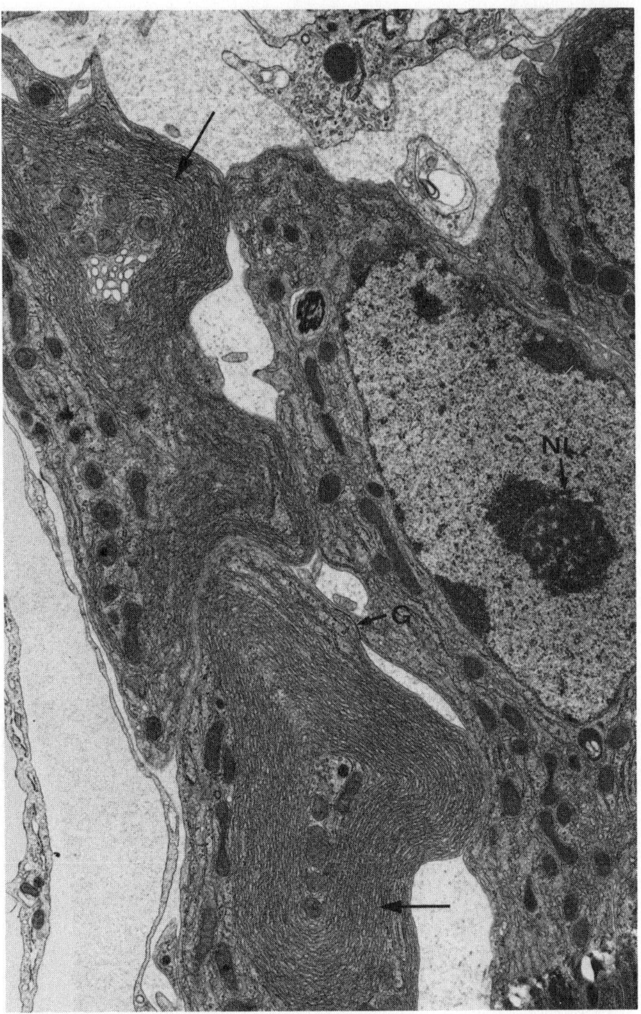

FIG. 95. Leydig cells from a 7-day experimentally cryptorchid rat testis, showing large concentric whorls of smooth endoplasmic reticulum. The Leydig cell nucleus contains a prominent nucleolus (NL), and a gap junction (G) is shown.

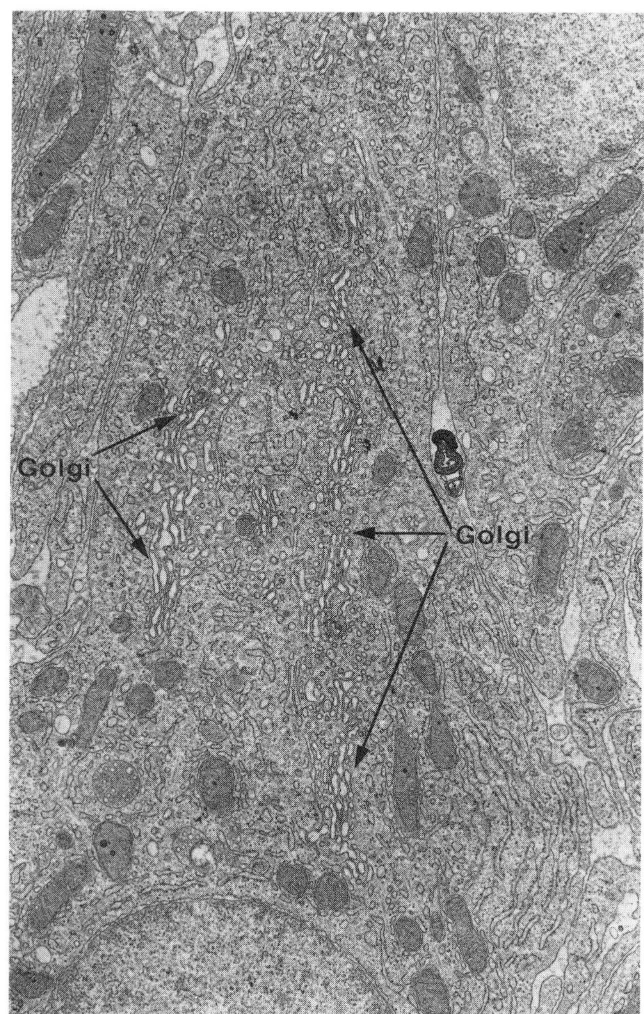

FIG. 96. Rat Leydig cell of the 4-week experimentally cryptorchid testis, illustrating proliferation of the Golgi apparatus and associated vesicles.

areas of the testis, destroy all the cells of the seminiferous epithelium. When the intertubular tissue was examined using morphometric techniques, the adjacent Leydig cells exhibited significant hyperplasia compared with saline-treated controls not experiencing seminiferous tubular damage. These observations emphasize that agents that disrupt the spermatogenic process also interfere with the Leydig cells.

The number of substances known to be specifically toxic to the intertubular tissue is large, and relevant reviews are available (588,732,742–744). Of particular interest are the influences of cadmium salts and the group of alkylating agents, diesters of methane sulfonic acid. For many years, cadmium administration, even in minute doses, has been recognized to cause acute testicular necrosis by rapid disturbance of the testicular circulation (488,742). Within several hours after cadmium exposure, morphological signs of intertubular disruption are noted, including edema, hemorrhage, and infiltration of mononucleated cells. Finally, complete testicular necrosis occurs, in which the seminiferous tubules degenerate totally, and the intertubular tissue resembles loose connective tissue mainly containing extracellular materials. A surprising long-term consequence of cadmium-induced testicular degeneration is the slow but unmistakable regeneration of Leydig cells within the intertubular tissue. The new generation of Leydig cells is functionally active, as indicated by restoration of previously reduced weights of seminal vesicles and prostate (488,588). It is of interest that regeneration of Leydig cells occurs initially just beneath the tunica albuginea and is accompanied by regeneration of blood vessels and intertubular macrophages. Continued proliferation of Leydig cells gives rise to interstitial cell tumors, but the seminiferous tubules remain permanently sclerosed. This observation raises the possibility that Leydig cell differentiation and hyperplasia may be dependent on vascular proliferation. The blood vessels that regenerate within these testes are evidently quite

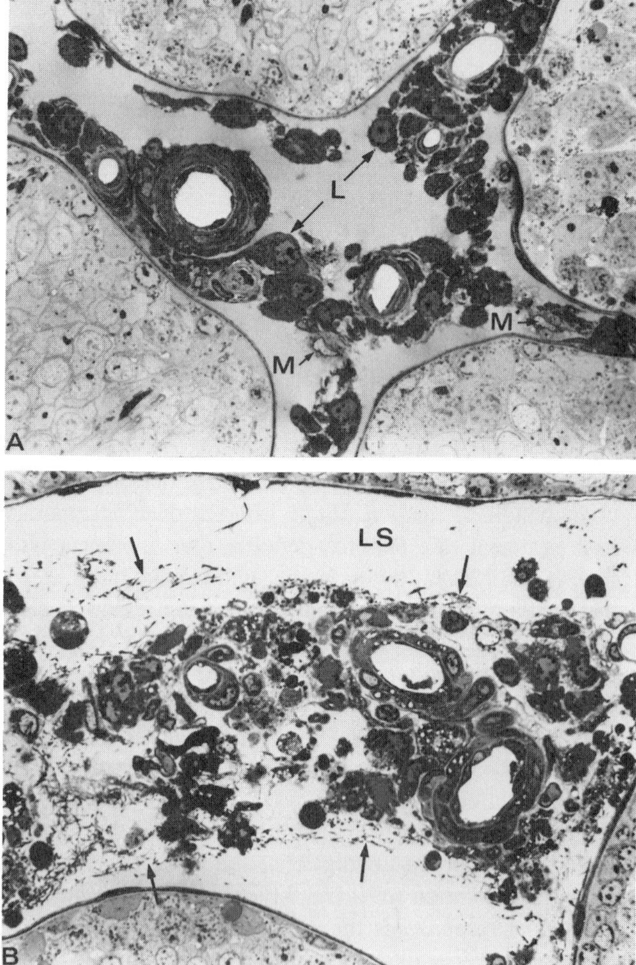

FIG. 97. A: Intertubular tissue of the normal rat testis, illustrating Leydig cells (L) and macrophages (M). **B:** Marked degeneration of Leydig cells of the rat testis 1 day after treatment with EDS. Widening of the lymphatic space (LS) and formation of fibrillar material (*arrows*) are noted.

different from those in the nontreated testis, because they do not react to a second cadmium treatment (745–747), thus conferring resistance on the regenerated Leydig cells to further cadmium insult.

In many respects, the toxic effects of ethane dimethane sulfonate (EDS) on the intertubular tissue of the rat testis bear some resemblance to those described for cadmium. EDS specifically destroys Leydig cells within 3 days after a single treatment (Figs. 97 and 98) (585–587,748–751). Macrophages phagocytose the degenerating Leydig cells and bring about complete elimination of Leydig cells from the testis (Figs. 99 and 100). However, beginning several weeks after initial treatment with EDS, new Leydig cells regenerate within the intertubular tissue and bear a striking morphological resemblance to Leydig cells seen in the fetal rat testis (Fig. 101). The fetal-type Leydig cells arise from perivascular and peritubular positions within the intertubular tissue (Fig. 98), and during 8 to 10 weeks after EDS treatment they transform into adult-type Leydig cells, occupying the previously mentioned positions and more central locations. However, it has also been shown (751) that the fetal-type Leydig cells are resistant to additional EDS exposure when given at weekly intervals for up to 6 weeks after initial treatment. Inability of EDS to destroy Leydig cells has also been shown for the Leydig cells of the immature rat testis (748), suggesting that only the adult type of Leydig cell is sensitive to the toxic effects of EDS. Data available from the responses of Leydig cells to indirect and direct assaults on them therefore indicate that although Leydig cells are sensitive to many agents causing testicular damage, the intertubular tissue retains the capacity to ensure their persistence in the testis.

Interesting results supporting the presence of paracrine regulation of Leydig cells are also available from studies using EDS. If given to cryptorchid rats, EDS causes destruction of Leydig cells as seen in normal animals, but the recovery of Leydig cells is more rapid in cryptorchid testes

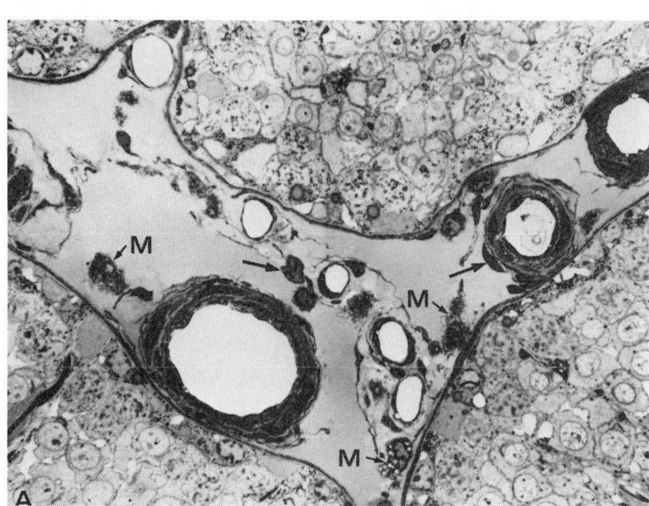

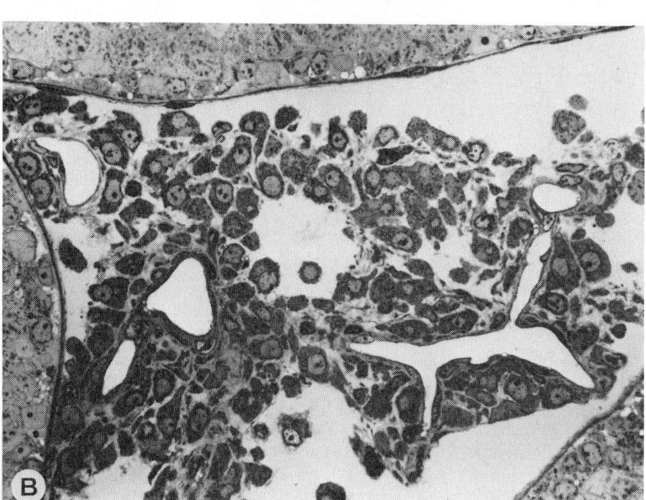

FIG. 98. A: Seven days after EDS treatment, illustrating macrophages (M) and irregularly shaped interstitial cells (*arrows*). **B:** Four weeks after EDS treatment, showing the regenerated population of Leydig cells.

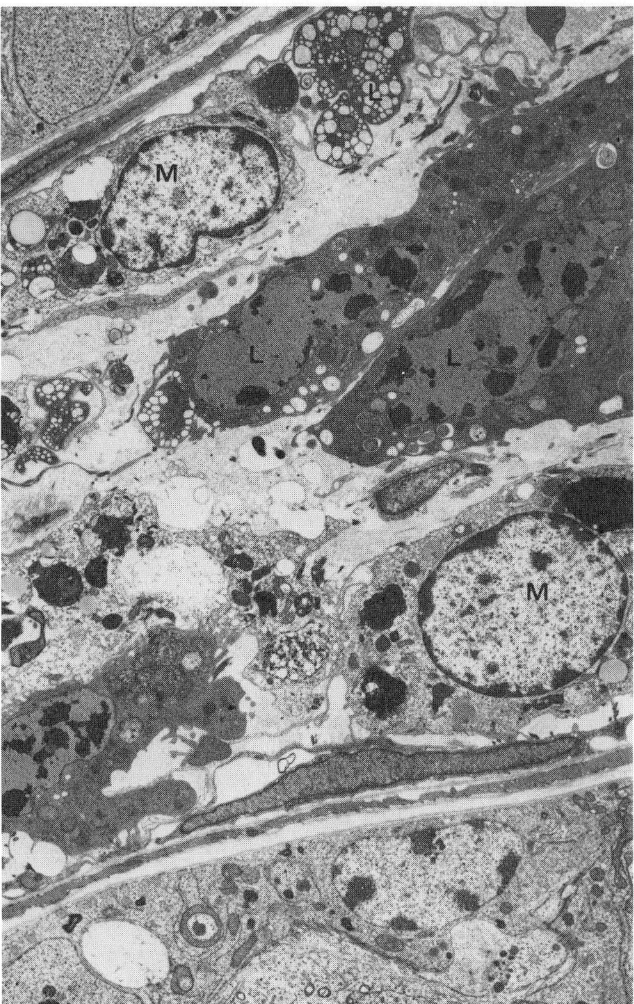

FIG. 99. Degenerative changes in Leydig cells (L) and accumulation of Leydig cell debris within the interstitial macrophages (M) 1 day after treatment with EDS.

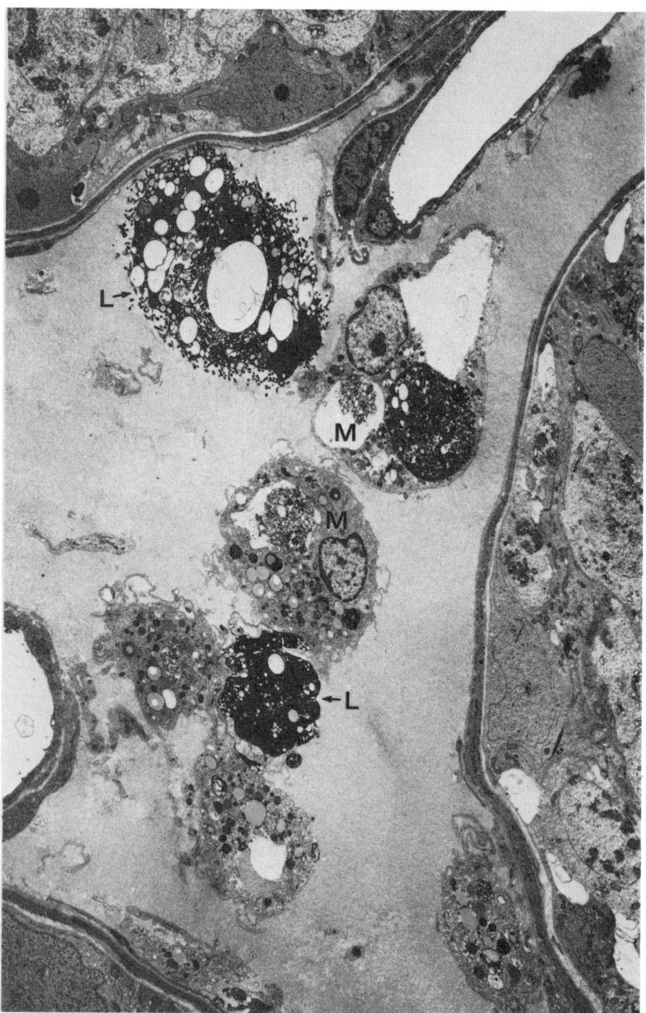

FIG. 100. Degeneration of Leydig cells (L) and their phagocytosis by macrophages (M) 2 days after treatment with EDS.

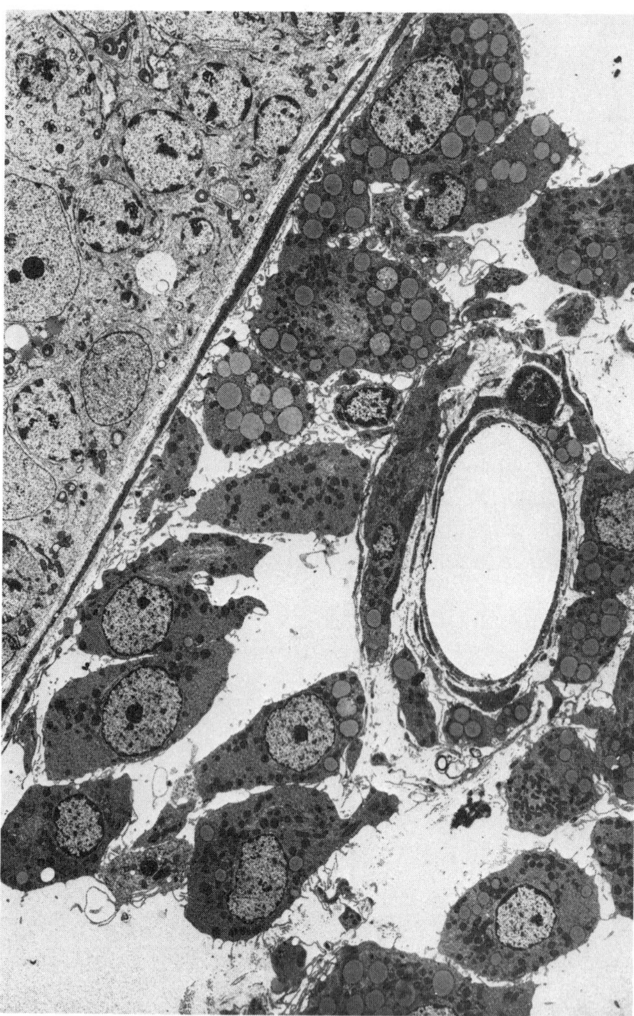

FIG. 101. Regeneration of fetal-type Leydig cells in the rat testis 4 weeks after treatment with EDS. Note the abundance of cytoplasmic lipid inclusions.

(752,753). These results are in accord with the observations of Rommerts and colleagues (*personal communication*), who noted a more rapid return of steroidogenesis following EDS treatment of rats with seminiferous tubule damage induced by fetal irradiation *in utero*. These results support the view that factors are present in testes with damaged seminiferous tubules that not only cause Leydig cell hypertrophy (603,735,736) but also stimulate a more rapid regeneration of Leydig cells following their destruction.

ACKNOWLEDGMENTS

We wish to acknowledge the help of our artist, Mrs. Sue Simpson, in developing some of the illustrations and Ms. Jenny McKervey for her excellent work in photography. The manuscript could not have been completed without the help of Mrs. S. Wainer, Ms. N. Jones, and the other secretaries of the Department of Anatomy. Aspects of this work were supported by grants from the National Health and Medical Research Council of Australia.

REFERENCES

1. Steinach, E. (1940): *Sex and Life: Forty Years of Biological and Medical Experiments*. Viking Press, New York.
2. Aristotle (1910): Aristotle historia animalium. In: *The Works of Aristotle, Vol. IV,* translated by D. W. Thompson. Clarendon Press, Oxford.
3. de Graaf, R. (1972): On the human reproductive organs, translated by N. D. Jocelyn and B. P. Setchell. *J. Reprod. Fertil.* [*Suppl. 17*].
4. van Leeuwenhoek, A. (1667): Observations de natis e semine genitali animaliulis. *Philos. Trans.,* 12:1040; cited by Bishop, M. W. H., and Walton, A. (1960): Spermatogenesis and the structure of mammalian spermatozoa. In: *Marshall's Physiology of Reproduction, Vol. 1,* pp. 1–129. Longmans Green, London.
5. von Kölliker, R. A. (1841): *Bertrage zur Kenntniss der Geschlechtverhaltsmisse und der Samen-flussigkeit wirbelloser Thiere und die Bedeutung de sogenannten Samenthiere*. Berlin.
6. Berthold, A. A. (1849): Transplantation der Hoden. *Arch. Anat. Physiol. Wiss. Med.,* 16:42–46.

7. Bouin, P., and Ancel, P. (1903): Recherches sur les cellules interstitielles der testicule des mammiferes. *Arch. Zool. (Stockh.) [Ser. IV]*, 1:437–523.
8. David, K., Dingemanse, E., Freud, J., and Laquer, E. (1935): Ueber krystallinisches mannliches Hormon aus Hoden (Testosteron), wirksamer als aus Harn oder aus Cholesterin bereites Androsteron. *Z. Physiol. Chem.*, 233:281–282.
9. Leeson, C. R., and Adamson, L. (1962): The mammalian tunica vaginalis testis and its fine structure and function. *Acta Anat.*, 51:226–240.
10. Holstein, A. F., and Weiss, C. (1967): Uber die Wirkung der glatten Muskulatur in der Tunica Albuginea in Hoden des Kaninchens Messungen des interstitiellen Druckes. *Z. Ges. Exp. Med.*, 142: 334–337.
11. Davis, J. R., and Langford, G. A. (1970): Pharmacological studies on the testicular capsule in relation to sperm transport. In: *The Human Testis*, edited by E. Rosenberg and C. A. Paulsen, pp. 495–514. Plenum, New York.
12. Clermont, Y., and Huckins, C. (1961): Microscopic anatomy of the sex cords and seminiferous tubules in growing and adult male albino rats. *Am. J. Anat.*, 108:79–97.
13. Bremer, J. L. (1911): Morphology of the tubules of the human testis and epididymis. *Am. J. Anat.*, 11:393–417.
14. Roosen-Runge, E. C. (1961): The rete testis in the albino rat; its structure, development and morphological significance. *Acta Anat.*, 45:1–30.
15. Scott, H. G., and Scott, P. P. (1956): Postnatal development of the testis and epididymis in the cat. *J. Physiol. (Lond.)*, 136:40.
16. Fawcett, D. W., Neaves, W. B., and Flores, M. N. (1973): Comparative observations on intertubular lymphatics and the organization of the interstitial tissue of the mammalian testis. *Biol. Reprod.*, 9:500–532.
17. Dym, M. (1974): The fine structure of monkey Sertoli cells in the transitional zone at the junction of the seminiferous tubules with the tubuli recti. *Am. J. Anat.*, 140:1–26.
18. Roosen-Runge, E. C., and Holstein, A. F. (1978): The human rete testis. *Cell Tissue Res.*, 189:409–433.
19. Bustos-Obregon, E., and Holstein, A. F. (1976): The rete testis in man: ultrastructural aspects. *Cell Tissue Res.*, 175:1–15.
20. Lincoln, G. A. (1981): Seasonal aspects of testicular function. In: *The Testis*, edited by H. Burger and D. de Kretser, pp. 255–302. Raven Press, New York.
21. Kerr, J. B., and Hedger, M. P. (1983): Spontaneous spermatogenic failure in the marsupial mouse *Antechinus stuartii* Macleay (Dasyuride: Marsupialia). *Aust. J. Zool.*, 31:445–466.
22. Setchell, B. P., and Waites, G. M. H. (1975): The blood-testis barrier. In: *Handbook of Physiology, Section 7, Vol. 5*, edited by D. W. Hamilton and R. O. Greep, pp. 143–172. Williams & Wilkins, Baltimore.
23. Wartenberg, H. (1981): Differentiation and development of the testes. In: *The Testis*, edited by H. Burger and D. de Kretser, pp. 39–80. Raven Press, New York.
24. Kirkham, W. B. (1915): The germ cell cycle in the mouse. *Anat. Rec.*, 10:217–219.
25. Allen, E. (1918): Studies on cell division in the albino rat. *J. Morphol.*, 31:133–185.
26. Hargitt, G. T. (1926): The formation of the sex glands and germ cells of mammals. I. The origin of the germ cells in the albino rat. *J. Morphol. Physiol.*, 40:517–558.
27. Regaud, C. (1901): Études sur la structure des tubes seminiférès et sur la spermatogenese chez les mammiférès. *Arch. Anat. Microsc.*, 4:101–156.
28. Clermont, Y., and Perey, B. (1957): Quantitative study of the cell population of the seminiferous tubules in immature rats. *Am. J. Anat.*, 100:241–267.
29. Black, V., and Christensen, A. K. (1969): Differentiation of interstitial cells and Sertoli cells in fetal guinea pig testes. *Am. J. Anat.*, 124:211–238.
30. Orth, J. (1982): Proliferation of Sertoli cells in fetal and postnatal rats: a quantitative autoradiographic study. *Anat. Rec.*, 203: 485–492.
31. Orth, J. M. (1984): The role of follicle stimulating hormone in controlling Sertoli cell proliferation in testes of fetal rats. *Endocrinology*, 115:1248–1255.
32. Magre, S., and Jost, A. (1980): The initial phases of testicular organogenesis in the rat. *Arch. Anat. Microsc. Morphol. Exp.*, 69:297–317.
33. Pelliniemi, L. J. (1975): Ultrastructure of the indifferent gonad in male and female pig embryos. *Tissue Cell*, 8:162–174.
34. Pelliniemi, L. J., (1975): Ultrastructure of the gonadal ridge in male and female pig embryos. *Anat. Embryol.*, 147:19–43.
35. Pelliniemi, L. J., and Niemi, M. (1969): Fine structure of the human foetal testis. *Z. Zellforsch.*, 99:507–522.
36. Jost, A., Vigier, B., Prepin, J., and Perchelet, J. P. (1973): Studies on sex differentiation in mammals. *Recent Prog. Horm. Res.*, 29:1–35.
37. Almond, G. D., and Singh, R. P. (1980): Development of the Sertoli cell in the fetal mouse. *Acta Anat.*, 106:276–280.
38. van Vorstenbosch, C. J. A. H. V., Spek, E., Colenbrander, B., and Wensing, C. J. G. (1984): Sertoli cell development of pig testis in the fetal and neonatal period. *Biol. Reprod.*, 31:565–577.
39. Kluin, P. M., Kramer, M. F., and de Rooij, D. G. (1984): Proliferation of spermatogonia and Sertoli cells in maturing mice. *Anat. Embryol.*, 169:73–78.
40. Clermont, Y., and Le Blond, C. P. (1953): Renewal of spermatogonia in the rat. *Am. J. Anat.*, 93:475–502.
41. Ortavant, R. (1959): Spermatogenesis and morphology of the spermatozoon. In: *Reproduction in Domestic Animals, Vol. 2*, edited by H. H. Cole and P. T. Cupps, 1–50. Academic Press, New York.
42. Hilscher, W., and Makoski, H. B. (1968): Histologisch und autoradiographische Untersuchungan zur 'Praspermatogenese' und 'Spermatogenese' der Ratte. *Z. Zellforsch.*, 86:327–350.
43. Steinberger, A., and Steinberger, E. (1971): Replication pattern of Sertoli cells in maturing rat testis *in vivo* and in organ culture. *Biol. Reprod.*, 4:84–87.
44. Steinberger, A., and Steinberger, E. (1977): The Sertoli cell. In: *The Testis, Vol. 4*, edited by A. D. Johnson and W. R. Gomes, pp. 371–399. Academic Press, New York.
45. Means, A. R., Fakunding, J. L., Huckins, C., Tindall, D. J., and Vitale, R. (1976): Follicle-stimulating hormone, the Sertoli cell, and spermatogenesis. *Recent Prog. Horm. Res.*, 32:477–522.
46. Chiappa, S., and Fink, G. (1977): Releasing factor and hormonal changes in the hypothalamic-pituitary-gonadotrophin and -adrenocorticotrophin systems before and after birth and puberty in male, female and androgenized female rats. *J. Endocrinol.*, 72:211–224.
47. Chowdhury, J., and Steinberger, E. (1976): Pituitary and plasma levels of gonadotropin in fetal and newborn male and female rats. *J. Endocrinol.*, 69:381–384.
48. Begeot, M., Dupouy, J. P., Dubois, M. P., and Dubois, P. M. (1981): Immunocytological determination of gonadotrophic and thyrotrophic cells in fetal rat anterior pituitary during normal development and under experimental conditions. *Neuroendocrinology*, 32:285–294.
49. Warren, D., Huhtaniemi, I., Tapanainen, J., Dufau, M., and Catt, K. (1984): Ontogeny of gonadotropin receptors in the fetal and neonatal rat testis. *Endocrinology*, 114:470–476.
50. Griswold, M., Solari, A., Tung, P., and Fritz, I. (1977): Stimulation by FSH of DNA synthesis and of mitosis in cultured Sertoli cells prepared from testes of immature rats. *Mol. Cell. Endocrinol.*, 7:151–165.
51. Solari, A. J., and Fritz, I. B. (1978): The ultrastructure of immature Sertoli cells. Maturation-like changes during culture and the maintenance of mitotic potentiality. *Biol. Reprod.*, 18:329–345.
52. Lording, D. W., and de Kretser, D. M. (1972): Comparative ultrastructural and histochemical studies of the interstitial cells of the rat testis during fetal and postnatal development. *J. Reprod. Fertil.*, 29:261–269.
53. Tapanainen, J., Kuopio, T., Pelliniemi, L. J., and Huhtaniemi, I. (1984): Rat testicular endogenous steroids and number of Leydig cells between the fetal period and sexual maturity. *Biol. Reprod.*, 31:1027–1035.
54. Weisz, J., and Ward, I. (1980): Plasma testosterone and progesterone titres of pregnant rats, their male and female fetuses and neonatal offspring. *Endocrinology*, 106:306–316.
55. Orth, J., and Weisz, J. (1980): Development of Δ^5-3β-hydroxysteroid dehydrogenase and glucose-6-phosphate dehydrogenase activity in Leydig cells of the fetal rat testis: a quantitative cytochemical study. *Biol. Reprod.*, 22:1201–1209.

56. Nomura, T., Weisz, J., and Lloyd, C. W. (1966): *In vitro* conversion of 7-^{3}H progesterone to androgens by the rat testis during the second half of fetal life. *Endocrinology,* 78:245–253.
57. Warren, D. W., Haltmeyer, G. C., and Eiknes, K. B. (1973): Testosterone in the fetal testis. *Biol. Reprod.,* 8:560–565.
58. Bishop, M. W. H., and Walton, A. (1960): Spermatogenesis and the structure of mammalian spermatozoa. In: *Marshall's Physiology of Reproduction, Vol. 1,* pp. 1–29. Longmans Green, London.
59. Attal, J., and Courot, M. (1963): Developpement testiculaire et establissement de la spermatogenese chez le taureau. *Ann. Biol. Anim. Biochim. Biophys.,* 3:219–241.
60. Sapsford, C. S. (1963): The development of the Sertoli cell of the rat and mouse: its existence as a mononucleate unit. *J. Anat.,* 97:225–238.
61. Ramos, A. S., and Dym, M. (1979): Ultrastructural differentiation of rat Sertoli cells. *Biol. Reprod.,* 21:909–922.
62. Flickinger, C. J. (1967): The postnatal development of the Sertoli cells of the mouse. *Z. Zellforsch.,* 78:92–113.
63. Nagano, T., and Suzuki, F. (1976): The postnatal development of the junctional complexes of the mouse Sertoli cells as revealed by freeze-fracture. *Anat. Rec.,* 185:403–418.
64. Vitale, R., Fawcett, D. W., and Dym, M. (1973): The normal development of the blood-testis barrier and the effects of clomiphene and estrogen treatment. *Anat. Rec.,* 176:333–344.
65. Kormano, M. (1967): Dye permeability and alkaline phosphatase activity of testicular capillaries in the postnatal rat. *Histochemie,* 9:327–338.
66. Gilula, W. B., Fawcett, D. W., and Aoki, A. (1976): The Sertoli cell occluding junctions and gap junctions in mature and developing mammalian testis. *Dev. Biol.,* 50:142–168.
67. Pelletier, R. M., and Friend, D. S. (1983): The Sertoli cell junctional complex: structure and permeability to filipin in the neonatal and adult guinea pig. *Am. J. Anat.,* 168:213–228.
68. Connell, C. J. (1980): Blood-testis barrier formation and the initiation of meiosis in the dog. In: *Testicular Development, Structure, and Function,* edited by A. Steinberger and E. Steinberger, pp. 71–78. Raven Press, New York.
69. Hagenas, L., Ploen, L., Ritzen, E. M., and Ekwall, H. (1977): Blood-testis barrier: maintained function of inter-Sertoli cell junctions in experimental cryptorchidism in the rat, as judged by a simple lanthanum-immersion technique. *Andrologia,* 9:250–254.
70. Vitale, R. (1975): The development of the blood-testis barrier in Sertoli-cell-only rats. *Anat. Rec.,* 181:501.
71. Bergh, A. (1981): Morphological signs of a direct effect of experimental cryptorchidism on the Sertoli cells in rats irradiated as fetuses. *Biol. Reprod.,* 24:145–152.
72. Rich, K. A., Kerr, J. B., and de Kretser, D. M. (1979): Evidence for Leydig cell dysfunction in rats with seminiferous tubule damage. *Mol. Cell. Endocrinol.,* 13:123–135.
73. Waites, G. M. H., and Gladwell, R. T. (1982): Physiological significance of fluid secretion in the testis and blood-testis barrier. *Physiol. Rev.,* 62:624–671.
74. Setchell, B. P., Voglmayr, J. K., and Waites, G. M. H. (1969): A blood-testis barrier restricting passage from blood into rete testis fluid but not into lymph. *J. Physiol. (Lond.),* 200:73–85.
75. Hägenas, L., Ploen, L., and Ekwall, H. (1978): Blood-testis barrier: evidence for intact inter-Sertoli cell junctions after hypophysectomy in the adult rat. *J. Endocrinol.,* 76:87–91.
76. Johnson, M. H. (1973): The role of the pituitary in the development of the blood-testis barrier in mice. *J. Reprod. Fertil.,* 32:509–511.
77. de Kretser, D. M., and Burger, H. G. (1972): Ultrastructural studies of human Sertoli cells in normal men and males with hypogonadotrophic hypogonadism before and after gonadotrophic treatment. In: *Gonadotropins,* edited by B. B. Saxena, C. G. Beling, and H. M. Gandy, pp. 640–656. Wiley, New York.
78. Fuss, A. (1912) Über die Geschlechtzellen des Menschen und der Säugetiere. *Arch. Mikrosk. Anat.,* 81:1–23.
79. Witschi, E. (1948): Migration of the germ cells of human embryos from the yolk sac to the primitive gonadal fold. *Carnegie Inst. Wash. Contrib. Embryol.,* 209:67–80.
80. Clark, J. M., and Eddy, E. M. (1975): Fine structural observations on the origin and associations of primordial germ cells of the mouse. *Dev. Biol.,* 47:136–155.
81. McKay, D. G., Hertig, A. T., Adams, E. C., and Danziger, S. (1953): Histochemical observations on the germ cells of human embryos. *Anat. Rec.,* 117:201–291.
82. Zamboni, L., and Upadhyay, S. (1983): Germ cell differentiation in mouse adrenal glands. *J. Exp. Zool.,* 228:173–193.
83. McLaren, A. (1983): Studies on mouse germ cells inside and outside the gonad. *J. Exp. Zool.,* 228:167–171.
84. Gondos, B., and Conner, L. A. (1973): Ultrastructure of developing germ cells in the fetal rabbit testis. *Am. J. Anat.,* 136:23–42.
85. Wartenburg, H. (1976): Comparative cytomorphologic aspects of the male germ cells especially of the "gonia." *Andrologia,* 8:117–130.
86. Hilscher, B., Hilscher, W., Bülthoff-Ohnolz, B., Krämer, U., Birke, A., Pelzer, H., and Gauss, G. (1974): Kinetics of gametogenesis. I. Comparative histological and autoradiographic studies of oocytes and transitional prospermatogonia during oogenesis and prespermatogenesis. *Cell Tissue Res.,* 154:443–470.
87. Roosen-Runge, E. C., and Leik, J. (1975): Gonocyte degeneration in the postnatal male rat. *Am. J. Anat.,* 122:275–300.
88. Gondos, B. (1977): Testicular development. In: *The Testis, Vol. IV,* edited by A. D. Johnson and W. R. Gomes, pp. 1–25. Academic Press, New York.
89. Gondos, B., and Hobel, C. J. (1971): Ultrastructure of germ cell development in the human fetal testis. *Z. Zellforsch.,* 119:1–20.
90. Clermont, Y. (1972): Kinetics of spermatogenesis in mammals: seminiferous epithelium cycle and spermatogonal renewal. *Physiol. Rev.,* 52:198–236.
91. Lee, V. W. K., de Kretser, D. M., Hudson, B. H., and Wang, C. (1975): Variations in serum FSH, LH and testosterone levels in male rats from birth to sexual maturity. *J. Reprod. Fertil.,* 42:121–126.
92. Müller, J., and Skakkebaek. N. E. (1983): Quantification of germ cells and seminiferous tubules by stereological examination of testicles from 50 boys who suffered from sudden death. *Int. J. Androl.,* 6:143–156.
93. von Ebner, V. (1871): Untersuchungen über den Bau der Samenkanalchen und die Entwicklung der Spermatozoiden bei den Sangentieren und beim Menschen. In: *Rollet's Untersuchunger aus dem Institut für Physiologie und Histologie, Vol. 2,* pp. 200–236. Graz, Leipzig.
94. von La Valette St. George, A. J. H. (1876): Uber die Genese der Samenkörper. *Arch. Mikrosk. Anat.,* 12:797–825.
95. Oakberg, E. F. (1956): A description of spermiogenesis in the mouse and its use in analysis of the cycle of the seminiferous epithelium and germ cell renewal. *Am. J. Anat.,* 99:391–413.
96. Hochereau, M. T. (1968): Etude des divisions spermatogiales et du renouvellement de la spermatogonie souche chez le taureau. In: *Sixth International Congress Animal Reproduction by Artificial Insemination,* 1:149–152.
97. Clermont, Y. (1960): Cycle of the seminiferous epithelium of the guinea pig. A method for identification of stages. *Fertil. Steril.,* 11:563–573.
98. Clermont, Y. (1962): Quantitative analysis of spermatogenesis of the rat: a revised model for the renewal of spermatogonia. *Am. J. Anat.,* 111:111–129.
99. Clermont, Y., and Bustos-Obregon, E. (1968): Re-examination of spermatogonial renewal in the rat by means of seminiferous tubules mounted "in toto." *Am. J. Anat.,* 122:237–247.
100. Branca, A. (1924): Les canilicules testiculaires et spermatogenese de l'homme. *Arch. Zool. Exp. Gen.,* 62:53–252.
101. Roosen-Runge, E. C., and Barlow, F. D. (1953): Quantitative studies on human spermatogenesis. I. Spermatogonia. *Am. J. Anat.,* 93:143–169.
102. Clermont, Y. (1966): Renewal of spermatogonia in man. *Am. J. Anat.,* 118:509–524.
103. Clermont, Y. (1966): Spermatogenesis in man. A study of the spermatogonial population. *Fertil. Steril.,* 17:705–721.
104. Clermont, Y., and Le Blond, C. P. (1959): Differentiation and renewal of spermatogonia in the monkey *Macacus rhesus. Am. J. Anat.,* 104:237–272.
105. Clermont, Y. (1969): Two classes of spermatogonial stem cells in the monkey (*Cercopithecus aethiops*). *Am. J. Anat.,* 126:57–72.
106. Fawcett, D. W., Ito, S., and Slautterback, D. B. (1959): The occurrence of intercellular bridges in groups of cells exhibiting synchronous differentiation. *J. Biophys. Biochem. Cytol.,* 5: 453–458.

107. Huckins, C. (1971): The spermatogonial stem cell population in adult rats. I. Their morphology, proliferation and maturation. *Anat. Rec.*, 169:533–558.
108. Dym, M., and Fawcett, D. W. (1971): Further observations on the numbers of spermatogonia, spermatocytes and spermatids connected by intercellular bridges in the mammalian testis. *Biol. Reprod.*, 4:195–215.
109. Vilar, O., Perez del Cerro, R., and Mancini, R. E. (1962): The Sertoli cell as a "bridge cell" between the basal membrane and the germinal cells. *Exp. Cell Res.*, 27:158–161.
110. Nicander, L., Abdel-Raouf, M., and Crabo, B. (1961): On the ultrastructure of the seminiferous tubules in bull calves. *Acta Morphol. Neerl. Scand.*, 4:127–135.
111. Rowley, M. J., Berlin, J. D., and Heller, C. G. (1971): The ultrastructure of four types of human spermatogonia. *Z. Zellforsch.*, 112:139–157.
112. Leeson, C. R. (1966): An electron microscopic study of cryptorchid and scrotal human testes, with special reference to pubertal maturation. *Invest. Urol.*, 3:498–511.
113. de Kretser, D. M. (1968): The fine structure of the immature human testis in hypogonadotrophic hypogonadism. *Virchows Arch.* [*Zellpathol.*], 1:283–296.
114. Watson, M. L. (1952): Spermatogenesis in the albino rat as revealed by electron microscopy. *Biochim. Biophys. Acta*, 8:369–374.
115. Moens, P. B., and Go, V. L. W. (1972): Intercellular bridges and division patterns of rat spermatogonia. *Z. Zellforsch.*, 127:201–208.
116. Fawcett, D. W. (1979): The cell biology of gametogenesis in the male. *Perspect. Biol. Med.*, 2:S56–S73.
117. Tres, L. L., and Solari, A. J. (1968): The ultrastructure of the nuclei and the behaviour of the sex chromosomes of human spermatogonia. *Z. Zellforsch.*, 91:75–89.
118. Schulze, W. (1978): Licht und elektronen-mikropische Studien an den A-Spermatogonien von Männern mit intakter Spermatogenese und bei Patienten nach Behandlung mit Antiandrogenen. *Andrologia*, 10:307–320.
119. Schulze, W. (1978): Zum Problem der morphologischen Characterisierung von Spermatogonien typen beim Erwachsenen. *Verh. Anat. Ges.*, 72:539–540.
120. Lubarsch, O. (1896): Über das Vorkommen krystallinischer und krystalloider Bildungen in den Zellen des menschlichen Hodens. *Virchows Arch.* [*Pathol. Anat.*], 145:316–338.
121. Sohval, A. R., Suzuki, Y., Gabrilove, J. L., and Churg, J. (1971): Ultrastructure of crystalloids in spermatogonia and Sertoli cells of normal human testis. *J. Ultrastruct. Res.*, 34:83–102.
122. Nagano, T. (1969): The crystalloid of Lubarsch in the human spermatogonium. *Z. Zellforsch.*, 97:491–501.
123. Fawcett, D. W. (1972): Observations on cell differentiation and organelle continuity in spermatogenesis. In: *Proceedings of an International Symposium on the Genetics of the Spermatozoon*, edited by R. A. Beatty and S. Gluecksohn-Waelsch, pp. 37–67. Bogtrykkeriet Forum, Copenhagen.
124. Brown, H. H. (1885): On spermatogenesis in the rat. *Q. J. Microsc. Sci.*, 25:343–370.
125. von Winiwater, H. (1901): Recherches sur l'ovogenese et l'organogenese de l'ovaire des mammiferes. *Arch. Biol.*, 17:33–199.
126. Montgomery, T. H. (1901): A study of the chromosomes of the germ cells of the Metazoa. *Trans. Am. Philos. Soc.*, 20:154–236.
127. Sutton, W. S. (1903): The chromosomes in heredity. *Biol. Bull.*, 4:231–251.
128. Swift, H. H. (1950): The desoxyribose nucleic acid content of animal nuclei. *Physiol. Zool.*, 23:169–200.
129. Wettstein, R., and Sotelo, J. R. (1967): Electron microscope serial reconstruction of the spermatocyte 1 nuclei at pachytene. *J. Microsc. (Oxf.)*, 6:557–576.
130. Painter, T. S. (1923): Studies in mammalian spermatogenesis. II. The spermatogenesis of man. *J. Exp. Zool.*, 37:291–338.
131. Moses, M. J. (1956): Chromosomal structures in crayfish spermatocytes. *J. Biophys. Biochem. Cytol.*, 12:215–218.
132. Fawcett, D. W. (1956): The fine structure of chromosomes in the meiotic prophase of vertebrate spermatocytes. *J. Biophys. Biochem. Cytol.*, 12:403–406.
133. Woolam, D. H. M., and Ford, E. H. R. (1964): The fine structure of the mammalian chromosome in meiotic prophase with special reference to the synaptinemal complex. *J. Anat.*, 98:163–173.
134. Moses, M. J. (1968): Synaptinemal complex. *Annu. Rev. Genet.*, 2:363–412.
135. Comings, D. E., and Okada, T. A. (1971): Fine structure of the synaptinemal complex. *Exp. Cell Res.*, 65:104–116.
136. Dresser, M. E., and Moses, M. J. (1979): Silver staining of synaptinemal complexes in surface spreads for light and electron microscopy. *Exp. Cell Res.*, 121:416–419.
137. Moses, M. J., and Solari, A. J. (1976): Positive contrast staining and protected drying of surface spreads: electron microscopy of the synaptonemal complex by a new method. *J. Ultrastruct. Res.*, 54:109–114.
138. Heyting, C., Dietrich, A. J., Redeker, E. J., and Vink, A. C. (1985): Structure and composition of synaptinemal complexes isolated from rat spermatocytes. *Eur. J. Cell Biol.*, 36:307–314.
139. Sachs, L. (1954): Sex linkage and sex chromosomes in man. *Ann. Eugen. (Lond.)*, 18:255–261.
140. Solari, A. J. (1964): The morphology and ultrastructure of the sex vesicle in the mouse. *Exp. Cell Res.*, 36:160–168.
141. Solari, A. J., and Tres, L. (1967): The ultrastructure of the human sex vesicle. *Chromosoma (Berl.)*, 22:16–31.
142. Solari, A. J. (1974): The behaviour of the XY pair in mammals. *Int. Rev. Cytol.*, 38:273–317.
143. Moses, M. J., Counce, S. J., and Paulson, D. F. (1975): Synaptonemal complex complement of man in spreads of spermatocytes with details of the sex chromosome pair. *Science*, 187:363–365.
144. Chandley, A. C., Gaetz, P., Hargreave, T. B., Joseph, A. M., and Speed, R. M. (1984): On the nature and extent of XY pairing at meiotic prophase in man. *Cytogenet. Cell Genet.*, 38:241–247.
145. Schultz, M. C., Hermo, L., and Le Blond, C. P. (1984): Structure, development and cytochemical properties of the nucleolus-associated "round body" in rat spermatocytes and early spermatids. *Am. J. Anat.*, 171:41–47.
146. Nicander, L., and Plöen, L. (1969): Fine structure of spermatogonia and primary spermatocytes in rabbits. *Z. Zellforsch.*, 99:221–234.
147. Andre, J. (1962): Contribution a la connaissance du chondriome. Etude de ses modifications ultrastructurales pendant la spermatogenese. *J. Ultrastruct. Res.* [*Suppl. 3*], 1–185.
148. Russell, L. D., and Frank, B. (1978): Ultrastructural characterization of nuage in spermatocytes in the rat testis. *Anat. Rec.*, 190:79–98.
149. Fawcett, D. W., Eddy, E., and Phillips, D. M. (1970): Observations on the fine structure and relationships of the chromatoid body in mammalian spermatogenesis. *Biol. Reprod.*, 2:129–153.
150. Rehbun, L. I. (1961): Some electron microscope observations on membranous basophilic elements of invertebrate eggs. *J. Ultrastruct. Res.*, 5:208–225.
151. Smith, F. E., and Berlin J. D. (1977): Cytoplasmic annulate lamellae in human spermatogenesis. *Cell Tissue Res.*, 176:235–242.
152. Chemes, H. E., Fawcett, D. W., and Dym, M. (1978): Unusual features of the nuclear envelope in human spermatogenic cells. *Anat. Rec.*, 192:495–512.
153. Russell, L. D. (1977): Desmosome-like junctions between Sertoli and germ cells in the rat testis. *Am. J. Anat.*, 148:301–312.
154. Kaya, M., and Harrison, R. G. (1976): The ultrastructural relationships between Sertoli cells and spermatogenic cells in the rat. *J. Anat.*, 121:279–290.
155. Russell, L. D. (1978): The blood-testis barrier and its formation relative to spermatocyte maturation in the adult rat: a lanthanum study. *Anat. Rec.*, 190:99–112.
156. von Ebner, V. (1888): Zur Spermatogenese bei den Säugethieren. *Arch. Mikrosk. Anat.*, 31:236–292.
157. Heller, C. G., and Clermont, Y. (1964): Kinetics of the germinal epithelium in man. *Recent Prog. Horm. Res.*, 20:545–575.
158. Montgomery, T. H. (1912): Human spermatogenesis, spermatocytes and spermiogenesis. A study in inheritance. *J. Acad. Nat. Sci. Phil.*, 15:1–22.
159. Nicander, L. (1967): An electron microscopical study of cell contacts in the seminiferous tubules of some mammals. *Z. Zellforsch.*, 83:375–397.
160. Holstein, A. F., and Roosen-Runge, E. C. (1981): *Atlas of Human Spermatogenesis*, pp. 1–224. Grosse Verlag, Berlin.
161. Gardner, P. J., and Holyoke, E. A. (1964): Fine structure of the seminiferous tubule of the Swiss mouse. I. The limiting membrane, Sertoli cell, spermatogonia and spermatocytes. *Anat. Rec.*, 150:391–404.

162. von La Valette St. George, A. J. H. (1885): Spermatologische Beitrage. *Arch. Mikrosk. Anat.*, 25:581–593.
163. Meves, F. (1898): Über das Verhalten der Zentralkörper bei der Histogenese der Samenfäden von Mensch und Ratte. *Arch. Mikrosk. Anat.*, 54:329–402.
164. Meves, F. (1898): Zur Entstehung der achsenfadën menschlicher Spermatozoen. *Anat. Anz.*, 14:168–170.
165. Gatenby, J. B., and Beams, H. W. (1936): The cytoplasmic inclusions in the spermatogenesis of man. *Q. J. Microsc. Sci.*, 78:1–33.
166. Le Blond, C. P., and Clermont, Y. (1952): Spermiogenesis of rat, mouse, hamster and guinea pig as revealed by the "periodic acid-fuchsin sulphurous acid" technique. *Am. J. Anat.*, 90: 167–206.
167. Le Blond, C. P., and Clermont, Y. (1952): Definition of the stages of the cycle of the seminiferous epithelium in the rat. *Ann. N.Y. Acad. Sci.*, 55:548–573.
168. Clermont, Y. (1963): The cycle of the seminiferous epithelium in man. *Am. J. Anat.*, 112:35–51.
169. Daoust, R., and Clermont, Y. (1955): Distribution of nucleic acids in germ cells during the cycle of the seminiferous epithelium in the rat. *Am. J. Anat.*, 96:255–283.
170. Bowen, R. H. (1922): On the idiosome, Golgi apparatus and acrosome in the male germ cells. *Anat. Rec.*, 24:158–180.
171. Bowen, R. H. (1924): On the acrosome of the animal sperm. *Anat. Rec.*, 28:1–13.
172. Burgos, M. H., and Fawcett, D. W. (1955): Studies of the fine structure of the mammalian testis. I. Differentiation of the spermatids in the cat (*Felis domestica*). *J. Biophys. Biochem. Cytol.*, 2:223–240.
173. Brökelmann, J. (1963): Fine structure of germ cells and Sertoli cells during the cycle of the seminiferous epithelium in the rat. *Z. Zellforsch.*, 59:820–850.
174. Gardner, P. (1966): Fine structure of the seminiferous epithelium of the Swiss mouse. The spermatid. *Anat. Rec.*, 155:235–250.
175. Holstein, A. F. (1976): Ultrastructural observations on the differentiation of spermatids in man. *Andrologia*, 8:157–165.
176. Hermo, L., Rambourg, A., and Clermont, Y. (1980): Three-dimensional architecture of the cortical region of the Golgi apparatus in the rat spermatids. *Am. J. Anat.*, 157:357–373.
177. Clermont, Y., and Tang, X. M. (1985): Glycoprotein synthesis in the Golgi apparatus of spermatids during spermiogenesis of the rat. *Anat. Rec.*, 213:33–43.
178. Sandoz, D. (1972): Etude autoradiographique de l'incorporation in vitro de galactose-^{3}H dans les spermatides de souris. *J. Microsc. (Oxf.)*, 15:403–408.
179. Lalli, M. F., Tang, X. M., and Clermont, Y. (1984): Glycoprotein synthesis in Sertoli cells during the cycle of the seminiferous epithelium of adult rats. A radioautographic study. *Biol. Reprod.*, 30:493–505.
180. Fawcett, D. W. (1975): The mammalian spermatozoon. *Dev. Biol.*, 44:394–436.
181. Pederson, H. (1972): The postacrosomal region of man and *Macaca artoides*. *J. Ultrastruct Res.*, 40:366–377.
182. Pederson, H. (1972): Further observations of the fine structure of the human spermatozoon. *Z. Zellforsch.*, 123:305–315.
183. Bedford, J. M. (1968): Ultrastructural changes in the sperm head during fertilization in the rabbit. *Am. J. Anat.*, 123:329–358.
184. Stefanini, M., Oura, C., and Zamboni, L. (1969): Ultrastructure of fertilization in the mouse. 2. Penetration of sperm into the ovum. *J. Submicrosc. Cytol.*, 1:1–23.
185. Fawcett, D. W., and Hollenberg, R. D. (1963): Changes in the acrosome of guinea pig spermatozoa during passage through the epididymis. *Z. Zellforsch.*, 60:276–292.
186. Harding, H. R., Carrick, F. N., and Shorey, C. D. (1976): Ultrastructural changes in spermatozoa of the brush-tailed possum *Trichosurus vulpecula* (Marsupialia) during epididymal transit. Part II. The acrosome. *Cell Tissue Res.*, 171:61–73.
187. Allison, A. C., and Hartree, E. F. (1970): Lysosomal enzymes in the acrosome and their possible role in fertilization. *J. Reprod. Fertil.*, 21:501–515.
188. Chang, M. C., and Hunter, R. H. F. (1975): Capacitation of mammalian sperm: biological and experimental aspects. In: *Handbook of Physiology, Section 7, Vol. 5, Male Reproductive System,* edited by D. W. Hamilton and R. O. Greep, pp. 339–352. Williams & Wilkins, Baltimore.
189. Bedford, J. M. (1967): Observations on the fine structure of spermatozoa of the bush baby (*Galago senegalensis*), the African green monkey (*Cercopithecus aethiops*) and man. *Am. J. Anat.*, 121:443–460.
190. Clermont, Y., Einberg, E., Le Blond, C. P., and Wagner, S. (1955): The perforatorium—an extension of the nuclear membrane of the rat spermatozoon. *Anat. Rec.*, 121:1–12.
191. Lalli, M. F., and Clermont, Y. (1981): Structural changes of the head components of the rat spermatid during spermatogenesis. *Am. J. Anat.*, 160:419–434.
192. Burgos, M. H., and Fawcett. D. W. (1956): An electron microscope study of spermatid differentiation in the toad, *Bufo arenarium Hensel*. *J. Biophys. Biochem. Cytol.*, 2:223–240.
193. Bedford, J. M. (1964): Fine structure of the sperm head in ejaculate and uterine spermatozoa of the rabbit. *J. Reprod. Fertil.*, 7:221–228.
194. Bane, A., and Nicander, L. (1963): The structure and formation of the perforatorium in mammalian spermatozoa. *Int. J. Fertil.*, 8:865–869.
195. Austin, C. R., and Bishop, M. W. H. (1958): Role of the rodent acrosome and perforatorium in fertilization. *Proc. R. Soc. Lond. [Biol.]*, 149:234–240.
196. Welch, J. E., and O'Rand, M. G. (1985): Identification and distribution of actin in spermatogenic cells and spermatozoa of the rabbit. *Dev. Biol.*, 109:411–417.
197. Horstmann, E. (1961): Elektronenmikroskopische Untersuchungen zur Spermiohistogenese beim Menschen. *Z. Zellforsch.*, 54:68–89.
198. de Kretser, D. M. (1969): Ultrastructural features of human spermiogenesis. *Z. Zellforsch.*, 98:477–505.
199. Gledhill, B. L., Gledhill, M. P., Rigler, R., and Ringertz, N. R. (1966): Changes in deoxyribonucleoprotein during spermatogenesis in the bull. *Exp. Cell Res.*, 41:652–665.
200. Vaughn, J. C. (1966): The relationship of the sphere chromatophile to the fate of displaced histones following histone transition in rat spermiogenesis. *J. Cell Biol.*, 31:257–278.
201. Bellve, A. R., Anderson, E., and Hanley-Bowdoin, L. (1975): Synthesis and amino acid composition of basic proteins in mammalian sperm nuclei. *Dev. Biol.*, 47:349–365.
202. Kistler, W. S., Nayes, C., Hsu, R., and Heinrikson, R. L. (1975): The amino acid sequence of a testis-specific basic protein that is associated with spermatogenesis. *J. Biol. Chem.*, 250:1847–1853.
203. Loir, M., and Lanneau, M. (1978): Partial characterization of ram spermatidal basic nuclear proteins. *Biochem. Biophys. Res. Commun.*, 80:975–982.
204. Fawcett, D. W., Anderson, W. A., and Phillips, D. M. (1971): Morphogenetic factors influencing the shape of the sperm head. *Dev. Biol.*, 26:220–251.
205. Bellve, A. R. (1979): The molecular biology of mammalian spermatogenesis. In: *Oxford Reviews in Reproductive Biology, Vol. 1*, edited by C. A. Finn, pp. 159–261. Clarendon Press, Oxford.
206. Fawcett, D. W. (1965): The anatomy of the mammalian spermatozoon with particular reference to the guinea pig. *Z. Zellforsch.*, 67:279–296.
207. McIntosh, J. R., and Porter, K. R. (1967): Microtubules in the spermatids of the domestic fowl. *J. Cell Biol.*, 35:153–173.
208. Clark, A. W. (1967): Some aspects of spermiogenesis in a lizard. *Am. J. Anat.*, 121:369–400.
209. Beatty, R. A. (1970): The genetics of the mammalian gamete. *Biol. Rev.*, 45:73–119.
210. Franklin, L. E. (1968): Formation of the redundant nuclear envelope in monkey spermatids. *Anat. Rec.*, 161:149–162.
211. Anberg, A. (1957): The ultrastructure of the human spermatozoon. *Acta Obstet. Gynaecol. Scand.* [*Suppl. 2*], 36:1–133.
212. Fawcett, D. W. (1958): The structure of the mammalian spermatozoon. *Int. Rev. Cytol.*, 7:195–234.
213. Sapsford, C. S., Rae, C. A., and Cleland, K. W. (1967): Ultrastructural studies on spermatids and Sertoli cells during early spermiogenesis in the bandicoot *Perameles nasuta Geoffroy* (Marsupialia). *Aust. J. Zool.*, 15:881–909.
214. Fawcett, D. W., and Phillips, D. M. (1969): The fine structure and development of the neck region of the mammalian spermatozoon. *Anat. Rec.*, 165:153–184.
215. Grimstone, A. V., and Klug, A. (1966): Observations on the substructure of flagella fibres. *J. Cell Sci.*, 1:351–362.

216. Warner, F. D. (1970): New observations on flagella fine structure: the relationship between matrix structure and the microtubule component of the axoneme. *J. Cell Biol.*, 47:159–182.
217. Tilney, L., Bryan, J., Bush, D. J., Fujievara, K., Mooseker, M. S., Murphy, B., and Snyder, D. H. (1973): Microtubules: evidence for 13 protofilaments. *J. Cell Biol.*, 59:267–275.
218. Gibbons, I. R. (1966): Studies on the ATP-ase activity of 14S and 30S dynein from cilia of tetrahymena. *J. Biol. Chem.*, 241:5590–5596.
219. Stephens, R. E. (1970): Isolation of nexin—the linkage protein responsible for the maintenance of the 9-fold configuration of flagellar axonemes. *Biol. Bull.*, 139:438–442.
220. Hopkins, J. M. (1970): Subsidiary components of the flagella of *Chlamydomonas reinhardtii*. *J. Cell Sci.*, 7:823–839.
221. Afzelius, B. A. (1976): A human syndrome caused by immotile cilia. *Science*, 193:317–319.
222. Sturgess, J. M., Chao, J., Wong, J., Aspin, N., and Turner, J. A. P. (1979): Cilia with defective radial spokes—a cause of human respiratory disease. *N. Engl. J. Med.*, 300:53–56.
223. Gerton, G. L., and Millette, C. F. (1984): Generation of flagella by cultured mouse spermatids. *J. Cell. Biol.*, 98:619–628.
224. Woolley, D. M., and Fawcett, D. W. (1973): The degeneration and disappearance of the centrioles during the development of the rat spermatozoon. *Anat. Rec.*, 177:289–301.
225. Fawcett, D. W. (1970): A comparative view of sperm ultrastructure. *Biol. Reprod.*, [*Suppl. 2*], 90–127.
226. Fawcett, D. W., and Ito, S. (1965): The fine structure of bat spermatozoa. *Am. J. Anat.*, 116:567–610.
227. Anderson, W. A., and Personne, P. (1967): The fine structure of the neck region of spermatozoa of *Helix aspersa*. *J. Microscopie*, 6:1033–1042.
228. Austin, C. R., and Sapsford, C. S. (1951): The development of the rat spermatid. *J. R. Microsc. Soc.*, 71:397–406.
229. Sud, B. N. (1961): Morphological and histochemical studies of the chromatoid body and related elements in spermatogenesis of the rat. *Q. J. Microsc. Sci.*, 102:495–505.
230. Maillet, P. L., and Gouranton, J. (1965) Sur l'expulsion de l'acide ribonucleique nucleaire par les spermatides de *Philaenus spumarius* L (Hamoptera, Cucopidae). *C. R. Acad. Sci.* [*D*] (*Paris*), 261:1417–1419.
231. Eddy, E. M. (1970): Cytochemical observations on the chromatoid body of the male germ cell. *Biol. Reprod.*, 2:114–128.
232. Walt, H., and Armbruster, B. L. (1984): Actin and RNA are components of the chromatoid body in spermatids of the rat. *Cell Tissue Res.*, 236:487–490.
233. Irons, M. J., and Clermont, Y. (1982): Formation of the outer dense fibres during spermiogenesis in the rat. *Anat. Rec.*, 202:463–471.
234. O'Brien, D. A., and Bellve, A. R. (1980): Protein constituents of the mouse spermatozoon. II. Temporal synthesis during spermatogenesis. *Dev. Biol.*, 75:405–418.
235. Telkka, A., Fawcett, D. W., and Christensen, A. K. (1961): Further observations on the structure of the mammalian sperm tail. *Anat. Rec.*, 141:231–246.
236. Bradfield, J. R. G. (1955): Fibre patterns in animal flagella and cilia. *Symp. Soc. Exp. Biol.*, 9:306–332.
237. Wartenberg, H., and Holstein, A. F. (1975): Morphology of the "spindle-shaped body" in the developing tail of human spermatids. *Cell Tissue Res.*, 159:435–443.
238. Nicander, L. (1962): Development of the fibrous sheath of the mammalian sperm tail. In: *Proceedings of the 5th International Conference for Electron Microscopy*, M-4.
239. Sapsford, C. S., Rae, C. A., and Cleland, K. W. (1970): Ultrastructural studies on the development and form of the principal piece sheath of the bandicoot spermatozoon. *Aust. J. Zool.*, 18:21–48.
240. Sotelo, J. R., and Trujillo-Cenoz, O. (1958): Electron microscope study of the kinetic apparatus in animal sperm cells. *Z. Zellforsch.*, 48:565–601.
241. Illison, L. (1968): Studies on the genetics and development of spermatozoon head shape in the house. Ph.D. thesis, University of Sydney, Australia.
242. Irons, M. J., and Clermont, Y. (1982): Kinetics of fibrous sheath formation in the rat spermatid. *Am. J. Anat.*, 165:121–130.
243. Jensen, O. S. (1887): Untersuchungen über die Samenkörper du Säugethiere, Vögel und Amphibien. I. Säugethiere. *Arch. Mikrosk. Anat.*, 30:379–425.
244. Benda, C. (1898): Über die Spermatogenese der Vertebraten und höherer Evertebraten. II. Die Histogenese der Spermien. *Arch. Physiol.*, pp. 385–393.
245. Yasuzumi, G. (1956): Spermatogenesis in animals as revealed by electron microscopy. I. Formation and submicroscopic structure of the middle-piece of the albino rat. *J. Biophys. Biochem. Cytol.*, 2:445–449.
246. Reed, C. I., and Reed, B. P. (1948): Comparative study of human and bovine sperm by electron microscopy. *Anat. Rec.*, 100:1–7.
247. Schultz-Larsen, J. (1958): The morphology of the human sperm. *Acta Pathol. Microbiol. Scand.* [*Suppl. 128*], 1–121.
248. Phillips, D. M. (1970): Development of spermatozoa in the woolly opossum with special reference to the shaping of the sperm head. *J. Ultrastruct. Res.*, 33:369–380.
249. von Lenhossek, M. (1898): Untersuchungen über Spermatogenese. *Arch. Mikrosk. Anat.*, 51:215–318.
250. Zlotnik, I. (1943): Nuclear ring in developing male germ cells of dog and cat. *Nature (Lond.)*, 151:670.
251. Gresson, R. A. R., and Zlotnik, I. (1945): A comparative study of the cytoplasmic components of the male germ cells of certain mammals. *Proc. R. Soc. Edinb.* [*Biol.*], 62:137–170.
252. Goodrowe, K. L., and Heath, E. (1984): Disposition of the manchette in the normal equine spermatid. *Anat. Rec.*, 290:177–183.
253. Kingsley-Smith, B. V., and Lacy, D. (1959): Residual bodies of seminiferous tubules of the rat. *Nature (Lond.)*, 184:249–251.
254. Lacy, D. (1960): Light and electron microscopy and its use in the study of factors influencing spermatogenesis in the rat. *J. Microsc. Soc.*, 79:290–295.
255. Dietert, S. E. (1966): Fine structure of the formation and fate of the residual bodies of mouse spermatozoa with evidence for the participation of lysosomes. *J. Morphol.*, 120:317–346.
256. Sapsford, C. S., Rae, C. A., and Cleland, K. W. (1969): The fate of residual bodies and degenerating germ cells and the lipid cycle in Sertoli cells in the bandicoot *Perameles nasuta Geoffroy* (Marsupialia). *Aust. J. Zool.*, 17:729–753.
257. Fouquet, J. P. (1974): La spermiation et la formation des corps residuels chez la hamster: role des cellules de Sertoli. *J. Microscopie*, 19:161–168.
258. Kerr, J. B., and de Kretser, D. M. (1975): Cyclic variations in Sertoli cell lipid content throughout the spermatogenic cycle in the rat. *J. Reprod. Fertil.*, 53:1–8.
259. Fawcett, D. W., and Phillips, D. M. (1969): Observations on the release of spermatozoa and on changes in the head during passage through the epididymis. *J. Reprod. Fertil.*, [*Suppl. 6*], 405–418.
260. Morales, C., and Clermont, Y. (1982): Evolution of Sertoli cell processes invading the cytoplasm of rat spermatids. *Anat. Rec.*, 203:233–244.
261. Holstein, A. F., and Schäfer, E. (1978): A further type of transient cytoplasmic organelle in human spermatids. *Cell Tissue Res.*, 192:359–361.
262. Breucker, H., Schafer, E., and Holstein, A. F. (1985): Morphogenesis and fate of the residual body in human spermiogenesis. *Cell Tissue Res.*, 240:303–309.
263. Russell, L. D., and Clermont, Y. (1976): Anchoring device between Sertoli cells and late spermatids in rat seminiferous tubules. *Anat. Rec.*, 185:259–278.
264. Vitale-Calpe, R. (1970): Ultrastructural studies of spontaneous spermiation in the guinea pig. *Z. Zellforsch.*, 105:222–223.
265. Burgos, M. H., and Vitale-Calpe, R. (1967): The fine structure of the Sertoli cell-spermatozoon relationship in the toad. *J. Ultrastruct. Res.*, 19:221–237.
266. Burgos. M. H., and Vitale-Calpe, R. (1967): The mechanism of spermiation in the toad. *Am. J. Anat.*, 120:227–252.
267. Russell, L. D., Lee, I. P., Ettlin, R., and Peterson, R. N. (1983): Development of the acrosome and alignment, elongation and entrenchment of spermatids in procarbazine-treated rats. *Tissue Cell*, 15:615–626.
268. Brökelmann, J. (1961): Surface modifications of Sertoli cells at various stages of spermatogenesis in the rat. *Anat. Rec.*, 139:211.
269. Nagano, T. (1968): Fine structure relation between the Sertoli cell and the differentiating spermatid in the human testis. *Z. Zellforsch.*, 89:39–43.
270. Flickinger, C. J., and Fawcett, D. W. (1967): The junctional specialization of Sertoli cells in the seminiferous epithelium. *Anat. Rec.*, 158:207–222.

271. Russell, L. D. (1979): Spermatid-Sertoli tubulobulbar complexes as devices for elimination of cytoplasm from the head region of late spermatids of the rat. *Anat. Rec.*, 194:233–246.
272. Russell, L. D. (1979): Further observations on tubulobulbar complexes formed by later spermatids and Sertoli cells in the rat testis. *Anat. Rec.*, 194:213–232.
273. Sertoli, E. (1865): Dell'esistenza di particulari cellule ramificate nei canalicoli seminiferi dell'testicolo umano. *Morgagni,* 7:31–39.
274. Sertoli, E. (1878): Sulla struttura dei canalicoli seminiferi dei testiculo. *Arch. Sci. Med. (Torino),* 2:267–295.
275. von Ebner, V. (1902): Mannliche Geschlechtsorgne. In: *Handbuch der Gewebelchre des Menschen,* edited by A. Kolliker, p. 402. Engelmann, Leipzig.
276. von La Valette St. George, A. J. H. (1878): Über die Genese der Samenkörper. *Arch. Mikrosk. Anat. Entwmech.*, 15:261–314.
277. Hoven, H. (1914): Histogenese du testicule des mammiferes. *Anat. Anz.*, 47:90–109.
278. Stieve, H. (1927): Die Entwicklung der Keimzellen und der Zwischenzellen in der Hodenaniage des Menschen. Ein Beitrag zur Keimbahufrage. *Z. Mikrosk. Anat. Forsch.*, 10:225–285.
279. Rolshoven, E. (1940): Die funktionelle Polymorphie des Sertolisyncytioms und ihr Zumsammenhang mit der Spermatogenese. *Z. Zellforsch.*, 31:156–164.
280. Elftman, H. (1950): The Sertoli cell cycle in the mouse. *Anat. Rec.*, 106:381–393.
281. Watson, M. L. (1952): Spermatogenesis in the albino rat as revealed by tissue sections in the electron microscope. University of Rochester Atomic Energy Project, Atomic Energy Report U.R. 185 (unclassified).
282. Challice, C. E. (1953): Electron microscope studies of spermiogenesis in some rodents. *J. R. Microsc. Soc.*, 73:115–127.
283. Fawcett, D. W. (1973): Interrelationships of cell types within the seminiferous epithelium and their implications for control of spermatogenesis. In: *The Regulation of Mammalian Reproduction,* edited by S. J. Segal, R. Crozier, P. A. Corfman, and P. G. Condliffe, pp. 116–138. Charles Thomas, Springfield, Ill.
284. Fawcett, D. W. (1973): Observations on the organization of the interstitial tissue of the testis and on the occluding cell junctions in the seminiferous epitheoium. *Adv. Biosci.*, 10:83–99.
285. Fawcett, D. W. (1975): Ultrastructure and function of the Sertoli cell. In: *Handbook of Physiology, Section 7, Endocrinology, Vol. 5, Male Reproductive System,* edited by D. W. Hamilton and R. O. Greep, pp. 21–55. Williams & Wilkins, Baltimore.
286. Fawcett, D. W. (1977): The ultrastructure and functions of the Sertoli cell. In: *Frontiers in Reproduction and Fertility Control,* edited by R. O. Green and M. A. Koblinsky, pp. 302–320. M.I.T. Press, Cambridge, Mass.
287. Fawcett, D. W. (1979): Comparative aspects of the organization of the testis and spermatogenesis. In: *Animal Models for Research on Contraception and Fertility,* edited by N. J. Alexander, pp. 84–104. Harper & Row, New York.
288. Schulze, C. (1974): On the morphology of the human Sertoli cell. *Cell Tissue Res.*, 153:339–355.
289. Schulze, C. (1984): Sertoli cells and Leydig cells in man. *Adv. Anat. Embryol. Cell Biol.*, 88:1–104.
290. Russell, L. D. (1980): Sertoli-germ cell interrelations: a review. *Gamete Res.*, 3:179–202.
291. Wong, V., and Russell, L. D. (1983): Three-dimensional reconstruction of a rat stage V Sertoli cell: I. Methods, basic configuration and dimensions. *Am. J. Anat.*, 167:143–161.
292. Weber, J. E., Russell, L. D., Wong, V., and Peterson, R. N. (1983): Three-dimensional reconstruction of a rat stage V Sertoli cell: II. Morphometry of Sertoli-Sertoli and Sertoli-germ cell relationships. *Am. J. Anat.*, 167:163–179.
293. Russell, L. D., Tallon-Doran, M., Weber, J. E., Wong, V., and Peterson, R. N. (1983): Three-dimensional reconstruction of a rat stage V Sertoli cell: III. A study of specific cellular relationships. *Am. J. Anat.*, 167:181–192.
294. Ploen, L., and Ritzen, E. M. (1984): Fine structural features of Sertoli cells. In: *Ultrastructure of Reproduction,* edited by J. Van Berkom and P. M. Motta, pp. 67–74. Martinus Nijhoff, The Hague.
295. Tindall, D. J., Rowley, D. R., Murthy, L., Lipshultz, L. I., and Chang, C. H. (1985): Structure and biochemistry of the Sertoli cell. *Int. Rev. Cytol.*, 94:127–149.
296. Elftman, H. (1963): Sertoli cells and testis structure. *Am. J. Anat.*, 113:25–33.
297. Lofts, B. (1972): The Sertoli cell. *Gen. Comp. Endocrinol. [Suppl. 3]*, 636–648.
298. Bergmann, M., Greven, H., and Schindelmeiser, J. (1983): Observations on the blood-testis barrier in a frog and a salamander. *Cell Tissue Res.*, 232:189–200.
299. Cooksey, E. J., and Rothwell, B. (1973): The ultrastructure of the Sertoli cell and its differentiation in the domestic fowl (*Gallus domesticus*). *J. Anat.*, 114:329–345.
300. Dufaure, J. P. (1971): L'ultrastructure du testicule de lezard vivipare (Reptile, Lacertilien). II. Les cellules de Sertoli. Etude du glycogene. *Z. Zellforsch.*, 115:565–578.
301. Baccetti, B., Bigliardi, E., Vegni Talluri, M., and Burrini, A. G. (1983): The Sertoli cells in lizards. *J. Ultrastruct. Res.*, 85:11–23.
302. Ross, M. H., and Dobler, J. (1975): The Sertoli cell junctional specializations and their relationship to the germinal epithelium as observed after efferent ductule ligation. *Anat. Rec.*, 183:267–292.
303. Rolshoven, E. (1945): Spermatogenese und Sertoli-Syncitium. *Z. Zellforsch.*, 33:439–460.
304. Vogl, A. W., and Soucy, L. J. (1985): Arrangement and possible function of actin filament bundles in ectoplasmic specializations of ground squirrel Sertoli cells. *J. Cell Biol.*, 100:814–825.
305. Kerr, J. B., Mayberry, R. A., and Irby, D. C. (1984): Morphometric studies on lipid inclusions in Sertoli cells during the spermatogenic cycle in the rat. *Cell Tissue Res.*, 236:699–709.
306. Wing, T. Y., and Christensen, A. K. (1982): Morphometric studies on rat seminiferous tubules. *Am. J. Anat.*, 165:13–25.
307. Roosen-Runge, E. C. (1955): Quantitative studies on spermatogenesis in the albino rat. III. Volume changes in the cells of the seminiferous tubules. *Anat. Rec.*, 123:385–398.
308. Johnson, L., Petty, C. S., and Neaves, W. B. (1980): A comparative study of daily sperm production and testicular composition in humans and rats. *Biol. Reprod.*, 22:1233–1243.
309. Cavicchia, J. C., and Dym, M. (1977): Relative volume of Sertoli cells in monkey seminiferous epithelium. *Am. J. Anat.*, 150:501–503.
310. Dym, M., and Cavicchia, J. C. (1978): Functional morphology of the testis. *Biol. Reprod.*, 18:1–15.
311. Chung, K. W. (1974): Fine structure of Sertoli cells and myoid cells in mice with testicular feminization. *Fert. Steril.*, 25:325–335.
312. Chung, K. W. (1974): A morphological and histochemical study of Sertoli cells in normal and XX sex reversed mice. *Am. J. Anat.*, 139:369–388.
313. Dym, M. (1973): The fine structure of the monkey (*Macaca*) Sertoli cell and its role in maintaining the blood-testis barrier. *Anat. Rec.*, 175:639–656.
314. Nagano, T. (1966): Some observations on the fine structure of the Sertoli cell in the human testis. *Z. Zellforsch.*, 73:89–106.
315. Bustos-Obregon, E., and Esponda, P. (1974): Ultrastructure of the nucleus of human Sertoli cells in normal and pathological testes. *Cell Tissue Res.*, 152:467–475.
316. Kerr, J. B., and de Kretser, D. M. (1981): The cytology of the human testis. In: *The Testis,* edited by H. Burger and D. M. de Kretser, pp. 141–170. Raven Press, New York.
317. Johnson, L., Zane, R. S., Petty, C. S., and Neaves, W. B. (1984): Quantification of human Sertoli cell population: its distribution, relation to germ cell numbers, and age-related decline. *Biol. Reprod.*, 31:785–795.
318. de Kretser, D. M., Kerr, J. B., and Paulsen, C. A. (1981): Evaluation of the ultrastructural changes in the human Sertoli cells in testicular disorders and the relationship of the changes to the levels of serum FSH. *Int. J. Andrology,* 4:129–144.
319. Dym, M., and Romrell, L. J. (1975): Intraepithelial lymphocytes in the male reproductive tract of rats and rhesus monkeys. *J. Reprod. Fertil.*, 42:1–7.
320. Chemes, H. E., Dym, M., Fawcett. D. W., Javadpour, N., and Sherins, R. J. (1977): Patho-physiological observations of Sertoli cells in patients with germinal aplasia or severe germ cell depletion. Ultrastructural findings and hormone levels. *Biol. Reprod.*, 17:108–123.
321. Kierszenbaum, A. L. (1974): RNA synthetic activities of Sertoli cells in the mouse testis. *Biol. Reprod.*, 11:365–376.

322. Mirre, C., and Knibiehler, B. (1982): A re-evaluation of the relationships between the fibrillar centres and the nucleolus-organizing regions in reticulated nucleoli: ultrastructural organization, number and distribution of the fibrillar centres in the nucleolus of the mouse Sertoli cell. *J. Cell Sci.*, 55:247–259.
323. Nicander, L. (1963): Some ultrastrutural features of mammalian Sertoli cells. *J. Ultrastruct. Res.*, 8:190–191.
324. Zibrin, M. (1971): Some ultrastructural aspects of nuclear morphology in developing spermatids and mature spermatozoa of the bull. *Mikroskopie*, 27:10–16.
325. Zibrin, M. (1972): Multivesicular nuclear body with nucleolar activity in Sertoli cells of bulls. An ultrastructural study. *Z. Zellforsch.*, 135:155–164.
326. Tersakis, J. A. (1965): The nucleolar channel system in the human endometrium. *J. Cell Biol.*, 27:293–304.
327. Nagano, T., and Suzuki, F. (1976): Freeze-fracture observations on the intercellular junctions of Sertoli cells and of Leydig cells in the human testis. *Cell Tissue Res.*, 166:37–48.
328. Ross, M. H. (1976): The Sertoli cell junctional specialization during spermiogenesis and at spermiation. *Anat. Rec.*, 186:79–104.
329. Vogl, A. W., Linck, R. W., and Dym, M. (1983): Colchicine-induced changes in the cytoskeleton of the golden mantled ground squirrel (*Spermophilus lateralis*) Sertoli cells. *Am. J. Anat.*, 168:99–108.
330. Rambourg, A., Clermont, Y., and Marrand, A. (1974): Three-dimensional structure of the osmium-impregnated Golgi apparatus as seen in the high voltage electron microscope. *Am. J. Anat.*, 140:27–46.
331. Rambourg, A., Clermont, Y., and Hermo, L. (1979): Three-dimensional architecture of the Golgi apparatus in Sertoli cells of the rat. *Am. J. Anat.*, 154:455–476.
332. Gunsalus, G. L., Musto, N. A., and Bardin, C. W. (1980): Bidirectional release of a Sertoli cell product, androgen binding protein, into the blood and seminiferous tubule. In: *Testicular Development, Structure, and Function*, edited by A. Steinberger and E. Steinberger, pp. 291–298. Raven Press, New York.
333. Wright, W. W., Parvinen, M., Musto, N. A., Gunsalus, G. L., Phillips, D. M., Mather, J. P., and Bardin, C. W. (1983): Identification of stage-specific proteins synthesized by rat seminiferous tubules. *Biol. Reprod.*, 29:257–270.
334. Ritzen, E. M., Boitani, C., and Parvinen, M. (1981): Cyclic secretion of proteins by the rat seminiferous tubule, depending on the stage of spermatogenesis. *Int. J. Androl.* [*Suppl.*], 3:57–58.
335. Robertson, D. M., Foulds, L. M., Leversha, L., Morgan, F. J., Hearn, M. T. W., Burger, H. G., Wettenhall, R. E. H., and de Kretser, D. M. (1985): Isolation of inhibin from bovine follicular fluid. *Biochem. Biophys. Res. Commun.*, 126:220–226.
336. Forage, R. G., Ring, J. M., Brown, R. W., McInerney, B. V., Cobon, G. S., Gregson, R. P., Robertson, D. M., Morgan, F. J., Hearn, M. T. W., Findlay, J. K., Wettenhall, R. E. H., Burger, H. G., and de Kretser, D. M. (1986): Cloning and sequence analysis of cDNA species coding for the two subunits of inhibin from bovine follicular fluid. *Proc. Natl. Acad. Sci. USA*, 83: 3091–3095.
337. Mason, A. J., Hayflick, J. S., Ling, N., Esch, F., Ueno, N., Ying, S. Y., Guillemin, R., Niall, H., and Seeburg, P. H. (1985): Complementary DNA sequences of ovarian follicular fluid inhibin show precursor structure and homology with transforming growth factor. B. *Nature*, 318:659–663.
338. McLachlan, R. I., Robertson, D. M., Burger, H. G., and de Kretser, D. M. (1986): The radioimmunoassay of bovine follicular fluid inhibin. *Mol. Cell. Endocrinol.*, 46:175–185.
339. Christensen, A. K. (1965): The fine structure of testicular interstitial cells in guinea pigs. *J. Cell Biol.*, 26:911–935.
340. Blanchette, E. J. (1966): Ovarian steroid cells: II. The lutein cell. *J. Cell Biol.*, 31:517–542.
341. Christensen, A. K., and Gillim, S. W. (1969): The correlation of fine structure and function in steroid-secreting cells, with emphasis on those of the gonads. In: *The Gonads*, edited by K. W. McKerns, pp. 415–488. Appleton-Century-Crofts, New York.
342. Abrunhosa, R. (1972): Microperfusion fixation of embryos for ultrastructural studies. *J. Ultrastruct. Res.*, 41:176–184.
343. Vogl, A. W., Lin, Y. C., Dym, M., and Fawcett, D. W. (1983): Sertoli cells of the golden-mantled ground squirrel (*Spermophilus lateralis*): a model system for the study of shape change. *Am. J. Anat.*, 168:83–98.
344. Kerr, J. B., and de Kretser, D. M. (1974): The role of the Sertoli cell in phagocytosis of the residual bodies of spermatids. *J. Reprod. Fertil.*, 36:439–440.
345. Olvik, N. M., and Dahl, E. (1981): Stage-dependent variation in volume density and size of Sertoli cell vesicles in the rat testis. *Cell Tissue Res.*, 221:311–320.
346. Welsh, M. J., and Wiebe, J. P. (1978): Sertoli cell capacity to metabolize C19 steroids. Variation with age and the effect of FSH. *Endocrinology*, 103:838–844.
347. Tcholakian, R. K., and Steinberger, A. (1978): Progesterone metabolism by cultured Sertoli cells. *Endocrinology*, 103: 1335–1343.
348. Lacy, D. (1962): Certain aspects of testis structure and function. *Br. Med. Bull.*, 18:205–208.
349. Lacy, D. (1967): The seminiferous tubules in mammals. *Endeavour*, 26:101–108.
350. Lacy, D., and Pettitt, A. J. (1969): Transmission electron microscopy and the production of steroids by the Leydig and Sertoli cells of the human testis. *Micron*, 1:15–33.
351. Lacy, D., and Pettitt, A. J. (1970): Sites of hormone production in the mammalian testis and their significance in the control of male fertility. *Br. Med. Bull.*, 26:87–91.
352. Johnson, A. D. (1970): Testicular lipids. In: *The Testis, Vol. II*, edited by A. D. Johnson, W. R. Gomes, and N. L. Van Demark, pp. 193–258. Academic Press, New York.
353. Kerr, J. B., Keogh, E. J., Hudson, B., Whipp, G. T., and de Kretser, D. M. (1980): Alterations in spermatogenic activity and hormonal status in a seasonally breeding rat, *Rattus fuscipes*. *Gen. Comp. Endocrinol.*, 40:78–88.
354. de Kretser, D. M., and Kerr, J. B. (1983): The effect of testicular damage on Sertoli and Leydig cell function. In: *The Pituitary and Testis. Clinical and Experimental Studies*, edited by D. M. de Kretser, H. G. Burger, and B. Hudson, pp. 133–154. Springer-Verlag, Berlin.
355. Collins, P. M., and Lacy, D. (1969): Studies on the structure and function of the mammalian testis. II. Cytological and histochemical observations on the testis of the rat after a single exposure of heat applied for different lengths of time. *Proc. R. Soc. Lond.* [*Biol.*], 172:17–38.
356. Posalaki, Z., Szabo, D., Bacsi, E., and Okros, I. (1968): Hydrolytic enzymes during spermatogenesis in rat. An electron microscopic and histochemical study. *J. Histochem. Cytochem.*, 16:249–262.
357. Beckman, J. K., and Conigliio, J. G. (1979): A comparative study of the lipid composition of isolated rat Sertoli and germinal cells. *Lipids*, 14:262–267.
358. Fleeger, J. L., Bishop, J. P., Gomes, W. R., and van Demark, N. L. (1968): Testicular lipids. I. Effect of unilateral cryptorchidism on lipid classes. *J. Reprod. Fertil.*, 15:1–7.
359. Stieve, H. (1930): Männliche Genitalorgane. In: *Handbuch der Mikroskopischen Anatomie des Menschen, Vol. 7, Part 2*, edited by W. Möllendorf, pp. 1–399. Springer, Berlin.
360. Spangaro, S. (1902): Über die histologischen Veranderungen des Hodens, Nebenhodens, und Samenleiters von Geburt an bis zum Griersalter, mit besonderer Berucksichtigung der Hodenatrophie, des elastischen Gewebes und des Vorkommens von Krystallen in Hoden. *Anat. Rec.*, 18:593–771.
361. Fawcett, D. W., and Burgos, M. H. (1956): The fine structure of Sertoli cells in the human testis. *Anat. Rec.*, 124:401.
362. Bawa, S. R. (1963): The fine structure of the Sertoli cell of the human testes. *J. Ultrastruct. Res.*, 9:459–474.
363. Toyama, Y. (1975): Ultrastructure study of crystalloids in Sertoli cells of the normal, intersex and experimental cryptorchid swine. *Cell Tissue Res.*, 158:205–213.
364. Toyama, Y., Obinata, T., and Holtzen, H. (1979): Crystalloids of actin-like filaments in the Sertoli cell of the swine testis. *Anat. Rec.*, 195:47–62.
365. von Bardeleben, K. (1897): Die Zwischenzellen des Saugetierhodens. *Anat. Anz.*, 13:529–536.
366. Benda, C. (1906): Die Spermiogenese der Marsupialier. *Denkschr. Mednaturn. Ges. Jena*, 6:441–458.
367. Greenwood, A. W. (1923): Marsupial spermatogenesis. *Q. J. Microsc. Sci.*, 64:203–218.

368. Duesberg, J. (1918): On the interstitial cells of the testicle in Didelphys. *Biol. Bull.*, 35:175–198.
369. Harding, H. R., Carrick, F. N., and Shorey, C. D. (1982): Crystalloid inclusions in the Sertoli cell of the koala, *Phascolarctos cinereus* (Marsupialia). *Cell Tissue Res.*, 221:633–642.
370. Maximow, A. (1899): Die histologische Vorgange bei der Heilung von Hodenvertetzungen und die Regenerationsfahigkeit des Hodengewebes. *Beitr. Pathol. Anat.*, 26:230–319.
371. Niemi, M., Harkonen, H., and Kokko, A. (1962): Localization and identification of testicular esterases in the rat. *J. Histochem. Cytochem.*, 10:186–193.
372. Posalaki, Z. (1964): Histochemische Untersuchungen der Spermiogenese. *Symp. Biol. Hung.*, 4:83–87.
373. Posalaki, Z. (1965): Activity of different dehydrogenases and diaphorases in the spermatogenesis of the rat and its relation to motility. *Acta Histochem.*, 20:86–90.
374. Niemi, M., and Kormano, M. (1965): Cyclical changes in and significance of lipids and acid phosphatase activity in the seminiferous tubules of the rat testis. *Anat. Rec.*, 157:159–170.
375. Parvinen, M., and Vanha-Pertulla, T. (1972): Identification and enzyme quantification of the stages of the seminiferous epithelial wave in the rat. *Anat. Rec.*, 174:435–450.
376. Barham, S. S., and Berlin, J. D. (1974): Fine structure and cytochemistry of testicular cells in men treated with testosterone propionate. *Cell Tissue Res.*, 148:159–182.
377. Clegg, E. J., and MacMillan, E. W. (1965): Uptake of vital dyes and particulate matter by the Sertoli cells of the rat testis. *J. Anat.*, 99:219–229.
378. Carr, I., Clegg, E. J., and Meek, G. A. (1968): Sertoli cells as phagocytes: an electron microscopic study. *J. Anat.*, 102:501–509.
379. Soares Pessoa, J. F., and David-Ferreira, J. F. (1980): Bidirectional transport of horseradish peroxidase by rat Sertoli cells. An *in vitro* study. *Biol. Cellulaire*, 39:301–304.
380. Reddy, J. K., and Svoboda, D. J. (1967): Lysosomal activity in Sertoli cells of normal and degenerating seminiferous epithelium of rat testis. *Am. J. Pathol.*, 51:1–17.
381. Morales, C., and Hermo, L. (1983): Demonstration of fluid phase endocytosis in epithelial cells of the male reproductive system by means of horseradish peroxidase colloidal gold complex. *Cell Tissue Res.*, 230:503–510.
382. Hinton, B. T., and Keefer, D. A. (1983): Evidence for protein absorption from the lumen of the seminiferous tubuli and rete testis of the rat testis. *Cell Tissue Res.*, 230:367–375.
383. Hermo, L., Morales, C. R., and Clermont, Y. (1982): Endocytic activity of Sertoli cells in the rat. *J. Cell Biol.*, 95:434a.
384. Morales, C., Clermont, Y., and Hermo, L. (1985): Nature and function of endocytosis in Sertoli cells of the rat. *Am. J. Anat.*, 173:203–217.
385. Gulyas, B. J. (1971): The rabbit zygote: formation of annulate lamellae. *J. Ultrastruct. Res.*, 35:112–126.
386. Maul, G. G. (1970): On the relationship between the Golgi apparatus and annulate lamellae. *J. Ultrastruct. Res.*, 30:368–384.
387. Wischnitzer, S. (1970): The annulate lamellae. *Int. Rev. Cytol.*, 27:65–100.
388. Sun, C. N., and White, H. J. (1979): Annulate lamellae in human tumor cells. *Tissue Cell*, 11:139–146.
389. Kessel, R. G. (1968): Annulate lamellae. *J. Ultrastruct. Res.* [*Suppl. 10*], 1–82.
390. Merkow, L., and Leighton, J. (1966): Increased numbers of annulate lamellae in myocardium of chick embryo incubated at abnormal temperatures. *J. Cell Biol.*, 28:127–137.
391. de Brabander, M., and Borgers, M. (1975): The formation of annulated lamellae induced by the disintegration of microtubules. *J. Cell Sci.*, 19:331–340.
392. Toyama, Y. (1976): Actin-like filaments in the Sertoli cell junctional specializations in the swine and mouse testis. *Anat. Rec.*, 186:477–492.
393. Franke, W. W., Grund, C., Fink, A., Weber, K., Jokusch, B. M., Zentgraf, H., and Osborn, M. (1978): Location of actin in the microfilament bundles associated with the junctional specializations between Sertoli cells and spermatids. *Biol. Cellulaire*, 31: 7–14.
394. Franke, W. W., Grund, C., and Schmid, E. (1979): Intermediate-sized filaments present in Sertoli cells are of the vimentin type. *Eur. J. Cell Biol.*, 19:269–275.
395. Russell, L. D. (1977): Observations on rat Sertoli ectoplasmic ('junctional') specializations in their association with germ cells of the rat testis. *Tissue Cell*, 9:475–498.
396. Aoki, A. (1980): Induction of sperm release by microtubule inhibitors in rat testis. *Eur. J. Cell Biol.*, 22:467.
397. Roosen-Runge, E. C. (1951): Quantitative studies on spermatogenesis in the albino rat. II. The duration of spermatogenesis and some effects of colchicine. *Am. J. Anat.*, 88:163–176.
398. Parvinen, L. M., Soderstrom, K. O., and Parvinen, M. (1978): Early effects of vinblastine and vincristine on the rat spermatogenesis: analysis by a new transillumination-phase contrast microscopic method. *Exp. Pathol.*, 15:85–96.
399. Russell, L. D., Malone, J. P., and MacCurdy, D. S. (1981): Effect of the microtubule disrupting agents, colchicine and vinblastine, on seminiferous tubule structure in the rat. *Tissue Cell*, 13:349–367.
400. Ribbert, H. (1904): Die abscheidung intravenos injizierten gelosten Karmins in den Geweben. *Z. Allg. Physiol.*, 4:201–214.
401. Bouffard, G. (1906): Injection des couters de benzidine aux animaux nomaux. *Annales de l'Institut Pasteur de Lille*, 20:539–546.
402. Pari, G. (1910): Über die Verwendbarkeit vitaler Karmineinspritzungen fur die pathologische Anatomie. *Frank. Z. Pathol.*, 4:1–29.
403. Goldacre, R. J., and Sylven, B. (1959): A rapid method for studying tumour blood supply using systemic dyes. *Nature*, 184:63–64.
404. Goldacre, R. J., and Sylven, B. (1962): On the access of blood-borne dyes to various tumor regions. *Br. J. Cancer*, 16:306–322.
405. Everett, N. B., and Simmons, B. (1958): Measurement and radioautographic localization of albumin in rat tissues after intravenous injection. *Circ. Res.*, 6:307–313.
406. Kormano, M. (1968): Penetration of intravenous trypan blue into the rat testis and epididymis. *Acta Histochem.*, 30:133–136.
407. Setchell, B. P. (1967): The blood-testicular fluid barrier in sheep. *J. Physiol. (Lond.)*, 189:63P–65P.
408. Cowie, A. T., Lascelles, A. K., and Wallace, J. C. (1964): Flows and protein content of testicular lymph in conscious rams. *J. Physiol. (Lond.)*, 171:176–187.
409. Waites, G. M. H., and Setchell, B. P. (1966): Changes in blood flow and vascular permeability of the testis, epididymis and accessory reproductive organs of the rat after administration of cadmium chloride. *J. Endocrinol.*, 34:329–342.
410. Waites, G. M. H., and Setchell, B. P. (1965): Some physiological aspects of the function of the testis. In: *The Gonads*, edited by K. W. McKerns, pp. 659–714. Appleton-Century-Crofts, New York.
411. Fawcett, D. W., Leak, L. V., and Heidger, P. M. (1970): Electron microscopic observations on the structural components of the blood-testis barrier. *J. Reprod. Fertil.*, [*Suppl. 10*], 105–122.
412. Ross, M. H. (1970): The Sertoli cell and the blood-testicular barrier: an electronmicroscopic study. In: *Morphological Aspects of Andrology*, edited by A. F. Hostein and E. Horstmann. pp. 83–86. Grosse Verlag, Berlin.
413. Dym, M., and Fawcett, D. W. (1970): The blood-testis barrier in the rat and the physiological compartmentation of the seminiferous epithelium. *Biol. Reprod.*, 3:308–326.
414. Russell, L. D., and Peterson, R. N. (1985): Sertoli cell junctions: morphological and functional considerations. *Int. Rev. Cytol.*, 94:177–211.
415. Nagano, T. (1980): Freeze-fracture observations on the rat Sertoli cell junctions by metal contact freezing. *J. Electron Microsc. (Tokyo)*, 29:250–255.
416. Connell, C. J. (1978): A freeze-fracture and lanthanum tracer study of the complex junction between the Sertoli cells of the canine testis. *J. Cell Biol.*, 76:57–75.
417. Dym, M., and Caviccia, J. C. (1977): Further observations on the blood-testis barrier in monkeys. *Biol. Reprod.*, 17:390–403.
418. Russell, L. D. (1977): Movement of spermatocytes from the basal to the adluminal compartment of the rat testis. *Am. J. Anat.*, 148:313–328.
419. Osman, D., Ekwall, H., and Ploen, L. (1980): Specialized cell contacts and the blood-testis barrier in the seminiferous tubules of the domestic fowl (*Gallas domesticus*). *Int. J. Androl.*, 3:553–562.
420. Franchi, E., Camatini, M., and de Curtis, I. (1982): Morphological evidence of a permeability barrier in urodele testis. *J. Ultrastruct. Res.*, 80:253–263.
421. Abraham, M., Rahamim, E., Tibika, H., Golenser, E., and Kieselstein, M. (1980): The blood-testis barrier in *Aphanius dispar* (Teleostei). *Cell Tissue Res.*, 211:207–214.

422. Marcaillou, C., and Szollosi, A. (1980): The blood-testis barrier in a nematode and a fish: a generalizable concept. *J. Ultrastruct. Res.*, 70:128–136.
423. Mattei, X., Mattei, C., Marcand, B., and Leung, T. K. D. (1982): Ultrastructure des cellules de Sertoli d'un poisson teleosteen: abudefduf marginatus. *J. Ultrastruct. Res.*, 81:333–340.
424. Billard, R. (1980): La spermatogenese de *Poecilia reticulata*. III. Ultrastructure des cellules de Sertoli. *Ann. Biol. Anim. Biochem. Biophys.*, 10:37–50.
425. Parmentier, H. K., van den Boogaart, J. G. M., and Timmermans, L. P. M. (1985): Physiological compartmentation in gonadal tissue of the common carp (*Cyprinus carpio* L). A study with horseradish peroxidase and monoclonal antibodies. *Cell Tissue Res.*, 242:75–81.
426. Szollosi, A., and Marcaillou, C. (1977): Electron microscope study of the blood-testis barrier in an insect *Locusta migratoria*. *J. Ultrastruct. Res.*, 59:158–172.
427. Szollosi, A., Reimann, J., and Marcaillou, C. (1980): Localization of the blood-testis barrier in the testis of the moth, *Anagasta kuehnilla*. *J. Ultrastruct. Res.*, 72:189–199.
428. Toshimori, K., Iwashata, T., and Oura, C. (1979): Cell junctions in the cyst envelope in the silkworm testis, *Bombyx mori Linne*. *Cell Tissue Res.*, 202:63–73.
429. Lane, N. J., and Skaer, H. L. (1980): Intercellular junctions in insect tissues. *Adv. Insect Physiol.*, 15:35–213.
430. O'Rand, M. G., and Romrell, L. J. (1977): Appearance of cell surface auto- and isoantigens during spermatogenesis in the rabbit. *Dev. Biol.*, 55:347–358.
431. Millette, C. F., and Bellve, A. R. (1977): Temporal expression of membrane antigens during mouse spermatogenesis. *J. Cell Biol.*, 74:86–97.
432. Romrell, L. J., and O'Rand, M. G. (1978): Capping and ultrastructural localization of sperm surface isoantigens during spermatogenesis. *Dev. Biol.*, 63:76–93.
433. Tung, P. S., and Fritz, I. B. (1978): Specific surface antigens on rat pachytene spermatocytes and successive classes of germ cells. *Dev. Biol.*, 64:297–315.
434. Tung, P. S., and Fritz, I. B. (1977): A maturation surface antigen of rat Sertoli cells. *J. Cell Biol.*, 75:165a.
435. Fritz, I. B. (1978): Sites of action of androgens and follicle-stimulating hormone on cells of the seminiferous tubule. In: *Biochemical Actions of Hormones, Vol. V*, edited by G. Litwak, pp. 249–281. Academic Press, New York.
436. Pelletier, R. M. (1986): Cyclic formation and decay of the blood-testis barrier in the mink (*Mustela vison*), a seasonal breeder. *Am. J. Anat.*, 175:91–117.
437. Russell, L. D. (1984): Spermiation—the sperm release process: ultrastructural observations and unresolved problems. In: *Ultrastructure of Reproduction*, edited by J. Van Berkom and P. M. Motta, pp. 46–66. Martinus Nijhoff, The Hague.
438. Russell, L. D., and Malone, J. P. (1980): A study of Sertoli-spermatid tubulobulbar complexes in selected mammals. *Tissue Cell*, 12:263–285.
439. Russell, L. D., Gardner, R. J., and Weber, J. E. (1986): Reconstruction of a type-B configuration monkey Sertoli cell: size, shapes and configurational and specialized cell-to-cell relationships. *Am. J. Anat.*, 175:73–90.
440. Russell, L. D., Myers, P., Ostenburg, J., and Malone, J. (1980): Sertoli ectoplasmic specializations during spermatogenesis. In: *Testicular Development, Structure, and Function*, edited by A. Steinberger and E. Steinberger, pp. 55–63. Raven Press, New York.
441. Gravis, C. J. (1979): Interrelationships between Sertoli cells and germ cells in the Syrian hamster. *Z. Mikrosk. Anat. Forsch.*, 93:321–342.
442. Romrell, L. J., and Ross, M. H. (1979): Characterization of Sertoli cell-germ cell junctional specialization in dissociated testicular cells. *Anat. Rec.*, 192:23–42.
443. Gravis, C. J. (1978): Inhibition of spermiation in the Syrian hamster using dibutyryl cyclic AMP. *Cell Tissue Res.*, 192:241–248.
444. Ross, M. H. (1977): Sertoli-Sertoli junctions and Sertoli-spermatid junctions after efferent ductule ligation and lanthanum treatment. *Am. J. Anat.*, 148:49–56.
445. Russell, L. D. (1979): Observations on the interrelationships of Sertoli cells at the level of the blood-testis barrier: evidence for formation and resorption of Sertoli-Sertoli tubulobulbar complexes during the spermatogenic cycle of the rat. *Am. J. Anat.*, 155:259–280.
446. Clermont, Y., McCoshen, J., and Hermo, L. (1980): Evolution of the enodplasmic reticulum in the Sertoli cell cytoplasm encapsulating the heads of late spermatids in the rat. *Anat. Rec.*, 196: 83–99.
447. Cooper, G. W., and Bedford, J. M. (1976): Asymmetry of spermiation and sperm surface charge patterns over the giant acrosome in the musk shrew *Suncus murinus*. *J. Cell Biol.*, 69:415–428.
448. Gravis, C. J. (1980): Ultrastructural observations on spermatozoa retained within the seminiferous epithelium after treatment with dibutyryl cyclic AMP. *Tissue Cell*, 12:309–322.
449. Altorfer, J., Fukuda, T., and Hedinger, C. (1974): Desmosomes in human seminiferous epithelium. *Virchows Arch. [Zellpathol.]*, 16:181–194.
450. Connell, C. J. (1974): The Sertoli cell of the sexually mature dog. *Anat. Rec.*, 178:333.
451. McGinley, D., Pozalaky, Z., and Porvaznik, M. (1977): Intercellular junctional complexes of the rat seminiferous tubules: a freeze-fracture study. *Anat. Rec.*, 189:211–232.
452. McGinley, D. M., Pozalaky, Z., Porvaznik, M., and Russell, L. D. (1979): Gap junctions between Sertoli and germ cells of rat seminiferous tubules. *Tissue Cell*, 11:741–754.
453. Lodge, J. R., and Salisbury, G. W. (1970): Seasonal variation and male reproductive efficiency. In: *The Testis, Vol. III*, edited by A. D. Johnson, W. R. Gomes, and N. L. Van Demark, pp. 139–167. Academic Press, New York.
454. Lofts, B., and Bern, H. A. (1972): The functional morphology of steroidogenic tissues. In: *Steroids in Non-Mammalian Vertebrates*, edited by D. R. Idler, pp. 37–125. Academic Press, New York.
455. Lofts, B., and Lam, W. L. (1973): Circadian regulation of gonadotrophin secretion. *J. Reprod. Fertil.*, 19:19–34.
456. Lincoln, G. A., and Short, R. V. (1980): Seasonal breeding: nature's contraceptive. *Recent Prog. Horm. Res.*, 36:1–52.
457. Hodgson, Y. M., Irby, D. C., Kerr, J. B., and de Kretser, D. M. (1979): Studies of the structure and function of the Sertoli cell in a seasonally breeding rodent. *Biol. Reprod.*, 21:1091–1098.
458. Irby, D. C., Kerr, J. B., Risbridger, G. P., and de Kretser, D. M. (1984): Seasonally and experimentally induced changes in testicular function of the Australian bush rat, *Rattus fuscipes*. *J. Reprod. Fertil.*, 70:657–666.
459. Zamboni, L., Conaway, C. H., and Van Pelt, L. (1974): Seasonal changes in production of semen in free-ranging rhesus monkeys. *Biol. Reprod.*, 11:251–267.
460. Pudney, J., and Lacy, D. (1977): Correlation between ultrastructure and biochemical changes in the testes of the American grey squirrel, *Sciurus carolinensis*, during the reproductive cycle. *J. Reprod. Fertil.*, 49:5–16.
461. Vendreley, E., Guerillot, C., and Da Lage, C. (1972): Variations saisonnieres des cellules de Sertoli et de Leydig dans le testicule der hamster dore. Etude caryometrique. *C. R. Acad. Sci. [D] Paris*, 275:1143–1146.
462. Berndston, W. E., and Desjardins, C. (1974): Circulating LH and FSH in hamsters during light deprivation and subsequent photoperiodic stimulation. *Endocrinology*, 95:195–205.
463. Lincoln, G. A. (1976): Seasonal variation in the episodic secretion of luteinizing hormone and testosterone in the ram. *J. Endocrinol.*, 69:213–226.
464. Michael, R. P., and Bonsall, R. W. (1977): A 3-year study of an annual rhythm in plasma androgen levels in male rhesus monkey (*Macaca mulatta*) in a constant laboratory environment. *J. Reprod. Fertil.*, 49:129–131.
465. Vilar, O. (1968): Ultrastructural changes observed after hypophysectomy in rat testis. In: *Gonadotrophins*, edited by E. Rosemberg, pp. 205–211. Geron-X, Los Angeles.
466. Gravis, C. J., and Weaker, F. J. (1977): Testicular involution following optic enucleation. *Cell Tissue Res.*, 184:67–77.
467. Nebel, B. R., and Murphy, C. J. (1960): Damage and recovery of mouse testis after 1000r acute localized X-irradiation, with reference to restitution cells, Sertoli cell increase, and type A spermatogonial recovery. *Radiat. Res.*, 12:626–641.
468. Clegg, E. J. (1963): Studies on artificial cryptorchidism: degenerative and regenerative changes in germinal epithelium of rat testis. *J. Endocrinol.*, 27:241–251.
469. Clegg, E. J. (1963): Studies on artificial cryptorchidism: degenerative and regenerative changes in germinal epithelium of rat testis. *J. Endocrinol.*, 26:567–574.

470. Felizet, G., and Branca, A. (1898): Histologie du testicule ectopique. *J. l'Anat. Physiol.*, 34:589–641.
471. Nagy, F. (1972): Cell division kinetics and DNA synthesis in the immature Sertoli cells of the rat testis. *J. Reprod. Fertil.*, 28:389–395.
472. Murphy, H. D. (1965): Sertoli cell stimulation following intratesticular injections of FSH in the hypophysectomized rat. *Proc. Soc. Exp. Biol. Med.*, 118:1202–1205.
473. Hochereau-de Reviers, M. T., and Lincoln, G. A. (1978): Seasonal variation in the histology of the testis of the red deer, *Cervus elaphus*. *J. Reprod. Fertil.*, 54:209–213.
474. Johnson, L., and Neaves, W. B. (1981): Age-related changes in the Leydig cell population, seminiferous tubules and sperm production in stallions. *Biol. Reprod.*, 24:703–712.
475. Johnson, L., and Thompson, D. L. (1983): Age-related and seasonal variation in the Sertoli cell population, daily sperm production and serum concentrations of follicle-stimulating hormone, luteinizing hormone and testosterone in stallions. *Biol. Reprod.*, 29:777–789.
476. Johnson, L. (1985): Increased daily sperm production in the breeding season of stallions is explained by an elevated population of spermatogonia. *Biol. Reprod.*, 32:1181–1190.
477. Hochereau-de Reviers, M. T. (1981): Control of spermatogonial multiplication. In: *Reproductive Processes and Contraception*, edited by K. W. McKerns, pp. 307–331. Plenum, New York.
478. Feig, L. A., Bellve, A. R., Erickson, N. H., and Klagsbrun, M. (1980): Sertoli cells contain a mitogenic polypeptide. *Proc. Natl. Acad. Sci. USA*, 77:4774–4778.
479. Harbitz, T. B. (1973): Morphometric studies of the Sertoli cells in elderly men with special reference to the histology of the prostate. *Acta Pathol. Microbiol. Scand.*, 81A:703.
480. Kerr, J. B., Rich, K. A., and de Kretser, D. M. (1979): Effects of experimental cryptorchidism on the ultrastructure and function of the Sertoli cell and peritubular tissue of the rat testis. *Biol. Reprod.*, 21:823–838.
481. Hoffer, A. P. (1983): Effects of gossypol on the seminiferous epithelium in the rat: a light and electron microscope study. *Biol. Reprod.*, 28:1007–1020.
482. Flickinger, C. J. (1981): Effects of clomiphene on the structure of the testis, epididymis and sex accessory glands of the rat. *Am. J. Anat.*, 149:533–562.
483. Krueger, P. M., Hodgen, G. D., and Sherins, R. J. (1974): New evidence for the role of the Sertoli cell and spermatogonia in feedback control of FSH secretion in male rats. *Endocrinology*, 95:955–962.
484. Chapin, R. E., Dutton, S. L., Ross, M. D., Sumrell, B. M., and Lamb, J. C. (1984): The effects of ethylene glycol monomethyl ether on testicular histology in F344 rats. *J. Andrology*, 5:369–380.
485. Hildebrandt-Stark, H. E., and Fawcett, D. W. (1978): Effects of deficiency of essential fatty acids and treatment with prostaglandin E_2 on the ultrastructure of the rat testis. *Biol. Reprod.*, 19:736–746.
486. Kierszenbaum, A. L. (1970): Effect of trenimon on the ultrastructure of Sertoli cells in the mouse. *Virchows Arch. [Zellpathol.]*, 5:1–12.
487. Zhuang, L. Z., Phillips, D. M., Gunsalus, G. L., Bardin, C. W., and Mather, J. P. (1983): Effects of gossypol on rat Sertoli and Leydig cells in primary culture and established cell lines. *J. Andrology*, 4:336–344.
488. Parizek, J. (1960): Sterilization of the male by cadmium salts. *J. Reprod. Fertil.*, 1:294–309.
489. Kerr, J. B., and Sharpe, R. M. (1986): Effects and interactions of LH and LHRH agonist on testicular morphology and function in hypophysectomized rats. *J. Reprod. Fertil.*, 76:175–192.
490. Vickery, B., McRae, G. I., Bergstrom, K., Briones, W., Worden, A., and Seidenberg, R. (1983): Inability of long-term administration of D-Nal(2)^6-LHRH to abolish fertility in male rats. *J. Andrology*, 4:283–291.
491. Schulze, W., and Schulze, C. (1981): Multinucleate Sertoli cells in aged human testis. *Cell Tissue Res.*, 217:259–266.
492. Schulze, C., Holstein, A. F., Schirren, C., and Korner, F. (1976): On the morphology of the human Sertoli cells under normal conditions and in patients with impaired fertility. *Andrologia*, 8:167–178.
493. Nistal, M., Paniagua, R., Abaurrea, M. A., and Santamaria, L. (1982): Hyperplasia and the immature appearance of Sertoli cells in primary testicular disorders. *Hum. Pathol.*, 13:1.
494. Paniagua, R., Amat, P., Nistal, M., and Martin, A. (1985): Ultrastructural changes in Sertoli cells in ageing humans. *Int. J. Androl.*, 8:295–312.
495. Benda, C. (1887): Untersuchunger über den Bau des funktionierenden Samenkanalchens einiger Saugetiere und Folgerungen für die Spermatogenese dieser Wirbeltierklasse. *Arch. Mikrosk. Anat.*, 30:49–110.
496. Curtis, G. M. (1918): The morphology of the mammalian seminiferous tubule. *Am. J. Anat.*, 24:339–394.
497. Roosen-Runge, E. C., and Giesel, L. O. (1950): Quantitative studies on spermatogenesis in the albino rat. *Am. J. Anat.*, 87:1–30.
498. Oakberg, E. F. (1956): Duration of spermatogenesis in the mouse and timing of stages of the cycle of the seminiferous epithelium. *Am. J. Anat.*, 99:507–516.
499. Ortavant, R. (1958): La cycle spermatogenetique chez le Belier. Thesis, Paris.
500. Chowdhury, A. K., and Marshall, G. (1980): Irregular pattern of spermatogenesis in the baboon (*Papio anubis*) and its possible mechanism. In: *Testicular Development, Structure, and Function*, edited by A. Steinberger and E. Steinberger, pp. 129–137. Raven Press, New York.
501. Schulze, W., and Rehder, U. (1984): Organization and morphogenesis of the human seminiferous epithelium. *Cell Tissue Res.*, 237:395–407.
502. Ortavant, R. (1954): Etude des generations spermatogoniales chez le Belier. *C. R. Soc. Biol. (Paris)*, 148:1958–1961.
503. Ortavant, R. (1956): Autoradiographie des cellules germinales du testicule de Belier. Duree des phenomenes spermatogenetiques. *Arch. Anat. Microsc. Morphol. Exp.*, 45:1–10.
504. Clermont, Y., and Harvey, S. G. (1965): Duration of the cycle of the seminiferous epithelium of normal hypophysectomized and hypophysectomized-hormone treated albino rats. *Endocrinology*, 76:80–89.
505. Desclin, J., and Ortavant, R. (1963): Influences des hormones gonadotropes sur la duree des processus spermatogenetiques chez le rat. *Ann. Biol. Anim. Biochem. Biophys.*, 3:329–342.
506. Russell, L. D., Lee, I. P., Ettlin, R., and Malone, J. P. (1983): Morphological pattern of response after administration of procarbazine: alteration of specific cell associations during the cycle of the seminiferous epithelium of the rat. *Tissue Cell*, 15:391–404.
507. Cleland, K. W. (1951): The spermatogenic cycle of the guinea pig. *Aust. J. Biol. Sci.*, 4:344–369.
508. Johnson, S. G. (1964): Studies on the testicular-hypophyseal feedback mechanism in man. *Acta Endocrinol. [Suppl. 90]*, 99–124.
509. Perey, B., Clermont, Y., and Le Blond, C. P. (1961): The wave of the seminiferous epithelium in the rat. *Am. J. Anat.*, 108:47–77.
510. Dym, M., and Clermont, Y. (1970): Role of spermatogonia in the repair of the seminiferous epithelium following X-irradiation of the rat testis. *Am. J. Anat.*, 128:265–282.
511. Moens, P. B., and Hugenholtz, A. D. (1975): The arrangement of germ cells in the rat seminiferous tubule: an electron microscopic study. *J. Cell Sci.*, 19:487–507.
512. Rolshoven, E. (1941): Zur Frage des "Alterns" de generativen Elemente in den Hodenkanalchen. *Anat. Anz.*, 91:1–8.
513. Huckins, C. (1971): Cell cycle properties of differentiating spermatogonia in adult Sprague-Dawley rats. *Cell Tissue Kinet.*, 4:139–154.
514. Huckins, C. (1971): The spermatogonial stem cell population in adult rats. III. Evidence for a long-cycling population. *Cell Tissue Kinet.*, 4:335–349.
515. Huckins, C. (1971): The spermatogonial stem cell population in adult rats. II. A radioautographic analysis of their cell cycle properties. *Cell Tissue Kinet.*, 4:313–334.
516. Oakberg, E. F. (1971): Spermatogonial stem-cell renewal in the mouse. *Anat. Rec.*, 169:515–531.
517. Huckins, C., and Oakberg, E. F. (1978): Morphological and quantitative analysis of spermatogonia in mouse testes using whole mounted seminiferous tubules. I. The normal testes. *Anat. Rec.*, 192:519–528.
518. Oud, J. L., and de Rooij, D. G. (1977): Spermatogenesis in the Chinese hamster. *Anat. Rec.*, 187:113–124.
519. de Rooij, D. G., Lok, D., and Weenk, D. (1985): Feedback regulation of the proliferation of the undifferentiated spermatogonia in the Chinese hamster by the differentiating spermatogonia. *Cell Tissue Kinet.*, 18:71–81.
520. Lok, D., Weenk, D., and de Rooij, D. G. (1982): Morphology, proliferation and differentiation of undifferentiated spermatogonia in the Chinese hamster and the ram. *Anat. Rec.*, 203:83–99.

521. Chowdhury, A. K., and Steinberger, E. (1971): A radioautography technique for human and rat seminiferous tubules mounted *in toto*. *Exp. Cell Res.*, 64:450–456.
522. Fuerst, C. (1887): Über die Entwicklung der Samenkoerperchen bei den Beteltieren. *Arch. Mikrosk. Anat.*, 81:1–23.
523. Hochereau, M. T. (1963): Constance des frequences relative des etudes du cycle de l'epithelium seminifere chez le taureau et chez le rat. *Ann. Biol. Anim. Biochem. Biophys.*, 3:93–102.
524. Tiba, T., Ishikawa, T., and Murakami, A. (1968): Histologische Untersuchung der Kinetik des Spermatogenes beim Mink. II. Samenepithelwelle in der Paarungszeit. *Jpn. J. Vet. Res.*, 16:159–187.
525. Parvinen, M. (1982): Regulation of the seminiferous epithelium. *Endocrine Rev.*, 3:404–417.
526. Jegou, B., Laws, A. O., and de Kretser, D. M. (1984): Changes in testicular function in the rat testis to heat: further evidence for interaction of germ cells, Sertoli cells and Leydig cells. *Int. J. Androl.*, 7:244–257.
527. Stieve, H. (1921): *Entwickelung Bau und Bedeutung der Keimdrusenzwichenzellen*. J. F. Bergmann, Munich.
528. Hanes, F. M. (1911): The relations of the interstitial cells of Leydig to the production of an internal secretion by the mammalian testis. *J. Exp. Med.*, 13:338–354.
529. Rasmusen, A. T. (1932): Interstitial cells of the testis. In: *Special Cytology, Vol. 3, Section XLII*, edited by E. V. Cowdrey, pp. 1675–1725. Hafner, New York.
530. Hooker, C. W. (1944): The postnatal history and function of the interstitial cells of the testis of the bull. *Am. J. Anat.*, 74:1–37.
531. Hooker, C. W. (1948): The biology of the interstitial cells of the testis. *Recent Prog. Horm. Res.*, 3:173–195.
532. Hooker, C. W. (1970): The intertubular tissue of the testis. In: *The Testis, Vol. 1*, edited by A. D. Johnson, W. R. Gomes, and N. L. Van Demark, pp. 483–550. Academic Press, New York.
533. Albert, A. (1961): The mammalian testis. In: *Sex and Internal Secretions, Vol. 1*, edited by W. C. Young, pp. 305–365. Williams & Wilkins, Baltimore.
534. Burgos, M. H., Vitale-Calpe, R., and Aoki, A. (1970): Fine structure of the testis and its functional significance. In: *The Testis, Vol. 1*, edited by A. D. Johnson, W. R. Gomes, and N. L. Van Demark, pp. 551–649. Academic Press, New York.
535. Fawcett, D. W., Heidger, D. M., and Leak, L. V. (1969): Lymph vascular system of the interstitial tissue of the testis as revealed by electron microscopy. *J. Reprod. Fertil.*, 19:109–119.
536. Connell, C. J., and Connell, G. M. (1977): The interstitial tissue of the testis. In: *The Testis, Vol. 4*, edited by A. D. Johnson and W. R. Gomes, pp. 333–370. Academic Press, New York.
537. Christensen, A. K. (1975): Leydig cells. In: *Handbook of Physiology, Section 7, Vol. 5, Male Reproductive System*, edited by D. W. Hamilton and R. O. Greep, pp. 57–94. Williams & Wilkins, Baltimore.
538. Leydig, F. (1850): Zur Anatomie der mannlichen Geschelechtsorgane und Analdrusen ser Saugetiere. *Z. Wiss. Zool.*, 2:1–57.
539. Hofmeister, H. (1872): Untersuchungen über die Zwischensubstanz im Hoden der Saugethiere. *Sitzungsb. Acad. Wissensch. Mathnaturw. Classe. Wien*, 5:77.
540. Plato, J. (1896): Die interstitiellen Zellen des Hodens und ihre physiologische Bedeutung. *Arch. Mikrosk. Anat.*, 48:280.
541. Lenhossek, M. (1897): Beitrage zur Kenntniss der Zwischenzellen des Hodens. *Arch. f. Anat. Physiol. Anat. Abt.*, 65:1–25.
542. Loisel, G. (1902): Etudes sur le spermatogenese chez le moineau domestique. *J. L'Anat. Physiol.*, 33:112.
543. Ganfini, C. (1902): Struttura e sviluppo delle cellule interstiziali del testicolo. *Arch. Ital. Anat. Embriol.*, 1:233.
544. Bouin, P., and Ancel, P. (1904): La glande interstitielle a seule dans le testicule une action generale sur l'organisme. *Demonstration Experimentale C. R. Acad. Sci. Paris*, 138:110.
545. Ancel, P., and Bouin, P. (1903): L'apparition des caracteres sexuels secondaires est sous la dependance de la gland interstitielle. *C. R. Acad. Sci. [D] Paris*, 138:168.
546. Ciaccio, C. (1910): Contributo alla distribuzione ed alla fisiopathologia cellulare dei lipoidi. *Arch. Zellforsch.*, 5:235.
547. Whitehead, R. H. (1912): On the chemical nature of certain granules in the interstitial cells of the testis. *Am. J. Anat.*, 14:63.
548. Lotz, A., and Jaffe, R. (1924): Die Hoden bei Allgemeiknerkrankungen. *Z. Konstit.*, 10:99.
549. McGee, L. C. (1927): Effect of injections of lipid fraction of bull testicle in capons. *Proc. Inst. Med. Chic.*, 6:242.
550. Gallagher, T. F., and Koch, F. C. (1929): The testicular hormone. *J. Biol. Chem.*, 84:495–500.
551. Butenandt, A., and Hanisch, G. (1935): Über Testosteron. Umwandlung des Dehydroandrosterons in Androstenediol und Testosteron: ein Weg zur Darstellung des Testosterons ans Cholesterin. *Z. Physiol. Chem.*, 237:89–97.
552. Ruzicka, L., and Wettstein, A. (1935): Kunstliche Herstellung des mannlichen Sexualhormones Transdehydro-androsten-3,17-dions. *Helv. Chim. Acta*, 18:986–994.
553. Wattenberg, L. W. (1958): Microscopic histochemical demonstration of steroid-3-ol dehydrogenase in tissue secretions. *J. Histochem. Cytochem.*, 6:225–232.
554. Levy, H., Deane, H. W., and Rubin, B. L. (1959): Visualization of steroid-3-ol-dehydrogenase activity in tissues of intact and hypophysectomized rats. *Endocrinology*, 65:932–943.
555. Baillie, A. H. (1964): Further observations on the growth and histochemistry of the Leydig tissue in the postnatal prepubertal mouse testis. *J. Anat.*, 98:403–419.
556. Christensen, A. K., and Mason, N. R. (1965): Comparative ability of seminiferous tubules and interstitial tissue of rat testes to synthesize androgens from progesterone-4-^{14}C *in vitro*. *Endocrinology*, 76:646–656.
557. Hall, P. F., Irby, D. C., and de Kretser, D. M. (1969): Conversion of cholesterol to androgens by rat testes: comparison of interstitial cells and seminiferous tubules. *Endocrinology*, 84:488–496.
558. Ludwig, C., and Tomsa, W. (1862): Die Lymphwege des Hodens und ihr Verhaltnis zu den Blut- und Samengefassen. *S. Ber. Akad. Wiss. Wein Math. Kl.*, 46:221.
559. Freg, H. (1963): Zur Kenntnis der Lymphbahnen in Hoden. *Virchows Arch.*, 28:563–569.
560. Regaud, C. (1897): Les vaisseaux lymphatiques de testicule. *C. R. Soc. Biol. (Paris)*, 14:695.
561. Testus, L. (1902): *Traite d'anatomie humanie*. Octave Doin, Paris.
562. Mihalkovics, V. (1873): Beitrage zur Anatomie und Histologie des Hodens. *Ber. Verbandl. K. Sachs. Gesellsch. Wiss. Math. Kl. (Leipzig)*, 25:217.
563. Gerster, R. (1876): Über die Lymphgefasse des Hodens. *Z. Anat. Entwicklungsgesch.*, 2:36.
564. Hasumi, S. (1930): Anatomische Untersuchungen über die Lymphgefasse des mannlichen Urogenital-systems. *Jpn. J. Med. Sci. Anat.*, 11:159–186.
565. Renyi Vamos, F. (1955): Das Lymphsystem des Hodens und Nebenhodens. *Z. Urol.*, 48:355–372.
566. Renyi Vamos, F. (1956): Beitrage und Richlinien zur Anatomie des Lymphgefassystems. *Virchows Arch. [Pathol. Anat.]*, 328:503.
567. Brzezinski, V. D. K. (1963): Nene Befunde mit einer verbesserten Darstellung experimentell anfgefullter Lymphkapillaren an Niere, Hoden-Nebenhoden, Darm- und Dickdaom. *Anat. Anz.*, 113:289–306.
568. Staudt, J., and Wenzel, J. (1965): Untersuchungen über das Lymphgefassystem des Kaninchenhodens. *Z. Mikrosk. Anat. Forsch.*, 73:60–72.
569. Clark, R. V. (1976): Three-dimensional organization of testicular interstitial tissue and lymphatic space in the rat. *Anat. Rec.*, 184:203–226.
570. Holstein, A. F., Orlandini, G. E., and Moller, R. (1979): Distribution and fine structure of the lymphatic system in the human testis. *Cell Tissue Res.*, 200:15–27.
571. Wagner, K. (1925): Sind die Zwischenzellen des Saugetierhodens Drusenzellen? Ein Beitrag zur Zytologie und Zygotogenese. *Biologia Generalis*, 1:22.
572. Hooker, C. W., Pfeiffer, C. A., and De Vita, J. (1946): The significance of the diameter of the interstitial cells of the testis in the aged dog. *Anat. Rec.*, 94:471–472.
573. Stein, A. A. (1931): Experimentelle Untersuchungen über die Zellformen des interstitiellen Hodengewebes. *Z. Zellforsch.*, 12:483.
574. Esaki, S. (1928): Über Kulturen des Hodengewebes der Saugthiere und über die Nater der interstitiellen Hodengewebes und des Zwischenzellen. *Z. Mikrosk. Anat. Forsch.*, 15:368–404.
575. Evans, H. M., and Schulemann, W. (1914): The action of vital stains belonging to the benzidine group. *Science*, 39:443.
576. Christensen, A. K., and Peacock, K. C. (1980): Increase in Leydig cell number in testis of adult rats treated chronically with an excess of human chorionic gonadotropin. *Biol. Reprod.*, 22: 383–392.

577. Ennist, D. L., and Jones, K. H. (1983): Rapid method for identification of macrophages in suspension by acid alpha-naphtyl acetate esterase activity. *J. Histochem. Cytochem.*, 31:960–963.
578. Molenaar, R., Rommerts, F. F. G., and van der Molen, H. J. (1986): Non-specific esterase: a specific and useful marker enzyme for Leydig cells from mature rats. *J. Endocrinol.* 108:329–335.
579. Miller, S. C., Bowman, B. M., and Rosland, H. G. (1983): Structure, cytochemistry, endocytic activity, and immunoglobulin (Fc) receptors of rat testicular interstitial-tissue macrophages. *Am. J. Anat.*, 168:1–13.
580. Miller, S. C. (1982): Localization of plutonium-241 in the testis. An interspecies comparison using light and electron microscope autoradiography. *Int. J. Radiat. Biol.*, 41:633–643.
581. Miller, S. C., and Bowman, B. M. (1983): Tissue, cellular and subcellular distribution of ^{241}Pu in the rat testis. *Radiat. Res.*, 94:416–426.
582. Orth, J., and Christensen, A. K. (1977): Localization of ^{125}I-labelled FSH in the testes of hypophysectomized rats by autoradiography at the light and electron microscope levels. *Endocrinology*, 101:262–278.
583. Christensen, A. K., Komorowski, T. E., Wilson, B., Ma, S.-F., and Stevens, R. W. (1985): The distribution of serum albumin in the rat testis, studies by electron micrscope immunocytochemistry on ultrathin frozen sections. *Endocrinology*, 116:1983–1996.
584. Bergh, A. (1985): Effect of cryptorchidism on the morphology of testicular macrophages: evidence for a Leydig cell-macrophage interaction in the rat testis. *Int. J. Andrology*, 8:86–96.
585. Kerr, J. B., Donachie, K. I., and Rommerts, F. F. G. (1985): Selective destruction and regeneration of rat Leydig cells *in vivo*. A new method for the study of seminiferous tubular-interstitial tissue interaction. *Cell Tissue Res.*, 242:145–156.
586. Jackson, A. E., O'Leary, P. O. I., Ayers, M. M., and de Kretser, D. M. (1986): The effects of ethylene dimethane sulphonate (EDS) on rat Leydig cells: evidence to support a connective tissue origin of Leydig cells. *Biol. Reprod.*, 35:425–437.
587. Kerr, J. B., Bartlett, J. M. S., and Donachie, K. (1986): Acute response of testicular interstitial tissue in rats to the cytotoxic drug ethane dimethanesulfonate. *Cell Tissue Res.*, 243:405–414.
588. Gunn, S. A., and Gould, T. C. (1975): Vasculature of the testes and adnexa. In: *Handbook of Physiology, Section 7, Endocrinology, Vol. 5, Male Reproductive System*, edited by D. W. Hamilton and R. O. Greep, pp. 117–142. Williams & Wilkins, Baltimore.
589. Maseki, Y., Miyake, K., Mitsuya, H., Kitamura, H., and Yamada, K. (1981): Mastocytosis occurring in the testes from patients with idiopathic male infertility. *Fertil. Steril.*, 36:814–817.
590. Nistal, M., Santamaria, L., and Paniagua, R. (1984): Mast cells in the human testis and epididymis from birth to adulthood. *Acta Anat.*, 119:155–160.
591. Pilsworth, L. M., and Setchell, B. P. (1981): Spermatogenic and endocrine functions of the testes of invertebrate and vertebrate animals. In: *The Testis*, edited by H. G. Burger and D. M. de Kretser, pp. 9–38. Raven Press, New York.
592. Roosen-Runge, E. C. (1977): *The Process of Spermatogenesis in Animals*. Cambridge University Press, Cambridge, U.K.
593. Lofts, B. (1968): Patterns of testicular activity. In: *Perspectives in Endocrinology. Hormones in the Lives of Lower Vertebrate*, edited by E. J. W. Barrington and C. B. Jorgensen, pp. 239–304. Academic Press, London.
594. Lofts, B. (1974): Reproduction. In: *Physiology of the Amphibia, Vol. II*, edited by B. Lofts, pp. 107–218. Academic Press, New York.
595. Pudney, J., Canick, J. A., Mak, P., and Callard, G. V. (1983): The differentiation of Leydig cells, steroidogenesis and the spermatogenic wave in the testis of *Necturus maculosus*. *Gen. Comp. Endocrinol.*, 50:43–66.
596. Ucci, A. A. (1982): A fine structural study of interstitial cell changes in the testis of *Necturus maculosus* during a portion of the annual cycle, and possible evidence for local feedback control by seminiferous epithelium. *Am. J. Anat.*, 165:22–38.
597. Schulze, C. (1973): Saisonbedingte Veranderungen in der Morphologie der Leydigzellen von *Rana esculenta*. *Z. Zellforsch.*, 142:367–386.
598. Terao, K. (1973): Annular nucleolus in Leydig cells of mouse. *Z. Zellforsch.*, 137:167–175.
599. Terao, L., Sakaibara, Y., Yamazaki, M., and Miyaki, K. (1971): Annular nucleolus in chicken embryonal hepatocyte induced by aflatoxin B_1. *Exp. Cell Res.*, 66:81–89.
600. Christensen, A. K., and Fawcett, D. W. (1966): The fine structure of testicular interstitial cells in mics. *Am. J. Anat.*, 118:551–572.
601. de Kretser, D. M. (1967): The fine structure of the testicular interstitial cells in men of normal androgenic status. *Z. Zellforsch.*, 80:594–609.
602. de Kretser, D. M. (1967): Changes in the fine structure of human testicular interstitial cells after treatment with human gonadotrophins. *Z. Zellforsch.*, 83:344–358.
603. Kerr, J. B., Rich, K. A., and de Kretser, D. M. (1979): Alteration of the fine structure and androgen secretion of the interstitial cells in the experimentally cryptorchid rat testis. *Biol. Reprod.*, 20:409–422.
604. Mori, H., and Christensen, A. K. (1980): Morphometric analysis of Leydig cells in the normal rat testis. *J. Cell Biol.*, 84:340–354.
605. Zirkin, B. R., Ewing, L. L., Kromann, N., and Cochran, R. C. (1980): Testosterone secretion by rat, rabbit, guinea pig, dog and hamster testes perfused *in vitro:* correlation with Leydig cell ultrastructure. *Endocrinology*, 107:1867–1874.
606. Mori, H., Kadota, A., Fukunishi, R., Kukita, H., Takeuchi, N., and Matsumoto, K. (1980): Effects of a cholesterol-rich-diet and a hypolipidemic drug (Clofibrate, CP1B) on Leydig cells in rats: stereological and biochemical analysis. *Andrologia*, 12: 271–291.
607. Mori, H., Hiromoto, N., Nakahara, M., and Shiraishi, T. (1982): Stereological analysis of Leydig cell ultrastructure in aged humans. *J. Clin. Endocrinol. Metab.*, 55:634–641.
608. Mori, H., Shimizu, D., Fukunishi, Y., and Christensen, A. K. (1982): Morphometric analysis of testicular Leydig cells in normal adult mice. *Anat. Rec.*, 204:333–339.
609. Connell, C. J., and Christensen, A. K. (1975): The ultrastructure of the canine testicular interstitial tissue. *Biol. Reprod.*, 12:368–382.
610. Weaker, F. J. (1977): The fine structure of the interstitial tissue of the testis of the nine-banded armadillo. *Anat. Rec.*, 187:11–28.
611. Camatini, M., Franchi, E., and De Curtis, I. (1981): Ultrastructure of Leydig cells in the African green monkey. *J. Ultrastruct. Res.*, 76:224–234.
612. Murakami, M., and Kitahara, Y. (1971): Cylindrical bodies derived from endoplasmic reticulum in Leydig cells of the rat testis. *J. Electron Microsc. (Tokyo)*, 20:318–323.
613. Christensen, A. K., and Fawcett, D. W. (1961): The normal fine structure of opossum testicular interstitial cells. *J. Biophys. Biochem. Cytol.*, 9:653–670.
614. Nakai, Y. (1974): Adult intersitial cell. In: *An Atlas of Electron Micrographs. Functional Morphology of Endocrine Glands*, edited by K. Kurosumi and H. Fujita, pp. 178–179. Igaku Shoin, Tokyo.
615. Emura, S. (1978): Electron microscopic studies on annulate lamellae in Leydig cells of rabbit. *Cell*, 10:752–756.
616. Ohata, M. (1979): Electron microscopic study on the testicular interstitial cells in the mouse. *Arch. Histol. Jpn.*, 42:51–79.
617. Ewing, L. L., Zirkin, B. R., Cochran, R. C., Kromann, N., Peters, C., and Ruiz-Bravo, N. (1979): Testosterone secretion by rat, rabbit, guinea pig, dog, and hamster testes perfused *in vitro:* correlation with Leydig cell mass. *Endocrinology*, 105:1135–1142.
618. Wing, T. Y., Ewing, L. L., and Zirkin, B. R. (1984): Effects of luteinizing hormone withdrawal on Leydig cell smooth endoplasmic reticulum and steroidogenic reactions which convert pregnenolone to testosterone. *Endocrinology*, 115:2290–2296.
619. Wing, T. Y., Ewing, L. L., Zegeye, B., and Zirkin, B. R. (1985): Restoration effects of exogenous luteinizing hormone on the testicular steroidogenesis and Leydig cell ultrastructure. *Endocrinology*, 117:1179–1787.
620. Russell, L. D., and Burguet, S. (1977): Ultrastructure of Leydig cells as revealed by secondary tissue treatment with a ferrocyanide-osmium mixture. *Tissue Cell*, 9:751–766.
621. Aoki, A., and Massa, E. M. (1972): Early responses of testicular interstitial cells to stimulation by interstitial cell stimulating hormone. *Am. J. Anat.*, 134:239–262.
622. Kerr, J. B., Robertson, D. M., and de Kretser, D. M. (1985): Morphological and functional characterization of interstitial cells from mouse testes fractionated on Percoll density gradients. *Endocrinology*, 116:1030–1043.

623. Wrobel, K. H., Sinowatz, F., and Mademann, R. (1981): Intertubular topography in the bovine testis. *Cell Tissue Res.*, 217:289–310.
624. Belt, W. D., and Cavazos, L. F. (1971): Fine structure of the interstitial cells of Leydig in the squirrel monkey during seasonal regression. *Anat. Rec.*, 169:115–128.
625. Russo, J., and Sacerdote, F. C. (1971): Ultrastructural changes induced by hCG in the Leydig cell of the adult mouse testis. *Z. Zellforsch.*, 112:363–370.
626. Nussdorfer, G. G., Robba, C., Mazzocchi, G., and Rebuffat, P. (1980): Effects of chorionic gonadotrophins on the interstitial cells of the rat testis: a morphometric and radioimmunological study. *Int. J. Andrology*, 3:319–332.
627. Neaves, W. B. (1978): The pattern of gonadotropin-induced changes in plasma testosterone, testicular esterified cholesterol and Leydig cell lipid droplets in immature mice. *Biol. Reprod.*, 19:864–871.
628. Aoki, A. (1970): Hormonal control of Leydig cell differentiation. *Protoplasma*, 71:209–225.
629. Merkow, L., Acevedo, H., Slifkia, M., and Caito, M. (1968): Studies on the interstitial cells of the testis: I. The ultrastructure of the immature guinea pig and the effect of stimulation with human chorionic gonadotropin. *Am. J. Pathol.*, 33:47–62.
630. Aoki, A., and Massa, E. M. (1975): Subcellular compartmentation of free and esterified cholesterol in the interstitial cells in the mouse testis. *Cell Tissue Res.*, 165:49–62.
631. Lalli, M. F., and Clermont, Y. (1975): Leydig cells and their role in the synthesis and secretion of glycoproteins. *Anat. Rec.*, 181:403–404.
632. Gemmell, R. T., and Stacy, B. D. (1979): Ultrastructural study of granules in the corpora lutea of several mammalian species. *Am. J. Anat.*, 155:1–14.
633. Gemmell, R. T., Laychock, S. G., and Rubin, R. P. (1977): Ultrastructural and biochemical evidence for a steroid-containing secretory organelle in the perfused cat adrenal gland. *J. Cell Biol.*, 72:209–215.
634. Loh, H. S., and Gemmell, R. T. (1980): Changes in the fine structure of the Leydig cells of the seasonally breeding bat, *Myotis adversus*. *Cell Tissue Res.*, 210:339–347.
635. Paavola, L. G., and Boyd, C. O. (1981): Cytoplasmic granules in luteal cells of pregnant and non-pregnant guinea pigs. A cytochemical study. *Anat. Rec.*, 201:127–140.
636. Porter, D. G. (1979): Relaxin: old hormone, new prospect. *Oxford Rev. Reprod. Endocrinol.*, 1:1–45.
637. Fields, P. A., Eldridge, R. K., Fuchs, A. R., Roberts, R. F., and Fields, M. J. (1983): Human placental and bovine corpora luteal oxytocin. *Endocrinology*, 112:1544–1546.
638. Hermo, L., Clermont, Y., and Lalli, M. (1985): Intracellular pathways of endocytosed tracers in Leydig cells of the rat. *J. Andrology*, 6:213–224.
639. Fawcett, D. W., and Burgos, M. H. (1960): Studies on the fine structure of the mammalian testis. II. The human interstitial tissue. *Am. J. Anat.*, 107:245–269.
640. Yamada, E. (1965): Some observations on the fine structure of the interstitial cells and Sertoli cells of the human testis. *Gunma Symp. Endocrinol.*, 2:1–17.
641. Nagano, T. (1965): Some observations on the structure of interstitial cells and Sertoli cells of the human testis. *Gunma Symp. Endocrinol.*, 2:19–28.
642. Reddy, J., and Svoboda, D. (1972): Microbodies (peroxisomes) in the interstitial cells of rodent testes. *Lab. Invest.*, 26:657–665.
643. Hruban, Z., Vigil, E. L., Steasers, A., and Hopkins, E. (1972): Microbodies, constituent organelles of animals. *Lab. Invest.*, 27:184–191.
644. Usui, N. (1976): Fine structure of interstitial cells and macrophages in immature rat testes. *J. Tokyo Womens Med. College*, 46: 809–825.
645. Tanuma, Y., and Ohata, M. (1978): Transmission electron microscopic observation of epithelial cells with single cilia in intrahepatic biliary ductules of bats. *Arch. Histol. Jpn.*, 41:367–376.
646. Temple, R., and Wolff, J. (1973): Stimulation of steroid secretion by antimicrotubular agents. *J. Biol. Chem.*, 248:2691.
647. Ray, P., and Strott, C. A. (1978): Stimulation of steroid synthesis by normal rat adrenocortical cells in response to antimicrotubular agents. *Endocrinology*, 103:1281–1288.
648. Clark, M. A., and Shay, J.-W. (1981): The role of tubulin in the steroidogenic response of murine adrenal and rat Leydig cells. *Endocrinology*, 109:2261–2263.
649. Laws, A. O., Kerr, J. B., and de Kretser, D. M. (1984): The role of the microtubular system in LH/hCG receptor downregulation in rat Leydig cells. *Mol. Cell. Endocrinol.*, 38:39–51.
650. Reinke, F. (1896): Beitrage zur Histologie des Menschen. *Arch. Mikrosk. Anat.*, 47:34–44.
651. Nagano, T., and Ohtsuki, I. (1971): Reinvestigation of the fine structure of Reinke's crystals in the human testicular interstitial cell. *J. Cell Biol.*, 51:148–161.
652. Yasuzumi, G., Nakai, Y., Tsubo, I., Yasuda, M., and Sugioka, T. (1967): The fine structure of nuclei as revealed by electronmicroscopy: IV. The intranuclear inclusion formation of Leydig cells of ageing human testes. *Exp. Cell Res.*, 45:261–276.
653. Janko, A. B., and Sandberg, E. C. (1970): Histochemical evidence for the protein nature of the Reinke crystalloid. *Obstet. Gynecol.*, 35:493–503.
654. Mori, H., Fukunishi, R., Fujii, M., Hataji, K., Shiraishi, T., and Matsumoto, K. (1978): Stereological analysis of Reinke crystals in human Leydig cells. *Virchows Arch. [Pathol. Anat.]*, 380:1–10.
655. Sohval, A. R., Gabrilove, J. L., and Chung, J. (1973): Ultrastructure of Leydig cell paracrystalline inclusions, possibly related to Reinke crystals, in the normal testis. *Z. Zellforsch.*, 142:13–26.
656. Kerr, J. B., Abbenhuys, D. C., and Irby, D. C. (1986): Crystalloid formation in rat Leydig cells. An ultrastructural and hormonal study. *Cell Tissue Res.*, 245:91–100.
657. Satoh, M. (1985): The histogenesis of the gonads in rat embryos. *J. Anat.*, 143:17–37.
658. Pelliniemi, L. J., and Dym, M. (1980): The fetal gonad and sexual differentiation. In: *Maternal-Fetal Endocrinology*, edited by D. Tulchinsky and K. J. Ryan, pp. 252–280. W. B. Saunders, Philadelphia.
659. Mancini, R. E., Vilar, O., Lavieri, J. C., Andrada, J. A., and Heinrich, J. J. (1963): Development of Leydig cells in the normal human testis. *Am. J. Anat.*, 112:203–214.
660. Pelliniemi, L., Dym, M., Crigler, J., Retik, A., and Fawcett, D. W. (1980): Development of Leydig cells in human fetuses and in patients with androgen insensitivity. In: *Testicular Development, Structure, and Function*, edited by A. Steinberger and E. Steinberger, pp. 49–54. Raven Press, New York.
661. Gondos, B. (1980): Development and differentiation of the testis and male reproductive tract. In: *Testicular Development, Structure, and Function*, edited by A. Steinberger and E. Steinberger, pp. 3–20. Raven Press, New York.
662. Gondos, B. (1981): Cellular interrelationships in the human foetal ovary and testis. *Prog. Clin. Biol. Res.*, 59:373–381.
663. Witschi, E. (1951): Embryogenesis of the adrenal and the reproductive gland. *Recent Prog. Horm. Res.*, 6:1–27.
664. Holstein, A. F., Wartenberg, H., and Vossmeyer, J. (1971): Zur Cytologie de pranatalen Gonadenentwicklung beim Menschen. III. Die Entwicklung der Leydig-zellen im Hoden von Embryonen und Feten. *Z. Anat. Entwicklungsgesch.*, 135:43–66.
665. Gondos, B., Paup, D., Ross, J., and Gorski, P. (1974): Ultrastructural differentiation of Leydig cells in the fetal and postnatal hamster testis. *Anat. Rec.*, 178:551–556.
666. Gondos, B., Renston, R., and Goldstein, D. (1976): Postnatal differentiation of Leydig cells in the rabbit testis. *Am. J. Anat.*, 145:167–182.
667. Gondos, B., Morrison, K., and Renston, R. (1977): Leydig cell differentiation in the prepubertal rabbit testis. *Biol. Reprod.*, 17:745–748.
668. Niemi, M., and Kormano, M. (1964): Cell renewal in the interstitial tissue of postnatal prepubertal rat testis. *Endocrinology*, 74: 996–998.
669. Prince, F. P. (1984): Ultrastructure of immature Leydig cells in the human prepubertal testis. *Anat. Rec.*, 209:165–176.
670. Chemes, H. E., Gottlieb, S. E., Pasqualini, T., Domenichini, E., Rivarola, M. A., and Bergada, C. (1985): Response to acute hCG stimulation and steroidogenic potential of Leydig cell fibroblastic precursors in humans. *J. Andrology*, 6:102–112.
671. Dierichs, R., Wrobel, K. H., and Schilling, E. (1973): Licht und elektronenmikroskopische Untersuchungen an den Leydigzellen des Schweines wahrend der postnatalen Entwicklung. *Z. Zellforsch.*, 143:207–227.

672. Dierichs, R., and Wrobel, K. H. (1973): Licht und elektronenmikroskopische Untersuchnugen an den peritubularen Zellen des Schwinhoden wahrend der postnatalen Entwicklung. *Z. Anat. Entwicklungsgesch.*, 143:49–64.
673. van Straaten, H. W. M., and Wensing, C. J. G. (1977): Histomorphometric aspect of testicular morphogenesis in the pig. *Biol. Reprod.*, 17:467–472.
674. van Straaten, H. W. M., and Wensing, C. J. G. (1978): Leydig cell development in the testis of the pig. *Biol. Reprod.*, 18:86–93.
675. Bressler, R. S., and Ross, M. H. (1972): Differentiation of peritubular myoid cells of the testis: effects of intratesticular implantation of newborn mouse testes into normal and hypophysectomized adults. *Biol. Reprod.*, 6:148–159.
676. Mori, H., Shiraishi, T., and Matsumoto, K. (1978): Leydig cells within the lamina propria of seminiferous tubules in four patients with azoospermia. *Andrologia*, 10:444–452.
677. Sniffen, R. C. (1950): The testis. I. The normal testis. *Arch. Pathol.*, 50:259–284.
678. Vilar, O. (1970): Histology of the human testis from neonatal period to adolescence. In: *The Human Testis*, edited by E. Rosenberg and C. A. Paulsen, pp. 95–108. Plenum, New York.
679. Hadziselimovic, F. (1977): Cryptorchidism: ultrastructure of normal and cryptorchid testis development. *Adv. Anat. Embryol. Cell Biol.*, 53:1–17.
680. Whitehead, R. H. (1904): The embryonic development of the interstitial cells of Leydig. *Am. J. Anat.*, 3:167.
681. Whitehead, R. H. (1905): Studies on the interstitial cells of Leydig. No. 2. Their post-embryonic development in the pig. *Am. J. Anat.*, 4:193.
682. Roosen-Runge, E. C., and Anderson, D. (1959): The development of the interstitial cells in the testis of the albino rat. *Acta Anat.*, 37:125–137.
683. Fouquet, J. P., Meusy-Dessolle, N., and Dang, D. G. (1984): Relationships between Leydig cell morphometry and plasma testosterone during postnatal development of the monkey, *Macaca fascicularis*. *Reprod. Nutr. Devel.*, 24:281–286.
684. Winter, J. S. D., Faiman, C., and Reyes, F. I. (1977): Sex steroid production by the human fetus: its role in morphogenesis and control by gonadotropins. In: *Birth Defects, Original Article Series, Vol. 13, No. 2: Morphogenesis and Malformation of the Genital System*, edited by R. J. Blandau and D. Bergsma, pp. 41–52. Alan R. Liss, New York.
685. Faiman, C., Winter, J. S. D., and Reyes, F. I. (1981): Endocrinology of the fetal testis. In: *The Testis*, edited by H. G. Burger and D. M. de Kretser, pp. 81–105. Raven Press, New York.
686. Niemi, M., Ikonen, M., and Hervonen, A. (1967): Histochemistry and fine structure of the interstitial tissue in the human foetal testis. In: *Endocrinology of the Testis*, edited by G. E. W. Wolstenholme and M. O'Connor, pp. 31–55. Churchill, London.
687. Gruenwald, P. (1946): Structure of the testis in infancy and in childhood. *Arch. Pathol.*, 42:35–48.
688. Ottowicz, J. (1963): The stadial development of Leydig cells. *Acta Med. Pol.*, 4:1–13.
689. Sharpe, R. M. (1982): The hormonal regulation of the Leydig cell. In: *Oxford Reviews of Reproductive Biology*, edited by C. A. Finn, pp. 241–317. Oxford University Press, Oxford.
690. Sharpe, R. M. (1983): Local control of testicular function. *Q. J. Exp. Physiol.*, 68:265–287.
691. Sharpe, R. M. (1984): Intratesticular factors controlling testicular function. *Biol. Reprod.*, 30:29–49.
692. Ichihara, I. (1970): The fine structure of testicular interstitial cells in mice during postnatal development. *Z. Zellforsch.*, 108:475–486.
693. Faiman, C., and Winter, J. S. D. (1974): Gonadotropins and sex hormone patterns in puberty: clinical data. In: *The Control of the Onset of Puberty*, edited by M. M. Grumbach, G. D. Grave, and F. E. Mayer, p. 32. Wiley, New York.
694. Swerdloff, R. S., and Heber, D. (1981): Endocrine control of testicular function from birth to puberty. In: *The Testis*, edited by H. G. Burger and D. M. de Kretser, pp. 107–126. Raven Press, New York.
695. Odell, W. D., and Swerdloff, R. S. (1974): The role of the gonads in sexual maturation. In: *The Control of the Onset of Puberty*, edited by M. M. Grumbach, G. D. Grave, and F. E. Mayer, p. 313. Wiley, New York.
696. Odell, W. D., and Swerdloff, R. S. (1976): Etiologies of sexual maturation: a model system based on the sexually maturing rat. *Recent Prog. Horm. Res.*, 32:245.
697. Lee, V. W. K., and Burger, H. G. (1983): Pituitary testicular axis during pubertal development. In: *The Pituitary and Testis. Clinical and Experimental Studies*, edited by D. M. de Kretser, H. G. Burger, and B. Hudson, pp. 44–83. Springer-Verlag, Berlin.
698. Charny, C., Conston, A., and Meranze, D. (1952): Development of the testis. *Fertil. Steril.*, 3:461–479.
699. de la Balze, F., Mancini, R., Arrillaga, F., Andrada, J., and Vilar, O. (1960): Pubertal maturation of the normal testis. A histologic study. *J. Clin. Endocrinol. Metab.*, 20:266–285.
700. Hayashi, H., and Harrison, R. (1971): The development of the interstitial tissue of the human testis. *Fertil. Steril.*, 22:351–355.
701. Forti, G., Santoro, S., Grisolia, G. A., Bassi, F., Boinnsegni, R., Fiorelli, G., and Serio, M. (1981): Spermatic and peripheral plasma concentrations of testosterone and androstenedione in prepubertal boys. *J. Clin. Endocrinol. Metab.*, 53:883–886.
702. Rivarola, M. A., Bergada, C., and Cullen, M. (1970): hCG stimulation test in prepubertal boys with cryptorchidism, in bilateral anorchia and in male pseudohermaphroditism. *J. Clin. Endocrinol. Metab.*, 31:526–530.
703. Chen, Y. D. I., Shaw, M. J., and Payne, A. P. (1977): Steroid and FSH action on LH receptors and LH-sensitive testicular responsiveness during sexual maturation of the rat. *Mol. Cell. Endocrinol.*, 8:291–299.
704. Odell, W. D., Swerdloff, R. S., Jacobs, H. S., and Hescox, M. A. (1973): FSH induction of sensitivity to LH: one cause of sexual maturation in the male rat. *Endocrinology*, 92:160–165.
705. van Beurden, W. M. O., Roodnat, B., de Jong, F. H., Mulder, E., and van der Molen, H. J. (1976): Hormonal regulation of LH stimulation of testosterone production in isolated Leydig cells of immature rats: the effects of hypophysectomy, FSH and estradiol-17. *Steroids*, 28:847–866.
706. Chen, Y. D. I., Payne, A. P., and Kelch, R. P. (1976): FSH stimulation of Leydig cell function in the hypophysectomized immature rat. *Proc. Soc. Exp. Biol. Med.*, 153:473–475.
707. Odell, W. D., and Swerdloff, R. S. (1975): The role of testicular sensitivity to gonadotrophins in sexual maturation of the male rat. *J. Steroid Biochem.*, 6:853–857.
708. Selin, L. K., and Moger, W. H. (1977): The effect of FSH on LH induced testosterone secretion in the immature hypophysectomized male rat. *Endocrine Res. Commun.*, 4:171–182.
709. Kerr, J. B., and Sharpe, R. M. (1985): Follicle-stimulating hormone induction of Leydig cell maturation. *Endocrinology*, 116:2592–2604.
710. Kerr, J. B., and Sharpe, R. M. (1985): Stimulatory effect of follicle-stimulating hormone on rat Leydig cells. A morphometric and ultrastructural study. *Cell Tissue Res.*, 239:405–415.
711. Neaves, W. B. (1973): Changes in testicular Leydig cells and in plasma testosterone levels among seasonally breeding rock hyrax. *Biol. Reprod.*, 8:451–466.
712. Neaves, W. B. (1979): The annual testicular cycle in an equatorial colony of lesser rock hyrax, *Heterohyrax brucei*. *Proc. R. Soc. Lond. [Biol.]*, 206:183–189.
713. Neaves, W. B. (1980): Asynchronous testicular cycles among equatorial colonies of rock hyrax (*Procavia habessinica*). In: *Testicular Development, Structure, and Function*, edited by A. Steinberger and E. Steinberger, pp. 411–418. Raven Press, New York.
714. Gustafson, A. W. (1975): Observations on the hydroxysteroid dehydrogenase and lipid histochemistry and ultrastructure of the Leydig cells in adult *Myotis lucifugus* during the annual reproductive cycle. *Anat. Rec.*, 181:366–367.
715. Wing, T. Y., and Lin, H. S. (1977): The fine structure of testicular interstitial cells in the adult golden hamster with special reference to seasonal changes. *Cell Tissue Res.*, 183:385–393.
716. Suzuki, F., and Racey, P. A. (1978): The organization of testicular interstitial tissue and changes in the fine structure of the Leydig cells of European moles (*Tulpa europaea*) throughout the year. *J. Reprod. Fertil.*, 52:189–194.
717. Wislocki, G. B. (1949): Seasonal changes in the testes, epididymides and seminal vesicles of deer investigated by histochemical methods. *Endocrinology*, 44:167–189.
718. Lofts, B. (1960): Cyclical changes in the distribution of the testis lipids of a seasonal mammal (*Talpa europaea*). *Q. J. Microsc. Sci.*, 101:199–205.

719. Kothari, L. K., and Gupta, A. S. (1974): Effect of ageing on the volume, structure and total Leydig cell content of the human testis. *Int. J. Fertil.*, 19:140–146.
720. Honore, L. H. (1978): Ageing changes in the human testis: a light microscopic study. *Gerontology*, 24:58–65.
721. Teem, M. V. B. (1935): The relation of the interstitial cells of the testis to prostatic hypertrophy. *J. Urol.*, 34:692–713.
722. Sargent, J. W., and McDonald, J. R. (1948): A method for the quantitative estimate of Leydig cells in the human testis. *Proc. Staff Meetings Mayo Clinic*, 23:249–254.
723. Sokal, Z. (1964): Morphology of the human testis in various periods of life. *Folia Morphol.*, 23:102–111.
724. Vermeulen, A. (1976): Leydig cell function in old age. In: *Hypothalamus, Pituitary and Ageing*, edited by A. V. Everitt and J. A. Burgess, pp. 458–463. Charles Thomas, Springfield, Ill.
725. Kaler, L. W., and Neaves, W. B. (1978): Attrition of the human Leydig cell population with advancing age. *Anat. Rec.*, 192:513–518.
726. Neaves, W. B., Johnson, L., Porter, J. C., Parker, C. R., and Petty, C. S. (1984): Leydig cell numbers, daily sperm production and serum gonadotropin levels in aging men. *J. Clin. Endocrinol. Metab.*, 59:756–763.
727. Neaves, W. B., Johnson, L., and Petty, C. S. (1985): Age-related change in numbers of other interstitial cells in testes of adult men: evidence bearing on the fate of Leydig cells lost with increasing age. *Biol. Reprod.*, 33:259–269.
728. Kaler, L. W., and Neaves, W. B. (1981): The androgen status of aging male rats. *Endocrinology*, 108:712–719.
729. Kerr, J. B., and de Kretser, D. M. (1983): Techniques for detecting and evaluating abnormalities in testicular function. In: *Methods for Assessing the Effects of Chemicals on Reproductive Functions*, edited by V. B. Vouk and P. J. Sheehan, pp. 247–262. Wiley, New York.
730. Russell, L. D. (1983): Normal testicular structure and methods of evaluation under experimental and disruptive conditions. In: *Reproductive and Developmental Toxicity of Metals*, edited by T. W. Clarkson, G. F. Nordberg, and P. R. Sager, pp. 227–252. Plenum, New York.
731. Mann, T., and Lutwak-Mann, C. (1981): *Male Reproductive Function and Semen. Themes and Trends in Physiology, Biochemistry and Investigative Andrology*. Springer-Verlag, Berlin.
732. Vermeulen, A. (1982): Effects of drugs on Leydig cell function. *Int. J. Andrology [Suppl. 5]*, 163:182.
733. de Kretser, D. M. (1982): Sertoli cell-Leydig cell interaction in the regulation of testicular function. *Int. J. Andrology [Suppl. 5]*, 11–17.
734. Wilton, L. J., and de Kretser, D. M. (1984): The influence of luteinizing hormone on the Leydig cells of cryptorchid rat testes. *Acta Endocrinol (Kbh.)*, 107:110–116.
735. Risbridger, G. P., Kerr, J. B., and de Kretser, D. M. (1981): Evaluation of Leydig cell function and gonadotrophin binding in unilateral and bilateral cryptorchidism: evidence for local control of Leydig cell function by the seminiferous tubule. *Biol. Reprod.*, 24:534–540.
736. Risbridger, G. P., Kerr, J. B., Peake, R. A., and de Kretser, D. M. (1981): An assessment of Leydig cell function after bilateral or unilateral efferent duct ligation: further evidence for local control of Leydig cell function. *Endocrinology*, 109:1234–1241.
737. Aoki, A., and Fawcett, D. W. (1978): Is there a local feedback from the seminiferous tubules affecting activity of the Leydig cell? *Biol. Reprod.*, 19:144–158.
738. Sharpe, R. M. (1985): Intragonadal hormones. *Bibl. Reprod.*, 133:C1–C15.
739. Sharpe, R. M. (1986): Paracrine control of the testis. *Clin. Endocrinol. Metab.*, 15:185–207.
740. Chemes, H. E., Rivarola, M. A., and Bergada, C. (1976): Effect of gonadotrophins and testosterone on the seminiferous tubules of the immature rat. *J. Reprod. Fertil.*, 46:283–288.
741. Rivier, C., Rivier, J., and Vale, W. (1979): Chronic effects of [D-Trp^6,Pro^9-NET] luteinizing hormone-releasing factor on reproductive processes in the male rat. *Endocrinology*, 105:1191–1201.
742. Johnson, A. D. (1977): The influence of cadmium on the testis. In: *The Testis, Vol. IV*, edited by A. D. Johnson and W. R. Gomes, pp. 565–576. Academic Press, New York.
743. Patanelli, D. J. (1975): Suppression of fertility in the male. In: *Handbook of Physiology, Section 7, Endocrinology, Vol. V, Male Reproductive System*, edited by D. W. Hamilton and R. O. Greep, pp. 245–258. Williams & Wilkins, Baltimore.
744. Jackson, H., and Ericsson, R. J. (1970): Effect of chemical agents and hormones on spermatogenesis and the epididymis. *Bibl. Reprod.*, 14:453–600.
745. Gunn, S. A., Gould, T. C., and Anderson, W. A. D. (1966): Loss of selective injurious vascular response to cadmium in regenerated blood vessels of testis. *Am. J. Pathol.*, 48:959–969.
746. Gunn, S. A., and Gould, T. C. (1970): Specificity of the vascular system of the male reproductive tract. *J. Reprod. Fertil. [Suppl. 10]*, 75–95.
747. Gunn, S. A., and Gould, T. C. (1970): Cadmium and other mineral elements. In: *The Testis, Vol. III*, edited by A. D. Johnson, W. R. Gomes, and N. L. Van Demark, pp. 377–481. Academic Press, New York.
748. Rommerts, F. F. G., Grootenhuis, A. J., Hoogerbrugge, J. W., and van der Molen, H. J. (1985): Ethane dimethane sulphonate specifically inhibits LH stimulated steroidogenesis in Leydig cells isolated from mature rats but not in cells from immature rats. *Mol. Cell. Endocrinol.*, 42:105–111.
749. Molenaar, R., de Rooij, D. G., Rommerts, F. F. G., Reuvers, P. J., and van der Molen, H. J. (1985): Specific destruction of Leydig cells in mature rats after *in vivo* administration of ethane dimethane sulfonate. *Biol. Reprod.*, 33:1213–1222.
750. Bartlett, J. M. S., Kerr, J. B., and Sharpe, R. M. (1986): The effect of selective destruction and regeneration of rat Leydig cells on seminiferous tubule morphology and the intratesticular distribution of testosterone. *J. Androl.*, 7:240–253.
751. Morris, I. D. (1985): Leydig cell resistance to the cytotoxic effect of ethylene dimethanesulphonate in the adult rat testis. *J. Endocrinol.*, 105:311–316.
752. O'Leary, P. O., Jackson, A. E., Averill, S., and de Kretser, D. M. (1986): The effects of ethane dimethanesulphonate (EDS) on bilaterally cryptorchid rat testes. *Mol. Cell. Endocrinol.*, 45:183–190.
753. Kerr, J. B., and Donachie, K. (1986): Regeneration of Leydig cells in unilaterally cryptorchid rats: evidence for stimulation by local testicular factors. *Cell Tissue Res.*, 243:405–414.
754. Mori, H., Shimizu, D., Takeda, A., Takioka, Y., and Fukuhishi, R. (1980): Stereological analysis of Leydig cells in normal guinea pig testes. *J. Electron Microsc. (Tokyo)*, 29:8–21.
755. Ewing, L. L., and Zirkin, B. R. (1983): Leydig cell structure and steroidogenic function. *Recent Prog. Horm. Res.*, 39:599.
756. Lin, H. S., and Wing, T. Y. (1979): A dense-cored filamentous body in Leydig cells of the golden hamster. *Cell Tissue Res.*, 201:369–376.
757. Payer, A. F., and Parkening, T. A. (1983): Membrane-bound intranuclear inclusions in the Leydig cell of the Chinese hamster (*Cricetulus griseus*). *J. Ultrastruct. Res.*, 84:317–325.
758. Mugisha-Girasi, H., Radke, B., and Schwarz, R. (1979): Observations on the Leydig cells in the male East African spring hare (*Pedetes surdaster larvalis*). *Z. Mikrosk. Anat. Forsch.*, 93: 65–73.
759. Stefan, Y., and Steimer, T. (1978): The Leydig cell of a hypogonadic rodent (*Ellobius lutescens, Th.*): correlation between ultrastructure and biosynthetic activity. *Biol. Reprod.*, 19:913–921.
760. Sinha, A. A., Erickson, A. W., and Seal, U. S. (1977): Fine structure of Leydig cells in crabeater, leopard and Ross seals. *J. Reprod. Fertil.*, 49:51–54.
761. Osman, D. J., and Ploen, L. (1978): The ultrastructure of Sertoli cells in the boar. *Int. J. Andrology*, 1:162–179.
762. Gotoh, M., Miyake, K., Mitsuya, H., Hoshino, T., and Yamada, K. (1983): Cytoplasmic inclusion bodies in Leydig cells from the testes of postpubertal cryptorchid patients. *Int. J. Andrology*, 6:221–228.
763. Clermont, Y., and Trott, M. (1969): Duration of the cycle of the seminiferous epithelium in the mouse and hamster determined by means of ^{3}H-thymidine and radioautography. *Fertil. Steril.*, 20:805–817.
764. de Rooij, D. G. (1968): Stem cell renewal and duration of spermatogonial cycle in the golden hamster. *Z. Zellforsch.*, 89: 133–136.
765. Swierstra, E. E. (1968): Cytology and duration of the seminiferous epithelium of the boar. Duration of spermatozoon transit through the epididymis. *Anat. Rec.*, 161:171–186.

766. Clermont, Y., Le Blond, C. P., and Messier, B. (1959): Duree du cycle de l'epithelium seminal du rat. *Arch. Anat. Microsc. Morphol. Exp.*, 48:37–56.

767. Hilscher, W. (1964): Beitrage zur Orthologie und Palhologie des "Spermatogoniogenes" der Ratte. *Beitr. Pathol. Anat.*, 130: 69–132.

768. Hochereau, M. T., Courot, M., and Ortavant, R. (1964): Marquage des cellules germinales du belier et du taureau par injection de thymidine tritee dans l'artere spermatique. *Ann. Biol. Anim. Biochim. Biophys.*, 2:157–161.

769. Orgebin-Crist, M. C. (1965): Passage of spermatozoa labelled with ^{3}H-thymidine through the ductus epididymidis of the rabbit. *J. Reprod. Fertil.*, 10:241–251.

770. Swierstra, E. E., and Foote, R. H. (1963): Cytology and kinetics of spermatogenesis in the rabbit. *J. Reprod. Fertil.*, 5:309–322.

771. Antar, M. (1971): Duration of the cycle of the seminiferous epithelium and of spermatogenesis in the monkey (*Macaca speciosa*). *Anat. Rec.*, 169:268–269.

772. Arsenieva, N. A., Dubinin, N. P., Orlova, N. N., and Bakulina, E. D. (1961): A radiation analysis of the duration of meiotic phases in the monkey (*Macaca mulatta*). *Dokl. Akad. Nauk. SSSR*, 141:1486–1489.

773. de Kretser, D. M., et al. (1982): Anatomical and functional aspects of the male reproductive organs. In: *Disturbances in Male Fertility*, pp. 1–131. Springer-Verlag, Berlin.

774. de Kretser, D. M. (1986): The light and electromicroscopic anatomy of the normal human testis. In: *Male Sexual Dysfunction: Diagnosis and Management of Hypogonadism, Infertility, and Impotence*, edited by R. J. Santen and R. J. Swerdloff, pp. 3–26. Marcel Dekker, New York.

The Physiology of Reproduction,
edited by E. Knobil and J. Neill *et al.*
Raven Press, Ltd., New York © 1988.

CHAPTER 21

The Sertoli Cell

C. Wayne Bardin, C. Yan Cheng, Neal A. Musto, and Glen L. Gunsalus

THE SERTOLI CELL

The testis can be divided functionally into interstitium and seminiferous tubules, which are responsible for the production of testosterone and spermatozoa, respectively. In the 1960s, assays for luteinizing hormone (LH) and testosterone as well as for other androgens were developed which permitted investigators to define the physiology and pathophysiology of Leydig cells, a major component of the interstitium. By contrast, an understanding of the function of cells in the seminiferous tubules did not advance as rapidly. This was due primarily to the complexity of spermatogenesis, a process involving interactions of multiple cells with several hormones over a relatively long period of time, which could be studied only *in vivo*. In addition, spermatozoa, the major product of the germinal epithelium, could be quantified only in testicular biopsies of the seminiferous tubular epithelium or after their appearance in the ejaculate following passage through the epididymis. In view of the difficulties in studying the seminiferous tubules, many investigators sought other products that could be measured more easily than spermatozoa. It was appreciated that Sertoli cells were the major secretory element of the germinal epithelium and that their proteins might be useful for studying this portion of the testis. Accordingly, a large number of Sertoli cell products were identified and used to monitor the function of Sertoli cells and intact seminiferous tubules, both *in vivo* and *in vitro* (Table 1). Identification of new Sertoli cell products also led to a better understanding of how testicular cells interact with each other.

A second major advance in the study of Sertoli cells was the development of procedures for *in vitro* studies, which involved the identification of factors required for their growth and differentiation (28–31). Although cells grown in this way do not mimic the morphological features of Sertoli cells *in vivo*, defined culture techniques provide a method for examining many aspects of Sertoli cell function not previously amenable to study. Techniques were also developed for culturing small segments of seminiferous tubules that corresponded to defined stages of the seminiferous tubular cycle (32). This permitted experiments on Sertoli cells with germ cells still attached. More recently, the growth of Sertoli cells on filters and matrices allowed media to be presented from the top and bottom (33,34). Cells grown in this way become confluent, establish junctional complexes, and assume an epithelial-like appearance reminiscent of Sertoli cells *in vivo*. These coupled cells appear to function as a polarized epithelium, which permits more complex studies of Sertoli cell biology.

Recent studies of the Sertoli cell focused on: (a) identification of Sertoli cell secretory products and investigation of their possible functions, both in the seminiferous tubule and in other parts of the testis; (b) definition of the humoral factors regulating Sertoli cell function *in vitro* and examination of their mechanisms of action; (c) determination of

TABLE 1. *Sertoli cell proteins*

Protein	Investigators (reference)
ABP	Hansson et al., 1975 (1) Bardin et al., 1981 (2) Ritzén et al., 1981 (3)
Inhibin	de Jong and Robertson, 1985 (4)
Growth factors	Feig et al., 1980 (5) Feig et al., 1983 (6) Brown et al., 1982 (7); Holmes et al., 1986 (8)
Somatomedin	Hall et al., 1983 (9)
Transferrin	Skinner and Griswold, 1980 (10) Skinner et al., 1984 (11)
Ceruloplasmin	Skinner and Griswold, 1983 (12)
Retinol-binding protein	Huggenvik and Griswold, 1981 (13) Carson et al., 1984 (14)
H-Y antigen	Brunner et al., 1984 (15)
Plasminogen activator	Lacroix et al., 1977 (16) Vihko et al., 1984 (17)
Clusterin	Fritz et al., 1983 (18) Blaschuk et al., 1984 (19) Tung and Fritz, 1985 (20)
Cyclic proteins	Wright et al., 1983 (21)
Dimeric acid glycoprotein	Sylvester et al., 1984 (22)
Scm proteins	DePhilip and Kierszenbaum, 1982 (23)
CMB proteins	Cheng et al., 1986 (24)
Testibumin	Cheng and Bardin, 1986 (25)
FSH- and testosterone-responsive protein (CMB-21)	Cheng, 1986 (26)
Testosterone-responsive proteins	Cheng et al., 1985 (27)

how other cells in the testis interact with and regulate Sertoli cells; and (d) definition of Sertoli cells as functional components of the seminiferous tubular epithelium *in vivo*. Although this review will focus on these recent studies, we will attempt to refer to earlier experiments covered in other reviews.

THE STRUCTURAL FEATURES OF SERTOLI CELLS

In his now classic review of Sertoli cell ultrastructure, Fawcett (35) point out that nuclei of these cells contain very little heterochromatin in comparison to other somatic cells. The nucleoplasm contains primarily euchromatin, consistent with the postulate that Sertoli cells express a large portion of their genome in accordance with their highly versatile functions. The structure of the multiple Golgi elements in this cell type is also consistent with a highly active mechanism for processing newly synthesized proteins; however, there appeared to be insufficient rough endoplasmic reticulum to account for appreciable protein synthesis. These observations, coupled with (a) the lack of large vacuoles or membrane-bound secretory granules in association with Golgi, (b) the paucity of morphologic evidence for exocytosis, and (c) the small number of vesicles opening into the lateral surfaces of Sertoli cells, suggested that this cell type did not release a significant amount of protein into the seminiferous tubular lumen. Although these morphological observations at first seemed contradictory to many investigators, they now appear to be consistent with the growing body of knowledge regarding Sertoli cell secretory products. That is, Sertoli cells may secrete up to 100 proteins, a finding consistent with the structures of nuclear chromatin and Golgi complex. It now appears that these proteins are not stored, but rather are secreted immediately after synthesis. This would account for the lack of obvious secretory granules. Even though Sertoli cells, like hepatocytes, synthesize multiple proteins, the total production per Sertoli cell per day may be much less than that produced by liver cells, especially when one considers the relative protein concentrations in seminiferous tubular fluid as compared to plasma (36).

In addition to the morphologic evidence for protein secretion, there are other structural features of Sertoli cells which relate to their function in the seminiferous tubular epithelium. These include: (a) numerous primary lysosomes, autophagic vacuoles, and heterophagic vacuoles, which are believed to participate in the phagocytosis and digestion of germ cells that degenerate during development; (b) large amounts of smooth endoplasmic reticulum in some species, suggestive of steroid synthesis; (c) specific alterations in Sertoli cell morphology along the length of the seminiferous tubule, suggesting that these cells participate, along with germinal elements, in forming the spermatogenic cycle; (d) unique junctional specializations between Sertoli cells which maintain the structural integrity of the tubular epithelium, provide low-resistance pathways for electrical coupling of adjacent cells, and constitute the epithelial component of the blood-testis barrier. These junctional complexes divide the epithelium of the seminiferous tubule into two separate physical compartments: (i) an exterior or basal compartment containing spermatogonia and preleptotene spermatocytes and (ii) an interior compartment containing the remaining spermatocytes and spermatids. The basal compartment is contiguous with the basal lamina, myoid cells, and the blood as well as with lymphatic vessels in the interstitial space. For the purposes of anatomical description, the interior compartment is further subdivided into two contiguous compartments: the adluminal and luminal compartments (see, e.g., ref. 35). The luminal space is continuous with the rete testis, efferent ducts, and epididymis. In general, substances present in the basal compartment can only enter the adluminal and luminal compartments by traversing Sertoli cell cytoplasm and vice versa. In the following discussion, we will emphasize the physical separation between the exterior and interior compartments of the seminiferous epithelium, which is provided by the Sertoli-Sertoli tight junctional complexes. These unique morphological features provide the background for present and future studies of Sertoli cell biology.

THE FUNCTIONS OF SERTOLI CELLS

Maintenance of the Blood-Testis Barrier and Secretion of Tubular Fluid

The seminiferous tubules compose the proximal portion of a continuous ductal system that comprises the male reproductive tract. Although there is considerable variation among different mammalian species, the general plan is similar for all. The seminiferous tubules of each testis empty by way of tubuli recti into the rete testis, which, in turn, empties by several efferent ducts into the proximal portion of the epididymis. The seminiferous tubule is a complex epithelium composed of Sertoli and germ cells which rests on the basal lamina. The junctional contacts between adjacent Sertoli cells form the structural basis of the most important portion of the blood-testis barrier (for a review see ref. 36) (37–40).

Part of the evidence indicating the existence of a blood-testis barrier is that the fluid composition inside the seminiferous tubule and rete testis is dramatically different from that found in testicular lymph and blood. The fluid secreted into the tubular epithelium by Sertoli cells contains five to seven times more potassium than does the fluid in the rete testis, which, in turn, contains two to three times more potassium than does the serum (41). Both testicular fluids contain proportionally less sodium and chloride (36). Seminiferous tubular fluid contains more protein than that of rete testis, but both have much less than serum (36,42,43). Fluid is produced in the testis of most species at a rate of 10 to 20 μl per gram of testis per hour (44–48) and is continuous without diurnal variation. This fluid drive provides a mechanism by which sperm are moved from the testis to the epididymis, where they become fully mature.

Fluid production begins when the first spermatozoa are released from the Sertoli cells (49). In immature animals, it is increased by follicle-stimulating hormone (FSH) but not by other pituitary hormones (50). Following hypophysectomy of adult animals, fluid secretion does not decrease until regression of the seminiferous tubule begins. Fluid secretion continues after the loss of germ cells, but at a reduced rate; the potassium concentration of such fluid is similar to that of plasma (51–53). Normal fluid production is dependent on the lower temperature found in the scrotum and a continuous supply of glucose (54,55). In his review on testicular fluid secretion, Setchell concluded that fluid production is dependent on hormones because of their ability to maintain the structural integrity of the seminiferous tubular epithelium (36).

In view of the unusual ion composition of tubular fluid, it is easy to understand that small molecules in lymph and serum do not readily enter into the seminiferous tubules and vice versa. This was first realized when it was noted that dyes injected into the blood did not enter into the lumen of the seminiferous tubules (56,57). The differential transport of various factors from the serum into tubular and rete testis fluids has been extensively reviewed (36). It would appear from a variety of studies that the rete testis is slightly more permeable to a variety of small molecules than are the seminiferous tubules. Furthermore, since protein concentrations in tubular and rete testis fluids are much lower than in blood, free movement of proteins into the testis does not occur. Thus, one functional consequence of the blood-testis barrier is to maintain a gradient of ions, small molecules, and proteins between blood and tubular fluid.

Although many studies suggest the potassium gradient is maintained by ion pumps, it is not clear how the complex protein composition of tubular fluid is maintained. It is possible that some proteins are moved into tubular fluid by selective transport mechanisms, analogous to those used to transport γ-globulins across epithelia in the gut (58). However, such transport mechanisms have not been demonstrated in Sertoli cells. As shall be discussed in the next section, it appears more likely that most of the proteins in tubular fluid are secreted by Sertoli cells (59). Thus, Sertoli cells secrete products that provide developing germ cells with a unique environment which is maintained by the blood-testis barrier (59). The ability to exclude small molecules allows the blood-testis barrier to protect developing germ cells from mutagenic agents. Since sperm are immunogenic, the blood-testis barrier also serves to sequester this population of cells from the immune system.

Secretion of Proteins, Peptides, and Other Products

Androgen-binding protein (ABP) was one of the first Sertoli cell-specific proteins to be identified and extensively studied (60–62). This product is important since it provides a prototype for other Sertoli cell secretory proteins. Studies in the rat indicate that approximately 80% of rABP is secreted into the lumen of the seminiferous tubule and then is transported to the epididymis, where it is taken into cells and degraded (1,63–65). The remaining 20% is released into the blood, probably from the base of Sertoli cells (66). These early observations gave rise to the concept that seminiferous tubular physiology can be monitored by measuring Sertoli cell secretory products in the peripheral blood and reproductive tract (66).

Another important concept regarding Sertoli cell secretory products derives from a series of observations in rats demonstrating that these cells secrete not only testis-specific proteins such as rABP, but also proteins that are normally found in the serum. Skinner and Griswold (10) first demonstrated that Sertoli cells secrete transferrin. Subsequently Wright et al. (67) showed that in addition to secreting transferrin, cultured Sertoli cells synthesize and secrete multiple serum proteins, including ceruloplasmin and acidic glycoprotein (Table 1).

It had long been known that serum-like proteins are present in tubular and rete testis fluids, and it had been proposed that these proteins are transported by some unknown mechanism across the seminiferous tubular epithelium. The demonstration that Sertoli cells can synthesize serum proteins provides an alternative explanation for the presence of such products in the adluminal compartment. These observations also set forth the concept that Sertoli cells can secrete the essential proteins necessary for maintenance and maturation of germ cells in the adluminal compartment. Thus, many proteins that are delivered to somatic cells by serum are provided to late spermatocytes and spermatids by tubular fluid.

Androgen-Binding Protein

This protein was first identified in the epididymis (60,61) and was later shown to be of testicular origin (68). The speculation that rABP is of Sertoli cell origin derives from observations that: (a) tubules depleted of germ cells by prenatal x-ray treatment secrete rABP; and (b) peritubular interstitial fluid contains little rABP compared to rete testis fluid, where the concentration is high (69). In addition, Sertoli cell-enriched cultures secrete large quantities of this binding protein into the media (70,71), confirming that rABP is derived from Sertoli cells. The development of methods for quantifying rABP by steady state polyacrylamide gel electrophoresis (SS-PAGE) (72), dextran-coated charcoal (73), and radioimmunoassay (74) allowed many investigators to study its hormonal regulation, tissue distribution, and physiologic function. The development of a photoaffinity ligand, $[^3H]$-Δ^6-testosterone, also facilitated studies of the physical properties of this protein in biological fluids without extensive purification (75–77). Studies with antibodies to ABP show that this protein is immunologically related to the testosterone-estradiol-binding globulin (TeBG) from the same species (78–81).

Rat ABP (rABP). The ability to obtain highly purified rABP in good yield depends on the development of a stable androgen-affinity chromatographic matrix, as well as a procedure for eluting the protein in high yield (82). The rat is an ideal species in which ABP can be identified unambiguously since there is no possibility of contaminating the purified protein with the serum protein, TeBG, because the latter protein is not present in serum of adult rats (83). Native rABP is a heterogeneous dimeric glycoprotein with a native molecular weight of 85,000. It is composed of two kinds of monomers with apparent molecular weights of 45,000 and 41,000. These monomers are designated heavy (H) and light (L), respectively ($rABP_H$; $rABP_L$), according to their electrophoretic mobilities in SDS-polyacrylamide gels. Since $rABP_H$ and $rABP_L$ are present in the native molecule in a ratio of 3:1, the dimer could not be composed of stoichiometric amounts of H and L. It was, therefore, concluded that H and L might be different forms, or protomers, of the same molecule. This conclusion is supported by observations that the H and L monomers have similar amino acid compositions, peptide maps, immunodeterminants, and binding sites (84–86). The structural basis for this size heterogeneity of protomers and how they are assembled to form the native molecule is not clearly understood, but there are several possibilities (59). Either variations in the lengths of the polypeptide chains or differences in glycosylation, or both, could be responsible for the size differences in $rABP_H$ and $rABP_L$. It is reasonable to suggest that $rABP_L$ is a proteolytic product of $rABP_H$, since this protein is usually isolated from the epididymis, a site of rABP degradation. If this were the case, then one would expect a preponderance of $rABP_H$ in rABP isolated from testes. This is not the case, however, since rABP purified from testes and rABP newly synthesized *in vitro* have H:L ratios of 3:1. These observations suggest that $rABP_L$ is not likely to be a degradation product of the H protomer (85). Thus, if one protomer is derived from the other, it is probably formed in Sertoli cells prior to secretion. This hypothesis is supported by recent studies showing that cDNA encoding for rABP hybridizes to a single-size mRNA species in testis and Sertoli cell poly(A) RNA (Fig. 1) (87). In addition to heterogeneity based on protomer size, the ABPs of rat and other species

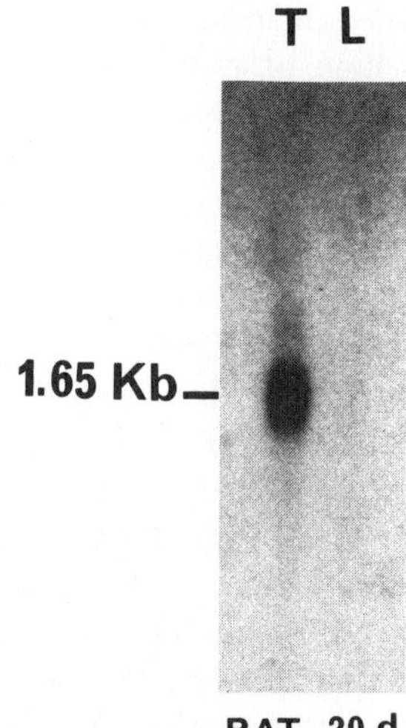

FIG. 1. Northern blot analysis of mRNA, isolated from testis and liver of a 20-day-old rat, probed with rABP cDNA. A single 1.65-kilodalton rABP mRNA is present in testis, but not in liver.

exhibit heterogeneity secondary to carbohydrate structure based on differential binding to Con A (88,89).

Further understanding of rABP structure will provide insight not only into this unique secretory product from rat testis, but also into ABP and TeBG of other species. The physical properties of all the androgen-binding proteins isolated to date are similar to rABP in that they all are dimeric glycoproteins which exhibit protomeric heterogeneity. In addition, within a given species, ABP and TeBG proteins bear strong resemblance to each other with regard to physicochemical and immunological properties. Furthermore, the amino acid sequence of rABP, recently predicted from a cDNA sequence, is greater than 65% homologous with the protein sequence of human TeBG (hTeBG) (P. H. Petra, *personal communication*). Because of the striking resemblance of ABPs to TeBGs, it is relevant to review the current knowledge of these latter proteins.

Rat TeBG (rTeBG). As noted previously, this protein is not detected in the serum of adult rats (83). However, a relatively large amount of rABP is secreted by Sertoli cells into the blood of male rats at the time of puberty, and this protein has been confused with TeBG (90). The basis for the distinction between these proteins rests upon the observation that rABP is present only in males and is clearly of testicular origin (74). By contrast, in those species that make TeBG, this protein is present in the serum of both males and females. Unexpectedly, an immunoreactive rABP-like material was detected in the serum and amniotic fluid of male and female fetuses (91–93). The concentrations of this material in these fluids decline during the last few days of fetal life and disappear from the blood of female rats by the fifth postnatal day. The fetal ABP-like material is in highest concentration in brain and liver. Studies using immunoprecipitation of radiolabeled proteins suggest that this material is synthesized in the liver but not the brain. Furthermore, the immunoprecipitated product produced by fetal hepatocytes contains two immunoreactive proteins in the ratio of 3:1; these proteins are slightly larger than the H and L protomers of rABP of testicular origin. When these observations are interpreted in light of extensive comparative studies performed on rabbit and human ABPs and TeBGs, they suggest that the protein of hepatic origin in fetal rats should be designated rTeBG. We conclude, therefore, that the rat does produce rTeBG and that this molecule, like rat alpha-fetoprotein, is synthesized during fetal life. Studies to date cannot distinguish whether rABP and rTeBG are the same or similar proteins.

Rabbit ABP and TeBG. In the rabbit, ABP (rbABP) is in the lumen of the male reproductive tract. In this species, studies of rbABP are complicated by the presence of another extracellular binding protein, rbTeBG, which is presumably of hepatic origin. Early studies using partially purified rbABP suggested that it shared immunodeterminants with rbTeBG (78). This observation, coupled with the desire to measure rbABP in the presence of rbTeBG, led to an extensive characterization of these proteins (79,94,95). Even though these two purified proteins have many similar physicochemical properties, including native molecular weights, isoelectric points, and binding constants, rbABP differs from rbTeBG with regard to the molecular weight and distribution of the two protomers, carbohydrate composition, and peptide composition. Similar results on the composition of these two proteins were obtained using unfractionated samples studied by photoaffinity labeling techniques (76,96). In addition, comparison of displacement curves using multiple dilutions of each protein in homologous and heterologous radioimmunoassays demonstrated that rbABP and rbTeBG have both common and unique immunodeterminants (81,97).

The above observations indicate that monospecific polyclonal antisera against rbABP and rbTeBG will recognize, but not distinguish between, the reciprocal protein. Monoclonal antibodies against highly purified rbABP do not interact with highly purified rbTeBG. It is of note, however, that this antibody does not distinguish between these proteins in freshly prepared tissue extracts. This suggests that highly purified rbABP has antigenic sites that are not exposed in biological fluids (N. A. Musto, *unpublished observations*). These latter observations suggest it may not be possible to produce antibodies that measure ABP in the presence of TeBG using highly purified proteins as antigens.

Studies using monospecific antiserum against rbTeBG localize the antigenic sites of this protein at the junction of the head and midpiece of ejaculated rabbit spermatozoa. By contrast, epididymal spermatozoa do not stain (98). The intracellular location of this protein is suggested, since the intensity of the staining is maximal following permeabilization of the plasma membrane with cold acetone. Such findings are used to support the postulate that rbABP and rbTeBG function as steroid carriers across the plasma membrane of the ejaculated spermatozoa (98).

Human ABP and TeBG. The presence of proteins in human serum that bind testosterone and estradiol was identified by Mercier et al. (99) and Rosenbaum et al. (100), respectively. Subsequent studies indicated that the same protein binds androgens as well as estrogens, and thus was designated testosterone-estradiol-binding globulin (hTeBG), sex steroid-binding globulin (SBG), or sex hormone-binding globulin (SHBG) by different groups of investigators (2,101). The highly purified protein is a dimer (102–106). Studies on purified photolabeled hTeBG indicate that it is composed of two types of monomers (Fig. 2), as is the case with the ABPs and TeBGs of other species (107). These monomers, designated $hTeBG_H$ and $hTeBG_L$ after the nomenclature established for rABP and rbABP, occur at a ratio of 10:1 (H:L) in multiple preparations using two different purification schemes (107–109). By contrast, protomers have many of the same epitopes because both polyclonal and monoclonal antibodies developed against hTeBG reacted with both protomers on immunoblots (110). Moreover, the size differences of the hTeBG protomers may not be entirely due to differential carbohydrate content, since removal of this moiety from the molecule, both by enzymatic and chemical treatment, did not abolish or alter the distribution of the protomeric forms of hTeBG (108).

The development of sensitive radioimmunoassays for hTeBG (111,112) not only enhanced the ability to study its physiology, but also allowed investigation of its relationship to similar proteins present in human testicular extracts. Soon after the identification of rABP, many investigators attempted to demonstrate the presence of a similar protein in primate testes. Studies using conventional fractionation procedures and binding assays were unable to conclusively distinguish the androgen-binding protein in human and monkey testes from primate TeBGs (113–115). However, these studies suggested that the androgen-binding activity in testicular cytosol was greater than might be expected from serum contamination (116). Subsequently, it was shown that hABP in testicular extracts could be distinguished from hTeBG in serum using Con A chromatography (117). The binding activity in testicular extracts resolves into two fractions: Form I hABP, which does not bind to Con A, and Form II hABP, which does (117,118). By contrast, hTeBG is bound quantitatively by this lectin (Fig. 3). In addition, both forms of hABP cross-react in a hTeBG radioimmunoassay (Fig. 4) using antiserum raised against hTeBG (80). Based on these studies, it was not possible to distinguish Form II hABP from hTeBG.

To further study the subtle differences between hABP and hTeBG, both proteins were purified, from testicular extracts and serum, respectively, by sequential androgen affinity and high-performance liquid chromatography. The two forms

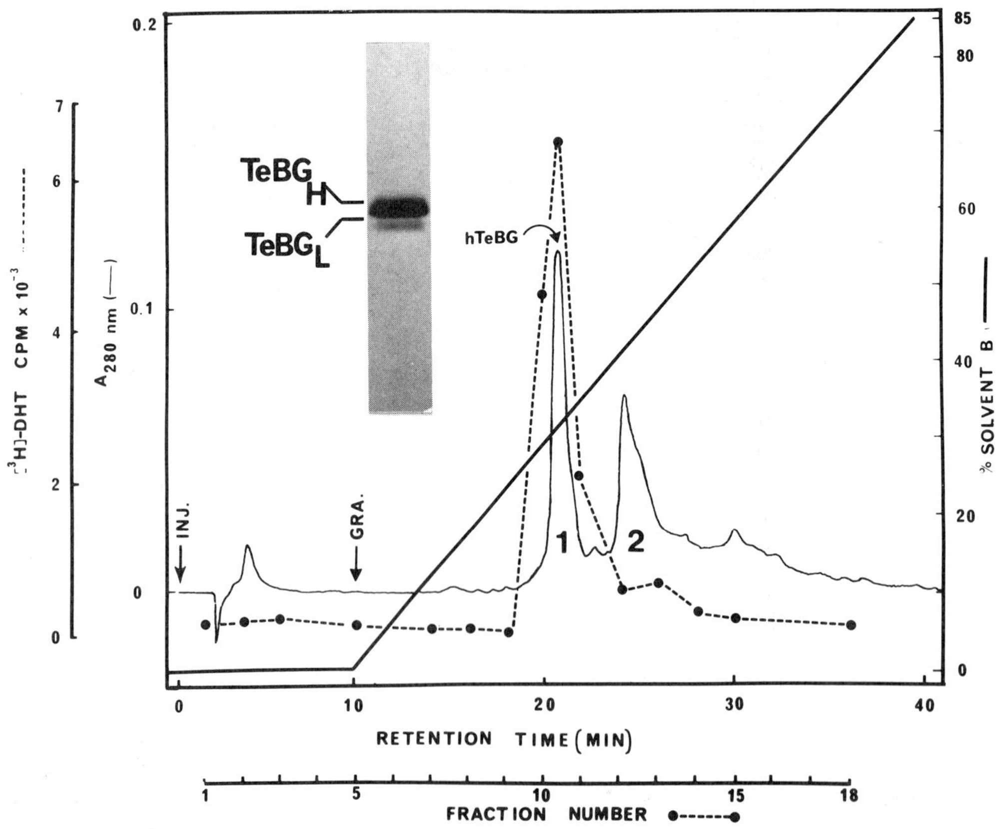

FIG. 2. Anion-exchange HPLC of partially purified hTeBG after affinity chromatography. INJ indicates where sample was loaded, GRA indicates beginning of gradient. The insert is a silver-stained SDS-polyacrylamide gel of the hTeBG purified by HPLC. The H and L indicate the relative mobility of $hTeBG_H$ and $hTeBG_L$. (Adapted from ref. 108.)

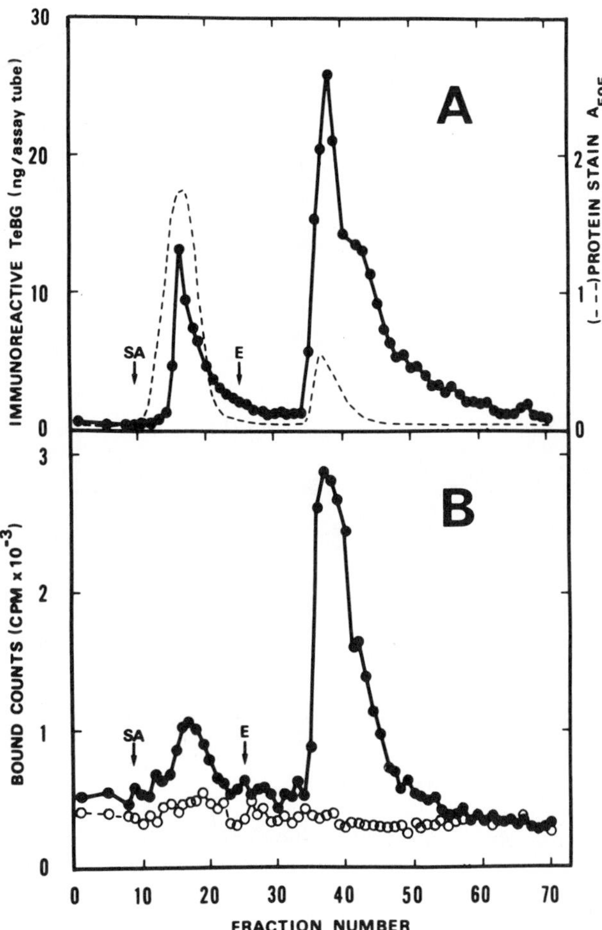

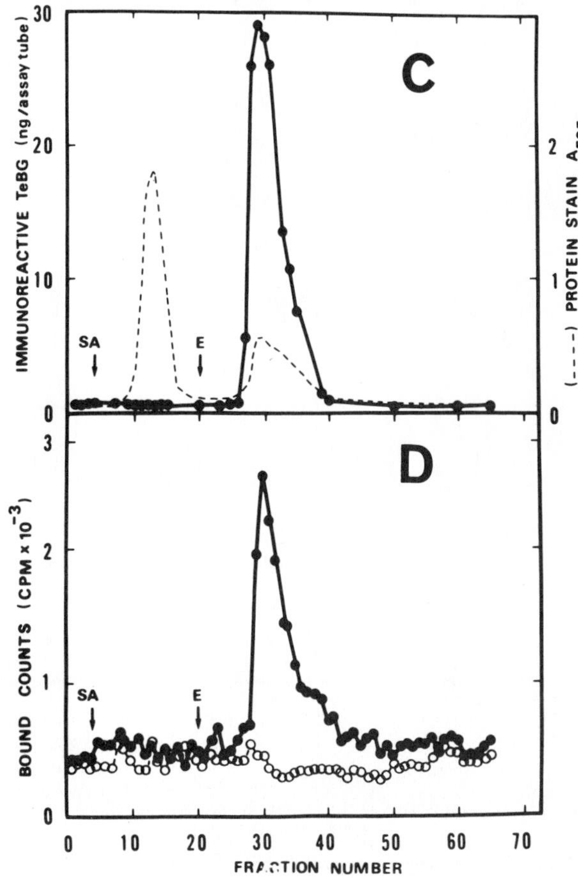

FIG. 3. Con A-Sepharose affinity chromatography of human testicular cytosol (**A,B**) and serum from a normal man (**C,D**). In A and C, the concentration of immunoreactive hTeBG-like material was measured by radioimmunoassay using an aliquot from each fraction; total protein was also estimated by dye binding. In B and D, an aliquot from each fraction was assayed for steroid binding by incubation with [^{3}H]DHT in the absence (●) or presence (○) of 2000-fold excess of nonradioactive DHT. SA indicates where sample was applied; E indicates elution of glycoproteins bound to Con A using methylglucoside. It is of note that human testicular cytosol contains two peaks showing immunoreactivity to hTeBG antiserum and binding, whereas human serum contains only one. (Adapted from ref. 80.)

of hABP were resolved on Con A-Sepharose. Form I hABP, like hTeBG, possesses heavy (H) and light (L) protomers after fractionation by SDS-PAGE (Fig. 5). The relative molecular weights of the individual protomers are: Form I $hABP_H$ > Form I $hABP_L \cong hTeBG_H > hTeBG_L$. The relative amounts of each protomer in both proteins also differ: hABP has more of the L component, whereas hTeBG has more of the H component. Peptide maps prepared from the H and L protomers of the two proteins suggest that they are similar but not identical (118). hTeBG and hABP photolabeled with [^{3}H]-Δ^6-testosterone both have a portion of the steroid-binding site on the H and L protomers (Fig. 5). Furthermore, the distribution of protomers seen with affinity labeling is identical to that observed by silver staining of the purified protein. These observations indicate that both the H and L protomers of the purified protein are components of native hABP. With the information available to date, it is not possible to know whether H:L in highly purified Form I hABP is the same (i.e., 2:3) as that secreted by Sertoli cells.

Form II hABP is similar to hTeBG with regard to Con A binding (80); on SDS-polyacrylamide gels, it migrates as a heterogeneous band with an average molecular weight greater than that of hTeBG (Fig. 5) (118). The peptide maps generated by Form II hABP are essentially the same as those of hTeBG when the peptide fragments are visualized by immunoblots using monospecific hTeBG antiserum, but slightly different from hTeBG when visualized by silver staining or lectin-blotting using Con A (118). Steroid-binding assays and an hTeBG radioimmunoassay demonstrated that both proteins have similar binding sites and shared immunodeterminants. The demonstration that the isoforms of hABP are distinct from hTeBG provides hope that both of these proteins may eventually be quantified in biological

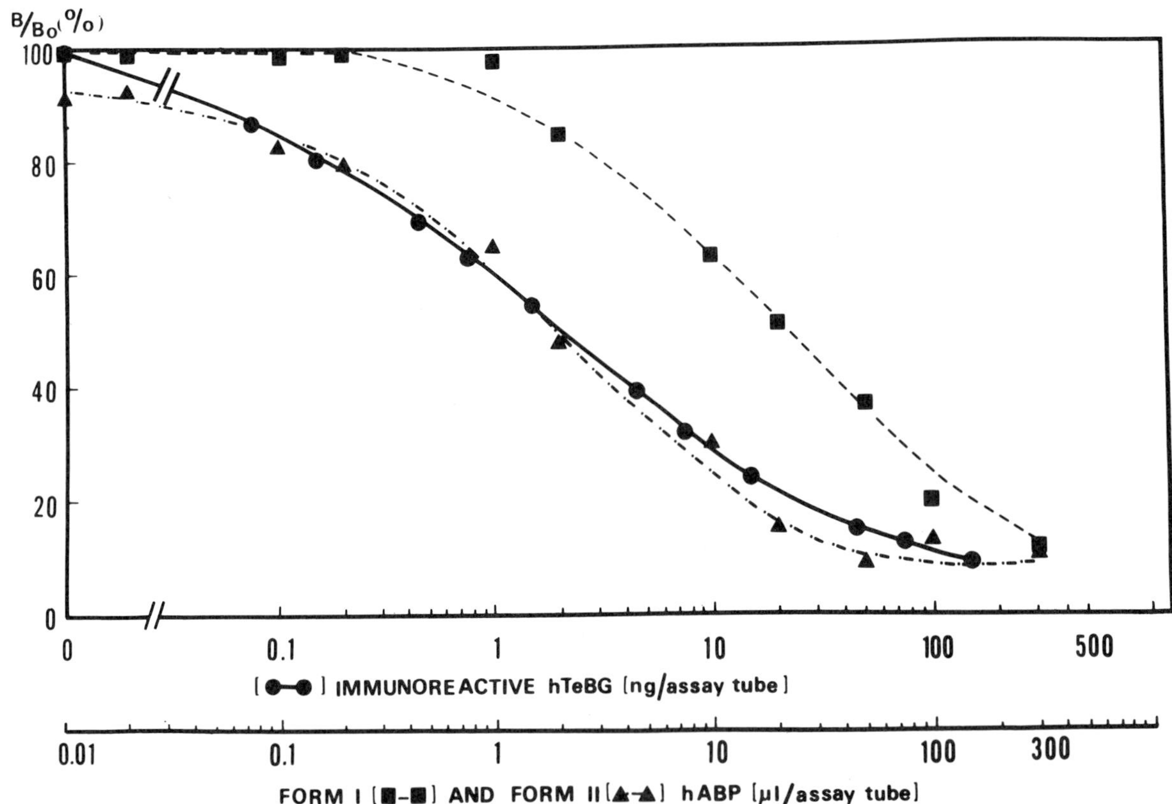

FIG. 4. Competition of [^{125}I]hTeBG binding to hTeBG antiserum by Form I and Form II hABP derived from human testicular extracts fractionated on Con A-Sepharose columns and by hTeBG from a pool of human pregnancy sera. The abscissa is the log dose of competitor. The ordinate is expressed as B/B_0, where B and B_0 are counts bound in the presence and absence of unlabeled competitor, respectively. (Adapted from ref. 80.)

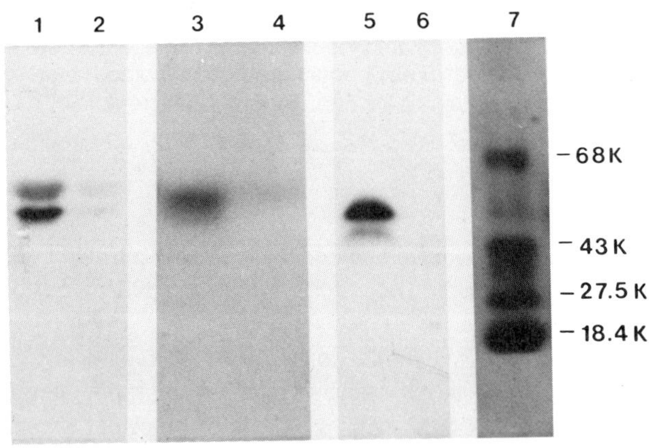

FIG. 5. SDS-polyacrylamide gel electrophoresis of photolabeled hABP and hTeBG. Highly purified Form I hABP (lanes 1 and 2), Form II hABP (lanes 3 and 4), and hTeBG (lanes 5 and 6) were photolyzed in the presence of Δ^6-[^{3}H]testosterone with or without nonradioactive DHT. After photolysis, samples were fractionated on an SDS-polyacrylamide slab gel, and the radioactive components were demonstrated by fluorography. Lanes 1, 3, and 5 indicate proteins photolyzed in the absence of competitor; lanes 2, 4, and 6 indicate samples that were photolyzed in the presence of competitor. Lane 7 is ^{14}C-labeled molecular-weight standards. (Adapted from ref. 118.)

fluids. However, the ability to distinguish how these isoforms differ from one another and from hTeBG must await their primary sequence analysis.

ABP in other species. In addition to being present in rat, rabbit, and human testes, ABPs are present in guinea-pig (77), monkey, and ovine testes. Since hTeBG shares immunodeterminants with monkey steroid-binding proteins (112,119,120), antiserum against this hTeBG can be used for studies in primates (120). Monkey ABP (mABP), like hABP, resolves into two forms on Con A chromatography, namely, two protomers of molecular weight (MW) 48,000 and 46,000, which are present in nonequivalent amounts. Purified ovine ABP differs from ovine TeBG in much the same way as rbABP differs from rbTeBG (C. Y. Cheng and C. W. Bardin, *unpublished observations*).

It has not been possible to detect androgen-binding activity in the reproductive tract of porcine and murine species using assays that could easily detect such binding sites in rat tissues. These observations raise some doubts as to the necessity for ABP in normal reproduction. It was of interest, therefore, to find immunostainable ABP-like activity (using anti-rABP) in mouse Sertoli cells, neural tissue, and epithelia of rete testis, efferent ductules, proximal caput epididymis, and vas deferens (S. D. Tsong, *unpublished ob-*

servations). In contrast, other cells in these tissues, as well as in 10 other control organs, were immunonegative. These observations suggest that there is a protein in the mouse that does not have a steroid-binding site detectable by conventional assays, but contains immunodeterminants similar to those of rABP. Since the tissue and cellular distribution of the immunostainable material in the mouse is exactly the same as the distribution of rABP in rat tissues using the same antisera, these observations suggest that the tissue distribution of this ABP-like immunoreactive protein in the mouse may not be dependent on the presence of a high-affinity testosterone-binding site. Whether similar ABP immunostainable activity exists in the same tissue of other species without steroid-binding sites remains to be established.

Functions of ABP. Although it is 10 and 20 years since the identification of rABP and hTeBG, respectively, their physiologic function is still not completely understood. It was once thought that ABP, like TeBG, could not be important because these proteins were not found in all species (2,83). Such a postulate was acceptable as long as it was believed that they served only as extracellular steroid transport proteins. Several observations suggest, however, that steroid-binding proteins are not just curiosities of evolution. First, ABP and TeBG have been found in several species that were originally thought not to have such proteins. Second, the conservation of a specific steroid-binding site for androgens and estrogens through philogeny suggests a selective advantage. Finally, it has become increasingly clear that ABP and TeBG are both present in cells other than those in which they are synthesized. For example, ABP and TeBG are localized immunocytochemically in selected cells that respond to, or metabolize, androgens. These observations suggest there may be a specific mechanism for transport of these proteins into such cells. Moreover, a specific saturable binding site for hTeBG has recently been demonstrated on prostatic cells (121). A similar binding site for rABP has also been postulated to occur on cells of the proximal caput epididymis, where the intracellular concentration of this protein is high (122).

The physiologic roles postulated for ABP have included: (a) a carrier of testosterone within the Sertoli cells; (b) a carrier to maintain high concentrations of androgens in seminiferous tubules and epididymides; and (c) a transporter of testosterone from the testis into the epididymis. Although data to support these functions are limited, they all are consistent with the steroid-binding activity exhibited by ABP (123,124). If binding of steroids by ABP is relevant, then this protein may influence androgen action or metabolism, particularly in the caput epididymis, where ABP is concentrated. This speculation is supported by studies indicating that the androgen concentrations in blood are not sufficient to maintain the function of this region once the entry of testicular androgens and proteins is limited by ligation of the efferent ductules (for a review see ref. 3). However, if ABP is the product of Sertoli cells that is important for the functioning of the caput epithelium, then the finding of immunoreactive ABP without demonstrable binding activity in the mouse questions whether all the functions postulated for this protein are related to its steroid-binding activity. In contrast to these speculations, it is clear that the Sertoli cells of many species produce ABP, presumably to serve the same function in the reproductive tract as TeBG serves in the systemic circulation.

Metal-Binding Proteins

As noted above, several investigators have demonstrated that Sertoli cells synthesize and secrete iron- and copper-transport proteins (10,12,67). These proteins have been called *testicular transferrin* and *ceruloplasmin,* respectively. The presence of both of these proteins in tubular fluid suggests a mechanism by which iron and copper can be transported to germ cells in the adluminal compartment (125).

A comparison of highly purified testicular transferrin to its homolog in serum using amino acid analysis and tryptic peptide patterns indicates that the only apparent difference between these two proteins is their carbohydrate content (11). This suggests that testicular and serum transferrin are the products of the same gene which have differential patterns of post-translational processing.

When serum-free culture media were developed for the growth of testicular cells, it was shown that Sertoli cells required transferrin for growth (126). It was postulated that this protein might serve as a specific mitogen for this cell type, independent of its ability to transport iron. Results of studies investigating this possibility demonstrate that in the absence of iron, transferrin has no growth-promoting activity (127). The proposed function of this protein on testicular cells is, therefore, to transport iron. It has been postulated that Sertoli cells synthesize and secrete this protein into the seminiferous tubular lumen to provide a mechanism for transport of Fe^{3+} to developing germ cells (10). The demonstration of transferrin's specific binding to spermatocytes (128) and of transferrin receptors on spermatids (M. Serio et al., *personal communication*) is consistent with this hypothesis.

Transferrin production by Sertoli cell cultures was stimulated by FSH, testosterone, retinol, and retinoic acid treatment (129). However, the effects of FSH on transferrin production by Sertoli cell-enriched cultures have not been routinely reproduced by other laboratories, probably because the concentration of some other factor(s) in the medium is critical for FSH action (24,127).

Thorbecke (130) surveyed several tissues with transferrin antiserum and observed that this protein is synthesized by both the testis and the ovary. Studies on seminal fluid of normal and vasectomized men suggest that more than 80% of seminal transferrin comes from the testes (or epididymides) (131), whereas seminal ceruloplasmin is from another part of the reproductive tract. More importantly, these studies show that seminal transferrin is a reliable index of seminiferous tubular function because levels of this protein are lower in patients with oligo- and azoospermia (131,132). These observations are important since they demonstrate that at least one Sertoli cell protein can pass through the epididymis and can be measured in semen. This is strikingly different from ABP that is quantitatively removed by the reproductive tract.

Clusterin

Fritz et al. (18) reported the presence of a macromolecule in ram rete testis fluid which elicited "clustering" of Sertoli cells from immature rats, TM_4 Sertoli cells, and erythrocytes of several species. Purified clusterin from ram rete testis fluid is a dimeric glycoprotein containing 36% carbohydrate (19,133). The protein is synthesized and secreted by Sertoli cells (19). The native dimer (MW 80,000) consists of two monomers of MW 40,000, each with different *N*-terminal amino acid sequences (C. Y. Cheng and C. W. Bardin, *unpublished observations*).

Recently, a glycoprotein that is responsive to FSH and testosterone was identified in primary Sertoli cell-enriched cultures prepared from rat testes (24), partially purified using sequential high-performance liquid chromatography (HPLC) columns, and designated CMB-21 (C. Y. Cheng and C. W. Bardin, *unpublished observations*). CMB-21 is a dimer of MW 90,000 consisting of two monomers of MW 45,000 with identical electrophoretic mobilities. A monospecific antiserum against this protein cross-reacts with ram clusterin and with a protein of similar size found in media from mouse Sertoli cell-enriched cultures (C. Y. Cheng and C. W. Bardin, *unpublished observations*). These observations suggest that the Sertoli cell protein, clusterin, is not limited to the ovine species.

Immunocytochemical studies using monoclonal antibodies against ram clusterin, in combination with indirect immunofluorescence microscopy, indicated that this protein is concentrated in the adluminal region of the seminiferous epithelium and in the epithelial cells of the rete testis and caput epididymides (20). The physiologic function of clusterin is unknown; however, it may act to facilitate cell-cell interactions (18). In this regard, immunoassayable clusterin has also been identified in the blood of rams, suggesting that it could have some actions outside the reproductive tract (C. Y. Cheng, J. P. Mather, and C. W. Bardin, *unpublished observations*).

Testicular Plasminogen Activators

The presence of serine proteases, plasminogen activators (PA), in Sertoli cell-enriched cultures was first reported in 1977 (16). The activity of this enzyme is stimulated by FSH or dibutyryl cAMP in the medium. It was proposed that PAs are involved in tissue restructuring and cell migration processes in normal tissues. In the reproductive tissue, PA may play a role in facilitating either the release of mature spermatids by Sertoli cells or the migration of germ cells (mainly preleptotene spermatocytes) from the basal compartment to the adluminal compartment of the seminiferous tubule by opening the occluding inter-Sertoli cell junctions, or both. The enzyme might also participate in remodeling the seminiferous epithelium (17,134,135).

More recent studies indicate that the secretion of PA is dependent on the stage of the seminiferous epithelium cycle (136,137). Secreted PA is of the urokinase type, which predominates in stages VII and VIII of the seminiferous epithelium cycle, whereas tissue-type PA is maximal in stages IX to XII of the cycle. Immunohistochemical analysis using specific antibodies revealed that urokinase-type PA is localized in Sertoli cells in stages VII and VIII; and tissue-type PA is in pachytene and diakinetic primary spermatocytes in stages VII to XIII. These studies suggest that the cyclic secretion of PA is related to the stages of the spermatogenic cycle. Thus, they provide insights into the relationship between the tissue-restructuring processes, such as movement of the preleptotene primary spermatocytes from basal lamina (134) and release of the spermatids from the seminiferous epithelium (138).

H-Y Antigen

H-Y antigen is a male-specific protein that binds to receptors on Sertoli cells of the primordial gonad. Specific receptors for H-Y antigen are found on testicular and ovarian cells but not on cells of extragonadal tissues (139,140). The coupling of H-Y antigen and its receptor is believed to elicit the formation of the testicular cords (141–143). There are two reports indicating that Sertoli cells secrete H-Y antigen. It has been shown that in Sertoli cell culture medium there is a product, similar to the H-Y antigen, which neutralizes the cytotoxicity of anti-H-Y serum against rat-tail epidermal cells (142). In another study, a monoclonal antibody developed against H-Y antigen shows that medium from both primary Sertoli cell-enriched cultures and TM_4 (a mouse Sertoli cell line) contain H-Y antigen (15). These observations, however, were not confirmed by another laboratory, where radiolabeled proteins secreted by rat Sertoli cells in primary culture were examined for specific interactions with polyclonal and monoclonal antibodies directed against serologically detectable H-Y antigen. It is of note that none of the Sertoli cell secretory proteins reacted specifically with H-Y antibodies as determined by immunoprecipitation (144). The reason for the discrepancies between these independent observations remains to be elucidated.

Growth Factors

It was first shown that mouse testes contain a potent mitogen that induces DNA synthesis and cell division in cultures of confluent, quiescent BALB/c 3T3 cells (5,7,145). This mitogen apparently originates from Sertoli cells because this component of the seminiferous epithelium from the prepubertal testis exhibits substantially higher levels of mitogenic activity than do components of other cell types (5). This growth factor is present in the seminiferous epithelium of several mammalian species, including rat, guinea pig, and calf (6). The partially purified growth factor has an MW of 15,700 and a pI between 4.8 and 5.8 (6). The physiologic function of this protein is not yet known; however, it is presumably involved in the regulation of cell proliferation in developing and adult testes (146).

An independent line of research showed that the fibroblast growth factor (FGF) originally isolated from pituitary fractions is a potent stimulator of ovarian cells in culture (147). Similar growth factors can be purified from a wide variety of tissues using heparin-Sepharose affinity chromatography (147,148). These growth factors have similar molecular weights and have relative affinities for heparin-Sepharose. Based on their isoelectric points, it appears that the majority of these endothelial cell mitogens fall into two general classes, namely, acidic and basic FGFs. Both of these peptides will stimulate proliferation of multiple endothelial cell types and both are potent angiogenic agents. Basic FGF is present in pituitary, brain, adrenal, retina, corpus luteum, and kidney, whereas acidic FGF is present in brain, retina, and testes. The cellular localization of FGF in the testis has not yet been established (149).

Recent completion of the amino acid sequences of both basic and acidic FGF has allowed comparison with each other, as well as with other potentially related proteins. Based on amino and carboxyl terminal sequences, there is homology between selected regions of interleukin I and the FGFs. This homology, however, is far less than between the two forms of FGF. For example, interleukin I has approximately 25% and 27% homology with bovine basic and acidic FGF, respectively. By contrast, there is a 53% homology between basic and acidic FGF, and up to 42 of the remaining 66 residues involve nucleotide substitution where a single base change could result in amino acid replacement (149–151). How FGF in the testis relates to the Sertoli cell growth factor of the same MW described above remains to be established.

Another growth factor that has been identified in Sertoli cell-enriched cultures is somatomedin C (9). Studies performed on ovarian cells indicate that this growth factor acts synergistically with FSH (152). It is highly likely that this factor has a similar effect on Sertoli cells. Epidermal growth factor has also been identified in testicular extracts and is known to bind to multiple testicular cells (153). Its site of origin is not known.

Testibumin

During a search for hormonally responsive products in media from Sertoli cell-enriched cultures, a protein that responds synergistically to FSH and testosterone was identified and designated *CMB-1* (154). Structural and immunological analyses, including *N*-terminal sequence determination and immunoblots, indicate that CMB-1 is related to albumin and alpha-fetoprotein (AFP) (25). Furthermore, CMB-1 is highly concentrated in the testicular and epididymal compartments in adult rats. In view of its localization and its similarity to albumin and AFP, we postulate that this may be the albumin homolog of the adluminal compartment of the testis and have called it *testibumin*. The fact that this protein is also found in the blood of adult female rats indicates that, unlike rABP, this protein is not synthesized exclusively in the testis.

Identification and Isolation of Other Sertoli Cell Proteins

As noted above, Sertoli cell products have been, and will continue to be, used as probes for studying Sertoli cells and their interactions with the multiple-germ cell types in the adluminal and basal compartments of the seminiferous tubules. The isolation of these proteins has been difficult because, in many instances, the procedures used to identify them, including one- or two-dimensional gel electrophoresis (21,67,155), have not been useful in subsequent purification as a result of their limited loading capacities. In addition, the use of radioactive amino acids to identify Sertoli cell proteins may confound a subsequent purification strategy because the intensity of labeling does not necessarily indicate which of the proteins in the medium are the major secretory products of Sertoli cells. This problem may be particularly pertinent in products having rapid turnover rates or a large number of the radiolabeled amino acid residues.

The recent application of newly developed HPLC columns to the rapid isolation of TeBGs from serum of human, rabbit, bull (156), and ram (C. Y. Cheng, *unpublished observations*) and of ABP from human testes (108) encouraged us to take a similar approach for the identification and isolation of major Sertoli cell secretory products. The first two steps of this procedure, anion-exchange HPLC and SDS-PAGE, applied to media from Sertoli cell-enriched cultures, are illustrated in Fig. 6. In such media there are more than 30 major acidic proteins (Fig. 6), which have been termed *CMB proteins* (24). When culture media are prepared from Sertoli cells grown with testosterone, FSH, or both hormones, these proteins are classified as those responding (a) to neither hormone, (b) primarily to testosterone, (c) primarily to FSH, or (d) to both hormones (24). It is now possible to isolate many of these proteins from 1 to 2 liters of medium using a variety of HPLC columns (25). It is of note that Sertoli cell-enriched cultures are likely to contain small amounts of peritubular cells and germ cells that can contribute directly or indirectly to the secreted proteins (157,158). Thus, proteins in the Sertoli cell media could be derived from peritubular and residual germ cells. In this regard, Sertoli cells do not secrete fibronectin or Type I collagen into the medium when maintained for up to 6 days

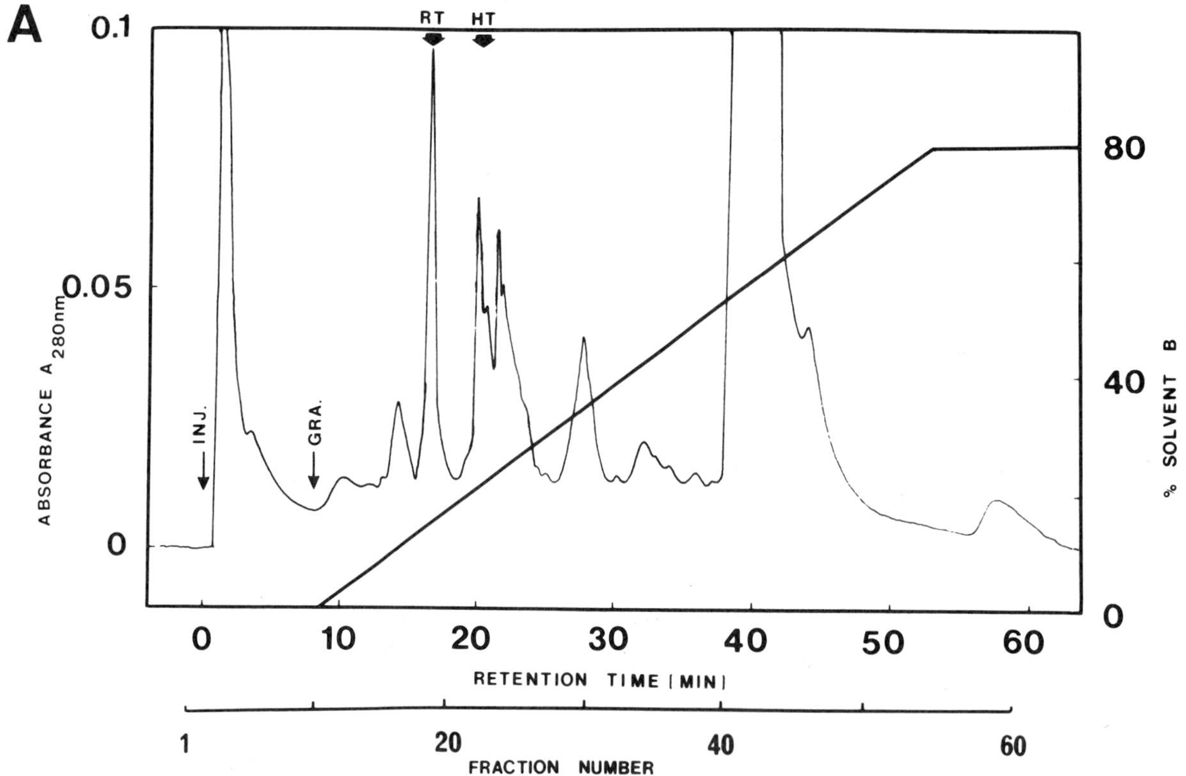

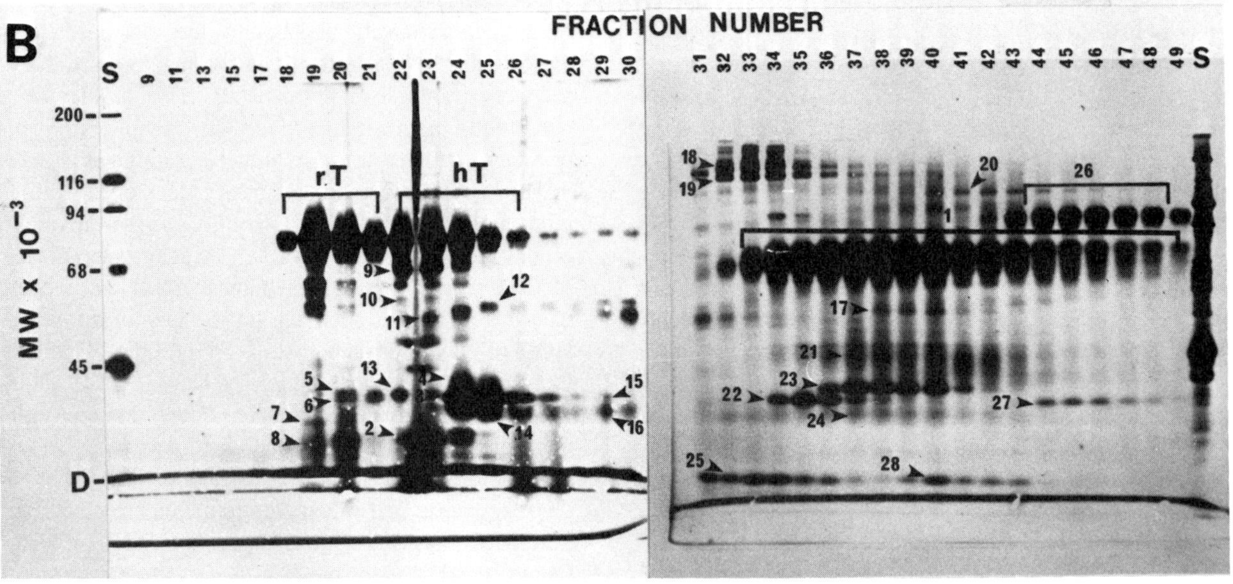

FIG. 6. Fractionation and identification of total secreted proteins, contained in Sertoli cell-enriched culture medium. **A:** Proteins in Sertoli cell-enriched culture medium. Spent medium obtained from Sertoli cells grown in the presence of FSH (300 ng/ml) and testosterone (2×10^{-7} M) was resolved by anion-exchange HPLC. After injection (INJ.) a gradient (GRA.) of 0–80% solvent B (20 mM Tris, 600 mM NaCl, pH 7.4 at 22°C) was applied to the column. Fractions were collected and proteins were monitored by UV absorbance at 280 nm. A total of 15 major protein peaks were resolved. **B:** Polyacrylamide gel electrophoresis of total proteins contained in the fractions resolved by HPLC as shown in A. The numbers indicate the tentative names for these Sertoli cell proteins. (Adapted from ref. 24.)

under serum-free conditions. By contrast, peritubular cells in culture secrete both of these proteins, and, when co-cultured with Sertoli cells, the secretion of both proteins is enhanced (159). Using a monospecific fibronectin antiserum, no fibronectin-like macromolecules were present by Western blotting in the Sertoli cell-enriched cultures used for the isolation of CMB proteins (C. Y. Cheng and C. W. Bardin, *unpublished observations*). This suggests that most of the CMB proteins are of Sertoli cell origin. Nonetheless, the origins of CMB proteins must be established with more direct methods following purification, assay development, and sequence analysis. The characterization of such proteins should show homology with Sertoli secretory products that have been identified by others (21,22,67,155,160–162).

Secretion of Sertoli Cell Hormones

Although many of the proteins and peptides produced by Sertoli cells have autocrine and paracrine effects on the testis, a few of these products are secreted into the blood and act as endocrine mediators on other tissues.

Inhibin

The existence of water-soluble substances of gonadal origin that selectively suppress FSH secretion has been suspected for more than five decades (163). The quest to chemically characterize these molecules, referred to as *inhibin,* proceeded slowly until 1985 (4,164). In the past few years, several investigators have isolated inhibin-like molecules from a variety of sources. Primary structures of a 31-peptide and 94-peptide with inhibin-like activities were reported by Ramasharma et al. (165) and Seidah et al. (166). These peptides were isolated from human seminal plasma. Subsequently, two additional peptides containing 52 and 92 amino acids were also reported (167). Studies using the synthetic 31-peptide demonstrated that it did not have the properties expected of inhibin, since it did not suppress the plasma levels of FSH in castrated rats (168). Robertson and colleagues reported on the isolation of inhibin, from bovine follicular fluid, that had an apparent MW of 56,000. This protein was characterized by two peptide chains of 14,000 and 46,000 MW connected by disulfide bonds (169). Inhibin from porcine follicular fluid was also isolated, but showed an apparent MW of 32,000 (150,170). This peptide consisted of dissimilar polypeptide subunits of 18,000 (α-inhibin) and 14,000 (β-inhibin) MW linked by disulfide bonds (168). A similar protein has also been isolated from ram rete testis fluid. All the preparations purified from ovarian and testicular fluids are several hundredfold more potent than any of the peptides isolated from seminal plasma.

Recently, the *N*-terminal amino acid sequence of α- and β-inhibin was determined, and the data were used to identify cloned complementary DNAs corresponding to the mRNA for pro-inhibin α and β (150,171,172). The complete amino acid sequences of these subunits were predicted from their nucleotide sequences, and it was found that β-inhibin shares a high homology with transforming growth factor β. It is of interest that molecules regulating reproduction and cell growth appear to be related. A more complete description of the history and biological activities of inhibin is given in Chapter 15 of this volume.

Steroids

In the 1930s, testosterone was first isolated from testicular tissue (173); however, it was not until the 1950s that *in vitro* studies using radiolabeled steroid precursors demonstrated that testicular tissue is capable of *de novo* synthesis of testosterone (174,175). *In vitro* studies showed that Leydig cells are responsible for the synthesis of most, if not all, of the androgens in the testis. This topic has been reviewed previously (176) and is also reviewed in another chapter in this volume.

The possibility that Sertoli cells are also involved in steroid biosynthesis has been raised by several observations over the years. One line of evidence is that tumors of Sertoli cell origin secrete steroids (177). In addition, electron microscopic studies show that Sertoli cells possess cytoplasmic organelles typical of steroid-secreting endocrine glands, including extensive smooth endoplasmic reticulum and cholesterol-containing lipid droplets (35). The ability to prepare various testicular cells for *in vitro* studies shows the extent to which various testicular cells are capable of secreting and metabolizing steroids (28,29,178). For example, isolated Sertoli cells exhibit 17β-hydroxysteroid oxidoreductase, 17α-hydroxylase, C17-C20 lyase, and 20α-hydroxysteroid oxidoreductase activities (179–182). In addition, Sertoli cell-enriched cultures from adult rats metabolize progesterone to testosterone, androstenedione, and 3α-hydroxy-5α-androstan-17-one (183). Primary Sertoli cell-enriched cultures from 10- to 20-day-old rats metabolize androstenedione to testosterone, dihydrotestosterone (DHT), and 5α-androstane-3α,17β-diol. The observation that these metabolic conversions are stimulated by FSH suggests that they occur in Sertoli cells rather than in another cell type present in the cultures. In addition, they are age-dependent because the conversion rate is higher in Sertoli cells cultured from 10- to 20-day-old rats than from rats after 20 days of age. This age-dependent pattern is the reverse of that seen in Leydig cells (180,182). Based on these studies it seems unlikely that Sertoli cells contribute significantly to the androgen pool in the blood of adult animals. However, it is possible that some of the steroids produced by Sertoli cells are important for the function of the seminiferous tubule, rete testis, or epididymis.

Following the demonstration that the prostate and seminal vesicles convert testosterone to DHT and the suggestion that the latter steroid may be the biologically active androgen in the male reproductive tract, many investigators measured the formation of DHT by testes (184–186). 5α-Reductase is higher in testes from younger animals and is stimulated by FSH and decreased by LH (187,188). Spermatocytes and Sertoli cells have a greater 5α-reductase activity than do spermatids, but there is very little of this enzyme in Leydig cells. In spermatocytes, the major 5α-reductase product of testosterone is DHT; however, in Sertoli cells, testosterone can be further metabolized to 5α-androstane-3α,17β-diol. In cells from intact testes, the formation of both 3α- and 3β-diol increases until puberty and then declines (189). Even though the testis shows 5α-reductase activity, it is important to compare its *in vivo* efficiency with that of the prostate and seminal vesicle. In prostate and seminal vesicle, the ratio of 5α-reduced metabolites to testosterone is 7:1 whereas in the testis it was 1:2 (190). These observations indicate that the pattern of testosterone metabolism in the seminiferous tubule is very different than that found in the accessory sex organs. Perfusion of the male reproductive tract with [^{3}H]testosterone indicates that dihydrotestosterone, the major androgen, binds to nuclear receptors in epididymis, prostate, and seminal vesicle, whereas testosterone is the major nuclear androgen in the testis (191). Taken together, these observations indicate that dihydrotestosterone is the major active androgen in the accessory sex organs, whereas in the mature testis it is testosterone.

Although Sertoli cell testosterone and androstenedione are not major components of the blood androgen pool, they are important substrates for estradiol and estrone produced in the seminiferous tubular epithelium of the developing animal. Aromatase is highest in young animals and is highly responsive to FSH (192,193). The estradiol production of cultured Sertoli cells in response to FSH has been used as a bioassay for this hormone (194). In the adult human, on whom the most extensive studies have been done, only a small fraction of the estradiol in blood is secreted by the testes; most of this steroid is derived from testosterone in extragonadal tissues. However, in patients with testicular disorders associated with elevated FSH levels, up to 40% of estradiol in blood is of testicular (and possibly of Sertoli cell) origin (195).

HUMORAL REGULATION OF SERTOLI CELL FUNCTION

The major hormonal regulators of the seminiferous epithelium *in vivo* are testosterone and FSH. From *in vitro* studies it is clear that the Sertoli cell is the principal site of action of these hormones and that the regulation of Sertoli cell function is more complex than could be appreciated from *in vivo* studies. The ability to maintain Sertoli cells under serum-free conditions permitted careful definition of the multiple hormones, growth factors, vitamins, metal transport proteins, and attachment factors that are required to maintain growth, protein secretion, and specific morphological features. Furthermore, various combinations of these humoral factors result in different patterns of growth and differentiated function of Sertoli cells *in vitro*. In addition, various cells of the testis regulate Sertoli cells either through direct contact or by modulating the environment of this cell through paracrine factors. These observations, coupled with those described above, indicate that the internal environment of the testis is controlled by Sertoli cells, whose function is, in turn, regulated by multiple humoral and cellular factors. The following is a compilation of some of the factors that have been shown to affect Sertoli cell function.

Polypeptide Hormones

FSH

FSH produces hypertrophy and changes in nuclear morphology of Sertoli cells when administered to hypophysectomized rats (196). In addition, FSH receptors are present on Sertoli cells, which constitute the major site of FSH binding in the testis (197–199). The actions of FSH on diverse functions such as energy metabolism, protein secretion, cell shape, and cell division are mediated via several second messengers, including cAMP and Ca^{2+}.

FSH receptor. Although the FSH receptor is located predominantly on Sertoli cells, recent observations suggest that some binding sites for this hormone may also be located on macrophages in the interstitium of the testis (200,201). The membrane-bound FSH receptor isolated from testis meets the requirements of a physiologically relevant receptor in that the binding of hormone results in activation of adenylate cyclase. This receptor can be detergent solubilized, and a variety of studies suggest that this represents the same molecular form as that present in the membrane. In addition, a cytoplasmic (buffer-soluble) FSH-binding component can be prepared from testes in the absence of detergent (202). The origin of the buffer-soluble binding component is not clear. However, FSH interacts with both forms of receptor in seemingly identical ways. Treatment with FSH produces a decline in the membrane receptor concentration which is coincident with an increase in the buffer-soluble component, suggesting that the latter may be derived from the membrane-bound form (203). It is, therefore, entirely possible that the FSH receptor-like material in cytoplasm is formed as a consequence of receptor processing or recycling. Until the membrane and cytoplasmic FSH-binding forms can be purified, their homologies cannot be confirmed.

Even though the receptor has not been purified to homogeneity, a considerable amount is known about its structure. It is of note that receptors for many peptides and protein hormones are glycoproteins. For example, receptors for growth hormone, insulin, epidermal growth factor, prolactin, TSH, and LH bind to concanavalin A (202). It is surprising, therefore, to find that the solubilized FSH receptor does not bind to this lectin. Evidence for the glycoprotein nature of the FSH receptor is derived from studies using neuraminidase. Removal of sialic acid from the receptor results in increased binding of [^{125}I]FSH which is secondary to a fivefold increase in binding affinity. The role of receptor-associated carbohydrates in hormone recognition and promotion of postbinding effects can be more clearly delineated once the structure of the receptor is known and mutations are produced with selected deletions of specific carbohydrates.

Phospholipids are believed to be components of a number of membrane receptors. Incubation of testicular membranes with phospholipase markedly reduces the specific binding of FSH to membrane-bound receptors. Treatment with this enzyme did not, however, reduce FSH binding to the detergent-solubilized receptor. These results suggest that phospholipids are important in maintaining the receptor in a conformation necessary for FSH binding when it is in the membrane (202).

The MW of the native FSH receptor has been estimated to be approximately 146,000 (204). Studies using cross-linking and photoaffinity-labeling reagents suggest that the FSH receptor may be multimeric, containing at least one 48,000-MW subunit plus other nonidentical subunits (204,205). Similar results have also been obtained for the LH receptor (206). Another interpretation of the presence of multiple nonidentical subunits is that they are produced by limited proteolysis during isolation of the cells or receptor. Such a possibility is suggested by recent studies showing only a single receptor subunit with an MW of 89,000 in the testis and in the ovary when protease inhibitors are used (207).

Large doses of FSH are known to induce the loss of FSH receptors from Sertoli cells both *in vivo* and *in vitro* (208,209). Although the exact mechanism by which FSH mediates this effect on its receptors is not established in detail, it is assumed, based on the large amount of data available on other hormones, that this occurs through receptor-mediated endocytosis. Under such conditions, virtually 100% of receptors are occupied as a result of excess hormone, thus the endocytotic route predominates and most of the surface receptor is depleted. If, however, cells are incubated with an amount of FSH to occupy only 35% of the available receptors, then only 8% of receptors are lost. If the same proportion of receptors are lost following the small and the large doses of FSH, then these observations are consistent with considerable receptor turnover and/or recycling (202). Studies using radioactive FSH indicate that much of the specifically bound hormone is removed from the cell surface within 15 min; following internalization, it is degraded to its component amino acids. Studies with inhibitors suggest that this latter process occurs in lysosomes (210). Receptors for other hormones have similar mechanisms of internalization, degradation, and repletion.

The interaction of FSH with its receptors is influenced by a wide variety of factors. Binding of FSH to membrane-bound receptor is stimulated by Mn^{2+}, Mg^{2+}, or Ca^{2+} and inhibited by Co^{2+} or Ni^{2+}. Binding is also inhibited by monovalent ions (211); bacitracin, polyamines (212), and low-MW factor(s) in seminal plasma (213) or serum (214). In the testes of several species, there are also factors with an MW of 10,000 to 33,000 which inhibit FSH binding to its receptor (215,216). The roles of all the above agents on receptor function and biological activity of FSH *in vivo* remain to be established.

Mediators of FSH action. It is well established that some of the actions of FSH are mediated via the adenylate cyclase-protein kinase system. FSH results in an increase of cAMP (217–222), and either cAMP or substances that elevate cAMP (i.e., cholera toxin) can mimic some of the actions of FSH. In addition to increasing the synthesis of cAMP, FSH also affects various components of this system such as phosphodiesterase and protein kinase inhibitor levels as well as protein phosphorylation per se (223–228).

Following the binding reaction, FSH stimulates adenylate cyclase activity (220). This results in an increase in the intracellular cAMP concentration (217), which, in turn, activates protein kinase (220,229). The phosphorylation of proteins is involved in stimulation and the cascade of subsequent events in the Sertoli cell which ultimately lead to altered function. The observations that FSH stimulates both RNA (230–234) and protein synthesis in the Sertoli cell (235–237) suggested that this hormone affects a number of specific differentiated functions by mechanisms other than modifying the activities of existing protein.

In addition to activating a variety of cellular functions, protein hormones also produce adaptive changes that tend to reduce the response of the cell to further stimulation. This is a general phenomenon that has been observed in many cell types (238–240). Refractoriness to continued hormonal stimulation is usually the result of receptor loss, impaired accumulation of the second messenger, cAMP, and/or alteration of other regulatory mechanisms. FSH-induced refractoriness of Sertoli cells is associated with a decreased number of FSH receptors (208,241), a reduced adenylate cyclase activity (242,243), and a large stimulation of high-affinity cAMP phosphodiesterase, both *in vivo* and *in vitro* (226,227,244). When refractory cells are treated with phosphodiesterase inhibitors, methyl-isobutyl-xanthine, or the nonxanthine phosphodiesterase inhibitor, RO20-1724, the FSH response returns to normal. Treatment of Sertoli cells with FSH also produces an impaired response to a secondary incubation with isoproterenol, cholera toxin, or forskolin. The responses of these compounds are also restored to normal in the presence of phosphodiesterase inhibitors. From these studies it is concluded that even though FSH treatment produces FSH-receptor down regulation and a desensitization of adenylate cyclase, these events are not sufficient to decrease the FSH response. The refractory state can be fully expressed only when adenylate cyclase desensitization is associated with the stimulation of high-affinity cAMP phosphodiesterase. These two regulatory mechanisms cooperate to decrease the intercellular cAMP level, which consequently blunts the subsequent actions of FSH (245).

The intercellular events mediated by peptide hormones are also regulated by calcium. Calmodulin can be thought of as the primary receptor for calcium in much the same way as the regulatory subunits of cAMP-dependent protein kinase are the predominant cAMP receptors in eukaryotic cells (246,247). The interaction of calcium with calmodulin causes a conformational change in this protein so that it can interact with a variety of enzymes to alter their activities (248,249). In some instances, the effects of calcium are antagonistic to those of cAMP, but there are examples of additive or synergistic effects of these intercellular mediators.

In Sertoli cells, widely divergent cellular processes are regulated by common phosphorylation-dephosphorylation reactions, as is the case in other cells. For example, in Sertoli cells, reactions that regulate energy generation involve glycogen synthetase, phosphorylase kinase, and phosphorylase. FSH markedly alters phosphorylase activity, leading to glycogen breakdown and energy production (250). The phosphorylase in these cells is activated by increased concentrations of either cAMP or calcium. The mechanism involves conversion of inactive phosphorylase-b to active phosphorylase-a by phosphorylation. The converting enzyme, phosphorylase kinase, is also activated by phosphorylation. In Sertoli cells, the phosphorylation occurs via the catalytic subunit of cAMP-dependent protein kinase in response to FSH-induced cAMP accumulation. In addition, increases in intercellular calcium also stimulate phosphorylase kinase. In addition to energy generation, calcium effects mediated via calmodulin are believed to affect functions as divergent as cell motility, protein secretion, and cell proliferation (251).

Effects of FSH on differentiated function. The hormonal control of protein secretion by Sertoli cells has been studied by many laboratories. Because rABP was the first specific Sertoli cell protein for which there was a specific immunoassay, it was extensively studied both *in vivo* and *in vitro*. Many studies confirm that rABP levels are increased by chronic FSH treatment both *in vivo* and *in vitro* (62,178,252). The acute effects of this hormone *in vivo* are somewhat more controversial. Tindall and Means (253) showed rapid increases in rABP within 2 hr following FSH treatment. These investigators suggested that this was attributed to the presence of LH contamination, which caused increased testicular testosterone levels. The increased testosterone levels, in turn, had a protective effect on rABP steroid-binding activity, resulting in increased amounts of measurable rABP. This line of reasoning is supported by the observation that enhanced recovery of rABP could be mimicked by the addition of calcium, testosterone, glycerol, or *p*-chloro-mercurophenylsulfonate to the homogenization medium. It was concluded that the rapid effects of FSH were not due to increased synthesis of rABP, but rather to better recovery of androgen-binding activity from testicular extracts. These conclusions are in contrast to those of Kotite et al. (254), who observed that FSH produced a rapid increase in rABP even when steps were taken to ensure maximum stabilization of rABP with glycerol and testosterone. This apparent dilemma has not been resolved. It is of note that it takes many hours before the *in vitro* effects of FSH on rABP accumulation in the culture medium can be observed (255).

In addition to rABP, the secretion of a number of other proteins is affected by FSH; this includes (a) several secretory proteins with unknown function (24,256), (b) plasminogen activator (16,257,258), and (c) the iron-carrier protein, transferrin (127,129,259). However, it is of note that FSH does not have a general effect on the secretion of all Sertoli cell products, since several secreted proteins are unaffected by treatment with this hormone (24).

The secretion of a Sertoli cell product, functionally identified as a *Leydig cell stimulatory factor* (LCSF), has also been shown to be increased *in vitro* by FSH (260,261). This factor has been shown to be a heat-labile, nondialyzable substance that stimulates steroidogenesis in Leydig cells and may be a paracrine substance that is a communication link between the Sertoli and Leydig cells (260,262,263). The existence of such a paracrine system is supported by several lines of evidence that are presented in more detail below.

In addition to protein secretion, several other aspects of Sertoli cell metabolism are regulated by FSH. There are changes in lipids in Sertoli cells that result from hypophysectomy, suggesting that FSH and/or testosterone influence lipid metabolism in this cell; however, the exact nature of the effect is not well established. Sertoli cell cholesterol esterase activity is also modulated by FSH. Two forms of cholesterol esterase are present in the testis: One is a heat-labile enzyme, found exclusively in the Sertoli cell, that increases 20-fold in response to FSH treatment of hypophysectomized rats; the other form is a heat-stable species that is located in Sertoli and Leydig cells and is increased by both LH and FSH. The role of this enzyme in the physiology of these cells is not known (264).

As noted above, FSH influences Sertoli cell energy metabolism. This includes the stimulation of glucose uptake (265), lactate production (266), and the activity of glycogen phosphorylase (250). Because it has been shown that germ cells depend heavily on lactate as an energy source (267), this mobilization of energy resources and the concomitant increase in lactate and pyruvate secretion may play a role in their nourishment.

In addition to affecting Sertoli cell secretory proteins, FSH also increases the synthesis of cell surface glycoproteins (268), which appear to be involved with one another in the interaction of Sertoli cells. FSH-induced cell-cell associations *in vitro* are blocked by specific lectins, inhibitors of protein synthesis, inhibitors of RNA synthesis, and cell surface modification (268,269). These results are consistent with the thesis that FSH increases the production of cell surface glycoproteins, which, in turn, serve as cell adhesion molecules.

Effects of FSH on cell division. In addition to its influence on differentiated function, FSH has a profound affect on the proliferation of Sertoli cells both in the pre- and postnatal period. Exogenous FSH stimulates thymidine incorporation into the DNA of Sertoli cells in fetal rats denied endogenous FSH by hypophysectomy (270). In addition, this hormone also regulates Sertoli cell proliferation in the neonate (271). Prior to 20 days of age in the rat, FSH increases DNA synthesis and mitotic activity (272,273). This response diminishes with increasing age and is not present in the adult. Indeed, this apparent change in FSH responsiveness of the Sertoli cells is observed with other endpoints as well (223,274,275) and may be a reflection of Sertoli cell differentiation prior to and during puberty. A more extensive discussion of Sertoli cell division is presented below with information about testicular hypertrophy.

Insulin and Insulin-Like Growth Factors

Although other polypeptide hormones such as insulin are not as extensively studied as FSH, they are known to play essential roles in regulating Sertoli cell function. Insulin is considered to be an essential factor for growth of these cells in serum-free medium, where it has effects on multiple metabolic parameters (28,276). Insulin appears to have an effect on uptake and incorporation of labeled orthophosphate into free nucleotide pools, which, in turn, is manifested by an increased rate of label incorporation into poly $(A)^+$ RNA (277). Moreover, it has been shown to increase thymidine incorporation into DNA, leucine incorporation into protein, lactate production (278), and hexose uptake (279). With regard to its effects on specific differentiated function in Sertoli cells, insulin has been shown to be essential for the secretion of both transferrin and rABP (276). All of the effects of insulin on Sertoli cells are observed *in vitro* at micromolar concentrations even though most of the actions that are thought to be mediated via the insulin receptor are believed to be maximally stimulated by nanomolar quantities of this hormone. Insulin-like effects are also observed with nanomolar concentrations of insulin-like growth factor I (DNA synthesis and hexose uptake) and insulin-like growth factor II (DNA and protein synthesis as well as lactate production) (278,279). It is, therefore, possible that many, if not all, of these responses of Sertoli cells to insulin may result from the binding of this hormone to insulin-like growth receptors. An alternative explanation for the requirement for supraphysiological amounts of insulin is that Sertoli cells produce insulinase *in vitro* which is particularly active in serum-free medium.

Glucagon. Another polypeptide hormone known to have an affect on the Sertoli cell is glucagon (280). This hormone increases cAMP levels and has a magnitude and kinetic response similar to that of FSH. One of the consequences of glucagon stimulation is an increase in the rate of testosterone aromatization, a response also produced by other substances, including FSH, that stimulate cAMP production by Sertoli cells (280).

Calcitonin. Receptors for calcitonin are present in membrane fractions of testes, and autoradiographic studies show these binding sites are located primarily on Leydig cells (281,282); however, examination of published autoradiographs suggests that binding sites for calcitonin are also present in seminiferous tubules, possibly on Sertoli cells. Although the physiologic functions of calcitonin receptors on testicular cells are not known, this hormone regulates (a) cAMP accumulation in the TM_4 Sertoli cell line and (b) rABP secretion by primary Sertoli cells (283). In addition, this peptide increases the total concentration of both androgen and estrogen receptors in TM_4 cells (283). The observation that 8-bromo-cAMP decreases androgen and estrogen receptor concentrations suggests that the calcitonin effect is not mediated by cAMP. The fact that calcitonin-induced increases in receptor levels can be reversed by lowering extracellular calcium concentrations suggests that the effects of calcitonin might be modulated by this cation. The effects of calcium channel blockers and calcium ionophores are consistent with this hypothesis (283). Thus, part of the effects of calcitonin on Sertoli cell function are mediated by cAMP and others by changes in intracellular calcium.

Pro-Opiomelanocortin (POMC)-derived peptides. Peptides derived from the hormone precursor POMC, including ACTH, α-MSH, and β-endorphin, have a variety of effects on Sertoli cells (284,285). This conclusion was reached after the demonstration of the presence of POMC-derived peptides in the male reproductive tract (286,287). In the testis, immunostainable β-endorphin and ACTH-like substances are in the cytoplasm of Leydig cells (288,289), suggesting that POMC-derived peptides are synthesized in this cell type. This postulate is supported by the demonstration of POMC mRNA in Leydig cells (290–292). The low concentrations of secreted peptides suggest that they might have autocrine and/or paracrine functions within the testis rather than effects via the general circulation (288).

Following the demonstration that all peptides with MSH-like activity, including ACTH, stimulate adenylate cyclase activity in the Sertoli cell (284,293,294), a detailed study was performed to determine the effects of α-MSH and des-acetyl-α-MSH on Sertoli cell function *in vitro* (295). Both peptides stimulate cAMP secretion and aromatase activity in primary Sertoli cell cultures when incubated in the presence of a phosphodiesterase inhibitor, FSH, or forskolin. Both peptides shift the FSH dose-response curve to the left, thus making the cells more sensitive to this gonadotropin. Furthermore, the apparent potencies of α-MSH and its des-acetyl derivative are similar when measured on Sertoli cells. In this regard, it is well known that *N*-acetylation has an important effect on the biological activities of POMC-derived peptides in the central nervous system. For example, in several behavioral actions such as arousal and expressive grooming, α-MSH is much more potent than des-acetyl-α-MSH (296,297). By contrast, only the des-acetylated form is able to block opiate analgesia and opiate receptor binding (298). In addition, the activity of α-MSH on melanosome dispersion in melanocytes of *Rana pipiens* is also influenced by *N*-acetylation because α-MSH is much more active than des-acetyl-α-MSH (299). In view of these observations, it is surprising that these peptides are equipotent in their actions on Sertoli cells (295).

To search for possible effects of β-endorphin on the testis, an investigation of its influence on testis growth in young animals was undertaken. Potent opiate antagonists, nalmefene or naloxone, injected intratesticularly in neonatal rats increased the compensatory hypertrophy following unilateral castration (300–302). Naloxone and β-endorphin antiserum increase Sertoli cell division in explants of neonatal testis (303). Treatment of hemicastrate male rats with the opiate antagonists was also associated with a marked rise in rABP secretion (284,302). The increase in testicular size and rABP secretion following antagonist administration is consistent with the hypothesis that β-endorphin or other endogenous opiates inhibit Sertoli cell growth and secretion during early testicular development and are antagonistic to gonadotropins during this time period. Recent studies have demonstrated the presence of receptors for β-endorphin on Sertoli cells (304). It is of note that other opiates in addition to β-endorphin are present in testes based on the results of peptide isolation and the presence of proenkephalin and prodynorphin mRNA (305).

Taken together, the results from *in vivo* and *in vitro* experiments suggest that peptides derived from various portions of the POMC molecule have differential effects on Sertoli cells. For example, ACTH stimulates proliferation and both ACTH and MSH-like peptides increase cAMP production by primary Sertoli cells and Sertoli cell lines. By contrast, β-endorphin or another endogenous opiate inhibits Sertoli cell proliferation and secretion of specific proteins. Opposing effects of different POMC-derived peptides in other tissues are also known. For example, ACTH-like peptides and β-endorphin have opposing effects on different types of behavior. β-Endorphin is a potent inhibitor of the lordosis response in rats, whereas α-MSH facilitates female sexual behavior (306). The interesting question raised by these observations is how two peptides, which can be produced in equimolar amounts from the same precursor, regulate opposite biological responses. The answer to this question is not known for any tissue where POMC is synthesized, but several possibilities may exist. First, there may be selective processing of POMC, as is the case for ACTH in anterior pituitary and α-MSH in intermediate pituitary. Second, the activity of a peptide can be altered by *N*-acetylation, as occurs for MSH and β-endorphin in the intermediate pituitary. Finally, there may be rapid turnover of a peptide from one portion of POMC by a locally produced protease which would allow a peptide from another part of the molecule to dominate (307). Thus, the biological consequences of POMC synthesis in the testis will depend not only on the amount of the precursor that is made but also on which of its component peptides are present in biologically active form. The autocrine effects of POMC-derived peptides on Leydig cells are reviewed elsewhere (308).

Steroid Hormones

A number of steroid hormones are known (or believed) to affect Sertoli cells because of either demonstrated effects or the presence of specific steroid receptors. The most extensively studied steroid is testosterone. In addition, other molecules, including estrogens, progestins, and glucocorticoids, also have effects on these cells. *In vitro* experiments permit detailed studies of the action of steroid hormones on Sertoli cells which are difficult to achieve with *in vivo* experiments.

Androgens

Sertoli cells have typical androgen receptors (309,310) that mediate the effects of testosterone. Some of the effects of this steroid mimic those of FSH. This can be observed on the secretion of selected proteins (24) and on the maintenance of spermatogenesis after hypophysectomy. In addition, some of the actions of testosterone appear to oppose those of FSH. For example, androgens inhibit FSH-induced "rounding up" of Sertoli cells in culture, presumably by enhancing actin organization, whereas FSH stimulates disorganization (311). In addition, testosterone inhibits FSH-induced inhibin secretion (P. Morris, *unpublished observations*). There are also morphological changes in Sertoli cells deprived of androgens. These include alteration in nuclear and mitochondrial morphology, increase in the amount of lipid droplets, and decreases in smooth endoplasmic reticulum (312).

Testosterone also has a general effect on transcriptional activity (232). The addition of this hormone to Sertoli cells in culture produces a rapid but transient (15 min) increase in RNA polymerase II activity followed by a further and more prolonged increase 3 to 6 hr later. This is in contrast to the response to FSH which increases polymerase, I, II, and III over a longer time period (232,233).

The effects of androgens on more terminally differentiated functions have also been studied using rABP as an endpoint both *in vivo* (313,314) and *in vitro* (255,315,316). Rat Sertoli cells cultured in serum-free medium survive longer and secrete more rABP when cultured with physiological concentrations of testosterone (255,317).

The *in vivo* effects of testosterone are dependent upon the stage of differentiation of the seminiferous epithelium. In immature long-term hypophysectomized animals, testicular but not epididymal levels of rABP increase following androgen treatment (91). This is consistent with the *in vitro* data outlined above. In mature animals, there is a slow decrease in testicular and epididymal rABP levels following hypophysectomy that can be prevented by the administration of androgen (318). If the testis is allowed to fully regress, subsequent androgen administration will increase rABP levels in the blood and testis but not in the epididymis (319). In this latter instance, FSH is required in order to facilitate secretion of rABP into the tubular lumen as well as facilitate its transport to the epididymis. These different effects of testosterone on the Sertoli cells of newly hypophysectomized and on fully regressed hypophysectomized animals are likely to be a function of the differentiated state of this cell. If Sertoli cells are fully differentiated, their function can be maintained by testosterone alone, whereas the acquisition of the differentiated state typical of intact adults occurs in response to FSH. Other explanations for these findings are also possible. For example, little is known about the *in situ* degradation of rABP during testicular regression and about the effects of testosterone on this process. It is, therefore, not known whether testosterone affects degradation as well as synthesis of rABP under these experimental conditions. It is possible that some effects of testosterone on maintaining the differentiated state may be to slow the turnover of rABP and other proteins as it is known to do in other organs (320).

Studies by Tsutsui and Ishii (321,322) suggest that, in some species, androgens play a role in regulating the number of FSH receptors. Testosterone administration to birds during photoperiod-induced testicular regression results in an increase in the density of FSH receptors. This response could also be observed with the administration of FSH, but combined treatment with both hormones caused a greater increase in these receptors. These authors suggest that testosterone and FSH act synergistically to induce FSH-receptor synthesis.

Finally, it should be noted that part of the effects of testosterone on Sertoli cells appear to be mediated by the action of this steroid on testicular myoid cells. An androgen-dependent product from these cells has marked effects on several Sertoli cell functions (157,158). These observations are perhaps similar to those in prostate, where mesenchyme cells appear to mediate most, if not all, of the actions of testosterone on the epithelium (323,324).

Estrogens

As noted above, Sertoli cells produce estradiol, which is under the influence of FSH. The observation that Sertoli cell lines have estrogen receptors and are growth inhibited by low levels of estradiol suggested that these cells might also respond to this class of hormones (31). Interestingly, estrogen receptors are present at or below the level of detection (12 $\pm$ 3 fmole/mg protein) in newly isolated Sertoli cells. However, following 15 days of culture, estrogen receptors rise to 50 $\pm$ 5 fmole/mg protein (325). The appearance of estrogen receptors in primary Sertoli cells with increasing time in culture suggests that these cells are capable of producing receptors even though they are undetectable in freshly isolated cells. There are many reasons why estrogen receptors may not be measurable in newly isolated Sertoli cells. One possibility is that these receptors are present in only a limited number of Sertoli cells along the length of the tubule as a result of interaction with germ cells of a specific stage of the cycle. The fact that estrogen receptors are not detectable in segments of tubules isolated and pooled according to stage of spermatogenic cycle argues against this possibility (326). An alternative possibility is that estrogen receptors are uniformly suppressed in all Sertoli cells by some testicular product(s). One candidate for such an agent is estradiol per se, since it is locally produced and causes translocation of receptors to the nucleus so that the content available in the cytoplasm at any one time is low. On the other hand, testosterone decreases estrogen receptors in a Sertoli cell line, suggesting that androgens may regulate this class of receptors in the seminiferous epithelium (325).

Other Steroid Hormones

There are limited studies on the effects of steroids other than androgens and estrogens on Sertoli cells. Both hydrocortisone and progesterone can be shown to increase ABP secretion *in vitro* (255). Progesterone also increases RNA polymerase II in Sertoli-enriched cultures, and Wagle et al. (327) suggested that these responses may be mediated through the androgen receptor.

Vitamins

Deficiencies of certain vitamins reduce fertility in male rats. Although reduced fertility in such animals could result from the systemic effects of the deficient states, the finding that at least two vitamins influence Sertoli cell function *in vitro* and that another has receptors in Sertoli cells suggests that these agents might directly influence testicular function.

Vitamin A

Vitamin A (retinol) is a lipid soluble vitamin known to be important in vision and fertility. Male animals made deficient in this vitamin cease production of spermatozoa, and several markers of Sertoli cell function also change. The production of at least two secretory proteins by Sertoli cells *in vitro* is influenced by retinol. This includes the increased secretion of transferrin in the presence of either retinol or retinoic acid (127,129). In addition, rABP is also influenced similarly by this vitamin (127,255,276). There is one report indicating that vitamin A also lowers uridine pools in Sertoli cells (328) but does not change either total protein synthesis or growth rate.

Retinoids exert their actions via an intracellular binding

protein much like the classic steroid hormone receptor. Vitamin A is concentrated by Sertoli cells (329); in addition, these cells contain an intracellular retinol-binding protein (13). This receptor has the same physical characteristics as the cellular retinol-binding protein found in the liver but is distinct from the cellular retinoic acid-binding protein found in germ cells (330). The amount of this cellular retinol-binding protein in the Sertoli cells is influenced by both FSH (13) and germ cell association (330).

Vitamin E

Another lipoidal vitamin that affects Sertoli cells is vitamin E. This substance appears to have no effect on transferrin production by Sertoli cells, but it does influence rABP secretion (127). In addition, vitamin E influences both plating efficiency and multiplication of immature Sertoli cells in culture (127).

Vitamin D

There are few studies on the effects of vitamin D_3 and its analogs on Sertoli cell function either *in vivo* or *in vitro*. There is, however, a high-affinity low-capacity receptor for this steroid. There is little or no vitamin D_3 receptor in testes from prepubertal rats, but there is a progressive increase as animals mature (331). Several studies suggest that these receptors are localized in a nongerminal component of seminiferous tubules, probably Sertoli cells (332). These findings support the postulate that the Sertoli cell is a site of action for vitamin D_3, but do not explain its role in testicular biology.

Cell Matrix and Attachment Factors

One of the more significant advances in cell biology in recent years has been the elucidation of how the insoluble extracellular matrix (ECM) which comprises the basal lamina influences the differentiated function of epithelial cells. This subject has been reviewed in detail by several groups of investigators (333–336). When Sertoli cells are grown *in vitro* on plastic, they form a flattened and well-spread monolayer. By contrast, the same cells grown on plastic covered by peritubular myoid cells (which produce ECM) (337), testicular extracellular matrix (338), or extracellular matrix derived from a tumor (339) attain a more cuboidal shape and spread more slowly. These morphological characteristics more closely resemble those of Sertoli cells *in vivo* (Fig. 7). Other characteristics of Sertoli cells grown on ECM are the formation of typical basolateral junctional complexes (338,339) and a decrease in the rate of DNA synthesis. These are also characteristics of Sertoli cells as they mature *in vivo* (273,339).

The effects of ECM on various differentiated functions revealed that the basal secretion of several proteins is enhanced when cells are grown on this substance. These include the well-established markers such as ABP and transferrin, as well as type-1 collagen. Furthermore, there is a substantial increase in total protein secretion (339). In addition to improving the basal secretion of proteins, ECM of all types markedly increases the response of Sertoli cells to FSH. The ECM formed by myoid cells had the most pronounced effect when compared to matrix components (337).

One poorly understood function of differentiated Sertoli cells is their ability to support the growth of germ cells. When Sertoli cells and their accompanying germ cells are plated on plastic surfaces, the germ cells degenerate over a period of several days. When comparable cultures are grown on ECM, viable germinal elements are retained in the Sertoli cell monolayer, but do not show signs of further development (339). These observations suggest that ECM contributes to Sertoli cell differentiation so as to allow them to maintain one component of Sertoli cell/germ cell interaction; however, contact alone is not sufficient to support further maturation. Germ cells can mature in culture in defined medium when a tubular segment is grown with intact basal lamina (ECM) and myoid cells (340).

One exciting observation is the demonstration that mixed Sertoli and germ cell cultures from 10-day-old rat testes are capable of reassociating into structures that resemble seminiferous tubules when grown on thick ECM layers. These cords of Sertoli cells are organized with spermatogonia embedded on their outer surfaces; junctional complexes form between adjacent Sertoli cells, and the interior of these cords becomes inaccessible to large molecules. With further time in culture, cells with morphological characteristics of late pachytene spermatocytes appear within the tubules (339). These results suggest that under appropriate conditions the native ability of Sertoli cells to form tubules occurs, thus producing an isolated environment that will allow the development of germ cells.

THE CELLULAR REGULATION OF SERTOLI CELLS

In addition to the effects of various humoral factors, Sertoli cells are also dramatically altered by the cells that surround them. These include germ, myoid, and Leydig cells. In some instances, these interactions require direct contact between cells, whereas other interactions depend upon paracrine factors. In many instances, the type of factor that mediates such interactions is not known.

Germ Cell/Sertoli Cell Interactions

The ability to examine Sertoli cell/germ cell interaction is based upon the observation that germ cells are not randomly distributed along the length of the seminiferous epithelium but are strictly arranged in defined cell associations or stages. The most commonly used classification of germ cell associations makes use of the "steps of spermatogen-

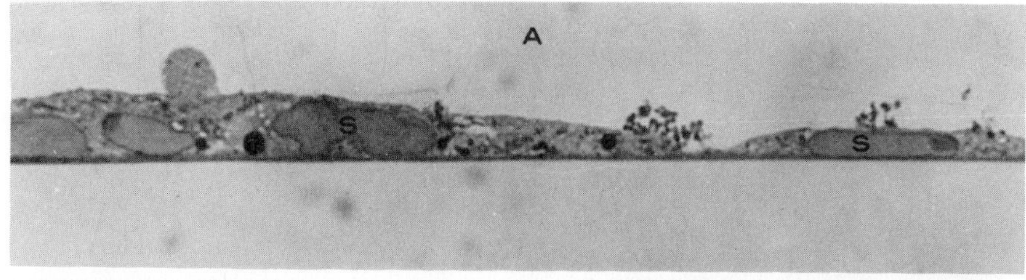

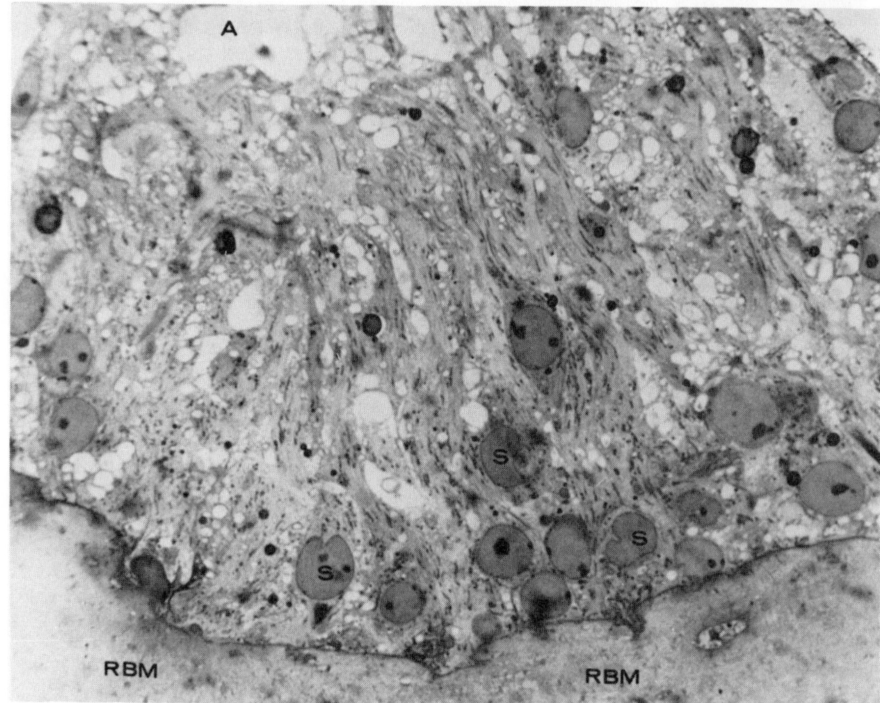

FIG. 7. Light micrographs (× 780) of Sertoli cells grown in serum-free media in the presence of various substrata. **Top:** Cells on plastic appear as low squamous cells with flattened nuclei. **Bottom:** Sertoli cells on reconstituted basement membrane (RBM) from the ETS tumor form tall monolayers with extensive cytoplasmic stalks. Sertoli cell nuclei (S) and apical surface (A) are indicated. (From ref. 339.)

esis," as seen in sections stained with periodic acid-Schiff reagent (138). In the rat, there are 14 morphologic stages, and each stage has a constant duration. The succession of different stages in time at a given point in the tubular epithelium is called the *spermatogenic cycle*. For each species, the duration of the cycle is constant and can be thought of as a biological clock for that species. In the rat, the complete cycle of stages lasts 12 days. Thus, at any site along the seminiferous tubule, the germ cells associated with a group of Sertoli cells are morphologically distinct from those associated with an adjacent group of Sertoli cells just a few millimeters away (Fig. 8) (32).

Sertoli cell morphology also varies along the length of the seminiferous tubule in conjunction with the changes in germ cells. These include changes in nuclear morphology, the quantity of cytoplasmic lipid, and the variation of the number of enzymes, as analyzed by histochemistry (138,341,342). These changes in Sertoli cells are coordinated with the spermatogenic cycle.

The different stages of the spermatogenic cycle in adjacent segments of the seminiferous tubular epithelium can be demonstrated by transillumination in freshly isolated, unstained, seminiferous tubules (Fig. 8) (343). Based on light transmission, tubular segments representing different stages can be isolated and studied *in vitro*. Using these segments, it is possible to demonstrate that many aspects of Sertoli cell function vary along the length of the tubule in concert with the stage of the cycle (32). For example, maximal FSH binding to receptors occurs on Sertoli cells in Stage I, whereas the maximal FSH-stimulated cAMP production occurs in stages I to III and cAMP phosphodiesterase is highest in stages VI and VII (32). In addition to the cyclic changes in constitutive Sertoli cell proteins, the secretion of a number of products by these cells is also enhanced during specific stages of the germ cell cycle (Fig. 9). For example, plasminogen activator is specifically secreted only in stages VII and VIII of the cycle (344). As noted above, this enzyme is believed to play a role in the release of maturing spermatids from the seminiferous tubular epithelium at stage VIII. Also at stage VIII, primary spermatocytes move from the basal compartment of the seminiferous tubular epithelium, through the junctional complexes between adjacent Sertoli cells, into the adluminal compartment. This process is also thought to involve plasminogen activator secreted by Sertoli cells. Androgen-binding protein is also secreted in a cyclic manner with a peak at stages IX to XI (318,345). The cyclic secretion of many other Sertoli cell products is known from *in vitro* studies

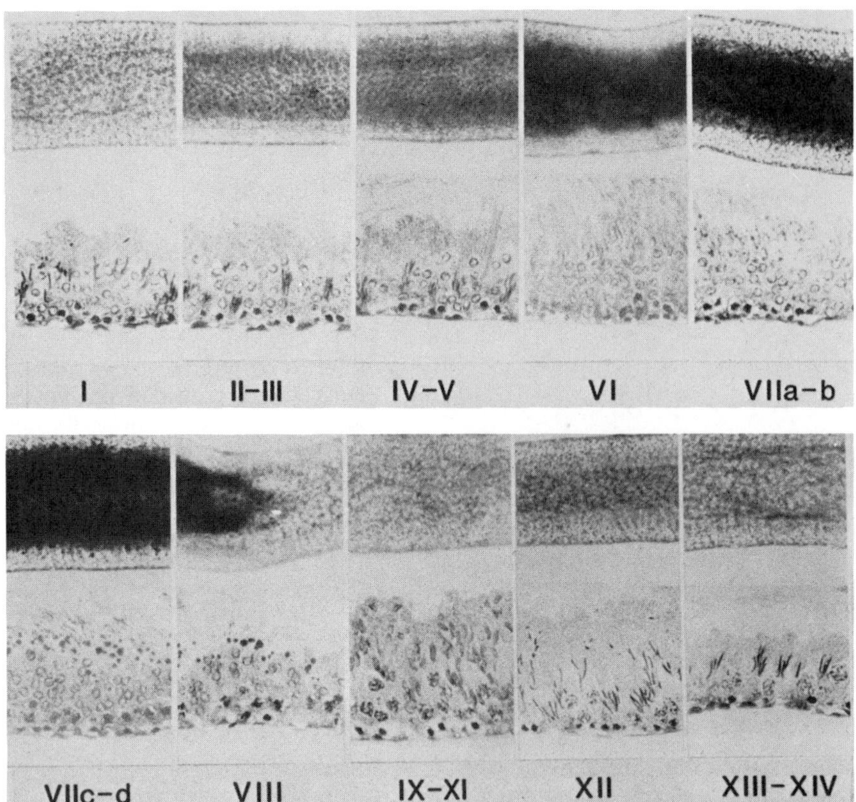

FIG. 8. Transillumination pattern of freshly isolated rat seminiferous tubule related to the stage of the cycle of the seminiferous tubule epithelium. The roman numerals indicate the stages of the cycle as defined by the fixed stained sections along the lower portion of the figure. These are correlated with the transillumination of the unfixed tubules in the upper portion of the figure. (From ref. 32.)

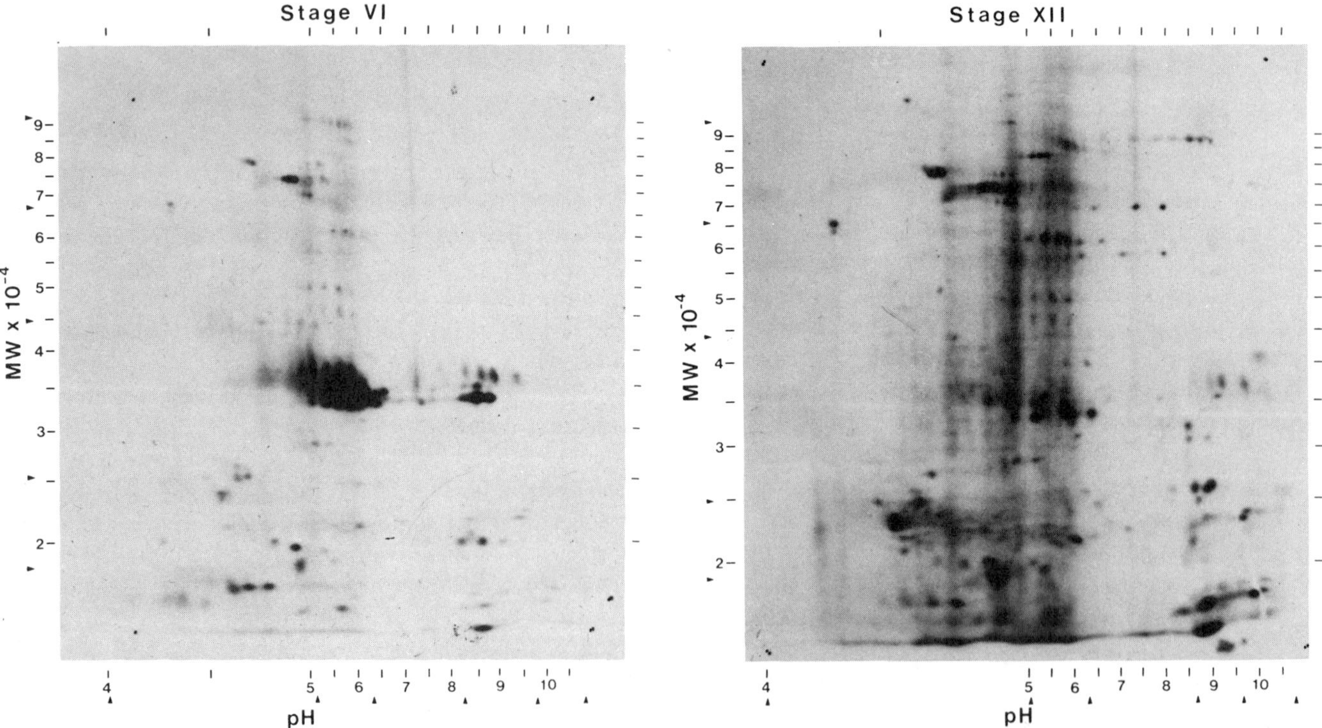

FIG. 9. Two-dimensional gel of electrophoresis of total ^{35}S-labeled secreted proteins at stage VI and stage XII of the cycle of the seminiferous tubular epithelium. Radiolabeled proteins were detected by fluorography. The position of the standards of each gel are indicated by the arrows next to the scales. The spots shown are believed to be proteins of Sertoli cell origin, because the segments were incubated in the absence of myoid cells. The pattern of secretion is reminiscent of those from two separate organs rather than from the same cells a few millimeters apart along the length of the seminiferous tubule. (From ref. 21.)

using tubular segments isolated by the transillumination technique. Results of these studies indicate that both the morphology and the biological functions of Sertoli cells cycle with the germinal components of the seminiferous tubular epithelium. Existing information suggests that germ and Sertoli cells are the minimal elements required to form the biological clock in the seminiferous tubule (21).

Myoid Cell/Sertoli Cell Interactions

In addition to the germ cell/Sertoli cell interaction, myoid cells also interact with Sertoli cells and influence their behavior. As noted above, a factor elicited by these cells influences the secretion of specific proteins (157,158,259) by Sertoli cells *in vitro*. The secretion of rABP and transferrin, but not plasminogen activator, are stimulated. In addition, it appears not to be a mitogenic factor (158). The induction of this putative paracrine factor by peritubular myoid cells is stimulated by androgens but not estrogens (157). This observation raises the question as to whether the testosterone effects on Sertoli cells are direct; they might be indirect through testosterone's action on peritubular myoid production of this factor (157,158,346).

The effects of myoid cell interaction with Sertoli cells are not confined to secreted proteins. Several enzymes (i.e., lactic dehydrogenase, succinic dehydrogenase, glucose-6-phosphate dehydrogenase, and nonspecific esterases) are maintained in Sertoli cells only when they are co-cultured with peritubular cells (347). In addition, there appears to be interaction between these two cell types with regard to the production and/or deposition of ECM (159,348). The presence of this ECM enhances plating efficiency and viability and accounts for the unique morphological characteristics seen in such co-cultures (346,348). Finally, myoid cells can modulate the cyclic secretion of Sertoli cell proteins that are entrained by the spermatogenic cycle. As noted above, rABP secretion is maximal at stages IX to XI. The peak secretion occurs at the same stages whether myoid cells are present or not. However, in the presence of myoid cells, rABP secretion is three to five times higher than in the absence of these cells (59). We conclude that myoid cells act as an amplifier of the clock created by the Sertoli cell/germ cell unit.

Leydig Cell/Sertoli Cell Interactions

Cellular interactions of Sertoli cells also affect Leydig cells, either directly or in their link between germ cells and myoid cells. Paracrine factors rather than cell-cell contacts are believed to be the important means of communication between Leydig cells and the seminiferous tubule (349). Leydig cells show a cyclic variation in size which is dependent on the stage of tubules adjacent to them (350). In this case, the cells adjacent to stages VII and VIII tubules are larger than those associated with other stages. These observations are further enhanced by the demonstration that rat (260,351) and pig (352,353) Sertoli cells secrete a product that can stimulate Leydig cell steroid production. Furthermore, the secretion of this factor is enhanced by FSH. Thus, it is tempting to speculate that there is a substance produced by Sertoli cells which is regulated by endocrine (FSH) and paracrine factors (germinal cell associations) and communicates with the adjacent Leydig cells to modulate the local production of testosterone. Inhibin is one possible candidate for such a substance, since its production by Sertoli cells is stimulated by FSH and it, in turn, stimulates steroidogenesis in Leydig cells (C. W. Bardin, *unpublished observations*).

In summary, it appears that Sertoli cell functions are controlled not only by humoral factors but also by a complex paracrine system that modulates this cell's responses and modifies its functions in a manner dependent on cell-cell interactions between Sertoli cells, germ cells, Leydig cells, and myoid cells.

THE SERTOLI CELL *IN VIVO*

The multiple factors implicated in control of Sertoli cell function are derived not only from the different cell types within the testis, but also from the circulation and possibly the nervous system. This complexity of control mechanisms, coupled with the implicit heterogeneity of the Sertoli cell population arising from the cycle of the seminiferous epithelium, cannot, as yet, be replicated for *in vitro* studies. Thus, there is impetus for studies of Sertoli cell function in the intact animal to complement the *in vitro* approach. The areas where significant advances have been made in recent years include: Sertoli cell differentiation; Sertoli cell proliferation; and the bidirectional release of Sertoli cell products in naturally occurring and experimentally induced pathophysiologic states.

Sertoli Cell Differentiation and Proliferation

The differentiation of Sertoli cells *in utero* and their subsequent proliferation during fetal and neonatal life are complex events involving presently unknown signals for the initiation of differentiation from within the testis as well as humoral factors from extratesticular sites. In the normal animal, this sequence of events results in the complement of mature Sertoli cells required to support spermatogenesis and fertility. Although there are, at present, several clearly identifiable factors modulating this progression, it appears that, once initiated, the process continues in an orderly fashion and is completed prior to puberty. In the rat, this occurs over a period of about 30 days of fetal and neonatal life. During this period a number of events are characterized by the appearance of clear markers that provide convenient indices for investigating the factors involved in modulating this developmental process. Recent morphological studies describe the developmental aspects of Sertoli cell ultrastructure in the rat (354), mouse (355), pig (356), and human (357). Specific reference to those aspects of ultrastructure development which have direct bearing on Sertoli cell function *in vivo* are noted below.

In mammals, the appearance of the primordial Sertoli cell is the first identifiable event in testicular differentiation. Early histological studies of the differentiating fetal rat testis (358), confirmed later by careful ultrastructural studies (359), indicate that these cells appear on day 13 post-fertilization and then aggregate and form seminiferous cords the following day. The signal responsible for eliciting the appearance of the primordial Sertoli cell has not been identified but presumably is related to gene products, encoded on the Y chromosome, that signal the bipotential fetal gonad to develop into a testis. The initial appearance of the differentiating Sertoli cell and subsequent organogenesis, that is, aggregation and formation of seminiferous cords, are apparently regulated independently, since early organogenesis is inhibited by factors present in fetal calf serum while morphologically distinct Sertoli cells are maintained (360,361).

Following the initial appearance of distinct Sertoli cells and the early stages of organogenesis, there is a period of rapid proliferation. In the rat this begins in fetal life, continues during early neonatal life, and is complete before closure of the blood-testis barrier (271,362). Since the Sertoli cell population in the adult animal is determined during this period, any disruption of the proliferative process will have a profound effect by reducing the ultimate Sertoli cell population, which will, in turn, influence testicular size of the adult animal. Recent studies confirm that inhibition of Sertoli cell proliferation in neonatal rats causes a decreased Sertoli cell population in the adult animal, with a commensurate decrease in germinal elements (363).

A number of investigators have studied this critical period in Sertoli cell development. Short-term uptake (2 hr) of [^{3}H]thymidine indicates that an appreciable fraction of Sertoli cells (~15%) are undergoing replication as early as day 16 post-conception (pc) (271). This fraction increases steadily to reach a peak value of about 27% on day 20 pc and then decreases monotonically to reach undetectable levels by day 21 post-partum. Thus, in the rat, maximum rates of Sertoli cell proliferation occur during fetal life. The cessation of Sertoli cell proliferation prior to puberty also occurs in other species. Studies of [^{3}H]thymidine uptake by Sertoli cell nuclei suggest that proliferation ceases by day 12 postpartum in the mouse (364) and does not occur in the post pubertal monkey (365). Histometric studies of the developing testis in the human indicated that a relatively constant Sertoli cell population may be achieved by as early as 3 years of age (366).

Based on proliferation rates found for Sertoli cells in the rat, it would appear that factors influencing this process in fetal animals have the greatest potential for affecting testicular function in adults, whereas events during late neonatal and prepubertal life may have a less dramatic affect on the adult Sertoli cell population.

Since FSH and androgens have long been considered to be of primary importance in regulation of Sertoli cell function *in vivo*, both in immature and adult animals, it is reasonable to expect them also to play a role in Sertoli cell function in the fetal animal. Recent studies employing *in utero* neutralization of FSH as well as ablation of the fetal pituitary by decapitation suggest that FSH is a major factor in controlling expansion of the Sertoli cell population in fetal rats (270). In addition, Sertoli cells from fetuses deprived of endogenous FSH are responsive to both FSH and cyclic nucleotides *in vitro*, and these agents can restore rates of Sertoli cell proliferation to those found in intact animals. Ablation studies performed in the fetal pig show that Sertoli cell ultrastructure develops normally, even in the absence of the fetal pituitary (356). These findings are consistent with the notion that a pattern for development of Sertoli cells is laid down early in fetal life and proceeds according to this intrinsic pattern.

The observation that FSH is essential for initiating spermatogenesis in immature animals, an event occurring near the end of the proliferative phase of Sertoli cell development, suggests the continued influence of FSH on Sertoli cells during this period (367). Studies using antibodies to neutralize FSH and LH in immature animals pointed out the importance of FSH to the normal developmental process (368). Further discussions of the *in vivo* effects of FSH as well as other modulating factors during the proliferative period are presented at several points later in this review.

Since FSH action on the Sertoli cell is dependent on its binding to surface receptors, the strong influence of this hormone on proliferation, as well as its continued action during prepubertal life, implies the existence of an adequate receptor population. Autoradiographic studies showing that Sertoli cells have most of the FSH-binding sites in the testis (369) are supported by binding studies using enriched Sertoli cell preparations and highly purified Leydig cells as negative controls (193). FSH binding is detectable in fetal rat testes shortly after the appearance of differentiated Sertoli cells (370). Thereafter, total testicular receptor content rises slowly until about 19 days pc, when there is a dramatic increase concomitant with the rapid rise in testis weight during the period of maximal Sertoli cell proliferation (271). Following birth, FSH binding per testis continues to increase, although there are conflicting data regarding the duration of the increase. One study shows a 10-fold increase, leading to a plateau on day 15, and then constant levels until at least day 60 of age (371), whereas other studies indicate a steady increase until well past puberty (372). Studies in the sheep (373) and mouse (372) also show that steady increases in total testicular FSH receptors continue through puberty. Experiments using isolated Sertoli cells confirm the early increase in FSH receptors, but do not resolve the question regarding FSH receptor numbers in nonproliferating Sertoli cells because the studies were not continued beyond 15 days of age (193). The attainment of a constant level of binding at about day 15, concomitant with cessation of Sertoli cell proliferation, would be consistent with a constant number of FSH receptors per Sertoli cell from day 15 through puberty, whereas continuously increasing FSH binding per testis would imply increasing numbers of FSH receptors per Sertoli cell during this period. Regardless of this problem, it appears that the number of FSH receptors per Sertoli cell does not change dramatically during the proliferative period, since the increase in total receptor content roughly parallels testicular growth during this time when the Sertoli cell is the dominant cell type in the testes.

During the period of rapid cell proliferation, Sertoli cells must begin to acquire the machinery required to support spermatogenesis in the mature animal. These changes include ultrastructural development of organelles and acquisition of metabolic and synthetic activities characteristic of the mature cell. Some of the morphological properties and expressed functions of these cells are held in common with other cell types in the animal, whereas others are unique to Sertoli cells. Although these general properties are important indices of Sertoli cell function, they can be used only when it can be verified that the responses originate in the Sertoli cell. Several of the secretory proteins synthesized by the Sertoli cell have been enumerated in previous sections of this review, as has their usefulness for *in vitro* studies of cell regulation. However, it is the Sertoli cell specific properties that provide the most convenient markers for the study of Sertoli cell function *in vivo*.

Concomitant with the morphological changes marking the differentiation of Sertoli cells *in utero* is the appearance of distinct Sertoli cell products. Of the known Sertoli cell proteins, the first to appear is anti-Müllerian hormone (AMH), or Müllerian duct inhibiting factor (MIF), the product responsible for causing regression of the Müllerian ducts in male fetuses (374). In addition to producing regression of normal fetal tissue, AMH also produces regression of carcinomas both *in vitro* (375–377) and *in vivo* (378). The appearance of AMH in the testis is associated with differentiating seminiferous cords in both fetal calves (379) and rats (380). Although cross-species bioreactivity provides a means for assay of bovine (381) and porcine (382) AMH using rat Müllerian ducts as target organs, there are species differences in molecular structure as evidenced by the inability of antibodies directed toward bovine AMH to cross-react with chicken, pig, mouse, rat, or human AMH (379,383). The expression of AMH in fetal rats occurs shortly after Sertoli cell differentiation and is not dependent on testicular organogenesis (380). Precise timing for the onset of AMH synthesis in the fetal rat awaits the development of sensitive species-specific probes. It has been shown that porcine (384) and bovine (379) Sertoli cells continue to secrete AMH during the postnatal period. AMH secretion drops sharply before any histological markers of puberty, including formation of the blood-testis barrier, are seen in the pig (384), and AMH levels drop to near the limit of detection in testes of 3-month-old calves (379).

One of the most striking morphologically and physiologically important features of Sertoli cells to develop in the prepubertal rat is the formation of Sertoli-Sertoli junctional complexes, which form an important part of the blood-testis barrier.

Although investigators have described several factors that can modulate formation of Sertoli-Sertoli junctional complexes, this process appears to proceed according to a predetermined pattern in much the same manner as seen in the proliferative phase. In normal rats the formation of the blood-testis barrier begins at about day 15 post-partum, just as Sertoli cell proliferation declines, and is completed between days 16 and 19. Junctional complexes do not form synchronously along the length of the developing seminiferous tubule, but rather seem to reflect the stage of spermatogenesis of the associated germ cells (385). Thus, although formation of the blood-testis barrier is modulated by germ cells, it is not dependent on their presence, since testes depleted of germinal elements by *in utero* irradiation still form junctional complexes (386,387). Although the junctional complexes in these Sertoli cell-enriched (SCE) testes appear about 10 days later than normal, they exclude electron opaque tracers and allow the formation of patent tubules capable of directing Sertoli cell secretory products to the epididymis. Competent blood-testis barriers also are formed in testes of several other animals with impaired fertility (367,388–390). The time of barrier formation seems also to be delayed in some of these animals.

Of the many Sertoli cell products characterized to date, androgen-binding protein remains the best marker of this cell *in vivo*. Measurement of this protein provides a useful index of Sertoli cell function during neonatal development and at puberty. However, studies in fetal rats are complicated by immunoreactive rABP-like material in the serum from fetuses of both sexes (2). This latter protein is produced by the fetal liver (391); synthesis by the liver commences prior to testicular differentiation, peaks at about 17 days pc, and then declines rapidly to undetectable levels prior to birth (Fig. 10) (92). This is associated with a decline of the levels of this protein in serum (Fig. 11). As noted above in the section on Sertoli cell proteins, this product of the fetal liver is believed to be the serum protein TeBG, which is present in adult animals of other species, but not in the adult rat.

Synthesis of rABP by the fetal testis is first detectable on day 18 pc, the time at which high synthetic rates are also observed in the liver (Fig. 10). Production of rABP by the testis increases rapidly, reaching a maximum at about day 21 pc, and then declines quickly before birth (392). Synthesis of rABP by the fetal testis corresponds to the time of maximum Sertoli cell proliferation (271) and the onset of the dramatic increase in total testicular FSH receptor levels

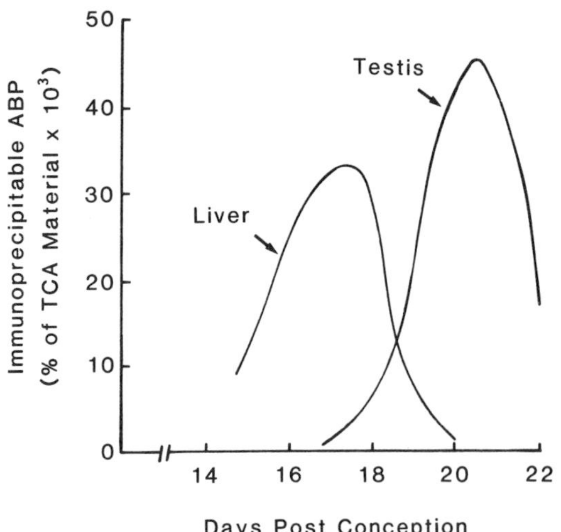

FIG. 10. Synthesis of immunoprecipitable ABP by liver and testes of fetal rats. Tissue minces of liver and testes, obtained from fetal rats at several times post-conception, were incubated for 17 hr in tissue culture medium supplemented with [^{35}S]methionine. Media were collected and centrifuged, and the ABP in the supernatants was immunoprecipitated with rabbit anti-rat ABP. Results are expressed as percentage of total TCA precipitable counts. (Adapted from ref. 392.)

(370). Except for this short burst of secretory activity late in fetal life, the Sertoli cell appears to be relatively quiescent during the remainder of the proliferative phase of development. Because of its small size, the fetal testis presumably contributes very little to rABP in blood at this time.

For the first few days following birth, immunoreactive rABP levels in blood are similar in both sexes and continue to decrease. This immunoreactive material is presumably the residual from the protein produced by the liver prior to birth, since the testes are quiescent with regard to rABP production during this period (Fig. 11). By day 4 postpartum, evidence for renewed synthetic activity by the Sertoli cell is marked by increasing levels of rABP in the blood of male rats, whereas those in females continue to decrease and reach undetectable levels by day 5 (92). During this time, and prior to formation of Sertoli-Sertoli junctional complexes, the entire surface of the Sertoli cell is in communication with the extracellular compartment. As a consequence, secretory products of Sertoli cells are released directly into the extracellular compartment and can presumably pass readily into blood. Thus, rABP levels in blood provide an index of the relative synthetic and secretory activity of the Sertoli cell over this time period. From days 4 through 10, serum rABP levels are maintained at a steady low level and then begin to rise slowly (Fig. 11). Then, at about the time Sertoli cell proliferation stops, serum rABP dramatically rises, increasing over 10-fold between days 12 and 20 (66). Testicular rABP concentration also shows a dramatic rise over this time period as a result of (a) increased synthesis and (b) retention following formation of the junctional complexes (Fig. 12, bottom panel) (388). Sometime between days 17 and 25 (the exact time depends on the animal strain or experimental manipulation), serum rABP levels peak and then begin to drop once the patent tubules form and direct the bulk of ABP to the epididymis. Prior to this time, low but detectable levels of rABP are in the epididymis (388). Nonetheless, the appearance of rABP, as measured by steroid binding, or the abrupt increase in immunoassayable rABP in the epididymis serves as a marker for formation of a patent tubule (386). Unlike serum rABP, testicular and epididymal ABP content continue to increase after day 25, then plateau at adult levels by day 60 (Fig. 12, top panel) (388,390).

Although it was known for several years that the testis was capable of synthesizing estrogen, there were conflicting views regarding the role of Sertoli cells in this process (394–397). It is now clear that in the immature rat, Sertoli cells express FSH-dependent aromatase activity (192,193). In the mature animal, aromatase activity in Sertoli cells declines as they become relatively refractory to the action of FSH, whereas Leydig cells are the major site of estrogen synthesis

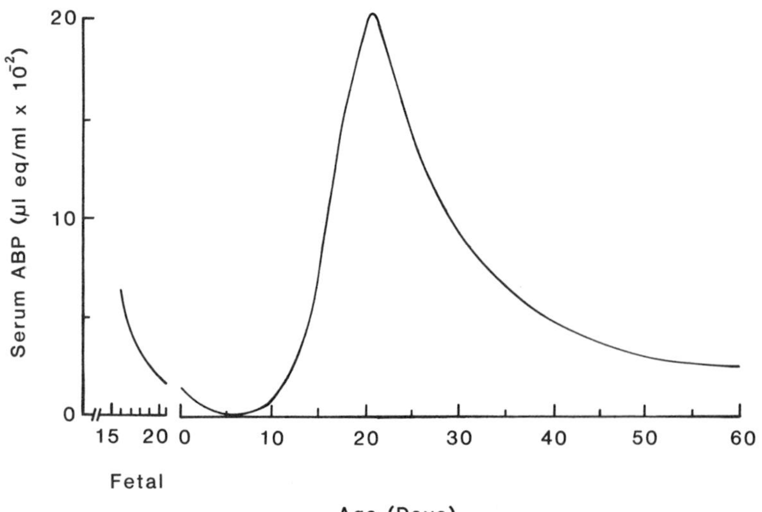

FIG. 11. Serum ABP levels in rats from 16 days post-conception to 60 days of age. Data are expressed as microliter equivalents (μl eq) of a standard rat epididymal cytosol measured in each assay (393). 1 μl eq, when measured by steady state polyacrylamide gel electrophoresis (72), is equivalent to 9.8 ± 0.9-fmole binding sites. Data are a composite from several studies: fetal and neonatal data (92), days 10–60 (388–390).

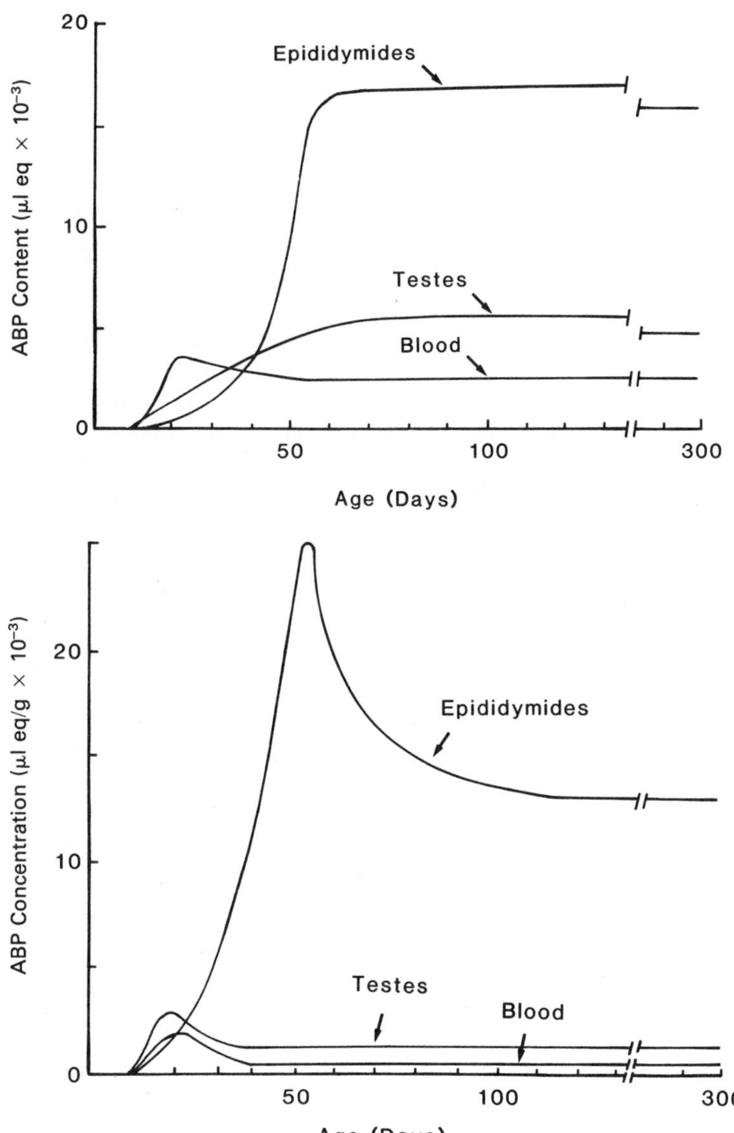

FIG. 12. Distribution of ABP in rat testes, epididymides and blood. **Top panel:** Total rABP content per organ pair or in the vascular compartment, expressed as μl eq (see legend of Fig. 11 for details). **Bottom panel:** rABP concentration in testes, epididymides, and blood. Tissue concentration is expressed as μl eq per g tissue (wet weight); serum concentration is expressed as μl eq per ml. Data are a composite of data from several studies (388–390).

in the adult (193). The physiological importance of aromatization by Sertoli cells in the immature animal has yet to be determined.

The Control of Testicular Size

Morphometric analysis of the adult rat testis shows the seminiferous tubule to comprise over 80% of testicular volume (398). Thus, the more important contributors to determination of adult testis size are Sertoli and germ cell populations. The highly irregular shape of the Sertoli cell relative to the germ cell makes it difficult to provide a quantitative measurement of the volume density of the former cell (399). However, careful measurement of the numerical density of both these cell types shows the ratio of germ cells to Sertoli cells to be about 16:1, with the distribution of cell types staying relatively constant throughout the cycle of the seminiferous epithelium (400). The ratio of volume density of germ cells to Sertoli cells is somewhat less than this figure because the germinal elements are smaller than Sertoli cells. A quantitative estimate based on comparison of testis weights of normal adult animals and of those in which germ cells were depleted by *in utero* irradiation (the SCE animal) puts this ratio at about 5:1 (386). This estimate does not take into consideration the possibility that Sertoli cells in these animals may not have the same volume as those in normal animals. A second estimation of this latter ratio can be made using the Sertoli cell volume of 6,012 μm^3 (derived from a completely reconstructed rat Sertoli cell) (401), the estimate of 22×10^6 Sertoli cells per adult testis, and the observation that the epithelium comprises 80% of the cross-sectional area of the seminiferous tubule (400). This yields a 10:1 ratio of volume density of germ cells to Sertoli cells. These calculations provide crude estimates at best and point to some of the problems that must be overcome if the quantitative aspects of testicular growth are to be understood. The most formidable problem is related to the complex structure of the Sertoli cell and the attendant problem of providing easily accessible number and volume densities of this cell type, as well as others in the testis, under a variety of experimental conditions. The effort involved in the elegant reconstructions of a single Sertoli cell in the rat (399,401,402), and more recently the monkey (403), emphasizes this point.

In spite of the difficulty in providing detailed quantitative measurement of the individual testicular cell types, it is still possible to approach the study of testis growth by other means. One approach is to focus on events occurring in the perinatal period, since this is a period of rapid Sertoli cell proliferation and testis growth. Factors affecting Sertoli cell proliferation, either positively or negatively, have a large potential for influencing testicular function in the adult animal. This notion is supported by the observation that, in the mouse, once Sertoli cell proliferation stops there is a constant numerical relationship between Sertoli cells and germ cells (364). This implies that the germ cell population in the adult animal is dependent on the number of Sertoli cells. The decision to study factors that influence Sertoli cell number during the neonatal period is bolstered by the observation that agents influencing this parameter during this period have permanent effects on testicular size in the adult animal, whereas the same treatments may be ineffectual or transitory when performed after puberty. Hemicastration and LH-releasing hormone (LHRH) antiserum are examples of such treatments that increase and decrease testicular size, respectively (388,404).

The fact that there is compensatory increase in weight by the testis remaining after hemicastration of prepubertal animals has been known for over 90 years (405). For a complete bibliography, see ref. 404. The weight increase has been fairly consistently referred to as *compensatory hypertrophy,* but there is evidence for both hypertrophy and hyperplasia. Compensatory increase in testicular size occurs only in rats hemicastrated before puberty, and the relative increase over that of a testis from an intact animal persists in the adult (404). The earlier the hemicastration is performed, the more pronounced its effect on testicular weight (404), an observation consistent with the finding that Sertoli cell proliferation after birth is programmed to continuously decrease, and thus there is presumably less time for the Sertoli cell population to respond before cell division is no longer possible (271). In rats hemicastrated on day 3, it is possible to see increased Sertoli cell proliferation, as measured by [^{3}H]thymidine incorporation into nuclei, as soon as 8 hr following surgery; however, this is not manifested as a significant weight increase until day 1 after surgery (406). In such animals, increasing Sertoli cell proliferation is observed for at least 4 days following hemicastration; however, 1 week following surgery, Sertoli cells in hemicastrated and intact animals showed comparable labeling, which became undetectable by 3 weeks following surgery. Thus, although the Sertoli cells in the testis remaining after hemicastration respond by increasing their proliferative rate relative to intact animals, the duration of the proliferative phase is not affected. This is consistent with the concept, noted earlier, that the temporal events influencing Sertoli cell development unfold according to a predetermined pattern, although the responses at a given time are subject to modulation. Increased Sertoli cell proliferation in the hemicastrated animal implies that a portion of the testis weight gain is attributable to Sertoli cell hyperplasia.

As noted before, FSH is implicated as a major factor in regulation of Sertoli cell proliferation. The hyperplasia noted following hemicastration in rats is associated with a doubling of serum FSH levels within 4 to 5 days of surgery (404,406) that is maintained throughout the proliferative phase (404). Similar studies in the hemicastrated lamb show serum FSH levels three to four times those found in intact animals (407,408). Serum FSH in hemicastrated lambs also remains elevated for several weeks and then returns, before lumen formation, to values found in intact animals. In addition to augmented cell division, Sertoli cells in these animals also show an increase in their cytoplasm (408), an observation consistent with both hypertropic and hyperplastic responses to hemicastration in some species. In contrast to serum FSH, LH levels in hemicastrated animals are either unaffected (406,407) or elevated only transiently (408). Whether this differential response in gonadotropin release is due to reduced inhibin levels secondary to the reduced Sertoli cell component in hemicastrated animals or due, instead, to other modulatory factors is not presently known. The fact that testis weight gain in hemicastrated rats can be inhibited by administration of testicular extracts, presumably containing inhibin, would be consistent with the former possibility (409).

The increased division of Sertoli cells seen in hemicastrated rats (406) and sheep (408) implies that Sertoli cell hypertrophy is an important factor in the increase in testicular weight observed immediately after surgery in these animals. This is supported by studies on animals with SCE testes in which hemicastration produced the same relative growth found in normal hemicastrates of the same age (404). Since animals with SCE testes are essentially devoid of germ cells, we can also conclude that the bulk of Sertoli cell hypertrophy is mediated by nongerminal elements.

Evidence presented thus far indicates that the FSH-provoked Sertoli cell proliferation in response to hemicastration in young animals is the major influence on testicular development at this time. In contrast, testosterone, a hormone known to be important for maintenance of spermatogenesis in the adult animal, plays an inhibitory role in this process. That is, the administration of testosterone to hemicastrated animals prevents the compensatory increase in testis weight (409). Studies using [^{3}H]thymidine as an index of Sertoli cell division indicate that this is due to suppression of Sertoli cell proliferation in the remaining testis (406). In addition, there is short-term suppression of Sertoli cell proliferation in intact animals that were administered testosterone. Whether testosterone has a direct effect on the Sertoli cell or is acting indirectly, perhaps via negative feedback on FSH levels, is not known.

The growth of the testes following hemicastration is in contrast to arrested or incomplete testicular development associated with hypogonadotropic hypogonadism, an inherited condition in humans (410) and other species, which is believed to be due, in most instances, to a deficiency of LHRH. In such animals, testicular size is reduced and spermatogenesis is incomplete, as expected, as a result of LH and FSH deficiency. Interestingly, testicular size increases but is never restored to normal when men with severe hypogonadotropic hypogonadism are treated for many months with FSH and hCG to restore spermatogenesis. Similarly, hypogonadotropic mice show an increase in testicular size to only 50% of normal following restoration of LH and FSH secretion by brain transplants, even though spermatogenesis was restored (292). It was suspected that the reason why testicular size was not restored following treatment for hypogonadotropism was that adequate replacement therapy was never achieved. Studies on transient hypogonadotropism provide an alternative explanation for these observations.

Transient hypogonadotropism can be produced in adult and immature animals by passive immunization with antiserum to LHRH (LHRH-AS) (for additional references see ref. 92). Male rats passively immunized at 5 days of age with a single injection of LHRH-AS have small testes and reduced fertility as adults despite normal serum concentrations of gonadotropins and testosterone (411,412). The LHRH-AS treatment results in a transient decrease of FSH, LH, and androgen levels during the period of Sertoli cell proliferation. This is associated with decreased testicular weights from day 10 onward to adult life (Fig. 13). In addition, altered Sertoli cell function is also apparent. There is a delay of 5 days in the peaks of serum and testicular rABP concentrations, suggesting that closure of the blood-testis barrier may also be retarded in animals treated with LHRH-AS. This was corroborated by a similar delay in the increase of epididymal rABP concentrations. A second effect is the decrease in secretory activity of Sertoli cells, which is reflected in reduced testicular, epididymal, and serum ABP levels from day 10 on. Testicular rABP and LH/hCG receptor content are commensurate with testis weight at all time points, a finding consistent with the fact that Sertoli and Leydig cell compartments are equally affected by LHRH-AS treatment. By contrast, at all ages, the cross sections of seminiferous tubules in animals that received LHRH-AS are normal, and spermatogenesis develops at the expected time (92). Since the seminiferous tubules appear to have a normal complement of germ cells when viewed in cross section, the most likely explanation for the marked reduction in testes size is that the length of the tubules is foreshortened by a decrease in the Sertoli cell number, which is accompanied by a parallel decrease in germ cells. Since FSH plays a central role in Sertoli cell proliferation, one possible explanation for the decreased testis size in animals treated with LHRH-AS would be the lack of adequate FSH to support the normal proliferative phase which occurs prior to puberty. Thereafter, the testes were unable to show a proliferative response to normal gonadotropin levels, which returned after the Sertoli cell proliferative phase was complete. This suggests a physiological basis for the inability of testes in adult mice and humans with hypogonadotropic hypogonadism to respond to seemingly adequate gonadotropin treatment with an increase to normal testicular size.

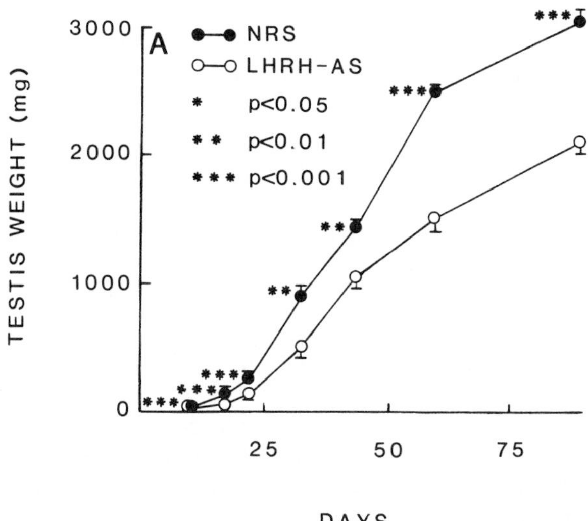

FIG. 13. Testis weight (organ pairs) in animals treated at 5 days of age with LHRH-AS or NRS. Values expressed as means ± SEM. (Data from ref. 388.)

Following neonatal hemicastration, testis size is permanently increased, probably because of the FSH-provoked proliferative response of Sertoli cells in the remaining testis; after LHRH-AS administration, testis size permanently decreases, possibly as a result of inadequate FSH during the proliferative phase. Since these two treatments produce opposite effects on adult testes, they were combined in a 2^2 factorial design to investigate whether they operate through a common factor. LHRH-AS treatment was found to decrease testis weights in both intact and hemicastrated animals, and there was an increase in testis size in response to hemicastration in both LHRH-AS-treated and control animals. Analysis of variance failed to show any interactive terms between the two treatments (413), a finding consistent with both affecting a common regulatory system. Whether these two treatments result in different distributions in cell volume and number density of the various cell types comprising the adult testis is not known. Resolution of this question requires a detailed morphometric study of the testes from these animals, a rather formidable undertaking. Although there is compelling evidence that FSH is the primary mediator of Sertoli cell proliferation, it is clear that factors other than FSH are important in determinating testis size in the adult animal. These include the complex interaction of the various cell types within the testis, mediated by paracrine function as well as by cell-cell contact.

The identification of β-endorphin-related and other peptides derived from pro-opiomelanocortin (POMC) in the male reproductive tract (286), and specifically in Leydig cells of hypophysectomized rats (287,288), suggested that opiate-like molecules were produced within the testis and, thus, could have direct action on testicular function. The presence of immunoreactive β-endorphin in testicular interstitial fluid, at levels severalfold higher than in peripheral blood, and the ability of hCG and LHRH analogs to modulate its levels in interstitial fluid (414) strongly support this hypothesis. Furthermore, the observation that Sertoli cells isolated from adult testes possess opiate receptors, coupled with the ability of naloxone to block the suppression of rABP synthesis by [D-Ala^2]-β-endorphin in Sertoli cells isolated from 18-day-old animals (304), are consistent with the direct action of opiates on the Sertoli cell.

Several lines of evidence suggest that testicular opiates may regulate Sertoli cell proliferation. A single intratesticular injection of opiate antagonist on day 5 was found to enhance testis weight gain and to promote testicular differentiation, which was evident in both hemicastrated and intact animals 5 to 6 days later (300); however, the effect of enhanced weight gain did not persist in hemicastrated animals (302). The inability to affect testis size by systemic administration of these antagonists, at dosages found to cause maximal weight gain by intratesticular delivery (302), supports the concept of a localized function for intratesticular opiates. Decreased serum testosterone levels (300) and tetosterone production (302) in animals treated with opiate antagonist suggest that intratesticular opiates also facilitate testosterone secretion by Leydig cells, whereas increased serum rABP levels in the same animals suggests that intratesticular opiates may exert a direct suppressive effect on Sertoli cell function. The correlation of decreased androgen levels and enhanced testicular weight gain in young hemicastrated animals treated with opiate antagonists may be related to consistent findings that administration of testosterone to young hemicastrated animals suppresses Sertoli cell proliferation and testis weight gain (406). Studies indicating that β-endorphin inhibits Sertoli cell proliferation in fetal (415) and in neonatal animals (303), when Sertoli cell proliferation is at a maximum (271), implies paracrine communication between Leydig and Sertoli cells. Whether the effect on Sertoli cells is a result of the direct action of intratesticular opiates or is the consequence of their action on Leydig cells remains to be elucidated.

The studies on testicular growth during fetal and neonatal life suggest that there are both positive and negative regulators of this process. FSH and possibly other agents that increase Sertoli cell cAMP production, such as β-adrenergic agonists and peptides with MSH activity, stimulate, whereas β-endorphin and other intratesticular opiates inhibit, Sertoli cell growth. Since total sperm production by a testis is limited by the number of Sertoli cells, the regulatory mechanisms that modulate Sertoli cell division are, in turn, determinants of testicular size and sperm output.

Bidirectional Secretion of Sertoli Cell Products into Seminiferous Tubules and Blood

Bidirectional Secretion by Normal Seminiferous Tubules

As outlined previously, in adult rats the majority of rABP is secreted into the lumen of the seminiferous tubule and subsequently transported, along with spermatozoa, to the epididymis via the rete testis and efferent ductules. In the epididymis a portion of rABP is taken up by the initial segment of the caput (63,64), and the remainder disappears during its passage through the epididymis (68), with minimal amounts being detectable in the vas deferens (416). Direct measurements of luminal fluid obtained by micropuncture from various points in the reproductive tract indicate that more than 95% of rABP is lost between the rete testis and cauda epididymis (43).

In the rat, extracellular proteins capable of binding androgens were considered to be confined to the reproductive tract because no specific binding activity could be found in serum (83). However, the development of a sensitive radioimmunoassay led to the discovery of rABP in the blood of mature male rats (74). Although serum rABP concentration is low compared to testicular and epididymal tissue concentrations, in the adult rat the total rABP content of the vascular compartment is equivalent to half the testicular content and accounts for an appreciable fraction of daily rABP production (Fig. 12). Evidence suggesting that proteins as large as rABP cannot pass from the lumen of the reproductive tract into blood, and the observation that several factors have differential effects on the rABP content of the testicular, epididymal, and blood compartments, gave rise to the concept of bidirectional release of this protein from the Sertoli cell (66). The major route of release is into the lumen of the seminiferous tubule, with subsequent transport to the epididymis; the minor route is from the basal aspect of the Sertoli cell into the interstitial space of the testis, with subsequent passage through the lymphatics to the vascular compartment. The decreasing gradient of rABP levels from the lumen of the seminiferous tubule to interstitial fluid, to peripheral blood, is consistent with this hypothesis (43). Calculations based on rABP pool sizes and half-lives in blood and epididymis of normal adult animals indicate that of the daily ABP production by the testes, 80% is transported to the epididymides and 20% is released into blood (66). More recent measurements permitting refinement of the values on which these calculations are based indicate no substantial changes in the conclusions drawn from the earlier studies (G. L. Gunsalus, *unpublished results*). An alternative calculation based on direct measurements of rABP levels in seminiferous tubular and interstitial fluid, as well as on flow rates of testicular lymph and of rete testis fluid to the efferent ducts, estimates rABP secretion to be 67% intratubular and 33% extratubular (43).

Several lines of evidence support the concept for basal release of Sertoli cell secretory proteins. As discussed briefly in a previous section of this review, the Sertoli-Sertoli junctional complexes separate the seminiferous tubule into the exterior and interior compartments (36,417). The inability of electron-opaque molecules (418) as well as proteins (419) and hormones (420), found normally in the blood, to move from the basal compartment past the Sertoli-Sertoli tight junctions and into the adluminal compartment implies that passage in the direction opposite the adluminal compartment would also be restricted. Indeed, the ability of the tight junctions in the seminiferous tubule and rete testis to withstand increased intraluminal pressure generated by efferent duct ligation and to restrict fluid loss from the lumen attests to the physical integrity of the barrier. A number of studies, in one or more species, have confirmed that, after ligation, tight junctions are maintained in both seminiferous tubules and rete testis under this condition (421–425). Although the tight junctions in the rest of the reproductive tract are not as extensively developed as in the testis, they are sufficient to maintain patent tubules and to prevent escape of luminal contents into the blood. Studies to determine whether rABP could escape from the epididymis and thus be an additional source of blood rABP showed that this pathway could, at best, contribute minimally (416). This also confirmed earlier studies (68) that indicated the epididymis to be the major site of ABP degradation. The site of blood ABP degradation is not known, but, by analogy to other serum glycoproteins, is presumed to be the liver (426).

The distribution and levels of rABP in the rat change dramatically between the appearance of Sertoli cells in the fetus and the achievement of sexual maturity in the adult. Over this time period, rABP levels in the various compartments correlate with several important events in the developmental process. In a previous section we described the distribution of rABP during the time of Sertoli cell proliferation (late fetal life to 15 days post-partum) and the temporal correlations with formation of the blood-testis barrier and arrival of mature spermatozoa in the epididymis (refer to Figs. 11 and 12). After 60 days of age, when the animal reaches full reproductive potential, rABP levels in the testes, epididymides, and serum achieve a steady state that is maintained throughout adult life. In the adult animal, the relative rABP contents are 2:6:1 (testes:epididymides:serum). In animals affected by genetic abnormalities, hormonal treatment, or surgical manipulation, the distribution of rABP is altered dramatically. Thus, it is possible to determine the factors that regulate the bidirectional release of Sertoli cell products. There are *in vitro* and *in vivo* studies that suggest bidirectional secretion of Sertoli cell transferrin and testibumin, respectively (25,34), but these proteins are not as useful as rABP because they are synthesized by extragonadal cells.

Bidirectional ABP Release by Abnormal Tubules

Animals homozygous for the *grc* complex or heterozygous for *Hre* have severe germ cell depletion and are infertile, as are rats depleted of germ cells by *in utero* X-irradiation (SCE testes). Although animals with both genetic defects have small testes, they are not genetically related to each other (427). These unrelated genes were both associated with markedly reduced rABP content of the testes and epididymides (389,390). By contrast, the serum rABP concentrations were normal or near normal in both groups at all ages. These observations are compatible with the hypothesis that both *grc* and *Hre* influence the secretion of rABP from the apical portion of Sertoli cells and its subsequent transport to the epididymis, but have little or no effect upon rABP secretion from the base of Sertoli cells into blood. Animals with SCE testes have patterns of rABP secretion similar to those shown by animals carrying the *grc* and *Hre* genes (390). It is possible, therefore, that abnormal ABP secretion into the tubular lumen of these animals is secondary to germ cell depletion, a feature common to *grc/grc*, *Hre/+*, and X-ray-treated rats.

The very low epididymal rABP content but normal serum rABP levels seen in animals with germ cell depletion implies that little of the blood rABP is derived from the epididymis, an observation consistent with the testicular origin of blood rABP. This hypothesis was further supported by data from a whole-body kinetic study performed to determine rABP half-life ($t_{1/2}$) and metabolic clearance rate using endogenous and exogenous protein (416). In studies performed using both intact rats and animals with testes removed but epididymides intact, it was possible to conclude that under androgen deprivation the epididymides are capable of releasing substantial amounts of rABP into the blood, but that the epididymides of normal animals contribute little, if any, rABP to the vascular compartment. These studies are consistent with the hypothesis that the testes release rABP directly into the lymph and/or blood. This is also confirmed by measurements of rABP in samples obtained from the testis by micropuncture that show that the concentration of rABP in the interstitial fluid is eight times higher than that present in thoracic duct lymph and four times higher than that in serum (428).

Several other studies provided corroborating evidence for differential control of the bidirectional release of rABP from the testis. For example, the ability to increase the release of rABP into blood, independent of that to the epididymides, by administration of medroxyprogesterone acetate (MPA) (but not potent androgens) (429) or the antispermatogenic compound, tolnidamine (430), is consistent with this concept. Knowledge about factors that alter bidirectional secretion of rABP provides insight into *in vivo* and *in vitro* approaches that can be used to examine intracellular sorting of Sertoli cell products between the basal and adluminal compartments. In addition, measurements of rABP and other Sertoli cell proteins in the blood and reproductive tract provide a means of studying the pathophysiology of the seminiferous tubule.

The Functional Basis for Bidirectional Secretion

Since the bidirectional secretion of Sertoli cells has been studied using rABP as an indicator, it is appropriate to determine whether there are structural features of this protein that favor secretion into the adluminal, rather than the basal, compartment. rABP can be fractionated into two forms by concanavalin A-Sepharose (Con A) chromatography: Form I, which does not bind, and Form II, which does. The ratio of the two forms of rABP is 1:1 in blood and cytosols prepared from the testes and epididymides of young rats before closure of the blood-testis barrier. After maturity, there is a fivefold decrease in the amount of Form I rABP relative to Form II secreted into the blood (i.e., a ratio of 1:5) (89). These observations led to a study of the heterogeneity of rABP in samples collected by micropuncture from the testes of adult rats; the ratio of Form I to Form II rABP was approximately 1:1 in seminiferous tubular and rete testis fluids. By contrast, this ratio was approximately 1:5 in interstitial fluid. These results indicate that Form I rABP is secreted preferentially into the adluminal compartment of the seminiferous tubule rather than into the interstitial fluid in the mature rat and suggest that partitioning of rABP between the basal and adluminal compartments may depend, in part, on its carbohydrate composition (428). These observations provide the first insight into a possible mechanism for how differential partitioning of rABP into blood and tubular fluid might occur. It is also possible that other structural features of rABP could contribute to this process, as is the case for proteins in other bipolar cells.

If a structural feature of rABP can account for differential secretion of this protein into basal and adluminal compartments of the normal adult animals, then this same mechanism could also explain changes in secretion during maturation or hormonal treatment. For example, there is a peak in the serum rABP between 20 and 25 days of age in developing rats. The rapid decline in the blood levels of this protein after the peak has been associated with formation of the blood-testis barrier (Fig. 11). There may be, however, a discrepancy between the formation of the barrier at age 19 days and the beginning of the decline in serum levels, at least in some strains of rats. One explanation is that different strains have a 4- to 5-day variation in the time of blood-testis barrier closure. An alternate possibility is that the sorting mechanism for this protein has not yet matured, resulting in continued secretion of rABP into blood after formation of the barrier. One test of this hypothesis is provided by measurement of serum testibumin over this time period. Serum levels of this protein do not rise or fall before or after day 25. This suggests that formation of the blood-testis barrier per se may not be responsible for the decline of serum rABP during puberty. At this point, such a possibility remains to be established because testibumin is synthesized by extragonadal cells in the rat; thus, a rise and fall in testicular secretion into blood may not have been detected if the contribution of extratesticular sources were large relative to that from the testes (25). Either closure of the barrier or maturation of a sorting process for ABP could also explain why secretion of form I rbABP does not occur past 24 weeks of age in rabbits (341).

The Study of Sertoli Cell Function in Humans

It is presumed that Sertoli cells in human testes are bipolar, as they appear to be in the rat. If an appropriate group of unique testicular proteins can be identified that are secreted into blood as well as the seminiferous tubular lumen, then Sertoli cell (and therefore tubular) function in humans can be studied in much the same way as in other bipolar cells, for example, hepatocytes. Deranged liver function can be monitored by measurement of hepatic products that partition abnormally between blood and bile ducts. It is hoped that, in the future, abnormalities of testicular function can be assessed by detecting deranged secretion of Sertoli cell proteins. At present, the only such test that is believed to be an index of Sertoli cell function in humans is semen transferrin (131).

REFERENCES

1. Hansson, V., Ritzén, E. M., French, F. S., and Nayfeh, S. N. (1975): Androgen transport and receptor mechanisms in testis and epididymis. In: *Handbook of Physiology, Section 7: Endocrinology, Volume V: Male Reproductive System,* edited by D. W. Hamilton and R. O. Greep, pp. 173–201. American Physiological Society, Washington, D.C.
2. Bardin, C. W., Musto, N., Gunsalus, G., Kotite, N., Cheng, S.-L., Larrea, F., and Becker, R. (1981): Extracellular androgen binding proteins. *Annu. Rev. Physiol.,* 43:189–198.
3. Ritzén, E. M., Hansson, V., and French, F. S. (1981): The Sertoli cell. In: *The Testis,* edited by H. Burger and D. de Kretser, pp. 171–197. Raven Press, New York.
4. de Jong, F. H., and Robertson, D. M. (1985): Inhibin: 1985 Update on action and purification. *Mol. Cell. Endocrinol.,* 42:95–103.
5. Feig, L. A., Bellve, A. R., Erickson, N. H., and Klagsbrun, M. (1980): Sertoli cells contain a mitogenic poly peptide. *Proc. Natl. Acad. Sci. USA,* 77:4774–4778.
6. Feig, L. A., Klagsbrun, M., and Bellve, A. R. (1983): Mitogenic polypeptide of the mammalian seminiferous epithelium: Biochemical characterization and partial purification. *J. Cell Biol.,* 97:1435–1443.
7. Brown, K. D., Blakeley, D. M., Henville, A., and Setchell, B. P. (1982): Rete testis fluid contains a growth factor for cultured fibroblasts. *Biochem. Biophys. Res. Commun.,* 105:391–397.
8. Holmes, S. D., Spotts, G., and Smith, R. G. (1986): Rat Sertoli cells secrete a growth factor that blocks epidermal growth factor (EGF) binding to its receptor. *J. Biol. Chem.,* 261:4076–4080.
9. Hall, K., Ritzén, E. M., Johnsonbaugh, R. E., and Parvinen, M. (1983): Secretion of somatomedin-like compound from Sertoli cells *in vitro.* In: *Insulin-Like Growth Factors/Somatomedins,* edited by E. M. Spencer, pp. 611–614. Walter de Gruyter, New York.
10. Skinner, M. K., and Griswold, M. D. (1980): Sertoli cells synthesize and secrete transferrin-like protein. *J. Biol. Chem.,* 255:9523–9525.
11. Skinner, M. K., Cosand, W. L., and Griswold, M. D. (1984): Purification and characterization of testicular transferrin secreted by rat Sertoli cells. *Biochem. J.,* 218:313–320.

12. Skinner, M. K., and Griswold, M. D. (1983): Sertoli cells synthesize and secrete a ceruloplasmin-like protein. *Biol. Reprod.*, 28:1225–1230.
13. Huggenvik, J., and Griswold, M. D. (1981): Retinol binding protein in rat testicular cells. *J. Reprod. Fertil.*, 61:403–408.
14. Carson, D. D., Rosenberg, L. I., Blaner, W. S., Kato, M., and Lennarz, W. J. (1984): Synthesis and secretion of a novel binding protein for retinol by a cell line derived from Sertoli cells. *J. Biol. Chem.*, 209:3117–3123.
15. Brunner, M., Moreira-Filho, C. A., Wachtel, G., and Wachtel, S. (1984): Secretion of H-Y antigen. *Cell*, 37:615–620.
16. Lacroix, M., Smith, F. E., and Fritz, I. B. (1977): Secretion of plasminogen activator by Sertoli cell enriched cultures. *Mol. Cell. Endocrinol.*, 9:227–236.
17. Vihko, K. K., Suominen, J. J. O., and Parvinen, M. (1984): Cellular regulation of plasminogen activator secretion during spermatogenesis. *Biol. Reprod.*, 31:383–390.
18. Fritz, I. B., Burdzy, K., Setchell, B., and Blaschuk, O. (1983): Ram rete testis fluid contains a protein clusterin which influences cell-cell interactions *in-vitro*. *Biol. Reprod.*, 28:1173–1188.
19. Blaschuk, O. W., and Fritz, I. B. (1984): Isoeletric forms of clusterin isolated from rate rete testis fluid and from secretions of primary cultures of ram and rat Sertoli cell enriched preparations. *Can. J. Biochem. Cell Biol.*, 62:456–461.
20. Tung, P. S., and Fritz, I. B. (1985): Immunolocalization of clusterin in the ram testis, rete testis, and excurrent ducts. *Biol. Reprod.*, 33:177–186.
21. Wright, W. W., Parvinen, M., Musto, N. A., Gunsalus, G. L., Phillips, D. M., Mather, J. P., and Bardin, C. W. (1983): Identification of stage-specific proteins synthesized by rat seminiferous tubules. *Biol. Reprod.*, 29:257–270.
22. Sylvester, S. R., Skinner, M. K., and Griswold, M. D. (1984): A sulfated glycoprotein synthesized by Sertoli cells and by epididymal cells is a component of the sperm membrane. *Biol. Reprod.*, 31:1087–1102.
23. DePhilip, R. M., and Kierszenbaum, A. L. (1982): Hormonal regulation of protein synthesis, secretion and phosphorylation in cultured rat Sertoli cells. *Proc. Natl. Acad. Sci. USA*, 79:6551–6555.
24. Cheng, C. Y., Mather, J. P., Byer, A. L., and Bardin, C. W. (1986): Identification of hormonally responsive proteins in primary Sertoli cell culture medium by high performance liquid chromatography. *Endocrinology*, 118:480–488.
25. Cheng, C. Y., and Bardin, C. W. (1986): Rat testicular testibumin is a glycoprotein responsive to FSH and testosterone that shares immunodeterminants with albumin. *Biochemistry*, 25:5276–5288.
26. Cheng, C. Y. (1986): A FSH and testosterone (T) responsive glycoprotein isolated from rat primary Sertoli cell-enriched cultures (SCCM) shares immunodeterminants with ram clusterin. *The Endocrine Society 68th Annual Meeting, June 25–27, 1986* (abstract 238).
27. Cheng, C. Y., Grima, J. G., and Bardin, C. W. (1985): Identification, purification and characterization of two testosterone (T) responsive glycoproteins from rat primary Sertoli cell culture medium (SCCM). *J. Cell Biol.*, 101:371a (abstract 1406).
28. Mather, J. P., and Sato, G. H. (1979): The use of hormone-supplemented serum-free media in primary cultures. *Exp. Cell Res.* 124:215–222.
29. Mather, J. P. (1980): Establishment and characterization of two distinct mouse testicular epithelial cell lines. *Biol. Reprod.*, 23:243–252.
30. Galdieri, M., Ziparo, E., Palombi, F., Russo, M. A. and Stefanini, M. (1981): Sertoli cell cultures: A new model for the study of somatic germ cell interactions. *J. Androl.*, 2:249–254.
31. Mather, J. P., Zhuang, L.-Z., Perez-Infante, V., and Phillips, D. M. (1982): Culture of testicular cells in hormone-supplemented serum-free medium. In: *The Cell Biology of the Testis, Vol. 383*, edited by C. W. Bardin and R. J. Sherins, pp. 44–68. New York Academy of Sciences, New York.
32. Parvinen, M. (1982): Regulation of the seminiferous epithelium. *Endocr. Rev.*, 3:404–417.
33. Byers, S. W., Hadley, M. A., Djakiew, D., and Dym, M. (1986): Growth and characterization of polarized monolayers of epididymal epithelial cells and Sertoli cells in dual environment culture chambers. *J. Androl.*, 7:59–68.
34. Janecki, A., and Steinberger, A. (1986): Polarized Sertoli cell function in a new two-component culture system. *J. Androl.*, 7:69–71.
35. Fawcett, D. W. (1975): Ultrastructure and function of the Sertoli cell. In: *Handbook of Physiology, Section 7: Endocrinology, Volume V: Male Reproductive System*, edited by D. W. Hamilton and R. O. Greep, pp. 21–55. American Physiological Society, Washington, D.C.
36. Setchell, B. P. (1978): *The Mammalian Testis*, Cornell University Press, Ithaca, New York.
37. Nicander, L. (1967): An electron microscopical study of cell contacts in the seminiferous tubules of some mammals. *Z. Zellforsch. Mikrosk. Anat.*, 83:375–397.
38. Dym, M., and Fawcett, D. W. (1970): The blood-testis barrier in the rat and the physiological compartmentation of the seminiferous epithelium. *Biol. Reprod.*, 3:308–326.
39. Dym, M. (1973): The fine structure of the monkey macaca Sertoli cell and its role in maintaining the blood-testis barrier. *Anat. Rec.*, 175:639–656.
40. Russell, L. D. (1978): The blood testis barrier and its formation relative to spermatocyte maturation in the adult rat: A lanthanum tracer study. *Anat. Rec.*, 190:99–112.
41. Mufly, K. E., Turner, T. T., Brown, M., and Hall, P. F. (1985): Contents of K^+ and Na^+ in seminiferous tubule and rete testis fluids from Sertoli cell-enriched testes. *Biol. Reprod.*, 33:1245–1251.
42. Johnson, M. H., and Setchell, B. P. (1968): Protein and immunoglobin content in rete testis fluid of rams. *J. Reprod. Fertil.*, 17:403–406.
43. Turner, T. T., Jones, C. E., Howards, S. S., Ewing, L. L., Zegeye, B., and Gunsalus, G. L. (1984): On the androgen microenvironment of maturing spermatozoa. *Endocrinology*, 115:1925–1932.
44. Voglmayr, J. K., Scott, T. W., Setchell, B. P., and Waites, G. M. H. (1967): Metabolism of testicular spermatozoa and characteristics of testicular fluid collected from the conscious ram. *J. Reprod. Fertil.*, 14:87–99.
45. Voglmayr, J. K., Larsen, L. H., and White, I. G. (1970): Metabolism of spermatozoa and composition of fluid collected from the rete testis of living bulls. *J. Reprod. Fertil.*, 21:449–460.
46. Tuck, R. R., Setchell, B. P., Waites, G. M. H., and Young, J. A. (1970): The composition of fluid collected by micropuncture and catheterization from the seminiferous tubules and rete testis of rats. *Eur. J. Physiol. (Pflugers Arch.)*, 129:225–243.
47. Waites, G. M. H., and Einer-Jensen, N. (1974): Collection and analysis of rete testis fluid from macaque monkeys. *J. Reprod. Fertil.*, 41:505–508.
48. Free, M. J., and Jaffee, R. A. (1979): Collection of rete testis fluid from rats without previous efferent duct ligation. *Biol. Reprod.*, 20:269–274.
49. Setchell, B. P. (1970): The secretion of fluid by the testis of rats, rams and goats with some observations on the effect of age, cryptorchidism and hypophysectomy. *J. Reprod. Fertil.*, 23:79–85.
50. Setchell, B. P., Duggan, M. C., and Evans, R. W. (1973): The effect of gonadotropins on fluid secretion and sperm production by the rat and hamster testis. *J. Endocrinol.*, 56:27–36.
51. Setchell, B. P. (1969): Do the Sertoli cells secrete the rete testis fluid? *J. Reprod. Fertil.*, 19:391–392.
52. Tuck, R. R. (1969): "An investigation of the fluid secreted by the seminiferous tubules and the rete testis of the rat." BSc. (Med.) thesis, University of Sydney, Sydney.
53. Levine, N., and Marsh, D. J. (1975): Micropuncture study of the fluid composition of 'Sertoli cell-only' seminiferous tubules in rats. *J. Reprod. Fertil.*, 43:547–550.
54. Linzell, J. L., and Setchell, B. P. (1969): Metabolism, sperm and fluid production of the isolated perfused testis of the sheep and goat. *J. Physiol.*, 201:129–143.
55. Setchell, B. P., Voglmayr, J. K., and Hinks, N. T. (1971): The effect of local heating on the flow and composition of rete testis fluid in the conscious ram. *J. Reprod. Fertil.*, 24:81–89.
56. Ribbert, H. (1904): Die abscheidung intravenos injizierten gelosten Karmins in den Geweben. *Z. Allgem. Physiol.*, 4:201–214.
57. Bouffard, G. (1906): Injection des couleurs de benzidine aux animaux normaux. *Ann. Inst. Pasteur*, 20:539–546.
58. Mostov, K. E., and Simister, N. E. (1985): Transcytosis. *Cell*, 43:389–390.
59. Mather, J. P., Gunsalus, G. L., Musto, N. A., Cheng, C. Y., Parvinen, M., Wright, W., Perez-Infante, V., Margioris, A., Liotta,

A., Becker, R., Krieger, D. T., and Bardin, C. W. (1983): The hormonal and cellular control of Sertoli cell secretion. *J. Steroid Biochem.,* 19:41–51.
60. Hansson, V., and Tveter, K. J. (1971): Uptake and binding *in vivo* of ^{3}H-labelled androgen in the rat epididymal and ductus deferens. *Acta Endocrinol.,* 66:745–755.
61. Ritzén, E. M., Nayfeh, S. N., French, F. S., and Dobbins, M. C. (1971): Demonstration of androgen binding components in rat epididymis cytosol and comparison with binding components in prostate and other tissues. *Endocrinology,* 89:143–151.
62. Vernon, R. G., Kopec, B., and Fritz, I. B. (1974): Observations on the binding of androgens by rat testis seminiferous tubules and testis extracts. *Mol. Cell. Endocrinol.,* 1:167–187.
63. Pelliniemi, L. J., Dym, M., Gunsalus, G. L., Musto, N. A., Bardin, C. W., and Fawcett, D. W. (1981): Immunocytochemical localization of androgen binding protein in the male rat reproductive tract. *Endocrinology,* 108:925–931.
64. Attramadal, A., Bardin, C. W., Gunsalus, G. L., Musto, N. A., and Hansson, V. (1981): Immunocytochemical localization of androgen binding protein in rat Sertoli and epididymal cells. *Biol. Reprod.,* 25:983–988.
65. Musto, N., Gunsalus, G., Cheng, C. Y., Tsong, S. D., Goldstein, M., Phillips, D., and Bardin, C. W. (1983): Identification of androgen-binding proteins and their localization in the testis and male reproductive tract. In: *Recent Advances in Male Reproduction: Molecular Basis and Clinical Implications,* edited by R. D'Agata, M. B. Lipsett, P. Polosa, and H. J. van der Molen, pp. 37–45. Raven Press, New York.
66. Gunsalus, G. L., Musto, N. A., and Bardin, C. W. (1980): Bidirectional release of a Sertoli cell product, androgen binding protein, into the blood and seminiferous tubule. In: *Testicular Development, Structure and Function,* edited by A. Steinberger and E. Steinberger, pp. 291–297. Raven Press, New York.
67. Wright, W. W., Musto, N. A., Mather, J. P., and Bardin, C. W. (1981): Sertoli cells secrete both testis-specific and serum proteins. *Proc. Natl. Acad. Sci. USA,* 78:7565–7569.
68. French, F. S., and Ritzén, E. M. (1973): A high affinity androgen binding protein (ABP) in rat testis: Evidence for secretion into efferent duct fluid and absorption by epididymis. *Endocrinology,* 93:88–95.
69. Hagenas, L., Ritzén, E. M., Ploen, L., Hansson, V., French, F. S., and Nayfeh, S. N. (1975): Sertoli cell origin of testicular androgen binding protein. *Mol. Cell. Endocrinol.,* 2:339–350.
70. Sanborn, B. M., Elkington, J. S. H., Steinberger, A., and Steinberger, E. (1975): Androgen binding in the testis: *In vivo* production of androgen binding protein (ABP) by Sertoli cell cultures and measurement of nuclear bound androgen by a nuclear exchange assay. In: *Hormonal Regulation of Spermatogenesis,* edited by F. S. French, V. Hansson, E. M. Ritzén, and S. N. Nayfeh, pp. 293–309. Plenum Press, New York.
71. Fritz, I. B., Rommerts, F. G., Louis, B. G., and Dorrington, J. H. (1976): Regulation by follicle stimulating hormone and dibutyryl cyclic AMP of the formation of androgen-binding protein in Sertoli cell-enriched cultures. *J. Reprod. Fertil.,* 46:17–24.
72. Ritzén, E. M., French, F. S., Weddington, S. C., Nayfeh, S. N., and Hansson, V. (1974): Steroid binding in polyacrylamide gels: Quantitation at steady state conditions. *J. Biol. Chem.,* 249:6597–6604.
73. Musto, N. A., and Bardin, C. W. (1976): Decreased levels of androgen binding protein in the reproductive tract of the restricted (H^{re}) rat. *Steroids,* 28:1–11.
74. Gunsalus, G. L., Musto, N. A., and Bardin, C. W. (1978): Immunoassay of androgen binding protein in blood: A new approach for the study of the seminiferous tubule. *Science,* 200: 65–66.
75. Taylor, C. A., Smith, H. E., and Danzo, B. J. (1980): Photoaffinity labeling of rat androgen binding protein. *Proc. Natl. Acad. Sci. USA,* 234–238.
76. Danzo, B. J., Taylor, C. A., Jr., and Eller, B. C. (1982): Some physicochemical characteristics of photoaffinity-labeled rabbit androgen-binding protein. *Endocrinology,* 111:1270–1277.
77. Danzo, B. J., Dunn, J. C., and Davies, J. (1982): The presence of androgen-binding protein in the guinea-pig testis, epididymis and epididymal fluid. *Mol. Cell. Endocrinol.,* 28:513–527.
78. Weddington, S. C., Brandtzaeg, P., Hansson, V., French, F. S., Petrusz, P., Nayfeh, S. N., and Ritzén, E. M. (1975): Immunological cross reactivity between testicular androgen-binding protein and serum testosterone-binding globulin. *Nature,* 258:257.
79. Musto, N. A., Larrea, F., Cheng, S.-L., Kotite, N., Gunsalus, G. L., and Bardin, C. W. (1982): Extracellular androgen binding proteins: Species comparison and structure-function relationships. *Ann. N.Y. Acad. Sci.,* 383:343–359.
80. Cheng, C. Y., Frick, J., Gunsalus, G. L., Musto, N. A., and Bardin, C. W. (1984): Human testicular androgen binding protein shares immunodeterminants with serum testosterone-estradiol-binding globulin. *Endocrinology,* 114:1395–1401.
81. Kotite, N. J., Cheng, S-L., Musto, N. A., and Gunsalus, G. L. (1986): Comparison of rabbit epididymal androgen binding protein and serum testosterone estradiol binding globulin. II. Immunological properties. *J. Steroid. Biochem.,* 25:171–176.
82. Musto, N. A., Gunsalus, G. L., Miljkovic, M., and Bardin, C. W. (1977): A novel affinity column for isolation of androgen binding protein from rat epididymis. *Endocr. Res. Commun.,* 4:147–157.
83. Corvol, P., and Bardin, C. W. (1973): Species distribution of testosterone binding globulin. *Biol. Reprod.,* 8:277–282.
84. Musto, N. A., Gunsalus, G. L., and Bardin, C. W. (1980): Purification and characterization of androgen binding protein from the rat epididymis. *Biochemistry,* 19:2853–2860.
85. Larrea, F., Musto, N. A., Gunsalus, G. L., Mather, J. P., and Bardin, C. W. (1981): Origin of the heavy and light protomers of androgen-binding protein from the rat testis. *J. Biol. Chem.,* 256:12566–12573.
86. Larrea, F., Musto, N. A., Gunsalus, G. L., and Bardin, C. W. (1981): The microheterogeneity of rat androgen binding protein from the testis, rete testis fluid, and epididymis as demonstrated by immunoelectrophoresis and photoaffinity labeling. *Endocrinology,* 109:1212–1220.
87. Joseph, D. R., Hall, S. H., and French, F. S. (1985): Identification of complementary DNA clones that encode rat androgen binding protein. *J. Androl.,* 6:392–395.
88. Hansson, V. (1981): Heterogeneity in end-terminal sugars of rabbit and rat androgen binding protein (ABP). *J. Androl.,* 4:220.
89. Cheng, C. Y., Gunsalus, G. L., Musto, N. A., and Bardin, C. W. (1984): The heterogeneity of rat androgen binding protein (rABP) in serum differs from that in testis and epididymis: Evidence for differential secretion. *Endocrinology,* 114:1386–1394.
90. Suzuki, Y., Ito, M., and Sinohara, H. (1981): Isolation and characterization of sex-steroid-binding protein from rat and rabbit plasma. *J. Biochem.,* 89:231–236.
91. Gunsalus, G. L., Musto, N. A., and Bardin, C. W. (1978): Factors affecting blood levels of androgen binding protein in the rat. *Int. J. Androl. (Suppl.),* 2:482–493.
92. Gunsalus, G. L., Carreau, S., Vogel, D. L., Musto, N. A., and Bardin, C. W. (1984): Use of androgen binding protein to monitor development of the seminiferous epithelium. In: *Sexual Differentiation: Basic and Clinical Aspects,* edited by M. Serio, M. Motta, M. Zanisi, L. Martini, pp. 53–64. Raven Press, New York.
93. Carreau, S., Musto, N. A., Bercu, B. B., Bardin, C. W., and Gunsalus, G. L. (1985): L'Androgen binding protein, un marqueur de la fonction Sertolienne chez le rat (The androgen binding protein as an index of the rat Sertoli cell function). In: *Recent Progress in Cellular Endocrinology of the Testis, Proceedings of the 3rd European Workshop on the Testis, Vol. 123,* pp. 157–162, INSERM.
94. Cheng, S.-L., and Musto, N. A. (1982): Purification and characterization of androgen binding protein from rabbit epididymis. *Biochemistry,* 21:2400–2405.
95. Kotite, N. J., and Musto, N. A. (1982): Subunit structure of rabbit testosterone estradiol-binding globulin. *J. Biol. Chem.,* 257:5118–5124.
96. Danzo, B. J., Taylor, C. A., Jr., and Eller, B. C. (1982): Some physicochemical characteristics of photoaffinity-labeled rabbit testosterone-binding globulin. *Endocrinology,* 111:1278–1285.
97. Cheng, S.-L., Wright, W. W., Musto, N. A., Gunsalus, G. L., and Bardin, C. W. (1982): Testicular proteins which can be used to study seminiferous tubular function: A study of ABP and other testis-specific markers. In: *Physiopathology of Hypophysial Disturbances and Diseases of Reproduction,* edited by A. de Micola, J. Blaquier, and R. J. Soto, pp. 193–216. Alan R. Liss, New York.

98. David, G. F. X., Koehler, J. K., Brown, J. A., Petra, P. H., and Farr, A. G. (1985): Light and electron microscopic studies on the localization of steroid-binding protein (SBP) in rabbit spermatozoa. *Biol. Reprod.*, 33:503–514.
99. Mercier, C., Alfsen, A., and Baulieu, E. E. (1966): A testosterone binding globulin. In: *Proceedings of the Second Symposium on the Steroid Hormones, International Congress Series 101*, 212. Excerpta Medica Foundation, Amsterdam.
100. Rosenbaum, W., Christy, N. P., and Kelly, W. G. (1966): Electrophoretic evidence for the presence of an estrogen-binding β-protein in human plasma. *J. Clin. Endocrinol.*, 26:1399–1403.
101. Siiteri, P. K., Murai, J. T., Hammond, G. L., Nisker, J. A., Raymoure, W. J., and Kuhn, R. W. (1982): The serum transport of steroid hormones. In: *Recent Progress in Hormone Research, Vol. 38*, pp. 457–510. Academic Press, New York.
102. Rosner, W., and Smith, R. N. (1975): Isolation and characterization of the testosterone-estradiol-binding globulin from human plasma. Use of a novel affinity column. *Biochemistry*, 14:4813–4820.
103. Mickelson, K. E., and Petra, P. H. (1975): Purification of the sex steroid binding protein from human serum. *Biochemistry*, 14:957–963.
104. Mercier-Bodard, C., Renoir, J. M., and Baulieu, E. E. (1979): Further characterization and immunological studies of human sex steroid binding plasma protein. *J. Steroid Biochem.*, 11:253–259.
105. Iqbal, M. J., and Johnson, M. W. (1979): Purification and characterization of human sex hormone binding globulin. *J. Steroid Biochem.*, 10:535–540.
106. Fernlund, P., and Laurell, C. B. (1981): A simple two-step procedure for the simultaneous isolation of corticosteroid binding globulin and sex hormone binding globulin from human serum by chromatography on cortisol-Sepharose and phenyl-Sepharose. *J. Steroid Biochem.*, 14:545–552.
107. Cheng, C. Y., Musto, N. A., Gunsalus, G. L., and Bardin, C. W. (1983): Demonstration of heavy and light protomers of human testosterone-estradiol-binding globulin. *J. Steroid Biochem.*, 19:1379–1389.
108. Cheng, C. Y., Musto, N. A., Gunsalus, G. L., and Bardin, C. W. (1985): The role of the carbohydrate moiety on the size heterogeneity and immunologic determinants of human testosterone-estradiol binding globulin. *J. Steroid Biochem.*, 22:127–134.
109. Petra, P. H., Stanczyk, F. Z., Senear, D. F., Namkung, P. C., Novy, M. J., Ross, J. B. A., Turner, E., and Brown, J. A. (1983): Current status of the molecular strucure and function of the plasma sex steroid binding protein (SBP). *J. Steroid Biochem.*, 19:699–706.
110. Khan, M. S., Ehrlich, P., Birkens, S., and Rosner, W. (1985): Size isomers of testosterone-estradiol-binding globulin exist in the plasma of individual men and women. *Steroids*, 45:463–472.
111. Khan, M. S. (1982): Radioimmunoassay for human testosterone-estradiol binding globulin. *J. Clin. Endocrinol.*, 54:705–710.
112. Cheng, C. Y., Bardin, C. W., Musto, N. A., Gunsalus, G. L., Cheng, S.-L., and Ganguly, M. (1983): Radioimmunoassay of testosterone-estradiol-binding globulin in humans: A reassessment of normal values. *J. Clin. Endocrinol. Metab.*, 56:68–75.
113. Vigersky, R. A., Loriaux, D. L., Howard, S. S., Hodgen, G. B., Lipsett, M. B., and Chrambach, A. (1976): Androgen binding protein of testis, epididymis and plasma in man and monkeys. *J. Clin. Invest.*, 58:1061–1068.
114. Lipshultz, L. I., Tsai, Y. H., Sanborn, B. M., and Steinberger, E. (1977): Androgen-binding activity in the human testis and epididymis. *Fertil. Steril.*, 28:947–951.
115. Purvis, K., Calandra, R., Sander, S., and Hansson, V. (1978): Androgen binding proteins and androgen levels in the human testis and epididymis. *Int. J. Androl.*, 1:531–548.
116. Burke, W. R., Aten, R. F., Eisenfeld, A. J., and Lytton, B. (1977): Androgen binding in human testis. *J. Urol.*, 118:52–57.
117. Hsu, A.-F., and Troen, P. (1978): An androgen binding protein in the testicular cytosol of human testis. Comparison with human plasma testosterone-estrogen binding globulin. *J. Clin. Invest.*, 61:1611–1619.
118. Cheng, C. Y., Musto, N. A., Gunsalus, G. L., Frick, J., and Bardin, C. W. (1985): There are two forms of androgen binding protein in human testes: Comparison of their protomeric variants with serum testosterone-estradiol-binding globulin. *J. Biol. Chem.*, 260:5631–5640.
119. Waheed, A., Winter, S. J., Farrow, G. M., Oshima, H., and Troen, P. (1985): Studies of the human testis. XIX. Preparation of an antibody to human testosterone-oestradiol-binding globulin and its application to the study of testicular androgen-binding protein. *Acta Endocrinol.*, 108:284–288.
120. Keeping, H. S., Winters, S. J., and Troen, P. (1985): Identification of androgen-binding protein from testis cytosol and Sertoli cell culture medium of the cynomolgus monkey, *Macaca fascicularis*. *Endocrinology*, 117:1521–1529.
121. Hryb, D. J., Khan, S. M., and Rosner, R. (1985): Testosterone-estradiol-binding globulin binds to human prostatic cell membranes. *Biochem. Biophys. Res. Commun.*, 128:432–440.
122. Byers, S. W., Musto, N. A., and Dym, M. (1985): Culture of ciliated and nonciliated cells from rat ductuli efferentes. *J. Androl.*, 6:271–278.
123. Lobl, T. J. (1981): Androgen transport proteins: Physical properties, hormonal regulation, and possible mechanism of TeBG and ABP action. *Arch. Androl.*, 7:133–151.
124. Campo, S., Pellizzari, E., Cigorraga, S., Monteagudo, C., and Nicolau, G. (1982): Androgen binding to subcellular particles of rat testis. *J. Steroid Biochem.*, 17:165–173.
125. Mather, J. P. (1982): Ceruloplasmin, a copper-transport protein, can act as a growth promoter for some cell lines in serum-free medium. *In Vitro*, 18:990–996.
126. Perez-Infante, V., and Mather, J. P. (1982): The role of transferrin in the growth of testicular cell lines in serum-free medium. *Exp. Cell Res.*, 142:325–332.
127. Perez-Infante, V., Bardin, C. W., Gunsalus, G. L., Musto, N. A., Rich, K. A., and Mather, J. P. (1986): Differential regulation of testicular transferrin and androgen-binding protein in primary cultures of rat Sertoli cells. *Endocrinology*, 118:383–392.
128. Holmes, S. D., Bucci, L. R., Lipshultz, L. I., and Smith, R. G. (1983): Transferrin binds specifically to pachytene spermatocytes. *Endocrinology*, 113:1916–1918.
129. Skinner, M. K., and Griswold, M. D. (1982): Secretion of testicular transferrin by cultured Sertoli cells is regulated by hormones and retinoids. *Biol. Reprod.*, 27:211–222.
130. Thorbecke, C. J., Liem, H. H., Knight, S., Cox, K., and Muller-Eberlard, U. (1973): Sites of formation of the serum proteins, transferrin and hemopexin. *J. Clin. Invest.*, 32:725–731.
131. Holmes, S. D., Lipshultz, L. I., and Smith, R. G. (1982): Transferrin and gonadal dysfunction in man. *Fertil. Steril.*, 38:600–604.
132. Orlando, C., Caldini, A. L., Barni, T., Wood, W. G., and Strasburger, C. J. (1985): Ceruloplasmin and transferrin in human seminal plasma: Are they an index of seminiferous tubular function. *Fertil. Steril.*, 43:280–284.
133. Blaschuk, O., Burdzy, K., and Fritz, I. B. (1983): Purification and characterization of a cell-aggregating factor (clusterin), the major glycoprotein in ram rete testis fluid. *J. Biol. Chem.*, 258:7714–7720.
134. Russell, L. (1977): Movement of spermatocytes from the basal to the adluminal compartment of the rat testis. *Am. J. Anat.*, 148:313–328.
135. Russell, L. D. (1980): Sertoli germ cell interrelations: a review. *Gamete Res.*, 3:179–202.
136. Vihko, K. K., Kristensen, P., Toppari, J., Saksela, O., Dano, K., and Parvinen, M. (1985): The function of plasminogen activator in the seminiferous epithelium. *J. Cell Biol.*, 101:367a (abstract 1392).
137. Toppari, J., Vihko, K. K., Rasanen, K. G. E., Eerola, E., and Parvinen, M. (1986): Regulation of stages VI and VIII of the rat seminiferous epithelial cycle *in vitro*. *J. Endocrinol.*, 108:417–422.
138. Leblond, C. P., and Clermont, Y. (1952): Definition of the stages of the cycle of the seminiferous epithelium in the rat. *Ann. NY Acad. Sci. USA*, 55:548–573.
139. Ohno, S., Nagai, Y., Ciccarese, S., and Iwata, H. (1979): Testis-organizing H-Y antigen and the primary sex determining mechanism of mammals. *Recent Prog. Horm. Res.*, 35:449–478.
140. Muller, U., Wolf, U., Siebers, J. W., and Gunther, E. (1979): Evidence for a gonad-specific receptor for H-Y antigen: Binding of exogenous H-Y antigen to gonadal cells is independent of β2-microglobulin. *Cell*, 17:331–335.
141. Ciccarese, S., and Ohno, S. (1978): 2 plasma membrane antigens of testicular Sertoli cells and h-2 restricted vs unrestricted lysis by female thymus derived cells. *Cell*, 13:643–650.

142. Zenzes, M. T., Wolf, U., Gunther, E., and Engel, W. (1978): Studies on the function of H-Y antigen: Dissociation and reorganization experiments on rat gonadal tissue. *Cytogenet. Cell Genet.*, 20:365–372.
143. Wachtel, S. S. (1983): *H-Y Antigen and the Biology of Sex Determination,* Grune and Stratton, New York.
144. Gore-Langton, R. E., Tung, P. S., and Fritz, I. B. (1983): The absence of specific interactions of Sertoli cell secreted proteins with antibodies directed against h-y antigen. *Cell,* 32:289–302.
145. Braunhut, S. J., Rufo, G. A., Jr., Ernisse, B. J., and Bellve, A. R. (1985): The seminiferous growth factor (SGF) stimulates the proliferation of transformed mouse Sertoli cells (TM_4) in a serum-free medium. *J. Cell Biol.,* 101:372a (abstract 1408).
146. Bellve, A. R., and Feig, L. A. (1984): Cell proliferation in the mammalian testis: Biology of the seminiferous growth factor (SGF). *Recent Prog. Horm. Res.,* 40:531–567.
147. Esch, F., Baird, A., Ling, N., Ueno, N., Hill, F., Denoroy, L., Klepper, R., Gospodarowicz, D., Böhlen, P., and Guillemin, R. (1985): Primary structure of bovine pituitary basic fibroblast growth factor (FGF) and comparison with the amino-terminal sequence of bovine brain acidic FGF. *Proc. Natl. Acad. Sci. USA,* 82:6507–6511.
148. Gospodarowicz, D., Baird, A., Cheng, J., Lui, G. M., Esch, F., and Böhlen, P. (1986): Isolation of fibroblast growth factor from bovine adrenal gland: Physiochemical and biological characterization. *Endocrinology,* 118:82–90.
149. Böhlen, P., Esch, F., Baird, A., and Gospodarowicz, D. (1985): Acidic fibroblast growth factor (FGF) from bovine brain: Amino-terminal sequence and comparison with basic FGF. *EMBO,* 4:1951–1956.
150. Ling, N., Ying, S.-Y., Ueno, N., Esch, F., Denoroy, L., and Guillemin, R. (1985): Isolation and partial characterization of a M_r 32,000 protein with inhibin activity from porcine follicular fluid. *Proc. Natl. Acad. Sci. USA,* 82:7217–7221.
151. Esch, F., Ueno, N., Baird, A., Hill, F., Denoroy, L., Ling, N., Gospodarowicz, D., and Guillemin, R. (1985): Primary structure of bovine brain acidic fibroblast growth factor (FGF). *Biochem. Biophys. Res. Commun.,* 133:554–562.
152. Adashi, E. Y., Resnick, C. E., Svoboda, M. E., and Van Wyk, J. J. (1986): Somatomedin-C as an amplifier of follicle-stimulating hormone action: Enhanced accumulation of adenosine 3′,5′-monophosphate. *Endocrinology,* 118:149–155.
153. Elson, S. D., Browne, C. A., and Thorburn, G. D. (1984): Identification of epidermal growth factor-like activity in human male reproductive tissue and fluids. *J. Clin. Endocrinol. Metab.,* 58:589–594.
154. Cheng, C. Y., Grima, J., Lee, W. M., and Bardin, C. W. (1987): The distribution of rat testibumin in the male reproductive tract. *Biol. Reprod. (in press).*
155. Kissinger, C., Skinner, M. K., and Griswold, M. D. (1982): Analysis of Sertoli cell-secreted proteins by 2 dimensional gel electrophoresis. *Biol. Reprod.,* 27:233–240.
156. Cheng, C. Y., Bardin, C. W., Nagendranath, N., Escobar, N., Han, A. C., Musto, N. A., and Gunsalus, G. L. (1985): Purification of testosterone-estradiol-binding globulins from mammalian sera by anion-exchange high-performance liquid chromatography. *Int. J. Androl.,* 8:1–12.
157. Skinner, M. K., and Fritz, I. B. (1985): Testicular peritubular cells secrete a protein under androgen control that modulates Sertoli cell functions. *Proc. Natl. Acad. Sci. USA,* 82:114–118.
158. Skinner, M. K., and Fritz, I. B. (1985): Androgen stimulation of Sertoli cell function is enhanced by peritubular cells. *Mol. Cell. Endocrinol.,* 40:115–122.
159. Skinner, M. K., Tung, P. S., and Fritz, I. B. (1985): Cooperativity between Sertoli cells and testicular peritubular cells in the production and deposition of extracellular matrix components. *J. Cell Biol.,* 100:1941–1947.
160. Spruill, W. A., Steiner, A. L., Tres, L. L., and Kierszenbaum, A. L. (1983): FSH dependent phosphorylation of vimentin in cultures of rat Sertoli cells. *Proc. Natl. Acad. Sci. USA,* 80:993–997.
161. Perrard, M. H., Saez, J. M., and Dazord, A. (1985): FSH stimulation of cytosolic protein synthesis in cultured pig Sertoli cells. *J. Steroid Biochem.,* 22:281–284.
162. Perrard-Sapori, M. H., Saez, J. M., and Dazord, A. (1985): Hormonal regulation of proteins secreted by cultured pig Sertoli cells: Characterization by two-dimensional polyacrylamide gel electrophoresis. *Mol. Cell. Endocrinol.,* 43:189–197.
163. McCullagh, D. D. (1932): Dual endocrine activity of the testis. *Science,* 76:19–20.
164. Channing, C. P., Gordon, W. L., Liu, V. K., and Ward, D. N. (1985): Minireview: Physiology and biochemistry of ovarian inhibin. *Biol. Med.,* 178:339–361.
165. Ramasharma, K., Sairam, M. R., Seidah, N. G., Chirtien, M., Manjunath, P., Schiller, P. W., Yamashiro, D., and Li, C. H. (1984): Isolation, structure and synthesis of a human seminal plasma peptide with inhibin-like activity. *Science,* 223:1199–1202.
166. Seidah, N. G., Ramasharma, K., Sairam, M. R., and Chretien, M. (1984): Partial amino acid sequence of a human seminal plasma peptide with inhibin-like activity. *FEBS Lett.,* 167:98–102.
167. Li, C. H., Hammonds, R. G., Ramasharma, K., and Chung, D. (1985): Human seminal α-inhibins: Isolation, characterization, and structure. *Proc. Natl. Acad. Sci. USA,* 82:4041–4044.
168. Rivier, J., McClintock, R., Vaughan, J., Yamamoto, G., Anderson, H., Spiess, J., Vale, W., Voglmayr, J., Cheng, C. Y., and Bardin, C. W. (1986): Partial purification of inhibin from ovine rete testis fluid. In: *Male Contraception: Advances and Future Prospects,* edited by G. Zatuchni, A. Goldsmith, and J. Sciarra, pp. 401–407. Harper and Row, Philadelphia.
169. Robertson, D. M., Foulds, L. M., Leversha, L., Moran, F. J., Hearn, M. T. W., Burger, H. G., Wettenhall, R. E. H., and de Kretser, D. M. V. (1985): Isolation of inhibin from bovine follicular fluid. *Biochem. Biophys. Res. Commun.,* 126:220–226.
170. Miyamoto, K., Hasegawa, Y., Fukuda, M., Nomura, M., Igarashi, M., Kangawa, K., and Matsuo, A. (1985): Isolation of porcine follicular fluid inhibin of 32K daltons. *Biochem. Biophys. Res. Commun.,* 128:396–403.
171. Mason, A. J., Hayflick, J. S., Ling, N., Esch, F., Ueno, N., Ying, S.-Y., Guillemin, R., Niall, H., and Seeburg, P. H. (1985): Complementary DNA sequences of ovarian follicular fluid inhibin show precursor structure and homology with transforming growth factor-β. *Nature,* 318:659–663.
172. Mason, A. J., Niall, H. D., and Seeburg, P. H. (1986): Structure of two human ovarian inhibins. *Biochem. Biophys. Res. Commun.,* 135:957–964.
173. David, K., Dingemanse, E., Freud, J., and Laqueur, E. (1935): Uber krystallinisches mannliches Hormon aus Hoden (Testosteron), Wirksamer als aus Harn oder aus Cholesterin bereitetes Androsteron. *Z. Physiol. Chem.,* 233:281–282.
174. Srere, P. A., Chaikoff, I. L., Treitman, S. S., and Burstein, L. S. (1950): The extrahepatic synthesis of cholesterol. *J. Biol. Chem.,* 182:629–634.
175. Brady, R. O. (1951): Biosynthesis of radioactive testosterone *in vitro. J. Biol. Chem.,* 193:145–148.
176. Steinberger, E., Steinberger, A., and Ficher, M. (1970): Study of spermatogenesis and steroid metabolism in cultures of mammalian testes. *Recent Prog. Horm. Res.,* 26:547–588.
177. Huggins, C., and Moulder, P. V. (1945): Estrogen production by Sertoli cell tumors of the testes. *Cancer Res.,* 5:510–514.
178. Steinberger, A., Elkington, J. S. H., Sanborn, B. M., Steinberger, E., Heindel, J., and Lindsey, J. N. (1975): Culture of FSH response of Sertoli cells isolated from sexually mature rat testes. In: *Hormonal Regulation of Spermatogenesis,* edited by F. S. French, V. Hansson, E. M. Ritzén, and S. N. Nayfeh, pp. 398–411. Plenum Press, New York.
179. Oshima, H. D., Fan, D. F., and Troen, P. (1975): Studies of the human testis. V. Properties of Δ^5-3β- and 17β-hydroxysteroid dehydrogenase in the biosynthesis of testosterone from dehydroepiandrosterone. *J. Clin. Endocrinol. Metab.,* 40:573–581.
180. Welsh, M. J., and Wiebe, J. P. (1976): Sertoli cells from immature rats: *in-vitro* stimulation of steroid metabolism by follicle stimulating hormone. *Biochem. Biophys. Res. Commun.,* 69:936–941.
181. Tcholakian, R. K., and Steinberger, A. (1979): Progesterone metabolism by cultured Sertoli cells. *Endocrinology,* 103:1335–1343.
182. Welsh, M. J., and Wiebe, J. P. (1978): Sertoli cell capacity to metabolize C-19 steroids: Variation with age and the effect of follicle-stimulating hormone. *Endocrinology,* 103:838–844.

183. Tcholakian, R. K., and Steinberger, A. (1979): *In vitro* metabolism of testosterone by cultured Sertoli cells and the effect of FSH. *Steroids,* 33:495–526.
184. Yamada, M., Yasue, S., and Matsumoto, K. (1972): Formation of 5α-reduced products from testosterone *in vitro* by germ cells from immature rats. *Acta Endocrinol. (Copenh.),* 71:383–400.
185. Payne, A. H., Kawano, A., and Jaffe, R. B. (1973): Formation of dihydrotestosterone and other 5α-reduced metabolites by isolated seminiferous tubules and suspension of interstitial cells in a human testis. *J. Clin. Endocrinol. Metab.,* 37:448–453.
186. Wiebe, J. P., Tilbe, K. S., and Buckingham, K. D. (1980): An analysis of the metabolites of progesterone produced by isolated Sertoli cells at the onset of gametogenesis. *Steroids,* 35:561–578.
187. Folman, Y., Sowell, J. G., and Eik-Nes, K. B. (1972): Presence and formation of 5α-dihydrotestosterone in rat testes *in vivo* and *in vitro*. *Endocrinology,* 91:702–709.
188. Dorrington, J. H., and Fritz, I. B. (1975): Cellular localization of 5-alpha reductase and 3-alpha hydroxy steroid dehydrogenase in the seminiferous tubule of the rat testis. *Endocrinology,* 96: 879–889.
189. Cochran, R. C., Schuetz, A. W., and Ewing, L. L. (1979): Age-related changes in conversion of 5α-androstan-17β-ol-3-one to 5α-androstane-3α,17β-diol and 5α-androstane-3β,17β-diol by rat testicular cells *in vitro*. *J. Reprod. Fertil.,* 57:143–147.
190. Kasai, H., Mizutani, S., and Matsumoto, K. (1973): Detection of [^{3}H]5α-androstane-3α,17β-diol and [^{3}H]17β-hydroxy-5α-androstan-3-one in mouse testes following administration of [^{3}H]testosterone. *Acta Endocrinol.,* 74:177–185.
191. Baker, H. W. G., Bailey, D. J., Feil, P. D., Jefferson, L. S., Santen, R. J., and Bardin, C. W. (1977): Nuclear accumulation of androgens in perfused rat accessory sex organs and testes. *Endocrinology,* 100:709–721.
192. Suarez-Quian, C. A., Dym, M., Makris, A., Brumbaugh, J., Ryan, K. J., and Canick, J. A. (1983): Estrogen synthesis by immature rat Sertoli cells *in-vitro*. *J. Androl.,* 4:203–209.
193. Tsai-Morris, C.-H., Aquilano, D. R., and Dufau, M. L. (1985): Cellular localization of rat testicular aromatase activity during development. *Endocrinology,* 116:38–46.
194. Ritzen, E. M., Van Damme, M. P., Froysa, B., Reuter, C., De La Torre, B., and Diczfalusy, E. (1981): Identification of estradiol produced by Sertoli cell enriched cultures during incubation with testosterone. *J. Steroid Biochem.,* 14:533–536.
195. Siiteri, P. K., and MacDonald, P. C. (1973): Role of extraglandular estrogen in human endocrinology. In: *Handbook of Physiology: Endocrinology, Section 7, Vol. 11,* edited by R. O. Greep and E. B. Astwood, pp. 615–629. American Physiological Society, Washington, D.C.
196. Murphy, H. D. (1965): Sertoli cell stimulation following intratesticular injection of FSH in the hypophysectomized rat. *Proc. Soc. Exp. Biol. Med.,* 118:1202–1205.
197. Means, A. R., and Vaitukaitis, J. (1972): Peptide hormone "receptors": Specific binding of ^{3}H-FSH T_4 testis. *Endocrinology,* 90:39–46.
198. Bhalla, V. K., and Reichert, L. E. (1974): Properties of follicle-stimulating hormone-receptor interaction. *J. Biol. Chem.,* 249:43–51.
199. Steinberger, E., and Chowdhury, M. (1974): Control of pituitary FSH in male rats. *Acta Endocrinol. (Copenh.),* 76:235–241.
200. Yee, J. B., and Hutson, J. C. (1983): Testicular macrophages: Isolation, characterization and hormonal responsiveness. *Biol. Reprod.,* 29:1319–1326.
201. Yee, J. B., and Hutson, J. C. (1985): *In vivo* effects of follicle-stimulating hormone on testicular macrophages. *Biol. Reprod.,* 32:880–883.
202. Reichert, L. E., Jr., Andersen, T. T., Dias, J. A., Fletcher, P. W., Sluss, P. M., O'Neill, W. C., and Smith, R. A. (1984): Studies on the molecular biology of the interaction of follicle-stimulating hormone with receptors from testis. In: *Hormone Receptors in Growth and Reproduction,* edited by B. B. Saxena et al. Raven Press, New York.
203. Dias, J. A., and Reichert, L. E., Jr. (1982): Characterization of a follicle-binding component prepared from immature bovine testis in the absence of detergent. *J. Biol. Chem.,* 257:613–620.
204. Branca, A. A., Sluss, P. M., Smith, R. A., and Reichert, L. E., Jr. (1985): The subunit structure of the follitropin receptor: Chemical cross-linking of the solubilized follitropin receptor complex. *J. Biol. Chem.,* 260:9988–9993.
205. Smith, R. A., Branca, A. A., and Reichert, L. E., Jr. (1985): The subunit structure of the follitropin (FSH) receptor: Photoaffinity labeling of the membrane-bound receptor follitropin complex *in situ*. *J. Biol. Chem.,* 260:14297–14303.
206. Dattatreyamurty, B., Rathnam, P., and Saxena, B. B. (1983): Isolation of the luteinizing hormone-chorionic gonadotropin receptor in high yield from bovine corpora lutea. *J. Biol. Chem.,* 258:3140–3158.
207. Ascoli, M., and Segaloff, D. L. (1986): Effects of 'collagenase' on the structure of the lutropin/choriogonadotropin (LH/CG) receptor. *J. Biol. Chem.,* 261:3807–3815.
208. Francis, G. L., Brown, T. J., and Bercu, B. B. (1981): Regulation by homologous hormone exposure. *Biol. Reprod.,* 24:995–961.
209. Francis, G. L., Triche, T. J., Brown, T. J., Brown, H. C., and Bercu, B. B. (1981): *In-vitro* gonadotropin stimulation of bovine Sertoli cell ornithine decarboxylase EC-4.1.1.17 activity. *J. Androl.,* 2:312–320.
210. Fletcher, P. W., and Reichert, L. E., Jr. (1984): Cellular processing of follicle-stimulating hormone by Sertoli cells in serum-free culture. *Mol. Cell. Endocrinol.,* 34:39–50.
211. Andersen, T. T., and Reichert, L. E., Jr. (1984): Correlation of β coefficient of viscosity for monovalent salts with effects on binding of human follitropin to receptor. *Mol. Cell. Endocrinol.,* 35:41–46.
212. Dias, J. A., Treble, D. H., and Reichert, L. E. (1983): Effect of bacitracin and polyamines on follicle-stimulating hormone binding to membrane-bound and detergent-solubilized bovine calf testis receptor. *Endocrinology,* 113:2029–2034.
213. Dias, J. A., Treble, D. H., Bennett, A. H., and Reichert, L. E., Jr. (1981): Follicle-stimulating hormone receptor binding inhibitors in human seminal plasma. *J. Androl.,* 5:259–268.
214. Sanzo, M. A., and Reichert, L. E., Jr. (1982): Gonadotropin receptor binding regulators in serum: Characterization and separation of follitropin binding inhibitor and lutropin binding stimulator. *J. Biol. Chem.,* 257:6033–6040.
215. Papkoff, H., Niswender, G. D., Murthy, H. M. S., and Wiebe, J. P. (1983): Properties of an ovine testicular peptide that inhibits the binding of FSH to gonadal tissues. *Endocrinology,* 112:267.
216. Dias, J. A., and Reichert, L. E., Jr. (1984): Evidence for a high molecular weight follicle-stimulating hormone binding inhibitor in bovine testis. *Biol. Reprod.,* 31:975–983.
217. Murad, F., Strauch, B. S., and Vaughn, M. (1969): The effect of gonadotrophins on testicular adenylate cyclase. *Biochim. Biophys. Acta,* 177:591–598.
218. Kuehl, F., Patanelli, D. J., Humes, J. L., and Tarnoff, J. (1970): Testicular adenylate cyclase: Stimulation by the pituitary gonadotrophins. *Biol. Reprod.,* 2:153–163.
219. Dorrington, J. H., Vernon, R. G., and Fritz, I. B. (1972): The effect of gonadotrophins on the 3′,5′-AMP levels of seminiferous tubules. *Biochem. Biophys. Res. Commun.,* 46:1523–1528.
220. Means, A. R. (1973): Early effects of FSH upon testicular metabolism. *Adv. Exp. Med. Biol.,* 36:431.
221. Dorrington, J. H., and Fritz, I. B. (1974): Effects of gonadotrophins on cyclic AMP production by isolated seminiferous tubules and interstitial cell preparations. *Endocrinology,* 94:395–403.
222. Heindel, J. J., Rothenberg, R., Robinson, G. A., and Steinberger, A. (1975): LH and FSH stimulation of cyclic AMP in specific cell types isolated from the testes. *J. Cyclic Nucleotide Res.,* 1:69–79.
223. Means, A. R. (1975): Biochemical effects of follicle-stimulating hormone on the testis. In: *Handbook of Physiology, Vol. V,* edited by R. O. Greep, pp. 203–218. American Physiological Society, Washington, D.C.
224. Beale, E. G., Dedman, J. R., and Means, A. R. (1977): Isolation and regulation of the protein kinase inhibitor and the calcium dependent cyclic nucleotide phosphodiesterase regulator in the Sertoli cell enriched testis. *Endocrinology,* 101:1621–1634.
225. Beale, E. G., Dedman, J. R., and Means, A. R. (1977): Isolation and characterization of a protein from rat testis which inhibits cyclic AMP dependent protein kinase EC-2.7.1.37 and phosphodiesterase. *J. Biol. Chem.,* 252:6322–6327.

226. Conti, M., Geremia, R., Adamo, S., and Stefanini, M. (1981): Regulation of Sertoli cell cyclic adenosine 3′:5′-monophosphate phosphodiesterase activity by follicle stimulating hormone and dibutyryl cyclic AMP. *Biochem. Biophys. Res. Commun.*, 98:1044–1050.
227. Conti, M., Toscano, M. V., Geremia, R., and Stefanini, M. (1983): Follicle-stimulating hormone regulates *in-vivo* testicular phosphodiesterase. *Mol. Cell. Endocrinol.* 29:79–90.
228. Ireland, M. E., Rosenblum, B. B., and Welsh, M. J. (1986): Two-dimensional gel analysis of Sertoli cell protein phosphorylation: Effect of short term exposure to follicle-stimulating hormone. *Endocrinology*, 118:526–532.
229. Means, A. R., MacDougall, E., Soderling, T., and Corbin, J. D. (1974): Testicular adenosine 3′:5′-monophosphate-dependent protein kinase. *J. Biol. Chem.*, 249:1231–1238.
230. Means, A. R. (1971): Concerning the mechanism of FSH action: Rapid stimulation of testicular synthesis of nuclear RNA. *Endocrinology*, 89:981–989.
231. Means, A. R., and Tindall, D. J. (1975): FSH-induction of androgen binding protein in testis of Sertoli cell-only rats. In: *Hormonal Regulation of Spermatogenesis*, edited by F. S. French, V. Hansson, S. H. Nayfeh, and M. Ritzén, pp. 383–398. Plenum, New York.
232. Lamb, D. J., Lee, A. L., Steinberger, A., and Sanborn, B. M. (1982): Correlation between androgen binding and stimulation of nuclear RNA polymerase II activity in cultured Sertoli cells. In: *Cell Biology of the Testis, vol. 383*, edited by C. W. Bardin and R. J. Sherins, pp. 470–471. New York Academy of Science, New York.
233. Lamb, D. J., Tsai, Y.-H., Steinberger, A., and Sanborn, B. M. (1981): Sertoli cell nuclear transcriptional activity. Stimulation by follicle stimulating hormone and testosterone *in vitro*. *Endocrinology*, 108:1020–1026.
234. Lamb, D. J., Wagle, J. R., Tsai, Y. H., Lee, A. L., Steinberger, A., and Sanborn, B. M. (1982): Specificity and nature of the rapid steroid stimulated increase in Sertoli cell nuclear RNA polymerase activity. *J. Steroid Biochem.*, 16:653–660.
235. Means, A. R., and Hall, P. F. (1967): Effect of FSH on protein biosynthesis in testis of the immature rat. *Endocrinology*, 81:1151–1160.
236. Abney, T. O., Skipper, J. K., and Williams, W. L. (1974): Gonadotropin stimulation of rat testicular protein synthesis. Polysome isolation and activity in a cell-free system. *Biochemistry*, 13:3956–3961.
237. Dorrington, J. H., Roller, N. F., and Fritz, I. B. (1975): Effects of follicle-stimulating hormone on cultures of Sertoli cell preparations. *Mol. Cell. Endocrinol.*, 3:57–70.
238. Terasaki, W. L., Brooker, G., de Vellis, J., Inglish, D., Hsu, C., and Moylan, R. D. (1978): Involvement of cyclic AMP and protein synthesis in catecholamine refractoriness. In: *Advances in Cyclic Nucleotide Research*, edited by W. J. George and L. J. Ignarro. Raven Press, New York.
239. Catt, K. T., Harwood, J. P., Aquilera, G., and Dufau, M. L. (1979): Hormonal regulation of peptide receptors and target cell response. *Nature*, 280:109–116.
240. Harden, T. (1983): Agonist-induced desensitization of the β-adrenergic receptor-linked adenylate cyclase. *Pharmacol. Rev.*, 35:5.
241. O'Shaughnessy, P. J. (1980): FSH receptor autoregulation and cyclic AMP production in the immature rat testis. *Biol. Reprod.*, 23:810.
242. Conti, M., Toscano, M. V., Petrelli, L., Geremia, R., and Stefanini, M. (1983): Involvement of phosphodiesterase in the refractoriness of the Sertoli cell. *Endocrinology*, 113:1845–1853.
243. Attramadal, H., Le Gac, F., Jahnsen, T., and Hansson, V. (1984): β-Adrenergic regulation of Sertoli cell adenylate cyclase: Desensitization by homologous hormone. *Mol. Cell. Endocrinol.*, 34:1–6.
244. Verhoeven, G., Cailleau, J., and De Moor, P. (1981): Hormonal control of phosphodiesterase activity in cultured rat Sertoli cells. *Mol. Cell. Endocrinol.*, 24:41–52.
245. Conti, M., Monaco, L., Geremia, R., and Stefanini, M. (1986): Effect of phosphodiesterase inhibitors on Sertoli cell refractoriness: Reversal of the impaired androgen aromatization. *Endocrinology*, 118:901–908.
246. Means, A. R. (1981): Calmodulin: Properties, intracellular localization and multiple roles in cell regulation. *Recent Prog. Horm. Res.*, 37:333–368.
247. Means, A. R., Tash, J. S., and Chafouleas, J. G. (1982): Physiological implications of the presence, distribution, and regulation of calmodulin in eukaryotic cells. *Physiol. Rev.*, 62:1–38.
248. LaPorte, D. C., Wierman, B. M., and Storm, D. R. (1980): Calcium-induced exposure of a hydrophobic surface on calmodulin. *Biochemistry*, 19:3814–3819.
249. Tanaka, T., and Hidaka, H. (1980): Hydrophobic regions function in calmodulin enzyme(s) interactions. *J. Biol. Chem.*, 255:11078–11080.
250. Slaughter, G. R., and Means, A. R. (1983): FSH activation of glycogen phosphorylase in the Sertoli cell enriched rat testis. *Endocrinology*, 113:1476–1485.
251. Means, A. R., Slaughter, G. R., and Putkey, J. A. (1984): Post-receptor signal transduction by cyclic adenosine monophosphate and the Ca^{2+}-calmodulin complex. *J. Cell Biol.*, 99:226s–231s.
252. Hansson, V., Reusch, E., Trygstad, O., Torgersen, O., French, F. S., and Ritzén, E. M. (1973): FSH stimulation of androgen binding protein (ABP). *Nature (New Biol.)*, 246:56–59.
253. Tindall, D. J., and Means, A. R. (1976): Concerning the hormonal regulation of androgen binding protein in rat testis. *Endocrinology*, 99:809–818.
254. Kotite, N. J., Nayfeh, S. N., and French, F. S. (1978): Follicle stimulating hormone and androgen regulation of Sertoli cell function in the immature rat. *Biol. Reprod.*, 18:65–73.
255. Rich, K. A., Bardin, C. W., Gunsalus, G. L., and Mather, J. P. (1983): Age-dependent pattern of androgen binding protein (ABP) secretion from rat Sertoli cells in primary culture. *Endocrinology*, 113:2284–2293.
256. Wilson, R. M., and Griswold, M. C. D. (1979): Secreted proteins from rat Sertoli cells. *Exp. Cell Res.* 123:127–135.
257. Lacroix, M., and Fritz, I. B. (1982): Control of synthesis and secretion of plasminogen activator by rat Sertoli cells in culture. *Mol. Cell. Endocrinol.*, 26:247–258.
258. Fritz, I. B., and Karmally, K. (1983): Hormonal influences on formation of plasminogen activator by cultured testis tubule segments at defined stages of the cycle of the seminiferous epithelium. *Can. J. Biochem. Cell Biol.*, 61:553–560.
259. Holmes, S. D., Lipshultz, L. I., and Smith, R. G. (1984): Regulation of transferrin secretion by human Sertoli cells cultured in the presence or absence of human peritubular cells. *J. Clin. Endocrinol. Metab.*, 59:1058–1062.
260. Verhoeven, G., and Cailleau, J. (1985): A factor in spent media from Sertoli cell-enriched cultures that stimulates steroidogenesis in leydig cells. *Mol. Cell. Endocrinol.*, 40:57–68.
261. Benahmed, M., Reventos, J., Tabone, E., and Saez, J. M. (1985): Cultured Sertoli cell-mediated FSH stimulatory effect on Leydig cell steroidogenesis. *Am. J. Physiol.*, 248:E176–E181.
262. Sharpe, R. M., and Bartlett, J. M. S. (1985): Stimulation of Leydig cell function by a polypeptide present in testicular interstitial fluid. *Med. Biol.*, 63:245–250.
263. Saez, J. M., Tabone, E., Perrard-Sapori, M. H., and Rivarola, M. A. (1985): Paracrine role of Sertoli cells. *Med. Biol.*, 63:225–236.
264. Durham, L. A., III, and Grogan, W. M. (1984): Characterization of multiple forms of cholesteryl ester hydrolase EC-3.1.1.13 in the rat testis. *J. Biol. Chem.*, 259:7433–7438.
265. Hall, P. F., and Mita, M. (1984): Influence of FSH on glucose transport by cultured Sertoli cells. *Biol. Reprod.*, 31:863–869.
266. Mita, M., Price, J. M., and Hall, P. F. (1982): Stimulation by FSH of synthesis of lactate by Sertoli cells from rat testis. *Endocrinology*, 110:1535–1541.
267. Mita, M., and Hall, P. F. (1982): Metabolism of round spermatids from rats lactate as the preferred substrate. *Biol. Reprod.*, 26:445–455.
268. Marzowski, J., Sylvester, S. R., Gilmont, R. R., and Griswold, M. D. (1985): Isolation and characterization of Sertoli cell plasma membranes and associated plasminogen activator activity. *Biol. Reprod.*, 32:1237–1246.
269. Bordy, M. J., Berger, S., Desjardins, C., and Davis, J. C. (1979): Active cell aggregation by immature rat Sertoli cells in primary culture: a role for cell surface glyco proteins. *J. Cell. Physiol.*, 99:175–182.
270. Orth, J. M. (1984): The role of FSH in controlling Sertoli cell proliferation in testes of fetal rats. *Endocrinology*, 115:1248–1255.

271. Orth, J. M. (1982): Proliferation of Sertoli cells in fetal and post natal rats: A quantitative autoradiographic study. *Anat. Rec.*, 203:485–492.
272. Griswold, M. D., Mably, E. R., and Fritz, I. B. (1976): Follicle stimulating hormone stimulation of DNA synthesis in Sertoli cells in culture. *Mol. Cell. Endocrinol.*, 4:139–149.
273. Griswold, M. D., Solari, A., Tung, P. S., and Fritz, I. B. (1977): Stimulation by follicle-stimulating hormone of DNA synthesis and of mitosis in cultured Sertoli cells prepared from testes of immature rats. *Mol. Cell. Endocrinol.*, 7:151–165.
274. Fakunding, J. L., Tindall, D. J., Dedman, J. R., Mena, C. R., and Means, A. R. (1976): Biochemical actions of follicle stimulating hormone in the Sertoli cell of the rat testis. *Endocrinology*, 98:392–402.
275. Means, A. R. (1977): Mechanisms of action of follicle-stimulating hormone (FSH). In: *The Testis, Vol. IV,* edited by A. D. Johnson and W. R. Gomes, pp. 163–188. Academic Press, New York.
276. Karl, A. F., and Griswold, M. D. (1980): Actions of insulin and vitamin A on Sertoli cells. *Biochem. J.*, 186:1001–1004.
277. Griswold, M. D., and Merryweather, J. (1982): Insulin stimulates the incorporation of inorganic phosphorus-32 into RNA in cultured Sertoli cells. *Endocrinology*, 111:661–667.
278. Borland, K., Mita, M., Oppenheimer, C. L., Blinderman, L. A., Massague, J., Hall, P. F., and Czech, M. P. (1984): The actions of insulin-like growth factors I and II on cultured Sertoli cells. *Endocrinology*, 114:240–246.
279. Mita, M., Borland, K., Price, J. M., and Hall, P. F. (1985): The influence of insulin and insulin-like growth factor-I on hexose transport by Sertoli cells. *Endocrinology*, 116:987–992.
280. Eikvar, L., Levy, F. O., Attramadal, H., Jutte, N. H. P. M., Froysa, A., Tvermyr, S. M., and Hansson, V. (1985): Glucagon-stimulated cyclic AMP production and formation of estradiol in Sertoli cell cultures from immature rats. *Mol. Cell. Endocrinol.*, 39:107–114.
281. Chausmer, A., Stuart, C., and Stevens, M. (1980): Identification of testicular cell plasma membrane receptors for calcitonin. *J. Lab. Clin. Med.*, 96:933.
282. Chausmer, A. B., Stevens, M. D., and Severn, C. (1982): Autoradiographic evidence for a calcitonin receptor on testicular Leydig cells. *Science*, 216:735.
283. Nakhla, A. M., Mather, J. P., Jänne, O. A., and Bardin, C. W. (1986): The action of calcitonin on cultured testicular cells. II. Changes in androgen binding protein secretion and sex steroid receptor concentrations in Sertoli cells. *J. Androl. (submitted for publication.)*
284. Bardin, C. W., Shaha, C., Mather, J., Salomon, Y., Margioris, A. N., Liotta, A. S., Gerendai, I., Chen, C.-L., and Krieger, D. T. (1984): Identification and possible function of pro-opiomelanocortin-derived peptides in the testis. *Ann. NY Acad. Sci.*, 438:346–364.
285. Krieger, D. T., Margioris, A. N., Liotta, A. S., Shaha, C., Gerendai, I., Pintar, J., and Bardin, C. W. (1984): Pro-opiomelanocortin (POMC)-derived peptides in the rodent male reproductive tract. In: *Opioid Modulation of Endocrine Function,* edited by G. Delitala, M. Motta and M. Serio, pp. 223–235. Raven Press, New York.
286. Sharpe, B., Pekary, A. E., Meyer, N. V., and Hersham, J. M. (1980): β-Endorphin in male rat reproductive organs. *Biochem. Biophys. Res. Commun.*, 95:618–623.
287. Tsong, S. D., Phillips, D. M., Halmi, N., Krieger, D., and Bardin, C. W. (1982): β-Endophin is present in the male reproductive tract of five species. *Biol. Reprod.*, 27:755–764.
288. Tsong, S.-D., Phillips, D. M., Bardin, C. W., Halmi, N., Liotta, A. J., Margioris, A., and Krieger, D. T. (1982): ACTH and β-endorphin related peptides are present in multiple sites in the reproductive tract of the rat. *Endocrinology*, 110:2204–2206.
289. Shaha, C., Liotta, A. S., Krieger, D. T., and Bardin, C. W. (1984): The ontogeny of immunoreactive β-endorphin in the fetal, neonatal, and pubertal testes from mouse and hamster. *Endocrinology*, 114:1584–1591.
290. Chen, C.-L., Mather, J. P., Morris, P. L., and Bardin, C. W. (1984): Expression of pro-opiomelanocortin-like gene in the testis and epididymis. *Proc. Natl. Acad. Sci. USA*, 81:5672–5675.
291. Melner, M. H., and Puett, D. (1984): Evidence for the synthesis of multiple pro-opiomelanocortin-like precursors in murine Leydig tumor cells. *Arch. Biochem. Biophys.*, 232:197–201.
292. Pintar, J. E., Schachter, B., Herman, A. B., Durgerian, S., and Krieger, D. T. (1984): Characterization and localization of pro-opiomelanocortin mRNA in the adult rat. *Science*, 225:632.
293. Shaha, C., Boitani, C., Hahn, E. F., Gerendai, I., Mather, J., Margioris, A. N., Liotta, A. S., Chen, C.-L., Krieger, D. T., and Bardin, C. W. (1984): The presence and possible function of proopiomelanocortin-derived peptides in the testis and ovary. In: *Opioid Peptides in Periphery,* edited by F. Fraioli, A. Isidori, and M. Mazzetti, pp. 53–59. Elsevier, Amsterdam.
294. Mather, J., Bardin, C. W., Byer, A., and Salomon, Y. (1985): Modulation of adenylate cyclase activity in Sertoli cells *in vitro*. In: *Recent Progress in Cellular Endocrinology of the Testis, Vol. 122,* edited by J. M. Saez, M. G. Forest, A. Dazord, and J. Bertrand, pp. 183–186. INSERM, Paris.
295. Boitani, C., Mather, J. P., and Bardin, C. W. (1986): Stimulation of cAMP production in rat Sertoli cells by α-MSH and des-acetyl α-MSH. *Endocrinology*, 118:1513–1518.
296. O'Donohue, T. L., Handelmann, T. L., Chaconas, T., Miller, R. L., and Jacobowitz, D. M. (1981): Evidence that *N*-acetylation regulates the behavioral activity of MSH in the rat and human central nervous system. *Peptides*, 2:333.
297. O'Donohue, T. L., Handelmann, G. E., Miller, R. L., and Jacobowitz, D. M. (1982): *N*-Acetylation regulates the behavioral activity of α-melanotropin in a multineurotransmitter neuron. *Science*, 215:1125.
298. Akil, H., Hewlitt, H., Barchas, J. D., and Ki, C. H. (1980): Binding of ^{3}H-β-endorphin to rat brain membranes: Characterization of opiate properties and interaction with ACTH. *Eur. J. Pharmacol.*, 64:1.
299. McCormack, A. M., Carter, R. J., Thody, A. J., and Shuster, S. (1982): Des-acetyl-α-MSH and α-MSH act as partial agonists to MSH on the Anolis melanophore. *Peptides*, 3:13.
300. Gerendai, I., Nemeskéri, A., and Csernus, V. (1983): Naloxone has a local effect on the testis of immature rats. *Andrologia*, 15:398–403.
301. Chen, C.-L.C., Margioris, A. N., Liotta, A. S., Morris, P. L., Boitani, C., Mather, J. P., Krieger, D. T., and Bardin, C. W. (1984): Pro-opiomelanocortin-derived peptides of Leydig cell origin may be modulators of testicular function. In: *Gonadal Proteins and Peptides and Their Biological Significance,* edited by M. R. Sairam and L. E. Atkinson, pp. 339–352. World Scientific, Singapore.
302. Gerendai, I., Shaha, C., Gunsalus, G. L., and Bardin, C. W. (1986): The effects of opioid receptor antagonists suggest that testicular opiates regulate Sertoli and Leydig cell function in the neonatal rat. *Endocrinology*, 118:2039–2044.
303. Orth, J. (1986): FSH-induced Sertoli cell proliferation in the developing rat is modified by β-endorphin produced in the testis. *Endocrinology*, 119:1876–1878.
304. Fabbri, A., Tsai-Morris, C. H., Luna, S., Fraioli, F., and Dufau, M. L. (1985): Opiate receptors are present in the rat testis. Identification and localization in Sertoli cells. *Endocrinology*, 117:2544–2546.
305. Kilpatrick, D. L., and Rosenthal, J. L. (1986): The proenkephalin gene is widely expressed within the male and female reproductive systems of the rat and hamster. *Endocrinology*, 119:370–374.
306. Thody, A. T., Wilson, C. A., and Everard, D. (1981): α-Melanocyte stimulating hormone stimulates sexual behaviour in the female rat. *Psychopharmacology*, 74:153.
307. Krieger, D. T., Liotta, A. S., Brownstein, M. J., and Zimmerman, E. A. (1980): ACTH, β-lipotropin, and related peptides in brain, pituitary, and blood. *Recent Prog. Horm. Res.*, 36:277–344.
308. Chen, C.-L., Mather, J. P., Morris, P. L., and Bardin, C. W. (1985): Expression of Pro-opiomelanocortin-like gene in the testis and Leydig cell lines. In: *Hormone Action and Testicular Function, Vol. 438,* edited by K. J. Catt and M. L. Dufau, pp. 659–662. Annals of the New York Academy of Science, New York.
309. Tindall, D. J., Miller, D. A., and Means, A. R. (1977): Characterization of androgen receptor in Sertoli cell enriched testis. *Endocrinology*, 101:13–23.
310. Sanborn, B. M., Steinberger, A., Tcholakian, R. K., and Steinberger, E. (1977): Direct measurement of androgen receptors in cultured Sertoli cells. *Steroids*, 29:493–502.
311. Chevalier, M., and Dufaure, J.-P. (1981): Effect of FSH testosterone and calcium on Sertoli cell micro filaments in the immature pig testis. *Biol. Cell*, 41:105–112.

312. Dym, M., and Raj, H. G. M. (1977): Response of adult rat Sertoli cells and Leydig cells to depletion of luteinizing hormone and testosterone. *Biol. Reprod.*, 17:676–696.
313. Elkington, J. S., Sanborn, B. M., and Steinberger, E. (1975): The effect of testosterone propionate on the concentration of testicular and epididymal androgen binding activity in hypophysectomized rat. *Mol. Cell. Endocrinol.*, 2:157–170.
314. Weddington, S. C., Hansson, V., Purvis, K., Varaas, T., Verjans, H. L., Eik-Nes, K. B., Ryan, W. H., French, F. S., and Ritzén, E. M. (1976): Biphasic effect of testosterone propionate on Sertoli cell secretory function. *Mol. Cell. Endocrinol.*, 5:137–145.
315. Louis, B. G., and Fritz, I. B. (1977): Stimulation by androgens of the production of androgen binding protein by cultured Sertoli cells. *Mol. Cell. Endocrinol.*, 7:9–16.
316. Louis, B. G., and Fritz, I. B. (1979): Follicle stimulating hormone and testosterone independently increase the production of androgen binding protein by Sertoli cells in culture. *Endocrinology*, 104:454–461.
317. Louis, B. G., and Fritz, I. B. (1976): Regulation by testosterone and follicle stimulating hormone of androgen binding protein production by Sertoli cells in culture. *Proc. Can. Fed. Biol. Soc.*, 19:148.
318. Gunsalus, G. L., Larrea, F., Musto, N. A., Becker, R. R., Mather, J. P., and Bardin, C. W. (1981): Androgen binding protein as a marker for Sertoli cell function. *J. Steroid Biochem.*, 15:99–106.
319. Elkington, J. S. H., Sanborn, B. M., Martin, M. W., Chowdhury, A. K., and Steinberger, E. (1977): Effect of testosterone propionate on ABP levels in rats hypophysectomized at different ages using individual sampling. *Mol. Cell. Endocrinol.*, 203–209.
320. Isomaa, V. V., Pajunen, A. E. I., Bardin, C. W., and Jänne, O. A. (1983): Ornithine decarboxylase in mouse kidney. Purification, characterization and radioimmunological determination of the enzyme protein. *J. Biol. Chem.*, 258:6735–6740.
321. Tsutsui, K., and Ishii, S. (1978): Effects of follicle stimulating hormone and testosterone on receptors of follicle stimulating hormone in the testis of the immature japanese quail. *Gen. Comp. Endocrinol.*, 36:297–305.
322. Tsutsui, K., and Ishii, S. (1980): Hormonal regulation of follicle stimulating hormone receptors in the testes of japanese quail. *J. Endocrinol.*, 85:511–518.
323. Cunha, G. R., Chung, L. W. K., Shannon, J. M., Taguchi, O., and Fujii, H. (1983): Hormone induced morphogenesis and growth: Role of mesenchymal-epithelial interactions. In: *Recent Prog. Horm. Res.*, 39:559–598.
324. Cunha, G. R., Bigsby, R. M., Cooke, P. S., and Sugimura, Y. (1985): Stromal-epithelial interactions in adult organs. *Cell Differ.* 17:137–148.
325. Nakhla, A. M., Mather, J. P., Jänne, O. A., and Bardin, C. W. (1984): Estrogen and androgen receptors in Sertoli, Leydig, myoid, and epithelial cells: Effects of time in culture and cell density. *Endocrinology*, 115:121–128.
326. Isomaa, V., Parvinen, M., Jänne, O. A., and Bardin, C. W. (1985): Nuclear androgen receptors in different stages of the seminiferous epithelial cycle and the interstitial tissue of rat testis. *Endocrinology*, 116:132–136.
327. Wagle, J. R., Steinberger, A., and Sanborn, B. M. (1983): Interaction of progestins with Sertoli cell androgen receptors. *J. Steroid Biochem.*, 18:253–256.
328. Carson, D. D., and Lennarz, W. J. (1983): Vitamin A deprivation selectively lowers uridine nucleotide pools in cultured Sertoli cells. *J. Biol. Chem.*, 258:1632–1636.
329. Rajguru, S. U., Kang, Y.-H., and Ahluwalia, B. S. (1982): Localization of retinol vitamin A in rat testes. *J. Nutr.*, 112:1881–1891.
330. Porter, S. B., Ong, D. E., Chytil, F., and Orgebin-Crist, M.-C. (1985): Localization of cellular retinol-binding protein and cellular retinoic-acid-binding protein in the rat testis and epididymis. *J. Androl.*, 6:197–212.
331. Levy, F. O., Eikvar, L., Jutte, N. H. P. M., Cervenka, J., Yoganathan, T, and Hansson, V. (1985): Appearance of the rat testicular receptor for calcitriol 1,25-dihydroxyvitamin d-3 during development. *J. Steroid Biochem.*, 23:51–56.
332. Merke, J., Huegel, U., and Ritz, E. (1985): Nuclear testicular 1,25-dihydroxyvitamin d-3 receptors in Sertoli cells and seminiferous tubules of adult rodents. *Biochem. Biophys. Res. Commun.*, 127:303–309.
333. Kleinman, H. K., Klebe, R. J., and Martin, G. R. (1981): Role of collagenous matrices in the adhesion and growth of cells. *J. Cell Biol.*, 88:473–485.
334. Gospodarowicz, D. J. (1984): Extracellular matrices and the control of cell proliferation and differentiation *in vitro*. In: *New Approaches to the Study of Benign Prostatic Hyperplasia*, edited by F. A. Kimball, A. E. Buhl, and D. B. Carter, pp. 103–128. Alan R. Liss, New York.
335. Hay, E. D. (1984): Cell-matrix interaction in the embryo: Cell shape, cell surface, cell skeletons, and their role in differentiation. In: *The Role of the Extracellular Matrix in Development*, edited by R. L. Trelstad, pp. 1–31. Alan R. Liss, New York.
336. Reid, L. M., and Jefferson, D. M. (1984): Cell culture studies using extracts of extracellular matrix to study growth and differentiation in mammalian cells. In: *Mammalian Cell Culture*, edited by J. P. Mather. Plenum, New York.
337. Mather, J. P., Wolpe, S. D., Gunsalus, G. L., Bardin, C. W., and Phillips, D. M. (1985): Effect of purified and cell-produced extracellular matrix components on Sertoli cell function. In: *Hormone Action and Testicular Function, Vol. 438*, edited by K. J. Catt and M. L. Dufau, pp. 572–575. Annals of the New York Academy of Science, New York.
338. Tung, P. S., and Fritz, I. B. (1984): Extracellular matrix promotes rat Sertoli cell histotypic expression *in-vitro*. *Biol. Reprod.*, 30:213–230.
339. Hadley, M. A., Byers, S. W., Suarez-Quian, C. A., Kleinman, H. K., and Dym, M. (1985): Extracellular matrix regulates Sertoli cell differentiation, testicular cord formation, and germ cell development *in vitro*. *J. Cell Biol.*, 101:1511–1522.
340. Parvinen, M., Wright, W. W., Phillips, D. M., Mather, J. P., Musto, N. A., and Bardin, C. W. (1983): Spermatogenesis *in vitro:* Completion of meiosis and early spermiogenesis. *Endocrinology*, 112:1150–1152.
341. Lacy, D. (1960): Light and electron microscopy and its use in the study of factors influencing spermatogenesis in the rat. *J. Microsc. Soc.*, 79:209.
342. Hilscher, B., Passia, D., and Hilscher, W. (1979): Kinetics of the enzymatic pattern in the testis. I. Stage dependence of enzymatic activity and its relation to cellular interactions in the testis of the Wistar rat. *Andrologia*, 11:169–181.
343. Parvinen, M., and Vanha-Perttula, T. (1972): Identification and enzyme quantitation of the stages of the seminiferous epithelial wave in the rat. *Anat. Rec.*, 174:435–450.
344. Lacroix, M., Parvinen, M., and Fritz, I. B. (1981): Localization of testicular plasminogen activator in discrete portions T stages VII and VIII of the seminiferous tubule. *Biol. Reprod.*, 25:143–146.
345. Ritzen, E. M., Boitani, C., Parvinen, M., French, F. C., and Feldman, M. (1982): Stage dependent secretion of androgen binding protein by rat seminiferous tubules. *Mol. Cell. Endocrinol.*, 25:25–34.
346. Tung, P. S., and Fritz, I. B. (1980): Interactions of Sertoli cells with myoid cells *in vitro*. *Biol. Reprod.*, 23:207–218.
347. Cameron, D. F., and Syndle, E. (1985): Selected enzyme histochemistry of Sertoli cells. 2. Adult rat Sertoli cells in co-culture with peritubular fibroblasts. *Andrologia*, 17:185–193.
348. Cameron, D. F., and Markwald, R. R. (1981): Structural response of adult rat Sertoli cells to peri tubular fibroblasts *in-vitro*. *Am. J. Anat.*, 160:343–358.
349. Parvinen, M., and Ruokonen, A. (1982): Endogenous steroids in the rat seminiferous tubules. Comparison of the stages of the epithelial cycle isolated by transillumination-assisted microdissection. *J. Androl.*, 3:211–220.
350. Bergh, A. (1983): Paracrine regulation of Leydig cells by the seminiferous tubules. *Int. J. Androl.*, 6:57–65.
351. Sharpe, R. M., Fraser, H. M., Cooper,, I., and Rommerts, F. F. G. (1981): Sertoli-Leydig cell communication via a luteinizing hormone releasing hormone like factor. *Nature*, 209:785–787.
352. Reventos, J., Benahmed, M., Tabone, E., and Saez, J. M. (1983): Modulation of Leydig cell functions by Sertoli cells: *in-vitro* studies. *C. R. Acad. Sci. III*, 296:123–126.
353. Tabone, E., Benahmed, M., Reventos, J., and Saez, J. M. (1984): Interactions between immature porcine Leydig and Sertoli cells *in-vitro:* An ultrastructural and biochemical study. *Cell Tissue Res.* 237:357–362.

354. Hatier, R., and Grignon, G. (1980): Ultrastructural study of Sertoli cells in rat seminiferous tubules during intra uterine life and post natal period. *Anat. Embryol.*, 160:11–28.
355. Almond, D. G., and Singh, R. P. (1980): Development of the Sertoli cell in the fetal mouse. *Acta Anat.*, 106:276–280.
356. Van Vorstenbosch, C. J. A. H. V., Spek, E., Colenbrander, B., and Wensing, C. J. G. (1984): Sertoli cell development of pig testis in the fetal and neonatal period. *Biol. Reprod.*, 31:565–578.
357. Nistal, M., and Paniagua, R. (1983): Post natal development of human Sertoli cells. *Z. Mikrosk. Anat. Forsch.*, 97:739–752.
358. Jost, A. (1972): Preliminary data on the initial stages of testicular differentiation in the rat. *Arch. Anat. Microsc. Morphol. Exp.*, 61:415–437.
359. Magre, S., and Jost, A. (1980): The initial phases of testicular organogenesis in the rat: an electron microscopic study. *Arch. Anat. Microsc. Morphol. Exp.*, 69:297–318.
360. Agelopoulou, R., Magre, S., Patsavoudi, E., and Jost, A. (1984): Initial phases of the rat testis differentiation *in-vitro*. *J. Embryol. Exp. Morphol.*, 83:15–32.
361. Jost, A., and Magre, S. (1984): Testicular development phases and dual hormonal control of sexual organogenesis. In: *Sexual Differentiation: Basic and Clinical Aspects, Vol. 11*, edited by M. Serio, M. Motta, M. Zanisi, and L. Martini, pp. 1–16. Raven, New York.
362. Steinberger A., and Steinberger, E. (1971): Replication pattern of Sertoli cells in maturing rat testis *in vivo* and in organ culture. *Biol. Reprod.*, 84:84–94.
363. Orth, J. M. (1985): Effect of Sertoli cell depletion during neonatal life on spermatid production in adults. *Anat. Rec.*, 211:144A (abstract).
364. Kluin, P. M., Kramer, M. F., and De Rooij, D. G. (1984): Proliferation of spermatogonia and Sertoli cells in maturing mice. *Anat. Embryol.*, 169:73–78.
365. Kluin, P. M., Kramer, M. F., and De Rooij, D. G. (1983): Testicular development in macaca-irus after birth. *Int. J. Androl.*, 6:25–43.
366. Nistal, M., Abaureea, M. A., and Paniagua, R. (1982): Morphological and histometric study on the human Sertoli cell from birth to the onset of puberty. *J. Anat.*, 134:351–363.
367. Chemes, H. E., Dym, M., and Raj, H. G. M. (1979): The role of gonadotropins and testosterone on initiation of spermatogenesis in the immature rat. *Biol. Reprod.*, 21:241–249.
368. Chemes, H. F., Dym, M., and Raj, H. G. M. (1979): Hormonal regulation of Sertoli cell differentiation. *Biol. Reprod.*, 21:251–262.
369. Orth, J., and Christensen, A. K. (1977): Localization of iodine-125 labeled follicle stimulating hormone in the testes of hypophysectomized rats by auto radiography at the light microscope and electron microscope levels. *Endocrinology*, 101:262–278.
370. Warren, D. W., Huhtaniemi, I. T., Tapanainen, J., Dufau, M. L., and Catt, K. J. (1984): Ontogeny of gonadotropin receptors in the fetal and neonatal rat testis. *Endocrinology*, 114:470–476.
371. Means, A. R., Fakunding, J. L., Huckins, C., Tindall, D. J., and Vitale, R. (1976): Follicle-stimulating hormone, the Sertoli cell, and spermatogenesis. *Recent Prog. Horm. Res.*, 32:477–528.
372. Tsutsui, K., Shimizu, A., Kawamoto, K., and Kawashima, S. (1985): Developmental changes in binding of follicle-stimulating hormone (FSH) to testicular preparations of mice and the effects of hypophysectomy and administration of FSH on the binding. *Endocrinology*, 117:2534–2543.
373. Barenton, B., Hochereau-De Reviers, M. T., Perreau, C., and Saumande, J. (1983): Changes in testicular gonadotropin receptors and steroid content through postnatal development until puberty in the lamb. *Endocrinology*, 112:1447–1453.
374. Tran, D., Meusy-Dessolle, N., and Josso, N. (1977): Anti-muellerian hormone is a functional marker of fetal Sertoli cells. *Nature*, 269:411–412.
375. Donahoe, P. K., Swann, D. A., Hayashi, A., and Sullivan, M. D. (1979): Mullerian duct regression in the embryo correlated with cytotoxic activity against a human ovarian cancer. *Science*, 205:913.
376. Fuller, A., Guy, S., and Donahoe, P., (1982): Mullerian inhibiting substance inhibits colony growth of a human ovarian carcinoma cell line. *J. Clin. Endocrinol. Metab.*, 54:1051–1055.
377. Fuller, A. F., Krane, I. M., Budzik, G. P., and Donahoe, P. K. (1985): Mullerian inhibiting substance reduction of colony growth of human gynecologic cancers in a stem cell assay. *Gynecol. Oncol.*, 2:135.
378. Donahoe, P., Fuller, A., Scully, R., and Guy, S. (1981): Mullerian inhibiting substance inhibits growth of a human ovarian cancer in nude mice. *Am. Surg.*, 194:472.
379. Tran, D., and Josso, N. (1982): Localization of antimuellerian hormone in the rough endoplasmic reticulum of the developing bovine Sertoli cell using immunocytochemistry with a monoclonal antibody. *Endocrinology*, 111:1562–1567.
380. Magre, S., and Jost, A. (1984): Dissociation between testicular organogenesis and endocrine cytodifferentiation of Sertoli cells. *Proc. Natl. Acad. Sci. USA*, 81:7831–7834.
381. Blanchard, M.-G., and Josso, N. (1974): Source of the anti-muellerian hormone synthesized by the fetal testis: Muellerian inhibiting activity of fetal bovine Sertoli cells in tissue culture. *Pediatr. Res.*, 8:968–971.
382. Josso, N., Picard, J. Y., Dacheaux, J. L., and Courot, M. (1979): Detection of anti-Müllerian activity in boar rete testis fluid. *J. Reprod. Fertil.*, 57:397–403.
383. Necklaws, E. C., LaQuaglia, M. P., MacLaughlin, D., Hudson, P., Mudgett-Hunter, M., and Donahoe, P. K. (1986): Detection of mullerian inhibiting substance in biological samples by a solid phase sandwich radioimmunoassay. *Endocrinology*, 118:791–796.
384. Tran, D., Meusy-Dessolle, N., and Josso, N. (1981): Waning of anti-muellerian activity: An early sign of Sertoli cell maturation in the developing pig. *Biol. Reprod.*, 24:923–932.
385. Bergmann, M., and Dierichs, R. (1983): Post natal formation of the blood testis barrier in the rat with special reference to the initiation of meiosis. *Anat. Embryol.*, 168:269–276.
386. Tindall, D. J., Vitale, R., and Means, A. R. (1975): Androgen binding protein as a biochemical marker of formation of the blood testis barrier. *Endocrinology*, 97:636–648.
387. Hatier, R., Grignon, G., and Touati, F. (1982): Ultrastructural study of seminiferous tubules in the rat after pre natal irradiation. *Anat. Embryol.*, 165:425–436.
388. Vogel, D. L., Gunsalus, G. L., Bercu, B. B., Musto, N. A., and Bardin, C. W. (1983): Sertoli cell maturation is impaired by neonatal passive immunization with antiserum to luteinizing hormone-releasing hormone. *Endocrinology*, 112:1115–1121.
389. Gunsalus, G. L., Musto, N. A., Bardin, C. W., Kunz, H. W., and Gill, T. J. III (1985): Rats homozygous for the *grc* complex have defective transport of androgen binding protein to the epididymis, but normal secretion into the blood. *Biol. Reprod.*, 33:1057–1063.
390. Gunsalus, G. L., Musto, N. A., Becker, R. R., and Bardin, C. W. (1986): The bidirectional secretion of androgen binding protein in rats with germ cell depletion secondary to the H^{re} gene and prenatal x-ray. *Endocrinology (in press)*.
391. Carreau, S., Musto, N. A., and Gunsalus, G. L. (1983): In fetal rats androgen binding protein (ABP) is synthesized by liver and testis. *Endocrinology*, 112:238 (abstract).
392. Carreau, S., Gunsalus, G. L., Musto, N. A., and Bardin, C. W. (1986): Sertoli rat androgen-binding protein is synthesized by liver and testis. *Endocrinology (submitted for publication)*.
393. Gunsalus, G. L., De Besi, L., Musto, N. A., and Bardin, C. W. (1986): Measurement of rat androgen-binding protein (rABP) by steroid binding, radioimmunoassay (RIA), and enzyme linked immunosorbent assay (ELISA). In: *Binding Proteins of Steroid Hormones*, INSERM, Paris, 149:227–236.
394. Dorrington, J. H., Fritz, I. B., and Armstrong, D. T. (1976): Site at which follicle stimulating hormone regulates estradiol 17-β biosynthesis in Sertoli cell preparations in culture. *Mol. Cell. Endocrinol.*, 6:117–122.
395. Steinberger, E., Tcholakian, R. K., and Steinberger, A. (1979): Steroidogenesis in testicular cells. *J. Steroid Biochem.*, 11:185–192.
396. Canick, J. A., Makris, A., Gunsalus, G. L., and Ryan, K. J. (1979): Testicular aromatization in immature rats: Localization and stimulation after gonadotropin administration *in vivo*. *Endocrinology*, 104:285–288.
397. Gore-Langton, R., Mckeracher, H., and Dorrington, J. (1980): An alternative method for the study of follicle stimulating hormone effects on aromatase activity in Sertoli cell cultures. *Endocrinology*, 107:464–471.
398. Mori, H., and Christensen, A. K. (1980): Morphometric analysis of Leydig cells in the normal rat. *J. Cell Biol.*, 84:340–354.

399. Wong, V., and Russell, L. D. (1983): Three-dimensional reconstruction of a rat stage V Sertoli cell. I. Methods, basic configuration, and dimensions. *Am. J. Anat.*, 167:143–162.
400. Wing, T.-Y., and Christensen, A. K. (1982): Morphometric studies on rat seminiferous tubules. *Am. J. Anat.*, 165:13–26.
401. Weber, J. E., Russell, L. D., Wong, V., and Peterson, R. N. (1983): Three-dimensional reconstruction of a rat stage V Sertoli cell. II. Morphometry of Sertoli-Sertoli and Sertoli germ cell relationships. *Am. J. Anat.*, 167:163–180.
402. Russell, L. D., Tallon-Doran, M., Weber, J. E., Wong, V., and Peterson, R. N. (1983): Three-dimensional reconstruction of a rat stage V Sertoli cell. III. A study of specific cellular relationships. *Am. J. Anat.*, 167:181–192.
403. Gardner, R., Weber, J. E., and Russell, L. D. (1985): Morphometric analysis of a reconstructed stage V monkey Sertoli cell. *J. Androl.*, 6:66-P (abstract).
404. Cunningham, G. R., Tindall, D. J., Huckins, C., and Means, A. R. (1978): Mechanisms for the testicular hypertrophy which follows hemicastration. *Endocrinology*, 102:16–22.
405. Ribbert, H. (1890): Ueber die compensatorische Hypertrophie der Geschlechtsdrusen. *Virchows Arch.*, 120:247.
406. Orth, J. M., Higginbotham, C. A., and Salisbury, R. L. (1984): Hemicastration causes and testosterone prevents enhanced uptake of tritium labeled thymidine by Sertoli cells in testes of immature rats. *Biol. Reprod.*, 30:263–270.
407. Walton, J. S., Evins, J. D., Hillard, M. A., and Waites, G. M. H. (1980): Follicle stimulating hormone release in hemicastrated prepubertal rams and its relationship to testicular development. *J. Endocrinol.*, 84:141–152.
408. Waites, G. M. H., Wenstrom, J. C., Crabo, B. G., and Hamilton, D. W. (1983): Rapid compensatory hypertrophy of the lamb testis after neonatal hemiorchiectomy: Endocrine and light microscopic morphometric analyses. *Endocrinology*, 112:2159–2167.
409. Hochereau-De Reviers, M.-T., and De Reviers, M. (1978): Inhibition de la croissance compensatrice du testicule restant chez le Raton Hemicastre par de la testosterone ou des extraits aqueux de testicule de Rat adulte. *C. R. Acad. Sci. (Paris)*, 287:1015–1018.
410. Santen, R. J., and Paulsen, C. A. (1973): Hypogonadotropic eunuchoidism. I. Clinical study of the mode of inheritance. *J. Clin. Endocrinol. Metab.*, 36:47–53.
411. Bercu, B. B., Jackson, I. M. D., Sawin, C. T., Safaii, H., and Reichlin, S. (1977): Permanent impairment of testicular development after transient immunological blockade of endogenous luteinizing hormone releasing hormone in the neonatal rat. *Endocrinology*, 101:1871.
412. Bercu, B. B., and Jackson, I. M. D. (1980): Response of adult male rats to LHRH after neonatal immunization with antiserum to LHRH. *J. Reprod. Fertil.*, 59:501–507.
413. Carreau, S., Bercu, B. B., Musto, N. A., Bardin, C. W., and Gunsalus, G. L. (1986): Rat Sertoli cell maturation: Effects of neonatal hemicastration and LHRH antiserum treatment. *Endocrinology (submitted for publication)*.
414. Valenca, M. C., and Negro-Vilar, N. (1986): Proopiomelanocortin-derived peptides in testicular interstitial fluid: Characterization and changes in secretion after human chorionic gonadotropin or luteinizing hormone-releasing hormone analog treatment. *Endocrinology*, 118:32–37.
415. Orth, J. M. (1984): Evidence that β-endorphin inhibits Sertoli cell proliferation in fetal rats. In: *7th International Congress of Endocrinology, Quebec, Canada*, pp. 1211. Excerpta Medica, Amsterdam (abstract 1902).
416. Becker, R. R., Gunsalus, G. L., Musto, N. A., and Bardin, C. W. (1984): The epididymis contributes minimally to serum androgen binding protein in the rat: A whole body kinetic study. *Endocrinology*, 114:2354–2360.
417. Setchell, B. P., and Waites, G. M. H. (1975): The blood-testis barrier. In: *Handbook of Physiology, Section 7: Endocrinology, Volume V: Male Reproductive System*, edited by D. W. Hamilton and R. O. Greep, p. 143. American Physiological Society, Washington, D. C.
418. Dym, M. (1976): The mammalian rete testis—A morphological examination. *Anat. Rec.*, 186:493–520.
419. Christensen, A. K., Komorowski, T. E., Wilson, B., Ma, S.-F., and Stevens, R. W. III (1985): The distribution of serum albumin in the rat testis studied by electron microscope immunocytochemistry on ultrathin frozen sections. *Endocrinology*, 116:1983–1996.
420. Setchell, B. P., Hinton, B. T., Jacks, F., and Davies, R. V. (1976): The restricted penetration of iodinated FSH and LH into the seminiferous tubules of the rat testis. *Mol. Cell. Endocrinol.*, 6:59.
421. Ross, M. H. (1977): Sertoli Sertoli junctions and Sertoli spermatid junctions after efferent ductule ligation and lanthanum treatment. *Am. J. Anat.* 148:49–56.
422. Osman, D. I., and Ploen, L. (1978): The terminal segment of the seminiferous tubules and the blood testis barrier before and after efferent ductule ligation in the rat. *Int. J. Androl.*, 1:235–249.
423. Nykanen, M., and Kormano, M. (1978): Early effects of efferent duct ligation on the rat rete testis. *Int. J. Androl.*, 1:225–234.
424. Osman, D. I. (1979): A comparative ultrastructural study on typical and modified Sertoli cells before and after ligation of the efferent ductules in the rabbit. *Anat. Histol. Embryol.*, 8:114–123.
425. Anton, E. (1982): Preservation of the rat blood testis barrier after ligation of the ductuli efferentes as demonstrated by intra-arterial perfusion with peroxidase. *J. Reprod. Fertil.*, 66:227–230.
426. Ashwell, G., and Morell, A. G. (1974): The role of surface carbohydrates in the hepatic recognition and transport of circulating glycoproteins. In: *Advances in Enzymology, Vol. 41*, edited by A. Meister, pp. 99–128. John Wiley & Sons, New York.
427. Gill, T. J. IV, Gill, T. J. III, Kunz, H. W., Musto, N. A., and Bardin, C. W. (1984): Genetic and morphometric studies of the heterogeneity in the testicular defect of the H^{re} rat and the interaction between the H^{re} and grc genes. *Biol. Reprod.*, 31:595–603.
428. Cheng, C. Y., Gunsalus, G. L., Morris, I. D., Turner, T. T., and Bardin, C. W. (1986): The heterogeneity of rat androgen binding protein (rABP) in the vascular compartment differs from that in the testicular tubular lumen: Further evidence for bidirectional secretion of rABP. *J. Androl.*, 7:175–179.
429. Lobl, T. J., Musto, N. A., Gunsalus, G. L., and Bardin, C. W. (1983): Medroxyprogesterone acetate has opposite effects on the androgen binding protein concentrations in serum and epididymis. *Biol. Reprod.*, 29:697–712.
430. Spitz, I. M., Gunsalus, G. L., Mather, J. P., Thau, R., and Bardin, C. W. (1985): The effects of the indazole carboxylic acid derivative, tolnidamine, on testicular function. I. Early changes in androgen binding protein secretion in the rat. *J. Androl.*, 6:171–178.
431. Escobar, N., and Musto, N. A. (1984): Assessing Sertoli cell function in the rabbit by measurement of serum androgen-binding protein. In: *7th International Congress of Endocrinology, Quebec, Canada*, p. 643. Excerpta Medica, Amsterdam (abstract 766).

The Physiology of Reproduction,
edited by E. Knobil and J. Neill *et al.*
Raven Press, Ltd., New York © 1988.

CHAPTER 22

Testicular Steroid Synthesis: Organization and Regulation

Peter F. Hall

The function of the Leydig cells of the testis is to secrete androgens in a regulated fashion. The principal regulating mechanism consists in the secretion of pulses of luteinizing hormone (LH) by the adenohypophysis (1). Androgens are responsible for the development and maintenance of the internal and external genitalia, the appearance of the secondary sexual characteristics, the development of the musculoskeletal system, feedback inhibition of the hypothalamopituitary axis, and stimulation of spermatogenesis. In addition, androgens stimulate a variety of other tissues including the skin and the kidneys. To a considerable extent, the difference between male and female mammalian organisms with respect to androgens is one of degree, so the male appearance can be induced in females by the administration of androgens.

The principal steroids secreted by the testis are androgens, and testosterone is by far the most important androgen because of its potency. Androstenedione and dehydroepiandrosterone are also secreted by the testis and show lesser degrees of androgenicity (2). These hormones are synthesized by the Leydig cells of the testis. This organ also secretes estrogens, which are synthesized by both Leydig cells and Sertoli cells (3).

SOURCE OF TESTICULAR ANDROGENS

Without doubt, almost all testicular androgens are formed and secreted by the Leydig cells (2,5). Some steroidogenic enzymes are found within the seminiferous tubule, which can convert progesterone to testosterone (4). It has been proposed that the seminiferous tubule can convert cholesterol to pregnenolone and is therefore capable of synthesizing androgens. Hall et al. (4) found no detectable production of [^{3}H]pregnenolone when seminiferous tubules of the rat were incubated with [7α-^{3}H]cholesterol. This failure could not be attributed to failure of the substrate to enter the germ cells or fibroblasts, first because cholesterol enters most cells freely so that labeled cholesterol would be expected to label intracellular cholesterol by exchange, if not by net uptake (6). Second, homogenate of seminiferous tubules incubated with [^{3}H]cholesterol does not produce detectable [^{3}H]pregnenolone or [^{3}H]androgens (7). On the one hand, it is never possible to say that there has been *no* conversion of one substance to another—only less than the minimal amount detected by the methods used. On the other hand, it is always difficult to exclude some contamination of seminiferous tubules by Leydig cells, and vice versa.

The problem is best considered functionally. There is no evidence that the seminiferous tubules can make a physiologically detectable contribution to androgen production, and there is no evidence that the seminiferous tubules can maintain spermatogenesis by their own production of androgens.

In addition to the secretion of androgens, the testis also produces small amounts of estrogens (3,8). Indirect evidence points to the Leydig cell as the source of such estrogens (9,10), although the Sertoli cell also contributes (3,11,12). It should be added that an important part of plasma estrogen in the male comes from extratesticular conversion of nonestrogenic steroids (13).

SYNTHESIS OF ANDROGENS BY LEYDIG CELLS

The synthesis of steroid hormones requires a substrate—that is, a source of the steroid ring system, a series of enzymes and cofactors that together constitute the biosynthetic pathway and a source of energy.

The Substrate

The immediate source of the steroid ring system used for the synthesis of steroid hormones consists of depots of cholesterol in the cytoplasm (14). Stores of cholesterol are to be seen in Leydig cells of various species in the form of conspicuous lipid droplets in the cytoplasm (15). Much work has been performed to determine whether this cholesterol is made in Leydig cells or brought from plasma in lipoproteins. It is clear that both sources are used (7,16). To determine the relative importance of these two sources of cholesterol, Chaikoff and co-workers studied the equilibration of plasma [^{14}C]cholesterol with testicular cholesterol and testosterone (17,18). They found that plasma cholesterol contributes no more than 13% to the total production of androgens in the guinea pig (17) and 40% in rat (18). Evidently the testis makes an important contribution to the steroidogenic cholesterol. When slices of testis are incubated *in vitro* with [^{14}C]acetate, the label is readily incorporated into testosterone in rabbit (19) but not demonstrably in rat (20). Unfortunately, the testis is complex in structure, and Leydig cells constitute no more than a small part of the organ. This limits the experimental approaches that can be used to answer such questions. Cultured Leydig cells offer a useful system for such studies. Clearly, the contribution of plasma cholesterol varies from species to species and is different in the adrenal (21). Future studies must evaluate each system individually. The relevant methods are now available (21), and, in the meantime, it must be concluded that steroidogenic cholesterol comes both from plasma and from local production in the Leydig cell.

The contribution of plasma cholesterol to the synthesis of steroid hormones comes from lipoproteins. Leydig tumor cells (MA-10) use low-density lipoprotein (LDL) as a source of steroidogenic cholesterol (22). The so-called classical pathway from LDL receptor to lysosomes, to cholesterol depots, is employed in these (22), as in other cells that import LDL from plasma (6). During stimulation by human chorionic gonadotropin (hCG), more than half of the steroidogenic cholesterol comes from LDL, and cholesterol stores are depleted within 4 hr (22). The pathway in these cells is unusual in that cholesterol from LDL does not inhibit the synthesis of cholesterol from acetate (6,22). On the other hand, rat testis has been shown to possess specific receptors for high-density lipoprotein (HDL) (23), so this form of lipoprotein may be important as a source of cholesterol for steroid synthesis as in rat adrenal (24).

The lipid droplets of Leydig cells are depleted during times of increased synthesis of androgens (15), in keeping with the well-accepted idea that the stored cholesterol is used for the synthesis of these hormones. The testis possesses a cholesterol ester hydrolase that is stimulated by hCG (25). Presumably, this enzyme serves to mobilize cholesterol for steroid synthesis as in the adrenal (26). From there on, no details are known concerning the steroid synthetic pathway in Leydig cells until cholesterol appears in the inner mitochondrial membrane, where the pathway continues with the conversion of cholesterol to pregnenolone. The adrenal cortex has been studied more intensely in this respect. Here, the cholesterol from LDL is reesterified for storage, and when cholesterol ester hydrolase releases free cholesterol, this substrate binds to sterol carrier protein (SCP_2), which accompanies it to mitochondria (21). This, or another protein, takes the cholesterol to the inner mitochondrial membrane (21,27). It is also clear that reesterificatiron of cholesterol for storage involves different fatty acids from those esterified to the cholesterol of LDL (21). Only future studies will reveal how closely the handling of cholesterol in Leydig cells resembles that in the adrenal. It seems reasonable to proceed with this discussion on the assumption that the two cells handle steroidogenic cholesterol in essentially the same way, provided the extent of this assumption is not overlooked.

The Pathway

The synthesis of androgens involves the conversion of cholesterol to testosterone, as illustrated below:

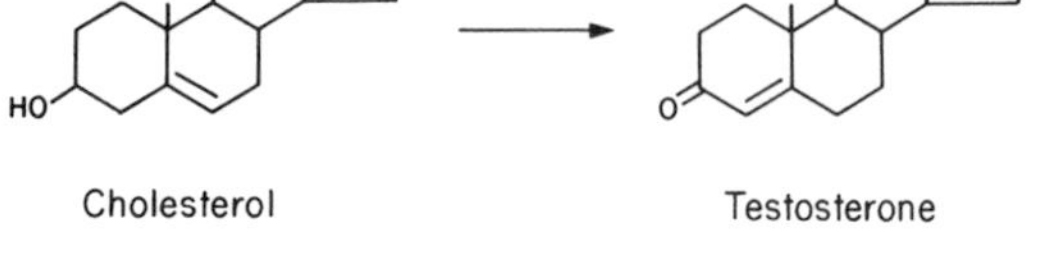

HO — Cholesterol → Testosterone — OH, O

The enzymatic reactions required for this conversion are as listed in Table 1.

TABLE 1. *Enzymatic reactions required for the conversion of cholesterol to testosterone*

Activity	C atom
Hydroxylation	17,20,22
Dehydrogenation	3β,17β
Isomerization	$\Delta^{4,5}$
C-C cleavage (lyase)	20,22 and 17,20

Hydroxylation and lyase activities require cytochromes P-450 (28). Dehydrogenation requires typical pyridine nucleotide dehydrogenases, and an isomerase moves the double bond to the more stable α,β-unsaturated ketone (16).

The pathway begins with the conversion of cholesterol to pregnenolone (C_{27} side-chain cleavage) which takes place in mitochondria. Pregnenolone is converted to testosterone by microsomal enzymes. Before discussing the individual enzymes involved, we must consider the general properties of cytochromes P-450, since two of these enzymes catalyze key reactions in the pathway to androgens—i.e., C_{27} side-chain cleavage (29) and C_{21} side-chain cleavage (30).

Cytochromes P-450

This remarkable family of enzymes is widely distributed in nature, where they are best known as enzymes for the disposal of lipophilic substrates by rendering these substances more soluble in water as the result of hydroxylation. The prototype for reactions catalyzed by these enzymes in the presence of $^{18}O_2$ can be summarized as follows (31):

$$\text{R—H} + \text{NADPH} + \text{H}^+ + {}^{18}\text{O}_2 \xrightarrow{[\text{P-450}]} \text{R-}{}^{18}\text{OH} + \text{H}_2{}^{18}\text{O} + \text{NADP}^+$$

This statement of the reaction indicates a number of important features of hydroxylation of substrates (RH) catalyzed by these enzymes. The enzyme uses atmospheric or molecular oxygen, one atom of which is attached to the substrate in a hydroxyl group, and the second is reduced to water. This type of oxidation is referred to as monooxygenation, since only one atom of oxygen appears in the product. The hydroxyl group in the product replaces a hydrogen atom in the substrate, so the product is more soluble in water than the substrate. This change facilitates the removal of the product from the body, because the more soluble product can be filtered by the kidney and because it is less able to dissolve in cell membranes to enter cells than the more lipophilic substrate. This mechanism provides a major defense against xenobiotics and drugs that are frequently lipophilic (32). In addition, the body uses this mechanism to remove such lipophilic substances as steroids and prostaglandins that are no longer required by the body; these substances are referred to as endogenous substrates to distinguish them from xenobiotics (exogenous substrates) (33). The reactions to be considered here fall into another category in which the changes produced in the substrate provide those features of the steroid hormones that are recognized by receptors and other intracellular molecules and which therefore enable the steroids to act as hormones.

The equation also shows the characteristic stoichiometry of monooxygenation—i.e., NADPH:O_2:RH of 1:1:1 (31,34). The above statement does not show the electron carriers used to convey electrons from reduced pyridine nucleotide to P-450. Microsomal cytochromes P-450 use a single flavoprotein reductase to discharge this function (35), whereas mitochondrial P-450 uses two carriers—a flavoprotein reductase and an iron-sulfur protein (36). The iron-sulfur proteins are referred to by the suffix "-oxin," e.g., adrenodoxin for the adrenal protein, and presumably testodoxin will be used for the testicular enzyme, which has not been studied in detail. The reductase proteins are referred to as adrenodoxin reductase, etc. It will be pointed out that the steroidogenic cytochromes P-450 are capable of reactions other than simple hydroxylation—e.g., cleavage of C–C bonds.

Cytochromes P-450 are heme proteins—each molecule of protein contains a heme moiety that is not covalently bound to the protein but that lies in a hydrophobic crevice. It turns out that all cytochromes P-450 show a number of important structural features, so it is useful to discuss this group of enzymes as a whole. The iron of the heme has the potential to engage in six bonds of which four are, of necessity, made to the four pyrrole nitrogens of the heme, and in P-450 one is to a cysteine in the protein. The four bonds with nitrogen lie in the plane of the pyrrole ring system, and the fifth and sixth bonds are at right angles to this plane and are thus called axial. The fifth bond takes the form of a thiolate bond with the sulfur of cysteine (37,38). The nature of the sixth ligand is uncertain. Finally, it should be pointed out that the iron may be hexacoordinate or pentacoordinate (6 or 5 bonds). The pentacoordinate iron is displaced from the plane of the ring, and the electrons of the d orbital of the iron are so arranged as to give the so-called high-spin form of this atom in contrast to the low-spin hexacoordinate form in which the iron lies in the plane of the heme ring system.

The conjugated double-bond system of heme gives rise to a striking property on absorption spectroscopy, namely a conspicuous peak at approximately 420 nm—the so-called Soret peak. The intensity and position of the Soret peak are influenced by the protein moiety of heme proteins. In the absence of bound substrate the heme moiety has a low-spin, hexacoordinate iron with a Soret peak in the vicinity of 420 nm. When substrate binds to P-450, the accompanying conformational change results in the formation of pentacoordinate high-spin iron displaced from the plane of the heme ring system. These changes are accompanied by a shift in the Soret peak to approximately 390 nm—the so-called substrate-induced spectral shift:

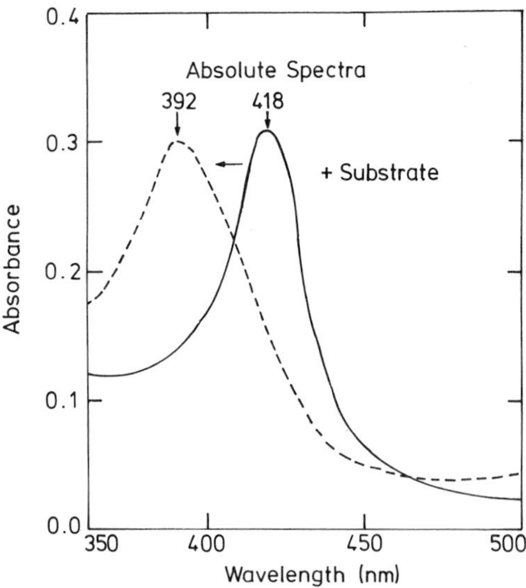

This shift is of great practical significance, because it can be measured by difference—i.e., substrate-induced difference spectroscopy. The spectrophotometer is set to subtract the absorbance of enzyme plus solvent (reference cuvette) from that of enzyme plus substrate (sample cuvette). The high-spin form (ES) gives a positive peak at 390 nm, and the low-spin form (no substrate) gives a negative peak, or trough, at 420 nm, because the absorbance in the reference cuvette is subtracted from that in the sample cuvette. The peak plus trough (A 390–420 nm) is proportional to the amount of enzyme present in the form ES, as illustrated below:

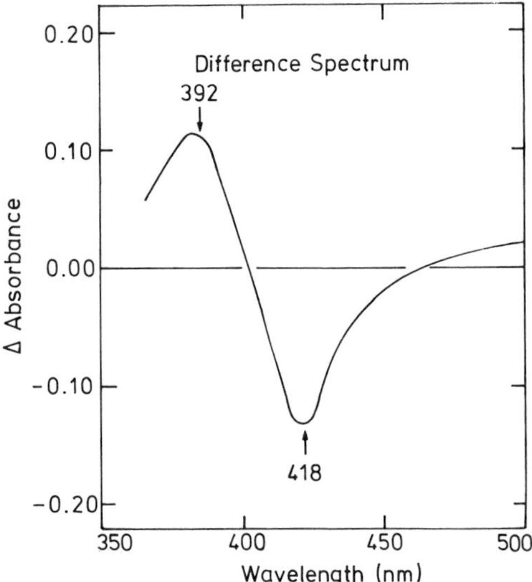

This provides a simple, rapid, direct, and nondestructive method of measuring binding as a function of substrate concentration. This difference spectrum (peak at 390 nm and trough at 420 nm) is referred to as a type I spectrum.

In the low-spin form of iron, all the *d* orbital electrons are of low-energy form called t_{2g}, and there is one unpaired electron. In short-hand nomenclature, this is referred to as 1/2. In the high-spin form of iron, all five electrons of the *d* orbitals are unpaired, and two have the high-energy form, eg. In short-hand nomenclature, this is referred to as 5/2. These spectral properties of P-450 are summarized in Table 2 (37–39).

TABLE 2. *Spectral properties of P - 450*

		Ferric iron		
Substrate	Coordination valence	Spin state	*d* Electrons	Soret band (nm)
Absent	6	low	1/2	420
Bound	5	high	5/2	390

We must consider one further spectral property which is also of practical importance since it is used to identify and measure all cytochromes P-450. Reduced heme proteins bind CO as the sixth ligand, and this shifts the Soret peak. The oxidized form does not bind CO. In most cases, the shift amounts to no more than a few nanometers. With P-450, the shift is unusually extensive (420–450 nm). The spectrum can be examined by difference: reduced P-450-CO minus oxidized P-450 plus CO (40). In addition to giving P-450 its name (pigment 450), this spectral property provides an accurate method for measuring P-450:

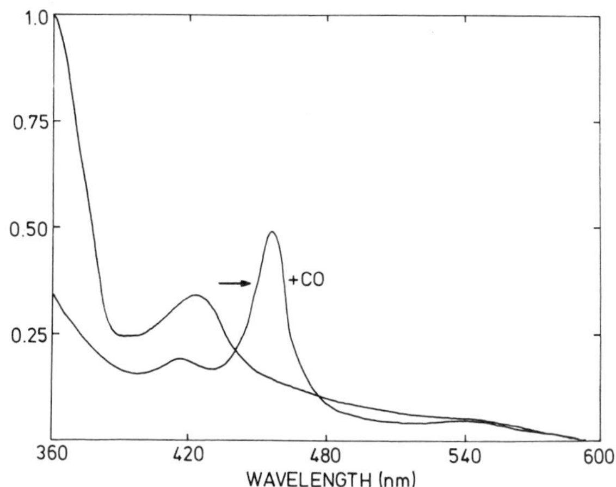

An important feature of all cytochromes P-450 is the so-called P-450 cycle by which the enzyme becomes reduced so that it can carry out its allotted function. The reduced (Fe^{2+}) enzyme must be reoxidized in readiness for the next cycle.

Since P-450 is reduced to the ferrous form by electrons from NADPH and reoxidized during catalytic activity, the enzyme must undergo cycles of oxidation and reduction. For descriptive purposes each cycle can be considered in five steps, although the steps flow rapidly into one another, and the last step is itself made up of several steps (37,38,41).

Step 1. Binding of substrate.

$$Fe^{3+} + RH \rightarrow Fe^{3+} - RH$$

where P-450 is represented by Fe. This step has two important consequences. First, it is associated with a conformational change which displaces the iron from the plane of the ring and produces the high-spin form of heme iron with a type I spectral shift. Second, binding of substrate promotes the passage of one electron (the so-called first electron) from adrenodoxin to the enzyme substrate complex.

Step 2. Reduction of the enzyme-substrate complex by the first electron.

$$Fe^{3+} - RH + e \rightarrow Fe^{2+} - RH$$

Step 3. Binding of oxygen. The reduced enzyme-substrate complex binds oxygen.

$$Fe^{2+} - RH + O_2 \rightarrow \begin{array}{c} Fe^{2+} - RH \\ | \\ O_2 \end{array}$$

Step 4. Activation of bound oxygen by second electron. The second electron activates oxygen bound to iron as the result of rearrangement of electrons.

$$\begin{array}{c} Fe^{2+} - RH \\ | \\ O_2 \end{array} + e + H^+ \rightarrow \begin{array}{c} Fe^{3+} - RH \\ | \\ O_2^{2-} \end{array} + OH^-$$

Step 5. Hydroxylation of substrate. This complex step results in the formation of the hydroxylated product.

$$\begin{array}{c} Fe^{3+} - RH \\ | \\ O_2^{2-} \end{array} \rightarrow Fe^{3+} + ROH$$

The hydroxyl group of the product produces repulsive forces at the hydrophobic active site of the enzyme, which facilitates removal of the product. The enzyme is now ready to start the cycle again. The cycle can be summarized as follows:

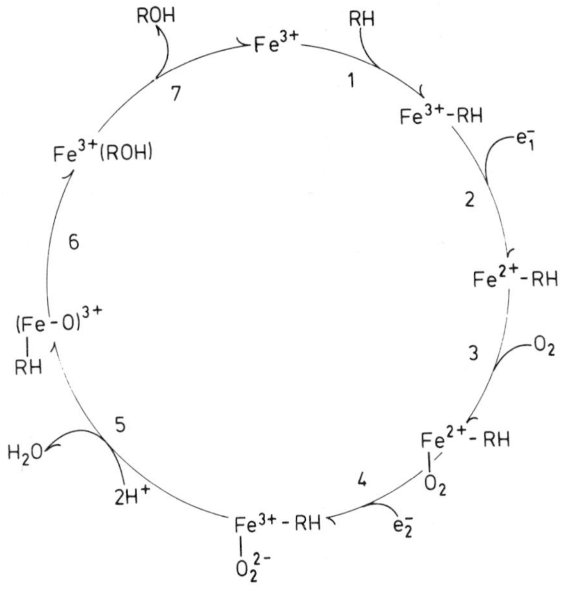

We can now consider the individual enzymes of the steroidogenic pathway beginning with the cytochromes P-450.

C_{27} Side-Chain Cleavage

The conversion of cholesterol to pregnenolone is catalyzed by a mitochondrial cytochrome P-450 in three steps:

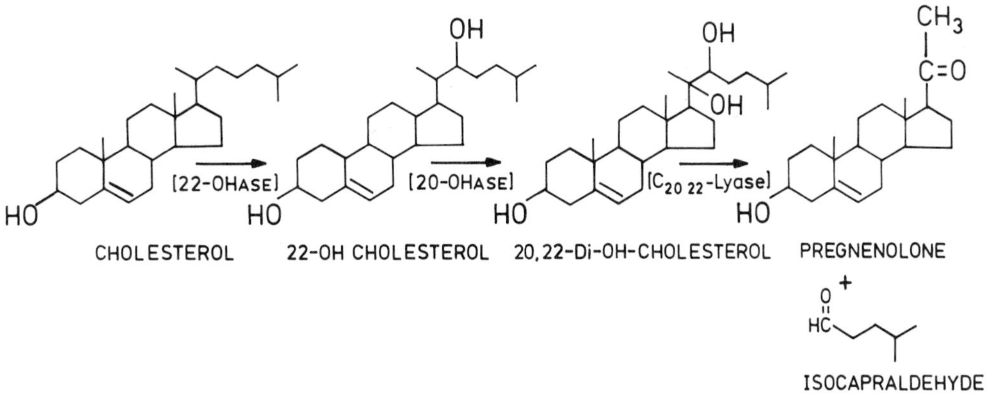

The classical hydroxylase activity of P-450 is used in the first two steps and the intervening C–C bond is cleaved to give two oxygenated products. This enzyme was the first cytochrome P-450 to be purified. It was isolated from mitochondria of bovine adrenal cortex using conventional chromatographic procedures (29,42,43). A variety of other methods have been used subsequently (44–47). Since the enzyme was shown to be homogeneous by gel electrophoresis and by double diffusion with an antibody raised against the pure enzyme showing the line of identity and by immunoelectrophoresis (29,43), we must conclude that all three steps in the above reaction are catalyzed by a single protein. The enzyme shows a single NH_2 terminal amino acid (namely glutamate) (43). Moreover, when the substrate used is [^{14}C]cholesterol, virtually all the disappearing cholesterol can be accounted for as [^{14}C]pregnenolone plus unused substrate (48,49). The existence of the two intermediates was demonstrated first by showing that the intermediates are rapidly converted to pregnenolone and later by the work of Burstein and Gut in which the kinetics of the conversion were studied using large-scale preparations of a crude enzyme system (50).

The next question to be raised was whether there is more than one active site on the enzyme. Kinetic and binding studies by Duque et al. (51) are consistent with a single binding site. Since the cleavage of a C–C bond is unusual for cytochrome P-450, it was important to demonstrate that the heme moiety of P-450 is involved in the last step of the conversion. This was accomplished by means of a photochemical action spectrum, which showed that CO inhibits the conversion of the dihydroxycholesterol to pregnenolone and that this inhibition is specifically reversed by light of wavelength 450 nm (52). This finding unequivocally established the involvement of the heme moiety in a classical P-450-catalyzed reaction. This conclusion was supported by measurement of the stoichiometry of the overall reaction and that of the individual steps. The overall reaction shows the following stoichiometry (53):

$$C_{27}H_{46}O + 3O_2 + 3\ NADPH + 3H^+ \rightarrow C_{21}H_{32}O_2 + C_6H_{12}O + 4H_2O$$

The stoichiometry of each step was found to be that of monooxygenation—i.e., 1 NADPH + 1 H^+ + 1 O_2 + 1 mole of substrate (31,53).

Evidently, the cleavage of the C_{21}–C_{22} bond involves a typical monooxygenation using the heme group of P-450. This finding established, for the first time, such C–C cleavage as a reaction catalyzed by P-450. A detailed study of the binding of substrate, intermediates, and product to the pure enzyme using electron spin resonance and absorption spectroscopy revealed a single binding site for each of these steroids (54). The values for the respective dissociation constants are as follows:

Steroid	Kd (nM)
22R-cholesterol	4.9
20R,22R-diOH cholesterol	81
Pregnenolone	2900

Moreover, 22R-OH cholesterol shows a dissociation frequency of $5S^{-1}$. It is therefore apparent that the two intermediates are tightly bound and that the product dissociates readily. It is also clear why the intermediates are so difficult to isolate: they are tightly bound to the enzyme, and one intermediate is rapidly converted to the next. The intermediates are therefore only present bound to the enzyme; i.e., virtually no free intermediates exist. It was for this reason that Burstein and Gut were forced to use large amounts of enzyme to recover measurable amounts of intermediates (50).

Evidently, the catalytic cycle of P-450 is modified for side-chain cleavage in such a way that a second cycle begins with the product of the first cycle still at the active site, and the same is true for the third cycle. When the third cycle is complete, the product (pregnenolone) dissociates from the active site, and the whole process starts again with the binding of cholesterol.

It should be pointed out that when pregnenolone is added to the pure C_{27} side-chain cleavage P-450, a spectral shift occurs that is the inverse of the usual shift produced by substrates—i.e., peak at 420 and trough at 390 nm, instead of vice versa (55). This shift (called inverse type I) results from the binding of pregnenolone to a site that differs from the active site (54–56). This binding is responsible for inhibition of the side-chain cleavage of cholesterol by pregnenolone (48).

In aqueous media, the C_{27} side-chain cleavage enzyme associates into oligomeric forms—tetramers, octomers, and hexadecamers (42). When the enzyme was centrifuged through buffered sucrose containing adrenodoxin, adrenodoxin reductase, cholesterol, and NADPH, it was found that only the hexadecamer form (16 subunits, MW 850,000) is enzymatically active (57). The nature of the active form in the inner mitochondrial membrane is unknown.

C_{21} Side-Chain Cleavage

The conversion of C_{21} steroids to C_{19} steroids proceeds in two steps—17α-hydroxylation and $C_{17,20}$-lyase:

PROGESTERONE → [17α-OHASE] → 17α-OH PROGESTERONE → [$C_{17,20}$-Lyase] → ANDROSTENEDIONE

In view of the mechanism of C_{27} side-chain cleavage just described, it might have been predicted that a single cytochrome P-450 is responsible for catalyzing both reactions. However, because the adrenal cortex synthesizes the 17α-hydroxy-C_{21}-steroid cortisol, it seemed clear that 17α-hydroxylation can proceed without $C_{17,20}$-lyase activity. This pointed to two separate enzymes, and some indirect evidence seemed to support this view (58).

However, when the testicular enzyme was purified to homogeneity, it was found that one enzyme catalyzes both reactions (59,60). The enzyme is microsomal, but otherwise it resembles the C_{27} side-chain cleavage enzyme to such an extent that they have been mistaken during purification (61). Evidence for homogeneity of the enzyme rests on gel electrophoresis, double diffusion, and immunoelectrophoresis with antibodies raised against the pure enzyme and extensive sequence determination with only one amino acid at each position in the molecule (59,60). Incidentally, the difference between the testicular adrenal enzymes provide a most unexpected result. The two enzymes are very similar (not quite identical) in almost every way (62,63). Binding and kinetic constants for the substrates are almost the same for both enzymes. The difference must lie in the microsomes, because in adrenal microsomes very little lyase activity is seen, yet the pure enzyme shows the same lyase activity as the pure testicular enzyme (62). This provides an intriguing example of microsomal regulation. One factor that promotes lyase activity is P-450 reductase, which is present in greater concentration in the microsomes of testis than in those of adrenal (64). In addition, cytochrome b_5 increases activity of lyase relative to hydroxylase (65), and testicular microsomes contain more cytochrome b_5 per milligram of protein than adrenal microsomes (64). However, there may be additional factors involved in microsomal regulation.

The next question to arise was whether there is one active site or two to catalyze the two steps in C_{21} side-chain cleavage. Studies with inhibition by antibody to the pure enzyme and competitive inhibition by two synthetic inhibitors, together with substrate-induced difference spectra and equilibrium dialysis, all support the idea of a single active site (59,60,66,67). An additional line of evidence proved important in support of the concept of a single active site. The enzyme was subjected to affinity alkylation by 17α-bromoacetoxyprogesterone. This substrate analogue binds covalently to a specific cysteine residue:

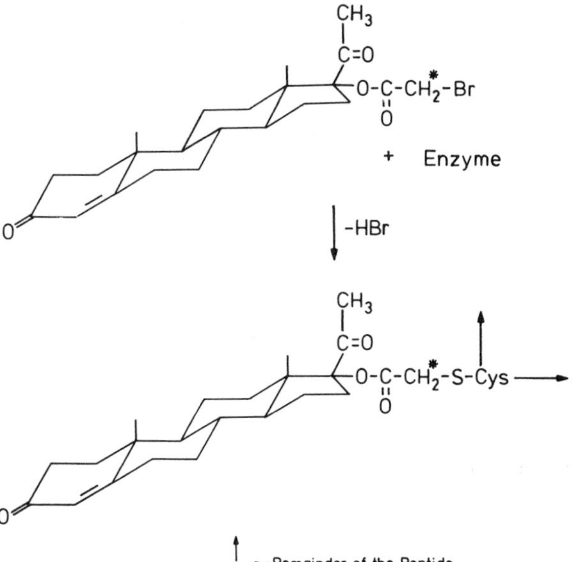

The process of affinity alkylation inactivates the enzyme. Inactivation proceeds by a first-order process that shows the same value for $t_{1/2}$ for both enzyme activities (hydroxylase and lyase) (67). Moreover, both substrates (progesterone and 17α-hydroxyprogesterone) protect both activities against inactivation (67). In other words, the substrate analogue and both substrates compete for a single active site (67).

The concept of one active site was confirmed by two additional observations. First, the $C_{17,20}$-lyase activity was shown to involve the heme moiety of the enzyme in a typical P-450-catalyzed reaction (68). Second, there is one heme group per peptide moiety. If heme is required for both reactions, it means that there is one active site or two overlapping sites both of which include the heme moiety.

Evidently, these two systems for C–C cleavage (C_{27} and C_{21}) use similar mechanisms. However, two important differences are seen between these enzymes: namely, the C_{27} system is mitochondrial whereas the C_{21} system is microsomal, and the C_{27} system requires three steps whereas the C_{21} substrate is already oxygenated at C_{20}, so only two steps are necessary.

Dehydrogenase-Isomerase

The A and B rings of pregnenolone are converted to the Δ^4-3-keto structure by a microsomal enzyme system that has not been purified to homogeneity:

PREGNENOLONE → PROGESTERONE

It remains uncertain whether both activities reside in a single enzyme or whether there are two enzymes. Partial purification failed to separate two enzymes (69). On the other hand, the organism *Pseudomonas testosteroni* has two separate enzymes, dehydrogenase and isomerase, each without the other activity (70,71). Only further purification will resolve this question. It has also been proposed that there are two enzyme systems—one for C_{21} substrates and one for C_{19} substrates. This view has been supported by recent work with acetylenic ketosteroids as inhibitors (72). Again, this problem must be resolved by purification.

If a single protein is shown to catalyze both reactions, more than one active site would seem likely, because the two reactions are so different: one is a typical pyridine nucleotide-linked dehydrogenase, and the other involves the rearrangement of a double bond. It should be pointed out, however, that whether there is one enzyme or two, no intermediate (i.e., no Δ^5-3-ketosteroid) has been detected when testicular microsomes are incubated with progesterone (73).

17β-Hydroxysteroid Dehydrogenase

The microsomal enzyme 17_{β}-hydroxysteroid dehydrogenase catalyzes the interconversion of androstenedione and testosterone with the aid of NAD^+:

Androstenedione [17β-OHSD] ⇌ Testosterone

OHSD: HYDROXYSTEROID DEHYDROGENASE

It is generally believed that the activity of this enzyme is not rate-limiting for the synthesis of testosterone (73). The enzyme shows the unusual property of product activation; i.e., testosterone promotes the formation of testosterone from androstenedione, and androstenedione does the same from testosterone (74). The reaction catalyzed is freely reversible, and the enzyme possesses two active sites (74,75). These remarkable properties suggest that the activity of the enzyme may be greatly influenced by the available concentrations of the two substrates and by the rate of removal of the products of the reaction. Special methods may be required to understand the regulation of this enzyme *in vivo*. The activity of the enzyme in the microsome is greatly decreased by the action of phospholipase C, indicating a stabilizing action of lipids on the enzyme (75,76). In addition, there appears to be a ketoreductase distinct from the dehydrogenase (76) and a separate enzyme within the seminiferous tubule—i.e., apart from that in Leydig cells (77). The details of this complex enzyme have been reviewed recently (78).

The Energy

Reactions catalyzed by cytochromes P-450 use NADPH. Energy is also presumably required for movement of substrate and intermediates through the cell, but the nature of these processes is not sufficiently understood to describe the sources of the energy required.

Organization of the Steroidogenic Pathway in the Cell

In discussing the performance of this pathway in the cell, it is important to consider the relationship between the mitochondrial and microsomal compartments, which is illustrated as follows:

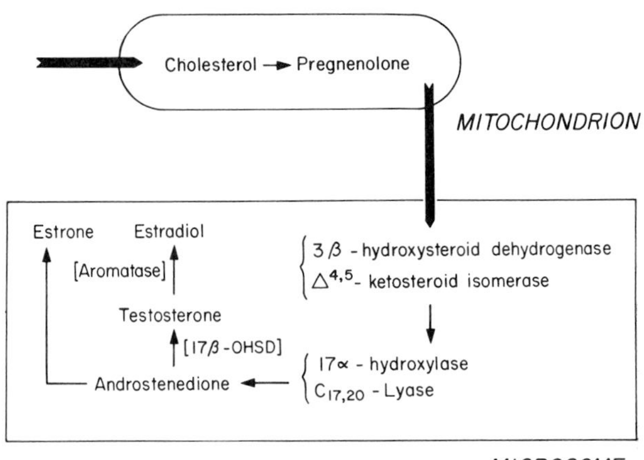

OHSD: hydroxysteroid dehydrogenase

It is clear that the pathway begins in the mitochondrion and that pregnenolone is transferred to microsomes to complete the synthesis of androgens.

Steroidogenic Inner Mitochondrial Membrane

The side-chain cleavage enzyme system is found only in the inner mitochondrial membrane, and immunoelectron microscopy with colloidal gold (79) showed that, at least in the adrenal cortex, all mitochondria contain the enzyme, and within each organelle the distribution is random (80). To study the enzyme in an environment that more closely resembles the mitochondrial membrane, it was incorporated into lipid vesicles prepared from an equal mixture of phosphatidylcholine and phosphatidylethanolamine with and without cholesterol (81). The entire side-chain cleavage system (adrenodoxin reductase, adrenodoxin, and P-450) can be incorporated into lipid vesicles so that on addition of NADPH, production of pregnenolone occurs. The enzyme is converted to the high-spin form and shows a great reduction in K_m for cholesterol (81).

The reconstituted side-chain cleavage system in lipid vesicles was studied in greater detail by Seybert et al. (82,83). These workers showed that P-450 in one vesicle does not use cholesterol incorporated into a different vesicle and that the binding site on P-450 for cholesterol is associated with the hydrophobic region of the bilayer, whereas the binding site on P-450 for adrenodoxin is on the surface of the vesicle facing the external water phase (82,83). The same group went on to show that adrenodoxin shuttles between the reductase and P-450 as follows. Oxidized adrenodoxin binds to reduced reductase, and, after transfer of one electron, the reduced adrenodoxin shows low affinity for the oxidized reductase and now binds to P-450. The binding of adrenodoxin to P-450 is promoted by the binding of substrate (cholesterol) to the P-450 (84,85). Adrenodoxin and P-450 are present in approximately equimolar amounts in the inner mitochondrial membrane, and reductase is present at a lower concentration (86).

As a result of the dissociation and reassociation of adrenodoxin and reductase, one molecule of reductase can serve numerous molecules of adrenodoxin and, hence, P-450 (84,85). Presumably, this mechanism explains the ability of the system to function *in vivo* with a low concentration of reductase. It is not clear at present whether this adrenodoxin shuttle regulates the rate of side-chain cleavage *in vivo*.

Steroidogenic Endoplasmic Reticulum

Less work has been performed with the organization of the endoplasmic reticulum than with the inner mitochondrial membrane. However, the homogeneous enzymes are available, and the same methods can be used. We can consider three problems associated with the microsomal system that have been investigated experimentally:

Sequence of Reactions

Since the product of C_{21} side-chain cleavage is androstenedione, the 17β-hydroxysteroid dehydrogenase must catalyze the last reaction in the pathway. If we consider the conversion of pregnenolone to androstenedione, and if we keep in mind that C_{21} side-chain cleavage is catalyzed by a single enzyme and that the dehydrogenase-isomerase acts as a single enzyme, we can see that there are two possible pathways for this conversion, depending on which enzyme acts first:

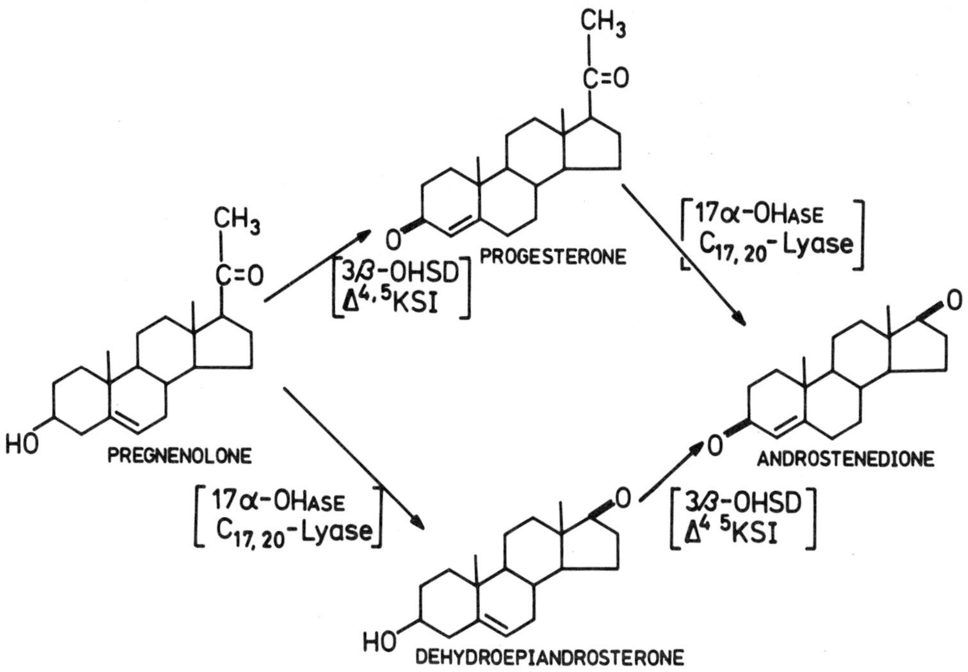

PROGESTERONE
PREGNENOLONE
ANDROSTENEDIONE
DEHYDROEPIANDROSTERONE
3β-OHSD $\Delta^{4,5}$KSI
17α-OHASE $C_{17,20}$-Lyase

The "upper" pathway is referred to as the progesterone, or Δ^4, pathway, in contrast to the "lower pathway," referred to as the Δ^5, or dehydroepiandrosterone, pathway. The choice of pathways is not random. For example, the rat uses the Δ^4 pathway largely if not exclusively (73). Pig (87), rabbit, and dog (88) use the Δ^5 pathway to varying degrees. In theory, regulation of the choice of pathway could arise either as the result of the properties of the enzymes or by their arrangement with the membrane. If, for example, the C_{21} side-chain cleavage enzyme has a higher affinity for pregnenolone than for progesterone, the Δ^5 pathway would prevail.

Similar considerations apply to the dehydrogenase-isomerase. The only evidence we have at present is consistent with that view, because the porcine C_{21} side-chain cleavage enzyme shows a considerably higher affinity for pregnenolone and 17α-hydroxypregnenolone than for the corresponding Δ^4 compounds (66). This affinity may help to explain the fact that, in pig testis, the Δ^5 pathway is extensively used (87). Clearly, much more information is needed before we can conclude that the sum of the properties of the individual enzymes accounts for the properties of the endoplasmic reticulum.

The alternative possibility is that the enzymes are arranged in a specific order and that pregnenolone enters the microsome at certain preferred points—entry ports established by the presence (for example) of a pregnenolone-binding protein. Preliminary evidence suggests that such a protein exists (28). The location of the binding protein relative to the two steroidogenic enzymes could influence the sequence of the reactions involved in the conversion of pregnenolone to androstenedione. There is no evidence for this concept, but recent advances in immunoelectron microscopy (79) and methods for chemical cross-linking of membrane proteins (89–91) make it possible to approach this question.

Location of Enzymes in the Lipid Bilayer

The endoplasmic reticulum *in situ* shows an external or cytoplasmic surface and an internal surface. When cells are disrupted by homogenization, fragments of endoplasmic reticulum form vesicles that are called right side out if the cytoplasmic surface remains outside and inside out if not. Membrane proteins may be associated with the bilayer by powerful hydrophobic forces which result in location of the protein deeply buried in the interior of the bilayer or by a mixture of hydrophobic and hydrophilic forces, in which case the proteins are predominantly on one or the other side of the membrane. Proteins may also be associated loosely with the surface of the membrane by hydrophilic forces; such proteins are, to a greater or lesser degree, removed during washing of the microsomes.

Since many enzymes cannot penetrate the bilayer, proteolytic enzymes and phospholipases can be used to determine whether the proteins in the membrane are accessible to these enzymes. Proteolytic enzymes can be used to demonstrate that a protein can be attacked from one surface or another, or whether it is buried in the bilayer and, hence, inaccessible to water-soluble proteolytic enzymes. Phospholipases can be used to show whether the enzyme in the microsomal membrane requires phospholipids for activity. It is then important to know whether the vesicles are right side out or not in order to relate these findings to the situation in the cell. This is usually easy, with rough endoplasmic reticulum, because ribosomes bind to the cytoplasmic surface of the membrane. It is generally assumed that the vesicles routinely produced from smooth endoplasmic reticulum are right side out, but this should be confirmed for each organ. It is likely that such questions will be successfully approached by immunoelectron microscopy, using second antibodies conjugated to gold particles (79).

Phospholipases A and C and trypsin were found by Samuels et al. to exert the following effects on testicular microsomes (75):

	Pregnenolone binding	3β-OHSD	Hydroxylase/ lyase activity
Phospholipase	↓	↓↓↓	No change
Trypsin	↓↓↓	↓↓↓	↓↓↓

Since it has been shown that, in hepatic microsomes, cytochrome P-450 is on the inside of microsomes (92), these results were taken to mean that hydroxylase/lyase activity is inhibited because the reductase is located on the outside of the microsome and trypsin inhibits the activity of P-450 by interfering with electron transport rather than by acting on P-450 itself. The activity of the dehydrogenase-isomerase apparently depends on the presence of phospholipid. Pregnenolone binding depends on a protein that faces the external (cytoplasmic) surface of the ribosome (75).

These findings should be considered in the light of earlier observations by Samuels which showed that microsomal P-450 acts on intramembrane steroid substrate, whereas the dehydrogenase-isomerase acts on substrate from the surrounding water phase (75). These observations can be summarized in diagrammatic form as follows:

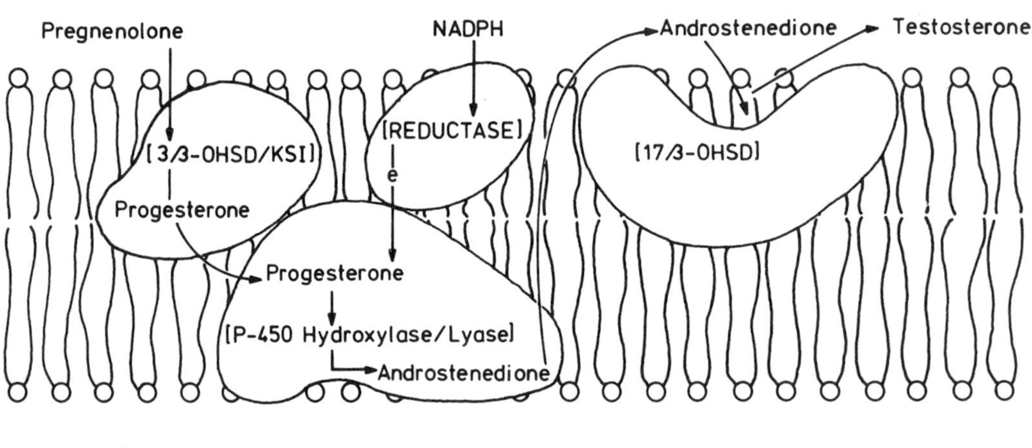

The diagram presents a schematic illustration of the findings of Samuels and colleagues (75). No doubt it will require repeated revision as more information becomes available.

Samuels et al. also showed that when testicular microsomes are incubated with [^{3}H]progesterone and 17α-hydroxy-[^{14}C]progesterone, the resulting androstenedione shows a higher ratio of [^{3}H]:[^{14}C] than the original mixture of substrates (93,94). This suggested that the access of progesterone to the active site of the hydroxylase/lyase is greater than that of 17α-hydroxyprogesterone. These workers also showed that the partition ratio of progesterone from water to microsomes was greater than that of the 17α-hydroxysteroid (93,94). We now know that the two steroids show the same affinity for the single active site on C_{21} side-chain cleavage P-450 (60,66) and that 17α-hydroxyprogesterone in the water phase exchanges freely with 17α-hydroxyprogesterone generated by the enzyme from progesterone (95).

It would seem, therefore, that the difference between the

two substrates lies in their respective rates of entry into the lipid bilayer. This presents us with a problem. We would expect progesterone to be formed from pregnenolone in the lipid bilayer. There would seem to be no reason for progesterone to leave the membrane only to return. Moreover, it was pointed out above that the hydroxylase/lyase allows immediate exchange between the intermediate 17α-hydroxyprogesterone generated by the enzyme and exogenous 17α-hydroxyprogesterone added to the surrounding water phase (95). We clearly cannot interpret these findings without more information. There may be proteins in the microsome that influence the affinity of the substrate for the hydroxylase/lyase. Although these studies have exposed rather than resolved these problems, such approaches provide our first insight into the organization of the steroidogenic microsome.

Influence of the Microsomal Environment

A comparison between the 17α-hydroxylase of adrenal microsomes and the hydroxylase/lyase of testicular microsomes proves instructive. As mentioned above, when progesterone is incubated with adrenal microsomes, only products of 17α-hydroxylation are found; no C_{19} steroids are isolated (62). On the other hand, testicular microsomes produce a mixture of steroids in which C_{19} steroids predominate (96). However, when the two enzymes are purified, they are indistinguishable, and both produce large amounts of C_{19} steroids (62,63). Clearly, the microsomal environment influences the behavior of the adrenal enzyme. Since the two enzymes behave in the same way when they are incorporated in liposomes prepared from lipids extracted from either adrenal or testicular microsomes, the difference cannot be attributed to the microsomal lipids (64). Testicular microsomes contain four times as much reductase relative to P-450 as adrenal microsomes, and addition of exogenous reductase to adrenal microsomes increases lyase activity (64). In addition, it was observed that cytochrome b_5 increases lyase activity relative to hydroxylase in both adrenal and testicular microsomes (64,65). Although it is generally believed that the rate of reduction of P-450 is not rate-limiting for the actions of cytochromes P-450, lyase is at a disadvantage relative to hydroxylase, because a second turn of the P-450 cycle (and therefore a second input from reductase) is required. Agents that facilitate reduction of P-450 may favor lyase activity (64).

Hepatic microsomes are known to contain much more P-450 than reductase (97). Attempts have been made to determine whether one molecule of reductase remains in a fixed cluster with many molecules of P-450 all served by the one molecule of reductase or whether P-450 can diffuse rapidly within the microsomal membrane so that each P-450 binds transiently to various reductase molecules in a random manner. Most available evidence concerning the mobility of proteins in membranes comes from studies with the more accessible plasma membrane in which proteins, even though restrained by attachment to the cytoskeleton, are sufficiently mobile to make the idea of a permanent cluster of molecules unthinkable (98). The concept has been extended, with less confidence, to mitochondrial membranes (99). If clusters of protein are possible in microsomal membranes, as the result of low mobility of proteins, these membranes must differ considerably from other cellular membranes. The relatively high content of protein in microsomal membranes would be a possible factor in accounting for such differences. Studies showing a break in the Arrhenius plots of microsomal membranes have been interpreted to favor the concept of a cluster of P-450 molecules associated with each molecule of reductase (100). On the other hand, spectroscopic studies suggest a high mobility of P-450 in microsomal membranes, so interaction with reductase may not require a long-lived complex (101). It has also been suggested that P-450 may not be active as a monomer but rather in the form of molecular aggregates (101). Similar studies need to be performed in the steroidogenic microsomes, where the number of molecules of P-450 is much closer to the number of molecules of reductase (unpublished).

REGULATION OF ANDROGEN SYNTHESIS BY LUTEINIZING HORMONE

In hypophysectomized animals, the synthesis of androgens by the testis proceeds at a greatly reduced rate (102). The pituitary owes its ability to stimulate the synthesis of androgens to the synthesis and secretion of LH. This hormone provides the most important physiological regulation of the production of androgens by the testes (1,103,104). Other regulatory agents will be discussed later.

Within recent years, it has become clear that most (perhaps all) cells use a limited number of molecular mechanisms all of which eventually involve proteins. When any cell responds to a stimulus, it does so by changing its proteins—either synthesizing new proteins, phosphorylating or otherwise modifying existing proteins, or both. Two messengers have been discovered to convert blood-borne stimuli into cellular responses, cyclic AMP and Ca^{2+}. These are the fundamental mechanisms used by cells to respond to various stimuli. The nature of the stimuli and the responses vary greatly from one cell type to another, but the underlying mechanisms are similar. These messengers, and the changes they produce in intracellular proteins, modify the functions of the various components of the cell which, in turn, provide the response to the original stimulus: the plasma membrane transduces stimuli and provides second messengers; the cytoskeleton organizes the compartments and surfaces of the cell, modifies its shape, and provides direction (i.e., vectors for movements inside the cell); the endoplasmic reticulum synthesizes proteins (rough) and steroids (smooth); the mitochondria provide energy; and the nucleus determines the nature and number of proteins synthesized by the cell.

With these mechanisms and these cellular components, LH stimulates the synthesis of testosterone by Leydig cells. We will now consider how this comes about. To do this, reference must be made to some studies that have been performed with ACTH and adrenal cells. It was pointed out above that studies with the adrenal cortex have proceeded more rapidly than those with the testis, largely for technical reasons. It is time that this disparity was put right, but, in the meantime, cautious extrapolation from studies with the adrenal will make the testicular system more readily interpretable.

Site of Action of LH

Early experiments with LH showed that stimulation of steroidogenesis by this hormone occurs in the steroidogenic pathway after cholesterol but before pregnenolone; in short, it appeared that the side-chain cleavage of cholesterol is stimulated by LH (14,105–107). When these experiments were performed, nothing was known about intracellular transport as a biological phenomenon. Although it was known that cholesterol is stored in cytoplasmic droplets and that the side-chain cleavage reaction occurs in mitochondria, little thought was given to the mechanism by which the enzyme is supplied with cholesterol. When Garren et al. observed that the action of ACTH is inhibited by cycloheximide at a step before side-chain cleavage of cholesterol, these workers proposed that ACTH stimulates the transport of cholesterol to mitochondria (108). This was confirmed directly by other studies (109,110).

When preparations of Leydig cells from rat testis became available (111), this idea was tested with the response to LH. It was found that this hormone, like ACTH, stimulates the transport of cholesterol to the inner mitochondrial membrane (112). On the other hand, the rate of conversion of cholesterol to pregnenolone by isolated mitochondria from Leydig cells incubated with and without LH is the same (112). At this point, it is important to consider the state of mitochondria in such experiments. It is difficult to prepare aerobic mitochondria unless special care is taken (113). If mitochondria become anaerobic, side-chain cleavage is inhibited, because this reaction requires oxygen (53), and cholesterol accumulates in the mitochondria (113).

When such mitochondria are incubated, they show a burst of synthesis of pregnenolone that is greater in mitochondria from cells incubated with LH, because these mitochondria are loaded with cholesterol (112). This point is crucial to the interpretation of such experiments, because the findings distinguish between an effect of LH on cholesterol transport, as opposed to an effect on the side-chain cleavage system per se (114). The problem has been more intensively studied in the adrenal, where it is now clear that the trophic hormone acts on cholesterol transport to the mitochondrial side-chain cleavage P-450 (114). Studies have not so far been reported with inner and outer mitochondrial membranes from Leydig cells to determine whether or not LH also stimulates the movement of cholesterol from the outer to the inner mitochondrial membrane, but it is clear that ACTH stimulates transport both to and within mitochondria (114). It seems likely that LH does the same.

Role of Cyclic AMP

It has long been known that cyclic AMP increases the synthesis of androgens by Leydig cells (115) and that LH increases the levels of cyclic AMP in these cells (116,117). In view of extensive evidence that cyclic AMP mediates the actions of various hormones, the idea has developed that the responses of Leydig cells to LH and hCG result from increased production of cyclic AMP as the result of the binding of LH to its receptor. Doubt concerning this as the *only* mechanism of action of the trophic hormones has arisen in the case of ACTH (118,119) and LH (120) and especially in the case of the steroidogenic action of LH on Leydig cells, because low concentrations of LH stimulate steroid synthesis without detectable change in total cell concentration of cyclic AMP (120). In considering this disparity between the level of cyclic AMP and the steroidogenic response, the reader must decide to what extent he accepts the concept of cytoplasmic pools. If one argues that since cyclic AMP can enter cells it must therefore be distributed uniformly throughout the cytoplasm, the evidence for cyclic AMP as an obligatory mediator of the action of LH will remain unconvincing. If, on the other hand, one accepts the growing evidence for inhomogeneity of the cytoplasm, one comes to expect that rather small changes in the total concentration of cyclic AMP can be compatible with local changes in the level of the cyclic nucleotide within reach of molecules of protein kinase. These local changes may be sufficient to amplify the original response to LH by activating the kinase.

Since cyclic AMP is metabolized by a phosphodiesterase, the cyclic AMP that does not immediately bind to protein kinase may be inactivated so that the duration of the response can be controlled by the cell. In restricting changes in cyclic AMP in this way, the cell can produce a local response without stimulating every cyclic AMP–dependent process in the cell. Such compartmentalization could permit a graded or submaximal response to LH and one that could be arrested when the original stimulus is withdrawn. In this situation, special approaches are needed to detect regional changes in cyclic AMP if the hypothesis is to be examined with meaningful results. Dufau et al. (121,122) have used the important approach of measuring the amount of cyclic AMP bound to the regulatory subunit (R) of protein kinase. The results were clear and justify confidence in the existence of local changes in the concentration of cyclic AMP within the cell that may not always be detected by measuring total levels of cyclic AMP. Low doses of LH cause an increase in the number of molecules of regulatory subunit with bound cyclic

AMP and a concomitant decrease in the number of free regulatory subunits (i.e., with no bound cyclic AMP). By measuring the binding of the cyclic nucleotide to the target molecule, the role of cyclic AMP in the response to low doses of LH is clearly revealed (121). These studies strongly suggest that cyclic AMP is an obligatory mediator of the action of LH. Partial inhibition of adenylate cyclase by various inhibitors cannot provide contradictory evidence (120)—it would be necessary to measure binding of cyclic AMP to R in the presence of the inhibitor to reveal the functionally significant fraction of total cyclic AMP.

In this connection, two terms used by proponents of local changes in the concentration of cyclic AMP in cells may not help their case—namely, "pools" and "cyclic AMP receptors" or binding sites. In spite of the intentions of the writer, the term pool suggests a local concentration of a metabolite—often in a defined or definable anatomical site, whereas what is intended is a specific proximity between one molecule and another which facilitates interaction, without necessarily implying an anatomical compartment. In this sense, a pool may be nothing more than a place in which, for example, the activity of phosphodiesterase is low enough to permit cyclic AMP to bind to R in significant amounts. Again, the term cyclic AMP receptor is apt to remind the reader of plasma membrane receptors. Although there is no guarantee at present that all bound cyclic AMP in the cell is associated only with the regulatory subunit of protein kinase, the discussion should indicate that this is a major component in the binding and that no other intracellular binding sites for cyclic AMP are known at this time. In addition, it may not prove helpful to consider R as a receptor; the term regulatory subunit is to be preferred in our present state of ignorance. In the meantime, measurement of cyclic AMP bound to R provides a value approach to the question of whether or not steroid synthesis in Leydig cells can be stimulated without the intervention of cyclic AMP.

In the case of the adrenal, Schimmer and co-workers have studied a series of mutant adrenal cells and shown that the ability of the various mutants to respond to ACTH is closely associated with the presence of a functional cyclic AMP–dependent protein kinase (123). Defects in the kinase are invariably accompanied by defective response to ACTH (123). This approach provides the strongest evidence for cyclic AMP as an obligatory messenger for the steroidogenic response to ACTH. It seems reasonable to assume that the same is true for LH until compelling evidence to the contrary is found.

Role of Protein Synthesis

In 1962, it was discovered that the steroidogenic response to LH is inhibited by puromycin (19). It was subsequently shown that LH increases incorporation of labeled amino acids into the total protein of Leydig cells (124). A detailed study by Janszen et al. revealed increased synthesis of two proteins in Leydig cells by LH (125). One of these (21K) appears 2 hr after addition of LH and shows a half-life greater than 30 min (125). The second protein (33K) has a short half-life (11 min). In both cases, the effect of LH on these proteins may be indirect. The authors propose that 33K may be an inactive precursor of short half-life that is activated in the presence of LH (125). The roles of these proteins in the response to LH deserve further study. These findings are disappointing when compared with the analogous studies with ACTH where proteins more closely related to the steroidogenic functions of the cell have been discovered (126,127). One of the adrenal proteins (2.2K) is relevant to the present discussion, because it has been found in the testis (127). This protein causes an increase in side-chain cleavage of cholesterol when it is added to mitochondria that have been loaded with cholesterol (127). It has been suggested that the protein promotes loading of the side-chain cleavage P-450 with substrate. Although the concept of loading with cholesterol remains to be proved, the idea is intriguing, and, if the effect of 2.2K proves to be specific, it may turn out to play an important role in the responses to LH and ACTH. It is therefore clear that new proteins are essential for the steroidogenic action of LH on Leydig cells. A major hurdle confronting investigators in this field is the identification of the responding proteins and the determination of their respective roles in the steroidogenic response.

Role of Ca^{2+}

Since most biological processes require Ca^{2+}, at least as a permissive agent, and since the steroidogenic response to ACTH requires Ca^{2+} (128), it is likely that the action of LH on Leydig cells also requires this cation. So far, the nature of the involvement of Ca^{2+} in the response to LH has not been clarified. However, it was found that trifluoperazine inhibits the steroidogenic action of LH (129). Moreover, when calmodulin is injected into Leydig cells by means of liposomes, the protein accelerates the synthesis of testosterone (129), and this acceleration is accompanied by increased transport of cholesterol to the inner mitochondrial membrane (129). Injection of Ca^{2+} alone is without effect, and the action of calmodulin is enhanced if it is first saturated with Ca^{2+} (129). These studies were interpreted to mean that in the unstimulated cell, insufficient Ca^{2+}-calmodulin is present in those regions of the cell at which the complex is required to accelerate steroid synthesis. The injected Ca^{2+}-calmodulin floods the cell and increases the concentration of this complex in various parts of the cell including those places in which it is required for increased steroid synthesis. This suggests that LH may cause redistribution of calmodulin and that this redistribution plays an important part in the stimulation of the synthesis of androgens by LH. Such an idea would be in keeping with observations made with luteinizing hormone–releasing hormone (LHRH), which causes redistribution of calmodulin in pituitary cells (130). Further studies are needed to characterize such redistribution of endogenous calmodulin.

Apart from this action of Ca^{2+}-calmodulin, Ca^{2+} may be involved elsewhere in the regulation of steroidogenesis. For example, Ca^{2+} is required for interaction of ACTH with its receptor (131). This and other aspects of the action of Ca^{2+} in Leydig cells remain to be investigated.

Role of Phosphorylation

Since cyclic AMP serves as a second messenger for LH and since the only known mechanism of action of cyclic AMP is to phosphorylate proteins (132), it follows that LH should promote phosphorylation of Leydig cell proteins. Indeed, Cooke et al. found that LH produces phosphorylation of three Leydig cell proteins, identified as 14K, 57K, and 78K (133). The extent of phosphorylation of these proteins showed some correlation with the steroidogenic response to LH (133). Some relevant information on the role of phosphorylation in the action of LH comes from studies in the ovary. Special attention has been paid to mitochondrial proteins because of the importance of the side-chain cleavage of cholesterol in that organelle. LH stimulates phosphorylation of two mitochondrial proteins in ovarian follicles, but the relationship of these changes to steroidogenesis is not clear (134). Studies by Inaba and Wiest (135) showed that the mitochondrial membrane prevents cyclic AMP–dependent protein kinase from stimulating the side-chain cleavage of cholesterol. However, disruption of the mitochondrial membrane by Ca^{2+} allows the protein kinase to stimulate side-chain cleavage of cholesterol—possibly by facilitating access of cholesterol to the enzyme (135). The problem in understanding the role of phosphorylation in this and other cellular responses lies in defining the change in the functions of a given protein when it is phosphorylated. So far, this has not proved possible with the response to LH.

The Possible Role of Phospholipids

One of the most interesting developments in our understanding of metabolic regulation in recent years has been the discovery of the role of phosphoinositides in a variety of cellular responses to various stimuli (136,137). Phosphoinositides undergo rapid breakdown and resynthesis in what may be regarded as a cyclic process:

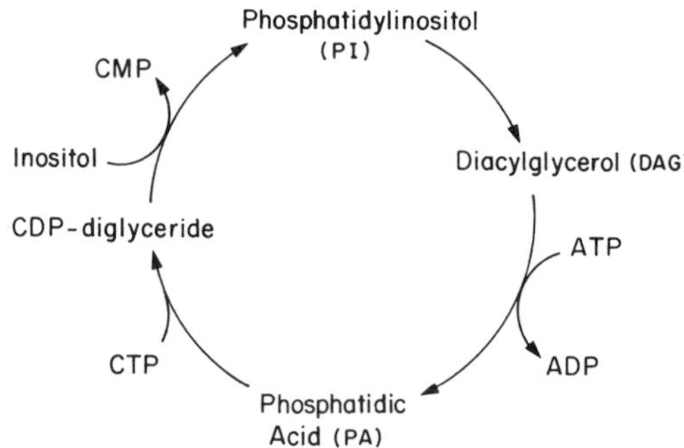

Moreover, a second cycle is superimposed on the first in which phosphatidylinositol is phosphorylated sequentially at the 4 and 5 positions on the inositol ring:

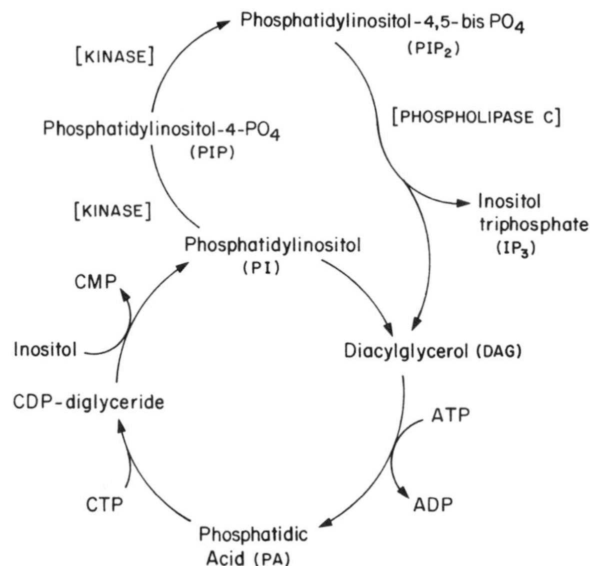

It is now believed that this polyphosphoinositide cycle is the key element in certain acute metabolic activities of these compounds. When phosphatidylinositol-4,5-bis PO_4 is subjected to the action of phospholipase C, two important products appear, namely, inositol triphosphate and diacylglycerol, as shown below:

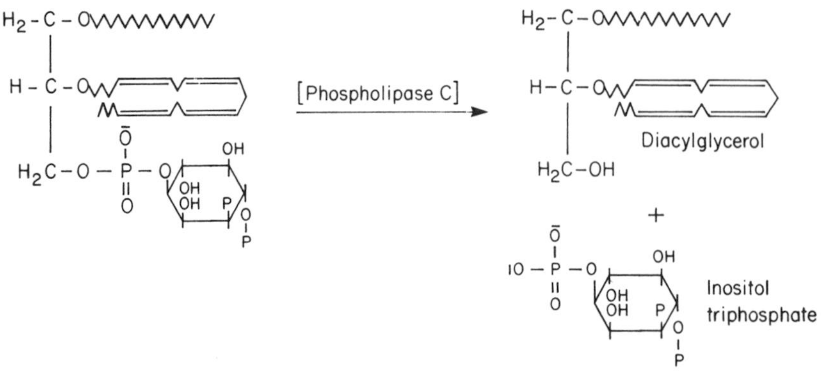

[Phospholipase C]

Diacylglycerol

\+

Inositol triphosphate

Inositol triphosphate (PIPP) is a Ca^{2+} ionophore (136,137), so increased production of this substance may result in raised intracellular concentrations of Ca^{2+}. The source of this Ca^{2+} is a subject of considerable interest. This may vary from cell to cell, and it may vary with time. For example, in some cells, the early response is microsomal, and later increases in intracellular Ca^{2+} may come from extracellular Ca^{2+} (reviewed in 138,139). Mitochondrial Ca^{2+} may be important in this connection, but recent studies have served to make this source of Ca^{2+} appear less important, if it contributes at all, to the responses under consideration (140). Meanwhile, the second product of the action of phospholipase C, namely, diacylglycerol, is capable of activating protein kinase C which also requires Ca^{2+} and phospholipid for activity (141); this activity is expressed in the form of phosphorylation of various proteins. Under some conditions, diacylglycerol can act as an ionophore, although the significance of this effect is uncertain (142).

One result of these changes is that PIPP emerges as a second messenger like cyclic AMP. In this formulation, protein kinase C (PKC) is to the phosphoinositide system what protein kinase A is to cyclic AMP. Ca^{2+} appears as an additional messenger in the phosphoinositide system, since an increase in intracellular Ca^{2+} can affect other cellular activities in addition to activating protein kinase C. Phospholipase is activated by or coupled to hormone receptors (143), and it has been proposed that a guanidine nucleotide–binding protein may be involved in this coupling (144). The two systems can be compared as illustrated below:

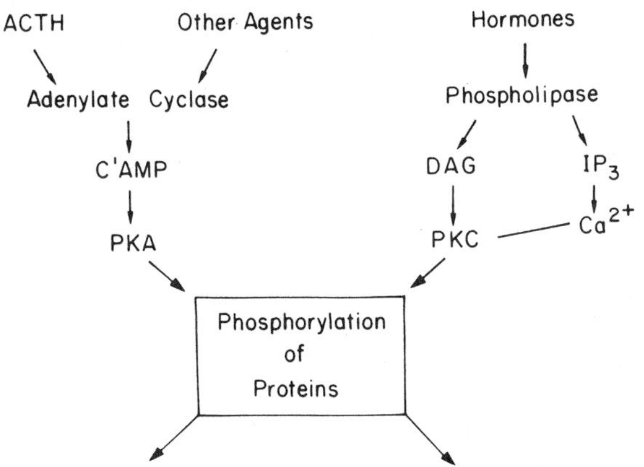

The arrows diverging from phosphorylation are intended to convey the idea that the two kinase enzymes may phosphorylate different substrates or different amino acids in the same substrate.

What remains uncertain is whether one hormone would use both kinase mechanisms—especially since the initial coupling to the receptor may be very similar, involving a GTP-binding protein in both systems. There would seem to be no reason for the cell to use two similar mechanisms. In general, it has been inferred that the phosphatidylinositide-Ca^{2+} mechanism may be an alternative to the cyclic AMP mechanism, one that is used by hormones such as vasopressin that clearly employ Ca^{2+}, but probably not cyclic AMP, as second messenger—at least not in the same cells as those using the former mechanism. Obviously, such a generalization cannot be used as evidence, and the question of one or two second messengers must be resolved case by case.

With this background, a series of publications from one laboratory reported that ACTH (145,146) and LH (147,148) administered *in vivo* promote synthesis of phosphoinositol in their respective target organs. The responses were studied in considerable detail, and it was proposed that the newly synthesized phospholipids acted on mitochondria to stimulate side-chain cleavage of cholesterol (146,148). The similarity between the changes reported in these studies and the phosphatidylinositide-Ca^{2+} mechanism proposed for other cells made it seem as though this mechanism or a variant of this mechanism is involved in the response to ACTH.

However, there are important differences. First, the work of Farese et al. does not directly demonstrate the occurrence of increased intracellular Ca^{2+} in response to the trophic hormones, although this could be inferred. Rather, it was conceived that the phosphoinositides themselves acted directly on mitochondria (148). Second, these responses involve increased synthesis of phosphatidylinositol, as opposed to increased turnover of polyphosphoinositides (145–148). Other workers have universally employed labeled precursors of phosphatidylinositol—^{32}Pi or [^{3}H]*myo*-inositol, to study the phosphoinositide mechanism in other cells (136,137). The use of labeled precursors makes the system more sensitive. On the other hand, attempts to measure net synthesis by measurement of mass must come close to the limit of sensitivity of the methods used. A reason for measuring mass as opposed to incorporation of labeled precursors may lie in the difficulty of establishing isotopic equilibrium in studies performed *in vivo*. However, it should be pointed out that adrenal cells and Leydig cells can be maintained in culture, which is ideal for such studies. Since the cultured cells respond well to ACTH, LH, and cyclic AMP, the phosphatidylinositol response should be demonstrable *in vitro* if it plays an important role in the action of LH. It is too early to assess the significance of the findings in the testis, but studies in the adrenal have shown that the phosphoinositide-Ca^{2+} mechanism does not apply in cultured adrenal cells (149). Under such circumstances, it is extremely important that findings in the rat be independently confirmed at every step. In the meantime, the role of a similar mechanism in the response to LH remains to be fully established.

The Possible Role of Protein Kinase C

Protein kinase has been shown to be present in rat testis (150), and phorbol ester has been found to stimulate synthesis of androgens by Leydig cells (151,152). The activity of protein kinase C in these cells may be dependent on external Ca^{2+}, since the effect of phorbol ester is blocked by nifedipine which blocks Ca^{2+} channels (151). It is difficult to relate these observations to the mechanism of action of LH. The evidence in the adrenal suggests that protein kinase C is unlikely to play a role in the mechanism of action of ACTH (153). It is possible that this enzyme plays an ancillary role in the regulation of steroid synthesis or in some other aspect of adrenal cell function. More information for the Leydig cell will be necessary before the role of protein kinase C in steroid synthesis can be evaluated.

Miscellaneous Factors

Although the principal regulatory mechanism for the production of androgens by Leydig cells is based on the secretion of pulses of LH by the adenohypophysis, other factors are capable of altering the rate of production of these steroids, and some of these factors may be important *in vivo*.

LHRH: The hypothalamic releasing factor or a testicular analogue of this factor appears to stimulate the production of androgens by Leydig cells (154). The factor does not act through adenylate cyclase and may form the basis of local interaction between Sertoli cells and Leydig cells (155). The idea is too new for final judgment, but the available evidence is reviewed in reference 154.

Prostaglandins: It has been shown that PGE_2 stimulates steroid synthesis in the Leydig cell (156). This substance also stimulates adenylate cyclase in the corpus luteum (157). On the other hand, $PGF_{2\alpha}$ inhibits the steroidogenic response to LH in corpus luteum (158). It is not clear at present whether PGE_2 is a second messenger for LH or the effects reported are only of pharmacological interest.

Blood flow: The rate of secretion of testosterone by the testis is closely related to the blood flow in the spermatic artery (159). However, it is not known whether or not LH directly influences the blood flow to the testis.

Nervous system: It remains uncertain whether the Leydig cell receives a direct nerve supply. Testicular nerves supply the vascular system of the testis, through which they may influence steroid synthesis indirectly by altering blood flow (160). Leydig cells possess β-adrenergic receptors that activate adenylate cyclase (161). Systemic administration of epinephrine decreases plasma testosterone presumably because of diminished blood flow to the testis (160). On the other hand, epinephrine stimulates the secretion of testosterone by the testis, provided the total volume of blood in the spermatic artery remains constant (160). This effect is believed to result from activation of β-adrenergic receptors (161). The physiological importance of these responses is unclear.

Roles of Components of the Leydig Cell

In the previous sections of this chapter, we have considered the molecular mechanisms that the Leydig cell uses in the synthesis of androgens. We must now turn to the morphology of the cell and the activities of those subcellular components of the cell in which these mechanisms are employed. The Leydig cell itself varies in appearance from species to species, although the functional significance of these variations is unclear. A detailed comparative approach to the morphology of the Leydig cell may prove rewarding. In the meantime, we will consider the human Leydig cell, because it has been thoroughly studied by Christensen (15), who has pointed out that the cell is typical of Leydig cells in general. The Leydig cell is polygonal and has a diameter of 15 to 20 μm. The surface area of the human Leydig cell has been estimated to be 800 μm^2 (15).

The Plasma Membrane

The plasma membrane is not unusual in appearance. In places it shows well-developed microvilli (15). This membrane contains the LH receptor coupled to adenylate cyclase.

The LH Receptor–Adenylate Cyclase

Each Leydig cell in the rat contains approximately 20,000 receptors, and the testis can bind about 1 pmole of LH per gram of wet weight (162). The receptor can bind both LH and hCG, so it is known as the LH/hCG receptor. For the sake of brevity, these receptors will be referred to here as LH receptors. The receptor has been partly purified and found to be a glycoprotein of MW 190,000 made up of two identical subunits of MW 90,000 (163). Attempts to remove all bound phospholipid result in loss of binding activity (163). The Leydig cell is said to show spare receptors, because maximal steroidogenesis can be obtained at concentrations of LH that are sufficient to occupy only a fraction of the total number of available LH receptors (164).

The LH receptor is coupled to adenylate cyclase, and, as in other cells, the cyclase contains GTP-binding or N proteins. Binding of GTP to the stimulatory N protein (Ns) results in activation of the cyclase, and activation is terminated by hydrolysis of GTP. An analogous inhibitory N protein (Ni) is also present in the adenylate cyclase complex. The process of activation can be studied with Gpp (NH)p, an analogue of GTP that is not hydrolyzed (165). Since the amount of Gpp (NH)p bound to Leydig cell membranes (p moles/mg protein) exceeds the number of LH receptors, it is concluded that one occupied receptor can activate many GTP-binding sites which results in a 20-fold amplification of the binding of LH (166). Moreover, binding of LH to its receptor results in phosphorylation of several membrane proteins, including one of MW 44,000. It has been suggested that this protein may be Ns (167).

Down-Regulation and Desensitization

When a single injection of LH or hCG is administered to a rat, a second injection produces a response that is quantitatively different from the first injection. Usually, the second injection produces a smaller response than the first (165). Since the administration of LH to a rat in any dose is unphysiological, the significance of the changes to be described is uncertain. Moreover, the field has been burdened with inappropriate colloquialisms which are not always adequately defined. It is common practice to refer to the diminished response to a second injection as down-regulation, if the full extent seen with the first response can be obtained with cyclic AMP—that is, if the limitation set on the second response results from a change in the LH receptor.

The confusion in nomenclature has been compounded with the terms homologous and heterologous down-regulation which refer respectively to altered responses produced by the same stimulating agent (e.g., LH and LH) or different agents (e.g., LH and forskolin). When the lesser second response cannot be corrected by cyclic AMP, the unfortunate term desensitization is used. This leaves an undefined group of responses in which the diminished second response results from changes in the cyclase itself. Under some conditions, which have not been fully studied, up-regulation, with the second response greater than the first, may be seen (168). This situation will not be discussed here.

The following changes have been reported in Leydig cells after an injection of LH: (a) decrease in number, but not affinity, of LH receptors (169,170); (b) alterations in the coupling and function of the cyclase (171,172); (c) depletion of substrate (173,174); (d) changes in the steroidogenic pathway at C_{21} side-chain cleavage (hydroxylase/lyase) (175,176) and, with larger doses, a decrease in C_{27} side-chain cleavage (177,178).

Decrease in number of receptors. The term down-regulation refers to a decrease in the number of receptors on the surface of the Leydig cell following an injection of LH. It appears that the receptors are internalized but not degraded (169,170). Presumably, the fate of occupied receptors includes internalization, dissociation of LH, and a regulated return of the free receptors to the surface of the cell. This cycle of receptors, from cell surface to the interior of the cell and back to the surface, has been studied intensely in other systems, and the findings have been reviewed (179,180). The binding of ligand (LH) to receptor influences the distribution of the receptor in the plasma membrane in such a way as to encourage internalization via coated vesicles. In the lysosome, the ligand is released and follows its own fate, which may be degradation (179,180). The receptor may be sorted in the Golgi apparatus and returned to the plasma membrane to function once again as a free receptor. The LH receptor acts in this respect like other receptors, and down-regulation should be seen in this light—as part of the normal cellular processing of receptors. It has been proposed that down-regulation may serve to limit the response to pulses of LH—one pulse could deplete receptors before later pulses appear (181). We are a long way from the sort of evidence necessary to discuss the physiological importance of the phenomenon of down-regulation, which has, however, prompted important research on the intracellular movement of receptors.

Alterations in adenylate cyclase. Studies with forskolin and cholera toxin, which stimulate adenylate cyclase, suggest that homologous and heterologous down-regulation result respectively from lesions before and after Ns in the process of activation of adenylate cyclase (182). Again, the physiological relevance of the findings is uncertain. It is also unclear whether these lesions are better referred to as down-regulation or desensitization.

Desensitization. Before reviewing the phenomena associated with desensitization, it is well to consider how far removed our best cell culture systems are from providing physiological conditions, because one of the most important contributions to come from the study of desensitization is the emphasis these investigations have given to the importance of the details of cell culture. Present systems of cell culture frequently use serum, almost always induce oxygen toxicity in the cells, and do not provide a regulated circulation of fresh medium. While serum-free medium is becoming commonplace, such media are still far removed from normal interstitial fluid, and perfusion is but a beginning of attempts to mimic circulatory conditions *in vivo*. The worst and least generally understood problem is that of oxygen toxicity. It is still necessary to point out that oxygen is highly toxic and that 20% O_2 is well above physiological levels for individual cells. Manufacturers of tissue culture apparatus have been slow to take up this challenge. We will see that availability of substrate and adverse effects of high O_2 tension may be important in desensitization.

Supply of cholesterol: It is clear that in some experimental studies, desensitization can be relieved by addition of LDL to cultured Leydig cells (173,174). The first injection causes sufficient stimulation of steroid synthesis to produce depletion of cholesterol. What is not clear is whether such depletion occurs *in vivo* under physiological circumstances.

Inhibition of the steroidogenic pathway: When the individual steps in the biosynthetic pathway to testosterone are examined in desensitized Leydig cells, C_{21} side-chain cleavage is seen to be depressed (175,176), and, with higher doses of LH at the first injection, side-chain cleavage of cholesterol (C_{27}) may be inhibited (177,178). It is no coincidence that these reactions are both catalyzed by cytochromes P-450. It will be recalled that binding of substrate to P-450 promotes the flow of the first electron to the cytochrome and that this is followed by activation of oxygen. The active oxygen is used to hydroxylate the substrate. Some steroids (e.g., the products of reactions catalyzed by P-450) can bind to the active site of P-450 but cannot be hydroxylated—for example, they may already be hydroxylated at the only accessible C atom. Such steroids are called pseudosubstrates. The binding of the pseudosubstrate will promote the activation of oxygen, and the active oxygen cannot be used for hydroxylation. Active oxygen can exist in a variety of forms—e.g., peroxide, hydroxyl radical, superoxide, etc. These forms of oxygen can attack heme and inactivate P-450 (183,184). Given the high oxygen tensions present in cell cultures, the question of active oxygen could be important in the inactivation of the two steroidogenic cytochromes P-450 involved in the synthesis of androgens. The topic of active oxygen has been extensively reviewed (183–185). Moreover, Payne and co-workers have shown that at low oxygen tension (1%), inhibition of P-450 during desensitization to LH is greatly diminished (175). Again, the physiological importance of these observations is not clear. It will be necessary to study the effects of more physiological conditions of oxygen tension between 1% and 20% before these findings can be interpreted.

Synthesis of estrogen: Yet another factor in the mechanism of desensitization appears to be the synthesis of estrogens by the Leydig cell. Desensitization can be diminished by treating Leydig cells with antiestrogen (Tamifoxen) (186). There are at least two ways in which estrogens can inhibit C_{21} side-chain cleavage. First, estradiol causes inhibition of the enzyme itself (187), and second, estradiol promotes the synthesis of a protein (24K) that can inhibit both C_{21} and C_{27} side-chain cleavage (188). The nature of this protein and the mechanism of inhibition are likely to be important. It is proposed that the first injection of LH increases the synthesis of estrogens as well as that of androgens, by the Leydig cell, and the estrogen inhibits the response to the second injection by one or both of the above mechanisms (189).

Endoplasmic Reticulum

The most conspicuous feature of the Leydig cell is an extensive endoplasmic reticulum (ER), most of which is smooth. The smooth ER is generally believed to be related to the synthesis of steroids. It has been proposed that the development of smooth ER is specifically related to the synthesis of cholesterol, which is consistent with the idea that the Leydig cell makes much of its own steroidogenic cholesterol. The smooth ER forms a network of tubules 800 to 1,200 Å in diameter, with an estimated surface area of 4,000 μm^2 (15). This enormous surface is used by the membrane-bound enzymes that synthesize cholesterol and steroid hormones. In addition, the Leydig cell contains rough ER with ribosomes. The rough ER interconnects with the smooth ER (15) and must be responsible for the synthesis of the proteins required for the response of Leydig cells to LH.

Cytoplasm

The most striking feature of Leydig cell cytoplasm is the presence of lipid droplets which are bounded by a membrane of 50 Å in width. This cannot be a typical bilayer structure, since the width of such a structure is approximately 75 Å (15). Presumably, cholesterol can pass freely through this membrane. Histochemical studies show that the droplets consist chiefly of cholesterol and neutral fats (190). In view of what is known of adrenal lipid stores, it seems reasonable to conclude that the droplets contain stores of cholesterol ester to be used in steroid synthesis. Christensen has pointed out that the content of lipid droplets varies greatly from cell to cell in one testis (15), and, since LH causes depletion of lipid droplets, these variations may reflect cycles of synthetic activity (15). This is a point of some importance in interpreting biochemical studies in which we may be examining the activity of a small number of cells at any one time in a given population, since many of the cells may not be in a phase of activity.

The functional contributions of the cytoplasm include the synthesis of new proteins, the storage of cholesterol, and the mobilization of this substrate. Mobilization includes cleavage of stored esters by cholesterol ester hydrolase and, presumably, binding to a carrier protein. It is also impossible to ignore the crystals of Reinke which are seen in the cytoplasm of human Leydig cells but in no other species. These structures consist largely of protein, but their functional significance remains obscure (15).

Mitochondria

In view of the importance of mitochondria in the synthesis of steroid hormones, it is disappointing that we learn so little from the morphology of those of the Leydig cell. These organelles vary considerably from species to species, but in all cases so far examined, some tubular, some lamellar, and some intermediate forms of cristae are seen (15). The mitochondria are responsible for the conversion of cholesterol to pregnenolone and for the transport of the cholesterol from the outer to the inner membrane (191,192). Evidence from the adrenal cortex shows that protein synthesis is necessary for this intramitochondrial transport (191,192). Mention has already been made of a 2.2K protein that may regulate this process (127). It is important that similar studies be performed with Leydig cells.

Cytoskeleton

Unfortunately, a systematic description of the cytoskeleton of the Leydig cell has not been reported, but the usual cytoskeletal elements are present in this cell (15). Although the full functional significance of the cytoskeleton in the economy of the cell is not known, some important functions deserve mention. The cytoskeleton provides surfaces and compartments within the cell that are responsible for the inhomogeneity of the cytoplasm (193). This inhomogeneity arises from subdivisions created by microtubules and perhaps by finer trabecular structures (194,195). Within the compartments, enzymatic activity takes place in bound water associated with the surfaces of the cytoskeleton (196). It is significant that the enzymes of glycolysis are associated with microtubules (197). In addition, the shape of the cell is determined by intermediate filaments (198). The presence of actin in microfilaments suggests the possibility of contractile activity that may be used for intracellular movements. The subject has been reviewed elsewhere (199).

The steroidogenic response of Leydig cells to LH is inhibited by antiactin injected into Leydig cells by fusion with liposomes (112). This inhibitory action of antiactin arises from inhibition of the transport of cholesterol to mitochondria (112). When these findings are considered in relation to the more detailed studies in the adrenal (200–202), we are left to conclude that LH requires a pool of G actin available for polymerization, and this, in turn, results in increased transport of cholesterol to mitochondria. This effect of LH is not inhibited by cycloheximide and does not, therefore, require newly synthesized proteins (unpublished). The mechanism by which actin is involved in cholesterol transport is not known. Microfilaments may promote bulk movement within the cytoplasm, they may provide direction and shortening, or they may construct new compartments within the cytoplasm which may constrain the movement of cholesterol in such a way as to increase the efficiency of the transfer of this substrate to mitochondria. These and other possibilities must be explored by new methods that can be used in the living cell, including videointensified Nomarski optics (203).

Nucleus

The Leydig cell possesses a large, round or oval nucleus which contains two nucleoli. The morphology of the Leydig cell nucleus can be regarded as typical of nuclei in general. Most of the nucleus consists of euchromatin with a peripheral ring of heterochromatin that is interrupted at nuclear pores (15). The pores are approximately 1,000 Å in diameter and are occluded by thin valves that may regulate the passage of substances to and from the nucleus (15). Following treatment with LH or hCG, the nucleus increases in size (204) and in content of DNA (205). It is very likely that long-term effects of LH include an action of the hormone on the synthesis of DNA, although such responses have yet to be studied in detail. Greater interest has been shown in the synthesis of RNA in response to LH. It is generally agreed that inhibitors of the synthesis of RNA (e.g., actinomycin and cordycepin) inhibit the steroidogenic response to LH *in vitro* (206,207). A direct demonstration of the effect of LH on the synthesis of RNA by Leydig cells has been proposed and questioned (208,209). However, Valladares and Ronco have reported that LH increases the incorporation of [^{3}H]uridine into Leydig cell RNA (210). Presumably, the new RNA is translated to give rise to the new proteins necessary for the response to LH (see above).

LH is known to promote synthesis of steroidogenic enzymes. For example, in hypophysectomized rats, hCG stimulates the synthesis of 3β-hydroxysteroid dehydrogenase (211). In cultured Leydig cells, LH promotes synthesis of both C_{21} (212) and C_{27} (213) side-chain cleavage enzymes. The latter responses apparently require new synthesis of RNA (212,213). It is noteworthy that, as in the adrenal, none of the newly synthesized proteins that appear within the first few minutes of administration of ACTH show a molecular weight like those of the enzymes just named (see above). It may be that hypophysectomy and cell culture result in cells that have undergone significant decline in steroidogenesis and that this decline permits an enhanced response to LH—i.e., the cell begins with a rate of steroid synthesis below the normal activity seen *in vivo*.

No doubt *in vivo* LH has a trophic or maintenance function as the result of which it keeps these enzymes at appropriate concentrations within the cell. In that case, the acute response to LH in intact animals *in vivo* may require the synthesis of small amounts of key proteins that, in turn, accelerate the synthesis of steroids with the existing levels of steroidogenic enzymes. The limiting factor in the unstimulated cell may be the availability of substrate rather than the levels of specific enzymes. The first proteins to appear may be those that have short half-lives and those that are involved in the transport of cholesterol. No doubt, the response to LH unfolds in a series of steps, the first of which lead to later changes and, at the same time, create the need for more of already existing enzymes as the cell begins to increase its output of androgens.

We can envisage a succession of rate-limiting steps each one accelerated in turn, as a result of the action of LH, so that a new step becomes rate-limiting, and so on, until the more chronic responses begin to appear in which many proteins must be synthesized and/or modified, until eventually, if the cell continues to be stimulated, hypertrophy and hyperplasia set in. Normal responses presumably stop short of these last extremes, which are seen in various disease states. The pulsatile nature of the stimulation by LH may provide a mechanism that permits return to prestimulation levels when the concentration of plasma LH returns to normal and the need for high output has passed. In any case, the pulsatile nature of the concentration of LH in plasma is likely to be a major determinant in shaping the response of the Leydig cell. The sooner we can imitate these pulses experimentally, the better for our understanding of LH and its effect on Leydig cells.

SUMMARY AND CONCLUSIONS

The synthesis of androgens in Leydig cells begins with the mobilization of cholesterol from depots of cholesterol esters in lipid droplets within the cytoplasm. The cholesterol is taken to the inner mitochondrial membrane in which it is converted to pregnenolone by C_{27} side-chain cleavage P-450. These events appear to include the slow step or steps in the steroidogenic pathway. Side-chain cleavage involves shuttling of adrenodoxin to-and-from between adrenodoxin reductase and P-450. The pregnenolone so formed moves to the microsomal compartment, in which it is attacked by membrane-bound enzymes including the C_{21} side-chain cleavage P-450 which converts the 21-carbon steroid to a 19-carbon androgen, androstenedione, or dehydroepiandrosterone, depending on whether the Δ^4 or Δ^5 pathway is used. Androstenedione is converted to the principal androgen, testosterone, by 17β-hydroxysteroid dehydrogenase.

The microsomal enzymes are organized in a specific arrangement in which some of the active sites are further removed from the aqueous surroundings of the microsomes than others. The two steroidogenic cytochromes P-450, especially the microsomal C_{21} side-chain cleavage system, are susceptible to degradation by various forms of active oxygen.

This pathway is chiefly regulated by pulses of LH from the pituitary. LH binds to a specific surface receptor, and binding activates a stimulatory GTP-binding protein which, in turn, stimulates neighboring adenylate cyclase. The resulting increase in cyclic AMP is probably responsible for all of the ensuing changes; if other second messengers exist, they have not been unequivocally identified at this time. The increased levels of cyclic AMP trigger a second "absolute" response—it appears that the *only* action of cyclic AMP is to phosphorylate proteins. Phosphorylation leads to altered functions of specific proteins. One protein affected by this form of posttranslational modification is cholesterol ester hydrolase that becomes active (or more active) on phosphorylation. The active hydrolase releases free cholesterol which is conveyed to the mitochondrion by a mechanism that involves microfilaments. To this point, the synthesis of new protein is not required—LH achieves these responses with the existing Leydig cell proteins.

As a result of the action(s) of one or more proteins synthesized at accelerated rates under the influence of LH, cholesterol is transported to the inner mitochondrial membrane where C_{27} side-chain cleavage takes place. The two processes of transport to and within the mitochondria appear to be points at which LH accelerates steroid synthesis. There may be, in addition, stimulation of the side-chain cleavage reaction itself.

Pregnenolone, formed as the result of C_{27} side-chain cleavage, proceeds to the microsomal system in which the remaining steps of the pathway take place. These reactions proceed more rapidly than the delivery of cholesterol to the C_{27} side-chain cleavage enzyme. However, the microsomal contribution to steroid synthesis is not without regulation. The degree to which the lyase activity of C_{21} side-chain cleavage is expressed, the relative activities of the Δ^4 and Δ^5 pathways, and the presence of a pregnenolone-binding protein are examples of regulation in the microsomal compartment.

The most pressing challenge in our attempts to understand the mechanism of action of LH appears to involve putting functions to bands or spots on polyacrylamide gels—bands or spots that change in amount and/or are subjected to posttranslational modification in response to LH.

ACKNOWLEDGMENTS

The preparation of this chapter was assisted by grants AM 28113, CA 29497, and AM 32236 from the National Institutes of Health.

REFERENCES

1. Dufau, M. L., Veldhuis, J., Fraioli, F., Johnson, M. H., and Catt, K. J. (1983): Mode of bioactive LH secretion in man. *J. Clin. Endocrinol. Metab.*, 57:993.
2. Eik-Nes, K. B., and Hall, P. F. (1965): Secretion of steroid hormones *in vivo*. *Vitam. Horm.*, 23:153.
3. Dorrington, J. H., and Armstrong, D. T. (1975): FSH stimulates estradiol-17β synthesis in cultured Sertoli cells. *Proc. Natl. Acad. Sci. USA*, 72:2677.
4. Hall, P. F., Irby, D. C., and De Kretser, D. M. (1969): Conversion of cholesterol to androgens by rat testes: Comparison of interstitial cells and seminiferous tubules. *Endocrinology*, 84:488.
5. Christensen, A. K., and Mason, N. R. (1965): Comparative ability of seminiferous tubules and interstitial tissue of rat testes to synthesize androgens from progesterone-4-^{14}C *in vitro*. *Endocrinology*, 76:646.
6. Brown, M. S., and Goldstein, J. L. (1976): Receptor-mediated control of cholesterol metabolism. *Science*, 191:150.
7. Hall, P. F. (1979): Testicular hormones: Synthesis and control. In: *Endocrinology*, edited by DeGroot et al., Vol. 3, p. 1511. Grune and Stratton, New York.
8. Nyman, M. A., Geiger, J., and Goldzieher, J. W. (1959): Biosynthesis of estrogen by the perfused stallion testis. *J. Biol. Chem.*, 234:16.
9. De Jong, F. H., Hey, A. H., and Van der Molen, H. J. (1974): Estradiol and testosterone in rat testis tissue: Localization and production *in vitro*. *J. Endocrinol.*, 60:409.
10. Tcholakian, R. K., and Steinberger, A. (1979): *In vitro* metabolism of testosterone by Sertoli cells and interstitial cells. In: *Testicular Development, Structure and Function*, edited by A. Steinberger and E. Steinberger, p. 177. Raven Press, New York.
11. Ritzen, E. M., Van Damme, M. P. Froysa, B., Reuter, C., De La Torre, B., and Dicafalusy, E. (1981): Identification of estradiol produced by Sertoli cell–enriched cultures. *J. Steroid Biochem.*, 14:533.
12. Camick, J. A., Makris, A., Gunsalus, G. L., and Ryan, K. J. (1979): Testicular aromatization in immature rats. *Endocrinology*, 104:285.
13. Fishman, L. M., Safarty, G. A., Wilson, H., and Lipsett, M. B. (1967): The role of the testis in oestrogen production. *Ciba Found. Colloq. Endocrinol.*, 16:156.
14. Hall, P. F. (1963): The effect of interstitial cell-stimulating hormone on the biosynthesis of testicular cholesterol from acetate-1-C^{14}. *Biochemistry*, 2:1232.
15. Christensen, A. K. (1975): Leydig cells. In: *Handbook of Physiology*, edited by R. O. Greep and E. B. Astwood, Sect. 7, Vol. V, p. 21. American Physiological Society, Washington.
16. Hall, P. F. (1970): Endocrinology of the testis. In: *Testicular Physiology and Biochemistry*, edited by A. D. Johnson, W. R. Gomes, and V. L. van Demnark, Vol. II, p. 1. Academic Press, New York.
17. Werbin, H., and Chaikoff, I. L. (1961): Utilization of adrenal gland cholesterol for the synthesis of cortisol. *Arch. Biochem. Biophys.*, 93:476.
18. Morris, M. D., and Chaikoff, I. L. (1959): The origin of cholesterol in liver, adrenal gland and testis of the rat. *J. Biol. Chem.*, 234:1095.
19. Hall, P. F., and Eik-Nes, K. B. (1962): The action of gonadotropic hormones upon rabbit testis *in vitro*. *Biochim. Biophys. Acta*, 63:411.
20. Sandler, R., and Hall, P. F. (1966): The response of rat testis to interstitial cell-stimulating hormone *in vitro*. *Comp. Biochem. Physiol.*, 19:833.
21. Vahouny, G. V., Chanderbhan, R., Noland, B. J., and Scallen, T. J. (1985): Cholesterol ester hydrolase and sterol carrier proteins. *Endocr. Res.*, 10:473.
22. Freeman, D. A., and Ascoli, M. (1983): The LDL pathway of cultured Leydig tumor cells. *Biochim. Biophys. Acta*, 754:72.
23. Chen, Y. I., Kraemer, F. B., and Reaven, G. M. (1980): Identification of specific HDL-binding sites in rat testis. *J. Biol. Chem.*, 255:9162–9169.
24. Gwynne, J. T., Hess, B., Hughes, T., Rountree, R., and Mahaffee, D. (1985): The role of high density lipoproteins in adrenal steroidogenesis. *Endocr. Res.*, 10:411.
25. Albert, D. H., Ascoli, M., Puett, D., and Coniglio, J. G. (1980): Lipid composition and gonadotropin-mediated lipid metabolism of the M5480 murine Leydig cell tumor. *J. Lipid Res.*, 21:862.

26. Naghshineh, S., Treadwell, C. R., Gallo, L. H., and Vahouny, G. V. (1978): Protein-kinase mediated phosphorylation of purified ester hydrolase from bovine adrenal cortex. *J. Lipid. Res.*, 19:561.
27. Conneely, O. M., Headon, D. R., Olson, C. D., Ungar, F., and Dempsey, M. E. (1984): Intramitochondrial movement of cholesterol carrier protein with cholesterol in response to corticotropin. *Proc. Natl. Acad. Sci. USA*, 81:2970.
28. Hall, P. F. (1984): Cellular organization for steroidogenesis. *Int. Rev. Cytol.*, 86:53.
29. Shikita, M., and Hall, P. F. (1973): Cytochrome P-450 from bovine adrenocortical mitochondria: An enzyme for the side-chain cleavage of cholesterol. I. Purification and properties. *J. Biol. Chem.*, 248:5598.
30. Nakajin, S., and Hall, P. F. (1981): Microsomal cytochrome P-450 from neonatal pig testis: Purification and properties of a C_{21} steroid side-chain cleavage system (17α-hydroxylase and $C_{17,20}$ lyase). *J. Biol. Chem.*, 256:3871.
31. Mason, H. S. (1957): Mechanisms of oxygen metabolism. *Science*, 125:1185.
32. Bresnick, E. (1980): The molecular biology of the induction of the hepatic mixed function oxidase. In: *Hepatic Cytochrome P-450 Monooxygenase System*, edited by J. B. Schenkman and D. Kupfer, p. 191. Pergamon Press, New York.
33. Hall, P. F. (1982): Microsomal metabolism of endogenous substrates: chairman's introduction. In: *Microsomal Metabolism of Endogenous Substrates*, edited by R. Sato and R. Kato. Fifth International Symposium on Microsomes, Drug Oxidations, and Drug Toxicity, Japan Societies Press, Tokyo. Wiley Interscience, New York.
34. Hayaishi, O. (1962): Oxygenases: History and scope. In: *Oxygenases*, p. 1. Academic Press, New York.
35. Masters, B. S. S., and Okita, R. T. (1982): The history, properties and function of NADPH-cytochrome P-450 reductase. In: *Hepatic Cytochrome P-450 Monooxygenase System*, edited by J. B. Schenkman and D. Kupfer, p. 343. Pergamon Press, New York.
36. Omura, T., Sanders, E., Estabrook, R. W., Cooper, D. Y., and Rosenthal, O. (1966): Isolation from adrenal cortex of a nonheme iron protein and a flavoprotein as a TPNH-cytochrome P-450 reductase. *Arch. Biochem. Biophys.*, 117:660.
37. Ullrich, V. (1979): Cytochrome P-450 and biological hydroxylation reactions. *Topics Current Chem.*, 83:68.
38. White, R. E., and Coon, M. J. (1980): Oxygen activation by cytochrome P-450. *Annu. Rev. Biochem.*, 49:315.
39. Rein, H., and Ristan, O. (1978): The importance of the high spin–low spin equilibrium existing in the cytochrome P-450 for the enzyme mechanism. *Pharmazie*, 33:325.
40. Omura, T., and Sato, R. (1964): The carbon monoxide–binding pigment of liver microsomes. *J. Biol. Chem.*, 239:2370.
41. Gunsalus, I. C., Meeks, J. R., Lipscomb, J. D., De Brunner, P., and Munck, E. (1974): Bacterial monooxygenase-the P-450 cytochrome system. In: *Molecular Mechanisms of Oxygen Activation*, edited by O. Hayaishi, p. 559. Academic Press, New York.
42. Shikita, M., and Hall, P. F. (1973): Cytochrome P-450 from bovine adrenocortical mitochondria: An enzyme for the side-chain cleavage of cholesterol. II. Subunit structure. *J. Biol. Chem.*, 248:5605.
43. Watanuki, M., Granger, G. A., and Hall, P. F. (1978): Cytochrome P-450 from bovine adrenocortical mitochondria: Immunochemical properties and purity. *J. Biol. Chem.*, 253:2927.
44. Tilley, B. E., Watanuki, M., and Hall, P. F. (1977): Preparation and properties of side-chain cleavage cytochrome P-450 from bovine adrenal cortex by affinity chromatography with pregnenolone as ligand. *Biochim. Biophys. Acta*, 493:260.
45. Takemori, S., Sato, H., Gomi, T., Suhara, K., and Katagiri, M. (1975): Purification and properties of cytochrome P-450 11β from adrenocortical mitochondria. *Biochem. Biophys. Res. Commun.*, 67:1151.
46. Ramseyer, J., and Harding, B. W. (1973): Solubilization of adrenal cortical cytochrome P-450 which cleave the cholesterol side-chain. *Biochim. Biophys. Acta*, 315:306.
47. Wang, H. P., and Kimura, T. (1977): Purification of adrenal cortex mitochondrial cytochrome P-450 specific for cholesterol side-chain cleavage activity. *J. Biol. Chem.*, 251:6068.
48. Koritz, S. B., and Hall, P. F. (1964): Feedback inhibition by pregnenolone: A possible mechanism. *Biochim. Biophys. Acta*, 93:215.
49. Hall, P. F., and Koritz, S. B. (1964): Inhibition of the biosynthesis of pregnenolone by 20α-hydroxycholesterol. *Biochim. Biophys. Acta*, 93:441.
50. Burstein, S., and Gut, M. (1976): Intermediates in the conversion of cholesterol to pregnenolone. *Steroids*, 38:115.
51. Duque, C., Morisaki, M., Ikekawa, N., and Shikita, M. (1978): The enzye activity of bovine adrenocortical cytochrome P-450 producing pregnenolone from cholesterol. *Biochem. Biophys. Res. Commun.*, 82:179.
52. Hall, P. F., Lee Lewes, J., and Lipson, E. D. (1975): The role of mitochondrial cytochrome P-450 from bovine adrenal cortex in side-chain cleavage of 20S 22R-dihydroxycholesterol. *J. Biol. Chem.*, 250:2283.
53. Shikita, M., and Hall, P. F. (1974): The stoichiometry of the conversion of cholesterol and hydroxycholesterols to pregnenolone (3β-hydroxypregn-5-en-20-one) catalyzed by adrenal cytochrome P-450. *Proc. Natl. Acad. Sci. USA*, 71:1441.
54. Orme-Johnson, N. R., Light, D. R., White-Stevens, R. W., and Orme-Johnson, W. H. (1979): Steroid-binding properties of beef adrenal cortical cytochrome P-450 which catalyzes conversion of cholesterol to pregnenolone. *J. Biol. Chem.*, 254:2103.
55. Young, D. G., Holroyd, J. D., and Hall, P. F. (1970): Enzymatic and spectral properties of solubilized cytochrome P-450 from bovine adrenocortical mitochondria. *Biochem. Biophys. Res. Commun.*, 38:184.
56. Kido, T., Arakawa, M., and Kimura, T. (1979): Adrenal cortex mitochondrial cytochrome P-450 specific to cholesterol side-chain cleavage reaction. *J. Biol. Chem.*, 254:8377.
57. Tagaki, Y., Shikita, M., and Hall, P. F. (1975): The active form of cytochrome P-450 from bovine adrenocortical mitochondria. *J. Biol. Chem.*, 250:845.
58. Betz, G., Tsai, P., and Weakley, R. (1976): Heterogeneity of cytochrome P-450 in rat testis microsomes. *J. Biol. Chem.*, 251:2839.
59. Nakajin, S., and Hall, P. F. (1981): Microsomal cytochrome P-450 from neonatal pig testis: Purification and properties of a C_{21} steroid side-chain cleavage system (17α-hydroxylase and $C_{17,20}$ lyase). *J. Biol. Chem.*, 256:3871.
60. Nakajin, S., Shively, J., Yuan, P.-M., and Hall, P. F. (1981): Microsomal cytochrome P-450 from neonatal pig testis: Two enzymatic activities (17α-hydroxylase and $C_{17,20}$-lyase) associated with one protein. *Biochemistry*, 20:4037.
61. Bumpus, J. A., and Dus, K. M. (1982): Bovine adrenocortical microsomal hemeproteins P-450 17α and P-450 C_{21}. *J. Biol. Chem.*, 257:12696.
62. Nakajin, S., Shinoda, M., and Hall, P. F. (1983): Purification and properties of 17α-hydroxylase from microsomes of pig adrenal: A second C_{21} side-chain cleavage system. *Biochem. Biophys. Res. Commun.*, 111:512.
63. Nakajin, S., Shinoda, M., Hanui, M., Shively, J. E., and Hall, P. F. (1984): The C_{21} steroid side-chain cleavage enzyme from porcine adrenal microsome: Purification and characterization of the 17α-hydroxylase $C_{17,20}$-lyase cytochrome P-450. *J. Biol. Chem.*, 259:3971.
64. Yanagabashi, K., and Hall, P. F. (1987): Role of electron transport in the regulation of lyase activity of C_{21} side-chain cleavage P-450 from porcine microsomes. *J. Steroid Biochem.* (*in press*).
65. Onoda, M., and Hall, P. F. (1982): Cytochrome b_5 stimulates purified testicular microsomal cytochrome P-450 (C_{21} side-chain cleavage). *Biochem. Biophys. Res. Commun.*, 108:454.
66. Nakajin, S., Hall, P. F., and Onoda, M. (1981): Testicular microsomal cytochrome P-450 for C_{21} steroid side-chain cleavage: Spectral and binding studies. *J. Biol. Chem.*, 256:6134.
67. Sweet, F., Onoda, M., Hall, P. F., Yanagabashi, K., and Shively, J. E. (1985): A P-450 enzyme from fetal pig testis converts progesterone to Δ^4-androstenedione via dual activity at its active site. *J. Biol. Chem.* (in press).
68. Nakajin, S., and Hall, P. F. (1983): Side-chain cleavage of C_{21} steroids by testicular microsomal cytochrome P-450 (17α-hydroxylase/lyase): Involvement of heme. *J. Steroid. Biochem.*, 1:1345.
69. Ford, H. C., and Engel, H. H. (1974): Purification of the Δ^5-3β-hydroxysteroid dehydrogenase-isomerase of sheep adrenal cortical microsomes. *J. Biol. Chem.*, 249:1363.
70. Goldman, A. S. (1968): Further studies of steroidal inhibitors of Δ^5-3β-hydroxysteroid dehydrogenase and Δ^5,Δ^4-3-ketosteroid isomerase

in *Pseudomonas testeroni* and in bovine adrenals. *J. Clin. Endocrinol.*, 18:1539.

71. Talalay, P., and Benson, A. M. (1972): Δ^5-3-Ketosteroid isomerase. In: *The Enzymes,* edited by P. D. Boyer, Vol. 6, p. 591. Academic Press, New York.
72. Penning, T. M., and Covey, D. F. (1982): Inactivation of Δ^5-3-ketosteroid isomerase(s) from beef adrenal cortex by acetylenic ketosteroids. *J. Steroid Biochem.*, 16:691.
73. Samuels, L. T. (1960): Metabolism of steroid hormones: In: *Metabolic Pathways,* edited by D. M. Greenberg, Vol. I, 2d Ed., Academic Press, New York.
74. Oshima, H., and Ochi, A. I. (1973): On testicular 17β-hydroxysteroid oxidoreductase: Product activation. *Biochim. Biophys. Acta,* 306:227.
75. Samuels, L. T., Bussman, L., Matsumoto, K., and Huseby, R. A. (1975): Organization of androgen biosynthesis in the testis. *J. Steroid Biochem.*, 6:291.
76. Bogovich, K., and Payne, A. H. (1980): Purification of rat testicular microsomal 17β-ketosteroid reductase. *J. Biol. Chem.*, 255:5552.
77. Murano, E. P., and Payne, A. H. (1976): Distinct testicular 17β-ketosteroid reductases, one in interstitial tissue and one in seminiferous tubules. *Biophys. Acta,* 450:89.
78. Ohba, H., Inano, H., and Tamaoki, B. (1982): Kinetic mechanism of porcine testicular 17β-hydroxysteroid dehydrogenase. *J. Steroid Biochem.*, 17:381.
79. Bendayan, M. (1984): Protein A–gold electron microscopic immunocytochemistry: Methods, applications and limitations. *J. Electron Microsc.*, 1:243.
80. Gueze, H. J., Slot, J. W., Yanagibashi, K., McCracken, J. A., and Hall, P. F. (1987): Immunoelectron microscopy of cytochromes P-450 in porcine adrenal cortex: Two enzymes (11β-hydroxylase and side-chain cleavage) are co-localized in the same mitochondria. *Histochemistry,* 86:551.
81. Hall, P. F., Watanuki, M., and Hamkalo, B. A. (1979): Adrenocortical cytochrome P-450 side-chain cleavage: Preparation of membrane-bound side-chain cleavage system from purified components. *J. Biol. Chem.*, 254:547.
82. Seybert, D. W., Lancaster, J. R., Lambert, J. D., and Kamin, H. (1979): Participation of the membrane in the side-chain cleavage of cholesterol. *J. Biol. Chem.*, 254:12088.
83. Seybert, D. W., Lambeth, J. D., and Kamin, H. (1978): The participation of a second molecule of adrenodoxin in cytochrome P-450 catalyzed 11β-hydroxylation. *J. Biol. Chem.*, 253:8355.
84. Lambeth, J. D., Seybert, D. W., and Kamin, H. (1979): Ionic effects on adrenal steroidogenic electron transport. *J. Biol. Chem.*, 254:7255.
85. Lambeth, J. D., Seybert, D. W., and Kamin, H. (1980): Phospholipid vesicle–reconstituted cytochrome P-450 SCC. *J. Biol. Chem.*, 255:138.
86. Kimura, T., Parcells, J. H., and Wang, H. (1978): Purification of adrenodoxin, adrenodoxin reductase and cytochrome P-450 from adrenal cortex. *Methods Enzymol.*, LII:132.
87. Ruokenen, A., and Vihko, R. (1974): Concentrations of unconjugated and sulfated neutral sterols in boar testis. *J. Steroid Biochem.*, 5:33.
88. Hall, P. F., Sozer, C. C., and Eik-Nes, K. B. (1964): Formation of dehydroepiandrosterone during *in vivo* and *in vitro* biosynthesis of testosterone by testicular tissue. *Endocrinology,* 74:35.
89. Baskin, L. S., and Yang, S. (1982): Cross-linking studies of the protein topography of rat liver microsomes. *Biochim. Biophys. Acta,* 684:263.
90. Nisimoto, Y., and Lambeth, J. D. (1985): NADPH–cytochrome P-450 reductase–cytochrome b_5 interactions: Crosslinking of the phospholipid vesicle–associated proteins by a water-soluble carbodiimide. *Arch. Biochem. Biophys.* 241:386.
91. Lambeth, J. D., Green, L. M., and Millett, F. (1984): Adrenodoxin interaction with adrenodoxin reductase and cytochrome P-450 SCC. *J. Biol. Chem.*, 259:10025
92. Welton, A. F., and Aust, S. D. (1974): The effects of 3-methylcholanthrene on the structure of the rat liver endoplasmic reticulum. *Biochim. Biophys. Acta,* 373:197.
93. Samuels, L. T., and Matsumoto, K. (1974): Localization of enzymes involved in testosterone biosynthesis in mouse testis. *Endocrinology,* 94:55.
94. Matsumoto, K., and Samuels, L. T. (1969): Influence of steroid distribution between microsomes and soluble fraction on steroid metabolism by microsomal enzymes. *Endocrinology,* 85:402.
95. Nakajin, S., and Hall, P. F. (1981): Side-chain cleavage of C_{21} steroids to C_{19} steroids by testicular microsomal cytochrome P-450: 17α-hydroxy C_{21} steroids as obligatory intermediates. *J. Steroid Biochem.*, 14:1249.
96. Tamaoki, B., and Shikita, M. (1966): Biosynthesis of steroids in testicular tissue *in vitro*. In: *Steroid Dynamics,* edited by G. Pincus, J. Tait, and T. Nakano, p. 493. Academic Press, New York.
97. Estabrook, R. W., Frankle, M. R., Cohen, B., Shigamatzu, A., and Hildebrandt, A. G. (1971): Influence of hepatic microsomal mixed function oxidation on cellular metabolism. *Metabolism,* 20:187.
98. Wu, E. S., Tank, D. W., and Webb, W. W. (1982): Unconstrained lateral diffusion of ConA receptos in bulbous lymphocytes. *Proc. Natl. Acad. Sci. USA,* 79:4962.
99. Hochman, J. H., Schindler, M., Lee, J. G., and Ferguson-Miller, S. (1982): Lateral mobility of cytochrome C in intact mitochondrial membranes as determined by fluorescence redistribution after photobleaching. *Proc. Natl. Acad. Sci. USA,* 79:6866.
100. Peterson, J. A., Ebel, R. E., O'Keefe, D. H., Matsubara, T., and Estrabrook, R. W. (1976): Temperature dependence of cytochrome P-450 reduction. *J. Biol. Chem.*, 251:4010.
101. Dean, W. L., and Gray, R. D. (1983): Relationship between state of aggregation and catalytic activity of P-450 LM_2 and P-450 reductase. *J. Biol. Chem.*, 257:14679.
102. Li, C. H., and Evans, H. M. (1948): Chemistry of anterior pituitary hormones. In: *The Hormones,* edited by G. Pincus and K. Thimann, Vol. 1, p. 631. Academic Press, New York.
103. Hall, P. F., and Eik-Nes, K. B. (1962): The action of gonadotropic hormones upon rabbit testis *in vitro*. *Biochim. Biophys. Acta,* 63:411.
104. Hall, P. F., and Eik-Nes, K. B. (1963): The influence of gonadotropins *in vivo* upon the biosynthesis of androgens by homogenate of rat testis. *Biochim. Biophys. Acta,* 71:438.
105. Hall, P. F. (1966): On the stimulation of testicular steroidogenesis in the rabbit by interstitial cell–stimulating hormone. *Endocrinology,* 78:690.
106. Hall, P. F., and Young, D. G. (1968): Site of action of trophic hormones upon the biosynthetic pathways to steroid hormones. *Endocrinology,* 82:559.
107. Mori, M., and Marsh, J. M. (1982): The site of LH stimulation of steroidogenesis in mitochondria of the rat corpus luteum. *J. Biol. Chem.*, 257:6178.
108. Garren, L. D., Ney, R. H., and Davis, W. W. (1965): Studies on the role of protein synthesis in the regulation of corticosterone production by ACTH *in vivo*. *Proc. Natl. Acad. Sci. USA,* 53:1443.
109. Hall, P. F., Charponnier, C., Nakamura, M., and Gabbiani, G. (1979): The role of microfilaments in the response of adrenal tumor cells to adrenocorticotropic hormone. *J. Biol. Chem.*, 254:9080.
110. Crivello, J. F., and Jefcoate, C. R. (1980): Intramitochondrial movement of cholesterol in rat adrenal cells. *J. Biol. Chem.*, 255:8144.
111. Dufau, M. L., and Catt, K. J. (1975): Gonadotropic stimulation of interstitial cell functions of the rat testis *in vitro*. In: *Methods in Enzymology XXXIX,* edited by J. G. Hardman and B. W. O'Malley, p. 252. Academic Press, New York.
112. Hall, P. F., Charponnier, C., Nakamura, M., and Gabbiani, G. (1979): The role of microfilaments in the response of Leydig cells to luteinizing hormone. *J. Steroid Biochem.*, 11:1361.
113. Bell, J. J., and Harding, B. (1974): The acute action of ACTH on adrenal steroidogenesis. *Biochim. Biophys. Acta,* 348:285.
114. Hall, P. F. (1985): Trophic stimulation of steroidogenesis. In: *Search of the Elusive Trigger,* edited by R. O. Greep, p. 41. Laurentian Hormone Conference, Academic Press, New York.
115. Sandler, R., and Hall, P. F. (1968): The influence of age upon the response of rat testis to intestitial cell–stimulating hormone *in vitro*. *Biochim. Biophys. Acta,* 164:445.
116. Marsh, J. M. (1976): The role of cyclic AMP in gonadal steroidogenesis. *Biol. Reprod.*, 14:30.
117. Schimmer, B. P. (1980): Cyclic nucleotides in hormonal regulation of adrenocortical function. *Adv. Cyclic Nucleotide Res.*, 13:181.
118. Moyle, W. R., Kong, Y. C., and Ramachandran, J. (1973): Steroidogenesis and cylic AMP accummulation in rat adrenal cells. *J. Biol. Chem.*, 248:2409.

119. Perchellet, J. P., Shanker, G., and Sharma, R. K. (1977): Regulatory role of cyclic GMP in ACTH-induced steroidogenesis. *Science,* 199:311.
120. Themen, A. P. N., Hoogerbrugge, J. W., Rommerts, F. F. G., and Van der Molen, H. J. (1985): Is cAMP the obligatory second messenger in the action of lutropin on Leydig cell steroidogenesis? *Biochem. Biophys. Res. Commun.,* 128:1164.
121. Dufau, M. L., Tsuruhara, T., Horner, K. A., Podesta, E., and Catt, K. J. (1977): Intermediate role of cyclic AMP and protein kinase during gonadotropin-induced steroidogenesis in Leydig cells. *Proc. Natl. Acad. Sci. USA,* 74:3419.
122. Dufau, M. L., Baukal, A. J., and Catt, K. J. (1980): Hormone-induced guanyl nucleotide binding and activation of adenylate cyclase in the Leydig cell. *Proc. Natl. Acad. Sci. USA,* 77:5837.
123. Schimmer, B. P., Tsao, J., Collie, G., Wong, M., and Schulz, P. (1984): Analysis of the mutation to forskolin-resistance in Y-1 adrenocortical tumor cells. *Endocr. Res.,* 10:365.
124. Irby, D. C., and Hall, P. F. (1971): Stimulation by ICSH of protein biosynthesis in isolated Leydig cells from hypophysectomized rats. *Endocrinology,* 89:1367.
125. Janszen, F. H. A., Cooke, B. A., and Van der Molen, H. J. (1977): Specific protein synthesis in isolated rat Leydig cells. Influence of LH and cycloheximide. *Biochem. J.,* 162:341.
126. Krueger, R. J., and Orme-Johnson, N. R. (1983): Active ACTH stimulation of adrenal corticosteroidogenesis. Discovery of a rapidly induced protein. *J. Biol. Chem.,* 258:10159.
127. Pedersen, R. C., and Brownie, A. C. (1983): Cholesterol side-chain cleavage in the rat adrenal cortex: Isolation of a cycloheximide-sensitive activator protein. *Proc. Natl. Acad. Sci. USA,* 80:1882.
128. Birmingham, M. K., Elliott, F. H., and Valere, P. H. L. (1953): The need for the presence of Ca^{2+} for the stimulation *in vitro* of rat adrenal glands by ACTH. *Endocrinology,* 53:687.
129. Hall, P. F., Osawa, S., and Mrotek, J. J. (1981): Influence of calmodulin on steroid synthesis in Leydig cells from rat testis. *Endocrinology,* 109:1677.
130. Conn, P. M., Chafouleas, J. G., Rogers, D., and Means, A. R. (1981): Gonadotropin releasing hormone stimulates calmodulin redistribution in rat pituitary. *Nature,* 292:264.
131. Cheitlin, R., Buckley, D. I., and Ramachandran, J. (1985): The role of extracellular calcium in corticotropin stimulated steroidogenesis. *J. Biol. Chem.,* 260:5327.
132. Kuo, J. F., and Greengard, P. (1969): Cyclic nucleotide–dependent kinase: Widespread occurrence of cyclic AMP–dependent protein kinase. *Proc. Natl. Acad. Sci. USA,* 64:1349.
133. Cooke, B. A., Lindh, M. L., and Janszen, F. H. A. (1977): Effect of lutropin on phosphorylation of endogenous proteins in testis Leydig cells. *Biochem. J.,* 168:43.
134. Neymark, M. A., Bieszczad, R. R., and Dimino, M. J. (1984): Phosphorylation of mitochondrial proteins in isolated porcine follicles after treatment with LH. *Endocrinology,* 114:588.
135. Inaba, T., and Wiest, W. G. (1985): Protein kinase stimulation of steroidogenesis in rat luteal cell mitochondria. *Endocrinology,* 117:315.
136. Michell, R. H. (1980): Phosphoinositide breakdown as the initiating reaction in receptor-stimulated inositol phospholipid metabolism. *Life Sci.,* 32:2083.
137. Berridge, M. J., Dawson, R. M. C., Downes, C. P., Heslop, J. P., and Irvine, R. F. (1983): Changes in levels of inositol phosphates after agonist-dependent hydrolysis of membrane phosphoinositide. *Biochem. J.,* 212:473.
138. Dawson, A. P., and Irvine, R. F. (1984): Inositol(1,4,5)triphosphate-promoted Ca^{2+} release from microsomal fractions of rat liver. *Biochem. Biophys. Res. Commun.,* 120:858.
139. Burgess, G. M., Godfrey, P. P., McKinney, J. S., Berridge, M. J., Irvine, R. F., and Putney, J. W. (1984): The second messenger linking receptor activation to internal Ca release in liver. *Nature,* 309:63.
140. Somlyo, A. P. (1984): Cellular site of calcium regulation. *Nature,* 309:516.
141. Mishizuka, Y., Takai, Y., Kishimoto, A., Kikkawa, Y., and Kaibuchi, K. (1984): Phospholipid turnover in hormone action. *Recent Prog. Horm. Res.,* 40:301.
142. Williamson, J. R., Cooper, R. H., Joseph, S. K. and Thomas, A. (1985): Inositol triphosphate and diacylglycerol as intracellular second messengers in liver. *Am. J. Physiol.,* 248:C203.
143. Nishizuka, Y. (1984): The role of protein kinase C in cell surface signal transduction and tumor promotion. *Nature,* 308:693.
144. Uhing, R. J., Jiang, H., Popic, V., and Exton, J. H. (1985): Regulation of a liver plasma membrane phosphoinositide by guanine nucleotides and calcium. *FEBS Lett.,* 188:317.
145. Farese, R. V., Sabir, M. A., Vendor, S. L., and Larson, R. E. (1980): Are phosphoinositides the cycloheximide-sensitive actions of ACTH and cyclic AMP? *J. Biol. Chem.,* 255:5728.
146. Farese, R. V., Sabir, M. A., Larson, R. E., and Trudeau, W. III. (1983): Further observations on the increases in inositide phospholipids after stimulation by ACTH, cyclic AMP and insulin. *Cell Calcium,* 4:195.
147. Lowitt, S., Farese, R. V., Sabir, M. A., and Root, A. W. (1982): Rat Leydig cell phospholipid content is increased by LH and 8-bromo-cyclic AMP. *Endocrinology,* 111:1415.
148. Farese, R. V. (1984): Phospholipids as intermediates in hormone action. *Mol. Cell. Endocrinol.,* 35:1.
149. Iida, S., Widmaier, E., and Hall, P. F. (1986): The phosphoinositide-Ca^{2+} hypothesis does not apply to the steroidogenic action of ACTH. *Biochem. J.,* 236:53.
150. Kimura, K., Katoh, N., Sakurada, K., and Kubo, S. (1984): Phospholipid-sensitive Ca^{2+}-dependent protein kinase system in testis. *Endocrinology,* 115:2391.
151. Lin, T. (1985): The role of Ca^{2+}/phospholipid-dependent protein kinase in Leydig cell steroidogenesis. *Endocrinology,* 117:119.
152. Moger, W. H. (1985): Stimulation and inhibition of Leydig cell steroidogenesis by the phorbol ester 12-0-tetradecanoylphorbol-13-acetate. *Life Sci.,* 37:869.
153. Widmaier, E. P., and Hall, P. F. (1985): Protein kinase C in adrenal cells: Possible role in regulation of steroid synthesis. *Mol. Cell. Endocrinol.,* 43:181.
154. Sharpe, R. M. (1984): Intratesticular factors controlling testicular function. *Biol. Reprod.,* 30:29.
155. Sharpe, R. M. (1985): Intratesticular regulation of testosterone secretion: Comparison of the effects and interactions of hCG and LHRH agonist and testicular interstitial fluid. *Mol. Cell. Endocrinol.,* 41:247.
156. Eik-Nes, K. B. (1969): Factors controlling the secretion of testicular steroids in the dog. *Gen. Comp. Endocrinol.* (Suppl.) 2:87.
157. Clark, M. R., Marsh, J. M., and LeMaire, W. J. (1978): Mechanism of LH regulation of prostaglandin synthesis in rat granulosa cells. *J. Biol. Chem.,* 253:7757.
158. Schramm, W., Bovaird, L., Glew, M. E., Schramm, G. S., and McCracken, J. (1983): Corpus luteal regression induced by ultra-low pulses of $PGF_{2\alpha}$. *Prostaglandins,* 26:347.
159. Eik-Nes, K. B. (1964): On the relationship between testicular blood flow and the secretion of testosterone in anesthetized dogs. *Can. J. Physiol. Pharmacol.,* 42:671.
160. Eik-Nes, K. B. (1969): An effect of isoproterenol on rates of synthesis and secretion of testosterone. *Am. J. Physiol.,* 217:1764.
161. Eik-Nes, K. B. (1971): Production and secretion of testicular steroids. *Rec. Prog. Horm. Res.,* 27:517.
162. Amsterdam, A., Naor, Z., Knecht, M., Dufau, M. L., and Catt, K. J. (1981): Hormone action and receptor redistribution in endocrine target cells. In: *Receptor Mediated Binding and Internalization of Toxins and Hormones,* edited by J. L. Middlebrook and L. D. Kohn, p. 61. Academic Press, New York.
163. Aubry, M., Collu, R., Ducharme, J. R., and Crine, P. (1982): Biosynthesis of a putative gonadotropin receptor component by rat Leydig cells. *Endocrinology,* 111:2129.
164. Dufau, M. L., Horner, K. A., Hayashi, K., Tsuruhara, T., Conn, P. M., and Catt, K. J. (1978): Actions of choleragen and gonadotropin in isolated Leydig cells. *J. Biol. Chem.,* 253:3721.
165. Dufau, M. L., Baukal, A. J., and Catt, K. J. (1980): Hormone-induced guanyl nucleotide binding and activation of adenylate kinase in the Leydig cell. *Proc. Natl. Acad. Sci. USA,* 77:5837.
166. Dufau, M. L., Winters, C. A., Hattori, M., Aquilano, D., Baranao, J. L. S., Nozu, K., Baukal, A., and Catt, K. J. (1984): Hormonal regulation of androgen production by the Leydig cell. *J. Steroid Biochem.,* 20:161.
167. Dufau, M. L., Baukal, A. J., Winters, C. A., and Catt, K. J. (1982): Guanyl nucleotide–induced phosphorylation of Leydig cell membrane protein. *Endocrinology,* 110:256.

168. Barano, J. L., and Dufau, M. L. (1983): Gonadotropin-induced changes in the LH receptors of cultured Leydig cells; evidence for up-regulation *in vitro*. *J. Biol. Chem.*, 258:7322.
169. Freeman, D. A., and Ascoli, M. (1981): Desensitization to gonadotropin receptors. *Proc. Natl. Acad. Sci. USA*, 75:6309.
170. Freeman, D. A., and Ascoli, M. (1982): Desensitization of steroidogenesis in cultured Leydig tumor cells: Role of cholesterol. *Proc. Natl. Acad. Sci. USA*, 79:7796.
171. Ezra, E., and Salomon, Y. (1980): Mechanism of desensitization of adenylate cyclase by lutropin. *J. Biol. Chem.*, 255:653.
172. Rebois, R. V., and Fishman, P. H. (1984): Down-regulation of gonadotropin receptors in a murine Leydig cell tumor. *J. Biol. Chem.*, 259:3096.
173. Quinn, P. G., Dombrausky, L. J., Chen, Y.-D. I., and Payne, A. H. (1981): Serum lipoproteins increase testosterone production in hCG-desensitized Leydig cells. *Endocrinology*, 109:1790.
174. Charreau, E. H., Calvo, J. C., Nozu, K., Pignataro, O., Catt, K. J., and Dufau, M. L. (1981): Hormonal modulation of HMG CoA reductase in desensitized Leydig cells. *J. Biol. Chem.*, 256:12719.
175. Quinn, P. G., and Payne, A. H. (1985): Steroid product–induced, oxygen-mediated damage of microsomal cytochrome P-450 enzymes in Leydig cell cultures. *J. Biol. Chem.*, 260:2092.
176. Chasalow, F., Marr, H., Haour, F., and Saez, J. M. (1979): Testicular steroidogenesis after hCG desensitization in rats. *J. Biol. Chem.*, 254:5613.
177. Cigorraga, S. B., Dufau, M. L., and Catt, K. J. (1978): Regulation of LH receptors and steroidogenesis in gonadotropin-desensitized Leydig cells. *J. Biol. Chem.*, 253:4297.
178. Catt, K. J., Harwood, J. P., Clayton, R. N., Davies, T. F., Chan, V., Katikineni, M., Nozu, K., and Dufau, M. L. (1980): Regulation of peptide hormone receptors and gonadal steroidogenesis. *Recent Prog. Horm. Res.*, 36:557.
179. Tycko, B., Keith, C. H., and Maxfield, F. R. (1983): Rapid acidification of endocytic vesicles containing asialoglycoprotein in cells of a human hepatoma line. *J. Cell. Biol.*, 97:1762.
180. Steinman, R. M., Mellman, I. S., Muller, W. A., and Cohn, Z. A. (1983): Endocytosis and the recycling of plasma membrane. *J. Cell Biol.*, 96:1.
181. Guillou, F., Martinat, N., and Combarnous, Y. (1985): Rapid *in vitro* desensitization in rat Leydig cells by subactive concentrations of porcine LH. *FEBS Lett.*, 184:6.
182. Dix, C. J., Habberfield, D., and Cooke, B. A. (1984): Characterization of the homologous and heterologous desensitization of rat Leydig-tumor-cell adenylate cyclase. *Biochem. J.*, 220:803.
183. Hornsby, P. J., and Crivello, J. F. (1983): The role of lipid peroxidation and biological antioxidants in the function of the adrenal cortex. Part 1. *Mol. Cell. Endocrinol.*, 30:1.
184. Hornsby, P. J., and Crivello, J. F. (1983): The role of lipid peroxidation and biological antoxidants in the function of the adrenal cortex. Part 2. *Mol. Cell. Endocrinol.*, 30:123.
185. Crivello, J. F., Hornsby, P. J., and Gill, G. N. (1982): Metyrapone and antioxidants are required to maintain aldosterone synthesis by cultured bovine adrenocortical zona glomerulosa cells. *Endocrinology*, 111:469.
186. Nozu, K., Dufau, M. L., and Catt, K. J. (1981): Estradiol-receptor mediated regulation of steroidogenesis in gonadotropin-desensitized Leydig cells. *J. Biol. Chem.*, 256:1915.
187. Onoda, M., and Hall, P. F. (1981): Inhibition of testicular microsomal cytochrome P-450 (17α-hydroxylase/$C_{17,20}$-lyase) by estrogens. *Endocrinology*, 109:763.
188. Nozu, K., Dehejia, A., Zawistowich, L., Catt, K. J., and Dufau, M. L. (1981): Gonadotropin-induced receptor regulation in cultured Leydig cells. *J. Biol. Chem.*, 256:12875.
189. Nozu, K., Dehejia, A., Zawistowich, L., Catt, K. J., and Dufau, M. L. (1982): Gonadotropin-induced desensitization of Leydig cells *in vivo* and *in vitro*. *Ann. N.Y. Acad. Sci.*, 383:230.
190. Johnson, A. D. (1979): Testicular lipids. In: *The Testis*, edited by A. D. Johnson, N. L. Gomes, and N. L. Van Demark, Vol. 2, p. 193. Academic Press, New York.
191. Ohno, Y., Yanagibashi, K., Yonezawa, Y., Ishiwatari, S., and Matsuba, M. (1983): Effect of ACTH, cycloheximide and aminoglutethimide on the content of cholesterol in the outer and inner mitochondrial membrane of rat adrenal cortex. *Endocrinol. Jpn.*, 30:335.
192. Privalle, C. T., Crivello, J. F., and Jefcoate, C. R. (1983): Regulation of intramitochondrial cholesterol side-chain cleavage P-450 in rat adrenal gland. *Proc. Natl. Acad. Sci. USA*, 80:702.
193. Clegg, J. S. (1982): Interrelationships between water and cell metabolism in Artemia cysts. *Cold Spring Harbor Symp. Quant. Biol.*, 46:23.
194. Wolosewick, J. J., and Porter, K. R. (1979): Microtrabecular lattice of the cytoplasmic ground substance. Artifact or reality. *J. Cell Biol.*, 82:114.
195. Gershon, N. D., Porter, K. R., and Trus, B. L. (1985): The cytoplasmic matrix: Its volume and surface area and the diffusion of molecules through it. *Proc. Natl. Acad. Sci. USA*, 82:5030.
196. Clegg, J. S. (1984): Properties and metabolism of the aqueous cytoplasm and its boundaries. *Am. J. Physiol.*, 246:R133.
197. Ottaway, J. H., and Mowbray, J. (1977): The role of compartmentation in the regulation of glycolysis. *Curr. Topics Cell. Regul.*, 12:108.
198. Lazarides, E. (1980): Intermediate filaments as mechanical integrates of cellular space. *Nature*, 283:249.
199. Hall, P. F. (1984): The role of cytoskeleton in hormone action. *Can. J. Biochem. Cell Biol.*, 62:653.
200. Hall, P. F. (1982): The role of the cytoskeleton in endocrine function. In: *Cellular Regulation of Secretion and Release*, edited by M. P. Conn, p. 195. Academic Press, New York.
201. Hall, P. F. (1984): The role of the cytoskeleton in the responses of target cells to hormones. In: *Regulation of Target Cell Responsiveness*, edited by K. W. McKerns, A. Aakvaag, and V. Hansson, Vol. 1, p. 205. Plenum, New York.
202. Osawa, S., Betz, G., and Hall, P. F. (1984): The role of actin in the responses of adrenal cells to ACTH and cyclic AMP: Inhibition by DNase I. *J. Cell Biol.*, 989:1335.
203. Allen, R. D., Travis, J. L., Allen, N. S., and Yilmaz, H. (1981): Video-enhanced contrast polarization (AVEC-POL) microscopy. *Cell Motil.*, 1:275.
204. Tonutti, E. (1954): Zur morphokinese sekretorisch tatiger Gewebe. *Verhndl. Anat. Ges.*, p. 125.
205. Liu, S. L. (1960): Histophotometrical study of the effect of 1CSH on the deoxyribonucleic acid content of the testicular interstitial cell nucleus. *Nature*, 186:475.
206. Reddy, P. R. K., and Villee, C. (1975): Messenger RNA synthesis in the testis of immature rats: Effect of gonadotropins and cyclic AMP. *Biochem. Biophys. Res. Commun.*, 63:1063.
207. Mendelson, C., Dufau, M. L., and Catt, K. J. (1975): Dependence of gonadotropin-induced steroidogenesis on RNA and protein synthesis in the interstitial cells of the rat testis. *Biochim. Biophys. Acta*, 411:222.
208. Williams, C. D., Horner, A. K., and Catt, K. J. (1979): Effects of methylxanthines on gonadotropin-induced steroidogenesis and protein synthesis in isolated testis interstitial cells. *Endocr. Res. Commun.*, 6:343.
209. Cooke, B. A., Janzen, F. H. A., and Van Oriel, M. J. A. (1978): Inhibition of Leydig cell steroidogenesis: Effect of actinomycin D before and after preincubation of Leydig cells *in vitro*. *Int. J. Androl.* (Suppl.) 2:1.
210. Valladares, L. E., and Ronco, A. M. (1984): Effect of LH on RNA synthesis in Leydig cells of immature rats. *J. Steroid Biochem.*, 21:443.
211. Samuels, L. T., and Helmreich, M. L. (1956): The influence of hCG on the 3β-ol dehydrogenase activity of testes and adrenals. *Endocrinology*, 58:435.
212. Anderson, C. M., and Mendelson, C. R. (1985): Regulation of steroidogenesis in rat Leydig cells in culture. *Arch. Biochem. Biophys.*, 238:378.
213. Funkenstein, B., Waterman, M. R., and Simpson, E. R. (1984): Induction of synthesis of cholesterol scc cytochrome P-450 and adrenodoxin by FSH, 8-bromocyclic AMP and LDL in cultured bovine adrenal cells. *J. Biol. Chem.*, 259:8572.
214. Payne, A. H., Quinn, P. G., and Rani, C. S. S. (1984): Regulation of microsomal cytochrome P-450 enzymes and testosterone production in Leydig cells. *Recent Prog. Horm. Res.*, 41:153.

The Physiology of Reproduction,
edited by E. Knobil and J. Neill *et al.*
Raven Press, Ltd., New York © 1988.

CHAPTER 23

Efferent Ducts, Epididymis, and Vas Deferens: Structure, Functions, and Their Regulation

Bernard Robaire and Louis Hermo

After the milestone contributions of Benoit in 1926 (1) and Young between 1929 and 1931 (2–4), relatively little attention, until the 1960s, was paid to studies of the structure and functions of the testicular excurrent duct system, i.e., efferent ducts, epididymis, and vas deferens. At this time, Mann (5) referred to the epididymis as the abandoned child of the reproductive system. In the mid- and late 1960s a resurgence of interest in the epididymis was spearheaded by Orgebin-Crist's (6,7) and Bedford's (8) demonstrations that spermatozoa did, in fact, mature, i.e., acquire the ability to swim and fertilize eggs, by passing through this tissue. These workers established the fact that the key event in spermatozoal maturation was not the passage of time, but rather exposure to the luminal environment of the epididymis. In 1972, one of the first detailed modern reviews on the structure of the mammalian epididymis was written (9). Research on the histological and functional properties of this tissue expanded rapidly so that by 1975 a series of major comprehensive reviews were published by Hamilton (10), Orgebin-Crist et al. (11), Bedford (12), and Neaves (13) in *Handbook of Physiology: Endocrinology, Male Reproductive System.* Since 1975 various other facets of the histology, physiology, biochemistry, and pharmacology of the excurrent ducts have appeared (14–21).

During the past decade an average of somewhat over 250 publications per year relating to the epididymis and vas deferens have been published. The objective of the present chapter is not to present a comprehensive review of all of the information about this tissue. Rather, we focus on some of the highlights of the structure of this tissue, at the light and electron microscopic levels, and emphasize facets of its functions and regulation of those functions that we perceive to be of more general importance, or particularly novel. A number of areas, e.g., pathological states of the epididymis, vasculature, and innervation of this tissue, are not discussed.

Although the excurrent duct systems of a large number of mammalian and nonmammalian species have been studied in the last decade, the rat has been used most frequently for histological, endocrinological, and biochemical studies. The differences between the rat and other mammals do not appear to be qualitative in nature. Hence, we have elected to describe, primarily, work done with the rat, unless explicitly stated otherwise. We begin with a brief description of Bedford's major contribution to our understanding of the evolution of the epididymis (22), and follow with a short description of the key facets of the development of this tissue.

EVOLUTIONARY PERSPECTIVES

In order to better understand the complex events taking place in the epithelium and in the lumen of the excurrent ducts of eutherian mammals, it is helpful to obtain an appreciation of when and how these functions evolved. Relatively little work has been done on comparative studies of the histology, biochemistry, and physiology of the epididymides in different species. However, in the mid- and late 1970s, Bedford and his colleagues (22–26) addressed themselves to the question of when, during evolution, the major functions that take place in the epididymal lumen, i.e., acquisition of motility and fertilizing ability of spermatozoa, were acquired. Though the available data remain scanty, some general conclusions about the evolution of certain epididymal functions have become clear.

A simple excurrent duct is found in fish (27). The apparent sole function of the excurrent ducts in most fish is that of transport of spermatozoa, since sperm coming out of the testis are fully functional (27). The skate, an elasmobranch, seems to be one of the first vertebrates where a function, i.e., the acquisition of sperm motility, occurs in the excurrent ducts (22). Birds (28–30) and reptiles, e.g., snakes (31), have a clearly defined structure that can be defined as an epididymis. In birds and reptiles, the epididymis also functions as a sperm transport duct and the site where motility of spermatozoa is acquired. Detailed studies on the lizard by Gigon and associates (32,33) have demonstrated that the epididymis actively secretes proteins under the control of androgens in this species. Because of the rapid passage of spermatozoa through the epididymis in these species, the acquisition of fertilizing potential has not been demonstrated to be dependent on the epithelial cell activity of the excurrent ducts.

In mammals, an increase in the complexity of the epididymis itself and of the functions it carries out has been reported (22). In monotreme mammals, such as the echidna (ant-eater), the epididymis is a fairly simple duct whose functions, like in birds, are limited to sperm transport and acquisition of sperm motility (25). The complex of epididymal functions that are described below appears first in marsupials (26) and is maintained in all higher mammals. Bedford suggests that the increase in epididymal functions coincides with the greater complexity of the spermatozoa themselves, and proposes the hypothesis that it is because of parallel changes in the females of the species that there is a need for this increase in complexity of epididymal function (22).

DEVELOPMENTAL PATTERN OF THE EXCURRENT DUCT SYSTEM

The efferent ducts, epididymis, vas deferens, and seminal vesicles are generally considered to be of mesonephric (Wolffian) duct origin, with the former two arising from the upper segment, the vas deferens from the middle segment, and the seminal vesicles from the lower segment (20). These tissues develop during gestation under the influence of testosterone and not dihydrotestosterone (34,35). A detailed description of the embryology of the reproductive system and of its hormonal control is in Chapters 1 and 8 (*these volumes*). There are, however, two facets of these tissues' development that should be highlighted here.

The first is that the common mesonephric origin of the epididymis and the kidney may, in large part, provide the necessary clues to allow us to understand the regulatory processes that create the highly complex and changing luminal constituents of the excurrent duct system. Recent studies have not only shown that there are ionic gradients in the epididymis analogous to those of the kidney (36,37) (see later section on ions in lumen), but also that hormones previously not thought to affect the epididymis but affecting the kidney, e.g., vitamin D (38,39) and prolactin (40), do have specific epididymal receptors and probably play a significant role in this tissue.

The second is based on studies using a strain of rats in which 10 to 15% of the animals are deficient in tissues arising from the mesonephric tubules: the ACI rats (41). On the side where these animals have no kidney, they are also expectedly missing the seminal vesicles, vas deferens, and part of the epididymis (42,43). It is interesting to note, however, that the efferent ducts and a proximal portion of the epididymis are still present in these animals; this led these investigators to propose that these regions of the excurrent system originate from the mesonephric tubules rather than the mesonephric ducts (43).

Thus, the common embryological origin of the kidney and epididymis should provide, thanks to the extensive studies that have been done on the kidney, clues to the normal functioning of parts of the testicular excurrent duct system.

After birth, in the rat, the epididymis goes though a phase of relatively slow growth (weight gain) followed by a rapid growth spurt associated with the onset of Leydig cell function and appearance of spermatozoa (44–48). The postnatal development of the epithelium of the epididymis of the rat has also been studied extensively (49–51). (These studies and the age at which spermatozoa first appear in the rat epididymis are discussed later.) The parallel changes in the chemical make-up of the epididymal lumen are largely unresolved with the notable exception of changes in the concentration of androgen-binding protein (ABP) (52–55). Though much less detailed information has been gathered about the postnatal development of the epididymis in other species, data on the cock (56), ram (57), calf (58), rabbit (59), and human (60) indicate that there are similar changes to those obtained with the rat.

BICOMPARTMENTAL NATURE OF THE EXCURRENT DUCT SYSTEM

The ductal nature of the excurrent duct system ideally lends itself to being divided into two compartments: the epithelium and the lumen.

The general histology of the epithelial lining of the duct followed by a detailed description at the electron microscopic level of each of the major cell types and of the blood-epididymis barrier is presented. The functions carried out by this epithelium, i.e., absorption, secretion, metabolism, and spermiophagy, are then discussed.

The constituents of the luminal compartment and how these constituents change as one moves from the efferent ducts through the different segments of the epididymis and finally into the vas deferens are described, as are the three functions taking place within the luminal compartment, i.e., sperm transport, acquisition of fertilizing ability (maturation), and storage.

Epithelial Compartment

Anatomy and Histology

Anatomy. The efferent ducts (ductuli efferentes) are a series of tubules that arise from the rete testis; depending on the species, the number varies from four to 20 (61,62). These tubules come together to form a single highly convoluted duct, the epididymis (from the Greek, meaning adjacent to the testis) that is extremely long and varies from 3 to 4 m in man to 80 m in horses (63).

The epididymis is usually divided into three gross anatomical segments: head (caput), body (corpus), and tail (cauda). Benoit (1) introduced the concept of an initial segment, between the efferent ducts and the caput epididymidis, that has a characteristic histological appearance; this region was found in an array of species (1). Subsequently, a number of other schemes has been proposed for dividing the epididymis into different segments (64–69). In the present chapter, we refer to the epididymis as being divided into an initial segment, the caput, the corpus, and the cauda. The extension of the epididymis is a straight tube, the vas deferens, which is surrounded by a very thick muscular layer. The vas deferens connects with the urethra which empties to the outside of the body. A schematic representation of the testis, efferent ducts, epididymis, and vas deferens is shown in Fig. 1.

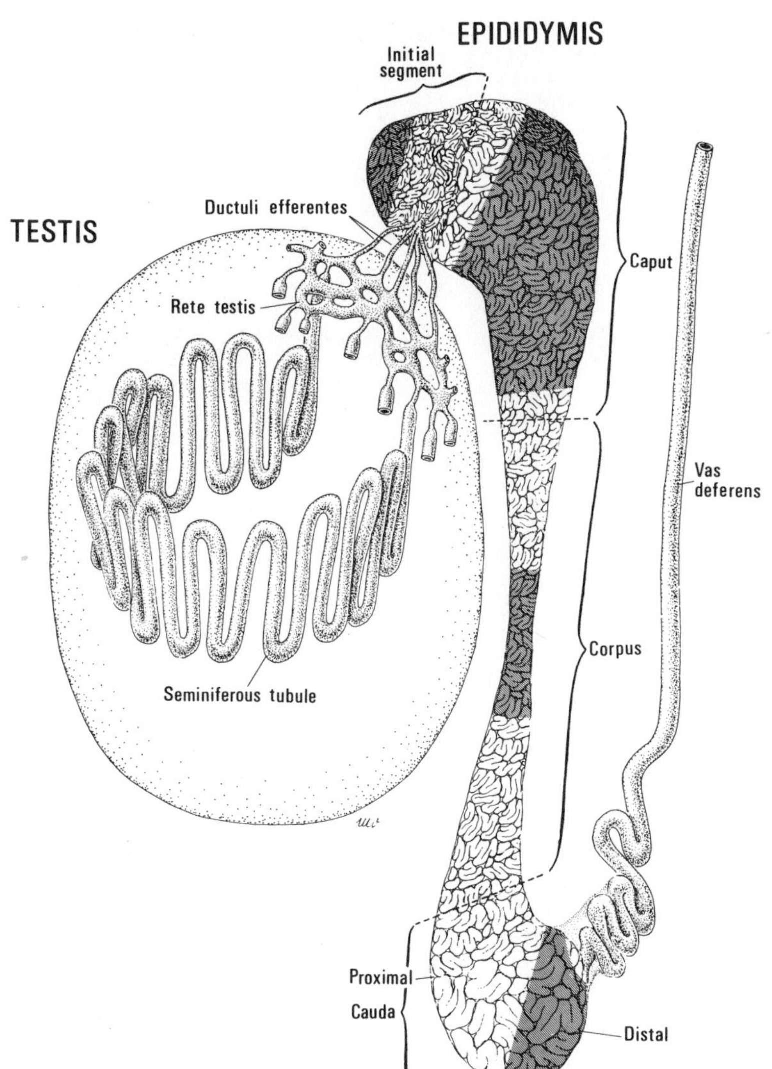

FIG. 1. Diagrammatic representation of the testis showing a seminiferous tubule and the rete testis, the ductuli efferentes, the epididymis, and vas deferens. The *shaded regions* indicate areas of the different segments of the epididymis, i.e., the initial segment, caput, corpus, and proximal and distal cauda, where data on the relative quantitative distribution of the major different epithelial cell types were obtained.

Histology: Light microscopy. Detailed descriptions of the appearance, at the light microscopic level, of the efferent ducts, the epididymis, and the vas deferens, for a number of species ranging from the mouse to man and including dog, camel, elephant, opossum, and monkey are available (1,10,57,61,66,69–86). There are few differences in the light microscopic appearance of the excurrent duct system of different mammalian species, and hence only a brief description of this tissue, as it appears in the adult rat, is given here.

Efferent Ducts: The delineation between the rete testis and the efferent ducts is a very sharp one (66) as can be seen in Fig. 2. The cell height increases dramatically from low cuboidal in the rete testis to tall columnar in the efferent ducts. Within the efferent ducts, there is a major difference in appearance between the initial and terminal zones (66). Though both regions contain columnar ciliated and nonciliated epithelial cells, the nonciliated cells of the initial zone have a supranuclear region filled with moderately stained granules (Fig. 3); in the terminal zone, the supranuclear region of these cells contains numerous dark granules (Fig. 4). The reasons for this difference are discussed below when the individual cell types are described. The ciliated cells are recognized by their deeper staining appearance, the apical position of their nuclei, and long cilia (Figs. 3 and 4). Halo cells are occasionally found in the epithelium of the efferent ducts.

Epididymis: The regional changes in the histology of the epididymis have been described, for the rat, by Reid and Cleland (66). Principal, narrow, clear, basal, and halo cells are present.

In the initial segment, principal cells show nuclei at different levels (Figs. 5,6); those with a nucleus in the upper half of the cell have been referred to as apical cells (10,66,87). Principal cells are moderately stained and show a few tall microvilli forming a brush border. These cells have a pale, round nucleus, showing a pronounced nucleolus and a few supranuclear dense granules. Longitudinal dense columns abide at the border between adjacent principal cells (Fig. 6). In the caput (Figs. 7,8), corpus (Figs. 9,10), and cauda (Figs. 11,12) epididymidis, principal cells show a moderately stained, irregularly shaped nucleus also having a prominent nucleolus; these cells are shorter than those of the initial segment. The supranuclear region contains many dense granules, while a typical brush border lines their luminal aspect (Figs. 7–12). Sparse dense granules are found in the basal region of all epididymal principal cells; however, selectively in the corpus epididymidis, moderately dense bodies fill the basal region of these cells (Figs. 9,10).

Narrow cells, found exclusively in the initial segment of the epididymis, are identified by a deep-staining cytoplasm, a dense elongated nucleus which is located in the upper half of the cell, and an ill-defined narrow base contacting the basement membrane (Fig. 6).

Clear cells found in the caput (Figs. 7,8), corpus (Figs. 9,10), and cauda (Figs. 11,12) epididymidis are identified

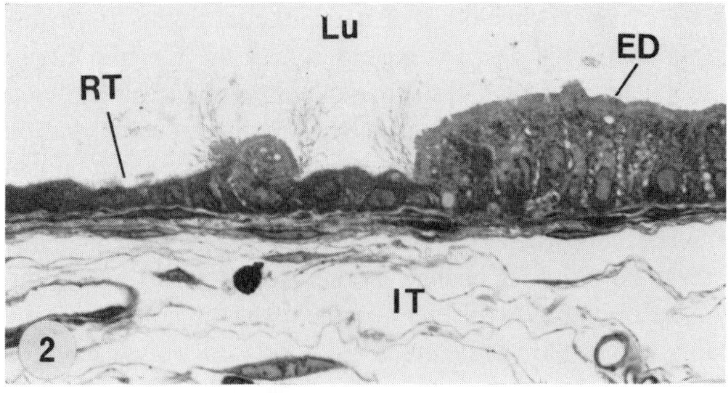

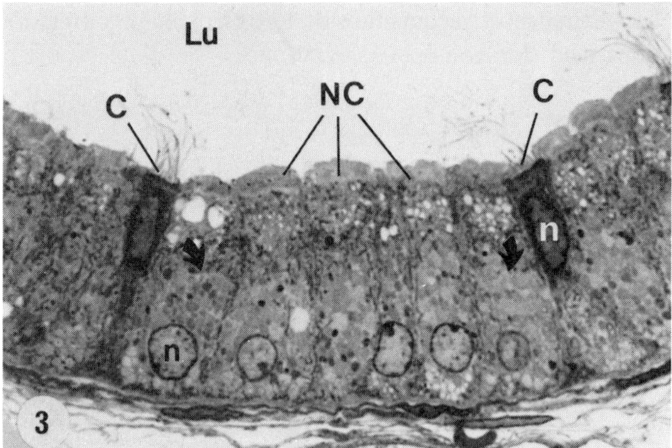

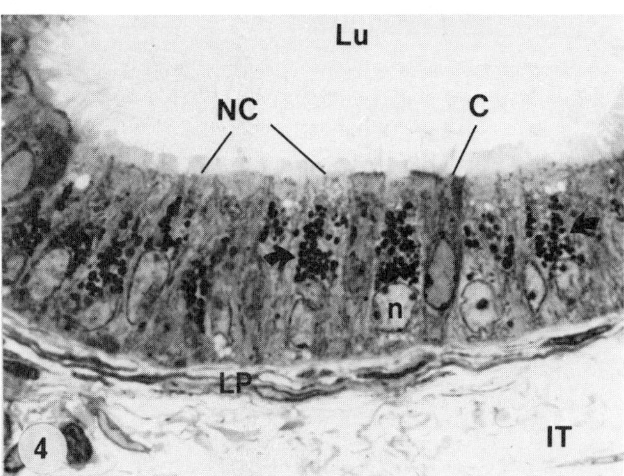

FIG. 2. Light microscope photograph showing the sharp demarcation between the cuboidal epithelial cells of the rete testis (RT) and the columnar epithelial cells of the efferent ducts (ED). Lu:lumen, IT:intertubular space. (×340.)

FIG. 3. Portion of the epithelium from the initial zone of an efferent duct at the light microscopic level showing numerous nonciliated cells (NC) and few ciliated cells (C). The nonciliated cells present a brush border, whereas long cilia extend into the lumen (Lu) from the ciliated cells. The nucleus (n) of the nonciliated cells is round, pale, and basally located, while that of the ciliated cells (n) is dark, elongated, and occupies the upper half of the cell. The supranuclear region of nonciliated cells is filled with moderately dense stained bodies (*arrows*). (×680.)

FIG. 4. Portion of the epithelium from the terminal zone of an efferent duct showing nonciliated (NC) and ciliated (C) cells. The supranuclear region of the nonciliated cells from this zone is occupied by numerous dense bodies (*arrows*). Lu:lumen, LP:lamina propria, IT:intertubular space. (×680.)

by a highly vacuolated apical region and the presence of numerous dense granules, above or below the nucleus. The basal region is usually filled with pale or moderately dense bodies (Figs. 7,8,10). The nucleus, variable in position, is round, pale-stained, and shows a prominent nucleolus.

Basal cells, found throughout the epididymis (Figs. 6,8,10,12), are flat elongated cells residing near the base of the epithelium where they contact the basement membrane; they have an elongated or spherical, moderately dense nucleus, showing peripheral patches of condensed chromatin enclosed by a pale-staining rim of cytoplasm.

Halo cells of the epididymis (Figs. 5,7,8) are similar to those of the efferent ducts. These cells are distributed at all levels of the epididymal epithelium and can be identified by a dense nucleus showing patches of peripheral condensed chromatin surrounded by a pale-staining cytoplasm.

The histogenesis of these different cell types has been studied by a number of investigators (49–51,88). In the rat, the principal cell, and the structurally related apical cell, derive from a cell defined by Sun and Flickinger as the columnar cell (50); this columnar cell also gives rise to the basal cell. The conversion of the columnar cell into principal and basal cells takes place at approximately day 28. The other major cell type in the immature rat (days 16–28) is the narrow cell; this cell is maintained in the initial segment of the adult rat, but in the rest of the epididymis, it gives rise to the clear (light) cell. Both the columnar and the narrow cell derive, at approximately day 16, from a common cell: the undifferentiated stem cell.

The proliferative activity of principal and basal cells has been examined by Clermont and Flannery (89). There was a progressive decline in the mitotic and labeling indices of principal and basal cells in rats aged 2.5, 4, and 12 months. These observations led the authors to suggest that the epididymal cell population (principal and basal) was expanding in adult animals and was not renewing itself. These results were further indicative of the fact that holocrine secretion, as proposed by Martan and collaborators (90–92), was not taking place in this tissue. In the hamster, Nagy and Edmonds (93) have reported that, after colchicine treatment, there is a diurnal cycle of proliferative activity of principal cells throughout the epididymis.

There are no data available on the relative quantitative distribution of these major different cell types—principal, narrow, clear, basal, and halo—as one moves from one segment of the epididymis to the next. Consequently, a study using glutaraldehyde-perfused-fixed rat epididymides was undertaken to determine their distribution in the initial segment, caput, corpus, and proximal and distal cauda epididymidis (at least 1,000 cells from three adult animals) (Fig. 13); because the patterns for the proximal and distal cauda were nearly identical, only one, that of the distal cauda, is shown. The exact areas used to quantitate the different cell types in each segment of the epididymis are indicated by the shaded areas in Fig. 1.

In the initial segment, the principal cells make up 80% of the total cells, while the basal cells contribute 12%, and halo cells make up just under 5%; the remaining 3% is made up by a cell type found only in this region of the epididymis—the narrow cell. As can be seen from Fig. 5, the principal cells are very tall in this segment, and the tubular and luminal diameters are relatively small (66).

The relative distribution of principal and basal cells is maintained in the caput epididymidis (Fig. 13). However, in this region, while no narrow cells are seen, clear cells (5%) are first encountered. The relative percentage of halo cells increases by 30%. By comparing cross-sections from the caput epididymidis (Fig. 7) and the initial segment (Fig. 5), it becomes apparent that the luminal diameter of the caput epididymidis is greatly increased and the height of the principal cells is decreased. As described by Reid and Cleland (66), the sparser density of spermatozoa in the lumen of the caput epididymidis coincides with the increase in luminal diameter.

The relative contribution of principal cells in the corpus epididymidis declines to 69%, while the basal cells' contribution increases to 21%; the relative contribution of the clear cells increases by 30% in the corpus, while that of the halo cells decreases from 6.5% (caput) to 3.8% in the corpus (Fig. 13). Neither the cell height nor the luminal diameter change markedly as one moves through the corpus (66).

The relative numbers of basal and halo cells remain nearly identical as one moves from the corpus to the cauda epididymidis. The further decrease in the relative distribution of the principal cells in the cauda epididymidis is accounted for entirely by an increase of clear cells, such that this number approaches 10% (Fig. 13). The tubular diameter increases substantially between the caput and cauda epididymidis, as does the density of spermatozoa (66). Using micropuncture techniques, it has been shown that the sperm density increases nearly 25-fold from the rete testis to the cauda of the epididymis, i.e., from 80 million/ml to 1,950 million/ml (94).

Vas Deferens: The regional differences in the lumen and epithelium of the vas deferens, as well as in the muscular layer surrounding it, have been described in detail by several investigators including Hamilton and Cooper (83), Kennedy and Heidger (84), and others (85,86,95,96). The histology of the proximal segment of the vas deferens closely resembles that of the cauda epididymidis. The epithelium is cuboidal and the lumen is highly distended; principal, basal, halo, and clear cells, similar to those of the cauda epididymidis, are present (Figs. 14,15).

As one moves from the proximal to the distal segment (Figs. 16,17) of the vas deferens, the height of the epithelium increases because of the tall columnar principal cells; basal and halo cells are still present, while clear cells are no longer seen (Figs. 16,17) (84). The lumen narrows and the distended appearance changes to one that is convoluted. Not surprisingly, there is a decrease in the content of spermatozoa as one progresses from the proximal to the distal end of the vas deferens (97). There is also a marked increase in the thickness of the smooth muscular layer surrounding

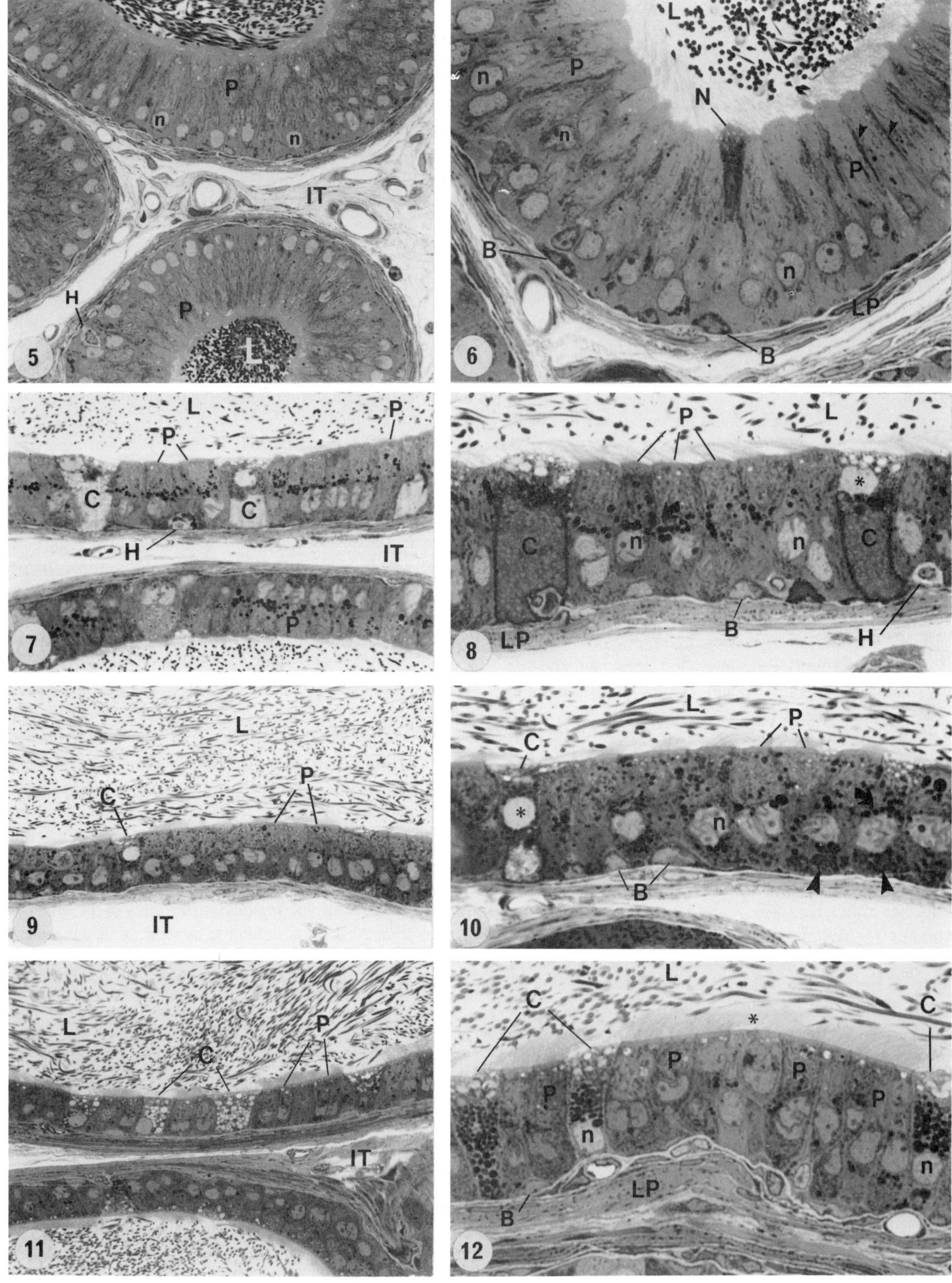
5
P
n
n
IT
H
P
L
6
L
P
n
N
n
P
B
n
LP
B
7
L
P
P
C
C
H
IT
P
8
P
L
*
C
n
n
C
B
H
LP
9
L
C
P
IT
10
L
P
C
*
n
B
11
L
C
P
IT
12
L
C
*
C
P
P
P
P
n
n
LP
B

this epithelium. The innervation of the vas deferens is extremely complex and has been reported to involve adrenergic (98–102), purinergic (103–105), and peptidergic (107–110) neurotransmission.

Histology: Electron microscopy. The main morphological features of each of the cell types introduced above are discussed at the electron microscopic level. Several fixation methods were employed which account for the different appearance of the images that are presented. In one case (Method A), rats were perfused with glutaraldehyde in sodium cacodylate buffer and then postfixed in a mixture of potassium ferrocyanide and osmium tetroxide (ferrocyanide-reduced osmium) to preserve intracytoplasmic membranes and reduce the density of the cytoplasmic matrix (111). In another instance (Method B), rats were perfused with glutaraldehyde in sodium cacodylate buffer containing tannic acid, and then postfixed in ferrocyanide-reduced osmium. In a third case (Method C), rats were fixed in a mixture of glutaraldehyde and paraformaldehyde in sodium cacodylate buffer and then postfixed in osmium tetroxide, followed by staining *en bloc* with uranyl acetate. The latter two methods were primarily employed to preserve the lattice coat of coated pits and vesicles, filaments, and ribosomes.

Nonciliated Cell of the Efferent Ducts: The electron microscopic appearance of the nonciliated cells of a wide variety of species, including the guinea pig (112), rat (9,10,113,114), hamster (71), ground squirrel (115), rabbit (116), opossum (117), bull (118–120), monkey (121), and human (122,123), has been studied by numerous investigators. By using a variety of electron-dense tracers introduced into the lumen of the ducts, it has been demonstrated that these cells readily incorporate material from the lumen (119,120,124–126) and that they are effective in performing both fluid phase and adsorptive endocytosis (83,114).

The structural features of the nonciliated cells have not been examined in detail in any of the species studied. Using the rat as our model, a detailed analysis is therefore presented. Although the nonciliated cells of the efferent ducts are more numerous than the neighboring ciliated cells, they also have a distinct morphological appearance that suggests they are specialized for the uptake of particulate material and fluid from the lumen.

A schematic representation of a nonciliated cell from the efferent ducts is shown in Fig. 18. In the apical region, the nonciliated cells, in addition to a few scattered cisternae of rough endoplasmic reticulum, filaments, microtubules, and mitochondria, contain several distinct membranous structures (Figs. 19–22).

Connected to the apical plasma membrane in areas between the bases of the microvilli, and extending for some distance into the apical cytoplasm, are large dilated tubular elements occasionally showing a bulbous extremity referred to as the tubular coated pits (Figs. 18,21). These membranous structures characteristically show a pale-stained lumen (Figs. 21,22). All of these tubular structures are lined on their luminal aspect with a uniform layer of fuzzy material, and on their cytoplasmic aspect with a clathrin-like lattice coat (Fig. 22). Although often seen subjacent to the cell

FIG. 5. Light microscope photograph showing several tubules of the initial segment of the epididymis. The epithelium is lined predominantly by tall columnar principal cells (P) showing a round, pale nucleus (n). A halo cell (H) is also visible in the epithelium. L:lumen, IT:intertubular space. (×360.)

FIG. 6. Portion of the epithelium lining the initial segment of the epididymis illustrating many tall columnar principal cells (P) with pale, round nuclei (n) located at different levels of the cell and showing a prominent nucleolus, a few elongated basal cells (B) at the base of the epithelium, and a deeply stained narrow cell (N). Longitudinal dense bands extend along the length of principal cells (*arrowheads*). L:lumen, LP:lamina propria. (×720.)

FIG. 7. Epithelium lining the epididymal duct of the caput epididymidis showing numerous principal cells (P) and a few clear cells (C). A halo cell (H) is also indicated. L:lumen, IT:intertubular space. (×360.)

FIG. 8. Principal (P) and clear (C) epithelial cells lining the caput epididymidis. The clear cells (C) show a frothy apical region below which abide dense and moderately dense bodies. The nucleus (*asterisk*) of one clear cell is pale, round, and located near the apical region. The principal cells show an irregular moderately dense nucleus (n) above which can be seen many dense bodies (*arrow*). B:basal cell, H:halo cell, LP:lamina propria, L:lumen. (× 720.)

FIG. 9. Epithelium lining the epididymal duct of the corpus epididymidis showing numerous principal (P) cells and a clear (C) cell. L:lumen, IT:intertubular space. (×360.)

FIG. 10. Principal (P) and clear (C) epithelial cells lining the corpus epididymidis. The clear cell presents a round, pale nucleus (*asterisk*), while principal cells have highly irregular, moderately dense nuclei (n). Dense bodies (*arrow*) occupy the supranuclear region of the principal cells while their base is filled with moderately stained masses (*arrowheads*). L:lumen, B:basal cells. (×720.)

FIG. 11. Epithelium lining the epididymal duct of the cauda epididymidis showing principal (P) and clear (C) cells. L:lumen, IT:intertubular space. (×360.)

FIG. 12. Principal (P) and clear (C) epithelial cells lining the cauda epididymidis. The clear cells have a frothy apical region below which can be found numerous dense bodies; their nucleus (n) is round and pale-stained. Principal cells (P) show an irregular nucleus, several dense bodies, and a uniform tall brush border (*asterisk*). Clear cells lack a brush border. B:basal cell, LP:lamina propria, L:lumen. (×720.)

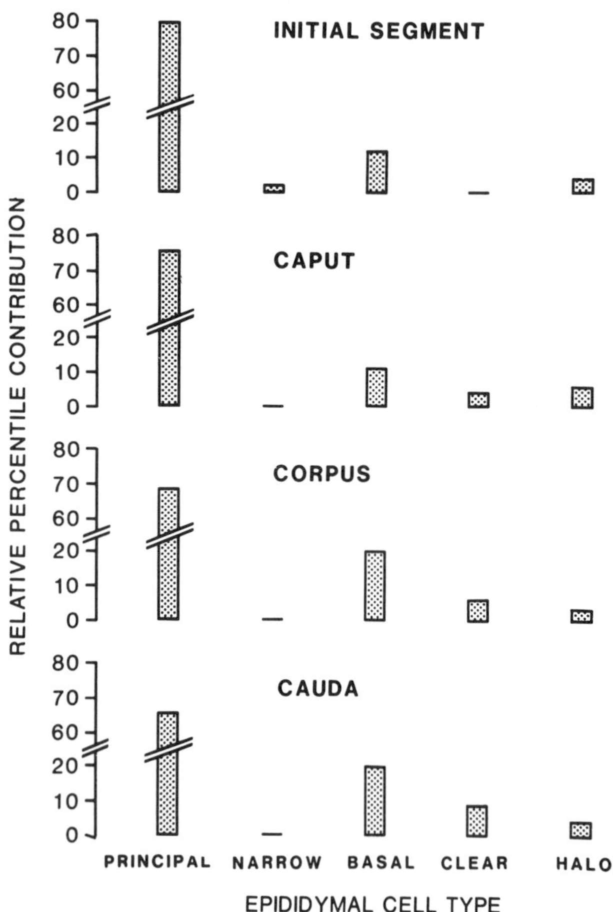

FIG. 13. Relative cell distribution in the initial segment, caput, corpus, and cauda epididymidis of the adult male rat. Rats were perfuse-fixed and the epididymides were embedded in Epon using standard methods. The area of tissue used for the cell counts for each of the four segments is indicated by the *shaded portions* of **Fig. 1.** Approximately 1,000 cells from at least three animals were counted in each of the four segments, and the relative number of principal, narrow, basal, clear, and halo cells was determined.

surface, they are probably still connected to the apical cell surface and are seen as detached, probably simply due to the plane of section.

Immediately beneath the cell surface are numerous membranous tubules varying in length and appearing as circular elements in cross-sectional profile (Figs. 18–22). Such elements have been identified in a wide variety of cell types including the kidney and are referred to as the apical tubules (128–131). These tubules have a constant diameter, are fairly straight, rarely branch, and have a uniform, moderately dense-staining content that fills their lumen (Figs. 21–23) (114). While apical tubules, sometimes showing dilated extremities (Fig. 23), are not seen to be continuous with the apical plasma membrane, images of transition between the tubular coated pits and apical tubules are present. This suggests that the tubular coated pits give rise to apical tubules (132).

Larger dilated membranous vacuoles, referred to as endosomes in other cell types (133), are also present in the apical region (Figs. 18,19,24). Such structures have a pale-stained lumen containing a fine flocculent material (Fig. 24). Several apical tubules are usually seen connected to these structures (Fig. 24).

Deeper in the apical region reside a number of multivesicular bodies showing either a pale, moderately dense, or dense-staining matrix (Figs. 18,25). Such bodies are often seen to be surrounded by many small vesicular profiles (Fig. 25). Small coated and uncoated vesicles of similar size (50–60 nm diameter) are also found in the apical region (Fig. 22).

The most conspicuous feature of the supranuclear region is the presence of an abundance of large membrane-bound bodies (Figs. 19,20). Such elements, more or less spherical in appearance, show a different staining intensity depending on whether initial or terminal zones of the efferent ducts are being analyzed, as observed in the guinea pig (112). In the case of nonciliated cells observed in the initial zone of the efferent ducts, these membrane-bound bodies appear stained in a uniformly pale manner and contain a fine flocculent material (Fig. 19). In the terminal zone, such bodies show a homogeneous deeply osmiophilic staining pattern (Figs. 18,20).

The large, membrane-bound elements from the terminal zone are acid-phosphatase-positive, and thus lysosomal in nature (114). Similar observations have been made on the large, pale-stained bodies of the supranuclear region of the initial zone (L. Hermo and C. Morales, *unpublished observations*).

Recent tracer studies have revealed that the nonciliated cells of the terminal zone of the efferent ducts are active endocytic cells. The tracers were found sequentially with time in the tubular coated pits; apical tubules; endosomes; pale, moderately dense, and dense multivesicular bodies; and lysosomes (114,127,132).

The presence of pale-stained lysosomes in the initial zone of the efferent ducts suggests that nonciliated cells from this region take up more fluid from the lumen, whereas the density of lysosomes from the terminal zone indicates that more particulate matter than fluid is taken up there.

In addition to the lysosomes, scattered mitochondria, and scanty cisternae of the rough endoplasmic reticulum, which in these cells appear in the form of an interconnected beaded chain, the supranuclear region contains the Golgi apparatus (Figs. 18,19). The latter, formed of several stacks of saccules and associated vesicular profiles, shows no evidence of secretory granule formation. Thus, at least in the rat, these cells do not appear to be active secretory cells; this is unlike the situation reported for the bull (119,120) and the goat (134). In light of the active endocytic activity of these cells, it would be of interest to analyze the Golgi saccules of a stack for the respective role of a given saccule in the formation of lysosomal enzymes, the manner by which they

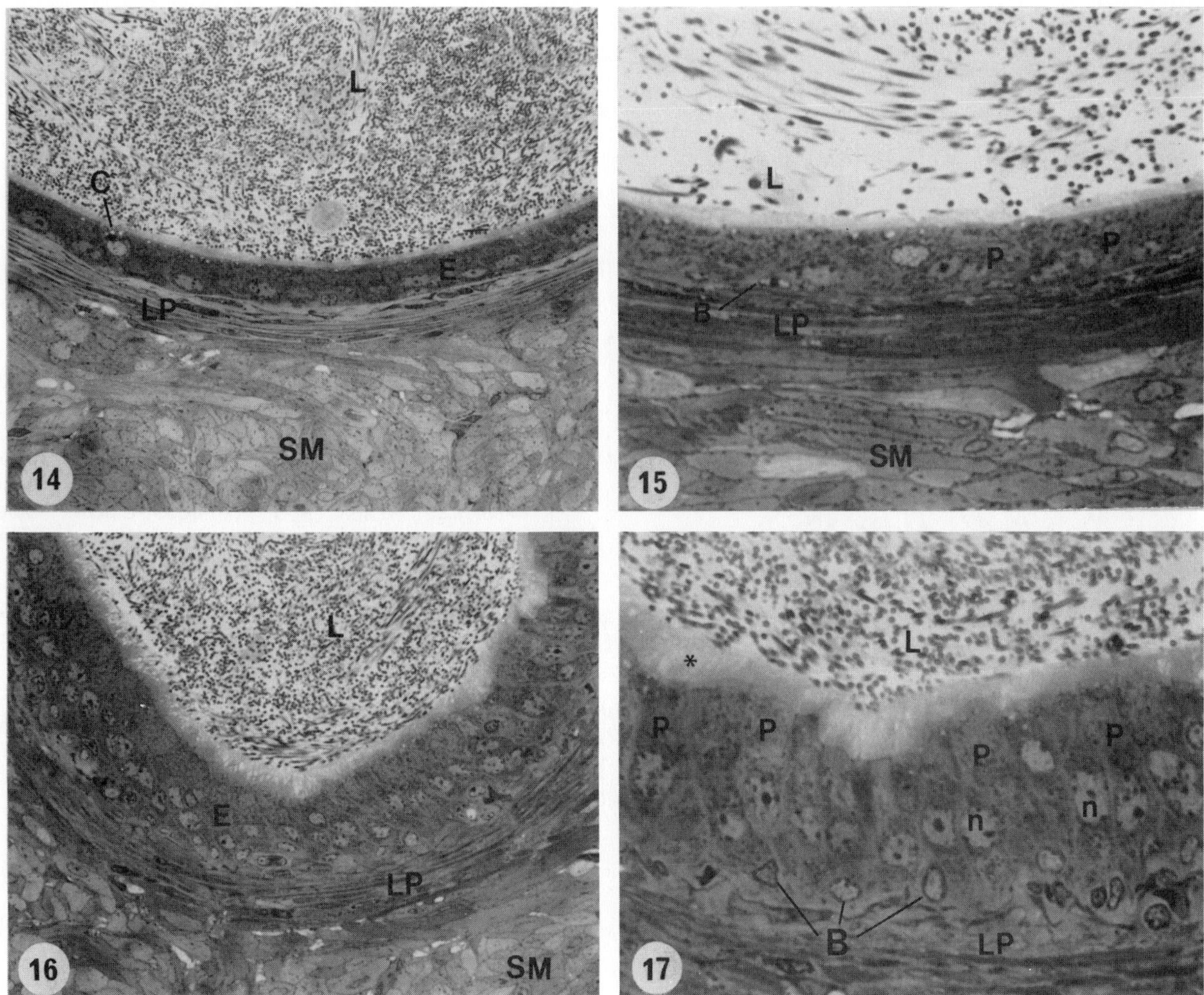

FIG. 14. Portion of the epithelium (E) lining the proximal segment of the vas deferens showing many cuboidal principal cells and a clear cell (C). L:lumen, LP:lamina propria, SM:smooth muscle. (×360.)

FIG. 15. Epithelium of the proximal segment of the vas deferens lined by cuboidal principal (P) cells and flattened basal (B) cells. L:lumen, LP:lamina propria, SM:smooth muscle. (×720.)

FIG. 16. Portion of the epithelium (E) lining the distal segment of the vas deferens. L:lumen, LP:lamina propria, SM:smooth muscle. (×360.)

FIG. 17. Tall columnar principal (P) epithelial cells lining the distal segment of the vas deferens showing a brush border (*asterisk*) and moderately stained nucleus (n) usually in the midregion of the cell. The basal cells (B) show a smaller roundish nucleus located at the base of the epithelium. L:lumen, LP:lamina propria. (×720.)

are delivered to endocytic organelles, and the location along the endocytic pathway where this occurs.

Also present in the supranuclear region are a number of membranous elements showing a lumen filled with a homogeneous, moderately stained, fine filamentous material (Fig. 26). Such elements are commonly found closely juxtaposed or completely surrounded by cisternae of the rough endoplasmic reticulum. Their morphological appearance and size as well as cytochemical tests for peroxidase [Fig. 26 (inset)] indicate that they are peroxisomes. The functional significance of peroxisomes in these cells is not known.

The basal region of the cell, containing a pale, indented nucleus, occasionally shows infranuclearly an abundance of lipid droplets, few cisternae of rough endoplasmic reticulum, and mitochondria (Fig. 18). Images of lysosomes and lipid forming a common body can be found in the basal region (Fig. 18) (114). In some cases, these structures appear to be completely enclosed by a common unit membrane (Fig. 27), whereas in other cases a unit membrane enclosing the lipidic portion is either incomplete or totally absent (Fig. 28). Such images suggest that a close relationship exists between the lysosomes and lipid of the nonciliated cells. Indeed Hermo and Morales (114) have shown that by 15 days after ligation of the efferent ducts, there was a dramatic

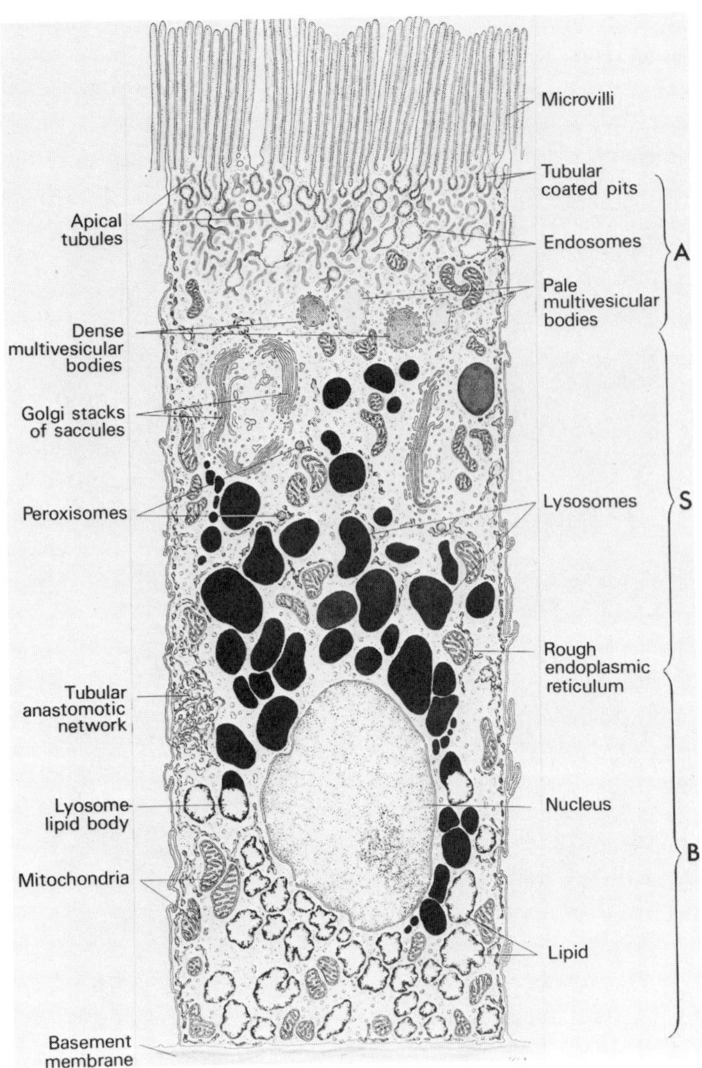

FIG. 18. A diagrammatic representation of a nonciliated cell from the terminal zone of the ductuli efferentes. A:apical region, S:supranuclear region, B:basal region. The apical region shows tubular coated pits connected to the cell surface, endosomes, pale and dense multivesicular bodies, and numerous apical tubules. Whereas the supranuclear region is filled with large dense lysosomes, the basal region is occupied by many lipid droplets. Note the location and appearance of the tubular anastomotic network. Also illustrated are a few peroxisomes and lysosome-lipid bodies.

loss of lysosomes from the supranuclear region of these cells, and that by day 30 after ligation only a few lipid droplets could be seen in the base of these cells. Further studies are required to understand the significance of these findings and the turnover of lysosomes and lipid.

Along the entire length of the cell, cisternae of rough endoplasmic reticulum often run parallel to the lateral plasma membrane (Fig. 18), and occasionally what appears to be the fusion of small vesicles with the lateral plasma membrane can also be observed (Fig. 29).

The lateral plasma membranes of adjacent nonciliated cells in the basal and supranuclear regions often show a few interdigitations with one another; it is not uncommon to find a close association of the lateral plasma membrane with an anastomosing well-localized tubular network (Figs. 18,29). Such networks are made up of short anastomosing tubes demarcating pores of various sizes, and are capped peripherally by a flattened membranous element that is continuous with the network (Fig. 29). Such anastomotic networks often show several points of direct continuity with the lateral plasma membrane. The lumen of this network is thus continuous with the lateral intercellular space (Fig. 29). Areas of close approximation between this network and cisternae of the rough endoplasmic reticulum are not uncommon,

FIG. 19. Apical and supranuclear regions of a nonciliated cell from the initial zone of the efferent ducts. Many large pale-stained, membrane-bound bodies identified as lysosomes (L) are seen above the nucleus (N) containing a fine flocculent material. The Golgi apparatus (G) is formed of several stacks of saccules and associated small vesicles. M:Mitochondrion, E:endosome, Lu:lumen. (×8,184.) (Method A.)

FIG. 20. Apical and supranuclear regions of a nonciliated cell from the terminal zone of the efferent ducts. Many large, homogeneous, electron-dense membrane-bound bodies identified as lysosomes (L) are present in the supranuclear region in addition to a moderately dense multivesicular body (*asterisk*). The apical region is filled with many apical tubules (*arrows*). m:Mitochondrion, Lu:lumen. (×7920.) (Method A.)

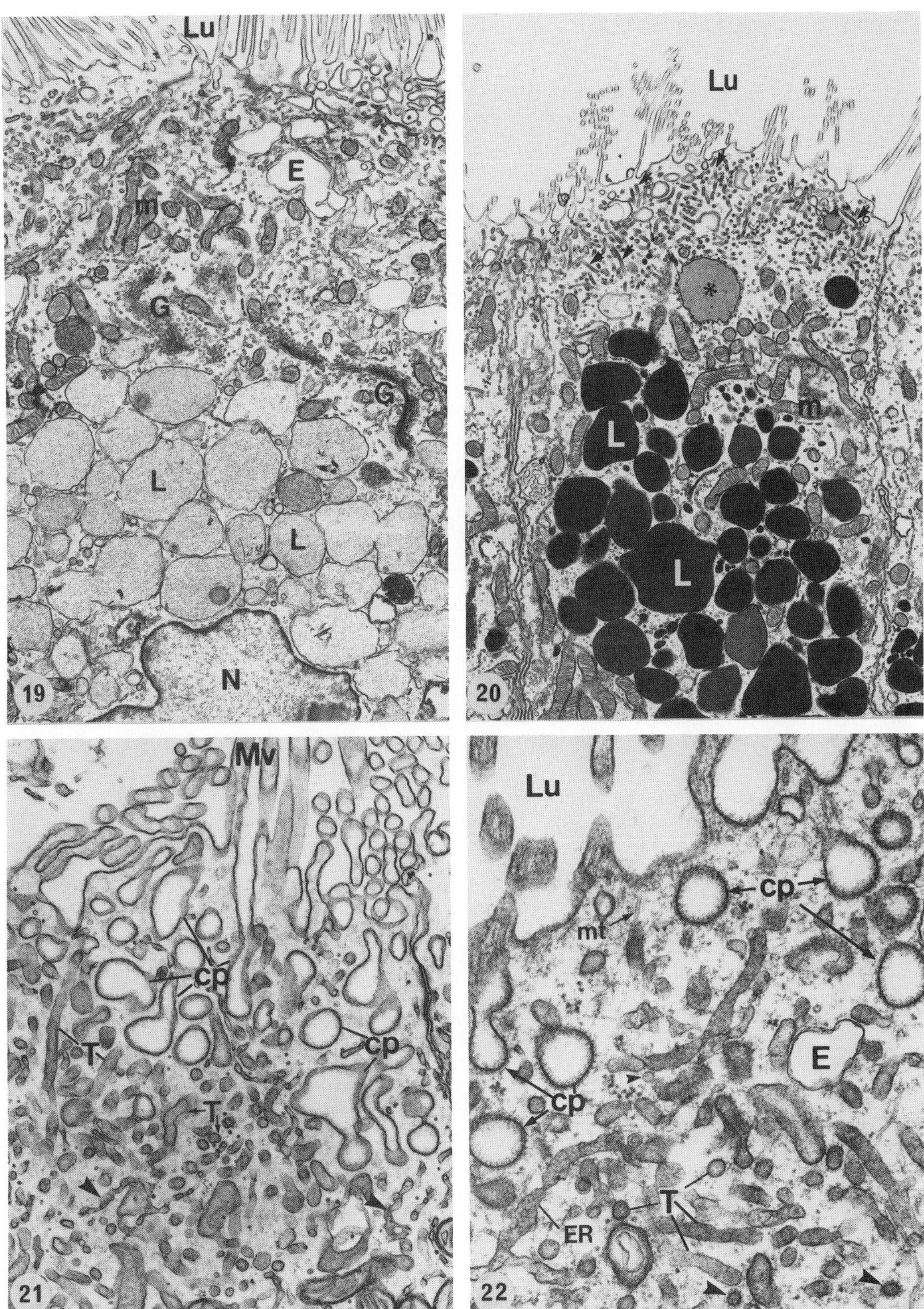

FIG. 21. High-power electron micrograph of the apical region of a nonciliated cell. Tubular coated pits (cp) connected to the apical plasma membrane can be seen extending into the cell cytoplasm from the bases of the microvilli (Mv). Such elements have a wide, pale-stained lumen and often end as bulbous extremities. Long narrow membranous tubules referred to as the apical tubules (T) are present. These have a moderately dense-staining content and are circular in cross-sectional profile (T). Cisternae of the rough endoplasmic reticulum (*arrowheads*) appear as a beaded chain showing occasional fenestrae. (×21,888.) (Method A.)

FIG. 22. High-power electron micrograph of the apical region of a nonciliated cell. Tubular coated pits (cp) presumed to be still connected to the cell surface are evident. Such elements showing a pale-stained lumen are lined on the luminal aspect of their delimiting membrane by a uniform fuzzy material and on their cytoplasmic aspect by a bristle clathrin-like coat. Also evident in this region are apical tubules (T), an endosome (E), and small uncoated (*small arrowhead*) and coated (*large arrowheads*) vesicles of similar size (50–60 nm). ER: cisterna of rough endoplasmic reticulum, Lu:lumen, mt:microtubule. (×40,000.) (Method C.)

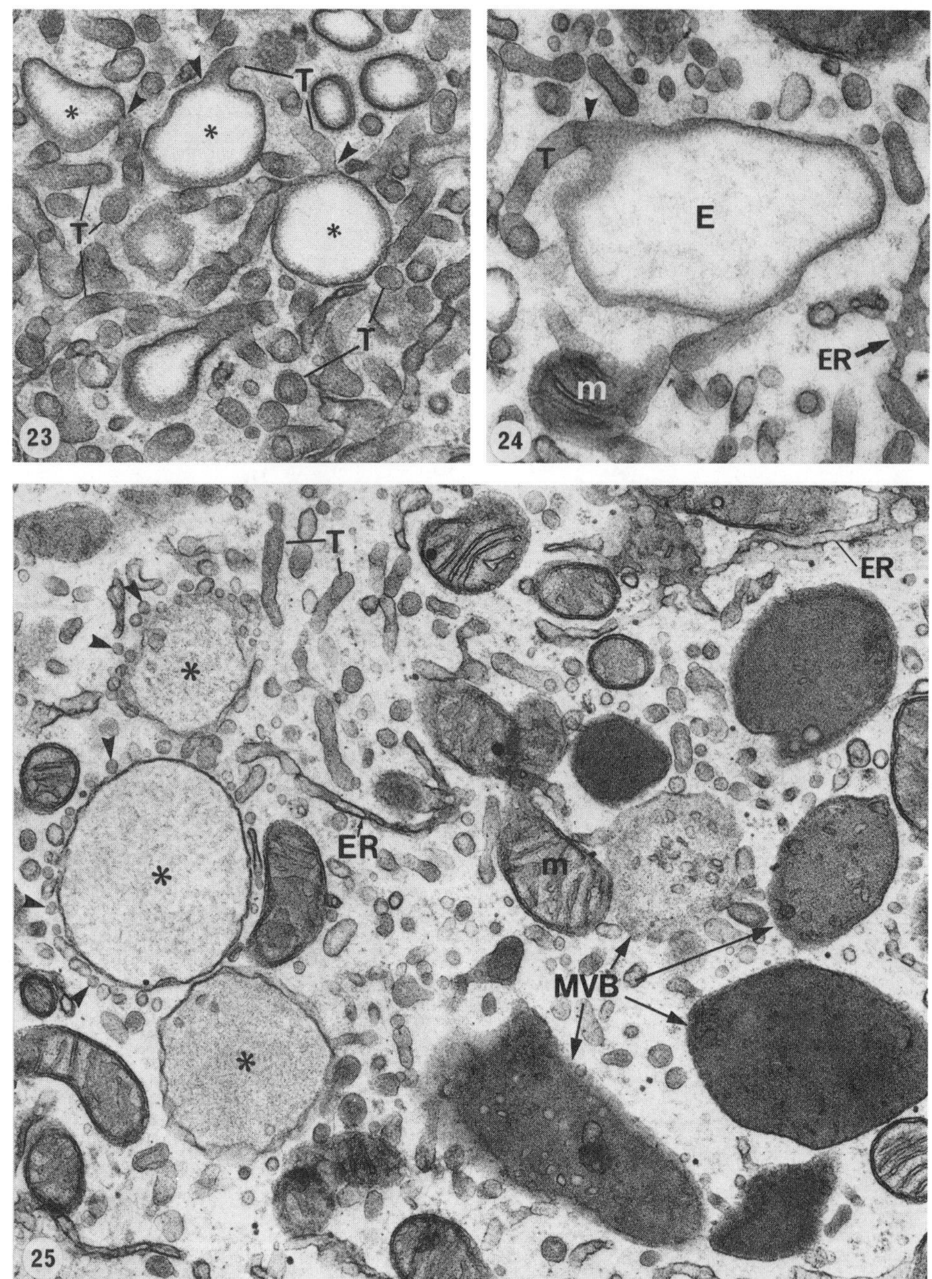

FIG. 23. High power of the apical region showing numerous apical tubules (T) with a uniform, moderately dense-staining content, some of which can be seen to be connected (*arrowheads*) to large dilated spherical membranous bodies (*asterisks*), showing an empty, pale-stained lumen lined by a fuzzy material. The latter are identical in size and appearance to the bulbous extremities of the tubular coated pits. (×35,490.) (Method A.)

FIG. 24. A large vacuole, containing a fine flocculent material, referred to as an endosome (E) is seen in the apical region to which is connected an apical tubule (T, *arrowhead*). m:Mitochondria, ER:rough endoplasmic reticulum. (×38,220.) (Method A.)

FIG. 25. Junction between the apical and supranuclear regions of a nonciliated cell of the terminal zone. Pale, multivesicular bodies with a matrix containing a fine flocculent material (*asterisks*) are seen in this region often surrounded by a corona of small vesicles (*arrowheads*) as well as multivesicular bodies with a moderate- or dense-staining matrix (MVB). T:apical tubules, ER:rough endoplasmic reticulum, m:mitochondria. (×29,790.) (Method A.)

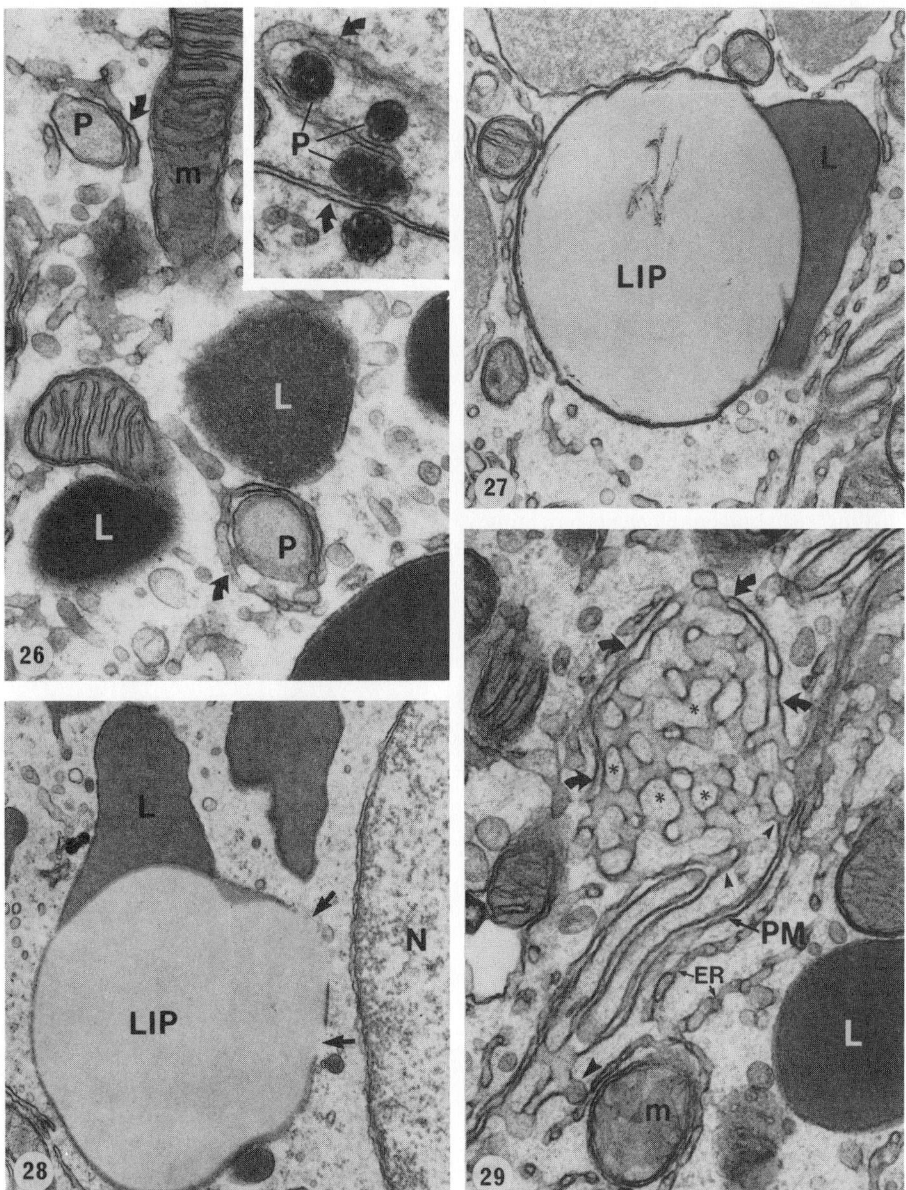

FIG. 26. Supranuclear region of a nonciliated cell showing several homogeneous dense lysosomes (L). Small membrane-bound bodies (P) containing a pale flocculent material are seen to be in close association with cisternae of the rough endoplasmic reticulum (*arrows*); m:mitochondria. (×35,000.) (Method A.)

FIG. 26 (inset). Such elements surrounded by cisternae of rough endoplasmic reticulum (*arrows*) can be shown cytochemically to be peroxisomes (P). (×32,760.)

FIG. 27. A membrane-bound body deep in the supranuclear region of a nonciliated cell showing features of a dense lysosome (L) and lipid (LIP) delimited by a common unit membrane. (×31,395.) (Method A.)

FIG. 28. A membrane-bound body next to the nucleus (N) of a nonciliated cell showing features of a dense lysosome (L) and lipid (LIP). The unit membrane over the lipid portion is not well defined and lacking in places (*arrows*). N:nucleus. (×21,420.) (Method A.)

FIG. 29. A well-defined tubular network of a nonciliated cell formed of short anastomosing tubes demarcating pores of various sizes (*asterisks*) is seen to be connected at several sites (*small arrowheads*) with the lateral plasma membrane (PM). The tubular network is delimited and continuous peripherally by flattened membranous elements (*arrows*) not found to be continuous with the rough endoplasmic reticulum. A small vesicle (*large arrowhead*) is connected with the lateral plasma membrane. ER:rough endoplasmic reticulum, L:lysosome, m:mitochondria. (×43,750.) (Method A.)

however, no direct continuity between these two structures is observed; its functional significance is unknown.

Ciliated Cells of the Efferent Ducts: The ciliated cells of the efferent ducts, like the nonciliated cells, are tall columnar cells reaching the lumen on the one hand and basement membrane on the other (Fig. 30). As observed in many species, such as the guinea pig (112), rat (10,113,135), hamster (71), ground squirrel (115), opossum (117), bull (118–120), monkey (121), and human (122), these cells are readily recognized by the presence of numerous cilia and a few microvilli extending from the cell surface into the lumen, a pale-stained elongated nucleus situated in the upper half of the cell, and an abundance of cytoplasmic filaments and mitochondria (Fig. 30).

In the rat, as in other species, the upper half of the cell, in addition to the basal bodies of the cilia, bundles of filaments, and several distinct membranous elements, contains a few delicate interconnected thread-like cisternae of rough endoplasmic reticulum, mitochondria, and the nucleus (Figs. 30–32). Occasional small uncoated and coated pits of the apical plasma membrane are present at the bases of the cilia or microvilli (Fig. 31). Subjacent to the cell surface are large uncoated and coated vesicles as well as membranous apical tubules (Fig. 31). The latter are similar in appearance to those found in the nonciliated cells, although they are smaller in size and much fewer in number (Fig. 31). A few larger vesicular elements (endosomes), as well as multivesicular bodies showing a pale-, moderate-, or dense-staining matrix, are scattered about in the apical region (Fig. 31).

Located at the upper pole of the nucleus is the Golgi apparatus showing the well-defined pattern of stacks of saccules and associated vesicular profiles (Fig. 32). Several membrane-bound bodies, often showing a homogeneous electron-dense periphery surrounding a paler, coarsely granulated region, are usually found above or alongside the nucleus. Such bodies have been shown to be acid-phosphatase-positive and are thus lysosomal in nature (135).

Ciliated cells of the rat efferent ducts are involved in the uptake of material from the lumen (135); an opposite conclusion had been drawn from earlier work (119,120,126). At early time intervals, tracers introduced into the lumen of the efferent ducts were found in uncoated and coated pits, apical tubules, endosomes, and subsequently in multivesicular bodies and lysosomes (135). Thus, in addition to their function of moving luminal fluids and sperm, ciliated cells also appear capable of modifying the composition of the luminal fluid by the process of endocytosis.

Subjacent to the nucleus, the cytoplasm contains polysomes, numerous bundles of filaments, mitochondria, a few cisternae of rough endoplasmic reticulum, and the occasional lysosome and lipid droplet. In the rat, glycogen granules are seen scattered throughout the entire cytoplasm (Figs. 31,32); this contrasts with the huge accumulation of such granules seen in ciliated cells of the ground squirrel (115).

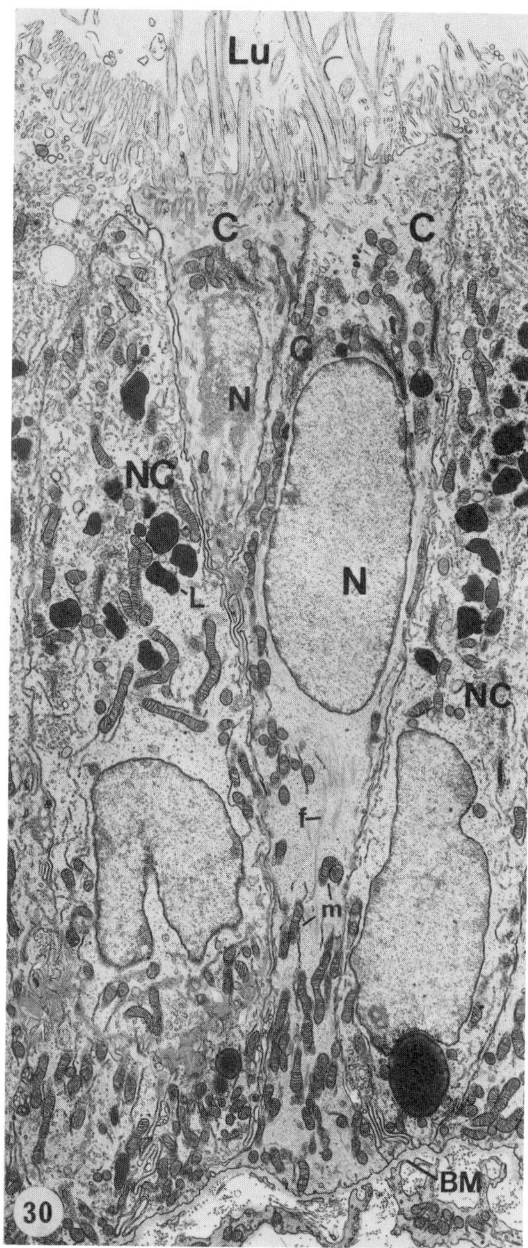

FIG. 30. Low-power electron micrograph showing tall columnar ciliated cells (C) and adjacent nonciliated cells (NC). The ciliated cells show cilia protruding into the lumen (Lu), a nucleus (N) located in the upper region of the cell, a Golgi apparatus (G) capping the nucleus, and numerous bundles of filaments (f) and mitochondria (m) below the nucleus. Numerous dense lysosomes (L) are present in the nonciliated cells. BM:basement membrane. ($\times$5,100.) (Method A.)

As in the case of the nonciliated cells, a single cisterna of endoplasmic reticulum can often be seen arranged in parallel with the lateral plasma membrane. Images of fusion of small vesicles with the lateral plasma membrane are also observed (Fig. 32). The possibility that such vesicles, observed in ciliated and nonciliated cells, are involved in transcytosis

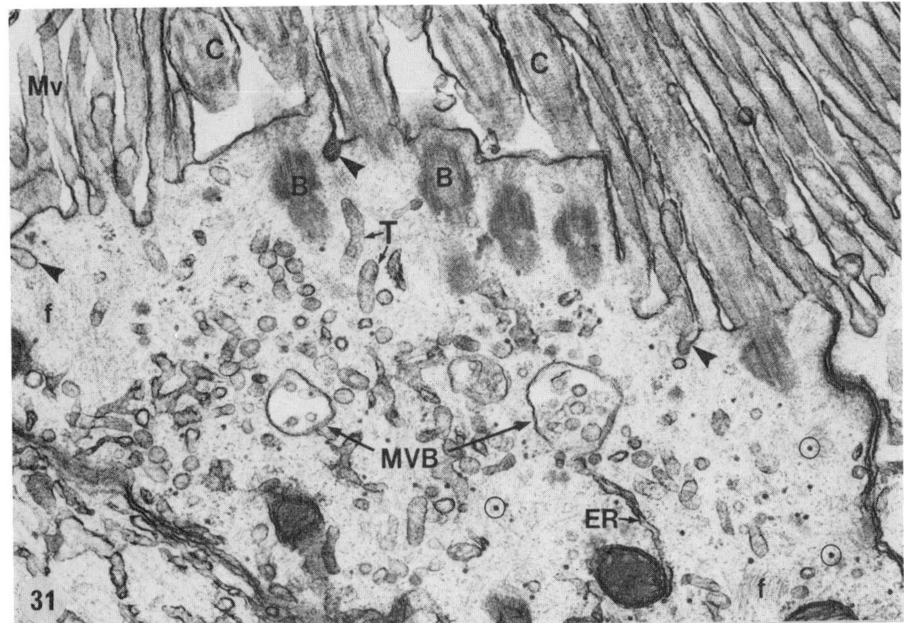

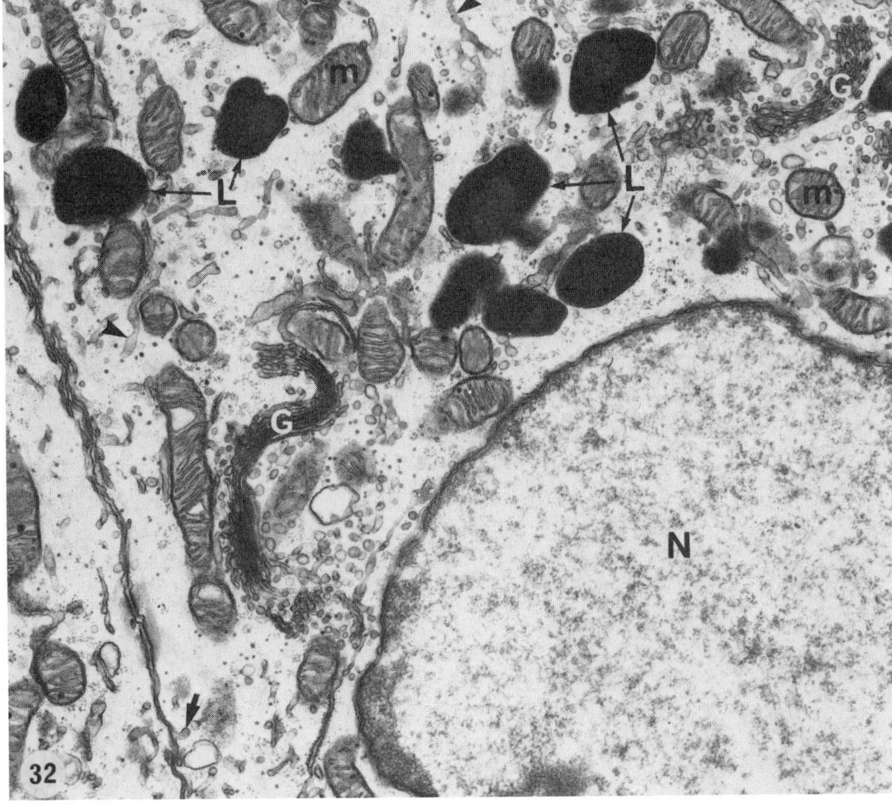

FIG. 31. High-power electron micrograph of the apical region of a ciliated cell presenting basal bodies (B), cilia (c), a few small coated and uncoated pits (*arrowheads*), apical tubules (T), numerous subsurface vesicular profiles, pale multivesicular bodies (MVB), glycogen granules (*circled*), and filaments (f). ER:rough endoplasmic reticulum, Mv:microvilli. (×29,640.) (Method A.)

FIG. 32. High power of the supranuclear region of a ciliated cell containing several membrane-bound dense bodies identified as lysosomes (L); such elements have a homogeneous electron-dense periphery enclosing a paler granulated region. A small vesicle is seen connected to the lateral plasma membrane (*arrow*). Sparse wavy strands of rough endoplasmic reticulum are visible (*arrowheads*). G:Golgi apparatus, N:nucleus, m:mitochondria. (×19,655.) (Method A.)

remains to be demonstrated. The basal plasma membrane, like that of the nonciliated cells, shows few coated or uncoated pits, and it has yet to be demonstrated that endocytosis occurs at the base of these cells.

Principal Cells: The tall columnar *principal cells of the initial segment of the epididymis,* while sharing some features with principal cells lining the remainder of the excurrent duct system, show remarkable differences, and hence are discussed separately. Some of the major features of these cells have been well described in several species (10,116,136–144).

A schematic representation of a principal cell of the initial segment is shown in Fig. 33. In the rat, the apical region, at times protruding into the lumen beyond the areas of the

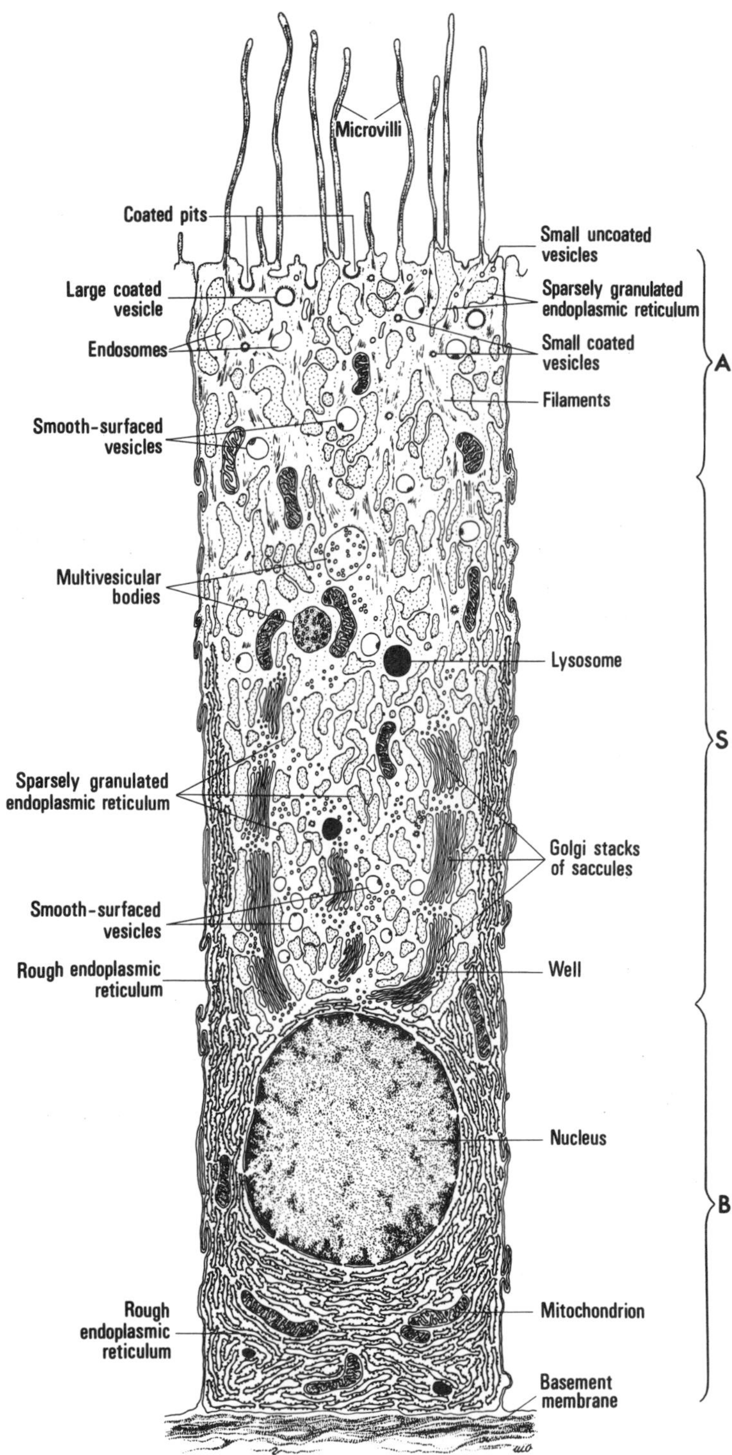

FIG. 33. Diagrammatic representation of a principal epithelial cell from the initial segment of the epididymis. A:apical region, S:supranuclear region, B:basal region. Note the abundance of the sparsely granulated endoplasmic reticulum in the apical and supranuclear regions and its close proximity to the apical plasma membrane. The rough endoplasmic reticulum is arranged along the lateral plasma membrane and fills the basal region. Smooth-surfaced vesicles are present in the Golgi region as well as in the apical region. Also indicated are coated pits, large coated vesicles, small coated and uncoated vesicles, endosomes, multivesicular bodies, lysosomes, and the Golgi stacks of saccules.

junctional specializations, contains numerous filaments, microtubules, glycogen, and mitochondria (Figs. 33–35). Large coated and uncoated pits of the apical plasma membrane can be seen at the bases of the microvilli (Figs. 33–35), and subjacent to the cell surface one can observe large spherical or elongated coated vesicular elements showing an electron lucent content (Fig. 35). Large spherical uncoated vesicles with a tail (endosomes) are also present (Fig. 33). Membranous apical tubules, although not abundant, are also seen in the apical region (Fig. 35). Several small coated and uncoated vesicles ranging in diameter between 50 and 60 nm are evident (Figs. 33–35).

Large uncoated vesicles (150–300 nm diameter), referred to as the smooth-surfaced vesicles, are conspicuous in variable numbers in the apical region. Such vesicles usually present either an electron lucent matrix, or a matrix con-

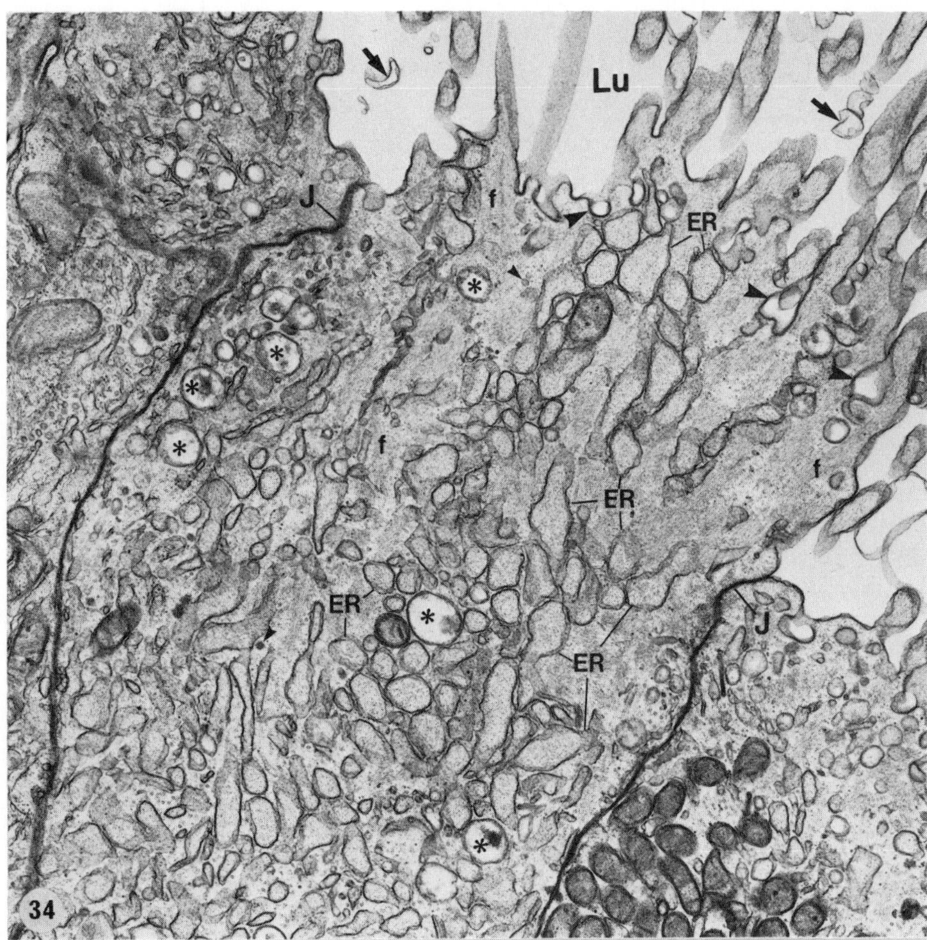

FIG. 34. Apical region of a principal cell from the initial segment of the epididymis showing large coated and uncoated pits of the cell surface (*large arrowheads*), numerous cisternae of the sparsely granulated endoplasmic reticulum (ER), several large smooth-surfaced vesicles showing a patchy flocculent material (*asterisks*), and the occasional small coated and uncoated vesicles (*small arrowheads*). Membranous elements (*arrows*) appear in the lumen (Lu). f:Filaments, J:area of junctional specialization between adjacent principal cells. (×15,225.) (Method B.)

taining a fine flocculent material, or patches of an electron-dense material usually adhering to the inner aspect of their membrane (Figs. 33–35).

The most prominent feature of the apical region is the presence of numerous large dilated irregularly shaped membranous elements referred to as the sparsely granulated endoplasmic reticulum (136,145). These elements present a lumen containing a uniform finely filamentous material; their outer surface shows an occasional ribosome (Figs. 33–35). As shown by Hoffer et al. (136), such cisternae of the endoplasmic reticulum can often be seen in close proximity to the apical plasma membrane at several sites (Figs. 33–35). However, points of continuity between these two structures are not observed. (The functional significance of such a close relationship between these cisternae of the endoplasmic reticulum and the apical plasma membrane is discussed in the section on secretion.)

In the large supranuclear region, long flattened cisternae of the rough endoplasmic reticulum make their appearance and are usually arranged in parallel rows along the lateral plasma membrane (Figs. 33,36). The central portion of this region is filled with cisternae of the sparsely granulated endoplasmic reticulum, mitochondria, and a few smooth-surfaced vesicles (150–300 nm) similar to those seen in the apical region (Fig. 36). Multivesicular bodies showing a pale-, moderate-, or dense-staining matrix (Figs. 33,36) are also seen in this region, as well as large membrane-bound bodies, identified as lysosomes, with a homogeneous electron-dense material [Fig. 36 (inset)].

Use of tracers, introduced into the lumen, allowed for the demonstration that these cells are involved in endocytosis. The endocytic route involved coated pits and vesicles, multivesicular bodies, and lysosomes (136).

The large Golgi apparatus, occupying the lower part of the supranuclear region, is formed of several stacks of saccules mainly running parallel to the long axis of the cell and associated small vesicles (Figs. 33,37). The saccules, up to as many as ten per stack, show on the immature, or

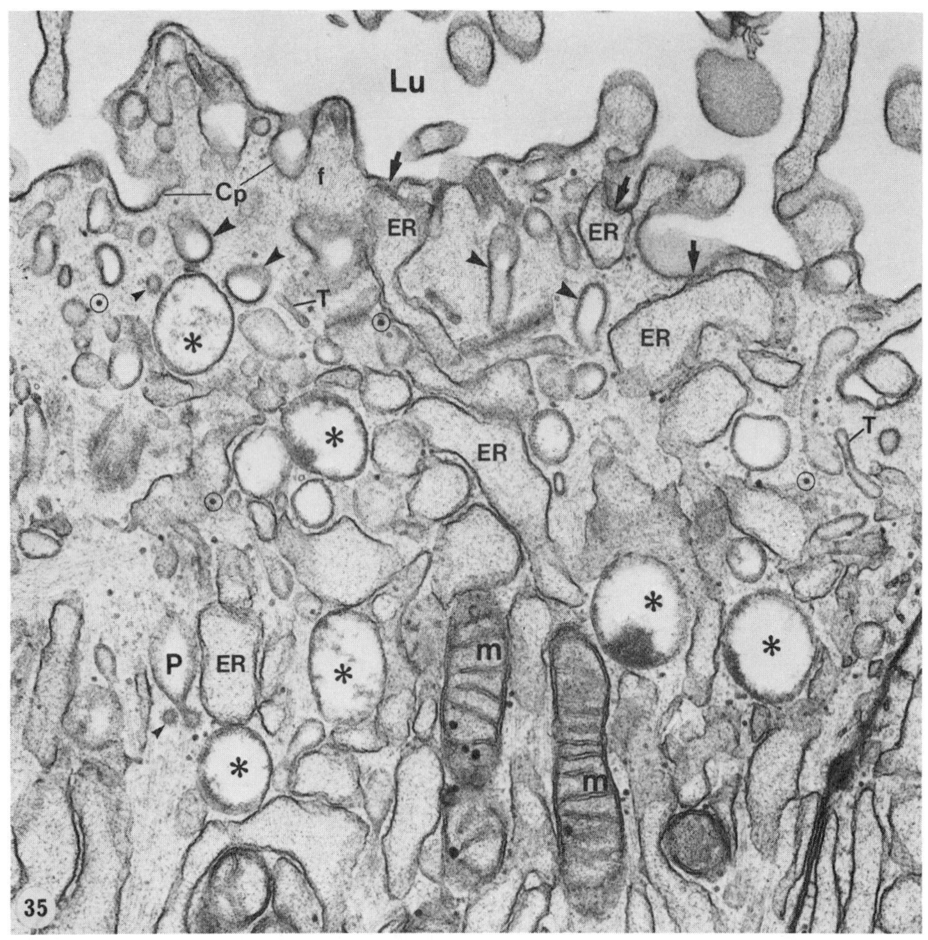

FIG. 35. High-power electron micrograph of the apical region of a principal cell from the initial segment of the epididymis. Numerous cisternae of the sparsely granulated endoplasmic reticulum (ER) containing a uniform filamentous material are evident, some of which can be seen in close proximity to the apical plasma membrane (*arrows*). Coated and uncoated pits of the cell surface (Cp) as well as subsurface spherical or elongated coated membranous elements (*large arrowheads*) are also present. Smooth-surfaced vesicles (150–300 nm) are scattered about and show a patchy electron-dense material (*asterisks*). Small coated vesicles (*small arrowheads*), glycogen granules (*circled*), filaments (f), and a few apical tubules (T) are also found in this region. A pear-shaped vesicle showing a bristle coat on its constricted end is also labeled (P). m:Mitochondria. (×35,490) (Method B.)

cis, face of the stack interruptions along their length which are in register with one another, forming characteristic wells (Figs. 37,38) similar to those described in spermatids (146) and other cell types (147,148). Such wells frequently show an accumulation of small vesicles (Fig. 38). The sparsely granulated endoplasmic reticulum is loosely distributed over the cis face of the Golgi stack. However, on the trans face it is often contiguous, but not continuous, with the trans-most Golgi saccule (Fig. 38). Although such an arrangement has also been described in the Golgi apparatus of spermatids (146) and acinar cells of the lacrimal gland (149), its functional significance is unknown.

Large smooth-surfaced vesicles similar in size (150–300 nm) and appearance to those present in the supranuclear and

FIG. 36. Supranuclear region of a principal cell of the initial segment of the epididymis. Numerous cisternae of the sparsely granulated endoplasmic reticulum (*stars*) occupy the central area, while elongated flattened cisternae of the rough endoplasmic reticulum (rER) are arranged in parallel rows along the lateral plasma membrane. Multivesicular bodies (MVB) showing a pale-stained or moderately dense matrix are labeled as are dense bodies identified as lysosomes (L). A smooth-surfaced vesicle is also seen in this region (*arrow*). m: Mitochondria. (×15,120.) (Method B.) **Inset**: High power of dense bodies of a principal cell of the initial segment identified cytochemically as lysosomes (L) showing a homogeneous electron-dense material. Also labeled: sparsely granulated endoplasmic reticulum (*stars*), Golgi apparatus (G). (×18,000.) Method B.)

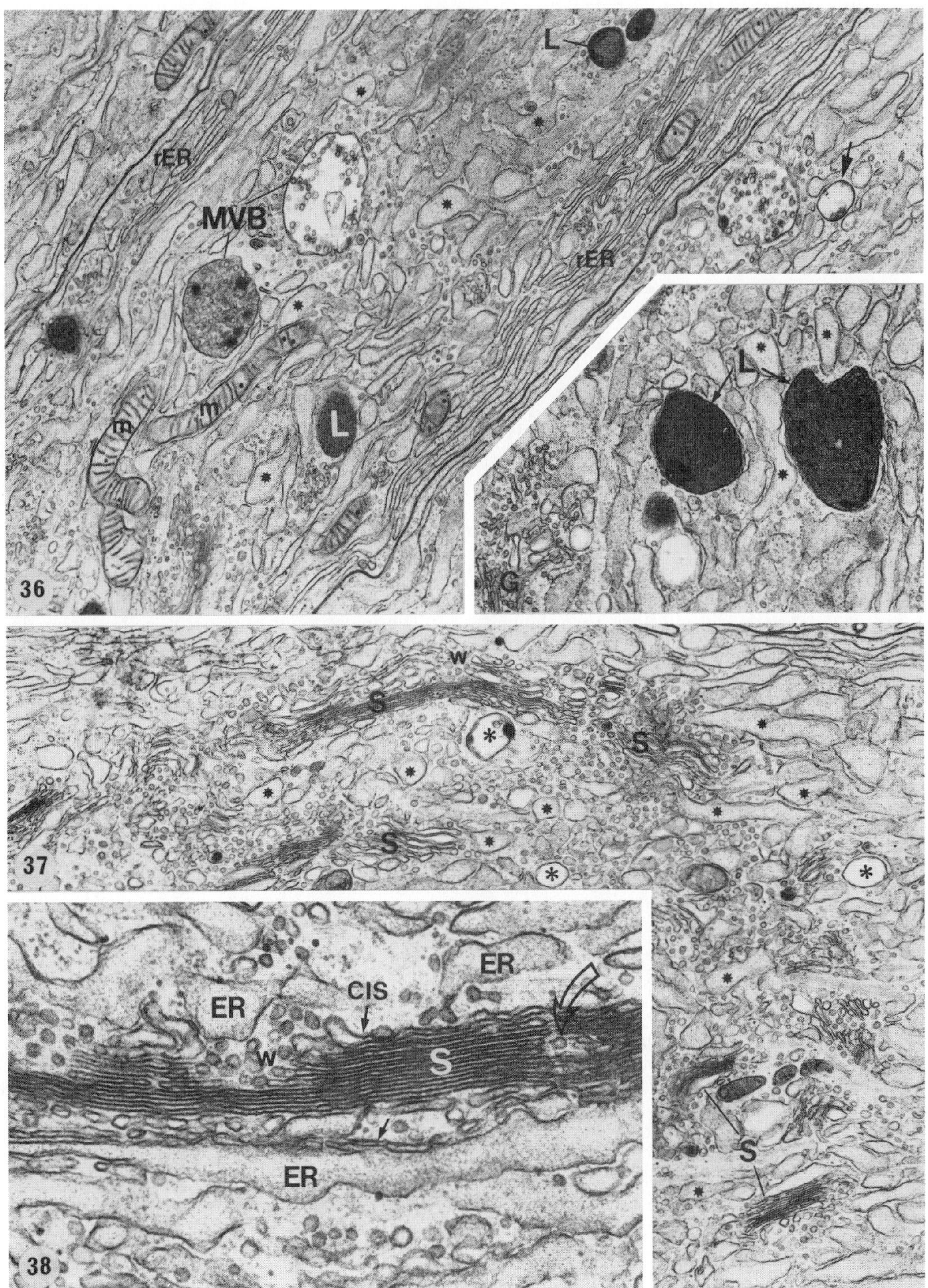

FIG. 37. Supranuclear region of a principal cell of the initial segment showing the Golgi apparatus formed of several stacks of saccules (S) seen in close association with the sparsely granulated endoplasmic reticulum (*stars*). The smooth-surfaced vesicles also appear in this region (*asterisks*). w: Well. (×16,800.) (Method B.)

FIG. 38. High power of a Golgi stack of saccules (S). On the cis face of the stack, the saccules show interruptions along their length which are in register with one another forming well defined gaps or "wells" (w) in which can be found small vesicles. On the cis face the sparsely granulated endoplasmic reticulum (ER) is loosely distributed, while on the opposite face (trans) it is closely applied to the transmost Golgi saccule (*small arrow*). Note the presence of a small vesicle in the middle of the Golgi stack (*large arrow*). (×44,000.) (Method B.)

apical regions are also evident in the Golgi region and in close proximity to the trans Golgi saccules (Fig. 37). (Their possible function is discussed in the section on secretion.)

The basal region of these cells is occupied by the nucleus and, infranuclearly, by numerous flattened cisternae of the rough endoplasmic reticulum, mitochondria, polyribosomes, and a few dense bodies identified cytochemically as lysosomes (L. Hermo and M. Lalli, *unpublished observations*) (Figs. 33,39). Lipid droplets are not a prominent feature of these cells. The ability of the principal cells to take up substances from their base has not been documented; coated or uncoated pits and vesicles, endosomes, or multivesicular bodies are not usually found in this region (Fig. 39).

Although cells with apically located nuclei have been identified in the initial segment of the epididymis and referred to as apical cells (66), morphological observations of such cells in the present work, as well as that of others (87,144,150), indicate that these cells are identical in appearance to the neighboring principal cells. The description of a separate population of apical cells may represent simply the topographical arrangement of the principal cells around the duct. In fact, in the mouse, apical cells have been shown to contact the underlying basement membrane (150).

Of all the various cell types in the male excurrent duct system, the ultrastructural features of the *principal cells of the head, body and tail of the epididymis* have been the most actively investigated over the last 10 years since the review of Hamilton (10). At the electron microscope level these cells have been studied by numerous investigators in a wide variety of species such as the rat (9,10,113,139, 151–155), mouse (141,142,150,156,157), guinea pig (69,143), hamster (67,71,158,159), rabbit (7,116,160), dog (81,161), bird (30,162), opossum (163), mole (164), tammar (144), echidna (25,140), bull (82), buffalo (165), armadillo (166,167), monkey (168–170), and human (77,123).

A schematic representation of the principal cell of the caput epididymidis of the rat is shown in Fig. 40. As found in other species, differences in the principal cells of other segments of the epididymis are relatively minor and will be discussed subsequently.

The principal epithelial cells of the caput, corpus, and cauda epididymidis are shorter than those of the initial segment; while they have a wide area of communication with the lumen, their basal plasma membrane may contact the underlying basement membrane by means of a wide (Fig. 40) or slender foot-like process (Fig. 51).

The apical region of principal cells of these three segments shows essentially the same structural features. Between the bases of the tall microvilli, small invaginations, or pits, of

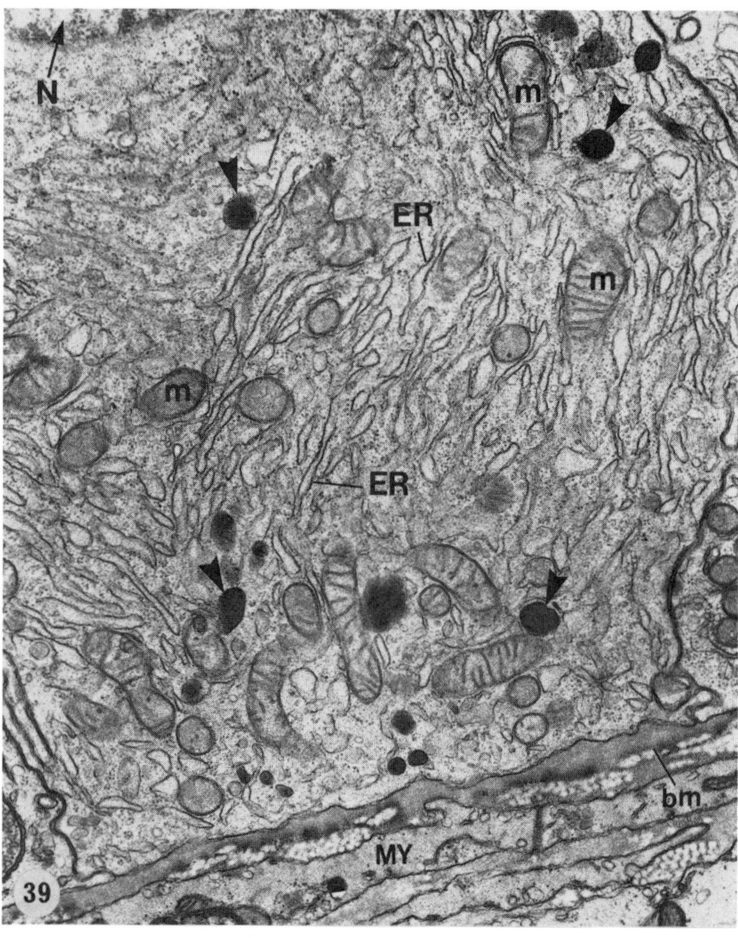

FIG. 39. Basal region of a principal cell of the initial segment. Numerous cisternae of the rough endoplasmic reticulum (ER) fill this region in addition to a few lysosomes (*arrowheads*) and mitochondria (m). N:nucleus, bm:basement membrane, MY:myoid cell of the lamina propria. (×16,850.) (Method B.)

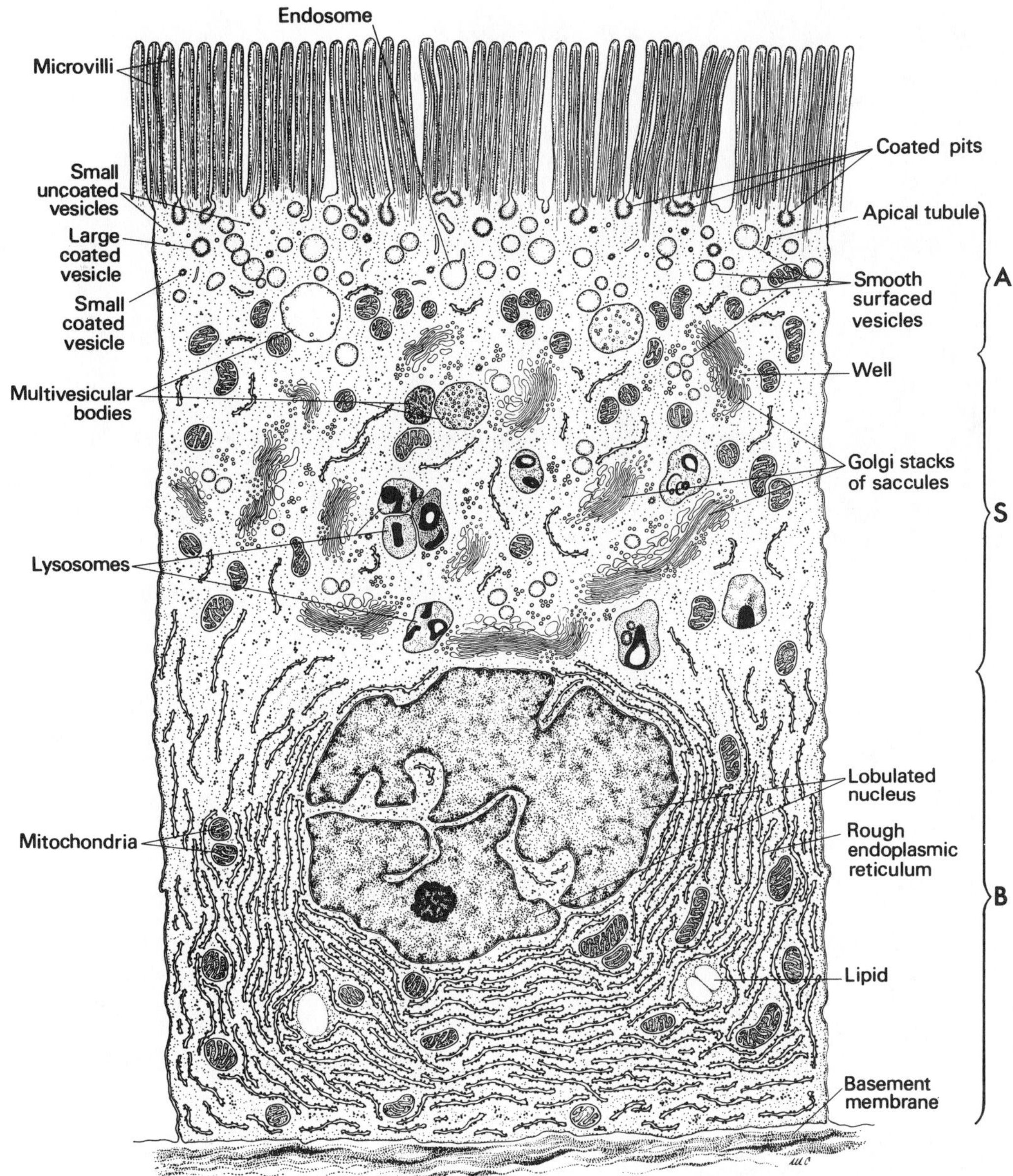

FIG. 40. Diagrammatic representation of a principal cell of the caput epididymidis. A:apical region, S:supranuclear region, B:basal region. The basal region shows an abundance of cisternae of rough endoplasmic reticulum, a few lipid droplets, and mitochondria. An elaborate Golgi apparatus occupies the supranuclear region in the company of lysosomes and multivesicular bodies. The apical region shows coated pits, large coated vesicles, endosomes, few apical tubules, small coated and uncoated vesicles, and smooth-surfaced vesicles also found next to the Golgi stacks of saccules.

the apical plasma membrane can be seen extending into the cytoplasm, often bearing a clathrin-like lattice coat (Figs. 41–43). Subjacent to the apical cell surface are a few large vesicles showing a uniform lattice coat referred to as the large coated vesicles (100 nm diameter) [Figs. 40,42,42(inset),43].

The most prominent feature of the apical region of these cells is the presence of numerous large uncoated vesicles (150–300 nm diameter). Such membranous elements, referred to as the smooth-surfaced vesicles, are more or less spherical in appearance and present an electron lucent or pale-stained lumen containing a wispy material (Figs. 40–43).

Small coated and uncoated vesicles of similar size (50–60 nm diameter) can be seen scattered about in the apical region and often in close proximity to the apical plasma membrane [Figs. 40,41,42 (inset),43]. Similar findings on the presence of small coated and uncoated vesicles and large coated vesicles have been made in principal cells of the rat (155) and mouse (142); in both cases, differences in their number were observed according to the different segments of the epididymis examined. Also evident in the apical re-

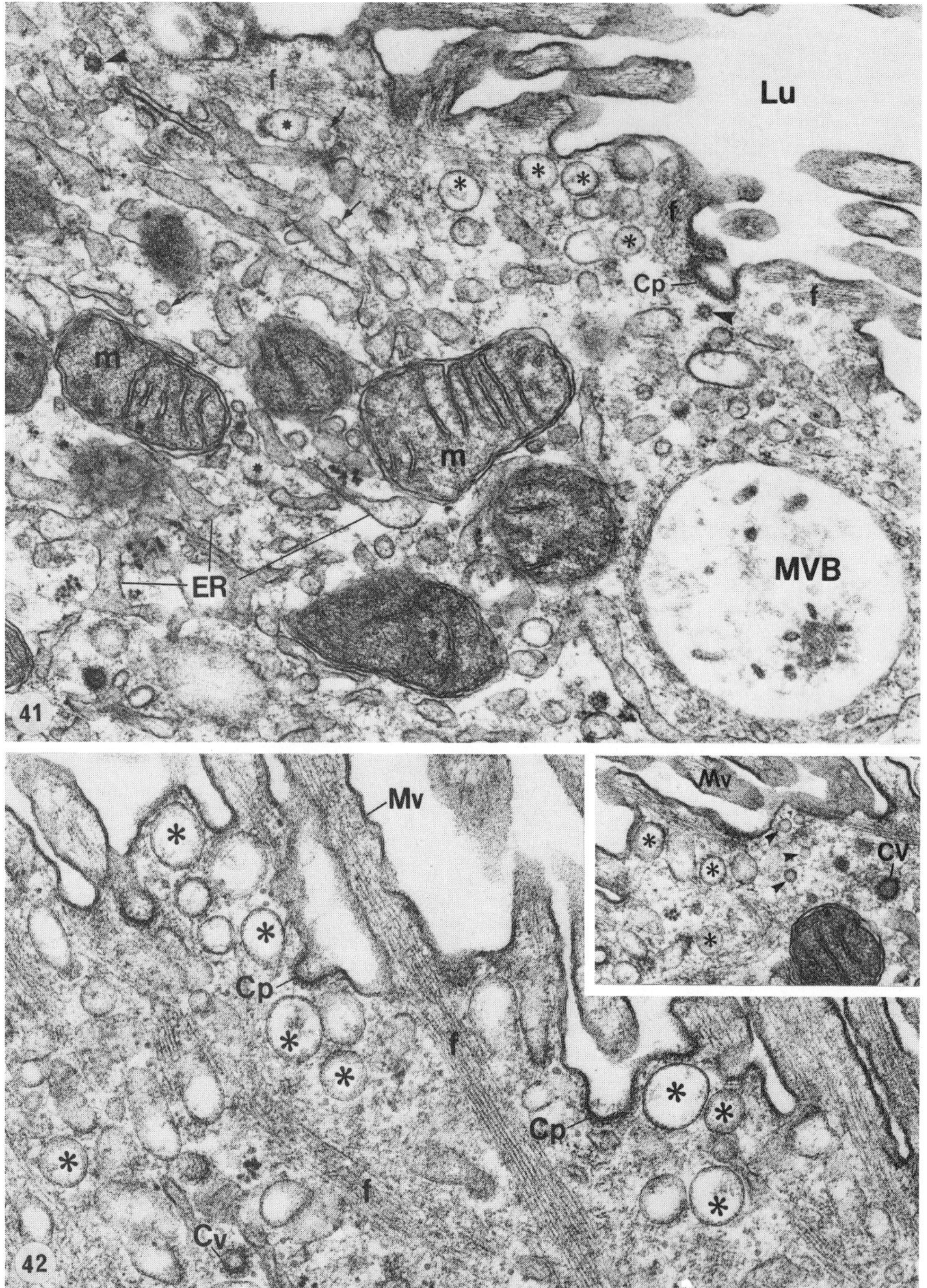

FIG. 41. High power of the apical region of a principal cell of the caput epididymidis. A coated pit (Cp) of the cell surface is present. Smooth-surfaced vesicles (*asterisks*) containing a flocculent material, small coated vesicles (*arrowheads*), small uncoated vesicles (*arrows*), and filaments (f) are labeled. An occasional smooth-surfaced vesicle shows a partial bristle coat (*stars*). Lu:lumen, MVB:pale multivesicular body, ER:rough endoplasmic reticulum, m:mitochondria. (×36,560.) (Method C.)

FIG. 42. High power of the apical region of a principal cell of the corpus epididymidis. Several smooth-surfaced vesicles containing a flocculent material are evident (*asterisks*), some of which are seen in close proximity to the apical plasma membrane although not in continuity with it. Coated pits (Cp) are seen in continuity with the apical plasma membrane. A large coated vesicle (100 nm) is also evident (Cv). Mv:microvillus, f:filaments. (×52,500.) (Method C.) **Inset**: Apical region of a principal cell of the cauda epididymidis showing smooth-surfaced vesicles (*asterisks*), a large coated vesicle (cv), and several small uncoated vesicles (*arrowheads*) close to the cell surface. Mv:microvillus. (×32,175.) (Method C.)

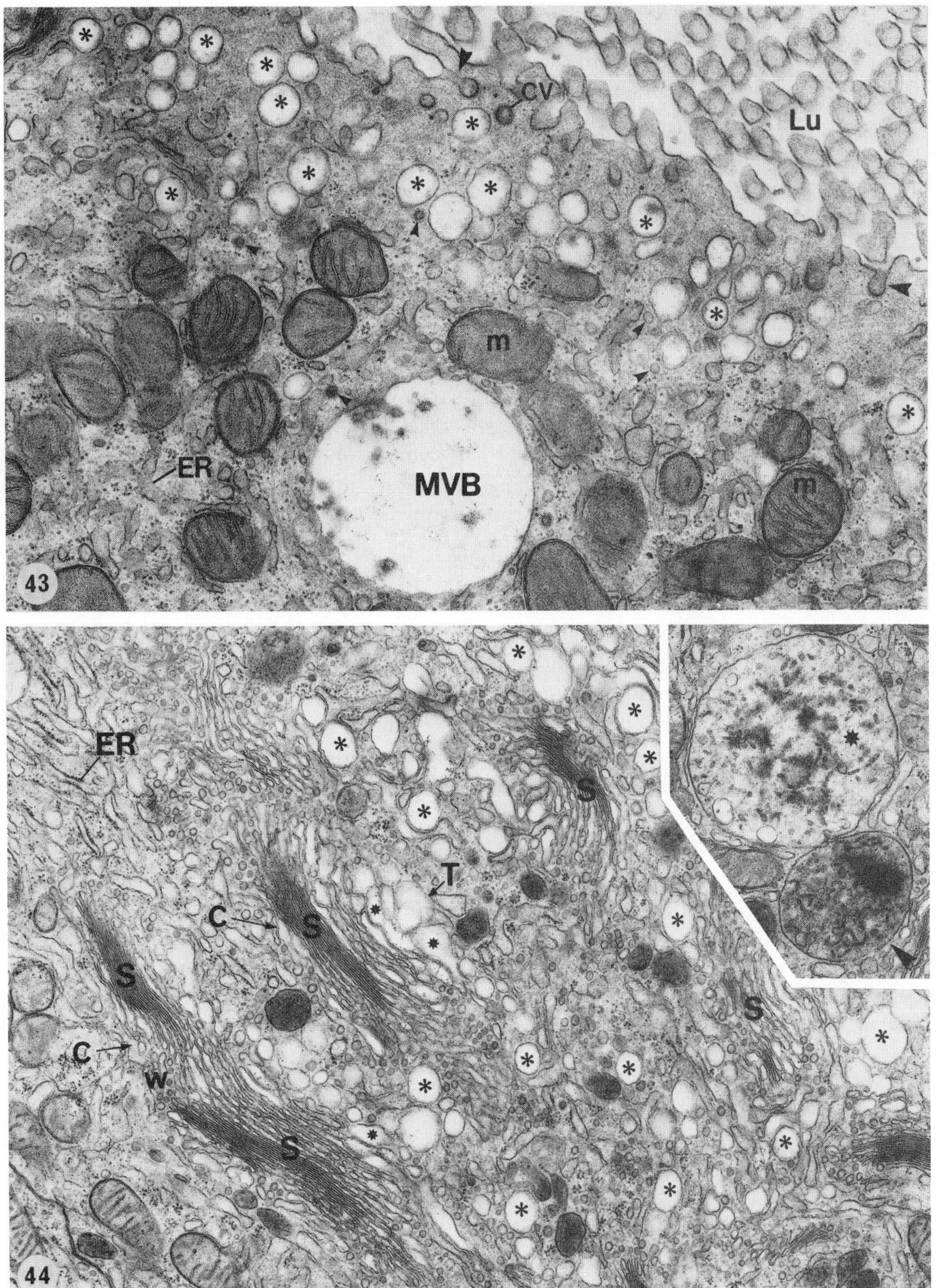

FIG. 43. Apical region of a principal cell of the cauda epididymidis. Numerous smooth-surfaced vesicles (*asterisks*) are present beneath the cell surface although not in continuity with it. Coated pits (*large arrowheads*), a large coated vesicle (CV), small coated and uncoated vesicles (*small arrowheads*) and a pale multivesicular body are also evident. Lu:lumen, ER:rough endoplasmic reticulum, m:mitochondria. (×23,400.) (Method B.)

FIG. 44. Supranuclear region of a principal cell of the cauda epididymidis showing an elaborate Golgi apparatus. The latter is formed of many stacks of saccules (S). On the cis face (C) of the stack, the saccules are flat and interrupted by wells (w) containing vesicles, while on the trans face (T) of the stack, the saccules are often dilated (*stars*). Numerous smooth-surfaced vesicles (*asterisks*) are present in relation to the Golgi stacks of saccules. ER:rough endoplasmic reticulum. (×18,430.) (Method B.) **Inset**: Multivesicular bodies in the supranuclear region of a principal cell of the cauda epididymidis containing spherical and flattened vesicular profiles embedded in a moderately dense (*star*) or dense (*arrowhead*) staining matrix presenting patches of densely stained material. (×19,305.) (Method B.)

gion, but less frequent, are elongated membranous elements identified as apical tubules.

The apical region also contains mitochondria, filaments, polysomes, microtubules, widely scattered cisternae of rough endoplasmic reticulum, endosomes, and pale multivesicular bodies (Figs. 40–43). Unlike principal cells of the initial segment, no large distended sparsely granulated cisternae of endoplasmic reticulum are present in these cells.

The most conspicuous feature of the supranuclear region of principal cells is the large Golgi apparatus formed of many stacks of saccules and associated vesicular elements of small size (Figs. 40,44,47,51). In appropriate planes of section, it can be seen that the individual stacks are composed of as many as 15 saccules; however, it has yet to be demonstrated whether the individual stacks are, in fact, interconnected.

On the cis face of the stack, well defined wells containing a few small vesicles can be identified (Fig. 44), as seen earlier for the Golgi apparatus of principal cells of the initial segment. While saccules on the cis face are flattened, those on the trans face of the stack show a dilated appearance; in this region large, smooth-surfaced vesicles, similar in size and appearance to those present in the apical region, can be found (Fig. 44). (The potential secretory function of these vesicles is discussed later.) Sporadic multivesicular bodies showing a moderately dense or dense-staining matrix are also evident in the supranuclear region [Figs. 40,44 (inset)]. These elements present a matrix in which are embedded spherical or flattened vesicular profiles and aggregates of an electron-dense material [Fig. 44 (inset)].

One major difference between principal cells of the head, body, and tail of the epididymis is in the appearance of a fair number of large, supranuclearly located, spherical membrane-bound bodies identified cytochemically as lysosomes (152) (L. Hermo and M. Lalli, *unpublished observations*). In the caput, these bodies are recognized by the presence of a pale lumen containing a flocculent material, loose membranous profiles, small vesicles, and electron-dense spherical or doughnut-shaped masses showing a linear periodicity (Figs. 40,45) (171). In the corpus, such large membrane-bound bodies, irregular or spherical in form, take on a different appearance; they characteristically contain a uniform homogeneous electron-dense material in which are embedded flattened membranous and vesicular profiles (Fig. 48). The equivalent structures in the cauda epididymis contain a moderate or dense-staining homogeneous material in which are embedded whorls of membranous profiles [Figs. 50,50 (inset)]. Similar observations on the differences in appearance and the amount of these dense bodies according to the various epididymal segments have been made in the mouse (142) and rabbit (116).

Aside from the difference in appearance in the supranuclear region between the lysosomal elements of the epididymis, one other dramatic difference can be found among principal cells of these three segments. In the corpus, but not in the other two segments of the epididymis, lipid droplets can be seen randomly distributed in the supranuclear region (Fig. 47).

Based on the work of several investigators, principal cells from the caput and cauda epididymidis have been shown to internalize tracers introduced into the lumen, which at early time intervals appeared in uncoated or coated pits and vesicles, and at later time intervals in multivesicular bodies and lysosomes (152,154).

The basal region of the principal cells of the caput, corpus, and cauda epididymidis shows a highly irregular nucleus (Figs. 40,50). In the caput (Figs. 40,46) and cauda (Figs. 50,51), this region contains numerous wavy thin strands of rough endoplasmic reticulum, often arranged in parallel, polysomes, a few lysosomes, mitochondria, and lipid droplets. In comparison, the basal region of the corpus epididymidis is often filled with lipid droplets (Fig. 49). These observations on abundance of lipid droplets in the corpus epididymidis coincide with those made on principal cells of region 2 of the guinea pig epididymis (69).

Along the basal plasma membrane, uncoated or coated pits are infrequently found (155). Unlike what has been reported for some species (116,143), the principal cells of the rat epididymis do not appear to contain profiles or whorls of smooth endoplasmic reticulum. Nor does the infranuclear region of the rat principal cells show accumulations of small dense granules suggested to be of endocrine (168,170) or exocrine function (143).

The lateral plasma membrane of principal cells is fairly smooth and does not show extensive interdigitation with neighboring cells (Fig. 51). Small vesicular profiles occasionally appear along the lateral plasma membrane in continuity with it, suggesting that these cells may be involved in transcytosis; this has recently been demonstrated for principal cells of the vas deferens (172).

While the electron microscopic appearance of the *principal epithelial cells lining the vas deferens* has been investigated in the monkey (85) and human (96,173–175) most studies have been performed on the rat (83,84,95, 156,176,177). Differences in the principal cells can be observed along the length of the vas deferens (6 cm), which can be divided into proximal, distal, and terminal segments (83).

Aside from a difference in height, principal cells from the proximal (cuboidal) and distal (columnar) (Fig. 52) segments show many features in common with principal cells of the caput, corpus, and cauda epididymidis. In the apical region, coated and uncoated pits, small coated and uncoated vesicles of similar size (50–60 nm), large coated vesicles (100 nm), and smooth-surfaced vesicles (150–300 nm) showing a wispy content and apical tubules are present (Fig. 55) (172). The most prominent feature of the supranuclear region is an elaborate Golgi apparatus formed of many stacks of saccules and associated small vesicles (Figs. 52,56,57). The stacks of Golgi saccules show on their trans face a close association with many smooth-surfaced vesicles containing a wispy material (Figs. 56,57), while wells containing a

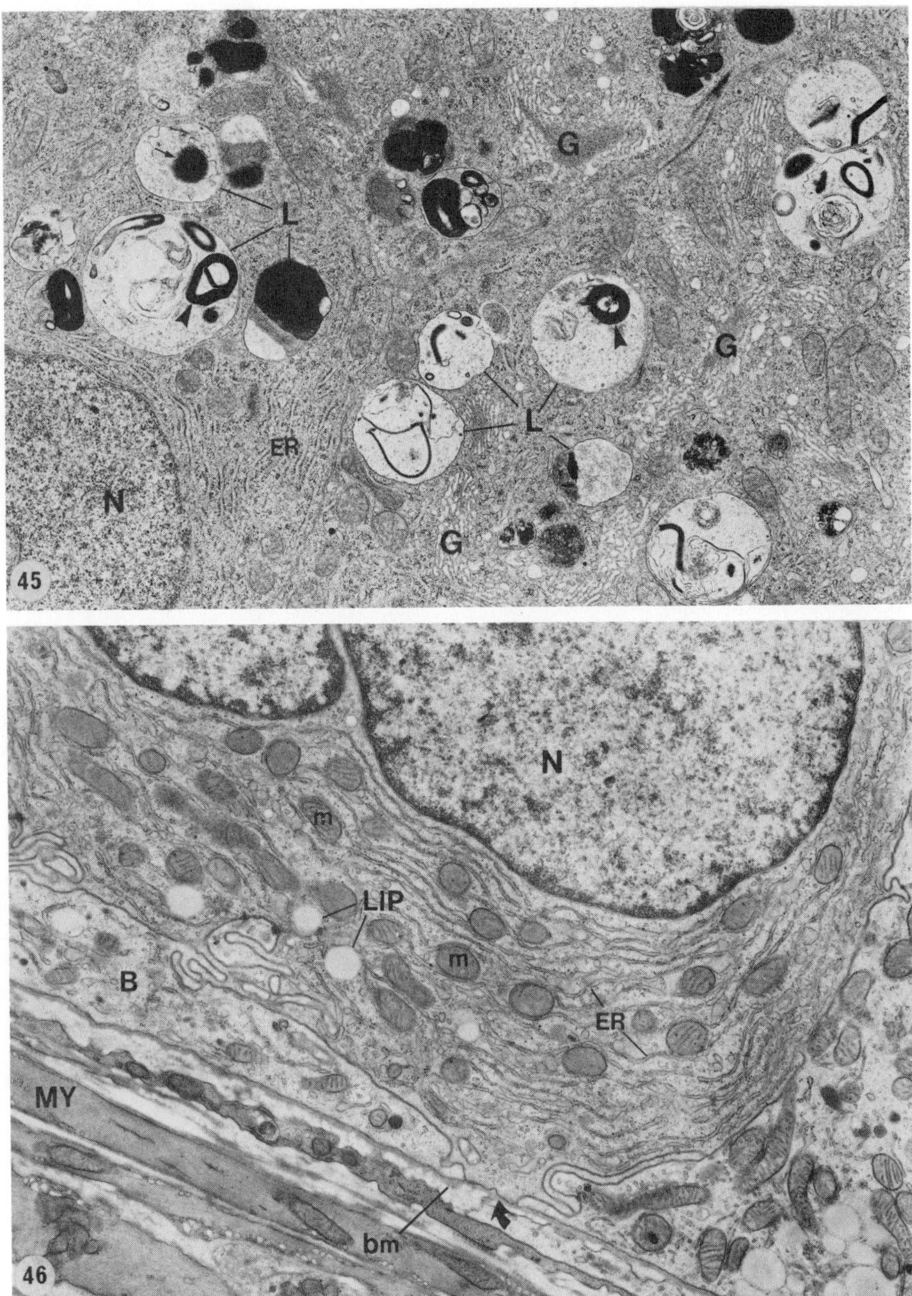

FIG. 45. Supranuclear region of a principal cell of the caput epididymidis. Numerous large membrane-bound bodies showing a pale-stained matrix containing a flocculent material in which are embedded electron-dense spherical (*arrows*) or doughnut-shaped (*arrowheads*) masses, small vesicles, and membranous profiles. Such elements are identified cytochemically as lysosomes (L). ER:rough endoplasmic reticulum, G:Golgi apparatus, N:nucleus. (×9,625.) (Method B.)

FIG. 46. Basal region of a principal cell of the caput epididymidis. Cisternae of rough endoplasmic reticulum (ER) fill this region. Also evident are mitochondria (m) and a few lipid droplets (LIP). Note the small area of contact of the principal cell (*arrow*) with the basement membrane (bm). N:nucleus, MY:myoid cell of lamina propria, B:basal cell cytoplasm. (×9,240.) (Method A.)

few vesicles can be found on their cis face (Fig. 57). Multivesicular bodies of variable density [Fig. 55 (inset)] and lysosomes (Fig. 52) are also evident (172,177). The latter clearly differ in appearance from those seen in epididymal cells; they show a homogeneous electron-dense central mass enclosed by a paler zone of finely granulated material (Fig. 53).

In the distal segment of the vas deferens, tracer studies have shown that the principal cells are involved in endocytosis (172,177). In these cells, the smooth-surfaced ves-

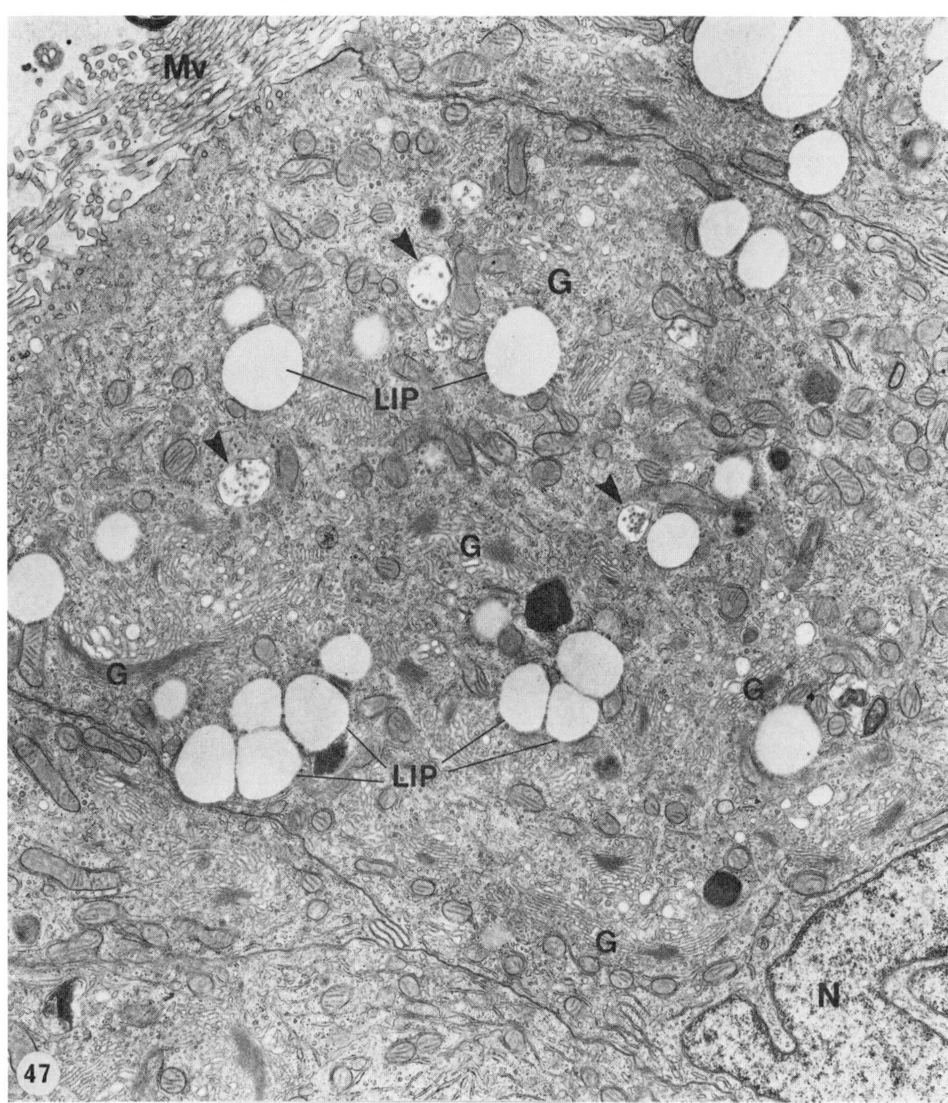

FIG. 47. Apical and supranuclear regions of a principal cell of the corpus epididymidis. Note the presence of lipid droplets (LIP) scattered about in the supranuclear region. Also indicated are pale, multivesicular bodies (*arrowheads*), the widely distributed Golgi apparatus (G), and the nucleus (N). Mv:microvilli. (×8,385.) (Method B.)

icles were never seen to become labeled with tracers injected into the lumen (172), thus indicating that these vesicles were not involved in endocytosis. (The possibility that they are involved in secretion is discussed later.)

In the basal region, the most conspicuous feature is the endoplasmic reticulum (Figs. 52,54). The endoplasmic reticulum of cells in the proximal segment is studded with ribosomes, but, as one approaches the terminal segment, a progressive development of smooth endoplasmic reticulum becomes evident (84,95). The base of principal cells often contacts the underlying basement membrane by means of only small foot-like processes (Fig. 54). Such a poor association of these cells with the basement membrane might therefore account for the numerous anchoring fibrils found associated with the basement membrane; these fibrils have been reported to hold principal cells in place during the vigorous contractions of the smooth muscle coat (178).

In the terminal segment of the vas deferens, a dramatic change occurs in the epithelium with the appearance of discrete clusters of cells that show blunt processes extending into the lumen (179). (Their function is discussed in the section on spermiophagy.)

The presence of goblet-shaped pencil cells in the epithelial lining of the rat vas deferens has been reported by Hamilton (10). These cells, few in number, present an apically located nucleus, numerous mitochondria, a few indented dense bodies, and multivesicular bodies (Fig. 58). The stacks of Golgi saccules surround the nucleus, while a few cisternae of rough endoplasmic reticulum are scattered about in the cytoplasm (Fig. 58). These cells are clearly different in ap-

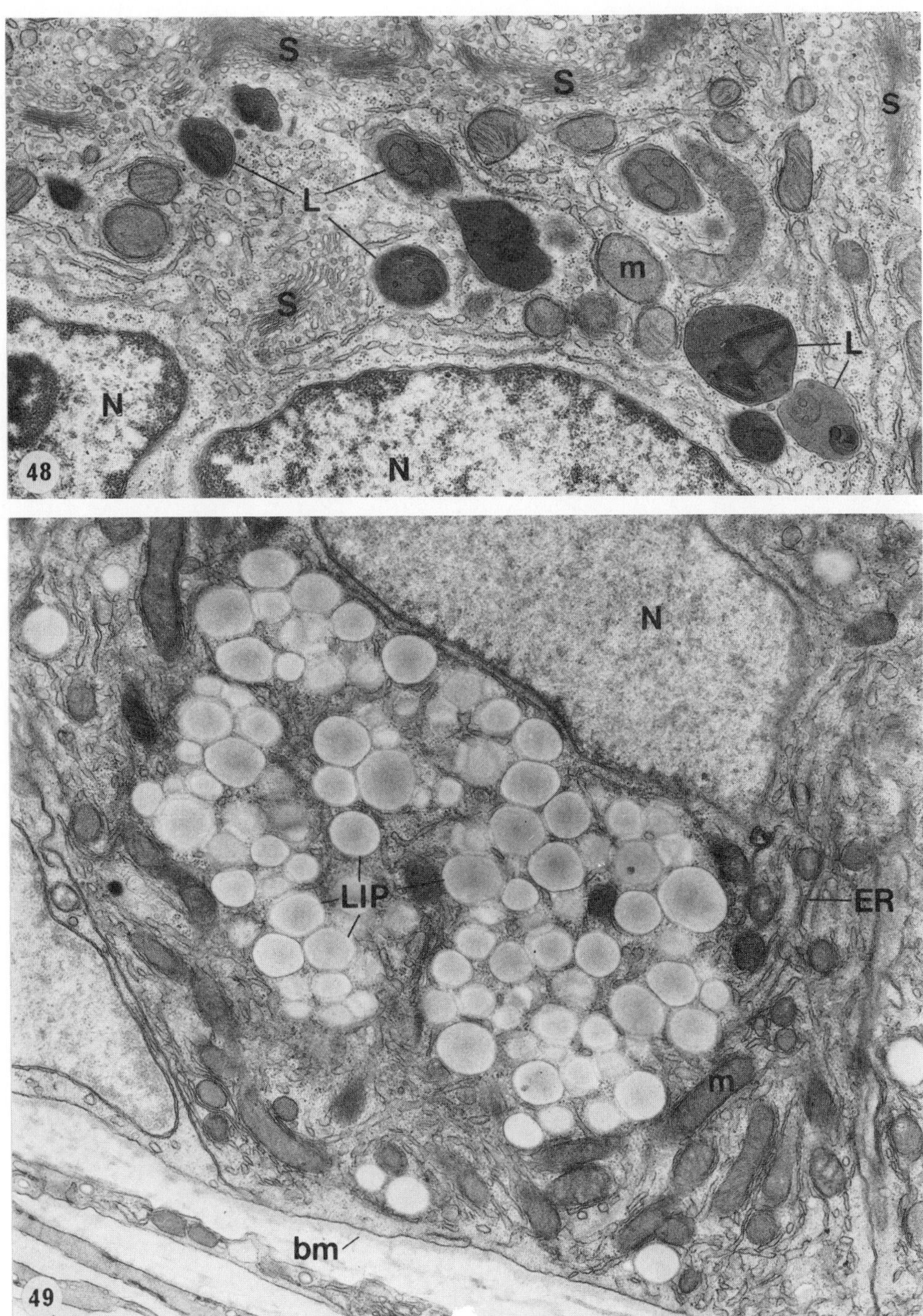

FIG. 48. Supranuclear region of a principal cell of the corpus epididymidis. Several membrane-bound bodies identified as lysosomes (L) present a homogeneous electron-dense material in which are embedded small vesicles and flat membranous profiles. Several stacks of saccules (S) of the Golgi apparatus are indicated. N:portions of a highly lobulated nucleus, m:mitochondria. (×13,950.) (Method B.)

FIG. 49. Basal region of a principal cell of the corpus epididymidis demonstrating an abundance of lipid droplets (LIP). The principal cell shows a wide area of contact with the basement membrane (bm). ER:cisternae of rough endoplasmic reticulum, m:mitochondria. N:nucleus. (×16,200.) (Method B.)

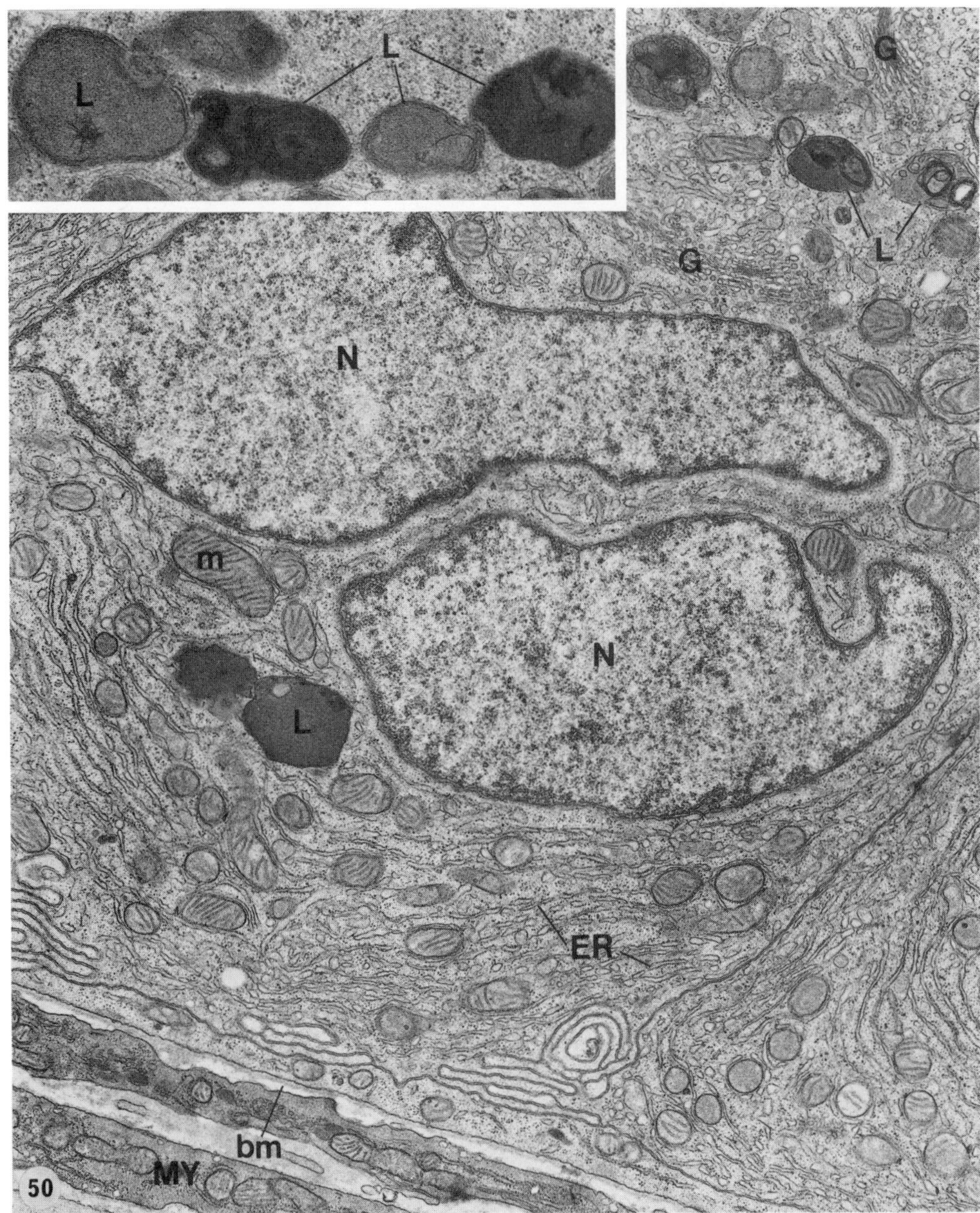

FIG. 50. Principal cell of the cauda epididymidis. The basal region contains numerous flattened cisternae of rough endoplasmic reticulum arranged in loose parallel rows, a few lysosomes (L), and mitochondria (m). Lysosomes (L) are also present above the nucleus (N) which is highly irregular in these cells. Since principal cells occasionally contact the basement membrane (bm) by means of only a small foot-like process, in some planes of section, as is the case here, no contact is observed. G:Golgi apparatus, MY:myoid cell. (×11,700.) (Method B.) **Inset**: High power of lysosomes (L) in the supranuclear region of a principal cell of the cauda epididymidis. Such elements have a homogeneous moderately dense or dense-staining matrix containing membranous whorls. (×21,940.) (Method B.)

pearance from the neighboring principal cells. In the human, pencil cells have been reported to be a dying epithelial cell (96); in the rat, their function is unknown but they certainly do not appear to be a dying cell type.

Narrow Cells: The narrow cells of the epididymis are tall columnar cells showing a narrower width than the adjacent principal cells (Fig. 59). These cells have been reported to be present only in the initial segment of the epididymis of the rat (82,87,139,180), mouse (141,150), hamster (71), and echidna (140). Narrow cells show many features in common with the so-called mitochondria-rich cells, described for other species, which are found in different segments of the epididymis [tammar (144), monkey (168)] or vas deferens [human (96)].

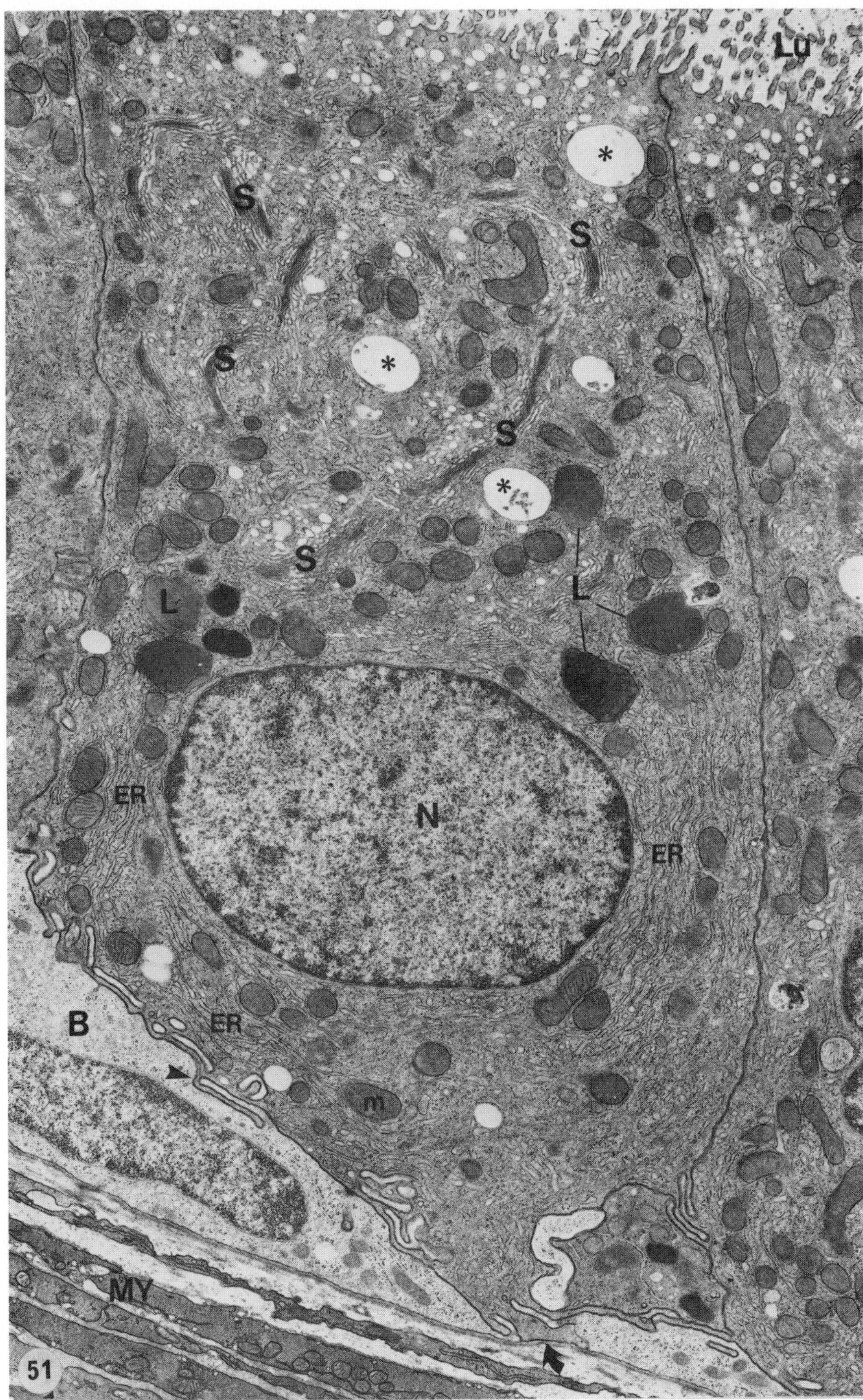

FIG. 51. A principal cell of the cauda epididymidis showing a slender foot-like process contacting the basement membrane (*arrow*) and interdigitations (*arrowhead*) with a basal cell (B). Also indicated are pale multivesicular bodies (*asterisks*), stacks of saccules (S) of the Golgi apparatus, lysosomes (L), cisternae of the rough endoplasmic reticulum (ER) arranged in parallel rows, mitochondria (m), and the nucleus (N). Lu:lumen, MY:myoid cell. (×8,640.) (Method B.)

In the rat these cells, as illustrated by Sun and Flickinger (87), are identified by the presence of an abundance of small, uncoated vesicular profiles in the apical region, and numerous mitochondria distributed throughout the cytoplasm, and a few cisternae of rough endoplasmic reticulum (Fig. 59). The former, completely filling the apical region, are predominantly C-shaped in appearance, and thus occasionally appear as spherical or double-walled structures, depending on their plane of section (Figs. 59–61). While seen close to the apical cell surface, no signs of continuity of these vesicles with the apical plasma membrane have been observed. Vesicles of similar size and appearance can also be found, although fewer in number, in the supranuclear region (Fig. 59). Although the function of these vesicles

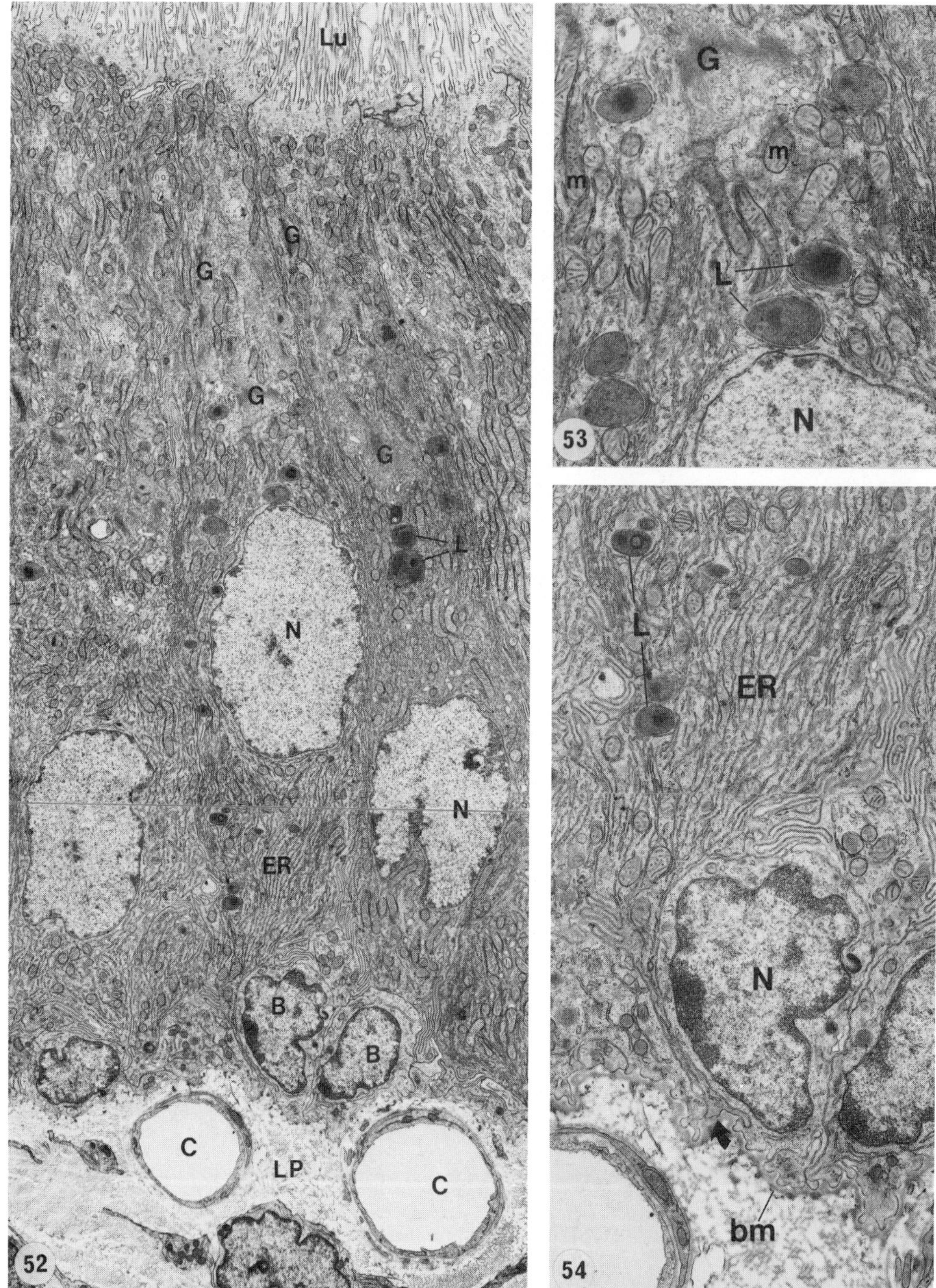

FIG. 52. A principal cell of the distal segment of the vas deferens. In this segment, these cells are tall columnar and show an elaborate Golgi apparatus (G), a few lysosomes (L), a pale nucleus (N), and basally located rough endoplasmic reticulum (ER). Two round basal cells (B) are indicated showing a small amount of cytoplasm surrounding their nuclei. C:capillaries, LP:lamina propria, Lu:lumen. (×4,455.) (Method A.)

FIG. 53. High power of the supranuclear region of a principal cell seen in Fig. 52. Note that the lysosomes (L) in these cells show a central homogeneous, electron-dense mass surrounded by a paler granulated material. G:Golgi apparatus, m:mitochondria, N:nucleus. (×10,640.) (Method A.)

FIG. 54. High power of the basal region of a principal cell seen in Fig. 52. A few lysosomes (L) and numerous parallel cisternae of rough endoplasmic reticulum (ER) fill this region. Note the small slender foot-like process of a principal cell (*arrow*) contacting the basement membrane (bm). Also indicated is the nucleus (N) of a round basal cell. (×9,405.) (Method A.)

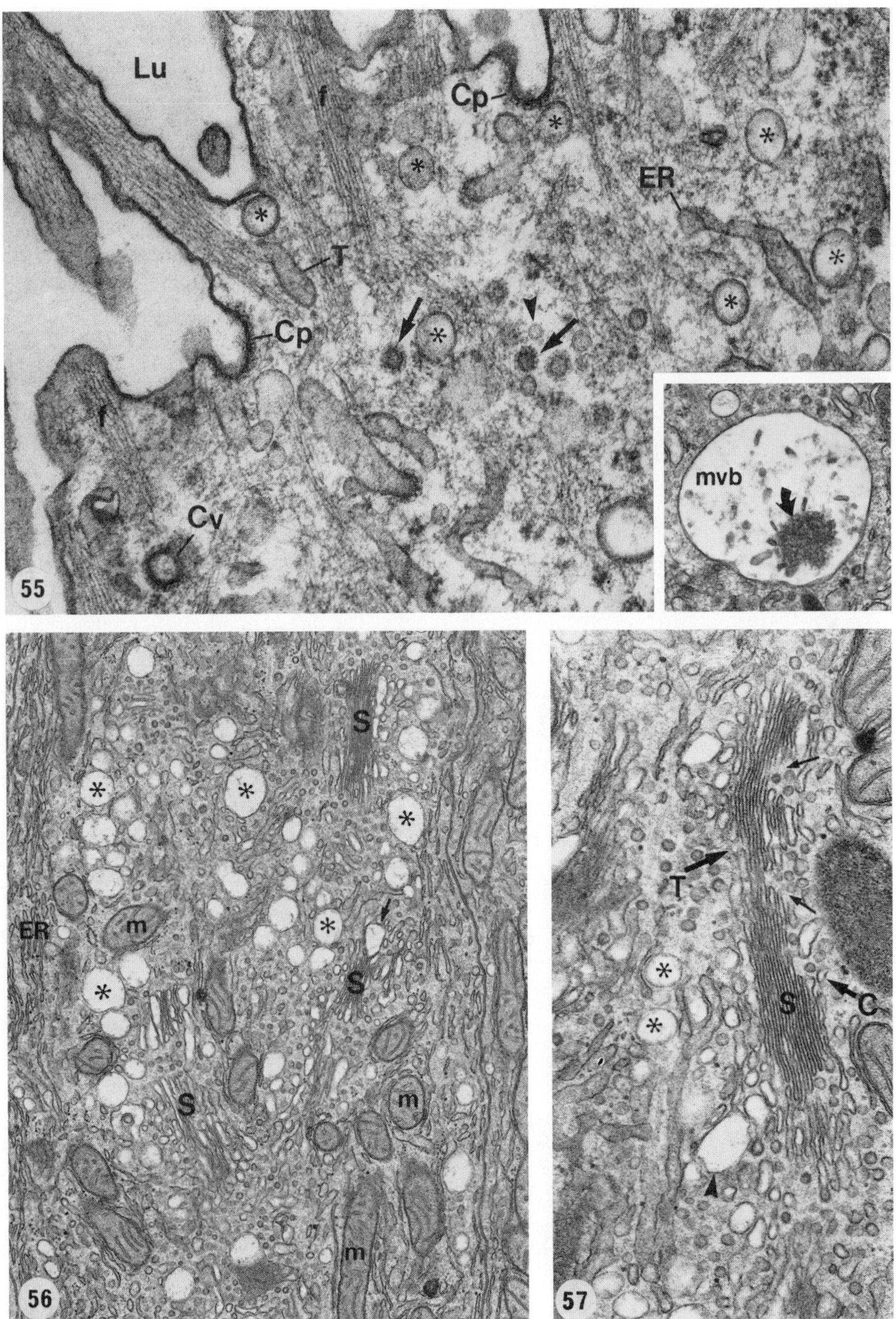

FIG. 55. Apical region of a principal cell of the vas deferens showing coated pits (Cp), large coated vesicles (Cv), smooth-surfaced vesicles (*asterisks*), and small coated (*arrows*), and uncoated (*arrowhead*) vesicles. Lu:lumen, ER:rough endoplasmic reticulum, f:filaments. (×54,375.) (Method C.) **Inset**: A multivesicular body (mvb) in the apical region of a principal cell showing a pale-stained matrix containing spherical and flattened vesicular profiles and a roundish mass of finely granular material (*arrow*). (×21,940.) (Method C.)

FIG. 56. The supranuclear region of a principal cell of the vas deferens. The elaborate Golgi apparatus is formed of many stacks of saccules (S) and associated small vesicles. Also evident in the Golgi region are numerous large smooth-surfaced vesicles (150–300 nm diameter), some of which can be seen in close proximity or in continuity (*arrow*) with the Golgi stacks. m:Mitochondria, ER:rough endoplasmic reticulum. (×15,225.) (Method A.)

FIG. 57. High power of a Golgi stack of saccules (S) showing on its cis face (C) interruptions of the saccules forming wells (*arrows*) in which are located small vesicles. Smooth-surfaced vesicles (*asterisks*) are seen on the trans face (T), one of which can be seen in continuity with a trans Golgi saccule (*arrowhead*). (×28,500.) (Method A.)

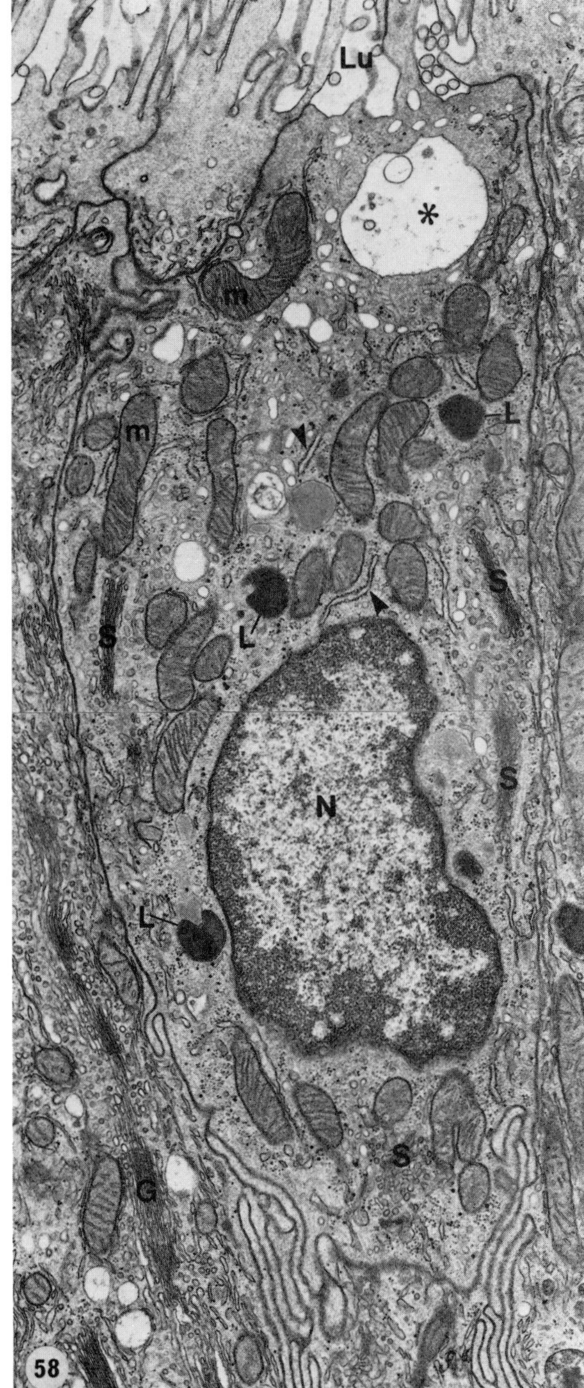

FIG. 58. A montage of a pencil cell within the epithelial lining of the vas deferens. These cells show a nucleus (N) in the upper half of the cytoplasm, numerous mitochondria (m), a few homogeneous dense bodies occasionally indented and presumed to be lysosomes (L), several scattered cisternae of rough endoplasmic reticulum (*arrowheads*), a multivesicular body (*asterisk*), and stacks of saccules (S) of the Golgi apparatus surrounding the nucleus. A portion of the elaborate Golgi apparatus (G) of an adjacent principal cell is also seen. (×14,040.) (Method A.)

has not been elucidated, it is reasonable to speculate that they are involved in endocytosis. The presence of vesicles of similar appearance has been reported in Leydig cells where it was shown that they are involved in adsorptive endocytosis (181).

Multivesicular bodies showing a pale, moderate- or dense-staining matrix are also evident in the supranuclear region in the company of a few dense membrane-bound bodies which are possibly lysosomes (Figs. 59,61). The role of the multivesicular bodies and lysosome-like bodies in endocytosis in the narrow cells has not been ascertained.

The Golgi apparatus is formed of several stacks of saccules and associated vesicles and is situated in the supranuclear region and alongside the nucleus (Fig. 59). The attenuated basal region shows, in addition to the nucleus which in this cell occupies the midregion of the cytoplasm, a few cisternae of rough endoplasmic reticulum, polysomes, and mitochondria (87). Scattered throughout the cytoplasm, one can find many glycogen granules often arranged in groups (Figs. 59,60) suggesting a high energy requirement for these cells. The differentiation of precursor cells into narrow cells seems to be androgen-independent, as demonstrated by the use of organ culture of immature rat epididymides (48). Narrow cells are the precursor cells to the clear cells (50). Despite the morphological studies performed on these cells, they have not as yet been given a function.

Clear Cells: Clear cells, also referred to as light or prominent cells, have been identified only in the rat (9,10,82, 113,139,153,154,182,183), hamster (71), mouse (141,150), and opossum (73).

In the rat, these cells are not found in the initial segment but are present in the caput, corpus, and cauda epididymidis, as well as in the proximal segment of the vas deferens.

The clear cells of the epididymis are characterized by an apical region containing numerous pale-stained vesicles of different sizes, a large supranuclear region packed with an abundance of large densely stained bodies of various shapes and sizes, and a basal region presenting the nucleus and a variable amount of lipid droplets (Fig. 62) (10,182).

Extending from the apical plasma membrane into the lumen are several unevenly distributed long, slender microvilli (Fig. 62) (113). Large coated invaginations or pits are seen in continuity with the apical plasma membrane (Fig. 63); subjacent to the cell surface, large coated vesicles, although few in number, can be found (Fig. 63). In the apical region, among a few scattered cisternae of the rough endoplasmic reticulum and mitochondria, are a plethora of small spherical, pale-stained vesicles (Figs. 63,64). Such vesicles are uncoated, and while they generally appear empty, a few contain one or more small particles of moderate density having a diffuse wall. Several larger uncoated vacuoles can also be found in the apical region; they often contain many of the small particles mentioned above (Figs. 62–64). Such vacuoles also contain flattened or dilated membranous elements of different sizes (Fig. 64). These large vacuoles

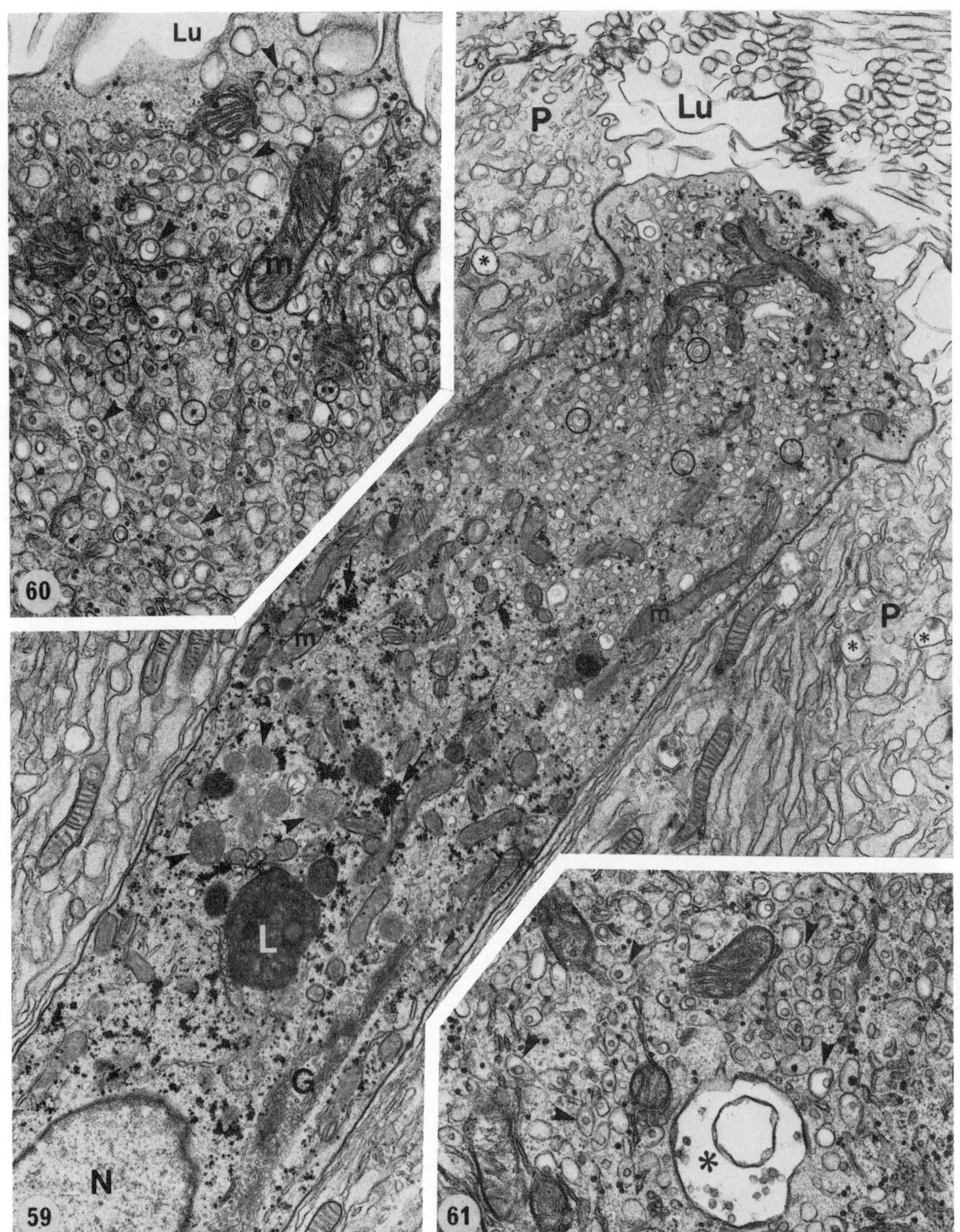

FIG. 59. Apical and supranuclear regions of a narrow cell of the initial segment of the epididymis. The apical region is filled with small C-shaped vesicles often appearing as a small vesicle enclosed by a larger vesicle due to the plane of section (*circles*), while the supranuclear region contains the Golgi apparatus (G), dense multivesicular bodies (*arrowheads*), a lysosome (L), and clumps of glycogen granules (*arrows*). m:Mitochondria, Lu:lumen, P:principal cells showing smooth-surfaced vesicles (*asterisks*). (×11,440.) (Method A.)

FIG. 60. High power of the apical region of a narrow cell showing numerous small C-shaped vesicles often appearing as double-walled structures (*arrowheads*) and glycogen granules (*circles*). Lu:lumen, m:mitochondria. (×23,760.) (Method A.)

FIG. 61. High power of the apical region of a narrow cell containing a pale multivesicular body (*asterisk*) and numerous small C-shaped vesicles (*arrowheads*). (×23,760.) (Method A.)

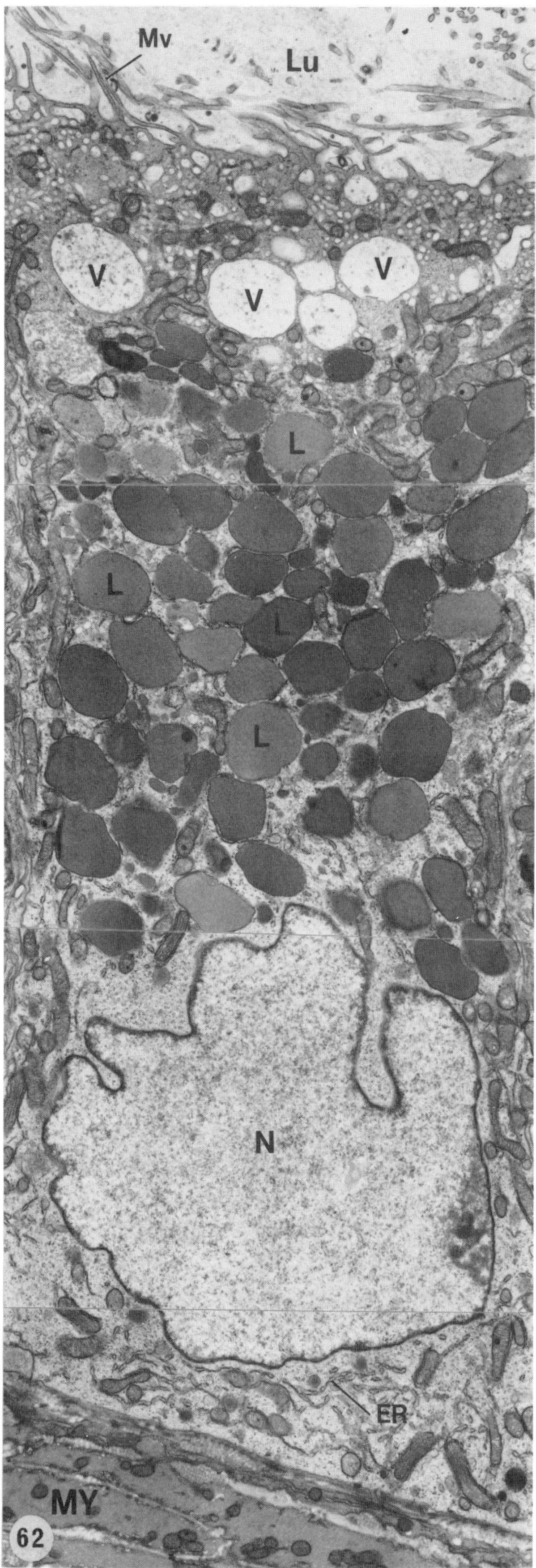

may also contain one or more small membrane-bound granules with an electron-dense core (Fig. 64). The apical cell surface also contains small coated and uncoated vesicles (50–60 nm diameter), free ribosomes, and several membranous apical tubules (Fig. 63).

By freeze-fracture studies, it has been found that the apical plasma membrane and the membrane delimiting the apical vesicles and vacuoles contain a higher density of intramembranous particles than that found in similar structures in principal cells of the epididymis (183); this is analogous to what has been reported for the narrow cell (180).

In the supranuclear region large membrane-bound bodies of different sizes and staining intensities can be observed (Figs. 62,65). Those with a moderate or densely stained intensity contain a homogeneous, finely filamentous material in which are embedded numerous particles of small size, as seen in the small vesicles and large vacuoles, the occasional small dense-core granule and membranous profiles [Figs. 65,65 (inset)]. Small vesicular profiles characteristic of multivesicular bodies are also present within these structures but are few in number (Fig. 65). These various elements are not seen in the very dense, homogeneous, membrane-bound bodies also found in the supranuclear region (Fig. 65). These latter structures are acid phosphatase-positive, and thus are lysosomal in nature (184).

After injection of tracers into the lumen of the cauda epididymidis, the apical vesicles and vacuoles of the clear cells were found labeled. This indicated an endocytic role for these cells; this endocytic activity was much greater in clear cells than in the adjacent principal cells, particularly in the cauda epididymidis (153,154). Mitochondria, a few cisternae of rough endoplasmic reticulum, and the Golgi apparatus are interspersed among these large bodies (Fig. 65).

The basal region containing the pale-stained nucleus is often filled in some cells with an abundance of lipid droplets (10), while in others only traces of lipid are present (Fig. 62). In all clear cells, a few cisternae of rough endoplasmic reticulum, polysomes, and mitochondria are present in the basal region (Fig. 62). The basal plasma membrane forms a uniform contact with the underlying basement membrane and shows few coated or uncoated pits and vesicles. (The possible role of these cells is discussed in the section on the lumen.)

Basal Cells: Basal cells, observed in all species studied to date, appear along the entire length of the male excurrent

FIG. 62. Montage of a clear cell of the cauda epididymidis. Unlike the neighboring principal cells, only a few microvilli (Mv) extend into the lumen (Lu) from the surface of these cells. In the apical region, small vesicles are seen as well as a few large vacuoles (V). Numerous lysosomes (L) fill the supranuclear region. A pale-stained nucleus (N) is located in the base of the cell as well as a few cisternae of rough endoplasmic reticulum (ER). MY:myoid cell. (×8,160.) (Method A.)

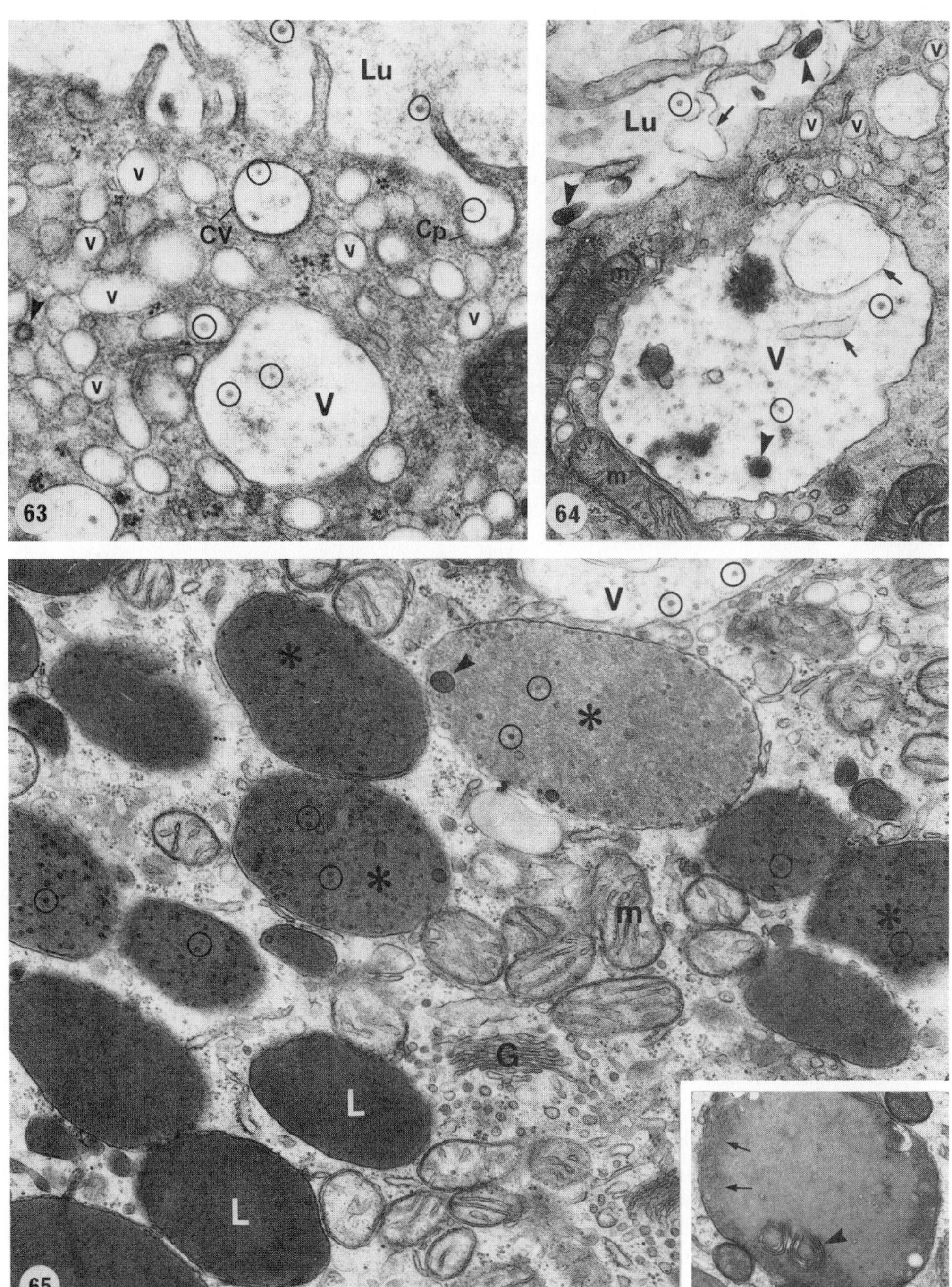

FIG. 63. High power of the apical region of a clear cell of the cauda epididymidis showing a large coated pit (Cp) and large coated vesicle (CV), numerous small uncoated vesicles (v), and a large vacuole (V). Note the presence of particles of small size with a diffuse wall (*circles*) in the lumen (Lu) and within the large coated pit, coated vesicle, small vesicle, and large vacuole. Also indicated is a small coated vesicle (50–60 nm) (*arrowhead*). (×34,200.) (Method B.)

FIG. 64. High power of the apical region of a clear cell of the cauda epididymidis. A large vacuole (V) is evident and contains membranous profiles (*arrows*), small particles (*circles*), and a small dense membrane-bound granule (*arrowhead*). The latter three structures are also found free in the lumen (Lu). v:Small uncoated vesicles, m:mitochondria. (×21,000.) (Method B.)

FIG. 65. Supranuclear region of a clear cell of the cauda epididymidis. Note the presence of a large vacuole (V) and membrane-bound bodies of increasing density (*asterisks*). The particles of small size (*circles*) as well as a small dense granule (*arrowhead*) can be seen in these various structures; however, they are no longer evident in the homogeneous electron-dense elements identified as lysosomes (L). G:Golgi apparatus, m:mitochondria. (×24,375.) (Method B.) **Inset**: A membrane-bound body of moderate density showing many particles (*arrows*) and membranous profiles (*arrowhead*). (×14,625.) (Method B.)

duct system with the exception of the efferent ducts. In the rat, basal cells are small, round, or elongated cells showing a large nucleus and a small amount of cytoplasm (Figs. 51,52,66,67). These cells, which do not reach the lumen, usually insinuate themselves between adjacent principal cells at the base of the epithelium where they show a large area of contact with the basement membrane (Figs. 66,67).

The remainder of their cell surface shows some interdigitation with the lateral plasma membrane of adjacent principal cells (Figs. 51,54,67). Desmosomes can be found between principal and basal cells (10). The cytoplasm, surrounding the nucleus, contains, in addition to the Golgi apparatus, mitochondria, and a few cisternae of rough endoplasmic reticulum, a few lysosomes, multivesicular bodies, and the occasional lipid droplet (Figs. 66,67). Though it is apparent that these cells are not very active, the presence of coated and uncoated pits along the cell surface together with multivesicular bodies and lysosomes suggests that these cells are capable of endocytosis (10). The functional role played by this population of cells is not known.

Halo Cells: The halo cells of the male excurrent duct system are found throughout the epithelial lining of the duct system as well as in the underlying lamina propria. These cells have been recognized in the epithelial lining of all species examined and have been frequently referred to as lymphocytes (10,71,82,96,136,139–141,144,168,185). These cells, which appear to migrate into the ductal epithelium during postnatal development (82), are remarkably similar in all species studied.

In the rat, halo cells are found in the underlying lamina propia (Figs. 67,68) and in the base of the epithelium (Fig. 69) or near the lumen. Their nucleus, often C-shaped, shows patches of condensed chromatin in association with the nuclear envelope (Figs. 68,69). The pale-staining cytoplasm, which is extensive in appropriate planes of section, shows in addition to a few cisternae of rough endoplasmic reticulum, mitochondria, free ribosomes, and a large Golgi apparatus in association with a pair of centrioles (Figs. 68,69). Characteristic of these cells, however, is the presence, throughout the cytoplasm, of many pale-stained vesicles and membrane-bound bodies showing an electron-dense core surrounded by a paler region (Figs. 68,69). These membrane-bound granules are acid-phosphatase-positive (L. Hermo and M. Lalli, *unpublished observations*) and hence are lysosomal in nature. Multivesicular bodies, although few in number, are also evident. No junctions of any sort are found between these cells and the neighboring epithelial cells.

Halo cells of the excurrent duct system are identical in appearance to the cells that have been described in the lamina propia (limiting membrane) surrounding normal seminiferous tubules of the rat (186) and man (187), where they have been shown to share many features in common with monocytes. Indeed, in the human, these cells were shown to be identical in appearance to circulating monocytes derived from human blood. However, unlike in the excurrent duct system, these cells were never found within the seminiferous epithelium (186,187). In the rat, based on their mitotic index and extent of labeling, these cells were shown to actively turn over in the limiting membrane (188). No such studies have as yet been done for halo cells in the male excurrent duct.

While halo cells have been referred to as lymphocytes, the possibility exists that they may, in fact, be monocytes. Since monocytes are well known precursors to macrophages (189), and since the latter have been well identified in the epithelial lining of the excurrent duct system as well as in the lumen of the duct (82,84,168,190–194), the possibility that these cells are in fact monocytes is well founded. Aside from their nature, their function is also unclear, although it has been suggested that they act as immunocompetent cells playing a role in segregating sperm antigens from the general circulation (185).

Blood-Epididymis Barrier

The anatomical and functional existence of a blood-testis barrier has been well established for a number of species [see review by Setchell and Waites (195)]. This topic is discussed in Chapter 19 (*these volumes*). Since the late 1970s there has been a growing body of evidence that there is also a blood-epididymis barrier. The probable functional existence of such a barrier was discussed as early as 1976 (196). Given the presence in spermatozoa of proteins that are recognized by the body as foreign, it only stands to reason that there should be a continuation beyond the testis of a functional barrier.

The first direct morphological evidence for such a barrier was presented in 1972 by Friend and Gilula (197), and subsequently confirmed by others (169,198–200). Friend and Gilula (197) have demonstrated the existence of extensive tight junctions between adjacent principal cells in the rat. Suzuki and Nagano (198) subsequently showed not only the existence of a belt-like series of tight junctions in the adluminal area of the principal cells of the epididymis, but also noted that the geometrical organization of this network varied along the duct; there was a general decrease in the number of tight junctional strands from proximal to distal segments of the epididymis. Similar observations were made for the epididymis of the guinea pig (199). Over the lateral cell surfaces of the principal cells of the vas deferens of the rat, many strands of tight junctions were seen, in addition to the belt-like network of tight junctional strands found in the adluminal area (198).

In the ductuli efferentes, however, a significantly lower number of tight junctional strands was found; based on a tracer study (201), it was concluded that this area was probably more "leaky." Belt-like gap junctions have been also found to be circumferentially distributed in the adluminal area between the nonciliated cells (201).

Hoffer and Hinton (200) further described the site of the

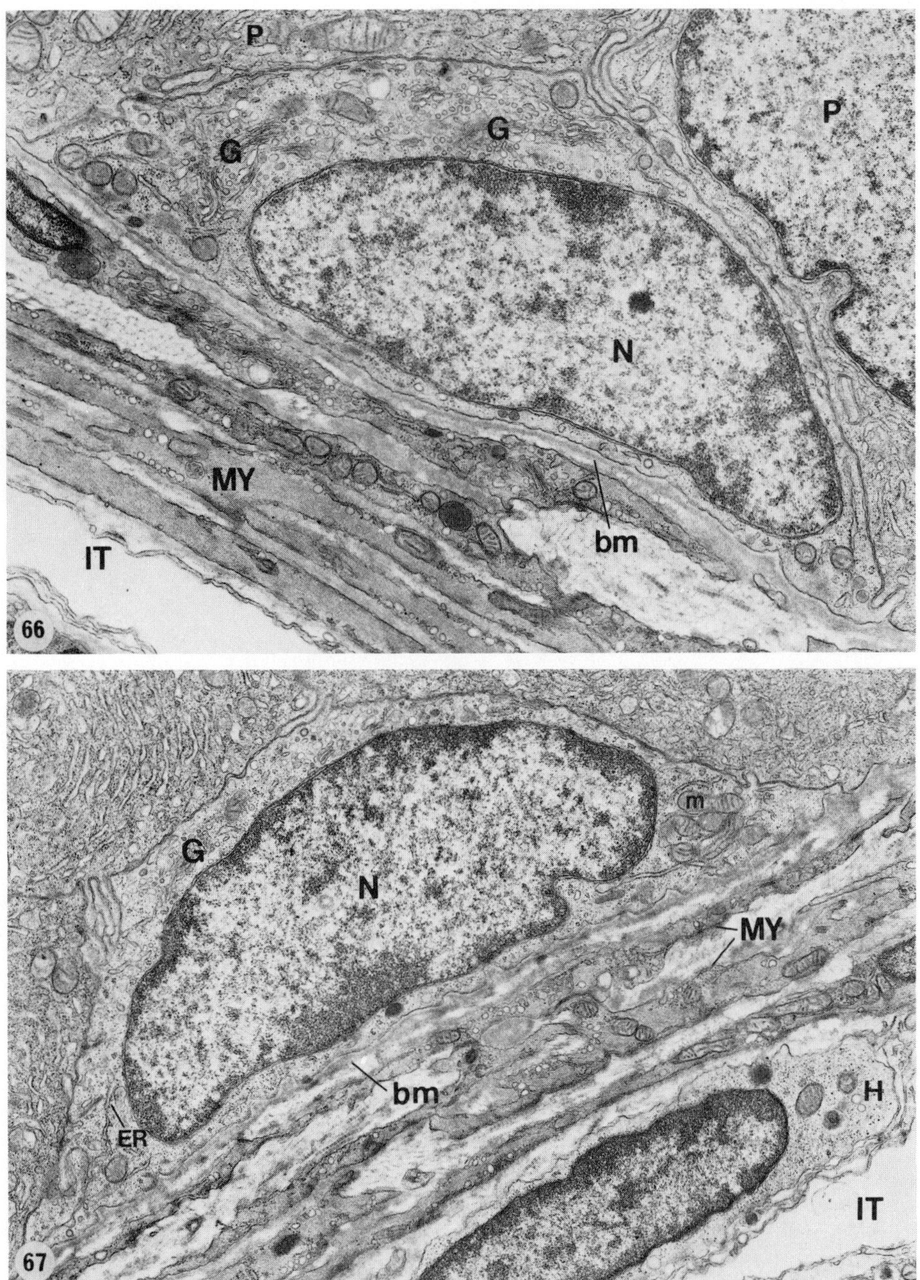

FIG. 66. A basal cell of the caput epididymidis, showing an elongated nucleus (N) enclosed by a small amount of cytoplasm containing a Golgi apparatus (G). This cell has a wide area of contact with the basement membrane (bm) and is capped above by two adjacent principal cells (P). MY:myoid cell, IT:intertubular space. (×12,740.) (Method A.)

FIG. 67. A basal cell of the cauda epididymidis. The cytoplasm shows a Golgi apparatus (G), mitochondria (m), and few cisternae of rough endoplasmic reticulum (ER). N:nucleus, bm:basement membrane, H:portion of a halo cell, MY:myoid cells, IT:intertubular space. (×10,780.) (Method A.)

blood-epididymis barrier; they demonstrated that neither the capillaries nor the peritubular myoid cell layer were effective in blocking the passage of the marker, lanthanum. Desmosomes were randomly distributed on the lateral surfaces of principal cells and occasional gap junctions were found between these cells in the base of the epithelium. However, the actual site of the blood-epididymis barrier was at the luminal surface of the principal cells where the typical tight junctional complexes (202) were found, preventing the entry of lanthanum into the lumen. Additional studies, with markers of varying molecular weight and charge, to better define the exact "tightness" of the barrier throughout the excurrent duct system from the efferent ducts to the vas deferens need to be done.

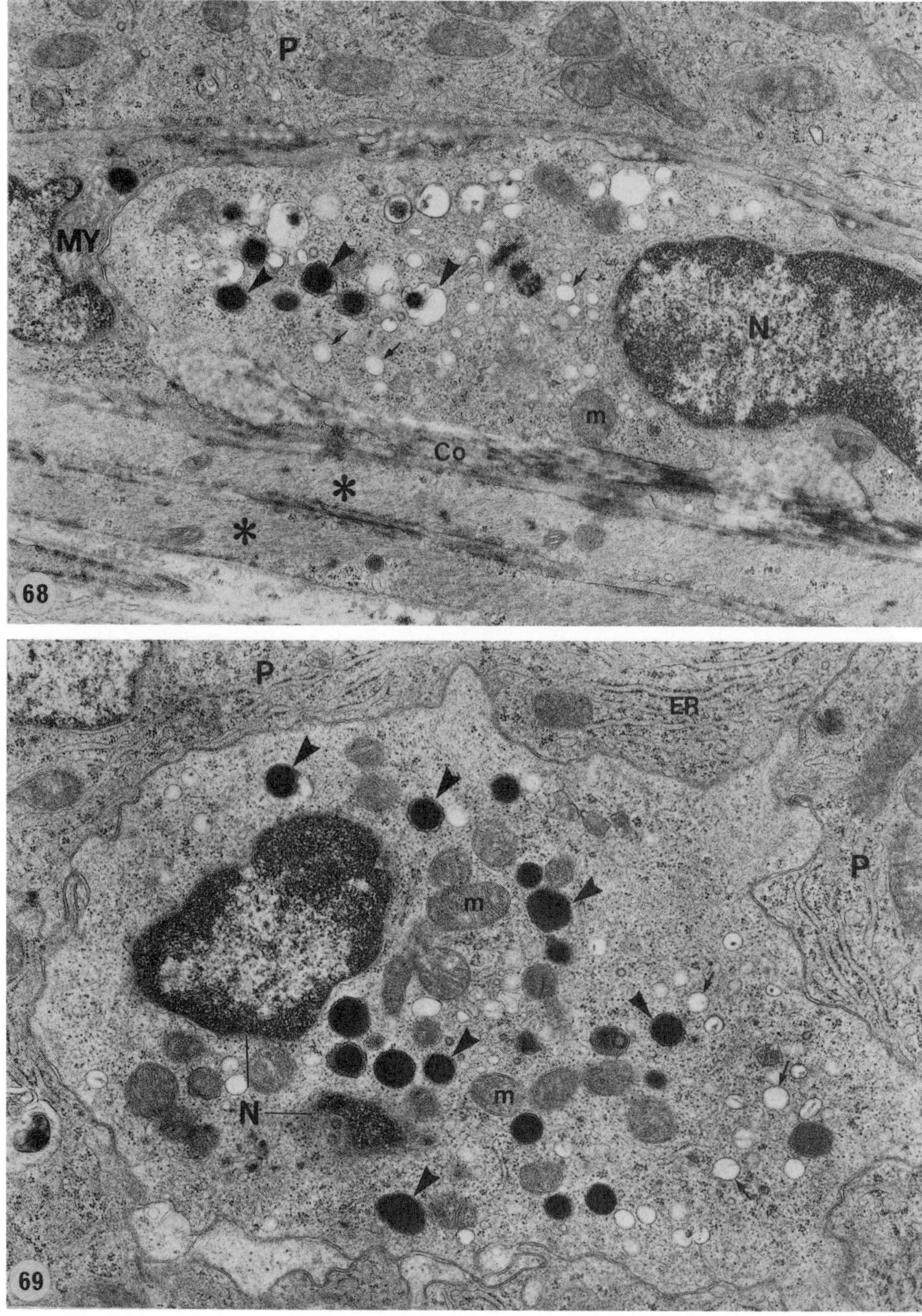

FIG. 68. A halo cell in the lamina propria of the epididymis enclosed by the arms of a myoid cell (MY). The cytoplasm of the halo cell contains small electron lucent vesicles (*arrows*) and membrane-bound bodies with an electron-dense homogeneous core surrounded by a paler region (*arrowheads*). Also indicated are the basal region of a principal cell (P), several myoid cells (*asterisks*), and collagen fibrils (Co) of the lamina propria. N:nucleus of halo cell, m: mitochondria. (×15,525.) (Method B.)

FIG. 69. A halo cell in the basal region of the epididymal epithelium. The halo cell shows an irregular nucleus (N) and a pale-stained cytoplasm containing numerous membrane-bound bodies showing an electron-dense core (*arrowheads*). Also indicated are small electron lucent vesicles (*arrows*) and mitochondria (m). ER:rough endoplasmic reticulum of the principal epithelial cells (P). (×16,200.) (Method B.)

In spite of the fairly recent morphological demonstration of the blood-epididymis barrier, there is extensive evidence that such a barrier does "functionally" exist because of the large differences in the concentration of inorganic and organic compounds between the luminal fluid and the blood. That luminal fluid has a different make-up than blood was suggested by the early studies of Crabo and Gustafsson (36), where differences between the ionic make-up of the lumen and blood were first demonstrated. A series of elegant micropuncture studies by Howards, Turner, Hinton, and collaborators (37,94,203–216) all pointed to a functionally active barrier (compartmentalization) between the fluid bathing spermatozoa in the excurrent duct system and that of the extracellular space.

Using inulin as a marker, the "tightness" of the blood-epididymis barrier was monitored under different conditions by collecting luminal fluid, over time, using *in vivo* micropuncture methods (214). It was found that high doses of estradiol (3 mg/day) given daily for 14 days (217), vasectomy, or induction of varicocele did not functionally alter the blood-epididymis barrier (214). Thus, this rather stable barrier is used for the creation of a highly defined environment where many ions and molecules are selectively excluded or concentrated. Hinton (213) has summarized some of the molecular gradients across this barrier (Fig. 70). It is apparent that some molecules such as inositol and carnitine can be concentrated ten- to 100-fold in the lumen of the caput epididymidis, while others such as inulin, L-glucose, and bovine serum albumin are effectively excluded (Fig. 70).

Studies on the blood-epididymis barrier are still very limited. For example, most of the evidence about this barrier has been obtained in the rat or the hamster. The existence of such a barrier in man has not yet been demonstrated. Though it would appear that this barrier is resistant to foreign substances [e.g., gossypol (200), estradiol (217)], little is known about the role played by this barrier in protecting spermatozoa from toxic substances and immunoglobulins. Indeed, the ability of this barrier to maintain its tightness under conditions of stress may play a pivotal role in allowing the epididymis to sustain its functions.

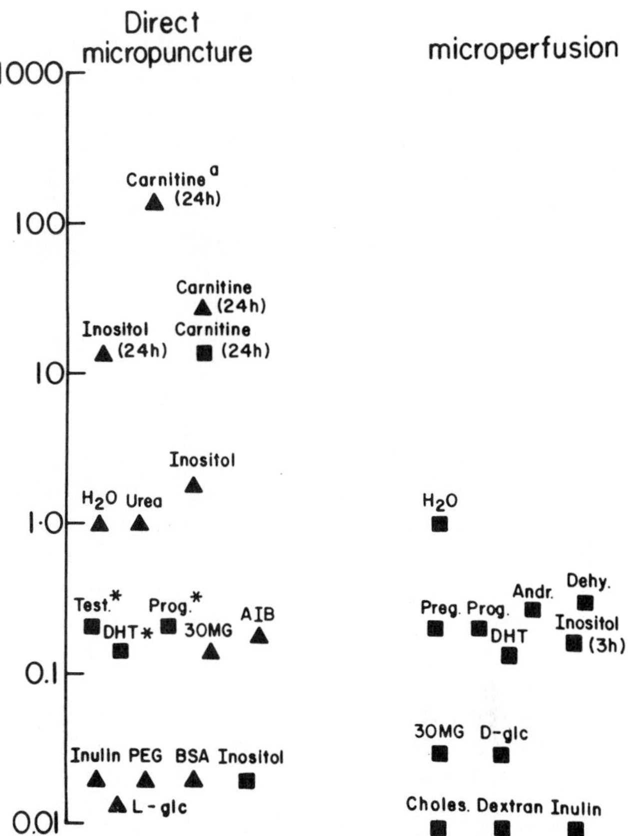

FIG. 70. Appearance of different organic solutes in the lumen of the rat and hamster (*) proximal caput, distal caput ([a]) epididymidis (▲), or cauda (■) epididymidis after systemic infusion of the radioactive compound, followed by direct micropuncture or microperfusion of the duct. Results are expressed in the logarithmic form of the ratio of the counts per minute per volume luminal fluid to the counts in the perfusate per minute per volume of blood plasma. Samples were collected after 2 hr unless indicated otherwise. D-glc: D-glucose, choles: cholesterol, 3-OMG: 3-*O*-methyl-D-glucose, L-glc: L-glucose, PEG: polyethylene glycol, AIB: α-aminoisobutyric acid, BSA: bovine serum albumin, H_2O: water, Test: testosterone, DHT: 5α-dihydrotestosterone, Prog: progesterone, Preg: pregnenolone, Andr: androstenedione, Dehy: dehydroepiandrosterone. (From ref. 213.)

Functions of the Epithelium of the Excurrent Duct System

A number of functions have been ascribed to the epithelium of the mammalian excurrent duct system. The first is the ability of the efferent ducts and the epididymis to absorb a large volume of fluid entering from the rete testis; this results in a multifold concentration of spermatozoa. This tissue can also internalize a number of molecules found in the luminal fluid. Secretion by the epididymis and vas deferens of proteins and other substances into the lumen of the duct is the second well-established function of this tissue; in some instances, this is associated with the related function of uptake of small organic molecules from the circulation and their secretion into the lumen of the duct system. Finally, a number of studies have addressed the ability of the epithelium of the excurrent duct system to: (a) support intermediary metabolism, (b) synthesize and metabolize steroids, and (c) synthesize and metabolize other compounds such as prostaglandins. In addition to these roles, another potential function may be deduced from data in the literature: the ability of this tissue to remove spermatozoa from the lumen (spermiophagy).

Absorption. The epithelia of the efferent ducts and epididymis are responsible for the absorption not only of large volumes of fluid secreted into the rete testis by the seminiferous tubules, but also of particulate matter.

Fluid, Ions, and Small Organic Molecules: In a variety of mammals, a large proportion of the fluid secreted from the rete testis has been found to be absorbed by the efferent ducts and/or the caput epididymidis. In the bull and the boar more than 90% of the fluid leaving the testis is taken up in this region (36), while in the rat this number has been estimated to be 50% (218). In the ram, the volume of fluid in the epididymis is approximately two orders of magnitude less than that entering the efferent ducts (219–222). Recent studies, using micropuncture techniques, on the different regions of the rat excurrent duct system indicate that the fluid absorption that takes place between the rete testis and the caput epididymidis accounts for an eightfold concentration of spermatozoa, while sperm are concentrated 20-fold by the time they reach the cauda epididymidis (94). The underlying mechanism responsible for the absorption of water in the rat epididymis, as proposed by Wong and his colleagues (223), is that of passive diffusion. According to their model, the driving molecule in the cauda epididymidis is sodium (224–226), while in the caput the responsible ion is chloride (223); they have further proposed that the transport of these ions is dependent on androgens (225). The similarities between these processes in the epididymis and those of the distal tubule of the kidney are striking.

Whether a functionally important amount of water is also taken up in the efferent ducts and epididymis by fluid phase endocytosis is not known. It is clear that this process does take place in this tissue (157), but the critical experiments that would distinguish between the uptake of water by fluid phase endocytosis or by passive diffusion remain to be done.

In addition to water, the absorption of ions has also been reported (15,36,218,223). The hypothesis put forth by Wong (223,225) mandates that both sodium and chloride be absorbed by the epididymis. This would certainly be consonant with the changes in ion concentrations found in different regions of the lumen of the epididymis (see below).

The absorption of the organic molecule, L-carnitine, from the proximal caput epididymidis was found to be saturable and primarily sodium-independent, whereas the absorption of this same substance in the cauda was purely passive (227).

Proteins and Other Particulate Matter: The ability of the epithelial cells of the excurrent duct system to take up nonspecific markers has been well demonstrated (114,136, 152,154,172,177). Using tracers such as cationic ferritin, native ferritin, horseradish peroxidase, or thorotrast, it has been established that, when injected into the lumen, these tracers were endocytosed by epithelial cells in a characteristic manner. At early time intervals, the tracers appeared in coated or uncoated pits, large coated vesicles, and endosomes; at later time intervals, they were found in multivesicular bodies of increasing density and eventually in lysosomes (Fig. 71).

While the endocytic pathway of epithelial cells of the efferent ducts, epididymis, and vas deferens has been mapped out, the nature of the proteins normally found in the lumen and taken up by these cells is largely unknown. Likewise, although the presence of coated structures attached to the cell surface implies that these cells may be involved in receptor-mediated endocytosis (for reviews see refs. 228,229), only a few studies have demonstrated this type of uptake in the epididymis.

Based on the disappearance of proteins that Turner (14) and Dacheux and Voglmayr (230) have reported between the initial segment and more distal segments of the epididymis, it becomes evident that specific proteins must be taken up by the epididymis. Indeed, androgen-binding protein has been shown to be localized, at the light microscopic level, within principal cells primarily in the efferent ducts and proximal segment of the caput epididymidis of the rat (231,232).

At the electron microscope level, it has been demonstrated that alpha-2-macroglobulin and transferrin are taken up by receptor-mediated endocytosis in rat caput principal cells (233,234). As in the case of nonspecific markers, both molecules were shown to be taken up initially in coated pits and vesicles, and subsequently internalized and sequestered within endosomes and multivesicular bodies. At later time intervals, alpha-2-macroglobulin, like the nonspecific tracers, was seen in lysosomes, while transferrin was reported to be recycled into the epididymal lumen (233,234). More recently Djakiew et al. (235) have shown that while transferrin is present in decreasing amounts in fluids taken from the caput to the cauda epididymidis, no significant difference in the net receptor-mediated endocytosis of transferrin was found between proximal caput and corpus epididymidis. As in the case of the epididymal principal cells (235), there is receptor-mediated uptake of transferrin by epithelial cells of the rete testis; after internalization, transferrin was demonstrated to be recycled back into the lumen by tubular extensions emanating from endosomes and multivesicular bodies (236). In addition to endocytosis, the rete epithelial cells (237) and principal cells of the vas deferens (Fig. 71) (172) have been reported to be involved in transcytosis; this phenomenon has been described for a variety of other cell types (129,238,239). No such activity has been demonstrated as yet for the principal epithelial cells of the epididymis.

Secretion. The ability of the epididymis and vas deferens to secrete into its lumen a variety of ions, small organic molecules, and glycoproteins has been studied extensively over the past 15 years. It has become clear that this tissue can take up from the circulation and transport and secrete an array of substances such as carnitine, inositol, and other sugars. In addition, the epididymis can synthesize and secrete small molecules such as glycerylphosphorylcholine as well as an array of glycoproteins.

Ions: Based on the concentrations of ions found in different regions of the epididymis (see below), it may be concluded that both potassium and phosphorus must be secreted by this tissue. The mechanisms responsible for the secretion of these ions have not yet been elucidated, but one may draw once again on the relationship between this

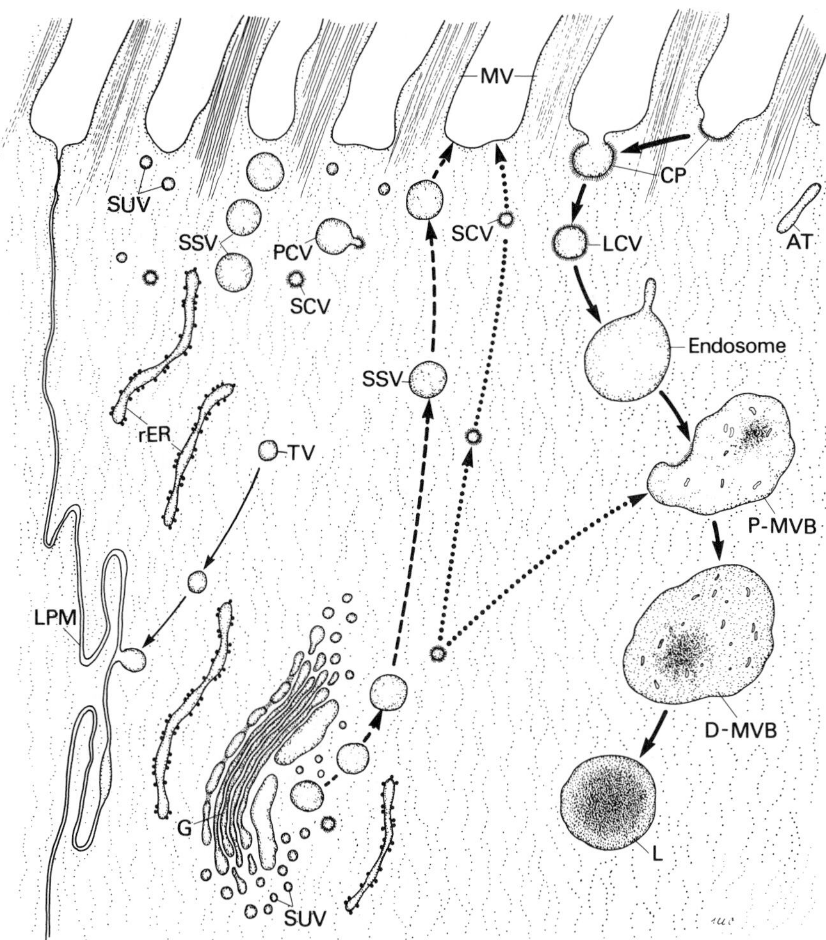

FIG. 71. Schematic representation of the probable steps in endocytosis, transcytosis, and secretion in principal cells of the epididymis and vas deferens. On the right, the endocytic pathway is depicted by the *solid heavy arrows;* CP:coated pit, LCV:large coated vesicle, P-MVB: pale multivesicular body, D-MVB: dense multivesicular body, L:lysosome. The *dotted arrows* represent the postulated fate of the small coated vesicles (SCV); the secretory pathway is that proposed by Flickinger (268), while the pathway to multivesicular bodies was proposed by Friend and Farquhar (177). The *dashed arrows* indicate the secretory pathway involving Golgi (G)-derived smooth-surfaced vesicles (SSV) as presented in the present study. The *solid light arrow* represents the pathway of the transcytotic vesicles (TV) to the lateral plasma membrane (LPM). The role of the small uncoated vesicles (SUV) and the pear-shaped partially coated vesicles (PCV) is unresolved. Also indicated are microvilli (MV), apical tubule (AT), and rough endoplasmic reticulum (rER).

tissue and the kidney. We propose that parathyroid hormone may play a role in regulating the flux of these ions in the epididymis, though no direct evidence for the action of this hormone is yet available.

Small Organic Molecules: The three small organic molecules that have been shown to be secreted by the epididymis are carnitine, inositol, and glycerylphosphorylcholine. The very high concentration of carnitine in the epididymis (up to 60 mM in the rat) was first reported by Marquis and Fritz in 1965 (240). It was established in the 1970s that this molecule could not be synthesized by the epididymis from precursors (241,242), nor did it enter the epididymis directly from the testis but, rather, it was actively taken up against a concentration gradient. The region with the highest ability to take up and secrete this molecule is the distal caput epididymidis (243). Carnitine is acetylated by both the epithelium and spermatozoa to acetylcarnitine (240,244). Yeung et al. (245) have proposed that the uptake of carnitine from extracellular fluid and its secretion into the lumen involve separate independent stereospecific mechanisms; the former is stimulated by the presence of choline, while the latter is choline-independent. The reasons for which the epididymis should need to concentrate such high amounts of carnitine are not clear, though a number of hypotheses have been put forth [see reviews by Hinton and Setchell (243) and by Brooks (244)].

Inositol is also found in very high concentrations in the epididymides of a number of species, reaching concentrations of 30 mM in the cauda epididymidis (15). The means by which these high concentrations are attained are threefold: (a) direct entry from the testis via the efferent ducts (246), (b) synthesis from glucose (247), and (c) uptake by the epididymal epithelium and secretion into the lumen via a selective and readily saturable process (248,249). The relative contribution of these three processes in bringing about this very high inositol concentration has not yet been worked out.

Glycerylphosphorylcholine and its metabolite, phosphorylcholine (250), are also found in the 30 to 50 and 10 mM range, respectively, in the epididymis (15). Glycerylphosphorylcholine is neither taken up by the epididymal epithelium nor does it directly enter the epididymis from the testis (251,252); rather, it is synthesized, primarily in the caput epididymidis, from blood lipoproteins (lecithin) (253).

Proteins and Glycoproteins: Suggestive evidence that proteins are secreted by the epididymis comes from a series of studies in the early 1970s where the electrophoretic patterns of protein bands from different regions of the excurrent duct system were studied and found to differ not only from plasma but also among different epididymal segments (230,254–259).

The first radioautographic evidence that sugars taken up by the epididymis can be synthesized into glycoproteins in this tissue came from early light microscope studies of Neutra and Leblond in 1966 (260). They found that, after administration of labeled galactose to adult rats, radioautographic silver grains first appeared over the Golgi apparatus and subsequently over the luminal surface of epididymal principal cells. Using labeled fucose, Kopecny and Peck (261) and Flickinger (262,263) confirmed that the epididymis could take up sugars and incorporate them into substances that are secreted into the lumen; this has also been found to be the case in the vas deferens (264).

The evidence that labeled amino acids could be incorporated into proteins by epididymal principal cells was presented by Venderly and Durliat (265), Kopecny (266), Kanka and Kopecny (267), and Flickinger and colleagues (145, 268,269). The path taken by labeled amino acids, after being synthesized in the rough endoplasmic reticulum, is their successive appearance over the Golgi apparatus, apical cell surface, and lumen. The relative protein synthetic ability in the initial segment and along the rest of the epididymis was also investigated (268). Flickinger (268) concluded that, in the mouse, it takes approximately 2 hr for the events involved in protein synthesis and secretion in epididymal principal cells, and that synthesis and intracellular transport of proteins were faster in the caput and corpus than in the cauda segments of the epididymis.

The mechanism by which proteins are secreted has been a subject of controversy. Although it was tempting for Hoffer et al. (136) to speculate that secretory proteins formed in the sparsely granulated endoplasmic reticulum might be directly released into the lumen and bypass the Golgi, since the latter were seen in close proximity to the apical cell surface (Figs. 33–35), the radioautographic work of Flickinger (145) did not support this idea. Though the cellular apparatus for the synthesis and packaging of proteins is evidently present in principal cells of the epididymis and vas deferens, Hoffer et al. (136), Hamilton (10), and Flickinger (145) have reported a lack of classical secretory granules.

In the present work, we have noted large smooth-surfaced vesicles (150–300 nm) in the Golgi, supranuclear, and apical regions of the principal cells of the epididymis and vas deferens (Figs. 34,35,37,42,43,44,55–57). Based on their close proximity to the trans (mature) face of the Golgi stacks, as well as their close proximity to the apical cell surface, it might be suggested that such vesicles represent secretory granules (Fig. 71). Although not previously described in the rat, structures similar in size, appearance, and distribution have been reported in principal cells of the initial segment of other species (67,137,270) where they were also considered as secretory vesicles. In the present work, such vesicles, although occasionally seen in close proximity to the apical cell surface, were not found to be continuous with it, nor were they readily observed in continuity with the trans Golgi saccules. Thus their identity as secretory granules is still speculative.

An alternative for the secretory granules of epididymal principal cells is the small coated vesicles (Fig. 71) (268,269). Such vesicles (50–60 nm) in the apical region (Figs. 35,41,43) could also be found in the Golgi region, and it has been suggested that they might serve to deliver hydrolytic enzymes to multivesicular bodies (Fig. 71) (152,177).

The identity of some of the specific proteins that are secreted has attracted much attention in the past decade. In 1978, Lea et al. (271) identified an acidic epididymal glycoprotein (AEG) having a molecular weight of 33,000; antibodies to this molecule reacted with a substance found selectively in principal cells. A number of other investigators have identified a similar or identical protein. Forward motility protein (FMP) of Acott and Hoskins (272) is of epididymal origin (273); it has a molecular weight of 35,000 to 40,000. Further examples include protein DE of Brooks and Higgins (274), protein IV of Jones et al. (275), DE protein of Garberi et al. (276), the 32K protein of Wong et al. (277), and the 37,000 dalton glycoproteins of Olson and co-workers (278,279). Whether these molecules represent a family of very similar glycoproteins or are, in fact, identical has not yet been resolved. Brooks described a protein—Protein F—which is primarily secreted by the caput epididymidis in organ culture (280). It has been proposed by Sylvester et al. (281) that this protein is identical to the dimeric acidic glycoprotein (DAG) that is secreted by both cultured Sertoli cells and the caput epididymidis.

In order to help resolve the confusion that is developing in the literature regarding the similarities and differences among all of these proteins or families of proteins secreted by the epididymis, an exchange of antibodies raised against these purified proteins between the concerned laboratories and verification of the identity or lack thereof of these substances would further the field. The proposed function of nearly all members of this "family" of proteins is linked with the maturation of spermatozoa.

Hamilton (282) established in 1981 that alpha-lactalbumin was present in the epididymis and proposed that it was synthesized by it. The presence in the epididymis of the mRNA for the alpha-lactalbumin specific DNA was reported by Qasba et al. (283); Byers et al. (284) demonstrated that it was selectively in the principal cells of the proximal caput epididymidis that immunoreactive alpha-lactalbumin could be found.

A large number of other proteins (both lighter and heavier), proposed to be secreted by the epididymis and identified by polyacrylamide gel electrophoresis in a number of laboratories (250,258,285–294), have been studied to a much lesser extent. The synthesis and secretion of at least many of these proteins is under androgenic control (250,274, 280,287,289,293). It is of interest to note, though, that a functional role for substances, other than androgens, secreted directly into the lumen of the epididymis via the rete testis and efferent ducts has been proposed. This hypothesis, as first presented by Robaire et al. in 1977 for the regulation of epididymal nuclear 5α-reductase (3-oxo-5α-steroid: $NADP^+$ 4-ene-oxidoreductase, EC 1.3.1.22) (295), also seems to apply to the regulation of the secretion of some proteins (296).

Metabolism. Various facets of biosynthesis and metabolism in the epididymis have been the subject of numerous studies. We discuss here those studies relating to certain facets of intermediary metabolism, steroid biosynthesis, and metabolism, and a few selected other substances. (The hormonal control of these metabolic processes is discussed in the section on regulation below.)

Intermediary Metabolism: As early as 1963, it was shown, using anesthetized rams, that glucose was a more effective metabolite for intermediary metabolism than acetate; all the acetate was metabolized to CO_2, whereas only approximately one-third of the glucose was broken down to CO_2 (297). The metabolism was found to be more glycolytic than oxidative in the mouse (298), rat (299), and rabbit (300); this differs markedly from what is found in most mammalian tissues.

The relative importance of glycolysis, the tricarboxylic acid cycle and the pentose cycle has been studied by a number of investigators (299,301–308) and has been reviewed by Brooks (309). Based on enzyme studies, it was established that, in both the caput and cauda epididymidis of rats, the potential flow of glucose is seven to ten times greater via glycolysis than via either the tricarboxylic acid cycle or the pentose phosphate pathway. This significant preference for glycolysis was not found, however, when tissue pieces were used to measure the conversion of metabolites; the rate of glycolysis decreased markedly under these conditions. Consequently, it can be assumed that the rate-limiting step in glycolysis is not the activity of the enzymes in the pathway but the availability of glucose (309). Indeed evidence has gathered to support the existence of a specific membrane-transport system for glucose (209,211, 307,309). This transport system is apparently situated on the baso-lateral membrane, cannot transport other hexoses, and can be inhibited by 3-*O*-methylglucose, a nonmetabolizable analog that is recognized by the transport system.

In the rat epididymis, oxidative metabolism has recently been reported to be high right after birth, to decline for the first 2 weeks of life, and then to rise in parallel with the increase in circulating androgens (310).

Steroids: One may most easily discuss the biosynthesis and metabolism of steroids in the epididymis by first considering evidence relating to the biosynthesis of testosterone and then its metabolism. Using acetate, cholesterol, pregnenolone, progesterone, or dehydroepiandrosterone, Frankel and Eik-Nes (311) were unable to demonstrate the biosynthesis of testosterone by slices of rabbit epididymides. Inano et al. (312) found that pregnenolone was not metabolized by the rat epididymis but that progesterone was readily converted, not to the traditional Δ-4 steroids and testosterone, as one would expect for androgen biosynthesizing tissues, but to a series of 5α-reduced metabolites. However, data from both of these studies indicated that there was low, but measurable, 17-hydroxylase, C 17-20 lyase and 17β-hydroxysteroid dehydrogenase activities; no evidence for the presence of 3β-hydroxysteroid dehydrogenase-Δ^4-Δ^5-isomerase enzyme was found. In contrast, Hamilton has presented evidence that the epididymis of a number of species including mouse (156), rat (313), rabbit and ram (314) can synthesize testosterone either *de novo* from acetate or cholesterol or from precursor steroids. Evans and Johnson (315) have also reported that cholesterol can be synthesized from acetate by bovine epididymis and that all the cholesterol is not esterified; this led them to propose that the epididymis can synthesize steroids *de novo*. Legault et al. (316) have shown that there is an 11-fold increase in desmosteryl sulfate as one progresses from the caput to the cauda epididymidis of hamsters without a commensurate decrease in desmosterol, cholesterol, or cholesteryl sulfate; the *de novo* synthesis of desmosteryl sulfate by this tissue was not demonstrated, however. Though this apparent conflict, potentially due to differences in methodologies used, has been in the literature for well over a decade, direct investigations of this question have not been pursued. In any case, it would appear that if the epididymis does have the ability to synthesize testosterone *de novo,* this activity must be minimal since epididymides atrophy after castration (1,295,317,318).

The discovery that testosterone is rapidly converted by the epididymis to 5α-reduced products was made almost simultaneously by two different groups (312,319). Inano et al. (312) demonstrated that cell-free homogenates converted either progestins or androgens to 5α-reduced metabolites, and subsequently could effectively further reduce these metabolites by converting the 3-keto to a 3α-hydroxy group. Gloyna and Wilson (318) found that 5α-reductase activity was present in the epididymal slices of all nine species studied and that in the rat, the only species where a large array of tissues was monitored for 5α-reductase activity, the epididymis was the tissue with the second highest level of activity. The structure of testosterone, dihydrotestosterone, and 3α-diol, as well as the enzymatic cofactor requirements and reversibility of the reactions, is indicated in Fig. 72.

Over the past 15 years a large number of studies have expanded on these early observations. These studies have involved measurements of steroid content in tissue homogenates, looking at the conversion of radioactive testosterone using a single point assay, measuring 5α-reductase activity using appropriately controlled enzyme assay conditions, and looking at testosterone conversion in cell and/or organ culture; these studies have been done in a wide variety of species (319) including mouse (320), rat (295,321–327), hamster (328), rabbit (329), dog (330), ram (R. Amann, *personal communication),* monkey (331,332), and man (333–

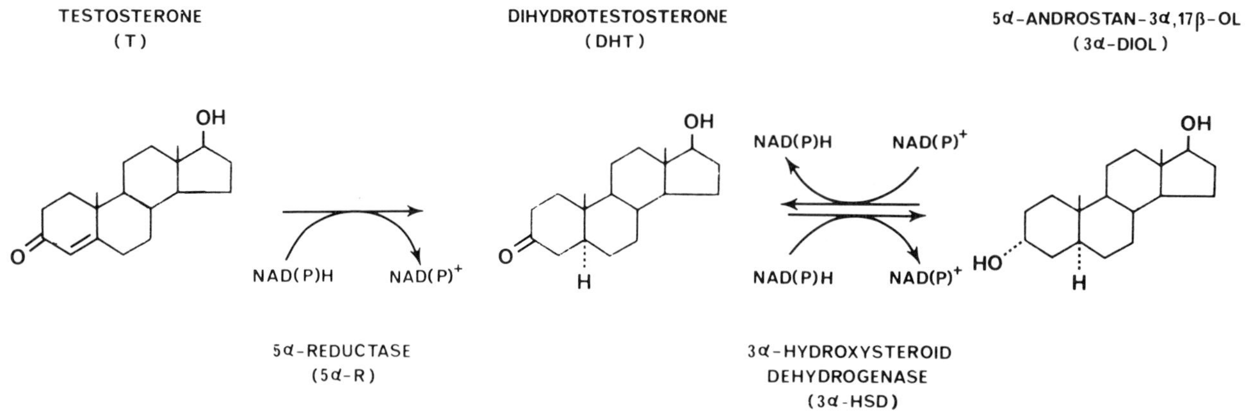

TESTOSTERONE (T)

DIHYDROTESTOSTERONE (DHT)

5α-ANDROSTAN-3α,17β-OL (3α-DIOL)

NAD(P)H NAD(P)$^+$

NAD(P)H NAD(P)$^+$

NAD(P)H NAD(P)$^+$

5α-REDUCTASE (5α-R)

3α-HYDROXYSTEROID DEHYDROGENASE (3α-HSD)

FIG. 72. Structure of testosterone, dihydrotestosterone, and 5α-androstan-3α,17β-ol and their enzymatic interconversion in the rat epididymis.

336). Unfortunately, in many studies where the activity of 5α-reductase is compared under different conditions, the requisite stipulations for such comparisons, i.e., linearity of product formation with respect to time and enzyme concentration and maintenance of substrate concentration to within ten times the $K_{m_{app}}$, have not been met.

It is, thus, perhaps not surprising that there are a number of apparent minor conflicts in this area. Despite these, some common features about the metabolism of testosterone by the mammalian epididymis have emerged: (a) the importance of the conversion of testosterone to dihydrotestosterone; (b) changes in 5α-reductase and 3α-hydroxysteroid dehydrogenase activities along the epididymis; (c) alterations in 5α-reductase activity during development and aging; and (d) further metabolism of 5α-reduced steroids in epididymal tissue.

When radioactive testosterone is administered peripherally, the radioactive steroid found in the epididymis is dihydrotestosterone (52,337,338). It has become clear that the mediation of androgen action in many target tissues, including the epididymis, requires the formation of dihydrotestosterone followed by its binding to a receptor specific for this androgen (339,340) (see review by D. S. Coffey, Chapter 24, *these volumes*).

Based on studies where the activity of 5α-reductase was measured either directly or indirectly (295,322,325–327,333) or where the concentration of different androgens in epididymal tissue was determined (94,324,341–344), it has become evident that, in many species, 5α-reductase activity changes markedly along the epididymis. There is a higher activity of 5α-reductase in the caput than in the cauda epididymidis in all species thus far examined, with the possible exception of the monkey (331) and man (335,336,345). It should be noted, however, that studies on human epididymal tissues have been limited to those obtained from individuals undergoing castration for treatment of prostatic cancer, and thus these tissues possibly are not representative of the normal young male. When the epididymis of the rat is further subdivided, 5α-reductase activity associated with the nuclear fraction is found to reside primarily in the initial segment of the epididymis. Further, the enzyme is located primarily in the epithelium, but not in the basal cells of the rat epididymal epithelium (323). In contrast, 3α-hydroxysteroid dehydrogenase activity is remarkably constant along this tissue, is apparently not localized in only one cell type, and has a much higher specific activity than 5α-reductase (295,322,326).

Since 1980, a number of studies have focused on the changes, during development (47,325,328,346,347) and aging (348), in epididymal 5α-reductase and 3α-hydroxysteroid dehydrogenase activities. In the rat, studies carried out over the first year of life, revealed that 5α-reductase activity is undetectable in the first 2 weeks of life, but is found in the epididymis well before spermatozoa first appear in this tissue (47). Surprisingly, a peak in 5α-reductase activity is found at either 6 or 11 weeks depending on whether the enzyme activity is expressed per tissue or per mg protein; this developmental pattern also varied with the segment of epididymis studied (347). In contrast, the specific activity of 3α-hydroxysteroid dehydrogenase does not change with age. Though other studies done on the rat epididymal testosterone metabolizing enzymes have generally supported these observations, in a recent study using golden hamsters from birth to 60 days, 5α-reductase activity was only found to increase with age (328). As rats age, the formation of total 5α-reduced metabolites decreased by nearly 50% from their adult value to that found at 28 months (348).

There are no reports, to date, on the purification of 5α-reductase from any source. The difficulty in purifying this enzyme is because it is membrane-bound and rapidly loses activity upon solubilization if not in the presence of emulsifying agents (349). 5α-Reductase is present in both nuclear and microsomal fractions (321,334,347,349,350), with the ratio of enzyme activity in these two fractions changing as a function of age (347). Studies on the characterization of this enzyme, either when membrane-bound or solubilized, have revealed that it has a pH optimum in the 6 to 7 range and has an absolute requirement for NADPH as cofactor

(321,334,349). The transfer of the proton from NADPH to testosterone is direct and not mediated by flavins or coenzyme Q (351). The mechanism of 5α-reductase enzyme activity is a rapid equilibrium, random bi-reactant process with a possible dead-end complex: testosterone-5α-reductase-NADP+ (679).

The purification and characterization of rat epididymal 3α-hydroxysteroid dehydrogenase, a soluble enzyme, has been accomplished by Hastings et al. (352,353). The enzyme has no remarkable physicochemical characteristics to distinguish it from 3α-hydroxysteroid dehydrogenase found in other tissues, but it has recently been reported that there may be two forms of the enzyme—one NADP-dependent, the other NADPH-dependent.

In both the dog and rat epididymides, 5α-reduced metabolites of testosterone have been shown to be further metabolized (354–358). Dihydrotestosterone and 3α-diol can be conjugated to form sulphated or glucuronidated metabolites (354,355). Alternatively, dihydrotestosterone can be reduced to 5α-androstan-3β,17β-diol, a biologically inactive androgen, and act as a substrate for the 7α-hydroxylase (358).

Other Compounds: In addition to the presence of enzymes involved in intermediary metabolism and steroid metabolism, a number of other enzymatic processes have been described for the epididymis. We limit our discussion here to three areas: glutathione metabolism and conjugation, prostaglandin biosynthesis, and vitamin D metabolism.

A number of enzymes involved in the biosynthesis, metabolism, and conjugation of glutathione are present in the epididymis. Chang and colleagues (359,360) reported the presence of a thiol oxidase, an enzyme that could convert 2 R-SH + O into an R-S-S-R and H_2O in the rat and hamster epididymis; enzyme activity was higher in the cauda than in the caput epididymidis. They proposed that such an enzyme could play a protective role for spermatozoa from endogenous free sulfhydryls. Exceptionally high concentrations of γ-glutamyl-transpeptidase have also been reported for the rat epididymis (361). This enzyme is involved in the transport of γ-glutamyl amino acids and can act as a glutathione oxidase, converting reduced to oxidized glutathione (362).

The family of enzymes involved in the conjugation of glutathione with electrophilic chemicals, the glutathione S-transferases, was first reported to be present in the epididymis in 1980 (363). This family of enzymes was resolved into six peaks, each having a characteristic isoelectric point and substrate specificity; one of the peaks, the most acidic, was very much higher in the epididymis than in other tissues and may be specific for this tissue. The longitudinal distribution of these enzymes was assessed in the epididymis and vas deferens (363). There was a general trend towards decreasing activity for each of the substrates as one moved from the caput to the cauda epididymidis and vas deferens; it is apparent from Fig. 73 that the different enzyme activities within this family, as determined by the use of different substrates and resolution by isoelectric point, exhibit different patterns in each segment of the epididymis-vas deferens.

Though it has not yet been established that prostaglandins are synthesized by the epithelial compartment of the epididymis, one may surmise that this is the case because these compounds have been found in epididymal homogenates and because they are fairly unstable. In the mid 1970s, Bartke and colleagues (364,365) found that prostaglandins of both the E and the F series were present in the rat epididymis and vas deferens; the concentration of both families of prostaglandins was greater in the vas than in the epididymis.

These observations were confirmed and further expanded by Gerozissis and Dray (366). They found that PGE_2 concentration in the vas deferens was more than 100-fold greater than that in the epididymis, while $PGF_{2\alpha}$ concentration only increased fourfold from the epididymis to the vas deferens of adult rats with the cauda epididymidis having selectively more PGE_2 than the caput. More recently, these authors (367) have found that 6-keto-PGF_1 and TXB_2 are also produced by the vas deferens of the rat with the prostacyclin pathway, as monitored by 6-keto-PGF_1 production, predominating only in prepubertal animals. A direct comparison of the concentration of PGE_2 and $PGF_{2\alpha}$ in the testis, caput, corpus, and cauda epididymidis and vas deferens of rat has clearly demonstrated that there is a dramatic stepwise increase; for both PGE_2 and $PGF_{2\alpha}$ the testis concentration is very low, the different segments of the epididymis are intermediate and the vas deferens concentration is very high (368).

Studies on the metabolism of vitamin D in the adult rat have revealed not only that the epididymis has, overall, a similar pattern of metabolites of vitamin D to that found in kidney, but that there is a specific accumulation of $24,25(OH)_2D_3$ in the cauda epididymidis (39). The specific enzymatic conversion of vitamin D metabolites by the epididymis has not yet been demonstrated; however, based on the metabolite pattern, one may surmise that a 24-hydroxylase is likely to be present selectively in the cauda of the epididymis.

Spermiophagy. The fate of spermatozoa that are not ejaculated has been and remains the subject of some controversy. In some species [man (369), ram (370), rabbit (12)] spermatozoa have been shown to be voided in the urine, but this phenomenon does not appear to account for the totality of nonejaculated spermatozoa in most mammals. An alternate and/or complimentary mechanism for disposing of unejaculated spermatozoa is their uptake and destruction by cells lining the excurrent duct system. Based on quantitative analysis, Amann and Almquist (371) and Orgebin-Crist (372) have proposed that a large proportion of spermatozoa are resorbed within the epididymis/vas deferens.

There is now morphological evidence, especially in the vas deferens, that spermiophagy does occur in a number of species under normal conditions, or after mechanical or

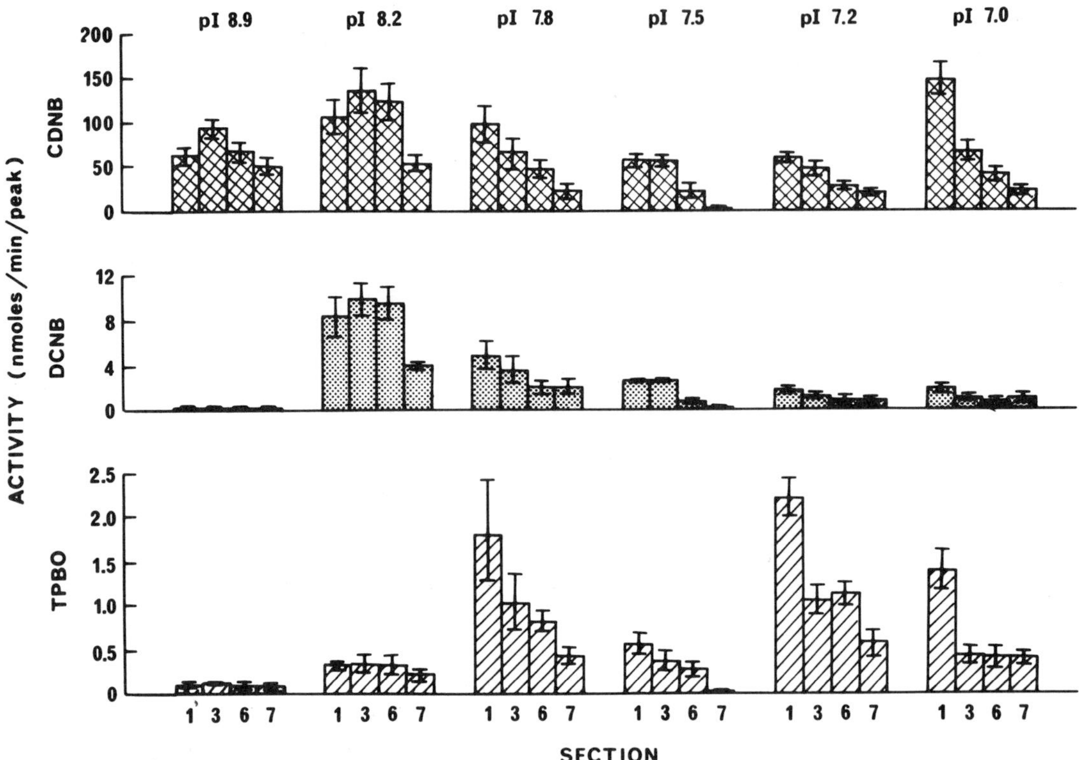

FIG. 73. Glutathione *S*-transferase activity in isoelectric focused peaks of sections of the epididymis-vas deferens. Glutathione *S*-transferase activity for each isoelectric focused peak was quantified by measuring peak height (nmol/min per gel piece). Values are means ± SEM for five replicates. Enzyme activity per peak toward 1-chloro-2,4-dinitrobenzene (CDNB), 1,2-dichloro-4-nitrobenzene (DCNB), and *trans*-4-phenylbut-3-en-2-one (TPBO) was measured in eluates of 3-mm pieces from isoelectric-focused polyacrylamide gels. Section numbers: 1 = initial segment; 3 = distal caput epididymidis; 6 = distal corpus epididymidis; 7 = proximal vas deferens. (From ref. 363.)

chemical manipulation. Such a process may involve the epithelial cells lining the excurrent duct system or the presence of luminal macrophages. In either case, spermatozoa in various stages of degeneration have been reported in these cells and it has been suggested that they are undergoing lysis. Discrete groups of epithelial cells lining the terminal region of the rat vas deferens (179), and epithelial cells lining the ampullary region of the vas deferens of the human, monkey, and cat (373,374,375,376) do phagocytose spermatozoa under normal conditions. Goyal (192) has suggested that the nonciliated cells of the ductuli efferentes of the bull can also phagocytose sperm. However, most observers have reached the conclusion (12,21) that the epithelial cells of the epididymis and most of the vas deferens are not involved in such activity under normal conditions.

Mechanical or chemical manipulation of the epididymis/vas deferens has been shown to cause epithelial cells of the different segments of the excurrent duct system to become phagocytic and engulf and digest spermatozoa (13,182,377–381). This would thus indicate that these cells do have the potential for sperm uptake, but that this function must be triggered by a specific stimulus. In a similar manner, spermiophagy by luminal macrophages has been shown to occur under abnormal (13,190,191,382,383) and only rarely under normal conditions (384).

It is interesting to speculate that the ability of the epithelial lining of the excurrent duct system to become active in the process of spermiophagy is dependent on either the presence of excess spermatozoa or on the presence of "abnormal" spermatozoa within the lumen. The mechanism by which either of these conditions could be recognized by the epithelial cells of the excurrent duct system is not clear. If one assumes that the first consequence of vasectomy is an increase in the concentration of spermatozoa in the lumen, then the data cited above certainly would support a role for an excess of these cells. Whether the presence of "abnormal" spermatozoa can, in fact, induce the epithelium to recognize and selectively engulf these spermatozoa remains to be determined.

Luminal Compartment

Luminal Composition

The lumen of the excurrent duct system contains water, ions, small organic molecules, proteins and glycoproteins, spermatozoa, and other particulate matter of undefined origin. From the efferent ducts all the way through to the vas deferens, numerous changes take place in the make-up of this complex of substances. Many of the chemical changes have been well described and are discussed below. Spermatozoa undergo a number of structural, chemical, and functional changes as they traverse the excurrent duct system. We briefly discuss some of these changes below. Another facet of these changes is presented in Chapter 2 (*these volumes*).

Ions. The first indication of the ionic make-up of the luminal compartment of the excurrent ducts came from studies in bulls (385). It was not until the study of Crabo and Gustafsson (36) that the regional distribution of sodium (decrease from caput to cauda epididymidis) and potassium (increase from initial segment to corpus followed by a small decrease) as well as the decrease in water content were well established. These studies, however, involved the homogenization of tissues and thus do not accurately represent what is actually happening within the luminal compartment.

In order to determine the actual changes in ionic make-up taking place within the lumen of the excurrent duct system, micropuncture methods, developed for studies in the kidney, were adapted for the male reproductive tract. These involved micropuncture of different segments of the duct and collection of fluid from the lumen for further analysis. Levine and Marsh (218) first applied these methods and showed that, in the rat epididymis-vas deferens, there is a precipitous fall in the concentration of chloride between the efferent ducts and the caput epididymidis, while a parallel fall in sodium is observed between the caput and cauda epididymidis; the rise in potassium was unable to account for the change in osmolarity and they proposed that the epididymis must therefore be involved in the secretion of organic ions (218).

Starting in 1976, Howards and his colleagues have presented a series of studies, using micropuncture methods (386), on the make-up, in a number of species, of the luminal composition of a large array of ions in the epididymis (37,196,205,387). Data taken from one of their studies (37) are represented in Fig. 74. It is apparent from this figure that there was nearly a 100 mM decrease in the concentration of sodium ions between the rete testis and cauda epididymidis, while the decline in chloride ions, although of similar magnitude, occurred between the rete testis and the caput epididymidis. The peak in potassium concentration of approximately 40 mM was reached in the corpus epididymidis, and, unlike the other ions in their study, potassium was the one whose peak concentration in the epididymis was similar to that in the seminiferous tubules. Phosphorus, whose serum level is usually in the 2 mM range, reached over 90 mM in the body of the epididymis. This high concentration was accounted for, in part, by the incorporation of phosphorus into glycerylphosphorylcholine and phosphocholine which make up approximately 50 and 20 mM, respectively; this

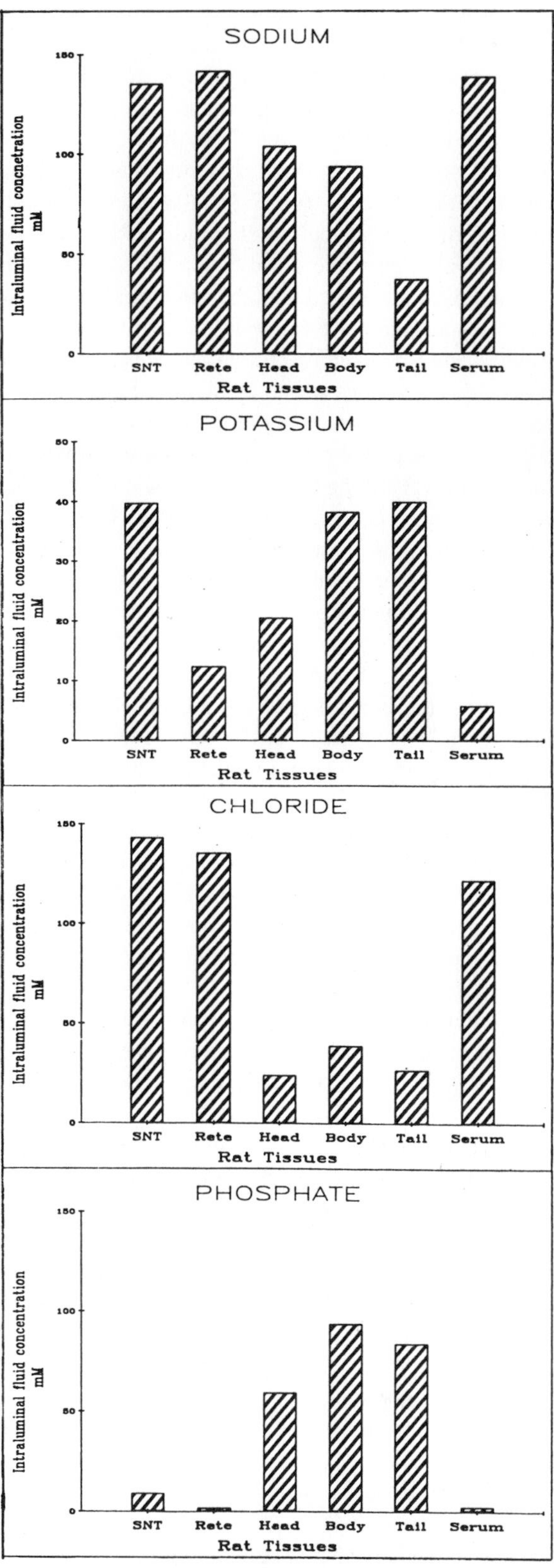

FIG. 74. Concentration (mM) of sodium, potassium, chloride, and phosphate in the luminal fluid of rat seminiferous tubules (SNT), rete testis, head (caput), body (corpus), and tail (cauda) of the epididymis. Serum concentrations of these chemicals are included for comparison. Data were obtained by micropuncture. (Adapted from ref. 37.)

left a concentration of over 10 mM of inorganic phosphorus in the cauda epididymidis and vas deferens (252). It would be of interest to determine whether this very high inorganic phosphorus concentration is maintained by the action of parathyroid hormone or vitamin D in this tissue.

The pH of the luminal fluid was shown by Levine and Marsh (218) to decrease from 7.31 in seminiferous tubules to 6.48 in the distal caput epididymidis and to rise again somewhat to 6.85 by the distal cauda. Most of the acidification initially associated with the cauda epididymidis was later shown to take place in the initial segment (388).

Small organic molecules. Based on the active absorptive and secretory activities of the epithelium lining the lumen of the male excurrent duct system, one would expect that the composition of the organic molecules found within the lumen would vary along the duct. Indeed, it has been noted for many years that certain molecules are in particularly high concentrations in the epididymal tissue in a number of species, but it is only in the past two decades that the actual concentration of individual organic molecules in the lumen of different regions of the epididymis and vas deferens have been ascertained. Carnitine, glycerylphosphorylcholine, phosphocholine, inositol, and steroids have been most extensively studied and are discussed below. Other substances such as sialic acid (389) and glycerol (390) have been reported to change in concentration as one moves along the excurrent duct system. However, it may be surmised, based on data obtained from tissue homogenates, that other compounds such as prostaglandins (365–367), glutathione (391), ascorbic acid (392,393), and vitamin D (39) will also be found to be differentially distributed along the excurrent duct system.

The luminal concentration of carnitine in the rat epididymis increased dramatically from less than 1 mM in rete testis fluid to 20 mM by the distal caput, and 52 mM by the proximal cauda epididymidis (243); these concentrations were greater than those found in any other mammalian tissue. Though often not as dramatic, increases in the concentration of this compound along the epididymis have been reported for many species including man, baboon, monkey, rabbit, hamster, and rat (206,243,394–396). Acetylcarnitine was also present in the lumen of the epididymis in concentrations similar to those found for carnitine (394,396). The physiological role of such high concentrations has not yet been resolved, but some of the proposed functions of carnitine are that it is present as a precursor to acetylcarnitine, which is then used as a source of energy by spermatozoa (396) or to promote the maturation of spermatozoa during epididymal transit (394).

Glycerylphosphorylcholine and phosphocholine were found in very low concentrations in rete testis fluid, rapidly rose in luminal fluid of proximal caput epididymidis to nearly 40 and 20 mM, respectively, and remained at about this very high concentration throughout the remainder of the excurrent duct system (15,252). Similarly, high concentrations of glycerylphosphorylcholine have been reported for the rabbit (206,251,397) but not for man (206), hence the universality of such high concentrations of this compound for normal functioning of the mammalian epididymis remains unclear.

Though several reports of the presence of inositol in the epididymis of mammals were made (398,399), the actual concentration of inositol in the lumen of the excurrent duct system, from the seminiferous tubules to the vas deferens, was not examined systematically using micropuncture techniques in a number of species until 1980 (400). In the rat there was a transitory increase of inositol in the initial segment (from 2.5 mM in rete testis fluid to 21 mM in initial segment fluid, and a decrease back to 9 mM of the proximal caput epididymidis), followed by a sustained increase in the cauda epididymidis and vas deferens to 30 and 50 mM, respectively (400). In the hamster, even higher concentrations of this sugar were found, reaching as high as 90 mM in the cauda epididymidis (400), but in many species, such as the ram or the baboon, inositol concentrations were in the low 1 to 10 mM range (400). Why the epididymis should accumulate in its lumen specifically inositol as a sugar, and no other sugars, is intriguing because, as of yet, no facet of intermediary metabolism of either spermatozoa or epididymal epithelium seems to have a preference for inositol as a source of energy.

A systematic study of the concentration of steroids, and of androgens in particular, in the luminal fluid of the excurrent duct system has, thus far, only been done for the bull (341) and the rat (94,338,343,401). In both species, testosterone was the most abundant androgen entering the epididymis, while dihydrotestosterone became the major androgen in the caput epididymidis (94,341).

In the bull (341), many other steroids were also measured; some of the more striking changes between rete testis fluid and cauda epididymal fluid steroid concentrations were a 50-fold increase in dihydrotestosterone to 20 ng/ml, a sevenfold increase in progesterone and a threefold increase in estradiol. The former observation is consistent with the well-established presence of 5α-reductase activity in this tissue (discussed above) (326), but the last two changes are particularly noteworthy in light of the scant evidence on the action of these hormones on the epididymis, as discussed below.

Micropuncture studies in the rat revealed that the concentration of testosterone declined from 18 to 5 ng/ml while that of dihydrotestosterone increased from 2.5 to 59 ng/ml between the rete testis and the caput epididymidis (94), once again demonstrating the major influence of epithelial 5α-reductase on the luminal steroid composition in this region. It is interesting to note that while testosterone remained essentially unchanged between caput and cauda epididymal fluid, dihydrotestosterone declined to 4.4 ng/ml; whether it was absorbed by the epididymis or further metabolized was not determined.

Proteins and glycoproteins. The observation that there are a number of specific proteins, separable by electrophoresis, that are present in the lumen of the excurrent duct system of mammals was made in the early 1970s for the ram (285), rat (402), and bull (255). Using micropuncture methods, Koskimies and Kormano (258) and Turner (14) demonstrated not only that the disc gel electrophoretic pattern of proteins obtained from different segments of the epididymis and vas deferens differed from those of serum or rete testis fluid, but also that they differed from each other, i.e., there were gradual changes in electrophoretic pattern from the caput to the corpus epididymidis and vas deferens.

Moore (286) demonstrated, using samples obtained by retrograde perfusion of the cauda epididymidis of the rabbit and the hamster, that there were specific luminal glycoproteins present in these fluids; further, he purified and used them to develop monospecific antibodies. These antibodies bound primarily to principal cells from the caput and corpus epididymidis, thus providing some direct evidence for the proposal that the change in protein make-up as one moves down the excurrent duct system is directly mediated by the secretory activity of the epithelium (see earlier section on secretion). Using similar microperfusion techniques, Wong et al. proposed in 1981 (277) that the changes in composition of luminal proteins, as determined by alterations in gel electrophoretic patterns, were due not only to absorption and secretion of proteins by the epithelium, but also to proteins "secreted" or adsorbed by spermatozoa as they pass through the epididymis (277).

From a study undertaken by Dacheux and Voglmayr (230), it is easy to appreciate the extent of the change in protein composition of different segments of the testicular excurrent duct system by following individual protein peaks, separated by electrophoresis, found in fluid obtained from the lumen of the rete testis or different segments of the ram epididymis (Fig. 75). These changes were also accompanied by changes in the cell surface proteins of spermatozoa obtained from different segments of the tissue (230). Similar observations have recently been made for the rat using micropuncture techniques (294).

The identity of most of these proteins has not yet been established. However, in the past few years, a few molecules, with specific physicochemical characteristics or identifiable biological activity found in the lumen of the epididymis, have been described. Albumin, α-2-macroglobulin, transferrin, and androgen-binding protein have been found in epididymal luminal fluid (94,255,403). Studies on the latter protein have demonstrated that this molecule exhibits a charge heterogeneity in different segments of the epididymis (404), and that its concentration clearly diminishes as one moves along the lumen of the excurrent ducts (94). Other proteins such as acidic epididymal glycoprotein (405), dimeric acidic glycoprotein (281), and forward motility protein (273) are also likely to be in the lumen of mammalian epididymides, but the evidence for their presence in the luminal compartment is indirect.

One of the first enzymes demonstrated to be present in

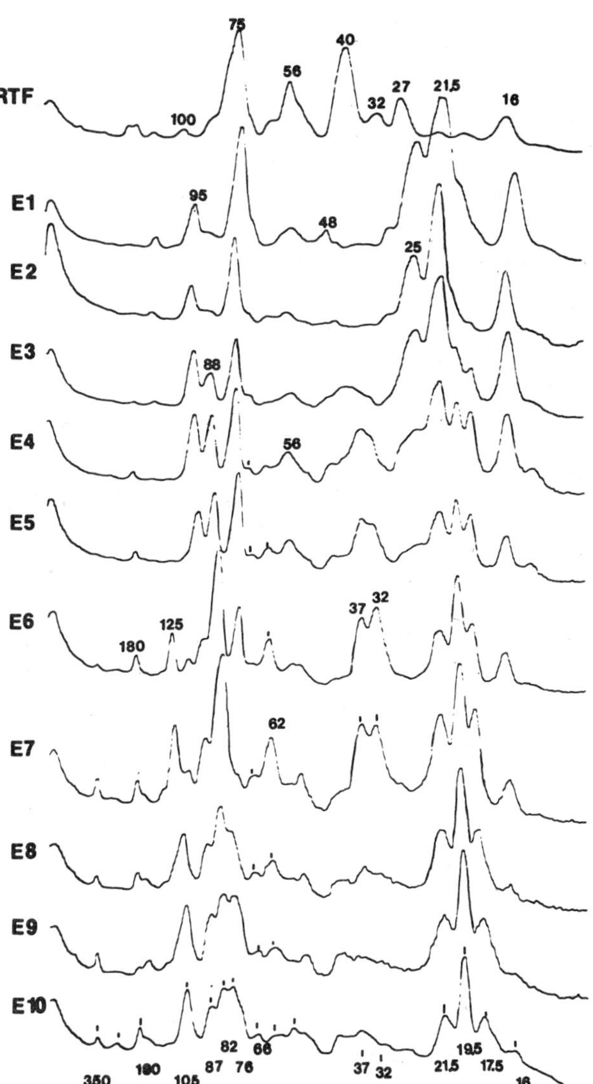

FIG. 75. Densitometric pattern of luminal proteins from the rete testis and epididymis of rams separated by one dimensional SDS polyacrylamide gel electrophoresis. RTF:rete testis fluid, E1: from the initial segment, E2–E4: from the caput, E5–E7: from the corpus, E8–E10: from the cauda epididymidis. The numbers at the bottom indicate the relative mobility of molecular weight markers. (From ref. 230.)

the lumen of the epididymis was galactosyltransferase (406). Though this enzyme had previously been reported to be in homogenates of the epididymis, its localization to the luminal compartment and its decrease in specific activity from the rete testis to the caput and cauda epididymidis, presumably due to its testicular origin, was not reported until 1980 (406). This was followed by a demonstration of the presence in rat epididymal luminal fluid of the regulatory component of the lactose synthetase complex, α-lactalbumin-like protein (282). Interestingly, this protein is not of testicular origin but, rather, seems to be synthesized in the epididymis (282); indeed, the mammary cDNA for α-lactalbumin hybridizes with epididymal mRNA (283). Jones and Brown (407) have further proposed that this α-lactalbumin-like luminal protein can bind to the membranes of spermatozoa during epididymal transit.

Another enzyme involved in carbohydrate metabolism, α-1,4-glucosidase, previously found in human epididymal homogenates (408), has recently been reported to be in the ram epididymal lumen (409). In the ram, enzyme activity was low in rete testis fluid and in the luminal fluid of the caput and corpus epididymidis, but it rose sharply in the fluid of the caudal segment paralleling the carnitine concentration.

Angiotensin I converting enzyme has also been found in the lumen of the rat epididymis (410,411). This enzyme cleaves angiotensin I by removal of a dipeptide to form angiotensin II and can also deactivate bradykinin; it was found in higher concentrations in the testis and epididymis than anywhere else in the body (410). Because of its decreasing activity along the testicular excurrent duct system (411), Hohlbrugger and Dahlheim (411) proposed that epididymal angiotensin-I-converting enzyme is of testicular origin, but more recent data have demonstrated that there is also a form of this enzyme that is specific to the epididymis (412).

Some of the other enzyme activities that have been found in fluids of the testicular excurrent duct system include acid phosphatase, *N*-acetyl-β-D-glucosaminidase, arylsulphatase, and β-glucuronidase (293). Much remains to be done on the characterization of these and other enzymes found in the fluids of the male excurrent duct system.

The presence, in the rat cauda epididymidis, of a glycoprotein of high molecular weight (> 1,000,000) whose proposed function was to act as an immobilization substance for spermatozoa was reported by Usselman and Cone (413). This substance, dubbed immobilin, was found to be the cause of the very high viscoelasticity of the fluid from rat cauda epididymidis (413). The high carbohydrate content of this glycoprotein (> 65%) led these investigators to propose that it was, in fact, a mucin (413). Recent studies from their laboratory have confirmed that this substance is a mucin but it is free of sialic acid, and two-thirds of the sugar residues are uncharged, rendering it less acidic than most other mucins (414).

In observing the lumen of the rat epididymis, it is interesting to note that it appears clear (electron lucent) in the caput region (71,415) (see Fig. 77), that a loosely distributed flocculent material starts to be seen in the corpus epididymidis (Fig. 78), and that by the cauda epididymidis the lumen is uniformly filled with this flocculent material (Fig. 80). It is enticing to speculate that this flocculent material may, in fact, be immobilin. By using appropriately tagged antibodies to immobilin, it should be relatively easy to test this hypothesis.

The viscoelasticity of cauda luminal fluid is, however, not universal among mammals. Turner and Reich (416) have demonstrated that while the viscoelasticity of the luminal fluid of the cauda epididymidis of the rat, guinea pig, and hamster is fairly high, that of the rabbit and of man is not, even though the protein concentration is similar. Hence, the means by which spermatozoa are maintained in an immobile state while in the cauda of the epididymis may not be ubiquitous among mammals.

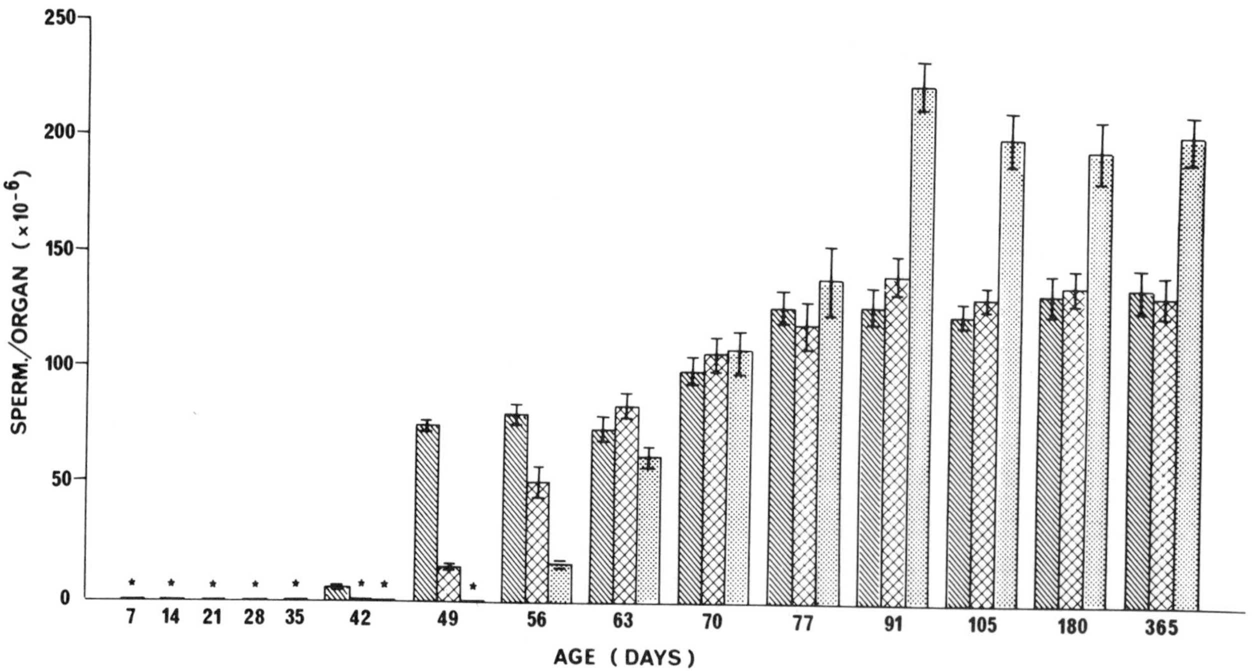

FIG. 76. Number of condensed sperm heads in the rat testis (▧), caput (▩), and cauda (▤) epididymidis as a function of age. Each *bar* represents mean ± SEM (n = 6). Ages where no sperm (condensed spermatids or spermatozoa) were detectable (< 50,000 sperm/organ) are indicated by a *star*.

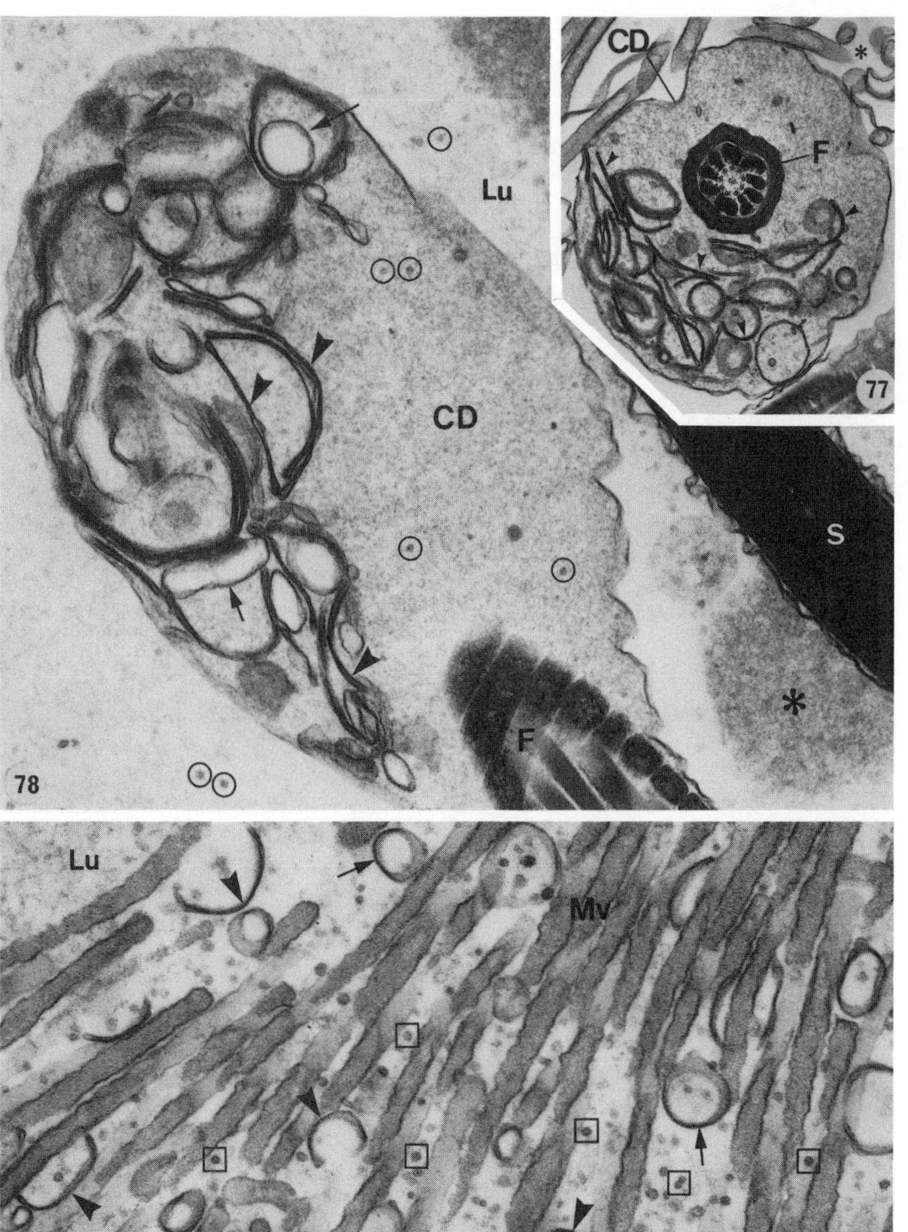

FIG. 77. Cross-section through the cytoplasmic droplet (CD) of a sperm located in the lumen of the caput epididymidis. Within the droplet one can observe the central position of the midpiece of the flagellum (F) and numerous flattened membranous elements (*arrowheads*) often seen in parallel to one another. Note the electron lucent appearance of the lumen of the duct of this segment (*asterisk*). (×16,380.) (Method A.)

FIG. 78. The cytoplasmic droplet (CD) of a sperm located in the lumen of the corpus epididymidis. In this case the droplet appears to be in the process of being shed from the flagellum (F). The contents of the droplet include small particles with a diffuse wall (*circles*) which also appear free in the lumen (Lu) and dilated (*arrows*), and flattened, often curved (*arrowheads*) membranous elements. A portion of the head of a sperm (S) is visible to which adheres a mass of moderately dense material (*asterisk*). Note that the lumen (Lu) of the epididymal duct from the segment of the corpus contains a hazy, loosely distributed flocculent material. (×29,750.) (Method A.)

FIG. 79. Lumen (Lu) of the cauda epididymidis. Among the microvilli (Mv) of the epididymal epithelial cells one can observe numerous particles of small size with a diffuse wall (*boxed in*); dilated (*arrows*); and flattened, often curved (*arrowheads*) membranous elements similar to those seen in the droplets still attached to sperm. (×30,030.) (Method A.)

Spermatozoa and other particulate matter. Spermatozoa are the major particulate material found within the luminal compartment of the excurrent duct system, although occasional residual bodies (Fig. 81) and germ cells can be found (375). Cooper and Hamilton (417) have also reported that, in the lumen of the cauda epididymidis and vas deferens of a variety of mammalian species, accumulations of a dense material can be seen in which are embedded vesicles, dense bodies, and spermatozoa undergoing degeneration.

Until puberty, the epididymal lumen is devoid of particulate matter. In the rat, the appearance of spermatozoa, as assessed by hemacytometric quantification of condensed sperm heads in tissue homogenates, was first noted in testes at 42 days of age, in the caput epididymidis at 49 days, and in the cauda epididymidis at 56 days (Fig. 76). In the caput epididymidis, the concentration of sperm did not reach a plateau until day 70, while, for the cauda epididymidis, such a plateau was not reached until the rats were 3 months old.

A number of morphological and biochemical changes reported to occur in spermatozoa during transit through the excurrent ducts have been reviewed (12,22,279). The most consistent morphological change that takes place in spermatozoa of different species during ductal transit is the migration of the cytoplasmic droplet from the neck region of the flagellum to the end of its midpiece (mitochondrial

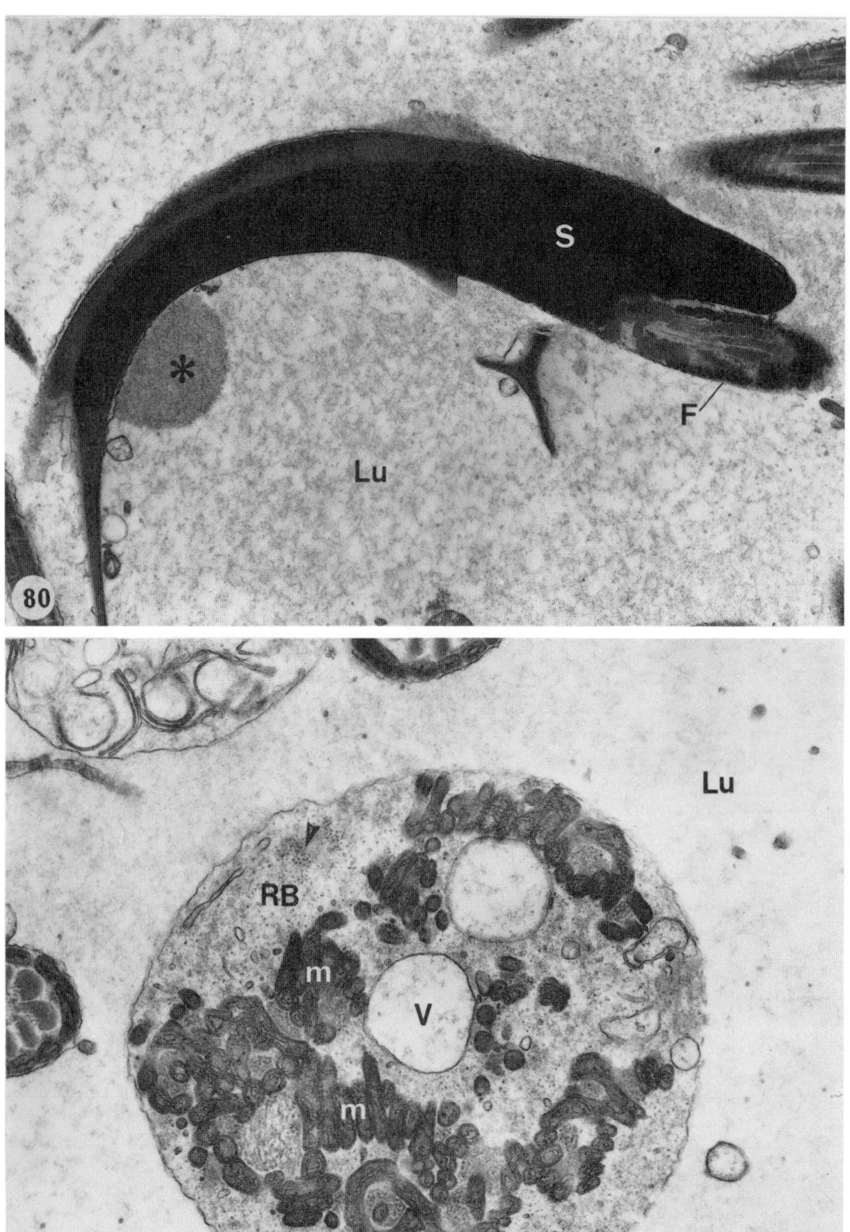

FIG. 80. A spermatozoon (S) present in the lumen (Lu) of the cauda epididymidis. Note that the lumen contains an evenly distributed flocculent material which is more abundant than that found in the corpus epididymidis. A mass of moderately dense material adheres to the plasma membrane of the sperm (*asterisk*). F:flagellum. (×10,725.) (Method A.)

FIG. 81. A residual body (RB) located in the lumen (Lu) of the corpus epididymidis, identified by the presence of many mitochondria (m), large vacuoles (V), and clusters of ribosomes (*arrowhead*). (×20,925.) (Method A.)

sheath) (418–421). This has been noted in snakes and birds (22), in many mammals (64,422), as well as in man (423). In the rat, lysosomal and other degradative enzymes are present within these droplets (424,425); however, the functional importance of these enzymes and of the droplets remains to be resolved.

A schematic representation of the movement, shedding and fate of the cytoplasmic droplet is shown in Fig. 82. In the rat, the droplet is usually not seen in different stages of transition between the neck and the end of the midpiece nor is it seen, intact, in the lumen after having been shed. A strong resemblance exists between the membranous elements and small particles with a diffuse wall that are seen within the droplets (Figs. 77,78) and those seen free in the lumen (Figs. 78,79). Selectively in clear cells, one can also observe the presence of these small particles and membranous elements within small apical vesicles, large vacuoles (Figs. 63,64) and membrane-bound bodies of increasing density [Figs. 65,65 (inset)]. This has led to the proposal that clear cells have, as a function, the recognition and

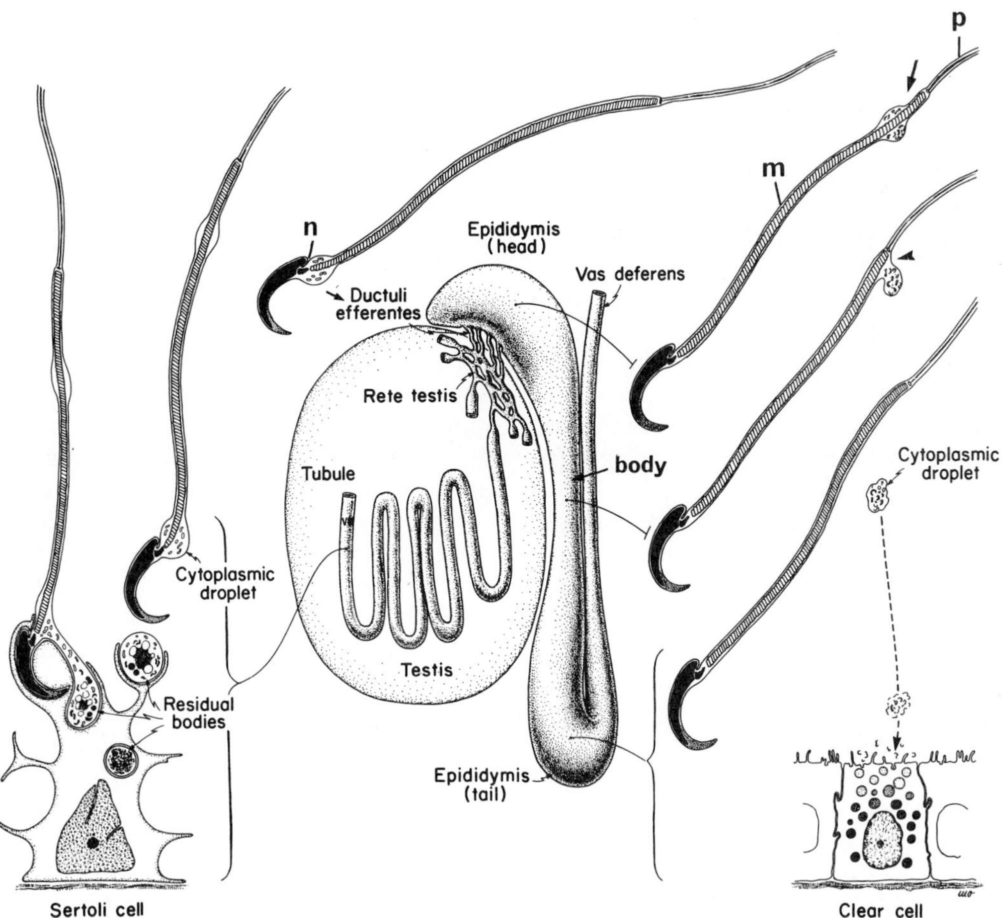

FIG. 82. Schematic representation showing the position of the cytoplasmic droplet of spermatozoa in the testis and various segments of the epididymis and its ultimate fate. The cytoplasmic droplet is a small mass of cytoplasm that is retained by the spermatozoa after its release into the lumen of the seminiferous tubule; the majority of its cytoplasm, however, referred to as the residual body, is taken up and phagocytosed by Sertoli cells lining the seminiferous epithelium. In the seminiferous tubules and efferent ducts, the droplet is seen surrounding the neck region (n) of the spermatozoon. In the head of the epididymis, the droplet is seen near the junction (*arrow*) between the middle (m) and principal (p) piece of the flagellum. In the body of the epididymis, the droplet shows a lateral displacement suggesting that it is being shed from the flagellum (*arrowhead*). In the tail of the epididymis most spermatozoa are devoid of droplets. While intact droplets are not found in the lumen of the cauda epididymidis, their contents can be observed free in the lumen of this segment of the duct as well as within the endocytic organelles of the clear cells. This suggests that after the droplets are released from spermatozoa, they break up in the lumen liberating their contents which are subsequently endocytosed by the population of clear cells to be sequestered and degraded within their numerous lysosomes.

internalization of remnants from cytoplasmic droplets (178) (Fig. 82). In the brush-tailed possum, Temple-Smith (426) has reported that cytoplasmic droplets are phagocytosed intact after being released from spermatozoa by a region of specialized principal cells of the epididymis.

In addition to the loss of the cytoplasmic droplet, spermatozoa, from a number of species, undergo a change in the size, shape, and/or internal structure of the acrosome as they go through the excurrent duct system. Fawcett and Hollenberg (427) first demonstrated dramatic changes in the acrosome of maturing spermatozoa of guinea pig. Similarly, the acrosome of the spermatozoa of chinchilla also undergoes marked alteration (419); in other species such as rabbit, elephant, hyrax, and monkey, acrosomal changes are also seen, but they are not as extensive (24,428,429), while in rodents they are very minor (22) and in man they seem to be absent (430).

An array of alterations in biochemically related parameters has been reported for spermatozoa as they traverse the excurrent ducts. Some extensive reviews on this topic are available (12,279,431). A partial list of some of these parameters is presented.

An increase in the relative number of disulfide bonds within the nucleus of spermatozoa as they reach the cauda epididymidis in many species has been observed (12,432–434). There is an increase in the anionic charge on spermatozoa as they reach the cauda epididymidis (12,435), which is probably acquired during passage through the corpus epididymidis (436).

The proteins of spermatozoa obtained from different segments of the epididymis of rats or rams have markedly different patterns after polyacrylamide gel electrophoresis (230,437–441). There is a decrease in the number of concanavalin A binding sites on the sperm membrane during epididymal transit (279,442,443). The ability of spermatozoa to activate complement also decreases during epididymal transit (444). The activity of protein methyltransferase in spermatozoa has been found to decrease dramatically during the transit through the epididymis (445). Echeverria et al. (446) have recently noted that the addition of a protein extract from hamster epididymides could increase the fertilizing ability of hamster spermatozoa.

The lipid composition of spermatozoa (447,448) and their plasma membrane in particular (449), has been reported to change dramatically during transit: there was a decrease in the amount of cholesterol while the amount of desmosterol and cholesterol sulfate increased (316,449); the relative distribution of the different polar lipids also changed, with some increasing while others decreased (449). This change in lipid composition has been proposed as the cause for the increased sensitivity to cold of caudal spermatozoa (449).

The changes in metabolic activity of spermatozoa during epididymal transit are numerous (309,450). Increases in the glycolytic and respiratory activity of spermatozoa during epididymal transit have been reported (451,452). The increase in cyclic AMP level associated with spermatozoa as they mature (453,454) has been attributed to both an increase in the synthesis of this second messenger as well as a decrease in its hydrolysis (455).

In spite of numerous detailed studies on how sperm change during epididymal transit, it is still not possible to dissociate those factors that are causal for the maturation of spermatozoa from those that are either consequential or incidental.

Functions Taking Place in the Luminal Compartment

There are three well-established spermatozoa-related functions taking place in the lumen of the mammalian excurrent duct system. The first, proposed over a century ago, and certainly the best established, is the role served by the epididymis as a conduit transporting spermatozoa from the efferent ducts to the vas deferens. Subsequently, it was hypothesized that spermatozoa acquire their swimming capacity while in the epididymis. Though debated for some time, the role of the epididymis as the site for maturation of spermatozoa, i.e., the acquisition of the abilities to fertilize eggs and to swim, has been put on a sound experimental base over the past two decades. The third function taking place in the lumen is the storage of mature spermatozoa in the cauda epididymidis. A proposed role of the epididymis related to this function is that this tissue acts as the "prime mover" (456,457) in bringing the testis-epididymis into the scrotum because of the necessity to store spermatozoa at a lower temperature than that of the body core.

Transport of spermatozoa. A number of methods have been used to evaluate the time it takes for spermatozoa to pass through different segments of the epididymis (16,458). Since the duration of transit in each segment of the epididymis is proportional to the size of the sperm reserve in that segment (459), it is possible to assess sperm transit time without the use of radioactively labeled spermatozoa. However, the ease and accuracy of using such labeled spermatozoa have rendered this the method of choice whenever possible (460,461).

There is an amazing consistency in the amount of time it takes for spermatozoa to traverse the epididymis in spite of the very large range in sperm production rate in different species (462). The time it takes for sperm transit through the epididymis of different mammals (Fig. 83) hovers at approximately 10 days (372,459,463–469). The time it takes for spermatozoa to pass through the epididymis in man appears, from the literature, to be highly variable (458, 462,470). Because of the unavailability of information on the transit time of spermatozoa in the caput and corpus epididymidis in man, this time has been represented as time in the caput epididymidis in Fig. 83. It is interesting to note, for all of the species shown in Fig. 83, that the relative amount of time spent in the cauda epididymidis is longer and more variable than that spent in any other segment. This is presumably because sperm transit in the caput and corpus epididymis is independent of ejaculatory frequency, while that of the cauda epididymidis is dependent on this frequency (371,471,472).

Using oil droplets that were microinjected into different segments of the epididymis, a variation in the rate of luminal flow in different segments has been demonstrated (473–475). This rate has been shown to decrease from 420 mm/2 hr in the initial segment to 64 mm/2 hr in the distal caput and 25 mm/2 hr in the cauda epididymidis and vas deferens (474).

The mechanism(s) responsible for driving the contents through the lumen of the epididymis include hydrostatic pressure, muscular contractions, and the action of cilia. A gradient of pressure has been found within the epididymal lumen of hamsters (476), guinea pigs (203), and rats (477), with highest pressure found in the cauda epididymidis. One should note, however, that most of the fluid secreted by the testis is resorbed in the initial part of the excurrent duct, as discussed above, and that consequently the "pressure head" is relatively small.

Talo and co-workers (473,475,478–481) have found that there is a low, regular electrical activity throughout the epididymis with frequencies hovering between seven and nine contractions per minute in the caput, corpus, and proximal cauda epididymidis, and declining precipitously to less than two contractions per minute by the distal cauda epi-

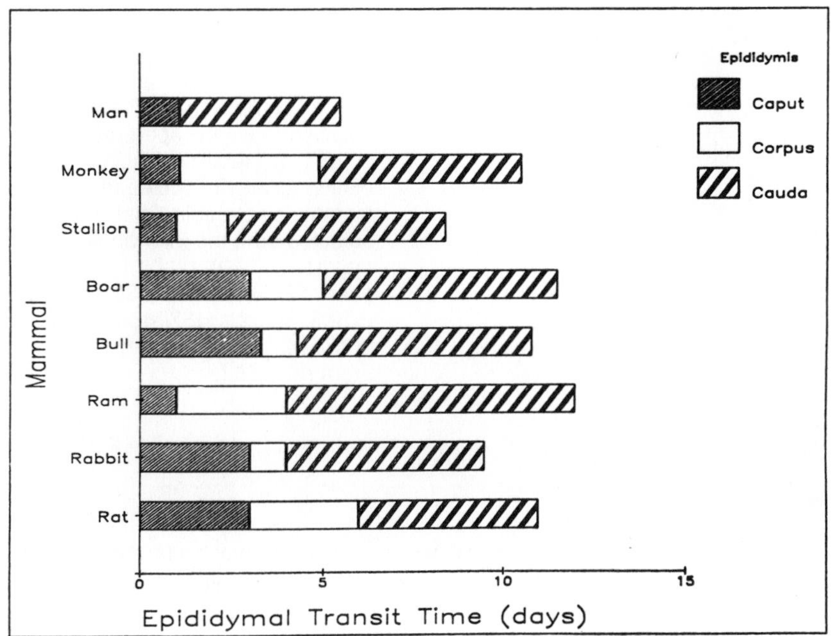

FIG. 83. Transit time in days for spermatozoa to traverse the caput (*shaded*), corpus (*clear*) and cauda (*striped*) epididymidis. For man, the *striped area* represents the combined transit time for the corpus and cauda epididymidis. [Data were obtained from the following sources: man (470), monkey (468), stallion (467), boar (463,466), bull (372), ram (459,465), rabbit (464), and rat (469).]

didymidis. However, the conduction velocity dramatically increases from 2.8 mm/sec in the cauda epididymidis to 890 mm/sec in the vas deferens. In the epididymis, electrical activity was associated with waves of intraluminal pressure which were dampened by the presence of spermatozoa (478). Though previous investigators had noted peristaltic activity in the epididymis (482,483), Talo's studies are the first clear demonstration of a functional role for epididymal electrical activity.

Both adrenergic and cholinergic mechanisms (484) as well as vasopressin (481) have been proposed to play a role in regulating this activity. In addition, the possibility that epididymal tubular contraction can be regulated by prostaglandins has recently been proposed by Cosentino et al. (368). They have shown that prostaglandin $F_{2\alpha}$ can increase the frequency and amplitude of epididymal tubule contractions while prostaglandin E_2, as well as acetylsalicylic acid (aspirin), decrease these contractions. It should be stressed that this electrical activity is distinct from that found in the cauda epididymidis and associated with ejaculation (see Chapter 19, *these volumes*).

The relative contribution of hydrostatic pressure, electrical activity, and ciliary action in driving luminal flow is still unresolved; it is unlikely that any single factor will fully account for luminal flow in all mammals.

Acquisition of fertilizing ability by spermatozoa. In mammals, spermatozoa leaving the testis do not have the ability to fertilize eggs, whereas those in the cauda of the epididymis have acquired this function. It has been debated whether the role of the epididymis in this function is passive, i.e., allowing enough time for spermatozoa to mature on their own by virtue of the long time needed to pass through the tissue, or active, i.e., functionally altering the environment of spermatozoa during epididymal transit in a way that permits for their acquisition of fertilizing potential. Thanks primarily to a series of elegant studies by Orgebin-Crist and colleagues (for review, see ref. 11) and by Bedford (485) from the mid-1960s onwards, it has become clear that the epididymis is not merely the site where spermatozoa mature, but that it plays an active role in the development of the acquisition of the fertilizing potential of spermatozoa in all mammals studied to date. Some excellent reviews on the maturation of spermatozoa in the epididymis are available (7,11,12,14,16,21,22,458).

A schematic summary of the site where spermatozoa acquire their fertilizing potential has recently been prepared by Orgebin-Crist (458) and is reproduced in Fig. 84. Though there is some species variation with respect to the exact site at which spermatozoa first gain their fertilizing potential, it is evident that passage through some part of the caput is essential for this function and that, in no species, is the entire length of the epididymis necessary for acquiring fertilizing potential.

It would appear that the acquisition of fertilizing potential is clearly not a simple "on" or "off" state. Studies with rabbits (486), rats (487–489), and rams (490) would suggest that spermatozoa first gain the ability to fertilize eggs, and only after further transit through the epididymis acquire the ability to produce complete litters of viable offspring. Spermatozoa from the ram corpus epididymidis have acquired the ability to fertilize eggs, yet these zygotes do not develop into viable offspring (491,492). Using rabbits, Orgebin-Crist noted an increase in both pre- and postimplantation loss when does were inseminated with corpus versus ejaculated spermatozoa (493); this is apparently due to a delay in the fertilization of eggs (493,494) and in the first zygotic division (495). In a subsequent study, Overstreet and Bedford (496) were unable to confirm these observations. In

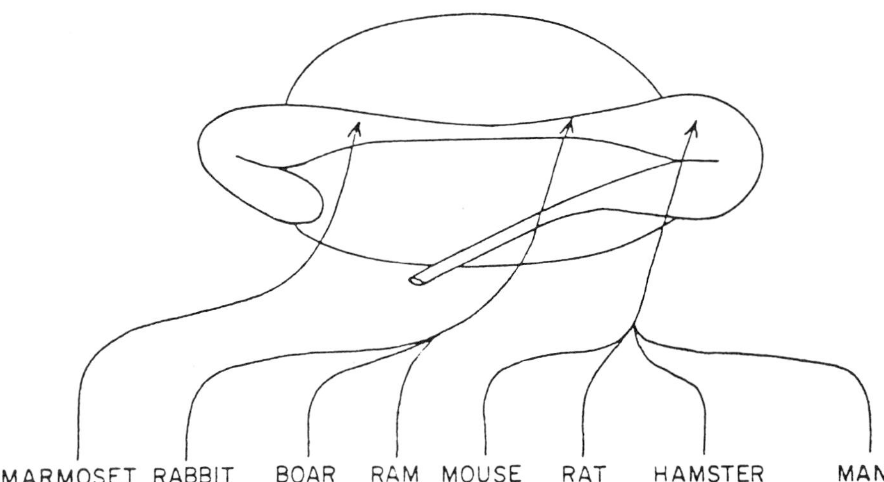

FIG. 84. Approximate site within the epididymis where spermatozoa acquire their fertilizing ability. [Information for each species, as brought together by Orgebin-Crist (458), was obtained from the following sources: marmoset (510), rabbit (6,485,486), boar (511), ram (490), mouse (512,513), rat (487–489), hamster (497,514,515), and man (516,517). From ref. 458.]

the rat, the decrease in litter size found after fertilization with spermatozoa that had just acquired their fertilizing potential is also presumably due to the presence of spermatozoa that can fertilize eggs, but that do not produce viable zygotes (489).

Associated with the acquisition by spermatozoa of the ability to fertilize eggs is a gain in potential for motility. This gain in motility potential is a required but not sufficient condition for spermatozoa to become fertile. In studies where different regions of the epididymis were ligated and spermatozoa were subsequently removed, it became apparent that spermatozoa could acquire the potential for motility, and yet not have acquired the ability to fertilize eggs (6,8,497).

Although, in the epididymis, spermatozoa are not motile, they acquire this capacity for movement as they traverse the epididymis. The cauda fluid composition prevents movement of spermatozoa, with the possible exception of the rabbit (see section above on secretion of proteins and glycoproteins and ref. 416). The underlying mechanism(s) for the acquisition of potential for motility is unknown; however, a number of potential factors have been proposed as regulators or mediators. These include forward-motility protein (498,499), acidic epididymal glycoprotein and albumin (500), carnitine (501,502), cyclic AMP (454,503), sperm-motility inhibiting factor (504), sperm-motility quiescence factor (505), immobilin (413), and ambient conditions (451). The underlying cellular and molecular mechanisms for this phasic acquisition of functionally mature spermatozoa have not yet been identified.

Storage of spermatozoa. The major site for storage of spermatozoa within the excurrent duct system of mammals is the cauda epididymidis. Though normal transit time in mammals through the cauda epididymidis is in the range of 3 to 10 days (Fig. 83), spermatozoa can be stored in this tissue for long periods of time extending beyond 30 days (11); in bats, spermatozoa may be stored in this tissue for many months and retain their function (506). Upon storage in the cauda epididymidis, a loss in fertilizing ability was found to occur before a loss in motility (507). Interestingly, spermatozoa that were aged in the male reproductive tract of rabbits, presumably in the cauda epididymidis, induced a tenfold higher incidence of chromosomal abnormalities in the resulting blastocysts than did their fresh counterparts (508).

Based on studies in a number of mammalian species, Amann (462) noted that 50 to 80% of spermatozoa present in the excurrent ducts were found in the cauda epididymidis (Fig. 76), and that approximately 50% of these spermatozoa were available for ejaculation (462). When animals (rabbits, stallions, and bulls) were at sexual rest, i.e., 7 or more days without ejaculation, the number of stored spermatozoa that were available for ejaculation was three- to fivefold greater than the daily sperm production rate and two- to threefold greater than that found in a "typical" ejaculate. Frequent ejaculation, i.e., one ejaculate every 1 to 2 days, did not result in a change in sperm production rate but did markedly decrease caudal epididymal sperm reserves and the number of spermatozoa in the ejaculate (462). In contrast, man, whose sperm production rate is well below that of most other mammals, has a sperm reserve that is only approximately equal to the number of spermatozoa found in an ejaculate, whether at sexual rest or not (462).

In a series of studies on the evolution of the scrotum, Bedford has proposed that the prime moving force behind the formation of the scrotum was the need to store spermatozoa at a low temperature (456,457,509). He suggested "that migration to a scrotal site has been ordained primarily by the sperm storage region—the cauda epididymidis—and that the function of the testis has only been an incidental factor in this evolutionary development" (457). This proposal was based on anatomical observations and on some physiological studies where the epididymis was placed abdominally while the testis remained in the scrotum; the rate of sperm passage through the cauda epididymidis was found to increase approximately twofold in the rabbit after such a procedure.

One would expect that the luminal environment required for the storage of spermatozoa in the cauda epididymidis versus that required for the acquisition of fertilizing ability would be different. Though many differences have been described in the luminal make-up of ions, small organic molecules, proteins, and glycoproteins between the cauda and the rest of the epididymis, those special conditions that allow for the storage of spermatozoa in a quiescent state for long time periods in this tissue have not yet been elucidated, with the possible exception of immobilin in the rat (413).

REGULATION OF EPIDIDYMAL AND VAS DEFERENS FUNCTIONS

Role of Circulating Hormones in Regulating Functions of the Excurrent Duct System

Regulation of both the epithelial and luminal functions is under complex hormonal control. Though androgens, and in particular the 5α-reduced metabolite of testosterone, 5α-dihydrotestosterone, are considered the primary modulators of epididymal functions, it has become apparent that many other regulatory molecules probably play specialized roles in maintaining normal functions within this tissue. Evidence has been gathered to indicate that, for at least some specific facets of epididymal function, there is, in addition to the endocrine regulation mediated by circulatory hormones, a paracrine regulation, i.e., regulation by factors entering the lumen of the epididymis directly from the efferent ducts.

Androgens

Effects of androgens. Even before the identification of testosterone as the major androgen produced by the testis, it was established, over 60 years ago, that epididymal histology was dependent on the presence of a testicular factor (1). A large number of studies during the last three decades have tested the effects of castration and replacement with testosterone on an immense array of parameters. Some specific facets of the androgen-dependence of epididymal functions have been thoroughly reviewed (11,309). A number of general conclusions regarding the androgen-dependence of the epididymis may be drawn. The epididymis atrophies when the testes are removed, and treatment with an amount of androgen that mimics the concentration found in the circulation can only partially maintain tissue epididymal weight; this is due to the large fractional coefficient (~ 40%) of epididymal weight attributable to luminal fluid and spermatozoa (295,318,521). In this respect, the excurrent duct system differs markedly from accessory tissues, such as the prostate and seminal vesicles. Nearly all the functions described above that take place in the epithelial or luminal compartment of the epididymis depend on the presence of androgens; the only function that has not yet been proven to directly depend on androgen is spermiophagy.

The effects of androgen withdrawal and its replacement on epididymal histology have been studied, since Benoit (1), by a number of investigators (153,522–524).

The regulation by androgens of intermediary metabolism in the epididymis has been studied extensively in the late 1970s by Brooks and reviewed by him in 1981 (309). He reported that, in the absence of androgens, epididymal intermediary metabolism is entirely dependent on carbohydrates for metabolic fuel; however, in the presence of androgens, the primary metabolic fuel becomes lipids. This switch in dependence on different substrates for energy was not found to be due to a depression in glycolysis, but rather to be due to an increase in lipid oxidation.

The transport of ions across the epididymal epithelium, an energy-dependent process, has been found by Wong and Yeung (224) to also be dependent on androgens. The systems responsible for transporting inositol and carnitine across the membranes of epididymal epithelial cells have also been shown to depend on androgens (244,245,525,526). Finally, the synthesis and secretion of a number of epididymal glycoproteins and the activity of a number of enzymes are to a large extent mediated by androgens (275,280,525,527–530). Whether any of these effects are directly mediated by androgens or must require the synthesis of new mRNA and consequently of new proteins is just being investigated now.

Transport of spermatozoa seems to be only indirectly dependent on the presence of androgens, since neuronal input to the epididymis is the apparent main driving force propelling the luminal content down the excurrent duct system. Both acquisition of fertilizing ability and storage of spermatozoa have been found to directly depend on androgens (11,12). Orgebin-Crist et al. (531) demonstrated, by using an *in vitro* organ culture system for monitoring sperm maturation, that only dihydrotestosterone and not its precursor, testosterone, or its metabolite, 3α-diol, was capable of permitting the development of fertilizing ability of spermatozoa.

Direct evidence that dihydrotestosterone is pivotal for spermatozoa to acquire their fertilizing potential has been obtained by assessing the effects of testosterone and dihydrotestosterone in the presence or absence of an inhibitor of 5α-reductase activity in adult, acutely castrated male mice (532). It was found that the presence of an inhibitor of 5α-reductase caused a decrease in the number of motile spermatozoa, in the percentage of oocytes fertilized, and in the number of blastocysts found even when given with testosterone. This was the first *in vivo* demonstration that fertilizing potential of spermatozoa in the epididymis is indeed acquired under the influence of 5α-reduced androgens.

Further evidence for the specificity of action of individual androgens on different functions carried out by the epididymis comes from a study by Lubicz-Nawrocki (519) on the effects of various androgens on the storage of spermatozoa in the golden hamster (Fig. 85). Spermatozoa kept in the ligated cauda epididymidis of golden hamsters for 7 days lose their ability to fertilize eggs; if different doses of androgens (testosterone, dihydrotestosterone, 3α-diol, or its 3β-epimer) are injected daily for 7 days and fertilization rates are then monitored, 3α-diol was found to be an order

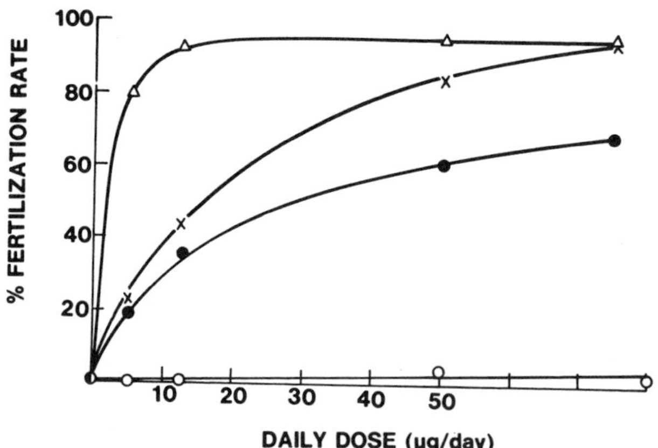

FIG. 85. Effect of increasing doses of testosterone (●), dihydrotestosterone (X), 5α-androstan-3α,17β-diol (△), and 5α-androstan-3β,17β-diol (○), injected daily, on the maintenance of the fertilizing ability of spermatozoa in the ligated hamster cauda epididymidis 1 week after castration. (Adapted from ref. 519.)

of magnitude more potent than testosterone and three to five orders of magnitude more potent than dihydrotestosterone in regulating the storage function of the epididymis.

The regulation of 5α-reductase in the epididymis is complex (47,295,326,329,347,533–535). This enzyme has been found associated with both the nuclear and microsomal fractions (Fig. 86); differential distribution of the enzyme with respect to both age and epididymal segment has also been observed (347). It is of interest to note that the specific activity in the nuclear fraction of the caput-corpus epididymidis reaches a peak at 7 weeks of age and steadily declines until 3 months. In contrast, microsomal 5α-reductase activity is relatively lower, but rises gradually so that by 3 months the specific activity in the microsomes is similar to that in the nuclear fraction (Fig. 86). The importance of the shift in the intracellular localization of 5α-reductase activity is not clear, but the coincidence between the high nuclear 5α-reductase activity and the age at which spermatozoa enter the epididymis is unlikely to be purely accidental.

Recently, it has been demonstrated that the microenvironment surrounding epididymal 5α-reductase is crucial for its activity (520). Removal from its membrane by solubilization or phospholipase treatment causes a reduction in the specific activity of the enzyme that can be reversed with the addition of phosphatidylcholines (Fig. 87). The exact chain length in the R1 and R2 positions in the phosphatidylcholine backbones proves to be crucial; twelve carbon chain lengths (dilaurylphosphatidylcholine) not only reverted the loss in activity that occurred upon solubilization

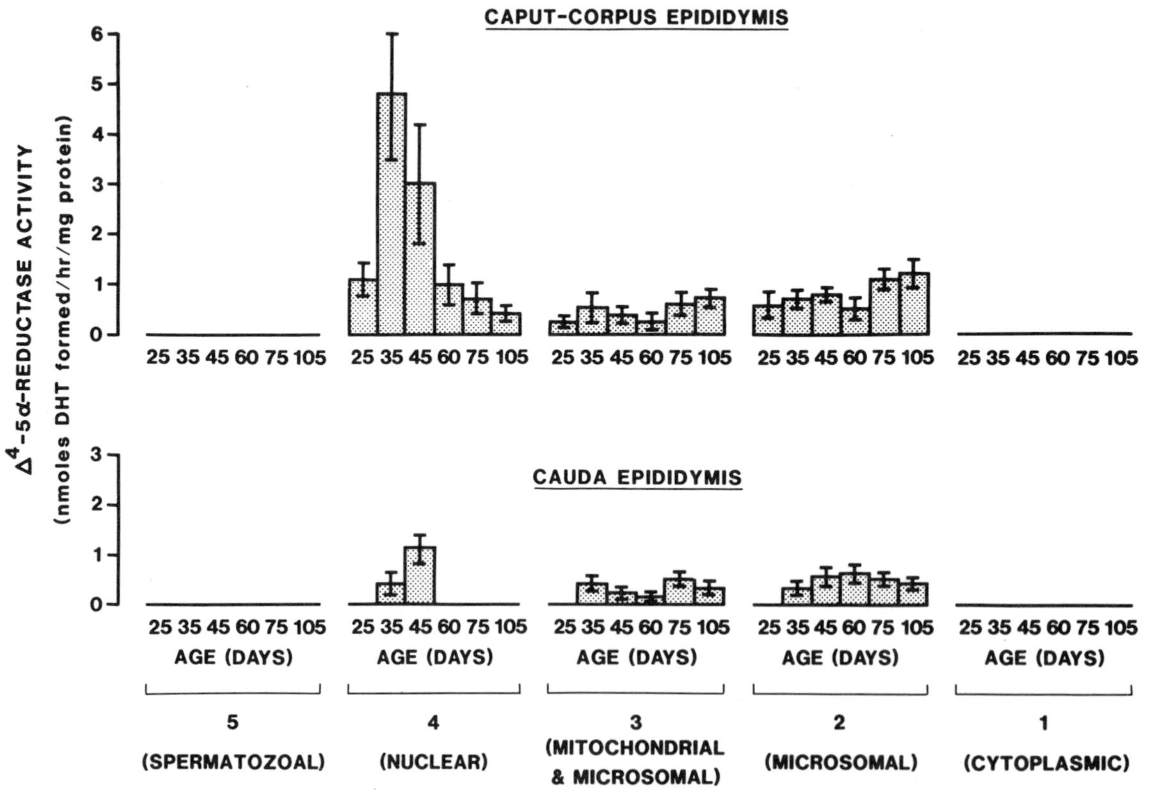

FIG. 86. Subcellular localization of 5α-reductase activity during development in the caput-corpus and cauda epididymidis. The horizontal axis represents the five different subcellular fractions obtained from discontinuous sucrose gradients; the tissues were obtained from animals of six different ages. The vertical axes represent 5α-reductase activity expressed as pmol dihydrotestosterone (DHT) formed/hr/mg protein. All values are expressed as mean ± SEM. (From ref. 347.)

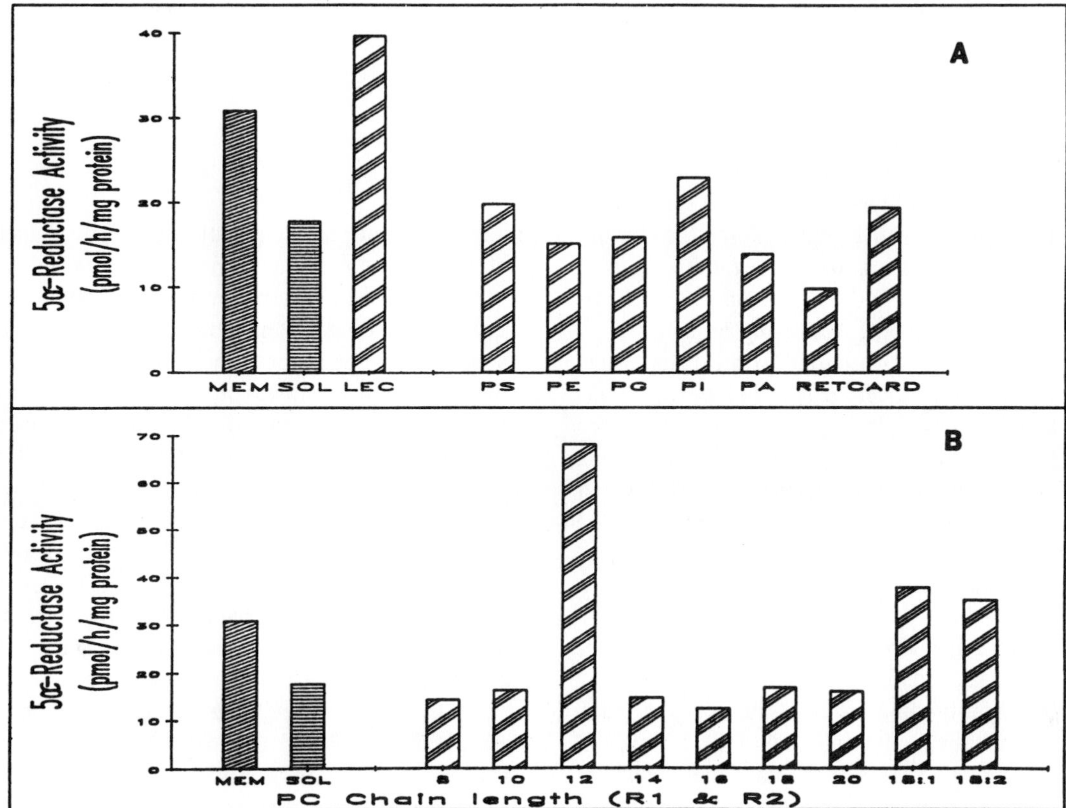

FIG. 87. Effects of various lipids (**A**) and phosphatidylcholines with defined acyl structure (**B**) on the specific activity of rat epididymal 5α-reductase. Membranes (MEM) were either assayed directly or solubilized, and the solubilized enzyme was assayed either alone (SOL) or in the presence of various lipids (500 μg/ml). LEC: egg lecithin, PS: phosphatidylserine, PE: phosphatidylethanolamine, PG: phosphatidylglycerol, PI: phosphatidylinositol, PA: phosphatidic acid, RET: retinol, CARD: cardiolipin. For panel **B**, the numbers 8, 10, 12, 14, 16, 18, and 20 refer to the length of the two unsaturated acyl chains of dicapryloyl, dicaproyl, dilauroyl, dimyristoyl, dipalmitoyl, distearoyl, and diarachidoyl phosphatidylcholine. The numbers 18.1 and 18.2 refer to the acyl chain lengths and degree of unsaturation of dioleoyl and dilinoleoyl phosphatidylcholines. (Adapted from ref. 520.)

but caused a greater than 100% increase in the specific activity of the 5α-reductase in the membrane preparation. The make-up of lipids in nuclear and microsomal fractions of epididymal principal cells has not yet been determined, but it is attractive to speculate that a potential rapid mechanism for regulating 5α-reductase activity within the epididymal cells may be via alterations in the microenvironment of the enzyme.

Though there is no debate that androgens do regulate epididymal function, the mechanism of androgen action is far less clear.

Mechanism of action-receptors. In order to identify a molecule as a biologically functional receptor for steroids, or other substances, it is essential to demonstrate not only that the proposed receptor molecule binds the agonist in a highly selective manner with strong affinity, but also that this proposed receptor actually mediates a response with a biological endpoint. In addition, the binding affinities of various agonists and antagonists should be parallel to their potency in a biological assay.

As we discuss below, two molecules with high affinity for the androgen agonist, dihydrotestosterone, have been found in the epididymis; these have been named "androgen receptor" and "androgen-binding protein." It must be stressed, however, that the conditions necessary to demonstrate that the proposed androgen receptor fulfills the above criteria have not been met. Specifically, no one has yet established that binding of dihydrotestosterone to the androgen receptor mediates the action of androgens in the epididymis. Consequently, it would have been preferable to designate the "androgen receptor" as an androgen-binding protein. But, for the sake of clarity, we will use the terms androgen receptor and androgen-binding protein to designate those two molecules described by Hansson and co-workers (52,536).

Little is known about the mechanism of androgen action in the epididymis, but it would appear that, in its general features, it resembles androgen action in the accessory sex glands such as the prostate and seminal vesicles. [The mechanism of action of androgens on their target tissues is discussed by D. S. Coffey (Chapter 24, *these volumes*)].

The first report that exogenously administered testosterone was transformed to dihydrotestosterone and found bound to a cytosolic protein in rat epididymides was made by Blaquier in 1971 (337). The presence of cytoplasmic receptors was confirmed for the rat (537,538), rabbit (539), dog (540,541), and ram (54,542). Epididymal cytoplasmic receptor seems to have many features in common with the androgen receptor found in the prostate (52,541,543). Although, in the rat (543), there are only minor changes in amount of androgen receptor as one moves from one segment to another of the epididymis (52,544), in ram epididymides striking differences have been reported (54) for different segments: The concentration in the caput and cauda epididymidis is 18 and 22 fmol/mg protein, respectively, while that in the corpus is only 4 fmol/mg protein.

The binding of dihydrotestosterone to the cytoplasmic receptor is blocked by antiandrogens such as cyproterone acetate and flutamide (543,545,546); it has been proposed (340) that antiandrogens mediate their action by preventing the translocation of the antagonist-receptor complex. However, in the light of the suggestion that steroid hormone receptors are only found in nuclei (547,548), the interpretation of these data on receptor translocation becomes questionable.

In 1971 Ritzen et al. (538) reported that rat epididymal cytosol contained a second high-affinity binding protein that was named androgen-binding protein. This protein, found in many species including guinea pig (549,550), rabbit (53), ram (552,581) and man (553), was shown to have a number of physicochemical properties that differed markedly from those of the cytoplasmic androgen receptor (537) [see review by V. Hansson et al. (52) and the chapter by C. W. Bardin et al. (Chapter 21, *these volumes*)].

Androgen-binding protein is synthesized by Sertoli cells and enters the epididymis via the efferent ducts (231,232,554–556). The function(s) of this protein are still unresolved, but it has been proposed that it acts as an androgen sink in seminiferous tubules (52), transports androgens to the epididymis (537), and/or is a regulator of epididymal nuclear 5α-reductase (326,327). A very strong resemblance between androgen-binding protein and the testosterone-estradiol-binding globulin present in blood has been established for both rat and rabbit (555,557,558). In a rat model, a correlation between the amount of epididymal androgen-binding protein and the fertilizing ability of spermatozoa has been established (559).

It is of particular interest to contrast two properties of androgen receptor and androgen-binding protein. The first is that the dissociation of ligand from androgen-binding protein is fairly rapid (half-time $\cong$ 6 min), whereas that from androgen receptor is very slow (half-time $>$ 2 days) (543). The second is that, though both proteins recognize dihydrotestosterone with high affinity, it would appear that the shape of the active site is different and that they recognize opposite faces of the planar steroid molecule (560–562); this has been taken advantage of in the design of drugs that will specifically bind to one protein (562,563). By taking these characteristics into account, as well as the observation that androgen-binding protein can be localized by the epithelium of the initial segment of the rat epididymis (231,232), it has been proposed that androgens are delivered directly to the cytoplasmic receptor by androgen-binding protein in the epididymis (561).

Other Hormones

In addition to the demonstrated actions of androgens on the excurrent duct system, there are a number of other hormones, e.g., estradiol, prolactin, and vitamin D, for which receptors (binding proteins) have been identified. Very little is currently known about the physiological functions mediated by such hormones in this tissue, yet our ability to unravel the fine regulatory mechanism of the excurrent duct system may well depend on our ability to understand more about these other regulators.

Estrogens. It has been known for many years that the administration of estrogens could affect the male reproductive system in general (564–573), and the epididymis in particular (574,575). Mediation of estrogen action was generally considered to take place via the hypothalamo-pituitary-gonadal axis resulting in a decreased luteinizing hormone (LH) secretion and a consequent decrease in testosterone production (567,569,572,576).

It was not until the last two decades that substantial evidence accumulated for the direct action of estrogens on androgen target tissues. Specific, high-affinity cytosolic and nuclear estrogen-binding proteins, presumably receptors, have been identified in epididymides from mice (518), rats (577,578), rabbits (579–582), dogs (540,583), and men (584). It is interesting to note that there is a fall in estradiol-binding sites in the epididymal cytosol of rabbits with age and that, looking at the entire tissue, there are more binding sites in the cauda than in the caput in both immature and mature rabbits (580).

Though the exact action of estrogen on male target tissues is still poorly understood, the proposal that estrogens have as their primary target, in male reproductive tissues, stromal as opposed to epithelial cells (585) is supported by studies where estrogen administration to young dogs (81) or rabbits (574) resulted in increases in weight of the epididymis that were almost entirely due to a hyperplasia of the stroma (lamina propria) of this tissue. Similar effects of estrogens on the adult epididymis have not yet been reported.

Estradiol administration to adult male mice has been shown to result in an increase in the rate of transport of spermatozoa through the epididymis (575). Whether this effect of estradiol on epididymal function was direct or indirect was not addressed experimentally, but the effect was clearly opposite to the effects observed with testosterone (575).

In a recent elegant study on the histo-localization of tritiated dihydrotestosterone and estradiol in the adult mouse epididymis, differential distribution of the presence of grains over nuclei in different segments of the excurrent duct system, as well as over different cell types, was noted (518). As can be seen from Fig. 88, the number of grains per

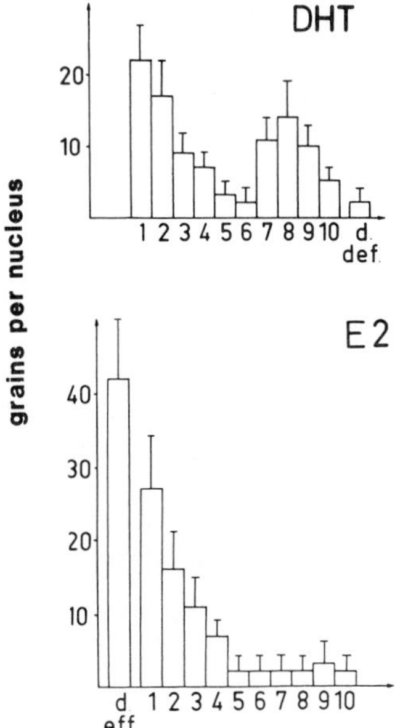

FIG. 88. Grain number over principal cell nuclei of mouse epididymis after injection of tritiated dihydrotestosterone (DHT) or tritiated estradiol (E2). Mean number of silver grains per nucleus from 50 nuclei per segment ± SEM is depicted for one DHT- and one E2-treated animal. The mean background of the photographic emulsion corresponding to nuclear area was approximately 1.5 silver grains. d. eff.: Ductulus efferens, d. def.: ductus (vas) deferens. Numbers 1 through 10 represent different segments of the epididymis: 1 = initial segment, 2–4 = caput, 5–6 = corpus, 7–9 = cauda, 10 = cauda, vas deferens. (Adapted from ref. 518.)

principal cell nucleus after dihydrotestosterone is relatively high in the initial segment and caput epididymidis (columns 1–3), declines markedly in the corpus epididymidis (columns 4–6), and rises again in the cauda epididymidis (columns 7–9). In marked contrast to this pattern, the number of grains over nuclei of principal cells after estradiol administration is highest in the efferent ducts, initial segment, and caput epididymidis and declines thereafter. These authors also noted that, particularly in the corpus and cauda epididymidis, there is a much denser labeling of the nuclei of clear cells with estradiol than with dihydrotestosterone. This is in sharp contrast to what was seen over nuclei of principal cells but similar to what was noted for connective tissue cells of the lamina propria.

A study such as that of Schleicher et al. (518) brings up the intriguing possibility that endogenous circulating, or potentially locally synthesized, estradiol may serve a specific function(s) in the epididymis, e.g., modulation of clear cell function. The difficulty in identifying estradiol receptors and aromatase activity in the epididymides of adult mammals may be due to the localization of activity to cells (clear cells) that are not abundant (see Fig. 13) in this tissue.

Aldosterone. Though it is clear that there are major changes in the concentration of ions along the excurrent duct system, the mechanism responsible for controlling these ion fluxes has not yet been elucidated. Because of the similarities between the ion fluxes seen in the epididymis and in the kidney, it has been proposed by Wong and Lee (586) and Jenkins et al. (587) that similar regulatory mechanisms may be operative. Indeed, specific binding sites for aldosterone, the adrenal mineralocorticosteroid, have been found located selectively by radioautography over clear cells (588), and this hormone, normally considered to have as its target site the kidney, has been shown to be involved in regulating the concentration of spermatozoa in the epididymis (589). Furthermore, spironolactone, an aldosterone antagonist, has been found to bring about a change in the intraluminal concentration of ions: Sodium was increased (587) and potassium was decreased (586); the regional sperm concentration within the epididymis was also modulated by this hormone analog (589). However, no change in fertility was found after treating rats with this drug (586). One should interpret these data cautiously, in view of the demonstrated antiandrogenic effect of this drug (590).

Prolactin. The two pituitary hormones that are the prime regulators of reproductive function are LH and follicle stimulating hormone (FSH). Prolactin is also synthesized and secreted by the pituitary and has been shown to modulate both testicular and prostatic processes (591,592). Recently, the hypothalamic peptide that is the precursor of luteinizing hormone releasing hormone (LHRH), has been found to also contain a fragment that can very effectively suppress prolactin secretion (593).

Specific binding proteins (receptors?) for prolactin have been found in homogenates of rat (594) and rabbit epididymides (40); the concentration of protein-binding sites in this tissue was higher than that found in any other tissue of the male reproductive tract of the rabbit but amongst the lowest of the rat. In light of the possible co-regulation of gonadotropin and prolactin release, of the apparent presence of prolactin "receptors" in the epididymis and of the proposal that prolactin regulates ion transport (see review, ref. 595), it is plausible that this hormone may play a major role in regulating certain facets of epididymal function.

Vitamin D. The known primary function of vitamin D is the homeostasis of calcium and phosphorus; the major sites of action of this vitamin (sterol hormone) are bone, intestine, and kidney (596). A number of complementary observations would suggest that the epididymis may also be a target for the action of this hormone. First, receptors for $1,25(OH)_2$ vitamin D have been found in the rat epididymis; the radiolabeled ligand was displaceable by excess unlabeled cold hormone, but not by the biologically inactive $25(OH)D_3$, or by progestins or estrogens (38). Second, the epididymis was found (39) to take up $25(OH)D_3$ and metabolize it to both $1,25(OH)_2D_3$ and $24,25(OH)_2D_3$; it is particularly interesting to note that the epididymis had a higher level of $24,25(OH)_2D_3$ than any other tissue studied, and that the cauda had three times more of this metabolite than the caput epididymidis. One of the ions known to be regulated by the metabolites of vitamin D is phosphorus; we have previously discussed that this element, in both organic and inorganic forms, is found in extraordinarily high concentrations in the cauda epididymidis (Fig. 74) (15). It is tempting to hypothesize that one of the vitamin D metabolites, potentially 24,25$(OH)_2D_3$, plays a pivotal role in regulating the flux of phosphorus into the epididymis.

Vitamin A. Vitamin A (retinol) is a fat-soluble vitamin that is essential for normal survival. It can be substituted for by retinoic acid in most tissues with the known exceptions of the retina and the testis. Selective binding proteins have been identified for both retinol and retinoic acid in most tissues of the male reproductive system (597–600). In 1983, Porter et al. (600) described the presence of high levels of cytoplasmic retinol-binding protein (CRBP) in the proximal cauda epididymidis. Using specific radioimmunoassays, Kato et al. (599) reported in 1985 that of all the tissues they studied throughout the body of the rat, the caput epididymidis had a 50% higher concentration of CRBP than the liver, the tissue with the next highest activity, and ten times more than in the cauda epididymidis. In contrast, cytoplasmic retinoic-acid-binding protein (CRABP) increased sevenfold between the caput and the cauda epididymidis, so that in the caput the ratio of CRBP to CRABP was nearly 100:1, while in the cauda it was approximately 1:1. The distribution of these molecules was apparently not affected by changes in the nutritional intake of vitamin A.

At nearly the same time, a report by Porter et al. (600) of the histochemical localization of CRBP and CRABP in the testis and throughout the epididymis appeared. Though their data are not quantitative, they did demonstrate that CRBP is found in the principal cells, and that the amount of staining was far greater in the proximal than in the distal caput epididymidis, with some staining over the stereocilia but no staining in the lumen of the tissue. No appreciable staining was found in the corpus or cauda epididymidis. In contrast, CRABP staining was very sparse over the principal cells but heaviest over the lumen and the stereocilia of the caput epididymidis, with a relatively small decrease of staining as one moved down the epididymis. In the vas deferens, CRABP staining over principal cells increased from the proximal to the distal segments.

The functional significance of the presence of these binding proteins is still unclear, however, given the fact that they are present in such high concentrations, and that their localization is so finely regulated, it is likely that vitamin A plays a significant role in the regulation of epididymal function. Vitamin A is a component of most of the vitamin supplements that are taken routinely by many people. It is worth noting that the 13-cis form of retinoic acid (Accutane®) is a drug that is now commonly used for the treatment of acne; the potential effects of such a drug on epididymal function have not yet been elucidated.

Relative Influence of Hormonal Exposure Via the Circulation and the Luminal Compartment

In addition to the well-established role for circulating hormones and, in particular, androgens in the regulation of epididymal functions, evidence has accumulated that certain epididymal functions are also regulated in a paracrine manner, i.e., by factor(s) coming from the testis that enter the epididymal lumen directly. A number of complementary lines of evidence have been developed in support of this hypothesis.

Studies on the regulation of rat epididymal nuclear 5α-reductase activity have demonstrated that testosterone administration, either at doses that matched those found in the circulation or in epididymal fluid, to castrated animals was unable to maintain this enzymatic activity (295); efferent duct transection also resulted in a fall of this enzymatic activity in the epididymis. This was in marked contrast to the situation reported for prostatic 5α-reductase (601) where circulating androgens were able to maintain this enzymatic activity. The possibility that some other serum factor(s) was responsible for regulating this enzymatic activity was excluded by demonstrating that, after unilateral orchidectomy, there was a fall in nuclear 5α-reductase activity selectively on the side where the testis had been removed (602). This inability of circulating androgens to maintain epididymal nuclear 5α-reductase activity is specific in that the subsequent enzyme in the metabolism of androgens, 3α-hydroxysteroid dehydrogenase, was not affected by castration and androgen replacement, efferent duct transection, or unilateral orchidectomy (295,602). Studies on rat (534), rabbit (329), and dog (V. K. Ganjam, *personal communication*) have confirmed these observations. Such observations led to the proposal that epididymal nuclear 5α-reductase is regulated by substance(s) entering the epididymis directly from the testis (295,326,601).

Histological observations of the initial segment of the epididymis in rats whose efferent ducts were ligated and were orchidectomized and treated with various doses of testosterone revealed that a number of characteristics were markedly altered by such treatments (138). In this study, Fawcett and Hoffer noted a decrease in duct diameter, epithelial cell height, endoplasmic reticulum, and Golgi complex, yet fluid phase pinocytosis was still evident. Consequently, a role for luminal factor(s), other than free testosterone, in the regulation of functions in the initial segment of the rat epididymis was proposed (138).

In a study on the protein biosynthetic ability of different segments of the rabbit epididymis, Jones et al. (296) found that, after castration and androgen replacement or efferent duct ligation, the protein synthesis ability of the corpus and cauda epididymidis was not affected, but that of the initial segment and caput epididymidis declined. This decline was not a general nonspecific effect; a group of three proteins having a molecular weight in the range of 22,000 could not be maintained when direct testicular input into the epididymal lumen was blocked. Once again, a role for direct, nonandrogenic, testicular regulation of epididymal function is apparent.

Orgebin-Crist et al. (11), using rabbits, studied the effects of castration and hypophysectomy on the ability to maintain spermatozoa fertile in the cauda epididymidis. They found that, over a 2-week period, hypophysectomy did not significantly affect sperm fertilizing ability, but that by 10 days after castration spermatozoa had reduced their fertilizing ability by 75%, and by 2 weeks it had become completely lost (Fig. 89). Such data could be viewed as supportive evidence for the hypothesis that factors present in the lumen are essential for maintaining epididymal function.

The testicular cell type responsible for elaborating the factor(s) having this paracrine regulatory role, at least for epididymal nuclear 5α-reductase, has been the subject of several investigations (47,326,535). Three complementary approaches were taken to differentiate between the potential role of the three major testicular cell types: hypophysectomy and androgen replacement (535), changes during development (47), and effects of testosterone administration to intact adult males (B. Robaire and L. L. Ewing, *unpublished observations*). Together these studies have led to the conclusion that epididymal nuclear 5α-reductase activity is not regulated by secretions from Leydig cells, advanced spermatids, or spermatozoa; rather, Sertoli cells, or, possibly, early germ cells, are the most likely cells to be synthesizing such substance(s) involved in paracrine regulation.

It has been proposed that androgen-binding protein may be the actual substance involved in regulating the activity of epididymal nuclear 5α-reductase (326). The rationale for this proposal is that the developmental pattern and longitudinal distribution along the epididymis for androgen-binding protein and 5α-reductase are very similar. The site where androgen-binding protein is internalized by the epididymis is nearly identical to that where maximal nuclear 5α-reductase activity is found (326,327). Further, the proposal discussed above, put forth by Lobl et al. (562), for the direct transfer of androgens from androgen-binding protein to the androgen receptor can logically be integrated with the present hypothesis. Hence, an androgen, testosterone or dihydrotestosterone, would enter the lumen of the epididymis bound to androgen-binding protein; the complex would be internalized and the androgen would be transferred to the androgen receptor; the receptor-hormone complex would cause, as a product of its interaction with chromatin, the synthesis of 5α-reductase, which would then be able to convert the high concentrations of testosterone that are entering the epididymis into dihydrotestosterone, the major androgen active in the epididymis and leaving the caput epididymidis (94). Though certain facets of this hypothesis have yet to be tested, Amann and collaborators (327,603) have been able to demonstrate, using cultured principal cells, that the conversion of testosterone to 5α-reduced metabolites is indeed regulated by a nonsteroidal factor, most probably androgen-binding protein, in rete testis fluid.

CELL AND ORGAN CULTURE OF THE EPIDIDYMIS

The intrinsic complexity of the functions carried out by the epididymis and the extent to which these different functions change in the various segments of this tissue have induced a number of laboratories to look at its properties in isolation. As far back as 1972 (604), efforts have been under way to culture epididymal tubules. Over the past few years, these efforts have intensified as an array of both organ and cell culture methods for different segments of the epididymis of different species have been published [organ (48,531,605–

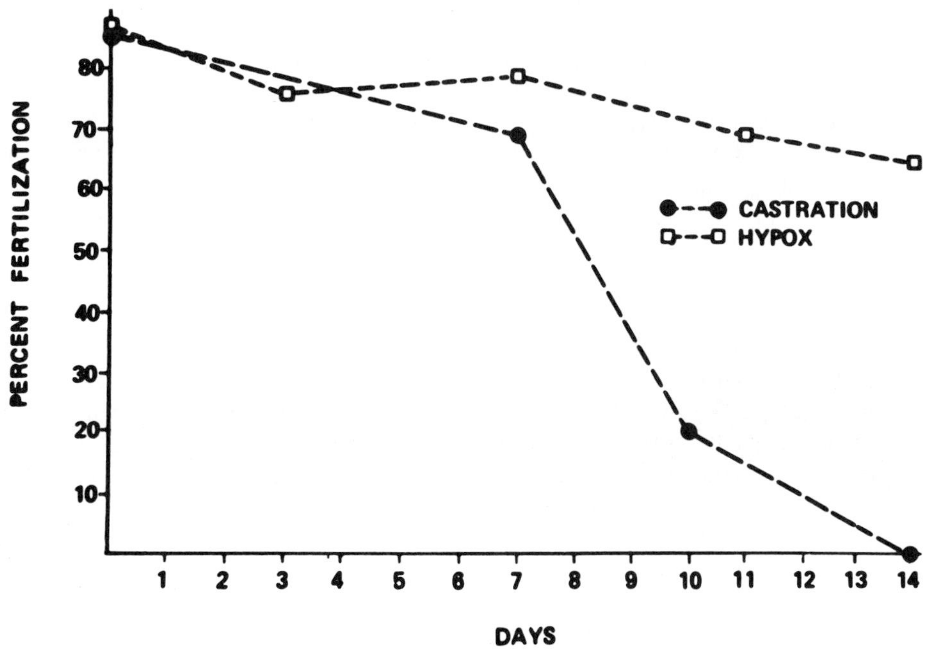

FIG. 89. Fertilizing ability of spermatozoa from the distal cauda epididymidis of the rabbit as a function of time after either castration or hypophysectomy (HYPOX). (From ref. 11.)

611, cell (612–619)]. Though there is still no standardized approach to this technically difficult problem, significant contributions have been made using these methods. A number of conclusions have emerged. Testosterone is not sufficient to maintain the tissue in a functionally "healthy" state in culture; it is necessary to have dihydrotestosterone in the culture medium (531,620). The ability of the cultured tissue to convert testosterone to its 5α-reduced metabolites cannot be maintained by the addition of testosterone or dihydrotestosterone to the medium; rather, it is essential that rete testis fluid be present (327). Thus, as in the *in vivo* situation (621), the necessity for factors of testicular origin, other than testosterone, for maintaining the activity of epididymal 5α-reductase is evident.

Epididymal Organ Culture

There are several advantages to using organ culture for the study of hormone-dependent tissues such as the epididymis (622). First, the endocrine environment of the tissue can be precisely defined and easily manipulated in organ culture. Thus, the direct effect of a single hormone, or the interaction of several compounds, can be studied under controlled and reproducible conditions. Second, tissues that are hormone-sensitive *in vivo* usually retain their hormone responsiveness in organ culture. Third, anatomic relationships between various cells are preserved in organ culture. Maintenance of the histological architecture may be of particular significance to studies of the epididymis.

Two main methods of organ culture have been used to study epididymal function and sperm maturation. The first is a static organ culture method, where a stainless steel grid is used to support segments of epididymal tubules at the gas-medium interface of the culture vessel; this method has been useful in studying the androgenic dependence of sperm maturation (531,604,622–624). However, this system has the inherent disadvantage that it relies solely on diffusion to supply nutrients and oxygen and eliminate waste products. Unfortunately, the morphological appearance of the tissue was not usually presented in these studies; yet, its appearance was often reported to be inconsistent, causing significant variability in the results. Moreover, the static organ culture method lacks the homeostasis present in vascularized tissue in which nutrients and oxygen are continually supplied and waste products are eliminated.

Using the organ culture static system, it was possible, however, to demonstrate in rabbits that the maturation of spermatozoa is androgen-dependent (604) and, more specifically, dependent on the presence of dihydrotestosterone (531,622); furthermore, the action of this steroid was demonstrated to be mediated via the synthesis of RNA and proteins (623). Also, in the rat, with a similar technique, Blaquier and colleagues demonstrated that dihydrotestosterone mediated the synthesis of RNA and proteins that were potentially important for the maturation of spermatozoa (606,607,624,625).

In order to overcome the inherent difficulties associated with a static organ culture system and to achieve conditions which more closely resemble the *in vivo* situation, Orgebin-Crist and Menezo (609) developed a second approach: a perfusion of isolated segments of epididymal tubules. In this system, epididymal tubules were submerged in a continuous flow chamber of oxygenated medium. Upon comparing the histology, metabolic activity, and ability to synthesize RNA and proteins in the continuous flow method with the static organ culture method, they found that the former was far superior with respect to all the parameters measured. Recently, Klinefelter and Hamilton (611) further refined this perifusion method. The synthesis and secretion of proteins by isolated tubules from rats (626) or blocks of tissue from mice (627) have been demonstrated. The morphology, at both the light and electron microscopic levels, remained essentially unchanged for up to 7 days in culture (611). Over 50% of spermatozoa, obtained from segments of caput epididymidis of rats, acquired progressive motility when tubules were cultured for 36 hr (611); the spermatozoa in epididymal tubules retained their fertilizing ability for at least 5 days, whereas the fertile span of spermatozoa in suspension was limited to hours.

Organ culture of the vas deferens has not yet been successfully developed. Recently, however, Wenstrom and Hamilton (628) have reported a method for observing functions in different regions of the vas deferens. Using epithelial strips, they showed that, at least over a 3-hr incubation period, morphological integrity of the tissue was maintained. The epithelium of the proximal vas was found to be more active in synthesizing and secreting proteins (glycoproteins) than the distal vas (628).

Epididymal Cell Culture

Although one loses organizational integrity by dissociating a tissue into isolated cells, it is possible to obtain more specific information with respect to the activity and functions of an individual cell type within the tissue. It is also possible to maintain the cells for longer periods of time and to study the hormonal regulation of the different cell types. Several attempts have been made to develop methods for the isolation of purified populations of viable epididymal epithelial cells. Disaggregation of the epididymis by enzymatic and/or mechanical methods has been successful in yielding viable, yet heterogeneous, suspensions of epididymal cells (612,613,629). Attempts have been made to purify these suspensions by unit gravity sedimentation (613,629), sequential enzyme treatment (615,630), and elutriation (614,631). However, the low epithelial or principal cell yield produced by the unit gravity method, and the length of time required for the separation seriously limit the use of this technique for physiological studies. Sequential enzyme treatment appears to yield highly enriched populations of epididymal epithelial cells; however, the efficacy of this procedure for removing nonepithelial cells, such as fibroblasts, is questionable. Primary cultures of cells derived from sequential enzyme treatment often require the use of medium containing D-valine, or the addition of cytosine arabinoside to inhibit fibroblast overgrowth (632). A novel method was recently developed for the isolation and culture of ciliated and nonciliated cells of the efferent ducts (633). Using collagenase, cell clumps (tubular fragments) were prepared and placed over Millipore filters coated with an extracellular matrix extract. Ciliary activity was maintained for at least 7 days and the cells were able to maintain their ability to take up androgen-binding protein (633).

Early studies were primarily designed at establishing an appropriate method for the preparation of principal and basal cells from the epididymis (612–614,616,629). Though the identification of isolated cells was possible after they were prepared for electron microscopy, a rapid method of recognizing principal cells in culture, without having to use a procedure that would prevent further studies on the cells, has proven very difficult because of the change in appearance of cells when they are isolated, i.e., rounding of nearly all epididymal cells (613–616,621,630). Autofluorescent granules and fluorescin isothiocyanate (FITC)-lectin binding protein have been proposed as useful "nonlethal" methods of identifying principal cells (630).

In an attempt to improve the yield of epididymal principal cells, a simple method based on the separation of cells by cell density using discontinuous Percoll gradient centrifugation was developed (621). This method provided a high yield of principal cells with > 90% viability that still maintained their ability to metabolize testosterone to its 5α-reduced metabolites.

Some clear observations on cell function have emerged using cell culture methods. Principal and not basal cells are the ones possessing most of the ability to convert testosterone to its 5α-reduced metabolites (323). It is interesting to note that 5α-reductase activity of rat epididymal principal cells is maximal when these cells are incubated at 31°C and not core temperature (Fig. 90); this is in support of Bedford's hypothesis that epididymal functions are carried out more effectively at temperatures lower than core (456).

It is also principal cells that, even in culture, seem to contain and secrete acidic epididymal glycoproteins (AEG) (615). From both caput and corpus epididymidis, glycerylphosphorylcholine is predominantly present in principal cells as opposed to basal cells or fibroblasts, while sialic acid is evenly distributed (631,634).

Upon isolation, the principal cells initially round up and have a spherical appearance (613–616,621,630). After plating on glass or plastic and maintenance in culture for a number of days, this appearance changes, at least in cells obtained from rat (617) and bull (619) epididymides; they initially flatten and then display projections that form desmosome-like contacts with adjacent cells (617). If, however, cell clumps, from either rat or ram, are cultured on a floating collagen matrix, the morphological characteristics, e.g., cell polarity, presence of microvilli, of cells kept over prolonged time periods are much better maintained (618,635). In fact, the reformation of junctional complexes between principal cells has been reported (618). The importance of the material on which epididymal cells are maintained in culture has recently been further demonstrated by Byers et al. (636). By coating a solid semipermeable support with an extract of rat epididymides, the "extracellular matrix," it was possible to maintain, as a confluent monolayer, the epididymal principal cells in a polarized state.

Brown et al. (327,603) have provided strong evidence for observations and hypotheses previously presented by Robaire's group (based on *in vivo* data) (295,326,535): The

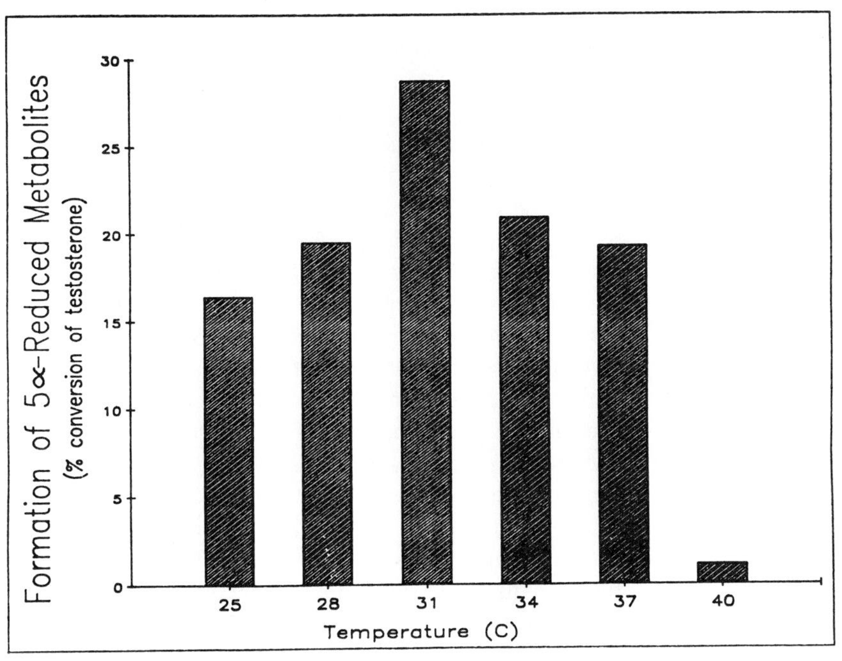

FIG. 90. Formation of 5α-reduced metabolites of testosterone by isolated rat caput epididymal principal cells incubated for 15 hr in serum-free medium at various temperatures ranging from 25 to 40°C. Activity is expressed as the percent of testosterone (5×10^{-7} M) converted to 5α-reduced metabolites per 100,000 principal cells per 15 hr.

ability of the epididymis to form 5α-reduced metabolites of testosterone is primarily found in cells from the caput epididymidis and this activity is dependent on a substance(s), other than steroids, found in rete testis fluid.

EFFECTS OF DRUGS ON THE EPIDIDYMIS AND VAS DEFERENS

It is apparent that the availability of drugs that would selectively modify functions carried out either in or by the epididymis should be of major value not only from the perspective of development of male contraceptives, but also for the treatment of male fertility problems whose etiology arises from the epididymis. The effects on the epididymis of a number of such potential drugs have been reviewed (15,637–639).

There has, to date, been no significant effort devoted toward the development of therapeutic agents that would be useful in the treatment of male infertility and would work via the epididymis. However, a number of studies have been undertaken with the goal of developing drugs that would be effective male contraceptive agents and would have as their target the epididymis.

A variety of approaches may be envisioned for the development of such drugs. These include modifying the action of the hormonal factors known to regulate epididymal function, altering the microenvironment of spermatozoa as they acquire their ability to fertilize eggs, or a direct alteration of the spermatozoa themselves, e.g., preventing the addition of or altering the glycoproteins that are added to the cell coat of the surface of sperm in the epididymis.

One obvious approach is to block the production of dihydrotestosterone within the epididymis, since it has been established (see above) that this androgen is essential for the maturation of spermatozoa and that there are specific receptors for dihydrotestosterone in the epididymis. A number of laboratories (640–644) have tested drugs such as cyproterone acetate or flutamide that are dihydrotestosterone receptor antagonists and found that these compounds successfully block epididymal function. However, as expected, the action of androgens in other target tissues was also blocked, and therefore these compounds had undesirable side effects.

An alternate approach to blocking the action of dihydrotestosterone in the epididymis is to prevent its synthesis by blocking the enzyme responsible for the production of this hormone, 5α-reductase. An array of compounds has been reported to block this enzyme in a variety of different tissues (645–654). However, reports on only three families of drugs have appeared on the ability of such compounds to block epididymal 5α-reductase (655–657). The first report is of a family of 5,10-secosteroids that are suicide substrates (irreversible inhibitors) of the enzyme *in vitro* and have been shown to inhibit the epididymal enzyme (655). These compounds have not yet been tested for their effect on fertility *in vivo* using a chronic low-dose regimen; however, a report has appeared that very high doses of the secosteroids do cause undesirable gastrointestinal side effects (658). It is interesting to note that the pregnane analog of this family of secosteroids does not inhibit the conversion of pregnenolone to testosterone by the testis (656) or the further metabolism of dihydrotestosterone by the epididymis (655).

One of the more extensively studied inhibitors of steroid-5α-reductase in the prostate and a variety of tissues is diethyl-4-methyl-3-oxo-4-aza-5α-androstane-17β-carboxamide (4-MA) (652–654); this compound has been found to be also a competitive inhibitor of the epididymal enzyme (656). There has been one study in which this compound has been shown not to alter the fertility of male rats; however, these investigators did not determine whether the dose used was, in fact, sufficient to inhibit epididymal 5α-reductase (659). The ability of 4-MA, at concentrations that inhibit the epididymal enzyme, to also inhibit the 3β-hydroxysteroid dehydrogenase-isomerase system makes it an unlikely candidate as a selective blocker of epididymal function.

The third family of compounds studied as inhibitors of 5α-reductase are the 17-chloroformate analogs of testosterone (657). These compounds can block the formation of dihydrotestosterone without significantly affecting its further metabolism by 3α-hydroxysteroid dehydrogenase. No studies of their efficacy as blockers of epididymal function *in vivo* have yet been done.

In the late 1960s a series of studies appeared on the ability of the drug α-chlorohydrin, a monochloro derivative of glycerol, to reversibly inhibit fertility in an array of species [see review by Jones (660), Jackson and Robinson (661), and Lobl (662)]. Subsequently, it was found that the action of this drug, at low doses, was to inhibit glyceraldehyde 3-phosphate dehydrogenase in spermatozoa that resided in the cauda epididymidis (663,664), and that the inhibition was selectively mediated by the levo (S) enantiomer (660,665). At higher doses, however, α-chlorohydrin caused the formation of spermatoceles in the caput epididymidis of rodents which result in the blockade of sperm transport through the tissue and consequent atrophy of the seminiferous tubules due to increases in back pressure (660,666,667); the mechanism responsible for the formation of these spermatoceles is not clear. Wong and colleagues (668–670) were able to demonstrate that α-chlorohydrin did block the resorption of sodium and water from the cauda epididymidis. Because of the severe toxicity (bone marrow depression) associated with this compound when tested in primates (671), it will not be developed as a male contraceptive in man, although, it is used to control the population in rodents. The possibility remains that structural analogs of α-chlorohydrin, devoid of these undesirable side effects and targeted at the epididymis, can be made.

In 1978, Ford and Waites (672) described another antifertility compound, 6-chloro-6-deoxyglucose, that has the ability to inactivate spermatozoa from the cauda epididymidis by blocking glyceraldehyde-3-phosphate dehydrogenase

(664). This compound was also found to affect different functions of the epididymis (667,670,673), but due to its neurotoxicity in primates (667) (associated with its effects on glucose transport), it is also unlikely to develop as an acceptable male contraceptive.

The discovery that gossypol was an effective antifertility agent in China elicited a large number of studies on the mechanism of action of this compound. A recent monograph deals with different facets of this drug in some detail (674). It would appear, though, that the early speculations that this compound selectively affected epididymal functions are not warranted; the blood-epididymis barrier and epididymal functions remain intact in the presence of this drug (675).

The epididymis has not usually been studied as one of the target tissues for the toxicological effects of drugs, and consequently little is known about the importance of this tissue as a target for toxic drug effects. In one recent study, however, it was found that the male-mediated teratogenic effect of cyclophosphamide (676,677), an anticancer and immunosuppressive drug, was associated with an increase in the number of clear cells and in the number of spermatozoa with abnormal tails in the epididymis of rats (678).

SUMMARY AND PERSPECTIVES

The growth of our knowledge about the histology, biochemistry, and physiology of the male excurrent duct system is impressive. Though we are now only beginning to appreciate the gaps in this knowledge, we have made major strides in elucidating the different structural components of the tissue, the functions carried out by it, and the regulation of these functions.

The cell types and their subcellular organelles are now well described. It has not only been unequivocally established that cells from different regions of the excurrent duct are involved in absorption and secretion, but mechanisms for these processes have been proposed.

The existence of many complex metabolic processes taking place within the efferent ducts, epididymis, and vas deferens is now widely accepted. These metabolic processes do not only include those facets of intermediary metabolism one might expect from any complex, active tissue, but also many other facets of metabolism are being uncovered in this tissue; these range from steroid metabolism to local conversion of vitamin D and prostaglandins.

Though it has been clearly demonstrated that hormonal regulation of events taking place in the excurrent duct system is under the control of androgens locally synthesized from testosterone, it has also become clear that additional regulatory processes almost certainly play a role in controlling the functions of this tissue. Over the next few years the precise role and importance of these other regulatory factors should be elucidated.

The application of methods developed in other fields, such as cell and organ culture, is now becoming more routine for studies of the epididymis and vas deferens. However, because of the complexity of this tissue it is becoming nec-
functions of the epididymis (667,670,673), but due to its
essary to develop novel approaches that are likely to find applications in other fields.

With our recent, tremendous increase in knowledge about the male excurrent duct system, we are now in a better position to assess the role of dysfunctions of this tissue in male infertility and to develop a wider spectrum of drugs that can selectively maintain or attack functions carried by this tissue.

In re-examining Mann's perception of 20 years ago, one can now perceive the epididymis and its adjacent tissues as having come a long way from being abandoned children. They could now be viewed as knowledgeable teen-agers.

ACKNOWLEDGMENTS

The assistance of Mrs. J. Duron in preparing the bibliography of this manuscript is deeply appreciated. Numerous helpful suggestions have been made by Dr. B. Hales. Various aspects of the electron microscopy work were carried out with the help of Drs. C. Morales and V. DeMelo. The technical assistance of Mrs. J. Mui and Ms. P. Hales is gratefully acknowledged. Dr. J. Trasler prepared tissues for light microscopy and collected the data presented in Fig. 13; light micrographs were prepared by Mr. T. Graham. Studies on cell isolation and enzyme activities were done by Dr. L. J. Buchanan. All line drawings were prepared by Mrs. M. Oeltzschner. Original studies presented in this manuscript were funded by grants to Drs. B. Robaire, L. Hermo, and Y. Clermont from the Medical Research Council of Canada (MRC) and the support of the Fonds pour la Formation de Chercheurs et l'Aide à la Recherche du Québec (FCAR).

REFERENCES

1. Benoit, J. (1926): Recherches anatomiques, cytologiques et histophysiologiques sur les voies excrétrices du testicule chez les mammifères. *Arch. Anat. Histol. Embryol. (Strasb)*, 5:175–412.
2. Young, W. C. (1929): A study of the function of the epididymis. I. Is the attainment of full spermatozoon maturity attributable to some specific action of the epididymal secretion? *J. Morphol. Physiol.*, 47:479–495.
3. Young, W. C. (1929): A study of the function of the epididymis. II. The importance of an aging process in sperm for the length of the period during which fertilizing capacity is retained by sperm isolated in the epididymis of the guinea-pig. *J. Morphol. Physiol.*, 48:475–491.
4. Young, W. C. (1931): A study of the function of the epididymis. III. Functional changes undergone by spermatozoa during their passage through the epididymis and vas deferens in the guinea pig. *J. Exp. Biol.*, 8:151–162.
5. Mann, T. (1964): *The Biochemistry of Semen and of the Male Reproductive Tract*. Methuen, London.
6. Orgebin-Crist, M.-C. (1967): Sperm maturation in rabbit epididymis. *Nature*, 216:816–818.
7. Orgebin-Crist, M.-C. (1969): Studies on the function of the epididymis. *Biol. Reprod.*, 1:155–175.
8. Bedford, J. M. (1967): Effects of duct ligation on the fertilizing ability of spermatozoa from different regions of the rabbit epididymis. *J. Exp. Zool.*, 166:271–282.

9. Hamilton, D. W. (1972): The mammalian epididymis. In: *Reproductive Biology,* edited by H. Balin and S. Glasser, pp. 268–337. Excerpta Medica, Amsterdam.
10. Hamilton, D. W. (1975): Structure and function of the epithelium lining the ductuli efferentes, ductus epididymidis and ductus deferens in the rat. In: *Handbook of Physiology, Sec. 7, Vol. 5,* edited by R. O. Greep and E. B. Astwood, pp. 259–301. American Physiological Society, Washington, D.C.
11. Orgebin-Crist, M.-C., Danzo, B. J., and Davies, J. (1975): Endocrine control of the development and maintenance of sperm fertilizing ability in the epididymis. In: *Handbook of Physiology, Sec. 7, Vol. 5,* edited by R. O. Greep and E. B. Astwood, pp. 319–338. American Physiological Society, Washington, D.C.
12. Bedford, J. M. (1975): Maturation, transport, and fate of spermatozoa in the epididymis. In: *Handbook of Physiology, Sec. 7, Vol. 5,* edited by R. O. Greep and E. B. Astwood, pp. 303–317. American Physiological Society, Washington, D.C.
13. Neaves, W. H. (1975): Biological aspects of vasectomy. In: *Handbook of Physiology, Sec. 7, Vol. 5,* edited by R. O. Greep and E. B. Astwood, pp. 383–404. American Physiological Society, Washington, D.C.
14. Turner, T. T. (1979): On the epididymis and its function. *Invest. Urol.,* 16:311–319.
15. Hinton, B. T. (1980): The epididymal microenvironment: A site of attack for a male contraceptive? *Invest. Urol.,* 18:1–10.
16. Courot, M. (1981): Transport and maturation of spermatozoa in the epididymis of mammals. *Prog. Reprod. Biol.,* 8:67–79.
17. Orgebin-Crist, M.-C. (1981): Epididymal physiology and sperm maturation. In: *Epididymis and Fertility: Biology and Pathology,* edited by C. Bollack and A. Clavert, pp. 80–89. Karger, Switzerland.
18. Brooks, D. E. (1982): Epididymal functions and their hormonal regulation. *Aust. J. Biol. Sci.,* 36:205–221.
19. Glover, T. D. (1982): The epididymis. In: *Scientific Foundations of Urology,* edited by G. D. Chisholm and D. I. Williams, pp. 544–555. Heinemann, London.
20. Howards, S. S. (1983): The epididymis, sperm maturation, and capacitation. In: *Infertility in the Male,* edited by L. I. Lipshultz and S. S. Howards, pp. 121–134. Churchill-Livingstone, New York.
21. Orgebin-Crist, M.-C. (1984): Epididymis physiology. In: *Médecine de la Reproduction Masculine,* edited by G. Schaison, P. Bouchard, J. Mahoudeau, and F. Labrie, pp. 51–61. Flammarion, Paris.
22. Bedford, J. M. (1979): Evolution of the sperm maturation and sperm storage functions of the epididymis. In: *The Spermatozoon,* edited by D. W. Fawcett and J. M. Bedford, pp. 7–21. Urban & Schwarzenberg, Baltimore.
23. Cooper, G. W., and Bedford, J. M. (1976): Asymmetry of spermiation and sperm surface charge patterns over the giant acrosome in the musk shrew, *Suncus murinus. J. Cell Biol.,* 69:415–428.
24. Bedford, J. M., and Millar, R. P. (1978): The character of sperm maturation in the epididymis of the acrotal hyrax, *Procarvia capensis* and armadillo, *Dasypus novemcinctus. Biol. Reprod.,* 19:396–406.
25. Bedford, J. M., and Rifkin, J. M. (1979): Evolutionary view of the male reproductive tract and sperm maturation in a monotreme mammal—the echidna, *Tachyglossus aculeatus. Am. J. Anat.,* 156:207–230.
26. Temple-Smith, P. D., and Bedford, J. M. (1980): Sperm maturation and the formation of sperm pairs in the epididymis of the opossum, *Didelphis virginiana. J. Exp. Zool.,* 214:161–171.
27. Henderson, N. E. (1962): The annual cycle in the testis of the eastern brook trout, *Salvelinus fontinalis mitchill. Can. J. Zool.,* 40:631–641.
28. Bailey, R. E. (1953): Accessory reproductive organs of male fringillid birds: Seasonal variations and response to various sex hormones. *Anat. Rec.,* 115:1–20.
29. Middleton, A. L. A. (1974): Spermiation and sperm transport in passerine birds. *J. Reprod. Fertil.,* 40:31–37.
30. Budras, K. D., and Meier, U. (1981): The epididymis and its development in ratite birds (Ostrich, Emu, Rhea). *Anat. Embryol. (Berl.),* 162:281–299.
31. Fox, W. (1952): Seasonal variation in the male reproductive system of Pacific coast garter snakes. *J. Morphol.,* 90:481–542.
32. Gigon, A., and Dufaure, J.-P. (1975): Mise en évidence par incorporation de leucine radioactive d'une élaboration protéique dans l'épididyme de Lézard. Etude au cours du cycle sexuel et après injection de testostérone chez l'animal entier et castré. *C. R. Seances Acad. Sci.* [III],280:2241–2244.
33. Gigon-Despeiges, A., and Dufaure, J.-P. (1977): Secretory activity of the lizard epididymis and its control by testosterone. *Gen. Comp. Endocrinol.,* 33:473–479.
34. Imperato-McGimley, J., Peterson, R. E., Gautier, T., and Sturla, E. (1979): Male pseudohermaphroditism secondary to 5α-reductase deficiency—A model for the role of androgens in both the development of the male phenotype and the evolution of a male gender identity. *J. Steroid Biochem.,* 11:637–645.
35. Wilson, J. D., George, F. W., and Griffin, J. E. (1981): The hormonal control of sexual development. *Science,* 211:1278–1284.
36. Crabo, B., and Gustafsson, B. (1964): Distribution of sodium and potassium and its relation to sperm concentration in the epididymal plasma of the bull. *J. Reprod. Fertil.,* 7:337–345.
37. Jenkins, A. D., Lechene, C. P., and Howards, S. S. (1980): Concentrations of seven elements in the intraluminal fluids of the rat seminiferous tubules, rete testis, and epididymis. *Biol. Reprod.,* 23:981–987.
38. Walters, M. R., Hunziker, W., and Norman, A. W. (1982): 1,25-dihydroxyvitamin D_3 receptors: Exchange assay and presence in reproductive tissues. In: *Vitamin D, Chemical, Biochemical and Clinical Endocrinology of Calcium Metabolism,* edited by A. W. Norman, K. Schaefer, D. V. Herrath, and H. G. Grigoleit, pp. 91–93. Walter de Gruyter, Berlin.
39. Kidroni, G., Harnir, T., Menczel, J., Frutkoff, I. W., Palti, Z., and Ron, M. (1983): Vitamin D_3 metabolites in rat epididymis: High 24,25-dihydroxy vitamin D_3 levels in the cauda region. *Biochem. Biophys. Res. Commun.,* 113:982–989.
40. Orgebin-Crist, M.-C., and Djiane, J. (1979): Properties of a prolactin receptor from the rabbit epididymis. *Biol. Reprod.,* 21:135–139.
41. Cramer, D. V., and Gill, T. J., III. (1975): Genetics of urogenital abnormalities in ACI inbred rats. *Teratology,* 12:27–32.
42. Marshall, F. F., Garcia-Bunuel, R., and Beisel, D. S. (1978): Hydronephrosis, renal agenesis, and associated genitourinary anomalies in ACI rats. *Urology,* 11:58–61.
43. Marshall, F. F., Reiner, W. G., and Goldberg, B. S. (1979): The embryologic origin of the caput epididymidis in the rat. *Invest. Urol.,* 17:78–82.
44. Flickinger, C. J. (1969): The fine structure of the Wolffian duct and cytodifferentiation of the epididymis in fetal rats. *Z. Zellforsch.,* 96:344–360.
45. Setty, B. S., and Jehan, Q. (1977): Functional maturation of the epididymis in the rat. *J. Reprod. Fertil.,* 49:317–322.
46. Schwartz, M., Hatier, R., and Grignon, G. (1978): Etude de la différentiation foetale et postnatale de l'épididyme de rat. *Biol. Cell.,* 32:2a.
47. Scheer, H., and Robaire, B. (1980): Steroid Δ4-5α-reductase and 3α-hydroxysteroid dehydrogenase in the rat epididymis during development. *Endocrinology,* 107:948–953.
48. Delongeas, J. L., and Gelly, J. L. (1985): Differentiation of the rat epididymis after withdrawal of androgen. *Cell Tissue Res.,* 241:657–662.
49. Reid, B. L. (1959): The structure and function of the epididymis. II. The histogenesis of the rat epididymis. *Aust. J. Zool.,* 7:22–38.
50. Sun, E. L., and Flickinger, C. J. (1979): Development of cell types and of regional differences in the postnatal rat epididymis. *Am. J. Anat.,* 154:27–55.
51. Sun, E.L., and Flickinger, C. J. (1982): Proliferative activity in the rat epididymis during postnatal development. *Anat. Rec.,* 203:273–284.
52. Hansson, V., Ritzen, E. M., French, F. S., and Nayfeh, S. N. (1975): Androgen transport and receptor mechanisms in testis and epididymis. In: *Handbook of Physiology, Sec. 7, Vol. 5,* edited by R. O. Greep and E. B. Astwood, pp. 173–201. American Physiological Society, Washington, D.C.
53. Danzo, B. J., Cooper, T. G., and Orgebin-Crist, M.-C. (1977): Androgen binding protein (ABP) in fluids collected from rete testis and cauda epididymidis of sexually mature and immature rabbit and observations on morphological changes in the epididymis following ligations of the ductuli efferentes. *Biol. Reprod.,* 17:64–77.
54. Carreau, S., Drosdowsky, M. A., and Courot, M. (1984): Androgen binding proteins in sheep epididymis: Age-related effects on androgen-binding protein, cytosolic androgen receptor and testosterone

concentrations. Correlations with histological studies. *J. Endocrinol.*, 103:281–286.
55. Becker, R. R., and Iles, D. J. (1985): Developmental pattern of androgen binding protein secretion during the critical period of sexual differentiation. *Arch. Androl.*, 14:107–114.
56. Croisille, Y., Gumpel-Pinot, M., and Gasc, J.-M. (1978): Transformation of the mesonephros into epididymis in the Cock: Fate of collecting and secretory tubule antigens. *Differentiation:* 11:39–49.
57. Nilnophakoon, N. (1978): Histological studies on regional postnatal differentiation of the epididymis in the ram. *Zentralbl. Veterinaermed. (A)*, 7:253–272.
58. Wildeus, S., and Entwistle, K. W. (1983): A quantitative histological study of testicular and epididymal development in bos-indicus cross bulls. *Anim. Reprod. Sci.*, 6:1–10.
59. Danzo, B. J., Orgebin-Crist, M.-C., and Eller, B. C. (1975): Changes in 5α-dihydrotestosterone binding to epididymal cytosol during sexual maturation in rabbits: Correlation with morphological changes in the testis and epididymis. *Mol. Cell. Endocrinol.*, 3:203–220.
60. Zondek, L. H., and Zondek, T. (1980): Normal and abnormal development of the epididymis of the fetus and infant. *Eur. J. Pediatr.*, 134:39–44.
61. Hemeida, N. A., Sack, W. O., and McEntee, K. (1978): Ductuli efferentes in the epididymis of boar, goat, ram, bull, and stallion. *Am. J. Vet. Res.*, 39:1892–1900.
62. Nistal, M., and Paniagua, R. (1984): Development of the male genital tract. In: *Testicular and Epididymal Pathology,* edited by M. Nistal and R. Paniagua, pp. 1–13. Thieme-Stratton, New York.
63. Maneely, R. B. (1959): Epididymal structure and function. A historical and critical review. *Acta Zool.*, 40:1–21.
64. Nicander, L. (1956–1958): On the regional histology and cytochemistry of the ductus epididymis in rabbits. *Acta Morphol. Neerl. Scand.*, 1:99–118.
65. Nicander, L. (1956–1958): Studies on the regional histology and cytochemistry of the ductus epididymis in stallions, rams, and bulls. *Acta Morphol. Neerl. Scand.*, 1:337–362.
66. Reid, B. L., and Cleland, K. W. (1957): The structure and function of the epididymis. I. The histology of the rat epididymis. *Aust. J. Zool.*, 5:223–246.
67. Nicander, L., and Glover, T. D. (1973): Regional histology and fine structure of the epididymal duct in the golden hamster (*Mesocricetus auratus*). *J. Anat.*, 114:347–364.
68. Holstein, A. F. (1969): Morphologische studien am nebenhoden des menschen. In: *Zwanglose Abhandlungen Ausdem Gebiet der Normalen un Pathologischen Anatomie,* edited by W. Bargmann and W. Doerr, p. 20. Georg Thieme Verlag, Stuttgart.
69. Hoffer, A. P., and Karnovsky, M. L. (1981): Studies on zonation in the epididymis of the guinea pig. I. Ultrastructural and biochemical analysis of the zone rich in large lipid droplets (Zone II). *Anat. Rec.*, 201:623–633.
70. Hoffer, A. P., and Greenberg, J. (1978): The structure of the epididymis, efferent ductules and ductus deferens of the guinea pig: A light microscope study. *Anat. Rec.*, 190:659–678.
71. Flickinger, C. J., Howards, S. S., and English, H. F. (1978): Ultrastructural differences in efferent ducts and several regions of the epididymis of the hamster. *Am. J. Anat.*, 152:557–586.
72. Tingari, M. D., and Moniem, K. A. (1979): On the regional histology and histochemistry of the epididymis of the camel (*Camelus dromedarius*). *J. Reprod. Fertil.*, 57:11–20.
73. Orsi, A. M., DeMelo, V. R., Ferreira, A. L., and Campos, V. J. M. (1980): Morphology of the epithelial cells of the epididymal duct of the South American opossum (*Didelphis azarae*). *Anat. Anz.*, 148:7–13.
74. Takano, H. (1980): Qualitative and quantitative histology and histogenesis of the mouse epididymis with special emphasis on the regional difference. *Acta Anat. Nippon,* 55:573–587.
75. Alsum, D. J., and Hunter, A. G. (1978): Regional histology and histochemistry of the ductus epididymis in the Rhesus monkey (*Macaca mulatta*). *Biol. Reprod.*, 19:1063–1069.
76. Jones, R. C., and Brosman, M. F. (1981): Studies of the deferent ducts from the testis of the African elephant, *Loxodonta africana*. I. Structural differentiation. *J. Anat.*, 132:376–386.
77. Vendrely, E. (1981): Histology of the epididymis in the human adult. In: *Epididymis and Fertility: Biology and Pathology,* edited by C. Bollack and A. Clavert, pp. 21–33. Karger, Switzerland.
78. Rogers, J. C. (1982): The testis and its excurrent ducts in American caenolestid and didelphid marsupials. *Am. J. Anat.*, 163:269–282.
79. Orsi, A. M. (1983): Regional histology of the epididymis of the dog. A light microscope study. *Anat. Anz.*, 153:441–445.
80. Abe, K., Takano, H., and Ito, T. (1984): Interruption of the luminal flow in the epididymal duct of the corpus epididymidis in the mouse, with special reference to differentiation of the epididymal epithelium. *Arch. Histol. Jpn.*, 47:137–147.
81. Connell, C. J., and Donjacour, A. M. (1985): A morphological study of the epididymides of control and estradiol-treated prepubertal dogs. *Biol. Reprod.*, 33:951–959.
82. Goyal, H. O. (1985): Morphology of the bovine epididymis. *Am. J. Anat.*, 172:155–172.
83. Hamilton, D. W., and Cooper, T. G. (1978): Gross and histological variations along the length of the rat vas deferens. *Anat. Rec.*, 190:795–810.
84. Kennedy, S. W., and Heidger, P. M. (1979): Fine structural studies of the rat vas deferens. *Anat. Rec.*, 194:159–180.
85. Ramos, A. S., Jr. (1979): Morphologic variations along the length of the monkey vas deferens. *Arch. Androl.*, 3:187–196.
86. Pal, C., and Bharadwaj, M. B. L. (1985): Anatomical studies on the vas deferens of buffalos (*Bubalus bubalis*) at different stages of maturity. I. Non-ampullated part. *Indian Vet. J.*, 62:668–674.
87. Sun, E. L., and Flickinger, C. J. (1980): Morphological characteristics of cells with apical nuclei in the initial segment of the adult rat epididymis. *Anat. Rec.*, 196:285–293.
88. Grignon, G., Hatier, R., and Malaprade, D. (1981): Histogenesis of the epididymis. In: *Epididymis and Fertility: Biology and Pathology,* edited by C. Bollack and A. Clavert, pp. 12–20. Karger, Switzerland.
89. Clermont, Y., and Flannery, J. (1970): Mitotic activity in the epithelium of the epididymis in young and old adult rats. *Biol. Reprod.*, 3:283–292.
90. Martan, J., and Risley, P. L. (1963): Holocrine secretory cells of the rat epididymis. *Anat. Rec.*, 146:173–190.
91. Martan, J., and Allen, J. M. (1964): Morphological and cytochemical properties of the holocrine cells in the epididymis of the mouse. *J. Histochem. Cytochem.*, 12:628–639.
92. Martan, J., Risley, P. L., and Hruban, Z. (1964): Holocrine cells of the human epididymis. *Fertil. Steril.*, 15:180–187.
93. Nagy, F., and Edmonds, R. H. (1975): Cellular proliferation and renewal in the various zones of the hamster epididymis after colchicine administration. *Fertil. Steril.*, 26:460–468.
94. Turner, T. T., Jones, C. E., Howards, S. S., Ewing, L. L., Zegeye, B., and Gunsalus, G. L. (1984): On the androgen microenvironment of maturing spermatozoa. *Endocrinology,* 115:1925–1932.
95. Flickinger, C. J. (1973): Regional variations in endoplasmic reticulum in the vas deferens of normal and vasectomized rats. *Anat. Rec.*, 176:205–224.
96. Hoffer, A. P. (1976): The ultrastructure of the ductus deferens in man. *Biol. Reprod.*, 14:425–443.
97. Prins, G. S., and Zaneveld, L. J. D. (1979): Distribution of spermatozoa in the rabbit vas deferens. *Biol. Reprod.*, 21:181–185.
98. Swedin, G. (1971): Studies on neurotransmission mechanisms in the rat and guinea-pig vas deferens. *Acta Physiol. Scand.*, [Suppl.369]:1–34.
99. Kasuya, Y., and Suzuki, N. (1978): Regional differences in the effects of denervation, cocaine and chronic reserpine administration on the responses of the rat vas deferens to norepinephrine and acetylcholine. *Arch. Int. Pharmacodyn. Ther.*, 236:202–213.
100. MacDonald, A., and McGrath, J. C. (1980): The distribution of adrenoreceptors and other drug receptors between the two ends of the rat vas deferens as revealed by selective agonists and antagonists. *Br. J. Pharmacol.*, 71:445–458.
101. Minneman, K. P., and Abel, P. W. (1984): "Spare" alpha 1-adrenergic receptors and the potency of agonists in rat vas deferens. *Mol. Pharmacol.*, 25:56–63.
102. Sneddon, P., and Burnstock, G. (1984): Inhibition of excitatory junction potentials in guinea pig vas deferens by alpha, beta-methylene-ATP. Further evidence for ATP and noradrenaline as cotransmitters. *Eur. J. Pharmacol.*, 100:85–90.
103. Muller, M. J., and Paton, D. M. (1979): Presynaptic inhibitory actions of 2-substituted adenosine derivatives on neurotransmission in rat vas deferens: Effects of inhibitors of adenosine uptake and deamination. *Naunyn Schmiedebergs Arch. Pharmacol.*, 306:23–28.

104. Sakai, K. K., Hymson, D. L., and Shapiro, R. (1979): The effects of adenosine and adenine nucleotides on the guinea-pig vas deferens: Evidence for existence of purinergic receptors. *Life Sci.*, 24:1299–1308.
105. French, A. M., and Scott, N. C. (1983): Evidence to support the hypothesis that ATP is a co-transmitter in rat vas deferens. *Experientia,* 39:264–266.
106. Ramaswamy, S., Nazimudeen, S. K., and Kameswaran, L. (1979): Effect of naloxone on the sensitivity of the vas deferens to various agonists. *J. Pharm. Pharmacol.*, 31:222–223.
107. Ronai, A. Z., Berzetei, I. P., and Kurgyis, J. (1981): Opioid effects in developing rat vas deferens. *Cell Mol. Neurobiol.*, 1:335–342.
108. Fauchère, J.-L. (1982): A quantitative structure-activity relationship study of the inhibitory action of a series of enkephalin-like peptides in the guinea pig ileum and mouse vas deferens bioassays. *J. Med. Chem.*, 25:1428–1431.
109. Huidobro-Toro, J. P., Caturay, E. M., Ling, N., Lee, N. M., Loh, H. H., and Way, E. L. (1982): Studies on the structural prerequisites for the activation of the β-endorphin receptor on the rat vas deferens. *J. Pharmacol. Exp. Ther.*, 222:262–269.
110. Lundberg, J. M., Hua, X. Y., and Franco-Cereceda, A. (1984): Effects of neuropeptide-Y (NPY) on mechanical-activity and neurotransmission in the heart, vas-deferens and urinary-bladder of the guinea-pig. *Acta Physiol. Scand.*, 121:325–332.
111. Karnovsky, M. J. (1971): Use of ferrocyanide-reduced osmium tetroxide in electron microscopy. *Proceedings: 11th American Society of Cell Biology,* 284:146 (abstract).
112. Ladman, A. J., and Young, W. C. (1958): An electron microscopic study of the ductuli efferentes and rete testis of the guinea pig. *J. Biophys. Biochem. Cytol.*, 4:219–226.
113. Hamilton, D. W., Olson, G. E., and Cooper, T. G. (1977): Regional variation in the surface morphology of the epithelium of the rat ductuli efferentes, ductus epididymidis and vas deferens. *Anat. Rec.*, 188:13–27.
114. Hermo, L., and Morales, C. (1984): Endocytosis in nonciliated epithelial cells of the ductuli efferentes in the rat. *Am. J. Anat.*, 171:59–74.
115. Pudney, J., and Fawcett, D. W. (1984): Seasonal changes in fine structure of the ductuli efferentes of the ground squirrel, *Citellus lateralis (Say)*. *Anat. Rec.*, 208:383–399.
116. Jones, R., Hamilton, D. W., and Fawcett, D. W. (1979): Morphology of the epithelium of the extratesticular rete testis, ductuli efferentes and ductus epididymidis of the adult male rabbit. *Am. J. Anat.*, 156:373–400.
117. Ladman, A. L. (1967): The fine structure of the ductuli efferentes of the opossum. *Anat. Rec.*, 157:559–576.
118. Wrobel, K.-H. (1973): On the morphology of the bovine ductuli efferentes. *Z. Zellforsch.*, 135:129–148.
119. Goyal, H. O., and Hrudka, F. (1980): The resorptive activity in the bull efferent ductules—A morphological and experimental study. *Andrologia,* 12:401–414.
120. Goyal, H. O., and Hrudka, F. (1981): Ductuli efferentes of the bull—A morphological, experimental and developmental study. *Andrologia,* 13:292–306.
121. Ramos, A. S., Jr., and Dym, M. (1977): Ultrastructure of the ductuli efferentes in monkeys. *Biol. Reprod.*, 17:339–349.
122. Morita, I. (1966): Some observations on the fine structure of the human ductuli efferentes testis. *Arch. Histol. Jpn.*, 26:341–365.
123. Goto, K. (1981): Surface morphology of the epithelium of human seminiferous tubules, rete testis, ductuli efferentes and ductus epididymidis. *Biochem. Res.*, [Suppl. 2]:361–374.
124. Burgos, M. H., Montes de Oca, H., and Montorzi, N. M. (1959): La incorporation de Fe_{59} en los conductos eferentes del hamster. *Rev. Soc. Argent. Biol.*, 35:26–39.
125. Montorzi, N. M., and Burgos, M. H. (1967): Uptake of colloidal particles by cells of the ductuli efferentes of the hamster. *Z. Zellforsch.*, 83:58–69.
126. Yokoyama, M., and Chang, J. F. (1971): An ultracytochemical and ultrastructural study of epithelial cells in ductuli efferentes of chinese hamster. *J. Histochem. Cytochem.*, 19:766–774.
127. Morales, C., and Hermo, L. (1983): Demonstration of fluid-phase endocytosis in epithelial cells of the male reproductive system by means of horseradish peroxidase-colloidal gold complex. *Cell Tissue Res.*, 230:503–510.
128. De Bruyn, P. P. H., Cho, Y., and Michelson, S. (1983): *In vivo* endocytosis by bristle coated pits of protein tracers and their intracellular transport in the endothelial cells lining the sinuses of the liver. I. The endosomal disposition. *J. Ultrastruct. Res.*, 85:272–289.
129. Gonnella, P. A., and Neutra, M. R. (1984): Membrane-bound and fluid-phase macromolecules enter separate prelysosomal compartments in absorptive cells of suckling rat ileum. *J. Cell Biol.*, 99:909–917.
130. Neiss, W. F. (1984): Invaginated apical vacuoles in the cells of the proximal convoluted tubule in the rat kidney. *Cell Tissue Res.*, 235:463–466.
131. Wilson, J. M., and King, B. F. (1985): Transport of horseradish peroxidase across monkey trophoblastic epithelium in coated and uncoated vesicles. *Anat. Rec.*, 211:174–183.
132. Hermo, L., De Melo, V., Harris, P. G., and Clermont, Y. (1986): The endocytic apparatus of non-ciliated epithelial cells of the ductuli efferentes of the rat. *Anat. Rec.*, 214:53A.
133. Helenius, A., Mellman, I., Wall, D., and Hubbard, A. (1983): Endosomes. *Trends Biochem. Sci.*, 8:245–250.
134. Gray, B. W., Brown, B. G., Ganjam, V. K., and Whitesides, J. F. (1983): Effect of deprival of rete testis fluid on the morphology of efferent ductules. *Biol. Reprod.*, 29:525–534.
135. Hermo, L., Clermont, Y., and Morales, C. (1985): Fluid-phase and adsorptive endocytosis in ciliated epithelial cells of the rat ductuli efferentes. *Anat. Rec.*, 211:285–294.
136. Hoffer, A. P., Hamilton, D. W., and Fawcett, D. W. (1973): The ultrastructure of principal cells and intraepithelial leucocytes in the initial segment of the rat epididymis. *Anat. Rec.*, 175:169–202.
137. Nicander, L., and Malmquist, M. (1977): Ultrastructural observations suggesting merocrine secretion in the initial segment of the mammalian epididymis. *Cell Tissue Res.*, 184:487–490.
138. Fawcett, D. W., and Hoffer, A. P. (1979): Failure of exogenous androgen to prevent regression of the initial segments of the rat epididymis after efferent duct ligation or orchidectomy. *Biol. Reprod.*, 20:162–181.
139. Zunke, V. U., and Gossrau, R. (1981): Morphology and zonal division of the ductus epididymidis of rats. *Anat. Anz.*, 149:409–424.
140. Djakiew, D., and Jones, R. C. (1982): Ultrastructure of the ductus epididymidis of the echidna, Tachyglossus aculeatus. *J. Anat.*, 135:625–634.
141. Soranzo, L., Dadoune, J.-P., and Fain-Maurel, M.-A. (1982): Segmentation of the epididymal duct in mouse: an ultrastructural study. *Reprod. Nutr. Dev.*, 22:999–1012.
142. Abe, K., Takano, H., and Ito, T. (1983): Ultrastructure of the mouse epididymal duct with special reference to the regional differences of the principal cells. *Arch. Histol. Jpn.*, 46:51–68.
143. Greenberg, J., and Forssmann, W.-G. (1983): Studies of the guinea pig epididymis. I. Ultrastructure and quantitative morphology of the principal cells. *Anat. Embryol. (Berl.)*, 168:173–194.
144. Jones, R. C., Hinds, L. A., and Tyndale-Biscoe, C. H. (1984): Ultrastructure of the epididymis of the tammar, Macropus eugenii, and its relationship to sperm maturation. *Cell Tissue Res.*, 237:525–535.
145. Flickinger, C. J. (1979): Synthesis, transport and secretion of protein in the initial segment of the mouse epididymis as studied by electron microscope radioautography. *Biol. Reprod.*, 20:1015–1030.
146. Hermo, L., Rambourg, A., and Clermont, Y. (1980): Three-dimensional architecture of the cortical region of the Golgi apparatus in rat spermatids. *Am. J. Anat.*, 157:357–373.
147. Rambourg, A., Segretain, D., and Clermont Y. (1984): Tridimensional architecture of the Golgi apparatus in the atrial muscle cell of the rat. *Am. J. Anat.*, 170:163–179.
148. Rambourg, A., and Clermont, Y. (1986): Tridimensional structure of the Golgi apparatus in type A ganglion cells of the rat. *Am. J. Anat.*, 176:393–409.
149. Hand, A. R., and Oliver, C. (1977): Relationship between the Golgi apparatus, GERL, and secretory granules in acinar cells of the rat exorbital lacrimal gland. *J. Cell Biol.*, 74:399–413.
150. Abou-Haila, A., and Fain-Maurel, M.-A. (1984): Regional differences of the proximal part of mouse epididymis: Morphological and histochemical characterization. *Anat. Rec.*, 209:197–208.
151. Flickinger, C. J. (1969): Fenestrated cisternae in the Golgi apparatus of the epididymis. *Anat. Rec.*, 163:39–54.

152. Friend, D. S. (1969): Cytochemical staining of multivesicular bodies and Golgi vesicles. *J. Cell Biol.*, 41:269–279.
153. Moore, H. D. M., and Bedford, J. M. (1979): Short-term effects of androgen withdrawal on the structure of different epithelial cells in the rat epididymis. *Anat. Rec.*, 193:293–312.
154. Moore, H. D. M., and Bedford, J. M. (1979): The differential absorptive activity of epithelial cells of the rat epididymis before and after castration. *Anat. Rec.*, 193:313–328.
155. Paulson, H. L., Byers, S. W., and Dym, M. (1985): Morphometric analysis of coated pits and vesicles in the proximal and distal caput epididymidis. *Biol. Reprod.*, 32:191–201.
156. Hamilton, D. W., Jones, A. L., and Fawcett, D. W. (1969): Cholesterol biosynthesis in the mouse epididymis and ductus deferens: A biochemical and morphological study. *Biol. Reprod.*, 1:167–184.
157. Glover, T. D., and Nicander, L. (1971): Some aspects of structure and function in the mammalian epididymis. *J. Reprod. Fertil.*, [Suppl.13]:39–50.
158. Vitale-Calpe, R., and Aoki, A. (1970): The hamster cauda epididymidis after coitus. *Acta Anat.* (*Basel*), 77:98–108.
159. Nagy, F., Pendergrass, P. B., and Scott, J. N. (1982): Structural features of a specialized region of the epididymis of the siberian hamster (*Phodopus-sungurus*). *J. Submicrosc. Cytol.*, 14:673–682.
160. Nicander, L., and Ploen, L. (1979): Studies on regional fine structure and function in the rabbit epididymis. *Int. J. Androl.*, 2:463–481.
161. Thomas, D., Gouranton, J., and Boujard, D. (1981): Nuclear inclusions in the epithelial cells of the caput epididymidis of the dog; Ultrastructure, nature and relations with androgens. *Biol. Cell*, 42:87–96.
162. Hess, R. A., and Thurston, R. J. (1977): Ultrastructure of the epithelial cells in the epididymal region of the turkey (*Meleagris gallopavo*). *J. Anat.*, 124:765–778.
163. De Melo, V. R., Orsi, A. M., Dias, S. M., and Oliveira, M. C. (1982): Fine-structure of principal and basal cells of the cauda epididymidis of the South American opossum (*Didelphis azarae*). *Anat. Anz.*, 151:497–502.
164. Suzuki, F., and Racey, P. A. (1976): Fine structural changes in the epididymal epithelium of moles (T. europaea) throughout the year. *J. Reprod. Fertil.*, 47:47–54.
165. Goyal, H. O., and Dhingra, L. D. (1975): The postnatal histology of the epididymis in buffalo (*Bubalus bubalis*). *Acta Anat.* (*Basel*), 91:573–582.
166. Edmonds, R. H., and Nagy, F. (1973): Some fine structural features of epididymal cells in an endentate, *Dasypus novemcinctus mexicanus*. *J. Reprod. Fertil.*, 32:105–107.
167. Edmonds, R. H., and Nagy, F. (1974): Fine structure of edentate (*Dasypus novemcinctus*) male reproductive system: The epididymis. *J. Anat.*, 118:337–351.
168. Ramos, A. S., and Dym, M. (1977): Fine structure of the monkey epididymis. *Am. J. Anat.*, 149:501–532.
169. Cavicchia, J. C. (1979): Fine structure of the monkey epididymis: A correlated thin-section and freeze-cleave study. *Cell Tissue Res.*, 201:451–458.
170. Ramos, A. S., Jr. (1980): Ultrastructural and histochemical observations on the principal cells of monkey epididymis. *Arch. Androl.*, 5:159–168.
171. Sawatzke, C. L., and Heidger, P. M. (1977): Ultrastructure of crystalloid inclusions in dog and rat epididymis. *Tissue Cell*, 9:733–744.
172. Hermo, L., and De Melo, V. (1987): The endocytic apparatus and transcytosis in epithelial cells of the vas deferens in the rat. *Anat. Rec.*, 217:153–163.
173. Popovic, N. A., McLeod, D. G., and Borski, A. A. (1973): Ultrastructure of the human vas deferens. *Invest. Urol.*, 10:266–277.
174. Orlandini, G. E. (1974): The fine structure of the vas deferens epithelium of man. *Verh. Anat. Ges.*, 68:213–218.
175. Paniagua, R., Regadera, J., Nistal, M., and Abaurrea, A. M. (1981): Histological, histochemical and ultrastructural variations along the length of the human vas deferens before and after puberty. *Acta Anat.* (*Basel*), 111:190–203.
176. Niemi, M. (1965): The fine structure and histochemistry of the epithelial cells of the rat vas deferens. *Acta Anat.* (*Basel*), 60:207–219.
177. Friend, D. S., and Farquhar, M. G. (1967): Functions of coated vesicles during protein absorption in the rat vas deferens. *J. Cell Biol.*, 35:357–376.
178. Clermont, Y., and Hermo, L. (1985): Ultrastructure of the lamina propria of the vas deferens in the rat. *Anat. Rec.*, 211:42A.
179. Cooper, T. G., and Hamilton, D. W. (1977): Phagocytosis of spermatozoa in the terminal region and gland of the vas deferens of the rat. *Am. J. Anat.*, 150:247–268.
180. Brown, D., and Montesano, R. (1980): Membrane specialization in the rat epididymis. I. Rod-shaped intramembrane particle in the apical (mitochondria-rich) cell. *J. Cell Sci.*, 45:187–198.
181. Hermo, L., Clermont, Y., and Lalli, M. (1985): Intracellular pathways of endocytosed tracers in Leydig cells of the rat. *J. Androl.*, 6:213–224.
182. Flickinger, C. J. (1972): Alterations in the fine structure of the rat epididymis after vasectomy. *Anat. Rec.*, 173:277–300.
183. Brown, D., and Montesano, R. (1981): Membrane specialization in the rat epididymis. II. The clear cell. *Anat. Rec.*, 201:477–483.
184. Hermo, L., and Clermont, Y. (1985): The role of the clear epithelial cells of the epididymis of the rat in the disposal of cytoplasmic droplets derived from spermatozoa. *J. Cell Biol.*, 101:420A.
185. Dym, M., and Romrell, L. J. (1975): Intraepithelial lymphocytes in the male reproductive tract of rats and rhesus monkeys. *J. Reprod. Fertil.*, 42:1–7.
186. Hermo, L., and Clermont, Y. (1976): Light cells within the limiting membrane of rat seminiferous tubules. *Am. J. Anat.*, 145:467–484.
187. Hermo, L., and Lalli, M. (1978): Monocytes and mast cells in the limiting membrane of human seminiferous tubules. *Biol. Reprod.*, 19:92–100.
188. Hermo, L., and Clermont, Y. (1981): Turnover of monocytoid cells within the limiting membrane of rat seminiferous tubules. *J. Androl.*, 2:321–325.
189. Van Furth, R. (1970): Origin and turnover of promonocytes, monocytes and macrophages in normal mice. In: *Mononuclear Phagocytes*, edited by R. Van Furth, pp. 151–165. Blackwell, Oxford.
190. Alexander, N. J. (1972): Vasectomy: Long-term effects in the rhesus monkey. *J. Reprod. Fertil.*, 31:399–406.
191. Phadke, A. M. (1975): Spermiophage cells in man. *Fertil. Steril.*, 26:760–774.
192. Goyal, H. O. (1982): Light microscopic and ultrastructural evidence of epithelial phagocytosis of sperm in the rete testis and ductuli efferentes in the bull. *Am. J. Vet. Res.*, 43:785–790.
193. Holstein, C. (1983): Morphology of free immature germ cells in human testis, epididymis, and ejaculate. *Andrologia*, 15:7–25.
194. Wang, Y. F., and Holstein, A. F. (1983): Intraepithelial lymphocytes and macrophages in the human epididymis. *Cell Tissue Res.*, 233:517–521.
195. Setchell, B. P., and Waites, G. M. H. (1975): The blood-testis barrier. In: *Handbook of Physiology, Sec. 7, Vol. 5*, edited by R. O. Greep and E. B. Astwood, pp. 143–172. American Physiological Society, Washington, D.C.
196. Howards, S. S., Jessee, S. J., and Johnson, A. L. (1976): Micropuncture studies of the blood-seminiferous tubule barrier. *Biol. Reprod.*, 14:264–269.
197. Friend, D. S., and Gilula, N. B. (1972): Variations in tight and gap junctions in mammalian tissues. *J. Cell Biol.*, 53:758–776.
198. Suzuki, F., and Nagano, T. (1978): Regional differentiation of cell junctions in the excurrent duct epithelium of the rat testis as revealed by freeze-fracture. *Anat. Rec.*, 191:503–520.
199. Greenberg, J., and Forssmann, W.-G. (1983): Studies of the guinea pig epididymis. II. Intercellular junctions of principal cells. *Anat. Embryol.*, 168:195–209.
200. Hoffer, A.P., and Hinton, B. T. (1984): Morphological evidence for a blood-epididymis barrier and the effects of gossypol on its integrity. *Biol. Reprod.*, 30:991–1004.
201. Nagano, T., and Suzuki, F. (1980): Belt-like gap junctions in the ductuli efferentes of some mammalian testes. *Arch. Histol. Jpn.*, 43:185–189.
202. Farquhar, M. G., and Palade, G. E. (1963): Junctional complexes in various epithelia. *J. Cell Biol.*, 17:374–412.
203. Johnson, A. L., and Howards, S. S. (1976): Intratubular hydrostatic pressure in testis and epididymis before and after long-term vasectomy in the guinea pig. *Biol. Reprod.*, 14:371–376.
204. Johnson, A. L., and Howards, S. S. (1977): Hyperosmolality in intraluminal fluids from hamster testis and epididymis: A micropuncture study. *Science*, 195:492–493.

205. Turner, T. T., Hartmann, P. K., and Howards, S. S. (1977): *In vivo* sodium, potassium, and sperm concentrations in the rat epididymis. *Fertil. Steril.,* 28:191–194.
206. Hinton, B. T., and Setchell, B. P. (1981): Micropuncture and microanalytical studies of rhesus monkeys and baboon epididymis and the human ductus deferens. *Am. J. Primatol.,* 1:251–256.
207. Hinton, B. T., and Howards, S. S. (1981): Permeability characteristics of the epithelium in the rat caput epididymis. *J. Reprod. Fertil.,* 63:95–99.
208. Turner, T. T., Cochran, R. C., and Howards, S. S. (1981): Transfer of steroids across the hamster blood testis and blood epididymal barriers. *Biol. Reprod.,* 25:342–348.
209. Hinton, B. T., and Howards, S. S. (1982): Rat testis and epididymis can transport [^{3}H] 3-*O*-Methyl-D-glucose, [^{3}H] inositol and [^{3}H] α-aminoisobutyric acid across its epithelia *in vivo. Biol. Reprod.,* 27:1181–1189.
210. Hinton, B. T. (1983): The epithelium of the caput epididymidis: Its permeability and its role in the formation of a specialized microenvironment. *Ann. NY Acad. Sci.,* 383:462–463.
211. Turner, T. T., D'Addario, D. A., and Howards, S. S. (1983): The transepithelial movement of ^{3}H-3-*O*-methyl-D-glucose in the hamster seminiferous and cauda epididymidal tubules. *Fertil. Steril.,* 40:530–535.
212. Turner, T. T. (1984): Resorption versus secretion in the rat epididymis. *J. Reprod. Fertil.,* 72:509–514.
213. Hinton, B. T. (1985): Physiological aspects of the blood-epididymis barrier. In: *Male Fertility and its Regulation,* edited by T. J. Lobl and E. S. E. Hafez, pp. 371–382. MTP Press, New York.
214. Turner, T. T., and Howards, S. S. (1985): The tenacity of the blood-testis and blood-epididymal barriers. In: *Male Fertility and its Regulation,* edited by T. J. Lobl and E. S. E. Hafez, pp. 383–393. MTP Press, New York.
215. Turner, T. T., Ewing, L. L., Jones, C. E., Howards, S. S., and Zebeye, B. (1985): Androgens in male rat reproductive tract fluids: hypophysectomy and steroid replacement. *Am. J. Physiol.,* 248:E274–E280.
216. Turner, T. T., Ewing, L. L., Jones, C. E., Howards, S. S., and Zegeye, B. (1985): Androgens in various fluid compartments of the rat testis and epididymis after hypophysectomy and gonadotropin supplementation. *J. Androl.,* 6:353–358.
217. Turner, T. T., Giles, R. D., and Howards, S. S. (1981): Effect of oestradiol valerate on the rat blood-testis and blood-epididymal barriers to [^{3}H] inulin. *J. Reprod. Fertil.,* 63:355–358.
218. Levine, N., and Marsh, D. J. (1971): Micropuncture studies of the electrochemical aspects of fluid and electrolyte transport in individual seminiferous tubules, the epididymis and vas deferens in rats. *J. Physiol.,* 213:557–570.
219. Crabo, B. (1965): Studies on the composition of epididymal content in bulls and boars. *Acta Vet. Scand.,* 6 [Suppl.5]:1–94.
220. Voglmayr, J. K., Waites, G. M. H., and Setchell, B. P. (1966): Studies on spermatozoa and fluid collected directly from the testis of the conscious ram. *Nature,* 210:861–863.
221. Voglmayr, J. K., Scott, T. W., Setchell, B. P., and Waites, G. M. H. (1967): Metabolism of testicular spermatozoa and characteristics of testicular fluid collected from conscious rams. *J. Reprod. Fertil.,* 14:87–99.
222. Waites, G. M. H., and Setchell, B. P. (1969): Physiology of the testis, epididymis and scrotum. In: *Advances in Reproductive Physiology,* edited by A. McLaren, pp. 1–63. Logos Press, London.
223. Wong, P. Y. D., Au, C. L., and Ngai, H. K. (1978): Electrolyte and water transport in rat epididymis; Its possible role in sperm maturation. *Int. J. Androl.,* [Suppl.2]:608–628.
224. Wong, P. Y. D., and Yeung, C. H. (1977): Hormonal regulation of fluid reabsorption in isolated rat cauda epididymis. *Endocrinology,* 101:1391–1397.
225. Wong, P. Y. D., and Yeung, C. H. (1978): Absorptive and secretory functions of the perfused rat cauda epididymidis. *J. Physiol.,* 275:13–26.
226. Cheung, Y. M., Hwang, J. C., and Wong, P. Y. D. (1978): Membrane potentials of epithelial cells in the epididymis of rats. Ionic and castration effects. *Comp. Biochem. Physiol.* [*A*], 59:403–407.
227. Hinton, B. T., and Hernandez, H. (1985): Selective luminal absorption of L-carnitine from the proximal regions of the rat epididymis. Possible relationships to development of sperm motility. *J. Androl.,* 6:300–305.
228. Goldstein, J. L., Anderson, R. G. W., and Brown, M. S. (1979): Coated pits, coated vesicles and receptor mediated endocytosis. *Nature,* 279:679–685.
229. Steinman, R. M., Mellman, I. S., Muller, W. A., and Cohn, Z. A. (1983): Endocytosis and recycling of plasma membrane. *J. Cell Biol.,* 96:1–27.
230. Dacheux, J. L., and Voglmayr, J. K. (1983): Sequence of sperm cell surface differentiation and its relationship to exogenous fluid proteins in the ram epididymis. *Biol. Reprod.,* 29:1033–1046.
231. Pelliniemi, L. J., Dym, M., Gunsalus, G. L., Musto, N. A., Bardin, C. W., and Fawcett, D. W. (1981): Immunocytochemical localization of androgen-binding protein in the male rat reproductive tract. *Endocrinology,* 108:925–931.
232. Attramadal, A., Bardin, C. W., Gunsalus, G. L., Musto, N. A., and Hansson, V. (1981): Immunocytochemical localization of androgen-binding protein in rat Sertoli and epididymal cells. *Biol. Reprod.,* 25:983–988.
233. Djakiew, D., Byers, S. W., and Dym, M. (1984): Receptor-mediated endocytosis of alpha-2-macroglobulin and transferrin in rat caput epididymal epithelial cells *in vitro. Biol. Reprod.,* 31:1073–1085.
234. Djakiew, D., Byers, S. W., Lewis, D. M., and Dym, M. (1985): Receptor-mediated endocytosis of alpha-2-macroglobulin by principal cells in the proximal caput epididymidis *in vivo. J. Androl.,* 6:190–196.
235. Djakiew, D., Griswold, M. D., Lewis, D. M., and Dym, M. (1986): Micropuncture studies of receptor-mediated endocytosis of transferrin in the rat epididymis. *Biol. Reprod.,* 34:691–699.
236. Morales, C., and Hermo, L. (1986): Intracellular pathways of endocytosed transferrin and non-specific tracers in epithelial cells lining the rete testis of the rat. *Cell Tissue Res.,* 245:323–330.
237. Morales, C., Hermo, L., and Clermont, Y. (1984): Endocytosis in epithelial cells lining the rete testis of the rat. *Anat. Rec.,* 209:185–195.
238. Herzog, V. (1983): Transcytosis in thyroid follicle cells. *J. Cell Biol.,* 97:607–617.
239. Simionescu, M., and Simionescu, N. (1984): Ultrastructure of the microvascular wall: Functional correlation. In: *Handbook of Physiology, Sec. 2, Vol. 4,* edited by E. M. Renkin and C. C. Michel, pp. 41–101. American Physiological Society, Washington, D.C.
240. Marquis, N. R., and Fritz, I. B. (1965): Effects of testosterone on the distribution of carnitine, acetylcarnitine, and carnitine acetyltransferase in tissues of the reproductive system of the male rat. *J. Biol. Chem.,* 240:2197–2200.
241. Brooks, D. E., Hamilton, D. W., and Mallek, A. H. (1973): The uptake of L-[methyl-^{3}H]carnitine by the rat epididymis. *Biochem. Biophys. Res. Commun.,* 52:1354–1360.
242. Casillas, E. R., and Erickson, B. J. (1975): Studies on carnitine synthesis in the rat epididymis. *J. Reprod. Fertil.,* 44:287–291.
243. Hinton, B. T., and Setchell, B. P. (1980): Concentration and uptake of carnitine in the rat epididymis: A micropuncture study. In: *Carnitine Biosynthesis, Metabolism, and Functions,* edited by R. A. Frankel and J. D. McGarry, pp. 237–249. Academic Press, New York.
244. Brooks, D. E. (1980): Carnitine in the male reproductive tract and its relation to the metabolism of the epididymis and spermatozoa. In: *Carnitine Biosynthesis, Metabolism, and Functions,* edited by R. A. Frankel and J. D. McGarry, pp. 219–235. Academic Press, New York.
245. Yeung, C. H., Cooper, T. G., and Waites, G. M. H. (1980): Carnitine transport into the perfused epididymis of the rat: regional differences, stereospecificity, stimulation by choline, and the effect of other luminal factors. *Biol. Reprod.,* 23:294–304.
246. Tuck, R. R., Setchell, B. P., Waites, G. M. H., and Young, J. A. (1970): The composition of fluid collected by micropuncture and catheterization from the seminiferous tubules and rete testis of rats. *Pfluegers Arch.,* 318:225–243.
247. Robinson, R., and Fritz, I. B. (1979): Myoinositol biosynthesis by Sertoli cells, and levels of myoinositol biosynthetic enzymes in testis and epididymis. *Can. J. Biochem.,* 57:962–967.
248. Cooper, T. G. (1982): Secretion of inositol and glucose by the perfused rat cauda epididymidis. *J. Reprod. Fertil.,* 64:373–379.

249. Lewin, L. M., Yannai, Y., Sulimovici, S., and Kraicer, P. F. (1976): Studies on the metabolic role of myo-inositol. Distribution of radioactive myo-inositol in the male rat. *Biochem. J.*, 156:375–380.
250. Bjerve, K. S., and Reitan, L. J. (1978): The presence of an androgen controlled phospholipase A in rat epididymis: Its possible function in the synthesis of sn-3-glycerophosphorylcholine and the supply of fatty acids to spermatozoa. *Int. J. Androl.*, [Suppl.2]:574–591.
251. Scott, T. W., Wales, R. G., Wallace, J. C., and White, I. G. (1963): Composition of ram epididymal and testicular fluid and the biosynthesis of glycerylphosphorylcholine by the rabbit epididymis. *J. Reprod. Fertil.*, 6:49–59.
252. Hinton, B. T., and Setchell, B. P. (1980): Concentrations of glycerophosphocholine, phosphocholine and free inorganic phosphate in the luminal fluid of the rat testis and epididymis. *J. Reprod. Fertil.*, 58:401–406.
253. Hammerstedt, R. H., and Rowan, W. A. (1979): Phosphatidylcholine of blood lipoprotein is the precursor of glycerophosphorylcholine found in seminal plasma. *Biochim. Biophys. Acta*, 710:370–376.
254. Barker, L. D. S., and Amann, R. P. (1971): Epididymal physiology. II. Immunofluorescent analyses of epithelial secretion and absorption, and of bovine sperm maturation. *J. Reprod. Fertil.*, 26:319–332.
255. Amann, R. P., Killian, G. J., and Benton, A. W. (1973): Differences in the electrophoretic characteristics of bovine rete testis fluid and plasma from the cauda epididymidis. *J. Reprod. Fertil.*, 35:321–330.
256. Jones, R. (1974): Absorption and secretion in the cauda epididymidis of the rabbit and the effects of degenerating spermatozoa on epididymal plasma after castration. *J. Endocrinol.*, 63:157–165.
257. Huang, H. F. S., and Johnson, A. D. (1975): Comparative study of protein pattern of epididymal plasma of mouse, rat, rabbit and sheep. *Comp. Biochem. Physiol. [B]*, 51:337–341.
258. Koskimies, A. I., and Kormano, M. (1975): Proteins in fluids from different segments of the rat epididymis. *J. Reprod. Fertil.*, 43:345–348.
259. Cameo, M. S., and Blaquier, J. A. (1976): Androgen-controlled specific proteins in rat epididymis. *J. Endocrinol.*, 69:47–55.
260. Neutra, M., and Leblond, C. P. (1966): Radioautographic comparison of the uptake of galactose-H3 and glucose-H3 in the Golgi region of various cells secreting glycoproteins or mucopolysaccharides. *J. Cell Biol.*, 30:137–150.
261. Kopecny, V., and Peck, V. (1977): An autoradiographic study of macromolecular synthesis in epithelium of ductus epididymidis in mouse. II. Incorporation of L-fucose-1-^{3}H. *Histochemistry*, 50:229–238.
262. Flickinger, C. J. (1983): Synthesis and secretion of glycoprotein by the epididymal epithelium. *J. Androl.*, 4:157–161.
263. Flickinger, C. J. (1985): Autoradiographic analysis of the secretory pathway for glycoproteins in principal cells of the mouse epididymis exposed to ^{3}H fucose. *Biol. Reprod.*, 32:377–389.
264. Bennet, G., Leblond, C. P., and Haddad, A. (1974): Migration of glycoprotein from the Golgi apparatus to the surface of various cell types as shown by radioautography after labelled fucose injection into rats. *J. Cell Biol.*, 60:258–284.
265. Vendrely, C., and Durliat, M. (1968): Etude autoradiographique de l'influence de l'hormone mâle sur l'incorporation de leucine dans le tractus génital de la souris blanche. *Arch. Anat.*, 51:735–740.
266. Kopecny, V. (1971): Epididymal luminal contents labelling after ^{14}C- or ^{3}H-lysine administration in the mouse. *Acta Histochem. (Jena)*, 40:116–122.
267. Kanka, J., and Kopecny, V. (1977): An autoradiographic study of macromolecular synthesis in the epithelium of the ductus epididymidis in the mouse. I. DNA, RNA, and protein. *Biol. Reprod.*, 6:421–427.
268. Flickinger, C. J. (1981): Regional differences in synthesis, intracellular transport, and secretion of protein in the mouse epididymis. *Biol. Reprod.*, 25:871–883.
269. Flickinger, C. J., Wilson, K. M., and Gray, H. D. (1984): The secretory pathway in the mouse epididymis as shown by electron microscope radioautography of principal cells exposed to monensin. *Anat. Rec.*, 210:435–448.
270. Nicander, L. (1979): Fine structure of principal cells in the initial segment of the epididymal duct in the ram. *Anat. Histol. Embryol.*, 8:318–330.
271. Lea, O. A., Petrusz, P., and French, F. S. (1978): Purification and localization of acidic epididymal glycoprotein (AEG): A sperm coating protein secreted by the rat epididymis. *Int. J. Androl.*, [Suppl.2]:592–607.
272. Acott, T. S., and Hoskins, D. D. (1978): Bovine sperm forward motility protein. Partial purification and characterization. *J. Biol. Chem.*, 253:6744–6750.
273. Brandt, H., Acott, T. S., Johnson, D. J., and Hoskins, D. D. (1978): Evidence for epididymal origin of bovine sperm forward motility protein. *Biol. Reprod.*, 19:830–835.
274. Brooks, D. E., and Higgins, S. J. (1980): Characterization and androgen-dependence of proteins associated with luminal fluid and spermatozoa in the rat epididymis. *J. Reprod. Fertil.*, 59:363–375.
275. Jones, R., Brown, C. R., Von Glos, K. I., and Parker, M. G. (1980): Hormonal regulation of protein synthesis in the rat epididymis. Characterization of androgen-dependent and testicular fluid-dependent proteins. *Biochem. J.*, 188:667–676.
276. Garberi, J. C., Kohane, A. C., Cameo, M. S., and Blaquier, J. A. (1979): Isolation and characterization of specific rat epididymal proteins. *Mol. Cell. Endocrinol.*, 13:73–82.
277. Wong, P. Y. D., Tsang, A. Y. F., and Lee, W. M. (1981): Origin of the luminal fluid proteins of the rat epididymis. *Int. J. Androl.*, 4:331–341.
278. Olson, G. E., and Hamilton, D. W. (1978): Characterization of the surface glycoproteins of rat spermatozoa. *Biol. Reprod.*, 19:26–35.
279. Olson, G. E., and Orgebin-Crist, M.-C. (1982): Sperm surface changes during epididymal maturation. *Ann. NY Acad. Sci.*, 383:372–391.
280. Brooks, D. E. (1983): Effect of androgens on protein synthesis and secretion in various regions of the rat epididymis as analysed by two-dimensional gel electrophoresis. *Mol. Cell. Endocrinol.*, 29:255–270
281. Sylvester, S. R., Skinner, M. K., and Griswold, M. D. (1984): A sulfated glycoprotein synthesized by Sertoli cells and by epididymal cells is a component of the sperm membrane. *Biol. Reprod.*, 31:1087–1101.
282. Hamilton, D. W. (1981): Evidence for α-lactalbumin-like activity in reproductive tract fluids of the male rat. *Biol. Reprod.*, 25:385–392.
283. Qasba, P. K., Hewlett, I. K., and Byers, S. (1983): The presence of the milk protein, alpha-lactalbumin and its mRNA in the rat epididymis. *Biochem. Biophys. Res. Commun.*, 117:306–312.
284. Byers, S. W., Qasba, P. K., Paulson, H. L., and Dym, M. (1984): Immunocytochemical localization of alpha-lactalbumin in the male reproductive tract. *Biol. Reprod.*, 30:171–178.
285. Alumot, E., Lensky, Y., and Schindler, H. (1971): Separation of proteins in the epididymal fluid of the ram. *J. Reprod. Fertil.*, 25:349–353.
286. Moore, H. D. M. (1980): Localization of specific glycoproteins secreted by the rabbit and hamster epididymis. *Biol. Reprod.*, 22:705–718.
287. Brooks, D. E. (1981): Secretion of proteins and glycoproteins by the rat epididymis: Regional differences, androgen-dependence, and effects of protease inhibitors, procaine, and tunicamycin. *Biol. Reprod.*, 25:1099–1117.
288. Dravland, E., and Joshi, M. (1981): Sperm-coating antigens secreted by the epididymis and seminal vesicle of the rat. *Biol. Reprod.*, 25:649–658.
289. Jones, R., Fournier-Delpech, S., and Willadsen, S. A. (1982): Identification of androgen-dependent proteins synthesized in vitro by the ram epididymis. *Reprod. Nutr. Dev.*, 22:495–504.
290. Toowicharanont, P., and Chulavatnatol, M. (1983): Characterization of sialoglycoproteins of rat epididymal fluid and spermatozoa by periodate-tritiated borohydride. *J. Reprod. Fertil.*, 67:133–141.
291. Mongkolsirikieat, S., and Chulavatnatol, M. (1984): Phosphorylated secretory proteins from rat epididymis and their androgenic control. *J. Reprod. Fertil.*, 72:423–428.
292. Brooks, D. E. (1985): Characterization of a 22 kDa protein with widespread tissue distribution but which is uniquely present in secretions of the testis and epididymis and on the surface of spermatozoa. *Biochim. Biophys. Acta*, 841:59–70.
293. Mayorga, L. S., and Bertini, F. (1985): The origin of some acid hydrolases of the fluid of the rat cauda epididymidis. *J. Androl.*, 6:243–245.

294. Olson, G. E., and Hinton, B. T. (1985): Regional differences in luminal fluid polypeptides of the rat testis and epididymis revealed by two-dimensional gel electrophoresis. *J. Androl.*, 6:20–34.
295. Robaire, B., Ewing, L. L., Zirkin, B. R., and Irby, D. C. (1977): Steroid Δ^4-5α-reductase and 3α-hydroxysteroid dehydrogenase in the rat epididymis. *Endocrinology,* 101:1379–1390.
296. Jones, R., Von Glos, K. I., and Brown, C. R. (1981): Characterization of hormonally regulated secretory proteins from the caput epididymidis of the rabbit. *Biochem. J.*, 196:105–114.
297. Annison, E. F., Scott, T. W., and Waites, G. M. H. (1963): The role of glucose and acetate in the oxidative metabolism of the testis and epididymis of the ram. *Biochem. J.*, 88:482–488.
298. Elliott, P. R. (1965): Metabolism of homogenates of the mouse epididymis. *J. Cell Comp. Physiol.*, 66:281–292.
299. Kraft, L. A., and Johnson, A. D. (1972): Epididymal carbohydrate metabolism. II. Substrates and pathway utilization of caput and cauda epididymal tissue from the rabbit, rat and mouse. *Comp. Biochem. Physiol. [B]*, 42:451–461.
300. Wallace, J. C., Wales, R. G., and White, I. G. (1966): Respiration of the rabbit epididymis and its synthesis of glycerylphosphorylcholine. *Aust. J. Biol. Sci.*, 19:849–856.
301. Johnson, A. D., and Turner, P. C. (1971): Epididymal carbohydrate metabolism. I. Glucose-1-^{14}C and glucose-6-^{14}C metabolism by mouse, rat, and rabbit tissues. *Comp. Biochem. Physiol. [A]*, 39:599–604.
302. Turner, T. T., and Johnson, A. D. (1973): The metabolic activity of the bovine epididymis. I. Utilization of glucose and fructose. *J. Reprod. Fertil.*, 34:201–213.
303. Turner, T. T., and Johnson, A. D. (1973): The metabolic activity of the bovine epididymis. II. Utilization of acetate, succinate, pyruvate, lactate, and glucose. *J. Reprod. Fertil.*, 35:445–451.
304. Brooks, D. E. (1976): Activity and androgenic control of glycolytic enzymes in the epididymis and epididymal spermatozoa of the rat. *Biochem. J.*, 156:527–537.
305. Brooks, D. E. (1978): Activity and androgenic control of enzymes associated with the tricarboxylic acid cycle, lipid oxidation and mitochondrial shuttles in the epididymis and epididymal spermatozoa of the rat. *Biochem. J.*, 174:741–752.
306. Brooks, D. E. (1978): Androgenic regulation of metabolic pathways in the rat epididymis. *Biol. Reprod.*, 18:629–638.
307. Brooks, D. E. (1979): Carbohydrate metabolism in the rat epididymis: Evidence that glucose is taken up by tissue slices and isolated cells by a process of facilitated transport. *Biol. Reprod.*, 21: 19–26.
308. Brooks, D. E. (1979): Influence of testicular secretions on tissue weight and on metabolic and enzyme activities in the epididymis of the rat. *J. Endocrinol.*, 82:305–313.
309. Brooks, D. E. (1981): Metabolic activity in the epididymis and its regulation by androgens. *Physiol. Rev.*, 61:516–555.
310. Delongeas, J. L., Gelly, J. L., Hatier, R., and Grignon, G. (1984): Postnatal evolution of epididymis oxidative metabolism in the rat. *C. R. Seances Acad. Sci. [III]*, 298:19–22.
311. Frankel, A. I., and Eik-Nes, K. B. (1970): Metabolism of steroids in the rabbit epididymis. *Endocrinology,* 87:646–652.
312. Inano, H., Machino, A., and Tamaoki, B.-I. (1969): *In vitro* metabolism of steroid hormones by cell-free homogenates of epididymides of adult rats. *Endocrinology,* 84:997–1003.
313. Hamilton, D. W., and Fawcett, D. W. (1970): *In vitro* synthesis of cholesterol and testosterone from acetate by rat epididymis and vas deferens. *Res. Soc. Exp. Biol. Med.*, 133:693–695.
314. Hamilton, D. W. (1971): Steroid function in the mammalian epididymis. *J. Reprod. Fertil.*, [Suppl.13]:89–97.
315. Evans, R. R., and Johnson, A. D. (1975): The metabolic activity of the bovine epididymis. III. Cholesterol and esterified cholesterol metabolism. *J. Reprod. Fertil.*, 43:527–530.
316. Legault, Y., Bouthillier, M., Bleau, G., Chapdelaine, A., and Roberts, K. D. (1979): The sterol and sterol sulfate content of the male hamster reproductive tract. *Biol. Reprod.*, 20:1213–1219.
317. Dinakar, N., Arora, R., and Prasad, M. R. N. (1974): Effects of microquantities of 5α-dihydrotestosterone on the epididymis and accessory glands of the castrated Rhesus monkey, *Macaca mulatta. Int. J. Fertil.*, 19:133–139.
318. Karkun, T., Rajalakshmi, M., and Prasad, M. R. N. (1974): Maintenance of the epididymis in the castrated golden hamster by testosterone and dihydrotestosterone. *Contraception,* 9:471–485.
319. Gloyna, R. E., and Wilson, J. D. (1969): A comparative study of the conversion of testosterone to 17β-hydroxy-5α-androstan-3-one (dihydrotestosterone) by prostate and epididymis. *J. Clin. Endocrinol.*, 29:970–977.
320. Hargreave, T. B., Busuttil, A., Elton, R. A., Harvey, J., Chan, A., and Chisholm, G. D. (1982): Studies of testicular and epididymal damage in relation to the occurrence of anti-sperm antibodies. *Br. J. Urol.*, 54:769–773.
321. Monsalve, A., and Blaquier, J. A. (1977): Partial characterization of epididymal 5α-reductase in the rat. *Steroids,* 30:41–51.
322. Pujol, A., and Bayard, F. (1978): 5α-reductase and 3α-hydroxysteroid oxidoreductase enzyme activities in epididymis and their control by androgen and the rete testis fluid. *Steroids,* 31:485–493.
323. Klinefelter, G. R., and Amann, R. P. (1980): Metabolism of testosterone by principal cells and basal cells isolated from the rat epididymal epithelium. *Biol. Reprod.*, 22:1149–1154.
324. Kumari, G. L., Allag, I. S., Das, R. P., and Datta, J. K. (1980): Regional differences in steroidogenesis and hormone levels in the epididymis and vas deferens of adult rats. *Int. J. Androl.*, 3:267–281.
325. Foldesy, R. G., and Leathem, J. H. (1981): Age-related changes in the metabolism of [^{3}H]testosterone *in vitro* by the epididymis of the immature rat. *J. Endocrinol.*, 91:43–51.
326. Robaire, B., Scheer, H., and Hachey, C. (1981): Regulation of epididymal steroid metabolizing enzymes. In: *Bioregulators of Reproduction,* edited by G. Jagiello and H. J. Vogel, pp. 487–498. Academic Press, New York.
327. Brown, D. V., Amann, R. P., and Wagley, L. M. (1983): Influence of rete testis fluid on the metabolism of testosterone by cultured principal cells isolated from the proximal or distal caput of the rat epididymis. *Biol. Reprod.*, 28:1257–1268.
328. Tsuji, M., Takeyama, M., Takatsuka, D., Yabumoto, H., Terada, N., and Matsumoto, K. (1984): 5α- and 5β-reductases for 4-ene-3-ketosteroids and 17β-ol-dehydrogenase in epididymis and testis of golden hamster during sexual development. *J. Steroid Biochem.*, 21:179–183.
329. Danzo, B. J., and Eller, B. C. (1980): Androgen metabolism by mature rabbit epididymal tissue: the effects of castration and androgen replacement. *J. Steroid Biochem.*, 13:661–667.
330. Boujard, D., Thomas, D., and Garnier, D. H. (1982): Regional distribution of steroids in the dog epididymis. *Reprod. Nutr. Dev.*, 22:931–939.
331. Arora-Dinakar, R., Dinakar, N., and Prasad, M. R. N. (1977): Metabolism in vitro of ^{3}H-testosterone in testis, epididymis and sex accessories of the rhesus monkey *Macaca mulatta:* Effects of cyproterone acetate on androgen metabolism. *Indian J. Exp. Biol.*, 15:953–958.
332. De Larminat, M. A., and Blaquier, J. A. (1978): Androgen concentration and partial characterization of 5α-reductase in the epididymis of the rhesus monkey. *Steroids,* 31:129–138.
333. De Larminat, M. A., Hinrichsen, M. J., Scorticati, C., Ghirlando, J. M., Blaquier, J. A., and Calandra, R. S. (1980): Uptake and metabolism of androgen by the human epididymis *in vitro. J. Reprod. Fertil.*, 59:397–402.
334. Kinoshita, Y., Hosaka, M., Nishimura, R., and Takai, S. (1980): Partial characterization of 5α-reductase in the human epididymis. *Endocrinol. Jpn.*, 27:277–284.
335. Leinonen, P., Hammond, G. L., and Vihko, R. (1980): Testosterone and some of its precursors and metabolites in the human epididymis. *J. Clin. Endocrinol. Metabol.*, 51:423–428.
336. Kinoshita, Y. (1981): Studies on the human epididymis: Partial characterization of 3α- and 3β-hydroxysteroid dehydrogenase, regional distribution of 5α-reductase and inhibitory effect of Δ^4-3-oxosteroids on 5α-reductase. *Endocrinol. Jpn.*, 28:499–513.
337. Blaquier, J. A. (1971): Selective uptake and metabolism of androgens by rat epididymis. The presence of a cytoplasmic receptor. *Biochem Biophys. Res. Commun.*, 45:1076–1082.
338. Back, D. J. (1975): The presence of metabolites of ^{3}H-testosterone in the lumen of the cauda epididymis of the rat. *Steroids,* 25:413–420.
339. Djøseland, O., Hastings, C. D., and Hansson, V. (1976): Androgen metabolism by rat epididymis. 5. Metabolic conversion and nuclear binding after injection of 5α-androstane-3α,17β-diol, *in vivo. Steroids,* 28:585–596.

340. Tezon, J. G., Vazquez, M. H., and Blaquier, J. A. (1982): Androgen-controlled subcellular distribution of its receptor in the rat epididymis: 5α-dihydrotestosterone-induced translocation is blocked by antiandrogens. *Endocrinology,* 111:2039–2045.
341. Ganjam, V. K., and Amann, R. P. (1976): Steroid content of fluids and sperm entering and leaving the bovine epididymis, in epididymidal tissue, and in accessory sex gland secretions. *Endocrinology,* 99:1618–1630.
342. Purvis, K., and Hansson, V. (1978): Androgens and androgen-binding protein in the rat epididymis. *J. Reprod. Fertil.,* 52:59–63.
343. Vreeburg, J. T. M. (1975): Distribution of testosterone and 5α-dihydrotestosterone in rat epididymis and their concentrations in efferent duct fluid. *J. Endocrinol.,* 67:203–210.
344. Jean-Faucher, C., Berger, M., Deturckheim, M., Veyssiere, G., and Jean, C. (1985): Testosterone and dihydrotestosterone levels in the epididymis, vas-deferens and preputial gland of mice during sexual maturation. *Int. J. Androl.,* 8:44–57.
345. Purvis, K., Calandra, R., Sander, S., and Hansson, V. (1978): Androgen binding proteins and androgen levels in the human testis and epididymis. *Int. J. Androl.,* 1:531–548.
346. De Larminat, M. A., Cuasnicu, P. S., and Blaquier, J. A. (1980): The *in vitro* metabolism of androgens in rat epididymis during sexual development. *J. Steroid Biochem.,* 13:1207–1213.
347. Scheer, H., and Robaire, B. (1983): Subcellular distribution of steroid Δ^4-5α-reductase and 3α-hydroxysteroid dehydrogenase in the rat epididymis during sexual maturation. *Biol. Reprod.,* 29:1–10.
348. Djøseland, O., Hoglo, S., Abyholm, T., and Haugen, H. N. (1981): Androgen metabolism by rat epididymis. 8. Age dependent changes in androgen metabolizing enzymes in rat accessory sex organs. *Arch. Androl.,* 6:229–238.
349. Scheer, H., and Robaire, B. (1983): Solubilization and partial characterization of rat epididymal Δ^4-steroid 5α-reductase (cholestenone 5α-reductase). *Biochem. J.,* 211:65–74.
350. Scheer, H., and Robaire, B. (1982): Characterization of epididymal Δ^4-5α-reductase. *Ann. NY Acad. Sci.,* 383:496–498.
351. Cooke, G. M., and Robaire, B. (1984): Mechanism of 4-ene-steroid 5α-reductase proton transfer in androgen target tissues. *J. Steroid Biochem.,* 20:1279–1284.
352. Hastings, C. D., Brekke, I., Purvis, K., Attramadal, A., and Hansson, V. (1980): Cofactor dependency of soluble 3α-hydroxysteroid oxidoreductase in rat testis, prostate, and epididymis. *Endocrinology,* 107:1762–1766.
353. Hastings, C. D., Brekke, I., Attramadal, A., and Hansson, V. (1980): Physico-chemical characterization of the soluble 3α-hydroxysteroid oxidoreductase in the rat testis and prostate. *Int. J. Androl.,* 3:72–81.
354. Ofner, P., Vena, R. L., and Martin, R. F. (1974): Acetylation and hydroxylation of 5α-androstane-3β,17β-diol by prostate and epididymis. *Steroids,* 24:261–279.
355. Djøseland, O. (1976): Androgen metabolism by rat epididymis. 4. The formation of conjugates. *Steroids,* 27:617–636.
356. Hastings, C. D., and Djøseland, O. (1977): Androgen metabolism by rat epididymis. Metabolic conversion of ^{3}H 5α-androstane-3α,17β-diol, *in vitro*. *Steroids,* 30:531–539.
357. Ofner, P., Vena, R. L., Leav, I., and Hamilton, D. W. (1979): Metabolism of C19-radiosteroids by explants of canine prostate and epididymis with disposition as hydroxylated products: A possible mechanism for androgen inactivation. *J. Steroid Biochem.,* 11:1367–1379.
358. Morfin, R. F., Leav, I., Orr, D., Piccart, D., and Ofner, P. (1980): C19 steroid metabolism by canine prostate, epididymis and perianal glands. *Eur. J. Biochem.,* 109:119–127.
359. Chang, T. S. K., and Morton, B. (1975): Epididymal sulfhydryl oxidase: A sperm-protective enzyme from the male reproductive tract. *Biochem. Biophys. Res. Commun.,* 66:309–315.
360. Chang, T. S. K., and Zirkin, B. R. (1978): Distribution of sulfhydryl oxidase activity in the rat and hamster male reproductive tract. *Biol. Reprod.,* 18:745–748.
361. DeLap, L. W., Tate, S. S., and Meister, A. (1977): γ-Glutamyl transpeptidase and related enzyme activities in the reproductive system of the male rat. *Life Sci.,* 20:673–680.
362. Tate, S. S., and Orlando, J. (1979): Conversion of glutathione to glutathione disulfide, a catalytic function of γ-glutamyl transpeptidase. *J. Biol. Chem.,* 254:5573–5575.
363. Hales, B. F., Hachey, C., and Robaire, B. (1980): The presence and longitudinal distribution of the glutathione *S*-transferases in rat epididymis and vas deferens. *Biochem. J.,* 189:135–142.
364. Bartke, A., and Koerner, S. (1974): Androgenic regulation of the concentration of prostaglandin F in the male reproductive system of rats and mice. *Endocrinology,* 95:1739–1743.
365. Badr, F. M., Barcikowski, B., and Bartke, A. (1975): Effect of castration, testosterone treatment and hereditary sterility on prostaglandin concentration in the male reproductive system of mice. *Prostaglandins,* 9:289–297.
366. Gerozissis, K., and Dray, F. (1977): Selective and age dependent changes in prostaglandin E-2 in the epididymis and vas deferens of the rat. *J. Reprod. Fertil.,* 50:113–115.
367. Gerozissis, K., and Dray, F. (1983): *In-vitro* prostanoid production by the rat vas deferens. *J. Reprod. Fertil.,* 67:389–394.
368. Cosentino, M. J., Takihara, H., Burhop, J. W., and Cockett, A. T. K. (1984): Regulation of rat caput epididymidis contractility by prostaglandins. *J. Androl.,* 5:216–222.
369. Baldwin, B. T. (1928): Determination of sex maturation in boys by laboratory method. *J. Comp. Psychol.,* 8:39–43.
370. Lino, B. F., Braden, A. W. H., and Turnbull, K. E. (1967): Fate of unejaculated spermatozoa. *Nature,* 213:594–595.
371. Amann, R.P., and Almquist, J. O. (1962): Reproductive capacity of dairy bulls. VI. Effect of unilateral vasectomy and ejaculation frequency on sperm reserves; aspects of epididymal physiology. *J. Reprod. Fertil.,* 3:260–268.
372. Orgebin-Crist, M.-C. (1962): Recherches expérimentales sur la durée de passage des spermatozoédes dans l'épididyme du taureau. *Ann. Biol. Animale Biochim. Biophys.,* 2:51–108.
373. Murakami, M., Sugita, A., and Hamasaki, M. (1982): Scanning electron microscopic observations of the vas deferens in man and monkey with special reference to spermiophagy in its ampullary region. *Scan. Electron Microsc.,* 3:1333–1339.
374. Murakami, M., Nishida, T., Iwanaga, S., and Shiromoto, M. (1984): Scanning and transmission electron microscopic evidence of epithelial phagocytosis of spermatozoa in the terminal region of the vas deferens of the cat. *Experientia,* 40:958–960.
375. Holstein, A. F. (1978): Spermatophagy in the seminiferous tubules and excurrent ducts of the testis in Rhesus monkey and in man. *Andrologia,* 10:331–352.
376. Murakami, M., Sugita, A., and Hamasaki, M. (1982): The vas deferens in man and monkey. Spermiophagy in its ampulla. In: *Atlas of Human Reproduction,* edited by E. S. E. Hafez and P. Kenemans, pp. 187–195. MTP Press, Lancaster, England.
377. Glover, T. D. (1969): Some aspects of function in the epididymis. *Int. J. Fertil.,* 14:215–221.
378. Alexander, N. J. (1973): Ultrastructural changes in rat epididymis after vasectomy. *Z. Zellforsch,* 136:177–182.
379. Hoffer, A. P., Hamilton, D. W., and Fawcett, D. W. (1973): The ultrastructural pathology of the rat epididymis after administration of α-chlorohydrin (U-5897). I. Effects of a single high dose. *Anat. Rec.,* 175:203–230.
380. Hoffer, A. P., and Hamilton, D. W. (1974): Phagocytosis of sperm by the epithelial cells in ductuli efferentes of experimental rats. *Anat. Rec.,* 178:376–377.
381. Hoffer, A. P., Hamilton, D. W., and Fawcett, D. W. (1975): Phagocytosis of spermatozoa by the epithelial cells of the ductuli efferentes after epididymal obstruction in the rat. *J. Reprod. Fertil.,* 44:1–9.
382. Bedford, J. M. (1976): Adaptations of the male reproductive tract and the fate of spermatozoa following vasectomy in the rabbit, rhesus monkey, hamster and rat. *Biol. Reprod.,* 14:118–142.
383. Flickinger, C. J. (1982): The fate of sperm after vasectomy in the hamster. *Anat. Rec.,* 202:231–239.
384. Bernard, R. T. F. (1984): The occurrence of spermiophagy under natural conditions in the cauda epididymidis of the Cape horseshoe bat (*Rhinolophus capensis*). *J. Reprod. Fertil.,* 71:539–543.
385. Salisbury, G. W., and Cragle, R. G. (1956): Freezing point depressions and mineral levels of fluids of the ruminant male reproductive tract. *Proceedings: 3rd International Congress on Animal Reproduction,* 1:25–28.
386. Hinton, B. T., and Howards, S. S. (1982): Micropuncture and microperfusion techniques for the study of testicular physiology. *Ann. NY Acad. Sci.,* 383:29–43.

387. Jessee, S. J., and Howards, S. S. (1976): A survey of sperm, potassium and sodium concentrations in the tubular fluid of the hamster epididymis. *Biol. Reprod.*, 15:626–631.
388. Levine, N., and Kelly, H. (1978): Measurement of pH in the rat epididymis *in vivo*. *J. Reprod. Fertil.*, 52:333–335.
389. Arora, R., Dinakar, N., and Prasad, M. R. N. (1975): Biochemical changes in the spermatozoa and luminal contents of different regions of the epididymis of the Rhesus monkey, *Macaca mulatta*. *Contraception*, 11:689–700.
390. Cooper, T. G., and Brooks, D. E. (1981): Entry of glycerol into the rat epididymis and its utilization by epididymal spermatozoa. *J. Reprod. Fertil.*, 61:163–169.
391. Li, T.-K. (1975): The glutathione and thiol content of mammalian spermatozoa and seminal plasma. *Biol. Reprod.*, 12:641–645.
392. Chinoy, N. J., Sharma, J. D., and Chinoy, M. R. (1983): Histochemical localization of ascorbic acid in the testis, epididymis and vas deferens of some rodents. *Z. Mikrosk. Anat. Forsch.*, 97:961–966.
393. Chinoy, N. J., Rao, M. V., and Kumar, R. A. (1984): Role of ascorbic acid in metabolism of rat testis and epididymis in relation to the onset of puberty. *J. Biosci.*, 6:857–863.
394. Casillas, E. R., and Chaipayungpan, S. (1979): The distribution of carnitine and acetylcarnitine in the rabbit epididymis and the carnitine content of rabbit spermatozoa during maturation. *J. Reprod. Fertil.*, 56:439–444.
395. Hinton, B. T., Snoswell, A. M., and Setchell, B. P. (1979): The concentration of carnitine in the luminal fluid of the testis and epididymis of the rat and some other mammals. *J. Reprod. Fertil.*, 56:105–111.
396. Casillas, E. R., Villalobos, P., and Gonzales, R. (1984): Distribution of carnitine and acetylcarnitine in the hamster epididymis and in epididymal spermatozoa during maturation. *J. Reprod. Fertil.*, 72:197–201.
397. Mann, T., and Lutwak-Mann, C. (1980): Epididymis and epididymal semen. In: *Male Reproductive Function and Semen*, edited by T. Mann and C. Lutwak-Mann, pp. 139–161. Springer-Verlag, New York.
398. Eisenberg, F., Jr., and Bolden, A. H. (1964): Reproductive tract as site of synthesis and secretion of inositol in the male rat. *Nature*, 202:599–600.
399. Voglmayr, J. K., and Amann, R. P. (1973): The distribution of free myo-inositol in fluids, spermatozoa, and tissues of the bull genital tract and observations on its uptake by the rabbit epididymis. *Biol. Reprod.*, 8:504–513.
400. Hinton, B. T., White, R. W., and Setchell, B. P. (1980): Concentrations of myo-inositol in the luminal fluid of the mammalian testis and epididymis. *J. Reprod. Fertil.*, 58:395–399.
401. Foldesy, R. G., and Leathem, J. H. (1981): Pubertal changes in androgen composition of rat rete testis and cauda epididymal fluid. *J. Steroid Biochem.*, 14:109–110.
402. Kormano, M., Koskimies, A. I., and Hunter, R. L. (1971): The presence of specific proteins, in the absence of many serum proteins in the rat seminiferous tubule fluid. *Experientia*, 27: 1461–1463.
403. Skinner, M. K., and Griswold, M. D. (1982): Secretion of testicular transferrin by cultured Sertoli cells is regulated by hormones and retinoids. *Biol. Reprod.*, 27:211–221.
404. Larrea, F., Musto, N., Gunsalus, G., and Bardin, C. W. (1981): The microheterogeneity of rat androgen-binding protein from the testis, rete testis fluid, and epididymis, as demonstrated by immunoelectrophoresis and photoaffinity labeling. *Endocrinology*, 109:1212–1220.
405. Lea, O. A., and French, F. S. (1981): Characterization of an acidic glycoprotein secreted by principal cells of the rat epididymis. *Biochim. Biophys. Acta*, 668:370–376.
406. Hamilton, D. W. (1980): UDP-galactose: *N*-Acetylglucosamine galactosyltransferase in fluids from rat rete testis and epididymis. *Biol. Reprod.*, 23:377–385.
407. Jones, R., and Brown, C. R. (1982): Association of epididymal secretory proteins showing α-lactalbumin-like activity with the plasma membrane of rat spermatozoa. *Biochem. J.*, 206:161–164.
408. Paquin, R., Chapdelaine, P., Dube, J. Y., and Tremblay, R. R. (1984): Similar biochemical properties of human seminal plasma and epididymal α-1,4-glucosidase. *J. Androl.*, 5:277–282.
409. Besancon, J., Dacheux, J. L., Paquin, R., Tremblay, R. R. (1985): Major contribution of epididymis to alpha-glucosidase content of ram seminal plasma. *Biol. Reprod.*, 33:296–301.
410. Hohlbrugger, G., Schweisfurth, H., and Dahlheim, H. (1982): Angiotensin I converting enzyme in rat testis, epididymis and vas deferens under different conditions. *J. Reprod. Fertil.*, 65:97–103
411. Hohlbrugger, G., and Dahlheim, H. (1983): The effect of age, mating and vasoligature on angiotensin I converting enzyme in rat testis and epididymis. In: *Kinins—III*, edited by H. Fritz, N. Back, G. Dietze, and G. L. Haberland, pp. 845–853. Plenum Press, New York.
412. Vanha-Perttula, T., Mather, J. P., Bardin, C. W., Moss, S. B., and Bellve, A. R. (1985): Localization of the angiotensin-converting enzyme activity in testis and epididymis. *Biol. Reprod.*, 33:870–877.
413. Usselman, M. C., and Cone, R. A. (1983): Rat sperm are mechanically immobilized in the caudal epididymis by "Immobilin," a high molecular weight glycoprotein. *Biol. Reprod.*, 29:1241–1253.
414. Usselman, M. C., Cone, R. A., and Rossignol, D. P. (1985): Rat cauda epididymal fluid is a mucus. *J. Androl.*, 6:315–320.
415. Suzuki, F.,and Nagano, T. (1980): Epididymal maturation of rat spermatozoa studied by thin sectioning and freeze-fracture. *Biol. Reprod.*, 22:1219–1231.
416. Turner, T. T., and Reich, G. W. (1985): Cauda epididymidal sperm motility: A comparison among five species. *Biol. Reprod.*, 32:120–128.
417. Cooper, T. G., and Hamilton, D. W.(1977): Observations on destruction of spermatozoa in the cauda epididymis and proximal vas deferens of non-seasonal male mammals. *Am. J. Anat.*, 149:93–110.
418. Bloom, G., and Nicander, L. (1961): On the ultrastructure and development of the protoplasmic droplet of spermatozoa. *Z. Zellforsch.*, 55:833–844.
419. Fawcett, D. W., and Phillips, D. H. (1969): Observations on the release of spermatozoa and on changes in the head during passage through the epididymis. *J. Reprod. Fertil.*, [Suppl. 6]:405–418.
420. Phillips, D. M. (1975): Mammalian sperm structure. In: *Handbook of Physiology, Sec. 7, Vol. 5*, edited by R. O. Greep and E. B. Astwood, pp. 405–419. American Physiological Society, Washington, D.C.
421. Kaplan, M., Russell, L. D., Peterson, R. N., and Martan, J. (1984): Boar sperm cytoplasmic droplets: their ultrastructure, their numbers, in the epididymis and at ejaculation and their removal during isolation of sperm plasma membranes. *Tissue Cell*, 16:455–468.
422. Branton, C., and Salisbury, G. W. (1947): Morphology of spermatozoa from different levels of the reproductive tract of the bull. *J. Anim. Sci.*, 6:154–160.
423. Hafez, E. S. E., and Prasad, M. R. N. (1976): Functional aspects of the epididymis. In: *Human Semen and Fertility Regulation in Men*, edited by E. S. E. Hafez, pp. 31–43. Mosby, St. Louis.
424. Dott, H. M., and Dingle, J. T. (1968): Distribution and lysosomal enzyme in the spermatozoa and cytoplasmic droplets of bull and ram. *Exp. Cell Res.*, 52:523–540.
425. Robert, M. L., Scouter, W. H., and Nyquisr, S. E. (1976): Isolation and characterization of the cytoplasmic droplet in the rat. *Biol. Reprod.*, 14:421–424.
426. Temple-Smith, P. D. (1984): Phagocytosis of sperm cytoplasmic droplets by a specialized region in the epididymis of the brushtailed possum. *Trichosurus vulpecula*. *Biol. Reprod.*, 30:707–720.
427. Fawcett, D. W., and Hollenberg, R. D. (1963): Changes in the acrosome of guinea pig spermatozoa during passage through the epididymis. *Z. Zellforsch.*, 60:276–292.
428. Bedford, J. M., and Nicander, L. (1971): Ultrastructural changes in the acrosome and sperm membranes during maturation of spermatozoa in the testis and epididymis of the rabbit and monkey. *J. Anat.*, 108:527–543.
429. Jones, R. C., Rowlands, I. W., and Skinner, J. D. (1974): Spermatozoa in the genital ducts of the african elephant: *Loxodonta africana*. *J. Reprod. Fertil.*, 41:189–192.
430. Bedford, J. M., Calvin, H., and Cooper, G. W. (1973): The maturation of spermatozoa in the human epididymis. *J. Reprod. Fertil.*, [Suppl. 18]:199–213.
431. Bedford, J. M., and Cooper, G. W. (1978): Membrane fusion events in the fertilization of vertebrate eggs. In: *Membrane Fusion*, edited by G. Poste and G. L. Nicolson, pp. 65–125. Elsevier North-Holland, Amsterdam.
432. Calvin, H., and Bedford, J. M. (1971): Formation of disulphide bonds in the nucleus and accessory structures of mammalian sper-

matozoa during maturation in the epididymis. *J. Reprod. Fertil.*, [Suppl.13]:65–75.
433. Bedford, J. M., Bent, M. J., and Calvin, H. (1973): Variations in structural character and stability of the nuclear chromatin in morphologically normal human spermatozoa. *J. Reprod. Fertil.*, 33:19–29.
434. Johnson, L., Amann, R. P., and Pickett, B. W. (1980): Maturation of equine epididymal spermatozoa. *Am. J. Vet. Res.*, 41:1190–1196.
435. Toowicharanont, P., and Chulavatnatol, M. (1983): Measurement of anionic sites of rat epididymal spermatozoa using tritiated polycationized ferritin. *J. Reprod. Fertil.*, 69:303–306.
436. Fain-Maurel, M. A., Dadoune, J. P., and Reger, J. F. (1983): Surface changes in monkey spermatozoa during epididymal maturation and after ejaculation. In: *The Sperm Cell,* edited by J. Andre, pp. 159–162. Martinus Nijhoff, Amsterdam.
437. Jones, R., Pholpramool, C., Setchell, B. P., and Brown, C. R. (1981): Labelling of membrane glycoproteins on rat spermatozoa collected from different regions of the epididymis. *Biochem. J.*, 200:457–460.
438. Chulavatnatol, M., Panyim, S., and Wititsuwannakul, D. (1982): Comparison of phosphorylated proteins in intact rat spermatozoa from caput and cauda epididymidis. *Biol. Reprod.*, 26:197–207.
439. Brown, C. R., Von Glos, K. I., and Jones, R. (1983): Changes in plasma membrane glycoproteins of rat spermatozoa during maturation in the epididymis. *J. Cell Biol.*, 96:256–264.
440. Jones, R., Von Glos, K. I., and Brown, C. R. (1983): Changes in the protein composition of rat spermatozoa during maturation in the epididymis. *J. Reprod. Fertil.*, 67:299–306.
441. Brooks, D. E., and Tiver, K. (1984): Analysis of surface proteins of rat spermatozoa during epididymal transit and identification of antigens common to spermatozoa, rete testis fluid and cauda epididymal plasma. *J. Reprod. Fertil.*, 71:249–257.
442. Lewin, L. M., Weissenberg, R., Sobel, J. S., Marcus, Z., and Nebel, L. (1979): Differences in concanavalin A-FITC binding to rat spermatozoa during epididymal maturation and capacitation. *Arch. Androl.*, 2:279–281.
443. Nicolson, G. L., and Yanagimachi, R. (1979): Cell surface changes associated with epididymal maturation of mammalian spermatozoa. In: *The Spermatozoon,* edited by D. W. Fawcett and J. M. Bedford, pp. 187–194. Urban & Schwarzenberg, Baltimore.
444. Witkin, S. S., Richards, J. M., and Bedford, J. M. (1983): Influence of epididymal maturation on the capacity of hamster and rabbit spermatozoa for complement activation. *J. Reprod. Fertil.*, 69:517–521.
445. Gagnon, C., Harbour, D., DeLamirande, E., Bardin, C. W., and Dacheux, J.-L. (1984): Sensitive assay detects protein methylesterase in spermatozoa: Decrease in enzyme activity during epididymal maturation. *Biol. Reprod.*, 30:953–958.
446. Echeverria, F. G., Cuasnicu, P. S., Piazza, A., Pineiro, L., and Blaquier, J. A. (1984): Addition of an androgen-free epididymal protein extract increases the ability of immature hamster spermatozoa to fertilize *in vivo* and *in vitro*. *J. Reprod. Fertil.*, 71:433–437.
447. Dacheux, J. L. (1977): Reinvestigation of the variation in total phospholipid content of the spermatozoa of the rat and the ram during epididymal transport. *IRCS Med. Sci.*, 5:18.
448. Evans, R. W., and Setchell, B. P. (1979): Lipid changes during epididymal maturation in ram spermatozoa collected at different times of the year. *J. Reprod. Fertil.*, 57:197–203.
449. Nikolopoulou, M., Soucek, D. A., and Vary, J. C. (1985): Changes in the lipid content of boar sperm plasma membranes during epididymal maturation. *Biochim. Biophys. Acta,* 815:486–498.
450. Voglmayr, J. K. (1975): Metabolic changes in spermatozoa during epididymal transit. In: *Handbook of Physiology, Sec. 7, Vol. 5,* edited by R. O. Greep and E. B. Astwood, pp. 437–451. American Physiological Society, Washington, D.C.
451. Dacheux, J. L., O'Shea, T., and Paquignon, M. (1979): Effects of osmolality, bicarbonate and buffer on the metabolism and motility of testicular, epididymal and ejaculated spermatozoa of boars. *J. Reprod. Fertil.*, 55:287–296.
452. Voglmayr, J. K., and White, I. G. (1979): Effects of rete testis and epididymal fluid on the metabolism and motility of testicular and post-testicular spermatozoa of the ram. *Biol. Reprod.*, 20:288–293.
453. Del Rio, A. G., and Raisman, R. (1978): cAMP in spermatozoa taken from different segments of the rat epididymis. *Experientia,* 34:670–671.
454. Amann, R. P., Hay, S. R., and Hammerstedt, R. H. (1982): Yield, characteristics, motility and cAMP content of sperm isolated from seven regions of ram epididymis. *Biol. Reprod.*, 27:723–733.
455. Purvis, K., Cusan, L., Attramadal, H., Ege, A., and Hansson, V. (1982): Rat sperm enzymes during epididymal transit. *J. Reprod. Fertil.*, 65:381–387.
456. Bedford, J. M. (1977): Evolution of the scrotum: The epididymis as the prime mover. In: *Reproduction and Evolution,* edited by J. H. Calaby, pp. 171–182. Australian Academy of Science, Canberra.
457. Bedford, J. M. (1978): Anatomical evidence for the epididymis as the prime mover in the evolution of the scrotum. *Am. J. Anat.*, 152:483–508.
458. Orgebin-Crist, M.-C., and Olson, G. E. (1984): Epididymal sperm maturation. In: *The Male in Farm Animal Reproduction,* edited by M. Courot, pp. 80–102. Martinus Nijhoff, Amsterdam.
459. Ortavant, R. (1959): Le cycle spermatogénétique chez le bélier. *Ann. Zootech.*, 8:183–244.
460. Monesi, V. (1962): Autoradiographic study of DNA synthesis and the cell cycle in spermatogonia and spermatocytes of mouse testis using tritiated thymidine. *J. Cell Biol.*, 14:1–18.
461. Amann, R.P., Koefoed-Johnson, H. H., and Levi, H. (1965): Excretion pattern of labelled spermatozoa and the timing of spermatozoa formation and epididymal transit in rabbits injected with thymidine-^{3}H. *J. Reprod. Fertil.*, 10:169–184.
462. Amann, R.P. (1981): A critical review of methods for evaluation of spermatogenesis from seminal characteristics. *J. Androl.*, 2:37–58.
463. Singh, G. (1962): Durée de passage dans l'épididyme des spermatozoides de verrats marqués au ^{32}P. *Ann. Biol. Anim. Biochim. Biophys.*, 2:43–46.
464. Orgebin-Crist, M.-C. (1965): Passage of spermatozoa labelled with thymidine ^{3}H through the ductus epididymis of the rabbit. *J. Reprod. Fertil.*, 10:241–251.
465. Amir, D., and Ortavant, R. (1968): Influence de la fréquence des collectes sur la durée du transit des spermatozoides dans le canal épididymaire du bélier. *Ann. Biol. Anim. Biochim. Biophys.*, 8:195–207.
466. Swierstra, E. E. (1968): Cytology and duration of the cycle of the seminiferous epithelium of the boar; duration of spermatozoa transit through the epididymis. *Anat. Rec.*, 161:171–186.
467. Gebauer, M. R., Pickett, B. W., and Swierstra, E. E. (1974): Reproductive physiology of the stallion. III. Extragonadal transit time and sperm reserves. *J. Anim. Sci.*, 39:737–742.
468. Amann, R. P., Johnson, L., Thompson, D. L., Jr., and Pickett, B. W. (1976): Daily spermatozoal production, epididymal spermatozoal reserves and transit time of spermatozoa through the epididymis of the rhesus monkey. *Biol. Reprod.*, 15:586–592.
469. Robb, G. W., Amann, R. P., and Killian, G. J. (1978): Daily sperm production and epididymal sperm reserves of pubertal and adult rats. *J. Reprod. Fertil.*, 54:103–107.
470. Rowley, M. J., Teshima, F., and Heller, C. G. (1970): Duration of transit of spermatozoa through the human male ductular system. *Fertil. Steril.*, 21:390–395.
471. Swierstra, E. E. (1971): Sperm production of boars as measured from epididymal sperm reserves and quantitative testicular histology. *J. Reprod. Fertil.*, 27:91–99.
472. Kirton, K. T., Desjardins, C., and Hafs, H. D. (1967): Distribution of sperm in male rabbits after various ejaculation frequencies. *Anat. Rec.*, 158:287–292.
473. Jaakkola, U. M., and Talo, A. (1982): Relation of electrical activity to luminal transport in the cauda epididymis of the rat *in vitro*. *J. Reprod. Fertil.*, 64:121–126.
474. Jaakkola, U. M. (1983): Regional variations in transport of the luminal contents of the rat epididymis *in vivo*. *J. Reprod. Fertil.*, 68:465–470.
475. Jaakkola, U. M., and Talo, A. (1983): Movements of the luminal contents in two different regions of the caput epididymidis of the rat *in vitro*. *J. Physiol.* (*Lond.*), 336:453–463.
476. Johnson, A. L., and Howards, S. S. (1975): Intratubular hydrostatic pressure in testis and epididymis before and after vasectomy. *Am. J. Physiol.*, 228:556–564.
477. Pholpramool, C., Triphom, N., and Dinudom, A. (1984): Intraluminal pressures in the seminiferous tubules and in different regions of the epididymis in the rat. *J. Reprod. Fertil.*, 71:173–179.

478. Markkula-Viitanen, M., Nikkanen, V., and Talo, A. (1979): Electrical activity and intraluminal pressure of the cauda epididymidis of the rat. *J. Reprod. Fertil.*, 57:431–435.
479. Talo, A., Jaakkola, U. M., and Markkula-Viitanen, M. (1979): Spontaneous electrical activity of the rat epididymis *in vitro*. *J. Reprod. Fertil.*, 57:423–429.
480. Jaakkola, U. M., and Talo, A. (1980): Effect of temperature on the electrical activity of the rat epididymis *in vitro*. *J. Therm. Biol.*, 5:207–210.
481. Jaakkola, U. M., and Talo, A. (1981): Effects of oxytocin and vasopressin on electrical and mechanical activity of the rat epididymis *in vitro*. *J. Reprod. Fertil.*, 63:47–51.
482. Muratori, G. (1953): Ulteriori observazioni sulla motilita spontanea dell epididimo del ratto. *Boll. Soc. Ital. Biol. Sper.*, 29:1026–1028.
483. Risley, P. L., and Turbyfill, C. (1957): Studies in vivo of the ductus epididymidis and vasa efferentia of the rat. *Anat. Rec.*, 128:607–608.
484. Pholpramool, C., and Triphrom, N. (1984): Effects of cholinergic and andrenergic drugs on intraluminal pressures and contractility of the rat testis and epididymis *in vivo*. *J. Reprod. Fertil.*, 71: 181–188.
485. Bedford, J. M. (1966): Development of the fertilizing ability of spermatozoa in the epididymis of the rabbit. *J. Exp. Zool.*, 163:319–329.
486. Nishikawa, Y., and Waide, Y. (1952): Studies on the maturation of spermatozoa. I. Mechanism and speed of transition of spermatozoa in the epididymis and their functional changes. *Bull. Natl. Inst. Agr. Sci.* [*G*], 3:69–81.
487. Blandau, R. J., and Rumery, R. E. (1964): The relationship of swimming movements of epididymal spermatozoa to their fertilizing capacity. *Fertil. Steril.*, 15:571–579.
488. Dyson, A. L. M. B., and Orgebin-Crist, M.-C. (1973): Effects of hypophysectomy, castration and androgen replacement upon the fertilizing ability of rat epididymal spermatozoa. *Endocrinology*, 93:391–402.
489. Paz (Frenkel), G., Kaplan, R., Yedwab, G., Homonnai, Z. T., and Kraicer, P. F. (1978): The effect of caffeine on rat epididymal spermatozoa: Motility, metabolism and fertilizing capacity. *Int. J. Androl.*, 1:145–152.
490. Fournier-Delpech, S., Colas, G., Courot, M., and Ortavant, R. (1977): Observations on the motility and fertilizing ability of ram epididymal spermatozoa. *Ann. Biol. Anim. Biochim. Biophys.*, 17:987–990.
491. Fournier-Delpech, S., Colas, G., Courot, M., Ortavant, R., and Brice, G. (1979): Epididymal sperm maturation in the ram: Motility, fertilizing ability and embryonic survival after uterine artificial insemination in the ewe. *Ann. Biol. Anim. Biochim. Biophys.*, 19:597–605.
492. Fournier-Delpech, S., Colas, G., and Courot, M. (1981): Observations sur les premiers clivages des oeufs intratubaires de brebis après fécondation avec des spermatozoides épididymaires ou éjaculés. *C. R. Seances Acad. Sci.* [*D*] (*Paris*), 292:515–517.
493. Orgebin-Crist, M.-C. (1967): Maturation of spermatozoa in the rabbit epididymis: Fertilizing ability and embryonic mortality in does inseminated with epididymal spermatozoa. *Ann. Biol. Anim. Biochim. Biophys.*, 7:373–389.
494. Orgebin-Crist, M.-C. (1968): Maturation of spermatozoa in the rabbit epididymis: Delayed fertilization in does inseminated with epididymal spermatozoa. *J. Reprod. Fertil.*, 16:29–33.
495. Orgebin-Crist, M.-C., and Jahad, N. (1977): Delayed cleavage of rabbit ova after fertilization by young epididymal spermatozoa. *Biol. Reprod.*, 16:358–362.
496. Overstreet, J. W., and Bedford, J. M. (1976): Embryonic mortality in the rabbit is not increased after fertilization by young epididymal spermatozoa. *Biol. Reprod.*, 15:54–57.
497. Cummins, J. M. (1976): Effects of epididymal occlusion on sperm maturation in the hamster. *J. Exp. Zool.*, 197:187–190.
498. Hoskins, D. D., Brandt, H., and Acott, S. (1978): Initiation of sperm motility in the mammalian epididymis. *Fed. Proc.*, 37:2534–2542.
499. Acott, T. S., Johnson, D. J., Brandt, H., and Hoskins, D. D. (1979): Sperm forward motility protein: Tissue distribution and species cross reactivity. *Biol. Reprod.*, 20:247–252.
500. Pholpramool, C., Lea, O. A., Burrow, P. V., Dott, H. M., and Setchell, B. P. (1983): The effects of acidic epididymal glycoprotein (AEG) and some other proteins on the motility of rat epididymal spermatozoa. *Int. J. Androl.*, 6:240–248.
501. Hinton, B. T., Brooks, D. E., Dott, H. M., and Setchell, B. P. (1981): Effects of carnitine and some related compounds on the motility of rat spermatozoa from the caput epididymis. *J. Reprod. Fertil.*, 61:59–64.
502. Inskeep, P. B., and Hammerstedt, R. H. (1982): Changes in metabolism of ram sperm associated with epididymal transit or induced by exogenous carnitine. *Biol. Reprod.*, 27:735–743.
503. Hoskins, D. D., and Casillas, E. R. (1975): Function of cyclic nucleotides in mammalian spermatozoa. In: *Handbook of Physiology, Sec. 7, Vol. 5*, edited by R. O. Greep and E. B. Astwood, pp. 453–460. American Physiological Society, Washington, D.C.
504. Turner, T. T., and Giles, R. D. (1982): Sperm motility-inhibiting factor in rat epididymis. *Am. J. Physiol.*, 242:R199–R203.
505. Carr, D. W., and Acott, T. S. (1984): Inhibition of bovine spermatozoa by caudal epididymidal fluid. I. Studies of a sperm motility quiescence factor. *Biol. Reprod.*, 30:913–925.
506. Gopalakrishna, A., and Bhatia, D. (1980): Storage of spermatozoa in the epididymis of the bat, *Hipposideros speoris* (*Schneider*). *Curr. Sci.*, 49:951–953.
507. Depeiges, A., Betail, G., Coulet, M., and Dufaure, J.-P. (1985): Histochemical study of epididymal secretions in the lizard, *Lacerta vivipara*. *Cell Tissue Res.*, 239:463–466.
508. Martin-DeLeon, P. A., Shaver, E. L., and Gammal, E. B. (1973): Chromosome abnormalities in rabbit blastocysts resulting from spermatozoa aged in the male tract. *Fertil. Steril.*, 24:212–220.
509. Bedford, J. M. (1978): Influence of abdominal temperature on epididymal function in rat and rabbit. *Am. J. Anat.*, 152:509–521.
510. Moore, H. D. M. (1981): An assessment of the fertilizing ability of spermatozoa in the epididymis of the marmoset monkey (*Callithrix jacchus*). *Int. J. Androl.*, 4:321–330.
511. Holtz, W., and Smidt, D. (1976): The fertilizing capacity of epididymal spermatozoa in the pig. *J. Reprod. Fertil.*, 46:227–229.
512. Pavlok, A. (1974): Development of the penetration activity of mouse epididymal spermatozoa *in vivo* and *in vitro*. *J. Reprod. Fertil.*, 36:203–205.
513. Hoppe, P. C. (1975): Fertilizing ability of mouse sperm from different epididymal regions and after washing and centrifugation. *J. Exp. Zool.*, 192:219–222.
514. Horan, A. H., and Bedford, J. M. (1972): Development of the fertilizing ability of spermatozoa in the epididymis of the syrian hamster. *J. Reprod. Fertil.*, 30:417–423.
515. Moore, H. D. M. (1981): Glycoprotein secretions of the epididymis in the rabbit and hamster: Localization on epididymal spermatozoa and the effects of specific antibodies on fertilization *in vivo*. *J. Exp. Zool.*, 215:77–85.
516. Hinrichsen, M. J., and Blaquier, J. A. (1980): Evidence supporting the existence of sperm maturation in the human epididymis. *J. Reprod. Fertil.*, 60:291–294.
517. Moore, H. D. M., Hartman, T. C., and Pryor, J. P. (1983): Development of the oocyte-penetrating capacity of spermatozoa in the human epididymis. *Int. J. Androl.*, 6:310–318.
518. Schleicher, G., Drews, U., Stumpf, W. E., and Sar, M. (1984): Differential distribution of dihydrotestosterone and estradiol binding sites in the epididymis of the mouse. An autoradiographic study. *Histochemistry*, 81:139–147.
519. Lubicz-Nawrocki, C. M. (1973): The effect of metabolites of testosterone on the viability of hamster epididymal spermatozoa. *J. Endocrinol.*, 58:193–198.
520. Cooke, G. M., and Robaire, B. (1985): Modulation of epididymal Δ^4-steroid 5α-reductase activity in vitro by the phospholipid environment. *J. Biol. Chem.*, 260:7489–7495.
521. Brooks, D. E. (1979): Influence of androgens on the weights of the male accessory reproductive organs and on the activities of mitochondrial enzymes in the epididymis of the rat. *J. Endocrinol.*, 82:293–303.
522. Brandes, D. (1974): Fine structure and cytochemistry of male accessory sex organs. In: *Male Accessory Sex Organs, Structure and Function in Mammals*, edited by D. Brandes, pp. 18–113. Academic Press, New York.
523. Orgebin-Crist, M.-C., and Davies, J. (1974): Functional and morphological effects of hypophysectomy and androgen replacement in the rabbit epididymis. *Cell Tissue Res.*, 148:183–201.
524. Flickinger, C. J. (1977): The influence of progestin and androgen on the fine structure of the male reproductive tract of the rat. II. Epididymis and sex accessory glands. *Anat. Rec.*, 187:431–462.

525. Bohmer, T., Weddington, S. C., and Hansson, V. (1977): Effect of testosterone propionate on levels of carnitine and testicular androgen binding protein (ABP) in rat epididymis. *Endocrinology,* 100:835–838.
526. Pholpramool, C., White, R. W., and Setchell, B. P. (1982): Influence of androgens on inositol secretion and sperm transport in the epididymis of the rat. *J. Reprod. Fertil.,* 66:547–553.
527. Rastogi, R. K., Milone, M., Di Meglio, M., Caliendo, M. F., and Chieffi, G. (1979): Effects of castration, 5α-dihydrotestosterone and cyproterone acetate on enzyme activity in the mouse epididymis. *J. Reprod. Fertil.,* 57:73–77.
528. Moore, H. D. M. (1981): Effects of castration on specific glycoprotein secretions of the epididymis in the rabbit and hamster. *J. Reprod. Fertil.,* 61:347–354.
529. Mayorga, L. S., and Bertini, F. (1982): Effect of androgens on the activity of acid-hydrolases in rat epididymis. *Int. J. Androl.,* 5:345–352.
530. Robaire, B., and Hales, B. F. (1982): Regulation of epididymal glutathione S-transferases: Effects of orchidectomy and androgen replacement. *Biol. Reprod.,* 26:559–565.
531. Orgebin-Crist, M.-C., Jahad, N., and Hoffman, L. H. (1976): The effects of testosterone, 5α-dihydrotestosterone, 3α-androstanediol, and 3β-androstanediol on the maturation of rabbit epididymal spermatozoa in organ culture. *Cell Tissue Res.,* 167:515–525.
532. Cohen, J., Ooms, M. P., and Vreeburg, J. T. M. (1981): Reduction of fertilizing capacity of epididymal spermatozoa by 5α-steroid reductase inhibitors. *Experientia,* 37:1031–1032.
533. De Larminat, M. A., Monsalve, A., Charreau, E. H., Calandra, R. S., and Blaquier, J. A. (1978): Hormonal regulation of 5α-reductase activity in rat epididymis. *J. Endocrinol.,* 79:157–165.
534. Foldesy, R. G., and Leathem, J. H. (1981): Effects of short-term bilateral and unilateral castration and androgen replacement on the metabolism of [^{3}H]testosterone *in vitro* by the epididymis of the immature rat. *J. Endocrinol.,* 91:53–60.
535. Robaire, B., and Zirkin, B. R. (1981): Hypophysectomy and simultaneous testosterone replacement: Effects on male reproductive tract and epididymal Δ^4-5α-reductase and 3α-hydroxysteroid dehydrogenase. *Endocrinology,* 109:1225–1233.
536. Hansson, V., Trygstad, O., French, F. S., McLean, W. S., Smith, A. A., Tindall, D. J., Weddington, S. C., Petrusz, P., Nayfeh, S. N., and Ritzen, E. M.(1974): Androgen transport and receptor mechanisms in testis and epididymis. *Nature,* 250:387–391.
537. Ritzen, E. M., Nayfeh, S. N., French, F. S., and Dobbins, M. C. (1971): Demonstration of androgen-binding components in rat epididymis cytosol and comparison with binding components in prostate and other tissues. *Endocrinology,* 89:143–151.
538. Hansson, V. Djøseland, O., Reusch, E., Attramadal, A., and Torgensen, O. (1973): Intracellular receptor for 5α-dihydrotestosterone in the epididymis of the adult rats. Comparison with the androgenic receptor in the ventral prostate and the androgen binding protein (ABP) in the testicular and epididymal fluid. *Steroids,* 22:19–33.
539. Danzo, B. J., Orgebin-Crist, M.-C., and Toft, D. O. (1973): Characterization of a cytoplasmic receptor for 5α-dihydrotestosterone in the caput epididymidis of intact rabbits. *Endocrinology,* 92:310–317.
540. Younes, M., Evans, B. A. J., Chaisiri, N., Valotaire, Y., and Pierrepoint, C. G. (1979): Steroid receptors in the canine epididymis. *J. Reprod. Fertil.,* 56:45–52.
541. Younes, M. A., and Pierrepoint, C. G. (1981): Androgen steroid-receptor binding in the canine epididymis. *Prostate,* 2:133–142.
542. Carreau, S., Drosdowsky, M. A., and Courot, M. (1984): Androgen-binding proteins in sheep epididymis: Characterization of a cytoplasmic androgen receptor in the ram epididymis. *J. Endocrinol.,* 103:273–279.
543. Tindall, D. J., Hansson, V., McLean, W. S., Ritzen, E. M., Nayfeh, S. N., and French, F. S. (1975): Androgen-binding proteins in rat epididymis: Properties of a cytoplasmic receptor for androgen similar to the androgen receptor in ventral prostate and different from androgen-binding protein (ABP). *Mol. Cell. Endocrinol.,* 3:83–101.
544. Pujol, A., and Bayard, F. (1979): Androgen receptors in the rat epididymis and their hormonal control. *J. Reprod. Fertil.,* 56:217–222
545. Tindall, D. J., Hansson, V., Sar, M., Stumpf, W. E., French, F. S., and Nayfeh, S. N. (1974): Further studies on the accumulation and binding of androgens in rat epididymis. *Endocrinology,* 95:1119–1128.
546. Danzo, B. J., and Eller, B. C. (1975): Androgen binding to cytosol prepared from epididymides of sexually mature castrated rabbits: Evidence for a cytoplasmic receptor. *Steroids,* 25:507–525.
547. King, W. J., and Greene, G. L. (1984): Monoclonal antibodies localize oestrogen receptor in the nuclei of target cells. *Nature,* 307:745–747.
548. Welshons, W. V., Lieberman, M. E., and Gorski, J. (1984): Nuclear localization of unoccupied oestrogen receptors. *Nature,* 307:747–749.
549. Fabre, F., Carreau, S., and Drosdowsky, M. A. (1979): Androgen binding protein (ABP) was demonstrated in testicular and epididymal cytosols of adult guinea pig. *Ann. Endocrinol.,* 40:15–16.
550. Danzo, B. J., Dunn, J. C., and Davies, J. (1982): The presence of androgen-binding protein in the guinea-pig testis, epididymis and epididymal fluids. *Mol. Cell. Endocrinol.,* 28:513–527.
551. Carreau, S., Drosdowsky, M. A., and Courot, M. (1979): Age related effects on androgen binding protein (ABP) in sheep testis and epididymis. *Int. J. Androl.,* 2:49–61.
552. Carreau, S., Drosdowsky, M. A., Pisselet, C., and Courot, M. (1980): Hormonal regulation of androgen-binding protein in lamb testes. *J. Endocrinol.,* 85:443–448.
553. Hsu, A. F., and Troen, P. (1978): An androgen-binding protein in the testicular cytosol of human testis: comparison with human testosterone estrogen binding globulin. *J. Clin. Invest.,* 61:1611–1619.
554. Gunsalus, G. L., Musto, N. A., and Bardin, C. W. (1978): Immunoassay of androgen binding protein in blood: A new approach for the study of the seminiferous tubule. *Science,* 200:65–66.
555. Musto, N. A., Larrea, F., Cheng, S.-L., Kotite, N., Gunsalus, G., and Bardin, C. W. (1982): Extracellular androgen-binding proteins: Species comparison and structure-function relationships. *Ann. NY Acad. Sci.,* 383:343–359.
556. Schmidt, W. N., Taylor, C. A., Jr., and Danzo, B. J. (1981): The use of the photoaffinity ligand to compare androgen-binding protein (ABP) present in rat Sertoli cell culture media with ABP present in epididymal cytosol. *Endocrinology,* 108:786–794.
557. Weddington, S. C., Brandtzaeg, P., Hansson, V., French, F. S., Petrusz, P., Nayfeh, S. N., and Ritzen, E. M. (1975): Immunological crossreactivity between testicular androgen binding protein and serum testosterone binding globulin. *Nature,* 258:257–259.
558. Danzo, B. J., and Eller, B. C. (1985): The ontogeny of biologically active androgen-binding protein in rat plasma, testis, and epididymis. *Endocrinology,* 117:1380–1388.
559. Anthony, C. T., Danzo, B. J., and Orgebin-Crist, M.-C. (1984): Investigations on the relationship between sperm fertilizing ability and androgen-binding protein in the restricted rat. *Endocrinology,* 114:1413–1418.
560. Tindall, D. J., Cunningham, G. R., and Means, A. R. (1978): 5α-Dihydrotestosterone binding to androgen binding protein. *J. Biol. Chem.,* 253:166–169.
561. Cunningham, G. R., Tindall, D. J., and Means, A. R. (1979): Differences in steroid specificity for rat androgen binding protein and the cytoplasmic receptor. *Steroids,* 33:261–276.
562. Lobl, T. J., Campbell, J. A., Tindall, D. J., Cunningham, G. R., and Means, A. R. (1980): A model for the mechanism of androgen binding, transport, and translocation to the nucleus. In: *Testicular Development, Structure, and Function,* edited by A. Steinberger and E. Steinberger, pp. 323–330. Raven Press, New York.
563. Kirchhoff, J., Soffie, M., and Rousseau, G. G. (1979): Differences in the steroid-binding site specificities of rat prostate androgen receptor and epididymal androgen-binding protein (ABP). *J. Steroid Biochem.,* 10:487–497.
564. Grayhack, J. T. (1965): Effect of testosterone-estradiol administration on citric acid and fructose content of rat prostate. *Endocrinology,* 76:1168–1174.
565. Steinberger, E., and Duckett, G. E. (1965): The effect of estrogen or testosterone on the initiation and maintenance of spermatogenesis in the rat. *Endocrinology,* 76:1184–1189.
566. Gay, V. L., and Dever, N. W. (1971): Effects of testosterone propionate and estradiol benzoate—alone or in combination—on serum LH and FSH in orchidectomized rats. *Endocrinology,* 89:161–168.
567. Oshima, H., Wakabayashi, K., and Tamaoki, I. (1967): The effect of synthetic estrogen on the biosynthesis *in vitro* of androgen and LH in the rat. *Biochim. Biophys. Acta,* 137:356–366.
568. Andersson, M., and Muntzing, J. (1972): The effect of a long-acting estrogen on the activity and distribution of some hydrolases in the

ventral prostate of intact, castrated, and androgen treated castrated adult rats. *Invest. Urol.,* 9:401–407.
569. Swerdloff, R. S., and Walsh, P. C. (1973): Testosterone and oestradiol suppression of LH and FSH in adult male rats: duration of castration, duration of treatment and combined treatment. *Acta Endocrinol.,* 73:11–21.
570. Chowdhury, M., Tcholakian, R., and Steinberger, E. (1974): An unexpected effect of oestradiol-17β on LH and testosterone. *J. Endocrinol.,* 60:375–376.
571. Karr, J. P., Kirdani, R. Y., Murphy, G. P., and Sandberg, A. A. (1974): Effects of testosterone and estradiol on ventral prostate and body weights of castrated rats. *Life Sci.,* 15:501–513.
572. Verjans, H. L., DeJong, F. H., Cooke, B. A., Van der Molen, H. J., and Eik-Nes, K. B. (1974): Effect of oestradiol benzoate on pituitary and testis function in the normal and adult male rat. *Acta Endocrinol.,* 77:636–642.
573. Ewing, L. L., Desjardins, C., Irby, D. C., and Robaire, B. (1977): Synergistic interaction of testosterone and oestradiol inhibits spermatogenesis in rats. *Nature,* 269:409–411.
574. Orgebin-Crist, M.-C., Eller, B. C., and Danzo, B. J. (1983): The effects of estradiol, tamoxifen, and testosterone on the weights and histology of the epididymis and accessory sex organs of sexually immature rabbits. *Endocrinology,* 113:1703–1715.
575. Meistrich, M. L., Hughes, T. J., and Bruce, W. R. (1975): Alteration of epididymal sperm transport and maturation in mice by oestrogen and testosterone. *Nature,* 258:145–147.
576. Robaire, B., Ewing, L. L., Irby, D. C., and Desjardins, C. (1979): Interactions of testosterone and estradiol-17β on the reproductive tract of the male rat. *Biol. Reprod.,* 21:455–463.
577. Van Beurden-Lamers, W. M. O., Brinkmann, A. L., Mulder, E., and Van der Molen, H. J. (1974): High-affinity binding of oestradiol-17β by cytosols from testis interstitial tissue, pituitary, adrenal, liver and accessory sex glands of the male rat. *Biochem. J.,* 140:495–502.
578. Danzo, B. J., Wolfe, M. S., and Curry, J. B. (1977): The presence of an estradiol binding component in cytosol from immature rat epididymides. *Mol. Cell. Endocrinol.,* 6:271–279.
579. Danzo, B. J., Sutton, W., and Eller, B. C. (1978): Analysis of [^{3}H] estradiol binding to nuclei prepared from epididymides of sexually immature intact rabbits. *Mol. Cell. Endocrinol.,* 9:291–301.
580. Danzo, B. J., and Eller, B. C. (1979): The presence of a cytoplasmic estrogen receptor in sexually mature rabbit epididymides: Comparison with the estrogen receptor in immature rabbit epididymal cytosol. *Endocrinology,* 105:1128–1134.
581. Danzo, B. J., Eller, B. C., and Hendry, W. J. (1983): Identification of cytoplasmic estrogen receptors in the accessory sex organs of the rabbit and their comparison to the cytoplasmic estrogen receptor in the epididymis. *Mol. Cell. Endocrinol.,* 33:197–209.
582. Hendry, W. J., Eller, B. C., Orgebin-Crist, M.-C., and Danzo, B. J. (1985): Hormonal effects on the estrogen receptor system in the epididymis and accessory sex organs of sexually immature rabbits. *J. Steroid Biochem.,* 23:39–49.
583. Younes, M. A., and Pierrepoint, C. G. (1981): Estrogen steroid-receptor binding in the canine epididymis. *Andrologia,* 13:562–572.
584. Murphy, J. B., Emmott, R. C., Hicks, L. L., and Walsh, P. C. (1980): Estrogen receptors in the human prostate, seminal vesicle, epididymis, testis, and genital skin: A marker for estrogen-responsive tissues. *J. Clin. Endocrinol. Metabol.,* 50:938–948.
585. Cunha, G. R., Chung, L. W. K., Shannon, J. M., and Reese, B. A. (1980): Stromal-epithelial interactions in sex differentiation. *Biol. Reprod.,* 22:19–42.
586. Wong, P. Y. D., and Lee, W. M. (1982): Effects of spironolactone (aldosterone antagonist) on electrolytes and water content of the cauda epididymidis and fertility of male rats. *Biol. Reprod.,* 27:771–777.
587. Jenkins, A. D., Lechene, C. P., and Howards, S. S. (1983): The effect of spironolactone on the elemental composition of the intraluminal fluids of the seminiferous tubules, rete testis and epididymis of the rat. *J. Urol.,* 129:851–854.
588. Hinton, B. T., and Keeper, D. A. (1985): Binding of [^{3}H] aldosterone to a single population of cells within the rat epididymis. *J. Steroid Biochem.,* 23:231–233.
589. Turner, T. T., and Cesarini, D. M. (1983): The ability of the rat epididymis to concentrate spermatozoa: Responsiveness to aldosterone. *J. Androl.,* 4:197–202.
590. Corvol, P., Michaud, A., Menard J., Freifeld, M., and Mahoudeau, J. (1975): Antiandrogenic effect of spirolactones: Mechanism of action. *Endocrinology,* 97:52–58.
591. Nicoll, C. S. (1975): Physiological actions of prolactin. In: *The Handbook of Physiology, Sec. 7, Vol. 4,* edited by R. O. Greep and E. B. Astwood. American Physiological Society, Washington, D. C.
592. Bartke, A., Smith, M. S., Michael, S. D., Peron, F. G., and Dalterio, S. (1977): Effects of experimentally induced chronic hyperprolactinemia on testosterone and gonadotropin levels in male rats and mice. *Endocrinology,* 100:182–186.
593. Nikolics, K., Mason, A. J., Szonyi, E., Ramachandran, J., and Seeburg, P. H. (1985): A prolactin-inhibiting factor within the precursor for human gonadotropin-releasing hormone. *Nature,* 316:511–517.
594. Aragona, C., and Friesen, H. G. (1975): Specific prolactin binding sites in the prostate and testis of rats. *Endocrinology,* 97:677–684.
595. Shiu, R. P. C., and Friesen, H. G. (1980): Mechanism of action of prolactin in the control of mammary gland function. *Annu. Rev. Physiol.,* 42:83–96.
596. De Luca, H. F. (1978): The hormonal nature of vitamin D function. In: *Hormones and Cell Regulation, Vol. 2,* edited by J. Dumont and J. Nunez, pp. 249–270. Elsevier/North-Holland, Amsterdam.
597. Ong, D. E., and Chytil, F. (1975): Retinoic acid-binding proteins in rat tissue. *J. Biol. Chem.,* 250:6113–6117.
598. Ong, D. E., Crow, J. A., and Chytil, F. (1982): Radioimmunochemical determination of cellular reinol- and cellular retinoic acid-binding proteins in cytosols of rat tissues. *J. Biol. Chem.,* 257:13385–13389.
599. Kato, M., Blaner, W. S., Mertz, J. R., Das, K., Kato, K., and Dewitt, S. (1985): Influence of retinoid nutritional status on cellular retinol- and cellular retinoic acid-binding protein concentrations in various rat tissues. *J. Biol. Chem.,* 260:4832–4838.
600. Porter, S. B., Ong, D. E., Chytil, F., and Orgebin-Crist, M.-C. (1985): Localization of cellular retinol-binding protein and cellular retinoic acid-binding protein in the rat testis and epididymis. *J. Androl.,* 6:197–212.
601. Wilson, J. D. (1975): Metabolism of testicular androgens. In: *Handbook of Physiology, Sec. 7, Vol. 5,* edited by R. O. Greep and E. B. Astwood, pp. 491–508. American Physiological Society, Washington, D.C.
602. Robaire, B. (1979): Effects of unilateral orchidectomy on rat epididymal Δ^4-5α-reductase and 3α-hydroxysteroid dehydrogenase. *Can. J. Physiol. Pharmacol.,* 57:998–1003.
603. Brown, D. V., and Amann, R. P. (1984): Influence of androgen binding protein (ABP) on testosterone metabolism in cultured ram epididymal principal cells. *Biol. Reprod.,* 30:[Suppl. 1]:82.
604. Orgebin-Crist, M.-C., and Tichenor, P. L. (1972): A technique for studying sperm maturation *in vitro. Nature,* 239:227–228.
605. Dufaure, J. P., Gigon, A., and Gathier, C. (1972): L'épididyme de lézard en culture *in vitro:* un nouveau système pour étudier le mode d'action des hormones androgènes. *CR Soc. Biol.,* 166: 366–379.
606. Blaquier, J. A. (1973): An *in vitro* action of androgens on protein synthesis by epididymal tubules maintained in organ culture. *Biochem. Biophys. Res. Commun.,* 52:1177–1183.
607. Blaquier, J. A., and Breger, D. (1974): The *in vitro* effects of androgens on RNA synthesis by cultured rat epididymal tubules. *Endocr. Res. Commun.,* 1:247–260.
608. Orgebin-Crist, M.-C., and Jahad, N. (1979): The maturation of rabbit epididymal spermatozoa in organ culture: Stimulation by epididymal cytoplasmic extracts. *Biol. Reprod.,* 21:511–515.
609. Orgebin-Crist, M.-C., and Menezo, Y. (1980): A continuous flow method for organ culture of rabbit epididymis: Morphology, amino acid utilization, glucose uptake, RNA, and protein synthesis. *J. Androl.,* 1:289–298.
610. Wong, P. Y. D., Au, C. L., and Ngai, H. K. (1980): The isolated duct of the rat cauda epididymidis as a model for isoosmotic transport studies. *Jpn. J. Physiol.,* 30:1–15.
611. Klinefelter, G. R., and Hamilton, D. W. (1984): Organ culture of rat caput epididymal tubules in a perifusion chamber. *J. Androl.,* 5:243–258.
612. Brooks, D. E. (1975): The isolation of epithelial cells from the rat epididymis. *Andrologia,* 7:241–253.

613. Killian, G. J., Snyder, J., and Amann, R. P. (1977): Unit gravity sedimentation separation of cells comprising the caput epididymidis of the rat. *Cell Tissue Res.*, 183:371–378.
614. Klinefelter, G. R., and Amann, R. P. (1980): Isolation of principal cells and basal cells by elutriation of suspensions of rat epididymal tissue. *Int. J. Androl.*, 3:287–300.
615. Kierzenbaum, A. L., Lea, O., Petrusz, P., French, F. S., and Tres, L. L. (1981): Isolation, culture, and immunocytochemical characterization of epididymal epithelial cells from pubertal and adult rats. *Proc. Natl. Acad. Sci. USA.*, 78:1675–1679.
616. Killian, G. J. (1981): A rapid and simple method for isolating principal cells from the rat caput epididymidis. *J. Androl.*, 5:255–258.
617. Olson, G. E., and Jonas-Davies, J., Hoffman, L. H., and Orgebin-Crist, M.-C. (1983): Structural features of cultured epithelial cells from the adult rat epididymis. *J. Androl.*, 4:347–360.
618. Wagley, L. M., Versluis, T. D., Brown, D. V., and Amann, R. P. (1984): Culture of principal cells from the ram epididymis. A comparison of the morphology of principal cells in culture and *in situ*. *J. Androl.*, 5:389–408.
619. Joshi, M. S. (1985): Isolation and cell culture of the epithelial cells of cauda epididymidis of the bull. *Biol. Reprod.*, 33:187–200.
620. Blaquier, J. A., Breger, D., Cameo, M. S., and Calandra, R. (1975): The activation of cultured epididymal tubules by androgens. *J. Steroid Biochem.*, 6:573–576.
621. Robaire, B., and Buchanan, L. J. (1985): The use of epididymal cell and organ culture in toxicology. In: *In Vitro Embryotoxicity and Teratogenicity Tests,* edited by F. Homburger and A. M. Goldberg, pp. 114–129. Karger, Basel.
622. Orgebin-Crist, M.-C., Jahad, N., and Hoffman, L. H. (1977): Effects of antiandrogens on 5α-dihydrotestosterone induced maturation of epididymal spermatozoa in organ culture. In: *Androgens and Antiandrogens,* edited by L. Martini and M. Motta, pp. 105–113. Raven Press, New York.
623. Orgebin-Crist, M.-C., and Jahad, N. (1978): The maturation of rabbit epididymal spermatozoa in organ culture: Inhibition by antiandrogens and inhibitors of ribonucleic acid and protein synthesis. *Endocrinology,* 103:46–53.
624. Cuasnicu, P. S., Echeverria, F. G., Piazza, A., and Blaquier, J. A. (1984): Addition of androgens to cultured hamster epididymis increases zona recognition by immature spermatozoa. *J. Reprod. Fertil.*, 70:541–547.
625. Blaquier, J. A. (1975): The influence of androgens on protein synthesis by cultured rat epididymal tubules. *Acta Endocrinol.*, 79:403–416.
626. Klinefelter, G. R., and Hamilton, D. W. (1985): Synthesis and secretion of proteins by perifused caput epididymal tubules, and association of secreted proteins with spermatozoa. *Biol. Reprod.*, 33:1017–1027.
627. Fain-Maurel, M.-A., Dadoune, J. P., and Jauzein-Leau, F. (1983): Protein secretion by the principal cells of mouse epididymis evidenced by *in vitro* incorporation of tritiated leucine. *Reprod. Nutr. Dev.*, 23:175–182.
628. Wenstrom, J. C., and Hamilton, D. W. (1984): Synthesis and secretion of proteins *in vitro* by isolated epithelial strips from the proximal and distal vas deferens of the rat. *Int. J. Androl.*, 7:215–235.
629. Killian, G. J., Amann, R. P., and Synder, J. (1976): Isolation of principal and basal cells from the epithelium of the hamster caput epididymidis by unit gravity sedimentation. *Biol. Reprod.*, 15:266–279.
630. Olson, G. E., Jonas-Davies, J., Hoffman, L. H., and Orgebin-Crist, M.-C. (1982): Structural characterization of isolated rat epididymal epithelial cells. *Gamete Res.*, 6:161–178.
631. Killian, G. J., and Chapman, D. A. (1980): Glycerylphosphorylcholine, sialic acid and protein in epithelial cells isolated from the rat caput epididymidis by elutriation. *Biol. Reprod.*, 22:846–850.
632. Orgebin-Crist, M.-C., Jonas-Davies, J., Storey, P., and Olson, G. E. (1984): Effect of D-valine and cytosine arabinoside on [^{3}H] thymidine incorporation in rat and rabbit epididymal epithelial cell cultures. *In Vitro,* 20:45–52.
633. Byers, S. W., Musto, N. A., and Dym, M. (1985): Culture of ciliated and nonciliated cells from rat ductuli efferentes. *J. Androl.*, 6:271–278.
634. Hoffmann, D. S., and Killian, G. J. (1981): Isolation of epithelial cells from the corpus epididymidis and analysis for glycerylphosphorylcholine, sialic acid, and protein. *J. Exp. Zool.*, 217:93–102.
635. Klinefelter, G. R., Amann, R. P., and Hammerstedt, R. H. (1982): Culture of principal cells from the rat caput epididymidis. *Biol. Reprod.*, 26:885–901.
636. Byers, S. W., Hadley, M. A., Djakiew, D., and Dym, M. (1986): Growth and characterization of polarized monolayers of epididymal epithelial cells and Sertoli cells in dual environment culture chambers. *J. Androl.*, 7:59–68.
637. Flickinger, C. J. (1977): Influence of antifertility agents on the fine structure of the male reproductive tract. In: *Male Reproductive System,* edited by R. D. Yates and M. Gordon, pp. 57–78. Masson, New York.
638. Nag, S., and Ghosh, J. J. (1979): Epididymal and testicular enzymes as monitors for assessment of male antifertility drugs. *J. Steroid Biochem.*, 11:681–686.
639. Ratnasooriya, W. D. (1982): Effects of drugs on the epididymis. *J. Sci. Industr. Res.*, 41:455–461.
640. Cummins, J. M., and Orgebin-Crist, M.-C. (1974): Effects of antiandrogen SK&F 7690 on the fertility of epididymal spermatozoa in the rabbit. *Biol. Reprod.*, 11:56–63.
641. Hib, J., and Ponzio, R. O. (1977): Effects of cyproterone acetate on spontaneous contractility of the rat epididymis. *Andrologia,* 9:329–331.
642. Rastogi, R. K. (1979): A critical appraisal of the effects of the antiandrogen, cyproterone acetate, on the epididymis in connection with fertility control in the male. *J. Steroid Biochem.*, 11:101–105.
643. Thampan, T. N. R. V., Dinakar, N., and Prasad, M. R. N. (1980): Anti-androgenic action of cyproterone acetate in the epididymis of the Rhesus monkey. *Experientia,* 36:361–362.
644. Agarwal, A., and Dominic, C. J. (1984): Effect of cyproterone acetate on the epididymis of the Indian palm squirrel, *Funambulus pennanti wroughton. Arch. Biol.*, 95:199–214.
645. Shimazaki, J., Ohki, Y., Koya, A., and Shida, K. (1972): Inhibition of nuclear testosterone 5α-reductase in rat ventral prostate by estrogens and anti-androgens. *Endocrinol. Jpn.*, 19:585–588.
646. Dupuy, G. M., Roberts, K. D., Bleau, G., and Chapdelaine, A. (1978): Steroidal inhibitors of prostatic 5α-reductase: Structure-activity relationships. *J. Steroid Biochem.*, 9:1043–1047.
647. Blohm, T. R., Metcalf, B. W., Laughlin, M. E., Sjoerdsma, A., and Schatzam, G. L. (1980): Inhibition of testosterone 5α-reductase by a proposed enzyme-activated, active site-directed inhibitor. *Biochem. Biophys. Res. Commun.*, 95:273–280.
648. Petrow, V., and Lack, L. (1981): Studies on a 5α-reductase inhibitor and their therapeutic implications. In: *Prostatic Cell: Structure and Function,* edited by G. P. Murphy, A. A. Sandberg and J. P. Karr, pp. 283–297. Liss, New York.
649. Rasmusson, G. H., Liang, T., and Brooks, J. R. (1983): Androgens: Pharmacodynamics and antagonists. Biochemical and biological studies with 4-aza-steroidal 5α-reductase inhibitors. *J. Steroid Biochem.*, 19:385–390.
650. Rasmusson, G. H., Liang, T., and Brooks, J. R. (1983): A new class of 5α-reductase inhibitors. In: *Gene Regulation by Steroid Hormones II,* edited by A. K. Roy and J. H. Clark, pp. 311–334. Springer-Verlag, New York.
651. Dean, H. J., and Winter, J. S. D. (1984): The effect of 5 synthetic progestational compounds on 5α-reductase activity in genital skin fibroblast monolayer. *Steroids,* 43:13–24.
652. Rasmusson, G. H., Reynolds, G. F., Utne, T., Jobson, R. B., Primka, R. L., Berman, C., and Brooks, J. R. (1984): Azasteroids as inhibitors of rat prostatic 5α-reductase. *J. Med. Chem.*, 27:1690–1701.
653. Liang, T., Brooks, J. R., Cheung, A., Reynolds, G. F., and Rasmusson, G. H. (1984): 4-Azasteroids as inhibitors of 5α-reductase. In: *Hormones and Cancer 2,* edited by F. Bresciani, J. B. K. King, M. E. Lippman, M. Namer, and J. P. Raynaud, pp. 497–505. Raven Press, New York.
654. Kadohama, N., Wakisaka, M., Kim, U., Karr, J. P., Murphy, G. P., and Sandberg, A. A. (1985): Retardation of prostate tumor progression in the noble rat by 4-methyl-4-aza-steroidal inhibitors of 5α-reductase. *J. Natl. Cancer Inst.*, 74:475–486.
655. Robaire, B., Covey, D. F., Robinson, C. H., Ewing, L. L. (1977): Selective inhibition of rat epididymal steroid Δ^4-5α-reductase by

conjugated allenic 3-oxo-5,10-secosteroids. *J. Steroid Biochem.*, 8:307–310.

656. Cooke, G. M., and Robaire, B. (1986): The effects of diethyl-4-methyl-3-oxo-4-aza-5α-androstane-17β-carboxamide (4-MA) and (4R)-5,10-seco-19-norpregna-4,5-diene-3,10,20-trione (SECO) on androgen biosynthesis in the rat testis and epididymis. *J. Steroid Biochem.* 24:877–886.
657. Robaire, B., Duron, J., and Lobl, T. J. (1986): Inhibition of epididymal 4-ene-5α-reductase (5α-R) and 3α-hydroxysteroid dehydrogenase (3α-HSD) by 17-substituted chloroformate androgen analogs. *J. Androl.*, 7:20P.
658. Batzold, F. H., Covey, D. F., and Robinson, C. H. (1977): Effects of novel acetylenic and allenic steroids on the rat prostate. *Cancer Treat. Rep.*, 61:255–257.
659. Brooks, J. R., Berman, C., Hichens, M., Primka, R. L., Reynolds, G. F., and Rasmusson, G. H. (1982): Biological activities of a new steroidal inhibitor of Δ^4-5α-reductase (41309). *Proc. Soc. Exp. Biol. Med.*, 169:67–73.
660. Jones, A. R. (1978): The antifertility actions of α-chlorohydrin in the male. *Life Sci.*, 23:1625–1646.
661. Jackson, H., and Robinson, B. (1976): The antifertility effects of α-chlorohydrins and their stereo-isomers in male rats. *Chem. Biol. Interact.*, 13:193–197.
662. Lobl, T. J. (1980): α-Chlorohydrin: Review of a model post-testicular antifertility agent. In: *Regulation of Male Fertility*, edited by G. R. Cunningham, W. B. Schill, and E. S. E. Hafez, pp. 109–122. Martinus Nijhoff, Netherlands.
663. Brown-Woodman, P. D. C., Mohri, H., Mohri, T., Suter, D., and White, I. G. (1978): Mode of action of α-chlorohydrin as a male anti-fertility agent. Inhibition of the metabolism of ram spermatozoa by α-chlorohydrin and location of block in glycolysis. *Biochem. J.*, 170:23–27.
664. Ford, W. C. L., and Harrison, A. (1983): The activity of glyceraldehyde 3-phosphate dehydrogenase in spermatozoa from different regions of the epididymis in laboratory rodents treated with α-chlorohydrin or 6-chloro-deoxyglucose. *J. Reprod. Fertil.*, 69: 147–156.
665. Ford, W. C. L., Harrison, A., and Waites, G. M. H. (1977): Effects of optical isomers of α-chlorohydrin on glycolysis by ram testicular spermatozoa and the fertility of male rats. *J. Reprod. Fertil.*, 51:105–109.
666. Reijonen, K., Kormano, M., and Ericsson, R. J. (1975): Studies on the rat epididymal blood vessels following alpha-chlorohydrin administration. *Biol. Reprod.*, 12:483–490.
667. Ford, W. C. L., and Waites, G. M. H. (1982): Activities of various 6-chloro-6-deoxysugars and (S)-α-chlorohydrin in producing spermatocoeles in rats and paralysis in mice and in inhibiting glucose metabolism in bull spermatozoa. *J. Reprod. Fertil.*, 65:177–183.
668. Wong, P. Y. D., Yeung, C. H., and Ngai, H. K. (1977): Effect of α-chlorohydrin on transport processes in perfused rat cauda epididymides. *Contraception*, 16:637–644.
669. Wong, P. Y. D., Yeung, C. H. (1977): Inhibition by α-chlorohydrin of fluid reabsorption in the rat cauda epididymidis. *J. Reprod. Fertil.*, 51:469–471.
670. Wong, P. Y. D., Au, C. L., Ngai, H. K. (1980): Effects of 6-chloro-6-deoxyglucose on electrolyte and water transport in the epididymis and fertility of male rats. *Int. J. Androl.*, 3:82–86.
671. Kirton, K. T., Ericsson, R. J., Ray, J. A., and Forbes, A. D. (1970): Male antifertility compounds: Efficacy of U-5897 in primates (*Macaca mulatta*). *J. Reprod. Fertil.*, 21:275–278.
672. Ford, W. C. L., and Waites, G. M. H. (1978): Chlorinated sugars: a biochemical approach to the control of male fertility. *Int. J. Androl.*, [Suppl.2]:541–564.
673. Ford, W. C. L., and Harrison, A. (1981): The effect of 6-chloro-6-deoxysugars on adenine nucleotide concentrations in and motility of rat spermatozoa. *J. Reprod. Fertil.*, 63:75–79.
674. Segal, S. J. (1985): *Gossypol: A potential contraceptive for men.* Plenum Press, New York.
675. Hoffer, A. P. (1985): Ultrastructural, biochemical, and endocrine studies on the effects of gossypol and its isomeric derivatives on the male reproductive tract. In: *Gossypol: A potential contraceptive for men*, edited by S. J. Segal, pp. 143–186. Plenum Press, New York.
676. Trasler, J. M., Hales, B. F., and Robaire, B. (1985): Paternal cyclophosphamide treatment of rats causes fetal loss and malformations without affecting male fertility. *Nature*, 316:144–146.
677. Trasler, J. M., Hales, B. F., and Robaire, B. (1986): Chronic low dose cyclophosphamide treatment of adult male rats: effect on fertility, pregnancy outcome and progeny. *Biol. Reprod.*, 34: 275–283.
678. Trasler, J. M., Hermo, L., and Robaire, B. (1985): Chronic paternal treatment of male rats with cyclophosphamide (CPA) affects epididymal and spermatozoal histology and pregnancy outcome. *Biol. Reprod.*, 32[Suppl.1]:76.
679. Cooke, G. M., and Robaire, B. (1987): The mechanism of rat epididymal 4-ene steroid 5α-reductase. *J. Steroid Biochem.*, 26: 361–368.

The Physiology of Reproduction,
edited by E. Knobil and J. Neill *et al.*
Raven Press, Ltd., New York © 1988.

CHAPTER 24

Androgen Action and the Sex Accessory Tissues

Donald S. Coffey

One of the leading frontiers in mammalian reproductive physiology is the requirement for more definitive studies and a clearer understanding of the role of the male sex accessory tissues such as the prostate, seminal vesicles, ampullary, and bulbourethral (Cowper's) glands (see Fig. 1). This need for further research is exemplified by the following five considerations:

1. Evolutionary Variation

Of the many different types of mammalian organs, the greatest variation between species is observed in the anatomy, biology, and function of the sex accessory tissues. For example, the seminal vesicles are large and prominent glands in the human and rat, but seminal vesicles are not present in the cat and dog. Although the presence of the prostate is universal in mammals, when compared between species the prostate is marked by tremendous variations in its anatomy, biochemistry, and pathology. For example, the rat prostate is characterized by distinct and separate anatomical lobes such as the dorsal, ventral, and lateral, each with separate functions; however, in the human and dog, these corresponding anatomical lobes are not apparent but may exist only as zones in what anatomically appears to be a single uniform prostate. The sex accessory tissues also produce secretions that form the ejaculate volume, and even this varies dramatically between species for no known reason. For example, the volume of boar ejaculate is approximately 250 ml, the stallion 70 ml, dog 9 ml, bull 4 ml, human 3 ml, and the ram only 1 ml. Human ejaculate clots and then lyses, whereas in many rodents a solid copulatory plug is ejaculated. Not only is there a vast variation in anatomical features and in secretion volumes, but this variation is also reflected in the biochemical composition of the glandular secretions and combined ejaculate. In the human ejaculate the major anion is citrate ion (4 mg/ml), whereas in the dog seminal plasma it is chloride ion. In summary, within mammals, no organ has such anatomical and biochemical diversity as the sex accessory tissues. The evolutionary and physiological reasons for this large variation might shed insight into the functions of these mysterious glands because it is difficult to understand why such changes should only be limited to sex accessory tissues. Although it might be argued that this variation has no biological meaning, this is difficult to accept and it might be suggested that the great diversity of environments and reproductive habits of mammals regulates different sex accessory functions to protect their genitourinary tracts from invasion by pathogens of external insult. Much speculation will always be generated until firm evidence is presented to explain these large biological differences between sex accessory tissues of various species.

2. Sex Accessory Tissues Are the Major Mammalian Organ with Unknown Functions

To date, we have no firm insight into the specific biological functions of the prostate, seminal vesicles, and bul-

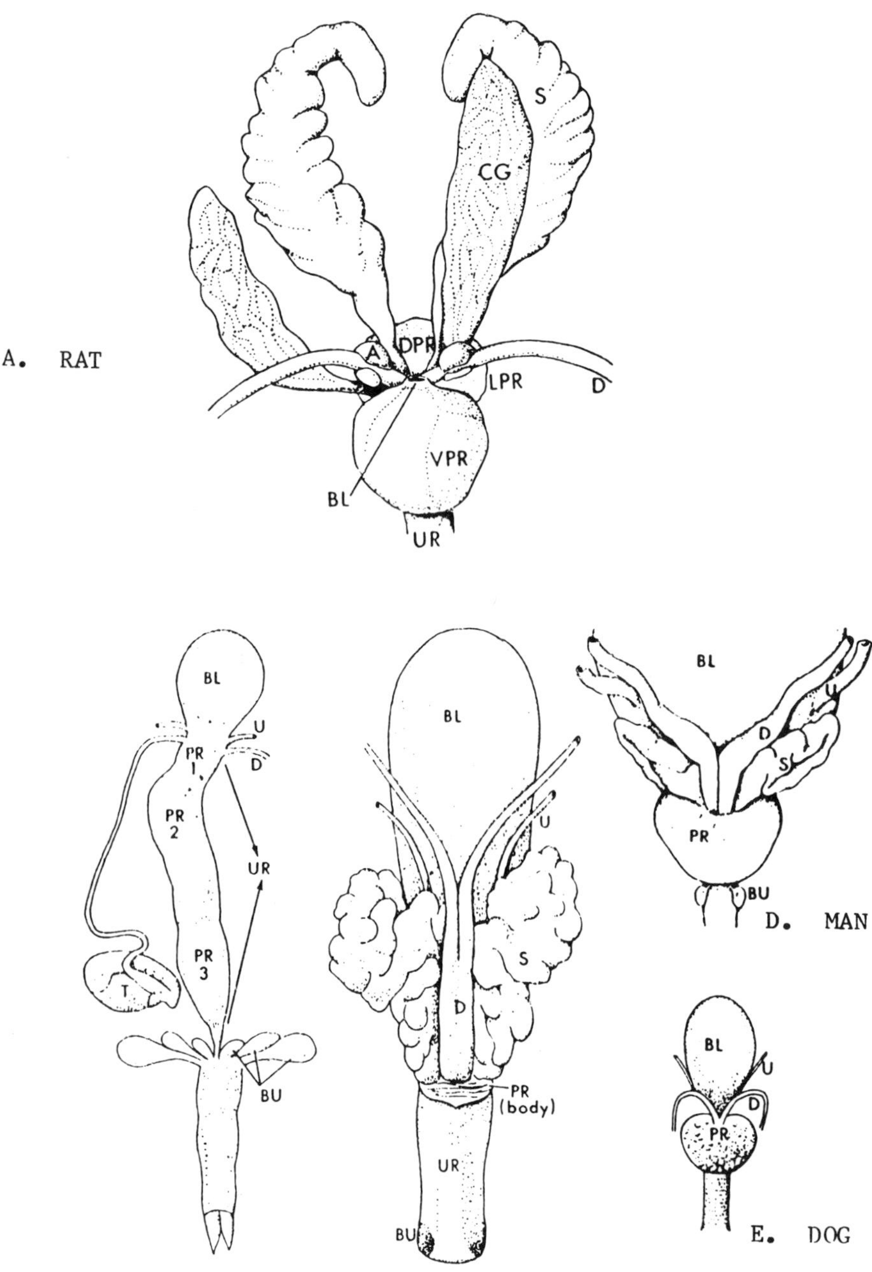

FIG. 1. Comparative anatomy of the sex accessory tissue from the: (**A**) rat; (**B**) opossum; (**C**) bull; (**D**) man; (**E**) dog. (BL) Bladder (which was removed in the rat schematic); (BU) bulbourethral gland; (D) ductus deferens; (DPR) dorsal prostate; (LPR) lateral prostate; (PR) prostate; (S) seminal vesicle; (T) testis; (U) ureter; (UR) urethra; (VPR) ventral prostate. (Adapted from ref. 310.)

bourethral (Cowper's) glands other than the simple observation that they produce the volume of the seminal plasma. The secretions of these glands constitute most of the volume and chemical composition of the seminal plasma; fluids from other parts of the male reproductive tract comprise less than 1% of the total semen volume. The sex accessory tissues produce extremely high concentrations of important and potent biological substances such as prostaglandins (now known to be from the seminal vesicle secretions, 200 μg/ml, but first mistakenly believed to be derived solely from the prostate gland—and thus the misnomer), fructose, citric acid, polyamines [such as spermine (3 mg/ml) and spermidine], and extremely high concentrations of zinc (150 μg/ml) and enzymes such as proteases and acid phosphatases at extremely high activities. At present, we have no clear knowledge of the physiological functions of any of these potent secretory products in the seminal plasma. Many investigators even question the necessity for these sex accessory secretions in the fertilization process, since in some mammals it has been observed that sperm removed from the epididymis are capable of fertilizing the ovum; therefore, the sperm are capable of fertilization without ever having made contact with the secretions of the prostate or seminal vesicles. In addition, the surgical removal of either the ventral prostate or seminal vesicles (but not both) in the rat does not abolish male fertility. Although the seminal plasma may not contain factors that are absolutely essential for fertilization, the secretions may nevertheless optimize conditions for sperm motility, survival, and transport in both the male and female reproductive tracts, but this has not been proven.

When we compare our ignorance of the function of these large sex accessory glands in mammals with our more complete knowledge of the function and biochemistry of the heart, kidney, and adrenal glands, the importance for more physiological and biochemical experiments on the sex accessory glands becomes apparent.

3. *Transport of Biological Components into and out of the Seminal Plasma*

What biological materials can be transported back and forth between the serum and the ejaculate? Our knowledge of the mechanisms and types of transport of ions, drugs, and natural products into and out of the secretions of the sex accessory tissues is very sparse. Of all the secretory glands in the body, the sex accessory gland has received the least study and yet may be one of the most important areas because this could be of great potential reproductive and therapeutic importance.

4. *Mechanism of Androgen Action*

A simple literature search will quickly demonstrate that there are almost an order of magnitude more research papers published on estrogen receptors than on androgen receptors. Indeed, compared to all of the published reports on steroid receptors, the androgen receptor has been the least studied and the least understood. Purification, cloning, and monoclonal antibodies to the androgen receptor are being eagerly awaited and should be available very soon. It is hard to understand why research on androgens has lagged so far behind estrogen, progesterone, and glucocorticoid studies. This past lack of emphasis on androgen-related research in almost every biological and physiological area is most surprising and difficult to rationalize, but it does need to be corrected by additional attention in the future.

5. *Pathology of the Prostate*

The diseases caused by pathology of one of the sex accessory tissues, the prostate, are some of the most common and devastating diseases in the male. For example, abnormal overgrowth (hyperplasia) of the human prostate will occur in over 80% of the male population before the age of 80, and 25% will require surgery at some time in their lives to alleviate urinary obstruction caused by this overgrowth (1). This enlargement, called benign prostatic hyperplasia (BPH), is the cause of over 300,000 surgical procedures each year in the United States, thus making BPH the *second leading cause of surgery* in the male. The surgically related costs of these operations exceed $1 billion per year in the United States. This high cost does not include the loss of time from work and the suffering of the millions with symptoms of BPH which are insufficiently severe to require surgery. As common as BPH is, the amount of research attention has been very small.

Prostate cancer is far less common than BPH but far more deadly. Prostate cancer is the second leading cause of cancer deaths in the American male, and there are 86,000 new cases each year and 26,000 deaths. This is small compared to the great potential that exists because 10% to 30% of all males over 50 years of age have pathological evidence of latent prostate cancer cells within their glands at the time of autopsy. It is apparent that over 11 million of these latent forms of prostate cancer that presently exist in the U.S. male will remain smoldering or silent and never manifest themselves within the lifetime of the patient. Why does this tremendous amount of latent prostate cancer remain dormant within our male population? Why is there so little prostate cancer clinically manifested in the Orient but almost the same amount of the dormant forms existing at autopsy?

Surprisingly, all of these abnormalities of prostate growth, including BPH and prostate cancer, are common only to humans and dogs (2). It is a mystery as to why the bull, horse, ram, cat, rodent, and all other species are essentially free of these prostate disease processes. In comparison, it is also not understood why in humans the prostate gland should be such a common site within the sex accessory tissues for these diseases, while the seminal vesicles are almost devoid of any significant incidence of abnormal growth such as benign or malignant hyperplasia. On first examination, it would appear that both the prostate and seminal vesicles receive the same endogenous hormones and, because of proximity, might be subjected to the same pathological insults by carcinogens and pathogens. Some believe the difference could be due to the embryonic origins: The prostate arises from the urogenital sinus, and the seminal vesicles arise from the Wolffian ducts. Whether the marked difference in pathology of the prostate and seminal vesicles also resides in intrinsic factors in the gland or within extrinsic physiological or pathological factors must obviously await further study and understanding.

In summary, the purpose of this general overview is to bring to the reader's attention some of the important problems with respect to the sex accessory tissues and to challenge them with regard to the importance of further studies of the sex accessory tissue to elucidate the normal and abnormal physiology of these most important glands. These are not only critical questions for reproduction and evolution, but also ones central to many important medical and social problems. The remainder of this chapter will attempt to provide the reader with a basic and selected review that will assist in the assessment of our present progress as well as areas that need further investigation. This chapter will be composed of the following two major sections: The first one will review the mechanism of androgen action on sex accessory tissue, and the second one will review the structure and function of the sex accessory tissues.

MECHANISM OF ANDROGEN ACTION ON SEX ACCESSORY TISSUES

Overview of the Biological Effects of Androgens

In 1786 John Hunter, the great English experimental surgeon, was the first to recognize that castration of an animal led to regression or involution in the size of the male sex accessory tissues (3). About 150 years passed before, in the 1930s, it could be shown that the substance that caused growth of the sex accessory tissue was an active factor from the testes called *testosterone*. When the substance was injected into a castrated animal, one could observe restoration of the size of the sex accessory tissues to that which had existed in intact animals. Indeed, any substance that is injected into a castrated animal that causes growth of the sex accessory tissue is defined as having *androgenic activity*. Essentially every compound thus far discovered that has androgenic activity has proven to be a steroid type of molecule. In contrast, the administration of any substance to an immature female that causes the uterus to grow is termed an *estrogen,* and there are many compounds, both natural and synthetic, that have estrogenic properties but that are not steroids. Why should androgenic activity be essentially limited to steroid-like structures whereas estrogenic activity can be present in a variety of structures?

It now appears that testicular functioning produces testosterone, which is the primary androgen that is metabolized to various forms in the body and that affects a wide range of virilization and hormone-induced changes. Androgens affect the embryonic development of the male sex accessory tissues and external genitalia *in utero* and then cause descent of the testes and later produce neonatal imprinting. This neonatal imprinting affects the brain and the aggressive nature of the animal as well as later functions of the sex accessory tissues. Androgens also feed back on the pituitary to regulate their own growth, and many of these brain functions involve the conversion of testosterone to estradiol through the aromatase reaction. At puberty and in adults, androgens also affect spermatogenesis as well as the growth and secretions of the sex accessory tissues such as the seminal vesicles, prostate, and bulbourethral gland. These glands, which require androgen for the maintenance of their size as well as their development, growth, and function, are called *secondary sex organs*. Androgens also function outside of the male reproductive tract in affecting the kidney, where they can induce modest growth and account for the fact that the male kidney is larger than the female kidney. Renal enzymes such as β-glucuronidase and ornithine decarboxylase can be induced by androgens in the mouse, where they affect certain cells that have specific responses. Androgens also affect the liver of many species, including the human, where they induce a wide variety of enzymes that are involved in steroid metabolism and overall drug processing such as the cytochrome P-450-containing enzymes. It appears that androgens can neonatally imprint the enzymatic profile of the liver and that androgens are also constantly involved in the liver for the maintenance of certain steroid hydroxylase enzymes. Therefore, androgens are involved in neonatal imprinting and, later, in producing the steroid pattern of metabolism that is associated with the male. Other proteins besides steroid-metabolizing enzymes are induced by androgens in the liver. These include α_2-macroglobulin, a protein that is found almost exclusively in male rat liver and is clearly regulated by androgen. Other nonreproductive tissues are affected by androgens. For example, the vocal cords are thickened at the time of puberty, and overall body muscle can be induced to increase its mass in the presence of androgens. This is termed the *anabolic action of androgens,* and great effort was devoted to the development of androgens that cause anabolic effect while minimizing the virilization effects. 19-Nortestosterone and its derivatives are examples of anabolic steroids. This is the basis for the steroids used by athletes, weight lifters, or football linemen that require heavy muscle mass or body weight. We do not know what the long-term impact of this practice of taking androgens in sports might be.

Androgens also affect erythropoiesis and have therefore been used to treat certain types of anemias. Many of these latter androgens are 5β metabolites of testosterone rather than the 5α metabolites that affect prostate growth. Androgens affect skin sebaceous secretions and the salivary glands in some species. Androgens stimulate long bone growth and subsequent induction of epiphyseal plate closure at puberty. The effects of androgens on the skeletal, connective tissue, and hair growth have also been related to reproductive processes such as growth of antlers, and, in birds, the growth of beaks and combs. The role of androgens in these many biological processes, as well as in the development of male aggressive behavior and libido, are complex issues that will not be addressed in this section on the mechanism of androgen action. Instead, we will focus our attention on androgen-induced growth of the male sex accessory tissues, with primary emphasis on the prostate because it is of such great medical importance; it will serve as a model for the way that androgens also affect other sex accessory tissues such as the seminal vesicles.

We will follow the fate of testicular testosterone, including its transport and metabolism on route to the prostate. Then we will examine the role of testosterone within the prostate by tracing its metabolism and androgen binding to receptors and its subsequent effects within the nucleus in altering gene function and in inducing DNA replication, both of which result in androgen-induced growth and function in sex accessory tissues.

Endocrine Control of Prostate Growth

Endocrine Overview

The human prostate weighs about 25 g and is located at the base of the bladder. The epithelial cells provide secretions that empty through ducts into the urethra to form a major component of the seminal plasma of the ejaculate. The prostate is stimulated to grow and is maintained in size and function by the presence of serum testosterone. The effect of the endocrine glands on the prostate is depicted in Fig. 2, where the hypothalamus releases a decapeptide referred to as LHRH (acronym for luteinizing-hormone-releasing hormone); it is alternatively called GnRH (acronym for gonadotropin-releasing hormone). Under the stimulation of LHRH, the pituitary releases the luteinizing hormone (LH) that acts directly on the testes to stimulate the steroid synthesis of testosterone, which is the major serum androgen stimulating prostatic growth. Most of the estrogen in the male is derived from peripheral conversion of testosterone to estrogens through an enzymatic aromatization reaction. Estrogens do not block androgen action on the prostate. The ability of therapeutic estrogens to diminish prostatic growth is not a direct effect, but indirect through blocking pituitary function and decreasing LH, which subsequently inhibits testicular testosterone production. Therapeutic estrogen is an effective "chemical castration," a term referring to the essential abolishment of circulatory androgen by estrogen administration. Other factors stimulating prostate growth include adrenal androgens formed from androstenedione; however, this is not a major pathway because, in animals and humans, castration leads to almost complete involution of the prostate, which means that adrenal androgens are not present in sufficient amounts to stimulate any meaningful growth of the prostate. Only when the adrenals are stimulated by adrenocorticotropic hormone (ACTH) or are overactive do they have any significant effect in stimulating prostatic growth.

Prolactin has often been postulated to enhance androgen-induced growth (4–9); however, several decades of study have failed to indicate the mechanism of this action, but it does not appear at present to be a major means of regulating normal prostatic growth.

Several protein-type growth factors have been reported to affect prostate growth. Of endocrine origin is insulin, and of paracrine and autocrine type is the prostatic growth factor (10–16).

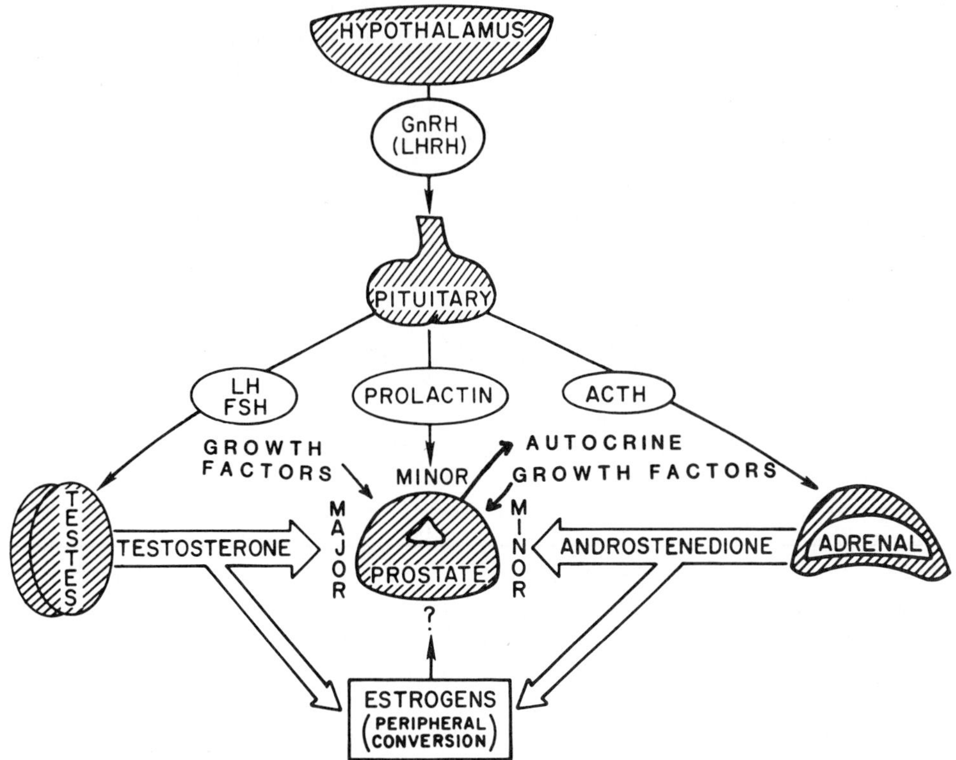

FIG. 2. A schematic of factors affecting the growth of the prostate. (GRH) Gonadotropin-releasing hormone; (LH) luteinizing hormone; (FSH) follicle-stimulating hormone; (ACTH) adrenocorticotropic hormone; growth factors are present in the serum; autocrine growth factors are protein factors released within the prostate that function either by autocrine or paracrine mechanisms. The schematic indicates that prolactin and the adrenal glands have only minor effects on prostate growth, whereas the effects of estrogens are still not established. (Adapted from ref. 309.)

Androgen Production by the Testes

Because the testes produce the major serum androgen supporting prostate and sex accessory tissue growth, it is important to briefly review this function. In the normal human male, the major circulating serum androgen is testosterone, which is almost exclusively (more than 95%) of testicular origin. Under normal physiological conditions the Leydig cells of the testis are the major source of the testicular androgens. The Leydig cells are stimulated by the gonadotropins (primarily LH) to synthesize testosterone from acetate and cholesterol. The spermatic vein concentration of testosterine is 40 to 50 μg/100 ml and is approximately 75 times more concentrated than the level detected in the peripheral venous serum (17), which is approximately 600 ng of testosterone/100 ml. Other androgens also leave the testes by the spermatic vein, and these include androstanediol, androstenedione (3 μg/100 ml), dehydroepiandrosterone (7 μg/100 ml), and dihydrotestosterone (at 0.4 μg/100 ml); therefore, the concentrations of these androgens are much lower than testosterone, with all being less than 15% of that of testosterone.

The total testosterone that enters the plasma is referred to as the *testosterone blood production rate* and is 6 to 7 mg/day in the human. Although other steroids, such as androstenedione from the adrenals, can be converted by peripheral metabolism to testosterone, they probably account for less than 5% of the overall production of plasma testosterone. The mean metabolic clearance rate for testosterone is around 1,000 liters per 24 hr and results in a plasma half-life of only 10 to 20 min.

The average testosterone concentration in the adult human male plasma is approximately 611 ng/100 ml ± 186 and is not greatly related to age between 25 and 70 years, although it does decline gradually to approximately 500 mg/100 ml after 70 years of age. It is recognized that plasma concentrations of testosterone can vary widely in an individual during the course of the day and may reflect both episodic and diurnal variations in the production rate of testosterone.

Only 2% of the total serum testosterone is not protein bound; this is termed the *free testosterone in the plasma,* and it is at a concentration of approximately 15 ng/100 ml or less than 1 nM. It is only this free testosterone that is available for metabolism by the liver and intestines, primarily to 17-ketosteroids, which are then secreted into the urine as final water-soluble conjugates of sulfuric acid and glucuronic acid (Fig. 3). The total 17-ketosteroids in the urine in adult males is from 4 to 25 mg per 24 hr and is not an accurate index of testosterone production, since other steroids from the adrenals as well as nonandrogenic steroids can be metabolized to 17-ketosteroids. Only small (25–160 μg/day) amounts of testosterone enter the urine without metabolism, and this urinary testosterone represents less than 2% of the daily testosterone production.

Although testosterone is the primary plasma androgen that induces growth of the prostate gland and other sex accessory tissues, it appears to function as a prohormone in that the active form of the androgen in the prostate is not testosterone but a metabolite (Fig. 3), *dihydrotestosterone* (DHT) (18–22). The formation of dihydrotestosterone involves the reduction of the double bond in the A ring of testosterone through the enzymatic action of the enzyme 5α-reductase. This conversion can take place directly in the prostate and seminal vesicles or in peripheral tissues. Dihydrotestosterone concentration in the plasma of normal men is very low, 56 ± 20 ng/100 ml, in comparison to testosterone, which is 11-fold higher at approximately 611 ng/100 ml (see Table 1). In summary, although dihydrotestosterone is a potent androgen (1.5 to 2.5 times as potent as testosterone in most bioassay systems), its low plasma concentration and tight binding to plasma proteins diminish its direct importance as a circulating androgen affecting prostate and seminal vesicle growth. In contrast, dihydrotestosterone is of paramount importance for growth within the prostate, where it is formed from testosterone. Dihydrotestosterone is the major form of androgen found within the prostate gland (5 ng/g tissue wet weight), and its concentration is fivefold higher than testosterone, whose concentration is 1 ng/g. In the prostate, DHT binds to specific androgen receptors and is transported into the nucleus, where approximately 100,000 DHT molecules reside per nucleus. In summary, DHT becomes the major androgen regulating the cellular events of growth, differentiation, and function in the prostate.

The plasma levels of some important steroids are summarized in Table 1. These values are derived as averages from several combined sources (23–26). The complete biologic importance of many of these steroids circulating in the plasma has not been determined.

Androgen Production by the Adrenals

There is evidence that hyperstimulation of the adrenal cortex causes the production of adrenal steroids that stimulate the growth of the prostate gland. For example, in humans, abnormal virilism has been observed in immature males with hyperfunction of the adrenal cortex resulting from neoplasia or hyperplasia of the adrenal gland. In rodents, overstimulation of the adrenals can also induce lim-

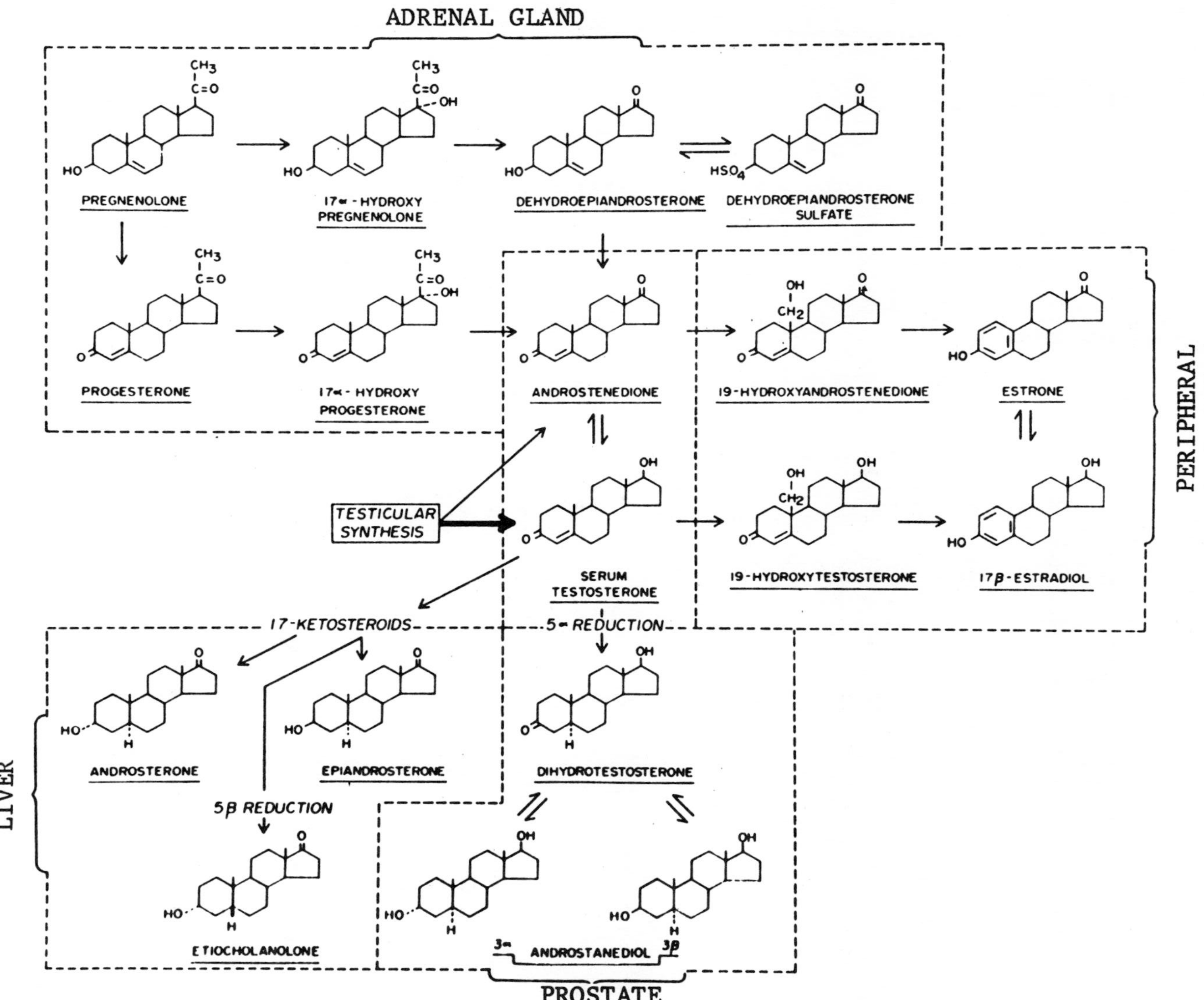

FIG. 3. The metabolism of testosterone in various organs and compartments. The adrenal gland contributes to androgens primarily through androstenedione. Both adrostenedione and serum testosterone are converted to estrogens by peripheral aromatase reactions. Serum testosterone enters the prostate gland, where it is metabolized to the androgens DHT, 3α-androstanediol, or 3β-androstanediol. Testosterone enters the liver, where it is converted to the 17-ketosteroids (309).

TABLE 1. *Average plasma levels of sex steroids in healthy human males*[a]

Steroid (common name)	Plasma concentration ng/100 ml	Plasma concentration Relative molarity	Daily blood production rate (mg/day)	Relative androgenicity rat VP assay[b]
Testosterone	611 ± 186	100	6.6 ± 0.5	100
Dihydrotesterone (DHT)	56 ± 20	9	0.3 ± 0.06	181
5α-Androstane-3α,17β-diol (3α-androstanediol)	14 ± 4	2	0.2 ± 0.03	126
5α-Androstane-3β,17β-diol (3β-androstanediol)	<2	<0.3		18
Androstenediol	161 ± 52	26		0.21
Androsterone	54 ± 32	9	0.28	53
Androstenedione	150 ± 54	25	1.4	39
Dehydroepiandrosterone (DHEA)	501 ± 98	81	29	15
Dehydroepiandrosterone sulfate (DHEAS)	135,925 ± 48,000	17,619		<1
Progesterone	30	4.5	0.75	
17β-Estradiol (E_2)	2.5 ± 0.8	0.4	0.045	
Estrone	4.6	0.8		

[a]Adapted from ref. 309.
[b]VP assay, ventral prostate growth in castrated rat.

ited prostate growth, even in the absence of testicular androgens. For example, administration of exogenous ACTH to castrated animals does significantly increase the growth of sex accessory tissue (27–29). Such ACTH stimulation of prostatic growth has been observed in both castrated and castrated-hypophysectomized animals, but does not occur in animals that are adrenalectomized (27).

The effect of normal levels of adrenal androgens on the prostate in noncastrated humans and adult male rats may not be significant because adrenalectomy has very little effect on prostate size, DNA, or morphology of the sex accessory tissue (30–32). Furthermore, following castration in animals, the prostate diminishes to a very small size (90% reduction in cell mass) without concomitant adrenalectomy. Finally, the small involuted ventral prostate in the castrated rat cannot be significantly reduced further by performing additional adrenalectomy or hypophysectomy (33). In rats that are castrated, the DHT level in the prostatic tissue is approximately 20% of that in normal intact animals. Adrenalectomy lowers the DHT to nondetectable levels without further diminution in prostate growth (33). This indicates that a threshold level of DHT is required in the prostate to stimulate growth and that the castrate level is below this threshold. It has also been concluded similarly that the human prostate does not restore itself following castration, indicating that adrenal androgens are insufficient to compensate for the loss of testicular function. Quantitative morphometry of the human prostate (30) also confirms that the adrenal gland has little effect on the prostate.

The adrenal steroids (dehydroepiandrosterone and the conjugate dehydroepiandrosterone sulfate) and androstenedione are androgens that are synthesized from acetate and cholesterol (Fig. 3) and that are secreted by the normal human adrenal glands. Essentially all of the dehydroepiandrosterone in the male plasma is of adrenal cortex origin, and the production rate in the human male is 10 to 30 mg/day. Less than 1% of the total testosterone in the plasma is derived from dehydroepiandrosterone (34–36).

The prostate and seminal vesicles of the rat, as well as the human prostate, can slowly hydrolyze dehydroepiandrosterone sulfate (DHEAS) to free steroids through a prostate sulfatase enzymatic activity, but the degree of 5α-conversion is low, thereby explaining why DHEAS is not a very potent androgen.

A second adrenal androgen is androstenedione, and the plasma concentration in adult males is approximately 150 ± 54 ng/100 ml (Table 1). The blood production rate of androstenedione in human males is about 2 to 6 mg/day, with approximately 20% of the androstenedione being generated by peripheral metabolism of other steroids. Androstenedione cannot be converted directly to DHT and therefore is a weak androgen. An important role for androstenedione in the male may be its peripheral conversion to estrogens through the aromatase reaction (see Fig. 3).

The adrenal gland also produces C_{21} steroids (e.g., progesterone). The plasma production rate (0.75 mg/day) is low, producing a low plasma progesterone concentration of 30 ng/100 ml. Although progesterone is weakly androgenic, it does not exert a significant effect on the prostate at the low concentrations present in normal male plasma. In summary, under normal conditions the adrenals do not support significant growth of prostatic tissue.

The Peripheral Production of Estrogens in Males

Only small amounts of estrogen are produced directly by the testes. Approximately 75% to 90% of the estrogens in the plasma of young healthy human males is derived from the peripheral conversion of androstenedione and testosterone to estrone and estradiol via the aromatase reaction (34,36). The pathways for the peripheral synthesis of the estrogens in the male are depicted in Fig. 3. The androgenic C_{19} steroids (testosterone and androstenedione) are converted to the estrogenic C_{18} steroids by removing the 19-methyl group and by subsequently forming an aromatic or phenolic steroid A ring (aromatase reaction), present in both estradiol and estrone. Estradiol is formed from testosterone, and estrone is formed from androstenedione; these two estrogens are then interconvertible. The daily production of estradiol in the human male is about 40 to 50 μg, and only 5 to 10 μg (10–25%) can be accounted for by direct testicular secretion (34,36,37). The dynamics of the synthesis of estrogens in human males have been quantitated by Siiteri and MacDonald (37), who showed that of 7.0 mg of testosterone produced in the human male each day, 0.35% was converted directly to estradiol, forming 24 μg/day. Of the 2.5 mg of androstenedione produced per day, 1.7% was converted to estrone, producing 42 μg/day. The interconversion of estrone and estradiol yielded a final total peripheral production of approximately 40 μg of estradiol per day. The exact location in the periphery where estrogen production occurs has not been elucidated on a quantitative basis, but it is believed that most of the daily production may involve adipose tissue. The small amount of estrogens secreted directly from the testes may originate, in part, from the Sertoli cells, since in culture these cells respond to follicle-stimulating-hormone (FSH) stimulation by producing small amounts of estradiol (38); in the adult rat the Leydig cell may be the source of estradiol.

Men over 50 years of age may have an increase in total plasma estradiol levels of approximately 50%, with minimal change (less than 10%) in the free estradiol levels because of increases in binding of the estradiol by elevated serum testosterone-estrogen-binding globulin (TeBG) levels, which are also age-related (39–41). An age-related decrease in the plasma free testosterone level, while the free estradiol level is maintained, produces a 40% increase in the free estradiol/free testosterone ratio (39–41). It is apparent that the availability of estrogens and androgens in the serum is regulated not only by their total level but also by the free level (i.e., unbound). Since the steroid-binding proteins in the serum can regulate the free levels, it is important to understand how they function.

Androgen-Binding Proteins in the Plasma

The great bulk of serum steroids do not circulate free in males but are reversibly bound to a variety of serum proteins. Less than 2% of the total testosterone in human plasma is free or unbound, and the remaining 98% is bound to several different types of plasma proteins (Fig. 4). The plasma proteins that bind steroids include human serum

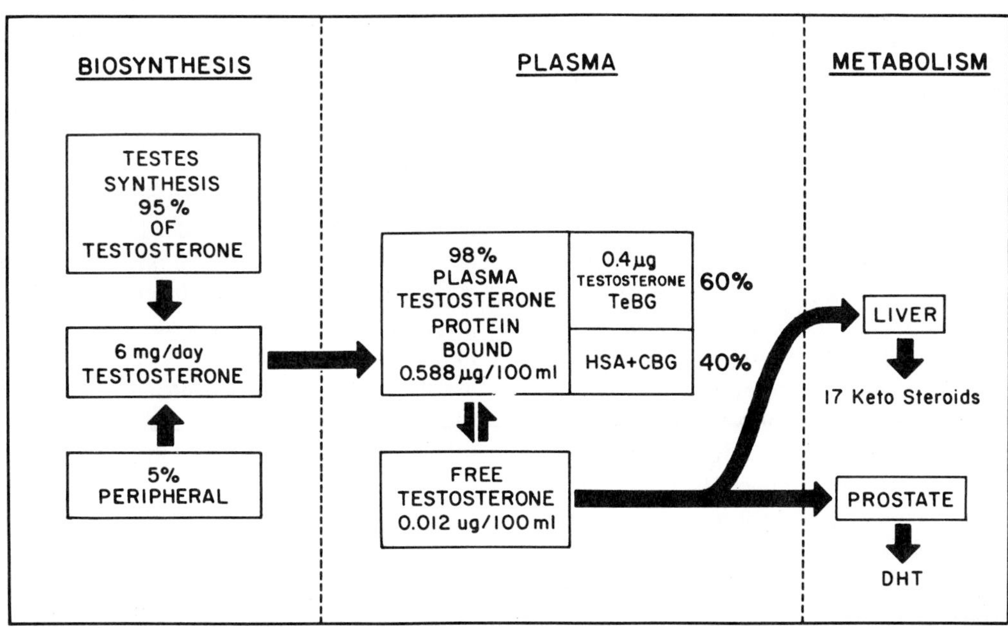

FIG. 4. The biosynthesis, plasma concentrations, and metabolism of testosterone. The left panel indicates the daily production of 6 mg/day of testosterone that is formed 95% by the testes and 5% by peripheral synthesis. This testosterone enters the plasma, where it is present at a circulating level of 600 ng/100 ml. This is equivalent to 0.6 μg/dl. Ninety-eight percent of serum testosterone is bound to plasma proteins. Free testosterone enters the liver and prostate for further metabolism to 17-ketosteroids and DHT, respectively.

albumin, testosterone-estrogen-binding globulin (denoted TeBG; also denoted SBG, the acronym for steroid-binding globulin), corticosteroid-binding globulin (CBG, also called *transcortin*), progesterone-binding globulin (PBG), and, to a lesser extent, the alpha-acid glycoprotein (AAG). The total amount of testosterone bound to PBG and AAG is not large and is usually ignored.

The regulation of the amount of androgen that is free is an important physiological variable and varies in different species. The total amount of bound steroid depends on two factors: (i) the *affinity* of the steroid to bind to a specific protein, and (ii) the *capacity,* which is the maximal potential binding when all of a binding protein is saturated with bound steroid; the capacity is governed by the amount of binding protein in the plasma. Serum albumin has a relatively low affinity for testosterone, but because albumin is at high concentration in the plasma, it can bind appreciable quantities of testosterone. Therefore, albumin is termed a low-affinity, high-capacity binding protein. In contrast, steroid-binding globulin (SBG or TeBG) that has been isolated from plasma has a high affinity for binding steroids, but the protein is present in relatively low concentrations; however, the plasma molarity of each binding protein exceeds the plasma molarity for total testosterone concentration. The majority of testosterone bound to plasma protein is associated with TeBG (39). For example, Vermeulen (40) has calculated that in the normal human male, 57% of testosterone in the plasma is bound to TeBG; 40% is bound to human serum albumin. Less than 1% is bound to CBG, and only 2% of the total testosterone is free (see Fig. 4). The normal plasma free testosterone level is therefore 12.1 $\pm$ 3.7 ng/100 ml or 0.42 nM; this non-protein-bound "free testosterone" is available to diffuse into the sex accessory tissue and into liver cells for metabolism. In addition, a large percentage of the TeBG is saturated, whereas only a small fraction of the total capacity of CBG and albumin is utilized under normal conditions. As testosterone levels increase in the plasma, the order of increasing saturation of the plasma proteins proceeds from TeBG to CBG to albumin (42). Therefore the binding of androgen is a dynamic equilibrium between various serum proteins.

The total plasma levels of TeBG can be altered by hormone therapy. Administration of testosterone decreases TeBG levels in the plasma, whereas estrogen therapy stimulates TeBG levels (39,43–47). Estrogen also competes with testosterone for binding to TeBG, but estrogen has only one-third the binding affinity of testosterone. Therefore, administration of small amounts of estrogen increases the total concentration of TeBG, and this effectively increases the binding of testosterone and thus lowers the free testosterone plasma concentration.

Testosterone enters sex accessory tissue (e.g., the prostate cell) in the free form, and the binding of testosterone to plasma proteins inhibits the uptake into the prostate (48). It is apparent that androgenic activity is regulated, in part, by the extent of binding of an androgen to the steroid-binding proteins in the plasma. Indeed, Anderson et al. (49) have postulated that altered testosterone binding to plasma proteins might produce amplified changes in free estrogen and androgen levels, and this could be an important factor in inducing gynecomastia and impotence.

The exact physiologic function of TeBG in the human male is not known, although the plasma concentration is inversely related to the rate of testosterone metabolism [metabolic clearance rate (MCR)]; this is because free testosterone is the form metabolized by the liver (311). In addition, estrogen therapy increases the level of TeBG and lowers the metastatic clearance rate of testosterone (50). This may be explained by the fact that estrogen treatment increases the amount of TeBG and thus increases the percentage of plasma testosterone that is protein bound; therefore, there is a reduction in the amount of free testosterone in the plasma that is available either to the liver for metabolism or to the prostate for androgenic stimulation.

The Effects of Prolactin on Growth

Exogenous androgens can restore 80% of the normal adult prostate size in hypophysectomized rats. To obtain full restoration with androgens in these hypophyectomized rats, supplements of exogenous prolactin were required (4,5). This observation has been confirmed in numerous animal experiments, in which prolactin was shown to be synergistic with androgens on prostate growth (6–8,51). In addition, prolactin increases zinc uptake in the tissue (52), alters androgen uptake and metabolism (6–8,53), and regulates citric acid and fructose levels. Prolactin receptors have been identified in prostatic tissue (9,54). Prolactin has a permissive effect on the growth of the lateral prostate of the rat, and this may be associated with increased nuclear androgen levels (6–8).

It is of interest that some cellular growth factors have homology with prolactin. Indeed, Lee and colleagues (7,55) have suggested that prolactin may enhance rat lateral prostate growth by an androgen-independent pathway, since hyperprolactin levels caused a decrease in the DHT levels in the lateral prostate while increasing growth. It is well known that the prostate contains an abundance of prolactin receptors (8,54). The direct action of prolactin on prostate epithelial cells has also been suggested through tissue and organ culture experiments (8,56).

The aforementioned evidence that prolactin affects prostatic growth in animals has led to much speculation about a similar role in humans. Prolactin levels in human blood are elevated with estrogens, some tranquilizing drugs, and stress, and can be decreased by L-DOPA and ergot derivatives. With improved assays, the levels are being monitored in patients of advanced age and in those with benign prostatic hyperplasia, but no clear correlation of cause of prostate pathology and prolactin effect is yet apparent (57).

Insulin

Many other common growth factors have been known to affect sex accessory tissue growth. For example, insulin has been reported to have synergistic or permissive effects on prostatic growth, but these data have been obtained previously in rodents and often in tissue or organ culture (8,56,58). Angervall et al. (59) and Sufrin and Prutkin (60) have demonstrated that diabetic castrated rats have a diminished response to exogenous androgens that can be restored with supplements of insulin, and these findings support the earlier conclusions of Calame and Lostroh (61) and Lostroh (62), who found that insulin was required for androgen response of the mouse prostate in organ culture. There is little information on the possible role of insulin in the growth of the human prostate. Recent focus on insulin-like growth factors in many tissues and cell types leaves open the importance of these factors on the growth of sex accessory tissue. In summary, most attention on endocrine factors regulating sex accessory tissue growth has focused on androgenic substances, and the above studies on prolactin and insulin force us to broaden our studies beyond steroids.

Regulation of Prostatic Growth at the Cellular Level

Overview

It now appears that direct cell-cell communication as well as growth and endocrine factors is at the forefront of biological regulation of sex accessory tissue. This is usually accomplished by several factors, as partly depicted in Fig. 5, and they include: (a) *endocrine factors* or long-range signals arriving at the prostate by serum transport from distant organs; this would include serum hormone-like steroids such as testosterone and estrogens, serum polypeptide hormones such as prolactin, and insulin, as discussed above; (b) *paracrine factors* or soluble tissue growth factors that stimulate or inhibit (chalones) growth that are elaborated over short ranges between cells within the prostate tissue compartment; (c) *autocrine factors,* which are soluble factors that are released by a cell and feed back on the same cell to regulate growth; and (d) *direct structural factors* that are insoluble and make direct and coupled contact between epithelial and stromal cells occurring through membrane junctions on intramembrane proteins attached to the basal membrane or extracellular matrix. These coupled and interlocking structural components form the important interacting system, termed the *tissue matrix,* that was first discussed by Isaacs et al. (63). Of the above four systems, the best understood have been the endocrine effects of androgenic steroid in the regulation of prostatic growth via changes in serum testosterone levels. Although we will concentrate on this latter system, it must be remembered that rapid progress is likely to be made in the autocrine, paracrine, and structural control of accessory sex organ growth and function in the near future.

In the serum, testosterone is bound to albumin and to the

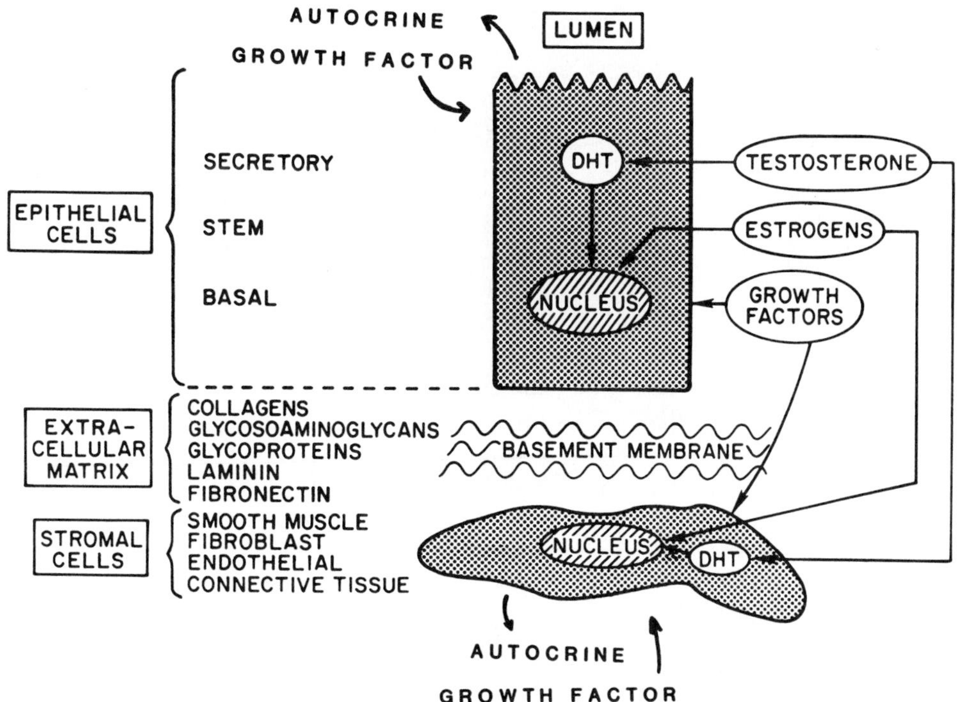

FIG. 5. The tissue organization of the epithelial and stromal cells separated by the basement membrane and extracellular matrix. The epithelial cells are made up of mature tall columnar secretory cells and stem cells that are located at the basement membrane and are called *basal cells.* Testosterone and estrogen affect both the epithelial and stromal cells as well as the production of growth factors that have both paracrine effects and autocrine effects on the same types of cells.

steroid-binding globulins, as depicted in Fig. 6. Only the free testosterone enters the prostate cell by diffusion, where it is then subjected to a variety of steroid metabolic steps that appear to regulate the activity and, finally, inactivation of the steroid hormone. The sequence of intracellular events is: (a) cellular uptake of testosterone; (b) steroid activation to DHT by metabolism; (c) DHT binding to specific androgen receptors; (d) translocation of steroid receptor to the nucleus, as well as binding to the nuclear matrix and specific sequences of DNA; (e) changes in DNA topology and chromatin; (f) the increased transcription and expression and regulation of specific genes; (g) the trimming and processing of the mRNA as it is transported through the nucleus to the nuclear pore complex; (h) the stability and transportation of mRNA into the cytoplasmic compartment to be translated into protein; (i) the transportation of the protein to specific cellular sites and its subsequent posttranslational modification; and, finally, (j) the storage of the protein in secretory granules poised for secretion into the lumen on neurological command during the process of ejaculation. The epithelial cell is the primary unit in secretion, but specific genes are also activated in the stromal cells, as depicted in Fig. 5, and these events are regulated by both testosterone and estrogens. Not all cells respond the same to androgens or estrogens. For simplicity, these steps will be discussed in relation to the epithelial cells because differences between the cell types have not been clearly established. Androgens and estrogens together and separately can affect prostate cells, and it appears that estrogens might have more effect on the stromal cells, but this is not fully established at the present time. We now will discuss the aforementioned events in androgen action in more detail.

Androgen Metabolism Within the Prostate

After the free testosterone in the plasma has entered the prostatic cells through diffusion, it is rapidly metabolized to other steroids by a series of prostatic enzymes (64–68). Over 90% of the testosterone is *irreversibly* converted to the main prostatic androgen, DHT (see Fig. 7) through the action of NADPH and the enzyme 5α-reductase (EC 1.3.1.22) located on the endoplasmic reticulum and on the nuclear membrane. The enzyme 5α-reductase reduces the unsaturated bond in testosterone between the 4 and 5 positions to form the 5α-reduced DHT (18–22). The enzyme is primarily localized to the stroma, the K_m for testosterone is 10 to 30 nM, and the serum level of testosterone is only in the range of 0.5 to 3.0 nM, indicating that the enzyme cannot be saturated because the substrate would be less than 10% of the K_m value (68). 5α-Reductase can also convert androstenedione or progesterone to the 5α-reduced form. After the DHT is formed from testosterone, it is subjected to a series of reversible reactions to form 3α-diol (5α-androstane

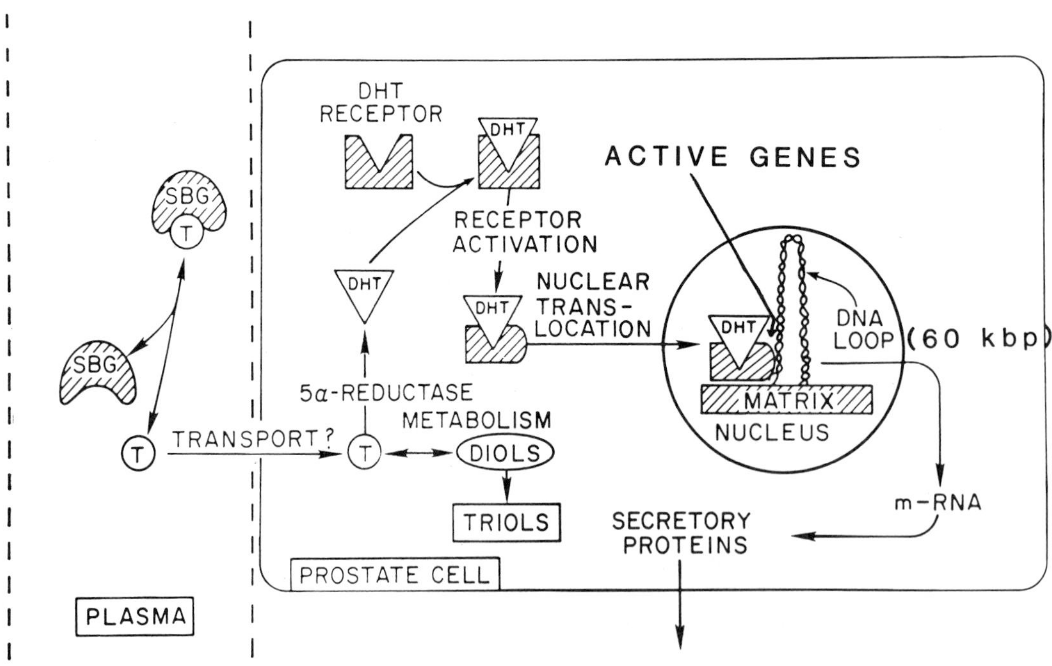

FIG. 6. A schematic of plasma testosterone bound to serum-binding globulin or TeBG. The free testosterone enters the prostatic epithelial cell and is converted by metabolism to DHT. The DHT then binds to the androgen receptor that is activated in the nucleus to bind to the nuclear matrix and DNA sequences present on the nuclear matrix. The DNA loop is approximately 60,000 base pairs and is equivalent in size to the replicon. There are approximately 20,000 of these loops per cell and only 2,000–5,000 charged DHT receptors. The receptors function by having domains that identify the DHT steroid, domains for binding the nuclear matrix, and domains of the receptor that have finger-like projections that interact with the DNA loop at its base in the vicinity of the gene.

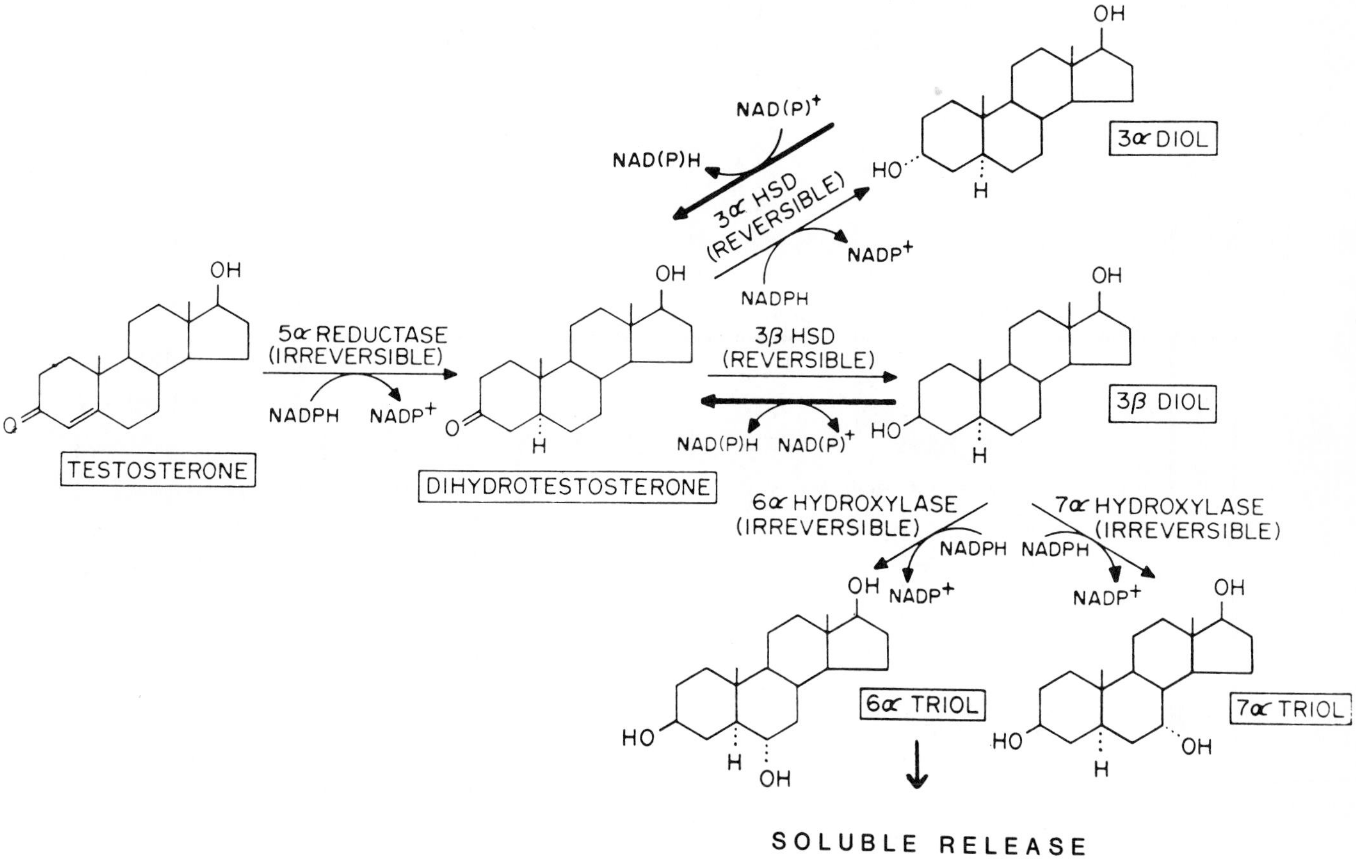

FIG. 7. The metabolic pathways of testosterone within the prostate. Testosterone is irreversibly converted to DHT, which is then reversibly converted to 3α-diol or 3β-diol. The diols are hydroxylated in either the 6α or 7α position in an irreversible manner, thus forming a triol. The triols are highly soluble and are released from the prostate in an inactive form.

3α,17β-diol) and 3β-diol (5α-androstane 3β,17β-diol) (see Fig. 7). The enzymes that perform this transformation of DHT are 3α- or 3β-hydroxysteroid oxidoreductases (3α-HSOR or 3β-HSOR). These enzymes utilize NADP as a cofactor, but, in contrast to 5α-reductase, they can also utilize NAD. The equilibrium for the metabolism of DHT favors the formation of DHT, i.e., the oxidation of the 3-hydroxy group of 3α- and 3β-diol to the 3-ketone that is present in DHT. It is known that administering 3α-diol to an animal is an effective androgen because of its rapid conversion to the effective DHT. On the other hand, 3β-diol is not very effective as an androgen because it is rapidly and irreversibly converted to the triol form by hydroxylation in the 6α or 7α- position (see Fig. 7). The triols are very water soluble and inactive as androgens and cannot reform DHT. In summary, testosterone is irreversibly metabolized to DHT that is in equilibrium with other reduced steroids primarily through oxidation and reduction at the 3 position. The steroids are inactivated by being irreversibly hydroxylated to the inactive triols. See Fig. 8 for more details on how these specific reactions of steroid biotransformation within the prostate are linked. The magnitude of activities in the prostates of humans, dogs, and rats have been discussed in more detail in several articles (64–68).

Steroid Receptors

The prostate and sex accessory tissue contain steroid-specific and high-affinity (10^{-9}–10^{-10} K_d) saturable (100–1,000 fmole of receptor per mg DNA equivalents of tissue) androgen receptors. There are 5,000 to 20,000 of these receptors per cell. The androgen receptors appear to be translocated into the nucleus, and they bind to specific nuclear acceptors that include chromatin and the nuclear matrix. The properties and hormonal regulation of androgen receptors have been discussed (69,70). The receptor is composed of three subunits for a total molecular weight of 80 to 120 kilodaltons and an *S* value of 4.5.

The problem in assessing the level of androgen receptors in the prostate is a methodological one because there are many binding globulins and plasma proteins that can interfere with the assay, and the labeled androgens that are utilized for these binding studies are often metabolized or transformed. To avoid many of these pitfalls, methyltrienolone R1881, a synthetic androgen, has been proposed and commonly used. This synthetic steroid does not bind well to many of the interfering proteins and is not actively metabolized. Another problem is that even highly specific steroid-binding ligands like R1881 can cross-bind to other ste-

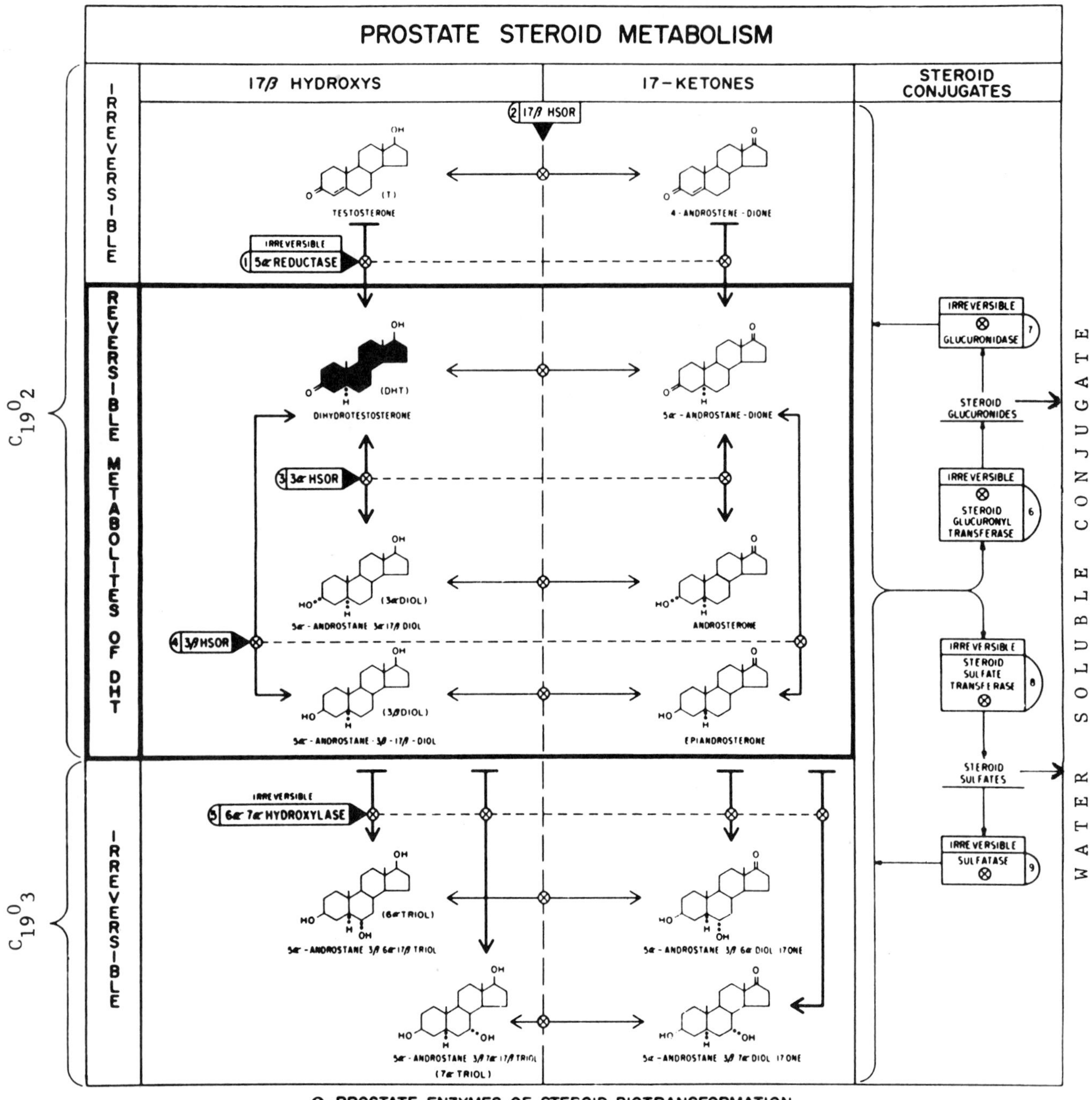

FIG. 8. A detail of the 12 major steroids located in the prostate gland that are synthesized from testosterone. The most prevalent steroid is DHT (*filled in black*). Each ⊗ indicates the common enzymatic pathway for the metabolism of the steroid substrates shown by the connecting arrows. There are nine major enzymes (*1–9*) involved in the metabolism of testosterone. The center box (*outlined in black*) indicates the reversible steroid metabolites of DHT. Outside the box are the irreversible reactions including the triols and conjugates that release the steroid from the prostate in a form that is more highly soluble.

roid receptors in the prostate such as the progesterone receptor. Care and attention must be given to ensure the investigator that the assay is both biochemically and kinetically correct. More recently, a new ligand, called *mibolerone*, has been used for studying androgen receptors. The androgen receptor is easily destroyed because the prostate is rich in protease enzymes that can rapidly degrade many enzymes and receptors. Quantitative recoveries are also limited because the prostatic connective tissue can also protect the disruption of many cells and can limit the extent of homogenization of individual cells.

Many investigators have focused their attention on the

cytoplasmic receptor instead of on the nuclear compartment, where the androgen action is believed to occur. In fact, the cytoplasmic receptor may be an extraction artifact, and most receptors may actually reside within the nucleus (71,72). For years it was believed that steroids get into the cell and bind specific cytoplasmic receptors and then, by a temperature sensitive step, these cytoplasmic receptors are activated and then translocated into the nucleus, where they bind to a mysterious nuclear acceptor. More recent studies (71,72) suggest that all of the receptor is in the nucleus; cytoplasmic receptor is only an artifact of nuclear receptor, which is extracted during the homogenization technique. This is primarily based on radioautographic studies of cellular location of labeled steroids and immunocytochemistry of receptor location. If this exclusive location of receptor within the nucleus proves true, the standard schematics representing this process (as shown in Fig. 6) must be altered to have the cytoplasmic receptor downplayed. Indeed, even within the nucleus, there appear to be several receptor compartments that can be assayed, including those that can be extracted in high salt concentrations of 0.4 to 0.6 M and those that resist the hypertonic salt extraction. These receptors are termed *salt-resistant receptors*. These salt-resistant receptors appear to be a reflection of receptor associated with the nonchromatin nuclear skeleton or nuclear matrix component of the nucleus (73–75). Barrack has recently shown that the nuclear matrix may contain the acceptor site, which is defined as the nuclear proteins that specifically bind steroid receptors within target tissues (75). The nuclear matrix is an important element in the organization of DNA structure and function and will be discussed in more detail in a subsequent section.

The most careful and informative studies carried out on receptor levels in normal, benign, and cancerous human prostates have been those of Walsh and Barrack (76–78). They have given careful attention to the development of highly specific receptor assay methods and have applied them to all of the known compartments of the cell, including cytoplasmic, nuclear salt-extractable, and salt-resistant binding. These considerations are of the utmost importance, since the use of steroid receptor assays has been proposed to correlate with the hormone responsiveness of the prostate.

In addition to the well-known androgen receptor, the prostate also contains estrogen receptors (78) and progesterone receptors (77,79,80). The radioligand used in the progesterone receptor assay is usually the synthetic progesterone R-5020. It is important to realize that these receptors may be distributed in various types of cells within the prostate, and, indeed, the estradiol concentration appears to be highest in the nuclei of stromal cells in human benign prostatic hyperplasia (81). Many of these steroid receptors might have multiple binding sites, and the high-affinity, low-capacity binding has usually been referred to as *type I,* whereas the moderate affinity and higher capacity estrogen receptor has been termed *type II sites* (78).

Other Factors That Modify Testosterone's Effect on the Cell

Estrogen/Androgen Synergism in Prostate Growth

Estrogens do not block androgen-induced growth of the prostate cell but, on the contrary, can synergize androgen effects. This has been well documented in the canine prostate, first by Walsh and Wilson (82) and subsequently by DeKlerk et al. (83). In the aforementioned studies the simultaneous administration of estradiol to castrated dogs receiving 5α-androstane metabolites such as DHT or 3α-diol produced a tremendous enhancement in the size of the prostate. The presence of estrogens more than doubled the androgen-induced growth, and this was associated with the development of a glandular hyperplasia. The mechanism of the androgen-estrogen synergism is not understood; however, it has been shown that estrogens increase the androgen nuclear receptor content in the prostate cell, which might be an important factor in this phenomenon (84).

The synergism of estrogens on androgen-induced growth in the dog prostate is observed only with the 5α-reduced androgens such as DHT or 3α-diol and is not observed when testosterone is administered (82–86). In addition, this synergism with androgens and estrogens in the dog does not occur in the rat prostate (87). The canine prostate is stimulated fourfold above normal by the combination of DHT and estradiol, but there is no similar enhanced stimulation by estradiol in the rat. Furthermore, the increase in wet weight of the dog prostate is paralleled by true hyperplasia, as measured by an increase in DNA content reflecting an increase in cell number. Whether this species difference occurs because the rat does not develop benign prostatic hyperplasia, and the dog does, is a matter of conjecture.

Stromal-Epithelial Interactions

Cell-cell interaction can modify the response of a cell to testosterone. There has been increasing interest in the role of stromal tissue elements (see Fig. 5) in inducing the growth of the sex accessory tissue since the early suggestions of Franks, in 1970, that epithelial cells require stroma for their growth. In addition, the classic experiments of Cunha, Chung, and co-workers (88,89) have clearly shown the direct importance of the embryonic mesenchyme in the induction of the differentiation of the normal prostatic epithelial cells. McNeal's proposal that in BPH the stroma may be reactivated in adult life to an embryonic state, thus stimulating the epithelial growth, has generated a great deal of interest and effort to understand these tissue components of the prostate.

The classic experiments of Cunha, Chung, and co-workers (88) have demonstrated that the mesenchyme of the urogenital sinus may have the director's role in inducing the growth and cytodifferentiation of prostatic epithelial cells.

In summary, they have shown that when heterografting sandwiches of mesenchyme cells in combination with epithelial cells, the mesenchyme dictates what the epithelial cell will differentiate into. For instance, placing bladder epithelia on urogenital sinus mesenchyme directs the bladder cells to form prostatic epithelial cells. More surprising, bladder epithelia from androgen-insensitive TfM mice explanted to normal wild-type mesenchyme developed normal prostatic epithelial cells from the bladder cells. In addition, in all combinations the number of mesenchymal cells determines the total overall size of the prostate, and the epithelial cells grow out until they cover the surface of the available mesenchyme. The opposite, an excess of epithelial cells, will not cause an overgrowth of the mesenchyme cells. In fact, Cunha and colleagues believe that the major cell target of androgen stimulation in the urogenital sinus is primarily the mesenchyme, not the epithelial cells.

Chung et al. (89) transplanted a fetal urogenital sinus into an adult rat prostate and induced a large overgrowth of adult prostatic tissue apparently stimulated by the presence of the fetal tissue. This has raised the question of whether direct contact with an insoluble embryonic extracellular matrix or with a soluble diffusible factor(s) is responsible for these observations. Muntzing (90) proposes that collagen of the prostate might limit prostate growth. Mariotti and Mawhinney (91) and Thornton et al. (92) have provided evidence that collagen synthesis and degradation can be important events in accompanying limitations on prostatic growth in animals. At present, a clear cause and effect of collagen on normal prostate growth has not been fully established.

The prostate stroma of animals does contain steroid receptors and does appear to respond to estrogens (92), and attempts to correlate enzyme levels with stromal composition (93) also indicates that the stroma has an androgen-metabolizing ability almost equal to that of the epithelium. Efforts to separate stroma and epithelia by mechanical means, as well as to study the isolated components, have supported these conclusions. It is still most difficult to obtain pure viable separations of high yields of stromal and epithelial components from the human prostate without excessive damage of the cells or poor yields. There is no doubt, however, that the interaction of stromal elements with the epithelium is an important part of the regulation of prostatic growth and development. It is also apparent that prostatic epithelial cells can metastasize elsewhere and establish growth in distant organs in the absence of prostatic stroma.

Prostatic Growth Factors

A search is underway by Chung, Cunha, and their associates (88,89) to identify soluble prostatic growth factors that may be proteinaceous and that are associated with the urogenital sinus mesenchyme. Because the normal adult prostate is not growing rapidly, one would not anticipate an abundance of active growth factors in the normal adult where the gland is not increasing in size. However, many adult tissues have growth factors that can be demonstrated using *in vitro* fibroblast assay systems. In 1979, Jacobs et al. (94) demonstrated the growth factor in crude extracts of normal, BPH, and cancerous human prostates. Efforts are underway to identify and isolate these prostatic growth factors (14–16).

There are some identified growth factors that originate in the prostate. One of them is urogastrone, a growth factor that is a 53-amino-acid polypeptide and belongs to the same family as mouse epidermal growth factor (EGF). It has recently been reported to be of high concentration (272 ng/ml) in human ejaculate and of prostate in origin (12). Recently, another prostate-derived growth factor has been purified, and partial characterization has been reported by Maehama (10). Bordoli and colleagues (11) have reported the complete primary structure of a prostate epithelial growth factor that they have termed *prostatropin*.

At present, much work will be required to pursue these potentially important observations and to eliminate contamination of other known growth factors and protease enzymes. There is little doubt that most tissues are susceptible to stimulation by growth factors and to inhibition of growth by tissue chalones. The balance between cell growth and cell death appears to be under some hormonal and growth factor control, and this remains one of the frontiers of understanding all tumor growth of the prostate.

Interaction of Steroid Receptors with Specific DNA Domains in Gene Regulation

In almost all cells in the body, steroids can enter the nucleus, but only a few cells can retain this steroid within their nucleus for any length of time. The cells that retain the steroid have receptors that are specific for binding the steroid and that, in some unknown way, appear to activate elements within the nucleus to increase the expression of certain specific genes that are under steroid control. Two cells can have the same androgen receptors present in their nuclei, but one will respond by making one type of androgen-induced protein while the other will produce a second type of androgen-induced protein. For example, in the rat the ventral prostate and the seminal vesicles both have androgen receptors and, in the presence of DHT bound to receptors in their nuclei, the prostate makes a pattern of androgen-controlled gene expression that is different from those induced in the seminal vesicles. How androgens specify gene response remains a mystery. Is it because the receptors are different in these two tissues in some subtle way or because certain DNA sequences have been slightly modified by methylation or changes in topology or chromatin structure? This is one of the major frontiers of endocrine molecular biology, and it has not been resolved for any tissue much less the androgen-sensitive sex accessory tissues where we have been unable to purify the receptor or to carry out precise molecular studies as has been done for estrogen, progesterone, and glucocorticoid sensitive tissues. For that reason, we will briefly describe the present understanding of hormone-regulated gene expression in other tissues, with the idea that homology to steroid reactions, in general, may exist.

It appears that steroid-receptor complex binds to specific regions of DNA and activates or inactivates specific genes by selectively effecting the transcription of the gene into RNA. The transcribed message is then processed in the nucleus to become messenger RNA (mRNA) to be shipped out of the nucleus. It appears that the mRNA is then transported to the ribosomes, where it is finally translated into protein. The problem in the specificity of this reaction of a receptor recognizing a small specific DNA sequence is like finding a needle in a haystack. This can be appreciated when it is considered that less than 0.01% of the protein in the sex accessory cell is an androgen-receptor molecule that must locate a small group of 12 or less nucleotides on the genome to be selected from a pool of three billion total nucleotides.

Part of the recognition of receptors and DNA may depend on the organization of the DNA within different nuclei. The steroid receptor complex can only interact with genes that are in regions that are "open" or in the transcriptionally active form, which means that they are susceptible to digestion by incubation with the enzyme DNase I. This means that the DNA in this region is in an accessible form to the DNase enzyme. Studies show that these open regions of chromatin with altered conformation extend up to 100,000 base pairs in length, or more than 10 times the size of a gene, which usually ranges from 1,000 to 10,000 base pairs. It is unknown how such a large range of DNA is altered in conformation, but it may be through binding to structures like the nuclear matrix, which can order large-loop domains in the region of 60,000 base pairs.

The genes in one of the open regions of DNA appear to be separated into two major areas: the structural DNA region, which is going to be transcribed and become part of the message; and a large regulatory region of DNA (adjacent to, and upstream toward, the 5′ end) that contains the control sites for this gene (see Fig. 9). The structural area is called the gene, and starting on its 5′ end, where it will initiate transcription, the nucleotide bases are numbered as +1 and increase as they move to the right into the gene and towards the 3′ end. Moving away from the gene and to the left of the initiation site and upstream in the 5′ direction, the nucleotide bases are numbered from right to left starting with −1 and increasing as you move to the left of the gene. We will first discuss the regulatory DNA regions lying next to, and upstream from, the gene (Fig. 9). The regulatory region is divided into a promoter element that is present in all

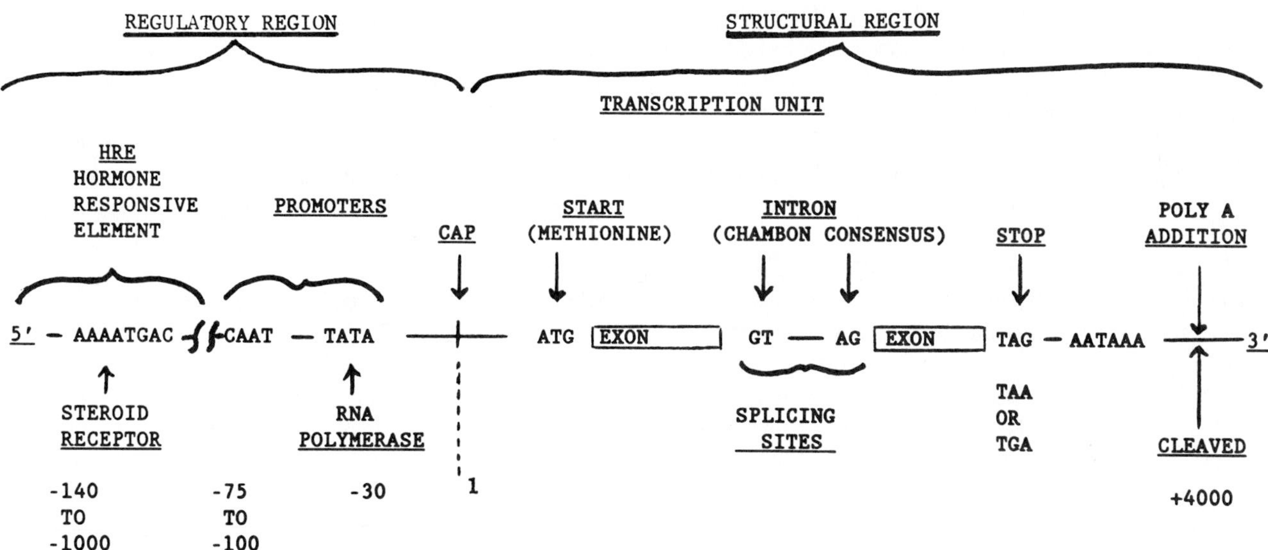

FIG. 9. Schematic of a typical gene structure that is activated by steroid-receptor complex. The structural region includes the coding sequences that will form the final messenger RNA, called *exons* (only two of many are shown). The exons are connected by intron sequences that will later be transcribed into RNA and that will ultimately be spliced out to form the final messenger RNA (mRNA). The reaction starts at the capping area, indicated by 1. The start of the transcription is at the binding of RNA polymerase at the TATA box and the equivalent of the first amino acid message at the ATG which codes for methionine. The stop sequence is TAG outside the last exon and is located further downstream in the 3′ direction; this is the area where polyA sequences will be added. Upstream to the left in the 5′ direction is the promoter and hormone responsive element (HRE), which contains the steroid-receptor binding region. This schematic represents typical information for a steroid-activated gene but is not specific in sequence for what might be activated by the androgen receptor. Until the androgen receptor is purified and its binding sequence identified, this drawing will have to be an estimate to illustrate the types of reactions that might be anticipated.

genes. This promoter element specifies the site to which RNA polymerase II will attach to the DNA and will determine the accuracy point for the initiation of transcription. This promoter starts at −16 to −32 nucleotides upstream from the gene initiation site. This region of −32 to −16 nucleotides was originally referred to as the *Goldberg-Hogness box* and has a consensus sequence of TATAAAAG; it also has homology to the functionally related Pribnow box (TATAAT) that is centered about 7 base pairs upstream from the start point in prokaryotic systems. The RNA polymerase II enzyme binds to this TATA box as one of the initial steps in transcription. Further upstream from the TATA box is a second gene control element, termed the *hormone responsive element* (HRE), that has been identified in many genes regulated by steroid hormones. This HRE area may contain several discrete sequences, but its overall role is to modulate the frequency of transcription initiation. In summary, the TATA box tells where the initiation of transcription is to start, and the HRE tells how frequently it is to be transcribed. Since the HRE element of DNA sequence has been shown to be independent of its position or its orientation, it resembles what has been called the transcription *enhancer element,* which has been found in many other types of genes. The HRE section can vary in its location upstream from the initiation of the gene, from −20 to −2,600 nucleotides for various types of hormones. With the steroid hormones it appears to reside about −140 nucleotides upstream from the initiation site. For example, in the glucocorticoid receptor system, the site is about −140 nucleotides upstream and contains a sequence of nucleotides of AAAATGGAC. This DNA sequence that binds a specific receptor may vary, depending on the type of steroid receptor, and a generalized sequence is presented in Fig. 9 as an example. Deletion mapping experiments have indicated that the receptor-binding domain located in the hormone-responsive element is indeed required for receptor binding and is necessary for steroid-mediated control of transcription. These experiments are carried out by making a fusion gene where the hormone-receptor-binding domain is ligated to a *reporter* gene that, when activated by the steroid receptor, can be activated and expressed; then the reporter gene product is assayed. This reporter gene is usually a steroid-induced molecule that brings about antibiotic resistance or expresses thymidine kinase. The fusion gene is placed in a cell that is usually not steroid-sensitive, and now the presence of the steroid will induce the transcription of the receptor gene. These experiments are valuable because not only the position but also the orientation and base substitutions of the steroid-receptor-binding sequence can be used to map out the biological activity of these areas.

Recently, the estrogen, glucocorticoid, and progesterone receptors have been cloned (95–98). It has been shown from these studies that primary protein sequences of these receptors have a homology in certain regions to v-erb-A of the oncogene family. Further work has established that the receptor contains a region that is highly conserved (with 50% to 60% homology between all receptor genes) and that is cysteine-rich. This region is structurally similar to the cysteine-rich sequence found in important transcription factor IIIA and other transcriptional regulatory proteins and seems to be able to form two small finger-like binding loops that are known to interact with DNA. It has been proposed that zinc may be bound to these cysteines to form a 13-amino-acid finger-like loop. This region determines the specificity of the receptor for binding to the nucleus and to specific gene areas. This region has been designated as region *C.* There is another region, called region *E,* that is part of the receptor domain and that encodes the hormone-binding domain of the receptor; this region is also a hydrophobic socket that may determine the specificity for the various steroids. Another region, called region *D,* is not heavily conserved amongst receptors and even between species, but is essential for nuclear binding.

With these new breakthroughs in understanding receptors, we can anticipate many new and exciting experiments on the androgen receptors to be forthcoming. At present we do not have the above type of experiment defined for the androgen receptor. As soon as the androgen receptor is isolated, purified, and cloned, one would propose that we would find many similar analogies to the progesterone, estrogen, and glucocorticoid systems.

The Role of the Nuclear Matrix in the Organization of DNA Structure and Function

More may be required than just a receptor and a DNA sequence to determine the high specificity of androgen hormone action. We know that there are great regions of at least 100 kilobases that are in an open conformation of chromatin, and this varies between cells with the same genome. In addition, in different cells, with both containing androgen receptors, one cell will express one type of protein while a second cell will express a second type of protein. The specificity between the two cells is difficult to visualize based only upon a common steroid receptor and a common genome sequence, and although DNA modification such as methylation might be involved in such processes, there is strong evidence to believe that structural components of the nucleus may organize the DNA into different topological constraints that permit specific steroid-receptor interactions among themselves. It is believed that these structural modifications of topology may be an integral part of differentiation. To show the complexity of organizing all of the cellular DNA, one must realize that if a nucleus were enlarged to 5 feet in diameter, the DNA would extend for 50 miles and would have to be wound in a highly organized manner into replicons, genes, and chromatin domains in the nucleus that could be completely copied and separated without entanglement. The nuclear matrix has been proposed to be an important structural element in this organization. It is the site that binds hormone-receptor complexes and organizes the location of the genes that can be expressed by the action of the steroid. For this reason, we will review the properties and describe the nuclear matrix structure in some detail.

The importance of the nuclear matrix as a target for androgen action. Barrack and Coffey (73) first showed that the nuclear matrix is a major target for androgen and estrogen action. Because the matrix has been implicated in many important nuclear events, it would provide an ideal target for androgen action. The matrix also organizes the structure of chromatin and DNA, which is known to be altered by hormonal action. It is therefore important to review the biological functions of the nuclear matrix.

The nuclear matrix has been defined as the dynamic structural subcomponent of the nucleus that directs the functional organization of DNA into loop domains and provides sites for the specific control of nucleic acids (99). Conceptually, it can be viewed as the nuclear equivalent to the cytomatrix or cytoskeleton. The nuclear matrix contains residual nuclear elements, including the pore-complex lamina, the residual nucleolus, and an internal ribonucleoprotein particle (RNP) network attached to a dynamic fibrous protein mesh (100,101). The nuclear matrix may be isolated by sequential extractions employing nonionic detergent (Triton X-100), brief digestion with DNase I, and a hypertonic salt buffer (e.g., 2 M NaCl). The residual nuclear matrix structures represent only 15%, or less, of the original nuclear mass. Over 98% of the DNA, 70% of the RNA, and 90% of the nuclear proteins have been extracted, and the remaining structure is essentially devoid of histones and lipids (99,102).

The nuclear matrix has been implicated as an important structural component in a wide variety of important biological functions (see Table 2). The nuclear matrix serves an important role in DNA organization. The DNA loop domains are attached to nuclear matrix at their bases (103,104), and this organization is maintained during interphase and metaphase (105–109). Topoisomerase II, an enzyme that modulates DNA topology, is associated with the nuclear matrix (110,111) and the mitotic chromosome scaffold (112). Hormones are known to activate genes and alter DNA structure, and many studies with a wide variety of systems have demonstrated that active genes are associated with the nuclear matrix, whereas transcriptionally inactive genes are not associated with the matrix. This location of active genes on the matrix provides further evidence that the matrix plays an important organizing role in DNA function (113–120).

Androgens can activate DNA replication in target tissues. The nuclear matrix also serves an important role in DNA replication. The matrix contains fixed sites for DNA synthesis (103,121–125) located at the base of the DNA loop. During DNA synthesis, the DNA loop domains are reeled down through the attached replicating complex that is fixed on the matrix. Therefore, the DNA replication fork, DNA polymerase, and newly replicated DNA have been shown to be associated with the nuclear matrix. The nuclear matrix is in a critical position to play an important role in the organization and control of DNA replication. It is easy to visualize how hormone action and alteration in the nuclear matrix structures could impinge on the androgen regulation of DNA synthesis and growth in a prostate cell.

TABLE 2. *Reported functions of the nuclear matrix*

Nuclear morphology: The nuclear matrix contains structural elements of the pore complexes, lamina, internal network, and nucleoli which give the nucleus its overall three-dimensional organization and shape.

DNA organization: DNA loop domains are attached to the nuclear matrix at their bases, and this organization is maintained during interphase and metaphase. The nuclear matrix shares proteins with the chromosome scaffold. Topoisomerase II, an enzyme that modulates DNA topology, is associated with the nuclear matrix and chromosome scaffolds. The matrix organizes chromatin structure.

DNA replication: The nuclear matrix has fixed sites for DNA replication, containing the DNA replication fork, DNA polymerase α, and newly replicated DNA.

RNA synthesis: The nuclear matrix contains transcriptional complexes, newly synthesized hnRNA, and snRNA. RNA processing intermediates are bound to the nuclear matrix. Actively transcribed genes are associated with the nuclear matrix; inactive genes are not.

Nuclear regulation: The nuclear matrix has specific sites for steroid hormone receptor binding. The nuclear matrix is a cellular target for transformation proteins, such as the large T antigen, E1A protein, and the myc gene product. The nuclear matrix proteins are phosphorylated.

The nuclear matrix is also associated with RNA synthesis. Transcriptional complexes have been identified on the nuclear matrix (126–128). O'Malley and his colleagues (129) observed that over 95% of the unprocessed mRNA precursor for ovalbumin was associated with nuclear matrix of the chick oviduct. When the intron portions of the RNA were processed out, the mature mRNA was released from the nuclear matrix. This led them to suggest that the nuclear matrix was involved in RNA processing. Mariman and van Venrooij have reported that all RNA cleavage products and RNA processing intermediates are firmly bound to nuclear matrix (130). Once again, alterations in nuclear matrix structures with steroid receptor interactions could alter important steps in transcription and RNA processing. Recently, Sharp has proposed an important role for the nuclear matrix in RNA splicing (131). The nuclear matrix contains the attachment sites for the small nuclear ribonucleoprotein particles (snRNP) that are part of the nuclear splicesome system that is central to the nuclear processing of hnRNA to the final mRNA that is transported out to the cytoplasm.

The nuclear matrix is an important modulator of nuclear regulation and is an ideal target for hormonal regulation. Indeed, the nuclear matrix is a major site of steroid-hormone receptor binding (73–76). In the prostate, over 60% of all nuclear androgen receptors are associated with the nuclear matrix. The matrix is also a target for many regulatory interactions including the products of oncogenes and viral proteins that can induce growth regulation similar to hormone-induced growth. For example, the nuclear matrix is reported to be a cellular target for the retrovirus myc oncogene protein (132,133), the adenovirus E1A transforming protein (134), and the polyoma large T antigen (135,136). All of these transformation proteins that bind to the nucleus are believed to be products of early molecular events in carcinogenesis or transformation. Therefore, the observation that androgen receptors interact with the matrix has precedence with the matrix as a common target in factors that regulate cell structure and function.

DNA loop domains organized by the nuclear matrix. Androgens alter DNA and chromatin structure in sex accessory tissue and produce DNase-sensitive regions in the range of 50 to 100 kilobase pairs of DNA. This is similar to the size of DNA loop domains. The organization of DNA within interphase chromatin, metaphase chromosomes, and the nucleus still remains largely unsolved. Three higher-order levels of DNA organization have been identified in the past decade: the nucleosome, the 30-nm chromatin fibers, and the DNA loop domain. Although controversy still exists with regard to the exact nature of each of these structures, each is well accepted as a basic unit of DNA organization. The DNA loop domain was first proposed by Cook et al. (137) in 1976; they suggested that loop structures are involved in the superhelical organization of eukaryotic DNA. In 1980, Vogelstein et al. (104) reported that DNA loop domains were attached at their base to the nuclear matrix and that these loops were topologically constrained by that attachment. This was accomplished by visualizing the DNA loop structures in the presence of ethidium bromide. In low concentrations of ethidium bromide, a large fluorescent halo was observed surrounding the periphery of the nuclear matrix. In high concentrations of ethidium bromide, this halo was supercoiled in the opposite direction and was observed to rewind. If the DNA was nicked, the halo structure could not rewind. This suggests that the nuclear matrix organizes DNA such that it has the topological properties equivalent to those of covalent closed circular DNA, with the matrix at the base of the loop providing the constraint. Furthermore, in finding that the nuclear matrix contained fixed sites for replication at DNA loops, Pardoll et al. (103) were able to show that these loops are the structural equivalents of the replicon units of DNA. The replicon is the unit of DNA that is replicated during androgen-induced DNA synthesis.

The DNA loop domain defines a basic unit of higher-order DNA structure that is present throughout the cell cycle in eukaryotic cells (138–140). These loops have been estimated to be between 10 and 180 kilobase pairs in length, with an average of 63 ± 14 kilobase pairs based on five independent studies (141). Warren and Cook (139) have noted that DNA loop domains appear to be the same size throughout the cell cycle. An average loop domain of 63 kilobase pairs would contain 21 μm of DNA double helix. Each loop would be large enough to contain a total of 315 nucleosomes. The nucleosomes form the filament of the loop that is wound with six nucleosomes per turn into a 30-nm solenoid fiber utilizing the fiber model proposed by Finch and Klug (142) and supported by observations by others (143). The 30-nm fiber forms the filament of a loop, a basic structure of interphase and metaphase DNA. If a diploid human nucleus contains a total of 6×10^9 base pairs, there would be approximately 100,000 of these 60-kilobase-pair DNA loop domains within a single nucleus. It is of importance that the androgen receptors bind to the nuclear matrix that is located at the base of the DNA loops.

The role of the nuclear matrix in chromosome structure. The higher-order structure of metaphase chromosomes is still a subject of controversy. Several different models have been described, including the radial-loop (144–146), the folded-fiber (147), the unit-fiber (148), and the coiled-coil models (149,150). We found that by comparing the amounts of DNA in a chromatid of the number 4 human chromosome with the chromatid dimensions, we could accommodate DNA loops into the actual chromatid dimensions only by utilizing a radial-loop model (see Fig. 10) (141). This radial-loop model features loops wrapped radially around the central axis of the chromatid as they stack to achieve overall chromosome length. Our analysis revealed that there would be 18 DNA loops per radial turn of the chromatid. Each of the 18 loops contained 60 kilobase pairs in a solenoid fiber of 30 nm. This18-loop unit composed of the 30-nm loop filament forms a new, higher-order structure of DNA organization that we have termed the "miniband" (141). The miniband is equivalent to one full radial turn of 18 loops around the central axis of the chromatid and contains approximately one million base pairs of DNA (18×63 kilobase pairs). The structural miniband–radial-loop model offers several insights into how biological functions may be occurring within the chromosome and nucleus.

The one million base pairs of DNA encompassed by a single miniband approximates the size of the genetic unit, the centimorgan, which is the common limit for DNA recombination events. Genetic recombination is caused by physical crossing over between different chromosome regions. The likelihood that crossing over will occur, i.e., that chiasma will form between two points between chromatids, depends on the base-pair distance in the DNA separating them. Genes located near one another will remain linked, but as the distance increases between them, the probability of crossing over between them increases. Genes on the same chromosome will be mapped to relative locations by their frequency of recombination. A centimorgan is the term assigned to the value of 1% recombination. The centimorgan is commonly referred to as the smallest length of DNA recombination usually observed in genetic cross-over experiments and, in the human genome, is equivalent to one million base pairs, which is similar to the base pairs in a miniband.

Therefore, the miniband may be a useful concept in pro-

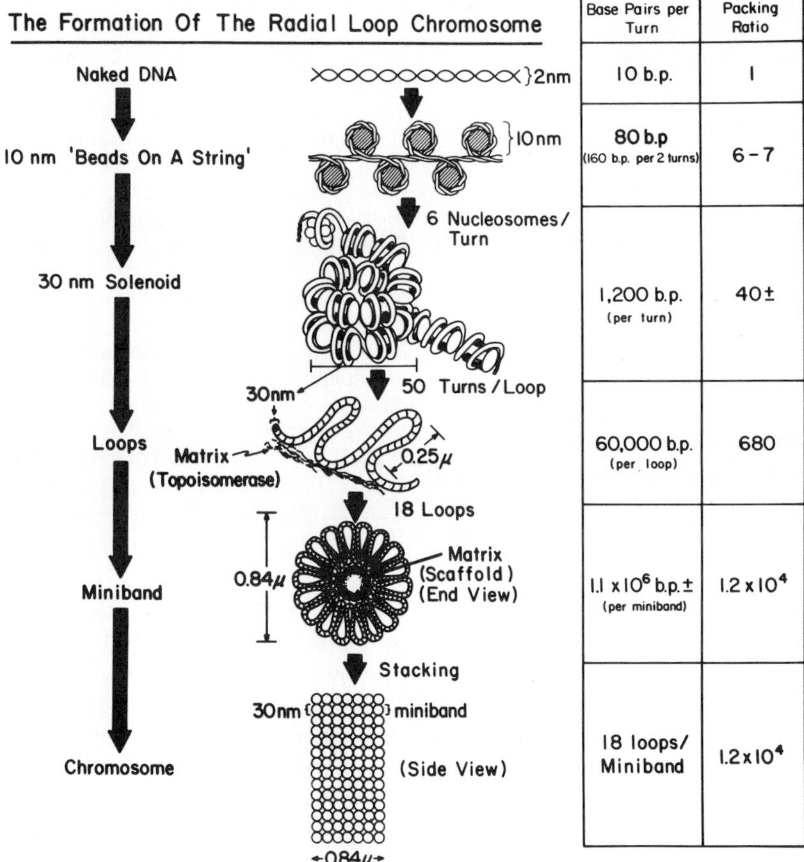

Base Pairs per Turn	Packing Ratio
10 b.p.	1
80 b.p (160 b.p. per 2 turns)	6 - 7
1,200 b.p. (per turn)	40±
60,000 b.p. (per loop)	680
1.1×10^6 b.p.± (per miniband)	1.2×10^4
18 loops/ Miniband	1.2×10^4

FIG. 10. A model of the way DNA is organized into the form of a chromosome. The DNA double strand is wrapped around a histone octamer to form nucleosomes, termed "beads-on-a-string." Six of these nucleosomes are wound into a solenoid to form a 30-nm chromatin fiber. The 30-nm fiber then becomes a ~0.25-μm loop that is attached at its base to the nuclear matrix. At the base is the enzyme topoisomerase II, which changes the topology of DNA. It is to this matrix region that the steroid receptors bind in their interaction with the active genes which are also located near the matrix. The ~60,000-base-pair DNA loops are each then wound into a radial loop model of 18 loops per turn (miniband), with the matrix located in the center as a chromosome scaffold. These loops are then wound up into a chromosome structure that resembles a Slinky toy.

viding a structure and mechanical model to the function of chromosomes. The thickness of an individual miniband, 30 nm, approaches that of the smallest bands seen in cytological Giemsa prophase banding of metaphase chromosomes.

We have just discussed the organization of the metaphase chromosome, and it is important to realize that the loops of the miniband are maintained in their organization, with the nuclear matrix as the internal structure of the nucleus. It is believed that the telomeres of the chromosome are attached to the peripheral lamina. As the nucleus approaches metaphase, the nuclear lamina proteins are phosphorylated and move into the cytoplasmic area as the nuclear envelope disintegrates. This leaves the chromosomes free to collapse into the condensed structures shown in Fig. 11. At the end of the telophase, the ends of the chromosome serve as an organizing center for the reformation of the lamina by condensing lamin proteins to these areas. In this model, it is apparent that some structures of the nuclear matrix that anchor the loops will be maintained as the core scaffolding or matrix of the chromosome (141). Recently, Earnshaw and Heck (112) have shown that the scaffold or matrix of the metaphase chromosome contains topoisomerase II, which is also a component of the interphase nucleus during the time of DNA synthesis. Nelson et al. (99) have recently reported that, in prostatic adenocarcinoma cells, newly synthesized DNA can be covalently attached to the topoisomerase II of the interphase nucleus and that this new label can be chased off in a manner indicating that the topoisomerase is firmly attached at the base of the loops and in close proximity to the replicating site on the matrix. This would be consistent with Reddy and Pardee's (151) observations that topoisomerase II is part of a large, 5-million-molecular-weight replitase particle that forms the replisome complex for a fixed site for DNA synthesis. In the future, much work will be needed to determine what DNA sequences are involved in the attachment of DNA loops to their base and how they interact with specific attachment proteins within the nuclear matrix and precisely where the androgen receptors bind. If, during steroid-hormone action, DNA loops are capable of moving on and off the matrix, it will be important to determine how this is accomplished in a dynamic manner. Insight into this process has been provided by fluorescent antibody studies of changes in the distribution of nuclear matrix antigens during the mitotic cell cycle (152,153). A series of antibodies developed against different components of the nuclear matrix clearly show the dynamic aspects of this structure throughout various phases of the cell cycle, including the formation of the metaphase chromosomes. Additional studies of this type are essential to further our understanding of the dynamic role of the nuclear matrix in hormone action. It is important to visualize the nuclear matrix not as a rigid skeleton but rather as a flexible

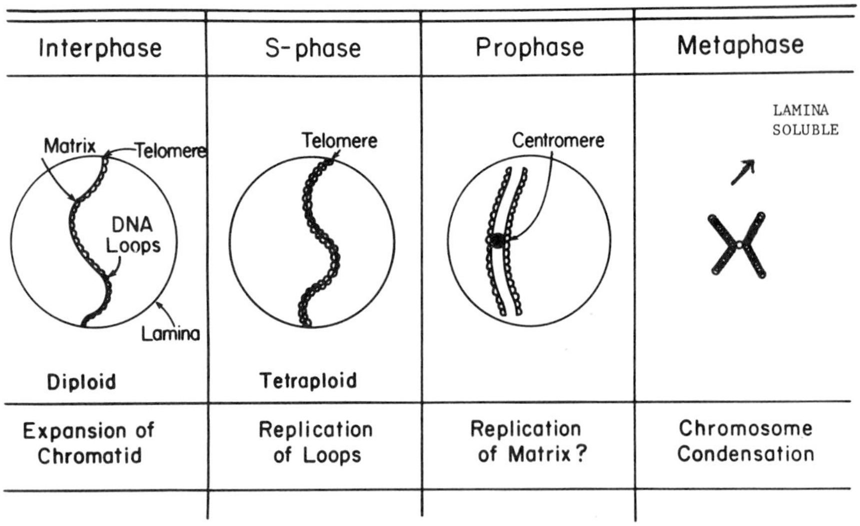

Interphase	S-phase	Prophase	Metaphase
Matrix, Telomere, DNA Loops, Lamina	Telomere	Centromere	LAMINA SOLUBLE
Diploid	Tetraploid		
Expansion of Chromatid	Replication of Loops	Replication of Matrix?	Chromosome Condensation

FIG. 11. The organization of DNA in the nucleus at various times in the cell cycle. During the interphase, the chromosome is expanded and invisible, with the telomeres bound to the lamina and the DNA loops attached to the matrix. During S phase, the loops are replicated by moving through the fixed replicating sites on the matrix to form a new set of loops. During prophase, the telomeres detach from the lamina and the centromeres form on the matrix, and this separates the newly replicated strands. The lamina proteins become phosphorylated and are solubilized and move into the cytoplasm, and the loops attached to the matrix condense to form the central scaffold of the metaphase chromosome. This condensation can be visualized by comparing this figure with Fig. 10.

dynamic interacting system that directs protein–nucleic-acid interactions and the transport of these components in and out of the nucleus.

The integration of the nuclear matrix within the tissue matrix. It is important to realize that the nuclear matrix actually forms an interlocking cellular matrix network by direct connection with the cytomatrix that extends throughout to the extracellular matrix (see Fig. 12). It has been proposed that a tissue matrix (63,154) provides a dynamic scaffolding system throughout the tissue. This concept has been well studied by Penman and his associates (155–157), who have proposed that the nuclear matrix is directly linked to an intermediate filament complex that functions as a structural unit within the cell. They provided convincing three-dimensional electron micrographs that showed that the nuclear matrix intermediate filaments were interconnected and extended via the desmosomes over the entire epithelial cell colony. Most important, they have shown that the nuclear-matrix intermediate filament scaffold retains proteins that are specific to its cell type and that this is unique to this

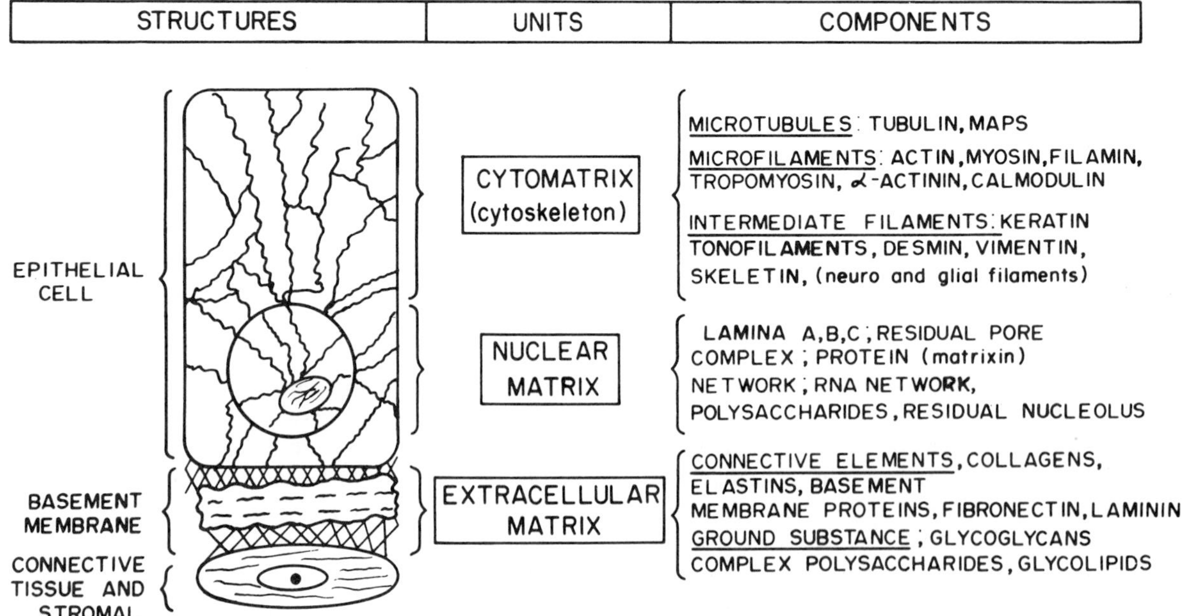

FIG. 12. The tissue matrix system. This schematic represents the interaction of the nuclear matrix with the cytomatrix and its coupling to the extracellular matrix. This provides a continuous solid-state support system between the stromal cells and the epithelial cells that comprises the overall tissue matrix. This tissue matrix is a highly dynamic structure and is involved in transport and organization of many important biological events that are under hormonal control.

substructure of the cell system (157). We still know very little about the integration and control of these cytoskeleton processes and how the information is transmitted to the nucleus. Ingber et al. (158) have suggested a tensegrity model to accompany this mechanical interaction. *Tensegrity* is defined by Buckminster Fuller as consisting of a dynamic interacting structural system that is composed of discontinuous compression elements hooked up by continuous-tension cables. It is important to recognize that the filaments making up the cytoskeleton in the nuclear matrix have very little resistance to bending, but a great deal of tensile strength. As construction elements, they would function much better in a tension-derived structure than in a compression-type system. A tensegrity system would provide this design. Indeed, our bodies, which have great chemomechanical flexibility, are composed of discontinuous compression elements in the form of our bones hooked together by continuous-tension cables in the formation of ligaments and muscle and are therefore a tensegrity model. Our time-lapse cinematography of prostate cancer cells indicates that one of their characteristics is the ability to undergo dynamic shape changes and motility, which includes ruffling, undulation, and translocation. It would appear that a tensegrity model would be far more conducive to rapid changes in structure than the more rigid skeleton system composed of a framework scaffolding that must be taken down and reconstructed for each change in shape and motility.

With additional information on how these matrix systems interact, we may have developed a new way of visualizing how hormones may regulate dynamic cellular functions.

Summary of Androgen Action

In summary, it is presently not known to what the androgen receptors bind within the nucleus; and, besides the possibility of binding to the nuclear matrix (73–76), it also appears that they may bind to specific sequences of the DNA. Through these interactions it is visualized that very specific nucleotide sequences within target tissues may directly bind steroid receptors and thus activate the genes to be expressed. The DNA appears to have topological constraints placed upon it by proteins and topoisomerase action, which winds the DNA into supercoiled loops. It is visualized that the presence of nuclear receptors somehow alters the chromatin and DNA conformation so that the DNA is in a new state that is more susceptible to being copied and transcribed into messenger RNA. In many target tissues this is measured by an increase in the sensitivity of the gene to DNase activity when it is in the activated state. Once the DNA is transcribed into RNA, the RNA is processed before it is transferred out of the nucleus. This involves removing pieces of RNA that will not become part of the final message. The action of steroids sets off a complex series of orderly and timed events starting with an increase in transcription initiation factors, messenger RNA and ribosomal RNA synthesis, cellular protein synthesis, and, finally, DNA synthesis and cell replication. These events are specific for all steroid target tissues that have been studied. It is unknown whether gene expression is increased by androgen-stimulated transcription, effects on RNA stability, processing, or translocation; all of these have been implicated. At present, much attention is being placed on hormone receptor binding to regulatory sequences upstream in enhancer sequences. Regardless of the complexity of the mechanism, the final results of androgen action are: dramatic change in chromatin structure, nuclear structure, and morphology, as well as dramatic effects on nuclear RNA and DNA synthesis, which are all interacted into a temporal pattern. These events almost surely will involve the many RNA components attached to the nuclear matrix.

STRUCTURE AND FUNCTION OF THE SEX ACCESSORY GLANDS

Overview

As stated earlier, the sex accessory tissues vary considerably between species and it is difficult to summarize a general concept of their structure and function. This section will therefore focus on the human sex accessory tissue, with emphasis on the prostate gland. A normal adult human prostate weighs approximately 20 g (1) and lies immediately below the base of the bladder surrounding the proximal portion of the urethra. The gland is located behind the inferior part of the symphysis pubis and rests directly above the urogenital diaphragm and in front of the rectal ampulla. The gland is composed of alveoli that are lined with tall columnar secretory epithelial cells. The acini of these alveoli drain, by a system of branching ducts and tubules, into the floor and lateral surfaces of the posterior urethra. The alveoli and ducts are embedded within a stroma of fibromuscular tissue.

The seminal vesicles in the human develop as large paired pouches forming from the vas deferens. The glands are 4 to 5 in. long and are located directly on the posterior side of the bladder, adjacent to the rectum. The glands are composed of tubular aveoli containing viscous secretions. The seminal vesicles were so named because it was erroneously believed that they stored semen and sperm. Their secretions contribute to semen, but they do not store secretions made elsewhere; also, the seminal vesicles do not store sperm. However, the ampulla at the distal end of the vas deferens does store sperm, and the seminal vesicles join the ampulla to form the beginning of ejaculatory ducts. The ejaculatory ducts pass through the prostate and finally terminate below the utricle within the prostate urethra at the verumontanum.

Other minor glands complete the list of sex accessory tissues in the human male; they include the Cowper's glands and glands of Littre. The Cowper's gland, or bulbourethral gland, is a paired, pea-sized, compound tubular gland located directly below the prostate within the urogenital sinus. This gland was named after its founder William Cowper, who first described it in 1698. The glands empty into the urethra, and the function and composition of their secretions are poorly understood. Very small urethral glands, termed glands of Littre, line the penile urethra. All of these sex accessory tissues depend on androgens for development, growth, and maintenance; their secretory products contribute to the composition of the seminal plasma of the ejaculate.

Tissue Organization of Sex Accessory Tissue

The organization of the human prostate is analogous to a bunch of grapes immersed in a fibrous gelatin. Each of these grapes would be equivalent to the alveoli, which are lined with tall columnar secretory epithelial cells that line the periphery of acini that drain by a system of branching ducts and tubules into the prostatic urethra. This permits the secretions of the prostate to be added to other seminal plasma components arriving through the ejaculatory ducts, which bring spermatozoa and secretions from the testes, epididymis, ampulla, and seminal vesicles. The ejaculatory ducts pass through the prostate posteriorly to the bladder neck and enter the prostatic urethra in the regions known as the *verumontanum*. The acini and ducts of the prostate are embedded in a tissue matrix composed of stromal components, including fibromuscular, vascular, and connective tissues.

Cell Types

The prostatic epithelium in the human is composed of three types of cells: the secretory epithelial cells, the basal cells, and/or the stem cells. In any cell-renewing population there is the flow of cells from reserve quiescent stem cells to a more rapidly dividing transient proliferating population and finally to the formation of the fully mature nondividing terminally differentiated secretory cell that will then die off. In the prostate the most common tall columnar epithelial cells are terminally differentiated and are easily distinguished by their morphology and abundant secretory granules and enzymes that stain abundantly with acid phosphatase and other enzymes such as leucine amino peptidase and prostatic-specific antigen. These tall columnar secretory cells appear like rows of a picket fence resting next to each other, with their base attached to a basement membrane and with their nuclei located at their base. Above the nucleus is a clear zone of abundant Golgi apparatus, and the upper cellular periphery is rich in secretory granules and enzymes. The apical plasma membrane facing the lumen possesses a microvilli, and secretions move out into the open collecting spaces of the acinus. These epithelial cells encircle the periphery of the acinus, and the acini drain into ducts that connect to the urethra.

Much smaller and less abundant in number are the basal cells, which are present in less than 10% of the number of secretory epithelial cells. These small cells are not columnar and are more round, with little cytoplasm and large irregularly shaped nuclei. They are less differentiated and almost devoid of secretory products such as acid phosphatase. These basal cells appear wedged between the bases of adjacent columnar epithelial cells and are always resting on the basement membrane. These basal cells are rich in tonofilaments and stain brightly with fluorescent antibodies to keratin (159). It was mistakenly believed that these cells were myoepithelial (160), but this is not true because they are not rich in actin or myosin. It is believed that these undifferentiated basal cells give rise to secretory epithelial cells and, as such, function as a type of stem cell (161). The importance of understanding the biology of these basal cells is realized because of the growing evidence that many neoplasias both benign and malignant are really stem-cell diseases.

The proper identification, in the prostate, of stem cells and transient proliferating cells has not been realized. Indeed, there may be several types of each of these cells as well as several types of secretory cells. Functional and immunological markers are needed to answer these questions.

Stroma and Tissue Matrix

The noncellular stroma and connective tissue of the prostate compose what is termed the *extracellular matrix* (Fig. 12). The extracellular matrix has long been recognized as one of the important inductive components during normal development of many different types of cells (154). A matrix system is defined as a biological scaffolding or residual skeleton structure that organizes cells as well as subcellular particles. The cellular matrix system is one of the most active areas of modern cell biology (i.e., extracellular matrix, cytoskeleton, and nuclear matrix). The extracellular matrix is far more than a supporting scaffolding because it has been shown to play a central role in development and the control of cellular function (162,163). It now appears that the extracellular matrix is just one of the three major matrix systems that interact and form the overall tissue matrix system of the prostate (164). In this concept the epithelial cell rests upon the basement membrane, which is connected by an extracellular matrix to the stromal cells. It is believed that phase shifts and communication through these structural matrix elements may play a central role in controlling prostatic development and function (164).

It is now established that all cells are composed of a cytomatrix or cytoskeleton network that is formed from microtubules, microfilaments, and intermediate filaments. Tubulin is ubiquitous in all cells as a microtubular protein and appears to anchor many cellular structures. The microfilaments are primarily actin, one of the major proteins in all cells. Actin has the ability to polymerize and depolymerize and, as such, constitutes one of the important structural chemomechanical systems within the cell that is involved in a central way with transport of particles and components within the cell.

The intermediate filaments of the cytomatrix are extremely important because they vary with differentiation and appear to define the various cell types within the body. For example, one of the intermediate filaments, called *desmin*, is a central component of all muscle cells, whereas the intermediate filament *vimentin* is found in all fibroblasts. Surprisingly, the intermediate filament *keratin* is universal as a major component of the tonofilaments of all epithelial cells. There is usually just one type of vimentin and desmin in the fibroblast or muscle cells. In contrast, in the epithelial cells the keratins represent 20 different molecular types that vary with the state of cellular differentiation and the types of epithelial cells ranging from stratified squamous to simple epithelial cells.

The cytomatrix (cell skeleton) just described terminates in the center of the cell by direct attachment to the nuclear matrix (Fig. 12). The prostatic epithelial cell therefore has direct structural linkage via the matrix systems from the DNA to the plasma membrane. The cytomatrix then makes direct contact to the basement membrane and extracellular matrix and ground substance of the stroma. This entire interlocking tissue scaffolding or superstructure is termed the *tissue matrix* (164) and may have dynamic properties in ordering biological processes and transport of the sex accessory tissues.

Understanding the biological components of the tissue matrix system within sex accessory tissues is of paramount importance. The epithelial cell is anchored to the basement membrane or basement lamina by an extracellular matrix protein called *laminin*. The laminin proteins are glycoproteins of the extracellular matrix that mediate attachment of cells to the collagen IV of the basement membrane. Laminin is produced by epithelial cells, but not by fibroblasts, and is a large molecule with molecular domains that interact with the type-IV collagen of the basement membrane and with the cell-surface glycocalyx of the epithelial cell. The basement membrane is not a membrane, but a complex structure containing type-IV collagen, glycosaminoglycans, complex polysaccharides, and glycolipids. The basement membrane forms the direct interface between the epithelial cells and the stroma.

A second type of important prostatic glycoprotein that is involved in cell adherence in the extracellular matrix is *fibronectin*. Fibronectin is secreted primarily by prostatic fibroblasts and forms an adhesive material binding mesenchymal and epithelial cells to various types of collagen and proteoglycans. This important protein has been proposed to play a key role in morphogenesis and control of cell growth.

The connective tissue of the prostate consists primarily of type-I and type-III collagen, which form the interstitial collagen (165), while type-IV and type-V collagen are found primarily in the basement membrane woven through the stroma and connective tissue of the extracellular matrix in a complex network of glycosaminoglycans and complex polysaccharides. Glycosaminoglycans are large negatively charged polymers (polyanions) that have proven to be critical factors in the signaling of extracellular matrix events in many different tissues (162,163). These latter polysaccharide polymers have long been proposed to play an important role in prostate growth (166); recently, DeKlerk (167) isolated these important glycosaminoglycans (GAGs) from the normal and benign human prostates and reported that dermatan sulfate is the predominant (40%) GAG, followed by heparin (20%), chondroitin (16%), and hyaluronic acid (20%). Fetal prostates are devoid of dermatan, and chondroitin sulfate increases with BPH. It will be of interest to determine the role of GAGs in sex accessory tissue function.

In the near future, one of the most active areas in unraveling the control of sex accessory tissue function will revolve around a clearer understanding of how all of these tissue matrix components interact. At present there have been several important studies (88,89,92,164,167) that all point to the importance of these structural elements. Of particular importance are: the work of Isaacs et al. (164), who have shown the localization of keratins, laminin, fibronectin, and actin within the various cell types of the prostate utilizing immunofluorescent studies, and the studies of Bartsch et al. (165) and Mawhinney and his colleagues (92) on the collagens of the prostate.

Function

Sex Accessory Gland Secretions

The average volume of the normal human ejaculate is 3 to 3.5 ml, ranging from 2 to 6 ml, and is composed of two components, spermatozoa and seminal plasma, which can be separated easily by centrifugation. The spermatozoa are present in the range of 100 million per milliliter, but because of the small volume of sperm (approximately 10 cubic mm per sperm), the volume of the spermatozoa component is insignificant in the volume of the total ejaculate (less than 1%). The seminal plasma is formed primarily from the secretions of the sex accessory tissues, which include the epididymis, vas deferens, ampullae, seminal vesicles, prostate, Cowper's (bulbourethral) gland, and glands of Littre. In an average ejaculate volume of 3 to 3.5 ml, the major contribution to the volume of the seminal plasma comes from the following: seminal vesicles, 1.5 to 2 ml; prostate, 0.5 ml; and Cowper's gland and glands of Littre, 0.1 to 0.2 ml (168,169). During ejaculation the secretions of these glands are released in a sequential manner (170–173).

The first fractions of the human ejaculate are rich in (a) sperm and (b) components from the prostatic secretion such as citric acid. The concentration of fructose represents a major secretory product from the seminal vesicles and is elevated in the later fractions of the ejaculate. The overall chemical composition of the normal human seminal plasma has been studied by many laboratories, and the results have been summarized in excellent reviews (174–176).

In relation to other body fluids, the seminal plasma is unusual because of its high concentrations of potassium, zinc, citric acid, fructose, phosphorylcholine, spermine, free amino acids, prostaglandins, and enzymes (most notably acid phosphatase, diamine oxidase, beta-glucuronidase, lactic dehydrogenase, alpha-amylase, and seminal proteinase).

Zinc. The high level of zinc in human seminal plasma appears to originate primarily from secretions of the prostate gland. In 1921, Bertrand and Vladesco (177) reported that the human prostate had the highest concentration of zinc (50 mg/100 g dry weight) of any organ tested. In 1962, Mackenzie et al. (312) reported that human seminal plasma contained 310 mg of zinc/100 g dry weight and that spermatozoa contained 200 mg/100 g dry weight. In comparison, prostatic secretions from eight normal subjects had 720 mg zinc/100 g dry weight. Animal studies on many species have confirmed these general observations as well as the high level of tissue uptake of administered radioactive zinc-65. Many of the early experiments and concepts related to zinc in the reproductive tract have been reviewed in detail by Byar (178). Zinc levels are elevated or stable in BPH, while there is a marked decrease in zinc content associated with prostatic adenocarcinoma. The localization of zinc in the human prostate by radioautography appears to be within the epithelial cells; however, in the lateral prostate of the rat, large quantities of zinc were also associated with the stroma and particularly with the basal membrane and the elastin protein component (179).

Many physiologic roles have been postulated for zinc since the classic studies of Gunn and Gould (180,181), who correlated endocrine effects on zinc uptake and concentration in the prostate of the rodent. There are many important zinc-containing metalloenzymes, but the concentration of zinc in the prostate probably exceeds that present in zinc-associated enzymes. Zinc is known to bind many proteins. Johnson et al. (182) characterized zinc-binding protein in the prostatic secretion of the dog, which contained only eight types of amino acids upon hydrolysis. Heathcote and Washington (183) described a zinc-binding protein in human BPH that was rich in histidine and alanine. There have been other studies on zinc-binding proteins from the prostate (184,185), and additional information on these interesting proteins is needed.

An important role for zinc in the prostatic secretion has been suggested in the studies of Fair and Wehner (184). The investigators show the direct role of zinc as a prostatic antibacterial factor. It had been known that the prostatic secretion contained antibacterial factors (184). One of the important factors has now been related to the zinc concentration in expressed prostatic fluid. In the study of 36 normal men free from bacterial prostatic infections, the mean value of zinc in the prostatic secretion was approximately 350 μg/ml, with a wide range of 150 to 1,000. In comparison, the prostatic fluid obtained from 61 specimens collected from 15 patients with documented chronic bacterial prostatis averaged only 50 μg/ml, with a range of 0 to 139. The authors (184) propose a lower limit of normal at 150 μg/ml. In addition, *in vitro* studies of zinc at concentrations normally found in prostatic fluid have confirmed the bactericidal activity of zinc against a variety of gram-positive and gram-negative bacteria.

The concentration of zinc in normal human seminal plasma (mean value: 140 g/ml) is less than half of that in the normal prostatic secretion. Earlier reports have commented on the association of decreased levels of zinc in seminal plasma of men with prostatitis (174). Although cause and effects are always difficult to resolve, the antibacterial properties of the zinc ion at physiologic concentrations suggest one possible role for high levels of zinc in the prostate gland and secretions. However, a considerable portion of the zinc in the prostate appears to be bound to unique proteins, and it is not certain how this might alter the biologic properties of zinc.

Citric acid. One of the major anions in the human seminal plasma is citrate (mean value: 376 mg/100 ml), which is in the range of 20 mM or 60 meq/liter. This is compared to the chloride ion (155 mg/100 ml) at 40 mM. Citrate is important in maintaining the osmotic equilibrium of the prostate (175). It is a potent binder of metal ions; the seminal plasma concentration of citrate, 20 mM, is comparable to that of the total divalent metals, 13.6 mM (calcium 7 mM; magnesium, 4.5 mM; zinc, 2.1 mM). Citric acid is localized in different sex accessory tissues according to species; however, in the human the prostate is the major source of citric acid that is present in the semen. This observation is based on the studies of Huggins (186), who studied nine samples of human prostatic secretion and recorded values ranging from 480 to 2,688 mg citric acid/100 ml. The values for two samples of seminal vesicle secretions were only 15 and 22 mg citric acid/100 ml, respectively. Assays of tissue levels of citric acid also implicate the prostate as the source of citric acid in the seminal plasma. Citric acid and acid phosphatase levels in semen have often been used as chemical indicators of prostatic function; however, citric acid seminal plasma levels cannot be equated directly to plasma levels of testosterone.

Fructose. The source of fructose in human seminal plasma is the seminal vesicles (175). Patients with congenital absence of the seminal vesicles also have an associated absence of fructose in their ejaculates (187). The seminal vesicle secretion contains smaller amounts of other free sugars such as glucose, sorbitol, ribose, and fucose, and these sugars usually amount to less than 10 mg/100 ml. In comparison, the concentration of the reducing sugar, fructose, is approximately 300 mg/100 ml in human seminal secretion and has a level of 200 mg/100 ml in seminal plasma. These levels of fructose are under androgenic regulation, but many factors such as storage, frequency of ejaculation, blood glucose levels, and nutritional status can also affect the seminal plasma concentration (175); these considerations may account for the wide variations encountered in different semen samples from the same patient. Furthermore, plasma levels of androgens do not always correlate with seminal plasma fructose levels (188), and these levels are therefore not a reliable index of the androgenic state of the subject.

The source of fructose in seminal vesicles appears to proceed from glucose by aldose reduction to sorbitol, followed by a ketone reduction to form fructose. The fructose of the seminal plasma appears to provide an anaerobic and aerobic source of energy for the spermatozoa (175). The cervical mucus has high concentrations of glucose and very low levels of fructose, and the sperm are capable of utilizing both types of sugars.

Phosphorylcholine and α-glycerophosphorylcholine. The semen of mammals is very rich in choline $[(CH_3)_3-N^+-(CH_2)_2-OH]$. In the human, phosphorylcholine predominates, whereas in most other species much higher levels of α-glycerophosphorylcholine are present, often exceeding 1 g/100 ml of seminal plasma. Seligman et al. (189) have demonstrated that phosphorylcholine is a highly specific substrate for prostatic acid phosphatase, which is also very active in seminal plasma. The result of this enzymatic activity is the rapid formation of free choline in the first ejaculate. In contrast, α-glycerophosphorylcholine is secreted primarily in the epididymis and is not readily hydrolyzed by acid phosphatase. For these reasons, Mann and Lutwak-Mann (175) have suggested that the level of α-glycerophosphorylcholine can be used as an index for assessing the contribution of the epididymal secretion to the ejaculate. The secretion from the epididymis is also under androgenic control (190). The function of these choline compounds is unknown; it appears that they are not metabolized by spermatozoa nor do they affect the respiration of the sperm (190).

Spermine. Spermine levels in the normal human seminal plasma range from 50 to 350 mg/100 ml and originate primarily from the prostate gland, which is the richest source of spermine in the body. Spermine $[NH_2-(CH_2)_3-NH-(CH_2)_4-(CH_2)_4-NH-(CH_2)_3-NH_2]$ is a very basic aliphatic polyamine and, because of its four positive charges, binds strongly to acidic or negatively charged molecules such as phosphate ions, nucleic acid, or phospholipids. When semen is allowed to stand at room temperature, acid phosphatase enzymatically hydrolyzes seminal phosphorylcholine to form free inorganic phosphate ions, which then interact with the positively charged spermine and precipitate as large translucent salt crystals of spermine phosphate. There has been much interest in spermine and other related polyamines such as spermidine and putrescine because of the rapid and dramatic changes in levels and ratios associated with many types of cells that have been induced into growth. Because polyamine metabolism is correlated with growth and because the potential of polyamines for interacting with DNA is documented, much speculation has resulted, but at present the biologic role of these polyamines has not been resolved.

Relationships between spermine levels in seminal plasma and sperm count and motility have also been suggested (191–193). Williams-Ashman and his colleagues have investigated in detail the biosynthesis and regulation of polyamines in the male reproductive tract and have characterized the enzymatic reactions that progress from ornithine to putrescine to spermidine to spermine (194–196). The polyamines are oxidized enzymatically by diamine oxidase (present in the seminal plasma) to form very reactive aldehyde compounds that can be toxic to both sperm and bacteria (197). The formation of these aldehyde products produces the characteristic odor of semen. It is also possible that these aldehydes or polyamines themselves may protect the genitourinary tract from infective agents. Polyamine can also form amide bonds to protein carboxylic groups (194,197).

Prostaglandins. The richest sources of prostaglandins in the human are the seminal vesicles. Prostaglandins are present in seminal plasma at a total concentration of approximately 100 to 300 μg/ml. Injected seminal plasma produces strong pharmacological effects. Goldblatt (198,199) and von Euler (200) independently reported the stimulatory and depressor effects of extracts of human seminal plasma on smooth muscle. In 1934, von Euler (200) proposed the name *prostaglandins* for the active components in seminal plasma in the belief that they originated from the prostate gland. Eliasson (201) established that the primary source of prostaglandin was the seminal vesicles, not the prostate. However, the original name has survived to the present. Prostaglandins have a wide distribution in mammalian tissues but at much lower concentrations than found in the seminal vesicles. Bergstrom et al. (202) recognized that there were many types of prostaglandins, and they purified and identified many of the chemical structures. There are 15 different prostaglandins present in human semen, and they are all 20-carbon hydroxy fatty acids containing a cyclopentane ring with two side chains; as such they are derivatives of prostanoic acid. The 15 types of prostaglandins are divided into four major groups, designated A, B, E, and F according to the structure of the five-membered cyclopentane ring, and each of these groups is further subdivided according to the position and number of double bonds in the side chain (therefore, PGE3 indicates prostaglandins of E type with three double bonds in the side chain). The E group of prostaglandins is the major component in the male reproductive tract, whereas the F predominates in the female system. Fuchs and Chantharaski (203) have summarized the reported levels of human seminal plasma prostaglandins and report the following mean values (μg/ml): PGE1, 20; PGE2, 15; (PGE1 + E2)-19-OH, 100; PGA1 + A2, 9; (PGA1 + A2)-19-OH1, 31; PGB1 + B2, 18; (PGB1 + B2)-19-OH, 13; PGF1a, 3; and PGF2a, 4. These compounds are very potent pharmacologic agents that have been implicated in a wide variety of biologic events in the male, including erection, ejaculation, sperm motility and transport, and testicular and penile contractions. In addition, prostaglandins from seminal fluid deposited in the vagina have been reported to affect cervical mucus, vaginal secretion, and sperm transport in the female genital tract. Not all of these effects have been established in a compelling manner.

Cholesterol and lipids. Scott (204) reported that human seminal plasma contained 185 mg/100 ml of total lipids, 103 mg/100 ml of cholesterol, and 83 mg/100 ml of phospholipids. In comparison, human prostatic secretion contained: total lipids, 186 mg/100 ml; cholesterol, 80 mg/100 ml; and phospholipids, 180 mg/100 ml. The lipids of semen have been further described (205), and the phospholipids of the seminal plasma are composed of 44% sphingomyelin, 12.3% ethanolamine plasmalogen, and 11.2% phosphatidylserine (206).

The reported levels of cholesterol in seminal plasma have varied considerably, from 11 to 103 mg/100 ml (201,204,206). White and colleagues (206) believe that the ratio of cholesterol to phospholipid in the seminal plasma stabilizes the sperm against temperature and environmental shock.

The prostate is a partial source of cholesterol in the seminal plasma (204). It has been reported that the human prostate can synthesize cholesterol and that the synthesis level is higher in benign prostatic hyperplasia; it has also been theorized that blocked secretion of cholesterol may be an etiologic factor in BPH.

Urinary cholesterol is reported to be elevated in about two-thirds of patients with prostatic adenocarcinoma (207,208). The source of urinary cholesterol has not been determined, and it remains to be established whether this elevated urinary cholesterol is unique to prostatic cancer.

Coagulation and liquefaction of semen. Human semen coagulates into a semisolid gel within 5 min following ejaculation; upon further standing, the clot spontaneously liquefies in a 5- to 20-min period to form a viscous liquid (175,209,210). Calcium-binding substances such as sodium citrate and heparin do not inhibit the coagulation process, nor is prothrombin, fibrinogen, or Factor XII required, since they are absent in seminal plasma (for review, see ref. 175). The seminal clot is formed of fibers 0.15 to 10 nm in width, and its morphology differs from that of a blood fibrin clot (175,209–212). From these observations and others, it appears that the coagulation of human semen is different from that of blood. In addition, factors affecting blood coagulation do not regulate semen viscosity (213).

Examination of split human ejaculates indicates that (a) the first fraction, originating primarily from Cowper's gland and the prostate, contains the liquefaction factors and (b) the final fraction, which is enriched by seminal vesicle secretions, is responsible for the coagulation of the ejaculate.

It has long been known that prostatic fluid has a dramatic fibrinolytic-like activity and that 2 ml of this secretion can liquefy 100 ml of clotted blood in 18 hr at 37°C (175,209). The factors involved in such proteolytic activity in semen have been resolved (175,209–211,214,215). Two types of seminal plasma proteolytic enzymes appear to be major factors in the liquefaction process: plasminogen activators and seminin.

Two plasminogen activators have been isolated from seminal plasma; they have molecular weights of 70,000 and 74,000 and appear to be related to urokinase (216). It is believed that the plasminogen activators originate from the prostatic secretions.

Seminin is a proteolytic enzyme (molecular weight 30,000) that appears in the first fraction of split ejaculates and is therefore believed to originate from the prostate gland (211,214,216–219). This seminal proteinase was first thought to have chymotrypsin-like properties, but this was proved incorrect upon further purification and characterization; furthermore, seminin does not have true fibrinolytic activity (214).

The seminal plasma contains a variety of other proteolytic enzymes, including pepsinogen, lysozyme, α-amylase, and hyaluronidase. In addition, human semen inhibits the activity of the proteolytic enzyme trypsin, and this is due to the presence in the seminal plasma of such proteinase inhibitors as α-1-antitrypsin and α-1-antichymotrypsin.

Coagulation and liquefaction vary in different species. For example, the semen of the bull or dog does not coagulate, whereas the semen of rodents such as the rat and guinea pig is ejaculated as a firm pellet that does not appear to liquefy (219,220). In rodents, the plugs form through the action of an enzyme called *vesiculase*, which comes from the anterior lobe of the prostate and reacts with seminal vesicle secretions. Because of this action, the anterior lobe of the rodent prostate is also called the *coagulating gland*. Vesiculase is not identical with thrombin, since it does not coagulate fibrinogen nor does thrombin clot the secretions of the seminal vesicles. Williams-Ashman et al. (221) have established that vesiculase has transamidase activity, catalyzing the formation of γ-glutamyl-ε-lysine cross-links in a clottable protein derived from the seminal vesicles. This seminal vesicle protein, which serves as a substrate for vesiculase, is a very basic substance with a molecular weight of 17,900; it has been characterized, with regard to its physical properties, by Notides and Williams-Ashman (222).

In the boar, the clot appears to result from a sialomucoprotein from the bulbourethral (Cowper's) gland interacting with two proteins secreted by the seminal vesicle (223). These species differences make it difficult to extrapolate mechanisms in animals to the human situation. In summary, it appears that seminal plasma coagulation and liquefaction are under enzymatic control, but the biologic purpose of this process has not been resolved. Enzymes and proteins of the seminal vesicles and prostate glands are involved in this system. There have been reports that some infertile men may have impairment of the liquefaction process (224–227).

Immunoglobulins. There are many reports establishing the presence of immunoglobulins in human seminal plasma. It is possible to measure levels of IgG from 7 to 22 mg/100 ml and IgA from 0 to 6 mg/100 ml; however, no IgM has been detected (228). The source of these antibodies is not known, although under certain conditions it appears that they are produced in the sex tissues. They are usually found at lower levels in seminal plasma than in blood, but the possibility of diffusion across the "blood/seminal-plasma barrier" has not been eliminated [see discussion by Friberg (228)].

Acid phosphatase. Because of the clinical and biological importance of prostatic acid phosphatase, it will be reviewed in more detail. Human semen contains a very high activity of acid phosphatase enzymes that originate from the secretions of the prostate gland. When prostatic cancer cells metastasize, they often continue to secrete acid phosphatases into the serum, producing elevated levels that are an important diagnostic aid in monitoring prostatic adenocarcinoma [see classic early studies of Gutman and Gutman (229) and Huggins and Hodges (230)].

Enzyme Assay: One of the most abundant enzymes in the ejaculate is acid phosphatase of prostatic origin. Phosphatases are very common enzymes in tissues but are extremely rich in the prostate. Phosphatase enzymes hydrolyze many types of organic monophosphate esters to yield inorganic phosphate ions and alcohol by the following reaction:

$$R—OPO_3H_2 + H_2O \rightarrow ROH + H_3PO_4$$

Many phosphatase enzymes exhibit optimal activity *in vitro* in the acid (pH 4–6) or alkaline (pH 8–11) ranges and are thus classified broadly as either acid or alkaline phosphatase. Both types of phosphatase appear to be ubiquitous in animal tissues.

Acid phosphatases may be further defined by factors that inhibit their enzymatic activity. For example, erythrocyte acid phosphatase is particularly sensitive to inhibition of 0.5% formaldehyde or copper ions (0.2 mM), whereas prostatic acid phosphatase activity is far more sensitive to inhibition by fluoride ions (1 mM) or L-tartrate (1 mM). These inhibitors have been utilized to improve the specificity of the assay, and the differential tartrate inhibition is often used to indicate the specific prostatic acid phosphatase fraction. This is often helpful in distinguishing the serum erythrocyte acid phosphatase that leaks from damaged or hemolyzed cells because the erythrocyte enzyme is not inhibited by tartrate.

Osteoclasts are also a rich source of tartrate-insensitive acid phosphatase, and this fact is useful because of the minor elevation in serum acid phosphatase levels that accompanies Paget's disease, osteoporosis, nonprostatic bone metastasis, and other conditions of increased bone resorption.

Platelets may also be a source of acid phosphatase, which, like the prostate enzyme, is also sensitive to tartrate ions; thus, tartrate inhibition is not entirely specific for prostatic acid phosphatase. Studies have been performed on the enzyme kinetics of the reaction of prostatic acid phosphatase with a variety of substrates.

Substrates for Acid Phosphatase: All acid phosphatases hydrolyze a wide range of natural and synthetic phosphomonoesters, and this has provided a wide variety of assay systems and the expression of many different units of activity. These synthetic substrates include, in part: phenylphosphate (229); phenolphthalein phosphate (231,232); para-nitrophenyl phosphate, also called Sigma 104; β-naphthyl phosphate (233); α-naphthyl phosphate (234); β-glycerophosphate (235); naphthol AS-B1 phosphate (236); and thymolphthalein phosphate (237). The specificity of these substrates varies with the type and source of acid phosphatase; it appears that thymolphthalein phosphate may be the most specific substrate for assaying serum levels of prostatic acid phosphatase because it is a very poor substrate for the erythrocyte enzyme that is often present as a contaminant in the serum (237). It should be emphasized, however, that activity with this substrate can be found with acid phosphatase from other tissues; therefore, although it is not entirely specific for the prostate enzyme, it is still the substrate of choice for serum assays. At present there is no agreed-upon standard method of assaying prostatic acid phosphatase or even of expressing the values. The natural substrate for prostatic acid phosphatase may be phosphorylcholine phosphate (see p. 1107), which is rapidly hydrolyzed in the semen. Seligman and his associates (233) have compared phosphorylcholine phosphate as a substrate for human acid phosphatase from both the prostate and the kidney and have shown that this substrate has a 1,000-fold greater specificity for the prostate enzyme. The biologic functions of this enzyme, as well as its reactions, are not known. It is also of interest that prostatic acid phosphatase will hydrolyze tyrosine phosphate esters, the natural products of many oncogene protein tyrosine kinases.

Isoenzymes of Acid Phosphatase: Many tissues contain several forms of acid phosphatase that can be resolved by electrophoretic techniques (238,239). Some of these enzyme forms can be separated by subfractionation of the tissue and may be associated primarily with either the lysosomes, secretions, or particular membrane fractions. Starch gel electrophoresis of prostate tissue extracts revealed 13 bands of activity, but only a single band was observed in seminal plasma (240). This observation suggested that these might be multiple forms of a common enzyme in various states of being processed for secretion. This was later supported by the observation that neuraminidase treatment, which removes sialic acid residues from the glycoprotein enzyme, converted the 13 bands to a single entity and that assay of the multiple forms could be accounted for by different amounts of sialic acid (241–243).

Human prostatic acid phosphatase is a 102,000-dalton glycoprotein and contains about 7% carbohydrate by weight; this carbohydrate is composed of 15 residues per mole of neutral sugars (fucose, galactose, and mannose); six residues per mole of sialic acid; and 13 residues of *N*-acetylglucosamine (241). The protein can be dissociated into two subunits. In summary, many secretory proteins and enzymes are glycosylated after they have been synthesized, and it appears that this accounts for some of the isoenzyme patterns of prostatic acid phosphatase. The secretory enzyme is probably the major form, and the lysosomal acid phosphatase may be similar in properties to that found in other tissue lysosomes.

The above discussion has pertained to human prostatic acid phosphatase. It is important to note that this high enzymatic activity is not characteristic of accessory tissues in many other species.

Leucine aminopeptidase. Aminopeptidases hydrolyze the *N*-terminal amino acid from small polypeptides Leucine aminopeptidases are particularly active against the substrate L-leucyl glycine, and some of these enzymes are referred to as *arylamidases* because the optimal substrate is L-leucyl β-naphthylamine. The human prostate is rich in the latter arylamidase type of leucine aminopeptidase. Mattila (244) demonstrated two forms of the enzyme in human prostatic tissue (molecular weights 107,000 and 305,000), only one of which was similar to that of the kidney. The kidney is one of the richest sources of leucine aminopeptidases, but at present the tissue-specific nature of any of these isoenzymes has not been established.

Leucine aminopeptidase is a product of the epithelial cells of the prostate (245) and is secreted into the lumen of the acini (246).

Lactic dehydrogenase. It has been reported that isoenzyme ratios of lactic dehydrogenases (LDH) in human semen may be altered if the patient has prostatic cancer (247–249). Lactic dehydrogenase (150,000 molecular weight) is composed of four subunits (each of 35,000 molecular weight) of only two different types of proteins, denoted M and H. The LDH of muscle has four M units and that of heart has four H units. Five isoenzymes of LDH can be found in tissues with a four-subunit composition as follows: LDH I, MMMM; LDH II, MMMH; LDH III, MMHH; LDH IV, MHHH; and LDH V, HHHH. The M and H subunits appear to be the same in all tissues, but the amounts of LDH I to V can vary. Denis and Prout (250) observed increased levels of LDH IV and V in prostatic cancer tissue. Several investigators have observed elevated ratios of LDH V/LDH I in human prostatic cancer (247,251,252). Belitsky et al. (253) measured serum levels of LDH V/LDH I after prostatic massage and believe this may be of diagnostic value. Assays of human prostatic fluid or semen for the isoenzyme ratio may become an important diagnostic tool.

Major proteins of sex accessory gland origin. There have been several studies to identify high-resolution two-dimensional electrophoresis profiles of major secretory protein markers from human ejaculate, seminal plasma, and prostatic secretions (254–257).

Prostatic Proteins: Prostatic-Specific Antigen and Prostatein: Isaacs and Shaper (258) have identified a major protein in the canine ejaculate that is of prostatic origin and is present at extremely high concentrations of 10 mg/ml in the seminal plasma. This protein accounts for the majority of soluble proteins in prostates of intact mature dogs, where its presence is androgen-dependent. The protein accounts for over 90% of the total protein found in prostatic fluid and is composed of two dissimilar subunits (~15,000 molecular weight) that are held together by disulfide bonds. This protein has also been studied extensively by Dube and his colleagues (259–263). Isaacs and Coffey (264) have shown two important functions for this secretory protein. The protein is an enzyme that is specifically an arginine esteroprotease (264) and is similar to one of the major esterases reported earlier in semen (265). The canine prostatic secretory protein, which is a protease, is present at 10 mg/ml in the canine ejaculate and rapidly hydrolyzes arginine esters; this enzyme also binds to canine sperm tails (264). Therefore, the secretory protein of the prostate can be identified on sperm tails that are collected from ejaculates but not on those from the epididymal sperm. It is unknown at present why the ejaculate should contain such a tremendous amount of protease activity or what its function is in binding to sperm tails. It is of interest that this secretory protein, which is the main component of the ejaculate protein in the dog, is a serine protease with kallikrein-like activities and has been shown to have sequence homology with an important protein in the human seminal plasma termed the *prostatic-specific antigen* (PA) (266). In addition, it may be similar to the glandular proteases that process pregrowth factors in the salivary gland (267).

In 1979, Wang et al. (268,269) reported the human prostate-specific antigen, which is becoming a very important marker of the prostate. This protein is a 33,000-dalton glycoprotein that contains 7% carbohydrate (266). This protein is detected only in the epithelial cells of the prostatic ductal elements by a specific antibody. Recently, prostatic antigen has been demonstrated to be clinically important for the detection and monitoring of prostate cancer (270,271). This protein has been used as a marker for postcoital detection in rape investigation (272). Watt et al. (266) have recently made an extensive study of this protein and have carried out the complete amino acid sequence. The single polypeptide chain contains 240 amino acids and an *O*-linked carbohydrate side chain attached to serine. The enzyme is a serine protease with trypsin-like activity. Recently, Lilja (273) reported that the structural protein of the seminal coagulum, the predominant seminal-vesicle-secreted protein, might be the physiological substrate for prostatic-specific antigen.

There has been a major secretory protein identified in the rat ventral prostate that has had a variety of different names, including α-protein, prostatic secretion protein, estramustine-binding protein, and prostatic binding protein, but the most common term and the one that is gaining popularity is *prostatein* [see review by Perry et al. (274)]. Prostatein is a protein composed of several chains, including one 6,000-dalton subunit referred to as C-1, one 10,000-dalton subunit termed C-2, and two 14,000-dalton subunits termed C-3. The gene for this protein has been sequenced and characterized, and it has been shown that the messenger RNA expression for this gene is under strict androgen control. This indicates that the gene is transcriptionally regulated.

It is believed that the receptor protein binds near to this gene during activation. Perry et al. (274) have shown that two regions of the androgen-regulated C-3 gene show preferential binding for the 4.5-S androgen receptor. The organization and expression of this prostatic gene for prostatein-binding protein have been studied in some detail by Parker and Needham (275).

Seminal-Vesicle Proteins: In 1983, Williams-Ashman wrote a classic review (276) on the regulatory features of the seminal vesicles' development and function. Besides the proteins and enzymes already discussed, several marker proteins have become active models for studying the way androgens activate and regulate specific genes. One of the best studied of these is the seminal-vesicle secretion IV and V gene. Many of these proteins share upstream sequence homologies with the androgen-regulated genes of the prostate (277). The sequence organization of the rat seminal-vesicle F gene has also been characterized by locating transcriptional start points as well as by performing sequence comparisons with six other androgen-regulated genes (278). Of considerable interest is the study of the methylation of the rat seminal-vesicle secretory protein IV gene, which undergoes extensive demethylation and may be a model system for many male sex accessory glands (279). DNA methylation has long been believed to be a regulatory step in gene expression, and the concept has been that demethylation allows the gene to be expressed; however, this has not been fully established. These proteins of the seminal vesicle not only serve as models for androgen regulation, but their enzymatic properties are of considerable interest. For example, androgen-regulated proteins of the rat seminal-vesicle secretion have been shown to constitute a structurally related family containing proteins that are present in a copulatory plug (280,281).

We are still not sure, beyond the coagulation reaction, what role these seminal vesicle proteins play, but their effect on fertility and uterine sperm motility has been studied in the mouse (282). Some of the proteins of the seminal vesicles also serve as substrates for the serine protease located in prostatic fluid (273). Other important enzymes that are seminal-vesicle proteins include the phospholipase C enzyme from sheep, which cleaves the phosphatidyl phosphoinositol system (283).

Involution of sex accessory tissue following castration and androgen deprivation. It was long believed that cell death following androgen withdrawal was simply the choking off of an important biological factor required to maintain the life of the cell. Recent studies have shown that this involution process is an active formation rather than a passive one. For example, Lee, Grayhack, and associates (284–287) were the first to report that if protein or RNA synthesis is blocked following castration, the ability of the prostate gland to involute was markedly reduced. This suggested that specific proteins derived from new messenger RNAs might be required to be activated to produce active cell death following androgen deprivation. This process is reminiscent of the system that occurs in bacteria, where bactericidal effects require the synthesis of over a dozen specific proteins required to kill the bacteria. Similar processes of specific protein synthesis also produce involution following androgen withdrawal. Several groups have studied the appearance of two-dimensional protein patterns that were altered by castration or androgen treatment (288–291). Liao and his colleagues (292) have shown that specific messages and products are required to be synthesized in the prostate during the process of involution. The most notable of these recent studies has been that of Saltzman, who showed that androgen withdrawal causes the production of a 29,000-dalton protein and its messenger RNA during the involution of the rat ventral prostate following castration (292). It will be interesting to follow this exciting work to learn how the growth of sex accessory tissues is regulated by both androgen-induced and androgen-repressed mechanisms. This is important because the final size of an organ's growth is a net balance of both proliferation and cell death.

Seminal plasma analysis and fertility. There have been several reviews related to semen analysis and fertility (224,293–295). Eliasson (293) emphasizes that decreased secretory function of the accessory genital glands is a common finding in men with acute and chronic infection or inflammation of the prostate or seminal vesicles; he further states that a decreased secretory capacity of the male sex accessory glands is not in itself a factor in infertility. Chemical alterations in the seminal plasma, however, may indicate abnormalities. Since seminal fructose is a secretory product of the seminal vesicles, it is often used as an index of the function of this gland. Fructose is absent from the semen in three situations (224): (1) Azoospermic males with congenital bilateral absence of the vas deferens and seminal vesicles do not produce seminal fructose. Embryologically, the seminal vesicles and vas deferens develop from the Wolffian ducts. Therefore, when the vas deferens is absent in development, so are the seminal vesicles; no fructose is present in the semen, and the ejaculate also does not coagulate. (2) The obstruction of both ejaculatory ducts prevents fructose from being added to the semen. (3) The presence of retrograde ejaculation leads to the absence of fructose in the semen. Fructose analysis of the semen is a simple test and should be performed routinely in every case of azoospermia (224). For additional details on obstructive occlusions in the reproductive tract and diagnostic approaches, see the review of Marina et al. (296).

Seminal fructose concentrations may also be lowered in vesiculitis. In addition, many authors have proposed the use of fructose levels in semen as a measurement of androgenic function, but there are serious limitations in such correlations (see earlier section on fructose). Moon and Bunge (297) have also discussed these limitations.

It seems probable that the sex accessory tissue secretions may enhance or protect functional properties of the sperm, but at present we do not know how these secretions interact with sperm under either normal or abnormal conditions.

Evaluation of the individual secretory components of the sex accessory glands is important in correlating glandular activity with fertility.

Transport of materials into the semen. Several natural products such as ergothioneine and other amino acids appear to be more highly concentrated in seminal plasma than in blood plasma (210). Some of these amino acids may have physiologic roles such as the conversion of arginine to ornithine by the action of the enzyme arginase. Ornithine then becomes the precursor for polyamines such as spermine and spermidine. Arginase is found at high concentrations in human prostatic tissues. Some of the amino acids may originate from proteolytic hydrolysis, but it seems apparent that a large portion is actually concentrated in the seminal plasma by an unknown mechanism (210). Other compounds are capable of entering the semen by simple diffusion, including ethanol (298), iodine (299), and antibiotics [see review of Reeves (300)].

Drugs entering prostatic secretions have been of interest because of the prevalence of prostatitis and the need for new modalities of chemotherapy. Stamey and his colleagues (301–303) have made extensive studies of the ability of chemotherapeutic agents to concentrate in the prostatic fluid of humans and dogs, and other laboratories have contributed to this knowledge (304,305). Few drugs reach concentrations in the prostatic secretion that approach or surpass their concentrations in blood, but some exceptions are the basic macrolides, erythromycin and oleandomycin; sulfonamides; chloramphenicol; tetracycline; clindamycin, and trimethoprim [see review of Reeves (300)]. In general, these drugs are assumed to pass across the membrane by nonionic diffusion, possibly by lipid solubility through the membrane; when they reach the more acidic prostatic fluid, they are protonated and acquire a more positive charge, thus becoming relatively trapped in the prostatic secretions. Several factors are critical, including the pK′ of the drug and the pH of the prostatic secretions, as well as the drug binding to proteins in each compartment. Basic drugs would be more ionized in acidic prostatic fluid than in blood. Slight changes in pH can have large effects on this nonionic diffusion. The pH of the prostatic secretion in the dog may be more acidic than in the human and may decrease with successive fractions during prostatic secretion collection under pilocarpine stimulation (302,303). Samples of prostatic secretions from humans varied widely in pH, from 6 to 8, with a mean value of 6.6; however, with prostatic inflammation the pH tended to be 7 or greater (306). Studies that are designed to avoid urine contamination and that utilize trimethoprim distribution agree, in general, with these values (304). Studies tend to indicate that nonionic diffusion may be the most critical factor in these processes (302,303). It should be realized that although prostatic secretions are slightly acidic, the pH of freshly ejaculated human semen is slightly alkaline (pH 7.3–7.7); on standing, semen first becomes more alkaline with the loss of carbon dioxide and then becomes acidic owing to accumulation of lactic acid.

Isaacs (65) has written a very well-prepared review of the concepts related to the transport properties of the prostate and seminal vesicles. He has compared the composition and volume of prostatic secretion under basal stimulation and under stimulation during ejaculation or pilocarpine stimulation. He shows an increase of 205-fold in the total potassium, chloride, and sodium output over the basal rate. He has shown that the prostate is capable of secreting five times its total content of sodium and chloride during active secretion. This obviously shows the tremendous transport powers of this system. Smith et al. (307) have looked at the transepithelial voltage changes during prostatic secretion in the dog and have concluded that sodium may move passively through the plasma in the prostatic fluid during ejaculation but that the movement of potassium and chloride ions involves active transcellular transport. Isaacs et al. (308) have shown that the androgen-induced secretions can be blocked in the presence of estrogen, although the growth properties and biological properties of the androgen on the prostate are not markedly altered. This would suggest a direct effect of estrogen in blocking a major transport system in the prostate.

It is conceivable that unique drugs may be developed that are transported into the semen to regulate fertility; however, more must be learned about the fundamental transport system in and out of the male reproductive tract before such an approach is feasible.

SUMMARY

The sex accessory tissues provide an excellent focus for future investigations because of their active role in the transport of sperm and the protection of the male reproductive tract. In addition, abnormal growth of the prostate represents one of the major medical problems facing the aging male. In light of their biological and medical importance, the sex accessory tissues deserve more study.

ACKNOWLEDGMENT

We wish to acknowledge the fine assistance and expertise of Ruth Middleton in the preparation of this manuscript.

REFERENCES

1. Berry, S. J., Coffey, D. S., Walsh, P. C., and Ewing, L. L. (1984): The development of human benign prostatic hyperplasia with age. *J. Urol.*, 132:474–479.
2. Berry, S. J., Coffey, D. S., and Ewing, L. L. (1985): A comparison of human and canine benign prostatic hyperplasia. In: *Regulation of Androgen Action in the Proceedings of an International Symposium, Montreal*, edited by N. Bruchovsky, A. Chapdelaine, and F. Neumann, pp. 59–68. Congressdruck R. Bruckner, Berlin.
3. Hunter, J. (1786): *Observations on Certain Parts of the Animal Oeconomy*, 1st edition: "Sold at 13 Castle Street," London; 2nd edition (1792). Nicol, London.
4. Grayhack, J. T., Bunce, P. K., Kearns, J. W., and Scott, W. W. (1955): Influence of the pituitary on prostatic response to androgen in the rat. *Bull. Johns Hopkins Hosp.*, 96:154.

5. Grayhack, J. T. (1963): Pituitary factors influencing growth of the prostate. *NCI Monogr.*, 12:189–199.
6. Manandhar, M. S. P., and Thomas, J. A. (1976): Effect of prolactin on the metabolism of androgens by the rat ventral prostate gland *in vitro*. *Invest. Urol.*, 14:20–22.
7. Assimos, D., Smith, C., Lee, C., and Grayhack, J. T. (1984): Action of prolactin in regressing prostate: Independent of action mediated by androgen receptors. *Prostate*, 5:589–595.
8. Sandberg, A. (1981): Experimental results with prolactin: An overview of the effect on the prostate. In: *The Prostate Cell: Structure and Function, Part B*, edited by G. P. Murphy, A. A. Sandberg, and J. P. Karr, pp. 55–62. Alan R. Liss, New York.
9. Witorsch, R. J., and Smith, J. P. (1977): Evidence for androgen-dependent intracellular binding of prolactin in rat ventral prostate gland. *Endocrinology*, 101:929–938.
10. Maehama, S., Lee, L. I. D., Nari, H., Leykam, J. F., and Duell, T. F. (1986): Purification and partial characterization of prostate-derived growth factor. *Proc. Natl. Acad. Sci., USA*, 83:8162–8166.
11. Crabb, J. W., Armes, L. G., Carr, S. A., Johnson, C. M., Roberts, G. D., Bordoli, R. S., and McKeehan, W. L. (1986): Complete primary structure of prostatropin, a prostate epithelial cell growth factor. *Biochemistry*, 25:4988–4993.
12. Gregory, H., Willshire, I. R., Kavanagh, J. P., Blacklock, N. J., Chowdury, S., and Richards, R. C. (1986): Urogastrone-epidermal growth factor concentration in prostatic fluid of normal individuals and patients with benign prostatic hypertrophy. *Clin. Sci.*, 70:359–363.
13. Shikita, H., Utsumi, N., Hiramatsu, M., Minami, N., Nemoto, N., and Shikita, T. (1984): Immunohistochemical localization of nerve growth factor and epidermal growth factor in guinea pig prostate gland. *Histochemistry*, 80:411–413.
14. Lawson, R. K., Storey, M. T., and Jacobs, S. C. (1981): In: *The Prostate Cell: Structure and Function*, Part A, edited by G. P. Murphy, A. A. Sandberg, and J. P. Karr, pp. 325–336. Alan R. Liss, New York.
15. Storey, M. T., Jacobs, S. C., and Lawson, R. K. (1983): Epidermal growth factor is not the major growth promoting agent in extracts of prostatic tissue. *J. Urol.*, 130:175–179.
16. Parrish, R. F., Heston, W. D. W., Pletscher, L. S., Tackett, R., and Fair, R. W. (1984): Prostate-derived growth factor. *Prog. Clin. Biol. Res.*, 145:181–195.
17. Hammond, G. L., Ruokonen, A., and Contturi, M. (1977): The simultaneous radioimmunoassay of seven steroids in human spermatic and peripheral venous blood. *J. Clin. Endocrinol. Metab.*, 45:16–24.
18. Bruchovsky, N., and Wilson, J. D. (1968): The conversion of testosterone to 5α-androstan-17β-ol-3-one by rat prostate *in vivo* and *in vitro*. *J. Biol. Chem.*, 243:2012–2121.
19. Shimazaki, J., Kurihara, H., Ito, Y., and Shida, K. (1965): Testosterone metabolism in prostate. Formation of androstane-17β-3-one and androst-4-ene-3,17-dione, and inhibitory effect of natural and synthetic estrogens. *Gunma J. Med. Sci.*, 14:313–325.
20. Shimazaki, J., Kurihara, H., Ito, Y., and Shida, K. (1965): Metabolism of testosterone in prostate. Separation of prostatic 17β-ol-dehydrogenase and 5α-reductase. *Gunma J. Med. Sci.*, 14:326–333.
21. Anderson, K. M., and Liao, S. (1968): Selective retention of dihydrotestosterone by prostatic nuclei. *Nature*, 219:277–279.
22. Farnsworth, W. E., and Brown, J. R. (1963): *Biology of the Prostate and Related Tissues, NCI Monograph, No. 12*, p. 323. NCI, Bethesda, Md.
23. Breuer, H., Hamel, D., and Kruskemper, H. L. (1976): *Methods of Hormone Analysis*. John Wiley & Sons, New York.
24. Dorfman, R. I. (1962): *Methods in Hormone Research, Vol. II, Bioassay*. Academic Press, New York.
25. Frieden, E. H. (1976): *Chemical Endocrinology*, Academic Press, New York.
26. Vida, J. A. (1969): *Androgens and Anabolic Agents*. Academic Press, New York.
27. Tisell, L. E. (1970): Effect of cortisone on the growth of the ventral prostate, the dorsolateral prostate, the coagulating gland and the seminal vesicles in castrated adrenalectomized and in castrated non-adrenalectomized rats. *Acta Endocrinol.*, 64:637–655.
28. Tullner, W. W. (1963): *Biology of the Prostate and Related Tissues, NCI Monograph, No. 12*, pp. 211–223. NCI, Bethesda, Md.
29. Walsh, P. C., and Gittes, R. F. (1970): Inhibition of extratesticular stimuli to prostatic growth in the castrate rat by antiandrogens. *Endocrinology*, 87:624–627.
30. Oesterling, J. E., Epstein, J. I., and Walsh, P. C. (1986): The inability of adrenal androgens to stimulate the adult prostate—An autopsy evaluation of men with hypogonadotropic hypogonadism and panhypopituitarism. *J. Urol.*, 136:103–104.
31. Arvola, I. (1961): The hormonal control of the amounts of the tissue components of the prostate. *Ann. Chir. Gynaecol. Fenn.*, 50(Suppl. 102):1–120.
32. Mobbs, B. J., Johnson, L. E., and Connolly, J. G. (1973): Influence of the adrenal gland on prostatic activity in adult rats. *J. Endocrinol.*, 59:335–343.
33. Kyprianou, N., and Isaacs, J. T. (1987): Biological significance of measurable androgen levels in the rat ventral prostate following castration. *Prostate*, 10:313–324.
34. Horton, R. J. (1976): In: *Benign prostatic hyperplasia. Proceedings of a Workshop Sponsored by the Kidney Disease and Urology Program of the NIAMDD*, pp. 183–190. U.S. Government Printing Office, Washington, D.C.
35. Wieland, R. G., Courcy, C. D., Levy, R. P., et al. (1965): $C_{19}O_2$ Steroids and some of their precursors in blood from normal adrenals. *J. Clin. Invest*, 44:159–168.
36. MacDonald, P. G. (1976): In: *Benign Prostatic Hyperplasia. Proceedings of a Workshop Sponsored by the Kidney Disease and Urology Program of the NIAMDD*, pp. 191–193. U.S. Government Printing Office, Washington, D.C.
37. Siiteri, P. K., and MacDonald, P. C. (1973): *Handbook of Physiology, Section 7, Endocrinology, Vol. II*, pp. 615–629. Williams & Wilkins, Baltimore, Md.
38. Dorrington, J. H., and Armstrong, D. T. (1975): Follicle stimulating hormone stimulates estradiol-17β synthesis in cultured Sertoli cells. *Proc. Natl. Acad. Sci. USA*, 72:2677–2681.
39. Vermeulen, A., Verdonck, L., Van der Straeten, M., and Orie, N. (1969): Capacity of the TeBG in human plasma and influence of specific binding of testosterone on its metabolic clearance rate. *J. Clin. Endocrinol.*, 29:1470–1480.
40. Vermeulen, A. (1973): The physical state of testosterone in plasma. In: *The Endocrine Function of the Human Testis, Vol. I*, pp. 157–170. Academic Press, New York.
41. Vermeulen, A. (1976): In: *Benign Prostatic Hyperplasia. Proceedings of a Workshop Sponsored by the Kidney Disease and Urology Program of the NIAMDD*, p. 177. U.S. Government Printing Office, Washington, D.C.
42. Rosner, W., and Deakins, S. M. (1968): Testosterone-binding globulins in human plasma: Studies on sex distribution and specificity. *J. Clin. Invest.*, 47:2109–2116.
43. August, G. P., Tkachuk, M., and Grumbach, M. M. (1969): Plasma testosterone-binding affinity and testosterone in umbilical cord plasma, late pregnancy, pre-pubertal children, and adult. *J. Clin. Endocrinol.*, 29:891–899.
44. Burton, R. M., and Westphal, U. (1972): Steroid hormone binding proteins in blood plasma. *Metabolism*, 21:253–276.
45. Westphal, U. (1975): Steroid binding to serum proteins. Some open questions. In: *Normal and Abnormal Growth of the Prostate*, pp. 616–631. Charles C Thomas, Springfield, Ill.
46. Forest, M. G., Rivarola, M. A., and Migeon, C. J. (1968): Percentage binding of testosterone, androstenedione and dehydroisoandrosterone in human plasma. *Steroids*, 12:323–343.
47. Forest, M. G., Cathiard, A., and Bertrand, J. A. (1973): Total and unbound testosterone levels in the newborn and in normal and hypogonadal children: Use of a sensitive radioimmunoassay for testosterone. *J. Clin. Endo. Metab.*, 36:1132–1142.
48. Lasnitzki, I., and Franklin, H. R. (1972): The influence of serum on uptake, conversion and action of testosterone in rat prostate glands in organ culture. *J. Endocrinol.*, 54:333–342.
49. Anderson, D. C., Marshall, J. C., and Galuao-Teles, A. (1972): Gynaecomastia and impotence associated with testosterone binding. *Proc. R. Soc. Med.*, 65:787–788.
50. Bardin, C. W., and Mahoudeau, J. A. (1970): Dynamics of androgen metabolism in women with hirsutism. *Ann. Clin. Res.*, 2: 251–262.
51. Danutra V., Harper, M. E., Bovns, A. K., Cole, E. N., Brownsey, B. G., and Griffith, K. (1973): The effect of certain stilbestrol an-

alogues on plasma prolactin and testosterone in the rat. *J. Endocrinol.*, 57:207–215.
52. Moger, W. H., and Geschwind, L. L. (1972): The action of prolactin on the sex accessory glands of the male rat. *Proc. Soc. Exp. Biol. Med.*, 141:1017–1021.
53. Lloyd, J. W., Thomas, J. A., and Mawhinney, M. G. (1973): A difference in the *in vitro* accumulation and metabolism by the rat prostate gland with prolactin. *Steroids*, 22:473–483.
54. Aragona, C., and Friesen, H. G. (1975): Specific prolactin binding sites in the prostate and testis of rat. *Endocrinology*, 97:677–684.
55. Lee, C., Hopkins, D., and Holland, J. M. (1985): Reduction in prostatic concentration of endogenous dihydrotestosterone in rats by hyperprolactinemia. *Prostate*, 6:361–367.
56. McKeehan, W. L., Adams, P. S., and Rosser, M. P. (1984): Direct mitogenic effects of insulin, epidermal growth factor, glucocorticoid, cholera toxin, unknown pituitary factors and possibly prolactin but not androgen on normal rat prostate epithelial cells in serum free, primary cell culture. *Cancer Res.*, 44:1998–2010.
57. Birkoff, J. D., Lattimer, J. K., and Frantz, A. G. (1974): Role of prolactin in benign prostatic hypertrophy. *Urology*, 4:557–561.
58. O'Connor, T., and Sinha, D. K. (1985): Characterization of rat ventral prostatic epithelial cells in collagen gel culture. *Prostate*, 7:305–319.
59. Angervall, L., Hesselsjo, R., Nilsson, S., and Tissel, L. E. (1967): Action of testosterone on ventral prostate, dorsolateral prostate, coagulating glands, and seminal vesicles of castrated alloxan-diabetic rats. *Diabetologia*, 3:395–401.
60. Sufrin, G., and Prutkin, L. (1974): Experimental diabetes and the response of the sex accessory organs on the castrate male rat to testosterone propionate. *Invest. Urol.*, 11:361–369.
61. Calame, S. S., and Lostroh, A. J. (1964): Effect of insulin and lack of effect of testosterone on the protein of ventral prostate from castrate mice maintained as organ cultures. *Endocrinology*, 75:451–454.
62. Lostroh, A. J. (1971): Effect of testosterone and insult *in vitro* on maintenance and repair of the secretory epithelium of the mouse prostate. *Endocrinology*, 88:500–503.
63. Isaacs, J. T., Barrack, E. R., Isaacs, W. B., and Coffey, D. S. (1981): The relationship of cellular structure and function: The matrix system. In: *The Prostatic Cell: Structure and Function, Vol. 75A*, edited by G. P. Murphy, A. A. Sandberg, and J. P. Karr, pp. 1–24. Alan R. Liss, New York.
64. Isaacs, J. T., and Coffey, D. S. (1981): Changes in dihydrotestosterone metabolism associated with the development of canine benign prostatic hyperplasia. *Endocrinology*, 108:445–453.
65. Isaacs, J. T. (1983): Prostatic structure and function in relation to the etiology of prostate cancer. *Prostate*, 4:351–366.
66. Isaacs, J. T., Brendler, C. B., and Walsh, P. C. (1983): Changes in the metabolism of dihydrotestosterone in the hyperplastic human prostate. *J. Clin. Endocrinol. Metab.*, 56:139–146.
67. Isaacs, J. T., and Berry, S. J. (1983): Changes in dihydrotestosterone metabolism in the development of benign prostatic hyperplasia in the aging beagle. *J. Steroid Biochem.*, 18:749–757.
68. Bruchovsky, N., and Dunstan-Adams, E. (1985): Regulation of 5α-reductase activity in stroma and epithelium of human prostate. In: *Regulation of Androgen Action. Proceedings of an International Symposium*, edited by N. Bruchovsky, A. Chapdelaine, and F. Neumann, pp. 31–34. Congressdruck R. Bruckner, Berlin.
69. Barrack, E. R., and Tindall, D. (1987): A critical evaluation of the use of androgen receptor assays to predict the androgen responsiveness of prostatic cancer. In: *Assessment of Current Concepts and Approaches to the Study of Prostate Cancer*, edited by J. P. Karr. Alan R. Liss, New York, p. 155–187.
70. Mulder, E., Brinkmann, A. O., and deBoer, W. (1985): Characterization and partial purification of different forms of the androgen receptor and their interaction with DNA and RNA. In: *Regulation of Androgen Action. Proceedings of an International Symposium, Montreal*, edited by N. Bruchovsky, A. Chapdelaine, and F. Neumann, pp. 141–147. Congressdruck R. Bruckner, Berlin.
71. King, W. J., and Greene, G. L. (1984): Monoclonal antibodies localize oestrogen receptor in the nuclei of target cells. *Nature*, 307:745–747.
72. Welshons, W. V., Lieberman, M. E., and Gorski, J. (1984): Nuclear localization of unoccupied oestrogen receptors. *Nature*, 307:747–749.
73. Barrack, E. R., and Coffey, D. S. (1980): Specific binding of estrogens and androgens to the nuclear matrix of sex hormone responsive tissue. *J. Biol. Chem.*, 2255:7265–7275.
74. Barrack, E. R., and Coffey, D. S. (1982): Biological properties of the nuclear matrix. Steroid hormone binding. *Recent Prog. Horm. Res.*, 38:133–195.
75. Barrack, E. R. (1983): The nuclear matrix of the prostate contains acceptor sites for androgen receptors. *Endocrinology*, 113:430–432.
76. Barrack, E. R., Bujnovszky, P., and Walsh, P. C. (1983): Subcellular distribution of androgen receptors in human normal, benign hyperplastic, and malignant prostatic tissues: Characterization of nuclear salt-resistant receptors. *Cancer Res.*, 43:1107–1116.
77. Ekman, P., Barrack, E. R., and Walsh, P. C. (1982): Simultaneous measurement of progesterone and androgen receptors in human prostate: A microassay. *J. Clin. Endocrinol. Metab.*, 55:1089–1099.
78. Ekman, P., Barrack, E. R., Greene, G. L., Jensen, E. V., and Walsh, P. C. (1983): Estrogen receptors in human prostate: Evidence for multiple binding sites. *J. Clin. Endocrinol. Metab.*, 57:166–176.
79. Belis, J. A., Lizza, E. F., and Tarry, W. F. (1984): Progesterone Receptors in the Prostate. In: *New Approaches to the Study of Benign Prostatic Hyperplasia*, edited by F. A. Kimball, A. E. Buhl, and D. B. Carter, pp. 345–361. Alan R. Liss, New York.
80. Gustaffson, J. A., Ekman, P., Pousette, A., Snochowski, M., and Hogberg, B. (1978): Demonstration of progesterone receptor in human benign prostatic hyperplasia and prostatic carcinoma. *Invest. Urol.*, 15:361–366.
81. Kozak, I., Bartsch, W., Krieg, M., and Voigt, K. (1982): Nuclei of stroma: Site of highest estrogen concentration in human benign prostatic hyperplasia. *Prostate*, 3:433–438.
82. Walsh, P. C., and Wilson, J. D. (1976): The induction of prostatic hypertrophy in the dog with androstanediol. *J. Clin. Invest.*, 57:1093–1097.
83. DeKlerk, D. P., Coffey, D. S., Ewing, L. L., McDermott, I. R., Reiner, W. G., Robinson, C. H., Scott, W. W., Strandberg, J. D. Talalay, P., Walsh, P. C., Wheaton, L. G., and Zirkin, B. R. (1979): Comparison of spontaneously and experimentally induced canine prostatic hyperplasia. *J. Clin. Invest.*, 64:842–849.
84. Trachtenberg, J., Hicks, L. L., and Walsh, P. C. (1981): Methods for the determination of androgen receptor concentration in human prostatic tissue. *Invest. Urol.*, 18:349–354.
85. Walsh, P. C. (1984): Human benign prostatic hyperplasia: Etiological consideration. In: *New Approaches to the Study of Benign Prostatic Hyperplasia*, edited by F. A. Kimball, A. E. Buhl, and D. B. Carter, pp. 1–25. Alan R. Liss, New York.
86. Moore, R. J., Gazak, J. M., Quebbeman, J. F., and Wilson, J. D. (1979): Concentration of dihydrotestosterone in 3α-androstanediol in naturally occurring and androgen induced prostatic hyperplasia in the dog. *J. Clin. Invest.*, 64:1003–1010.
87. Ehrlichman, R. J., Isaacs, J. T., and Coffey, D. S. (1981): Differences in the effects of estradiol on dihydrotestosterone induced growth of the castrate rat and dog. *Invest. Urol.*, 18:466–470.
88. Cunha, G. R., Chung, L. W. K., Shannon, J. M., Toguchi, O., and Fujii, H. (1983): Hormonal induced morphogenesis and growth: Role of the mesenchymal-epithelial interactions. *Recent Prog. Horm. Res.*, 39:559–598.
89. Chung, L. W. K., Matsuura, J., Rocco, A. K., Thompson, T. C., Miller, G. H., and Runner, M. N. (1984): A new mouse model for prostatic hyperplasia: Induction of adult prostatic overgrowth by fetal urogenital sinus implants. In: *New Approaches to the Study of Benign Prostatic Hyperplasia*, edited by F. A. Kimball, A. E. Buhl, and D. B. Carter, pp. 291–306. Alan R. Liss, New York.
90. Muntzing, J. (1980): Androgen and collagen as growth regulators of the rat ventral prostate. *Prostate*, 1:71–78.
91. Mariotti, A., and Mawhinney, M. G. (1981): Hormonal control of accessory sex organ fibromuscular stroma. *Prostate*, 2:397–408.
92. Thornton, M. O., Frederickson, R., Matal, J., and Mawhinney, M. (1984): Preliminary studies on the relationship between collagen and the growth of male accessory sex organ epithelial cells. In: *New Approaches to the Study of Benign Prostatic Hyperplasia*, edited by F. A. Kimball, A. E. Buhl and D. A. Carter, pp. 143–158. Alan R. Liss, New York.
93. Bartsch, G., and Rohr, H. P. (1983): Endocrinological basis and clinical experience in conservative therapy in benign prostatic hy-

perplasia. In: *Androgens and Antiandrogens,* edited by F. H. Schroder, pp. 69–94. Schering, The Netherlands.

94. Jacobs, S. C., Pikna, D., and Lawson, R. K. (1979): Prostatic osteoblastic factor. *Invest. Urol.,* 17:195–198.
95. Green, S., Walter, P., Kumar, V., Krust, T. A., Bornert, J. M., Argos, P., and Chambon, T. (1986): Human estrogen receptors cDNA sequence expression and homology to v-erb A. *Nature,* 320:134–139.
96. Krust, A., Green, S., Argos, P., Kumar, V., Walter, P., Bornert, J. M., and Chambon, P. (1986): The chicken estrogen receptor sequence: Homology with v-erb A and the human estrogen and glucocorticoid receptors. *EMBO J.,* 5:891–897.
97. Weinberger, C., Hollenberg, S. M., Rosenfeld, M. G., and Evans, R. M. (1985): The main structure of human glucocorticoid receptor and its relationship to v-erb A oncogene product. *Nature,* 318:670–672.
98. Maxwell, B. L., McDonnell, D. P., Conneely, O. M., Schulz, T. Z., Greene, G. L., and O'Malley, B. W. (1987): Structural organization and regulation of the chicken estrogen receptor. *Mol. Endocrinol.,* 1:25–35.
99. Nelson, W. G., Pienta, K. J., Barrack, E. R., and Coffey, D. S. (1986): The role of the nuclear matrix in the organization and function of DNA. *Annu. Rev. Biophys. Biophys. Chem.,* 15:457–475.
100. Berezney, R., and Coffey, D. S. (1974): Identification of a nuclear protein matrix. *Biochem. Biophys. Res. Commun.,* 60:1410–1417.
101. Berezney, R., and Coffey, D. S. (1977): Nuclear matrix: Isolation and characterization of a framework structure from rat liver nuclei. *J. Cell Biol.,* 73:616–637.
102. Shaper, J. H., Pardoll, D. M., Kaufmann, S. H., Barrack, E. R., Vogelstein, B., and Coffey, D. S. (1979): The relationship of the nuclear matrix to cellular structure and function. *Adv. Enzyme Regul.,* 17:213–248.
103. Pardoll, D. M., Vogelstein, B., and Coffey, D. S. (1980): A fixed site of DNA replication in eucaryotic cells. *Cell,* 19:527–536.
104. Vogelstein, B., Pardoll, D. M., and Coffey, D. S. (1980): Supercoiled loops and eucaryotic DNA replication. *Cell,* 22:79–85.
105. Razin, S. V., Chernokhvostov, V. V., Roodyn, A. V., Zbarsky, I. B., and Georgiev, G. P. (1981): Proteins tightly bound to DNA in the regions of DNA attachment to the skeletal structures of interphase nuclei and metaphase chromosomes. *Cell,* 27:65–73.
106. Detke, S., and Keller, J. M. (1982): Comparison of the proteins present in HeLa cell interphase nucleoskeletons and metaphase chromosome scaffolds. *J. Biol. Chem.,* 257:3905–3911.
107. Peters, K. E., Okada, T. A., and Comings, D. E. (1982): Chinese hamster nuclear proteins: An electrophoretic analysis of interphase, metaphase, and nuclear matrix preparations. *Eur. J. Biochem.,* 129:221–232.
108. Pieck, A. C. M., van der Velden, H. M. W., Rijken, A. A. M., Neis, J. M., and Wanka, F. (1985): Protein composition of the chromosomal scaffold and interphase nuclear matrix. *Chromosoma,* 91:137–144.
109. Bekers, A. G. M., Gijzen, H. J., Taalman, R. D. F. M., and Wanka, F. (1981): Ultrastructure of the nuclear matrix from physarum-polycephalum during the mitotic cycle. *J. Ultrastruct. Res.,* 75:352–362.
110. Berrios, M., Osheroff, N., and Fisher, P. A. (1985): *In-situ* localization of DNA topoisomerase II: A major polypeptide component of the *Drosophila-melanogaster* nuclear matrix fraction. *Proc. Natl. Acad. Sci. USA,* 82:4142–4146.
111. Halligan, B. D., Small, D., Vogelstein, B., Hsieh, T. -S., and Liu, L. F. (1984): Localization of type II DNA topoisomerases in nuclear matrix. *J. Cell Biol.,* 99:128a.
112. Ernshaw, W. C., and Heck, M. M. S. (1985): Localization of topoisomerase II in mitotic chromosomes. *J. Cell Biol.,* 100:1716–1725.
113. Intres, R., and Donady, J. J. (1985): A constitutively transcribed actin gene is associated with the nuclear matrix in a Drosophila cell line. *In Vitro Cell. Dev. Biol.,* 21:641–648.
114. Robinson, S. I., Nelkin, B. D., and Vogelstein, B. (1982): The ovalbumin gene is associated with the nuclear matrix of chicken oviduct cells. *Cell,* 28:99–106.
115. Robinson, S. I., Small, D., Izerda, R., McKnight, G. S., and Vogelstein, B. (1983): The association of transcriptionally active genes with the nuclear matrix of the chicken oviduct. *Nucl. Acids Res.,* 11:5113–5130.
116. Pardoll, D. M., and Vogelstein, B. (1980): Sequence analysis of nuclear matrix associated DNA from rat liver. *Exp. Cell Res.,* 128:466–470.
117. Ciejek, E. M., Nordstromn, J. L., Tsai, M., and O'Malley, B. W. (1982): Ribonucleic acid precursors are associated with the chick oviduct nuclear matrix. *Biochemistry,* 21:4945–4953.
118. Hentzen, P. C., Rho, J. H., and Bekhor, I. (1984): Nuclear matrix DNA from chicken erythrocytes contains β-globin gene sequences. *Proc. Natl. Acad. Sci. USA,* 81:304–307.
119. Jost, J. P., and Seldran, M. (1984): Association of transcriptionally active vitellogenin II gene with the nuclear matrix of chicken liver. *EMBO J.,* 3:2005–2008.
120. Cook, P. R., Langa, J., Mayday, A., Lania, L., Fried, M., Chiswell, P. and Wyke, J. A. (1982): Active viral genes in transformed cells lie close to the nuclear cage. *EMBO J.,* 1:447–452.
121. Berezney, R., and Coffey, D. S. (1975): Nuclear protein matrix: Association with newly synthesized DNA. *Science,* 189:291–293.
122. Berezney, R., and Buchholtz, L. A. (1981): Dynamic association of replicating DNA fragments with the nuclear matrix of regenerating liver. *Exp. Cell Res.,* 132:1–13.
123. van der Velden, H. M. W., van Willigan, G., Wetzels, R. H. W., and Wanka, F. (1984): Attachment of origins of replication to the nuclear matrix and the chromosomal scaffold. *FEBS,* 171:13–16.
124. Dijkwel, P. A., Mullenders, L. M. F., and Wanka, F. (1979): Analysis of the attachment of replicating DNA to a nuclear matrix in mammalian interphase nuclei. *Nucl. Acids Res.,* 6:219–230.
125. Tubo, R. A., and Berezney, R. (1987): Pre-replicative association of multiple replicative enzyme activities with the nuclear matrix during rat liver regeneration. *J. Biol. Chem.,* 262:1148–1154.
126. Jackson, D. A., McCready, S. J., and Cook. P. R. (1981): RNA is synthesized at the nuclear cage. *Nature,* 292:552–555.
127. Jackson, D. A., Caton, A. J., McCready, S. J., and Cook, P. R. (1982): Influenza virus RNA is synthesized at fixed sites in the nucleus. *Nature,* 296:366–368.
128. Abulafia, R., Ben-Ze'ev, A., Hay, N., and Aloni, Y. (1984): Control of the simian virus 40 transcription by the attenuation mechanism and transcriptionally active ternary complexes are associated with the nuclear matrix. *J. Mol. Biol.,* 172:467–487.
129. Ciejek, E., Tsai, M. H., and O'Malley, B. W. (1983): Actively transcribed genes are associated with the nuclear matrix. *Nature,* 307:607–609.
130. Mariman, E. C., and van Venrooij, W. J. (1985): The nuclear matrix and RNA-processing: Use of human antibodies. In: *Nuclear Envelope Structure and RNA Maturation,* edited by E. G. Smuckler and G. A. Clawson, pp. 315–319. Alan R. Liss, New York.
131. Sharp, P. (1987): Splicing of messenger RNA precursors. *Science,* 235:766–771.
132. Eisenman, R. N., Tachibana, C. Y., Abrams, M. D., and Mann, S. R. (1985): V-myc and C-myc encoded proteins are associated with the nuclear matrix. *Mol. Cell. Biol.,* 5:114–126.
133. Moelling, K., Benter, T., Bunte, T., Pfaff, E., Deppert, W., Egly, J. M., and Miyamoto, N. B. (1984): Properties of the myc-gene product: Nuclear association, inhibition of transcription and activation in stimulated lymphocytes. In: *Current Topics in Microbiology and Immunology,* pp. 198–207. Springer-Verlag, Berlin.
134. Sarnow, P., Mearing, P., Anderson, C. W., Reich, N., and Levine, A. J. (1982): Identification and characterization of an immunologically conserved adenovirus early region 11,000 m_r protein and its association with the nuclear matrix. *J. Mol. Biol.,* 162:565–583.
135. Staufenbiel, M., and Deppert, W. (1983): Different structural systems of the nucleus are targets for SV40 large T antigen. *Cell,* 33:173–181.
136. Verdame, M. F., Kohtz, D. S., and Pollack, R. E. (1983): 94,000- and 100,000-molecular-weight simian weight simian virus 40 T-antigens are associated with the nuclear matrix in transformed and revertant mouse cells. *J. Virol.,* 46:575–583.
137. Cook, P. R., Brazell, I. A., and Jost, E. (1976): Characterization of nuclear structures containing superhelical DNA. *J. Cell. Sci.,* 22:303–324.
138. Huberman, J. A., and Riggs, A. D. (1968): On the mechanism of DNA replication in mammalian chromosomes. *J. Mol. Biol.,* 32:327–341.

139. Warren, A. C., and Cook, P. R. (1978): Supercoiling of DNA and nuclear conformation during the cell cycle. *J. Cell. Sci.*, 30:211–226.
140. Paulson, J. R., and Laemmeli, U. K. (1977): The structure of histone-depleted metaphase chromosomes. *Cell*, 12:817–828.
141. Pienta, K. J., and Coffey, D. S. (1984): A structural analysis of the role of the nuclear matrix and DNA loops in the organization of the nucleus and chromosome. *J. Cell Sci. (Suppl.)*, 1:123–135.
142. Finch, J. T., and Klug, A. (1976): Solenoid model for superstructure in chromatin. *Proc. Natl. Acad. Sci. USA*, 73:1897–1901.
143. Butler, P. J. G. (1984): A defined structure of the 30 nm chromatin fiber which accommodates different nucleosomal repeat lengths. *EMBO J.*, 3:2599–2604.
144. Laemmli, U. K. (1978): Levels of organization of the DNA in eukaryotic chromosomes. *Pharmacol. Rev.*, 30:469–476.
145. Marsden, M. P. F., and Laemmli, U. K. (1979): Metaphase chromosome structure: Evidence for a radial loop model. *Cell*, 17:848–858.
146. Adolph, K. W., and Kreisman, L. R. (1983): Surface structure of isolated metaphase chromosomes. *Exp. Cell Res.*, 147:155–166.
147. Dupraw, E. (1970): *DNA and Chromosomes*. Holt, Rinehart & Winston, New York.
148. Bak, A. L., Zeuthen, J., and Crick, F. H. C. (1977): Higher-order structure of human mitotic chromosomes. *Proc. Natl. Acad. Sci. USA*, 74:1595–1599.
149. Ohnuki, Y. (1968): Structure of chromosomes. I. Morphological studies of the spiral structure of human somatic chromosomes. *Chromosoma*, 25:402.
150. Sedat, J., and Manuelidis, L. (1978): A direct approach to the structure of eukaryotic chromosomes. *CSHSQB*, XII:331–350.
151. Reddy, G. P. V., and Pardee, A. B. (1980): Multienzyme complex for metabolic channeling in mammalian DNA replication. *Proc. Natl. Acad. Sci. USA*, 77:3312–3316.
152. Chaly, N., Bladon, T., Setterfield, G., Little, J. E., Kaplan, J. G., and Brown, D. L. (1984): Changes in distribution of nuclear matrix antigens during the mitotic cell cycle. *J. Cell. Biol.*, 99:661–671.
153. Setterfield, G., Bladon, T., Hall, R., Chaly, N., Brasch, K., El Ansary, M., and Brown, D. L. (1985): Extrachromatin nuclear components and structural changes in nuclei. In: *Nuclear Envelope Structure and RNA Maturation*, edited by E. A. Smuckler and G. A. Clawson, pp. 63–86. Alan R. Liss, New York.
154. Bissell, M. J., Hall, M. G., and Parry, G. (1982): How does the extracellular matrix direct gene expression? *J. Theor. Biol.*, 99:31–68.
155. Fey, E. G., and Penman, S. (1984): Tumor promoters induce a specific morphological signature in the nuclear matrix-intermediate filament scaffold of Madin-Darby canine kidney (MDCK) cell colonies. *Proc. Natl. Acad. Sci. USA*, 81:4409–4413.
156. Fey, E. G., Wan, K. M., and Penman, S. (1984): Epithelial cytoskeletal framework and nuclear matrix-intermediate filament scaffold: Three-dimensional organization and protein composition. *J. Cell Biol.*, 98:1973–1984.
157. Fey, E. G., Wan, K. M., and Penman, S. (1984): Nuclear matrix-intermediate filament scaffold subfraction of the skeletal framework that retains proteins specific to cell type. In: *Molecular Biology of the Cytoskeleton*, edited by G. G. Borisy, D. W. Cleveland, and D. B. Murphy, pp. 87–98. Cold Spring Harbor Laboratory, New York.
158. Ingber, D. E., Madri, J. N., and Jamieson, J. D. (1981): Role of basal lamina in neoplastic disorganization of tissue architecture. *Proc. Natl. Acad. Sci. USA*,78:3901–3905.
159. Isaacs, W. B. (1984): Structural and functional components in normal and hyperplastic canine prostate. *Prog. Clin. Biol. Res.*, 145:307–332.
160. Franks, L. M. (1954): Benign nodular hyperplasia of the prostate: A review. *Ann. R. Coll. Surg. Engl.*, 14:92–106.
161. Merk, F. B., Ofner, P., Qwann, P. W. L., Leav, I., and Venar, L. (1982): Ultrastructure and biochemical expression of divergent differentiation in prostates of castrate dogs treated with estrogens and androgen. *Lab. Invest.*, 47:437–450.
162. Hay, E. D. (1981): *The Cell Biology of the Extracellular Matrix*, Plenum Press, New York.
163. Hay, E. D. (1982): Interaction of embryonic cell surfaces and cytoskeleton with extracellular matrix. *Am. J. Anat.*, 165:1–12.
164. Isaacs, J. T., Barrack, E. R., Isaacs, W. B., and Coffey, D. S. (1981): The relationship of cellular structure and function: The matrix system. In: *The Prostate Cell Structure and Function, Part A*, edited by G. P. Murphy, A. A. Sandberg, and J. P. Karr, pp. 1–24. Alan R. Liss, New York.
165. Bartsch, G., Brungger, A., Schweikert, U., Hinter, H., Stanzlu, J., Marth, C., Daxenbichler, G., and Rohr, H. P. (1984): The importance of stromal tissue in benign prostatic hyperplasia: Morphological, immunofluorescence and endocrinological investigations. In: *New Approaches to the Study of Benign Prostatic Hyperplasia*, edited by F. A. Kimball, A. E. Buhl, and D. A. Carter, pp. 159–180. Alan R. Liss, New York.
166. Arcadi, J. A. (1954): Role of ground substance in atrophy of normal and malignant prostatic tissue following estrogen administration and orchiectomy. *J. Clin. Endocrinol.*, 14:1113–1125.
167. DeKlerk, D. P. (1983): Glycosaminoglycans of normal and hyperplastic prostate. *Prostate*, 4:73–81.
168. White, I. J. (1958): Mammalian semen. *Anim. Breeding*, 26:709–711 (*abstract*).
169. Perry, E. J. (1968): Factors influencing the quality and quantity of semen. In: *The Artificial Insemination of Farm Animals*, 4th edition, edited by E. J. Perry, p. 76. Rutgers University Press, New Brunswick, N.J.
170. Amelar, R D., and Hotchkiss, R. S. (1965): The split ejaculate: Its use in the management of male infertility. *Fertil. Steril.*, 16: 46–60.
171. Tauber, P. F., Zaneveld, L. J. D., Propping, D., and Schumacher, G. F. B. (1976): Components of human split ejaculate. II. Enzymes and proteinase inhibitors. *J. Reprod. Fertil.*, 46:165–171.
172. Tauber, P. F., Zaneveld, L. J. D., Propping, D., and Schumacher, G. F. B. (1975): Components of human split ejaculate. *J. Reprod. Fertil.*, 43:249–267.
173. Zaneveld, L. J. D., and Tauber, P. F. (1981): Contributions of prostatic fluid components to the ejaculate. In: *Prostatic Cell: Structure and Function, Part A, Progress in Clinical and Biological Res., Vol. 75A*, edited by G. P. Murphy, A. A. Sandberg, and J. P. Carr, pp. 265–277. Alan R. Liss, New York.
174. Eliasson, R. (1977): Seminal plasma accessory genital glands and fertility. In: *Male Infertility: Workup, Treatment and Research*, edited by A. T. K. Cockett and R. L. Urry, pp. 189–204. Grune & Stratton, New York.
175. Mann, T., and Lutwak-Mann, C. L. (1981): *Male Reproductive Function and Semen*. Springer-Verlag, New York.
176. Polakoski, K. L., and Kopta, M. (1982): Seminal plasma. In: *Biochemistry of Mammalian Reproduction*, edited by L. J. D. Zaneveld and R. T. Chatterton, p. 89–117. John Wiley & Sons, New York.
177. Bertrand, G., and Vladesco, R. (1921): Prostatic zinc concentration. *C. R. Acad. Sci. (III)*, 173:176–179.
178. Byar, D. P. (1974): Zinc in male sex accessory organs: Distribution and hormonal response. In: *Male Sex Accessory Organs, Structure and Function in Mammals*, edited by D. Brandes, pp. 161–171. Academic Press, New York.
179. Chandler, J. A., Timms, B. G., and Morton, M. S. (1977): Subcellular distribution of zinc in rat prostates studied by x-ray microanalysis. I. Normal prostate. *Histochem. J.*, 9:103–120.
180. Gunn, S. A., and Gould, T. C. (1956): The relative importance of androgen and estrogen in the selective uptake of zinc 65 by the dorsolateral prostate of the rat. *Endocrinology*, 58:443–452.
181. Gunn, S. A., Gould, T. C., and Anderson, W. A. (1965): The effect of growth hormone and prolactin preparations on the control by interstitial cell stimulating hormone of uptake of 65 zinc by the rat dorsolateral prostate. *J. Endocrinol.*, 32:205–214.
182. Johnson, L., Wickstrom, S., and Nylander, G. (1969): The vehicle of zinc in the prostatic secretion of dog. *Scand. J. Urol. Nephrol.*, 3:9–11.
183. Heathcote, J. G., and Washington, R. J. (1973): Analysis of the zinc binding protein derived from the human benign hypertrophic prostate. *J. Endocrinol.*, 58:421–423.
184. Fair, W. R., and Wehner, N. (1976): The prostatic antibacterial factor: Identity and significance. *Prog. Clin. Biol. Res.*, 6:383–403.
185. Reed, M. J., and Stitch, S. R. (1973): The uptake of testosterone and zinc *in vitro* by the human benign hypertrophic prostate. *J. Endocrinol.*, 58:405–419.
186. Huggins, C. (1947): The prostatic secretion. *Harvey Lect.*, 42:148.

187. Phadke, A. M., Samant, N. R., and Deval, S. P. (1973): Significance of seminal fructose studies in male fertility. *Fertil. Steril.*, 24:894–903.
188. Moon, A. K. H., and Bunge, R. G. (1971): Seminal fructose as an indicator of androgenic activity: Critical analysis. *Invest. Urol.*, 8:373–376.
189. Seligman, A. M., Sternberger, N. J., and Paul, B. D. (1975): Design of spindle poisons activated specifically by prostatic acid phosphatase and new methods for prostatic acid phosphatase cytochemistry. *Cancer Chemother. Rep.*, 59:233–242.
190. Dawson, R. M. C., Mann, T., and White, L. G. (1957): Glycerophosphorylcholine and phosphorylcholine in semen and the relationship to choline. *Biochemistry*, 65:627–631.
191. Fair, W. R., and Parrish, R. T. (1981): Antibacterial substance in prostatic fluid. In: *Prostatic Cell: Structure and Function, Part A*, edited by G. P. Murphy, A. A. Sandberg, and J. P. Karr, pp. 247–264. Alan R. Liss, New York.
192. Stamey, T. A., Fair, W. R., Timothy, M. M., and Wehner, N. (1968): Antibacterial nature of prostatic fluid. *Nature*, 218:44–415.
193. Fair, W. R., Couch, J., and Wehner, N. (1973): The purification and assay of the prostatic antibacterial factor (PAF). *Biochem. Med.*, 8:329–339.
194. Williams-Ashman, H. G., Corti, A., and Sheth, A. R. (1975): Formation and functions of aliphatic polyamines in the prostate gland and its secretions. In: *Normal and Abnormal Growth of the Prostate*, edited by M. Goland, pp. 222–239. Charles C Thomas, Springfield, Ill.
195. Williams-Ashman, H. G., Janne, J., Coppoe, G. C., Geroch, M. E., and Schenone, A. (1972): New aspects of polyamine biosynthesis in eukaryotic organisms. *Adv. Enzyme Regul.*, 10:225–245.
196. Williams-Ashman, H. G., Pegg, A. E., and Lockwood, D. H. (1969): Mechanisms and regulation of polyamine and putrescine biosynthesis in male genital glands and other tissues of mammals. *Adv. Enzyme Regul.*, 1:291–323.
197. Falk, J. E., Park, M. H., Chung, S. I., et al. (1980): Polyamines as physiological substrates for transglutaminases. *J. Biol. Chem.*, 255:3695–3700.
198. Goldblatt, M. W. (1935): Properties of human seminal plasma. *J. Physiol. (Lond.)*, 84:202–218.
199. Goldblatt, M. W. (1933): A depressor substance in seminal fluid. *J. Soc. Chem. Ind. (Lond.)*, 52:1056.
200. von Euler U. S. (1934): Zur kenntnis der pharmakologischen wirkungen von natirsekreten und extrackten mammlicher accessorischer geschlechtsdrusen. *Arch. Pathol. Pharmacol.*, 175:78–84.
201. Eliasson, R. (1959): Studies on prostaglandins. Occurrence, formation, and biological actions. *Acta Physiol. Scand.* 158(Suppl. 46):1.
202. Bergstrom, S., Carlson, L. A., and Weeks, L. R. (1968): The prostaglandins: A family of biologically active lipids. *Pharmacol. Rev.*, 20:1–48.
203. Fuchs, A. R., and Chantharaski, U. (1976): Prostaglandins and male fertility. In: *Human Semen and Fertility Regulation in Men*, edited by E. S. E. Hafez, pp. 187–197. C. V. Mosby, St. Louis.
204. Scott, W. W. (1945): Lipids of prostatic fluid, seminal plasma and enlarged prostate gland of man. *J. Urol.*, 53:712–718.
205. White, I. G., Darin-Bennett, A., and Poulos, A. (1976): Lipids of human semen. In: *Human Semen and Fertility Regulation in Men*, edited by E. S. E. Hafez, pp. 144–152. C. V. Mosby, St. Louis.
206. Poulos, A., and White, L. G. (1973): Phospholipids of human spermatozoa and seminal plasma. *J. Reprod. Fertil.*, 35:265–272.
207. Acevedo, H. F., Campbell, E. A., Saier, E. L., et al. (1973): Urinary cholesterol. V. Its excretion in men with testicular and prostatic neoplasms. *Cancer*, 32:196–205.
208. Chu, T. M., Shukia, S. K., Mittelman, A., and Murphy, G. P. (1975): Comparative evaluation of serum acid phosphatase, urinary cholesterol, and androgens in diagnosis of prostatic cancer. *Urology*, 6:291–294.
209. Huggins, C., and Neal, W. (1942): Coagulation and liquefaction of semen. Proteolytic enzymes and citrate in prostatic fluid. *J. Exp. Med.*, 76:527–541.
210. Tauber, P. F., and Zaneveld, L. J. D. (1976): Coagulation and liquefaction of human semen. In: *Human Semen and Fertility Regulation in Men*, edited by E. S. E. Hafez, pp. 153–166. C. V. Mosby, St. Louis.
211. Tauber, P. F., Zaneveld, L. J. D., Propping, D., and Schumacher, G. F. B. (1976): Components of human split ejaculates. II. Enzymes and proteinase inhibitors. *J. Reprod. Fertil.*, 46:165–171.
212. Oettle, A. G. (1954): Morphologic changes in normal human semen after ejaculation. *Fertil. Steril.*, 5:227–240.
213. Amelar, R. D. (1962): Coagulation, liquefaction and viscosity of human semen. *J. Urol.*, 87:187–190.
214. Syner, F. N., Moghissi, K. S., and Yanez, J. (1975): Isolation of a factor from normal human semen that accelerates dissolution of abnormally liquefying semen. *Fertil. Steril.*, 26:1064–1069.
215. Zaneveld, L. J. D., and Chatterton, R. T. (1982): *Biochemistry of Mammalian Reproduction*. John Wiley & Sons, New York.
216. Propping, D., Tauber, P. F., Zaneveld, L. J. D., and Schumacher, G. F. B. (1974): Purification and characterization of two plasminogen activators from human seminal plasma. *Fed. Proc.*, 33:289.
217. Fritz, H., Arnhold, M., Forg-Brey, B., Zaneveld, L. J. D., and Schumacher, G. F. B. (1972): Zerhalten der chymotrypsin-ahnlichen proteinase aus humansperma gegnuber protein-proteinase-inhibitoren. *Hoppe-Seylers Z. Physiol. Chem.*, 353:1651–1653.
218. Lundquist, F., Thorsteinsson, T., and Buus, O. (1955): Purification and properties of some enzymes in human seminal plasma. *Biochem. J.*, 56:69–79.
219. Tauber, P. F., Zaneveld, L. J. D., Propping, D., and Schumacher, G. F. B. (1975): Components of human split ejaculate. *J. Reprod. Fertil.*, 43:249–267.
220. Tauber, P. F., and Zaneveld, L. J. D. (1976): Coagulation and liquefaction of human semen. In: *Human Semen and Fertility Regulation in Men*, edited by E. S. E. Hafez, pp. 153–166. C. V. Mosby, St. Louis.
221. Williams-Ashman, H. G., Wilson, J., Beil, R., and Lorand, L. (1977): Transglutaminase reactions associated with the rat semen clotting system. *Biochem. Biophys. Res. Commun.*, 79: 1192–1198.
222. Notides, A. C., and Williams-Ashman, H. G. (1967): The basic protein responsible for clotting of guinea pig semen. *Proc. Natl. Acad. Sci. USA*, 58:1991–1995.
223. Boursnell, J. C., Hartree, E. F., and Briggs, P. A. (1970): Studies on the bulbourethral (Cowper's) gland mucin and seminal gel of the boar. *Biochem. J.*, 117:981–988.
224. Amelar, R. D. and Dubin, L. (1977): Semen analysis. In: *Male Infertility*, edited by R. D. Amelar, L. Dubin, and P. C. Walsh, pp. 105–140. W. B. Saunders, Philadelphia.
225. Eliasson, R. (1973): Parameters of male fertility. In: *Human Reproduction*, edited by E. S. E. Hafez and T. N. Evans, pp. 39–51. Harper and Row, New York.
226. Bunge, R. G. (1970): Some observations on the male ejaculate. *Fertil. Steril.*, 21:639–644.
227. Bunge, R. G., and Sherman, J. K. (1954): Liquefaction of human semen by alpha-amylase. *Fertil. Steril.*, 5:353–356.
228. Friberg, J., and Tilly-Friberg, I. (1976): Antibodies in human seminal fluid. In: *Human Semen and Fertility Regulation in Men*, edited by E. S. E. Hafez, pp. 258–264. C. V. Mosby, St. Louis.
229. Gutman, A. B., and Gutman, E. B. (1938): "Acid" phosphatase occurring in serum of patients with metastasizing carcinoma of the prostate gland. *J. Clin. Invest.*, 17:473–478.
230. Huggins, C., and Hodges, C. V. (1941): Studies on prostatic cancer; effect of castration, of estrogen and of androgen injection on serum phosphatases in metastatic carcinoma of the prostate. *Cancer Res.*, 1:293–297.
231. Huggins, C., and Talalay, P. (1945): Sodium phenolphthalein phosphate as a substrate for phosphatase tests. *J. Biol. Chem.*, 159:399–410.
232. Bessey, O. A., Lowry, O. H., and Brock, M. J. (1946): Method for rapid determination of alkaline phosphatase with five cubic millimeters of serum. *J. Biol. Chem.*, 164:321–329.
233. Seligman, A. M. (1951): The colorimetric determination of phosphatases in human serum. *J. Biol. Chem.*, 190:7–15.
234. Babson, A. L., and Read, P. A. (1959): A new assay for prostatic acid phosphatase in serum. *Am. J. Clin. Pathol.*, 32:88–91.
235. Woodard, H. Q. (1959): The clinical significance of serum acid phosphatase. *Am. J. Med.*, 27:902–910.

236. Vaughan, A., Guilbault, G. G., and Hackney, D. (1971): Fluorometric methods for analysis of acid and alkaline phosphatase. *Anal. Chem.*, 43:721–724.
237. Roy, A. V., Brower, M. E., and Hayden, J. E. (1971): Sodium thymolphthalein monophosphate: A new acid phosphatase substrate with greater specificity for the prostatic enzyme in serum. *Clin. Chem.*, 17:1093–1102.
238. Moncure, C. W., and Prout, G. R. Jr. (1970): Antigenicity of human prostatic acid phosphatase. *Cancer*, 25:463–467.
239. Moncure, C. W. (1977): Isoenzymes in prostatic carcinoma. In: *Urologic Pathology: The Prostate*, edited by M. Tannenbaum, pp. 141–156. Lea & Febiger, Philadelphia.
240. Sur, B. K., Moss, D. W., and King, E. J. (1962): Apparent heterogeneity of prostatic acid phosphatase. *Biochem. J.*, 84:55P.
241. Chu, T. M., Wang, M. C., Kuciel, L., Valenzuela, L., and Murphy, G. P. (1977): Enzyme markers in human prostatic carcinoma. *Cancer Treat. Rep.*, 61:193–200.
242. Ostrowski, W., Wasyl, Z., and Weber, M. (1970): The role of neuraminic acid in the heterogeneity of acid phosphomonoestrase from the human prostate gland. *Biochim. Biophys. Acta*, 221:297–306.
243. Smith, J. K., and Whitby, L. G. (1968): The heterogeneity of prostatic acid phosphatase. *Biochim. Biophys. Acta*, 151:607–618.
244. Mattila, S. (1969): Further studies on the prostatic tissue antigens. Separation of two molecular forms of aminopeptidase. *Invest. Urol.*, 7:1–9.
245. Niemi, M., Harkonen, M., and Larmi, T. K. (1963): Enzymic histochemistry of human prostate. *Arch. Pathol.*, 75:528–537.
246. Kirchheim, D., Gyorkey, F., Brandes, D., and Scott, W. W. (1964): Histochemistry of the normal, hyperplastic, and neoplastic human prostate gland. *Invest. Urol.*, 4:403–421.
247. Oliver, J. A., el-Hilali, M. M., and Belitsky, P. (1970): LDH isoenzymes in benign and malignant prostate tissue. The LDH/VI ratio as an index of malignancy. *Cancer*, 25:863–866.
248. Hein, R. C., Grayhack, J. T., and Goldberg, E. (1975): Prostatic fluid-lactic dehydrogenase isoenzyme patterns of prostatic cancer and hyperplasia. *J. Urol.*, 13:511–516.
249. Grayhack, J. T., Wendel, E. F., Lee, C., Oliver, L., and Choen, E. (1977): Lactate dehydrogenase isoenzymes in human prostatic fluid: An acid in recognition of malignancy. *J. Urol.*, 118:204–208.
250. Denis, L. J., and Prout, G. R. Jr. (1963): Lactic dehydrogenase in prostatic cancer. *Invest. Urol.*, 1:101–111.
251. Elhilali, M. M., Oliver, J. A., Sherwin, A. L., and Mackinnon, K. J. (1968): Lactate dehydrogenase isoenzymes in hyperplasia and carcinoma of the prostate: A clinical study. *J. Urol.*, 98:686–692.
252. Flocks, R. H., and Schmidt, J. D. (1972): Lactate dehydrogenase isoenzyme patterns of prostatic cancer and hyperplasia. *J. Surg. Oncol.*, 4:161–167.
253. Belitsky, P., Elhilali, M. M., and Oliver, J. A. (1970): The effect of stilbestrol on the isoenzymes of lactic dehydrogenase in benign and malignant prostatic tissue. *J. Urol.*, 104:453–456.
254. Tsai, Y. C., Harrison, H. H., Lee, C., Daufeld, T., Oliver, L., and Grayhack, J. T. (1984): Systematic characterization of human prostatic fluid proteins with 2-dimensional electrophoresis. *Clin. Chem.*, 30:2026–2030.
255. Carter, D. B., and Resnick, M. I. (1982): High resolution analysis of human prostatic fluid by 2-dimensional electrophoresis. *Prostate*, 3:27–33.
256. Forsgren, B., Bjork, P., Carlstrom, K., Gustafsson, J. A., Pousette, A., and Hogberg, B. (1979): Purification and distribution of a major protein in rat prostate that binds estramustine, a nitrogen mustard derivative of estradiol. *Proc. Natl. Acad. Sci., USA*, 76:3149–3153.
257. Johnson, A. H., Merchant, D. J., Lee, C., Norman, J., and Bourgeois, S. N. (1985): A search for differentiation markers in prostatic fluid components with 2-dimensional electrophoresis and multiple protein detectors. *Prostate*, 7:429–439.
258. Isaacs, W. B., and Shaper, J. H. (1983): Isolation and characterization of the major androgen-dependent glycoprotein of canine prostatic fluid. *J. Biol. Chem.*, 258:6610–6615.
259. Chapdelaine, P., Dube, J. Y., Frenette, G., and Tremblay, R. R. (1984): Identification of arginine esterase as the major androgen-dependent protein secreted by dog prostate and preliminary molecular characterization in seminal plasma. *J. Androl.*, 5:206–210.
260. Dube, J. Y., Chapdelaine, P., and Tremblay, R. R. (1983): Effects of testicular hormones on synthesis of soluble proteins by dog prostate slices. *Can. J. Biochem. Cell Biol.*, 61:756–763.
261. Frenette, G., Dube, J. Y., and Tremblay, R. R. (1985): Enzymatic characterization of arginine esterase from seminal plasma. *Biochim. Biophys. Acta*, 838:270–276.
262. Frenette, G., Dube, J. Y., Marcotte, J. R., and Tremblay, R. R. (1985): Arginine esterase from isolated dog prostate secretory granules is fully active enzymatically. *Can. J. Physiol. Pharmacol.*, 63:1603–1607.
263. Frenette, G., Dube, J. Y., and Tremblay, R. R. (1983): Effect of castration and steroid treatments on the activity of some hydrolytic enzymes in the dog prostate. *Prostate*, 4:383–390.
264. Isaacs, W. B., and Coffey, D. S. (1984): The predominant protein of canine seminal plasma is an enzyme. *J. Biol. Chem.*, 259:11520–11526.
265. Gotterer, G., Banks, J., and Williams-Ashman, H. G. (1956): Hydrolysis of arginine esters by male sex accessory tissues. *Proc. Soc. Exp. Biol. Med.*, 92:58–61.
266. Watt, K. W. K., Lee, P. J., Mtimkulu, T., Chang, W. P., and Loor, R. (1986): Human prostate specific antigen: Structural and functional similarity with serine proteases. *Proc. Natl. Acad. Sci., USA*, 83:3166–3170.
267. Isaacs, W. B., and Shaper, J. H. (1985): Immunological localization and quantitation of the androgen-dependent secretory protease of the canine prostate. *Endocrinology*, 117:1512–1520.
268. Wang, M. C., Valenzuela, L. A., Murphy, G. P., and Chu, T. M. (1979): Purification of a human prostate specific antigen. *Invest. Urol.*, 17:159–163.
269. Wang, M. C., Papsidero, L. M., Kuriyama, M., Valenzuela, L. A., Murphy, G. P., and Chu, T. M. (1981): Prostate antigen: A new potential marker for prostatic cancer. *Prostate*, 2:89–96.
270. Kuriyama, M., Wang, M. C., Lee, C. L., Killian, C. S., Papsidero, L. D., Inaji, H., Loor, R. M., Lin, M. F., Nishiura, T., Slack, N. H., Murphy, G. P., and Chu, T. M. (1982): Multiple marker evaluation in human prostate cancer with the use of tissue specific antigens. *J. Natl. Cancer Inst.*, 68:99–105.
271. Kuriyama, M., Wang, M. C., Lee, C. L., Papsidero, L. M., Killian, C. S., Inaji, H., Slack, N. H., Nishiura, T., Murphy, G. P., and Chu, T. M. (1981): Use of human prostate-specific antigen in monitoring prostate cancer. *Cancer Res.*, 41:3874–3876.
272. Graves, H. C. B., Sensabaugh, G. F., and Blake, R. T. (1985): Postcoital detection of a male-specific semen protein. Application to the investigation of rape. *N. Engl. J. Med.*, 312:338–343.
273. Lilja, H. (1985): A kallikrein-like serum protease in prostatic fluid cleaves the predominant seminal vesicle protein. *J. Clin. Invest.*, 76:1899–1903.
274. Perry, S. T., Viskochil, D. H., Ho, K. C., Fong, K., Stafford, D. W., Wilson, E. M., and French, F. S. (1985): Androgen receptor binding to the C3 (1) subunit gene of rat prostatein. In: *Regulation of Androgen Action*, edited by N. Bruchovsky, A. Chapdelaine, and F. Neumann, pp. 167–173. Congressdruck R. Bruckner, Berlin.
275. Parker, M., and Needham, M. (1985): Organization and expression of prostatic steroid binding protein. In: *Regulation of Androgen Action*, edited by N. Bruchovsky, A. Chapdelaine, and F. Neumann, pp. 175–183. Congressdruck R. Bruckner, Berlin.
276. Williams-Ashman, H. G. (1983): Regulatory features of the seminal vesicle development and function. *Curr. Top. Cell. Regul.*, 22:201–275.
277. Kandall, J. C., Kistler, M. K., and Kistler, W. S. (1985): Androgen regulated genes from prostate and seminal vesicles share upstream sequence homologies. *Biochem. Biophys. Res. Commun.*, 126:948–952.
278. Williams, L., McDonald, C., and Higgins, S. (1985): Sequence organization of rat seminal vesicle F gene: Location of transcriptional start point and sequence comparison with 6 other androgen-regulated genes. *Nucleic Acids Res.*, 13:659–672.
279. Kandall, J. C., Kistler, W. S., and Kistler, M. K. (1985): Methylation of the rat seminal vesicle secretory protein IV gene. Extensive demethylation occurs in several male sex accessory glands. *J. Biol. Chem.*, 260:15959–15964.
280. Fawell, S. E., Pappin, D. J., McDonald, C. J., and Higgins, S. J. (1986): Androgen regulated proteins of rat seminal vesicle secretions

constitute a structurally related family present in the copulatory plug. *Mol. Cell. Endocrinol.*, 45:205–213.

281. Limpaseni, T., and Chulavatnatol, M. (1986): A new sialoglycoprotein from rat seminal vesicles and its association with semen coagulum. *Biochem. Biophys. Res. Commun.*, 136:753–759.
282. Peitz, B., and Olds-Clark, E. P. (1986): Effects of seminal vesicle removal on fertility and uterine sperm motility in the house mouse. *Biol. Reprod.*, 35:608–617.
283. Wilson, D. B., Bross, T. E., Sherman, W. R., Berger, R. A., and Majerus, P. W. (1985): Inositol cyclic phosphates are produced by cleavage of a phosphatidylphosphoinositol with purified sheep seminal vesicle phospholipase C enzyme. *Proc. Natl. Acad. Sci., USA*, 82:4013–4017.
284. Stanisic, T., Sadlowski, R., Lee, C., and Grayhack, J. T. (1978): Partial inhibition of castration-induced ventral prostate regression with actinomycin D and cycloheximide. *Invest. Urol.*, 16:19–22.
285. Sharer, W. C., Lee, C., and Grayhack, J. T. (1979): Partial inhibition of castration-induced involution of rat prostate by chloroquine. A preliminary observation. *Invest. Urol.*, 17:135–137.
286. Engel, G., Lee, C., and Grayhack, J. T. (1980): Acid ribonuclease in rat prostate during castration-induced involution. *Biol. Reprod.*, 22:827–831.
287. Lee, C. (1981): Physiology of castration-induced regression in rat prostate. In: *The Prostatic Cell: Structure and Function, Part A*, edited by G. P. Murphy, A. A. Sandberg, and J. P. Karr, pp. 145–159. Alan R. Liss, New York.
288. Anderson, K. M., Baranowski, J, Economou, S. G., and Rubenstein, M. (1983): A qualitative analysis of acidic proteins associated with regression, growing, or dividing rat ventral prostate cells. *Prostate*, 4:151–165.
289. Carter, D. B., Silverberg, A. B., and Harris, S. E. (1980): Effects of spirolactone on androgen-dependent proteins in the ventral prostate of the rat. *J. Endocrinol.*, 86:471–476.
290. Lee, C., Tsai, Y., Harrison, H. H., and Sensabar, J. (1985): Proteins of the prostate: I. Preliminary characterization by 2-dimensional electrophoresis. *Prostate*, 7:171–182.
291. Wada, F., Nishi, N., Muguruma, Y., Tanaka, Y., and Matuo, Y. (1985): Changes of cytosol proteins in the ventral and dorsolateral prostates of rats during sexual maturation: Immature prostate-abundant proteins as detected by polyacrylamide gel electrophoresis. *Prostate*, 7:395–408.
292. Saltzman, A. G., Hiipakka, R. A., Chang, C., and Liao, S. (1987): Androgen regression of the production of a 29-kilodalton protein and its mRNA in the rat ventral prostate. *J. Biol. Chem.*, 262:432–437.
293. Eliasson, R. (1973): Parameters of male fertility. In: *Human Reproduction: Conception and Contraception*, edited E. S. E. Hafez and T. N. Evans, pp. 39–51. Harper & Row, New York.
294. Freund, M., and Peterson, R. (1976): Semen evaluation and fertility. In: *Human Semen and Fertility Regulation in Men*, edited by E. S. E. Hafez, pp. 344–354. C. V. Mosby, St. Louis.
295. Walsh, P. C., and Amelar, R. (1977): Embryology, anatomy and physiology of the male reproductive system. In: *Male Infertility*, edited by R. D. Amelar, L. Dubin, and P. C. Walsh, pp. 3–32. W. B. Saunders, Philadelphia.
296. Marina, S., Pomerol, J. M., and Zungri, E. R. (1976): Occlusions in the male reproductive tract: Diagnostic radiology. In: *Human Semen and Fertility Regulation in Men*, edited by E. S. E. Hafez, pp. 404–410. C. V. Mosby, St. Louis.
297. Moon, K. H., and Bunge, R. G. (1971): Seminal fructose as an indicator of androgenic activity: Critical analysis. *Invest. Urol.*, 8:373–376.
298. Farrell, J. L. (1938): The secretion of alcohol by the genital tract. *J. Urol.*, 40:62–65.
299. Mroueh, A. M. (1971): The excretion of radioiodine in human semen. *Fertil. Steril.*, 22:61–63.
300. Reeves, D. S. (1982): Pharmacology of the prostate. In: *Scientific Foundations of Urology*, 2nd edition, edited by G. D. Chisholm and D. I. Williams, pp. 514–520. Heinemann Medical Books, London.
301. Hessl, J. M., and Stamey, T. A. (1971): The passage of tetracyclines across epithelial membranes with special reference to prostatic epithelium. *J. Urol.*, 106:253–256.
302. Stamey, T. A. (1980): Urinary infections in males. In: *Pathogenesis and Treatment of Urinary Tract Infections*, edited by T. Stamey, pp. 342–429. Williams & Wilkins, Baltimore.
303. Stamey, T. A., Bushby, S. R. M., and Bragonje, J. (1973): The concentration of trimethoprim in prostatic fluid: Nonionic diffusion or active transport? *J. Infect. Dis.* (*Suppl.*), 128:686.
304. Fowle, A. S. E., and Bye, A. (1972): *Advances in Antimicrobial and Antineoplastic Chemotherapy*, p. 1289. Urban & Schwarzenberg, Munich.
305. Madsen, P. O., Baumueller, A., and Hoyne, U. (1978): Experimental models for determination of antimicrobials in prostatic tissue, interstitial fluid and secretion. *Scand. J. Infect. Dis.* (*Suppl.*), 14:145.
306. White, M. A. (1975): Changes in pH of expressed prostatic secretion during the course of prostatitis. *Proc. R. Soc. Med.*, 68:511–513.
307. Smith, E. R., Miller, T. B., and Pebler, R. S. (1983): Transepithelial voltage changes during prostatic secretion in the dog. *Am. J. Physiol.*, 245:F470–F477.
308. Isaacs, J. T., Isaacs, W. B., Wheaton, L. G., and Coffey, D. S. (1980): Differential effects of estrogen treatment on canine seminal plasma components. *Invest. Urol.*, 17:495–498.
309. Coffey, D. S. (1985): Biochemistry and Physiology of the prostate and seminal vesicles. In: *Campbell's Urology*, 5th ed., edited by P. C. Walsh et al. W. B. Saunders, Philadelphia.
310. Price, D. (1962): Comparative aspects of development and structure in the prostate. In: *Biology of the Prostate and Related Tissues*. National Cancer Institute Monograph 12, p. 2.
311. Bardin, C. W., and Lipsett, M. B. (1967): Estimation of testosterone and androstenedione in human peripheral plasma. *Steroids*, 9:71–84.
312. MacKenzie, A. R., Hall, T., and Whitmore, W. F. Jr. (1962): Zinc content of expressed human prostatic fluid. *Nature*, 193:72–73.

The Physiology of Reproduction,
edited by E. Knobil and J. Neill *et al.*
Raven Press, Ltd., New York © 1988.

Chapter 25

Male Sexual Function: Erection, Emission, and Ejaculation

George S. Benson

Our knowledge of the physiologic mechanisms that control male sexual function is rapidly expanding. In the past decade the development of successful therapy, both surgical and pharmacological, for impotence has been primarily responsible for stimulating the considerable research effort presently being undertaken to better understand both the normal physiology of penile erection and the pathophysiology of disease states leading to sexual dysfunction. Although significant progress has been made, many basic questions remain unanswered.

Three components of male sexual function will be discussed in this chapter: erection, emission, and ejaculation. Erection is defined as penile rigidity or tumescence. What is generally referred to as the "ejaculatory process" is, in fact, two distinct events: emission and ejaculation. Emission, by definition, is the deposition of seminal fluid components from the vasa deferentia, seminal vesicles, and prostate gland into the posterior urethra, while ejaculation refers to the passage of seminal fluid through the urethra and its expulsion from the urethral meatus (1).

ERECTION

Our understanding of the mechanisms involved in the production of penile erection remains incomplete. Much of the data is derived from clinical observation and is subjective. Recently, however, several new approaches to obtaining objective data in humans have been developed and have been instrumental in redirecting our thinking and correcting widely accepted misconceptions. The lack of a universally accepted animal model for penile erection has also hampered research efforts in the past, but recent *in vivo* data obtained in the dog and monkey have nevertheless clarified much of our misunderstanding.

Penile Anatomy

Unlike several animal species the human does not possess an os penis (like the canine) or a retractor penis muscle (multiple animal species) (2–4). Anatomic and physiologic data obtained from much animal work to explain the complex events responsible for human penile erection is therefore suspect. In the human, erectile tissue is contained within three corporal bodies, two dorsally positioned corpora cavernosa, and a ventrally positioned corpus spongiosum, which also contains the urethra (Fig. 1). Each of the three corpora is surrounded by a thick layer of fibrous tissue (tunica albuginea) which separates the corpora from each other. Buck's fascia lies superficial to the tunica albunginea and surrounds all three corporal bodies.

Following the realization that the erectile tissue of the corpora not only acts as a reservoir for blood, but also plays an active role in the development of erection, this tissue has been the subject of much recent anatomic, physiologic, and pharmacologic investigation. Anatomically, the erectile tissue of both the corpora cavernosa and corpus spongiosum is composed of numerous cavernous spaces separated by trabeculae. The trabeculae are composed not only of fibroblasts, collagen, and elastic fibers, but also of significant amounts of smooth muscle. Endothelial cells, which resemble those found in blood vessels, cover the surfaces of the trabeculae. In general, the corpus spongiosum differs from

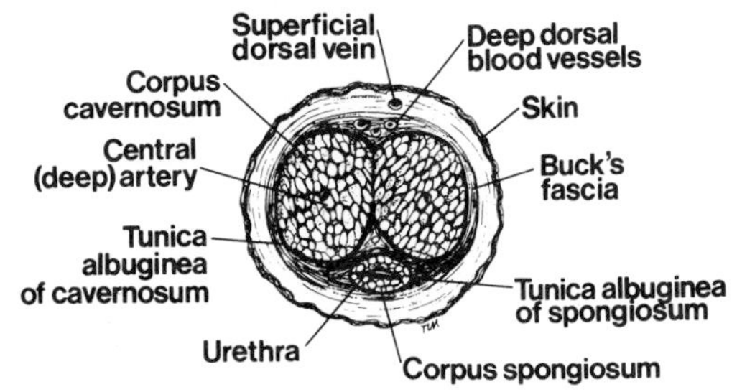

FIG. 1. Cross-sectional anatomy of the human penis.

the corpus cavernosum in that the spongiosum contains larger cavernous spaces and the trabeculae are smaller and contain fewer smooth muscle cells (5).

Penile Vasculature

It has long been recognized that penile erection is primarily a vascular event. The basis for increasing penile blood flow (and pressure) is, however, incompletely understood.

Arterial Supply

In the human, penile arterial blood supply is derived from the pudendal arteries, which are branches of the internal iliac (hypogastric) arteries (Fig. 2). Each of the paired internal pudendal arteries supplies two arteries to the corpus spongiosum: (i) a bulbar branch, which supplies the proximal corpus spongiosum; and (ii) the urethral artery, which courses from the perineum to the glans penis. Prior to entering the crus of the penis, the internal pudendal artery divides into two terminal branches: the deep penile and the dorsal penile artery.

The dorsal penile artery anatomically does not enter the corpora cavernosa. It courses distally between the tunica

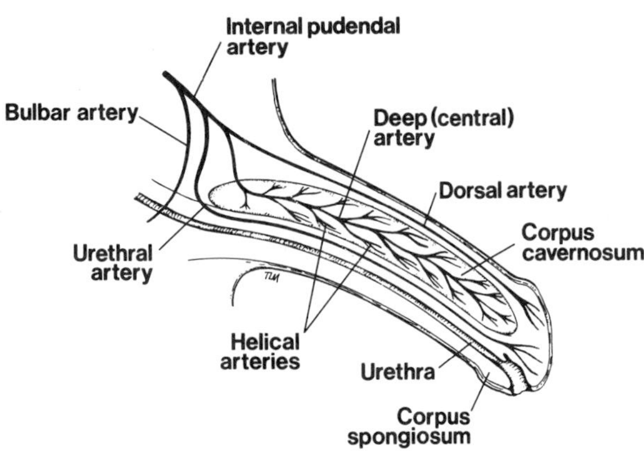

FIG. 2. Arterial blood supply to the human penis.

albuginea of the corpora cavernosa and Buck's fascia. Each of the paired deep arteries enters the crus of the penis in the perineum and then courses distally through each corpus cavernosum as the central (deep) artery. The central arteries supply nutrient vessels to the corpora cavernosa and numerous small vessels (helical arteries), which further divide into end arteries as they open directly into the cavernous spaces (6). In the human, the central artery also sends anastomotic branches to the opposite corpus cavernosum; the result of these anastomoses is that the two human corpora cavernosa act as one functional unit (7,8). In the dog, however, such anastomoses do not exist, and the two corpora are capable of functioning independently (9). Although it would appear that the arterial supply to the corpora cavernosa is derived solely from the deep arteries, numerous anastomotic channels interconnect all arteries of the penis. In addition, "shunt arteries," which connect the central arteries in the corpora cavernosa with arteries in the corpus spongiosum, have been described (10). The significance of these arterial interconnections and specifically their role in the production of penile erection is not understood.

Venous Drainage

The venous drainage of the penis is anatomically more complex than the arterial supply. Although numerous anastomotic interconnections exist in the penile venous system, at least four major components have been identified (11). The superficial dorsal vein is formed by the confluence of multiple superficial veins and lies subcutaneously superficial to Buck's fascia. Bulbar and urethral veins provide drainage for the proximal corpus spongiosum. The major venous systems draining the primary erectile bodies, the corpora cavernosa, are the deep dorsal veins and the deep veins (venae profundae). The deep dorsal vein receives veins from the glans penis and also receives emissary and circumflex veins from the corpora cavernosa. These anastomosing vessels, as well as the deep dorsal vein itself, course between the tunica albuginea of the corpora and Buck's fascia. The deep penile veins (venae profundae) exit the corpora cavernosa proximally in the area of the penile crura and drain into the internal pudendal venous system.

The anatomy and significance of the venous drainage of the penis require much further investigation. For years, the venous drainage systems were thought to contribute minimally, if at all, to the physiology of normal erection. The differences in venous drainage between the corpora cavernosa and the corpus spongiosum/glans penis were appreciated and formed the basis for "shunting" operations (cavernosum-spongiosum and cavernosum-glans penis shunts) used to divert blood from the corpora cavernosa in patients with priapism. Recently, however, the importance of increased corporal outflow resistance in attaining normal erection has been demonstrated in animals (9), and impotence secondary to "venous leakage" has been observed clinically

(12). This data and its significance will be discussed subsequently.

Penile Innervation

The penis is innervated by both divisions of the autonomic nervous system (sympathetic and parasympathetic) as well as by the somatic nervous system (Fig. 3). The innervation of the penis and its vasculature is complex and controversial.

The penis, and presumably its vasculature, receives its autonomic innervation from the pelvic plexus. In humans, this ganglionic plexus is located retroperitoneally near the rectum (13). The pelvic plexus receives autonomic nerve input from both the sympathetic and parasympathetic systems. Sympathetic nerves originate in the low thoracic and upper lumbar regions of the spinal cord and course retroperitoneally to condense into the superior hypogastric plexus (presacral nerve) located just inferior to the aortic bifurcation. Nerve fibers leave the superior hypogastric plexus as the paired hypogastric nerves which fuse distally and then enter the pelvic (inferior hypogastric) plexus (14). The parasympathetic contribution to the pelvic plexus is derived from nerves whose cell bodies are located in the sacral (S2–4) spinal cord. Parasympathetic fibers fuse to form the pelvic nerve, which courses in the endopelvic fascia prior to reaching the pelvic plexus (13).

Anatomically, it is extremely difficult to trace nerve fibers leaving the pelvic plexus and more difficult (if not impossible) to determine the origin of specific nerve fibers leaving the pelvic plexus. Nerve fibers leaving the pelvic plexus innervate not only the penis, but also other pelvic viscera, including the urinary bladder, prostate, and rectum. Significant recent anatomic studies have clarified the gross anatomy of the autonomic nerves that supply the corpora cavernosa. These cavernosal nerves leave the pelvic plexus, course between the rectum and urethra, enter the urogenital diaphragm in proximity to the muscular wall of the urethra, and finally enter the dorsal medial aspect of the corpora cavernosa. These nerves presumably innervate the smooth musculature and vasculature located within the corpora cavernosa (13).

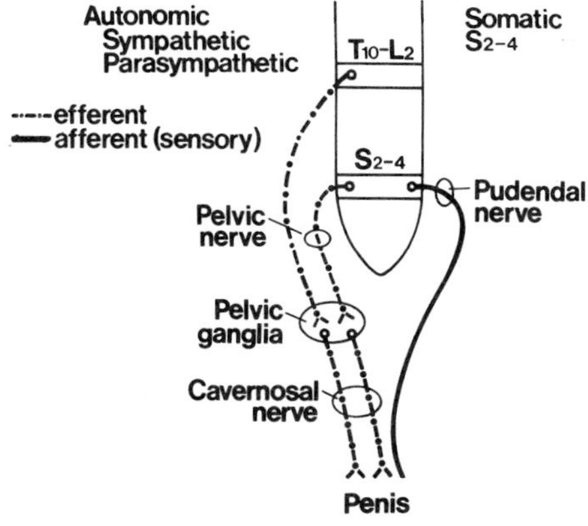

FIG. 3. Innervation of the human penis.

The somatic innervation to the penis is carried via the pudendal nerve; periurethral striated muscles as well as the sensory innervation of the penis are supplied by this system. The pudendal nerve, like the parasympathetic autonomic fibers, arises from the sacral (S2–4) spinal cord. The pudendal nerve accompanies the internal pudendal blood vessels along the lateral wall of the ischiorectal fossa (13). Penile sensation is carried in the dorsal nerve of the penis, a branch of the pudendal nerve.

Histochemical techniques have been utilized to study the autonomic innervation of the smooth musculature of the corpora cavernosa and the penile vasculature. Adrenergic nerves, whose neurotransmitter is by definition a catecholamine, have been studied by histofluorescent techniques. Initial studies in humans described a sparse adrenergic innervation to the smooth muscle of the corpora (15); subsequent investigation demonstrated a considerable adrenergic innervation (5).

Adrenergic nerves can be identified coursing through trabeculae of the corpora cavernosa and approaching the walls of the cavernous spaces (Fig. 4). In addition, the blood vessels within the corpora contain dense aggregations of nerve varicosities in the outer tunic (16,17). Adrenergic nerves are also found in the corpus spongiosum. Unlike the corpora cavernosa, however, the density of innervation in the spongiosum is sparse. Electron microscopic evaluation of the corpora is consistent with the light microscopic data; nerves containing small (400–600 Å), electron-dense vesicles that are considered to be adrenergic have been identified (17).

Cholinergic nerves, whose neurotransmitter by definition is acetylcholine, have also been anatomically identified. Although acetylcholinesterase staining may not be specific for only cholinergic neurons (18), this technique has classically been utilized to demonstrate cholinergic innervation. Although cholinergic (acetylcholinesterase positive) nerves have been found in the trabeculae of the corpora cavernosa, their density is controversial. Like the adrenergic innervation, the corpora cavernosa contains more cholinergic nerves than the corpus spongiosum, and cholinergic nerves are found in the outer tunic of most penile arterioles (16,17) (Fig. 5).

Neuropharmacologically, penile erection does not appear to be entirely dependent upon classic adrenergic and cholinergic mechanisms. This will be discussed below. Anatomically, nerves containing other putative neurotransmitters have been described in penile tissue from animals and humans. Vasoactive intestinal polypeptide (VIP) has been identified at both the light and electron microscopic levels utilizing histochemical techniques (19,20) (Fig. 6). Electron microscopically, in addition to VIP immunopositive vesicles, a variety of large vesicles that are not VIP positive have also been seen and are hypothesized to contain other peptides that may act as neurotransmitters (21).

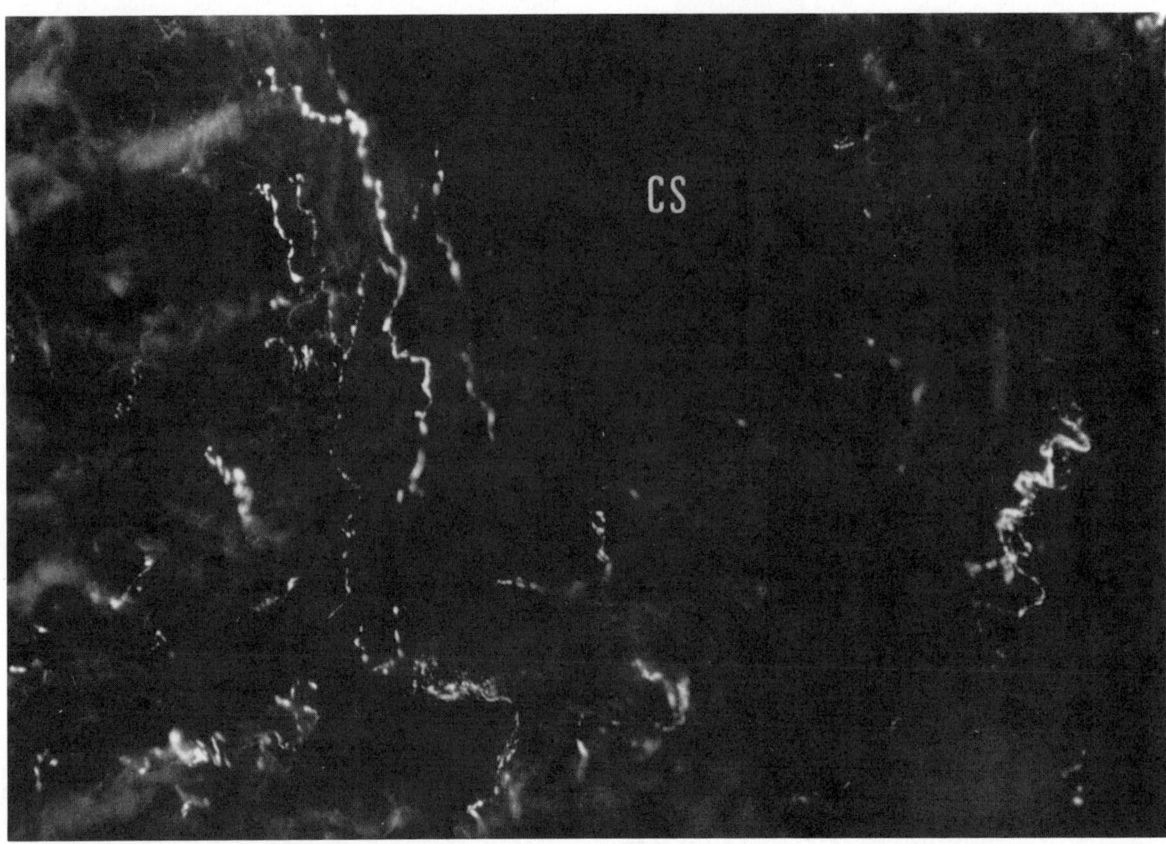

FIG. 4. Histofluorescent (adrenergic) nerve fibers in the human corpus cavernosum. The nerve fibers are located in the trabeculae, which surround the cavernous space (CS). × 80. (From ref. 1.)

Hemodynamic Aspects of Penile Erection

Penile erection is clearly dependent upon vascular events. The importance of increased arterial flow was demonstrated experimentally by Semans and Langworthy in their classic experiments in cats (22). Aortic occlusion prevented the development of penile erection produced by sacral nerve root stimulation. Furthermore, after an erection had been produced by nerve stimulation, aortic occlusion resulted in prompt detumescence. The importance of arterial flow was recognized clinically by Leriche and Morel (23). Patients with aortoiliac occlusive vascular disease were recognized

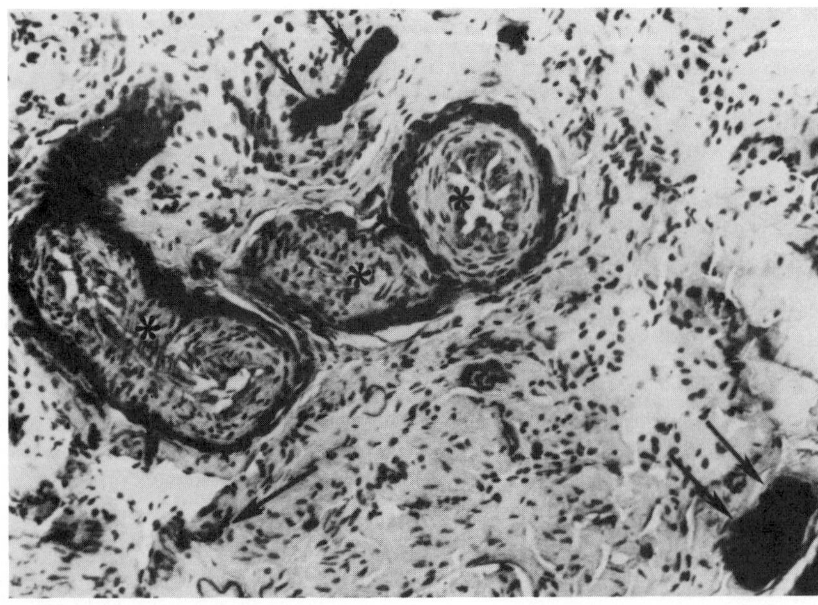

FIG. 5. Acetylcholinesterase-positive fibers in corpus cavernosum in the outer tunic of tortuous arteriole (*asterisks*). Nerve bundles containing acetylcholinesterase are also seen (*arrows*). × 126. (From ref. 17.)

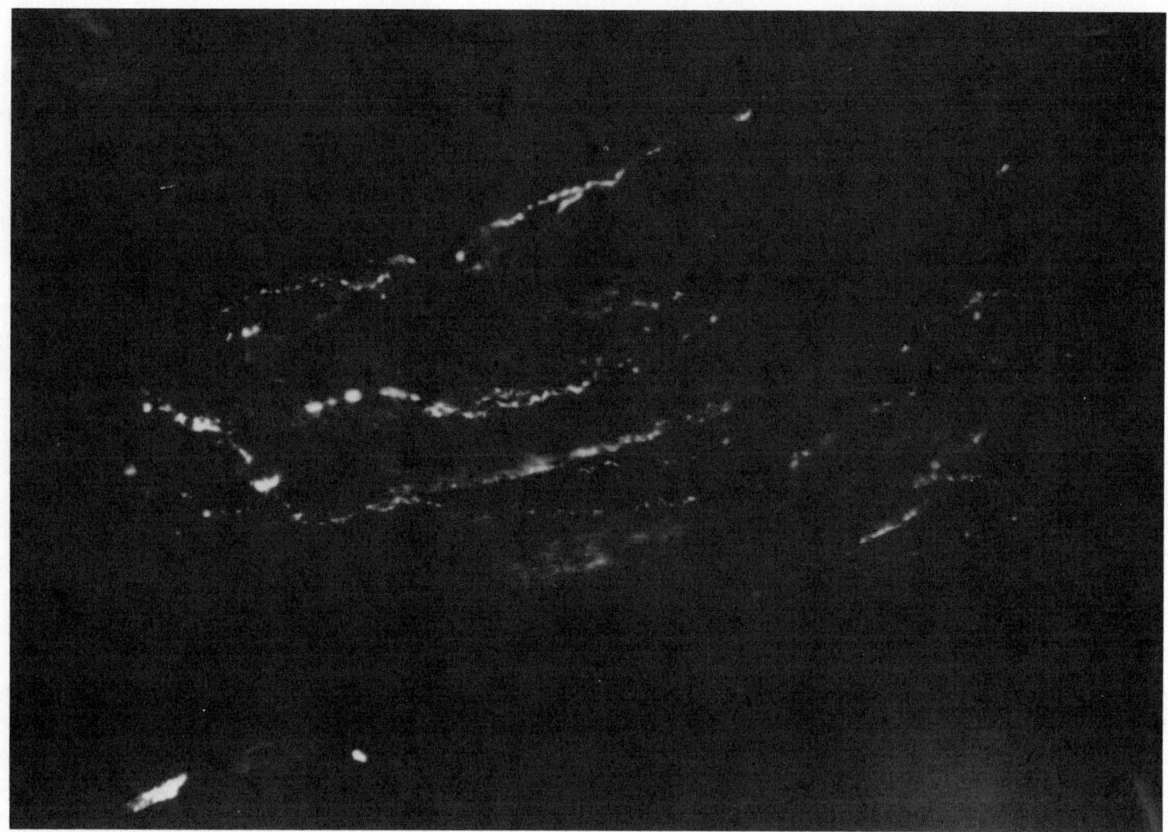

FIG. 6. VIP fluorescent nerve fibers in trabeculae of corpus cavernosum in the monkey penis. × 100. (From ref. 21.)

to suffer not only from intermittent claudication of the lower extremities, but also from impotence.

Although general agreement exists concerning the importance of increased arterial blood flow in the production and maintenance of erection, the role of the venous drainage system, despite extensive investigation, is still controversial. In 1967, Dorr and Brody extensively studied the hemodynamic aspects of erection in the canine (24). With erection produced by pelvic nerve stimulation, these investigators demonstrated that dorsal artery perfusion pressure fell while venous pressure rose. Blood flow through not only the dorsal artery, but also the dorsal vein, markedly increased. To ascertain whether a venous occlusive mechanism was, at least in part, responsible for the production and maintenance of erection, pressures were measured at multiple venous sites from the corpora cavernosa distally to the internal pudendal vein proximally. No venous pressure gradient could be found, and these investigators concluded that increased arterial inflow was of primary importance in the production of erection and that increased venous outflow resistance was of little, if any, significance.

In other animal experiments performed in several species, however, data exist which do implicate the obstruction of venous flow from the penis as being mechanistically important in the production of erection. In dogs, the highest recorded pressures in the corpora cavernosa occur during intromission and coincide with electromyographically demonstrable contraction of the ischiocavernosus muscle (25). A plausible explanation for this observation is that skeletal muscle contraction produces compression and, therefore, blockade of venous flow. An equally plausible explanation, however, is that the skeletal muscle is simply compressing the corpora cavernosa in an already erect, high pressure state. In goats, bulls, and stallions, anesthesia of the ischiocavernosus muscles prevents these animals from copulating because of their inability to achieve erection (26). In humans, however, the importance of striated perineal muscle activity in the production of erection appears to be insignificant. Human erection can occur with no increase in electromyographic activity of the bulbocavernosus, deep transverse perineal, or urethral sphincter muscles (27).

In the early 1980s, xenon washout techniques were utilized to study hemodynamic changes in penile erection in humans. This technique appeared ideal to resolve the question of whether increased venous resistance significantly contributes to the production of penile erection. Blood flow through the corpora cavernosa in the flaccid state is minimal. If ^{133}Xe were injected into the corpora cavernosa, with penile erection produced by visual sexual stimulation, the rate of ^{133}Xe "washout" in the flaccid and erect states should determine whether venous flow was increased or decreased with erection. ^{133}Xe "washout" techniques have been utilized by two groups of investigators, with remarkably conflicting results. Shirai and Ishii reported an increase in the "washout" of ^{133}Xe and therefore concluded that venous flow increases with erection and that no increase in venous vascular resistance, therefore, occurs (28). Utilizing similar techniques, however, Wagner found that the rate of "washout" of ^{133}Xe decreased with erection (29). Wagner concluded that decreased venous flow, and therefore increased resistance, was an important physiologic event occurring with erection.

Recently, more sophisticated animal experimentation and clinical laboratory techniques have emerged; these data, in general, support the necessity for increased venous resistance in the production and maintenance of erection. In the canine model, Lue et al. determined that with electrical stimulation of the cavernosal nerve, arterial flow through the internal pudendal artery increased by 250% (9). With erection, pressure within the corpora cavernosa is approximately 10 mm Hg below the systolic arterial blood pressure, and blood flow into and out of the corpora cavernosa, although present, is markedly reduced. Utilizing a technique of saline infusion into the corpora with the aorta clamped, an initial drop in cavernosal pressure as well as decreased venous flow was observed during erection produced by cavernosal nerve stimulation. Thus, these investigators conclude that erection is the result of increased arterial inflow, active relaxation of the smooth muscle of the trabeculae of the corpora cavernosa, and active increase in venous outflow resistance. The mechanism responsible for the increase in venous outflow resistance is unclear, but may be related to relaxation of the trabeculae of the corpora cavernosa and increased intracavernosal pressure rather than to active constriction of veins and venules per se.

Clinical studies utilizing cavernosography also support the concept of increased venous resistance. When an erection is produced pharmacologically in humans, contrast agents infused into the corpora cavernosa can be radiologically observed to remain in the corpora cavernosa; venous drainage systems of the penis are not normally visualized. In fact, a new etiology for impotence, "venous leak" impotence, has been proposed (30). The pathological event in these patients is probably dysfunction of the smooth muscle of the corpora cavernosa rather than dysfunction of the veins themselves; this new concept will be discussed in further detail in the section on neuropharmacology. Although the controversy concerning the importance of increased venous resistance in the production of penile erection remains unresolved, current evidence supports the concept that both increased arterial inflow and decreased venous outflow contribute to normal erectile physiology.

An equally controversial area concerns the mechanism(s) by which blood is shunted into the penis during the development of erection. In the flaccid state, blood flow through the corpora cavernosa is low. With erection, the cavernous spaces are dilated and filled with blood and the pressure within the corpora cavernosa increases. For years, extremely complex shunt mechanisms were believed to be responsible for increasing blood flow within the corpora cavernosa. In 1939, Deysach hypothesized that "venous sluices" opened and closed and produced erection by altering venous outflow resistance (8). In 1952, Conti, in an anatomic study performed on cadavers, described "polsters," which consist of columns of smooth muscle within the intima of penile arteries and veins (31). Conti proposed that relaxation and contraction of "polsters" could divert blood into and away from the corpora cavernosa and thereby control erection and detumescence. Conti's "polster theory" was widely accepted until evidence was presented that "polsters" are not specialized anatomic structures, but rather arterosclerotic changes in penile blood vessels (32,33). In addition, no innervation to these structures has ever been identified.

Recently, another "shunt theory" has been proposed based on "shunt arteries" (10). According to this hypothesis, the helicine arteries that supply the corpora cavernosa are constricted during detumescence, and blood is diverted to the corpus spongiosum through "shunt arteries." With appropriate stimuli for erection, "shunt arteries" constrict and the helicine arteries dilate, and the net result is that blood flow is increased to the corpora cavernosa. All theories concerning specialized structures that shunt blood away from the corpora in detumescence and into the corpora with erection are speculative. There are no physiologic data to support such mechanisms. In all probability, dilation of the arterial supply to the penis, the helicine arteries, and the trabeculae of the corpora cavernosa is all that is required to shunt blood into the corpora cavernosa.

Neurophysiology

The fact that penile erection is under neurologic control cannot be disputed; the neural pathways involved and the neurophysiologic events responsible for penile erection have been studied since the mid-nineteenth century. The importance of the pelvic parasympathetic nerve was first recognized by the classic observations of Eckhard (34). In the canine, stimulation of these nerves ("nervi erigentes") resulted in penile erection; stimulation of the hypogastric nerve (a sympathetic nerve) did not produce erection.

Similar, but refined, experiments were performed by Muller in the dog (35) and Root and Bard in the cat (36). The results of these two classic experiments are similar. Two types of stimuli are capable of producing penile erection in these species: (i) tactile genital stimulation and (ii) psychogenic stimulation through proximity to a bitch in heat or cat in estrous. When the entire sacral and most of the lumbar spinal cord are surgically excised, these animals no longer develop erection with genital stimulation. These animals are, however, still capable of developing psychogenic erections. In Root and Bard's study, when cats, in addition to having the lumbosacral spinal cord ablated, also underwent spinal cord transection between T11 and T12 or T13, and L1, no erectile activity could be seen with either tactile or psychogenic stimuli. In addition, in those animals that had undergone lumbosacral ablation, removal of the hypogastric nerves also resulted in cessation of psychogenically stimulated erection. With the lumbosacral cord intact, however, resection of the hypogastric nerves or inferior mesenteric ganglion had no effect on erections produced by either tactile or psychic stimuli. The results of these studies can be summarized as follows. In the dog and cat, two peripheral neural pathways are capable of producing penile erection. The lumbosacral portion of the spinal cord appears to be capable of mediating erection by both tactile and psychic stimuli, and the lower thoracic cord and peripheral sympathetic nerves appear to be capable of mediating erection secondary to psychic stimuli.

Other animal data exist, however, which do not support such relatively simplistic neurologic control mechanisms. In all animal studies performed in the dog, cat, and rabbit, parasympathetic nerve or nerve root stimulation produces erection. Results obtained with sympathetic nerve stimulation have not been so consistent. With hypogastric nerve stimulation, Eckhard reported erection in rabbits, but not in dogs. Other investigators have indicated that hypogastric nerve stimulation in the canine results in a slight increase in penile volume (37). In the feline, Semans and Langworthy did not find penile erection upon hypogastric nerve stimulation; in fact, stimulation of these sympathetic nerves produced contraction of penile arteries and actually caused an erect penis to become flaccid (22). In animal experimentation, therefore, parasympathetic nerve stimulation consistently results in penile erection. Although the sympathetic nervous system may be capable of mediating psychogenic erection, experimental evidence supporting this concept is not conclusive.

Available human data, although scant, is generally consistent with the results of animal experimentation. However, two major flaws exist in most studies in humans. First, the completeness of the neurologic lesion can rarely be accurately defined by clinical testing. Secondly, much of the data is retrospective and has been obtained by interview technique. There are few, if any, convincing studies available because of the lack of objective clinical data pertaining to potency in the presence of neurologic injury or neurologic disease.

The largest study dealing with sexual function in spinal-cord-injured patients was published by Bors and Comarr (38). No patient with a complete lower motor neuron lesion achieved an erection with genital stimulation. Twenty-four percent of these patients, however, reported penile erection with psychogenic stimulation. Most patients with spinal cord lesions above the level of the sacral spinal cord did report erections with genital tactile stimulation. Patients with spinal cord injuries above the level of the sacral spinal cord also reported erections with psychic stimulation; the percentage of patients achieving psychogenic erection, however, depended on the level of the injury. Psychogenic erections were reported by 4% with cervical lesions; 0% with thoracic, T1 to T6 lesions; 8% with thoracic, T7 to T12 lesions; and 56% with lumbar lesions. These human data are, in general, consistent with the previously described animal data. In humans, penile erection produced by tactile genital stimulation appears to be dependent upon an intact sacral spinal reflex arc. The sympathetic nervous system does appear, at least in some patients, to be capable of mediating psychogenic erection through pathways that connect the cerebral cortex, thoracolumbar spinal cord, and peripheral sympathetic pathways to the penis and its vasculature.

In human and animal studies, the importance of the parasympathetic nervous system in erectile physiology appears clear. Clinical data relating to importance of the sympathetic innervation of the penis are obtained from young male patients undergoing retroperitoneal lymph node dissection for testis cancer. In these patients, the periaortic sympathetic chain and the entire sympathetic innervation to the pelvis are removed from the level of the renal vein to the aortic bifurcation. These patients almost uniformly develop symptoms referable to peripheral sympathetic denervation (lack of seminal fluid emission or retrograde ejaculation), but they do not experience impotence (39,40). Sympathetic innervation, therefore, does not appear to be necessary for the development of erection from tactile or psychogenic stimulation in humans. In some patients with sacral spinal cord lesions, the sympathetic nervous system may be responsible for psychogenically induced erections. The overall importance of the sympathetic nervous system in the neurologically normal patient requires better definition.

Supraspinal neurologic control of penile erection undoubtedly is of major importance. Psychogenic impotence is a well-recognized clinical phenomenon. Our understanding of the specific significant central neural pathways is limited. There are some animal data that describe the results of central nervous system ablation and stimulation experiments. Human data are scarce and are based primarily on isolated case reports of patients with central nervous system diseases or patients following ablative neurosurgical procedures.

Experimentally, the importance of the supraspinal nervous system in regulating penile erection was emphasized by Kluver and Bucy (41). These investigators reported hypersexual behavior in monkeys following removal of both temporal lobes, including the uncus and part of the hippocampus. Even under nonstimulated conditions, these monkeys exhibited frequent penile erections. Other experiments utilizing stereotaxic electrical stimulation of various parts of the brain, particularly the limbic system, have demonstrated that the supraspinal central nervous system is capable of mediating penile erection (42–44). Cortical lesions in humans are also associated with impotence (45,46).

Neuropharmacology

A significant amount of recent research has concentrated on the peripheral neuropharmacology of penile erection.

Humankind has been searching for an effective aphrodisiac for centuries; recent reports of possibly effective oral therapy for impotence have emphasized the importance of better definition of the end-organ neuropharmacology (47). In addition, effective intracorporal injection therapy has emerged and will be subsequently discussed. Despite concentrated research efforts, the identification of the neurotransmitter(s) responsible for the production of penile erection remains elusive.

As previously discussed, in animals and humans, the parasympathetic nervous system (specifically the pelvic nerve) is the primary neural pathway responsible for mediating penile erection. Since the parasympathetic nervous system has been classically thought to be composed of cholinergic neurons, acetylcholine would appear to be the logical candidate for the neurotransmitter that is responsible for penile erection. Acetylcholine should, therefore, dilate penile blood vessels and relax the smooth muscle of the corpora cavernosa.

Available experimental data, however, do not support the fact that acetylcholine is the primary neurotransmitter, or the only neurotransmitter, responsible for penile erection (16). In animals, erection produced by pelvic nerve stimulation can be prevented by pretreatment with the ganglionic blocking agent hexamethonium, but not by pretreatment with atropine (24,48). Available studies in humans also support that concept that penile erection is at least partially atropine resistant (49). If acetylcholine is the neurotransmitter responsible for penile erection, infusion of this agent should produce erection. In animal models, however, penile erection does not follow the intravascular injection of acetylcholine (24,50). Furthermore, corporal smooth muscle relaxation is thought to be of primary importance in producing erection, and, in *in vitro* experiments, strips of corporal smooth muscle respond minimally, if at all, to acetylcholine stimulation (5). Relevant criticisms of these experiments have been forwarded, including the possibility that acetylcholine infused intravascularly may be hydrolyzed before it reaches the smooth-muscle receptor and that, in these experimental situations, acetylcholine and atropine do not reach the vascular and corporal receptors. An alternative explanation is that penile erection is not a cholinergically (or exclusively cholinergically) mediated event.

If acetylcholine is not the neurotransmitter responsible for penile arterial dilation and corporal smooth muscle relaxation, could a catecholamine be responsible for the physiologic events leading to penile erection? Adrenergic neurons are carried in the pelvic parasympathetic nerves of rats and cats (51,52), and this could conceivably also be true in humans. Stimulation of the pelvic parasympathetic nerve could perhaps, therefore, activate adrenergic as well as cholinergic neurons. As previously discussed, the penile vasculature and corporal smooth muscle are anatomically richly supplied by adrenergic neurons, and high norepinephrine levels in the corpora cavernosa have been demonstrated (53). In addition, in humans, radioligand binding studies have demonstrated high alpha-adrenergic receptor density in corporal preparations (54).

In the cat, the intravenous infusion of the beta-adrenergic agonist salbutamol and the alpha-adrenergic blocker phenoxybenzamine produces penile erection (50). In addition, isolated strips of human corpora cavernosa relax when exposed to isoproterenol and salbutamol (55). Beta-adrenergic stimulation or alpha-adrenergic blockade would appear, therefore, to promote erection. Stimulation of isolated human corporal strips with norepinephrine, however, results in contraction; this contractile response can be blocked by pretreating the strips with phentolamine (5). The infusion of norepinephrine in the dog (24) and cat (50) does not cause erection. Epinephrine infusion, in fact, causes contraction of canine penile arteries (56). The oral administration of large doses of alpha- and beta-adrenergic antagonists (phenoxybenzamine and propranolol) has no effect on erections produced by mechanical or visual sexual stimulation in humans (49). The evidence concerning the possibility that a catecholamine is the neurotransmitter responsible for erection appears to favor the conclusion that adrenergic stimulation promotes penile detumescence (vascular constriction and corporal contraction) rather than penile erection. Further, more convincing evidence is presented below in the discussion of the intracorporal injection of vasoactive agents.

Thus, the neuropharmacology of penile erection cannot be totally explained by classic adrenergic and cholinergic mechanisms (16). Numerous putative nonadrenergic, noncholinergic neurotransmitters have been neuropharmacologically investigated. Available evidence indicates that prostaglandins (PGE_1, PGE_2, and $PGF_{2\alpha}$), bradykinin, 5-hydroxytryptamine, histamine, and several amino acids are not the neurotransmitter responsible for the vascular and corporal smooth-muscle relaxation that are necessary for the production of penile erection (3,4). Adenosine triphosphate (ATP, a putative purinergic neurotransmitter) has not been physiologically linked to the erectile process.

The search for a nonadrenergic, noncholinergic mechanism to explain the neuropharmacology of penile erection has in recent years been concentrated on possible peptidergic mechanisms. VIP is the polypeptide that has been most extensively investigated. As previously discussed, nerves containing VIP have been anatomically demonstrated in the trabeculae of the corpora cavernosa and in the outer tunic of penile blood vessels at both the light and electron microscopic levels. VIP not only causes vasodilation (57,58), but also has been demonstrated *in vitro* to cause relaxation of strips of rabbit, cat, monkey, and human corpora cavernosa (20,21,59,60). Other animal experiments have yielded conflicting results. In *in vitro* experiments, VIP has been reported to have little or no effect on the corpora cavernosa urethra of the rabbit, guinea pig, dog, or cat. In addition, VIP stimulation also did not produce relaxation of penile blood vessels in the bull (61). In strips of human corpora cavernosa, VIP exerts no effect unless the strips have been previously contracted via norepinephrine stimulation. After norepinephrine stimulation, a weak relaxant effect is noted (21).

A major reason for the interest in a peptidergic mechanism being responsible for penile erection deals with the issue of atropine resistance. As previously discussed, atropine does not completely block the erectile response elicited by pelvic nerve stimulation. A similar situation has been shown to occur in the cat submandibular gland. Specifically, the vasodilation seen with nerve stimulation in this organ is also atropine resistant. VIP has been demonstrated to be responsible for the atropine-resistant vasodilation; both VIP and acetylcholine are present in the same neuron, and both are released with nerve stimulation (62). If similar mechanisms exist in the penis, many basic questions concerning the neuropharmacology of erection could be answered.

A breakthrough in our understanding of the neuropharmacology and neurophysiology of erection occurred with the description of the intracorporal injection of vasoactive agents. In 1984, Virag et al. reported that papaverine injected directly into the corpora cavernosa caused penile erection (63). This agent produces smooth-muscle relaxation by direct action(s) on the smooth-muscle cell and does not act through neuroreceptors. Brindley's observation that the intracorporal injection of phenoxybenzamine (an alpha-adrenergic blocking agent) also results in penile erection in humans clarified the situation further (64). As previously discussed, norepinephrine causes the smooth muscle of the corpora cavernosa to contract; this effect is alpha-adrenergic-receptor mediated and is prevented by the alpha-adrenergic blocking agents phenoxybenzamine and phentolamine. Although both of these agents probably also increase arterial blood flow into the penis, the importance of relaxation of the trabeculae of the corpora cavernosa in initiating and maintaining penile erection is now appreciated. A variety of other agents, including imipramine and verapamil (a calcium channel blocker), also produce erection when they are injected intracorporally (65). Since agents that cause smooth-muscle relaxation produce erection, pharmacologic agents that cause the corporal smooth muscle to contract should produce detumescence. Norepinephrine, the postganglionic sympathetic neurotransmitter, causes both penile vasoconstriction and contraction of the corporal smooth muscle. The sympathetic nervous system, therefore, appears to be responsible for penile detumescence. The use of intracorporal injection is not only an important research method, but is also a valuable diagnostic and therapeutic modality in the patient with impotence. This will be discussed below.

Although significant advances have been made in clarifying the neuropharmacology of the peripheral nervous system as it relates to erection, our knowledge of central nervous system mechanisms is limited. Serotonin has been demonstrated to inhibit, and dopamine to stimulate, male sexual activity in the rat (66). In male patients with Parkinson's disease treated with L-DOPA, increased sexual activity has been reported (67,68). Trazodone, an antidepressant commonly used clinically, is associated with the occurrence of priapism (69). Trazodone is thought to act primarily by blocking the reuptake of serotonin into nerve terminals. In addition, chlorophenylpiperazine, a metabolite of trazodone, causes erection in monkeys when this agent is injected intravenously (70,71).

Summary and Clinical Correlation

The description of acceptable penile prostheses in the mid-1970s (72,73) not only popularized the evaluation and treatment of impotence, but also emphasized how little was actually known about the basic physiology of erection. Currently, both semirigid prostheses (Fig. 7) and inflatable prostheses (Fig. 8) are commonly implanted with low complication and high patient-satisfaction rates (74,75).

The two major events responsible for penile erection are (i) increased arterial flow to the penis and (ii) relaxation of the smooth muscle of the trabeculae, which allows blood to be shunted into the corpora cavernosa. As previously discussed, increased venous outflow resistance probably also occurs, not by active constriction of the venous outflow, but by passive occlusion caused by increased intracorporal pressure.

Although erectile difficulty secondary to atherosclerotic disease has been recognized for years (23), the standardization of techniques to measure penile blood flow has significantly clarified our understanding of the importance of arterial flow in several disease processes.

The simplest and most commonly used method to assess penile arterial blood flow is the measurement of arterial pressure in the dorsal penile and cavernosal arteries. These measurements are obtained by utilizing a 10-mHz Doppler probe positioned over the penile arteries. A pneumatic cuff is placed around the base of the penis and is inflated to the point where arterial flow ceases. The cuff is then slowly deflated, and the pressure at which arterial flow is reestablished is the penile systolic blood pressure. The penile systolic blood pressure divided by the brachial artery systolic blood pressure gives the penile-brachial index (PBI). The PBI yields valuable information regarding the status of the

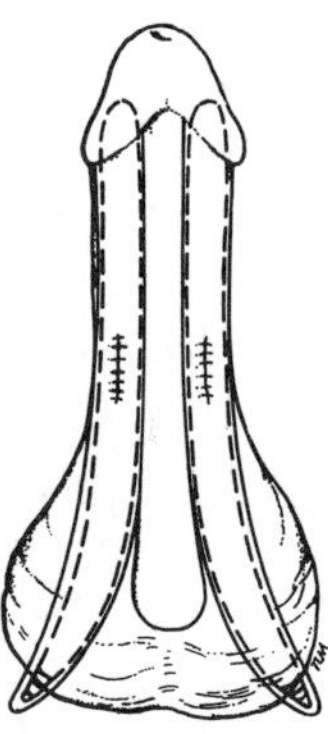

FIG. 7. Semirigid penile prosthesis. Paired cylinders have been surgically implanted into the corpora cavernosa.

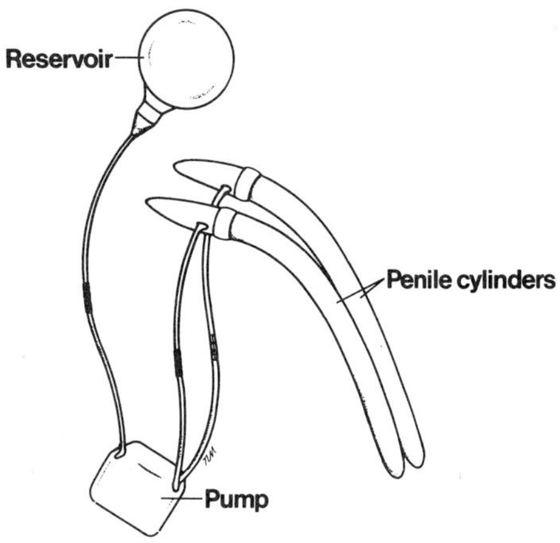

FIG. 8. Inflatable penile prosthesis.

arterial supply to the penis; values of <0.6 are strongly suggestive of vasculogenic impotence (76). Recently, the use of the duplex ultrasound scanner in the measurement of arterial blood flow has been reported (77). This technique shows promise in evaluating arterial flow in the flaccid and erect penis, but further studies are needed to ascertain its accuracy in measuring flow through small vessels.

The use of objective measurements of penile arterial flow has allowed description of several clinical entities. For example, patients who initially develop a good erection and then experience difficulty maintaining it during intercourse may demonstrate the "external iliac" or "pelvic steal" syndrome (78,79). In these patients, with exercise, blood is shunted from the pelvis to the buttocks and legs. A normal PBI that drops to less than 0.6, or a drop of greater than 0.15 after exercise, is strongly suggestive of this syndrome.

Impotence in patients who have undergone successful renal transplantation may also be secondary to vascular factors. In renal transplantation, often the internal iliac (hypogastric) artery is transected and used in an end-to-end anastomosis to the transplant renal artery. If a second transplant is performed utilizing the opposite internal iliac artery in a similar fashion, impotence secondary to decreased arterial flow to the penis is likely to occur (80). Second renal transplants can be performed by an end-to-side technique on the external iliac or common iliac artery, with penile blood flow preserved.

Although much experimental information concerning the neuroanatomy and neurophysiology of erection has been recently generated, clinical studies to assess the integrity of sensory and motor pathways are less than adequate. The integrity of neural pathways can be ascertained by measuring evoked potentials. The sacral evoked potential (sacral latency time) is performed by stimulating penile skin and recording from a needle electrode placed in the bulbocavernosus muscle (81). The time from stimulation to the first electrical response in the bulbocavernosus muscle is measured and is the sacral latency time. The neural reflex controlling penile erection consists of pudendal afferent (sensory) fibers and parasympathetic efferent (motor) fibers. The sensory portion of the sacral reflex that governs erection, and the sensory portion of the reflex that is measured by sacral evoked potential testing, are, therefore, identical. This sensory portion of the reflex arc can also be evaluated by measuring dorsal penile nerve conduction velocity (82). The efferent part of the reflex that controls erection is, however, different from the efferent innervation that is measured by sacral evoked-potential testing. This study measures pudendal sensory afferent nerves and pudendal (somatic) motor efferent nerves. At present, no methodology exists which can directly measure the efferent (parasympathetic) portion of the reflex controlling erection. Measurement of sacral latency times provides some information concerning reflex activity through the sacral spinal cord, but does not directly test efferent penile innervation.

Neurologic testing of central nervous system pathways that control erection is even less precise. Genitocerebral evoked potentials can be measured; the penis is stimulated as in the sacral evoked response examination, and recordings are taken from electroencephalographic leads placed on the scalp (83). The clinical significance of such studies is not yet clear. Methods to clinically directly evaluate penile innervation are needed.

The recent description of the anatomy of the corporal nerves in humans has allowed the technique of several surgical procedures to be modified. Previously, most patients undergoing radical prostatectomy for prostate cancer experienced postoperative impotence. Following the precise anatomic description of the cavernosal nerves, Walsh and Donker concluded that impotence in these patients results from injury to the autonomic innervation during transection of the prostatic apex and the urethra, or during division of the lateral pelvic fascia and lateral pedicle (13). After modification of the surgical technique to preserve these nerves, 86% of patients who have undergone radical prostatectomy are potent 1 year after surgery (84).

Recent advances in our understanding of erectile neuropharmacology have already become clinically useful. The intracorporal injection of various drugs causes penile erection. In humans, the injection of papaverine alone and papaverine combined with phentolamine has been utilized both diagnostically and therapeutically (77,85). These injection techniques have been combined with cavernosometry and cavernosography as diagnostic studies in humans. Pressure responses to drug injection and the physiologic measurements of blood flow under various test situations can be measured. Both arterial and venous channels can be visualized in both the tumescent and flaccid states. These techniques, however, have been only recently described, and drug dosage, indications, and interpretation of these studies require further definition. Intracorporal injection therapy for impotence has been reportedly successful in large numbers of patients (85,86). Self-injection with combinations of papaverine and phentolamine is thought to be relatively free of side effects (86); the long-term effects of such therapy in humans, however, are not known.

A significant complication of the intracorporal injection of the drugs that produce erection is priapism (87). In the past, priapism has been treated primarily by surgical procedures that shunt blood out of the corpora cavernosa and into either the saphenous vein, glans penis, or corpus spongiosum (88,89). By applying new knowledge of the neuropharmacology of the penis, it is now possible to treat some patients with priapism by pharmacologic methods. Laboratory studies have demonstrated that catecholamines cause the smooth muscle of the corpora to contract and constrict penile arteries. Since erection is produced by corporal dilation and vasodilation, the intracorporal injection of catecholamines into an already erect penis should, theoretically, produce detumescence. This, in fact, is the case, and some patients with priapism, particularly those patients whose priapism is secondary to the prolonged effects of intracorporally injected papaverine and phentolamine, can be successfully treated by the intracavernosus injection of norepinephrine (87).

The ultimate goal of pharmacologic therapy of impotence is the discovery and development of a drug that can be taken orally and that would reproducibly result in the development of penile erection. Various agents have been utilized for this purpose in the past; none have yielded satisfactory results. Testosterone therapy in impotent patients with normal serum testosterone levels is no more efficacious than placebo (90). Recently, renewed interest in yohimbine has emerged. For many years this agent was considered an aphrodisiac and, in combination with testosterone and nux vomica extract, was widely used for the therapy of impotence in the 1960s. Clinical trials with yohimbine have again emerged. Morales et al. reported that 6 of 23 patients treated with this drug note the reappearance of full, sustained erections (47). Further controlled studies utilizing a placebo control group and the measurement of objective parameters are necessary to ascertain whether yohimbine is indeed efficacious.

An equally important pharmacologic question concerns the incidence and mechanisms by which many commonly used drugs cause erectile dysfunction. Medication may be the single most common cause of impotence in the United States. Objective evidence is so limited, however, that very few conclusions can be reached. Virtually every class of drugs has been implicated as being causally related to impotence; the theoretical mechanisms for these adverse drug effects include central nervous system sedation or depression, drug-related hyperprolactinemia, direct antiandrogen effects, and anticholinergic or antiandrenergic effects (91). An example of the complexity of drug effects on erectile function is cimetidine, a histamine (H_2)-receptor antagonist widely used in the treatment of duodenal ulcer disease. This agent has been associated with diminished libido and impotence in up to 50% of male patients taking this drug (92). The mechanisms, however, by which cimetidine causes impotence are unclear. Cimetidine has been associated with elevated prolactin levels and gynecomastia (93,94). In addition, peripheral H_2-receptor blockade in corporal smooth muscle may also be responsible (95). The pharmacologic central effects of most medications are unknown. There are few, if any, well-controlled studies that have utilized objective parameters to evaluate the adverse effects of the most commonly used medications on penile erection.

In summary, a significant amount of new basic laboratory information concerning the physiology of erection has been obtained during the past decade. Much of this information has been directly applicable to clinical practice. Many important questions remain unanswered. What neurotransmitters control vascular dilatation and corporal smooth-muscle relaxation? What role does the sympathetic nervous system play in humans? What are the mechanisms by which the central nervous system controls erection? What are the mechanisms by which commonly prescribed drugs adversely affect erection? In contrast to a decade ago, a significant number of laboratories are now currently involved in basic science and clinical research in the areas of penile erection and impotence. Answers to many questions concerning male erectile dysfunction should be available in the near future.

EMISSION AND EJACULATION

In recent years, research in the area of erectile dysfunction has produced a significant amount of new clinical information. The study of erectile dysfunction is presently achieving much attention primarily because of the high incidence of impotence and public awareness that satisfactory therapy exists. Fewer patients experience primary disorders of emission and ejaculation. The physiology of these events is understood to some extent, and treatment is available for some patients with disorders of seminal fluid emission and ejaculation. Emission, the deposition of seminal fluid into the posterior urethra, is dependent upon the integrity of the vasa deferentia, seminal vesicles, prostate gland, and bladder neck. Ejaculation is dependent primarily upon the function of the striated perineal musculature.

Anatomy

Spermatozoa are transported from the testes and epididymides to the posterior urethra by the vasa deferentia. The tubular vas deferens in approximately 35 cm long in the human adult. It extends from the tail of the epididymis to the region of the verumontanum in the posterior urethra (Fig. 9). The vas deferens joins the duct of the seminal vesicle to form the ejaculatory duct. Anatomically, the vas deferens in humans can be divided into five parts: (i) the sheathless epididymal portion contained within the tunica vaginalis, (ii) the scrotal portion, (iii) the inguinal portion, (iv) the retroperitoneal portion, and (v) the ampulla.

Embryologically, the vas deferens is derived from the Wolffian ductal system. On physical examination, the vas

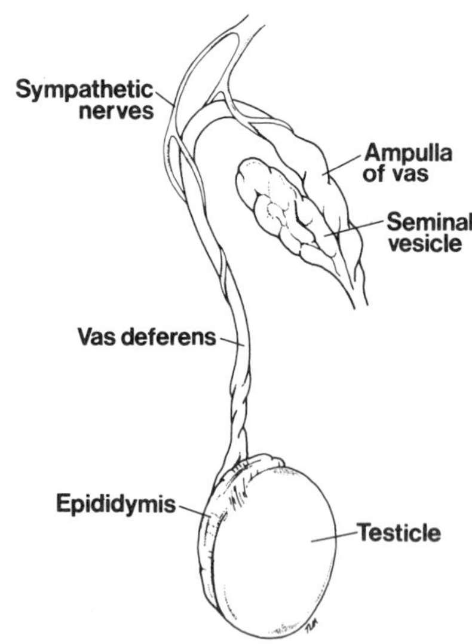

FIG. 9. Anatomy of the human vas deferens.

deferens is easily palpable as a thick cord-like structure in the scrotum. The vas is not present in patients with cystic fibrosis and in some patients with renal agenesis. Histologically, the thick wall of the vas surrounds a very narrow lumen (approximately 0.05 cm). The wall is composed of three layers: (i) a mucosal layer; (ii) a thick muscular layer consisting of inner longitudinal, middle circular, and outer longitudinal layers; and (iii) an adventitial layer composed of a sheath of connective tissue containing numerous small blood vessels and nerves (96).

At the time of seminal fluid emission and ejaculation, the bladder neck closes to prevent the retrograde ejaculation of seminal fluid into the bladder (97). The anatomy of the bladder neck is controversial, and the anatomic basis for bladder neck closure in preventing not only retrograde ejaculation, but also urinary incontinence, is unclear. Most investigators agree that no anatomic sphincter consisting of circular smooth-muscle fibers exists in the area of the bladder outlet (98,99). A physiologic sphincter, however, does exist. The bladder neck probably remains collapsed because of (a) tension created by the large amount of elastic tissue in this area and (b) smooth-muscle contraction under alpha-adrenergic control (100). Following transurethral resection of the prostate, the bladder neck closure mechanism is destroyed. Patients remain continent because of a second, more distal, continence mechanism that is present in the region of the membranous urethra (101) (Fig. 10). Most patients who have undergone transurethral resection of the prostate, however, do experience retrograde ejaculation.

Following emission, the seminal fluid that has been deposited in the posterior urethra is expelled out the urethral meatus by the process of ejaculation. Clonic contractions of the perineal striated musculature, primarily the bulbocavernosus and ischiocavernosus muscles, are primarily responsible for this event (102). The bulbocavernosus muscle takes its origin from the central tendon, encircles the corpus spongiosum, and inserts into the corpus cavernosum. The ischiocavernosus muscle arises from the inner surface of the ischial tuberosity and inserts into the penile crura. In humans, the experience of orgasm occurs simultaneously with the clonic contractions of these striated muscles during ejaculation (27).

Neuroanatomy of the Vas Deferens, Bladder Neck, and Perineal Musculature

The vas deferens and bladder neck, like the penis, are supplied by nerves from the pelvic plexus. For reasons that will be subsequently discussed, the innervation to these organs is thought to be primarily sympathetic in origin. In humans, the cell bodies of the sympathetic neurons are located in the lateral column of gray matter in the thoracic and upper lumbar segments of the spinal cord. Sympathetic nerve fibers exit the spinal cord via the ventral roots. These preganglionic sympathetic fibers synapse with either (a) paravertebral sympathetic chain ganglia, (b) abdominal or pelvic plexuses, or (c) ganglia located near or in the end organ. The anatomy of the abdominal and pelvic sympathetic nervous system is complex and variable, and its nomenclature is poorly standardized. Peripheral sympathetic nerves are extremely difficult to anatomically trace, and individual variability of even the paravertebral sympathetic chain is marked. Pick and Sheehan carefully dissected the paravertebral sympathetic chain in 25 cadavers (103). They found the first lumbar ganglion to be independent in 11, fused with other ganglia in 10, and separated into two parts in two. The second lumbar ganglion was absent in two, independent in 12, fused in 7, and split in four.

Sympathetic nerve fibers exiting the thoracolumbar spinal cord synapse in all of the abdominal and pelvic plexuses (celiac, superior mesenteric, aortic, inferior mesenteric, superior hypogastric, inferior hypogastric, and pelvic). In humans, the paired hypogastric nerves exit the superior hypogastric ganglion, which is also called the *presacral nerve* (14). The superior hypogastric ganglion anatomically extends from approximately the fourth lumbar to the first sacral vertebra. The pelvic plexus is located retroperitoneally beside the rectum and receives input from both the sympathetic and parasympathetic nervous systems. Autonomic nerves leaving the pelvic plexus supply the penis, prostate, seminal vesicle, vas deferens, and bladder (Fig. 11).

The perineal striated musculature (including the bulbocavernosus and ischiocavernosus muscles) is innervated by the pudendal nerve. The pudendal nerve is a somatic nerve that emanates from the sacral spinal cord (S2–4). Peripherally, the pudendal nerve does not enter the pelvic plexus, but exits the pelvis through the greater sciatic foramen, crosses the spine of the ischium, and reenters the pelvis through the lesser sciatic foramen (13).

Histologically, striated-muscle fibers can be seen periurethrally as far cephalad as the area of the bladder neck

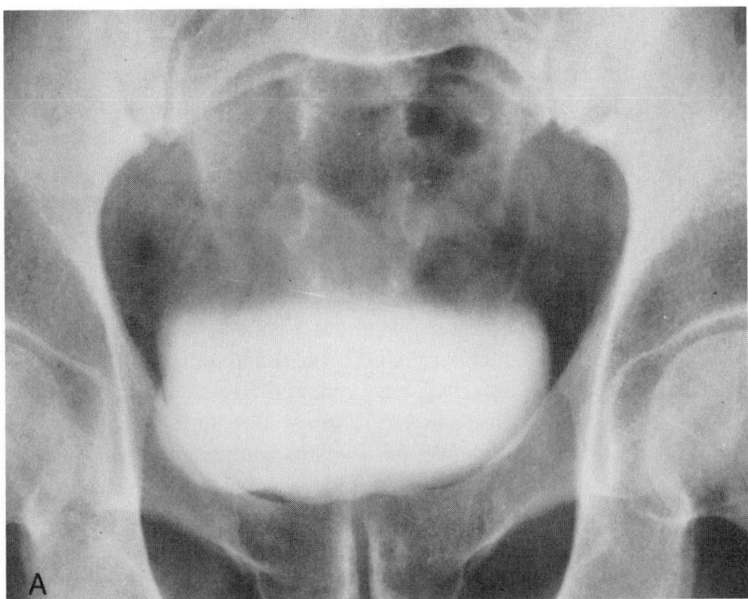

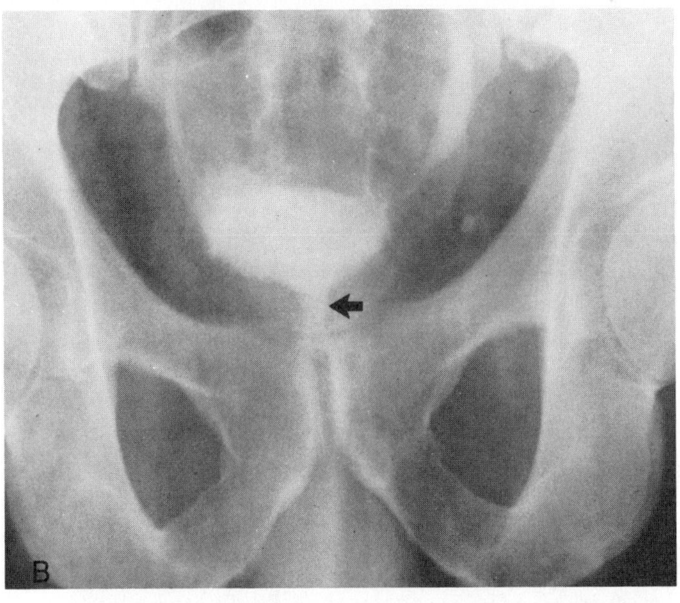

FIG. 10. Cystogram before (**A**) and after (**B**) transurethral resection of prostate (TURP). Note that contrast in A is contained within bladder by competent bladder neck. After TURP, contrast is seen past the area of the bladder neck in the region of the prostatic urethra (*arrow*).

(104). Anatomic evidence has been presented that this periurethral striated musculature is composed of two distinct types of muscle fibers: fast twitch and slow twitch (105). Evidence has also been presented that this periurethral striated musculature is innervated not by the pudendal (somatic) nerve, but by autonomic fibers from the pelvic plexus (106). In addition, Elbadawi and Shenk have reported finding a "triple innervation" (somatic, adrenergic, and cholinergic) to the periurethral striated musculature (107). Other studies, however, have failed to demonstrate an autonomic innervation to this striated musculature (108,109). At present, most anatomic evidence supports the concept that the innervation of the musculature responsible for ejaculation is somatic and not autonomic (Fig. 11).

Microscopically, utilizing histofluorescent techniques, the vas deferens in animals (cat, rat, dog, and monkey), as well as in humans, is heavily innervated by adrenergic nerves (110) (Fig. 12). High concentrations of norepinephrine determined by fluorimetric techniques have also been demonstrated (111). The inguinal portion of the vas deferens appears to be more densely adrenergically innervated and to possess a higher norepinephrine content than that portion of the vas nearer the testicle (112). Electron microscopic studies relating to the adrenergic innervation of the vas deferens are consistent with the light microscopic data. Nerve varicosities containing small (400–600 Å) dense-core vesicles have been identified. Utilizing a gluteraldehyde-dichromate technique, these small vesicles have been shown to contain catecholamine (113).

Although, anatomically, the primary innervation to the vas appears to be adrenergic, other types of nerve fibers have been demonstrated. A sparse cholinergic component

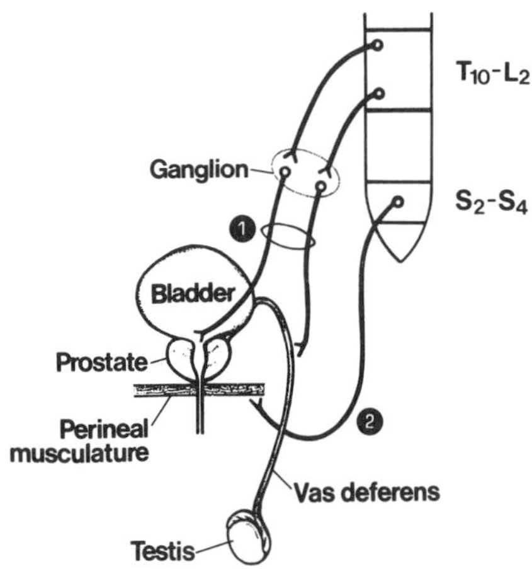

FIG. 11. Innervation of bladder neck, vas deferens, and perineal striated musculature: (*1*) Sympathetic innervation to bladder neck and vas deferens; (*2*) somatic innervation to striated perineal musculature.

was observed by Baumgarten et al. (112). Recent light and electron microscopic studies have confirmed the presence of a cholingeric innervation and also demonstrated a peptidergic innervation. Presumptive cholinergic vesicles (400–600 Å small clear vesicles) are present in the vas (113). VIP immunoreactive nerve fibers have been seen closely beneath the basement membrane of the epithelium, but only occasionally in the smooth musculature of the vas. In addition, avian pancreatic polypeptide immunoreactive nerves are particularly dense in the muscular coat of the vas deferens, and somatostatin has been demonstrated to be present in the vas by radioimmunoassay (20). The physiologic significance of this peptidergic innervation is unclear.

Morphologically, in animal models, the bladder base is richly innervated by both adrenergic and cholinergic nerves. In the dog, the bladder base contains a much more dense adrenergic innervation than does the bladder body (100). Human data are, in general, consistent with that obtained in animals. Acetylcholinesterase-positive (presumptive cholinergic) and histofluorescent (adrenergic) nerve fibers are reported to be numerous in the trigone and less dense in the anterior bladder base in both males and females (114). Gosling et al., however, have reported a sexual difference and describe a dense adrenergic innervation throughout the bladder base in the male and a sparse adrenergic innervation in this area in the female (115). In considering the neuroanatomical basis for bladder neck closure during emission and ejaculation, however, there is general agreement that, in the male, this region possesses a significant adrenergic innervation.

Neurophysiology and Neuropharmacology

Electrical stimulation of either the superior hypogastric ganglion (presacral nerve) or the hypogastric nerves in humans results in contraction of the bladder neck, prostatic musculature, seminal vesicles, and ejaculatory ducts (14). Similar results have been obtained from experiments in the cat (22). The exact spinal cord level from which these sym-

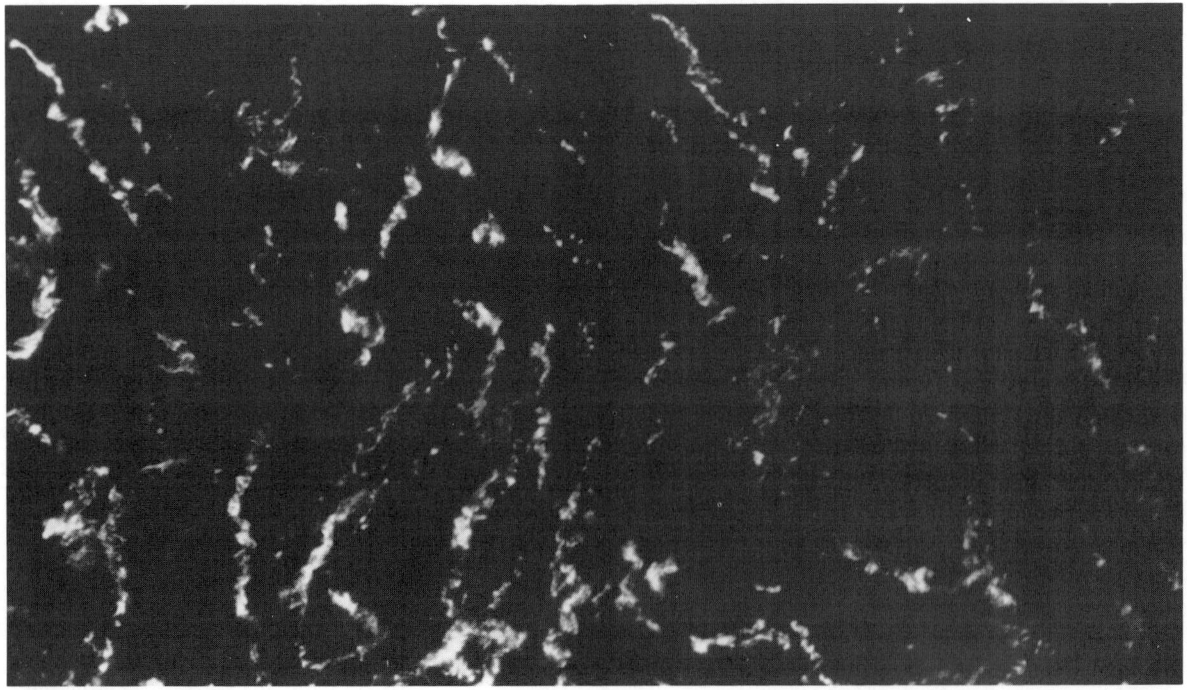

FIG. 12. Micrograph of human vas deferens demonstrating abundant histofluorescent (adrenergic) nerves. × 80.

pathetic nerves originate is difficult to ascertain because of the previously discussed marked anatomic variability.

The neuropharmacology of the vas deferens in several animal species has been extensively studied. Although the importance of the sympathetic nervous system and adrenergic innervation to the vas is well recognized, evidence has accumulated which indicates that nonadrenergic neurotransmission may be responsible for part of the contraction of the vas deferens in several animal species, including the guinea pig and the rat (116–118). In humans, however, norepinephrine is most probably the only significant neurotransmitter responsible for vasal contraction. Norepinephrine causes a marked contractile response in *in vitro* preparations of the human vas deferens. These norepinephrine-induced contractions can be blocked by phentolamine, phenoxybenzamine, and prazocin (119–121). The smooth muscle of the vas deferens exhibits spontaneous motility unless it has been exposed to local anesthetic agents. Local anesthetics also inhibit the response of the vas to norepinephrine stimulation. Other pharmacologic agents (acetylcholine, isoproterenol, histamine, and serotonin) exert little or no effect on the human vas deferens (122). In summary, in humans the primary neurologic control of the contractility of the vas deferens is the sympathetic nervous system; adrenergic nerves release norepinephrine and act via stimulation of alpha$_1$-adrenergic receptors.

Strips of muscle from the bladder base (bladder neck) also contract when stimulated *in vitro* with norepinephrine. Like the vas deferens, these contractile responses are blocked by pretreating the tissue with alpha-adrenergic antagonists (123). To the contrary, strips of bladder body, the part of bladder circumferentially above the level of the ureteral orifices, respond to adrenergic stimulation with norepinephrine by exhibiting beta-adrenergic receptor-mediated relaxation (100). Radioligand-binding studies in animals have shown that alpha-adrenergic receptors outnumber beta-adrenergic receptors in the bladder base (bladder neck). Beta-adrenergic receptors outnumber alpha receptors in the bladder body (124). It therefore appears that increased sympathetic (adrenergic) nerve activity causes contraction of the vas deferens (emission) and also closure of the bladder neck to prevent retrograde ejaculation.

The neurophysiology and neuropharmacology of ejaculation are less well understood. In humans, ejaculation is associated with rhythmic contractions of the periurethral and anal sphincter muscles (102,125). Some animal data concerning central nervous system control of emission and ejaculation have been generated. Seminal fluid emission in rats occurs after stimulation of parts of the hypothalamus (126), and ejaculation in monkeys has been produced by stimulating the preoptic area (127). In humans, both erection and ejaculation have occurred following the intrathecal injection of prostigmine, a drug that blocks cholinesterase (128). This technique has been utilized clinically to obtain semen in patients with neurologic injury. Its usefulness is limited by the fact that significant hypertension commonly occurs. The physiologic and pharmacologic basis for the central nervous system actions of this drug are not known.

Summary and Clinical Correlation

Clinical observation has significantly contributed to our understanding of the basic physiologic mechanisms involved in emission and ejaculation. Following retroperitoneal lymph-node dissection (RLND) for testicular cancer, many patients report that, although penile erection and orgasm are unchanged postoperatively, they experience a "dry ejaculate" or "shoot blanks." RLND is an extensive retroperitoneal dissection that includes removal of the sympathetic nerves and ganglia lying on the aorta and vena cava as well as removal of the paravertebral ganglia. For years the "dry ejaculate" was thought to be secondary to retrograde ejaculation of seminal fluid into the bladder; the extensive "sympathectomy" had presumably rendered the bladder unable to close during emission and ejaculation. Further study of these patients revealed that this explanation for the "dry ejaculate" was incomplete. Examination of postmasturbation bladder washings in these patients failed to demonstrate any sperm or fructose (39,40). The most reasonable explanation for the occurrence of a "dry ejaculate" following RLND is not retrograde ejaculation, but rather the absence of seminal fluid emission. Although lack of emission is the most common cause of sexual dysfunction following RLND, some patients do exhibit retrograde ejaculation. The etiology of these disorders appears to be interruption of the sympathetic innervation of the vas deferens and/or bladder neck.

Except for the previously mentioned efforts to produce emission and ejaculation with the intrathecal administration of prostigmine, efforts to pharmacologically manipulate these processes are directed at the end organ. No specific therapy for disturbances of ejaculation per se is available. Attempts to pharmacologically alter ejaculation are actually directed toward seminal fluid emission and bladder neck closure.

Since seminal fluid emission and bladder neck closure are controlled by the sympathetic innervation acting through alpha-adrenergic receptors, rational drug therapy directed toward correcting vas deferens and bladder neck dysfunction is at least theoretically possible. The sequence of events at the adrenergic nerve terminal is depicted in Fig. 13. With adrenergic nerve stimulation, norepinephrine is released from the nerve terminal and then interacts with alpha$_1$-adrenergic receptors located on the smooth-muscle membrane. Norepinephrine reuptake into the nerve terminal, as well as degradation by monamine oxidase and catechol-*O*-methyltransferase, then occurs. In addition, norepinephrine interacts with presynaptic alpha$_2$-adrenergic receptors on the nerve terminal in a "negative-feedback" fashion, whereby stimulation of the alpha$_2$ receptors decreases the amount of norepinephrine released by the nerve terminal. Pharmacologic

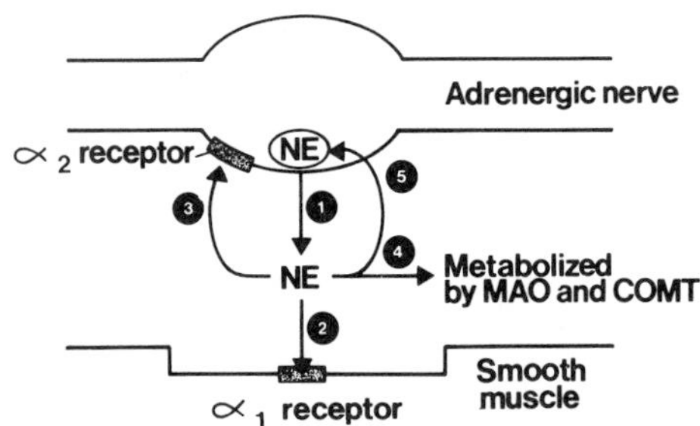

FIG. 13. Physiologic events at adrenergic nerve terminal: (*1*) With nerve stimulation, norepinephrine is released from the nerve terminal; (*2*) norepinephrine stimulates alpha$_1$-adrenergic receptors on smooth muscle membrane; (*3*) norepinephrine also stimulates presynaptic alpha$_2$-adrenergic receptors; (*4*) norepinephrine is degraded by monamine oxidase and catechol-*O*-methyl-transferase; (*5*) remaining norepinephrine undergoes reuptake into the nerve terminal.

agents that can influence several of these events at the nerve terminal are available.

A number of adrenergic-receptor agonists have been used clinically to stimulate contraction of the vas deferens, prostate, seminal vesicle, and bladder neck. Ephedrine sulfate directly stimulates both alpha- and beta-adrenergic receptors and also causes norepinephrine to be released from nerve terminals. Prolonged usage of this drug results in tachyphylaxsis, probably because of depletion of norepinephrine in the nerve terminal (129). Pseudoephedrine hydrochloride (a stereoisomer of ephedrine) exerts similar pharmacologic effects. Phenylpropanolamine hydrochloride, an ingredient in many commonly used nasal decongestants, also directly stimulates alpha-adrenergic receptors. These agents have been used to treat patients with both urinary incontinence and lack of seminal fluid emission and retrograde ejaculation (130).

Imipramine, a tricyclic antidepressant, has also been clinically utilized to treat disorders of emission (131). Imipramine probably potentiates peripheral adrenergic activity by blocking the reuptake of norepinephrine into the nerve terminal. This "cocaine-like" effect occurs in the central nervous system; the peripheral effects of this drug are less clear. Imipramine does possess both anticholinergic and direct smooth-muscle depressant properties (132,133). It is not known whether the clinical benefits of this drug on the urogenital tract are primarily from central or peripheral nervous system effects.

Clinical disorders of emission and ejaculation can be broadly categorized into four groups: (i) anatomic (e.g., secondary to transurethral resection of the prostate or Y-V plasty of the bladder neck), (ii) neuropathic (e.g., secondary to diabetes or RLND), (iii) psychogenic ("ejaculatory incompetence"), or (iv) idiopathic (130). Exogenous drugs possessing alpha-adrenergic blocking properties, e.g., phenoxybenzamine, can also result in failure of seminal fluid emission and/or retrograde ejaculation. Surgical and medical management of patients with "ejaculatory dysfunction" is improving, but major breakthroughs will be contingent upon a better understanding of the physiologic, particularly central nervous system, mechanisms involved.

REFERENCES

1. Benson, G. S., Lipshultz, L. I., and McConnell, J. A. (1981): Mechanisms of human erection, emission, and ejaculation: Current clinical concepts. In: *Sexual Rehabilitation of the Urologic Cancer Patient,* edited by A. C. von Eschenbach and D. B. Rodriguez, pp. 54–68. G. K. Hall, Boston.
2. Benson, G. S. (1981): Mechanisms of penile erection. *Invest. Urol.,* 19:65–69.
3. Klinge, E., and Sjostrand, N. O. (1974): Contraction and relaxation of the retractor penis muscle and the penile artery of the bull. *Acta Physiol. Scand. (Suppl),* 420:1–88.
4. Klinge, E., and Sjostrand, N. O. (1977): Comparative study of some isolated mammalian smooth muscle effectors of penile erection. *Acta Physiol. Scand.,* 100:354–367.
5. Benson, G. S., McConnell, J. A., Lipshultz, L. I., Corriere, J. N. Jr., and Wood, J. (1980): Neuromorphology and neuropharmacology of the human penis. *J. Clin. Invest,* 65:506–513.
6. Newman, H. F., and Northup, J. D. (1981): Mechanism of human penile erection: An overview. *Urology,* 17:399–408.
7. Reiss, H. F., Northup, H. F., and Zorngiotti, A. (1982): Artificial erection by perfusion of penile arteries. *Urology,* 20:284–288.
8. Deysach, L. J. (1939): The comparative morphology of the erectile tissue of the penis with especial emphasis on the probable mechanism of erection. *Am. J. Anat.,* 64:111–131.
9. Lue, T. F., Takamura, T., Umraiya, M., Schmidt, R. A., and Tanagho, E. A. (1984): Hemodynamics of canine corpora cavernosa during erection. *Urology,* 24:347–352.
10. Wagner, G., Bro-Rasmussen, F., Willis, E. A., Neilsen, M. H. (1982): New theory on the mechanism of erection involving hitherto undescribed vessels. *Lancet,* 1:416–418.
11. Van Arsdalen, K. N., Malloy, T. R., and Wein, A. J. (1983): Erectile physiology, dysfunction and evaluation. Part 1: Physiology of erection. In: *1983 Monographs in Urology,* edited by T. A. Stamey, p. 137. Custom Publishing Services, Princeton.
12. Wespes, E., and Shulman, C. C. (1985): Venous leakage: Surgical treatment of a curable cause of impotence. *J. Urol.,* 133:796–798.
13. Walsh, P. C., and Donker, P. J. (1982): Impotence following radical prostatectomy: Insight into etiology and prevention. *J. Urol.,* 128:492–497.
14. Learmonth, J. R. (1931): A contribution to the neurophysiology of the urinary bladder in man. *Brain,* 54:147–176.
15. Shirai, M., Sasaki, K., and Rikimaru, A. (1972): Histochemical investigation on the distribution of adrenergic and cholinergic nerves in the human penis. *Tohoku J. Med.,* 107:403–404.
16. Benson, G. S. (1983): Penile erection: In search of a neurotransmitter. *World J. Urol.,* 1:209–212.
17. McConnell, J. A., and Benson, G. S. (1982): Innervation of human penile blood vessels. *Neurourol. Urodynam.,* 1:199–210.
18. Chubb, I. W., Hodgson, A. J., and White, G. H. (1980): Acetylcholinesterase hydrolyzes substance P. *Neuroscience,* 5:2065–2072.
19. Polak, J. M., Gu, J., Mina, S., and Bloom, S. R. (1981): Vipergic nerves in the penis. *Lancet,* 2:217–219.
20. Gu, J., Polak, J. M., Probert, L., Islam, K. N., Marangos, P. J., Mina, S., Adrian, T. E., McGregor, G. P., O'Shaughnessy, D. J., and Bloom, S. R. (1983): Peptidergic innervation of the human male genital tract. *J. Urol.,* 130:386–391.
21. Steers, W. D., McConnell, J. A., and Benson, G. S. (1984): Anatomical localization and some pharmacologic effects of vasoactive intestinal polypeptide in human and monkey corpus cavernosum. *J. Urol.,* 132:1048–1053.
22. Semans, J. H., and Langworthy, O. R. (1939): Observations on the neurourophysiology of sexual function in the male cat. *J. Urol.,* 40:836–846.
23. Leriche, R., and Morel, A. (1948): Syndrome of thrombotic obliteration of the aortic bifurcation. *Ann. Surg.,* 127:193–206.
24. Dorr, L. D., and Brody, M. J. (1967): Hemodynamic mechanism of erection in the canine penis. *Am. J. Physiol.,* 213:1526–1531.

25. Purohit, R. C., and Beckett, S. D. (1976): Penile pressures and muscle activity associated with erection and ejaculation in the dog. *Am. J. Physiol.*, 231:1343–1348.
26. Beckett, S. D., Hudson, R. S., Walker, D. F., Vachon, R. I., and Reynolds, T. M. (1972): Corpus cavernosum penis pressure and external penile muscle activity during erection in the goat. *Biol. Reprod.*, 7:359–364.
27. Kollberg, S., Peterson, I., and Stener, I. (1962): Preliminary results of an electromyographic study of ejaculation. *Acta Chir. Scand.*, 123:478–483.
28. Shirai, M., and Ishii, N. (1981): Hemodynamics of erection in man. *Arch. Androl.*, 6:27–32.
29. Wagner, G. (1981): Erection, physiology and endocrinology. In: *Impotence*, edited by G. Wagner and R. Green. pp. 29–30. Plenum Press, New York.
30. Lue, T. F., Hricak, H., Schmidt, R. A., and Tanago, E. A. (1986): Functional evaluation of penile veins by cavernosography in papaverine-induced erection. *J. Urol.*, 135:479–482.
31. Conti, G. (1952): L'erection du penis humain et ses bases morphologico-vascularies. *Acta Anat. (Basel)*, 14:217–262.
32. Benson, G. S., McConnell, J. A., and Schmidt, W. A. (1981): Penile "polsters": Functional structures or atherosclerotic changes? *J. Urol.*, 125:800–803.
33. McConnell, J. A., Benson, G. S., and Schmidt, W. A. (1982): The vasculature of the human penis: A reexamination of the morphological basis for the polster theory of erection. *Anat. Rec.*, 203:475–484.
34. Eckhard, C. (1863): Untersuchungen uber die erection des penis beim hunde. In: *Beitrage zur Anatomie und Physiologie*, edited by C. Eckhard, III Band. Giessen.
35. Muller, L. R. (1902): Klinische und experimentelle studien uber die innervation der blase, des mastdarms, und des genitalapparates. *Deutsch. Z. Nervenheilk*, 21:86–154.
36. Root, W. S., and Bard, P. (1947): The mediation of feline erection through sympathetic pathways with some remarks on sexual behavior after deafferentiation of the genitalia. *Am. J. Physiol.*, 151:80–90.
37. Bacq, Z. M. (1934): Recherches sur la physiologie et la pharmacologie du systeme nerveux anatonome: XII Nature cholinergique et adrenergique des diverses innervations vasomotrices du penis chez le chren. *Arch. Int. Physiol.*, 40:311–321.
38. Bors, E., and Comarr, A. E. (1960): Neurologic disturbances of sexual function with special reference to 529 patients with spinal cord injury. *Urol. Survey*, 10:191–222.
39. Kedia, K. R., Markland, C., and Fraley, E. E. (1975): Sexual function following high retroperitoneal lymphadenectomy. *J. Urol.*, 114:237–239.
40. Kom, C., Mulholland, S. G., and Edson, M. (1971): Etiology of fertility after retroperitoneal lymphadenectomy. *J. Urol.*, 105:528–530.
41. Kluver, H., and Bucy, P. C. (1939): Preliminary analysis of functions of the temporal lobes in monkeys. *Arch. Neurol. Psychiatry*, 42:979–1000.
42. Dua, S., and MacLean, P. D. (1964): Localization for penile erection in medial frontal lobe. *Am. J. Physiol.*, 207:1425–1434.
43. MacLean, P. D. (1955): The limbic system ("visceral brain") in relation to central gray and reticulum of the brain stem. Evidence of interdependence in emotional processes. *Psychosom. Med.*, 17:355–366.
44. MacLean, P. D., and Ploog, D. W. (1962): Cerebral representation of penile erection. *J. Neurophysiol.*, 25:29–55.
45. Hierons, R., and Saunders, M. (1966): Impotence in patients with temporal-lobe lesions. *Lancet*, 2:761–763.
46. Meyers, R. (1962): Three cases of myoclonus alleviated by bilateral ansotomy, with a note on postoperative alibido and impotence. *J. Neurosurg.*, 19:71–81.
47. Morales, A., Surridge, D. H. C., Marshall, P. G., and Fenemore, J. (1982): Nonhormonal pharmacological treatment of organic impotence. *J. Urol.*, 128:45–47.
48. Henderson, V. E., and Roepke, M. H. (1933): On the mechanism of erection. *Am. J. Physiol.*, 106:441–448.
49. Wagner, G., and Brindley, G. S. (1980): The effect of atropine, alpha and beta blockers on human penile erection: A controlled pilot study. In: *Vasculogenic Impotence. International Symposium on Corporal Revascularization*, edited by A. Zorgniotti and J. Rossi, pp. 77–81. Charles C Thomas, Springfield, Ill.
50. Domer, F. R., Wessler, G., Brown, R. L., and Charles, H. C. (1978): Involvement of the sympathetic nervous system in the urinary bladder internal sphincter and in penile erection in the anesthetized cat. *Invest. Urol.*, 15:404–407.
51. Alm, P., and Elmer, M. (1975): Adrenergic and cholinergic innervation of the rat urinary bladder. *Acta Physiol. Scand.*, 94:36–45.
52. Sundin, T., and Dahlstrom, A. (1973): The sympathetic innervation of the urinary bladder and urethra in the normal state and after parasympathetic denervation at the spinal root level: An experimental study in cats. *Scan. J. Urol. Nephrol.*, 7:131–149.
53. Melman, A., and Henry, D. (1979): The possible role of the catecholamines of the corpora in penile erection. *J. Urol.*, 121:419–421.
54. Levin, R. M., and Wein, A. J. (1980): Adrenergic alpha receptors outnumber beta receptors in human penile corpus cavernosum. *Invest. Urol.*, 18:225–226.
55. Adaikan, P. G., and Karim, S. M. M. (1981): Adrenoreceptors in the human penis. *J. Auton. Pharmacol.*, 1:199–203.
56. Elliott, T. R. (1905): The action of adrenalin. *J. Physiol. (Lond.)*, 32:401–467.
57. Said, S. I., and Rosenberg, R. N. (1976): Vasoactive intestinal polypeptide: Abundant immunoreactivity in neural cell lines and normal nervous tissue. *Science*, 192:907–908.
58. Uddman, R., Alumets, J., Efvinsson, L., Hakanson, R., and Sundler, F. (1981): VIP nerve fibers around peripheral vessels. *Acta Physiol. Scand.*, 112:65–70.
59. Willis, E., Ottesen, B., Wagner, G., Sundler, R., and Fahrenkrug, J. (1981): Vasoactive intestinal polypeptide (VIP) as a possible neurotransmitter involved in penile erection. *Acta Physiol. Scand.*, 113:545–547.
60. Larsson, L. I., Fahrenkrug, J., and Schaffalitzky de Muckadell, O. B. (1977): Occurrence of nerves containing vasoactive intestinal polypeptide immunoactivity in the male genital tract. *Life Sci.*, 21:503–508.
61. Sjostrand, N. O., Klinge, E., and Himberg, J. J. (1981): Effects of VIP and other putative neurotransmitters on smooth muscle effectors of penile erection. *Acta Physiol. Scand.*, 113:403–405.
62. Lundberg, J. M., Anggard, A., Fahrenkrug, J., Hokfelt, T., and Mutt, V. (1980): Vasoactive intestinal polypeptide in cholinergic neurons of exocrine glands: Functional significance of coexisting transmitters for vasodilation and secretion. *Proc. Natl. Acad. Sci. USA*, 77:1651–1655.
63. Virag, R., Frydman, D., Legman, M., and Virag, H. (1984): Intravenous injection of papaverine as a diagnostic and therapeutic method in erectile failure. *Angiology*, 35:79–87.
64. Brindley, G. S. (1983): Cavernosal alpha blockade: A new technique for investigating and treating penile impotence. *Br. J. Psychiatry*, 143:332–337.
65. Brindley, G. S. (1986): Pilot experiments on the actions of drugs injected into the human corpus cavernosum penis. *Br. J. Pharmacol.* 87:495–501.
66. Gessa, G. L., and Tagliamonte, A. (1974): Role of brain monoamines in male sexual behavior. *Life Sci.*, 14:425–436.
67. Barbeau, A. (1969): L-DOPA therapy in Parkinson's disease: A critical review of nine years' experience. *Can. Med. Assoc. J.*, 101:791–799.
68. Jenkins, R. B., and Groh, R. H. (1970): Mental symptoms in Parkinsonian patients treated with L-DOPA. *Lancet*, 2:177–179.
69. Medical Letter (1984): Priapism with trazodone. *Medical Letter*, 26:35.
70. Caccia, S., Ballabio, M., Samanin, R., Zanini, M. G., and Garattini, S. (1981): (−)-*m*-Chlorophenyl-piperazine, a central 5-hydroxytryptamine agonist, is a metabolite of trazodone. *J. Pharm. Pharmacol.*, 33:477–478.
71. Aloi, J. A., Insel, T. R., Mueller, E. A., and Murphy, D. L. (1984): Neuroendocrine and behavioral effects of *m*-chlorophenylpiperazine administration in rhesus monkeys. *Life Sci.*, 34:1325–1331.
72. Scott, F. B., Bradley, W. E., and Timm, G. W. (1973): Management of erectile impotence: Use of implantable inflatable prosthesis. *Urology*, 2:80–82.
73. Small, M. P., Carrion, H. M., and Gordon, J. A. (1975): Small-Carrion penile prosthesis: New implant for management of impotence. *Urology*, 5:479–486.

74. Malloy, T. R., Wein, A. J., and Carpiniello, V. L. (1983): Revised surgical technique to improve survival of penile cylinders for the inflatable penile prosthesis. *J. Urol.*, 130:1105–1106.
75. Fallon, B., Rosenberg, S., and Culp, D. A. (1984): Long-term follow-up in patients with an inflatable penile prosthesis. *J. Urol.*, 132:270–271.
76. Gewertz, B. L., and Sarins, C. K. (1985): Vasculogenic impotence. In: *Diagnosis and Treatment of Erectile Disturbances: A Guide for Clinicians*, edited by R. T. Seagraves and H. W. Schoenberg, pp. 105–113. Plenum Press, New York.
77. Lue, T. F., Hricak, H., Marick, K. W., and Tanagho, E. A. (1985): Vasculogenic impotence evaluated by high-resolution ultrasonography and pulsed Doppler spectrum analysis. *Radiology*, 155:777–781.
78. Michal, V., Kramar, R., and Pospichal, J. (1978): External iliac "steal syndrome." *J. Cardiovas. Surg.*, 19:355–357.
79. Goldstein, I., Siroky, M. B., Nath, R. L., McMillian, T. N., Menzoian, J. O., and Krane, R. J. (1982): Vasculogenic impotence; role of the pelvic steal test. *J. Urol.*, 128:300–306.
80. Gittes, R. F., and Waters, W. B. (1979): Sexual impotence: The overlooked complication of a second renal transplant. *J. Urol.*, 121:719–720.
81. Krane, R. J., and Siroky, M. B. (1980): Studies on sacral evoked potentials. *J. Urol.*, 124:872–876.
82. Gerstenberg, T. C., and Bradley, W. E. (1983): Nerve conduction velocity measurement of dorsal nerve of penis in normal and impotent males. *Urology*, 21:90–92.
83. Haldeman, S., Bradley, W. E., and Bhatia, N. N. (1982): Pudendal evoked responses. *Arch. Neurol.*, 39:280–283.
84. Walsh, P. C., and Mostwin, J. L. (1984): Radical prostatectomy and cystoprostatectomy with preservation of potency. Results utilizing a new nerve sparing technique. *Br. J. Urol.*, 56:694–697.
85. Sidi, A. A., Cameron, J. S., Duffy, L. M., and Lange, P. H. (1986): Intracavernous drug-induced erections in management of male erectile dysfunction: Experience with 100 patients. *J. Urol.*, 135:704–706.
86. Zorgniotti, A. W., and Lefleur, R. S. (1985): Autoinjection of the corpus cavernosum with a vasoactive drug combination for vasculogenic impotence. *J. Urol.*, 133:39–41.
87. Lue, T. F., Hellstrom, W. J. G., McAninch, J. W., and Tanagho, E. A. (1986): Priapism: a refined approach to diagnosis and treatment. *J. Urol.*, 136:104–108.
88. Grayhack, J. T., McCullough, W., O'Connor, V. J. Jr., and Trippel, O. (1964): Venous bypass to control priapism. *Invest. Urol.*, 1:509–513.
89. Winter, C. C. (1976): Cure of idiopathic priapism: New procedure for creating fistula between glans penis and corpora cavernosa. *Urology*, 8:389–391.
90. Benkert, O., Witt, W., Adam, W., and Leitz, A. (1979): Effects of testosterone undecanoate on sexual potency and the hypothalamic-pituitary-gonadal-axis of impotent males. *Arch. Sex. Behav.*, 8:471–479.
91. Horowitz, J. D., and Gobel, A. J. (1979): Drugs and impaired male sexual function. *Drugs*, 18:206–217.
92. Jensen, R. T., Collen, M. J., Pandol, S. J., Allende, H. J., Raufman, J. P., Bissoneette, B. M., Duncan, W. C., Durgin, P. L., Gillin, J. C., and Gardner, J. D. (1983): Cimetidine-induced impotence and breast changes in patients with gastric hypersecretory states. *N. Engl. J. Med.*, 308:883–887.
93. Hall, W. H. (1976): Breast changes in males on cimetidine. *N. Engl. J. Med.*, 295:841.
94. Carlson, H. E., and Ippoliti, A. F. (1977): Cimetidine, an H_2-antihistamine, stimulates prolactin secretion in man. *J. Clin. Endocrinol. Metab.*, 45:367–370.
95. Adaikan, P. G., and Karim, S. M. M. (1979): Male sexual dysfunction during treatment with cimetidine (Letter to Editor). *Br. Med. J.*, 1:1282.
96. Hackett, R. E., and Waterhouse, K. (1973): Vasectomy—Reviewed. *Am. J. Obstet. Gynecol.*, 116:438–455.
97. Koraitim, M., Schafer, W., Melchior, H., and Lutzeyer, W. (1977): Dynamic activity of bladder neck and external sphincter in ejaculation. *Urology*, 10:130–132.
98. Woodburne, R. G. (1968): Anatomy of the bladder and bladder outlet. *J. Urol.*, 100:474–487.
99. Tanagho, E. A., and Smith, D. R. (1966): The anatomy and function of the bladder neck. *Br. J. Urol.*, 38:54–71.
100. Raezer, D. M., Wein, A. J., Jacobowitz, D., and Corriere, J. N. Jr. (1973): Autonomic innervation of canine urinary bladder: Cholinergic and adrenergic contributions and interaction of sympathetic and parasympathetic nervous systems in bladder function. *Urology*, 2:211–221.
101. Turner-Warwick, R., Whiteside, C. G., Arnold, E. P., Bates, C. P., Worth, P. H. L., Milroy, E. G. J., Webster, J. R., and Weir, J. (1973): A urodynamic view of prostatic obstruction and the results of prostatectomy. *Br. J. Urol.*, 45:631–645.
102. Peterson, I., and Stener, I. (1970): An electromyographic study of the striated urethral sphincter, the striated anal sphincter, and the levator ani muscle during ejaculation. *Electromyography*, 1:23–44.
103. Pick, J., and Sheehan, D. (1946): Sympathetic rami in man. *J. Anat.*, 80:12–20.
104. Wesson, M. B. (1920): Anatomical, embryological, and physiological studies of the trigone and neck of the bladder. *J. Urol.*, 4:279–307.
105. Gosling, J. A., Dixon, J. S., Critchley, H. O. D., and Thompson, S. A. (1981): A comparative study of the human external sphincter and periurethral levator ani muscles. *Br. J. Urol.*, 53:35–41.
106. Donker, D. J., Droes, J. Th. P. M., and Van Ulden, B. M.: Anatomy of the musculature and innervation of the bladder and urethra. In: *Scientific Foundations of Urology, Vol. 2*, edited by D. E. Williams and G. D. Chisholm, p. 32. Year Book Medical Publishers, Chicago.
107. Elbadawi, A., and Schenk, E. A. (1974): A new theory of the innervation of the bladder musculature. Part 4. Innervation of vesicourethral junction and external urethral sphincter. *J. Urol.*, 111:613–615.
108. Wein, A. J., Benson, G. S., and Jacobowitz, D. (1979): Lack of evidence for adrenergic innervation of the external urethral sphincter. *J. Urol.*, 121:324–326.
109. Lincoln, J., Crowe, R., Bokor, J., Light, J. K., Chilton, C. P., and Burnstock, G. (1986): Adrenergic and cholinergic innervation of the smooth and striated muscle components of the urethra from patients with spinal cord injury. *J. Urol.*, 135:402–408.
110. McConnell, J. A., Benson, G. S., and Wood, J. G. (1982): Autonomic innervation of the urogenital system: Adrenergic and cholinergic elements. *Brain Res. Bull.*, 9:679–694.
111. Baumgarten, H. G., Falck, B., Holstein, A. F., Owman, C., and Owman, T. (1968): Adrenergic innervation of the human testis, epididymis, ductus deferens, and prostate: A fluorescence microscopic and fluorimetric study. *Z. Zellforsch.*, 90:81–85.
112. Baumgarten, H. G., Holstein, A. F., and Rosengren, E. (1971): Arrangement, ultrastructure, and adrenergic innervation of smooth musculature of the ductuli efferentes, ductus epididymis, and ductus deferens of man. *Z. Zellforsch.*, 120:37–79.
113. McConnell, J. A., Benson, G. S., and Wood, J. (1978): Distribution of autonomic fibers to pelvic/perineal viscera of the human male. *Anat. Rec.*, 190:475.
114. Ek, A., Alm, P., Andersson, D. E., and Persson, C. G. A. (1977): Adrenergic and cholinergic nerves of the human urethra and urinary bladder. A histochemical study. *Acta Physiol. Scand.*, 99: 345–352.
115. Gosling, J. A., Dixon, J. S., and Lendon, R. G. (1977): The autonomic innervation of the human male and female bladder neck and proximal urethra. *J. Urol.*, 118:302–305.
116. Ambache, N., and Aboo Zar, M. (1971): Evidence against adrenergic motor transmission in the guinea-pig vas deferens. *J. Physiol.*, 216:359–389.
117. Jenkins, D. A., Marshall, I., and Nasmyth, P. A. (1976): Is noradrenaline the motor transmitter in the mouse vas deferens? *J. Physiol.*, 254:49P–50P.
118. McGrath, J. C. (1978): Adrenergic and "non-adrenergic" components in the contractile response of the vas deferens to a single indirect stimulus. *J. Physiol.*, 283:23–39.
119. Anton, P. G., and McGrath, J. C. (1977): Further evidence for adrenergic transmission in the human vas deferens. *J. Physiol.*, 273:45–55.
120. Birmingham, A. T. (1968): The human isolated vas deferens: Its response to electrical stimulation and to drugs. *Br. J. Pharmacol.*, 34:692P–693P.
121. Hedlund, H., Andersson, K. E., and Larson, B. (1985): Effect of drugs interacting with adrenoceptors and muscarinic receptors in the

epididymal and prostatic parts of the isolated human vas deferens. *J. Auton. Pharmacol.,* 5:261–270.
122. McLeod, D. G., Reynolds, D. G., and Demaree, G. E. (1973): Some pharmacologic characteristics of the human vas deferens. *Invest. Urol.,* 10:338–341.
123. Benson, G. S., Wein, A. J., Raezer, D. M., and Corriere, J. N. Jr. (1976): Adrenergic and cholinergic stimulation and blockade of the human bladder base. *J. Urol.,* 116:174–175.
124. Levin, R. M., and Wein, A. J. (1979): Distribution and function of adrenergic receptors in the urinary bladder of the rabbit. *Mol. Pharmacol.,* 16:441–448.
125. Mitsuya, H., Asai, J., Suyama, K., Ushida, T., and Hosoe, K. (1960): Application of x-ray cinematography in urology. I. Mechanism of ejaculation. *J. Urol.,* 83:86–92.
126. Herberg, L. J. (1963): A hypothalamic mechanism causing seminal ejaculation. *Nature,* 198:219–220.
127. Robinson, B. W., and Mishkin, M. (1966): Ejaculation evoked by stimulation of the preoptic area in monkey. *Physiol. Behav.,* 1:269–272.
128. Guttmann, L., and Walsh, J. J. (1971): Prostigmin assessment test of fertility in spinal man. *Paraplegia,* 9:39–51.
129. Innes, I. R., and Nickerson, M. (1975): Norephinephrine, epinephrine and the sympathomimetic amines. In: *The Pharmacological Basis of Therapeutics,* edited by L. S. Goodman and A. Gilman, p. 477. Macmillan, New York.
130. Lipshultz, L. I., McConnell, J. A., and Benson, G. S. (1981): Current concepts of the mechanisms of ejaculation. *J. Reprod. Med.,* 26(10):499–507.
131. Kelly, M. E., and Needle, M. A. (1979): Imipramine for aspermia after lymphadenectomy. *Urology,* 13:414–415.
132. Benson, G. S., Sarshik, S. A., Raezer, D. M., and Wein, A. J. (1977): Bladder muscle contractility: Comparative effects and mechanisms of action of atropine, propantheline, flavoxate, and imipramine. *Urology,* 9:31–35.
133. Gregory, J. G., Wein, A. J., and Schoenberg, H. W. (1974): A comparison of the action of tofranil and probanthine on the urinary bladder. *Invest. Urol.,* 12:233–235.

The Pituitary and the Hypothalamus

The Physiology of Reproduction,
edited by E. Knobil and J. Neill *et al.*
Raven Press, Ltd., New York © 1988.

CHAPTER 26

Pituitary and Hypothalamus: Perspectives and Overview

John W. Everett

Nearly all that we know about the hypothalamic-pituitary system has been gathered during the 20th century, building on fragmentary notions from earlier times. Galen regarded the pituitary as a sump for waste products (phlegm = *pituita*) derived in the brain from distillation of "animal spirit." Supposedly the phlegm then would filter through openings in the ethmoid bone into the nasal passages. That notion held without question until 1655 when Conrad Victor Schneider of Wittenburg concluded, on anatomical grounds, that the openings in the cribriform plate of the ethmoid bone are for the olfactory nerves and that fluids cannot pass from the cranial cavity into the nose (1). Richard Lower of Oxford confirmed this in 1670 with a case of hydrocephalus and with a series of experiments in cadavers. Although intraventricular fluid was greatly increased after injection of water into the jugular veins, no fluid appeared in the nasal cavities. Lower envisioned substances to be conducted from the ventricles through the infundibulum to the pituitary, there to be "distilled" into the blood stream (1).

Recognition of the dual embryonic origin of the pituitary from the diencephalon and the buccal epithelium awaited disclosure in 1838 by Martin Heinrich Rathke of Königsberg, an embryologist noted for discovering the embryonic gill slits and gill arches (2). Rathke described a dorsal outpocketing from the roof of the stomodeum extending to meet a ventral process from the diencephalic floor. Knowledge of the histological structure of the respective components was many years in the future, however. Only the same year of Rathke's report, the cell theory was proposed for plants by Schleiden and extended the following year by Schwann to include animals. Methods for fixing tissues were in use, but histology did not come into its own until the latter part of the 19th century. Staining with hematoxylin (Waldeyer) and with aniline dyes (Beneke) was described in 1863, and the microtome was introduced by His in 1870. Although the distinction between glands with and without ducts was apparent by older methods, the identification of ductless glands structurally specialized for internal secretion required the microscopic observations made possible by these procedures and improved lens systems.

Claude Bernard first conceptualized "internal secretion," noting that all tissues and organs influence the body as a whole by discharging substances into the blood (3). The idea was extended by Brown-Séquard and d'Arsonval (3) with the view that internal secretions serve to coordinate body functions. The concept of control of specific target tissues by circulating messengers ("hormones") was stated by Bayliss and Starling in their Croonian Lecture (4) relating their discovery of secretin.

Although histology of the pituitary complex (Table 1) clearly showed the glandular features of the pars distalis, the neural lobe did not appear to be a secretory organ. Silver-staining methods devised by Golgi and modified by Ramón y Cajal disclosed a rich content of nerve fibers in the neural

TABLE 1. *Terminology of the subdivisions of the hypophysis*

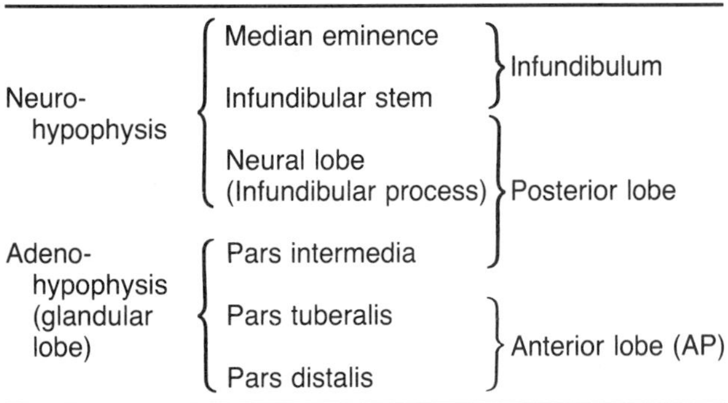

Neuro-hypophysis	Median eminence	Infundibulum
	Infundibular stem	
	Neural lobe (Infundibular process)	Posterior lobe
Adeno-hypophysis (glandular lobe)	Pars intermedia	
	Pars tuberalis	Anterior lobe (AP)
	Pars distalis	

lobe which Cajal (5) judged to be sensory fibers with terminals in the surrounding epithelium of the pars intermedia. Camus and Roussy (6), on the other hand, considered the neural lobe to be merely a "fragment nerveux atrophié." Bailey and Bremer (7), as late as 1921, agreed with that, after observing that experimental removal of the neural lobe had no evident effect. They interpreted pituitrin as nothing more than a "pharmacologically interesting extract." They also noted with respect to the pars distalis that in spite of its obviously glandular structure there was "little actual knowledge of its functional significance." Nonetheless, Evans and Long (8) had already produced gigantism in rats by long-term daily treatment with extracts of beef anterior pituitary (AP).

In retrospect, the functional relationship between the pars distalis and body growth is apparent in clinical reports beginning in 1864. The syndrome of acromegaly described by Pierre Marie (9) was shown by Minkowski (9) to be accompanied consistently by the presence of a pituitary tumor. Unfortunately, he wrongly assumed that a tumor must represent loss of function and, hence, that the syndrome must be due to impaired pituitary activity. That notion persisted into the 20th century and led to various attempts at experimental hypophysectomy. Most notable of these attempts were reported by Paulesco (9), Cushing and associates (10–12), and Aschner (13,14). Because Paulesco had been unable to obtain survival of hypophysectomized dogs for more than a few days, the concept at first arose that the pituitary is essential for life. There were also arguments about complications from possible damage to the hypothalamus. However, Aschner by operating on puppies obtained survival for several months in the total absence of the hypophysis and without damage to the brain. The puppies failed to grow. It was by no means clear, however, that this failure represented specific loss of a particular hormone, for there were metabolic defects in the cachectic animals, and the thyroids and adrenal cortex were obviously impaired. Impairment of the reproductive organs could similarly have been due to the general debility. Questions of specificity also applied to the early AP extracts alleged to contain growth hormone. The sorting out of the specific trophic hormones present in the gland and their eventual purification were to occupy investigators for many years to come.

Several other lines of evidence stand in the background of present awareness of the central position of the hypothalamic-pituitary apparatus in regulating gonadal functions. Seasonal influences of the environment on animal reproduction in temperate zones were well known from time immemorial (15,16). Especially noteworthy is the fact that in some species ovulation and corpus luteum formation require the stimulus of copulation. This was demonstrated in domestic rabbits by both Haighton (17) and Cruikshank (18) in presentations to the Royal Society of London in 1797, confirmed later by Barry (19), Heape (20) and many others. By mating rabbits after cutting the fallopian tubes, Haighton showed that the effect could not be due to contact of the semen with the ovary. Provoked ovulation was later described in ferrets (21) and domestic cats (22). Numerous other species have been added in recent years (1).

Retroactive influence of the gonads on the AP was recognized by Fichera (23), who reported that in several species gonadectomy was followed by AP enlargement and, in the rat, by the occurrence of many enlarged, vacuolated cells having a signet-ring appearance. Such "castration cells" were identified by Addison (24) as belonging to the basophil cell class. Other phenomena now recognized as reflecting the influence of the gonads on the AP were the suppression of estrous and menstrual cycles during pregnancy and the prompt return of cycles after removal of corpora lutea (25). The tendency for lactation to suppress cycles, likewise a hypothalamic-pituitary effect, was well known from early times.

The period from 1916 to 1926 was marked by a series of discoveries fundamental for modern endocrinology and reproductive biology. Development of the vaginal smear method by Stockard and Papanicolaou (26) to reveal the estrous cycle of the guinea pig was a breakthrough that led eventually to the isolation and synthesis of the estrogens. The method was soon applied to the rat by Long and Evans (27), and to the mouse by Edgar Allen (28). Allen and Doisy (28a) and Allen et al. (29) soon reported that oily extracts of porcine follicular fluid when injected into spayed mice brought about full cornification of the vagina; the Allen-Doisy test became a basic procedure for the biochemical studies that followed.

Procedures for hypophysectomy received continuing attention. Both Allen (30,31) and Smith (32) investigated effects of hypophysectomy (removal of Rathke's pouch) in amphibian larvae, noting atrophy of the adrenals and thyroids and failure to metamorphose. Smith and Smith (33,34) counteracted these losses by intraperitoneal administration of bovine AP material. Smith (35–37) subsequently devised the parapharyngeal technique for pituitary ablation in rats, a breakthrough that enabled isolation, purification, and chemical characterization of the various AP hormones. Smith and Engle (38) promptly demonstrated maintenance and repair of gonads by repeated intramuscular implants of fresh AP tissue in hypophysectomized rats.

No less important was the classic monograph by Long and Evans (27) detailing many aspects of reproduction in the rat. The usual length of the estrous cycles was shown to be either 4 or 5 days, not 10 days or longer as most earlier reports had indicated. Stages of the vaginal cycle were defined and correlated with events in the ovary, reproductive tract, and mammary glands. Pseudopregnancy was described and named as the result of infertile copulation or mechanical stimulation of the cervix. The production of deciduomata by uterine trauma was described, and the importance of the critical timing of traumatization was noted. Since pseudopregnancy occurred readily in animals whose ovaries had been transplanted, it did not involve the ovarian innervation. In the correlated investigation by Evans and Long (8) of the effects of prolonged daily intraperitoneal administration of bovine AP substance, in addition to gigantism the females showed marked enlargement of the ovaries with masses of corpora lutea, together with suppression of estrous cycles. Here was the first demonstration of the presence of both growth-promoting and gonad-stimulating substances in the anterior lobe.

Evans et al. (39,40) succeeded in separating fractions of AP extracts having these respective activities. Separation of thyroid-stimulating and gonadotropic fractions was achieved by Greep (41). Eventually, by the late 1930s the existence of six AP hormones had been established: hormones controlling body growth, the gonads, mammary glands, thyroids, and adrenal cortex. The advances toward their eventual isolation and determination of their chemical structures required progressive sophistication of *in vitro* techniques. This was accompanied by progressive refinement of definitions of the biological actions of the respective hormones.

In the case of the gonadotropins, progress was delayed from time to time by certain faulty assumptions, sometimes engendered by impurities in the substances administered. The existence of two gonadotropic principles was first proposed by Zondek (42,43), who had obtained a follicle-stimulating material (Prolan A) from the urine of ovariectomized or postmenopausal women and a luteinizing material (Prolan B) from human pregnancy urine. He assumed both to be secreted by the AP. Although Prolan B was later shown to originate from the placenta (44–47), the idea of a separate luteinizer led to intensive search for distinct pituitary principles having potencies resembling the two Prolans. The dual hormone concept was championed by Fevold, Hisaw, and associates in Wisconsin. Fevold et al. (48) were first to succeed in separating the respective fractions from pyridine extracts. Details of the efforts leading to eventual isolation and determination of the chemical structure of follicle-stimulating hormone (FSH) and luteinizing hormone (LH) have been admirably reviewed by Greep (49). A major misapprehension not emphasized was the early failure to distinguish formation, *per se,* of corpora lutea (luteinization) and maintenance of their function (luteotropic action). In rats and mice the principal luteotropin is prolactin, a fact unknown until demonstrated in 1941 by Astwood (50) and Evans et al. (51).

Prolactin research stems from an observation by Stricker and Grueter (52,53) after induction of ovulation in rabbits by administration of AP extract. In rabbits that received the material for several days after ovulation the mammary glands were distended with milk. The effect was confirmed by Corner (54) who also obtained it in ovariectomized estrous rabbits. Evans and Simpson (55) saw mammary glands distended with milk in rats that had received an AP extract for 20 to 30 days. A series of studies by Riddle and associates (56–59) between 1931 and 1935 disclosed that, in the pigeon and ring-dove, secretion of crop milk was governed by the AP and that the same hormone, which they named prolactin, caused milk secretion in mammals. It suppressed gonadal function by inhibiting FSH secretion. In both mice and rats, daily treatment interrupted estrous cycles for approximately 2 weeks (60,61). Although Lahr and Riddle (61) saw large corpora lutea, demonstration of the luteotropic action of prolactin was 5 years in the future, as noted above. The growth-promoting power of prolactin was shown in hypophysectomized pigeons, as for years Riddle, Bates, and others questioned "the concept of a growth hormone as an individual entity." The disagreement was finally resolved by Bates et al. (62) through use of highly purified AP hormones. Optimal metabolic effects were obtained in hypophysectomized pigeons by giving a combination of ovine prolactin, bovine growth hormone, thyroxine, and prednisone.

ANTERIOR PITUITARY CYTOLOGY

From the very beginning of microscopic observation of the pituitary, considerable variation was evident in size, shape, and granule content of pars distalis cells. Application of dyes disclosed coloration differences as well. Schönemann (63) is credited with having made the original distinction among basophils ("cyanophils"), acidophils ("eosinophils"), and "chromophobes" as seen in human pituitaries stained with alum hematoxylin and eosin. Holmes and Ball (64) present a useful summary of the complex story of efforts in this century to subdivide these classes and to relate the subclasses to particular hormones and functional states. Underlying these efforts was the developing knowledge of the number of AP hormones, coupled with the feeling that the number of cell types ought to correspond.

Early confusion arose from the finding that in most animals other than man the basophil cells cannot be stained by hematoxylin. Staining of ergastoplasm by basic dyes like toluidin blue added further confusion. The use of multiple acid dyes introduced by Mallory (65) produced an array of tinctorial cell types. Modifications of the Mallory procedure were especially useful in some species and appeared to distinguish cells with granules containing simple proteins from the cells having granules of glycoprotein. Application of the McManus (66) periodic acid (PAS) histochemical method provided a generally useful distinction between "serous" cells (67) and "mucoid" cells (68). The latter types are those producing FSH, LH, melanocyte-stimulating hormone (MSH) and thyroid-stimulating hormone (TSH), all of which are glycoproteins.

The eventual availability of highly purified AP hormones and antibodies and the advent of immunocytochemical methods (69) in both light microscopy and electron microscopy have led far in recent years toward the ideal of a functional classification. The older terminologies have given way largely to the naming of cells according to the hormone produced, whenever known. Some problems remain, as when a gonadotropic cell contains granules that react with both FSH and LH antibodies. Special difficulties attend the localization of ACTH, MSH, and the related peptides, several of which may be contained within a parent molecule in some cells (70).

Pituitary histology and cytology have moved hand-in-hand with progress in pituitary physiology and biochemistry. Regional variations of cell types in the bovine AP made it possible for Smith and Smith (33) to distinguish the selective growth-promoting power of the acidophilic lateral portions from the thyrotropic power of the anteromedial portion containing basophils and chromophobes. AP enlargement and castration-cell formation after gonadectomy provided means for testing the feedback actions of gonadal hormones. The lack of castration cells in rat AP transplants to sites away from the brain was an early sign of the importance of the brain for regulating of AP secretions (71).

EVIDENCE FOR NEURAL CONTROL OF PARS DISTALIS SECRETION

Frölich's (72) original description of the syndrome termed urogenital dystrophy was the start of prolonged controversy about the respective roles of damage to the hypothalamus or the pituitary gland in causing the disease. An intracranial cystic tumor thought to be a craniopharyngeoma was surgically drained, after which there was satisfactory recovery. Eventually, following experimental studies by Camus and Roussy (6), Bailey and Bremer (7), Smith (36), and Hetherington and Ranson (73–75), it became clear that both obesity and genital atrophy can result from injury to the hypothalamus without direct involvement of the AP. Among 60 clinical cases of hypothalamic pathology assembled by Bauer (76), 43 manifested either hypogonadism or sexual precocity, five showing obesity. Precocity was commonly associated with basal tuberal lesions, while hypogonadism accompanied lesions located more rostrally.

Smith's observations of the effects of hypothalamic damage were made as he developed his method for parapharyngeal hypophysectomy (36). One attempt to ablate the gland was to inject chromic acid into the pituitary capsule, with the result that some of the acid passed beyond and damaged the brain. He then found that selective damage to the hypothalamus itself produced genital atrophy and obesity. Soon afterward Grafe and Grünthal (77) reported similar results. During the following 25 years, paralleling the progressive purification of the several AP secretions and determination of their actions, there was growing interest in the possible control of these secretions by the nervous system. Although the Moore and Price hypothesis (78) of pituitary-gonad reciprocity did not seem to take the nervous system into account, the authors recognized the modifying influences of environmental factors.

There was also strong implication of neural participation in the special case of the coitally induced ovulation in rabbits. Fee and Parkes (79,80) demonstrated two important features of that process; since the hypophysis must remain in place for only an hour after copulation, the necessary release of hormone must be relatively acute, and since anesthesia of the vagina prevented the ovulation, the nervous system must be directly involved. Participation of the brain was more directly indicated by Marshall and Verney (81), who obtained ovulation in estrous rabbits by passing an electric current through the head. With greater precision, Harris (82) and Haterius and Derbyshire (83) produced the same effect by local stimulation of the hypothalamus. The importance of the pituitary stalk to complete the reflex connection to the pars distalis was shown by Westman and Jacobsohn (84). Ovulation failed when the stalk had been cut and a metal foil barrier had been placed between the hypothalamus and pituitary gland, supposedly interrupting neural connections. The result also seemed to eliminate participation of autonomic fibers directly innervating the pars distalis.

Several workers had described autonomic fibers within the pars distalis parenchyma. However, a careful study by Rasmussen (85) of the pituitaries of man, rat, guinea pig, rabbit, dog, cat, and monkey led him to conclude that the only nerve fibers present in the AP must be vasomotor. Many parts of the gland were free of nerves. This view has been widely corroborated.

Meanwhile, the concept of a "sexual center" in the hypothalamus arose from the studies in rats by Hohlweg and associates (71,86), confirmed and amplified by Westman and Jacobsohn (87–89). As noted above, Hohlweg and Junkmann (71) saw that gonadectomy failed to produce castration cells in hypophyses that had been transplanted to a site away from the brain. Searching for effects of estrogen on the AP, Hohlweg and Chamorro (86) discovered that a single injection of estradiol benzoate into prepuberal rats induced formation of a set of corpora lutea within 7 days, presumptive evidence of increased LH secretion and ovulation. Luteinization was prevented by hypophysectomy 2 days after injection, but not at 4 days. Westman and Jacobsohn (87–89), after confirming the Hohlweg effect, examined the results of stalk section and insertion of a barrier of metal foil. Stalk section less than 2 and one-half days after estrogen injection prevented luteinization, but not when performed later on. As in the rabbit reflex, the estrogen stimulus was thought to operate through an essential neural link from the hypothalamus. The pituitary portal vessels were not yet generally recognized.

Pituitary Portal Vessels

Prominent vessels on the pituitary stalk were first well described by Pietsch (90) and Popa and Fielding (91,92). The latter authors described them as *portal vessels connecting capillary beds in the median eminence and pars distalis*. Erroneously they concurred with Pietsch that blood moves "upward" from the gland toward the brain. That conclusion was based partly on the experimental observation in rabbits that when a clamp was placed on the stalk the vessels distended below the clamp. Unknown at the time was the fact that rabbits, unlike most mammals, have a direct arterial supply to the pars distals.

Evidence for "downward" flow in the portal vessels was first reported by Houssay et al. (93) from direct microscopic observation of the exposed vessels in South American toads. Furthermore, lesioning of the infundibulum caused infarction of the pars distalis. On histologic grounds, Wislocki and King (94) and Wislocki (95) reached the conclusion that the primary capillary bed occupies the median eminence and the infundibular stem, whence blood is transported by the portal vessels to the secondary capillaries in the pars distalis. They further recognized the median eminence as a part of the neurohypophyis, not of the hypothalamus. Direct observation of downward blood flow was later reported in several species [amphibia: Green (96); duck: Benoit and Assenmacher (97); rat: Green and Harris (98,99) and others; mouse: Worthington (100,101); dog and cat: Török (102,103); baboon and monkey: Daniel (104)]. Although the possibility of some recurrent flow was indicated recently (105–107), the present view is that the principal flow is downward, transmitting hypophysiotropic agents to the AP.

Considerable territorial specificity exists in the origins of the various portal vessels from the primary capillaries and distributions of the secondary capillaries within the pars distalis. After stalk sectioning in the rat, sheep, goat, monkey, and man the extent of the infarcted area in the AP depends on the number and location of portal vessels interrupted (108). Daniel (104) proposed that the territorial specificity may explain the regional variation of cell types. An experimental basis for such a view was shown by Pasteels (109). In the amphibian *Pleurodeles waltlii,* he removed the hypophysis and reimplanted it in the original location, but inverted and rotated 180°. The cytology of the gland became regionally reversed in accord with the relationship to the portal circulation. A contrary view has been expressed by Porter et al. (110) after they found in rats that when the portal vessels were exposed and a colored fluid was injected into a single vessel through a microcannula, the distribution of the dye in the AP was greatly varied, sometimes reaching the entire gland. One may suggest, however, that under physiological conditions of balanced pressure territorial specificity would be maintained.

Neurohumoral Regulation

The concept of neurohumoral control of the pars distalis can be traced back to a paper by Hinsey and Markee (111). Failing to prevent postcoital ovulation in rabbits by severing the cervical sympathetic trunks, they suggested that the reflex involves a humoral link, transmitting some substance from the "posterior lobe" to the pars distalis. After Wislocki and King (94) presented their strong evidence for downward movement of blood in the portal vessels, there was speculation that these channels might constitute the humoral pathway (see ref. 112 and accompanying discussions). Resistance to the idea continued for awhile, partly because in avian and cetacean forms a heavy connective tissue septum separates the neural lobe from the pars distalis. However, it has been fully demonstrated that in such cases a "portotuberal tract" transmits the portal vessels rostral to that septum (97,113). Green (114) concluded from his comparative study that the pituitary portal vessels or their equivalent are a constant feature of all vertebrates.

Green and Harris (98), reversing Harris' earlier view (82), presented several strong arguments in favor of the humoral transmission via the portal vessels. They proposed that the variable effects others had encountered from cutting the stalk may have resulted from ability of the vessels to regenerate. Harris (115) conclusively demonstrated in stalk-sectioned rats that recovery of reproductive function was directly proportional to the extent of portal vessel regeneration. Regeneration was also demonstrated in monkeys (116) and rabbits (117). Thus, to fully interrupt hypothalamic influence on the AP by stalk section, an impermiable barrier is mandatory.

These findings seemed to explain the restoration of function in the pars distalis grafts that Greep (118) placed in the original site after hypophysectomy. Yet there remained some uncertainty, since it would be difficult to distinguish remnants of the gland left *in situ*. To avoid this, Harris and Jacobsohn (119) modified the experiment with a dual operation, hypophysectomizing female rats by the parapharyngeal route and implanting pars distalis tissue by the transtemporal approach to a location beneath the median eminence. Donors of the grafts were either several of the subjects' own male or female young, adult females, or adult males. Control subjects received the grafts under the temporal lobe. Estrous cycles returned in all rats bearing infantile grafts under the median eminence, often within a week. Several became pregnant and delivered normal young. Adrenals and thyroids were histologically normal. Significantly, similar results appeared in the few subjects bearing adult male grafts, one having a successful pregnancy. No traces of AP tissue were microscopically detectable in the original sites. These highly significant findings were confirmed and supplemented by Nikitovitch-Winer and Everett (120,121) in a two-stage experiment. The pars distalis of adult female rats was first autografted to the renal capsule where capacity for secretion of FSH, LH, adrenocorticotropin (ACTH), and TSH was largely lost. Several weeks later, the graft was retransplanted by the transtemporal route beneath the median eminence. Controls either received the graft under the temporal lobe or were left with the graft on the kidney. Estrous cycles reappeared in most rats having grafts revascularized from the median eminence, and in many cases the animals became pregnant when mated. Secretion of ACTH and TSH appeared to be moderately restored, whereas the control grafts continued to secrete mostly prolactin. Grafts under the median eminence contained many large gonadotrophs and thyrotrophs, which were absent from the controls. Thus, in spite of the double surgical insult with considerable loss of tissue due to infarction at each operation, the gland could rapidly renew its several trophic secretions once it received blood from the median eminence. Smith (122,123) contributed a further confirmatory variation of Greep's experiment. In both male and female rats, months after hypophysectomy he introduced homografts of pars distalis tissue near the median eminence through the reopened pituitary capsules. Fertility was restored along with significantly improved thyrotropic and adrenotropic functions. During the long intervals after hypophysectomy the typical apituitary syndrome had shown the essential completeness of that operation. Since hypophysectomy was performed in young subjects around 40 days of age, the return of somatotropin secretion was demonstrable after the grafts were introduced.

Thus it became fully evident that the hypophysial portal circulation is essential for stimulating the pars distalis to secrete FSH, LH, TSH, ACTH, and somatotropin (GH, STH). Although Green and Harris (98) had suggested that there might be separate transmitter agents, excitatory or inhibitory, controlling these respective secretions, there were alternative possibilities (124). A single agent might act permissively or its different concentrations in the portal blood might selectively influence particular secretions. Nevertheless, the territorial variations in cell types argued strongly for multiple stimulative factors. Saffran et al. (125) coined the term "releasing factor" and the acronym "RF."

Although inhibitory neural action on the pars intermedia was known, the first evidence of inhibitory neurohumoral control of a pars distalis secretion emerged in experiments involving autotransplantation of the gland to the renal capsule (126,127). When the operation was performed in female rats on the day after ovulation, the newly forming corpora lutea were activated and continued to secrete progesterone for weeks or months until the experiment concluded. Since the principal luteotropin in rats is prolactin, the results demonstrated enhancement of prolactin secretion by removal of the pars distalis from hypothalamic influence. Although not recognized at the time, this effect had previously been obtained by Westman and Jacobsohn (89) after separating the gland from the hypothalamus by stalk section and placement of an impermeable barrier; they interpreted the result as being due to stimulation of the cervix. Desclin (128) also had evidence of prolactin secretion by transplanted pars distalis, but thought it due to the direct stimulative effect of treatment with estrogen. Nikitovitch-Winer (129), repeated the stalk-sectioning experiment of Westman and Jacobsohn, but omitting the cervical stimulation, showed clearly that the enhanced prolactin secretion must be due to removal from hypothalamic inhibition. *In vitro* organ cultures and tissue cultures of pars distalis from several mammals show autonomous secretion of prolactin, increasing with time, while other secretions diminish (130–134). Addition of hypothalamic tissue or extract to the cultures reduces prolactin output, extracts of cerebral cortex having no such effect.

Hypothalamic Hormones

Several different releasing (and inhibiting) factors are recognized today as hypothalamic hormones transmitted to the pars distalis via the portal vessels, each factor having more or less selective action on pituitary secretions. The agents of primary importance for reproduction include first and foremost the luteinizing hormone-releasing hormone LHRH (or GnRH, since it stimulates both FSH and LH secretion). TRH, the releasing agent for the thyroid-stimulating hormone, has the added capacity for stimulating prolactin secretion. The chemical structures of both LHRH, a decapeptide, and TRH, a tripeptide, are known and both are available in synthetic form. The remarkable story of the elucidation of their chemistry and their synthesis has been fully told by Wade (135). PIF, inhibitor of prolactin, remains to be fully characterized. Dopamine, a potent inhibitor (136), appears in the arcuate nuclei-median eminence and portal vessels (137), but may not be the only inhibiting agent.

Hypothalamic-Pituitary Control of Ovulation

Pharmacologic Blockade

In rabbits, the sequence of events provoked by the copulatory stimulus and culminating in ovulation begins with a very brief triggering period during which the process can be blocked by the intravenous injection of certain drugs (138–140). The α-adrenergic blockers, Dibenamine or a congener SKF-501, when injected intravenously within 1 min after coitus, prevented ovulation in 80% of the subjects. Atropine sulphate or another cholinergic blocker, Banthine, also blocked, but they had to be injected more rapidly still, indicating that a cholinergic mechanism precedes the adrenergic trigger. That was further indicated by ovulation induced by injecting a high dose of Adrenaline (Parke-Davis) to estrous rabbits protected from the lethal effects by atropine. The initial postulate that the neurohumoral transmitter carried to the pars distalis by the portal vessels is a catecholamine was later abandoned. Sawyer (141) determined that ovulation could be induced in rabbits by intraventricular injection of either epinephrine or norepinephrine (see also ref. 142). Thus, both the cholinergic and adrenergic links in the rabbit ovulatory reflex are central neural processes, completed within a very few minutes *post coitum*. Although no means has been devised for sampling the portal blood content after the mating stimulus, indirect evidence indicates that LHRH rises rapidly during the first hour, then remains high for several hours (143). The LHRH rise is thought to slightly precede the LH surge, which peaks at 60 to 90 min, remains high for approximately an hour, and then declines (143–146). The prolonged high level of LHRH recalls a report by Westman (147) who placed clamps on the pituitary stalks of estrous rabbits, mated them, and removed the clamps 50 to 60 min later; ovulation followed unless the pituitaries were also removed. A related observation by Westman and Jacobsohn (84) was that, while hypophysectomy 30 min *post coitum* prevented ovulation, exsanguination and replacement with blood from another rabbit at that time allowed ovulation to take place. But it failed if exsanguination and replacement were delayed until 75 to 90 min *post coitum*. In the first instance, the continuing LH surge surely added enough for ovulation, whereas in the latter case any added LH was inadequate.

Reflex ovulators. During the interval between the LH surge and ovulation, in both reflex ovulators and spontaneous ovulators, certain maturation changes take place in the Graafian follicles and ova: follicular hyperemia and swelling, appearance of "secondary liquor," dispersal of cells in the cumulus oophorus, formation of a prominent corona, production of the first polar body (typically), and formation of the second polar division spindle. In retrospect, the relatively brief preovulatory spurt of follicle enlargement described in the guinea pig by Dempsey (148) was an early indication of a spontaneous abrupt increase of gonadotropin secretion.

Spontaneous ovulators. Clear demonstration of acute timing of a preovulatory gonadotropin surge in the spontaneously ovulating rat was presented in a series of studies by Everett, Sawyer, and associates (149–155) employing a number of drugs including those that blocked the rabbit reflex. In addition to Dibenamine and atropine, drugs effective in rats included several barbiturates, chlorpromazine, reserpine, morphine, and urethane. Their use defined a "critical period" of 2 to 3 hours on the afternoon of proestrus, beginning predictably at approximately 1400 hr. Analysis by injecting atropine sulphate or pentobarbital or by hypophysectomy at progressively later times during the critical period indicated temporal variation in the beginning of LH release among different individuals (156–158). Hormone release could be interrupted while in progress as readily by the drugs as by hypophysectomy. Hence, although an atropine-sensitive mechanism controls the spontaneous surge in rats, the action is essential throughout the surge rather than like the brief trigger in the rabbit reflex. The analysis also indicated that the time needed to release the minimal ovulation quota of LH in rats is approximately 30 min. There were indications that the normal surge continues much longer, however. Modern data from radioimmunoassay confirm that and show that the full amount of LH released is far greater than the minimum quota. The surge begins during the critical period, but reaches peak level later, remaining high for 2 to 3 hours and returning to base line typically by 1800 hr to 1900 hr (159). It is provoked by a rise of LHRH in the pituitary-portal blood (160).

The occurrence of acute preovulatory surges of LH and FSH is now recognized as universal among spontaneous and reflex ovulators alike. The duration of the surges tends to be considerably longer in larger mammals; in the human female and other large primates it exceeds 24 hours.

The use of barbiturates for blocking spontaneous ovulation in rats led to three discoveries: (a) Circadian periodicity of the neural stimulus for release of the LH surge. (b) "Delayed pseudopregnancy." (c) The fact that rats pharmacologically blocked from ovulating spontaneously can nevertheless be made to release an ovulatory surge of LH by stimulating the brain.

Circadian periodicity of the LH surge mechanism. Rats that were blocked with pentobarbital on the proestrus afternoon presented a similar critical period on the next day; if they were blocked at that time, the critical period was repeated on the third afternoon (152). Blockade for 3 days produced an anovulatory cycle, followed by a short diestrus and return of cyclic ovulation. Thus, circadian rhythmicity was clearly evident. This had been implied by the 24-hr advance of ovulation through treatment of rats with progesterone (161), by the fact that this advance could be blocked pharmacologically on the preceding afternoon (151), and by the temporal dependency of the LH surge on regularity of environmental lighting (162). As noted later (*this chapter*) although the close relationship of the spontaneous ovulatory surge of LH to time of day has been amply demonstrated in rats and hamsters, this feature appears to be limited to the small polyestrous rodents.

Delayed Pseudopregnancy

A serendipitous finding occurred during experiments that were intended to search for reflex ovulation in rats blocked with pentobarbital (163,164). They were caged with fertile bucks overnight, and proof of copulation was shown next morning by presence of vaginal plugs and spermatozoa. A few had ovulated, but when similarly treated rats were blocked again on the second afternoon, the usual result was early follicular atresia, a short diestrus of 2 to 3 days, then a new proestrus and estrus with spontaneous ovulation, followed by pseudopregnancy of normal duration. The influence of the copulatory stimulus had been retained for over a week, supposedly through some functional change in the central nervous system. Such a long-delayed effect could not be obtained by stimulating the cervix, but shorter delay had been shown by Greep and Hisaw (165) when cervical stimulation during late diestrus caused pseudopregnancy beginning 2 days later, after completion of the cycle. Quinn and Everett (166) produced delayed pseudopregnancy by electrically stimulating the dorsomedial-ventromedial hypothalamus, a stimulation site not conducive to ovulation. As with genital stimulation, there was a quantitative effect, depending in this case on duration of the stimulus: 10-min stimulation was adequate for short-term delay, but 30-min stimulation was needed for long-term delay. This was confirmed by Beach et al. (167,168) who also recorded twice-daily surges of prolactin secretion during the long-delay interval. It is known, however, that these surges during the interval are not essential to the subsequent pseudopregnancy (169). The mnemonic influence of genital or hypothalamic stimulation suggests a protracted change in brain chemistry somehow expressed in the prolactin surges.

Brain Stimulation of Gonadotropin in Rats

In spite of the strong indirect evidence that the central nervous system controls spontaneous as well as reflex ovulation, until 1957 there were no reports of gonadotropin release induced in spontaneous ovulators by brain stimulation. In that year, Anand et al. (170) appear to have had some success from daily hypothalamic stimulation of monkeys early in their menstrual cycles. Bunn and Everett (171), using rats in constant estrus under continuous illumination, consistently induced ovulation and luteinization by electrical stimulation of the amygdala and, in one case, the lateral septum. Critchlow (172) discovered that rats blocked during the proestrus critical period with pentobarbital can be ovulated by stimulating the medial basal tuber (MBT) close to the median eminence. Such pharmacologically blocked rats have become favorite experimental subjects for artificial stimulation of gonadotropin release.

Attempts in the writer's laboratory to repeat Critchlow's work led to the demonstration that the medial preoptic area (MPOA) is an especially useful stimulation site. In contrast to the MBT, electrode placement in the MPOA is much less restricted. Everett and Radford (173) encountered the fact that passage of anodic direct current or anodic pulse trains through electrodes containing iron will produce an irritative focal lesion. Such an *electrochemical stimulus* in the MPOA or anterior hypothalamus can induce ovulation, its effectiveness being determined by the amount of iron deposited. A dose-response relationship between size of the electrochemical (EC) focus and the amount of LH released has been well documented, initially by its ovulatory effectiveness (174–177), and later by radioimmunoassay of the LH surge. Large bilateral EC foci involving most of the MPOA may produce enough gonadotropin within 30 min for full ovulation, as shown by hypophysectomy at that time (174). The amount of LH in the complete surge produced by the large bilateral stimulus reportedly resembles the normal proestrous surge in magnitude and duration (176).

EC stimulation is especially useful because of the very short time required for the passage of current (< 60 sec) and the long period of the stimulative action. Plasma LH typically rises slowly at first, then rapidly to reach peak concentration at 90 to 120 min, falling gradually thereafter. The stimulative processes near the EC lesion are poorly understood, but increased electrical activity in zones 0.4 to 0.8 mm from center of EC lesions has been reported (178). Spiking activity has also been observed 1 mm behind the MPOA, rising sharply after some 15 min and continuing for several hours (179). Although on the day after stimulation the EC lesion consists of a coagulated core of damaged tissue surrounded by an extensive halo devoid of nerve cells and fibers, on the preceding day soon after the passage of current, the region of the eventual halo shows no apparent neuronal damage. It is likely that this outlying region is the site of the increased neural activity. Although there has been some controversy over the possibility that EC lesions act by disinhibition rather than by direct neuronal excitation (180,181), the weight of evidence favors the latter alternative. After Hillarp et al. (182) placed electrolytic lesions with nichrome electrodes in the lateral preoptic areas of male rats there were pronounced behavioral manifestations for as long a 6 hr. Recent investigations by Willmore et al. (183,184) of the effects of ferrous ions introduced into the cerebral cortex indicate that the resulting epileptiform focus is produced by transient formation of free radical oxygen, hydroxyl radicals, and peroxides, causing neural lipid peroxidation.

A major limitation of electrochemical stimulation, aside from uncertainties about how it acts, is that a bulk of tissue is destroyed. That precludes repeated stimulation at the same site and may eliminate neurons important for effective stimulation elsewhere. When EC stimulation is applied near the median eminence, the damage itself may confound the experiment nonspecifically by emptying LHRH into the portal vessels. Knife cuts across the basal tuber (185) or radiofrequency lesions in the arcuate nucleus-median eminence (186) can cause release of an ovulatory quantity of LH. A further limitation of EC stimulation is that the duration of stimulation cannot be controlled.

Such problems are avoided by *electrical stimulation,* especially with platinum electrodes and nonlesioning current, such as matched biphasic pulse pairs. As with EC stimulation, electrical stimulation can induce ovulation in rats under blockade with pentobarbital (and several other drugs), except that it must continue much longer. The amount of LH released and the proportionate numbers of rats ovulating vary with microamperage of the pulses, overall duration of the stimulus, pulse frequency, and other features (187–192). The amount of LH released in a given time by MPOA electrical stimulation is less than expected after electrochemical stimulation, perhaps because of involvement of fewer components of the preoptic-tuberal neuronal system, judged to be diffuse at that level (187–189). Where that system converges upon the arcuate nucleus-median eminence (ARC-ME), electrical stimulation consistently produces more LH than stimulation of the MPOA (174).

Curvilinear Pattern of Ovulatory Gonadotropin Surges

Comparison of the patterns of LH secretion induced by MPOA and ARC-ME stimulations (189) presents a distinct curvilinear parallel, with relatively slow increase during the first 30 to 60 min, followed by rapid increase thereafter. The greater amount of LH discharged during the second hour corresponds to the great excess commonly produced in the spontaneous proestrus surge and undoubtedly reflects the self-priming action of LHRH on the pars distalis (193–195). Aiyer et al. (193) disclosed that if two identical amounts of LHRH were injected intravenously 1 hr apart, plasma LH rose sixfold after the second injection. Comparable priming occurred *in vitro* (195). Fink et al. (194) noted a similar response pattern when the MPOA was electrically stimulated with two 15-min pulse trains at a 45-min interval. Grieg and Weisz (196) calculated that only approximately 15% of the normal surge is needed for ovulation. This conforms with the minimal ovulation quota released in the first 20 to 40 min as estimated from the results of hypophysectomy or atropine block during the critical period (156,157).

The curvilinear pattern of the ovulatory surge of LH (and FSH) is apparent in other species, both reflex ovulators and spontaneous ovulators, provided that frequent blood samples are assayed. Note, for example, the characteristic surges at midcycle in rhesus monkeys shown by Weick et al. (197). From beginning to end, the LH surge in monkeys lasts for 48 hr. But how much of this constitutes the minimal ovulation quota? That information is available for only the rat and, from the pioneer hypophysectomy experiments of Fee and Parkes (79,80) and others (198), in rabbits. While the quota is released within 60 min *post coitum* in rabbits, peak levels of plasma LH may be reached later and are said to continue 1 hr or 2 hr longer (199). The function of the great excess is not understood, although one effect was noted in rats (156). After hypophysectomy or atropine blockade during the critical period, rats that had ovulated by the next morning characteristically lacked the depletion of cholesterol from the interstitial tissue normally shown at that time.

ACTIONS OF GONADAL SECRETIONS ON PITUITARY SECRETION

Functional mammalian corpora lutea suppress estrous cycles and ovulation. This view, expressed by Beard late in the 19th century (200), was supported experimentally by Loeb (201), who noted the early return of estrus and ovulation in guinea pigs after removal of corpora lutea during pregnancy or during the luteal phase of the cycle. Luteectomy in the pregnant goat (202) and cow (203) had the same effect. After confirming Loeb's finding in cyclic guinea pigs (204), Papanicolaou (205) determined that administration of a lipid extract of corpora lutea had the same inhibitory action as the active luteal tissue. Similar findings were reported for the mouse (206) and the rat (207). Once progesterone became available, its daily administration gave the same result (208,209). According to Kennedy (210) and Mahnert (211) corpus luteum extracts prevented ovulation in rabbits if injected before coitus; that effect was later shown by Makepeace et al. (212) with pure progesterone. Mahnert, in fact, speculated on the possibility of female sterilization with luteal extracts, apparently the first expression of an idea that would emerge 30 years later as a primary means of population control, the Pincus Pill. Inhibition of gonadotropic potency of the AP by gonadal hormones was the basis for the Moore and Price (213) hypothesis of pituitary-gonadal reciprocity. The idea of negative feedback control was so firmly entrenched by the early 1930s, that the equally important stimulative actions were slow to emerge.

The first indication of a positive stimulative influence of estrogen lay in its induction of early puberty (214). As mentioned earlier, Hohlweg and Chamorro (86) induced corpus luteum formation in prepubertal rats by treating them with estradiol benzoate, a result that could be prevented by hypophysectomy 2 days later. Confirming that, Westman and Jacobsohn (87–89) noted that the effect could also be prevented by pituitary stalk section. In adult rats, Hohlweg (215) observed that daily, month-long injections of estrogen resulted in great enlargement of the corpora lutea, an effect that can now be ascribed to the luteotropic action of prolactin. Although he states (216) that he observed estrogen-induced ovulation in adult rats, I am not aware of a published record.

Induction of ovulation by estrogen treatment of adult mammals was first recorded by Hammond et al. (217) for anestrous ewes and confirmed by Hammond (218) and Casida (219). Everett (220) reported that in rats having regular 5-day cycles ovulation was advanced 24 hr by administering estradiol benzoate or implanting an estradiol crystal on the second day of diestrus. In pregnant (221) or pseudopregnant rats (222), treatment with estradiol benzoate on day 4 or 5 of vaginal leukocytosis resulted in renewed ovulation and formation of new corpora lutea. These stimulative effects in the rat were subject to pharmacologic blockade with either atropine or Dibenamine (222,223).

The first indication that progesterone has a positive as well as a negative influence on gonadotropin secretion arose from Everett's observation that in rats persistently presenting spontaneous vaginal estrus and polycystic ovaries, ovulation could be induced by certain progesterone treatments. It was known that in normal rats the minimal daily subcutaneous dose for suppressing estrous cycles is 1.5 mg in oil. That was confirmed in the persistent-estrous rats, but daily injection of smaller amounts induced sequences of ovulatory cycles (224). Further study showed progesterone to be primarily important each time that the animal returned to proestrus-estrus, whereupon a single injection of 0.5 mg or more consistently induced ovulation (225). The positive action was next demonstrated in normal rats having 5-day cycles. Progesterone injection on diestrus day 3 induced 24-hr advancement of ovulation. As with advancement by estrogen, the progesterone effect was subject to pharmacologic blockade (226).

Biphasic Action of Progesterone: Interaction with Estrogen

There is an obvious interaction between progesterone and estrogen to produce the positive influence on gonadotropin secretion. In most such cases, progesterone acts acutely against a background of elevated estrogen. The action is biphasic (220): stimulation during the first several hours, followed by inhibition. Daily administration thereafter of a large amount of progesterone will suppress the next cyclic proestrus day-to-day until after treatment stops, thus reproducing the effect of functional corpora lutea. For example, injection for 2 days on diestrus days 1 and 2 of the rat cycle extends the normal diestrus exactly 2 days, proestrus occurring 3 days thereafter. However, omission of one daily injection allows the next injection of progesterone to exert its stimulative effect.

The timing of a progesterone injection on the day of proestrus is critical for determining whether it will stimulate or inhibit an ovulatory LH surge (227–229). Injection at 0200 hr will inhibit ovulation (227), whereas injection between 0900 hr and 1200 hr will produce an ovulatory surge of hormone in advance of the normal critical period (227–229). Comparable temporal relationships are seen in estrogen-primed ovariectomized rats (230). Progesterone's biphasic influence is well documented in the rabbit also (231), where for a few hours it enhances but later inhibits the coital ovulation reflex. Correlated biphasic effects were recorded (232) on behavior and on thresholds for the EEG afterreactions to electrical stimulation of the hypothalamus or the rhinencephalon.

In the special case of ovulation induced in pregnant or pseudopregnant rats by estrogen administration, progesterone serves as a background for the stimulative action of acutely rising estrogen. It is of some interest that the induced gonadotropin release occurs during an afternoon critical period like that in proestrus (222). The progesterone produced by the corpora lutea does not apparently advance the time of release under these circumstances.

Episodic Gonadotropin Release

Gonadectomized animals of either sex are valuable subjects in these inquiries. The finding of highly variable plasma levels of LH in ovarectomized rhesus monkeys led to the first demonstration that gonadotropins tend to be released in pulsatile fashion (233). Pulsatile (episodic, ultradian) release is now recognized as a general phenomenon of AP physiology in many species, including humans (234–237). The concentrations of circulating gonadotropins are known to depend on the frequency and amplitude of LHRH pulses discharged into the pituitary portal vessels and these, in turn, upon the endocrine status. The extensive studies of rhesus monkeys by Knobil and associates (236) show that while continuous infusion of LHRH fails to release LH, pulsatile infusion is effective, optimal results being obtained with a pulse frequency of 1/hr. In rats, while continuous infusion of LHRH will stimulate LH release (237), pulsatile infusion is nevertheless more effective (238). Castration of either sex increases the magnitude of episodic LHRH release, resulting in a rise of circulating gonadotropins (239–243). Replacement with gonadal steroids reduces the pulse frequency of LH at first, thus depressing plasma LH and FSH, but prolonged exposure to estrogen in gonadectomized females reverses the inhibition. There are correlated changes in electrical activity in the medial basal hypothalamus. Dufy et al. (244) recorded pronounced pulsatile multiunit events in the arcuate nuclei of ovariectomized monkeys immediately preceding each LH pulse.

Since LHRH promotes secretion of both LH and FSH, and no specific FSH releaser has been identified, the means for differential regulation of these two secretions has been a mystery. A suggestion of an answer comes from observations that the LH/FSH ratios are influenced by changes in the LHRH pulse frequency (239,243), LH secretion being favored by higher frequencies and FSH by lower frequencies. Controls of the respective gonadotropins may thus be served entirely by the one neurohumor. (There is some evidence that certain regions of the hypothalamus contain a specific releaser for FSH and the search for such an agent continues.)

Steroids and the Phasic Release of Gonadotropins

Whereas the episodic discharge of LH appears universally to be determined by hypothalamic signals mediated by LHRH, the relative involvement of the hypothalamus and the AP itself in the phasic (preovulatory) surge of gonadotropins varies greatly from species to species. In the rat, mouse, and hamster, whose reproductive processes are closely attuned to the photoperiod, the hypothalamus has the leading role. Under the influence of the gonadal steroids there is a rapid increase of LHRH content in the medial basal hypothalamus just before the critical afternoon period of proestrus (245). Multiple pulses of LHRH in the portal blood follow, accompanied by increased frequency of pulsatile LH release, at intervals of 16 to 25 sec (246). The magnitude of these LH pulses is governed initially by the responsiveness of the AP after being primed by estrogen. As the plasma

LH concentration rises, the responsiveness is enhanced, partly by the self-priming action of LHRH and probably also by the increased exposure of the gonadotrophs to progesterone. Whether progesterone or some other progestin is active at the very start of the surge has long been debated.

At the other extreme from the rat is the rhesus monkey, in which the role of the hypothalamus is judged to be more permissive and the timing of the LH surge is determined directly by the response of the AP to the rising tide of estrogen (236,247). Knobil et al. (248) have shown that in female monkeys bearing long-term lesions of the arcuate nuclei, the month-long infusion of the LHRH pulses once per hour sustained complete menstrual cycles. In long-term ovariectomized females having similar hypothalamic lesions and similarly treated with LHRH, administration of estrogen invoked LH surges. No relationship to the time of day was evident in such responses. Nevertheless, the amount of LHRH in the portal blood does vary in the rhesus monkey, being relatively high during the estrogen-induced LH surge (249). A modulating, though nonessential, influence of the hypothalamus has been suggested (247), and others have proposed a specific hypothalamic message (250).

The guinea pig is intermediate between the rat and monkey, such that in ovariectomized subjects the time of an LH surge induced by estrogen depends not only on the time of injection, but also on the time of day and dosage (251,252); the surge is larger in the dark than in the light phase of the daily rhythm. In intact animals, spontaneous surges are also more frequent in the dark phase. Furthermore, unlike the rat and hamster, the ovariectomized guinea pig receiving estrogen fails to present repeated daily surges of LH.

The ovariectomized rat, chronically supplied with estrogen, either by repeated injection of estradiol benzoate (253) or by implanted silastic capsules containing estradiol (254,255), displays daily proestrus-like surges of LH secretion, confirming that there is an innate circadian periodicity in the control mechanism in this species. When progesterone is introduced into such a preparation early in the day, the amount of LH released is enhanced, but release on the days following is diminished or prevented (230,256). Both effects are dose-dependent (257).

The female hamster presents interesting variations on the circadian manifestations displayed by the rat (258–260). During the anestrus induced by short photoperiods, when estrogen levels are low and progesterone is high, there are daily afternoon surges of LH (261,262). Estrogen treatment of long-day subjects intensifies the surges at first, but later suppresses them; that inhibition is hastened by progesterone.

Investigation of the positive and negative actions of the sex steroids on the hypothalamic-pituitary complex proceeds apace, resulting already in a voluminous literature that defies balanced analysis. A recent review (245) addressed selectively to the control of LH secretion in the laboratory rat cites over 400 articles, of which over 300 were published during the last decade. The broad perspective embraces similarities and differences among species, sex differences, developmental aspects, changes during pregnancy, and the influences of old age. There are concerns with anatomy of the LHRH nerve cells and fibers and their physical connections with steroid-concentrating neurons and other neural systems. Much interest focuses on influence of the steroids on hypothalamic neurochemistry, on the participation of several neurotransmitters and hypothalamic enzymes that affect LHRH synthesis, transport, and release.

Nonsteroid Gonadal Feedback

The participation of nonsteroidal gonadal secretions in modulating the pars distalis responses to LHRH assumes increasing significance for the differential regulation of FSH and LH synthesis and discharge. Such material obtained from ovarian follicular fluid or testis extracts (inhibin, folliculostatin, gonadostatin) selectively inhibits FSH secretion *in vivo* and *in vitro* (263,264). On the other hand, inhibin is said to enhance the secretion *in vitro* of LH in response to LHRH, adding to the stimulative action of estradiol (265).

CONCLUSION

This chapter focuses primarily on background studies of the regulation of gonadotropin and prolactin secretion in adult female mammals. Little or no attention is given to a number of important subjects such as the pars intermedia and the classical neurosecretory system terminating in the neural lobe. Present knowledge of the mammalian hypothalamo-pars distalis apparatus is necessarily limited to a few readily available species. For the vast majority, distributed through more than 900 genera, the details of reproductive physiology are poorly known and for practical reasons will probably remain so. One can only assume that the range of specializations recognized among familiar species is representative. Each has contributed importantly in its own way. Thus, as principal representative of the reflex ovulators, the rabbit gave the first clues to the importance of the central nervous system and the hypothalamic-pars distalis connection for the ovulation process. The guinea pig gave the initial evidence that the corpora lutea suppress ovulation. The mouse, through the Allen-Doisy test, was influential in the purification and synthesis of estrogens. The rat, through the technique of hypophysectomy, greatly facilitated the isolation and purification of the several pars distalis hormones. From the rat also came the first proof of the regenerative capacity of the pituitary portal vessels and demonstration of the importance of the vascular supply to the gland from the median eminence, as well as the evidence for neurohumoral inhibition of prolactin secretion. The ovulation-blocking action of certain drugs in rabbits and rats gave the first clear evidence for an acute preovulatory surge of gonadotropins in spontaneous ovulators. The predictable time of this surge in rats, its dependence on the lighting rhythm, and failure of the surge in old rats led to disclosure of the biphasic action of progesterone and its interaction with estrogen in promoting the surge. Blockage of the surge pharmacologically or by exposure to continuous lighting fostered various studies of the central neural apparatus controlling spontaneous ovulation. Critical comparisons among rats, hamsters, guinea pigs, sheep, and monkeys, facilitated by radioimmunoassay and other modern techniques, have yielded interpretations that seem generally applicable to human subjects, a major goal of all research in reproductive biology.

ACKNOWLEDGMENTS

This research was supported in part by grants from the Research Council of Duke University and, since 1957, from the National Science Foundation. The author is also grateful to John Graves for typing the manuscript.

REFERENCES

1. Harris, G. W. (1972): Humours and hormones, the Sir Henry Dale lecture for 1971. *J. Endocrinol.*, 53:ii–xxii.
2. Rathke, M. H. (1838): Über die Entstehung der Glandula pituitaria. *Arch. Anat. Physiol. Wiss. Med.*, pp. 482–485. Cited by Medvei, V. C. (1982): *A History of Endocrinology*. MTP Press, Boston.
3. Bayliss, W. M. (1915): *Principles of General Physiology*. Longmans, Green, London.
4. Bayliss, W. M., and Starling, E. H. (1904): The chemical regulation of the secretory process. *Proc. R. Soc. Lond. (Biol.). B.*, 73:310–322.
5. Ramón y Cajal, S. (1894): Algunas contribuciónes conociamento de los ganglios del encéfale. *Anal. Soc. Espan. Hist. Nat.*, 23:214–215.
6. Camus, J., and Roussy, G. (1920): Experimental researches on the pituitary body. Diabetes insipidus, gycosuria, and those dystrophies considered as hypohysial in origin. *Endocrinology*, 4:507–522.
7. Bailey, P., and Bremer, F. (1921): Experimental diabetes insipidus. *Arch. Intern. Med.*, 28:773–803.
8. Evans, H. M., and Long, J. A. (1921): Effect of anterior lobe of hypophysis administered intraperitoneally upon growth, maturity, and oestrous cycles in the rat. *Anat. Rec.*, 21:61 (abstract).
9. Anderson, E. (1969): Earlier ideas of hypothalamic function, including irrelevant concepts. In: *The Hypothalamus*, edited by W. Haymaker, E. Anderson, and W. J. H. Nauta, pp. 1–12. Thomas, Springfield, Illinois.
10. Cushing, H. (1909): The hypophysis cerebri: chemical aspects of hyperpituitarism and hypopituitarism. *JAMA* 53:249–255.
11. Crowe, S. J., Cushing, H., and Homans, J. (1910): Experimental hypophysectomy. *Bull. Johns Hopkins Hosp.*, 21:127–169.
12. Cushing, H. (1912): *The Pituitary and Its Disorders*. Lippincott, Philadelphia.
13. Aschner, B. (1909): Demonstration von Hunden nach Extirpation der Hypophyse. *Wien. Klin. Wochenschr.*, 22:1730–1732.
14. Aschner, B. (1912): Ueber die Function der Hypophyse. *Pflügers Arch. Ges. Physiol.*, 146:1–147.
15. Marshall, F. H. A. (1936): Sexual periodicity and the causes which determine it. The Croonian lecture. *Philos. Trans. R. Soc. Lond. (Biol.)*, 226:423–456.
16. Marshall, F. H. A. (1942): Exteroceptive factors in sexual periodicity. *Biol. Rev.*, 17:68–90.
17. Haighton, J. (1797): An experimental study concerning animal impregnation. *Philos. Trans. R. Soc.*, 87:157–196.
18. Cruikshank, W. (1797): Experiments in which, on the third day after impregnation, the ova of rabbits were found in the Fallopian tubes; and on the fourth day after impregnation in the uterus itself; with the first appearance of the foetus. *Philos. Trans. R. Soc.*, 87:197–214.
19. Barry, M. (1839): Researches in embryology. *Philos. Trans. R. Soc.*, 129:307–380.
20. Heape, W. (1905): Ovulation and degeneration of ova in rabbit. *Proc. Roy. Soc. Lond. (Biol.)*, 76:266–268.
21. Marshall, F. H. A. (1904): The oestrous cycle of the common ferret. *Q. J. Microsc. Sci.*, 48:323–345.
22. Longley, W. H. (1911): Maturation of the egg and ovulation in the domestic cat. *Am. J. Anat.*, 12:139–172.
23. Fichera, G. (1905): Sur l'hypertrophie de la gland pituitaire consecutive à la castration. *Arch. Ital. Biol.*, 43:405–426.
24. Addison, W. H. F. (1917): The cell changes of the hypophysis of the albino rat after castration. *J. Comp. Neurol.*, 28:441–461.
25. Loeb, L. (1911): Über die Bedeutung des Corpus luteum für die Periodizität des sexuellen Zyklus beim weiblichen Säugetier-organismus. *Dtsch. Med. Wochenschr.*, 37:17–21.
26. Stockard, C. R., and Papanicolaou, G. N. (1917): The existence of a typical oestrous cycle in the guinea pig—with a study of its histological and physiological changes. *Am. J. Anat.*, 22:225–283.
27. Long, J. A., and Evans, H. M. (1922): The oestrous cycle in the rat and its associated phenomena. *Mem. Univ. Calif.*, 6:1–111.
28. Allen, E. (1922): The oestrous cycle in the mouse. *Am. J. Anat.*, 30:297–371.

28a. Allen, E., and Doisy, E. A. (1923): An ovarian hormone; a preliminary report on its localization, extraction and partial purification, and action in test animals. *JAMA*, 81:819–821.

29. Allen, E., Pratt, J. P., and Doisy, E. A. (1925): The ovarian follicular hormone. Its distribution in human genital tissues, *JAMA*, 85:399–405.
30. Allen, B. M. (1916): The results of extirpation of the anterior lobe of the hypophysis and of the thyroid of *Rana pipiens* larvae. *Science*, 44:755–757.
31. Allen, B. M. (1920): Experiments in the transplantation of the hypophysis of adult *Rana pipiens* to tadpoles. *Science*, 52:274–276.
32. Smith, P. E. (1916): The effect of hypophysectomy in the early embryo upon growth and development of the frog. *Anat. Rec.*, 11:57–64.
33. Smith, P. E., and Smith, I. P. (1922): The effect of intraperitoneal injection of fresh anterior lobe substance in hypophysectomized tadpoles. *Anat. Rec.*, 23:38–39.
34. Smith, P. E., and Smith, I. P. (1922): The repair and activation of the thyroid in the hypophysectomized tadpole by the parenteral administration of fresh anterior lobe of the bovine hypophysis. *J. Med. Res.*, 43:267–283.
35. Smith, P. E. (1926): Ablation and transplantation of the hypophysis in the rat. *Anat. Rec.*, 32:221 (abstract).
36. Smith, P. E. (1927): The disabilities caused by hypophysectomy and their repair. *JAMA*, 88:158–161.
37. Smith, P. E. (1930): Hypophysectomy and replacement therapy in the rat. *Am. J. Anat.*, 45:205–274.
38. Smith, P. E., and Engle, E. T. (1927): Experimental evidence regarding the role of the anterior pituitary in the development and regulation of the genital system. *Am. J. Anat.*, 40:159–217.
39. Evans, H. M., Meyer, K., and Simpson, M. E. (1933): The growth and gonad-stimulating hormones of the anterior hypophysis. *Mem. Univ. Calif.*, 11:67–229.
40. Evans, H. M., Pencharz, R. I., Meyer, K., and Simpson, M. E. (1933): The growth and gonad-stimulating hormones of the anterior hypophysis. *Mem. Univ. Calif.*, 11:315–334.
41. Greep, R. O. (1935): Separation of a thyrotropic from the gonadotropic substances of the pituitary. *Am. J. Physiol.*, 110:692–699.
42. Zondek, B. (1930): Über die Hormone des Hypophysenvorderlappens. I. Wachstumshormon, Follikelreifungshormon (Prolan A), Luteinisierungshormon (Prolan B), Stoffwechselhormon. *Klin. Wochenschr.*, 9:245–248.
43. Zondek, B. (1930): Über die Hormone des Hypophysenvorderlappens. II. Follikelreifungshormon Prolan A-Klamakterium-Kastration. *Klin. Wochenschr.*, 9:393–396.
44. Reichert, F. L., Pencharz, R. I., Simpson, M. E., Meyer, K., and Evans, H. M. (1932): Relative ineffectiveness of Prolan in hypophysectomized animals. *Am. J. Physiol.*, 100:157–161.
45. Leonard, S. M., and Smith, P. E. (1934): Responses of the reproductive system of hypophysectomized rats to injections of pregnancy-urine extracts. II. The female. *Anat. Rec.*, 58:175–200.

46. Gey, G. O., Seegar, G. E., and Hellman, L. M. (1938): The production of gonadotropic substance (Prolan) by placental cells in tissue culture. *Science,* 88:306–307.
47. Jones, G. E. S., Gey, G. O., and Cey, M. K. (1943): Hormone production by placental cells maintained in continuous culture. *Bull. Johns Hopkins Hosp.,* 72:26–38.
48. Fevold, H. L., Hisaw, F. L., and Leonard, S. L. (1931): The gonad-stimulating and the luteinizing hormones of the anterior lobe of the hypophysis. *Am. J. Physiol.,* 97:291–301.
49. Greep, R. O. (1974): History of research on anterior hypophysial hormones. In: *Handbook of Physiology, Section 7, Endocrinology, Vol. IV,* part 2, pp. 1–27.
50. Astwood, E. B. (1941): The regulation of corpus luteum function by hypophysial luteotropin. *Endocrinology,* 28:309–320.
51. Evans, H. M., Simpson, M. E., Lyons, W. R., and Turpeinen, K. (1941): Anterior pituitary hormones which favor production of traumatic uterine placentoma. *Endocrinology,* 28:933–945.
52. Stricker, P., and Grueter, F. (1928): Action du lobe antérieur de l'hypophyse sur la montée laiteuse. *C. R. Soc. Biol. (Paris),* 99:1978–1980.
53. Stricker, P., and Grueter, F. (1929): Fonctions du lobe antérieur de l'hypophyse: Influence des extraits du lobe antérieur sur l'appareil génitale de la lapine et sur la montée laiteuse. *Presse Med.,* 37:1268–1271.
54. Corner, G. W. (1930): The hormonal control of lactation. I. Non-effect of the corpus luteum. II. Positive action of extracts of the hypophysis. *Am. J. Physiol.,*95:43–55.
55. Evans, H. M., and Simpson, M. E. (1929): Hyperplasia of the mammary apparatus of adult virgin females induced by anterior hypophyseal hormones. *Proc. Soc. Exp. Biol. Med.,* 26:598.
56. Riddle, O. (1937): Physiological responses to prolactin. *Cold Spring Harbor Symp. Quant. Biol.,* 5:218–228.
57. Riddle, O. (1938): Prolactin. *Assoc. Res. Nerv. Mental Dis.,* 17:287–297.
58. Riddle, O., and Braucher, P. F. (1931): Studies on the physiology of reproduction in birds. XXX. Control of the special secretion of the crop gland in pigeons by an anterior pituitary hormone. *Am. J. Physiol.,* 97:617–625.
59. Riddle, O., Bates, R. W., and Dykshorn, S. W. (1933): The preparation, identification and assay of prolactin—a hormone of the anterior pituitary. *Am. J. Physiol.,* 105:191–216.
60. Dresl, L. (1935): The effect of prolactin on the estrus cycle of non-parous mice. *Science,* 82:173.
61. Lahr, L., and Riddle, O. (1936): Temporary suppression of estrous cycles in the rat by prolactin. *Proc. Soc. Exp. Biol. Med.,* 34:880–893.
62. Bates, R. W., Miller, R. A., and Garrison, M. M. (1962): Evidence in the hypophysectomized pigeon of a synergism among prolactin, growth hormone, thyroxine and prednisone upon weight of the body, digestive tract, kidney and fat stores. *Endocrinology,* 71:345–360.
63. Schönemann, A. (1892): Hypophysis und Thyroidea. *Virchows Arch. (Pathol. Anat.),* 129:310–336.
64. Holmes, R. L., and Ball, J. N. (1974): *The Pituitary Gland—A Comparative Account.* Cambridge University Press, Cambridge.
65. Mallory, F. B. (1900): A contribution to staining methods. *J. Exp. Med.,* 5:15–20.
66. McManus, J. F. A. (1946): Histological demonstration of mucin after periodic acid. *Nature,* 158:202.
67. Herlant, M. (1960): Étude critique de deux techniques nouvelles destinées à mettre en evidence les différentes catégories cellulaires présente dans la glands pituitaire. *Bull. Microsc. Appl.,* 10:37–44.
68. Pearse, A. G. E. (1953): Cytological and cyto-chemical investigations on the foetal and adult hypophysis in various physiological and pathological states. *J. Pathol. Bacteriol.,* 65:355–370.
69. Coons, A. H. (1956): Histochemistry with labelled antibody. *Int. Rev. Cytol.,* 5:1–23.
70. Halmi, N. S., and Krieger, D. (1983): Immunocytochemistry of ACTH-related peptides in the hypophysis. In: *The Anterior Pituitary Gland,* edited by A. S. Bhatnagar, pp. 1–15. Raven Press, New York.
71. Hohlweg, W., and Junkmann, K. (1932): Die hormonal-nervöse Regulierung der Funktion des Hypophysenvorderlappens. *Klin. Wochenschr.,* 11:321–323.
72. Fröhlich, A. (1901): Ein Fall von Tumor der Hypophysis cerebri ohne Akromegalie. *Wien. Klin. Rundschau,* 15:883–886; 906–908.
73. Hetherington, A. W., and Ranson, S. W. (1939): Experimental hypothalamico-hypophyseal obesity in the rat. *Proc. Soc. Exp. Biol. Med.,* 41:465–466.
74. Hetherington, A. W., and Ranson, S. W. (1940): Hypothalamic lesions and adiposity in the rat. *Anat. Rec.,*78:149–172.
75. Hetherington, A. W., and Ranson, S. W. (1942): The relation of various hypothalamic lesions to adiposity in the rat. *J. Comp. Neurol.,* 76:475–499.
76. Bauer, H. G. (1954): Endocrine and other clinical manifestations of hypothalamic disease. *J. Clin. Endocrinol.,* 14:13–31.
77. Grafe, E., and Grünthal, E. (1929): Über isolierte Beinflussung des Gesamtstoffwechsels vom Zwischenhirn aus. *Klin. Wochenschr.,* 8:1013–1016.
78. Moore, C. R., and Price, D. (1932): Gonad hormone functions and the reciprocal influence between gonads and hypophysis with its bearing on the problem of sex-hormone antogonisms. *Am. J. Anat.,* 50:13–71.
79. Fee, A. R., and Parkes, A. S. (1929): The relation of the anterior pituitary body to ovulation in the rabbit. *J. Physiol. (Lond.),* 67:383–388.
80. Fee, A. R., and Parkes, A. S. (1930): Effects of vaginal anesthesia on ovulation in the rabbit. *J. Physiol. (Lond.),* 70:385–388.
81. Marshall, F. H. A., and Verney, E. B. (1936): The occurrence of ovulation and pseudopregnancy in the rabbit, as a result of central nervous stimulation. *J. Physiol. (London),* 86:327–336.
82. Harris, G. W. (1937): The induction of ovulation in the rabbit by electrical stimulation of the hypothalamo-hypohysial mechanism. *Proc. R. Soc. Lond. (Biol.),* 122:374–394.
83. Haterius, H. O., and Derbyshire, A. J., Jr. (1937): Ovulation in the rabbit upon stimulation of the hypothalamus. *Am. J. Physiol.,* 119:329–330.
84. Westman, A., and Jacobsohn, D. (1937): Experimentelle Untersuchungen über die Bedeutung des Hypophysen-Zwischenhirnsystems für die Produktion gonadotroper Hormone des Hypophysenvorderlappens. *Acta Obstet. Gynecol. Scand.,* 17:235–265.
85. Rasmussen, A. T. (1938): Innervation of the hypophysis. *Endocrinology,* 23:263–278.
86. Hohlweg, W., and Chamorro, A. (1937): Über die luteinisierende Wirkung des Follikelhormons durch Beinflussung der endogenen Hypophysenvorderlappensekretion. *Klin. Wochenschr.,* 16: 196–197.
87. Westman, A., and Jacobsohn, D. (1938): Endokrinologische Untersuchungen an Ratten mit durchtrenntem Hypophysenstiel. I. Hypophysenveränderungen nach Kastration und nach Oestrinbehandlungen. *Acta Obstet. Gynecol. Scand.,* 18:99–108.
88. Westman, A., and Jacobsohn, D. (1938): Endokrinologische Untersuchungen an Ratten mit durchtrenntem Hypophysenstiel. III. Über die luteinisierende Wirkung des Follikelhormons. *Acta Obstet. Gynecol. Scand.,* 18:115–123.
89. Westman, A., and Jacobsohn, D. (1938): Endokrinologische Untersuchungen an Ratten mit durchtrenntem Hypophysenstiel. VI. Produktion und Abgabe der gonadotropen Hormone. *Acta Pathol. Microbiol. Scand.,* 15:445–453.
90. Pietsch, K. (1930): Aufbau und Entwicklung der Pars tuberalis des menschlichen Hirnanhangs in ihren Beziehung zu den übrigen Hypophysenteilen. *Z. Mikrosk. Anat. Forsh.,* 22:227–257.
91. Popa, G. T., and Fielding, U. (1930): A portal circulation from the pituitary to the hypothalamic region. *J. Anat. (Lond.),* 65:88–91.
92. Popa, G. T., and Fielding, U. (1933): Hypophysio-portal vessels and their colloid accompaniment. *J. Anat. (Lond.),* 67:227–232.
93. Houssay, B. A., Biosotti, A., and Sammartino, R. (1935): Modifications fonctionelles de l'hypophyse après les lésions infundibulotubériennes chez le crapaud. *C. R. Soc. Biol. (Paris),* 120:725–727.
94. Wislocki, G. B., and King, L. S. (1936): The permeability of the hypophysis and the hypothalamus to vital dyes, with a study of the hypophysial vascular supply. *Am. J. Anat.,* 58:421–472.
95. Wislocki, G. B. (1938): The vascular supply of the hypophysis cerebri of the rhesus monkey and man. *Res. Publ. Assoc. Nerv. Ment. Dis.,* 17:48–68.

96. Green, J. D. (1947): Vessels and nerves of the amphibian hypophysis: a study of the living circulation and of the histology of the hypophysial vessels and nerves. *Anat. Rec.*, 99:21–54.
97. Benoit, J., and Assenmacher, I. (1955): Le controle hypothalamique de l'activité préhypophysaire gonadotrope. *J. Physiol. (Paris)*, 47:427–567.
98. Green, J. D., and Harris, G. W. (1947): The neurovascular link between the neurohypophysis and adenohypophysis. *J. Endocrinol.*, 5:136–146.
99. Green, J. D., and Harris, G. W. (1949): Observations of the hypophysial portal vessels of the living rat. *J. Physiol. (Lond.)*, 108:359–361.
100. Worthington, W. C., Jr. (1955): Some observations on the hypophyseal portal system in the living mouse. *Bull. Johns Hopkins Hosp.*, 97:343–357.
101. Worthington, W. C., Jr. (1960): Vascular responses in the pituitary stalk. *Endocrinology*, 66:19–31.
102. Török, B. (1954): Lebendbeobachtung des Hypophysenkreislaufes an Hunden. *Acta Morphol. Hungarica*, 4:83–89.
103. Török, B. (1962): Neue Angaben zum Blutkreislauf der Hypophyse. *Anat. Anz.*, 109(Suppl.):622–629.
104. Daniel, P. M. (1966): The anatomy of the hypothalamus and pituitary gland. In: *Neuroendocrinology, Vol. I*, edited by L. Martini and W. F. Ganong, pp. 15–80. Academic Press, New York.
105. Page, R. B., and Bergland, R. M. (1977): The neurophysial capillary bed. I. Anatomy and arterial supply. *Am. J. Anat.*, 148:345–358.
106. Bergland, R. M., and Page, R. B. (1978): Can the pituitary secrete directly to the brain? (Affirmative anatomical evidence). *Endocrinology*, 102:1325–1338.
107. Oliver, C., Mical, R. S., and Porter, J. C. (1977): Hypothalamic-pituitary vasculature: evidence for retrograde blood flow in the pituitary stalk. *Endocrinology*, 101:598–604.
108. Daniel, P. M., and Prichard, M. M. L. (1975): Studies of the hypothalamus and the pituitary gland with special reference to the effects of transection of the pituitary stalk. *Acta Endocrinol.*, 80(Suppl. 201):1–216.
109. Pasteels, J. L. (1960): Étude expérimentale des différentes catégories d'éléments chromophiles de l'hypophyse adulte de *Pleurodeles waltlii* et de leur controle par l'hypothalamus. *Arch. Biol. (Paris)*, 71:409–471.
110. Porter, J. C., Kamberi, I. A., and Grazia, Y. A. (1971): Pituitary blood flow and portal vessels. In: *Frontiers in Neuroendocrinology*, edited by L. Martini and W. F. Ganong, pp. 145–175. Oxford University Press, New York.
111. Hinsey, J. C., and Markee, J. E. (1933): Pregnancy following bilateral section of the cervical sympathetic trunks in the rabbits. *Proc. Soc. Exp. Biol. Med.*, 31:270–271.
112. Hinsey, J. C. (1937): The relationship of the nervous system to ovulation and other phenomena of the female reproductive tract. *Cold Spring Harbor Symp. Quant. Biol.*, 5:269–279.
113. Wingstrand, K. G. (1966): Comparative anatomy and evolution of the hypophysis. In: *The Pituitary Gland, Vol. 1*, edited by G. W. Harris and B. T. Donovan, pp. 58–126. Butterworths, London.
114. Green, J. D. (1951): The comparative anatomy of the hypophysis, with special reference to its blood supply and innervation. *Am. J. Anat.*, 88:225–312.
115. Harris, G. W. (1950): Oestrous rhythm, pseudopregnancy and the pituitary stalk in the rat. *J. Physiol. (Lond.)*, 111:347–360.
116. Harris, G. W., and Johnson, R. T. (1950): Regeneration of the hypophysial portal vessels after section of the hypophysial stalk, in the monkey *Macaca rhesus*. *Nature*, 165:819–820.
117. Jacobsohn, D. (1954): Regeneration of hypophysial portal vessels and grafts of anterior pituitary glands in rabbits. *Acta Endocrinol. (Copenhagen)*, 17:187–197.
118. Greep, R. O. (1936): Functional pituitary grafts in rats. *Proc. Soc. Exp. Biol. Med.*, 34:754–755.
119. Harris, G. W., and Jacobsohn, D. (1952): Functional grafts of the anterior pituitary gland. *Proc. R. Soc. Lond. (Biol.)*, 139:263–276.
120. Nikitovitch-Winer, M., and Everett, J. W. (1958): Functional restitution of pituitary grafts re-transplanted from kidney to median eminence. *Endocrinology*, 63:916–930.
121. Nikitovitch-Winer, M., and Everett, J. W. (1959): Histo-cytologic changes in grafts of rat pituitary on the kidney and upon retransplantation under the diencephalon. *Endocrinology*, 65:357–368.
122. Smith, P. E. (1961): Postponed homotransplants of the hypophysis into the region of the median eminence in hypophysectomized male rats. *Endocrinology*, 68:130–143.
123. Smith, P. E. (1963): Postponed pituitary homotransplants into the region of the hypophysial portal circulation in hypophysectomized female rats. *Endocrinology*, 73:793–806.
124. Harris, G. W. (1955): *Neural Control of the Pituitary Gland*. Arnold, London.
125. Saffran, M., Schally, A. V., and Benfry, B. G. (1955): Stimulation of the release of corticotropin from the adenohypophysis by a neurohypophysial factor. *Endocrinology*, 57:439–444.
126. Everett, J. W. (1954): Luteotrophic function of autografts of the rat hypophysis. *Endocrinology*, 54:685–690.
127. Everett, J. W. (1956): Functional corpora lutea maintained for months by autografts of rat hypophyses. *Endocrinology*, 58:786–796.
128. Desclin, L. (1950): A propos du méchanisme d'action des oestrogènes sur le lobe antérieur de l'hypophyse chez le Rat. *Ann. Endocrinol.*, 11:656–659.
129. Nikitovitch-Winer, M. B. (1965): Effect of hypophysial stalk transection on luteotropic hormone secretion in the rat. *Endocrinology*, 77:658–666.
130. Nicoll, C. S., and Meites, J. (1962): Prolactin secretion *in vitro:* comparative aspects. *Nature*, 195:606–607.
131. Nicoll, C. S. (1965): Neural regulation of adenohypophysial prolactin secretion in tetrapods: indications from *in vitro* studies. *J. Exp. Zool.*, 158:203–210.
132. Meites, J. (1967): Control of prolactin secretion. *Arch. Anat. Microsc. Morphol. Exp.*, 56(Suppl.):516–529.
133. Pasteels, J. L. (1961): Sécrétion de prolactine par l'hypophyse en culture de tissus. *C. R. Acad. Sci. (Paris)*, 253:2140–2142.
134. Pasteels, J. L. (1961): Premiers résultats de culture combinée *in vitro* d'hypophyis et d'hypothalamus dans le but d'en apprécier la sécrétion de prolactine. *C. R. Acad. Sci. (Paris)*, 253:3074–3075.
135. Wade, N. (1981): *The Nobel Duel*. Anchor Press/Doubleday, New York.
136. MacLeod, R. M. (1976): Regulation of prolactin secretion. In: *Frontiers in Neuroendocrinology*, edited by L. Martini and W. F. Ganong, pp. 169–194. Raven Press, New York.
137. Ben-Jonathan, N., Oliver, C., Weiner, H. J., Mical, R. S., and Porter, J. C. (1977): Dopamine in hypophysial portal plasma of the rat during the estrous cycle and throughout pregnancy. *Endocrinology*, 100:452–458.
138. Sawyer, C. H., Markee, J. E., and Hollinshead, W. H. (1947): Inhibition of ovulation in the rabbit by the adrenergic-blocking agent Dibenamine. *Endocrinology*, 41:395–402.
139. Markee, J. E., Sawyer, C. H., and Hollinshead, W. H. (1948): Adrenergic control of the release of luteinizing hormone from the hypophysis of the rabbit. *Recent Prog. Horm. Res.*, 2:117–151.
140. Sawyer, C. H., Markee, J. E., and Townsend, B. F. (1949): Cholinergic and adrenergic components in the neurohumoral control of the release of LH in the rabbit. *Endocrinology*, 44:18–37.
141. Sawyer, C. H. (1952): Stimulation of ovulation in the rabbit by the intraventricular injection of epinephrine or norepinephrine. *Anat. Rec.*, 112:385 (abstract).
142. Sawyer, C. H. (1979): The Seventh Stevenson Lecture. Brain amines and pituitary gonadotrophin secretion. *Can. J. Physiol. Pharmacol.*, 57:667–680.
143. Tsou, R. C., Dailey, R. A., McLanahan, C. S., Parent, A. D., Tindall, G. T., and Neill, J. D. (1977): Luteinizing hormone releasing hormone (LHRH) levels in pituitary stalk plasma during the preovulatory gonadotropin surge of rabbits. *Endocrinology*, 101:534–539.
144. Dufy-Barbe, L., Franchimont, P., and Faure, J. M. A. (1973): Time courses of LH and FSH release in the female rabbit. *Endocrinology*, 92:1318–1321.
145. Kanematsu, S., Scaramuzzi, R. J., Hilliard, J., and Sawyer, C. H. (1974): Patterns of ovulation-inducing LH release following coitus, electrical stimulation and exogenous LH-RH in the rabbit. *Endocrinology*, 95:247–252.
146. Goodman, A. L., and Neill, J. D. (1976): Ovarian regulation of postcoital gonadotropin release in the rabbit: reexamination of a functional role for 20α dihydro-progesterone. *Endocrinology*, 99:852–860.

147. Westman, A. (1942): Der Einfluss des Hypophysenzwishchenhirnsystems auf die Sexualfunktionen. *Schweiz. Med. Wochenschr.*, 72:113–116.
148. Dempsey, E. W. (1937): Follicular growth rate and ovulation after various experimental procedures in the guinea pig. *Am. J. Physiol.*, 120:126–132.
149. Everett, J. W., Sawyer, C. H., and Markee, J. E. (1949): A neurogenic timing factor in control of the ovulating discharge of luteinizing hormone in the cyclic rat. *Endocrinology*, 44:234–250.
150. Sawyer, C. H., Everett, J. W., and Markee, J. E. (1949): A neural factor in the mechanism by which estrogen induces the release of luteinizing hormone in the rat. *Endocrinology*, 44:218–233.
151. Everett, J. W., and Sawyer, C. H. (1949): A neural timing factor in the mechanism by which progesterone advances ovulation in the cyclic rat. *Endocrinology*, 45:581–595.
152. Everett, J. W., and Sawyer, C. H. (1950): A 24-hour periodicity in the "LH-release apparatus" of female rats, disclosed by barbiturate sedation. *Endocrinology*, 47:198–218.
153. Barraclough, C. A., and Sawyer, C. H. (1955): Inhibition of the release of pituitary ovulatory hormone in the rat by morphine. *Endocrinology*, 57:329–337.
154. Barraclough, C. A., and Sawyer, C. H. (1957): Blockade of the release of pituitary ovulating hormone in the rat by chlorpromazine and reserpine: possible mechanisms of action. *Endocrinology*, 61:341–351.
155. Blake, C. A., and Sawyer, C. H. (1972): Ovulation blocking actions of urethane in the rat. *Endocrinology*, 91:87–94.
156. Everett, J. W., and Sawyer, C. H. (1953): Estimated duration of the spontaneous activation which causes release of ovulating hormone from the rat hypophysis. *Endocrinology*, 52:83–92.
157. Everett, J. W. (1956): The time of release of ovulating hormone from the rat hypophysis. *Endocrinology*, 59:580–585.
158. Everett, J. W., and Tejasen, T. (1967): Time factor in ovulation blockade in rats under differing lighting conditions. *Endocrinology*, 80:790–792.
159. Blake, C. A. (1976): A detailed characterization of the proestrous luteinizing hormone surge. *Endocrinology*, 98:445–450.
160. Sarkar, D. K., Chiappa, S. A., Fink, G., and Sherwood, N. M. (1976): Gonadotropin-releasing hormone surge in pro-oestrous rats. *Nature*, 264:461–463.
161. Everett, J. W. (1948): Progesterone and estrogen in the experimental control of ovulation time and other features of the estrous cycle in the rat. *Endocrinology*, 43:389–405.
162. Everett, J. W. (1970): Photoregulation of the ovarian cycle in the rat. In: *La Photorégulation de la Reproduction chez les Oiseaux et les Mammifères*, edited by J. Benoit and I. Assenmacher, pp. 387–403. C.N.R.S., Paris.
163. Everett, J. W. (1952): Presumptive hypothalamic control of spontaneous ovulation. *Ciba Foundation Colloquia Endocrinol.*, 4:167–178.
164. Everett, J. W. (1967): Provoked ovulation or long-delayed pseudopregnancy from coital stimuli in barbiturate-blocked rats. *Endocrinology*, 80:145–154.
165. Greep, R. O., and Hisaw, F. L. (1938): Pseudopregnancies from electrical stimulation of the cervix in the diestrum. *Proc. Soc. Exp. Biol. Med.*, 39:359–360.
166. Quinn, D. L., and Everett, J. W. (1967): Delayed pseudopregnancy induced by selective hypothalamic stimulation. *Endocrinology*, 80:155–162.
167. Beach, J. E., Tyrey, L., and Everett, J. W. (1975): Serum prolactin and LH in early phases of delayed versus direct pseudopregnancy in the rat. *Endocrinology*, 96:1241–1246.
168. Beach, J. E., Tyrey, L, and Everett, J. W. (1978): Prolactin secretion preceding delayed pseudopregnancy in rats after electrical stimulation of the hypothalamus. *Endocrinology*, 103:2247–2251.
169. de Greef, W. J., and Zeilmaker, G. H. (1976): Prolactin and delayed pseudopregnancy in the rat. *Endocrinology*, 98:305–310.
170. Anand, B. K., Malkani, P. K., and Dua, S. (1957): Effect of electrical stimulation of the hypothalamus on menstrual cycle in monkey. *Indian J. Med. Res.*, 45:499–502.
171. Bunn, J. P., and Everett, J. W. (1957): Ovulation in persistent-estrous rats after electrical stimulation of the brain. *Proc. Soc. Exp. Biol. Med.*, 96:369–371.
172. Critchlow, V. (1958): Ovulation induced by hypothalamic stimulation in the anesthetized rat. *Am. J. Physiol.*, 195:171–174.
173. Everett, J. W., and Radford, H. M. (1961): Irritative deposits from stainless steel electrodes in the preoptic rat brain causing release of pituitary gonadotropin. *Proc. Soc. Exp. Biol. Med.*, 108: 604–609.
174. Everett, J. W. (1964): Preoptic stimulative lesions and ovulation in the rat: "thresholds" and LH-release time in late diestrus and proestrus. In: *Major Problems in Neuroendocrinology*, edited by E. Bajusz and G. Jasmin, pp. 346–366. Karger, Basel.
175. Everett, J. W., Krey, L. C., and Tyrey, L. (1973): The quantitative relationship between electrochemical preoptic stimulation and LH release in proestrous *versus* late diestrous rats. *Endocrinology*, 93:947–953.
176. Turgeon, J., and Barraclough, G. A. (1973): Temporal patterns of LH release following graded preoptic electrochemical stimulation in proestrous rats. *Endocrinology*, 92:755–761.
177. Velasco, M. E., and Rothchild, I. (1973): Factors influencing the secretion of luteinizing hormone and ovulation in response to electrochemical stimulation of the preoptic area in rats. *J. Endocrinol.*, 58:163–176.
178. Colombo, J. A., Whitmoyer, D. I., and Sawyer, C. H. (1974): Local changes in multiple unit activity induced by electrochemical means in preoptic and hypothalamic areas in the female rat. *Brain Res.*, 71:1175–1183.
179. van der Schoot, P., Lincoln, D. W., and Clark, J. S., (1978): Activation of hypothalamic neuronal activity by electrolytic deposition of iron into the preoptic area. *J. Endocrinol.*, 79:107–120.
180. Dyer, R. G., and Burnet, F. (1976): Effects of ferrous ions on preoptic area neurons and luteinizing hormone secretion in the rat. *J. Endocrinol.*, 69:247–254.
181. Dyball, R. E., Dyer, R. G., MacLeod, N. K., Wright, R. J., and Yates, J. O. (1976): Effects of ferrous ions on secretion from incubated nerve terminals. *J. Endocrinol.*, 72:73P.
182. Hillarp, N. A., Olivecrona, H., and Silferskiöld, W. (1954): Evidence for the participation of the preoptic area in male mating behaviour. *Experientia*, 10:224–225.
183. Willmore, L. J., Hurd, R. W., and Sypert, G. W. (1978): Epileptiform activity initiated by pial iontophoresis of ferrous and ferric chloride on rat cerebral cortex. *Brain Res.*, 152:406–410.
184. Willmore, L. J., Hiramatsu, M., Kochi, H., and Mori, A. (1983): Formation of superoxide radicals after $FeCl_3$ injection into rat isocortex. *Brain Res.*, 277:393–396.
185. Tejasen, T., and Everett, J. W. (1967): Surgical analysis of the preoptico-tuberal pathway controlling ovulatory release of gonadotropins in the rat. *Endocrinology*, 81:1387–1396.
186. Everett, J. W., and Tyrey, L. (1977): Induction of LH release and ovulation in rats by radiofrequency lesions of the medial basal tuber cinereum. *Anat. Rec.*, 187:575 (abstract).
187. Everett, J. W., Quinn, D. L., and Tyrey, L. (1976): Comparative effectiveness of preoptic and tuberal stimulation for luteinizing hormone release and ovulation in two strains of rats. *Endocrinology*, 98:1302–1308.
188. Gosden, R. G., Everett, J. W., and Tyrey, L. (1976): Luteinizing hormone requirement for ovulation in the pentobarbital-treated proestrous rat. *Endocrinology*, 99:1046–1053.
189. Everett, J. W., and Tyrey, L. (1981): Comparative increments of circulating luteinizing hormone in rats with increasing duration of electrical stimulation in medial preoptic or medial basal tuberal sites. *Endocrinology*, 109:691–696.
190. Fink, G., and Jamieson, M. G. (1976): Immunoreactive luteinizing hormone releasing factor in rat pituitary stalk blood: effects of electrical stimulation of the medial preoptic area. *J. Endocrinol.*, 68:71–87.
191. Cramer, O. M., and Barraclough, C. A. (1971): Effect of electrical stimulation of the preoptic area on plasma LH concentrations in proestrous rats. *Endocrinology*, 88:1175–1183.
192. Everett, J. W., and Tyrey, L. (1982): Similarity of luteinizing hormone surges induced by medial preoptic stimulation in female rats blocked with pentobarbital, morphine, chlorpromazine, or atropine. *Endocrinology*, 111:1979–1985.
193. Aiyer, M. S., Chiappa, S. A., and Fink, G. (1974): A priming effect of luteinizing hormone releasing factor on the anterior pituitary gland in the female rat. *J. Endocrinol.*, 62:573–588.

194. Fink, G., Chiappa, S. A., and Aiyer, M. S. (1976): Priming effect of luteinizing hormone releasing factor elicited by preoptic stimulation and by intravenous infusion and multiple injections of the synthetic peptide. *J. Endocrinol.*, 69:359–372.
195. Pickering, A. J. M. C., and Fink, G. (1979): Priming effect of luteinizing hormone releasing factor *in vitro:* role of protein synthesis, contractile elements, Ca^{++} and cyclic AMP. *J. Endocrinol.*, 81:223–234.
196. Grieg, F., and Weisz, J. (1973): Preovulatory levels of luteinizing hormone, the critical period and ovulation in rats. *J. Endocrinol.*, 57:235–245.
197. Weick, R. F., Dierschke, D. J., Karsch, F. J., Butler, W. R., Hotchkiss, J., and Knobil, E. (1973): Periovulatory time courses of circulating gonadotropic and ovarian hormones in the rhesus monkey. *Endocrinology*, 93:1140–1147.
198. Westman, A., and Jacobsohn, D. (1936): Über Ovarialveränderungen beim Kaninchen nach Hypophysektomie. *Acta Obstet. Gynecol. Scand.*, 16:483–508.
199. Hilliard, J., Haywood, J. N., and Sawyer, C. H. (1964): Postcoital patterns of secretion of pituitary gonadotropin and ovarian progestin in the rabbit. *Endocrinology*, 75:957–963.
200. Beard, J. (1898): The rhythm of reproduction in animals. *Anat. Anz.*, 14:97–102.
201. Loeb, L. (1911): Über die Bedeutung des Corpus luteum für die Periodizität des sexuellen Zyklus beim weiblichen Säugetierorganismus. *Dtsch. Med. Wochenschr.*, 37:17–21.
202. Drummond-Robinson, G., and Asdell, S. A. (1926): The relation between the corpus luteum and the mammary gland. *J. Physiol. (Lond.)*, 61:608–614.
203. Hammond, J. (1927): *The Physiology of Reproduction in the Cow.* Cambridge University Press, Cambridge.
204. Papanicolaou, G. N. (1920): Effect of removal of corpora lutea and ripe follicles on oestrous periodicity in guinea pigs. *Anat. Rec.*, 19:251 (abstract).
205. Papanicolaou, G. N. (1926): A specific inhibitory hormone of the corpus luteum. *JAMA*, 86:1422–1424.
206. Parkes, A. S., and Bellerby, C. W. (1928): Studies on the internal secretion of the ovary. V. The oestrus-inhibiting function of the corpus luteum. *J. Physiol. (Lond.)*, 64:233–245.
207. Gley, P. (1928): Sur l'inhibition de l'ovulation par le corps jaune. *C. R. Soc. Biol. (Paris)*, 98:504–505.
208. Selye, H., Browne, J. S. L., and Collip, J. B. (1936): Effects of large doses of progesterone in the female rat. *Proc. Soc. Exp. Biol. Med.* 34:472–474.
209. Dempsey, E. W. (1937): Follicular growth rate and ovulation after various experimental procedures in the guinea pig. *Am. J. Physiol.*, 120:126–132.
210. Kennedy, W. P. (1925): Corpus luteum extracts and ovulation in the rabbit. *Q. J. Exp. Physiol.*, 15:103–112.
211. Mahnert, A. (1930): Weitere Untersuchungen über die Beziehungen zwischen Hypophysenvorderlappen und Ovarium. Zugleich ein Beitrag zur Frage der hormonalen Sterilisierung. *Zentralbl. Gynaekol.*, 54:2883–2887.
212. Makepeace, A. W., Weinstein, G. L., and Friedman, M. H. (1937): The effect of progestin and progesterone on ovulation in the rabbit. *Am. J. Physiol.*, 119:512–516.
213. Moore, C. R., and Price, D. (1932): Gonad hormone functions and the reciprocal influence between gonads and hypophysis. *Am. J. Anat.*, 50:13–72.
214. Engle, E. T. (1931): The pituitary gonadal relationship and the problem of precocious sexual maturity. *Endocrinology*, 15:405–420.
215. Hohlweg, W. (1934): Veränderungen des Hypophysenvorderlappens und des Ovariums nach Behandlungen mit grossen Dosen von Follikelhormonen. *Klin. Wochenschr.*, 13:92–95.
216. Hohlweg, W. (1975): The regulatory centers of endocrine glands in the hypothalamus. In: *Pioneers in Neuroendocrinology, Vol. 1,* edited by J. Meites, B. Donovan, and S. M. McCann, pp. 161–172. Plenum Press, New York.
217. Hammond, J., Jr., Hammond, J., and Parkes, A. S. (1942): Hormonal augmentation of fertility in sheep. I. Induction of ovulation, superovulation, and heat in sheep. *J. Agric. Sci.*, 32:308–323.
218. Hammond, J., Jr. (1945): Induced ovulation and heat in anestrous sheep. *J. Endocrinol.*, 4:169–180.
219. Casida, L. E. (1946): Induction of ovulation and subsequent fertility in domestic animals. In: *The Problem of Fertility,* edited by E. T. Engle, pp. 49–59. Princeton University Press, Princeton.
220. Everett, J. W. (1948): Progesterone and estrogen in the experimental control of ovulation time and other features of the estrous cycle in the rat. *Endocrinology*, 43:389–405.
221. Everett, J. W. (1947): Hormonal factors responsible for deposition of cholesterol in the corpus luteum of the rat. *Endocrinology*, 41:364–377.
222. Everett, J. W., and Nichols, D. C. (1968): The timing of ovulatory release of gonadotropin induced by estrogen in pseudopregnant and diestrous cyclic rats. *Anat. Rec.*, 160:346 (abstract).
223. Everett, J. W., Sawyer, C. H., and Markee, J. E. (1949): A neurogenic timing factor in control of the ovulatory discharge of luteinizing hormone in the cyclic rat. *Endocrinology*, 44:234–250.
224. Everett, J. W. (1940): The restoration of ovulatory cycles and corpus luteum formation in persistent-estrous rats by progesterone. *Endocrinology*, 27:681–686.
225. Everett, J. W. (1943): Further studies on the relationship of progesterone to ovulation and luteinization in the persistent-estrous rat. *Endocrinology*, 32:285–292.
226. Everett, J. W., and Sawyer, C. H. (1949): A neural timing factor in the mechanism by which progesterone advances ovulation in the cyclic rat. *Endocrinology*, 45:581–595.
227. Zeilmaker, G. H. (1966): The biphasic effect of progesterone on ovulation in the rat. *Acta Endocrinol.*, 51:461–468.
228. Everett, J. W. (1951): Effects of estrogen-progesterone synergy on thresholds and timing of the "LH-release apparatus" of the female rat. *Anat. Rec.*, 109:291 (abstract).
229. Redmond, W. C. (1968): Ovulatory response to brain stimulation or exogenous luteinizing hormone in progesterone-treated rats. *Endocrinology*, 83:1013–1022.
230. Caligaris, L., Astrada, J. J., and Taleisnik, S. (1971): Biphasic effect of progesterone on the release of gonadotropin in rats. *Endocrinology*, 89:331–337.
231. Sawyer, C. H., and Everett, J. W. (1959): Stimulatory and inhibitory effects of progesterone on the release of pituitary ovulatory hormone in the rabbit. *Endocrinology*, 65:644–651.
232. Kawakami, M., and Sawyer, C. H. (1959): Neuroendocrine correlates of changes in brain activity thresholds by sex steroids and pituitary hormones. *Endocrinology*, 65:652–668.
233. Dierschke, D. J., Bhattacharya, A. N., Atkinson, L. E., and Knobil, E. (1970): Circhoral oscillations of plasma LH levels in the ovariectomized monkey. *Endocrinology*, 87:850–853.
234. Brinkley, H. J. (1981): Endocrine signaling and female reproduction. *Biol. Reprod.*, 24:22–43.
235. Knobil, E. (1981): Patterns of hypophysiotropic signals and gonadotropin secretion in the rhesus monkey. *Biol. Reprod.*, 24:44–49.
236. Knobil, E. (1980): The neuroendocrine control of the menstrual cycle. *Recent Prog. Horm. Res.*, 36:53–88.
237. Blake, C. A. (1976): Simulation of the proestrous luteinizing hormone (LH) surge after infusion of LH-releasing hormone in phenobarbital-blocked rats. *Endocrinology*, 98:451–460.
238. Weick, R. F. (1981): The pulsatile nature of luteinizing hormone secretion. *Can. J. Physiol. Pharmacol.*, 59:779–785.
239. Wise, P. M., Rance, N., Barr, G. D., and Barraclough, C. A. (1979): Further evidence that luteinizing hormone-releasing hormone also is follicle-stimulating hormone-releasing hormone. *Endocrinology*, 104:940–947.
240. Carmel, P. W., Araki, S., and Ferin, M. (1976): Pituitary stalk portal blood collection in rhesus monkeys: evidence for pulsatile release of gonadotropin-releasing hormone. *Endocrinology*, 99:243–248.
241. Nett, T. M., Akbar, A. M., and Niswender, G. D. (1974): Serum levels of luteinizing hormone and gonadotropin-releasing hormone in cycling, castrated and anestrous ewes. *Endocrinology*, 94:713–718.
242. Savoy-Moore, R. T., and Schwartz, N. B. (1980): Differential control of FSH and LH secretion. In: *Reproductive Physiology III, International Review of Physiology, Vol. 22,* edited by R. O. Greep, pp. 203–248. University Park Press, Baltimore.
243. Wildt, L., Häusler, A., Marshall, G., Hutchison, J. S., Plant, T. M., Belchetz, P. E., and Knobil, E. (1981): Frequency and ampli-

tude of gonadotropin-releasing hormone stimulation and gonadotropin secretion in the rhesus monkey. *Endocrinology,* 109:376–385.

244. Dufy, B., Dufy-Barbe, L., Vincent, J. D., and Knobil, E. (1979): Étude électrophysiologique des neurones hypothalamiques et régulation gonadotrope chez de singe rhesus. *J. Physiol. (Paris),* 75:105–108.
245. Kalra, S. P. (1986): Neural circuitry involved in the control of LHRH secretion: a model for preovulatory LH release. In: *Frontiers in Neuroendocrinology,* edited by W. F. Ganong and L. Martini, pp. 203–246. Raven Press, New York.
246. Gallo, R. V. (1981): Pulsatile LH release during the ovulatory LH surge on proestrus in the rat. *Biol. Reprod.,* 24:100–104.
247. Cogen, P. H., Antunes, J. L., Louis, K. M., Dyrenfurth, I., and Ferin, M. (1980): The effects of anterior hypothalamic disconnection on gonadotropin secretion in the female rhesus monkey. *Endocrinology,* 107:677–683.
248. Knobil, E., Plant, T. M., Wildt, L., Belchetz, P. E., and Marshall, G. (1980): Control of the rhesus monkey menstrual cycle: permissive role of hypothalamic gonadotropin-releasing hormone. *Science,* 207:1371–1373.
249. Neill, J. D., Patton, J. M., Dailey, R. A., Tsou, R. C., and Tindall, G. T. (1977): Luteinizing hormone releasing hormone (LHRH) in pituitary stalk blood of rhesus monkeys: relationship to level of LH release. *Endocrinology,* 101:430–434.
250. Norman, R. L., Gliessman, P., Lindstrom, S. A., Hill, J., and Spies, H. G. (1982): Reinitiation of ovulatory cycles in pituitary stalk-sectioned rhesus monkeys: evidence for a specific hypothalamic message for the preovulatory release of luteinizing hormone. *Endocrinology,* 111:1874–1882.
251. Terasawa, E., Rodriguez, J. S., Bridson, W. E., and Wiegand, S. J. (1979): Factors influencing the positive feedback action of estrogen upon the luteinizing hormone surge in the ovariectomized guinea pig. *Endocrinology,* 104:680–686.
252. Terasawa, E., King, M. K., Wiegand, S. J., Bridson, W. E., and Goy, R. W. (1979): Barbiturate anesthesia blocks the positive feedback effect of progesterone, but not of estrogen, on luteinizing hormone release in ovariectomized guinea pigs. *Endocrinology,* 104:687–692.
253. Caligaris, L., Astrada, J. J., and Taleisnik, S. (1971): Release of luteinizing hormone induced by estrogen injection into ovariectomized rats. *Endocrinology,* 88:810–815.
254. Legan, S. J., Coon, G. A., and Karsch, F. J. (1975): Role of estrogen as initiator of daily LH surges in the ovariectomized rat. *Endocrinology,* 96:50–56.
255. Wise, P. M., Camp-Grossman, P., and Barraclough, C. A. (1981): Effects of estradiol and progesterone on plasma gonadotropins, prolactin, and LHRH in specific brain areas of ovariectomized rats. *Biol. Reprod.,* 24:820–830.
256. Banks, J. A., and Freeman, M. E. (1978): The temporal requirement of progesterone on proestrus for extinction of the estrogen-induced daily signal controlling luteinizing hormone release in the rat. *Endocrinology,* 102:426–432.
257. DePaolo, L. V., and Barraclough, C. A. (1979): Dose-dependent effects of progesterone on the facilitation and inhibition of spontaneous gonadotropin surges in estrogen treated ovariectomized rats. *Biol. Reprod.,* 21:1015–1023.
258. Norman, R. L., Blake, C. A., and Sawyer, C. H. (1973): Estrogen-dependent twenty-four-hour periodicity in pituitary LH release in the female hamster. *Endocrinology,* 93:965–970.
259. Norman, R. L., and Spies, H. G. (1974): Neural control of the estrogen-dependent twenty-four-hour periodicity of LH release in the golden hamster. *Endocrinology,* 95:1367–1372.
260. Stetson, M. H., Watson-Whitmyre, M., and Matt, K. S. (1978): Cyclic gonadotropin release in the presence and absence of estrogenic feedback in ovariectomized golden hamsters. *Biol. Reprod.,* 19:40–50.
261. Seegal, R. F., and Goldman, B. D. (1975): Effects of photoperiod on cyclicity and serum gonadotropins in the Syrian hamster. *Biol. Reprod.,* 12:223–231.
262. Bridges, R. D., and Goldman, B. D. (1975): Diurnal rhythms in gonadotropins and progesterone in lactating and photoperiod induced acyclic hamsters. *Biol. Reprod.,* 13:617–622.
263. Schwartz, N. B. (1982): Role of ovarian inhibin (folliculostatin) in regulating FSH secretion in the female rat. In: *Intraovarian Control Mechanisms,* edited by C. P. Channing and S. J. Segal, pp. 15–36. Plenum Press, New York.
264. Thomas, C. L., Jr., and Nikitovitch-Winer, M. B. (1984): Complete suppression of plasma follicle-stimulating hormone in castrated male and female rats during continuous administration of porcine follicular fluid. *Biol. Reprod.,* 30:427–433.
265. Miller, W. L., and Huang, E. S. R. (1985): Secretion of ovine luteinizing hormone *in vitro:* differential positive control by 17β-estradiol and a preparation of porcine ovarian inhibin. *Endocrinology,* 117:907–911.

The Physiology of Reproduction,
edited by E. Knobil and J. Neill *et al.*
Raven Press, Ltd., New York © 1988.

CHAPTER 27

The Anatomy of the Hypothalamo-Hypophyseal Complex

Robert B. Page

Consider the pituitary gland as did Harvey Cushing 75 years ago (1). The pituitary gland that Cushing saw differed from that seen by others. It was defined by a dictionary of the time as ". . . a small bilobed body of unknown function attached to the infundibulum at the base of the brain" (2). Common wisdom of the day held it to be a vestigial organ. Cushing saw a structure composed of neural and epithelial elements lying in the sella turcica in the base of the skull. He realized that the epithelial component developed from an oral pouch that was derived from the ectoderm of the primitive mouth (3) and not from the entoderm of the primitive foregut as initially proposed by Rathke. Cushing further realized that the epithelial portion, the anterior lobe, was organized in a glandular pattern (4,5) and that its cells could be differentiated into chromophobes and chromophiles on the basis of their staining affinity for hematoxylin and eosin dyes (1). He observed that the anterior lobe of the gland was very vascular and that its glandular cells assumed an intimate relationship with its sinusoids. His understanding of the blood supply to the pituitary was based on the studies of Dandy and Goetsch (6), which were carried out under his direction. They described an arterial supply to the canine anterior lobe that arose from the vessels of the circle of Willis and coursed centripetally over the tuber cinereum to supply it at its junction with the anterior lobe. They saw the venous drainage of the anterior lobe to be directed toward the base of the brain (6). Based upon the writings of Claude Bernard (1853) and of Brown-Sequard (1856), who had proposed that one cell could secrete "on its own account certain products or special ferments which influence all other cells of the body by a mechanism other than the central nervous system," and upon his experience with patients suffering from acromegaly (7), Cushing (1) came to believe that the anterior lobe of the pituitary body was a gland of internal secretion and that a tumor of this apparently insignificant organ might cause profound changes in body habitus and metabolism because it released its secretion into the bloodstream in excessive amounts.

Cushing recognized that acromegaly was not the uniform result of a tumor of the anterior lobe of the pituitary. Some patients with pituitary tumors developed adiposal-genital dystrophy and died (8). To test the hypothesis that this syndrome might be due to destruction of the gland, with a consequent reduction or cessation of its secretions, he began a series of ablative experiments on dogs in the newly established Hunterian Laboratory at the Johns Hopkins Hospital (9). He was able to demonstrate that the anterior lobe was necessary to support the structure and function of the gonads, adrenals, and thyroid, to support the normal growth of the young animal, and to support even life itself. The injection or ingestion of pituitary extracts did not reverse the effect of hypophysectomy. His attempt to reverse the deficits produced by hypophysectomy by transplanting the pituitary gland (to the rectus sheath, to bone marrow, or to brain) met with only limited success (10). He was able to establish that in cases of partial ablation of the gland, the transplant seemed to support the dog (which otherwise would have died) until the remaining fragments could recover and hypertrophy. Although it was not until almost 20 years later that P. E. Smith (11) was able to reverse all the deficits caused by hypophysectomy in rats by the injection of pituitary extract, Cushing (1) in 1912 clearly saw the anterior lobe of the pituitary as a ductless gland that synthetized hormones and secreted them into the bloodstream that carried them toward the brain. These secretions of the anterior lobe of the pituitary gland supported the function of the other ductless glands and permitted normal body growth.

In 1912 Cushing (1) realized that most of the posterior lobe (the neural portion of the pituitary gland) was derived from the brain (3), but he included the pars intermedia with the neural lobe under the rubric of the "posterior lobe." He saw colloid in the posterior lobe as had Herring (4) when he examined the posterior lobe histologically (1) (Fig. 1). He proposed, on the basis of the analogy with the thyroid, that colloid, now called "Herring bodies," was a secretion of the posterior lobe; but he believed it was a secretion of the pars intermedia, not of the pars nervosa. The pars nervosa (along with the cervical sympathetics) served to innervate the pars intermedia (1,12). His visualization of colloid on microscopic examination within the pars intermedia, the neural lobe, beneath the ependyma of the diencephalic floor, and apparently bursting into the third ventricle convinced him that the posterior lobe secreted directly to the brain (13). The paucity of blood vessels in the posterior lobe (6) reinforced his belief that the secretions of the neural lobe entered the third ventricle, not the circulation.

To determine the function of the posterior lobe, he performed either hypophysectomies, selective ablation of the anterior or posterior lobes, or selective stimulations of these regions of the pituitary gland in dogs. On the basis of these experiments, Cushing proposed that the posterior lobe secretions caused glucosuria, whereas their absence resulted in a rise in glucose tolerance (14). This surmise was strengthened by his finding that stimulation of the pars nervosa or of the superior cervical ganglion, both of which structures he envisioned as innervating the intermediate lobe (1,12), caused glucosuria (15). He was aware that a vasopressor effect of posterior lobe extract had been reported (16,17) as had an oxytotic effect (18). He accepted these observations as true, but thought these roles were subordinate to the role of the posterior lobe in glucose metabolism. He did not accept the proposal that the posterior lobe secreted an antidiuretic substance. As late as 1930 he stated "too much attention has been paid to the symptoms of thirst and polyuria, and too little to the symptoms of the opposite of these, oliguria having been observed not infrequently as a sequel of our early (1908–1910) canine hypophysectomies" (2). In 1912 Cushing (1) saw the posterior lobe as a gland (the pars intermedia) that was innervated principally

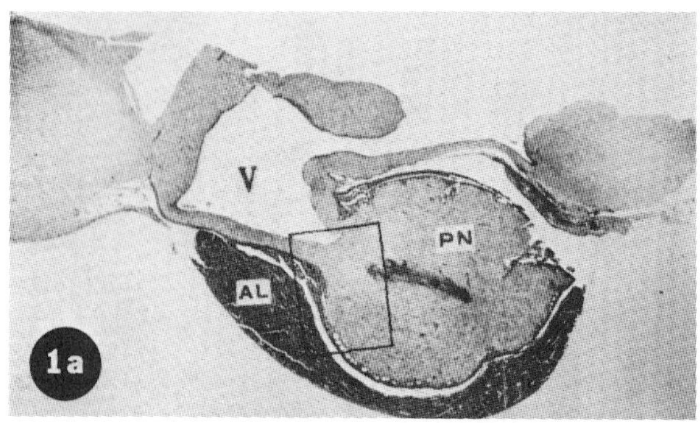

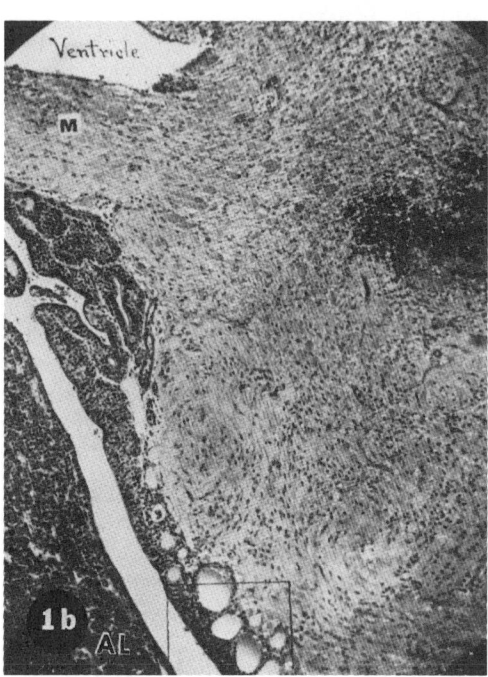

FIG. 1. (a) Midsagittal section of canine pituitary gland. Note layer of colloid globules arising from the epithelial investment of the pars nervosa (PN). Anterior lobe (AL) is separated from posterior lobe by cleft. (V) Third ventricle. **(b)** Enlargement of squared-off area in Fig. 1a. Anterior lobe (AL) is separated by cleft from investment of pars nervosa containing colloid masses. (Reprinted from ref 1.)

by the pars nervosa. Hormones synthesized in the pars intermedia were carried through the pars nervosa to the third ventricle and functioned to regulate glucose metabolism, vascular tone, and uterine contractions.

In the intervening years from 1912 to 1930, when he delivered the Lister Memorial Lecture (2), Cushing clung to these two tenets: that the anterior lobe released its secretions into blood vessels draining toward the brain, and that the posterior lobe released its secretions into the third ventricle. The discovery of a portal system in the pituitary gland by Popa and Fielding (19,20) did not alter his convictions. It was based upon his concept that the anterior and posterior lobes each received an independent blood supply and the posterior lobe drained to the cavernous sinus (6); but, it supplied a (portal) route by which anterior pituitary secretions could be delivered to the brain prior to being delivered to the remainder of the body (see ref. 21 for review). He continued to believe that the posterior lobe was a special brain gland whose secretory cells in the pars intermedia were innervated by the pars nervosa and that it released its secretions into the brain's ventricular system (22).

In those intervening years, he had become aware that in some unknown fashion the hypothalamus and the pituitary gland are inextricably joined. The accepted belief at that time held that the secretions of the posterior lobe were synthesized there in glial cells of the pars nervosa (23,24), in epithelial cells of the pars intermedia (22), or in glandular cells in the neural lobe (25) (for review, see ref. 26). As early as 1912, Cushing had been aware of the report of Cajal (1894) describing a neural tract that originated in the hypothalamus and ended in the neural lobe (1). He cited reports of Greving (1926) and of Pines (1928) describing a fiber tract passing from the supraoptic nuclei (SON) and paraventricular nuclei (PVN) to the neural lobe, but he persisted in thinking that this tract innervated the pars intermedia (2). The function of the supraoptico-hypophyseal tract (SOHT) remained unsuspected (27,28). He acknowledged that diabetes insipidus could be caused by making tuberal lesions in rats which interrupted the SOHT and could be cured by giving the rats posterior lobe extract; but he did not accept the significance of this observation. Although he misunderstood the means by which the hypothalamus-regulated posterior lobe functions, he realized that "it is highly improbable that two corresponding effects should be produced, the one by a hypothalamic lesion, the other by removing the source of chemical messages, in the absence of any functional interaction" (2).

Cushing also noted that the brain apparently controlled certain aspects of anterior lobe function, such as ovulation in the rabbit, because it regularly follows 10 hr after copulation in that species and hence resembles a reflex act. He became further aware of the role of the diencephalon in regulating sympathetic tone, alertness, body temperature, body habitus, and sexual function from caring for patients with tumors that invaded the third ventricle and hypothalamus, such as gliomas of the optic chiasm and craniopharyngiomas, but spared the pituitary gland. Their occurrence brought home to Cushing the realization that there is an "interdependence of the diencephalon and the pituitary body," which he explained in the following manner. Nerves in the diencephalon projecting to the pituitary gland through the SOHT stimulate the release of substances from the pars intermedia in the posterior lobe that are transported directly into the third ventricle, where they influence neural centers in its walls. Discharge from these diencephalic centers activates sympathetic mechanisms that stimulate glandular cells in the anterior lobe through the cervical sympathetic plexus. In his picture the peripheral sympathetic nervous system was the final common pathway to the epithelial cells of the anterior lobe of the pituitary and to the epithelial cells of the adrenal medulla, as well as to the smooth muscle cells of the intestines and the blood vessels (2). Unknown to Cushing, forces were marshaling which would undo many of his concepts and change the way investigators see the pituitary gland.

To see the gland as most see it today, it is necessary to start with a consideration of the work of Wislocki and King (29). Published 6 years after Cushing's last public lecture on the pituitary gland, their work challenged several of his basic concepts. They stressed the observation that the pituitary gland and viscera stained after the intravascular injection of acid vital dyes into monkeys, cats, and rabbits, whereas the brain (with the exception of the choroid plexus and several small regions surrounding the third ventricle and the area postrema of the IV ventricle) did not. The contents of the third ventricle were not stained following the intravascular injection with acid dyes, even when the neural lobe was heavily stained. They thus demonstrated that substances could enter, and presumably leave, the neural portion of the hypophysis by vascular routes, but that it was unlikely that substances in the neurohypophysis were discharged into the third ventricle. Wislocki and King (29) also studied the vascular anatomy of the pituitary. They made intravascular injections of monkeys, rabbits, and rats with India ink and examined either serial sections of the injected gland or whole mounts after clearing the tissue. They concluded that they could not corroborate Popa and Fielding's (19,20) observations that a large artery arising from each supraclinoid carotid artery supplies the pars distalis and that large venules connect the pars distalis to the hypothalamus. Their report erased a picture of the pituitary gland that had been held for almost 30 years. Neither the neural nor the glandular portion of the pituitary could discharge their contents directly to the brain. A new concept had to be developed.

Wislocki and King (29) provided the basis for it. First, they noted that the eminentia saccularis (the median eminence of the tuber cinereum or the infundibulum) was stained, as were the anterior and posterior lobes, after the intravascular injection of acid dyes, whereas the tuber cinereum was not. They proposed that the median eminence should, as a consequence of this similarity with the pituitary gland, be classified as part of it. In this schema, based upon the observation that the hypophysis lacks a blood-brain barrier, the neurohypophysis is composed of the infundibulum (median eminence, eminentia saccularis), infundibular stem, and infundibular process (neural lobe). The adenohypophysis is composed of the pars tuberalis (applied to the infundibulum and infundibular stem), the pars intermedia (applied to the infundibular stem and infundibular process), and the pars distalis (anterior lobe) (29,30). This classification recognizes that the pituitary gland lies not only within the sella turcica (the lower infundibular stem and infundibular process with the pars intermedia and the pars distalis) but also in the subarachnoid space and is applied to the base of the brain (the median eminence and upper infundibular stem with the pars tuberalis). Wislocki and King (29) observed, after the intravascular injection of vital dyes, that the boundary of the stained pituitary gland with the unstained hypothalamus is located at the level of the tubero-infundibular sulcus. This sulcus, which separates the tuber cinereum of the hypothalamus from the infundibulum, not from the diaphragm sella, forms the rostral boundary of the pituitary gland (Fig. 2).

Second, they correctly surmised the direction of blood flow in the portal system and suggested its role in control of anterior pituitary function. They described superior hypophyseal arteries in the monkey that arose from the supraclinoid internal carotid arteries and the vessels of the circle of Willis. These vessels approached the eminentia saccularis (median eminence) and pituitary stalk (pars tuberalis and infundibular stem) and the rostral pole of the pars distalis. The superior hypophyseal arteries bifurcated, sending one branch to the pars distalis and one branch to the infundibular stem and median eminence. The capillary bed in the median eminence and upper part of the infundibular stem was fed by the superior hypophyseal arteries. It was drained by portal vessels that discharged their contents into a secondary capillary bed in the pars distalis. The pars distalis, in turn, drained into the adjacent cavernous sinuses

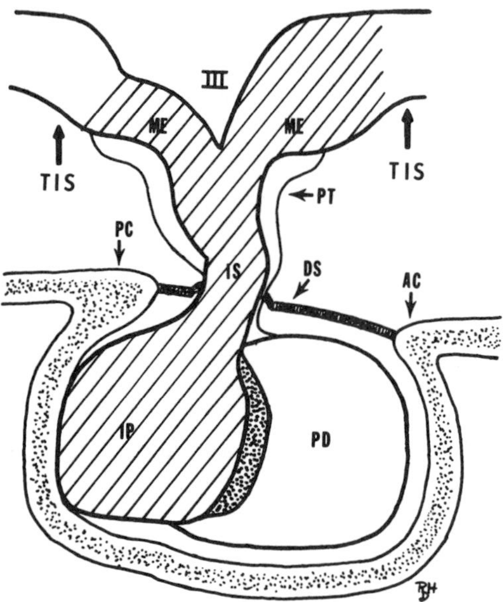

FIG. 2. Diagrammatic midsagittal section of the human pituitary gland. The neurohypophysis (hatching) consists of the median eminence (ME) (or infundibulum), infundibular stem (IS) and infundibular process (IP) (or neural lobe). The adenohypophysis consists of the pars tuberalis (PT), which is applied to the ME and IS and lies in the subarachnoid space above the diaphragm sella (DS) and the pars distalis (PD), which lies within the sella turcica beneath the DS. The region corresponding to the pars intermedia of other forms is indicated by the stippled area between the PD and the IP. (AC) Anterior clinoid; (PC) posterior clinoid; (III) third ventricle; (TIS) tubero-infundibular sulcus. (From ref. 872.)

via lateral hypophyseal veins. The pars distalis, according to the account of Wislocki and King (29), resembled the liver receiving both an arterial and a venous blood supply. They surmised that the direction of blood flow through the portal vessels had to be from the median eminence to the pars distalis, since they could demonstrate no significant outflow routes from the median eminence to the vessels at the base of the brain. The only apparent outflow was from the median eminence to the pars distalis, which could, in turn, drain to the adjacent cavernous sinuses via lateral hypophyseal veins (Fig. 3).

Third, they saw the circulation of the neural lobe as isolated from that of the portal system. They described the origin and course of the inferior hypophyseal arteries from the intracavernous segment of the carotid arteries to the infundibular process and the paired venous structures (inferior hypophyseal veins) that drained it. The function of the neural lobe had been clarified by 1936. In 1924 Starling and Verney (31) had reported that posterior-lobe extract corrected diabetes insipidus, reduced urinary flow, and raised urinary solute concentration. The posterior (neural) lobe was also recognized to play a role in the regulation of blood pressure (16) and to stimulate uterine contractions (18). Its structure was by then clear. The neural lobe contained axons and terminals of the SOHT, specialized glial cells called *pituicytes,* and blood vessels (27,28). With the demonstration, by Ingram and his co-workers (32–34), that lesions of the SOHT caused diabetes insipidus, atrophy of the neural lobe, and degeneration of cell bodies in the supraoptic nucleus, it became apparent that the SOHT regulated, in some unknown manner, the release of hormones from the neural lobe.

Ernest and Berte Scharrer provided the answer to this puzzle, explaining not only how the brain regulates neural lobe function (35,36), but (by extension of their ideas) also how it regulates adenohypophyseal function. The concept of neurosecretion, first promulgated by E. Scharrer, received support from the observations of Palay (37), who found the presence of a colloid material, stainable with silver or Masson's trichrome technique, that was unique to the preoptico-hypophyseal tract of the goldfish (a tract analogous to the SOHT of mammals). Bargmann and Hild (38) found that the chrome-alum-hematoxylin technique of Gomori selectively stained neurosecretory (colloid) material within the SOHT, as it selectively stained secretory material in the islet cells of the pancreas. One the basis of finding stainable neurosecretory material in the cell bodies of large cells in the supraoptic nucleus and of finding this material in the axons of these cells and in their terminals in the neural lobe, Bargmann and Scharrer (39) proposed that hormones released from the posterior lobe of the pituitary were not synthesized there. They were synthesized in the supraoptic nucleus of the hypothalamus, transported down their axons to their terminals in the posterior lobe, and were released from these terminals into the bloodstream. Cushing had seen stainable (colloid) material in the neural lobe and proposed,

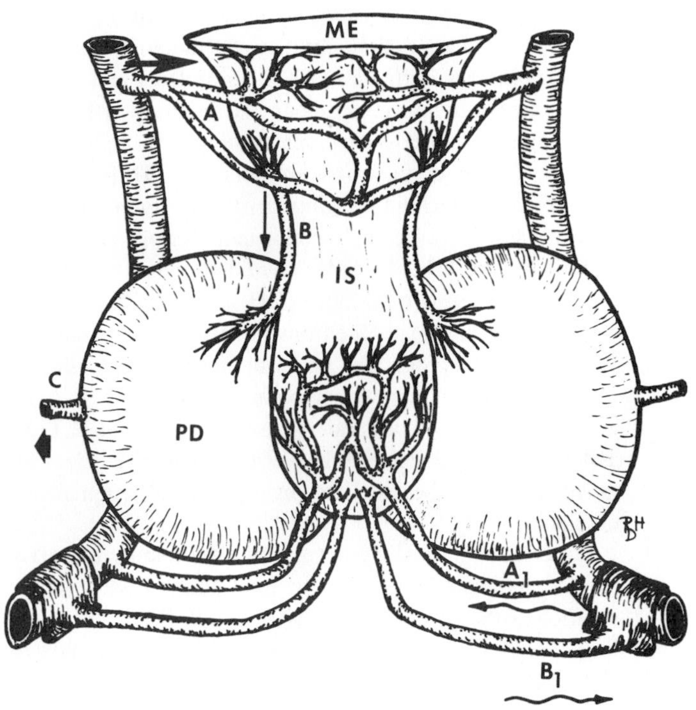

FIG. 3. Classical schema of pituitary blood flow proposed by Wislocki and King (29). Blood enters the median eminence (ME) at point A through superior hypophyseal arteries (*large arrow*). It passes through the ME primary capillary plexus and drains (*small arrow*) through portal vessels (B) to the secondary capillary plexus in the pars distalis (PD). From the PD, blood drains through lateral hypophyseal veins (C) to the cavernous sinus (*arrowhead*). Blood enters the neural lobe through inferior hypophyseal arteries (A_1). It drains from the neural lobe through inferior hypophyseal veins (B_1). (IS) Infundibular stem. (From ref. 558.)

on the basis of analogy with the thyroid, that it was a secretion of the pars intermedia in the posterior lobe. Because he saw few vessels in the posterior lobe and because he saw colloid bursting into the third ventricle, he came to believe that the neural lobe secreted to the brain. Scharrer saw similar material within nerves lying in the hypothalamus and in their terminals in the neural lobe. Based upon the analogy with the neurosecretory system of insects and the knowledge that the neural lobe lacked a blood-brain barrier but possessed direct venous connections to the cavernous sinuses, he proposed the (correct) mechanism by which the brain controls pituitary function. He saw that secretions of the neural lobe were made in the hypothalamus, transported to the neural lobe, and released into the circulation. Each looked at the pituitary and saw a different organ.

Scharrer broadened the scope of his histological observations (40–42), but it was the biochemical and physiological investigations of others that confirmed his seminal concept. The neural lobe hormone responsible for uterine contraction and for milk injection was identified as oxytocin (OT) (43,44). The neural lobe hormone responsible for antidiuresis was identified as arginine vasopressin (AVP) (45–47). They were found not only in the neural lobe of the pituitary but also in the hypothalamic supraoptic (and paraventricular) nuclei (48). Subsequent anatomical and physiological studies have demonstrated that oxytocin and vasopressin are synthesized in separate cell bodies lying in the supraoptic and paraventricular nuclei, transported down the axons of the SOHT to their axon terminals in the neural lobe, and released into the systemic circulation in response to appropriate stimulation (49–64).

Harris (65) pursued the observation that, in the rabbit, ovulation reflexly follows copulation. He induced ovulation by stimulation of the hypothalamus but not the pituitary. The mechanism could not be a direct neural innervation of glandular cells because the pars distalis lacked nerves other than those terminating on vessels (66). In 1947 Green and Harris (67) proposed that there was a neurovascular link between axons terminating in the median eminence and glandular cells in the pars distalis. This link was provided by the portal vessels on the anterior surface of the pituitary stalk. Green and Harris supported their proposal with the following observations: (a) Nerves terminating in the median eminence and upper infundibular stem are in close contact with capillaries that drain into portal vessels (67,68); (b) blood flowed through portal vessels of living animals (frogs and rats) from the median eminence to the pars distalis (69,70); (c) stimulation of the hypothalamus caused ovulation in the anesthetized (65) and unanesthetized rabbit (71); (d) stalk section disrupted trophic function of gland and disrupted estrous cycles, but trophic function and estrous cycles returned if portal vessels were permitted to regenerate (72–74); (e) functional grafting of the excised pituitary gland only occurred if the excised portion was replaced beneath the median eminence and the portal vessels were permitted to regenerate (75,76). Harris (21,77), in monographs published in 1948 and 1955, summarized the extant evidence that the anterior pituitary is regulated by the brain.

The findings of Green and Harris gained more significance when it was appreciated that a portal vascular system characteristically links the median eminence with the pars distalis in vertebrates (66,78–80), including humans (81–83). Although Harris (84) reported there was an independent arterial supply to the pars distalis of the rabbit [in addition to the portal (venous) supply], Green (66) could not identify a separate arterial supply to the pars distalis in 76 other species. Reexamination of the vascular supply of the rabbit pituitary, employing scanning electron microscopy of vascular casts (85), failed to confirm Harris's findings. Contrary to Wislocki's belief (29,86–89), the pars distalis does not appear to have a dual blood supply as does the liver. It appears to be bathed entirely by blood that has passed through the neurohypophysis.

Stalk-section experiments strengthened the case for a neurovascular link and further weakened the case for a separate arterial supply to the pars distalis. Such sections divided the SOHT, which linked cells of the supraoptic nucleus with their terminals in the neural lobe; they also divided the portal vessels, which linked terminals in the median eminence with glandular cells in the pars distalis. Stalk section transiently disrupts neural-lobe function until regeneration of divided axons, or establishment of new neurohemal contacts, can occur (90–94). With interruption of the portal vessels, the pars distalis atrophies, but the degree of atrophy depends on the species studied and the extent to which channels from the neural lobe to the adjacent pars distalis are available (95–99). Estrous cycles are abolished (73), and trophic anterior pituitary function is destroyed (74,75,93).

Halasz sought to evaluate the neural influences on pituitary function by separating the pituitary gland, with its attachment to the medial basilar hypothalamus, from the rest of the brain. Reasoning that the only portion of the brain that could support a pituitary transplant is located in the region of the tuber cinereum (76,100,101), he set out to study this hypophysiotropic area (HTA) (102). He was able to isolate this region, which included the infundibulum and entire pituitary gland as well as the arcuate nuclei, a portion of the ventromedial nuclei, the periventricular nuclei, the ventral premammillary, the median mammillary nuclei, and the retrochiasmatic area from the remainder of the brain. The supraoptico-hypophyseal and paraventriculo-hypophyseal tracts were divided, as was all other neural input into the HTA. However, neural input to the median eminence from the arcuate nucleus (the tubero-infundibular tract) (103) was spared (102). Isolation of the HTA and the pituitary gland from the brain produced (in the rat) a different picture than did isolation of the pars distalis from the median eminence by stalk section. Trophic pituitary function was not seriously disturbed (102). Basal thyroid function, adrenal output of corticosteroids, and testicular sperm production were maintained. The histologic picture of the thyroid, adrenals, and testis was not markedly altered, and compensatory hypertrophy of the remaining adrenal gland occurred after unilateral adrenalectomy (104–108). Modulating neural influences on pituitary function were disrupted, however, because the estrous cycle was abolished and an increased secretion of adrenal corticosteroids in response to stress did not occur (see ref. 107 for summary). These observations focused attention on the HTA, and particularly on the median eminence, as the focal point of converging neural systems for the humoral relay of information from the brain to the anterior pituitary gland.

The median eminence was found to contain substances that were capable of stimulating or inhibiting the release of anterior pituitary hormones (109,110). Saffran and Schally (111) and Guillemin (112) incubated pituitary tissue with hypothalamic tissue *in vitro* and were able to demonstrate support of adenocorticotropic hormone (ACTH) production using bioassay techniques. Further studies employing such *in vitro* assays revealed hypothalamic factors capable of stimulating ACTH (113,114), thyroid-stimulating hormone (TSH) (115), growth hormone (GH) (116), and luteinizing hormone (LH) (117) release from incubated pituitary glands. Prolactin (PRL) production from anterior pituitary cells was inhibited by incubation with hypothalamic tissue (118–121). Anterior pituitary hormone release of ACTH (122,123), TSH (124), GH (125), FSH (126,127), and LH (128,129) *in vivo* could also be stimulated by injection of hypothalamic extracts.

Porter et al. (130,131) developed a technique for perfusion of, and sampling from, the long portal vessels on the anterior surface of the rat's pituitary stalk. Perfusion of the long portal vessels with hypothalamic extract stimulated FSH and LH release from the anterior pituitary (132,133). TSH release was also stimulated by infusion of hypothalamic extracts into portal vessels (134). Gonadotropin-releasing activity (135) has been found in portal blood collected from the severed pituitary stalk, and GH- and TSH-releasing activity (136) and gonadotropin-releasing activity (133) were found in blood sampled by cannulation of portal vessels.

The chemical composition of thyrotropin-releasing hormone (TRH) was the first of the hypothalamic releasing hormones to be discovered (137–139) and to have its function verified. TSH was released from the anterior pituitary following the infusion of TRH into a portal vessel on the surface of the rat pituitary stalk (140). The structures of gonadotropin-releasing hormone (GnRH) (141–143), corticotropin-releasing hormone (CRH) (144,145), somatostatin (SRIF) (146), and growth-hormone-releasing factor (GRF) (147–150) have been subsequently elucidated. There is an increasing body of evidence supporting the role of dopamine as a prolactin-inhibiting factor (151–158).

The chemical characterization of some hypothalamic hypophysiotropic hormones has permitted their localization within hypothalamic neurons by means of immunohistochemical techniques (159,160). The pattern revealed by their localization is one of convergence of axons containing peptide hormones (peptidergic neurons) upon the median eminence from diverse hypothalamic loci (161,162). Immunohistochemistry, when combined with transmission electron microscopy, permitted the subcellular localization of hypothalamic hormones (163,164). GnRH-containing cells were believed by early investigators to originate in the hypothalamus and terminate in the median eminence of the rat. In the median eminence, GnRH was localized within granular vesicles in axon terminals (165) that are located in the perivascular space of median eminence capillaries. In cell bodies in the hypothalamus, GnRH was identified in granular vesicles associated with the Golgi apparatus. On the basis of morphologic evidence, it was proposed that GnRH is synthesized on polysomes in the cell body, packaged into dense core vesicles in the Golgi apparatus, and transported within vesicles down the axon, by axoplasmic flow, to be stored within axon terminals and released upon appropriate stimulation (163–167). The process of the synthesis of a hypothalamic releasing (or inhibiting) hormone in cell bodies lying in diverse hypothalamic nuclei, as well as its delivery to, and its release from, neural terminals in the median eminence, was generally held to be analogous to the synthesis of AVP or OT in cell bodies lying in the supraoptic nuclei, as well as its delivery to, and release from, axon terminals in the neural lobe.

Cushing (1) saw an organ composed of a neural and an epithelial portion lying in the sella turcica. His pars anterior released its secretions under regulation of the peripheral sympathetic system into veins that carried them to the brain and then to distant glands that they supported. His posterior lobe released its secretions, which were synthesized in the pars intermedia, under the regulation of the SOHT. They were carried through the neural lobe to the third ventricle, which they entered to influence periventricular hypothalamic centers. These, in turn, regulated the sympathetic system that controlled the tone of smooth muscle in the intestines and arteries, regulated adrenal medullary function, and controlled the function of the anterior lobe of the pituitary. Some 75 years later we see a different organ. The rostral end of its neural region lies on the base of the brain and is the site where protein secretions manufactured outside the pituitary and behind the blood-brain barrier in the hypothalamus are released from nerve terminals and are carried by restricted portal routes to the epithelial region of the pituitary gland (pars distalis within the sella turcica) to regulate its function. The caudal end of the neural region lies within the sella turcica and is the site where secretions (synthesized in the hypothalamus) are released from terminals of the SOHT and are carried by systemic routes to regulate the function of the kidneys, breast, and uterus. The objective of this review is to explore, in further detail, (a) the structures employed by the brain to control pituitary function and (b) the organization employed by the diencephalon to coordinate endocrine and neural responses to changes in the internal milieu and external environment.

THE ADENOHYPOPHYSIS

Epithelial Cells of the Adenohypophysis

Epithelial cells and smooth-muscle cells are the motor elements of the neuroendocrine and autonomic nervous systems which arise in the diencephalon. The epithelial cells of the neuroendocrine system are found in the adenohypophysis, the glandular portion of the pituitary body. These epithelial cells carry out their role as effector elements of the neuroendocrine system by synthesizing protein hormones and secreting them into nearby capillaries (Fig. 4). They are round to polygonal in shape and are characterized by the presence of electron-dense granules, lucent vesicles, rough endoplasmic reticulum, and a Golgi apparatus in their cytoplasm. The electron-dense granules are round to ovoid in shape and range from about 100 to 700 nm in diameter. They are the site of storage of pituitary hormones (168–170). The electron-lucent vesicles are about 40 nm in diameter and are believed to "shuttle" nascent proteins from the endoplasmic reticulum to the Golgi apparatus. The Golgi apparatus in these cells is made up of a half-moon-shaped system of stacked parallel cisternae. The cis face of the Golgi apparatus is the convex surface that faces the rough endoplasmic reticulum. The trans face is the concave surface that faces the cell nucleus or the plasmalemma. The small lucent vesicles are most frequently found between the rough endoplasmic reticulum and the convex cis face of the Golgi apparatus, whereas the large electron-dense granules are usually aggregated near the concave trans face as well as dispersed throughout the cytoplasm. Cytochemical staining techniques reveal specific enzymes localized to specific cisternae of the Golgi stacks (see ref. 171 for review). The ultrastructural elements necessary for protein synthesis, storage, and release into the extracellular space (rough endoplasmic reticulum, vesicles, Golgi apparatus, and secretory granules) are present in the endocrine cells of the adenohypophysis and resemble those found in the exocrine cells of the pancreas (172).

Farquhar and Wellings (173) first presented transmission electron-microscopic (TEM) evidence which suggested that secretory granules were formed within the Golgi apparatus. Electron micrographs revealed small granules surrounded by membranes at the end of the Golgi lamellae, with progressive enlargement of the granules with increasing distance from the Golgi (173,174). Pulse labeling experiments employing labeled amino acids reveal a path from rough endoplasmic reticulum via vesicles to the Golgi apparatus and then to secretory granules (175–178). With stimulation of the cells (such as stimulation of lactotrophs by suckling), the rough endoplasmic reticulum becomes more pronounced, vesicles increase in number, and the granules discharge their contents by exocytosis (179). TEM examination of ultrathin sections and of freeze-fracture material demonstrates exocytosis with membrane retrieval by endocytosis of coated membrane (180,181). There is, at this time, debate as to whether the only pathway employed in the synthesis and release of protein is from rough endoplasmic reticulum to vesicles to Golgi to granules to discharge (182) (Fig. 5), or whether, under conditions of stimulation, the Golgi may be short circuited and accompanied by release of newly synthesized peptide hormone from cytoplasmic sites such as the channels of the endoplasmic reticulum (183).

Biochemical evidence suggests that at least two pituitary hormones (GH and PRL) are assembled on polyribosomes as prohormones with an excess 27 amino acids at the amino terminus. This segment serves as a signal sequence to permit passage of the hormone being assembled from the polysome through the membranous lamellae of the rough endoplasmic

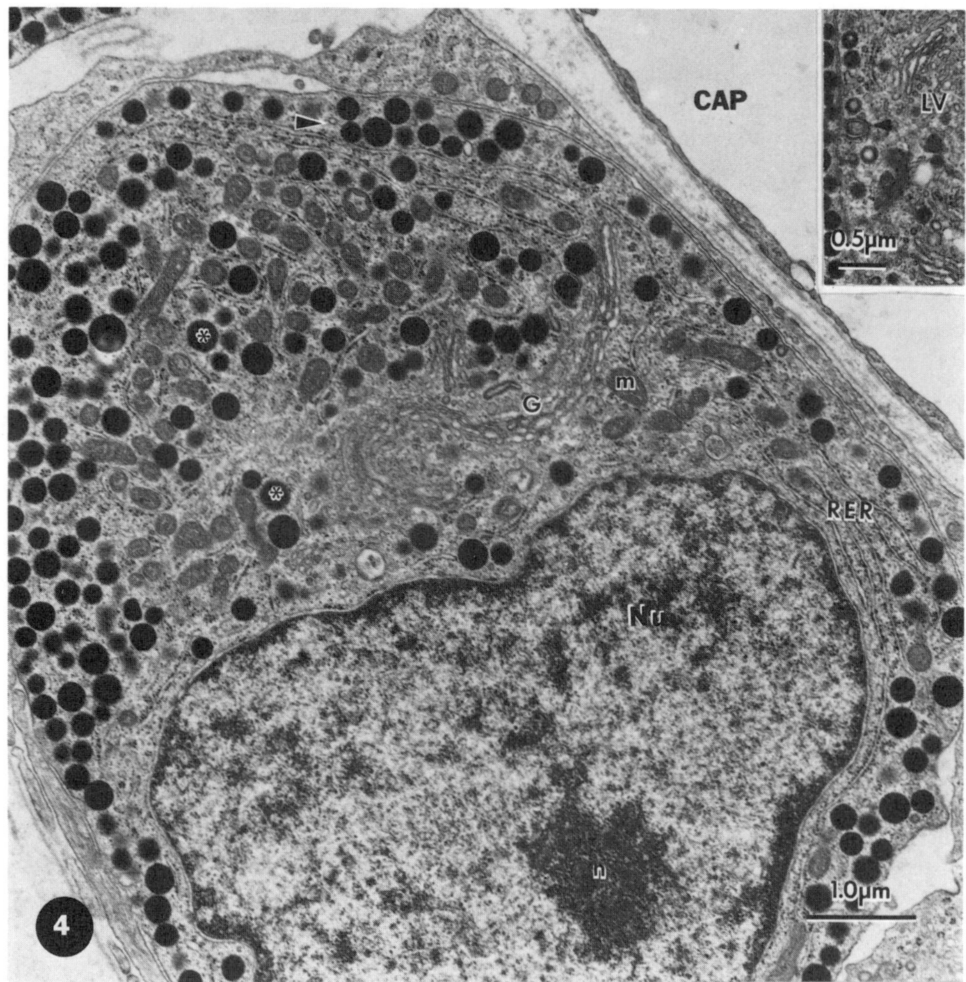

FIG. 4. Transmission electron micrograph of a rabbit pars distalis epithelial cell. The large nucleus (Nu) contains a single nucleolus (n). Nuclear chromatin is homogenously dispersed except at the nuclear membrane, where it is aggregated. The cytoplasm contains many electron-dense granules (*). Mitochondria (m) are abundant. The rough endoplasmic reticulum (RER) is plentiful. The Golgi apparatus (G) is found close to the nucleus. The cis border faces the nucleus. The trans (concave) border is associated with dense granules of varying size. A coated vesicle is indicated by the small arrowhead. (CAP) Capillary. Note fenestra in capillary endothelial tube. (*Inset*) Extrusion of granule with formation of omega figure at arrowhead. Both dense granules and coated vesicles are present at cell plasmalemma. (LV) Lucent vesicles.

reticulum into its channels (184,185). Membrane, pinched off from the channels of the endoplasmic reticulum, is believed to form the lucent vesicles that transport the protein to the Golgi apparatus for packaging (or alternatively to the plasmalemma for discharge under conditions of stimulation). In the Golgi apparatus, hormones are packaged into granules. In addition to packaging of hormone, post-translational modification of prohormones by enzymatic cleavage of peptide bonds is initiated in the Golgi apparatus, which is also the site of sulfonation and of glycosylation of proteins (186).

The release of protein hormones from adenohypophyseal cells can be regulated by the amine or steroid secretions of other endocrine glands such as the adrenal medulla or the target organs of the pituitary: the adrenal cortex, the gonads, or the thyroid. Catecholamines, thyroid hormone, and adrenal and gonadal steroids are carried to the adenohypophyseal cells from distant sites through the systemic circulation and regulate (trophic) hormone secretion from these cells. Current evidence suggests that glucocorticoids react with receptors at the cell surface and are incorporated into the cell nucleus to influence protein hormone synthesis at the transcriptional level (187–190). The release of hormones from some adenohypophyseal cells can be regulated by catecholamines released from local axon terminals or carried to the adenohypophysis through the systemic circulation (191–193). Current evidence suggests that these catecholamines interact with receptors at the cell surface and activate second messenger systems in the cell's interior. Dopamine receptors at the surface of melanotroph cells in the pars intermedia of the rat are negatively coupled to the adenyl cyclase second messenger system (194), whereas β-adrenergic receptors on these cells are positively coupled to the adenyl cyclase system (192,195). Dopamine receptors on the surface of lac-

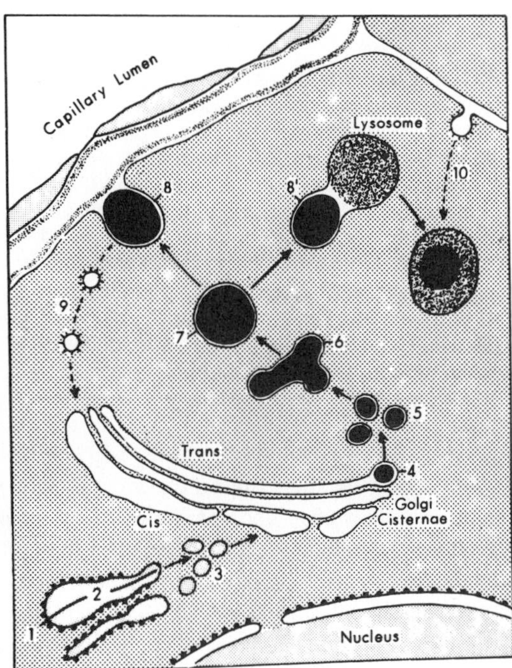

FIG. 5. Diagram illustrating the intracellular traffic that takes place in connection with the synthesis, packaging, and secretion of prolactin, as documented by work from many laboratories. Protein is synthesized on ribosomes (*1*), segregated into rough ER (*2*), and transported by small vesicles (*3*) to the Golgi complex; then it passes through the Golgi complex and is concentrated into small granules on the trans side of the stack (*4*). Several of these aggregate (*5* and *6*) to form the mature secretory granule (*7*). During active secretion, the latter fuses with the cell membrane by exocytosis (*8*), its content is discharged into the perivascular spaces, and the granule membrane recycles back to the Golgi cisternae (*9*). When secretory activity is suppressed and the cell must dispose of excess stored hormone, some granules fuse with lysosomes (*8'*) and their content is degraded. Besides these routes, an endocytic pathway from the cell surface to lysosomes has been demonstrated. (From ref. 182.)

totrophs appear to be internalized (in conjunction with dopamine) to become associated with secretory granules (196), but whether they function via modulation of adenyl cyclase activity is debated (157,196–198). The release of hormones from adenohypophyseal cells is also regulated by peptide secretions of nerves that terminate in the neurohypophysis. These hypothalamic releasing and inhibiting hormones are carried to the adenohypophyseal cells through a restricted portal circulation. There is ample evidence that peptide hypothalamic-hypophysiotropic releasing hormones cause degranulation of target adenohypophyseal cells, with consequent hormone release (199–203). Hypothalmic releasing hormones interact with receptors at the cell surface and may be internalized by endocytosis (204). Cyclic AMP, calcium, and phosphatidylinositol have each been implicated as the second messengers mediating exocytosis stimulated by releasing factors (205–212) and are the subjects of more in-depth discussion in later chapters.

Development of the Adenohypophysis

The adenohypophysis arises from the ectodermal tissue of the primitive mouth (3,213,214). The pouch of Rathke, which evaginates from the stomadeum, migrates dorsally. The floor of the diencephalon, the saccus infundibuli, migrates ventrally. This hollow diverticulum of brain is made up of a ventral (pituitary) and dorsal (saccular) wall. Caudally, these walls fuse to form the lower infundibular stem and infundibular process. As the pouch of Rathke migrates dorsally, its aboral (posterior) wall becomes apposed to the caudal region of the saccus infundibuli (the presumptive lower infundibular stem and infundibular process). It will become the pars intermedia. According to Herring (3), the anterior (oral) wall of Rathke's pouch grows massively, whereas the posterior (aboral) wall does not. Hence, the pars intermedia (aboral lobe) remains a thin band of glandular tissue, separated from the expanded pars anterior (oral lobe) by Rathke's cleft, except at the apex of the pouch, where the oral and aboral walls are united. Wingstrand (79) agrees that the aboral wall becomes apposed to the lower infundibular stem and infundibular process to form the pars intermedia. However, he proposes that the aboral wall of Rathke's pouch enlarges to form most of the pars distalis. The rostral region of the ventral diencephalic floor develops into the median eminence or infundibulum. The oral wall makes contact with the presumptive median eminence and becomes the site where portal connections between the median eminence and the pars distalis develop—the zona tuberalis. From the oral lobe two lateral buds develop which enlarge. These lateral lobes migrate cranially to approach the rostral portion of the ventral (or pituitary) surface of the evaginating saccus infundibuli. They become applied to it, fuse together, and develop into the pars tuberalis. It lies on the remaining surface of the median eminence and on the external and posterior surfaces of the infundibular. The zona tuberalis of the pars distalis (derived from the oral lobe), which is continuous with the median eminence and pars tuberalis, lies on the anterior surface of the infundibular stem surrounded by the remainder of the pars distalis, which is derived from the aboral lobe (Fig. 6).

Takor and Pearse (215) proposed that the entire hypophysis (neural and glandular) is of neuroectodermal origin. They reported that the ventral neural ridge of the white leghorn chick embryo is the origin of both pituitary components. Because some adenohypophyseal cells demonstrate amine precursor uptake and decarboxylation (APUD) activity, and because such cells are held to be of neural origin, their theory is consistent. However, immunohistochemical staining of pars distalis cells for neurofilament protein is negative (216), and hence their neural origin is unlikely.

The adenohypophysis is applied to the neurohypophysis in all chordates. The pars tuberalis is applied to the median eminence (the infundibulum) and the upper infundibular stem, and the pars intermedia is applied to the lower infundibular stem and infundibular process (78). There is con-

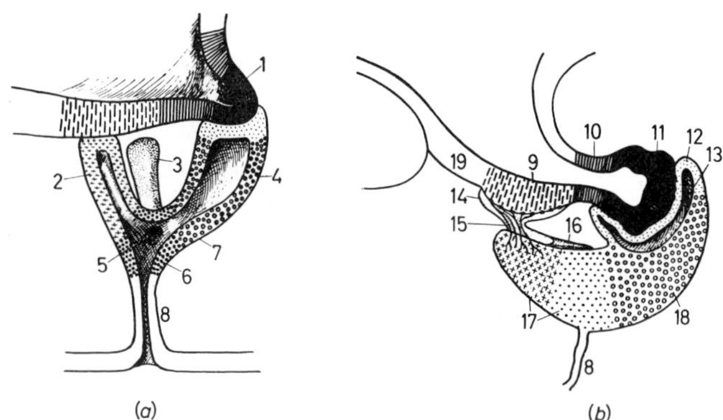

FIG. 6. Diagrams showing the structure of a generalized amniote pituitary (**b**) and its embryonic origin (**a**) as seen, particularly, in reptiles. (*1*) Saccus infundibuli; (*2*) anterior process; (*3*) lateral lobe; (*4*) aboral lobe; (*5*) opening of the lateral lobe cavity; (*6*) oral lobe; (*7*) constriction of Rathke's pouch; (*8*) epithelial stalk; (*9*) median eminence; (*10*) infundibular stem; (*11*) neural lobe; (*12*) pars intermedia; (*13*) hypophyseal cleft; (*14*) juxtaneural pars tuberalis; (*15*) portotuberal tract; (*16*) pars tuberalis interna; (*17*) cephalic lobe of the pars distalis; (*18*) caudal lobe of the pars distalis; (*19*) pars oralis tuberis. (From ref. 79.)

siderable variation in the development of the neurohypophysis and in the relationship of the neurointermediate lobe to the pars distalis among classes of animals. For example, in fishes and in some birds, the saccus vasculosus is well developed. In birds the intermediate lobe does not develop, and the neural lobe is separated from the pars distalis by connective tissue (in some cases even by bone) of variable thickness. Neither neural nor vascular structures cross between the pars distalis and the infundibular process in birds. Furthermore, there is some dispute as to whether the pouch of Rathke is the analog of the pituitary in all classes of vertebrates. Some feel that the pituitary may arise from Hatschek's pit in cyclostomes or from the nasal placode or dorsal lip in other lower species (79,80,217).

Even among mammals, species differences (e.g., the degree of persistence of Rathke's cleft or amount of coaptation of the saccular and ventral surfaces of the saccus infundibuli and hence the depth of the infundibular recess) exist. Nevertheless, the apposition of glandular tissue to the rostral region of the evolving neurohypophysis with the consequent trapping of an interposed layer of vascular mesenchyme which will supply both the glandular and neural tissue at the base of the brain is a common characteristic of the (fetal) pituitary body in vertebrates (79). The pouch of Rathke develops into the adenohypophysis, which consists of a pars tuberalis applied to the median eminence at the base of the brain, a pars intermedia applied to the neural lobe (infundibular process) within the sella turcica, and a pars distalis, which lies in the sella turcica separated from the neurohypophysis (Fig. 2).

Organization of the Adenohypophysis

Pars Distalis

Upon the completion of its development, the pars distalis is comprised of glandular epithelial cells, a connective tissue stroma, and many capillaries. Nerves do not terminate on or near pars distalis cells (78). There is no blood-brain barrier in the adenohypophysis (29,218). The capillaries in the adenohypophysis are not sinusoids (as believed by early investigators) because there are no phagocytic elements or large gaps in their walls. The capillaries of the adenohypophysis are fenestrated. Interposed between the epithelial cells and the fenestrated capillary tubes is a double basement membrane, which on occasion is widely split with the space between the basal lamina containing connective tissue elements (219). The epithelial cells are arranged in cords (4,5). Adjacent epithelial cells are united by desmosomes and gap junctions (220,221). This anatomical organization has the obvious consequence that hormones released into the extracellular space of the adenohypophysis from any epithelial cell can reach nearby capillaries by diffusion or bulk flow and enter them through fenestrations in their endothelial tubes (Fig. 7). However, three other consequences can also be foreseen: (a) Hormones can reach adenohypophyseal cells from the brain as easily as those from distant glands such as the thyroid, gonads, adrenal cortex, or adrenal medulla; (b) hormones released by one epithelial cell are free to interact with neighboring cells that contain appropriate receptors in their cell membranes (222); and (c) intercellular communication between adjacent cells is possible by electrotonic means through gap junctions (220).

The structure of eight hormones secreted by the adenohypophysis has been identified. Although species differences occur frequently, TSH, FSH, LH (223), PRL (224–228), GH (229,230), ACTH (231–233), MSH (234–239), beta endorphin (β-End) (240–244), and β-lipotropin (β-LPH) have been isolated from several species and sequenced. That each hormone secreted by the pituitary gland is synthesized in, and released from, a functionally specific group of cells (i.e., TSH by thyrotrophs, ACTH by corticotrophs, etc.) has long been postulated. This hypothesis was initially explored by attempting to correlate clinical syndromes produced by pituitary tumors with pituitary histology. Subsequent attempts have employed histochemistry (245), immunohistochemistry (246), transmission electron microscopy (247), and radioautographic localization of messenger RNA by light-microscopic examination of histological sections after *in situ* hybridization (248); however, to date, not every pituitary hormone has been housed in its own cell.

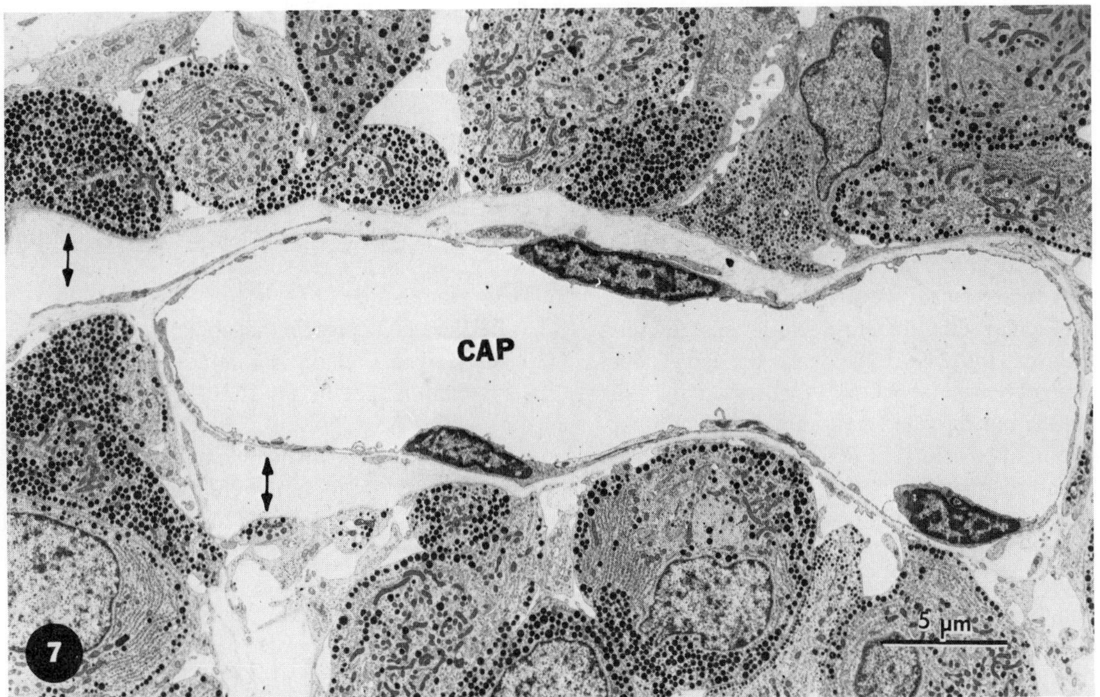

FIG. 7. Transmission electron micrograph of rabbit pars distalis. A fenestrated capillary (CAP) is surrounded by a double basement membrane (*arrows*) that defines the perivascular space upon which epithelial cells abut. Note occasional wide expansions of the perivascular space (↔) in which cell processes of connective tissue elements are seen. Glandular epithelial cells, identified by the presence of secretory granules, are closely related to the perivascular space and closely apposed to each other.

The attempt to relate structure to function began with light-microscopic examination of stained pituitary sections. The human male gland was reported to be composed of 52% chromophobes, 37% acidophils, and 11% basophils (249). In females the proportions differed in different stages of the menstrual cycle and with pregnancy (250). Acidophils are located in the lateral wings of the human pars distalis, and basophils are located in the central (mucoid) wedge (249). It was recognized early that the staining of chromophils occurred as a result of the staining of granules in their cytoplasm (251,252). The belief that these granules represented a stored source of hormone was based upon the observed depletion of granules following castration, thyroidectomy, or adrenalectomy of experimental animals, and it has been subsequently substantiated (168–170). Cushing (253,254) had noted a preponderance of acidophils in the pituitary tumors associated with acromegaly, and he proposed that the substance responsible for excess growth in these individuals was released from these cells. His finding of a predominance of basophils in tumors associated with bilateral adrenal cortical hyperplasia (subsequently called *Cushing's disease*) convinced him that the hormone responsible for the support of the adrenal glands (ACTH) was made in, and released from, basophils (255).

This picture became muddied when it was found that the number of acidophils increased in female animals at the time of parturition and that this increase was maintained during lactation (252). It was not known if acidophils secrete two hormones (one to support lactation and one to support growth) or just one. In addition, changes in the morphology of both acidophils and basophils occurred during the estrous cycle, during pregnancy, and following castration (for review, see refs. 251 and 252). Further, thyroidectomy produced a decrease in the number of acidophils and degranulation of basophils, while adrenalectomy also produced degranulation of basophils. In order to clarify the situation, more histochemical techniques were employed based upon modifications of the use of an acid dye such as eosin or orange G to stain acidophils and of the periodic acid-Schiff (PAS) reaction to stain basophils. The result has been a chaotic picture adding little to the knowledge of the problem at hand—the localization of specific hormones within specific cell types as defined by histochemical staining. Confusion arose because of the vagaries of staining by different lots of aniline dyes, the lack of knowledge of the chemical reaction between the dye and the cellular or hormone elements, species differences in staining patterns, and the use of the same terminology to describe cells stained by different dyes and so of different appearance. The subject is reviewed in detail by Romeis (256), Pearse (257), Herlant (258), Pearse and Noorden (245), and Purves (259). From the light-microscopic examination of stained sections, the following firm conclusions were reached: (a) Hormones are stored in granules in pituitary epithelial cells; (b) the hormone (or hormones) responsible for growth and lactation is found in eosinophils; (c) these eosinophils are localized predominantly in the lateral wings of the gland (249,260); (d) basophilic cells can be thyrotrophic, gonadotrophic, or adrenocorticotrophic, and they lie predominantly in the middle of the gland (245,249,258–261); (e) the positive PAS reaction that characterizes basophils indicates glycosylation of the protein hormone molecule in these cells (245,257).

Observation of adenohypophyseal cells with the electron microscope revealed that all the glandular cells, with the exception of follicular cells, contain electron-dense granules in their cytoplasm (179,247,262). Hence the large population of chromophobes (about 50%) observed by light microscopy in the human gland could not represent a population of uncommitted cells (251,252). The granules in the cytoplasm of chromophobes were too small, or too few, to be observed by light microscopy.

The eosinophils were divided by light microscopists into two groups [alpha cells and eta (or epsilon) cells (256) or orangophiles and carminophils (258)]. The color of the granules differs with the stain employed and the species studied, but appropriate techniques reveal two types of acidophil: one type is found predominantly in the lateral wings of the pars distalis and does not vary with pregnancy; the other type also lies in the lateral wings and becomes much more frequent at the time of pregnancy and parturition (259,262). Purves and Greisbach (263) further classified these two classes of acidophils in rats. Acidophils found on the interior of cell cords became degranulated after castration or estrogen therapy and were believed to be lactotrophs. Columnar acidophils arranged radially about capillaries became prominent following castration or estrogen therapy, but became degranulated after thyroidectomy and were classified as somatotrophs. On electron-microscopic examination, putative somatotrophs meeting these criteria were described as containing secretory granules of about 350 nm in their cytoplasm which lined up along the plasmalemma in a single row (264). These cells became more prominent after castration (264) and less prominent (degranulated) after thyroidectomy (265). The somatotroph in the rat pituitary is described by Kurosumi (247) as a round, oval, or polygonal cell with distinctive short clubbed mitochondria and round dense secretory granules with a maximum diameter of 350 nm. Injection of a stalk median eminence extract rich in GRF activity results in rapid degranulation of these cells (199). The use of immunohistochemistry (246) further strengthened the argument that growth hormone is produced by a functionally specific and morphologically identifiable line of cells and is stored within cytoplasmic secretory granules (262,266–268).

The presumptive lactotroph meeting the criteria of Purves and Greisbach (263) was found by Farquhar and Rinehart (264,265) to contain elliptical, rather than round, secretory vesicles that were as large as 600 to 900 mm in their longest diameter. Such cells became degranulated and developed large laminar areas of rough endoplasmic reticulum under the stimulus of suckling (179). Similar cells were identified by Kurosumi (247) as lactotrophs. Nakane (266,267) localized immunoreactive PRL within their granules. Growth hormone and PRL are thus present in morphologically distinct cell lines. These cells are acidophilic on light-microscopic examination, but can be separated by the coloration of their granules following staining with selected acid dyes. Their shape, granular size, and the development of their rough endoplasmic reticulum serve to differentiate them on TEM examination (179,262).

TSH is a glycoprotein that contains two chains designated α and β. The α chain is common to TSH, LH, and FSH; the β chain is specific for TSH (223). TSH-containing cells stain with PAS (256,269,270). Small angular cells in the rat's pituitary gland, which contained granules with a maximal diameter of 140 nm, were found on TEM examination by Farquhar and Rinehart (265) to exhibit a depletion of cytoplasmic dense granules and a marked increase in the number of lucent cytoplasmic vesicles following thyroidectomy. Using antibodies to TSH, preabsorbed with β-human chorionic gonadotropin and without cross-reaction with FSH or LH, Baker et al. (271) were able to localize immunoreactive TSH to cells in the rat pituitary which corresponded to thyroidectomy cells (265). Moriarty and Tobin (272,273) employed antibodies to the β chain of TSH and obtained similar results. They (272) found granules in the cytoplasm of TSH-containing cells to be of the same size as those in the presumptive thyrotropes of Farquhar and Rinehart (265). Kawarai (274) localized immunoreactive TSH within a specific cell population in the rat pituitary, but stated that the cells and their cytoplasmic granules are larger than those described by either Farquhar and Rinehart (265) or Kurosumi (247).

FSH and LH are also glycoproteins that contain (a) an α chain common to TSH, FSH, and LH and (b) a β chain specific for each gonadotropin (223). PAS-staining pituitary cells that become hyalinized following castration are termed "signet ring" or "castration cells" and are presumed to be gonadotrophs. Attempts have been made to distinguish FSH- and LH-containing cells from other pituitary cell types and from each other based upon their coloration after staining with different histochemical procedures. On the basis of their reaction with such stains as Alcian Blue, Aldehyde Fuchsin, and Resorcin Fuchsin and their staining characteristics with such dyes following oxidation with potassium permanganate, PAS-positive cells have been subclassified into FSH-, LH-, TSH-, and ACTH-containing cells (245,256–259,262). Such schemes are complex, with patterns of staining which vary from species to species, and they have never gained wide acceptance.

Based on their TEM observations, Farquhar and Rinehart (264) described two types of castration cell in the rat. The first appeared soon after castration and contained ovoid cytoplasmic vesicles. The second did not appear until later and contained irregularly shaped vesicles separated by cytoplasmic strands. It was described as resembling a filigree.

The authors proposed that the former cells were "FSH producers" and that the latter were "LH producers." Kurosumi and Oota (275) proposed that FSH gonadotrophs are large and round, with two populations of granules in their cytoplasm—one of 200 nm diameter and the second as large as 700 nm in diameter. LH gonadotrophs were described as being smaller than FSH gonadotrophs and frequently located along blood vessels (a site presumptively not occupied by FSH gonadotrophs). LH gonadotrophs were said to be polygonal, with secretory vesicles measuring 250 nm, and situated at the periphery of the cell. In contrast to the FSH cell, the LH cell was said to have a small Golgi apparatus with little development of the rough endoplasmic reticulum. However, Moriarty (276) demonstrated the presence of immunoreactive LH-β in each of these cell types. Immunoreactive FSH and LH have been localized in the same cells in the human pituitary (277). In male rats, 80% of gonadotrophs contained both FSH and LH, 10% contained only LH, and 10% contained only FSH (278). Cells containing immunoreactive FSH or LH only were randomly distributed among putative FSH and LH cell types, as predicted by ultrastructural criteria. Some cells containing FSH or LH resembled corticotrophs (278). In male rats, "castration cells" are indeed gonadotrophs, but the localization of hormone(s) within a gonadotrope is not predicted by its morphology alone (279). In female rats, there are twice as many cells that stain for FSH-β as LH-β in all phases of the estrous cycle. The ultrastructure of the gonadotrophs in female rat pituitaries is no more predictive of the hormone stored by the cell than that in male rats (280). As opposed to somatotrophs, lactotrophs, and thyrotrophs, gonadotrophs may contain one or two hormones and may assume one of several appearances upon TEM examination or upon light-microscopic (LM) examination following staining with PAS and basic dyes. Basophils (thyrotrophs and gonadotrophs) aggregate in the central region of the pars distalis, i.e., the *mucoid wedge* (so named because its cells contain glycoproteins). The mucoid wedge occupies the zona tuberalis, which, with the pars tuberalis, arises from the oral lobe of Rathke's pouch (79).

ACTH is not a glycoprotein in humans and in most species (281). It is a single-chain protein hormone that is 39 amino acids in length. However, in rats and mice, both glycosylated and nonglycosylated forms of ACTH 1-39 have been identified (282). ACTH-containing cells have been described as basophilic as well as acidophilic, amphophilic, and chromophobic (see refs. 258,259,262, and 268 for reviews). ACTH cells in the human are described by Baker (262) as being intensely basophilic. His description of ACTH-containing basophil cells is consistent with the finding of basophils in adenomas of the human pituitary that secrete ACTH and cause Cushing's disease (255). The source of the positive reaction obtained with PAS staining of human corticotrophs has been attributed to glycolipids (such as phosphatidylinositol), glycoproteins, or mucoproteins in the secretory granules or in their membranes (245,247,262). Pro-opiomelanocortin (POMC) (281,283), the 31-kilodalton prohormone from which ACTH (and MSH) is derived, is glycosylated; and POMC, not ACTH, may be the source of PAS positivity in corticotrophs that contain the nonglycosylated form of ACTH in their granules (268).

In the rat, ACTH cells have been reported to be basophilic by Purves (259) and Baker (262) but acidophilic by Herlant (258). Siperstein (284) reported that adrenalectomy cells in the rat were chromophobic and morphologically distinct (by LM appearance) from castration and thyroidectomy cells. Adrenalectomy cells were described as large, irregular in outline, and with a tendency "to insinuate cytoplasmic projections between neighboring cells in the direction of sinusoids" (285). Their cytoplasm contained many vesicles, and their granules measured 200 nm on average. Following the administration of cortisol to normal rats, dense granules accumulated in the cytoplasm in large angular cells believed to be corticotrophs. Following the administration of cortisol to adrenalectomized rats, an increase in the number of cytoplasmic granules was accompanied by a decrease in the number of clear cytoplasmic vesicles that are found in adrenalectomy cells of untreated rats (286,287). While employing an antibody to 17-39 or 25-39 ACTH, Moriarty and Halmi (288) were able to localize immunoreactive ACTH within granules in the cytoplasm of cells that resembled those identified as corticotrophs by Siperstein and Miller (286,287).

ACTH shares a common sequence of amino acids with β-MSH (ACTH 4-10), and ACTH 1-13 is α-MSH (231–239). Furthermore, ACTH, α-MSH, β-MSH, β-LPH, β-End, and α-End are all derived from the same parent hormone (POMC) by enzymatic cleavage of peptide bonds (281,289–291). Pars distalis corticotrophs process this parent hormone principally to ACTH and β-LPH, whereas pars intermedia melanotrophs further process (a) ACTH to α-MSH and corticotropin-like-intermediate-peptide (CLIP) and (b) β-LPH to β-End and α-LPH (which, in turn, can be processed to β-MSH) (281). Immunohistochemical studies of "corticomelanotrophs" must be done with particular care with respect to controls because (for example) an antibody to ACTH 4-9 could stain ACTH, α-MSH, and β-MSH as well as POMC; and antibodies to β-LPH may react with β-End as well as with the 31-kilodalton prohormone. Immunohistochemical study of the human pars distalis with antibody against ACTH 17-39 demonstrates ACTH-containing cells in the pars distalis which are basophilic (PAS positive) (292). These same cells also stain β-MSH (293), but this reaction may reflect LPH, rather than β-MSH, activity (294). β-LPH has been localized in the same secretory granules of corticotrophs in the pars distalis as has ACTH by TEM examination of human, monkey, ox, pig, and rat pituitaries (295). It appeared that ACTH and β-End are found in the same granules of corticotrophs in the rat pars distalis (296). Because corticotrophs in the rat's pars distalis only rarely stain for melanotropin (297), it seems more likely that ACTH is colocalized with β-LPH in the same secretory granules of corticotrophs of the rat pars distalis and not with β-End. This supposition is heightened by the recent finding of Tanaka and Kurosumi (298), who localized ir-α-MSH and ir-ACTH in different granules in the same corticotroph in the rat's pars distalis.

The pars distalis contains somatotrophs, lactotrophs, thyrotrophs, gonadotrophs, and corticomelanotrophs. Somatotrophs and lactotrophs have a distinctive morphology on TEM examination, are acidophilic on LM examination, and have a predilection for the lateral wings of the pars distalis. Thyrotrophs may resemble corticotrophs in the eyes of some (280), but not all (299), electron microscopists; however, they are identified with immunohistochemical techniques employing antibodies to TSH-β as a unique line of basophils. Unlike lactotrophs and somatotrophs and thyrotrophs, gonadotrophs and corticotrophs may synthesize and store more than one hormone. The majority of gonadotrophs contain both LH and FSH and are predominantly found in the central (mucoid) wedge of the gland. Corticotrophs contain cleavage products of pro-opiomelanocortin in addition to ACTH and, in humans, predominate in the anterior medial portion of the mucoid wedge. These epithelial cells are not innervated. In some cases they are regulated by the interaction with the hormonal secretions of target organs that have reached receptors on the cell surface through the systemic circulation, but in all cases they are regulated by hypothalamic releasing and inhibiting hormones that reach receptors on their cell surface through the restricted portal circulation.

Pars Intermedia

This structure is prominent in many mammalian species, including the rat, but is lacking in others, such as adult humans (with the exception of the pregnant female). The pars intermedia is also present in the human fetus. Although neither α-MSH nor β-MSH is a glycoprotein, pars intermedia cells have long been recognized as being intensely basophilic and the source of a hormone that regulates skin color in amphibians (261). As in corticomelanotrophs in the pars distalis, the source of this PAS positivity may be the presence of POMC, a glycosylated protein, in the storage granules of pars intermedia cells.

The (rat) pars intermedia is lobulated. Capillaries separate adjacent lobules but are sparse. The cells, with the exception of those that line the lumen of the hypophyseal cleft, are polygonal. Light and dark cells can be distinguished by LM (on the basis of their staining affinity for PAS) and by TEM. There are more light cells than dark ones. Light cells have large ovoid nuclei. Their cytoplasm contains many clear vesicles that are round and measure 200 to 300 nm. Round, dense granules measuring 200 to 300 nm in diameter lie in the Golgi region, which is well developed and lies near the nucleus. Apparent transition forms from empty vesicles to electron-dense granules can be found in the Golgi region. Dark cells are irregular in outline and contain lobulated nuclei. The cytoplasm contains closely packed particles, measuring 20 nm in diameter, that give the cells their dark appearance. The endoplasmic reticulum is well developed, but vesicles are scant (300).

α-MSH is localized in pars intermedia cells of the human fetus and pregnant female (301). Both light and dark cells in the pars intermedia of the rat contain immunoreactive β-melanotropin (302). In cows, pigs, rabbits, and rats, immunoreactive ACTH 17-39 was found in pars intermedia cells (303), although the concentration of ACTH is believed to be much less than β-MSH in these cells (297). Moriarty and Halmi (304) localized immunoreactive ACTH 17-39 to granules of dark and light cells, and subsequently Moriarty and Garner (294) found that the granules in corticomelanotrophs in the rat intermediate lobe stain both for ACTH 17-39 and for β-MSH. Similar findings have been reported in the mouse (302). β-MSH staining may also have indicated the presence of β-lipotropin because the entire sequence of β-MSH is found in β-LPH; and ACTH 17-39 staining may be due to binding with POMC, but not with ACTH 1-39.

The pars intermedia is less well vascularized than the pars distalis. Capillaries are few in number. The extracellular space is well developed and communicates with the hypophyseal cleft and the extracellular space of the adjacent infundibular process (neural lobe) and pars distalis (305). Axons terminate in the pars intermedia and make synaptoid contact with its epithelial cells (300,306–308). Pars intermedia cells can be regulated by direct neural contact. β-Adrenergic (195,309) and serotonergic fibers (310) innervate pars intermedia cells in the rat and putatively stimulate MSH release. Dopaminergic (311) and GABAergic (312–314) also terminate in the pars intermedia and inhibit MSH release from melanotrophs. The side chain of oxytocin, Pro-Leu-Gly-NH_2, has been proposed as a melanocyte hormone-inhibiting factor (315) and can reach melanotrophs from the extracellular spaces of the neural lobe. In the rabbit and hare, Pro-Leu-Gly-NH_2 may reach melanotrophs directly by synaptoid contact between oxytocinergic fibers and melanotrophs in the pars intermedia (316). CRH, which releases melanotropin from pars intermedia cells as well as corticotropin from pars distalis corticotrophs (317,318), can reach melanotrophs from the extracellular spaces of the pars distalis. Although relatively avascular, the pars intermedia can be regulated by three different mechanisms and has an ample extracellular space into which it can release its secretions.

Pars Tuberalis

The pars tuberalis, as described in the rabbit, is comprised of glandular epithelial cells arranged in cords and containing dense cytoplasmic granules and interstitial cells that may encircle the glandular epithelial cells. These cells contain many microfilaments in their cytoplasm. In addition, ciliated cells and connective tissue elements are present as are many (fenestrated) capillaries. Occasionally, an axon terminal is found adjacent to a glandular epithelial cell (319). Gonadotrophs have been localized within the pars tuberalis of the rat (320). In the pars tuberalis of the monkey (*Macacca mulatta*), gonadotrophs and thyrotrophs have been found (321). However, Girod et al. (322) reported localization of only LH-β in scattered cells of the pars tuberalis in *Macacca irus*. With hypophysectomy of rats, there is an increase in the number and size of immunoreactive gonadotrophs and an increase in their gonadotrophin hormone production (323,324), which are presumably regulated by feedback mechanisms and hypothalamic hypophysiotropic hormones.

THE NEUROHYPOPHYSIS

Nerve Terminals of the Neurohypophysis

Nerve terminals in the neurohypophysis release hormones [employed by other organs and organisms, at perhaps other times, to perform other tasks (325–327)] into blood vessels to be carried to the adenohypophysis or to distant target organs to regulate their function. Three basic types of terminals can be recognized by TEM. The first is found predominantly in the neural lobe and, in the rat, measures 1.5 to 7.0 μm in diameter. These terminals of the hypothalamo-hypophyseal tract contain mitochondria, large dense-core vesicles that measure 180 nm on average, and small lucent synaptic vesicles of 50-nm average diameter. The second type of terminal lies predominantly in the median eminence and is smaller, measuring 0.3 to 1.4 μm in the rat. It contains mitochondria, large granular vesicles measuring 90 nm on average, and small lucent vesicles about 50 nm in diameter. The third type of terminal contains only lucent vesicles measuring about 50 nm in diameter (328). In the rabbit, terminals of the hypothalamo-hypophyseal tract contain (a) large dense-core vesicles that are 250 to 300 nm in diameter and (b) small lucent vesicles with an average diameter of 50 nm. In the rabbit's median eminence, some axon terminals contain (a) large granular vesicles that average 120 nm in diameter and (b) small lucent vesicles, whereas others contain only small lucent vesicles with an average diameter of 50 nm (329,330). Similar observations have been made by others in the rat (331,332) and in the human (333,334), and even in submammalian species, for example, the toad (335,336). However, the number of groups into which the terminals are classified by the authors, based upon the size of their vesicles, varies with the author and with the species (Fig. 8).

Terminals of axons in the hypothalamo-hypophyseal tract arise from large neurons in the hypothalamic supraoptic and paraventricular nuclei (33,34,337–339). This magnocellular neurosecretory system can also be classified as peptidergic because it synthesizes, stores, and secretes oxytocin and vasopressin with their associated neurophysins (I and II, respectively) (62,340). These hormones are stored in the dense-core vesicles in terminals of the hypothalamo-hypophyseal tract (63). Oxytocin and vasopressin have been isolated from bovine dense-core vesicles (341). Vasopressin and neurophysin have been localized in terminals of the

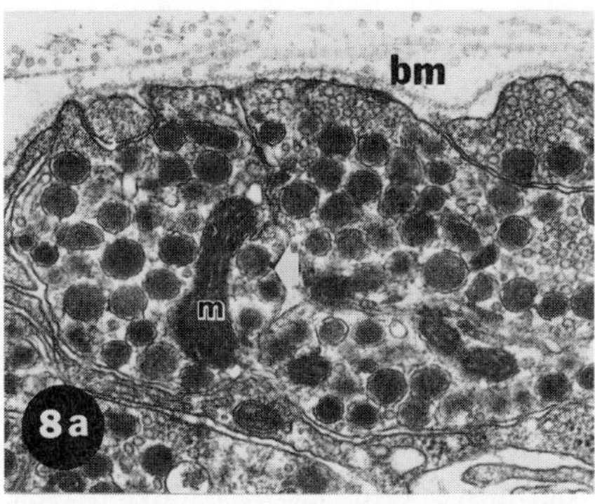

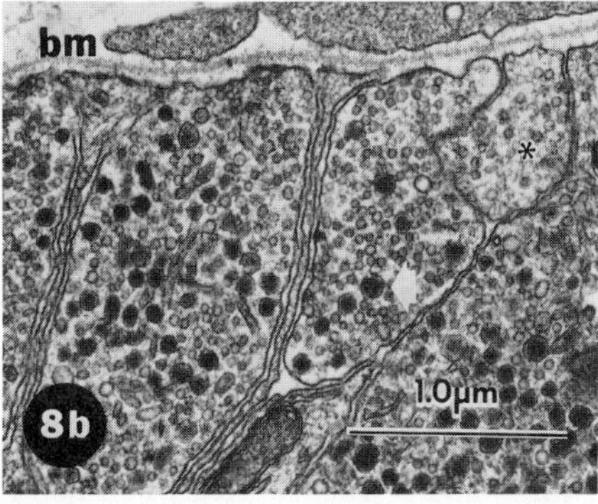

FIG. 8. Transmission electron micrograph of neural terminals in the rat neurohypophysis. (**a**) Neural lobe. Large dense-core vesicles (*white arrowhead*) and small lucent vesicles fill neural terminals. (bm) Basement membrane; (m) mitochondria. (**b**) Median eminence. Smaller terminals contain large granular vesicles (*white arrowhead*) and lucent vesicles. One terminal (*) contains only lucent vesicles. Dense-core vesicles (Fig. 8a) are larger than large granular vesicles (Fig. 8b). Lucent vesicles in Fig. 8a resemble those in Fig. 8b.

hypothalamo-hypophyseal tract of the guinea pig by combining TEM and immunohistochemical techniques (342). The large dense-core vesicles containing peptide hormones are transported from cell bodies in the hypothalamus by axoplasmic flow to terminals in the neural lobe (55,58).

The contents of the dense-core vesicles are released from the nerve terminal by exocytosis (343). Transmission electron microscopy of thin sections (343) and of freeze-fracture preparations (344) demonstrates fusion of the dense-core vesicles with the terminal membrane and then demonstrates the formation of omega figures (Ω) with opening of the membrane at the fusion site and release of the contents of the vesicles. Hormone is preferentially released by exocytosis from nerve terminals that abut the basement membrane; and calculations based on the estimated hormone content of a single vesicle and the decrease in the number of dense-core vesicles in terminals following stimulation suggest that all the hormone released can be accounted for by this mechanism (345).

Large vesicles in the terminals of the SOHT of a single specimen are not always uniform in appearance when viewed by TEM (328,333,346–350). Frequently, large vacuoles the same size as large dense-core vesicles, but devoid of osmophilic material, are found in terminals. Following the injection of histamine (346) or following ether treatment (347), the number of large dense-core vesicles decreased and the number of large empty vacuoles increased. Such observations led to the concept that hormone release from magnocellular terminals was a result of its escape through the membranes of dense-core vesicles into the axoplasm, leaving behind an empty vesicle; and, from the axoplasm in the nerve terminal, through a process of molecular dispersion, hormone was released into the extracellular space. This theory is at odds with the concept that hormones are secreted from nerve terminals by exocytotic release from dense-core vesicles. Douglas et al. (343) stated that with optimal fixative techniques, empty vacuoles were few in number and were most probably a fixation artifact. They reported that with stimulation the number of large empty vacuoles remained unchanged, but that the number of small "synaptic" vesicles increased.

The role of these small "synaptic" vesicles in large axon terminals of the SOHT is not clear. They resemble synaptic vesicles in size and shape, but do not contain neurotransmitters. Douglas et al. (343) proposed that these clear vesicles, about 50 nm in diameter, were involved in membrane retrieval. Morris and Nordmann (345) disputed the observation of Douglas et al. (343)—that the number of microvesicles increases after stimulation—and reported that the number of vacuoles increased. They proposed that vacuoles are responsible for membrane retrieval, and, on the basis of experiments that demonstrated ATP-dependent Ca^{2+} binding in microvesicles, proposed that these vesicles are involved in calcium homeostasis within the nerve terminal (351,352). Broadwell et al. (353) presented evidence, based on TEM observations of endocytosis of wheat-germ agglutinin by terminals of the SOHT, that microvesicles as well as vacuoles participate in the neurosecretory process by endocytosis and recycling of neurohypophyseal membrane.

Axon terminals that contain large granular and small lucent vesicles may be aminergic or peptidergic (354–356). As is the case in trying to differentiate between certain types of adenohypophyseal cells, the use of TEM alone cannot permit differentiation of aminergic from peptidergic parvicellular terminals. TRH (357,358), SRIF (359,360), and GnRH (360,361) have been localized, by immunohistochemical techniques, to large granular vesicles in the terminals of parvicellular peptidergic systems. Exocytosis characterized by fusion of the large granular vesicles with a terminal membrane and release of their granular material has been demonstrated (362,363). The role of small lucent vesicles in parvicellular peptidergic systems remains elusive. Ajika (364) employed antibodies to luteinizing-hormone-releasing hormone (LHRH) and to tyrosine hydroxylase to identify LHRH- and dopamine-containing cells in the same sections. LHRH was preferentially localized over large granular vesicles. Tyrosine hydroxylase was localized over small lucent vesicles of different cells. Small lucent vesicles in LHRH-containing cells did not stain. A similar study localized TRH by immunohistochemistry and monoamines by autoradiography (after injection with tritiated monoamines) and demonstrated similar findings (365). Broadwell et al. (353) proposed that small lucent vesicles in the terminals of parvicellular peptidergic neurons play the same role in endocytosis and terminal membrane recycling that they proposed in magnocellular neurosecretory systems.

Aminergic terminals may also contain large granular and small lucent vesicles (355). Uptake of the false neurotransmitter 5-hydroxydopamine (5-OH-DA) occurs in both the large granular and the small lucent vesicles in aminergic terminals (330,355,366–368). Autoradiographic techniques (364–368), as well as immunohistochemical techniques employing antibodies against specific enzymes in the biosynthetic pathway (369–371), localize amines to small lucent vesicles. Although an amine (serotonin) and a peptide (substance P) have been colocalized in the same neuron in several systems (see ref. 372 for review), they have not as yet been colocalized in neurohypophyseal terminals containing large granular and small lucent vesicles. Thureson-Klein (373) proposed that exocytosis of amines occurs from both large and small vesicles in aminergic terminals. Schwab and Thoenen (374) proposed that large granular vesicles in aminergic terminals return used synaptic vesicle membrane and associated transmitter to the cell body.

Terminals containing only small lucent vesicles are also found on TEM examination of the neurohypophysis after aldehyde fixation (330). While some of these neurons may be aminergic, systems containing other neurotransmitters terminate in the neurohypophysis (312–314,375). The full spectrum of neurotransmitters and neurohormones, as well as their subcellular localization in terminals of the neurohypophysis, remains to be clarified.

Nerve terminals in the neurohypophysis are organized to release their contents into the perivascular space of fenestrated capillaries and not into a synaptic cleft between neuronal elements. Although terminals in the hypothalamus and other regions of the brain may contain peptides or amines, the distribution of vesicles within their terminals differs from that in the terminals in the neurohypophysis. In brain regions organized for neurotransmission, lucent synaptic vessels are aggregated within aminergic terminals near a presynaptic thickening of the terminal membrane that borders a synaptic cleft. In the cerebrum, presynaptic TRH (peptidergic) neurons are characterized by the presence of small lucent vesicles aggregated near the thickening of the presynaptic terminals, whereas the large granular vesicles are randomly distributed throughout the terminal (357). In the neurohypophysis, this organizational pattern is seldom seen. The axon terminals are remarkably free of synaptic specializations, and synapses are not frequently found on TEM examination. Both large and small vesicles are randomly distributed within the axon terminals. Thickening of an axon terminal, when present, occurs at its free surface facing the outer basal lamina and the perivascular space. The peptidergic systems in the neurohypophysis are not organized for neurotransmission but are organized for neurosecretion. Even the aminergic systems in the neurohypophysis release their transmitters into the extracellular space of the neurohypophysis or the perivascular space of its fenestrated capillaries. The termination of a secretory neuron near a blood vessel without an interposed blood-brain barrier constitutes the fundamental organizational pattern of the neurohypophysis.

Development of the Neurohypophysis

The saccus infundibuli is discernible on the 15th day of gestation in the fetal rat (376). At that time, the floor of the third ventricle is made up only of six to 10 layers of round or oval cells. The presumptive infundibular process is an oval mass of cells, with its long axis directed perpendicular (not parallel as in the adult case) to the floor of the diencephalon. By this time, the aboral wall of Rathke's pouch has become apposed to the presumptive neural lobe, and the oral wall has become apposed to the presumptive median eminence. However, it is unlikely that migration of Rathke's pouch was induced by the presence of neurosecretory terminals, because none are present in the saccus infundibuli at this time (376,377). The capillaries, entrapped between the anterior (oral) wall of Rathke's pouch and the presumptive median eminence, display only a few fenestrations, but pinocytotic vesicles are present in their endothelial cells. Ependymal terminals, not neural terminals, lie in the perivascular space of this developing tuberal (mantle) plexus.

On the 16th fetal day, neuronal processes can be clearly identified in the ventral region of the developing median eminence in the rat. These neurites contain only a few electron-dense granules and neurotubules, and hence their site of origin in the hypothalamus cannot be deduced (376). They are oriented parallel to the ventral (oral) surface of the median eminence and lie between extended processes of ependymal cells (tanycytes) that stretch between the ventricular surface and the external surface of the median eminence. The nuclei of these stretched ependymal cells are indistinguishable from the nuclei of the primitive matrix cells found in abundance in the median eminence on day 15.

During the next 2 days (days 17 and 18) in the fetal life of the rat, the median eminence thickens as more axons enter it. The stretched ependymal cells lengthen in response to the thickening of the median eminence. In the endothelial tubes of the tuberal plexus, the number of fenestra increase and the number of pinocytotic vesicles decrease. Surface vascular connections are established by this plexus between the developing median eminence and the pars distalis. In the adenohypophysis, mitotic figures are frequently found and the Golgi apparatus becomes prominent in many of the developing glandular epithelial cells. Nerve fibers arrive in the neural lobe on the 17th day of gestation, 1 day after they were first demonstrated in the median eminence. Neurosecretory granules are first noted in axon terminals in the neural lobe on the 18th fetal day, but do not attain the size found in adults until the 9th postnatal day (378).

Neurohemal contact can be first demonstrated by TEM in the rat and in the mouse median eminence 2 to 3 days before birth. Abundant numbers of large granular and small clear vesicles and of mitochondria are found within the enlarged neural terminals that have displaced ependymal terminals and lie next to the outer basal lamina in the perivascular space of fenestrated capillaries near the surface of the median eminence (376,379–381). Concurrently, dense-core granules first appear in the cytoplasm of adenohypophyseal cells (376). Immunoreactive (ir) GnRH-, SRIF-, and CRH-containing terminals are first identified in the rat median eminence on the 19th fetal day by TEM examination of immunostained material (382–384). Setalo et al. (385) could not detect ir-GnRH in the median eminence of the rat with LM techniques until the day of birth. However, TEM examination has demonstrated ir-GnRH-containing fibers in the median eminence when LM examination of immunostained sections failed (382). Similar findings are reported in mice where ir-GnRH is first detected in the median eminence on day 17 of gestation 3 days prior to birth (386). Both neurohemal contact in the median eminence and the presence of immunoreactive LH in adenohypophyseal cells can first be demonstrated on that day (379,387). The functional significance of these observations for the rodent fetus was questioned by Monroe and Paull (381), who demonstrated that neurohemal contact, although begun, was not "well established" until the day of birth. Freeze-fracture studies first demonstrated configurations suggesting exocytosis from nerve terminals on the third postnatal day. However, the number of adequate preparations from earlier time periods was limited, and exocytosis may have been initiated at an earlier stage (388). Aminergic terminals appear later in the development of the rat's median eminence than do peptidergic terminals, becoming evident only several days after birth (389,390). In light of these limited and sometimes conflicting observations, it is not clear when the pituitary gland of the rat is first able to function under the direction of the brain.

The epithelium lining the saccus infundibuli also changes markedly with development. The infundibular recess in the rat brain is slit-like on the 15th and 16th days of gestation when viewed in coronal section. The ependymal cells of the saccus infundibuli are several layers thick and cannot be distinguished from the matrix cells. The floor of the ventricle is formed by round cells and by cells with apical processes, ovoid parikaryia, and basal processes (391). The apical processes of these tanycytes line the ventricular surface and are bathed by ventricular fluid. Their basal processes abut the outer basal lamina and lie in the perivascular space of capillaries of the tuberal plexus which are interposed between the rostral region of the saccus infundibuli and the oral lobe of Rathke's pouch. The tanycytes demonstrate polarity with the Golgi apparatus and mitochondria gathered in the apical process of each cell between the nucleus and the ventricular surface. The rough endoplasmic reticulum and ribosomes are poorly developed.

Between the 16th and 18th day, the number of these cells (relative to the thickness of the median eminence) decreases with the ingrowth of axons from the hypothalamus. The median eminence becomes thicker; and the floor of the infundibular recess widens, thus increasing its ventricular surface. The apical processes of tanycytes shorten, bringing the nuclei closer to the surface. A second type of ependymal cell, which is cuboidal and without apical or basal processes, appears in the expanding epithelial lining. The number and types of organelles in the cytoplasm of the tanycytes (mitochondria, polysomes, lipid bodies, lysosomes, and laminated dense bodies) increase until the cells come to resemble those seen in adult animals (381). Gap junctions between ependymal cells are numerous on day 17, while the development of tight junctions is rudimentary. Tight junctions between ependymal cells of the ventricular floor in the infundibular recess are not mature until birth (392). The surface of the floor of the third ventricle remains flat without microvilli or apical blebs throughout gestation. The specializations at the ventricular surface which are characteristic of some tanycytes in the adult median eminence do not appear until after birth.

By the 18th day of gestation, 3 days before birth, the median eminence has attained half the thickness of that of the adult rat. Further differentiation of the median eminence will occur prior to and after birth, and the median eminence will not assume its adult morphology for several weeks (376,379,381,393,394). However, in the rat by the 18th day of gestation, the basic organizational pattern of the adult neurohypophysis has been established. The neurohypophysis has differentiated into an infundibular process (neural

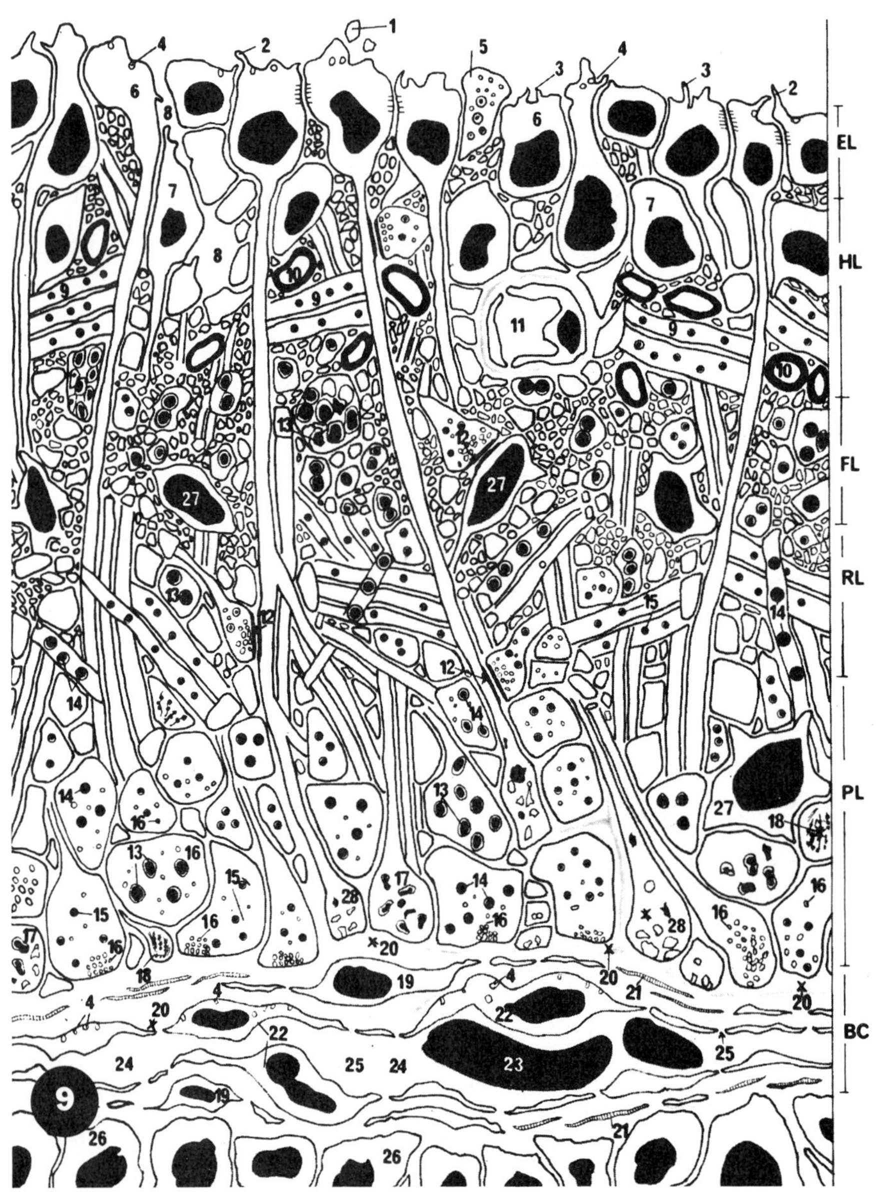

FIG. 9. Diagram of the fine structure of the rat median eminence. (BC) Capillaries of the primary plexus; (EL) ependymal layer; (FL) fiber layer; (HL) hypendymal layer; (PL) palisade layer; (RL) reticular layer. (*1*) Cytoplasmic masses released from ependymal cells into the third ventricle; (*2*) marginal fold; (*3*) finger-like microvilli; (*4*) pinocytotic vesicles; (*5*) monoaminergic axon terminals protruding into the third ventricle; (*6*) ependymal cell; (*7*) hypendymal cell; (*8*) intercellular cavity; (*9*) commissure of monoaminergic axons; (*10*) myelinated axon; (*11*) capillaries (note thin pericapillary space); (*12*) synaptoid contact; (*13*) large granule; (*14*) intermediate granule; (*17* and *18*) two types of unidentified processes; (*19*) fibroblast; (*20*) basement membranes; (*21*) collagen fiber; (*22*) endothelial cell; (*23*) red cell; (*24*) capillary lumen; (*25*) fenestration; (*26*) pars tuberalis cell; (*27*) glial cell; (*28*) terminal of ependymal, hypendymal, or glial process. (From ref. 396.)

lobe), an infundibular stem, and an infundibulum (median eminence). Neurohemal contact has been initiated. The median eminence has further differentiated into an ependymal zone, an internal layer defined by the presence of the hypothalamo-hypophyseal tract, and an external layer of small axons and terminals (395–397) (Fig. 9).

Organization of the Neurohypophysis

Infundibular Process

The principal elements of the neural lobe, as ascertained by light microscopy, are nerve terminals, glial cells called *pituitcytes,* and capillaries (27). Transmission electron-microscopic studies of the neural lobe have been performed in the rat (328,346), mouse (398), rabbit (347), and human (333,334), as well as in submammalian species (349). A basic picture of nerve terminals in the perivascular space of fenestrated capillaries is maintained, and differences between mammalian species at the ultrastructural level are not marked. The axons of the SOHT in the neural lobe are not uniform in diameter. Discrete swellings along the course of these axons give them a varicose appearance. Swellings contain dense-core vesicles but not lucent vesicles, a feature which helps to differentiate them from terminals. Large swellings, filled with dense-core vesicles, are called *Herring bodies*. Pulse labeling experiments suggest that newly synthesized hormone is first transported in dense-core vesicles to terminals, but subsequently the hormone is transported to the axon swellings if the hormone newly arrived at the axon terminal is not released (399). Swellings are viewed as a mechanism for storage of hormones.

Most of the terminals are large and contain dense-core and lucent vesicles (Type 3; 349). OT and AVP are stored in separate terminals of the SOHT, which terminates in the neural lobe (400). In the rat, AVP-containing fibers are congregated centrally in the neural lobe, whereas OT-containing fibers lie peripherally (401). Whitnall et al. (402) have reported that dynorphin-A-(1-8) is colocalized with AVP in terminals in the rat neural lobe. Met- and leu-enkephalin have been isolated from the rat neural lobe. Immunohistochemical LM studies demonstrate ir-leu-enkephalin (leu-Enk) in varicose fibers in the neural lobe. Their cell bodies in the paraventricular and supraoptic nuclei have the characteristics of magnocellular neurons (403). Zamir (404) concluded, on the basis of lesioning experiments, that met- and leu-enkephalin have different cells of origin and that separate populations of magnocellular neurons contribute to the met- and leu-enkephalin content of the posterior pituitary. However, differences of opinion persist as to whether there is a separate enkephalinergic system or whether the enkephalins are colocalized with the classical neurohypophyseal hormones. VanLeeuwen et al. (405) proposed that enkephalins are localized in large granular vesicles of about 120 nm in diameter and hence not in the terminals of magnocellular neurons that contain AVP or OT. Martin and Voigt (406) presented LM studies which suggest (from examination of serial sections) that met-Enk is colocalized with OT and that leu-Enk is colocalized with AVP. Martin et al. (407) subsequently reported co-localization of ir-OT and met-Enk in dense core vesicles within magnocellular terminals. Met-Enk, proenkephalin and OT have been localized by immunohistochemistry within the same magnocellular neurons in the bovine hypothalamus (408). Leu-Enk was colocalized in dense-core vesicles with ir-AVP, but, because staining was enhanced by Trypsin pretreatment, the leu-Enk was believed to be incorporated into a larger prohormone. Because α-neoendorphin and dynorphin have also been colocalized with AVP and because the sequence of leu-Enk is found at the *N*-terminus of these peptides, the sequence of leu-Enk demonstrated in the AVP-containing terminals was believed to be incorporated into these larger molecules (407). Opiate systems terminating in the neural lobe are believed to play an inhibitory role in the regulation of AVP and OT secretion (409,410). Neurons containing immunoreactive gastrin-like and cholecystokinin-like peptide have been demonstrated to arise in the paraventricular and supraoptic nuclei and to terminate in the neural lobe of the rat (411). Based on LM examination of immunostained sections of the rat hypothalamus, Kiss et al. (412) concluded that immunoreactive cholecystokinin is colocalized with OT. In addition, substance P is present in terminals in the mouse neural lobe in the same distribution as AVP-containing terminals (413). Large terminals of the magnocellular system could thus contain: AVP with its associated neurophysin II (414); AVP, neurophysin II, and/or dynorphin and/or substance P; OT with its associated neurophysin I (414); and OT, neurophysin I, and met-enkephalin (or OT, neurophysin I, and gastrin-like, cholecystokinin-like peptide).

The parvicellular peptidergic terminals in the (rat) neural lobe are found far less frequently than are magnocellular peptidergic terminals. Their terminals contain large granular and small lucent vesicles (Type II; 349). Such terminals may contain TRH because TRH-containing fibers are abundant in the rat neural lobe (415). Somatostatin-containing fibers are also present in the rat neural lobe but are in fewer number (401). Aminergic terminals resemble peptidergic ones on TEM examination (Type II; 349). The dopaminergic tuberohypophyseal tract terminates in the neural lobe (308,416) in close proximity to AVP terminals (417). Norepinephrine or epinephrine is also present in aminergic terminals located in the neural lobe, but these terminals are not closely related to AVP terminals (418). The content of terminals in the neural lobe containing only lucent vesicles (Type I; 349) has not been determined. Catecholamines can be found in such terminals (355). Immunoreactive GABA-containing terminals have been demonstrated in the neural lobe by LM (312–314), but immunoelectron microscopic studies of these terminals in the neural lobe have not yet been reported.

Species variations in the distribution and content of the

peptidergic and dopaminergic systems terminating in the neural lobe, of course, exist. In fishes, vasotocin and isotocin are released from magnocellular terminals; however, in amphibians, vasotocin and mesotocin are released from these terminals. Even among mammals, differences are present. GnRH, not present in the neural lobe of the rat (401), is present in the neural lobe of bats, ferrets, monkeys, and humans (419). In the pig, CRH terminals are reported to lie in the perivascular space of the neural lobe in the same distribution as do vasopressin-containing fibers (420).

Glial cells of the neural lobe have received little attention since the 1930s, when they were considered to be the parenchymous elements of the neural lobe and the source of its secretions (24). Takei et al. (421) classified pituicytes into five major types. "Major pituicytes" resembled cerebral astrocytes, and their processes were frequently found in the perivascular space of capillaries. "Dark pituicytes" resembled major pituicytes but were more electron dense. "Ependymal pituicytes" contained cilia. "Oncocytic pituicytes" contained abundant numbers of mitochondria in their cytoplasm and were only occasionally observed. "Granular pituicytes" contained numerous cytosegresomes (electron-dense granules that are round or irregular in shape and are usually surrounded by a single membrane). These authors postulated that granular pituicytes are involved in the uptake and catabolism of extracellular material. The significance of ependymal and oncocytic pituicytes is not known (421).

The role of "major and dark" pituicytes has been evaluated by Hatton and Tweedle (422–428). They have shown that the relationship between terminals of the hypothalamo-hypophyseal tract and glial cells is not static (426,427). Under resting conditions, glial processes enclose terminals of the hypothalamo-hypophyseal tract and lie interposed between these terminals and the perivascular space of capillaries. Synaptoid contact between nerve terminals and glial cells was occasionally found (422). With dehydration (deprivation of water for 24 hr), the number of enclosed axons decreased and more exposed terminals were present in the perivascular space (423). If the neural lobe was removed and incubated in hyperosmotic medium (as compared with incubation in a medium of low osmotic strength), the number of enclosed neurons was similarly decreased (428). In an analogous manner the number of enclosed neurons was decreased in postpartum and lactating rats when compared with control females (424,425). These interactions between glial cells and nerve terminals, along with an increase in the release of hormone from nerve terminals, an increase in neural lobe blood flow (429), and an increase in the permeability of the neural lobe (430), serve to facilitate the movement of neurohypophyseal hormones from the nerve terminal to the bloodstream in response to specific physiologic stimuli.

Infundibular Stem

The principal elements of the infundibular stem are axons of the magnocellular peptidergic systems as well as axons and terminals of the parvicellular peptidergic and aminergic systems which pass into the neural lobe. There is considerable variation in the length of the infundibular stem among mammals: For example, the length of the infundibular stem of the cat is very short, whereas that of the ferret or human is very long (78). In addition to axon terminals containing TRH and SRIF, the rat's infundibular stem contains terminals that stain for GnRH (161), CRH (431), GRH (432), and neurotensin (433).

Infundibulum (Median Eminence)

The ependymal layer of the median eminence lines the infundibular recess. It is interposed between the neuropil of the median eminence and the fluid of the third ventricle. The ependymal cells comprising the epithelial lining of the infundibular recess differ in appearance from the extrachoroidal ependymal cells that comprise the epithelial lining of the remainder of the ventricular system. The ependymal layer of the median eminence is not ciliated. Scanning electron-microscopic (SEM) studies of the third ventricular surface and of the infundibular recess have been carried out in frogs (434,435), birds (436), rats (437,438), mice (439), cats (440), rabbits (441), mink (442), sheep (443), monkeys (444), humans (439,445), and even in armadillos (446). The basic pattern is similar in each of these species. Ependyma overlying the dorsal third ventricle is ciliated. In the ventral regions of the third ventricle, the number of ciliated cells decreases at about the level of the ventromedial hypothalamic nuclei. As the infundibular recess is approached (at the level of the arcuate nuclei), ciliated cells become widely separated and sparse. The ventricular surface is lined by cells with abundant microvilli. This region between the ciliated ependyma of the dorsal third ventricle and the ependyma overlying the infundibular recess is called the *transition zone*. It overlies the ventromedial and arcuate hypothalamic nuclei. Beneath the level of the tubero-infundibular recess, the surface of the ventricular lining again changes. In the walls of the lateral recess, the cell surfaces become elevated and take on the appearance of cobblestones. Apical excrescences or blebs are seen at the cell surface.

The floor of the infundibular recess shows regional variation in its appearance. Studies in the rabbit (447) demonstrate that the ependymal lining in the anterior third ventricular recess is a flattened squamous epithelium with a smooth surface. In the middle third the surface of the cells is covered by microvilli. In the posterior third the surface of each cell is raised. Many apical blebs protrude from the elevated surface and give the cell a riveted appearance. A somewhat different regional variation is reported in the rat (448), but flat smooth cells, microvillated cells, and riveted cells with apical excrescences are also present. These blebs contain few organelles (437,449–451) and no secretory granules. Supraependymal cells (neurons and macrophages) lie on the ependymal surface in the floor of the infundibular recess (450–453).

Tanycytes contribute to the ependymal lining that overlies the hypothalamus in the ventral region of the third ventricle and the median eminence in the infundibular recess. Light-microscopic studies of the distribution and morphology of tanycytes have been reported in the rat (454–457) as well as in the quail (458). Tanycytes are bipolar ependymal cells with a soma, a short apical process that extends to the ventricular surface, and a long basal process. The basal process is subdivided into a neck, a tail, and a terminal. Akmayev and Popov (459) designated tanycytes in the transition zone that overlie the hypothalamus of the rat as α-tanycytes. β-Tanycytes are found in the ependyma overlying the lateral recess (β_1) or lining the floor of the infundibular recess (β_2).

α-Tanycytes are present in the transition zone of the third ventricle, and they stretch between the ventricular surface and the ventromedial or arcuate hypothalamic nuclei, where they terminate on neurons or capillaries in these hypothalamic regions (454,458) or on the pial surface of the tuber cinereum (455). Their apical processes are located between ciliated ependymal cells in the epithelium lining the transition zone. The ventricular surface of the apical processes contains many microvilli. Occasional apical protrusions are present. Mitochondria, ribosomes, and numerous tubules are present in their apical cytoplasm of α-tanycytes. Adjacent apical processes are interdigitated and linked by gap junctions and desmasomes. Zonulae occludens are not found in the transition zone (400,401). The soma of α-tanycytes contains the same complement of organelles and inclusions as do epithelial cells in general. Their ovoid nucleus contains a single large nucleolus. The Golgi apparatus, free ribosomes, and mitochondria are present in the soma. Vesicles associated with the Golgi and lysosomes are also found. The basal process contains a distinctive array of microtubules that are oriented parallel to the long axis of the process. In the neck, the endoplasmic reticulum elaborates "concentric shells of smooth cisternae" (460). The neck and tail of the basal processes contain a varied collection of inclusions and organelles, including short tubules of endoplasmic reticulum and vesicles of differing shapes and sizes. Ependymal processes have been found to terminate on the basement membrane in the perivascular space of capillaries in the arcuate nucleus (460).

β-Tanycytes in the ependymal layer of the median eminence are stretched between the ventricular surface and the perivascular space of fenestrated capillaries on the oral surface of the median eminence (454) (Fig. 10). Akmayev and Popov (459) cited several ultrastructural differences between tanycytes in the epithelium lining of the hypothalamus (α-tanycytes) and tanycytes in the ependymal layer of the median eminence (β-tanycytes). At the surface of the β-tanycytes are apical blebs that are granular on TEM examination and contain no secretory granules or organelles. The β-tanycytes lining the infundibular recess are more fibrillar in appearance than α-tanycytes lining the third ventricular walls because of the striking number of microtubules in their cytoplasm. They contain a well-developed system of membranous cavities and cisterns and a system of mitochondrion-borne tubules (462). Spine-like protrusions project from the basal process, which differs from that of an α-tanycyte process because it contains polysomes, lipid droplets, and a unique collection of vesicles. Smooth, dense-core vesicles 40 to 50 nm in diameter lie in the Golgi area. Coated vesicles in the soma and in terminals form omega figures with the plasmalemma in these regions. Dense-core vesicles about 100 nm in diameter also lie in the soma, neck, tail, or terminal. Frequently, rosettes or arrays of vesicles about 100 nm in diameter are found in terminals where glycogen bodies and lipid inclusions are prominent (463). Terminals of the β-tanycytes lie in the perivascular space of fenestrated capillaries on the surface of the median eminence. Their apical processes, along with squamous and cuboidal ependymal cells, form the ependymal layer of the median eminence.

Adjacent epithelial cells in the ependymal layer of the median eminence are joined by zonulae occludens as well as by gap junctions and desmasomes (464–466). Brightman et al. (465) found that junctions become increasingly tight (exhibit more particles per row and more rows per junction) as the infundibular floor is approached from the transition zone. They proposed that the lining of the ventricle formed a graded sieve, more porous at the periphery than at the center. Gotow and Hashimoto (461) divided the ventral region of the third ventricle (the transition zone) into two regions: one is dorsal to the level of the arcuate nucleus, and the other is ventral to the level of the arcuate nucleus. In the dorsal region, tight junctions were not found on transmission electron-microscopic examination of freeze-fracture replicas. Ventral to the level of the arcuate nucleus, tight junctions were found. They increased in number in the lateral recess and in the floor of the infundibular recess over the median eminence. Furthermore, the number of rows of particles that comprise the tight junctions in freeze-fracture replicas and the density of particles per row increased from the transition zone through the lateral recess onto the floor of the infundibular recess. Horseradish peroxidase could pass between ependymal cells in the transition zone but not between ependymal cells lining the lateral recess of the third ventricle. In this region, microperoxidase could pass between the ependymal cells. In the floor of the infundibular recess, microperoxidase could not pass between ependymal cells, but 5-hydroxydopamine could pass by circumventing tight junctions. These findings indicate an increasing tightness of the intercellular junctions in a centripetal pattern centered on the floor of the infundibular recess.

Kobayashi and co-workers (467,468) reported that horseradish peroxidase passed between the third ventricle and the neuropil of the median eminence. This passage was presumably accomplished by "active" pinocytotic transport (469). The observation of synaptoid contact between neurosecretory terminals and tanycyte processes (470,471) encouraged the concept that such transport could be controlled by hypothalamic (neural) projections. The observation that the surface of the ependymal lining changed concurrent with

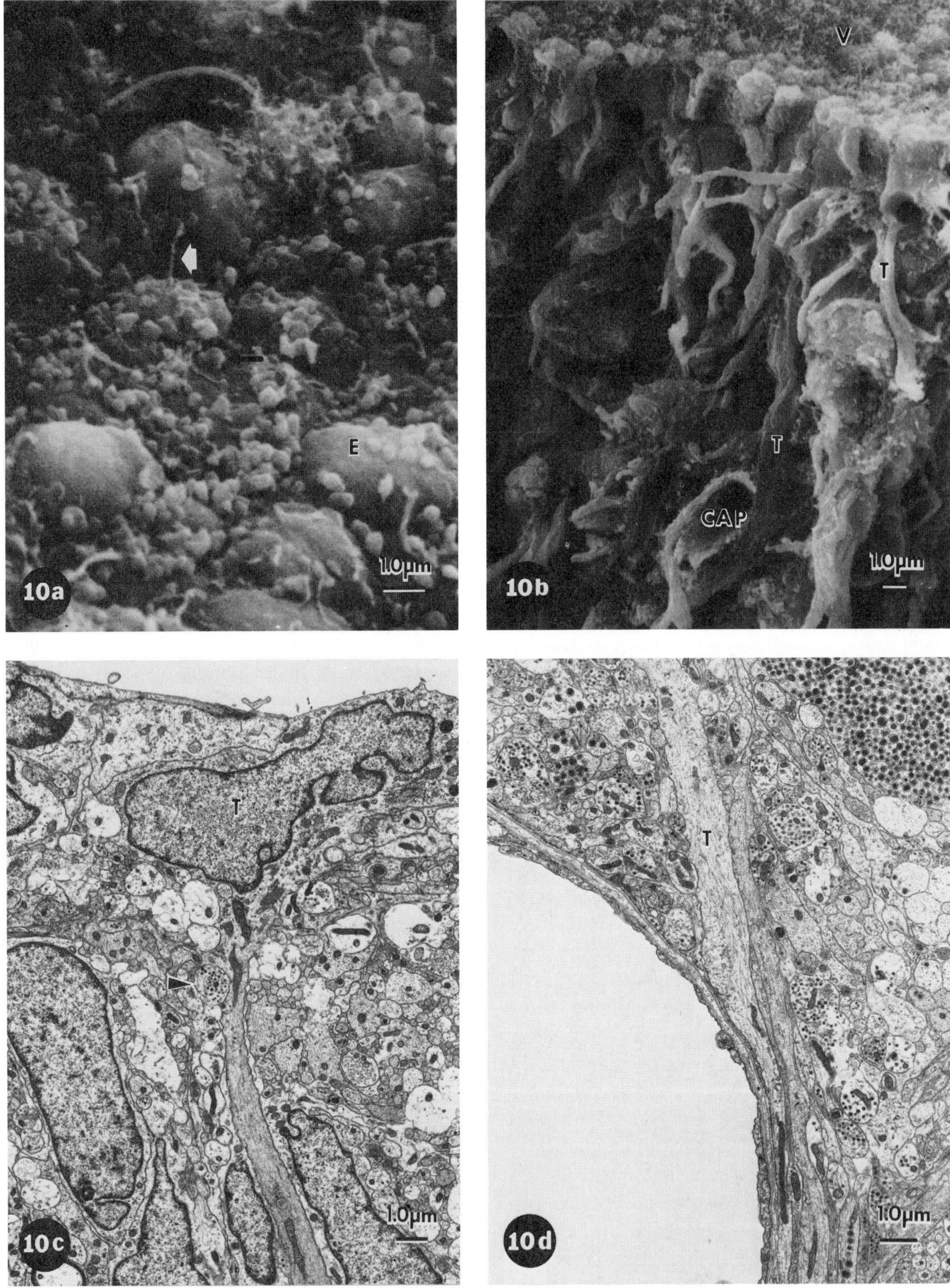

FIG. 10. (a) Scanning electron micrograph of the floor of the rabbit third ventricle overlying the median eminence. White arrowhead points to microvilli. Black arrow points to an apical bleb. E designates the surface of one ependymal cell. Note the profusion of apical blebs in this (posterior) region of the infundibular recess. (From ref. 873). **(b)** Scanning electron micrograph of median eminence neuropil. Median eminence has been broken, thus exposing tissue between ventricular lumen (V) at top of picture and pial surface (not shown) at bottom. Tanycytes (T) lining the rabbit infundibulum extend from the ventricular surface (V) to median eminence capillaries (CAP). Apical surface of tanycytes contains microvilli. (From ref. 874.) **(c)** Transmission electron micrograph of rabbit median eminence. Tanycyte (T) sends basal process vertically through neuropil to the oral surface. In this region of the infundibular recess the ependymal cells are smooth. The organelles are concentrated in the cell body. A neurite (*at arrowhead*) contacts the basal process at its neck. Aggregates of microtubules give the basal process a filamentous appearance. **(d)** Transmission electron micrograph of rabbit median eminence. A tanycyte terminal (T) as well as neural terminals lies in the perivascular space of a fenestrated capillary. (From ref. 875.)

the reproductive cycles of the monkey (472) had previously rekindled the idea of a humoral link between the third ventricle and the pituitary gland (1).

Ependymosecretion was proposed as a mechanism to supplement neurosecretion. Hypothalamic hormones released into the ventricular system (it was proposed) are transported from the ventricular lumen to portal capillaries and carried to the median eminence to regulate anterior pituitary function (473,474). Pilgram (475) pointed out that the intensity of horseradish peroxidase staining of tanycytes reported by Kobayashi et al. (467) indicated cellular damage. He found no evidence of pinocytic transport. Enzyme systems indicative of active transport are not found in β-tanycytes in the median eminence but are found in α-tanycytes in the hypothalamus (476,477). The evidence against a role for the ependymal layer of the median eminence in hypothalamo-hypophyseal interactions is summarized by Pilgram (475).

Although the transport role of tanycytes in the ependymal layer of the median eminence remains speculative, one role of this ependymal layer seems quite clear. This ependymal layer effectively separates the extracellular fluid of the median eminence from the ventricular fluid of the third ventricle. This epithelial layer prohibits either the unregulated loss of hypothalamic hormones into the ventricular system or their dilution within the extracellular spaces of the median eminence (478). Rodriguez et al. (462) demonstrated that the basal processes of β-tanycytes in the rostral and postinfundibular palisade regions, as well as in the lateral palisade region of the preinfundibular median eminence, form a continuous cuff at the ventral (oral) surface of the rat's median eminence, which abuts the basal lamina about the fenestrated capillaries. This cuff is composed of ependymal terminals linked by gap junctions and desmasomes that are interposed between neuronal terminals near the surface of the lateral palisade zone and the basal lamina. Only in the medial palisade zone of the rat median eminence do neurosecretory terminals directly contact fenestrated capillaries. The significance of this finding is not yet fully understood. Given the active role of pituicyte processes in neurosecretion in the neural lobe, an analogous role may be played by ependymal processes (479) in the median eminence.

The internal zone lies beneath the ependymal layer of the vertebrate median eminence (79). In some species [e.g., the rat (395) or the rabbit (330)], it can be subdivided into a hypendymal layer and a fiber layer (396). The hypendymal layer lies directly beneath the ependymal layer and contains subependymal cells and pituicytes. In the rat, parvicellular peptidergic axons projecting from the hypothalamus (356,480), as well as aminergic terminals of the reticulo-infundibular tract projecting from the brain stem, are present in the hypendymal layer of the internal zone (356,416). The fiber layer is defined by axons of the hypothalamo-hypophyseal tract (79,481). Although axon terminals of the magnocellular hypothalamo-hypophyseal tract are not found in the fiber layer, terminals of other systems are present (330). The noradrenergic reticulo-infundibular tract terminates in the internal zone of the rat's median eminence, principally in its medial third (161,356,482). Peptidergic neurons that contain the processed products of POMC, including ACTH, α-MSH, β-LPH and β-End, terminate in the internal zone of the rat's median eminence (483,484).

The external zone is comprised of nerve terminals, pituicytes, ependymal (tanycyte) terminals, and capillaries (395–397,485). Transmission electron-microscopic studies of the external zone have been performed in the rat (328,332), rabbit (329), and human (334), as well as in submammalian species (335,486). The external zone of the rat median eminence has been divided into a reticular layer and a palisade layer (395). The reticular layer lies between the fiber layer of the internal zone and the palisade layer of the external zone. It contains ependymal and glial processes as well as axons of aminergic and peptidergic systems. The palisade layer lies between the reticular layer and the ventral surface of the median eminence. It is recognized, on light-microscopic examination, by the presence of glial and tanycytic processes oriented at right angles to the ventricular surface of the infundibular recess (79,481) and, on transmission electron-microscopic examination, by fascicles of axons and terminals (separated by tanycytic processes) in the perivascular space of median eminence capillaries (395,396,485). In the rat, the palisade layer may be further subdivided into a medial palisade zone (medial third) and a lateral palisade zone (lateral third). The medial palisade zone lies beneath the floor of the infundibular recess. The lateral palisade zone lies lateral to it and extends to the tubero-infundibular sulcus (335).

Aminergic fibers in the median eminence can be identified by LM using formaldehyde fluorescence (487–489) or glyoxylic-acid-induced fluorescence (490,491). Fluorescence LM studies demonstrate catecholamines in the palisade layer of the external zone and in the hypendymal layer of the internal zone (487–489). Combining the fluorescence LM technique with the use of selective enzyme inhibitors to halt synthesis of norepinephrine or dopamine, Loftstrom et al. (482) concluded that amine fibers in the hypendymal layer of the internal zone were predominantly noradrenergic, fibers in the lateral palisade zone were predominantly dopaminergic, and fibers in the medial palisade zone were both dopaminergic and noradrenergic. Ajika and Hokfelt (492) estimated the number of monaminergic terminals to be one-third the total number of terminals in the median eminence. Over twice as many dopaminergic terminals are present in the lateral palisade zone as in the medial palisade zone of the rat's median eminence. A similar distribution of fluorescence has been found in the rabbit (493,494) and cat (495). As in the rat, fluorescence was maximal in the palisade layer of the external zone and the hypendymal layer of the internal zone in these animals. The distribution of catecholamine terminals is presumed to be analogous to that in the rat. Neurotensin has been identified in the palisade layer of the rat's median eminence (433), and it has been colocalized with dopamine and hypothalamic neurons (496).

Immunohistochemical studies demonstrated two other neurotransmitters in the median eminence—acetylcholine (375) and GABA (312,313)—by demonstrating the presence of ir-acetylcholine esterase or glutamic acid decarboxylase in nerve terminals.

Several peptidergic systems terminate in the palisade layer of the external zone. Their distribution has been reviewed extensively (161), and this discussion will concentrate primarily on more recent findings. GnRH has been localized within large granular vesicles in terminals that, at infundibular levels, lie in the lateral palisade zone in the rat's median eminence. In the pre- and postinfundibular median eminence, GnRH fibers are more uniformly distributed between the medial and lateral palisade zones (161,360). If pre-embedding immunohistochemical techniques are employed on vibrotome sections, more GnRH is found in the medial palisade zone than is found in paraffin-embedded thick sections, and the difference between the medial and lateral palisade zones is less striking (497). Simultaneous localization of GnRH- and dopamine-containing terminals demonstrates GnRH fibers preferentially in the lateral palisade zone of the rat's median eminence in close relationship to dopamine-containing fibers (498,499). On examination of their light-microscopic preparations, which are fluorescence stained for dopamine terminals and immunohistochemically stained for GnRH, McNeill and Sladek (498) found one population of aminergic terminals closely associated with portal vessels and a second population of aminergic terminals closely related to GnRH-containing terminals. They proposed that dopaminergic terminals inhibit GnRH released from peptidergic terminals through axo-axonic synapses. Dopamine-containing terminals have been found closely apposed to GnRH-containing terminals on transmission electron-microscopic studies (500). Although synapses were not reported, an interaction between dopamine and GnRH-containing terminals seems certain. In agreement with the findings of Rodriguez et al. (462), Ohtsuka et al. (360) found that GnRH terminals did not reach the basal lamina at the surface of the lateral palisade zone. Most are located at a distance greater than 0.5 μm from the perivascular space and were separated from it by a "glio-ependymal cuff."

Species differences in the distribution of GnRH terminals have been stressed by Anthony et al. (419). In primates, GnRH-staining fibers were found in the internal zone of the median eminence and could be followed into the infundibular stem and process. The authors pointed out that GnRH terminals in the neural lobe are juxtaposed to regions in the pars distalis that are rich in gonadotrophs and that "short portal" vascular connections between the neural lobe and pars distalis are ample in these animals. It is not clear whether a relationship of GnRH terminals to dopamine terminals is maintained in the neural lobe of these animals.

TRH terminals are aggregated in the medial palisade zone (161,415,501). These terminals lie in the perivascular space of capillaries in the median eminence (358). Somatostatin-containing fibers are found throughout the external and internal zones of the median eminence in the rat (161). These terminals, like those that contain TRH, lie in the perivascular space of capillaries (360). GRH-immunostained fibers are distributed in a pattern similar to somatostatin fibers in the rat median eminence (502,503). CRH terminals also lie principally in the medial palisade layer of the external zone (504–506) in the rat and in an analogous site in the monkey (507).

Vasopressin- and oxytocin-containing neurons also terminate in the palisade layer of the median eminence, principally in its medial region (508–512). In the guinea pig these terminals contain large granular vesicles (90–110 nm in diameter), not the large dense-core vesicles (>150 nm in diameter) in which hormones are localized in terminals in the neural lobe (342,513). In the pre- and postinfundibular region of the rat's median eminence, there is considerable overlap between the distribution of immunoreactive CRH, AVP, and OT. In the infundibular region, only a few AVP or OT fibers were found in the palisade zone, whereas CRH-containing fibers were plentiful there (514). However, AVP-containing neurons have adequate access to capillaries in the median eminence because portal vessels contain high concentrations of AVP and neurophysin (515) as well as of CRH (516). AVP-containing neurons were described as coursing ventrally, at right angles to the fiber layer, to gain access to capillaries in the external zone in this region. This pattern was accentuated after adrenalectomy (514). AVP (517,518) and OT (519) potentiate CRH-stimulated ACTH release from corticotrophs. Terminals containing angiotensin II have recently been identified by immunohistochemistry in the palisade zone of the rat's median eminence, and their staining is selectively enhanced by adrenalectomy (520). In general, it may be said of the (rat) median eminence that those neurosecretory systems necessary for survival and maintenance of the individual are found in the medial palisade zone, whereas those neurosecretory systems necessary for survival and maintenance of the species (reproduction) lie in the lateral palisade zone.

POMC derivatives are primarily localized, by immunohistochemical techniques and LM, to the external zone of the median eminence in several species other than the rat. In the sheep and ox, β-LPH "projects to portal capillaries" (521). Bloch et al. (522) found that in humans, fibers containing immunoreactive β-End terminate "close to vessels in the median eminence." Such neurons are also reactive to antisera against ACTH, MSH, and β-LPH (523). Although species differences in the distribution of terminals containing the derivatives of POMC may be present, there seems to be general agreement that terminals in the median eminence are closely related to capillaries of the portal system because ACTH and β-End are present in portal blood (524,525).

Enkephalins have been localized within the external zone of the (rat's) median eminence with antibodies that do not cross-react with POMC, β-LPH, or β-End (526). Substance

P has been localized to the external zone of the rat (161), the mouse (413), the monkey, and the human (527) median eminence. Immunoreactive vasoactive intestinal peptide (161), neurotensin (433), cholecystokinen (412), and gastrin (161) have been identified in the palisade layer of the rat's median eminence. Immunoreactive PRL (528) and GH (529,530) have also been identified in the external zone of the rat's median eminence and persist after hypophysectomy. GH is colocalized with TRH (530).

The pattern of regional segregation of neurosecretory systems within the neurohypophysis has been most clarified in the rat. The temptation to regard this pattern as a prototype for the mammalian hypophysis should be resisted because species differences may be marked. The distinction between the internal zone and the external zone is blurred in some mammalian species, including the human, by invasion of the palisade layer into the internal zone (481). The site of termination of a particular neurosecretory system can also vary with the species studied (419). However, the basic organizational pattern of the mammalian neurohypophysis stands out clearly from the blurred background of differences in species detail. This pattern involves the relationship of individual axon terminals to capillaries and the regional segregation of systems of neurosecretory terminals within the neurohypophysis. Blood vessels, not other nerves, will carry the messages released from these axon terminals in the median eminence and neural lobe and will contribute to the organization of the neurohypophysis.

THE PORTAL SYSTEM

Capillaries of the Hypophysis

The capillaries and portal vessels of the pituitary gland carry blood from which oxygen, nutrients, and amino acids have been removed and to which metabolic waste products and peptide hormones have been added from the neurohypophysis to the adenohypophysis. These peptide hormones leave the blood to interact with receptors at the cell's surface and to regulate their release of protein hormones that, in turn, enter the capillaries and are carried away from the gland. A single capillary bed extends throughout the entire neurohypophysis (29,532) (Fig. 11). It communicates, via capillary or portal routes, with similar-appearing capillaries in the pars tuberalis and pars distalis of the adenohypophysis (66,532), and its perivascular space communicates extensively with the extracellular space of the pars intermedia (305). Hypophyseal capillaries do not exclude acid vital dyes from the pituitary that lacks a blood-brain barrier (29). Neurohypophyseal (328,329,332,346) and adenohypophyseal (219) capillaries are fenestrated, as are the portal vessels that unite them (329,532). These fenestrated capillaries are surrounded by a double basement membrane. The inner basal lamina lies next to each fenestrated endothelial tube, whereas the outer basal lamina is separated from it and lies

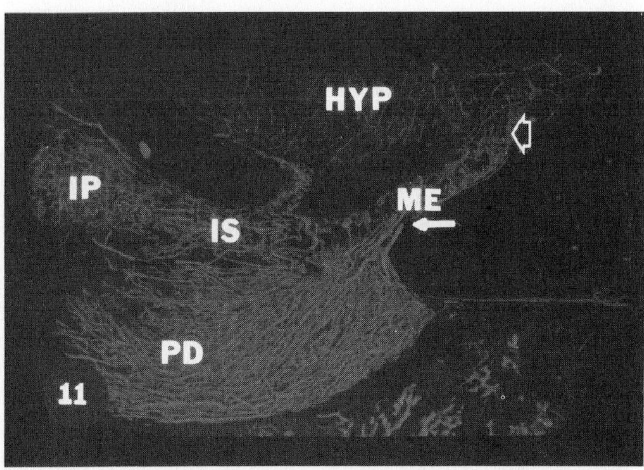

FIG. 11. Rabbit median eminence in sagittal section. A confluent capillary bed unites the median eminence (ME), infundibular stem (IS), and infundibular process (IP). Within the median eminence an external and an internal plexus may be discerned. Connections between median eminence and hypothalamic capillaries are seen far rostrally at hollow arrowhead. Portal connections between median eminence and pars distalis (PD) are indicated by white arrow. ×25. (HYP) Hypothalamus. (From ref. 532.)

next to the parenchymal elements (Figs. 7,12). In the adenohypophysis, these parenchymal elements are epithelial cells arranged in cords. Because their capillaries are linearly arrayed (532), the configuration of the perivascular space is not complex (219). In the neurohypophysis these parenchymal elements are axons and their terminals, ependymal terminals, and glial cells, and the configuration of the perivascular space can be complex. The inner and outer basal lamina define the perivascular space, which, in the neural lobe of the mouse, is 0.3 to 0.5 μm in width and contains reticular fibers (533). In the median eminence of the rabbit, it surrounds entire vascular formations (330) that have invaginated from the surface into the neuropil. The perivascular space forms an extensive system of channels that are revealed with tannic acid staining (533) or silver impregnation (398). In the neural lobe these channels form an extensive system of connections between neighboring capillaries. Pericytes, histiocytes, fibroblasts, and mast cells have been identified between the basal lamina in the perivascular space of human neural lobes (350). In both the median eminence and neural lobe, extensions of the perivascular space increase the surface area available for neurohemal contact, with a minimal increase in neurohypophyseal volume.

Secretory elements in the hypophysis, neural or glandular, are disposed along the outer basal lamina of the perivascular space. Fenestrated capillaries are disposed along the inner basal lamina. Large protein molecules in the blood are relatively free to pass through fenestrae in the endothelial tube and interact with receptors at the cell's surface. Protein molecules sequestered in vesicles in the cell's cytoplasm are relatively free (after release into the perivascular space) to pass through the fenestrations in the capillaries into the

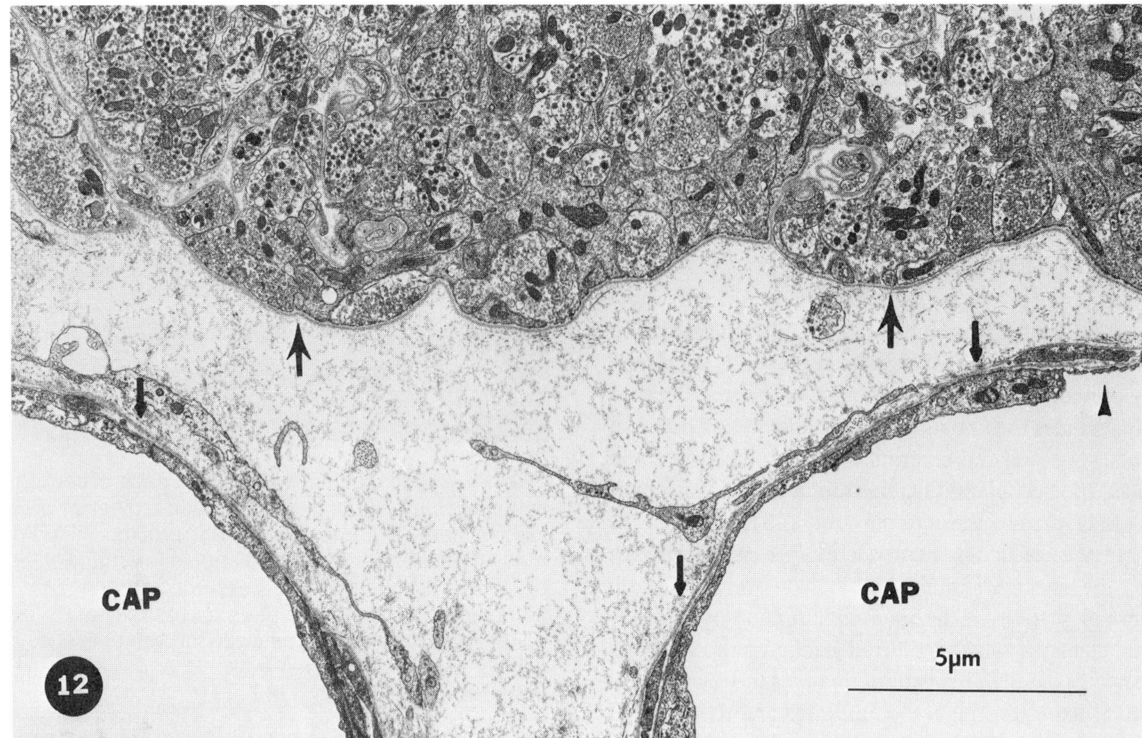

FIG. 12. Transmission electron micrograph of rabbit median-eminence–internal-zone–horizontal section. Two limbs of a capillary loop in the median eminence floor (CAP) are cut in horizontal section. One limb is fenestrated (*arrowhead*). The perivascular space is common to both. The outer basement membrane material is condensed at the margin of the contact zone common to both capillaries (*vertical large arrows*). The inner basement membrane is condensed about each individual capillary component (*vertical small arrows*). (From ref. 330.)

bloodstream. This freedom of passage is not absolute, however, because (for example) basic dyes do not enter the hypophysis easily. Simionescu et al. (534,535) demonstrated the presence of microdomains in fenestrated endothelial cells of mouse pancreatic capillaries and "expected that these structures will select permeant molecules according to charge, in addition to size." Similar findings can be anticipated in the fenestrated endothelial cells of the hypophysis.

Development of the Portal System

Vessels of the hypophysis develop from the mesenchyme that is entrapped between the advancing saccus infundibuli and Rathke's pouch and that invades both structures according to Wislocki (536). Enemar (537) proposed that a (primary) plexus of capillaries lines the surface of the saccus infundibuli and that another (secondary) plexus of capillaries lies on the surface of the Rathke's pouch in the mouse by the 14th fetal day. They are united by "linking" capillaries at the junction of the rostral portion of the saccus infundibuli and the oral wall of Rathke's pouch. These linking capillaries become more numerous by the 15th fetal day, and by the 16th fetal day in the mouse the primary plexus of capillaries overlying the saccus infundibuli has become very dense. As the saccus infundibuli enlarges and differentiates over the next 2 days, the continuous capillary network over the presumptive median eminence, infundibular stem, and infundibular process increases in thickness and begins to invade the developing neurohypophysis. Concurrently, the presumptive pars distalis becomes more densely vascularized by invasion of capillaries from its surface. By the 19th fetal day, portal vessels on the ventral surface of the median eminence (which unite the primary and secondary capillary plexuses) have become distinct. This appearance is unchanged on the 20th (birth) day of the mouse. The capillary loops of the internal (deep) plexus in the median eminence do not appear until 2 to 3 days after birth and do not complete their development for 2 weeks. The deep system of long capillary loops and subependymal vessels is completed by 7 days, but the system of short capillary loops is not completed until 14 days of age.

The development of the pituitary vessels is similar in the rat (538). On the 15th fetal day, capillaries of the primary plexus on the surface of the saccus infundibuli and on the surface of the remainder of the neural tube are nonfenestrated endothelial tubes that lie free in the mesenchyme. On that day, fenestrae have been found only in capillaries entrapped between the presumptive median eminence and pars distalis (376). Fenestrae did not attain the size, density, or distribution of those found in the adult rat neurohypophyseal and adenohypophyseal capillary beds until the 20th fetal day (380,388). Ugrumov et al. (539) identified some short capillary loops in the rat's median eminence on the 18th fetal day. Few mitotic figures were found at this time. He explained the formation of capillary loops by the growth and attenuation of preexisting cells on the oral surface of the median eminence with buckling of the capillaries inward from the surface and invasion of the neuropil. A similar mechanism was proposed by Page and Dovey-Hartman (330). In the rat, development of the internal plexus in the median eminence is delayed until after birth as it is in the mouse (538); but this pattern is not representative of all mammals because in the rabbit it is completed before birth (540).

Organization of the Portal System

The neurohypophyseal capillary bed extends from the median eminence to the neural lobe. It is supplied rostrally by superior hypophyseal arteries and caudally by inferior hypophyseal arteries (531). A third source of arterial supply has been identified and variously named the "anterior hypophyseal artery" (84), "peduncular artery" (541), "loral artery" (542), or "trabecular artery" (81,99). The name "middle hypophyseal artery" seems appropriate because this vessel arises from the internal carotid artery between the origins of the inferior and superior hypophyseal arteries. The inferior hypophyseal arteries arise as a pair of vessels from the intracavernous segment of the internal carotid arteries and supply the neural lobe (infundibular process). Frequently they unite to form an anastomosis between the left and right internal carotid arteries prior to supplying the neural lobe. The middle hypophyseal arteries also arise from the intracavernous segment of the internal carotid arteries. They frequently unite (as in the rabbit, rat, and cat) to form a single artery that then supplies the infundibular stem (531). The superior hypophyseal arteries arise from the intracranial carotid arteries and from the circle of Willis. These (multiple) arteries approach the median eminence centripetally to form an anastomotic ring about it and to supply the rostral region of the neurohypophysis (the median eminence) (531,537,543). The arterial supply to the pituitary gland thus represents three ascending levels of anastomotic channels between the paired carotid arteries whose branches supply the neurohypophyseal capillary bed.

Superior and inferior hypophyseal arteries are innervated by postganglionic sympathetic nerves. Innervation of the middle hypophyseal artery by these nerves is expected but has not as yet been reported. Arterioles that supply the neural lobe of the pig and rat (544) are also innervated by sympathetic fibers, but a similar innervation of arterioles supplying the rat (487,488) or rabbit (545) median eminence has not been found. Precapillary arterioles do lie on the surface of the median eminence near catecholamine-secreting terminals of central aminergic systems and near fenestrated capillaries on the surface of the median eminence (330).

The venous drainage of the caudal region of the neurohypophyseal capillary bed mirrors its arterial supply. Paired inferior hypophyseal veins course from the neural lobe to the posterior intercavernous sinus and to the posterior regions of the paired cavernous sinuses that lie lateral to the midline (543). A less prominent route of drainage is from the neural lobe to the adjacent pars distalis via capillary and "short portal" routes. Short portal veins uniting the neural lobe with the pars distalis are abundant in some species (i.e., rat, mouse, and rabbit) but few in others (i.e., pig, dog, and monkey) (85,532). The hypophyseal cleft limits the number and disposition of vascular connections between the pars distalis and the neuro-intermediate lobe. The neural lobe has ample venous drainage routes to the systemic circulation and limited venous drainage routes to the pars distalis (543).

There are no direct venous drainage routes of the territory supplied by the middle hypophyseal artery, except for the short portal vessels that connect the infundibular stem with the pars distalis.

Venous drainage of the rostral region of the neurohypophyseal capillary bed (the median eminence) does not mirror its arterial supply (29,66,81,82) (Fig. 13). The primary plexus in the median eminence is drained by fenestrated long portal vessels that course to the pars distalis and then arborize into a secondary capillary plexus. Direct capillary connections may also be plentiful depending on the length of the infundibular stem and the species being examined (66,328,329,532). Drainage routes from the primary capillary plexus in the median eminence to veins at the surface of the brain were denied by Wislocki (29,86–89). However, Duvernoy et al. (546) demonstrated systemic drainage routes from the postinfundibular median eminence in humans, and Ambach et al. (547) have demonstrated venous channels from the preinfundibular median eminence to the tuberal and chiasmatic veins in the rat. In both cases, drainage routes from the median eminence to these systemic sites were poorly developed, and they probably represent a regression of the ample venous connections between the saccus infundibuli and the remainder of the neural tube which were present prior to the apposition of the saccus infundibuli and Rathke's pouch and the development of portal vessels. Venous drainage routes from the rostral region of the neurohypophyseal capillary bed, the median eminence, to the secondary capillary bed in the pars distalis are ample, whereas venous drainage routes to the systemic circulation are not.

The adenohypophysis, contrary to the belief of Wislocki (29,86–89), does not appear to receive a direct arterial supply (66,81,82,85,532). Blood destined for the adenohypophysis passes through the neurohypophysis. Capillaries and veins bring blood to the pars tuberalis and pars distalis.

Veins from the pars distalis to the paired cavernous and

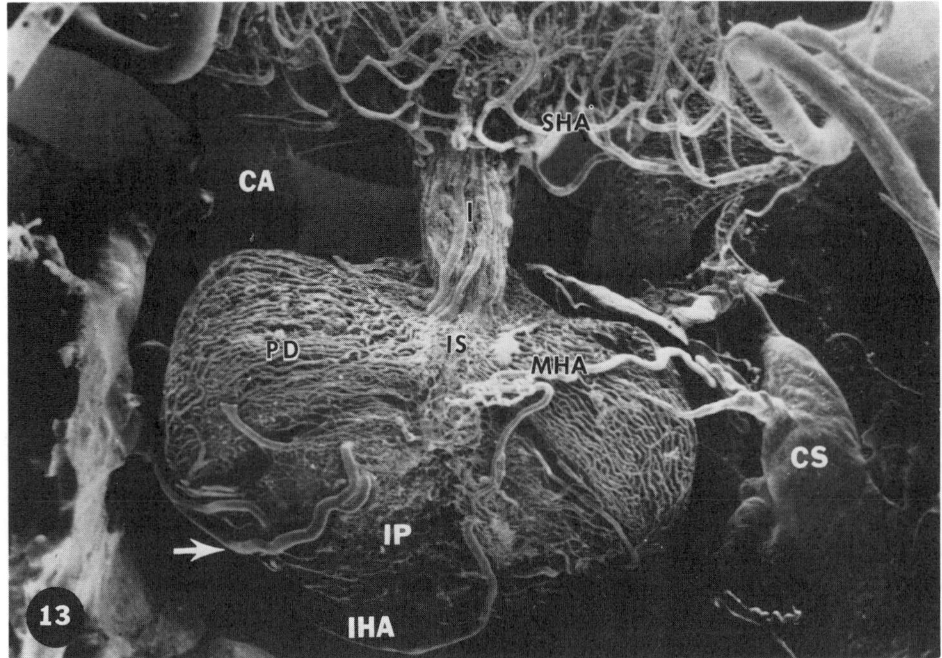

FIG. 13. Scanning electron micrograph of hypothalamic-pituitary vascular cast of the monkey as seen from behind. A common capillary bed extends throughout the infundibulum (I), infundibular stem (IS), and infundibular process (IP). It is supplied rostrally by superior hypophyseal arteries (SHA) and caudally by inferior hypophyseal arteries (IHA). Long portal vessels are present on the surface of the infundibulum. Lateral hypophyseal veins from the pars distalis to the cavernous sinus (CS) are few in number. Y-shaped inferior hypophyseal veins (*arrow*) drain both the pars distalis (PD) and the infundibular process. (MHA) Middle hypophyseal artery; (CA) carotid artery. (From ref. 543.)

posterior intercavernous sinuses provide routes of egress for blood in the pars distalis. There are only scant venous drainage routes from the pars distalis to the adjacent cavernous sinus. Named lateral hypophyseal veins by Wislocki (29,86–89), they were believed by him to be sufficient in size and number to drain the entire pars distalis. Green (548) also believed them to be sufficient. However, Torok (549,550) and Bergland and Page (543) felt that such venous drainage routes appeared inadequate for the task of draining the pars distalis. The latter authors demonstrated the presence of large paired Y-shaped inferior hypophyseal veins. One limb drained the pars distalis, whereas the other limb drained the neural lobe; the common trunk passed to the posterior intercavernous sinus or to the posterior regions of the cavernous sinuses.

The pattern of neural traffic is determined by the connectivity of neurons. The direction of information flow and the destination of that information can be deduced from a study of the neuronal circuitry of interest. The available patterns of blood flow are also determined by the vascular anatomy, but the patterns of blood flow employed in living animals are not easily deduced from anatomical studies of blood vessels. Observations of blood flow in the portal vessels of living animals leave no doubt that blood flows from the median eminence to the pars distalis (69,70,549–555). The hypothalamic hypophysiotrophic releasing factors in the terminals of neurons in the median eminence are carried to the pars distalis over restricted vascular routes.

Observation of blood flow in the neurohypophysis reveals blood flow between adjacent neurohypophyseal regions (between the neural lobe and lower infundibular stem and between the median eminence and the upper infundibular stem). It also reveals a major drainage route from the rostral neurohypophysis (the median eminence) to the pars distalis and reveals that the major drainage route of the caudal neurohypophysis (neural lobe) is the cavernous sinus. However, some blood does flow from the neural lobe to the adjacent pars distalis and neural hormones released in the neural lobe have access to glandular epithelium in this region (555). In addition, neural lobe hormones (e.g., OT and its side chain [Pro-Leu-Gly-NH_2]) have access to the pars intermedia through extensive connections between the perivascular space of the neural lobe and the extracellular space of the pars intermedia (305).

Rostrally, in the median eminence, the neurohypophyseal capillary bed is specialized (Fig. 11). The primary plexus is subdivided into an external and an internal plexus (85,532). The external plexus corresponds to the superficial network of Duvernoy (556) and the mantle plexus of Romeis (256). The external plexus lies on the surface of the median eminence and is continuous with the capillaries of the infundibular stem and process. It receives the arterial supply to the median eminence. Its morphology differs little from species to species [compare the external plexus of the toad (557) to that of the rabbit (85) (Fig. 14)]. The external plexus forms a reticular network of fenestrated capillaries that lie

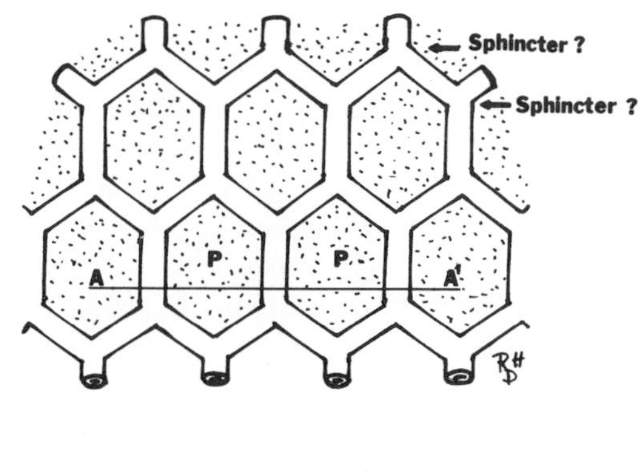

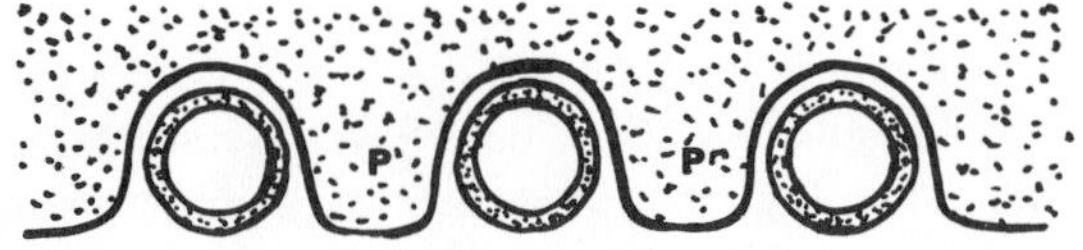

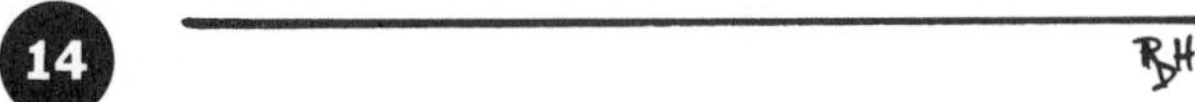

FIG. 14. Top: Schematic view of external plexus from below. Hexagonal arrays of capillaries are separated by posts (P) of median eminence tissue. **Bottom:** Schematic cross-sectional view of median eminence external plexus along plane A-A′ in top panel. Capillaries lie embedded in neuropil separated by posts (P) of median eminence tissue. (From ref. 558.)

partially buried within the oral (ventral) surface of the median eminence (85,330,532,558). These capillaries form a mosaic, made up of multiple hexagonal units, that is oriented parallel to the surface of the median eminence. TEM studies (330,558) demonstrate that the capillaries are partially embedded within the external zone such that their oral surface is flush with the oral surface of the palisade layer. The central region of each hexagonal capillary unit is filled with "posts" of median eminence tissue. This capillary pattern resembles that found in two other organs where the exchange of materials between the blood and tissue is rapid—the gastric mucosa and the lung (559,560). Sobin et al. (561) described the pulmonary vascular space as resembling "an underground garage consisting of a floor, a ceiling, and supportive pillars, all covered with endothelium", and they argued that blood flows as a sheet through an essentially continuous space lined by endothelium. In the median eminence a similar pattern of flow may be present because the angioarchitecture of the external plexus resembles that in the lung.

The organization of the palisade layer and of the external plexus has functional consequences of importance to the regulation of the adenohypophysis. Each hexagonal capillary unit (microvascular module) encloses a post (microdomain) of neurosecretory axon terminals and glial tissue. With increased functional demand, glial processes can be expected to retract from positions interposed between axon terminals and capillaries to make more surface area available for the release of hypothalamic peptides and amines into the portal system to be carried to the pars distalis (562). Within each microdomain, amines and peptides released from one terminal are free to act upon neighboring terminals if appropriate receptors are present: A paracrine action of secretions released by terminals in the palisade layer upon neighboring terminals is possible as well as an endocrine action upon the epithelial cells of the pars distalis. If sheet flow should occur across the surface of the median eminence, the secretions of one microdomain would be free to interact with the terminals in other microdomains. The microcirculation in the palisade layer could permit interactions between microdomains separated from one another on the surface of the median eminence. If future TEM studies should reveal smooth-muscle sphincters arrayed at the entrance to each hexagonal microvascular module, the opportunities to permit very regional adjustments in the distribution of blood flow at the surface of the palisade layer would be present, and the capacity for neurons terminating in one microdomain to influence neurons terminating in another could be limited or regulated.

Whereas the external plexus receives the arterial blood supply from the superior hypophyseal arteries, it distributes blood into portal vessels coursing to the pars distalis or into the internal plexus that invades the median eminence.

The internal plexus arises from the external plexus (537,538,540). There is considerable variability in the anatomy of the internal plexus between species (compare the rat, the rabbit, and the monkey) (85,532). Viewed from within the ventricle, the median eminence forms a bowl or a funnel, and hence the term *infundibulum* is employed to describe it. The bowl has a floor and walls. The basic pattern

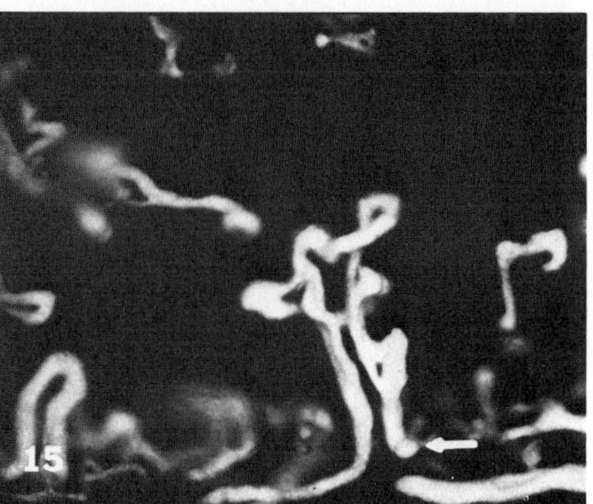

FIG. 15. Light-microscopic photograph of rabbit median eminence in sagittal section. Microfil injection. An internal-plexus capillary loop arises from the external plexus (*small arrow*) to arborize beneath the ventricular surface and then drain to a portal vessel. Ependymal processes terminate about the apex of the loop, whereas small neurons make neurohemal contact along the limbs of these formations. If sphincters are present at the origin of these modules, a mechanism for regional control of blood flow within small (functional) regions of the median eminence will be present. ×100. (From ref. 532.)

of the internal plexus is one of capillary loops in the floor of the infundibulum, and, in some animals, capillary coils in its walls. The capillary loops in the floor of the median eminence (of the rat) have been subdivided into (a) long capillary loops that stretch into the hypendymal layer and (b) short capillary loops that extend from the surface of the palisade layer, only as far as the reticular layer.

The capillary loops of the internal plexus are well seen when the median eminence has been sectioned in the mid-sagittal plane following the intravascular injection of India ink (29,66,556,563–565), neoprene latex (99), or Microfil (532) and viewed with a light microscope or by examining corrosion casts of the median eminence with the SEM (85,532). Such techniques revealed the loops of the internal plexus to be made up of an ascending limb, an apex, and a descending limb (Fig. 15). The ascending limb arises from the external plexus and passes through the palisade layer and reticular layer into the internal zone, where it may pass as deep as the hypendymal layer. There may be extensive arborization beneath the ependyma at the apex of the long loops. The descending limb is larger than the ascending limb and passes back through the internal zone, the reticular layer, and the palisade layer to the surface of the median eminence, where it joins either an external plexus capillary or a portal vessel (564).

The capillary loops of the internal plexus also form a series of microvascular modules which is best appreciated on sagittal section (Fig. 11). They arise from the external plexus phylogenetically (they are not present in amphibians but are present in mammals) (557) and embryologically (537,538,540). As a loop invaginates into the median eminence, it carries with it an expanded perivascular space that surrounds the entire formation (330,539). Hence on serial sections, elements of a single vascular module can be identified in light or TEM studies (330). The perivascular space between the ascending and descending limbs of each loop is continuous with the perivascular space on the surface of the palisade layer. It lies between the widely split basal lamina, whose inner layer is applied to the convoluted endothelial tube and whose outer layer invests the entire formation in a fashion analogous to the disposition of the visceral and parietal peritoneum. Neurohemal contact has recently been documented along the course of these loops in the external and in the internal zone of the rabbit median eminence (330). Columns of capillary loops surrounded by parvicellular axon terminals thus stand upon a base comprised of hexagonal arrays of capillaries, each of which encloses a microdomain of neurosecretory terminals (Fig. 16). Because each loop invaginated from the surface into the depths of the median eminence, it can be expected to

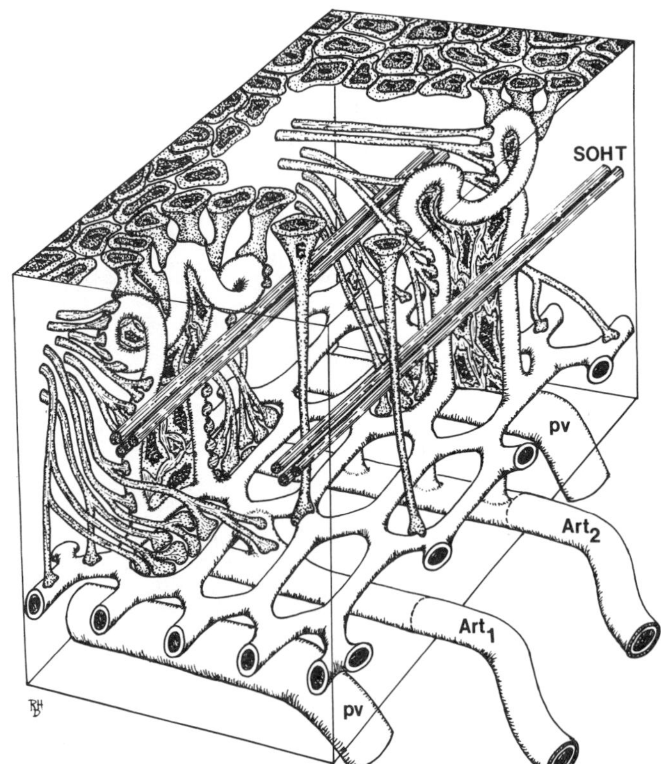

FIG. 16. Diagram of neurovascular organization in the medial third of the rabbit median eminence. The external plexus forms a hexagonal array oriented parallel to the median eminence external surface and receives arterial blood from arteriolar branches of the superior hypophyseal arteries (Art$_1$, Art$_2$). Internal plexus capillary loops arise from the external plexus and arborize in the subependymal zone. Connective tissue fills the spaces between the ascending and descending limbs of the internal plexus loops and the ventral aspect of the median eminence between the surface of the external zone and the pars tuberalis. Nonciliated ependymal cells line the infundibular recess (E). The basal process of some ependymal cells end in the perivascular space about the apex of capillary loops and form an ependymal cuff about them in the hypendymal layer. Some ependymal processes extend to the external plexus. Parvicellular axons terminate on external plexus capillaries and about internal plexus capillary loops to form axonal cuff about them deep in the fiber layer and in the palisade zone. These axons are peptidergic and aminergic. Magnocellular systems (SOHT) pass through the fiber layer and do not send collaterals to the capillary loops. Arterioles that originate from superior hypophyseal arteries lie on the median eminence surface and supply the external plexus by tapering down from terminal arterioles to precapillary arterioles (Art$_1$) and/or by sending small (precapillary arteriolar) branches at right angles from the terminal arterioles (Art$_2$). Arterioles lie in close proximity to the external plexus and to posts (microdomains) of neurosecretory and aminergic terminals. Portal vessels (pv) are fenestrated and do not contain a continuous layer of smooth muscles in their walls. (Modified from ref. 330.)

have carried with it axon terminals from the surface of the palisade layer. Each vertical column should then be expected to contain terminals functionally similar to those at its base. The area for neurohemal contact will be increased, but the endocrinotopic organization of the median eminence (356) will be preserved by such an arrangement. In this regard it is of interest that a regional difference in the dopamine concentration in portal vessels has been reported, with the dopamine concentration higher in medial than in lateral long portal vessels of the rat (566). It is not known at present whether smooth-muscle cells are arrayed at the origin of each capillary loop, and thus it is not known if the flow into these capillary loops can be regulated by sphincters. The recruitment of vascular columns in functionally specific regions of the median eminence would markedly enhance the neuroendocrine response to a functional demand. Coupled with such mechanisms as an increase in neurosecretion, an increase in blood flow, an increase in the permeability of the median eminence, and a retraction of the glial processes located between axon terminals and capillaries, the recruitment of microvascular modules would significantly add to the ability of the median eminence to respond to demands placed upon it.

A subependymal system of capillaries is present in the median eminence of some species, and, in addition to the external and internal plexuses, forms a third capillary network in the median eminence that unites it with the hypothalamus in mammals. In birds these capillaries appear to be hypothalamic vessels that unite the left and right sides of the hypothalamus and appear to be spatially separated from the capillaries of the primary plexus (458). In mammals, their relationship to capillaries in the median eminence is quite different. They unite the apices of adjacent long capillary loops in the median eminence and pass to the arcuate nucleus (532,547). Ambach et al. (547) employed LM to examine serial sections of the rat's hypothalamus and pituitary gland after the intravascular injection of India ink. To differentiate arteries from veins and capillaries, they first injected the animals with a blue India ink mixed in a gelatin solution of low viscosity and then injected the animal with a red India ink in a gelatin solution of high viscosity. Vessels containing the red (high-viscosity) mixture were identified as arteries because the high-viscosity mixture was not expected to pass into smaller capillaries and thence to veins. Vessels containing the blue dye were identified as capillaries or veins. They employed this technique to identify subependymal vessels in the median eminence of the rat which united the apices of internal plexus capillary loops. They stated that the subependymal plexus had an independent arterial supply in the median eminence and drained to the hypothalamus. Page et al. (532) employed SEM to study the angioarchitecture of the rat, dog, cat, sheep, and monkey median eminence. The subependymal plexus was found in the rat, dog, and sheep median eminence and was continuous with the subependymal capillaries in the hypothalamus, but a direct arterial supply was not found. It arose from the apices of capillary loops. In the rabbit, cat, and monkey, a subependymal plexus was not present, but connections between the internal plexus of the median eminence and subependymal capillaries in the walls of the third ventricle over the hypothalamic arcuate nucleus were present (Fig. 17). Akmayev (567,568) had previously stressed the presence of these capillary connections between the median eminence and the arcuate nucleus. Ambach et al. (547) argued that the capillary beds of the arcuate nucleus and the neurohypophysis should be considered as a single unit. The hypophyseal vascular system is not as isolated from the hypothalamus as originally proposed and subsequently defended by Wislocki (29,86–89).

Torok (549,550) reported that blood flowed from the external plexus into capillary loops of the internal plexus and then into subependymal vessels and then to the hypothalamus. He further reported that upon dissection of the pituitary stalk with separation of the infundibular stem from the pars distalis, he found some deep portal vessels in which blood appeared to be flowing from the pars distalis to the median eminence. This observation has not been independently verified. Neither the observation nor its obvious consequences have been widely accepted. However, they cannot be easily dismissed. A labeled analog of ACTH [^{3}H]ACTH4-9 and of [^{3}H]β-LPH have been injected into the pars distalis of the rat, with subsequent recovery of label in the hypothalamus. If the pituitary stalk was severed just prior to injection, the label was not recovered in the hypothalamus. If 8 days were permitted to pass following stalk section (sufficient time for vascular but not neural regeneration), label was again recovered from the hypothalamus after injection into the pituitary (569,570). Injection of neurotensin into the rat pituitary produced a profound decrease in core body temperature. This effect is only seen if neurotensin reaches the hypothalamus in adequate amounts. The effect was abolished by prior stalk section but was regained if the vessels were permitted to regenerate (571). Although it is possible that the act of injection of substances into the pars distalis could have reversed the normal direction of pituitary blood flow, the possibility of "two-way transport in the hypothalamo-hypophyseal system" (570) remains open.

The arterial supply to the median eminence is to its external plexus. Arterioles that supply the median eminence lie close to axon terminals and fenestrated capillaries of the external plexus containing vasoactive catecholamines and peptides (545). Hence they will be exposed to high levels of dopamine and neurohormones released at the ventral surface of the median eminence. In addition, the descending limbs of capillary loops carry blood to the external plexus capillaries from deep in the internal zone. Aminergic as well as peptidergic terminals contact these loops in the internal zone (330). The noradrenergic reticulo-infundibular tract terminates in that zone. Blood returning to the external plexus through the internal plexus may contain norepinephrine and epinephrine (572) as well as dopamine. The resistance vessels lying at the surface of the median eminence regulate blood flow into its external plexus, but they are, in turn, exposed to vasoactive amines and peptides secreted

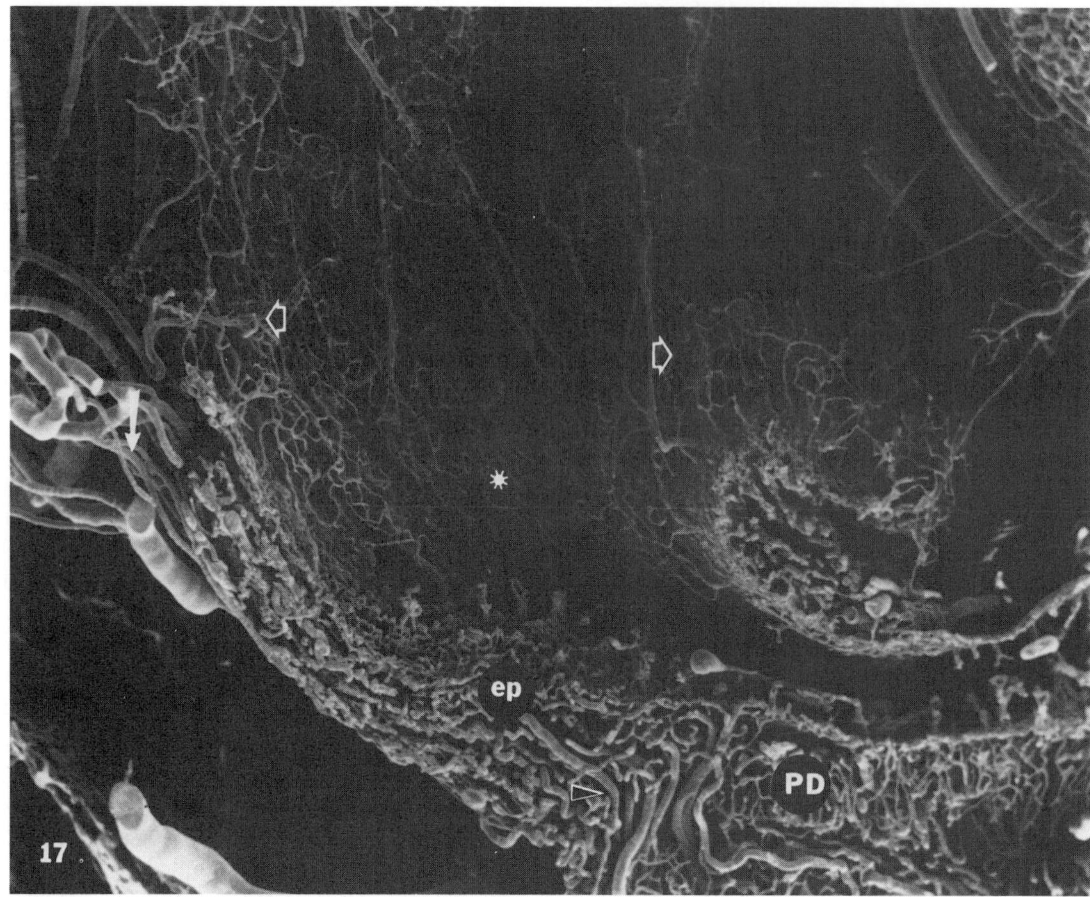

FIG. 17. Scanning electron micrograph of cat hypothalamus and median eminence, sagittal view. The rostral position is to the reader's left. The median eminence external plexus (ep) lies interposed between pars distalis (PD) capillaries below and internal plexus capillary loops above. Vertical arrow designates superior hypophyseal arteries, which vascularize external plexus. External plexus capillaries unite to form portal vessels coursing to the pars distalis (*black arrowhead*). Capillary connections between the median eminence and hypothalamus are present anteriorly and posteriorly at hollow arrowheads and in the periventricular zone at the asterisk. Note that periventricular capillary connections uniting the lateral wall of the median eminence with the hypothalamus cannot be appreciated on Microfil section (compare with Fig. 11). (From ref. 532.)

by the median eminence (545). The neurosecretory systems terminating in the median eminence may regulate blood flow into it (Fig. 16).

THE HYPOTHALAMUS

Cell Bodies of the Hypothalamus

Peptidergic neurons synthesize protein hormones in their cell bodies in the hypothalamus behind the blood-brain barrier and transport them to nerve terminals in the neurohypophysis outside the blood-brain barrier. Magnocellular peptidergic neurons have large cell bodies measuring 12 to 30 μm in diameter in the goldfish (51), 25 to 50 μm in diameter in the rabbit (573), and about 25 μm in diameter in the rat (574). Their cell bodies are oval or pear shaped and contain an eccentrically placed nucleus that contains a single nucleolus. LM examination of cresyl violet preparations reveals (a) a cytoplasm with a granular marginal zone rich in Nissl substance and (b) a clear central zone. These cells are multipolar or bipolar. Golgi-Cox preparations reveal the soma of multipolar (but not bipolar) neurons to be spiny (573). Many of them have a "rough shaggy surface" (575). A single axon and three to five (primary) dendrites emerge from the cell body. The primary dendrites bifurcate into secondary dendrites shortly after emerging. Spines are prominent on both primary and secondary dendrites, which are bulbous and varicose. Tertiary branching is not frequent. Bipolar neurons are fusiform in shape, with a single spiny dendrite arising from each pole of a smooth cell body. Axons typically emerge from a primary or a secondary dendrite (573) or from the cell body (576). Axons are thinner than dendrites and frequently have a beaded appearance (575–577). Axon collaterals have been identified (575,576) and are presumed to be inhibitory on the basis of physiological studies (578). Immunohistochemical preparations reveal that OT and AVP, with their associated neurophysins (I and II), are present in the cell bodies of separate magnocellular neurons (59,62,340,579–581) as well as in their axons and dendrites (576). The significance of the finding that dendrites contain peptide hormones is unknown at present.

The ultrastructural appearance of these magnocellular neurons was first described by Palay (51), who studied the preoptic nucleus of the goldfish. Subsequent descriptions of their ultrastructure in other species are not significantly different, although they are perhaps more complete (582–584). These cells are found in the supraoptic (SON) and paraventricular (PVN) nuclei of mammals, and their ultrastructural appearance is similar in the two locations (585,586) (Fig. 18). The eccentrically placed nucleus contains a prominent nucleolus. The nucleus is folded, and it presents a smooth convex surface to the marginal zone and an indented folded surface to the central zone. The marginal zone is rich in rough endoplasmic reticulum (RER), with flattened cisternae that may be arrayed, in places, parallel to the surface of the neuron. The central zone contains a random assortment of organelles, including mitochondria, (shuttle) vesicles, Golgi, dense-core vesicles, lysosomes, smooth endoplasmic reticulum (SER), and ribosomes. Occasional Golgi cisternae can sometimes be seen to pinch off a (new) dense-core vesicle (neurosecretory granule).

Pulse labeling experiments suggest that labeled amino acids are incorporated first into the rough endoplasmic reticulum, then into the Golgi, and then into dense-core vesicles (587). Broadwell et al. (588) employed TEM and immunohistochemistry to localize neurophysin to sites of protein synthesis and storage (the nuclear envelope, RER, saccules of the Golgi apparatus, and dense-core vesicles). Subsequently, Broadwell and Oliver (589) examined dense-core-vesicle formation in neurosecretory cells of the SON in mice under normal conditions and after water deprivation for 5 to 8 days. With water deprivation, the Golgi apparatus became hypertrophied and dense-core vesicles budded off from saccules of both the trans and cis regions. Kozlowski et al. (590) could localize neurophysin only to dense-core vesicles in the neurons of the rat's SON, whereas Piekut et al. (591) could localize AVP only to the dense-core vesicles of the PVN of the rat. Events related to protein synthesis in the magnocellular peptidergic somata are similar to the events in the epithelial cells in the pars distalis. Unlike the adenohypophyseal glandular cell, which releases the hormone locally, the neuron transports the hormone to a distant terminal for release. Biochemical and immunohistochemical findings demonstrate that newly synthesized hormone in magnocellular neurons is incorporated within a larger prohormone molecule, which undergoes posttranslational modification and cleavage as it is carried within the dense-core vesicle by axoplasmic flow to an axon terminal in the neural lobe (58,61,63,64,592,593).

With stimulation, the changes in the ultrastructural morphology of AVP- and OT-containing neurons are similar. Kalimo (594) reported that in rats deprived of water for 4 to 6 days or suckled for 13 to 24 days, the magnocellular neurons in the PVN and SON increased in size. The nucleus and nucleolus also enlarged. The RER increased, as did the number of flattened cisternae. Many cisternae became dilated. The Golgi apparatus hypertrophied. Increased numbers of small vacuoles were found at both the cis and trans faces of the Golgi, and dense-core vesicles could be seen budding off from the Golgi in both the cis and trans regions. If suckling was prolonged, large vacuoles filled the cytoplasm in a fashion analogous to the

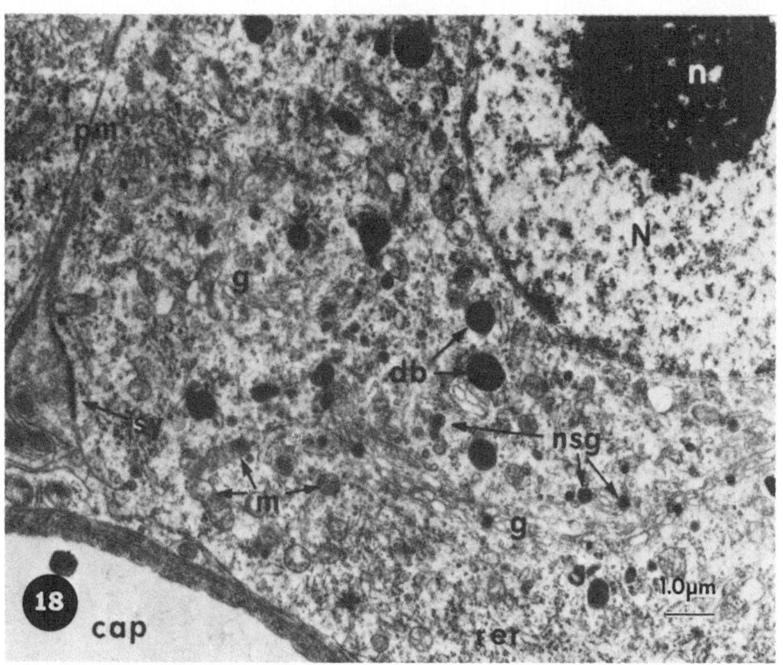

FIG. 18. A low-power electron micrograph of a typical large PVN neuron. The nucleus (N) is large, with a very prominent nucleolus (n). Around the nucleus there are extensive Golgi complexes (g). Rough-surfaced endoplasmic reticulum (rer) is situated mainly at the periphery of the neuron. Many mitochondria (m), neurosecretory granules (nsg), and lysosomal dense bodies (db) are seen in the cytoplasm. The neuron is separated from the lumen of a capillary (cap) by a thin rim of neuropil. On the left the neuron makes a close contact with another neuron, and below this there is a synapse (sy). (pm) Plasma membrane. (From ref. 585.)

"castration" or "thyroidectomy" cells in the adenohypophysis.

The percentage of magnocellular neurons in the rat's PVN that demonstrated dilatation of the cisternae of the RER rose from 12% to 24% after 12 hr of dehydration and remained elevated at 21% after 24 hr of dehydration (595). The number of cytoplasmic small dense-core vesicles (<160 nm) per cell was decreased 4 and 12 hr after the start of dehydration but returned to normal levels at 24 hr. The number of large dense-core vesicles (>160 nm) was decreased at 4 hr but then returned to normal values (596), suggesting that after an initial decrease the addition of new dense-core vesicles to the cytoplasm is balanced by their removal into the axon and transport to, and release from, the terminal. However, radioimmune assay studies show that the hypothalamic content of AVP decreases by 60% and that the pituitary content decreases by 88% in the mouse after 3 days of dehydration (597). Increasing numbers of cells are progressively recruited over the duration of the stimulus, although electrophysiologic studies suggest that all cells do not increase their (electrical) activity equally or in synchrony throughout a period of dehydration (598). Based on these studies, one would have expected to find progressively larger numbers of cells that show the morphological characteristics of increased protein synthesis. Perhaps new neurons are added to the population of active cells as old ones drop out to recover, thus keeping the percentage of cells showing morphological changes commensurate with active protein synthesis constant.

Krisch (599) found that in control rats, reaction product localizing ir-AVP was only present over dense-core vesicles in magnocellular somata and axons of the hypothalamo-hypophyseal tract. After 9 days of dehydration, reaction product was found over the RER in the marginal zone as well as over the Golgi apparatus and nearby small dense-core vesicles. In addition, reaction product was found in the intercellular space separating neighboring somata. The frequency of contact between capillaries and the cell somata was increased. In the internal zone of the median eminence, axons of the hypothalamo-hypophyseal tract were dilated and contained amorphous collections of reaction product that were not associated with dense-core vesicles that were absent from the axons in the median eminence or the terminals in the neural lobe. Krisch (600) proposed (a) that AVP could be released from the cell soma into the neuropil, where it could enter the ventricular fluid by passing between ependymal cells, and then be transported to the floor of the infundibular recess to be carried by the ependyma of the median eminence to blood vessels or (b) that AVP could be transported down the axon through channels of the endoplasmic reticulum, incorporated into small vesicles that budded off these channels in axon terminals, and released. However, Kozlowski (601) cautions that reaction product not associated with dense-core vesicles may be artifactual. A specialized system of channels in the smooth endoplasmic reticulum has been independently identified in the soma, axons, and terminals of magnocellular neurons; and Alonso and Assenmacher (602) have described electron-dense material in vesicles budding off from its channels in the axon terminals. Broadwell and Brightman (603) also identified a system of channels in the magnocellular neurons of mice that was associated with a smooth endoplasmic reticulum. It was involved in anterograde transport of lysosomes from the cell body to the axon terminals, as demonstrated by its movement of horseradish peroxidase (HRP) from the soma to the terminal and its association with acid-phosphatase positive-staining small vesicles. These vesicles contained a dense core that could not be distinguished from neurosecretory material. Because the dense material in the vesicles identified by Alonso and Assenmacher (602) was not immunostained, their presumption that they contain hormones is not justified. The case for extragranular transport of hormone from the soma to the terminal is not strong.

Additional hormones are synthesized in magnocellular neurons. Dynorphin has been colocalized with AVP in cell bodies (604) as well as in terminals (402) of magnocellular neurons. Bilateral destruction of the PVN reduced the levels of immunoreactive dynorphin as well as immunoreactive OT and AVP in the neuro-intermediate lobe of the rat (605). Enkephalin has also been identified by immunohistochemistry in magnocellular neurons. Reaves and Hayward (606) localized ir-Enk to a population of neurons in the preoptic nucleus of the goldfish separate from those that contain isotocin or vasotocin. Vanderhaeghen et al. (408) reported colocalization of met-Enk and pro-Enk in the same cells as OT in the magnocellular nuclei of the bovine hypothalamus. Gastrin-like, cholecystokinin-like peptide may also be colocalized with oxytocin (411,412). Substance P is present in some magnocellular neurons (413). Immunoreactive angiotensin II has also been localized in magnocellular neurons (340,520).

Parvicellular peptidergic neurons are found in, but are not restricted to, the arcuate, suprachiasmatic, and paraventricular hypothalamic nuclei and in preoptic and hypothalamic periventricular area in mammals. A given parvicellular neuron in a hypothalamic nuclear group may or may not be peptidergic. Optimal preparation for ultrastructural studies is not optimal for immunohistochemical studies. Hence identification and description of parvicellular peptidergic neurons at the ultrastructural level have been difficult, and studies of the ultrastructural correlates of hormone synthesis are lacking.

Flament-Durand (583) described a population of parvicellular neurons, present in the PVN of the rat, with a large nucleus that contained a large nucleolus. In the cytoplasm the endoplasmic reticulum was less well developed than in magnocellular neurons of the same animals. Only a few dense-core vesicles were present in the cytoplasm, and they averaged 75 nm in diameter. Their axons contained many microtubules and dense-core vesicles 75 nm in diameter. Gross et al. (607) described neurons of the arcuate nucleus as having a lobulated nucleus with an evenly dispersed chromatin. The RER was well developed, and free ribosomes and polysomes were abundant. The Golgi apparatus was frequently associated with a few dense-core vesicles whose diameter was 80 to 120 nm. In a more detailed study, Brawer et al. (608) characterized the neurons of the arcuate nucleus as being ellipsoid-shaped cells with an average diameter of 15 μm. Each nucleus contained a prominent nucleolus, and its profile varied from smooth and round to highly folded. The Nissl substance was prominent in the cytoplasm. The RER was not confined to the Nissl substance, where the cisternae were stacked in parallel rows, but was found in other regions as a loosely arranged reticulum. Dense-core vesicles ranging from 100 to 150 nm in diameter were few in number. The Golgi apparatus was not distinctive. Mitochondria, lysosomes, multivesicular bodies, and microtubules were also present in the cytoplasm. Golgi impregnation demonstrated unipolar or bipolar neurons with fusiform-shaped perikaryia. The dendrites were varicose but were not well endowed with regular spines. Except for two features, neurons in the arcuate nucleus conformed to textbook descriptions of cerebral neurons: (a) The nucleolus was frequently associated with the nuclear envelope at a location where the heterochromatin had formed into a large dense tuft, (b) a round "clump of densely intermeshed filaments" containing a central clear spot was frequently found in the cytoplasm. Bugnon et al. (609) studied the ultrastructure of cells in the arcuate nucleus that were first identified as peptidergic by positive immunohistochemical staining for ACTH 17-39 and/or β-End. In order to obtain adequate immunostaining, they had to pretreat the rats with colchicine; the ultrastructure was adversely affected by this drug. The peptide-secreting cells resembled those described by Brawer et al. (608) because they contained a large nucleolus, tufts of heterochromatin along the wall of the nuclear envelope, and whorls of filaments in the cytoplasm as well as small dense-core vesicles associated with the Golgi apparatus. Pre-embedding colloidal gold immunostaining of similar neurons in the arcuate nucleus with antibodies against β-End localized the reaction product to the dense-core vesicles (610).

Laminar whorls were found to be increased in the cytoplasm of arcuate neurons in rats that were either treated with morphine for 2 weeks or castrated (611). King et al. (612) had previously correlated the number of these structures, which they called "ribbon rolls," to the stages of the estrous cycle in female rats. However, similar findings were not reproduced in a study of the mouse arcuate nucleus (613). The ribbon rolls were described as being made up of two to eight lamellae with a central core of cytoplasm devoid of organelles or granules. The outer lamellae were associated with the RER. Their appearance and description resembled the "whorls" described by Brawer (608). Naik (163,164) claimed to localize GnRH in arcuate neurons that, on ultrastructural examination, were found to contain "whorls" or "ribbon rolls" and that resembled the cells described by Brawer (608). King and Gerall (614) described cells with similar ultrastructural features in the region of the arcuate nucleus, where the concentration of GnRH (measured by radioimmune assay) was high and where the population of GnRH-containing cells was reported as being dense. However, the population of cells containing POMC and its derivatives is also dense in this region (compare Fig. 9 in ref. 614, or Fig. 5 in ref. 616), and the presence of GnRH-containing neurons in the arcuate nucleus of the rat is not generally accepted (876). High levels of GnRH assayed in this region could have been due to the presence of GnRH in fibers of passage.

Jennes et al. (617) have recently employed TEM to study ir-GnRH-containing cells in the medial septum, the nucleus

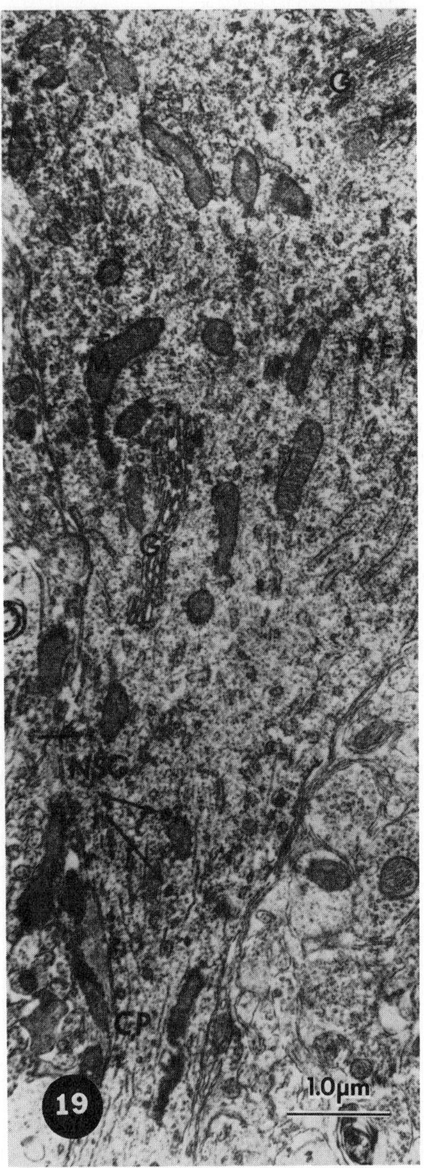

FIG. 19. Transmission electron micrograph of GnRH nerve cell bodies showing well-developed rough endoplasmic reticulum (RER), Golgi apparatus (G), and mitochondria (M) in basis of cell process that contains neurosecretory granules (NSG) and a coated pit (CP). (From ref. 617.)

of the diagonal band of Broca, and the medial preoptic area (Fig. 19). The ultrastructure of their perikaryia does not differ markedly from that of POMC- or putative GnRH-containing cells in the arcuate nucleus. Of considerable interest is the authors' description of two populations of neurons: spiny and smooth. Spiny neurons also have spiny axons that synapse with the soma and dendrites of other neurons. Synapsis involving smooth axons (which arise from smooth perikaryia) are only occasionally found. The authors suggest that smooth neurons make neurohemal contact with vessels in the median eminence, whereas spine neurons make synaptic contact with other neurons. TRH- and SRIF-secreting neurons may be similar in appearance to POMC- and (smooth) GnRH-containing neurons, but in the reported studies (which localized the hormone of interest to dense-core vesicles about 100 nm in diameter) the neurons were not sufficiently well preserved for ultrastructural analysis (618,619).

Development of Neurosecretory Systems

The basic neuroanatomic organization of the hypothalamus has been presented by Crosby and Showers (620), Nauta and Haymaker (621), and Knigge and Silverman (397). The development of the mammalian hypothalamus has been presented by Papez (622) and Christ (623). A detailed description of diencephalic development in the rat is provided by Coggeshall (624). This discussion will focus on the development of peptidergic neurosecretory systems in the hypothalamus.

Hyyppa (625) stated that on postcoital day 15, the rat diencephalon was composed of a germinal layer (lining the third ventricle), a mantle layer, and a marginal layer. Fiber systems such as the fasciculus retroflexus, the mammillotegmental tract, the medial forebrain bundle, and the stria medullaris are present in the mantle and marginal layers at this time (624). Hyyppa (625) reported, on the basis of LM examination of histologic sections, that nuclear groups, which are now known to contain peptidergic neurons, such as the SON, PVN, periventricular nucleus (PvN), arcuate nucleus (AN), and suprachiasmatic nucleus (ScN), originated from the germinal layer. A more detailed study was reported by Altman and Bayer (626). Employing pulse labeling with tritiated thymidine, they were able to define the time at which cells in a given nuclear group ceased dividing (i.e., the birthday of these cells). They reasoned that all cells (and hence all nuclear groups) originated in the germinal layer. By labeling separate animals with thymidine pulses on successive postcoital days, they could trace the migration of cells from the germinal layer to their final nuclear location. They determined that (in general) there was a lateral to medial pattern of migration. Cells destined for lateral nuclear sites migrated before cells destined for medial sites. Four classes of cells were established. In Class 1 were cells contributing to nuclear groups in the lateral zone (lateral preoptic, dorsal preoptic, lateral hypothalamic, and lateral mammillary nuclei). In Class 2 were large cells of the SON and PVN as well as those of the medial preoptic area (MPOA). Also in this second wave were the cells destined for the premammillary nuclei, the posterior hypothalamic nucleus, and the ventral portion of the ventromedial nuclei. Within Class 2 there was a rostrocaudal gradient such that the first three nuclear groups formed before the second three. In Class 3 were the dorsal portion of the ventromedial nucleus (VMN), the dorsal medial nucleus, the anterior arcuate nucleus, the preoptic periventricular area, and the suprachiasmatic nucleus. The anterior arcuate nucleus, preoptic periventricular area, and the suprachiasmatic nucleus all contain parvicellular peptidergic neurons at maturation. In Group 4, the last group to migrate, were the cells of the posterior arcuate (infundibular) nucleus and the tuberomammillary nucleus. This last group also will contain peptidergic cells.

The peptidergic cells contributing to the magnocellular components of the SON and PVN as well as the cells contributing to the preoptic nuclei migrate concurrently but not from the same site. Large neurons of the preoptic area originate from the germinal epithelium of the inferior horns of the lateral ventricles. Cells contributing to the magnocellular supraoptic nucleus and the magnocellular portion of the PVN were documented to arise from a single specialized locus of germinal epithelium located adjacent to the third ventricle at the level of the "adult" PVN. Internuclear magnocellular neurons (between the PVN and SON) were found along the course taken by migrating cells from this germinal region to the site of the adult SON over the optic tract. The neurons forming the SON were "born" on the 13th through the 15th fetal days. They were recognized over the optic tract on postcoital day 16 and were found in moderate numbers on day 17. Paraventricular large neurons were "born" on the same days and were first seen on fetal day 16 in their adult locus. More cells appeared on day 17; by day 18, growth into magnocellular neurons was discernible (627). Neurophysin was first localized in developing neurons of the PVN and SON on the 18th fetal day. AVP was identified in these nuclear groups on the 19th fetal day, but OT was not detectable until the 4th postnatal day. Neurophysin was also detected in the median eminence and in the neural lobe on the 19th fetal day (628). It is of interest that Fink and Smith (376) first noted neural processes in the developing median eminence on the 16th fetal day, at a time when magnocellular neurons first arrive in the region of the SON and PVN nuclei. Altman and Bayer (627) proposed that the cells of tuberomammillary nucleus and those of the caudal arcuate (infundibular) nucleus also share a common site of origin—the inferior lobule at the anterior margin of the mammillary recess—and that they may comprise part of the parvicellular peptidergic system. Similar studies have been performed in the mouse (629,630) and in the cat (631) with analogous, but less detailed, results.

Gonadotropin-producing neurons may, in contrast, have an extracerebral origin (632). GnRH was first detected by immunohistochemistry in the 15-day rat fetus in the nervus terminalis. In the 17-day fetus (where immunopositive cells were first present in the rhinencephalon, limbic lobe, and preoptic area), gonadotropins were first detected in the pars distalis. About 60% of the total GnRH-containing cell population was localized in the ganglion cells of the nervus terminalis on that day. By the 19th fetal day, immunoreactive nerve terminals had appeared in the organum vasculosum of the lamina terminalis (OVLT) and in the median eminence. Immunopositive cells in the nervus terminalis accounted for only about 30% of the total population. The number of cells in the septum, olfactory tubercle, and preoptic area had doubled when compared with fetal day 17. The findings suggest that GnRH-containing cells originate outside the CNS and migrate inward.

Although a common locus and concurrent migration of magnocellular neurons to their final destination seems apparent, a common locus or a common date of origin for cells that contribute from diverse nuclear groups to the parvicellular neurosecretory system has not as yet been revealed. The PVN, which contains parvicellular as well as magnocellular elements, may be an example of "sequential generation of nuclear components" to form a complex system, as is the case for the mammillary body, which contains cells from several sites which migrate at different times (626). Birth does not mark the end of development of hypothalamic nuclei of the rat (633,634) or hamster (394). Maturation of structure and a synaptic organization continues into the second postnatal week.

Organization of Neurosecretory Systems

Cell bodies of neurosecretory neurons are arranged in nuclear groups. These peptidergic neurons form neurosecretory systems not only by virtue of the location of their cell bodies and the site of their terminals, but also by virtue of the hormone(s) they synthesize. Difficulties arise because there is seldom a strict correspondence between a given nuclear group and specific cell type containing a single hormone. Further, a single nuclear group is seldom the unique location of cells synthesizing a given hormone. The difficulties are compounded by the observation that a hypothalamic nuclear group may project to several different sites and that any given peptide may play one role at one site and a different role at another. Finally, a particular cell in a nuclear group may contain more than one peptide. However, it appears that Dale's hypothesis still holds and that the same substance(s) secreted from one terminal of a neuron is (are) released from all terminals of that neuron (635).

The SON is composed of magnocellular neurons (340,573,620,636,637). Their cell bodies are closely related to the soma of other magnocellular neurosecretory cells. Adjacent cells are separated by glial processes, which in many instances are very attenuated (51,585). Actual somasomatic contact was found in 4% of cells examined in the rat's supraoptic nucleus, and the percentage of cells that directly contacted their neighbors increased with dehydration (586). This increased contact is presumably due to retraction of interposed glial processes. The vascularity of the SON is dense (567,568), and neurosecretory cells occasionally are found to lie in direct contact with the basement membrane about nonfenestrated capillaries (599). This arrangement is a fitting one for a nuclear group whose cells must transport amino acids across the blood-brain barrier and incorporate them in order to synthesize proteins for excretion into fenestrated neurohypophyseal capillaries.

The SON "surmounts the lateral border of the optic tract" in mammals (620). It extends from the lamina terminalis at the level of the organum vasculosum of the lamina terminalis (OVLT) to midtuberal levels. In the mouse, the SON is divided into an anterior, as well as a retrochiasmatic, portion. The anterior nucleus lies dorsolateral to the optic tract, whereas the retrochiasmatic portion lies ventromedial to it (638). A similar parcellation was made in the rat by Peterson (639) and Rhodes et al. (640), except that the latter called the anterior nucleus the "principal nucleus" and the former considered the retrochiasmatic portion to be one of the accessory supraoptic nuclei. Three subdivisions of the SON were described in the monkey. The dorsolateral, dorsomedial and ventromedial subdivisions are all described by their relationship to the optic tract (62). OT and AVP, with their associated neurophysins and colocalized hormones, are synthesized in different cells in the supraoptic nuclei (59,62,414,579–581). Within the principal portion of the rat's SON, OT-producing cells are aggregated in the dorsal and rostral portions of the nucleus (640). In the monkey, OT-producing cells are present in the dorsal and medial regions of the SON (62).

The major projection of the SON is to the neural lobe (infundibular process) via the SOHT. Up to 90% of its neurons degenerate after (high) section of the SOHT (641,642). Injection of horseradish-peroxidase (HRP) into the neural lobe of the rat results in a dense accumulation of HRP in cell bodies lying in the SON for several hours (643,644). Examination of autoradiographs of the rat's hypothalamus and hypophysis after injection of tritiated leucine into the SON revealed the principal projection to be through the SOHT to the neural lobe, where it tended to be concentrated in the internal region (602). Nerve fibers in the SOHT display irregular swellings, and many have a beaded appearance in Golgi preparations. Collateral axons are present. Fibrous astrocytes and their processes abound and give the tract a "striking appearance" (575). Projections to neural as well as to neurohypophyseal sites have been identified by several authors employing immunohistochemistry. Labeled axons of magnocellular neurons course dorsally toward the stria medullaris (645). Zimmerman (340) described a projection from the rostral region of the SON to the OVLT, a circumventricular organ implicated in the regulation of (a) salt and water homeostasis and (b) drinking behavior (646). Brownfield and Kozlowski (647) described a hypothalamic-choroidal tract on the basis of LM examination of immunohistochemically stained sections of the rat hypothalamus. However, the major accepted pathway emerging from the SON is the SOHT to the neural lobe.

Other magnocellular neurosecretory centers are present in the hypothalamus. Crosby and Showers (620) named these scattered small cell groups of neurosecretory cells that lie, for the most part, between the PVN and the SON—the "pars diffusa" of the PVN. These nuclear groups, with two exceptions, appear to lie very close to the SON or PVN, or to lie along the course taken by cells migrating from the germinal matrix in the periventricular region to their final location over the optic tract. The anterior commissural nucleus lies immediately posterior to the anterior commissure near the midline just rostral to the PVN. The nucleus circularis lies halfway between the SON and the PVN. The retrochiasmatic nucleus lies just ventral to the SON. The anterior and posterior fornical nuclei and the nucleus of the medial forebrain bundle are disposed more laterally than the presumed path of migration of the magnocellular neurons from the periventricular germinal epithelium to their site over the optic chiasm and tract (639). The retrochiasmatic nucleus was classified by Broadwell and Bleier (638) and by Rhodes et al. (640) as part of the SON. The anterior commissural nucleus was included by Swanson and Kuypers (648) as part of the PVN. All these nuclear groups are labeled after HRP injection into the neural lobe of the rats (643,644,649). OT or AVP has been localized in all of the accessory nuclear groups, and they project to the neural lobe (574,576,640).

The PVN contains not only magnocellular neurons (620,636,650), but also parvicellular neurons (637,648,650). The territory of the PVN, however, is described differently by different authors. Crosby and Showers (620) described a triangular-shaped nuclear group lying in the dorsal hypothalamic zone on either side of the third ventricle with its base parallel and adjacent to the third ventricle. Its anterior border lay in the plane of the posterior border of the anterior commissure and the posterior border of the optic chiasm. Its posterior extent was described as differing with different species. Swanson and Kuypers (648) described a nuclear group in the dorsal zone of the hypothalamus adjacent to the third ventricle that, on coronal sections, is polygonal in shape anteriorly and that becomes triangular posteriorly. Their periventricular cluster of parvicellular neurons is the periventricular nucleus of other authors (30). Their anterior and medial magnocellular divisions are in the anterior commissural nucleus of Peterson (639). Defendini and Zimmerman (637) described the PVN as fusiform in shape and oriented almost at right angles to the SON. It lies next to the wall of the third ventricle and extends from the inferior boundary of the nucleus reuniens of the thalamus to the superior border of the arcuate nucleus of the hypothalamus. Although it is not clear from their description how this ventral extension relates to the periventricular nucleus, the reader must assume that it lies next to the third ventricle surrounded anteriorly and posteriorly by the periventricular nucleus [compare Fig. 4 of Defendini and Zimmerman (639) with Figs. 7, 9, 10, and 17 of Rioch et al. (30)]. (This periventricular territory seems to be the source of considerable dispute because it is reported, by various authors, to be part of the periventricular, paraventricular, and arcuate nuclei.) Midway along the dorsoventral course of this nucleus is a swelling directed laterally and posteriorly [the PVN of Crosby and Showers (620)], extending from the level of the optic chiasm and the anterior commissure to the anterior (639) or midtuberal (30) regions.

The manner in which the PVN is parcellated by different investigators varies. Swanson and Kuypers (648) described three magnocellular clusters in the PVN surrounded by five clusters of parvicellular neurons. Their anterior magnocellular and medial magnocellular clusters, along with the anterior parvicellular cluster, correspond to the anterior commissural nucleus of Peterson (639). Their posterior magnocellular division is partially surrounded by the periventricular, medial, lateral, and dorsal parvicellular divisions of the PVN, and this entire group corresponds to the PVN of other authors (638,640). Van Den Pol (651) found that magnocellular neurons tended to be aggregated in the lateral region of the PVN on coronal section. His Fig. 3a corresponds to Fig. 1b of Swanson and Kuypers (648) and suggests that he, as others, considered the posterior magnocellular division of Swanson and Kuypers (648) to represent the magnocellular region of the PVN. Armstrong et al. (652) arranged the magnocellular clusters of neurons into the anterior commissural nucleus, the medial and lateral paraventricular nuclei, and the posterior subnucleus of the PVN. Their medial and lateral paraventricular nuclei seem to correspond to the posterior magnocellular division of Swanson and Kuypers (648). The anterior commissural nucleus of Armstrong et al. (652) is the anterior magnocellular division of Swanson and Kuypers (648). It is difficult for me to find a homology of the posterior subnucleus of the paraventricular nucleus (PVPO) (652) in the schema of Swanson and Kuypers (648). It corresponds in position to their medial and lateral parvicellular divisions but contains magnocellular as well as parvicellular neurons. A common terminology and agreement about the boundaries and subdivisions of the nucleus is needed now that attempts are being made to localize different projections and different receptive fields to specific subdivisions of the nucleus.

As in the SON, in the PVN the magnocellular neurons are closely packed, being separated from each other only by slender glial processes. As in the SON, cells in the PVN are occasionally seen to lie adjacent to each other without an intervening glial process (594,595). As in the SON, OT and AVP with their associated neurophysins are found in separate neurons in the PVN (59,62,414,579–581). Hatton et al. (653) described two populations of magnocellular neurons in the rat's PVN which could be distinguished on the basis of their size. Smaller cells were found in the anteromedial region of the PVN (652), whereas in the dorsolateral region the cells were larger and rounder. Their prediction that cells in the anteroventromedial region would contain OT whereas those in the dorsolateral region would contain AVP was subsequently confirmed with immunohistochemical techniques (640,654). Defendini and Zimmerman (637), on the basis of their own experience and on review of the extant literature, did not confirm the presence of a regional segregation of OT and AVP neurons in the PVN in humans, although segregation of these neurons was acknowledged in other animals.

The magnocellular neurons of the (posterior magnocellular division of the) PVN project to the neurohypophysis. Their axons leave the PVN at its apex (651) and then course laterally and then ventrally to the level of the SON (574). There the fiber tract is joined by projections from the SON (SOHT) to form the hypothalamo-hypophyseal tract. This fascicle of magnocellular axons approaches the median eminence through the lateral retrochiasmatic area and passes from lateral to medial as it moves caudally to enter the median eminence from its anterior aspect (Fig. 20). In the median eminence, its fibers lie in the internal zone. They pass on to the infundibular stem and process, where they terminate (in the rat) near the ventral surface adjacent to the pars tuberalis and pars intermedia (602,652).

The projection of the magnocellular neurons to the neural lobe is not at this time believed to be very substantial. Stalk section, even at high levels, resulted in the degeneration of only about 20% of large neurons in the PVN (641). However, following HRP injection into the neural lobe of the rat, Sherlock et al. (643) found that cells in "the magnocellular (i.e. lateral) part of the PVN were loaded with HRP reaction product." It seems unlikely that the injection spilled into the median eminence, because cells in the adjacent arcuate nucleus did not contain HRP. Ono et al. (655) also found labeling of magnocellular neurons in the rat PVN after injection of HRP into the neural lobe. Again the arcuate nucleus was not labeled. Perhaps the old idea that collaterals leave the hypothalamo-hypophyseal tract at the level of the median eminence (21) should be reexplored, because it would reconcile the apparently contradictory conclusions drawn from stalk section and HRP injection protocols.

Neurons in the PVN project to the median eminence (656,657). Destruction of the PVN of the monkey resulted in loss of ir-AVP and ir-OT as well as their associated neurophysins from the external zone of the median eminence (656). The projections from the PVN to the external zone are ipsilateral and arranged topographically. Following adrenalectomy the intensity of immunohistochemical staining for NP or AVP increased. This increase was blocked by pretreatment with dexamethasone (658). Following unilateral ablation of the PVN, bilateral adrenalectomy induced collateral sprouting of fibers of the hypothalamo-hypophyseal tract from the intact side of the median eminence to the denervated side (659). Coupled with the evidence that AVP and CRH act synergistically to stimulate corticotrophs (660), these anatomical observations leave little doubt that the projections to the median eminence from the PVN play a role in the regulation of the pituitary-adrenal axis and in the response mounted by the animal to stress.

The source of OT and AVP terminals in the median eminence is the PVN, but it has not been clarified which group of cells in the PVN project there. The parvicellular divisions of the PVN contain 31% of OT-stained cells and 20% of the AVP-stained cells in the PVN of the rat (654). The OT and AVP terminals and their neurosecretory granules are smaller in the external zone of the (guinea-pig) median eminence than they are in the neural lobe (57,513), suggesting that terminals in the external zone arise from parvicellular neurons. Retrograde tracer studies employing injection of HRP or WGA injection into the median eminence have revealed heavier labeling in the parvicellular than in the magnocellular divisions (649,661,662). Labeling of magnocellular neurons could have resulted from migration of tracer into the internal zone from the site of injection in the external zone. Because only 20% of the magnocellular neurons in the PVN project to the neural lobe, it has been presumed by some authors that the other 80% project to the median eminence (637,663). Others presume that the parvicellular neurons containing AVP or OT in the medial parvicellular nuclear group, along with other parvicellular neurons containing hypothalamic releasing and inhibiting hormones, project to the median eminence (664,665). More direct evidence is needed before the matter can be settled.

Although the parvicellular components of the (rat's) PVN partially surround the magnocellular components (648), the largest aggregation of parvicellular neurons lies medial to the (posterior) magnocellular division (648,651). Parvicellular neurons are not as tightly packed together as are the magnocellular neurons. Immunohistochemical staining demonstrates OT- and AVP-containing parvicellular neurons. All five parvicellular divisions contained both OT and AVP neurons, but AVP-containing cells are concentrated in the medial parvicellular division (648,651). Somatostatin-containing cells have been identified in the periventricular division (nucleus) (161,666–669) as have TRH-containing cells, which are also present in the medial parvicellular division (415). Cells that contain the presumptive precursor of TRH (670) and its mRNA (671) are present in the medial parvicellular division of the PVN in the same distribution as the TRH-containing cells. This observation is compatible with the postulate that TRH is synthesized in neurons in this location. Although cell bodies stain well for TRH precursor, axons do not, suggesting that the TRH precursor molecule (which contains five copies of TRH) is rapidly processed in the Golgi apparatus or in the secretory granules into TRH. Processing of the peptide in the granules as they are transported down the axon (as is the case with AVP synthesis) appears unlikely in the case of TRH synthesis. Immunoreactive GH has been colocalized in TRH-synthesizing cells (672). CRH has been found by immunohistochemical techniques in parvicellular neurons of the PVN of the cow (673) and sheep (674) as well as the rat (506,675–678). Several reports of colocalization of CRH with OT and/or AVP in magnocellular neurons have appeared (679–681), but the accuracy of these observations has been challenged by Taniguchi (682). Kiss et al. (683) reported that parvicellular CRH-containing cells in the PVN became AVP-positive after adrenalectomy. Leu-enkephalin-containing cells have been described in the parvicellular neurons in the rat's PVN (516). Neurotensin (433) and cholesystokinin (412) have also been found in the parvicellular divisions of the PVN as have dopamine-containing cells (684). Angiotensin II has also been identified in PVN cells (both large and small) by immunohistochemical techniques. A projection to the internal zone and to the external zone of the median eminence has been identified and related to fluid balance and pituitary-adrenal function, respectively (520). Hokfelt et al. (685) described cell bodies in the parvicellular regions of the PVN which contained immunoreactive CRH, enkephalin, and PHI-27 (a peptide with prolactin-stimulating activity that is closely related to VIP), and they envisioned that release of these peptides from the same terminals in the median eminence could provide a mechanism for a coordinated response to stress. In their proposal, CRH stimulates ACTH release from corticotrophs in the pars distalis, PHI-27 stimulates PRL release from lactotrophs in the pars distalis, and enkephalin inhibits dopamine release from neighboring neurons by a paracrine action to further enhance PRL stimulation in lactotrophs and it also inhibits SRIF release from neighboring terminals to promote GH release from somatotrophs in the pars distalis.

Axons of hormone-containing cells in the medial and lateral parvicellular divisions leave the PVN laterally, at its apex, to follow the course of magnocellular axons in the hypothalamo-hypophyseal tract and to pass by the SON, where fibers from the SON are added. This fascicle of axons containing peptidergic projections from the hypothalamus enters the median eminence anterolaterally through the lateral retrochiasmatic zone (686) (Fig. 20). This projection brings together two systems that stimulate ACTH release (the vasopressinergic and oxytocinergic systems and the CRH systems) with the system that regulates thyroid function. Additional SRIF and TRH neurons in the periventricular division (nucleus) course ventrally in the periventricular zone to enter the median eminence at its lateral margin. In the rat, systems related to survival of the individual are aggregated (a) in the medial palisade zone in the median eminence and (b) in the PVN and adjacent periventricular regions in the hypothalamus.

Parvicellular neurons in the PVN also project to the brain stem and spinal cord regions. These neurons are not the same neurons that project to the median eminence (687). Most such neurons contain OT or AVP and originate from parvicellular neurons in the caudal region of the PVN (652,688). Cells that project to the spinal cord lie in the dorsal and ventral regions of the medial parvicellular division, whereas cells that project to the dorsal vagal complex lie in the ventral region of the medial parvicellular division (689). Small numbers of SRIF and enkephalin-labeled (690) and of tyrosine hydroxylase-labeled cells (684) in the posterior parvicellular division of the PVN also project to the brain stem and spinal cord. Identified neurons account for only 10% to 20% of the fibers projecting from the PVN to brain stem and spinal cord levels, suggesting that other, unknown, peptidergic systems participate in this projection (688,689). Descending neural projections to the dorsal vagal complex (the nucleus of the solitary tract and the dorsal motor nucleus) and to the intermediolateral cell column of the spinal cord have been identified by immunohistochemical techniques (690). OT-containing fibers predominate (688). Injection of different markers at medullary and spinal levels demonstrated that about 15% of the labeled cells in the PVN were double-labeled and hence that these cells sent collaterals to both the dorsal vagal complex and the spinal cord (689). Electrophysiologic studies also provide evidence of a direct pathway from the medial regions of the PVN to the

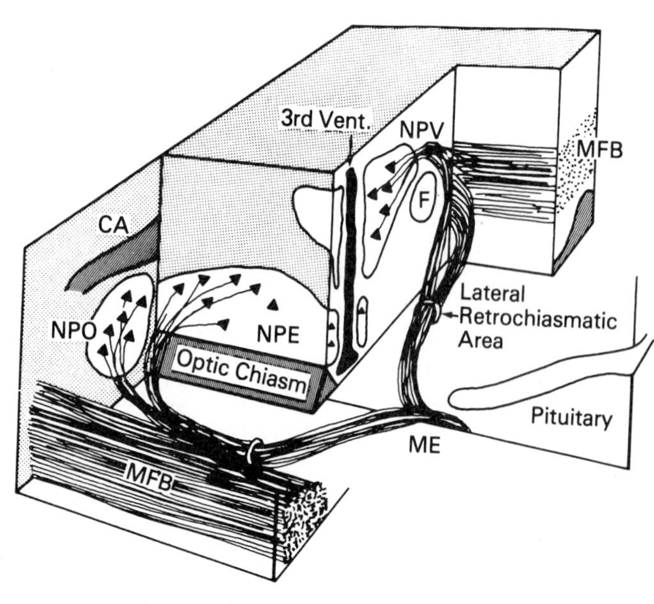

FIG. 20. Schematic drawing of the topography of the lateral retrochiasmatic area and cell groups that project axons through it to the median eminence. (NPO) Medial preoptic nucleus; (NPE) periventricular nucleus; (NPV) paraventricular nucleus; (MFB) medial forebrain bundle; (ME) median eminence; (CA) anterior commissure. (From ref. 686.)

TABLE 1. *Efferents from MPOA-HTA*[a]

	SON	PVN(m)	PVN(p)	PVN	AN	MPOA
NL	+	+				
ME		?	+	+	+	+
OVLT						+
SON		+			+	
PVN(m)	+				+	
PVN(p)					+	
PVN					+	
AN				+		
MPOA				+	+	
VMN				+	+	
Habenula				+		+
Hipp.			+	+		
Septum			+	+	+	+
BNST			+	?	+	+
Amygdala			+	?	+	+
Ol.Tub.				+		+
IPN				+		
SN			+			
Teg.				+		+
PbN			+			+
LC			+			+
LRN			+			+
PVC			+			+

[a]SON, supraoptic nucleus; PVN(m), magnocellular paraventricular nucleus; PVN(p), parvicellular paraventricular nucleus; PVN, periventricular nucleus; AN, arcuate nucleus; MPOA, medial preoptic area; NL, neural lobe; ME, median eminence; OVLT, organum vasculosum of the lamina terminalis; VMN, ventromedial nucleus; Hipp., hippocampus; BNST, bed nucleus of the stria terminalis; Ol.Tub., olfactory tubercle; IPN, interpeduncular nucleus; SN, substantia nigra; Teg., midbrain tegmentum; PbN, parabrachial nucleus; LC, locus ceruleus; LRN, lateral reticular nucleus; DVC, dorsal vagal complex.

spinal cord (691). Additional descending projections of OT- and AVP-containing neurons in the PVN to the substantia nigra, the parabrachial nucleus, the locus ceruleus, the lateral reticular nucleus, and the commissural nucleus have been described (692).

Paraventricular parvicellular neurons also project rostrally. OT-containing cells project over the fornix to the hippocampus and also project to the septal area and to the bed nucleus of the stria terminalis and the medial nucleus of the amygdala (693–695). Additional projections to the medial preoptic area (MPOA) and the periventricular nucleus of the thalamus have been revealed by autoradiographic studies following injection of labeled amino acids into the PVN (696) (Table 1).

Axons of parvicellular neurons also project to sites within the paraventricular nucleus. Whereas intrinsic axons were found not to arise from magnocellular neurons, they were found to arise from parvicellular neurons. Local axons terminated in both the medial parvicellular and lateral magnocellular regions of the PVN (651). The dendritic arbors of parvicellular neurons remain within the confines of the nucleus. They are oriented horizontally, parallel to the floor of the ventricle and to the intrinsic axons in the medial portion of the nucleus. In the periventricular regions, the dendritic arbors are oriented vertically, parallel to the ascending input from the suprachiasmatic and arcuate nuclei. The dendrites of parvicellular neurons peripherally surrounding the (posterior) magnocellular division are oriented parallel to the surface of the nucleus, forming a network of dendrites about it. The parvicellular neurons are thus arrayed to serve as receptor sites for incoming afferent axons, as interneurons relaying afferent input to large and small peptidergic neurons, as neurosecretory cells releasing hormones in the median eminence to control anterior pituitary function, and as neurons projecting to limbic regions in the forebrain and to autonomic centers in the brain stem and in the spinal cord to coordinate pituitary and endocrine function (651).

The periventricular nucleus (PvN) is included by Rioch et al. (30) as a part of the periventricular region that includes the arcuate nucleus (AN) and the periventricular preoptic nucleus. Ingram (636) states that it is characterized by "the presence of small cells arranged in vertical rows as seen in transverse sections stained with Nissl stain." It extends through the rostrocaudal extent of the hypothalamus and encircles the third ventricle. Anteriorly it is continuous with the preoptic periventricular system (30). At the level of the paraventricular nucleus, it is sometimes ceded to the paraventricular nucleus (648). In the region between the AN and the PVN, several peptides have been localized within cells in the periventricular nucleus. A substantial proportion of somatostatin neurons (SRIF-containing cells) lie in this region (161,666–669,697,698). Somatostatin neurons in the periventricular nucleus of the rat project (a) to the median eminence, (b) to the preoptic and arcuate nuclei in the periventricular zone, (c) to the VMN, ScN, and premammillary nuclei in the hypothalamus, and (d) to the habenular nuclei of the epithalamus via the stria medullaris. They further project to the midbrain tegmentum through the stria medullaris via the fasciculus retroflexus to the interpeduncular nucleus and via the periventricular gray into the midbrain tegmentum (667,699). Ascending projections carrying ir-SRIF to the olfactory tubercle, septum, and hippocampus have also been demonstrated (667,686). In addition, immunohistochemical techniques have localized leu-Enk- (700), thyrosine hydroxylase- (701), neurotensin- (702), and CRH-containing (428) cells in this region of the rat's hypothalamus and have identified their projections to the median eminence (Table 1).

The AN (nucleus infundibularis) is a paired lateral expansion of the periventricular gray that lies juxtaposed to the most ventral region of the third ventricle at its entrance into the infundibular recess (623,638). It is bounded inferiorly by the tubero-infundibular recess and the median eminence and superiorly by the dorsal medial nucleus of the hypothalamus. Crosby and Woodburne (703), Crosby and Showers (620), Rioch et al. (30), Ingram (636), Papez (622), Christ (623), and Nauta and Haymaker (621) all consider the AN to be part of the periventricular system of neurons that, except at the level of the median eminence, encircles the third ventricle. The superior boundary of the arcuate nucleus in the periventricular zone is somewhat arbitrary because it is defined by the region where the condensation of neurons in the arcuate nucleus meets the less dense population of neurons in the periventricular hypothalamic nucleus, and it is regarded differently by different authors in different species. Van Den Pol and Cassidy (704) described a triangular-shaped nucleus (in the rat) with the side parallel to the third ventricle, the base parallel to the dorsal border of the median eminence and the tubero-infundibular sulcus, and the hypotenuse (dorsolateral border) defined by the cell-poor zone that separates the arcuate nucleus from the ventromedial nucleus of the hypothalamus. Others see a more pear-shaped nucleus with its concave lateral border defined by the cell-poor zone separating the arcuate nucleus from the ventromedial nucleus. The nucleus extends as a column of cells from the anterior margin of the infundibular recess to a position slightly caudal to the posterior pole of the ventromedial nucleus (i.e., through the tuberal and mammillary regions of the median eminence) and can thus be divided into a tuberal and a mammillary division (620,623). The nucleus is arcuate in shape anterior to the infundibulum in the rat (704) but not in the human (621), but it changes from a paired to a single arcuate nucleus behind the infundibulum in the human (621). Retrograde transport of HRP and WGA has demonstrated the arcuate nucleus to be the source of many afferent fibers to the rostral region of the neurohypophysis—the median eminence (649,661,662).

Cells of the AN were described by Szentagothai et al. (103) as small fusiform or triangular cells with several dendrites. The axons originated from the cell body or from the proximal portion of a dendrite. The ultrastructure of the neurons in the arcuate nucleus appears to be uniform (394,607,608,705) and does not differ from the description given for parvicellular neurons in the section on development of neurosecretory systems. LM examination of Golgi preparations, however, reveals three different kinds of neurons in the arcuate nucleus (704,706). Fusiform neurons with one apical dendrite lie medially in a juxtaventricular position. Fusiform neurons with two sparsely arborizing dendrites lie mainly in the medial and dorsal parts of the nucleus. Polygonal neurons with four to five repeatedly branching stem dendrites lie in the ventral and lateral regions of the nucleus. Dendritic morphology exhibits considerable variability, with some dendrites containing many spines, some containing none, and some dendrites having a beaded appearance. The pattern of dendritic arborization in the arcuate nucleus differs from that in the adjacent hypothalamus (103,704,706). Cell bodies in the dorsal (and hence, of necessity, in the medial) region of the nucleus possess vertically oriented dendritic trees, while the cell bodies localized ventrally have horizontally oriented dendritic trees. The center of mass of the cell body and its dendritic tree lies lateral to, and beneath, the cell body of a neuron in the lateral (and hence, of necessity, in the ventral) region of the nucleus and dorsal to the cell body of a neuron in the medial region. In horizontal section, the course of dendrites in the periventricular zone is parallel to the third ventricle and orthogonal to the course of tanycytic processes. Immediately above the infundibular recess, the dendrites (in the medial portion of the nucleus) are oriented rostrocaudally, whereas more dorsally they are oriented dorsoventrally. In the periventricular zone of the AN, the neuropil is not separated from the ventricular system by a subependymal glial layer (454,460,704). Dendrites and axons course between laterally extending tanycytic processes.

Axons may terminate locally within the nucleus or leave the nucleus to terminate at distant sites. Recurrent collaterals may arise from these latter axons (103,704). Axons of the tubero-infundibular tract leave the tuberal division of the AN and project to the internal and external zones of the median eminence, where they may collateralize (103). Arcuate neurons that project to the median eminence appear to be clustered in the dorsomedial and basolateral regions of the arcuate nucleus (649,662). Axons also project beneath the anterior third ventricle (rostral to the infundibulum of the rat) to terminate in the contralateral AN. Other axons are seen to project dorsolaterally through the cell-poor zone toward the ventromedial nucleus (704,706), although a knife cut in the cell-poor zone between the arcuate nucleus and the ventromedial nucleus of the rat produced axonal degeneration in the ventromedial nucleus (706). HRP injection into the medial and central nuclei of the amygdala demonstrates labeling in the AN of the rat and cat (707). These latter observations suggest that the AN sends projections to the ventromedial nucleus of the hypothalamus and to the amygdala. In addition, axons project dorsomedially to terminate in the periventricular division of the PVN (704).

Dopaminergic neurons in the AN project through the tubero-infundibular tract to the median eminence. The presence of these neurons was first revealed in the AN by the formaldehyde fluorescence technique (161,487–489,708–712). Fluorescence of dopaminergic cell bodies in the AN and of dopaminergic terminals in the median eminence was preserved if the AN was surgically isolated from the remainder of the brain but not if it was lesioned (416,713–716). Dopamine, as well as other catecholamines, has been identified in the AN by enzymatic assay (717). Tyrosine-hydroxylase-containing (presumably dopaminergic) cells have also been localized in the AN (701). Neither dopamine as identified by enzymatic assay (717) nor dopamine-containing cells as identified by formaldehyde fluorescence (718) are homogeneously distributed in the rodent's AN. Some dopaminergic neurons also contain ir-neurotensin (753). Dopamine-containing cells were scarce in the medial aspect of the nucleus rostrally and in the ventral region of the tuberal division of the nucleus in the mouse (718). Bugnon et al. (719) localized dopamine (by using fluorescence techniques) and ACTH (by means of immunohistochemistry) in different neurons. Dopaminergic neurons were aggregated medially and dorsally (in the distribution of the fusiform neurons) (Fig. 21), and ACTH-containing fibers were concentrated ventrally and laterally (in the distribution of the polygonal neurons). Chan-Palay et al. (701) reported that tyrosine-hydroxylase-containing cells in the AN were fusiform in shape and that cells near the ventricle were oriented vertically, whereas more ventral (and lateral) cells were oriented horizontally. Tyrosine-hydroxylase-containing cells were not frequently found in the ventromedial portions of the AN. Some dopaminergic neurons also contain ir-neurotensin (753). In addition to dopaminergic neurons, the AN also contains cholinergic (375) and GABAergic (312,313) neurons that project through the tuberohypophyseal tract to the median eminence.

Peptidergic neurons also reside in the AN and project to the median eminence through the tubero-hypophyseal tract. GnRH has been found in the AN of the rat by means of microdissection and radioimmune assay (720) but may be in axons of passage rather than in cell bodies. Immunohistochemistry has been difficult to employ to localize GnRH-containing cells within the AN of the rat because the same antibodies that revealed GnRH in preoptic sites often failed to do so in hypothalamic sites (161,721). Immunoreactive GnRH has been identified in arcuate neurons in the mouse and rat (161,163,164,721–723), monkey (721,724), rabbit (725), guinea pig, bat, and human (726–730). (The relationship between dopamine- and GnRH-containing cell bodies in the arcuate nucleus has not been studied and might be of interest in view of the close relationship of their terminals in the median eminence.)

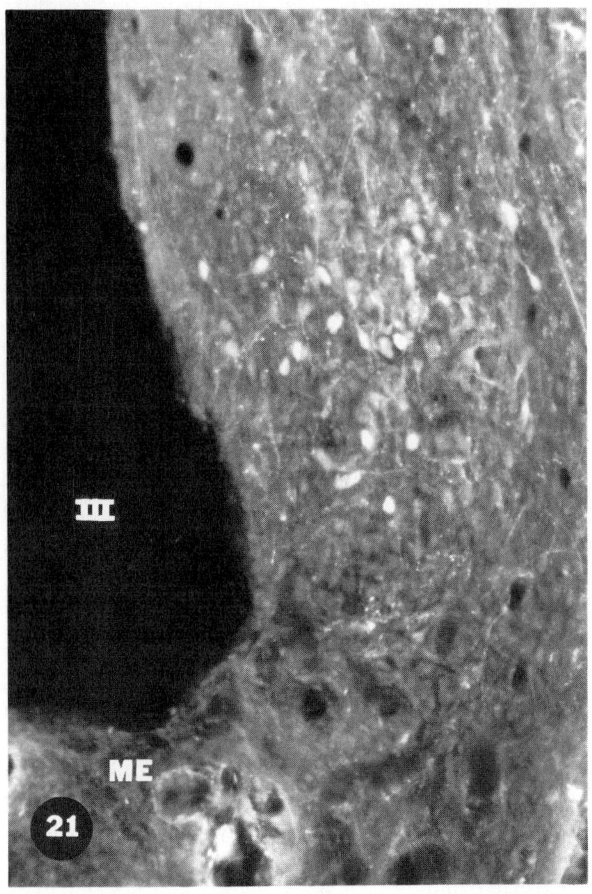

FIG. 21. Fluorescent dopaminergic neurons in the dorsal region of the rabbit arcuate nucleus. Glyoxylic acid treatment. (III) Third ventricle; (ME) median eminence.

POMC-derived peptides have been isolated from the hypothalamus and identified by radioimmunoassay (483,731–733). *In vitro* synthesis of ir-POMC and ir-β-End by hypothalamic tissue has been reported (734). The highest hypothalamic concentrations of α-MSH, β-End, and ACTH were found in the AN (483). The AN of the sheep and ox contained cells staining for β-LPH (521). Immunoreactive β-LPH has been found in the arcuate neurons of the rat (735). ACTH and β-LPH, as well as ACTH and β-End, were localized in the same arcuate neurons by immunohistochemical techniques (736,737). Immunoreactive ACTH and β-End were found in the same cells in the rat's AN (738). β-LPH, ACTH, β-End, and MSH have been localized in the same cells in the AN of the rat (739) and human (740–742). Cells containing POMC-derived peptides were localized ventrally in the rat's AN, whereas dopaminergic cells were localized dorsally (719). Cells containing POMC-derived peptides project to the median eminence (521,736,739). In addition, cells containing POMC-derived peptides make synaptic contact with other cells in the AN (521,738) and innervate other hypothalamic regions. Eskay et al. (733) demonstrated that lesions which destroyed the arcuate nucleus abolished immunostaining of hypothalamic fibers for α-MSH and resulted in a significant reduction in radioimmunoassayable intra- and extrahypothalamic α-MSH. Sawchenko et al. (743) demonstrated ir-ACTH fibers leaving the rat's arcuate nucleus dorsomedially to course vertically in the periventricular zone and to enter the dorsal parvicellular division and the ventromedial aspect of the medial parvicellular division of the PVN. These regions contain a cluster of OT-containing cells that project to the spinal cord and dorsal vagal complex. The ir-ACTH projection also terminated in the anterior magnocellular division of the PVN that contains only OT neurons, as well as in the anteroventral region of the posterior magnocellular divison—an area with a high concentration of OT neurons. Similar results were reported by Mezey et al. (483). With retrograde labeling of the arcuate nucleus by injection of true blue into the ACTH-innervated regions of the PVN, double-labeled (ir-ACTH and true-blue-containing) cells were found in the ventrolateral regions of the AN. Interestingly, true-blue-labeled cells were also found in the dorsomedial region of the AN, where fusiform dopaminergic neurons with vertically oriented dendritic trees are found (743).

Growth-hormone-releasing factor (GRF) has been localized by immunohistochemical techniques within arcuate neurons of the monkey (744,745), cat (746), and rat, ox, and monkey (747,748). Merchenthaler et al. (749) also found ir-GRF in cells in the rat's arcuate nuclei and demonstrated that these cells project to the median eminence. In addition, these authors found immunoreactive cell bodies which projected to the median eminence and which were scattered in the perifornical region of the lateral hypothalamus. Bloch et al. (750) reported that GRF immunostaining of the arcuate nucleus and median eminence was abolished after treatment of neonatal rats with monosodium glutamate, a drug thought to specifically affect arcuate neurons (751,752), thus suggesting that most of the GRF innervation to the median eminence comes from the AN in the rat. Sawchenko et al. (432) also reported the presence of cells in the AN which contained ir-GRF. They were distributed in the nucleus in the same pattern as POMC derivatives. An additional group of GRF-containing cells was found in the ventromedial nucleus. GRF projections to the periventricular nucleus and to the anterior and ventromedial regions of the medial parvicellular division of the PVN were described by Sawchenko et al. (432). A second projection of GRF fibers from the arcuate nucleus ascended and descended through the ventromedial hypothalamus just dorsal to the base of the brain. It projected into the anterior hypothalamic area, the preoptic region, the bed nucleus of the stria terminalis, the medial nucleus of the amygdala, and the lateral septum. The descending tract projected to the posterior hypothalamus. A contribution to the tubero-infundibular tract was also identified and is the pathway by which GRF fibers reach the median eminence. In 20% to 40% of GRF-containing cells in the anterior arcuate nucleus, neurotensin could be colocalized. Neurotensin has been identified in the arcuate nucleus by Ibata et al. (702) and Hokfelt et al. (754) and colocalized with dopamine by these authors.

Other peptides have been found in AN cells using immunohistochemistry. Substance P (755), leu-Enk (526,700, 756), and scattered cells containing SRIF (666) have been identified and demonstrated to project to the external zone of the rat's median eminence. It is of interest that the leu-Enk-containing cells also stain for a fragment of the adrenal enkephalin precursor fragment (BAM-22P). The precursor staining is restricted to the cell bodies, suggesting that, unlike AVP (but like TRF), processing of the enkephalin prohormone occurs rapidly in the Golgi or soon after packaging of the hormone in secretory granules (757).

Perhaps it would be advantageous to consider the parvicellular neurosecretory system from another point of view. Consider the periventricular gray as being composed of the periventricular (hypothalamic) nucleus along the border of the third ventricle. From this vertically oriented column of cells arise two lateral projections. The ventrolateral projection is the arcuate nucleus. The dorsolateral projection is the parvicellular cluster of paraventricular neurons. In the AN are cells containing dopamine, GnRH, POMC derivatives, GRF, neurotensin, substance P, and leu-Enk. In the periventricular nucleus are cells containing dopamine, SRIF, leu-Enk, neurotensin, and CRH. In the parvicellular divisions of the PVN are cells containing dopamine, TRH, CRH, SRIF, OT, and AVP. These periventricular cell groups are unique because they are retrogradely labeled by the application of HRP or wheat-germ agglutinin–horseradish peroxidase (WGA-HRP) on the median eminence (649,661,662), i.e., these nuclear groups send projections to the median eminence. Cells located medially project to the median eminence by descending periventricular paths. Cells located more laterally in the PVN take a lateral and then a descending pathway with projections from the posterior magnocellular division of the PVN and from the region of the SON, where they are joined by fibers of the SOHT. This fiber bundle comprised of axons from the SON and PVN passes through the lateral retrochiasmatic area to enter the median eminence anterolaterally (Fig. 20).

In addition to the arcuate, the periventricular, and the parvicellular divisions of the PVN, one might arguably include the suprachiasmatic nucleus and the ventromedial nucleus among the parvicellular neurosecretory groups. Cells in the ScN contain immunoreactive vasopressin (758) but project to neural targets (645,693,759,760), not to the median eminence (649,661,662). The ventromedial nucleus (VMN) was included by Halasz and Pupp (102) in the HTA, but the evidence in support of a direct projection from the VMN to the median eminence is not strong. HRP applied to, or injected into, the median eminence is not transported to the VMN (649,661), and only scant labeling is found in the VMN after the application of WGA-HRP (662). One study employing anterograde autoradiographic techniques after ^{3}H-amino acid injection into the VMN demonstrated a projection to the median eminence from the VMN (761), whereas others have not (762–764). Peptidergic neurons in the VMN have not been demonstrated to project to the median eminence (432). Peptidergic cells in the hypothalamic periventricular gray made up of the AN, PvN, and PVN truly constitute a "hypophysiotropic area" in the hypothalamus. However, their cells project not only to the median eminence to regulate neuroendocrine function in response to changes in the environment or internal milieu but also to autonomic centers in the medulla and spinal cord to reticular regions in the mesencephalon and to limbic and rhinencephalic regions of the forebrain (Table 1).

The median eminence is believed to be the terminus of the noradrenergic reticular infundibular tract arising in the brain stem (713,714). On the basis of lesioning and deafferentation experiments, it has been proposed that noradrenergic fibers arising in the lower brain stem ascend in the central tegmental tract, enter the medial forebrain bundle, and then turn medially to terminate in the internal zone of the median eminence (416,482). However, retrograde labeling experiments involving application or injection of HRP or WGA-HRP onto (into) the median eminence failed to label brain stem sites in the rat (649,661,662). Perhaps the HRP did not reach the parvicellular terminals in the hypendymal zone because of the presence of the fiber layer but instead remained confined to the palisade layer.

The preoptic area (POA) does contain cells that are labeled following the topical application of wheat-germ agglutinin (WGA) to the surface of the median eminence (662). Although the POA has been considered by different authors to be a diencephalic or a telencephalic derivative, it is intimately related to the hypothalamus (620). It has been implicated in temperature regulation (765,766), thirst and the maintenance of fluid balance (646,767,768), integration of adrenocortical response with autonomic responses (769), cardiovascular regulation (768,770), sexual differentiation (771), masculine sexual behavior (772), scent-marking behavior (773), and cyclicity of gonadotropin secretions in female rodents (but not in primates) (774,775). The basis for considering this functionally important region to be a diencephalic derivative is reviewed by Christ (623). It is considered to work in conjunction with the hypothalamus by Crosby and Woodburne (703), Rioch et al. (30), and Crosby and Showers (620) and is considered to be part of the hypothalamus by Nauta and Haymaker (621). Papez (622) viewed the preoptic area as the gateway through which rostral innervation to the hypothalamus and to the epithalamus must pass.

The anterior border to the POA is defined by the lamina terminalis and by the diagonal band of Broca (DBB). It is bordered inferiorly by the optic chiasm and the suprachiasmatic nucleus and superiorly by the anterior commissure. Posteriorly the boundary between the POA and the (remainder of) the hypothalamus in the adult mammal is difficult to define (620–623,703). A line drawn from the posterior border of the anterior commissure to the posterior border of the optic chiasm or the rostral extremity of the PVN would appear to be a good operational definition. The POA is continuous dorsomedially with the bed nucleus of the stria terminalis, which actually enters the POA in its most anterior extent. It is continuous anteriorly with the olfactory tubercle and anteriorly and superiorly with the septal region (621).

The POA is divided, on cytoarchitectonic grounds, into a periventricular zone, a medial zone, a lateral zone, and a magnocellular preoptic nucleus (776). The periventricular zone [periventricular preoptic nucleus area (PVPOA)] is a thin band of cells lying beneath the ependyma of the third ventricle that is continuous caudally with the periventricular zone of the hypothalamus (620). Its cells are often oriented parallel to the third ventricle (776).

The medial preoptic zone [medial preoptic area (MPOA)] stretches the length of the POA bordered dorsally by the anterior commissure and ventrally by the optic chiasm. Its rostral tip merges with the bed nucleus of the stria terminalis. The cells are of medium size and are densely packed (776). TEM examination has revealed light and dark neurons in the MPOA (777). In light neurons the cytoplasm is the same density as the surrounding neuropil. The RER is dispersed throughout the cytoplasm. Free ribosomes and polysomes are numerous. The Golgi apparatus is well developed and is associated with clear vesicles 40 to 80 nm in diameter and dense-core vesicles about 100 nm in diameter. "Coated vesicles" are often seen. The RER extends into the dendrites. Occasional structures resembling the "whorls" or "ribbon rolls" in the cells of the arcuate nucleus are found. In dark neurons, some of the increased electron density is due to an increase in the number of free ribosomes. Free ribosomes lie between stacks of dilated endoplasmic reticulum. Many vesicles are associated with the Golgi apparatus. Both myelinated and unmyelinated axons are present in the neuropil of the MPOA, with myelinated axons typically occurring in small clusters. A few axons contain dense-core vesicles with diameters ranging from 125 to 165 nm. Dendrites are frequently beaded in appearance, with large varicosities joined by narrow necks. Both symmetrical and asymmetrical synapses on dendritic shafts, dendritic spines, axons, and cell bodies are found. Greenough et al. (778) reported that sex differences were present in the dendritic field patterns of the MPOA in hamsters. Dendrites in the MPOA of males tended to be clustered centrally, whereas the dendrites in the MPOA of females were distributed more irregularly. These observations suggested to them that a differential input may occur in the MPOA of male and female animals.

The MPOA of the rat contains a sexually dimorphic nucleus (SDN-MPOA) that can be identified by visual inspection of Nissl-stained sections (779). In males, the central region of the MPOA is more darkly stained and has sharper borders than in females. Its volume is larger in males than in females. The different staining pattern is secondary to an increase in cell density in the SDN-MPOA. Differences can be found between male and female rats as early as the first day of (extrauterine) life (780). The cells of the SDN-MPOA migrate there from more ventral regions of the MPOA. A male pattern can be induced in females by exposure to androgens on the day of birth. Gonadectomy of males on postnatal day 1 reduced the size of the SDN-MPOA by more than 50% (781). A similar sexual dimorphism has been found in the MPOA of the guinea pig (782), gerbil (773), toad (783), and human (784). The role of this developmental difference between males and females is unknown. It is of interest that the sexually dimorphic region of the MPOA in the male toad is considered to be the center for mate calling and that its nuclear volume varies with the breeding season (783).

Stimulation of the preoptic area of proestrus female rats causes an increase in plasma LH concentration and ovulation (785). The integrity of the posterior region of the preoptic area is necessary for the exhibition of male sexual behavior in the rat (772). It is to be expected then that this region (in the rodent) is related to ovulation, and hence to the feedback relationships of estrogen on GnRH-containing neurons, and to sexual behavior. Testosterone-concentrating neurons have been localized in the arcuate and preoptic regions of adult rats (786). Estrogen-concentrating neurons have also been identified by autoradiographic means in the preoptic area (787–789).

The bed nucleus of the stria terminalis enters the dorsal region of the MPOA and has been extensively studied in the rat. A sexual dimorphism of the pattern of nonstrial synapses in the bed nucleus of the stria terminalis was first reported by Raisman and Field (790). Female rats had more nonstrial synapses on dendritic spines than did males. This pattern, along with the cyclic pattern of gonadotropin release and behavioral estrus, was abolished if the females were treated on postnatal day 4 with testosterone. Males castrated within 12 hr of birth developed a female pattern of cyclic gonadotropin release and a female pattern of nonstrial synapses in the bed nucleus of the stria terminalis. Cells in the lateral subdivision of the bed nucleus of the stria terminalis contain two or three dendrites that branch sparingly but that may extend 300 to 400 μm across the field of incoming strial neurons; these dendrites are oriented perpendicular to these neurons to form a reticular grid (791). This arrangement should maximize contact between neurons of the bed nucleus and axons entering through the stria terminalis.

The magnocellular preoptic nucleus lies in the lateral zone, lateral to the diagonal band of Broca. Saper (792) believed this nuclear group to be part of a system of large neurons, 20 to 30 μm in diameter, that are grouped into clusters in the medial septal nucleus, the magnocellular preoptic nucleus, substantia inominata, and globus pallidus. These neurons stain immunohistochemically for acetylcholine transferase. The lateral zone [lateral preoptic area (LPOA)] is characterized by the presence of medium-sized neurons scattered among the fibers of the medial forebrain bundle (MFB).

Peptide hormones have been localized by immunohistochemistry within cells making up the nuclear groups of the POA of the rat. Somatostatin has been found within cells of the PVPOA (668,669,697,793). Immunoreactive human growth hormone has been localized within cells of the PVPOA and MPOA (529). Cells containing ir-CRH (506,675) and ir-enkephalin (526) have been identified in the PVPOA and MPOA. Cells containing ir-TRH have been localized within the MPOA and the diagonal band of Broca (415). Cells in the bed nucleus of the stria terminalis have been identified which contain immunoreactive vasoactive intestinal peptide (VIP) (794), AVP (795), and CRH (506,675). Cells containing substance P (794), met-Enk (794), and leu-Enk (796) have been identified in the MPOA and LPOA.

GnRH is also found in the MPOA of the rat (720), but the cells containing this peptide are not confined within its borders (797,798). Immunoreactive cells are also present in the olfactory bulb, olfactory tubercle, nucleus of the diagonal band of Broca, medial septum, and lateral hypothalamus (797,798). Unlike earlier investigators (163,164,721–723), recent investigators have failed to confirm the presence of GnRH in the arcuate nucleus of the rat (797,798). King et al. (797) suggested that previous studies employed antibodies that reacted against ACTH. The presence of GnRH in cells of the arcuate nucleus of the rabbit (725), guinea pig (726), monkey (724), and human (730) is generally accepted.

The projections of the POA have been studied by autoradiography following the injection of labeled amino acids into the preoptic area of the rat brain (776,799) and following the injection of WGA-HRP (800). The PVPOA projections were principally descending ones in the periventricular zone; these projected to the "hypophysiotrophic area" of the medial basilar hypothalamus and the median eminence (799). Swanson (766) stated that dorsal, intermediate, and ventral parts of the PVPOA project to "characteristically different terminal fields." A lesser projection courses laterally to join the medial region of the medial forebrain bundle to terminate in the hypophysiotrophic area of the hypothalamus and the internal zone of the median eminence.

Neurons in the PVPOA and in the MPOA project to the OVLT (801). A projection of GnRH-containing neurons from the MPOA to the OVLT has been identified in the rat (797). Immunoreactive TRH- (415), somatostatin- (669), and HGH-containing (529) fibers in the OVLT also originate in the MPOA (801). AVP-containing fibers that terminate in the OVLT probably arise from the suprachiasmatic nucleus (760) and not from the supraoptic nucleus (340). The function of this circumventricular organ is unknown. The relationship of its fenestrated capillaries to its neurosecretory terminals is analogous to that found in the median eminence. Yet its venous drainage does not lead to a gland but instead leads to the great vessels at the base of the brain (801). Palkovits et al. (801) speculate that terminals on blood vessels on the OVLT might be sensing the state of blood passing through the organ or it might be the site where peptides are released into blood to be transported by ependymal cells into the ventricular fluid.

Ascending projections of the MPOA are to the stria medullaris (and hence via the habenular nuclei and fasciculus retroflexus to the midbrain tegmentum), to the diagonal band of Broca (and hence to the medial septum) and to the medial forebrain bundle (799). Projections of the guinea-pig MPOA are similar to those in the rat described by Conrad and Pfaff (799) except that the guinea pig's MPOA projects to the neural lobe (802). Chiba and Murata (800) have reported more-extensive ascending projections to the bed nucleus of the stria terminalis, nucleus of the diagonal band of Broca, medial amygdaloid nucleus, and septal regions. (The interested reader is referred to refs. 764,776, 799,800, and 803.)

The descending projections of the MPOA resemble those of the PVPOA, except that the contribution to the lateral pathway through the MFB is more robust. Neither Conrad and Pfaff (764) nor Swanson (776) could trace descending pathways further caudally than the mesencephalon. Chiba and Murata (800) were able to follow descending fibers from the MPOA to the lateral parabrachial nucleus of the pons as well as to the locus ceruleus and to the nucleus and tractus solitarius and the vagal complex of the medulla in the rat by using WGA-HRP as a tracer. They propose that these projections are the basis of the functional relationship between the MPOA and autonomic control of blood pressure, of thermoregulation, and of angiotensin-II-induced drinking behavior (Table 1).

The efferent pathways of specific peptidergic systems from the MPOA and PVPOA are being investigated. Somatostatin fibers have been demonstrated, by lesioning experiments, to course along a basically periventricular path from the PVPOA to the median eminence, although the fibers course slightly lateral to the third ventricle, just anterior to the median eminence, to enter it from its lateral aspect (793). Whether other peptide-containing cells in the PVPOA—such as ir-CRH-, ir-met-Enk-, and ir-HGH-containing cells—also project along such pathways to the median eminence is as yet unsettled.

GnRH pathways from the preoptic and septal regions of the rat brain have been established, and the basic schema has been agreed upon by several investigators. GnRH-containing perikaryia are arranged across the region of the rat's basilar forebrain in the shape of an inverted V. The apex is directed at midline nuclear groups such as the OVLT and the PVPOA, and the diverging wings are bisected by the third ventricle. Two systems project caudally and ventrally to the median eminence: a periventricular system originating medially and a lateral system originating laterally and descending in the MFB. Although some differences exist with regard to detail, the systems following this basic pattern are described by King et al. (797), Hoffman and Gibbs (804), and Merchenthaler et al. (805). Analogous systems are described in the guinea pig (726,806), monkey (807), baboon (808), and human (730), except that GnRH-containing cells in the arcuate nucleus as well as in the MPOA project to the median eminence.

GnRH cells in the preoptic area of the baboon project to stria medullaris and to the ME and the OVLT. Cells in the PVPOA project to the median eminence. GnRH cells were also found in the medial septum, bed nucleus of the stria terminalis, lateral hypothalamus, and lateral preoptic area, but these cells did not project to the median eminence. They were believed to be involved with reproductive behavior other than endocrine function (808). In the hamster, projections from the septum are reported to gain access to the hippocampus and to reach the amygdala via the stria terminalis. Projections from the medial septum also reach the OVLT and subfornical organ (SFO). Projections from the olfactory tubercle reach the amygdala and piriform cortex via the ventroamygdalofugal pathway. Supracallosal projections reach the indiseum griseum. Descending projections to the midbrain course along the stria medullaris and fasciculus retroflexus, and some continue caudally into the pons (809). A similar pattern of GnRH projections in the rhinencephalon and limbic system and brain stem is found in the rat (810), bat (727), and guinea pig (726). The GnRH cells project to cerebral and brain-stem regions that could promote sexual behavior as well as to diencephalic regions that can promote reproductive function.

In summary, concepts of the hypophysiotrophic area, first proposed by Harris (73–77) on the basis of his transplantation experiments and developed by Halaz and Pupp (102) on the basis of their hypothalamic islands, have been recast. Cells that contain hypophysiotrophic peptides and terminate in the median eminence are found (principally) in nuclear groups that extend along the periventricular area from the lamina terminalis to the mammillary body. Smaller populations of cells are dispersed laterally (in the lateral septum, lateral preoptic area, and anterior hypothalamic area). Peptidergic cells project to the median eminence, but they also project to nuclear groups in the brain stem and spinal cord, to other circumventricular organs, mainly the OVLT, and to terminal fields in the rhinencephalon and the limbic midbrain and forebrain. The dispersion of functional hypophysiotrophic cell types along the rostrocaudal axis in the periventricular zone permits each cell type to become closely related to several different cell types at specific sites. For example, SRIF-containing cells are in close proximity to GnRH-containing cells in the rat's MPOA but not in the rat's arcuate nucleus. Disparate peptidergic cells in a nuclear group frequently project to the same terminal fields. For example, OT, SRIF, and enkephalin-containing cells project to common sites in the brain stem and spinal cord from a common site in the PVN. CRH- and AVP-containing fibers from a common locus in the PVN project to a common site in the median eminence. In the MPOA, GnRH, SRIF, and AVP, fibers project to the olfactory tubercle and to the central and medial nuclei of the amygdala; these fibers project rostrally into the stria medullaris and thence to the mesencephalic tegmentum. Perhaps more importantly, the dispersion of functional cell groups brings clusters of hypophysiotrophic cells into the terminal fields of specific ascending and descending afferent fiber systems to permit appropriate regulation of endocrine function in response to neural stimuli; and because a cell's location will determine its projections, this organization will permit the integration of endocrine, autonomic, and (higher) cerebral function.

INPUT TO THE PERIVENTRICULAR HYPOTHALAMUS

Afferent systems from the rhinencephalon, from limbic structures, and from the brain stem project to specific preoptic and hypothalamic sites where neurosecretory neurons reside. These sites may be occupied by clusters of homogeneous neurons that manufacture the same peptide(s), by clusters of heterogeneous neurons that manufacture different peptides, or by clusters of heterogeneous neurons in which only a few manufacture peptides but most do not. Neurons in cell groups thus defined need not share a common peptide but share a common pattern of afferent input. They represent a terminal field upon which converge axons from diverse sites unique to each cell group.

Afferents enter the periventricular hypothalamus by one of four routes: the medial forebrain bundle, the periventricular system, the fornix, and the stria terminalis. The medial forebrain (MFB) lies in the lateral zone of the hypothalamus and extends from preoptic to mammillary levels. The cells within the lateral zone are called "path neurons" by Millhouse (811). These cells are oriented perpendicular to the plane of the fibers running in a rostrocaudal direction, and each dendritic tree radiates like a fan in the path of the fibers in the MFB. Their axons project medially into the medial and periventricular zones and innervate the nuclear groups in the MPOA-HTA (812). Collaterals from MFB neurons branch at right angles to the parent axon and course parallel to the dendrites of path neurons. Hence, one axon of a fiber in the MFB passes through the dendritic arbor of several path neurons in series, with the opportunity to send collaterals to each (811).

Ascending and descending inputs enter into, and pass through, the MFB. Millhouse (811) proposed that descending input tended to project collaterals to rostral regions (the MPOA and anterior hypothalamic area), whereas ascending input tended to send collaterals preferentially to caudal regions (the tuberomammillary region). He also proposed that the fascicles of the MFB maintained constant and characteristic positions in the MFB that were related to their origin. Both these concepts were based on LM study of degenerating fibers after placement of lesions in presumptive afferent sites. They have received support from recent autoradiographic studies on the injection of ^{3}H-amino acids into sites projecting to the MFB in the rat (813,814). Ascending components are confined to the dorsal half of the bundle, and descending components are confined to the ventral half. Major fiber groups that descend in the MFB (a) arise in the olfactory tubercle, amygdala, basal ganglia, and MPOA and lie in its ventral and ventrolateral regions and (b) arise in the septum and are confined to the ventromedial region of the bundle. Ascending systems are probably similarly arranged, with the ventral tegmental component near the center of the bundle and the ascending fibers from the parabrachial area in the dorsal and dorsolateral regions. Further ascending systems have yet to be studied (815).

There is disagreement regarding the nature of catecholaminergic fibers in the MFB. These fibers arise in the brain stem and ascend in the MFB to reach diencephalic and telencephalic terminal fields (815). The dorsal tegmental bundle is held to arise from the locus ceruleus (A6) catecholaminergic (CA) cell group (816) and to ascend in the central tegmental tract. According to the account of Lindvall and Bjorklund (815), rendered on the basis of fluorescence following glyoxylic acid treatment, fibers of the dorsal tegmental bundle enter the MFB. On the basis of immunohistochemical staining for DBH, Swanson and Hartman (817) concluded that noradrenergic fibers from the locus ceruleus traveled with other ascending noradrenergic systems in the "principal noradrenergic system" in the central tegmental tract and entered the hypothalamus from a lateral position in a discrete bundle in the zona inserta lateral to the MFB. CA fibers innervated the PVN by passing from lateral to medial and then innervated the AN by passing down through the periventricular area. The MPOA was innervated both from the periventricular area and from fibers coursing medially from the anterior extension of the noradrenergic bundle in the zona inserta.

The ventral tegmental noradrenergic bundle in the pons and mesencephalon receives input from A1 (lateral reticular nucleus), A2 (dorsal medullary complex), A5 and A7 (parabrachial nucleus) (816), and from the subceruleus region (815). This projection ascends in the central tegmental tract, and, according to the account of Lindvall and Bjorklund (815), contributes to the MFB at the level of the tegmental radiations. Swanson and Hartman (817) disputed this interpretation on the basis of their DBH studies and stated that the dorsal and ventral tegmental bundles form the principal ascending noradrenergic bundle, which enters the hypothalamus as a discrete system in the region of the zona inserta. They believed that the fluorescent fibers seen in the MFB by Lindvall and Bjorklund (815) are dopaminergic and arise from the ventral tegmental region to ascend in the MFB to hypothalamic and limbic forebrain sites (818,819). Palkovits et al. (820) appear to accept the account of Lindvall and Bjorklund (815) because lesions separating the MFB from the MPOA-HTA reduced the norepinephrine content in that region. However, these lesions would have also separated the zona incerta from the MPOA-HTA. At this time one can conclude that the MFB contains dopaminergic neurons, but the matter of noradrenergic neurons is unsettled. The presence of adrenergic neurons in the MFB has yet to be carefully addressed.

The periventricular nucleus (650) extends around the third ventricle. Axon terminals are oriented in a dorsal-ventral plane as are the axons and dendritic fields of neurons in this region (103,650). This region also carries fibers that project rostrally and caudally. Major descending input enters from the MPOA (776,799,802). Within the MPOA-HTA, the PVN also contributes to this system (764). Outside the periventricular region, the ventral median nucleus of the hypothalamus sends ascending and descending fibers into the periventricular system (761–763). Input also enters via the stria terminalis. Ascending input from the brain stem is through the dorsal longitudinal fasciculus, which receives input from the A2 cell group in the dorsal medullary complex and, to a lesser extent, from the locus ceruleus and the subceruleus area (815,820–822).

The fornix also projects to the MPOA-HTA, but the hippocampal fibers destined for hypothalamic terminals originate in the prosubiculum, not in Ammon's horn (823). Fibers originating in field CA1 of Ammon's horn project through the fornix to terminate (with or without relay in the mammillary nuclei) in the anterior nucleus of the thalamus. Field CA3 of Ammon's horn sends projections through the fimbria to the precommissural fornix, where they terminate principally in the septal nuclei. Fibers destined for the hypothalamus arise in the subiculum and course in the dorsal region of the fornix behind the anterior commissure, where they depart from the postcommissural fornix to form the medial cortical hypothalamic tract, which terminates in the arcuate nucleus. The dentate gyrus and Ammon's horn both receive a massive input from the rhinencephalon and sensory regions of the forebrain. The dentate gyrus projects to Ammon's horn, which, in turn, projects to the prosubiculum and thence to the AN (824,825). The medial cortical-hypothalamic tract, which is prominent in rodents, is not found in primates (621). The pathway from the hippocampus to the hypothalamus in humans has not been established with certainty.

The stria terminalis carries projections from the amygdala to the bed nucleus of the stria terminalis and the preoptic area (794) as well as to the ventromedial nucleus of the hypothalamus (826). Several different peptidergic fiber systems are present in this tract, but their relationship to neurosecretory cells in the MPOA remains to be evaluated.

The SON receives input from the MPOA, the SFO, and the OVLT as determined from retrograde HRP studies on the injections of small amounts of HRP into loci contained entirely within the SON of the rat (827) (Table 2). This observation is compatible with the accepted role of the anteroventral third ventricular region (AV3V region) in fluid and electrolyte balance (646,767,768). The AN sends a projection of ir-ACTH-containing axons to the SON, which is distributed to regions where OT cells predominate (743).

TABLE 2. *Afferents to MPOA-HTA*[a]

	SON	PVN(m)	PVN(p)	PVN	AN	MPOA
OVLT	+	+				+
SFO	+	+				+
SON		+				
PVN(m)						
PVN(p)						
PVN					+	
AN	+	+	+	+		+
MPOA	+	+	+	+		+
VMN			?	+	+	
Hipp.	+	+	?			
Septum	+	+	?			+
BNST		?	+			+
Amygdala		?	+			+
Ol. Tub.						
IPN						
SN						
Teg.	?					
PbN			+		?	+
LC	+			?		
Raphe	+					+
LRN	+	+	+	+	+	
PVC	+		+	+	+	

[a]Abbreviations are the same in Table 1. Also: SFO, subfornical organ.

Descending input to the SON is revealed by larger injections of HRP which extend slightly beyond the borders of the SON; this reveals a more extensive input from hypothalamic regions outside the MPOA-HTA to regions about the SON (827). Fibers, descending from the subiculum, septum, and nucleus of the diagonal band of Broca were labeled. Although Swanson and Cowan (803) did not report labeling of the SON following injection of labeled amino acids into the septal region, Tribbolet et al. (827) noted labeling in the region immediately surrounding the SON following the injection of tritiated amino acids into the septum and subiculum. This pattern of labeling signifies a functional connection between these limbic regions and the SON because (a) the dendritic field of the SON is not limited to the confines of the nucleus but extends beyond it particularly in the ventral glial lamina (828), (b) TEM studies on the SON region following placement of septal lesions demonstrate degeneration of terminals (829), (c) TEM studies on anterograde transport of HRP from the septum demonstrate labeled terminals synapsing on neurites at the border of the SON which stain immunohistochemically for either OT or AVP (830), and (d) electrophysiologic studies demonstrated antidromic activation of septal neurons after stimulation of the SON (831).

The ascending input to the SON from the brain stem enters the hypothalamus through the periventricular dorsal longitudinal fasciculus or the medial forebrain bundle (621). Both norepinephrine and dopamine are present in the SON (717,821,832). Catecholamine-containing terminals have been demonstrated in the SON of the rat (708), cat (833), and monkey (834), and several sources have been suggested. Small injections of HRP confined within the locus of the SON of the rat label the A1 (lateral reticular nucleus) and the A2 (nucleus of the solitary tract and the dorsal vagal complex) noradrenergic cell groups (827). Similar observations were made in the rabbit, where, after SON injection, HRP labeling of catecholaminergic cells identified by fluoroscopic methods was demonstrated in the A1 and A2 cell groups (835). Anterograde labeling of the SON followed the injection of tritiated amino acids into the A1 (but not the A2) cell group (835). Similar findings were also noted in the rat (822). Electrophysiologic studies demonstrate that stimulation of the carotid sinus nerves or baroreceptors activates neurons in the location of the A1 cell group and that stimulation of these noradrenergic neurons selectively facilitates activity of phasic vasopressin-secreting neurons in the SON (836,837). Evidence that the A2 cell group directly innervates the SON is less compelling. Anterograde labeling experiments in the rat (822,838) and in the rabbit (835) failed to confirm the presence of a direct innervation of the SON by the A2 cell group. Stimulation of the nucleus of the solitary tract excited some neurons by "slow," presumably polysynaptic, pathways.

Injections of HRP which extend beyond the SON's borders also label cells in the A6 (locus ceruleus) and A7 (parabrachial nucleus) cell groups. However, anterograde injection studies do not confirm a projection from A7 to the SON (839–841). They do show descending fiber systems from the lateral parabracheal nucleus passing through the region of the A1 cell group (840), which, in turn, projects to the SON. Lindvall and Bjorklund (842) stated that the A6 cell group innervates the SON but that most of the innervation of the SON arises from the dorsal medulla and the lateral tegmentum of the brain stem. This finding is confirmed by Sawchenko and Swanson (822), who demonstrated that less than 10% of the noradrenergic terminals in the SON arise from the A6 cell group. Thus there is strong evidence that the SON is principally innervated by cells arising from the A1 cell group in the lateral reticular nucleus. The A1 cell group also projects to A2, A6, and A7 and in return receives non-noradrenergic reciprocal innervation from these cell groups (843).

Noradrenergic terminals within the SON are found aggregated in its ventromedial region, where cells containing AVP are clustered (684,844,845). Noradrenergic axons terminate on cell bodies or proximal dendrites (684,844,845). McNeill and Sladek (844) noted that in the rat, CA terminals are most frequently found surrounding the SON and are particularly abundant in the ventral glial lamina (828), where they contact dendrites of SON neurons. These anatomic observations nicely complement Day and Renaud's (837) physiologic findings that stimulation of the A1 cell groups selectively activates phasic AVP-secreting neurons.

Dopamine terminals are also present in the SON. They are homogeneously distributed throughout the nucleus and terminate on the soma of OT- and AVP-containing cells (846). In view of the close relationship of AVP terminals in the neural lobe of the rat to terminals of the dopaminergic tuberohypophyseal tract (417), it is of interest to determine the site of origin of dopaminergic terminals about the magnocellular neurons in the SON. Buijs et al. (846) have suggested that they arise in the arcuate nucleus. Simon et al. (818) identified a projection from the A10 dopaminergic cell group in the ventral tegmental area of Tsai to the SON using anterograde and retrograde tracing techniques. Further work is necessary before the origin of the dopaminergic terminals in the SON can be considered established.

Serotonin-containing terminals in the SON originate in the raphe nuclei and enter the hypothalamus through the medial forebrain bundle (847). The distribution of serotonin fibers within the SON and their mode of termination (axosomatic, axodendritic, or axoaxonic) is not presently known.

The PVN receives input from several structures in the MPOA-HTA region of the rat's hypothalamus. On the basis of studies employing retrograde transport of HRP following its injection into the PVN, input from the MPOA, AN, and SON has been demonstrated (848,849), as has input from the OVLT and SFO (849). Anterograde autoradiographic tracer studies on the injection of [^{3}H]proline into the MPOA of the guinea pig demonstrate a projection into the PVN (802). Anterograde studies in the rat have not been definitive. Conrad and Pfaff (799) found that [^{3}H]proline or [^{3}H]leucine injected into the POA revealed fibers that entered the MFB and labeled the periventricular region of the hypothalamus. "A few" silver grains were seen over the PVN. Swanson (776) stated that it was difficult to tell if the few silver grains found over the PVN after injection of ^{3}H-amino acids into the MPOA were localized in terminals or in axons of passage. Chiba and Murata (800) injected WGA-HRP into the MPOA of the rat and found labeling in multiple hypothalamic nuclei, including the PVN. Sawchenko et al. (743) employed immunohistochemistry to demonstrate an ACTH projection from the AN of the rat to the magnocellular regions of the PVN, where OT fibers predominated. The pattern resembled that of the arcuate ACTH projection to the OT-rich regions in the SON. Arcuate ACTH fibers also terminated about parvicellular neurons. They were found to project to the ventromedial region of the medial parvicellular division and to the dorsal parvicellular division of the PVN. These regions contain OT-synthesizing neurons that project to the dorsovagal complex and to the spinal cord. GRF cells in the arcuate nucleus also project to the anterior, periventricular, and ventromedial parvicellular regions of the PVN (432). Silverman et al. (849) proposed that input to the PVN from the SON arises from collaterals of the SOHT. The pattern of input into the PVN from nuclear groups within the MPOA-HTA of the hypothalamus resembles that into the SON, with the obvious addition of input into the parvicellular divisions.

Hypothalamic regions outside the MPOA-HTA also project to the PVN. Projections from the dorsomedial nucleus (DMN), ventromedial nucleus (VMN), and suprachiasmatic nucleus (ScN) have been revealed by studies of retrograde transport of HRP following its injection into the PVN (848,849). Anterograde tracer studies with labeled amino acids have been carried out to determine the efferent pathways of the VMN, but the authors do not mention a projection from VMN to PVN in the rat (761,762,799). Saper et al. (762) stated that the anterograde labeling studies revealed no projection from the VMN to the PVN in the monkey. However, following placement of an electrolytic lesion in the VMN of the cat, Kaelber and Leeson (850) found degenerating terminals in the PVN. If confirmed, the projection from hypothalamic areas outside the MPOA-HTA such as the VMN marks a major difference in input to the PVN when compared with the SON.

The PVN, like the SON, receives descending input from the septum and subiculum (848,849). Swanson and Cowan (803) could not demonstrate a projection from the lateral septum or subiculum to the PVN with anterograde tracing techniques using LM examination of autoradiographs after injection of labeled amino acids. However, Oldfield et al. (830) employed TEM techniques to examine the PVN after injection of HRP into the subiculum or septum and immunohistochemical staining of the PVN for OT and AVP. A projection from these limbic regions onto AVP- and OT-containing neurites just lateral or ventrolateral to the PVN was demonstrated. Unlike the SON, the PVN receives a projection from the medial and central nuclei of the amygdala (848,849) and from the bed nucleus of the stria terminalis (803,849,851). TEM studies demonstrate that the input from the amygdala is to the AVP-containing neurites just lateral and ventrolateral to the nucleus. Projections from the amygdala, from the bed nucleus of the stria terminalis, and from the ventromedial nucleus of the hypothalamus, which receives input from the amygdala (826,852,853), are unique to the PVN when compared with the SON. It is tempting to relate these projections from rhinencephalic regions that contain glucocorticoid receptors to the parvicellular regions of the PVN that (a) contain AVP, CRH, and Ang II, (b) project to the median eminence (or to the medulla and spinal cord), (c) are implicated in the regulation of the pituitary adrenal and autonomic neural axes (849).

The PVN receives a much more elaborate ascending innervation than does the SON. Catecholamines are present in the PVN (717,821,832), and CA terminals have been demonstrated in the PVN of the rat (708), cat (833), and monkey (834). In the magnocellular divisions of the rat (844) and monkey (845), CA fibers are more abundant in regions rich in AVP cells than in regions where cells containing OT predominate. Swanson et al. (684) employed immunohistochemistry to demonstrate that noradrenergic terminals containing dopamine-β-hydroxylase (DBH) but not phenylethanolamine-*N*-methyltransferase (PNMT) were present predominantly in regions where AVP-containing magnocellular neurons were found. However, these observations must be interpreted cautiously because Silverman et al. (854) demonstrated, on TEM study of the PVN, that CA terminals primarily innervated the dendritic processes of nonvasopressinergic neurons. When noradrenergic terminals contacted AVP-containing neurons, contact was axodendritic, not axosomatic. Because the dendrites of peptidergic cells within the PVN have a large medial-to-lateral extension (651), the specific location of noradrenergic terminals within subdivisions of the PVN may not be predictive of the type of cell innervated.

Retrograde tracing experiments demonstrate that the lateral reticular nucleus (A1 cell group) projects to the PVN in rats (822,848) and rabbits (835) (Fig. 22). Anterograde labeling experiments confirm this pattern in the rabbit (835) and rat (822,855) and further demonstrate that the A1 projection is preferential to the magnocellular regions in the nucleus. However, the caution noted by Silverman et al. (854)—that noradrenergic innervation of AVP neurons is to their dendrites, which may extend far from the region where the cell bodies are grouped—is again applicable. The principle that A1 neurons do preferentially innervate magnocellular neurons in the PVN which contain AVP is supported by the observation that stimulation in the region of the A1 cell group activates phasic (AVP) neurons in the PVN (856–858) as it activates phasic (AVP) neurons in the SON (837). It is difficult not to place functional significance upon the observation that large cells in the PVN and SON arise from the same germinal cell group, migrate to their final destinations at the same time, receive input from the same limbic,

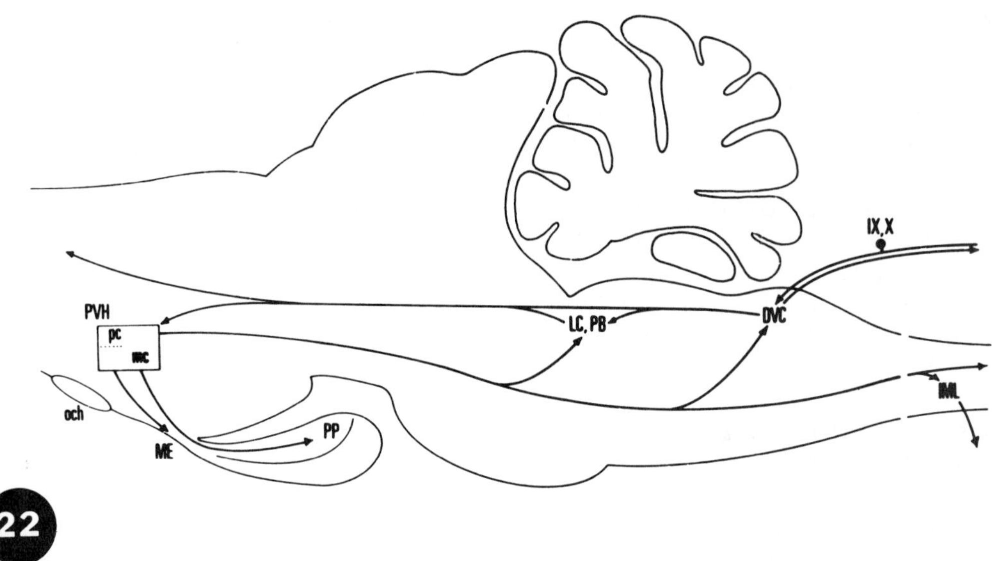

FIG. 22. A summary of the major longer connections of PVH in the rat. In this diagram, relationships between the PVH and cell groups associated with the autonomic nervous system are emphasized. (DVC) Dorsal vagal complex; (IML) intermediolateral column; (LC) locus ceruleus; (mc) magnocellular division of PVH; (ME) median eminence; (och) optic chiasm; (PB) parabrachial nucleus; (pc) parvocellular division of PVH; (PP) posterior pituitary; (PVH) paraventricular nucleus; (IX) glossopharyngeal nerve; (X) vagus nerve. (From ref. 859.)

circumventricular, preoptic, and brain-stem structures, and project to the same terminal field—the neural lobe.

Catecholaminergic terminals are also found in the parvicellular divisions of the PVN in the rat, where they are aggregated in the periventricular, dorsal, and medial parvicellular regions (844). Swanson et al. (684) demonstrated that these fibers are most likely adrenergic, since positive staining for PNMT and DBH characterized terminals in these regions. Anterograde tracer experiments reveal projections from the A2 cell group to the medial and dorsal parvicellular divisions and from the A6 (locus ceruleus) to the medial parvicellular division. These brain-stem catecholaminergic sites project via different pathways (the ventral and dorsal tegmental bundles), first in the central tegmental area to the medial forebrain bundle and then to the PVN (665,859,860). Further studies demonstrate an additional projection from the "pontine taste area" (the parabrachial-nucleus-A7-noradrenergic cell group) to the PVN (839,841). Anterograde tracing studies demonstrate that the A7 cell group projects to the parvicellular divisions of the PVN, particularly to the dorsal and medial parvicellular regions (which project back to the dorsovagal region in the medulla and to the intermediolateral cell column in the spinal cord) (840,855). In addition, the A7 cell group projects heavily to the central nucleus of the amygdala (839), which, in turn, projects to the PVN (848,849) and to the A1-region, which, in turn, projects to PVN (840). Neurophysiologic studies demonstrate that stimulation of the PVN antidromically activates units in the A1 region to which the PVN projects, as confirmed by HRP injection. These same A1 neurons are activated (presumably by polysynaptic pathways passing through the nucleus of the solitary tract) by stimulation of carotid sinus and aortodepressor nerves (691,861). Non-noradrenergic pathways have been identified from the nucleus of the solitary tract to the A1 cell group, as have noradrenergic pathways from A1 to A2 and A6 (822). A2 and A6, in turn, project to the parvicellular region of the PVN while A1 projects preferentially to magnocellular regions of the PVN and SON.

Other amine systems reportedly project to the PVN. Buijs et al. (846) reported that dopaminergic fibers innervate the nucleus homogeneously, although DA fibers were not identified in the nucleus by Swanson et al. (684) employing an antibody against DBH and TH. The serotonin innervation of the PVN is sparse (847).

The PVN differs from the SON, not only because it is located in a different place but because it is quite simply the SON and more. It contains another population of small neurons that (one would predict) arises from a different germinal site. It projects to additional terminal fields in the dorsal medulla and spinal cord as well as to a different terminal field in the neurohypophysis (the median eminence). It receives additional rhinencephalic and brain-stem input. The aggregation of peptidergic parvicellular neurons (which receive input from the rhinencephalic and brain-stem centers related to steroid feedback and regulation of cardiovascular status) about magnocellular elements that receive input concerning the osmolality of the blood and the regulation cardiovascular status is presumably more than fortuitous. These functions are not carried out independently but are integrated by the axodendritic contacts within the nucleus between the magnocellular and parvicellular populations (651).

The periventricular nucleus (PvN) receives ACTH-containing fibers from the arcuate nucleus as they pass on to the PVN (Table 2). GRF-containing fibers from the arcuate nucleus terminate in the preoptic and hypothalamic periventricular sites, which are rich in SRIF-containing neurons (432). The descending projections from the MPOA to the periventricular nucleus by periventricular routes as well as by the MFB have been documented in the rat and guinea pig (776,799,802), as have projections from the bed nucleus of the stria terminalis in the rat (803). Other hypothalamic regions, the VMN (761–763), and the anterior hypothalamic area (696) outside the MPOA-HPA project to the periventricular nucleus. Catecholamine terminals have been demonstrated by fluorescence techniques in the periventricular region (708,833,834). Although they presumably arise in the brain stem (815), perhaps from the A1, A2, and A6 cell groups (822), and ascend into the hypothalamus through the periventricular system and the MFB (818), the ascending fiber pathways to the narrow periventricular region of the hypothalamus have not been worked out in detail.

The AN receives input from other regions in the MPOA-HTA. Immunoreactive SRIF-containing neurons in the periventricular nucleus have been shown to project to the AN (667). Further input from the periventricular nucleus has not as yet been revealed by immunohistochemical techniques but may be expected. The MPOA has been shown to project to the AN in HRP retrograde tracing experiments (799).

The VMN, which lies outside the MPOA-HTA, is believed to project to the arcuate nucleus. Szentagothai et al. (103) reported that "even very small foci in this region produced abundant signs of degeneration in all parts of the ipsilateral hypothalamus." Golgi studies by the same group revealed axon projections to the periventricular gray. HRP injection of the median eminence labeled the VMN if the injection spread into the arcuate nucleus (649). Saper et al. (763) described a projection from the VMN to the AN in the monkey and the cat after injecting the VMN with labeled amino acids and employing autoradiography to study anterograde transport. On the other hand, Suten and Eager (862) did not describe any degeneration in the AN of the cat following placement of discrete lesions in the VMN. The axonal projections from the VMN are described by both Szentagothai et al. (103) and Millhouse (863) as being primarily directed dorsally and posteriorly on the basis of studying Golgi preparations, although abundant collaterals were noted by both authors. Anterograde autoradiographic studies with tritriated amino acids have not demonstrated a projection between the VMN and the AN in the rat because the distances between them are small (761,762,764).

The VMN is an oval-shaped hypothalamic cell group that lies dorsal and lateral to the AN (103,863). It is characterized by the presence of a cell-rich core and a cell-poor capsule (863). Dendrites from axons in the VMN extend into the cell-poor capsule. In the cell-poor zone between the AN and VMN lie dendrites of both nuclear groups (863). The VMN is made up of two compact cellular aggregates; this permits its subdivision into dorsolateral and ventromedial regions (762). Immunohistochemical techniques have revealed GRF in cells that encapsulate (but do not lie within) the nucleus and do not project to the median eminence or to the arcuate nucleus (432).

Heimer and Nauta (826) studied the pattern of degeneration in the rat's hypothalamus following transection of the stria terminalis. They described three projections over the stria terminalis from the ipsilateral amygdala: one to the bed nucleus of the stria terminalis, one to a field immediately caudal to the anterior commissure, and a third (supracommissural) component to the cell-poor zone about the VMN. Raisman (825) transected the stria terminalis and demonstrated that the degenerating supracommissural axons terminated on the dendritic spines of VMN neurons in the cell-poor zone. McBride and Sutin (852) injected HRP into the tuberal hypothalamus after ipsilateral transection of the stria terminalis and demonstrated that the cortical nucleus of the amygdala projected to the VMN solely by the stria terminalis. The medial nucleus employed both the ventral amygdalofugal pathway and the stria terminalis to reach the hypothalamus, and the basal nucleus projected to the VMN solely by the ventral amygdalofugal pathway. Krettek and Price (853) employed anterograde autoradiographic studies to trace the path of tritiated amino acids injected into different nuclear groups in the amygdala. While they agreed with previous authors that the VMN was a target of a large projection from the amygdala, they disagreed with the pattern of innervation. They found that both the medial and basal medial nuclei of the amygdala projected to the core of the VMN and not to its outer shell. The outer shell received a projection only from the subiculum via the dorsal fornix. Perhaps earlier experiments lesioned the dorsal fornix in the attempt to transect the stria terminalis. The evidence that the VMN sends descending projections through the posterior periventricular region to the central gray of the brain stem, through the medial forebrain bundle to the capsule about the mammillary complex, and through the ventral supraoptic commissure to the contralateral hemisphere is fairly strong, as is the evidence for ascending projections in the periventricular gray and medial forebrain bundle to the preoptic area and lateral septum (761–763). In addition, long reciprocal connections to the medial amygdaloid nucleus originate principally from the VMN (762,864,865). The anatomic evidence suggests that the VMN serves as a gateway by which projections from the amygdala can influence the AN and hence median eminence function, but that evidence is far from strong. On firmer footing is the supposition that projections from the amygdala to the PVN provide the route by which this structure influences median eminence function (803,848,849,851).

Within the hypothalamus, the anterior hypothalamic area projects to the AN (799). Descending cortical input into the AN from the subiculum to the hypothalamus is carried via fibers in the dorsal fornix that leave the postcommissural fornix as a discrete bundle, in the rat and rabbit, to form the medial corticohypothalamic tract, which terminates in the AN (824,825). This fiber pathway is not evident in the brains of cats, monkeys, and humans (621).

Ascending projections to the AN have been identified and are believed to be principally noradrenergic (842,866). The norepinephrine content of the AN was reduced 75% by hypothalamic deafferentation (821). Terminals containing ir-DBH were found in the AN of the rat (817). Lesion experiments (820) and anterograde tracing experiments (838) suggest that the AN is, like the SON, the PVN, and the PvN, predominantly innervated by the A1 and A2 cell groups in the medulla. Saper and Loewy (840) described labeling of the AN following injection of ^{3}H-amino acids into the A7 cell group in the parabracheal nucleus of the rat. However, such injections could have spread into the ventral tegmental system, and further confirmatory studies are indicated. Palkovits (820) pointed out that "the median eminence and any of the hypothalamic nuclei may receive NA fibers from any of the NA cell groups, as monosynaptic communication between them have already been proved." Fibers from the raphe nuclei, believed to be indolaminergic, reach the AN via the medial forebrain bundle (867).

The MPOA receives input from several hypothalamic nuclei in the MPOA-HTA periventricular complex. Retrograde HRP studies demonstrate afferents from the AN and PVN (800). Afferents from hypothalamic nuclear groups outside the HPA have also been demonstrated and include projections from the VMN (761), the DMN, and the mammillary complex (800). Descending input from the lateral septal nucleus via the medial forebrain bundle and from the medial septal nucleus via the periventricular system have been demonstrated by ^{3}H-amino acid autoradiographic studies (803). Afferents from the bed nucleus of the stria terminalis (800) and from the medial and central nuclei of the amygdala have also been demonstrated (868). Ascending input from the A1 and A2 CA cell groups in the medulla was demonstrated by double labeling with HRP injection into the MPOA and fluorescent staining for catecholamines of brain-stem nuclear groups (856). Input from the A7 area of the parabracheal nucleus [the "pontine taste area" of Norgren (839)] has been demonstrated by retrograde transport of HRP (800). This input is peptidergic, not aminergic, because some fibers contain ir-CRH and others contain ir-leu-Enk (869). The authors noted that the parabracheal nucleus is involved with cardiovascular control (as demonstrated by its activation upon stimulation of baroreceptors or the carotid sinus nerve through connections with the nucleus of the solitary tract) and that the MPOA is related to cardiovascular control and fluid balance as part of the "AV3V" region, and the authors stated that the input from the parabracheal nucleus is appropriate (869). However, the MPOA is also sexually dimorphic and is related to sexual behavior and a site where GnRH cell bodies are found. Projections from the pontine taste area are appropriate in this context also. The B7, B8, and B9 (816) raphe cell groups also project to the MPOA (867). The projection is serotonergic and sexually dimorphic (870). GnRH cells are present in the MPOA as well as in the nucleus of the diagonal band of Broca and the septum. The study of the afferent input into the scattered GnRH-containing cells in these regions has begun with the demonstration that synaptic contact with GnRH-containing cells in the MPOA is made by GABA-containing terminals (871). The details of the afferent input into GnRH cells will be the subject of later chapters.

REFERENCES

1. Cushing, H. (1912): *The Pituitary Body and Its Disorders*. J. B. Lippincott, Philadelphia.
2. Cushing, H. (1930): Neurohypophyseal mechanisms from a clinical standpoint. Parts I and II. *Lancet,* 2:119, 175.
3. Herring, P. T. (1908): The development of the mammalian pituitary and its morphological significance. *Q. J. Exp. Physiol.,* 1:161.
4. Herring, P. T. (1908): The histological appearances of the mammalian pituitary body. *Q. J. Exp. Physiol.,* 1:121.
5. Tilney, F. (1911): Contribution to the study of the hypophysis cerebri with especial reference to its comparative histology. *Mem. Wistar Inst. Anat. Biol.,* no. 2.
6. Dandy, W. E., and Goetsch, E. (1910): The blood supply of the pituitary body. *Am. J. Anat.,* 11:137.
7. Marie, P. (1886): Sur deux d'acromegaly; hypertropic singuliere non congenitale des extremites superieures, inferieurs et cephalique. *Rev. Med.,* VI:297, cited by Cushing (1).
8. Frolich, A. (1901): Ein fall von tumor der hypophysis cerebri ohne akromegalie. *Wein. Klin. Rundschau,* XV:883, cited by Cushing (1).
9. Crowe, S. J., Cushing, H., and Homans, J. (1910): Experimental hypophysectomy. *Bull. Johns Hopkins Hosp.,* 21:127.
10. Crowe, S. J., Cushing, H., and Homans, J. (1908): Effects of hypophyseal transplantation following hypophysectomy in the canine. *Q. J. Exp. Physiol.,* 1:121.
11. Smith, P. E. (1930): Hypophysectomy and a replacement therapy. *Am. J. Anat.,* 45:205.
12. Dandy, W. E. (1913): The nerve supply to the pituitary body. *Am. J. Anat.,* 15:333.
13. Cushing, H., and Goetsch, E. (1910): Concerning the secretion of the infundibular lobe of the pituitary body and its presence in the cerebrospinal fluid. *Am. J. Physiol.,* 27:60.
14. Goetsch, E., Cushing, H., and Jacobson, C. (1911): Carbohydrate tolerance and the posterior lobe of the hypophysis cerebri. An experimental and clinical study. *Bull. Johns Hopkins Hosp.,* 22:165.
15. Weed, L. H., Cushing, H., and Jacobson, C. (1913): Further studies on the role of the hypophysis in the metabolism of carbohydrates. The autonomic control of the pituitary gland. *Johns Hopkins Hosp. Bull.,* 24:40.
16. Oliver, G., and Schafer, E. A. (1895): On the physiological action of extracts of pituitary body and certain other glandular organs. *J. Physiol.,* 18:277.
17. Howell, W. H. (1898): The physiologic effects of extracts of the hypophysis cerebri and infundibular body. *J. Exp. Med.,* 3:254.
18. Dale, H. H. (1909): The action of extracts of the pituitary body. *Biochem. J.* 4:427.
19. Popa, G., and Fielding, U. (1931): A portal circulation from the pituitary to the hypothalamic region. *J. Anat.,* 65:88.
20. Popa, G., and Fielding, U. (1930): The vascular link between the pituitary and the hypothalamus. *Lancet,* 2:238.
21. Harris, G. W. (1948): Neural control of the pituitary gland. *Physiol. Rev.,* 28:139.
22. Cushing, H. (1933): Posterior pituitary activity from an anatomical standpoint. *Am. J. Pathol.,* 9:539.
23. Gersh, I. (1938): Relation of histological structure to the active substances extracted from the posterior lobe of the hypophysis. *Res. Publ. Assoc. Res. Nerv. Ment. Dis.,* 17:433.
24. Gersh, I. (1939): The structure and function of the parenchymatous glandular cells in the neurohypophysis of the rat. *Am. J. Anat.,* 64:407.
25. Lewis, D., and Lee, F. C. (1927): On the glandular elements in the posterior lobe of the human hypophysis. *Bull. Johns Hopkins,* 41:241.
26. Rioch, D. (1938): Paths of secretion from the hypophysis. *Res. Publ. Assoc. Res. Nerv. Ment. Dis.,* XVII:151.
27. Bucy, P. C. (1930): The pars nervosa of the bovine hypophysis. *J. Comp. Neurol.,* 50:505.
28. Bucy, P. C. (1932): The hypophysis cerebri. In: *Cytology and Cellular Pathology of the Central Nervous System, Vol. 2,* edited by W. Penfield, p. 705. Hoeber, New York.
29. Wislocki, G. B., and King, L. S. (1936): The permeability of the hypophysis and hypothalamus to vital dyes, with a study of the hypophyseal vascular supply. *Am. J. Anat.,* 58:421.
30. Rioch, D., Wislocki, G., and O'Leary, J. (1940): A precis of preoptic, hypothalamic and hypophyseal terminology with atlas. *Res. Publ. Assoc. Res. Nerv. Ment. Dis.,* 20:3.
31. Starling, E. H., and Verney, E. B. (1924): The secretion of urine as studied on the isolated kidney. *Proc. R. Soc. Lond. (B),* 97:321.
32. Fisher, C., Ingram, W. R., Hare, W. K., and Ranson, S. W. (1935): The degeneration of the supraoptico-hypophyseal system in diabetes insipidus. *Anat. Rec.,* 63:29.
33. Fisher, C., Ingram, W. R., Ranson, S. W. (1935): The relation of the hypothalamo-hypophyseal system to diabetes insipidus. *Arch. Neurol. Psychiatry,* 34:124.
34. Ingram, W. R., Fisher, C., and Ranson, S. W. (1936): Experimental diabetes insipidus in the monkey. *Arch. Int. Med.,* 57:1067.
35. Scharrer, E., and Scharrer, B. (1940): Secretory cells within the hypothalamus. *Res. Publ. Assoc. Res. Nerv. Ment. Dis.,* 20:170.
36. Scharrer, B., and Scharrer, E. (1944): Neurosecretion VI. A comparison between the intercerebralis-cardiacum-allatum of the insects and the hypothalamohypophyseal system of the vertebrates. *Biol. Bull.,* 87:242.
37. Palay, S. L. (1945): Neurosecretion. VII. The preoptico-hypophysial pathway in fishes. *J. Comp. Neurol.,* 82:129.
38. Bargmann, W., and Hild, W. (1949): Uber die morphologie der neurosekretorischen verknupfung von hypothalamus und neurohypophyse. *Acta Anat.,* 8:264.
39. Bargmann, W., and Scharrer, E. (1951): The site of origin of the hormones of the posterior pituitary. *Am. Scientist,* 39:255.
40. Scharrer, E., and Scharrer, B. (1954): Hormones produced by neurosecretory cells. *Recent Prog. Horm. Res.,* 10:183.
41. Scharrer, E. (1965): The final common path in neuroendocrine integration. *Arch. Anat. Microsc.,* 54:359.
42. Scharrer, B. (1967): The neurosecretory neuron in neuroendocrine regulatory mechanisms. *Am. Zool.,* 7:161.
43. Pierce, J. G., and du Vignaud, V. (1950): Studies on high potency oxytotic materials from beef posterior pituitary lobes. *J. Biol. Chem.,* 186:77.
44. du Vignaud, V., Ressler, C., Swan, J. M., Roberts, W., Katsoyannis, P. G., and Gordon, S. (1953): The synthesis of an octapeptide amide with the hormonal activity of oxytocin. *J. Am. Chem. Soc.,* 75:4879.
45. Turner, R. A., Pierce, J. G., du Vignaud, V. (1951): The purification and the amino acid content of vasopressin preparations. *J. Biol. Chem.,* 191:21.
46. du Vignaud, V., Lawler, H. C., and Papenea, E. A. (1953): Enzymatic cleavage of glycinamide from vasopressin and a proposed structure for this pressor-antidiuretic hormone of the posterior pituitary. *J. Am. Chem. Soc.,* 75:4880.

47. du Vignaud, V., Gish, D., and Katsayannis, P. G. (1954): A synthetic preparation possessing biological properties associated with arginine vasopressin. *J. Am. Chem. Soc.*, 76:4751.
48. Van Dyke, H. B., Adamsons, K., Engel, S. L. (1955): Aspects of the biochemistry and physiology of the neurohypophyseal hormones. *Recent Prog. Horm. Res.*, XI:1.
49. Verney, E. B. (1947): The antidiuretic hormone and the factors which determine its release. *Proc. R. Soc. Lond. (B)*, 135:25.
50. Palay, S. L. (1955): An electron microscope study of the neurohypophysis in normal, hydrated, and dehydrated rats. *Anat. Rec.*, 121:348.
51. Palay, S. L. (1960): The fine structure of secretory neurons in the preoptic nucleus of the goldfish (*Carassius auratus*). *Anat. Rec.*, 138:417.
52. Sloper, J. C., Arnott, D. J., and King, B. C. (1960): Sulphur metabolism in the pituitary and hypothalamus of the rat: A study of radioisotope-uptake after the injection of ^{35}S *dl*-cysteine, methionine, and sodium sulphate. *J. Endocrinol.*, 20:9.
53. Sloper, J. C. (1972): The validity of current concepts of hypothalamo-neurohypophyseal neurosecretion. *Prog. Brain Res.*, 38:123.
54. Bargmann, W. (1966): Neurosecretion. *Int. Rev. Cytol.*, 19:183.
55. Norstrom, A., Hansson, H.-A., Sjostrand, J. (1971): Effects of colchicine on axonal transport and ultrastructure of the hypothalamo-neurohypophyseal system of the rat. *Z. Zellforsch.*, 113:271.
56. Lederis, K. (1974): Neurosecretion and the functional structure of the neurohypophysis. In: *Handbook of Physiology. Chapt. 4, Sec. 7: Endocrinology, Vol. IV. The Pituitary Gland and Its Neuroendocrine Control. Pt. 1*, edited by R. O. Greep and E. B. Astwood, p. 81. American Physiological Society, Washington, D.C.
57. Silverman, A. J., and Zimmerman, E. A. (1975): Ultrastructural immunocytochemical localization of neurophysin and vasopressin in the median eminence and posterior pituitary of the guinea pig. *Cell Tissue Res.*, 159:291.
58. Flament-Durand, J., Couck, A. M., and Dustin, P. (1975): Studies on the transport of secretory granules in the magnocellular hypothalamic neurons of the rat. II. Action of vincrestine on axonal flow and neurotubules in the paraventricular and supraoptic nuclei. *Cell Tissue Res.*, 164:1.
59. Vandersande, F., and Dierickx, K. (1975): Identification of the vasopressin-producing and of the oxytocin-producing neurons in the hypothalamic magnocellular neurosecretory system of the rat. *Cell Tissue Res.*, 164:153.
60. Weitzman, R. E., and Fisher, D. A. (1977): Log linear relationship between plasma arginine vasopressin and plasma osmolality. *Am. J. Physiol.*, 233:E37.
61. Gainer, H., Sarne, Y., and Brownstein, M. J. (1977): Biosynthesis and axonal transport of rat neurohypophysial proteins and peptides. *J. Cell Biol.*, 73:366.
62. Antunes, J. L., and Zimmerman, E. A. (1978): The hypothalamic magnocellular system of the rhesus monkey: An immunocytochemical study. *J. Comp. Neurol.*, 181:539.
63. Brownstein, M. J., Russell, J. T., and Gainer, H. (1980): Synthesis, transport, and release of posterior pituitary hormones. *Science*, 207:373.
64. Russell, J. T., Brownstein, M. J., and Gainer, H. (1980): Biosynthesis of vasopressin, oxytocin, and neurophysins: Isolation and characterization of two common precursors (propressophysin and prooxyphysin). *Endocrinology*, 107:1880.
65. Harris, G. W. (1937): The induction of ovulation in the rabbit by electrical stimulation of the hypothalamo-hypophyseal mechanism. *Proc. R. Soc. Lond. (B)*, 122:374.
66. Green, J. D. (1951): The comparative anatomy of the hypophysis, with special reference to its blood supply and innervation. *Am. J. Anat.*, 88:225.
67. Green, J. D., and Harris, G. W. (1947): The neurovascular link between the neurohypophysis and adenohypophysis. *J. Endocrinol.*, 5:136.
68. Green, J. D. (1948): The histology of the hypophyseal stalk and median eminence in man with special reference to blood vessels, nerve fibers and a peculiar neurovascular zone in this region. *Anat. Rec.*, 100:273.
69. Green, J. D. (1947): Vessels and nerves of amphibian hypophyses. *Anat. Rec.*, 99:21.
70. Green, J. D., and Harris, G. W. (1949): Observation of the hypophysio-portal vessels of the living rat. *J. Physiol.*, 108:359.
71. Harris, G. W. (1948): Electrical stimulation of the hypothalamus and the mechanism of neural control of the adenohypophysis. *J. Physiol.*, 107:418.
72. Harris, G. W. (1949): The relationship of the nervous system to (a) the neurohypophysis and (b) the adenohypophysis. *J. Endocrinol.*, 6:xvii.
73. Harris, G. W. (1950): Oestrous rhythm pseudopregnancy and the pituitary stalk in the rat. *J. Physiol. (Lond.)*, 111:347.
74. Harris, G. W., and Johnson, R. T. (1950): Regeneration of the hypophyseal portal vessels, after section of the hypophyseal stalk in the monkey (*Macacus rhesus*). *Nature*, 165:819.
75. Harris, G. W. (1949): Regeneration of the hypophysial portal vessels. *Nature*, 163:70.
76. Harris, G. W., and Jacobson, D. (1952): Functional grafts of the anterior pituitary gland. *Proc. R. Soc. Lond. (B)*, 139:263.
77. Harris, G. W. (1955): *Neural Control of the Pituitary Gland*. Edward Arnold, London.
78. Green, J. D. (1966): The comparative anatomy of the portal vascular system and of the innervation of the hypophysis. In: *The Pituitary Gland, Vol. 1*, edited by G. W. Harris and B. T. Donovan, Chapter 3, p. 27. University of California Press, Berkeley.
79. Wingstrand, K. G. (1966): Comparative anatomy and evaluation of the hypophysis. In: *The Pituitary Gland, Vol. 1*, edited by G. W. Harris and B. T. Donovan, Chapter 2, p. 58. University of California Press, Berkeley.
80. Jorgensen, C. B., and Larsen, L. O. (1967): Neuroendocrine mechanisms in lower vertebrates. In: *Neuroendocrinology, Vol. II*, edited by L. Martini and W. F. Ganong, p. 485. Academic Press, New York.
81. Xuereb, G. P., Prichard, M., and Daniel, P. M. (1954): The arterial supply and venous drainage of the human hypophysis cerebri. *Am. J. Exp. Physiol.*, 39:199.
82. Xuereb, G. P., Prichard, M. M., and Daniel, P. M. (1954): The hypophysial portal system of vessels in man. *Q. J. Exp. Physiol.*, 39:219.
83. Daniel, P. M. (1966): The blood supply of the hypothalamus and pituitary gland. *Br. Med. Bull.*, 22:202.
84. Harris, G. W. (1947): The blood vessels of the rabbit's pituitary gland, and the significance of the pars and zona tuberalis. *J. Anat.*, 81:343.
85. Page, R. B., Munger, B. L., and Bergland, R. M. (1976): Scanning microscopy of pituitary vascular casts: The rabbit pituitary portal system revisited. *Am. J. Anat.*, 146:273.
86. Wislocki, G. B. (1937): The vascular supply of the hypophysis cerebri of the cat. *Anat. Rec.*, 69:361.
87. Wislocki, G. B. (1938): Further observations on the blood supply of the hypophysis cerebri of the rhesus monkey. *Anat. Rec.*, 72:137.
88. Wislocki, G. B. (1938): The vascular supply of the hypophysis cerebri of the rhesus monkey and man. *Res. Publ. Assoc. Res. Nerv. Ment. Dis.*, 17:48.
89. Wislocki, G. B. (1938): Further observations on the blood supply of the hypophysis cerebri of the rhesus monkey. *Anat. Rec.*, 72:137.
90. Moll, J. (1957): Regeneration of the supraoptico-hypophyseal and paraventriculo-hypophyseal tracts in the hypophysectomized rat. *Z. Zellforsch.*, 46:686.
91. Moll, J., and DeWied, D. (1962): Observations on the hypothalamo-posthypophyseal system of the posterior lobectomized rat. *Gen. Comp. Endocrinol.*, 2:215.
92. Adams, J. H., Daniel, P. M., and Prichard, M. M. (1969): Degeneration and regeneration of hypothalamic nerve fibers in the neurohypophysis after pituitary stalk section in the ferret. *J. Comp. Neurol.*, 135:121.
93. Daniel, P. M., and Prichard, M. M. (1970): Regeneration of hypothalamic nerve fibers after hypophysectomy in the goat. *Acta Endocrinol.*, 64:696.
94. Raisman, G. (1973): Electron microscopic studies of the development of new neurohemal contacts in the median eminence of the rat after hypophysectomy. *Brain Res.*, 55:245.
95. Daniel, P. M., and Prichard, M. M. (1958): The effects of pituitary stalk section in the goat. *Am. J. Pathol.*, 34:433.
96. Daniel, R. M., Duchen, L. W., and Prichard, M. M. (1964): The effect of transection of the pituitary stalk on the cytology of the pituitary gland of the rat. *Q. J. Exp. Physiol.*, 49:235.

97. Adams, J. H., Daniel, P. M., and Prichard, M. M. (1969): The blood supply of the pituitary gland of the ferret with special reference to infarction after stalk section. *J. Anat.*, 104:209.
98. Daniel, P. M., and Prichard, M. M. (1972): The human hypothalamus and pituitary stalk after hypophysectomy or pituitary stalk section. *Brain*, 95:813.
99. Daniel, P. M., and Prichard, M. M. (1975): Studies of the hypothalamus and the pituitary gland. With special reference to the effects of transection of the pituitary stalk. *Acta Endocrinol.*, 80(Suppl. 201):1.
100. Nikitovitch-Winer, M., and Everett, J. W. (1959): Histologic changes in grafts of rat pituitary on the kidney and upon re-transplantation under the diencephalon. *Endocrinology*, 65:357.
101. Nikitovitch-Winer, M., and Everett, J. W. (1958): Functional restitution of pituitary grafts retransplanted from kidney to median eminence. *Endocrinology*, 63:916.
102. Halasz, B., and Pupp, L. (1965): Hormone secretion of the anterior pituitary gland after physical interruption of all nervous pathways to the hypophysiotropic area. *Endocrinology* 77:553.
103. Szentagothai, J., Flerko, B., Mess, B., and Halasz, B. (1968): *Hypothalamic Control of Anterior Pituitary Function*. Akademiai Kiado, Budapest.
104. Halasz, B., and Gorski, R. A. (1967): Gonadotropic hormone secretion in female rats after partial or total interruption of neural afferents to the medial basal hypothalamus. *Endocrinology*, 80:608.
105. Halasz, B., Slusher, M., and Gorski, R. A. (1967): Adrenocorticotropic hormone secretion in rats after partial or total deafferentation of the medial basal hypothalamus. *Neuroendocrinology*, 2:43.
106. Halasz, B., Florsheim, W. H., Cocorran, N. L., and Gorski, R. A. (1967): Thyrotrophic hormone secretion after partial or total interruption of neural afferents to the medial basal hypothalamus. *Endocrinology*, 80:1075.
107. Halasz, B. (1969): The endocrine effects of isolation of the hypothalamus from the rest of the brain. In: *Frontiers of Neuroendocrinology*, p. 307. Oxford University Press, New York.
108. Halasz, B. (1973): Neural control of pituitary ACTH secretion under resting conditions. *Acta Med.*, 29:71.
109. Guillemin, R. (1964): Hypothalamic factors releasing pituitary hormones. *Recent Prog. Horm. Res.*, 20:89.
110. Schally, A. V., Arimura, A., Bowers, C. Y., Kastin, A. J., Sawano, S., and Redding, T. W. (1968): Hypothalamic neurohormones regulating anterior pituitary function. *Recent Prog. Horm. Res.*, 24:497.
111. Saffran, M., and Schally, A. V. (1955): Release of corticotropin by anterior pituitary tissue *in vitro*. *Can. J. Biochem. Physiol.*, 33:408.
112. Guillemin, R. (1955): Hypothalamic control of anterior pituitary study with tissue cultures techniques. *Fed. Proc.*, 14:65.
113. Guillemin, R., and Rosenberg, B. (1955): Humoral hypothalamic control of anterior pituitary: A study with combined tissue cultures. *Endocrinology*, 57:599.
114. Guillemin, R., Hearn, W. R., Cheek, W. R., and Housholder, D. E. (1957): Control of corticotropin release: Further studies with *in vitro* methods. *Endocrinology*, 60:488.
115. Schreiber, V., Rybak, M., Eckertova, A., Jirgl, V., Koci, J., Franc, Z., and Kmentova, V. (1962): Isolation of a hypothalamic peptide with TRF (thyrotrophin releasing factor) activity *in vitro*. *Experientia*, 18:338.
116. Deuben, R. R., and Meites, J. (1964): Stimulation of pituitary growth hormone release by a hypothalamic extract "*in vitro*." *Endocrinology*, 74:408.
117. Schally, A. V., and Bowers, C. Y. (1964): *In vitro* and *in vivo* stimulation of the release of luteinizing hormone. *Endocrinology*, 75:312.
118. Gala, R. R., Reece, R. P. (1965): *In vitro* lactogen production by anterior pituitaries from various species. *Proc. Soc. Exp. Biol. Med.*, 120:263.
119. Meites, J., Kahn, R. H., and Nicoll, C. S. (1961): Prolactin production by rat pituitary *in vitro*. *Proc. Soc. Exp. Biol. Med.*, 108:440.
120. Pastels, J. L. (1962): Administration d'extraits hypothalamiques à l'hypophyse de rat *in vitro*, dans le but d'en controler la secretion du prolactaire. *C. R. Acad. Sci. (III)*, 254:2664.
121. Talwaker, P. K., Ratner, A., and Meites, J. (1963): *In vitro* inhibition of pituitary prolactin synthesis and release by hypothalamic extract. *Am. J. Physiol.*, 205:213.
122. Porter, J. C., and Jones, J. C. (1956): Effect of plasma from hypophyseal-portal vessel blood on adrenal-ascorbic acid. *Endocrinology*, 58:62.
123. Porter, J. C., Dhariwal, A. P. S., and McCann, S. M. (1967): Response of the anterior pituitary—Adrenocortical axis to purified CRF. *Endocrinology*, 80:679.
124. Guillemin, A., Yamazaki, E., Jutisz, M., and Sakig, E. (1962): Presence dans un extrait de tissus hypothalamiques d'une substance stimulant le secretion de l'hormone hypophysaire threotrope 1962. *C. R. Acad. Sci. (III)*, 255:1018.
125. Garcia, J. F., and Geschwind, I. (1966): Increase in plasma growth hormone levels in the monkey following the administration of sheep hypothalamic extracts. *Nature*, 211:372.
126. Dhariwal, A. P. S., Nallar, R., Batt, M., and McCann, S. M. (1965): Separation of follicle stimulating hormone-releasing factor from luteinizing hormone releasing factors. *Endocrinology*, 76:290.
127. Igarashi, M., and McCann, S. M. (1964): A hypothalamic follicle stimulating hormone-releasing factor. *Endocrinology*, 74:446.
128. McCann, S. M., Taleisnik, S., and Friedman, H. M. (1960): LH-releasing activity in hypothalamic extracts. *Proc. Soc. Exp. Biol. Med.*, 104:432.
129. McCann, S. M. (1962): A hypothalamic leuteinizing-hormone-releasing factor. *Am. J. Physiol.*, 202:395.
130. Porter, J. C., Mical, R. S., Kamberi, I. A., and Grazia, Y. R. (1970): A procedure for the cannulation of a pituitary stalk portal vessel and perfusion of the pars distalis in the rat. *Endocrinology*, 87:197.
131. Porter, J. C., Mical, R. S., Ondo, J. G., and Kamberi, I. A. (1972): Perfusion of the rat anterior pituitary via a cannulated portal vessel. *Acta Endocrinol. (Suppl.)*, 158:249.
132. Kamberi, I., Mical, R., and Porter, J. C. (1971): Pituitary portal infusion of hypothalamic extract and release of LH, FSH and prolactin. *Endocrinology*, 88:1294.
133. Kamberi, I. A., Mical, R. S., and Porter, J. C. (1971): Hypophysial portal vessel infusion: *In vivo* demonstration of LRF, FRF, and PIF in pituitary stalk plasma. *Endocrinology*, 89:1042.
134. Averill, R. L. W., and Kennedy, T. H. (1967): Elevation of thyrotropin release by intrapituitary infusion of crude hypothalamic extracts. *Endocrinology*, 81:113.
135. Fink, G., Nallar, R., and Worthington, W. C. (1967): The demonstration of luteinizing hormone releasing factor in hypophyseal portal blood of pro-estrus and hypophysectomized rats. *J. Physiol. (Lond.)*, 191:407.
136. Wilber, J., and Porter, J. C. (1970): Thyrotropin and growth hormone releasing activity in hypophyseal portal blood. *Endocrinology*, 87:807.
137. Boler, J., Enzmann, F., and Folkers, K. (1969): The identity of chemical and hormonal properties of the thyrotropin releasing hormone and pyroglutamyl-histidylproline amide. *Biochem. Biophys. Res. Commun.*, 37:705.
138. Burgus, R., Dunn, T. F., Desiderio, D. M., Ward, D. N., Vale, W., and Guillemin, R. (1970): Characterization of ovine hypothalamic hypophysiotropic TSH releasing factor. *Nature*, 226:321.
139. Burgus, R., Dunn, T. F., Desiderio, D. M., Ward, D. N., Vale, W., Guillemin, R., Felix, A. M., Gillessen, D., and Stader, R. O. (1970): Biological activity of synthetic polypeptide derivatives related to the structure of hypothalamic TRF. *Endocrinology*, 86:573.
140. Porter, J. C., Vale, W., Burgus, R., Mical, R. S., and Guillemin, R. (1971): Release of TSH by TRF infused directly into a pituitary stalk portal vessel. *Endocrinology*, 89:1054.
141. Arimura, A., Matsuo, H., Baba, Y., Debeljuk, L., Sandow, J., and Schally, A. V. (1972): Stimulation of release of LH by synthetic LH-RH *in vivo*. I. A comparative study of natural and synthetic hormones. *Endocrinology*, 90:163.
142. Geiger, R., Konig, W., Wissmann, H., Geisen, K., and Enzmann, F. (1971): Synthesis and characterization of a decapeptide having LH-RH/FSH-RH activity. *Biochem. Biophys. Res. Commun.*, 45:767.
143. Schally, A. V., Arimura, A., Baba, Y., Nair, R. M. G., Matsuo, H., Redding, T. W., Debeljuk, L., and White, W. F. (1971): Isolation and properties of FSH and LH releasing hormone. *Biochem. Biophys. Res. Commun.*, 43:393.
144. Spiess, J., Rivier, J., Rivier, C., and Vale, W. (1981): Primary structure of corticotropin-releasing factor from ovine hypothalamus. *Proc. Natl. Acad. Sci. USA*, 78:5617.
145. Vale, W., Spiess, J., Rivier, C., and Rivier, J. (1981): Characterization of a 41-residue ovine hypothalamic peptide that stimulates secretion of corticotropin and β-endorphin. *Science*, 213:1394.
146. Brazeau, P., Vale, W., Burgus, R., Ling, N., Butcher, M., Rivier, J., and Guillemin, R. (1973): Hypothalamic polypeptide that inhibits

the secretion of immunoreactive pituitary growth hormone. *Science,* 179:77.
147. Rivier, J., Spiess, J., Thorner, M., and Vale, W. (1982): Characterization of a growth hormone-releasing factor from a human pancreatic islet tumor. *Nature,* 300:276.
148. Thorner, M. O., Spiess, J., Vance, M. L., Rogol, A. D., Kaiser, D. L., Webster, J. D., Rivier, J., Borges, J. L., Bloom, S. R., Cronin, M. J., Evans, W. S., MacLeod, R. M., and Vale, W. (1983): Human pancreatic growth-hormone-releasing factor selectively stimulates growth-hormone secretion in man. *Lancet,* 1:24–28.
149. Spiess, J., Rivier, J., and Vale, W. (1983): Characterization of rat hypothalamic growth hormone-releasing factor. *Nature,* 303:532.
150. Wehrenberg, W. B., and Ling, N. (1983): *In vivo* biological potency of rat and human growth hormone-releasing factor and fragments of human growth hormone releasing factor. *Biochem. Biophys. Res. Commun.,* 115:525.
151. Shaar, C. J., and Clemens, J. H. (1974): The role of catecholamines in the release of anterior pituitary prolactin *in vitro. Endocrinology,* 95:1202.
152. Neill, J. D., Patton, J. M., Dailey, R. A., Tsou, R. C., and Tindall, G. T. (1977): Luteinizing hormone releasing hormone (LHRH) in pituitary stalk blood of rhesus monkeys: Relationship to level of LH release. *Endocrinology,* 101:430.
153. Gibbs, D. M., and Neill, J. D. (1978): Dopamine levels in hypophyseal stalk blood are sufficient to inhibit prolactin secretion *in vivo. Endocrinology,* 102(6):1895.
154. Pilotte, N. S., Gudelsky, G. A., and Porter, J. C. (1980): Relationship of prolactin secretion to dopamine release into hypophyseal portal blood and dopamine turnover in the median eminence. *Brain Res.,* 193:284.
155. Gudelsky, G. A., and Porter, J. C. (1980): Release of dopamine from tubero-infundibular neurons into pituitary stalk blood after prolactin or haloperidol administration. *Endocrinology,* 106:526.
156. Selmanoff, M. (1981): The lateral and medial median eminence: Distribution of dopamine, norepinephrine, and luteinizing hormone-releasing hormone and the effect of prolactin on catecholamine turnover. *Endocrinology,* 108:1716.
157. Foord, S. M., Peters, J. R., Dieguez, C., Scanlon, M. F., and Hall, R. (1983): Dopamine receptors on intact anterior pituitary cells in culture: Functional association with the inhibition of prolactin and thyrotropin. *Endocrinology,* 112:1567.
158. Frawley, L. S., and Neill, J. D. (1984): Brief decreases in dopamine result in surges of prolactin secretion in monkeys. *Am. J. Physiol.,* 247:E778.
159. Nakane, P. K., and Pierce, G. B. (1967): Enzyme-labeled antibodies for the light and electron microscopic localization of tissue antigens. *J. Cell Biol.,* 33:307.
160. Sternberger, L. (1979): *Immunocytochemistry.* John Wiley & Sons, New York.
161. Hokfelt, T., Elde, R., Fuxe, K., Johansson, O., Ljungdahl, A., Goldstein, M., Luft, R., Efendic, S., Nilsson, G., Terenius, L., Ganten, D., Jeffcoate, S. L., Rehfeld, J., Said, S., Perez de la Mora, M., Possani, L., Rapia, R., Teran, L., and Palacios, R. (1978): Aminergic and peptidergic pathways in the nervous system with special reference to the hypothalamus. In: *The Hypothalamus,* edited by S. Reichlin, R. J. Baldessarini, and J. B. Martin, p. 69. Raven Press, New York.
162. Fink, G., and Geffen, L. B. (1978): The hypothalamo-hypophysial system: Model for central peptidergic and monoaminergic transmission. *Int. Rev. Physiol.,* 17:1.
163. Naik, D. V. (1975): Immunoreactive LH-RH neurons in the hypothalamus identified by light and fluorescent microscopy. *Cell Tissue Res.,* 157:423.
164. Naik, D. V. (1975): Immunoelectron microscopic localization of luteinizing hormone-releasing hormone in the arcuate nuclei and median eminence of the rat. *Cell Tissue Res.,* 157:437.
165. Styne, D. M., Goldsmith, P. C., Brustein, S. R., Kaplan, S. L., and Grumbach, M. M. (1977): Immunoreactive somatostatin and luteinizing hormone releasing hormone in median eminence synaptosomes of the rat: Detection by immunohistochemistry and quantification by radioimmunoassay. *Endocrinology,* 101:1099.
166. Barry, J., Dubois, M. P., and Poulain, P. (1973): LRF producing cells of the mammalian hypothalamus. A fluorescent antibody study. *Z. Zellforsch.,* 146:351.
167. Barry, J., Dubois, M. P., Poulain, P., and Leonardelli, J. (1973): Neuroendocrinologie—Caracterisation et topographic des neurones hypothalamiques immunoreactifs avec des anticorps anti-LRH de synthese. *C. R. Acad. Sci. Ser. D,* 276:3191.
168. Hymer, W. C., and McShan, W. H. (1962): Isolation of cytoplasmic pituitary granules by column chromatography. *J. Cell Biol.,* 13:350.
169. Hymer, W. C., and McShan, W. H. (1963): Isolation of rat pituitary granules and the study on their biological properties and hormonal activities. *J. Cell Biol.,* 17:67.
170. Hymer, W. C. (1975): Separation of organelles and cells from the mammalian adenohypophysis. In: *The Anterior Pituitary. Ultrastructure in Biological Systems, Vol. 7,* edited by A. Tixier-Vidal and M. G. Farquhar, p. 137. Academic Press, New York.
171. Farquhar, M. G., and Palade, G. E. (1981): The golgi apparatus (complex)—1954–1981—From artifact to center stage. *J. Cell Biol.,* 91:77s.
172. Palade, G. (1975): Intracellular aspects of the process of protein synthesis. *Science,* 189:347.
173. Farquhar, M. G., and Wellings, S. R. (1957): Electron microscopic evidence suggesting secretory granule formation within the Golgi apparatus. *J. Biophys. Biochem. Cytol.,* 3:319.
174. Farquhar, M. G. (1961): Origin and fate of secretory granules in cells of the anterior pituitary gland. *Trans. NY Acad. Sci.,* 23:346.
175. Racadot, J., Olivier, L., Porcile, E., and Droz, B. (1965): Appareil de golgi et origine des graines de secretion dans les cellules adenohypophysaires chez le rat. Etude radioautographique en microscopie electronique après injection de leucine tritiée. *C. R. Acad. Sci. (Paris),* 261:2972.
176. Tixier-Vidal, A., and Picart, R. (1967): Etude quantitative par radioautographie au microscope electronique de l'utilisation de la DL-leucine-^{3}H par les cellules de l'hypophyse du canard en culture organotypique. *J. Cell Biol.,* 35:501.
177. Howell, S. L., and Whitfield, M. (1973): Synthesis and secretion of growth hormone in the rat anterior pituitary. I. The intracellular pathway, its time course and energy requirements. *J. Cell Sci.,* 12:1.
178. Farquhar, M. G., Reid, J. J., and Daniell, L. W. (1978): Intracellular transport and packaging of prolactin: A quantitative electron microscope autoradiographic study of mammotrophs dissociated from rat pituitaries. *Endocrinology,* 102:296.
179. Farquhar, M. G. (1971): Processing of secretory products by cells of the anterior pituitary cell. *Mem. Soc. Endocrinol.,* 19:79.
180. Farquhar, M. G. (1978): Recovery of surface membrane in anterior pituitary cells. *J. Cell Biol.,* 77:R35.
181. Ishimura, K., Egawa, K., and Fujita, H. (1980): Freeze-fracture images of exocytosis and endocytosis in anterior pituitary cells of rabbits and mice. *Cell Tissue Res.,* 206:233.
182. Farquhar, M. G. (1985): Membrane tissue in prolactin and other secretory cells. In: *Prolactin, Basic and Clinical Correlates,* edited by R. M. MacLeod, M. O. Thorner, and U. Scapagnini, *Fidia Research Series, Vol. 1,* p. 3. Liviana Press, Padova.
183. Nikitovitch-Winer, M. B., Yu, S. M., and Papka, R. E. (1985): Soluble prolactin may be directly released from cellular compartments other than secretory granules. In: *Prolactin, Basic and Clinical Correlates,* edited by R. M. MacLeod, M. O. Thorner, and U. Scapagini, *Fidia Research Series, Vol. 1,* p. 17. Liviana Press, Padova.
184. Blobel, G., and Dobberstein, B. (1975): Transfer of proteins across membranes. *J. Cell Biol.,* 67:835.
185. Lingappa, V. R., Devillers-Thiery, A., and Blobel, G. (1977): Nascent prehormones are intermediates in the biosynthesis of authentic bovine pituitary growth hormone and prolactin. *Proc. Natl. Acad. Sci. USA,* 74:2432.
186. Rosenzweig, L. J., and Farquhar, M. G. (1980): Sites of sulfate incorporation into mammotrophs and somatotrophs of the rat pituitary as determined by quantitative electron microscopic autoradiography. *Endocrinology,* 107:422.
187. Watanabe, H., Orth, D. N., and Toft, D. O. (1973): Glucocorticoid receptors in pituitary tumor cells. *J. Biol. Chem.,* 248:7625.
188. Watanabe, H., Orth, D. N., and Toft, D. O. (1974): Glucocorticoid receptors in mouse pituitary tumor cells. II. Nuclear binding. *Biochemistry,* 13:332.
189. Nakanishi, S., Kita, T., Tah, S., Imura, H., and Numa, S. (1977): Glucocorticoid effect on the level of corticotropin messenger RNA activity in rat pituitary. *Proc. Natl. Acad. Sci. USA,* 74:3283.
190. Birnberg, N. C., Lissitzky, J.-C., Hinman, M., and Herbert, E. (1983): Glucocorticoids regulate proopiomelanocortin gene expres-

sion *in vivo* at the levels of transcription and secretion. *Proc. Natl. Acad. Sci. USA,* 80:6982.

191. Vermes, I., Mulder, G. H., Smelik, P. G., and Tilders, F. J. H. (1980): Differential control of β-endorphin/β-lipotropin secretion from anterior and intermediate lobes of the rat pituitary gland *in vitro*. *Life Sci.,* 27:1761.
192. Tilders, F. J. H., Post, M., Jackson, S., Lowry, P. J., and Smelik, P. G. (1981): Beta-adrenergic stimulation of the release of ACTH- and LPH-related peptides from the pars intermedia of the rat pituitary gland. *Acta Endocrinol.,* 97:343.
193. Gibbs, D. M., Stewart, R. D., Liu, J. H., Vale, W., Rivier, J., and Yen, S. S. C. (1982): Effects of synthetic corticotropin-releasing factor and dopamine on the release of immunoreactive β-endorphin/β-lipotropin and α-melanocyte-stimulating hormone from human fetal pituitaries *in vitro*. *J. Clin. Endocrinol. Metab.,* 55:1149.
194. Meunier, H., and Labrie, F. (1982): The dopamine receptor in the intermediate lobe of the rat pituitary gland is negatively coupled to adenylate cyclase. *Life Sci.,* 30:963.
195. Cote, T., Munemura, M., Eskay, R. L., and Kebabian, J. W. (1980): Biochemical identification of the β-adrenoceptor and evidence for the involvement of an adenoside 3′,5′-monophosphate system in the β′-adrenergically induced release of α-melanocyte-stimulating hormone in the intermediate lobe of the rat pituitary gland. *Endocrinology,* 107:108.
196. Nansel, D. D., Gudelsky, G. A., and Porter, J. C. (1979): Subcellular localization of dopamine in the anterior pituitary gland of the rat: Apparent association of dopamine with prolactin secretory granules. *Endocrinology,* 105:1073.
197. Rosenzweig, L. J., and Kanwar, Y. S. (1982): Dopamine internalization by and intracellular distribution within prolactin cells and somatotrophs of the rat anterior pituitary as determined by quantitative electron microscopic autoradiography. *Endocrinology,* 111:1817.
198. Schettini, G., Cronin, M. J., and MacLeod, R. M. (1983): Adenosine 3′,5′-monophosphate (cAMP) and calcium-calmodulin interrelation in the control of prolactin secretion: Evidence for dopamine inhibition of cAMP accumulation and prolactin release after calcium immobilization. *Endocrinology,* 112:1801.
199. Couch, E. F., Arimura, A., Schally, A. V., Saito, M., and Sawano, S. (1969): Electron microscope studies of somatotrophs of rat pituitary after injection of purified growth hormone releasing hormone factor (GRF). *Endocrinology,* 85:1084.
200. Coates, P. W., Ashby, E. A., Krulich, L., Dhariwal, A. P. S., McCann, S. M. (1970): Morphologic alterations in somatotrophs of the rat adenohypophysis following administration of hypothalamic extracts. *Am. J. Anat.,* 128:389.
201. Shiino, M., Arimura, A., Schally, A. V., and Rennels, E. G. (1972): Ultrastructural observations of granule extrusion from rat anterior pituitary cells after injection of LH-releasing hormone. *Z. Zellforsch.,* 128:152.
202. Stratmann, I. E., Ezrin, C., Kovacs, K., and Sellers, E. A. (1973): Effect of TRH on the fine structure and replication of TSH and prolactin cells in the rat. *Z. Zellforsch.,* 145:23.
203. Westlund, K. N., Aguilera, G., and Childs, G. V. (1985): Quantification of morphological changes in pituitary corticotropes produced by *in vivo* corticotropin-releasing factor stimulation and adrenalectomy. *Endocrinology* 116:439.
204. Posner, B. I., Bergeron, J. J. M., Jofesberg, Z., Kahn, M. N., Kahn, R. J., Patel, B. A. Sikstrom, R. A., and Verma, A. K. (1981): Polypeptide hormones: Intracellular receptors and internalization. *Recent Prog. Horm. Res.,* 37:539.
205. Samli, M. H., Geschwind, I. I. (1968): Some effects of energy transfer inhibitors and of Ca^{++}-free or K^{+} enhanced media on the release of luteinizing hormone (LH) from rat anterior pituitaries *in vitro*. *Endocrinology,* 82:225.
206. Parsons, J. A. (1969): Calcium ion requirement for prolactin secretion by rat adenohypophyses *in vitro*. *Am. J. Physiol.,* 217:1599.
207. Giguere, V., and Labrie, F. (1982): Vasopressin potentiates cyclic AMP accumulation and ACTH release induced by corticotropin-releasing factor (CRF) in rat anterior pituitary cells in culture. *Endocrinology,* 111:1752.
208. Sutton, C. A., and Martin, T. F. J. (1982): Thyrotropin-releasing hormone (TRH) selectively and rapidly stimulates phosphatidylinositol turnover in GH pituitary cells: A possible second step of TRH action. *Endocrinology,* 110:1273.
209. Labrie, F., Veilleux, R., Lefevre, G., Coy, D. H., Sueiras-Diaz, J., and Schally, A. V. (1982): Corticotropin-releasing factor stimulates accumulation of adenosine 3′,5′-monophosphate in rat pituitary corticotrophs. *Science,* 216:1007.
210. MacLeod, R. M., Judd, A. M., Koike, K., Canonico, P. L., and Login, I. S. (1984): The role of phospholipid hydrolysis in the release of prolactin from anterior pituitary cells. In: *Endocrinology,* edited by F. Labrie and L. Proulx, *International Congress Series No. 655,* p. 195. Excerpta Medica/Elsevier, New York.
211. Murakami, K., Hashimoto, K., and Ota, Z. (1985): Calmodulin inhibitors decrease the CRF- and AVP-induced ACTH release *in vitro:* Interaction of calcium-calmodulin and the cyclic AMP system. *Neuroendocrinology,* 41:7.
212. Catt, K. J., Loumaye, E., Synn, P., Suarez-Wuian, C., Kiesel, L., Iwashita, M., Hirota, K., Morgan, R., and Chang, J. (1984): Receptor-mediated activation mechanisms in the hypothalamic control of pituitary-gonadal function. In: *Endocrinology,* edited by F. Labrie and L. Proulx, p. 57. Excerpta Medica, New York.
213. Atwell, W. J. (1926): The development of the hypophysis cerebri in man, with special reference to the pars tuberalis. *Am. J. Anat.,* 37:159.
214. Tilney, F. (1938): The glands of the brain with especial reference to the pituitary gland. *Res. Publ. Assoc. Res. Nerv. Ment. Dis.,* 17:3.
215. Takor, T. T., and Pearse, A. G. E. (1975): Neuroectodermal origin of avian hypothalamo-hypophyseal complex: The role of the ventral neural ridge. *J. Embryol. Exp. Morphol.,* 34:311.
216. Trojanowski, J. Q., Gordon, D., Obrocka, M., and Lee, V. M. Y. (1984): The developmental expression of neurofilament and glial filament proteins in the human pituitary gland: An immunohistochemical study with monoclonal antibodies. *Dev. Brain Res.,* 13:229.
217. Farner, D. S., Wilson, F. E., and Oksche, A. (1967): Neuroendocrine mechanisms in birds. In: *Neuroendocrinology, Vol. II,* edited by L. Martini and W. F. Ganong, Chapter 30, p. 529. Academic Press, New York.
218. Dempsey, E. W., and Wislocki, G. B. (1955): An electron microscopic study of the blood-brain barrier in the rat, employing silver nitrate as a vital stain. *J. Biophys. Biochem. Cytol.,* 1:245.
219. Farquhar, M. G. (1961): Fine structure and function in capillaries of the anterior pituitary gland. *Angiology,* 12:270.
220. Fletcher, W. H., Anderson, N. C., and Everett, J. W. (1975): Intercellular communication in the rat anterior pituitary gland. *J. Cell Biol.,* 67:469.
221. Herbert, D. C. (1979): Intercellular junctions in the rhesus monkey pars distalis. *Anat. Rec.,* 195:1.
222. Denef, C., and Andries, M. (1983): Evidence for paracrine interaction between gonadotrophs and lactotrophs in pituitary cell aggregates. *Endocrinology,* 112:813.
223. Pierce, J. G., and Parsons, T. F. (1981): Glycoprotein hormones: Structure and function. *Annu. Rev. Biochem.,* 50:465.
224. Shome, B., and Parlow, A. F. (1977): Human pituitary prolactin (hPRL): The entire linear amino acid sequence. *J. Clin. Endocrinol. Metab.,* 45:1112.
225. Li, C. H., Dixon, J. S., Lo, T.-B., Pankov, Y. A., and Schmidt, K. D. (1969): Amino-acid sequence of ovine lactogenic hormone. *Nature,* 224:695.
226. Li, C. H., Dixon, J. S., Lo, T.-B., Schmidt, K. D., and Pankov, Y. A. (1970): Studies on pituitary lactogenic hormone. XXX. The primary structure of the sheep hormone. *Arch. Biochem. Biophys.,* 141:705.
227. Li, C. H. (1976): Studies on pituitary lactogenic hormone. The primary structure of the porcine hormone. *Int. J. Pept. Protein Res.,* 8:205.
228. Wallis, M. (1974): The primary structure of bovine prolactin. *FEBS Lett.,* 44:205.
229. Li, C. H., Hayashida, T., Doneen, B. A., and Rao, A. J. (1976): Human somatotropin: Biological characterization of the recombinant molecule. *Proc. Natl. Acad. Sci. USA,* 73:3463.
230. Lewis, U. J., Singh, R. N. P., Tutwiler, G. F., Sigel, M. B., VanderLaan, E. F., and VanderLaan, W. P. (1980): Human growth hormone: A complex of proteins. *Recent Prog. Horm. Res.,* 36:377.
231. Howard, K. S., Shepherd, R. G., Eigner, E. A., Davies, D. S., and Bell, P. H. (1955): Structure of β-corticotropin: Final sequence. *J. Am. Chem. Soc.,* 77:3419.

232. Li, C. H., Geschwind, I. I., Cole, R. D., Raacke, I. D., Harris, J. I., and Dixon, J. S. (1955): Amino-acid sequence of alpha-corticotropin. *Nature,* 176:687.
233. Li, C. H. (1959): Proposed system of terminology for preparations of adrenocorticotropic hormone. *Science,* 129:969.
234. Harris, J. I., and Roos, P. (1956): Amino-acid sequence of a melanophore stimulating hormone. *Nature,* 178:90.
235. Harris, J. I., and Roos, P. (1959): Studies on pituitary polypeptide hormones. 1. The structure of β-melanocyte-stimulating hormone from pig pituitary gland. *Biochem. J.,* 71:434.
236. Geschwind, I. I., Li, C. H., and Barnafi, L. (1956): Isolation and structure of melanocyte-stimulating hormone from porcine pituitary glands. *J. Am. Chem. Soc.,* 78:4494.
237. Harris, J. I., and Lerner, A. B. (1957): Amino-acid sequence of the α-melanocyte stimulating hormone. *Nature,* 179:1346.
238. Geschwind, I. I., and Li, C. H. (1957): The isolation and characterization of a melanocyte stimulating hormone (β-MSH) from hog pituitary glands. *J. Am. Chem. Soc.,* 79:615.
239. Geschwind, I. I., Li, C. H., and Barnafi, L. (1957): The structure of the β-melanocyte stimulating hormone. *J. Am. Chem. Soc.,* 79:620.
240. Li, C. H., and Chung, D. (1976): Isolation and structure of an untriakontapeptide with opiate activity from camel pituitary glands. *Proc. Natl. Acad. Sci. USA,* 73:1145.
241. Li, C. H., and Chung, D. (1976): Primary structure of human β-lipotropin. *Nature,* 260:622.
242. Li, C. H., Tan, L., and Chung, D. (1977): Isolation and primary structure of beta-endorphin and beta-lipotropin from bovine pituitary gland. *Biochem. Biophys. Res. Commun.,* 77:1088.
243. Teschemacher, H., Opheim, K. E., Cox, B. M., and Goldstein, A. (1975): A peptide-like substance that acts like morphine. 1. Isolation. *Life Sci.,* 16:1771.
244. Teschemacher, H., Opheim, K. E., Cox, B. M., and Goldstein, A. (1975): A peptide-like substance that acts like morphine. 2. Purification and properties. *Life Sci.,* 16:1777.
245. Pearse, A. G., and Van Noorden, S. (1963): The functional cytology of the human adenohypophysis. *Can. Med. Assoc. J.,* 88:462.
246. Nakane, P. K. (1968): Simultaneous localization of multiple tissue antigens using the peroxidase-labeled antibody method: A study on pituitary glands of the rat. *J. Histochem. Cytochem.,* 16:557.
247. Kurosumi, K. (1968): Functional classification of cell types of the anterior pituitary gland accomplished by electron microscopy. *Arch. Histol. Jpn.,* 29:329.
248. Pochet, R., Brocas, H., Vassart, G., Toubeau, G., Seo, H., Refetoff, S., Dumont, J. E., and Pasteels, J. L. (1981): Radioautographic localization of prolactin messenger RNA on histological sections by *in situ* hybridization. *Brain Res.,* 211:433.
249. Rasmussen, A. T. (1929): The percentage of the different types of cells in the male human hypophysis. *Am. J. Pathol.,* 5:263.
250. Rasmussen, A. T. (1933): The percentage of different types of cells in the anterior lobe of the hypophysis of the adult female. *Am. J. Pathol.,* 9:459.
251. Severinghaus, A. E. (1938): The cytology of the pituitary gland. *Res. Publ. Assoc. Res. Nerv. Ment. Dis.,* 17:69.
252. Severinghaus, A. E. (1939): Anterior hypophyseal cytology in relation to the reproductive hormones. In: *Sex and Internal Secretions,* edited by M. B. Allen, p. 1045. Wood & Co., New York.
253. Cushing, H. (1927): Acromegaly from a surgical standpoint. *Br. Med. J.,* 2:1.
254. Cushing, H., and Davidoff, L. (1927): The pathologic findings in four cases of acromegaly with a discussion of their significance. *Monogr. Rockefeller Inst. Med. Res.,* 22.
255. Cushing, H. (1932): The basophile adenomas of the pituitary body and their clinical manifestations. *Bull. Johns Hopkins Hosp.,* 50:137.
256. Romeis, B. (1940): Hypophyse. In: *Handbuch der Mikroskopischen Anatomie des Menschen,* edited by W. Van Mollendorff. Springer, Berlin.
257. Pearse, A. G. E. (1952): Observations on the localisation, nature and chemical constitution of some components of the anterior hypophysis. *J. Pathol. Bacteriol.,* 64:791.
258. Herlant, M. (1960): Etude critique de deux techniques nouvelles destinées à mettre en evidence les differentes categories cellulaires présent dans la glande pituitaire. *Bull. Microsc. Appl.,* 10:37.
259. Purves, H. D. (1966): Cytology of the adenohypophysis. In: *The Pituitary Gland, Vol. 1. Anterior Pituitary,* edited by G. W. Harris and B. T. Donovan, p. 147. University of California Press, Berkeley.
260. Smith, P. E., and Smith, I. P. (1923): The topographical separation in the bovine anterior hypophysis of the principle reacting with the endocrine system from that controlling general body growth, with suggestions as to the cell types elaborating these encrations. *Anat. Rec.,* 25:150.
261. Smith, P. E., and Smith, I. P. (1923): The response of the hypophysectomized tadpole to the intraperitoneal injection of the various lobes and colloid of the bovine hypophysis. *Anat. Rec.,* 25:150.
262. Baker, B. (1974): Functional cytology of the hypophyseal pars distalis and pars intermedia. In: *Handbook of Physiology, Vol. 7. The Pituitary Gland and Its Neuroendocrine Control, Part 1,* edited by E. Knobil and W. H. Sawyer, p. 45. Williams & Wilkins, Baltimore.
263. Purves, H. D., and Greisbach, W. E. (1952): Functional deafferentation in the acidophil cells and the gonadotropic basophil cells of the rat pituitary. *Proc. Univ. Otago Med. School,* 30:27 (cited in refs. 264 and 265).
264. Farquhar, M. G., and Rinehart, J. F. (1954): Electron microscope studies of the anterior pituitary gland of castrate rats. *Endocrinology,* 54:516.
265. Farquhar, M. G., and Rinehart, J. F. (1954): Cytologic alterations in the anterior pituitary gland following thyroidectomy: An electron microscope study. *Endocrinology,* 55:857.
266. Nakane, P. K. (1970): Classifications of anterior pituitary cell types with immunoenzyme histochemistry. *J. Histochem. Cytochem.,* 18:9.
267. Nakane, P. K. (1971): Application of peroxidase-labelled antibodies to the intracellular localization of hormones. *Acta Endocrinol. (Suppl.),* 153:190.
268. Moriarty, G. (1973): Adenohypophysis: ultrastructural cytochemistry. *J. Histochem. Cytochem.,* 21:855.
269. Phifer, R. F., and Spicer, S. S. (1973): Immunohistochemical and histologic demonstration of thyrotropic cells of the human adenohypophysis. *J. Clin. Endocrinol. Metab.,* 36:1210.
270. Girod, C., and Trouillas, J. (1980): Individualisation immunohistochimique des cellules thyreotropes antehypophysaires chez le Singe *Macacus irus,* à l'aide d'un anticorps anti-β-TSH humaine. *C. R. Acad. Sci. (Paris),* 291:261.
271. Baker, B. L., Pierce, J. G., and Cornell, J. S. (1972): The utility of antiserums to subunits of TSH and LH for immunochemical staining of the rat hypophysis. *Am. J. Anat.,* 135:251.
272. Moriarty, G. C., and Tobin, R. B. (1976): Ultrastructural immunocytochemical characterization of the thyrotroph in rat and human pituitaries. *J. Histochem. Cytochem.,* 24:1131.
273. Moriarty, G. C., and Tobin, R. B. (1976): An immunocytochemical study of TSH_B storage in rat thyroidectomy cells with and without D or L thyroxine treatment. *J. Histochem. Cytochem.,* 24:1140.
274. Kawarai, Y. (1980): Identification of ACTH cells and TSH cells in rat anterior pituitary with the unlabeled antibody enzyme method on adjacent thin and thick sections. *Acta Histochem. Cytochem.,* 13: 627.
275. Kurosumi, K., and Oota, Y. (1968): Electron microscopy of two types of gonadotrophs in the anterior pituitary gland of persistent estrous and diestrous rats. *Z. Zellforsch.,* 85:34.
276. Moriarty, G. C. (1975): Electron microscopic-immunocytochemical studies of rat pituitary gonadotrophs: A sex difference in morphology and cytochemistry of LH cells. *Endocrinology,* 97:1215.
277. Phifer, R. F., Midgley, A. R., and Spicer, S. S. (1973): Immunohistologic and histologic evidence that follicle-stimulating hormone and luteinizing hormone are present in the same cell type in the human pars distalis. *J. Clin. Endocrinol. Metab.,* 36:125.
278. Childs (Moriarty), G. V., Ellison, D. G., and Gardner, L. (1980): An immunocytochemist's view of gonadotropin storage in the adult male rat. Cytochemical and morphological heterogeneity in serially stained gonadotropes. *Am. J. Anat.,* 158:397.
279. Childs, G. V., Ellison, D. G., Lorenzen, J. R., Collins, T. J., and Schwartz, N. B. (1982): Immunocytochemical studies of gonadotrophin storage in developing castration cells. *Endocrinology,* 111:1318.
280. Moriarty, G. C. (1976): Ultrastructural-immunocytochemical studies of rat pituitary gonadotrophs in cycling female rats. *Gunma Symp. Endocrinol.,* 13:207.
281. Eipper, B. A., and Mains, R. E. (1980): Structure and biosynthesis of pro-ACTH/endorphin and related peptides. *Endocr. Rev.,* 1:1.

282. Eipper, B. A., and Mains, R. E. (1977): Peptide analysis of glycoprotein form of adrenocorticotropic hormone. *J. Biol. Chem.*, 252:8821.
283. Hope, J., and Lowry, P. J. (1981): Pro-opiocortin: The ACTH/LPH common precursor protein. *Front. Horm. Res.*, 8:44.
284. Siperstein, E. R. (1963): Identification of the adrenocorticotropin producing cells in the rat hypophysis by autoradiography. *J. Cell Biol.*, 17:521.
285. Siperstein, E. R., and Allison, V. F. (1965): Fine structure of the cells responsible for the secretion of adrenocorticotrophin in the adrenalectomized rat. *Endocrinology,* 76:70.
286. Siperstein, E. R., and Miller, K. J. (1970): Further cytophysiologic evidence for the identity of the cells that produce adrenocorticotrophic hormone. *Endocrinology,* 86:451.
287. Siperstein, E. R., and Miller, K. J. (1973): Hypertrophy of the ACTH-producing cell following adrenalectomy: A quantitative electron microscopic study. *Endocrinology,* 93:1257.
288. Moriarty, G. C., and Halmi, N. S. (1972): Electron microscopic study of the adrenocorticotropin producing cell with the use of unlabeled antibody and the soluble peroxidase-antiperoxidase complex. *J. Histochem. Cytochem.*, 20:590.
289. Mains, R. E., Eipper, B. A., and Ling, N. (1977): Common precursor to corticotropins and endorphins. *Proc. Natl. Acad. Sci. USA,* 74:3014.
290. Roberts, J. L., Seeburg, P. H., Shine, J., Herbert, E., Baxter, J. D., and Goodman, H. M. (1979): Corticotropin and β-endorphin: Construction and analysis of recombinant DNA complementary to mRNA for the common precursor. *Proc. Natl. Acad. Sci. USA,* 76:2153.
291. Nakanishi, S., Inoue, A., Kita, T., Nakamura, M., Chang, A. C. Y., Cohne, S. N., and Nuima, S. (1979): Nucleotide sequence of cloned cDNA for bovine corticotropin-β-lipotropin precursor. *Nature,* 278:423.
292. Phifer, R. F., Spicer, S. S., and Orth, D. N. (1970): Specific demonstration of the human hypophyseal cells which produce adrenocorticotropic hormone. *J. Clin. Endocrinol. Metab.*, 31:347.
293. Phifer, R. F., Orth, D. N., and Spicer, S. S. (1972): Immunohistologic evidence that β-melanocyte stimulating hormone (β-MSH) and adrenocorticotropin (ACTH) are produced in the same human hypophyseal cells. Excerpta Medica, Amsterdam.
294. Moriarty, G. C., and Garner, L. L. (1977): Immunoelectronmicroscopical localization of ACTH/MSH peptides in rat and human pituitaries. *Front. Horm. Res.*, 4:26.
295. Pelletier, G., Leclerc, R., Labrie, F., Cote, J., Chretien, M., and Lis, M. (1977): Immunohistochemical localization of β-lipotropic hormone in the pituitary gland. *Endocrinology,* 100:770.
296. Weber, E., Voigt, K. H., and Martin, R. (1978): Concomitant storage of ACTH and endorphin-like immunoreactivity in the secretory granules of anterior pituitary corticotrophs. *Brain Res.*, 157:385.
297. Baker, B. L., and Drummond, T. (1972): The cellular origins of corticotropin and melanotropin as revealed by immunochemical staining. *Am. J. Anat.*, 134:395.
298. Tanaka, S., and Kurosumi, K. (1986): Differential subcellular localization of ACTH and α-MSH in corticotropes of the rat anterior pituitary. *Cell Tissue Res.*, 243:229.
299. Girod, C. (1984): Fine structure of the pituitary pars distalis. In: *Ultrastructure of Endocrine Cells and Tissues,* edited by P. M. Motta, p. 12. Nijhoff, Boston.
300. Kurosumi, K., Matsuzawa, T., and Shibasaki, S. (1961): Electron microscope studies on the fine structures of the pars nervosa and pars intermedia, and their morphological interrelation in the normal rat hypophysis. *Gen. Comp. Endocrinol.*, 1:433.
301. Visser, M., and Swaab, D. F. (1977): αMSH in the human pituitary. *Front. Horm. Res.*, 4:42.
302. Naik, D. V. (1973): Electron microscopic-immunocytochemical localization of adrenocorticotropin and melanocyte stimulating hormone in the pars intermedia cells of rats and mice. *Z. Zellforsch.*, 142:305.
303. Phifer, R. F., and Spicer, S. S. (1970): Immunohistologic and immunopathologic demonstration of adrenocorticotropic hormone in the pars intermedia of the adenohypophysis. *Lab. Invest.*, 23:543.
304. Moriarty, G. C., and Halmi, N. S. (1972): Adrenocorticotropin production by the intermediate lobe of the rat pituitary. An electron microscopic-immunocytochemical study. *Z. Zellforsch.*, 132:1.
305. Saland, L. C. (1980): Extracellular spaces of the rat pars intermedia as outlined by lanthanum tracer. *Anat. Rec.*, 196:355.
306. Kobayashi, Y. (1965): Functional morphology of the pars intermedia of the rat hypophysis as revealed with the electron microscope. II. Correlation of the pars intermedia with the hypophyseo-adrenal axis. *Z. Zellforsch.*, 68:155.
307. Naik, D. V. (1970): Pituitary-adrenal relationships in mice with hereditary nephrogenic diabetes insipidus, with special emphasis on the neurohypophysis and pars intermedia. *Z. Zellforsch.*, 107:317.
308. Baumgarten, H. G., Bjorklund, A., Holstein, A. F., and Nobin, A. (1972): Organization and ultrastructural identification of the catecholamine nerve terminals in the neural lobe and pars intermedia of the rat pituitary. *Z. Zellforsch.*, 126:483.
309. Tilders, F. J. H., Post, M., Jackson, S., Lowry, P. J., and Smelik, P. G. (1981): Beta-adrenergic stimulation of the release of ACTH and LPH-related peptides from the pars intermedia of the rat pituitary gland. *Acta Endocrinol.*, 97:343.
310. Westlund, K. N., and Childs, G. V. (1982): Localization of serotonin fibers in the rat adenohypophysis. *Endocrinology,* 111:1761.
311. Tilders, F. J. H., and Smelik, P. G. (1977): Direct neural control of MSH secretion in mammals: The involvement of dopaminergic tubero-hypophysial neurones. *Front. Horm. Res.*, 4:80.
312. Vincent, S. R., Hokfelt, T., and Wu, J.-Y. (1982): GABA neuron systems in hypothalamus and the pituitary gland. *Neuroendocrinology,* 34:117.
313. Tappaz, M. L., Wassef, M., Oertel, W. H., Paut, L., and Pujol, J. F. (1983): Light- and electron-microscopic immunocytochemistry of glutamic acid decarboxylase (GAD) in the basal hypothalamus: Morphological evidence for neuroendocrine γ-Aminobutyrate (GABA). *Neuroscience,* 9:271.
314. Verburg-Van Kemenade, B. M., Tappaz, M., Paut, L., and Jenks, B. G. (1986): GABAergic regulation of melanocyte-stimulating hormone secretion from the pars intermedia of *Xenopus laevis:* Immunocytochemical and physiological evidence. *Endocrinology,* 118:260.
315. Celis, M. E. (1977): Hypothalamic peptides involved in control of MSH secretion: Identity, biosynthesis and regulation of their release. *Front. Horm. Res.*, 4:69.
316. Schimchowitsch, S., Stoeckel, M. E., Klein, M. J., Garaud, J. C., Schmitt, G., and Porte, A. (1983): Oxytocin-immunoreactive nerve fibers in the pars intermedia of the pituitary in the rabbit and hare. *Cell Tissue Res.*, 228:255.
317. Sakly, M., Schmitt, G., and Koch, B. (1982): CRF enhances release of both αMSH and ACTH from anterior and intermediate pituitary. *Neuroendocrinol. Lett.*, 4:289.
318. Proulx-Ferland, L., Labrie, F., Dumont, D., Cote, J., Coy, D. H., and Sveiraf, J. (1982): Corticotropin-releasing factor stimulates secretion of melanocyte-stimulating hormone from the rat pituitary. *Science,* 217:62.
319. Cameron, E., and Foster, C. L. (1972): Some light- and electron-microscopical observations on the pars tuberalis of the pituitary gland of the rabbit. *J. Endocrinol.*, 54:505.
320. Baker, B. L., and Yu, Y. Y. (1975): Immunocytochemical analysis of cells in the pars tuberalis of the rat hypophysis with antisera to hormones of the pars distalis. *Cell Tissue Res.*, 156:443.
321. Baker, B. L., Karsch, F. J., Hoffman, D. L., and Beckman, W. C. (1977): The presence of gonadotropic and thyrotropic cells in the pituitary pars tuberalis of the monkey (*Macaca mulatta*). *Biol. Reprod.*, 17:232.
322. Girod, C., Dubois, M. P., and Trouillas, J. (1980): Immunohistochemical study of the pars tuberalis of the adenohypophysis in the monkey, *Macaca irus. Cell Tissue Res.*, 210:191.
323. Gross, D. S., and Page, R. B. (1979): Luteinizing hormone and follicle stimulating hormone production in the pars tuberalis of hypophysectomized rats. *Am. J. Anat.*, 156:285.
324. Gross, D. S. (1983): Hormone production in the hypophysial pars tuberalis of intact and hypophysectomized rats. *Endocrinology,* 112:733.
325. Grimmelikhuijzen, C. J. P., Dierickx, K., and Boer, G. J. (1982): Oxytocin/vasopressin-like immunoreactivity is present in the nervous system of hydra. *Neuroscience,* 7:3191.
326. LeRoith, D., Liotta, A. S., Roth, J., Shiloach, J., Lewis, M. E., Pert, C. B., and Krieger, D. T. (1982): Corticotropin and β-endorphin-like materials are native to unicellular organisms. *Proc. Natl. Acad. Sci. USA,* 79:2086.

327. Krieger, D. T. (1983): Brain peptides: What, where and why? *Science,* 222:975.
328. Monroe, B. G. (1967): A comparative study of the ultrastructure of the median eminence, infundibular stem and neural lobe of the hypophysis of the rat. *Z. Zellforsch.,* 76:405.
329. Duffy, P. E., and Menefee, M. (1965): Electron microscopic observations of neurosecretory granules, nerve and glial fibers and blood vessels in the median eminence of the rabbit. *Am. J. Anat.,* 117:251.
330. Page, R. B., and Dovey-Hartman, B. J. (1984): Neurohemal contact in the internal zone of the rabbit median eminence. *J. Comp. Neurol.,* 226:274.
331. Kobayashi, H., Oota, Y., Uemura, H., and Hirano, T. (1966): Electron microscopic and pharmacological studies on the rat median eminence. *Z. Zellforsch.,* 71:387.
332. Rinne, U. K. (1966): Ultrastructure of the median eminance of the rat. *Z. Zellforsch.,* 74:98.
333. Lederis, K. (1965): An electron microscopical study of the human neurohypophysis. *Z. Zellforsch.,* 65:847.
334. Bergland, R. M., and Torack, R. M. (1969): An electron microscopic study of the human infundibulum. *Z. Zellforsch.,* 99:1.
335. Rodriguez, E. M. (1969): Ultrastructure of the neurohemal region of the toad median eminence. *Z. Zellforsch.,* 93:182.
336. Rodriguez, E. M. (1969): Ependymal specializations. I. Fine structure of the neural (internal) region of the toad median eminence, with particular reference to the connections between the ependymal cells and the subependymal capillary loops. *Z. Zellforsch.,* 102:153.
337. Magoun, H. W., and Ranson, S. W. (1939): Retrograde degeneration of the supraoptic nuclei after section of the infundibular stalk in the monkey. *Anat. Rec.,* 75:107.
338. Rasmussen, A. T. (1940): Effects of hypophysectomy and hypophysial stalk resection of the hypothalamic nuclei of animals and man. *Res. Publ. Assoc. Res. Nerv. Ment. Dis.,* 20:245.
339. Sherlock, D. A., Field, P. M., and Raisman, G. (1975): Retrograde transport of horseradish peroxidase in the magnocellular neurosecretory system of the rat. *Brain Res.,* 88:403.
340. Zimmerman, E. A. (1981): The organization of oxytocin and vasopressin pathways. In: *Neurosecretion and Brain Peptides,* edited by J. B. Martin, S. Reichlin, and K. L. Bick, p. 63. Raven Press, New York.
341. Barer, R., Heller, H., and Lederis, K. (1963): The isolation, identification and properties of the hormonal granules of the neurohypophysis. *Proc. R. Soc. Lond. Biol.,* 158:388.
342. Silverman, A. J., and Zimmerman, E. A. (1975): Ultrastructural immunocytochemical localization of neurophysin and vasopressin in the median eminence and posterior pituitary of the guinea pig. *Cell Tissue Res.,* 159:291.
343. Douglas, W. W., Nagasawa, J., and Schulz, R. (1971): Electron microscopic studies on the mechanism of secretion of posterior pituitary hormones and significance of microvesicles (synaptic vesicles): Evidence of secretion by exocytosis and formation of microvesicles as a by-product of this process. *Mem. Soc. Endocrinol.,* 19:353.
344. Theodosis, D. T., Dreifuss, J. J., and Orci, L. (1978): A freeze-fracture study of membrane events during neurohypophysial secretion. *J. Cell Biol.,* 78:542.
345. Morris, J. F., and Nordmann, J. J. (1980): Membrane recapture after hormone release from nerve endings in the neural lobe of the rat pituitary gland. *Neuroscience,* 5:639.
346. Hartmann, J. F. (1958): Electron microscopy of the neurohypophysis in normal and histamine-treated rats. *Z. Zellforsch.,* 48:291.
347. Barer, R., and Lederis, K. (1966): Ultrastructure of the rabbit neurohypophysis with special reference to the release of hormones. *Z. Zellforsch.,* 75:201.
348. Barer, R., Heller, H., and Lederis, K. (1963): The isolation, identification and properties of the hormonal granules of the neurohypophysis. *Proc. Roy. Soc. B,* 158:388.
349. Rodriguez, E. M. (1971): The comparative morphology of neural lobes of species with different neurohypophysial hormones. *Mem. Soc. Endocrinol.,* 19:263.
350. Seyama, S., Pearl, G. S., and Takei, Y. (1980): Ultrastructural study of the human neurohypophysis. I. Neurosecretory axons and their dilatations in the pars nervosa. *Cell Tissue Res.,* 205:253.
351. Nordmann, J. J., and Chevallier, J. (1980): The role of microvesicles in buffering (Ca^{2+}) in the neurohypophysis. *Nature,* 287:54.
352. Shaw, F. D., and Morris, J. F. (1980): Calcium localization in the rat neurohypophysis. *Nature,* 287:56.
353. Broadwell, R. D., Cataldo, A. M., and Balin, B. J. (1984): Further studies of the secretory process in hypothalamo-neurohypophysial neurons: An analysis using immunocytochemistry, wheat germ agglutinin-peroxidase, and native peroxidase. *J. Comp. Neurol.,* 228:155.
354. Bloom, F. E., and Aghajanian, G. K. (1968): An electron microscopic analysis of large granular synaptic vesicles of the brain in relation to monoamine content. *J. Pharm. Exp. Ther.,* 159:261.
355. Bloom, F. E. (1970): The fine structural localization of biogenic monoamines in nervous tissue. *Int. Rev. Neurobiol.,* 13:27.
356. Ajika, K. (1980): Relationship between catecholaminergic neurons and hypothalamic hormone-containing neurons in the hypothalamus. In: *Frontiers of Neuroendocrinology, Vol. 6,* edited by L. Martini and W. F. Ganong, p. 1. Raven Press, New York.
357. Johansson, O., Hokfelt, T., Jeffcoate, S. L., White, N., and Sternberger, L. A. (1980): Ultrastructural localization of TRH-like immunoreactivity. *Exp. Brain Res.,* 38:1.
358. Shioda, S., and Nakai, Y. (1983): Immunocytochemical localization of TRH and autoradiographic determination of ^{3}H-TRH-binding sites in the arcuate nucleus-median eminence of the rat. *Cell Tissue Res.,* 228:475.
359. Pelletier, G., Labrie, F., Arimura, A., and Schally, A. V. (1974): Electron microscopic immunohistochemical localization of growth hormone-release inhibiting hormones (somatostatin) in the rat median eminence. *Am. J. Anat.,* 140:583.
360. Ohtsuka, M., Yamamoto, Y., and Daikoku, S. (1983): Topography and ultrastructure of LHRH- and somatostatin-containing axonal terminals in the median eminence of rats. *Arch. Histol. Jpn.,* 46:203.
361. Silverman, A. J., and Desnoyers, P. (1976): Ultrastructural immunocytochemical localization of luteinizing hormone-releasing hormone (LH-RH) in the median eminence of the guinea pig. *Cell Tissue Res.,* 169:157.
362. Stoeckart, R., Jansen, H. G., and Kreike, A. J. (1972): Ultrastructural evidence for exocytosis in the median eminence of the rat. *Z. Zellforsch.,* 131:99.
363. Daikoku, S., Takahashi, T., Kojimoto, H., and Watanabe, Y. G. (1973): Secretory surface phenomena in freeze-etched preparations of the adenohypophysial cells and neurosecretory fibers. *Z. Zellforsch.,* 136:207.
364. Ajika, K. (1979): Simultaneous localization of LHRH and catecholamines in rat hypothalamus. *J. Anat.,* 128:331.
365. Nakai, Y., Shioda, S., Ochiai, H., Kudo, J., and Hashimoto, A. (1983): Ultrastructural relationship between monoamine- and TRH-containing axons in the rat median eminence as revealed by combined autoradiography and immunocytochemistry in the same tissue section. *Cell Tissue Res.,* 230:1.
366. Tranzer, J. P., and Thoenen, H. (1967): Electronmicroscopic localization of 5-hydroxydopamine (3,4,5-trihydroxyphenyl-ethylamine), a new "false" sympathetic transmitter. *Experientia,* 23:743.
367. Richards, J. G., and Tranzer, J.-P. (1970): The ultrastructural localisation of amine storage sites in the central nervous system with the aid of a specific marker, 5-hydroxydopamine. *Brain Res.,* 17:463.
368. Tranzer, J.-P., and Richards, J. G. (1976): Ultrastructural cytochemistry of biogenic amines in nervous tissue: Methodologic improvements. *J. Histochem. Cytochem.,* 24:1178.
369. Pickel, V. M., Joh, T. H., and Reis, D. J. (1975): Ultrastructural localization of tyrosine hydroxylase in noradrenergic neurons of the brain. *Proc. Natl. Acad. Sci. USA,* 72:659.
370. Pickel, V. M., Joh, T. H., Field, P. M., Becker, C. G., and Reis, D. J. (1975): Cellular localization of tyrosine hydroxylase by immunohistochemistry. *J. Histochem. Cytochem.,* 23:1.
371. Pickel, V. M., Joh, T., and Reis, D. J. (1976): Monoamine-synthesizing enzymes in central dopaminergic, noradrenergic and serotonergic neurons. Immunocytochemical localization by light and electron microscopy. *J. Histochem. Cytochem.,* 24:792.
372. Hokfelt, T., Lundberg, J. M., Schultzberg, M., Johansson, O., Ljungdahl, A., and Rehfeld, J. (1980): Coexistence of peptides and putative transmitters in neurons. In: *Neural Peptides and Neuronal Communication,* edited by E. Costa and M. Trabucchi, p. 1. Raven Press, New York.
373. Thureson-Klein, A. (1983): Commentary: Exocytosis from large and small dense core vesicles in noradrenergic nerve terminals. *Neuroscience,* 10:245.

374. Schwab, M., and Thoenen, H. (1983): Mechanism of uptake and retrograde axonal transport of noradrenaline in sympathetic neurons in culture: Reserpine-resistant large dense-core vesicles as transport vehicles. *J. Cell. Biol.*, 96:1538.
375. Carson, K. A., Nemcroff, C. B., Rone, M. S., Youngblood, W. W., Prange, A. J., Hanber, J. S., and Kizer, J. S. (1977): Biochemical and histochemical evidence for the existence of a tubero-infundibular cholinergic pathway in the rat. *Brain Res.*, 129:169.
376. Fink, G., and Smith, G. C. (1971): Ultrastructural features of the developing hypothalamo-hypophysial axis in the rat. *Z. Zellforsch.*, 119:208.
377. Paull, W. K. (1973): A light and electron microscopic study of the development of the neurohypophysis of the fetal rat. *Anat. Rec.*, 175:407.
378. Dellmann, H.-D., Castel, M., and Linner, J. G. (1978): Ultrastructure of peptidergic neurosecretory axons in the developing neural lobe of the rat. *Gen. Comp. Endocrinol.*, 36:477.
379. Eurenius, L., and Jarskar, R. (1971): Electron microscope studies on the development of the external zone of the mouse median eminence. *Z. Zellforsch.*, 122:488.
380. Monroe, B. G., Newman, B. L., and Schapiro, S. (1972): Ultrastructure of the median eminence of neonatal and adult rats. In: *Brain-Endocrine Interaction. Median Eminence: Structure and Function*, edited by K. M. Knigge, D. E. Scott, and A. Weindl, p. 7. Karger, New York.
381. Monroe, B. G., and Paull, W. K. (1974): Ultrastructural changes in the hypothalamus during development and hypothalamic activity: The median eminence. *Prog. Brain Res.*, 41:185.
382. Kawano, H., Watanabe, Y. G., and Daikoku, S. (1980): Light and electron microscopic observation on the appearance of immunoreactive LHRH in perinatal rat hypothalamus. *Cell Tissue Res.*, 213:465.
383. Adachi, T., Ohtsuka, M., Hisano, S., Tsuruo, Y., and Daikoku, S. (1984): Ontogenetic appearance of somatostatin-containing nerve terminals in the median eminence of rats. *Cell Tissue Res.*, 236:47.
384. Bugnon, C., Fellmann, D., Gouget, A., and Cardot, J. (1982): Immunocytochemical study of the ontogenesis of the CRF-containing neuroglandular system in the rat. *C. R. Acad. Sci. (III)*, 294:599.
385. Setalo, G., Antalicz, M., Saarossy, K., Arimura, A., Schally, A. V., and Flerko, B. (1978): Ontogenesis of the LH-RH containing neuronal elements in the hypothalamus of the rat. *Acta Biol. Acad. Sci. Hung.*, 29:285.
386. Gross, D. S., and Baker, B. L. (1977): Immunohistochemical localization of gonadotropin-releasing hormone (GnRH) in the fetal and early postnatal mouse brain. *Am. J. Anat.*, 148:195.
387. Gross, D. S., and Baker, B. L. (1979): Developmental correlation between hypothalamic gonadotropin-releasing hormone and hypophysial luteinizing hormone. *Am. J. Anat.*, 154:1.
388. Monroe, B. G., and Holmes, E. M. (1983): The freeze-fractured median eminence. II. Developmental changes in the neurohemal contact zone of the median eminence of the rat. *Cell Tissue Res.*, 233:81.
389. Bjorklund, A., Enemar, A., and Falck, B. (1968): Monoamines in the hypothalamo-hypophyseal system of the mouse with special reference to the ontogenetic aspects. *Z. Zellforsch.*, 89:590.
390. Ibata, Y., Tani, N., Obata, H. L., Tanaka, M., Kubo, S., Fujui, K., Fujimoto, M., Kinoshita, H., Watanabe, K., Sano, Y., Hashimura, E., Sin, S., and Imagawa, K. (1981): Correlative ontogenetic development of catecholamine- and LHRH-containing nerve endings in the median eminence of the rat. *Cell Tissue Res.*, 216:31.
391. Ugrumov, M. V., Chandrasekhar, K., Borisova, N. A., and Mitsekevich, M. S. (1979): Light and electron microscopical investigations on the tanycyte differentiation during the perinatal period in the rat. *Cell Tissue Res.*, 201:295.
392. Monroe, B. G., and Holmes, E. M. (1982): The freeze-fractured median eminence. 1. Development of intercellular junctions in the ependyma of the 3rd ventricle of the rat. *Cell Tissue Res.*, 222:389.
393. Silverman, A. J., and Desnoyers, P. (1975): Post-natal development of the median eminence of the guinea pig. *Anat. Rec.*, 183:459.
394. Lamperti, A., and Mastovich, J. (1983): Morphological changes in the hypothalamic arcuate nucleus and median eminence in the golden hamster during the neonatal period. *Am. J. Anat.*, 166:173.
395. Kobayashi, H., and Matsui, T. (1969): Fine structure of the median eminence and its functional significance. In: *Frontiers in Neuroendocrinology*, edited by W. F. Ganong and L. Martini, p. 3. Oxford University Press, New York.
396. Kobayashi, H., Matsui, T., and Ishii, S. (1970): Functional electron microscopy of the hypothalamic median eminence. *Int. Rev. Cytol.*, 29:281.
397. Knigge, K. M., and Silverman, A.-J. (1974): Anatomy of the endocrine hypothalamus. In: *Handbook of Physiology. Section 7: Endocrinology. Vol. IV. The Pituitary Gland and Its Neuroendocrine Control*, edited by R. O. Greep and E. B. Astwood, p. 1. American Physiological Society, Washington, D.C.
398. Enemar, A., and Eurenius, L. (1979): Organization and development of the perivascular space system in the neurohypophysis of the laboratory mouse. *Cell Tissue Res.*, 199:99.
399. Heap, P. F., Jones, C. W., Morris, J. F., and Pickering, B. T. (1975): Movement of neurosecretory product through the anatomical compartments of the neural lobe of the pituitary gland. (An electron microscopic autoradiographic study). *Cell Tissue Res.*, 156:483.
400. Aspeslagh, M.-R., Vandesande, F., and Dierickx, K. (1976): Electron microscopic immunocytochemical demonstration of separate neurophysin-vasopressinergic and neurophysin-oxytocinergic nerve fibres in the neural lobe of the rat hypophysis. *Cell Tissue Res.*, 171:31.
401. VanLeeuwen, F. W., de Raay, C., Swaab, D. F., and Fisser, B. (1979): The localization of oxytocin, vasopressin, somatostatin and luteinizing hormone releasing hormone in the rat neurohypophysis. *Cell Tissue Res.*, 202:189.
402. Whitnall, M. H., Gainer, H., Cox, B. M., and Molineaux, C. J. (1983): Dynorphin-A-(1-8) is contained within vasopressin neurosecretory vesicles in rat pituitary. *Science*, 222:1137.
403. Rossier, J., Pittman, Q., Bloom, F., and Guillemin, R. (1980): Distribution of opioid peptides in the pituitary: A new hypothalamic-pars nervosa enkephalinergic pathway. *Fed. Proc.*, 39:2555.
404. Zamir, N. (1985): On the origin of leu-enkephalin and met-enkephalin in the rat neurohypophysis. *Endocrinology*, 117:1687.
405. VanLeeuwen, F. W., Pool, C. W., and Sluiter, A. A. (1983): Enkephalin immunoreactivity in synaptoid elements on glial cells in the rat neural lobe. *Neuroscience*, 8:229.
406. Martin, R., and Voigt, K. H. (1981): Enkephalins co-exist with oxytocin and vasopressin in nerve terminals of rat neurohypophysis. *Nature*, 289:502.
407. Martin, R., Geis, R., Holl, R., Schafer, M., and Voigt, K. H. (1983): Co-existence of unrelated peptides in oxytocin and vasopressin terminals of rat neurohypophyses: Immunoreactive methionine^5-enkephalin-, leucine^5-enkephalin- and cholecystokinin-like substances. *Neuroscience*, 8:213.
408. Vanderhaeghen, J. J., Lotstra, F., Liston, D. R., and Rossier, J. (1983): Proenkephalin, (Met)enkephalin, and oxytocin immunoreactivities are colocalized in bovine hypothalamic magnocellular neurons. *Proc. Natl. Acad. Sci. USA*, 80:5139.
409. Rossier, J., Battenberg, E., Pittman, Q., Bayon, A., Koda, L., Miller, R., Guillemin, R., and Bloom, F. (1979): Hypothalamic enkephalin neurones may regulate the neurohypophysis. *Nature*, 277:653.
410. Clarke, G., Wood, P., Merrick, L., and Lincoln, D. W. (1979): Opiate inhibition of peptide release from the neurohumoral terminals of hypothalamic neurones. *Nature*, 282:746.
411. Vanderhaeghen, J. J., Lotstra, F., DeMey, J., and Gilles, C. (1980): Immunohistochemical localization of cholecystokinin and gastrin-like peptides in the brain and hypophysis of the rat. *Proc. Natl. Acad. Sci. USA*, 77:1190.
412. Kiss, J. Z., Williams, T. H., and Palkovits, M. (1984): Distribution and projections of cholecystokinin-immunoreactive neurons in the hypothalamic paraventricular nucleus of rat. *J. Comp. Neurol.*, 227:173.
413. Stoeckel, M. E., Porte, A., Klein, M. J., and Cuello, A. C. (1982): Immunocytochemical localization of substance P in the neurohypophysis and hypothalamus of the mouse compared with the distribution of other neuropeptides. *Cell Tissue Res.*, 223:533.
414. Zimmerman, E. A., Robinson, A. G., Husain, M. K., et al. (1974): Neurohypophysial peptides in the bovine hypothalamus: The relationship of neurophysin I to oxytocin, and neurophysin II to vasopressin, in supraoptic and paraventricular regions. *Endocrinology*, 95:931.

415. Lechan, R. M., and Jackson, I. M. D. (1982): Immunohistochemical localization of thyrotropin-releasing hormone in the rat hypothalamus and pituitary. *Endocrinology,* 111:55.
416. Bjorklund, A., Moore, R. Y., Nobin, A., and Stenevi, U. (1973): The organization of tubero-hypophyseal and reticulo-infundibular catecholamine neuron systems in the rat brain. *Brain Res.,* 51:171.
417. Pelletier, G. (1983): Identification of endings containing dopamine and vasopressin in the rat posterior pituitary by a combination of radioautography and immunocytochemistry at the ultrastructural level. *J. Histochem. Cytochem.,* 31:562.
418. Saavedra, J. M. (1985): Central and peripheral catecholamine innervation of the rat intermediate and posterior pituitary lobes. *Neuroendocrinology,* 40:281.
419. Anthony, E. L. P., King, J. C., and Stopa, E. G. (1984): Immunocytochemical localization of LHRH in the median eminence, infundibular stalk, and neurohypophysis. (Evidence for multiple sites of releasing hormone secretion in humans and other mammals). *Cell Tissue Res.,* 236:5.
420. Kawata, M., Hashimoto, K., Takahara, J., and Sano, Y. (1983): Immunohistochemical identification of the corticotropin releasing factor (CRF)-containing nerve fibers in the pig hypophysis, with special reference to the relationship between CRF and posterior lobe hormones. *Arch. Histol. Jpn.,* 46:183.
421. Takei, Y., Seyama, S., Pearl, G. S., Tindall, G. T. (1980): Ultrastructural study of the human neurohypophysis. II. Cellular elements of neural parenchyma, the pituicytes. *Cell Tissue Res.,* 205:273.
422. Tweedle, C. D., and Hatton, G. I. (1980): Glial cell enclosure of neurosecretory endings in the neurohypophysis of the rat. *Brain Res.,* 192:555.
423. Tweedle, C. D., and Hatton, G. I. (1980): Evidence for dynamic interactions between pituicytes and neurosecretory axons in the rat. *Neuroscience,* 5:661.
424. Hatton, G. I., and Tweedle, C. D. (1982): Magnocellular neuropeptidergic neurons in hypothalamus: Increases in membrane apposition and number of specialized synapses from pregnancy to lactation. *Brain Res. Bull.,* 8:197.
425. Tweedle, C. D., and Hatton, G. I. (1982): Magnocellular neuropeptidergic terminals in the neurohypophysis: rapid glial release of enclosed axons during parturition. *Brain Res. Bull.,* 8:205.
426. Tweedle, C. D. (1983): Ultrastructural manifestations of increased hormone release in the neurohypophysis. *Prog. Brain Res.,* 60:259.
427. Hatton, G. I., Perlmutter, L. S., Salm, A. K., and Tweedle, C. D. (1984): Dynamic neuronal-glial interactions in hypothalamus and pituitary: Implications for control of hormone synthesis and release. *Peptides* 5(Suppl. 1).
428. Perlmutter, L. S., Hatton, G. I., and Tweedle, C. D. (1984): Plasticity in the *in vitro* neurohypophysis: Effects of osmotic changes on pituicytes. *Neuroscience,* 12:503.
429. Ziedonis, D. M., Severs, W. B., Brennan, R. W., and Page, R. B. (1986): Blood flow and functional responses correlate in the ovine neural lobe. *Brain Res.,* 373(1–2):27.
430. Gross, P. M., Blasberg, R. G., Fenstermacher, J. D., and Patlak, C. S. (1985): Rapid amino acid uptake in rat pituitary neural lobe during functional stimulation by chronic dehydration. *J. Cereb. Blood Flow Metab.,* 5:151.
431. Merchenthaler, I., Vigh, S., Petrusz, P., and Schally, A. V. (1982): Immunocytochemical localization of corticotropin-releasing factor (CRF) in the rat brain. *Am. J. Anat.,* 165:385.
432. Sawchenko, P. E., Swanson, L. W., Rivier, J., and Vale, W. W. (1985): The distribution of growth-hormone-releasing factor (GRF) immunoreactivity in the central nervous system of the rat: An immunohistochemical study using antisera directed against rat hypothalamic GRF. *J. Comp. Neurol.,* 237:100.
433. Kahn, D., Abrams, G. M., Zimmerman, E. A., Carraway, R., and Leeman, S. E. (1980): Neurotensin neurons in the rat hypothalamus: An immunohistochemical study. *Endocrinology,* 107:47.
434. Dierickx, K., and DeWaele, G. (1975): Scanning electron microscopy of the wall of the third ventricle of the brain of Rana temporaria III. Electron microscopy of the ventricular surface of the median eminence. *Cell Tissue Res.,* 161:343.
435. Nakai, Y., Ochiai, H., and Uchida, M. (1977): Fine structure of ependymal cells in the median eminence of the frog and mouse revealed by freeze-etching. *Cell Tissue Res.,* 181:311.
436. Mikami, S.-I. (1975): A correlative ultrastructural analysis of the ependymal cells of the third ventricle of Japanese quail, *Coturnix japonica*. In: *Brain-Endocrine Interaction. II. The Ventricular System,* edited by K. M. Knigge, D. E. Scott, H. Kobayashi, and S. Ishii, p. 80. Karger, Basel.
437. Martinez, P. M., and DeWeerd, H. (1977): The fine structure of the ependymal surface of the recessus infundibularis in the rat. *Anat. Embryol.,* 151:241.
438. Paull, W. K., Martin, H., and Scott, D. E. (1977): Scanning electron microscopy of the third ventricular floor of the rat. *J. Comp. Neurol.,* 175:301.
439. Bruni, J. E., Montemurro, D. G., Clattenburg, R. E., and Singh, R. P. (1972): A scanning electron microscopic study of the ependymal surface of the third ventricle of the rabbit, rat, mouse and human brain. *Anat. Rec.,* 174:407.
440. Climenti, F., Marini, D. (1972): The surface fine structure of the walls of cerebral ventricles and of choroid plexus in cat. *Z. Zellforsch.,* 123:82.
441. Bruni, J. E., Clattenburg, R. E., and Montemurro, D. G. (1974): Ependymal tanycytes of the rabbit third ventricle: a scanning electron microscopic study. *Brain Res.,* 73:145.
442. Scott, D. E. (1973): A comparative ultrastructural analysis of the third cerebral ventricle of the North American mink. *Anat. Rec.,* 175:155.
443. Kozlowski, G. P., Scott, D. E., and Dudley, G. (1973): Scanning electron microscopy of the 3rd ventricle of sheep. *Z. Zellforsch.,* 136:169.
444. Scott, D. E., Krobisch-Dudley, G., Paull, W. K., Kozlowski, G. P., and Ribas, J. (1975): The primate median eminence. I. Correlative scanning-transmission electron microscopy. *Cell Tissue Res.,* 162:61.
445. Scott, D. E., Paull, W. K., Dudley, G. K. (1972): A comparative scanning electron microscopic analysis of the human cerebral ventricular system. I. The third ventricle. *Z. Zellforsch.,* 132:203.
446. Jacobs, J. J., and Monroe, K. D. (1977): A scanning electron microscopic survey of the brain ventricular system of the female armadillo. *Cell Tissue Res.,* 183:531.
447. Bruni, J. E., Montemurro, D. G., and Clattenburg, R. E. (1977): Morphology of the ependymal lining of the rabbit third ventricle following intraventricular administration of synthetic luteinizing hormone-releasing hormone (LH-RH): A scanning electron microscopic investigation. *Am. J. Anat.,* 150:411.
448. Paull, W. K., Martin, H., and Scott, D. E. (1977): Scanning electron microscopy of the third ventricular floor of the rat. *J. Comp. Neurol.,* 175:301.
449. Matsui, T., and Kobayashi, H. (1968): Surface protrusions from the ependymal cells of the median eminence. *Arch. Anat.,* 51:429.
450. Dierickx, K., and DeWaele, G. (1975): Scanning electron microscopy of the wall of the third ventricle of the brain of *Rana temporara*. III. Electron microscopy of the ventricular surface of the median eminence. *Cell Tissue Res.,* 161:343.
451. Scott, D. E., Krobisch-Dudley, G., Paull, W. K., and Kozlowski, G. P. (1977): The ventricular system in neuroendocrine mechanisms. III. Supraependymal neuronal networks in the primate brain. *Cell Tissue Res.,* 179:235.
452. Bleier, R., Albrecht, R., and Cruce, J. A. F. (1975): Supraependymal cells of hypothalamic third ventricle: identification as resident phagocytes of the brain. *Science,* 189:299.
453. Bleier, R. (1977): Ultrastructure of supraependymal cells and ependyma of hypothalamic third ventricle of mouse. *J. Comp. Neurol.,* 174:359.
454. Bleier, R. (1971): The relations of ependyma to neurons and capillaries in the hypothalamus: A Golgi-Cox study. *J. Comp. Neurol.,* 142:439.
455. Millhouse, O. E. (1971): A Golgi study of the third ventricle tanycytes in the adult rodent brain. *Z. Zellforsch.,* 121:1.
456. Millhouse, O. E. (1972): Light and electron microscopic studies of the ventricular wall. *Z. Zellforsch.,* 127:149.
457. Card, J. P., and Rafols, J. A. (1978): Tanycytes of the third ventricle of the neonatal rat: A Golgi study. *Am. J. Anat.,* 151:173.
458. Sharp, P. J. (1972): Tanycyte and vascular patterns in the basal hypothalamus of corturnix quail with reference to their possible neuroendocrine significance. *Z. Zellforsch.,* 127:552.

459. Akmayev, I. G., and Popov, A. P. (1977): Morphological aspects of the hypothalamic-hypophyseal system. VII. The tanycytes: Their relation to the hypophyseal adrenocorticotrophic function. An ultrastructural study. *Cell Tissue Res.*, 180:263.
460. Brawer, J. R. (1972): The fine structure of the ependymal tanycytes at the level of the arcuate nucleus. *J. Comp. Neurol.*, 145:25.
461. Gotow, T., and Hashimoto, P. H. (1981): Graded differences in tightness of ependymal intercellular junctions within and in the vicinity of the rat median eminence. *J. Ultrastruct. Res.*, 76:293.
462. Rodriguez, E. M., Gonzalez, C. B., and Delannoy, L. (1979): Cellular organization of the lateral and postinfundibular regions of the median eminence in the rat. *Cell Tissue Res.*, 201:377.
463. Brawer, J. R., and Walsh, R. J. (1982): Response of tanycytes to aging in the median eminence of the rat. *Am. J. Anat.*, 163:247.
464. Brightman, M. W., and Reese, T. S. (1969): Junctions between intimately apposed cell membranes in the vertebrate brain. *J. Cell Biol.*, 40:648.
465. Brightman, M. W., Prescott, L., and Reese, T. S. (1975): Intercellular junctions of special ependyma. In: *Brain-Endocrine Interaction II. The Ventricular System,* edited by K. M. Knigge, D. E. Scott, H. Kobayashi, and S. Ishii, p. 146. Karger, Basel.
466. Nakai, Y., Ochiai, H., and Uchida, M. (1977): Fine structure of ependymal cells in the median eminence of the frog and mouse revealed by freeze-etching. *Cell Tissue Res.*, 181:311.
467. Kobayashi, H., Wada, M., and Uemura, H. (1972): Uptake of peroxidase from the 3rd ventricle by ependymal cells of the median eminence. *Z. Zellforsch.*, 127:545.
468. Kobayashi, H. (1975): Absorption of cerebrospinal fluid by ependymal cells of the median eminence. In: *Brain-Endocrine Interaction II. The Ventricular System,* edited by K. M. Knigge, D. E. Scott, H. Kobayashi, and S. Ishii, p. 109. Karger, Basel.
469. Nakai, Y., and Naito, N. (1975): Uptake and bidirectional transport of peroxidase injected into the blood and cerebrospinal fluid by ependymal cells of the median eminence. In: *Brain-Endocrine Interaction II. The Ventricular System,* edited by K. M. Knigge, D. E. Scott, H. Kobayashi, and S. Ishii, p. 94. Karger, Basel.
470. Guldner, F.-H., and Wolff, J. R. (1973): Neurono-glial synaptoid contacts in the median eminence of the rat: Ultrastructure, staining properties and distribution on tanycytes. *Brain Res.*, 61:217.
471. Scott, D. E., and Paull, W. K. (1979): The tanycyte of the rat median eminence. I. Synaptoid contacts. *Cell Tissue Res.*, 200:329.
472. Knowles, F., and Kumar, T. C. A. (1969): Structural changes, related to reproduction, in the hypothalamus and in the pars tuberalis of the rhesus monkey. *Philos. Trans. R. Soc. Lond. (Biol.),* 256: 357.
473. Knowles, F. (1972): Ependyma of the third ventricle in relation to pituitary function. *Prog. Brain Res.*, 38:255.
474. Knigge, K. M., Joseph, S. A., Sladek, J. R., et al. (1976): Uptake and transport activity of the median eminence of the hypothalamus. *Int. Rev. Cytol.*, 45:383.
475. Pilgram, Ch. (1978): Commentary: Transport function of hypothalamic tanycyte ependyma: How good is the evidence? *Neuroscience,* 3:277.
476. Luppa, H., Feustel, G., Weiss, J., and Luppa, D. (1975): Localization of ATPase activity in IIIrd ventricle ependyma of the rat. A contribution to the function of ependyma. *Brain Res.*, 83:15.
477. Firth, J. A., and Bock, R. (1976): Distribution and properties of an adenosine triphosphatase in the tanycyte ependyma of the IIIrd ventricle of the rat. *Histochemistry,* 47:145.
478. Krisch, B., Leonhardt, H., and Buchheim, W. (1978): The functional and structural border of the neurohemal region of the median eminence. *Cell Tissue Res.*, 192:327.
479. Wittkowski, W., and Scheuer, A. (1974): Functional changes of the neuronal and glial elements at the surface of the external layer of the median eminence. *Z. Anat. Entwickl-Gesch.*, 143:255.
480. Bugnon, C., Fellmann, D., Gouget, A., and Cardot, J. (1982): Corticoliberin in rat brain: Immunocytochemical identification and localization of a novel neuroglandular system. *Neurosci. Lett.*, 30:25.
481. Hanstrom, B. (1953): The neurohypophysis in the series of mammals. *Z. Zellforsch.*, 39:241.
482. Lofstrom, A., Jonsson, G., and Fuxe, K. (1976): Microfluorimetric quantitation of catecholamine fluorescence in rat median eminence. I. Aspects on the distribution of dopamine and noradrenaline nerve terminals. *J. Histochem. Cytochem.*, 24:415.
483. Mezey, E., Kiss, J. Z., Mueller, G. P., Eskay, R., O'Donohue, T. L., and Palkovits, M. (1985): Distribution of the pro-opiomelanocortin derived peptides, adrenocorticotrope hormone, α-melanocyte-stimulating hormone and β-endorphin (ACTH, α-MSH, β-End) in the rat hypothalamus. *Brain Res.*, 328:341.
484. Kiss, J. Z., Mezey, E., Cassell, M. D., Williams, T. H., Mueller, G. P., O'Donohue, T. L., and Palkovits, M. (1985): Topographical distribution of pro-opiomelanocortin-derived peptides (ACTH/β-End/α-MSH) in the rat median eminence. *Brain Res.*, 329:169.
485. Knigge, K. M., and Scott, D. E. (1970): Structure and function of the median eminence. *Am. J. Anat.*, 129:223.
486. Rodriguez, E. M. (1972): Comparative and functional morphology of the median eminence. In: *Brain-Endocrine Interaction: Structure and Function,* edited by K. M. Knigge, D. E. Scott, and A. Weindl, p. 319. Karger, Basel.
487. Fuxe, K. (1963): Cellular localization of monoamines in the median eminence and infundibular stem of some mammals. *Acta Physiol. Scand.*, 58:383.
488. Fuxe, K. (1964): Cellular localization of monoamines in the median eminence and infundibular stem of some mammals. *Z. Zellforsch.*, 61:710.
489. Fuxe, K. (1965): Evidence for the existence of monoamine neurons in the central nervous system. IV. The distribution of monoamine nerve terminals in the central nervous system. *Acta Phys. Scand. (Suppl.),* 247:39.
490. Lindvall, O., and Bjorklund, A. (1974): The glyoxylic acid fluorescence histochemical method. A detailed account of the methodology for the visualization of central catecholamine neurons. *Histochemistry,* 39:97.
491. Chiba, T., Hwang, B. H., and Williams, T. H. (1976): A method for studying glyoxylic acid induced fluorescence and ultrastructure of monoamine neurons. *Histochemistry,* 49:95.
492. Ajika, K., and Hokfelt, T. (1973): Ultrastructural identification of catecholamine neurons in the hypothalamic periventricular-arcuate nucleus-median eminence complex with special reference to quantitative aspects. *Brain Res.*, 57:97.
493. Bensch, C., Lescure, H., Dufy, B., and Gross, C. (1979): Histofluorometrie des catecholamines de la couche externe de l'eminence mediane hypothalamique de la lapine. *Ann. Endocrinol.*, 39:281.
494. Bensch, C., Lescure, H., Robert, J., and Faure, J. (1975): Catecholamine histofluorescence in the median eminence of female rabbits activated by mating. *J. Neural. Transm.*, 36:1.
495. Nojyo, Y., Ibata, Y., and Sano, Y. (1976): Demonstration of tuberinfundibular tract of the cat. Fluorescence histochemistry and electron microscopy. *Cell Tissue Res.*, 168:289.
496. Ibata, Y., Fukui, K., Okamura, H., Kawakami, T., Tanaka, M., Obata, H. L., Tsuto, T., Terubayashi, H., Yanaihara, C., and Yanaihara, N. (1983): Coexistence of dopamine and neurotensin in hypothalamic arcuate and periventricular neurons. *Brain Res.*, 269:177.
497. Joseph, S. A., Piekut, D. T., and Knigge, K. M. (1981): Immunocytochemical localization of luteinizing hormone-releasing hormone (LHRH) in vibratome-sectioned brain. *J. Histochem. Cytochem.*, 29:247.
498. McNeill, T. H., and Sladek, J. (1978): Fluorescence-immunocytochemistry. Simultaneous localization of catecholamines and gonadotropin-releasing hormone. *Science,* 200:72.
499. Ibata, Y., Watanabe, K., Kinoshita, H., Kubo, S., Sano, Y., Sin, S., Hashimura, E., and Imagewa, K. (1979): Detection of catecholamine and luteinizing hormone-releasing hormone (LH-RH) containing nerve endings in the median eminence and the organum vasculosum laminae terminalis by fluorescence histochemistry and immunohistochemistry on the same microscopic sections. *Neurosci. Lett.*, 11:181.
500. Ajika, K. (1979): Simultaneous localization of LHRH and catecholamines in rat hypothalamus. *J. Anat.*, 128:331.
501. Johansson, O., and Hokfelt, T. (1980): Thyrotropin releasing hormone, somatostatin, and enkephalin: Distribution studies using immunohistochemical techniques. *J. Histochem. Cytochem.*, 28:364.
502. Merchenthaler, I., Vigh, S., Schally, A. V., and Petrusz, P. (1984): Immunocytochemical localization of growth hormone-releasing factor in the rat hypothalamus. *Endocrinology,* 114:1082.
503. Sawchenko, P. E., Swanson, L. W., Rivier, J., and Vale, W. W. (1985): The distribution of growth-hormone-releasing factor (GRF)

immunoreactivity in the central nervous system of the rat: An immunohistochemical study using antisera directed against rat hypothalamic GRF. *J. Comp. Neurol.*, 237:100.
504. Fellmann, D., Bugnon, C., Gouget, A., and Cardot, J. (1982): Les neurones à corticoliberine (CRF) du cerveau de rat. *C. R. Soc. Biol. (Paris)*, 176:511.
505. Bugnon, C., Fellmann, D., Gouget, A., Cardot, J. (1982): Immunocytochemical detection of the CRF-containing neurons in the rat brain. *C. R. Acad. Sci. (III)*, 294:279.
506. Swanson, L. W., Sawchenko, P. E., Rivier, J., and Vale, W. W. (1983): Organization of ovine corticotropin-releasing factor immunoreactive cells and fibers in the rat brain: An immunohistochemical study. *Neuroendocrinology*, 36:165.
507. Kawata, H., Hashimoto, K., Takahara, J., and Sano, Y. (1982): Immunohistochemical demonstration of corticotropin releasing factor containing nerve fibers in the median eminence of the rat and monkey. *Histochemistry*, 76:15.
508. Vandesande, F., Dierickx, K., and DeMey, J. (1975): Identification of separate vasopressin-neurophysin II and oxytocin-neurophysin I containing nerve fibres in the external region of the bovine median eminence. *Cell Tissue Res.*, 158:509.
509. Dierickx, K., Vandesande, F., and DeMey, J. (1976): Identification, in the external region of the rat median eminence, of separate neurophysin-vasopressin and neurophysin-oxytocin containing nerve fibers. *Cell Tissue Res.*, 168:141.
510. Dierickx, K., and Vandesande, F. (1977): Immunocytochemical demonstration, in the external region of the amphibian median eminence, of separate vasotocinergic and mesotocinergic nerve fibres. *Cell Tissue Res.*, 177:47.
511. Zimmerman, E. A., and Antunes, J. L. (1976): Organization of the hypothalamic-pituitary system: Current concepts from immunohistochemical studies. *J. Histochem. Cytochem.*, 24:807.
512. Antunes, J. L., Carmel, P. W., Zimmerman, E. A. (1977): Projections from the paraventricular nucleus to the zona externa of the median eminence of the rhesus monkey: An immunohistochemical study. *Brain Res.*, 137:1.
513. Silverman, A. J. (1976): Ultrastructural studies on the localization of neurohypophyseal hormones and their carrier proteins. *J. Histochem. Cytochem.*, 24:816.
514. Kawata, M., Hashimoto, K., Takahara, J., and Sano, Y. (1983): Differences in the distributional pattern of CRF-, oxytocin-, and vasopressin-immunoreactive nerve fibers in the median eminence of the rat. *Cell Tissue Res.*, 230:247.
515. Zimmerman, E. A., Carmel, P. W., Husain, M. K., et al. (1973): Vasopressin and neurophysin: High concentrations in monkey hypophyseal portal blood. *Science*, 182:925.
516. Gibbs, D. M., and Vale, W. (1982): Presence of corticotropin releasing factor-like immunoreactivity in hypophysial portal blood. *Endocrinology*, 111:1418.
517. Gillies, G. E., Linton, E. A., and Lowry, P. J. (1982): Corticotropin releasing activity of the new CRF is potentiated several times by vasopressin. *Nature*, 299:355.
518. Rivier, C., Rivier, J., Mormede, P., and Vale, W. (1984): Studies of the nature of the interaction between vasopressin and corticotropin-releasing factor on adrenocorticotropin release in the rat. *Endocrinology*, 115:882.
519. Gibbs, D. M., Vale, W., Rivier, J., and Yen, S. S. C. (1984): Oxytocin potentiates the ACTH-releasing activity of CRF (41) but not vasopressin. *Life Sci.*, 34:2245.
520. Lind, R. W., Swanson, L. W., Bruhn, T. O., and Ganten, D. (1985): The distribution of angiotensin II-immunoreactive cells and fibers in the paraventriculo-hypophysial system of the rat. *Brain Res.*, 338:81–89.
521. Zimmerman, E. A., Liotta, A., and Krieger, D. T. (1978): β-Lipotropin in brain: Localization in hypothalamic neurons by immunoperoxidase technique. *Cell Tissue Res.*, 186:393.
522. Bloch, B., Bugnon, C., Lenys, D., and Fellmann, D. (1978): Description des neurones immunoreactifs à un immunoserum anti β-endorphin present dans le noyau infundibulaire chez l'homme. *C. R. Acad. Sci. (III)*, 287:309.
523. Bugnon, C., Bloch, B., Lenys, D., and Fellmann, D. (1979): Infundibular neurons of the human hypothalamus simultaneously reactive with antisera against endorphins, ACTH, MSH, and β-LPH. *Cell Tissue Res.*, 199:177.
524. Newman, C. B., Wardlaw, S. L., Van Vugt, D. A., Ferin, M., and Frantz, A. G. (1984): Adrenocorticotropin immunoactivity in monkey hypophyseal portal blood. *J. Clin. Endocrinol. Metab.*, 59:108.
525. Wardlow, S. L., Wehrenberg, W. B., Ferin, M., Carmel, P. W., and Frantz, A. G. (1980): High levels of β-endorphin in hypophyseal portal blood. *Endocrinology*, 106:1323.
526. Hokfelt, T., Elde, R. P., Johansson, O., Terenius, L., and Stein, L. (1977): Distribution of enkephalin-like immunoreactivity in the rat central nervous system. *Neurosci. Lett.*, 5:25.
527. Hokfelt, T., Pernow, B., Nilsson, G., Wetterberg, L., Goldstein, M., and Jeffcoate, S. L. (1978): Dense plexus of substance P immunoreactive nerve terminals in eminentia medialis of the primate hypothalamus. *Proc. Natl. Acad. Sci. USA*, 75:1013.
528. Fuxe, K., Hokfelt, T., Eneroth, P., Gustaffsson, J.-A., and Skett, P. (1977): Prolactin-like immunoreactivity: Localization in nerve terminals of rat hypothalamus. *Science*, 196:899.
529. Lechan, R. M., Nestler, J. L., and Molitch, M. E. (1981): Immunohistochemical identification of a novel substance with human growth hormone-like immunoreactivity in rat brain. *Endocrinology*, 109:1950.
530. Lechan, R. M., King, J. C., Molitch, M. E., and Aalberg, J. (1982): Immunohistochemical localization of human growth hormone-like material in the median eminence of the rat: Light and electron microscopic observations. *Neurosci. Lett.*, 30:229.
531. Page, R. B., and Bergland, R. M. (1977): The neurohypophyseal capillary bed. Part I. Anatomy and arterial supply. *Am. J. Anat.*, 148:345.
532. Page, R. B., Leure-duPree, A. E., and Bergland, R. M. (1978): The neurohypophyseal capillary bed. Part II. Specializations within median eminence. *Am. J. Anat.*, 153:33.
533. Livingston, A., and Wilks, P. N. (1976): Perivascular regions of the rat neural lobe. *Cell Tissue Res.*, 174:273.
534. Simionescu, N., Simionescu, M., and Palade, G. E. (1981): Differentiated microdomains on the luminal surface of the capillary endothelium. I. Preferential distribution of anionic sites. *J. Cell Biol.*, 90:605.
535. Simionescu, M., Simionescu, N., Silbert, J. E., and Palade, G. E. (1981): Differentiated microdomains on the luminal surface of the capillary endothelium. II. Partial characterization of their anionic sites. *J. Cell Biol.*, 90:614.
536. Wislocki, G. B. (1937): The meningeal relations of the hypophysis cerebri. II. An embryological study of the meninges and blood vessels of the human hypophysis. *Am. J. Anat.*, 61:95.
537. Enemar, A. (1961): The structure and development of the hypophysial portal system in the laboratory mouse, with particular regard to the primary plexus. *Arkh. Zool.*, 13:203.
538. Glydon, R. St. J. (1957): The development of the blood supply of the pituitary in the albino rat, with special reference to the portal vessels. *J. Anat.*, 91:237.
539. Ugrumov, M. V., Ivanova, I. P., and Mitskevich, M. S. (1983): Light- and electron-microscopic study on the maturation of the primary portal plexus during the perinatal period in rats. *Cell Tissue Res.*, 234:179.
540. Campbell, H. J. (1966): The development of the primary portal plexus in the median eminence of the rabbit. *J. Anat.*, 100:381.
541. Landsmeer, J. M. E. (1951): Vessels of the rat's hypophysis. *Acta Anat.*, 12:82.
542. McConnell, E. M. (1953): The arterial blood supply of the human hypophysis cerebri. *Anat. Rec.*, 115:175.
543. Bergland, R. M., and Page, R. B. (1978): Can the pituitary secrete directly to the brain? (Affirmative anatomical evidence). *Endocrinology*, 102:1325.
544. Bjorklund, A. (1968): Monamine-containing fibers in the neuro-intermediate lobe of the pig and rat. *Z. Zellforsch.* 89:573.
545. Page, R. B., and Dovey-Hartman, B. J. (1984): Resistance vessels in the tuber cinereum of the rabbit, rat and cat. *Anat. Rec.*, 210:647.
546. Duvernoy, H., Koritke, J. G., and Monnier, G. (1971): Sur la vascularisation du tuber posterieur chez l'homme et sur les relations vasculaires tubero-hypophysaires. *J. Neuro-Visc. Relations*, 32:112.
547. Ambach, G., Palkovits, M., and Szentagothai, J. (1976): Blood supply of the rat hypothalamus. IV. Retrochiasmatic area, median eminence, arcuate nucleus. *Acta Morphol. Acad. Sci. Hung.*, 24:93.
548. Green, H. T. (1957): The venous drainage of the human hypophysis cerebri. *Am. J. Anat.*, 100:435.

549. Torok, B. (1954): Lebendbeobachtung des hypophysenkreis-laufes an hunden. *Acta Morphol. Acad. Sci. Hung.*, 4:83.
550. Torok, B. (1964): Structure of the vascular connections of the hypothalamo-hypophyseal region. *Acta Anat.*, 59:84.
551. Houssay, B. A., Biasotti, A., and Sammartino, R. (1935): Modifications fonctionnelles du l'hypophyse apres les lesions infundibulo-tuberiennes chez le crapaud. *C. R. Soc. Biol. (Paris)*, 120:725.
552. Barnett, R. J., and Greep, R. O. (1951): The direction of blood flow in the blood vessels of the infundibular stalk. *Science*, 113:185.
553. Worthington, W. C. (1955): Some observations on the hypophyseal portal system in the living mouse. *Bull. Johns Hopkins Hosp.*, 97:343.
554. Worthington, W. C. (1960): Vascular responses in the pituitary stalk. *Endocrinology*, 66:19.
555. Page, R. B. (1983): Directional pituitary blood flow: A microcine-photographic study. *Endocrinology*, 112:157.
556. Duvernoy, H. (1972): The vascular architecture of the median eminence. In: *Brain-Endocrine Interaction. Median Eminence; Structure and Function*, edited by K. M. Knigge, D. E. Scott, and A. Weindl, p. 79. Karger, Basel.
557. Lametschwandtner, A., and Simonsberger, P. (1975): Light and scanning electron microscopical studies of the hypothalamo-adeno-hypophysial portal vessels of the toad *Bufo bufo* (L). *Cell Tissue Res.*, 162:131.
558. Page, R. B. (1982): Pituitary blood flow. *Am. J. Physiol.*, 243:E427.
559. Baez, S. (1977): Skeletal muscle and gastrointestinal microvascular morphology. In: *Microcirculation, Vol. 1*, edited by G. Kalsz and B. Altura, p. 69. University Park Press, Baltimore.
560. Sobin, S. S., and Tremer, H. M. (1977): Three-dimensional organization of microvascular beds as related to function. In: *Microcirculation, Vol. 1*, edited by G. Kalsz and B. Altura, p. 43. University Park Press, Baltimore.
561. Sobin, S. S., Tremer, H. M., and Fung, Y. C. (1970): The morphometric basis of the sheet-flow concept of the pulmonary alveolar microcirculation in the cat. *Circ. Res.*, 26:397.
562. Wittkowski, W., and Scheuer, A. (1974): Functional changes of the neuronal and glial elements at the surface of the external layer of the median eminence. *Z. Anat. Entwickl.-Gesch.*, 143:255.
563. Duvernoy, H. (1969): Considerations sur la vascularisation de l'hypophyse. *Acta Neurol. Belg.*, 69:469.
564. Duvernoy, H., and Koritke, J. G. (1964): Contribution de l'etude de l'angioarchitectonie des organes circumventriculaires. *Arch. Biol. (Suppl.)*, 75:849.
565. Duvernoy, H., and Koritke, J. G. (1968): Les vaisseaux sous-ependymaires due recessus hypophysaire. *J. Hirnforsch.*, 10:227.
566. Reymond, M. J., Speciale, S. G., and Porter, J. C. (1983): Dopamine in plasma of lateral and medial hypophysial portal vessels: Evidence for regional variation in the release of hypothalamic dopamine into hypophysial portal blood. *Endocrinology*, 112:1958.
567. Akmayev, I. G. (1971): Morphological aspects of the hypothalamic-hypophyseal system II. Functional morphology of pituitary microcirculation. *Z. Zellforsch.*, 116:178.
568. Akmayev, I. G. (1971): Morphological aspects of the hypothalamic-hypophyseal system. III. Vascularity of the hypothalamus, with special reference to its quantitative aspects. *Z. Zellforsch.*, 116:195.
569. Mezey, E., Palkovits, M., deKloet, E. R., Verhoef, J., and deWied, D. (1978): Evidence for pituitary-brain transport of a behaviorally potent ACTH analog. *Life Sci.*, 22:831.
570. Mezey, E., Palkovits, M. (1982): Two way transport in the hypothalamo-hypophysial system. In: *Frontiers in Neuroendocrinology, Vol. 7*, edited by W. F. Ganong and L. Martini, p. 1. Raven Press, New York.
571. Dorsa, D. M., deKloet, E. R., Mezey, E., and deWied, D. (1979): Pituitary-brain transport of neurotensin: Functional significance of retrograde transport. *Endocrinology*, 104:1663.
572. Gibbs, D. M. (1985): Hypothalamic epinephrine is released into hypophysial portal blood during stress. *Brain Res.*, 335:360.
573. Felten, D. L., and Cashner, K. A. (1979): Cytoarchitecture of the supraoptic nucleus. A Golgi study. *Neuroendocrinology*, 29:221.
574. Fisher, A. W. F., Price, P. G., Burford, G. D., and Lederis, K. (1979): A 3-dimensional reconstruction of the hypothalamo-neuro-hypophysial system of the rat. The neurons projecting to the neuro-intermediate lobe and those containing vasopressin and somatostatin. *Cell Tissue Res.*, 204:343.
575. LuQui, I. J., and Fox, C. A. (1976): The supraoptic nucleus and the supraoptico-hypophysial tract in the monkey *(Macaca mulatta)*. *J. Comp. Neurol.*, 168:7.
576. Sofroniew, M. V., and Glasmann, W. (1981): Golgi-like immuno-peroxidase staining of hypothalamic magnocellular neurons that contain vasopressin, oxytocin or neurophysin in the rat. *Neuroscience*, 6:619.
577. Dyball, R. E. J., Howard, M., and Kemplay, S. K. (1979): A Golgi study of the neurosecretory neurons in the supraoptic nucleus of the rat. *J. Anat.*, 128:417.
578. Renaud, L. P. (1978): Neurophysiological organization of the endocrine hypothalamus. In: *The Hypothalamus*, edited by S. Reichlin, R. J. Baldessarini, and J. B. Martin, p. 269. Raven Press, New York.
579. DeMey, J., Vandesande, F., and Dierickx, K. (1974): Identification of neurophysin producing cells. II. Identification of the neurophysin I and the neurophysin II producing neurons in the bovine hypothalamus. *Cell Tissue Res.*, 153:531.
580. Dierickx, K., and Vandesande, F. (1979): Immunocytochemical demonstration of separate vasopressin-neurophysin and oxytocin-neurophysin neurons in the human hypothalamus. *Cell Tissue Res.*, 196:203.
581. Kawata, M., and Sano, Y. (1982): Immunohistochemical identification of the oxytocin and vasopressin neurons in the hypothalamus of the monkey *(Macaca fuscata)*. *Anat. Embryol.*, 165:151.
582. Sloper, J. C., and Bateson, R. G. (1965): Ultrastructure of neurosecretory cells in the supraoptic nucleus of the dog and rat. *J. Endocrinol.*, 31:139.
583. Flament-Durand, J. (1971): Ultrastructural aspects of the paraventricular nuclei in the rat. *Z. Zellforsch.*, 116:61.
584. Morris, J. F., and Dyball, R. E. J. (1974): A quantitative study of the ultrastructural changes in the hypothalamo-neurohypophysial system during and after experimentally induced hypersecretion. *Cell Tissue Res.*, 149:525.
585. Kalimo, H. (1971): Ultrastructural studies on the hypothalamic neurosecretory neurones of the rat. I. The paraventricular neurones of the non-treated rat. *Z. Zellforsch.*, 122:283.
586. Tweedle, C. D., and Hatton, G. I. (1976): Ultrastructure comparisons of neurons of supraoptic and circularis nuclei in normal and dehydrated rats. *Brain Res. Bull.*, 1:103.
587. Nishioka, R. S., Zambrano, D., and Bern, H. A. (1970): Electron microscope radioautography of amino acid incorporation by supraoptic neurons of the rat. *Gen. Comp. Endocrinol.*, 15:477.
588. Broadwell, R. D., Oliver, C., and Brightman, M. W. (1979): Localization of neurophysin within organelles associated with protein synthesis and packaging in the hypothalamo-neurohypophysial system: An immunocytochemical study. *Proc. Natl. Acad. Sci. USA*, 76:5999.
589. Broadwell, R. D., and Oliver, C. (1981): Golgi apparatus, GERL, and secretory granule formation within neurons of the hypothalamo-neurohypophysial system of control and hyperosmotically stressed mice. *J. Cell Biol.*, 90:474.
590. Kozlowski, G. P., Frenk, S., and Brownfield, M. S. (1977): Localization of neurophysin in the rat supraoptic nucleus. I. Ultrastructural immunocytochemistry using the post-embedding technique. *Cell Tissue Res.*, 179:467.
591. Piekut, D. T. (1983): Ultrastructural characteristics of vasopressin-containing neurons in the paraventricular nucleus of the hypothalamus. *Cell Tissue Res.*, 234:125.
592. Lu, C.-L., Cantin, M., Seidah, N. G., and Chretien, M. (1982): Distribution pattern in the human pituitary and hypothalamus of a new neuropeptide: The *C*-terminal glycoprotein-fragment of human pro-pressophysin (CPP). *Histochemistry*, 75:319.
593. Pickering, B. T., Swann, R. W., Birkett, S. D., O'Shaughnessy, P., Wathes, D. C., and Porter, D. G. (1984): Precursors and products in the formation of neurohypophysial hormones. In: *Endocrinology*, edited by F. Labrie and L. Proulx, p. 653. Elsevier, New York.
594. Kalimo, H. (1975): Ultrastructural studies on the hypothalamic neurons of the rat. III. Paraventricular and supraoptic neurons during lactation and dehydration. *Cell Tissue Res.*, 163:151.
595. Gregory, W. A., Tweedle, C. D., Hatton, G. I. (1979): Ultrastructure of neurons in the paraventricular nucleus of normal, dehydrated and rehydrated rats. *Brain Res. Bull.*, 5:301.

596. Tweedle, C. D., and Hatton, G. I. (1977): Ultrastructural changes in rat hypothalamic neurosecretory cells and their associated glia during minimal dehydration and rehydration. *Cell Tissue Res.*, 181:59.
597. Epstein, Y., Castel, M., Glick, S. M., Sivan, N., and Ravid, R. (1983): Changes in hypothalamic and extra-hypothalamic vasopressin content of water-deprived rats. *Cell Tissue Res.*, 233:99.
598. Wakerley, J. B., Poulain, D. A., and Brown, D. (1978): Comparison of firing patterns in oxytocin- and vasopressin-releasing neurones during progressive dehydration. *Brain Res.*, 148:425.
599. Krisch, B. (1977): Electronmicroscopic immunocytochemical study on the vasopressin-containing neurons of the thirsting rat. *Cell Tissue Res.*, 184:237.
600. Krisch, B. (1979): Indication for a granule-free form of vasopressin in immobilization-stressed rats. *Cell Tissue Res.*, 197:95.
601. Kozlowski, G. P. (1983): Comparative ultrastructure of neuropeptide-containing cells of the parvo- and magnocellular neurosecretory system. In: *Structure and Function of Peptidergic and Aminergic Neurons*, edited by Y. Sano, Y. Ibata, and E. A. Zimmerman, p. 73. Japanese Scientific Society Press, Tokyo.
602. Alonso, G., and Assenmacher, I. (1979): The smooth endoplasmic reticulum in neurohypophysial axons of the rat: Possible involvement in transport, storage and release of neurosecretory material. *Cell Tissue Res.*, 199:415.
603. Broadwell, R. D., and Brightman, M. W. (1979): Cytochemistry of undamaged neurons transporting exogenous protein *in vivo*. *J. Comp. Neurol.*, 185:31.
604. Watson, S. J., Akil, H., Fischli, W., Goldstein, A., Zimmerman, E., Nilaver, G., and Greidanus, T. B. V. W. (1982): Dynorphin and vasopressin: Common localization in magnocellular neurons. *Science*, 216:85.
605. Millan, M. H., Millan, M. J., and Herz, A. (1984): The hypothalamic paraventricular nucleus: Relationship to brain and pituitary pools of vasopressin and oxytocin as compared to dynorphin, β-endorphin and related opioid peptides in the rat. *Neuroendocrinology*, 38:108.
606. Reaves, T. A., and Hayward, J. N. (1980): Functional and morphological studies of peptide-containing neuroendocrine cells in goldfish hypothalamus. *J. Comp. Neurol.*, 193:777.
607. Gross, J. H., Knigge, K. M., and Sheridan, M. N. (1976): Fine structure of neurons of the arcuate nucleus and median eminence of the hypothalamus of the golden hamster following immobilization. *Cell Tissue Res.*, 168:385.
608. Brawer, J. R. (1971): The role of the arcuate nucleus in the brain-pituitary-gonad axis. *J. Comp. Neurol.*, 143:411.
609. Bugnon, C., Bloch, B., and Lenys, D. (1981): Ultrastructural study of presumptive pro-opiocortin producing neurons in the rat hypothalamus. *Neuroscience*, 6:1299.
610. Lamberts, R., and Goldsmith, P. C. (1985): Preembedding colloidal gold immunostaining of hypothalamic neurons: light and electron microscopic localization of β-endorphin-immunoreactive perikaryia. *J. Histochem. Cytochem.*, 33:499.
611. Price, M. T., Olney, J. W., and Cicero, T. J. (1976): Proliferation of lamellar whorls in arcuate neurons of the hypothalamus of castrated and morphine-treated male rats. *Cell Tissue Res.*, 171:277.
612. King, J. C., Williams, T. H., and Gerall, A. A. (1974): Transformation of hypothalamic arcuate neurons. I. Changes associated with stages of the estrous cycle. *Cell Tissue Res.*, 153:497.
613. Nishizuka, M., and Kawashima, S. (1979): The neurons containing dense core vesicles in the mouse hypothalamic arcuate nucleus: Distribution and influence of ovarian activity. *Acta Anat.*, 105:452.
614. King, J. C., and Gerall, A. A. (1976): Localization of luteinizing hormone-releasing hormone. *J. Histochem. Cytochem.*, 24:829.
615. Hisano, S., Kawano, H., Nishiyama, T., and Daikoku, S. (1982): Immunoreactive ACTH/β-endorphin neurons in the tuber-infundibular hypothalamus of rats. *Cell Tissue Res.*, 224:303.
616. Pelletier, G., and Leclerc, R. (1979): Immunohistochemical localization of adrenocorticotropin in the rat brain. *Endocrinology*, 104: 1426.
617. Jennes, L., Stumpf, W. E., and Sheedy, M. E. (1985): Ultrastructural characterization of gonadotropin-releasing hormone (GnRH)-producing neurons. *J. Comp. Neurol.*, 232:534.
618. Johansson, O., Hokfelt, T., Jeffcoate, S. L., White, N., and Sternberger, L. A. (1980): Ultrastructural localization of TRH-like immunoreactivity. *Exp. Brain Res.*, 38:1.
619. Ibata, Y., Obata, H. L., Kubo, S., Fukui, K., Okamura, H., Ishigami, T., Imagawa, K., and Sin, S. (1983): Some cellular characteristics of somatostatin neurons and terminals in the periventricular nucleus of the rat hypothalamus and median eminence. Electron microscopic immunohistochemistry. *Brain Res.*, 258:291.
620. Crosby, E. C., and Showers, M. J. C. (1969): Comparative anatomy of the preoptic and hypothalamic areas. In: *The Hypothalamus*, edited by W. Haymaker, E. Anderson, and W. J. H. Nauta, p. 61. Charles C Thomas, Springfield, Ill.
621. Nauta, W. J. H., and Haymaker, W. (1969): Hypothalamic nuclei and fiber connections. In: *The Hypothalamus*, edited by W. Haymaker, E. Anderson, and W. J. H. Nauta, p. 136. Charles C Thomas, Springfield, Ill.
622. Papez, J. W. (1940): The embryologic development of the hypothalamic area in mammals. *Res. Publ. Assoc. Res. Nerv. Ment. Dis.*, 20:31.
623. Christ, J. F. (1969): Derivation and boundaries of the hypothalamus with atlas of hypothalamic grisea. In: *The Hypothalamus*, edited by W. Haymaker, E. Anderson, and W. J. H. Nauta, p. 13. Charles C Thomas, Springfield, Ill.
624. Coggeshall, R. E. (1964): A study of diencephalic development in the albino rat. *J. Comp. Neurol.*, 122:241.
625. Hyyppa, M. (1969): Differentiation of the hypothalamic nuclei during ontogenetic development in the rat. *Z. Anat. Entwickl.-Gesch.*, 129:41.
626. Altman, J., and Bayer, S. A. (1978): Development of the diencephalon in the rat. I. Autoradiographic study of the time of origin and settling patterns of neurons of the hypothalamus. *J. Comp. Neurol.*, 182:945.
627. Altman, J., and Bayer, S. A. (1978): Development of the diencephalon in the rat. II. Correlation of the embryonic development of the hypothalamus with the time of origin of its neurons. *J. Comp. Neurol.*, 182:973.
628. Choy, V. J., and Watkins, W. B. (1979): Maturation of the hypothalamo-neurohypophysial system. I. Localization of neurophysin, oxytocin and vasopressin in the hypothalamus and neural lobe of the developing rat brain. *Cell Tissue Res.*, 197:325.
629. Karim, M. A., and Sloper, J. C. (1980): Histogenesis of the supraoptic and paraventricular neurosecretory cells of the mouse hypothalamus. *J. Anat.*, 130:341.
630. Okamura, H., Fukui, K., Koyama, E., Tsutou, H. L. O., Tsutou, T., Terubayashi, H., Fujisawa, H., and Ibata, Y. (1983): Time of vasopressin neuron origin in the mouse hypothalamus: Examination of combined technique of immunocytochemistry and (^{3}H)thymidine autoradiography. *Dev. Brain Res.*, 9:223.
631. Wyss, J. M., Sripanidkulchai, B. (1985): An autoradiographic analysis of the time of origin of neurons in the hypothalamus of the cat. *Dev. Brain Res.*, 21:89.
632. Schwanzel-Fukuda, M., Morrell, J. I., Pfaff, D. W. (1985): Ontogenesis of neurons producing luteinizing hormone-releasing hormone (LHRH) in the nervus terminalis of the rat. *J. Comp. Neurol.*, 238:348.
633. Krisch, B. (1980): Electron microscopic immunocytochemical investigation on the postnatal development of the vasopressin system in the rat. *Cell Tissue Res.*, 205:453.
634. Koritsanszky, S. (1979): Cyto- and synaptogenesis in the arcuate nucleus of the rat hypothalamus during fetal and early postnatal life. *Cell Tissue Res.*, 200:135.
635. Dale, H. (1935): Pharmacology and nerve-endings. *Proc. R. Soc. Med.*, 28:319.
636. Ingram, W. R. (1940): Nuclear organization and chief connections of the primate hypothalamus. *Proc. Assoc. Res. Nerv. Ment. Dis.*, 20:195.
637. Defendini, R., and Zimmerman, E. A. (1978): The magnocellular neurosecretory system of the mammalian hypothalamus. In: *The Hypothalamus*, edited by S. Reichlin, R. J. Baldessarini, and J. B. Martin, p. 137. Raven Press, New York.
638. Broadwell, R. D., and Bleier, R. (1976): A cytoarchitectonic atlas of the mouse hypothalamus. *J. Comp. Neurol.*, 167:315.
639. Peterson, R. P. (1966): Magnocellular neurosecretory centers in the rat hypothalamus. *J. Comp. Neurol.*, 128:181.
640. Rhodes, C. H., Morrell, J. I., Pfaff, D. W. (1981): Immunohistochemical analysis of magnocellular elements in rat hypothalamus: Distribution and numbers of cells containing neurophysin, oxytocin and vasopressin. *J. Comp. Neurol.*, 198:45.

641. Rasmussen, A. T. (1940): Effects of hypophysectomy and hypophysial stalk resection on the hypothalamic nuclei of animals and man. *Proc. Assoc. Res. Nerv. Ment. Dis.*, 20:245.
642. Raisman, G. (1973): An ultrastructural study of the effects of hypophysectomy on the supraoptic nucleus of the rat. *J. Comp. Neurol.*, 147:181.
643. Sherlock, D. A., Field, P. M., and Raisman, G. (1975): Retrograde transport of horseradish peroxidase in the magnocellular neurosecretory system of the rat. *Brain Res.*, 88:403.
644. Price, P., and Fisher, A. W. F. (1978): Electron microscopical study of retrograde transport of horseradish peroxidase in the supraoptico-hypophyseal tract in the rat. *J. Anat.*, 125:137.
645. DeVries, G. J., Buijs, R. M., VanLeeuwen, F. W., Caffe, A. R., and Swaab, D. F. (1985): The vasopressinergic innervation of the brain in normal and castrated rats. *J. Comp. Neurol.*, 233:236.
646. Simpson, J. B. (1981): The circumventricular organs and the central actions of angiotensin. *Neuroendocrinology*, 32:248.
647. Brownfield, M. S., and Kozlowski, G. P. (1977): The hypothalamo-choroidal tract. I. Immunohistochemical demonstration of neurophysin pathways to telencephalic choroid plexuses and cerebrospinal fluid. *Cell Tissue Res.*, 178:111.
648. Swanson, L. W., and Kuypers, H. G. J. M. (1980): The paraventricular nucleus of the hypothalamus: Cytoarchitectonic subdivisions and organization of projections to the pituitary, dorsal vagal complex, and spinal cord as demonstrated by retrograde fluorescence double-labeling methods. *J. Comp. Neurol.*, 194:555.
649. Wiegand, S. J., and Price, J. L. (1980): Cells of origin of the afferent fibers to the median eminence in the rat. *J. Comp. Neurol.*, 192:1.
650. Krieg, W. J. S. (1932): The hypothalamus of the albino rat. *J. Comp. Neurol.*, 55:19.
651. Van Den Pol, A. N. (1982): The magnocellular and parvocellular paraventricular nucleus of rat: intrinsic organization. *J. Comp. Neurol.*, 206:317.
652. Armstrong, W. E., Warach, S., Hatton, G. I., and McNeill, T. H. (1980): Subnuclei in the rat hypothalamic paraventricular nucleus: A cytoarchitectural, horseradish peroxidase and immunocytochemical analysis. *Neuroscience*, 5:1931.
653. Hatton, G. I., Hutton, U. E., Hoblitzell, E. R., and Armstrong, W. E. (1976): Morphological evidence for two populations of magnocellular elements in the rat paraventricular nucleus. *Brain Res.*, 108:187.
654. Sawchenko, P. E., and Swanson, L. W. (1982): Immunohistochemical identification of neurons in the paraventricular nucleus of the hypothalamus that project to the medulla or to the spinal cord in rat. *J. Comp. Neurol.*, 205:260.
655. Ono, T., Nishino, H., Sasaka, K., Muramoto, K., Yano, I., and Simpson, A. (1978): Paraventricular nucleus connections to spinal cord and pituitary. *Neurosci. Lett.*, 10:141.
656. Antunes, J. L., Carmel, P. W., and Zimmerman, E. A. (1977): Projections from the paraventricular nucleus to the zona externa of the median eminence of the rhesus monkey: An immunohistochemical study. *Brain Res.*, 137:1.
657. Vandesande, F., Dierickx, K., and DeMey, J. (1977): The origin of the vasopressinergic and oxytocinergic fibres of the external region of the median eminence of the rat hypophysis. *Cell Tissue Res.*, 180:443.
658. Silverman, A. J., Hoffman, D., Gadde, C. A., Krey, L. C., and Zimmerman, E. A. (1981): Adrenal steroid inhibition of the vasopressin-neurophysin neurosecretory system to the median eminence of the rat. *Neuroendocrinology*, 32:129.
659. Silverman, A. J., and Zimmerman, E. A. (1982): Adrenalectomy increases sprouting in a peptidergic neurosecretory system. *Neuroscience*, 7:2705.
660. Rivier, C., and Vale, W. (1983): Interaction of corticotropin-releasing factor and arginine vasopressin on adrenocorticotropin secretion *in vivo*. *Endocrinology*, 113:939.
661. Lechan, R. M., Nestler, J. L., Jacobson, S., and Reichlin, S. (1980): The hypothalamic "tuberoinfundibular" system of the rat as demonstrated by horseradish peroxidase (HRP) microiontophoresis. *Brain Res.*, 195:13.
662. Lechan, R. M., Nestler, J. L., and Jacobson, S. (1982): The tuberoinfundibular system of the rat as demonstrated by immunohistochemical localization of retrogradely transported wheat germ agglutinin (WGA) from the median eminence. *Brain Res.*, 245:1.
663. Zimmerman, E. A., Hou-Yu, A., Nilaver, G., Valiquette, G., and Silverman, A.-J. (1983): Organization of the oxytocin and vasopressin systems of the hypothalamus: Intra- and extra-hypothalamic projections. In: *Structure and Function of Peptidergic and Aminergic Neurons*, edited by Y. Sano, Y. Ibata, and E. A. Zimmerman, p. 1. Japanese Scientific Society Press, Tokyo.
664. Armstrong, W. E., and Hatton, G. I. (1980): The localization of projection neurons in the rat hypothalamic paraventricular nucleus following vascular and neurohypophysial injections of HRP. *Brain Res. Bull.*, 5:473.
665. Swanson, L. W., and Sawchenko, P. E. (1983): Hypothalamic integration: Organization of the paraventricular and supraoptic nuclei. *Annu. Rev. Neurosci.*, 6:269.
666. Dierickx, K., and Vandesande, F. (1979): Immunocytochemical localization of somatostatin-containing neurons in the rat hypothalamus. *Cell Tissue Res.*, 201:349.
667. Krisch, B. (1978): Hypothalamic and extrahypothalamic distribution of somatostatin immunoreactive elements in the rat brain. *Cell Tissue Res.*, 195:499.
668. Elde, R. P., and Parsons, J. A. (1975): Immunocytochemical localization of somatostatin in cell bodies of the rat hypothalamus. *Am. J. Anat.*, 144:541.
669. Bennett-Clarke, C., Romagnano, M. A., and Joseph, S. A. (1980): Distribution of somatostatin in the rat brain: Telencephalon and diencephalon. *Brain Res.*, 188:473.
670. Jackson, I. M. D., Wu, P., and Lechan, R. M. (1985): Immunohistochemical localization in the rat brain of the precursor for thyrotropin-releasing hormone. *Science*, 229:1097.
671. Lechan, R. M., Wu, P., Jackson, I., Wolf, H., Cooperman, S., Mandel, G., and Goodman, R. H. (1986): Thyrotropin-releasing hormone precursor: characterization in rat brain. *Science*, 231:159.
672. Lechan, R. M., Molitch, M. E., and Jackson, I. M. D. (1983): Distribution of immunoreactive human growth hormone-like material and thyrotropin-releasing hormone in the rat central nervous system: evidence for their coexistence in the same neurons. *Endocrinology*, 112:877.
673. Paull, W. K., Scholer, J., Arimura, A., Meyers, C. A., Chang, J. K., Chang, D., and Shimizu, M. (1982): Immunocytochemical localization of CRF in the ovine hypothalamus. *Peptides*, 1:183.
674. Kolodziejczyk, E., Baertschi, A. J., and Tramu, G. (1983): Corticoliberin-immunoreactive cell bodies localised in two distinct areas of the sheep hypothalamus. *Neuroscience*, 9:261.
675. Merchenthaler, I., Vigh, S., Petrusz, P., and Schally, A. V. (1982): Immunocytochemical localization of corticotropin-releasing factor (CRF) in the rat brain. *Am. J. Anat.*, 165:385.
676. Joseph, S. A., Knigge, K. M. (1983): Corticotropin releasing factor: Immunocytochemical localization in rat brain. *Neurosci. Lett.*, 35:135.
677. Tilders, F. J. H., Schipper, J., Lowry, P. J., Vermes, I. (1982): Effect of hypothalamus lesions on the presence of CRF-immunoreactive nerve terminals in the median eminence and on the pituitary-adrenal response to stress. *Regul. Pept.*, 5:77.
678. Paull, W. K., and Gibbs, F. P. (1983): The corticotropin releasing factor (CRF) neurosecretory system in intact, adrenalectomized, adrenalectomized-dexamethasone treated rats. *Histochemistry*, 78:303.
679. Roth, K. A., Weber, E., and Barchas, J. D. (1982): Immunoreactive corticotropin releasing factor (CRF) and vasopressin are colocalized in a subpopulation of the immunoreactive vasopressin cells in the paraventricular nucleus of the hypothalamus. *Life Sci.*, 31:1857.
680. Kawata, M., Hashimoto, K., Takahara, J., and Sano, Y. (1982): Immunohistochemical demonstration of the localization of corticotropin releasing factor-containing neurons in the hypothalamus of mammals including primates. *Anat. Embryol.*, 165:303.
681. Kawata, M., Hashimoto, K., Takahara, J., and Sano, Y. (1983): Immunohistochemical identification of neurons containing corticotropin-releasing factor in the rat hypothalamus. *Cell Tissue Res.*, 230:239.
682. Taniguchi, Y. (1984): Immunohistochemical evidence against the coexistence of a corticotropin-releasing factor and oxytocin or vasopressin in the rat paraventricular nucleus. *Arch. Histol. Jpn.*, 47:475.
683. Kiss, J. Z., Mezey, E., and Skirboll, L. (1984): Corticotropin-releasing factor-immunoreactive neurons of the paraventricular nucleus become vasopressin positive after adrenalectomy. *Proc. Natl. Acad. Sci. USA*, 81:1854.

684. Swanson, L. W., Sawchenko, P. E., Berod, A., Hartman, B. K., Helle, K. B., and Vanorden, D. E. (1981): An immunohistochemical study of the organization of catecholamine cells and terminal fields in the paraventricular and supraoptic nuclei of the hypothalamus. *J. Comp. Neurol.*, 196:271.
685. Hokfelt, T., Fahrenkrug, J., Tatemoto, K., Mutt, V., Werner, S., Hulting, A.-L., Terenius, L., and Chang, K. J. (1983): The PHI (PHI-27)/corticotropin-releasing factor/enkephalin immunoreactive hypothalamic neuron: Possible morphological basis for integrated control of prolactin, corticotropin, and growth hormone secretion. *Proc. Natl. Acad. Sci. USA*, 80:895.
686. Palkovits, M. (1982): Neuropeptides in the median eminence: Their sources and destinations. *Peptides*, 3:299.
687. Swanson, L. W., Sawchenko, P. E., Wiegand, S. J., and Price, J. L. (1980): Separate neurons in the paraventricular nucleus project to the median eminence and to the medulla or spinal cord. *Brain Res.*, 198:190.
688. Sofroniew, M. V., and Schrell, U. (1981): Evidence for a direct projection from oxytocin and vasopressin neurons in the hypothalamic paraventricular nucleus to the medulla oblongata: Immunohistochemical visualization of both the horseradish peroxidase. *Neurosci. Lett.*, 22:211.
689. Sawchenko, P. E., and Swanson, L. W. (1982): Immunohistochemical identification of neurons in the paraventricular nucleus of the hypothalamus that project to the medulla or to the spinal cord in the rat. *J. Comp. Neurol.*, 205:260.
690. Swanson, L. W. (1977): Immunohistochemical evidence for a neurophysin-containing autonomic pathway arising in the paraventricular nucleus of the hypothalamus. *Brain Res.*, 128:346.
691. Caverson, M. M., Ciriello, J., and Calaresu, F. R. (1984): Paraventricular nucleus of the hypothalamus: An electrophysiological investigation of neurons projecting directly to intermediolateral nucleus in the cat. *Brain Res.*, 305:380.
692. Sofroniew, M. V. (1980): Projections from vasopressin, oxytocin and neurophysin neurons to neural targets in the rat and human. *J. Histochem. Cytochem.*, 28:475.
693. Buijs, R. M. (1978): Intra- and extrahypothalamic vasopressin and oxytocin pathways in the rat. *Cell Tissue Res.*, 192:423.
694. Buijs, R. M., and Swaab, D. F. (1979): Immuno-electron microscopical demonstration of vasopressin and oxytocin synapses in the limbic system of the rat. *Cell Tissue Res.*, 204:355.
695. DeVries, G. J., Buijs, R. M. (1983): The origin of the vasopressinergic and oxytocinergic innervation of the rat brain with special reference to the lateral septum. *Brain Res.*, 273:307.
696. Conrad, L. C. A., and Pfaff, D. W. (1976): Efferents from medial basal forebrain and hypothalamus in the rat. II. An autoradiographic study of the anterior hypothalamus. *J. Comp. Neurol.*, 169:221.
697. Alpert, L. C., Brawer, J. R., Patel, Y. C., and Reichlin, S. (1976): Somatostatinergic neurons in anterior hypothalamus: Immunohistochemical localization. *Endocrinology*, 98:225.
698. Crowley, W. R., and Terry, L. C. (1980): Biochemical mapping of somatostatinergic systems in rat brain: Effects of periventricular hypothalamic and medial basal amygdaloid lesions on somatostatin-like immunoreactivity in discrete brain nuclei. *Brain Res.*, 200:283.
699. Krisch, B. (1981): Somatostatin-immunoreactive fiber projections into the brain stem and the spinal cord of the rat. *Cell Tissue Res.*, 217:531.
700. Finley, J. C. W., Maderdrut, J. L., and Petrusz, P. (1981): The immunocytochemical localization of enkephalin in the central nervous system of the rat. *J. Comp. Neurol.*, 198:541.
701. Chan-Palay, V., Zaborszky, L., Kohler, C., Goldstein, M., and Palay, S. L. (1984): Distribution of tyrosine-hydroxylase-immunoreactive neurons in the hypothalamus of rats. *J. Comp. Neurol.*, 227:467.
702. Ibata, Y., Kawakami, F., Fukui, K., Obata-Tsuto, H. L., Tanaka, M., Kubo, T., Okamura, H., Morimoto, N., Yanaihara, C., and Yanaihara, N. (1984): Light and electron microscopic immunocytochemistry of neurotensin-like immunoreactive neurons in the rat hypothalamus. *Brain Res.*, 302:221.
703. Crosby, E. C., and Woodburne, R. T. (1966): The comparative anatomy of the preoptic area and the hypothalamus. *Res. Publ. Assoc. Res. Nerv. Ment. Dis.*, 20:52.
704. Van Den Pol, A. N., and Cassidy, J. R. (1982): The hypothalamic arcuate nucleus of rat—A quantitative Golgi analysis. *J. Comp. Neurol.*, 204:65.
705. Walsh, R. J., and Brawer, J. R. (1979): Cytology of the arcuate nucleus in newborn male and female rats. *J. Anat.*, 128:121.
706. Bodoky, M., and Rethelyi, M. (1977): Dendritic arborization and axon trajectory of neurons in the hypothalamic arcuate nucleus of the rat. *Exp. Brain Res.*, 28:543.
707. Ottersen, O. P. (1980): Afferent connections to the amygdaloid complex of the rat and cat. II. Afferents from the hypothalamus and the basal telencephalon. *J. Comp. Neurol.*, 194:267.
708. Fuxe, K. (1965): Evidence for the existence of monoamine neurons in the central nervous system. III. The monoamine nerve terminal. *Z. Zellforsch.*, 65:573.
709. Fuxe, K., and Hokfelt, T. (1966): Further evidence for the existence of tubero-infundibular dopamine neurons. *Acta Physiol. Scand.*, 66:245.
710. Lichthensteiger, W., and Langemann, H. (1966): Uptake of exogenous catecholamines by monoamine-containing neurons of the central nervous system: Uptake of catecholamines by arcuato-infundibular neurons. *J. Pharm. Exp. Ther.*, 151:400.
711. Fuxe, K., and Hokfelt, T. (1969): Catecholamines in the hypothalamus and the pituitary gland. In: *Frontiers in Neuroendocrinology*, edited by W. F. Ganong and L. Martini, p. 47. Oxford University Press, New York.
712. Bjorklund, A., and Nobin, A. (1973): Fluorescence histochemical and microspectrofluorometric mapping of dopamine and noradrenaline cell groups in the rat diencephalon. *Brain Res.*, 51:193.
713. Bjorklund, A., Falck, B., Hromek, F., Owman, C., and West, K. A. (1970): Identification and terminal distribution of the tubero-hypophyseal monoamine fibre systems in the rat by means of stereotaxic and microspectrofluorimetric techniques. *Brain Res.*, 17:1.
714. Jonsson, G., Fuxe, K., and Hokfelt, T. (1972): On the catecholamine innervation of the hypothalamus, with special reference to the median eminence. *Brain Res.*, 40:271.
715. Smith, G. C., and Fink, G. (1972): Experimental studies on the origin of monoamine-containing fibres in the hypothalamo-hypophysial complex of the rat. *Brain Res.*, 43:37.
716. Nojyo, Y., Ibata, Y., and Sano, Y. (1976): Demonstration of tuberoinfundibular tract of the cat. *Cell Tissue Res.*, 168:289.
717. Palkovits, M., Brownstein, M., Saavedra, J. M., and Axelrod, J. (1974): Norepinephrine and dopamine content of hypothalamic nuclei of the rat. *Brain Res.*, 77:137.
718. Nishizuka, M. (1979): Topography of the dopamine neurons in the arcuate nucleus of the mouse hypothalamus. *Acta Anat.*, 103:34.
719. Bugnon, C., Bloch, B., Lenys, D., Gouget, A., and Fellmann, D. (1979): Comparative study of the neuronal populations containing β-endorphin, corticotropin and dopamine in the arcuate nucleus of the rat hypothalamus. *Neurosci. Lett.*, 14:43.
720. Selmanoff, M. K., Wise, P. M., and Barraclough, C. A. (1980): Regional distribution of luteinizing hormone-releasing hormone (LH-RH) in rat brain determined by microdissection and radioimmunoassay. *Brain Res.*, 192:421.
721. Silverman, A. J., and Zimmerman, E. A. (1978): Pathways containing luteinizing hormone-releasing hormone (LHRH) in the mammalian brain. In: *Brain-Endocrine Interaction. III. Neural Hormones and Reproduction*, edited by D. E. Scott, G. P. Kozlowski, and A. Weindl, p. 83. Karger, Basel.
722. Kozlowski, G. P., Nett, T. M., and Zimmerman, E. A. (1975): Immunocytochemical localization of gonadotropin-releasing hormone (Gn-RH) and neurophysin in the brain. In: *Anatomical Neuroendocrinology*, edited by W. E. Stumpf, and L. D. Grant, p. 185. Karger, Basel.
723. Kawano, H., and Daikoku, S. (1981): Immunohistochemical demonstration of LHRH neurons and their pathways in the rat hypothalamus. *Neuroendocrinology*, 32:179.
724. Silverman, A. J., Antunes, J. L., Ferin, M., and Zimmerman, E. A. (1977): The distribution of luteinizing hormone-releasing hormone (LHRH) in the hypothalamus of the rhesus monkey. Light microscopic studies using immunoperoxidase technique. *Endocrinology*, 101:134.
725. Barry, J. (1976): Characterization and topography of LH-RH neurons in the rabbit. *Neurosci. Lett.*, 2:201.

726. Silverman, A. J., and Krey, L. C. (1978): The luteinizing hormone-releasing hormone (LH-RH) neuronal networks of the guinea pig brain. I. Intra- and extrahypothalamic projections. *Brain Res.*, 157:233.
727. King, J. C., Anthony, E. L. P., Gustafson, A. W., and Damassa, D. A. (1984): Luteinizing hormone-releasing hormone (LH-RH) cells and their projections in the forebrain of the bat *Myotis lucifugus lucifugus*. *Brain Res.*, 298:289.
728. Barry, J. (1976): Characterization and topography of LH-RH neurons in the human brain. *Neurosci. Lett.*, 3:287.
729. Barry, J. (1977): Immunofluorescence study of LRF neurons in man. *Cell Tissue Res.*, 181:1.
730. King, J. C., Anthony, E. L. P., Fitzgerald, D. M., and Stopa, E. G. (1985): Luteinizing hormone-releasing hormone neurons in human preoptic/hypothalamus: Differential intraneuronal localization of immunoreactive forms. *J. Clin. Endocrinol. Metab.*, 60:88.
731. Rossier, J., Vargo, T. M., Minick, S., Ling, N., Bloom, F. E., and Guillemin, R. (1977): Regional distribution of β-endorphin and enkephalin contents in rat brain and pituitary. *Proc. Natl. Acad. Sci. USA*, 74:5162.
732. Oliver, C., and Porter, J. C. (1978): Distribution and characterization of α-melanocyte-stimulating hormone in the rat brain. *Endocrinology*, 102:697.
733. Eskay, R. L., Giraud, P., Oliver, C., and Brownstein, M. J. (1979): Distribution of α-melanocyte-stimulating hormone in the rat brain: Evidence that α-MSH-containing cells in the arcuate region send projections to extrahypothalamic areas. *Brain Res.*, 178:55.
734. Liotta, A. S., Gildersleeve, D., Brownstein, M. J., and Krieger, D. T. (1979): Biosynthesis *in vitro* of immunoreactive 31,000-dalton corticotropin/β-endorphin-like material by bovine hypothalamus. *Proc. Natl. Acad. Sci. USA*, 76:1448.
735. Watson, S. J., Barchas, J. D., and Li, C. H. (1977): β-Lipotropin: Localization of cells and axons in rat brain by immunocytochemistry. *Proc. Natl. Acad. Sci. USA*, 74:5155.
736. Nilaver, G., Zimmerman, E. A., Defendini, R., Liotta, A. S., Krieger, D. T., and Brownstein, M. J. (1979): Adrenocorticotropin and β-lipotropin in the hypothalamus. Localization in the same arcuate neurons by sequential immunocytochemical procedures. *J. Cell Biol.*, 81:50.
737. Sofroniew, M. V. (1979): Immunoreactive β-endorphin and ACTH in the same neurons of the hypothalamic arcuate nucleus in the rat. *Am. J. Anat.*, 154:283.
738. Hisano, S., Kawano, H., Nishiyama, T., and Daikoku, S. (1982): Immunoreactive ACTH/β-endorphin neurons in the tubero-infundibular hypothalamus of rats. *Cell Tissue Res.*, 224:303.
739. Bloch, B., Bugnon, C., Fellmann, D., Lenys, D., and Gouget, A. (1979): Neurons of the rat hypothalamus reactive with antisera against endorphins, ACTH, MSH and β-LPH. *Cell Tissue Res.*, 204:1.
740. Bloch, B., Bugnon, C., Fellmann, D., and Lenys, D. (1978): Immunocytochemical evidence that the same neurons in the human infundibular nucleus are stained with anti-endorphins and antisera of other related peptides. *Neurosci. Lett.*, 10:147.
741. Bloch, B., Bugnon, C., Fellmann, D., and Lenys, D. (1978): Presence de determinants antigeniques de la β-LPH, de la β-MSH, de l'α-endorphine, de l'ACTH et de l'α-MSH dans les neurones reveles par l'anti-β-endorphine au niveau du noyau infundibulaire de l'Homme. *C. R. Acad. Sci. (III)*, 287:1019.
742. Bugnon, C., Bloch, B., Lenys, D., and Fellmann, D. (1979): Infundibular neurons of the human hypothalamus simultaneously reactive with antisera against endorphins, ACTH, MSH and β-LPH. *Cell Tissue Res.*, 199:177.
743. Sawchenko, P. E., Swanson, L. W., and Joseph, S. A. (1982): The distribution and cells of origin of ACTH(1-39)-stained varicosities in the paraventricular and supraoptic nuclei. *Brain Res.*, 232:365.
744. Bloch, B., Brazeau, P., Bloom, F., and Ling, N. (1983): Topographical study of the neurons containing hpGRF immunoreactivity in monkey hypothalamus. *Neurosci. Lett.*, 37:23.
745. Lechan, R. M., Lin, H. D., Ling, N., Jackson, I. M. D., Jacobson, S., and Reichlin, S. (1984): Distribution of immunoreactive growth hormone releasing factor (1-44) NH_2 in the tuberoinfundibular system of the rhesus monkey. *Brain Res.*, 309:55.
746. Bugnon, C., Gouget, A., Fellmann, D., and Clavequin, M. C. (1983): Immunocytochemical demonstration of a novel peptidergic neurone system in the cat brain with an anti-growth hormone-releasing factor serum. *Neurosci. Lett.*, 38:131.
747. Bloch, B., Brazeau, P., Ling, N., Bohlen, P., Esch, F., Wehrenberg, W. B., Benoit, R., Bloom, F., and Guillemin, R. (1983): Immunohistochemical detection of growth hormone-releasing factor in brain. *Nature*, 301:607.
748. Fellmann, D., Bugnon, C., and Lavry, G. N. (1985): Immunohistochemical demonstration of a new neurone system in rat brain using antibodies against human growth hormone-releasing factor (1-37). *Neurosci. Lett.*, 58:91.
749. Merchenthaler, I., Vigh, S., Schally, A. V., and Petrusz, P. (1984): Immunocytochemical localization of growth hormone-releasing factor in the rat hypothalamus. *Endocrinology*, 114:1082.
750. Bloch, R., Ling, N., Benoit, R., Wehrenberg, W. B., and Guillemin, R. (1984): Specific depletion of immunoreactive growth hormone-releasing factor by monosodium glutamate in rat median eminence. *Nature*, 307:272.
751. Holzwarth-McBride, M. A., Hurst, E. M., and Knigge, K. M. (1976): Monosodium glutamate induced lesions of the arcuate nucleus. I. Endocrine deficiency and ultrastructure of the median eminence. *Anat. Rec.*, 186:185.
752. Holzwarth-McBride, M. A., Sladek, J. R., and Knigge, K. M. (1976): Monosodium glutamate induced lesions of the arcuate nucleus. II. Fluorescence histochemistry of catecholamines. *Anat. Rec.*, 186:197.
753. Ibata, Y., Fukui, K., Okamura, H., Kawakami, T., Tanaka, M., Obata, H. L., Tsuto, T., Terubayashi, H., Yanaihara, C., and Yanaihara, N. (1983): Coexistence of dopamine and neurotensin in hypothalamic arcuate and periventricular neurons. *Brain Res.*, 269:177.
754. Hokfelt, T., Everitt, B. J., Theodorsson-Norheim, E., and Goldstein, M. (1984): Occurrence of neurotensinlike immunoreactivity in subpopulations of hypothalamic, mesencephalic, and medullary catecholamine neurons. *J. Comp. Neurol.*, 222:543.
755. Tsuruo, Y., Kawano, H., Nishiyama, T., Hisano, S., and Daikoku, S. (1983): Substance P-like immunoreactive neurons in the tuberinfundibular area of rat hypothalamus, light and electron microscopy. *Brain Res.*, 289:1.
756. Johansson, O., and Hokfelt, T. (1980): Thyrotropin-releasing hormone, somatostatin, and enkephalin: distribution studies using immunohistochemical techniques. *J. Histochem. Cytochem.*, 28:364.
757. Khachaturian, H., Lewis, M. E., and Watson, S. J. (1983): Enkephalin systems in diencephalon and brainstem of the rat. *J. Comp. Neurol.*, 220:310.
758. Sofroniew, M. V., and Weindl, A. (1980): Identification of parvocellular vasopressin and neurophysin neurons in the suprachiasmatic nucleus of a variety of mammals including primates. *J. Comp. Neurol.*, 193:659.
759. Sofroniew, M. V., and Weindl, A. (1978): Projections from the parvocellular vasopressin- and neurophysin-containing neurons of the suprachiasmatic nucleus. *Am. J. Anat.*, 153:391.
760. Hoorneman, E. M. D., and Buijs, R. M. (1982): Vasopressin fiber pathways in the rat brain following suprachiasmatic nucleus lesioning. *Brain Res.*, 243:235.
761. Krieger, M. S., Conrad, L. C. A., and Pfaff, D. W. (1979): An autoradiographic study of the efferent connections of the ventromedial nucleus of the hypothalamus. *J. Comp. Neurol.*, 183:785.
762. Saper, C. B., Swanson, L. W., and Cowan, W. M. (1976): The efferent connections of the ventromedial nucleus of the hypothalamus of the rat. *J. Comp. Neurol.*, 169:409.
763. Saper, C. B., Swanson, L. W., and Cowan, W. M. (1979): Some efferent connections of the rostral hypothalamus in the squirrel monkey (*Saimiri sciureus*) and cat. *J. Comp. Neurol.*, 184:205.
764. Conrad, L. C. A., and Pfaff, D. W. (1976): Efferents from medial basal forebrain and hypothalamus in the rat. II. An autoradiographic study of the anterior hypothalamus. *J. Comp. Neurol.*, 169:221.
765. Hammel, H. T. (1968): Regulation of internal body temperature. *Annu. Rev. Physiol.*, 30:641.
766. Squires, R. D., and Jacobson, F. H. (1968): Chronic deficits of temperature regulation produced in cats by preoptic lesions. *Am. J. Physiol.*, 214:549.
767. Ramsay, D. J., Thrasher, T. N., and Keil, L. C. (1983): The organum vasculosum laminae terminalis: A critical area for osmoreception. *Prog. Brain Res.*, 60:91.
768. Brody, M. J., and Johnson, A. K. (1980): Role of the anteroventral third ventricle region in fluid and electrolyte balance, arterial pressure regulation, and hypertension. In: *Frontiers in Neuroendocrinology,*

Vol. 6, edited by L. Martini and W. F Ganong, p. 249. Raven Press, New York.
769. Saphier, D., and Feldman, S. (1986): Effects of stimulation of the preoptic area on hypothalamic paraventricular nucleus unit activity and corticosterone secretion in freely moving rats. *Neuroendocrinology,* 42:167.
770. Struyker-Boudier, H. S., Smeets, G., Brouwer, G., and Van Rossum, J. M. (1975): Central nervous system a-adrenergic mechanisms and cardiovascular regulation in rats. *Arch. Int. Pharmacodyn.,* 213:285.
771. Gorski, R. A. (1984): Critical role for the medial preoptic area in the sexual differentiation of the brain. *Prog. Brain Res.,* 61:129.
772. Arendash, G. W., and Gorski, R. A. (1983): Effects of discrete lesions of the sexually dimorphic nucleus of the preoptic area or other medial preoptic regions on the sexual behavior of male rats. *Brain. Res. Bull.,* 10:147.
773. Commins, D., Yahr, P. (1984): Adult testosterone levels influence the morphology of a sexually dimorphic area in the mongolial gerbil brain. *J. Comp. Neurol.,* 224:132.
774. Masken, J. F., Kragt, C. L., Gallo, R. V., and Ganong, W. F. (1974): Release of luteinizing hormone by electrical stimulation of the medial preoptic area and arcuate nucleus in the male rate. *Neuroendocrinology,* 15:249.
775. Knobil, E., Plant, T. M., Wildt, L., Belchetz, P. E., and Marshall, G. (1980): Control of the rhesus monkey menstrual cycle: Permissive role of hypothalamic gonadotropin-releasing hormone. *Science,* 207:1371.
776. Swanson, L. W. (1976): An autoradiographic study of the efferent connections of the preoptic region in the rat. *J. Comp. Neurol.,* 167:227.
777. Prince, F. P., Jones-Witters, P. H. (1974): The ultrastructure of the medial preoptic area of the rat. *Cell Tissue Res.,* 153:517.
778. Greenough, W. T., Carter, C. S., Steerman, C., and DeVoogd, T. J. (1977): Sex differences in dendritic patterns in hamster preoptic area. *Brain Res.,* 126:63.
779. Gorski, R. A., Harlan, R. E., Jacobson, C. D., Shryne, J. E., and Southam, A. M. (1980): Evidence for the existence of a sexually dimorphic nucleus in the preoptic area of the rat. *J. Comp. Neurol.,* 193:529.
780. Jacobson, C. D., Shryne, J. E., Shaprio, F., and Gorski, R. A. (1980): Ontogeny of the sexually dimorphic nucleus of the preoptic area. *J. Comp. Neurol.,* 193:541.
781. Dohler, K.-D., Coquelin, A., Davis, F., Hines, M., Shryne, J. E., and Gorski, R. A. (1982): Differentiation of the sexually dimorphic nucleus in the preoptic area of the rat brain is determined by the perinatal hormone environment. *Neurosci. Lett.,* 33:295.
782. Hines, M., Davis, F. C., Coquelin, A., Goy, R. W., and Gorski, R. A. (1985): Sexually dimorphic regions in the medial preoptic area and the bed nucleus of the stria terminalis of the guinea pig brain: A description and an investigation of their relationship to gonadal steroids in adulthood. *J. Neurosci.,* 5:40.
783. Takami, S., and Urano, A. (1984): The volume of the toad medial amygdala-anterior preoptic complex is sexually dimorphic and seasonally variable. *Neurosci. Lett.,* 44:253.
784. Swaab, D. F., and Fliers, E. (1985): A sexually dimorphic nucleus in the human brain. *Science,* 228:1112.
785. Cramer, O. M., and Barraclough, C. A. (1971): Effect of electrical stimulation of the preoptic area on plasma LH concentrations in proestrous rats. *Endocrinology,* 88:1175.
786. Sar, M., and Stumpf, W. E. (1973): Autoradiographic localization of radioactivity in the rat brain after the injection of 1,2-^{3}H-testosterone. *Endocrinology,* 92:251.
787. Stumpf, W. E. (1970): Estrogen-neurons and estrogen-neuron systems in the periventricular brain. *Am. J. Anat.,* 129:207.
788. Pfaff, D., and Keiner, M. (1973): Atlas of estradiol-concentrating cells in the central nervous system of the female rat. *J. Comp. Neurol.,* 151:121.
789. Pfaff, D. W., Gerlach, J. L., McEwen, B. S., Ferin, M., Carmel, P., and Zimmerman, E. A. (1976): Autoradiographic localization of hormone-concentrating cells in the brain of the female rhesus monkey. *J. Comp. Neurol.,* 170:279.
790. Raisman, G., and Field, P. M. (1973): Sexual dimorphism in the neuropil of the preoptic area of the rat and its dependence on neonatal androgen. *Brain Res.,* 54:1.
791. McDonald, A. J. (1983): Neurons of the bed nucleus of the stria terminalis: A golgi study in the rat. *Brain Res. Bull.,* 10:111.
792. Saper, C. B. (1984): Organization of the cerebral cortical afferent systems in the rat. II. Magnocellular basal nucleus. *J. Comp. Neurol.,* 222:313.
793. Epelbaum, J., Arancibia, L. T., Herman, J. P., Kordon, C., and Palkovits, M. (1981): Topography of median eminence somatostatinergic innervation. *Brain Res.,* 230:412.
794. Woodhams, P. L., Roberts, G. W., Polak, J. M., and Crow, T. J. (1983): Distribution of neuropeptides in the limbic system of the rat: The bed nucleus of the stria terminalis, septum and preoptic area. *Neuroscience,* 8:677.
795. DeVries, G. J., and Buijs, R. M. (1983): The origin of vasopressinergic and oxytocinergic innervation of the rat brain with special reference to the lateral septum. *Brain Res.,* 273:307.
796. Khachaturian, H., Lewis, M. E., and Watson, S. J. (1983): Enkephalin systems in diencephalon and brainstem of the rat. *J. Comp. Neurol.,* 220:310.
797. King, J. C., Tobet, S. A., Snavely, F. L., and Arimura, A. A. (1982): LHRH immunopositive cells and their projections to the median eminence and organum vasculosum of the lamina terminalis. *J. Comp. Neurol.,* 209:287.
798. Merchenthaler, I., Gorcs, T., Setalo, G., Petrusz, P., and Flerko, B. (1984): Gonadotropin-releasing hormone (GNRH) neurons and pathways in the rat brain. *Cell Tissue Res.,* 237:15.
799. Conrad, L. C. A., and Pfaff, D. W. (1976): Efferents from medial basal forebrain and hypothalamus in the rat. I. An autoradiographic study of the medial preoptic area. *J. Comp. Neurol.,* 169:185.
800. Chiba, T., and Murata, Y. (1985): Afferent and efferent connections of the medial preoptic area in the rat: A WGA-HRP study. *Brain Res. Bull.,* 14:261.
801. Palkovits, M., Mezey, E., Ambach, G., Kivovics, P. (1978): Neural and vascular connections between the organum vasculosum laminae terminalis and preoptic nuclei. In: *Brain-Endocrine Interaction III. Neural Hormones and Reproduction,* edited by D. E. Scott, G. P. Kozlowski, and A. Weindl, p. 302. Karger, Basel.
802. Anderson, C. H., and Shen, C. L. (1980): Efferents of the medial preoptic area in the guinea pig: An autoradiographic study. *Brain Res. Bull.,* 5:257.
803. Swanson, L. W., and Cowan, W. M. (1979): The connections of the septal region in the rat. *J. Comp. Neurol.,* 186:621.
804. Hoffman, G. E., and Gibbs, F. P. (1982): LHRH pathways in rat brain: Deafferentiation spares a sub-chiasmatic LHRH projection to the median eminence. *Neuroscience,* 7:1979.
805. Merchenthaler, I., Gorcs, T., Setalo, G., Petrusz, P., and Flerko, B. (1984): Gonadotropin-releasing hormone (GNRH) neurons and pathways in the rat brain. *Cell Tissue Res.,* 237:15.
806. Krey, L. C., and Silverman, A. J. (1978): The luteinizing hormone-releasing hormone (LH-RH) neuronal networks of the guinea pig brain. II. The regulation of gonadotropin secretion and the origin of terminals in the median eminence. *Brain Res.,* 157:247.
807. Silverman, A. J., Antunes, J. L., Abrams, G. M., Nilaver, G., Thau, R., Robinson, J. A., Ferin, M., and Krey, L. C. (1982): The luteinizing hormone-releasing hormone pathways in rhesus (*Macaca mulatta*) and pigtailed (*Macaca nemestrina*) monkeys: New observations on thick, unembedded sections. *J. Comp. Neurol.,* 211:309.
808. Marshall, P. E., and Goldsmith, P. C. (1980): Neuroregulatory and neuroendocrine GnRH pathways in the hypothalamus and forebrain of the baboon. *Brain Res.,* 193:353.
809. Jennes, L., and Stumpf, W. E. (1980): LHRH-systems in the brain of the golden hamster. *Cell Tissue Res.,* 209:239.
810. Witkin, J. W., Paden, C. M., and Silverman, A.-J. (1982): The luteinizing hormone-releasing hormone (LHRH) systems in the rat brain. *Neuroendocrinology,* 35:429.
811. Millhouse, O. E. (1969): A golgi study of the descending medial forebrain bundle. *Brain Res.,* 15:341.
812. Van Cuc, H., Leranth, C., and Palkovits, M. (1980): Light and electron microscopic studies on the medial forebrain bundle in rat: III. Degenerated nerve elements in the medial hypothalamic nuclei following surgical transections of the medial forebrain bundle. *Brain Res. Bull.,* 5:13.
813. Nieuwenhuys, R., Geeraedts, L. M. G., and Veening, J. G. (1982): The medial forebrain bundle of the rat. I. General introduction. *J. Comp. Neurol.,* 206:49.

814. Veening, J. G., Swanson, L. W., Cowan, W. M., Nieuwenhuys, R., and Geeraedts, L. M. G. (1982): The medial forebrain bundle of the rat. II. An autoradiographic study of the topography of the major descending and ascending components. *J. Comp. Neurol.*, 206:82.
815. Lindvall, O., and Bjorklund, A. (1974): The organization of the ascending catecholamine neuron systems in the rat brain (as revealed by the glyocylic acid fluorescence method). *Acta Phys. Scand. (Suppl.)*, 412:1.
816. Dahlstrom, A., and Fuxe, K. (1964): Evidence for the existence of monoamine-containing neurons in the central nervous system. I. Demonstration of monoamines in the cell bodies of brain stem neurons. *Acta Phys. Scand.*, 62(Suppl. 232):1.
817. Swanson, L. W., and Hartman, B. K. (1975): The central adrinergic system. An immunofluorescence study of the location of cell bodies and their efferent connections in the rat utilizing dopamine-β-hydroxylase as a marker. *J. Comp. Neurol.*, 163:467.
818. Simon, H., LeMoal, M., and Calas, A. (1979): Efferents and afferents of the ventral tegmental-A10 region studied after local injection of (^{3}H)leucine and horseradish peroxidase. *Brain Res.*, 178:17.
819. Moore, K. E., and Demarest, K. T. (1982): Tuberoinfundibular and tuberohypophyseal dopaminergic neurons. In: *Frontiers in Neuroendocrinology, Vol. 7,* edited by W. F. Ganong, and L. Martini, p. 161. Raven Press, New York.
820. Palkovits, M., Zaborszky, L., Feminger, A., Mezey, E., Fekete, M. I. K., Herman, J. P., Kanyicska, B., and Szabo, D. (1980): Noradrenergic innervation of the rat hypothalamus: Experimental biochemical and electron microscopic studies. *Brain Res.*, 191:161.
821. Palkovits, M., Fekete, M., Makara, G. B., and Herman, J. P. (1977): Total and partial hypothalamic deafferentations for topographical identification of catecholaminergic innervations of certain preoptic and hypothalamic nuclei. *Brain Res.*, 127:127.
822. Sawchenko, P. E., and Swanson, L. W. (1981): Central noradrenergic pathways for the integration of hypothalamic neuroendocrine and autonomic responses. *Science*, 214:685.
823. Swanson, L. W., Cowan, W. M. (1975): Hippocampo-hypothalamic connections: Origin in subicular cortex, not Ammon's horn. *Science*, 189:303.
824. Raisman, G., Cowan, W. M., and Powell, T. P. S. (1966): An experimental analysis of the efferent projection of the hippocampus. *Brain*, 89:83.
825. Raisman, G. (1970): An evaluation of the basic pattern of connections between the limbic system and the hypothalamus. *Am. J. Anat.*, 129:197.
826. Heimer, L., and Nauta, W. J. H. (1969): The hypothalamic distribution of the stria terminalis in the rat. *Brain Res.*, 13:284.
827. Tribollet, E., Armstrong, W. E., Dubois-Dauphin, M., and Dreifuss, J. J. (1985): Extra-hypothalamic afferent inputs to the supraoptic nucleus area of the rat as determined by retrograde and anterograde tracing techniques. *Neuroscience*, 15:135.
828. Armstrong, W. E., Scholer, J., and McNeill, T. H. (1982): Immunocytochemical, golgi and electron microscopic characterization of putative dendrites in the ventral glial lamina of the rat supraoptic nucleus. *Neuroscience*, 7:679.
829. Zaborszky, L., Leranth, C. S., Makara, G. B., and Palkovits, M. (1975): Quantitative studies on the supraoptic nucleus in the rat. II. Afferent fiber connections. *Exp. Brain Res.*, 22:525.
830. Oldfield, B. J., Hou-Yu, A., Silverman, A.-J. (1985): A combined electron microscopic HRP and immunocytochemical study of the limbic projections to rat hypothalamic nuclei containing vasopressin and oxytocin neurons. *J. Comp. Neurol.*, 231:221.
831. Poulain, D. A., Lebrun, C. J., and Vincent, J. D. (1981): Electrophysiological evidence for connections between septal neurones and the supraoptic nucleus of the hypothalamus of the rat. *Exp. Brain Res.*, 42:260.
832. Versteeg, D. H. G., Van der Gugten, J., De Jong, W., and Palkovits, M. (1976): Regional concentrations of noradrenaline and dopamine in rat brain. *Brain Res.*, 113:563.
833. Cheung, Y., and Sladek, J. R. (1975): Catecholamine distribution in feline hypothalamus. *J. Comp. Neurol.*, 164:339.
834. Hoffman, G. E., Felten, D. L., and Sladek, J. R. (1976): Monoamine distribution in primate brain. III. Catecholamine-containing varicosities in the hypothalamus of *Macaca mulatta*. *Am. J. Anat.*, 147:501.
835. Blessing, W. W., Jaeger, C. B., Ruggiero, D. A., and Reis, D. J. (1982): Hypothalamic projections of medullary catecholamine neurons in the rabbit: A combined catecholamine fluorescence and HRP transport study. *Brain Res. Bull.*, 9:279.
836. Ciriello, J., and Caverson, M. M. (1984): Direct pathway from neurons in the ventrolateral medulla relaying cardiovascular afferent information to the supraoptic nucleus in the cat. *Brain Res.*, 292:221.
837. Day, T. A., and Renaud, L. P. (1984): Electrophysiological evidence that noradrenergic afferents selectively facilitate the activity of supraoptic vasopressin neurons. *Brain Res.*, 303:233.
838. Ricardo, J. A., and Koh, E. T. (1978): Anatomical evidence of direct projections from the nucleus of the solitary tract to the hypothalamus, amygdala, and other forebrain structures in the rat. *Brain Res.*, 153:1.
839. Norgren, R. (1976): Taste pathways to hypothalamus and amygdala. *J. Comp. Neurol.*, 166:17.
840. Saper, C. B., and Loewy, A. D. (1980): Efferent connections of the parabrachial nucleus in the rat. *Brain Res.*, 197:291.
841. Takeuchi, Y., and Hopkins, D. A. (1984): Light and electron microscopic demonstration of hypothalamic projections to the parabrachial nuclei in the cat. *Neurosci. Lett.*, 46:53.
842. Lindvall, O., and Bjorklund, A. (1983): Dopamine- and norepinephrine-containing neuron systems: their anatomy in the rat brain. In: *Chemical Neuroanatomy,* edited by P. C. Emson, p. 229. Raven Press, New York.
843. Morris, J. F. (1983): Organization of neural inputs to the supraoptic and paraventricular nuclei: anatomical aspects. *Prog. Brain Res.*, 60:3.
844. McNeill, T. H., and Sladek, J. R. (1980): Simultaneous monoamine histofluorescence and neuropeptide immunocytochemistry: II. Correlative distribution of catecholamine varicosities and magnocellular neurosecretory neurons in the rat supraoptic and paraventricular nuclei. *J. Comp. Neurol.*, 193:1023.
845. Sladek, J. R., and Zimmerman, E. A. (1982): Simultaneous monoamine histofluorescence and neuropeptide immunocytochemistry: VI. Catecholamine innervation of vasopressin and oxytocin neurons in the rhesus monkey hypothalamus. *Brain Res. Bull.*, 9:431.
846. Buijs, R. M., Geffard, M., Pool, C. W., and Hoorneman, E. M. D. (1984): The dopaminergic innervation of the supraoptic and paraventricular nucleus: A light and electron microscopical study. *Brain Res.*, 323:65.
847. Moore, R. Y., Halaris, A. E., and Jones, B. E. (1978): Serotonin neurons of the midbrain raphe: Ascending projections. *J. Comp. Neurol.*, 180:417.
848. Tribollet, E., and Dreifuss, J. J. (1981): Localization of neurones projecting to the hypothalamic paraventricular nucleus area of the rat: A horseradish peroxidase study. *Neuroscience*, 6:1315.
849. Silverman, A. J., Hoffman, D. L., and Zimmerman, E. A. (1981): The descending afferent connections of the paraventricular nucleus of the hypothalamus (PVN). *Brain Res. Bull.*, 6:47.
850. Kaelber, W. W., and Leeson, C. R. (1967): A degeneration and electron microscopic study of the nucleus hypothalamicus ventromedialis of the cat. *J. Anat.*, 101:209.
851. Sawchenko, P. E., and Swanson, L. W. (1983): The organization and biochemical specificity of afferent projections to the paraventricular and supraoptic nuclei. *Prog. Brain Res.*, 60:19.
852. McBride, R. L., and Sutin, J. (1977): Amygdaloid and pontine projections to the ventromedial nucleus of the hypothalamus. *J. Comp. Neurol.*, 174:377.
853. Krettek, J. E., and Price, J. L. (1978): Amygdaloid projections to subcortical structures within the basal forebrain and brainstem in the rat and cat. *J. Comp. Neurol.*, 178:225.
854. Silverman, A.-J., Oldfield, B., Hou-Yu, A., and Zimmerman, E. A. (1985): The noradrenergic innervation of vasopressin neurons in the paraventricular nucleus of the hypothalamus: An ultrastructural study using radioautography and immunocytochemistry. *Brain Res.*, 325:215.
855. McKellar, S., and Loewy, A. D. (1981): Organization of some brain stem afferents to the paraventricular nucleus of the hypothalamus in the rat. *Brain Res.*, 217:351.
856. Day, T. A., Blessing, W., and Willoughby, J. O. (1980): Noradrenergic and dopaminergic projections to the medial preoptic area of the rat. A combined horseradish peroxidase/catecholamine fluorescence study. *Brain Res.*, 193:543.

857. Kannan, H., Yamashita, H., and Osaka, T. (1984): Paraventricular neurosecretory neurons: synaptic inputs from the ventrolateral medulla in rats. *Neursci. Lett.*, 51:183.
858. Tanaka, J., Kaba, H., Saito, H., and Seto, K. (1985): Inputs from the A1 noradrenergic region to hypothalamic paraventricular neurons in the rat. *Brain Res.*, 335:368.
859. Swanson, L. W., and Sawchenko, P. E. (1980): Paraventricular nucleus: A site for the integration of neuroendocrine and autonomic mechanisms. *Neuroendocrinology*, 31:410.
860. Sawchenko, P. E., and Swanson, L. W. (1982): The organization of noradrenergic pathways from the brain stem to the paraventricular and supraoptic nuclei in the rat. *Brain Res. Rev.*, 4:275.
861. Ciriello, J., and Caverson, M. M. (1984): Ventrolateral medullary neurons relay cardiovascular inputs to the paraventricular nucleus. *Am. J. Phys.*, 246:R968.
862. Sutin, J., and Eager, R. P. (1969): Fiber degeneration following lesions in the hypothalamic ventromedial nucleus. *Ann. NY Acad. Sci.*, 157:610.
863. Millhouse, O. E. (1973): The organization of the ventromedial hypothalamic nucleus. *Brain Res.*, 55:71.
864. Ottersen, O. P. (1980): Afferent connections to the amygdaloid complex of the rat and cat. II. Afferents from the hypothalamus and the basal telencephalon. *J. Comp. Neurol.*, 194:267.
865. Amaral, D. G., Veazey, R. B., and Cowan, W. M. (1982): Some observations on hypothalamo-amygdaloid connections in the monkey. *Brain Res.*, 252:13.
866. Ajika, K., and Hokfelt, T. (1975): Projections to the median eminence and the arcuate nucleus with special reference to monoamine systems: Effects of lesions. *Cell Tissue Res.*, 158:15.
867. Steinbusch, H. W. M., and Nieuwenhuys, R. (1983): The raphe nuclei of the rat brain stem: A cytoarchitectonic and immunohistochemical study. In: *Chemical Neuroanatomy*, edited by P. C. Emson, p. 131. Raven Press, New York.
868. Berk, M. L., and Finkelstein, J. A. (1981): Afferent projections to the preoptic area and hypothalamic regions in the rat brain. *Neuroscience*, 6:1601.
869. Lind, R. W., and Swanson, W. (1984): Evidence for corticotropin releasing factor and leu-enkephalin in the neural projection from the lateral parabrachial nucleus to the median preoptic nucleus: A retrograde transport, immunohistochemical double labeling study in the rat. *Brain Res.*, 321:217.
870. Simerly, R. B., Swanson, L. W., and Gorski, R. A. (1984): The cells of origin of a sexually dimorphic serotonergic input to the medial preoptic nucleus of the rat. *Brain Res.*, 324:185.
871. Leranth, C., MacLusky, N. J., Sakamoto, H., Shanabrough, M., and Naftolin, F. (1985): Glutamic acid decarboxylase-containing axons synapse on LHRH neurons in the rat medial preoptic area. *Neuroendocrinology*, 40:536.
872. Page, R. B. (1985): In: *Hypothalamic Control of Anterior Pituitary Function: Surgical Implications*, edited by R. Wilkins and S. Rengachary, p. 791. McGraw-Hill, New York.
873. Page, R. B. (1975): Scanning electron microscopy of the ventricular system in normal and hydrocephalic rabbits. *J. Neurosurg.*, 42:646.
874. Page, R. B., and Leure-duPree, A. E. (1983): Ependymal alterations in hydrocephalus. In: *Neurobiology of Cerebrospinal Fluid*, edited by J. Wood, Chapter 51, p. 789. Plenum Press, New York.
875. Page, R. B. (1986): The pituitary portal system. In: *Current Topics in Neuroendocrinology, Vol. 7*, edited by D. Pfaff and D. Ganten. Springer-Verlag, New York.
876. King, J. E., Tobet, S. A., Snavely, F. L., and Arimura, A. A. (1982): LHRH immunopositive cells and their projections to the median eminence and organum vasculosum of the lamina terminalis. *J. Comp. Neurol.*, 209:287.

The Physiology of Reproduction,
edited by E. Knobil and J. Neill *et al.*
Raven Press, Ltd., New York © 1988.

CHAPTER 28

Role of Classic and Peptide Neuromediators in the Neuroendocrine Regulation of LH and Prolactin

Richard I. Weiner, Paul R. Findell, and Claude Kordon

This chapter will attempt to review the extensive literature on the role of neuromediators (i.e., monoamines and peptides) in the regulation of luteinizing hormone (LH) and prolactin (PRL) secretion. The classic neurotransmitters to be studied include: norepinephrine, epinephrine, dopamine, serotonin, histamine, and γ-aminobutyric acid (GABA). Peptides to be reviewed include: somatostatin, luteinizing-hormone-releasing hormone (LHRH), tachykinins, neurotensin, atrial natriuretic factor, neuropeptide Y (NPY), peptide YY (PYY), pancreatic peptide, galanin, oxytocin, vasopressin, thyrotropin-releasing hormone (TRH), corticotropin-releasing factor (CRF), cholecystokinins, angiotensin II, bradykinin, bombesin, vasoactive intestinal polypeptide (VIP), peptide histidine isoleucine (PHI), gastrin inhibitory peptide (GIP), glucagon, growth-hormone-releasing hormone (GRH), and opioid peptides. This chapter will summarize our knowledge on the action of neuromediators that encode neural information essential for neuroendocrine integration of the activity of the neurosecretory neurons regulating LH and PRL secretion. These include: the LHRH neurons for LH and follicle-stimulating-hormone (FSH) regulation; neurons for the PRL inhibitory hormone, dopamine; and the putative PRL-releasing-factor neurons VIP and TRH.

At this point it is worth briefly considering the potential strengths and weaknesses of various general approaches that have been employed. Clearly the further understanding of neuroendocrine control rests firmly on the rapidly evolving fabric of neuroanatomy. For the most part, the topography of the neurosecretory neurons has been carefully described, while studies regarding neuromediator-containing neurons are still underway. Newly developed techniques for the double staining of the contents of neuronal processes at the light and electron-microscopic level have begun to furnish us with insights into the layered patchwork of neuroendocrine integration. For example, it is quite clear that GABA-containing axonal terminals directly synapse on LHRH-containing neurons in rodents (1), as do opioid neurons in primates (2). These techniques, in conjunction with anterograde and retrograde staining of the projections of neurons, offer us considerable promise that we will shortly know (a) the major projections to the neurosecretory neurons and (b) the identity of neuromediators involved.

Information concerning anatomical connections must be integrated with data on the receptors involved in mediating (a) the action of the neuromediators and (b) the activity patterns of the neurons. In some instances, considerable neurochemical data are available concerning discrete regional changes in the metabolism or release of neuromediators that reflect changes in activity of the neurons. If the density of neuronal processes and the duration of these signals are sufficient, then these techniques are of value. In this regard, the activity of norepinephrine(NE)-containing neurons in the hypothalamus has been extensively characterized in microdissected brain regions during the estrous cycle of the rat (3).

Recently developed techniques, such as microdialysis probing, offer further promise in monitoring ongoing neuromediator release. A well-used approach for evaluating the activity of various neuromediators has been the use of pharmacological agents that potentiate or inhibit the action of these neuromediators. This approach was pioneered by the work of Sawyer and colleagues in studying the regulation of ovulation (4). However, each drug involves many potential problems, including the specificity of its action and the realization that observed physiological effects represent the summation of actions at multiple sites. These considerations are particularly worrisome when studying small numbers of neurons which contain a neuromediator and which project to much of the brain, e.g., NE (5,6). Secondly, it is clear that multiple receptors are involved in mediating the action of the neuromediators, and therefore highly specific pharmacological agents are necessary to design meaningful experiments; e.g., NE injected into the third ventricle likely acts at several sites in the hypothalamus, possibly each mediated by different adrenergic receptors.

Finally, the understanding of the coding of this complexity of neurochemical information into some integrated effect on the activity of neurosecretory neurons is essential. Neuromediators can generally be thought of as acting as neurotransmitters or neuromodulators, i.e., respectively affecting the resting potential of target neurons or altering the responsiveness of the target neurons without affecting the resting potential. It is clear that multiple systems are simultaneously involved in coding information and that the intensity, duration, and sequence of these signals play important roles in this so-called "pleotropic regulation." Advances in electrophysiological techniques, i.e., patch clamping in conjunction with advances in nerve culture technique, open new approaches to unraveling these questions.

CATECHOLAMINES

We will not attempt to review the extensive literature in this area accumulated over the past 35 years. Several previous reviews have made this attempt (4,7–11). The diversity of models studied, the use of drugs with questionable specificity, and the complexities of the neuroanatomical organization render much of the literature contradictory and difficult to interpret. Instead we will highlight experiments that have yielded interpretable data that support a series of supportable hypotheses.

Neuroanatomy of Catecholaminergic Neurons

Anatomy of Noradrenergic Neurons

Noradrenergic innervation of the hypothalamus is extrinsic, as demonstrated by the dramatic decline in NE content following surgical isolation of the medial basal hypothalamus (12,13). Norepinephrine-containing terminals have a wide, but uneven, distribution throughout the hypothalamus (14). Terminals in the hypothalamus are projections from cell bodies in the brainstem first described by Dahlstrom and Fuxe (15) and termed A_1, A_2, A_5, A_6, and A_7. A_1 cell bodies are located in the caudal ventrolateral medulla, A_2 cell bodies are in the caudal nucleus of the solitary tract, A_5 cell bodies are in the ventrolateral corner of the pons, A_6 cell bodies are in the locus coeruleus, and A_7 cell bodies are in the mesencephalic reticular formation. Fibers from these neurons project to the hypothalamus via several pathways. The major projection to the hypothalamus is via the ventral bundle, which receives fibers from all the noradrenergic cell groups but predominantly A_1 (6). The dorsal noradrenergic bundle is composed mainly of fibers from the locus coeruleus, and it innervates the dorsal hypothalamic nuclei. The best characterized hypothalamic region receiving noradrenergic innervation is the paraventricular nucleus (PVN). Approximately 70% of the noradrenergic innervation of the PVN arises from A_1 cell bodies, 20% arises from the A_2 cell bodies, and the balance arises from the locus coeruleus (16). Noradrenergic projections to the preoptic area also appear to exclusively arise from A_1 and A_2 cell bodies (17).

Axon terminals containing dopamine-β-hydroxylase, which

is present in both noradrenergic and adrenergic neurons, were shown to end in close proximity to LHRH-containing neurons in the preoptic area (18). However, ultrastructural studies were not able to demonstrate any synaptic specializations between NE- and LHRH-containing neurons (19). However, noradrenergic neurons appeared to form synapses with GABA neurons in the region. Furthermore, the action of catecholamine-containing neurons appear to be mediated in the central nervous system, in part, by so-called nonsynaptic interactions (20).

The anatomical data leaves one with conflicting views concerning the noradrenergic innervation of the hypothalamus. The majority of findings support a system in which several thousand neurons have a global integrative function and make synaptic contact with every region of the neuroaxis. The small number of neurons, their vast terminal projections, and the lack of discrete postsynaptic specializations support this notion. However, a second level of organization could exist within specific groups of noradrenergic neurons that either receive discrete afferent inputs, project to defined areas of the brain, or terminate on neurons whose postsynaptic receptors determine the response (16). We will attempt to discuss these possibilities when reviewing evidence for the role of noradrenergic neurons in gonadotropin and PRL regulation.

Anatomy of Adrenergic Neurons

Separate groups of adrenergic cell bodies have been identified: the C_1 group in the rostral ventrolateral medulla; the C_2 group in the rostromedial part of the nucleus of the solitary tract; and the C_3 group in the rostromedial medulla (21,22). The pathway by which fibers reach the hypothalamus is not clear, although they don't appear to run in the ventral noradrenergic bundle as first believed (6). High concentrations of epinephrine (E) are found in the dorsomedial, paraventricular, periventricular, arcuate, and supraoptic nuclei (23). Some evidence for selectivity of adrenergic versus noradrenergic innervation exists, since in the paraventricular nucleus the parvicellular region receives both types of terminals while the magnocellular region receives mainly noradrenergic terminals (24).

Anatomy of Dopaminergic Neurons

Dopamine(DA)-containing neurons that innervate the hypothalamus have their cell bodies concentrated in three brain regions: the so-called A_{11}, A_{12}, A_{13}, and A_{14} cell groups. The largest group of neurons is the A_{12} or tuberoinfundibular neurons (25), which constitute 3% to 5% of the cell bodies of the arcuate nucleus (6). The terminals of these neurons are found in the median eminence in close apposition to the primary capillaries of the hypophyseal portal plexus. These neurons function as neurosecretory neurons releasing large amounts of DA into portal blood (26) and play a central role in the regulation of PRL (9). The regulation of the A_{12} DA-containing neurons will be discussed in detail in Chapter 33.

The function of these neurons in the control of the release of LHRH has been repeatedly proposed. Numerous authors have suggested that these interactions would occur via nonsynaptic axo-axonal interactions in the median eminence. We observed few, if any, D_2 dopamine receptors in the bovine stalk median eminence (27). In agreement with the findings in bovine tissue, there were relatively few dopaminergic sites labeled by [^{3}H]spiroperidol in the median eminence of the rat (28). However, there were significant numbers of dopaminergic sites labeled with the D_1 ligand [^{3}H]ADTN. Therefore the possibility exists that DA may act through D_1 rather than D_2 receptors in the median eminence. However, it seems unlikely that a neurosecretory neuronal system that is tonically active in the suppression of PRL secretion should somehow be involved in regulating phasic changes in LH secretion.

Neurons with their cell bodies in the caudal thalamus, posterior hypothalamic area, and the medial zona incerta (A_{11} and A_{13}) project periventricularly in the dorsal part of the hypothalamus (29). The A_{14} cell group, located more rostrally in the anterior periventricular nucleus, project to the preoptic nucleus (30). Interestingly, synaptic contacts have been described in this area between LHRH- and possibly DA-containing neurons (19). These intrahypothalamic dopaminergic pathways are scattered, which has made it difficult to study their role in the regulation of LH and prolactin secretion.

Role of Catecholaminergic Neurons in the Control of LH Secretion

Pulsatile LH Release

In ovariectomized animals, frequent large-amplitude LH pulses are observed. Several lines of evidence have shown that pulses of LH secretion are driven by the pulsatile release of LHRH. Therefore, ovariectomized animals have frequently been used to determine if a neurotransmitter is involved in the regulation of the so-called LHRH pulse generator. Inhibition of noradrenergic activity by inhibition of NE synthesis (31–33), blockade of α-adrenergic receptors (34), or destruction of the ventral noradrenergic bundle with 6-hydroxydopamine (35) all result in suppression of pulsatile LH release in the ovariectomized rat. Blockade of β-adrenergic receptors with propranolol had no effect (34). In ovariectomized monkeys, blockade of α-receptors with phenoxybenzamine and phentolamine inhibited pulsatile LH release, whereas treatment with propranolol was ineffective (36). That the stimulatory action of NE is mediated via α-receptors was supported by the observations that administration of the α-agonist clonidine overrode the blockade of pulsatile LH release caused by treatment with the NE synthesis inhibitor FLA-63 (37). Although clonidine is generally thought of as an α_2-agonist, sufficient dose and pharmacological manipulations were not performed to determine the subclass of α-receptors involved in mediation of this response.

It does not appear that E-containing neurons are involved in regulation of pulsatile LH release, since specific inhibition of E synthesis did not affect pulsatile release (38). However, it is impossible to be certain that α-adrenergic antagonists, which inhibit pulsatile LH release, are not partly blocking the action of E as well as NE.

Although observations in which endogenous noradrenergic activity is blocked are consistent with an ongoing stimulatory action of noradrenergic neurons on pulsatile LH release, the administration of NE into the third ventricle causes inhibition (39). Intraventricular administration of NE predominantly inhibits LH pulse frequency (40), an action mediated at least partly at sites in the medial preoptic area (41). This action of administered NE was not affected by the simultaneous administration of serotonin or DA antagonists (40). Furthermore, electrical stimulation of the major ascending noradrenergic pathway also inhibits pulsatile LH release in ovariectomized rats (42). These observations, rather than a demonstration that noradrenergic neurons are normally involved in mediating pulsatile LH release, only show that there are adrenergic receptors on some neuronal element which, when activated, inhibit pulsatile LH release.

It does not appear that dopaminergic neurons are involved in pulsatile LH release in ovariectomized rats, since blockade of DA receptors with specific antagonists has no effect (32,34,43). However, if DA agonists are administered via the third ventricle, pulsatile LH release is inhibited (32,33,43). The effects of the DA agonists can be reversed by administration of DA antagonists (32).

In conclusion, in the absence of steroid feedback it appears that noradrenergic neurons are involved in the stimulation of pulsatile LH release. The release of NE in the medial preoptic nucleus, as measured via push-pull cannulae, is pulsatile; however, there is a lack of correlation between the pulses of NE and LH (44). This action of NE is mediated via adrenergic receptors, although it is unclear whether α_1- or α_2-receptors are involved. Neither E- nor DA-containing neurons appear to play a role in regulation of pulsatile LH release. A question still to be answered is the site(s) on which the α-adrenergic receptors are located. Noradrenergic neurons do not appear to be the pulse generator in rats or in monkeys. Complete deafferentation of the hypothalamus destroys all of the noradrenergic neurons innervating the circumscribed region, since the cell bodies of the noradrenergic neurons are outside the island. This procedure does not block pulsatile LH release in the rhesus monkey (45).

Ovulatory Surge of LH

To consider the question of the role of catecholamine-containing neurons in regulation of the ovulatory surge of LH, a logical first step is to summarize the actions of gonadal steroids on activity of these neurons. It is clear that the major signals for the synchronization of the ovulatory surge are the positive and negative feedback actions of estradiol (E_2) and progesterone.

In ovariectomized rats the implantation of E_2-filled silastic capsules results in ovulatory-like LH surges every 24 hr. Associated with the LH surge, the turnover rate (an index of neuronal activity) of NE increased in the medial preoptic, arcuate, and suprachiasmatic nuclei and median eminence (46). Furthermore, an increase in the episodic release of NE was measured via push-pull cannulae in the medial preoptic area from the morning to the afternoon of the LH surge (47). In animals treated with E_2 plus progesterone, the LH surge was advanced, as was the increase in NE turnover rate (46). These observations are in close agreement with findings in cycling rats. An increase in the turnover rate of NE occurs in the same hypothalamic areas around the time of the ovulatory surge of LH on the afternoon of proestrus (3). No changes in NE turnover rate were seen in these areas on the afternoon of diestrous day 1.

Relative to the negative feedback action of E_2, the turnover rate of NE in a large preoptic area fragment increased 3 days post-ovariectomy (48). Three hours following the administration of E_2, the NE turnover rate was suppressed in the preoptic area and median eminence. In another study utilizing a more precise dissection, the NE turnover rate was only observed to decrease in the periventricular nucleus 3 hr after treatment with E_2 (49). Estradiol administration for 3 hr also decreased the release rate of NE collected via a push-pull cannulue implanted in the medial basal hypothalamus (44).

The action of estrogen on NE turnover could be mediated directly on the noradrenergic neurons, since they appear to contain estrogen receptors (50). However, the possibility also exists that the steroid effect on noradrenergic activity could be mediated through opiate or GABA-containing interneurons that contain steroid receptors. These interactions will be discussed later in the chapter.

The turnover rate of E-containing neurons also appears to increase in some areas of the hypothalamus simultaneous with the ovulatory surge of LH. Increases in E turnover were observed in the medial basal hypothalamus (51) or the medial preoptic area (52) on the afternoon of proestrus. Increases in E turnover were also reported in the medial basal hypothalamus following E_2-plus-progesterone-induced LH surges (53). However, one group was unable to measure a change in E turnover in the medial preoptic nucleus on the afternoon of proestrus (3). Discrepancies in these findings could be due to the difficulty in measuring the relatively low levels of E in these areas.

Data on effects of ovarian steroids on the number and affinity of α- and β-adrenergic receptors in the hypothalamus is not extensive. No changes in hypothalamic β-adrenergic receptors were seen throughout the estrous cycle of the rat (54). However, treatment of ovariectomized rats with E_2 (or E_2 plus progesterone) increased the number of receptors. No changes were seen in the number of α-adrenergic receptors labeled with [^{3}H]dihydroergocryptine either during the estrous cycle or following steroid treatment of ovariectomized rats (54).

The significance of effects of ovarian steroids on the activity of dopaminergic neurons is less clear than with noradrenergic neurons. Changes in the activity of the tuberoinfundibular DA neurons are closely coupled to the secretion of PRL. Estrogen treatment increases PRL levels; PRL, in turn, increases the turnover of the dopaminergic neurons (55). However, dopaminergic cell bodies in the arcuate nucleus contain E_2 receptors (56,57), and E_2 (or E_2 plus progesterone) could affect the activity of these neurons directly (58).

In the rat the turnover rate of DA in the median eminence and arcuate nucleus increases on the afternoon of proestrus between 12:00 p.m. and 2:00 p.m. and then decreases between 3:00 p.m. and 5:00 p.m. (3). No change is seen in dopaminergic activity in the medial preoptic nucleus at that time. In ovariectomized rats in which LH surges were induced with E_2 plus progesterone, no changes in DA turnover rate were seen in the arcuate and medial preoptic nuclei and median eminence from morning to afternoon (46).

Ovariectomy had little effect on the turnover of DA in several hypothalamic areas (47). Estradiol administration for 3 hr caused a small, but statistically significant, decrease in DA turnover in the preoptic area (47) and median eminence (48) and an increase in the medial basal hypothalamus (47).

There is extensive literature regarding the effect of catecholaminergic agents on (a) the ovulatory surge of LH on proestrus and (b) estrogen(or estrogen plus progesterone)-induced LH surges. The literature has followed the trail blazed in 1950 by Sawyer et al. (59), who showed that α-adrenergic antagonists would block ovulation in the rat (59). The studies have been refined over the years by our increasing knowledge concerning hormonal changes during the periovulatory period and the use of more specific pharmacological agents. Clearly, noradrenergic and adrenergic neurons are involved in the generation of the ovulatory LH surge in the rat.

Drugs that inhibit catecholamine synthesis [e.g., α-methyl-*p*-tyrosine (α-MPT)] or NE and E synthesis [e.g., diethyldithiocarbamate (DDC)] inhibit the ovulatory surge of LH (60–62). Blockade of α-adrenergic receptors also interrupts ovulation (59,63,64). The α_1-subtype selective antagonist prazosin was capable of inhibiting the ovulatory surge of LH, whereas the α_2-antagonist piperoxane was ineffective (62). Destruction of the ventral noradrenergic bundle by the neurotoxin 6-hydroxydopamine (65) or by surgical transection (61) caused only a temporary interruption of ovulation. The return of ovulation was surprising, considering the 83% decrease seen in the NE content of the hypothalamus following surgical transection (61). The development of denervation supersensitivity or the possible sparing of E-containing neurons can only partially explain the return of function post-surgery, since treatment of these animals with DDC was found to block ovulation only 40% of the time (61). This finding supports the existence of multiple control mechanisms for ovulation, thereby allowing other systems to compensate for the loss of noradrenergic regulation.

Similarly, blockade of catecholamine synthesis with α-MPT or NE and E synthesis with DDC (66) or FLA-63 (53), also inhibits E_2-plus-progesterone-induced LH surges. The inhibitory effects of these agents could be reversed by the simultaneous repletion of NE and E with dihydroxyphenylserine. Blockade of α-adrenergic receptors, but not β-adrenergic receptors, also inhibited the steroid-induced LH surges (66,67). The receptors mediating this response appear to be α_1-receptors, since the α_1-selective antagonist prasozin was more effective than the α_2-selective antagonist yohimbine (67).

On close inspection it is difficult to separate whether drugs affecting the ovulatory surge of LH work through NE- or E-containing neurons or both. Both the actions of NE and E are mediated via α- and β-adrenergic receptors, with only small differences in their potency at these receptors. Previously, catecholamine synthesis inhibitors that were used (i.e., DDC and FLA-63) had been found to deplete both NE and E, since they inhibited the activity of dopamine β-hydroxylase. With the advent of relatively specific inhibitors of phenylethanolamine *N*-methyltransferase (PNMT), which selectively depletes E, this question has been restudied.

Several laboratories have shown that inhibition of E synthesis will block the ovulatory surge of LH (62,68). These findings are difficult to assess because several of the drugs used to inhibit E synthesis also have α-adrenergic blocking properties, e.g., SKF 64139 and LY7835 (69). Furthermore, treatment with LY134046, an E synthesis inhibitor that has no antagonist activity, was not capable of inhibiting ovulation (69). The drug was ineffective when given for 1 or 5 days even though the long-term treatment resulted in a 95% depletion of E in the medial preoptic nucleus. Unfortunately no assessment of LH levels was made in this study. LH levels could have been partially suppressed without affecting ovulation.

In animals treated with E_2 plus progesterone to induce an LH surge, both the less specific PNMT inhibitors LY 78335 and SKF 64139 (53,70) as well as the one without α-antagonist properties, SKF 83593 (38), blocked the induced LH surge.

In numerous studies the effects of NE and E have been studied *in vivo* by intraventricular administration to circumvent the blood-brain barrier. Previously we discussed the inhibitory actions of NE on pulsatile LH release in ovariectomized animals. However, when ovariectomized animals are primed with E_2 or E_2 plus progesterone for several days, NE and E administration stimulates LH release (39,71,72). Also, NE administration to estrogen-primed rabbits stimulates an ovulatory surge of LH (73). In rats in which ovulation was blocked with pentobarbitol E (but not NE) was able to induce ovulation (74). The mechanism by which steroid priming reverses the response to intraventricular catecholamines is not clear.

Consistent with the above findings, when NE is added to median eminence fragments from male rats *in vitro,* the release of LHRH is stimulated (75,76). The response is dose dependent and can be blocked by the α-adrenergic antagonist phentolamine. The stimulatory action of NE appears to be mediated by α_2-receptors, since it is blocked by yohimbine but not prazosin (77). The response to NE is not blocked by DA or β-adrenergic antagonists. These findings are of interest because a large number of α_2-adrenergic receptors have been described in the median eminence (27). The physiological role of these α_2-adrenergic receptors in the control of LHRH release from nerve terminals in the median eminence is unclear, since the limited data with subtype-selective drugs supports the idea that the stimulatory role of NE or E in the ovulatory surge or pulsatile release of LH is mediated by α_1-adrenergic receptors (62,67).

The data we have summarized strongly supports the concept that NE- and E-containing neurons are involved in the stimulation of the ovulatory surge of LH in rodents. The action appears to be mediated via α_1-adrenergic receptors most likely located in the medial preoptic area. Clearly there is an increase in noradrenergic neuronal activity in this area on the afternoon of proestrus.

However, in primates there are little data that support a role for noradrenergic pathways in the regulation of ovulation, since normal menstrual cycles are seen in monkeys with complete deafferentation of the medial basal hypothalamus (45,78).

Before concluding the discussion regarding the role of NE and E on LH release, it is of interest to review data suggesting that NE can inhibit LH release via β-adrenergic receptors (11). Electrical stimulation of the noradrenergic neurons of the locus coeruleus inhibits the LA surge on proestrus (79). This inhibition could be blocked by the local injection in the premammillary nuclei of the β-adrenergic blocker propranolol but not the α-adrenergic antagonist phenoxybenzamine (80). Intraventricular injection of the β-agonist isoproterenol was also capable of inhibiting the steroid-induced LH surge (81). Furthermore, the release of LH induced by administration of NE to steroid-primed rats was potentiated by pretreating the animals with propranolol (84). Interestingly, a recent study showed that not only intraventricular administration of NE or isoproterenol but also two α_1-adrenergic agonists phenylephrine and methoxamine inhibited LH release when administered after the initiation of steroid-induced LH surges (83).

These data clearly show that NE can inhibit LH release. However, as with the inhibitory effect of NE seen on pulsatile LH in ovariectomized rats, none of these inhibitory effects were seen during the normal regulation of LH. These effects are only seen after electrical stimulation of noradrenergic pathways or the intraventricular administration of NE or related agonists. In fact, in every instance when the β-antagonist propranalol was given to ovariectomized, proestrous, or steroid-treated ovariectomized rats, not only did it not interfere with LH release but it also did not potentiate it. Therefore, inhibition of LH secretion, by NE via β-adrenergic neurons, doesn't appear to occur during these physiological states. The physiological function of what appears to be a distinct inhibitory noradrenergic pathway is yet to be elucidated.

The role of DA-containing neurons in the regulation of the ovulatory surge of LH is controversial (4,9). The administration of the relatively specific DA antagonist pimozide on the morning of proestrus greatly reduced the afternoon LH surge (84). Effects of less specific DA antagonists (e.g., haloperidol and chlorpromazine), which have significant α-adrenergic antagonist properties, will not be discussed. Pimozide treatment for 2 days before or after the expected midcycle surge of LH in women also reduced the LH levels (85).

Consistent with a stimulatory role of DA on LH release, the intraventricular administration of DA to proestrous rats was reported to increase LH levels (86). Both the intraventricular administration of DA and the DA agonist apomorphine stimulated LH secretion in ovariectomized steroid-primed rats (87). However, other laboratories have seen no effect on LH after the administration of DA to E_2- or E_2-plus-progesterone-primed rats (39,71,88).

Intravenous infusion of DA to women causes a significant decrease in resting LH levels only around midcycle (89). This finding suggests that DA is acting at the level of the median eminence, since DA does not cross the blood-brain barrier and does not act directly on the gonadotrophs. Apomorphine administration had no effect on LH secretion in humans (90).

In-vitro studies have also given conflicting results. Most recently, perifusion with DA was shown to increase LHRH release from medial basal hypothalamic fragments from male rats (91). However, the effect was blocked by the α-adrenergic antagonist phentolamine but not the DA antagonist pimozide. DA was shown not to be acting by uptake and conversion to NE, i.e., since it worked in the presence of DDC. However, DA treatment was shown to displace NE from terminals in the median eminence. This study demonstrates the difficulty in interpreting studies following administration of exogenous amines. Incubation with DA has previously been reported to inhibit LHRH release from median eminence fragments (75). However, in these studies, treatment with pimozide inhibited the action of DA.

In conclusion, there are changes in the activity of dopaminergic neurons correlated with the estrous cycle of the rat. Clearly, changes in the activity of the tuberoinfundibular neurons will directly affect the secretion of PRL through DA receptors on lactotrophs. However, that these neurons play an important role in the regulation of the ovulatory surge or pulsatile release of LH in ovariectomized animals is unclear.

Role of Catecholamines in the Control of Prolactin Secretion

Unlike LH secretion, the secretion of PRL is under tonic inhibitory control by the hypothalamic hormone DA (92).

Prolactin secretion appears to be regulated by inhibition of DA release and/or the release of PRL-releasing factors. Although the identity of the PRL-releasing factors is unknown, there is experimental data supporting this role for VIP and TRH. In the rat, changes in PRL secretion include: a large surge on the afternoon of proestrus just preceding the LH surge; nocturnal increases during pregnancy; diurnal changes; and stress-induced release and suckling-induced release during lactation (93). In primates there is no increase in PRL secretion associated with the midcycle surge of LH. During the night, irregular episodes of PRL secretion are observed which may or may not be correlated with stages of sleep (94). In all mammals, suckling induces large increases in PRL secretion.

There is not a great deal of evidence describing the role of brain catecholamines in the neural regulation of PRL secretion, although the catecholamine DA is the major hypothalamic hormone regulating PRL secretion. Norepinephrine-containing neurons appear to play an important role in the regulation of PRL secretion under a variety of physiological conditions.

Dopaminergic Neurons

The tuberoinfundibular DA neurons are neurosecretory neurons that are responsible for the production of high levels of DA in the hypophyseal portal blood (26). The discussion of the regulation of these neurons and their role in the regulation of PRL secretion from lactotrophs are covered in detail in Chapter 33.

Noradrenergic Neurons

Basal PRL secretion is pulsatile in nature. The administration of the NE- and E-synthesis inhibitor DDC completely inhibited pulsatile PRL secretion in ovariectomized rats (95). However, in male rats, treatment with the NE- and E-synthesis inhibitor FLA-63 had no effect on pulsatile or basal PRL release (96).

Administration of α-adrenergic antagonist phenoxybenzamine in high doses to ovariectomized rats treated with E_2 was found to stimulate PRL release, whereas phentolamine had no effect (97). However, administration of both phentolamine and phenoxybenzamine to ovariectomized monkeys stimulated PRL release (98). In male rats (99,100) and male monkeys (101) the administration of the α_2-adrenergic blocker, yohimbine, stimulated basal levels of PRL. However, no effect of yohimbine was observed on basal PRL levels in men (102). Stimulation of PRL secretion by yohimbine was reversed by the administration of the α_2-agonist clonidine (99,101).

These data on the role of noradrenergic neurons in the regulation of basal PRL secretion are paradoxical. Inhibition of the synthesis of NE inhibits pulsatile PRL release, whereas blockade of α_2-adrenergic receptors increases basal PRL secretion. One possible explanation is that pulsatile PRL secretion is controlled by neurosecretory neurons receiving a stimulatory noradrenergic innervation mediated via α_1-adrenergic neurons, whereas basal PRL secretion is controlled by separate neurosecretory neurons receiving a noradrenergic input mediated via α_2-adrenergic receptors. Clearly, multiple inhibitory and stimulatory neurosecretory neuronal systems that regulate PRL have been described. One note of caution in terms of the importance of a noradrenergic innervation on basal PRL secretion comes from findings with complete deafferentated female rats. Complete deafferentation, which destroys all of the noradrenergic input to the medial basal hypothalamus, does not elevate basal PRL levels (103,104).

The surge in PRL on the afternoon of proestrus can be inhibited by the injection of the neurotoxin 6-hydroxydopamine into the ventral noradrenergic tract (105). Afternoon surges in PRL induced by the treatment of ovariectomized rats with E_2 plus progesterone could be blocked by the NE- and E-synthesis inhibitor DDC (106). Estrogen-induced surges in ovariectomized animals were blocked by the α-adrenergic antagonists phenoxybenzamine and phentolamine but not by the β-adrenergic antagonist propranolol (107).

A noradrenergic pathway does not appear to be involved in the suckling-induced release of PRL. The synthesis of hypothalamic norepinephrine does not change following suckling (108), and the suckling-induced release of PRL is not affected by the blockade of NE and E synthesis with DDC (109).

The role of noradrenergic neurons in the stress-induced release of PRL has not been well studied; however, the data available suggest that blockade of noradrenergic activity with 6-hydroxydopamine and DDC blocked stress-induced prolactin release in rats. This area should be more carefully studied, since the cell bodies of two putative prolactin releasing factors, TRH and VIP, are located in the PVN nucleus, an area with a dense noradrenergic innervation (24). This area is also known to be involved in the control of the stress-induced release of adrenocorticotropic hormone (ACTH).

In conclusion, it appears that a stimulatory noradrenergic component is involved in the regulation of the afternoon surge of LH. The role of noradrenergic neurons in the regulation of basal PRL secretion is unclear and deserves further study. Existing data suggest that noradrenergic neurons are involved in the stress-induced release of PRL. Lastly, no work has been done to determine that the observed effects were mediated via NE-containing neurons and not E-containing ones. This possibility should be clarified.

SEROTONIN

Anatomy of Serotonergic Neurons

The basic organization of the central serotonin [5-hydroxytryptamine (5-HT)] neuronal system consists of a population of brainstem neurons arising mainly from the midbrain raphe nuclei (110–112). Their axons project with a high degree of collateralization and multidirectionality to innervate most areas of the forebrain, with the hypothalamus receiving extensive innervation. Fibers mainly from the dorsal and median raphe nuclei project to the hypothalamus via the medial forebrain bundle, a dorsal raphe arcuate tract, and a dorsal raphe periventricular tract (113). Fibers may also originate from serotonergic cell bodies located within the hypothalamus, since total deafferentation of the hypothalamus does not completely deplete the rat hypothalamus of 5-HT (114). A group of cells in the pars ventralis of the nucleus dorsomedialis hypothalami has been shown to concentrate intraventricularly administered 5-HT (115,116). Some caution should be taken in the interpretion of these results because both dopaminergic and noradrenergic neurons possess a low-affinity 5-HT uptake mechanism (117). Frankfurt et al. (118), using a specific anti-5-HT antiserum, failed to detect cell bodies containing 5-HT immunoreactivity in this area unless the rats were pretreated with L-tryptophan and pargyline, which stimulate 5-HT synthesis and inhibit 5-HT degradation, respectively. According to these authors, if there is indeed a serotonergic cell group present in the hypothalamus, its turnover of 5-HT is slow and its synthesis is limited by availability of substrate.

The arcuate nucleus receives a dense serotonergic innervation (110,111,119). There is a close approximation of 5-HT-containing fibers to dopaminergic cell bodies in the arcuate nucleus and in the medial zona incerta, which also provides dopaminergic input to the hypothalamus (120,121). Synaptic junctions between serotonergic terminals and cell bodies were observed (121). However, these synapses were infrequent, suggesting that 5-HT action is mediated via nonsynaptic interactions.

There is extensive anatomical overlap in the distribution of LHRH- and serotonin-containing neurons in the hypothalamus. Close appositions of neuronal elements containing 5-HT and LHRH immunoreactivity were demonstrated in the septo-preoptic region (122) as well as in the median eminence and organum vasculosum of the lamina terminalis (123,124). Synaptic contacts between serotonergic terminals and immunoreactive LHRH elements were described in the medial preoptic area (125). Again, only a small percentage of terminals were seen in contact with immunoreactive LHRH neurons.

These 5-HT/DA and 5-HT/LHRH interactions provide a neuroanatomical basis for 5-HT neurons in the regulation of PRL and gonadotropin release. The final link in demonstrating the basis for these interactions is the localization of the receptors mediating the action of 5-HT.

Histofluorescent and immunocytochemical techniques have been utilized to identify endogenous 5-HT in the mammalian pituitary gland, although there is some disagreement as to its localization. Serotonin was reported to be present only in nerve terminals located in the intermediate lobe of the pituitary (126,127), in the posterior lobe (128), or in both the intermediate and posterior lobes of the pituitary (129–131). Westlund and Childs (132) also reported 5-HT in the anterior lobe in fine nerve fibers localized around major blood vessels and at the capsule of the gland.

In the anterior pituitary of submammalian vertebrates, the presence of 5-HT neurons is common (133,134), whereas in mammalian anterior pituitary, 5-HT appears to be mainly localized in secretory granules of gonadotrophs (129). The source of the endogenous 5-HT in gonadotrophs is still unclear. The presence of significant amounts of tryptophan hydroxylase (the rate-limiting enzyme in the synthesis of 5-HT) in the anterior pituitary may reflect *de novo* synthesis of 5-HT (135). Alternatively, the immunoreactive 5-HT in these cells may be the result of an uptake and accumulation of 5-HT synthesized elsewhere and delivered to these cells. Secretory granules of gonadotrophs become radioautographically labeled when exposed to low concentrations of exogenous [^{3}H]5-HT (136,137). Uptake is saturable and inhibited by the selective 5-HT uptake blocker fluoxitine (137).

Direct radioligand binding studies with [^{125}I]lysergic acid and indirect binding studies with cinanserin-displaced [^{3}H]spiperone binding have identified stereoselective, saturable, and high-affinity 5-HT-binding sites in the rat pituitary gland (138). As determined by quantitative light-microscopic autoradiography, the highest concentration of the sites was found in the intermediate lobe, with progressively decreasing concentrations in the posterior and anterior lobes of the pituitary.

Role of Serotonin in the Control of Prolactin Secretion

Serotonergic input was first implicated in the control of PRL release when the intraventricular infusion of 5-HT or its metabolites was observed to elevate plasma PRL in rats (139–141). The systemic administration of 5-hydroxytryptophan (5-HTP), the immediate precursor of 5-HT, also was effective in producing a rapid and pronounced increase in serum PRL in intact rats and in hypophysectomized rats with pituitary grafts under the kidney capsule (142). Since 5-HT was shown not to act directly at the pituitary to release PRL (143), these studies led to the belief that intraventricularly placed 5-HT or systemically administered 5-HTP liberates a PRL-releasing factor. These studies must be interpreted with some caution because the direct infusion of 5-HT or its metabolites into the ventricle may not mimic the endogenous activation of 5-HT neurons and may not provide an accurate assessment of 5-HT as a physiological regulator of PRL (144). Additionally, 5-HTP administered at high doses can be taken up by catecholamine terminals, can become decarboxylated, and can displace the neurotransmitter present in the terminal (145).

The acute depletion of central 5-HT by *p*-chlorophenylalanine (PCPA) treatment does not alter baseline PRL levels in castrated male rats (146) or in ovariectomized (147) or postpartum female rats (148). In normal male rats (149,150) or ovariectomized E_2-primed rats (151), PCPA treatment was accompanied by a marked reduction in baseline circulating PRL levels. Frequently used high doses of PCPA (>100 mg/kg body weight) may not selectively act on serotonergic neurons. Neutral amino acids, such as PCPA, can compete with tyrosine for uptake into catecholamine neurons (152). When PCPA was administered with desmethylimipramine (DMI), an inhibitor of uptake into catecholaminergic neurons, for the most part PCPA was without effect on baseline or stress-induced PRL release (150).

Whereas the involvement of 5-HT in the regulation of basal PRL secretion is unclear, more clear-cut findings have been obtained during episodes of stimulated PRL release. For example, suckling-induced pituitary PRL release in lactating rats almost certainly involves 5-HT. Kordon et al. (148) demonstrated that an acute blockade of 5-HT biosynthesis with PCPA can completely abolish the suckling-induced increase in circulating PRL. The blockade of 5-HT receptors with methysergide also inhibited the suckling-induced increase in PRL (147). The suckling-induced PRL release is accompanied by a rapid fall in hypothalamic 5-HT levels and a corresponding increase in its major metabolite, 5-hydroxyindoleacetic acid (5-HIAA) (153). Parisi et al. (154) demonstrated that the 5-HIAA increase during suckling occurs in the terminals in the rostral part of the anterior hypothalamic nucleus. These changes in hypothalamic 5-HT activity occur immediately after the onset of suckling and continue until the suckling stimulus is stopped (153). The 5-HT response to suckling does not occur when pups have been separated from their mother for over 24 hr (i.e., under weaning conditions). Prolactin is not released under these same conditions (153,135).

Other conditions of evoked PRL release also appear (at least in part) to be dependent upon central 5-HT activity. The PRL-releasing effects of ether (156) and restraint stress (157) are blocked in normal male rats pretreated with methysergide. Treating male rats with PCPA and/or electrolytic destruction of the midbrain raphe nuclei abolishes their diurnal and nocturnal PRL surges (158). Electrolytic destruction of the dorsal raphe, but not of the median raphe nuclei, attenuates the E_2-induced afternoon PRL surge in female rats (159). Treatment with PCPA or ketanserin, a 5-HT antagonist, is also effective in blocking this PRL surge (159).

In summary, 5-HT neurons appear to be important in the modulation of PRL secretory responses but not important in the control of basal PRL release. The mechanism(s) whereby 5-HT influences PRL secretion is still unclear, but, as mentioned previously, its site of action is not at the anterior pituitary. The incubation of anterior pituitary tissue with 5-HT (143,165) fails to alter PRL release. Serotonin's effects on PRL release have been linked to the modulation of inhibitory dopaminergic inputs to the pituitary. The 5-HT agonist, quipazine, increases serum PRL when administered to ovariectomized rats (161). Concomitant with this increase is a decrease in the turnover rate of dopaminergic neurons. Furthermore, DA levels in hypophyseal portal blood were decreased in male rats receiving intraventricular 5-HT (162). However, when DA was infused intravenously into these rats, elevating the concentration of DA severalfold, 5-HT-induced PRL release was not prevented. This introduces an alternate explanation for 5-HT's effects on PRL release, namely that 5-HT directly liberates a PRL-releasing factor (PRF). Clemens et al. (163) found that pharmacological potentiation of serotonergic pathways always released considerably more PRL than did the removal of dopaminergic inhibition. These authors concluded that 5-HT releases PRL not by inhibiting dopaminergic neurons but rather by stimulating the liberation of PRF. The intermediate lobe of the rat pituitary may also play an as-yet poorly understood role in the mediation of 5-HT's regulation of PRL. Removal of the neurointermediate lobe in male rats can completely abolish the increase in plasma PRL levels normally observed following 5-HTP administration (164).

Serotonin appears to be involved in the negative-feedback control of PRL. Decreasing circulating PRL levels via hypophysectomy of ovariectomized rats was shown to be accompanied by an increased rate of 5-HT synthesis in the median eminence and mediobasal hypothalamus (165). This effect was reversed if exogenous PRL was given to these animals. Furthermore, the blockade of DA receptors reversed the ability of exogenous PRL to inhibit the increased rate of 5-HT synthesis, indicating that this feedback mechanism apparently involves an intermediary DA component. Hyperprolactinemia produced by pituitary homografts implanted beneath the kidney capsule in ovariectomized rats attenuated ovarian-steroid-stimulated 5-HT synthesis in the preoptic area of the hypothalamus, an area involved in the regulation of gonadotropin release (166). The steroid-induced increase in serum LH was also attenuated in the hyperprolactinemic animals. Further investigations are required to elucidate the mechanism(s) through which 5-HT regulated PRL release. These investigations may also help elucidate the poorly understood mechanism(s) whereby high levels of circulating PRL inhibit gonadotropin release.

Role of Serotonin in the Control of LH Secretion

An abundance of evidence, largely pharmacological, supports a participatory role for 5-HT in gonadotropin regulation. Reminiscent of the action of NE, serotonergic neurons may play facilitatory or inhibitory roles in LH secretion, depending on the steroid environment. Initial studies generally concentrated on (a) the effects of the systemic administration of large amounts of 5-HT or its precursor 5-HTP, which blocked spontaneous ovulation in mature rats (169), and (b) ovulation induced in immature rats by the administration of pregnant mare serum gonadotropin (PMSG) (168–170). These data met with some skepticism in view of the inability of 5-HT to cross the blood-brain barrier (171) and because 5-HTP was effective only when given in combination with a monoamine oxidase inhibitor (167). The suppression of ovulation was also counteracted by treatment with a vasodilator (172). However, data supporting an inhibitory role continued to accumulate. The pharmacological elevation of hypothalamic 5-HT levels with monoamine oxidase inhibitors suppressed both PMSG-induced (144) and spontaneous ovulation (167) in rats. In sheep (173) and rabbits (174), infusion of 5-HT into the medial basal hypothalamus blocked the ovulatory discharge of LH and ovulation. Intraventricular 5-HT blocked the release of LH induced by electrochemical stimulation of the preoptic hypothalamic area, an effect antagonized by 5-HT receptor blockade (175). Direct electrochemical stimulation of 5-HT neurons in the dorsal raphe nuclei inhibited LH secretion in ovariectomized rats and blocked spontaneous ovulation in normal rats (176,177). The inhibitory effect was reversed in ovariectomized rats by the 5-HT receptor antagonist metergoline (177). However, administration of metergoline alone to ovariectomized rats had no effect on pulsatile LH release (177). Therefore, it does not appear that 5-HT is involved in the regulation of pulsatile LH release in the absence of ovarian steroids.

Contrary to the above, several lines of evidence support a permissive or facilitatory role for 5-HT in ovulation. Decreased endogenous 5-HT levels, induced by the inhibition of 5-HT synthesis with PCPA, block ovulation (167) and the proestrous rise in LH (178) in rats. Several 5-HT antagonists have been reported to block spontaneous ovulation (179) and PMSG-induced ovulation in immature rats (180). Lesioning the dorsal and median raphe nuclei with the neurotoxin 5,7-DHT produced a dose-dependent inhibition of the incidence of PMSG-induced ovulation (181). Correlated with the suppression of ovulation was a significant decrease in the uptake of 5-HT in the suprachiasmatic and arcuate-median eminence hypothalamic regions of the rats. Thus 5-HT input to these regions appears to be essential for ovulation. The functional recovery of gonadotropin secretion was shown to be well correlated with the 5-HT axon regeneration and reinnervation of the hypothalamus following 5,7-DHT lesioning (150). As a possible explanation of the above contradictory roles for 5-HT in ovulation, Kordon and Glowinski (144) proposed the existence of (a) an inhibitory serotonergic center located in the medial basal hypothalamus and (b) a stimulatory or permissive center located in the preoptic-suprachiasmatic region. There is evidence to support the existence of such centers. The stereotaxic microinjection of the 5-HT neurotoxin 5,7-DHT into the medial basal hypothalamus elevates resting levels of LH, whereas similar injections into the preoptic hypothalamic area lowers circulating LH levels (182).

The hormonal environment of the animal is likely to be critical to the expression of 5-HT actions on gonadotropin secretion and ovulation. Gonadal steroids have been shown to exert considerable influence on the actions of 5-HT. The intraventricular administration of 5-HT has been shown to inhibit LH release in castrated female rats (86) but stimulates LH release in intact male rats (118) and is without effect on LH levels in intact female rats (86). Systemically administered 5-HT effectively increases circulating LH levels (a) when ovariectomized rats are pretreated with E_2 and (b) in normal cycling rats during estrus (183). A diurnal afternoon surge of LH occurs in estrogen-treated, ovariectomized rats (184); this appears to be dependent upon 5-HT input. Properly timed administration of PCPA, which caused a marked decrease in brain tryptophan hydroxylate activity and 5-HT levels, blocks the E_2-induced afternoon LH surge (184). This effect is reversed with 5-HTP administered to these rats either intraventricularly or systemically (185,186). Serotonin levels in the suprachiasmatic nucleus display a transitory peak concurrent with the LH surge (187). This peak is absent in both male rats and untreated, ovariectomized female rats, suggesting that the facilitatory action of 5-HT on LH release is E_2-dependent. The sequential administration of E_2 and progesterone produces significant increases in both 5-HT concentration and 5-HT synthesis in the dorsal raphe nuclei, the site of the serotonergic cell bodies (188). These nuclei give rise to a major portion of the serotonergic innervation within the hypothalamus. Consequentially, steroid administration also produces significant increases in 5-HT levels in the median eminence (189,190), the preoptic-anterior hypothalamus (191), and other related hypothalamic regions (182). Estradiol injections cause a selective increase in the density of serotonin (5-HT) receptors in the preoptic area, anterior hypothalamus, lateral septum, and arcuate-median eminence regions in ovariectomized rats (192). The increase in 5-HT receptors may be relevant, since these anatomical structures are known to be important in the control of ovulation. The density of 5-HT receptors in the basal forebrain, which includes the hypothalamus, septum, and preoptic area, has been shown to undergo regular changes during the estrous cycle of the rat (193). A significantly lower density was found on proestrus and estrus than on diestrus. Significant changes were not observed in other brain regions, i.e., hippocampus, cortex, and caudate.

It is likely that the actions of 5-HT on LH secretion and ovulation are expressed via changes in the outflow of LHRH from neurosecretory neurons rather than direct actions at the pituitary gland. Leonardelli et al. (194) provided evidence that 5-HT can act directly on hypothalamic LHRH-releasing structures. These investigators induced neurons in the preoptic-suprachiasmatic region to stain immunocytochemically for LHRH by infusing 5-HT into the lateral ventricle of rats. The 5-HT neuronal system is potentially one of several neurotransmitter systems intimately related to the gonadotropin-regulating functions of the preoptic-anterior hypothalamus, medial basal hypothalamus, and median eminence. Gonadal steroid modulation of the activity of these neurotransmitter systems is a central mechanism through which these hormones affect cyclic gonadotropin secretion and control ovulation (195). It is not surprising, then, that gonadal steroids have been shown to exert actions on 5-HT neuronal activity. Thus during the periovulatory period, 5-HT-containing neurons are involved in the stimulation of LH secretion, whereas in the absence of high E_2 levels, the converse is true.

γ-AMINOBUTYRIC ACID

Neuroanatomy of GABA Neurons

The levels of GABA and the rate-limiting enzyme for its synthesis, glutamate decarboxylase (GAD), are found in high levels in the hypothalamus (196). A fivefold difference in GAD activity levels was seen among the hypothalamic nuclei of the rat. High levels were seen in the preoptic, anterior, and dorsomedial nuclei, with low levels in the arcuate and supraoptic nuclei and median eminence. Levels of GABA were fairly uniform among hypothalamic nuclei. Deafferentation studies suggest that there are GABA neurons intrinsic to the hypothalamus (197). Using [^{3}H]GABA uptake studies in conjunction with autoradiography, GABA-concentrating cells were seen in the medial basal hypothalamus (198) and in nerve fibers in the external layer of the median eminence (199). Immunohistochemical studies with a purified GAD antibody revealed numerous GABA neurons within the nuclei of the hypothalamus (200). A dense plexus of GAD-containing nerve terminals was seen in the external layer of the median eminence.

Interestingly, immunohistochemically identified GAD neurons in the medial-preoptic/anterior-hypothalamic regions were shown to contain estrogen receptors (201). In this same region, GAD-containing terminals have been shown to synapse on LHRH-containing neurons (1).

The rich GABAergic innervation of the hypothalamus is consistent with the data (which we will now discuss) that show that GABA is involved in the neural regulation of LH and PRL. However, several lines of evidence also suggest that GABA may be a hypothalamic hormone involved in the inhibitory regulation of PRL. The presence of significant numbers of GAD-staining terminals in the external layer of the median eminence is consistent with this hypothesis.

Role of GABA in the Control of LH Secretion

The administration of either GABA (202) or the GABA agonist muscimol (202,203) inhibits the pulsatile release of LH in ovariectomized rats. Treatment with aminooxyacetic acid, a blocker of GABA degradation, also inhibited pulsatile LH release (204). In ovariectomized rats primed with E_2 plus progesterone, the GABA agonists baclofen and muscimol, as well as aminooxyacetic acid, blocked the surge of LH (204,205). The action of muscimol could be partially blocked with the GABA antagonist bicuculline; however, the action of baclofen was not affected (205).

Correlated with these inhibitory effects of GABA on both pulsatile and steroid-induced surges of LH, changes in the activity of noradrenergic neurons have been reported. Systemic injection of muscimol and baclofen into ovariectomized, steroid-primed rats decreased the turnover rate of NE in the medial preoptic area and medial basal hypothalamus (205). No effects on DA turnover were seen in either structure. In ovariectomized rats the intraventricular injection of muscimol also inhibited the turnover rate of NE in the medial-preoptic/anterior-hypothalamic area (203). In this study the turnover rate of DA was decreased in the anterior medial basal hypothalamus and medial-preoptic/anterior-hypothalamic area. In ovariectomized E_2-primed rats the release of GABA, as measured via push-pull cannulae, decreased in the afternoon of the LH surge, whereas that of NE increased (47). In the morning, when LH levels were suppressed by the steroid-priming relative to ovariectomized animals, the levels of GABA release were high compared to those seen in the ovariectomized animals. It has been proposed that GABA neurons in the preoptic area mediate the negative feedback action of E_2 (47,201). This is substantiated by the following findings: (a) GABA neurons in this region contain estrogen receptors; (b) estrogen increases the activity of these neurons during negative feedback. The increase in GABA activity is closely correlated with a decrease in noradrenergic activity, which is implicated in the stimulation of LH release. The possibility also exists that GABAergic neurons may directly inhibit LHRH release, since GABA-containing terminals synapse with LHRH-containing neurons.

Role of GABA in the Control of Prolactin Secretion

As we have discussed, a relatively dense innervation of GABA terminals exists in the external layer of the median eminence. GABA has been measured in the hypophyseal portal blood but with conflicting results. One laboratory using a radioreceptor assay found equivalent levels of GABA in the portal and peripheral blood of diestrous rats (206). In a subsequent report, GABA levels in portal blood also measured by a radioreceptor assay were found to be twice that in peripheral blood of male rats (207). However, data indicated that a significant portion of this GABA-like activity was not GABA but possibly a metabolite of GABA. Electrical stimulation of the median eminence caused an eightfold increase in GABA levels, demonstrating the ability of median eminence neurons to release GABA in large amounts into portal blood. Treatment of ovariectomized rats with ethanolamine-*O*-sulfate, an inhibitor of GABA metabolism, caused a three- to fourfold increase in GABA levels in portal blood (208). This increase in GABA levels was closely correlated with a decrease in circulating PRL levels.

Clearly, there are GABA receptors in the anterior pituitary (208), and they suppress PRL secretion (209) and synthesis (210). However, one disturbing aspect of GABA's role as an inhibitory modulator of PRL secretion is that administration of the GABA antagonists bicuculline and picrotoxin does not elevate PRL secretion in male or ovariectomized E_2-treated rats (211). Administration of DA antagonists, on the other hand, has been universally found to elevate PRL secretion (9). Therefore it appears that an inhibitory GABAergic neurosecretory system is present in the rat; however, it does not appear to tonically regulate PRL secretion at the pituitary level. Under what physiological circumstances it does is still unclear.

Besides this potential action of GABA as a PRL inhibitory hormone, there is also evidence that it acts centrally to stimulate PRL release. Intraventricular administration of GABA (211,213) or the GABA agonist muscimol stimulates PRL release in male rats as well as in both ovariectomized and ovariectomized E_2-primed female rats (203,211). One possible mechanism for this stimulatory action of GABA could be by the inhibition of the activity of tuberoinfundibular DA neurons. In one study the turnover rate of DA neurons was decreased following administration of muscimol (203); however, in a second study there was no effect (205).

HISTAMINE

Histamine-containing neurons have been implicated in the neuroendocrine regulation of both LH and PRL secretion. The actions of histamine are mediated through pharmacologically well-characterized H_1 and H_2 receptors. The availability of subtype-selective agonists and antagonists has greatly aided recent studies. As with other amines, histamine does not cross the blood-brain barrier; therefore it is necessary to inject it into the ventricular system to study its central effects.

Anatomy of Histaminergic Neurons

Histamine is found in high concentrations in the hypothalamus (214). The content of histamine varies throughout the hypothalamus, with the highest levels observed in the median eminence; the arcuate, suprachiasmatic, and mammillary nuclei also contain high levels (215). The regional distribution of histidine decarboxylase, the enzyme that converts histidine to histamine, follows closely with that of histamine content except in the median eminence (216). It appears that a portion of the histamine in the median eminence is in mast cells, which are not capable of synthesizing histamine. However, in a recent immunocytochemical study using antibodies to histamine, large numbers of histamine-containing nerve terminals were observed in both the external and internal zones of the median eminence (217). Histamine-containing cell bodies were observed in the lateral hypothalamus, an observation consistent with the finding that lesions of the lateral hypothalamus decreased hypothalamic histidine decarboxylase activity by approximately 50% (218). Further suggesting that hypothalamic histamine-containing nerve processes are projections from intrahypothalamic cell bodies is the observation that complete deafferentation of the medial basal hypothalamus does not decrease histamine levels in the median eminence as well in the ventromedial and dorsomedial nuclei (197).

Role of Histamine in the Regulation of LH Secretion

Sawyer (219), in 1955, first demonstrated that the intraventricular (but not intravenous) administration of histamine induced ovulation in estrogen-primed rabbits. The intraventricular administration of histamine increases LH secretion in ovariectomized E_2-primed rats (220) and proestrous rats (222) but not in male rats (222,223). Intravenous histamine was shown to have no effect (220).

In men (224) and women (225) the systemic administration of histamine did not affect LH levels. However, the administration of histamine did potentiate the response to LHRH. The potentiation by histamine of the response to LHRH in men could be blocked by both the H_1 antagonist mepyramine and the H_2 antagonist cimetidine (224). The significance of this effect is unclear because histamine has been shown to have no direct effect *in vitro* on the secretion of LH or the stimulation of LH secretion by LHRH in the rat anterior pituitary (226). Since histamine does not cross the blood-brain barrier and does not affect basal LH secretion, it is unclear how it is acting to potentiate the action of LHRH.

The central stimulating effects of histamine may be mediated via an H_1 receptor that regulates the release of LHRH. Perifusion of medial basal hypothalamic fragments from diestrous female rats with histamine or the H_1 agonist 2-methylhistamine causes a significant increase in the release of LHRH (226). The effect was blocked by simultaneous administration of the H_1 antagonist mepyramine. No effect of histamine was observed on the basal or LHRH-stimulated release of LH from the anterior pituitary. However, in another *in-vitro* study using medial basal hypothalamic fragments from male rats, histamine had no effect on LHRH release (227).

The role of histamine in the physiological regulation of LH secretion is unclear. Few experiments to determine the effects of histamine antagonists on LH secretion have been reported. The fragmentary data that exist suggest that histamine might play a role in LH regulation; however, further data are needed for a convincing argument to be made.

Role of Histamine in the Regulation of PRL Secretion

Substantially more data exist showing that the central activation of histaminergic neurons results in the release of PRL. This effect is not mediated at the level of the anterior pituitary because neither the injection of histamine into the pituitary (220) nor the incubation of primary cultures of anterior pituitary cells with histamine (226) affects PRL secretion.

Intraventricular injection of histamine releases PRL in both male (221–223) and female rats (220,222). Intraventricular administration of the H_2 antagonists cimetidine and metamide, but not the H_1 antagonist diphenhydramine, blocked the stimulation of PRL by histamine in male rats (227,229,230). The effect of histamine could be mimicked by the intraventricular administration of the H_2 agonists 4-methylhistamine and dimaprit, whereas the H_1 agonists 2,2-pyridylethylamine and 2-thiazolylethylamine have no effect (229,230).

When histamine is administered systemically it also stimulates PRL release in male rats; however, the response appears to be mediated via an H_1 receptor (230). The H_1 agonist 2-thiazolylethylamine mimics the action of systemic histamine, and the systemic action of histamine is blocked by the H_1 antagonist mepyramine (230). No effect of histamine was seen on PRL release when incubated with anterior pituitaries or when administered to stalk-sectioned rats. In normal men the infusion of histamine also stimulated PRL release, and the response was inhibited by the H_1 blocker mepyramine (231); however, in women the systemic administration of histamine had no effect (225).

The stimulatory effect of histamine could be mediated either via the inhibition of DA release or the stimulation of the release of TRH. Intraventricular histamine decreases the portal blood levels of DA in male rats by 26% (232). However, this change in DA could only account for a portion of the sixfold increase in PRL secretion. Incubation of hypothalamic slices (233) or hypothalamic synaptosomes (234) with histamine stimulated the release of TRH. Systemic administration of histamine to women also potentiated TRH-induced PRL secretion; however, as with the potentiating effect of histamine on LHRH, the mechanism of this response is unclear (225).

Administration of histamine antagonists have been reported to have little or no effect on basal PRL secretion (234). The H_2 antagonist cimetidine has been reported to increase PRL levels when administered systemically to rats; however, this effect does not appear to be mediated by histamine receptors (236).

Interestingly, the H_1 antagonist diphenhydramine has been reported to inhibit increases in PRL and decreases in LH caused by restraint stress (220). The suckling-induced release of PRL was dramatically suppressed by the intraventricular administration of the H_1 antagonists diphenhydramine and mepyramine but not the H_2 antagonist metiamide (237). However, metiamide administration increased PRL levels in nonsuckling mothers, whereas diphenhydramine had no effect. Therefore in lactating rats it appears that histaminergic neurons are involved in the tonic suppression of resting levels of PRL via H_2 receptors but that, during suckling, histaminergic neurons partially mediate the stimulation of PRL release via H_1 receptors.

Further studies will be necessary to determine the physiological role of histaminergic neurons in PRL secretion. Clearly, there are multiple histaminergic effects mediated by both H_1 and H_2 receptors. An important step in the understanding of the action of histamine will be the careful elucidation of the neuroanatomy of histaminergic neurons and their connectivity with other neuroendocrine elements.

NEUROPEPTIDES

Recent improvements in neuropeptide characterization and localization methods have resulted in an in-depth reappraisal of our understanding of neuroendocrine control. In addition to "conventional" neurotransmitters, over 30 peptides have recently been shown to regulate pituitary reproductive hormones. Less than five of them were known in 1969. Most of them have been found in significant amounts in the mediobasal hypothalamus and are released into the hypophyseal portal system. In the pituitary they affect not one, but usually several, adenohypophyseal cell types. In addition, they can interact with each other's release or modulate nonpeptide neurotransmission at hypothalamic synapses or in the median eminence. These properties endow them with both direct and indirect effects on hormone control.

Hypothalamic-peptide-producing neurons exhibit a common organization pattern. Despite their apparent scattering throughout the hypothalamus, most of their cell bodies (over 90%) are located in the paraventricular nucleus, the medial periventricular area, or the arcuate nucleus. Smaller populations of neurons are found in the medial preoptic area (sometimes also referred to as the anterior periventricular area) and the suprachiasmatic nucleus (238,239).

Irrespective of the location of their cell bodies, major projections of all those neurons exhibit a common final pathway. In rodents, for instance, medial preoptic neurons follow an initial dorsolateral course, proceed caudally with the medial forebrain bundle, and leave it to enter the median eminence from an anterolateral direction. As they come close to the paraventricular and the arcuate nucleus, these fibers merge with axons proceeding from those areas (240).

The distribution area of hypothalamic neurosecretory neurons has widened in the course of evolution. In fishes, neurosecretory neurons are concentrated in the periventricular space around the medial hypothalamus. They progressively invade more rostral areas in birds and reptiles. Diversity is also observed in the pattern in mammals: In primates, the deeper funnel-like shape of the tuber cinereum caused a few preoptic neurons to migrate closer to arcuate-periventricular structures as compared with migration observed in rodents (241).

According to mapping studies based on neuron labeling or electrophysiological methods, the median eminence is only one of several projection sites for neurosecretory neurons. Their axon collaterals innervate several hypothalamic, as well as extrahypothalamic, structures. Paraventricular and arcuate neurons, in particular, are in contact with a large number of brain structures (240). This strategic position accounts for their role in coordinating hormone regulation, other autonomic functions, and behavior.

Techniques of functional neuroanatomy have recently permitted formal identification of a few neuropeptide synapses. Most of them represent articulations of nerve endings with perikarya elaborating a different transmitter, but synapses connecting homologous neurons (e.g., LHRH fibers on LHRH cell bodies, or oxytocin fibers on oxytocin cell bodies) have also been described. In addition, juxtaposition of nerve endings within the median eminence seems to account for axo-axonal interactions, even in the absence of identifiable synaptic specialization.

In this section, five groups of neuropeptide-producing neurons will be considered separately, because each of them shares common anatomical or functional properties: (a) those that predominantly originate in the preoptic area, namely somatostatin or somatotropin-release-inhibiting factor (SRIF), LHRH, tachykinins, neurotensin, atrial natriuretic factor (ANF); (b) peptides produced in the arcuate nucleus, namely peptides from the pancreatic family (NPY, PYY, pancreatic polypeptide, and galanin); (c) those mainly produced in perikarya of the paraventricular or supraoptic nuclei, namely TRH, CRF, cholecystokinin, vasopressin, oxytocin, angiotensin, bradykinin, and bombesin; (d) gastrointestinal peptides of the secretin-glucagon family (GRF, VIP, PHI, secretin, gastric inhibitory peptide, oxyntomodulin); (e) the opioid peptide family. In each case, we will briefly review the anatomical organization, the biosynthetic pathways, the distribution of receptors in the brain, and general effects of each peptide. We will then review their direct effects on pituitary cells (most of which are discussed at length in other chapters of these volumes) and describe the hypothalamic mechanisms by which they can modulate secretion of gonadotropins, PRL, and oxytocin or exert other actions on reproductive functions. In summary tables, we will attempt to distinguish effects or interactions that appear reasonably well characterized from a pharmacological point of view from those that should still be considered preliminary.

HYPOTHALAMIC PEPTIDES PRODUCED IN THE PREOPTIC-PERIVENTRICULAR AREA

Major neuropeptides with hypothalamic perikarya of neuroendocrine relevance located in this area are somatostatin, LHRH, tachykinins, neurotensin, and atrial natriuretic peptide. Although a somewhat denser mass of neurons is found in the central portion of the area (242), most cell bodies of the preoptico-infundibular system are scattered throughout the anterior hypothalamus, with a few perikarya located as far rostrally as the organum vasculosum of the lamina terminalis. Distribution of their projections presents several commonalities. Most of them innervate the olfactory tubercules, basal nuclei, periaqueductal gray, and suprachiasmatic nucleus and many are also found in the amygdala, the septum, and the cortex.

Somatostatin

Biochemistry, Distribution, and Pharmacology

Somatostatin, characterized in 1972 (243), is processed from a 210-amino-acid precursor (244). The nucleotide sequence of the gene coding for the precursor was originally characterized in the fish pancreas (245). The rat (244) and human genes (246) were subsequently described. Somatostatin is widely distributed throughout the brain, particularly in the hypothalamus, the limbic system, the septum, the hippocampus, the cortex, and the medulla (247,248). Somatostatin-producing neurons can be put into three categories. The first includes hypothalamic projections, most of which derive from the anterior periventricular portion of the diencephalon (249–254). Electrical stimulation of this area is most effective in releasing the peptide into the portal system (255). A second group of long extrahypothalamic neurons originates in the amygdala (256–258), whereas the last group consists of short interneurons present in several brain structures (258,259). Connections between hypothalamic and extrahypothalamic somatostatin neurons are scarce, but a few hypothalamic neurons project to the locus coeruleus and the substantia nigra (260), whereas hypothalamic projections from the amygdala have been postulated on the basis of indirect experiments (261). In addition, homologous somatostatin synapses have been described in the periventricular area (262). They may account for the "ultrashort" somatostatin-to-somatostatin feedback observed after intraventricular infusion of the peptide (263,264).

Post-translational processing can generate two distinct molecules endowed with somatostatin activity, somatostatin 14, and somatostatin 28 (265). Both forms (266), as well as somatostatin 28(1–12), the C-terminal residue of the longer peptide, can be released from the median eminence and have been assayed in hypophyseal portal blood (267). The distribution of somatostatin 14 and 28 does not completely overlap in the central nervous system (268), but their occurrence in different neurons is still unsettled (258). Differential production of either one has been obtained in populations of neurons in culture (269).

Somatostatin-binding sites are present in several brain areas, particularly those rich in endogenous peptide (270). In the adenohypophysis (271), receptors are located on somatotrophs as well as on thyrotrophs and lactotrophs (272). They have also been identified on growth-hormone (GH) and on PRL-producing human tumor cells (273). In the brain, the existence of subsets of receptors for somatostatin 14 and 28 has been reported (274), but their kinetic properties show only minor differences (275). So far, only one subset of binding sites has been found in the pituitary (274,275).

Somatostatin has a wide range of effects on brain functions. For instance, it may be involved in neuropathologic disorders such as Alzheimer's senile dementia (258).

Effects of Somatostatin on Adenohypophyseal Hormones

Somatostatin is a most potent inhibitor of GH secretion (243); under discrete endocrine conditions, it also inhibits TSH (276) and PRL secretion (277). These effects involve direct actions of the peptide on the pituitary and are discussed in other chapters of these volumes. We will thus only summarize them briefly. Somatostatin inhibition of plasma PRL levels is most effective in hypothyroid animals (277) and after treatment with estrogens (278), which results in an increase in the number of pituitary somatostatin receptors (278). Somatostatin may directly inhibit PRL release under these conditions or, alternatively, decrease the sensitivity of lactotrophs to PRL-releasing factors such as TRH and VIP (279). In fasting rats, passive immunization with anti-somatostatin antibodies results in an increased secretion of PRL (280), an observation that suggests that endogenous somatostatin is functionally involved in controlling that hormone (264).

Effects of Somatostatin Mediated by the Hypothalamus

In addition to the classic pituitary action of somatostatin, release of the peptide from nerve endings modulates several neurotransmitter systems. Norepinephrine release is inhibited by somatostatin in hypothalamus (281), but it is stimulated in the cortex (282). The peptide also facilitates DA turnover in the diencephalon when infused intraventricularly (283). *In vitro* it releases serotonin from cortical, hippocampal, and hypothalamic slices (284). Other *in-vitro* effects of the peptide include inhibition of LHRH (285) and TRH release from superfused hypothalamic fragments (286,287). Finally, somatostatin has been shown to exhibit weak antagonistic properties on opiate receptors (288).

Hypothalamic somatostatin synaptic transmission appears episodic (289) and correlates with the release of GRH, slightly preceding it (290). Paraventricular projections to the arcuate nucleus (291) probably account for the correlation and play a role in the regulation of the frequency of GH ultradian rhythms (290).

These interactions are summarized in Table 1. They show a certain degree of agreement with the overall hormonal consequences of somatostatin administration. Somatostatin-induced inhibition of gonadotropins is consistent with its inhibitory actions on both hypothalamic NE (281) and LHRH (285). Decreased TRH (286,287) and increased DA release (283) can be assumed to act synergistically with the direct negative action of somatostatin on lactotrophs.

Luliberin or LHRH

The structure of the LHRH precursor has been deduced from the DNA sequence of the gene coding for the peptide (292). It consists of 92 amino acids. The major, if not the exclusive, brain localization of the corresponding neurons is the periventricular area of the hypothalamus and a circumventricular organ, the organum vasculosum of the lamina terminalis (293–295). In addition to their major projec-

TABLE 1. *Reproductive actions of medial-preoptic–periventricular and arcuate peptide-containing neurons*[a]

	Overall neuroendocrine effect						
	Prolactin		Gonadotropins				
Peptide	Direct (1)	Indirect (2)	Direct (1)	Indirect (2)	Effects at hypothalamic level	Other reproductive actions	Physiological relevance
SRIF	↓	↓		↓	↓ NA, ↓ LHRH, ↓ TRH		Hypothyroidism, high E_2 fasting stress
DA							
LHRH		↑	↑			↑ Sexual behavior	
SP	↑			↑ ?			
NPY			↑	(3) ↓ or ↑ (4)	LHRH pulsatility	↓ Sexual behavior	
NT	↑	↓			↓ SRIF, suprachiasmatic rhythmicity		
Galanin	↑				↓ DA		

[a](1) Direct actions on pituitary cells; (2) by indirect effects on hypothalamic neurons; (3) only in castrated animals; (4) only in intact or in sex-steroid-treated animals; (↑ ↓) increases or decreases hormone or transmitter release; (↑ ↓) effect not fully characterized yet.

tions to the median eminence, which they reach from a dorsolateral course (296), LHRH neurons project to several extrahypothalamic structures, particularly the mesencephalic central gray, the midbrain (297), the hippocampus, the amygdala (298), and the olfactory tubercules (299). Immunocytochemical studies with antibodies raised against a non-LHRH-containing portion of the precursor sequence gave comparable results (300). Extrahypothalamic projections are believed to proceed from subsets of neurons distinct from those innervating the median eminence (298). Coordination between both subsets is probably achieved by the numerous collateral synaptic contacts between LHRH-producing preoptic neurons (301). This may represent the anatomical basis of the synchronous electrical activation of those neurons (302), which is presumably involved in pulsatile release of massive amounts of the decapeptide.

A fairly dense population of LHRH receptors has recently been visualized in the hippocampus by autoradiographic studies (303,304). But most LHRH receptors are located in the pituitary (305), where they stimulate gonadotrophs with apparent biphasic affinities for the peptide (306).

LHRH is able to modulate the activity of discrete neurons (307). Some of these actions are dependent upon levels of sex steroids (308), which is suggestive of a possible coordination with reproductive functions. But the major extrapituitary effect of the peptide is undoubtedly to facilitate sex behavior and lordosis (309,310). The action involves mostly LHRH projections to the mesencephalic central gray matter (311). Participation of the endogenous peptide is suggested by experiments in which local administration of anti-LHRH antisera suppressed sex behavior (312).

In addition, interesting actions of an LHRH precursor sequence [GnRH-associated peptide (GAP)] have been reported on PRL inhibition (313) as well as on FSH and LH stimulation from pituitary cells in rats and monkeys (314). In the latter case, a 13-amino-acid fragment of GAP increased gonadotropin secretion by a mechanism of action distinct from that of LHRH, since LHRH antagonists did not prevent the action of GAP and the GAP fragment did not displace [^{3}H]LHRH bound to pituitary membranes (314). However, only fairly high concentrations of the peptide (10^{-5} M) were found active. Therefore, the relevance of GAP effects still awaits confirmation.

Atypical stimulation of PRL by administration of LHRH was initially reported in acromegalic patients (315) and was subsequently confirmed under various pathological conditions and in normal human subjects (316). Increased PRL secretion was also observed in the rat (317) and can be induced *in vitro* by addition of LHRH to pituitary-cell aggregates (318). Effects of LHRH on PRL are not believed to involve a direct effect of the decapeptide on lactotrophs (318). They are probably mediated by LHRH-induced release of an intermediate paracrine factor from gonadotrophs. Hypothetically, candidates for the paracrine effect are dynorphin, angiotensin II, or substance P, three peptides that coexist with gonadotropins in the same cell (319,320,330) and that are able to affect pituitary lactotrophs (see below). Alternately, alpha subunits of LH, cosecreted with the hormone but devoid, by themselves, of gonadotropic activity, were shown to stimulate PRL (321) and could thus qualify as a paracrine intermediate between LHRH and PRL responses.

Tachykinins

Tachykinins are a class of peptides consisting of substance P [a very early discovered peptide (322)] and the neurokinins A and B (or substance K). Neurokinins A and B are derived from cleavage of the closely related precursor molecules, beta and alpha protachykinin A, whereas substance P is derived from gamma protachykinin (323). Three subsets of receptors with preferential affinities for substance P and neurokinins A and B have been characterized pharmacologically (323). Neurokinin A receptors have mainly been described in peripheral tissues.

Tachykinins are widely distributed throughout the brain, mainly in the septum, the amygdala, the hippocampus, the cortex, and the medulla (324). As somatostatin, they are produced either by neurons located in the hypothalamus or amygdala with long projections, or by short interneurons (325). Substance P is a potent stimulator of locomotor activity and plays an important role in nociception (323). Tachykinin receptors are widely distributed in the brain (326) and are present in the pituitary (327).

The major site of synthesis of substance P (like that of somatostatin and LHRH) within the hypothalamus is the periventricular area, but it is produced by different neurons. These project mainly to the median eminence and the septum (328), and their distribution pattern within the hypothalamus resembles that of somatostatin (329). Substance-P-like immunoreactivity is also found in pituitary lactotrophs and gonadotrophs (330,331).

Intraventricular administration of substance P stimulates PRL and inhibits GH release in rats (332,333) and primates (334). The effect on PRL was also observed after intravenous administration of the peptide to intact rats (333) or to animals bearing a hypothalamic lesion (334), as well as on pituitary cells *in vitro* (333). These data are suggestive of a direct effect at the pituitary level.

The action of substance P on gonadotropins is more controversial. It was initially reported to stimulate LH when infused into the third ventricle (333,335) of rats but was found ineffective under the same conditions in monkeys (334). In contrast, incubation of pituitary cells in the presence of substance P was reported to decrease the responsiveness of LH cells to LHRH (336). A role of endogenous substance P in LH regulation was postulated on the basis of passive immunization experiments with anti-substance-P antisera, but those led either to increased FSH and LH plasma levels (337) or, on the contrary, to decreased LH without a change in FSH (338). Endogenous levels of substance P in discrete hypothalamic areas fluctuate during the estrous cycle of rat (339,340), as do receptors for the peptide in the pituitary, with maximal binding in late proestrus (340).

Neurotensin

Neurotensin is a 13-amino-acid peptide. Its precursor has not been characterized as yet (341). The neuronal distribution of neurotensin is comparable to that of other neuropeptides described in this section. Most of its hypothalamic cell bodies are found in the anterior periventricular system, although some perikarya are also present in the paraventricular and the arcuate nuclei (342–344). Some periventricular and arcuate neurons colocalize neurotensin and DA (345,346). As with LHRH neurons, those elaborating neurotensin project to the olfactory tubercules (347). Similarly to somatostatin, neurotensin is abundant in cell bodies of the amygdala and the septum (343). Fibers originating in the medial nucleus of the amygdaloid complex project to the hypothalamic ventromedial nucleus (348). Other densely innervated structures are the periaqueductal gray, the caudate putamen, the locus coeruleus, the septum, and the suprachiasmatic nucleus (343). A few cells in the anterior pituitary also stain with anti-neurotensin antibodies (343).

Two classes of binding sites have been described in the brain, with 1 or 5 nM affinity for their ligand (349). Their distribution, for the most part, follows along with the anatomical localizations of the peptide (350). In addition, receptors are also found in the suprachiasmatic nucleus (351).

The major nonreproductive endocrine functions of neurotensin are: stimulation of insulin secretion (352), inhibition of glucagon secretion (352), and modulation of gastrointestinal motility (347). Neurotensin receptors have been found on cholinergic cell bodies in the nucleus basalis (353). Since the concentration of neurotensin receptors is reduced in Alzheimer's senile dementia, the peptide may be associated with somatostatin and NPY in the cholinergic dysfunctions observed in that disease (354).

Intraventricular administration of relatively large doses of neurotensin has been shown to inhibit plasma LH. The effect is not mimicked by systemic administration and is not observed when pituitary cells are exposed to neurotensin *in vitro* (332). The peptide was thus assumed to modulate as-yet unknown hypothalamic components of gonadotropic control. When infused directly into the preoptic area, the region where most neurotensin cell bodies are located, the peptide stimulates LH release (355). Similar conflicting effects on GH secretion have been observed after the intraventricular or systemic administration of neurotensin (335,356).

The effect of neurotensin on PRL secretion appears complex. The intraventricular administration of relatively high doses of neurotensin inhibits plasma PRL levels with a rather poor dose-dependent relationship (332). In contrast, it has a strong PRL-releasing activity when administered intravenously (332,335), an effect shown to correspond to a demonstrated direct action on the lactotroph (357). The action of neurotensin on pituitary hormone secretion is highly dependent upon sex steroids (358) (Table 1).

Several direct effects of neurotensin on brain transmitters have been described, with emphasis on DA turnover in nigrostriatal neurons (359) and on ascending cholinergic neurons (360). In the hypothalamus the peptide has been claimed to inhibit somatostatin release *in vitro* (361). This effect could account for the decreased PRL and GH secretion observed after the intraventricular infusion of neurotensin.

High concentrations of neurotensin and neurotensin receptors are found in the suprachiasmatic nucleus (350). In addition, concentrations of a subpopulation of these receptors, located in the anteromedial portion of the nucleus, decrease to a marked extent after treatment with E_2 (351). Neurotensin thus may play a role in the regulation of circadian rhythms. Other E_2-dependent processes within the suprachiasmatic nucleus have been shown to participate in the regulation of reproductive hormone cyclicity (362).

Atrial Natriuretic Factor

Atrial natriuretic factor, which was initially discovered in the heart, is a 28-amino-acid peptide containing a single disulfide bond and is derived from a 152-amino-acid preprohormone sequence (363). The peptide and its receptors have been identified in several brain structures, particularly those concerned with control of water balance (364) and circumventricular organs, including the organum vasculosum of the lamina terminalis and the median eminence (365). Most hypothalamic cell bodies containing atrial natriuretic factor are located in the medial preoptic area, but a few are also found in the paraventricular and the arcuate nuclei (366). Atrial natriuretic factor in relatively high concentrations (10–1,000 nM) has been reported to stimulate the release of LH from pituitary cells *in vitro* and to prolong the effect of LHRH (367). But it is still unclear whether the action is due to the peptide itself or to a possible contaminant (368). Atrial natriuretic factor is also able to act directly at the testicular level to increase testosterone synthesis (369). Actions on both pituitary and testis are thought to involve the activation of guanylate cyclase (368,369).

Atrial natriuretic factor is predominantly inhibitory to neuronal activity upon direct local application (370). One of its major neuroendocrine roles is to inhibit vasopressin release (371), particularly after dehydration (372).

HYPOTHALAMIC NEUROPEPTIDES SYNTHESIZED IN THE ARCUATE NUCLEUS

The arcuate nucleus is the major hypothalamic source of several neurohormones important for neuroendocrine control: DA, beta-endorphin and other POMC-related peptides, peptides from the pancreatic family (neuropeptide Y, peptide YY, and pancreatic peptide), GRF, and galanin. In addition to the external layer of the median eminence and the posterior pituitary, arcuate neurons project to the periventricular and supraoptic nucleus as well as to the medial preoptic area. The major projections relevant to the scope of this chapter are neurons containing POMC-derived peptides, which establish contacts with LHRH neurons in the preoptic area (373) and with cell bodies in the paraventricular nucleus (374,375). Additionally, neurons containing neuropeptide Y also provide input to the paraventricular nucleus (376). Intrinsic connections between arcuate POMC-producing neurons have also been demonstrated (377,378).

Peptides from the Pancreatic Family: Neuropeptide Y, Peptide YY, and Pancreatic Peptide

Peptides belonging to this family are closely related. Both NPY and PYY contain 36 amino acids (379) and differ only by nine amino-acid substitutions (380,381). They are derived from related 97-amino-acid precurors (pre-pro-NPY).

Neuropeptide Y is widely distributed in the brain, particularly in the amygdala, the septum, the bed nucleus of the stria terminalis, the cortex, and the hippocampus (382–384). Its distribution resembles that of somatostatin (385–387). Both peptides have been shown to colocalize in various extrahypothalamic structures (387). Several neurons also contain both NPY and catecholamines (388). In many regions, NPY overlaps with peptide YY and the pancreatic polypeptide.

Neuropeptide Y is particularly abundant in the arcuate nucleus (382), but scattered NPY neurons are also found in the preoptic-periventricular area of the ventromedial hypothalamus (389,390). Neuropeptide Y and PYY neurons send numerous projections to the suprachiasmatic nucleus (382,389,390), a structure important for cyclic endocrine control (362).

Two subsets of receptors for the pancreatic polypeptide family have been described. One exhibits the highest affinity for NPY and is widely distributed in the brain (391). The other has a greater affinity for PYY, but also recognizes NPY at 10-fold higher concentrations, and is mainly present in peripheral organs (391).

NPY has a paradoxical action on gonadotropins. Several authors have found that it inhibits LH release when administered to castrated male (392) or female rats (393,394) or rabbits (395). In contrast, in male and female intact animals or in estrogen-treated castrates, the peptide elevates LH levels (393). Both the inhibitory and stimulatory effects of NPY could be reproduced by administration of pancreatic polypeptide to ovariectomized rats or estrogen-supplemented ovariectomized rats, respectively (396,397).

Perfusion of NPY into the median eminence in conscious castrated rabbits has been found to decrease the frequency of LHRH pulses (395). This suggests that the primary action of the peptide is on hypothalamic structures outside the blood-brain barrier, i.e., on the median eminence or organum vasculosum of the lamina terminalis (392), since intravenous and intraventricular administration were equally effective. In addition, the stimulatory action of NPY could involve a direct, steroid-dependent action on pituitary gonadotrophs, since it was observed to potentiate the LH response to LHRH in incubated hemipituitaries (Table 1).

In discrete brain regions, immunoreactive NPY concentrations have been found to correlate with median eminence LHRH and plasma LH concentrations (399).

Inhibition of sex behavior could represent an additional function of NPY in reproductive function (400). The peptide is also a good stimulator of feeding behavior, and it might play a role in the coordination of both functions.

Galanin

Galanin, a 29-amino-acid peptide (401), is widely distributed in the central nervous system (402,403). It has recently been identified in the lateral portion of the arcuate nucleus colocalized with GRF, neurotensin, GABA, and tyrosine hydroxylase (404). The major neuroendocrine effect of galanin described thus far is a stimulation of GH upon intraventricular infusion of low (50 pM) concentrations of the peptide (405). This effect could involve the activation of GRF neurons, which colocalize galanin (405). Galanin has an inhibitory effect on the turnover rate of tuberoinfundibular DA neurons (406), a finding that may suggest an interesting short-loop feedback mechanism for neurons colocalizing both transmitters. No presynaptic DA autofeedback has been found in the tuberoinfundibular DA neurons. This function could thus be fulfilled by colocalized galanin. Effects of galanin on PRL have not been reported yet. Galanin is not believed to have direct actions on the pituitary (405) (Table 1).

HYPOTHALAMIC NEUROPEPTIDES SYNTHESIZED IN THE PARAVENTRICULAR NUCLEUS

The paraventricular nucleus of the hypothalamus is among the most dense neuronal masses of the diencephalon. It contains a medial magnocellular portion as well as a large number of parvocellular neurons located in more lateral parts of the nucleus (407). Vasopressin and oxytocin, together with the additional sequences of their precursor molecules, neurophysins I and II, were the two earliest characterized neuropeptides (409,410). Another important source of both peptides is provided by neurons located in the supraoptic nucleus (411). Parvocellular suprachiasmatic cell bodies also contain large concentrations of vasopressin (412). More recent studies have shown that several other peptides of neuroendocrine relevance are also produced in paraventricular perikarya: TRH (413), CRF (414) partially colocalized with vasopressin (415), cholecystokinin (416), angiotensin (417), bradykinin (418), bombesin (419), and VIP (420).

The periventricular nucleus receives a very rich innervation. Over 2,500 axon terminals appear to be associated with each magnocellular neuron (421). The nucleus is also extremely rich in axon collaterals (422). In addition to its projections to the median eminence and the posterior pituitary, the paraventricular nucleus contributes fibers to the medial preoptic area, the suprachiasmatic nucleus, and the arcuate nucleus (291). The nucleus also sends projections to several extrahypothalamic structures, such as the lower brain stem, the nucleus of the solitary tract, and the spinal cord (423). It is a major relay of stress-induced hormonal responses (424) (see Figs. 1 and 2).

Oxytocin and Vasopressin

Both neuropeptides are coded for by related genes with large structural homologies. They are processed from their respective precursors to give rise to nonapeptides with a disulfide bond (the active hormones), neurophysins (from which they are separated by an intermediary tripeptide), and a glycopeptide of unknown function. The C-terminal end of vasopressin consists of Arg-Gly-NH_2 in most mammals, and of Lys-Gly-NH_2 in porcine species (for a review see ref. 425).

Vasopressin (426–429) and oxytocin (426) are also widely distributed in extrahypothalamic structures. Both peptides are released into the hypophyseal portal system (430,431).

Only one class of oxytocin receptors is known, but three subsets of vasopressin receptors have been described (432). For the most part, two of them (Vla and Vlb) have been found in the central nervous system and pituitary gland (432,433).

The most conspicuous effect of vasopressin on the pituitary is the stimulation of ACTH release and the potentiation of CRF effects (434–437). These actions are mediated by vasopressin-binding sites on anterior pituitary corticotrophs (433). Oxytocin has been shown to potentiate the CRF-induced stimulation of ACTH in rat cells *in vitro* (438,439). The evidence appears more controversial in humans, since oxytocin was reported instead to inhibit the potentiated effects of CRF by vasopressin (440). Both peptides have also been shown to stimulate PRL secretion in the rat (441–443). This effect has been reported to involve a direct action of oxytocin on the pituitary (443,444) and perhaps also for arginine vasotocin (445,446). These results have been challenged by other authors, who reported inhibitory actions of posterior pituitary hormones on PRL (447). The major mode of action of vasopressin on PRL seems to involve an increased turnover of DA in tuberoinfundibular neurons (448). Dopamine metabolism is also affected by vasopressin in other brain nuclei (449). In addition, the stimulation of PRL by vasopressin may involve opiate neurons, since the effect is counteracted by naloxone (450). Participation of endogenous neurohypophyseal peptides in the regulation of PRL secretion is suggested by observed changes in PRL secretion after removal of the posterior pituitary (451).

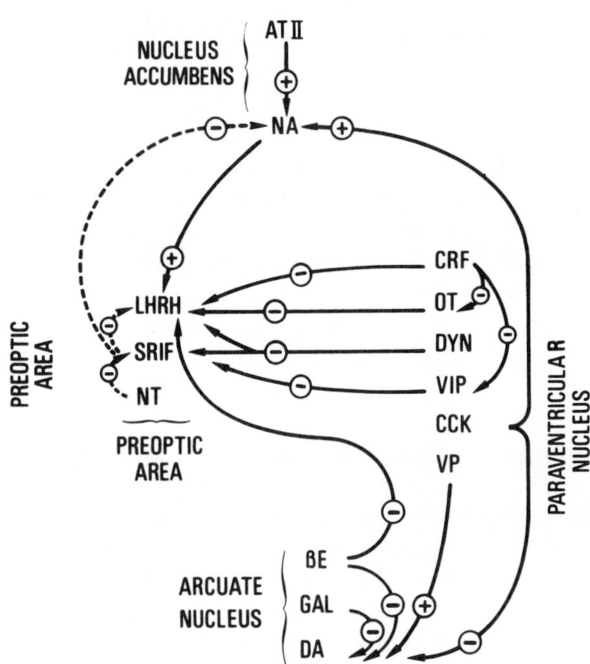

FIG. 1. Schematic representation of major hypothalamic transmitter and peptide interactions involved in the regulation of gonadotropins and prolactin. Several peptides that are produced in the paraventricular nucleus and that are concerned with processing stress, corticotropin-releasing factor (CRF), oxytocin (OT), dynorphin (DYN), as well as β-endorphin (βE), are produced in the arcuate nucleus, and are inhibitory to luteinizing-hormone-releasing hormone (LHRH). Activation of LHRH neurons is mostly achieved by noradrenergic (NA) projections. Norepinephrine release from these projections can be activated by cholecystokinin (CCK) and angiotensin II (AI II), as well as inhibited by somatostatin. Inhibition of dopamine (DA) by β-E, CCK, and galanin (GAL) represents the major indirect input to prolactin regulation. Corresponding evidence is presented in the text; it is derived mainly from *in-vitro* experiments or from experiments involving intraventricular infusion of agonists or antagonists of those peptides. Neuroanatomical studies have demonstrated the existence of synapses between βE-containing projections from the arcuate nucleus and LHRH neurons. In addition, they have shown that CRF-, OT-, and DYN-containing projections from the paraventricular nucleus are abundant in those areas, where most LHRH and somatotropin-release inhibiting-factor (SRIF) cell bodies are located. NT, neurotensin; VIP, vasoactive intestinal polypeptide; VP, vasopressin.

Effects of vasopressin and oxytocin on PRL are more pronounced under conditions of stress (452). Both peptides (452) [or, according to other authors, oxytocin only (453)] are believed to act as modulators of stress responses. Vasopressin (454) or oxytocin (455) can temper the stress-induced stimulation of ACTH. Increased oxytocin activity is also thought to play a role in the inhibition of gonadotropins observed during stress or lactation, since LH levels increase following ablation of the neural lobe (451). Subnanomolar concentrations of oxytocin inhibit basal or depolarization-induced LHRH release from the median eminence *in vitro*.

Oxytocin may facilitate the onset of estrogen-induced maternal behavior (457). The estrogen dependency of this action may involve an increase in the density of oxytocin receptors in discrete brain areas, such as the ventromedial nucleus, the organum vasculosum of the lamina terminalis, the nucleus accumbens, and, to a lesser extent, the amygdala (458). Several other nonendocrine actions of vasopressin and oxytocin have been documented and reviewed (459).

Thyrotropin-Releasing Hormone

Thyrotropin-releasing hormone (TRH) (*p*-Glu-His-Pro-NH_2), a tripeptide, was first described in 1969 (460,461). The peptide is derived from a 30-kilodalton precursor, and the corresponding gene has been characterized (462). High concentrations of TRH were initially described in the median eminence, the paraventricular nucleus, and the arcuate nucleus (463). Most TRH cell bodies were subsequently identified in the paraventricular nucleus (413, 464,465). Their nerve terminals project to the arcuate nucleus and the median eminence, since paraventricular lesions lead to a large decrease in TRH levels in these structures (413). Axons of paraventricular neurons also project to the septum (466). A large number of TRH neurons are also found in a number of extrahypothalamic structures, particularly the amygdala, the nucleus accumbens, the bed nucleus of the stria terminalis, the cortex, and the spinal cord (467). In the human hypothalamus, the distribution of TRH was reported to be asymmetrical, with a predominance on the left side (468). Significant concentrations of TRH were also found in the pituitary (465), where the peptide is believed to be internalized and stored within anterior pituitary cells (469).

Thyrotropin-releasing-hormone receptors have been localized in several brain structures and in the pituitary (470), where they may exist under two forms, each with a different affinity for their ligand (471).

In addition to its eponymal action on thyrotropin release (460,461,472), TRH has been shown to directly stimulate the release of PRL (472,474) and GH (475). The action of TRH on somatotrophs is inconsistent and more controversial (476) than its actions on PRL and TSH. Effects of TRH on GH have primarily been reported in rats after the removal of other hypothalamic influences, either by mediobasal hypothalamic lesions (477), by placing the pituitary *in vitro* (477), or in humans associated with pathological conditions (478).

Prolactin release by TRH is enhanced by E_2, presumably by an action of the steroid on the number of TRH-binding sites of lactotrophs (479). Pituitary TRH receptor number and efficacy on PRL release fluctuate during the estrous cycle (480). An endogenously formed dipeptide metabolite of TRH, His-Pro-diketopiperazine, has been shown to inhibit PRL release (481), but the relevance of that action is still unclear.

Thyrotropin-releasing hormone is able to affect transmitter turnover in various brain structures. It modulates acetylcholine release (360), antagonizes neurotensin-induced antinociception (482), and enhances NE turnover in extrahypothalamic structures (483–485). Effects on NE may participate in the antidepressive action attributed to the tripeptide (486). An interaction between TRH and serotonin at the level of the spinal cord has been postulated to play a role in the control of sex behavior in male rats (487).

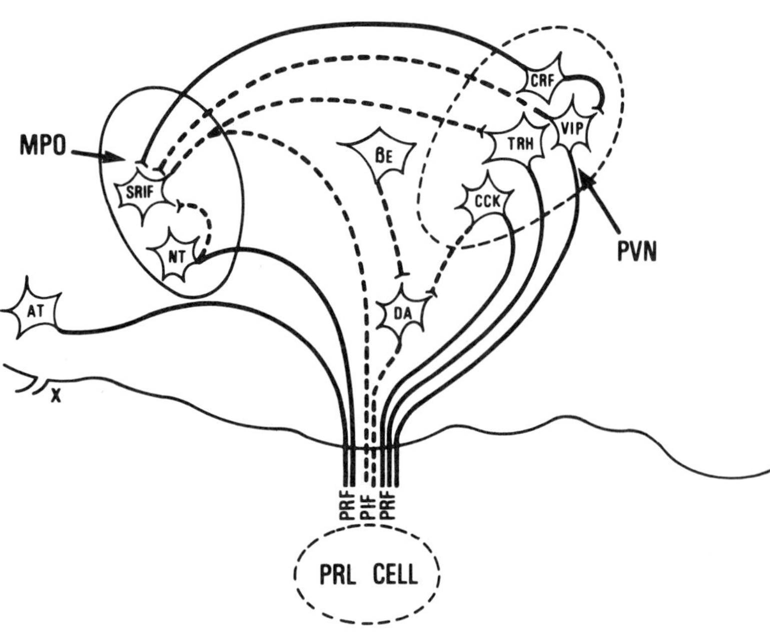

FIG. 2. Major factors regulating prolactin secretion [namely, thyrotropin-releasing hormone (TRH), vasoactive intestinal polypeptide (VIP), cholecystokinin (CCK), neurotensin (NT), and angiotensin II (AT)] can be released into the hypothalamo-hypophyseal portal system to stimulate pituitary lactotrophs. Dopamine is the predominant prolactin-inhibiting factor (PIF), but endogenous somatostatin can also inhibit prolactin secretion under discrete physiological conditions. Tuberoinfundibular dopamine can be inhibited by β-endorphin (βE) and cholecystokinin (CCK); somatotropin-release inhibiting-factor (SRIF) release is stimulated by corticotropin-releasing factor (CRF), inhibited by VIP, and is itself inhibitory to TRH. Solid lines refer to stimulatory inputs, whereas dotted lines refer to inhibitory ones. Corresponding evidence is presented in the text. MPO, medial preoptic area; PVN, paraventricular nucleus; X, optic chiasm; DA, dopamine; PRF, prolactin-releasing factors; PRL, prolactin.

Corticotropin-Releasing Factor

Corticotropin-releasing factor (CRF) is a 41-amino-acid peptide (488) derived from a 196-amino-acid precursor (489). Its main source in the hypothalamus is the paraventricular nucleus. Most of the CRF there is produced by parvocellular neurons (414,490), where CRF is found colocalized with oxytocin (491) as well as vasopressin (415). A few scattered cells located more rostrally, in the periventricular area and in the suprachiasmatic nucleus, can also be stained with CRF antisera (491). Paraventricular neurons project to the median eminence and to the posterior pituitary (491), a structure in which the presence of corticotropin activity was suspected for some time (492). A relatively dense CRF innervation of the anterior preoptic area, with numerous varicosities, has also been described (490).

Corticotropin-releasing-factor neurons in the paraventricular nucleus project to the basal telencephalon and the brain stem, areas important in autonomic control (493). In addition, the amygdala, the bed nucleus of the stria terminalis, the central gray, and some caudal catecholamine-rich nuclei (A1 and A5) also receive a dense CRF innervation, presumably via the medial forebrain bundle, which interconnects these areas with the hypothalamus (490). Scattered CRF interneurons are also present throughout the cortex (490).

Different subsets of CRF cell bodies within the paraventricular nucleus, as well as in other structures, appear regulated in an independent manner. Adrenalectomy, for instance, only affects the metabolism of the peptide in parvocellular neurons, which also contain neurohypophyseal hormones and project to the median eminence and the posterior pituitary (490).

The major endocrine action of CRF is to stimulate the release of proopiomelanocortin-derived hormones (494). The peptide also affects the release of reproductive hormones. Plasma levels of LH are inhibited by CRF administration (495), an effect likely to involve a direct action on LHRH release. Ten to 100 nM CRF added to fragments of median eminence inhibit both basal and K^+-stimulated LHRH release (496,497). The effect is reversed by CRF antagonists (496). Intraventricular administration of CRF was also shown to inhibit PRL secretion (498), as does sauvagine (499), a peptide that exhibits structural analogies with CRF (500). Under the same conditions, CRF also inhibits GH release (498), presumably by a direct stimulation of somatostatin release, as observed with brain neurons in culture (501).

In addition, CRF infused intraventricularly stimulates the release of oxytocin into the hypophyseal portal system (502,503). It is also a potent inhibitor of sexual receptivity in female rats (504,505).

Corticotropin-releasing factor is considered an important factor in mediating stress-induced inhibitory effects on reproductive functions (506). The peptide also excites hippocampal neurons (507), facilitates behavioral activation (508), decreases slow-wave sleep, and has anxiogenic effects (509). Behavioral activation by CRF is independent of pituitary-adrenal stimulation by the peptide (510) and may involve direct effects on central noradrenergic neurons (511,512).

Cholecystokinins

Cholecystokinins (CCK) represent a family of peptides of variable length (active forms range from 4 to 58 amino acids) derived from a 114-amino-acid precursor. The most common forms are CCK4 (Trip-Met-Asp-Phe-NH_2) and CCK8 (Asp-Tyr [SO_3H] Met-Gly extension of the N-terminus of CCK4). They are present in several brain structures (416,513). In the cortex, the octapeptide is produced by neurons with a distribution quite comparable to that of CRF and somatostatin interneurons (514). The major hypothalamic source of the peptide is from both magnocellular and parvocellular neurons of the paraventricular nucleus (513,515), where they have been shown to be colocalized with oxytocin and neurophysin (515). Cholecystokinin's colocalization with DA, serotonin, and GABA has also been reported in other brain areas (516). In addition, the ventromedial nucleus of the hypothalamus receives long ascending projections from the CCK-containing neurons in the brain stem (517).

Central and peripheral CCK receptors are believed to exhibit slightly different properties (518). Brain CCK receptors are widely distributed (519) and show high densities in the ventromedial hypothalamic nucleus, supraoptic and paraventricular nuclei (520), and also in the pituitary. In ventromedial and paraventricular nuclei, receptors are down-regulated by estrogens (521) and are increased by ovariectomy (522).

Cholecystokinin stimulates PRL and GH release by direct actions on the pituitary (523). It elevates plasma gonadotropin levels after intraventricular infusion (524) or direct implantation into the medial preoptic area (525). In contrast to intravenous administration, intraventricular treatment with the peptide inhibits PRL release (523), a paradoxical effect that we already mentioned for other neuropeptides such as neuropeptide Y or neurotensin. Prolactin inhibition, and possibly also LH stimulation, could be mediated by effects of CCK on tuberoinfundibular DA activation (525). Furthermore, the peptide is able to induce electrical activation of a large population of tuberoinfundibular neurons in an estrogen-dependent manner (526). Midbrain DA neurons colocalizing CCK can also be activated by the peptide (527).

Cholecystokinin has been reported to influence noradrenergic neurons in the ventromedial hypothalamus (528), an effect possibly related to the control of feeding behavior (529). In view of its dual role on feeding behavior and neuroendocrine parameters in closely related hypothalamic structures, CCK could be involved in the synchronization of both events (530), which has been observed under certain hormonal conditions. Sexual behavior in female rats has also been shown to be altered by CCK8 as well as by CRF (531).

Angiotensin II

Angiotensin is an octapeptide (Asn-Arg-Val-Tyr-Ile-His-Pro-Phe) formed by cleavage of a larger precursor, angiotensinogen, by renin (532). It is present in several brain structures (533,534). In the hypothalamus, it is mostly found in paraventricular and supraoptic nuclei (417), where it is colocalized with vasopressin in parvocellular neurons (535). The peptide is also synthesized in pituitary gonadotrophs (320). Angiotensin-converting enzyme (536) and angiotensin receptors have been localized in discrete brain areas (537) and in the pituitary (538).

The earliest documented neuroendocrine effect of angiotensin was the stimulation of ACTH *in vivo* (539) and *in vitro* (540). It was subsequently discovered that the peptide was also capable of stimulating LH release upon its intraventricular administration to rats (541). The effect is steroid-dependent and is seen in ovariectomized rats treated with estrogen and progesterone. Contrary to the above, in untreated ovariectomized animals, angiotensin decreases the frequency and amplitude of LH circhoral pulses (542). A physiological role for endogenous angiotensin is supported by the observation that administration of saralasin, an angiotensin antagonist, decreases or delays the proestrous surge of LH (541). Angiotensin convertase inhibitors induce the same effect (541).

Angiotensin also enhances PRL release by a direct action on pituitary lactotrophs (543–551). The effect is sensitive to E_2, since the hormone decreases the number of pituitary receptors for angiotensin (546,547). The action of the peptide on adenylate cyclase also appears to be sensitive to E_2 (547). Surprisingly, these changes are not paralleled by a decreased efficacy of angiotensin to release PRL (546,547). This discrepancy could be due to the existence of multiple postreceptor coupling mechanisms for angiotensin, which uses phosphoinositides and cAMP as second messengers (545).

When infused into the ventricle, angiotensin II tends, paradoxically, to decrease plasma PRL levels. The action is blocked by domperidone, suggesting it involves a direct action on tuberoinfundibular DA neurons (548).

Brain receptors to the neuropeptide also fluctuate during the estrous cycle of the rat and reach maximal concentrations in the preoptic area during proestrus (549). These changes appear also to correlate with fluctuations in drinking behavior (550). In addition, angiotensin II receptors are sensitive to mineralocorticoids (551).

Angiotensin increases catecholamine turnover in discrete brain areas (552). This effect might underlie the LH-stimulating effects of the peptide (542,548). Angiotensin was also reported to stimulate release of vasopressin (553).

Other Paraventricular Peptides

Bradykinin and bombesin are abundant in the rat hypothalamus (419). Their actions are still poorly understood. Bradykinin (554) and bombesin, at relatively high doses (555,556), inhibit PRL by an indirect hypothalamic action, since they produce the effect after intraventricular, but not after intravenous, administration. Inhibition of GH was also reported (554,556). In the case of bombesin, this effect may involve a parallel increase in hypothalamic tyrosine hydroxylase activity (555). *In vitro,* bombesin was reported to stimulate somatotrophs (557). Under these conditions, bradykinin seems to affect only the secretion of ACTH (558) and other POMC-derived hormones (559).

Conclusion

Many neuropeptides produced in the paraventricular nucleus thus seem to share common PRL-stimulating properties at the pituitary level (Fig. 2, p. 1254). This is the case with TRH (472,474), cholecystokinin (523), angiotensin II (609–617), and VIP (642,646). A similar action has been attributed to oxytocin (443,444) and vasopressin (445,446), but the evidence remains controversial (447). In addition, most of these peptides can also interact with the release of neurohormones from the median eminence, mainly by elevating concentrations of PRL-inhibiting factors in portal blood. Vasopressin (448), cholecystokinin (523,525,526), and angiotensin II (548) have all been shown to increase tuberoinfundibular DA neuron activity. Bombesin might do the same (555), although the evidence is not as convincing. Parallel effects of CRF are believed to involve, instead, stimulation of somatostatin release from the median eminence (501). These paradoxical effects at both anatomical levels probably account for the opposite results obtained after systemic or intraventricular administration of these peptides (Fig. 2).

Actions of the paraventricular peptides on gonadotropin secretion appear exclusively mediated by the hypothalamus. They involve the indirect stimulation of LH by CCK (524,525) and angiotensin II (541) as well as the indirect inhibition of that hormone by CRF (495) and oxytocin (456). Corresponding data are summarized in Table 2.

NEUROPEPTIDES OF THE GLUCAGON SUPERFAMILY

The family consists of several related peptides with considerable structural homologies. They are glucagon, gastrin-inhibitory peptide (GIP), secretin, vasoactive intestinal peptide (VIP), histidine-isoleucine (PHI) and histidine methionine (PHM) peptides, and GH-releasing factor (GRH). In the central nervous system, VIP and PHI are very abundant in a number of brain structures, whereas other members of the family are more highly concentrated in the hypothalamus. Hypothalamic cell bodies producing the peptides belong to the so-called medial hypothalamic systems. Neurons containing VIP and PHI are mostly found in the paraventricular nucleus (561,562), whereas GRH neurons are lo-

TABLE 2. *Reproductive actions of peptide-containing neurons in the paraventricular nucleus*[a]

	Overall neuroendocrine effect						
	Prolactin		Gonadotropins				
Peptide	Direct (1)	Indirect (2)	Direct (1)	Indirect (2)	Effects at hypothalamic level	Other reproductive actions	Physiological relevance
Vasopressin	↓	↓			↑ DA		Stress
Oxytocin	↓	↓		⇣			Stress, lactation
TRH	↑					Male sexual behavior	
CRF		↓		↓	↓ LHRH, ↑ SRIF, ↓ VIP, ↓ OT	↓ Female receptivity	Stress
CCK	↑	⇣		↑	⇡ DA*, ↑ NA	↓ Sexual behavior	
Angiotensin II	↑			(3) ↓ or ↑ (4)	↑ VP, ↑ NA		↑ LH surge amplitude
Bradykinin		⇣	⇣ (FSH)				
Bombesin	↑						

[a](1) Direct actions of pituitary cells; (2) by indirect effects on hypothalamic neurons; (3) only in castrated animals; (4) only in intact or in sex-steroid-treated animals; (↑ ↓) increases or decreases hormone or transmitter release; (⇡ ⇣) effect not fully characterized yet; (*) indirect evidence only.

cated in the arcuate nucleus and adjacent parts of the ventromedial nucleus (563).

Representatives of the family most important for neuroendocrine functions are VIP (a 22-amino-acid peptide) and GRH (a 27–44-amino-acid peptide). These molecules show over 30% homology at their N-terminus. Growth-hormone-releasing factor is further extended by 16 additional C-terminal amino acids (564,565). In humans, PHI (566) and PHM are coded by adjacent exons of the pre-pro-VIP gene (567). Secretin, glucagon, and GIP also belong to the family but have predominantly pancreatic and gastrointestinal functions.

VIP, PHI, GIP, and Glucagon

In the brain, VIP, unlike GRF, is widely distributed. It is particularly conspicuous in hippocampal structures (568) and in cortical interneurons (569). In the hypothalamus, cell bodies are mainly located in the paraventricular nucleus (561). About 20% of the suprachiasmatic neurons also elaborate the peptide, as do a few supramamillary cells (569,570). Paraventricular neurons project to the median eminence (571) and the posterior pituitary, whereas suprachiasmatic neurons project to the periventricular preoptic area (570).

In the paraventricular nucleus, some VIP cell bodies contain vasopressin (562). Histidine-isoleucine is also found with VIP in the same neurons (562). Histidine-isoleucine was reported also to colocalize with CRF and enkephalins in the paraventricular nucleus (570). This observation, however, was challenged by other authors as being an artifact (572). Glucagon is also found in hypothalamic neurons (573). Immunocytochemical evidence for the presence of VIP in pituitary PRL cells has been reported (574). The peptide could be synthesized there or reach the gland via the hypophyseal portal system (575).

A single class of VIP receptors has been described. Receptors were initially solubilized from liver membranes and shown to be a glycoprotein (576). These receptors are present in several brain areas and in the pituitary. They also recognize other peptides of the family, particularly PHI and, with lower affinity, secretin and GRF (576).

The major neuroendocrine action of VIP is to stimulate PRL secretion (577). A direct action on pituitary lactotrophs was shown by *in-vitro* experiments with pituitary tissue (578–581) or dispersed cells (581). Prolactin cells express binding sites for the peptide (582). A direct stimulation of VIP on GH (583,584) and on TSH (585) has been documented. Glucagon is also able to stimulate GH secretion (586). Interestingly, VIP and TRH may act synergically on lactotrophs to release PRL, whereas their combined action has been shown to antagonize each other with regard to GH and TSH secretion (583).

Functionally, endogenous VIP is probably involved in suckling (587) and the stress-induced stimulation of PRL secretion (588). Passive immunization with anti-VIP antisera was shown to attenuate the elevation of plasma PRL during suckling (587) or after exposure to ether stress (588). The PRL response to the administration of 5-HTP is also attenuated by passive immunization against VIP as well as against PHI (589). A role for endogenous VIP is also supported by observations that suckling increases VIP immunoreactivity in neurons of the paraventricular nucleus and the median eminence (590). In addition, lactating animals show higher hypothalamic concentrations of mRNA corresponding to the VIP precursor (591). This suggests that the suckling stimulus may increase transcription of the gene coding for the peptide. Finally, PRL, as with E_2, is able to modify VIP concentrations in the hypothalamus and anterior pituitary (592). Hypophyseal VIP could also act as an autocrine factor to directly trigger PRL secretion. Immunoneutralization of the peptide in the medium of dispersed pituitary cells has been shown to lower basal PRL release (593).

In addition to its effect on PRL, VIP has been reported to stimulate LH and GH secretion (594). Gastrin-inhibitory peptide, another member of the glucagon superfamily, has been shown to have similar actions (595). The effect of GIP on LH appears to involve the potentiation of LHRH stimulation of LH but apparently not of FSH (595). Effects on LH (and, in part, effects on GH and PRL) have been implicated to involve a hypothalamic site of action (594). This could involve an inhibition of somatostatin release, as observed when mediobasal hypothalamic tissue was treated with VIP *in vitro* (596). A negative effect on presynaptic somatostatin release could thus account for GH and PRL responses to intraventricular VIP administration. Other examples of dual pituitary hormone control by a peptide are known and are mediated through redundant actions at the hypothalamic and pituitary levels.

Interactions between VIP and somatostatin have also been observed on primary cultures of fetal cortical and diencephalic neurons. In that case, VIP appeared to enhance somatostatin release rather than to lower it (598).

Vasoactive intestinal peptide affects serotonin turnover in the suprachiasmatic nucleus, a major component of the central clock regulating endocrine rhythms (362). The effects are estrogen-dependent (599). Along with neurotensin, VIP could thus play a role in the circadian control of LH and PRL secretion. Vasoactive intestinal peptide seems also able to induce the release of ACTH from human corticotropin-producing tumors (600) or from a corticotropic clone (601). In this case, high-affinity receptors for VIP were postulated to coexist with receptors with a low affinity for several peptides of the glucagon family, i.e., PHI, GRF, GIP, secretin, and glucagon itself (602). It this were also true in the case of normal pituitary cells, it would account for the potentiation of CRF-induced ACTH secretion by relatively large concentrations of VIP (603) and would possibly account also for the PHI potentiation of GRF-stimulated GH release (604).

Finally, glucagon enhances somatostatin release into the hypophyseal portal system (597). This could account for the opposite effects of VIP and glucagon on GH secretion (586).

Growth-Hormone-Releasing Hormone

Human GRH is comprised of peptides that range from 37 to 44 amino acids (564,565) and that are derived from a 108-amino-acid precursor (560). Some structural variability exists between human and murine forms of the molecule, which differ by as many as 14 amino acids (605). Unlike other members of the glucagon family, GRF has a relatively limited distribution in the brain. It is mainly produced by neurons located in the arcuate nucleus and adjacent areas (606–609). These neurons colocalize neuropeptide Y (610). Their main projections are to the median eminence, where GRH is released into the hypophyseal portal system (609). A few paraventricular neurons also contain GRH (290). In addition to the median eminence, immunoreactive fibers have been traced to the periventricular area and the suprachiasmatic nucleus (607). Outside the hypothalamus, fibers are found in the stria terminalis and the amygdala (607). The major documented action of GRH is its stimulation of GH release (564,565) mediated by pituitary GRH receptors (611). Effects of high doses of GRH on PRL release or potentiation of PRL responses to TRH (612) are believed to act via an interaction with VIP receptors, for which GRH has a low affinity (576,613). In addition, some synthetic analogs of GRH, i.e., Ac-Tyr hGRH or *N*-Ac-Tyr DPhe2-GRH(1–29)-NH_2, have been shown to act as weak antagonists of VIP receptors (576).

OPIOID PEPTIDES

Anatomical Organization, Biosynthesis, and Receptors of Brain Opioid Pathways

Opioid peptides are derived from three different precursors: proenkephalin A, prodynorphin or proenkephalin B, and proopiomelanocortin. These three are coded by distinct genes and are expressed in distinct neuron systems.

Proenkephalin

Proenkephalin A is a 241-amino-acid sequence (614) predominantly produced by interneurons found throughout the brain and the medulla (615). In the brain, post-translational maturation of the precursor molecule results in four molecules of metenkephalin (Tyr-Gly-Gly-Phe-Met) and one molecule each of leu-enkephalin (Tyr-Gly-Gly-Phe-Leu), enkephalin heptapeptide (Tyr-Gly-Gly-Phe-Met-Arg-Phe), and enkephalin octapeptide (Tyr-Gly-Gly-Phe-Met-Arg-Gly-Leu) (616). These peptides are preferential ligands for delta opiate receptors (616).

Prodynorphin

Hypothalamic prodynorphin, a 234-amino-acid sequence, is mostly synthesized in neurons of the paraventricular nucleus (617,618), in which it is partially colocalized with CRF (570) and vasopressin (619). It has also been found in pituitary gonadotrophs (319,620). Corresponding projections innervate the median eminence [from which dynorphin can be released into the hypophyseal portal system (619)] and the posterior pituitary [where dynorphin is colocalized in oxytocin- and vasopressin-containing nerve terminals (621)]. A large number of nonhypothalamic structures, such as the hippocampus, basal nuclei, and the nucleus of the solitary tract, also contain high concentrations of dynorphin and of opiate receptors (622). Post-translational cleavage generates alpha and beta neo-endorphins (Tyr-Gly-Gly-Phe-Leu-Arg-Lys-Tyr-Pro, the alpha form having an additional lysine at the C-terminal), dynorphin A and B, and possibly leu-enkephalin. These peptides are preferential agonists for the kappa receptor subclass (616).

Proopiomelanocortin

Proopiomelanocortin contains 241 amino acid residues (623). It is mainly synthesized in POMC cells of the anterior and intermediate lobes of the pituitary (623). It is also produced in large amounts by neurons of the arcuate nucleus (624), which project to the median eminence and to a wide spectrum of other brain structures (625,626). The major opioid product of POMC processing is beta-endorphin. The precursor also gives rise to ACTH and beta-LPH in the anterior pituitary (623), as well as to alpha- and beta-MSH and CLIP (corticotropin-like intermediary peptide) in the intermediate lobe and in the central nervous system (623). Here they colocalize in the same neurons (627–630). Colocalization with DA has also been observed in some arcuate neurons (631). Hypothalamic beta-endorphin has been measured in the hypophyseal portal blood (632). The peptide is highly active on delta and mu opiate receptors (616).

Major Hormonal Effects of Opiates

Under appropriate conditions, opiates have been shown to have effects on the secretion of all hormones of the anterior and posterior lobes of the pituitary. They markedly increase PRL (633–640), as well as GH (633–637), release; however, in the latter case, this is done more conspicuously in rats than in humans (639). In contrast, they inhibit the secretion of LH (635,641), FSH, and TSH (635). The complete literature documenting these effects has been reviewed (634,642).

Opiates and Secretion of Gonadotropins

Morphine and opioid peptides inhibit the ovulatory surge of LH in rats (635,641) and, in general, inhibit gonadotropin release in many species, including monkeys (643). The action is more pronounced on LH than on FSH (644). Opiate antagonists, among which naloxone has been used most extensively, are able to elevate plasma levels of LH in many species (645,646) including humans (647,648). Thus, endogenous opiates may act as tonic inhibitors of LH secretion. Infusion of antisera to beta-endorphin or to dynorphin into the third ventricle elevates plasma LH (649).

A major impact of opiates on gonadotropic secretion concerns the regulation of amplitude and, more conspicuously, the frequency of the pulsatile pattern of LH secretion. Administration of beta-endorphin reduces the LH pulsatility in conscious, castrated rats (645,650). This likely involves a modulation of the hypothalamic pacemaker controlling the periodic activation of LHRH neurons, since the frequency of LHRH pulses in the hypophyseal portal blood of monkeys is also reduced by opiates (643). Morphine also inhibits the firing frequency of hypothalamic neurons associated with the release of LHRH in the monkey (651). On the other hand, administration of naloxone increases LH pulse frequency in normal men (647,648,652,653) as well as in women (654–656), especially during the late follicular and the luteal phases of the menstrual cycle (657). This treatment also reverses the decreased LH pulse frequency induced by the administration of sex steroids to men (658).

The gonadotropin response to naloxone has been proposed to be used as a functional test in reproductive pathology. The response is blunted in delayed puberty (659) and in anorexic patients (660). However, there is no general agreement on these observations (661).

Opiate effects on LH secretion are generally believed to involve the mu receptor subtype (662–665). However, the observation that ethylketocyclazocine (666) and bremazocine (667), two preferential kappa agonists, are as potent as morphine to lower LH secretion in immature female rats led to the conclusion that both types of receptors could be involved in mediating the response (668). This interpretation is also supported by experiments using kappa antagonists (669).

The importance of endogenous opiates in hypothalamic mechanisms controlling LH secretion seems highly dependent upon the endocrine condition of experimental animals (670,671). In spite of an increased episodic rhythm of LH pulses (672), the naloxone-induced elevation of mean levels of LH is extremely reduced, or absent, in gonadectomized rats (670,671). It can be restored by pretreatment with testosterone (670) or estrogens (673) and further enhanced by progesterone (673). Conversely, chronic morphine treatment has been reported to sensitize LH feedback mechanisms to testosterone (674) and estrogens (675). These effects are consistent with the change in hypothalamic opiate activity observed after treatment with sex steroids. Estrogens decrease hypothalamic concentrations of beta-endorphin (676) and increase its release into the hypophyseal portal blood (632,677). Concentrations of the neuropeptide also fluctuate during the estrous cycle in discrete hypothalamic nuclei (678). Beta-endorphin immunoreactivity increases from diestrus to estrus (678). During late pregnancy and early postpartum, beta-endorphin concentrations in the hypothalamus have also been reported to increase in parallel with the elevated plasma levels of estrogens during the period (679).

At any rate, estrogen modulation of hypothalamic beta-endorphin levels could result from a direct effect of the steroid on a subset of neurons producing the peptide. A few (but not all) beta-endorphin neurons identified immunocytochemically within, or close to, the arcuate nucleus accumulate E_2 (680) and express receptors for the hormone (681). Naloxone-induced LH responses seem to correlate with circadian fluctuations of hypothalamic opiate-binding sites (682). In addition, some authors report that sex steroids affect the number of opiate-binding sites in the brain (683–685), but this finding has been challenged (686). Corticosteroid hormones may also modulate the effect of opiates on gonadotropin secretion (687).

Gonadotropin responses to opiates are dependent upon maturation and sexual differentiation of the hypothalamus and the onset of puberty. In infantile male rats, LH responses appear insensitive to opiate antagonists (688) and show marked differences during the prepubertal period in both male and female rats (689,690). The LH response is also affected by androgen sterilization during the early postnatal period (691). This observation may be correlated with the dimorphic distribution of opiate peptides in the preoptic area of the hypothalamus in males, or in females treated neonatally with testosterone (392). Interestingly, neonatal administration of naloxone has been reported to induce precocious puberty in the female rat (693,694). In parallel, gonadotropin regulation by opiates shows marked differences in seasonal breeders relative to age (695,696).

Hyperprolactinemia interferes with the opiate regulation of LH. In ovariectomized rats that were rendered hyperprolactinemic by ectopic pituitary grafts, administration of naloxone results in a greater increase of plasma LH than that observed in ungrafted controls (697). The effect is due to an increased pulsatile release of LHRH into the hypophyseal portal blood (698). Naloxone is more effective in elevating plasma LH in women with PRL-secreting microadenomas than in normoprolactinemic control patients (699,700). A discrepant observation was reported, however, in intact male rats (701). Taken together, these observations suggest that opiates exert a stronger tonic inhibition on LHRH in the presence of elevated PRL levels. This conclusion is also supported by increased hypothalamic levels of beta-endorphin and metenkephalin in hyperprolactinemic animals (702). Opiates also appear to be involved in other central consequences of hyperprolactinemia—for instance, those influencing thermoregulation (703).

Opiates are likely to play a role in the decreased gonadotropin secretion observed during both acute and chronic stress (704), since this response is counteracted by opiate antagonists (705–707). Elevated beta-endorphin brain concentrations have been reported in foot-shock-stressed animals (708).

Opiates and Secretion of Prolactin

Morphine (635) and several opioid peptides induce a marked stimulation of plasma PRL levels (636,638). Beta-endorphin enhances the suckling-induced stimulation of PRL in lactating animals (702). Naloxone, alone, induces a slight decrease in basal circulating concentrations of PRL (635,637,640). However, it is quite effective in lowering stimulated PRL levels, especially during suckling (710,711) or stress (710). A single injection of the antagonist, which has a relatively short half-life, delays the rise of PRL observed under these conditions, whereas repeated injections prevent it completely (710). These data indicate that endogenous opiates are involved in the stress- and suckling-induced release of PRL, a conclusion substantiated by the increased biosynthesis and processing of enkephalins in lactating animals (712). Prolactin stimulation by cervicovaginal stimulation in the rat is also dependent upon endogenous opiates (713). As in the case of gonadotropic regulation, sex steroids are able to modulate the amplitude of PRL responses to opiates and to naloxone, in rats as well as in postmenopausal women (714).

Opiate receptors involved in PRL regulation are generally believed to belong to the mu class (715,716) and possibly to the mu-1 subclass (717). Administered intraventricularly, dermorphin, a potent mu-1 agonist, is quite effective in elevating plasma PRL in the rat (715,718,719) as well as in humans (720). The same class of opiate receptors thus seems to regulate both LH and PRL, in contrast to GH release, which is reportedly dependent upon delta receptors (716). A few reports, however, support the contention that, as in the case of LH, kappa receptors could be involved concurrently with mu receptors. Dynorphin A (721–723) and neoendorphin (721), preferential kappa agonists, are both potent stimulators of PRL release in rats (721), primates (722,723), and in humans (724). Kappa agonists bremazocine and U50488 stimulate PRL at fairly low doses (725), but the amplitude of the hormonal responses that they elicit is significantly smaller than than that elicited with the mu agonists (726).

Opiates and Oxytocin Release

Release of oxytocin from the neurohypophyseal lobe is inhibited by opiates (727,728). The effect is particularly marked in rats during pregnancy or parturition and involves mainly an action on oxytocin-containing nerve terminals (728). Naloxone reverses the effect and amplifies oxytocin responses to suckling (729). The participation of opiate neurons has been postulated to account for the central inhibition of oxytocin induced by relaxin during parturition (730).

Site of Opiate Modulation of Reproductive Hormones

Only a few dissenting observations report a direct opiate effect on gonadotrophs (731); the effect, however, might involve nonopiate receptors, since it is not reversed by naloxone (732). Most authors agree that the major site of the LH inhibition by opiates is at the hypothalamic level (733). Morphine suppresses the proestrous release of GnRH into hypophyseal portal blood (734). In parallel, it inhibits the firing frequency of hypothalamic neurons associated with the release of LHRH (651). Opiate peptides have also been shown to decrease LHRH concentrations in the hypophyseal portal blood (697). In addition, they inhibit depolarization-induced release of LHRH from mediobasal hypothalamic slices *in vitro* (735,736). Inhibition of LHRH by the mu agonist DAGO is suppressed by orchidectomy and is restored by the administration of testosterone (737). Opiate-binding sites have been measured on median eminence nerve terminals originating apparently from the preoptic periventricular system, since deafferentation of corresponding projections markedly reduced binding (738). The authors of this study concluded that the opiate receptors were very likely present on LHRH and/or somatostatin nerve endings, which represent the major input to the median eminence from the preoptic periventricular system (736).

In addition to a direct, presynaptic inhibitory action on LHRH neurons, opiates are also believed to affect gonadotropin secretion by interfering with catecholaminergic neurotransmission in the hypothalamus (739) and to inhibit stimulatory noradrenergic inputs to the anterior preoptic area (740,741). An inhibition of tuberoinfundibular DA turnover (742,743) and release into the hypophyseal portal system (744) are the best-documented effects of opiates on hypothalamic catecholamines. These effects account for the PRL-stimulating effect of opioid peptides (745). In parallel, a decrease in portal blood DA concentrations correlates well with morphine-induced PRL secretion (746).

Opiates also appear to modulate reproductive hormone control by parallel effects on a number of other hypothalamic transmitters and peptides. They stimulate the release of 5-HT (747), a process that has been postulated to account partially for the opiate gonadotropic interaction (748). Opiates inhibit the synaptic release of TRH, both *in vitro* under depolarizing conditions (749) and *in vivo* in anesthetized rats submitted to a cold stress (750). In addition, a direct interaction on TRH-binding sites in the brain has been reported (751,752).

Other neuropeptides affected by opiates within the hypothalamus are somatostatin and CRF. The release of somatostatin from median eminence slices *in vitro* induced by high extracellular K^+ concentrations is antagonized by morphine and opioid peptides. This effect is reversed by naloxone (736,753). The release of corticotropin-releasing hormone *in vitro* is enhanced by beta-endorphin in subnanomolar concentrations. This is consistent with an action on mu receptors (754). At higher (micromolar) concentrations, however, an inhibition of basal as well as stimulated CRF release is observed. This response, however, is not suppressed by naloxone and is thus unlikely to involve opiate receptors (755).

Except for the CRF-releasing action of low doses of endorphin, the positive interaction with 5-HT, and a possible positive interaction with the release of GRH (756), most actions of opiates on hypothalamic neurotransmitters or peptides appear to involve an inhibition of presynaptic release (728,736). This mechanism seems to be a prevalent mode of action of morphinomimetic drugs throughout the brain. Hypothetically, the few instances of opiate stimulation of transmitter release could involve inhibition of inhibitory influences on these neurons. Simultaneous monitoring of release and electrical activity of oxytocin neurons suggests that presynaptic inhibition involves uncoupling of action potentials from the resultant exocytosis (728). This conclusion agrees with data obtained after experimental depolarization of neurons (736). This effect might involve a presynaptic blockade of Ca^{2+} channels (757). Activation of GTPase activity has been proposed as an alternate mechanism of action for the peptides (758).

As summarized in Table 3, effects of endogenous or exogenous opiates are mediated by several parallel hypothalamic pathways. The most important ones involve direct inhibition of LHRH release, tonic activation of LHRH neurons by noradrenergic projections, and inhibition of tuberoinfundibular DA release into portal blood. Alternate mechanisms may also be involved in the overall hormonal

TABLE 3. *Effect of morphine, opioid peptides, or their antagonists (relative to the inferred agonist effect) on hypothalamic transmitters and neuropeptides*

Transmitter	Hypothalamic		*In-vivo* release measured		Presynaptic release *in vitro*	Portal blood concentration	Interaction with receptors
	content	turnover	Directly	Indirectly			
Dopamine		↓	↓	↓	↓	↓	No
Noradrenalin		↓		↓			
5-HT		↑					
LHRH				↓	↓	↓	
TRH			↓		↓		+
SRIF			↓				
CRF					↑		
GRH				↑			
Oxytocin			↓	↓		↓*	
Vasopressin			↓			↓*	

[a](↑) Elevated by agonists (or decreased by antagonists); (↓) decreased by agonists (or elevated by antagonists); (+) interaction; (*) measurement in peripheral plasma. Detailed explanations are given in the text.

responses, although their physiological relevance is less clearly established. Increased levels of 5-HT and CRF may act synergically, with a decreased norepinephrine turnover to suppress LHRH secretion. An inhibition of TRH and somatostatin could participate in PRL modulation under appropriate conditions.

Finally some studies suggest that, in addition to the major impact of opiates at the hypothalamic level, pituitary cells may also respond directly to the peptides. On the basis of indirect experiments, an opiate effect on human gonadotrophs has been postulated (759). Morphine (760) and endogenous opiates do not affect PRL release from incubated pituitaries (761,762) or cultured pituitary cells (763). They have been reported, however, to antagonize the PRL-inhibitory action of DA *in vitro* (760,761). These effects do not involve a direct competition of opiates at DA receptors (762). Direct opiate effects on PRL release have also been observed in both normal (764) and in pituitary tumor cells (768). The direct opiate effects on hormone release are not widely accepted. Morphine administration has failed to elicit a hormonal response after section of the pituitary stalk in female monkeys (766). In stalk-sectioned rats, however, opiates were shown to reverse the PRL inhibition induced by constant intravenous infusion of DA (767). Most investigators have been unsuccessful in characterizing opiate-binding sites in the anterior pituitary. Pituitary opiate receptors are restricted to the neural lobe and belong to the kappa subclass (768). A recent report contends, however, that the failure to identify anterior pituitary opiate-binding sites may be due to the presence of endogenous beta-endorphin in the membrane preparations. After appropriate treatment of the membranes to remove beta-endorphins, a relatively small, but significant, number of naloxone displaceable etorphin-binding sites has been reported (769).

If confirmed, a direct action of opiates on lactotrophs would be consistent with the finding of higher levels of enkephalins in hypophyseal portal circulation. This implies that pituitary endorphins and/or dynorphin might exert an additional paracrine effect over PRL regulation. This hypothesis could also account for the paradoxical stimulation of PRL by LHRH, since gonadotrophs have been shown to contain large, estrous-cycle-dependent (319) amounts of dynorphin (620).

Other Opiate-Related Effects

Intratesticular opiates have been claimed to affect Sertoli and Leydig cells (770). In addition, nonopiate peptides derived from a common opiate precursor could also interface with brain or neuroendocrine mechanisms. Brain muscarinic receptors in the rat interact with ACTH *in vitro* (771); MSH, another cleavage product of proopiomelanocortin, interacts with beta-endorphin to modulate pituitary hormone secretion (772).

GENERAL CONCLUSIONS

This review of the abundant literature concerning the action of various peptide and amine neuromediators on hypothalamic regulation of LH and PRL highlights a multitude of unanswered questions. Reading the staccato litany of substance by substance effects leaves one with little sense of how these diverse mechanisms concordantly result in regulation of reproductive processes. Clearly the administration of agonists into the interstitial space of neurons and other non-neuronal elements via the ventricular system does not address these questions. With many of the neuropeptides, antagonists are not yet available, precluding one's ability to study the effects of inhibiting endogenous activity. Much of the early experimentation on the role of neuromediators was hampered by our lack of knowledge concerning the final common pathways of neuroendocrine regulation, the neurosecretory neurons. Our increased knowledge in this area is now permitting investigators to determine the neuroanatomical connectivity of the neuroendocrine systems at this second level of integration. Clearly the recent work concerning the neuroanatomy of the paraventricular nucleus (16,407) hallmarks the potential insights to be gained from this approach. In this spirit we will attempt to make a few generalizations concerning peptide-transmitter interactions involved in controlling reproductive function.

Several transmitters exhibit redundant actions within the hypothalamus, or at both the hypothalamus and pituitary. In some cases, these actions are synergistic and potentiate each other (see Fig. 2, p. 1254). VIP, for instance, stimulates PRL release (578–581) and, at the same time, inhibits the hypothalamic release of SRIF (596). Somatostatin is known to inhibit PRL secretion, at least in some instances (264,280). At the hypothalamic level, SRIF inhibits TRH release (286,287) and also tempers the PRL-releasing capacity of the tripeptide on the lactotroph (279).

Somatostatin can also inhibit the release of LHRH *in vitro* (285) as well as inhibit hypothalamic noradrenergic activity (281). Clearly noradrenergic neurons are involved in the stimulation of LHRH. On the other hand, CRF can inhibit both the release of LHRH from the median eminence (496,497) and LHRH-dependent stimulation of sex behavior (504,505).

In other cases, actions at the hypothalamic and pituitary levels appear antagonistic. Vasopressin, CCK, or angiotensin II can directly stimulate lactotrophs (445,523,545) as well as simultaneously activate dopamine-mediated inhibition of PRL release (448,525,548). These paradoxical effects reviewed in the concluding subsection of the section on hypothalamic neuropeptides synthesized in the paraventricular nucleus account for the discrepant responses obtained after intravenous or intraventricular administration of these peptides. They suggest that transmitter signaling to the neurosecretory neurons does not involve straightforward stimulatory or inhibitory messages. Instead it depends on complex interactions within hypothalamic networks, which transfer information to the gland over several alternate neurohormonal signals. A few transmitters can even induce a partial interruption of hypothalamo-hypophyseal communication, by inhibiting the presynaptic release of several hypothalamic neuromediators. For example, opiates presynaptically inhibit the release of several hypothalamic peptides (728,735) as well as of catecholamines (740,742).

Many transmitters affect gonadotropin secretion in a steroid-dependent manner. They usually inhibit LH release in castrated animals but, on the other hand, are ineffective or even stimulatory in steroid-primed animals. The action of NPY (393), neurotensin (332), and angiotensin II (541,542) exhibit this property. Conversely, opiate inhibition of LH is attenuated by castration. Two of these transmitters (β-endorphin and NPY) have their cell bodies in the arcuate nucleus. Others, e.g., angiotensin II, are believed to act mainly by modulating noradrenergic inputs to LHRH neurons (548). Noradrenergic neurons are, themselves, steroid sensitive (50). In parallel, endogenous levels and receptors of these peptides are affected by steroids; endogenous NPY (399) and β-endorphin (678) are increased in the mediobasal hypothalamus by E_2. The number of neurotensin receptors are decreased by the steroid in the suprachiasmatic nucleus (351).

Different peptides produced in the same anatomical structure often have parallel effects on the secretion of pituitary hormones. This suggests that hypothalamic regional organization may exhibit a certain degree of functional homogeneity with regard to neuroendocrine processes. For instance, transmitters found in the the arcuate nucleus (β-endorphin, NPY) have been reported to affect the hypothalamic-oscillator-regulating circhoral episodes of LH (395,643,645,650). The arcuate nucleus may thus be considered a key structure for this function. This is consistent with the observation that pulsatile LH release is not affected by hypothalamic deafferentation in the monkey (45).

Neurons located in [VIP (569)], or projecting to [5-HT, NPY, PYY, neurotensin (119,351,382,386)], the suprachiasmatic nucleus appear important for the control of circadian rhythmicity. Endogenous levels or receptor numbers of these peptides are affected by estrogens (351,399), which play an important role in maintaining high-amplitude circadian fluctuations of LH in the rat (362). VIP can modulate 5-HT turnover (599) and is a possible candidate for the transfer of rhythmic information from the suprachiasmatic nucleus to the medial preoptic area, to which VIP neurons supply numerous projections (510).

The paraventricular nucleus plays a key role in processing visceral afferent information (424). Most peptides elaborated in that nucleus appear to participate in stress-induced changes of gonadotropins and PRL secretion (see Table 2, and Figs. 1 and 2). CRF (495), oxytocin (669), and dynorphin (452) inhibit LH, probably by decreasing LHRH release (456,496,497). VIP (577), dynorphin (721), and CCK (523) stimulate PRL. Those effects are all consistent with the hormonal profiles characteristic of stress responses, particularly elevation of PRL and inhibition of LH. The paraventricular nucleus also receives a dense noradrenergic innervation, which is a major pathway for the transfer of visceral afferent information (16).

Colocalization in gonadotrophs or lactotrophs of neuropeptides able to affect PRL secretion suggests that integration of neuroendocrine information involves paracrine and autocrine effects. Stimulation of PRL by dynorphin (319), angiotensin II (320), or substance P (330), three peptides produced in gonadotrophs, could represent an important instance of paracrine regulation. Stimulation of PRL by VIP (574) and substance P (330) could also be mediated via an autocrine pathway.

Finally, a few hypotheses can be proposed for the functional role of some endogenous peptides. In addition to the involvement of peptides in ultradian or circadian rhythms and in paracrine synchronization, which has been discussed above, experiments using peptide antagonists or passive immunization suggest that hypothalamic CRF (506), oxytocin (451), VIP (587), and opiates (705,710) are involved in mediating stress signals to the pituitary. In addition, VIP (587) and opiate peptides (711) play a role in suckling-induced stimulation of PRL secretion and, in the latter case, of oxytocin (729). Angiotensin II may regulate the amplitude of LH bursts (541). Endogenous somatostatin, which does not seem to have conspicuous effects on LH or PRL under normal conditions, appears able to compensate for the loss of tonic dopaminergic inhibition observed under conditions of long-term high levels of estrogen (278). In view of the negative effect of hyperprolactinemia on reproductive function, this compensatory relationship represents a potential fail-safe mechanism.

Currently, rapid progress is being made concerning the chemistry and neuroanatomy of the neurosecretory neurons as well as the neurons containing peptides and amines that regulate their function. As discussed, this information will permit a clearer picture of the role of individual neuromediatory systems. However, the real challenge still lies in our ability to understand how this information is integrated into coherent patterns of regulation. Unraveling the complexity of the interactions involved in LH and PRL regulation will take considerable effort, and whether or not it will be resolved with a reductionist approach into a simple intuitively obvious code is still in question.

REFERENCES

1. Leranth, C., Maclusky, N., Salamoto, H., Shanabrough, M., and Naftolin, F. (1985): Glutamic acid decarboxylase-containing axons synapse on LHRH neurons in the rat medial preoptic area. *Neuroendocrinology,* 40:536–539.
2. Thind, K., and Goldsmith, P. (1987): GnRH "pulsegenerator" neurons receive direct inhibition from arcuate opioid neurons in juvenile primates. *Neuroendocrinology (in press).*
3. Rance, N., Wise, P., Selmanoff, M., and Barraclough, C. (1981): Catecholamine turnover rates in discrete hypothalamic areas and as-

sociated changes in median eminence luteinizing hormone-releasing hormone and serum gonadotropins on proestrus and diestrous day 1. *Endocrinology,* 108:1795–1802.
4. Ramirez, D., Feder, H., and Sawyer, C. (1984): The role of brain catecholamines in the regulation of LH secretion: A critical inquiry. In: *Frontiers in Neuroendocrinology, vol. 8,* edited by L. Martini and W. Ganong, pp. 27–84. Raven Press, New York.
5. Moore, R., and Bloom, F. (1979): Central catecholamine neuron systems: Anatomy and physiology of the norepinephrine and epinephrine systems. *Annu. Rev. Neurosci.,* 2:113–168.
6. Palkovits, M. (1981): Catecholamines in the hypothalamus: An anatomical review. *Neuroendocrinology,* 33:123–128.
7. Barraclough, C., Wise, P., and Selmanoff, M. (1984): A role for hypothalamic catecholamines in the regulation of gonadotropin secretion. *Recent Prog. Horm. Res.,* 40:487–529.
8. Barraclough, C., and Wise, P. (1982): The role of catecholamines in the regulation of pituitary luteinizing hormone and follicle-stimulating hormone secretion. *Endocr. Rev.,* 3:91–119.
9. Weiner, R., and Ganong, W. (1978): Role of brain monoamines and histamine in regulation of anterior pituitary secretion. *Physiol. Rev.,* 58:905–976.
10. Gallo, R. (1980): Neuroendocrine regulation of pulsatile luteinizing hormone release in the rat. *Neuroendocrinology,* 30:122–131.
11. Taleisnik, S., and Sawyer, C. (1986): Activation of the CNS noradrenergic system may inhibit as well as facilitate pituitary luteinizing hormone release. *Neuroendocrinology,* 44:265–268.
12. Weiner, R., Shryne, J., Gorski, R., and Sawyer, H. (1972): Changes in the catecholamine content of the rat hypothalamus following deafferentation. *Endocrinology,* 90:867–873.
13. Brownstein, M., Palkovits, M., Tappaz, M., Saavedra, J., and Kizer, J. (1976): Effect of surgical isolation of the hypothalamus on its neurotransmitter content. *Brain Res.,* 117:287–296.
14. Palkovits, M., Brownstein, M., Saavedra, J., and Axelrod, J. (1974): Norepinephrine and dopamine content of hypothalamic nuclei of rat. *Brain Res.,* 77:137–149.
15. Dahlstrom, A., and Fuxe, K. (1964): Evidence for the existence of monoamine-containing neurons in the central nervous system. I. Demonstration of monoamine in cell bodies of brain stem neurons. *Acta Physiol. Scand. (Suppl.),* 232:1–55.
16. Swanson, L. and Sawchenko, P., and Lind, R. (1986): Regulation of multiple peptides in CRF parocellular neurosecretory neurons: Implications for the stress response. *Brain Res.,* 68:169–190.
17. Day, T., Blessing, W., and Willoughby, J. (1980): Noradrenergic and dopaminergic projections to the medial preoptic area of the rat. A combined hoseradish peroxidase/catecholamine fluorescence study. *Brain Res.,* 193:543–548.
18. Jennes, L., Beckman, W., Stumpf, W., and Grzanna, R. (1982): Anatomical relationships of serotoninergic and noradrenalinergic projections with the GnRH system in septum and hypothalamus. *Exp. Brain Res.,* 46:331–338.
19. Naftolin, F., Leranth, C., and Machusky, N. (1986): Norepinephrine (NE) and dopamine (DA) innervation of medial preoptic area (MPO) LHRH and GABA neurons in the rat. *Soc. Neurosci. Abstr.,* 12:1152.
20. Descarries, L., Walkins, K., and Lapierre, Y. (1977): Noradrenergic axon terminals in cerebral cortex of the rat. III. Topographic ultrastructural analysis. *Brain Res.,* 133:197–222.
21. Hökfelt, T., Fuxe, K., Goldstein, M., and Johansson, O. (1974): Immunohistochemical evidence for the existence of adrenaline neurons in the rat brain. *Brain Res.,* 66:239–251.
22. Howe, P., Costa, M., Furness, J., and Chalmers, J. (1980): Simultaneous demonstration of phenylethanolamine-*N*-methyltransferase immunofluorescent and catecholamine fluorescent nerve cell bodies in the rat medulla oblongata. *Neuroscience,* 5:2229–2238.
23. Gugten, J., Palkovits, M., Wijnen, H., and Versteg, D. (1976): Regional distribution of adrenaline in rat brain. *Brain Res.,* 107:171–175.
24. Swanson, L., and Mogenson, G. (1981): Neural mechanisms for the functional coupling of autonomic, endocrine and somatomotor responses and adaptive behavior. *Brain Res. Rev.,* 31:1–34.
25. Fuxe, K., and Hokfelt, T. (1966): Further evidence for the existence of tuberoinfundibular dopamine neurons. *Acta Physiol. Scand.,* 66:245–246.
26. Ben-Jonathan, N., Oliver, C., Weiner, H., Mical, R., and Porter, J. (1977): Dopamine in hypophysial portal plasma of the rat during the estrous cycle and throughout pregnancy. *Endocrinology,* 100:452–458.
27. Chen, H., Roberts, J., and Weiner, R. (1981): Binding of ^{3}H-dihydroergocryptine to an α-adrenergic site in the stalk median eminence of the steer. *Endocrinology,* 109:2138–2143.
28. Leibowitz, S., Jhanwar-Uniyal, M., Dvorkin, B., and Makman, M. (1982): Distribution of α-adrenergic, β-adrenergic and dopaminergic receptors in discrete hypothalamic areas of the rat. *Brain Res.,* 233:97–114.
29. Bjorklund, A., Lindvall, O., and Nobin, A. (1975): Evidence of an incerto-hypothalamic dopamine neuron system in the rat. *Brain Res.,* 89:29–42.
30. Day, T., Blessing, W., and Willoughby, J. (1980): Noradrenergic and dopaminergic projections to the medial preoptic area of the rat. A combined horseradish peroxidase/catecholamine fluorescence study. *Brain Res.,* 193:543–548.
31. Negro-Vilar, A., Advis, J., Ojeda, S., and McCann, S. (1982): Pulsatile luteinizing hormone (LH) patterns in ovariectomized rats: Involvement of norepinephrine and dopamine in the release of LH-releasing hormone and LH. *Endocrinology,* 111:932–938.
32. Drouva, S., and Gallo, R. (1976): Catecholamine involvement in episodic luteinizing hormone release in adult ovariectomized rats. *Endocrinology,* 99:651–658.
33. Gnodde, H., and Schuling, G. (1976): Involvement of catecholaminergic and cholinergic mechanisms in the pulsatile release of LH in the long term ovariectomized rat. *Neuroendocrinology,* 20:212–223.
34. Weick, R. (1978): Acute effects of adrenergic receptor blocking drugs and neuroleptic agents on pulsatile discharges of luteinizing hormone in the ovariectomized rat. *Neuroendocrinology,* 26:108–117.
35. Hancke, J., Berk, W., Baumgarten, H., Hohn, K., and Wuttke, W. (1977): Modulatory effect of noradrenaline and serotonin on circhoral LH release in adult ovariectomized rats. *Acta Endocrinol. (Suppl.) (Copenh.),* 208:22–23.
36. Bhattacharya, A., Dierschke, D., Yamaji, J., and Knobil, E. (1972): The pharmacologic blockade of the circhoral mode of LH secretion in the ovariectomized rhesus monkey. *Endocrinology,* 90:778–786.
37. Estes, K., Simpkins, J., and Kalra, S. (1982): Resumption with clonidine of pulsatile LH release following acute norepinephrine depletion in ovariectomized rats. *Neuroendocrinology,* 35:56–62.
38. Crowley, W., Terry, L., and Johnson, M. (1982): Evidence for the involvement of central epinephrine systems in the regulation of luteinizing hormone, prolactin, and growth hormone release in female rats. *Endocrinology,* 110:1102–1107.
39. Gallo, R., and Drouva, S. (1979): Effect of intraventricular infusion of catecholamines on luteinizing hormone release in ovariectomized and ovariectomized, steroid primed rats. *Neuroendocrinology,* 29:149–162.
40. Gallo, R. (1984): Further studies on norepinephrine-induced suppression of pulsatile luteinizing hormone release in ovariectomized rats. *Neuroendocrinology* 39:120–125.
41. Leipheimer, R., and Gallo, R. (1985): Medial preoptic area involvement in norepinephrine-induced suppression of pulsatile luteinizing hormone release in ovariectomized rats. *Neuroendocrinology,* 40:345–351.
42. Leung, P., Arendash, G., Whitmoyer, D., Gorski, R., and Sawyer, C. (1981): Electrical stimulation of mesencephalic noradrenergic pathway: Effects on luteinizing hormone levels in blood of ovariectomized and ovariectomized, steroid-primed rats. *Endocrinology,* 109:720–728.
43. Drouva, S., and Gallo, R. (1977): Further evidence for inhibition of episodic luteinizing hormone release in ovariectomized rats by stimulation of dopamine receptors. *Endocrinology,* 100:792–798.
44. Jarry, H., Sprenger, M., and Wuttke, W. (1986): Rates of release of GABA and catecholamines in the mediobasal hypothalamus of ovariectomized and ovariectomized estrogen-treated rats: Correlation with blood prolactin levels. *Neuroendocrinology,* 44:422–428.
45. Krey, L., Butler, W., and Knobil, E. (1975): Surgical disconnection of the medial basal hypothalamus and pituitary function in the rhesus monkey. I. Gonadotropin secretion. *Endocrinology,* 96:1073–1087.
46. Wise, P., Rance, N., and Barraclough, C. (1981): Effects of estradiol and progesterone on catecholamine turnover rates in discrete hypothalamic regions in ovariectomized rats. *Endocrinology,* 108:2186–2193.

47. Demling, J., Fuchs, E., Baumert, M., and Wuttke, W. (1985): Preoptic catecholamine, GABA, and glutamate release in ovariectomized and ovariectomized estrogen primed rats utilizing a push-pull cannula technique. *Neuroendocrinology,* 41:212–218.
48. Advis, J., McCann, S., and Negro-Vilar, A. (1980): Evidence that catecholaminergic and peptidergic (luteinizing hormone-releasing hormone) neurons in suprachiasmatic-medial preoptic, medial basal hypothalamus and median eminence are involved in estrogen-negative feedback. *Endocrinology,* 107:892–901.
49. Crowley, W. (1982): Effects of ovarian hormones on norepinephrine and dopamine turnover in individual hypothalamic and extrahypothalamic nuclei. *Neuroendocrinology,* 34:381–386.
50. Heritage, A., Grant, L., and Stumpf, W. (1977): ^{3}H-estradiol in catecholamine neurons of rat brain stem: Combined localization by autoradiography and formaldehyde-induced fluorescence. *J. Comp. Neurol.,* 176:607–630.
51. MacKinnon, P., Clement, E., Clark, C., and Sheares, R. (1983): Hypothalamic adrenergic activity precedes the preovulatory luteinizing hormone surge in the rat. *Neurosci. Lett.,* 43:221–226.
52. Coombs, M., and Coen, C. (1983): Adrenaline turnover rates in the medial preoptic area and mediobasal hypothalamus in relation to the release of luteinizing hormone in female rats. *Neuroscience,* 10:207–210.
53. Adler, B., Johnson, M., Lynch, C., and Crowley, W. (1983): Evidence that norepinephrine and epinephrine systems mediate the stimulatory effects of ovarian hormones on luteinizing hormone and luteinizing hormone-releasing hormone. *Endocrinology,* 113:1431–1438.
54. Wilkinson, M., Herdon, H., Pearce, M., and Wilson, C. (1979): Radioligand binding studies on hypothalamic noradrenergic receptors during the estrous cycle or after steroid injection in ovariectomized rats. *Brain Res.,* 168:652–655.
55. Gudelsky, G., and Porter, J. (1980): Release of dopamine from tuberoinfundibular neurons into pituitary stalk blood after prolactin or haloperidol administration. *Endocrinology,* 106:526–529.
56. Grant, L., and Stumpf, W. (1973): Localization of ^{3}H-estradiol and catecholamines in identical neurons in the hypothalamus. *J. Histochem. Cytochem.,* 21:404.
57. Sar, M. (1983): Estradiol is concentrated in tyrosine hydroxylase-containing neurons of the hypothalamus. *Science,* 223:938–940.
58. Wang, P., and Porter, J. (1986): Hormonal modulation of the quantity and *in situ* activity of tyrosine hydroxylase in neurites of the median eminence. *Proc. Natl. Acad. Sci. USA,* 83:9804–9806.
59. Sawyer, C., Markee, J., and Everett, J. (1950): Further experiments on blocking pituitary activity in the rabbit and rat. *J. Exp. Zool.* 113:659–682.
60. Kalra, S., and McCann, S. (1974): Effects of drugs modifying catecholamine synthesis on plasma LH and ovulation in the rat. *Neuroendocrinology,* 15:79–91.
61. Clifton, D., and Sawyer, C. (1979): LH release and ovulation in the rat following depletion of hypothalamic norepinephrine: Chronic vs. acute effects. *Neuroendocrinology,* 28:442–449.
62. Coen, C., and Coombs, M. (1983): Effects of manipulating catecholamines on the incidence of the preovulatory surge of luteinizing hormone and ovulation in the rat: Evidence for a necessary involvement of hypothalamic adrenaline in the normal or "midnight" surge. *Neuroscience,* 10:187–206.
63. Ratner, A. (1971): Effect of phenoxybenzamine on luteinizing hormone release in the female rat. *Proc. Soc. Exper. Biol. Med.,* 138:995–998.
64. Clifton, D., and Sawyer, C. (1980): Positive and negative feedback effects of ovarian steroids on luteinizing hormone release in ovariectomized rats following chronic depletion of hypothalamic norepinephrine. *Endocrinology,* 106:1099–1102.
65. Nicholson, G., Greeley, G., Humm, J., Youngblood, W., and Kizer, J. (1978): Lack of effect of noradrenergic denervation of the hypothalamus and medial preoptic area on the feedback regulation of gonadotropin secretion and the estrous cycle. *Endocrinology,* 103:539–566.
66. Kalra, P., Kalra, S., Krulich, L., Fawcett, C., and McCann, S. (1972): Involvement of norepinephrine in transmissions of the stimulatory influence of progesterone on gonadotropin release. *Endocrinology,* 90:1168–1176.
67. Drouva, S., Laplante, E., and Kordon, C. (1982): α_1-Adrenergic receptor involvement in the LH surge in ovariectomized estrogen-primed rats. *Eur. J. Pharmacol.,* 81:341–344.
68. Kalra, S. (1985): Catecholamine involvement in preovulatory LH release: Reassessment of the role of epinephrine. *Neuroendocrinology,* 40:139–144.
69. Sheaves, R., Laynes, R., and MacKinnon, P. (1985): Reduction of central epinephrine concentration is consistent with continued occurrence of ovulation in rats treated with an inhibitor (LY 134046) of phenylethanolamine *N*-methyltransferase. *Neuroendocrinology,* 41:432–436.
70. Crowley, W., and Terry, C. (1981): Effects of an epinephrine synthesis inhibitor, SKF64139, on the secretion of luteinizing hormone in ovariectomized female rats. *Brain Res.,* 204:231–235.
71. Krieg, R., and Sawyer, C. (1976): Effects of intraventricular catecholamines on luteinizing hormone release in ovariectomized-steroid-primed rats. *Endocrinology,* 99:411–419.
72. Leung, P., Arendash, G., Whitmoyer, D., Gorski, R., and Sawyer, C. (1982): Differential effects of central adrenoceptor agonists on luteinizing hormone release. *Neuroendocrinology,* 34: 207–214.
73. Sawyer, C., Hilliard, J., Kanematsu, S., Scaramuzzi, R., and Blake, C. (1974): Effects of intraventricular infusions of norepinephrine and dopamine on LH release and ovulation in the rabbit. *Neuroendocrinology,* 15:328–337.
74. Rubinstein, L., and Sawyer, C. (1970): Role of catecholamines in stimulating the release of pituitary ovulating hormone(s) in rats. *Endocrinology,* 86:988–995.
75. Negro-Vilar, A., Ojeda, S., and McCann, S. (1979): Catecholamine modulation of luteinizing hormone-releasing hormone release by median eminence terminals *in vitro. Endocrinology,* 104: 1749–1757.
76. Ojeda, S., Negro-Vilar, A., and McCann, S. (1982): Evidence for involvement of α-adrenergic receptors in norepinephrine-induced prostaglandin E^2 and luteinizing hormone-releasing hormone release from median eminence. *Endocrinology,* 110:409–412.
77. Negro-Vilar, A. (1982): The median eminence as a model to study presynaptic regulation of neural peptide release. *Peptides,* 3:305–310.
78. Knobil, E. (1980): The neuroendocrine control of the menstrual cycle. *Recent Prog. Horm. Res.,* 36:53–88.
79. Dotti, C., and Taleisnik, S. (1982): Inhibition of the release of LH and ovulation by activation of the noradrenergic system. Effect of interrupting the ascending pathways. *Brain Res.,* 249:281–290.
80. Dotti, C., and Tabeisnik, S. (1984): Beta-adrenergic receptors in the premammillary nucleus mediate the inhibition of LH release evoked by the locus ceruleus stimulation. *Neuroendocrinology,* 38:6–11.
81. Leung, P., Whitmoyer, D., Garland, K., and Sawyer, C. (1982): β Adrenergic suppression of progesterone-induced luteinizing hormone surge in ovariectomized, estrogen-primed rats. *Proc. Soc. Exp. Biol. Med.,* 169:161–164.
82. Caceras, A., and Taleisnik, S. (1980): Inhibition of secretion of luteinizing hormone induced by electrochemical stimulation of the anterior cingulate cortex mediated by a β-adrenergic mechanism. *J. Endocrinol.,* 87:419–429.
83. Bergen, H., and Leung, P. (1986): Suppression of progesterone-induced gonadotropin surge by adrenergic agonists in estrogen-primed ovariectomized rats. *Neuroendocrinology,* 43:397–403.
84. Choudhury, S., Sharpe, R., and Brown, P. (1974): The effect of pimozide, a dopamine antagonist, on pituitary gonadotrophic function in the rat. *J. Reprod. Fertil.,* 39:275–283.
85. Leppäluoto, J., Männistö, P., Ranta, T., and Linnoila, M. (1976): Inhibition of mid-cycle gonadotrophin release in healthy women by pimozide or fusaric acid. *Acta Endocrinol.,* 81:455–460.
86. Schneider, H., and McCann, S. (1970): Monoamine and indolamines and control of LH secretion. *Endocrinology,* 86:1127–1133.
87. Vijayan, E., and McCann, S. (1978): Re-evaluation of the role of catecholamines in control of gonadotropin and prolactin release. *Neuroendocrinology,* 25:150–165.
88. Ojeda, S., Harms, P., and McCann, S. (1974): Possible role of cyclic AMP and prostaglandin E_1 in the dopaminergic control of prolactin release. *Endocrinology,* 95:1694–1703.
89. Judd, S., Rakoff, J., and Yen, S. (1978): Inhibition of gonadotropin and prolactin release by dopamine: effect of endogenous estradiol levels. *J. Clin. Endocrinol. Metab.,* 47:494–498.
90. Lal, S., DeLa Vega, C., Sourkes, T., and Friesen, H. (1973): Effect of apomorphine on growth hormone, prolactin, luteinizing hormone

and follicle-stimulating hormone levels in human serum. *J. Clin. Endocrinol. Metab.*, 37:719–724.
91. Jarjour, L., Handelsman, D., Raum, W., and Swerdloff, R. (1986): Mechanism of action of dopamine on the *in vitro* release of gonadotropin-releasing hormone. *Endocrinology*, 119:1726–1732.
92. Ben-Jonathan, N. (1985): Dopamine: A prolactin-inhibiting hormone. *Endocr. Rev.*, 6:564–589.
93. Neill, J. (1980): Neuroendocrine regulation of prolactin secretion. In: *Frontiers in Neuroendocrinology, Vol. 6,* edited by L. Martini and W. Ganong, pp. 129–155. Raven Press, New York.
94. Yen, S. (1986): Prolactin human reproduction. In: *Reproductive Endocrinology*, edited by S. Yen and R. Jaffe, pp. 237–263. W. B. Saunders, Philadelphia.
95. Negro-Vilar, A., Ojeda, S., Advis, J., and McCann, S. (1979): Evidence for noradrenergic involvement in episodic prolactin and growth hormone release in ovariectomized rats. *Endocrinology*, 105:86–91.
96. Terry, L., and Martin, J. (1981): Evidence for α-adrenergic regulation of episodic growth hormone and prolactin secretion in the undisturbed male rat. *Endocrinology*, 108:1869–1873.
97. Lawson, D., and Gala, R. (1975): The influence of adrenergic, dopaminergic, cholinergic and serotoninergic drugs on plasma prolactin levels in ovariectomized, estrogen treated rats. *Endocrinology*, 96:313–318.
98. Quardri, S., Pierson, C., and Spies, H. (1978): Effects of centrally acting drugs on serum prolactin levels in Rhesus monkey. *Neuroendocrinology*, 27:136–147.
99. Lien, E., Morrison, A., Kassarich, J., and Sullivan, D. (1986): Alpha-2-adrenergic control of prolactin secretion. *Neuroendocrinology*, 44:184–189.
100. Meltzer, H., Simonovic, M., and Gudelsky, G. (1983): Effect of yohimbine on rat prolactin secretion. *J. Pharmacol. Exp. Ther.*, 224:21–27.
101. Gold, M., Donabedian, R., and Redmond, D. (1979): Further evidence for alpha-2-adrenergic receptor mediated inhibition of prolactin secretion: The effect of yohimbine. *Psychoneuroendocrinology*, 3:253–260.
102. Tatar, P., and Vigas, M. (1984): Role of $alpha_1$- and $alpha_2$-adrenergic receptors in the growth hormone release and prolactin response to insulin-induced hypoglycemia in man. *Neuroendocrinology*, 39:275–280.
103. Weiner, R., Shyrne, J., Gorski, R., and Sawyer, C. (1972): Changes in the catecholamine content of the rat hypothalamus following deafferentation. *Endocrinology*, 90:867–873.
104. Blake, C., Weiner, R., and Sawyer, C. (1972): Pituitary prolactin secretion in female rats made persistently estrous or diestrous by hypothalamic deafferentation. *Endocrinology*, 90:862–866.
105. Langelier, P., and McCann, S. (1977): The effects of interruption of the ventral noradrenergic pathway on the proestrous discharge of prolactin in the rat. *Proc. Soc. Exp. Biol. Med.*, 154:553–557.
106. Kalra, S., Kalra, P., Chen, C., and Clemens, C. (1978): Effect of norepinephrine synthesis inhibitors and a dopamine agonist on hypothalamic LHRH, serum gonadotrophin and prolactin levels in gonadal steroid treated rats. *Acta Endocrinol.*, 89:1–9.
107. Subramanian, M., and Gala, R. (1976): The influence of cholinergic, adrenergic, and serotoninergic drugs on the afternoon surge of plasma prolactin in ovariectomized, estrogen treated rats. *Endocrinology*, 98:842–848.
108. Voogt, J., and Carr, L. (1974): Plasma prolactin levels and hypothalamic catecholamine synthesis during suckling. *Neuroendocrinology*, 16:108–118.
109. Carr, L., Conway, P., and Voogt, J. (1977): Role of norepinephrine in the release of prolactin induced by suckling and estrogen. *Brain Res.*, 133:305–314.
110. Parent, A., Descarries, L., and Beaudet, A. (1981): Organization of ascending serotonin systems in the adult rat brain. A radioautographic study after intraventricular administration of [^{3}H]5-hydroxytryptamine. *Neuroscience*, 6:15–138.
111. Steinbusch, H. W. M. (1981): Distribution of serotonin-immunoreactivity in the central nervous system of the rat-cell bodies and terminals. *Neuroscience*, 6:557–618.
112. Steinbusch, H. W. M. (1984): Serotonin-immunoreactive neurons and their projections in the CNS. In: *Handbook of Chemical Neuroanatomy. Vol. 3, Classical Transmitters and Transmitter Receptors in the CNS. Part II,* edited by A. Bjorklund, T. Hokfelt, and M. J. Kuhar, pp. 68–125. Elsevier, Amsterdam.
113. Azmita, E. C., and Segal, M. (1970): An autoradiographic analysis of the differential ascending projections of the dorsal and median raphe nuclei in the rat. *J. Comp. Neurol.*, 179:641–668.
114. Palkovits, M. (1979): Effect of surgical deafferentation on the transmitter and hormone content of the hypothalamus. *Neuroendocrinology*, 29:140–148.
115. Beaudet, A., and Descarries, L. (1979): Radioautographic characterization of a serotonin accumulating nerve cell group in the adult rat hypothalamus. *Brain Res.*, 160:231–243.
116. Fuxe, K., and Ungerstedt, V. (1968): Histochemical studies on the distribution of catecholamine and 5-hydroxytryptamine after intraventricular injections. *Histochemia*, 13:16–28.
117. Shaskan, E. G., and Snyder, S. H. (1970): Kinetics of serotonin accumulation into slices from rat brain: Relationship to catecholamine uptake. *J. Pharmacol. Exp. Ther.*, 175:404–418.
118. Frankfurt, M., Lauder, J. M., and Azimitia, E. C. (1981): The immunocytochemical localization of serotonergic neurons in the rat hypothalamus. *Neurosci. Lett.*, 24:227–232.
119. Descarries, L., and Beaudet, A. (1978): The serotonin innervation of adult rat hypothalamus. In: *Cell Biology of Hypothalamic Neurosecretion,* edited by J.D. Vincent and C. Kordon, pp. 135–153. CNRS, Paris.
120. Bosler, C., Joh, T. H., and Beaudet, A. (1984): Ultrastructural relationships between serotonin and dopamine neurons in the rat arcuate nucleus and medial zona incerta: A combined radioautographic and immunocytochemical study. *Neurosci. Lett.*, 48:279–285.
121. Kiss, J., and Halasz, B. (1986): Synaptic connections between serotonergic axon terminals and tyrosine hydroxylase-immunoreactive neurons in the arcuate nucleus of the rat hypothalamus. A combination of electron microscopic autoradiography and immunocytochemistry. *Brain Res.*, 364:284–294.
122. Jennes, L., Beckman, W. C., Stumph, W. E., and Grzanna, R. (1982): Anatomical relationships of serotoninergic and noradrenalingeric projections with the GnRH system in septum and hypothalamus. *Exp. Brain Res.*, 46:331–338.
123. Pelletier, G., Leclerc, R., and Dube, D. (1976): Immunocytochemical localization of hypothalamic hormones. *J. Histochem. Cytochem.*, 24:864–871.
124. Mazzuca, M. (1977): Immunocytochemical and ultrastructural identification of luteinizing hormone-releasing hormone (LH-RH)-containing neurons in the vascular organ of the lamina terminalis (OVLT) of the squirrel monkey. *Neurosci. Lett.*, 5:123–127.
125. Kiss, J., and Halasz, B. (1985): Demonstration of serotoninergic axons terminating on luteinizing hormone-releasing hormone neurons in the preoptic area of the rat using a combination of immunocytochemistry and high resolution autoradiography. *Neuroscience*, 14:69–78.
126. Friedman, E., Krieger, D. T., Mezey, E., Leranth, C. S., Brownstein, M. J., and Palkovits, M. (1983): Serotonergic innervation of the rat pituitary intermediate lobe: Decrease after stalk section. *Endocrinology*, 112:1943–1947.
127. Mezey, E., Leranth, C., Brownstein, M. J., Friedman, E., Krieger, D. T., and Palkovits, M. (1984): On the origin of serotonergic input to the intermediate lobe of the rat pituitary. *Brain Res.*, 294:231–237.
128. Steinbusch, H. W. M., and Nieuwenhuys, R. (1982): Localization of serotonin-like immunoreactivity in the central nervous system and pituitary of the rat, with special reference to the innervation of the hypothalamus. In: *Serotonin: Current Aspects of Neurochemistry and Function,* edited by B. Haber, S. Gabay, M.R. Issidorides, and S.G.A. Alivijatos, pp. 7–35. Plenum Press, New York.
129. Payette, R. F., Gershon, M. D., and Nunez, E. A. (1985): Serotonergic elements of the mammalian pituitary. *Endocrinology*, 116:1933–1942.
130. Bjorklund, A., and Falck, B. (1969): Pituitary amines of the cat with special reference to the presence of an unidentified monoamine-like substance in the adenohypophysis. *Z. Zellforsch. Mikrosk. Anat.*, 93:254–264.
131. Sano, Y., Takeuchi, Y., Matsuura, T., Kawata, M., and Yamada, H. (1982): Immunohistochemical demonstration of serotonin nerve fibers in the cat neurohypophysis. *Histochemistry*, 75:293–299.

132. Westlund, K. N., and Childs, G. V. (1982): Localization of serotonin fibers in the rat adenohypophysis. *Endocrinology,* 111:1761–1763.
133. Kah, O., and Chambolle, P. (1983): Serotonin in the brains of goldfish, *Carassius auratus:* An immunocytochemical study. *Cell Tissue Res.,* 234:319–333.
134. Kondo, Y., Nagatsu, I., Yoshida, M., Karadawa, N., and Nagatsu, T. (1983): Existence of Noradrenalin cells and serotonin cells in the pituitary gland of *Rana catesbeiana. Cell Tissue Res.,* 228:405–408.
135. Saavedra, J. M., Palkovits, M., Kizer, J. S., Brownstein, J. M., and Zwin, J. A. (1975): Distribution of biogenic amines and related enzymes in the rat pituitary gland. *J. Neurochem.,* 25:257–260.
136. Nunez, E. A., Gershon, M. D., and Silverman, A. J. (1981): Uptake of 5-hydroxytryptamine by gonadotrophs of the bat's pituitary: A combined immunocytochemical radioautographic analysis. *J. Histochem. Cytochem.,* 29:1336–1346.
137. Johns, M. A., Azmita, E. C., and K. Rieger, D. T. (1982): Specific *in vitro* uptake of serotonin by cells in the anterior pituitary of the rat. *Endocrinology,* 110:754–760.
138. DeSouza, E. B. (1986): Serotonin and dopamine receptors in the rat pituitary gland: Autoradiographic identification, characterization, and localization. *Endocrinology,* 119:1534–1542.
139. Porter, J. C., Mical, R. S., and Cramer, O. M. (1971): Effect of serotonin and other indoles on the release of LH, FSH and prolactin. *Gynecol. Invest.,* 2:13–22.
140. Caligaris, L., and Taleisnek, S. (1974): Involvement of neurons containing 5-hydroxytryptamine in the mechanism of prolactin release induced by estrogen. *J. Endocrinol.,* 62:25–33.
141. Meltzer, H. Y., Fang, V. S., Paul, S. M., and Kaluskar, R. (1976): Effect of quipazine on rat plasma prolactin levels. *Life Sci.,* 1:1073–1078.
142. Lu, K. H., and Meites, J. (1973): Effects of serotonin precursors and melatonin on serum prolactin release in rats. *Endocrinology,* 93:152–155.
143. Talwalker, P. K., Ratner, A., and Meites, J. (1963): *In vitro* inhibition of pituitary prolactin synthesis and release by hypothalamic extract. *Am. J. Physiol.,* 205:213–218.
144. Kordon, C., and Glowinski, J. (1972): Role of hypothalamic monoaminergic neurons in the gonadotrophin release-regulating mechanisms. *Neuropharmacology,* 11:153–162.
145. Ng, L. K. Y., Chase, N., Colburn, R., and Kopin, I. (1972): Release of [^{3}H] dopamine by L-5-hydroxytryptophan. *Brain Res.,* 45:499–506.
146. Donoso, A. O., Bishop, W., Fawcett, C. P., Krulich, L., and McCann, S. M. (1971): Effects of drugs that modify brain monoamine concentrations on plasma gonadotropin and prolactin levels in the rat. *Endocrinology,* 89:774–784.
147. Gallo, R. V., Rabii, J., and Moberg, G. P. (1975): Effect of methysergide, A blocker of serotonin receptors on plasma prolactin levels in lactating and ovariectomized rats. *Endocrinology,* 97:1096–1105.
148. Kordon, C., Blake, C. A., Terkel, J., and Sawyer, C. H. (1973): Participation of serotonin-containing neurons in the suckling-induced rise in plasma prolactin levels in lactating rats. *Neuroendocrinology,* 13:213–223.
149. Gil, A. D., Zambotti, F., Carruba, M. O., Vicentini, L., and Muller, E. E. (1976): Stimulatory role for brain serotonergic system on prolactin secretion in the male rat. *Proc. Soc. Exp. Biol. Med.,* 151:512–518.
150. Wuttke, W., Bjorklund, A., Baumgarten, H. G., Lachenmayer, L., Fenske, M., and Klemm, H. P. (1977): De- and regeneration of brain serotonin neurons following 5,7-dihydroxytryptamine treatment: Effects on serum LH, FSH and prolactin levels in male rats. *Brain Res.,* 134:317–331.
151. Chen, H. J., and Meites, J. (1975): Effects of biogenic amines and TRH on release of prolactin and TSH in the rat. *Endocrinology,* 96:10–14.
152. Wurtman, R. J., Larin, F., Mostafapour, S., and Fernstrom, J. D. (1974): Brain catechol synthesiss: Control by brain tyrosine concentration. *Science,* 185:183–184.
153. Mena, F., Enjalbert, A., Carbonell, A., Priam, M., and Kordon, C. (1976): Effect of suckling on plasma prolactin and hypothalamic monoamine levels in the rat. *Endocrinology,* 99:445–452.
154. Parisi, M. N., Vitale, M. L., Villar, M. J., Estivas, F. E., Chiocchio, S. R., and Tramezzani, J. H. (1987): Serotonergic terminals in the anterior hypothalamic nucleus involved in the prolactin release during suckling. *Endocrinology,* 120:2404–2412.
155. Grosvenor, C. E., Mena, F., and Schaefgen, D. A. (1967): Effects of nonsuckling interval and duration of suckling on the suckling induced fall in pituitary prolactin concentration in the rat. *Endocrinology,* 81:449–453.
156. Marchlewska-Koj, A., and Krulich, L. (1975): The role of central monoamines in the stress-induced prolactin release in rats. *Fed. Proc. Fed. Am. Soc. Exp. Biol.,* 34:252.
157. Meltzer, H. Y., Fang, V. S., and Daniels, S. (1976): Biogenic amines and serum prolactin levels during stress in male rats. *Fed. Proc. Fed. Am. Soc. Exp. Biol.,* 35:554.
158. Mulloy, A. L., and Moberg, G. P. (1975): Effects of *p*-chlorophenylalanine and raphe lesions on diurnal prolactin release in the rat. *Fed. Proc. Fed. Am. Soc. Exp. Biol.,* 34:251.
159. Pan, J., and Gala, R. R. (1987): The influence of raphe lesions, *p*-chlorophenylalanine, and ketanserin on the estrogen-induced afternoon prolactin surge. *Endocrinology,* 120:2070–2077.
160. Lamberts, S. W. J., and MacLeod, R. M. (1978): The interaction of the serotonergic and dopaminergic systems on prolactin secretion in the rat. *Endocrinology,* 105:287–295.
161. Clemens, J. A., Sawyer, B. D., and Cerimele, B. (1975): Further evidence that serotonin is a neurotransmitter involved in the control of prolactin secretion. *Endocrinology,* 100:692–698.
162. Pilotte, N. S., and Porter, J. C. (1981): Dopamine in hypophysial portal plasma and prolactin in systemic plasma of rats treated with 5-hydroxytryptamine. *Endocrinology,* 108:2137–2141.
163. Clemens, J. A., Roush, M. E., and Fuller, R. W. (1978): Evidence that serotonin neurons stimulate secretion of prolactin releasing factor. *Life Sci.,* 22:2209–2214.
164. Johnston, C. A., Fagin, K. D., Alper, R. H., and Negro-Vilar, A. (1986): Prolactin release after 5-hydroxytryptophan treatment requires an intact neurointermediate pituitary lobe. *Endocrinology,* 118:805–810.
165. King, T. S., Steger, R. W., and Morgan, W. W. (1985): Effect of hypophysectomy and subsequent prolactin administration of hypothalamic 5-hydroxytryptamine synthesis in ovariectomized rats. *Endocrinology,* 116:485–491.
166. King, T. S., Carrillo, A. J., and Morgan, W. W. (1986): Hyperprolactinemia attenuates ovarian steroid stimulation of region-specific hypothalamic serotonin synthesis and luteinizing hormone release in ovariectomized rats. *Neuroendocrinology,* 42:351–357.
167. Labhsetwar, A. P. (1972): Role of monoamines in ovulation: Evidence for a serotonergic pathway for inhibition of spontaneous ovulation. *J. Endocrinol.,* 54:269–275.
168. Kordon, C. (1969): Effect of selective experimental changes in regional hypothalamic monoamine levels of superovulation in the immature rat. *Neuroendocrinology,* 4:129–138.
169. O'Steen, W. K. (1964): Serotonin suppression of luteinizition in gonadotrophin-treated, immature rats. *Endocrinology,* 74: 885–888.
170. O'Steen, W. K. (1965): Suppression of ovarian activity in immature rats by serotonin. *Endocrinology,* 75:937–939.
171. Axelrod, J., and Inscoe, J. K. (1963): The uptake and binding of circulating serotonin and the effect of drugs. *J. Pharmacol. Exp. Ther.,* 141:161–165.
172. Wilson, C. A., and McDonald, P. G. (1974): Inhibitory effect of serotonin on ovulation in adult rats. *J. Endocrinol.,* 60:253–260.
173. Domanski, E., Przekop, F., Skubiskewski, B., and Wolinska, E. (1975): The effect and site of action of indoleamines on the hypothalamic centers involved in the control of LH release and ovulation in sheep. *Neuroendocrinology,* 17:265–273.
174. Przekop, F., Skubiskewski, B., and Domanski, E. (1975): The effects of indolamines (serotonin and melatonin) on induction of ovulation in rabbits. *Acta Physiol. Pol.,* 26:395–343.
175. Cramer, O. M., and Barraclough, C. A. (1978): The actions of serotonin, norepinephrine, and epinephrine on hypothalamic processes leading to adenohypophysial luteinizing hormone release. *Endocrinology,* 103:694–703.
176. Carrer, H. F., and Taleisnik, S. (1972): Neural pathways associated with the mesencephalic inhibitory influence on gonadotropin secretion. *Brain Res.,* 38:299–313.
177. Arendash, G. W., and Gallo, R. V. (1978): Serotonin involvement in the inhibition of episodic luteinizing hormone release during elec-

trical stimulation of the midbrain dorsal raphe nucleus in ovariectomized rats. *Endocrinology,* 102:1199–1206.
178. Hery, M., Laplante, E., and Kordon, C. (1976): Participation of serotonin in the phasic release of LH. Evidence from pharmacological experiments. *Endocrinology,* 99:496–503.
179. Marko, M., and Fluckiger, E. (1980): Role of serotonin in the regulation of ovulation. *Neuroendocrinology,* 30:228–231.
180. Wilson, C. A., Horth, C. E., McNeilly, A., and McDonald, P. C. (1975): Effect of serotonin and progesterone on induced ovulation in immature rats. *J. Endocrinology,* 64:337–347.
181. Meyer, D. C. (1978): Hypothalamic and raphe serotonergic systems in ovulation control. *Endocrinology,* 103:1067–1074.
182. Johnson, M. D., and Crowley, W. R. (1983): Acute effects of estradiol on circulating luteinizing hormone and prolactin concentrations and on serotonin turnover in individual brain nuclei. *Endocrinology,* 113:1934–1941.
183. Becu de Villalobos, D., Lux, V. A. R., Lacau DeMengido, L., and Libertun, C. (1984): Sexual differences in the serotonergic control of prolactin and luteinizing hormone secretion in the rat. *Endocrinology,* 115:84–89.
184. Hery, M., Laplante, E., Pattou, E., and Kordon, C. (1975): Interaction de la serotonine cerebrale avec la liberation cyclique de LH chez la ratte. *Ann. Endocrinol. (Paris),* 36:123–130.
185. Coen, C. W., and MacKinnon, P. C. B. (1979): Serotonin involvement in the control of phasic luteinizing hormone release in the rat: Evidence for a critical period. *J. Endocrinol.,* 82: 105–113.
186. Hery, M., Laplante, E., and Kordon, C. (1978): Participation of serotonin in the phasic release of luteinizing hormone. II. Effects of lesions of serotonin-containing pathways in the central nervous system. *Endocrinology,* 102:1019–1025.
187. Hery, M., Faudon, M., Dusticier, G., and Hery, F. (1982): Daily variations in serotonin metabolism in the suprachiasmatic nucleus of the rat: Influence of oestradiol impregnation. *J. Endocrinol.,* 94:157–166.
188. Cone, R. I., Davis, G. A., and Goy, R. W. (1981): Effects of ovarian steroids on serotonin metabolism within grossly dissected and microdissected brain regions of the ovariectomized rat. *Brain Res. Bull.,* 7:639–644.
189. Crowley, W. R., O'Donohue, T. L., Muth, E. A., and Jacobowitz, D. M. (1979): Effects of ovarian hormones on levels of luteinizing hormone in plasma and on serotonin concentrations in discrete brain nuclei. *Brain Res. Bull.,* 4:571–574.
190. Munaro, N. I. (1978): The effect of ovarian steroids on hypothalamic 5-hydroxytryptamine neuronal activity. *Neuroendocrinology,* 26:270–276.
191. King, T. S., Steger, R. W., and Morgan, W. W. (1986): Effect of ovarian steroids to stimulate region-specific hypothalamic 5-hydroxytryptamine synthesis in ovariectomized rats. *Neuroendocrinology,* 42:344–350.
192. Biegon, A., Fischette, C. T., Rainbow, T. C., and McEwen, B. S. (1983): Serotonin receptor modulation by estrogen in discrete brain nuclei. *Neuroendocrinology,* 35:287–291.
193. Biegon, A., Bercovitz, H., and Samuel, D. (1980): Serotonin receptor concentration during the estrous cycle of the rat. *Brain Res.,* 187:221–225.
194. Leonardelli, J., Dubois, M. P., and Poulain, P. (1974): Effect of exogenous serotonin on LH-RH secreting neurons in the guinea pig hypothalamus as revealed by immunofluorescence. *Neuroendocrinology,* 15:69–72.
195. McEwen, B. S., and Parsons, B. (1982): Gonadal steroid action on the brain: Neurochemistry and neuropharmacology. *Annu. Rev. Pharmacol. Toxicol.,* 22:555–598.
196. Tappaz, M., Braunstein, M., and Kopin, I. (1977): Glutamate decarboxylase (GAB) and γ-aminobutyric acid (GABA) in discrete nuclei of hypothalamus and *substantia nigra. Brain Res.,* 125:109–121.
197. Browstein, M., Palkovits, M., Tappaz, M., Saavedra, J., Kizer, J. (1976): Effect of surgical isolation of the hypothalamus on its neurotransmitter content. *Brain Res.,* 117:287–295.
198. Makara, G., Rappay, G., and Stark, E. (1975): Autoradiographic localization of ^{3}H-gamma-amino-butyric acid in medial hypothalamus. *Exp. Brain Res.,* 22:449–455.
199. Tappaz, M., Aguera, M., Belin, M., and Pujol, F. (1980): Autoradiography of GABA in the rat hypothalamic median eminence. *Brain Res.,* 186:379–391.
200. Vincent, S., Hokfelt, T., and Wu, J. (1982): GABA neuron system in hypothalamus and the pituitary gland. *Neuroendocrinology,* 34:117–125.
201. Flugge, G., Oertel, W., and Wuttke, W. (1986): Evidence for estrogen-receptive GABAergic neurons in the preoptic/anterior hypothalamic area of the rat brain. *Neuroendocrinology,* 43:1–5.
202. Lamberts, R., Mansky, T., Stock, K., Vijayan, E., and Wuttke, W. (1984): Involvement of preoptic-anterior hypothalamic GABA neurons in the regulation of pituitary LH and prolactin release. *Exp. Brain Res.,* 52:356–362.
203. Fuchs, E., Mansky, T., Stock, K., Vijayan, E., and Wuttke, W. (1984): Involvement of catecholamines and glutamate in GABAergic mechanisms regulatory to luteinizing hormone and prolactin secretion. *Neuroendocrinology,* 38:484–489.
204. Donoso, A., and Banzan, A. (1984): Effects of increase of brain GABA levels on the hypothalamic-pituitary-luteinizing hormone axis in rats. *Acta Endocrinol.,* 106:298–304.
205. Adler, B., and Crowley, W. (1986): Evidence for γ-aminobutyric acid modulation of ovarian hormonal effects on luteinizing hormone secretion and hypothalamic catecholamine activity in the female rat. *Endocrinology,* 118:91–97.
206. Mulchahey, J., and Neill, J. (1982): Gamma amino butyric acid (GABA) levels in hypophyseal stalk plasma of rats. *Life Sci.,* 31:453–456.
207. Mitchell, R., Grieve, G., and Fink, G. (1983): Endogenous GABA receptor ligands in hypophysial portal blood. *Neuroendocrinology,* 37:169–176.
208. Gudelsky, G., Apud, J., Masotto, C., Locatelli, V., Cocchi, D., Racagui, G., and Muller, E. (1983): Ethanolamine-*O*-sulfate enhances γ-aminobutyric acid secretion into hypophyseal portal blood and lowers serum prolactin concentrations. *Neuroendocrinology,* 37:397–399.
209. Grandison, L., and Guidotti, A. (1979): γ-Amino-butyric acid receptor functions in rat anterior pituitary: Evidence for control of prolactin release. *Endocrinology,* 105:754–759.
210. Loeffler, J., Kley, N., Pittius, C., Almeida, O., and Hollt, V. (1986): *In vivo* and *in vitro* studies of GABAergic inhibition of prolactin biosynthesis. *Neuroendocrinology,* 43:504–510.
211. Locatelli, V., Cocchi, D., Frigerio, C., Betti, R., Krogsgaard-Larsen, P., Racagri, G., and Muller, E. (1979): Dual γ-aminobutyric acid control of prolactin secretion in the rat. *Endocrinology,* 105:778–785.
212. Pass, K., and Ondo, J. (1977): The effects of γ-aminobutyric acid on prolactin and gonadotropin secretion in the unanesthetized rat. *Endocrinology,* 100:1437–1442.
213. Mioduszewski, R., Grandison, L., and Meites, J. (1976): Stimulation of prolactin release in rats by GABA. *Proc. Soc. Exp. Biol. Med.,* 151:44–46.
214. Schwartz, J. (1977): Histaminergic mechanisms in brain. *Annu. Rev. Pharmacol. Toxicol.,* 17:325–339.
215. Brownstein, M., Saavedra, J., Palkovits, M., and Axelrod, J. (1974): Histamine content of hypothalamic nuclei of the rat. *Brain Res.,* 77:151–156.
216. Pollard, H., Bischoff, S., Llorens-Cortes, C., and Schwartz, J. (1976): Histidine decarboxylase and histamine in discrete nuclei of rat hypothalamus and the evidence for mast-cells in the median eminence. *Brain Res.,* 118:509–513.
217. Wilcox, B., and Seybold, V. (1982): Localization of neuronal histamine in rat brain. *Neurosci. Lett.,* 29:105–110.
218. Garbarg, M., Barbin, G., Bischoff, S., Pollard, H., and Schwartz, J. (1976): Dual localization of histamine in an ascending neuronal pathway and in non-neuronal cells evidenced by lesions in the lateral hypothalamic area. *Brain Res.,* 106:333–348.
219. Sawyer, C. (1955): Rhinencephalic involvement in pituitary activation by intraventricular histamine in the rabbit under nembutal anesthesia. *Am. J. Physiol.,* 180:37–46.
220. Libertun, C., and McCann, S. (1976): The possible role of histamine in the control of prolactin and gonadotropin release. *Neuroendocrinology,* 20:110–120.
221. Rivier, C., and Vale, W. (1977): Effects of γ-aminobutyric acid and histamine on prolactin secretion in the rat. *Endocrinology,* 101:506–511.
222. Donoso, A. (1978): Induction of prolactin and luteinizing hormone

release by histamine in male and female rats and the influence of brain transmitter antagonists. *J. Endocrinol.*, 76:193–202.
223. Donoso, A., and Bannza, A. (1976): Acute effects of histamine on plasma prolactin and luteinizing hormone levels in male rats. *J. Neurol. Transmission*, 39:95–101.
224. Knigge, U., Wollesen, F., Dejgaard, A., Larsen, K., and Christiansen, P. (1984): Modulation of basal and LRH-stimulated gonadotrophan secretion by histamine in normal men. *Neuroendocrinology*, 38:93–96.
225. Knigge, U., Thuesen, B., Wollesen, F., Svenstsrup, B., and Christiansen, P. (1985): Effect of histamine on basal and TRH/LHRH stimulated PRL and LH secretion during different phases of the menstrual cycle in normal women. *Neuroendocrinology*, 41:337–341.
226. Miyake, A., Ohtsuka, S., Nishizaki, J., Tasaka, K., Aono, T., Tanizawa, O., Yamatodani, A., Watanabe, T., and Wada, H. (1987): Involvement of H_1 histamine receptor in basal and estrogen-stimulated luteinizing hormone-releasing hormone secretion in rats *in vitro*. *Neuroendocrinology*, 45:191–196.
227. Charli, J., Rotsztejn, W., Pattou, E., and Kordon, C. (1978): Effect of neurotransmitters on *in vitro* release of luteinizing-hormone-releasing hormone from the mediobasal hypothalamus of male rats. *Neurosci. Lett.*, 159:163.
228. Reynolds, L., Rubel, A., and Nikitovich-Winer, M. (1980): Cimetidine inhibits the histamine-induced prolactin release in male rats. *Proc. Soc. Exp. Biol. Med.*, 163:322–325.
229. Donoso, A., Zarate, M., and Seltzer, A. (1983): Histamine-induced prolactin release: Pharmacological characterization of receptors in male rats. *Neuroendocrinology*, 36:436–442.
230. Knigge, U., Matzen, S., and Warbeg, J. (1986): Histaminergic stimulation of prolactin secretion mediated via H_1- and H_2-receptors: Dependence on routes of administration. *Neuroendocrinology*, 44:41–48.
231. Knigge, U., Dejaard, A., Wollesen, F., Thuesen, B., and Christiansen, P. (1982): Histamine regulation of prolactin secretion through H_1 and H_2 receptors. *J. Clin. Endocrinol. Metab.*, 58:118–122.
232. Gibbs, D., Plotsky, P., deGreef, W., and Neill, J. (1979): Effect of histamine and acetylcholine on hypophysial stalk plasma dopamine and peripheral plasma prolactin levels. *Life Sci.*, 24:2063–2070.
233. Charli, J., Joseph-Bravo, P., Palacios, J., and Kordon, C. (1978): Histamine-induced release of thyrotropin releasing hormone from hypothalamic slices. *Eur. J. Pharmacol.*, 52:401–403.
234. Bennet, G., and Keeling, M. (1981): H_2-mediated histamine-induced release of thyrotropin releasing hormone (TRH) from hypothalamic synaptosomes: A neuroendocrine role for histamine. *Br. J. Pharmacol.*, 72:151–152.
235. Donoso, A., and Banzan, A. (1980): H_1- and H_2-histamine receptor antagonists and induced release of prolactin in male rats. *Neuroendocrinology*, 30:11–14.
236. Sibilia, V., Nettic, C., Guidobono, F., Pagani, F., and Pecile, A. (1985): Cimetidine-induced prolactin release: Possible involvement of the GABAergic system. *Neuroendocrinology*, 40:189–192.
237. Akakelian, M., and Libertum, C. (1977): H_1 and H_2 histamine receptor participation in the brain control of prolactin secretion in lactating rats. *Endocrinology*, 100:890–895.
238. Palkovits, M. (1984): Distribution of neuropeptides in the central nervous system: A review of biochemical mapping studies. *Prog. Neurobiol.*, 23:151–189.
239. Palkovits, M., and Brownstein, M. J. (1985): Distribution of neuropeptides in the central nervous system using biochemical micromethods. In: *Handbook of Chemical Neuroanatomy, Vol. 4*, edited by A. Björklund and T. Hökfelt, pp. 1–70. Elsevier, Amsterdam.
240. Palkovits, M. (1987): Organization of the stress response at the anatomical level. In: *Progress in Brain Research, Vol. 72*, edited by F. R. de Kloet, V. M. Wiegant, and D. de Wied, pp. 47–56. Elsevier, Amsterdam.
241. Kordon, C., Rotten, D., Durand, D., and Bluet-Pajot, M. T. (1987): Neuroendocrine control of episodic hormone secretion. In: *Episodic Hormone Secretion*, edited by T. O. F. Wagner and M. Filicori, pp. 25–36. T. M. Verlag, Hameln.
242. Simerly, R. B., Gorski, R. A., and Swanson, L. W. (1986): Neurotransmitter specificity of cells and fibers in the medial preoptic nucleus: An immunohistochemical study in the rat. *J. Comp. Neurol.*, 246:343–363.
243. Brazeau, P., Vale, W., Burgus, R., Ling, N., Butcher, M., Rivier, J., and Guillemin, R. (1972): Hypothalamic polypeptide that inhibits the secretion of immunoreactive pituitary growth hormone. *Science*, 129:77–79.
244. Tavianini, M., Hayest, T., Magazin, M., Minth, C., and Dixon, J. (1984): Isolation, characterization and DNA sequence of the rat somatostatin gene. *J. Biol. Chem.*, 259:11798–11803.
245. Goodman, R. H., Jacobs, J. W., Chin, W., Lund, P. K., Dee, P. C., and Habener, J. F. (1980): Nucleotide sequence of a cloned structural gene coding for a precursor of pancreatic somatostatin. *Proc. Natl. Acad. Sci. USA*, 77:5869–5873.
246. Shen, L. P., and Rutter, W. S. (1984): Sequence of human somatostatin gene. *Science*, 274:168–171.
247. Brownstein, M., Arimura, A., Sato, H., Schally, A. V., and Kizer, J. S. (1975): The regional distribution of somatostatin in the rat brain. *Endocrinology*, 96:1456–1461.
248. Palkovits, M., Brownstein, M. J., Arimura, A., Sato, H., Schally, A. V., and Kizer, J. S. (1976): Somatostatin content of the hypothalamic ventromedial and arcuate nuclei and the circumventricular organ in the rat. *Brain Res.*, 109:430–434.
249. Elde, R. P., and Parsons, J. A. (1975): Immunocytochemical localization of somatostatin in cell bodies of the rat hypothalamus. *Annu. J. Anat.*, 144:541–548.
250. Alpert, L. C., Brawer, J. R., Patel, Y. C., and Reichlin, S. (1976): Somatostatin neurons in anterior hypothalamus: Immunocytochemical localization. *Endocrinology*, 98:255–258.
251. Epelbaum, J., Willouhby, J. O., Brazeau, P., and Martin, J. B. (1977): Effect of brain lesions and hypothalamic deafferentation on somatostatin distribution in rat brain. *Endocrinology*, 101:1495–1502.
252. Epelbaum, J., Tapia-Arancibia, L., Herman, J. P., Kordon, C., and Palkovitis, M. (1981): Topographical distribution of median eminence somatostatinergic innervation. *Brain Res.*, 250:412–416.
253. Makara, G. B., Palkovits, M., Antoni, F. A., and Kiss, J. Z. (1983): Topography of the somatostatin immunoreactive fibers to the stalk median eminence of the rat. *Neuroendocrinology*, 37:1–8.
254. Kita, T., Chihara, J., Abe, H., Mihamitani, H., Kaji, H., Kodama, H., Chiba, T., Fujika, T., and Kanaihara, N. (1986): Regional distribution of gastrin releasing peptide and somatostatin like immunoreactivity in the rabbit hypothalamus. *Brain Res.*, 398:18–22.
255. Chihara, K., Arimura, A., Kubli-Garfias, C., and Schally, A. V. (1979): Enhancement of immunoreactive somatostatin release into hypophyseal blood by electrical stimulation in the preoptic area in the rat. *Endocrinology*, 105:1416–1419.
256. Bennett-Clark, C., Romagnamo, M. A., and Joseph, S. A. (1980): Distribution of somatostatin in the rat brain: Telencephalon and diencephalon. *Brain Res.*, 188:473–486.
257. Johansson, O., Hökfelt, T., and Elde, R. P. (1984): Immunohistochemical distribution of somatostatin like immunoreactivity in the central nervous system of the adult rat. *Neuroscience*, 13:265–339.
258. Epelbaum, J. (1986): Somatostatin in the central nervous system: physiology and pathological modifications. *Prog. Neurobiol.*, 27:63–100.
259. Krisch, B. (1978): Hypothalamic and extrahypothalamic distribution of somatostatin immunoreactive elements in the rat brain. *Cell Tissue Res.*, 195:495–513.
260. Palkovits, M., Tapia-Arancibia, L., Kordon, C., and Epelbaum, J. (1982): Somatostatin connections between the hypothalamus and the limbic system of the rat brain. *Brain Res.*, 250:223–228.
261. Terry, L. C., and Crowley, W. R. (1986): Regulation of growth hormone and thyrotropin secretion by somatostatin systems in rat brain. *Neuroendocrinology*, 42:218–225.
262. Alonso, G., Tapia-Arancibia, L., and Assenmacher, I. (1985): Electron microscopic immunocytochemical study of somatostatin neurons in the periventricular nucleus of the rat hypothalamus with special reference to their relationships with homologue neuronal processes. *Neuroscience*, 16:297–306.
263. Lumpkin, M. O., Negro-Vilar, A., and McCann, S. M. (1981): Paradoxical elevation of growth hormone by intraventricular somatostatin: Possible ultrashort feedback. *Science*, 211:1072.
264. Epelbaum, J., Tapia-Arancibia, L., Alonso, G., Astier, H., and Kordon, C. (1986): The anterior periventricular hypothalamus is the site of somatostatin inhibition on its own release: An *in vitro* and immunocytochemical study. *Neuroendocrinology*, 44:255–259.
265. Pradayrol, L., Jörvall, H., Mutt, V., and Ribet, A. (1980): N-terminally extended somatostatin: The primary structure of somatostatin 28. *FEBS Lett.*, 109:55–58.

266. Millar, R., Sheward, W., Wegener, I., and Fink, G. (1983): Somatostatin 28 is an hormonally active peptide secreted into hypophyseal ported vessel blood. *Brain Res.*, 260:334–337.
267. Sheward, J., Benoit, R., and Fink, G. (1984): Somatostatin 28 (1–12)-like immunoreactive substance is secreted into hypophyseal portal vessel blood in the rat. *Neuroendocrinology*, 38:88–90.
268. Morrison, J., Benoit, R., Magistretti, P., and Bloom, F. (1983): Immunocytochemical distribution of prosomatostatin related peptides in cerebral cortex. *Brain Res.*, 262:344–351.
269. Lewis, M. D., Foord, S. M., Lewis, M. B., Hall, R., and Scanlon, M. F. (1986): Differential production of SRIF 14 and 28 by fetal rat hypothalamic cells enriched by velocity sedimentation. *Neuroendocrinology*, 44:125–131.
270. Epelbaum, J., Tapia-Arancibia, L., Kordon, C., and Enjalbert, A. (1982): Characterization, regional distribution and subcellular distribution of 125I-Tyr, somatostatin binding sites in rat brain. *J. Neurochem.*, 38:1515–1523.
271. Schonbrunn, A., and Tashjian, A. (1978): Characterization of functional receptors for somatostatin in rat pituitary cells in culture. *J. Biol. Chem.*, 253:6473–6483.
272. Morel, G., Leroux, P., and Pelletier, G. (1985): Localization and characterization of somatostatin 14 and 28 receptors in the rat pituitary as studied by slide mounted frozen sections. *Neuropeptides*, 6:41–52.
273. Moyse, E., Le Dafniet, M., Epelbaum, J., Pagesy, P., Peillon, F., Kordon, C., and Enjalbert, A. (1984): Somatostatin receptors in human growth hormone and prolactin secreting pituitary adenomes. *J. Clin. Endocrinol. Metab.*, 61:98–103.
274. Srikant, C., and Patel, Y. (1981): Receptor binding of somatostatin 28 is tissue specific. *Nature*, 294:259–260.
275. Moyse, E., Benoit, R., Enjalbert, A., Gautron, J. P., Kordon, C., Ling, N., and Epelbaum, J. (1984): Subcellular distribution of somatostatin 14 and 28 in rat brain cortex and comparison of their respective binding sites in brain and pituitary. *Regul. Pept.*, 9:129–137.
276. Ferland, L., Labrie, F., Jobin, M., Arimura, A., and Schally, A. V. (1976): Physiological role of somatostatin in the control of growth hormone and thyrotropin secretion. *Biochem. Biophys. Res. Commun.*, 68:149.
277. Vale, W., Rivier, C., Brazeau, P., and Guillemin, R. (1974): Effects of somatostatin on the secretion of thyrotropin and prolactin. *Endocrinology*, 95:968–977.
278. Kimura, N., Hayafuji, C., Konagaya, H., and Takahashi, K. (1986): 17β estradiol induces somatostatin inhibition of prolactin release and regulates SRIF receptors in rat anterior pituitary cells. *Endocrinology*, 119:1028–1036.
279. Enjalbert, Z., Epelbaum, J., Arancibia, S., Tapia-Arancibia, L., Bluet-Pajot, M. T., and Kordon, C. (1982): Reciprocal interactions of somatostatin with thyrotropin releasing hormone and vasoactive intestinal peptide on prolactin and growth hormone secretion *in vitro*. *Endocrinology*, 111:42–47.
280. Enjalbert, A., Bertrand, P., Le Dafniet, M., Epelbaum, J., Hugues, J. N., Kordon, C., Moyse, E., Peillon, F., and Shu, C. (1986): Somatostatin and regulation of prolactin secretion. *Psychoneuroendocrinology*, 11:155–165.
281. Göthert, M. (1980): Somatostatin selectively inhibits noradrenaline release from hypothalamic neurons. *Nature*, 288:86–88.
282. Tsujimoto, A., and Tanaka, S. (1981): Stimulatory effect of somatostatin on norepinephrine release from rat cortex slices. *Life Sci.*, 28:903–910.
283. Garcia-Sevilla, J. A., Magnusson, T., and Carlsson, A. (1978): Effect of intracerbroventricularly administered somatostatin on brain monoamine turnover. *Brain Res.*, 155:159–164.
284. Tanaka, S., and Tsujimoto, A. (1981): Somatostatin facilitates the serotonin release from rat cerebral cortex hippocampus and hypothalamus slices. *Brain Res.*, 208:219–222.
285. Rotsztejn, W. H., Drouva, S. V., Epelbaum, J., and Kordon, C. (1982): Somatostatin inhibits *in vitro* release of luteinizing hormone releasing hormone from rat mediobasal hypothalamic slices. *Experientia*, 38:974–975.
286. Hirooka, Y., Hollander, C. S., Suzuki, S., Ferdinand, F., and Juan, S. I. (1978): Somatostatin inhibits release of thyrotropin releasing factor from organ cultures of rat hypothalamus. *Proc. Natl. Acad. Sci.*, 75:4509–4513.
287. Tapia-Arancibia, L., Arancibia, S., and Astier, H. (1984): K^+ induced thyrotropin releasing hormone release from superfused mediobasal hypothalami in rats; inhibition by somatostatin. *Neurosci. Lett.*, 45:47–52.
288. Terenius, L. (1976): Somatostatin and ACTH are peptides with partial antagonist like selectivity for opiate receptors. *Eur. J. Pharmacol.*, 38:211–213.
289. Arancibia, S., Epelbaum, J., Alonso, G., and Assenmacher, I. (1983): Mise en évidence d'une sécrétion pulsatile de somatostatine (SRIF) dans le troisième ventricule cérébral chez le rat non anesthésié. *C. R. Acad. Sci. (Paris)*, 296:47–52.
290. Plotsky, P. M., and Vale, W. (1985): Patterns of growth hormone releasing factor and somatostatin secretion into the hypophyseal portal circulation of the rat. *Science*, 230:461.
291. Conrad, C. C. A., and Pfaff, D. W. (1976): Efferents from medial basal forebrain and hypothalamus in the rat. I. An autoradiographic study of the medial preoptic area. *J. Comp. Neurol.*, 169: 185–220.
292. Seeburg, P. H., and Adelman, J. P. (1984): Characterization of cDNA for precursor of human luteinizing hormone releasing hormone. *Nature*, 311:666–668.
293. Barry, J., Dubois, M. P., and Poulain, P. (1973): LRF producing cells in the mammalian hypothalamus. A fluorescent antibody study. *Z. Zellforsch.*, 146:351–366.
294. Barry, J., and Dubois, M. P. (1975): Immunofluorescence study of LRH producing neurons in the rat and the dog. *Neuroendocrinology*, 18:290–298.
295. Setalo, G., Vigh, S., Schally, A. V., Arimura, A., and Flerko, B. (1976): Immunohistochemical study of the origin of LHRH containing nerve fibers of the rat hypothalamus. *Brain Res.*, 103:597–602.
296. Palkovits, M., Pattou, E., Herman, J. P., and Kordon, C. (1984): Mapping of LHRH containing projections to the mediobasal hypothalamus by differential deafferentation experiments. *Brain Res.*, 298:283–288.
297. Liposits, Z., and Sétalo, G. (1980): Descending luteinizing hormone releasing hormone (LHRH) nerve fibers to the midbrain of the rat. *Neurosci. Lett.*, 20:1–4.
298. Jennes, L. (1987): Sites of origin of gonadotropin releasing hormones containing projections to the amygdala and the interpeduncular nucleus. *Brain Res.*, 404:339–344.
299. Jennes, L. (1986): The olfactory gonadotropin releasing hormone immunoreactive system in mouse. *Brain Res.*, 396:351–363.
300. Phillips, H. S., Nikolics, K., Brando, D., and Seeburg, P. H. (1985): Immunocytochemical localization in rat brain of a prolactin release inhibiting sequence of gonadotropin releasing hormone prohormone. *Nature*, 316:542–545.
301. Léranth, C. S., Segwa, L. M., Palkovits, M., McLusky, M. J., and Naftolin, F. (1985): The LHRH containing neuronal network in the preoptic area of the rat: Demonstration of LHRH containing nerve terminals in synaptic contact with LHRH neurons. *Brain Res.*, 345:332–336.
302. Wilson, R. C., Kesner, J. S., Kaufman, J. M., Uemura, T., Akema, T., Knobil, E. (1984): Central electrophysiologic correlates of pulsatile luteinizing hormone secretion in the rhesus monkey. *Neuroendocrinology*, 39:256–260.
303. Reubi, J. C., and Maurer, R. (1985): Visualization of LHRH receptors in the rat brain. *Eur. J. Pharmacol.*, 106:453–454.
304. Haour, F., Dusaillant, M., Leblanc, P., and Rostène, W. (1987): Mise en évidence et répartition topographique des récepteurs du LHRH chez le rat mâle normal et castré au niveau du système nerveux central. *C. R. Acad. Sci.* (Paris), 305:41–44.
305. Clayton, R. N., Catt, K. J. (1981): Gonadotropin releasing hormone receptors: Characterization, physiological regulation and relationship to reproductive function. *Endocr. Rev.*, 2:186.
306. Leblanc, P., Pattou, E., L'Heritier, A., Gogan, F., Slama, A., and Kordon, C. (1983): Biphasic pattern of follicle stimulating and luteinizing hormone responses to gonadotropic releasing hormone *in vitro*. *Neuroendocrinology*, 36:88–94.
307. Hsueh, A. J. W., and Jones, P. B. C. (1981): Extrapituitary actions of gonadotropin releasing hormone. *Endocr. Rev.*, 2:437.
308. Chan, A., Dudley, C. A., and Moss, R. I. (1983): Hormonal modification of the responsiveness of midbrain central gray neurons to LHRH. *Neuroendocrinology*, 41:163–168.
309. Pfaff, D. W. (1973): Luteinizing hormone releasing factor potentiates lordosis behaviour in hypophysectomized ovariectomized female rats. *Science*, 182:1148–1149.

310. Moss, R. L., and McCann, S. M. (1973): Induction of mating behavior in rats by luteinizing hormone releasing factor. *Science,* 181:177–179.
311. Sakuma, Y., and Pfaff, D. W. (1980): LHRH in the mesencephalic central grey can potentiate lordosis reflex of female rats. *Nature,* 283:566–567.
312. Sakuma, Y., and Pfaff, D. W. (1983): Modulation of the lordosis reflex of female rats by LHRH, its antiserum and analogs in the mesencephalic central gray. *Neuroendocrinology,* 36:218–224.
313. Nikolics, K., Mason, A. J., Szonyi, E., Ramachandran, J., and Seeburg, P. H. (1985): A prolactin inhibiting factor within the precursor for human gonadotropin releasing hormone. *Nature,* 316:511–517.
314. Millar, R. P., Wormald, P. J., and Milton, R. C. (1986): Stimulation of gonadotropin release by a non GnRH peptide sequence of the GnRH precursor. *Science,* 232:68–70.
315. Catania, A., Cantalamessa, L., and Reschini, E. (1976): Plasma prolactin response to luteinizing hormone releasing hormone in acromegalic patients. *J. Clin. Endocrinol. Metab.,* 43:689–691.
316. Mais, V., Melis, G. B., Paoletti, A. M., Strigini, F., Antonori, D., and Fioretti, D. (1986): Prolactin releasing action of a low dose of exogenous gonadotropin releasing hormone throughout the human menstrual cycle. *Neuroendocrinology,* 44:326–330.
317. Yen, S. S. C., Hoff, J. D., Lasley, B. L., Casper, R. F., and Sheehan, K. (1980): Induction of prolactin release by LRF and LRF agonist. *Life Sci.,* 26:1963–1967.
318. Denef, C., and Andries, M. (1983): Evidence for paracrine interaction between gonadotrophs and lactotrophs in pituitary cell aggregates. *Endocrinology,* 112:813–821.
319. Knepel, N., Schwaninger, M., Helm, C., and Kiesel, L. (1986): Top concentration of dynorphin like immunoreactivity in fractions of rat anterior pituitary cells enriched in gonadotrophs. *Life Sci.,* 38:2363.
320. Steele, M. K., Brownfield, M. S., and Ganong, W. F. (1982): Immunocytochemical localization of angiotensin immunoreactivity in gonadotropes and lactotropes of the rat anterior pituitary gland. *Neuroendocrinology,* 35:155–158.
321. Bégeot, M., Hemming, F. J., Dubois, P. M., Combarnous, Y., and Aubert, M. L. (1984): Induction of pituitary lactotrope differentiation by luteinizing hormone subunit. *Science,* 226:566–568.
322. Vou Euler, U. S., and Gaddum, J. H. (1931): An unidentified depressor substance in certain tissue extracts. *J. Physiol.,* 72:74–87.
323. Jordan, C. C., and Gehme, P. (1985): *Substance P, Metabolism and Biological Actions.* Taylor and Francis, London and Philadelphia.
324. Brownstein, M. J., Mroz, E. A., Kizer, J. S., Palkovits, M., and Leeman, S. E. (1976): Regional distribution of substance P in the brain of the rat. *Brain Res.,* 116:299–311.
325. Ljungdahl, A., Hökfelt, T., Nilsson, G., and Goldstein, M. (1978): Distribution of substance P like immunoreactivity in the central nervous system of the rat. *Neuroscience,* 3:861–944.
326. Danks, J. A., Rothman, R. B., Carcieri, M. A., Chicchi, G. G., Liang, T., and Herdenham, M. (1986): A comparative autoradiographic study of the distributions of substance P and eledoisin binding sites in rat brain. *Brain Res.,* 385:273–281.
327. Kerdelhué, B., Tartar, A., Lenoir, V., El Abed, A., Hublau, P., and Millar, R. P. (1985): Binding studies of substance P anterior pituitary binding sites; changes in substance P binding sites during the rat estrous cycle. *Regul. Pept.,* 10:133–143.
328. Hökfelt, T., Pernow, B., Nilsson, G., Wetterberg, M., Goldstein, M., and Jeffcoate, S. L. (1978): Dense plexus of substance P immunoreactive nerve terminals in eminentia medialis of the primate hypothalamus. *Proc. Natl. Acad. Sci. USA,* 75: 1013–1015.
329. Stoeckel, M. E., Porte, A., Klein, M. J., and Cuello, A. C. (1982): Immunocytochemical localization of substance P in the neurohypophysis and the hypothalamus of the mouse compared with the distribution of other neuropeptides. *Cell Tissue Res.,* 223:544–553.
330. Morel, G., Chayvialle, J. A., Kerdelhué, B., and Dubois, P. M. (1982): Ultrastructural evidence for endogenous substance P like immunoreactivity in the rat pituitary gland. *Neuroendocrinology,* 35:86–92.
331. De Palavis, L. R., Khorram, O., Ho, R. H., Negro-Vilar, A., and McCann, S. M. (1984): Partial characterization of immunoreactive substance P in the rat pituitary gland. *Life Sci.,* 34:225–238.
332. Vijayan, E., and McCann, S. M. (1979): *In vivo* and *in vitro* effects of substance P and neurotensin on gonadotropin and prolactin release. *Endocrinology,* 105:64–68.
333. Kato, Y., Chiara, K., Ohgo, S., Ivasak, Y., Abe, H., and Imura, H. (1976): Growth hormone and prolactin release by substance P in rats. *Life Sci.,* 19:441–446.
334. Eckstein, N., Wehrenberg, W. B., Louis, K., Carmel, P. V., Zimmerman, E. A., and Ferin, M. (1980): Effects of substance P on the anterior pituitary secretion in the female rhesus monkey. *Neuroendocrinology,* 31:338–342.
335. Rivier, C., Braun, M., and Vale, W. (1977): Effect of neurotensin, substance P and morphine sulfate on the secretion of prolactin and growth hormone in the rat. *Endocrinology,* 100:751–754.
336. Kerdelhué, B., Khar, A., Dennay, D., Langlois, Y., Bernardo, T., Linska, J., and Jutisz, M. (1979): Inhibition *in vitro* par la substance P de l'excretion des gonadotropines induites par la LHRH à partir de cellules antehypophysaires de rat en culture. *C. R. Acad. Sci. (Paris),* 287:879–882.
337. Kerdelhué, B., Valens, M., and Langlois, Y. (1978): Stimulation de la sécrétion de LH et TSH hypophysaires après immunoneutralisation de la substance P endogène chez le rat cyclique. *C. R. Acad. Sci. (Paris),* 286:977–979.
338. Dees, W. L., Skelley, C. W., and Kozlowski, G. P. (1985): Central effects of an antagonist and an antiserum to substance P on serum gonadotropin and prolactin secretion. *Life Sci.,* 37:1627–1631.
339. Kerdelhué, B., Palkovits, M., Kerteszi, K., and Reinberg, A. (1981): Circadian variations in substance P, luliberin (LHRH) and thyroliberin (TRH) contents in hypothalamic and extrahypothalamic brain nuclei of adult male rats. *Brain Res.,* 206:405–413.
340. Frankfurt, M., Siegel, R. A., Sim, I., and Wuttke, W. (1986): Estrous cycle variations in cholecystokinin and substance P concentrations in discrete areas of the rat brain. *Neuroendocrinology,* 42:226–231.
341. Carraway, R., and Leeman, S. E. (1973): The isolation of a new hypotensive peptide, neurotensin, from bovine hypothalami. *J. Biol. Chem.,* 248:6854.
342. Kahn, D., Abrams, G., Zimmerman, F. A., Carraway, R., and Leeman, S. E. (1980): Neurotensin neurons in the rat hypothalamus: An immunohistochemical study. *Endocrinology,* 107:47–54.
343. Jennes, L., Stumpf, W. E., and Kalivas, P. W. (1982): Neurotensin: Topographical distribution in rat brain by immunocytochemistry. *J. Comp. Neurol.,* 210:211–224.
344. Ibata, Y., Kawakami, F., Fujui, K., Okamura, H., Obata-Tsuto, H. L., Tsuto, T., and Terubayashi, H. (1984): Morphological survey of neurotensin-like immunoreactive neurons in the hypothalamus. *Peptides,* 5:109–120.
345. Ibata, Y., Fukui, K., Okamura, H., Kawakami, T., Tanaka, M., Obata, H. L., Tsuto, T., Terabayashi, H., Yanaihara, C., and Yanaihara, N. (1983): Coexistence of dopamine and neurotensin in hypothalamic arcuate and periventricular neurons. *Brain Res.,* 269:177–179.
346. Hökfelt, T., Everitt, B. H., Theodorsson-Norheim, E., and Goldstein, M. (1984): Occurrence of neurotensin like immunoreactivity in subpopulations of hypothalamic, mesencephalic and medullary catecholamine neurons. *J. Comp. Neurol.,* 222:543–559.
347. Saint-Pierre, S. A., Kerouac, R., Quirion, R., Jolicoeur, F. B., and Rioux, F. (1984): Neurotensin. In: *Peptide and Protein Review, Vol. 2,* edited by M. T. Hearn, pp. 83–171. Marcel Dekker, New York.
348. Inagaki, S., Yamano, M., Shiosaka, S., Takagi, H., and Tohyama, M. (1983): Distribution and origins of neurotensin containing fibers in the nucleus ventromedialis hypothalami of the rat: An experimental immunohistochemical study. *Brain Res.,* 273:229–235.
349. Goedert, M., Lightman, S. L., Mantyh, P. W., Hunt, S. P., and Emson, P. C. (1985): Neurotensin like immunoreactivity and neurotensin receptors in the rat hypothalamus and in the neurointermediate lobe of the pituitary gland. *Brain Res.,* 358:59–69.
350. Moyse, E., Rostène, W. H., Vial, M., Leonard, K., Mazella, J., Kitabgi, P., Vincent, J. P., and Beaudet, A. (1987): Radioautographic distribution of neurotensin binding sites in the rat brain: A light microscopic study using monoiodo-^{125}I-Tyr3-neurotensin. *Neuroscience* (in press).
351. Moyse, E., Miller, M. M., Kitabgi, P., Rostène, W., and Beaudet, A. (1986): Effects of gonadal steroids on the binding of ^{125}I neurotensin in rat suprachiasmatic nucleus. *Soc. Neurosci.,* 614.
352. Brown, M., and Vale, W. (1976): Effects of neurotensin and substance P on plasma insulin glucagon and glucose levels. *Endocrinology,* 98:819.

353. Szigethy, E., and Beaudet, A. (1987): Neurotensin receptors are selectively associated with cholinergic neurons in the rat basal forebrain. *Neurosci. Lett.* (*in press*).
354. Lamour, Y., and Epelbaum, J. (1987): Interactions between cholinergic and peptidergic systems in the cerebral cortex and hippocampus. *Prog. Neurobiol.* (*in press*).
355. Ferris, C. F., Pan, J., Singer, E., Boyd, W., Caraway, R., and Leeman, S. (1984): Stimulation of luteinizing hormone release after stereotaxic microinjection of neurotensin into the medial preoptic area of rats. *Neuroendocrinology,* 3:145–151.
356. Madea, K., and Frohman, L. A. (1978): Dissociation of systemic and central effects of neurotensin on the secretion of growth hormone, prolactin and thyrotropin. *Endocrinology,* 103:1903.
357. Enjalbert, A., Arancibia, S., Priam, M., Bluet-Pajot, M. T., and Kordon, C. (1982): Neurotensin stimulation of prolactin secretion *in vitro. Neuroendocrinology,* 34:95–98.
358. Goedert, M., Lightman, S. L., and Emson, P. C. (1984): Neurotensin in the rat anterior pituitary gland: Effects of endocrinological manipulations. *Brain Res.,* 299:160–163.
359. Fuxe, K., Agnati, L. F., Andersson, K., Eneroth, P., Harfstrand, A., Goldstein, M., and Zoli, M. (1984): Studies on neurotensin catecholamine interactions in the hypothalamus and in the forebrain of male rat. *Neurochem. Int.,* 6:737–750.
360. Malthe-Sorenssen, D., Wood, P. L., Cheney, D. L., and Costa, E. (1978): Modulation of the turnover rate of acetylcholine in rat brain by intraventricular injection of thyrotropin releasing hormone, somatostatin, neurotensin and angiotensin II. *J. Neurochem.,* 31:685–692.
361. Shimatsu, A., Kato, Y., Matsuhita, N., Katakami, H., Yanahaira, N., and Imura, H. (1982): Effects of glucagon, neurotensin and vasoactive intestinal peptide in somatostatin release from perifused rat hypothalamus. *Endocrinology,* 110:2113–2117.
362. Raisman, G., and Brown-Grant, K. (1977): The "suprachiasmatic syndrome": Endocrine and behavioural abnormalities following lesions of the suprachiasmatic nuclei in the female rat. *Proc. R. Soc. Lond.,* 198:297–314.
363. De Bold, A. J. (1985): Atrial natriuretic factor: A hormone produced by the heart. *Science,* 230:767–770.
364. Quirion, R., Dalpe, M., De Léan, A., Gutkowska, J., Cantin, M., and Genest, J. (1984): Atrial natriuretic factor (ANF) binding sites in brain and related structures. *Peptides,* 5:1167–1172.
365. Bianchi, C., Gutkowska, J., Ballak, M., Thibault, G., Garcia, R., Genest, J., and Cantin, M. (1986): Radioautographic localization of ^{125}I. atrial natriuretic factor binding sites in the brain. *Neuroendocrinology,* 44:365–372.
366. Jacobowitz, D. M., Skofitsch, G., Keiser, H. R., Eskay, R. L., and Zamir, N. (1984): Evidence for the existence of atrial natriuric factor containing neurons in rat brain. *Neuroendocrinology,* 40:92–94.
367. Harvath, J., Ertl, T., and Schally, A. V. (1986): Effect of atrial natriuretic peptide on gonadotropin release in superfused rat pituitary cells. *Proc. Natl. Acad. Sci. USA,* 83:3444–3446.
368. Abou-Samra, A. B., Catt, K. J., and Aguilera, G. (1987): Synthetic atrial natriuretic factors (ANFs) stimulate guanine 3′5′-monophosphate production but not hormone release in rat pituitary cells: Peptide contamination with a gonadotropin releasing hormone agonist explains luteinizing hormone releasing activity of certain ANFs. *Endocrinology,* 120:18–24.
369. Pandey, K. N., Pavlow, S. N., Kovacs, W. J., and Inagami, T. (1986): Atrial natriuretic factor regulates steroidogenic responsiveness and cyclic nucleotide levels in mouse Leydig cells *in vitro. Biochem. Biophys. Res. Commun.,* 138:399–404.
370. Wong, M., Samson, W. K., Dudley, C. A., and Moss, R. L. (1986): Direct neuronal action of atrial natriuretic factor in rat brain. *Neuroendocrinology,* 44:49–53.
371. Crandall, M. E., and Gregg, C. M. (1986): *In vitro* evidence for an inhibitory effect of atrial natriuretic peptide on vasopressin release. *Neuroendocrinology,* 44:439–445.
372. Samson, W. K. (1985): Atrial natriuretic factor inhibits dehydration and hemorrhage induced vasopressin release. *Neuroendocrinology,* 40:277–279.
373. Léranth, C. S., McLusky, M. J., and Naftolin, F. (1985): Proopiomelanocortin derived neuropeptide immunoreactive cells of the ventromedial arcuate nucleus establish direct synaptic connections with LHRH neurons of the medial preoptic area in the rat. *Proc. Neurosci. Soc.,* 15:146.
374. Sawchenko, P. E., Swanson, L. W., and Joseph, S. A. (1982): The distribution and cells of origin of ACTH (1–39) stained varicosities in the paraventricular and supraoptic nuclei. *Brain Res.,* 232:365–374.
375. Kiss, J. Z., Cassel, M. D., and Palkovits, M. (1984): Analysis of the ACTH/BEND/MSH immunoreactive afferent input to the hypothalamic paraventricular nucleus of the rat. *Brain Res.,* 324:91–99.
376. Bai, F. L., Yamano, M., Shiotani, Y., Emson, P. C., Smith, A. D., Powell, J. F., and Tohyama, M. (1985): An arcuato-paraventricular and dorsomedial hypothalamic neuropeptide Y containing system which lacks noradrenaline in the rat. *Brain Res.,* 331:172–175.
377. Chen, Y. Y., and Pelletier, G. (1983): Demonstration of contacts between proopiomelanocortin neurons in the rat hypothalamus. *Neurosci. Lett.,* 43:261–272.
378. Kiss, J. Z., and Williams, T. H. (1983): ACTH immunoreactive boutons form synaptic contacts in the hypothalamic arcuate nucleus of rat: Evidence for local opiocortin connections. *Brain Res.,* 263:142–146.
379. Tatemoto, K. (1982): Neuropeptide Y: Complete amino acid sequence of the brain peptide. *Proc. Natl. Acad. Sci. USA,* 79:5485–5489.
380. Tatemoto, K., Carlquist, M., and Mutt, V. (1982): Neuropeptide Y, a novel brain peptide with structural similarities to peptide YY and pancreatic polypeptide. *Nature,* 296:659–660.
381. Solomon, T. E. (1985): Pancreatic polypeptide, peptide YY and neuropeptide Y family of regulatory peptides. *Gastroenterology,* 88:838–844.
382. Allen, Y. S., Adrian, T. E., Allen, J. M., Tatemoto, K., Crow, T. J., Bloom, S. R., and Polak, J. M. (1983): Neuropeptide Y distribution in the brain. *Science,* 221:877.
383. Gray, T. S., and Marley, J. E. (1986): Neuropeptide Y: Anatomical distribution and possible functions in mammalian nervous system. *Life Sci.,* 38:389–400.
384. Chronwall, B. M., Di Maggio, D. A., Massari, V. J., Pickel, D. A., Ruggiko, D. A., and O'Donohue, T. L. (1985): The anatomy of neuropeptide Y containing neurons in the rat brain. *Neuroscience,* 15:1159–1181.
385. Beal, M. F., Chattha, G. K., and Martin, J. B. (1986): A comparison of regional somatostatin and neuropeptide Y distribution in rat striatum and brain. *Brain Res.,* 377:240–245.
386. Lundberg, J. M., Terenius, L., Hökfelt, T., and Tatemoto, K. (1984): Comparative immunohistochemical and biochemical analyses of pancreatic polypeptide-like peptides in central and peripheral neurons. *J. Neurosci.,* 4:2376–2386.
387. Hendry, S. H., Jones, E. G., and Emson, P. (1984): Morphology, distribution and synaptic relations of somatostatin and neuropeptide Y immunoreactive neurons in rat and monkey neocortex. *J. Neurosci.,* 4:2497–2517.
388. Everitt, B. J., Hökfelt, T., Terenius, L., Tatemoto, K., Mutt, V., and Goldstein, M. (1984): Differential coexistence of neuropeptide Y-like immunoreactivity with catecholamines in the central nervous system of the rat. *Neuroscience,* 11:443–462.
389. O'Donohue, T., Chronwall, B. M., Pruss, R. M., Mezey, E., Kiss, J. Z., Eiden, L. E., Massari, V. J., Tesset, J. G., Pickel, V. M., Di Maggio, D. A., Hotchkiss, A. J., Crowley, W. R., and Zuckowska-Grojec, Z. (1985): Neuropeptide Y and peptide YY neuronal and endocrine systems. *Peptides,* 6:755–768.
390. Moore, R. Y., Gustofson, E. L., and Card, J. P. (1984): Identical immunoreactivity of afferents to the rat suprachiasmatic nucleus with antisera against pancreatic polypeptide, molluscan cardioexcitatory peptide and neuropeptide Y. *Cell Tissue Res.,* 236:41–46.
391. Laburthe, P. (1986): Interaction of peptide YY with rat intestinal epithelial plasma membranes. *Endocrinology,* 118:1910–1917.
392. Kerkerian, L., Guy, J., Lefèvre, C., and Pelletier, G. (1985): Effects of neuropeptides Y (NPY) on the release of anterior pituitary hormones in the rat. *Peptides,* 6:1201–1204.
393. Kalra, S. P., and Crowley, W. R. (1984): Norepinephrine-like effects of neuropeptide Y on LH release in the rat. *Life Sci.,* 35:1173.
394. McDonald, J. K., Lumpkin, M. D., Samson, W. K., and McCann, S. M. (1985): NPY affects secretion of luteinizing hormone and growth hormone in ovariectomized rats. *Proc. Natl. Acad. Sci. USA,* 82:561.

395. Khorram, O., Pau, F. K. Y., and Spiess, H. G. (1987): Bimodal effects of neuropeptide Y or hypothalamic release of gonadotropin releasing hormone in conscious rabbits. *Neuroendocrinology,* 45:290–297.
396. Kalra, S. P., and Crowley, W. R. (1984): Differential effects of pancreatic polypeptide on luteinizing hormone release in female rats. *Neuroendocrinology,* 38:511–513.
397. McDonald, J. K., Lumpkin, M. D., Samson, W. K., and McCann, S. M. (1985): Pancreatic polypeptides affect luteinizing and growth hormone secretion in rats. *Peptides,* 6:79–84.
398. Crowley, W. R., Hassid, A., and Kalra, S. P. (1987): Neuropeptide Y enhances the release of luteinizing hormone induced by LH releasing hormone. *Endocrinology,* 120:941–945.
399. Crowley, W. R., Tessel, R. E., O'Donohue, T. L., Adler, B. A., and Kalra, S. P. (1985): Effect of ovarian hormones on the concentrations of immunoreactive neuropeptide Y in discrete brain regions of the female rat: Correlation with serum luteinizing hormone (LH) and median eminence LH releasing hormone. *Endocrinology,* 117:1151–1155.
400. Clark, J. T., Kalra, P. S., and Kalra, S. P. (1985): Neuropeptide Y stimulates feeding but inhibits sexual behavior in rats. *Endocrinology,* 117:2435–2442.
401. Tatemoto, K., Rökaeus, A., Jörnvall, H., McDonald, T. J., and Mutt, V. (1983): Galanin—A novel biologically active peptide from porcine intestine. *FEBS Lett.,* 164:124–128.
402. Melander, T., Hökfelt, T., and Rökaeus, A. (1986): Distribution of galanin-like immunoreactivity in the rat central nervous system. *J. Comp. Neurol.,* 248:475–517.
403. Skofitsch, G., and Zacobowitz, D. M. (1985): Immunocytochemical mapping of galanin-like neurons in the rat central nervous system. *Peptides,* 6:509–546.
404. Melander, T., Hökfelt, T., Rökaeus, A., Cuello, A. C., Oertel, W. H., Verhofstad, A., and Goldstein, M. (1986): Coexistence of galanin-like immunoreactivity with catecholamines, 5-hydroxytryptamine GABA and neuropeptides in the rat CNS. *J. Neurosci.,* 6:3640–3654.
405. Ottlecz, A., Samson, W. K., and McCann, S. M. (1986): Galanin: Evidence for a hypothalamic site of action to release growth hormone. *Peptides,* 7:51–53.
406. Nordsfröm, O., Melander, T., Hökfelt, T., Bartfai, T., and Goldstein, M. (1987): Evidence for an inhibitory effect of the peptide galanin on dopamine release from the rat median eminence. *Neurosci. Lett.,* 73:21–26.
407. Swanson, L. W., and Kuypers, H. G. (1980): The paraventricular nucleus of the hypothalamus: Cytoarchitectonic subdivisions and the organization of projections to the pituitary, dorsal vagal complex and spinal cord as demonstrated by retrograde fluorescence double labelling methods. *J. Comp. Neurol.,* 194:555–570.
408. Bargenann, W., and Scharrer, E. (1951): The site of origin of the hormones of the posterior pituitary. *Am. Sci.,* 39:255–259.
409. Katsoyannis, P. G., and Du Vigneaud, V. (1958): Arginine vasotocine, a synthetic analogue of the posterior pituitary hormones containing the ring of oxytocin and the side chain of vasopressin. *J. Biol. Chem.,* 233:1352–1354.
410. Sachs, H., and Lajtha, A. (1969): Neurosecretion. In: *Handbook of Neurochemistry, Vol. 4,* pp. 323–428. Plenum Press, New York.
411. Vandesande, F., Dierickx, K., and De Mey, J. (1975): Identification of the vasopressin-neurophysin producing neurons of the rat suprachiasmatic nuclei. *Cell Tissue Res.,* 56:377–380.
412. Sofroniew, M. V., and Weindl, A. (1980): Identification of parvocellular vasopressin and neurophysin neurons in the suprachiasmatic nucleus of a variety of mammals including primates. *J. Comp. Neurol.,* 193:659–675.
413. Brownstein, M. J., Eskay, R. L., and Palkovits, M. (1982): Thyrotropin releasing hormone in the median eminence is in processes of paraventricular nucleus neurons. *Neuropeptides,* 2:197–201.
414. Pelletier, G., Desy, I., Cote, J., Lefèvre, G., Vaudry, H., and Labrie, F. (1982): Immunoelectron microscopic localization of corticotropin releasing factor in the rat hypothalamus. *Neuroendocrinology,* 35:402–404.
415. Roth, K. A., Weber, E., and Barchas, J. D. (1982): Immunoreactive corticotropin releasing factor (CRF) and vasopressin are colocalized in a subpopulation of immunoreactive vasopressin cells in the paraventricular nucleus of the hypothalamus. *Life Sci.,* 31:1857–1860.
416. Beinfeld, M. C. (1983): Cholecystokinin in the central nervous system: A minireview. *Neuropeptides,* 3:411–427.
417. Lind, R. W., Swanson, L. W., Bruhn, T. O., and Ganten, D. (1985): The distribution of angiotensin II immunoreactive cells and fibers in the paraventriculo-hypophyseal system of the rat. *Brain Res.,* 338:81–89.
418. Carrea, F. M., Innes, R. B., Uhl, G. R., and Snyder, S. H. (1979): Bradykinin-like immunoreactive neuronal system localized histochemically in rat brain. *Proc. Natl. Acad. Sci. USA,* 76:1489–1493.
419. Moudy, T. W., O'Donohue, T. L., and Jacobowitz, D. M. (1982): Biochemical localization and characterization of bombesin-like peptides in discrete regions of the brain. *Peptides,* 2:75–79.
420. Mezey, E. (1986): Vasoactive intestinal polypeptide immunopositive neurons in the rat paraventricular nucleus of the homozygous Brattleboro rat. *Neuroendocrinology,* 42:88–90.
421. Kiss, J. Z., Palkovits, M., Zaborsky, L., Tribollet, E., Szabo, D., and Makara, G. B. (1983): Quantitative histological studies on the hypothalamic paraventricular nucleus in rats. I. Number of cells and synaptic boutons. *Brain Res.,* 262:217–224.
422. Van den Pol, A. N. (1982): The magnocellular and parvocellular paraventricular nucleus of the rat: Intrinsic organization. *J. Comp. Neurol.,* 206:317–345.
423. Nilaver, G., Zimmerman, E. A., Wilkins, J., Michaels, J., Hoffman, D., and Silverman, A. J. (1980): Magnocellular hypothalamic projections to the lower brain stem and spinal cord of the rat. *Neuroendocrinology,* 30:150–158.
424. Doris, P. A. (1984): Vasopressin and central integrative processes. *Neuroendocrinology,* 38:75–85.
425. Ivell, R., and Richter, D. (1984): Structure and comparison of the oxytocin and vasopressin genes from the rat. *Proc. Natl. Acad. Sci. USA,* 81:2006–2010.
426. Dogterom, J., Suijdewint, F. G., and Buijs, R. M. (1978): The distribution of vasopressin and oxytocin in the rat brain. *Neurosci. Lett.,* 9:341–346.
427. Hawthorn, J., Aug, V. T., and Jenkins, J. S. (1980): Localization of vasopressin in the rat brain. *Brain Res.,* 197:75–81.
428. Glick, S. M., and Brownstein, M. J. (1980): Vasopressin content of rat brain. *Life Sci.,* 27:1103–1110.
429. Rossor, M. N., Iversen, L. L., Hawthorn, J., Aug, V. T., and Jenkins, J. S. (1981): Extrahypothalamic vasopressin in human brain. *Brain Res.,* 214:349–355.
430. Zimmerman, E. A., Carmel, P., Husain, M. K., Férina, M., Tannerbaum, M., Frantz, A. G., and Robinson, A. G. (1973): Vasopressin and neurophysin high concentration in monkey hypophysial portal blood. *Science,* 182:925–927.
431. Gibbs, D. M. (1984): High concentrations of oxytocin in hypophysial portal plasma. *Endocrinology,* 114:1216–1218.
432. Jard, S. (1986): Vasopressin antagonists allow demonstration of a novel type of vasopressin receptors in the rat adenohypophysis. *Mol. Pharmacol.,* 30:171–177.
433. Koch, B., and Lutz-Bucher, B. (1985): Specific receptors for vasopressin in the pituitary gland: Evidence for down-regulation and desensitization to adrenocorticotropin releasing factor. *Endocrinology,* 116:671–676.
434. Yates, F. E., Russel, S. M., Dallman, M. R., Hedge, C. A., McCann, S. M., and Dhariwal, A. P. (1971): Potentiation by vasopressin of corticotropin release induced by CRF. *Endocrinology,* 88:3–15.
435. Buckingham, J. L. (1980): The influence of vasopressin on hypothalamic corticotropin releasing activity in rats with inherited diabetes insipidus. *J. Physiol.,* 312:9–16.
436. Gillies, G. E., Linton, E. A., and Lowry, P. J. (1982): Corticotropin releasing activity is potentiated several times by vasopressin. *Nature,* 399:355–357.
437. Rivier, C., and Vale, W. (1983): Interaction of corticotropin releasing factor and arginine vasopressin on adrenocorticotropin secretion *in vivo*. *Endocrinology,* 113:939–942.
438. Antoni, F. A., Holmes, M. C., and Jones, M. T. (1983): Oxytocin as well as vasopressin potentiates ovine CRF *in vitro*. *Peptides,* 4:411–415.
439. Gibbs, D. M., Vale, W., Rivier, J., and Yen, S. S. C. (1984): Oxytocin potentiates the ACTH releasing activity of CRF 41 but not vasopressin. *Life Sci.,* 34:2245–2249.
440. Suh, B. Y., Liu, J. H., Rasmussen, D. D., Gibbs, D. M., Steinberg, J., and Yen, S. S. C. (1986): Role of oxytocin in the modulation of ACTH release in women. *Neuroendocrinology,* 44:309–313.

441. Vaughan, M. K., Blask, D. E., Vaughan, G. M., and Reiter, R. J. (1976): Dose dependent prolactin releasing activity of arginine vasotocin in intact and pinealectomized estrogen progesterone treated adult male rats. *Endocrinology,* 99:1319–1322.
442. Johnson, L. Y., Vaughan, M. F., Reiter, R. J., Petterborg, L. J., and Chen, H. J. (1980): Acute effects of arginine vasopressin on plasma and pituitary levels of prolactin in the male rat: Influence of urethane anesthesia. *Horm. Res.,* 13:109–120.
443. Lumpkin, M. D., Samson, W. K., and McCann, S. M. (1983): Hypothalamic and pituitary sites of action of oxytocin to alter prolactin secretion in the rat. *Endocrinology,* 112:1711–1717.
444. Gala, R. R., and Rice, R. P. (1965): Influence of neurohumors on anterior pituitary lactogen production *in vitro. Proc. Soc. Exp. Biol. Med.,* 120:220.
445. Vaughan, M. K., Blask, D. E., Johnson, L. Y., and Reiter, R. J. (1975): Prolactin releasing activity of arginine vasopressin *in vitro. Horm. Res.,* 6:342–350.
446. Chin, S. H. (1982): Vasopressin has a direct effect on prolactin release in male rats. *Neuroendocrinology,* 34:55–58.
447. Marmède, P., Vincent, J. D., and Kerdelhué, B. (1986): Vasopressin and oxytocin reduce plasma prolactin levels of conscious rats in basal and stress conditions. Study of the characteristics of the receptor involved. *Life Sci.,* 39(19):1737–1743.
448. De Paolo, L. V., Berardo, P. V., and Carillo, A. J. (1986): Intraventricular administration of arginine vasopressin suppresses prolactin release via a dopaminergic mechanism. *Peptides,* 7:541.
449. Tanaka, M., De Kleet, E. R., De Wied, D., and Versteeg, D. H. (1977): Arginine vasopressin affects catecholamine metabolism in specific brain nuclei. *Life Sci.,* 20:1799–1808.
450. Blask, D. E., and Vaughan, M. K. (1980): Naloxone inhibits arginine vasopressin (AVT) induced prolactin release in urethane anesthetised male rats *in vivo. Neurosci. Lett.,* 18:184.
451. Ben-Jonathan, N., and Peters, L. L. (1982): Posterior pituitary lobectomy: Differential elevation of plasma prolactin and luteinizing hormone in estrous and lactating rats. *Endocrinology,* 110:1861–1865.
452. Gibbs, D. M. (1986): Vasopressin and oxytocin: Hypothalamic modulators of the stress response: A review. *Psychoneuroendocrinology,* 11:131–140.
453. Lang, R. E., Heil, J. W. E., Ganten, D., Hermann, K., Unger, T., and Rascher, W. (1983): Oxytocin unlike vasopressin is a stress hormone in the rat. *Neuroendocrinology,* 37:314–316.
454. Rivier, C., and Vale, W. (1983): Modulation of stress induced ACTH release by corticotropin releasing factor, catecholamines and vasopressin. *Nature,* 305:325–327.
455. Gibbs, D. M. (1986): Stress specific modulation of ACTH secretion by oxytocin. *Neuroendocrinology,* 42:456–458.
456. Gambacciani, M., Yen, S. S. C., and Rasmussen, D. D. (1986): GnRH release from mediobasal hypothalamus *in vitro:* Regulation by oxytocin. *Neuroendocrinology,* 42:181–183.
457. Fahrbach, S. E., Morrell, J. I., and Pfatt, D. W. (1985): Possible role for endogenous oxytocin in estrogen facilitated maternal behavior in rats. *Neuroendocrinology,* 40:526–532.
458. Kleet, E. R., Voarhuis, D. A. M., Boschma, Y., and Elands, J. (1986): Estradiol modulates density of putative oxytocin receptors in discrete rat brain regions. *Neuroendocrinology,* 44:415–421.
459. De Wied, D., and Gispen, W. H. (1977): Behavioral effects of peptides. In: *Peptides in Neurobiology,* edited by H. Gainer, pp. 397–448. Plenum Press, New York.
460. Burgus, R., Dunn, T. F., Desiderio, D., and Guillemin, R. (1969): Structure moléculaire du facteur hypothalamique TRF d'origine bovine: Mise en évidence par spectrométrie de masse de la séquence PCA-his-pro-NHe. *C. R. Acad. Sci. (Paris),* 269:1870–1873.
461. Boler, J., Enzmann, F., Folkers, K., Bowers, C. Y., and Shally, A. V. (1969): The identity of chemical and hormonal properties of the thyrotropin releasing hormone and pyroglotamyl-histidyl-proline amide. *Biochem. Biophys. Res. Commun.,* 37:705–710.
462. Richter, D., Kawashina, E., Egger, R., and Kreil, R. (1984): Biosynthesis of thyrotropin releasing hormone in the skin of *xenopus laevis:* Partial sequence of the precursor deduced from cloned DNA. *EMBO J.,* 3:617–621.
463. Brownstein, M. J., Palkovits, M., Saavedra, J. M., Bassiri, R. M., and Utiger, R. D. (1974): Thyrotropin releasing hormone in specific nuclei of the brain. *Science,* 185:267–269.
464. Bassiri, R. M., and Utiger, R. D. (1977): Thyrotropin releasing hormone in the hypothalamus of the rat. *Endocrinology,* 94:188.
465. Lechan, R., and Jackson, I. (1982): Immunohistochemical localization of thyrotropin releasing hormone in the rat hypothalamus and pituitary. *Endocrinology,* 111:55–65.
466. Ishikawa, K., Taniguchi, Y., Kurosumi, K., and Suzuki, M. (1986): Origin of septal thyrotropin releasing factor in the rat. *Neuroendocrinology,* 44:54–58.
467. Lechan, R. M., Wu, P., and Jackson, I. M. D. (1986): Immunolocalization of the thyrotropin releasing hormone prohormone in the rat central nervous system. *Endocrinology,* 119:1210–1216.
468. Borson-Chazot, F., Jordan, D., Fèvre-Montange, M., Kopp, N., Tourniaire, N., Rouzioux, J. M., Vesseyre, M., and Mornex, R. (1986): TRH and LHRH distribution in discrete nuclei of the human hypothalamus: Evidence for a left prominence of TRH. *Brain Res.,* 382:433–436.
469. Brunet, N., Gourdgi, D., Tixier-Vidal, A., Pradelles, Ph., Morgat, J. L., and Fromafeut, P. (1974): Chemical evidence for associated TRF with subcellular fractions after incubation of intact rat prolactin cells (GH3) with ^{3}H-labelled TRF. *FEBS Lett.,* 38:129–133.
470. Pazos, A., Cortès, R., and Palacios, J. (1985): Thyrotropin releasing hormone receptor binding sites: Autoradiographic distribution in the rat and guinea pig brain. *J. Neurochem.,* 45:1448–1463.
471. Horita, A., Carino, M. A., and Lai, H. (1986): Pharmacology of thyrotropin releasing hormone. *Annu. Rev. Pharmacol. Toxicol.,* 26:311–332.
472. Chen, H. T., and Meites, J. (1975): Effects of biogenic amines and TRH on the release of prolactin and TSH in the rat. *Endocrinology,* 96:10.
473. Tashjian, A. R., Borowsky, N. J., and Jensen, D. K. (1971): Thyrotropin releasing hormone: Direct evidence for stimulation of prolactin production by pituitary cells in culture. *Biochem. Biophys. Res. Commun.,* 43:516.
474. Vale, W., Blackwell, R., Grant, G., and Guillemin, R. (1973): TRF and thyroid hormones in prolactin secretion by rat anterior pituitary cells *in vitro. Endocrinology,* 93:26.
475. Bluet-Pajot, M. T., Durand, D., Drouva, S. V., Pressac, M., and Kordon, C. (1986): Further evidence that thyrotropin releasing hormone participates in the regulation of growth hormone secretion in the rat. *Neuroendocrinology,* 44:70–75.
476. Chihara, K., Kato, Y., Ohgo, S., Iwasaki, Y., Abe, H., Maeda, K., and Imura, H. (1976): Stimulating and inhibiting effects of thyrotropin releasing hormone on growth hormone release in rats. *Endocrinology,* 98:1047.
477. Müller, E. E., Panerai, A. E., Cocchi, D., Gril-Ad, I., Rossi, G. L., and Olgiati, V. R. (1977): Growth hormone releasing activity of thyrotropin releasing hormone in rats with hypothalamic lesions. *Endocrinology,* 100:1663–1677.
478. Irie, M., and Tsushima, T. (1972): Increase of serum growth hormone concentration following thyrotropin releasing hormone injection in patients with acromegaly or gigantism. *J. Clin. Endocrinol. Metab.,* 35:97–100.
479. Gerschengorn, M. C., Marcus-Samuels, B. E., and Geras, E. (1979): Estrogens increase the number of thyrotropin releasing hormone receptors on mammotropic cells in culture. *Endocrinology,* 105:171.
480. De Léan, A., Garon, M., Kelly, P. A., and Labrie, F. (1977): Changes in pituitary thyrotropin releasing hormone (TRH) and prolactin response to TRH during the rat estrous cycle. *Endocrinology,* 100:1505.
481. Enjalbert, A., Ruberg, M., Arancibia, S., Priam, M., Bauer, K., and Kordon, C. (1979): Inhibition of *in vitro* prolactin secretion by histidyl-proline diketoperazine, a degradation product of TRH. *Eur. J. Pharmacol.,* 58:97–98.
482. Osbahr, A. J., Neureroff, C. B., Luttinger, D., Mason, G. A., and Prange, A. J. (1981): Neurotensin induced antinociception in mice: Antagonism by thyrotropin releasing hormone. *J. Pharmacol. Exp. Ther.,* 217:645–651.
483. Keller, H. H., Bartholini, G., and Pletscher, A. (1974): Enhancement of cerebral noradrenalin turnover by thyrotropin releasing hormone. *Nature,* 248:528–529.
484. Reigle, T. C., Avni, J., Platz, P. A., Schildkrant, J. J., and Plotnikoff, N. P. (1974): Norepinephrine metabolism in the rat brain following acute and chronic administration of thyrotropin releasing hormone. *Psychopharmacologia,* 37:1–6.

485. Lotti, V. J., Yarbrough, G. G., and Clineschmidt, B. V. (1980): Investigations in the interactions on thyrotropin releasing hormone (TRH) and MK771 with central noradrenergic mechanisms. *Psychopharmacology,* 70:145–148.
486. Prange, A. J., Wilson, I. C., Lara, P. P., Alltop, L. B., and Breese, G. R. (1972): Effects of thyrotropin releasing hormone in depression. *Lancet,* 11:999–1002.
487. Hansen, S., Svensson, L., Hökfelt, T., and Everitt, B. J. (1983): 5-Hydroxytryptamine-thyrotropin releasing hormone interactions in the spinal cord: Effects on parameters of sexual behaviour in the male rat. *Neurosci. Lett.,* 42:299–304.
488. Vale, W., Spiess, J., Rivier, C., and Rivier, J. (1981): Characterization of 41 residue ovine hypothalamic peptide that stimulates secretion of corticotropin and β-endorphin. *Science,* 213: 1394–1397.
489. Shibahara, S., Moromoto, Y., Furutani, Y., Notake, M., Takahashi, H., Shimiza, S., Horikawa, S., and Numa, S. (1983): *EMBO J.,* 2:775–779.
490. Swanson, L. W., Sawchenko, P. E., Rivier, J., and Vale, W. (1983): Organization of ovine corticotropin releasing factor immunoreactive cells and fibers in the rat brain: An immunocytochemical study. *Neuroendocrinology,* 36:165–186.
491. Burlet, A., Tonon, M. C., Taukosic, P., Coy, D., and Vaudry, H. (1983): Comparative immunocytochemical localization of corticotropin releasing factor (CRF 41) and neurohypophysial peptides in the brain of Brattleboro and Long-Evans rats. *Neuroendocrinology,* 37:64–72.
492. McCann, S. M., and Haberland, P. (1959): Relative abundance of vasopressin and corticotropin releasing factor in neurohypophyseal extracts. *Proc. Soc. Exp. Biol. Med.,* 102:319–325.
493. Nakane, T., Andhya, T., Hollander, C. S., Schlesinger, D. H., Kardor, P., Brown, C., and Passarelli, I. (1986): Corticotropin releasing factor in extrahypothalamic brain of the mouse: Demonstration by immunoassay and immunoneutralization of bioassayable activity. *J. Endocrinol.,* 111:143–149.
494. Vale, W., Rivier, C., Yang, L., Minick, S., and Guillemin, R. (1978): Effects of purified hypothalamic corticotropin releasing factor and other substances on the secretion of adrenocorticotropin and β-endorphin-like immunoreactivities *in vitro. Endocrinology,* 103:1910–1915.
495. Rivier, C., and Vale, W. (1984): Influence of corticotropin releasing factor on reproductive functions in the rat. *Endocrinology,* 114:914.
496. Gambacciani, M., Yen, S. S. C., and Rasmussen, D. D. (1986): GnRH release from the mediobasal hypothalamus: *in vitro* inhibition by corticotropin releasing factor. *Neuroendocrinology,* 43: 533–536.
497. Nikolarakis, K. E., Almeida, O. F., and Herz, A. (1986): Corticotropin releasing factor (CRF) inhibits gonadotropin releasing hormone (GnRH) release from superfused rat hypothalami *in vitro. Brain Res.,* 377:388–390.
498. Ono, N., Lumpkin, M. D., Samson, W. K., McDonald, J. K., and McCann, S. M. (1984): Intrahypothalamic action of corticotropin releasing factor (CRF) to inhibit growth hormone and LH release in the rat. *Life Sci.,* 35:1117–1123.
499. Motta, M. (1985): Neuroendocrine effects of some amphibian peptides. *Peptides,* 6(Suppl. 3):131–135.
500. Brown, M. R., Fisher, L. A., Spiess, J., Rivier, J., Rivier, C., and Vale, W. (1982): Comparison of the biologic actions of corticotropin releasing factor and sauvagine. *Regul. Pept.,* 4:107.
501. Peterfreund, R., and Vale, W. (1983): Ovine corticotropin releasing factor stimulates somatostatin secretion from cultured brain cells. *Endocrinology,* 112:1275–1279.
502. Ilotzky, P. M., Bruhn, T. O., and Otto, S. (1984): Central modulation of immunoreactive arginine vasopressin and oxytocin secretion into the hypophyseal portal circulation by corticotropin releasing factor. *Endocrinology,* 116:1669–1671.
503. Bruhn, T. O., Sulton, S. W., Plotsky, P. M., and Vale, W. W. (1986): Central administration of corticotropin releasing factor modulates oxytocin secretion in the rat. *Endocrinology,* 119:1558–1563.
504. Sirinathsinghji, D. J., Rees, L. H., Rivier, J., and Vale, W. (1983): Corticotropin releasing factor is a potent inhibitor of sexual receptivity in the female rat. *Nature,* 305:15.
505. Sirinathsinghji, D. J. (1985): Modulation of lordosis behaviour in the female rat by corticotropin releasing factor, β endorphin and gonadotropin releasing hormone in the mesencephalic central gray. *Brain Res.,* 336:45–55.
506. Rivier, C., Rivier, J., and Vale, W. (1986): Stress induced inhibition of reproductive functions: Role of endogenous corticotropin releasing factor. *Science,* 231:607.
507. Aldenhoff, J. B., Gruol, D. L., Rivier, J., Vale, W., and Siggins, G. R. (1983): Corticotropin releasing factor decreases post-burst hyperpolarizations and excites hippocampal neurons. *Science,* 221:875–877.
508. Sutton, R. E., Koob, G. F., Le Moal, M., Rivier, J., and Vale, W. (1982): Corticotropin releasing factor produces behavioural activation in rats. *Nature,* 297:331–333.
509. Ehlers, C. L., Reed, T. K., and Henriksen, S. J. (1986): Effect of corticotropin releasing factor and growth hormone releasing factor on sleep and activity in rats. *Neuroendocrinology,* 42:467–474.
510. Britton, K. T., Lee, G., Dana, R., Risch, S. C., and Koob, G. F. (1986): Activating and anxiogenic effects of CRF are not inhibited by blockade of the pituitary adrenal system with dexamethasone. *Life Sci.,* 39:1281–1286.
511. Valentino, R. J., Foote, S. L., and Aston-Jones, G. (1983): Corticotropin releasing factor activates noradrenergic neurons of the *locus coeruleus. Brain Res.,* 270:363–367.
512. Valentino, R. J., and Foote, S. L. (1987): Corticotropin releasing factor disrupts sensory responses of brain noradrenergic neurons. *Neuroendocrinology,* 45:28–36.
513. Beinfeld, M. C., Meyer, D. K., Eskay, R. L., Jensen, R. T., and Brownstein, M. J. (1981): The distribution of cholecystokinin immunoreactivity in the central nervous system of the rat as determined by radioimmunoassay. *Brain Res.,* 212:51–57.
514. Iunis, R. B., Correa, F. M., Uhl, G. R., Schneider, B., and Snyder, S. H. (1979): Cholecystokinin octapeptide-like immunoreactivity: Histochemical localization in rat brain. *Proc. Natl. Acad. Sci. USA,* 76:521–525.
515. Vanderhaegben, J. J., Lostra, F., Vandesande, F., and Dierickx, K. (1981): Coexistence of cholocystokinin and oxytocin-neurophysin in some magnocellular hypothalamo-hypophyseal neurons. *Cell Tissue Res.,* 221:227–231.
516. Hökfelt, T., Holets, V. R., Staines, W., Meister, B., Melander, T., Schalling, M., Schutzberg, M., Freedman, J., Björklund, H., Olson, L., Lindh, B., Elfvin, L. G., Lundberg, J. M., Lindgren, J. A., Samuelsson, B., Penow, B., Terenius, L., Post, C., Everitt, B., and Goldstein, M. (1986): Coexistence of neuronal messengers—An overview. In: *Progress in Brain Research,* edited by T. Hökfelt, K. Fuxe, and B. Pernow, *Vol. 68,* pp. 33–70. Elsevier, Amsterdam.
517. Zaborszky, L., Beinfeld, M. C., Palkovits, M., and Heimer, L. (1984): Brainstem projections to the hypothalamic ventricular nucleus in the rat: A CCK containing long ascending pathway. *Brain Res.,* 303:225–231.
518. Saito, A., Sankaran, H., Godfine, L. D., and Williams, J. A. (1980): Cholecystokinin receptors in the brain: Characterization and distribution. *Science,* 208:1155–1156.
519. Zarbin, M. A., Iunis, R. B., Wamsley, J. K., Snyder, S. H., and Kuhar, M. J. (1983): Autoradiographic localization of cholecystokinin receptors in rodent brain. *J. Neurosci.,* 3:877–906.
520. Day, N. C., Hall, M. D., Clark, C. R., and Hughes, J. (1986): High concentrations of cholecystokinin receptor binding sites in the ventromedial hypothalamus. *Neuropeptides,* 8:1–18.
521. Akesson, T. R., Mantyh, P. W., Mantyh, C. R., Matt, D. W., and Micewych, P. E. (1987): Estrous cyclicity of ^{125}I cholecystokinin octapeptide binding in the ventromedial hypothalamic nucleus. Evidence for down modulation by estrogen. *Neuroendocrinology,* 45:257–262.
522. Akesson, T. R., and Micevych, P. E. (1986): Binding of ^{125}I cholecystokinin octapeptide in the paraventricular but not the supraoptic nucleus is increased by ovariectomy. *Brain Res.,* 385:165–168.
523. Vijayan, E., Samson, W. K., and McCann, S. M. (1979): *In vitro* and *in vivo* effects of cholecystokinin on gonadotropin, prolactin, growth hormone and thyrotropin release in the rat. *Brain Res.,* 172:295–302.
524. Kimura, F., Hashimoto, R., and Kawakami, M. (1983): The stimulatory effect of cholecystokinin implanted in the medial preoptic area on luteinizing hormone secretion in the ovariectomized estrogen primed rat. *Endocrinol. Jpn.,* 30:305–309.
525. Haghimoto, R., and Kimura, F. (1986): Inhibition of gonadotropin

secretion induced by cholecystokinin implants in the medial preoptic area by a dopamine receptor blocker, pimozide, in the rat. *Neuroendocrinology,* 42:32–37.
526. Pau, J. T., Kow, L. M., and Pfaff, D. W. (1986): Single unit activity of hypothalamic arcuate neurons in brain tissue slices. Effect of anterior pituitary hormones, cholecystokinin octapeptide and neurotransmitters. *Neuroendocrinology,* 43:189–196.
527. Skirboll, L. R., Grace, A. A., Homer, D. W., Rehfeld, J., Goldstein, M., Hökfelt, T., and Bunney, B. S. (1981): Peptide monoamine coexistence: Studies on the action of cholecystokinin-like peptide on the electrical activity of midbrain dopamine neurons. *Neuroscience,* 6:2111–2124.
528. McCaleb, M. L., and Lyers, R. D. (1980): Cholecystokinin acts on the hypothalamic noradrenergic system involved in feeding. *Peptides,* 1:47–49.
529. Kow, L. M., and Pfaff, D. W. (1986): CCK8 stimulation of ventromedial hypothalamic neurons *in vitro:* A feeding relevant event? *Peptides,* 7:473–480.
530. Fulwiler, C. E., and Saper, C. B. (1985): Cholecystokinin immunoreactive innervation of the ventromedial hypothalamus in the rat: Possible substrate for autonomic regulation of feeding. *Neurosci. Lett.,* 53:289–296.
531. Mendelson, S. D., and Gorzalka, B. B. (1984): Cholecystokinin octapeptide produces inhibition of lordosis in the female rat. *Pharmacol. Biochem. Behav.,* 21:755–759.
532. Campbell, D. J., Bochnik, J., Ménard, J., and Corvol, P. (1984): Identity of angiotensinogen precursors of rat brain and liver. *Nature,* 308:206–208.
533. Lind, R. W., Swanson, L. W., and Ganten, D. (1985): Organization of angiotensin II immunoreactive cells and fibers in the rat central nervous system. An immunohistochemical study. *Neuroendocrinology,* 40:2–24.
534. Philips, M. I., Weyhenmeyer, J., Felix, D., Ganten, D., and Hoffman, W. E. (1979): Evidence for an endogenous brain renin angiotensin system. *Fed. Proc.,* 38:2260–2266.
535. Kilcoyne, M. M., Hoffman, D. L., and Zimmerman, E. A. (1980): Immunocytochemical localization of angiotensin II and vasopressin in the rat hypothalamus: Evidence for production in the same neuron. *Clin. Sci.,* 59:57–60.
536. Saavedra, J. M., Fernandez-Pardal, J., and Chevillard, C. (1982): Angiotensin converting enzyme in discrete areas of the rat forebrain and pituitary gland. *Brain Res.,* 245:317–326.
537. Healy, D. P., Maciejewski, A. R., and Printz, M. P. (1986): Localization of central angiotensin II receptors with (^{125}I) ser ile 8 angiotensin II: Periventricular sites of the anterior third ventricle. *Neuroendocrinology,* 44:22–28.
538. Hauger, R. L., Aguilera, G., Baukol, A., and Catt, K. (1982): Characterization of angiotensin II receptors in the pituitary gland. *Mol. Cell. Endocrinol.,* 25:203–212.
539. Steele, M. K., Negro-Vilar, A., and McCann, S. M. (1981): Effect of angiotensin II on *in vivo* and *in vitro* release of anterior pituitary hormones in the female rat. *Endocrinology,* 109:893–899.
540. Gaillard, R. C., Grossman, A., Gillies, G., Rees, L., and Besser, G. M. (1981): Angiotensin II stimulates the release of ACTH from dispersed rat anterior pituitary cells. *Clin. Endocrinol.,* 15:573–578.
541. Steele, M. K., Gallo, R. V., and Ganong, W. F. (1983): A possible role for the brain renin-angiotensin system in the regulation of LH secretion. *Am. J. Physiol.,* 245:R805–R810.
542. Steele, M. K., Gallo, R. V., and Ganong, W. F. (1985): Stimulatory and inhibitory effects of angiotensin II upon LH secretion in ovariectomized rats: A function of gonadal steroids. *Neuroendocrinology,* 40:210–216.
543. Aguilera, R. A., Hyde, C., and Catt, K. (1982): Angiotensin II receptors and prolactin release in pituitary lactotrophs. *Endocrinology,* 111:1045–1050.
544. Schramme, C., and Denef, C. (1983): Stimulation of prolactin release by angiotensin II in superfused rat anterior pituitary cell aggregates. *Neuroendocrinology,* 36:483–485.
545. Enjalbert, A., Sladeczek, F., Guillon, G., Bertrand, P., Shu, C., Epelbaum, J., Garcia-Saenz, J. A., Jard, C., Lombard, C., Kordon, C., and Bockaert, J. (1986): Angiotensin II and dopamine modulate both cAMP and inositol phosphate production in anterior pituitary cells. Involvement in prolactin secretion. *J. Biol. Chem.,* 261:4071–4075.
546. Platia, M. P., Catt, K. J., and Aguilera, G. (1986): Effect of 17β estradiol on angiotensin II receptors and prolactin release in cultured pituitary cells. *Endocrinology,* 119:2768–2772.
547. Enjalbert, A., Bertrand, P., Bockaert, J., Drouva, S., and Kordon, C. (1987): Multiple coupling of neurohormone receptors with cyclic AMP and inositol phosphate production in anterior pituitary cells. *Biochimie,* 69:271–279.
548. Steele, M. K., Negro-Vilar, A., and McCann, S. M. (1982): Modulation by dopamine and estradiol of the central effects of angiotensin II on anterior pituitary hormone release. *Endocrinology,* 11:722–729.
549. Chen, M. F., Hawkins, R., and Printz, M. P. (1982): Evidence for a functional, independent brain angiotensin system: Correlation between regional distribution of brain ATII receptors, brain angiotensinogen and drinking during the estrous cycle of the rat. In: *The Renin-Angiotensin System in the Brain,* edited by D. Ganten, M. Printz, M. Phillips, and B. A. Scholkens, pp. 157–168. Raven Press, New York.
550. Findlay, A. L., Fitzimmons, J. T., and Kucharczyk, J. (1979): Dependence of spontaneous and angiotensin induced drinking in the rat upon the estrous cycle and gonadal hormones. *J. Endocrinol.,* 82:215–225.
551. Wilson, K. M., Summers, C., Hathaway, S., and Fregly, M. J. (1986): Mineralocorticoids modulate central angiotensin II receptors in rats. *Brain Res.,* 382:87–96.
552. Fuxe, K., Andersson, K., Ganten, D., Hökfelt, T., and Enroth, P. (1980): Evidence for the existence of an angiotensin II like immunoreactive central system and its interactions with the central catecholamine pathways. In: *Enzymatic Release of Vasoactive Peptides,* edited by F. Gross, and G. Vogel. Raven Press, New York.
553. Keil, L. C., Summy-Long, J., and Severs, W. B. (1975): Release of vasopressin by angiotensin II. *Endocrinology,* 96:1063–1065.
554. Steele, M. K., Negro-Vilar, A., and McCann, S. M. (1980): Effect of central injection of bradykinin and bradykinin potentiating factor upon release of anterior pituitary hormones in ovariectomized female rats. *Peptides,* 1:201–205.
555. Babu, G. N., and Viajayan, E. (1983): Plasma gonadotropin, prolactin levels and hypothalamic tyrosine hydroxylase activity following intraventricular bombesin and secretin in ovariectomized conscious rats. *Brain Res. Bull.,* 11:25–29.
556. Karashima, T., Okajima, T., Kato, K., and Ibayashi, H. (1984): Suppressive effects of cholecystokinin and bombesin on growth hormone and prolactin secretion in urethane anesthetized rats. *Endocrinol. Jpn.,* 31:539–547.
557. Bicknell, R. J., and Chapman, C. (1983): Bombesin stimulates growth hormone secretion from cultured bovine pituitary cells. *Neuroendocrinology,* 36:33–38.
558. Okajima, T., and Hertting, G. (1986): Bradykinin induced ACTH release from rat pituitary tissue *in vitro. Neuroendocrinology,* 43:336–339.
559. Matsumura, M., Ohura, M., Shimizu, I., Yamonoi, A., Iwaskai, A., and Saito, S. (1985): *In vivo* and *in vitro* effects of bradykinin on the release of β-endorphin-like immunoreactivity. *Neuroendocrinology,* 41:101–106.
560. Bell, G. I. (1986): The glucagon superfamily precursor structure and gene organization. *Peptides,* 7(Suppl. 1):27–36.
561. Mezey, E. (1986): Vasoactive intestinal polypeptide immunopositive neurons in the rat paraventricular nucleus of the homozygous Brattleboro rat. *Neuroendocrinology,* 42:88–90.
562. Okamura, H., Murakami, S., Fukui, K., Uda, K., Kawamoto, K., Kawashima, S., Yanaihara, N., and Ibata, Y. (1986): Vasoactive intestinal peptide and peptide histidine isoleucine amide-like immunoreactivity colocalize with vasopressin-like immunoreactivity in the canine hypothalamus neurohypophyseal neuronal system. *Neurosci. Lett.,* 69:227–232.
563. Panula, P., Yang, H., and Costa, E. (1982): Neuronal location of the bombesin-like immunoreactivity in the central nervous system of the rat. *Regul. Pept.,* 4:275–283.
564. Guillemin, R., Brazeau, P., Bohlen, P., Esch, F., Ling, N., and Wehrenberg, W. B. (1982): Growth hormone releasing factor from a human pancreatic tumor that caused acromegaly. *Science,* 218:585–587.
565. Rivier, J., Speiss, J., Thorner, M., and Vale, W. (1982): Characterization of a growth hormone releasing factor from a human pancreatic tumor. *Nature,* 300:276–278.
566. Tatemoto, K., and Mutt, V. (1981): Isolation and characterization

of the intestinal peptide porcine PHI (PHI 27), a new member of the glucagon secretin family. *Proc. Natl. Acad. Sci. USA,* 78:6603–6607.

567. Itoh, N., Obota, K., Yanaihara, N., and Okamoto, H. (1983): Human preprovasoactive intestinal polypeptide contains a novel PHI-like peptide, PHM 27. *Nature,* 304:547–549.
568. Hökfelt, T., Schultzberg, M., Lundberg, J. M., Fuxe, K., Mutt, V., Fahrenkrug, J., and Said, S. I. (1980): Distribution of the vasoactive intestinal peptide in the central and the peripheral nervous systems as revealed by immunocytochemistry. In: *Vasoactive Intestinal Peptide, Vol. 65,* edited by S. I. Said, p. 90. Raven Press, New York.
569. Fuxe, K., Hökfelt, T., Said, S. I., and Mutt, V. (1977): Vasoactive intestinal polypeptide and the nervous system: Immunohistochemical evidence for localization in central and peripheral neurons, particularly intracortical neurons of the cerebral cortex. *Neuroscience,* 5:241–246.
570. Hökfelt, T., Fahrenkrug, J., Tatemoto, K., Mutt, V., Werner, S., Hulting, A. L., Terenius, K., and Chang, K. J. (1983): The PHI (PHI 27)/corticotropin releasing factor/enkephalin immunoreactive hypothalamic neuron: Possible morphological basis for integrated control of prolactin, corticotropin, and growth hormone secretion. *Proc. Natl. Acad. Sci. USA,* 80:895–898.
571. Besson, J., Rotsztejn, W., Laburthe, M., Epelbaum, J., Beaudet, A., Kordon, C., and Rosselin, G. (1979): Vasoactive intestinal peptide (VIP): Brain distribution subcellular localization and effect of deafferentation of the hypothalamus in male rats. *Brain Res.,* 165:79–85.
572. Berkenbosch, F., Linton, E. A., and Tilders, F. J. (1986): Colocalization of peptide histidine isoleucine amine and corticotropin releasing factor immunoreactivity in neurons of the rat hypothalamus: A surprising artefact. *Neuroendocrinology,* 44:338–346.
573. Tager, H., Hobenboken, M., Markese, J., and Dinerstein, R. J. (1980): Identification and localization of glucagon related polypeptides in rat brain. *Proc. Natl. Acad. Sci. USA,* 77:6229.
574. Morel, G., Besson, J., Rosselin, G., and Dubois, P. M. (1982): Ultrastructural evidence for endogenous vasoactive intestinal peptide-like immunoreactivity in the pituitary gland. *Neuroendocrinology,* 34:85–89.
575. Said, S. I., and Porter, J. C. (1979): Vasoactive intestinal peptide: Release into hypophyseal blood. *Life Sci.,* 24:227–230.
576. Rosselin, G. (1986): The receptors of the VIP family (VIP, secretin, GRF, PHI, PHM, GIP, glucagon and oxyntomodulin), specificities and identity. *Peptides* 7(Suppl. 1):89–100.
577. Kato, Y., Iwasaki, I., Iwasaki, J., Abe, H., and Yanahara, N. (1978): Prolactin release by vasoactive intestinal polypeptide in rats. *Endocrinology,* 103:554–558.
578. Ruberg, M., Rotsztejn, W. H., Arancibia, S., Besson, J., and Enjalbert, A. (1978): Stimulation of prolactin release by vasoactive intestinal peptide (VIP). *Eur. J. Pharmacol.,* 51:319–320.
579. Enjalbert, A., Arancibia, S., Ruberg, M., Priam, M., Bluet-Pajot, M. T., Rotsztejn, W. H., and Kordon, C. (1980): Stimulation of *in vitro* prolactin release by vasoactive intestinal peptide. *Neuroendocrinology,* 31:200–204.
580. Shaar, C. J., Clemens, J. A., and Dininger, N. B. (1979): Effect of vasoactive intestinal peptide on prolactin release *in vitro. Life Sci.,* 25:2071–2074.
581. Samson, W. K., Said, S. I., Snyder, G., and McCann, S. M. (1980): *In vitro* stimulation of prolactin release by vasoactive intestinal peptide. *Peptides,* 1:325.
582. Gourdji, D., Bataille, D., Vauclin, N., Grouselle, D., Rosselin, G., and Tixier-Vidal, A. (1979): Vasoactive intestinal peptide (VIP) stimulates prolactin (PRL) release and cAMP production in a rat pituitary cell line (GH3B6). *FEBS Lett.,* 104:165–168.
583. Denef, C., Schramme, C., and Baes, M. (1985): Stimulation of growth hormone release by vasoactive intestinal peptide and peptide PHI in rat anterior pituitary aggregates. Permissive action of a glucocorticoid and inhibition by thyrotropin releasing hormone. *Neuroendocrinology,* 40:88–91.
584. Bluet-Pajot, M. T., Mounier, F., Léonard, J. F., Kordon, C., and Durand, D. (1987): Vasoactive intestinal peptide induces a transient release of growth hormone in the rat. *Peptides,* 8:35–38.
585. Mitsuma, T., Nogimori, T., and Choya, M. (1984): Effect of vasoactive intestinal polypeptide on hypothalamic pituitary thyroid axis in rats. *Endocrinol. Exp.,* 18:93–100.
586. Takahara, J., Yunoki, S., Yamancki, J., Yakshihi, W., Hosogi, H., and Ofuji, T. (1978): Effect of glucagon on growth hormone secretion in rats. *Horm. Metab. Res.,* 10:227.
587. Abe, H., Engler, D., Molitch, M. E., Bollinger, J., and Reichlin, S. (1985): Vasoactive intestinal peptide is a physiological mediator of prolactin release in the rat. *Endocrinology,* 116:1383–1390.
588. Kaji, H., Chihara, K., Kita, T., Kashio, Y., Okimura, Y., and Fujita, T. (1985): Administration of antisera to vasoactive intestinal polypeptide and peptide histidine isoleucine attenuates ether induced prolactin secretion in rats. *Neuroendocrinol.,* 41:529–531.
589. Kaji, H., Chihara, K., Abe, H., Kita, T., Kashio, Y., Okimura, Y., and Fjuita, T. (1985): Effect of passive immunization with antisera to vasoactive intestinal peptide and peptide histidine isoleucine amide on 5-hydroxy-l-trytophan induced prolactin release in rats. *Endocrinology,* 117:1914–1919.
590. Mezey, E., and Kiss, J. Z. (1984): Vasoactive intestinal peptide containing neurons in the paraventricular nucleus may participate in regulation of prolactin secretion. *Proc. Natl. Acad. Sci. USA,* 82:245–247.
591. Gozes, I., and Shani, Y. (1986): Hypothalamic vasoactive intestinal peptide messenger ribonucleic acid is increased in lactating rats. *Endocrinology,* 119:2497–2501.
592. Maletti, M., Rostène, W. H., Carr, L., Scherrer, H., Rotten, D., Kordon, C., and Rosselin, G. (1982): Interaction between estradiol and prolactin on vasoactive intestinal peptide (VIP) concentrations in the hypothalamus and in the anterior pituitary of the female rat. *Neurosci. Lett.,* 32:307–314.
593. Hogen, T. C., Arnaout, M. A., Scherzer, W. J., Martinson, D. R., and Garthwaite, A. C. (1986): Antisera to vasoactive intestinal polypeptide inhibit basal prolactin release from dispersed anterior pituitary cells. *Neuroendocrinology,* 43:641–645.
594. Vijayan, E., Samson, W. K., Said, S. J., and McCann, S. M. (1979): Vasoactive intestinal peptide. Evidence for a hypothalamic site of action to release growth hormone, luteinizing hormone and prolactin in conscious ovariectomized rats. *Endocrinology,* 104:53–57.
595. Ottlecz, A. W., Samson, K., and McCann, S. M. (1985): The effects of gastric inhibitory polypeptide (GIP) on the release of anterior pituitary hormones. *Peptides,* 6:115–119.
596. Epelbaum, J., Tapia-Arancibia, L., Besson, J., Rotsztejn, W. H., and Kordon, C. (1979): Vasoactive intestinal peptide inhibits release of somatostatin from hypothalamus *in vitro. Eur. J. Pharmacol.,* 58:493–495.
597. Abe, H., Kato, Y., Taminato, H., Chiba, T., and Imura, H. (1978): Plasma immunoreactive somatostatin levels in rat hypophyseal portal blood: Effect of glucagon administration. *Life Sci.,* 23:1647.
598. Tapia-Arancibia, L., and Reichlin, S. (1985): Vasoactive intestinal peptide and PHI stimulate somatostatin release from rat cerebral cortical and diencephalic cells in dispersed cell culture. *Brain Res.,* 336:67–72.
599. Héry, M., Faudon, M., and Héry, F. (1984): Effect of vasoactive intestinal peptide on serotonin release in the suprachiasmatic area of the rat: Modulation by estradiol. *Peptides,* 5:313–317.
600. Oliva, D., Nicosia, S., Spada, A., and Giannattasio, G. (1982): VIP stimulates ACTH release and adenylate cyclase in human ACTH secreting pituitary adenomas. *Eur. J. Pharmacol.,* 83:101–105.
601. White, M. C., Adams, E. F., Loizon, M., and Mashiter, K. (1982): Vasoactive intestinal peptide stimulates adrenocorticotropin release from human corticotropin cells in culture: Interaction with arginine vasopressin and hydrocortisone. *J. Clin. Endocrinol. Metab.,* 55:967–972.
602. Westendorf, T. M., and Schonbrunn, A. (1985): Peptide specificity for stimulation of corticotropin secretion: Activation of overlapping pathways by the vasoactive intestinal peptide family and corticotropin releasing factor. *Endocrinology,* 116:2528–2535.
603. Tilders, F. J., Tatemoto, K., and Berkenbosch, F. (1984): The intestinal peptide PHI 27 potentiates the action of corticotropin releasing factor on ACTH release from pituitary fragments *in vitro. Endocrinology,* 115:1633–1635.
604. Vigh, S., and Schally, A. V. (1984): Interaction between hypothalamic peptides in a superfused pituitary cell system. *Peptides,* 5(Suppl. 1):241–247.
605. Spiess, J., Rivier, J., and Vale, W. (1982): Characterization of rat hypothalamic growth hormone releasing factor. *Nature,* 303:532.
606. Bloch, B., Ling, N., Benoit, R., Wehrenberg, W. B., and Guillemin, R. (1984): Specific depletion of immunoreactive growth hormone

releasing factor by monosodium glutamate in rat median eminence. *Nature,* 307:272–273.

607. Sawchenko, P. E., Swanson, L. W., Rivier, J., and Vale, W. (1985): The distribution of growth hormone releasing factor (GRF) immunoreactivity in the central nervous system of the rat: An immunohistochemical study using antisera directed against rat hypothalamic GRF. *J. Comp. Neurol.,* 237:100–115.
608. Kita, T., Chihara, K., Abe, H., Minamitani, N., Kaji, H., Kashio, Y., Okimura, Y., Fujita, T., and Ling, N. (1985): Regional distribution of rat growth hormone releasing factor-like immunoreactivity in rat hypothalamus. *Endocrinology,* 116:259–262.
609. Vandepol, C. J., Leidy, J. W., Finger, T. E., Robbins, R. J. (1986): Immunohistochemical localization of GRF containing neurons in rat brain. *Neuroendocrinology,* 42:143–147.
610. Ciofi, P., Croix, D., and Tramu, G. (1987): Coexistence of hGHRH and NPY immunoreactivities in neurons of the arcuate nucleus of the rat. *Neuroendocrinology,* 45:425–428.
611. Seifert, H., Perrin, M., Rivier, J., and Vale, W. (1985): Binding sites for growth hormone releasing factor on rat anterior pituitary cells. *Nature,* 317:487–489.
612. Law, G. H., Ray, K. P., and Wallis, M. (1984): Effects of growth hormone releasing factor, somatostatin and dopamine on growth hormone and prolactin secretion from cultured ovine pituitary cells. *FEBS Lett.,* 166:189.
613. Laburthe, M., Amiranoff, B., Boige, N., Rouyer-Fessard, C., Tatemoto, K., and Moroder, L. (1983): Interaction of GRF with VIP receptors and stimulation of adenylate cyclase in rat and human intestinal epithelial membranes. Comparison with PHI and secretin. *FEBS Lett.,* 159:89.
614. Gubler, U., Seeburg, P., Hoffman, B. J., Gage, L. P. and Udenfriend, S. (1982): Molecular cloning establishes proenkephalins as precursors of enkephalin containing peptides. *Nature,* 295:206–208.
615. Fallon, J. H., and Leslie, F. M. (1986): Distribution of dynorphin and enkephalin peptides in the rat brain. *J. Comp. Neurol.,* 249:293–336.
616. Udenfriend, S., and Meienhofer, J. (1984): Opioid peptides: Biology, chemistry and genetics. In: *The Peptides, Vol. 6,* Academic Press, New York.
617. Code, R. A., and Fallon, J. H. (1986): Some projections of dynorphin immunoreactive neurons in the rat central nervous system. *Neuropeptides,* 8:165–172.
618. Palkovits, M., Brownstein, M. J., and Zamir, N. (1983): Immunoreactive dynorphin and neo-endorphin in rat hypothalamo-neurohypophyseal system. *Brain Res.,* 278:258–261.
619. Watson, S. J., Akil, H., Frichli, W., Goldstein, A., Zimmerman, E. A., and Nilever, F. (1982): Dynorphin and vasopressin: Common localization in magnocellular neurons. *Nature,* 216:85–87.
620. Khatchaturian, H., Sherman, T. G., Lloyd, R. V., Civelli, O., Douglas, J., Herbert, E., Akil, H., and Watson, J. J. (1986): Prodynorphin is endogenous in the anterior pituitary and is colocalised with LH and FSH in the gonadotrophs. *Endocrinology,* 119:409.
621. Martin, R., and Voigt, K. H. (1981): Enkephalin coexists with oxytocin and vasopressin in nerve terminals of the rat neurohypophysis. *Nature,* 289:502–504.
622. Slater, P., and Cross, A. J. (1986): Autoradiographic distribution of dynorphin 1-9 binding sites in primate brain. *Neuropeptides,* 8:71–76.
623. Mains, R. E., Eipper, B., and Ling, N. (1977): Common precursor to corticotropin and endorphins. *Proc. Natl. Acad. Sci. USA,* 74:3014.
624. Bloch, B., Bugnon, C., Lenys, D., and Fellmann, D. (1978): Description des neurones immunoréactifs à un antisérum anti-β endorphine présents dans le noyau infundibulaire chez l'Homme. *C. R. Acad. Sci. (Paris),* 287D:309–312.
625. Finlay, J. C. W., Lindshon, P., and Petrusz, P. (1981): Immunocytochemical localization of β endorphin containing neurons in the rat brain. *Neuroendocrinology,* 33:28–42.
626. Emrson, P. C., Corder, R., Ratter, S. J., Tomlin, S., Lowry, P. J., Rees, L., Arregui, A., and Rosser, M. N. (1984): Regional distribution of proopiomelanocortin derived peptides in the human brain. *Neuroendocrinology,* 38:45–50.
627. Sofroniew, M. V. (1979): Immunoreactive β endorphin and ACTH in the same neurons of the hypothalamic arcuate nucleus in the rat. *Annu. J. Anat.,* 154:283–289.
628. Krieger, D. T., Liotta, A. S., and Brownstein, M. J. (1977): Presence of corticotropin in brain of normal and hypophysectomized rats. *Proc. Natl. Acad. Sci. USA,* 74:648–652.
629. Dubé, D., Lissitzky, J. C., Leclere, R., and Pelletier, G. (1978): Localization of melanocyte stimulating hormone in rat brain and pituitary. *Endocrinology,* 102:1283–1291.
630. Bloch, B., Bugnon, C., Fellmann, D., and Lenys, D. (1978): Immunocytochemical evidence that the same neurons in the human infundibular nucleus are stained with anti-endorphins and antisera of other related peptides. *Neurosci. Lett.,* 10:147–152.
631. Bugnon, C., Bloch, B., Lenys, D., Goubet, A., and Fellmann, D. (1979): Comparative study of the neuronal populations containing β endorphin, corticotropin and dopamine in the arcuate nucleus of the rat hypothalamus. *Neurosci. Lett.,* 14:43–48.
632. Wardlaw, S. L., Wehrenberg, W. B., Férin, M., Antunes, J. L., and Frank, A. G. (1982): Effect of sex steroids on β endorphin in hypophyseal portal blood. *J. Clin. Endocrinol. Metab.,* 55:877–881.
633. Meites, J., Bruni, J. F., Van Vugt, D. A., and Smith, A. C. (1979): Relation of endogenous peptides and morphine to neuroendocrine functions. *Life. Sci.,* 24:1325–1336.
634. Morley, J. (1981): The endocrinology of opiates and opioid peptides. *Metabolism,* 30:195–209.
635. Bruni, J. F., Van Vugt, D., Marshall, S., and Meites, J. (1977): Effects of naloxone, morphine and methionine enkephalin of serum prolactin, luteinizing hormone, follicle stimulating hormone, thyroid stimulating hormone and growth hormone. *Life Sci.,* 21:461–466.
636. Rivier, C., Vale, W., Ling, N., Brown, M., and Guillemin, R. (1977): Stimulation *in vivo* of the secretion of prolactin and growth hormone by β endorphin. *Endocrinology,* 100:238–241.
637. Shaar, C. J., Frederickon, R. C., Dininger, N. B., and Jackson, L. (1977): Enkephalin analogues and naloxone modulate the release of growth hormone and prolactin: Evidence for regulation by an endogenous opioid brain peptide. *Life Sci.,* 21:853–860.
638. Grossmann, A., and Rees, L. H. (1983): The neuroendocrinology of opioid peptides. *Br. Med. Bull.,* 39:83–88.
639. Dupont, A., Cusan, L., Labrie, F., Loy, D. H., and Li, C. H. (1977): Stimulation of prolactin release in the rat by intraventricular injection of β endorphin and methionin enkephalin. *Biochem. Biophys. Res. Commun.,* 75:76–82.
640. Grandison, L., and Guidotti, A. (1977): Regulation of prolactin release by endogenous opiates. *Nature,* 270:357–359.
641. Barraclough, C. A., and Sawyer, C. H. (1955): Inhibition of the release of pituitary ovulatory hormone in the rat by morphine. *Endocrinology,* 57:329–336.
642. Millan, M. J., and Herz, A. (1985): The endocrinology of the opioids. In: *International Review of Neurobiology, Vol. 26,* pp. 1–83. Academic Press, New York.
643. Gilbeau, P. H., Almirez, R. G., Holaday, J. W., and Smith, C. G. (1985): Opioid effects on plasma concentrations of luteinizing hormone and prolactin in the adult rhesus monkey. *J. Clin. Endocrinol. Metab.,* 60:299–305.
644. Pang, C. N., Zimmermann, E., and Sawyer, C. H. (1977): Morphine inhibition of the preovulatory surges of plasma luteinizing hormone and follicle stimulating hormone in the rat. *Endocrinology,* 101:1726.
645. Van Vugt, D. A., Sylvester, P. W., Aylsworth, C. F., and Meites, J. (1982): Counteraction of gonadal steroid inhibition of LH by naloxone. *Neuroendocrinology,* 34:274.
646. Cicero, T. J., Schainker, B. A., and Meyer, E. R. (1979): Endogenous opioids participate in the regulation of the hypothalamic pituitary luteinizing hormone axis and testosterone negative feedback control of luteinizing hormone. *Endocrinology,* 104:1286–1291.
647. Morley, J. E., Baranetsky, N. G., Wingert, T. D., Carlson, H. E., Hershman, J. M., Melmed, S., Levin, S. R., Jamison, K. R., Weitzman, R., Chang, R. J., and Varner, A. A. (1980): Endocrine effects of naloxone induced opiate receptor blockade. *J. Clin. Endocrinol. Metab.,* 50:251.
648. Delitala, G., Devilla, L., and Arata, L. (1981): Opiate receptors and anterior pituitary hormone secretion in man. *Acta Endocrinol. (Copenh.),* 97:150–156.
649. Schultz, R., Wilhelm, A., Pirke, K. M., Gramsch, C., and Herz, A. (1981): Endorphin and dynorphin control serum luteinizing hormone level in immature female rats. *Nature,* 294:757–759.
650. Kinashita, F., Nakai, I., Katakami, H., Kato, G., Yajima, H., and Imura, H. (1980): Effect of β endorphin on pulsatile luteinizing hormone release in conscious castrated rats. *Life Sci.,* 27:843.

651. Kesner, J. S., Kaufman, J. M., Wilson, R. C., Kuroda, G., and Knobil, E. (1986): The effect of morphine on the electrophysiological activity of the hypothalamic luteinizing hormone releasing hormone pulse generator in the rhesus monkey. *Neuroendocrinology,* 43:686–688.
652. Moult, P. J., Grossman, A., Evans, J. M., Rees, L. H., and Besser, G. M. (1981): The effect of naloxone on pulsatile gonadotrophin release in normal subjects. *Clin. Endocrinol.,* 14:321–324.
653. Ellingboe, J., Veldhuis, J. D., Mendelson, J. H., Kuehule, J. C., and Mello, N. K. (1982): Effect of endogenous opioid blockade on the amplitude and frequency of pulsatile luteinizing hormone secretion in normal men. *J. Clin. Endocrinol. Metab.,* 54:854.
654. Baranowska, B., Rozbicka, G., Jeske, W., and Abdel-Fattah, M. H. (1984): The role of endogenous opiates in the mechanism of inhibited luteinizing hormone (LH) secretion in women with anorexia nervosa: The effect of naloxone on LH, follicle stimulating hormone, prolactin and β endorphin secretion. *J. Clin. Endocrinol. Metab.,* 59:412.
655. Férin, M., Van Vugt, D., and Wasdlaw, S. (1984): The hypothalamic control of the menstrual cycle and the role of endogenous opioid peptides. *Recent Prog. Horm. Res.,* 40:411–485.
656. Rupert, J. F., Quigley, M. E., and Yen, S. S. C. (1981): Endogenous opiates modulate pulsatile luteinizing hormone release in humans. *J. Clin. Endocrinol. Metab.,* 52:583–587.
657. Quigley, M. E., and Yen, S. S. C. (1980): The role on endogenous opiates on LH secretion during the menstrual cycle. *J. Clin. Endocrinol. Metab.,* 51:179.
658. Veldhuis, J. D., Rogol, A. D., Samojik, E., and Ertel, N. H. (1984): Role of endogenous opiates in the expression of negative feedback actions of androgen and estrogen on pulsatile properties of luteinizing hormone secretion in man. *J. Clin. Invest.,* 74:47–55.
659. Petraglia, F., Bernasconi, S., Lughetti, L., and Loche, S. (1986): Naloxone induced luteinizing hormone secretion in normal, precocious, and delayed puberty. *J. Clin. Endocrinol. Metab.,* 63:1112–1116.
660. Quigley, M. E., Shechan, K. L., Casper, R. F., and Yen, S. S. C. (1980): Evidence for increased dopaminergic and opioid activity in patients with hypothalamic hypogonadotropic amenorrhea. *J. Clin. Endocrinol. Metab.,* 50:949.
661. Lightman, S. L., Jacobs, H. S., Maguire, A. K., McGarrick, G., and Jeffcoate, S. L. (1981): Constancy of opioid control of luteinizing hormone in different pathophysiological states. *J. Clin. Endocrinol. Metab.,* 52:1260.
662. Cicero, T. J., Owens, D. P., Schmoeker, P. F., and Meyer, E. R. (1983): Morphine induced enhancement of the effects of naloxone on serum luteinizing hormone levels in the male rat: Specificity for mu antagonists. *J. Pharmacol. Exp. Ther.,* 226:770–774.
663. Pfeiffer, D. G., Pfeiffer, A., Shimahigashi, K., Merriam, G. R., and Loriaux, D. L. (1983): Predominant involvement of mu rather than delta or kappa opiate receptors in LH secretion. *Peptides,* 4:647–649.
664. Panerai, A., Petraglia, F., Sacerdote, P., and Genazzani, A. R. (1985): Mainly mu opiate receptors are involved in luteinizing hormone and prolactin secretion. *Endocrinology,* 117:1096–1099.
665. Leadem, C. A., and Kalra, S. P. (1985): Effects of endogenous opioid peptides and opiates on luteinizing hormone and prolactin secretion in ovariectomized rats. *Neuroendocrinology,* 41: 342–352.
666. Pfeiffer, D. G., Pfeiffer, A., Shimohigashi, Y., Merriam, G. R., and Loriaux, D. L. (1983): Predominant involvement of mu rather than delta or kappa opiate receptors in LH secretion. *Peptides,* 4:647.
667. Goodman, R. R., Snyder, S. H., Kuhar, M. J., and Young, W. S. (1980): Differentiation of delta and mu opiate receptor localization by light microscopic autoradiography. *Proc. Nat. Acad. Sci. USA,* 77:6239.
668. Schulz, Wilhelm, A., Pirke, K. M., and Herz, A. (1982): Regulation of luteinizing hormone secretion in prepubertal male and female rats. *Life Sci.,* 31:2167–2170.
669. Markó, M., and Römer, M. (1983): Inhibitory effect of a new opioid agonist on reproductive endocrine activity in rats of both sexes. *Life Sci.,* 33:233–240.
670. Bhanot, R., and Wilkinson, M. (1983): Opiatergic control of LH secretion is eliminated by gonadectomy. *Endocrinology,* 112:399–401.
671. Piva, F., Limonta, P., Maggi, R., and Martini, L. (1986): Stimulatory and inhibitory effect of the opioids on gonadotropic secretion. *Neuroendocrinology,* 42:504–512.
672. Kalra, P. S., and Kalra, S. P. (1982): Discriminating effects of testosterone on hypothalamic luteinizing hormone releasing hormone levels and luteinizing hormone secretion in castrated male rats: Analyses of dose and duration characteristics. *Endocrinology,* 111:24–29.
673. Gabriel, S. M., Simkins, J. W., Kalra, S. P. (1983): Modulation of endogenous opioid influence on luteinizing hormone secretion by progesterone and estrogen. *Endocrinology,* 113:1806–1811.
674. Gabriel, S. M., Simpkins, J. W., Kalra, S. P., and Kalra, P. S. (1985): Chronic morphine treatment induces hypersensitivity to testosterone negative feedback in castrated male rats. *Neuroendocrinology,* 40:39–44.
675. Gabriel, S. M., Berglund, I. A., Kalra, S. P., Kalra, P. S., and Simpkins, J. W. (1986): The influence of chronic morphine treatment on the negative feedback regulation of gonadotropin secretion by gonadal steroids. *Endocrinology,* 119:2762–2767.
676. Wardlaw, S. L., Thoron, L., and Frank, A. G. (1982): Effects of sex steroids on brain β endorphin. *Brain Res.,* 245:327–331.
677. Sarkar, D. H., and Yen, S. S. (1985): Changes in β endorphin-like immunoreactivity in pituitary portal blood during the estrous cycle and after ovariectomy in rats. *Endocrinology,* 116:2075–2079.
678. Barden, N., Mérand, Y., Rouleau, D., Garon, M., and Dupont, A. (1981): Changes in the β endorphin content of discrete hypothalamic nuclei during the estrous cycle of the rat. *Brain Res.,* 204:441.
679. Wardlaw, S. L., and Frank, A. G. (1983): Brain β endorphin during pregnancy, parturition and the post partum period. *Endocrinology,* 113:1664–1668.
680. Morrell, J. L., McGinty, J. F., Pfaff, D. W. (1985): A subset of β endorphin or dynorphin containing neurons in the medial basal hypothalamus accumulates estradiol. *Neuroendocrinology,* 41:417–426.
681. Jirikowski, G. F., Merchenthaler, I., Rieger, G. E., and Stumpf, W. E. (1986): Estradiol target sites immunoreactive for β endorphin in the arcuate nuclei of rat and mouse hypothalamus. *Neurosci. Lett.,* 65:121–126.
682. Jacobson, W., and Wilkinson, M. (1986): Association of diurnal variations in hypothalamic but not cortical opiate (3H naloxone) binding sites with the activity of naloxone to induce LH release in the prepubertal female rat. *Neuroendocrinology,* 44:132.
683. Hahn, F. F., and Fishman, J. (1979): Changes in rat brain opiate receptor content upon castration and testosterone replacement. *Biochem. Biophys. Res. Commun.,* 90:819–823.
684. Wilkinson, M., Herdon, H., and Wilson, C. A. (1981): Gonadal steroid modification of adrenergic and opiate receptor binding in the central nervous system. In: *Steroid Hormone Regulation of the Brain,* edited by K. Fuxe, J. A. Gustaffsson, and L. Wetterby, pp. 253–263. Pergamon Press, New York.
685. Hahn, E. E., and Fishman, J. (1985): Castration affects male rat brain opiate receptor content. *Neuroendocrinology,* 41:60–63.
686. Cicero, T. J., Newman, K. S., and Meyer, E. R. (1982): Testosterone does not influence opiate binding sites in the male rat brain. *Biochem. Biophys. Res. Commun.,* 108:1313–1319.
687. Kalra, S. P., and Kalra, P. S. (1984): Opioid adrenergic steroid connection in regulation of luteinizing hormone secretion in the rat. *Neuroendocrinology,* 38:418–426.
688. Valenca, M. M., and Negro-Vilar, A. (1986): Lack of a functional coupling between endogenous opiate system and LHRH neurons during the infantile period in the male rat. *Neuroendocrinol. Lett.,* 8:165–172.
689. Sylvester, P. W., Sarkar, D. K., Briski, K. P., and Meites, J. (1985): Relation of gonadal hormones to differential LH responses to naloxone in prepubertal male and female rats. *Neuroendocrinology,* 40:165–170.
690. Blank, M. S., Panerai, A. E., and Friesen, H. G. (1979): Opioid peptide modulate luteinizing hormone secretion during sexual maturation. *Science,* 203:1129–1131.
691. Petersen, S. L., and Barraclough, C. A. (1986): Effects of morphine and naloxone on LH and prolactin release in androgen sterilized rats. *Neuroendocrinology,* 44:84–88.
692. Watson, R. E., Hoffmann, G. E., and Wiegand, S. J. (1986): Sexually dimorphic opioid distribution in the preoptic area: manipulation by gonadal steroids. *Brain Res.,* 398:157–163.
693. Lira, S. A., Phipps, D. W., and Sarkar, D. K. (1986): Loss of

estradiol positive feedback action on LH release during prepubertal period in rats treated postnatally with an opiate antagonist. *Neuroendocrinology,* 44:331–337.
694. Sirinathsinghji, D. J., Motta, M., and Martini, L. (1985): Induction of precocious puberty in the female rat after chronic naloxone administration during the neonatal period: The opiate "brake" on prepubertal gonadotropin secretion. *J. Endocrinol.,* 104:299–307.
695. Chen, H. J., Targovnik, J., McMillan, L., and Randall, S. (1984): Age difference in endogenous opiate modulation of short photoperiod induced testicular regression in golden hamsters. *J. Endocrinol.,* 101:1–6.
696. Ebling, F. J., and Lincoln, G. A. (1985): Endogenous opioids and the control of seasonal LH secretion in Soay rams. *J. Endocr.,* 107:341–353.
697. Sarkar, D. K., and Yen, S. S. C. (1985): Hyperprolactinemia decreases the luteinizing hormone releasing hormone concentration in pituitary portal plasma: A possible role for β endorphin as a mediator. *Endocrinology,* 116:2080–2084.
698. Carter, D. A., Cooper, J. S., Inkster, S. E., and Whitehead, S. A. (1984): Evidence for an increased opioid inhibition of LH secretion in hyperprolactinemic ovariectomized rats. *J. Endocrinol.,* 101:57.
699. Quigley, M. E., Sheehan, K. L., Casper, R. F., and Yen, S. S. C. (1980): Evidence for an increased opioid inhibition of luteinizing hormone secretion in hyperprolactinemic patients with pituitary microadenomas. *J. Clin. Endocrinol. Metab.,* 50:427.
700. Seki, K., Kato, K., and Shima, K. (1986): Parallelism in the luteinizing hormone responses to opioid and dopamine antagonists in hyperprolactinemic women with pituitary adenomas. *J. Clin. Endocrinol. Metab.,* 63:1225–1228.
701. Sweeney, C. A., Morgan, W. W., Smith, M. S., and Bartke, A. (1985): Altered sensitivity to an opiate antagonist, naloxone, in hyperprolactinemic male rats. *Neuroendocrinology,* 41:1–6.
702. Panerai, A. E., Sawynok, J., La Bella, F. S., and Friesen, H. G. (1980): Prolonged hyperprolactinemia influences β endorphin and metenkephaline in the brain. *Endocrinology,* 106:1804.
703. Simpkins, J. W., Taylor, S. T., Gabriel, S. M., Katovich, M. J., and Millard, W. J. (1984): Evidence that chronic hyperprolactinemia affects skin temperature regulation through an opioid mechanism. *Neuroendocrinology,* 39:321.
704. Enker, J. J., Meites, J., and Riegle, C. D. (1973): Effects of acute stress on serum LH and prolactin in intact, castrated and dexamethasone treated male rats. *Endocrinology,* 96:85.
705. Brisky, K. P., Quigley, K., and Meites, J. (1984): Endogenous opiate involvement in acute and chronic stress induced changes in plasma LH concentrations in the male rat. *Life Sci.,* 34:2485.
706. Gilbeau, P. M., and Smith, C. G. (1985): Naloxone reversal of stress induced reproductive effects in the male rhesus monkey. *Neuropeptides,* 5:335.
707. Petraglia, F., Vale, W., and Rivier, C. (1986): Opioids act centrally to modulate stress induced decrease in luteinizing hormone in the rat. *Endocrinology,* 119:2445–2450.
708. Rossier, J., French, E. D., Rivier, C., Ling, N., Guillemin, R., and Bloom, F. E. (1977): Foot shock induced stress increases β endorphin levels in brain. *Nature,* 270:618.
709. Selmanoff, M., Gregerson, K. A., (1986): Suckling induced prolactin release is suppressed by naloxone and stimulated by β endorphin. *Neuroendocrinology,* 42:255–259.
710. Ferland, L., Kledzik, G. S., Cusan, L., and Labrie, F. (1978): Evidence for a role of endorphins in stress-induced and suckling-induced prolactin release in the rat. *Mol. Cell. Endocrinol.,* 12:267.
711. Knight, P. G., Howles, C. M., and Cunningham, E. J. (1986): Evidence that opioid peptides and dopamine participate in the suckling induced release of prolactin in the ewe. *Neuroendocrinology,* 44:29–35.
712. White, J. D., and McKelvy, J. F. (1986): Enkephalin biosynthesis and processing during lactation. *Neuroendocrinology,* 43:377–382.
713. Sirinathsinghji, D. J., and Audsley, A. R. (1985): Endogenous opioid peptides participate in the modulation of prolactin release in response to cervicovaginal stimulation in the female rat. *Endocrinology,* 117:549–556.
714. Melis, G. B., Gambacciani, M., Paoletti, A. M., Mais, V., Cagnacci, A., Petacchi, F. D., and Fioretti, P. (1985): Sex steroids modulate prolactin response to naloxone in postmenopausal women. *Neuroendocrinology,* 41:138–141.
715. Rossi, A., Disalle, E., Briatico, G., Arcari, G., De Castigliane, R., and Perseo, G., (1983): Antinociceptive, prolactin releasing and intestinal motility inhibiting activities of dermorphin and analogues after subentaneous administration in the rat. *Peptides,* 4:577–580.
716. Koenig, J. J., Mayfield, M. A., McCann, S. M., and Kruhlich, L. (1984): Differential role of the opioid μ and κ receptors in the activation of prolactin and growth hormone secretion of morphine in the male rat. *Life Sci.,* 34:1829–1837.
717. Spiegel, K., Konrid, G. W., and Pasternak, G. W. (1982): Prolactin and growth hormone release by morphine in the rat: Different receptor mechanism. *Science,* 217:745–747.
718. Rossi, A., Disalle, E., Briatico, G., Arcari, G., De Castigliane, R., and Perseo, G. (1983): Antinociceptive, prolactin releasing and intestinal motility inhibiting activities of dermorphin and analogues after subentaneous administration in the rat. *Peptides,* 4:577–580.
719. Erspamer, V., Melchiorri, P., Broccardo, M., Erspamer, G. F., Falaschi, P., Improta, G. Negri, L., and Renda, T. (1981): The brain-gut-skin triangle: New peptides. *Peptides (Suppl.),* 2:7–16.
720. Uberti, E. C., Trasforini, G., Salvadori, S., Margutti, A., Tomatis, R., and Pansini, R. (1985): The effects of dermorphin in the endocrine system in man. *Peptides (Suppl.),* 3:171–175.
721. Matsushita, N., Kato, Y., Shimatsu, A., Katakami, H., Fujino, M., Matsuo, H., and Imura, H. (1982): Stimulation of prolactin secretion in the rat by α-neo-endorphin β neo-endorphin and dynorphin. *Biochem. Biophys. Res. Commun.,* 107:735–741.
722. Gilbeau, P. M., Hosobuchi, Y., Lee, N. M. (1986): Dynorphin effects on plasma concentration of anterior pituitary hormones in the nonhuman primate. *J. Pharmacol. Exp. Ther.,* 238:974–978.
723. Gilbeau, P., Hosobuchi, Y., and Lee, N. M. (1987): Consequence of dynorphin A administration on anterior pituitary hormone concentrations in the adult male rhesus monkey. *Neuroendocrinology,* 45:284–289.
724. Pfeiffer, A., Braun, S., Mann, K., Meyer, H. D., and Brantl, V. (1986): Anterior pituitary hormone responses to a κ opioid agonist in man. *J. Clin. Endocrinol. Metab.,* 62:181–185.
725. Kruhlich, L., Koenig, J. E., Conway, S., McCann, S. M., and Mayfield, M. A. (1986): Opioid K receptors and the secretion of prolactin (PRL) and growth hormone (GH) in the rat. Effects of opioid κ receptor agonists bremazocine and U50488 on secretion of PRL and GH; comparison with morphine. *Neuroendocrinology,* 42:75–81.
726. Kruhlich, L., Koenig, J. E., Conway, S., McCann, S. M., and Mayfield, M. A. (1986): GH and PRL release inhibiting effects of the opioid κ receptor agonists bremazocine and U50488. *Neuroendocrinology,* 42:82–87.
727. Hartman, R. D., Rosella-Dampman, L. M., Emmert, S. E., Summy-Long, J. Y. (1986): Inhibition of release of neurohypophyseal hormones by endogenous opioid peptides in pregnant and parturient rats. *Brain Res.,* 382:352–359.
728. Clarke, G., Wood, P., Merrick, L., and Lincoln, D. W. (1979): Opiate inhibition of peptide release from the neurohumoral terminals of hypothalamic neurons. *Nature,* 282:746–748.
729. Samson, W. K., McDonald, J. K., and Lumpkin, M. D. (1985): Naloxone induced dissociation of oxytocin and prolactin releases. *Neuroendocrinology,* 40:68–71.
730. Jones, S. A., and Summerlee, A. J. S. (1986): Relaxin acts centrally to inhibit oxytocin release during parturition: An effect that is reversed by naloxone. *J. Endocrinology,* 111:99–102.
731. Blank, M. S., Fabbri, A., Catt, K. J., and Dufau, M. I. (1986): Inhibition of luteinizing hormone release by morphine and endogenous opiates in cultured pituitary cells. *Endocrinology,* 118:2097.
732. Sanchez-Franco, F., and Cacicedo, L. (1986): Inhibitory effect of β endorphin on gonadotropin releasing hormone and thyrotropin releasing hormone activity in cultured rat anterior pituitary cells. *Hormone Res.,* 24:55–61.
733. Cicero, T. J., Badger, T. M., Wilcox, C. E., Bell, R. D., and Meyer, E. R. (1977): Morphine decreases luteinizing hormone by an action on the hypothalamic pituitary axis. *J. Pharmacol. Exp. Ther.,* 203:548–554.
734. Ching, M. (1983): Morphine suppresses the proestrous surge of GnRH in pituitary portal plasma of rats. *Endocrinology,* 112:2209–2211.
735. Drouva, S. V., Epelbaum, J., Tapia-Arancibia, L., Laplante, E., and Kordon, C. (1980): Met enkephalin inhibition of K^+ induced LHRH and SRIF release from rat mediobasal hypothalamic slices. *Eur. J. Pharmacol.,* 61:411–412.
736. Drouva, S. V., Epelbaum, J., Tapia-Arancibia, L., Laplante, E.,

and Kordon, C. (1981): Opiate receptors modulate LHRH and SRIF release from mediobasal hypothalamic neurons. *Neuroendocrinology,* 32:163–167.
737. Nikolarakis, K. E., Pfeiffer, D. G., Almeida, O. F., and Herz, A. (1986): Opioid modulation of LHRH release *in vitro* depends upon levels of testosterone *in vivo*. *Neuroendocrinology,* 44:314–319.
738. Rotsztejn, W. H., Drouva, S. V., Pollard, H., Sokoloff, P., Pattou, E., and Kordon, C. (1982): Further evidence for the existence of opiate binding sites on neurosecretory LHRH mediobasal hypothalamic nerve terminals. *Eur. J. Pharmacol.,* 80:139–141.
739. Leadem, C. A., Crowley, W. R., Simpkins, J. W., and Kalra, S. P. (1985): Effects of naloxone on catecholamine and LHRH release from the perifused hypothalamus of the steroid primed rat. *Neuroendocrinology,* 40:497–500.
740. Van Vugt, D. A., Aylswarth, C. F., Sylvester, P. W., Leung, F. C., and Meites, J. (1981): Evidence for hypothalamic noradrenergic involvement in naloxone induced stimulation of luteinizing hormone release. *Neuroendocrinology,* 33:261.
741. Petersen, S. L., and Barraclough, C. A. (1986): Interaction between the hypothalamic opiate and catecholamine systems in the regulation of LH and prolactin secretion. In: *Neuroendocrine Perspectives, Vol. 5,* edited by E. E. Muller and R. M. McLeod, pp. 283–290. Elsevier, Amsterdam.
742. Ferland, L., Fuxe, K., Eneroth, P., Gustafsson, J. A., and Skett, P. (1977): Effects of methionine enkephalin on prolactin release and catecholamine levels and turnover in the median eminence. *Eur. J. Pharmacol.,* 43:89–90.
743. Van Loon, G. R., Ho, D., and Kim, C. (1980): β Endorphin induced decrease in hypothalamic dopamine turnover. *Endocrinology,* 106:76–80.
744. Gudelsky, G. A., and Porter, J. C. (1979): Morphine and opioid peptide induced inhibition of the release of dopamine from tuberoinfundibular neurons. *Life Sci.,* 25:1697–1702.
745. Wood, P. L. (1983): Opioid regulation of CNS dopaminergic pathways: A review of methodology, receptor types, regional variations and species differences. *Peptides,* 4:595–601.
746. Arita, J., and Porter, J. C. (1984): Relationship between dopamine release and prolactin after morphine treatment in rats. *Neuroendocrinology,* 38:62–67.
747. Van Loon, G. R., and De Souza, E. B. (1978): Effects of β endorphin on brain serotonin metabolism. *Life Sci.,* 23:971–978.
748. Leiri, T., Chen, H. T., and Meites, J. (1980): Naloxone stimulation of luteinizing hormone release in prepubertal female rats; role of serotonergic system. *Life Sci.,* 26:1269–1274.
749. Tapia-Arancibia, L., and Astier, H. (1983): Opiate inhibition of K^+ induced TRH release from superfused mediobasal hypothalamus in rats. *Neuroendocrinology,* 37:166–168.
750. Arancibia, S., Tapia-Arancibia, L., Roussel, J. P., Assenmacher, I., and Astier, H. (1986): Effects of morphine on cold induced TRH release from the median eminence of unanesthetized rats. *Life Sci.,* 38:59–66.
751. Bhargawa, H. N., and Das, S. (1986): Evidence for opiate action at the brain receptors for thyrotropin releasing hormone. *Brain Res.,* 368:262–267.
752. Das, S., and Bhargawa, H. N. (1987): Unidirectional interaction between thyrotropin hormone and opiates at the level of their brain receptors. *Gen. Pharmacol.,* 18:99–102.
753. Sheppard, M. C., Kronhein, S., and Pimstone, B. L. (1979): Effect of substance P, neurotensin and the enkephalins on somatostatin release from the rat hypothalamus *in vitro*. *J. Neurochem.,* 32:647–649.
754. Buckingham, J. C., and Cooper, T. A. (1986): Pharmacological characterisation of the opioid receptors influencing the secretion of corticotropin releasing hormone in the rat. *Neuroendocrinology,* 44:36–40.
755. Buckingham, J. C. (1986): Stimulation and inhibition of corticotropin releasing factor secretion by β-endorphin. *Neuroendocrinology,* 42:148–152.
756. Ferland, L., Labrie, F., Arimura, A., and Schally, A. V. (1977): Stimulated release of hypothalamic growth hormone releasing activity by morphine and pentobarbital. *Mol. Cell. Endocrinol.,* 6:247–252.
757. Drouva, S. V., Epelbaum, J., Hery, M., Tapia-Arancibia, L., Laplante, E., and Kordon, C. (1981): Ionic channels involved in the LHRH and SRIF release from rat mediobasal hypothalamus. *Neuroendocrinology,* 32:155–162.
758. Clark, M. J., Levenson, S. D., and Medzihradsky, F. (1986): Evidence for coupling of the opioid receptor to brain GTPase. *Life Sci.,* 39:1721–1728.
759. Grossman, A., Moult, D. A., Cunnal, D., and Besser, M. (1986): Different opioid mechanisms are involved in the modulation of ACTH and gonadotropin release in man. *Neuroendocrinology,* 42:357–360.
760. Enjalbert, A., Ruberg, M., Fiore, L., Arancibia, S., Priam, M., and Kordon, C. (1979): Effect of morphine on the dopamine inhibition of pituitary prolactin release *in vitro*. *Eur. J. Pharmacol.,* 53:211–212.
761. Enjalbert, A., Ruberg, M., Arancibia, S., Priam, M., and Kordon, C. (1979): Endogenous opiates block dopamine inhibition of prolactin secretion *in vitro*. *Nature,* 280:595–597.
762. Lugin, I. S., MacLeod, R. M. (1979): Failure of opiates to reverse inhibition of prolactin secretion *in vitro*. *Eur. J. Pharmacol.,* 60:253–255.
763. Grandison, L., Fratta, W., and Guidotti, A. (1980): Location and characterisation of opiate receptors regulating pituitary secretion. *Life Sci.,* 26:1633.
764. Bentley, A. M., and Wallis, M. (1986): Effects of two enkephalin analogues, morphine sulfate, dopamine and naloxone on prolactin secretion from rat anterior pituitary glands *in vitro*. *J. Endocrinol.,* 109:313–320.
765. Cheung, C. Y. (1984): Does β-endorphin modulate basal and dopamine inhibited prolactin release by an action at the anterior pituitary? *Neuroendocrinology,* 39:489–495.
766. Férin, M., Wehrenberg, W. B., Lam, N. Y. Alston, E. F., and Vandewiele, R. L. (1982): Effects and site of action of morphine on gonadotropin secretion in the female rhesus monkey. *Endocrinology,* 111:1652.
767. Wuttke, W., Duker, E., Control of pituitary prolactin release. E. Endröczi, ed., *Interactive neurohormonal mechanisms,* Elsevier, Amsterdam.
768. Herkenham, M., Rice, K. C., Jacobson, A. E., and Rothman, R. B. (1986): Opiate receptors in rat pituitary are confined to the neural lobe and are exclusively kappa. *Brain Res.,* 382: 365–371.
769. Rotten, D., Leblanc, P., Kordon, C., Weiner, R. I., Enjalbert, A. (1986): Interference of endogenous β-endorphin with opiate binding in the anterior pituitary. *Neuropeptides,* 8:377–392.
770. Gerendai, I., Shala, C., Gumsalus, G. L., and Bardin, C. W. (1986): The effects of opioid receptor antagonists suggest that testicular opiates regulate sertoli and Leydig cell function in the neonatal rat. *Endocrinology,* 118:2039–2044.
771. Tonaer, J. A., Van Vugt, M., and De Graaf, J. S. (1986): *In vitro* interaction of ACTH with rat brain murcarinic receptors. *Peptides,* 7:425–430.
772. Khorram, O., McLann, S. M. (1986): Interaction of alpha melanocyte stimulating hormone with β-endorphin to influence anterior pituitary hormone secretion in the female rat. *Endocrinology,* 119:1071–1075.
773. Lichtensteiger, W., and Monnet, F. (1979): Differential response of dopamine neurons to α-melanotropin and analogues in relation to their endocrine and behavioural potency. *Life Sci.,* 25:2070–2087.

The Physiology of Reproduction,
edited by E. Knobil and J. Neill *et al.*
Raven Press, Ltd., New York © 1988.

CHAPTER 29

The Gonadotropin-Releasing Hormone (GnRH) Neuronal Systems: Immunocytochemistry

Ann-Judith Silverman

The purification, sequencing, and synthesis of the decapeptide luteinizing-hormone-releasing hormone (LHRH, now usually referred to as GnRH for gonadotropin-releasing hormone) by laboratories headed by Guillemin (1) and Schally (2,3) can now be seen as an important transition point in the study of the neuroendocrinology of reproduction. It was the culmination of the research efforts of Hohlweg, Harris, McCann, Everett, and Sawyer, work that spanned five decades and implicated the central nervous system in the control of luteinizing hormone (LH) and follicle-stimulating hormone (FSH) secretion. Such regulation of anterior pituitary function is mediated by the release of the now well-characterized neurohormone into the portal capillaries in the median eminence and its delivery to the target via the hypophysial portal veins. The availability of the decapeptide and antibodies directed against it has provided the tools for the anatomical dissection of the neurosecretory pathways. It is our premise that knowledge of the unique anatomy of the GnRH neuronal networks and the integration of these neurons into the wiring of the CNS must provide the critical underpinnings of physiological and neuropharmacological research. We shall see that this neurosecretory system is very diffuse; it contains individual neurons, located in vastly different regions of the brain, presumably integrating different kinds of information. Determining how this system is coordinated will be one of the major anatomical challenges during this decade.

In this chapter we will review the advances made in the last decade on the anatomy of GnRH neuronal networks. We stand, however, on the threshold of the next transition. The characterization and sequencing of the gene for precursor protein that contains GnRH (4) will soon allow us to apply anatomical procedures, such as *in situ* hybridization (cf. ref. 5), to study the regulatory mechanisms at the level of the individual neuron.

IMMUNOCYTOCHEMICAL PROCEDURES

Before discussing the findings based on immunocytochemical techniques, we should first examine the nature of the procedure from which we obtain such important data. Immunocytochemistry represents a variety of techniques that permit the localization of an antigen in tissue sections. Its validity is based on the premise that the antibody-antigen two molecules can be visualized. Criteria for specificity have become more complex, because the field has become more sophisticated. In general, antibodies are first tested for their binding specificities in either liquid- or solid-phase radioimmunoassay. Such approaches permit one to test large numbers of antigens and to examine the modifications of the parent molecule that are compatible with antigen recognition. It is, however, essential that absorption tests using tissue sections also be carried out. Here antisera are incubated with test ligand prior to the use of those antisera in the immunocytochemical procedure. Comparison of staining intensity is then made among sections reacted with untreated antiserum, antiserum absorbed with native antigen (e.g., GnRH), and antiserum absorbed with a modified antigen. It has frequently been observed that antisera which can be used effectively in radioimmunoassay are not always applicable to anatomical studies.

In addition to controls for antibody specificity, one also performs tests on the specificity of the immunocytochemical procedure itself. In this case, one wishes to ensure that any staining seen in the tissue is ultimately dependent on the binding of primary antibody to tissue antigen and not either to the nonspecific attachment of reagents or to endogenous fluorescent or enzymatic activities.

Since the introduction of the unlabeled antibody procedure by Sternberger (6), several methodological advances to enhance the signal derived from immunocytochemical procedures have been introduced. Two major advances have been made. One is the use of fixed but unembedded sections, a procedure that reduces the loss of antigen that occurs during tissue preparation for paraffin or epoxy embedding. The second is the increased ratio of enzyme or other detection molecule to the binding of a single-antibody molecule to the tissue. We shall also see that the development of many double-label procedures is now in use to examine the synaptology of the neurosecretory cell.

DISTRIBUTION OF GnRH NEURONS AND THEIR PROJECTIONS IN THE MAMMALIAN BRAIN

The Septo-Preoptico-Infundibular Pathway

The distribution of GnRH neurons and their axonal projections has been studied by applying light microscopic immunocytochemical techniques to tissue sections. Anatomical studies were first carried out by Barry and his colleagues (7,8); a similar approach to their questions continues to the present, with more recent studies refining and extending the initial observations. This topic has been the subject of many recent reviews that have stressed comparative aspects (9–13). This chapter will emphasize data from species most frequently used in research on reproduction.

In all mammals studied in detail, several distinct subpopulations of GnRH neurons can be identified within the CNS. GnRH cells are not segregated into nuclear clusters, but instead appear as loose networks spread through many classic cytoarchitectonic divisions. The most prominent of these networks, and the one most likely to contribute directly to the regulation of gonadotropin secretion, is composed of those neurons forming a loose continuum from the telencephalic diagonal band of Broca and more dorsal septal nuclei (including the medial and triangular septal nuclei), the bed nucleus of the stria terminalis, and the diencephalic areas [including the periventricular, medial, and lateral preoptic areas, anterior hypothalamic areas, and retrochiasmatic zone (medial to optic tract)]. Also to be included in this continuum are clusters of cells in the lateral hypothalamus and those lying dorsal to, and occasionally within, the supraoptic nucleus. Diagrammatic representations of the distribution of these neuronal groups are shown in Fig. 1 (rat) and Fig. 2 (sheep).

One of the major controversies in the localization of GnRH neurons has been whether they are present or absent from the medial basal hypothalamus. It is now agreed by the majority of workers (14–18) that GnRH cells are not found in the arcuate nucleus of the rat, although a few positive neurons may be present in the cell-poor zone that separates the arcuate nucleus from the ventromedial region (17,19,20). Treatment of neonatal rats with monosodium glutamate (21,22), which destroys 80% to 90% of the neurons in the arcuate nucleus, does not significantly reduce the amount of GnRH in the median eminence. Small numbers of GnRH neurons in the basal hypothalamic area are also present in the hamster (23), mouse (24; and E. A. Zimmerman, *unpublished observations*) and sheep (25). In other species, GnRH neurons are found throughout the medial basal hypothalamus, including the arcuate nucleus, the dorsal median eminence, and premammillary nuclei. Such species include the guinea pig (26–28); rhesus, pigtailed, and squirrel monkeys (29,30); humans, bats, and ferrets (31); and new world monkey, cows, horse, cat, dog, and rabbit (see refs. 10 and 13 for further references). In all such species the absolute number of cells within these more caudal regions is usually a small proportion of the total (cf. refs. 25 and 28), although this is apparently not true of the human (32).

The projections of the neurons in this telencephalic/diencephalic continuum have been studied both by reconstructing pathways from tissue sections and/or by an analysis of fiber loss following placement of CNS lesions. The most prominent projection is to the median eminence, which is the final common pathway for regulation of anterior pituitary function. GnRH fibers reach the median eminence by more than one route (see Fig. 2 and refs. 10,18,19,30, and 33–37). The major septo-preoptico-infundibular pathway(s), common to most species, begins as a midline bundle of GnRH processes anteriorly near the level of the diagonal band of Broca, originating from septal components rostrally. This bundle divides in two near the preoptic recess of the third ventricle. Both bundles travel near the midline, one along the dorsal and the other along the ventral surface of

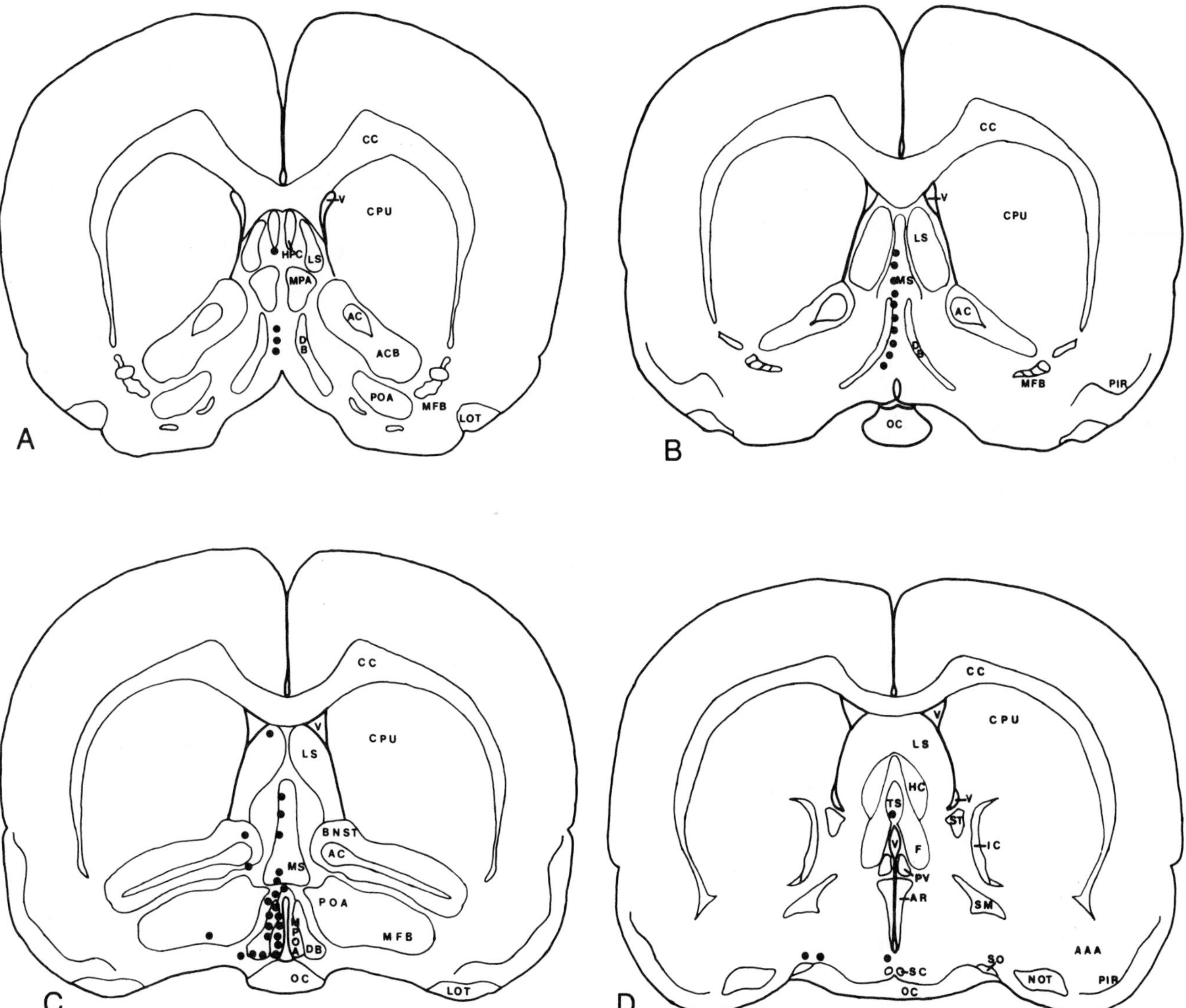

FIG. 1. (**A–D**) Diagrammatic representation of the distribution of GnRH neurons in the rat brain (exclusive of olfactory-related structures). The number of filled circles gives an approximation of the density of cells in a particular region. Note how widely scattered in the forebrain are GnRH cells. (AAA) anterior amygdaloid area; (AC) anterior commissure; (ACB) nucleus accumbens; (AR) arcuate nucleus; (BNST) bed nucleus of the stria terminalis; (CC) corpus callosum; (CPU) caudate and putamen; (DB) diagonal band of Broca; (F) fornix; (HC) hippocampal commissure; (HPC) hippocampus; (IC) internal capsule; (LOT) lateral olfactory tract; (LS) lateral septum; (MPA) medial parolfactory area; (MFB) medial forebrain bundle; (MPOA) medial preoptic area; (MS) medial septum; (NOT) nucleus of the olfactory tract; (OC) optic chiasm; (PIR) piriform cortex; (POA) preoptic area; (SC) suprachiasmatic nucleus; (SM) stria medullaris; (SO) supraoptic nucleus; (ST) stria terminalis; (TS) triangular septal nucleus; (V) ventricle.

the optic chiasm. The ventral bundle tends to run close to the surface of the brain, being covered only by the pia (18,34; see Fig. 3). Axons of GnRH neurons in the more caudal and lateral aspects of the preoptic area and hypothalamus travel in or near to the medial forebrain bundle. These turn medially near the level of the median eminence (Fig. 2). Additional fibers from the pericommissural region pass through the dorsomedial hypothalamus, forming a periventricular subependymal GnRH network (Fig. 2). The use of the ependymal processes as tunnels through which the fibers course has been demonstrated ultrastructurally (38). These periventricular fibers contribute to the median eminence innervation and possibly to innervation of more caudal structures. In those species in which GnRH cells are also present in the arcuate nucleus, GnRH axons extend from these cells into the median eminence, and fibers often continue down the infundibular stalk (10) to enter the posterior pituitary (39).

It is essential that all such pathways to the median eminence are taken into account when using paradigms involving surgical interruption of pathways or placement of lesions. Particular attention should be paid to the difficult-

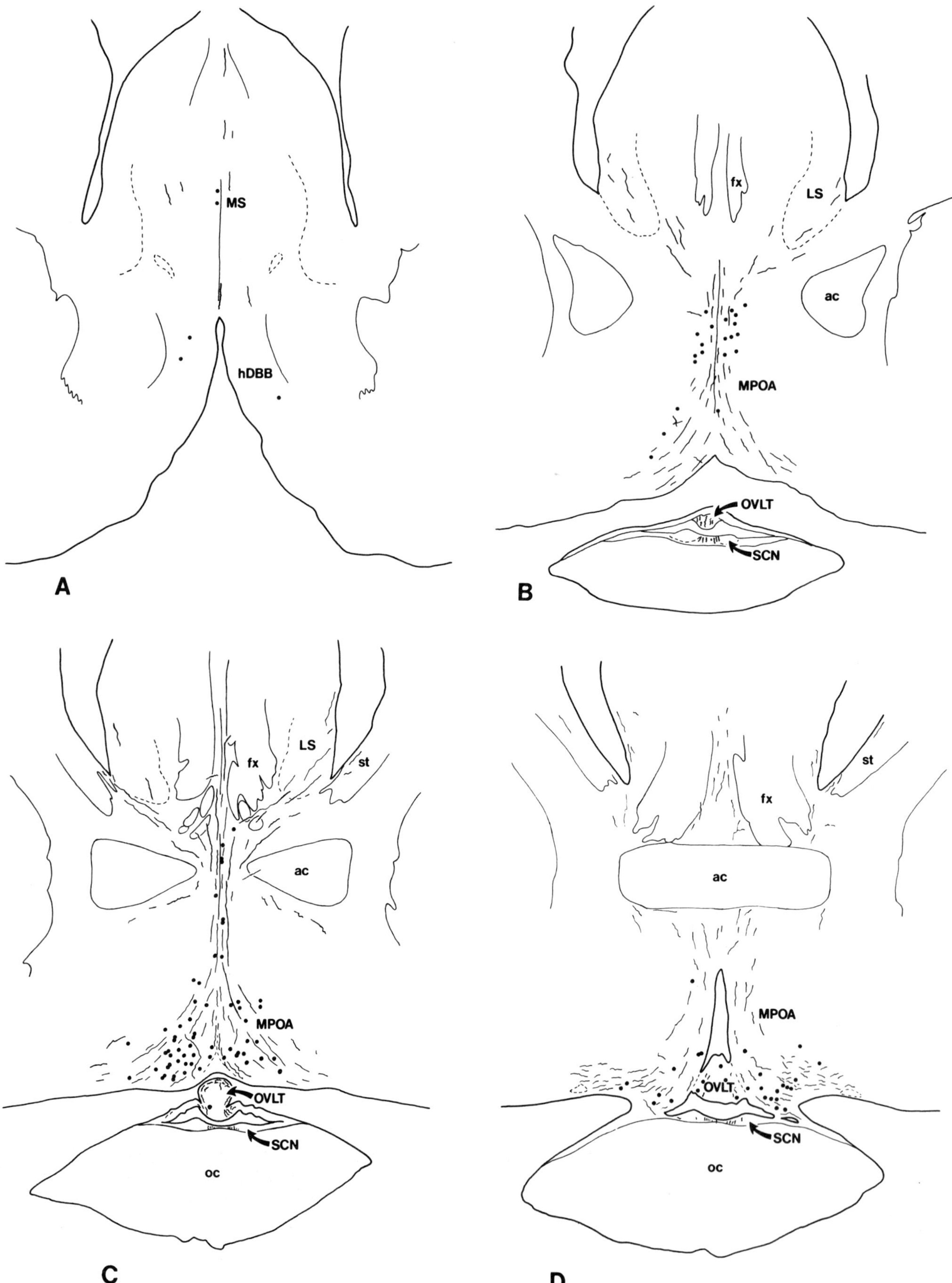

FIG. 2. See legend on facing page.

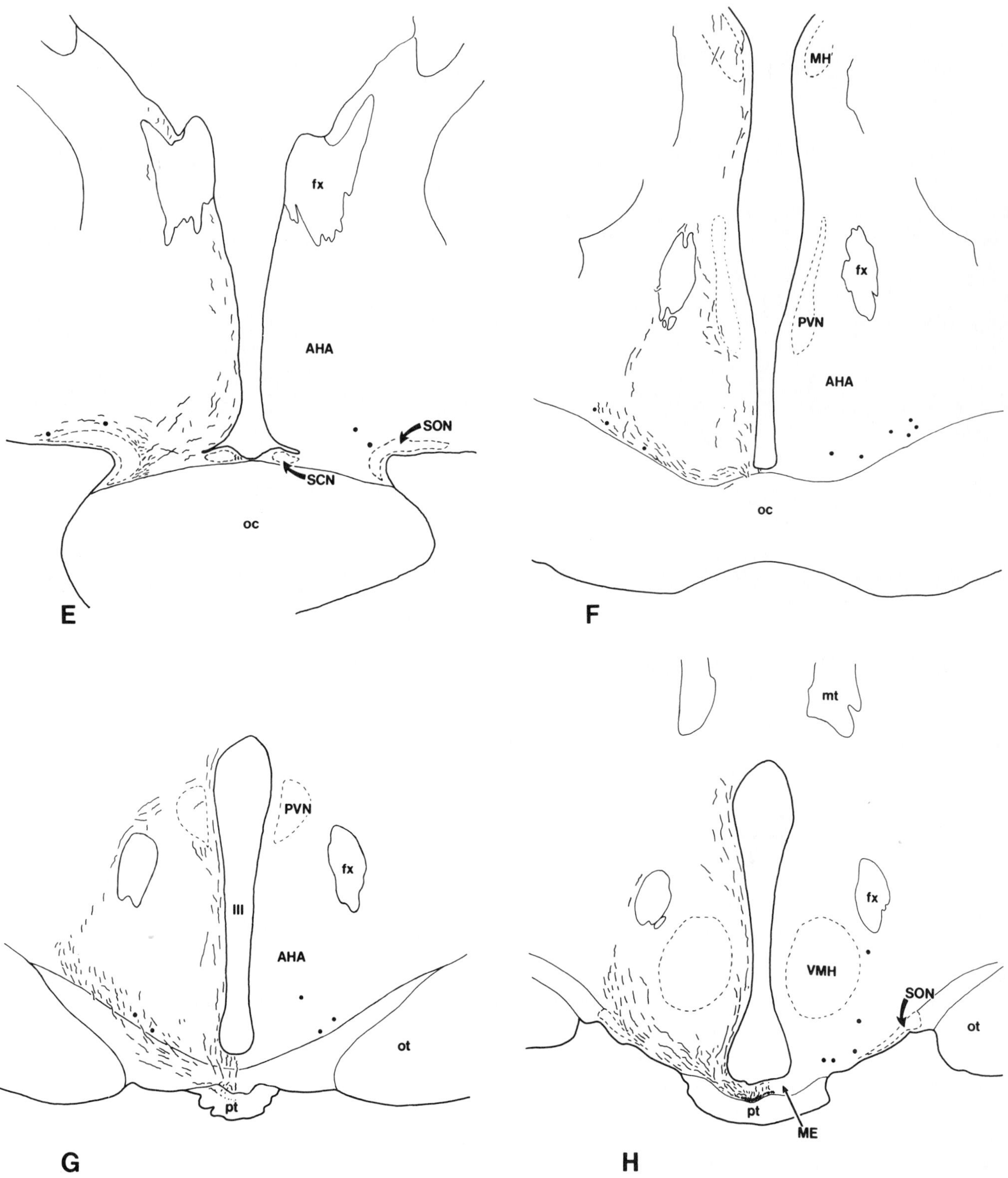

FIG. 2. The distribution of GnRH cells (●) and fibers (short solid lines) in drawings of coronal brain sections, rostral to caudal (**A–L**), through the preoptic area and hypothalamus of the ewe. Immunoreactive fibers are represented bilaterally in A–D, but, for clarity, only unilaterally on the left side of E–L. Note that more than one trajectory brings GnRH axons to the median eminence. (ac) Anterior commissure; (AHA) anterior hypothalamic area; (ARC) arcuate nucleus; (fx) fornix; (hDBB) horizontal limb of the diagonal band of Broca; (ir) infundibular recess; (is) infundibular stalk; (LS) lateral septum; (MB) mammillary body, medial division; (ME) median eminence; (MH) medial habenula; (MPOA) medial preoptic area; (MS) medial septum; (mt) mammillothalamic tract; (oc) optic chiasm; (ot) optic tract; (OVLT) organum vasculosum of the lamino terminalis; (pd) pars distalis; (pt) pars tuberalis; (PVN) paraventricular nucleus; (SCN) suprachiasmatic nucleus; (SON) supraoptic nucleus; (st) stria terminalis; (ti) tuberoinfundibular recess; (VMH) ventromedial nucleus; (ze) zona externa of the median eminence; (zi) zona interna of the median eminence; (III) third ventricle.

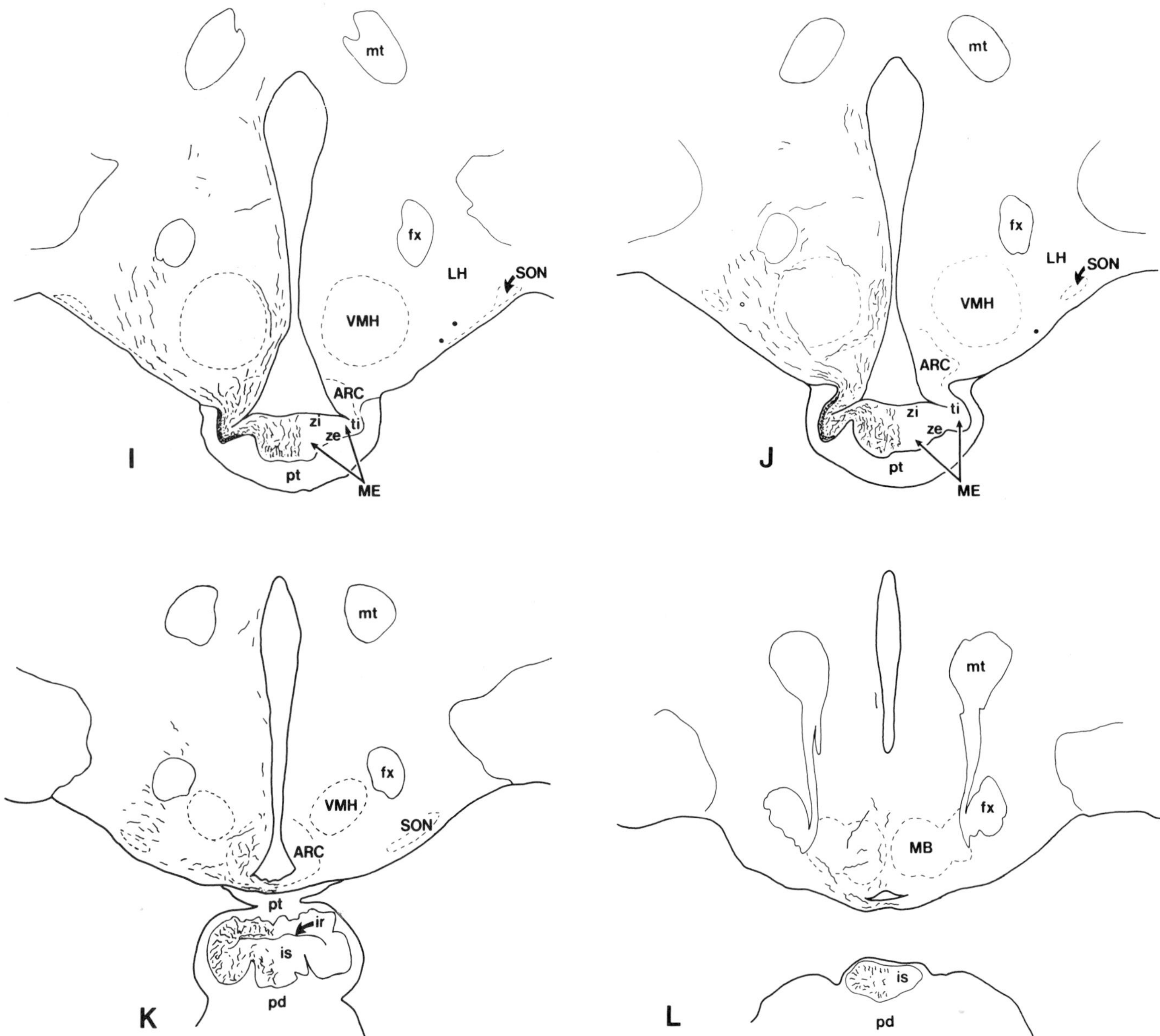

FIG. 2. See legend on page 1287.

to-sever subchiasmatic fibers (Fig. 3) found in rodents (34) and primates, including humans (40). It should also be noted in this context that GnRH fibers are capable of considerable sprouting. Tissue at the edge of a lesion will become invested with numerous GnRH axons (Silverman, *personal observation;* Lehman and Jackson, *unpublished observations*). The age at which lesions are made is also a critical factor. Medial basal hypothalamic (MBH) deafferentation in the early neonatal period results in regrowth of GnRH axons across the cut, but surgical interruption of axonal pathways in older animals leads to a depletion of GnRH fibers in the median eminence and to anovulatory cycles (41).

Although GnRH cells in many regions contribute to the axonal bundles that project to the median eminence, all cells do not participate in this pathway. Knowing which cells form the neurosecretory connection is clearly a central issue in understanding the nature of the neuronal pathways that regulate gonadotropin secretion. Initial observations in the rat indicated that complete surgical isolation of the MBH eliminated or very substantially reduced the number of GnRH fibers in the median eminence (35,37,42–45), suggesting an anterior origin for such fibers. Deafferentations, when complete (i.e., include the ventral pathway), coincide with failure of pulsatile and tonic gonadotropin secretion. By inference, similar deafferentations of MBH of the rhesus monkey must not disrupt all GnRH input to the median eminence, since MBH islands can support pulsatile and

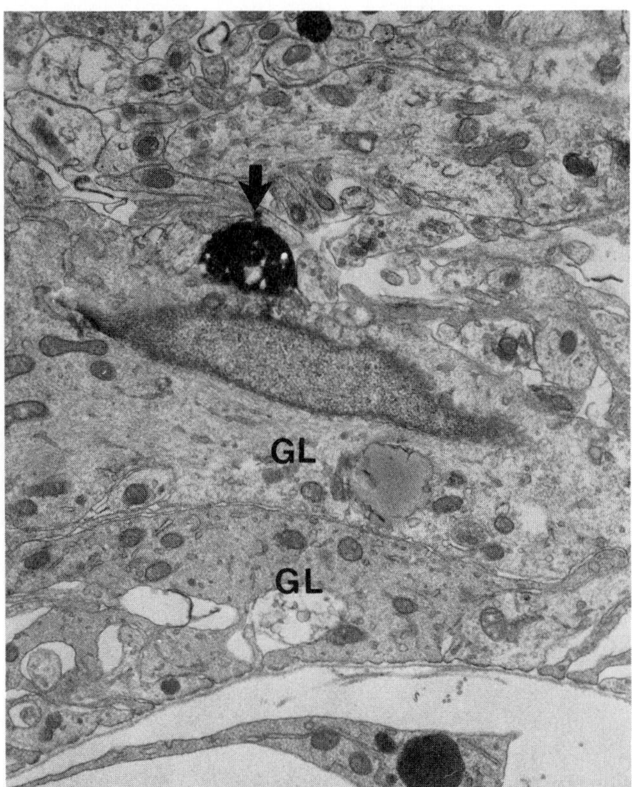

FIG. 3. In Fig. 2, GnRH fibers are illustrated coursing close to the surface of the brain. At the ultrastructural level, as shown here, an immunoreactive axon (*arrowhead*) can be found next to the limiting glial lamina (GL). × 15,000.

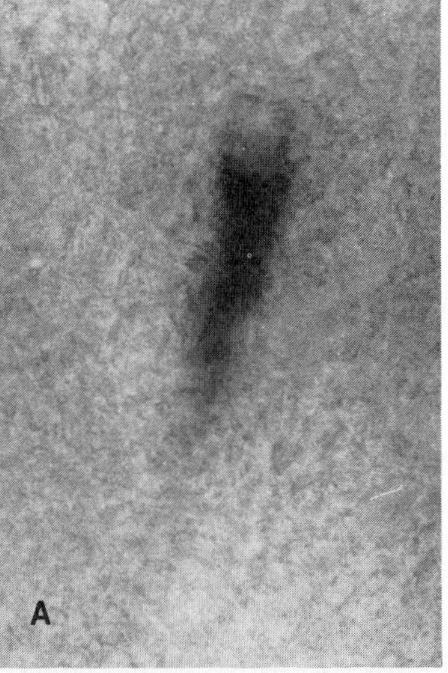

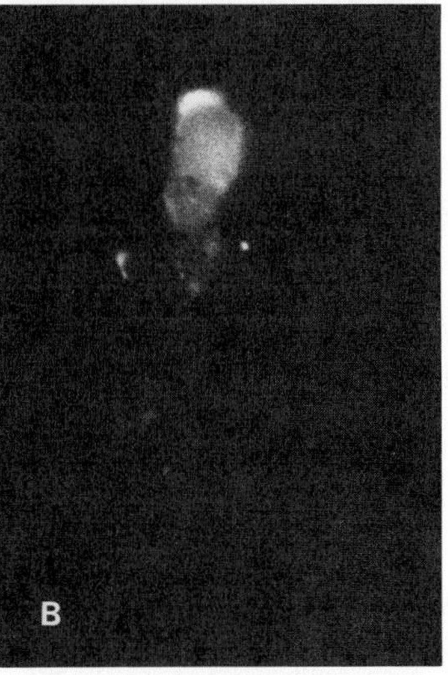

FIG. 4. To determine which GnRH neurons project to the median eminence the lectin, wheat-germ agglutinin was applied to the ventral surface of the median eminence and then localized in vesicular structures by immunocytochemistry and photographed with bright field optics (**A**). The same tissue section was subsequently incubated in antiserum to GnRH, which was localized by a fluorescent label and photographed with phloem epifluorescent optics (**B**). Thus A and B are two micrographs of a doubly labeled cell. The presence of the dark material (reaction product) tends to reduce the intensity of fluorescence, hence the apparent absence of GnRH from the dendrite.

estrogen-induced surges of gonadotropins (46). In the guinea pig the preoptic area and pericommissural regions as well as the arcuate nucleus contribute inputs to the median eminence, with each region forming a different terminal field within the median eminence (47). However, only the arcuate input is essential for tonic and cyclic gonadotropin release (47,48). Septal GnRH cells do not appear to make a substantial contribution to the median eminence in this species (47).

Recently a more direct approach has been taken to determine which GnRH neurons actually supply the innervation of the median eminence [rat (49); mouse (50)]. In these experiments, tracer proteins are applied either directly to the surface of the median eminence (49) or injected into the peripheral circulation (50). Such tracers are taken up by nerve terminals in the median eminence (or in the case of the mouse experiments, by all terminals located outside of the blood-brain barrier) and transported in vesicles back to the cell bodies. Both the tracer and GnRH are localized in the same tissue section, and the cells are identified as being afferent to the median eminence (doubly labeled; see Fig. 4A and B) are mapped and counted. Neurons found containing both labels are located as far rostrally as the diagonal band of Broca and are present within all of the architectonic regions cited above. Fifty to sixty percent of all GnRH neurons in the septal, preoptic, and hypothalamic areas contribute to the median eminence projection. No morphological characteristics distinguish median eminence afferent neurons from those that do not project to this neural-hemal organ. Furthermore, cells that are truly neurosecretory (doubly labeled) are frequently located immediately next to those whose function is currently unknown (GnRH positive only). It can be argued that tracer uptake, because it is dependent on neuronal activity, did not occur in all the terminals. However, in the mouse experiments, neuronal activity was increased by prior castration of the animals. No significant differences were noted between castrates and intacts (50). It is my suggestion that the cells which do not project to the median eminence instead innervate other preoptic or hypothalamic regions and/or send fibers to extrahypothalamic sites (see below). This hypothesis must be tested by similar tracing studies (see 50a). Experiments must also be carried out in those species with GnRH neurons in the arcuate nucleus to determine the contribution made by such cells to the median eminence innervation. In the guinea pig (47) the GnRH neurons in the arcuate nucleus, although few in number, are a major source of GnRH axons to the median eminence. This strongly suggests that cells may project to the median eminence but may not play a critical role in gonadotropin secretion. This hypothesis is supported by recent findings, in the rat, that bilateral knife cuts which sever the septal projection to the median eminence and cause a 30% reduction in median eminence GnRH do not interfere with ovulation. Similarly, unilateral knife cuts that interrupt all GnRH input ipsilaterally as measured by radioimmunoassay also do not interfere with ovulation (50b).

At the ultrastructural level, numerous investigators have described GnRH axon profiles within the median eminence and their proximity to the fenestrated capillaries of the portal plexus (cf. refs. 51–53). It is interesting to note that in most instances, GnRH axons are separated from the perivascular space by ependymal foot processes (51,52). Whether changes in access to the vasculature during times of increased secretion by contraction of glial elements occur, as it does in the posterior pituitary (54), is not known.

GnRH Pathways to Other Circumventricular Organs

Circumventricular organs are sites within the CNS in which the ependymal lining of the ventricular space are highly specialized and where the capillaries forming the blood supply are fenestrated, thereby permitting access to blood-borne substances into the nervous tissue. In addition to the dense GnRH innervation of the median eminence, cells of the septal-preoptic area also contribute to the GnRH innervation of the organum vasculosum of the lamina terminalis (OVLT), the second most densely innervated structure in the CNS (Fig. 5) in most species. This pathway was originally termed the *septo-preoptico terminal tract* by Barry and co-workers (10), and its role, if any, in the regulation of gonadotropin function is unknown. In the rat, no changes in OVLT staining were observed with gonadectomy with or without steroid replacement therapy, treatments which altered the amount of GnRH staining in the median eminence (17,55). However, in the squirrel monkey, changes in GnRH staining intensity occur both in the median eminence (56) and in the OVLT (29) during the estrous cycle. Evaluation of experiments in which lesions are placed in the area of the OVLT (cf. ref. 57) are difficult to interpret, since such lesions would inevitably destroy numerous GnRH neurons, including many that project to the median eminence.

Many fibers, presumably from cells within the septum itself, ramify within the septal region, with some converging on the lateral ventricular wall, whereas others innervate the subfornical organ. This circumventricular organ, like the OVLT, also contains a few GnRH cells of its own. However, the organization of the fibers at the lateral edges of the structure suggests that the majority of fibers are of extrinsic origin.

The posterior pituitary, though not a true circumventricular organ, is nonetheless a CNS component that is outside of the blood-brain barrier. In some species, GnRH fibers extend for varying lengths down the infundibular stalk and into the neural lobe (39). The role of these terminals in reproductive function is unknown.

Extrahypothalamic Projections

The cells in the septum and preoptic areas also contribute to many of the extrahypothalamic terminals of GnRH axons as first described by Barry (for a review see ref. 10; also

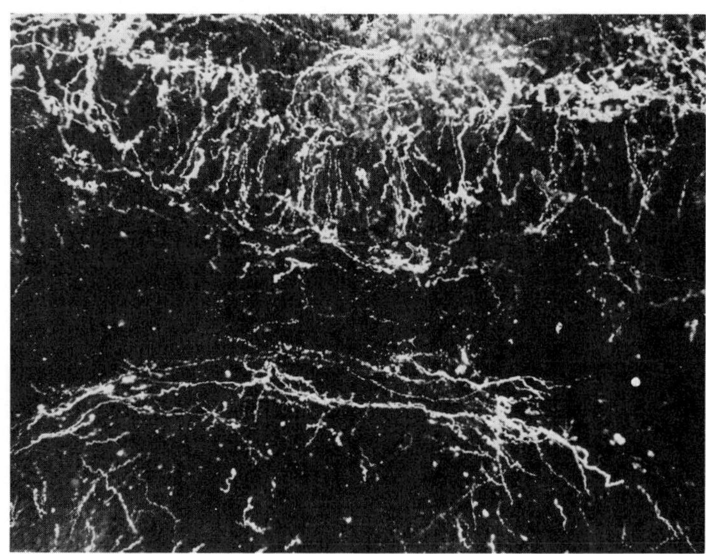

FIG. 5. GnRH fibers in the OVLT-supraoptic organ of the rhesus monkey. The sheep has a similarly complex OVLT. The OVLT of rodents is a much simpler structure, but is also well innervated by GnRH fibers.

see refs. 18,23,36, and 48 and Fig. 6). Some cells, especially from the medial and triangular septal nuclei and pericommissural region, send fibers into the stria medullaris to innervate the epithalamus (habenula and possibly the pineal) and continue into the fasciculus retroflexus to terminate in the midbrain region near blood vessels of the posterior perforated substance. Others, especially from the bed nucleus of the stria terminalis and preoptic area, enter the stria terminalis and project into the medial amygdala. A ventral pathway into the amygdala (30,58) has also been observed in some species. Finally, cells in this region contribute to a much more diffuse periventricular pathway whose fibers enter the mammillary complex and then converge on the mammillary peduncle and proceed into the ventral tegmental area of the midbrain. There they mingle with fibers derived from the fasciculus retroflexus. Some of these fibers have been postulated to enter the subarachnoid space, though this observation requires ultrastructural confirmation. Fibers continue caudalward, coursing the dorsal border of the interpeduncular nucleus, and, in the rat (18), but not the guinea pig (36), continue into the raphe nuclei. Fibers from this periventricular source also extend into the periaqueductal region.

DISTRIBUTION OF GnRH NEURONS AND AXONS IN OLFACTORY-RELATED STRUCTURES

The Nervus Terminalis

Barry and his colleagues initially identified GnRH neurons in rostral regions, termed the *parolfactory area* (10). Similar observations were made by Silverman and Krey (36) when they noted in the guinea pig that small clusters of these neurons were associated with the blood vessels of the anterior perforated substance (also see ref. 59). These cell groups were finally recognized to be part of the nervus terminalis (60). In the guinea pig, this nerve (sometimes referred to as the *zero cranial nerve*) has peripheral, intracranial, and intracerebral components (Fig. 7). The peripheral portion is comprised of neurons and their processes below the cribiform plate that are associated with the ol-

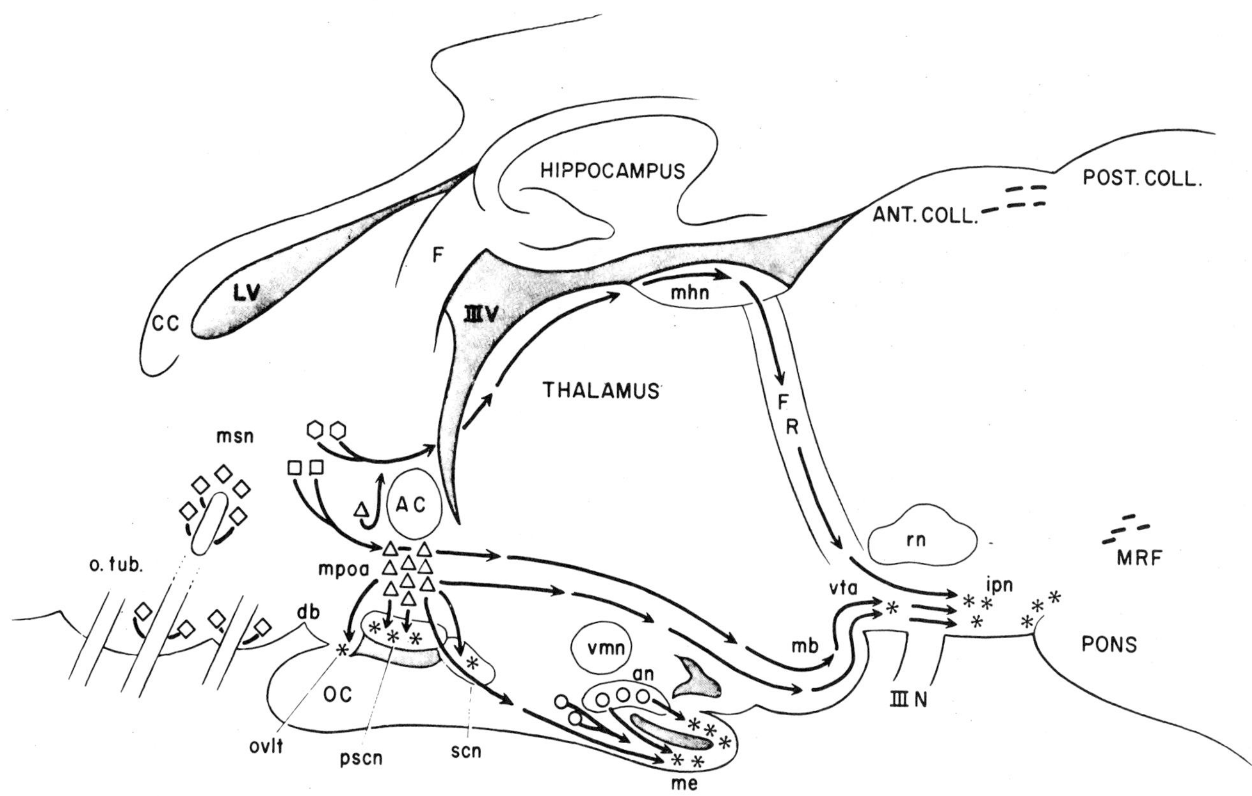

FIG. 6. Midsagittal plane of the guinea pig brain from the level of the septum rostrally to the pons posteriorly. Different groups of GnRH cells are indicated by the geometric symbols, fiber pathways are indicated by arrows, and terminal fields are indicated by asterisks. The subchiasmatic pathway is not indicated. It is not known if any GnRH cells have more than one projection. (AC) Anterior commissure; (an) arcuate nucleus; (CC) corpus callosum; (db) diagonal band of Broca; (F) fornix; (FR) fasciculus retroflexus; (ipn) interpeduncular nucleus; (LV) lateral ventricle; (mb) mammillary body, medial division; (me) median eminence; (mhn) medial habenula; (mpoa) medial preoptic area; (msn) medial septum; (OC) optic chiasm; (o. tub) olfactory tubercle; (ovlt) organum vasculosum of the lamino terminalis; (pscn) preoptic suprachiasmatic nucleus; (rn) red nucleus; (scn) suprachiasmatic nucleus; (vmn) ventromedial nucleus; (vta) ventral tegmental area; (IIIV) third ventricle; (IIIN) occulomotor nerve.

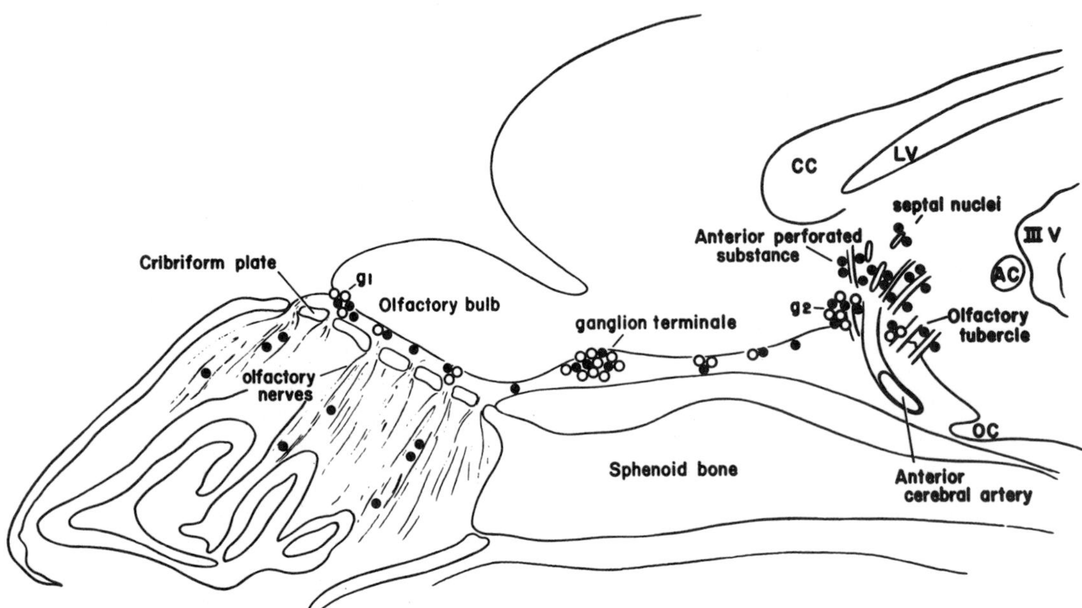

FIG. 7. The nervus terminalis of the guinea pig based on composite camera lucida drawings of a 45-day fetal guinea-pig brain. GnRH immunoreactive cell bodies (●) are seen throughout the course of this ganglionated nerve. In the periphery they accompany the olfactory and vomeronasal nerves below in cribiform plate. Intracranially, GnRH and nonimmunoreactive neurons (○) form ganglia along the ventromedial surface of the brain. The major ganglia are indicated. Neurons of the nervus terminalis penetrate the CNS along with the branches of the anterior cerebral artery and extend into the olfactory tubercle and septal nuclei. Not illustrated is the network of GnRH fibers that connects all portions of the nervus terminalis.

factory and vomeronasal nerves. In the rat (61,62) and hamster (M. N. Lehman, *personal communication*) GnRH fibers have been identified in the sensory epithelium of the vomeronasal organ. The intracranial portion consists of several ganglia that lie in the pial layer of the pia mater (in the guinea pig) and contain both GnRH-positive and GnRH-negative neurons. The ganglia are found on the ventromedial surface of the olfactory bulbs and forebrain. The largest are the ganglion terminale at the caudal pole of the olfactory bulbs: g1 is located at the frontal pole of the olfactory bulbs, and g2 is located at the level of the olfactory tubercle where the anterior cerebral artery enters the CNS. Each of these ganglia and other smaller clusters of cells are connected by fiber bundles, e.g., the terminal nerve. The organization of the nervus terminalis of the hamster is similar to that of the guinea pig (63). In the rat, scattered cells are seen in this region, but no large ganglia are observed. Given the location of these cells, they or their processes might have access both to blood-borne substances and to the cerebrospinal fluid in the subarachnoid space. Within the CNS, GnRH cells and fibers follow the course of the anterior cerebral artery and its branches through the olfactory tubercle and septal regions.

The nervus terminalis also contains non-GnRH-containing neurons that have a morphology similar to sympathetic ganglion cells (60). In the hamster, two distinct populations of cells have been distinguished: those that are GnRH positive and those that contain acetylcholine esterase (63). In the rat, non-GnRH-positive cells, at least in the intracerebral portion, are cholinergic (i.e., contain choline acetyltransferase) and/or contain VIP (M. Schwanzel-Fukuda, *personal communication*). In both the guinea pig (28) and the rat (62), the GnRH cells of the nervus terminalis are the first GnRH neurons to appear during development (see below).

The nervus terminalis is also found in nonmammalian species. Tracing studies in teleosts have shown that this complex nerve projects peripherally to the retina and centrally to the preoptic and supracommissural nuclei of the area ventralis of the forebrain (64–66). This nerve then is in a position to coordinate olfactory and visual cues and has a clear sensory component. Demski et al. (67) have shown that injection of GnRH into the preoptic area of goldfish results in the sustained release of sperm; these workers have suggested that, under normal conditions, GnRH derived from the nervus terminalis may be released in this area. The GnRH neurons of the teleost nervus terminalis also contain the molluscan cardioexcitatory peptide (FRMFamide) (68). GnRH/FMRFamide axons are present in the goldfish inner nuclear and inner plexiform layers of the retina, which originate from the nervus terminalis (68). These peptides have quite dramatic effects on the "on-off"-center double-color-opponent ganglion cells. This has led Stell and his colleagues to postulate that olfactory-related cues influence the output of the retinal ganglion cells that respond to color contrast. The numbers of neurons positive for either peptide change with the reproductive status of the goldfish, being most numerous during the season of reproductive activity

(W. K. Stell, *personal communication*). No such changes have been reported in mammals.

Less work has been done on the direction of information flow in the mammalian terminal nerve. Recently, Wirsig and Leonard (63) carried out a series of experimental disconnections at different levels of the nerve in neonatal hamsters, examining the brain for GnRH immunoreactivity at short intervals thereafter. Lesions placed below the cribriform plate reduced or eliminated GnRH axons in the nerve along the olfactory bulbs, including all immunoreactive processes running in the vomeronasal nerve and entering the accessory olfactory bulb. This suggests that a portion of the GnRH cells in the peripheral component are sensory in nature and are afferent to the accessory olfactory bulb. In these animals, the ganglion terminale persists and contains immunoreactive neurons, but the dense fiber plexus in the ganglion is much reduced, indicating that the peripheral neurons innervate this intracranial component. Lesions at the level of the olfactory bulbs do not change the number of cells seen in the vomeronasal nerve, but result in a buildup of GnRH proximal to the cut and again reduce staining in the intracranial ganglia. Disruption at the level of the forebrain results in depletion of GnRH central to the cut, as well as a buildup proximal to the cut. All of these data indicate that the GnRH portion of the nervus terminalis of the hamster is centripetal, presumably sensory. In this species, transection of the nervus terminalis results in failure to mate in half of the treated animals; in those that do mate, there is an increase in the number of intromissions prior to ejaculation, when compared to intact controls (69). These effects are similar to those reported following destruction of the vomeronasal system (70). Determining the interplay of the nervus terminalis and the vomeronasal system in the coordination of olfactory stimuli that are important for reproductive behavior and physiology will be an exciting area of experimentation in the future.

Other Olfactory-Related Pathways

It is quite clear that olfactory cues play a critical role in the reproductive physiology and behavior of many mammalian species. In addition to the nervus terminalis discussed above, olfactory information enters the central nervous system via either the olfactory projection to the main olfactory bulb or via the vomeronasal organ's projection (VNO) into the accessory olfactory bulb (70). Within the CNS, the secondary and tertiary projections of each of these systems remain segregated, both anatomically and functionally. Recent data suggest that the VNO system is the system most intimately related to reproduction (70). The degree of development of GnRH neuronal networks in the main and accessory olfactory bulbs, anterior olfactory nucleus, and olfactory portions of the limbic system varies considerably across species, being underdeveloped in the guinea pig (28), highly developed in the hamster (23,59) and of intermediate prominence in the rat (Fig. 8). In the latter species (18,61), GnRH neurons are present in the accessory olfactory bulb, and these most likely contribute to some of the GnRH processes in this structure. In the hamster (59) and the neonatal rat (61), the main olfactory bulbs may contain their own small complement of GnRH neurons. The innervation of the bulbs in both species is derived, in part, from neurons in the nervus terminalis (see above). An input to the main olfactory bulb from cells in the anterior olfactory nucleus and anterior hippocampal rudiment are also likely. It has been suggested that olfactory bulb input may also originate from septal structures (18), but this has not been observed by other investigators (61). Within both the main and accessory bulbs, GnRH fibers ramify primarily in the external plexiform layer.

The olfactory bulbs of three primate species have been

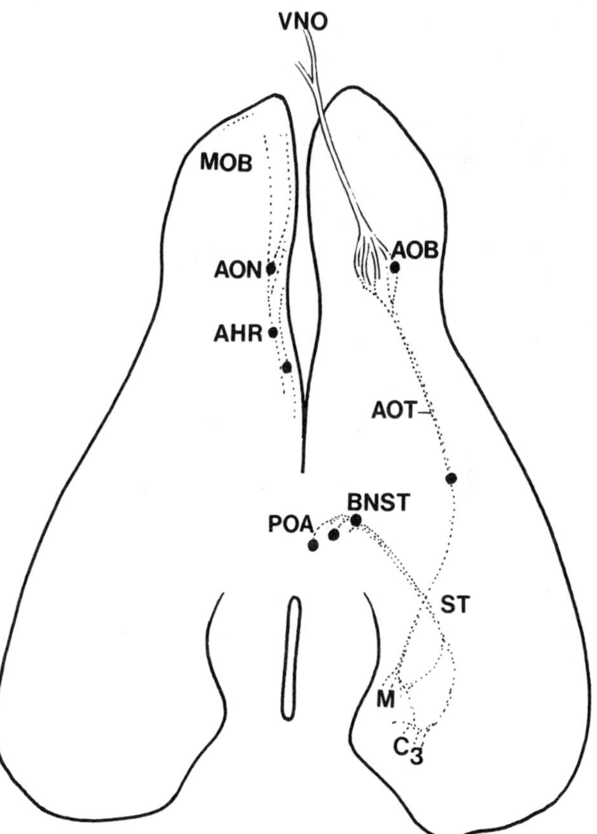

FIG. 8. A dorsal view of the rat brain showing a portion of the GnRH innervation of intracerebral olfactory-related structures. GnRH cells (dots) found in the anterior hippocampal rudiment (AHR) and anterior olfactory nucleus (AON) innervate the main olfactory bulb (MOB). Cells are present within the accessory olfactory bulb (AOB), and this structure also receives an input from nervus terminalis neurons (not illustrated). Cells in the preoptic area/bed nucleus of the stria terminalis project to the medial (M) and posteromedial cortical (C_3) amygdala, which may also receive a GnRH input from the accessory olfactory bulb. (BNST) Bed nucleus of stria terminalis; (ST) stria terminalis; (POA) preoptic area; (AOT) accessory olfactory terminalis; (VNO) vomeronasal organ.

studied (71). Old world monkeys lack a distinct accessory olfactory bulb, but in *Macaca fascicularis* a few GnRH neurons and axons are present in the main bulb, with a few fibers entering the lateral olfactory tract. In the squirrel monkey (new world, *Saimiri sciureus*), GnRH neurons are found in the main olfactory bulb, and fibers are ramified within both the main and accessory bulbs, mostly in the external plexiform layer. Finally, in the owl monkey (*Aotus trivirgatus*), GnRH neurons are seen in the accessory bulb, and fibers are present in both bulbs and in the vomeronasal nerve.

In the rat, groups of GnRH neurons have been identified (18): (a) extending from the genu of the corpus callosum (anterior hippocampal rudiment) to the medial division of the anterior olfactory nucleus; (b) in the hippocampus, primarily in the indusium griseum, loosely dispersed between the genu and splenium of the corpus callosum; and (c) in Ammon's horn. A small number of cells are found dorsal to the corpus callosum and innervate the cingulate cortex.

The question still remains as to whether the GnRH neurons present in olfactory regions of the mammalian CNS play any direct role in reproduction. Change in levels of GnRH in the posterior aspect of the olfactory bulbs of female voles exposed to male urine has been reported (72), and these changes in the content could be due to either changes in the nervus terminalis or in the CNS proper. Clearly, continued experimentation in this field is essential.

CYTOLOGY OF GnRH NEURONS

For neurons, upon which the continuation of the species depends, the morphology is surprisingly simple. In most species, the vast majority of GnRH neurons are oval or fusiform in shape, with a maximum diameter of 10 to 20 μm. Simple, unbranched dendritic processes extend from one or both poles of the cell. Axons emerge either directly from the cell body (Fig. 9A) or from a dendrite, and the dendrite may assume a beaded appearance and become axonal. Although this simple cell is found in all species examined to date, it is now clear, from work using thick unembedded sections, that some of these neurosecretory cells have a greater range of shape and complexity than previously appreciated. In the rat, two major categories of cells have been recognized: those with a smooth contour, as described above, and those with a more ragged outline (73–76). This latter subset may be further subdivided by the number of spinous processes (77). It has been suggested (75,76) that such thorny cells receive a more dense innervation than smooth cells. Even more complex shapes have been seen in the sheep (25; Fig. 9B) and rhesus monkey (Fig. 9C). In the former, especially in the anestrous state, GnRH cells are larger than those reported for other species and possess a complex, branching dendritic arbor. Somatic protuberances can cover the entire surface of the cell body. Similar encrusted appearances are also seen in the rhesus monkey hypothalamus (Fig. 9C).

GnRH neurons have a large, centrally placed nucleus and a thin rim of cytoplasm, the latter then extending into the tapering cones of the principal dendrites (Fig. 10). Nuclei contain one or two large nucleoli, and the nuclear envelope is frequently indented. The cytoplasm contains many stacks of rough endoplasmic reticulum, one or more prominent Golgi stacks, and neurosecretory granules. Cilia have been observed in the rat (75,78), but have not been reported in other species. Immunoreactivity is frequently associated with some, but not all, cisternae of the rough endoplasmic reticulum (79; see Fig. 11A) as well as with neurosecretory granules, but rarely with the Golgi lamellae (80; see Fig. 11B). The subcellular distribution may depend on the epitopes recognized by the antiserum employed, since antisera that recognize precursor forms of GnRH may react with material in the Golgi apparatus (81).

Examination of light microscopic material has suggested that several types of GnRH/GnRH interactions are possible. Such interactions were first suggested by Marshall and Goldsmith (82) and were based on examination of GnRH neurons and their processes in baboons. Ultrastructural studies have recently lent support to this hypothesis. Axosomatic or axodendritic synapses between GnRH elements have now been reported in the rat by two laboratories (83,84; see Fig. 12), although they disagree as to the frequency of such occurrences. These findings, if substantiated and extended to other species, are particularly exciting. It is well known that gonadotropin secretion occurs in a pulsatile manner, and this pulsatility is presumably driven by pulses of GnRH. Indeed, bursts of multiunit activity that correlate one for one with pulses of LH can be recorded from the CNS (of rhesus monkeys) (85). Yet, as we have seen, the GnRH neurosecretory system is very diffuse. It is possible that the synaptic connections between GnRH neurons as well as between GnRH neurons and their nonimmunoreactive neighbors (see below) form a part of the substrate for the coordination of the GnRH signal.

Given the significance of such synaptic interactions in our eventual understanding of the organization and regulation of the GnRH neurosecretory system, the strictest morphological criteria for a synapse should be applied when discussing GnRH/GnRH interactions or synaptic input to GnRH cells and their processes. The criteria include (a) the presence of a well-defined synaptic cleft, (b) the clustering of synaptic vesicles in the presynaptic element, and (c) membrane specializations on the pre- and postsynaptic side.

Somatic apposition between GnRH cells has also been suggested, again on the basis of light microscopic data. Tantalizing hints of such appositions have been found (albeit rarely) in hamster (80; see Fig. 13); however, in hamster and mouse, GnRH cells are seen in close apposition to nonimmunoreactive neighbors (Fig. 14). In these cases, the soma plasma membranes are not separated from each other

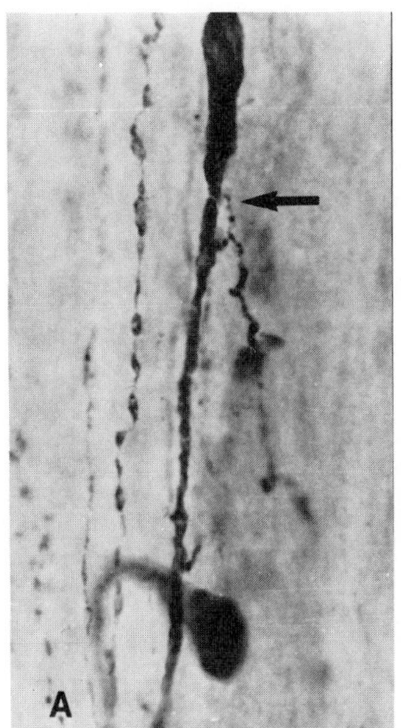

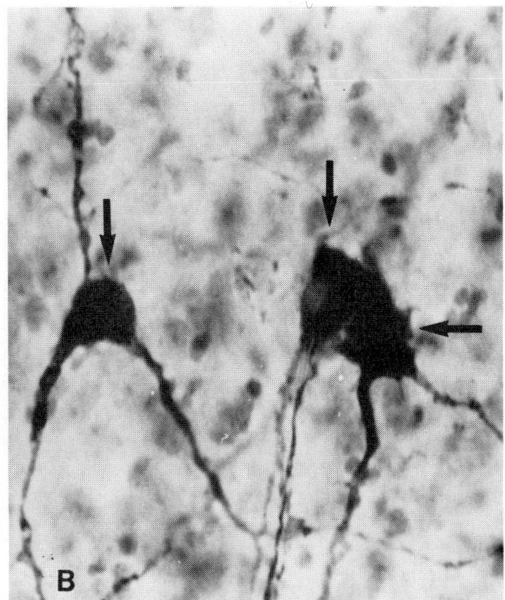

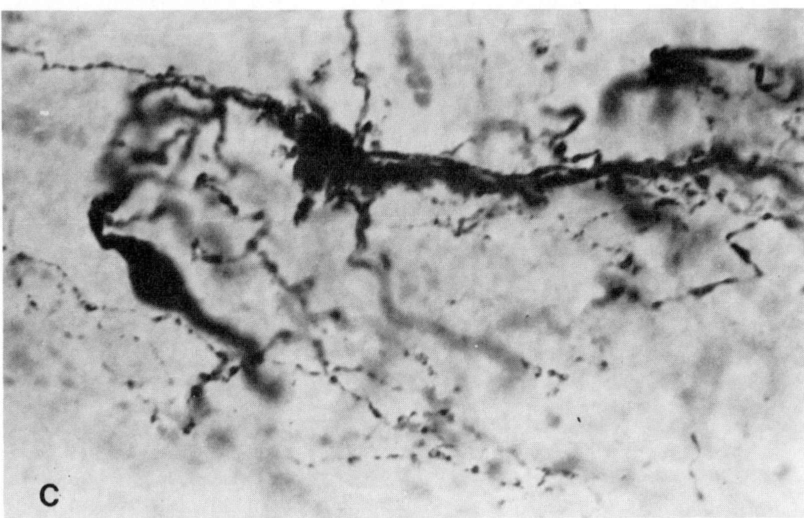

FIG. 9. Three fields showing GnRH neurons of differing morphology. In **A**, two very simple, smooth cells from the vertical limb of the diagonal band of Broca of the rhesus monkey are shown. The arrow indicates the point of emergence of the axon of this cell. In **B**, three cells (each indicated by an arrow) from the ewe preoptic area are shown. These cells have numerous primary dendrites and a more triangular appearance. The two cells on the right appear to be in close contact. Ultrastructural studies (M. N. Lehman, *unpublished results*) indicate that glial processes separate these neurons from each other. In **C**, taken from the ventral preoptic area of the rhesus monkey, two neurons are in the field of view. On the left is a relatively smooth surfaced cell with primary dendrites extending from each pole. On the right, oriented horizontal to the surface of the brain, is a thorny cell with many irregularities on the surface. This cell is also in close proximity to many GnRH fibers in the vicinity.

by intervening glial processes. However, no examples of clear synaptic contact have been found. It should be noted that gap junctions would be particularly difficult to identify in such material, but one might hypothesize that the coordination of the "pulse" of GnRH release might be coordinated by interactions between cells of the neurosecretory unit.

One possible site of GnRH interactions not yet studied in sufficient detail are those that may occur among axons along the pathway to the median eminence or within the neurohemal structure itself. In the hamster (80), GnRH axons travel in tight bundles through the anterior aspect of the arcuate/median eminence before diverging toward the lateral aspects over the tuberoinfundibular sulci. Are there interactions within such bundles? Are there axo-axonic contacts between axons near their terminus? These are among the critical anatomical questions whose resolution might help in unraveling the mechanism by which GnRH release is coordinated.

SYNAPTIC INPUT AND OUTPUT

In ultrastructural immunocytochemical studies of the median eminence, GnRH is found in membrane-bound granules within axon profiles and neurosecretory terminals (51,52,86,87). Granules range in size from 40 to 130 nm. Some of the variability in size of the granules may stem from the location of the granule (i.e., cell body, axon, terminus) (52,87) or from the difficulty in measuring gran-

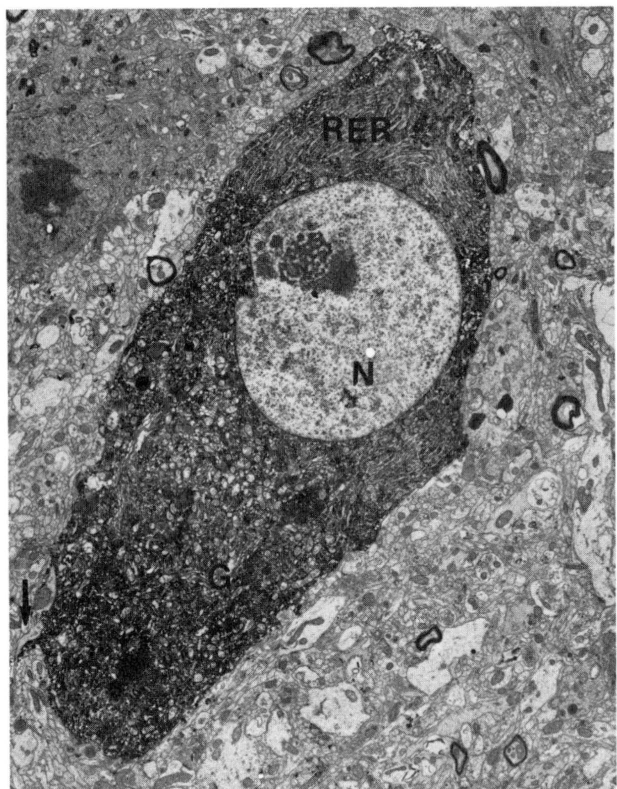

FIG. 10. Low-power electron micrograph of a GnRH cell from the preoptic area of a guinea pig. The nucleus (N) has a single nucleolus, and the nuclear envelope is slightly indented. The cytoplasm is filled with stacks of rough endoplasmic reticulum (RER) and has a prominent Golgi apparatus (G). Note the small somatic protuberance (*arrow*). Frequently the use of detergent in the immunocytochemical procedure results in reaction product artifactually spread throughout the cytoplasm. × 4,500.

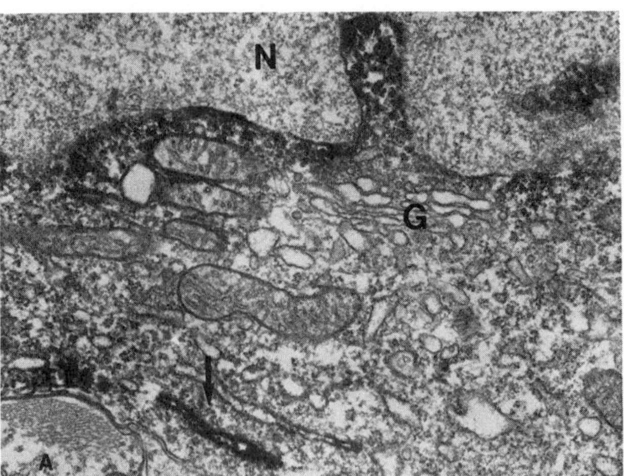

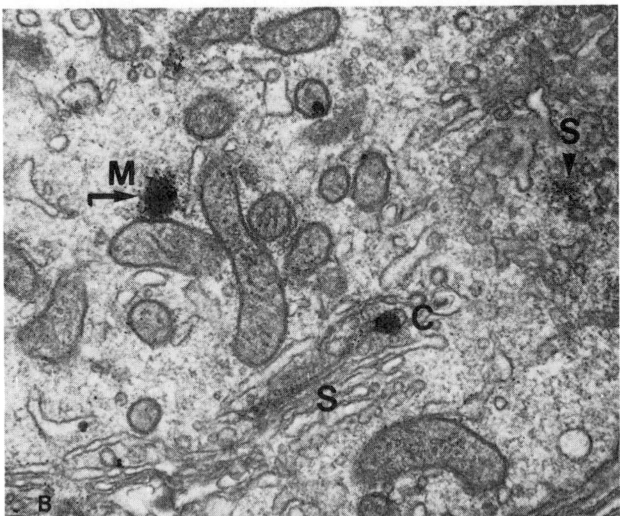

FIG. 11. Two electron micrographs showing the subcellular distribution of immunoreactivity as demonstrated with the LR-1 antiserum (83,100). **A**: Mouse cell. Reaction product is localized to one stack of the rough endoplasmic reticulum (*arrow*) and to the rough endoplasmic reticulum associated with the nuclear envelope. (G) Golgi apparatus. **B**: Hamster cell. A silver intensification of the DAB reaction (80) was applied to the tissue sections. This reduced silver is associated with Golgi saccules (S), a condensing granule (C), and a more mature neurosecretory granule (M).

ules in material with ill-preserved biological membranes. Similar granules have been found in the GnRH terminals of the OVLT (88,89) and subfornical organ (90).

Recent studies have concentrated on the synaptic input to GnRH cells. Although GnRH neurons in the preoptic area of the rat were initially reported not to receive a synaptic input (78), both axosomatic and axodendritic inputs do occur (75,76,83,91; see Fig. 15A and B). However, at least in the male rat, the density of innervation of these cells is considerably lower than that observed for other preoptic-area neurons in the same electron micrographs. In measurements of approximately 1,000 μm^2 of tissue, 0.38% of GnRH dendritic membrane was in synaptic apposition, whereas 6.61% of non-GnRH dendritic membrane was occupied (83). Since the lengths of synaptic specializations did not vary, these measurements indicate that the absolute number of inputs to GnRH cells is smaller when compared to their neighbors.

That the degree of innervation may be species specific is suggested by studies now being conducted in the hamster (80), the sheep (M. N. Lehman, *unpublished observations*), and the guinea pig (92). In the hamster, only one axosomatic synapse and three axodendritic synapses have been found on GnRH structures, after examination of several sections through approximately 20 cells. In contrast, synapses onto GnRH neurons in the diagonal band/preoptic area in both the sheep and the guinea pig are frequently encountered, though quantitative analysis of synaptic density onto GnRH cells and their nonimmunoreactive neighbors has yet to be carried out. These apparent species differences in the arrangement of synaptic input suggest that caution must be exercised in generalizing findings in the rat to other species.

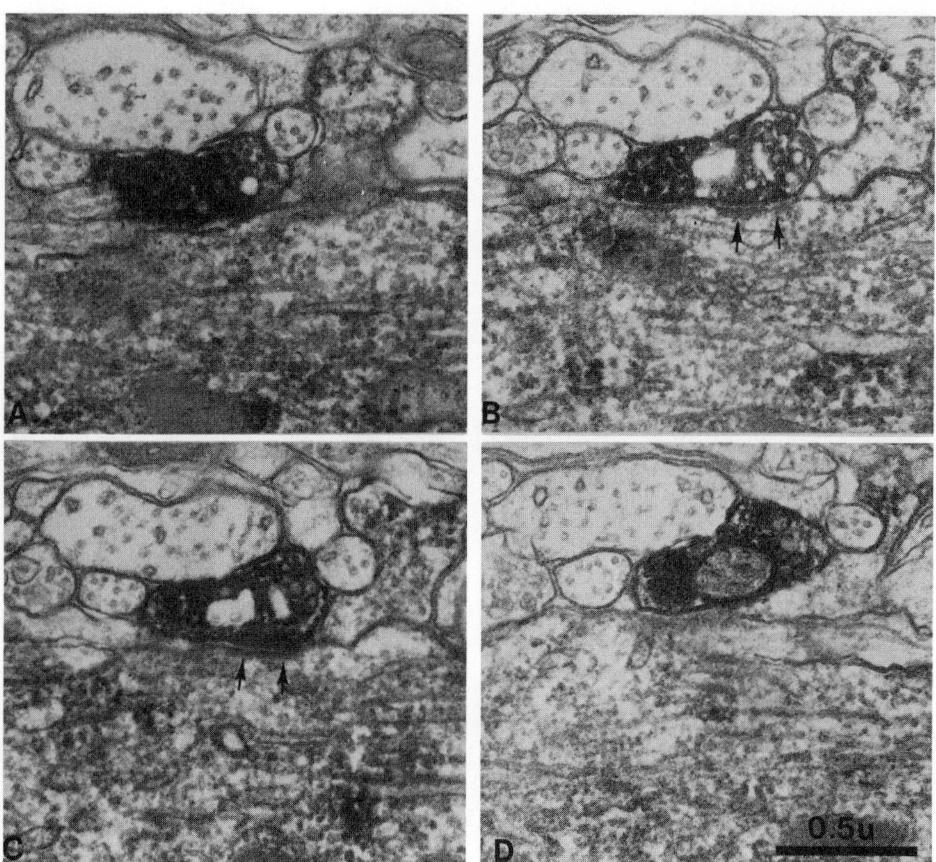

FIG. 12. A series of four sections through a GnRH axon that forms a synapse with a GnRH neuron. Arrows indicate the region of the synaptic cleft and active zone of the synapse.

In addition to species differences, there are also quite dramatic changes in input to the GnRH cell body with age in the male rat (92a). Quite surprisingly, this quantitative study has revealed that the number of synapses per unit of membrane and as observed in any random thin section of a perikaryon is increased from youth to middle age and from middle age to old age. This suggests that the changes that occur in the CNS vis-à-vis the aging process need not be degenerative. Instead, this may reflect an increase in the ratio of inhibitory inputs. Such a hypothesis clearly requires physiological testing.

Studies have now been initiated in several laboratories to examine the nature of the neurotransmitter systems that innervate the GnRH neurons and their processes. The majority of these studies have involved double-labeling procedures for GnRH and a transmitter (or its synthetic enzymes) and analysis at the light microscopic level. Since synaptic contacts can only be verified ultrastructurally, these data must be regarded as provisional. Such studies indicate a possible association between GnRH neurons (or their processes) and serotonin, dopamine beta-hydroxylase (93), tyrosine hydroxylase (93,94), glutamic acid decarboxylase (93), and neurotensin and substance P (95) terminals. All such possible associations must be confirmed at the ultrastructural level, and three such studies have been published to date. Using anterograde degeneration to identify a population of axon terminals following surgical interruption of the ventral noradrenergic pathway, Palkovits et al. (96) found evidence for a catecholaminergic input to GnRH processes in the arcuate nucleus. Kiss and Halasz (97) recently published evidence for a serotonergic input to GnRH cells and dendrites in the preoptic area. In this study, tritiated serotonin and ultrastructural radioautography were used to mark the serotonin terminals. Unfortunately no statistical analysis of the autoradiograms was presented (98). A study that found glutamic acid decarboxylase-positive terminals on GnRH cells and processes (99) suffered from poor morphological preservation of the tissue, so that a final acceptance of this input must await further study. A clear understanding of the nature of the systems impinging on the GnRH neuron requires further work.

In addition to receiving an input, GnRH neurons also form synapses. This was first suggested in studies by Krisch in the rat preoptic area (73) and has now been demonstrated conclusively in the preoptic area of the guinea pig (92,100) and the rat (83,84). These axodendritic synapses were characterized by a well-defined synaptic cleft, as well as accumulations of both large immunoreactive granules and small

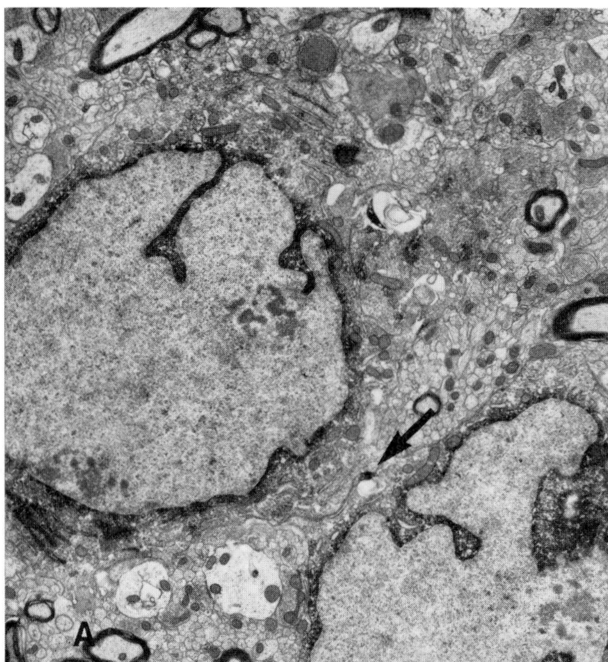

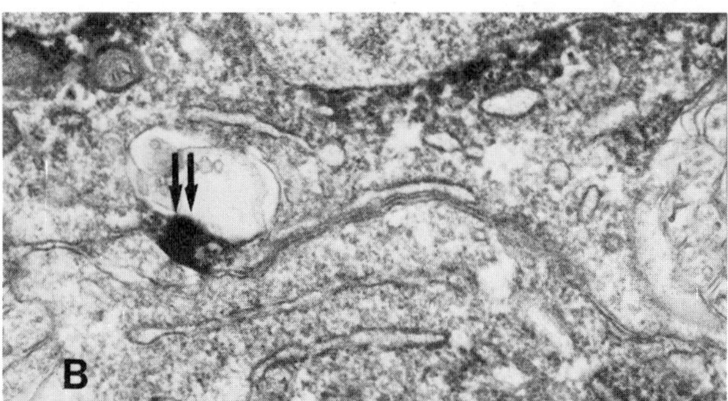

FIG. 13. Two GnRH cells in the hamster preoptic area in close apposition. The arrow in **A** indicates the region of higher magnification shown in **B**. There are no glial processes between the plasma membranes of the two cells. An immunoreactive granule is seen at the cell surface in B (*double arrow*), but it cannot be proven that this represents a release site.

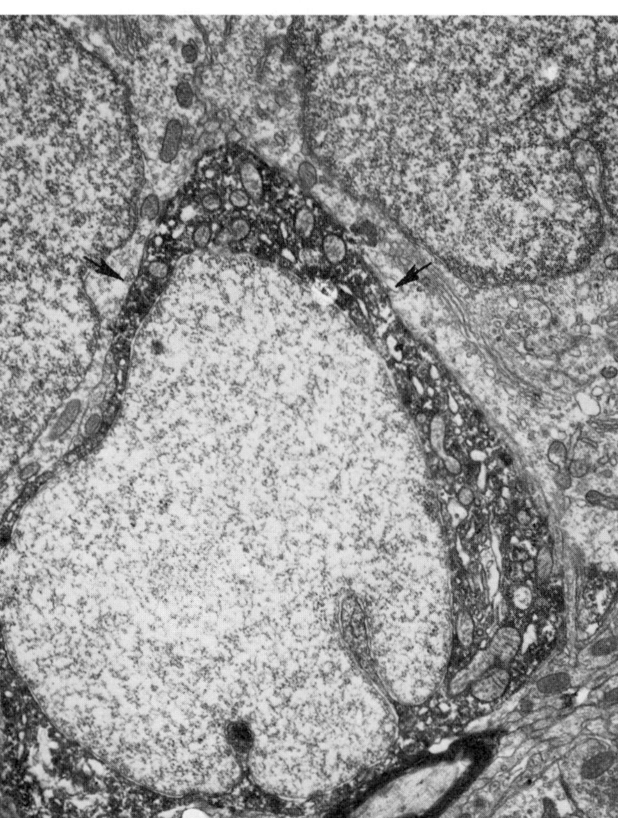

FIG. 14. In the mouse preoptic area, some GnRH neurons are found tightly packed, without intervening glial processes, with neighboring nonimmunoreactive cells. To date, no synaptic specializations have been found. Arrows indicate regions of cell-to-cell apposition. × 9,000.

lucent nonimmunoreactive vesicles. In the guinea pig (92) there was also evidence for other varieties of local circuit interactions, including dendrodendritic and somatodendritic interactions (Fig. 15B), with the GnRH component participating as either the pre- or postsynaptic element.

GnRH synapses have also been observed in the accessory olfactory bulb of the hamster (101), and it is likely that examination of other extrahypothalamic sites will reveal additional evidence for such interactions.

DO GnRH NEURONS CONTAIN OTHER NEUROPEPTIDES OR NEUROTRANSMITTERS?

In GnRH neurons in the preoptic area of the guinea pig, a second peptide that cross-reacts with an antiserum directed against ACTH 17-39 has been identified (102,103). Similarly, beta-endorphin-like immunoreactivity has been reported in human GnRH neurons in both the preoptic area and arcuate nucleus (104). Given the importance of opiate peptides in the regulation of gonadotropin secretion, these observations need to be extended and confirmed. Proof that the proopiomelanocortin gene is transcribed in these cells must await analysis combining *in situ* hybridization and immunocytochemistry (cf. ref. 105). Whether the colocalization of these peptides and GnRH is common to all species is not known.

RELATIONSHIP OF GnRH NEURONS TO ESTRADIOL-CONCENTRATING NEURONS

Gonadal steroids are the major regulatory substances controlling the release of gonadotropins. They also play an essential role during the perinatal period in the development of the anatomical sexual dimorphisms of the CNS, including those that relate to the sex differences in the control of gonadotropin secretion. Presumably these substances act within the CNS as well as at the level of the pituitary via the nuclear receptors visualized by radioautrography. If go-

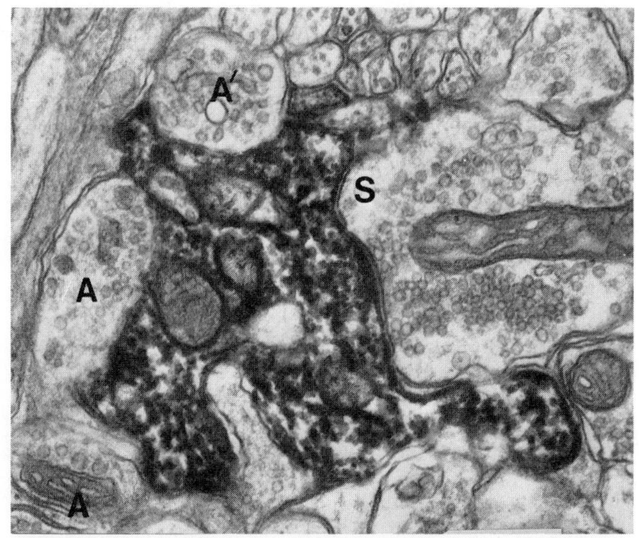

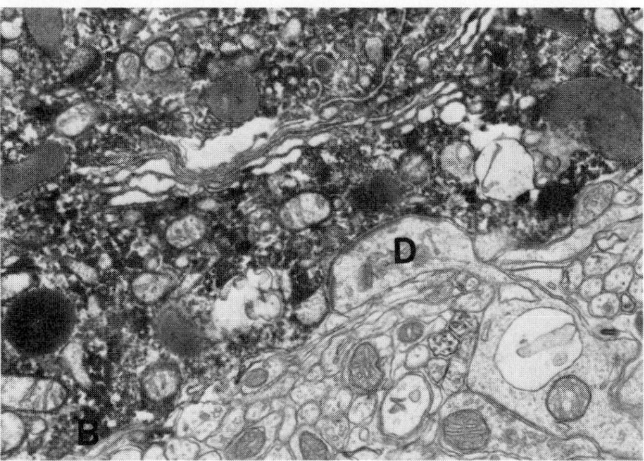

FIG. 15. Two examples of synaptic input to GnRH neurons in the guinea-pig preoptic area. **A** is an axodendritic input (S indicates a presynaptic element). Note the synaptic cleft and the clustering of round, clear synaptic vesicles. Axon profiles (A and A′) cannot be said to be in synaptic contact with the GnRH dendrite, since no synaptic specializations are seen in this plane. × 35,000. In **B**, a dendrosomatic input to a GnRH neuron is illustrated. D indicates the presynaptic non-immunoreactive dendrite. At the dendrosomatic synapse a clear synaptic cleft is present as well as presynaptic membrane thickenings. In this plane, only a few synaptic vesicles are evident. × 15,000.

nadal hormones regulate the synthesis, processing, or release of GnRH within the CNS, one might have predicted that the GnRH neuron would contain estradiol receptors. It was therefore surprising and of considerable interest that in the rat (106) the neurons in the preoptic area that concentrate estradiol (as determined by radioautography following accumulation of [^{3}H]estradiol) and those that contain GnRH do not overlap. Of 435 GnRH cells counted, only one doubly labeled cell was found. This would suggest that regulation of the GnRH neuron by gonadal steroids occurs mainly, if not entirely, via interneurons, adding a layer of complexity to this circuitry.

Colocalization of [^{3}H]estradiol and GnRH was reported in both arcuate and preoptic-area neurons of the fetal guinea pig (107), but these authors did not indicate the frequency of such overlap, so one does not know if this represents a significant population. The photomicrographs presented as data for the double label show immunocytochemical staining that is too pale to permit conclusive identification of the cells as GnRH-containing. A definitive resolution of this problem awaits the application of a monoclonal antibody to the estradiol receptor to localize estradiol-sensitive neurons (108).

CAN IMMUNOCYTOCHEMISTRY BE USED TO EXAMINE CHANGES IN GnRH CONTENT IN NEURONAL STRUCTURES?

Radioimmunoassay can provide a precise quantitative measure of changes in GnRH content in a cytoarchitectonic area. Such procedures cannot, however, determine the neuronal compartment or subset of neurons within which these changes occur. Quantitative anatomical approaches can theoretically add substantially to our understanding of these neuronal networks in animals of differing reproductive status. Can such immunocytochemical procedures be truly quantitative? As will be seen in studies discussed below, immunocytochemistry, when coupled with careful morphometric procedures, can provide quantitative answers to certain questions. However, such data, no matter how consistent and reproducible, present problems in interpretation. Do changes in staining intensity, fiber density, cell number, etc., represent changes in synthesis, processing, or release of the peptide? In many cases, answers to these questions are inferred from physiological data (e.g., LH release), but such inferences may not always be legitimate. Nonetheless, such studies may provide insight into both the development of GnRH systems and their regulation by steroidal and synaptic input.

Development of the GnRH Neuronal Networks

The earliest developing GnRH neurons in both the guinea pig (28) and the rat (62) appear in the nervus terminalis. The onset of synthesis of GnRH in these neurons, as determined by immunocytochemistry (day 28 and day 15, respectively), coincides with the onset of the immunoreactivity for the beta LH subunit, though a causal relationship has not been established. Aubert et al. (109) were able to detect GnRH by radioimmunoassay in the rat brain on day 12 of gestation. These investigators ascribe the immunoreactivity to the hypothalamus; however, whole brain GnRH content was measured at this time point. On fetal day 17, which coincides with the appearance of rat GnRH neurons in the septo-preoptico-hypothalamic continuum (62), Aubert et al. (109) observed the first high-affinity, low-capacity GnRH-receptor sites in the anterior pituitary. The innervation of the median eminence (ME) and of the OVLT [which was initially thought to precede that for the ME (110)] are evident by day 19 of gestation in the rat, whereas in the guinea pig they appear at days 30 and 35, respectively. Whether axons contain the peptide while they are growing toward their target(s) is not known.

The morphology of the GnRH neuron has also been observed to change both during development and with changes in reproductive status. Wray and Hoffman (74) and Wray and Gainer (77) have observed an increase in the proportion of the thorny GnRH cells in the rat through to the pubertal period, after which the ratio of smooth versus thorny stabilizes. Such shifts in population were not observed in the hypothalamic GnRH cells of female rhesus monkeys aged 1 to 25 years (111). Changes in the shape of GnRH cells, as measured by the complexity of branching of the dendritic arbor, were studied quantitatively in anestrous and estrous ewes. Although no statistically significant differences were found, there was clearly a trend toward more complex shapes during the nonbreeding season (25). Since the degree of complexity of the neuronal shape may reflect the complexity of synaptic input, such changes may provide clues to changes in the mechanisms of regulation of these cells at different times in the life history of the animal.

Effects of Sex Steroids on the Anatomy of the GnRH System

Immunocytochemical procedures have also been used to examine the GnRH neuronal networks for sex differences and the effects of gonadectomy and/or steroid treatment in both adults and developing animals. In the perinatal period, there are more GnRH neurons in the male than in the female (15). Treatment on day 2 with estradiol reduced the number of GnRH neurons in the male, but increased them in the female. These investigators also reported differences in the amount of fiber staining in the OVLT and median eminence, but this study, like many preceding it, utilized nonquantitative approaches to the analysis of fiber distribution. More recently, quantitative morphometric techniques using computer image analysis systems and/or optical density recordings have been applied to similar problems (17,55,112). In adult males, gonadectomy decreased (a) the number of GnRH neurons and the intensity with which they stained and (b) the area of the median eminence but not the OVLT that was covered with GnRH fibers (17). In this same study, gonadectomized females were compared to gonadectomized, estrogen-replaced animals. The number of GnRH cells was similar in these two groups, but the density of staining was greater in the steroid-treated animals. Estrogen treatment also increased the area of the median eminence occupied by GnRH axons. Breski et al. (112) compared the concentration of GnRH, as measured by radioimmunoassay, with the volume of the median eminence occupied by GnRH fibers, as measured with quantitative morphometric techniques. Long-term, but not short-term, gonadectomy reduced median eminence staining as well as assayable GnRH.

As stated above, quantification of anatomical material is both laudable and critical to the precision of this science, but problems in interpretation persist. Does decreased perikaryal staining reflect a more rapid egress of GnRH neurosecretory granules into the axon? Is there a change in processing of the GnRH precursor that causes a change in the detectability of the antigen? These and many other questions are still to be addressed.

Although immunocytochemistry has also been used to examine changes in the median eminence during the estrous/menstrual cycle, all reports to date have used qualitative impressions of changes in intensity of staining rather than the quantitative methods cited above. In the squirrel monkey (29,56), the rat (113) and the guinea pig (33,114), there is a maximum of GnRH staining in the median eminence during late diestrus, with a minimum (emptying of fibers?) in the periovulatory period. Such a pattern would suggest (not surprisingly) that there is a periovulatory release of GnRH.

THE *hpg* MOUSE AND THE USE OF CNS IMPLANTS TO REVERSE AN ENDOCRINE DEFICIENCY

The hypogonadal mutant (*hpg*) mouse, discovered at Harwell, England, has an infantile reproductive tract because of a deficiency in GnRH (115). Immunocytochemical analysis has shown that no GnRH neurons are found in the brain of this mutant (116), and data from molecular biology indicate that the defect in the gene results in a deletion in the mRNA of two exons (116a). The absence of GnRH from all brain regions in the *hpg* mouse strongly suggests that in mammals, all of the GnRH immunoreactivity from olfactory bulb caudalward is the decapeptide and is derived from the same gene product. This is in contrast to the amphibian, where CNS GnRH immunoreactivity is the decapeptide, but the material in the sympathetic ganglion (117) is not (118).

The endocrine deficiency of the *hpg* mouse can, at least in part, be overcome in adults by the implantation of normal fetal or neonatal septal-preoptic tissue into the third ventricle. Such a procedure results in the recovery of testicular and seminal vesicle weights and the onset of spermatogenesis in males (119), increased ovarian and uterine weights in females (120), and the ability of females to mate, ovulate following mating, become pregnant, successfully give birth, and nurture their offspring (120,121).

The number of GnRH neurons in the transplants and the distribution of GnRH axons in the hosts displaying these reproductive activities were determined. These immunocytochemical analyses of the transplants have provided astounding information in that reproductive function can be subserved by a very small number of GnRH cells and their axons on the portal capillaries in the median eminence. The cells visualized by immunocytochemistry in females showing postcopulatory ovulations, successful pregnancy, and maternal behavior (121) ranged from one to 16, and immunoreactive fibers were found in the host primarily in the arcuate nucleus and median eminence. Since the studies were carried out on thick sections that exceeded the diameter of the GnRH neuron, it is possible that the number of cells were underestimated by two- to threefold. Even so, such numbers are far fewer than the estimated 500 to 1,500 cells in the septal-preoptic-hypothalamic continuum that innervates the median eminence in normal animals. It is possible that the neurosecretory unit—that minimum number of cells which can support at least some aspects of reproductive function—can be very few in number. The fact that GnRH axons did not innervate any additional targets strongly suggests that only the GnRH in the portal blood is essential for reproduction. Is it possible that in the normal animal, only a very small number of cells at any one time drives the pituitary gonadal axis and that the remainder of cells provide a redundancy that protects the individual in case of neuronal cell death? Do different subpopulations provide for tonic versus bursting release of LH? Such intriguing questions will hopefully be solved by combining anatomical and physiological approaches to the problems of CNS regulation of reproduction.

ACKNOWLEDGMENTS

The research for this chapter as well as the research at my laboratory cited in this chapter have been supported by USPHS grants HD 10665 and NS 20337. I would also like to thank Drs. Joan Witkin and Michael Lehman for critical readings of the manuscript, for providing me with excellent illustrations and micrographs, and for allowing me to cite unpublished work. I would also like to thank Ms. Kate Bock for assistance with the photomicrography.

REFERENCES

1. Amoss, M., Burges, R., Blackwell, R., Vale, W., Fellows, R., and Guillemin, R. (1971): Purification, amino acid composition and *n*-terminus of the hypothalamic luteinizing hormone releasing hormone factor (LRF) of ovine origin. *Biochem. Biophys. Res. Commun.*, 44:205–210.
2. Schally, A. V., Arimura, A., Baker, Y., Nair, R. M. G., Matsuo, H., Redding, T. W., Debeljuk, L., and White, W. F. (1971): Isolation and properties of the FSH and LH-releasing hormone. *Biochem. Biophys. Res. Commun.*, 43:393–399.
3. Matsuo, H., Baba, Y., Nau, R. M. G., Arimura, A., and Schally, A. V. (1971): Structure of the porcine LH and FSH releasing hormone. I. Proposed amino acid sequence. *Biochem. Biophys. Res. Commun.*, 43:1334–1339.
4. Seeburg, P. H., and Adelman, J. P. (1984): Characterization of cDNA for precursor of human luteinizing hormone releasing hormone. *Nature*, 311:666–668.
5. Shiver, B. D., Harlan, R. E., Hejtmancik, J. F., Conn, P. N., and Pfaff, D. W. (1985): Localization of cell containing LHRH-like mRNA in rat brain. *Soc. Neurosci. Abstracts*, 11:143.
6. Sternberger, L. A. (1974): *Immunocytochemistry*, pp. 129–171. Prentice-Hall, Englewood Cliffs, N.J.
7. Barry, J., DuBois, M. P., and Poulain, P. (1973): LRF producing cells of the mammalian hypothalamus. *Z. Zellforsch.*, 146:351–366.
8. Barry, J., DuBois, M. P., Poulain, P., and Leonardelli, J. (1973): Caracterisation et topographie des neurones hypothalamiques immunoréactifs avec des anticorps anti-LRF de synthèse. *C. R. Acad. Sci. (Paris)*, 276:3191–3193.
9. Barry, J. (1976): Immunohistochemical localization of hypothalamic hormones (especially LRF) at the light microscopic level. In: *Hypothalamus and Endocrine Functions*, edited by F. Labrie, J. Meites, and G. Pelletier, pp. 451–471. Plenum Press, New York.
10. Barry, J. (1979): Immunohistochemistry of luteinizing hormone releasing hormone-producing neurons of vertebrates. *Int. Rev. Cytol.*, 60:179–219.
11. Sternberger, L. A., and Hoffman, G. E. (1978): Immunocytology of luteinizing hormone releasing hormone. *Neuroendocrinology*, 25:111–128.
12. Silverman, A. J., Krey, L. C., and Zimmerman, E. A. (1979): A comparative study of the luteinizing hormone releasing hormone (LHRH) neuronal networks in mammals. *Biol. Reprod.*, 20:98–110.
13. Krey, L. C., and Silverman, A. J. (1983): Luteinizing hormone releasing hormone. In: *Brain Peptides*, edited by D. T. Krieger, M. Brownstein, and J. Martin, pp. 687–709. John Wiley & Sons, New York.
14. Setalo, G., Vigh, S., Schally, A. V., Arimura, A., and Flerko, B. (1976): Immunohistological study of the origin of the LHRH containing nerve fibers of the rat hypothalamus. *Brain Res.*, 103:597–602.
15. Elkind-Hirsch, K., King, J. C., Gerall, A. A., and Arimura, A. A. (1981): The luteinizing hormone releasing hormone system in normal and estrogenized neonatal rats. *Brain Res. Bull.*, 7:645–654.
16. Witkin, J. W., Paden, C. M., and Silverman, A. J. (1982): The luteinizing hormone-releasing hormone (LHRH) systems in the rat brain. *Neuroendocrinology*, 35:429–438.
17. Shivers, B. D., Harlan, R. E., Morrell, J. I., and Pfaff, D. W. (1983): Immunocytochemical localization of luteinizing hormone-releasing hormone in male and female rat brains. *Neuroendocrinology*, 36:1–12.
18. Merchanthaler, I., Gorcs, T., Setalo, G., Petrusz, P., and Flerko, B. (1984): Gonadotropin-releasing hormone (GnRH) neurons and pathways in the rat brain. *Cell Tissue Res.*, 237:15–29.
19. King, J. C., Tobet, S. A., Snavely, F. L., and Arimura, A. (1982): LHRH immunopositive cells and their projections to the median eminence and organum vasculosum of the lamina terminalis. *J. Comp. Neurol.*, 209:287–300.
20. Ellinwood, W. K., Ronnekleiv, O. K., Kelly, M. J., and Resko, J. A. (1985): A new antiserum with conformational specificity for LHRH: Usefulness for radioimmunoassay and immunocytochemistry. *Peptides*, 6:45–52.
21. Nemeroff, C. B., Konkol, R. J., Bissette, G., Youngblood, W., Martin, J. B., Brazeau, P., Rone, M. S., Prange, A. J. Jr., Breese, G. R., and Kizer, J. S. (1977): Analysis of the disruption in hypothalamic-pituitary regulation in rats treated neonatally with monosodium L-glutamate (MSG): Evidence for the involvement of tuberoinfundibular cholinergic and dopaminergic systems in neuroendocrine regulation. *Endocrinology*, 101:613–622.
22. Jennes, L., Stumpf, W. E., Bissette, G., and Nemeroff, C. B. (1984): Monosodium glutamate lesions in rat hypothalamus studied by immunohistochemistry for gonadotropin releasing hormone, neurotensin, tyrosine hydroxylase and glutamic acid decarboxylase and by autoradiography for [^{3}H]estradiol. *Brain Res.*, 308:245–253.
23. Jennes, L., and Stumpf, W. E. (1980): LHRH-systems in the brain of the golden hamster. *Cell Tissue Res.*, 209:239–256.
24. Hoffman, G. E., Knigge, K. M., Moynihan, J. A., Nelnyk, V., and Arimura, A. (1978): Neuronal fields containing luteinizing hormone releasing hormone. *Neuroscience*, 3:219–231.
25. Lehman, M. N., Robinson, J., Karsch, F., and Silverman, A. J. (1986): Immunocytochemical localization of luteinizing hormone releasing hormone (LHRH) pathways in sheep brain during anestrus and the mid-luteal phase of the estrous cycle. *J. Comp. Neurol.*, 244:19–35.
26. Barry, J. and DuBois, M. P. (1976): Immunoreactive LRF neurosecretory pathways in mammals. *Acta Anat.*, 94:497–503.
27. Silverman, A. J. (1976): Distribution of luteinizing hormone releasing hormone (LHRH) in the guinea pig brain. *Endocrinology*, 99:30–41.
28. Schwanzel-Fukuda, M., Robinson, J. A., and Silverman, A. J. (1981): The fetal development of the luteinizing hormone releasing hormone

(LHRH) neuronal systems of the guinea pig brain. *Brain Res. Bull.*, 7:293–315.
29. Barry, J. (1979): Immunofluorescence study of the preoptico-terminal LRH tract in the female squirrel monkey during the estrous cycle. *Cell Tissue Res.*, 198:1–13.
30. Silverman, A. J., Antunes, J. L., Abrams, G. M., Nilaver, G., Thau, R., Ferin, M., and Krey, L. C. (1982): The luteinizing hormone releasing hormone pathways in rhesus (Macaca mulatta) and pigtailed (*Macaca nemestrina*) monkeys: New observations on thick, unembedded sections. *J. Comp. Neurol.*, 211:309–317.
31. King, J. C., and Anthony, E. L. P. (1984): LHRH neurons and their projections in humans and other mammals: Species comparisons. *Peptides*, (Suppl. 1):195–207.
32. King, J. C., Anthony, E. L. P., Fitzgerald, D. M., and Stopa, E. G. (1985): LHRH neurons in human preoptic/hypothalamus: Differential intraneuronal localization of immunoreactive forms. *J. Clin. Endocrinol.*, 60:88–97.
33. Barry, J., DuBois, M. P., and Carette, B. (1974): Immunofluorescence study of the preoptico-infundibular LRF neurosecretory pathway in the normal, castrated or testosterone-treated male guinea pig. *Endocrinology*, 95:1416–1423.
34. Hoffman, G. E., and Gibbs, F. P. (1982): LHRH pathways in rat brain: 'Deafferentation' spares a sub-chiasmatic LHRH projection to the median eminence. *Neuroscience*, 7:1979–1993.
35. Merchanthaler, I., Kovacs, G., and Setalo, G. (1980): The preoptico-infundibular LHRH tract of the rat. *Brain Res.*, 198:63–74.
36. Silverman, A. J., and Krey, L. C. (1978): The luteinizing hormone releasing hormone (LHRH) neuronal networks of the guinea brain. I. Intra- and extra-hypothalamic projections. *Brain Res.*, 157:233–246.
37. Kawano, H., and Daikoku, S. (1981): Immunohistochemical demonstration of LHRH neurons and their pathways in the rat hypothalamus. *Neuroendocrinology*, 32:179–186.
38. Kozlowski, G. P., and Coates, P. W. (1985): Ependymoneuronal specializations between LHRH fibers and cells of the cerebroventricular system. *Cell Tissue Res.*, 242:301–311.
39. Anthony, E. L. P., King, J. C., and Stopa, E. G. (1984): Immunocytochemical localization of LHRH in the median eminence, infundibular stalk and neurohypophysis. Evidence for multiple sites of releasing hormone secretion in humans and other mammals. *Cell Tissue Res.*, 236:5–14.
40. Coen, C., Howe, P. R. C., and C. DeLanerolle, N. (1985): Immunohistochemical evidence for a subchiasmatic pathway containing luteinizing hormone releasing hormone, somatostatin, neuropeptide Y and tyrosine hydroxylase. *Soc. Neurosci. Abstracts*, 11:351.
41. Liposits, Z., Nagy, L., and Setalo, G. (1982): Frontal deafferentation of the mediobasal hypothalamus in the neonatal rat and its effects on the preoptico-infundibular LHRH-tract. *Cell Tissue Res.*, 225:179–187.
42. Brownstein, M. J., Arimura, A., Palkovits, M., Kizer, J. S., and Schally, A. V. (1976): The effect of surgical isolation of the hypothalamus on its luteinizing hormone releasing hormone content. *Endocrinology*, 98:662–665.
43. Setalo, G., Vigh, S., Schally, A. V., Arimura, A., and Flerko, B. (1976): Immunohistological study of the origin of LHRH-containing nerve fibers of the rat hypothalamus. *Brain Res.*, 103:597–602.
44. Ibata, Y., Watanabe, K., Konishita, H., Kubo, S., and Sano, Y. (1979): The location of LHRH neurons in the rat hypothalamus and their pathways to the median eminence. Experimental immunohistochemistry and radioimmunoassay. *Cell Tissue Res.*, 198:381–395.
45. Wise, P. M., Rance, N., Selmanoff, M., and Barraclough, C. A. (1981): Changes in radioimmunoassayable luteinizing hormone releasing hormone in discrete brain areas of the rat at various times on proestrus, diestrous day 1, and after phenobarbital administration. *Endocrinology*, 108:2179–2185.
46. Krey, L. C., Butler, W. R., and Knobil, E. (1975): Surgical disconnection of the medial basal hypothalamus and pituitary function in the rhesus monkey. I. Gonadotropin secretion. *Endocrinology*, 96:1073–1087.
47. Krey, L. C., and Silverman, A. J. (1978): The luteinizing hormone releasing hormone (LHRH) neuronal networks of the guinea pig brain. II. The regulation of gonadotropin secretion and the origin of terminals in the median eminence. *Brain Res.*, 157:247–255.
48. Krey, L. C., and Silverman, A. J. (1981): The luteinizing hormone releasing hormone (LHRH) neuronal networks of the guinea pig brain. III. The regulation of cyclic gonadotropin secretion. *Brain Res.*, 229:429–444.
49. Silverman, A. J., Jamandas, J., and Renaud, L. P. (1987): Localization of LHRH neurons that project to the median eminence. *J. Neurosci.*, 7:2312–2319.
50. Jennes, L., and Stumpf, W. E. (1986): GnRH immunoreactive neurons with access to fenestrated capillaries in mouse brain. *Neuroscience*, 18:403–416.
50a. Lehman, M. N., Winans-Newman, S., and Silverman, A. J. (1987): Luteinizing hormone releasing hormone (LHRH) in the vomeronasal system and terminal nerve of the hamster. *Ann. N.Y. Acad. Sci. (in press)*.
50b. Koves, K., and Molnar, J. (1986): Effects of various hypothalamic deafferentations injuring different parts of the GnRH pathway on ovulation, GnRH content of the median eminence and plasma LH and FSH levels. *Neuroendocrinology*, 44:172–183.
51. Goldsmith, P. C., and Ganong, W. F. (1975): Ultrastructural localization of luteinizing hormone releasing hormone in the median eminence of the rat. *Brain Res.*, 97:181–193.
52. Silverman, A. J., and Desnoyers, P. (1976): Ultrastructural immunocytochemical localization of LHRH in the median eminence of the guinea pig. *Cell Tissue Res.*, 169:157–166.
53. Krisch, B. (1978): The distribution of LHRH in the hypothalamus of the thirsting rat. A light and electron microscopic immunocytochemical study. *Cell Tissue Res.*, 186:135–148.
54. Hatton, G. I., Perlmutter, L. S., Salm, A. K., and Tweedle, C. D. (1984): Dynamic neuronal-glial interactions in hypothalamus and pituitary: Implications for control of hormone synthesis and release. *Peptides*, 5(Suppl. 1):121–138.
55. Rothfield, J. M., and Gross, D. S. (1985): GnRH within the organum vasculosum of the lamina terminalis in ovariectomized, estrogen/progesterone treated rat: Quantitative immunocytochemical study using image analysis. *Brain Res.*, 338:309–315.
56. Barry, J., and Croix, D. (1978): Immunofluorescence study of the hypothalamo-infundibular LRH tract and serum gonadotropin levels in the female squirrel monkey during the estrous cycle. *Cell Tissue Res.*, 192:215–226.
57. Samson, W. K., and McCann, S. M. (1979): Effects of lesions in the organum vasculosum lamina terminalis on the hypothalamic distribution of luteinizing hormone releasing hormone and gonadotropin secretion in the ovariectomized rat. *Endocrinology*, 105:939–946.
58. Leonardelli, J., and Poulain, P. (1977): About a ventral LHRH preoptico-amygdaloid pathway in the guinea pig. *Brain Res.*, 124:538–543.
59. Jennes, L., and Stumpf, W. E. (1980): LHRH neuronal projections to the inner and outer surfaces of the brain. *Neurosci. Lett.*, 2:241–246.
60. Schwanzel-Fukuda, M., and Silverman, A. J. (1980): The nervus terminalis of the guinea pig: A new luteinizing hormone releasing hormone neuronal system. *J. Comp. Neurol.*, 191:213–225.
61. Witkin, J. W., and Silverman, A. J. (1983): Luteinizing hormone releasing hormone (LHRH) in rat olfactory systems. *J. Comp. Neurol.*, 218:426–432.
62. Schwanzel-Fukuda, M., Morrell, J. I., and Pfaff, D. W. (1985): Ontogenesis of neurons producing luteinizing hormone releasing hormone in the nervus terminalis of the rat. *J. Comp. Neurol.*, 238:348–364.
63. Wirsig, C. R., and Leonard, C. M. (1986): The terminal nerve projects centrally in the hamster. *Neuroscience*, 19:709–718.
64. Demsky, L. S., and Northcutt, R. G. (1983): The terminal nerve: A new chemosensory system in vertebrates? *Science*, 220:435–437.
65. Springer, A. D. (1982): Centrifugal innervation of goldfish retina from ganglion cells of the nervus terminalis. *J. Comp. Neurol.*, 214:404–415.
66. Munz, H., Claas, B., Stumpf, W. E., and Jennes, L. (1982): Centrifugal innervation of the retina by luteinizing hormone releasing hormone (LHRH)-immunoreactive telencephalic neurons in teleostean fishes. *Cell Tissue Res.*, 222:313–323.
67. Demski, L. S., Dluka, J. G., and Northcutt, R. G. (1982): Chemosensory control of spawning mechanism in goldfish. *Soc. Neurosci. Abstracts*, 8:611.

68. Stell, W. K., Walker, S. E., Chohan, K. S., and Ball, A. K. (1984): The goldfish nervus terminalis: A luteinizing hormone releasing hormone and molluscan cardioexcitatory peptide immunoreactive olfactoretinal pathway. *Proc. Natl. Acad. Sci. USA,* 81:940–944.
69. Wirsig, C. R., and Leonard, C. (1985): Terminal nerve damage affects hamster mating behavior. *Assoc. Chemoreception Sci. Abstract VII,* No. 184.
70. Wysocki, C. J. (1979): Neurobehavioral evidence for the involvement of the vomernasal system in mammalian reproduction. *Neurosci. Biobehav. Rev.,* 3:301–342.
71. Witkin, J. W. (1985): Luteinizing hormone releasing hormone in olfactory bulbs of primates. *Am. J. Primatol.,* 8:309–315.
72. Dluizen, D. E., Ramirez, V. D., Carter, C. S., and Getz, L. L. (1981): Male vole urine changes LHRH and norepinephrine in female olfactory bulb. *Science,* 212:573–575.
73. Krisch, B. (1980): Two types of luliberin-immunoreactive perikarya in the preoptic area of the rat. *Cell Tissue Res.,* 212:443–455.
74. Wray, S., and Hoffman, G. (1986): Postnatal morphological changes in rat LHRH neurons correlated with sexual maturity. *Neuroendocrinology,* 43:93–97.
75. Jennes, L., Stumpf, W. E., and Sheedy, M. E. (1985): Ultrastructural characterization of gonadotropin-releasing hormone (GnRH)-producing neurons. *J. Comp. Neurol.,* 232:534–547.
76. Liposits, Zs., Setalo, Gy., and Flerko, B. (1984): Application of the silver-gold intensified 3,3′-diaminobenzidine chromagen to the light and electron microscopic detection of the luteinizing hormone releasing hormone system of the rat brain. *Neuroscience,* 13:513–525.
77. Wray, S., and Gainer, H. (1985): Post-natal development of "smooth" and "spiny" LHRH cells: Effect of neonatal gonadectomy. *Soc. Neurosci. Abstracts,* 11:901.
78. Kozlowski, G. P., Chu, L., Hostetter, G., and Kerdelhue, B. (1980): Cellular characteristics of immunolabeled luteinizing hormone releasing hormone (LHRH) neurons. *Peptides,* 1:37–46.
79. Silverman, A. J., Zimmerman, E. A., Kokoris, G. J., and Gibson, M. J. (1986): Ultrastructure of GnRH neuronal structures derived from normal fetal preoptic area and transplanted into hypogonadal mutant (hpg) mice. *J. Neurosci.,* 6:2090–2096.
80. Lehman, M. N., and Silverman, A. J. (1985): Ultrastructure of LHRH neurons in intact and castrate male hamsters. *Soc. Neurosci. Abstracts,* 11:351.
81. King, J. C., and Anthony, E. L. P. (1983): Biosynthesis of LHRH: Inferences from immunocytochemical studies. *Peptides,* 4:963–970.
82. Marshall, P. E., and Goldsmith, P. C. (1980): Neuroregulatory and neuroendocrine GnRH pathways in the hypothalamus and forebrain of the baboon. *Brain Res.,* 193:353–372.
83. Witkin, J. W., and Silverman, A. J. (1985): Synaptology of LHRH neurons in rat preoptic area. *Peptides,* 6:263–271.
84. Leranth, C., Seguraum, L. M. G., Palkovits, M., MacLusky, N. J., Shanabrough, M., and Naftolin, F. (1985): The LH-RH containing neuronal network in the preoptic area of the rat: Demonstration of LH-RH containing nerve terminals in synaptic contact with LHRH neurons. *Brain Res.,* 345:332–336.
85. Wilson, R. C., Kesner, J. S., Kaufman, J. M., Uemura, T., Akena, T., and Knobil, E. (1984): Central electrophysiologic correlates of pulsatile LH secretion in the rhesus monkey. *Neuroendocrinology,* 39:256–260.
86. Pelletier, G., Labrie, F., Puviani, R., Arimura, A., and Schally, A. V. (1974): Immunohistochemical localization of luteinizing hormone releasing hormone in the rat median eminence. *Endocrinology,* 95:554–558.
87. Bugnon, G., Bloch, B., Lenys, D., and Fellmann, D. (1977): Ultrastructural study of LHRH containing neurons in the human fetus. *Brain Res.,* 137:175–180.
88. Mazzuca, M. (1977): Immunocytochemical and ultrastructural identification of luteinizing hormone releasing hormone (LH-RH) containing neurons in the vascular organ of the lamina terminalis (OVLT) of the squirrel monkey. *Neurosci. Lett.,* 5:123–127.
89. Pelletier, G., LeClerc, R., Dube, D., Arimura, A., and Schally, A. C. (1977): Immunohistochemical localization of LHRH and somatostatin in the organum vasculosum of the lamina terminalis of the rat. *Neurosci. Lett.,* 4:27–31.
90. Krisch, B., and Leonhardt, H. (1980): Luliberin and somatostatin fiber terminals in the subfornical organ of the rat. *Cell Tissue Res.,* 210:33–45.
91. Hisano, S., Kawano, H., Maki, Y., and Daikoku, S. (1981): Electron microscopic study of immunoreactive perikarya with special reference to neuronal regulation. *Cell Tissue Res.,* 220:511–518.
92. Silverman, A. J., and Witkin, J. W. (1985): Synaptic interactions of LHRH neurons in the guinea pig preoptic area. *J. Histochem. Cytochem.,* 33:66–72.
92a. Witkin, J. W. (1987): Ageing changes in synaptology of LHRH neurons in male rat preoptic area. *Neuroscience (in press).*
93. Jennes, L., Stumpf, W. E., and Tappaz, M. L. (1983): Anatomical relationships of dopaminergic and GABAergic systems with the GnRH-systems in the septo-hypothalamic area. *Exp. Brain Res.,* 50:91–99.
94. Hoffman, G. E., Wray, S., and Goldstein, M. (1982): Relationship of catecholamines and LHRH: Light microscopic study. *Brain Res. Bull.,* 9:417–430.
95. Hoffman, G. E. (1985): Organization of LHRH cells: Differential apposition of neurotensin, substance P and catecholamine axons. *Peptides,* 6:439–461.
96. Palkovits, M., Leranth, C., Jew, J. Y., and Williams, T. (1982): Simultaneous characterization of pre- and postsynaptic neuron contact sites in brain. *Proc. Natl. Acad. Sci. USA,* 79:2705–2708.
97. Kiss, J., and Halasz, B. (1985): Demonstration of serotonergic axons terminating on luteinizing hormone-releasing hormone neurons in the preoptic area of the rat using a combination of immunocytochemistry and high resolution autoradiography. *Neuroscience,* 14:69–78.
98. Williams, A. (1969): The assessment of electron microscopic autoradiograms. *Adv. Opt. Microsc.,* 3:219–229.
99. Leranth, C., MacLusky, N. J., Sakamoto, H., Ganabrough, M., and Naftolin, F. (1985): Glutamic acid decarboxylase containing axons synapse on LHRH neurons in the rat medial preoptic area. *Neuroendocrinology,* 40:536–539.
100. Silverman, A. J. (1984): Luteinizing hormone releasing hormone containing synapses in the diagonal band and preoptic area of the guinea pig. *J. Comp. Neurol.,* 227:452–458.
101. Phillips, H. S., Ho, B. T., and Linner, J. G. (1982): Ultrastructural localization of LHRH immunoreactive synapses in the hamster accessory olfactory bulb. *Brain Res.,* 246:193–204.
102. Tramu, G., Leonardelli, J., and DuBois, M. P. (1977): Immunohistochemical evidence for an ACTH-like substance in hypothalamic LHRH neurons. *Neurosci. Lett.,* 6:305–309.
103. Beauvillain, J. C., Tramu, G., and DuBois, M. P. (1981): Ultrastructural immunocytochemical evidence of the presence of a peptide related to ACTH in granules of LHRH nerve terminals in the median eminence of the guinea pig. *Cell Tissue Res.,* 218:1–6.
104. Leonardelli, J., and Tramu, G. (1979): Immunoreactivity for b-endorphin in LHRH neurons of the fetal human hypothalamus. *Cell Tissue Res.,* 203:201–207.
105. Wolfson, B., Manning, R. W., Davis, L. G., Arentzen, R., and Baldwin, F. Jr. (1985): Colocalization of CRF and VP mRNA in neurons after adrenalectomy. *Nature,* 315:59–61.
106. Shivers, B. D., Harlan, R. E., Morrell, J. I., and Pfaff, D. W. (1983): Absence of oestradiol concentration in cell nuclei of LHRH immunoreactive neurones. *Nature,* 304:345–347.
107. Tardy, J., and Pasqualini, J. R. (1983): Localization of [^{3}H] estradiol and gonadotropin releasing hormone (GnRH) in the hypothalamus of the fetal guinea pig. *Exp. Brain Res.,* 49:77–83.
108. Press, M. F., Nousek-Goebl, N. A., and Greene, G. L. (1985): Immunoelectron microscopic localization of estradiol receptor with a monoclonal estrophilin antibody. *J. Histochem. Cytochem.,* 33:915–924.
109. Aubert, M. L., Bigeat, M., Winiger, B. P., Morel, G., Sizonenko, P. C., and Dubois, P. M. (1985): Ontogeny of hypothalamic gonadotropin releasing hormone (GnRH) and pituitary GnRH receptors in fetal and neonatal rat. *Endocrinology,* 116:1565–1576.
110. Watanabe, K. (1980): Regional differences in the development of LHRH nerve endings in rat. *Endocrinology,* 106:133–144.
111. Witkin, J. W. (1986): Luteinizing hormone releasing hormone (LHRH) neurons in aging female rhesus macaques. *Neurobiol. Aging,* 7:259–263.
112. Briski, K. P., Baker, B. L., and Christensen, A. K. (1983): Effect of ovariectomy on the hypothalamic content of immunoreactive gonadotropin releasing hormone in female mouse as revealed by quantitative immunocytochemistry and radioimmunoassay. *Am. J. Anat.,* 166:187–208.
113. Kobayashi, R. M., Lu, K. H., Moore, R. Y., and Yen, S. S. C. (1978): Regional distribution of hypothalamic LHRH in proestrous

rats: Effects of ovariectomy and of estrogen replacement. *Endocrinology,* 102:98–105.

114. Barry, J., and DuBois, P. M. (1974): Immunofluorescence study of the preoptico-infundibular LHRH neurosecretory pathway of the guinea pig during the estrous cycle. *Neuroendocrinology,* 15: 200–208.
115. Cattanach, H. M., Iddon, C. A., Charlton, H. M., Chiappa, S. A., and Fink, G. (1977): Gonadotropin-releasing hormone deficiency in a mutant mouse with hypogonadism. *Nature,* 269:338–340.
116. Silverman, A. J., Zimmerman, E. A., Gibson, M. J., Perlow, M. J., Charlton, H. M., and Krieger, D. T. (1985): Implantation of normal fetal preoptic area into hypogonadal mutant mice: Temporal relationships of the growth of gonadotropin-releasing hormone neurons and the development of the pituitary/testicular axis. *Neuroscience,* 16:69–84.

116a. Mason, A. J., Hayflick, J. S., Zoeller, R. T., Young, W. S., Phillips, H. S., Nikoliks, K., and Seeburg, P. (1986): A deletion truncating the GnRH gene is responsible for hypogonadism in the hpg mouse. *Science,* 234:1366–1371.

117. Jan, Y. N., Jan, L. Y., and Kuffler, S. W. (1979): A peptide as a possible transmitter in sympathetic ganglia of the frog. *Proc. Natl. Acad. Sci. USA,* 76:1501–1505.
118. Eiden, L. E., and Eskay, R. L. (1980): Characterization of LRF-like immunoreactivity in the frog sympathetic ganglia: Non-identify with LRF decapeptide. *Neuropeptides,* 1:29–37.
119. Krieger, D. T., Perlow, M. J., Gibson, M. J., Davies, D. T., Zimmerman, E. A., Ferin, M., and Charlton, H. M. (1982): Brain grafts reverse hypogonadism of gonadotropin releasing hormone deficiency. *Nature,* 298:1–3.
120. Gibson, M. J., Perlow, M. J., Charlton, H. M., Zimmerman, E. A., Davies, T. F., and Krieger, D. T. (1984): Preoptic area brain grafts in hypogonadal (hpg) female mice abolish effects of congenital hypothalamic gonadotropin releasing hormone (GnRH) deficiency. *Endocrinology,* 114:1938–1940.
121. Gibson, M. J., Krieger, D. T., Charlton, H. M., Zimmerman, E. A., Silverman, A. J., and Perlow, M. J. (1984): Mating and pregnancy can occur in genetically hypogonadal mice with preoptic area brain grafts. *Science,* 225:949–951.

The Physiology of Reproduction,
edited by E. Knobil and J. Neill *et al.*
Raven Press, Ltd., New York © 1988.

CHAPTER 30

Lactotropes and Gonadotropes

Claude Tougard and Andrée Tixier-Vidal

Lactotropes and gonadotropes are two glandular cell types of the anterior pituitary which are specialized for the synthesis and release of three hormones that play key roles in the physiology of reproduction: a protein hormone, called prolactin (PRL), and two glycoprotein hormones, known as luteinizing hormone (LH) and follicle-stimulating hormone (FSH). The study of these cells involves three objectives: (i) to localize, within a heterogeneous glandular tissue, the cells that are responsible for the secretion of each of these hormones; (ii) to follow their morphological modifications in relation to the control of reproduction; and (iii) to analyze, at the cellular and subcellular levels, the mechanisms involved in the secretion and release of these hormones. This review has been organized with these three objectives in mind and is limited to studies performed on mammals. For studies involving the other classes of vertebrates, the readers may refer to ref. 1.

The elucidation of the cellular origin of PRL, LH, and FSH was lengthy and particularly difficult to attain because of the functional and structural heterogeneity of the anterior pituitary gland. It took 50 years of research to solve this problem, and the studies over this time period followed three successive steps. First, cytologists described several classes of cells at the light-microscopic level, on the basis of tinctorial affinities (2) and cytochemical properties, and attributed to each of them a functional significance using histophysiological indirect correlations (see refs. 3 and 4 for reviews). Then the use of conventional electron microscopy, which originated with the pioneering work of Farquhar and Rinehart (5), helped to establish the ultrastructural characteristics of such presumptive cell types and to describe their functional changes at the subcellular level [see reviews by Herlant (3,4) and Farquhar et al. (6)]. However, the usefulness of electron-microscope criteria to identify the cell types was questionable in light of findings obtained by the third, most conclusive, approach: immunocytochemistry. Indeed, progress in the chemistry and purification of anterior pituitary hormones, together with the preparation of specific antibodies and the technical improvements of immunocytochemistry at the light- and electron-microscopic levels, allowed the assignment of a specific hormonal function, with better accuracy than before (7–9), to each cell type. However, it should be noted that the identifications formerly proposed by conventional methods were often confirmed with the advent of immunocytochemistry.

These three approaches clearly revealed that, depending on the physiological and pathological situations, the number, size, shape, staining affinities, intensity of immunostaining, and ultrastructural features greatly vary. Such variations, together with the use of sophisticated methods such as high-resolution autoradiography and electron-microscopic immunocytochemistry, have permitted access to the understanding of the secretory pathway and its regulation. Moreover, this was favored by the development of anterior pituitary cell cultures, which offered simplified situations in which to analyze the direct effect of a single agent and to correlate morphological data to hormonal secretion. Such a reductionist approach, however, does not represent an end in itself, but rather a necessary step toward the understanding of the highly integrated events involved at the pituitary level in the physiology of reproduction.

MORPHOLOGICAL FEATURES AND FUNCTIONAL SIGNIFICANCE

Lactotropes

Identification and Morphological Heterogeneity

The identification of PRL cells in the anterior pituitary tissue was first performed at the light-microscopic level as a result of their affinity for erythrosine following Herlant's tetrachrome (3) and then confirmed by immunocytochemistry using specific antibodies in the rat (7,10), the mouse (11), and the human (12–14), as well as in several other mammalian species (1). In the rat, PRL-containing cells are sparsely distributed in the lateroventral portion of anterior lobe and are present near the pars intermedia (7). Their shape and size are heterogeneous. They are frequently angular or polyhedral but are sometimes oval, rounded, and small. In the rat, "cup cells" with long cytoplasmic processes have been shown to surround gonadotropes (7,15). The number of PRL cells greatly varies in a given species, depending on the physiological situation and on the method used to determine their number (see below).

At the electron-microscopic level the identification of PRL cells was first based on cytophysiological studies using conventional electron-microscopic methods. They were characterized by a well-developed rough endoplasmic reticulum (RER), a large Golgi zone, and large polymorphic secretory granules, at least in the rat (16,17) and in the human (3,16,18). The advent of immunoelectron-microscopic methods (7,9) confirmed such identification (Fig. 1) but also emphasized the risk of identifying PRL cells using ultrastructural criteria only, without the help of immunocytochemistry. Indeed, the presence of polymorphic secretory granules as a criterion to identify lactotropes was reconsidered in light of the electron-microscopic immunocytochemical findings. For example, in the same species (the rat), PRL secretory granules are sometimes spherical and of variable diameter (130–300 nm) (Fig. 2). Moreover, in the same pituitary gland, some PRL cells may contain only small rounded secretory granules, whereas others contain either large polymorphic granules or a mixed population of granules (19,20) (Figs. 1–3). Such diversity, which could not be related to a cell shape, has helped to distinguish three types of PRL cells in the rat pituitary: type I, having small spherical granules (130–200 nm in diameter); type II, having medium-sized spherical or polymorphic granules (250–300 nm in diameter); and type III, having large polymorphic granules (up to 700 nm in diameter) (15,21). A diversity in the shape and size of secretory granules was also observed in other mammalian species, such as the guinea-pig pituitary (22) and the bovine and porcine pituitaries (23,24). The functional meaning of

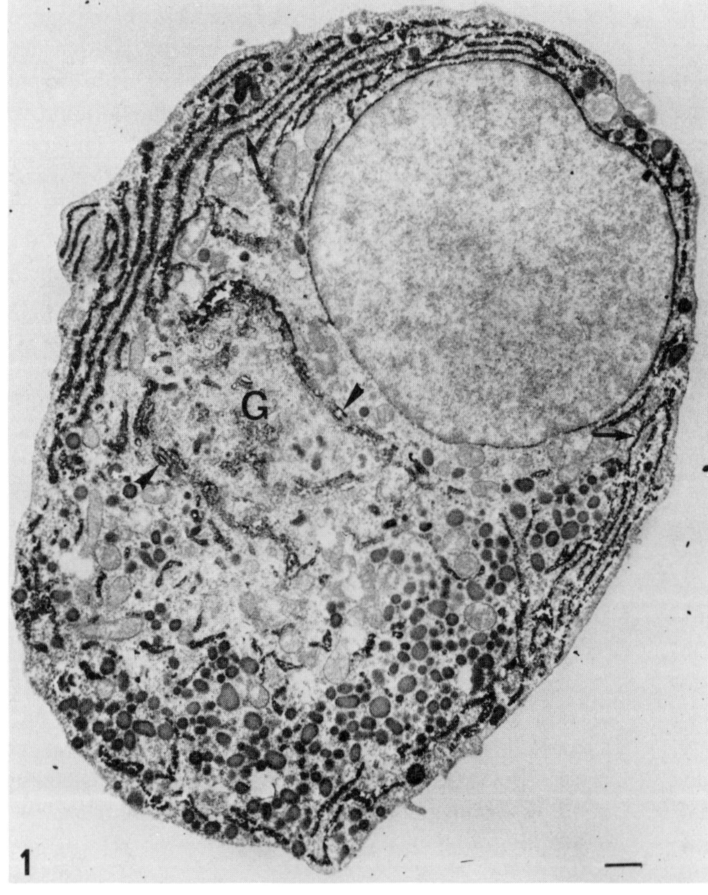

FIG. 1. A lactotrope in a primary culture of dispersed rat anterior pituitary cells is immunochemically stained with an antiserum against rat PRL using a preembedding immunoperoxidase method. This immunoreactive cell is characterized by flattened and parallel RER cisternae (*arrows*), a large Golgi zone (G), and polymorphic secretory granules. PRL is detected within RER cisternae and Golgi saccules (*arrowheads*). With this method, the large secretory granules are only outlined with reaction product. Bar represents 1 μm. × 5,500.

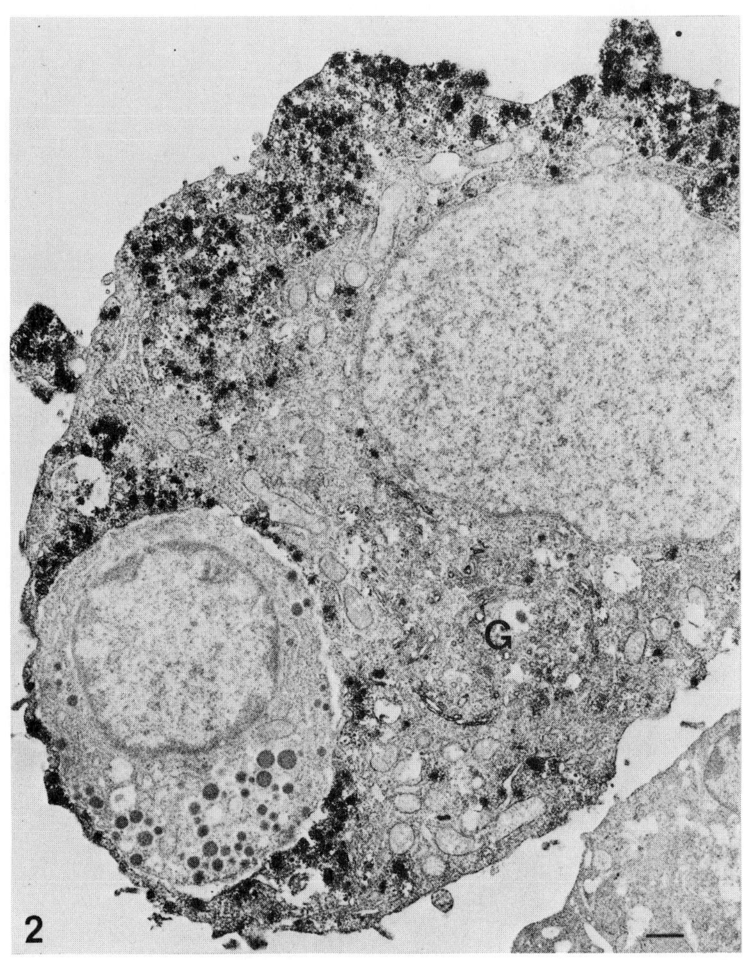

FIG. 2. Same material as Fig. 1. This immunoreactive PRL cell is characterized by its small and rounded secretory granules, which are strongly labeled. (G) Golgi zone. Bar represents 1μm. × 5,500.

the morphological heterogeneity of PRL cells is discussed later on in this chapter (see section on functional heterogeneity of lactotropes).

Distinction from Somatotropes

The fact that PRL and GH are each secreted by a different cell type was clearly established through the use of immunocytochemistry and by the availability of antisera specific for each of these two hormones in several species: the rat (7,8,10), the mouse (11), the human (12,14,25), the cow (23), the monkey (26), the guinea pig (22), and the pig (24). These methods confirmed previous conclusions based on the selective affinity of GH cells for Orange G and of PRL cells for erythrosine (see ref. 3). At the light-microscope level, GH cells differ from lactotropes mostly by their ovoid or rounded shape. They are generally more numerous than lactotropes, and, at least in the rat, they are similarly distributed, except near the intermediate lobe, where they are rarely found (7). At the electron-microscopic level the identification previously proposed by cytophysiological studies (see ref. 3) was confirmed by immunocytochemical methods (7,8). Like PRL cells, they possess a well-developed endoplasmic reticulum, but their secretory granules are always rounded and with an average diameter of 300 to 350 nm.

However, the existence of mixed cells containing both PRL and GH remains controversial in the case of pituitary adenomas of the rat and the human being, as well as for rat GH3 cell lines that derive from a rat mammosomatotropic tumor (27). The controversy originated from functional observations showing a frequent association of hyperprolactinemia with acromegaly. Similarly, most of the subclones of the GH cell lines produce both PRL and GH in variable amounts, depending on the clones and the culture conditions. However, the attempt to colocalize GH and PRL in the same cells either failed or was considered doubtful or controversial because of technical limitations (27). Convincing data concerning human pituitary adenomas were recently reported by Halmi (28), who showed, at the light-microscopic level using double immunostaining of individual sections or comparison of adjacent sections, a "partial to almost complete identity of the cell populations containing GH and PRL" in 5 of 6 human somatotropic pituitary adenomas. In contrast, Trouillas et al. (29) found such a colocalization in only one tumor.

Regarding "normal" nontumoral pituitaries, the existence of cells containing both PRL and GH was again recently

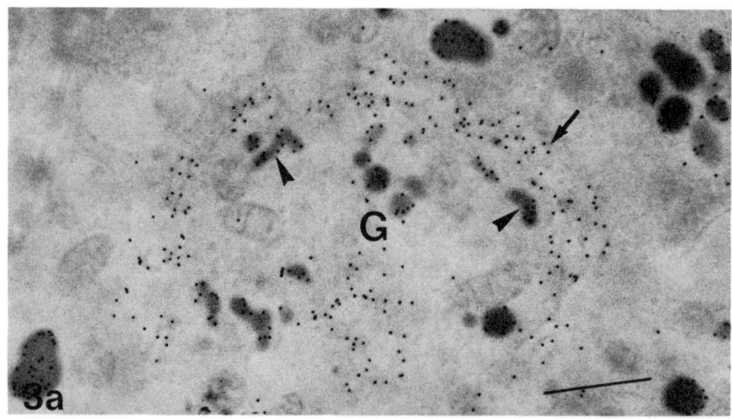

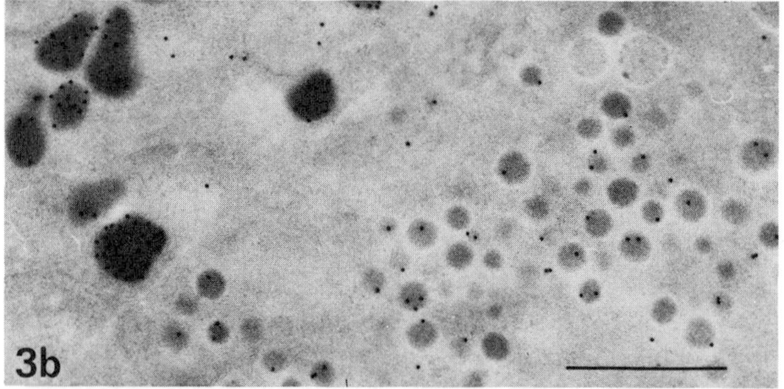

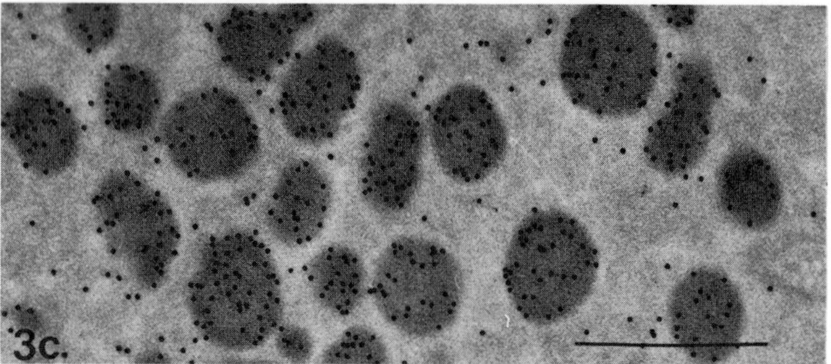

FIG. 3. Details of lactotropes of normal male rat pituitary immunochemically stained with an antiserum against rat PRL using a postembedding method (embedding in Lowicryl) and protein-A–gold complex (15 nm gold). (Courtesy of Dr. E. Vila-Porcile.) (**a**) Detail of a Golgi zone (G). With this method, PRL is detected within all Golgi saccules (*arrows*) and on newly formed secretory granules (*arrowheads*). Bar represents 1 μm. × 17,000. (**b**) The secretory granules of two adjacent lactotropes are immunolabeled. One cell contains large polymorphous secretory granules, whereas the other contains small rounded secretory granules. Bar represents 1 μm. × 24,000. (**c**) High magnification of the large polymorphous secretory granules that display, with this method, a strong immunostaining. Bar represents 1 μm. × 27,200.

put forward. Fumagalli and Zanini (30), using double immunostaining with specific antibodies and protein-A gold particles of different sizes, found in the bovine pituitary a population of multinucleated cells containing both PRL and GH. In these somatomammotropic cells, PRL and GH were mostly localized in separate granules, although the coexistence of the two hormones in the same granules was observed in a few cells. The authors mentioned that these mutinucleated mammosomatotropes, which they described, for the first time, in a lactating cow, were also present in a virgin cow, but in lower number. The fact that such dual cells were not found by Dacheux and Dubois in the same species (23) suggests that they might represent a minor population, the proportion of which may depend on the functional state. In the rat, contradictory results were reported depending on the authors, although the same immunogold method but different antibodies were used. PRL and GH were colocalized in the same granules of PRL cells by Papka et al. (31), whereas Smets et al. (32) could not find PRL and GH in the same cells.

From a functional point of view the hemolytic plaque assay method of Neill and Frawley (33) allows the analysis of hormone release at the individual cell level and provides another approach to the problem of the dual-versus-separate origin of GH and PRL. However, the data reported so far are partially controversial. The existence of a minor proportion of mammosomatotropes (5%) in adult Sprague-Dawley male and female rat pituitaries was deduced from careful statistical studies and was found only in the presence of hGRF (34). On the other hand, Frawley et al. (35), using a sequential plaque assay, observed a far greater proportion of mammosomatotropes in adult Holtzman male rat pituitaries, where they represented one-third of GH and/or PRL secretors; this was confirmed by double immunostaining of cells treated with dopamine.

In conclusion, the present state of the literature indicates that PRL and GH are, in most cases, stored in, and released from, separate cell types. However, one should keep in mind that, depending on the pathological and possibly physiological situation, both hormones can be secreted by the same cell. This may reflect an interconversion from one cell type to the other as speculated by Stratman et al. (36) in the normal rat pituitary, as well as by Boockfor et al. (37) for GH3 cells. This might also represent variations in the respective level of expression of the two genes which would be switched on in the same cells. In that respect it is worth mentioning that PRL and GH genes are believed to derive from a common ancestral gene (38) and are subject to reciprocal controls. However, Nelson et al. (39) have recently reported that the cell-specific expression of the GH and PRL genes appears to be controlled by structurally distinct cis-active sequences. Progress in the analysis of the cellular and molecular mechanisms involved in the storage and secretion of PRL and GH, respectively, is needed to clarify this intriguing question.

Subcellular Distribution of PRL Immunostaining. Relationship to Secretory Pathway

PRL cells have been often used as an archetype to analyze the secretory process in anterior pituitary cells (40–42). In particular, quantitative electron-microscopic autoradiographic studies performed on cultured mammotropes (43,44) have shown that the newly synthesized proteins undergo an intracellular transit analogous to that primarily established for the exocrine pancreas (45), involving the following steps: (a) synthesis on attached polysomes and transfer into the RER, (b) concentration and packaging into membrane-bound secretory granules in the Golgi zone, (c) storage in mature secretory granules, and (d) extracellular discharge of secretory granules by exocytosis or, alternatively, intracellular degradation of secretory granules in excess following their fusion with lysosomes. However, the chemical nature of the intraluminal secretory product could only be determined by electron-microscope immunocytochemistry.

In fact, the results greatly vary depending on the technical conditions (postembedding versus preembedding, fixative permeabilization). In most cases, and whatever the technical conditions, the staining was observed on secretory granules, whatever their size or shape (Fig. 3). In contrast, the immunocytochemical detection of PRL within the RER cisternae and Golgi saccules and vesicles could be achieved only with the preembedding method and with the aid of permeabilizing agents in primary cultures of rat pituitary cells (19) (Fig. 4) and in GH3 cells (46) (Fig. 5). Similar results were observed in PRL cells *in vivo,* without the aid

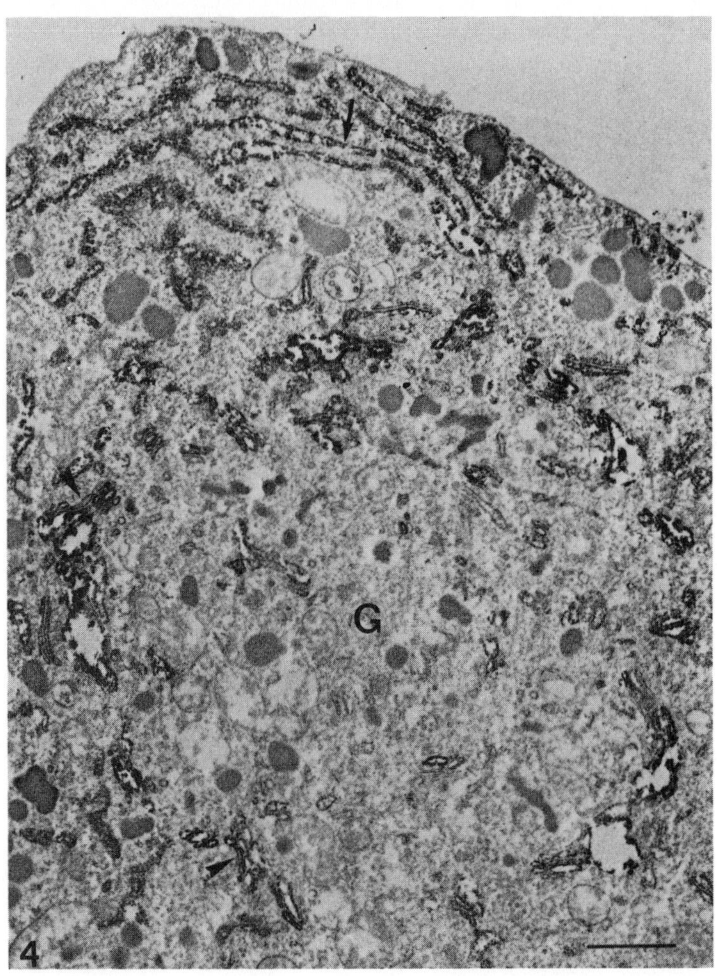

FIG. 4. Same material as Fig. 1. Detail of a Golgi zone (G) of an immunoreactive PRL cell. PRL is detected on the luminal surface of all Golgi saccules (*arrowheads*) and within RER cisternae (*arrow*). Bar represents 1 μm. × 14,000.

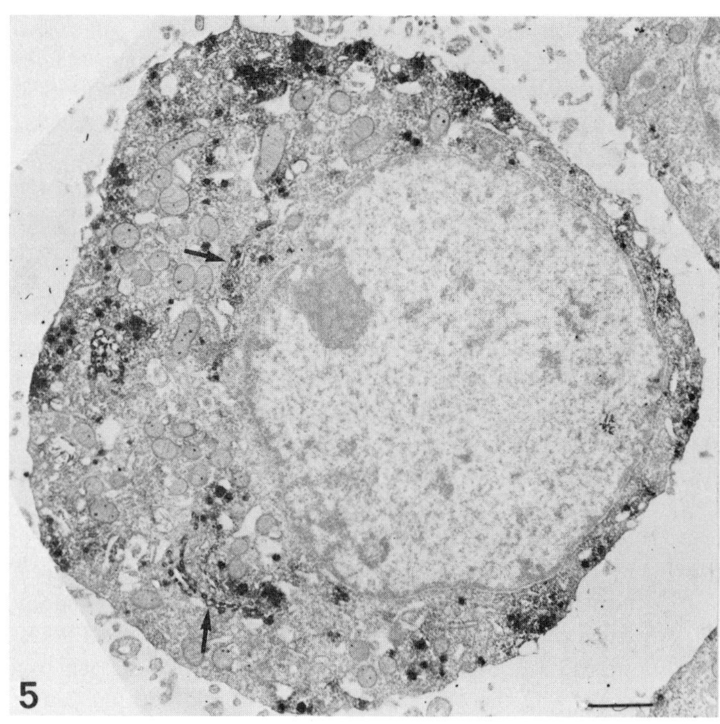

FIG. 5. A GH3B6 cell grown for 6 days in a chemically defined medium (189) and immunochemically stained with an antiserum against rat PRL. PRL is detected within Golgi saccules (*arrows*) and in the numerous small secretory granules. Bar represents 1 μm. × 10,000. (Courtesy of Dr. N. De Carvalho-Brunet and R. Picart.)

of a permeabilizing agent (47) or after lowicryl embedding (Vila Porcile, *unpublished observation*) (Fig. 3). The features of the reaction deposit differed along the two compartments of the endoplasmic reticulum: it was heterogeneous, or granular, in the RER cisternae, including the perinuclear cisternae, and more homogeneous and dense on the luminal face of the Golgi cisternae (Fig. 4). Moreover, the respective intensity of the staining of these two compartments also varied from one cell to another, which may be related to functional heterogeneity (see below). The preembedding approach also revealed an immunostaining of the cytoplasm. The possibility that this staining represents an artifact, caused by displacement of the reaction product from other antigenic sites, cannot be completely ruled out. However, the fact that it was also observed in GH3 cells, which have very few secretory granules (46), suggests that it may represent a cytoplasmic material immunologically related to PRL (see below).

In conclusion, because of technical improvements, immunoelectron methods have helped to localize PRL at the main subcellular steps delineating its intracellular pathway. This has raised the possibility of detecting variations in the distribution of subcellular PRL staining, depending on physiological conditions *in vivo* and *in vitro* (see below).

In addition to PRL, other components were immunocytochemically detected in lactotropes. The major tyrosine-sulfated protein of the bovine anterior pituitary, TSP 86/84, or secretogranine II, was found in a subpopulation of granules in lactotropes (48). This component could also be localized by the preembedding immunoperoxidase method in GH3 cells (Tougard et al., *unpublished observations*). The acidic nature of this component suggested that it might play a role in the sorting and specific routing of protein hormones (48). These findings allow the development of important new insights into the understanding of the secretory process. Thyroliberin-like immunoreactivity was also detected in PRL secretory granules (49,50). Laminin, a major component of the basement membrane of anterior pituitary tissue, was recently localized in the endoplasmic reticulum of normal PRL cells *in vivo* (51) and in culture (52).

Functional Heterogeneity

The first indication of a link between structural heterogeneity and functional heterogeneity was provided by studies performed with rat lactotropes separated by velocity sedimentation at unit gravity (53). Using this method, subgroups of lactotropes were isolated on the basis of their size and secretory granule content. This study revealed that the intracellular PRL content varies along with the cell fractions and according to different patterns, depending on the physiological state of the donor rat. Moreover, when the sorted cells were cultured for 14 days, the amount of PRL released into the medium during 14 days was positively correlated with their initial PRL content.

Further convincing evidence for the functional heterogeneity of PRL cells was then obtained by two independent approaches: (i) pulse-chase experiments with labeled amino acids and (ii) the hemolytic plaque assay method for the detection of hormone secretion by individual cells. Both methods were applied to cultured cells: that is, primary cultures as well as GH3 cells.

The development of pulse-chase experiments to analyze

functional heterogeneity in PRL cells began with the study of Swearingen (54), which revealed the first evidence for a heterogeneous turnover of PRL in the rat, *in vivo* and *in vitro,* and thus raised the question of the cellular origin of this heterogeneity. After an interval of 10 years this question could be reexamined because of the use of high-resolution autoradiography associated with immunoprecipitation methods applied in parallel. Using 2-day primary cultures of dispersed rat pituitary cells, Walker and Farquhar (55) confirmed that newly synthesized PRL was preferentially released under basal conditions. Moreover, the analysis of the distribution of total silver grains per cell in mammotropes identified by their ultrastructural features revealed the existence of several functional subpopulations that differed in the rapidity of loss of silver grains during the chase period. This suggested that some cells have a faster turnover time of PRL than others, which could result in the rapid release of newly synthesized PRL observed after 15 to 30 min of chase. Whether this corresponded to differences in the cell ultrastructural organization or in the size of the intracellular PRL pool was not determined. The existence of several functional subpopulations of PRL cells in primary culture was further corroborated by pulse-chase experiments where the chase was followed for up to 24 hr and was conducted in the presence of cycloheximide to prevent the dilution of labeled PRL by newly synthesized unlabeled PRL. This study clearly revealed an asynchrony of the release of labeled PRL in the medium, which occurred in successive waves (56).

GH3 cells, which differ from normal PRL cells by their very small intracellular PRL store and possess very few small secretory granules, were submitted to the same protocol of pulse-chase experiments and compared to normal PRL cells. This study revealed both similarities and differences between the two cell systems. In both cases, newly synthesized PRL was rapidly and preferentially released in basal conditions, and the pattern of the decay of specific radioactivity of PRL released into the medium suggested the existence of at least two PRL pools. Thus, whatever the size of the intracellular PRL store, the following events occur: (a) Newly synthesized PRL is rapidly released under basal conditions and (b) the turnover of PRL in a randomized cell population is heterogeneous. However, the turnover time of the two PRL pools was eight times greater in normal cells than in GH3 cells (56,57). These findings suggest that functional heterogeneity may be linked to variations in the size of the intracellular PRL store in normal cells, as well as in GH3 cells. The latter cells, indeed, also display individual variations of PRL intracellular content, as previously revealed by immunostaining (46,58).

The reverse hemolytic plaque assay (RHPA) offers a unique approach to the analysis of the cellular release capacity at the individual cell level and thus allows direct access to the question of functional heterogeneity (33). Indeed, it allows the determination of two parameters of functional heterogeneity within a cell monolayer: (i) the percentage of plaque-forming cells, which is the percentage of secretors in a given population, and (ii) the plaque area, which was found to be linearly related to the release of radioimmunoassayable PRL (33,59). Measurement of plaque areas on lactotropes derived from proestrous rats and cultured under basal conditions revealed a bimodal frequency distribution indicating the existence of two functional subpopulations of lactotropes (59). Moreover, the combination of RHPA with autoradiography has revealed that the large plaque-forming cells secrete most of the unlabeled and labeled hormones (60). Effects of secretagogues on these parameters have also been investigated (see section on morphological correlates of PRL cell responses to stimulating agents). The RHPA was also applied to GH3 cells. A close agreement was found between the percentage of immunostained PRL cells and the percentage of PRL plaque-forming cells. This study suggested a direct link between the storage and release capacity of GH3 cells, at least under basal conditions (37).

In conclusion, the functional heterogeneity of PRL cells, in terms of PRL turnover, is now well established. The existence of an inverse relationship between the size of the intracellular store and the turnover time, as well as a direct relationship between the intracellular content and the release capacity, seems rather well supported. This suggests an autoregulation of PRL secretion, as documented by Kadowaki et al. (61) and by Frawley and Clark, using RHPA (62). Whether there are subpopulations of PRL cells specialized for the release of newly synthesized PRL and for the response to secretagogues, respectively, will be examined in the following section. However, the exact link between morphological heterogeneity (as defined by ultrastructural criteria) and functional heterogeneity remains unclear and requires further study at the single cell level. Whatever the meaning, the structural heterogeneity of PRL cells represents a great obstacle in analyzing the ultrastructural correlates of pituitary function *in vivo* as well as *in vitro* (see section on morphological correlates of physiological regulation of lactotropes and gonadotropes).

Gonadotropes

Identification and Morphological Heterogeneity

The problem of establishing the cellular origin of LH and FSH has been a subject of controversy for many years. A separate cellular origin for these two hormones was postulated long ago on the basis of (a) nonparallel secretion of LH and FSH and (b) histophysiological correlations (3,6). The classic tinctorial methods more or less failed to completely solve the problem of gonadotrope identification. The introduction of cytochemical methods provided a better means of identifying glycoprotein-producing cells, but permitted only an indirect distinction between thyrotropic and gonadotropic basophils. This last category was further subdivided into FSH and LH gonadotropes (63). Definitive progress was made with the advent of immunocytochemistry. The earliest immunocytochemical studies, carried out using antisera directed against whole hormones that share a common α subunit (see Chapter 31), showed that LH and FSH were present in the same cells (7). This was later confirmed with the use of antibodies against the specific β subunit of each hormone which permitted a more accurate identification of LH and FSH containing cells. Therefore, the concept of "one hormone, one cell" does not hold for gonadotropes.

At the light-microscopic level, the cells containing LH and FSH, which were identified by immunocytochemistry in the rat anterior pituitary using antibodies specific to rat β-LH and rat β-FSH, are distributed in an identical manner scattered throughout the glandular parenchyma, including the areas adjacent to the intermediate lobe. Two cell types can be distinguished by their shape and localization: large rounded or oval cells, which are abundant in the lateral and anterior regions of the pars distalis, and small oval cells, which are more numerous in the posterior portion. Using Alcian blue–periodic acid-Schiff staining (AB-PAS) (3,64,65), all of these cells displayed the same violet color, indicating that they were AB and PAS positive (66,67). Gonadotropes were also detected in the pars tuberalis of the rat, as well as in other mammals (68–72). Combining immunocytochemistry with light-microscopic morphometry, gonadotropes represent approximately 14% of the cell population of normal adult rats (73) and normal female rats (74). These morphometric analyses confirmed a great variability in the size of gonadotropes, ranging from 30 to 160 μm^2 in area for male rat pituitaries (73) and from 130 to 170 μm^2 for female rat pituitaries (74).

A considerable morphological heterogeneity of rat gonadotropes has also been described at the electron-microscopic level. The first classification of gonadotropes was established on the basis of cytophysiological studies using conventional electron microscopy. Following the classic studies of Farquhar and Rinehart (5) and Barnes (75,76), Kurosumi and Oota (77) distinguished two types of gonadotropes in rats, one producing FSH and one producing LH, according to the criteria described by Barnes (75) in mice. With the advent of immunocytochemical techniques, this classification has been questioned since it was discovered that the two cell types contain both gonadotropic hormones. The original Kurosumi-Oota FSH cell, characterized by a large and rounded shape, slightly dilated RER cisternae, and two types of secretory granules (200 nm and 300–700 nm in diameter, respectively), was named type-A gonadotrope by Nakane (7,9) and Tougard et al. (67,78) and type-I gonadotrope by Moriarty (79) and Childs (Moriarty) et al. (80) (Fig. 6). This cell type, the most abundant in the normal male rat, contained both gonadotropic hormones, since it was labeled by antisera specific to the beta chain of LH and FSH. The original Kurosumi-Oota LH cell, characterized by an ovoid shape, flattened RER cisternae, and secretory granules of uniform size (200–250 nm in diameter), was named type-B gonadotrope by Tougard et al. (67,78) and type-II gonadotrope by Moriarty (79) and Childs (Moriarty) et al. (80) (Fig. 7). This cell type, less abundant in the normal male rat, also contained both gonadotropic hor-

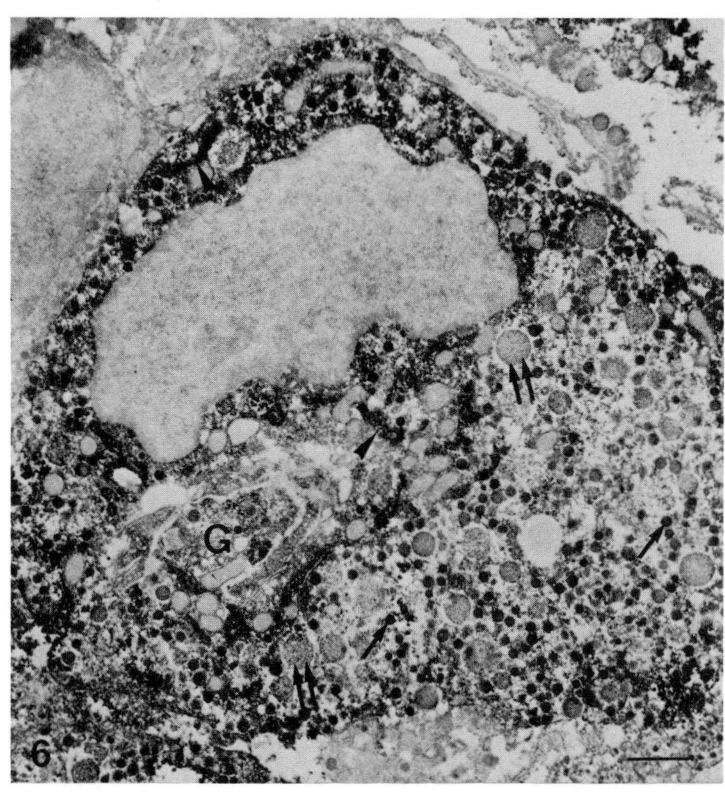

FIG. 6. A type-I gonadotrope (two classes of rounded secretory granules) from a normal male rat pituitary is immunochemically stained with an antiserum against rat β-LH using a preembedding immunoperoxidase method. With this method, the immunocytochemical staining is more abundant over the small secretory granules (*arrows*) than over the large ones (*double arrows*). The reaction product is also observed in slightly dilated RER cisternae (*arrowheads*). In the Golgi zone (G), the saccules are negative, but some immunoreactive secretory granules can be seen. Bar represents 1 μm. × 10,000.

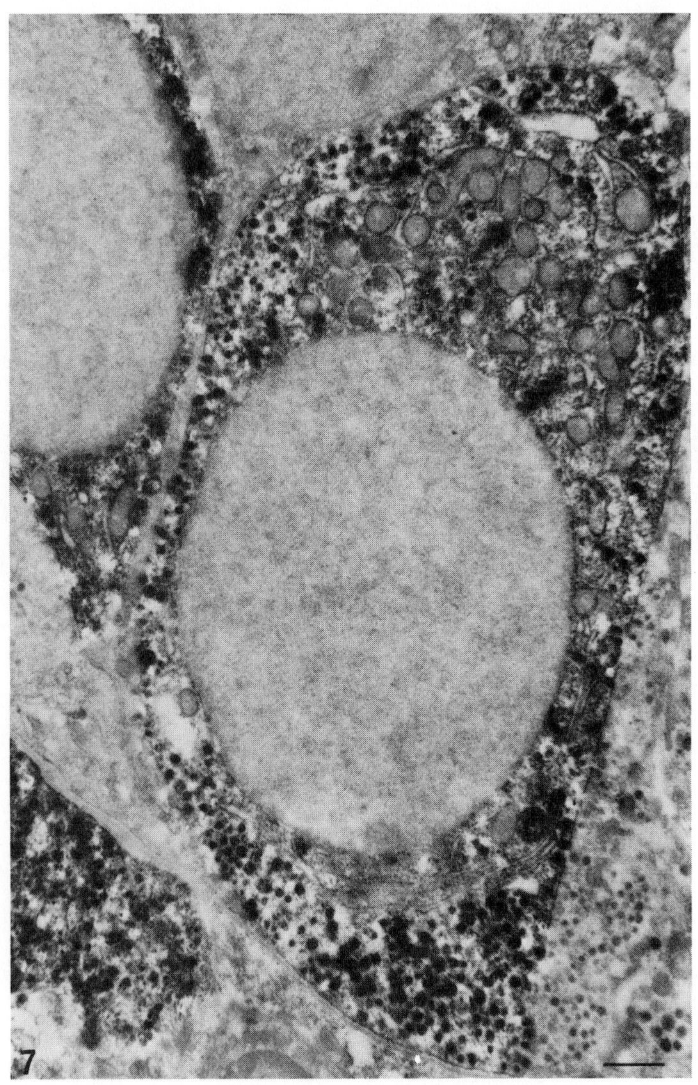

FIG. 7. A type-II gonadotrope (one class of small secretory granules) from a normal male rat pituitary is immunochemically stained with an antiserum against rat β-LH using a preembedding immunoperoxidase method. The small secretory granules are strongly labeled. Bar represents 1 μm. × 9,900. (From ref. 67.)

mones. Numerous intermediate forms of these two cell types were observed (66,78,81) (Fig. 8). A third type of gonadotrope, far less numerous, has been described by Nakane (7), Moriarty (79), Moriarty and Garner (82), and Childs (Moriarty) et al. (80): it was called type-III gonadotrope by Moriarty and her co-workers, and it displayed the morphological features of ACTH-producing cells, i.e., an angular and stellate shape, as well as peripherally distributed secretory granules of 220 to 250 nm in diameter. Moreover, it was stained by antisera against ACTH (ACTH 17–39) as well as antisera against the β chain of FSH or LH. Such angularly shaped cells were found only after using the postembedding method involving an antiserum against β-LH by Tougard et al. (67) and by Inoue and Hagino (83). These cells were not stained by an antiserum against ACTH (83). The significance of these cells will be discussed below (see the section on neonatal development).

In the human (84) and in other mammalian species (85,86), only one type of gonadotrope was found which contained both gonadotropic hormones. Moreover, an FSH-ACTH cell resembling a corticotrope was also described by Dacheux (87,88) in the pig.

In all species, the concentration of FSH and LH seems to vary from cell to cell, as suggested by variations in the intensity of immunostaining. When serial sections were stained for β-LH or β-FSH, respectively, or when double staining was applied to the same sections, it appeared that LH and FSH were stored in the same cells in the rat (7,9,67,78, 79,81,89–93) (Figs. 9,10), the human being (84,94), the monkey (95,96,97), the dog (71), the mouse (11), and the pig (86,98). However, some of these authors found cells containing only FSH or LH (7,71,73,79,80,84,86,87,96,99–102). The number of these monohormonal cells varied, depending on the authors, according to physiological or experimental conditions. In the rat, the range of the percentages of monohormonal gonadotropes was from 40% to 10% in all the gonadotropes examined. As recently discussed by Childs (74), most of these studies were performed on serial sections of fixed-embedded tissue, and, since the size of gonadotropes greatly varies, the thickness of the section can

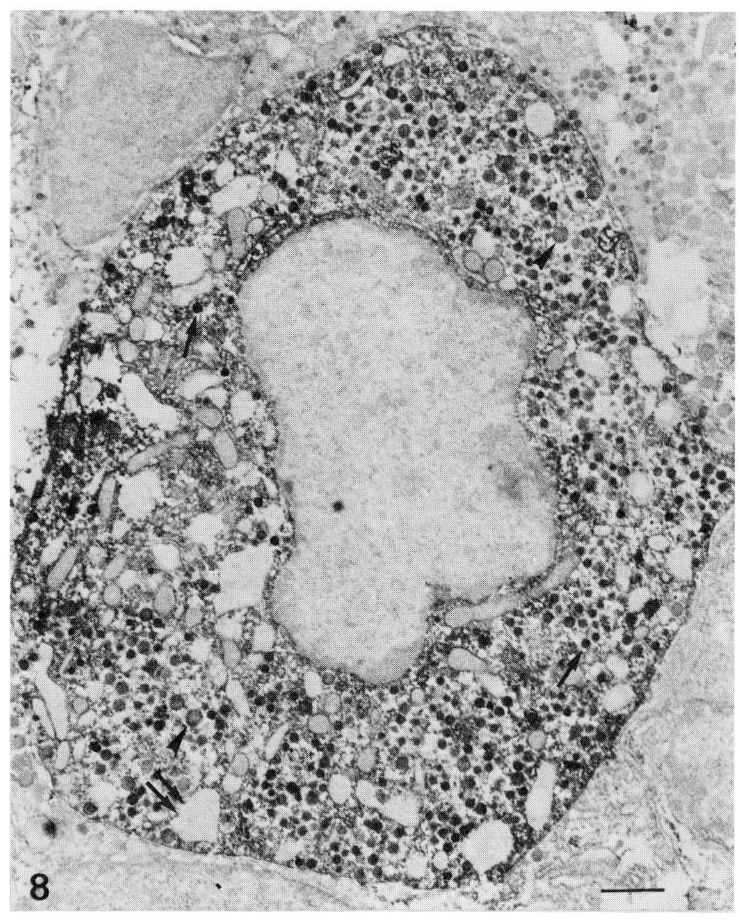

FIG. 8. An intermediate form between type-I and type-II gonadotropes from a normal male rat pituitary is immunochemically stained with an antiserum against rat β-LH using a preembedding immunoperoxidase method. This cell displays numerous small immunoreactive secretory granules (*arrows*), a few large secretory granules (*arrowheads*), and dilated RER cisternae (*double arrows*). Bar represents 1 μm. × 10,000.

shift the relative percentages of multihormonal and monohormonal gonadotropes. Moreover, extensive studies of Childs and her colleagues showed that under various experimental conditions (see the following sections) the number of multihormonal cells varied. This indicates clearly a certain fluidity of the gonadotrope population, as shown by the variability in their storage capacity (80). Therefore, it is clear that most gonadotropes are multihormonal. The monohormonal cells are, in fact, multipotential and, under specific conditions (see section on morphological correlates of phys-

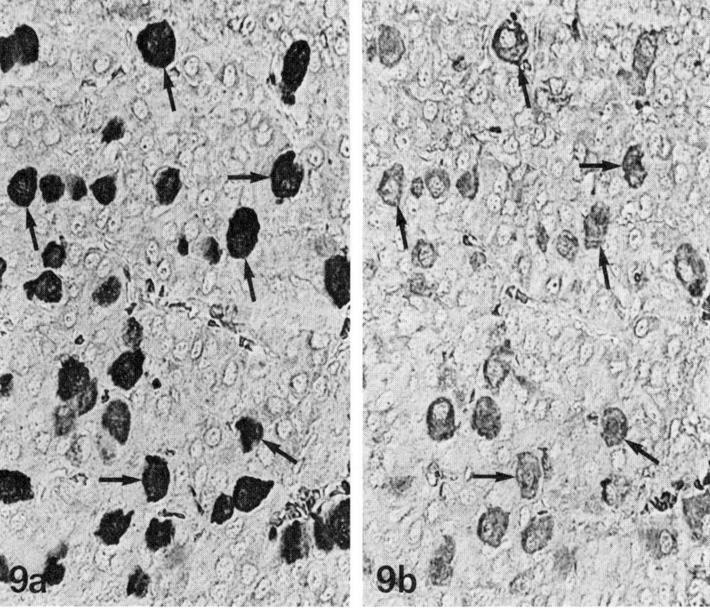

FIG. 9. Adjacent 3-μm paraffin sections of a normal male rat pituitary are immunochemically stained with antisera against rat β-LH (**a**) and against rat β-FSH (**b**) using a postembedding immunoperoxidase method. Same cells are stained by the two antisera (*arrows*) and, therefore, contain both hormones. The staining intensity is weaker with A-β-rFSH. × 425. (From ref. 67.)

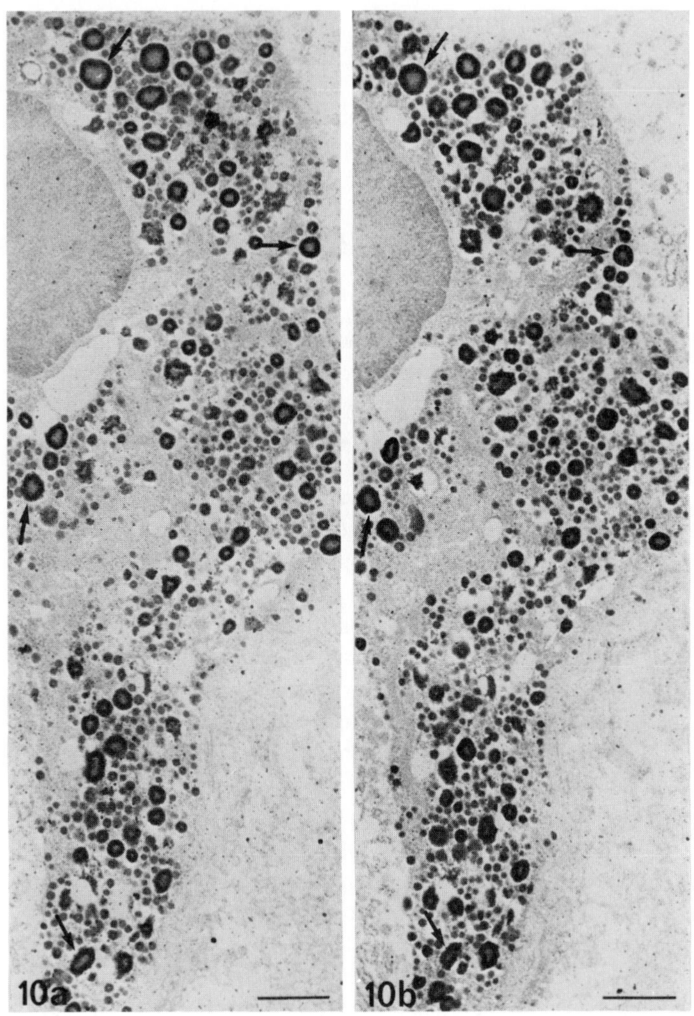

FIG. 10. Adjacent ultrathin araldite sections of a normal male rat pituitary are immunochemically stained with antisera against rat β-LH (**a**) and against rat β-FSH (**b**), using a postembedding immunoperoxidase method. Details of the staining of secretory granules of type-I gonadotrope are shown. Some of the large secretory granules (*arrows*) are stained by the two antisera and, therefore, contain both hormones. Bar represents 1 μm. × 12,000. (From ref. 67.)

iological regulation of lactotropes and gonadotropes), bihormonal.

An important conclusion can be drawn from these immunocytochemical studies using highly specific antibodies applied to homologous species: The structural heterogeneity of gonadotropes does not reflect a biochemical specialization. Therefore, what is the physiological significance of the morphological heterogeneity of gonadotropes? It has been proposed that the structural heterogeneity of gonadotropes may reflect several stages of the secretory cycle of one single cell type capable of storing or releasing LH and FSH in different proportions, depending on physiological conditions (66). Thus, structural heterogeneity might correspond to a functional heterogeneity, which will be discussed at a later point in this chapter (see section on functional heterogeneity).

Subcellular Distribution of Gonadotropic Hormones

LH and FSH are glycoprotein hormones consisting of two different noncovalently linked α and β subunits. These subunits are synthesized as precursors that undergo posttranslational maturation. Glycosylation occurs both on the α subunit and the β subunit (see Chapter 31). As indicated above, the autoradiographic approach provides data related to the migration of neosynthesized proteins and glycoproteins, but not to the specific secretory product. Electron-microscopic immunocytochemistry should help to identify, within a given cell, the specific secretory product, among the other exported proteins at the successive steps of the secretory pathway. In fact, as mentioned above for PRL, the results for gonadotropic hormones vary greatly, depending on the methods (preembedding versus postembedding staining) and the fixative used (67,100,103).

The presence of an immunoreactive material within RER cisternae was only observed in some gonadotropes with an anti-β-LH antiserum in normal rats, and exclusively with the preembedding method (66,67), whereas β-LH and β-FSH were frequently observed in dilated RER of highly stimulated castration cells with both the preembedding and postembedding methods in rats (78,101,104) and in pigs (105).

In most studies, the Golgi saccules and vesicles were devoid of immunoreactive material, with the exception of some positive secretory granules in the core of the Golgi zone in gonadotropes (67,78,101) (Fig. 6). This may result from either a low level of hormonal content, a masking of antigenicity during the addition of carbohydrate components, or an inadequate entry of immunological probes into the membrane of this compartment. Indeed, Dacheux (105) has recently reported, with the use of the preembedding method and permeabilization with saponin, a strong labeling of saccules, small vesicles, and condensed material in the Golgi zone of highly active castration cells in pigs.

In all studies, secretory granules display the strongest staining intensity, which is in agreement with the data on hormone-storing cells. On ultrathin serial sections of rat (66,67,80) and pig pituitaries (86,98) β-LH and β-FSH were detected in the same granules (Fig. 10), clearly implying that the two hormones are simultaneously present in, at least, some granules. However, some authors have described granules containing either LH or FSH in LH/FSH gonadotropes using immunoperoxidase, immunoferritin, or immunogold techniques (86,93,104,106–108). Recent dual preembedding staining of gonadotropins in pituitary cell monolayers also suggests that LH and FSH can be stored in different regions of the same cell (109,110). Moreover, until recently, there was no conclusive evidence for the different subcellular localization of α and β subunits of LH or FSH. Both classes of secretory granules (large and small) were stained with an anti-α-LH, as well as with an anti-β-LH (67). This is of a great importance because it suggests that there is no compartmentalization of both subunits during their intracellular transport until storage in the secretory granule occurs, when they are found colocalized. However, we cannot exclude the possibility that secretory granules might contain different amounts of LH and FSH subunits.

Recently, the presence of other molecules in the secretory granule matrix of gonadotropes has been reported: secretogranin II, an acidic tyrosine-sulfated secretory protein (48) that is released concomitantly with LH under gonadotropin-releasing hormone (GnRH) stimulation (111), and laminin, a major component of basement membranes (51,52). These proteins may play a role in the sorting and packaging of gonadotropic hormones.

Several studies have reported a subcellular localization of GnRH, the hypothalamic decapeptide that controls the secretion of both LH and FSH in gonadotropes. Endogenous immunoreactive GnRH was observed in the matrix of secretory granules, which also contained β-LH and/or β-FSH immunoreactivity (88,112–114).

As described for lactotropes, a slight cytoplasmic staining was only observed with the preembedding method (67,78, 85,105). The meaning of such a localization has been discussed in the earlier section on lactotropes. As concerns gonadotropes, to our knowledge, no experimental data exist to determine whether this is an artifact or not.

In conclusion, it appears that immunocytochemistry allows us to delineate the secretory pathway of gonadotropic hormones within a given cell. However, until immunological probes that discriminate respectively between the precursor forms of gonadotropic subunits, the glycosylated or unglycosylated molecules, and the quaternary structure of mature hormones are available and applicable, this technique does not allow us to follow with precision the post-translational maturation of gonadotropic hormones during the successive steps of the secretory process.

Functional Heterogeneity

To investigate the significance of the morphological heterogeneity of gonadotropes, several attempts to separate cell types have been performed using techniques based mainly on the variability of cell size.

Using sedimentation techniques at unit gravity, Denef et al. (115) separated gonadotropes from 14-day-old male or female rats and found that irrespective of cell size, the majority of the cells contained both FSH and LH, but that FSH and, to a lesser extent, LH were also stored in separate cells. These authors demonstrated that gonadotropes also differ in terms of their relative content and release of FSH and LH. The proportion of these two hormones differed according to cell size as well as sex and age of the rats (115). In small and medium-sized gonadotropes from 14-day-old rats, the FSH/LH ratio was lower than in large gonadotropes, and the release was in favor of LH. In adult males, the small and medium-sized gonadotropes released more FSH than LH, and, inversely, the release in favor of LH was observed in large gonadotropes. These gonadotrope subtypes also differed in their response to GnRH, as well as in the effects of androgen treatment on differential FSH and LH release (116–118). Moreover, Denef et al. (118) demonstrated that the majority of the largest gonadotropes corresponded to the type-A gonadotrope containing 200- and 700-nm secretory granules, whereas the small cells corresponded mainly to gonadotropes with 200-nm secretory granules. However, cells displaying numerous intermediate ultrastructural features were also found in the different cell populations. When placed in culture for 6 days, both subgroups of gonadotropes evolved toward a single cell type with small secretory granules (Tougard and Denef, *unpublished results*). Thus, the morphological heterogeneity of the gonadotrope disappears in culture, whereas the functional heterogeneity persists (117,119).

Using centrifugal elutriation to separate subtypes of gonadotropes from pituitaries of a mixed group of cycling female rats, Childs et al. (102) also demonstrated a heterogeneous LH and FSH storage pattern, related to cell size, on serially sectioned and immunocytochemically stained cells: Smaller gonadotropes appeared to store only one of the hormones, whereas most of the larger cells either stored LH and FSH together, or FSH alone. This heterogeneous storage pattern persisted for up to 3 days in culture (102). Moreover, these gonadotrope subtypes differed in their capacity to bind GnRH; the small monohormonal cells contained little or no GnRH-binding activity (120).

Using the reverse hemolytic plaque assay (33) for the measurement of secretion by individual cells, Smith et al. (121) demonstrated a heterogeneity in the release capacity of gonadotropes that contain immunoreactive LH. However, no link was observed between this functional heterogeneity and the morphological heterogeneity.

Taken together, these findings strongly suggest that the selective modulation of FSH or LH release *in vivo* is linked to the functional heterogeneity of the gonadotrope subtypes. However, the gonadotrope subtypes do not appear to correspond to different classes of cells, but rather to several stages of the secretory cycle (66,102). In the future, a direct correlation of the ultrastructure and secretory activity at the single cell level, using the very promising reverse hemolytic plaque assay, would allow confirmation of this interpretation.

Topographical Relationship Between Lactotropes and Gonadotropes

In early studies, similar distribution and preferential association of lactotropes and gonadotropes were observed by Nakane (7) in his pioneering immunocytochemical study of the anterior pituitary, which suggested some physiological relationship between them. In later work, gap junctions (122) and small adherent junctions between lactotropes and gonadotropes (123) were reported. Such a topographical relationship between the two cell types was also observed *in vitro* after dissociation of the pituitary cells and reassociation during cell culture. *In vivo,* cup-shaped or angular PRL cells surrounded large gonadotropes using long cytoplasmic processes (7,15). *In vitro,* lactotropes surrounding gonadotropes and, inversely, gonadotropes surrounding lactotropes were frequently observed (Fig. 11).

This selective topographical relationship suggested the existence of a functional interaction between these two cell types. This exciting hypothesis has been extensively investigated for several years by Denef (119,124) using co-cultures or reaggregated cell cultures of lactotrope- and gonadotrope-enriched populations, obtained by unit gravity sedimentation. This author has demonstrated that these cell types are functionally coupled and that gonadotropes can activate the secretory activity of lactotropes through the release of a paracrine factor (125).

MORPHOLOGICAL CORRELATES OF PHYSIOLOGICAL REGULATION OF LACTOTROPES AND GONADOTROPES

The morphological correlates of the physiological regulation involved in the control of reproduction have been studied *in vivo* and *in vitro*. In the first case, the morphological observations were correlated with biological responses that represent a series of integrated events involving multifactorial interactions and a cascade of events ranging from variations in the circulating levels of PRL and gonad-

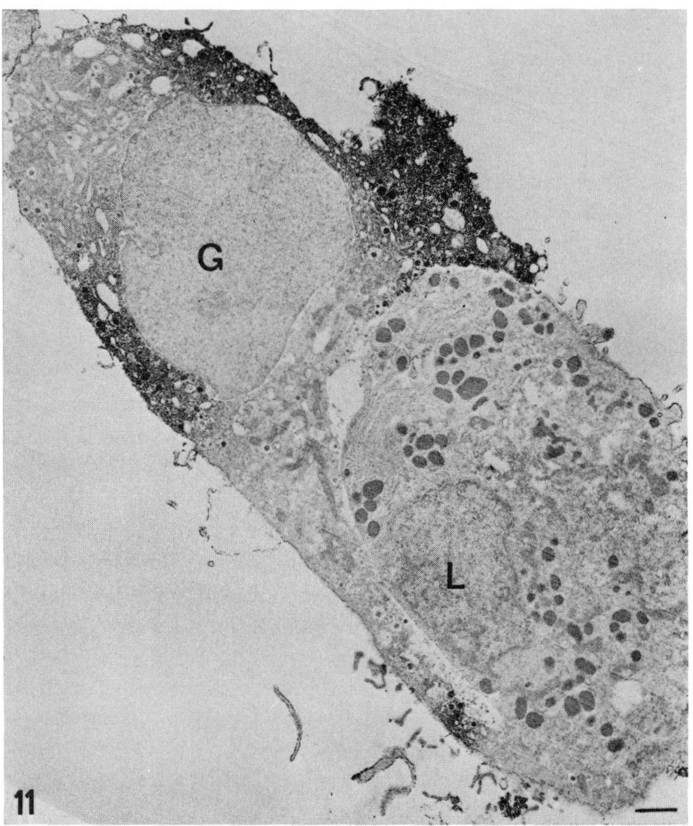

FIG. 11. A 7-day monolayer of rat anterior pituitary cells is immunochemically stained with an antiserum against ovine LH. An immunoreactive gonadotrope (G) surrounds a negative lactotrope (L) that is characterized by its polymorphic secretory granules. Bar represents 1 μm. × 7,000.

otropins, to lactation and gonadal activity. In the second case, the morphological observations could be better correlated to the pituitary cell response, sometimes at the individual cell level. Thus, these studies provided deeper insight into the understanding of cellular and subcellular mechanisms underlying the control of the physiology of reproduction at the anterior pituitary level.

Lactotropes

In-Vivo *Studies on Lactotropes*

Morphological modifications of lactotropes were observed in relation to lactation, castration, and estrogen treatment in adenomas, as well as in relation to development and aging. Various parameters were taken into account, depending on the studies: cell number, cell shape, and immunostaining at the light-microscopic level; and cell ultrastructure and subcellular sites of immunostaining at the electron-microscopic level. The present review pays particular attention to results obtained from cells identified immunocytochemically, which provide more reliable information.

The number of PRL cells is known to vary according to physiological conditions. The data are often semiquantitative or based on subjective evaluation. More precise evaluations were recently made using either RHPA (34,59,62,126) or immunostaining of freshly dissociated cells (127). In basal conditions, however, the percentage of PRL cells varies, depending on the studies or the methods used: from 10% to 30% in the male rat, and from 30% to 50% in the female.

Gestation and lactation. The increase in number and size of acidophils during gestation and lactation was correlated long ago with PRL secretion in the rat and the human (16,128). This observation was then reexamined with the immunostaining of PRL. In the rat, Merchant (129) distinguished two types of cells among immunostained lactotropes: type-I cells, which are small and polyhedral; and type-II cells, also polyhedral, but much larger than type-I cells. Type-I cells, which are the most numerous, do not change much in size, staining, and number during gestation and lactation. In contrast, type-II cells, which are less numerous than type-I cells and have a limited distribution, become prominent during gestation. Their staining greatly increases during late gestation, only to decline rapidly on day 1 of lactation and remain low during continuous lactation (129).

At the ultrastructural level and without the aid of immunocytochemistry, PRL cells were identified in lactating rats separated from their litters according to the conditions defined by Grosvenor and Turner (130). After a 10-hr separation, a striking accumulation of secretory granules in the cytoplasm was first described by Pasteels (16) and later confirmed by others. Simultaneously, secretory granules were seen fusing with lysosomes according to the process described as *crinophagy* by Smith and Farquhar (17), thus revealing the role of lysosomes in the regulation of PRL secretion. Suckling for 5 to 15 min, following removal of litters, resulted in a dramatic increase in granule extrusion (16,131,132). Such variations are consistent with variations in intracellular and serum PRL levels under similar conditions (130).

In the human pituitary, hypertrophy and hyperplasia of immunostained PRL cells have been observed in pituitaries of postpartum and lactating women (12,13).

Sex-related differences—Steroid treatments and castration. In the human (14) as well as in the rat (21) the number of immunostained PRL cells is only slightly greater in the female. However, when the cellular releasing capacity is taken into account using the RHPA, their proportion is greater in the female rat according to Leong et al. (34). In the mouse, a sexual dimorphism of PRL cells has been described and correlated with differences in amino acid composition (133).

The stimulating effect of long-term estrogen treatment on PRL secretion was correlated long ago with the hyperplasia and hypertrophy of acidophils in the rat (16) as well as in several mammalian species (see ref. 1 for a review). This was confirmed at the electron-microscopic level in the rat (134–136). More recently, interesting observations were reported following treatments (5–15 days) with testosterone or 17-β-estradiol of young male and female rats. PRL cells were immunocytochemically identified by a superimposition technique, and the relative proportions of cells grouped into the three classes previously defined by these authors (see above) were determined as a function of treatment for each sex (21). This suggested an interconversion from type-I to type-II and type-III cells, concomitant with an increase in pituitary PRL content and serum PRL levels as a result of estradiol treatment in females, and, to a lesser extent, in males. Testosterone treatment, which slightly decreased the serum level of PRL and did not change pituitary PRL content, mostly increased the percentage of type-II cells. This interesting study suggests that a sustained stimulation of PRL synthesis and release leads to an enlargement of secretory granules (type-III cells were characterized by very large pleomorphic secretory granules).

In contrast to estrogen treatment, castration has been shown to induce a marked decrease of PRL cell size, an accumulation of small secretory granules (47), and a decrease in cell number in the female rat after 4 weeks (137). Treatment of castrated rats with estrogen induced, within 4 days, cell hypertrophy, the disappearance of secretory granules, and a considerable development of RER cisternae containing PRL, whereas the Golgi zone remained small and almost unstained. Interestingly, the RER cisternae were often perpendicular to, and in contact with, the plasma membrane, suggesting the possibility of direct secretion from the RER (47).

Pituitary adenomas.

Experimental Tumors: It is well known that massive and prolonged (for months) administration of natural or synthetic estrogens gives rise to pituitary adenomas and eventually transplantable tumors, which can be serially transferred and lose their estrogen dependency (see refs. 138 and 139 for reviews). In general, the development of adenoma coincides with the reduction in size and number of secretory granules. PRL has been immunocytochemically localized in small secretory granules, and GH has been localized in larger granules, but these have been found in separate cell types in transplantable rat mammosomatotropic tumors (140). The appearance of tumors depends on several factors such as age, sex, and species. For example, in the dog and the monkey, estrogens stimulate PRL secretion without inducing tumors (141).

Human Prolactinomas: Variability in the size and structure of cells in human prolactinomas has been widely described at the electron-microscopic level (139,142) and can also be observed after PRL immunostaining. At the light-microscopic level, the intensity of the immunostaining greatly varies from cell to cell (143,144), suggesting again a functional heterogeneity of tumor cells.

The effects of bromocriptine (a dopamine agonist that is widely used to reduce PRL secretion in patients with prolactinomas) on PRL cell morphology were analyzed in order to explain the cellular mechanisms involved in the reduction of tumor size and secretory activity (145–147). These studies revealed a reduction in cell size (by about 50%), mostly involving the whole cytoplasm, whereas the number of secretory granules tended to increase. Depending on the reports, or on the tumors, the PRL cell immunoreactivity was either lowered or unchanged. Such analyses, however, are hampered by the considerable heterogeneity of structure among tumors, as well as among cells for a given tumor.

Ontogenesis and postnatal development. The appearance of immunoreactive PRL cells during the ontogenesis of the anterior pituitary has been determined in several mammalian species. They are generally one of the last cell types to appear. In the ovine fetus and the bovine fetus, PRL cells appear later than GH cells: not before 80 days in the ovine (148) and not before 100 days in the bovine (149). In the rat, PRL cells only appear within the last days of gestation and, depending on the authors, on the 17th gestation day (150), the 21st day (151,152), or only in the newborn (153). These differences might be related to rat strains or experimental conditions. In the human fetus, PRL cells are detected at 14 weeks of gestation but remain few in number up to 23 weeks (14). This time course was confirmed by Begeot et al. (154), who detected the first cells at 18 weeks. Moreover, these authors have shown that in anencephalic fetuses, PRL cells were more numerous and larger than in normal fetuses, which suggests that their development does not require a hypothalamic influence and might even be under an inhibitory control during fetal life. Several authors reached a similar conclusion by using cultures of hypophyseal primordia taken at different ages; in all cases, PRL cells differentiated *de novo in vitro* at different time intervals (155,156). However, when hypophyseal primordia are taken at very early stages (10–12 days) and cultured in a serum-free medium, PRL cells fail to differentiate. Under these conditions, GnRH mediates the release of the α-LH subunit, which plays a role in the differentiation of lactotropes (157).

The ultrastructural features of immuno-identified PRL cells undergo marked changes during postnatal development of the rat. At birth, the cells contain very few small granules. In immature (4–6 weeks) rats of both sexes only one class of PRL cells with small spherical (200 nm) granules was observed. The diversity of ultrastructural organization, as reported above, was found in the adult rat only (32).

The mitotic index of immunohistochemically stained PRL cells is maximal at 1 month in male and female rats and then decreases throughout the remainder of life; however, in young females, it steeply increases at estrus (158).

The development of the secretory capacity of PRL cells was investigated using the RHPA. This study revealed that the first secretors appeared in cultures obtained from 4-day-old animals. Moreover, only 1.7% of the cells released PRL alone, whereas 35.8% released both GH and PRL (159), suggesting again that both hormones are secreted by the same cells.

Aging. In the human, immunocytochemically identified lactotropes have been found to considerably decrease in number and size with advancing age (48, 65, and 76 years) in both sexes (14).

In the rat, the spontaneous occurrence of prolactinomas associated with repeated pseudogestations has been reported in senile female Wistar rats by Ascheim (160). The predominant cell type in these tumors was observed by Pasteels (16) to display the characteristic affinity of PRL cells for erythrosine. These pioneering observations were thereafter largely confirmed (see ref. 127 for a review). Spontaneous tumors, which often consist solely of PRL cells, have now been described in several rat strains (161–163).

The cellular mechanisms of these age-related hyperprolactinemias were recently examined by Chuknyiska et al. (127) using short-term cultures of dissociated anterior pituitary cells taken from either (a) adult (6 months) Wistar rats at estrus or diestrus or (b) old (22–24 months) rats in constant estrus or diestrus. This study revealed that aging is associated with a significant but small increase (30–35%) in cell number and a tremendous increase (80–120%) in the secretory response to estradiol treatment *in vitro* for 4 days. This suggests that the control of PRL gene expression may be altered by aging.

In-Vitro *Functional Studies on Lactotropes*

Lactotropes in culture have been extensively studied within the last 20 years to analyze the cellular and molecular mechanisms involved in the control of PRL secretion. Such studies took advantage of the availability of two model systems that were described in the section on morphological features and functional significance: (i) primary cultures of enzymatically dispersed, normal rat anterior pituitary cells in which the proportion of PRL cells rapidly increases (up to 70%) concomitantly with a rise in PRL release (see refs. 164–166 for reviews); and (ii) PRL cell lines, primarily GH3 cells and their subclones that derive from a transplantable rat mammosomatotropic tumor (167).

The secretion of PRL *in vivo* is subject to a multifactorial control that results in either a decrease or an increase in PRL plasma level. *In vitro,* primary cultures and clonal GH3 cells respond equally well to all of the factors that stimulate *in vivo* PRL secretion, which are neuropeptides (TRH, VIP, PHI, and bombesin) and estrogen (see refs. 168 and 169 for reviews). Concerning inhibitory agents, GH3 cells differ from PRL cells in primary cultures by their lack of response to one of the most potent inhibitors of PRL secretion *in vivo* (dopamine) and its agonists. However, they do respond to some inhibitory peptides (somatostatin, histidyl-prolyl-diketopiperazin) (see ref. 169 for a review). Because of these two systems, great progress has been made in the analysis of the major steps involved in the mode of action of neuropeptides: binding to specific receptors, transduction mechanisms, and gene transcription. Although the morphological correlates of these regulations have been, so far, less extensively investigated, significant progress has been made in the analysis of the secretory process in PRL cells.

Morphological correlates of response to inhibitory agents. Following the pioneering work of Smith and Farquhar (17), who demonstrated *in vivo* the role of lysosomes in regulating PRL secretion (see section on morphological features and functional significance), a few morphological studies have dealt with the analysis of intracellular events associated with the arrest of PRL release in response to a defined inhibitory agent.

In normal rat PRL cells in primary culture, bromocriptine treatment for a period ranging from 4 hr to 24 hr induced the accumulation of large secretory granules and the formation of acid-phosphatase-positive dense bodies and autophagic vacuoles. These effects were accompanied by a transient increase in cell immunoreactivity, followed by a decrease occurring after several days. These events are concomitant with a transient increase in intracellular PRL which lasts for up to 24 hr (166). A delayed decrease of PRL content in culture has also been observed after long-term treatment (170). Biochemical studies have shown that this decrease is the consequence, at least in part, of PRL degradation. Attempts to detect an increase in lysosomal enzyme activities following treatment with dopamine or bromocriptine *in vivo* led to contradictory results (170,171).

The heterogeneity of the PRL cell response to dopamine was investigated using the RHPA. This study revealed that dopamine induces, in a dose-dependent manner, a shift in the percentage of large plaque-forming cells to the percentage of small plaque-forming cells. This suggests that dopamine preferentially inhibits the lactotropes that secrete large amounts of PRL. The reasons for such effects are still unknown (59). When the rate of plaque formation was used as an index of the rate of PRL secretion, dopamine was found to transiently inhibit the proportion of plaque-forming cells, and this effect was reversed by TRH (62). Interestingly, exposure to the lysosomotropic drug chloroquine largely overrode dopamine inhibition, indicating the participation of lysosomes in the inhibitory response. Under the same experimental conditions, ovine PRL also inhibited the rate of plaque formation, but this effect was not additive to that of dopamine, suggesting that the same subpopulation of PRL cells was involved (62). These interesting findings support dopamine action on a subpopulation of PRL cells, although they do not identify the responsive cells.

Human pituitary adenomas *in vitro* also respond to treatment with L-DOPA by the formation of lysosomes. Interesting observations were recently reported on monolayers obtained from three human PRL adenomas cultured on an extracellular matrix in serum-free medium and treated with 10^{-10} M bromocriptine (172). Cells were examined after 24 hr and 16 days and subjected to morphometric analysis and immunostaining at the electron-microscopic level. This study clearly showed that morphological alterations are delayed with respect to the rapid decrease of PRL release (66–88% after 24 hr). The first evidence of this consisted of a dramatic decrease in exocytosis. After 16 days the cytoplasmic surface was greatly decreased and the number of secretory granules was considerably augmented, although their diameter was decreased. This accumulation of granules accounted for the increase in cellular immunostaining. However, in contrast to control cells, PRL could not be detected in RER and Golgi cisternae. This suggested a delayed inhibition of PRL synthesis. As compared to data observed with normal rat PRL cells, the induction of lysosomes seems very limited or quite delayed in this system (172).

On the whole, the most intriguing aspect of dopamine agonist action appears to reside in the long delay prior to the decrease in PRL intracellular content.

Morphological correlates of PRL cell responses to stimulating agents. The morphological correlates of the stimulation of PRL secretion in culture have been studied with only two factors—thyroliberin (TRH) and 17β-estradiol—which induce a different pattern of response. TRH has been shown to exert a rapid action (within minutes) on the release of intracellularly stored hormone, as well as a delayed effect (hours and days) on the synthesis of prolactin (see ref. 168 for a review). A similar pattern of activity has been observed for most hypophysiotropic neuropeptides *in vitro,* as well as *in vivo,* although the first phase remains the most documented so far (see refs. 173 and 174 for reviews). Thus, the morphological correlates of TRH effects may be of general value. In contrast, estrogens primarily exert a long-term action on PRL synthesis, which requires at least 1 or 2 days of treatment, *in vivo,* as well as *in vitro,* in normal, as well as clonal, PRL cells (175,176).

Acute PRL Release in Response to TRH:

GH3 cells. The morphological correlates of acute PRL release following exposure to TRH for up to 30 min were analyzed at the electron-microscopic level, mostly for GH3 cells. Because these cells possess very few secretory granules, granule exocytosis was rarely observed. However, at 5 to 15 min onwards, TRH induced the appearance, in the Golgi zone and beneath the plasma membrane, of numerous vesicles, and exocytosis of such vesicles was frequently observed (164). Electron-microscopic immunostaining using a preembedding method revealed that these vesicles contained PRL reaction product localized on their luminal surface. Once the vesicles fused with the plasma membrane they lost their reaction product. At the same time, the immunostaining of RER cisternae disappeared and that of Golgi saccules greatly decreased. These findings suggest that TRH transiently accelerates the intracellular transit of PRL and induces the formation of vesicles that serve as carriers for PRL release (46). It should be emphasized that these early effects of TRH were first detectable in a small number of cells, and, after 1 hr, in 57% of immunoreactive cells (46). This reveals the heterogeneity of the cell response. Moreover, when a 135-Kd Golgi antigen was immunocytochemically localized using similar experimental conditions, TRH also induced a flow of Golgi-derived vesicles toward the plasma membrane; the exocytosis of these vesicles led to the insertion of patches of Golgi antigen into the plasma membrane (177).

The rapid effect of TRH on PRL release by GH3 cells has been recently found to be composed of two phases: (i) The first phase involves a burst of PRL release, which occurs within 15 sec and peaks at 1 to 2 min; (ii) the second is a sustained phase of PRL release at a lower level (178–180). A similar pattern was observed in primary cultures (181). Preliminary observations suggest that the burst of PRL release results from exocytosis of a population of secretory granules already positioned next to the plasma membrane (Tougard, *unpublished observations*).

Another interesting morphological effect of short-term exposure to TRH is an increased mobility of the plasma membrane, as revealed by stretching of the plasma membrane (182), formation of blebs visible with the scanning electron microscope (183), and stimulation of endocytosis (184). Under the phase-contrast microscope, the cells are spread out over their substratum in a manner rather specific to TRH treatment [not observed with VIP (Gourdji, *unpublished observations*)]. This change in cell shape suggests an involvement of cytoskeletal components in the cell response to TRH. This cytoskeletal effect has received little attention so far, except for studies involving colchicine which enhanced PRL content in GH3 cells (58).

Primary cultures. After 1 hr of treatment with TRH, a distribution of the granules along the cell membrane was observed in some cells, whereas after 4 hr, most cells were significantly degranulated. At the same time, numerous blebs and microvilli were seen at the cell surface (166). Using electron-microscopic immunostaining with the preembedding approach, we have found that, as in GH3 cells, within 1 hr, TRH induces the formation of PRL-loaded vesicles in the Golgi zone and near the plasma membrane, as well as the insertion of Golgi antigen-labeled vesicles into the plasma membrane. Destaining of the RER occurs simultaneously. Some granule exocytosis could be seen. Although these modifications were seen in a small number of cells and after 4 hr of exposure to TRH, many cells still contained numerous large polymorphic secretory granules whereas others contained a few small rounded secretory granules (Tougard, *unpublished observations*). In fact, the structural heterogeneity of normal PRL cells in culture greatly hampered this morphological analysis. This problem deserves particular attention.

Heterogeneity of the cell response. The relationship between the structural heterogeneity of PRL cells and their acute response to TRH was analyzed in GH3 cells and/or in primary cultures by the following approaches: PRL immunostaining, reverse hemolytic plaque assay, and pulse-chase experiments.

As previously emphasized, GH3 cells display a strong heterogeneity of intracellular PRL content, as revealed by PRL immunostaining (46,58,185) (Fig. 12). The cells are organized into small colonies that contain a mixture of weakly, moderately, or heavily stained cells in variable proportions (Fig. 12). Within the first 30 min of exposure to TRH, there is a considerable loss of PRL immunostaining in all cell populations, with a shift toward an increased proportion of weakly stained cells (46,185) (Fig. 12). Such destaining could be correlated with changes in the subcellular distribution of PRL as described above, due to the experimental conditions used, i.e., *in-situ* embedding of the monolayers and selection of small colonies prior to thick sectioning (46). Without these technical improvements, the rapid effects of TRH on the subcellular distribution of PRL would probably have been underestimated or missed entirely.

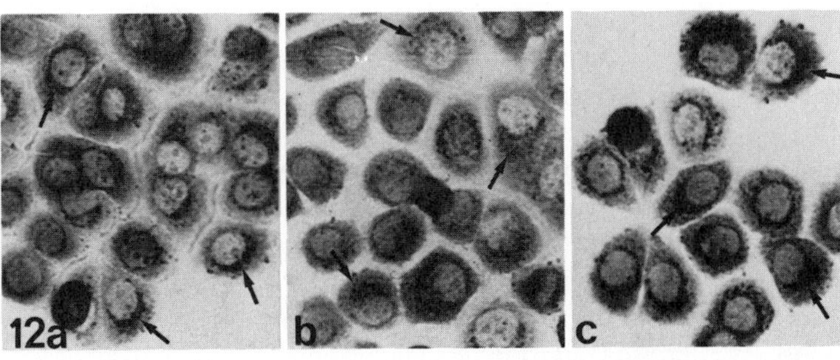

FIG. 12. GH3B6 cells immunocytochemically stained with an antiserum against rat PRL. (**a**) The PRL immunostaining of GH3B6 is strongly heterogeneous. A prominent crescent-shaped positive zone (*arrows*) is detected near the nucleus and corresponds to the Golgi zone. (**b**) After 1 hr of TRH treatment, the cells are spread out, with a decrease of PRL immunostaining, particularly in the Golgi zone (*arrows*). (**c**) After 2 hr of TRH treatment, the Golgi zone is reloaded with immunoreactive PRL (*arrows*). × 400. (From ref. 46.)

The RHPA has provided direct evidence that TRH preferentially stimulates the release of PRL by a subpopulation of PRL cells forming large plaque areas. However, the features of the responsive subpopulation are not well-defined (59). The rate of plaque formation, which reveals another aspect of the heterogeneity of the cell response to TRH, is transiently accelerated (126). Thus it appears that TRH stimulates, in a time-dependent manner, an increasing number of PRL cells; however, it is unable to recruit additional cells to secrete. These findings are in excellent agreement with previous immunocytochemical studies involving GH3 cells (46,185).

Pulse-chase experiments have been used to ascertain an effect of TRH on the heterogeneous turnover of PRL. Consistent results were obtained with both normal PRL cells (55,56) and GH3 cells (57); in both cases TRH induced the preferential release of stored PRL, which was synthesized prior to the pulse. These findings are in agreement with those obtained from immunocytochemistry, which suggests that the TRH-mobilizable PRL pool is located in secretory granules, as well as in the endoplasmic reticulum. However, this raises the question of the subcellular origin of the newly synthesized PRL, which is preferentially released under basal conditions. Two alternative hypotheses have been proposed. According to Walker and Farquhar (55), the two PRL pools are located in different cells. TRH would then act on a subpopulation of PRL cells, which differ from the others by their slow turnover of PRL and by their greater number of TRH-binding sites. Alternatively, the existence of two intracellular routes for the nonregulated basal release of PRL and the regulated release of PRL cannot be ruled out, in accordance with the concept of Kelly (186). In accordance with the latter hypothesis are the effects of monensin on GH3 cells. Monensin has been shown to induce an accumulation of PRL in large Golgi-derived vacuoles; this was correlated with a decrease in basal PRL release, without inducing an alteration of the percent stimulation of PRL release in response to TRH (187). Pulse-chase experiments have revealed that monensin, in fact, decreases PRL basal release without affecting that of the newly synthesized PRL, whereas it does not affect the release of unlabeled PRL in response to TRH. This supports the existence of two intracellular routes arising from an early Golgi subcompartment, located upstream from the monensin blockade, for the release of newly synthesized PRL, and from a late Golgi subcompartment, located downstream from the monensin blockade, for the release of stored PRL. The latter may consist of both secretory granules and vesicles (57). The two hypotheses may not be mutually exclusive. Preliminary studies performed with the RHPA technique suggest that, whatever the individual basal rate of PRL release, normal PRL cells respond to TRH by releasing unlabeled PRL (60).

In conclusion, if one compares the patterns of acute morphological responses to TRH in GH3 cells and normal PRL cells, one is surprised to see many similarities between two cell models, which greatly differ by their intracellular store of secretory granules. Recently, a similar conclusion was reached by a comparison of the patterns of PRL release by perifused GH4C1 cells and primary cultures in response to several agents, including TRH (181). Thus, the capacity to store a greater or smaller number of secretory granules does not seem to determine the pattern of the acute response.

Long-term Responses to Stimulatory Agents:

GH3 cells. At the light-microscopic level, treatment with 30 nM TRH for 48 hr has been shown to slightly increase the percentage of immunoreactive cells, as well as the intensity of their immunostaining. Moreover, the difference between the small increase in the percentage of immunopositive cells (from 35% to 45%) and the large increase in PRL cellular content (450% of control value) supports the assumption that TRH acts on GH3 cells "principally by raising the mean hormonal content of individual positive cells rather than by increasing the proportion of cells committed to PRL production" (58). Consistent data were recently obtained concerning the percentage of PRL-releasing cells, as determined by RHPA; the number of cells increased from 20% to 35%, by chronic treatment for 6 days with a pharmacological dose of TRH (37).

At the electron-microscopic level, long-term treatment with TRH was found to induce an obvious extension of the Golgi zone, which contained, in addition to stacks of saccules, many vesicles and often newly formed secretory granules. Moreover, the number of secretory granules was increased (164,182). Subcellular localization of PRL using electron-microscopic immunocytochemistry revealed the involvement of the RER, which recommenced PRL reloading after 2 to 4 hr of exposure to TRH. This was accompanied by the reloading of Golgi cisternae and vesicles. This reloading was totally blocked by simultaneous exposure to cycloheximide, indicating that it reflects a neosynthesis of PRL (46). Under these conditions, the intensity of the cytoplasmic immunostaining was not affected, indicating that the cytoplasmic material was not mobilizable by TRH (46). Biochemical studies have shown that this immobile material is immunologically related to PRL but consists of larger PRL molecules (57).

Chronic treatment with estradiol has been shown to induce an increase in both intracellular and medium PRL levels in GH3 cells under various culture conditions (188,189). This effect was recently correlated with an increase in the number and size of secretory granules in GH3 cells that were simultaneously exposed to 17β estradiol, insulin, and EGF (190).

Primary cultures. To our knowledge, the only study concerning the morphological correlates of long-term treatment with 17β estradiol (10^{-8} M) was carried out for up to 8 days. In this system, estradiol induced an increase of PRL secretion and morphological changes, which became maximal between 4 and 8 days of treatment. The morphological changes consisted of hypertrophy and increased immunostaining of PRL cells without modification of PRL cell number. At the electron-microscopic level, the treated cells displayed an enlarged Golgi zone containing an increased number of vesicles and immature secretory granules, as well as a distension of Golgi cisternae. An "increase in the RER" was also noticed. With regard to secretory granules, "large secretory granules were seldomly seen up to 4 days of treatment but could be seen in some cells between days 4 and 8." In addition, the cell surface was also modified in the same manner as by TRH, i.e., an increase in number of microvilli (166) was observed.

In conclusion, a comparison between the *in vivo* and *in vitro* data is possible for a limited number of factors, including dopamine or bromocriptine, 17β estradiol, and TRH, although the effects *in vivo* of the latter were reported for TSH cells but not for PRL cells, to our knowledge (27). Moreover, the *in-vitro* models are not always the same, and the morphological approaches vary greatly; in particular, electron-microscopic immunostaining has been used in a limited number of cases. This obviously limits the number of general conclusions that can be drawn.

One is reminded that the effects of a given factor on cellular ultrastructure are quite similar *in vivo* and *in vitro,* provided that the time course of treatment is similar. An acute or sustained stimulation of PRL secretion is always correlated with an enlargement of the Golgi zone, an increased number of forming secretory granules, and an association of secretory granules with the plasma membrane. The accumulation of PRL in the RER and the development of RER cisternae are, in general, signs of a sustained stimulation. The observations concerning secretory granules are not always clear or consistent. An increase in number and size is sometimes reported, whereas a decrease in diameter and a scarcity occur in other cases. The analysis of the data is hampered by the structural heterogeneity of the cells, as well as the interaction of several unidentified factors *in vivo* and *in vitro*.

Concerning the morphological correlates of the inhibition of PRL secretion, the precise comparison of *in vivo* and *in vitro* data remains difficult because of a limited number of studies. An accumulation of secretory granules, which lasts for several days, seems to be a common feature, whereas an induction of lysosomes is not always observed.

An important difference between *in vivo* and *in vitro* data resides in the control of cell proliferation. Long-term estradiol treatment induces *in vivo,* but not *in vitro,* a hyperplasia of immunoreactive PRL cells. Similarly, the growth of GH3 tumor cells *in vivo* is dependent on circulating estrogens, whereas *in vitro,* estradiol does not stimulate GH3 cell proliferation, under most conditions (189), except in the presence of gelding serum (191).

Gonadotropes

In-Vivo *Studies on Gonadotropes*

Morphological modifications or numerical variations of gonadotropes have been reported in relation to sex, estrous cycle, castration, GnRH treatment, adenomas, ontogenesis, and postnatal development. These observations, primarily obtained on the basis of immunocytochemical studies performed at the light- and electron-microscopic levels, will be examined successively.

Sex-related differences—Estrous cycle. From quantitative immunocytochemical analyses performed at the light-microscopic level on rat pituitary, it was clear that: (a) the percentage of multihormonal LH/FSH cells varied in relation to sex, i.e., in the female rat 37% to 40% of gonadotropes contained both hormones, as compared with 70% in the male rat (74); and (b) the absolute number of gonadotropes did not change in the adenohypophysis of the adult female rat throughout the estrous cycle (74,192). Moreover, according to Childs (74) there are changes in the storage pattern of the gonadotropes, which vary with the stage of the estrous cycle and which can be correlated with the respective level of circulating gonadotropins. Indeed, a decrease in the percentage of monohormonal LH cells at proestrus suggests that these cells may be responsible for the LH surge. The multihormonal LH/FSH cells may then become responsive during estrus (74). Using the reverse hemolytic plaque assay, Smith et al. (121) demonstrated that nonsecretory gonadotropes were found in the pituitary of diestrous rats, whereas nearly all of the gonadotropes were secretory at proestrus.

At the electron-microscopic level, the number of each gonadotropic cell type, characterized by its ultrastructural features, also varies during the estrous cycle (67,78,89). Type-II cells, which are scarce in the male rat, increase in number during proestrus and estrus in female rats, concomitantly with a decrease in the number of type-I cells (79,89). There is a similar shift from type-I to type-II cells for the anti-β-LH-stained cell population and for the anti-β-FSH-stained cell population indicating, once more, that these two gonadotrope subtypes correspond to different stages of secretory activity in the same cell.

Castration. Morphological changes induced in the pituitary after castration have been described in early studies at the light-microscopic level (193), with the appearance of so-called "castration cells" or "signet-ring cells," each of which contains a large vacuole. Such castration cells were later described by conventional electron microscopy, first by Farquhar and Rinehart (5), followed by Yoshimura and Harumiya (194) in the rat, by Barnes (75,76) in the mouse, and more recently by Kurosumi et al. (195) in the rat. Hypertrophied castration cells are characterized by dilation of the endoplasmic reticulum inducing either round vacuoles or irregularly shaped and dilated cisternae resembling filigree. Progressively, with increasing time after castration, the typical signet-ring cells appear, characterized by a very large vacuole induced by the gradual expansion and confluence of the endoplasmic reticulum cisternae.

The coexistence of LH and FSH within castration cells was clearly demonstrated in castrated male and female rats (78,101,196), as well as in castrated pigs (101). The castration cells did not stain for ACTH (101,105). The percentage of gonadotropes that stored both LH and FSH, which was determined by morphometric analysis of immunoreactive cells, increased in developing castration cells, from 70% to 91% in the male rat and from 50% to 75% in the female (101). This suggested (a) that an early response to castration consists of the stimulation of dual hormone production and (b) that all gonadotropes are bipotential. Three months after castration, there was a threefold increase in the percentages of LH and FSH cells, followed by a decrease by 6 months (137). The increased number of gonadotropes during the first 3 months is probably due to cell division (197,198). Simultaneous adrenalectomy and castration result in a significant decrease in the percentage of castration cells (199).

In many studies (66,78,195) the castration cells were derived mainly from the type-I gonadotrope, which progressively displayed a dilation of the RER and a decrease and eventual disappearance of large secretory granules. The small secretory granules persisted and were mainly localized at the cell periphery along the cell membrane. At the same time, type-II gonadotropes remained scarce and unmodified (78). In highly degranulated cells, the content of the dilated RER cisternae was stained with anti-β-LH and, to a lesser extent, with anti-LH.

GnRH treatment. Gonadotropin-releasing hormone (GnRH) exerts a biphasic stimulatory effect on LH/FSH secretion (see Chapter 32). This effect involves the rapid release of a previously formed hormonal pool, as well as a delayed stimulation of hormone synthesis. The respective ultrastructural correlates of these two phases have been studied mainly *in vivo* using conventional electron microscopy.

A rapid and obvious extrusion of secretory granules via exocytosis occurs within minutes in response to GnRH in gonadotropes of persistent estrous rats (200) or in intact or gonadectomized male and female rats pretreated (or not) with estrogen and/or progesterone (201–203). The diameter and electron density of secretory granules of gonadotropes decrease rapidly after GnRH injection (204). Moreover, along with granule exocytosis, a progressive extension of the RER and of the Golgi zone occurs in gonadotropes after infusion of GnRH into the portal vessels (205). All these observations suggest that the acute hormonal release is rapidly correlated with modifications of the entire ultrastructural organization of the cell.

The effects of chronic injection or prolonged infusion with GnRH or TRH, or both, in male rats have been extensively analyzed by Yoshimura and his colleagues (206–210). All of these studies revealed similar features of the continuously stimulated cells, including development and dilation of the RER, extension of the Golgi zone, and a decrease in the size and number of secretory granules concomitant with hypertrophy of the cell, all of which induce the appearance of gonadectomized or thyroidectomized cells. The sequential ultrastructural transformation of anterior pituitary basophils (gonadotropes and thyrotropes), identified on the basis of conventional electron microscopy, suggested to these authors a theory involving the secretory cycle of a single basophilic cell type that would successively secrete TSH, FSH, and LH (206).

Gonadotropic adenomas. According to Kovacs et al. (142), no convincing studies of experimental gonadotropic adenomas have been reported so far.

Gonadotropes can give rise to neoplasia. However, in great contrast to prolactinomas, gonadotropic adenomas are rare in human beings and difficult to identify at the light-microscopic level because they appear to be chromophobic (144,211,212). The cells can only be identified through the use of immunocytochemistry and have been shown to contain either FSH alone or FSH and LH (212). At the electron-microscopic level, human gonadotropic adenomas display well-developed RER cisternae, a prominent Golgi zone, and sparse small secretory granules (142,144).

Ontogenesis and postnatal development. The appearance of gonadotropes during the ontogenesis of the anterior pituitary has been extensively studied using immunocytochemistry at the light-microscopic level. In the rat fetus, some immunoreactive LH cells, localized in the ventral part of the gland, appear on the 17th day of gestation, are more numerous at 18 days of gestation, and their number continues to increase until the end of gestation (150,153,213,214). Immunoreactive FSH cells appear later on, depending on the study, between days 19 and 20 of gestation, and their distribution is similar to that of immunoreactive LH cells. Gonadotropes appear on the 49th day of gestation in the sheep fetus (215), on the 45th day of gestation in the pig fetus (216,217), and not before the 53rd day of gestation in the monkey fetus (218). In the human fetus, only subunits are detected by the 8th week of intra-uterine life, followed by LH during the third month, and FSH by the beginning of the fourth month (219,220). LH and FSH were present in the same cells, which were more numerous in the female fetus. At birth, the gonadotropes are scarce and are located at the ventromedial zone of the anterior pituitary. From all of these immunocytochemical studies performed with specific antisera, it is clear that (a) α and β subunits of LH and FSH are not synthesized at the same time (the α subunit generally appears earlier than the β subunit or the complete hormone) and (b) LH appears earlier than FSH. Gross and Baker (221) have shown that LH gonadotropes and GnRH-containing neurons appear concomitantly in the mouse fetus at the 17th day of gestation, suggesting a neuroendocrine control of gonadotropin differentiation. This hypothesis has been the subject of several studies. Morphological studies performed either after experimental encephalectomy (214) or with cultures of adenohypophysial primordia explanted at different ages of gestation support the hypothesis of an autodifferentiation of gonadotropes, independent of hypothalamic GnRH (155,156,214,222). However, contradictory conclusions were reported by several groups. Recent studies performed *in vitro* by Begeot et al. (223,224) suggested that GnRH can stimulate the differentiation of gonadotropes at a very early fetal stage (11 days) in synergy with insulin. Clonal cells (2A8), derived from the epithelium of Rathke's pouch of fetal rat (11–13 days) (225), which did not contain gonadotropes when grown *in vitro,* were able to differentiate into all pituitary cell types after implantation into the hypothalamus of hypophysectomized rats (226,227) or when the culture medium was supplemented with fresh serum from hypophysectomized rats (228). This suggests that factors present in the serum are necessary for cytodifferentiation of gonadotropes.

At the electron-microscopic level, using conventional methods, the first granulated cells are detected between the 16th and 17th days of gestation in the fetal rat pituitary. They do not display the ultrastructural features of mature adult cells and cannot be identified on this basis. Morphological analogy with adult cells begins to occur between the 18th and 19th days of gestation (229–231). Electron-microscopic immunocytochemistry allowed the identification of the first immunoreactive gonadotropes on day 16 in the rat fetus (213) and on day 40 in the pig fetus (232). These cells initially display the ultrastructural features of immature cells with a few small secretory granules and then, with increasing time of gestation, they undergo progressive morphological differentiation involving the development of RER cisternae and the Golgi zone, as well as an increased number and size of secretory granules. At the end of gestation in the pig, gonadotropes possess the ultrastructural features of mature cells (232), whereas in the rat they still differ from adult gonadotropes (213).

During postnatal development of the rat pituitary, gonadotropes undergo important changes in number, size, and structure. They increase in number during the first week of postnatal life (233,234). Thereafter, their percentage is greater than that in the adult, with an increased cell number in females as compared to males. Matsumura and Daikoku (235) demonstrated that sex steroids may be responsible for the sexual differences in the morphological development (cell number and cell size) of LH cells in newborn rats. As in adult cells, most of the gonadotropes of the young rats contained both LH and FSH (234). However, according to Childs and her colleagues (234,236) a great number of gonadotropes contain ACTH-like immunoreactivity during postnatal development and might subserve a function related to that of adrenal-gonadal maturation. This observation was a subject of controversy because according to Inoue and Hogino (83), angular-shaped gonadotropes in neonatal and immature rats did not contain ACTH. At the electron-microscopic level, the morphological maturation of the gonadotropes in the rat pituitary occurs during the first 7 days of postnatal life; after 1 to 2 weeks of age, most of the cells resemble adult cell types (234). All of these morphological observations clearly emphasize the importance of the first 2 to 3 weeks of life for the functional maturation of the gonadotropic population (237).

In-Vitro *Functional Studies on Gonadotropes*

Most recently, *in vitro* functional studies on gonadotropes have been performed either on newly dispersed anterior pituitary cells or on dissociated cells grown in monolayers or in reaggregate cell cultures. Such models represent the available tools to examine the cell response to various physiological stimuli. Indeed, it has been shown that just after enzymatic dispersion, and at least for the first days in culture, gonadotropes from adult rat pituitaries retain their morphological heterogeneity (6,164,238,239) and their capacity to respond to specific regulatory agents (164). After the first week of culture, FSH and LH secretion progressively declines with time whereas immunoreactive gonadotropes still remain present (165,239) (Fig. 13), even in long-term primary cultures (35 or 56 days) (239). Progressive modifications of the ultrastructural organization of immunoreactive cells occur with increasing time in culture; finally, a single gonadotropic cell type remains, characterized by immature features: small secretory granules (125–150 nm), a few RER cisternae, and an inconspicuous Golgi complex (239). Gonadotropes in aggregates of cells from dispersed rat anterior pituitaries, as well as from enriched populations of gonadotropes, also retain their ultrastructural characteristics and respond selectively to various agents in a superfusion system (240).

Whereas modifications of hormonal secretion under specific regulatory agents have been extensively studied *in vitro* (see Chapter 32), the morphological modifications following stimulation of the secretory activity of gonadotropes are far less numerous and primarily concern the response to GnRH.

Morphological correlates of gonadotropes in response to GnRH. Short-term Effects of GnRH: In 7-day primary cultures of dispersed rat anterior pituitary cells exposed to GnRH for 15 to 30 min, classic exocytotic profiles were not observed in gonadotropes, but many secretory granules were lined up along the plasma membrane and, after immunocytochemical staining, displayed structural changes. This suggests that GnRH simultaneously induced a rapid migration of secretory granules toward the plasma membrane, with a structural reorganization of their matrix visualized by a decrease in electron density (164). Using other culture conditions and immunocytochemical methods, Childs has also found that GnRH stimulation results in the formation of cellular processes that contain monohormonal secretory granules in multihormonal cells (104). In addition, these processes also stained for releasing hormone (104,110,241). From these observations, Childs (110) postulates that these "processes provide attractive morphological correlates for potential sites of local control of nonparallel LH and FSH release from multihormonal cells." The mechanisms involved in such a dissociation of gonadotropin stores, as well as the mechanisms involved in its control, have not yet been determined.

Similar observations concerning the rapid migration of secretory granules were recorded by Lewis et al. (242,243) with mouse hemipituitaries incubated for two consecutive hours with GnRH. This treatment induces a priming effect of GnRH on gonadotropin secretion (see *these volumes*). Under these experimental conditions, the initial exposure to GnRH induced a translocation of gonadotrope secretory

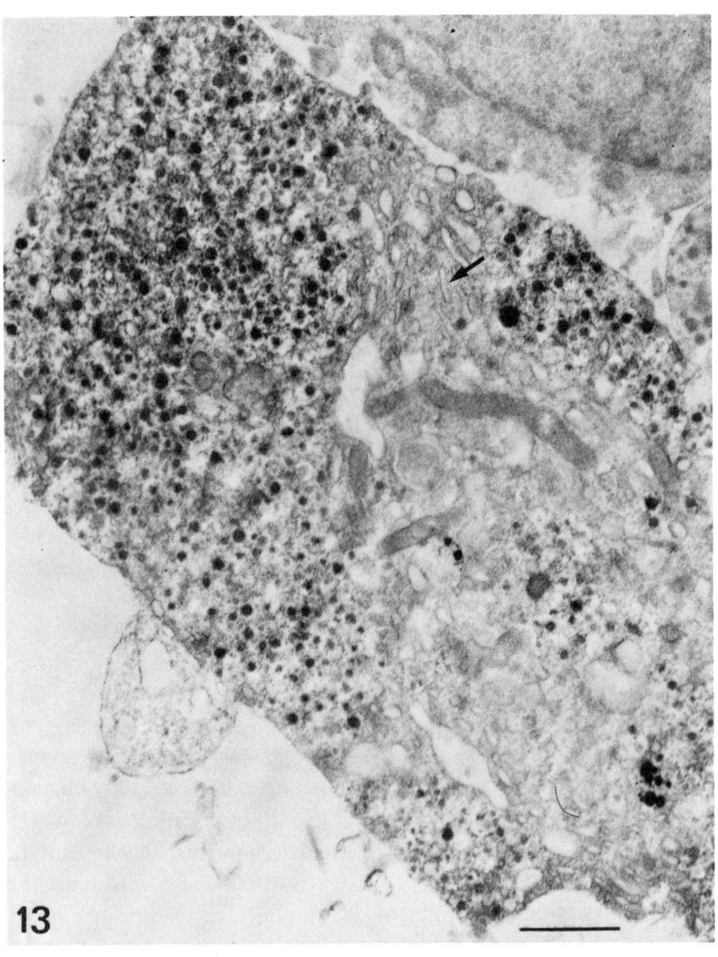

FIG. 13. A 12-day monolayer of rat anterior pituitary cells is immunochemically stained with an antiserum against rat β-LH. This immunoreactive gonadotrope displays small secretory granules and slightly dilated RER cisternae (*arrows*). Bar represents 1 μm. × 16,200.

granules toward the plasmalemma, as well as a decrease in granule size. Granules adjacent to the plasma membrane may therefore represent a readily releasable pool of hormone that responds to a second exposure to GnRH and that can sustain the priming effect of GnRH (243). The migration of the secretory granules appears to be reversible following GnRH withdrawal (244). Concomitant with these ultrastructural modifications, these authors have shown that the GnRH priming effect is associated with an increase in length and a change in the orientation of microfilaments in gonadotropes, suggesting a role for cytoskeletal components in granule translocation (242).

Another important rapid morphological modification of stimulated cells involves modifications of the plasma membrane, which results in the formation of microvilli and branched cytoplasmic processes (164). This modification was reported only for *in vitro* systems. Near the cell periphery, numerous small vesicles or canaliculi appear, which are sometimes labeled with exogenous horseradish peroxidase, indicating an increase in endocytotic activity (184). Simultaneously, a progressive extension of the Golgi zone occurs, in addition to an increase in the number of small vesicles and multivesicular bodies in this area. Condensing (164). These ultrastructural observations suggest that GnRH may stimulate membrane traffic in gonadotropes at the same time as secretory activity.

GnRH has also been found to rapidly modify the relative proportion of LH and FSH in gonadotropes. Indeed, Childs (110,241) has shown that it increases the proportion of gonadotropes containing both hormones while causing a corresponding decrease in monohormonal cells, indicating once more that monohormonal gonadotropes are, in fact, bipotential.

The heterogeneity of the gonadotropic response to GnRH was recently investigated in depth by Neill et al. (245) using RHPA. This study indicated that not all gonadotropes respond in the same manner to GnRH, as assessed by several functional parameters. The differences between the smallest and largest individual cell responses were up to 500- to 1000-fold. Some cells did not respond, although they contained an ample store of immunodetectable LH. Thus, there are nonreleasable stores of LH, particularly at diestrus, a stage when gonadotropes are the largest (244) and display an increased number of secretory granules (89,244). Surprisingly, there was no direct correlation between the amount of labeled GnRH bound by a given cell and the size of the secretory material was found inside some Golgi cisternae plaque area, suggesting that only a fraction of receptors are functional (245).

Long-term Effects of GnRH: Morphological studies on chronic stimulation with GnRH have been performed in organ cultures of rat pituitary exposed for up to 24 hr (246). These studies also revealed a decrease in the size and number of secretory granules, an extension of the Golgi zone, and a development and dilation of the RER cisternae inducing hypertrophy of stimulated gonadotropes. Indeed, cells similar to the so-called "castration cells" may appear in cultures exposed to high doses of GnRH for 3 to 6 hr.

Chronic treatment of primary cultures of rat anterior pituitary cells with GnRH for a month induced hypertrophy and degranulation of gonadotropes, which, at this late stage of culture, displayed only one class of very small (100 nm) rounded secretory granules and the development of parallel and flattened RER cisternae (164). In addition, chronic treatment with GnRH did not increase the number of immunoreactive gonadotropes nor did it prevent the fall in LH and FSH secretion (164).

In conclusion, the morphological correlates of the stimulation of LH and FSH secretion by GnRH are quite similar *in vivo* and *in vitro*. They always correspond to (a) a migration of secretory granules toward the plasma membrane, (b) an enlargement of the RER cisternae, and (c) an extension of the Golgi zone. The size of secretory granules decreases in highly stimulated cells, with a concomitant disappearance of the large secretory granules. Simultaneously, change in the hormonal storage pattern of gonadotropes occurs, which is revealed by an increase in the percentage of multihormonal cells.

GENERAL CONCLUSIONS

The identity of the cell types responsible for the secretion of the three anterior pituitary hormones that control reproduction in mammals is well established because of the availability of specific immunological probes. With certain exceptions, one may maintain that PRL and GH are generally contained and secreted by different cells, whereas LH and FSH are found mainly in the same cells.

The functional adaptation of these cells to the complexity of the physiological regulation of the control of reproduction is achieved by diversification of the ultrastructural organization of both lactotropes and gonadotropes. Such a diversity is progressively established during postnatal development and clearly corresponds to a functional heterogeneity. However, the exact link between a given type of ultrastructural organization and the corresponding secretory activity is still unclear. This question deserves further study at the single cell level. It seems, *a priori,* easier to solve for lactotropes than for gonadotropes because of the complexity of synthetic machinery of LH and FSH, from genes to post-translational maturation.

The morphological response of these cell types to specific agents has been more thoroughly analyzed *in vitro* because of the development of culture methods. Again the significance of morphological changes is better defined for lactotropes than for gonadotropes. This is the consequence of two occurrences: (i) the considerable difference between the long-term secretory ability in culture of lactotropes and gonadotropes and (ii) the absence of a model of a responsive gonadotrope cell line, when compared to GH3 prolactin cells. Attempts to immortalize differentiated gonadotropes are likely to result in great progress in the future. In addition, the present data suggest that similar cellular mechanisms might be involved in the rapid effect of stimulating hypothalamic peptides, such as rapid migration of secretory granules toward the plasma membrane and concomitant reorganization of the Golgi complex. Future studies will involve the elucidation of the biochemical mechanisms of such membrane traffic.

ACKNOWLEDGMENTS

We gratefully acknowledge Miss A. Bayon for her valuable help in typing this manuscript, Mr. C. Pennarun for his skillful competence in the preparation of photomicrographs, Dr. E. Vila-Porcile and R. Picart for their helpful assistance in the final preparation of illustrations, and Dr. A. Weisman for correcting the English of the manuscript.

Part of our work reported in this review was supported by grants from the Centre National de la Recherche Scientifique (grant ER 89, UA 041115, ATP) and from the Direction Générale à la Recherche Scientifique et Technique (contract 72 7 0100).

REFERENCES

1. Girod, C. (1983): Immunocytochemistry of the vertebrate adenohypophysis. In: *Handbuch der Histochemie, Vol. VIII, Sup. Part 5,* edited by W. Graumann and K. Neumann, Fischer Verlag, Jena.
2. Romeis, B. (1940): Hypophyse. In: *Handbuch der mikroskopischen Anatomie des Menschen, Vol. 6,* Part 3, edited by W. von Möllendorff, 625 pages, Springer, Berlin.
3. Herlant, M. (1964): The cells of the adenohypophysis and their functional significance. *Int. Rev. Cytol.,* 17:299–382.
4. Herlant, M. (1975): Introduction. In: *The Anterior Pituitary Gland,* edited by M. G. Farquhar and A. Tixier-Vidal, pp. 1–19, Academic Press, New York.
5. Farquhar, M. G., and Rinehart, J. F. (1954): Electron microscope studies of the anterior pituitary of castrate rats. *Endocrinology,* 54:516–541.
6. Farquhar, M. G., Skutelsky, E. H., and Hopkins, C. R. (1975): Structure and function of the anterior pituitary and dispersed pituitary cells. *In vitro* studies. In: *The Anterior Pituitary,* edited by M. G. Farquhar and A. Tixier-Vidal, pp. 83–135. Academic Press, New York.
7. Nakane, P. K. (1970): Classifications of anterior pituitary cell types with immunoenzyme histochemistry. *J. Histochem. Cytochem.,* 18:9–21.
8. Moriarty, G. (1973): Adenohypophysis: Ultrastructural cytochemistry. A review. *J. Histochem. Cytochem.,* 21:855–894.
9. Nakane, P. K. (1975): Identification of anterior pituitary cells by immunoelectron microscopy. In: *The Anterior Pituitary,* edited by

M. G. Farquhar and A. Tixier-Vidal, pp. 45–61. Academic Press, New York.

10. Baker, B. L., Midgley, A. R. Jr., Gersten, B. E., and Yu, Y. Y. (1969): Differentiation of growth hormone and prolactin containing acidophils with peroxidase-labeled antibody. *Anat. Rec.*, 164:163–171.
11. Baker, B. L., and Gross, D. S. (1978): Cytology and distribution of secretory cell types in mouse hypophysis as demonstrated with immunocytochemistry. *Am. J. Anat.*, 153:193–215.
12. Pasteels, J. L., Gausset, P., Danguy, A., Ectors, F., Nicoll, C. S., and Varavudhi, P. (1972): Morphology of the lactotropes and somatotropes of man and rhesus monkeys. *J. Clin. Endocrinol. Metab.*, 34:959–967.
13. Halmi, N. S., Parsons, J. A., Erlandsen, S. L., and Duello, T. (1975): Prolactin and growth hormone cells in the human hypophysis: A study with immunoenzyme histochemistry and differential staining. *Cell Tissue Res.*, 158:497–507.
14. Baker, B. L., and Yu, Y. Y. (1977): An immunocytochemical study of human pituitary mammotropes from fetal life to old age. *Am. J. Anat.*, 148:217–240.
15. Nogami, H., and Yoshimura, F. (1982): Fine structural criteria of prolactin cells identified immunohistochemically in the male rat. *Anat. Rec.*, 202:261–274.
16. Pasteels, J. L. (1963): Recherches morphologiques et expérimentales sur la sécrétion de prolactine. *Arch. Biol. Liège*, 74:439–453.
17. Smith, R. E., and Farquhar, M. G. (1966): Lysosome function in the regulation of the secretory process in cells of anterior pituitary gland. *J. Cell Biol.*, 31:319–347.
18. Pasteels, J. L., Ectors, F., Danguy, A., Robyn, C., L'Hermite, M., and Dujardin, M. (1973): Histological immunofluorescent and electron microscopic identification of prolactin producing cells in the human pituitary. *IVth International Congress of Endocrinology, Excerpta Medica International Congress, Series No. 273*, pp. 616–621. Excerpta Medica, Amsterdam.
19. Tougard, C., Picart, R., and Tixier-Vidal, A. (1980): Electron microscopic cytochemical studies on the secretory process in primary culture. *Am. J. Anat.*, 158:471–490.
20. Nogami, H., and Yoshimura, F. (1980): Prolactin immunoreactivity of acidophils of the small granule type. *Cell Tissue Res.*, 211:1–4.
21. Nogami, H. (1984): Fine structural heterogeneity and morphological changes in rat pituitary prolactin cells after estrogen and testosterone treatment. *Cell Tissue Res.*, 237:195–202.
22. Beauvillain, J. C., Mazzuca, M., and Dubois, M. P. (1977): The prolactin and growth hormone producing cells of the guinea pig pituitary. Electron microscopic study using immunocytochemical means. *Cell Tissue Res.*, 184:343–358.
23. Dacheux, F., and Dubois, M. P. (1976): Ultrastructural localization of prolactin, growth hormone and luteinizing hormone by immunocytochemical techniques in the bovine pituitary. *Cell Tissue Res.*, 174:245–260.
24. Dacheux, F. (1980): Ultrastructural immunocytochemical localization of prolactin and growth hormone in the porcine pituitary. *Cell Tissue Res.*, 207:277–286.
25. Martin-Comin, J., and Robyn, C. (1976): Comparative immunoenzymatic localization of prolactin and growth hormone in human and rat pituitaries. *J. Histochem. Cytochem.*, 24:1012–1016.
26. Girod, C., and Dubois, M. P. (1976): Immunofluorescent identification of somatotropic and prolactin cells in the anterior lobe of the hypophysis (pars distalis) of the monkey *Macacus irus*. *Cell Tissue Res.*, 172:145–148.
27. Tixier-Vidal, A., Tougard, C., Dufy, B., and Vincent, J. D. (1982): Morphological, functional and electrical correlates in anterior pituitary cells. In: *Neuroendocrine Perspectives, Vol. 1*, edited by E. E. Müller and R. M. MacLeod, pp. 211–251. Elsevier Biomedical Press, Amsterdam.
28. Halmi, N. S. (1982): Occurrence of both growth hormone and prolactin immunoreactive material in the cells of human somatotropic pituitary adenomas containing mammotropic elements. *Virchows Arch. A.*, 398:19–31.
29. Trouillas, J., Girod, C., Lheritier, M., Claustrat, B., and Dubois, M. P. (1980): Morphological and biochemical relationships in 31 human pituitary adenomas with acromegaly. *Virchows Arch. A.*, 389:127–142.
30. Fumagalli, G., and Zanini, A. (1985): In cow anterior pituitary, growth hormone and prolactin can be packed in separate granules of the same cell. *J. Cell Biol.*, 100:2019–2024.
31. Papka, R. E., Yu, S. M., and Nikitovitch-Winer, (1986): Use of immunoperoxidase and immunogold methods in studying prolactin secretion and application of immunogold labeling for pituitary hormones and neuropeptides. *Am. J. Anat.*, 175:289–306.
32. Smets, G., Welkeniers, B., Finne, E., Baldys, A., Gepts, W., and Vanhaelst, L. (1987): Postnatal development of growth hormone and prolactin cells in male and female pituitary. An immunocytochemical light and electron microscopic study. *J. Histochem. Cytochem.*, 35:335–342.
33. Neill, J. D., and Frawley, L. S. (1983): Detection of hormone release from individual cells in mixed populations using a reverse hemolytic plaque assay. *Endocrinology*, 112:1135–1137.
34. Leong, D. A., Lau, S. K., Sinha, Y. N., Kaiser, D. L., and Thorner, M. O. (1985): Enumeration of lactotropes and somatotropes among male and female pituitary cells in culture: Evidence in favor of a mammosomatotrope subpopulation in the rat. *Endocrinology*, 116:1371–1378.
35. Frawley, L. S., Boockfor, F. R., and Hoeffler, J. P. (1985): Identification by plaque assays of a pituitary cell type that secretes both growth hormone and prolactin. *Endocrinology*, 116:734–737.
36. Stratman, I. E., Ezrin, C., and Sellers, E. A. (1974): Estrogen induced transformation of somatotrophs into mammotrophs in the rat. *Cell Tissue Res.*, 152:229–238.
37. Boockfor, F. R., Hoeffler, J. P., and Frawley, L. S. (1985): Cultures of GH3 cells are functionally heterogeneous: Thyrotropin-releasing hormone, estradiol and cortisol cause reciprocal shifts in the proportions of growth hormone and prolactin secretors. *Endocrinology*, 117:418–420.
38. Cooke, N. E., Coit, D., Weiner, R. I., Baxter, J., and Martial, J. A. (1980): Structure of cloned DNA complementary to rat prolactin messenger RNA. *J. Biol. Chem.*, 255:6502–6510.
39. Nelson, C., Crenshaw, E. B., Franco, R., Lira, S. A., Albert, V. R., Evans, R. M., and Rosenfeld, M. G. (1986): Discrete cis-active genomic sequences dictate the pituitary cell type specific expression of rat prolactin and growth hormone genes. *Nature*, 322:557–562.
40. Farquhar, M. G. (1977): Secretion and crinophagy in prolactin cells. In: *Comparative Endocrinology of Prolactin*, edited by H. D. Dellman, J. A. Johnson, and D. M. Klachko, pp. 37–91. Plenum Press, New York.
41. Tixier-Vidal, A. (1980): Structural basis of adenohypophyseal secretory processes. In: *Synthesis and Release of Adenohypophyseal Hormones*, edited by M. Jutisz and K. W. McKerns, pp. 1–14. Plenum Press, New York.
42. Zanini, A., Giannattasio, G., and Meldolesi, J. (1980): Intracellular events in prolactin secretion. In: *Synthesis and Release of Adenohypophyseal Hormones*, edited by M. Jutisz and K. W. McKerns, pp. 105–124. Plenum Press, New York.
43. Tixier-Vidal, A., and Picart, R. (1967): Etude quantitative par radioautographie au microscope électronique de l'utilisation de la DL-Leucine ^{3}H par les cellules de l'hypophyse du Canard en culture organotypique. *J. Cell Biol.*, 35:501–519.
44. Farquhar, M. G., Reid, J., and Daniell, L. W. (1978): Intracellular transport and packaging of prolactin: A quantitative electron microscope autoradiographic study of mammotrophs dissociated from rat pituitaries. *Endocrinology*, 102:296–311.
45. Palade, G. E. (1975): Intracellular aspects of the process of protein secretion. *Science*, 189:347–358.
46. Tougard, C., Picart, R., and Tixier-Vidal, A. (1982): Immunocytochemical localization of prolactin in the endoplasmic reticulum of GH3 cells. Variations in response to thyroliberin. *Biol. Cell.*, 43:89–102.
47. Osamura, R. Y., Komatsu, N., Izumi, S., Yoshimura, F., and Watanabe, K. (1982): Ultrastructural localization of prolactin in the rat anterior pituitary glands by preembedding peroxidase-labeled antibody method. *J. Histochem. Cytochem.*, 30:919–925.
48. Rosa, P., Fumagalli, G., Zanini, A., and Huttner, W. B. (1985): The major tyrosine-sulfated protein of the bovine anterior pituitary is a secretory protein present in gonadotrophs, thyrotrophs, mammotrophs and corticotrophs. *J. Cell Biol.*, 100:928–937.

49. Childs (Moriarty), G. V., Cole, D. E., Kubek, M., Tobin, R. B., and Wilber, J. F. (1978): Endogenous thyrotropin-releasing hormone in the anterior pituitary: Sites of activity as identified by immunocytochemical staining. *J. Histochem. Cytochem.*, 26:901–908.
50. Morel, G., Gourdji, D., Grouselle, D., Brunet, N., Tixier-Vidal, A., and Dubois, P. M. (1985): Immunocytochemical evidence for *in vivo* internalization of thyroliberin into rat pituitary target cells *Neuroendocrinology*, 41:312–320.
51. Vila-Porcile, E., Picart, R., Tixier-Vidal, A., and Tougard, C. (1987): Cellular and subcellular distribution of laminin in adult rat anterior pituitary. *J. Histochem. Cytochem.*, 35:287–299.
52. Tougard, C., Louvard, D., Picart, R., and Tixier-Vidal, A. (1985): Immunocytochemical localization of laminin in rat anterior pituitary cells *in vivo* and *in vitro*. *In Vitro Cell. Dev. Biol.*, 21:57–61.
53. Snyder, J. M., Wilfinger, W., and Hymer, W. C. (1976): Maintenance of separated rat pituitary mammotrophs in cell culture. *Endocrinology*, 98:25–32.
54. Swearingen, K. C. (1971): Heterogeneous turnover of adenohypophysial prolactin. *Endocrinology*, 89:1380–1388.
55. Walker, A. M., and Farquhar, M. G. (1980): Preferential release of newly synthesized prolactin granules is the result of functional heterogeneity among mammotrophs. *Endocrinology*, 107:1095–1104.
56. Morin, A., Rosenbaum, E., and Tixier-Vidal, A. (1984): Effects of thyrotropin-releasing hormone on prolactin compartments in normal rat pituitary cells in primary cultures. *Endocrinology*, 115:2278–2284.
57. Morin, A., Rosenbaum, E., and Tixier-Vidal, A. (1984): Effects of thyrotropin releasing hormone on prolactin compartments in clonal rat pituitary tumor cells. *Endocrinology*, 115:2271–2277.
58. Hoyt, R. F., and Tashjian, A. H. (1980): Immunocytochemical analysis of prolactin production by monolayer cultures of GH3 rat anterior pituitary tumor cells. I. Long term effects of stimulation with thyrotropin-releasing hormone (TRH). *Anat. Rec.*, 197:153–162.
59. Luque, E. H., Munoz de Toro, M., Smith, P. F., and Neill, J. D. (1986): Subpopulations of lactotropes detected with the reverse hemolytic plaque assay show differential responsiveness to dopamine. *Endocrinology*, 118:2120–2124.
60. Luque, E. H., Munoz de Toro, M., and Neill, J. D. (1985): Measurement of pulse labeled prolactin release from individual lactotropes using the reverse hemolytic plaque assay. *Endocrinology*, abstract, no. 234.
61. Kadowaki, J., Ku, N., Oetting, W. S., and Walker, A. M. (1984): Mammotroph autoregulation: Uptake of secreted prolactin and inhibition of secretion. *Endocrinology*, 114:2060–2067.
62. Frawley, L. S., and Clark, C. L. (1986): Ovine prolactin and dopamine preferentially inhibit PRL release from the same subpopulation of rat mammotropes. *Endocrinology*, 119:1462–1466.
63. Purves, H. D., and Griesbach, W. E. (1955): Changes in the gonadotrophs of the rat pituitary after gonadectomy. *Endocrinology*, 56:374–386.
64. Herlant, M. (1960): Etude critique de deux techniques nouvelles destinées à mettre en évidence les différentes catégories cellulaires présentes dans la glande pituitaire. *Bull. Microsc. Appl.*, 10:37–44.
65. Pasteels, J. L., and Herlant, M. (1962): Notions nouvelles sur la cytologie de l'antéhypophyse chez le Rat. *Z. Zellforsch.*, 56:20–39.
66. Tougard, C. (1980): Immunocytochemical identification of LH and FSH secreting cells at the light and electron microscope levels. In: *Synthesis and Release of Adenohypophyseal Hormones*, edited by M. Jutisz and K. W. McKerns, pp. 15–37. Plenum Press, New York.
67. Tougard, C., Picart, R., and Tixier-Vidal, A. (1980): Immunocytochemical localization of glycoprotein hormones in the rat anterior pituitary. A light and electron microscope study using antisera against rat β subunits: A comparison between preembedding and postembedding methods. *J. Histochem. Cytochem.*, 28:101–114.
68. Baker, B. L., and Yu, Y. Y. (1975): Immunocytochemical analysis of cells in the pars tuberalis of the rat hypophysis with antisera to hormones of the pars distalis. *Cell Tissue Res.*, 156:443–449.
69. Baker, B. L. (1977): Cellular composition of the human pituitary pars tuberalis as revealed by immunocytochemistry. *Cell Tissue Res.*, 182:151–163.
70. Herbert, D. C. (1978): Identification of the LH and TSH secreting cells in the pituitary gland of the rhesus monkey. *Cell Tissue Res.*, 190:151–161.
71. El Etreby, M. F., and Fath El Bab, M. R. (1977): Localization of gonadotropic hormones in the dog pituitary gland. *Cell Tissue Res.*, 183:167–175.
72. Stoëckel, M. E., and Porte, A. (1984): Fine structure and development of the pars tuberalis in mammals. In: *Ultrastructure of Endocrine Cells and Tissues*, edited by P. M. Motta, pp. 29–38. Martinus Nijhoff, The Hague.
73. Fellmann, D., Bresson, J. L., Clavequin, M. C., and Bugnon, C. (1982): Quantitative immunocytochemical studies on the gonadotrophs isolated from the pituitary of the male rat. *Cell Tissue Res.*, 224:137–144.
74. Childs, G. V. (1984): Fluidity of gonadotropin storage in cycling female rats. In: *Hormonal Control of the Hypothalamo-Pituitary-Gonadal Axis*, edited by K. W. McKerns and Z. Naor, pp. 181–198. Plenum Press, New York.
75. Barnes, B. G. (1962): Electron microscope studies on the secretory cytology of the mouse anterior pituitary, *Endocrinology*, 71:618–628.
76. Barnes, B. G. (1963): The fine structure of the mouse adenohypophysis in various physiological states. In: *Cytologie de l'Adénohypophyse*, edited by J. Benoit and C. Da Lage, pp. 91–109. CNRS, Paris.
77. Kurosumi, K., and Oota, Y. (1968): Electron microscopy of two types of gonadotrophs in the anterior pituitary glands of persistent estrous and diestrous rats. *Z. Zellforsch.*, 85:34–46.
78. Tougard, C., Kerdelhué, B., Tixier-Vidal, A., and Jutisz, M. (1973): Light and electron microscope localization of binding sites against ovine luteinizing hormone and its two subunits in rat adenohypophysis using peroxidase-labeled antibody technique. *J. Cell Biol.*, 58:503–521.
79. Moriarty, G. V. (1976): Immunocytochemistry of the pituitary glycoprotein hormones. *J. Histochem. Cytochem.*, 24:846–863.
80. Childs (Moriarty), G. V., Ellison, D. G., and Garner, L. L. (1980): An immunocytochemist's view of gonadotropin storage in the adult male rat: Cytochemical and morphological heterogeneity in serially sectioned gonadotropes. *Am. J. Anat.*, 158:397–409.
81. Yoshimura, F., Nogami, H., Shirasawa, N., and Yashiro, T. (1981): A whole range of fine structural criteria for immunohistochemically identified LH cells in rats. *Cell Tissue Res.*, 217:1–10.
82. Moriarty, G. V., and Garner, L. L. (1977): Immunocytochemical studies of cells in the rat adenohypophysis containing both ACTH and FSH. *Nature*, 265:356–358.
83. Inoue, K., and Hagino, N. (1984): Comparative immunocytochemical demonstration of ACTH, LH and FSH-containing cells in the pituitary of neonatal immature and adult rats. *Cell Tissue Res.*, 235:71–75.
84. Pelletier, G., Leclerc, R., and Labrie, F. (1976): Identification of gonadotropic cells in the human pituitary by immunoperoxidase technique. *Mol. Cell. Endocrinol.*, 6:123–128.
85. Beauvillain, J. C., Tramu, G., and Dubois, M. P. (1975): Characterization by different techniques of adrenocorticotropin and gonadotropin producing cells in Lerot pituitary (*Eliomys quercinus*). A superimposition technique and an immunocytochemical technique. *Cell Tissue Res.*, 158:301–317.
86. Dacheux, F. (1978): Ultrastructural localization of gonadotrophic hormones in the porcine pituitary using the immunoperoxidase technique. *Cell Tissue Res.*, 191:219–232.
87. Dacheux, F. (1981): Proportions of FSH/LH cells, LH cells and FSH cells in the porcine anterior pituitary. *IRCS Med. Sci.*, 9: 952–953.
88. Dacheux, F. (1981): Ultrastructural localization of gonadotropin-releasing hormone in the porcine gonadotropic cells. *Cell Tissue Res.*, 216:143–150.
89. Moriarty, G. C. (1975): Electron microscopic-immunocytochemical studies of rat pituitary gonadotrophs: A sex difference in morphology and cytochemistry of LH cells. *Endocrinology*, 97:1215–1225.
90. Herbert, D. C. (1975): Localization of antisera to LHβ and FSHβ in the rat pituitary gland. *Am. J. Anat.*, 144:378–385.
91. Bugnon, C., Fellmann, D., Lenys, D., and Bloch, B. (1977): Etude cyto-immunologique des cellules gonadotropes et des cellules thy-

réotropes de l'adénohypophyse du rat. *C. R. Soc. Biol. (Paris)*, 907–913.

92. Kofler, R. (1982): Immunofluorescence localization of glycoprotein hormones in the rat anterior pituitary gland using monoclonal antibodies and polyclonal antisera. *J. Histochem. Cytochem.*, 30:645–649.
93. Inoue, K., and Kurosumi, K. (1984): Ultrastructural immunocytochemical localization of LH and FSH in the pituitary of the untreated male rat. *Cell Tissue Res.*, 235:77–83.
94. Phifer, R. F., Midgley, A. R., and Spicer, S. S. (1973): Immunohistologic and histologic evidence that follicle-stimulating hormone and luteinizing hormone are present in the same cell type in the human pars distalis. *J. Clin. Endocrinol. Metab.*, 36:125–141.
95. Herbert, D. C. (1976): Immunocytochemical evidence that luteinizing hormone (LH) and follicle-stimulating hormone (FSH) are present in the same cell type in the rhesus monkey pituitary gland. *Endocrinology*, 98:1554–1557.
96. Girod, C., Dubois, M. P., and Trouillas, J. (1980): Mise en évidence de cellules gonadotropes de l'adénohypophyse (pars distalis et pars tuberalis) du Singe *Macacus irus*. Etude en immunogluorescence à l'aide d'anticorps anti-β FSH humaine et anti-β LH ovine. *C. R. Soc. Biol. (Paris)*, 174:304–313.
97. Girod, C., Dubois, M. P., and Trouillas, J. (1981): Immunohistochemical localization of FSH and LH in the pars distalis of Vervet (*Cercopithecus aethiops*) and Baboon (*Papio hamadryas*) pituitaries. *Cell Tissue Res.*, 217:245–257.
98. Batten, T. F. C., and Hopkins, C. R. (1978): Discrimination of LH, FSH, TSH and ACTH in dissociated porcine anterior pituitary cells by light and electron microscope immunocytochemistry. *Cell Tissue Res.*, 192:107–120.
99. Purandare, T. (1978): Immunohistochemical localization of FSH and LH in rat pituitary. *Mol. Cell. Endocrinol.*, 10:57–62.
100. Childs, G. V. (1983): The use of multiple methods to validate immunocytochemical stains. *J. Histochem. Cytochem.*, 31:168–176.
101. Childs (Moriarty), G. V., Ellison, D. G., Lorenzen, J. R., Collins, T. J., and Schwartz, N. B. (1982): Immunocytochemical studies of gonadotropin storage in developing castration cells. *Endocrinology*, 111:1318–1328.
102. Childs, G. V., Hyde, C., Naor, Z., and Catt, K. (1983): Heterogeneous luteinizing hormone and follicle stimulating hormone storage patterns in subtypes of gonadotropes separated by centrifugal elutriation. *Endocrinology*, 113:2120–2128.
103. Childs, G. V., Unabia, G., and Tibolt, R. (1985): How the fixation-embedding protocol affects the specificity and efficiency of immunocytochemical stains for gonadotropin subunits. *Am. J. Anat.*, 174:409–417.
104. Childs, G. V. (1986): Differential sites of gonadotropin storage in multihormonal gonadotropes. In: *Pars Distalis of the Pituitary Gland—Structure, Function and Regulation*, edited by F. Yoshimura and A. Gorbman, pp. 115–124. Elsevier, Amsterdam.
105. Dacheux, F. (1984): Subcellular localization of gonadotropic hormones in pituitary cells of the castrated pig with the use of pre- and post-embedding immunocytochemical methods. *Cell Tissue Res.*, 236:153–160.
106. Dacheux, F. (1979): Are FSH and LH contained in the same granules? *IRCS Med. Sci.*, 7:280–281.
107. Dacheux, F. (1980): Ultrastructural localization of LH and FSH in the porcine pituitary. In: *Synthesis and Release of Adenohypophyseal Hormones*, edited by M. Jutisz and K. W. McKerns, pp. 187–195. Plenum Press, New York.
108. Childs, G. V., Unabia, G., and Ellison, D. (1986): Immunocytochemical studies of pituitary hormones with PAP, ABC, and immunogold techniques: Evolution of technology to best fit the antigen. *Am. J. Anat.*, 175:307–330.
109. Childs, G. V. (1983): Application of dual preembedding stains for gonadotropins to pituitary cell monolayers with avidin-biotin (ABC) and peroxidase antiperoxidase (PAP) complexes: Light microscopic studies. *Stain Technol.*, 58:281–289.
110. Childs, G. V. (1985): Shifts in gonadotropin storage in cultured gonadotropes following GnRH stimulation, *in vitro*. *Peptides*, 6:103–107.
111. Cozzi, M. G., and Zanini, A. (1986): Sulfated LH subunits and a tyrosine-sulfated secretory protein (secretogranin II) in female rat adenohypophyses: Changes with age and stimulation of release by LH-RH. *Mol. Cell. Endocrinol.*, 44:47–54.
112. Sternberger, L. A., Petrali, J. P., Joseph, S. A., Meyer, H. C., and Mills, K. R. (1978): Specificity of the immunocytochemical luteinizing hormone-releasing hormone receptor reaction. *Endocrinology*, 102:63–73.
113. Childs, G. V., and Ellison, D. G. (1980): A critique of the contributions of immunoperoxidase cytochemistry to our understanding of pituitary cell function, as illustrated by our current studies of gonadotropes, corticotropes and endogenous pituitary GnRH and TRH. *Histochem. J.*, 12:405–418.
114. Bauer, T. W., Moriarty, C. M., and Childs, G. V. (1981): Studies of immunoreactive gonadotropin releasing hormone (GnRH) in the rat anterior pituitary. *J. Histochem. Cytochem.*, 29:1171–1178.
115. Denef, C., Hautekeete, E., De Wolf, A., and Vanderschueren, B. (1978): Pituitary basophils from immature male and female rats: Distribution of gonadotrophs and thyrotrophs as studied by unit gravity sedimentation. *Endocrinology*, 103:724–735.
116. Denef, C., Hautekeete, E., and Dewals, R. (1978): Monolayer cultures of gonadotrophs separated by velocity sedimentation: Heterogeneity in response to luteinizing hormone releasing hormone. *Endocrinology*, 103:736–747.
117. Denef, C., Hautekeete, E., Dewals, R., and De Wolf, A. (1980): Differential control of luteinizing hormone and follicle-stimulating hormone secretion by androgens in rat pituitary cells in culture: Functional diversity of subpopulations separated by unit gravity sedimentation. *Endocrinology*, 106:724–729.
118. Denef, C., Swennen, L., and Andries, M. (1982): Separated anterior pituitary cells and their response to hypophysiotropic hormones. *Int. Rev. Cytol.*, 76:225–244.
119. Denef, C. (1980): Functional heterogeneity of separated dispersed gonadotropic cells. In: *Synthesis and Release of Adenohypophyseal Hormones*, edited by M. Jutisz and K. W. McKerns, pp. 659–676. Plenum Press, New York.
120. Naor, Z., Childs, G. V., Leifer, A. M., Clayton, R. N., Amsterdam, A., and Catt, K. J. (1982): Gonadotropin-releasing hormone binding and activation of enriched populations of pituitary gonadotrophs. *Mol. Cell. Endocrinol.*, 25:85–97.
121. Smith, P. F., Frawley, L. S., and Neill, J. D. (1984): Detection of LH release from pituitary cells by the reverse hemolytic plaque assay: Estrogen increases the fraction of gonadotropes responding to GnRH. *Endocrinology*, 115:2484–2486.
122. Fletcher, W. H., Anderson, N. C. Jr., and Everett, J. W. (1975): Intercellular communication in the rat anterior pituitary gland. *J. Cell Biol.*, 67:469–476.
123. Horvath, E., Kovacs, K., and Ezrin, C. (1977): Junctional contact between lactotrophs and gonadotrophs in the rat pituitary. *IRCS Med. Sci.*, 5:511.
124. Denef, C. (1984): Functional interrelationships between pituitary cells. In: *Trends in Diagnosis and Treatment of Pituitary Adenomas*, edited by S. W. J. Lamberts, F. J. H. Tilders, E. A. Van der Veen, and J. Assies, pp. 25–35. Free University Press, Amsterdam.
125. Denef, C. (1985): Paracrine interaction in anterior pituitary. In: *Prolactin. Basic and Clinical Correlates, Fidia Research Series, Vol. I*, edited by R. M. MacLeod, M. O. Thorner, and U. Scapagnini, pp. 53–57. Liviana Press, Padova.
126. Boockfor, F. R., Hoeffler, J. P., and Frawley, L. S. (1986): Analysis by plaque assays of GH and prolactin release from individual cells in cultures of male pituitaries. *Neuroendocrinology*, 42:64–70.
127. Chuknyiska, S. R., Blackman, M. R., Hymer, W. C., and Roth, S. R. (1986): Age related alterations in the number and function of pituitary lactotropic cells from intact and ovariectomized rat. *Endocrinology*, 118:1856–1862.
128. Everett, N. B., and Baker, B. L. (1945): The distribution of cell types in the anterior hypophysis during late pregnancy and lactation. *Endocrinology*, 37:83–88.
129. Merchant, F. W. (1974): Prolactin and luteinizing hormone cells of pregnant and lactating rats as studied by immunohistochemistry and radioimmunoassay. *Am. J. Anat.*, 139:245–268.
130. Grosvenor, C. E., and Turner, C. W. (1958): Pituitary lactogenic hormone and milk secretion in lactating rats. *Endocrinology*, 63:535–539.

131. Shiino, M., Williams, G., and Rennels, E. G. (1972): Ultrastructural observation of pituitary release of prolactin in the rat by suckling stimulus. *Endocrinology,* 90:176–181.
132. Vila-Porcile, E., and Olivier, L. (1980): Exocytosis and related membrane events. In: *Synthesis and Release of Adenohypophyseal Hormones,* edited by M. Jutisz and K. W. McKerns, pp. 67–104. Plenum Press, New York.
133. Harigaya, T., Kohmoto, K., and Hoshino, K. (1983): Immunohistochemical identification of prolactin producing cells in the mouse adenohypophysis. *Acta Histochem. Cytochem.,* 16:51–58.
134. Pantic, V. R., and Genbacev, O. (1969): Ultrastructure of pituitary lactotropic cells of oestrogen treated male rats. *Z. Zellforsch.,* 95:280–287.
135. Gersten, B. E., and Baker, B. L. (1970): Local action of intrahypophyseal implants of estrogen as revealed by staining with peroxidase-labelled antibody. *Am. J. Anat.,* 128:1–19.
136. Shiino, M., and Rennels, E. G. (1976): Recovery of rat prolactin cells following cessation of estrogen treatment. *Anat. Rec.,* 185:31–48.
137. Ibrahim, S. N., Moussa, S. M., and Childs, G. V. (1986): Morphometric studies of rat anterior pituitary cells after gonadectomy: Correlation of changes in gonadotropes with the serum levels of gonadotropins. *Endocrinology,* 119:629–637.
138. Furth, J., Clifton, K. H., Gadsden, E. L., and Buffet, R. F. (1956): Dependent and autonomous mammotropic pituitary tumors in rats: Their somatotropic features. *Cancer Res.,* 16:608–616.
139. Olivier, L., Vila-Porcile, E., Racadot, O., Peillon, F., and Racadot, J. (1975): Ultrastructure of pituitary tumor cells. A critical study. In: *The Anterior Pituitary,* edited by A. Tixier-Vidal and M. G. Farquhar, pp. 231–276. Academic Press, New York.
140. Baskin, D. G., Erlandsen, S. L., and Parsons, J. A. (1980): Functional classification of cell types in the growth hormone and prolactin-secreting rat MtTW 15 mammosomatotropic tumor with ultrastructural immunocytochemistry. *Am. J. Anat.,* 158:455–461.
141. El Etreby, M. F. (1980): The role of steroid hormones in the pathogenesis of pituitary tumors in various experimental animals. In: *Pituitary Adenomas,* edited by P. J. Derome, C. P. Jedynak, and F. Peillon, pp. 39–48. Asclepios Publishers, France.
142. Kovacs, K., McComb, D. J., and Horvath, E. (1983): Subcellular investigation of experimental and human pituitary adenomas. In: *Neuroendocrine Perspectives, Vol. 2,* edited by E. E. Muller and R. M. MacLeod, pp. 251–291, Elsevier, Amsterdam.
143. Halmi, N. S. (1978): Immunostaining of growth hormone and prolactin in paraffin-embedded and stored or previously stained materials. *J. Histochem. Cytochem.,* 26:486–495.
144. Girod, C., Mazzuca, M., Trouillas, J., Tramu, G., Lhéritier, M., Beauvillain, J. C., Claustrat, B., and Dubois, M. P. (1980): Light microscopy, fine structure and immunohistochemistry studies of 278 pituitary adenomas. In: *Pituitary Adenomas,* edited by P. J. Derome, C. P. Jedynak, and F. Peillon, pp. 3–18. Asclepios Publishers, Paris.
145. Tindall, G. R., Kovacs, K., Horvath, E., and Thorner, M. O. (1982): Human prolactin-producing adenomas and bromocriptine: A histological, immunocytochemical, ultrastructural and morphometric study. *J. Clin. Endocrinol. Metab.,* 55:1178–1184.
146. Landolt, A. M., Minder, H., Osterwalder, V., and Landolt, T. A. (1983): Bromocriptine reduces the size of cells in prolactin-secreting adenomas. *Experientia,* 39:625–627.
147. Bassetti, M., Spada, A., Pizzo, G., and Giannattasio, G. (1984): Bromocriptine treatment reduces the cell size in human macroprolactinomas: A morphometric study. *J. Clin. Endocrinol. Metab.,* 58:268–276.
148. Stokes, H., and Boda, J. M. (1968): Immunofluorescent localization of growth hormone and prolactin in the adenohypophysis of fetal sheep. *Endocrinology,* 83:1362–1366.
149. Dubois, M. P. (1971): Mise en évidence par immunofluorescence des cellules somatotropes et des cellules à prolactine dans l'hypophyse foetale des bovins. *C. R. Acad. Sci. Ser. D (Paris),* 272:433–435.
150. Setalo, G., and Nakane, P. K. (1976): Functional differentiation of the fetal anterior pituitary cells in the rat. *Endocrinol. Exp.,* 10:155–166.
151. Chatelain, A., Dubois, M. P., and Dupouy, J. P. (1977): Les cellules à prolactine chez la ratte gestante, le foetus, le nouveau-né et le jeune. *Ann. Biol. Anim. Biochim. Biophys.,* 17:403–412.
152. Chatelain, A., Dupouy, J. P., and Dubois, M. P. (1979): Ontogenesis of cell producing polypeptide hormones (ACTH, MSH, LPH, GH, prolactin) in the fetal hypophysis of the rat: influence of the hypothalamus. *Cell Tissue Res.,* 196:409–427.
153. Watanabe, Y. G., and Daikoku, S. (1979): An immunohistochemical study on the cytogenesis of adenohypophysial cells in fetal rats. *Dev. Biol.,* 68:557–567.
154. Begeot, M., Dubois, M. P., and Dubois, P. M. (1984): Evolution of lactotropes in normal and anencephalic human fetuses. *J. Clin. Endocrinol. Metab.,* 58:726–730.
155. Nemeskery, A., Németh, A., Sétalo, G., Vigh, S., and Halasz, B. (1976): Cell differentiation of the fetal rat anterior pituitary *in vitro. Cell Tissue Res.,* 170:263–273.
156. Watanabe, Y. G., and Daikoku, S. (1976): Immunohistochemical study on adenohypophysial primordia in organ culture. *Cell Tissue Res.,* 166:407–412.
157. Begeot, M., Hemming, F. J., Dubois, P. M., Combarnous, Y., Dubois, M. P., and Aubert, M. L. (1984): Induction of pituitary lactotrope differentiation by luteinizing hormone α-subunit. *Science,* 226:566–568.
158. Kawashima, S., and Takahashi, S. (1986): Morphological and functional changes of prolactin cells during aging in the rat. In: *Pars Distalis of the Pituitary Gland—Structure, Function and Regulation,* edited by F. Yoshimura and A. Gorbman, pp. 51–56. Elsevier, Amsterdam.
159. Hoeffler, J. P., Boockfor, F. R., and Frawley, L. S. (1985): Ontogeny of prolactin cells in neonatal rats: Initial prolactin secretors also release growth hormone. *Endocrinology,* 117:187–195.
160. Ascheim, P., and Pasteels, J. L. (1963): Etude histophysiologique de la sécrétion de prolactine chez les rattes séniles. *C. R. Acad. Sci. (Paris),* 257:1373–1375.
161. Kovacs, K., Horvath, E., Ilse, R. G., Ezrin, C., and Ilse, D. (1977): Spontaneous pituitary adenomas in aging rats. A light microscopic immunocytochemical and fine structural study. *Beitr. Pathol.,* 161:1–16.
162. Berkvens, J. M., Van Nesslrooy, J. H. J., and Kroes, R. (1980): Spontaneous tumors in the pituitary gland of old Wistar rats. A morphological and immunocytochemical study. *J. Pathol.,* 130:179–191.
163. Trouillas, J., Girod, C., Claustrat, B., Curé, M., and Dubois, M. P. (1982): Spontaneous pituitary tumors in Wistar/Furth/Ico rat strain: An animal model of human prolactin adenoma. *Am. J. Pathol.,* 109:57–70.
164. Tixier-Vidal, A., Gourdji, D., and Tougard, C. (1975): A cell culture approach to the study of the anterior pituitary. *Int. Rev. Cytol.,* 41:173–239.
165. Baker, B. L., Reel, J. R., Van Dewark, S. D., and Yu, Y. Y. (1974): Persistence of cell types in monolayer cultures of dispersed cells from the pituitary pars distalis as revealed by immunocytochemistry. *Anat. Rec.,* 179:93–106.
166. Antakly, T., Pelletier, G., Zeytinoglu, F., and Labrie, F. (1980): Changes of cell morphology and prolactin secretion induced by 2-Br-α-ergocryptine, estradiol, and thyrotropin-releasing hormone in rat anterior pituitary cells in culture. *J. Cell. Biol.,* 86:377–387.
167. Tashjian, A. H. Jr., Bancroft, F. C., and Levine, L. (1970): Production of both prolactin and growth hormone by clonal strains of rat pituitary tumor cells. *J. Cell Biol.,* 47:61–70.
168. Gourdji, D., Tougard, C., and Tixier-Vidal, A. (1982): Clonal prolactin strains as a tool in neuroendocrinology. In: *Frontiers in Neuroendocrinology, Vol. 7,* edited by W. F. Ganong and L. Martini, pp. 317–357. Raven Press, New York.
169. Gourdji, D. (1985): Multihormonal regulation of the pituitary gland binding and secretory responses to hypothalamic neuropeptides in rat GH pituitary strains in culture. *Neurochem. Int.,* 7:979–994.
170. Nagy, I., Rappay, G., Makara, G. B., Horvath, G., Bacsy, E., and MacLeod, R. M. (1983): Is there a direct correlation between the activities of various lysosomal enzymes and prolactin secretion in the rat anterior pituitary? *Endocrinology,* 112:470–475.
171. Nansel, D. D., Gudelsky, G. A., Reymond, M. J., Neaves, W. B., and Porter, J. C. (1981): A possible role for lysosomes in the inhibitory action of dopamine on PRL release. *Endocrinology,* 108:896–902.
172. Hassoun, J., Jaquet, P., Devictor, B., Andonian, C., Grisoli, F., Gunz, G., and Toga, M. (1985): Bromocriptine effects on cultured

human prolactin producing pituitary adenomas: *In vitro* ultrastructural, morphometric and immunoelectron microscopic studies. *J. Clin. Endocrinol. Metab.*, 61:686–692.
173. Vale, W., Rivier, C., and Brown, M. (1977): Regulatory peptides of the hypothalamus. *Annu. Rev. Physiol.*, 39:473–527.
174. Tixier-Vidal, A., and Gourdji, D. (1981): Mechanism of action of synthetic hypothalamic peptides on anterior pituitary cells. *Physiol. Rev.*, 61:974–1001.
175. Haug, E., and Gautvik, K. M. (1976): Effects of sex steroids on prolactin secreting rat pituitary cells in culture. *Endocrinology*, 99:1482–1489.
176. Brunet, N., Gourdji, D., Moreau, M. F., Grouselle, D., Bournaud, F., and Tixier-Vidal, A. (1977): Effects of 17-β estradiol on prolactin secretion and thyroliberin responsiveness in two rat prolactin continuous cell lines. *Ann. Biol. Anim. Biochim. Biophys.*, 17:413–424.
177. Tougard, C., Louvard, D., Picart, R., and Tixier-Vidal, A. (1983): The rough endoplasmic reticulum and the Golgi apparatus visualized using specific antibodies in normal and tumoral prolactin cells in culture. *J. Cell Biol.*, 96:1197–1207.
178. Albert, P. R., and Tashjian, A. H. Jr. (1984): Thyrotropin-releasing hormone-induced spike and plateau in cytosolic free Ca^{2+} concentrations in pituitary cells. *J. Biol. Chem.*, 259:5827–5832.
179. Aizawa, T., and Hinkle, P. M. (1985): Thyrotropin-releasing hormone rapidly stimulates a biphasic secretion of prolactin and growth hormone in GH4C1 rat pituitary tumor cells. *Endocrinology*, 116:73–82.
180. Martin, T. F. J., and Kowalchik, J. A. (1984): Evidence for the role of calcium and diacylglycerol as dual second messengers in TRH-releasing hormone action. *Endocrinology*, 115:1517–1526, 1527–1536.
181. Delbeke, D., Kojima, I., and Dannies, P. S. (1985): Comparison of patterns of prolactin release in GH4C1 cells and primary pituitary cultures. *Mol. Cell. Endocrinol.*, 43:15–22.
182. Gourdji, D., Kerdelhué, B., and Tixier-Vidal, A. (1972): Ultrastructure d'un clone de cellules hypophysaires sécrétant de la prolactine (clone GH3). Modifications induites par l'hormone hypothalamique de libération de l'hormone thyréotrope (TRF). *C. R. Acad. Sci. Ser. D (Paris)*, 274:437–440.
183. Tashjian, A. H. Jr., and Hoyt, R. F. Jr. (1972): Transient controls of organ specific functions in pituitary cells in culture. In: *Molecular Genetics and Developmental Biology*, edited by S. Sussman, pp. 353–387, Prentice-Hall, Englewood Cliffs, N.J.
184. Tixier-Vidal, A., Moreau, M. F., and Picart, R. (1976): Endocytose et sécrétion dans les cellules antéhypophysaires en culture. Action des hormones hypothalamiques. *J. Microsc. Biol. Cell.*, 25:159–172.
185. Hoyt, R. F., and Tashjian, A. H. Jr. (1980): Immunocytochemical analysis of prolactin production by monolayer cultures of GH3 rat anterior pituitary tumor cells. II. Variation in prolactin content of individual cell colonies and dynamics of stimulation with thyrotropin-releasing hormone (TRH). *Anat. Rec.*, 197:163–181.
186. Kelly, R. B. (1985): Pathways of protein secretion in eukaryotes. *Science*, 230:25–32.
187. Tougard, C., Picart, R., Morin, A., and Tixier-Vidal, A. (1983): Effect of monensin on secretory pathway in GH3 prolactin cells. A cytochemical study. *J. Histochem. Cytochem.*, 31:745–754.
188. Kiino, D. R., Burger, D. E., and Dannies, P. S. (1982): Prolactin storage in a clonal strain of rat pituitary tumor cells is cell-cycle dependent. *J. Cell Biol.*, 93:459–462.
189. De Carvalho, N., Picart, R., and Tixier-Vidal, A. (1985): 17β-estradiol regulates prolactin secretion but not cell proliferation of GH3/B6 cells in chemically defined medium. *Mol. Cell. Endocrinol.*, 39:49–60.
190. Scammell, J. G., Burrage, T. G., and Dannies, P. S. (1986): Hormonal induction of secretory granules in a pituitary tumor cell line. *Endocrinology*, 119:1543–1546.
191. Amara, J. F., Van Itallie, C., and Dannies, P. S. (1987): Regulation of prolactin production and cell growth by estradiol: Difference in sensitivity to estradiol occurs at the level of messenger ribonucleic acid accumulation. *Endocrinology*, 120:264–271.
192. Dada, M. O., Campbell, G. T., and Blake, C. A. (1983): A quantitative immunocytochemical study of the luteinizing hormone and follicle stimulating hormone cells in the adenohypophysis of adult male rats and adult female rats throughout the estrous cycle. *Endocrinology*, 113:970–984.
193. Severinghaus, A. E. (1933): A cytological study of the anterior pituitary of the rat, with special reference to the Golgi apparatus and to cell relationship. *Anat. Rec.*, 57:149–175.
194. Yoshimura, F., and Harumiya, K. (1965): Electron microscopy of the anterior lobe of pituitary in normal and castrated rats. *Endocrinol. Jpn.*, 12:119–152.
195. Kurosumi, K., Kawarai, Y., Yukitake, Y., and Inoue, K. (1976): Electron microscopic morphometry of the rat castration cells. *Gunma Symp. Endocrinology*, 13:221–236.
196. Tougard, C., Kerdelhué, B., Tixier-Vidal, A., and Jutisz, M. (1971): Localisation par cytoimmunoenzymologie de la LH, de ses sous-unités, α et β et de la FSH dans l'adénohypophyse de la ratte castrée. *C. R. Acad. Sci. (Paris)*, 273:897–900.
197. Smith, P. F., and Keefer, D. A. (1982): Immunocytochemical and ultrastructural identification of mitotic cells in the pituitary gland of ovariectomized rats. *J. Reprod. Fertil.*, 66:383–389.
198. Sakuma, S., Shirasawa, N., and Yoshimura, F. (1984): A histochemical study of immunohistochemically identified mitotic adenohypophysial cells in immature and mature castrated rats. *J. Endocrinol.*, 100:322–328.
199. Childs, G. V., Ellison, D. G., Lorenzen, J. R., Collins, T. J., and Schwartz, N. B. (1983): Retarded development of castration cells after adrenalectomy or sham adrenalectomy. *Endocrinology*, 113:166–177.
200. Shiino, M., Arimura, A., Schally, A. V., and Rennels, E. G. (1972): Ultrastructural observations of granule extrusion from rat anterior pituitary cells after injection of LH-releasing hormone. *Z. Zellforsch.*, 128:152–161.
201. Mendoza, D., Arimura, A., and Schally, A. V. (1973): Ultrastructural and light microscopic observations of rat pituitary LH-containing gonadotrophs following injection of synthetic LH-RH. *Endocrinology*, 92:1153–1160.
202. Soji, T., Taya, K., Igarashi, M., and Yoshimura, F. (1974): Acute and subacute effect of LH-RH upon LH- and FSH-gonadotrophs in castrated female rats with short-term estrogen-progesterone pretreatment. *Endocrinol. Jpn.*, 21:407–428.
203. Shiino, M. (1982): Ultrastructural evidence of gonadotrophin release from castration cells following injection of LH-RH in the rat. *Cell Tissue Res.*, 222:213–222.
204. Nakamura, F., and Yoshimura, F. (1986): Morphological characterization of LH secretory granule response to LH-RH and calmodulin inhibitor. *Mol. Cell. Endocrinol.*, 44:11–15.
205. Wilbur, D. L., and Spicer, S. S. (1980): Pituitary secretory activity and endocrinophagy. In: *Synthesis and Release of Adenohypophyseal Hormones*, edited by M. Jutisz and K. W. McKerns, pp. 167–186. Plenum Press, New York.
206. Yoshimura, F., Soji, T., Yachi, H., and Ishikawa, H. (1974): Life stage and secretory cycle of anterior pituitary basophils. *Endocrinol. Jpn.*, 21:217–249.
207. Soji, T., Yashiro, T., and Yoshimura, F. (1976): TRH and LRH and their target cells with special reference to secretory cycle of basophils. In: *Gunma Symp. Endocrinol.*, 13:237–257.
208. Yoshimura, F., Soji, T., Kumagai, T., and Yokoyama, M. (1977): Secretory cycle of the pituitary basophils and its morphological evidence. *Endocrinol. Jpn.*, 24:185–202.
209. Soji, T. (1978): Cytological changes of the pituitary basophils in rats slowly infused with thyrotropin-releasing hormone (TRH). *Endocrinol. Jpn.*, 25:245–258.
210. Soji, T. (1978): Cytological changes of the pituitary basophils in rats slowly infused with LRH and with LRH and TRH in combination. *Endocrinol. Jpn.*, 25:259–274.
211. Kovacs, K., Horvath, E., Van Loon, G. R., Rewcastle, N. B., Ezrin, C., and Rosenbloom, A. A. (1978): Pituitary adenomas associated with elevated blood follicle-stimulating hormone levels. A histologic, immunocytologic and electron microscopic study of two cases. *Fertil. Steril.*, 29:622–628.
212. Trouillas, J., Girod, C., Sassolas, G., Claustrat, B., Lheritier, M., Dubois, M. P., and Goutelle, A. (1981): Human pituitary gonadotropic adenoma: Histological, immunocytochemical and ultrastructural studies with hormonal relationships in eight cases. *J. Pathol.*, 135:315–336.

213. Tougard, C., Picart, R., and Tixier-Vidal, A. (1977): Cytogenesis of immunoreactive gonadotropic cells in the fetal rat pituitary at light and electron microscope levels. *Dev. Biol.*, 58:148–163.
214. Begeot, M., Dupouy, J. P., Dubois, M. P., and Dubois, P. M. (1981): Immunocytological determination of gonadotropic and thyrotropic cells in fetal rat anterior pituitary during normal development and under experimental conditions. *Neuroendocrinology,* 32:285–294.
215. Dubois, M. P., and Mauléon, P. (1969): Mise en évidence par immunofluorescence des cellules à activité gonadotrope LH dans l'hypophyse du foetus de brebis. *C. R. Acad. Sci. Ser. D (Paris)*, 269:219–222.
216. Danchin, E., and Dubois, M. P. (1982): Immunocytochemical study of the chronology of pituitary cytogenesis in the domestic pig (*Sus scrofa*) with special reference to the functioning of the hypothalamo-pituitary-gonadal axis. *Reprod. Nutr. Dev.*, 22:135–151.
217. Dacheux, F., and Martinat, N. (1983): Immunocytochemical localization of LH, FSH and TSH in the fetal porcine pituitary. *Cell Tissue Res.*, 228:277–295.
218. Danchin, E., Dang, D. C., and Dubois, M. P. (1981): An immunocytochemical study of the adult crab-eating macaque (*Macaca fascicularis*) pituitary and its cytological differentiation during fetal life. *Reprod. Nutr. Dev.*, 21:441–454.
219. Bugnon, C., Bloch, B., and Fellmann, D. (1977): Cytoimmunological study of the ontogenesis of the gonadotropic hypothalamo-pituitary axis in the human fetus. *J. Steroid Biochem.*, 8:565–575.
220. Dubois, P. M., Begeot, M., Dubois, M. P., and Herbert, D. C. (1978): Immunocytological localization of LH, FSH, TSH and their subunits in the pituitary of normal and anencephalic human fetuses. *Cell Tissue Res.*, 191:249–265.
221. Gross, D. S., and Baker, B. L. (1979): Developmental correlation between hypothalamic gonadotropin-releasing hormone and hypophysial luteinizing hormone. *Am. J. Anat.*, 154:1–10.
222. Daikoku, S., Kawano, H., Matsumura, H., and Saito, S. (1978): *In vivo* and *in vitro* studies on the appearance of LH-RH neurons in the hypothalamus of perinatal rats. *Cell Tissue Res.*, 194:433–445.
223. Begeot, M., Dubois, M. P., and Dubois, P. M. (1983): Comparative study *in vivo* and *in vitro* of the differentiation of immunoreactive gonadotropic cells in fetal rat anterior pituitary. *Neuroendocrinology,* 37:52–58.
224. Begeot, M., Morel, G., Rivest, R. W., Aubert, M. L., Dubois, M. P., and Dubois, P. M. (1984): Influence of gonadoliberin on the differentiation of rat gonadotrophs: an *in vivo* and *in vitro* study. *Neuroendocrinology,* 38:217–225.
225. Ishikawa, H., Shiino, M., Arimura, A., and Rennels, E. G. (1977): Functional clones of pituitary cells derived from Rathke's pouch epithelium of fetal rats. *Endocrinology,* 100:1227–1230.
226. Shiino, M., Ishikawa, H., and Rennels, E. G. (1977): *In vitro* and *in vivo* studies on cytodifferentiation of pituitary clonal cells derived from the epithelium of Rathke's pouch. *Cell Tissue Res.*, 181:473–485.
227. Bowie, E. P., Ishikawa, H., Shiino, M., and Rennels, E. G. (1978): An immunocytochemical study of a rat pituitary multipotential clone. *J. Histochem. Cytochem.*, 26:94–97.
228. Shiino, M., Ishikawa, H., and Rennels, E. G. (1978): Accumulation of secretory granules in pituitary clonal cells derived from the epithelium of Rathke's pouch. *Cell Tissue Res.*, 186:53–61.
229. Yoshimura, F., Harumiya, K., and Hiyama, H. (1970): Light and electron microscopic studies of the cytogenesis of anterior pituitary cells in perinatal rats in reference to the development of target organs. *Arch. Histol. Jpn.*, 31:333–369.
230. Dupouy, J. P., and Magre, S. (1973): Ultrastructure des cellules granulées de l'hypophyse foetale du rat. Identification des cellules corticotropes et thyréotropes. *Arch. Anat. Microsc.*, 62:185–205.
231. Svalander, C. (1974): Ultrastructure of the fetal rat adenohypophysis. *Acta Endocrinol.*, 76:1–114.
232. Dacheux, F. (1984): Functional differentiation of the anterior pituitary cells in the fetal pig. An ultrastructural immunocytochemical study. *Cell Tissue Res.*, 235:623–633.
233. Matsumura, H., and Daikoku, S. (1977): Sexual difference in LH-cells of the neonatal rats as revealed by immunocytochemistry. *Cell Tissue Res.*, 182:541–548.
234. Childs (Moriarty), G. V., Ellison, D., Foster, L., and Ramaley, J. A. (1981): Postnatal maturation of gonadotropes in the male rat pituitary. *Endocrinology,* 109:1683–1692.
235. Matsumura, H., and Daikoku, S. (1978): Quantitative observations of the effect of sex-steroids on the postnatal development of LH cells. An immunohistochemical study. *Cell Tissue Res.*, 188:491–496.
236. Childs (Moriarty), G. V., Ellison, D. G., Ramaley, J. A., and Unabia, G. (1982): Storage of anterior lobe adrenocorticotropin in corticotropes and a subpopulation of gonadotropes during the stress nonresponsive period in the neonatal male rat. *Endocrinology,* 110:1676–1692.
237. Döhler, K. D., Von zur Mühlen, A., and Döhler, U. (1977): Pituitary luteinizing hormone (LH), follicle stimulating hormone (FSH) and prolactin from birth to puberty in female and male rats. *Acta Endocrinol.*, 85:718–728.
238. Tixier-Vidal, A. (1975): Ultrastructure of anterior pituitary cells in culture. In: *The Anterior Pituitary,* edited by M. G. Farquhar and A. Tixier-Vidal, pp. 181–224. Academic Press, New York.
239. Tougard, C., Tixier-Vidal, A., Kerdelhué, B., and Jutisz, M. (1977): Etude immunocytochimique de l'évolution des cellules gonadotropes dans des cultures primaires de cellules antéhypophysaires de rat: Aspects quantitatifs et ultrastructuraux. *Biol. Cell.*, 28:251–260.
240. Van der Schueren, B., Denef, C., and Cassiman, J. J. (1982): Ultrastructural and functional characteristics of rat pituitary cell aggregates. *Endocrinology,* 110:513–523.
241. Childs, G. V. (1985): Studies of hormone storage and secretion in the multipotential gonadotrope. *Excerpta Med. Int. Congr. Ser.*, 655:499–502.
242. Lewis, C. E., Morris, J. F., and Fink, G. (1985): The role of microfilaments in the priming effect of LH-releasing hormone: An ultrastructural study using cytochalasin B. *J. Endocrinol.*, 106:211–218.
243. Lewis, C. E., Morris, J. F., Fink, G., and Johnson, M. (1986): Changes in the granule population of gonadotrophs of hypogonadal (hpg) and normal female mice associated with the priming effect of LH-releasing hormone in vitro. *J. Endocrinol.*, 109:35–44.
244. Morris, J. F., Lewis, C. E., and Fink, G. (1986): LH-RH priming in gonadotrophs: A model system for the analysis of neuroendocrine mechanisms at the cellular level. In: *Neuroendocrine Molecular Biology,* edited by G. Fink, A. J. Harmar, and K. W. McKerns, pp. 341–352. Plenum Press.
245. Neill, J. D., Smith, P. F., Luque, E. H., Munoz de Toro, M., Nagy, G., and Mulchahey, J. J. (1986): Analysis of hormone secretion from individual pituitary cells. In: *Neuroendocrine Molecular Biology,* edited by G. Fink, A. J. Harmar, and K. W. McKerns, pp. 325–340. Plenum Press.
246. Zambrano, D., Cuerdo-Rocha, S., and Bergmann, I. (1974): Ultrastructure of rat pituitary gonadotrophs following incubations of the gland with synthetic LH-RH. *Cell Tissue Res.*, 150:179–192.

The Physiology of Reproduction,
edited by E. Knobil and J. Neill *et al.*
Raven Press, Ltd., New York © 1988.

CHAPTER 31

Gonadotropins: Chemistry and Biosynthesis[1]

John G. Pierce

Among the chemical messengers (hormones) necessary for the initiation and maintenance of reproductive processes are three structurally related glycoproteins: follicle-stimulating hormone (FSH) and luteinizing hormone (LH) from the pituitary and, in primates and some other species, a chorionic or placental gonadotropin. Of the latter, human chorionic gonadotropin (hCG) has been the best studied; its structure and overall biological properties are very similar to those of pituitary LH. As with many hormones, the existence of these substances was first postulated from observations of physiological changes that occurred (a) after injection of crude, or partially purified, extracts of pregnancy urine or of the pituitary or (b) after hypophysectomy. The effects of pituitary extracts on estrus and ovulation were described by Evans and Long (1) in 1922, and the ability of pituitary implants to stimulate the function and development of the gonads was described by Smith (2) and by Zondek and Ascheim (3). The separation of pituitary extracts into two fractions, one of which promotes primarily the growth of ovarian follicles and the other luteinization of follicles, was first reported by Fevold et al. (4) in 1931—thus we can see how these gonadotropins were named. Because of overlap in biological effects of many early preparations of FSH and LH, the older literature contains many discussions concerning whether or not two distinct chemical entities existed, the overlap being due both to impure preparations and to synergism in bioassay systems.

Gonadotropin activity was also found in human pregnancy urine in 1927 by Ascheim and Zondek (5). In the early 1930s it was shown that this gonadotropin was not identified with the pituitary gonadotropins; it was designated as human chorionic gonadotropin. Postmenopausal urine also contains gonadotropins; these are almost certainly of pituitary origin. Concentrates have been made for many years and have widespread clinical use, but their chemistry is not well defined in terms of how they may have been modified either during their secretion, circulation in the blood, or excretion. The designation HMG (human menopausal gonadotropin) refers to concentrates of postmenopausal urine; a common commercial preparation is Pergonal.

Thyroid-stimulating hormone has a chemical structure similar to those of the gonadotropins (6), and the genes for the four hormones are thought to have evolved from a single precursor gene (7).

Beginning in the 1930s many routes toward the isolation of the gonadotropins were tried, but progress including precise biological characterization was slow. It was impeded by overlapping activities in some assays, uncertainties in correlation of bioassays involving different species, and, early on, by different laboratory standards against which activity was measured. It also was not until the 1950s and 1960s that ion-exchange chromatography and gel filtration of proteins were developed together with better methods for analysis of the extent of chemical purification (including gel electrophoresis and quantitative amino acid analysis). Purification of each hormone has been achieved by a variety of approaches; some were more successful with animal hor-

[1]The very large increase in the literature concerning the gonadotropins precludes citation of all original articles, and the author has cited what he hopes are representative papers, together with reviews that can direct the reader to the original literature. For excellent summaries of early work, the reader is referred to *Handbook of Physiology, Series 7, Endocrinology*, edited by R. O. Greep and E. B. Astwood, American Physiology Society, Washington, D.C. (1974).

mones, e.g., LH, others with material from human pituitaries, e.g., FSH (see refs. 8 and 9 for descriptions of gonadotropins from diverse species).

PURIFICATION OF GONADOTROPINS

Present methods of purification differ depending on the species studied and the objectives of a particular laboratory. Usually, hCG is obtained from commercial concentrates of first-trimester pregnancy urine that contain about 25% of hCG (10). The hormone is then further purified by gel filtration and anion-exchange chromatography. Microheterogeneity of hCG is found, with much of it being caused by the presence of different numbers of neuraminic acid residues at the termini of its oligosaccharides. Very small amounts of hCG or hCG-like material have been detected by immunological means in many tissues and have been partially purified from the pituitary (see refs. 11 and 12 for references and purification). An extensive and excellent purification scheme for the human pituitary gonadotropins is that of Stockell-Hartree (13); a fraction containing glycoproteins after separation from growth-hormone-rich fractions is utilized. All procedures are performed at 4°C, and after aqueous acid-ethanol extraction of an acetone powder of pooled human pituitaries, supernatants are precipitated by increasing the ethanol concentration. FSH is then separated from LH and TSH by ion-exchange chromatography on carboxylmethyl (CM) cellulose. LH and TSH are separated by anion exchange chromatography, and each is further purified by additional chromatography.

A relatively simple scheme for obtaining bovine LH (and TSH) in good yield is that of Bloomfield et al. (14), in which, after extraction from minced pituitaries and a series of precipitations, the glycoproteins are absorbed to a column of Sepharose-linked concanavalin A and, after washing the column, the glycoproteins are eluted with a buffer containing α-methyl mannoside or α-methyl glucoside. Anion-exchange chromatography on diethylaminoethyl (DEAE) cellulose then separates LH from TSH. Although bovine pituitaries are not a good source for FSH, its purification has been accomplished (see, e.g., refs. 15 and 16). Ovine and equine LH and FSH have been purified in several laboratories, and detailed protocols for purification are given in refs. 17 to 19.

Affinity procedures have been used to purify very small amounts of gonadotropins for radioreceptor studies and to determine whether a given hormone possesses intrinsic biological activities unrelated to its main hormonal function (20,21).

Purification of gonadotropins has always been complicated by polymorphism, which is most readily revealed by gel electrophoresis. In addition, constancy of biological response in terms of activity per milligram dry weight of protein, both of individual preparations and from preparation to preparation, has also been a particular problem for FSH (and for TSH). The reasons for the instability are still not clear. With FSH, most success in isolation of material of high purity and reasonable stability has been with the human hormone; amino acid sequences are known for human, porcine, ovine, and equine FSH (see refs. 22 and 23 for reviews). Luteinizing-hormone preparations from sheep, cattle, and humans have been the most studied; amino acid sequences are known for these species as well as for pig, horse, carp (partial), rabbit, mouse, and rat. The latter two are derived from nucleotide sequences (see ref. 24 for a review).

THE SUBUNIT NATURE OF GONADOTROPINS

The subunit nature of these hormones was first recognized for LH in the 1960s (25,26), and in the early 1970s the striking relationships between its subunits and those of TSH (and subsequently for FSH and hCG) were observed (27). Each hormone consists of two dissimilar peptide chains (α and β); both are rich in intrachain disulfide bonds and are glycosylated at specific amino acid residues. One subunit (α) is common to all four hormones, and hormone activity is formed by the association of an α subunit with a hormone-specific β subunit. In the laboratory an α subunit isolated from any of the four hormones (or from a different species) will reassociate to yield the activity represented by the β subunit. Differences in amino acid sequence between the subunits of the hormones from the same species are confined to the region from the NH_2-terminus to the first half-cystine residue and are due to additional proteolysis (probably artifactual) after removal of a signal peptide from newly synthesized α subunit. Although they are obviously different in sequence, the β subunits also exhibit considerable homology between each other (22). Both subunits contain oligosaccharides *N*-linked to asparagine residues. It has been found that hCG-β also contains, in a COOH terminal extension, vis-à-vis hLH, four additional oligosaccharides that are *O*-linked through hydroxyl groups of serine side chains. That the gonadotropins were glycoproteins was long suspected because of the relatively high carbohydrate content of partially purified preparations. High-performance liquid chromatography (HPLC) has been most useful for the rapid purification of the subunits of these hormones. In a single procedure the subunits of bovine LH or TSH can be readily isolated from purified preparations in amounts of 1 to 100 mg (28). A preliminary dissociation is carried out in 6 M guanidine hydrochloride, and the subunits are separated on reverse-phase columns. The method works equally well for the human pituitary gonadotropins. Reverse-phase chromatography has not, as yet, been extensively used in the purification of intact hormones because the interaction of the hormones with column packings results, in many systems, in considerable dissociation.

The amino acid sequences of TSH, LH, and hCG were determined in the early 1970s; that of FSH was determined somewhat later. Typical sequences are given in Figs. 1 and 2, along with the location of the oligosaccharides. Differences are also found between the peripheral sugars of the several hormones and from one subunit to another (22,23). For example, LH contains *N*-acetylgalactosamine residues in its *N*-linked oligosaccharides in addition to *N*-acetylglucosamine, but galactosamine is absent in hCG except in its *O*-linked oligosaccharides. The oligosaccharides of bovine LH contain negligible amounts of galactose and neuraminic (sialic) acids, and they terminate with *O*-sulfated *N*-acetylgalactosamine residues (35). FSH has neuraminic acid residues at its oligosaccharide termini and its β subunit probably does not contain *N*-acetylgalactosamine (36). The *N*-linked oligosaccharides of hCG also do not contain galactosamine. The oligosaccharides of human LH are partially sulfated; they also contain significant amounts of galactose and neuraminic acid. Typical carbohydrate structures are given in Fig. 3.

In 1975, gel filtration of human pituitary extracts showed the presence of a considerable amount of material that had the properties of uncombined α subunits (see, e.g., ref. 43), and such material was subsequently isolated from bovine pituitary extracts (44). It is not found in combination with any β subunits, and its biological function is unknown, although there have been a few reports of possible functions such as influence on lactotope differentiation (45). It is almost certainly a product of the same gene that is responsible for the α subunit found in intact hormones, but it contains an *O*-linked oligosaccharide at position 43 of the α sequence (Fig. 1) in addition to the usual two *N*-linked oligosaccharides. An excess of a similar "α-like material" is also produced by various tumor cell lines derived from humans, e.g., trophoblast tumor cell lines (see, e.g., refs. 46 and 47; see also ref. 48 for further references); in some instances, free β subunit is produced (49). The α-amino acid sequence is presumably that of hCG-α, and, here again, the presence of an additional *O*-linked sugar is likely (see below).

Thus, to date, the following picture of gonadotropin structure is available. Each hormone is a compact, glycosylated, globular protein whose molecular weight is 28,000 to 29,000 for LH and FSH and 37,000 for hCG. Each subunit, within itself, is internally cross-linked and stabilized by disulfide bonds (five in α subunits, six in β subunits). In my opinion, the locations of the disulfide bonds in each subunit have not all been unequivocally determined, although several proposals have been made (see refs. 22–24 and 50–52). In the α subunit, bonds between half-cystine 11 and 35 (see Fig. 1) and 14-36 are most likely correct. Correct assignments of β-subunit disulfides are those between positions 93-100, 26-110, and 23-72. Two laboratories have proposed that the other three disulfides are 9-90, 34-88, and 38-57. The uncertainty of some of these assignments is because disulfide exchange cannot be ruled out with the techniques used for determination of the bonds.

In almost all assay systems, individual subunits have little, if any, biological activity. The two subunits are associated by noncovalent forces with, in all probability, mul-

```
                                            10                                      20
human   Ala Pro Asp Val Gln-----------------Asp Cys Pro Glu Cys Thr Leu Gln Glu Asn Pro Phe Phe Ser Glu
bovine  Phe         Gly Glu Phe Thr Met Gln Gly                 Lys     Lys         Lys Tyr         Lys

                            30                                      40
human   Pro Gly Ala Pro Ile Leu Gln Cys Met Gly Cys Cys Phe Ser Arg Ala Tyr Pro Thr Pro Leu Arg Ser Lys
bovine                      Tyr                                                         Ala

            50                   *                  60                                      70
human   Lys Thr Met Leu Val Gln Lys Asn Val Thr Ser Glu Ser Thr Cys Cys Val Ala Lys Ser Tyr Asn Arg Val
bovine                      Pro  *  Ile                 Ala                         Ala Phe Thr Lys Ala

                                    80       *                              90
human   Thr Val Met Gly Gly Phe Lys Val Glu Asn His Thr Ala Cys His Cys Ser Thr Cys Tyr Tyr His Lys Ser COOH
bovine                  Asn Val Arg          *          Glu
```

FIG. 1. Amino acid sequences of the α subunits of human and bovine glycoprotein hormones. The human sequence is used as reference, and only the amino acid differences are shown for the bovine sequence; a blank space indicates the same residues as in human. The dashed line shows the position of the deletion of four residues in the human versus the bovine sequence. Asterisks show the point of attachment of oligosaccharides. Heterogeneity (i.e., loss of one or more residues) is often found at the amino termini. Extensive sequence compilations and references of sequence determination can be found in refs. 22,23, and 29. The sequence of ovine FSH can be found in refs. 30 and 31; that of rabbit can be found in refs. 32 and 33.

```
                                              10                                      20
hLHβ      Ser Arg Glu Pro Leu Arg Pro Trp Cys His Pro Ile Asn Ala Ile Leu Ala Val Glu Lys Glu Gly Cys Pro
hCGβ      Ser Lys                     Arg     Arg         *       Thr
b,oLHβ    Ser     Gly                 Leu     Gln         *       Thr         Ala             Ala
hFSHβ                         NH2-Asn Ser     Glu Leu Thr *   Ile Thr Ile     Ile             Glu     Arg-
oFSHβ                             NH2 Ser     Glu Leu Thr *   Ile Thr Ile Thr                 Glu     Ser-

                              30                                      40
hLHβ      Val Cys Ile Thr Val Asn*Thr Thr Ile Cys Ala Gly Tyr Cys Pro Thr Met Met Arg Val Leu Gln Ala Val
hCGβ                             *                                        Thr                     Gly
b,oLHβ                    Phe Thr     Ser                             Ser     Lys             Pro Val Ile
hFSHβ     Phe     Ile Ser Ile    *        Trp                     Tyr     Arg Asp Leu     Tyr Lys Asp Pro
oFSHβ     Phe         Ser Ile    *        Trp                     Tyr         Asp Leu     Tyr Lys Asx Pro

              50                                      60                                      70
hLHβ      Leu Pro Pro Leu Pro Gln Val Val Cys Thr Tyr Arg Asp Val Arg Phe Glu Ser Ile Arg Leu Pro Gly Cys
hCGβ              Ala                         Asn
b,oLHβ                Met             Arg             His Glu Leu         Ala     Val
hFSHβ     Ala Arg     Lys Ile     Lys Thr         Phe Lys Glu Leu Val Tyr     Thr Val     Val
oFSHβ     Ala     Pro Asx Ile     Lys Thr         Phe Lys Glu Leu Val Tyr     Thr Val Lys Val Pro Gly

                                      80                                      90
hLHβ      Pro Arg Gly Val Asp Pro Val Val Ser Phe Pro Val Ala Leu Ser Cys Arg Cys Gly Pro Cys Arg Arg Ser
hCGβ                      Asn                 Tyr Ala                     Gln     Ala Leu
b,oLHβ        Pro                 Met                                     His                     Leu
hFSHβ     Ala His His Ala     Ser Leu Tyr Thr Tyr             Thr Gln     His         Lys     Asp Ser Asp
oFSHβ     Ala His His Ala Asp Ser Leu Tyr Thr Tyr             Thr Glu     His         Lys     Asp Ser Asp

                      100                                     110                                     120
hLHβ      Thr Ser Asp Cys Gly Gly Pro Lys Asp His Pro Leu Thr Cys Asp His Pro Gln Leu Ser Gly Leu Leu Phe
hCGβ          Thr                                                     Asp     Arg Phe Gln Asp Ser Ser Ser
b,oLH     Ser Thr             Pro Gly Arg Thr Gln         Ala                 Pro     Pro Asp Ile COOH
hFSHβ     Ser Thr         Thr Val Arg Gly Leu Gly     Ser Tyr     Ser Phe Gly Glu Met Lys Glu COOH
oFSHβ     Ser Thr Asp     Thr Val Arg Gly Leu Gly     Ser Tyr     Ser Phe Ser Asp Ile Glu Arg Glx COOH

                                              130                                     140
hLHβ      Leu COOH
           *                       *                   *                       *
hCGβ      Ser Lys Ala Pro Pro Pro Ser Leu Pro Ser Pro Ser Arg Leu Pro Gly Pro Ser Asp Thr Pro Ile Leu Pro
b,oLH
hFSHβ
oFSHβ

hCGβ      Gln COOH
```

FIG. 2. Amino acid sequence of β subunits of gonadotropins. See legend of Fig. 1 for key. Recent studies (34) on the sequence of the bovine LH-β gene show the bovine sequence (and perhaps the ovine) to be Pro-Gly at positions 102-103. Two additional residues, Phe-Leu, at the COOH terminus are also predicted by the genomic sequence. There are discrepancies in the FSH-β sequences reported (see refs. 22 and 23). The sequence shown is derived from a cDNA clone for FSH-β (courtesy of Integrated Genetics, Framingham, Mass.).

tisite interactions. It has been shown recently (53,54) that the hormones do not inactivate quickly at the low concentrations found in blood (10^{-9}–10^{-11} M) because of slow dissociation rates rather than because of an unusually high affinity between subunits. For example, at physiological pH, hCG has a half-life of about 37 days and ovine LH has one of 11 days.

THREE-DIMENSIONAL STRUCTURE OF THE GONADOTROPINS

The positions of the half-cystine residues in the several sequences are very analogous (22), but because the hormones have not been crystallized, no detailed three-dimensional structures from X-ray diffraction studies are avail-

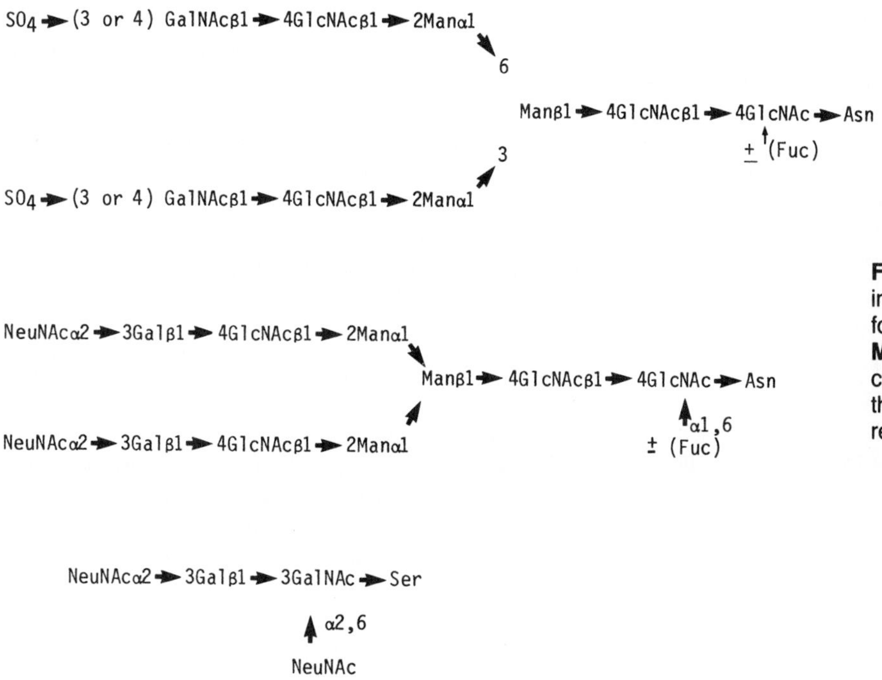

```
SO4 → (3 or 4) GalNAcβ1 → 4GlcNAcβ1 → 2Manα1
                                            ↘ 6
                                              Manβ1 → 4GlcNAcβ1 → 4GlcNAc → Asn
                                            ↗ 3                      ↑
SO4 → (3 or 4) GalNAcβ1 → 4GlcNAcβ1 → 2Manα1                         ± (Fuc)

NeuNAcα2 → 3Galβ1 → 4GlcNAcβ1 → 2Manα1
                                      ↘
                                        Manβ1 → 4GlcNAcβ1 → 4GlcNAc → Asn
                                      ↗                         ↑ α1,6
NeuNAcα2 → 3Galβ1 → 4GlcNAcβ1 → 2Manα1                          ± (Fuc)

NeuNAcα2 → 3Galβ1 → 3GalNAc → Ser
                     ↑ α2,6
                   NeuNAc
```

FIG. 3. Typical oligosaccharide structures in glycoprotein hormones. **Top**: A structure for *N*-linked oligosaccharides in bovine LH. **Middle**: A structure for *N*-linked oligosaccharides in hCG. **Bottom**: A structure for the *O*-linked oligosaccharides of hCG. See refs. 37–42.

able. Thus, model building of three-dimensional structures has not yet been productive. Numerous indirect physical studies indicate low helix content together with a relatively large amount of β structure and β turns, which is consonant with their high disulfide and proline content. The best evidence (other than sequence homology) of similar overall conformations of β subunits is that each can interact with high affinity with the common α subunit to give an active hormone. The presence of carbohydrate contributes to solubility in aqueous solution. Although the disulfide bonds confer considerable stability and rigidity to the three-dimensional structure of these hormones, as do other secondary interactions, there is almost certainly flexibility of structure as now thought to be the case with all compact globular proteins [e.g., insulin (55)]. Changes in conformation during interaction of subunits have been detected by numerous physicochemical measurements, including nuclear magnetic resonance, spectrophotometric titrations, circular dichroism, and measurement of fluorescence, as well as by changes in reactivity of amino acid side chains (see refs. 22 and 56–58 for reviews of the literature).

STRUCTURE-FUNCTION RELATIONSHIPS: THE EFFECTS OF STRUCTURE MODIFICATION

Lacking detailed knowledge of three-dimensional structure, what can one say concerning structural features necessary for interaction with receptor, including what regions of amino acid side chains determine specificity, i.e., distinguish LH or hCG actions from those of FSH? Also, what structural requirements are needed for subsequent steps in hormone action? Some provisional answers have been provided by a large number of investigations on the effects of chemical or enzymatic modifications to intact hormones. These studies have been well reviewed (see, e.g., refs. 22,23,29, and 56–60; the reader is referred to these for original literature citations). Individual subunits have also been modified, and their ability to reassociate, plus the ability of the reassociated molecule to elicit a biological response, has been determined. Three types of assay systems involving three different aspects of gonadotropin activity—the ability to compete with radiolabeled hormone in binding to receptor preparations (competitive binding assays), stimulation of adenylate cyclase activity, and stimulation of steroidogenesis—have been used in such studies.

Results of modification must be interpreted with caution because a number of experiments have shown that the high-affinity interaction of a gonadotropin with its receptor is dependent on conformation even though some conformational flexibility is present. Even if a reagent is fully specific for a particular amino acid or sugar, the effects of a modified group may be to induce changes in conformation in another domain of the molecule. These cautions are magnified with the gonadotropins because a modification can also lead to an increased rate of dissociation of the subunits. In considering the effects of modifications as well as other factors influencing biological activity, it is also well to remember that many competitive binding assays (as well as others) are done with heterologous systems. An excellent example of misleading information is that equine chorionic gonadotropin (eCG), whose structure is similar to that of hCG (in that both have carboxyl-terminal extensions not seen in LH from all species), was long thought to have a predominately FSH activity rather than an LH-type activity, as does hCG. However, the assay system used to come to this conclusion was derived from rats, and when a homologous assay (i.e., one with equine receptor material) was employed, PMSG was found to closely resemble LH in its activity (see, e.g., refs. 61–63). Similarly, statements about the relative potency of, for example, ovine LH versus hCG, when assayed in a radioreceptor assay utilizing rat receptors, should be viewed cautiously.

With the above caveats in mind, modification studies have indicated a number of residues or regions of the structure which seem to be important in hormone receptor interaction and subsequent response. One region is the carboxyl-terminal pentapeptide of the α subunit. This sequence also contains a tyrosine residue at position 92 in all species thus far studied (see Fig. 1), and its modification, together with that of Tyr 93 (present in most species), leads to inactivation, as does removal of the entire pentapeptide by treatment with carboxypeptidase (22,29,59). Thus Tyr 92 is almost surely a point of interaction with receptor. One study has indicated that this domain has a role in determining the final conformation of LH or hCG (others have not). Integrity of the disulfide bonds of each subunit is also necessary, other than the 11-35 bond in the α subunit. This bond can be specifically reduced and appropriately derivitized with retention of activity (64). Less-specific information concerning precise areas of interaction with receptor is available for the three β subunits. Neither LH nor hCG contains as many tyrosines as the α subunit, and, when modified by some reagents, receptor binding can (after recombination with unmodified α) still occur. The single tryptophan of human FSH-β, at position 33, is inaccessible to *N*-bromosuccinimide; that at position 8 in human LH-β is reactive, with a loss in binding activity.

Numerous modifications of charged groups, e.g., ε-lysine groups, carboxyl groups of glutamic and aspartic acid residues, and the guanido group of arginine, have also been made. A variety of results have been obtained, depending on which subunits and which hormones were investigated, and generalizations concerning specific charged residues vital to receptor interactions do not appear feasible. Less-specific studies have been made with FSH (65).

With respect to what amino acid side chains are directly involved in receptor interaction, the lack of receptor binding activity after a number of different types of modifications, as well as immunological data (66,67), imply direct α-subunit-receptor interaction. Interpretation of the more limited modification data available for β subunits is more difficult because of the three different β sequences. Nevertheless there is good reason to believe that the β subunit, which does confer a specificity of interaction, also interacts directly with receptor. Strong chemical evidence for direct participation of β subunit is also provided by cross-linking of hCG and LH via photoaffinity labeling to membrane proteins that are most probably part of the receptor structure (68,69).

One of the more interesting questions posed by the existence of two subunits is: What happens to them after interaction with receptor? Does the hormone dissociate, and does the common α subunit then become the vehicle through which the cyclase system is stimulated? As previously stated, no significant effect of α subunits alone can be demonstrated in most systems (see ref. 23), which may well be because as an individual subunit their conformation is different. Certainly they do not bind as free subunits to receptor with any great affinity, and many studies show marked changes in conformation during interaction with β. Chemical cross-linking between the subunits with bifunctional reagents has provided excellent evidence that, after receptor interaction, the α subunit need not be translocated from the β in order for cyclase stimulation or steroid production to occur (70,71). Lysine α-49 and aspartic acid α-111 were found as the linked residues (72); obviously these residues are not interacting significantly with receptor.

Other modifications have indicated regions of both subunits interacting to form active hormone (22,29); the latter reference gives excellent detail and interpretation of the data, including conclusions concerning the functions of residues that have been found, so far, to be invariant in the sequences presently known.

The most interesting modification of the gonadotropins has been with regard to their oligosaccharides. The sugar residues in these hormones, i.e., mannose, *N*-acetyl glucosamine, *N*-acetyl galactosamine, galactose, fucose, and *N*-acetyl neuraminic (sialic) acid, are not easily modified in a specific fashion, and, until recently, sugars could not be removed easily from LH by enzymatic means, although hCG and FSH are more susceptible to glycosidase action, apparently because their terminal sugars are not sulfated. It has been known for many years that the removal of neuraminic acid residues from hCG and FSH (with exposure of vicinal galactose residues) results in a drastically reduced half-life in the blood, thus giving apparent inactivation in long-term *in vivo* assays; short-term *in vitro* responses are retained. There have also been numerous studies showing differences in the ratio of biological to immunological activity in forms of FSH, LH, and hCG that contain different amounts of neuraminic acid (see, e.g., refs. 73–75); any physiological significance remains to be determined. Moyle et al. (76) initially carried out a series of graded enzymatic hydrolyses of hCG in which residues further into the oligosaccharide structure were removed. The resulting preparations, while binding to receptor, showed a progressive loss of ability to reduce cyclic AMP and stimulate steroidogenesis as the sugars were removed. Later studies, first carried out by Sairam and colleagues (77) and continued in many laboratories (see, e.g., refs. 78–83), have clearly shown that, after chemical deglycosylation or after enzymatic deglycosylation, the ability to bind to receptor is *enhanced* as much as two- to threefold (*N*-acetyl glucosamines adjacent to an asparagine residue in the peptide chain are not removed). However, the potency of the deglycosylated preparations in stimulation of cyclic AMP production and steroid production, as well as the maximum amount of steroid that can be made, is drastically reduced. All the data strongly point to a major functional role for the carbohydrate, particularly that of the α subunit, in the coupling of the receptor-hormone complex to the adenylate cyclase system (see ref. 78a for a review). The deglycosylated hormone also can act as an antagonist against the unmodified hormone under appropriate conditions, and inhibition by a given deglycosylated preparation is consistent with its β subunit specificity. Experiments have also been done with only one, or the other, subunit deglycosylated with subsequent reassociation with native counterpart subunit. The ensuing reduction in potency, i.e., stimulation of steroid production, is greater when α, as opposed to β, is deglycosylated, again implying a direct role of the α subunit in the expression of hormone activity after receptor interaction. The idea is intriguing and intellectually satisfying, since the activity of all glycoprotein hormones is mediated via cyclase activation and the α subunit is common to all, and it is possible that removal of the carbohydrate alters the lateral mobility of the hormone-receptor complex in the membrane (84). Recent studies have shown that binding of deglycosylated hCG to receptor does not result in aggregation of receptors (85) and that the presence of antibody against hCG partially restores the activity of deglycosylated hormone (86). Deglycosylation of the subunits does not interfere with *in vitro* reassociation; it is of interest that a recent report (87) describes a markedly increased rate of reassociation of deglycosylated LH-α with native β subunit (10 min versus 24 hr for maximum recovery of receptor binding activity).

The carbohydrate moieties of the gonadotropins are also involved in the folding of newly biosynthesized peptide chains, as described in the following section.

BIOSYNTHESIS OF THE GONADOTROPINS

During the past 10 years, a remarkable amount of information concerning the biosynthesis of the gonadotropins has been acquired. The process is a complex one, consisting of transcription and translation, via messenger RNA, of the genetic information and of extensive posttranslational modifications, including addition and modification of oligosaccharides. Any step in the process is a potential locus for physiological control of hormone formation and secretion; research in this area is increasing rapidly. The subject has been reviewed recently in detail (22,24,88–91).

The new information has resulted primarily from application of the techniques of biochemistry and molecular biology, including cell-free translation of mRNA and analyses of gene structure and expression. Many of the experimental studies involved with the protein portion are similar to earlier work on the synthesis of parathyroid hormone and insulin (see ref. 92 for a review of earlier studies). A major contribution to an understanding of posttranslational events with the gonadotropins comes from studies on the synthesis of the structurally related glycoprotein, mouse TSH, in transplantable TSH-producing tumors (93–95). Message for all the pituitary glycoprotein hormones is only a small percentage of the total mRNA in the pituitary (0.1–1%), and the availability of mRNA enriched in TSH message was extremely useful in many early studies. Choriocarcinoma cell lines and human placental tissue explants have been a medium for studying posttranslational events in hCG synthesis (see, e.g., refs. 96 and 97), but, to date, no cell line producing only FSH or LH has been described.

It is now known that each subunit is coded by a different gene or set of genes and that the genes for α and β subunits are located on different chromosomes (in humans α is on 7, β is on 19). For the present discussion the biosynthetic process can be divided into three phases. One is the transcription of the genetic information into RNA and processing to form mature message; the second is the translation of the coding regions (exons) to produce nascent polypeptide including the "signal" or "leader" sequence characteristic of most secreted proteins (98). The third phase is the processing of the two translated subunit peptide chains. This phase includes: cleavage of the signal peptide sequence as each peptide passes through the endoplasmic reticulum; attachment of the *N*-linked mannose-rich oligosaccharides via their dolichol phosphate intermediates (see ref. 99 for a review); and folding of each subunit into its three-dimensional structure, including disulfide formation, formation of the α-β complex, attachment of *O*-linked oligosaccharides (where found), and further processing of the *N*-linked, mannose-rich oligosaccharides, which includes "trimming" of this moiety followed by addition of the peripheral sugar components.

With respect to gene structure, the α gene from humans and cattle has been cloned and characterized, as have the copy DNAs (cDNA) from cattle, rat, and mouse. The overall structure of the α genes from humans and cattle is given in Fig. 4a. In both species, only a single gene, which contains four coding regions (exons), is present. The intervening sequences (introns) are in identical positions, but the first is considerably larger (13,500 nucleotides) in cattle than in humans (6,400 nucleotides); otherwise the organization is similar. Three variants of the human α gene have been found (100,101), depending on the individual from which the DNA is obtained. The three do not differ in their coding regions, but do differ either in intron A or in the region distal to the 3′ end of the coding region. The structures of the human and cattle α genes, as well as those of their "copy DNAs," confirm the earlier studies of protein sequence, including the fact that the human α subunit has four amino acids deleted as compared to bovine α. The deleted codons correspond to positions 6 through 9 of the bovine sequence (see Fig. 1), and the deletion is at the splice junction between the first coding region and intron B. The heterogeneity observed at the amino terminus of bovine and other α subunits (see Fig. 1) (22) thus appears to be caused by additional proteolysis after signal peptide cleavage. Knowledge of the gene structure confirms earlier ideas that considerable variation can be present at the NH_2 terminus without significant effects on biological activity. The homology between the

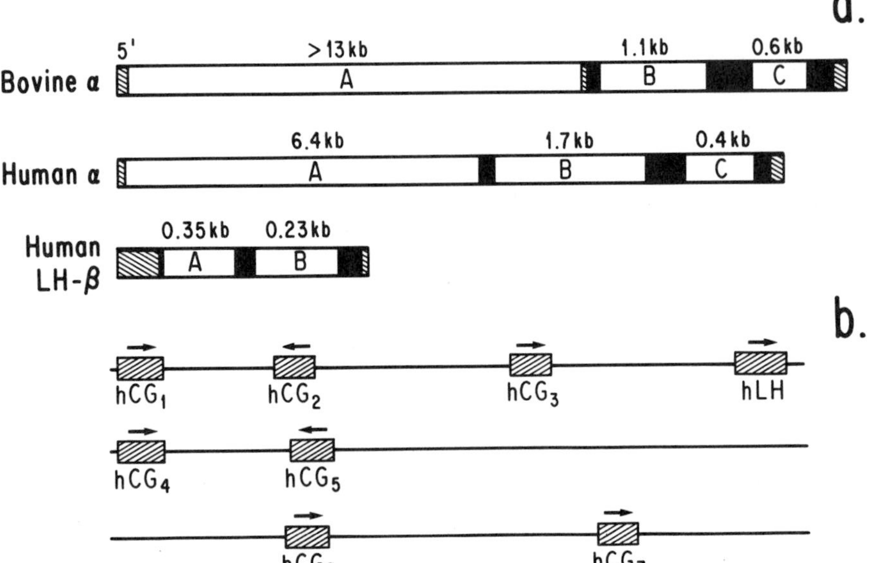

FIG. 4. (**a**) Overall gene structure of bovine and human α subunits (100–102) and human LH-β subunit (103). The dark areas represent the sequences coding for protein, including the pre- or signal sequence; the light areas represent the intervening sequences (introns), whose size is indicated in kilobases (kb) above each diagram. The untranslated 5′ and 3′ regions (found in the mRNA) are crosshatched. The bovine gene contains approximately 16,500 base pairs; the mRNA is 730 nucleotides long. Intron A interrupts the 5′-untranslated region of the mRNA, B splits the codon for residue number 10 (Fig. 1), and C is between residues 71 and 72. The human gene is smaller (9,400 base pairs). Intron A is between residues −16 and −15 in the signal or prepeptide (cf. Fig. 5 for analogous numbering) and B is between residues 41 and 42. The hCG-β gene is very similar to the hLH-β gene in terms of intron and exon positions, except that much of the 3′-untranslated region has been converted to a coding sequence (see text). The structure of the bovine and rat LH-β genes is similar to the human β genes, except that their mRNAs contain unusually short 5′-untranslated regions [seven nucleotides for rat and six to 11 for cattle (34)]. (**b**) The general organization of the genes (and pseudogenes) of hCG-β and the hLH-β gene in chromosome 19. Crosshatched areas indicate transcribed, but untranslated, regions. Arrows indicate the direction of presumed transcription (103 and 104).

bovine and human α subunits extends to the 5′ and 3′ untranslated regions of the mRNAs. Much less homology exists between either bovine or human α genes when compared with that of the rat, whose sequence is given in Fig. 5. Unexpected homology (69%) was also found between nucleotide positions 44 and 68 of the 5′ region of human α and positions 1-26 of the 5′ region (also untranslated) of human growth hormone. The bovine α gene also contains two regions of homology with a region of the chicken ovalbumin gene which has been proposed to be the site of progesterone binding with its receptor complex.

Concerning β-subunit genes, a different situation presents itself (103,104). There appears to be, as for the α gene, only a single gene for human, rat, cattle, and mouse LH-βs (34,89,90). As of this writing, reports concerning the structure of the cDNA or the gene for FSH-β have not appeared. With TSH-β there is evidence of a single gene in rat and perhaps two in mouse. However, in the human, seven hCG-β genes or pseudogenes (i.e., nucleotide sequences with great similarity to those of expressed hCG-β genes) have been identified and are found together with the hLH-β gene on chromosome 19. The organization of these genes is given in Fig. 4, together with the structure of the LH-β gene (that of the expressed hCG-β is very similar). Detailed examination of the structures, both in coding and noncoding regions, indicates that only three of them, namely hCG-β 1, 3, and 5, have the potential of being expressed to yield β subunit; present evidence is that at least two of the three are expressed. Examination of the gene structure also provides a rationale for the carboxyl-terminal extension of hCG-β versus human (or bovine, ovine, or porcine) LH-β (89). A deletion in the hCG-β gene of a single nucleotide (position 114) results in a frame shift thus bypassing a stop codon. Translation proceeds for a total of 24 additional amino acid residues before reaching the next termination point (two nucleotides not in the LH-β gene have also been introduced in the region that is being translated). Recent studies of equine LH-β and PMSG-β (equine chorionic gonadotropin) have shown that both of them contain the carboxyl-terminal extension (see, e.g., ref. 105) and that their entire amino acid sequences, but not their sugar moieties, are most probably the same (D. N. Ward, *personal communication*). Copy DNAs for rat LH-β, hLH-β, and hCG-β have been cloned, and amino acid sequences have been derived from them. The sequence of the rat gene is given in Fig. 6. The sequences of the hLH-β gene show seven additional residues to be at their carboxyl termini in comparison with the sequence determined for isolated hLH-β by traditional chemical methods (106,107) [similar carboxyl-terminal extensions have also been found for TSH-β (108) and bovine LH-α (34)]. Whether processing ("trimming") of these extensions has physiological significance or whether an artifactual proteolytic cleavage has occurred during storage, extraction and purification of the LH and TSH is not known.

Translation of gonadotropin mRNA has been studied in several laboratories, with very similar conclusions reached for each of the four glycoprotein hormones (see, e.g., refs. 93–95 and 109–111). There are three major elements in these systems: messenger RNA from the tissue source; wheat-

```
                                                                    -20                                      -10
CACATCCTTCCAAGATCCAGAGTTTGCAGGAGAGCT ATG GAT TGC TAC AGA AGA TAT GCG GCT GTC ATT CTG GTC ATG CTG
                                     Met Asp Cys Tyr Arg Arg Tyr Ala Ala Val Ile Leu Val Met Leu

                                    -1  +1                                      +10
TCC ATG GTC CTG CAT ATT CTT CAT TCT CTT CCT GAT GGA GAC CTT ATT ATT CAG GGT TGT CCA GAA TGT AAA CTA
Ser Met Val Leu His Ile Leu His Ser Leu Pro Asp Gly Asp Leu Ile Ile Gln Gly Cys Pro Glu Cys Lys Leu

            +20                                     +30                                     +40
AAG GAA AAC AAA TAC TTC TCC AAG CTG GGT GCC CCC ATC TAT CAG TGT ATG GGC TGT TGC TTC TCC AGG GCA TAC
Lys Glu Asn Lys Tyr Phe Ser Lys Leu Gly Ala Pro Ile Tyr Gln Cys Met Gly Cys Cys Phe Ser Arg Ala Tyr

                                    +50                                     +60
CCG ATC CCC GCA AGG TCC AAG AAG ACA ATG TTG GTT CCA AAG AAT ATT ACC TCG GAG GCC ACG TGC TGT GTG GCC
Pro Thr Pro Ala Arg Ser Lys Lys Thr Met Leu Val Pro Lys Asn Ile Thr Ser Glu Ala Thr Cys Cys Val Ala

            +70                                     +80                                     +90
AAA TCA TTT ACT AAG GCC ACA GTG ATG GGA AAC GCC AGA GTG GAG AAC CAC ACG GAC TGC CAC TGT AGC ACT TGT
Lys Ser Phe Thr Lys Ala Thr Val Met Gly Asn Ala Arg Val Glu Asn His Thr Asp Cys His Cys Ser Thr Cys

TAC TAC CAC AAG TCG stop
Tyr Tyr His Lys Ser TAG CTTCCATGTGTGCCAAGGGCTGCGCTGACGACT---
```

FIG. 5. Nucleotide sequence of copy DNA of rat LH-α (90) and derived amino acid sequence including the pre- or signal peptide. The numbers indicate the signal peptide (−20 to −1) and the mature LH-β protein (+1 to +121). Codons, and thus residues 6 through 9, are the segments deleted in the human structure (see text). "Stop" is the signal for termination of translation.

germ extract, or mouse ascites tumor cells, or rabbit reticulocytes, which contain the ribosomes, enzymes, and cofactors necessary for protein synthesis; and a microsomal or membrane fraction that can remove the signal peptide and initiate glycosylation (see, e.g., ref. 109). The translation products are labeled by addition of a radioactive amino acid ([^{35}S] cysteine or methionine) in the mixture of amino acids used and are immunoprecipitated by antisera against the subunit of interest. The products are then subjected to polyacrylamide gel electrophoresis in the presence of sodium dodecyl sulfate and visualized by fluorography. Two types of antisera have been used. One is directed against the "sequential" immunogenic determinants of a subunit (i.e., against a "random" or linear conformation). The immunogen usually used is an isolated subunit with its disulfide bonds reduced and *S*-carboxymethylated. The other type consists of antisera generated against isolated subunits whose structures are not modified (thus containing "conformational" determinants) (112). Three major translation products can be recognized, depending on the system used, the "prepeptide" (subunit chain) containing its own signal or leader sequence, the subunit chain minus the signal peptide, and subunit chains that have been *N*-glycosylated. The initial glycosylation is believed to be cotranslational, i.e., it occurs before the entire nascent polypeptide chain is released from the ribosome, as does, most probably, the removal of the signal peptide. If the translations are carried out in the absence of a crude membrane or microsome fraction (which can be from one of several mammalian sources), only the prepeptide is formed; it is precipitated by antisera against sequential determinants. The signal peptides of the α subunits of LH from several species consist of 24 amino acid residues; those of hCG-β and LH-β consist of 20 residues (22,88,89). In each, many of the residues are hydrophobic and, for both subunits, are highly conserved from species to species. Sequences are given in Figs. 5 and 6 for the rat peptides.

Addition of a membrane fraction to the system results in the cleavage of the signal peptide and *N*-glycosylation. In the case of α subunits, some experiments reveal two glycosylated forms which, by their relative apparent molecular weights (as determined by gel electrophoresis), represent glycosylation of one or both of the potential sites at positions 56 and 82 (see Fig. 1).

Formation of three-dimensional structures, assembly of the folded α and β subunits into dimers, trimming of the mannose-rich *N*-linked oligosaccharides, addition of distal sugars, and *O*-glycosylation occur during translocation of the newly glycosylated chains to the Golgi apparatus or while they are transversing the compartments of the Golgi (99,113). The exact timing and locations of all of these events are not known; pulse-chase labeling, together with immunoprecipitation and gel electrophoresis, particularly with hCG and rat LH [as well as with TSH systems (114)],

```
            -20                                     -10                                     -1  1
5' --AA    ATG GAG AGG CTC CAG GGG CTG CTG CTG TGG CTG CTG CTG AGC CCA AGT GTG GTG TGG GCC TCC AGG GGC
           Met Glu Arg Leu Gln Gly Leu Leu Leu Trp Leu Leu Leu Ser Pro Ser Val Val Trp Glu Ser Arg Gly

                                   10              *                   20
           CCC CTT CGG CCA CTG TGC CGG CCT GTC AAC GCA ACC CTG GCT GCA GAG AAT GAG TTC TGC CCA GTC TGC
           Pro Leu Arg Pro Leu Cys Arg Pro Val Asn Ala Thr Leu Ala Ala Glu Asn Glu Phe Cys Pro Val Cys

                               30                                      40
           ATC ACC TTC ACC ACC AGC ATC TGT GCC GGC TAC TGT CCT AGC ATG GTT CGA GTA CTG CCA GCT GCC TTG
           Ile Thr Phe Thr Thr Ser Ile Cys Ala Gly Tyr Cys Pro Ser Met Val Arg Val Leu Pro Ala Ala Leu

           50                                      60                                      70
           CCT CCC GTG CCT CAG CCA GTG TGC ACC TAC CGT GAG CTG CGC TTC GCC TCT GTC CGC CTC CCT GGC TGC
           Pro Pro Val Pro Glu Pro Val Cys Thr Tyr Arg Glu Leu Arg Phe Ala Ser Val Arg Leu Pro Gly Cys

                                       80                                      90
           CCA CCT GGT GTA GAC CCC ATA GTC TCC TTT CCT GTG GCC CTC AGC TGC CGC TGT GGG CCC TGC CGT CTC
           Pro Pro Gly Val Asp Pro Ile Val Ser Phe Pro Val Ala Leu Ser Cys Arg Cys Gly Pro Cys Arg Leu

                               100                                     110
           AGT AGC TCT GAC TGT GGG GGT CCC AGG ACT CAA CCA ATG ACC TGT GAC CTT CCC CAC CTC CCC GGC CTT
           Ser Ser Ser Asp Cys Gly Gly Pro Arg Thr Glu Pro Met Thr Cys Asp Leu Pro His Leu Pro Gly Leu

               120     stop
           CTC CTC TTC TGA TGCCCACCCACTAACTCCCCATTCTTCTGGAGCCAGCAGGTGTTCTAACCATCCCTCCCAATAAAGGCTTT
           Leu Leu Phe

           ACAACTGG-----polyA---3'
```

FIG. 6. Nucleotide sequence of copy DNA of rat LH-β (90) and derived amino acid sequence, including the pre- or signal peptide. Numbers indicate the signal peptide (−20 to −1) and the mature rat LH-β protein (+1 to +118). "Stop" is the signal for termination of translation.

has given the following picture. Correct folding, and therefore assembly into α-β dimers, requires at least some glycosylation. There is evidence that assembly may begin at the rough endoplasmic reticulum rather than later in the pathway of synthesis, but it cannot be excluded that a major site of assembly is within the Golgi (115). Based on work with other systems, it is likely that late processing events, including (a) addition of the distal carbohydrate components (such as galactose) and the more peripheral amino sugars and neuraminic (sialic) acids and (b) sulfate ester formation, occur in the Golgi or before entrance into secretory granules.

Two *O*-glycosylation reactions occur during the biosynthesis of the gonadotropins. One of these reactions is the glycosylation of serine residues in the carboxyl-terminal region of the β subunit of hCG, PMSG, and equine LH. Any function of β-subunit *O*-glycosylation is unknown. In the other reaction, the "free" or uncombined α subunit, which is produced on both the pituitary and the placenta, is *O*-glycosylated and perhaps otherwise modified. There are several intriguing possible functions for this reaction. An obvious and attractive hypothesis is that the synthesis of "combinable" α subunits is under regulation. Neither human nor bovine "free α" can form α-β complexes, but, in experiments with bovine α, enzymatic removal of the *O*-linked oligosaccharide at Thr 43 (see Fig. 1) allows α-β dimer to form (116). Because *O*-glycosylation blocks association with β subunits, it is thus possible that the *O*-glycosylation plays a role in the control of dimer formation. If this were the case, *O*-glycosylation would have to occur early in the pathway of biosynthesis rather than in the Golgi. It is also possible that in the case of cells that produce both LH and FSH, the conversion of excess α subunit to a form that will not associate with β may play a role in determining the relative amounts of FSH and LH formed (117). Recently Corliss and Boime (48) have found that differential secretion of *O*-glycosylated free α and intact LH occurs in the presence of LH-releasing hormone. Two secretory pathways are postulated based on an experiment in which the addition of LHRH to bovine pituitary slices results in a 14-fold increase in LH secretion and only a twofold increase of free α material. In the similar *O*-glycosylation that has been reported for uncombined hCG-α secreted during pregnancy or by a variety of tumor cells (see, e.g., ref. 97), all of the secreted free α may not be *O*-glycosylated (which may also be true in the pituitary, although all the free α seems to have a larger molecular weight than does the α in α-β combination). There are also tumor cell lines in which an excess of β subunit is found (118).

Carbohydrates appear to have an important function in the correct folding of each subunit into its three-dimensional structure. With α subunits complete reduction and reoxidation of their disulfide bonds (analogous to the classic experiments with ribonuclease) result in a product indistinguishable from isolated LH-α in a variety of tests, including reassociation with β subunits to give active hormone (119). Similar results are obtained with chemically or enzymatically deglycosylated α (note however, that amino sugars vicinal to the peptide chain remain).

Experiments in which completely aglyco α was expressed from *E. coli* after insertion of its transcriptionally functional cDNA into the bacterium lead to the conclusion that although carbohydrate is not obligatory for correct folding, its presence greatly facilitates the process (120). Bovine α subunit synthesized in a cell-free translation system also folds poorly prior to the glycosylation step, whereas glycosylated subunits fold to native structures (112).

With β subunits, surprisingly the same results of *in vitro* refolding have not been obtained, and the only successful recovery of activity with reduced and reoxidized β has been with the enzymatically deglycosylated hCG-β, albeit with a relatively low yield (83). Data from the cell-free translation and processing of β-subunit mRNA show, as with α, that only a subunit with an oligosaccharide moiety attached can form a correct tertiary structure (121). The expression of biologically active hCG and LH and of functional α subunits after insertion of the appropriate subunit genes or cDNA into mammalian cell lines has also been achieved (122–124). In these cases the products were almost certainly glycosylated. In summary, the data strongly suggest, together with data concerning TSH (125), that formation of correct tertiary structure may require some carbohydrate attached to the peptide chain and, more importantly, that the folding of the subunit begins during the formation of the nascent peptide chains.

PROSPECTS: PRESENT AND FUTURE

Although much has been learned in the past 20 years concerning the chemistry of gonadotropins, a major problem, that of three-dimensional structures, remains unsolved. Crystals suitable for X-ray diffraction studies have not been obtained, and, because no related three-dimensional structures are known, modeling via computer techniques does not appear to have been successful. A promising approach to the solution of a three-dimensional structure would be the *in vitro* production of gonadotropins that might readily crystallize if microheterogeneity, of both amino termini and oligosaccharides, is not present. In terms of determining precisely what domains of the structure are needed for interaction with receptor and stimulation of subsequent biochemical events, site-directed mutations via genetic engineering offer great promise and will allow one to build on the often somewhat tenuous conclusions afforded by chemical modification studies (see ref. 126 for review). Site-directed mutations of key half-cystine residues in which, for example, an alanine or serine residue is substituted for a half-cystine, coupled with subsequent investigation of correct or incorrect folding of a subunit, is another intriguing possibility. The results of such experiments might help to solve the disulfide placements in each subunit and thus permit computer-assisted development of models of three-dimensional structure. The physiological significance of the carboxyl-terminal extension of CG-like molecules and their distribution are also interesting points to ponder. CG-like molecules in appreciable amounts are found in primates, in horses (where there seems to be only the hCG type of β subunit in both equine LH and CG), and in guinea pigs and related species (see, e.g., ref. 127). There are conflicting reports concerning CG-like molecules in rats, but no evidence of G-β-like genes has been found in the placenta of this species (see, e.g., ref. 128).

Another area where chemical knowledge is imprecise is that of what significant structural modifications, if any, from the originally secreted hormones are found in the gonadotropins obtained from postmenopausal urine. A considerable effort concerning the separation and purification of urinary LH and FSH was made in the 1970s (see, e.g., refs. 129–131), but, as best as I can determine, subsequent definitive structural studies have not been carried out. Certainly other directions have been more promising for protein and carbohydrate chemists. However, as so clearly shown by their structures and by the many steps in their biosynthesis, the gonadotropins are complex molecules, and the significance of metabolic alterations of their structures remains to be determined.

ACKNOWLEDGMENTS

The author acknowledges, with many thanks, the sequence data compilation made available by Dr. Anne Stockell-Hartree, Cambridge, England. Dr. Bruce Weintraub and Dr. William Chin are thanked for preprints of articles, and grateful appreciation is expressed to many colleagues whose fruitful interactions made possible the extraordinary increase in information concerning gonadotropin chemistry.

REFERENCES

1. Evans, H., and Long, J. (1922): Characteristic effects upon growth, oestrus and ovulation induced by the introperitoneal administration of fresh anterior hypophyseal substance. *Proc. Natl. Acad. Sci. USA*, 8:38–39.
2. Smith, P. E. (1926): Hastening development of female genital system by daily hymoplastic pituitary transplants. *Proc. Soc. Explt. Biol.*, 24:131–132.
3. Zondek, B., and Ascheim, S. (1926): Über die funkion des ovariums. *Z. Geburtshilfe Gynaekol.*, 9:372–376.
4. Fevold, H. L., Hisaw, F. L., and Leonard, S. L. (1931): The gonad-stimulating and the luteinizing hormones of the anterior lobe of the hypophysis. *Am. J. Physiol.*, 97:291–301.

5. Ascheim, S., and Zondek, B. (1927): Hypophysenvononderlappenhormon und ovarialhormone im harn von schwangeren. *Klin. Wochenschr.*, 6:1322.
6. Pierce, J. G. (1971): Eli Lilly Lecture: The subunits of pituitary thyrotropin—Their relationship to other glycoprotein hormones. *Endocrinology*, 89:1331–1334.
7. Fontaine, Y. A., and Burzawa-Gerard, E. (1977): Esquisse de l'evolution des hormones gonadotropes et tyréotropes des vertébrés. *Gen. Comp. Endocrinol.*, 32:341–347.
8. Licht, P., Papkoff, H., Farmer, S., Muller, C., Tsui, H.-W., and Crews, D. (1977): Evolution of gonadotropin structure and function. *Recent Prog. Horm. Res.*, 33:169–218.
9. Farmer, S., and Papkoff, H. (1979): Comparative biochemistry of pituitary growth hormone, prolactin and the glycoprotein hormones. In: *Hormone and Evolution, Vol. 2*, edited by E. J. W. Barrington, pp. 525–559. Academic Press, London.
10. Canfield, R. E., and Morgan, F. J. (1974): Human chorionic gonadotropin (hCG) 1-purification and biochemical characterization. In: *The Methods in Investigative and Diagnostic Endocrinology*, edited by S. A. Berson and R. S. Yalow, pp. 727–744. North-Holland, Amsterdam.
11. Stockell-Hartree, A., Shownkeen, R., Stevens, V., Matsuura, S., Ohashi, M., and Chen, H-C. (1983): Studies on the human chorionic gonadotropin-like substance of human pituitary glands and its significance. *J. Endocrinol.*, 96:115–126.
12. Braunstein, G. (1982): Chorionic gonadotropin (hCG) and hCG-like substances in human tissues and bacteria. In: *Pregnancy Proteins, Biology, Chemistry and Clinical Application*, edited by J. G. Grudzinskas, B. Teisner, and M. Suppälä, pp. 39–49. Academic Press, Syndey.
13. Stockell-Hartree, A. (1975): Purification of human pituitary glycoprotein hormones. In: *Methods in Enzymology, Vol. XXXVII, Hormone Action, Part B, Peptide Hormones*, edited by B. W. O'Malley and J. G. Hardman, pp. 380–389. Academic Press, New York.
14. Bloomfield, G., Faith, M. R., and Pierce, J. G. (1978): Sepharose-linked concanavalin A in the purification and characterization of glycoprotein hormones of the bovine pituitary. *Biochim. Biophys. Acta*, 533:371–372.
15. Cheng, K. W. (1976): Purification and properties of bovine pituitary follitropin. *Biochem. J.*, 159:651–659.
16. Grimek, H., Gorski, J., and Wentworth, B. (1979): Purification and characterization of bovine follicle stimulating hormone: Comparison with ovine follicle-stimulating hormone. *Endocrinology*, 104:140–147.
17. Ward, D. N., Adams-Mayne, M., Ray, N., Balke, D., Coffey, J., and Showalter, M. (1967): Comparative studies of luteinizing hormones from beef, pork and sheep pituitaries. 1. Purification and physical properties. *Gen. Comp. Endocrinol.*, 8:44–53.
18. Papkoff, H., Gospodarowicz, D., and, Li, C. H. (1967): Purification and properties of ovine follicle-stimulating hormone. *Arch. Biochem. Biophys.*, 120:434–439.
19. Bousfield, G., and Ward, D. (1984): Purification of lutropin and follitropin on high yield from horse pituitary glands. *J. Biol. Chem.*, 259:1911–1921.
20. Dufau, M., Tsuruhara, T., and Catt, K. J. (1972): Interaction of glycoprotein hormones with agarose-concanavalin A. *Biochim. Biophys. Acta*, 278:281–292.
21. Williams, T. F., Davies, T., Catt, K. J., and Pierce, J. G. (1980): Receptor-binding activity of highly purified bovine luteinizing hormone and thyrotropin, and their subunits. *Endocrinology*, 106:1353–1359.
22. Pierce, J. G., and Parsons, T. F. (1981): Glycoprotein hormones: Structure and function. *Annu. Rev. Biochem.*, 50:465–495.
23. Sairam, M. (1983): Gondadotropin hormones: Relationship between structure and function with emphasis on antagonists. In: *Hormonal Proteins and Peptides, Vol. XI*, edited by C.H. Li, pp. 1–79. Academic Press, New York.
24. Strickland, T. W., Parsons, T. F., and Pierce, J. G. (1985): Structure of LH and hCG. In: *Luteinizing Hormone Action and Receptors*, edited by Mario Ascoli, pp. 2–15. CRC Press, Boca Raton, Fl.
25. de la Llosa, P., and Jutisz, M. (1969): Reversible dissociation with subunits and biological activity of ovine luteinizing hormone. *Biochim. Biophys. Acta*, 181:426–436.
26. Papkoff, H., and Samy, T. S. A. (1967): Isolation and partial characterization of polypeptide chains of ovine interstitial cell stimulating hormone. *Biochim. Biophys. Acta*, 147:175–177.
27. Pierce, J. G., Liao, T.-H., Howard, S. M., Shome, B., and Cornell, J. S. (1971): Studies on the structure of thyrotropin: Its relationship to luteinizing hormone. *Recent Prog. Horm. Res.*, 27:165–212.
28. Parsons, T. F., Strickland, T. W., and Pierce, J. G. (1984): Rapid and easy separation of the subunits of bovine and human glycoprotein hormones by use of high performance liquid chromatography. *Endocrinology*, 114:2223–2227.
29. Gordon, W. L., and Ward, D. N. (1985): Structural aspects of luteinizing hormone actions. In: *Luteinizing Hormone Action and Receptors*, edited by Mario Ascoli, pp. 173–197. CRC Press, Boca Raton, Fl.
30. Sairam, M. (1981): Primary structure of the ovine pituitary follitropin alpha subunits. *J. Biochem.*, 197:535–539.
31. Sairam, M. (1981): The primary structures of the ovine pituitary follitropin beta subunits. *J. Biochem.*, 197:541–552.
32. Glenn, S., Nahm, H., and Ward, D. (1984): The amino acid sequence of the rabbit glycoprotein hormone α subunit. *J. Prot. Chem.*, 3:143–156.
33. Glenn, S., Nahm, H., and Ward, D. (1984): The amino acid sequence of the rabbit lutropin β subunit. *J. Protein Chem.*, 3:259–273.
34. Virgin, J., Silver, B., Thomason, A., and Nilson, J. (1985): The gene for the β subunit of bovine luteinizing hormone encodes a gonadotropin mRNA with an unusually short 5′ untranslated region. *J. Biol. Chem.*, 260:7072–7077.
35. Hortin, G., Natowicz, M., Pierce, J. G., Baenziger, J., Parsons, T., and Boime, I. (1981): Metabolic labeling of lutropin with [^{35}S]sulfate. *Proc. Natl. Acad. Sci. USA*, 78:7468–7472.
36. Parsons, T. F., and Pierce, J. G. (1984): Carbohydrate compositions of the human pituitary glycoprotein hormone subunits (isolated by high performance liquid chromotography) indicate different oligosaccharide processing. *Abstracts of the 7th International Congress of Endocrinology*, p. 1134. Excerpta Medica, Elsevier, Amsterdam.
37. Kessler, M., Reddy, M. S., Shah, R., and Bahl, O. (1979): Structure of *N*-glycosidic carbohydrate units of human chorionic gonadotropin. *J. Biol. Chem.*, 254:7901–7908.
38. Kessler, M., Mise, T., Ghai, R., and Bahl, O. (1979): Structure and location of the *O*-glycosidic carbohydrate units of human chorionic gonadotropin. *J. Biol. Chem.*, 254:7908–7914.
39. Endo, Y., Yamashita, K., Tachibana, Y., Tojo, S., and Kobata, A. (1979): Structure of the asparagine-linked sugar chains of human choriogonadotropin. *J. Biochem. (Tokyo)*, 85:669–679.
40. Mizuochi, T., Nishimura, R., Derappe, C., Taniguchi, T., Hamamoto, T., Michizuki, M., and Kobata, A. (1983): Structure of the asparagine-linked sugar chains of human chorionic gonadotropin produced in choriocarcinoma. *J. Biol. Chem.*, 218:14126–14129.
41. Bedi, G., French, W., and Bahl, O. (1982): Structure of carbohydrate units of ovine luteinizing hormone. *J. Biol. Chem.*, 247:4345–4555.
42. Green, E., van Halbeck, H., Boime, I., and Baenziger, J. (1985): Structural elucidation of the disulfated oligosaccharide from bovine lutropin. 260:15623–15630.
43. Kourides, I., Weintraub, B., Ridgway, E., and Maloof, F. (1975): Pituitary secretion of free alpha and beta subunits of human thyrotropin patients with thyroid disorders. *J. Clin. Endocrinol. Metab.*, 40:872–885.
44. Parsons, T. Bloomfield, G., and Pierce, J. G. (1983): Purification of an alternate form of the α-subunit of the glycoprotein hormones from bovine pituitaries oligosaccharide. *Biol. Chem.*, 218:240–244.
45. Begeot, M., Hemming, F., Dubois, P., Combarnous, Y., Dubois, M., and Aubert, M. (1984): Induction of pituitary lactotrope differentiation of luteinizing hormone α subunit. *Science*, 226:566–568.
46. Ruddon, R. W., Hartle, R. J., Peters, B. P., Anderson, C., Haot, R. I., and Stromberg, K. (1981): Biosynthesis and secretion of chorionic gonadotropin subunit by organ cultures of first trimester human placenta. *J. Biol. Chem.*, 256:11389–11392.
47. Cole, L. A., Perini, F., Birken, S., and Ruddon, R. W. (1984): An oligosaccharide of the *O*-linked type distinguishes the free from the combined form of HCGα subunit. *Biochem. Biophys. Res. Commun.*, 122:1260–1267.
48. Corliss, C., and Boime, I. (1985): Differential secretion of *O*-glycosylated gonadotropin α-subunit and luteinizing hormone (LH) in

the presence of LH-releasing hormone. *Endocrinology*, 117:1699–1706.

49. Peters, B., Krzesicki, R., Hartle, R., Perini, F., and Ruddon, R. (1984): A kinetic comparison of the processing and secretion of the αβ dimer and the uncombined α and β subunits of chorionic gonadotropin synthesized by human choriocarcinoma cells. *J. Biol. Chem.*, 259:15123–15130.
50. Pierce, J. G. (1981): Problems in the determination of disulfide bonds in the glycoprotein hormones of the pituitary and placenta. In: *Chemical Synthesis and Sequencing of Peptides and Proteins*, edited by P. Liu, A. Schechter, R. Heinrikson, and P. Condliffe, pp. 221–229. Elsevier/North Holland.
51. Mise, T., and Bahl, O. (1980): Assignment of disulfide bonds in the α subunit of human chorionic gonadotropin. *J. Biol. Chem.*, 255:8516–8522.
52. Mise, T., and Bahl, O. (1981): Assignment of disulfide bonds in the β subunit of human chorionic gonadotropin. *J. Biol. Chem.*, 256:6587–6592.
53. Strickland, T., and Puett, D. (1982): The kinetic and equilibrium parameters of subunit association and gonadotropin dissociation. *J. Biol. Chem.*, 257:2954–2960.
54. Forasteiri, H., and Ingham, K. (1982): Thermal stability of human chorionic gonadotropin: Reversible dissociation of subunits at neural pH. *J. Biol. Chem.*, 257:7976–7981.
55. Blundell, T., and Wood, S. (1982): The conformation, flexibility, and dynamics of polypeptide hormones. *Annu. Rev. Biochem.*, 51:123–154.
56. McKerns, K., editor (1978): *Structure and Function of Gonadotropins*, p. 628. Plenum Press, New York.
57. Bishop, W., Nureddin, A., and Ryan, R. J. (1976): Pituitary luteinizing and follicle stimulating hormones. In: *Peptide Hormones*, edited by J. A. Parsons, pp. 273–298. Park Press, Baltimore.
58. Parsons, T. F., and Pierce, J. G. (1983): Studies of the histidine residues of human and bovine glycoprotein hormones by nuclear magnetic resonance. *Int. J. Pept. Protein Res.*, 21:522–535.
59. Ward, D. N. (1978): Chemical approaches to the structure function relationships of luteinizing hormone (lutropin). In: *Structure and Function of the Gonadotropins*, edited by K. W. McKerns, pp. 31–45. Plenum Press, New York.
60. Bahl, O., and Kalyan, N. (1983): Chemistry and biology of placenta choriogonadotropin and related proteins. In: *Role of Proteins and Peptides in Reproduction*, edited by S. M. McCann and D. S. Dhindsa, pp. 293–327. Elsevier, Amsterdam.
61. Licht, P., Bono Gallo, A., Agzarwahl, B., Farmer, S., Castellano, J., and Papkoff, H. (1979): Biological and binding activities of equine gonadotropins and PMSG. *J. Endocrinol.* 83:311–322.
62. Moore, W., Burleigh, B., and Ward, D. N. (1980): Chorionic gonadotropins: Comparation studies and comments on relationships to other glycoprotein hormones. In: *The Proceedings of the Lake Como Conference on the Chorionic Gonadotropin Molecule*, edited by S. Siegel, pp. 713–792. Plenum Press, New York.
63. Moore, W., and Ward, D. (1980): Pregnant mare serum gonadotropin: An *in vitro* biological characterization of the lutropin-follitropin dual activity. *J. Biol. Chem.*, 255:6930–6966.
64. Giudice, L., and Pierce, J. G. (1979): Studies on the disulfide bonds of glycoprotein hormones: Formation and properties of 11,35-bis(*S*-alkyl) derivatives of the α subunit. *J. Biol. Chem.*, 254:1164–1169.
65. Rathnam, P, and Saxena, B. (1979): Studies on modification of tryptophan, methionine, tyrosine, and arginine residues of human follicle stimulating hormone and its subunits. *Biochim. Biophys. Acta*, 576:81–87.
66. Moyle, W., Ehrlich, P., and Canfield, R. (1982): Use of monoclonal antibodies to subunits of human chorionic gonadotropin to examine the orientation of the hormone in its complex with receptor. *Proc. Natl. Acad. Sci. USA*, 70:2245–2249.
67. Milias, P., Midgley, A., and Birken, S. (1983): Differential masking by the receptor of immunoreaction sites on the α subunit of human chorionic gonadotropin. *Proc. Natl. Acad. Sci. USA*, 80: 7375–7379.
68. Ji, I., Buck, J., and Ji, T. (1985): Composition and peptide maps of cross-linked human choriogonadotropin cells. *J. Biol. Chem.*, 260:12815–12821.
69. Rebois, R., Omedo-Sale, F., Brody, R., and Fishman, P. (1981): Covalent cross-linking of human chorionic gonadotropin to its receptor in rat testes. *Proc. Natl. Acad. Sci. USA*, 78:2086–2089.
70. Weare, J. A., and Reichert, L. E. Jr. (1979): Studies of the carbodimide-cross-linked derivatives of bovine lutropin. I. The efforts of specific group modifications on receptor site binding in testes. *J. Biol. Chem.*, 254:6964–6971.
71. Parsons, T. F., and Pierce, J. G. (1979): Biologically active covalently cross-linked glycoprotein hormones and the effects of modification of the COOH-terminal region of their α subunits. *J. Biol. Chem.*, 254:6010–6015.
72. Weare, J. A., and Reichert, L. E. Jr. (1979): Studies with carbodimide-cross-linked derivations of bovine lutropin. II. Function of the cross-linked and replication for interaction with receptor in testes. *J. Biol. Chem.*, 254:6972–6979.
73. Chappel, S., Ulloa-Aguirre, A., and Contijanis, C. (1983): Biosynthesis and secretion follicle-stimulating hormone. *Endocrinol. Rev.*, 4:179–211.
74. Sharpe, R., Shahmanesh, M., Ellwood, M., Hartog, M., and Brown, P. (1979): A comparison of activity of luteinizing hormone stored in and released *in vitro* from pituitary glands of rats under various gonadal states. *Endocrinology*, 104:925–931.
75. Van Hall, E., Vaitakaitis, J., Ross, G., Hickman, J., and Ashwell, G. (1971): Immunological and biological activity of hCG following progressive desialylation. *Endocrinology*, 88:456–464.
76. Moyle, W. R., Bahl, O. P., and Marz, L. (1975): Role of the carbohydrate of human chorionic gonadotropin in the mechanism of hormone action. *J. Biol. Chem.*, 250:9163–9169.
77. Sairam, M. R., and Schiller, P. W. (1979): Receptor binding, biological and immunological properties of clinically deglycosylated pituitary lutropin. *Arch. Biochem. Biophys.*, 197:294–310.
78. Sairam, M. (1985): Protein glycosylation and receptor-ligand interactions. In: *The Receptors, Vol. II*, edited by M. Conn, pp. 307–340.
78a. Kalgan, N., and Bahl, O. (1983): Role of carbohydrate in human chorionic gonadotropin. Effect of deglycosylation on the subunit interaction and on its *in vitro* and *in vivo* biological properties. *J. Biol. Chem.*, 258:67–74.
79. Keutman, H., McIlroy, P., Bergert, E., and Ryan, R. (1983): Chemically deglycosylated human chorionic gonadotropin subunits: Characterization and biological properties. *Biochemistry*, 22:3067–3072.
80. Chen, H.-C., Shimohgashi, Y., Dufau, M., and Catt, K. (1982): Characterization and biological properties of chemically deglycosylated human chorionic gonadotropin. *J. Biol. Chem.*, 257:14446–14452.
81. Sairam, M. R., and Manjunath, P. (1983): Hormonal antagonistic properties of chemically deglycosylated human choriogonadotropin. *J. Biol. Chem.*, 258:445–449.
82. Liu, W-L., Young, J., and Ward, D. (1984): Deglycosylated ovine lutropin: Preparation and characterization by *in vitro* binding and steroidogenesis. *Mol. Cell. Endocrinol.*, 37:29–39.
83. Goverman, J. M., Parson, T. F., and Pierce, J. G. (1982): Enzymatic deglycosylation of the subunits of chorionic gonadotropin. *J. Biol. Chem.*, 257:15059–15064.
84. Amsterdam, A., Berkowitz, A., Nimrod, A., and Kohen, F. (1980): Aggregation of luteinizing hormone receptors in granulosa cells: A possible mechanism of desensitization to the hormone. *Proc. Natl. Acad. Sci. USA*, 77:5837–5841.
85. Bahl, O. Thotakura, N., and Anumula, K. (1984): Biological role of carbohydrates in gonadotropins. In: *Hormone Receptors in Growth and Reproduction*, edited by B. B. Saxena, K. J. Catt, L. Birnbaumer, and L. Martini, pp. 165–183. Raven Press, New York.
86. Rebois, R., and Fishman, R. (1984): Antibodies against human chorionic gonadotropin convert the deglycosylated hormone from an antogonist to an agonist. *J. Biol. Chem.*, 219:8087–8090.
87. Sairam, M., and Bhargavi, G. (1985): A role for glycosylation of the α subunit on transduction of biological signal in glycoprotein hormones. *Science*, 229:6567.
88. Chin, W. (1984): Biosynthesis of the glycoprotein hormones. In: *Secretory Tumors of the Pituitary Gland: Progress in Endocrine Research and Therapy, Vol. 1*, edited by Peter McL. Black et al., pp. 327–342. Raven Press, New York.

89. Chin, W. (1986): Glycoprotein hormone genes. In: *Genes Encoding Hormones and Regulatory Peptides*, edited by J. F. Habener. Humana Press, Clifton, New Jersey.
90. Chin, W. (1985): Organization and expression of glycoprotein hormone genes. In: *The Pituitary Gland*, edited by H. Imura, pp. 103–125. Raven Press, New York.
91. Hussa, R. (1980): Biosynthesis of hCG. *Endocr. Rev.*, 1:268–293.
92. Porter, R., and Fitzsimons, editors (1976): *Polypeptide Hormones: Molecular and Cellular Aspects. Ciba Foundation Symposium 41 (New Series)*. Elsevier/Excerpta Medica/North-Holland, Amsterdam.
93. Magner, J. A., and Weintraub, B. D. (1986): Thyroid-stimulating hormone biosynthesis. In: *The Thyroid*, 2nd ed., edited by S. Ingber and L. Braverman, pp. 271–287. Lippincott, New York.
94. Weintraub, B., Stannard, B. Mayner, J. A., Ronin, C., Taylor, T., Joshi, L., Constant, R., Monezes-Ferrira, M., Petrick, P., and Geshandheit, N. (1985): Glycosylation and posttranslational processing of thyroid stimulating hormones—Clinical implications. *Recent Prog. Horm. Res.*, 44:577–606.
95. Kourides, I., Gurr, J., and Wolf, O. (1984): The regulation and organization of thyroid stimulating hormone genes. *Recent Prog. Horm. Res.*, 40:79–120.
96. Ruddon, R., Hanson, C., Bryan, A., Pattermen, G., White, E., Perini, F., Mead, K., and Aldenderfer, P. (1980): Synthesis and secretion of human chorionic gondadotropin subunits by cultured human malignant cells. *J. Biol. Chem.*, 255:1000–1007.
97. Dean, D., Weintraub, B., and Rosen, S. (1980): *De novo* synthesis and secretion of heterogeneous forms of hCG and its free α-subunit in human choriocarcinoma clonal cell line JE G-3. *Endocrinology*, 106:849–858.
98. Wickner, W., and Lodish, H. (1985): Multiple mechanisms of protein insertion into and across membranes. *Science*, 230:400–407.
99. Kornfeld, R., and Kornfeld, S. (1985): Assembly of asparagine linked oligosaccharides. *Annu. Rev. Biochem.*, 54:631–664.
100. Fiddes, J., and Goodman, H. (1981): The gene encoding the common alpha subunit of the four human glycoprotein hormones. *J. Mol. Appl. Genet.*, 1:3–18.
101. Boothby, M., Rudden, R., Anderson, C., McWilliams, D, and Boime, I. (1981): A single gonadotropin α-subunit gene in normal tissue and tumor-derived cell lines. *J. Biol. Chem.*, 256:5121–5127.
102. Goodwin, R., Moreman, C., and Nilson, J. (1986): Characterization and nucleotide sequence of the gene for the common α subunit of the bovine pituitary glycoprotein hormones. *Nucleic Acids Res.*, 11:6873–6883.
103. Fiddes, J., and Talmadge, K. (1984): Structure, expression and evolution of the gene for the human glycoprotein hormones. *Recent Prog. Horm. Res.*, 40:43–78.
104. Bornstein, W., Vamvakopoulos, N., and Fiddes, J. (1982): Human chorionic gonadotropin β-subunit is encoded by at least eight genes arranged in tandem and inverted pairs. *Nature*, 300:419–422.
105. Bousfield, G., Sugino, H., and Ward, D. N. (1985): Demonstration of a COOH-terminal extension on equine lutropin by means of a common acid-labile bond in equine lutropin and equine chorionic gonadotropin. *J. Biol. Chem.*, 260:9531–9533.
106. Talmadge, K., Vamvakopoulos, N., and Fiddes, J. (1984): Evolution of the genes for the β-subunit of human chorionic gonadotropin and luteinizing hormone. *Nature*, 307:37–40.
107. Chin, W., Godine, T., Klein, D., Chang, A., Tan, L., and Habener, J. (1983): Nucleotide sequence of the cDNA encoding the precursor of the beta subunit of rat lutropin. *Proc. Natl. Acad. Sci. USA*, 80:4649–4653.
108. Maurer, R., Croyle, M., and Donelson, J. (1984): The sequence of a cloned cDNA for the β-subunit of bovine thyrotropin predicts a protein containing both NH_2- and COOH-terminal extensions. *J. Biol. Chem.*, 259:5024–5027.
109. Daniels-McQueen, S., McWilliams, D., Birkens, S., Canfield, R., Landefeld, T., and Boime, I. (1978): Identification of mRNAs encoding the α and β subunits of human choriogonadotropin. *J. Biol. Chem.*, 253:7109–7114.
110. Alexander, D., and Miller, W. (1982): Regulation of ovine follicle stimulating hormone β-chain mRNA by 17 β-estradiol *in vivo* and *in vitro*. *J. Biol. Chem.*, 257:2282–2286.
111. Landefeld, T. (1979): Identification of an *in vitro* synthesized pituitary glycoprotein α subunit translation of a possible precursor. *J. Biol. Chem.*, 258:3685–3688.
112. Strickland, T., and Pierce, J. G. (1983): The α-subunit of pituitary glycoprotein hormones: Formation of three-dimensional structure during cell-free biosynthesis. *J. Biol. Chem.*, 258:5927–5932.
113. Hanover, T., Elting, J., Mintz, G., and Lennarz, W. (1982): Temporal aspects of the *N*- and *O*-glycosylation of human chorionic gonadotropin. *J. Biol. Chem.*, 257:10172–10177.
114. Weintraub, B., Stannard, B., Linnekin, D., and Marshall, M. (1980): Relationship of glycosylation to *de novo* thryroid-stimulating hormone biosynthesis and secretion by mouse pituitary tumor cells. *J. Biol. Chem.*, 255:5715–5723.
115. Hoshina, H., and Boime, I. (1982): Combination of rat lutropin subunits occurs early in the secretory pathway. *Proc. Natl. Acad. Sci. USA*, 79:7649–7653.
116. Parsons, T. F., and Pierce, J. G. (1984): Free alpha like material from bovine pituitaries; removal of its *O*-linked oligosaccharide permits combination with lutropin-alpha. *J. Biol. Chem.*, 259:2662–2666.
117. Green, E., Baenziger, J., and Boime, I. (1985): Cell-free sulfation of human and bovine pituitary hormones—comparison of the sulfated oligosaccharides of lutropin, follitropin and thyrotropin. *J. Biol. Chem.*, 260:15631–15638.
118. Cole, L., Hutle, R., Laferla, J., and Ruddon, R. (1983): Detection of the free beta subunit of human chorionic gonadotropin (hCG) on culture of normal and malignant trophoblast cells, pregnant sera, and sera of patients with choriocarcinoma. *Endocrinology*, 113:1176–1178.
119. Giudice, L., and Pierce, J. G. (1976): Studies on the disulfide bonds of glycoprotein hormones. Complete reductions and reoxidation of the disulfide bonds of that subunit of bovine luteinizing hormone. *J. Biol. Chem.*, 251:6392–6399.
120. Strickland, T. W., Thomason, A. R., Nilson, J. H., and Pierce, J. G. (1986): The common α-subunit of bovine pituitary glycoprotein hormones: Characterization of the gene product expressed in *E. coli*. *J. Cell. Biochem.*, 29:225–237.
121. Strickland, T. W., and Pierce, J. G. (1985): The β-subunits of glycoprotein hormones: Formation of three-dimensional structure during cell free biosynthesis of lutropin β. *J. Biol. Chem.*, 260:5816–5819.
122. Romabadron, T., Reitz, B., and Tiemeier, D. (1984): Synthesis and glycosylation of the common α-subunit of human glycoprotein hormones in mouse cells. *Proc. Natl. Acad. Sci. USA*, 81:6701–6705.
123. Reddy, V., Beck, A., Garramore, A., Vellucci, V., Lustbader, J., and Bernstine, E. (1985): Expression of human choriogonadotropin in monkey cells using a single simian virus 40 vector. *Proc. Natl. Sci. USA*, 82:3644–3648.
124. Kaetzel, D., Browne, J., Wondisford, F., Nett, T., Thomason, A., and Nilson, J. (1985): Expression of biologically active bovine luteinizing hormone in Chinese hamster cells. *Proc. Natl. Acad. Sci. USA*, 82:7280–7283.
125. Weintraub, B., Stannard, B., and Meyers, L. (1983): Glycosylation of thyroid-stimulating hormone in pituitary tumor cells: Influence of high mannose oligosaccharide units on subunit aggregation, combination and intracellular degradation. *Endocrinology*, 112:1331–1345.
126. Ackers, G., and Smith, F. (1985): Effects of site-specific amino acid modification on protein interactions and biological function. *Annu. Rev. Biochem.*, 54:597–629.
127. Bambra, C., Lynch, S., Foxcroft, G., Robinson, G., and Amoroso, E. (1984): Purification and characterization of guinea-pig chorionic gonadotropin. *Reprod. Fertil.*, 71:227–233.
128. Carr, F., and Chin, W. (1985): Absence of detectable chorionic gonadotropin subunit messenger ribonucleic acids in the rat placenta throughout gestation. *Endocrinology*, 116:1151–1157.
129. Van Hell, H., Schuurs, A., and den Hollander, F. (1972): Purification and some properties of human urinary FSH and LH. In: *Gonadotropins*, edited by B.B. Saxena, C.G. Beling, and H.M. Gandy, pp. 185–199. Wiley-Interscience, New York.
130. Beitens, I., Derfel, R., O'Loughlin, K., and McArthur, J. (1977): Immunoreaction luteinizing hormone, follicle stimulating hormone and their subunits in human urine following gel filtration. *J. Clin. Endocrinol. Metab.*, 44:149–159.
131. Van Damme, M.-P., Robertson, D., and Diczfalusy, E. (1977): Biological and immunological characterization of human luteinizing hormone: III. Biological and immunological profiles of urine preparations after electrofocusing. *Mol. Cell. Endocrinol.*, 9:69–79.

The Physiology of Reproduction,
edited by E. Knobil and J. Neill *et al.*
Raven Press, Ltd., New York © 1988.

CHAPTER 32

Gonadotropin Secretion and Its Control

George Fink

Gonadotropin secretion in mammals is controlled by feedforward and feedback mechanisms that involve the central nervous system (CNS), the anterior pituitary gland, and the gonads. The pituitary-gonadal system is influenced by factors in the external environment by way of the CNS, and this ensures that gonadotropin secretion is appropriate in relationship to factors such as day length, temperature, availability of food, and the sexual receptivity of the opposite sex (Fig. 1). Factors in the "internal" environment, such as body metabolism, weight, and fat, also influence the secretion of gonadotropins partly by way of the nervous system (1). The historical basis for our understanding of the control of gonadotropin secretion has been reviewed extensively (2–4). Briefly, the major landmarks were (a) the observation that ovulation in the rabbit occurred reflexly in response to mating (5–8), (b) the dramatic effect of light on reproductive function (9–12), (c) the technique of parapharyngeal hypophysectomy devised by P. E. Smith (13), and (d) the description of the hypophysial portal vessels (14). Experimental proof that gonadotropin secretion is controlled by the CNS was shown by the fact that electrical stimulation of the hypothalamus produced ovulation in rabbits (15). The absence of a significant number of nerve fibers in the anterior pituitary gland and the presence of the hypophysial portal vessels led to the view that the CNS control of the anterior pituitary gland (particularly gonadotropin control) was mediated by a neurohumoral mechanism (2,16). The neurohumoral hypothesis of anterior pituitary control was not readily accepted by all workers, but during the 1940s compelling physiological evidence in favor of the hypothesis was obtained mainly from the laboratory of G. W. Harris (2). Of particular importance were experiments in which Harris and Jacobsohn (17) showed that in hypophysectomized rats, pituitary grafts vascularized by the hypophysial portal, but not by cerebral systemic vessels, restored gonadal function. Final proof that gonadotropin secretion was controlled by a neurohumoral mechanism came from studies which showed that the brain synthesizes a decapeptide, luteinizing-hormone-releasing hormone (LHRH) (18–20), which is released into the hypophysial portal vessels (21,22) and is capable of releasing luteinizing hormone (LH) and follicle-stimulating hormone (FSH) (23).

Attention will be focused here on the female, in which "basal" gonadotropin secretion, which occurs during most of reproductive life, is punctuated by massive ovulatory surges of gonadotropin secretion which are produced by a precise and intricate positive feedback cascade. In both male and female, basal gonadotropin secretion is pulsatile, and the physiological significance of this mode of secretion, and the way in which gonadal steroids can exert both negative and positive effects on the hypothalamic-pituitary system, will also be considered.

THE OVULATORY SURGE OF LUTEINIZING HORMONE

Ovulation is brought about by a positive feedback cascade that involves the ovary, the CNS, and the anterior pituitary

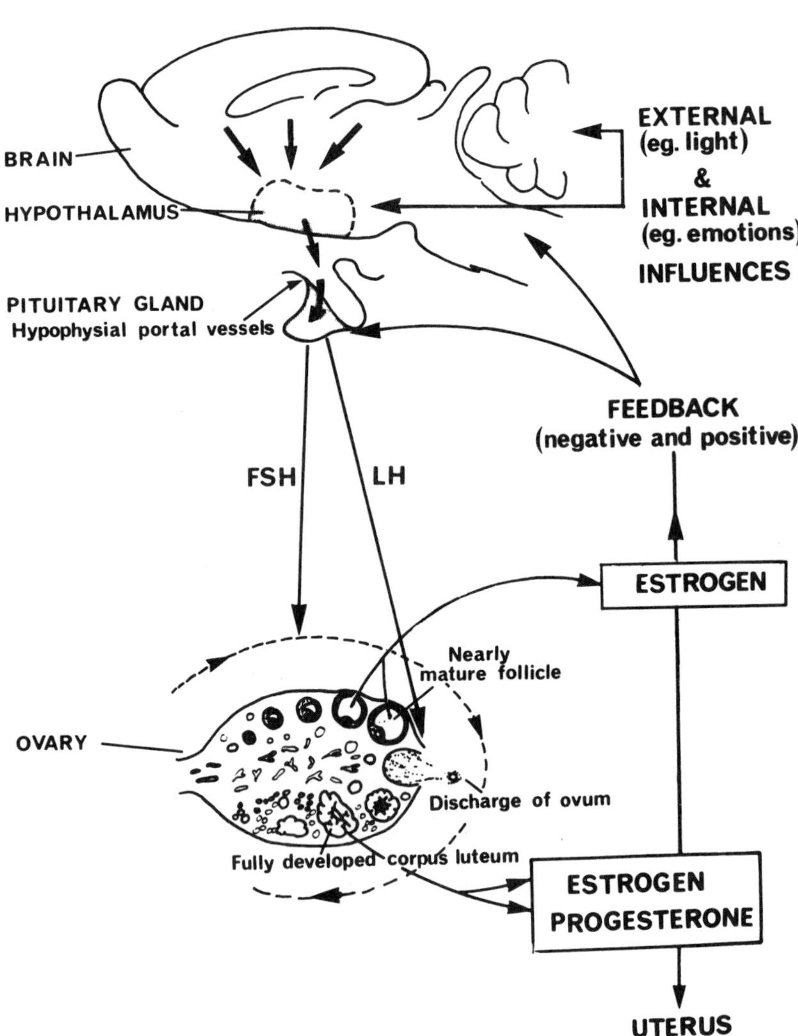

FIG. 1. Schematic diagram of the control of the ovarian cycle by follicle-stimulating hormone (FSH) and luteinizing hormone (LH) released from the anterior pituitary gland. The secretion of LH and FSH is controlled by the brain by way of luteinizing-hormone-releasing hormone (LHRH), a decapeptide that is released from hypothalamic neurons into the hypophysial portal vessels. The release of LHRH from hypothalamic neurons is influenced by external and internal factors acting by way of central nervous pathways, and the system is regulated by positive- and negative-feedback control involving estrogen and progesterone secreted by the ovary. Estrogen and progesterone act on the uterus to prepare the endometrium for implantation of the zygote should fertilization occur. Not shown, for the sake of simplicity, is the protein inhibition that is secreted by ovarian follicles and inhibits FSH release (see ref. 205).

gland and results in the massive release of LH, the ovulatory hormone. In some mammals such as the rabbit, cat, ferret, short-tailed tree shrew, 13-lined ground squirrel, and vole, ovulation occurs as a reflex to mating; however, in the majority of mammals, ovulation occurs spontaneously. Superimposed on this broad division of mammals into reflex and spontaneous ovulators, species can be further classified on the basis of whether they are seasonal breeders and whether they have estrous or menstrual cycles (2,3,11,24–26). Seasonal breeding is determined mainly by day length. Sheep and deer, for example, are short-day breeders: that is, their breeding season occurs in the autumn. Other species such as the hamster and the vole are long-day breeders, with their breeding season occurring in the spring. Humans show no prominent seasonality in breeding. The term *estrous cycle* refers to the cyclical occurrence of the receptivity of the female to the sexual advances of the male; the term *estrum* (Greek for "gadfly") refers to the increased activity shown by females during the period of increased receptivity. The term *menstrual cycle* refers to the shedding of the uterine endometrium and the accompanying bleeding that occurs at approximately monthly intervals in the human and other primates. Human females do not show any obvious estrum, but many nonhuman primates do show a period of increased sexual receptivity, as well as seasonal changes in reproductive behavior (27,28). There is no direct association between the mechanism of ovulation and the type and length of reproductive cycle. Thus, the female rabbit, a reflex ovulator, usually has two periods of estrum in the year. The length of the estrous cycle also varies considerably between species; e.g., they last 4 to 5 days in the rat and mouse and 17 days in sheep (29).

Our understanding of the gonadotropin control of spontaneous ovulation is based mainly on the rat, sheep, rhesus monkey, and human, and therefore attention will be focused on data obtained from studies on these species.

General Overview of the Mechanism of the Spontaneous Gonadotropin Surge

Follicle-stimulating hormone (FSH) stimulates the growth and maturation of ovarian follicles, whereas LH causes rupture of the follicle (Fig. 1). Under the influence of basal levels of FSH and LH, the granulosa cells of the follicle secrete estrogen, mainly estradiol-17β, and after follicular rupture, the granulosa cells proliferate and undergo structural and biochemical changes that result in the formation of the corpus luteum, which secretes large amounts of progesterone as well as estradiol-17β. The synthesis and release of LH and FSH are regulated by LHRH (30), which is synthesized by neurons in the hypothalamus (31), released into the hypophysial portal vessels, and thereby conveyed to the anterior pituitary gland (Fig. 2). The synthesis and release of LHRH are modulated by neurons in forebrain, midbrain, and hindbrain (Fig. 2) and by steroid hormones acting either directly on LHRH neurons or by way of other neurons that modulate the activity of LHRH neurons.

It was generally assumed that, like other neuropeptides, LHRH is synthesized as part of a larger precursor. This assumption was supported by gel filtration studies of hypothalamic extracts (32,33) and by immunoprecipitation of *in vitro* translation products of mRNA (34,35). The mRNA for the precursor was not found (as assessed by *in vitro* translation) in extracts of hypothalamus from hypogonadal (*hpg*) mice (35), a mutant strain totally deficient in hypothalamic LHRH (36,37). More recently Seeburg and Adelman (38) and Nikolics et al. (39) showed, on the basis of the cDNA to human placental mRNA, that the LHRH precursor in human placenta has a molecular weight of about 10,000 (Fig. 3). The hypothalamic LHRH precursor in the rat and mouse is similar to the human placental precursor, as assessed by immunohistochemistry (40) and recent studies of the gene and cDNA for LHRH in the rat and mouse (41,268). The mutation in the *hpg* mouse involves a massive deletion of a region of the gene comprising two exons that encode most of the precursor distal to LHRH (268), which Seeburg and associates have termed the *gonadotropin-releasing-hormone-associated peptide* (GAP; see below). In contrast to the somatostatin precursor from which somatostatin 28, somatostatin 28(1–12), and somatostatin 14 are all released into hypophysial portal blood (42,43), most, if not all, of the LHRH that is released into hypophysial portal blood, as measured by radioimmunoassay (21,44,45), is in the form of the decapeptide (37).

Until the early 1970s, it was assumed that the LH surge was produced by a massive surge of LHRH (then called *LH-releasing factor*) acting on a pituitary gland whose responsiveness to LHRH remained unchanged. However, experiments with LHRH and its agonists showed that: (a) massive changes occur in responsiveness of the anterior pituitary gland during estrous and menstrual cycles, and the increase in pituitary responsiveness to LHRH is essential for the occurrence of the ovulatory surge; (b) LHRH has the unique capacity to increase pituitary responsiveness to itself, i.e., the priming effect of LHRH; (c) the pituitary becomes refractory to continuous exposure to LHRH; and (d) LHRH plays a key role in the regulation of LH and FSH synthesis.

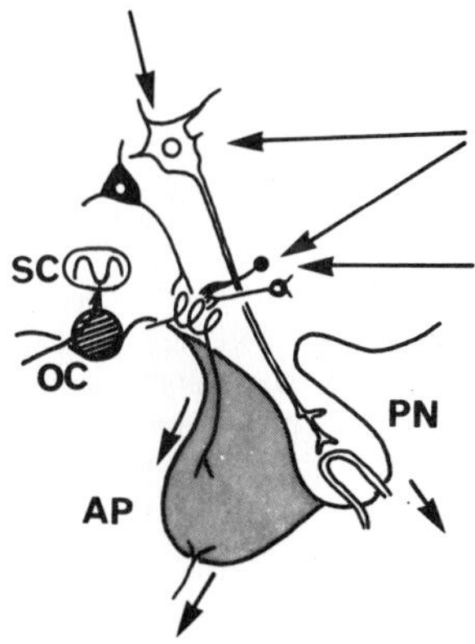

FIG. 2. A schematic diagram of the hypothalamic-pituitary system showing the magnocellular (white) projections directly to the systemic vessels of the pars nervosa (PN); also shown are parvocellular (black) projections to the primary plexus of the hypophysial portal vessels, which convey transmitters to the pars distalis of the anterior pituitary gland (AP). Dorsal to the optic chiasm (OC) are the suprachiasmatic nuclei (SC), which receive direct projections from the retina and play a key role in the control of circadian and other rhythms (indicated by the sinusoidal curve). The activity of the intrinsic neurons of the hypothalamus is greatly influenced by projections *(arrows)* from numerous areas of the forebrain and hindbrain, particularly the limbic system, as well as by hormones, mainly estrogen, progesterone, and prolactin, in the case of the hypothalamic-pituitary-gonadal system.

Detailed Physiological Mechanisms of the Spontaneous Preovulatory Gonadotropin Surge

The LH surge is the most dramatic spontaneous signal emitted by the hypothalamic-pituitary system and depends on resonance between neural and ovarian oscillators. The mechanism of the LH surge has been studied most extensively in the rat, which, allowing for a much shorter cycle length, has hormonal profiles that resemble those that occur during the menstrual cycle in women (Fig. 4). The cascade of events that leads to the LH surge is initiated by the increased secretion of estradiol-17β (46–48) (Fig. 5). Elevated concentrations of estradiol permit the expression of a neural signal for LH release in the form of a surge of LHRH and an increase in the responsiveness of the pituitary gonadotropes to LHRH (Fig. 5). The LH surge reaches a peak when increased concentrations of LHRH in hypophysial portal blood act upon an anterior pituitary gland whose responsiveness has been further augmented by the priming effect of LHRH and by progesterone secreted during the LH surge. The probable role of the priming effect of LHRH is to coordinate increasing pituitary responsiveness with increasing concentrations of LHRH in hypophysial portal vessel blood so that both reach a peak at about the same time. The termination of the LH surge is due mainly to the fall in portal plasma LHRH concentrations (44,49) and, to a

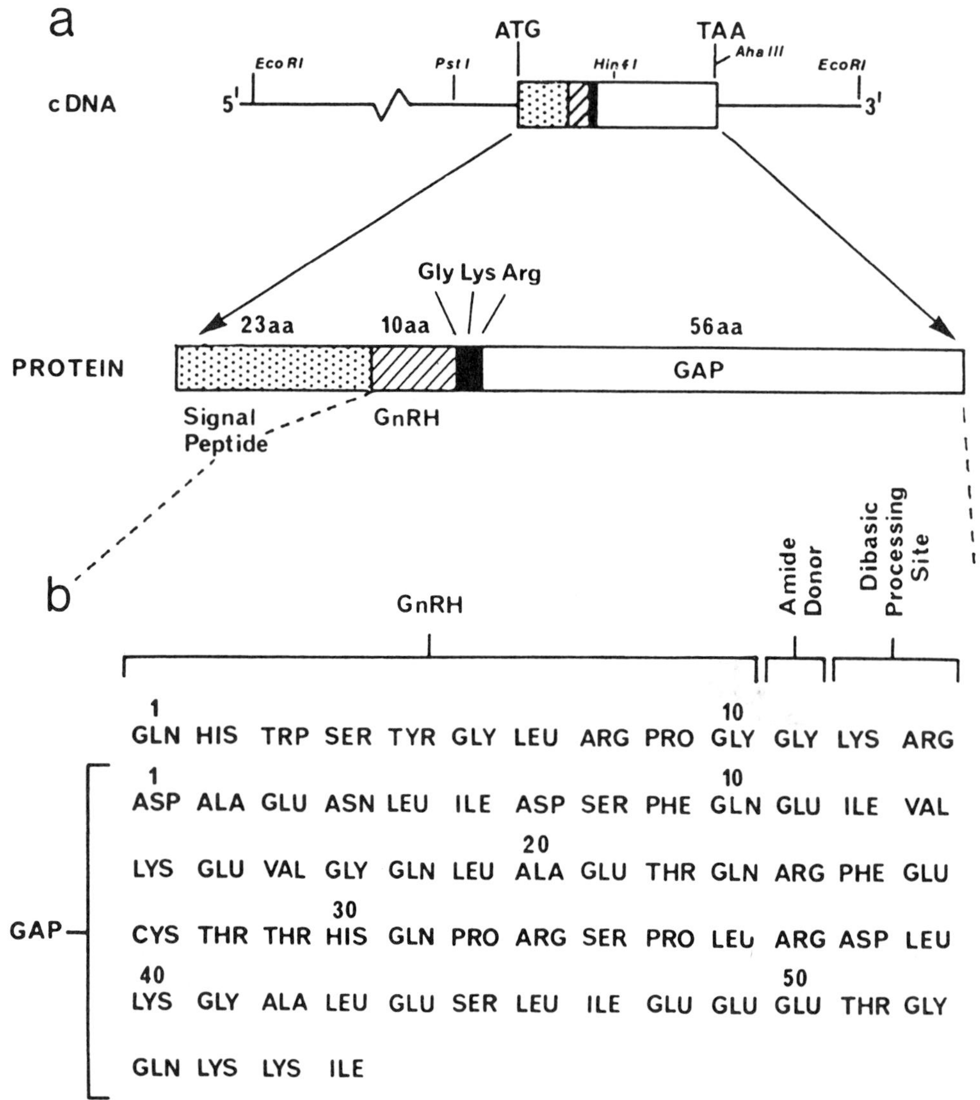

FIG. 3. Complementary DNA and precursor protein for human LHRH. The structure and encoded amino-acid sequence of human placental cDNA for prepro-LHRH are shown. (**a**) Partial restriction endonuclease map. The coding region is located between the initiation codon for protein synthesis ATG and the termination codon TAA. Schematic representation of the encoded protein identifies the three domains, namely, signal peptide, LHRH (GnRH in the figure), and GAP (gonadotropin-releasing-hormone-associated peptide) with the respective sizes in amino-acid (aa) residues. (**b**) Amino-acid sequences of LHRH and GAP with an enzymatic processing site separating the two moieties. Numbers refer to the respective positions within $LHRH_{1-10}$ or GAP_{1-56}. (From ref. 39.)

lesser extent, to the decline in pituitary responsiveness to LHRH, which is not due simply to exhaustion of pituitary LH stores (50).

The Ovarian Signal

The hormonal events surrounding the first (pubertal) surge of LH in the rat constitute important evidence for the assertion that the estradiol surge is the first event in the cascade (Fig. 6). As in the adult, the first LH surge is due to a surge of LHRH and a marked increase in pituitary responsiveness to LHRH (51). Both are preceded by an increase in plasma estradiol concentration which occurs in the absence of any major change in the mean plasma gonadotropin concentrations (52), but which may depend on pulsatile LH release (53; also see below). The brain-pituitary mechanism that subserves the positive gonadotropin response to estradiol is capable of functioning about 20 days before the first LH surge (53), and, therefore, the time of occurrence of the first LH surge may depend mainly on the capacity of the ovary to secrete estradiol-17β in a cyclical manner (54; see also Fig. 6).

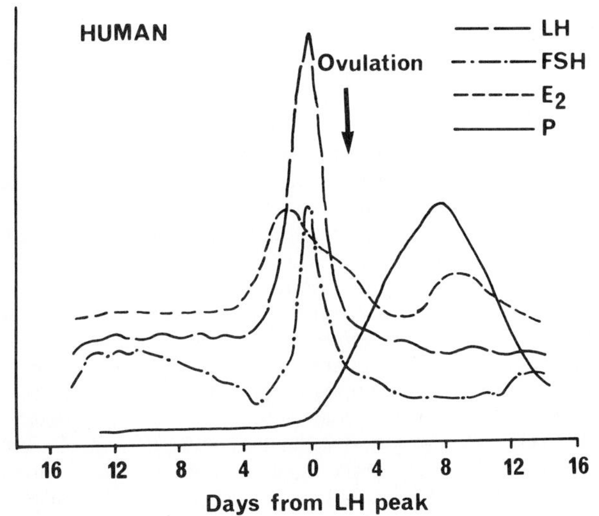

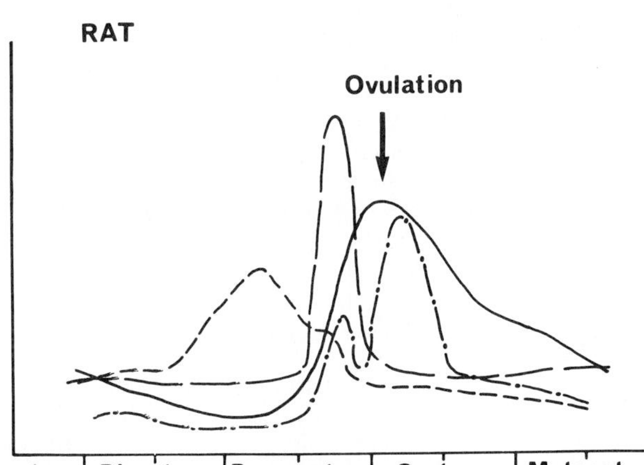

FIG. 4. Schematic diagram of the key hormonal changes during the human menstrual cycle and rat estrous cycle. Ovulation is preceded by a surge of luteinizing hormone (LH), which is triggered by a surge of estradiol-17β (E_2) and accompanied and followed by a surge of progesterone (P). Most of the progesterone is secreted by the ovary in response to LH, but in the rat a small amount of progesterone is secreted by the adrenal gland just before the onset of the LH surge. In the human, the timing and magnitude of the FSH surge are less consistent than that of the LH surge, and in the rat the major peak of the FSH surge occurs on the morning of estrus (after or about the time of ovulation).

The Neural Signal

The LHRH neurons of the hypothalamus constitute the final common pathway for the neural signal (Fig. 2). Studies in the rat have shown that the neural signal occurs daily (47,55,56), but is only expressed as a surge of LHRH in the presence of high plasma concentrations of estradiol (44,45,49,51) (Figs. 7 and 8). A similar mechanism operates in the rhesus monkey (57). Depending upon dosage, progesterone was found either to have no effect or to reduce the facilitatory effect of estradiol on LHRH release (58), and this suggests that the facilitatory effect of progesterone on the LH surge is exerted mainly at the level of the pituitary gland. It must be stressed that the LHRH surge in hypophysial portal blood can only be detected under certain anesthetics. In the rat the surge could only be detected under alphaxalone anesthesia: The surge was blocked by sodium pentobarbitone, ketamine hydrochloride, urethane, and α-chloralose (49). In the experiments by Neill et al. (57) the rhesus monkeys were anesthetized with phencyclidine hydrochloride.

The site in the brain in which the neural signal for LHRH release is generated has not yet been determined; however, an area known to be crucial for the surge is the anterior hypothalamus (Fig. 9), which encompasses the medial preoptic area and suprachiasmatic nuclei and contains the cell bodies of many hypothalamic LHRH neurons (31,59–65). Studies in which the anterior hypothalamus was systematically separated by knife cuts from the rest of the brain and the medial basal hypothalamus (Fig. 9) suggest that the region of the preoptic area and suprachiasmatic nuclei is capable of generating surges of LH. However, the estrous cycles in animals in which the connections between the preoptic area and hypothalamus were kept intact but in which these areas were disconnected from the rest of the brain were neither regular nor did they correspond in frequency to those estrous cycles in normal intact animals (66). Thus the regular activity of the LHRH surge generator may depend on the integrity of one or more of the major inputs to the anterior hypothalamus from the midbrain and forebrain limbic systems (67,68). For many years the hypothalamus and amygdala, the anatomically most prominent components of the forebrain limbic system, were thought to play a major role in controlling the ovulatory surge of LH, but rats in which the major connections between hippocampus and amygdala and the hypothalamus have been severed show regular estrous cycles (69). However, this does not exclude a possible synchronizing or inhibitory influence of the limbic system on the LHRH surge generator. The limbic system has long been thought to play a major role in the generation of emotions and certainly conveys olfactory signals that are so important for reproductive behavior. Studies on the turnover of central monoaminergic neurons, or on the effects of lesions or the administration of pharmacological agents, suggest that ascending noradrenergic (NA) projections to the hypothalamus from the midbrain and hindbrain may play an important role in triggering the LHRH surge by way of a mechanism that involves postsynaptic (α_1) adrenoreceptors (70–74; also see below).

The potent effects of visual and auditory stimuli on ovulation could be mediated by the multisynaptic pathways that link the neocortex of the brain with the hypothalamus (75). Light, in addition to affecting ovulation by way of the multisynaptic connections between the visual cortex and the hypothalamus, could affect ovulation by a direct pathway

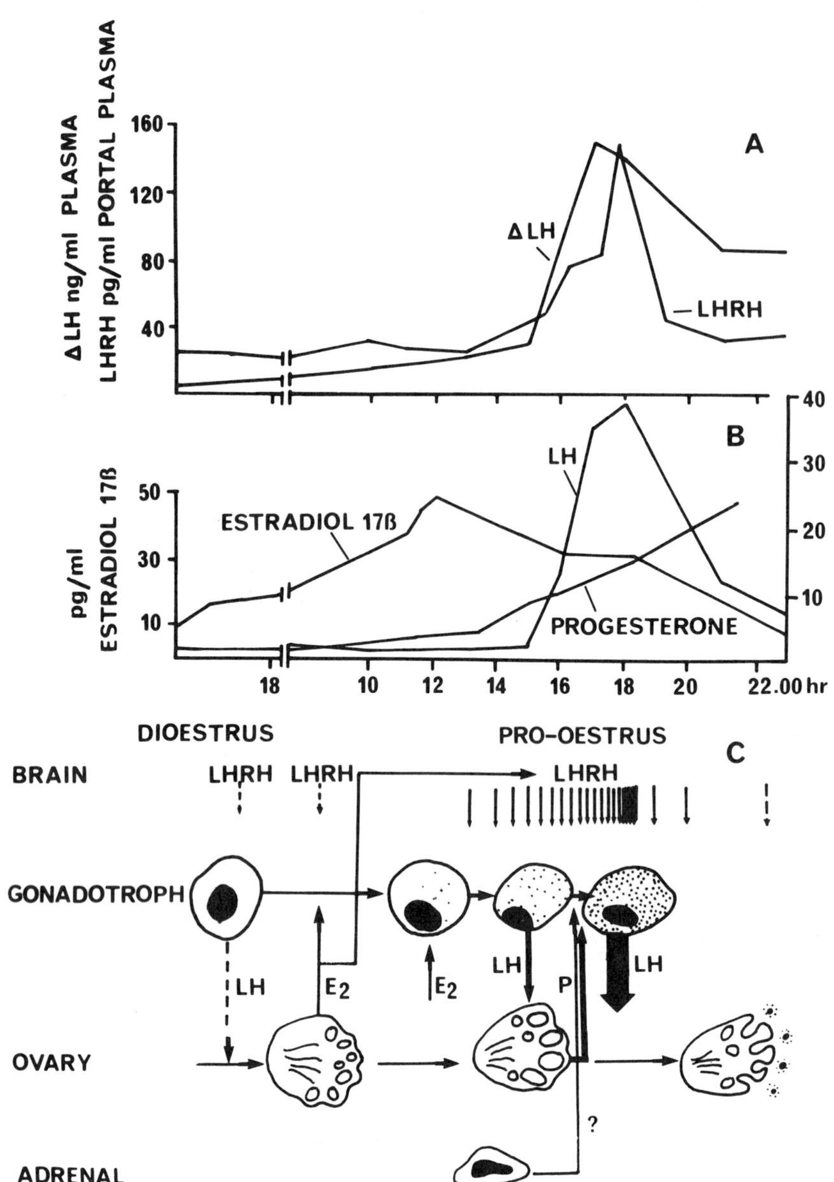

FIG. 5. Cascade of events leading to the spontaneous ovulatory surge in the rat. **A:** Changes in pituitary responsiveness (curve labeled ΔLH) and mean concentrations of luteinizing-hormone-releasing hormone (LHRH) in hypophysial portal plasma during diestrus and proestrus. ΔLH: Mean maximal increments in peripheral plasma LH after intravenous injection of 50 ng LHRH/100 g body weight. **B:** Mean concentrations of estradiol-17β, LH, and progesterone during diestrus and proestrus. **C:** Schematic diagram which shows that the increase in the plasma concentrations of estradiol-17β (the ovarian signal) increases the responsiveness of the pituitary gonadotropes (as indicated by increased stippling) to LHRH and also triggers the surge of LHRH. Pituitary responsiveness to LHRH is further increased by progesterone secreted from the ovary in response to the LH released during the early part of the LH surge and by the priming effect of LHRH. The priming effect of LHRH coordinates the surge of LHRH with increasing pituitary responsiveness so that the two events reach a peak at the same time. The conditions are thereby made optimal for a massive surge of LH. This cascade, which represents a form of positive feedback, is terminated by the rupture of the ovarian follicles (ovulation). For source of data see ref. 23.

that links the retina with the suprachiasmatic nuclei, as well as by another multisynaptic pathway, which involves the retina, the suprachiasmatic nuclei, the superior cervical ganglia, and the pineal gland. The latter pathway is especially important in species such as the hamster, vole, and sheep, in which the reproductive cycle is under photoperiodic control (76–81).

The pineal gland plays a particularly fascinating role in the wallaby, in which reproduction is controlled by a seasonal mechanism, which involves the retinal-superior cervical ganglion-pineal pathway, as well as by a lactational mechanism (82). Although the pineal contains several putative neurotransmitters such as vasotocin, it is generally thought that the inhibitory effects of increased pineal activity (which occurs in the dark) on the hypothalamic pituitary gonadal system are mediated by its major secretory product, melatonin (81,83,84). The evidence for a major role of the pineal-melatonin system in the adult rat is not compelling, but recent studies suggest that melatonin may play a role in the timing of sexual maturation in the rat (83). Similarly, melatonin has been implicated in the onset of puberty in humans on the basis of the measurement of melatonin concentrations in peripheral plasma (85). Studies on dispersed pituitary cells from prepubertal female rats have shown that melatonin can inhibit LH release induced by LHRH or Ca^{2+} ionophores but not by K^+ (86).

Site of Action of Estrogen in Triggering the LHRH Surge

Evidence against a direct action on LHRH neurons. The site of action of estrogen in triggering the surge of LHRH has not been determined. Recent studies in which LHRH

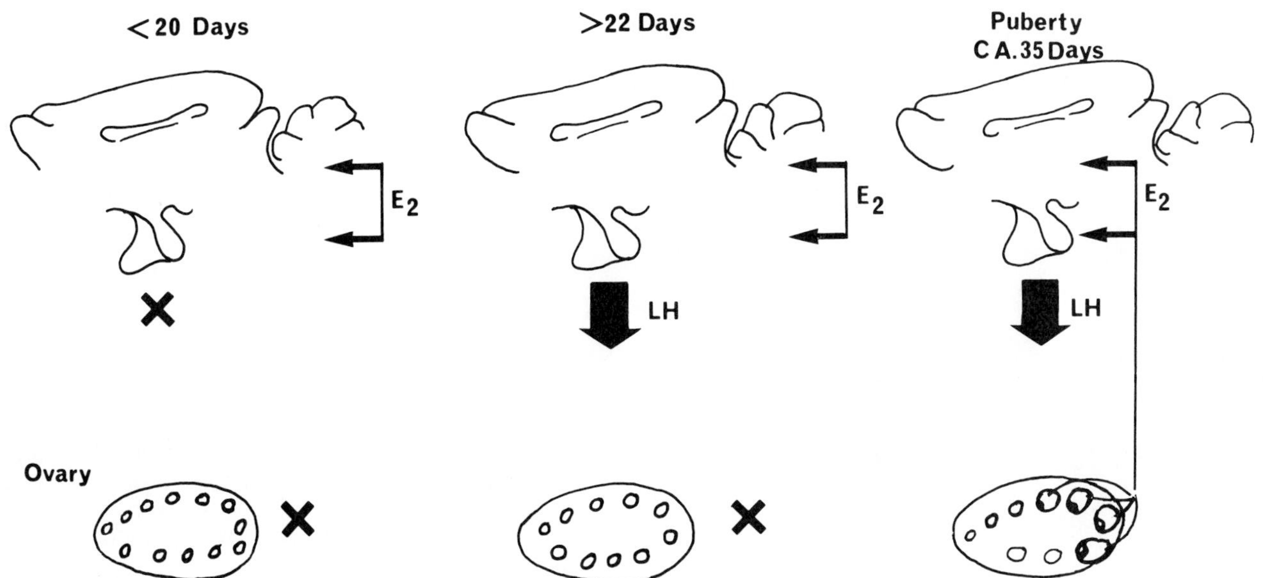

FIG. 6. Schematic diagram to show the ontogeny of the positive-feedback system leading to the first pubertal surge of luteinizing hormone (LH) in the rat. Before the 20th postnatal day the hypothalamic-pituitary system is not responsive to estradiol-17β (E_2). After 22 days of life the hypothalamic-pituitary system becomes responsive to the stimulating effects of E_2, but the enzymatic mechanisms necessary to produce estrogen have not yet developed in the ovary. With time and under the influence of "basal" (probably pulsatile) gonadotropin levels, the first batch of ovarian follicles grow and at the same time develop the capacity to synthesize and secrete E_2 in the form of a surge which then triggers the surge of LH. A similar mechanism probably operates in the human but takes about 12 yr to develop. In humans (and nonhuman primates) the hypothalamic-pituitary system is active during the first 4 yr of life and then becomes refractory before the developmental changes that lead to puberty (25,53).

neurons were identified by immunocytochemistry and nuclear receptors for estrogen were identified by autoradiography showed that in the rat hypothalamus only 1 of 435 LHRH neurons contained estrogen receptors (87). Observations in normal intact animals as well as in ovariectomized rats have shown that estrogen takes about 26 to 28 hr to trigger the surges of LHRH and LH (23,48,58), a period of time that would be more than sufficient for RNA and protein synthesis (88,89) and structural changes to occur in neurons and anterior pituitary cells. However, the fact that few, if any, LHRH neurons have estrogen receptors, taken together with other data, suggests that estrogen does not have a direct action on LHRH neurons, but rather triggers the LHRH surge by an action on other types of neurons that terminate on, and affect the activity of, LHRH neurons.

Possible actions through monoaminergic and opioid neurons. It has been known for several decades that gonadotropin secretion is stimulated by adrenaline (A) and NA, and possibly acetylcholine (2,90,91), and inhibited by morphine (91,92) and possibly dopamine (DA) (93). The hypothalamic monoaminergic and opioid neuronal cell bodies and processes have been traced by fluorescence histochemistry and immunocytochemistry, and a picture has emerged of the neurons that could conceivably interact with LHRH neurons and thereby mediate the effects of estrogen and other steroids (71–74,93). Most NA and A nerve terminals in the hypothalamus are derived from ascending projections from nuclei in the midbrain and hindbrain. The most prominent group of DA neurons are the tuberoinfundibular group (the so-called TIDA neurons), which have their cell bodies in the arcuate and ventromedial nuclei (Fig. 9) and project to the primary plexus of hypophysial portal vessels, where they form close axo-axonic relationships with the terminals of LHRH neurons. Although there are no structures that resemble classical synapses between the LHRH and TIDA terminals, it is generally assumed that DA released at TIDA terminals could inhibit LHRH release by a direct action on LHRH terminals (an action comparable to presynaptic inhibition in other parts of the CNS). Other DA nerve terminals in the hypothalamus which could also influence the activity of LHRH neurons are derived from cell groups in the zona incerta as well as the midbrain and hindbrain (94).

Enkephalin and endorphin-containing neurons are situated in several hypothalamic nuclei, but predominate in the region of the arcuate nucleus (95–97). As in the case of DA neurons, it is conceivable that the endorphin-containing neurons in the arcuate nucleus could influence LHRH release by an axo-axonic mechanism as well as by way of their terminals on the soma and/or dendrites of the LHRH neurons (72,73).

The hypothalamic nuclei, and, in particular, the suprachiasmatic nuclei, both of which are the most important components of the central circadian pacemaker system (98), also receive a dense innervation from serotonergic (5-HT)

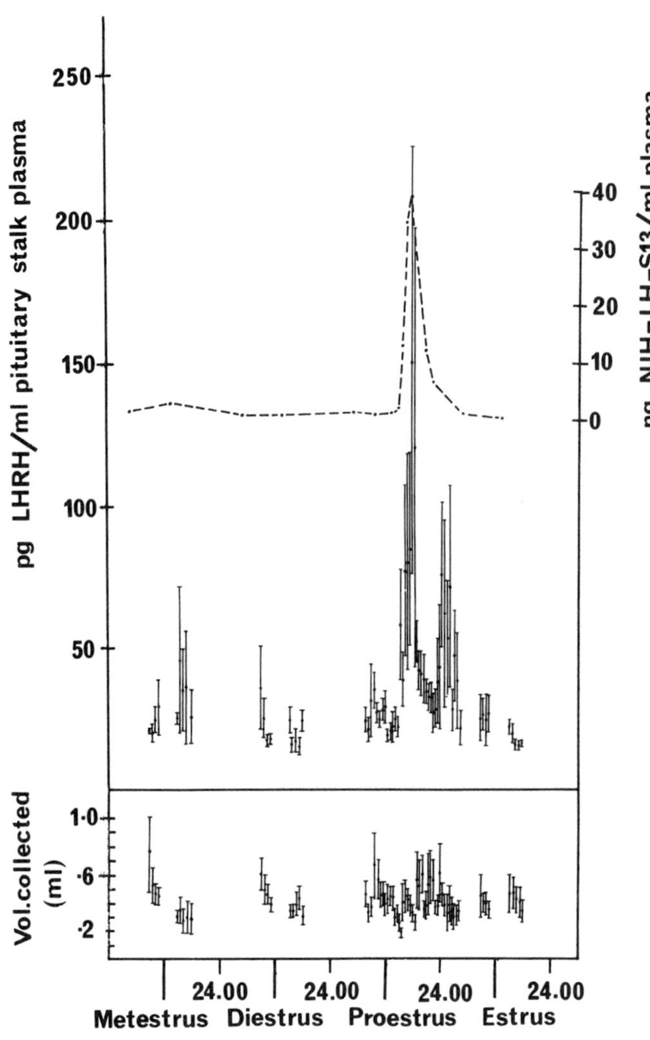

FIG. 7. Mean (± SEM) concentrations of LHRH (**top panel**) and volumes (**bottom panel**) of 30-min collections of pituitary stalk blood. Most means are based on five to 15 samples; a few are based on three to four samples. (-·-) Mean concentrations of plasma LH. (From ref. 44.)

neurons located in the midbrain. As assessed by the effects of blocking 5-HT synthesis with parachlorophenylalanine (PCPA), the 5-HT neurons play an important role in maintaining the circadian rhythm of LH release that occurs in long-term ovariectomized rats treated with estrogen, presumably by virtue of the 5-HT modulation of the suprachiasmatic nuclei (99). Blockade of 5-HT synthesis by administration of PCPA also blocks the spontaneous ovulatory surge of LH, but because manipulation of 5-HT also affects ovarian blood flow and the secretion of estradiol, it is not clear whether central 5-HT neurons play a crucial role in triggering the LHRH surge or whether some of the effects of manipulating 5-HT are due to interference with the stimulatory surge of estradiol (99). It is now also known that, in addition to blocking 5-HT synthesis, PCPA affects synthesis and turnover of the other monoamines (100).

Thus, the present data suggest that LHRH release is stimulated by central NA (and possibly A) mechanisms and is inhibited by central opioid and DA mechanisms; these data also suggest that the stimulatory effect of estrogen on LHRH release could be brought about by stimulation of the facilitatory mechanisms, inhibition of the inhibitory mechanisms, or both. Recent pharmacological studies suggest that there may be important interactions between opioid and NA neurons in producing the LHRH surge (101,102). Estrogen and other steroids are known to exert potent effects on both the production of enzymes, by way of genomic mechanisms, and the activity of enzymes by allosteric mechanisms. An action of estrogen on the synthesis and/or activity of the enzymes responsible for synthesizing and/or degrading monoamines and peptides could underlie the mechanism by which estrogen triggers the LHRH surge. This scheme is outlined diagrammatically in Fig. 10, which, it must be stressed, is necessarily oversimplified and does not take account of the facts that other transmitters [such as γ-aminobutyric acid (103,104) or neurotensin], substance P, and other neuropeptides (97,105–107) may influence the activity of LHRH neurons and/or the gonadotropes. Furthermore, lesions of the ascending NA systems do not lead to permanent loss of estrous cycles (108,109). However, the effects of such lesion studies do not exclude the importance of NA in stimulating LHRH release because: (a) about 20%

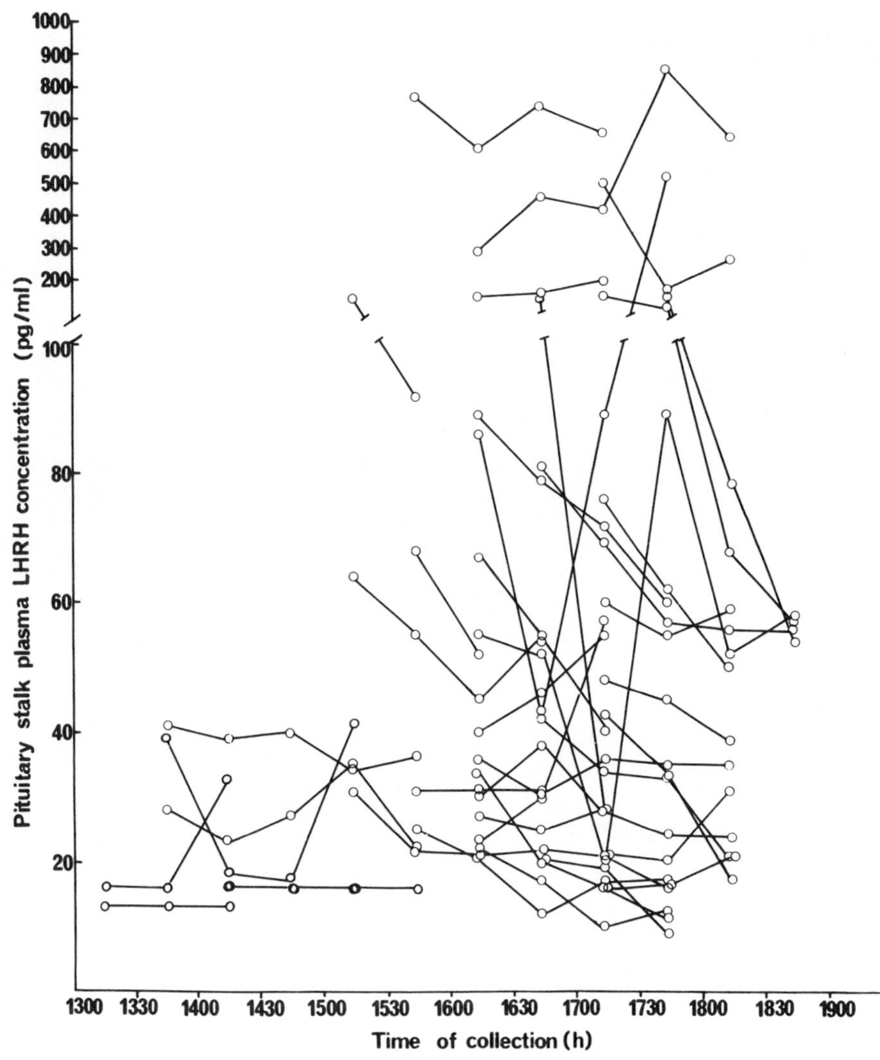

FIG. 8. Concentrations of LHRH in hypophysial portal plasma in individual rats anesthetized with Althesin on the day of proestrus. The figure illustrates that the large variations around the mean in Fig. 7 are due to individual variations in the timing and magnitude of the proestrous LHRH surge. Nonetheless, when considered in the context of 96 hr (the cycle length in the animals used for this study), a between-animal variation of onset of the LHRH surge of only about 2 hr shows remarkable precision. (From ref. 49.)

NA remained in the median eminence after the lesion (108); (b) the lesions may lead to NA supersensitivity, and, as a consequence, the NA remaining in the hypothalamus might be sufficient to drive the system; and (c) the lesions may have also destroyed systems antagonistic to the facilitatory actions of the ascending NA system and thereby counterbalanced the effect of the NA lesion.

Electrophysiological correlates. In spite of several decades of study, no clear picture has emerged with regard to the electrophysiological correlates of the action of steroids in triggering the LHRH surge. In the rat, estrogen enhances spontaneous or evoked firing of hypothalamic units (110–112), and on the afternoon of proestrus an increase in single-unit activity has been reported in various hypothalamic nuclei (110,111). As assessed by the release of LHRH into hypophysial portal vessel blood, estrogen also increases the responsiveness of the preoptic-LHRH release system to electrical stimulation (21,112). In ovariectomized rhesus monkeys primed with estrogen, progesterone increased the firing rate of units in the ventral hypothalamus and concomitantly induced a surge of LH (113). Yeoman and Terasawa (113) speculate that the increased firing occurred in "interneurons" and that this is consistent with early studies in the rat (114) which showed that increased firing in the preoptic-anterior hypothalamic region on the afternoon of proestrus occurred only in units that were not antidromically identified to project to the medial basal hypothalamus. Estrogen also increases the firing of (a) units which are within the hypothalamus, but which may be concerned with mating behavior rather than the LH surge (115), and (b) units in other areas remote from the hypothalamus, such as the neostriatum (116). These apparently disparate actions of estrogen could be linked in that it is conceivable that the action of estrogen on neurons ("interneurons") that modulate the activity of LHRH neurons, neurons of the ventromedial nucleus that stimulate mating behavior, and neurons of the neostriatum involved in motor behavior could underlie the proestrous surge of LHRH, mating, and increased motor activity, all of which occurs in the 12 hr between the afternoon of proestrus and the early morning of estrus. However, sophisticated

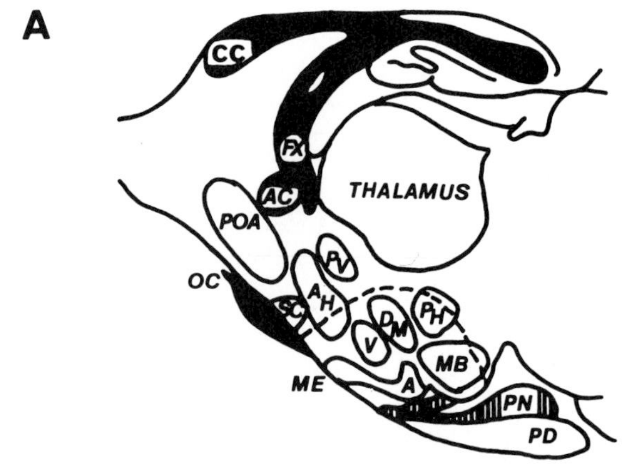

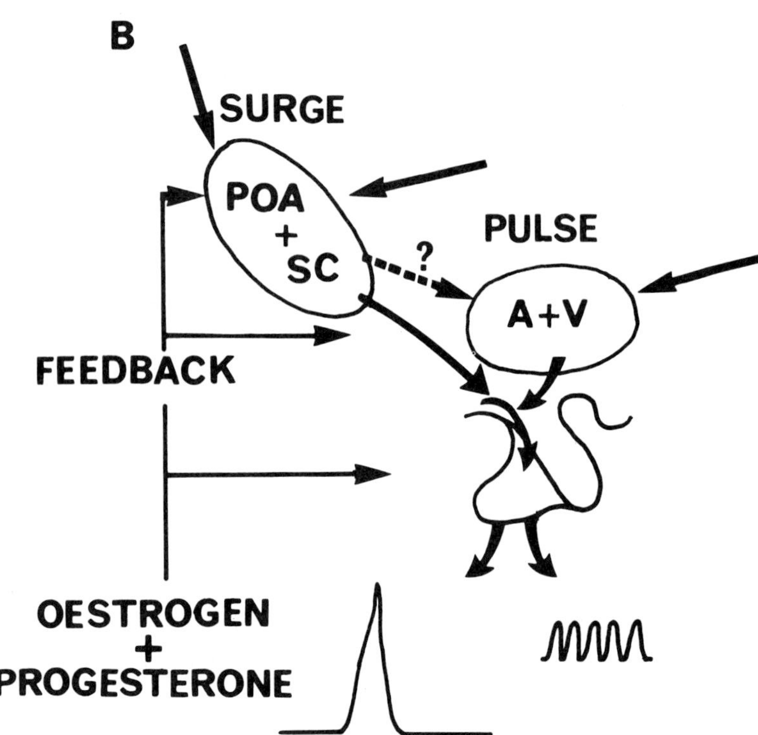

FIG. 9. A: Schematic diagram of a sagittal section of the rat brain and pituitary gland showing the main hypothalamic nuclei. The medial basal hypothalamus is enclosed by the dashed line. **B:** Schematic diagram of the LH surge and pulse generators. The LH surge generator appears to be located in the region of the preoptic and suprachiasmatic nuclei, whereas the pulse generator is thought to be in the medial basal hypothalamus. Both generators are influenced by neurons extrinsic and intrinsic to the hypothalamus. It is not clear whether and, if so, how the generators are linked. Arrows indicate controlled inputs from exhypothalamic regions of the central nervous system and the positive- and negative-feedback systems. The important abbreviations are: POA, preoptic area; SC, suprachiasmatic nuclei; AC, anterior commissure; CC, corpus callosum; FX, fornix; A, arcuate nuclei; V, ventromedial hypothalamic nucleus; ME, median eminence; OC, optic chiasm; PD, pars distalis of the pituitary gland; PN, pars nervosa of the pituitary gland.

and meaningful interpretation of the effects of estrogen on LHRH release will not be possible until the detailed circuitry of the LHRH surge generator has been determined.

Changes in Pituitary Responsiveness to LH-Releasing Hormone

Pituitary responsiveness to LHRH increases significantly before and during the spontaneous LH surge in women, monkeys, sheep, hamsters, and rats (23,48; Fig. 11). Experimental studies show that the spontaneous preovulatory surge of LHRH (above) would be far too small to produce the ovulatory surge of LH without the massive increase in pituitary responsiveness to LHRH which precedes ovulation (117; Fig. 12). In women, as in rats, the increase occurs in two phases: gradually during the 2 days before the midcycle LH surge, and then abruptly (10-fold) on the day of the surge (118), resulting in an overall increase of about 50-fold between the early follicular and the ovulatory phases in women and diestrus and proestrus in rats. In both humans and rats, the preovulatory increase in the plasma estradiol concentration is essential for initiating and maintaining the increase in pituitary responsiveness to LHRH. Estradiol, at its peak physiological concentration, takes about 8 to 12 hr to enhance responsiveness; in the first few hours the effect of estradiol is inhibitory (119–121). The abrupt rise in re-

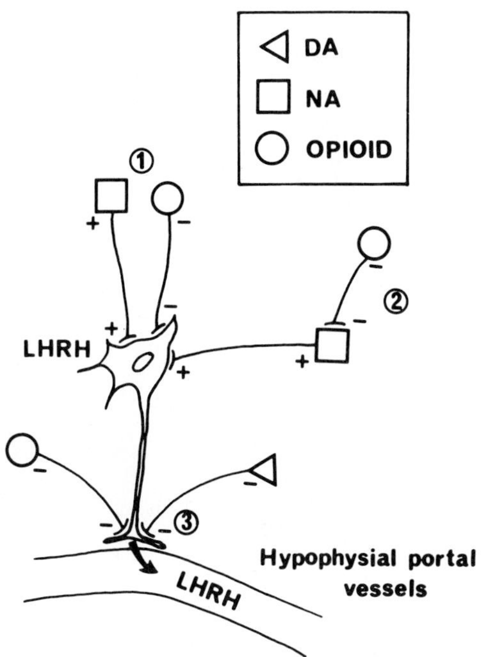

FIG. 10. Schematic diagram of how estrogen could trigger the LHRH surge. It is unlikely that estrogen has a direct effect on LHRH neurons, since the latter have no estrogen receptors (87). The steroid probably triggers the LHRH surge by acting on neurons that terminate on, and affect the activity of, LHRH neurons. The plus and minus signs indicate stimulatory and inhibitory effects, respectively, of estrogen at the cell bodies and of the neurons at synapses or points of contact. Three of many different possible mechanisms are shown. Scheme 1 shows that estrogen could stimulate noradrenergic (NA) neurons that stimulate LHRH neurons, or could inhibit opioid neurons that inhibit LHRH neurons. Scheme 2 shows that estrogen could inhibit opioid neurons that could inhibit NA neurons: This disinhibition of NA neurons would effect an increase in the firing of LHRH neurons. Scheme 3 shows that estrogen could inhibit the inhibitory actions of dopaminergic (DA) and opioid neurons whose terminals in the median eminence may be juxtaposed to, and thereby have a presynaptic effect on, LHRH neurons. It must be stressed that this diagram is highly oversimplified and does not take into account the many other types of neurons that may influence LHRH release (see text) or the other types of circuits by which the activity of LHRH neurons could be altered.

sponsiveness at the time of the LH surge is caused by the priming effect of LHRH [i.e., the capacity of LHRH to increase (by direct action) the responsiveness of the gonadotropes (122–124)] and by the increase in plasma progesterone concentration that accompanies the LH surge (125,126). Progesterone also augments the effect of estradiol in women (118,123), but because of the timing of increased progesterone secretion it is not certain whether this plays a major role in the midcycle LH surge (127). Steroids do not mediate the priming effect of LHRH, but they do affect significantly the magnitude of the effect (122). Consequently, the response to the second of two injections of LHRH is highest at the proestrus in rats (122) and at the midcycle and the midluteal phase in humans (123).

In rats, because of increased adrenal secretion, the plasma progesterone concentration rises before the beginning of the LH surge (Fig. 4). However, though important for ensuring full sexual receptivity, the early increase in plasma progesterone is not essential for the occurrence of the LH surge (128). The limited surveys of steroids other than estradiol and progesterone have shown that progesterone is more potent than any of its major metabolites in facilitating pituitary responsiveness and that androgens reduce the LH response, but have either no, or only a slight, facilitatory effect on the FSH response to LHRH (126,129).

The mechanism by which steroids increase pituitary responsiveness to LHRH is not clear. During the 24 hr before the LH surge there is an increase in pituitary LH content (130), and this is compatible with the possibility that estrogen may stimulate LH synthesis and thereby increase the amount of LH available for release. However, steroids also alter the sensitivity of the gonadotropes, as shown by the marked increase in the response to LHRH which occurs in the absence of a significant change in pituitary LH content in long-term ovariectomized rats treated with estrogen and progesterone (131).

The nuclear and total concentrations of estradiol-receptor complexes in the pituitary are greater at proestrus than at other times of the cycle (132), and progesterone receptors in the pituitary are estrogen dependent (133). Studies using dispersed rat pituitary cells, or rats in which the pituitary stalk has been cut, show that estrogen and progesterone can facilitate pituitary responsiveness by a direct action on the gonadotropes (129,134,135). Estradiol also stimulates gonadotropin release in rhesus monkeys bearing lesions of the arcuate nuclei and infused intermittently with LHRH (136). However, there are several facts which suggest that at least part of estradiol's action in increasing pituitary responsiveness to LHRH may depend upon "normal" or increased concentrations of LHRH in hypophysial portal blood, which increase pituitary responsiveness by way of the priming effect of LHRH. These facts are: (a) Estradiol can stimulate LHRH release in the rat (58) and rhesus monkey (57); (b) the fall in portal LHRH concentrations that occurs after ovariectomy on diestrus can be prevented by implanting an estradiol-containing capsule (137); (c) sodium pentobarbitone administration, which blocks LHRH release into portal blood, blocked the facilitatory action of estradiol on the LH response to LHRH (119); and (d) estradiol implants in the preoptic area were more effective than estradiol implants in the median eminence [from which estrogen would diffuse mainly to the anterior pituitary gland (138)] in inducing an LH surge in the rat (139). Early studies (126,140) showed that there was a marked sex difference in the effect of estrogen on the LH response to LHRH. This was initially puzzling, since there is good evidence that, in the rat, sexual differentiation of the hypothalamic-pituitary-ovarian system

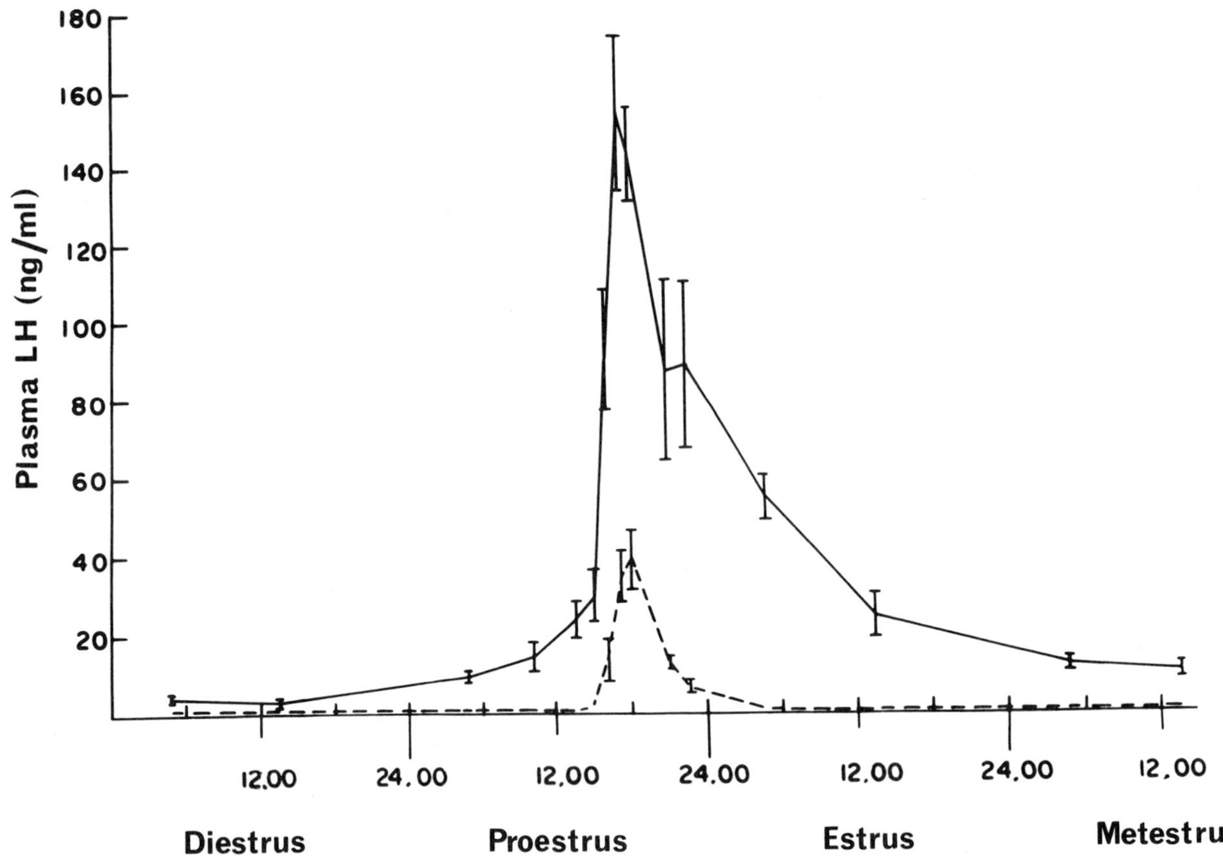

FIG. 11. Changes in pituitary responsiveness to LHRH during the estrous cycle of the rat. The figure shows the mean (± SEM) preinjection concentrations (---) and mean maximal increments (—) in plasma LH concentrations (ng NIH-LH-S13/ml) in animals anesthetized with sodium pentobarbitone 30–60 min before the injection of 50 ng LHRH/100 g body weight at different stages of the estrous cycle. (From ref. 143.)

is due to changes predominantly in the brain (127,141,142). However, if at least part of the action of estrogen in increasing pituitary responsiveness to LHRH requires normal function of the hypothalamic LHRH system, this could explain why there is a marked sex difference in the effect of estrogen on pituitary responsiveness to LHRH.

The Priming Effect of LHRH

Two observations raised the possibility that LHRH increases the responsiveness of the pituitary gland to itself, the priming effect of LHRH (122). First, studies in humans and the rat (122,143) showed that there was a positive correlation between the basal plasma concentrations of LH and the magnitude of the increment in plasma LH concentrations in response to LHRH. Second, the magnitude of the LH response to LHRH in proestrous rats could be reduced significantly by injecting sodium pentobarbitone, which is known to block LH release by blocking the release of LHRH (44,49,143). *In vivo* studies showed that in proestrous rats the magnitude of the LH response to the second of two injections of LHRH separated by various time intervals was always significantly greater than the response to the first LHRH injection; these studies also showed that the difference between the first and second response was greatest when the two injections were separated by an interval of 60 min (Fig. 13). Steroids affect the magnitude but do not mediate the priming effect of LHRH (122,144). The priming effect of LHRH could also be elicited by continuous infusions of LHRH in female, but not male, rats, or by applying two short electrical stimuli to the preoptic area of the brain, which showed that endogenous LHRH was as effective as exogenous LHRH in eliciting the priming effect (145).

A point that is often overlooked is that low levels of LHRH secreted continuously or in the form of pulses can also prime the anterior pituitary gland (Fig. 14). This was shown in experiments on rats in which pulses of LHRH were administered every 15 min (145). The dose of each pulse by itself was far too small to produce a detectable increase in the plasma concentration of LH, but after a period of about 60 min this regimen produced a fairly sudden and massive surge of LH (145,146). Similarly, the continuous infusion of small doses of LHRH, far too low to produce a detectable increase in plasma LH or LHRH, nonetheless primed the anterior pituitary gland so that a subsequent

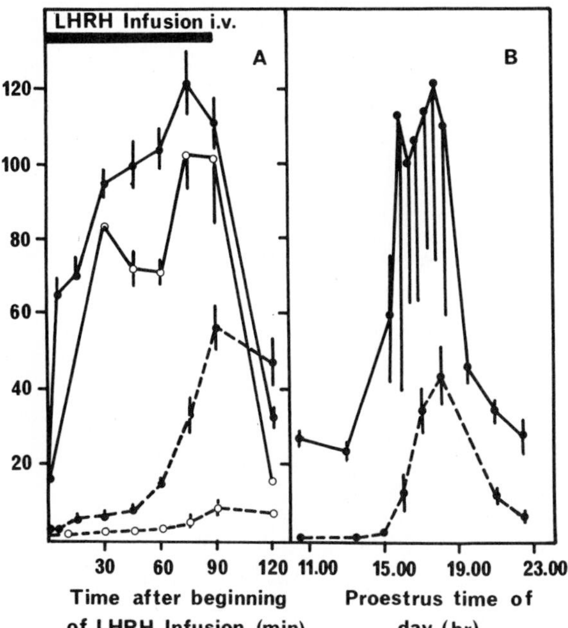

FIG. 12. Demonstration that the spontaneous surge of LHRH is too small to produce a spontaneous surge of LH except on proestrus, when the responsiveness of the anterior pituitary gland is 20 to 50 times greater than on diestrus. Units on the ordinate are nanograms for LH and picograms for LHRH per ml plasma. **A:** The mean (± SEM) peripheral plasma concentrations of LH (ng NIH-LH-S18) (---) and LHRH (—) in either proestrous (●; n = 11) or diestrous (○; n = 5) rats that were infused intravenously with synthetic LHRH at a rate of 0.167 ng/100 g/min for a period of 90 min after anesthesia with sodium pentobarbitone at 13.30 hr (1:30 p.m.). The data were obtained from ref. 145. **B:** The mean (± SEM) concentrations of LHRH in hypophysial portal plasma (—; n = 9–52) and LH (NIH-LH-S13) in peripheral plasma (---; n = 6–9) during the day of proestrus. The concentrations of LHRH are from refs. 44 and 49, and the LH concentrations are from ref. 143.

larger pulse of LHRH resulted in a surge of LH with a magnitude equivalent to that of the spontaneous LH surge (137). It is important to bear this in mind in terms of understanding the hypothalamic actions of estrogen (see above) and how relatively small surges or pulses of LHRH could conceivably produce an ovulatory surge of LH. Although the spontaneous LH surge in the rhesus monkey may be less dependent than the LH surge in the rat on the integrity of the hypothalamic connections (147,148), it must be stressed that in the rat, as in the rhesus monkey, the surge of LH is not dependent upon a massive surge of LHRH. Pulses of LHRH are sufficient to produce an ovulatory surge of LH in both species (Fig. 14). This does not mean that an LHRH surge does not normally occur: The physiological significance of the LHRH surge in the rat is probably that it serves to ensure that the LH surge occurs at a relatively precise time in relationship to the light-dark periods of the environment and sleep-wake cycle of the animal (Figs. 4,5,7, and 8).

So far, no other neuropeptide or nonpeptide transmitter has been shown to exert a priming effect on pituitary or other types of effector cells. Why LHRH has the apparently unique capacity to increase the responsiveness of its effector cells to itself is not clear, but perhaps it is related to the fact that apart from the uterine contraction-oxytocin release system that operates during parturition, the LH surge is the only endocrine positive-feedback system that is known to occur under physiological conditions.

The mechanism of the priming effect of LHRH. The mechanism of the priming effect has been studied *in vitro* mainly using short-term incubation of hemipituitary glands (149,150). The results of these studies and the similar studies carried out by other groups (151,152) revealed major differences between the priming and the releasing action of LHRH, which are summarized in Table 1. Several experiments showed that the new protein synthesized as part of LHRH priming (Table 1, g) is not gonadotropin (150), but rather a protein with a molecular weight (MW) of about 69,000 (153). Whether this new protein is related to a hypothalamic, estrogen-stimulated 70,000-MW protein, postulated to be of the heat shade type (269), or to the LHRH-stimulated synthesis of an 87,000-MW protein in dispersed pituitary cells (154) remains to be established. In addition to new protein synthesis, LHRH priming is associated with changes in the isoelectric points of two other proteins, possibly due to phosphorylation (153). While normal concentrations of extracellular Ca^{2+} are not essential for LHRH priming, experiments with cold conditions suggested that the priming effect involves the release of Ca^{2+} from endoplasmic reticulum (153). Quantitative ultrastructural studies showed that LHRH priming is associated with a change in orientation and length of the microfilaments (intracellular contractile elements) and a significant migration of secretory granules of the gonadotropes to a "marginal" zone, close to the plasmalemma, from which the granules can easily be released as a consequence of a second exposure to a secretagogue such as K^+ depolarization, Ca^{2+} ionophores, or LHRH itself (155). This migration of secretory granules (Fig. 15), due presumably to changes in the contractile elements of the cell, probably explains the increase in the readily releasable pool of LH that occurs before and during the spontaneous ovulatory LH surge (156; Fig. 16).

The Role of LHRH Receptors

The role of LHRH receptors in the changes in pituitary responsiveness to LHRH that occur around the time of the LH surge remains unclear. In the intact rat the numbers of pituitary LHRH receptors increase on the evening of diestrus and are maintained until just before the LH surge on proestrus, at which time they fall (157–159). Whatever the mechanism of the decline in LHRH receptor number, which was also found to accompany the LH surge induced by estrogen in juvenile female rats (160), these data suggest that although an increase in LHRH receptors may contribute to the early increase in pituitary responsiveness to LHRH, the

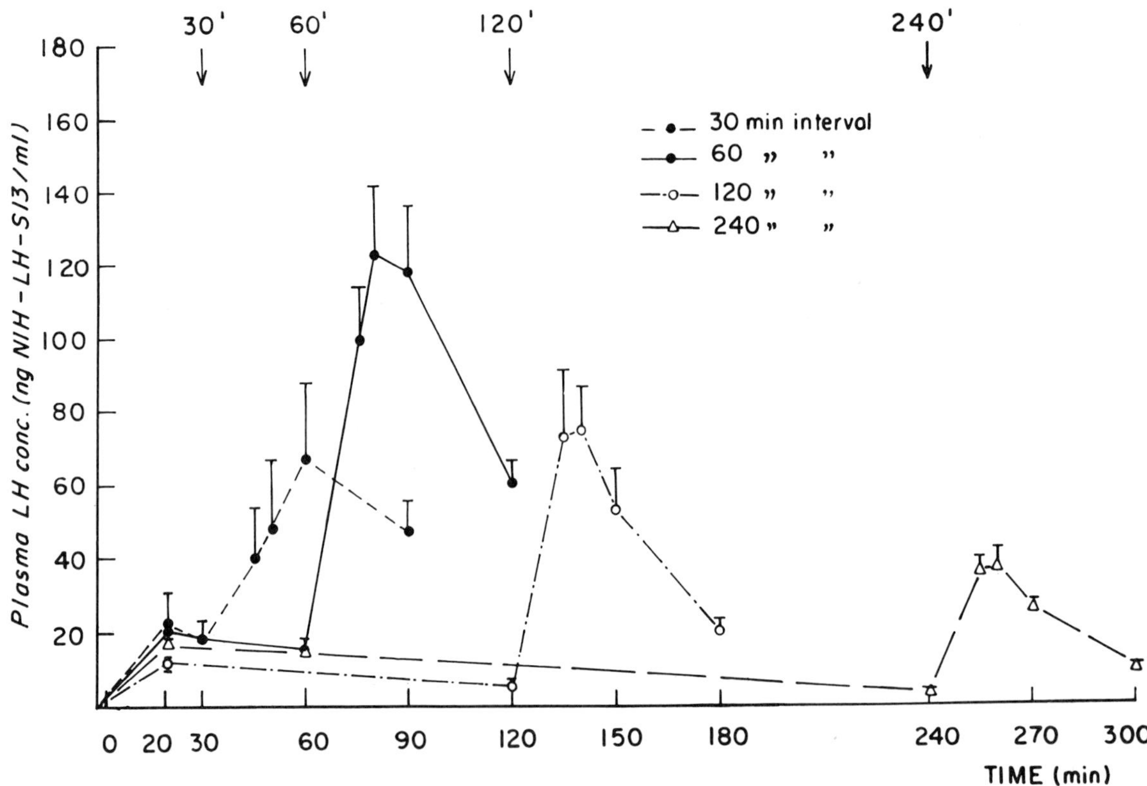

FIG. 13. The priming effect of LHRH in the rat. Mean (± SEM) plasma LH concentrations (ng NIH-LH-S13/ml) after two successive intravenous injections of 50 ng LHRH/100 g body weight. The first dose of LHRH was injected 30–60 min after the administration of sodium pentobarbitone at 13.30 hr (1:30 p.m.) of proestrus; the second dose of LHRH was injected either 30, 60, 120, or 240 min after the first. (From ref. 122.)

massive increase in responsiveness that occurs during the LH surge is not dependent upon an increase in the number of LHRH receptors. The link between gonadotropin secretion and the number of LHRH receptors is tighter in gonadectomized rats, in which there is an increase both in gonadotropin secretion and LHRH receptor number (161). Experimental studies suggest that the increase in LHRH receptor number in gonadectomized rats is brought about by increased LHRH release into hypophysial portal vessel blood (161) (so-called "up-regulation" of receptors). Gonadectomy in mice, however, results in a 50% decrease in pituitary LHRH receptors, and so the finding in gonadectomized rats cannot be adopted as a universal principle (162). Indeed, for reasons reviewed by Smith and Ojeda (160), our understanding of the factors that determine the number of LHRH-binding sites which are presumed to be receptors is far from complete.

It has long been known that for many ligands only a relatively small proportion of receptors is required for a maximum biological response [concept of "spare receptors" (163)], and, therefore, it is not surprising that in intact animals there is no tight association between gonadotropin secretion, LHRH release, and pituitary responsiveness to LHRH. The changes in pituitary responsiveness that occur during the estrous cycle can be elicited in dispersed pituitary cells by K^+ depolarization equally as well as by a pulse of LHRH (164), and this suggests that as in the case of LHRH priming (see above), changes in the amount of LH available for release [due to margination of the secretory granules in the gonadotropes (155)] and in the "release" apparatus itself may be more important than receptor number in determining the responsiveness of the anterior pituitary gland to LHRH.

THE FSH SURGE AND THE APPARENT DISSOCIATION BETWEEN LH AND FSH SECRETION

In women, the midcycle surge of LH is usually accompanied by a surge of FSH, but the relative magnitude of the FSH surge and its consistency and precision are much less than that of the LH surge. In the rat, the peak of the spontaneous FSH surge occurs about 11 hr after the spontaneous proestrous LH surge (143,165), and dissociation between LH and FSH secretion also occurs during development (166–168) and experimental manipulation of sex steroids (125,169,170). Clear-cut dissociation between LH and FSH secretion in women also occurs during the follicular phase of the menstrual cycle and during pregnancy (171,172), as well as after the administration of estradiol (173).

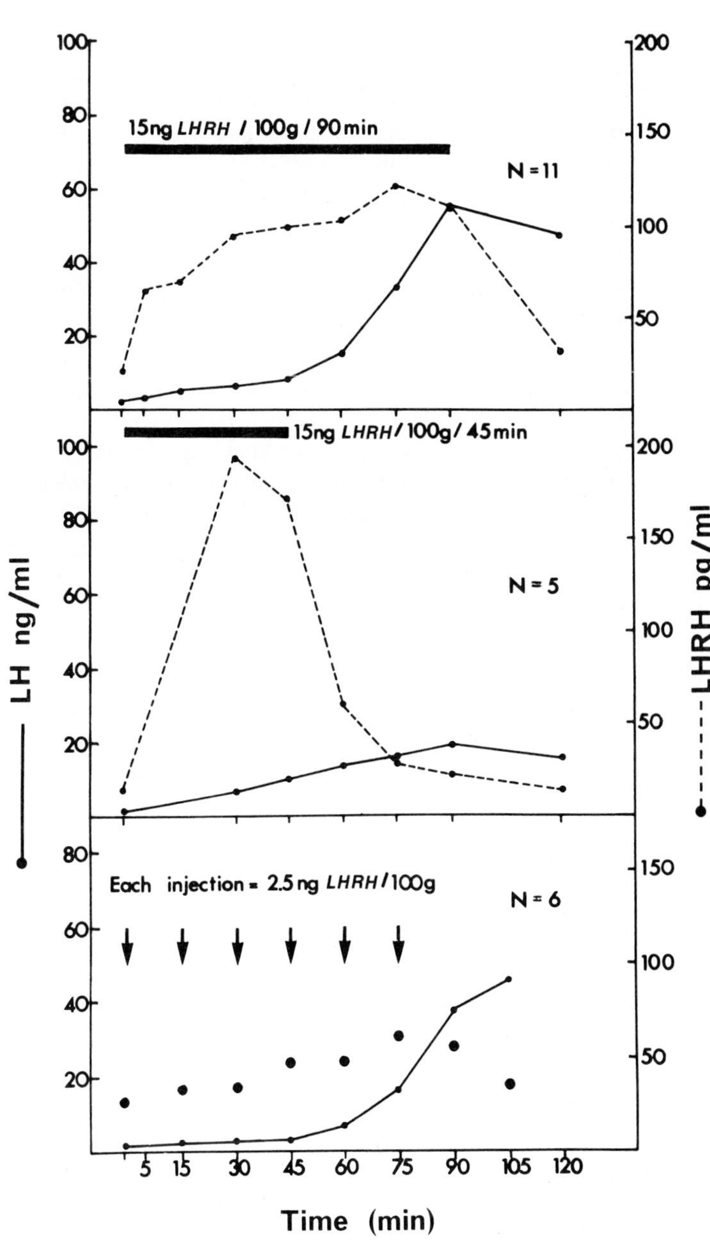

FIG. 14. Demonstration of the fact that exposure of the rat pituitary gland *(in vivo)* to low continuous concentrations of LHRH or to small pulses of LHRH can result in a surge of LH which is similar in magnitude to the spontaneous ovulatory surge of LH. Mean plasma LH concentrations are shown before and during either continuous intravenous infusions **(top panel)** or multiple small intravenous injections of LHRH **(bottom panel).** Note that the effect is time dependent in that infusion of the same total dose of LHRH **(middle panel)** for 45 rather than 90 min failed to produce a surge of LH. In the bottom panel the plots represent LHRH concentrations in plasma measured before, and 15 min after, each LHRH injection. (From ref. 146.)

TABLE 1. *Comparison of releasing and priming actions of LHRH in the female rat.*[a]

Action	Releasing	Priming
(a) Ontogenetic development	Early as day 5	Only after day 17[b]
(b) Can be repeated frequently	Yes	No (once only in 11-hr period)[c]
(c) Enhanced by estrogen	Yes	Yes
(d) Dependent on extracellular Ca^{2+}	Yes	No
(e) Mimicked by high extracellular K^{+}	Yes	No
(f) Mimicked by Ca^{2+} ionophores	Yes	No
(g) Dependent on protein synthesis	No	Yes
(h) Dependent on integrity of microfilaments	No	Yes
(i) Cyclic AMP acts as second messenger	No	No
(j) Elicited in dispersed cells	Yes	Not so far[d]

[a]Data based mainly on ref. 150.
[b]Ref. 144.
[c]Ref. 265.
[d]But has been demonstrated in cells obtained from bovine pituitary glands (266,267)

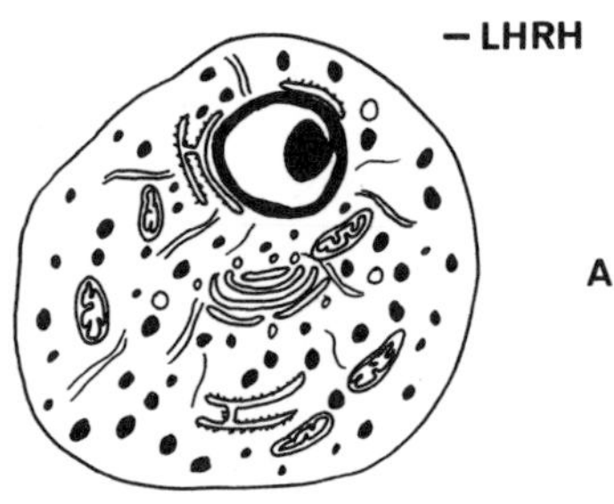

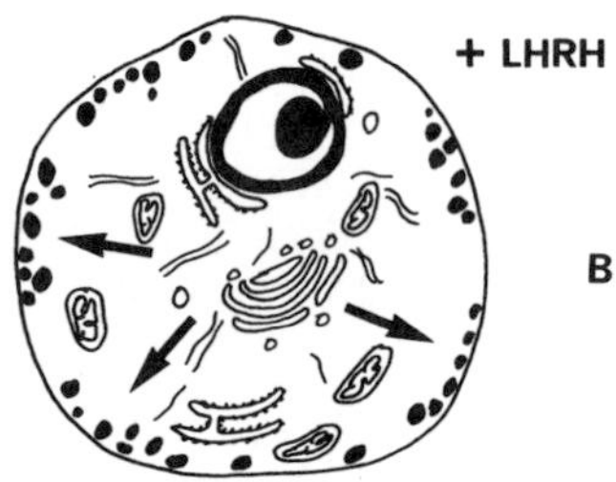

FIG. 15. Sketches of pituitary gonadotrophs as seen under the electron microscope (from ref. 155). **A:** Gonadotroph has not been exposed to LHRH. Note that the secretory granules are scattered randomly throughout the cytoplasm. **B:** Gonadotroph has been exposed to LHRH for 2 hr: The granules are fewer in number (presumably because of release) and have moved close to the plasmalemma. The movement of granules to the plasmalemma, which is probably due to the activation of contractile elements of the cell, is the basis for the priming effect of LHRH. That is, LHRH stimulates "margination" of the secretory granules so that much more gonadotropin is available for release when the cells are exposed to another pulse of LHRH or to another secretagogue such as K^+ depolarization.

Dissociation between LH and FSH could be due to three major factors. First, there may be a separate FSH-releasing hormone (FSH-RH). Experimental evidence for a separate FSH-RH comes from studies of the effects of hypothalamic lesions and stimulation (174,175). Early gel-filtration studies also suggested that hypothalamic FSH-releasing activity was distinct from LH-releasing activity, but this separate FSH-releasing activity was subsequently found to be due mainly to polyamines (176). Until there is firm biochemical proof for a distinct hypothalamic FSH-RH, it will generally be accepted that LHRH is a (if not "the") neuropeptide that stimulates FSH as well as LH secretion. Indeed, in the *hpg* mouse, LHRH would appear to be more potent in stimulating the synthesis of FSH than that of LH (177).

Secondly, steroids, inhibin, or other factors may differentially alter pituitary responsiveness to LHRH with respect to FSH, as compared with LH. Although such a mechanism might explain dissociation between the secretion of the two gonadotropins under some circumstances, it does not explain the dissociation between the LH and FSH surge in the rat, since the changes in the LH and FSH responses to exogenous and endogenous LHRH are coincident around the time of the ovulatory surge of LH.

Thirdly, dissociation between LH and FSH secretion may be due to differences between the degree to which the release of the two gonadotropins is dependent upon exposure of the pituitary gland to LHRH. Brown-Grant and Greig (178) showed, for example, that in the rat the spontaneous LH surge could be blocked immediately and completely by the injection of sodium pentobarbitone at any time during the rising phase of the surge, but, once established, the FSH surge was not interrupted by the injection of sodium pentobarbitone. In the human, it also appears that, once established, FSH release continues for much longer than LH release (179,180). These observations suggest that the secretion of LH, but not FSH, is dependent upon the minute-by-minute exposure of the pituitary gland to LHRH. Once FSH secretion is initiated by LHRH, it may continue to be secreted, perhaps autonomously, at least for several hours. Conceivably, termination of the FSH surge in the rat may be brought about by inhibin rather than by cessation of the LHRH surge, which is a major factor in the case of LH.

Further research is required to determine which of these three possibilities is correct.

WHY IS THERE NO SURGE OF LH IN THE MALE?

In the rodent the absence of an LH surge is because the male does not have an ovary; of equal importance is the fact that sexual differentiation of the brain, due presumably to neonatal exposure to androgen, results in an anatomical and/or functional change in the brain which leads to an absence, in the male, of a central LHRH surge apparatus that is sensitive to estrogen (127,141,142). In castrated men and rhesus monkeys, however, an LH surge can be evoked by estrogen (46,181), and this suggests that the absence of an LH surge in the primate is due mainly to the absence of an ovary that can secrete surges of estrogen, rather than to the absence of an estrogen-sensitive surge mechanism in the brain.

THE REFLEX-INDUCED GONADOTROPIN SURGE

Intuitively it might be thought that reflex ovulators would provide better models than spontaneous ovulators for studying the neural mechanisms involved in triggering the ovulatory gonadotropin surge. However, in spite of much extensive research, our understanding of the mechanism of the reflex gonadotropin surge induced by mating is significantly less than our understanding of the spontaneous surge. Many of the studies on reflex gonadotropin release have been carried out on rabbits, rats exposed to continuous illumination, and the vole, and here the data relating to these species will be briefly reviewed.

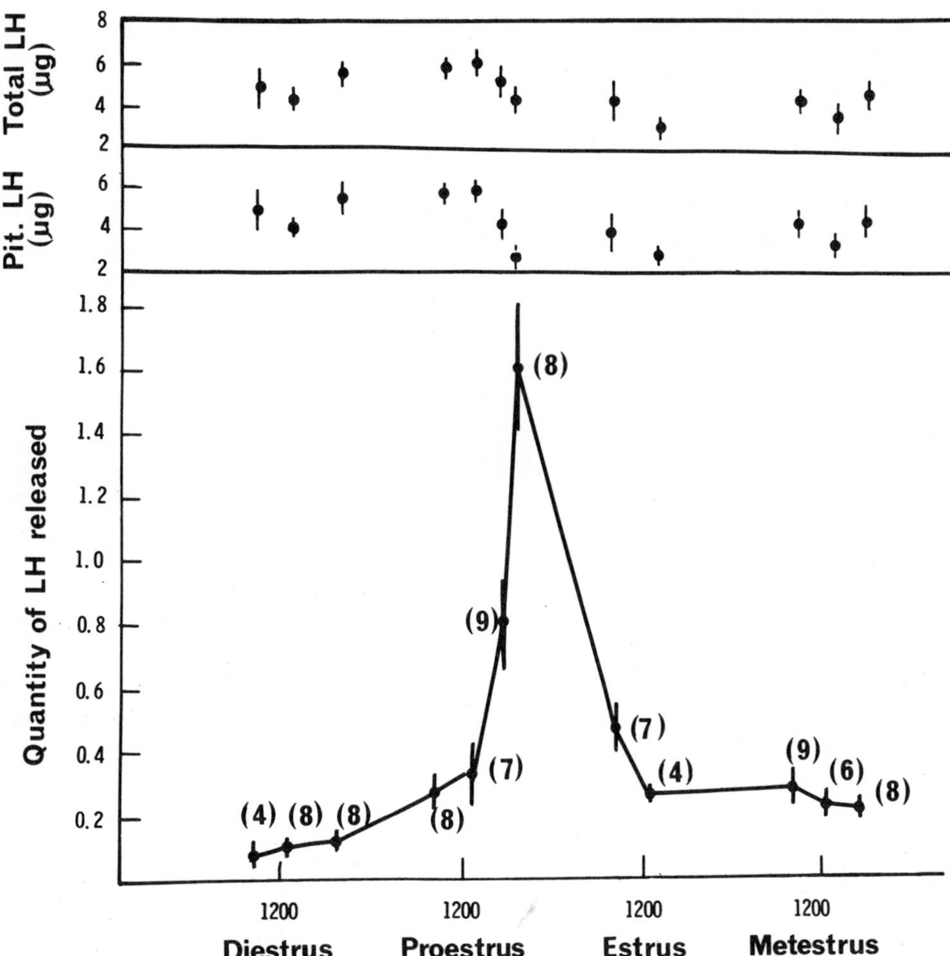

FIG. 16. Demonstration of the 20-fold increase in the amount of LH available for release in response to LHRH between diestrus and proestrus. The quantity of LH released (μg) **(bottom panel)** was calculated from the plasma LH concentrations before, and at intervals up to 120 min after, the intravenous injection of a supramaximal dose of LHRH (1,000 ng/100 g body weight) and the clearance rate of LH from blood. Pituitary LH content **(middle panel)** and total LH **(top panel)** in the system (pituitary LH content plus amount of LH released) are also shown. The animals (the quantity of which are represented by numbers in parentheses) were anesthetized with sodium pentobarbitone and, in order to block protein synthesis, given an intravenous injection of cyclohexamide 100 μg/100 g body weight 30 min before the injection of LHRH. (Data from ref. 156.)

The Rabbit

Many early studies carried out without direct measurement of plasma gonadotropin concentrations (i.e., using ovulation as the endpoint) predicted that coitus in the rabbit would be followed by a rapid and massive surge of LH (182), and indeed this was proved to be the case in that coitus is followed by a massive (~ 60%) drop in pituitary LH content (183) and a concomitant surge of LH (184–186). The peak of the LH surge is reached 1 to 2 hr after mating, when plasma LH concentrations are increased by as much as 100 times that of the precoital values (184–186). Dufy-Barbe et al. (185) reported that in contrast to spontaneous ovulators, the LH surge in the rabbit was not accompanied by a surge of FSH; Goodman and Neill (187), however, did find a small, but significant, postcoital FSH surge. Electrical stimulation of the median eminence and amygdala stimulated LH release, as assessed by ovarian progesterone release (188) or by LH radioimmunoassay (189), but the rate of LH increase produced by stimulation of the amygdala was not as rapid as that which follows mating (189). As assessed by the measurement of LHRH surges in rabbit portal plasma that were induced by cupric acetate, it can be assumed with reasonable certainty that LHRH probably mediates the neural control of the reflex LH surge (190). The magnitude of the cupric-acetate-induced LHRH surges was similar to that of the spontaneous LHRH surge in the rat (44,45,49).

The main progestin secreted by the rabbit ovary is 20α-hydroxy-pregn-4-en-3-one, and Hilliard et al. (191) proposed that this progestin acted in a positive-feedback manner to potentiate the reflex LH surge in the rabbit. However, although there is no doubt that progestin secretion increases almost immediately after mating, the positive-feedback hypothesis was not supported by extensive studies carried out with the aid of LH radioimmunoassay (187).

Early studies suggested that an adrenergic mechanism was involved in the coital stimulation of the ovulatory hormone, and indeed infusion of NA into the third ventricle of the rabbit resulted in a massive surge of LH, which, for reasons that are not clear, was inhibited by infusion of DA (192). Injection of α-methyl-*p*-tyrosine (α-MPT), an inhibitor of tyrosine hydroxylase, at a dosage sufficient to deplete most of the catecholamine histofluorescence in the median eminence, did not reduce either the magnitude of the postcoital surge of LH or the number of follicles that had ruptured (186). However, mating did reduce significantly the number of catecholamine-fluorescent cell bodies in the arcuate nuclei of the female rabbits that had been treated with α-MPT (186), which suggests that during or after mating the release of DA had occurred. This is puzzling in view of the results of Sawyer et al. (192).

In sum, as was predicted long ago, mating in the rabbit is followed by a massive ovulatory surge of LH which is probably mediated by a surge of LHRH. Monoamines appear to be involved in the surge, as does the amygdala, but the precise neuroanatomy and neurochemistry of the reflex gonadotropin surge in the rabbit remain to be elucidated.

Rats Exposed to Continuous Illumination

Exposure of rats to continuous illumination (LL rats) soon abolishes the regular estrous cycles that occur in rats exposed to a summer lighting regime (LD) and results in persistent vaginal cornification. The ovaries of LL rats develop large follicles, and the animals undergo a switch from spontaneous to reflex ovulators (for review see ref. 193). The effects of LL occur rapidly in that in rats exposed to LL from the day of estrus to the next proestrus, the onset of the LH surge is delayed by about 6 hr, the height of the LH surge is reduced by about 50%, and pituitary responsiveness to LHRH is markedly reduced (194). In contrast to LD rats, treatment of LL rats with estrogen and progesterone after ovariectomy failed to restore normal pituitary responsiveness to LHRH, which is markedly reduced by ovariectomy. Pituitary responsiveness in ovariectomized LL rats was also not enhanced by implanting a silicone elastomer capsule containing estradiol-17β, a regime that causes a significant increase in the LH response to LHRH in LD rats (194).

Plasma concentrations of estradiol-17β are raised in LL rats, as compared with the basal levels in LD rats (130,195). Copulation in LL rats is followed by a rapid increase in plasma LH concentrations, which can be mimicked in about 50% of LL rats by injecting progesterone (195,196). This reflex LH surge is accompanied by a significant loss of LH-releasing activity (as assessed by the ovarian ascorbic acid depletion method) in hypothalamic extracts (197), and injection of progesterone induces a surge of LHRH into hypophysial portal vessel blood (58). Progesterone also increases pituitary responsiveness, and especially the priming effect of LHRH (195). The amplitude and frequency of LH pulses in long-term ovariectomized LL rats are similar to those in androgen-sterilized rats and are significantly lower than the amplitude and frequency of pulses in LD rats (198). Exposure to LL produces effects similar to those of anterior deafferentation of the medial basal hypothalamus or lesions of the suprachiasmatic nuclei in that both types of animal develop persistent vaginal cornification, do not ovulate spontaneously, and have ovaries that are comprised mainly of large follicles (199). As in the LL rat, an injection of progesterone will produce a surge of LH in about 40% of animals with lesions of the suprachiasmatic nucleus (199).

The LL rat, therefore, should, in principle, provide an excellent model for studying the mechanism of gonadotropin control. It seems that exposure to LL produces an early shift in phase of the LH surge and a dramatic decrease in pituitary responsiveness. The LL rat is insensitive to the facilitatory effects of estrogen, but a surge of LH can be evoked in about half the animals, in an all-or-none fashion, by injecting progesterone. Several of the neuroendocrine characteristics of the LL rat resemble those of the androgen-sterilized rat and animals with anterior hypothalamic lesions. Thus exposure to LL blocks the activity of the LHRH surge generator, alters the frequency and amplitude of the LHRH-LH pulse generator, and disrupts circadian rhythms. As assessed by the changes that occur during early response to LL, it would appear that the timing of the surge generator is altered first. Overall, the data derived from the LL rat provide further evidence that suprachiasmatic and preoptic nuclei are major components of the neural circuitry for sexual differentiation and the generation of the LHRH surge in the rodent.

The Vole

The short-tailed field vole *(Microtus agrestis)* and the Montana vole *(Microtus montanus)* are both reflex ovulators, with LH surges occurring shortly after copulation (200,201). The reflex LH surge in *Microtus agrestis* is accompanied by a 56% drop in the hypothalamic content of immunoreactive LHRH, suggesting that the LH surge is caused by a massive reflex release of LHRH (202). Because of these dramatic changes induced by mating, and because of its small size, we thought that the vole would be an excellent model for studying, with the aid of the [^{14}C]2-deoxyglucose (2DG) method (203), the pathways associated with the reflex surges of LHRH and LH. However, although copulation produced dramatic LH surges in mated, as compared with sham-mated or nonmated, female voles (36.9 ± 9.6, as compared with < 2.5 ng NIH-LH-S18/ml plasma, respectively) no significant difference in 2DG uptake could be detected in 30 different regions of the brain, with the exception of the midbrain central gray, in which 2DG uptake was significantly increased after mating or sham-mating (exposed to the male, but having vagina taped) (203). Since plasma LH concentrations did not increase in the sham-mated females, the increase in 2DG uptake of the midbrain central gray might be related to the role that the midbrain central gray plays in lordosis (204), rather than to the mechanism of the reflex LHRH-LH surge.

CONTROL OF BASAL GONADOTROPIN RELEASE

For most of the reproductive life of both females and males, plasma gonadotropin levels are kept within a relatively low range by the negative feedback of gonadal steroids and, in the case of FSH, inhibin (for review see ref. 205). The effects of implantation of estrogen into the rat brain or pituitary gland (138) and the placement of lesions in the arcuate nuclei in the rhesus monkey (136,206) suggested that the inhibitory effect of estrogen is exerted at the pituitary gland. However, in the rat, at least, a hypothalamic site of action cannot be excluded, because after ovariectomy there is a steady increase in the mean concentration of LHRH in portal vessel blood which parallels the increase in peripheral plasma LH concentration (207). Twenty-four days after ovariectomy the mean concentration of LHRH in hypophysial portal vessel blood was about 60 pg/ml plasma. Although this is low compared with 150 pg LHRH/ml of portal blood at the peak of the LHRH surge (Fig. 4), the anterior pituitary gland in ovariectomized rats is exposed almost continuously to concentrations of LHRH which are much higher than in intact rats in which concentrations of about 100 pg LHRH/ml plasma are capable of producing a 20-fold increase in plasma LH concentration after 75 min (145; Fig. 14). Furthermore, the release of LHRH into portal blood of the rat is pulsatile, with some pulses reaching as high as 1,000 pg/ml. The situation in the rhesus monkey is not yet clear. The concentrations of LHRH in portal plasma were significantly elevated above those in the follicular phase in two of four ovariecomized monkeys (57), and the amplitude of LHRH oscillations, but not the mean concentration of LHRH, in portal plasma was higher in ovariectomized animals than in animals in the follicular phase (208). Acute administration of estradiol reduced the LHRH concentrations in portal plasma from long-term ovariectomized rats (207), but not in that from rhesus monkeys (208).

Pulsatile Release of LH

Gonadectomy in the rhesus monkey (208a) and in the rat (209) was found to produce pulsatile LH secretion with each pulse, having a duration of about 1 hr. Subsequently, it was shown that pulses occur also in intact rats, sheep, and humans. In the human female the frequency and amplitude of the pulses change during the menstrual cycle (210). The LHRH/LH pulse generator, at least in rodents, differs from the LHRH/LH surge generator in that the pulse, but not the surge, generator is active in male rats, female rats in which the neuroendocrine brain has been masculinized by neonatal exposure to androgen, and in female rats exposed to constant illumination (198). Deafferentation of the medial basal hypothalamus blocks surges of LH, but does not inhibit pulsatile LH release (211). In contrast to the ovulatory LHRH surge, LHRH/LH pulses are inhibited by increased central NA activity; however, the surge and the pulse generators are both inhibited by opioids in the rat (212) and the monkey (97). The different properties of the two generators are summarized in Fig. 9. The apparent location of the pulse generator in the rat medial basal hypothalamus (211) prompts us to ask about the location of the LHRH neurons that secrete the pulses, since some workers have found it difficult to demonstrate many (and, in some cases, any) LHRH neurons within the medial basal hypothalamus (31). In the rhesus monkey, however, there are relatively many LHRH neurons in the medial basal hypothalamus (31).

Why is the "basal" secretion of LH and FSH pulsatile? Since many neurotransmitters and hormones are secreted in a pulsatile nature, pulsatile LHRH and gonadotropin secretion may simply reflect an inherent property of neuroendocrine and endocrine cells, and indeed one early study suggested that this might be the case for the gonadotropes (213). However, the changing frequency and amplitude of the gonadotropin pulses during the menstrual and estrous cycles (210,212,214) suggest that pulsatile gonadotropin release serves a physiological purpose in that control within the hypothalamic-pituitary gonadal system may depend as much on frequency as on amplitude modulation. This applies especially to seasonal breeders, such as the sheep, where the frequency and amplitude of the LH pulses vary considerably with the time of year and appear to play a crucial role in switching the gonads on and off (215). It has been postulated that the frequency and amplitude of LH pulses may, as in the case of switching-on the gonads during the breeding season, switch-on the gonads at puberty (53,215). In humans, LH pulses associated with rapid eye movement sleep occur selectively at puberty, and the same phenomenon occurs in anorexia nervosa as the patients pass into and out of the crisis phase of the disease (216).

These observations, which suggest that pulsatile gonadotropin release is physiologically important, receive support from several sets of experimental data. First, pulsatile release of LHRH has been found in rhesus monkeys (208), rats (207), and sheep (217). Secondly, in the hypogonadal mouse (177) and rhesus monkey (147) the pulsatile administration of LHRH at frequencies of 1 to 2 hr is much more effective than either continuous infusions or a single large bolus injection of LHRH in stimulating gonadotropin synthesis and release and thereby establishing and/or maintaining the normal function of the gonads. Thirdly, the frequency and, in some species, amplitude of LHRH and LH pulses are increased by castration and reduced by testosterone administration, suggesting that the inhibitory (negative-feedback) effects of testosterone on the hypothalamic-pituitary system may be exerted by way of reducing gonadotropin pulse frequency (218,219). Fourthly, continuous exposure to relatively high concentrations of LHRH results in a decrease ("down-regulation") of receptor number, probably due to massive internalization and then processing of the LHRH-receptor complex (220–223), which, in turn, leads to a reduction in gonadotropin output. In sum, pulsatile LHRH and gonadotropin release may serve as a signaling device that allows for frequency and amplitude modulation of hormone effects, as well as prevents receptor down-regulation and the consequent development of refractoriness in the hypothalamic-pituitary-gonadal system.

The Apparent Paradox of Negative-Positive Feedback of Estrogen and Progesterone

Whether estrogen and progesterone inhibit or stimulate gonadotropin output depends upon the duration, timing, and level of exposure to the steroid. Thus, progesterone will stimulate LH release only when acting on a hypothalamic-pituitary system that has been exposed for many hours to elevated plasma concentrations of estrogen. In the rat, the switch from an inhibitory to a facilitatory action of progesterone occurs relatively precisely during the early hours of proestrus, when the anti-estrogens also cease to be effective in blocking ovulation (125,224). During most of the cycle, plasma estrogen concentrations are low. In the monkey (46) an LH surge will occur only if estradiol concentrations are maintained at about 200 to 400 pg/ml plasma for at least 36 hr. Basal concentrations, or increments of less than 100 pg/ml, or of a duration shorter than 36 hr, reduce LH output. The magnitude of the plasma estradiol concentrations and the duration of exposure at which a switch from an inhibitory to a facilitatory effect occurs in the human is similar to that in the monkey (118,225). In the rat (226,227), sheep (228), and human (229), progesterone and estrogen act synergistically to inhibit gonadotropin release. Thus, in the presence of relatively high plasma progesterone concentrations, basal or elevated concentrations of estrogen will inhibit gonadotropin output. Progesterone by itself has little effect, but this may be because the abundance of progesterone receptors in the hypothalamus and pituitary depends on estrogen (133).

SUPPRESSION OF THE HYPOTHALAMIC-GONADOTROPIN SYSTEM BY HIGH PLASMA PROLACTIN CONCENTRATIONS

It has long been known that, in humans and some other species of mammal, fertility is reduced or completely blocked during suckling and that this is due mainly to a blockade of ovulation by high concentrations of prolactin in plasma. The precise mechanism of action of prolactin in blocking ovulation remains to be established. However, it seems clear that the hormone either inhibits the release of LHRH [either by a direct action on LHRH neurons or by increasing DA release from the TIDA neurons (230,231)] or reduces pituitary responsiveness to LHRH, or both (232–238). Hyperprolactinemia also inhibits the priming effect of LHRH in normal, but not *hpg*, mice (239). Studies by Nikolics et al. (39) on the human placental cDNA for the LHRH precursor showed that a 56-amino-acid component (GAP) of the precursor immediately following the LHRH peptide (Fig. 3) inhibited prolactin release from pituitary cells in culture. Nikolics et al. postulated that this association between LHRH and a prolactin-inhibiting peptide could explain the apparent inverse relationship that occurs between plasma LH and prolactin concentrations during lactation and other states of hyperprolactinemia (e.g., as a consequence of prolactin-secreting tumors). However, the control of prolactin release involves complex interactions between hypothalamic factors that stimulate and inhibit prolactin release (240,241) and, therefore, although the simplicity of the hypothesis advanced by Nikolics et al. (39) is attractive, it is unlikely to explain the complex and intriguing interactions between prolactin and the hypothalamic-pituitary-ovarian system.

THE MECHANISM OF ACTION OF LHRH

The precise mechanism of action of LHRH remains to be determined, but a working hypothesis has emerged which may explain the three major actions of the decapeptide, which are gonadotropin release, gonadotropin synthesis, and the priming effect. Although cyclic AMP may be involved in some of the later actions of LHRH, it does not serve as a second messenger for LHRH (150,223). Figure 17 shows schematically that when LHRH binds to its receptor [apparently a 60,000-MW glycoprotein (242)], calcium channels are opened, resulting in the influx of extracellular Ca^{2+}, and phosphatidylinositol (PI) is hydrolyzed by phosphodiesterase to form diacylglycerol (DG) and inositol triphosphate (IP_3), which further increases cytosolic Ca^{2+} concentrations by releasing Ca^{2+} from endoplasmic reticulum (243). Increased cellular concentrations of Ca^{2+} interact with calmodulin and activate phospholipase A_2, leading to the formation of arachidonic acid (AA) and, as a consequence, the derivatives of AA, the prostaglandins (by the cyclooxygenase pathway), and the HETEs and leukotrienes (by the lipoxygenase pathway). Diacylglycerol activates protein kinase C (which is involved in protein phosphorylation and cell proliferation) (243–246). Increased intracellular Ca^{2+} and activation of PI turnover may lead to activation of actin (a major intracellular contractile element) (247,248); increased PI turnover, by activating protein kinase C, may enhance the Ca^{2+} current (249). There is considerable experimental evidence that supports the assertion that Ca^{2+} and the PI cascade act as second messenger systems for the action of LHRH (223,250–253). Evidence from the *hpg* mouse shows that although it is not crucial for either

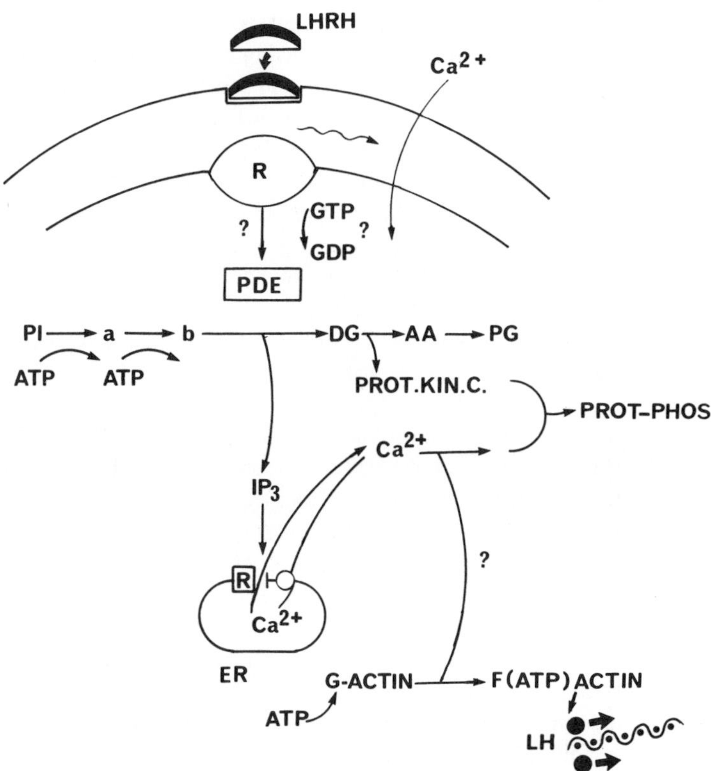

FIG. 17. Shows the mechanism of action of LHRH by stimulating Ca^{2+} influx and the phosphatidylinositol (PI) cascade. The hydrolysis of PI is initiated by activation of phosphodiesterase (PDE), consequent upon the interaction between LHRH and its receptor. The latter process probably involves GTP. The main product of PI hydrolysis is diacylglycerol (DG), which is further metabolized to arachidonic acid (AA), which in turn can be metabolized to form the prostaglandins (PG), leukotrienes, and HETEs. DG activates protein kinase C, which stimulates protein phosphorylation, an important step in protein (including gonadotropin) synthesis. The other major derivative of PI is inositol triphosphate (IP_3), which releases Ca^{2+} from the endoplasmic reticulum (ER). The increased Ca^{2+} in cytosol has several actions, including stimulation of protein phosphorylation and activation of actin, which are likely to be involved in gonadotropin release and the priming effect of LHRH. (For details see text.)

the differentiation of the gonadotropes or the synthesis of small amounts of immunoreactive as well as bioactive LH and FSH, LHRH is a potent stimulus for gonadotropin synthesis (36,177,254). It may be added parenthetically that ultrastructural (255) and immunoassay (167) studies suggested that differentiation of gonadotropes and the synthesis of gonadotropins followed differentiation of, as well as the appearance of, LHRH in the median eminence; the *hpg* mouse suggests that the anterior pituitary gland has some degree of autonomy in terms of gonadotrope differentiation and gonadotropin synthesis. The studies in the *hpg* mouse confirm earlier findings in the rat that LHRH stimulates LH synthesis (256) and the glycosylation of LH (257,258). The activation of actin may, to a large extent, be responsible for the movement of LH secretory granules toward the plasmalemma of the gonadotropes (155) and, as a consequence, the massive increase in the readily releasable pool of LH that parallels the increase in pituitary responsiveness (Fig. 15). In addition to the effects of LHRH outlined above, a recent report suggests that LHRH stimulates an increase in nuclear estrogen receptors in the anterior pituitary gland (259).

Thus, it is reasonable to propose that LHRH increases Ca^{2+} influx into the gonadotropes and increases the turnover of PI, which, in turn, leads to the release of Ca^{2+} from intracellular Ca^{2+} stores. This cascade stimulates the immediate release of gonadotropin granules that are close to the plasmalemma *(the releasing action of LHRH),* brings more gonadotrope granules toward the plasmalemma so that subsequent exposure to a secretagogue leads to heightened release of gonadotropin *(the priming effect of LHRH),* and stimulates *gonadotropin synthesis*. For many obvious reasons the above account is, no doubt, highly oversimplified. For example, it is likely that several intermediary steps are involved, of which one might be the synthesis of a "priming protein." The interactions between ion channels in membranes are probably also more complex than outlined here; for example, pharmacological studies suggest a sex difference in the LH response to LHRH in that Ca^{2+} channel opening and potassium-A current blockade play a major role in the male pituitary, whereas potassium-M current blockade and, to a lesser extent, Ca^{2+} opening are important in the female (260). Nonetheless, the present outline provides a basis for further detailed investigation of the several actions of LHRH.

How estrogen and progesterone potentiate the gonadotropin response to LHRH also remains unclear, but these steroids could, by their genomic effects, increase the number of LHRH receptors or stimulate the production of proteins/enzymes involved in the activation of the cytoskeleton and, in addition, exert extragenomic allosteric effects on enzyme action.

An alternative or an additional action of estrogen has been revealed by J. D. Neill, who has recently applied the reverse hemolytic plaque assay to the study of pituitary cells (261). With the aid of this elegant method, which allows study of the secretory activity of single pituitary cells, Neill and associates have shown that, at diestrus, many gonadotropes identified by immunocytochemistry are totally unresponsive to LHRH (262). Incubation of the cells with estrogen for

24 hr before the plaque assay almost doubled the number of secretory gonadotropes (262). Conceivably, LHRH can itself exert similar effects in that the subcutaneous injection of male *hpg* mice with 2 μg LHRH daily for 20 days produced a twofold increase in pituitary LH content, a 63-fold increase in pituitary FSH content, a 1.6-fold increase in the number of immunoreactive gonadotropes, a 1.9-fold increase in the size of the gonadotropes, and a 2.3-fold increase in the number of secretory granules in gonadotropes (263). It remains to be determined whether, like estrogen, LHRH can convert nonsecretory to secretory gonadotropes. By the same token it is possible that factors which inhibit gonadotropin release, such as hyperprolactinemia (see above), might exert at least part of their action by converting secretory to nonsecretory gonadotropes. The concept of changing populations of active and inactive cells in the anterior pituitary gland is not new and was proposed on the basis of early light microscopy observations (264). However, the importance of the finding by Neill and associates is that even though a cell is fully replete with hormone, it may not necessarily respond to its specific secretagogue; that is, the readily releasable pool of hormone is defined as much by the operational state of the receptor-release apparatus as by hormone content.

CONCLUSIONS

The physiology of the control of gonadotropin secretion has broadly been established, and the key points may be summarized as follows:

(a) Basal gonadotropin secretion is kept in check by the negative feedback of gonadal steroids. Secretion is pulsatile, and this facilitates frequency as well as amplitude modulation in the hypothalamic-pituitary-gonadal system and also prevents down-regulation of hormone receptors.

(b) The spontaneous ovulatory gonadotropin surge is produced by a dramatic positive-feedback cascade, which is initiated by estrogen release from the ovary. The surge of estrogen, the timing of which depends on the interaction of appropriate gonadotropin signals with intrinsic ovarian mechanisms, initiates an increase in pituitary responsiveness to LHRH and triggers a surge of LHRH. Both actions of estrogen take a relatively long time (many hours). Responsiveness of the anterior pituitary gland is further increased by the priming effect of LHRH and, in some species, by progesterone. The priming effect of LHRH coordinates the increased release of LHRH (during the LHRH surge) into hypophysial portal vessel blood with the increase in pituitary responsiveness so that both events reach a peak at the same time and thereby produce a massive surge of LH.

(c) Reflex ovulation is also produced by a massive surge of LH, which has been measured in the rabbit, rats exposed to continuous illumination, and the vole, but the detailed mechanism of the reflex LH surge in these species is not known other than that it is mediated by a surge of LHRH. The effects of exposing female rats to continuous illumination are similar to those of placing a lesion in the anterior hypothalamus (and in the suprachiasmatic nucleus, in particular) or injecting testosterone during the early neonatal period. This provides further evidence for the existence in the preoptic-suprachiasmatic region of the neural circuitry involved in sexual differentiation and generation of the LHRH surge.

(d) As well as stimulating gonadotropin release and increasing pituitary responsiveness (priming), LHRH also stimulates gonadotropin synthesis and the recruitment of pituitary cells into the gonadotrope pool.

(e) The secretion of FSH is dissociated from LH secretion under several physiological and experimental circumstances. The possible factors that underlie this dissociation include: differences in the secretory mechanism of the two gonadotropes (secretion of LH, but not of FSH, depends on the minute-by-minute exposure of gonadotropes to LHRH); the action of inhibin on the secretion of FSH, but not of LH; and the possible existence of a separate FSH-RH.

(f) High plasma concentrations of prolactin inhibit gonadotropin secretion by reducing pituitary responsiveness to, and the priming effect of, LHRH and, possibly, by inhibiting LHRH release.

The questions that now remain are the most interesting and difficult to answer. For example, can a unitary hypothesis involving the influx of Ca^{2+} and the phosphatidylinositol cascade really explain the three major actions of LHRH? How do steroids modulate the action of LHRH? How does estrogen and possibly LHRH convert nonsecretory to secretory gonadotropes? What is the precise neural circuitry of LHRH pulse and surge generators, and how are these generators linked to the circuitry responsible for circadian rhythmicity? Where and how does estrogen act to trigger the surge of LHRH? The answers to these and other obvious questions, which will occupy the attention of several more generations of endocrinologists, are important not only for our understanding of the gonadotropin system per se, but also for our general understanding of how neurons and endocrine cells function.

ACKNOWLEDGMENT

I am most grateful to Jo Donnelly for her excellent assistance in preparing this manuscript.

REFERENCES

1. Warren, M. P. (1983): Effects of undernutrition on reproductive function in the human. *Endocr. Rev.*, 4:363–377.
2. Harris, G. W. (1955): *Neural Control of the Pituitary Gland*. Edward Arnold, London.
3. Harris, G. W. (1972): Humours and hormones. *J. Endocrinol.*, 53:ii–xxiii.
4. Everett, J. W. (1987): Pituitary and hypothalamus: perspectives and overviews. Chapter 26, these volumes.

5. Haighton, J. (1797): An experimental enquiry concerning animal impregnation. *Philos. Trans. R. Soc. Lond. (Biol.),* 87:159–196.
6. Cruikshank, W. (1797): Experiments in which, on the third day after impregnation, the ova of rabbits were found in the Fallopian tubes; and on the fourth day after impregnation in the uterus itself, with the first appearance of the foetus. *Philos. Trans. R. Soc. Lond. (Biol.),* 87:197–214.
7. Barry, M. (1839): Researches in embryology—Second series. *Philos. Trans. R. Soc. Lond. (Biol.),* 129:307–380.
8. Heape, W. (1905): Ovulation and degeneration of ova in rabbit. *Proc. R. Soc. Lond. (Biol.),* 76:260–268.
9. Benoit, J. M. (1934): Activation sexuelle obtenue chez le canard par l'eclairement artificial pendant la periode de repas genital. *C. R. Hebd. Seanc. Acad. Sci. (Paris),* 199:1671–1673.
10. Bissonette, T. H. (1937): Photoperiodicity in birds. *Wilson Bull.,* 49:241–270.
11. Marshall, F. H. A. (1936): The Croonian lecture: Sexual periodicity and the causes which determine it. *Philos. Trans. R. Soc. Lond. (Biol.),* 226:423–456.
12. Rowan, W. (1928): Reproductive rhythm in birds. *Nature,* 122:11–12.
13. Smith, P. E. (1932): The secretory capacity of the anterior hypophysis as evidenced by the effect of partial hypophysectomies in rats. *Anat. Rec.,* 52:191–208.
14. Popa, G. T., and Fielding, U. (1930): A portal circulation from the pituitary to the hypothalamic region. *J. Anat.,* 65:88–91.
15. Harris, G. W. (1937): The induction of ovulation in the rabbit, by electrical stimulation of the hypothalamo-hypophysial mechanism. *Proc. R. Soc. Lond. (Biol.),* 122:374–394.
16. Hinsey, J. C. (1937): The relation of the nervous system to ovulation and other phenomena of the female reproductive tract. *Cold Spring Harbor Symp. Quant. Biol.,* 5:269–279.
17. Harris, G. W., and Jacobsohn, D. (1952): Functional grafts of the anterior pituitary gland. *Proc. R. Soc. Lond. (Biol.),* 139:263–276.
18. Matsuo, H., Baba, Y., Nair, R. M. G., Arimura, A., and Schally, A. V. (1971): Structure of the porcine LH- and FSH-releasing hormone. I. The proposed amino acid sequence. *Biochem. Biophys. Res. Commun.,* 43:1334–1339.
19. Schally, A. V., Arimura, A., Baba, Y., Nair, R. M. G., Matsuo, H., Redding, T. W., Debeljuk, L., and White, W. F. (1971): Isolation and properties of the FSH- and LH-releasing hormone. *Biochem. Biophys. Res. Commun.,* 43:393–399.
20. Burgus, R., Butcher, M., Amoss, M., Ling, N., Monahan, M., Rivier, J., Fellows, R., Blackwell, R., Vale, W., and Guillemin, R. (1972): Primary structure of the ovine hypothalamic luteinising hormone-releasing factor (LRF). *Proc. Natl. Acad. Sci. USA,* 69:278–282.
21. Fink, G., and Jamieson, M. G. (1976): Immunoreactive luteinizing hormone releasing factor in rat pituitary stalk blood: Effects of electrical stimulation of the medial preoptic area. *J. Endocrinol.,* 68:71–87.
22. Eskay, R. L., Mical, R. S., and Porter, J. C. (1977): Relationship between luteinizing hormone releasing hormone concentration in hypophysial portal blood and luteinizing hormone release in intact, castrated, and electrochemically-stimulated rats. *Endocrinology,* 100:263–270.
23. Fink, G. (1979): Neuroendocrine control of gonadotrophin secretion. *Br. Med. Bull.,* 35,2:155–160.
24. Marshall, F. H. A. (1942): Exteroreceptive factors in sexual periodicity. *Biol. Rev.,* 17:68–90.
25. Lamming, G. E., editor (1984): *Marshall's Physiology of Reproduction Vol. 1,* 4th ed. Churchill Livingstone, Edinburgh.
26. Lipner, H. (1987): Mechanism of mammalian ovulation. Chapter 12, these volumes.
27. Dixson, A. F. (1983): The hormonal control of sexual behaviour in primates. In: *Oxford Review of Reproductive Biology, Vol. 5,* pp. 131–219. Oxford University Press, Oxford.
28. Spies, H. G., and Chappel, S. C. (1984): Mammals: Nonhuman primates. In: *Marshall's Physiology of Reproduction,* edited by G. E. Lamming, pp. 659–712. Churchill Livingstone, Edinburgh.
29. Rowlands, I. W., and Weir, B. J. (1984): Mammals, Non-primate eutherians. In: *Marshall's Physiology of Reproduction, Vol. 1,* 4th ed., edited by G. E. Lamming, pp. 455–658. Churchill Livingstone, Edinburgh.
30. Schally, A. V., Arimura, A., and Kastin, A. J. (1973): Hypothalamic regulatory hormones. *Science,* 179:341–350.
31. Silverman, A. J. (1987): The gonadotropin-releasing hormone (GnRH) neuronal systems: Immunocytochemistry. Chapter 29, these volumes.
32. Millar, R. P., Aehnelt, C., and Rossier, G. (1977): Higher molecular weight immunoreactive species of luteinizing hormone releasing hormone: Possible precursors of the hormone. *Biochem. Biophys. Res. Commun.,* 74:720–731.
33. Gautron, J. P., Pattou, E., and Kordon, C. (1981): Occurrence of higher molecular forms of LHRH in fractionated extracts from rat hypothalamus, cortex and placenta. *Mol. Cell. Endocrinol.,* 24:1–15.
34. Curtis, A., and Fink, G. (1983): A high molecular weight precursor of luteinizing hormone releasing hormone from rat hypothalamus. *Endocrinology,* 112:390–392.
35. Curtis, A., Lyons, V., and Fink, G. (1983): The human hypothalamic LHRH precursor is the same size as that in rat and mouse hypothalamus. *Biochem. Biophys. Res. Commun.,* 117:872–877.
36. Cattanach, B. M., Iddon, C. A., Charlton, H. M., Chiappa, S. A., and Fink, G. (1977): Gonadotrophin-releasing hormone deficiency in a mutant mouse with hypogonadism. *Nature,* 269:338–340.
37. Sheward, W. J., Harmar, A. J., and Fink, G. (1985): LH-RH in the rat and mouse hypothalamus and rat hypophysial portal blood: Confirmation of identity by high performance liquid chromatography. *Brain Res.,* 345:362–365.
38. Seeburg, P. H., and Adelman, J. P. (1984): Characterization of cDNA for precursor of human luteinizing hormone releasing hormone. *Nature,* 311:666–668.
39. Nikolics, K., Mason, A. J., Szonyi, E., Ramachandran, J., and Seeburg, P. H. (1985): A prolactin-inhibiting factor within the precursor for human gonadotropin-releasing hormone. *Nature,* 316:511–517.
40. Phillips, H. S., Nikolics, K., Branton, D., and Seeburg, P. H. (1985): Immunocytochemical localization in rat brain of a prolactin release-inhibiting sequence of gonadotropin-releasing hormone prohormone. *Nature,* 316:542–545.
41. Adelman, J. P., Mason, A. J., Hayflick, J. S., and Seeburg, P. H. (1986): *Proc. Natl. Acad. Sci. USA,* 83:179–183.
42. Millar, R. P., Sheward, W. J., Wegener, I., and Fink, G. (1983): Somatostatin 28 is a hormonally active peptide released into hypophysial portal vessel blood. *Brain Res.,* 260:334–337.
43. Sheward, W. J., Benoit, R., and Fink, G. (1984): Somatostatin-28(1-12)-like immunoreactive substance is secreted into hypophysial portal vessel blood in the rat. *Neuroendocrinology,* 38:88–90.
44. Sarkar, D. K., Chiappa, S. A., Fink, G., and Sherwood, N. M. (1976): Gonadotropin-releasing hormone surge in pro-oestrous rats. *Nature,* 264:461–463.
45. Ching, M. (1982): Correlative surges of LHRH, LH and FSH in pituitary stalk plasma and systemic plasma of rat during proestrus. *Neuroendocrinology,* 34:279–285.
46. Knobil, E. (1974): On the control of gonadotropin secretion in the Rhesus monkey. *Recent Prog. Horm. Res.,* 30:1–36.
47. Legan, S. J., and Karsch, F. J. (1975): A daily signal for the LH surge in the rat. *Endocrinology,* 96:57–62.
48. Fink, G. (1979): Feedback actions of target hormones on hypothalamus and pituitary with special reference to gonadal steroids. *Annu. Rev. Physiol.,* 41:571–585.
49. Sherwood, N. M., Chiappa, S. A., Sarkar, D. K., and Fink, G. (1980): Gonadotropin-releasing hormone (GnRH) in pituitary stalk blood from proestrous rats: Effects of anesthetics and relationship between stored and released GnRH and luteinizing hormone. *Endocrinology,* 107:1410–1417.
50. Blake, C. A. (1976): Simulation of the proestrous luteinizing hormone (LH) surge after infusion of LH-releasing hormone in phenobarbital-blocked rats. *Endocrinology,* 98:451–460.
51. Sarkar, D. K., and Fink, G., (1979): Mechanism of the first spontaneous gonadotrophin surge and that induced by pregnant mare serum and effects of neo-natal androgen in rats. *J. Endocrinol.,* 83:339–354.
52. Meijs-Roelofs, H. M. A., Uilenbroek, J. Th. J., de Greef, W. J., de Jong, F. H., and Kramer, P. (1975): Gonadotrophin and steroid levels around the time of first ovulation in the rat. *J. Endocrinol.,* 67:275–282.

53. Mackinnon, P. C. B., Puig-Duran, E., and Laynes, R. (1978): Reflections on the attainment of puberty in the rat: Have circadian signals a role to play in its onset? *J. Reprod. Fertil.*, 52:401–412.
54. Ojeda, S. R., and Urbanski, H. F. (1987): Puberty in the rat. Chapter 39, these volumes.
55. Everett, J. W., and Sawyer, C. H. (1950): A 24-hour periodicity in the 'LH-release apparatus' of female rats, disclosed by barbiturate sedation. *Endocrinology*, 47:198–218.
56. Henderson, S. R., Baker, C., and Fink, G. (1977): Effects of oestradiol-17β exposure on the spontaneous secretion of gonadotrophins in chronically gonadectomized rats. *J. Endocrinol.*, 73: 455–462.
57. Neill, J. D., Patton, J. M., Dailey, R. A., Tsou, R. C., and Tindall, G. T. (1977): Luteinizing hormone releasing hormone (LHRH) in pituitary stalk blood of Rhesus monkeys: Relationship to level of LH release. *Endocrinology*, 101:430–434.
58. Sarkar, D. K., and Fink, G. (1979): Effects of gonadal steroids on output of luteinizing hormone releasing factor into pituitary stalk blood in the female rat. *J. Endocrinol.*, 80:303–313.
59. Barraclough, C. A. (1966): Modifications in the CNS regulation of reproduction after exposure of prepubertal rats to steroid hormones. *Recent Prog. Horm. Res.*, 22:503–529.
60. Halasz, B., and Pupp, L. (1965): Hormone secretion of the anterior pituitary gland after physical interruption of all nervous pathways to the hypophysiotrophic area. *Endocrinology*, 77:553–562.
61. Halasz, B., and Gorski, R. A. (1967): Gonadotrophic hormone secretion in female rats after partial or total interruption of neural afferents to the medial basal hypothalamus. *Endocrinology*, 80:608–622.
62. Raisman, G., and Brown-Grant, K. (1977): The 'suprachiasmatic syndrome': Endocrine and behavioural abnormalities following lesions of the suprachiasmatic nuclei in the female rat. *Proc. R. Soc. Lond. (Biol.)*, 198:297–314.
63. Rethelyi, M., Vigh, S., Setalo, G., Merchenthaler, I., Flerko, B., and Petrusz, P. (1981): The luteinizing hormone releasing hormone-containing pathways and their co-termination with tanacyte processes in and around the median eminence and the pituitary stalk of the rat. *Acta Morphol. Acad. Sci. Hung.*, 29(2–3):259–283.
64. Kelly, M. J., Ronnekleiv, O. K., and Eskay, R. L. (1982): Immunocytochemical localization of luteinizing hormone-releasing hormone in neurons in the medial basal hypothalamus of the female rat. *Exp. Brain Res.*, 48:97–106.
65. Kozlowski, G. P., and Les Dees, W. (1984): Immunocytochemistry for LHRH neurons in the arcuate nucleus area of the rat. *J. Histochem. Cytochem.*, 32:83–91.
66. Koves, K., and Halasz, B. (1970): Location of the neural structures triggering ovulation in the rat. *Neuroendocrinology*, 6:180–193.
67. Nauta, W. J. H. (1963): Central nervous organization and the endocrine motor system. In: *Advances in Neuroendocrinology*, edited by A. V. Nalbandov, pp. 5–12. University of Illinois Press, Urbana.
68. Raisman, G. (1966): Neural connexions of the hypothalamus. *Br. Med. Bull.*, 22:197–201.
69. Chiappa, S. A., Fink, G., and Sherwood, N. M. (1977): Immunoreactive luteinizing hormone releasing factor (LRF) in pituitary stalk plasma from female rats: Effects of stimulating diencephalon, hippocampus and amygdala. *J. Physiol.*, 267:625–640.
70. Sarkar, D. K., and Fink, G. (1981): Gonadotropin-releasing hormone surge: Possible modulation through postsynaptic α-adrenoreceptors and two pharmacologically distinct dopamine receptors. *Endocrinology*, 108:862–867.
71. Barraclough, C. A., and Wise, P. M. (1982): The role of catecholamines in the regulation of pituitary luteinizing hormone and follicle-stimulating hormone secretion. *Endocr. Rev.*, 3:91–119.
72. Fink, G., Stanley, H. F., and Watts, A. G. (1983): Central nervous control of sex and gonadotropin release: Peptide and nonpeptide transmitter interactions. In: *Brain Peptides*, edited by D. Krieger, M. Brownstein, and J. Martin, pp. 413–435. John Wiley & Sons, New York.
73. Kalra, S. P., and Kalra, P. S. (1983): Neural regulation of luteinizing hormone secretion in the rat. *Endocr. Rev.*, 4:311–351.
74. Barraclough, C. A., Wise, P. M., and Selmanoff, M. K. (1984): A role for hypothalamic catecholamines in the regulation of gonadotropin secretion. *Recent Prog. Horm. Res.*, 40:487–529.
75. Jones, E. G., and Powell, T. P. S. (1970): An anatomical study of converging sensory pathways within the cerebral cortex of the monkey. *Brain*, 93:793–820.
76. Klein, D. C. (1978): The pineal gland: A model of neuroendocrine regulation. In: *The Hypothalamus*, edited by S. Reichlin, R. J. Baldessarini, and J. B. Martin, pp. 303–327. Raven Press, New York.
77. Moore, R. Y. (1978): Central neural control of circadian rhythms. In: *Frontiers in Neuroendocrinology, Vol. 5*, edited by W. F. Ganong and L. Martini, pp. 185–206. Raven Press, New York.
78. Reiter, R. J. (1981): The mammalian pineal gland: structure and function. *Am. J. Anat.*, 62:287–313.
79. Versi, E., Chiappa, S. A., Fink, G., and Charlton, H. M. (1983): Pineal influences hypothalamic GnRH content in the vole, *Mictrotus agrestis*. *J. Reprod. Fertil.*, 67:365–368.
80. Karsch, F. J., Bittman, E. L., Foster, D. L., Goodman, R. L., Legan, S. J., and Robinson, J. E. (1984): Neuroendocrine basis of seasonal reproduction. *Recent Prog. Horm. Res.*, 40:185–225.
81. Bittman, E. L., Kaynard, A. H., Olster, D. H., Robinson, J. E., Yellow, S. M., and Karsch, F. J. (1985): Pineal melatonin mediates photoperiodic control of pulsatile luteinizing hormone secretion in the ewe. *Neuroendocrinology*, 40:409–418.
82. Renfree, M. B. (1981): Marsupials: alternative mammals. *Nature*, 293:100.
83. Lang, U., Aubert, M. L., Rivest, R. W., Viras-Bradtke, J. C., and Sizonenko, P. C. (1984): Daily afternoon administration of melatonin does not irreversibly inhibit sexual maturation in the male rat. *Endocrinology*, 115:2303–2310.
84. Tamarkin, L., Baird, C. J., and Almeida, O. F. X. (1985): Melatonin: A coordinating signal for mammalian reproduction? *Science*, 227:714–720.
85. Waldhauser, F., Frisch, H., Waldhauser, M., Weiszenbacher, G., Zeitlhuber, U., and Wurtman, R. J. (1984): Fall in nocturnal serum melatonin during prepuberty and pubescence. *Lancet*, i:362–365.
86. Symons, A. M., Arendt, J., and Pryde, S. J. (1985): Differential effects of melatonin on the stimulated release of LH from dispersed pituitary cells of the prepubertal female rat. *J. Endocrinol.*, 107:107–112.
87. Shivers, B. D., Harlan, R. E., Morell, J. I., and Pfaff, D. W. (1983): Absence of oestradiol concentration in cell nuclei of LHRH-immunoreactive neurones. *Nature*, 304:345–347.
88. Jackson, G. L. (1972): Effect of actinomycin D on estrogen-induced release of luteinizing hormone in ovariectomized rats. *Endocrinology*, 91:1284–1287.
89. Jackson, G. L. (1973): Time interval between injection of estradiol benzoate and LH release in the rat and effect of actinomycin D or cycloheximide. *Endocrinology*, 93:887–892.
90. Taubenhaus, M., and Soskin, S. (1941): Release of luteinizing hormone from the anterior hypophysis by an acetylcholine-like substance from the hypothalamic region. *Endocrinology*, 29:958–964.
91. Sawyer, C. H. (1963): Neuroendocrine blocking agents: Discussion. In: *Advances in Neuroendocrinology*, edited by A. V. Nalbandov, pp. 444–457. University of Illinois, Urbana.
92. Barraclough, C. A., and Sawyer, C. H. (1955): Inhibition of the release of pituitary ovulatory hormone in the rat by morphine. *Endocrinology*, 57:329–337.
93. Fuxe, K., and Hokfelt, T. (1970): Participation of central monoamine neurons in the regulation of anterior pituitary function with special regard to the neuro-endocrine role of tuberoinfundibular dopamine neurons. In: *Aspects of Neuroendocrinology*, edited by W. Bargmann and B. Sharrer, pp. 192–205. Springer, Berlin.
94. Sarkar, D. K., Smith, G. C., and Fink, G. (1981): Effect of manipulating central catecholamines on puberty and the surge of luteinizing hormone and gonadotropin releasing hormone induced by pregnant rare serum gonadotropin in female rats. *Brian Res.*, 213:335–349.
95. Roberts, J. L., Chen, C-L. C., Eberwine, J. H., Evinger, M. J. Q., Gee, C., Herbert, E., and Shacter, B. S. (1982): Glucocorticoid regulation of proopiomelanocortin gene expression in rodent pituitary. *Recent Prog. Horm. Res.*, 38:227–256.
96. Gee, C. E., Chen, C. C., Roberts, J. L., Thompson, R., and Watson, S. J. (1983): Identification of proopiomelanocortin neurones in rat hypothalamus by *in situ* cDNA-mRNA hybridization. *Nature*, 306:374–376.

97. Ferin, M., Van Vugt, D., and Wardlaw, S. (1984): The hypothalamic control of the menstrual cycle and the role of endogenous opioid peptides. *Recent Prog. Horm. Res.*, 40:441–480.
98. Rusak, B., and Zucker, I. (1979): Neural regulation of circadian rhythms. *Physiol. Rev.*, 59:449–526.
99. Horn, A. M., and Fink, G. (1985): Parachlorophenylalanine blocks the spontaneous pro-oestrous surge of prolactin as well as LH and affects the secretion of oestradiol-17β. *J. Endocrinol.*, 104:415–418.
100. Coen, C. W., and Coombs, M. C. (1983): Effects of manipulating catecholamines on the incidence of the preovulatory surge of luteinizing hormone and ovulation in the rat: Evidence for a necessary involvement of hypothalamic adrenaline in the normal or 'midnight' surge. *Neuroscience*, 10:187–206.
101. Akabori, A., and Barraclough, C. A. (1986): Gonadotropin responses to naloxone may depend upon spontaneous activity in noradrenergic neurons at the time of treatment. *Brain Res.*, 362:55–62.
102. Akabori, A., and Barraclough, C. A. (1986): Effects of morphine on luteinizing hormone secretion and catecholamine turnover in the hypothalamus of estrogen-treated rats. *Brain Res.*, 362:221–226.
103. Mitchell, R., Grieve, G., Dow, R., and Fink, G. (1983): Endogenous GABA receptor ligands in hypophysial portal blood. *Neuroendocrinology*, 37:169–176.
104. Negro-Vilar, A., Vijayan, E., and McCann, S. M. (1980): The effect of intraventricular gamma aminobutyric acid (GABA) on hypothalamic catecholamines and LHRH and on pituitary hormone release. *Brain Res. Bull.*, 5:239–244.
105. Vijayan, E., Samson, W. K., Said, S. I., and McCann, S. M. (1979): Vasoactive intestinal peptide (VIP): Evidence for a hypothalamic site of action to release growth hormone, luteinizing hormone and prolactin in conscious ovariectomized rats. *Endocrinology*, 104:53–57.
106. Kerdelhue, B., Tartar, A., Lenoir, V., El Abed, A., Hublau, P., and Millar, R. P. (1985): Binding studies of substance P anterior pituitary binding sites: Changes in substance P binding sites during the rat estrous cycle. *Regul. Pept.*, 10:133–143.
107. McCann, S. M., Samson, W. K., Aguila, M. C., Bedran de Castro, J., Ono, N., Lumpkin, M. D., and Khorram, O. (1986): The role of brain peptides in the control of anterior pituitary hormone secretion. In: *Neuroendocrine Molecular Biology*, edited by G. Fink, A. J. Harmar, and K. W. McKerns, Plenum Press, New York.
108. Clifton, D. K., and Sawyer, C. H. (1980): Positive and negative feedback effects of ovarian steroids on luteinizing hormone release in ovariectomized rats following chronic depletion of hypothalamic norepinephrine. *Endocrinology*, 106:1099–1102.
109. Nicholson, G., Greeley, G., Humm, J., Youngblood, W., and Kizer, J. S. (1978): Lack of effect of noradrenergic denervation of the hypothalamus and the medial preoptic area on the feedback regulation of gonadotropin secretion and the estrous cycle of the rat. *Endocrinology*, 103:559–566.
110. Cross, B. A. (1973): Unit responses in the hypothalamus. In: *Frontiers in Neuroendocrinology*, edited by W. F. Ganong and L. Martini, pp. 133–171. Oxford University Press, Oxford.
111. Hayward, J. N. (1977): Functional and morphological aspects of hypothalamic neurons. *Physiol. Rev.*, 57:574–658.
112. Sherwood, N. M., Chiappa, S. A., and Fink, G. (1976): Immunoreactive luteinizing hormone releasing factor in pituitary stalk blood from female rats; sex steroid modulation of response to electrical stimulation of preoptic area or median eminence. *J. Endocrinol.*, 70:501–511.
113. Yeoman, R. R., and Terasawa, E. (1984): An increase in single unit activity of the medial basal hypothalamus occurs during the progesterone-induced luteinizing hormone surge in the female rhesus monkey. *Endocrinology*, 115:2445–2452.
114. Dyer, R. G. (1973): An electrophysiological dissection of the hypothalamic regions which regulate the pre-ovulatory secretion of luteinizing hormone in the rat. *J. Physiol.*, 234:421–442.
115. Pfaff, D. W. (1983): Impact of estrogens on hypothalamic nerve cells: Ultrastructural, chemical and electrical effects. *Recent Prog. Horm. Res.*, 39:127–175.
116. Tansey, E. M., Arbuthnott, G. W., Fink, G., and Whale, D. (1983): Oestradiol-17β increases the firing rate of antidromically identified neurones of the rat neostriatum. *Neuroendocrinology*, 37:106–110.
117. Fink, G., Aiyer, M., Chiappa, S., Henderson, S., Jamieson, M., Levy-Perez, V., Pickering, A., Sarkar, D., Sherwood, N., Speight, A., and Watts, A. (1982): Gonadotropin-releasing hormone: Release into hypophyseal portal blood and mechanism of action. In: *Hormonally Active Brain Peptides: Structure and Function*, edited by K. McKerns, pp. 397–426. Plenum Press, New York.
118. Yen, S. S. C., Lasley, B. L., Wang, C. F., Leblanc, H., and Siler, T. M. (1975): The operating characteristics of the hypothalamic pituitary system during the menstrual cycle and observations of biological action of somatostatin. *Recent Prog. Horm. Res.*, 31:321–357.
119. Henderson, S. R., Baker, C., and Fink, G. (1977): Oestradiol-17β and pituitary responsiveness to luteinizing hormone releasing factor in the rat; a study using rectangular pulses of oestradiol-17β monitored by nonchromatographic radioimmunoassay. *J. Endocrinol.*, 73:441–453.
120. Vilchez-Martinez, J. A., Arimura, A., Debeljink, L., and Schally, A. V. (1974): Biphasic effect of estradiol benzoate on the pituitary responsiveness to LHRH. *Endocrinology*, 94:1300–1303.
121. Cooper, K. J., Fawcett, C. P., and McCann, S. M. (1974): Inhibitory and facilitatory effects of estradiol-17β on pituitary responsiveness to a luteinizing hormone-follicle stimulating hormone releasing factor (LH-RF/FSH-RF) preparation in the ovariectomized rat. *Proc. Soc. Exp. Biol. Med.*, 145:1422–1426.
122. Aiyer, M. S., Chiappa, S. A., and Fink, G. (1974): A priming effect of luteinizing hormone releasing factor on the anterior pituitary gland in the female rat. *J. Endocrinol.*, 62:573–588.
123. Wang, C. F., Lasley, B. L., Lein, A., and Yen, S. S. C. (1976): The functional changes of the pituitary gonadotrophs during the menstrual cycle. *J. Clin. Endocrinol. Metab.*, 42:718–728.
124. Fink, G., and Pickering, A. J. M. C. (1980): Modulation of pituitary responsiveness to gonadotropin-releasing hormone. In: *Synthesis and Release of Adenohypophyseal Hormones*, edited by M. Jutisz and K. W. McKerns, pp. 617–638. Plenum Press, New York.
125. Aiyer, M. S., and Fink, G. (1974): The role of sex steroid hormones in modulating the responsiveness of the anterior pituitary gland to luteinizing hormone releasing factor in the female rat. *J. Endocrinol.*, 62:553–572.
126. Fink, G., and Henderson, S. R. (1977): Steroids and pituitary responsiveness in female, androgenized female and male rats. *J. Endocrinol.*, 73:157–164.
127. Fink, G. (1977): The hypothalamic pituitary ovarian axis. In: *Recent Advances in Obstetrics and Gynaecology*, 12th ed., edited by J. Stallworthy and G. Bourne, pp. 3–54. Churchill Livingstone, London.
128. Feder, H. H., Brown-Grant, K., and Corker, C. S. (1971): Pre-ovulatory progesterone, the adrenal cortex and the 'critical period' for luteinizing hormone release in rats. *J. Endocrinol.*, 50: 29–39.
129. Drouin, J., and Labrie, F. (1976): Selective effect of androgens on LH and FSH release in anterior pituitary cells in culture. *Endocrinology*, 98:1528–1534.
130. Naftolin, F., Brown-Grant, K., and Corker, C. S. (1972): Plasma and pituitary luteinizing hormone and peripheral plasma oestradiol concentrations in the normal oestrous cycle of the rat and after experimental manipulation of the cycle. *J. Endocrinol.*, 53:17–30.
131. Aiyer, M. S., Sood, M. D., and Brown-Grant, K. (1976): The pituitary response to exogenous luteinizing hormone releasing factor in steroid treated gonadectomized rats. *J. Endocrinol.*, 69:255–262.
132. Sen, K. K., and Menon, K. M. J. (1978): Oestradiol receptors in the rat anterior pituitary gland during the oestrous cycle: Quantitation of receptor activity in relation to gonadotrophin releasing hormone-mediated luteinizing hormone release. *J. Endocrinol.*, 76:211–218.
133. MacLusky, N. J., and McEwen, B. S. (1978): Oestrogen modulates progestin receptor concentrations in some rat brain regions but not in others. *Nature*, 274:276–278.
134. Fink, G., and Henderson, S. R. (1977): Site of modulatory action of oestrogen and progesterone on gonadotrophin response to luteinizing hormone releasing factor. *J. Endocrinol.*, 73:165–170.
135. Hsueh, A. J. W., Erickson, G. F., and Yen, S. S. C. (1978): Sensitization of pituitary cells to luteinizing hormone releasing hormone by clomiphene citrate *in vitro*. *Nature*, 273:57–59.
136. Nakai, Y., Plant, T. M., Hess, D. L., Keogh, E. J., and Knobil, E. (1978): On the sites of the negative and positive feedback actions

of estradiol in the control of gonadotropin secretion in the Rhesus monkey. *Endocrinology,* 102:1008–1014.
137. Speight, A., Popkin, R., Watts, A. G., and Fink, G. (1981): Oestradiol-17β increases pituitary responsiveness by a mechanism that involves the release and the priming effect of luteinizing hormone releasing factor. *J. Endocrinol.,* 88:301–308.
138. Bogdanove, E. M., Nolin, J. M., and Campbell, G. T. (1975): Qualitative and quantitative gonad-pituitary feedback. *Recent Prog. Horm. Res.,* 31:567–619.
139. Goodman, R. L. (1978): The site of the positive feedback action of estradiol in the rat. *Endocrinology,* 102:151–159.
140. Turgeon, J. L., and Barraclough, C. A. (1974): Further studies of the hypothalamo-hypophysial-gonadal axis of the androgen-sterilized rat. In: *Endocrinolgie sexuelle de la periode perinatale,* edited by M. G. Forrest and J. Bertrand, pp. 339–356. INSERM, Paris.
141. Harris, G. W. (1970): Hormonal differentiation of the developing central nervous system with respect to patterns of endocrine function. *Philos. Trans. R. Soc. Lond. (Biol.),* 259:165–177.
142. Brown-Grant, K. (1973): In: *Foetal and Neonatal Physiology,* edited by R. S. Comline, K. W. Cross, G. S. Dawes, and P. W. Nathanielsz, pp. 527–545 (Proceedings of The Sir Joseph Barcroft Centenary Symposium held at Cambridge, 25–27 July 1972), Cambridge University Press, Cambridge.
143. Aiyer, M. S., Fink, G., and Grieg, F. (1974): Changes in the sensitivity of the pituitary gland to luteinizing hormone releasing factor during the oestrous cycle of the rat. *J. Endocrinol.,* 60:47–64.
144. Meidan, R., Fink, G., and Koch, Y. (1981): Ontogeny of the sensitizing effect of oestradiol and luteinizing hormone releasing hormone on the anterior pituitary gland of the female rat. *J. Endocrinol.,* 91:347–351.
145. Fink, G., Chiappa, S. A., and Aiyer, M. S. (1976): Priming effect of luteinizing hormone releasing factor elicited by preoptic stimulation and by intravenous infusion and multiple injections of the synthetic decapeptide. *J. Endocrinol.,* 69:359–372.
146. Fink, G. (1976): The development of the releasing factor concept. *Clin. Endocrinol.,* 5(Suppl.):245–260.
147. Knobil, E. (1980): The neuroendocrine control of the menstrual cycle. *Recent Prog. Horm. Res.,* 36:53–88.
148. Knobil, E. (1987): Chapter 47, these volumes.
149. Pickering, A. J. M. C., and Fink, G. (1976): Priming effect of luteinizing hormone releasing factor; *in vitro* and *in vivo* evidence consistent with its dependence upon protein and RNA synthesis. *J. Endocrinol.,* 69:373–379.
150. Pickering, A. J. M. C., and Fink, G. (1979): Priming effect of luteinizing hormone releasing factor *in vitro:* Role of protein synthesis, contractile elements, Ca^{2+} and cyclic AMP. *J. Endocrinol.,* 81:223–234.
151. Waring, D. W., and Turgeon, J. L. (1980): Luteinizing hormone-releasing hormone-induced luteinizing hormone secretion *in vitro:* Cyclic changes in responsiveness and self-priming. *Endocrinology,* 106:1430–1436.
152. Turgeon, J. L., and Waring, D. W. (1981): Acute progesterone and 17β-estradiol modulation of luteinizing hormone secretion by pituitaries of cycling rats superfused *in vitro. Endocrinology,* 108:413–419.
153. Curtis, A., Lyons, V., and Fink, G. (1985): The priming effect of LH-releasing hormone: Effects of cold and involvement of new protein synthesis. *J. Endocrinol.,* 105:163–168.
154. Hubert, J-F., de Monti, M., and Duval, J. (1985): Le LHRH stimule la secretion d'une proteine 87 K par les cellules gonadotropes en culture. *C. R. Acad. Sci. (Paris),* 300:613–616.
155. Lewis, C. E., Morris, J. F., and Fink, G. (1985): The role of microfilaments in the priming effect of LH-releasing hormone: An ultrastructural study using cytochalasin B. *J. Endocrinol.,* 106:211–218.
156. Pickering, A. J. M. C., and Fink, G. (1979): Variation in size of the 'readily releasable pool' of luteinizing hormone during the oestrous cycle of the rat. *J. Endocrinol.,* 83:53–59.
157. Savoy-Moore, R. T., Schwartz, N. B., Duncan, J. A., and Marshall, J. C. (1980): Pituitary gonadotropin releasing hormone receptors during the rat estrous cycle. *Science,* 209:942–944.
158. Clayton, R. N., Solano, A. R., Garcia-Vela, A., Dufau, M. L., and Catt, K. J. (1980): Regulation of pituitary receptors for gonadotropin-releasing hormone during the rat estrous cycle. *Endocrinology,* 107:699–706.
159. Clayton, R. N., and Catt, K. J. (1981): Gonadotropin-releasing hormone receptors: Characterization, physiological regulation and relationship to reproductive function. *Endocr. Rev.,* 2:186–209.
160. Smith, S. S., and Ojeda, S. R. (1985): Estradiol induced LH release in juvenile female rats: Nembutal blocks both the decline and the exposure of nonavailable pituitary LHRH receptor sites. *Neuroendocrinology,* 41:246–251.
161. Clayton, R. N., Naik, S. I., Young, L. S., and Charlton, H. M. (1984): Physiological regulation of pituitary GnRH receptors. In: *Hormonal Control of the Hypothalamo-Pituitary-Gonadal Axis,* edited by K. W. McKerns and Z. Naor, pp. 141–151. Plenum Press, New York.
162. Clayton, R. N., Young, L. S., Naik, S. I., Detta, A., and Abbot, S. D. (1986): Pituitary GnRH receptors—Recent studies and their functional significance. In: *Neuroendocrine Molecular Biology,* edited by G. Fink, A. J. Harmar, and K. W. McKerns. Plenum Press, New York.
163. Catt, K. J., Harwood, J. P., Aguilera, G., and Dufau, M. L. (1979): Hormonal regulation of peptide receptors and target cell responses. *Nature,* 280:109–116.
164. Speight, A., and Fink, G. (1981): Changes in responsiveness of dispersed pituitary cells to luteinizing hormone releasing hormone at different times of the oestrous cycle of the rat. *J. Endocrinol.,* 89:129–134.
165. Daane, T. A., and Parlow, A. F. (1971): Periovulatory patterns of rat serum follicle-stimulating hormone and luteinizing hormone during the normal estrous cycle: Effects of pentobarbital. *Endocrinology,* 88:653–663.
166. Swerdloff, R. S., Walsh, P. C., Jacobs, H. S., and Odell, W. D. (1971): Serum LH and FSH during sexual maturation in the male rat: Effects of castration and cryptorchidism. *Endocrinology,* 88:120–128.
167. Chiappa, S. A., and Fink, G. (1977): Releasing factor and hormonal changes in the hypothalamic-pituitary-gonadtrophin and -adrenocorticotrophin systems before and after birth and puberty in male, female and androgenized female rats. *J. Endocrinol.,* 72:211–224.
168. Brown-Grant, K., Fink, G., Greig, F., and Murray, M. A. F. (1975): Altered sexual development in male rats after oestrogen administration during the neonatal period. *J. Reprod. Fertil.,* 44:25–42.
169. Zanisi, M., Motta, M., and Martini, L. (1973): Recent findings of the physiology of the gonadotropin-releasing factors. In: *Hypothalamic Hypophysiotropic Hormones,* edited by C. Gual and E. Rosenberg, pp. 24–32. Excerpta Medica, Amsterdam.
170. Bowers, C. Y., Chang, J. K., and Folkers, K. (1973): Studies on the LH and FSH releasing activity of the hypothalamic hormone, P·Glu-His-Trp-Ser-Tyr-Gly-Leu-Arg-Pro-Gly-HH_2 (decapaptide), its analogs and other small peptides. In: *Hypothalamic Hypophysiotropic Hormones,* edited by C. Gual and E. Rosenberg, pp. 68–88. Excerpta Medica, Amsterdam.
171. Jaffe, R. B., Lee, P. A., and Midgley, A. R. Jr. (1969): Serum gonadotropins before, at the inception of, and following human pregnancy. *J. Clin. Endocrinol. Metab.,* 29:1281–1283.
172. Parlow, A. F., Daane, T. A., and Dignam, W. J. (1970): On the concentrations of radioimmunoassayable FSH circulating in blood throughout human pregnancy. *J. Clin. Endocrinol. Metab.* 31:213–214.
173. Nillius, S. J., and Wide, L. (1971): Induction of a midcycle-like peak of luteinizing hormone in young women by exogenous oestradiol-17β. *J. Obstet. Gynaecol. Br. Commonwealth,* 78:822–827.
174. Jamieson, M. G., and Fink, G. (1976): Parameters of electrical stimulation of the medial preoptic area for release of gonadotropins in male rats. *J. Endocrinol.,* 68:57–70.
175. Lumpkin, M. D., and McCann, S. M. (1984): Effect of destruction of the dorsal anterior hypothalamus on follicle-stimulating hormone secretion in the rat. *Endocrinology,* 115:2473–2480.
176. Schally, A. V., Kastin, A. J., and Arimura, A. (1972): FSH-releasing hormone and LH-releasing hormone. *Vitam. Horm.,* 30:83–164.
177. Charlton, H. M., Halpin, D. M. G., Iddon, C., Rosie, R., Levy, G., McDowell, I. F. W., Megson, A., Morris, J. F., Bramwell, A., Speight, A., Ward, B. J., Broadhead, J., Davey-Smith, G., and Fink, G. (1983): The effects of daily administration of single and

multiple injections of gonadotropin-releasing hormone on pituitary and gonadal function in the hypogonadal *(hpg)* mouse. *Endocrinology,* 113:535–544.

178. Brown-Grant, K., and Greig, F. (1975): A comparison of changes in the peripheral plasma concentrations of luteinizing hormone and follicle stimulating hormone in the rat. *J. Endocrinol.,* 65:389–397.
179. Yen, S. S. C., Rebar, R., Vandenberg, G., Naftolin, F., Ehara, Y., Englbom, S., Ryan, K. J., Benirscke, K., Rivier, J., Amoss, M., and Guillemin, R. (1972): Synthetic luteinsing hormone-releasing factor: A potent stimulator of gonadotropin in man. *J. Clin. Endocrinol. Metab.,* 34:1108–1111.
180. Yen, S. S. C., Vandenberg, G., Rebar, R., and Ehara, Y. (1972): Variation of pituitary responsiveness to synthetic LRF during different phases of the menstrual cycle. *J. Clin. Endocrinol. Metab.,* 35:931–934.
181. Stearns, E. L., Winter, J. S. D., and Fairman, C. (1973): *J. Clin. Endocrinol. Metab.,* 37:635–638.
182. Sawyer, C. H. (1975): Some recent developments in brain-pituitary-ovarian physiology. *Neuroendocrinology,* 17:97–124.
183. Brown-Grant, K., El Kabir, D. J., and Fink, G. (1968): The effect of mating on pituitary luteinizing hormone and thyrotrophic hormone content in the female rabbit. *J. Endocrinol.,* 41:91–94.
184. Scaramuzzi, R. J., Blake, C. A., Papkoff, H., Hilliard, J., and Sawyer, C. H. (1972): Radioimmunoassay of rabbit luteinizing hormone: Serum levels during various reproductive states. *Endocrinology,* 90:1285–1291.
185. Dufy-Barbe, L., Franchimont, P., and Faure, J. M. A. (1973): Time courses of LH and FSH release after mating in the female rabbit. *Endocrinology,* 92:1318–1321.
186. Fink, G., Smith, G. C., McMaster, R., Osborne, L. W., and Chiappa, S. A. (1975): The catecholamine-containing tubero-infundibular system and the control of luteinizing hormone release in the rabbit. *Brain Res.,* 89:71–80.
187. Goodman, A. L., and Neill, J. D. (1976): Ovarian regulation of postcoital gonadotropin release in the rabbit: Reexamination of a functional role for 20α dihydroprogesterone. *Endocrinology,* 99:852–860.
188. Hayward, J. W., Hilliard, J., and Sawyer, C. H. (1964): Time of release of pituitary gonadotropin induced by electrical stimulation of the rabbit brain. *Endocrinology,* 74:108–113.
189. Kanematsu, S., Scaramuzzi, R. J., Hilliard, J., and Sawyer, C. H. (1974): Patterns of ovulation-inducing LH release following coitus, electrical stimulation and exogenous LH-RH in the rabbit. *Endocrinology,* 95:247–252.
190. Tsou, R. C., Dailey, R. A., McLanahan, C. S., Parent, A. D., Tindall, G. T., and Neill, J. D. (1977): Luteinizing hormone releasing hormone (LHRH) levels in pituitary stalk plasma during the preovulatory gonadotropin surge of rabbits. *Endocrinology,* 101:534–539.
191. Hilliard, J., Penardi, R., and Sawyer, C. H. (1967): A functional role for 20α-hydroxypregn-4-en-3-one in the rabbit. *Endocrinology,* 80:901–909.
192. Sawyer, C. H., Hilliard, J., Kanematsu, S., Scaramuzzi, R., and Blake, C. A. (1974): Effects of intraventricular infusions of norepinephrine and dopamine on LH release and ovulation in the rabbit. *Neuroendocrinology,* 15:328–337.
193. Critchlow, V. (1963): The role of light in the neuroendocrine system. In: *Advances in Neuroendocrinology,* edited by A. V. Nalbandov, pp. 337–402. University of Illinois Press, Urbana.
194. Watts, A. G., and Fink, G. (1981): Effects of short-term constant light on the proestrous luteinizing hormone surge and pituitary responsiveness in the female rat. *Neuroendocrinology,* 33:176–180.
195. Watts, A. G., and Fink, G. (1985): Effects of progesterone on the pituitary responsiveness to, and the priming effect of, luteinizing hormone releasing hormone in female rats exposed to constant light. *Neuroendocrinology,* 40:152–159.
196. Brown-Grant, K., Davidson, J. M., and Greig, F. (1973): Induced ovulation in albino rats exposed to constant light. *J. Endocrinol.,* 57:7–22.
197. Smith, E. R., and Davidson, J. M. (1974): Luteinizing hormone releasing factor in rats exposed to constant light: Effects of mating. *Neuroendocrinology,* 14:129–138.
198. Watts, A. G., and Fink, G. (1984): Pulsatile luteinizing hormone release, and the inhibitory effects of estradiol-17β in gonadectomized male and female rats: Effects of neonatal androgen or exposure to constant light. *Endocrinology,* 115:2251–2259.
199. Brown-Grant, K., and Raisman, G. (1977): Abnormalities in reproductive function associated with the destruction of the suprachiasmatic nuclei in female rats. *Proc. R. Soc. Lond. (Biol.),* 198:279–296.
200. Charlton, H. M., Naftolin, F., Sood, M. C., and Worth, R. W. (1975): The effect of mating upon LH release in male and female voles of the species *Microtus agrestis. J. Reprod. Fertil.,* 42:167–170.
201. Gray, G. D., Davis, H. N., Kenney, A. McM., and Dewsbury, D. A. (1976): Effects of mating on plasma levels of LH and progesterone in Montana voles *(Microtus montanus). J. Reprod. Fertil.,* 47:89–91.
202. Versi, E., Chiappa, S. A., Fink, G., and Charlton, H. M. (1982): Effect of copulation on the hypothalamic content of gonadotrophic hormone-releasing hormone in the vole, *Microtus agrestis. J. Reprod. Fertil.,* 64:491–494.
203. Sutherland, R. C., Fink, G., and Charlton, H. M. (1984): Effect of mating on the metabolic activity of the brain and pituitary gland assessed by [^{14}C]2-deoxyglucose in a reflex ovulator, the vole *(Microtus agretis). Brain Res.,* 311:317–322.
204. Sakuma, Y., and Pfaff, D. W. (1983): Modulation of the lordosis reflex of female rats by LHRH, its antiserum and analogs in the mesencephalic central gray. *Neuroendocrinology,* 36:218–224.
205. Steinberger, A., and Ward, D. N. (1987): Inhibin. Chapter 15, these volumes.
206. Plant, T. M., Nakai, Y., Belchetz, P., Keogh, E., and Knobil, E. (1978): The sites of action of estradiol and phentolamine in the inhibition of the pulsatile, circhoral discharges of LH in the Rhesus monkey *(Macaca mulatta). Endocrinology,* 102:1015–1018.
207. Sarkar, D. K., and Fink, G. (1980): Luteinizing hormone releasing factor in pituitary stalk plasma from long-term ovariectomized rats: Effects of steroids. *J. Endocrinol.,* 86:511–524.
208. Carmel, P. W., Araki, S., and Ferin, M. (1976): Pituitary stalk portal blood collection in Rhesus monkeys: Evidence for pulsatile release of gonadotropin-releasing hormone (GnRH). *Endocrinology,* 99:243–248.
208a. Dierschke, D. J., Bhattacharya, A. N., Atkinson, L. E., and Knobil, E. (1970): Circhoral oscillations of plasma LH levels in the ovariectomized rhesus monkey. *Endocrinology* 87:850–853.
209. Gay, V. L., and Sheth, N. A. (1972): Evidence for a periodic release of LH in castrated male and female rats. *Endocrinology* 90:158–162.
210. Yen, S. S. C., Tsai, C. C., Naftolin, F., Vandenberg, G., and Ajabor, L. (1972): Pulsatile patterns of gonadotropin release in subjects with and without ovarian function. *J. Clin. Endocrinol. Metab.,* 34:671–675.
211. Blake, C. A., and Sawyer, C. H. (1974): Effects of hypothalamic deafferentation on the pulsatile rhythm in plasma concentrations of luteinizing hormone in ovariectomized rats. *Endocrinology,* 94:730–736.
212. Fox, S. R., and Smith, M. S. (1985): Changes in the pulsatile pattern of luteinizing hormone secretion during the rat estrous cycle. *Endocrinology,* 116:1485–1492.
213. Mortimer, C. H., Besser, G. M., Hook, J., and McNeilly, A. S. (1974): Intravenous, intramuscular, subcutaneous and intranasal administration of LH/FSH-RH: The duration of effect and occurrence of asynchronous pulsatile release of LH and FSH. *Clin. Endocrinol.,* 3:19–25.
214. Crowley, W. F. Jr., Filicari, M., Spratt, D. I., and Santaro, N. F. (1985): The physiology of gonadotropin-releasing hormone (GnRH) secretion in men and women. *Recent Prog. Horm. Res.,* 41:473–526.
215. Lincoln, G. A., and Short, R. V. (1980): Seasonal breeding: Nature's contraceptive. *Recent Prog. Horm. Res.,* 36:1–43.
216. Boyar, R. M., Finkelstein, J., Roffwarg, H., Kapen, S., Weitzman, E. D., and Hellman, L. (1973): Twenty-four-hour luteinising hormone and follicle-stimulating hormone secretory patterns in gonadal dysgenesis. *J. Clin. Endocrinol. Metab.,* 37:521–525.
217. Clarke, I. J., and Cummins, J. T. (1982): The temporal relationship between gonadotropin releasing hormone (GnRH) and luteinizing

hormone (LH) secretion in ovariectomized ewes. *Endocrinology*, 111:1737–1739.

218. Steiner, R. A., Bremner, W. J., and Clifton, D. K. (1982): Regulation of luteinizing hormone pulse frequency and amplitude by testosterone in the adult male rat. *Endocrinology*, 111:2055–2061.
219. Plant, T. M., and Dubey, A. K. (1984): Evidence from the rhesus monkey *(Macaca mulatta)* for the view that negative feedback control of luteinizing hormone secretion by the testis is mediated by a deceleration of hypothalamic gonadotropin-releasing hormone pulse frequency. *Endocrinology*, 115:2145–2153.
220. Schuiling, G. A., and Gnodde, H. P. (1976): Secretion of luteinizing hormone caused by continuous infusions of luteinizing hormone releasing hormone in the long-term ovariectomized rat: Effect of oestrogen pretreatment. *J. Endocrinology*, 71:1–11.
221. Sandow, J., von Rechenberg, W., Jerzabek, G., Engelbort, K., Kuhl, H., and Fraser, H. (1980): Hypothalamic-pituitary-testicular functions in rats after supraphysiological doses of highly active LRH analogue (buserelin). *Acta Endocrinol.* 94:489–497.
222. Schuiling, G. A., Pols-Valkhof, N., van der Schaaf-Verdonk, G. C. J., and Koiter, T. R. (1984): Blockade of LH and FSH secretion by LH-releasing hormone, by the LH-releasing hormone analogue, buserelin, and by combined treatment with LH-releasing hormone and oestradiol benzoate. *J. Endocrinol.*, 103:301–309.
223. Naor, Z., Amsterdam, A., and Catt, K. J. (1984): Binding and activation of gonadotrophin-releasing hormone receptors in pituitary gonadotrophs. In: *Hormone Receptors in Growth and Reproduction*, edited by B. B. Saxena et al., pp. 1–19. Raven Press, New York.
224. Brown-Grant, K. (1969): The effects of progesterone and of pentobarbitone administered at the dioestrous stage on the ovarian cycle of the rat. *J. Endocrinol.*, 43:539–552.
225. Bogumil, R. J. (1977): The human menstrual cycle. In: *Endocrinology, Vol. 1*, edited by V. H. T. James, pp. 250–255 (International Congress Series, No. 402). Excerpta Medica, Amsterdam.
226. McCann, S. M. (1962): Effect of progesterone on plasma luteinizing hormone activity. *Am. J. Physiol.*, 202:601–604.
227. Goodman, R. L. (1978): A quantitative analysis of the physiological role of estradiol and progesterone in the control of tonic and surge secretion of luteinizing hormone in the rat. *Endocrinology*, 102:142–150.
228. Hauger, R. L., Karsch, F. J., and Foster, D. L. (1977): A new concept for control of the estrous cycle of the ewe based on the temporal relationship between luteinizing hormone, estradiol and progesterone in peripheral serum and evidence that progesterone inhibits tonic LH secretion. *Endocrinology*, 101:807–817.
229. Van Look, P. F. A. (1976): Failure of positive feedback. *Clin. Obstet. Gynaecol.*, 3:555–578.
230. Weber, R. F. A., de Greef, W. J., de Koning, J., and Vreeburg, J. T. M. (1983): LH-RH and dopamine levels in hypophysial stalk plasma and their relationship to plasma gonadotrophins and prolactin levels in male rats bearing an prolactin- and adrenocorticotrophin-secreting pituitary tumor. *Neuroendocrinology*, 36:205–210.
231. Yen, S. S. C., and Lein, G. E. (1984): Mammals: Man. In: *Marshall's Physiology of Reproduction, Vol. 1*, 4th ed., edited by G. E. Lamming, pp. 713–788. Churchill Livingstone, Edinburgh.
232. Brar, A. K., McNeilly, A. S., and Fink, G. (1985): Effects of hyperprolactinaemia and testosterone on the release of LH-releasing hormone and the gonadotrophins in intact and castrated rats. *J. Endocrinol.*, 104:35–43.
233. Cheung, C. Y. (1983): Prolactin suppresses luteinizing hormone secretion and pituitary responsiveness to luteinizing hormone-releasing hormone by a direct action at the anterior pituitary. *Endocrinology*, 113:632–638.
234. Lu, K. H., Chen, H. T., Grandison, L., Huang, H. H., and Meites, J. (1976): Reduced luteinizing hormone-releasing hormone (LHRH) in postpartum lactating rats. *Endocrinology*, 98:1235–1240.
235. Marchetti, B., and Labrie, F. (1982): Prolactin inhibits pituitary luteinizing hormone-releasing hormone receptors in the rat. *Endocrinology*, 111:1209–1216.
236. McNeilly, A. S., Sharpe, R. M., and Fraser, H. M. (1983): Increased sensitivity to the negative feedback effects of testosterone induced by hyperprolactinaemia in the adult male rat. *Endocrinology*, 112:22–28.
237. Smith, M. S. (1982): Effect of pulsatile gonadotropin-releasing hormone on the release of luteinizing hormone and follicle-stimulating hormone *in vitro* by anterior pituitaries from lactating and cycling rats. *Endocrinology*, 110:882–891.
238. Smith, M. S. (1985): Release of luteinizing hormone and follicle-stimulating hormone from pituitaries of lactating rats by gonadotropin-releasing hormone and high potassium concentration. *Endocrinology*, 116:1826–1834.
239. Lewis, C. E., Fink, G., Dow, R. C., and Morris, J. F. (1986): Hyperprolactinaemia induced by pituitary isografts suppresses the priming effect of LH-releasing hormone in normal and hypogonadal mice. *Neuroendocinology*, 43:584–589.
240. Leong, D. A., Frawley, L. S., and Neill, J. D. (1983): Neuroendocrine control of prolactin secretion. *Annu. Rev. Physiol.*, 45:109–127.
241. Neill, J. D. (1987): Prolactin secretion and its control. Chapter 33, these volumes.
242. Hazum, E. (1982): GnRH-receptor of rat pituitary is a glycoprotein: Differential effect of neuraminidase and lectins on agonists and antagonists binding. *Mol. Cell. Endocrinol.*, 26:217–222.
243. Berridge, M. J., and Irvine, R. F. (1984): Inositol triphosphate, a novel second messenger in cellular signal transduction. *Nature*, 312:315–321.
244. Nishizuka, Y., Takai, Y., Kishimoto, A., Kikkawa, U., and Kaibuchi, K. (1984): Phospholipid turnover in hormone action. *Recent Prog. Horm. Res.*, 40:301–341.
245. Truneh, A., Albert, F., Golstein, P., and Schmitt-Verhulst, A-M. (1985): Early steps of lymphocyte activation bypassed by synergy between calcium ionophores and phorbol ester. *Nature*, 313:318–320.
246. Wolf, M., Le Vine, H. III, May, W. S. Jr., Cuatrecasas, P., and Sakyoun, N. (1985): A model for intracellular translocation of protein kinase C involving synergism between Ca^{2+} and phorbol esters. *Nature*, 317:546–549.
247. Burn, P., Rotman, A., Meyer, R. K., and Burger, M. M. (1985): Diacylglycerol in large α-actinin/actin complexes and in the cytoskeleton of activated platelets. *Nature*, 314:469–472.
248. Lassing, I., and Lindberg, U. (1985): Specific interaction between phosphatidylinositol 4,5-biphosphate and profilactin. *Nature*, 314:472–474.
249. DeRiemer, S. A., Strong, J. A., Albert, K. A., Greengard, P., and Kaczmarek, L. K. (1985): Enhancement of calcium current in *Aplysia* neurones by phorbol ester and protein kinase C. *Nature*, 313:313–316.
250. Conn, P. M., Marian, J., McMillan, M., Stern, J. E., Rogers, D. R., Hamby, M., Penna, A., and Grant, E. (1981): Gonadotropin-releasing hormone action in the pituitary: A three step mechanism. *Endocr. Rev.*, 2:174–185.
251. Conn, P. M., Rogers, D. C., and Seay, S. G. (1983): Structure-function relationship of calcium ion channel antagonists at the pituitary gonadotrope. *Endocrinology*, 113:1592–1595.
252. Catt, K. J., Loumaye, E., Wynn, P., Suarez-Quian, C., Kiesel, L., Iwashuta, M., Hirota, K., Morgan, R., and Chang, J. (1984): Receptor-mediated activation mechanisms in the hypothalamic control of pituitary-gonadal function. In: *Endocrinology*, edited by F. Labrie and L. Proulx (International Congress Series, No. 655). Excerpta Medica, Amsterdam.
253. Mason, W. T., and Waring, D. W. (1985): Electrophysiological recording from gonadotrophs: Evidence for Ca^{2+} channels mediated by gonadotrophin-releasing hormone. *Neuroendocrinology*, 41:258–268.
254. Fink, G., Sheward, W. J., and Plant, T. M. (1984): The hypogonadal mouse pituitary contains bioactive LH. *J. Reprod. Fertil.*, 70:277–280.
255. Fink, G., and Smith, G. C. (1971): Ultrastructural features of the developing hypothalamo-hypophysial axis in the rat: A correlative study. *Z. Zellforsch.*, 119:208–226.
256. Liu, T.-C., and Jackson, G. L. (1979): Comparison of the biosynthesis and release of luteinizing hormone by rat pituitaries *in vitro* in response to gonadotropin-releasing hormone analogs. *Endocrinology*, 104:962–966.
257. Liu, T.-C., and Jackson, G. L. (1978): Modifications of luteinizing hormone biosynthesis and release by gonadotropin-releasing hormone, cycloheximide and actinomycin D. *Endocrinology*, 103:1253–1263.
258. Azhar, J., Reel, J. R., Pastushok, C. A., and Menon, K. M. J.

(1978): LH biosynthesis and secretion in rat anterior pituitary cell cultures: Stimulation of LH glycosylation and secretion by GnRH and an agonistic analogue and blockade by an antagonistic analogue. *Biochem. Biophys. Res. Commun.*, 80:659–666.
259. Singh, P., Bhalla, V. K., and Muldoon, T. G. (1985): Apparent lack of involvement of cAMP as a mediator of LHRH stimulation of nuclear estrogen receptor activity in the rat anterior pituitary. *Neuroendocrinology,* 40:430–437.
260. Mitchell, R., Ogier, S-A., Johnson, M., Cleland, A., Bennie, J., and Fink, G. (1986): Evidence for sex differences in GnRH receptors and mechanism of action. In: *Neuroendocrine Molecular Biology,* edited by G. Fink, A. J. Harmar, and K. W. McKerns. Plenum Press, New York.
261. Neill, J. D., and Frawley, L. S. (1983): Detection of hormone release from individual cells in mixed populations using a reverse haemolytic plaque assay. *Endocrinology,* 112:1135–1137.
262. Smith, P. F., Frawley, L. S., and Neill, J. D. (1984): Detection of LH release from individual cells by the reverse haemolytic plaque assay: Estrogen increases the fraction of gonadotropes responding to GnRH. *Endocrinology*, 115:2484–2486.
263. McDowell, I. F. W., Morris, J. F., Charlton, H. M., and Fink, G. (1982): Effects of luteinizing hormone releasing hormone on the gonadotrophs of hypogonadal (*hpg*) mice. *J. Endocrinol.*, 95:331–340.
264. Purves, H. D. (1966): Cytology of the adenohypophysis. In: *The Pituitary Gland, Vol. 1*, edited by G. W. Harris and B. J. Donovan, pp. 147–232. Butterworths, London.
265. Speight, A., and Fink, G. (1981): Comparison of steroid and LH-RH effects on the responsiveness of hemipituitary glands and dispersed pituitary cells. *Mol. Cell. Biol.*, 24:267–281.
266. Padmanabhan, V., Kesner, J. S., and Convey, E. M. (1981): A priming effect of luteinizing hormone releasing hormone on bovine pituitary cells *in vitro*. *J. Anim. Sci.,* 52:1137–1142.
267. Padmanabhan, V., Leung, K., and Convey, E. M. (1982): Ovarian steroids modulate the self-priming effect of luteinizing hormone-releasing hormone on bovine pituitary cells *in vitro*. *Endocrinology*, 110:717–721.
268. Mason, A. J., Hayflick, J. S., Zoeller, R. T., Scott-Young, W., Phillips, H. S., Nikolics, K., and Seeburg, P. H. (1986): A deletion truncating the gonadotropin-releasing hormone gene is responsible for hypogonadism in the *hpg* mouse. *Science,* 234:1366–1381.
269. Mobbs, C. V., and Pfaff, D. W. (1987): Estrogen-regulated behaviour: possible roles of synaptosomal secretory-vesicle-uncoating protein, enkephalin and protein kinase. In *Brain and Female Reproductive Function: Basic and Clinical Aspects,* edited by A. R. Genazzani (in press).

The Physiology of Reproduction,
edited by E. Knobil and J. Neill *et al.*
Raven Press, Ltd., New York © 1988.

CHAPTER 33

Prolactin Secretion and Its Control

Jimmy D. Neill

INTRODUCTION

Prolactin is the most versatile pituitary hormone in both the number and diversity of physiological processes it regulates (1,2). The decisive role it plays in the preparation, maintenance, and secretory activity of the mammary gland during lactation is of utmost importance (2). Indeed, prolactin is essential to the survival of most mammalian young after birth. During lactation, the stimulus for prolactin secretion is triggered as the young suckle the mother's nipple. Neural impulses generated by suckling are conveyed to the central nervous system, where they impinge upon specialized secretory neurons located in the hypothalamus. These neurons release the hypophysiotropic hormones into the hypophyseal portal vessels that connect the nervous system and the adenohypophysis. Thus the neurogenic message engendered by suckling is finally conveyed to the pituitary in the form of hypophysiotropic hormones that stimulate or inhibit prolactin secretion (2).

This account of prolactin secretion and its control will emphasize the hypophysiotropic control of suckling-induced prolactin secretion. Such a restricted view is taken because lactation is the only well-studied function of prolactin that is universal in mammals. The role of prolactin as a stimulator of progesterone secretion, although well studied, is probably restricted to rodents and perhaps to a few other species. A definitive physiological role for prolactin released in response to stress, though ubiquitous, is not established.

HYPOTHALAMIC CONTROL

Background

The development of the neurohumoral hypothesis for hypothalamic control of adenohypophysial secretion by Geoffrey Harris and colleagues (3) led to the expectation that prolactin secretion would be regulated by a stimulatory hypothalamic hypophysiotropic factor. Nevertheless, Everett (4,5) demonstrated that separation of the pituitary gland from the hypothalamus was sufficient by itself to initiate a prolonged elevation of prolactin secretion, as evidenced by the induction and maintenance of an essentially permanent pseudopregnancy in the rat. Everett (4,5) postulated the existence of a factor in the hypothalamus that was released into the hypophyseal portal blood to inhibit prolactin secretion. Subsequently, Pasteels and colleagues (6,7) showed that hypothalamic pieces or extracts reduced the release of prolactin from pituitary glands incubated *in vitro*. Soon thereafter, Meites and colleagues (8,9) confirmed the existence of a prolactin-inhibiting factor (PIF) and demonstrated that the active substance in hypothalamic extracts was not identical with neurohumoral agents thought to reside in the brain. Based on the observations that drugs disrupting catecholamine metabolism altered prolactin secretion (10–13) and that dopamine was present in the median eminence in high concentrations (14), several investigators found that dopamine inhibited prolactin release from the pituitary gland (15,16). MacLeod, in particular, championed this view and provided much experimental evidence to support dopamine as the PIF (17). Acceptance of a nonpeptidic hypothalamic-inhibiting factor (dopamine) was delayed (a) by the bias that PIF should be peptidic since other hypophysiotropic factors were peptides, (b) by the numerous reports that such peptide PIFs existed, and (c) by the fact that large doses of dopamine seemed to be required for inhibition of prolactin secretion.

Control of Spontaneous Prolactin Secretion

The secretion of prolactin is viewed as being spontaneous (i.e., occurs without stimulation by the hypothalamus) (2) since prolactin secretion occurs at a high rate for prolonged periods when the pituitary gland is transplanted to a site distant from the hypothalamus or when cultured *in vitro* (18,19). *In vivo,* prolactin secretion appears to be severely restrained by the hypothalamus, since serum prolactin levels remain low in the absence of prolactin-releasing stimuli (19). A large amount of work has established that dopamine is the hypothalamic hypophysiotropic agent that holds spontaneous prolactin secretion in check (17,19,20). This work includes the demonstration that spontaneous prolactin secretion is inhibited by small amounts of dopamine (21,22), that dopamine receptors are present on lactotropes (23–25), and that dopamine is secreted into hypophysial stalk blood in amounts sufficient to inhibit prolactin release (26–29).

Is dopamine sufficient to account for the inhibition of prolactin secretion to the levels normally observed in animals in the basal state, or do other PIFs exist? In early studies of this issue, investigators reported that the amount of dopamine in stalk blood was sufficient to account for only about two-thirds of the prolactin inhibition normally observed (19,27,30). This conclusion was based on quantitative studies in which dopamine was infused into rats depleted of endogenous dopamine with the false neurotransmitter, α-methyl-*p*-tyrosine; the rate of dopamine infusion was set to mimic the levels measured in stalk blood (19). However, subsequent developments strongly suggest that such studies failed to account for an important dopamine contribution to the anterior pituitary gland from the posterior pituitary gland reaching the adenohypophysis by way of the short portal vessels (20,31–33). Such dopamine would not be present in pituitary stalk blood; i.e., dopamine concentrations reaching the adenohypophysis apparently were underestimated. Removal of the posterior pituitary gland elevates basal prolactin secretion, which can be blocked by dopamine treatment (32–35). Consistent with this finding is the report that electrochemically detectable dopamine in the anterior pituitary gland is reduced after surgical removal of the posterior lobe (36). Subsequent surgical sectioning of the hypophysial stalk reduced the electrochemical signal representing dopamine to low levels as did treatment with α-methyl-*p*-tyrosine; amounts of dopamine given by infusion that were sufficient to inhibit the elevated prolactin levels were also sufficient to return the dopamine levels in the anterior pituitary to pretreatment levels (36). Thus, dopamine of hypothalamic origin which is delivered to the adenohypophysis by way of the long and the short portal vessels seems quantitatively sufficient to account for inhibition of prolactin release.

Despite the seeming sufficiency of dopamine to fully inhibit prolactin release, other PIFs have been reported to exist, but their physiologic role remains undetermined. γ-Aminobutyric acid (GABA) directly inhibits the release of prolactin (37–39), its receptors are present on adenohypophysial cells (40,41), and GABA-containing neurons are present in the median eminence (42,43); these findings require consideration of GABA in the economy of prolactin secretion. GABA appears to be a secretory product of the median eminence, at least during electrical stimulation of the hypothalamus (44); basal secretion of GABA into hypophysial stalk blood has been reported to occur (44) or not occur (45) depending on the source. At all events, micromolar quantities are required to inhibit prolactin release *in vitro* (38,39). Thus, a role for GABA in regulating prolactin secretion cannot be rationalized at present.

Another reported PIF is gonadotropin-releasing-hormone-associated peptide (GAP) (46). This 56-amino-acid peptide is the carboxy-terminal portion of the peptide precursor for gonadotropin-releasing hormone (GnRH), which itself resides in the amino-terminal 10 amino acids of the precursor. This peptide is reported to be exceedingly potent at inhibiting prolactin secretion (46); also, since it is associated with GnRH, its secretion into hypophysial stalk blood would be expected. The prolactin-inhibiting activity of this peptide is not yet confirmed, so that a role for it in prolactin economy must be considered unsettled.

The pattern of prolactin secretion by the pituitary gland restrained by dopamine is not constant and unvarying as might have been expected. Instead, it is pulsatile, occurring as discrete bursts of prolactin release (47,48). Pulsatile release of prolactin was thought to reflect an overlying hypothalamic hypophysiotropic control, but Shin and Reifel (49) reported that such prolactin pulses originate within the pituitary gland itself. These observations were made on hypophysectomized rats bearing renal grafts of anterior pituitary tissue. Similar observations of pulsatile prolactin secretion *in vitro* have also been reported (33,50). The existence of spontaneously pulsatile prolactin release suggests a communicating network of lactotropes (2). However, such a network is hard to envision if direct cell-cell communication is required, since lactotropes are distributed more or less evenly within two layers of the pituitary gland (51,52).

Control of Evoked Prolactin Secretion

The stimuli of apparent universal importance that elevate prolactin secretion above baseline are suckling (18), stress (53), and the ovarian hormones (18), primarily estrogen. The first two of these are neurogenic stimuli arising from the environment, whereas the last, estrogen, is endogenous. Although the many elements of the final common pathway for the increase in prolactin by these two classes of stimuli are similar, they are sufficiently different to warrant separate discussions. In addition, only the suckling stimulus will be considered here, since it is the only one to have been sufficiently studied to permit detailed analysis.

Prolactin-Inhibiting Factors

Suckling is a powerful stimulus for prolactin release into the circulation. Large increases in plasma prolactin levels begin within 2 to 5 min after suckling starts; if suckling continues, levels 60 times higher than baseline accumulate in the circulation within 20 to 30 min (54–56). Such increases may be viewed as being superimposed upon the low baseline values of prolactin, held there by tonic hypothalamic inhibition (2).

The simplest explanation for increases in prolactin release would be that stimuli such as suckling reduce the tonic inhibition exerted by the hypothalamus, freeing the pituitary gland to express its inherent capacity to secrete prolactin spontaneously at a very high rate (2,19,57). Indeed, treatment of lactating rats with sufficient amounts of α-methyl-*p*-tyrosine to completely suppress dopamine secretion into hypophysial stalk blood leads to increases in prolactin secretion quantitatively similar to those observed after suckling (58). Similar results are obtained *in vitro:* Removal of a dopamine infusion results in a rapid elevation of prolactin release (59). Thus, disinhibition is a potential explanation for the neurogenic stimulation of prolactin release if prolactin-releasing stimuli could be shown to dramatically alter dopamine release.

Numerous studies of catecholamine metabolism using a variety of approaches have been made during experimental alterations in prolactin release. However, the results are mixed. Dopamine concentration in the median eminence during suckling is reported to be depleted (60–62) or unchanged (63–65). In other studies, dopaminergic impulse flow in the median eminence during suckling was thought to increase (66), decrease (64,67,68), or remain unchanged (63) depending on the study. The most direct studies of suckling-induced alterations in dopamine release are those in which the mammary nerve was stimulated electrically to simulate suckling and dopamine release measured in hypophysial stalk blood (69,70) or in the median eminence with an electrochemical probe (71). Although a mirror-image relationship between dopamine secretion and prolactin secretion might have been anticipated, only a brief (3–5 min), 60% to 70% decline in dopamine release was observed (69–71). This decline was followed by a series of rapid pulses of dopamine above the baseline which lasted for the duration of mammary nerve stimulation (71).

Simulation of the brief decrease in dopamine secretion both *in vivo* (72) and *in vitro* (59) has led to the conclusion that it is insufficient to account for suckling-induced prolactin secretion. In the *in-vivo* studies (72), endogenous dopamine secretion was inhibited with α-methyl-*p*-tyrosine after a dopamine infusion was started that was sufficient to hold prolactin levels at baseline; then, the dopamine infusion was stopped for 5 min. Small increases in prolactin secretion occurred, but they were small fractions of the amount secreted after mammary nerve stimulation (72).

Prolactin-Releasing Factors

Many prolactin-releasing factors (PRFs) have been described, some as identified peptides and some as activities in hypothalamic extracts. However, it has been difficult to demonstrate a requirement for a prolactin-releasing factor in a physiologic context until recently. One argument for the existence of a PRF is the observation described earlier of a seeming inertia of dopamine secretion in response to prolactin-releasing stimuli (69–71). A second, more compelling, argument is the recent observation that surgical removal of the posterior pituitary lobe blocks suckling-induced prolactin release without evoking major alterations in baseline prolactin secretion; i.e., apparently dopamine secretion was not greatly altered by the surgical procedure (35). Posterior lobe extracts will stimulate major prolactin releases from pituitary cells cultured *in vitro;* the identity of the activity was not identified but probably was not vasoactive intestinal peptide (VIP), thyrotropin-releasing hormone (TRH), oxytocin, or any other identified compound (73).

Two peptides that have gathered popular support as prolactin-releasing factors in recent years are TRH and VIP. Both are stimulatory to prolactin release by direct actions on the pituitary gland (74–78), they are secreted into hypophysial stalk blood (79–82), their antisera administered systemically will suppress prolactin secretion (83–85), and the responsiveness of the pituitary gland to their prolactin-releasing effects is increased during suckling (56,86). Similar evidence has been presented recently for oxytocin (87–89). However, none seems to fulfill quantitative criteria demanded of prolactin-releasing factors. Large amounts of VIP exceeding those found in hypophysial stalk blood evoke only relatively small increases in prolactin secretion—even during suckling, when the responsiveness of the pituitary is heightened (56). Similar observations have been made for TRH (74), but, in addition, much larger increases in thyroid-stimulating hormone (TSH) secretion occur after TRH administration than after suckling (2,90). Finally, most investigators report difficulties in evoking prolactin secretion *in vitro* with oxytocin (91).

Passive-immunization studies are generally viewed with favor as specific approaches to accepting or ruling out candidate peptides as hypothalamic-hypophysiotropic factors. Thus, it has been concluded that VIP, TRH, and oxytocin are "physiological" prolactin-releasing factors (83–86). Yet for each hormone, the antisera only delayed or reduced prolactin secretion after suckling. This contrasts with the complete inhibition observed after posterior lobectomy (35). One interpretation of the passive immunization studies is that they are not as specific to neutralization of the hormone in portal blood as is commonly supposed. For instance, VIP is a demonstrated autocrine regulator of prolactin secretion (92,93), and it is not abundantly clear that such a source of VIP would remain unaffected during *in-vivo* passive-neutralization studies. Similar comments apply to paracrine factors that affect prolactin secretion (94). In summary then, a convincing PRF bearing the same relationship to prolactin that (a) GnRH bears to leuteinizing hormone, (b) corticotropin-releasing factor bears to adrenocorticotropic hormone, (c) growth-hormone-releasing factor bears to growth hormone, or (d) TRH bears to TSH has not been demonstrated. Such an authentic PRF should potently stimulate prolactin release both *in vivo* and *in vitro,* be effective in the presence of inhibitory doses of dopamine, and be secreted in increased amounts in response to suckling; also, passive neutralization studies should block suckling-induced prolactin secretion. The posterior pituitary gland as a source of such an authentic PRF currently holds the greatest promise (35,73).

A firm definition of the criteria needed to define a physiological PRF assumes importance in the face of a growing list of naturally occurring compounds that will release prolactin by a direct action on the pituitary gland. TRH, VIP, and oxytocin have already been mentioned. To the list can be added serotonin (95), β-endorphin (96,97), met-enkephalin (96,98), leu-enkephalin (98), neurotensin (99,100), bombesin (101), GnRH (102,103), angiotensin II (104,105), vasopressin (106), substance P (100,107), epidermal growth factor (108,109), fibroblast growth factor (108,109), cholecystokinin (110), peptide PHI-27 (111–114), bradykinin (115), neurophysin II (116), leumorphin (117), α-neoendorphin (118,119), β-neoendorphin (118,119), dynorphin (118,119), α subunit of LH (119–121), and probably others. The appearance of VIP, GnRH, and the α subunit of LH on this list may be particularly instructive regarding the growing confusion about the identify of a PRF. VIP is an established autocrine stimulator of prolactin secretion (93), GnRH is a paracrine regulatory agent (94), and the LH α subunit apparently plays a role in stimulating differentiation of the lactotrope (118–120). Indeed, a long list of neuropeptides that reside within the pituitary gland and that apparently play a local role in regulating hormone secretion, including prolactin, is accumulating (94). Thus, the definition of PRF requires sharpening.

LACTOTROPES: PROLACTIN-SECRETING CELLS

Prolactin-secreting cells of the anterior pituitary gland have been called *mammotrophs* or *lactotrophs* in reference to the primary function of prolactin in the first case or in reference to the name of the hormone produced in the second case (prolactin was formerly called *lactogenic hormone*) (123). Most recently, prolactin-secreting cells have been called *lactotropes* (124,125) rather than lactotrophs to update the nomenclature of cells to match that used for the hormones; i.e., cells producing gonadotropins are called *gonadotropes,* cells producing thyrotropin are called *thyrotropes,* etc., so that for consistency lactotrophs have been renamed *lactotropes* (124,125).

Morphology, Abundance, and Topography

The prolactin-secreting cell has classically been described at the electron-microscopic level as containing large polymorphic secretory granules (500–900 nm in diameter) (126–128). This description has been amply confirmed by electron-microscopic immunocytochemical studies (129). However, lactotropes apparently take other forms as well. In male rats, some lactotropes have small granules in the range of 250 to 350 nm in diameter (129), whereas others are cup-shaped cells and are closely associated with gonadotropes (130,131). Lactotropes are generally described as being scattered throughout the anterior pituitary gland without special localization, although, on occasion, small clusters of 5 to 10 lactotropes are formed (130). Recently, however, two zones of concentrated lactotropes were reported to occur in the pituitary glands of lactating rats: One was a thin peripheral rim of cells separated from a thick central zone of lactotropes (51). Cells located in the outer zone were depleted of immunocytochemically detectable prolactin more quickly after suckling than were those located centrally (51).

Estimates of the fraction of pituitary cells constituted by lactotropes have varied widely, depending on the methods used for estimation. Early studies reported that 30% to 40% of all cells in the pituitary gland were lactotropes in females, whereas in males the reported percentage was lower, namely, in the range of 25% (132,133). However, after more recent studies using higher-affinity prolactin antisera for immunocytochemistry and the reverse-hemolytic plaque assay that detects prolactin secretion from individual cells, these fractions have been revised upward (125). Several investigators have reported now that lactotropes constitute 40% to 50% of all cells in the pituitary gland of both females and males (125,134,135). Since some of these estimates are derived from studies of trypsin-dispersed cells, the recovery of cells during dispersion either must be estimated or, alternatively, must be complete. The total number of cells in the pituitary gland of the adult rat on the basis of DNA measurements has been estimated as approximately 4.5×10^6 (136). On the basis of counts of cell nuclei recovered after homogenization of whole pituitary glands in sucrose with a loose-fitting pestle, the total number of pituitary cells was estimated to be approximately 6×10^6 (137). The studies reporting lactotropes in males and females to be 40% to 50% of all pituitary cells presented evidence for recovery in the range of 5×10^6 to 7×10^6 pituitary cells (125,134). Thus, apparently complete recovery of all pituitary cells was obtained in those studies, requiring no correction for cell losses.

Functional Heterogeneity

In addition to morphological heterogeneity, adenohypophysial lactotropes show functional heterogeneity (138–140). Using the reverse hemolytic plaque assay for measurement of prolactin secretion by individual lactotropes derived from the pituitary of a single female rat, Luque et al. (125) and Neill et al. (141) reported a 150-fold range in the amount of prolactin secreted by individual cells. When such cells were examined in frequency distributions according to the amount of hormone secreted per cell, two subpopulations were found: one secreting "small" amounts of prolactin and one secreting "large" amounts. The cells secreting large amounts of prolactin were preferentially responsive to the inhibitory effects of dopamine. No such preferential responsiveness to TRH was found (125). More indirect evidence of functional lactotrope heterogeneity was reported earlier by Hymer et al. (132) and by Walker and Farquhar (139). Hymer et al. (132) reported (a) that lactotropes could be separated into several fractions based on cell size and (b) that more prolactin per cell was secreted by the larger lactotropes. Estrogen treatment increased the number of large, heavily granulated lactotropes that secreted more prolactin per cell; however, not all lactotropes were affected to the same degree by the estrogen treatment (132). Walker and Farquhar (139) reported that, after [^{3}H]leucine pulse-labeling of lactotropes, three waves of [^{3}H]prolactin release occur as measured by electron-microscopic, autoradiographic studies. They attributed these differences to variations in prolactin turnover rates among different types of lactotropes.

The question of the origin of such functional differences among lactotropes thus becomes a matter of considerable importance. Globally, the differences could be either intrinsic or extrinsic. Intrinsic differences could arise if the stage of the cell cycle influenced hormone secretion, but this possibility is difficult to assess because (a) normal lactotropes divide only very slowly and (b) little investigation has been done on this topic (142,143). Another possible intrinsic origin for lactotrope heterogeneity is a cell secretory cycle (144). Such a cycle was considered likely in the older literature based on histological observation of pituitary tissue, and it was said to be a cycle of secretion, exhaustion, and restoration (144). However, no contemporary description of such a process is available, but only recently has the technology for its direct study at the single-cell level become available. Extrinsic differences might arise from local cell interactions such as has been observed with the "cup cell" wherein some lactotropes partially surround, and closely adhere to, gonadotropes (131). Such differences may arise from topographic location within the gland, where a greater vascularity might exist or where hypothalamic releasing or inhibiting factors might be delivered. Indeed, cells derived from the outer zone of the pituitary gland are reported to be highly responsive to TRH but only moderately so to dopamine; the reverse situation occurred for cells derived from the inner pituitary zone (145).

In summary, it is apparent that functional lactotrope heterogeneity is large and that location within the pituitary gland is one of its determinants. Whether this reflects a true extrinsic influence remains unknown. It is impressive that adenohypophysial lactotropes can remain in culture for at least a week and continue to show heterogeneity in the amount of prolactin secretion (141). Indeed, cells of a clonally derived pituitary cell line (GH_3) plated at densities in the hemolytic plaque assay that preclude cell-cell interaction still show large heterogeneity in the amount of hormone secreted per cell (Neill, *unpublished observation*). Thus, this cell line may provide the model required to distinguish between intrinsic and extrinsic control of cell variation.

Paracrine Control

Paracrine interactions between pituitary cell types have been studied extensively by Denef and colleagues (94). Paracrine interactions with lactotropes have been described for two cell types: gonadotropes (146) and folliculostellate cells (147). With respect to gonadotropes, the intimate contacts occurring with lactotropes *in vivo* (131,148,149) do not seem necessary (94). The agent mediating this effect appears to be angiotensin II (AII), released from gonadotropes in response to GnRH treatment (94). AII stimulates prolactin release (94,150,151); the effect of AII can be blocked with specific AII antagonists (150); AII receptors have been found on pituitary cells (152), presumably lactotropes (151–154); and AII is localized in anterior pituitary cells (155,156). The physiologic significance of this paracrine regulation of prolactin secretion by gonadotropes is unknown. However, it probably operates *in vivo,* since GnRH has been reported to release prolactin in hypothalamic-lesioned, ovariectomized monkeys (103) and in women during the menstrual cycle (157,158). Folliculostellate cells (identified as containing S-100 protein) inhibit the secretion of prolactin when they are cultured with lactotropes as cell aggregates (147). The prolactin secretory response to AII and TRH was also inhibited in such coaggregates (147). As observed with paracrine interactions between gonadotropes and lactotropes (94), intimate contacts between lactotropes and folliculostellate cells were not required for this inhibition, since it was still observed after dispersion of the coaggregates into single cells (147). Thus, an inhibitory paracrine factor of folliculostellate cell origin seems indicated but its identity is unknown.

The findings of paracrine interactions between lactotropes and other cell types is difficult to place in a physiologic perspective. It seems unlikely that such interactions are important for acute release of prolactin but seems more likely for chronic changes in prolactin secretion such as that occurring after estrogen treatment.

Autocrine Control

Autocrine control of prolactin secretion is the latest mode of hormone regulation to be demonstrated in the pituitary gland (93). Vasoactive intestinal peptide (VIP), a known hypothalamic, hypophysiotropic stimulator of prolactin release (81–84), also has been reported to be synthesized by the anterior pituitary gland (159) and to be present in lactotropes, as assessed by immunocytochemical procedures (160). Recently, Hagen et al. (92) have shown that VIP antiserum, but not another hyperimmune serum, blocked basal (unstimulated) or spontaneous secretion of prolactin *in vitro* and suggested that the high spontaneous rate of prolactin secretion observed in the absence of hypothalamic influence was due to paracrine or autocrine stimulation of prolactin secretion by locally produced VIP. Nagy et al. (93) have shown, using the reverse hemolytic plaque assay for measurement of prolactin secretion by individual lactotropes in which the cells were plated at sufficiently low density to preclude paracrine interactions, that VIP antiserum or a VIP antagonist would indeed suppress prolactin secretion by about 65% to 70%. Hence, autocrine control of prolactin secretion by VIP was demonstrated. Thus, this endocrinologically unprecedented conclusion demonstrates that the peculiar ability of lactotropes to secrete prolactin spontaneously may be due to a positive feedback if VIP can be shown to stimulate its own secretion simultaneously with prolactin; i.e., if VIP is packaged and secreted in prolactin secretory granules. The action of dopamine to suppress prolactin secretion must occur either by way of antagonizing the stimulatory effect of VIP or by inhibiting VIP secretion, or both. VIP, thus, is both an autocrine and an endocrine (secretion by the hypothalamus and delivery to the pituitary gland by way of hypophysial portal blood) stimulator of prolactin secretion (93).

The discovery of paracrine (94) and autocrine (93) regulatory mechanisms for prolactin secretion raises the interesting question of whether peptides other than AII and VIP will be found to act in similar manners. Numerous other peptides have been described as residing in anterior pituitary cells; there is reason to believe that these peptides are synthesized locally rather than being taken up after delivery in the portal circulation. These include: substance P (161–163), neurotensin (161,164), GnRH (165,166), TRH (167), corticotropin-releasing factor (168), growth-hormone releasing factor (169), somatostatin (170), motilin (171), gastrin (172), secretin (173), peptides of the proenkephalin A and B families (174–177), and vasopressin (178). It probably is significant that a majority of the members on this list have been described as stimulating prolactin secretion by a direct action on the pituitary gland (96,98–100,106,107,117–119) but were considered PRF candidates. Such peptides may be shown to play paracrine or autocrine regulatory roles in prolactin secretion and, if so, will confirm an earlier prediction (2) that lactotropes "show a regulatory complexity commonly accorded only to neurons."

CELLULAR MECHANISMS IN THE CONTROL OF PROLACTIN SECRETION

Lactotropes synthesize, package, and release prolactin by standard mechanisms for all secretory cells (179). Indeed, lactotropes are frequently used as the prototype for secretion by adenohypophysial cells (128). The main steps in the synthesis/secretory cycle are: (a) transcription of the prolactin gene into RNA; (b) processing of this pre-RNA within the nucleus into mature mRNA; (c) translocation of the mRNA to the cytoplasm; (d) attachment of the mRNA to ribosomes and translation into pre-prolactin; (e) discharge into the lumen of the rough endoplasmic reticulum during which the leader sequence of pre-prolactin is removed; (f) concentration and packaging of prolactin into secretory granules surrounded by membranes within the Golgi apparatus; (g) storage of prolactin in secretory granules; and (h) movement of the secretory granules into the cortical cytoplasm and extracellular discharge by exocytosis.

Synthesis (steps a–g) and release (step h) are distinct processes that can be experimentally separated (180); that is, the physiologically relevant secretagogues that evoke prolactin secretion (TRH, VIP, and dopamine) affect both processes probably by way of the same second messenger, acting in the cytoplasm on release of stored hormone on the one hand but acting in the nucleus to alter synthesis of prolactin on the other (181,182). Receptors for TRH (183), VIP (184), and dopamine (185) are membrane-bound and, upon binding to their ligand, generate second messengers such as cAMP, calcium, and members of the phosphoinositide family.

The GH_3 clonal cell line frequently is used for studies of the cellular mechanisms in the control of prolactin secretion (183). This cell line was derived originally from an estrogen-induced pituitary tumor and repeatedly cloned to produce a theoretically homogeneous group of cells (183). Thus, it offers advantages over pituitary lactotropes that are always mixed with other pituitary cell types even after cell purification. The GH_3 cell line has a number of disadvantages, however. It does not respond to dopamine (183), it may not be as functionally homogeneous as originally believed (186), it secretes both growth hormone and prolactin, and it stores only small amounts of hormone in the cytoplasm in organelles that are more vesicular than granular (183). Nevertheless, several important functional characteristics of pituitary lactotropes were discovered originally in this cell line (183).

Dopamine

Dopamine suppresses both the synthesis and release of prolactin by lactotropes (17). Although calcium may participate (187), the primary mechanism of dopamine action appears to be inhibition of cAMP production (188). Dopamine or its agonists inhibit pituitary adenylate cyclase (189) and, in lactotrope-rich cell fractions, will suppress cAMP levels within minutes (188,190). Conversely, cAMP stimulates large increases in prolactin release (188) and in prolactin gene transcription (191).

Receptors for dopamine are located in the plasma membrane of lactotropes, where they are negatively coupled to adenylate cyclase (185). Such receptors are classified as D-2—in contrast to D-1—receptors, which stimulate cAMP production and are located primarily in the caudate nucleus and parathyroid gland (33,185). The D-2 dopamine receptors have been studied in anterior pituitary membranes of several species, where they have been characterized as having high affinity, being saturable, and showing stereoselectivity among dopamine agonists and antagonists (33,185). Apomorphine and ergots (bromocryptine, lisuride, and lergotrile) are dopamine agonists, show high binding affinity to the anterior pituitary cell membranes, and are strong inhibitors of prolactin release both *in vitro* and *in vivo* (33,185). Spiperone, haloperidol, and domperidone are examples of D-2 receptor antagonists; they do not affect prolactin release when tested alone but increase prolactin release when they are administered *in vivo,* presumably by antagonizing endogenous dopamine (33).

The anterior pituitary dopamine receptor appears to exist in two different affinity states as a result of interacting with a guanine-nucleotide-binding protein (185,193). The agonist high-affinity form of the receptor is involved in inhibiting adenylate cyclase and hence prolactin release, since there is a high correlation between high-affinity agonist binding and biological activity (185,192). The effect of guanine nucleotides is to decrease the proportion of the receptor existing in the high-affinity form. Thus, the model developed for D-2 dopamine receptor envisions dopamine binding to the receptor, forming a complex that couples to a guanine-nucleotide-regulatory protein (185,193). This complex is responsible for the high-affinity state of the receptor and also presumably accounts for inhibiting the catalytic subunit of adenylate cyclase (185,193).

VIP

As described earlier, VIP is an autocrine stimulator of the apparent "spontaneous" prolactin secretion that is peculiar to lactotropes (93), but it also acts as a hypothalamic hypophysiotropic stimulator of prolactin release (75–78,81–84). Less experimental attention has been paid to its mechanism of action to release prolactin, probably because its importance in regulating prolactin secretion has only recently become apparent. VIP stimulates anterior pituitary adenylate cyclase and production of cAMP. VIP receptors were reported in one study to be present on pituitary cells, presumably lactotropes (184).

Dopamine's mechanism of action to inhibit prolactin release will have to be reconsidered in light of the finding of an autocrine stimulatory role for VIP (93). Since the actions of both dopamine and VIP appear to be cAMP-dependent (see above), the most conservative hypothesis would be that dopamine and VIP receptors regulate a common adenylate cyclase through separate guanyl-nucleotide-binding proteins (195,196): an inhibitory one (G_i) for dopamine and a stimulatory one (G_3) for VIP. Alternatively, or perhaps additionally, dopamine might inhibit VIP synthesis and secretion, which are, themselves, cAMP-dependent. To illustrate the latter mechanism, studies will need to establish the mode of VIP and VIP-receptor synthesis, packaging, and delivery to the cell surface of lactotropes. That is, if VIP is packaged in prolactin secretory granules and its receptors are present in the granule's limiting membrane, then dopamine simultaneously would inhibit prolactin and VIP secretion.

TRH

Despite its problematic role as a physiologic regulator of prolactin secretion (see above), TRH is the best studied among prolactin secretagogues (183). Extensive investigations have examined the characteristics of its receptor (183) and have produced compelling evidence that calcium and phosphoinositides act as second messengers in its action (180,183,197,198). cAMP also may be involved, but its role remains unclarified (199). The action of TRH to release prolactin was originally discovered in the GH_3 cell line, and thus most of the studies of its mechanism of action have been done there (183). The prolactin-stimulating effect of TRH is extremely rapid, with increases in prolactin release occurring within seconds and increases in prolactin transcription occurring at about 2 min (180). Newly synthesized prolactin does not appear until about an hour after application of TRH (183).

TRH receptors are well-characterized (183). They are located on the cell surface and show binding affinities in the nanomolar range (183). TRH binding to cell membranes meets the standard criteria required to be considered receptors: They show specificity with respect to their appropriate target cells; with respect to hormone and structural analogs displaying varying levels of biological activity, they have limited capacity and high affinity, consistent with the dose-response relationship to biological activity; and finally, they show reversibility (183).

Early work seemed to indicate that cAMP served as the second messenger for TRH-induced prolactin secretion (200). Later investigations, however, have produced substantial evidence against such a role (197–199,201). Instead, the focus of much recent research has shifted toward possible roles of calcium and lipids as the second messengers for TRH action (180,197,198). This rapidly progressing area of research is in such a state of flux that summaries of its current state are doomed to be outdated rapidly.

REFERENCES

1. Nicoll, C. S. (1974): Physiological actions of prolactin. In: *Handbook of Physiology, Section 7, Endocrinology, Vol. 4*, edited by E. Knobil and W. H. Sawyer, p. 253. American Physiological Society, Washington, D. C.
2. Leong, D. A., Frawley, S. L., and Neill, J. D. (1983): Neuroendocrine control of prolactin secretion. *Annu. Rev. Physiol.*, 45:109.
3. Harris, G. W. (1955): *Neural Control of the Pituitary Gland*. Edward Arnold, London.
4. Everett, J. W. (1954): Luteotropic function of autografts of the rat hypophysis. *Endocrinology*, 54:685.
5. Everett, J. W. (1956): Functional corpora lutea maintained for months by autografts of rat hypophysis. *Endocrinology*, 58:786.
6. Pasteels, J. L. (1961): Secretion de prolactine par l'hypophyse en culture de tissus. *C. R. Acad. Sci. Ser. D*, 253:2140.
7. Pasteels, J. L. (1963): Recherches morphologiques et experimentales sur la sécrétion de prolactine. *Arch. Biol.*, 74:439.
8. Meites, J., Nicoll, C. S., and Talwalker, P. K. (1963): The central nervous system and the secretion and release of prolactin. *In: Advances in Neuroendocrinology*, edited by A. V. Nalbandov. University of Illinois Press, Urbana. p. 238.
9. Talwalker, P. K., Ratner, A., and Meites, J. (1963): *In vitro* inhibition of pituitary prolactin synthesis and release by hypothalamic extract. *Am. J. Physiol.*, 205:213.
10. Barraclough, C. A., and Sawyer, C. H. (1959): Induction of pseudopregnancy in the rat by reserpine and chlorpromazine. *Endocrinology*, 65:563.
11. Kanematsu, S., Hillard, J., and Sawyer, C. H. (1963): Effect of reserpine on pituitary prolactin content and its hypothalamic site of action in the rabbit. *Acta Endocrinol.*, 44:467.
12. Coppola, J. A., Leonardi, R. G., Lippman, W., Perrine, J. W., and Ringler, I. (1965): Induction of pseudopregnancy in rats by depletors of endogenous catecholamines. *Endocrinology*, 77:485.
13. Coppola, J. A. (1968): The apparent involvement of the sympathetic nervous system in the gonadotropin secretion of female rats. *J. Reprod. Fertil.* (Suppl.), 4:35.
14. Fuxe, K. (1965): Evidence for the existence of monoamine neurons in the central nervous system. *Acta Physiol. Scand. (Suppl.)*, 247:39.
15. MacLeod, R. M. (1969): Influence of norepinephrine and catecholamine-depleting agents on the synthesis and release of prolactin and growth hormone. *Endocrinology*, 85:916.
16. Birge, C. A., Jacobs, L. S., Hammeo, C. T., and Daughaday, W. H. (1970): Catecholamine inhibition of prolactin secretion by isolated rat adenohypophyses. *Endocrinology*, 86:120.
17. MacLeod, R. M. (1976): Regulation of prolactin secretion. In: *Frontiers in Neuroendocrinology, Vol. 4*, edited by L. Martini and W. F. Ganong, p. 169. Raven Press, New York.
18. Neill, J. D. (1974): Prolactin: Its secretion and control. In: *Handbook of Physiology, Section 7, Endocrinology, Vol. 4*, edited by E. Knobil and W. H. Sawyer, American Physiological Society, Washington, D. C.
19. Neill, J. D. (1980): Neuroendocrine regulation of prolactin secretion. In: *Frontiers in Neuroendocrinology*, edited by L. Martini and W. F. Ganong, p. 129. Raven Press, New York.
20. Ben-Jonathan, N. (1980): Catecholamines and pituitary prolactin release. *J. Reprod. Fertil.*, 58:501.
21. Shaar, C. J., and Clemens, J. A. (1974): The role of catecholamines in the release of anterior pituitary prolactin *in vitro*. *Endocrinology*, 95:1202.
22. Takahara, J., Arimura, A., and Schally, A. V. (1974): Suppression of prolactin release by a purified porcine PIF preparation and catecholamines infused into a rat hypophysial portal vessel. *Endocrinology*, 95:462.
23. Brown, G. M., Seeman, P., and Lee, T. (1976): Dopamine/neuroleptic receptors in basal hypothalamus and pituitary. *Endocrinology*, 99:1407.
24. Creese, I. R., Schneider, P., and Snyder, S. H. (1977): ^{3}H-spiroperidol labels dopamine receptors in pituitary and brain. *Eur. J. Pharmacol.*, 46:377.
25. Goldsmith, P. C., Cronin, M. J., and Weiner, R. I. (1979): Dopamine receptor sites in the anterior pituitary. *J. Histochem. Cytochem.*, 27:1205.
26. Ben-Jonathan, N., Oliver, C., Weiner, H. J., Mical, R. S., and Porter, J. C. (1977): Dopamine in hypophysial portal plasma of the rat during the estrous cycle and throughout pregnancy. *Endocrinology*, 100:452.
27. Gibbs, D. M., and Neill, J. D. (1978): Dopamine levels in hypophysial stalk blood in the rat are sufficient to inhibit prolactin secretion *in vivo*. *Endocrinology*, 102:1895.
28. Plotsky, P. M., Gibbs, D. M., and Neill, J. D. (1978): Liquid chromatographic-electrochemical measurement of dopamine in hypophysial stalk blood of rats. *Endocrinology*, 102:1887.
29. Neill, J. D., Plotsky, P. M., de Greef, W. (1979): Catecholamines, the hypothalamus and neuroendocrinology—Applications of electrochemical methods. *Trends Neurosci.*, 2:60.
30. de Greef, W. J., and Neill, J. D. (1979): Dopamine levels in hypophysial stalk plasma of the rat during surges of prolactin secretion induced by cervical stimulation. *Endocrinology*, 105:1093.
31. Ben-Jonathan, N., and Peters, L. L. (1982): Posterior pituitary lobectomy: Differential elevation of plasma prolactin and luteinizing hormone in estrous and lactating rats. *Endocrinology*, 110:1861.
32. Peters, L. A., Hoefer, M. T., and Ben-Jonathan, N. (1981): The posterior pituitary: Regulation of anterior pituitary prolactin secretion. *Science*, 213:659.
33. Ben-Jonathan, N. (1985): Dopamine: A prolactin-inhibiting hormone. *Endocr. Rev.*, 6:564.
34. Murai, I., and Ben-Jonathan, N. (1986): Chronic posterior pituitary lobectomy: Prolonged elevation of plasma prolactin and interruption of cyclicity. *Neuroendocrinology*, 43:453.
35. Murai, I., and Ben-Jonathan, N. (1987): Posterior pituitary lobectomy abolishes the suckling-induced rise in prolactin (PRL): Evidence for a PRL-releasing factor in the posterior pituitary. *Endocrinology*, 121:205.
36. Mulchahey, J. J., and Neill, J. D. (1986): Dopamine levels in the anterior pituitary gland monitored by *in vivo* electrochemistry. *Brain Res.*, 386:332.
37. Schally, A. V., Redding, T. W., Arimura, A., Dupont, A., and Linthicum, G. L. (1977): Isolation of gamma-amino butyric acid from pig hypothalami and demonstration of its prolactin release-inhibiting (PIF) activity *in vivo* and *in vitro*. *Endocrinology*, 100:681.
38. Enjalbert, A., Ruberg, M., Arancibia, S., Fiore, L., Priam, M., and Kordon, C. (1979): Independent inhibition of prolactin secretion by dopamine and γ-aminobutyric acid *in vitro*. *Endocrinology*, 105:823.
39. Racagni, G., Apud, J. A., Locatelli, V., Cocchi, D., Nistico, G., di Giorgio, R. M., and Muller, E. E. (1979): GABA of CNS origin in the rat anterior pituitary inhibits prolactin secretion. *Nature*, 281:575.
40. Grandison, L., and Guidotti, A. (1979): γ-Aminobutyric acid receptor function in rat anterior pituitary: Evidence for control of prolactin release. *Endocrinology*, 105:754.
41. Grandison, L., Cavagnini, F., Schmid, R., Invitti, C., and Guidotti, A. (1982): γ-Aminobutyric acid- and benzodiazepine-binding sites in human anterior pituitary tissue. *J. Clin. Endocrinol. Metab.*, 54:597.
42. Tappaz, M. L., Brownstein, M. J., and Kopin, I. J. (1977): Glutamate decarboxylase (GAD) and γ-aminobutyric acid (GABA) in discrete nuclei of hypothalamus and *substantia nigra*. *Brain Res.*, 125:109.
43. Vincent, S. R., Hokfelt, T., and Wu, J. Y. (1982): GABA neuron systems in hypothalamus and the pituitary gland: Immunohistochemical demonstration using antibodies against glutamate decarboxylase. *Neuroendocrinology*, 34:117.
44. Mitchell, R., Grieve, G., Dow, R., and Fink, G. (1983): Endogenous GABA receptor ligands in hypophysial portal blood. *Neuroendocrinology*, 37:169.
45. Mulchahey, J. J., and Neill, J. D. (1982): Gamma amino butyric acid (GABA) levels in hypophyseal stalk plasma of rats. *Life Sci.*, 31:453.

46. Nikolics, K., Mason, A. J., Szonyi, E., Ramachandran, J., and Seeburg, P. H. (1985): A prolactin-inhibiting factor within the precursor for human gonadotropin-releasing hormone. *Nature,* 316:511.
47. Saunders, A., Terry, L. C., Audet, J., Brazeau, P., and Martin, J. B. (1976): Dynamic studies of growth hormone and prolactin secretion in the female rat. *Neuroendocrinology,* 21:193.
48. Leighton, P. C., McNeilly, A. S., and Chard, T. (1976): Short-term variation in blood levels of prolactin in women. *J. Endocrinol.,* 68:177.
49. Shin, S. H., and Reifel, C. W. (1981): Adenohypophysis has an inherent property for pulsatile prolactin secretion. *Neuroendocrinology,* 32:139.
50. Stewart, J. K., Clifton, D. K., Koerker, D. J., Rogol, A. D., Jaffee, T., and Goodner, C. J. (1985): Pulsatile release of growth hormone and prolactin from the primate pituitary *in vitro. Endocrinology,* 116:1.
51. Papka, R. E., Yu, S. M., and Nikitovitch-Winer, M. B. (1986): Use of immunoperoxidase and immuno-gold labelling for pituitary hormones and neuropeptides. *Am. J. Anat.,* 175:289.
52. Boockfor, F. R., Frawley, S. L. (1987): Functional variations among prolactin cells from different pituitary regions. *Endocrinology,* 120:874.
53. Neill, J. D. (1970): Effect on stress on serum prolactin and luteinizing hormone levels during the estrous cycle of the rat. *Endocrinology,* 87:1192.
54. Grosvenor, C. E., Mena, F., and Whitworth, N. S. (1979): The secretion rate of prolactin in the rat during suckling and its metabolic clearance rate after increasing intervals of nonsuckling. *Endocrinology,* 104:372.
55. Mattheij, J. A. M., Gruisen, E. F. M., and Swarts, J. J. M. (1979): The suckling-induced rise of plasma prolactin in lactating rats. Its dependence on stage of lactation and litter size. *Horm. Res.,* 11:325.
56. Leong, J. A., and Neill, J. D. (1987): Regulation of prolactin release in lactating rats: An increase in prolactin secretory responsiveness to TRH and VIP during suckling. *J. Endocrinol. (in press).*
57. Neill, J. D., Frawley, L. S., Plotsky, P. M., Peck, J. D., and Leong, D. A. (1982): Hypothalamic regulation of prolactin secretion. In: *Pituitary Hormones and Related Peptides,* edited by M. Motta, M. Zanisi, and F. Piva, p. 223. Academic Press, New York.
58. Leong, D. A., and Neill, J. D. (1987): The role of hypophysiotropic dopamine during suckling-induced prolactin secretion. *Am. J. Physiol. (in press).*
59. Fagin, K. D., and Neill, J. D. (1981): The effect of dopamine on thyrotropin-releasing hormone-induced prolactin secretion *in vitro. Endocrinology,* 109:1835.
60. Chiocchio, S. R., Cannata, M. A., Cordero Funes, J. R., and Tramezzani, J. H. (1979): Involvement of adenohypophysial dopamine in the regulation of prolactin release during suckling. *Endocrinology,* 105:544.
61. Mena, F., Enjalbert, A., Carbonell, L., Priam, M., and Kordon, C. (1976): Effects of suckling on plasma prolactin and hypothalamic monoamine levels in the rat. *Endocrinology,* 99:445.
62. Moore, K. E., and Demarest, K. T. (1982): Tuberoinfundibular and tuberohypophyseal dopaminergic neurons. In: *Frontiers in Neuroendocrinology,* edited by W. F. Ganong and L. Martini, p. 161. Raven Press, New York.
63. Moyer, J. A., O'Donohue, T. L., Herrenkohl, L. R., Gala, R. R., and Jacobowitz, D. M. (1979): Effects of suckling on serum prolactin levels and catecholamine concentrations and turnover in discrete brain regions. *Brain Res.,* 176:125.
64. Selmanoff, M., and Wise, P. M. (1981): Decreased dopamine turnover in the median eminence in response to suckling in the lactating rat. *Brain Res.,* 212:101.
65. Voogt, J. L., and Carr, L. A. (1974): Plasma prolactin levels and hypothalamic catecholamine synthesis during suckling. *Neuroendocrinology,* 16:108.
66. Fuxe, K., Hokfelt, T., and Nilsson, O. (1969): Factors involved in the control of the activity of tuber-infundibular dopamine neurons during pregnancy and lactation. *Neuroendocrinology,* 5:257.
67. McKay, D. W., Demarest, K. T., Riegle, G. D., and Moore, K. E. (1980): Lactation alters the activity of tuberoinfundibular dopaminergic neurons. Program of the 10th Annual Meeting of Society of Neuroscience, Cincinnati, Ohio, p. 152 (abstract).
68. Selmanoff, M., and Gregerson, K. A. (1982): Suckling-induced decreases in dopamine turnover occur in both medial and lateral aspects of the median eminence of the lactating rat. *Fed. Proc.,* 41:1100.
69. deGreef, W. J., Plotsky, P. M., and Neill, J. D. (1981): Dopamine levels in hypophysial stalk plasma and prolactin levels in peripheral plasma of the lactating rat: Effects of a simulated suckling stimulus. *Neuroendocrinology,* 32:229.
70. Plotsky, P. M., and Neill, J. D. (1982): The decrease in hypothalamic dopamine secretion induced by suckling: Comparison of voltammetric and radioisotopic methods of measurement. *Endocrinology,* 110:691.
71. Plotsky, P. M., deGreef, W. J., and Neill, J. D. (1982): *In situ* voltammetric microelectrodes: Application to the measurement of the median eminence catecholamine release during simulated suckling. *Brain Res.,* 250:251.
72. Plotsky, P. M., and Neill, J. D. (1982): Interactions of dopamine and thyrotropin releasing hormone (TRH) in the regulation of prolactin release in lactating rats. *Endocrinology,* 111:168.
73. Andrews, P. C., Hyde, J. F., and Ben-Jonathan, N. (1987): Fractionation by HPLC of prolactin-releasing factor (PRF) from rat and bovine posterior pituitaries. Program of the 69th Annual Meeting of the Endocrine Society, Indianapolis, Indiana, p. 179 (abstract).
74. Blake, C. A. (1974): Stimulation of pituitary prolactin and TSH release in lactating and proestrous rats. *Endocrinology,* 94:503.
75. Shaar, C. J., Clemens, J. A., Dininger, N. B. (1979): Effect of vasoactive intestinal polypeptides on prolactin release *in vitro. Life Sci.,* 25:2071.
76. Samson, W. K., Said, S. I., Snyder, G., and McCann, S. M. (1980): *In vitro* stimulation of prolactin release by vasoactive intestinal peptide. *Peptides,* 1:425.
77. Ruberg, M., Rotszten, W. H., Arancibia, S., Besson, J., and Enjalbert, A. (1978): Stimulation of prolactin release by vasoactive intestinal peptide (VIP). *Eur. J. Pharmacol.,* 51:319.
78. Gourdji, D., Bataille, D., Vauclin, N., Grouselle, D., Rosselin, G., and Tixier-Vidal, A. (1979): Vasoactive investinal peptide (VIP) stimulates prolactin (PRL) release and cAMP production in rat pituitary cell line (GH3/B6). Additive effects of VIP and TRH on PRL release. *FEBS Lett.,* 104:165.
79. deGreef, W. J., and Visser, T. J. (1981): Evidence for the involvement of hypothalamic dopamine and thyrotropin-releasing hormone in suckling-induced release of prolactin. *J. Endocrinol.,* 91:213.
80. Fink, G., Koch, Y., and Ben Aroya, N. (1982): Release of thyrotropin releasing hormone into hypophysial portal blood is high relative to other neuropeptides and may be related to prolactin secretion. *Brain Res.,* 243:186.
81. Said, S. I., and Porter, J. C. (1979): Vasoactive intestinal polypeptide: Release into hypophysial portal blood. *Life Sci.,* 24:227.
82. Shimatsu, A., Kato, Y., Matsushita, N., Katakami, H., Yanaihara, N., and Imura, H. (1981): Immunoreactive vasoactive intestinal polypeptide in rat hypophysial portal blood. *Endocrinology,* 108:395.
83. Abe, H., Engler, D., Molitch, M., Bollinger-Gruber, J., and Reichlen, S. (1985): Vasoactive intestinal peptide is a physiological mediator of prolactin release in the rat. *Endocrinology,* 116:1383.
84. Kaji, H., Chihara, K., Abe, H., Kita, T., Kashio, Y., Okimura, Y., and Fujita, T. (1985): Effect of passive immunization with antisera to vasoactive intestinal peptide and peptide histidine isoleucine amide on 5-hydroxy-L-tryptophan induced prolactin release in rats. *Endocrinology,* 117:1914.
85. deGreef, W. J., Voogt, J. L., Visser, T. J., Lamberts, S. W. J., and van der Schoot, P. (1987): Control of prolactin release induced by suckling. *Endocrinology,* 121:316.
86. Grosvenor, C. E., and Mena, F. (1980): Evidence that thyrotropin-releasing hormone and a hypothalamic prolactin-releasing factor may function in the release of prolactin in the lactating rat. *Endocrinology,* 107:863.
87. Lumpkin, M. D., Samson, W. K., and McCann, S. M. (1983): Hypothalamic and pituitary sites of action of oxytocin to alter prolactin secretion in the rat. *Endocrinology,* 112:1711.
88. Samson, W. K., Lumpkin, M. D., and McCann, S. M. (1986): Evidence for a physiological role for oxytocin in the control of prolactin secretion. *Endocrinology,* 119:554.
89. Gibbs, D. M. (1984): High concentrations of oxytocin in hypophysial portal plasma. *Endocrinology,* 114:1216.

90. Riskind, P. N., Millard, W. J., and Martin, J. B. (1984): Evidence that thyrotropin-releasing hormone is not a major prolactin-releasing factor during suckling in the rat. *Endocrinology,* 115:312.
91. Frawley, L. S., Leong, D. A., and Neill, J. D. (1985): Oxytocin attenuates TRH-induced TSH release from rat pituitary cells. *Neuroendocrinology,* 40:201.
92. Hagen, T. C., Arnaout, M. A., Scherzer, W. J., Martinson, D. R., and Garthwaite, T. L. (1986): Antisera to vasoactive intestinal peptide inhibit basal prolactin release from dispersed anterior pituitary cells. *Neuroendocrinology,* 43:641.
93. Nagy, G., Mulchahey, J. J., and Neill, J. D. (1987): Autocrine control of hormone secretion in anterior pituitary cells (*submitted for publication*).
94. Denef, C., Baes, M., and Schramme, C. (1986): Paracrine interactions in the anterior pituitary: Role in the regulation of prolactin and growth hormone secretion. In: *Frontiers in Neuroendocrinology, Vol. 9,* edited by W. F. Ganong and L. Martini, p. 115. Raven Press, New York.
95. Wehrenberg, W. B., McNicol, D., Frantz, A. G., and Ferin, M. (1980): The effects of serotonin on prolactin and growth hormone concentrations in normal and pituitary stalk-sectioned monkeys. *Endocrinology,* 107:1747.
96. Enjalbert, A., Ruberg, M., Arancibia, S., Priam, M., and Kordon, C. (1979): Endogenous opiates block dopamine inhibition of prolactin secretion *in vitro*. *Nature,* 280:595.
97. Grandison, L., and Guidotti, A. (1977): Regulation of prolactin release by endogenous opiates. *Nature,* 270:357.
98. Lien, E. L., Fenichel, R. L., Garsky, V., Sarantakis, D., and Grant, N. H. (1976): Enkephalin-stimulated prolactin release. *Life Sci.,* 19:837.
99. Enjalbert, A., Arancibia, S., Priam, M., Eluet-Pajot, M. T., and Kordon, C. (1982): Neurotensin stimulation of prolactin secretion *in vitro*. *Neuroendocrinology,* 34:95.
100. Vijayan, E., and McCann, S. M. (1979): *In vivo* and *in vitro* effects of substance P and neurotensin on gonadotropin and prolactin release. *Endocrinology,* 105:64.
101. Westendorf, J. M., and Schonbrunn, A. (1982): Bombesin stimulates prolactin and growth hormone release by pituitary cells in culture. *Endocrinology,* 110:352.
102. Denef, C. (1981): LHRH stimulates prolactin release from rat pituitary lactotrophs co-cultured with a highly purified population of gonadotrophs. *Ann. Endocrinol. (Paris),* 42:65.
103. Wildt, L., Hausler, A., Marshall, G., and Knobil, E. (1980): GnRH has prolactin-releasing activity. *Fed. Proc.,* 39:372 (abstract).
104. Steele, M. K., Negro-Vilar, A., and McCann, S. M. (1981): Effect of angiotensin II on *in vivo* and *in vitro* release of anterior pituitary hormones in the female rat. *Endocrinology,* 109:893.
105. Schramme, C., and Denef, C. (1983): Stimulation of prolactin release by angiotensin II in superfused rat anterior pituitary cell aggregates. *Neuroendocrinology,* 36:483.
106. Shin, S. H. (1982): Vasopressin has a direct effect on prolactin release in male rats. *Neuroendocrinology,* 34:55.
107. Kato, Y., Chihara, K., Ohgo, S., Iwasaki, Y., Abe, H., and Imura, H. (1976): Growth hormone and prolactin release by substance P in rats. *Life Sci.,* 19:441.
108. Johnson, L. K., Baxter, J. D., Vlodavsky, I., and Gospodarowicz, D. (1980): Epidermal growth factor and expression of specific genes: Effects on cultured rat pituitary cells are dissociable from the mitogenic response. *Proc. Natl. Acad. Sci. USA,* 77:394.
109. Schonbrunn, A., Krasnoff, M., Westendorf, J. M., and Tashjian, A. H., Jr. (1980): Epidermal growth factor and thyrotropin-releasing hormone act similarly on a clonal pituitary cell strain: Modulation of hormone production and inhibition of cell proliferation. *J. Cell Biol.,* 85:786.
110. Malarkey, W. B., O'Dorisio, T. M., Kennedy, M., and Cataland, S. (1981): The influence of vasoactive intestinal polypeptide and cholecystokinin on prolactin release in rat and human monolayer cultures. *Life Sci.,* 28:2489.
111. Hokfelt, T., Fahrenkrug, J., Tatemoto, K., Mutt, V., Werner, S., Hulting, A. L., Terenius, L., and Chang, K. J. (1983): The PHI (PHI-27)/corticotropin releasing factor/enkephalin immunoreactive neuron: Possible morphological basis for integrated control of prolactin, corticotropin, and growth hormone secretion. *Proc. Natl. Acad. Sci. USA,* 80:895.
112. Samson, W. K., Lumpkin, M. D., McDonald, J. K., and McCann, S. M. (1983): Prolactin releasing activity of porcine intestinal peptide (PHI-27). *Peptides,* 4:817.
113. Werner, S., Hulting, A. L., Hokfelt, T., Eneroth, P., Tatemoto, K., Mutt, V., Moroder, L., and Wunsch, E. (1983): Effect of the peptide PHI-27 on prolactin release *in vitro*. *Neuroendocrinology,* 37:476.
114. Kaji, H., Chihara, K., Abe, H., Minamitani, N., Kodama, H., Kita, T., Fujita, T., and Tatemoto, K. (1984): Stimulatory effect of peptide histidine isoleucine amide-27 on prolactin release in the rat. *Life Sci.,* 35:641.
115. Jones, T. H., Brown, B. L., and Dobson, P. R. M. (1987): Bradykinin stimulates inositol phosphate production and prolactin release in rat anterior pituitary cells. Program of the 6th Joint Meeting of British Endocrine Societies, Warwick, England (abstract 155).
116. Shin, S. H., Obonsawin, M. C., Vincent, S. (1985): The major prolactin releasing activity from bovine posterior pituitary is identified as neurophysin II. In: *Prolactin: Basic and Clinical Correlates,* edited by R. M. MacLeod, M. O. Thorner, and U. Scapagnini, p. 95. Liviana Press, Padova.
117. Tojo, K., Kato, Y., Ohto, H., Shimatsu, A., Matsushita, N., Kabayama, Y., Inoue, T., Yanaihara, N., and Imura, H. (1985): Potent stimulatory effect of leumorphin on prolactin secretion from the pituitary in rats. In: *Prolactin: Basic and Clinical Correlates,* edited by R. M. MacLeod, M. O. Thorner, and U. Scapagnini, p. 552. Liviana Press, Padova.
118. Matsushita, N. Kato, Y., Shimatsu, A., Katakami, H., Fugino, M., Matsuo, H., and Imura, H. (1982): Stimulation of prolactin secretion in the rat by α-neo-endorphin, β-neo-endorphin and dynorphin. *Biochem. Biophys. Res. Commun.,* 107:735.
119. Kato, Y., Matsushita, N., Katakami, H., Shimatsu, A., and Imura, H. (1981): Stimulation by dynorphin of prolactin and growth hormone secretion in the rat. *Eur. J. Pharmacol.,* 73:353.
120. Begeot, M., Hemming, F. J., Dubois, P. M., Combarnous, Y., Dubois, M. P., and Aubert, M. L. (1984): Induction of pituitary lactotrope differentiation by luteinizing hormone α subunit. *Science,* 226:566.
121. Begeot, M., Hemming, F. J., Martinat, N., Dubois, M. P., and Dubois, P. M. (1983): Gonadotropin releasing hormone (GnRH) stimulates immunoreactive lactotrope differentiation. *Endocrinology,* 112:2224.
122. Begeot, M., Morel, G., Rivest, R. W., Aubert, M. L., Dubois, M. P., and Dubois, P. M. (1984): Influence of gonadoliberin on the differentiation of rat gonadotrophs: An *in vivo* and *in vitro* study. *Neuroendocrinology,* 38:217.
123. Baker, B. L. (1974): Functional cytology of the hypophysial pars distalis and pars intermedia. In: *Handbook of Physiology, Section 7, Endocrinology, Vol. 4,* edited by E. Knobil and W. H. Sawyer, p. 45. American Physiological Society, Washington, D. C.
124. Neill, J. D., and Frawley, L. S. (1983): Detection of hormone release from individual cells in mixed populations using a reverse hemolytic plaque assay. *Endocrinology,* 112:1135.
125. Luque, E. H., Munoz de Toro, M., Smith, P. F., and Neill, J. D. (1986): Subpopulations of lactotropes detected with the reverse hemolytic plaque assay show differential responsiveness to dopamine. *Endocrinology,* 118:2120.
126. Hedinger, C. E., and Farquhar, M. G. (1957): Electronenmikroskopische untersuchungen von zwei typen acidophiler hypophysenvorderlappenzellen bei der ratte. *Schweiz. Z. Allgem. Pathol. Bakteriol.,* 20:766.
127. Kurosumi, K. (1968): Functional classification of cell types of the anterior pituitary gland accomplished by electron microscopy. *Saibo Kaku Byorigaku Zasshi,* 29:329.
128. Farquhar, M. G., Skutelsky, E. H., and Hopkins, C. R. (1975): Structure and function of the anterior pituitary and dispersed pituitary cells: *In vitro* studies. In: *The Anterior Pituitary,* edited by A. Tixier-Vidal and M. G. Farquhar, p. 84. Academic Press, New York.
129. Nakane, P. K. (1975): Identification of anterior pituitary cells by immunoelectron microscopy. In: *The Anterior Pituitary,* edited by A. Tixier-Vidal and M. G. Farquhar, p. 45. Academic Press, New York.
130. Nogami, H., and Yoshimura, F. (1982): Fine structural criteria of prolactin cells identified immunohistochemically in the male rat. *Anat. Rec.,* 202:261.

131. Sato, S. (1980): Postnatal development, sexual difference and sexual cycle variation of prolactin cells in rats: Special reference to the topographic affinity to a gonadotroph. *Endocrinol. Jpn.,* 27:573.
132. Hymer, W. C., Snyder, J., Wilfinger, W., Swanson, N., and Davis, J. (1974): Separation of pituitary mammotrophs from the female rat by velocity sedimentation at unit gravity. *Endocrinology,* 95:107.
133. Hymer, W. C., and Hatfield, J. M. (1983): Separation of cells from the rat anterior pituitary gland. *Methods Enzymol.,* 103:257.
134. Smith, P. F., Luque, E. H., and Neill, J. D. (1986): Detection and measurement of secretion from neuroendocrine cells using a reverse hemolytic plaque assay. *Methods Enzymol.,* 124:443.
135. Dada, M. O., Campbell, G. T., and Blake, C. A. (1984): Pars distalis cell quantification in normal adult male and female rats. *J. Endocrinol.,* 101:87.
136. Leavitt, W. W., Kimmel, G. L., and Friend, J. P. (1973): Steroid hormone uptake by anterior pituitary cell suspensions. *Endocrinology,* 92:94.
137. Friend, J. P. (1979): Cell size and cell division of the anterior pituitary: Time course in the growing rat. *Experientia,* 35:1517.
138. Hymer, W. C., Page, R., Kelsey, R. C., Augustine, E. C., Wilfinger, W., and Ciolkosz, M. (1980): Separated somatotropes: Their use *in vitro* and *in vivo*. In: *Synthesis and Release of Adenohypophysial Hormones,* edited by M. Jutisz and K. W. McKerns, p. 125. Plenum Press, New York.
139. Walker, A. M., and Farquhar, M. G. (1980): Preferential release of newly synthesized PRL granules is the result of functional heterogeneity among mammotrophs. *Endocrinology,* 107:1095.
140. Merchant, F. W. (1974): PRL and luteinizing hormone cells of pregnant and lactating rats as studied by immunohistochemistry and radioimmunoassay. *Am. J. Anat.,* 139:245.
141. Neill, J. D., Smith, P. F., Luque, E. H., Munoz de Toro, M., Nagy, G., Mulchahey, J. (1987): Detection and measurement of hormone secretion from individual pituitary cells. *Recent Prog. Horm. Res.,* 43:175.
142. Snyder, J., Wilfinger, W., and Hymer, W. C. (1976): Maintenance of separated rat pituitary mammotrophs in culture. *Endocrinology,* 98:25.
143. Snyder, J., Hymer, W. C., and Wilfinger, W. (1978): Culture of human pituitary prolactin and growth hormone cells. *Cell Tissue Res.,* 191:379.
144. Severinghaus, A. E. (1937): Cellular changes in the anterior hypophysis with special reference to its secretory activities. *Physiol. Rev.,* 17:556.
145. Boockfor, F. R., Frawley, S. L. (1987): Functional variations among prolactin cells from different pituitary regions. *Endocrinology,* 120:874.
146. Denef, C., and Andries, M. (1983): Evidence for paracrine interaction between gonadotrophs and lactotrophs in pituitary cell aggregates. *Endocrinology,* 112:813.
147. Baes, M., Allaerto, W., and Denef, C. (1987): Evidence for functional communication between folliculo-stellate cells and hormone secreting cells in perifused anterior pituitary cell aggregates. *Endocrinology,* 120:685.
148. Horvath, E., Kovacs, K., and Ezrin, C. (1977): Functional contact between lactotrophs and gonadotrophs in rat pituitary. *ICRS Med. Sci.,* 5:511.
149. Nakane, P, K. (1970): Classification of pituitary cell types with immunoenzyme histochemistry. *J. Histochem. Cytochem.,* 18:9.
150. Schramme, C., and Denef, C. (1983): Stimulation of prolactin release by angiotensin II in superfused rat anterior pituitary aggregates. *Neuroendocrinology,* 36:483.
151. Aguilera, G., Hyde, C. L., and Catt, K. J. (1982): Angiotensin II receptors and prolactin release in pituitary lactotrophs. *Endocrinology,* 111:1045.
152. Capponi, A. M., Favrod-Coune, C. A., Gaillard, R. C., and Muller, A. F. (1982): Binding and activation properties of angiotensin II in dispersed rat anterior pituitary cells. *Endocrinology,* 110:1043.
153. Hauger, R. L., Aguilera, G., Baukal, A. J., and Catt, K. J. (1982): Characterization of angiotensin II receptors in the anterior pituitary gland. *Mol. Cell. Endocrinol.,* 25:203.
154. Mukherjee, A., Kulkarni, P., McCann, S. M., and Negro-Vilar, A. (1982): Evidence for the presence and characterization of angiotensin II receptors in rat anterior pituitary membranes. *Endocrinology,* 110:665.
155. Naruse, K., Takii, Y., and Inagami, T. (1981): Immunohistochemical localization of renin in luteinizing hormone-producing cells of rat pituitary. *Proc. Natl. Acad. Sci. USA,* 78:7579.
156. Steele, M. K., Brownfield, M. S., and Ganong, W. F. (1982): Immunocytochemical localization of angiotensin immunoreactivity in gonadotrophs and lactotrophs of the rat anterior pituitary gland. *Neuroendocrinology,* 35:155.
157. Yen, S. C. C., Hoff, J. D., Lasley, B. L., Casper, R. J., and Sheehan, K. (1980): Induction of prolactin release by LRF and LRF agonist. *Life Sci.,* 26:1963.
158. Casper, R. F., and Yen, S. C. C. (1981): Simultaneous pulsatile release by prolactin and luteinizing hormone induced by luteinizing hormone releasing factor agonist. *J. Clin. Endocrinol. Metab.,* 52:934.
159. Arnaout, M. A., Garthwaite, T. L., Martinson, D. R., and Hagen, T. C. (1986): Vasoactive intestinal peptide is synthesized in anterior pituitary tissue. *Endocrinology,* 119:2052.
160. Morel, G., Chayvialle, J. A., Kerdelhue, B., and Dubois, P. M. (1982): Ultrastructural evidence for endogenous substance P-like immunoreactivity in the rat pituitary gland. *Neuroendocrinology,* 35:86.
161. Aronin, N., Coslovsky, R., and Leeman, S. E. (1986): Substance P and neurotensin: Their roles in the regulation of anterior pituitary function. *Annu. Rev. Physiol.,* 48:537.
162. Jonassen, J. A., Mulliken-Kilpatrick, D., McAdam, A., and Leeman, S. E. (1986): Thyroid hormone regulates substance P and substance K gene expression in the rat anterior pituitary gland. Program of the 68th Annual Meeting of the Endocrine Society, Anaheim, Cal. p. 262 (abstract).
163. Jonassen, J. A., Mulliken-Kilpatrick, D., and Leeman, S. E. (1986): Thyroid hormone status and sex steroid hormones regulate preprotachykinin gene expression in female rat anterior pituitary gland. Program of the 16th Annual Meeting of the Society for Neuroscience, Washington, D. C., p. 691 (abstract).
164. Goedert, M., Lightman, S. L., Nagy, J. I., Marley, P. D., and Emson, P. C. (1982): Neurotensin in the rat anterior pituitary gland. *Nature,* 298:163.
165. Bauer, T. V., Moriarty, C. M., and Childs, G. V. (1981): Studies of immunoreactive gonadotropin-releasing hormone (GnRH) in the rat anterior pituitary gland. *J. Histochem. Cytochem.,* 29:1171.
166. Morel, G., and Dubois, P. M. (1982): Immunocytochemical evidence for gonadoliberin in rat anterior pituitary gland. *Neuroendocrinology,* 34:197.
167. Childs (Moriarty), G. V., Cole, D. E., Kubek, M., Tobin, R. B., and Wilber, J. F. (1978): Endogenous thyrotropin-releasing hormone in the anterior pituitary: Sites of activity as identified by immunocytochemical staining. *J. Histochem. Cytochem.,* 26:901.
168. Morel, G., Hemming, F., Tonon, M. C., Vaudry, H., Dubois, M. P., Coy, D., and Dubois, P. M. (1982): Ultrastructural evidence for corticotropin-releasing factor (CRF)-like immunoreactivity in the rat pituitary gland. *Biol. Cell,* 44:89.
169. Morel, G., Mesguich, P., Dubois, M. P., and Dubois, P. M. (1984): Ultrastructural evidence for endogenous growth hormone-releasing factor (GRF)-like immunoreactivity in the monkey pituitary gland. *Neuroendocrinology,* 38:123.
170. Morel, G., Mesguich, P., Dubois, M. P., and Dubois, P. M. (1983): Ultrastructural evidence for endogenous somatostatin immunoreactivity in the pituitary gland. *Neuroendocrinology,* 36:291.
171. Loftus, C. M., Nilaver, G., Defendini, P., Post, K. D., and Beinfeld, M. D. (1983): Program of the 13th Annual Meeting of the Society for Neuroscience, p. 1015 (abstract).
172. Rehfield, J. F. (1978): Localization of gastrins to neuro- and adenohypophysis. *Nature,* 271:771.
173. O'Donohue, T. L., Charlton, C. G., Miller, R. L., Boden, G., and Jacobowitz, D. M. (1981): Identification, characterization, and distribution of secretin immunoreactivity in rat and pig brain. *Proc. Natl. Acad. Sci. USA,* 78:5221.
174. Weber, E., Voigt, K. H., and Martin, R. (1978): Pituitary somatotropes contain [Met] enkephalin-like immunoreactivity. *Proc. Natl. Acad. Sci. USA,* 75:6134.
175. Tramu, G., and Leonardelli, J. (1979): Immunohistochemical localization of enkephalins in median eminence and adenohypophysis. *Brain Res.,* 168:457.
176. Kitamura, K., Minamino, N., Hayashi, Y., Kanagawa, K., and Matsuo, H. (1982): Regional distribution of β-neoendorphin in rat brain and pituitary. *Biochem. Biophys. Res. Commun.,* 109:966.

177. Seizinger, B. R., Grimna, C., Hollt, V., and Herz, A. (1984): Evidence for a selective processing of proenkephalin β into different opioid peptide forms in particular regions of rat brain and pituitary. *J. Neurochem.*, 42:447.
178. Clements, J. A., and Funder, J. W. (1986): Arginine vasopressin (AVP) and AVP-like immunoreactivity in peripheral tissues. *Endocr. Rev.*, 7:449.
179. Habener, J. (1985): Genetic control of hormone formation. In: *Textbook of Endocrinology,* 7th edition, edited by J. D. Wilson and D. W. Foster, p. 9. WB Saunders, Philadelphia.
180. Martin, T. J. F. (1985): Dual intracellular signaling by Ca^{+2} and lipids mediates the actions of TRH. In: *Prolactin: Basic and Clinical Correlates,* edited by R. M. MacLeod, M. O. Thorner, and U. Scapagnini, p. 165. Liviana Press, Padova.
181. Rosenfeld, M. G., Amara, S. G., Birnberg, N. C., Mermod, J.-J., Murodoch, G. H., and Evans, R. M. (1983): Calcitonin, prolactin, and growth hormone gene expression as model systems for the characterization of neuroendocrine regulation. *Recent Prog. Horm. Res.*, 39:305.
182. Murodoch, G. H., Evans, R. M., and Rosenfeld, M. G. (1985): Polypeptide hormone regulation of prolactin gene transcription. In: *Biochemical Actions of Hormones, Vol. 12,* edited by G. Litwack, p. 37. Academic Press, New York.
183. Martin, T. F. J., and Tashjian, A. H., Jr. (1977): Cell culture studies of thyrotropin-releasing hormone action. In: *Biochemical Actions of Hormones, Vol. 4,* edited by G. Litwack, p. 270. Academic Press, New York.
184. Bataille, D., Peillon, F., Besson, J., and Rosselin, G. (1979): Vasoactive intestinal peptide (VIP): Receptors specifique et activation de l'adenylate cyclase dans une tumeur hypophysaire a prolactin. *C. R. Acad. Sci. Ser. D (Paris)*, 288:1315.
185. Caron, M. G., Kilpatrick, B. F., McDonald, W. M. (1985): The dopamine receptor of the anterior pituitary gland: Involvement of a guanine nucleotide-sensitive agonist high affinity form of the receptor in the mechanism of action of dopamine. In: *Catecholamines as Hormone Regulators,* edited by N. Ben-Jonathan, J. M. Bahr, and R. I. Weiner, p. 89. Raven Press, New York.
186. Boockfor, F. J., Hoeffler, J. P., and Frawley, L. C. (1985): Cultures of GH_3 cells are functionally heterogeneous: Thyrotropin-releasing hormone, estradiol and cortisol cause reciprocal shifts in the proportions of growth hormone and prolactin secretors. *Endocrinology,* 117:418.
187. Thorner, M. O., Hackett, J. T., Murad, F., and MacLeod, R. M. (1980): Calcium rather than cyclic AMP as the physiological intracellular regulator of prolactin release. *Neuroendocrinology,* 31:390.
188. Swennen, L., and Denef, C. (1982): Physiological concentrations of dopamine decrease adenosine 3′5′-monophosphate levels in cultured rat anterior pituitary cells and enriched populations of lactotrophs: Evidence for a causal relationship to inhibition of prolactin release. *Endocrinology,* 111:398.
189. Giannattasio, G., DeFerrari, M. E., and Spada, A. (1981): Dopamine inhibits adenylate cyclase in female rat adenohypophysis. *Life Sci.*, 28:1605.
190. Barnes, G. D., Brown, B. L., Gard, T. C., Atkinson, D., Ekins, R. P. (1978): Effect of TRH and dopamine on cyclic AMP levels in enriched mammotroph and thyrotroph cells. *Mol. Cell. Endocrinol.*, 12:273.
191. Maurer, R. A. (1981): Transcriptional regulation of the prolactin gene by ergocryptine and cyclic AMP. *Nature,* 294:94.
192. Creese, I., Sibley, D. R., and Leff, S. E. (1984): Agonist interactions with dopamine receptors: Focus on radioligand binding studies. *Fed. Proc.*, 43:2779.
193. Kilpatrick, B. F., and Caron, M. G. (1984): Dopamine receptor of the porcine anterior pituitary gland: Solubilization and characterization. *Biochem. Pharmacol.*, 22:1981.
194. Gourdji, D., Bataille, D., Vauclin, N., Grouselle, D., Rosselin, G., and Tixier-Vidal, A. (1979): Vasoactive intestinal peptide (VIP) stimulates prolactin (PRL) release and cAMP production in a rat pituitary cell line (GH_3/B6): Additive effects of VIP and TRH on PRL release. *FEBS Lett.*, 104:165.
195. Gilman, A. G. (1984): G proteins and dual control of adenylate cyclase. *Cell,* 36:577.
196. Helmreich, E. J. M., and Pfeuffer, T. (1985): Regulation of signal transduction of β-adrenergic hormone receptors. *Trends Pharmacol. Sci.*, 6:438.
197. Gershengorn, M. C. (1982): Thyrotropin releasing hormone: A review of the mechanisms of acute stimulation of pituitary hormone release. *Mol. Cell. Biochem.*, 45:163.
198. Gershengorn, M. C. (1985): Thyrotropin-releasing hormone: Mechanism of calcium-mediated stimulation of prolactin secretion. *Recent Prog. Horm. Res.*, 41:607.
199. Drust, D. S., Sutton, C. A., and Martin, T. F. J. (1982): Thyrotropin-releasing hormone and cyclic AMP activate distinctive pathways of protein phosphorylation in GH pituitary cells. *J. Biol. Chem.*, 257:3306.
200. Poirer, G., Labrie, F., Barden, N., and Lemaire, S. (1972): Thyrotropin-releasing hormone receptor: Its partial purification from bovine anterior pituitary gland and its close association with adenylyl cyclase. *FEBS Lett.*, 20:283.
201. Hinkle, P. M., Tashjian, A. H., Jr. (1977): Adenylyl cyclase and cyclic nucleotide phosphodiesterases in GH strains of rat pituitary cells. *Endocrinology,* 100:934.

Subject Index

D

E

F

G

I

J

K

O